W9-APK-021

# KIRK'S
# CURRENT
# VETERINARY
# THERAPY
# XII

## SMALL ANIMAL PRACTICE

# KIRK'S
# CURRENT
# VETERINARY
# THERAPY

# XII

# SMALL ANIMAL PRACTICE

## W. B. SAUNDERS COMPANY
*A Division of Harcourt Brace & Company*

Philadelphia London Toronto Montreal Sydney Tokyo

**W. B. SAUNDERS COMPANY**
*A Division of Harcourt Brace & Company*

The Curtis Center
Independence Square West
Philadelphia, PA 19106

**Library of Congress Cataloging-in-Publication Data**

Current veterinary therapy. 1964/65—
Philadelphia, W. B. Saunders
v. 26 cm.
"Small animal practice."
Editor: 1964/65- R. W. Kirk.
Key title: Current veterinary therapy, ISSN 0070-2218.
1. Veterinary medicine—Periodicals.        2. Pets—Diseases—
    Periodicals.      I. Kirk, Robert Warren, ed.
    [DNLM: W1 CU823]
SF 745.C8      636.0896      64–10489
                                    MARC-S
Library of Congress      [8308]

Kirk's Current Veterinary Therapy XII                                    ISBN   0-7216-5188-7

Printed in the United States of America.

Last digit is the print number:      9      8      7      6      5      4      3      2

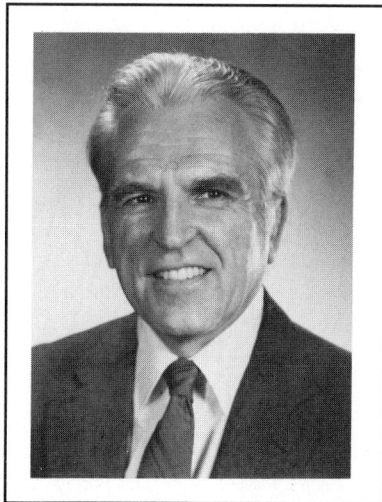

This edition of *Current Veterinary Therapy* is dedicated to Dr. Robert W. Kirk. Bob Kirk has been an outstanding leader and friend of veterinary medicine for almost five decades. His strong desire to help practicing veterinarians and students provide the best possible care for their patients has been the impetus behind the book that bears his name. That *Current Veterinary Therapy*, or "Kirk" as most call his textbook, is the most widely read veterinary textbook in the world is a tribute to his vision and accomplishments.

JDB

# CONTRIBUTORS

**JONATHAN A. ABBOTT, D.V.M., Dipl. A.C.V.I.M. (Cardiology)**
Consultant, Cardiopet Incorporated, Floral Park, New York
*Traumatic Myocarditis*

**KENNETH L. ABRAMS, D.V.M., Dipl. A.C.V.O.**
Veterinary Ophthalmologists; Veterinary Ophthalmology Services, Inc., Warwick, Rhode Island
*Ocular Drug Reactions and Toxicities*

**ROBERTO F. AGUILAR, D.V.M.**
Staff Veterinarian, Audubon Park Zoo, New Orleans, Louisiana
*Diagnosis and Treatment of Avian Aspergillosis*

**ALBERT H. AHN, D.V.M.**
Resident, Small Animal Medicine, Tufts University School of Veterinary Medicine, North Grafton, Massachusetts
*Approach to the Hypothermic Patient; Approach to the Anemic Patient*

**JANET ALDRICH, D.V.M.**
Staff Veterinarian, Emergency/Critical Care Service, University of California, Davis, California
*Monitoring the Critically Ill Patient*

**TIMOTHY A. ALLEN, D.V.M., Dipl. A.C.V.I.M.**
Veterinary Fellow, Mark Morris Institute, Topeka, Kansas; Adjunct Faculty, Veterinary Teaching Hospital, Kansas State University, Manhattan, Kansas
*Medical Implications of Fasting and Starvation*

**NANCY L. ANDERSON, D.V.M., B.S.E., Dipl. A.B.V.P. (Avian)**
Clinical Instructor, The Ohio State University College of Veterinary Medicine, Columbus, Ohio
*Intraosseous Fluid Therapy in Small Exotic Animals*

**MAX J. G. APPEL, D.V.M., Ph.D.**
Professor, Cornell University College of Veterinary Medicine, Ithaca, New York
*CVT Update: Canine Lyme Disease*

**CLARKE E. ATKINS, D.V.M., Dipl. A.C.V.I.M. (Internal Medicine Cardiology)**
Professor of Medicine and Cardiology, College of Veterinary Medicine, North Carolina State University; Veterinary Teaching Hospital, North Carolina State University, Raleigh, North Carolina
*Supraventricular Tachycardia Associated with Accessory Atrioventricular Pathways in Dogs*

**HELIO S. AUTRAN DE MORAIS, D.V.M., M.S., Dipl. A.C.V.I.M. (Internal Medicine Cardiology)**
Clinical Instructor, Department of Veterinary Clinical Sciences, The Ohio State University, Ohio; Associate Professor, Departamento de Clínicas Veterinárias, Universidade Estadual de Londrina, Londrina, Paraná, Brazil
*Strong Ions and Acid-Base Disorders*

**E. MURL BAILEY, D.V.M., Ph.D.**
Professor of Toxicology, Department of Veterinary Physiology and Pharmacology, College of Veterinary Medicine, Texas A&M University, College Station, Texas
*Toxic Ornamental and Garden Plants*

**JOAN BARRIE, D.V.M.**
Resident in Clinical Pathology, New York State College of Veterinary Medicine, Cornell University, Ithaca, New York; Clinical Pathologist, Grange Laboratories, Wetherby, West Yorkshire, United Kingdom
*Hyperlipidemia*

**JEANNE A. BARSANTI, D.V.M., M.S., DIPL. A.C.V.I.M.**
Professor, College of Veterinary Medicine, University of Georgia; Internist, Veterinary Medical Teaching Hospital, University of Georgia, Athens, Georgia
*Section 10, Consulting Editor; The Role of Dimethyl Sulfoxide and Glucocorticoids in Lower Urinary Tract Diseases; CVT Update: Treatment of Canine Bacteria Prostatitis, Medical Management of Canine Prostatic Hyperplasia*

**JOSEPH W. BARTGES, D.V.M., Ph.D.**
Assistant Professor, Department of Small Animal Medicine, College of Veterinary Medicine, University of Georgia; Small Animal Clinical Nutritionist, University of Georgia, Athens, Georgia
*Ten Guiding Principles to Enhance the Benefit of Current Veterinary Therapy; Influence of Fasting and Eating on Laboratory Values*

**CATHERINE J. BATY, D.V.M.**
Graduate Research Associate, College of Veterinary Medicine, North Carolina State University, Raleigh, North Carolina
*Warfarin Therapy of the Cat at Risk of Thromboembolism*

**BONNIE V. BEAVER, D.V.M., M.S., Dipl. A.C.V.B.**
Professor and Chief of Medicine, Department of Small Animal Medicine and Surgery, Texas A&M University, College Station, Texas
*Nonpharmacologic Management of Common Behavioral Disorders*

**ELLEN N. BEHREND, V.M.D., M.S.**
Resident in Small Animal Medicine, Department of Clinical Sciences, College of Veterinary Medicine and Biomedical Sciences, Colorado State University, Fort Collins, Colorado
*Clinical Applications of Glucocorticoid Therapy in Nonendocrine Diesease; Corticosteroid Withdrawal Syndrome*

**FORD W. BELL, D.V.M.**
Clinical Assistant Professor, Oncology, University of Minnesota, Lewis Hospital for Companion Animals, University of Minnesota, St. Paul, Minnesota
*Canine Prostatic Disorders*

**DAVID BENNETT, B.Sc., B.V.Med., Ph.D.**
Reader in Veterinary Clinical Science, University of Liverpool, Liverpool, United Kingdom
*Treatment of the Immune-Based Inflammatory Arthropathies of the Dog and Cat*

**R. AVERY BENNETT, D.V.M., M.S., Dipl. A.C.V.S.**
Assistant Professor of Zoo and Wildlife Medicine, University of Florida, Gainesville, Florida; Formerly: Chief Veterinarian, San Francisco Zoo, San Francisco, California
*Reptile Anesthesia*

**CLIFFORD R. BERRY, D.V.M., Dipl. A.C.V.R.**
Assistant Professor, Veterinary Radiology, College of Veterinary Medicine, North Carolina State University, Raleigh, North Carolina
*Recognition of Congenital Heart Disease in the Adult Dog and Cat*

**ELIZABETH HERST BERTOY, D.V.M.**
Resident, Small Animal Internal Medicine, University of California Veterinary Medical Teaching Hospital, University of California, Davis, California
*Diagnosis and Treatment of Macrotumors in Dogs with Pituitary-Dependent Hyperadrenocorticism*

**DAVID S. BILLER, D.V.M., Dipl. A.C.V.R.**
Associate Professor, Radiology, Department of Clinical Sciences, Kansas State University; Head of Radiology, Veterinary Teaching Hospital, Kansas State University, Manhattan, Kansas
*Ultrasonographic Findings in Renal Disease; Familial Renal Disease in Cats*

**STEPHEN J. BIRCHARD, D.V.M., M.S., Dipl. A.C.V.S.**
Associate Professor, The Ohio State University College of Veterinary Medicine, Columbus, Ohio
*Definitive Surgical Treatment for Cancer*

**DALE E. BJORLING, D.V.M., M.S., Dipl. A.C.V.S.**
Professor and Chair, Department of Surgical Sciences, School of Veterinary Medicine, University of Wisconsin, Madison, Wisconsin
*Laryngeal Paralysis*

**MARK S. BLOOMBERG, D.V.M., M.S., Dipl. A.C.V.S.**
Collins Professor and Chairman, Department of Small Animal Clinical Sciences, University of Florida, Chief of Staff, Veterinary Medical Teaching Hospital, College of Veterinary Medicine, University of Florida, Gainesville, Florida
*Early Neutering of the Dog and Cat*

**GÖRAN BÖLSKE, D.V.M.**

Head of Mycoplasma Section, The National Veterinary Institute, Uppsala, Sweden

*Canine Genital Mycoplasmas and Ureaplasmas*

**JOHN D. BONAGURA. D.V.M., Dipl. A.C.V.I.M (Cardiology, Internal Medicine)**

Professor, Department of Veterinary Clinical Sciences, Head, Small Animal Medicine Veterinary Teaching Hospital, The Ohio State University, Columbus, Ohio

*Therapy of Heart Failure; CVT Update: Canine Subvalvular Aortic Stenosis; Restrictive Cardiomyopathy*

**DAWN MERTON BOOTHE, D.V.M., Ph.D., Dipl. A.C.V.I.M., A.C.V.C.P.**

Assistant Professor of Veterinary Physiology and Pharmacology, College of Veterinary Medicine, Texas A&M University; Attending Clinician, Veterinary Teaching Hospital, Small Animal Clinic, Texas A&M University, College Station, Texas

*Principles of Drug Therapy for the Practicing Veterinarian; Effects of Drugs on Endocrine Tests; Effects of Hepatic Disease on Drug Disposition*

**DAVID R. BOSTWICK, D.V.M., M.S., Dipl. A.C.V.I.M. (Internal Medicine)**

Resident, Small Animal Medicine, Veterinary Teaching Hospital, Colorado State University, Fort Collins, Colorado; Internal Medicine Staff, Critical Care Associates of Seattle, Seattle, Washington

*Bilirubin and Bile Acids in the Diagnosis of Hepatobiliary Disease*

**THOMAS H. BOYER, D.V.M.**

Clinical Instructor in Wildlife and Zoological Medicine, College of Veterinary Medicine and Biomedical Sciences, Colorado State University, Fort Collins, Colorado

*Clinical Reptilian Microbiology*

**WILLIAM F. BRAUN, JR., D.V.M., Dipl. A.C.T.**

Associate Professor, Theriogenology, Department of Veterinary Medicine and Surgery, College of Veterinary Medicine, University of Missouri, Columbia, Missouri

*Potbellied Pigs: General Medical Care*

**KYLE G. BRAUND, B.V.Sc., M.V.Sc., Ph.D., F.R.C.V.S., Dipl. A.C.V.I.M. (Neurology)**

Professor, Department of Small Animal Medicine and Surgery, College of Veterinary Medicine, Auburn University; Director, Neuromuscular Laboratory, College of Veterinary Medicine, Auburn University, Auburn, Alabama

*Section 12, Consulting Editor; Laryngeal Paralysis-Polyneuropathy Complex in Young Dalmatian Dogs*

**P. WALTER BRAVO, D.V.M., M.S., Ph.D.**

Postgraduate Research, Department of Population Health and Reproduction, School of Veterinary Medicine, University of California, Davis, California

*Reproductive Physiology of South American Camelids*

**CORY F. BRAYTON, D.V.M.**

Director, Facility for Comparative Studies, Assistant Scientist, The Hospital for Special Surgery; Attending Veterinarian, The New York Blood Center, New York, New York

*Use and Misuse of DMSO*

**EDWARD B. BREITSCHWERDT, D.V.M., Dipl. A.C.V.I.M. (Internal Medicine)**

Professor of Medicine and Infectious Diseases, Department of Companion Animal and Special Species Medicine, College of Veterinary Medicine, North Carolina State University; Veterinary Teaching Hospital, College of Veterinary Medicine, North Carolina State University, Raleigh, North Carolina

*Section 4, Consulting Editor; CVT Update: Zinc Toxicity; Feline Rickettsial Diseases, CVT Update: Rocky Mountain Spotted Fever*

**WILLIAM G. BREWER, JR., D.V.M., A.C.V.I.M Dipl. (Internal Medicine, Oncology)**

Assistant Professor, College of Veterinary Medicine, Auburn University; Section Chief, Internal Medicine, Department of Small Animal Surgery and Medicine, College of Veterinary Medicine, Auburn University, Auburn, Alabama

*Drug Interactions with Antineoplastic Agents*

**JOHN D. BROUSSARD, D.V.M.**

Staff Doctor, MedVet-Columbus, Columbus, Ohio

*Insulin Treatment of Diabetes Mellitus in the Dog and Cat*

**SCOTT A. BROWN, V.M.D., Ph.D., Dipl. A.C.V.I.M.**

Associate Professor, Department of Physiology and Pharmacology, College of Veterinary Medicine, University of Georgia; Department of Small Animal Medicine, Veterinary Medical Teaching Hospital, College of Veterinary Medicine, University of Georgia, Athens, Georgia

*Inappropriate Dietary Protein and Mineral Restriction in Dogs and Cats; Reassessment of the Use of Calcitriol in Chronic Renal Failure; The Role of Dimethyl Sulfoxide and Glucocorticoids in Lower Urinary Tract Diseases*

**WILLIAM A. BROWN, D.V.M.**

Cardiology Research Instructor, University of Veterinary Medicine, University of Illinois, Urbana, Illinois,

*Ventricular Septal Defects in the English Springer Spaniel*

**CINDY J. BRUNNER, D.V.M., Ph.D.**

Associate Professor, Department of Pathobiology, College of Veterinary Medicine, Auburn University, Auburn, Alabama

*Autoimmunity*

**DAVID S. BRUYETTE, D.V.M., Dipl. A.C.V.I.M.**

Assistant Professor, Department of Clinical Sciences, College of Veterinary Medicine, Kansas State University; Head, Small Animal Medicine, Veterinary Medical Teaching Hospital, Kansas State University, Manhattan, Kansas

*Alternatives in the Treatment of Hyperadrenocorticism in Dogs and Cats*

**JORG BÜCHELER, D.V.M., Dr. Med. Vet., FTA., Dipl. A.C.V.I.M.**

Clinical Assistant Professor, Tufts University School of Veterinary Medicine, Department of Medicine, Tufts University, North Grafton, Massachusetts

*Canine Immune-Mediated Hemolytic Anemia*

**WILLIAM B. BUCK, D.V.M., M.S., A.B.V.T.**

Professor of Toxicology, College of Veterinary Medicine, University of Illinois; Director National Animal Poison Control Center, Urbana, Illinois

*Top 25 Generic Agents Involving Dogs and Cats Managed by the National Animal Poison Control Center in 1992*

**ROBERT G. BUERGER, D.V.M., Dipl. A.C.V.D.**

Private Referral Practice, Veterinary Dermatology Center, Baltimore, Maryland

*Insect and Arachnid Hypersensitivity Disorders of Dogs and Cats*

**C. A. TONY BUFFINGTON, D.V.M., Ph.D., Dipl. A.C.V.N.**

Associate Professor, The Ohio State University; Chief, Nutrition Support Service, The Ohio State University Veterinary Hospital, The Ohio State University, Columbus, Ohio

*Does Interstitial Cystitis Occur in Cats?*

**SUSAN E. BUNCH, D.V.M., Dipl. A.C.V.I.M.**

Associate Professor of Medicine, College of Veterinary Medicine, North Carolina State University; Companion Animal Internist, Veterinary Teaching Hospital, College of Veterinary Medicine, North Carolina State University, Raleigh, North Carolina

*Feline Portosystemic Vascular Shunts*

**MARY JO BURKHARD, D.V.M.**

Resident, Clinical Pathology, College of Veterinary Medicine and Biomedical Sciences, Colorado State University, Fort Collins, Colorado

*Causes and Effects of Interference with Clinical Laboratory Measurements and Examinations*

**THOMAS J. BURKE, D.V.M., M.S.**

Professor, University of Illinois College of Veterinary Medicine, Urbana, Illinois; Clinical Consultant, Capitol Illinois Veterinary Hospital, Springfield; Research Associate, Lincoln Park Zoo, Chicago, Illinois

*"Wet Tail" in Hamsters and Other Diarrheas of Small Rodents*

**ROY B. BURNS, D.V.M.**

Staff Veterinarian, Louisville Zoological Garden, Louisville, Kentucky

*Euthanasia Methods for Ectothermic Vertebrates*

**CAROLYN BUTLER, M.S.**

Co-Director, Changes: The Support for People and Pets Program, Department of Veterinary Clinical Services, College of Veterinary Medical and Biomedical Sciences, Veterinary Teaching Hospital, Colorado State University, Fort Collins, Colorado

*Facilitating Owner-Present Euthanasia*

**JANICE L. CAIN, D.V.M. Dipl. A.C.V.I.M**

Staff Internist, Norris Canyon Veterinary Center, San Ramon, California

*The Use and Misuse of Reproductive Hormones in Canine Reproduction*

**CLAY A. CALVERT, D.V.M., B.S.**

Associate Professor, Department of Small Animal Medicine, College of Veterinary Medicine, University of Georgia, Athens, Georgia

*Diagnosis and Management of Ventricular Tachyarrhythmias in Doberman Pinschers with Cardiomyopathy*

**KAREN L. CAMPBELL, D.V.M., M.S., Dipl. A.C.V.I.M., A.C.V.D.**

Associate Professor, Department of Veterinary Clinical Medicine, College of Veterinary Medicine, University of Illinois Veterinary Medical Teaching Hospital, University of Illinois, Small Animal Clinic, University of Illinois, Urbana, Illinois

*The Effect of Potentiated Sulfonamides on Canine Thyroid Function*

**MARCIA A. CAROTHERS, D.V.M., Dipl. A.C.V.I.M.**

Staff Internist, Veterinary Referral Clinic, Cleveland, Ohio; Adjunct Clinical Instructor, Department of Veterinary Clinical Sciences, College of Veterinary Medicine, The Ohio State University, Columbus, Ohio

*Utility of Diagnostic Assays in the Evaluation of Hypercalcemia and Hypocalcemia: Parathyroid Hormone, Vitamin D Metabolites, Parathyroid Hormone-Related Peptide, and Ionized Calcium*

**SHARON A. CENTER, D.V.M., Dipl. A.C.V.I.M.**

Associate Professor, New York State College of Veterinary Medicine, Cornell University, Ithaca, New York

*Chronic Hepatitis: Therapeutic Considerations*

**C. B. CHASTAIN, D.V.M., M.S., Dipl. A.C.V.I.M.**

Professor, Small Animal Medicine, Associate Dean of Academic Affairs, College of Veterinary Medicine, University of Missouri; Professor, Small Animal Medicine, Veterinary Medical Teaching Hospital, University of Missouri, Columbia, Missouri

*Uses and Misuses of Aspirin; Monitoring Long-Term Control in the Diabetic Patient*

**MATTHEW J. CHAVKIN, D.V.M., M.S.**

Veterinary Referral Center of Colorado, Denver, Colorado

*Feline Uveitis*

**DENNIS J. CHEW, D.V.M., Dipl. A.C.V.I.M.**

Professor, Department of Clinical Sciences, College of Veterinary Medicine, The Ohio State University; Internist, Attending Staff-Internal Medicine, The Ohio State University Veterinary Medical Teaching Hospital, College of Veterinary Medicine, The Ohio State University, Columbus, Ohio

*Utility of Diagnostic Assays in the Evaluation of Hypercalcemia and Hypocalcemia: Parathyroid Hormone, Vitamin D Metabolites, Parathyroid Hormone-Related Peptide, and Ionized Calcium; Does Interstital Cystitis Occur in Cats?*

**TERRENCE P. CLARK, D.V.M., Ph.D.**

Assistant Professor, St. Norbert College, De Pere, Wisconsin

*CVT Update: Sample Collection and Testing Protocols in Endocrinology*

**SUSAN L. CLUBB, D.V.M., Dipl., A.B.V.P. (Avian)**

Parrot Jungle and Gardens, Miami, Florida

*Nonsurgical Means of Sex Determination in Psittacine Birds*

**JOAN R. COATES, D.V.M., M.S., Dipl. A.C.V.I.M. (Neurology)**

Assistant Professor-Clinical Neurology, Department of Small Animal Medicine, College of Veterinary Medicine, University of Georgia, Athens, Georgia

*Congenital and Inherited Neurologic Disorders in Dogs and Cats*

**ROBERT D. COHEN, D.V.M.**

Clinical Instructor, Staff Veterinarian, Tufts University School of Veterinary Medicine, Tufts University, North Grafton, Massachusetts

*Systemic Anaphylaxis*

**PATRICK W. CONCANNON, M.S., Ph.D.**

Senior Research Associate, College of Veterinary Medicine, Cornell University, Ithaca, New York

*Ultrasonography of the Reproductive Tract of the Female Dog and Cat; Use of Progesterone-Suppressing Drugs for Termination of Unwanted Pregnancy in Dogs*

**PETER D. CONSTABLE, B.V.Sc., M.S., Ph.D., Diplomate, A.C.V.I.M**

Assistant Professor and Head, Food Animal Medicine and Surgery Section. College of Veterinary Medicine, University of Illinois, Urbana, Illinois

*Preventive Medicine in Llamas*

**DANIEL L. COSTA, Sc.D., Dipl. A.B.T.**

Chief, Pulmonary Toxicology Branch of the Health Effects Research Laboratory of the United States Environmental Protection Agency, Research Triangle Park, North Carolina

*A Brief Guide to Indoor Air Pollutants and Relevance to Small Animals*

**SUSAN M. COTTER, D.V.M., Dipl. A.C.V.I.M (Internal Medicine, Oncology)**

Professor of Medicine, Tufts University School of Veterinary Medicine, North Grafton, Massachusetts

*Canine Immune-Mediated Hemolytic Anemia; Approach to the Anemic Patient*

**C. GUILLERMO COUTO, D.V.M., Dipl. A.C.V.I.M. (Internal Medicine, Oncology)**

Associate Professor, Department of Veterinary Clinical Sciences, College of Veterinary Medicine, The Ohio State University, Columbus, Ohio

*Spontaneous Bleeding Disorders; Nonsurgical Management of Soft Tissue Sarcomas*

**LAINE A. COWAN, D.V.M., M.S., Dipl. A.C.V.I.M. (Internal Medicine)**

Assistant Professor, Small Animal Internal Medicine, Department of Clinical Sciences, Kansas State University, Manhattan, Kansas

*Immune Function in Renal Failure*

**ANNETTE K. COWELL, D.V.M., Dipl. A.B.V.P.**

The Cat Clinic of Stillwater, Stillwater, Oklahoma

*Management of Bee and Other Hymenoptera Stings*

**RICK L. COWELL, D.V.M., M.S., Dipl. A.C.V.P.**

Professor of Clinical Pathology, College of Veterinary Medicine, Oklahoma State University, Stillwater, Oklahoma

*Management of Bee and Other Hymenoptera Stings*

**LARRY D. COWGILL, D.V.M., Ph.D., Diplomate A.C.V.I.M**

Associate Professor, Department of Medicine and Epidemiology, School of Veterinary Medicine, University of California, Davis, California

*CVT Update: Use of Recombinant Human Erythropoietin; CVT Update: Veterinary Applications of Hemodialysis*

**KATHY L. CRENSHAW, D.V.M.**

Research Associate, The Rogosin Institute, New York, New York

*Complications and Concurrent Disease Associated with Diabetic Ketoacidosis and Other Severe Forms of Diabetes Mellitus*

**DENNIS T. (TIM) CROWE, JR., D.V.M., Dipl. A.C.V.S., A.C.V.E.C.C., N.R.E.M.T.**

Director of Research, Professor of Surgery, Veterinary Institute of Trauma, Emergency and Critical Care, Chief of Surgery, The Animal Emergency Center, Milwaukee, Wisconsin

*Doppler Assessment of Blood Flow and Pressure in Surgical and Critical Care Patients; Counterpressure Use in Shock and Hemorrhage*

**JOHN F. CUMMINGS, D.V.M., Ph.D.**

Professor of Anatomy, College of Veterinary Medicine, Cornell University, Ithaca, New York

*Canine Neurodegenerative Disease Involving Motor Neurons*

**PETER G. G. DARKE, B.V.Sc., Ph.D., D.V.R., D.V.C., M.R.C.V.S.**

Head of Cardiopulmonary Services, Royal School of Veterinary Studies, University of Edinburgh, Edinburgh, United Kingdom

*Mitral Valve Disease in Cavalier King Charles Spaniels*

**AUTUMN P. DAVIDSON, D.V.M., Dipl. A.C.V.I.M.**

Staff Veterinarian, Small Animal Medicine, University of California, Davis, California; Staff Internist, Encina Veterinary Hospital, Walnut Creek, California

*Treatment of Nasal Aspergillosis with Topical Clotrimazole; Medical Treatment of Pyometra with Prostaglandin $F_{2a}$ in the Dog and Cat*

**GIGI DAVIDSON, B.S., R.Ph.**

Director of Pharmacy, Veterinary Teaching Hospital, North Carolina State, Director of Pharmacy, Veterinary Teaching Hospital, College of Veterinary Medicine, North Carolina State University, Raleigh, North Carolina

*Unapproved Use of Drugs in Small Animals*

**HARRIET J. DAVIDSON, D.V.M., M.S., Dipl. A.C.V.O.**

Animal Eye Consultants, Fayetteville, North Carolina

*Bacterial keratitis*

**DOUGLAS J. DEBOER, D.V.M., Dipl. A.C.V.D.**

Assistant Professor, Department of Medical Sciences, School of Veterinary Medicine, University of Wisconsin, Faculty Dermatologist, Veterinary Medical Teaching Hospital, University of Wisconsin, Madison, Wisconsin

*Management of Chronic and Recurrent Pyoderma in the Dog*

**TERESA DEFRANCESCO, D.V.M., B.S. (Biology)**

Cardiology Resident, College of Veterinary Medicine, North Carolina State University, Raleigh, North Carolina

*Twenty-Four-Hour Ambulatory Electrocardiography (Holter Monitoring)*

**ALEXANDER DE LAHUNTA, D.V.M., Ph.D., Dipl. A.C.V.I.M. (Neurology, Internal Medicine)**

James Law Professor of Anatomy, College of Veterinary Medicine, Cornell University; Clinical Neurologist, Teaching Hospital, College of Veterinary Medicine, Cornell University, Ithaca, New York

*Canine Neurodegenerative Disease Involving Motor Neurons*

**ROBERT C. DENOVO, D.V.M., M.S., Dipl. A.C.V.I.M. (Internal Medicine)**

Associate Professor of Medicine, Department of Small Animal Clinical Sciences, College of Veterinary Medicine, University of Tennessee, Knoxville, Tennessee

*Selecting a Gastrointestinal Endoscope*

**NISHI DHUPA, B.V.M., Cert. SAC, M.R.C.V.S., Dipl. A.C.V.E.C.C.**

Staff Consultant, Cardiopet Incorporated, Floral Park, New York

*Magnesium Therapy*

**SHARON M. DIAL, D.V.M., Ph.D., Dipl. A.C.V.P.**

Staff Pathologist, Southwest Veterinary Diagnostics, Incorporated, Phoenix, Arizona

*Antifreeze Poisoning*

**STEPHEN P. DIBARTOLA, D.V.M., Diplomate, A.C.V.I.M**

Professor, Small Animal Internal Medicine, Department of Veterinary Clinical Sciences, The Ohio State University, Columbus, Ohio

*Familial Renal Disease in Cats*

**KRISTA L. DICKINSON, A.H.T.**
Head Oncology Nurse, Comparative Oncology Unit, Department of Clinical Sciences, College of Veterinary Medicine and Biomedical Sciences, Colorado State University, Fort Collins, Colorado
*Safe Handling and Administration of Chemotherapeutic Agents in Veterinary Medicine*

**DONNA S. DIMSKI, D.V.M., M.S., Dipl. A.C.V.I.M.**
Associate Professor, Department of Veterinary Clinical Sciences, Louisiana State University; Veterinary Internist, Veterinary Teaching Hospital and Clinics, Louisiana State University, Baton Rouge, Louisiana
*Therapy of Inflammatory Bowel Disease*

**MARK DORFMAN, D.V.M., M.S., Dipl. A.C.V.I.M.**
Internist, Veterinary Internal Medicine Specialty Practice, Roswell, Georgia
*CVT Update: Treatment of Canine Bacterial Prostatitis*

**DAVID C. DORMAN, D.V.M., Ph.D., Dipl. A.B.V.T., Dipl. A.B.T.**
Neurotoxicologist, Chemical Industry Institute of Toxicology, Research Triangle Park, North Carolina; Adjunct Assistant Professor, Department of Anatomy, Physiological Sciences, and Radiology, College of Veterinary Medicine, North Carolina State University, Raleigh, North Carolina
*Emergency Treatment of Toxicosis; Neurotoxic Drugs in Dogs and Cats*

**STEVEN W. DOW, Dipl. A.C.V.I.M.**
Instructor, Department of Medicine, National Jewish Center for Immunology and Respiratory Medicine, Denver, Colorado
*Diagnosis of Bacteremia in Critically Ill Dogs and Cats; Immunopathologic Consequences of Infectious Disease*

**KENNETH J. DROBATZ, D.V.M., Dipl. A.C.V.I.M., A.C.V.E.C.**
Assistant Professor, Section of Medicine, Director, Emergency Service, Veterinary Hospital of the University of Pennsylvania, School of Veterinary Medicine, University of Pennsylvania, Philadelphia, Pennsylvania
*Oxygen Supplementation*

**CYNTHIA A. DUESBERG, D.V.M.**
Clinical Instructor, Veterinary Medical Teaching Hospital, University of California, Davis, California
*Diagnosis and Treatment of Macrotumors in Dogs with Pituitary-Dependent Hyperadrenocorticism*

**GENEVIEVE A. DUMONCEAUX, D.V.M.**
Resident, Zoologic Medicine, University of California, Davis, California
*Illicit Drug Intoxication in Dogs*

**ROBERT W. DUNSTAN, D.V.M., M.S., Dipl. A.C.V.P.**
Professor, Department of Pathology and Animal Health, Diagnostic Laboratory, College of Veterinary Medicine, Michigan State University, East Lansing, Michigan
*The Diagnosis of Sebaceous Adenitis in Standard Poodle Dogs*

**JANICE A. DYE, D.V.M., M.S., Dipl. A.C.V.I.M.**
Postdoctoral Fellow, Center for Environmental Medicine and Lung Biology, University of North Carolina, Chapel Hill, North Carolina
*A Brief Guide to Indoor Air Pollutants and Relevance to Small Animals*

**DAVID A. DZANIS, D.V.M., Ph.D., Dipl. A.C.V.N.**
Center for Veterinary Medicine, U.S. Food and Drug Administration, Rockville, Maryland
*Appendices*

**MARC S. ELIE, D.V.M.**
Lecturer in Medicine, Veterinary Hospital of the University of Pennsylvania, University of Pennsylvania, Philadelphia, Pennsylvania
*Antiemetic Therapy*

**ROBERT V. ENGLISH, D.V.M., Ph.D.**
Visiting Assistant Professor, College of Veterinary Medicine, North Carolina State University, Raleigh, North Carolina
*Feline Immunodeficiency Virus*

**RICHARD H. EVANS, D.V.M., M.S.**
Veterinary Pathology Services, Laguna Niguel, California
*Nutritional and Environmental Considerations in Neonatal Medicine*

**GEORGE E. EYSTER, V.M.D., M.S., Dipl. A.C.V.S.**
Professor, Department of Small Animal Clinical Sciences, College of Veterinary Medicine, Michigan State University, East Lansing, Michigan
*Patent Ductus Arteriosus*

**DANIEL A. FEENEY, D.V.M., M.S., Dipl. A.C.V.R.**
Professor of Radiology, College of Veterinary Medicine, University of Minnesota, Staff Radiologist, Veterinary Teaching Hospital, College of Veterinary Medicine, University of Minnesota, St Paul, Minnesota
*Imaging the Reproductive Tract in the Male Dog*

**EDWARD C. FELDMAN, D.V.M., Dipl. A.C.V.I.M.**

Professor and Chief of Service, Small Animal Medicine, Department of Medicine, School of Veterinary Medicine, University of California, Davis, California

*Diagnosis and Treatment of Macrotumors in Dogs with Pituitary-Dependent Hyperadrenocorticism; Transplantation as a Means of Treating Diabetes Mellitus; Treatment of Feline Diabetes Mellitus with the Oral Sulfonylurea Glipizide*

**LAWRENCE J. FELICE, Ph.D.**

Associate Professor, College of Veterinary Medicine, University of Minnesota, St. Paul, Minnesota

*CVT Update: Anticoagulant Rodenticides*

**WILLIAM R. FENNER, D.V.M., Dipl. A.C.V.I.M. (Neurology)**

Associate Professor, Veterinary Clinical Sciences, College of Veterinary Medicine, The Ohio State University, Columbus, Ohio

*Uremic Encephalopathy*

**DUNCAN C. FERGUSON, V.M.D., Ph.D., Dipl. A.C.V.I.M.**

Professor Physiology and Pharmacology and of Small Animal Medicine, The University of Georgia College of Veterinary Medicine, The University of Georgia, Athens, Georgia

*Free Thyroid Hormone Measurements in the Diagnosis of Thyroid Disease*

**DELMAR R. FINCO, D.V.M., Ph.D., Dipl. A.C.V.I.M.**

Professor, Department of Physiology, College of Veterinary Medicine, University of Georgia, Athens, Georgia

*Inappropriate Dietary Protein and Mineral Restriction in Dogs and Cats; Reassessment of the Use of Calcitriol in Chronic Renal Failure; The Role of Dimethyl Sulfoxide and Glucocorticoids in Lower Urinary Tract Diseases; Medical Management of Canine Prostatic Hyperplasia*

**JAMES M. FINGEROTH, D.V.M., Dipl. A.C.V.S.**

Chief of Surgery, Veterinary Specialists of Rochester, Rochester, New York

*Treatment of Canine Intervertebral Disk Disease: Recommendations and Controversies*

**ROGER B. FINGLAND, D.V.M., M.S., Dipl. A.C.V.S.**

Associate Professor, Chief, Small Animal Surgery, Kansas State University; General Surgeon, Veterinary Medical Teaching Hospital, College of Veterinary Medicine, Kansas State University, Manhattan, Kansas

*Temporary Tracheostomy*

**RICHARD B. FORD, D.V.M., M.S., Dipl. A.C.V.I.M.**

Associate Professor of Medicine, College of Veterinary Medicine, North Carolina State University, Raleigh, North Carolina

*Infectious Tracheobronchitis*

**THERESA W. FOSSUM, D.V.M., M.S., Ph.D., Dipl. A.C.V.S.**

Associate Professor, Texas A&M University; Staff Surgeon, Texas Veterinary Medical Center, College of Veterinary Medicine, Texas A&M University, College Station, Texas

*Lung Lobe Torsion*

**JAMES G. FOX, D.V.M., Dipl.. A.C.L.A.M.**

Professor and Director, Division of Comparative Medicine, Massachusetts Institute of Technology, Cambridge, Massachusetts; Adjunct Professor, Tufts University School of Veterinary Medicine, Tufts University, North Grafton, Massachusetts; Adjunct Professor, University of Pennsylvania School of Veterinary Medicine, University of Pennsylvania, Philadelphia, Pennsylvania

*Helicobacter-Associated Gastric Disease in Ferrets, Dogs, and Cats; Desulfovibrio-Associated Proliferative Colitis in Ferrets*

**LESLIE E. FOX, D.V.M., M.S., Dipl. A.C.V.I.M (Internal Medicine)**

Assistant Professor, University of Florida College of Veterinary Medicine, Gainesville, Florida

*The Paraneoplastic Disorders*

**PHILIP R. FOX, D.V.M., M.Sc., Dipl. A.C.V.I.M. (Cardiology)**

Chairman, Department of Clinical Services, The Animal Medical Center; Staff Cardiologist, Department of Medicine, The Animal Medical Center, New York, New York

*Angiotensin-Converting Enzyme Inhibitors; Myocarditis in the Dog and Cat; Restrictive Cardiomyopathy*

**DEBORAH S. FRIEDMAN, D.V.M., Dipl. A.C.V.O.**

Animal Eye Care, Fremont, California

*Infectious Feline Keratoconjunctivitis*

**TAM GARLAND, D.V.M., Ph.D., Dipl. A.B.V.T.**

Research Associate, Department of Veterinary Physiology and Pharmacology, College of Veterinary Medicine, Texas A&M University, College Station, Texas

*Toxic Ornamental and Garden Plants*

**DIANE F. GERKEN, D.V.M., Ph.D., Dipl. A.B.V.T.**

Associate Professor, Department of Veterinary Biosciences The Ohio State University, Columbus, Ohio

*Lawn Care Products*

**LAUREL J. GERSHWIN, D.V.M., Ph.D., Dipl. A.C.V.M.**

School of Veterinary Medicine, University of California, Davis; Director of Clinical Immunology and Virology Laboratory, Veterinary Medicine Teaching Hospital. University of California, Davis, California

*Monoclonal Antibodies: Applications in Diagnosis and Treatment*


**STEPHEN D. GILSON, D.V.M.**

Surgeon and Owner, Sonora Veterinary Surgery and Oncology, Scottsdale, Arizona

*Transitional Cell Carcinoma: Surgical Limitations*


**HELEN GLOBUS, D.V.M.**

Resident in Comparative Dermatology, University of Minnesota, St. Paul, Minnesota

*Canine Otitis Externa*


**NEIL T. GORMAN, B.V.Sc., Ph.D., F.R.C.U.S., Dipl. A.C.V.I.M**

Head of Research, Waltham Centre for Pet Nutrition, Melton Mowbray, Leceistershire, United Kingdom

*Tumor Immunology and Tumor Immunotherapy*


**GREGORY F. GRAUER, D.V.M., M.S., Dipl. A.C.V.I.M. (Internal Medicine)**

Associate Professor, Department of Clinical Sciences, College of Veterinary Medicine and Biomedical Sciences, Colorado State University, Staff Internist, Veterinary Teaching Hospital, College of Veterinary Medicine and Biomedical Sciences, Colorado State University, Fort Collins, Colorado

*Antifreeze Poisoning; Prevention of Hospital-Acquired Acute Renal Failure*


**THOMAS K. GRAVES, D.V.M.**

Instructor, Department of Small Animal Clinical Sciences, College of Veterinary Medicine, Michigan State University, Resident in Internal Medicine, Small Animal Hospital, Michigan State University, East Lansing, Michigan

*Complications of Treatment and Concurrent Illness Associated with Hyperthyroidism in Cats*


**DEBORAH S. GRECO, D.V.M., Ph.D., Dipl. A.C.V.I.M.**

Assistant Professor, Department of Clinical Sciences, College of Veterinary Medicine and Biomedical Sciences, Colorado State University, Fort Collins, Colorado

*Pediatric Endocrinology; Clinical Applications of Glucocorticoid Therapy in Nonendocrine Disease; Corticosteroid Withdrawal Syndrome*


**CRAIG E. GREENE, D.V.M., M.S., Dipl. A.C.V.I.M. (Internal Medicine, Neurology)**

Professor, Department of Small Animal Medicine, College of Veterinary Medicine, University of Georgia; Veterinary Medical Teaching Hospital, University of Georgia, Athens, Georgia

*Pet Ownership for Immunocompromised People*


**RUSSELL T. GREENE, D.V.M., Ph.D., Dipl. A.C.V.I.M. (Internal Medicine), A.C.V.M. (Bacteriology and Mycology)**

Staff Veterinarian at Southwest Diagnostics, Inc., and Phoenix Veterinary Internal Medicine Services, Phoenix, Arizona

*Canine Ehrlichiosis: Clinical Implications for Humoral Factors*


**WILLIAM F. GREENTREE, D.V.M.**

Ophthalmology Resident, Iowa State University, College of Veterinary Medicine, Department of Veterinary Clinical Sciences, Ames, Iowa; *formerly*, Staff Veterinarian, National Animal Poison Control Center, University of Illinois, College of Veterinary Medicine, Urbana, Illinois

*Iron Toxicosis*


**CLARE R. GREGORY, D.V.M.**

Associate Professor, Department of Surgical and Radiological Sciences, School of Veterinary Medicine, University of California; Chief, Small Animal Surgical Sciences, Veterinary Medical Teaching Hospital, School of Veterinary Medicine, University of California, Davis, California

*Transplantation Immunology*


**AMY M. GROOTERS, D.V.M.**

Clinical Assistant Professor, Department of Veterinary Medicine and Surgery, University of Missouri; Internist, Veterinary Teaching Hospital, University of Missouri, Columbia, Missouri

*Budd-Chiari–Like Syndromes in Dogs; Ultrasonographic Findings in Renal Disease*


**THELMA LEE GROSS, D.V.M., Dipl. A.C.V.P.**

Pathologist, California Dermatopathology Service, Consulting Pathologist, Consolidated Veterinary Diagnostics, West Sacramento, California

*Hereditary Lupoid Dermatosis of the German Shorthaired Pointer; Canine Mucocutaneous Pyoderma; Ulcerative Dermatosis of Shetland Sheepdogs and Collies*


**W. GRANT GUILFORD, B.V.Sc., B.Phil. Ph.D., F.A.C.U.Sc., Dipl. A.C.V.I.M.**

Senior Lecturer, Massey University; Internist, Small Animal Veterinary Clinic, Massey University, Palmerston North, New Zealand

*Breed-Associated Gastrointestinal Disease*

**TIMOTHY B. HACKETT, D.V.M., M.S.**

Resident, Emergency Medicine and Critical Care, Colorado State University, Fort Collins, Colorado; Staff Internist, VCA West Los Angeles Animal Hospital, Los Angeles, California

*Cardiopulmonary Resuscitation*

**SUSAN HACKNER, B.V.Sc., M.R.C.V.S., Dipl. A.C.V.I.M.**

Director, Intensive Care Unit, Veterinary Referral Associates, Incorporated, Gaithersburg, Maryland

*Oxygen Supplementation*

**JAN A. HALL, B.V.M. & S., M.S., Dipl. A.C.V.D., M.R.C.V.S.**

Clinical Dermatologist, College of Veterinary Medicine and Biomedical Sciences, Colorado State University Veterinary Teaching Hospital, Colorado State University, Fort Collins, Colorado

*The Effect of Potentiated Sulfonamides on Canine Thyroid Function*

**JEFFREY O. HALL, D.V.M., Dipl. A.B.V.T.**

Associate Director, National Animal Poison Control Center, College of Veterinary Medicine, University of Illinois, Urbana, Illinois

*Iron Toxicosis*

**ROBERT L. HAMLIN, D.V.M., Ph.D., Dipl. A.C.V.I.M.**

Professor, Department of Physiology and Pharmacology, College of Veterinary Medicine, The Ohio State University College of Veterinary Medicine, Columbus, Ohio

*Recognition and Treatment of Pulmonary Hypertension*

**ALAN S. HAMMER, D.V.M., Dipl. A.M.V.I.M., (Internal Medicine Oncology)**

Director of Medicine, Criticare Veterinary Services, Louisville, Kentucky

*Nonsurgical Management of Soft Tissue Sarcomas*

**BERNIE HANSEN, D.V.M., M.S., Dipl. A.C.V.I.M., A.C.V.E.C.C.**

Visiting Assistant Professor, College of Veterinary Medicine, North Carolina State University, Raleigh, North Carolina

*Blood Pressure Measurement*

**STEVEN R. HANSEN, D.V.M., M.S., Dipl. A.B.T.**

Manager, Technical Services, Sandoz Animal Health, Des Plaines, Illinois

*Management of Adverse Reactions to Pyrethrin and Pyrethroid Insecticides; Management of Organophosphate and Carbamate Insecticide Toxicoses*

**ANN M. HARGIS, D.V.M., M.S., Dipl. A.C.V.P.**

Affiliate Associate Professor, Department of Comparative Medicine, University of Washington, Seattle, Washington; Owner, DermatoDiagnostics, Edmonds, Washington, Consultant, Phoenix Central Laboratory, Everett, Washington

*The Diagnosis of Sebaceous Adenitis in Standard Poodle Dogs*

**NEIL K. HARPSTER, V.M.D., Dipl. A.C.V.I.M. (Cardiology)**

Adjunct Professor, Tufts University School of Veterinary Medicine, Tufts University, North Grafton; Director of Cardiology, Angell Memorial Animal Hospital, Boston, Massachusetts

*Warfarin Therapy of the Cat at Risk of Thromboembolism*

**JOHN W. HARVEY, D.V.M., Ph.D., Dipl. A.C.V.P.**

Professor of Clinical Pathology, University of Florida College of Veterinary Medicine; Chief, Clinical Pathology Service, Veterinary Medicine Teaching Hospital, University of Florida College of Veterinary Medicine, Gainesville, Florida

*Methemoglobinemia and Heinz-Body Hemolytic Anemia*

**STEVE C. HASKINS, D.V.M., M.S. Dipl. A.C.V.E.C.C.**

Professor, Department of Surgery and Radiology, School of Veterinary Medicine, University of California; Director, Small Animal Intensive Care Unit, Veterinary Medical Teaching Hospital, School of Veterinary Medicine, University of California, Davis, California

*Monitoring the Critically Ill Patient*

**ELEANOR C. HAWKINS, D.V.M., Dipl. A.C.V.I.M.**

Associate Professor of Medicine, Department of Companion Animal and Special Species Medicine, College of Veterinary Medicine, North Carolina State University; Internist, Veterinary Teaching Hospital, North Carolina State University, Raleigh, North Carolina

*Aspiration Pneumonia*

**R. GAYMEN HELMAN, Ph.D. Dipl. A.C.V.P.**

Clinical Assistant Professor, Department of Veterinary Pathobiology, College of Veterinary Medicine, Texas A&M University, College Station, Texas

*Canine Chagas' Myocarditis*

**JOAN C. HENDRICKS, V.M.D., Ph.D., Dipl. A.C.V.I.M.**

Associate Professor of Medicine, School of Veterinary Medicine, University of Pennsylvania; Vice Chair, Department of Clinical Studies, Veterinary Hospital of the University of Pennsylvania, Philadelphia, Pennsylvania

*Pulse Oximetry; End-Tidal Carbon Dioxide Monitoring; Recognition and Treatment of Congenital Respiratory Tract Defects in Brachycephalics*

**CAROLYN J. HENRY, D.V.M., M.S. Dipl. A.C.V.I.M. (Oncology)**

Assistant Professor, College of Veterinary Medicine, Washington State University, Pullman, Washington

*Drug Interactions with Antineoplastic Agents*

**KAREN HICKS-ALLDREDGE, D.V.M.**

Sweetwater Veterinary Hospital, Sweetwater, Texas

*Ostrich Management*

**STEVEN L. HILL, D.V.M.**

Resident, Small Animal Medicine, Department of Clinical Sciences, College of Veterinary Medicine and Biomedical Sciences, Colorado State University, Fort Collins, Colorado

*Cryptosporidiosis in the Dog and Cat*

**ELIZABETH V. HILLYER, D.V.M.**

Hillyer Medical Writing and Editing, Oldwick, New Jersey

*Blood Collection and Transfusion in Ferrets*

**DWIGHT C. HIRSH, D.V.M., Ph.D.**

Professor of Microbiology, Department of Pathology, Microbiology, Immunology, School of Veterinary Medicine, University of California, Davis; Chief, Microbiology Service, Veterinary Medical Teaching Hospital, School of Veterinary Medicine, University of California, Davis, California

*Optimizing Laboratory Diagnosis of Infectious Diseases*

**MARK E. HITT, D.V.M., M.S., Dipl. A.C.V.I.M.**

Chesapeake Veterinary Referral Center, Annapolis, Maryland

*Biopsy of the Gastrointestinal Tract*

**HEIDI L. HOEFER, D.V.M., Dipl., A.B.V.P.**

Staff Veterinarian, Department of Avian and Exotic Pets, The Animal Medical Center, New York, New York

*Antimicrobials in Pet Birds*

**ANN E. HOHENHAUS, D.V.M., Dipl. A.C.V.I.M. (Oncology)**

The Animal Medical Center, Staff Oncologist, The Donaldson-Atwood Cancer Clinic, New York, New York

*Syndromes of Hyperglobulinemia: Diagnosis and Therapy*

**MOLLYANN HOLLAND, D.V.M.**

Small Animal Medicine Resident, College of Veterinary Medicine, University of Missouri; Small Animal Medicine Resident, Veterinary Medical Teaching Hospital, University of Missouri, Columbia, Missouri

*Uses and Misuses of Aspirin*

**PETER E. HOLT, B.V.M.S., Ph.D., C.Biol., M.I.Biol., Dipl. E.C.V.S., F.R.C.V.S.**

Senior Lecturer, University of Bristol, Bristol, Avon, United Kingdom

*Feline Urinary Incontinence*

**CARL S. HORNFELDT, M.S., Dipl., A.B.A.T.**

Clinical Assistant Professor, College of Pharmacy, University of Minnesota; Veterinary Service Coordinator, Hennepin Regional Poison Center, Hennepin County Medical Center, Minneapolis, Minnesota

*Incidence of Small Animal Poison Exposures in a Major Metropolitan Area*

**JOHNNY D. HOSKINS, D.V.M., Ph.D., Dipl., A.C.V.I.M.**

Professor, Department of Veterinary Clinical Medicine, School of Veterinary Medicine, Louisiana State University, Baton Rouge, Louisiana

*Fading Puppy and Kitten Syndrome; Fluid Therapy in the Puppy and Kittens*

**MICHAEL J. HUERKAMP, D.V.M., Dipl. A.C.L.A.M.**

Assistant Professor, Department of Pathology and Laboratory Medicine, Emory University School of Medicine; Chief, Laboratory Animal Medicine, Division of Animal Resources, Medical Administration, Emory University School of Medicine, Atlanta, Georgia

*Anesthesia and Postoperative Management of Rabbits and Pocket Pets*

**KARYL J. HURLEY, D.V.M.**

Resident, Internal Medicine, North Carolina State University, Raleigh, North Carolina

*Proteinuria in Dogs and Cats: A Diagnostic Approach*

**PETER J. IHRKE, V.M.D., Dipl. A.C.V.D.**

Professor of Dermatology, School of Veterinary Medicine, University of California, Davis, California; Adjunct Clinical Professor of Dermatology, School of Medicine, Stanford University, Palo Alto, California; Chief of Dermatology Service, Veterinary Medical Teaching Hospital, School of Veterinary Medicine, University of California, Davis, California

*The Use of Synthetic Retinoids in Veterinary Medicine; Canine Mucocutaneous Pyoderma; Ulcerative Dermatosis of Shetland Sheepdogs and Collies*

**RAMIRO ISAZA, D.V.M., M.S.**

Clinical Instructor, Department of Small Animal Clinical Sciences, College of Veterinary Medicine, University of Florida, Gainesville, Florida

*Non-Nutritional Bone Diseases in Reptiles*

**RANDALL J. ITKIN, D.V.M., M.S.**

Research Associate, Department of Veterinary Biosciences, University of Illinois, Urbana, Illinois

*When and How to Measure Glomerular Filtration Rate and Effective Renal Plasma Flow*

**ROBERT M. JACOBS, D.V.M., Ph.D., Dipl. A.C.V.P.**

Professor of Pathology Chief, Clinical Pathology Service, Department of Pathology, Ontario Veterinary College, University of Guelph, Guelph, Ontario, Canada

*Appendices, Consulting Editor*

**R. H. JACOBSON, Ph.D., M.S.**

Associate Professor, College of Veterinary Medicine, Cornell University, Ithaca, New York

*CVT Update: Canine Lyme Disease*

**ELLIOTT R. JACOBSON, D.V.M., Ph.D., Dipl. A.C.Z.M.**

Professor, Wildlife and Zoological Medicine, College of Veterinary Medicine, University of Florida; Chief of Service, Wildlife and Zoological Medicine, Gainesville, Florida

*Non-Nutritional Bone Diseases in Reptiles*

**KATHERINE M. JAMES, D.V.M.**

Resident, Small Animal Internal Medicine, University of Minnesota College of Veterinary Medicine, St. Paul, Minnesota

*Metabolic Acidosis in Renal Failure: Consequences, Diagnosis, and Treatment*

**ALBERT E. JERGENS, D.V.M., M.S., Dipl., A.C.V.I.M.**

Assistant Professor, Department of Veterinary Clinical Sciences, College of Veterinary Medicine, Iowa State University, Ames, Iowa

*Acute Diarrhea*

**CHERI A. JOHNSON, D.V.M., M.S., Dipl., A.C.V.I.M. (Internal Medicine)**

Professor, Department of Small Animal Clinical Sciences, College of Veterinary Medicine, Michigan State University, East Lansing, Michigan

*Management of Brucella Canis Outbreaks in Breeding Kennels*

**KENNETH A. JOHNSON, M.V.Sc., Ph.D., FACVSc, Dipl. A.C.V.S.**

Associate Professor of Surgery, Department of Surgical Sciences, School of Veterinary Medicine, University of Wisconsin-Madison, Madison, Wisconsin

*Treatment of Osteomyelitis, Discospondylitis, and Septic Arthritis*

**LYNELLE R. JOHNSON, D.V.M., Dipl., A.C.V.I.M. (Internal Medicine)**

Post-Doctoral Fellowship in Radiation Oncology, College of Veterinary Medicine and Biomedical Sciences, Colorado State University, Fort Collins, Colorado

*Recognition and Treatment of Pulmonary Hypertension*

**GARY R. JOHNSTON, D.V.M., M.S., Dipl. A.C.V.R.**

Professor, Department of Small Animal Clinical Sciences, College of Veterinary Medicine, University of Minnesota; Professor of Radiology, Veterinary Teaching Hospital, University of Minnesota, St. Paul, Minnesota

*Imaging the Reproductive Tract in the Male Dog*

**SHIRLEY D. JOHNSTON, D.V.M., Ph.D., Dipl. A.C.T.**

Professor, Department of Small Animal Clinical Sciences, College of Veterinary Medicine, University of Minnesota, St. Paul, Minnesota

*Pregnancy Termination in the Bitch Using Prostaglandin $F_{2\alpha}$; Complications of Noncopulatory Ovulation in Queens; Canine Prostetic Disorders*

**SPENCER A. JOHNSTON, V.M.D., Dipl. A.C.V.S.**

Assistant Professor, Department of Small Animal Clinical Sciences, Virginia-Maryland Regional College of Veterinary Medicine, Virginia Tech, Blacksburg, Virginia

*Patent Ductus Arteriosus*

**BOYD R. JONES, B.V.Sc., F.A.C.V.Sc., M.R.C.V.S.**

Associate Professor in Small Animal Medicine, Palmerston North, New Zealand

*Hyperchylomicronemia in the Cat*

**LENNART H. JÖNSSON, D.V.M., Ph.D.**

Professor of Pathology, Faculty of Veterinary Medicine, Swedish University of Agricultural Sciences, Uppsala, Sweden

*Pathogenic Aspects of Chronic Liver Disease in the Dog*

**HOLLY L. JORDAN, D.V.M.**

College of Veterinary Medicine, North Carolina State University, Raleigh, North Carolina

*Canine and Feline Mycobacterial Infection*

**SANJAY KAPIL, D.V.M., M.S., Ph.D., A.C.V.M.**

Assistant Professor, College of Veterinary Medicine, Veterinary Diagnostic Investigation, Manhattan, Kansas

*Laboratory Diagnosis of Canine Viral Enteritis*

**BRUCE W. KEENE, D.V.M., M.S., Dipl. A.C.V.I.M. (Cardiology)**

Associate Professor, College of Veterinary Medicine, North Carolina State University, Raleigh, North Carolina

*Section 9, Consulting Editor; Therapy of Heart Failure; Myocarditis in the Dog and Cat*

**ROBERT J. KEMPPAINEN, D.V.M., Ph.D.**

Professor of Physiology and Pharmacology, Director of Endocrine Diagnostic Laboratory, Auburn University College of Veterinary Medicine, Auburn University, Auburn, Alabama

*CVT Update: Sample Collection and Testing Protocols in Endocrinology*

**THOMAS J. KERN, D.V.M., Dipl. A.C.V.O.**

Associate Professor of Ophthalmology, College of Veterinary Medicine, Cornell University, Ithaca, New York

*Canine Uveitis*

**STEPHEN J. KERPSACK, D.V.M., M.S.**

Clinical Instructor, Small Animal Surgery, College of Veterinary Medicine, The Ohio State University, Columbus, Ohio

*Management of Feline Chylothorax*

**LESLEY G. KING, M.V.B., M.R.C.V.S., Dipl. A.C.V.I.M., A.C.V.E.C.C.**

Assistant Professor, Seciton of Medicine, Department of Clinical Studies, School of Veterinary Medicine, University of Pennsylvania; Director, Intensive Care Unit, Veterinary Hospital of the University of Pennsylvania, University of Pennsylvania, Philadelphia, Pennsylvania

*Outcome Prediction in Emergency and Critical Care Patients*

**PETER P. KINTZER, D.V.M., Dipl. A.C.V.I.M.**

Clinical Assistant Professor, Department of Medicine, Assistant Director, Division of Laboratory Animal Medicine, Tufts University School of Veterinary Medicine, Tufts University; Clinician, Foster Hospital for Small Animals, Tufts New England Veterinary Medical Center, Tufts University, North Grafton, Massachusetts

*Mitotane (o,p'-DDD) Treatment of Hyperadrenocorticism in Dogs; Hypoadrenocorticism in Dogs*

**REBECCA KIRBY, D.V.M., Dipl. A.C.V.I.M., A.C.V.E.C.C.**

Director of Education, Veterinary Institute of Trauma, Emergency and Critical Care; Chief of Medicine, Animal Emergency Center, Milwaukee, Wisconsin

*Septic Shock*

**BARBARA E. KITCHELL, D.V.M., Ph.D., Dipl. A.C.V.I.M. (Internal Medicine, Oncology)**

Assistant Professor, College of Veterinary Medicine, University of Illinois, Urbana, Illinois

*Mammary Tumors*

**MARK D. KITTLESON, D.V.M., Ph.D.**

Professor of Medicine, Department of Medicine, School of Veterinary Medicine, University of California, Davis, California

*CVT Update: Feline Hypertrophic Cardiomyopathy*

**JEFFREY S. KLAUSNER, D.V.M., M.S., Dipl. A.C.V.I.M. (Internal Medicine, Oncology)**

Professor and Chair, Department of Small Animal Clinical Sciences, College of Veterinary Medicine, University of Minnesota, St. Paul, Minnesota

*Clinical Epidemiology for the Veterinary Practitioner: The Diagnostic Process; Canine and Feline Calcium Phosphate Urolithiasis; Canine Prostatic Disorders*

**MARY KAY KLEIN, D.V.M., M.S., Dipl. A.C.V.I.M. (Oncology)**

Clinical Lecturer, College of Medicine, University of Arizona, Tucson, Arizona

*Anticancer Drugs: Dose Schedule and Guidelines*

**KAREN L. KLINE, B.S., D.V.M., Dipl. A.C.V.I.M. (Neurology)**

Clinical Instructor in Neurology, College of Veterinary Medicine, University of Missouri, Columbia, Missouri

*Congenital and Inherited Neurologic Disorders in Dogs and Cats*

**DEBORAH W. KNAPP, D.V.M., M.S., Dipl. A.C.V.I.M. (Oncology)**
Assistant Professor in Comparative Oncology, Department of Veterinary Clinical Sciences, Purdue University, West Lafayette, Indiana
*Medical Therapy of Canine Transitional Cell Carcinoma of the Urinary Bladder*

**DAVID H. KNIGHT, D.V.M., Dipl. A.C.V.I.M. (Cardiology)**
Professor of Cardiology, School of Veterinary Medicine, University of Pennsylvania; Chief, Section of Cardiology, Veterinary Hospital, University of Pennsylvania, Philadelphia, Pennsylvania
*Guidelines for Diagnosis and Management of Heartworm (Dirofilaria Immitis) Infection*

**JAN KOMTEBEDDE, D.V.M.**
Staff Surgeon, Solano Veterinary Consultants, Cordelia, California
*Feline Portosystemic Vascular Shunts*

**DORSEY L. KORDICK, B.S.**
Graduate Student, North Carolina State University, Raleigh, North Carolina
*Feline Rickettsial Diseases*

**DONALD R. KRAWIEC, D.V.M., M.S., Ph.D., Dipl. A.C.V.I.M.**
Associate Professor of Clinical Veterinary Medicine, Department of Veterinary Clinical Medicine, University of Illinois; Chief, Small Animal Medicine Section, Department of Veterinary Clinical Medicine, University of Illinois, Urbana, Illinois
*When and How to Measure Glomerular Filtration Rate and Effective Renal Plasma Flow*

**STEPHEN A. KRUTH, D.V.M., Dipl. A.C.V.I.M (Internal Medicine)**
Professor, Department of Clinical Studies, Ontario Veterinary College, University of Guelph, Guelph, Ontario, Canada
*Cytokines and Biologic Response Modifiers in Small Animal Practice*

**BARBARA A. KUMMEL, D.V.M.**
Staff Dermatologist/Allergist, Veterinary Referral Associates, Gaithersburg, Maryland
*Medical Treatment of Canine Pemphigus-Penphigoid*

**KENNETH W. KWOCHKA, D.V.M., Dipl. A.C.V.D.**
Associate Professor of Dermatology, Department of Veterinary Clinical Sciences, College of Veterinary Medicine, The Ohio State University; Chief of Dermatology Service, Veterinary Teaching Hospital, College of Veterinary Medicine, The Ohio State University, Columbus, Ohio
*Shampoos and Moisturizing Rinses in Veterinary Dermatology*

**MARY ANNA LABATO, D.V.M., Dipl. A.C.V.I.M.**
Clinical Assistant Professor, Department of Medicine, Tufts University School of Veterinary Medicine; Staff Veterinarian, Foster Hospital for Small Animals, Tufts University School of Veterinary Medicine, Tufts University, North Grafton, Massachusetts
*Nutritional Support in Uremia*

**JERRY LABONDE, M.S., D.V.M.**
Colorado State University, Fort Collins; Avian and Exotic Animal Hospital, Englewood, Colorado
*Household Poisonings in Caged Birds*

**LAUREL LAGONI, M.S.**
Co-Director, Changes: The Support for People and Pets Program, Department of Veterinary Clinical Sciences, College of Veterinary Medicine and Biomedical Sciences, Veterinary Teaching Hospital, Colorado State University, Fort Collins, Colorado
*Facilitating Owner-Present Euthanasia*

**INDIA F. LANE, D.V.M., M.S., Dipl. A.C.V.I.M.**
Assistant Professor, Department of Companion Animals, Atlantic Veterinary College, University of Prince Edward Island; Internist, University of Prince Edward Island, Charlottetown, Prince Edward Island, Canada
*Urinary Incontinence and Congenital Urogenital Anomalies in Small Animals*

**GARY C. LANTZ, D.V.M., Dipl. A.C.V.S.**
Professor of Surgery, School of Veterinary Medicine, Purdue University, West Lafayette, Indiana
*Oxygen Free Radicals and Reperfusion Injury*

**MICHAEL R. LAPPIN, D.V.M., Ph.D., Dipl. A.C.V.I.M.**
Associate Professor, Department of Clinical Sciences, College of Veterinary Medicine and Biomedical Sciences, Colorado State University, Fort Collins, Colorado
*Immunopathologic Consequences of Infectious Diseases; Feline Rickettsial Diseases; CVT Update: Feline Toxoplasmosis; Cryptosporidiosis in the Dog and Cat; Urinary Incontinence and Congenital Urogenital Anomalies in Small Animals*

**SUSAN M. LARUE, D.V.M., Ph.D.**
Assistant Professor of Radiation Oncology, Department of Radiological Health Sciences, Colorado State University; Radiation Oncologist, Colorado State University Veterinary Teaching Hospital, Colorado State University, Fort Collins, Colorado
*Radiation Therapy for Pituitary Tumors*

**KENNETH S. LATIMER, D.V.M., Ph.D., Dipl. A.C.V.P.**

Professor of Pathology, The University of Georgia College of Veterinary Medicine, Athens, Georgia

*Avian Polyomavirus; Psittacine Beak and Feather Disease Virus*

**DENNIS F. LAWLER, D.V.M.**

Senior Research Veterinarian, Ralston Purina Company, St. Louis, Missouri

*Nutritional and Environmental Considerations in Neonatal Medicine; Complications of Noncopulatory Ovulation in Queens*

**ALFRED M. LEGENDRE, D.V.M., M.S., Dipl. A.C.V.I.M.**

Professor of Medicine, University of Tennessee, Knoxville, Tennessee

*Antimycotic Drug Therapy*

**LINDA B. LEHMKUHL, D.V.M., M.S., Dipl. A.C.V.I.M.**

Assistant Professor, The Ohio State University; Cardiologist, Veterinary Teaching Hospital, The Ohio State University, Columbus, Ohio

*CVT Update: Canine Subvalvular Aortic Stenosis*

**MICHAEL S. LEIB, D.V.M., M.S., Dipl. A.C.V.I.M.**

Professor, Small Animal Medicine, Virginia-Maryland Regional College of Veterinary Medicine, Virginia Tech; Staff Internist, Virginia Tech, Blacksburg, Virginia

*Giardia: Diagnosis and Treatment*

**CYNTHIA R. LEVEILLE-WEBSTER, D.V.M., Dipl. A.C.V.I.M.**

Clinical Assistant Professor, Tufts University School of Veterinary Medicine, Tufts University, North Grafton, Massachusetts

*Chronic Hepatitis: Therapeutic Considerations*

**JULIE K. LEVY, D.V.M., Dipl. A.C.V.I.M.**

Research Assistant, Department of Microbiology, Pathology, and Parasitology, College of Veterinary Medicine, North Carolina State University, Raleigh, North Carolina

*Feline Portosystemic Vascular Shunts*

**GREGORY A. LEWBART, M.S., V.M.D.**

Assistant Professor of Aquatic Medicine, North Carolina State University College of Veterinary Medicine, Raleigh, North Carolina; Adjunct Associate Professor, University of Pennsylvania School of Veterinary Medicine (Pathology), Philadelphia, Pennsylvania

*Emergency Pet Fish Medicine*

**CATHARINA LINDE-FORSBERG, D.V.M., Ph.D.**

Associate Professor of Small Animal Reproduction, Department of Obstetrics and Gynaecology, Faculty of Veterinary Medicine, Swedish University of Agricultural Sciences, Uppsala, Sweden

*Canine Genital Mycoplasmas and Ureaplasmas*

**GERALD V. LING, D.V.M.**

Professor of Medicine, Urinary Stone Analysis Laboratory, Department of Medicine, School of Veterinary Medicine, University of California, Davis, California

*Nephrolithiasis: Prevalence of Mineral Type; CVT Update: Management and Prevention of Urate Urolithiasis*

**WILLIAM D. LISKA, D.V.M., Dipl. A.C.V.S.**

Referral Surgeon, Gulf Coast Veterinary Specialists, Houston, Texas

*The Roles of the Veterinarian and the Veterinary Specialist in Management of Neurologic and Musculoskeletal Problems*

**SI-KWANG LIU, D.V.M., Ph.D.**

Professor of Comparative Pathology, New York Medical College, Visiting Professor of Pathology, National Taiwan University, Taiwan, Republic of China; Senior Pathologist, The Animal Medical Center, New York, New York; Senior Researcher and Consultant, Pig Research Institute, Taiwan, Republic of China; Scientific Fellow, New York Zoological Society, Consultant, Molecular Cardiology Studies, Cornell Medical Center, New York, New York

*Myocarditis in the Dog and Cat*

**CLINTON D. LOTHROP, JR., D.V.M., Ph.D., Dipl. A.C.V.I.M**

Professor, Auburn University College of Veterinary Medicine, Department of Small Animal Surgery and Medicine, Scott Ritchey Research Program, Auburn, Alabama

*Congenital Adrenal Hyperplasia-Like Syndrome*

**JODY P. LULICH, D.V.M., Ph.D., Dipl. A.C.V.I.M.**

Assistant Professor, Department of Small Animal Clinical Sciences, College of Veterinary Medicine, University of Minnesota, St. Paul, Minnesota

*Ten Guiding Principles to Enhance the Benefit of Current Veterinary Therapy; Treatment of Uremic Anorexia; Canine and Feline Nephroliths; Feline Calcium Oxalate Uroliths; Canine Calcium Oxalate Uroliths; Canine and Feline Calcium Phosphate Urolithiasis; Voiding Urohydropropulsion: A Nonsurgical Technique for Removal of Urocystoliths*

**JOHN H. LUMSDEN, D.V.M., M.Sc., Dipl. A.C.V.P.**

Professor, Department of Pathology, Ontario Veterinary College, University of Guelph, Guelph, Ontario, Canada

*Appendices*

**ELIZABETH M. LUND, D.V.M., M.P.H.**

Postdoctoral Fellow, College of Veterinary Medicine, University of Minnesota, St. Paul, Minnesota

*Clinical Epidemiology for the Veterinary Practitioner: The Diagnostic Process*

**NANCY P. LUNG, V.M.D., M.S.**

Director of Animal Health, Fort Worth Zoological Association, Forth Worth, Texas

*Current Approaches to Feather Picking*

**ROSLYN G. MACHON, B.V.Sc. (Hona), M.V.Sc.**

Resident, Comparative Anesthesiology, Department of Small Animal Clinical Sciences, College of Veterinary Medicine, University of Minnesota, St. Paul, Minnesota

*Propofol: A New Sedative-Hypnotic Anesthetic Agent*

**DOUGLASS K. MACINTIRE, D.V.M., M.S., Dipl. A.C.V.I.M., Dipl. A.C.V.E.C.C.**

Assistant Professor, Small Animal Internal Medicine, Auburn University; Director, Intensive Care Unit, Small Animal Clinic, College of Veterinary Medicine, Auburn University, Auburn, Alabama

*The Practical Use of Constant-Rate Infusions*

**JILL E. MADDISON, B.V.Sc., Ph.D., F.A.C.U.Sc.**

Senior Lecturer, Department of Pharmacology, The University of Sydney, New South Wales, Australia

*Medical Management of Chronic Hepatic Encephalopathy*

**BRUCE R. MADEWELL, V.M.D., M.S., Dipl. A.C.V.I.M. (Oncology, Internal Medicine)**

Professor, Department of Veterinary Surgery and Radiological Sciences, University of California; Chief, Oncology Service, Veterinary Medical Teaching Hospital, University of California, Davis, California

*Section 6, Consulting Editor; Treatment of Skin Cancer*

**ORLA M. MAHONY, M.V.B., M.R.C.V.S.**

Clinical Instructor, Tufts University School of Veterinary Medicine, North Grafton, Massachusetts

*Treatment of Feline Malignant Lymphoma*

**PAUL A. MANLEY, D.V.M., M.Sc., Dipl. A.C.V.S.**

Associate Professor, Department of Surgical Sciences, University of Wisconsin-Madison School of Veterinary Medicine, Madison, Wisconsin

*Treatment of Degenerative Joint Disease*

**CRAIG H. MARETZKI, V.M.D.**

Resident, Small Animal Internal Medicine, Veterinary Teaching Hospital, School of Veterinary Medicine, University of California, Davis, Davis, California

*CVT Update: Veterinary Applications of Hemodialysis*

**SANDRA MANFRA MARRETTA, D.V.M., Dipl. A.C.V.S., A.V.D.C.**

Assistant Professor, Small Animal Surgery and Dentistry, Department of Veterinary Clinical Medicine, College of Veterinary Medicine, University of Illinois; Veterinary Medical Teaching Hospital, Small Animal Clinic, University of Illinois, Urbana, Illinois

*Current Concepts in Canine and Feline Dentistry*

**LINDA G. MARTIN, D.V.M., M.S.**

Resident, Emergency Medicine and Critical Care, Colorado State University, Fort Collins, Colorado

*Magnesium and the Critically Ill Patient*

**MICHAEL E. MATZ, D.V.M., Dipl. A.C.V.I.M.**

Internist, Southwest Veterinary Specialties, Tucson, Arizona

*Gastrointestinal Ulcer Therapy*

**JOHN V. MAUTERER, JR., D.V.M., Dipl. A.C.V.S.**

Staff Surgeon, MedVet Incorporated, Columbus, Ohio

*Endoscopic and Nonendoscopic Percutaneous Gastrostomy Tube Placement*

**MELBA L. MCGEE, R.R.T., C.V.T.**

Critical Care Nurse, Colorado State University; Critical Care Unit, Colorado State University Veterinary Teaching Hospital, Colorado State University, Fort Collins, Colorado

*Critical Care Nursing*

**PATRICK F. MCKEEVER, D.V.M., M.S., Dipl. A.C.V.D.**

Professor of Veterinary and Comparative Dermatology, University of Minnesota, St. Paul, Minnesota

*Canine Otitis Externa*

**PAMELA J. MCKELVIE, B.S., V.M.D.**

Penn Hip Associate, Havertown, Pennsylvania

*Current Concepts in the Diagnosis of Canine Hip Dysplasia*

**WILLIAM MCMAHAN**
Curator of Ectotherms, Louisville Zoological Garden, Louisville, Kentucky
*Euthanasia Methods for Ectothermic Vertebrates*

**SCOTT MCVEY, D.V.M., Ph.D., Dipl. A.C.V.M.**
Associate Professor, Immunology, Department of Pathology and Microbiology, Kansas State University, Manhattan, Kansas
*Immune Function in Renal Failure*

**KATHRYN M. MEURS, D.V.M.**
Veterinary Clinical Associate, Department of Small Animal Medicine and Surgery, College of Veterinary Medicine, Texas A&M University; Veterinary Clinical Associate, Texas Veterinary Medical Center, Texas A&M University, College Station, Texas
*CVT Update: Zinc Toxicity; Canine Chagas' Myocarditis*

**D. J. MEYER, D.V.M., Dipl. A.C.V.I.M., Dipl. A.C.V.P.**
Professor, Department of Pathology, College of Veterinary Medicine and Biomedical Sciences, Colorado State University; Chief, Clinical Pathology Service Veterinary Teaching Hospital, Colorado State University, Fort Collins, Colorado
*Causes and Effects of Interference with Clinical Laboratory Measurements and Examinations; Bilirubin and Bile Acids in the Diagnosis of Hepatobiliary Disease*

**VICKI N. MEYERS-WALLEN, V.M.D., Ph.D., Dipl. A.C.T.**
Associate Professor, Department of Anatomy, J. A. Baker Institute for Animal Health, College of Veterinary Medicine, Cornell University; Chief-of-Service, Small Animal Fertility and Infertility Clinic, Veterinary Medical Teaching Hospital, Cornell University, Ithaca, New York
*Section 11, Consulting Editor; The Elective Cesarean Section*

**ELLEN MILLER, D.V.M., M.S., Dipl. A.C.V.I.M.**
Associate Professor, College of Veterinary Medicine and Biomedical Sciences, Colorado State University; 60% Clinical Appointment, Veterinary Teaching Hospital, Colorado State University, Fort Collins, Colorado
*Diagnostic Studies and Sample Collection in Neonatal Dogs and Cats*

**MATTHEW W. MILLER, D.V.M., M.S., Dipl. A.C.V.I.M. (Cardiology)**
Associate Professor, Department of Small Animal Medicine and Surgery, College of Veterinary Medicine, Texas A&M University; Staff Cardiologist, Texas Veterinary Medical Center, Texas A&M University, College Station, Texas
*Canine Chagas' Myocarditis*

**R. ERIC MILLER, D.V.M., Dipl. A.C.Z.M.**
Adjunct Assistant Professor, College of Veterinary Medicine, University of Missouri; Director of Animal Health and Research, St. Louis Zoological Park, St. Louis, Missouri
*Section 14, Consulting Editor; Appendices*

**PAUL E. MILLER, D.V.M., Dipl. A.C.V.O.**
Assistant Clinical Professor of Ophthalmology, School of Veterinary Medicine, University of Wisconsin-Madison, Madison, Wisconsin
*Glaucoma*

**THOMAS R. MILLER, D.V.M., M.S., Dipl. A.C.V.O.**
Attending Ophthalmologist, Tampa Bay Veterinary Referral, Incorporated, Largo, Florida
*Anti-Inflammatory Therapy of the Eye*

**WILLIAM H. MILLER, JR., V.M.D., Dipl. A.C.V.D.**
Associate Professor of Medicine (Dermatology), College of Veterinary Medicine, Cornell University, Ithaca, New York
*Section 7, Consulting Editor; Epidermal Dysplastic Disorders of Dogs and Cats; Treatment of Generalized Demodicosis in Dogs*

**NICHOLAS J. MILLICHAMP, B.Vet.Med., Ph.D., Dipl. A.C.V.O.**
Associate Professor, Department of Small Animal Medicine and Surgery, College of Veterinary Medicine, Texas A&M University, College Station, Texas
*Reptile Ophthalmology*

**N. SYDNEY MOISE, D.V.M., Dipl. A.C.V.I.M. (Internal Medicine, Cardiology)**
Associate Professor of Medicine, Cornell University, Adjunct Associate Professor of Pediatric Cardiology, Department of Pediatrics, State University of New York Health Science Center, Ithaca, New York
*Twenty-Four Hour Ambulatory Electrocardiography (Holter Monitoring); Tricuspid Valve Dysplasia in the Dog*

**MARTHA MOON, D.V.M., M.S., Dipl. A.C.V.R.**
Associate Professor, Radiology, Virginia-Maryland Regional College of Veterinary Medicine, Virginia Tech; Radiologist, Virginia-Maryland Regional College of Veterinary Medicine, Veterinary Teaching Hospital, Virginia Tech, Blacksburg, Virginia
*Lung Lobe Torsion*

**ANTONY S. MOORE, B.V.Sc., M.V.Sc., Dipl. A.C.V.I.M. (Oncology)**
Assistant Professor of Medicine and Surgery, Tufts University School of Veterinary Medicine, North Grafton, Massachusetts
*Treatment of Feline Malignant Lymphoma*

**WILLIAM W. MUIR, D.V.M., Ph.D., Dipl. A.C.V.A., A.C.V.E.C.C.**
Professor, Department of Veterinary Clinical Sciences, The Ohio State University, Columbus, Ohio
*Strong Ions and Acid-Base Disorders*

**ALAN C. MUNDELL, D.V.M., Dipl. A.C.V.D.**
Animal Dermatology Service, Seattle, Washington
*Mycobacterial Skin Diseases in Small Animals*

**MICHAEL J. MURPHY, D.V.M. Ph.D., Dipl. A.B.V.T.**
Associate Professor, Department of Veterinary Diagnostic Medicine, College of Veterinary Medicine, University of Minnesota, St. Paul, Minnesota
*Incidence of Small Animal Poison Exposures in a Major Metropolitan Area; CVT Update: Anticoagulant Rodenticides*

**ROBERT J. MURTAUGH, D.V.M., M.S., Dipl. A.C.V.I.M., A.C.V.E.C.C.**
Associate Professor, Department of Medicine, Tufts University School of Veterinary Medicine, Tufts University, North Grafton, Massachusetts
*Section 2, Consulting Editor; Use of Catecholamines in Critical Care Patients*

**RAYMOND F. NACHREINER, D.V.M., Ph.D.**
Professor, Animal Health Diagnostic Laboratory, Departments of Large Animal Clinical Sciences and Physiology, College of Veterinary Medicine, Michigan State University, East Lansing, Michigan
*Monitoring Thyroid Hormone Replacement Therapy*

**LARRY A. NAGODE, D.V.M., Ph.D.**
Associate Professor, Department of Veterinary Pathobiology, College of Veterinary Medicine, The Ohio State University, Columbus, Ohio
*Utility of Diagnostic Assays in the Evaluation of Hypercalcemia and Hypocalcemia: Parathyroid Hormone, Vitamin D Metabolites, Parathyroid Hormone-Related Peptide, and Ionized Calcium*

**MARK P. NASISSE, D.V.M., Dipl. A.C.V.O.**
Associate Professor, College of Veterinary Medicine, North Carolina State University, Raleigh, North Carolina
*Innovations in Cataract Surgery*

**RICHARD W. NELSON, D.V.M., Dipl. A.C.V.I.M.**
Associate Professor, Department of Medicine and Epidemiology, School of Veterinary Medicine, University of California, Davis, California
*Insulin Resistance in Diabetic Dogs and Cats; Transplantation as a Means of Treating Diabetes Mellitus; Treatment of Feline Diabetes Mellitus with the Oral Sulfonylurea Glipizide*

**RHETT NICHOLS, D.V.M., Dipl. A.C.V.I.M.**
Director of Internal Medicine, Veterinary Research, Farmingdale, New York
*Complications and Concurrent Disease Associated with Diabetic Ketoacidosis and Other Severe Forms of Diabetes Mellitus*

**E. E. OETTLÉ, B.V.Sc., Ph.D.**
Fisantekuil Animal Clinic, Wellington; Previously: Lecturer, Department of Theriogenology, University of Pretoria, Onderstepoort; Senior Medical Natural Scientist, Groote Schuur Hospital Observatory, Cape Town, South Africa
*Sperm Abnormalities and Fertility in the Dog*

**GREGORY K. OGILVIE, D.V.M., Dipl. A.C.V.I.M. (Internal Medicine, Oncology)**
Associate Professor of Oncology/Internal Medicine, Comparative Oncology Unit, Department of Clinical Sciences, College of Veterinary Medicine and Biomedical Sciences, Colorado State University; Medical Oncologist, Veterinary Teaching Hospital, Colorado State University, Fort Collins, Colorado
*Safe Handling and Administration of Chemotherapeutic Agents in Veterinary Medicine*

**BARBARA L. OGLESBEE, D.V.M., Dipl. A.B.V.P. (Avian)**
Clinical Assistant Professor, Small Animal Medicine, The Ohio State University College of Veterinary Medicine, Columbus, Ohio
*Emergency Medicine for Pocket Pets*

**CARL A. OSBORNE, D.V.M., Ph.D., Dipl. A.C.V.I.M.**
Professor, Department of Small Animal Clinical Sciences, College of Veterinary Medicine, University of Minnesota, St. Paul, Minnesota
*Section 1, Consulting Editor; Ten Guiding Principles to Enhance the Benefit of Current Veterinary Therapy; Diagnosis by Rule-Out: Judgment in the Absence of Certainty; Influence of Fasting and Eating on Laboratory Values; Metabolic Acidosis in Renal Failure: Consequence, Diagnosis, and Treatment; Treatment of Uremic Anorexia; Canine and Feline Nephroliths; Feline Calcium Oxalate Uroliths; Canine Calcium Oxalate Uroliths; Canine and Feline Calcium Phosphate Urolithiasis; Voiding Urohydropropulsion: A Nonsurgical Technique for Removal of Urocystoliths; Medical Management of Urethral Prolapse in Male Dogs*

**GARY D. OSWEILER, D.V.M., Ph.D.**
Professor of Veterinary Toxicology; Director, Veterinary Diagnostic Laboratory, College of Veterinary Medicine, Iowa State University, Ames, Iowa
*Section 3, Consulting Editor; Toxicologic Disorders*

**JERRY M. OWENS, D.V.M., Dipl. A.C.V.R.**

Staff Radiologist, Special Veterinary Services, Berkeley, California, Staff Radiologist, Madera Pet Hospital, Corte Madera, California, President, Veterinary Telerad, San Rafael, California

*Gastrointestinal Diagnostic Imaging*

**PHILIP PADRID, D.V.M.**

Assistant Professor of Medicine, Section of Pulmonary and Critical Care Medicine, Committee on Comparative Medicine and Pathology, University of Chicago, Chicago, Illinois

*Diagnosis and Therapy of Canine Chronic Bronchitis*

**RODNEY L. PAGE, D.V.M., Dipl. A.C.V.I.M., (Internal Medicine, Oncology)**

Professor, Oncology, College of Veterinary Medicine, North Carolina State University, Raleigh, North Carolina

*Canine and Feline Oropharyngeal Neoplasms*

**MARK G. PAPICH, B.S., D.V.M., M.S., Dipl. A.C.V.C.P.**

Associate Professor of Clinical Pharmacology, Advisor of Clinical Pharmacology Laboratory, North Carolina State University; Clinical Pharmacologist, College of Veterinary Medicine, North Carolina State University, Raleigh, North Carolina

*Unapproved Use of Drugs in Small Animals; Incompatible Critical Care Drug Combinations; Empiric Antibiotic Therapy; Appendices, Consulting Editor*

**DEMOSTHENES PAPPAGIANIS, M.D., Ph.D.**

Professor, Department of Medical Microbiology and Immunology, School of Medicine, University of California, Davis, California

*Treatment of Nasal Aspergillosis with Topical Clotrimazole*

**ALAN J. PARKER, B.Sc., B.V.Sc., M.S., Ph.D., M.R.C.V.S., Dipl. A.C.V.I.M. (Neurology)**

Professor of Medicine/Neurology, Chief of Staff, Small Animal Hospital, College of Veterinary Medicine, University of Illinois, Urbana, Illinois

*"Little White Shakers" Syndrome: Generalized, Sporadic, Acquired, Idiopathic Tremors of Adult Dogs*

**DOMINIQUE PENNINCK, D.V.M., Dipl. A.C.V.R.**

Assistant Professor, School of Veterinary Medicine, Tufts University, North Grafton, Massachusetts

*Renal Biopsy Using An Automated Biopsy Device*

**MARK E. PETERSON, D.V.M., Dipl. A.C.V.I.M.**

Head, Division of Endocrinology, Department of Medicine, The Animal Medical Center, New York, New York

*Section 5, Consulting Editor; Radioactive Iodine (Radioiodine) Treatment for Hyperthyroidism in Cats; CVT Update: Insulin and Insulin Syringes; Mitotane (o,p') Treatment of Hyperadrenocorticism in Dogs; Hypoadrenocorticism in Dogs*

**DAVID J. POLZIN, D.V.M., Ph.D., Dipl. A.C.V.I.M.**

Professor of Veterinary Internal Medicine, University of Minnesota College of Veterinary Medicine, St. Paul, Minnesota

*Chronic Renal Failure: Improving Therapeutic Response with Patient Monitoring; Metabolic Acidosis in Renal Failure: Consequences, Diagnosis, and Treatment; Treatment of Uremic Anorexia*

**ROBERT H. POPPENGA, D.V.M., Ph.D., Dipl. A.B.V.T.**

Assistant Professor, Clinician-Educator Track, School of Veterinary Medicine, University of Pennsylvania, Kennett Square, Pennsylvania

*Risks Associated with Herbal Remedies*

**SALLY POWELL, A.H.T.**

Animal Health Technician, Nursing Supervisor of Emergency Service, Veterinary Hospital of the University of Pennsylvania, School of Veterinary Medicine, University of Pennsylvania, Philadelphia, Pennsylvania

*Oxygen Supplementation*

**HELEN T. POWER, D.V.M., Dipl. A.C.V.D.**

Dermatology for Animals, Los Gatos, California

*The Use of Synthetic Retinoids in Veterinary Medicine*

**JACQUELINE S. RAND, B.V.Sc., D.V.Sc., Dipl. A.C.V.I.M.**

Senior Lecturer, Department of Companion Animal Medicine and Surgery, School of Veterinary Science, The University of Queensland, St. Lucia, Queensland, Australia

*The Analysis of Cerebrospinal Fluid in Cats*

**PATRICK T. REDIG, D.V.M., Ph.D.**

Associate Professor, Department of Small Animal Clinical Services, College of Veterinary Medicine, University of Minnesota; Director, The Raptor Center at the University of Minnesota, St Paul, Minnesota

*Diagnosis and Treatment of Avian Aspergillosis*

**KENT R. REFSAL, D.V.M., Ph.D.**

Associate Professor, Animal Health Diagnostic Laboratory, Department of Small Animal Clinical Sciences, College of Veterinary Medicine, Michigan State University, East Lansing, Michigan

*Monitoring Thyroid Hormone Replacement Therapy*

**CRAIG, R. REINEMEYER, D.V.M., Ph.D.**

Associate Professor, Department of Comparative Medicine, College of Veterinary Medicine, University of Tennessee, Knoxville, Tennessee

*Canine Gastrointestinal Parasites; Parasites of the Respiratory System*

**KAREN HELTON RHODES, D.V.M., Dipl. A.C.V.D.**

Head, Dermatology Service, The Animal Medical Center, New York, New York; Clinical Instructor, Department of Dermatology, New York University Hospital; Clinical Instructor, Comparative Dermatology, Faculty, Department of Dermatology, Ronald C. Perelman Dermatology Department, New York University Hospital, New York, New York

*Feline Immunomodulators*

**YASUKO RIKIHISA, Ph.D.**

Professor, Department of Veterinary Pathobiology, College of Veterinary Medicine, The Ohio State University, Columbus, Ohio

*Salmon Poisoning Disease*

**BRANSON W. RITCHIE, D.V.M., Ph.D.**

Associate Professor, Avian/Zoologic Medicine, University of Georgia College of Veterinary Medicine, Athens, Georgia

*Avian Polyomavirus; Psittacine Beak and Feather Disease Virus*

**STEVEN M. ROBERTS, D.V.M., M.S., Dipl. A.C.V.O.**

Associate Professor, Ophthalmology, Department of Clinical Sciences, College of Veterinary Medicine and Biomedical Sciences, Colorado State University, Fort Collins, Colorado

*Pannus*

**ELAINE P. ROBINSON, B.V.M., M.V.Sc., M.R.C.V.S., Dipl. A.C.V.A.**

Associate Professor, Department of Small Animal Clinical Sciences, College of Veterinary Medicine, University of Minnesota; Head, Section of Anesthesiology, University of Minnesota Veterinary Teaching Hospital, University of Minnesota, St. Paul, Minnesota

*Propofol: A New Sedative-Hypnotic Anesthestic Agent*

**RICHARD A. ROCKAR, V.M.D.**

Robert S. Brodey Resident in Soft Tissue Surgery, Department of Clinical Sciences, School of Veterinary Medicine, University of Pennsylvania, Philadelphia, Pennsylvania; VCA Veterinary Care Animal Hospital, Albuquerque, New Mexico

*Outcome Prediction in Emergency and Critical Care Patients*

**APRIL ROMAGNANO, D.V.M., Ph.D.**

Resident, Avian Medicine, North Carolina State University, College of Veterinary Medicine, Raleigh, North Carolina

*Current Approaches to Feather Picking*

**MARGARET V. ROOT, D.V.M.**

Resident, Department of Small Animal Clinical Sciences, College of Veterinary Medicine, University of Minnesota, St. Paul, Minnesota

*Pregnancy Termination in the Bitch Using Prostaglandid $F_{2a}$*

**SØREN ROSENDAL, D.V.M., Ph.D.**

Professor of Veterinary Microbiology, Ontario Veterinary College, University of Guelph, Guelph, Ontario, Canada

*Mycoplasma Infections of Dogs and Cats*

**WAYNE S. ROSENKRANTZ, D.V.M., Dipl. A.C.V.D.**

Veterinary Dermatologist, Animal Dermatology Clinic, Garden Grove, California

*Congenital Adrenal Hyperplasia-Like Syndrome*

**THOMAS J. ROSOL, D.V.M., Ph.D., Dipl. A.C.V.P.**

Associate Professor, Department of Veterinary Pathobiology, College of Veterinary Medicine, The Ohio State University, Columbus, Ohio

*Utility of Diagnostic Assays in the Evaluation of Hypercalcemia and Hypocalcemia: Parathyroid Hormone, Vitamin D Metabolites, Parathyroid Hormone-Related Peptide, and Ionized Calcium*

**LINDA A. ROSS, D.V.M., M.S., Dipl. A.C.V.I.M.**

Associate Dean for Clinical Programs and Hospital Director, Tufts University School of Veterinary Medicine, Tufts University, North Grafton, Massachusetts

*Renal Biopsy Using an Automated Biopsy Device*

**ROD A. W. ROSYCHUK, D.V.M., Dipl. A.C.V.I.M.**

Assistant Professor, Colorado State University, Fort Collins, Colorado

*Diseases of the Claw and Claw Fold*

**JAMES A. ROTH, D.V.M., Ph.D.**

Professor, Department of Microbiology, Immunology and Preventive Medicine, College of Veterinary Medicine, Iowa State University, Ames, Iowa

*Immunosuppression and Immunodeficiency*

**PHILIP ROUDEBUSH, D.V.M., Dipl. A.C.V.I.M. (Internal Medicine)**

Veterinary Fellow, Hill's Science and Technology Center, Director of Professional Education, Mark Morris Institute, Topeka, Kansas; Adjunct Professor, Department of Clinical Sciences, College of Veterinary Medicine, Kansas State University, Manhattan, Kansas

*Diagnosis and Management of Adverse Food Reactions*

**STANLEY I. RUBIN, D.V.M., M.S., Dipl. A.C.V.I.M. (Internal Medicine)**

Professor, Department of Veterinary Internal Medicine, Western College of Veterinary Medicine, University of Saskatchewan; Staff Internist, Small Animal Clinic, Veterinary Teaching Hospital, Western College of Veterinary Medicine, University of Saskatchewan, Saskatoon, Saskatchewan, Canada

*Management of Fluid and Electrolyte Disorders in Uremia*

**JOHN E. RUSH, D.V.M., M.S., Dipl. A.C.V.I.M. (Cardiology), A.C.V.E.C.C.**

Assistant Professor, Tufts University School of Veterinary Medicine, Tufts University; Head Clinical Cardiologist and Co-director of Intensive Care Unit and Emergency Services, Tufts University School of Veterinary Medicine, Tufts University, North Grafton, Massachusetts

*Cardiac Arrhythmias in Systemic Disease*

**LISA C. RUSSELL, D.V.M.**

Resident in Critical Care and Emergency, Tufts University School of Veterinary Medicine, Tufts University, North Grafton, Massachusetts

*Cardiac Arrhythmias in Systemic Disease*

**G. R. RUTTEMAN, D.V.M., Ph.D.**

Assistant Professor, Veterinary Oncology, Department of Clinical Sciences of Companion Animals, Faculty of Veterinary Medicine, Utrecht University, Utrecht, The Netherlands

*Mammary Tumors in the Dog*

**M-A SALISBURY, D.V.M., Dipl. A.C.V.O.**

President, Animal Eye Care. Inc., Sarasota, Florida

*Keratoconjunctivitis Sicca*

**KATHARINE R. SALMERI, D.V.M., Dipl. A.C.V.S.**

Staff Surgeon, Red Bank Veterinary Referral Services, Red Bank, New Jersey

*Early Neutering of the Dog and Cat*

**GARY R. SAMPSON, B.S., D.V.M.**

Private Practice; Limited to Cat and Dog Behavior Modification, Indianapolis, Indiana

*CVT Update: Insulin and Insulin Syringes*

**SHERRY L. SANDERSON, D.V.M.**

Resident in Clinical Nutrition, University of Minnesota Veterinary Teaching Hospital, University of Minnesota, St. Paul, Minnesota

*Treatment of Uremic Anorexia; Propofol: A New Sedative-Hypnotic Anesthetic Agent; Medical Management of Urethral Prolapse in Male Dogs*

**WILLIAM D. SCHALL, D.V.M., Dipl. A.C.V.I.M.**

Professor, College of Veterinary Medicine, Michigan State University; Veterinary Teaching Hospital, Michigan State University, East Lansing, Michigan

*Use of Zinc Acetate for the Treatment and Prevention of Canine Copper Hepatotoxicosis*

**PATRICIA SCHENCK, D.V.M., Ph.D.**

Post-Doctoral Fellow, Department of Veterinary Pathobiology, College of Veterinary Medicine, The Ohio State University, Columbus, Ohio

*Utility of Diagnostic Assays in the Evaluation of Hypercalcemia and Hypocalcemia: Parathyroid Hormone, Vitamin D Metabolites, Parathyroid Hormone-Related Peptide, and Ionized Calcium*

**LYNN P. SCHMEITZEL, D.V.M., Dipl. A.C.V.D.**

Associate Professor, University of Tennessee College of Veterinary Medicine, Department of Small Animal Clinical Sciences, Knoxville, Tennessee

*Congenital Adrenal Hyperplasia-Like Syndrome*

**STEVEN C. SCHRADER, D.V.M., Dipl. A.C.V.S.**

Associate Professor, College of Veterinary Medicine, The Ohio State University, Columbus, Ohio

*Section 12, Consulting Editor; The Use of the Laboratory in the Diagnosis of Joint Disorders of Dogs and Cats; Differential Diagnosis of Nontraumatic Causes of Lameness in Young Growing Dogs*

**KEVIN T. SCHULTZ, D.V.M., Ph.D.**

Associate Professor, Department of Pathobiological Sciences, School of Veterinary Medicine, University of Wisconsin at Madison, Madison, Wisconsin, Staff Allergist, VCA Berwyn Veterinary Hospital, Berwyn, Illinois

*The Current Immunology of Allergy*

**WAYNE SCHWARK, D.V.M., Ph.D.**

Professor of Pharmacology, College of Veterinary Medicine, Cornell University; Director of Clinical Pharmacology, College of Veterinary Medicine, Cornell University, Ithaca, New York

*Use and Misuse of DMSO*

**DANNY W. SCOTT, B.S., D.V.M., Dipl. A.C.V.D.**

Professor of Medicine, College of Veterinary Medicine, Cornell University, Ithaca, New York

*Rational Use of Glucocorticoids in Dermatology*

**HOWARD B. SEIM III, D.V.M., Dipl. A.C.V.S.**

Associate Professor, Small Animal Surgery, Colorado State University, Head of Small Animal Surgery, Colorado State University, Fort Collins, Colorado

*Management of Peritonitis*

**BARBARA A. SELCER, D.V.M., Dipl. A.C.V.R.**

Associate Professor, College of Veterinary Medicine, University of Georgia, Athens, Georgia

*Ultrasonographic Findings in Feline Lower Urinary Tract Diseases*

**RANCE K. SELLON, D.V.M., Dipl. A.C.V.I.M. (Internal Medicine)**

Department of Microbiology, Pathology, and Parasitology, College of Veterinary Medicine, North Carolina State University, Raleigh, North Carolina

*CVT Update: Rocky Mountain Spotted Fever*

**DAVID F. SENIOR, B.V.Sc., Dipl. A.C.V.I.M**

Professor and Head, Veterinary Clinical Sciences, School of Veterinary Medicine, Louisiana State University, Baton Rouge, Louisiana

*Lithotripsy in Companion Animals*

**EWA SEVELIUS, V.M.D.**

Chief of Staff, Specialist in Small Animal Diseases, Small Animal Clinic, Animal Hospital of Helsingborg, Helsingborg, Sweden

*Pathogenic Aspects of Chronic Liver Disease in the Dog*

**GLENN A. SEVERIN, D.V.M., M.S., Dipl. A.C.V.O.**

Professor of Ophthalmology, College of Veterinary Medicine and Biomedical Sciences, Colorado State University, Fort Collins, Colorado

*Feline Uveitis*

**KEVIN J. SHANLEY, D.V.M., Dipl. A.C.V.D.**

Assistant Professor of Dermatology, University of Pennsylvania, Philadelphia, Pennsylvania; Staff Dermatologist, Metropolitan Veterinary Associates, Valley Forge, Pennsylvania; Staff Dermatologist, Delaware Veterinary Specialty Group, Newark, Delaware

*Acquired, Nonendocrine Alopecias of the Dog and Cat*

**LINDA SHELL, D.V.M.**

Associate Professor, Department of Small Animal Clinical Sciences, Virginia-Maryland Regional College of Veterinary Medicine, Virginia Tech, Blacksburg, Virginia

*Otitis Media and Interna*

**G. DIANE SHELTON, D.V.M., Ph.D., Dipl. A.C.V.I.M.**

Associate Clinical Professor, Department of Pathology, School of Medicine, University of California, San Diego; Director, Comparative Neuromuscular Laboratory, School of Medicine, University of California, San Diego, La Jolla, California

*Canine Lipid Storage Myopathies*

**D. DAVID SISSON, D.V.M., Dipl. A.C.V.I.M. (Cardiology)**

Staff Cardiologist Veterinary Medical Teaching Hospital, University of Illinois; Assistant Professor, College of Veterinary Medicine, University of Illinois, Urbana, Illinois

*Angiotensin-Converting Enzyme Inhibitors*

**DANIEL D. SMEAK, D.V.M., Dipl. A.C.V.S.**

Associate Professor, Small Animal Surgery, College of Veterinary Medicine, The Ohio State University; Section Head, Small Animal Surgery, The Ohio State University, Columbus, Ohio

*Budd-Chiari–Like Syndromes in Dogs; Management of Feline Chylothorax*

**GAIL K. SMITH, V.M.D., Ph.D.**

Associate Professor and Chief of Surgery, University of Pennsylvania School of Veterinary Medicine; Director, Penn HIP^R, Philadelphia, Pennsylvania

*Current Concepts in the Diagnosis of Canine Hip Dysplasia*

**PATRICK SOON-SHIONG, M.D.**

Director, Islet Transplant Center, Wadsworth Medical Center, Los Angeles, California

*Transplantation as a Means of Treating Diabetes Mellitus*

**JULIE L. SORENSON, D.V.M.**

Post Graduate Researcher, Urinary Stone Analysis Laboratory, Department of Medicine, School of Veterinary Medicine, University of California, Davis, California

*CVT Update: Management and Prevention of Urate Urolithiasis*

**CHERYL L. SPENCER, C.V.T.**

Critical Care Nurse, Colorado State University Veterinary Teaching Hospital, Colorado State University, Fort Collins, Colorado

*Critical Care Nursing*

**GARY J. SPODNICK, D.V.M., Dipl. A.C.V.S.**

Assistant Professor, Surgery, College of Veterinary Medicine, North Carolina State University, Raleigh, North Carolina

*Canine and Feline Oropharyngeal Neoplasms*

**DAVID E. SPRENG, D.V.M.**

Research Fellow, Veterinary Institute of Trauma, Emergency and Critical Care; Surgeon, The Animal Emergency Center, Milwaukee, Wisconsin
*Doppler Assessment of Blood Flow and Pressure in Surgical and Critical Care Patients*

**GARY L. STAMP, D.V.M., M.S., Dipl. A.B.V.P., A.C.V.E.C.C.**

Director, Department of Defense Military Dog Medical Center, Lackland Air Force Base, San Antonio, Texas
*Disaster Medicine: Meeting the Needs of the Small Animal Patient*

**KIMBERLY M. STANZ, D.V.M.**

Resident in Veterinary and Comparative Ophthalmology, University of Wisconsin-Madison School of Veterinary Medicine, Madison, Wisconsin
*Antibiotic Therapy of the Eye*

**REBECCA L. STEPIEN, D.V.M., M.S., Dipl. A.C.V.I.M. (Cardiology)**

Assistant Professor, University of Wisconsin; Cardiologist, School of Veterinary Medicine, Veterinary Medical Teaching Hospital, University of Wisconsin, Madison, Wisconsin
*Sedation for Cardiovascular Procedures*

**ELIZABETH A. STONE, D.V.M., M.S., M.P.P., Dipl. A.C.V.S.**

Professor and Department Head, Department of Companion Animal and Special Species Medicine, College of Veterinary Medicine, North Carolina State University; Surgeon, North Carolina State University, Raleigh, North Carolina
*Transitional Cell Carcinoma: Surgical Limitations*

**MICHAEL K. STOSKOPF, D.V.M., Ph.D., Dipl. A.C.Z.M.**

Professor of Wildlife and Aquatic Medicine, College of Veterinary Medicine, North Carolina State University, Raleigh, North Carolina
*Anesthesia of Pet Fishes*

**RODNEY C. STRAW, B.V.Sc., Dipl. A.C.V.S.**

Associate Professor of Oncology, Veterinary Teaching Hospital, Colorado State University, Fort Collins, Colorado
*Treatment of Canine Osteosarcoma*

**W. PRESTON STUBBS, D.V.M.**

Clinical Instructor, Small Animal Surgery, University of Florida, Gainesville, Florida
*Early Neutering of the Dog and Cat*

**JOSEPH TABOADA, D.V.M., Dipl. A.C.V.I.M. (Internal Medicine)**

Associate Professor, School of Veterinary Medicine, Louisiana State University; Chief, Companion Animal Medicine Service, Veterinary Teaching Hospital and Clinics, School of Veterinary Medicine, Louisiana State University, Baton Rouge, Louisiana
*Canine Babesiosis*

**MICHELLE M. TAYLOR, D.V.M., Dipl. A.C.V.S.**

Clinical Associate, Ontario Veterinary College, University of Guelph, Guelph, Ontario, Canada
*Indolent Corneal Erosions*

**ROBERT A. TAYLOR, D.V.M., M.S., Dipl. A.C.V.S.**

Alameda East Veterinary Hospital, Denver, Colorado
*Physical Therapy and Rehabilitation*

**ALAIN P. THÉON, D.V.M., M.S.**

Assistant Professor, School of Veterinary Medicine, University of California, Davis; Radiation Oncologist, Veterinary Medical Teaching Hospital, University of California, Davis, California
*Indications and Applications of Radiation Therapy*

**WILLIAM P. THOMAS, D.V.M., Dipl. A.C.V.I.M. (Cardiology)**

Professor, Department of Medicine and Epidemiology, University of California; Chief, Cardiology Service, Veterinary Medical Teaching Hospital, University of California, Davis, California
*Therapy of Congenital Pulmonic Stenosis*

**MARY ANNA THRALL, D.V.M., M.S., Dipl. A.C.V.P.**

Professor, Department of Pathology, College of Veterinary Medicine and Biomedical Sciences, Colorado State University; Clinical Pathologist, Colorado State University Veterinary Teaching Hospital, Colorado State University, Fort Collins, Colorado
*Antifreeze Poisoning*

**ROSAMA THUMCHAI, D.V.M., M.S., Dipl. A.C.V.P.**

Research Assistant, Department of Small Animal Clinical Sciences, College of Veterinary Medicine, University of Minnesota, St. Paul, Minnesota
*Feline Calcium Oxalate Uroliths*

**PHILIP W. TOLL, D.V.M., M.S.**

Senior Scientist, Mark Morris Institute, Topeka, Kansas; Adjunct Faculty, Department of Anatomy and Physiology, Kansas State University, Manhattan, Kansas
*Medical Implications of Fasting and Starvation*

**DAVID C. TWEDT, D.V.M., Dipl. A.C.V.I.M.**
Professor and Head, Small Animal Medicine Section, College of Veterinary Medicine and Biomedical Sciences, Colorado State University, Fort Collins, Colorado
*Section 8, Consulting Editor*

**LISA K. UNGER, C.V.T.**
Principal Veterinary Technician, Department of Small Animal Clinical Sciences, College of Veterinary Medicine, University of Minnesota, St. Paul, Minnesota
*Canine and Feline Nephroliths; Canine and Feline Uroliths*

**SHELLY L. VADEN, D.V.M., Ph.D., Dipl. A.C.V.I.M.**
Assistant Professor, Internal Medicine, College of Veterinary Medicine, North Carolina State University, Raleigh, North Carolina
*Cyclosporine; Empiric Antibiotic Therapy; Proteinuria in Dogs and Cats: A Diagnostic Approach*

**DAVID M. VAIL, D.V.M., M.S., Dipl. A.C.V.I.M. (Oncology)**
Assistant Professor of Oncology, Department of Medical Sciences, School of Veterinary Medicine; Associate Member, Wisconsin Comprehensive Cancer Center, Department of Human Oncology, School of Medicine, University of Wisconsin-Madison, Madison, Wisconsin
*Treatment and Prognosis of Canine Malignant Lymphoma*

**DEBORAH R. VAN PELT, D.V.M., M.S., Dipl. A.C.V.E.C.C.**
Assistant Professor, Emergency Medicine and Critical Care, Colorado State University, Fort Collins, Colorado
*Critical Care Nursing; Magnesium and the Critically Ill Patient; Cardiopulmonary Resuscitation*

**WILLIAM VERNAU, B.V.M.S., D.V.Sc., Dipl. A.C.V.P.**
Staff Pathologist, Veterinary Pathology Services, Sydney, New South Wales, Australia
*Appendices*

**EMILY J. WALDER, V.M.D., Dipl. A.C.V.P.**
An Independent Biopsy Service (Private Pathology Lab)
*Fibropruritic Nodules in the Dog*

**ROBIN E. WALL, D.V.M., Dipl. A.C.V.E.C.C**
Staff Critical Clinician, Mission MedVet, Mission, Kansas
*Monitoring Gastrointestinal Mucosal pH in Critical Care Patients*

**MELISSA S. WALLACE, D.V.M., Dipl. A.C.V.I.M.**
Staff Veterinarian, Division of Nephrology, Endocrinology and Reproductive Services, Department of Medicine, The Animal Medical Center, New York, New York
*Insulin Treatment of Diabetes Mellitus in the Dog and Cat*

**PATRICIA A. WALTER, D.V.M., M.S., Dipl. A.C.V.R.**
Associate Professor, Department of Small Animal Clinical Sciences, College of Veterinary Medicine, University of Minnesota, St. Paul, Minnesota
*Imaging the Reproductive Tract in the Male Dog*

**DANIEL A. WARD, D.V.M., Ph.D.**
Assistant Professor of Ophthalmology, Department of Small Animal Clinical Medicines, College of Veterinary Medicine, University of Tennessee, Knoxville, Tennessee
*Oculomycosis*

**WENDY A. WARE, D.V.M., M.S., Dipl. A.C.V.I.M. (Cardiology)**
Associate Professor, Departments of Veterinary Clinical Sciences and Veterinary Physiology and Pharmacology, Iowa State University; Staff Cardiologist, Veterinary Teaching Hospital, Iowa State University, Ames, Iowa
*Cardiac Neoplasia*

**ROBERT J. WASHABAU, V.M.D., Ph.D. Dipl. A.C.V.I.M.**
Assistant Professor of Medicine, Department of Clinical Studies, School of Veterinary Medicine, University of Pennsylvania, Philadelphia, Pennsylvania
*Antiemetic Therapy*

**TIMOTHY D. G. WATSON, B.V.M.S., Ph.D., M.R.C.V.S.**
Senior Postdoctoral Research Fellow, Departments of Veterinary Medicine and Pathological Biochemistry (Royal Infirmary), Glasgow University Veterinary School, University of Glasgow, Glasgow, United Kingdom
*Hyperlipidemia*

**RALPH C. WEICHSELBAUM, D.V.M.**
Resident-Veterinary Radiology, University of Minnesota; Resident-Veterinary Teaching Hospital, University of Minnesota, St. Paul, Minnesota
*Imaging the Reproductive Tract in the Male Dog*

**GLADE WEISER, D.V.M., Dipl. A.C.V.P.**
Professor and Chairman, Department of Pathology, Colorado State University, Fort Collins, Colorado
*Hematologic Technology for Diagnosing Anemias*

**DOUGLAS J. WEISS, D.V.M., PH.D., Dipl. A.C.V.P.**
Professor of Clinical Pathology, University of Minnesota; Veterinary Teaching Hospital, University of Minnesota, St. Paul, Minnesota
*Leukocyte Disorders and Their Treatment*

**STEPHEN D. WHITE, D.V.M., Dipl. A.C.V.D.**
Associate Professor, College of Veterinary Medicine and Biomedical Sciences, Colorado State University; Veterinary Teaching Hospital, Colorado State University, Fort Collins, Colorado
*Hereditary Lupoid Dermatosis of the German Shorthaired Pointer*

**WAYNE O. WHITNEY, D.V.M., Dipl. A.C.V.S.**
Referral Surgeon, Gulf Coast Veterinary Specialists, Houston, Texas
*The Roles of the Veterinarian and the Veterinary Specialist in Management of Neurologic and Musculoskeletal Problems*

**DAVID A. WILLIAMS, M.A., Vet M.B., Ph.D., M.R.C.V.S., Dipl. A.C.V.I.M.**
Head, Small Animal Medicine, Purdue University, West Lafayette, Indiana
*Feline Exocrine Pancreatic Insufficiency*

**DAVID L. WILLIAMS, M.A., Vet M.B., Cert.V. Ophthal., M.R.C.V.S.**
Wellcome Research Scholar, Royal Veterinary College, London, England
*Amphibian Dermatology*

**MICHELLE WILLETTE-FRAHM, D.V.M.**
Staff Veterinarian, Gladys Porter Zoo, Brownsville, Texas
*Blood Collection Techniques in Amphibians and Reptiles*

**WAYNE E. WINGFIELD, M.S., D.V.M.**
Professor of Medicine; Chief, Emergency and Critical Care Medicine, Department of Clinical Sciences, College of Veterinary Medicine and Biomedical Sciences, Fort Collins, Colorado
*Magnesium and the Critically Ill Patient*

**STEPHEN J. WITHROW, D.V.M., Dipl. A.C.V.S., A.C.V.I.M. (Oncology)**
Professor of Surgical Oncology, Colorado State University; Chief, Clinical Oncology Service, Comparative Oncology Unit, College of Veterinary Medicine, Colorado State University, Fort Collins, Colorado
*Risks Associated with Biopsies for Cancer; Treatment of Canine Osteosarcoma*

**JAMES S. WOHL, D.V.M.**
Resident, Small Animal Medicine/Critical Care, Department of Medicine, Tufts University School of Veterinary Medicine, Tufts University, North Grafton, Massachusetts
*Use of Catecholamines in Critical Care Patients*

**ALICE M. WOLF, D.V.M., Dipl. A.C.V.I.M.**
Associate Professor, Department of Small Animal Medicine and Surgery, College of Veterinary Medicine, Texas A&M University, College Station, Texas
*Opportunistic Fungal and Algal Infections*

**KATHY N. WRIGHT, D.V.M.**
Resident, Small Animal Internal Medicine and Cardiology, College of Veterinary Medicine, University of Tennessee, Knoxville, Tennessee
*Supraventricular Tachycardia Associated with Accessory Atrioventricular Pathways in Dogs*

**AMY E. YEAGER, D.V.M., Dipl. A.C.V.R.**
Staff Veterinarian–Radiology Section, College of Veterinary Medicine, Cornell University, Ithaca, New York
*Ultrasonography of the Reproductive Tract of the Female Dog and Cat*

**ANNE M. ZAJAC, D.V.M.**
Associate Professor, Department of Pathobiology, Virginia-Maryland Regional College of Veterinary Medicine, Virginia Tech, Blacksburg, Virginia
*Giardia: Diagnosis and Treatment*

**GARY ZIMMERMAN, D.V.M., M.S., Ph.D.**
Zimmerman Research, Livingston, Montana
*Salmon Poisoning Disease*

# PREFACE

This newest edition of Kirk's *Current Veterinary Therapy* continues the tradition established by Dr. Kirk 11 editions ago. Essential to the success of this work has been the publication of concise, clinically useful, and timely chapters in an easy-to-read format. This volume follows that formula and contains over 300 new articles, each written by an author active in his or her respective clinical specialty. The volume draws increasingly on the expertise of clinical specialists from outside of North America, and provides the reader with a global perspective regarding up-to-date management of medical and surgical problems in small animal practice. As always, each section is edited by an internationally respected Consulting Editor; these individuals are largely responsible for assuring that *CVT* stays "current." We are hopeful that this 12th edition really lives up to its name.

We continue our policy of integrating this edition with prior editions of *Current Veterinary Therapy*, thereby minimizing the duplication of articles that are "still current" in prior editions. Veterinary medical information is too extensive to fit into a single volume, and reprinting all articles from prior editions would add an unnecessary expense to the reader. As I have stated before, Dr. Kirk and I believe that our readers will be best served by receiving a textbook that is updated frequently (about every 3 years) and that does not waste page space. I believe the articles found in this edition are very complementary to those found in *CVT XI*, and that the reader will find information that is both current and very practical. The book continues to be organized in 14 sections, beginning with "Special Therapy," Critical Care Therapy," "Toxicologic Disorders," and "Infectious Diseases," and followed by eight sections organized on an organ system basis. The final section, "Diseases of Birds and Exotic Pets," has been expanded with many new authors to emphasize this increasingly important area of companion animal practice. The Appendices, including the "Table of Common Drugs," have been updated to keep pace with the other advances described in this edition.

The best way to gain information from *Current Veterinary Therapy* is to first consult the index, which is cumulative and includes "still current" articles found in the prior two editions. Using this method, the reader will be able to find a brief and accurate article about most clinical problems. We have made every attempt to extensively cross-index information, including article references in the "Table of Common Drugs." Each section begins with a table of contents that indicates that section's articles, related articles located "Elsewhere in CVT," and articles that are "Still Current" and found in prior editions. Section tables of contents give the reader an opportunity to peruse the information that can be found in the "family" of *CVT* editions.

I am very thankful to the hundreds of excellent veterinarians and scientists who have contributed to this book. This edition would not be possible without the expertise and diligent work of Consulting Editors who supervise their respective sections. Dr. Bob Kirk is still an active participant in this volume, and I continue to benefit from his guidance. I am especially appreciative of Mr. David Kilmer, Developmental Editor at WB Saunders for his organizational skills and help in the preparation of manuscripts for production. Ray Kersey, Lee Walton, and Lorraine B. Kilmer at Saunders have provided general supervision for this edition of *CVT*. I am grateful to my students, Dr. Theresa Austin and Mr. Matt Ehrsmann, who ably organized manuscripts and kept the editorial process moving in Columbus. Thanks to Dr. Debra Primovic, for her help in cross-referencing this volume, and to Berta Steiner and associates at Bermedica Production, for so capably copyediting and producing this edition.

*Current Veterinary Therapy* is a book for veterinary practitioners and students of veterinary medicine. I would be very grateful to receive any comments from our readership, including your concerns about possible errors or omissions, as well as your ideas to improve this textbook. Dr. Kirk and I are most appreciative of your acceptance of this book, and hope the volumes of *Current Veterinary Therapy* will continue to be a useful reference.

JOHN D. BONAGURA, D.V.M.
*Columbus, Ohio*

# CONTENTS

Section 2
## CRITICAL CARE
Robert J. Murtaugh, *Consulting Editor*

Section 4
# INFECTIOUS DISEASES
Edward B. Breitschwerdt, *Consulting Editor*

Section 5
# ENDOCRINE AND METABOLIC DISORDERS
Mark E. Peterson, *Consulting Editor*

Section 6
# HEMATOLOGY, ONCOLOGY, AND IMMUNOLOGY
Bruce R. Madewell, *Consulting Editor*

Section 7

# DERMATOLOGIC DISEASES
William H. Miller, Jr., *Consulting Editor*

Section 8
# GASTROINTESTINAL DISORDERS
David C. Twedt, *Consulting Editor*

Section 9

# CARDIOPULMONARY DISEASE
Bruce W. Keene, *Consulting Editor*

Section 11

# REPRODUCTIVE DISORDERS

Vicki N. Meyers-Wallen, *Consulting Editor*

Section 12
## NEUROLOGIC AND MUSCULOSKELETAL DISORDERS
Kyle G. Braund and Steven C. Schrader, *Consulting Editors*

Section 13

# OPHTHALMOLOGIC DISEASES
Thomas J. Kern, *Consulting Editor*

Section 14

# DISEASES OF BIRDS AND EXOTIC PETS
R. Eric Miller, *Consulting Editor*

## APPENDICES
Robert M. Jacobs and Mark G. Papich, *Consulting Editors*

# NOTICE

Companion animal practice is an ever-changing field. Standard safety precautions must be followed, but as new research and clinical experience grow, changes in treatment and drug therapy become necessary or appropriate. The authors and editors of this work have carefully checked the generic and trade drug names and verified drug dosages to assure that dosage information is precise and in accord with standards accepted at the time of publication. Readers are advised, however, to check the product information currently provided by the manufacturer of each drug to be administered to be certain that changes have not been made in the recommended dose or in the contraindications for administration. This is of particular importance in regard to new or infrequently used drugs. Recommended dosages for animals are sometimes based on adjustments in the dosage that would be suitable for humans. Some of the drugs mentioned here have been given experimentally by the authors. Others have been used in dosages greater than those recommended by the manufacturer. In these kinds of cases, the authors have reported on their own considerable experience. It is the responsibility of those administering a drug, relying on their professional skill and experience, to determine the dosages, the best treatment for the patient, and whether the benefits of giving a drug justify the attendant risk. The editors cannot be responsible for misuse or misapplication of the material in this work.

THE PUBLISHER

# Section
# 1

# SPECIAL
# THERAPY

CARL A. OSBORNE
*Consulting Editor*

***Still Current Information Found in Current Veterinary Therapy XI:***

# TEN GUIDING PRINCIPLES TO ENHANCE THE BENEFIT OF CURRENT VETERINARY THERAPY

CARL A. OSBORNE,
JODY P. LULICH,
*St. Paul, Minnesota*
*and* JOSEPH W. BARTGES
*Athens, Georgia*

## WHAT IS EMPIRIC THERAPY?

Webster's Dictionary defines an empiric remedy as one chosen on the basis of practical (uncontrolled) experience, without reference to scientific principle. Empiric therapy is a common phenomenon. Why is this true? Could it be that empiric acceptance of the apparent value of various therapeutic modalities is unconsciously reinforced by the fact that most diseases are self-limiting? Isn't it true that the severity of most disorders declines within a day or two? In this situation, any form of treatment may appear to be beneficial, as long as it is not overtly harmful. Because a desired clinical response often occurs coincidentally with the administration of a therapeutic agent, many interpret the outcome as a cause-and-effect relationship.

Empiricism may also thrive because all of us have a tendency to generalize prematurely, owing to our eagerness to formulate conclusions. Too frequently we offer opinions based on one or two uncontrolled observations. Even though our intentions may be good, in reality this is a form of intellectual dishonesty. Rather than forcing conclusions on facts, we must be alert to allow reproducible observations (facts) to force conclusions.

Empiricism is also rooted in a culture where the veterinary profession, the medical profession, and the manufacturers and distributors of drugs have often promulgated an unrealistic concept of efficacy of therapeutic agents. The public has responded by demonstrating its belief that most diseases and disorders can be resolved or helped by administration of drugs or by surgery. Rather than ask, "How do you diagnose the problem?" too many individuals begin with the question, "How do you treat the problem?" We often hear that individuals are too busy to diagnose problems in their patients. Very few state that they are too busy to treat the problems. This is analogous to utilizing this sequence of events when using a gun: "Ready! Fire! . . . Aim!" There has been misplaced emphasis on what drug to prescribe rather than whether to prescribe.

How can we place a balanced perspective on the concept of empiricism? The limitations of simple clinical observations must be understood by all deliverers of health care if they are to consistently help, rather than harm, their patients. However, the ability to recognize true cause-and-effect relationships is not an innate characteristic—it must be learned! The ability to understand the enormous conceptual difference between random clinical observations and results of controlled clinical trials should be a prerequisite for every veterinarian. Rational scientific treatment, rather than empiric therapy, emerged when clinical research changed from anecdotal documentation to prospective, randomized, controlled, double-blind studies. We recognize that randomized trials are not methods of discovery, but rather a means of validation. Empiric observations are extremely important. The therapist who accepts the results of uncontrolled studies in lieu of properly controlled ones may, however, be responsible for perpetuation of medical myths. Lacking acceptable evidence of therapeutic efficacy, the occasional dramatic result is vividly remembered, the failures are forgotten, and folklore therapy often becomes established.

## TEN GUIDING PRINCIPLES OF THERAPY

In order for therapy to reach its maximum potential in each patient, the right reasons based on the right knowledge must be utilized to prescribe the right drug for the right patient at the right time in the right amount using the right dosage form and the right route of administration to bring about a right (or desired) response, and the right results must be recorded in the right record in a timely fashion.

### The Right Reasons

This edition of *Current Veterinary Therapy* is filled with information about the right reasons to select various types of therapy. When utilizing this information, however, we should also use proper reasoning to provide the quality of care that we would desire if we were the patients. The reason is that there are some patients we cannot help, but there are none we cannot harm. No patient should be the worse for having seen the doctor. Thus, we would use caution not to develop the unempathetic mindset encompassed by the often-used cliché, "A chance to cut is a chance to cure." Why not?

3

Because thoughtful veterinarians would not opt for cures based merely on chance. Ethics demand that we not let ill-conceived empiric treatment jeopardize the welfare of our patients.

Why do some veterinarians offer some form of therapy to clients who seek their advice, irrespective of whether a logical rationale for therapy has been established? Perhaps they feel that interaction with their clients must include some tangible form of treatment. Perhaps they reason that failure to prescribe some form of treatment will be interpreted as an admission of their inefficiency or fallibility. Perhaps they want to avoid being criticized of being ignorant or disinterested in the patient's welfare. Some defend the practice of mandatory treatment with the comment that clients expect it. We hope that if one of your clients wants some type of medicine that you know is not needed, or that is unlikely to be effective, you will not prescribe it on the premise that if you do not, your client will visit one of your colleagues who will. In some instances, a better alternative would be to dispense reassurance that self-limiting diseases do not require treatment. To paraphrase Hippocrates, it is a good remedy sometimes to do nothing. However, a decision to withhold treatment should be accompanied by an explanation as to why drugs are not prescribed, or why surgery is unlikely to benefit the patient.

## The Right Knowledge

The dictum *primum non nocere*—first do no harm—is attributed to Hippocrates. *Primum non nocere* infers that therapeutic intervention must be based on accurate scientific knowledge and rationale. Each patient should be evaluated with regard to the degree of necessity of therapy. Drugs should not be administered without a working knowledge of their pharmacokinetics and pharmacodynamics. Pharmacokinetics refers to how the body absorbs, distributes, metabolizes, and eliminates drugs and their metabolites from the body. Pharmacodynamics refers to the body's physiologic or psychologic response to a drug or a combination of drugs. In addition, knowledge of (1) species differences in drug actions and interactions, (2) possible effects of disease states on drug pharmacokinetic parameters and pharmacodynamic processes, and (3) possible interactions of combinations of drugs should be considered. Before prescribing drugs for the first time, the package insert that accompanies the drug should be reviewed.

Therapeutic plans should state the expected outcome (or goal) by indicating whether the therapeutic intervention is specific, supportive, or symptomatic in nature. Goal-setting forces precision, and precision forces logical plans.

## The Right Drug

Drugs may be given with the goal of providing specific, supportive, or symptomatic therapy. Specific treatment is given to eliminate, destroy, or modify the primary cause(s) of the disease process. Examples of specific treatment include use of antibiotics to eliminate bacterial infections, use of antidotes to counteract toxins, and replacement hormone therapy. Supportive treatment consists of therapy that modifies or eliminates abnormalities that occur secondary to the primary disease. Treatment designed to correct deficits and excesses in fluid, electrolyte, acid-base, endocrine, and nutrient balance caused by primary renal failure is an example of supportive therapy. Successful specific therapy is often dependent on successful supportive therapy. Symptomatic treatment consists of therapy given to eliminate or suppress clinical signs. Examples of symptomatic treatment include use of antiemetics to control vomiting, and use of glucocorticoids to control pruritis.

Choice of the right drug should also be based on knowledge of previous history of adverse drug events (e.g., rash, anxiety, tremors, anorexia, vomiting, diarrhea). To minimize adverse drug interactions, it is best to avoid unnecessary use of multiple combinations of drugs.

Unfortunately, selection of the right form of specific, supportive, or symptomatic therapy is not always associated with expected results. Drugs used to prevent, control, or eliminate various diseases also have the potential to induce disease. It is unfortunate that many pharmacokinetic and toxicity studies designed to minimize adverse drug events have been performed in normal animals, despite the fact that many drugs are given to patients with disease and perhaps dysfunction of one or more body systems. This phenomenon is important because these organs may play a vital role in the absorption, biotransformation, and elimination of drugs. If doses of pharmacologic agents designed for patients with normal organ function are repeatedly given to patients with organ dysfunction, the likelihood of adverse drug events is enhanced. To the unsuspecting therapist and patient, such adverse drug events may be erroneously attributed to progression of the underlying disease, or may be regarded as an unusual manifestation of the underlying disorder.

## The Right Patient

Giving the right drug chosen for the right reasons based on the right knowledge to the wrong patient is of little benefit, and sometimes harmful. When a team approach to dispensing and administering various types of medication is utilized, drugs and prescribing information for in-hospital use should be identified by patient name, not just patient location. Likewise, clients should be advised of the hazards of giving medications prescribed for one patient to another dog or cat that develops an illness with similar signs.

## The Right Time

The effectiveness or toxicity or both of many drugs is influenced by the frequency with which they are administered (so-called maintenance intervals). For example, one of the most significant reasons that antimicrobial therapy is ineffective in eliminating infections is that clients are unwilling or unable to follow recommended dosing intervals. Rather than following directions to give the total daily dose of the antibiotic in two equally spaced subdoses, they may only give one half the total daily dose once per day. Thus, the right drug is ineffective because it does not attain therapeutic concentrations in body fluids or tissues.

Failure to consistently administer drugs at the right times is especially common when multiple drugs are given at frequent or varying time intervals. Improper dosage intervals may also be associated with inability of clients to administer drugs by the oral or parenteral route. Before prescribing complicated therapeutic regimens, the client should be asked if they are willing and able to comply with the therapeutic plan.

## The Right Amount

A variety of factors influence selection and administration of the right amount of drug. They include counteracting or potentiating effects of multiple drugs. The influence of organ function or dysfunction on the absorption, biotransformation, and excretion of drugs is also of paramount importance. For example, in addition to the effect of kidney diseases on reduced renal clearance of drugs, decreased intake of dietary protein may also reduce renal plasma flow, creatinine clearance, and the clearance of drugs by the kidneys. Likewise, hypoalbuminemia may have a profound effect on the dosage of drugs that normally bind to plasma proteins.

Even though manufacturers specify therapeutic dosage ranges for drugs, drug dosages must be individualized for each patient. In addition to considering body weight, proper dosage may be influenced by such factors as magnitude of weight loss, state of hydration, presence of ascites, or degree of obesity. For example, highly fat-soluble drugs may have an increased duration of effect in obese patients. Likewise, drugs that are safe in normal adults may create problems in pediatric or aged patients. If dosages are calculated for patients at one body weight, but not subsequently adjusted if substantial weight gain or weight loss occurs, underdosing or overdosing may be an adverse consequence. Pharmacokinetic studies of different drugs indicate that drug absorption, protein binding, drug metabolism, and drug clearance may be altered by protein calorie malnutrition (Williams, Davis, and Lowenthal, 1993).

The effect of food on the absorption of orally administered drugs should also be considered. Absorption of drugs may be decreased, delayed, increased, or unaffected by physiologic changes that occur in the gastrointestinal tract in fed and fasting states. In general, food reduces the bioavailability of drugs. Likewise, the administration of drugs through nasogastric tubes or gastrostomy tubes containing various types of enteral nutrition formulas may affect their bioavailability.

## The Right Dosage Form

Drugs are available in a variety of forms, including powders, capsules, tablets, liquids, lotions, ointments, suppositories, nebulizers, and injectables. Numerous factors influence choice of dosage form, including ease of administration, patient tolerance, rate of absorption, state of hydration, status of the gastrointestinal tract, and desired timing and duration of effect. Clients should be advised not to crush tablets that have special coatings, as this will negate the purpose of the coating. They should also be advised of the action to take if they are unable or unwilling to administer drugs in the dosage form prescribed.

## The Right Route of Administration

As with dosage forms, numerous factors influence choice of the route of administration of the drugs. Vomiting, diarrhea, or inability to swallow all have an impact on whether to choose orally administered medications. Likewise, inability of a client to give a cat or dog the proper dosage and frequency of oral medications will have an impact on the route of administration of a drug. The magnitude of dehydration influences whether rehydrating fluids will be administered by the intravenous, subcutaneous, oral, or a combination of routes. Desired onset and duration of action, as well as cost of drugs, are also important.

## The Right Response

The definition of the right response is that which accomplishes a therapeutic goal. The question remains: How will achievement of this goal be monitored and recognized?

The problem-oriented medical system emphasizes the need to obtain pertinent clinical data before proceeding with an unprejudiced analysis of the facts. Diagnostic data bases (minimum data bases and problem-specific data bases) have been developed to permit systematic and consistent collection of data that are not unduly biased by premature establishment of a tentative diagnosis (Osborne et al., 1983). Whereas minimum data bases were designed as screening protocols that aid in identification of important problems, problem-specific data bases were designed as searching protocols that aid in evaluation of a problem in sufficient depth to characterize it adequately. Following this line of reasoning, we recommend development and use of therapeutic-specific data bases (Tables 1 and 2) (Lulich et al., 1992). The simplicity or complexity of the therapeutic-specific data base is influenced by the nature of the disease being treated, as well as the safety and efficacy of the drug(s) being used. Following development of therapeutic-specific data bases, they should be reexamined periodically for important omissions and redundancies. They must be updated as new information about drugs is discovered. Once a therapeutic-spe-

**Table 1.** *Therapeutic-Specific Data Base for Treatment of Bacterial UTI*

I.   Has bacterial UTI been confirmed?
     A.  Simple or complicated?
     B.  First episode or recurrent episode?
II.  Select appropriate drug
     A.  Antimicrobial susceptibility test?
     B.  Upper or lower UTI? Prostatitis?
     C.  Status of renal function?
III. Select appropriate dose and maintenance interval
     A.  Client compliance?
     B.  Status of renal function?
IV.  Select appropriate duration of treatment
     A.  Upper or lower UTI? Prostatitis?
     B.  First episode or recurrent episode?
         1.  Relapse?
         2.  Reinfection?
     C.  Simple or complicated UTI?
V.   Consider need for ancillary treatment
VI.  Monitor response
     A.  Clinical signs
     B.  Urinalysis
     C.  Urine culture
VII. Consider prevention
     A.  Status of host defenses?
     B.  Preventative antibiotic treatment (reinfections)
     C.  Suppressive antibiotic treatment (persistent infections)

Abbreviation: UTI = urinary tract infection.

cific data base has been defined, it should be written down. The strongest memory is weaker than the palest ink!

Using a therapeutic-specific data base as a reference point may help in education of clients about the nature of the problem(s) identified in their animals, the probable future course of events (prognosis), and the reasons and schedule for therapy. Owners must be informed about the veterinarian's predictions of the progress of the case so that they will be able to recognize deviations from the expected, and so that they will have some perspective of the significance of deviations. Veterinarians should convey to their clients that their judgments, opinions, and management plans are not infallible, and that if significant changes from the expected occur, they should call for help or return for reevaluation.

We would like to emphasize one more point. The fact that our patients get well does not prove that our diagnosis and treatment were correct. The greater the knowledge and experience of the doctor, the less (s)he is likely to interpret the results of the therapeutic recommendations as completely successful.

**Table 2.** *Therapeutic-Specific Data Base for Monitoring Renal Failure in Cats[*]*

| Minimum Follow-up Data | Problem-Specific Considerations |
| --- | --- |
| A.  History checklist<br>  1.  Diet: Type? Compliance?<br>      Frequency of feeding? Willingness to eat?<br>      Quantity consumed? Supplements?<br>  2.  Water consumption: Increased? Decreased?<br>      No change? Unknown?<br>  3.  Micturition: Frequency? Quantity? Color?<br>      Odor?<br>  4.  Amelioration of polysystemic signs:<br>      a.  Anorexia?    d.  Weight Loss?<br>      b.  Vomiting?    e.  Constipation?<br>      c.  Diarrhea?    f.  Others?<br>  5.  Medication history: Medications given?<br>      When given? Dosage? Compliance?<br>      Response?<br>B.  Physical examination checklist<br>  1.  Temperature, pulse, and respiratory rate?<br>  2.  Amelioration of clinical signs:<br>      a.  Dehydration?<br>      b.  Gastrointestinal signs?<br>          (1)  Mucosal ulcers?<br>          (2)  Discoloration of tongue?<br>      c.  Cardiovascular signs:<br>          (1)  Pale mucous membrane color?<br>          (2)  Abnormal pulse rate and<br>               character?<br>          (3)  Delayed capillary refill time?<br>          (4)  Venous distention?<br>          (5)  Elevated arterial blood pressure?<br>      d.  Abnormal kidney size, shape, consistency, contour, pain?<br>C.  Laboratory data checklist<br>  1.  Urinalysis<br>  2.  Kidney function tests (serum creatinine and urea nitrogen)<br>  3.  Hematocrit, total plasma protein concentration (CBC?) | A.  Urinary tract infection<br>  1.  Quantitative urine culture<br>B.  Protein-losing glomerulonephropathy<br>  1.  Urine protein creatinine ratio<br>  2.  Serum albumin concentration<br>C.  Obstructive uropathy<br>  1.  Ultrasonography or contrast radiography<br>      (e.g., intravenous urography, cystography) to<br>      verify continued patency of urinary tract.<br>D.  Divalent ion disorders<br>  1.  Serum concentrations of phosphorus, calcium, parathyroid hormone (?), and 1,25 vitamin D (?).<br>  2.  Evaluate for signs of osteodystrophy:<br>      a.  Loose or missing teeth?<br>      b.  Enlargement of maxillary tissues?<br>      c.  "Rubber jaw"<br>E.  Acidosis<br>  1.  Serum concentrations of total $CO_2$, $HCO_3$, and hydrogen ion (pH)<br>F.  Anemia<br>  1.  Hematocrit<br>  2.  Total plasma protein concentration<br>G.  Hypertension<br>  1.  Arterial blood pressure<br>  2.  Ophthalmoscopic examination for retinopathies (detachment? hemorrhage? others?)<br>H.  Potassium disorders<br>  1.  Serum concentration of potassium<br>  2.  Evaluate for signs of hypokalemia<br>      a.  Muscle weakness<br>      b.  Renal concentration<br>  3.  Evaluate for signs of hyperkalemia<br>      a.  Auscultate heart rate and rhythm<br>      b.  Electrocardiogram |

[*]Data derived from Lulich et al., 1992.

## Recording the Right Results in the Right Record

Medical records are an important tool in the practice of veterinary medicine. They serve as a basis for planning patient care and as a means of communication between members of the hospital staff. They furnish documentary evidence of the patient's illness, care, and treatment. They serve as a basis for review, study, and evaluation of medical care rendered by the hospital (Saidla et al., 1978).

This concise statement in the *Medical Records Manual* of the American Animal Hospital Association summarizes the vital role medical records play in the practice of veterinary medicine. The key concepts encompassed in this paragraph are (1) planning of patient care; (2) communication between the doctor and all other individuals involved with patient care; (3) written accounts that will aid in assessment of the progress of the patient; and (4) review (or audit), which serves as an excellent source of continuing self-education. Properly constructed medical records provide important reminders that foster effective and efficient medical action. Notes about therapeutic plans and drugs that have been dispensed should be entered into a medical record in a timely fashion, in a legible and reproducible form that is readily retrievable. Hospitals that cannot retrieve medical records in a timely fashion have no advantage over hospitals that do not keep medical records.

## SUMMARY

The common denominator of the ten guiding principles to enhance the benefit of current veterinary therapy is to strive to provide the quality of care that we would desire if we were the patients. This can best be accomplished if we envision ourselves in their situation. We must avoid the mindset of "a pill for every ill." Remember the admonition of Hippocrates: "To help, or at least do no harm." No patient should be worse for having seen the doctor.

## References and Suggested Reading

Lulich JP, Osborne CA, O'Brien TD, and Polzin DJ: Feline renal failure: Questions, answers, questions. Compend Cont Educ 14:127, 1992.

Osborne CA, et al: The problem-oriented medical system. Vet Clin North Am 13:745, 1983.

Saidla JE, Jeffrey KL, Lorenz MD, et al: *Medical Records Manual.* Denver, CO, American Animal Hospital Association, 1978.

Williams L, Davis JA, and Lowenthal DT: The influence of food on the absorption and metabolism of drugs. Med Clin North Am 77:815, 1993.

# CLINICAL EPIDEMIOLOGY FOR THE VETERINARY PRACTITIONER: THE DIAGNOSTIC PROCESS

ELIZABETH M. LUND
*and* JEFFREY S. KLAUSNER
*St. Paul, Minnesota*

Although veterinary practitioners make diagnostic decisions every day, it is important to remember that the diagnostic process is imperfect. Rarely do animals develop diseases that can be diagnosed on the basis of one or more pathognomonic findings. Typically, a combination of the historic, physical, and laboratory findings determine the most probable cause of illness.

Because of the nature of the process, all diagnoses are expressed with some degree of uncertainty. For example, a veterinarian may express to a client the certainty of a diagnosis of feline leukemia infection as, "It is likely that your cat has feline leukemia virus infection" or, "There is a 50% chance that your cat has feline leukemia virus infection." Establishing a diagnosis is a process of removing uncertainty until the veterinarian believes, with a high degree of confidence, that the suspected diagnosis is correct. Results of history, physical examination, radiographic studies, and clinical chemistry studies aid in elimination of uncertainty.

Uncertainty regarding diagnosis exists because of biologic variability between individuals and within individuals from time to time. Uncertainty is often expressed in terms of probability (i.e., the odds of feline leukemia are 3:1 or, the probability of feline leukemia virus infection is 33%). The concepts of probability may seem to be more appropriate to blackjack than to clinical diagnosis, but the laws of probability are as integral to the activity of a veterinarian as to a blackjack dealer.

In this article, we review, through examples, some concepts of clinical epidemiology that will help practitioners understand the probabilities inherent to the diagnostic process. With this knowledge, practitioners can better determine which diagnostic tools to utilize and how to improve their interpretation of diagnostic test results.

### Clinical Example

A 6-year-old male intact domestic shorthair cat is admitted to your clinic because of decreased appetite and weight loss. The cat has been losing weight for 3 weeks. Physical examination reveals a very thin cat with pale mucous membranes. The owners noted that the cat had been allowed to go out of doors most of the summer months. Although you are unsure of the diagnosis at this point, you believe that feline leukemia virus infection (FeLV) is a possibility.

*How can knowledge of sensitivity and specificity aid in deciding between two diagnostic tests?*

## SENSITIVITY AND SPECIFICITY

Knowledge of sensitivity and specificity of diagnostic tests aids in determining whether one test may be preferred in a given clinical situation. Sensitivity and specificity are properties of diagnostic tests that reflect the ability of a certain test to identify a truly diseased or nondiseased individual. Sensitivity and specificity can be calculated for diagnostic tests as well as physical signs or historic findings; however, a "gold standard" must exist. A gold standard is a definitive marker for a disease—a valid indicator of the disease in question. For example, histopathologic confirmation of a cancer diagnosis often serves as a gold standard. Without a gold standard, there is no reference to evaluate the diagnostic test in question.

Feline leukemia virus is high on our diagnostic "rule-out" list. A simple test to screen for this disease would be appropriate at this point; the enzyme-linked immunosorbent assay (ELISA) test is quick and can be done in the practice setting. You wish to perform an ELISA test for FeLV, but you are uncertain whether it would be better to perform the test using saliva or serum.

To evaluate the sensitivity and specificity of the two ELISA tests, the immunofluorescent antibody test (IFA) will be used as a gold standard (virus isolation could be used as well [Hardy, 1981]). The results of the IFA and both the saliva and serum ELISA tests will be compared for a hypothetical population of cats.

Sensitivity represents the percentage of individuals with the disease who have a positive test (i.e., the "true"-positive rate). This can be calculated from 2 X 2 tables (Figs. 1 and 2), and is shown in Figure 1 by dividing the number of individuals with the disease who tested positive (cell A) by the number of individuals with the disease who tested both positive and negative (A + C). Those with the disease who tested negative are referred to as false negatives; the false negative rate = 1 − sensitivity. As can be seen from the calculations in Figures 3 and 4, the sensitivity (SE) for the serum ELISA test is 95% and the sensitivity for the ELISA test performed on saliva is 86%.

Specificity represents the percentage of individuals without the disease who tested negative (i.e., the "true"-negative rate). Specificity is calculated by dividing the number of individuals without the disease who tested negative (cell D) by the number of all the individuals who are truly disease free (B + D). Those without the disease who test positive are referred to as false positives; the false-positive rate = 1 − specificity. As can be seen from the calculations in Figures 3 and 4, the specificity (SP) of the serum ELISA test is 90%, and 40% for the salivary ELISA test.

How can this information help us choose between the saliva and serum ELISA? If given a choice between a very sensitive or very specific test, which should be selected? A sensitive test is most appropriate for use as a screening test, a tool to identify all those who are positive to go on for more definitive testing. A sensitive test will minimize the false negative rate so that the diagnosis (and therefore treatment) will be missed in as few truly diseased individuals as possible based on this particular test. When ruling out a disease, sensitivity is more important than specificity, a negative result is relied on more heavily at this point in the diagnostic

Figure 1. Sensitivity and specificity.

$$\text{Sensitivity} = \frac{A}{A + C}$$

$$\text{Specificity} = \frac{D}{B + D}$$

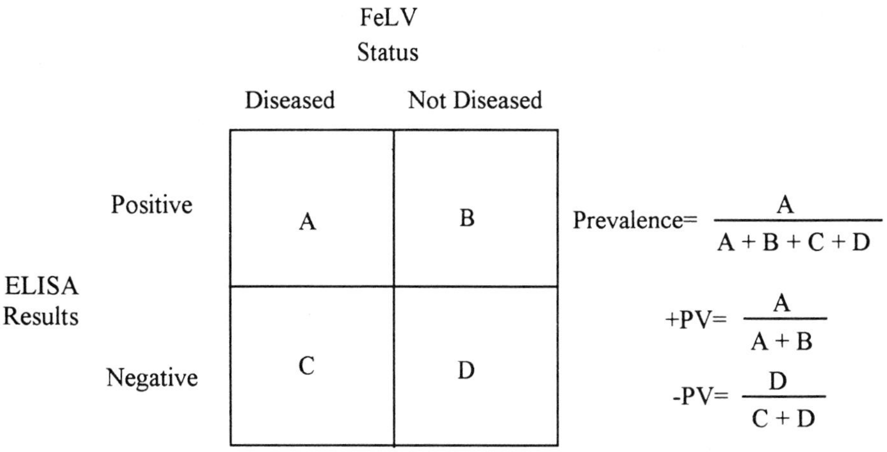

FeLV
Status

Diseased    Not Diseased

**Figure 2.** Positive and negative predictive value. Abbreviations: +PV = positive predictive value, −PV = negative predictive value.

Positive | A | B

ELISA
Results

Negative | C | D

$$Prevalence = \frac{A}{A+B+C+D}$$

$$+PV = \frac{A}{A+B}$$

$$-PV = \frac{D}{C+D}$$

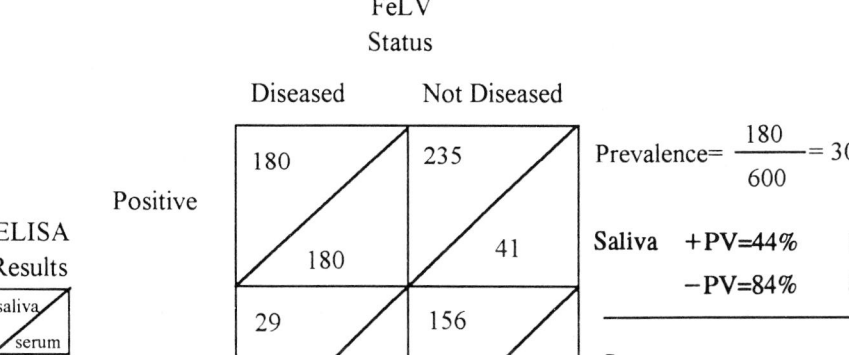

FeLV
Status

Diseased    Not Diseased

Positive | 180 | 235 |
| 180 | 41 |

ELISA
Results

saliva/serum

Negative | 29 | 156 |
| 10 | 369 |

$$Prevalence = \frac{180}{600} = 30\%$$

Saliva  +PV=44%    SE=86%
        −PV=84%    SP=40%

Serum   +PV=81%    SE=95%
        −PV=97%    SP=90%

**Figure 3.** Example using 30% FeLV prevalence. Abbreviations: +PV = positive predictive value, −PV = negative predictive value, SE = sensitivity, SP = specificity.

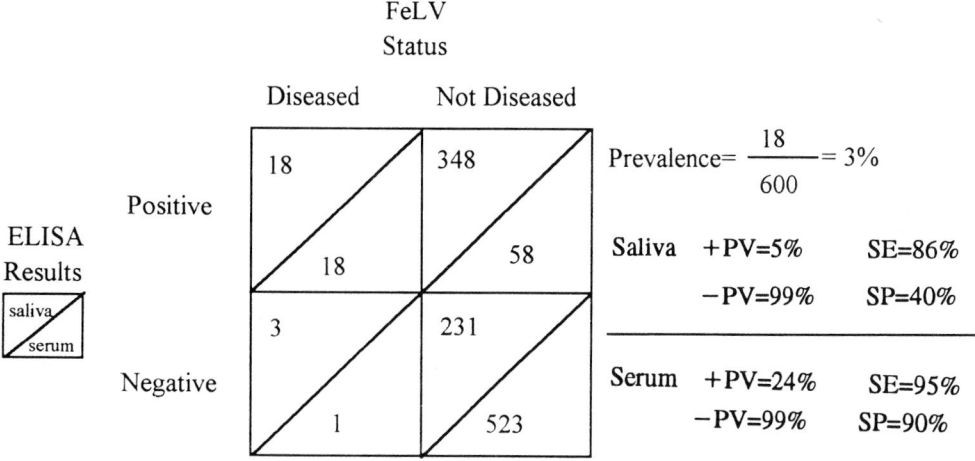

FeLV
Status

Diseased    Not Diseased

Positive | 18 | 348 |
| 18 | 58 |

ELISA
Results

saliva/serum

Negative | 3 | 231 |
| 1 | 523 |

$$Prevalence = \frac{18}{600} = 3\%$$

Saliva  +PV=5%     SE=86%
        −PV=99%    SP=40%

Serum   +PV=24%    SE=95%
        −PV=99%    SP=90%

**Figure 4.** Example using 3% FeLV prevalence. Abbreviations: +PV = positive predictive value, −PV = negative predictive value, SE = sensitivity, SP = specificity.

process. Alternatively, when it is important to confirm a diagnosis or to "rule-in" a disease, a more specific test should be used to minimize the false-positive rate. Otherwise, a treatment course/medical management strategy could be used based on a result that incorrectly indicates that a patient is diseased.

Based on the calculated sensitivity and specificity of the two ELISA tests, we might be tempted to choose to perform just the serum test, as both the sensitivity and specificity are higher compared to the saliva test. However, the cat is very debilitated and it would be easier to do a saliva test. Could *either* the saliva or the serum test be used in this patient as a rule-out test for FeLV, since the sensitivity for both is high? Is the serum ELISA test appropriate as a rule-in test as well? Since we are unsure, we decide to do the ELISA on both serum and saliva; the results for both tests are positive for this patient.

Although sensitivity and specificity help us to understand how well the two ELISA tests perform in general compared to the IFA, more information is needed to interpret the results for this particular individual.

*How can knowledge of predictive value aid in determining if a positive test result is likely to be a true positive?*

## PREDICTIVE VALUE

Although sensitivity and specificity can be useful in comparing and evaluating tests, knowing the probability that a certain test result is indicative of a truly diseased or nondiseased state is even more pertinent to the clinical decision-making process. In other words, given a positive or negative result for a specific test, what is the likelihood that the patient does or doesn't have the disease in question?

Unlike sensitivity and specificity, the determination of predictive value is dependent on the *prevalence of disease* in the population being tested (the percentage of individuals with existing disease). Prevalence is also referred to as the pretest probability (i.e., the probability an individual in a defined population is diseased before any additional diagnostic information is obtained). Since our patient comes from a multiple-cat household and was ill prior to evaluation, the pretest probability is approximately 30%.

The prevalence of disease in a population affects the ability of a specific test to predict whether an individual animal is truly diseased or not. If a disease is relatively common in a population, there is a more likely probability that a test will be able to predict a truly diseased individual (i.e., there will be few false-positives). Alternatively, if a disease is relatively rare, the ability of the test to identify a truly diseased individual will be diminished, and more false-positives will be identified.

Positive predictive value (+PV) is calculated (Fig. 2) by dividing the number of truly diseased individuals with a positive test by all the individuals with a positive test (A/A + B). Negative predictive value (−PV) is determined by dividing the number of truly non diseased

individuals with negative test results by all the individuals with a negative test result (D/C + D). Using a prevalence of 30%, the +PV=81% and the −PV=97% for the serum ELISA; the +PV=44% and the −PV=84% for the ELISA test on saliva (Fig. 3). The negative predictive values are high for both tests in this example, exactly what is needed for a rule-out test. If the test results had been negative, our confidence in the "truth" of the results would have been greater. However, the results were positive for the patient in our example. How can the positive predictive values be interpreted? Eighty-one per cent of the individuals with a positive serum ELISA test actually have FeLV, whereas the likelihood of FeLV infection for an individual with a positive saliva test is only 44%. The positive predictive value is low for both ELISA tests as a result of the relatively low prevalence of FeLV in this population, and the relatively low specificity of the ELISA tests.

Does the cat have FeLV infection (can FeLV infection be ruled in)? The positive predictive value for the better of the two tests, the serum ELISA, was only 81%. Thus, with a relatively sensitive and specific test and a 30% prevalence of disease, there is still a one in five chance that the positive result is false. For the ELISA test performed using saliva, there is less than a 50% chance that the positive result represents a true-positive. This highlights the importance of interpreting test results in conjunction with the rest of the clinical findings (such as historic, physical examination, and radiographic indicators of the disease in question) and the need to use a more specific test, such as the IFA, to rule in a diagnosis.

If our patient was healthy and had been living in a single-cat household, the pretest probability (the prevalence of FeLV) would have been lower, approximately 3%. Using a prevalence of 3% for our example, the +PV=24% and the −PV=99% for the serum ELISA; the +PV=5% and the −PV=98% for the ELISA on saliva (Fig. 4). Again, we would have more confidence in the negative results. As the prevalence decreased between our two examples, the negative predictive values increased. As the pretest probability of disease decreases so does the likelihood of falsely identifying negative individuals. As the prevalence of disease decreased from 30% to 3%, the positive predictive values decreased as well; there is a far greater chance of an incorrect diagnosis based on a positive result.

Would either the serum or salivary ELISA tests ever be specific enough to use for ruling in a diagnosis (i.e., would the positive predictive value be great enough to make a definitive diagnosis)? As the specificity increases, the false-positive rate decreases and the positive predictive value increases. If we use the serum ELISA as an example, to achieve a +PV=91% (approximately nine out of every ten cats tested positive are really positive), the prevalence of FeLV must be 50% in the population tested. Alternatively, if we had an improved ELISA test for serum with a specificity of 99% (sensitivity=95%), the probability of a correct diagnosis of FeLV increases to 98% in a population with a prevalence of 30%.

## SUMMARY

Equipped with an understanding of sensitivity and specificity, practitioners can make more informed decisions about the most appropriate diagnostic tools to use for ruling in and ruling out diagnoses. With additional knowledge of the prevalence of disease in their veterinary population, practitioners can use predictive values to better quantify the likelihood of disease for a particular patient. Thus, application of clinical epide-miology to medical decision making enhances the quality of patient care.

## References and Suggested Reading

Fletcher RH, Fletcher SW, and Wagner EH: *Clinical Epidemiology. The Essentials*, 2nd edition. Baltimore, Williams & Wilkins, 1988.
Greenberg RS: *Medical Epidemiology*. Norwalk, CT, Appleton & Lange, 1993.
Hardy WD Jr: The feline leukemia virus. J Am Anim Hosp Assoc 17:951, 1981.
Sackett DL, Haynes RB, Guyatt GH, and Tugwell P: *Clinical Epidemiology. A Basic Science for Clinical Medicine*, 2nd edition. Boston, Little, Brown and Company, 1991.
Smith RD: *Veterinary Clinical Epidemiology. A Problem-Oriented Approach*. Boston, Butterworth's, 1991.
Sox HC, Blatt MA, Higgins MC, and Marton KI: *Medical Decision Making*. Boston, Butterworth's, 1988.

# DIAGNOSIS BY RULE-OUT: JUDGMENT IN THE ABSENCE OF CERTAINTY

CARL A. OSBORNE

*St. Paul, Minnesota*

## PATIENT CARE FROM THE CLIENT'S VIEWPOINT

From a client's point of view, the antemortem differentiation of potentially reversible from irreversible disease is the single most important unknown related to clinical assessment of disease. Clients typically ask, "Can you help, doctor?" Our clients are concerned about the probability of recovery of their animals from disease states with or without therapy, the nature and cost of therapy, and whether recovery will be partial or complete. In order for the veterinarian to make this distinction logically and consistently in the living patient, establishment of the underlying cause of the disease, knowledge of its biologic behavior, and an understanding of the body's compensatory response to organ disease and organ failure are essential.

## PATIENT CARE FROM THE VETERINARIAN'S VIEWPOINT

The concept of a "key" (pathognomonic finding) that will unlock the barrier to a specific diagnosis is misleading. Rarely will a single historic event, a single physical finding, a single laboratory test result, or a single radiograph provide information of sufficient specificity to permit establishment of a definitive diagnosis. Nor will memorization of the key clinical manifestations of a specific disease described in textbooks be effective in detecting it, since the same disease typically induces a variety of manifestations of different degrees of severity in different patients. Most textbook descriptions are abstracts of prototypical features of diseases that uncommonly coexist in each patient. To quote Sir James Paget: "As no two individuals are exactly alike in health, so neither are any two in disease."

A more realistic analogy is to consider that a combination lock must be opened before one can determine the underlying cause of a problem. The history is one numeral of the combination; the physical examination is another. Proper selection of laboratory tests, radiographic or ultrasonographic techniques, and biopsy procedures are additional numerals to the combination. Response to pharmacologic agents and exploratory surgery are additional examples that may be a part of the combination leading to the specific diagnosis of some disease states. As in the case with any combination lock, the bolt will not be released unless one has knowledge and understanding of the proper sequence of the numerals in addition to their specific identity.

## PROBLEM DEFINITION VERSUS PROBLEM SOLUTION

One of the fundamental steps in the diagnostic process is the capacity to define the patient's medical problems without overstating them. This is a crucial first step in the diagnostic process, since one must be able to define problems before they can be solved. No veterinarian has or ever will be trained to single-handedly solve all types of medical problems. No one can ever memorize enough knowledge and master enough techniques to guarantee the best care of every patient. Veterinarians can be trained to identify problems, however. They can and should be master "problem definers." Accurate definition of all of a patient's problems will permit the diagnostician to utilize available resources, such as journals, books, consultations, and referrals, to solve diagnostic and therapeutic problems. A problem well defined is half solved.

In the process of defining problems, one must use care not to mix observations with interpretations randomly. Observations and interpretations represent distinctly separate facets of diagnosis. Although observations are often correct, interpretations of observations are frequently erroneous. If misinterpretations are accepted as facts, the ultimate result may be misdiagnosis and formulation of inappropriate or contraindicated therapy.

## DIAGNOSIS BY RULE-OUT

Traditionally, diagnostic plans encompass formulation of differential or tentative diagnoses (called rule-outs [R/O] or rule-ins [R/I]) and choice of tests to prove or disprove these hypotheses. However, consideration of tentative diagnoses is premature unless the problems have been accurately defined, verified, and if possible, localized. These beginning steps of diagnosis are a part of an overall priority of clinical investigation (Table 1).

It is often necessary to verify the presence and nature of problems detected by clients. Errors in verification of clinical problems are among the most common and fundamental causes of misdiagnosis. Clients often make inaccurate observations that, if accepted without verification, may lead to a great deal of nonproductive activity in pursuit of nonexistent disorders. They may also result in a costly and time-consuming series of diagnostic and therapeutic plans before errors are identified. For example, if polyuria is identified as an owner's complaint in the problem list, the first diagnostic plan should be to "confirm polyuria" by observation and/or evaluation of urine specific gravity or osmolality. In other situations, clients' observations may be accurate (e.g., "My male cat has been straining to eliminate"), but their interpretation may be erroneous (e.g., "My cat is constipated," when in reality the cat has urethral obstruction). Once again, diagnostic consideration should be given to verifying the owner's statement about constipation.

Localization of problems should follow their verification (Table 1). For example, if a patient is examined because of gross hematuria, but no other abnormalities are initially identified, the problem should be listed as gross hematuria. Additional information is required to determine its location(s) (kidneys, ureters, urinary bladder, urethra, or genital tract) and cause(s) (anomalies,

**Table 1.** *The Four Priorities of Clinical Investigation*

I.  **First Priority: Verification of Problems**
    A. Especially important for historic problems such as polyuria, tenesmus, vomiting, diarrhea, and so forth
    B. Also of importance for transient or intermittent problems

II. **Second Priority: Localization of Problems**
    A. Strive to localize problem to a body system or organ
    B. Localization may also be utilized to categorize the underlying pathophysiology of the disease
    C. Examples include:
       1. Prerenal, primary renal, and postrenal azotemia
       2. Primary or secondary gastrointestinal disease
       3. Small-bowel or large-bowel diarrhea
       4. Regenerative or nonregenerative anemia
       5. Preglomerular, glomerular, or postglomerular proteinuria
       6. Peripheral nervous versus central nervous system disease
       7. Neurogenic versus non-neurogenic incontinence
       8. Physiologic versus pathologic versus pharmacologic polyuria

III. **Third Priority: Consideration of Probable Pathophysiologic Cause(s) of Disease (DAMN IT)**
    A. D = Degenerative; developmental; demented (psychologic)
    B. A = Anomaly; Allergic; autoimmune
    C. M = Metabolic; mechanical
    D. N = Nutritional; neoplastic (benign or malignant)
    E. I = Inflammatory (infectious or noninfectious); immune; iatrogenic; ischemic; idiopathic
    F. T = Toxicity (endogenous or exogenous); trauma (internal or external)

IV. **Fourth Priority: Establishing Specific Cause(s) of Disease**

neoplasia, infection, uroliths, exogenous or endogenous toxins, coagulopathies, and so on). In contrast, if hematuria occurs independent of micturition and is associated with a palpable lesion of the urethra, the problem might be defined as a urethral lesion associated with gross hematuria.

Following localization of problems to a body system or organ, it is useful to think of basic pathophysiologic mechanisms when trying to determine probable (rather than possible) causes of each problem (Table 1). The acronym "DAMN IT" (see Table 1) may be useful for this purpose. One of the most frequent errors made by inexperienced diagnosticians is the premature consideration of specific disease entities without verifying the existence of problems (especially those identified by owners), without localizing problems to the appropriate body system or organ, and without considering basic pathophysiologic disease mechanisms that might be involved. If one habitually bypasses these important components of problem solving, one will become overly dependent on establishing diagnoses on the basis of previous experience, rather than developing the capacity to diagnose disease processes that he or she has never personally encountered.

Following consideration of basic pathophysiologic mechanisms of disease, one may consider the most probable cause(s) of the problem (i.e., the specific diagnoses) (Table 1). They should be arranged in order of priority so that the most probable causes are evaluated first, while the least possible causes are considered last (if they are considered at all). At this phase of clinical investigation, the diagnostic plans should state what cause(s) is to be ruled-out or ruled-in and by what tests or procedures (laboratory data, radiographic data, biopsy data, exploratory surgery, and so forth). The specific tests and procedures chosen to evaluate each problem and the rate and frequency with which they are determined are dependent on the status of the patient. If the problem is life threatening, several diagnostic probabilities (rule-outs) may have to be investigated simultaneously; that is, in parallel. For example, if a critically ill patient is admitted because of rapidly progressing vomiting, dehydration, polyuria, and extreme depression, it will be necessary to select laboratory and radiographic data to simultaneously (in parallel) prove or disprove primary renal failure, diabetic ketoacidosis, hepatic failure, and pyometra. If an individual priority list is established and each problem is evaluated one at a time, the patient may die before a specific diagnosis is established. In contrast, if these problems are not as severe, are not life threatening, and do not appear to be progressing at a rapid rate, the most probable hypothesized cause (e.g., primary renal failure) should be pursued first (i.e., in series). If clinical data rule out the disease that the clinician considered to be the most probable cause (e.g., primary renal failure), the second most probable cause (e.g., diabetic ketoacidosis) should be pursued, and so on.

## DIAGNOSIS OF A DIAGNOSIS

Confusion and misunderstanding often occur when two people attempt to communicate using two different languages. More commonly, confusion arises between individuals using the same language, but each attaching a different meaning or a different definition for what appears to be a universally accepted term.

The noun "diagnosis" is derived from Greek words meaning to distinguish or to discern. Establishment of a diagnosis encompasses determination of the cause of disease(s) by detection and evaluation of its manifestations. The diagnostic process often involves complex cognitive activities. Knowledge of the specific cause of the patient's disease(s) is important because it often

permits (1) an accurate forecast of the biologic behavior of the disease, (2) assessment of the availability of specific therapy, (3) assessment of the need for supportive or symptomatic therapy or both, and (4) assessment of the ability of the body to compensate for irrevocable damage to various biologic functions.

Interpretation of the term diagnosis often is difficult and confusing because it is used to convey a variety of different meanings. Clarification of intended meaning often can be achieved by use of appropriate adjectives, including anatomic, bacteriologic, clinical, definitive, differential, exclusion, final, necropsy, pathologic, physiologic, physical, probable, radiographic, specific, tentative, and so forth.

Although most would agree that establishment of a specific diagnosis is an important component of current veterinary therapy, the diagnosis is often a matter of opinion rather than a matter of fact. Most clinical diagnoses require judgment in the absence of certainty. If a specific diagnosis has been established on the basis of insufficient evidence, it is an overdiagnosis. It also may represent a misdiagnosis. In many situations diagnosis of a clinical problem(s) does not represent unequivocal identification of the cause(s) of disease. The fact that a patient gets well does not prove that the diagnosis was correct or that the treatment given was beneficial.

Too often, veterinary students and veterinarians have been trained to become proficient in making diagnoses on the basis of insufficient clinical information. This mode of medical action tends to become increasingly prevalent when veterinarians are subjected to the pressures of a busy hospital or client economic limitations. This approach to diagnosis overemphasizes the memorization, the need for experience, and educated guesswork. Teachers of this concept unwittingly encourage students to become intellectually dishonest. It is one thing to make a diagnosis and another to substantiate it. If diagnoses are never audited for accuracy, there is no way of detecting and correcting errors. Soon one begins to rely less and less on data and more and more on intuition. Diagnosis by intuition is a rapid method of reaching the wrong conclusion. This activity is best viewed as a form of intellectual brownian movement. In fact, it often represents activity without accomplishment. For most diagnoses, what is needed is an ounce of knowledge, an ounce of intelligence, and a pound of thoroughness.

# CAUSES AND EFFECTS OF INTERFERENCE WITH CLINICAL LABORATORY MEASUREMENTS AND EXAMINATIONS

MARY JO BURKHARD
*and* D. J. MEYER

*Fort Collins, Colorado*

*Primum non nocere (First do no harm).*

Hippocrates

Laboratory medicine complements the clinical examination of the veterinary patient. Normal and abnormal laboratory results provide objective information for differential diagnosis, formulation of a prognosis, and monitoring treatment. Abnormal laboratory measurements and examinations are defined clinically as values that lie outside the limits of the reference range. Reference ranges are obtained by sampling a representative population and statistically eliminating outliers. The resultant data are commonly used to define health. What is normal? The answer is more difficult than it superficially appears. It should be specific for species, and in some cases for breed, geographic locale, and laboratory methodology. Since abnormal is predicated by the reference range, it becomes a critical data base.

Interpretation of laboratory data derived from properly collected specimens appears to be a straightforward process. However, interpretation of laboratory data becomes problematic when artifact is suspected. The objective of this article is to provide guidance in identifying and recognizing factitious laboratory data. Problems, pitfalls, limitations of laboratory medicine, and drug interactions are discussed.

An artifact is suspected when the laboratory data do not "fit" the patient, or an inappropriate relationship is observed. For example, lipemia frequently causes an increased serum bilirubin value determined by commonly used methods. A serum concentration greater than 1.0 mg/dl should be associated with a concomitant bilirubinuria. If absent, the serum bilirubin value is suspect. Some laboratories provide numeric indices of lipemia, hemolysis, and icterus to help determine if the magnitude is sufficient to alter laboratory measurements (also see Appendix this volume, p 1404).°

---

°The consequences of spurious laboratory results are of great importance to clinicians. Many of the interferences discussed in this chapter have been documented in animals, while others have thus far been reported only in human patients or using specific reagents or methods. The potential of laboratory interferences should always be considered, however, and laboratory tests interpreted in light of relevant clinical and laboratory findings. The reader should find the information in this chapter, and that in the Appendix pages 1396–1417, useful in their assessment of clinical laboratory studies.
R. Jacobs and J. Bonagura

## SPECIMEN INTERFERENCES

### Lipemia

By scattering light, lipemia causes a number of changes in hematology and chemistry measurements made by spectrophotometric methods (Meyer, Coles, and Rich, 1992; Statland and Winkel, 1991; Willard, Tredten, and Turnwald, 1989; Tietz, 1990) (Table 1). Refractometer readings of plasma protein will be increased, and thus cause a discrepancy between plasma protein and total serum protein values measured biochemically. Electrolytes measured by flame photometry are decreased, while those measured by ion-specific electrodes (ISE) are not affected. This type of information can be obtained by calling the laboratory.

Lipemia can be partially cleared by ultracentrifugation techniques or precipitating agents (polyethylene glycol, liposol, lipoclear); however, clearing agents themselves may induce artifacts. A 12-hr fast will usually provide a clear serum sample. Persistence of lipemia following an overnight fast may suggest a pathologic process (hypothyroidism, diabetes mellitus, hyperadrenocorticism, pancreatitis, primary lipid disorder).

### Hemolysis

Hemolysis causes interference by several mechanisms: direct influence on absorbance readings determined spectrophotometrically, and alteration of the pH of enzymatic reactions (Meyer, Coles, and Rich, 1992; O'Neill and Feldman, 1989; Willard, Tvedten, and Turnwald, 1989; Tietz, 1990). Constituents that are higher in concentration in erythrocytes than in serum will be increased (e.g., aspartate aminotransferase [AST] and lactate dehydrogenase [LDH] activities).

Many laboratory changes are associated with hemolysis (Table 1). Thrombin time, plasminogen concentration, and antithrombin III measurements are increased. Rocket immunoelectrophoresis measurements of von Willebrand's factor are decreased, and fibrinogen values are increased (O'Neill and Feldman, 1989). Thyroxine ($T_4$) and adrenocorticotrophic hormone (ACTH) determinations are not usually affected by hemolysis,

**Table 1.** *Patient/Collection Variables*

| | BUN | Creatinine | ALT | AST | ALP | GGT | T. Bilirubin | Bile Acids | Glucose | Cholesterol | Triglycerides | Calcium | Phosphorus | Total Protein | Globulins | Albumin | Sodium | Chloride | Potassium | Magnesium | Amylase | Lipase | CK | SDH | Iron | PCV | Hemoglobin | MCV | MCHC |
|---|---|---|---|---|---|---|---|---|---|---|---|---|---|---|---|---|---|---|---|---|---|---|---|---|---|---|---|---|---|
| Lipemia | v | ⇑ | ⇑ | ⇑ | ⇑ | v | ⇑ | ⇑ | ⇑ | v | | ⇑ | ⇑ | ⇑7 | | ⇓ | ⇓1 | ⇓1 | ⇓1 | | ⇓ | | | | | | ⇑ | | ⇑ |
| Hemolysis | | ⇓ | ⇑ | ⇑ | ⇓ | | ⇑ | ⇓2 | ⇑ | | | ⇑ | ⇑ | ⇑7 | | ⇑ | | v | ⇑34 | ⇑ | ⇑ | ⇑ | ⇑ | | ⇑ | ⇓ | ⇑ | ⇓ | ⇑ |
| Icterus | | ⇓ | | | ⇑ | | | | v | v | ⇓ | | ⇑ | ⇑ | | | | ⇑ | | ⇓ | | v | | | | | | | |
| Hyperglycemia | | | | | | | | | | | | | | | | | ⇓1 | | | | | | | | | | | | |
| Hyperproteinemia | | | | | | | | | | ⇑ | | | | ⇑7 | | | ⇓1 | | ⇓3 | | | | | | | | | | |
| Ketonemia | | ⇑ | | ⇑ | | | ⇑ | | ⇑ | | | | | | | | ⇓13 | | ⇓13 | | | | | | | | | | |
| Severe azotemia | | | | | | | | | | | | | | ⇑7 | | | | | ⇓3 | | | | | | | | | | |
| Immature animals | ↓ | ↓ | | | ↑ | ↑9 | | | | | | | ↑ | ↓ | ↓ | ↓ | | | ↑ | | | | | | | ↑ | | ↑ | ↑ |
| Aging changes (3–12 yr) | ↓ | ↓ | | | | ↓ | | | | | | | | ↑ | ↑ | | | | | | | | | | ↓ | | | | |
| Anticoagulants EDTA | | | | | ⇓ | | | | | | | ⇓ | v | | | | ⇑6 | | | ⇓ | ⇓ | ⇓ | ⇓ | ⇓ | ⇓ | | | | |
| Oxalate | ⇑8 | ⇓ | | | ⇓ | | | | | | | ⇓ | v | | | | ⇑6 | | ⇑5 | ⇓6 | ⇓ | ⇓ | ⇓ | ⇓ | ⇓ | | | | |
| Citrate | ⇓6 | | | | ⇓ | | | | | | | ⇓ | v | | | | ⇑6 | | | ⇓6 | ⇓ | ⇓ | ⇓ | ⇓ | ⇓6 | | | | |
| Fluoride | ⇓ | ⇓ | | | ⇓ | | | | ⇓6 | ⇑ | | ⇓ | | | | | | | ⇑5 | | ⇓ | | | | ⇓ | | | | |
| Heparin | ⇑8 | | | | | | | ⇑ | | | | | | | | | | | ⇑5 | | | | | | | | | | |
| Sample Dehydration | | | | | | | | | | | | | | ⇑ | | | ⇑ | | ⇑ | | | | | | | ⇑ | | | |
| UV Light | | | | | | | ⇓ | | | | | | | | | | | | | | | | ⇓ | | | | | | |

Key: ↑ = value increased due to physiologic change, ↓ = value decreased due to physiologic change, ⇑ = value increased due to interference with methodology or collection changes, ⇓ = value decreased due to interference with methodology or collection changes, v = variable change depending on methodology, 1 = flame photometric methods only, ISE not affected, 2 = RIA not affected, 3 = dry reagent methods, 4 = Akita dogs, 5 = potassium salt, 6 = sodium salt, 7 = refractometer, 8 = ammonium, 9 = if nursing.

but insulin values are decreased. Since methodologies vary, it is prudent to consult the laboratory.

## Hyperbilirubinemia and Hyperglobulinemia

Bilirubin increases the serum concentrations of albumin assayed by the HABA (2-(p-hydroxyphenyl-azo)-benzoic acid) procedure, cholesterol using ferric chloride reagents, glucose using o-toluidine method, and total protein measured by the biuret method. Severe hyperbilirubinemia can artifactually decrease the serum creatinine concentration (Jaffe reaction). Marked hyperglobulinemia can falsely increase the serum concentration of inorganic phosphate, and falsely decrease serum electrolyte measurements obtained by flame photometry. Hyperglobulinemia does not affect ISE measurements of these values (Table 1).

## Anticoagulants

Anticoagulants can alter measurements of a variety of analytes (Table 1). Values are increased if the anticoagulant contains the analyte being measured, or if it activates enzymes, but decreases the value if it binds the analyte. Ethylenediaminetetraacetic acid (EDTA) alters the morphology of neutrophils, with prolonged storage making them appear "toxic." An improper EDTA/blood ratio causes shrinkage of red blood cells, decreasing the packed cell volume (PCV) and mean corpuscular volume (MCV), but increasing the mean corpuscular hemoglobin concentration (MCHC). Heparin causes poor staining quality of white blood cells but is acceptable for most plasma chemistry, blood gas, and ammonia determinations. Notable exceptions include ammonium heparin for measurement of plasma ammonia concentrations, sodium and potassium heparin for measurement of those respective electrolytes, and heparinized plasma for bile acid determinations (slight increase).

## PHYSIOLOGIC CONSIDERATIONS

### Age

Selected laboratory results that are normal for immature animals are often outside the reference range of mature animals (Table 1). Maturity is attained by 6 to 8 months for dogs (although giant breeds may take longer), and by 4 to 6 months for cats. Growth hormone appears to play a role in the increased serum phosphorous and decreased serum urea nitrogen concentrations of juvenile animals. Between 3 and 14 years of age, most hematologic and biochemical values are relatively constant (although increases and decreases have been noted; Lowseth et al., 1990) (Table 1).

***Table 2.*** *Comparison of Hematologic Changes Seen with Stress/Corticosteroids, Epinephrine Response, and Inflammation*

| Stress/Steroid | Epinephrine Response | Inflammation |
| --- | --- | --- |
| Leukocytosis | Leukocytosis | Leukocytosis |
| Mature neutrophilia | Mature neutrophilia | Neutrophilia ± left shift |
| | | Toxic neutrophils |
| Lymphopenia | Lymphocytosis[†] | |
| Monocytosis[°] | | |
| Eosinopenia[°] | | |

[°]Most consistent in the dog.
[†]More common in the cat.

### Stress and Epinephrine Responses

Stress and increased epinephrine release cause a physiologic leukocytosis that must be differentiated from inflammation (Table 2). The stress response is associated with the release of endogenous glucocorticoids, or the administration of exogenous corticosteroids. The response, particularly monocytosis, is more consistent in dogs.

Excitement- or exercise-induced epinephrine release causes a demargination of neutrophils in blood vessels. The response is more prominent in cats because of a greater marginated neutrophil "pool." Another prominent feature in cats is a marked lymphocytosis, probably as a consequence of temporary alteration of lymphocyte recirculation. Transient hyperglycemia, with or without a transient glucosuria, can occur because of epinephrine-stimulated hepatic glycogenolysis and corticosteroid-induced insulin resistance.

### Hydration and Diet

The hydration state will affect the expressed concentration or activity of an analyte in body fluids. Because of wide reference ranges, this is not usually a clinical concern. One should appreciate that rehydration of a severely dehydrated patient will, in itself, decrease the measured analyte value. Severe dehydration can alter the blood/anticoagulant ratio for the activated partial thromboplastin time (APTT) sample and cause an increased value.

Diet can alter several biochemical measurements. A high-protein diet can increase the serum urea nitrogen concentration. Prolonged use of a low-protein diet can cause decreased serum albumin and urea nitrogen concentrations and increased serum alkaline phosphatase (ALP) and alanine aminotransferase (ALT) activities.

## PHARMACOLOGIC AND THERAPEUTIC AGENTS

Numerous families of drugs alter urine dipstick, specific gravity, and sulfosalicylic acid measurements (Statland and Winkel, 1991; Willard, Tvedten, and Turnwald, 1989; Tietz, 1990) (Table 3). Endogenous metabolites (e.g., nitrites and ascorbic acid) can also adversely affect urine reagent strip measurements (Table 3).

Drug-induced alterations of laboratory test results are numerous (Meyer, Coles, and Rich, 1992; Statland and Winkel, 1991; Willard, Tvedten, and Turnwald, 1989; Tietz, 1990). Mechanisms include enzyme induction, direct interference with test methodology, and indirect systemic influences caused by changes in blood pressure or acid-base status.

Selected categories of drugs are discussed below. Commonly used medications and their potential effects are listed in Table 4.

### Corticosteroids

Corticosteroids (topical, oral, and parenteral) cause changes in the hemogram, biochemistry profile, urinalysis, and endocrine and immunologic tests (Table 4). Although the changes are usually predictable, the magnitude of change is not.

Corticosteroids cause an increase in the serum activities of hepatic enzyme tests in dogs. Most frequently and of greatest magnitude are increases in the serum ALP and γ-glutamyltransferase (GGT) activities. Increases in serum ALT and AST activities occur less commonly. Although uncommon, corticosteroids and megestrol acetate can cause small increases in serum hepatic enzyme tests in cats. Megestrol acetate can cause hyperglycemia, and glucosuria in cats. Hypercholesterolemia, hyperglycemia, and hypertriglyceridemia can develop in association with hypercortisolemia. Glucocorticoids may also alter renal tubular concentrating mechanisms resulting in low or inappropriate urine specific gravity values despite dehydration.

Some corticosteroids (such as prednisone) are measured as cortisol by certain assays, while dexamethasone is not. Corticosteroids suppress the hypothalamic-pituitary-adrenal axis, adversely affecting its assessment. Thyroid function in dogs is also impaired as a result of corticosteroid administration. The Coombs' test and antinuclear antibody (ANA) test may become negative in patients with immune-mediated diseases if measured after treatment with corticosteroids has been initiated (usually 2 to 3 days' duration is necessary).

### Nonsteroidal Anti-inflammatory Drugs

Nonsteroidal anti-inflammatory drugs (NSAIDs) can alter laboratory test results (Table 4). Aspirin causes platelet dysfunction and increases the bleeding time. Aspirin and acetaminophen artificially decrease serum glucose values measured by the oxidase system. Intravenous dipyrone can negatively interfere with measurement of creatine kinase (CK), LDH, triglyceride, cholesterol, and creatinine concentrations (Gascón et al., 1993). Hepatocellular damage resulting in increased serum ALT and AST activities has been associated with several NSAIDs. They also can cause inappropriate antidiuretic hormone (ADH) secretion and hyponatremia.

### Antibiotics

Antibiotics can directly interfere with chemistry methodologies (Table 4). Examples of changes in bio-

***Table 3.*** *Uroanalytical Alterations*

| | Specific Gravity | Urine pH | Proteinuria | Glucosuria (Dipstick) | Ketonuria | Bulirubinuria | Urobilinogen | Hemo/Myoglobinuria | Nitrituria | Pyuria |
|---|---|---|---|---|---|---|---|---|---|---|
| Acetazolamide | | ↑ | ⇑[1] | | | | ⇑ | | | |
| Aminoglycosides | | | ⇑[2] | ↑ | | | | | | ⇑[1] |
| Ascorbic acid | | ↓ | | ⇓ | | ⇓ | ↓ | ⇓ | ⇓ | |
| Cephalosporins | | | ⇑[2] | | | | | | | ⇑[1] |
| Chlorpromazine | | | ⇑[2] | | | ⇓ | | | | |
| Colchicine | ↓ | | | | | | | | | |
| Corticosteroids | ↓ | | | | | | | | | |
| Dipyrone | | | | ⇓ | | | | | | |
| Diuretics | ↓ | | | | | | | | | |
| Methionine | | ↓ | | | ↑ | | | | | |
| Penicillins | | | ⇑[2] | | | | | | | |
| Phenazopyridine | | | ⇑[1] | | ⇑ | ⇑ | ⇑ | | ⇑ | |
| Phenolphthalein | | | | | | ⇑ | | | | |
| Phenothiazines | | | | | | ⇑ | ⇑ | | | |
| Procaine | | | | | | | ⇑ | | | |
| Radiographic contrast media | ⇑ | | ⇑[2] | | | | | | | |
| Salicylates | | | ⇑[2] | ⇓ | | | ⇓ | | | |
| Sodium bicarbonate | | ↑ | ⇑[1] | | | | ↑ | | | |
| Sulfobromophthalein (BSP) | | | | | ⇑ | | ⇑ | | | |
| Sulfonamides | | | ⇑[2] | | | | ⇑ | | | |
| Urinary acidifiers | | ↓ | | | | | ↓ | | | |
| Acetoacetate (ketonuria) | | | | ⇓ | | | | | | |
| Alkaline urine | ⇓[1] | | ⇑[1]⇓[2] | | | | | | | ⇓[3] |
| Bilirubinuria | | | | | | | ⇑ | | | |
| Highly concentrated urine | | | | | | | | ⇓ | | |
| Nitrituria | | | | | | ⇓ | ⇓ | ⇓ | | |
| Proteinuria | ⇑[1] | | | | | | | | | |
| Refrigerated urine | | | | ⇓ | | | | | | |
| Time | | | | ⇑ | | | | | | |
| UV light | | | | | | ⇓ | ⇓ | | | |

Key: ↑ = value increased due to physiologic change, ↓ = value decreased due to physiologic change, ⇑ = value increased due to interference with methodology, ⇓ = value decreased due to interference with methodology, 1 = dipstick, 2 = sulfosalicyclic acid method, 3 = sediment.

## Table 4. Biochemical Alterations

| | BUN | Creatinine | ALT | AST | ALP | GGT | T. Bilirubin | Bile Acids | Glucose | Cholesterol | Triglycerides | Calcium | Phosphorus | Total Protein | Albumin | Sodium | Chloride | Potassium | Magnesium | Amylase | Lipase | CK | Thyroxine | ACTH | Cortisol | Gastrin |
|---|---|---|---|---|---|---|---|---|---|---|---|---|---|---|---|---|---|---|---|---|---|---|---|---|---|---|
| Corticosteroids | ↑ | | ↑ | ↑ | ↑ | ↑ | | | ↑ | ↑ | ↑ | ↓ | | ↑ | | ↑ | | ↓ | | ↓ | ↑ | ↑ | ↓ | ↓ | v | |
| Mineralocorticoids | | | | | | | | | | | | | | | | ↑ | | ↓ | | | | | | | | |
| Anabolic steroids | | | ↑ | | ↑ | | | | | | v | ↑ | v | ↑ | | | | | | | | | | | | |
| NSAIDs | ↑ | ↑ | | | | | | | | | | | | | | ↓ | | ↑ | | | | | | | | |
|   Acetaminophen | | | ↑ | | | | ↑ | | ⇓ | | | | | | | | | | | | | | | | | |
|   Aspirin | ↑ | ↑ | ↑ | | | | | | ⇓ | | | | | | | | | ↓ | | | | | | | | |
|   Dipyrone | | ⇓ | | | | | | | | ⇓ | ⇓ | | | | | | | | | | ⇓ | | | | | |
|   Ibuprofen | ↑ | ⇑ | ↑ | | | | | | | | | | | | | | | | | | | | | | | |
|   Phenylbutazone | ↑ | | ↑ | | | | ↑ | | | | | | | | | ↑ | | | | | | | ↓ | | | |
| Antibiotics<br>  Aminoglycosides | ↑ | ↑ | | | | | | | | | | | | | | | | | ↓ | | | | | | | |
|   Cephalosporins | | ⇑ | | | | | ↑ | | | | | | | | | | | | | | | | | | | |
|   Chloramphenicol | v | | | | | | | | | | | | | | | | | | | | | | | | | |
|   Penicillins | | ⇑ | | | | | | | | | | | | | | | | | | | | | | | | |
|   Sulfonamides | | | ↑ | | ↑ | | ↑ | | | | | | | | | | | | | ↑ | ↑ | | ↓ | | | |
|   Tetracycline | | | | | | | | | | | | | v | | | | | | | ↑ | ↑ | | | | | |
| Anticonvulsants | | | | | | | | | | | | ↓ | ↓ | | | | | | | | | | | | ↑ | |
|   Phenobarbital | | | ↑ | | ↑ | ↑ | ↓ | | | | | | | | | | | | | | | | ↓ | | | |
|   Phenytoin | | | ↑ | | ↑ | | | | ↑ | ↑ | | | | | | | | | | | | | ↓ | | | |
|   Potassium bromide | | | | | | | | | | ⇑ | | | | | | | ⇑ | | | | | | | | | |
|   Primidone | | | ↑ | | ↑ | | | | | | | | | | | | | | | | | | ↓ | | | |
| Hormones<br>  Androgens | | | | | | | | | | | | ↑ | | | | ↑ | ↑ | | | | | | ↓ | | | |
|   Estrogen | | | | | | | ↑ | | | | ↑ | ↑ | | | ↓ | | | | | ↑ | | | | | ↑ | |
|   Insulin | | | | | | | | | ↓ | | | | ↓ | | | | | ↓ | | | | | ↑ | ↑ | | ↑ |
|   Progesterone | | | | | | | ↑ | | | | | ↑ | | | | | | | ↑ | | | | | | | |
|   Thyroxine | | | | | | | | | ↑ | ↓ | | | | | | | | | | | | | ↑ | | | |
| Amphotericin B | ↑ | ↑ | | | | | | | | | | | | | | | | ↓ | ↓ | | | | | | | |
| Ascorbic acid | | ⇑ | | v | | ⇓ | | | ⇓ | | ↓ | | | | | | | | | | | | | | | |
| Asparaginase | | | ↑ | | | | | | ↑ | ↓ | ↑ | | | | | | | | | ↑ | ↑ | | | | ↓ | |
| Azathioprine | | | ↑ | | ↑ | | | | | | | | | | | | | | | ↑ | ↑ | | | | | |
| Barbiturates | | ⇑ | ↑ | | ↑ | | | | | | | | | | | | | | | | | | | | | |
| B-Adrenergics | | | | | | | | | ↑ | | | | | | | | | | | | | | | | | |
| Captopril | ↑ | ↑ | | | | | | | | | | | | | | | | ↑ | | | | | | | | |
| Cholestyramine | | | | | | | | ↓ | | ↓ | ↑ | | | | | | ↑ | | | | | | | | | |
| Cimetidine | | | ↑ | | | | | | | | | | | | | | | | | ↑ | | | | | | ↑ |
| Cisplatin | ↑ | ↑ | | | | | | | | | | | | | | | | | ↓ | | | | | | | |
| Colchicine | | | | | | | | | | ↓ | | | | | | | | | | | | | | | | |
| Flucytosine | | ⇑ | | | | | | | | | | | | | | | | | | | | | | | | |
| Furosemide | ↑ | | | | | | | | ↑ | | | ↑ | | | | ↓ | ↓ | ↓ | ↓ | ↑ | | | | | | |
| Glucose | | ⇑ | | | | | | | ↑ | | | | | | | | | | | ↑ | | | | | | |
| Heparin | | | | | | | | | ↑ | | ↓ | | | | | | | ↑ | | | | ↑ | ↓ | | | |
| Methimazole | | | | ↑ | | | | | ⇑ | ↑ | | | | | | | | | | | | | ↓ | | | |
| Metronidazole | | | | ⇓ | | | | | | | | | | | | | | | | ↑ | ↑ | | | | | |
| Phenothiazines | | | | | ↑ | | | | ↑ | ↑ | | | ⇓ | | | | | | | | | | ↓ | | | |
| Propranolol | | | | | | | | ⇑ | ↓ | | | | | | | | | ↑ | | | | | ↑ | | | |
| Radiographic contrast media | ↑ | ↑ | | | | | | | | | | | | | | | | | | | | | ↑ | | | |
| Salicylates | ↑ | ↑ | ↑ | ↑ | | | | | v | | | | ↓ | | | | | | | | | | ↓ | | | |
| Sodium bicarbonate | | | | | | | | | | | | | | | | ↑ | ↓ | ↓ | | | | | | | | |
| Sulfobromophthalein (BSP) | | ⇑ | | | | | | | | | | | | | | | | | | | | | | | | |
| Theophylline | | | | | | ⇓ | | ⇓ | | ↑ | | | | | | | | | | | | | | | | |
| Thiacetarsamide | | | ↑ | | | | | | | | | | | | | | | | | | | | | | | |

Key: ↑ = value increased due to physiologic change, ↓ = value decreased due to physiologic change, ⇑ = valued increased due to interference with methodology or collection changes, ⇓ = value decreased due to interference with methodology or collection changes, v = variable change depending on methodology.

chemical measurements caused by antibiotics include an increase in the serum creatinine concentration using the Jaffe reaction, and alterations in serum glucose and phosphorous concentrations caused by tetracycline. Changes in serum urea nitrogen concentration may be associated with administration of chloramphenicol. Certain antibacterial agents, such as sulfa drugs, cause changes by enzyme induction. Trimethoprim-sulfa has been shown to decrease thyroid function in dogs (Hall et al., 1993; see this volume, p 595). Many antibiotics cause false-positive reactions for protein measured by urine reagent strips and by the sulfosalicylic acid procedure (Table 3).

### Anticonvulsants

Anticonvulsant medications, particularly phenobarbital, can increase serum liver enzyme activities and may decrease serum thyroxine concentrations. Patients on potassium bromide may have increased serum chloride concentrations; bromide is measured as chloride by flame photometry and ISE methods. Bromide also interferes with the cholesterol measurement (Table 4).

### Blood Transfusions

The use of citrate blood transfusion products has been associated with decreased serum ionized calcium concentrations in dogs, especially with greater than 40% blood replacement (Dhupa et al., 1993).

### Radiographic Contrast Media

Cerebrospinal fluid measurements are altered by contrast media used for myelograms. The specific gravity and Pandy score may be falsely increased. Protein concentrations and white blood cell counts can be increased (Wider et al., 1992).

Radiographic contrast media can also increase urine specific gravity values and urine protein values. (Table 3). Radiographic contrast media can form pleomorphic crystals in acid urine up to 3 days following administration.

### Hormones

Numerous *in vivo* effects are mediated by hormones, which in turn can affect laboratory test results (Table 4). For example, the administration of insulin not only decreases the plasma glucose concentration, but also plasma potassium and phosphorous concentrations.

### Vitamins

Ascorbic acid decreases serum glucose concentration (oxidase method), increases serum creatinine concentration (Table 4) and causes false-negative glucose and nitrate reactions measured by urine reagent strip (Table 3).

## COLLECTION AND STORAGE

Most biochemical parameters are stable (as serum or plasma) at 4°C for at least 24 hr. The serum or plasma should be removed from red cells within 20 to 30 min, and refrigerated or frozen for storage. Prolonged contact of erythrocytes with serum will decrease the serum glucose concentration at a rate of about 10% per hour. Decreased stability of certain analytes occurs with exposure to ultraviolet (UV) light (Table 1). Urine bilirubin is rapidly oxidized to biliverdin by exposure to fluorescent lights. As a consequence, the urine color can appear green and the reagent strip test for bilirubin is negative. Likewise, fluorescent lighting can cause oxidation of colorless urobilinogen to urobilin, resulting in a negative reagent strip test and imparting a greenish color. EDTA-anticoagulated blood can be stored at 4°C; the MCV will increase and the MCHC will decrease after approximately 12 hr.

Several hormones are storage sensitive. ACTH, insulin, and gastrin degrade quickly at room temperature and should be immediately placed on ice following collection. Since plasma ACTH adheres to glass surfaces, previous analysis methods involved collection of blood in a plastic container. However, recent work suggests that samples can be collected in an EDTA-coated glass tube and placed on ice, as long as the plasma is separated and stored in a plastic container within 15 minutes from the time of collection. The laboratory performing the assay should be contacted for current recommendations.

Dehydration can cause increases in PCV, plasma protein concentration, and white blood cell counts in mail-in samples. Biochemical changes are usually limited to increases in the serum sodium and potassium concentrations. In our experience, clinically important increases in the serum sodium and potassium concentrations can occur if the measurements are delayed by as little as 1 hr in an arid environment.

As Dr. A. L. Bloomfield stated, *"There are some patients whom we cannot help, there are none whom we cannot harm."* To help, but not harm, patients interpretation of laboratory data should begin with proper sample management and development and use of reliable reference ranges. As laboratory medicine for the assessment of veterinary patients becomes more sophisticated, knowledge of the nuances associated with potential interferences becomes more critical. Dry reagent technology has opened a new era in clinical chemistry analysis. It is critical that the methodologies are validated and references ranges established for use in veterinary medicine. There are disparate values for some measurements when comparisons are made to wet reagent methodologies. While the novel technology will provide the convenience of "in-house" measurements, it will also bring an added responsibility of quality control to ensure accuracy of the data in patient management. The role of the veterinary clinical pathologist in these areas will have greater importance in the future.

ACKNOWLEDGMENT: This work supported in part by funds provided through the Iris M. McGee Foundation and Dr. David J. Smith, Bay Road Animal Hospital, Sarasota, FL.

## References and Suggested Reading

Dhupa N, Holt D, Hendricks J, et al: Ionized hypocalcemia induced by citrated blood product transfusion in dogs (abstr). J Vet Intern Med 7:129, 1993.
   *Measurement of pre- and post-transfusion concentration of ionized calcium.*
Gascón N, Otal C, Martens-Bru C, et al: Dipyrone interference on several common biochemical tests. Clin Chem 39:1033, 1993.
   *Study of the interference of intravenous dipyrone on human biochemical profiles utilizing two methods.*
Hall IA, Campbell KL, Chambers MD, and Davis CN: Effect of trimethoprim/sulfamethoxazole on thyroid function in dogs with pyoderma. J Am Vet Med Assoc 202:1959, 1993.
   *Evaluation of thyroid tests in euthyroid dogs given trimethoprim-sulfamethoxazole.*
Lowseth LA, Gillett NA, Gerlach RF, and Muggenburg BA: The effects of aging on hematology and serum chemistry values in the beagle dog. Vet Clin Pathol 19:12, 1990.
   *Consecutive laboratory data following age-related changes from 3 to 14 years in beagles.*

Meyer DJ, Coles EH, and Rich LJ: Laboratory tests, clinical enzymology. Hepatic test abnormalities. In *Veterinary Laboratory Medicine, Interpretation and Diagnosis.* Philadelphia, WB Saunders Co, 1992, pp 3, 55.
   *Discussion of the potential causes of laboratory test variability. Drug-induced hepatic test alterations.*
O'Neill SL and Feldman BF: Hemolysis as a factor in clinical chemistry and hematology of the dog. Vet Clin Pathol 18:58, 1989.
   *Effects of hemolysis on selected parameters using various methodologies with the development of interferographs.*
Statland BE and Winkel P: Preparing patients and specimens for laboratory testing. In Henry JB (ed): *Clinical Diagnosis and Management by Laboratory Methods,* 18th edition. Philadelphia, WB Saunders Co, 1991, p 68.
   *Drug and patient interferences of biochemical laboratory tests.*
Wider WR, DeNicola DB, Blevins WE, et al: Cerebrospinal fluid changes after iopamidol and metrizamide myelography in clinically normal dogs. Am J Vet Res 53:396, 1992.
   *Study of the alterations of CSF measurements secondary to myelographic contrast media.*
Willard MD, Tvedten H, and Turnwald GH: *Small Animal Clinical Diagnosis by Laboratory Methods.* Philadelphia, WB Saunders Co, 1989.
   *Discussion of biochemical alterations, includes sections on artifact- and drug induced alterations for each analyte.*
Tietz NW: *Clinical Guide to Laboratory Tests,* 2nd edition. Philadelphia, WB Saunders Co, 1990.
   *Laboratory test alterations, including artifact and drug induced. Also, discusses effects on variable methodologies.*

# INFLUENCE OF FASTING AND EATING ON LABORATORY VALUES

JOSEPH W. BARTGES

*Athens, Georgia*

*and* CARL A. OSBORNE

*St. Paul, Minnesota*

The goal of clinical *in vitro* laboratory tests is to determine the concentrations of measured analytes as they were *in vivo*. The validity of information provided by a clinical laboratory test is determined by the accuracy, precision, analytical sensitivity, and analytical specificity of the test. However, factors such as diet, patient preparation, medications, and sample handling may substantially influence laboratory test values (Galen and Peters, 1986). Veterinarians use laboratory tests to screen for disease in seemingly healthy individuals, to diagnose disease, to monitor biologic behavior of diseases, and to monitor the response of disease to treatment. For most veterinarians, emphasis is placed on the effect of diseases and treatment protocols on various test results. However, other factors, especially diets, have considerable influence on the composition of blood, plasma, serum, urine, and feces (Young and Bermes, 1986).*

---

*The consequences of spurious laboratory results are of great importance to clinicians. Many of the dietary and nutritional interferences and influences described in this chapter have been documented in animals, while others have thus far been reported only in human patients or using specific reagents or methods. The potential of laboratory interferences should always be considered, however, and laboratory tests interpreted in light of relevant clinical and laboratory findings. The reader should find the information in this chapter, and that in the Appendix pages 1396–1417, useful in their assessment of clinical laboratory studies.
R. Jacobs and J. Bonagura

Following consumption of a meal, food is digested, absorbed, and metabolized. Metabolism occurs primarily in the liver. Digested dietary components are used to provide energy for metabolic processes (adenosine triphosphate [ATP]), replenish energy stores (glycogen and adipose tissue), and provide substrates necessary for cell regeneration and tissue growth. Between meals, energy for metabolic processes is derived primarily from glycogen. However, when food is withheld for prolonged periods, energy sources such as fat are utilized to conserve protein. During periods of anorexia and stress due to trauma or illness, protein and fat are utilized at an accelerated rate.

## INFLUENCE OF FASTING ON LABORATORY VALUES

When food is withheld, there is a decrease in blood glucose concentration and insulin secretion, but a reciprocal increase in glucagon secretion to promote glycogen mobilization and gluconeogenesis (Young and Bermes, 1986). If food is withheld for longer than 24 to 48 hr, lipolysis predominates, resulting in production of ketones (acetone, acetoacetic acid, and β-hydroxybuteric acid) (Rapoport, From, and Husdan, 1965; Young and Bermes, 1986). Although ketogenesis occurs in dogs and cats, these species apparently utilize ketones so efficiently that ketoacidemia rarely occurs (Lemieux and Plante, 1968). If ketoacidemia and ketoaciduria are detected in an anorexic patient, diabetes mellitus or hepatic failure may be the underlying cause.

Because the liver is the primary site for gluconeogenesis during periods of food deprivation, serum bilirubin concentration, alanine transaminase (ALT) activity, aspartate transaminase (AST) activity, and sulfobromophthalein (BSP) retention time may be increased (Young and Bermes, 1986). Therefore, if animals are anorexic for prolonged periods, caution must be used in interpreting these tests in patients suspected of having hepatic dysfunction. Likewise, detection of normal plasma ammonia and serum bile acid concentrations in anorexic patients does not exclude hepatic failure (Center, 1989).

Serum urea nitrogen (SUN) and serum phosphorus concentrations decrease during periods of decreased protein consumption. Therefore, if patients in renal failure are anorexic, SUN and serum phosphorus concentrations may underestimate the degree of renal dysfunction. Because renal medullary urea concentration is important in production of concentrated urine, decreased protein consumption is also associated with decreased urine specific gravity (Edgren and Wester, 1971). If a patient is azotemic due to dehydration and has been anorexic, renal failure may be inappropriately diagnosed. Likewise, reduction in consumption in dietary protein will reduce glomerular filtration rate, and therefore the blood, plasma, and serum concentrations of solutes dependent on glomerular filtration for excretion may increase.

Following food deprivation, aldosterone secretion increases. Increased aldosterone secretion promotes renal tubular sodium reabsorption and potassium excretion. As a consequence, plasma potassium concentration decreases, urinary potassium excretion increases, and urinary sodium and chloride excretion decrease (Lulich et al., 1991; Young and Bermes, 1986). During fasting, urinary calcium, magnesium, and uric acid excretions are reduced. However, urinary excretion of phosphorus, oxalate, and citrate are apparently not affected by fasting (Lulich et al., 1991). In dogs, urinary ammonia, titratable acid, and hydrogen ion excretions decrease, and urine pH values rise when food is withheld (Lemieux and Plante, 1968; Lulich et al., 1991). Therefore, measurement of 24-hr urinary solute excretions may be different when measured following food consumption compared to periods when food is withheld.

**Table 1.** *Potential Influences of Fasting on Laboratory Values in Selected Diseases*

| System | Laboratory Value | Influence |
|---|---|---|
| **Endocrine** | | |
| Hypoadrenocorticism | Serum sodium, potassium, urea nitrogen, total carbon dioxide concentrations | Decrease |
| | Urine pH | Increase |
| Hyperadrenocorticism | Serum triglyceride, cholesterol concentrations | Decrease |
| Hypothyroidism | Serum triglyceride, cholesterol concentrations | Decrease |
| Hyperthyroidism | Serum ALT, AST activities | Increase |
| | Serum urea nitrogen concentration | Decrease |
| Diabetes mellitus | Serum glucose concentration | Increase |
| | Serum and urine ketone concentrations | Decrease |
| Hypoglycemia | Serum glucose concentration | Decrease |
| Hyperparathyroidism | Serum calcium, phosphorus concentrations | Decrease |
| Hypoparathyroidism | Serum calcium, phosphorus concentrations | Decrease |
| **Liver** | | |
| Failure | Serum ALT, AST activities; serum bilirubin concentration | Increase |
| | Serum total protein, albumin, glucose concentrations | Decrease |
| | Plasma ammonia concentration | Decrease |
| **Urinary** | | |
| Renal failure | Serum urea nitrogen, creatinine, phosphorus, potassium, calcium concentrations | Decrease |
| Urolithiasis—struvite | Urine magnesium, ammonia, phosphorus concentrations | Decrease |
| Urolithiasis—calcium | Urine calcium concentrations | Decrease |
| Urolithiasis—urate | Urine uric acid, ammonia concentrations | Decrease |
| Urolithiasis—cystine | Urine cystine concentration | Decrease |
| **Cardiovascular** | | |
| Congestive failure | Serum sodium concentration, serum potassium concentration | Decrease |
| **Intestinal** | | |
| Pancreatitis | Serum lipase, amylase activities | Decrease |
| Malabsorption/ maldigestion | Serum total protein, albumin, triglyceride, cholesterol concentrations | Decrease |

Water consumption and hydration status must be considered when interpreting laboratory results. Serum urea nitrogen concentration may be increased in healthy patients or be disproportionately increased in patients with renal failure if dehydration is present. Likewise, decreased water consumption and dehydration is associated with decreased rate of formation of glomerular filtrate and urine production resulting in increased urine specific gravity and urine solute concentrations (Tabaru et al., 1993). Caution must be used in interpreting 24-hr excretions of solutes in the diagnosis and therapy of urolithiasis if hospitalized animals consume less water than in the home environment.

## INFLUENCE OF EATING ON LABORATORY VALUES

Following digestion of a meal, nutrients are metabolized by the liver. In humans, serum bilirubin concentration, ALT activity, AST activity, and BSP retention time increase 2 hr after a meal (Young and Bermes, 1986). There is also an increase in postprandial serum alkaline phosphatase (ALP) activity in humans. The increase in ALP activity is due to circulating intestinal isoenzyme (Young and Bermes, 1986). However, since the serum half-life of canine and feline intestinal ALP isoenzyme is less than 6 min, intestinal ALP isoenzyme does not influence total serum ALP activity in these species (Duncan and Prasse, 1986). In dogs and cats, serum glucose concentration increases 2 to 4 hr after consumption of food (Duncan and Prasse, 1986). Therefore, caution must be used in interpreting postprandial serum glucose concentrations during periods of stress.

After a meal, plasma concentration of total lipids increases. If large quantities of fat are contained in the diet, visible lipemia may occur. Lipemia enhances hemolysis *in vitro*. Hemolyzed serum in turn may alter test results such as serum lipase and ALT activities. Turbidity of serum due to lipemia may interfere with spectrophotometric determinations (e.g., serum glucose concentrations) and flame photometric determinations (e.g., serum sodium and potassium concentrations). Also, lipemia results in false elevations of plasma protein concentrations measured by refractometry (Duncan and Prasse, 1986). To minimize lipemia, a patient may be fasted for 10 to 24 hr prior to collection of blood samples for chemical analysis (Meyer et al., 1992).

Following digestion of a meal, particularly one that is not restricted in protein, plasma ammonia levels increase. This fact should be considered when measuring blood ammonia concentrations to diagnose and monitor therapy of hepatic dysfunction.

Provocative serum bile acid tests are used to detect hepatic dysfunction or hepatic perfusion abnormalities. Dietary fat and protein and duodenal acidification by gastric juices cause numerous neurohumoral and hormonal factors to induce bile secretion and gallbladder contraction. However, gastric emptying may be delayed by consumption of a meal containing only fat. Therefore, normal serum bile acid concentrations may occur with abnormal hepatic function (Center, 1989).

Consumption of food stimulates gastric secretion of hydrochloric acid. As a result, a decrease in plasma chloride concentration and an increase in bicarbonate concentration occurs in venous blood draining the stomach. Serum total carbon dioxide concentration and plasma bicarbonate concentration increase. The resulting metabolic alkalosis is commonly called the postprandial alkaline tide (Young and Bermes, 1986). Urine pH will increase unless acidifying substances are contained in the diet. In a study of healthy beagles, eating was associated with increased urinary excretion of hydrogen ions, ammonia, sodium, potassium, calcium, magnesium, and uric acid (Lulich et al., 1991).

The form of solutes in food, and their metabolism once absorbed from the gastrointestinal tract, affect plasma and urine concentrations of metabolites. For example, inorganic phosphorus is more readily absorbed from the intestines of cats than organic forms, resulting in marked increases in plasma concentrations after consumption. Likewise, urinary phosphorus excretion is increased following consumption of inorganic phosphorus (Finco et al., 1992).

Laboratory results may be substantially affected by changes in diets fed in a home environment compared to different diets fed in a hospital environment. Urine crystals that form while animals are consuming diets fed in the hospital may be different from urine crystals formed by animals eating at home. This factor should be considered when interpreting crystalluria. To determine the influence of home-fed diets on laboratory test results, consider asking clients to bring home-fed diets for use during periods of diagnostic hospitalization (Osborne et al., 1990).

Diets may be reformulated as new information concerning nutrition and health or disease processes is discovered. Therefore, effects of diet on laboratory values may change even when the same brand name of diet is consumed. For example, a diet formulated in 1985 to induce canine struvite urolith dissolution was associated with decreases in albumin concentrations and increases in serum ALT and ALP activities (Osborne et al., 1985). Today the same brand of diet has been reformulated to contain a greater quantity of protein, and its consumption by dogs is not associated with these serum chemical changes.

## INFLUENCE OF SPECIFIC DIETARY COMPONENTS ON LABORATORY VALUES

### Protein

Following consumption of a protein-rich meal, serum and urine concentrations of urea nitrogen, phosphorus, and uric acid increase (Young and Bermes, 1986). Likewise, plasma ammonia concentration and urinary ammonia excretion increase. Urine pH decreases. Because consumption of a protein-rich meal stimulates insulin production, a decrease in serum glucose concentration occurs. Consumption of large quantities of meat containing creatinine and noncreatinine chromagens results in increased serum creatinine concentration (Schuster and Seldin, 1985). Glomerular filtration rate is increased following consumption of large quantities of protein.

## Fat

Consumption of a high-fat meal results in increases in serum triglyceride and cholesterol concentrations. Serum uric acid concentrations and urinary excretions of uric acid are decreased. Serum urea nitrogen concentrations are also decreased. In order to maintain acid-base homeostasis during consumption of a high-fat diet, the body nitrogen pool is depleted to meet the requirement for excretion of ammonium ions (Young and Bermes, 1986).

## Carbohydrate

The influence of a carbohydrate-rich meal is not as profound as that of a protein-rich meal (Young and Bermes, 1986). Following consumption of a high-carbohydrate meal, blood glucose concentrations increase. However, serum phosphorus concentrations decrease due to cellular uptake of phosphorus for phosphorylation of glycolytic enzymes (Young and Bermes, 1986). A high-carbohydrate meal stimulates insulin production, which in turn promotes movement of potassium into cells and sodium out of cells. Urine pH increases following a high-carbohydrate meal. Consumption of a high-carbohydrate diet is associated with decreased serum concentrations of very-low-density lipoproteins (VLDL), low-density lipoproteins (LDL), triglyceride, and cholesterol. Bran impedes absorption of dietary calcium, triglyceride, and cholesterol, thereby lowering their serum concentrations.

## Vitamins and Minerals

Consumption of excessive amounts of vitamins and minerals may influence results of laboratory tests. Vitamin D, in part, regulates calcium metabolism. Excess vitamin D consumption may be associated with increases in serum and urine calcium and phosphorus concentrations. Vitamin C given in high doses is a weak urine acidifying agent. Also, vitamin C is a precursor of oxalic acid, and its consumption may enhance the likelihood of formation of calcium oxalate crystals (Osborne et al., 1992). Increased urine concentrations of minerals occur with excessive dietary consumption (Finco et al., 1985).

## RECOMMENDATIONS

- Information concerning feeding, diet consumed, or length of fasting should be recorded on laboratory submission forms or in patients' records.
- If possible, hospitalized patients should be fed diets that are fed at home to establish baseline laboratory data prior to dietary change.
- To evaluate the influence of dietary modification on a disease process, blood, plasma, serum, and urine samples should be collected 2 to 6 hr after food consumption.
- To minimize unwanted postprandial influence on laboratory test results, a patient should be fasted at least 12 hr prior to collection of blood, serum, and plasma samples. Because dietary solutes may be excreted in urine for at least 8 hr and possibly longer following consumption of a meal, the urinary bladder should be emptied at that time and urine samples collected to determine the influence of fasting or eating on urinary solute concentrations.
- Diets substantially influence urine pH values and urine solute concentrations. This should be considered when collecting urine for diagnostic purposes, or for monitoring response to therapy.

## References and Suggested Readings

Center SA: Pathophysiology and laboratory diagnosis of liver disease. In Ettinger SJ (ed): Veterinary Internal Medicine. Philadelphia, WB Saunders Co, 1989, p 1421.

Duncan JR and Prasse KW: Veterinary Laboratory Medicine: Clinical Pathology. Ames, IA, Iowa State University Press, 1986.

Edgren B and Wester PO: Impairment of glomerular filtration in fasting for obesity. Acta Med Scand 190:389, 1971.

Finco DR, et al: Characterization of magnesium-induced urinary disease in the cat and comparison with feline urologic syndrome. Am J Vet Res 46:391, 1985.

Finco DR, Barsanti JA, and Brown SA: Solute fractional excretion rates. In Kirk RW and Bonagura JD (eds) Current Veterinary Therapy XI. Philadelphia, WB Saunders Co, 1992, p 818.

Galen RS and Peters TJ: Analytical goals and clinical relevance of laboratory procedures. In Tietz NW (ed): Textbook of Clinical Chemistry. Philadelphia, WB Saunders Co, 1986, p 387.

Lemieux G and Plante GE: The effect of starvation in the normal dog including the Dalmatian coach hound. Metabolism 17:620, 1968.

Lulich JP, Osborne CA, Polzin DJ, et al: Urine metabolite values in fed and nonfed clinically normal beagles. Am J Vet Res 52:1573, 1991.

Meyer DJ, Coles EH, and Rich LJ: Veterinary Laboratory Medicine: Interpretation and Diagnoses. Philadelphia, WB Saunders Co, 1992.

Osborne CA, Lulich JP, Bartges JW, et al: Medical dissolution and prevention of canine and feline uroliths: Diagnostic and therapeutic caveats. Vet Rec 127:369, 1990.

Osborne CA, Lulich JP, Unger LK, et al: Canine and feline urolithiasis: Relationship of etiopathogenesis to treatment and prevention. In Bojrab MJ (ed): Disease Mechanisms in Small Animal Surgery. Philadelphia, Lea & Febiger, 1992, p 464.

Osborne CA, Polzin DJ, Abdullahi SU, et al: Struvite urolithiasis in animals and man: Formation, detection, and dissolution. Adv Vet Sci Comp Med 29:1, 1985.

Rapoport A, From GLA, and Husdan H: Metabolic studies in prolonged fasting: II. Organic metabolism. Metabolism 14:47, 1965.

Schuster VL and Seldin DW: Renal clearance. In Seldin DW and Giebisch G (ed) The Kidney: Physiology and Pathophysiology. New York, Raven Press, 1985, p 365.

Tabaru H, Finco DR, Brown SA, et al: Influence of hydration state on renal functions of dogs. Am J Vet Res 54:1758, 1993.

Young DS and Bermes EWJ: Specimen collection and processing: Sources of biological variation. In Tietz NW (eds): Textbook of Clinical Chemistry. Philadelphia, WB Saunders Co, 1986, p 478.

# RISKS ASSOCIATED WITH BIOPSIES FOR CANCER

STEPHEN J. WITHROW

*Fort Collins, Colorado*

A biopsy is the cornerstone of diagnosis for many disease states, including cancer. Thousands of biopsies are performed on a daily basis in this country, yet many misconceptions exist as to the risks associated with these procedures. The risks of biopsy can be roughly divided into whole body risks, body cavity risks, and local tissue risks.

## WHOLE BODY RISKS

A longstanding misconception about biopsy of a malignancy is the possible spread of cancer cells through the vascular or lymphatic system that will result in an increase in the metastatic rate. Cancer cells are frequently leaving the primary tumor and entering the vascular system. The ability of an individual cancer cell to proceed on to a metastatic focus is a very complex event and requires an intricate interaction between the cell itself and the host (Fidler, 1990). It is likely that many thousands or even millions of tumor cells must leave the primary tumor before a metastasis can take place. It is also likely that a biopsy can and does result in a transient increase in circulating tumor cells. In spite of that increase, there are no published clinical trials in humans or animals that have shown an increase in distant metastasis or a decrease in survival after a properly performed biopsy. The value of the information obtained from the biopsy far outweighs the theoretic risk of distant tumor dissemination.

## BODY CAVITY RISKS

Lesions or masses within the thoracic or abdominal cavities present unique diagnostic and therapeutic dilemmas. In spite of great advances in noninvasive diagnostic procedures, it is often impossible to distinguish neoplastic from non-neoplastic conditions with 100% accuracy. The specific disease state as well as the extent of disease (stage) is the most important step in formulating a rational treatment plan.

Many forms of cancer occur within the thoracic and abdominal cavities. A tissue diagnosis can be simplistically divided into open surgical approaches (thoracotomy or laparotomy), or closed cavity tissue procurement (fine-needle aspirate [FNA], needle core biopsy, or laparoscopic techniques). All of the above-mentioned techniques can provide diagnostic material. The choice of a technique will be influenced by your personal expertise and experience, the availability of equipment, and the owner's wishes. If all staging studies reveal a *solitary* mass in the thorax or abdomen, we prefer to approach both the diagnosis and possible surgical therapy via thoracotomy or laparotomy. Notable exceptions include anterior mediastinal masses (usually lymphoma and treated with chemotherapy) or sublumbar masses (usually lymphoma or metastasis and not treated with curative intent surgery).

A quote from a recent paper on peritoneal seeding of a tumor after FNA summarizes our concerns and philosophy regarding preoperative biopsy of solitary masses within body cavities.

> Peritoneal contamination and tumor seeding can occur with FNA and they probably do occur more often than is recognized clinically. Therefore, we caution against the use of FNA in the assessment of potentially curable intra-abdominal tumors, and recommend that this technique be used only when a cytologic diagnosis is required before initiation of palliative therapy.
>
> Pasieka JL and Thompson, 1992

The advantages of open exploration over closed techniques are: more accurate staging, more accurate biopsy positioning, better control of hemorrhage or fluid leakage, larger tissue samples, and the hope of a curative or palliative resection.

Closed biopsies offer several theoretic and practical advantages over open surgical techniques. These advantages include: rare need for general anesthesia, speed, and cost effectiveness. The disadvantages include: small sample size, generally poor visualization of the tissue to be sampled, inability to immediately manage hemorrhage or fluid leakage, and potential seeding or implantation of tumor cells into the body cavity. Although it is very difficult to document with certainty, the risk of iatrogenic tumor seeding of the body cavity has to be considered a risk of closed procedures.

In a study of human patients with pancreatic carcinoma, it was determined the peritoneal washings were positive in 75% of patients undergoing preoperative FNA and only 19% of patients who did not undergo FNA. Iatrogenic implantation of tumor cells (Warshaw, 1991) has also been reported after aspiration of ovarian "cysts" (Trimbos and Hacker, 1993), renal carcinoma (Kiser, Totonchy, and Barry, 1986), prostate carcinoma (Haddad and Somsin, 1987), and pulmonary carcinoma (Sinner and Zajicek, 1976). In one experiment, mice with established lung tumors underwent percutaneous transthoracic FNAs and 89% of the needle tracks were found to contain tumor cells (Struve-Christensen, 1978).

Anyone who has explored the abdomen of a dog with a ruptured hemangiosarcoma knows how well this tumor type can implant and grow on serosal surfaces, rendering it unsuitable for complete removal. Other tumor types may also implant and become unresectable. The ability of a given tumor cell to implant is undoubtedly a complicated event and is influenced by tumor type, cell number, site of implantation, and probably tumor cell and host growth factors. Iatrogenic tumor cell implantation is difficult to document but has been reported in humans and should not be ignored in animals.

Although not unique to cancer contamination, closed needle biopsies in the abdomen certainly carry the risk of rupture and leakage of fluid-filled organs such as urinary bladder, gallbladder, bowel, or uterus (pyometra) (Leveille et al., 1993). Uncontrolled hemorrhage is also a possibility with any closed technique (Leveille et al., 1993). Transthoracic lung aspiration can also result in serious complications such as pneumothorax, hemorrhage, and death (Teske, 1991).

## LOCAL TISSUE RISKS

Any cancer is surrounded by or contiguous with normal tissue. When normal tissue is disturbed via the biopsy procedure (incisional, needle core, or fine-needle aspirate), it is possible to iatrogenically implant tumor cells in the biopsy tract (Meller and Mozes, 1991). This may not pose a serious problem if the biopsy tract is completely excised with the tumor, radiated with the main tumor bed, or treated with known effective chemotherapeutics. Biopsy tract contamination is well documented in people and animals and may drastically alter the necessary treatment plan. In one human study that looked at biopsy complications for malignant primary bone and soft-tissue sarcomas, it was noted that the optimal treatment plan had to be changed in 18% of cases due to a poorly performed biopsy (Mankin, Lange, and Spanier, 1982). In an ideal world, the person who performs the biopsy should be the same person who will perform the definitive treatment. It is likely that the greatest risk (and probably accuracy) is associated with incisional biopsy followed by needle core, and lastly, FNA (Enneking and Maale, 1988; Gilson and Stone, 1990; Smith, 1984; Fornari et al., 1989; Eriksson, Hagman, and Ryd, 1984).

## WHAT'S THE BOTTOM LINE?

Biopsies are necessary for an accurate diagnosis but are not free of risk. The true incidence of tumor dissemination in body cavities or locally is unknown and poorly documented but is undoubtedly higher than that reported in the literature. The diagnosis of any disease, including cancer, requires a careful consideration of the risks and benefits of the diagnostic tests performed.

Spreading cancer cells into the vascular or lymphatic system has little known clinical significance. Release of cancer cells into body cavities that cannot be excised is a real concern and we believe that most solitary intrathoracic (especially pulmonary) or intra-abdominal masses should be managed by excisional biopsy. Local tissue contamination by FNA, needle core biopsy, or incisional biopsy does occur both experimentally and clinically. Local biopsy sites should be resected *en bloc* or irradiated with the main mass to decrease chances of local tumor recurrence.

## References and Suggested Reading

Enneking WF and Maale GE: The effect of inadvertent tumor contamination of wounds during the surgical resection of musculoskeletal neoplasms. Cancer 62:1251, 1988.
*Showed a 39% local recurrence rate when a tumor is broken into at surgery even if a wider excision was undertaken.*

Eriksson O, Hagmar B, and Ryd W: Effects of fine-needle aspiration and other biopsy procedures on tumor dissemination in mice. Cancer 54:73, 1984.
*Tumor cell seeding and tumor outgrowth by way of the needle track may occur under "extreme" test conditions.*

Fidler IJ: Critical factors in the biology of human cancer metastasis: Twenty-eighth GHA Clowes Memorial Award Lecture. Cancer Res 50:6130, 1990.
*Explains the clinical and experimental basis of cancer metastasis.*

Fornari F, Civardi G, Cavanna L, DiStasi M, Rossi S, Sbolli G, Buscarini L, and The Cooperative Italian Study Group: Complications of ultrasonically guided fine-needle abdominal biopsy. Scand J Gastroenterol 24:949, 1989.
*Reports a 0.18% major complication rate after fine-needle biopsy of the abdomen in over 10,000 people.*

Gilson SD and Stone EA: Surgically induced tumor seeding in eight dogs and two cats. J Am Vet Med Assoc 196:1811, 1990.
*Documents iatrogenic tumor implantation in previously noninvolved tissue after surgery.*

Haddad FS and Somsin AA: Seeding and perineal implantation of prostatic cancer in the track of the biopsy needle: three case reports and a review of the literature. J Surg Oncol 35:184, 1987.
*Reports a 0.34% rate of needle track seeding after perineal biopsy of the prostate.*

Kiser GC, Totonchy M, and Barry JM: Needle tract seeding after percutaneous renal adenocarcinoma aspiration. J Urol 136:1292, 1986.
*Reports a case of iatrogenic needle tract seeding of renal carcinoma and reviews the false-negative and false-positive rate of 4 to 8% by needle biopsy.*

Leveille R, Partington BP, Biller DS, and Miyabayashi T: Complications after ultrasound-guided biopsy of abdominal structures in dogs and cats: 246 cases (1984–1991). J Am Vet Med Assoc 23:413, 1993.
*Describes a 1.2% major complication rate after needle biopsy of the abdomen.*

Mankin HJ, Lange TA, and Spanier SS: The hazards of biopsy in patients with malignant primary bone and soft-tissue tumors. J Bone Joint Surg 64A:1121, 1982.
*Reviewed 329 patients biopsied for sarcomas and showed a high complication rate including 15 patients undergoing an unnecessary amputation.*

Meller I and Mozes M: Tumor existence in biopsy scar tissue as seen after definitive resection of soft tissue and bony tumors. Soft Tiss Prob Treatment VI. In Brown KLB (ed): Complications of Limb Salvage, 6th International Symposium. Montreal, ISOLS, 1991, p 335.
*Showed a 37% incidence of biopsy track tumor growth that varied with tumor type and biopsy technique in humans.*

Pasieka JL and Thompson NW: Fine-needle aspiration biopsy causing peritoneal seeding of a carcinoid tumor. Arch Surg 127:1248, 1992.
*Describes a case report of a carcinoid tumor growing in a needle track and warns against fine-needle aspirates of localized masses in the abdomen.*

Sinner WN and Zajicek J: Implantation metastasis after percutaneous transthoracic needle aspiration biopsy. Acta Radiol Diagn 17:473, 1976.
*Suggests a low incidence of transthoracic aspiration biopsy and suggest that needle size and type may make a difference.*

Smith EH: The hazards of fine-needle aspiration biopsy. Ultrasound Med Biol 10:629, 1984.
*Suggests that fine-needle aspiration is generally safe but that serious and even fatal complications do occur.*

Struve-Christensen E: Iatrogenic dissemination of tumour cells. Dan Med Bull 25:82, 1978.
*Demonstrated an 89% incidence of needle track contamination in mice with lung cancer but probable rare incidence in humans.*

Teske E, Stokhof Aa, ven den Ingh TSGAM, Wolvekamp WThC, Slappendel RJ, and de Vries HW: Transthoracic needle aspiration biopsy of the lung in dogs with pulmonic diseases. J Am Anim Hosp Assoc 27:289–294, 1991. *Reports five deaths after transthoracic needle biopsy in 43 animals.*

Trimbos JB and Hacker NF: The case against aspirating ovarian cysts. Cancer 72:828, 1993.

*Aspiration of ovarian "cysts" is potentially dangerous and should not be regarded as routinely acceptable clinical practice.*

Warshaw AL: Implications of peritoneal cytology for staging of early pancreatic cancer. Am J Surg 161:26, 1991. *This study shows that even "localized" pancreatic cancer is often not contained and suggests caution with biopsy of potentially curable lesions.*

# DIAGNOSTIC STUDIES AND SAMPLE COLLECTION IN NEONATAL DOGS AND CATS

ELLEN MILLER

*Fort Collins, Colorado*

The development of the pediatric veterinary patient is often divided into the neonatal period (birth to 2 weeks of age), the transition period (2 to 4 weeks of age), the socialization period (4 to 12 weeks), and the juvenile period (12 weeks to 6 months). By the time the socialization and juvenile periods start, most pediatric patients are smaller versions of adults with respect to sample collection. This article will therefore discuss acquiring diagnostic samples from the puppy or kitten from birth to 4 weeks of age.

## GENERAL CONSIDERATIONS

The history and physical examination are extremely important in the assessment of sick neonates. The history should include information on the mother, littermates, and potentially other members of the pedigree, as well as the patient. The physical examination should be done with the developmental stage of the neonate in mind. Accurate recording of body weight is especially important. If any littermates have died, information gained by necropsy may be beneficial to the diagnosis of the patient. Knowledge of the normal differences in necropsy findings in the adult and the neonate is useful (Haskins, 1985).

## INTEGUMENTARY SYSTEM

Most skin diseases affecting young puppies or kittens are either infectious in nature due to the immunologically naive state, or due to congenital defects. Common problems include pyodermas, external parasite infestation, and dermatophyte infection. Skin scrapings, plucking hairs for fungal culture, and skin biopsies may be approached as in the adult animal.

## URINARY SYSTEM

Congenital defects are a common cause of urinary tract disease in the young puppy or kitten, although clinical signs may not develop or be noticed until weaning or later. Infectious diseases and trauma also account for a portion of disorders. A complete blood count; serum urea nitrogen, creatinine, electrolytes, calcium and phosphorous concentrations (normal reference ranges are given in Tables 1 through 3); and crystals, white blood cells, bacteria, and glucose in the urine may indicate urinary tract involvement. However, glucosuria can be normal in puppies up to 8 weeks of age (Crawford, 1990). Urine concentration must be interpreted in light of the age of the neonate, as puppies are not able to fully concentrate their urine until 8 weeks of age (Crawford, 1990). Blood and urine collection techniques will be covered below. Radiography and ultrasonography may also supply important diagnostic information regarding kidney architecture, ureteral anomalies, vaginal or penile anomalies, and bladder or urachal anomalies. Poor abdominal detail due to lack of intra-abdominal and retroperitoneal fat may hamper the diagnostic usefulness of plain radiography. Contrast studies, when necessary, can be completed following adult guidelines. Since renal development is not complete until approximately 8 weeks of age, modifications of the contrast media dosage may be indicated.

## CARDIOVASCULAR SYSTEM

Congenital heart anomalies are the most common cause of cardiovascular disease in pediatric dogs and cats and are frequently manifested in the form of cardiac murmurs auscultated during physical examination (Bright and Holmberg, 1990). The location, grade, character, timing, and radiation of the murmur can help identify the cardiac defect. However, chest radiography,

**Table 1.**  *Normal Hematologic Parameters in the Neonatal Dog and Cat*

| Parameter | Canine[*] 0–2 Weeks | Canine[*] 2–4 Weeks | Feline[†] 0–2 Weeks | Feline[†] 2–4 Weeks |
|---|---|---|---|---|
| RBC$_s$(X 10$^6$/µl) | 3.6–5.9 | 3.4–4.9 | 5.0–5.5 | 4.6–4.8 |
| Hb (gm/dl) | 14.0–17.5 | 8.5–11.6 | 11.5–12.7 | 8.5–8.9 |
| PCV (%) | 33–52.5 | 27–37 | 33.6–37 | 25.7–27.3 |
| MCV (fl) | 89–93 | 73–83 | 65.5–69.3 | 52.7–55.1 |
| MCH (pg) | 28–30 | 23–25.5 | 22.4–23.6 | 18–19.6 |
| MCHC (%) | 32 | 32 | 33.7–35.3 | 32.5–33.5 |
| WBC$_s$(X 10$^3$/µl) | 6.8–23 | 23–25.5 | 9.1–10.2 | 14.1–16.5 |
| Bands | 0–4.8 | 0.3–1.2 | 0.04–0.08 | 0.07–0.15 |
| Neutrophils | 3.8–15.8 | 1.4–12.8 | 5.3–6.7 | 6.2–7.7 |
| Lymphocytes | 0.5–9.4 | 1.0–10.1 | 3.2–4.2 | 6.0–7.1 |
| Monocytes | 0.2–2.5 | 0.1–1.5 | 0–0.02 | 0–0.04 |
| Esosinophils | 0–2.8 | 0–1.8 | 0.5–1.4 | 1.2–1.6 |
| Basophils | 0–0.2 | 0–0.2 | 0.01–0.03 | 0 |

[*]Adapted from Earl FL, Melvegar BA, and Wilson RL: The hemogram and bone marrow profile of normal neonatal and weanling beagle dogs. Lab Animal Sci 23:630, 1971, with permission.
[†]Adapted from Meyers-Wallen VN, Haskins ME, and Patterson DF: Hematologic values in healthy neonatal, weaning, and juvenile kittens. Am J Vet Res 45:1322, 1984, with permission.
Abbreviations: RBC = red blood cells, HB = hemoglobin, PCV = packed cell volume, MCV = mean corpuscular volume, MCH = mean corpuscular hemoglobin, MCHC = mean corpuscular hemoglobin concentration, WBC = white blood cells. (Also see pp 1397–1400)

**Table 2.**  *Normal Serum Biochemical Parameters of the Neonatal Dog and Cat[*]*

| Parameter | Canine 0–2 Weeks | Canine 4 Weeks | Feline 0–2 Weeks | Feline 4 Weeks |
|---|---|---|---|---|
| Bilirubin (mg/dl) | 0.1–1.0 | 0–0.1 | 0.1–1.0 | 0.1–0.2 |
| ALT (IU/L) | 10–337 | 9–24 | 11–24 | 14–26 |
| AST (IU/L) | 10–194 | 14–23 | 8–48 | 12–24 |
| ALP (IU/L) | 176–8760 | 135–201 | 68–269 | 90–135 |
| Total protein (gm/dl) | 3.4–5.2 | 3.9–4.2 | 4.0–5.2 | 4.6–5.2 |
| Albumin (gm/dl) | 1.5–2.8 | 1.0–2.0 | 2.0–2.4 | 2.2–2.4 |
| Cholesterol (mg/dl) | 112–344 | 266–352 | 164–443 | 222–434 |
| Glucose (mg/dl) | 52–146 | 86–115 | 76–129 | 99–112 |

[*]Adapted from Center SA, et al: New York State College of Veterinary Medicine–1987. Cornell University, Ithaca, NY, with permission.
Abbreviations: ALT = alanine transaminase, AST = aspartate transaminase, ALP = alkaline phosphatase.

**Table 3.**  *Normal Serum Biochemical Parameters of the Neonatal Dog and Cat*

| Parameter | Canine[*] 5 Weeks | Feline[†] 4–6 Weeks |
|---|---|---|
| BUN (mg/dl) | 11.7–18.7 | Not available |
| Creatinine (mg/dl) | 0.36–0.49 | 0.5–0.7 |
| Na (mEq/L) | 149.9–143.9 | 147–158 |
| Cl (mEq/L) | 104.4–112.2 | 118–127 |
| K (mEq/L) | 4.9–6.4 | 3.7–5.6 |
| Ca (mg/dl) | 10.6–11.7 | 8.4–11.0 |
| Phosphorous (mg/dl) | 8.2–9.4 | 5.0–9.9 |

[*]From Chandler ML, Miller EM, and Olson PN: Colorado State University, Fort Collins, CO.
[†]From Crawford MA: The urinary system. In Hoskins JD (ed): *Veterinary Pediatrics*. Philadelphia, WB Saunders Co, 1990, p 274, with permission.
Abbreviations: BUN = blood urea nitrogen, Na = sodium, Cl = chlorine, K = potassium, Ca = calcium.

echocardiography, and electrocardiography are often necessary to make the definitive diagnosis. These procedures are noninvasive and can be performed on the neonate as in the adult. Acquired heart diseases, including myocarditis and endocarditis, are most often caused by infectious agents (i.e., canine distemper or parvoviruses, bacteria). Serum virus-specific antibody titers in the neonate and bitch or queen may be helpful in the diagnosis. Immunofluorescence of conjunctival or tonsillar scrapings for canine distemper virus may be used to investigate distemper virus infection. An ophthalmic spatula held at a 90-degree angle to the conjunctiva or tonsil is lightly moved over the surface with enough pressure to obtain epithelial cells. The collected material is then gently smeared over the surface of a glass microscope slide.

Bacterial endocarditis may occur as a result of entry of organisms through the umbilicus or skin wounds. Although blood cultures may confirm the diagnosis of bacterial endocarditis, the volume of blood removed is the limiting factor in the neonate. Because blood volume correlates with the rate of positive blood cultures (Dow and Jones, 1989), it is better to take a high volume (5 ml) once on neonates less than 0.5 kg or twice from neonates greater than 0.5 kg than to get three small (1 ml) samples. The timing is not critical and blood collection does not need to be temporally related to temperature spikes, especially because neonates may not respond as adults in generating a fever. Commercial multipurpose nutrient broths are recommended for blood culture collection and transport (Dow and Jones, 1989).

Blood pressure is lower in the neonate than in the adult animal. The mean systolic blood pressure for newborn and 1- to 4-week-old beagle puppies as determined by indirect (Doppler) methods is 61±5 mm Hg and 82±6 mm Hg, respectively (Adelman and Wright, 1985). Blood pressure can be most efficiently and noninvasively monitored in neonates by the Doppler method. Cuff size has been a problem in the author's experience with indirect methods that do not use the Doppler sensing device (see this volume, p 113).

## RESPIRATORY SYSTEM

As with other systems, respiratory disease in the neonate most commonly is related to infectious and congenital causes. Aspiration pneumonia and bacterial pneumonia secondary to bacteremia from umbilical or skin infections result in dyspnea and sometimes cyanosis. Chest radiographs can aid in differentiation of cardiovascular from respiratory diseases, and in distinguishing the various types of respiratory disease.

Because collection of arterial blood in the neonate is technically difficult or impossible, pulse oximetry, a noninvasive means to monitor oxygen saturation of arterial blood, can be used. The hairless skin on the ventral abdomen works well for pulse oximetry (Fig. 1). Normal neonates without supplemental oxygen have oxygen saturations above 90% in the author's experience. Pulse oximetry is limited in that it cannot be used to assess oxygen delivery to the tissues, ventilation, or acid-base status (Aughey et al., 1991).

Collection of fluid samples from the lungs for culture and cytology is difficult in the neonate. Endotracheal intubation and wash can be accomplished on the anesthetized patient; however, sick neonates are a high anesthetic risk. Perhaps the best method is a transthoracic fine-needle aspirate; however, this should be done with extreme caution. The patient should be restrained in ventral or lateral recumbancy. While an assistant holds the mouth and nose closed for 1 to 2 sec to stop respiratory movements, a 23-gauge needle with a 6 ml syringe attached is advanced into the chest at the cranial edge of the rib in the eighth to ninth interspace or a location determined by radiography. Two or three quick 3- to 4-ml aspirations are made and the needle is removed from the chest. The fluid obtained can be placed on a sterile swab, which is then placed in transport media for culture, or smeared onto glass microscope slides for cytologic evaluation. If viral infections such as distemper or feline rhinotracheitis virus are suspected, conjunctival scrapings for fluorescent antibody staining can be obtained from neonates with open eyes (technique is described under "Cardiovascular System" above). Congenital defects can often be diagnosed by physical examination and radiography. In a recent case

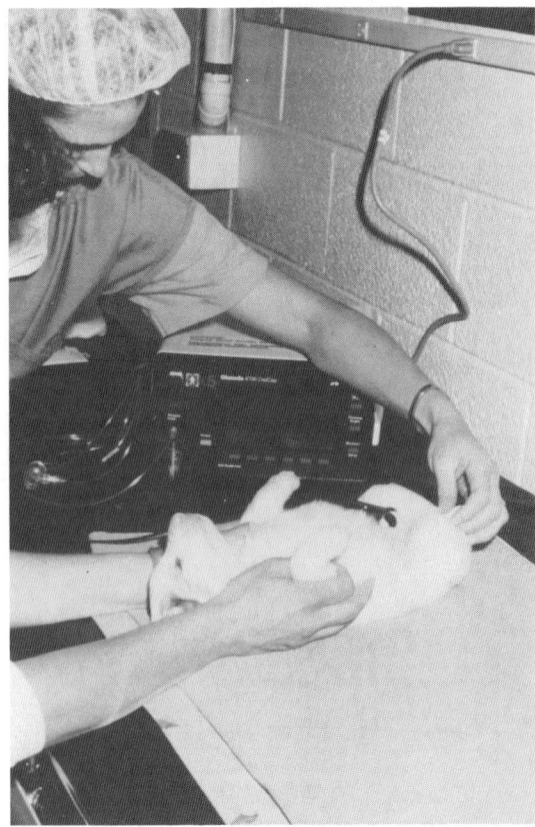

**Figure 1.** Pulse oximetry can be utilized to assess arterial oxygen saturation in the neonate.

of inspiratory stridor in a 10-day-old puppy, laryngoscopy was key in the diagnosis of laryngeal paralysis.

## HEPATOBILIARY SYSTEM

At this age, one is concerned most with congenital anomalies of the liver or portal vascular system; however, clinical signs generally do not develop until after weaning. Bacterial hepatitis can be a sequela to septicemia. Certain viral infections such as feline infectious peritonitis infection can also cause liver disease in neonates.

Routine serum chemical analyses of liver enzymes, blood urea nitrogen, albumin, bilirubin, and glucose may be helpful in the diagnosis of liver disease in the neonate, keeping in mind that at this age urea nitrogen and albumin concentrations are normally lower than adult values (Tables 2 and 3). Fasting and postprandial serum bile acids can be assessed at this age; normal values are the same as for adult animals. Other tests of liver function such as blood ammonia concentrations and sulfobromophthalein (BSP) clearance can also be utilized in the neonate. Shortly after birth of puppies, clearance of BSP is within the adult normal range while by 2 months of age blood ammonia concentrations are within the normal adult range (Center, Hornbuckle, and Hoskins, 1990). By 2 months of age, coagulation tests are usually in the normal adult range. Radiographic and ultrasonographic procedures to evaluate liver architecture and blood flow can be performed as in the adult.

## GASTROINTESTINAL SYSTEM

When vomiting, regurgitation, diarrhea, or loss of appetite occur in the neonate, assessment of the gastrointestinal tract is in order. Visual inspection of the oral cavity may reveal congenital anomalies of the palate and teeth. Feces may be utilized for visual inspection, fecal flotation for parasites, and cytologic and microbiologic evaluation. Collection can be accomplished easily in the neonate by gently stimulating the perineal area with a warm, moist cloth. This is usually more productive if the patient has been separated from the mother for a period of time such that she has not recently stimulated defecation. Feces may also be examined for fat, starch, or trypsin activity if pancreatic exocrine insufficiency is suspected. Other means of gastrointestinal tract assessment includes abdominal or thoracic survey and contrast radiography; however, detail may be poor due to lack of intra-abdominal fat.

## MUSCULOSKELETAL SYSTEM

Congenital anomalies of the skeletal system and traumatic fractures or dislocations may be detected by physical examination. Radiography may confirm the diagnosis in these instances. Skeletal deformities can be a result of inborn errors of metabolism. Screening for such diseases is available (Medical Genetics Laboratory at the University of Pennsylvania). Urine collected on a filter paper, dried, and mailed to the lab.

Infectious joint disease can be a sequela to septicemia. Using care to maintain aseptic technique, fluid from swollen joints may be collected for cytology and culture as in the adult. Inherited myopathies usually become manifest at a later stage in life; however, they can show up as early as 4 to 6 weeks of age. Muscle biopsies and electromyography can be utilized to help with the diagnosis (consult your pathologist for proper handling). Congenital myasthenia gravis typically becomes apparent at 5 to 8 weeks of age. Electromyography is useful in the diagnosis. Infection with *Toxoplasma gondii* in utero or in the newborn may cause myelitis or myositis. Because serum antibody titers are not consistently elevated in early infections, demonstration of organisms in muscle biopsies is considered diagnostic.

## NERVOUS SYSTEM AND SPECIAL SENSES

Developmental anomalies and infectious disease again are the primary causes of neurologic disease in the neonate. Physical examination and complete neurologic examination of the patient is needed for diagnosis. Neurologic examination of the neonate has been reviewed (Shores, 1983). Aids in the diagnosis of neurologic disease might include fundic exam after the eyes are open, ultrasonography through an open fontanel to detect hydrocephalus, serum titers and conjunctival scrapings for viral infections, cerebrospinal fluid collection for infectious or inherited metabolic disease, and computed tomography. Cerebrospinal fluid collection must be obtained while the patient is anesthetized. The technique and landmarks are the same as for adults; however, only 0.25 ml of cerebrospinal fluid can be removed. This procedure is not recommended in toy breeds due to their small size.

Inborn errors of metabolism may be manifested as central nervous system disease in young animals. A urine sample collected on a filter paper can be analyzed for products of abnormal metabolism (see above). Electroencephalography is not routinely done in the neonate due to the difficulties in interpretation.

The ears open at approximately 2 weeks of age. The newborn can respond to loud noises; however, auditory evoked potentials attain adult patterns by 3 to 4 weeks of age (Breazile, 1978). By 10 to 14 days of age, the eyes of most neonates are open. Pupillary light responses are sluggish until 4 weeks of age. At this time the electroretinogram attains a normal adult pattern; therefore it might be a useful diagnostic tool (Breazile, 1978). Tear production in neonates has not been studied to the author's knowledge, but Schirmer tear testing may be helpful in ruling out keratoconjunctivitis sicca.

## IMMUNE SYSTEM

Even in adult animals the immune system is difficult to assess. Specific tests of immune function may only be available at referral centers. However, crude tests such as complete blood cell counts, immunoglobulin and complement quantitation, and antibody response to vaccination may indicate immunologic status. Keep in mind that the neonate is born immunologically incompetent and develops immunologic maturity between 6 weeks and 6 months of age (Felsburg, 1990).

## BLOOD AND URINE COLLECTION

In the author's experience, the easiest method of blood collection is via jugular venipuncture. The patient is placed in lateral recumbancy with the neck in moderate dorsiflexion and the forelimbs pulled caudally. Pressure across the thoracic inlet with the thumb will result in distention of the jugular vein, which is then readily visible. Wet the skin over the vein with alcohol. A 22-gauge needle and 3-ml syringe is then directed caudally and inserted through the skin at a 30- to 45-degree angle. The angle is gradually reduced as the needle is threaded into the vein all the way to the needle hub. Gentle aspiration to avoid collapse of the vein will allow withdrawal of blood. If no blood is obtained because the other side of the vein was penetrated, slowly back out the needle with negative pressure on the syringe. If unsuccessful, remove the needle from the patient and start over. The blood collected should be immediately transferred to appropriate sample collection tubes. In tubes containing anticoagulants, a minimum volume of blood is needed to obtain reliable results. Collection tubes designed for small volumes (300 to 500 $\mu$l-liters; Microtainer, Becton-Dickinson) are ideal for puppies and kittens.

Urine is easily collected by gently stimulating the perineal area with a warm, moist cloth. This is usually more successful if the neonate has been separated from the mother for an hour or so. Be ready to catch the urine with a collection device.

## References and Suggested Reading

Adelman RD and Wright J: Systolic blood pressure and heart rate in the growing beagle puppy. Dev Pharmacol Ther 8:396, 1985.
  *A comparison of direct and indirect blood pressure measurement in the developing beagle dog.*
Aughey K, Hess D, Eitel D, et al: An evaluation of pulse oximetry in pehospital care. Ann Emerg Med 20:887, 1991.
  *A comparison of arterial oxygen saturation to pulse oximetry oxygen saturation in human patients.*
Breazile JE: Neurologic and behavioral development in the puppy. Vet Clin North Am 8:31, 1978.
  *A review of normal neurologic development of the puppy.*
Bright JM and Holmberg DL: The cardiovascular system. *In* Hoskins JD (ed): *Veterinary Pediatrics.* Philadelphia, WB Saunders Co, 1990, p 43.
  *A review of diseases, diagnostics, and treatments of the cardiovascular system in the pediatric veterinary patient.*
Center SA, Hornbuckle WE, and Hoskins JD: The liver and pancreas. *In* Hoskins JD (ed): *Veterinary Pediatrics.* Philadelphia, WB Saunders Co, 1990, p 205.
  *A review of the diseases, diagnostics, and treatments of the liver in the pediatric veterinary patient.*
Crawford MA: The urinary system. *In* Hoskins JD (ed): *Veterinary Pediatrics.* Philadelphia, WB Saunders Co, 1990, p 271.
  *A review of the diseases, diagnostics, and treatments of the urinary system in pediatric veterinary patients.*
Dow SW and Jones RL: Bacteremia: Pathogenesis and diagnosis. Compend Cont Educ 11:432, 1989.
  *A review of the pathophysiology of bacteremia and methods for diagnosis.*
Felsburg PJ: The immune system. *In* Hoskins JD (ed): *Veterinary Pediatrics.* Philadelphia, WB Saunders Co, 1990, p 325.
  *A review of the diseases, diagnostics, and treatments of the immune system in the pediatric veterinary patient.*
Haskins M: Neonatal and pediatric pathology. *Proceedings of Eastern States Veterinary Conference,* January, 1985, p 23.
  *A review of the value and methods of performing necropsies on pediatric patients.*
Shores A: Neurologic examination of the canine neonate. Compend Cont Educ 5:1033, 1983.
  *A review of the techniques of neurologic examination of the pediatric patient and the normal responses expected.*

# FADING PUPPY AND KITTEN SYNDROME

JOHNNY D. HOSKINS
*Baton Rouge, Louisiana*

Puppy and kitten losses during the first 12 weeks of life usually approximate 15 to 40%, although precise figures from well-established kennels and catteries may vary (Lawler and Monti, 1984; Norworthy, 1979; Scott and Geissinger, 1978). Most losses occur during the following specific periods: *in utero* (abortions and fetal resorptions); at the time of birth (stillbirths); immediately after the birth period (birth to 2 weeks of age); or in the immediate postweaning period (5 to 12 weeks of age). Losses after these periods are generally low.

Puppy and kitten deaths during the period immediately after birth are often referred to as the "fading puppy syndrome," or "fading kitten syndrome." Affected puppies or kittens are apparently healthy at birth but fail to survive beyond 2 weeks of age. This age distinctness is arbitrary; it might be more appropriate to consider the period from birth to 12 weeks of age.

## ETIOLOGY

Puppy and kitten losses during the period between birth and 12 weeks of age usually result from problems acquired *in utero*, during the birth process (birth to 2 weeks of age), or in the postweaning period (5 to 12 weeks of age) (Pedersen, 1991). Death losses during the latter period are primarily attributed to infectious diseases potentiated by weaning stress, exposure to pathogenic organisms in the immediate environment, and underdeveloped local and/or systemic immunity (see "Nutritional and Environmental Considerations in Neonatal Medicine," this volume, p 37). Puppy and kitten losses generally occur because of congenital anomalies, teratogenic effects, nutritional diseases resulting from improper diets fed to the dam or young, abnormally low birth weights, traumatic insults during or after the birth process (dystocia, cannibalism, or maternal neglect), neonatal isoerythrolysis, infectious diseases, and other (miscellaneous) factors (Pedersen, 1991).

### Congenital Anomalies

Congenital anomalies are disorders of unspecified cause that are present at birth. Although they are of genetic origin in many situations, teratogenic factors may be responsible. Some congenital anomalies (particularly those that involve the central nervous, cardiovascular, and respiratory systems) may be immediately incompatible with life, resulting in death at birth or within 2 weeks of an apparently normal birth. Other anomalies might remain unnoticed until the animal is fully ambulatory. Often, these congenital anomalies are first diagnosed during the initial clinical examination before vaccination, or as the result of limited exercise tolerance or failure to thrive.

Anatomic anomalies include cleft palates, cranial deformities, agenesis of the small or large intestines, cardiac anomalies, extensive umbilical or diaphragmatic hernias, anomalies of the kidneys and lower urinary tract, and musculoskeletal anomalies. Microanatomic or biochemical congenital anomalies probably account for an equal number of puppy and kitten losses (Pedersen, 1991). Such defects go unreported and are usually included under the general heading of stillbirths, fading puppy or kitten syndrome (so-called faders), or undetermined cause of death.

### Teratogenic Effects

The extent to which puppy and kitten losses may be attributed to teratogenic effects is unclear. There are authenticated reports of the teratogenic potential of some drugs and chemicals that contribute to congenital anomalies or faders. It is generally best to avoid the administration or application of any drug or chemical during pregnancy. Although specific information for canine and feline species may be lacking, it is advisable to avoid the use of any drug or chemical, such as corticosteroids and griseofulvin, with known adverse teratologic effects in animals.

### Nutrition

Bitches and queens fed poor-quality diets during pregnancy may produce diseased or weak puppies and kittens. The most serious dietary problem documented in the last decade has been taurine deficiency in cats. Deficiencies of dietary taurine are known to cause fetal resorptions, abortions, stillbirths, and poor-growing kittens (Sturman and Gargano, 1986). Malnutrition of a puppy or kitten also may be the result of severe maternal malnutrition or a lack of adequate maternal blood supply, possibly because of competition for placental space.

### Low Birth Weight

Low birth weights are associated with higher puppy and kitten losses. The cause of abnormally low birth weights has not been determined but probably involves several factors. The birth weight of puppies and kittens is not affected by sex, litter size, or weight of the dam (Festing and Bleby, 1970; Lawler and Monti, 1984). Although low birth weight is often attributed to prematurity, most abnormally small puppies and kittens are born at term. The small stature is probably caused by congenital anomalies or poor nutrition.

Low birth weight is associated with a greater likelihood of stillbirths and deaths during the first 6 weeks of life (Lawler and Monti, 1984). In addition, a disproportionate number of underweight puppies and kittens tend to be chronic "poor doers" and tend to die young. Many faders that die in the first weeks of life are of normal size, but their growth is slow and they are below normal weight at the time of death. It is thus important to weigh puppies and kittens not only at birth, but also at frequent intervals until they are completely weaned (at least 6 weeks of age).

### Traumatic Insult

Puppy and kitten deaths caused by traumatic insults during birth or the first 5 days of life are usually associated with dystocia, cannibalism, or maternal neglect. Cannibalism often involves nervous or high-strung mothers. Because cannibalism of sickly puppies and kittens is common, it is incorrect always to incriminate trauma as the direct cause of death. It is not always possible to differentiate maternal neglect of otherwise normal puppies and kittens from maternal neglect of sickly puppies and kittens. The latter is a programmed maternal response that is akin to cannibalism.

## Neonatal Isoerythrolysis

Neonatal isoerythrolysis occurs infrequently among domestic shorthair kittens, but may be relatively common in certain purebred kittens (Giger, 1992 in *CVT XI*, p 470). Unlike puppies, kittens have naturally occurring antibodies against the other blood types in their plasma, commonly referred to as alloantibodies. Kittens acquire maternal alloantibodies of the IgG class, and to a lesser extent of the IgM class, via colostrum.

Kittens with blood type A have weak anti-B alloantibodies. Kittens with blood type B have strong anti-A alloantibodies with hemagglutinin and hemolysin titers of 1:64 or higher. At 6 to 10 weeks of age, kittens begin to produce their own alloantibodies; these titers may reach peak levels by a few months of age. Prior blood transfusion or pregnancy is thus not necessary for the production of alloantibodies in kittens. These alloantibodies, particularly anti-A alloantibodies, are responsible for the major incompatibility reactions. Colostral anti-A alloantibodies from blood type B queens may cause neonatal isoerythrolysis in blood type A (or blood type AB) kittens. Blood type AB mismatched blood transfusions have a short half-life (and are thus ineffective) and cause life-threatening transfusion reactions in blood type B cats.

During the first 24 hr of life, maternal antibodies are normally transferred to the kitten via colostrum. If the kitten has blood type A (or AB) and the queen has blood type B, these colostral alloantibodies will bind to and lyse erythrocytes in the kitten. The destruction of erythrocytes may be intravascular and extravascular, and cause severe anemia, chromoproteinuric nephropathy, and other organ failures, as well as disseminated intravascular coagulation. Because all blood type B cats have high alloantibody titers, even primiparous queens can have litters with neonatal isoerythrolysis.

Clinical signs of neonatal isoerythrolysis often develop in blood type A (or AB) kittens born to blood type B queens. Because the feline fetus is protected from maternal antibodies, kittens that are at risk are born healthy and usually start nursing vigorously. After intake of colostrum, which contains high titers of maternal alloantibodies, the kittens exhibit the first clinical signs within hours to days.

The clinical course may vary. The following are common:

- Kittens that die suddenly during the first day of life without clinical signs.
- Kittens that stop nursing during the first 3 days of life and fail to thrive. Clinical findings may include dark brownish red urine caused by severe hemoglobinuria, icterus and severe anemia, continued fading and death during the first week of life, and (rarely) tail-tip necrosis between first and second weeks of life.
- Kittens that continue to nurse, thrive, and demonstrate no clinical signs of illness except tail-tip necrosis, but that have laboratory abnormalities such as a positive direct Coombs' test and a moderately responsive anemia.

## Infectious Diseases

Infectious diseases account for a substantial proportion of puppy and kitten losses, especially bacterial infections during the postweaning period (5 to 12 weeks of age). During this time, most deaths are attributed to primary infection of the respiratory tract or the gastrointestinal tract and peritoneal cavity. If puppies and kittens are exposed to bacteria in nonstressful conditions, mild and self-limiting or clinically inapparent infections are typical. When host and environmental factors are unfavorable, immediate illnesses are more apt to be severe, and puppy and kitten losses are high. If bacterial infections exceed the immune system's ability to protect against infectious agents, neonatal sepsis occurs.

If overwhelming sepsis develops in puppies and kittens 5 to 12 weeks of age, the severity of illness usually influences survival. Factors that predispose puppies and kittens of this age group to septicemic conditions include the coexistence of inadequate nutrition, inadequate thermoregulation, viral infections, parasitism, and developmental and heritable defects of the immune system.

Neonatal sepsis is usually caused by common bacteria (e.g., *Staphylococcus, Escherichia, Klebsiella, Enterobacter, Streptococcus, Enterococcus, Pseudomonas, Clostridium, Bacteroides, Fusobacterium, Pasteurella, Brucella, and Salmonella*). Of these, gram-negative bacilli are the most common. They enter the bloodstream from the gastrointestinal tract and peritoneal cavity, respiratory tract, skin and associated wounds, and urinary tract.

Several viral groups (i.e., parvovirus, coronavirus, herpesvirus, adenovirus, calicivirus, retrovirus, and morbillivirus) have been implicated in puppy and kitten losses. Clinical signs of viral infections vary according to the route and time of infection, and the degree of passively derived antibody protection of the individual puppy or kitten. Even against a background of routine vaccine protection of breeding stock, there are situations in which passive immunity protection is inadequate (possibly because of colostral deprivation) and in which puppies and kittens are susceptible to viral infections that are normally considered to be well controlled.

Canine herpesvirus infection is a common cause of puppy losses (Carmichael and Greene, 1990). Most canine herpesvirus infections are acquired during late pregnancy and during the first 3 weeks of life. Clinical signs manifested by puppies with canine herpesvirus infection may vary from mild to severe, depending upon the age, maternal herpesvirus antibody titers, stress, and concurrent bacterial infections. If canine herpesvirus infection is acquired *in utero*, fetal death, mummification, abortion, or neonatal death can result. Most puppy losses occur between the 9th and 14th days of life. Severe clinical disease in a puppy older than 4 weeks is unlikely. Affected puppies suddenly develop severe illness characterized by depression, anorexia, persistent crying, abdominal discomfort, bloating, rapid and shallow respiration, hypothermia, and profound weakness. The clinical course commonly ends in death in 18 to 24 hr.

## Miscellaneous Factors

Roundworm and hookworm infections have been implicated in puppy and kitten losses. The intestinal worm burden is detrimental to the puppy's or kitten's growth. Although deaths attributable to ectoparasitism are uncommon, newly weaned puppies and kittens frequently have well-established flea or tick burdens.

Fatty liver syndrome, especially of 4- to 16-week-old toy breeds, may cause ill-thriving puppies (van der Linde-Sipman et al., 1990). Affected puppies suddenly develop severe illness characterized by depression, anorexia, persistent crying, diarrhea, rapid and shallow respiration, hypothermia, seizures, and profound weakness. The clinical course usually ends in death in 1 to 6 days.

There are other, poorly understood causes of kitten loss. Losses are lowest in fifth litters; first litters and litters after the fifth parity have higher kitten losses (Lawler and Monti, 1984). Medium-sized queens tend to have lower kitten losses than large or small queens. Kitten losses are twice as high in one-kitten litters as in larger litters. The lowest kitten losses occur in litters with five kittens.

## DIAGNOSIS

Puppy and kitten losses are apparently common and often unavoidable in breeding establishments. However, preweaning losses (live-born deaths and stillbirths) exceeding 20% and postweaning losses (weaning to 7 months of age) exceeding 10% are reasons for serious concern (Pedersen, 1991). Disproportionate losses to a single cause (e.g., congenital anomaly or specific infectious disease) and percentages greater than those described here are additional reasons for concern, regardless of the overall percentage.

The clinical approach to identifying the cause of fading puppy or kitten syndrome should be based on thorough clinical evaluation, which includes history, physical examination, routine laboratory tests (p 26), EKG and possibly lead-II electrocardiography strip, radiography, or ultrasonography (Hoskins, 1990). A thorough physical examination should always be performed. It is advisable to obtain a complete blood count, plasma chemistry profile, urinalysis, urine or blood culture or both, and culture of suspected sources of infection. It is imperative to conduct a thorough search for the primary sources of infection and to collect appropriate bacterial culture samples before initiating antimicrobial therapy.

Hemograms are particularly helpful in the diagnosis of septicemic puppies and kittens. Normochromic normocytic anemia, thrombocytopenia, and mild to moderate immature neutrophilia may be present. Hypoglycemia is another laboratory finding that is consistent with, but not specific for, septicemic "faders." The remaining laboratory values from the plasma chemistry profile and urinalysis may reflect a specific organ failure.

Complete and accurate necropsy is one of the most expensive and crucial aspects of identifying the cause of fading puppy and kitten syndrome in breeding establishments (Pedersen, 1991). It is advisable to euthanize the puppy or kitten and perform a fresh necropsy as soon as it becomes apparent that death is inevitable. Puppies and kittens that die before euthanasia should be immediately refrigerated; freezing should be avoided because it ruins tissue for gross and light microscopic examination. Necropsy must be performed by competent personnel. Gross abnormalities are often subtle and may go unnoticed by untrained eyes.

Representative tissue should be taken as aseptically as possible and, if necessary, frozen for microbiologic (viral, bacterial, and fungal cultures) or toxicologic studies. In addition, representative samples of tissue should be preserved in formalin for light microscopic examination. Formalin-fixed tissues, along with detailed descriptions of gross lesions and the clinical history, should then be forwarded to veterinary pathologists for evaluation. If tissue indicates that an infectious or toxic disease is the cause of death, samples of frozen tissues can be submitted to microbiologists or toxicologists for further study.

## MANAGEMENT

A certain number of puppy and kitten losses is unavoidable. Nevertheless, it may be possible to identify the specific cause of a fading puppy syndrome or fading kitten syndrome and initiate appropriate management measures. When the primary cause is determined, a concerted effort is necessary to eliminate the causative factors before the next breeding or purchase.

## References and Suggested Reading

Carmichael LE and Greene CE: Canine herpesvirus infection. *In* Greene CE (ed): *Infectious Diseases of the Dog and Cat*. Philadelphia: WB Saunders, 1990, p 252.

Festing MFW and Bleby J: Breeding performance and growth of SPF cats (*Felis catus*). J Small Anim Pract 11:533, 1970.

Giger U: The feline AB blood group system and incompatibility reactions. *In* Kirk RW and Bonagura JD (eds): *Current Veterinary Therapy XI*. Philadelphia, WB Saunders Co, 1992, p 470.

Hoskins JD: Examination of the young dog and cat: Birth to four months. Proc Am Coll Vet Intern Med 8:631, 1990.

Lawler DF and Monti KL: Morbidity and mortality in neonatal kittens. Am J Vet Res 45:1455, 1984.

Norsworthy GD: Kitten mortality complex. Feline Pract 9:57, 1979.

Pedersen NC: Common infectious diseases of multiple-cat environments. *In* Pedersen NC (ed): *Feline Husbandry: Diseases and Management in the Multiple-Cat Environment.* Goleta, CA, American Veterinary Publications, Inc, 1991, p 177.

Scott FW and Geissinger C: Kitten mortality survey. Feline Pract 8:31, 1978.

Sturman JA and Gargano AD: Feline maternal taurine deficiency effects on mother and offspring. J Nutrition 116:655, 1986.

van der Linde-Sipman JS, van den Ingh TSGAM, van Toor AJ: Fatty liver syndrome in puppies. J Am Anim Hosp Assoc 26:9, 1990.

# FLUID THERAPY IN THE PUPPY AND KITTEN

### JOHNNY D. HOSKINS
*Baton Rouge, Louisiana*

Puppies and kittens younger than 6 weeks of age are predisposed to hydration deficit because extracellular fluid is increased, renal capacity to conserve water is decreased, the surface area/body weight ratio is large, and fluid loss through immature skin is greater (Kerner and Sunshine, 1979). Brain volume normally decreases during the first 2 days of life in puppies and kittens; hypovolemic hypotension at this age predisposes to neonatal hemorrhage, particularly if followed by rapid volume replacement or administration of hyperosmolar fluids.

The primary purpose of fluid therapy in the puppy and kitten is to induce a positive fluid balance (DiBartola, 1992). For patients, in need of medical care, the need for fluid therapy depends on assessment of the animal's state of dehydration. For surgical patients additional indications for fluid therapy include maintenance of venous access for emergencies and establishment of diuresis to maintain renal perfusion during anesthesia. The hydration status of the adult dog or cat is estimated by evaluation of the history, physical examination findings, and the results of a few simple laboratory tests (packed cell volume, total plasma protein concentration, and urine specific gravity). Similar principles for effective fluid therapy also apply to puppies and kittens (Table 1).

Historic information about lack of fluid intake and routes of fluid loss may suggest the puppy's or kitten's hydration, electrolyte, and acid-base needs. Physical examination findings associated with fluid losses vary from no clinically detectable changes (5% loss of body weight) to signs of hypovolemic shock and impending death (15% loss of body weight). The veterinarian may estimate the hydration deficit by evaluating skin turgor or pliability, moistness of the mucous membranes, the position of the eyes in their orbits, heart rate, the character of peripheral pulses, capillary refill time, and extent of peripheral venous distention (DiBartola, 1992). In puppies and kittens younger than 6 weeks of age, skin turgor and probably the percentage estimation of dehydration (5 to 15%) does not apply. A more accurate estimation of dehydration may be obtained by evaluating the moistness of mucous membranes and color of urine. The urine of puppies and kittens younger than 6 weeks of age is normally clear and colorless. Any color tint of their urine indicates dehydration.

## FLUID PREPARATIONS

Fluid preparations may be classified as crystalloids or colloids. *Crystalloids* are solutions containing electrolyte and nonelectrolyte solutes capable of entering all body fluid compartments (e.g., 5% dextrose in water, 0.9% saline solution, lactated Ringer's solution, Ringer's solution). *Colloids* are large-molecular-weight substances restricted to the plasma compartment; they include plasma, dextrans, and hydroxyethyl starch (hetastarch). Colloids may be used to treat shock and severe hypoalbuminemia.

Crystalloid solutions are further classified as either replacement or maintenance solutions. The composition of *replacement* solutions (e.g., lactated Ringer's solution, Ringer's solution) resembles that of extracellular fluid. *Maintenance* solutions contain less sodium (40 to 60 mEq/L) and more potassium (15 to 30 mEq/L) than replacement fluids. A simple maintenance solution can be formulated by mixing one part 0.9% saline solution with two parts 5% dextrose solution and adding 20 mEq potassium chloride per liter of final solution. The approximate composition of such a fluid would be 51 mEq/L sodium, 20 mEq/L potassium, 71 mEq/L chloride, and 16.7 gm/L dextrose. This fluid provides 67 kcal/L and has an osmolality of 235 mOsm/kg (DiBartola, 1992). Manufactured maintenance solutions, such as Pedialyte and Rehydralyte (Ross Laboratories, Columbus, OH), contain similar electrolyte and dextrose composition.

The most useful crystalloid solutions for routine use are replacement solutions, such as Ringer's or lactated Ringer's solution, 0.9% saline solution, and 5% dextrose in water. Supplementation of crystalloid solutions with potassium chloride may be necessary if losses include large amounts of potassium. An empiric scale routinely

### Table 1. Medical Management of an Ill Puppy or Kitten

I. External warming procedure
   A. Use circulating hot water blanket and hot water bottle
   B. Take at least 20 to 30 minutes for gradual warming of the patient
   C. Turn the patient every hour
   D. Record rectal temperature every hour

II. Parenteral fluid therapy
   A. Use multiple electrolyte solution (Ringer's solution) supplemented with 5% dextrose solution
   B. Supplement the fluids with potassium chloride solution if plasma potassium concentration is less than 2.5 mmol/L
   C. Administer warm fluids slowly by intravenous or intraosseous route

III. Glucose replacement therapy
   A. Administer 5% dextrose solution intravenously or intraosseously, to effect
   B. Administer 1 to 2 ml/kg of a 10 to 25% dextrose solution to the patient that is profoundly depressed or having seizures
   C. Maintain plasma glucose concentration at 80 to 200 mg/dl for euglycemia

IV. Provide nutritional therapy: encourage food and water intake once patient is normothermic and adequately hydrated

V. Monitor the effectiveness of medical management
   A. Observe for improvement in the patient's general demeanor
   B. Regularly assess the cardiopulmonary status: it is extremely easy to overhydrate the ill puppy and kitten so attentive monitoring of breathing pattern is helpful for early recognition of overhydration
   C. Weigh the patient three to four times a day to record weight gain
   D. Observe for moistness of mucous membranes in assessing for adequate hydration

used for adult dogs and cats to estimate the amount of potassium to add to parenterally administered fluids can also be used for puppies and kittens (Greene and Scott, 1975) (Table 2). Before use, crystalloid solutions should be stored at room temperature or preferably warmed near body temperature in a 37°C (98.6°F) water bath or incubator. Warming minimizes decreases in body temperature caused by administering fluids with a temperature less than 37°C.

The choice of fluid to administer depends on the underlying disease, and the composition of the fluid lost. Fluid losses should be replaced with fluids similar

### Table 2. Sliding Scale for Potassium Supplementation°

| Serum Potassium (mmol/L) | Potassium Chloride Added to 250 ml Fluid |
|---|---|
| Below 2.0 | 20 mEq |
| 2.0–2.5 | 15 mEq |
| 2.6–3.0 | 10 mEq |
| 3.1–3.5 | 7 mEq |

°From Green RW and Scott RC: Lower urinary tract disease. In Ettinger SJ (ed): *Textbook of Veterinary Internal Medicine*, 3rd edition. Philadelphia, WB Saunders Co, 1989, p 1928, with permission.

in volume and electrolyte composition to that lost from the body. If clinical assessment of hydration suggests hypovolemia, a replacement fluid should be administered rapidly. If there are no clinical signs of hypovolemia, the combined hydration deficit and maintenance fluid needs may be combined and administered over the next 12 to 24 hr. Most patients treated with lactate-containing replacement fluid solutions respond well, probably as a result of extracellular fluid volume expansion and improved tissue perfusion (DiBartola, 1992). In puppies and kittens (younger than 6 weeks of age that require fluid therapy), Ringer's solution is often a better replacement fluid solution. At this age, puppies and kittens may not effectively metabolize lactate to bicarbonate.

Benzoic acid derivatives (e.g., benzyl alcohol, ethylparaben, methylparaben, propylparaben) are added to some crystalloid solutions for their antimicrobial effect. However, crystalloid solutions with preservatives must be avoided in kittens. Crystalloid solutions with preservatives given to kittens may result in behavioral changes, hypersalivation, ataxia, muscle fasciculations, seizures, dilated nonresponsive pupils, coma, and even death (Cullison, Menard, and Buck, 1983).

## ROUTES OF ADMINISTRATION

INTRAVENOUS. Intravenous administration by means of an indwelling catheter is recommended when puppies and kittens are very ill, when there has been severe fluid loss, or when fluid loss has been acute. Intravenous administration is also used during anesthesia to maintain renal perfusion and vascular access for emergencies. Use of the intravenous route requires close monitoring during infusion to avoid complications such as overhydration, infection, thrombosis, phlebitis, embolism, and impaired fluid delivery (e.g., obstruction of the catheter by change in the patient's position). Vascular access for puppies and kittens younger than 6 weeks of age are generally restricted to the jugular and cephalic veins. The jugular vein is preferred because it allows uniform delivery of fluids in small uncooperative patients with small veins.

SUBCUTANEOUS. The subcutaneous route is convenient for maintenance fluid therapy in puppies and kittens. Volume overload is unlikely to occur when fluids are administered by this route. The subcutaneous route is inadequate for puppies and kittens with acute or chronic fluid losses (e.g., shock) and is not recommended for extremely dehydrated or hypothermic patients.

ORAL. Fluids with a wide variety of compositions may be given by oral route. Oral fluids can be administered rapidly with minimal side effects. However, the oral route should not be used in the patient with gastrointestinal dysfunction (e.g., vomiting). The oral route also is inadequate for puppies and kittens that have sustained acute or extensive fluid losses.

INTRAOSSEOUS. The intraosseous route is useful in very ill puppies and kittens in which vascular access is difficult (see *CVT XI*, p 107). This route provides quick vascular access via bone marrow sinusoids and medullary venous channels, and thus facilitates rapid dispersion of fluids. Intraosseous sites suitable for administration of fluids include the tibial tuberosity, trochanteric fossa of the femur, wing of the ilium, and the greater tubercle of the humerus. In most puppies and kittens younger than 6 weeks of age, the femoral trochanteric fossa is the preferred site for intraosseous administration of warm fluids. Fluid flow rates up to 11 ml/min can be achieved with gravity. An 18- or 20-gauge spinal needle (depending on the size of the animal) is aseptically inserted parallel to the long axis of the femur; the stylet is removed from the needle immediately before fluid infusion. The catheter is then secured to the skin. Routine catheter care is required; catheters can be left in place for 72 hr. Potential risks include osteomyelitis, and pain during administration of fluids. Pain generally results from injecting cold or irritating solutions, placing too much weight on the needle inserted in the marrow cavity, or administering a large fluid volume too rapidly.

INTRAPERITONEAL. Intraperitoneal administration of fluids allows for rapid absorption of large volumes; however, only isotonic fluids can be used. The intraperitoneal route is not commonly recommended because of the risk of peritonitis in potentially immunocompromised puppies or kittens.

## FLUID ADMINISTRATION

The rate of fluid administration is dictated by the magnitude and rate of the fluid loss. Acute, severe losses in puppies and kittens with hypotension or shock demand rapid replacement. If necessary, fluids can be given safely to young puppies and kittens at a rate of 40 to 45 ml/kg/hr. However, when fluids are given this rapidly, cardiopulmonary and renal function should be monitored.

It usually is unnecessary and undesirable to rapidly replace hydration deficit in chronic disease states. Instead, the maintenance fluid requirement (40 to 50 ml/kg/day) can be administered over a 24 hr period. This approach allows adequate time for equilibration of fluid and electrolytes within the intracellular compartment, and thus minimizes complications such as edema or effusion due to increased hydrostatic pressure, diuresis, and loss of electrolytes in urine. An alternative approach is to replace the maintenance fluid requirement over the first 4 to 8 hr of treatment, followed by maintenance therapy.

Whenever possible, fluid deficits should be replaced before anesthesia and surgery. During the induction and maintenance of anesthesia, prevention of hypovolemia and maintenance of renal perfusion is essential. Inducing diuresis in this situation may be an important factor in the prevention of intraoperative acute renal failure. A basal fluid administration rate of 4 to 10 ml/kg/hr is recommended during anesthesia and surgery (Hosgood, 1992). During major surgery (e.g., exploratory laparotomy, thoracotomy), fluid administration at twice the basal rate is recommended.

## FAILURE TO ACHIEVE REHYDRATION

Repeated assessment of clinical signs and determination of body weight of the puppy and kitten is mandatory in making appropriate readjustments of fluid therapy. Reasons for failure to achieve satisfactory rehydration include underestimation of the amount of fluids needed, losses greater than first appreciated (e.g., vomiting, diarrhea), and infusion of fluids at an excessively rapid rate with obligatory urinary loss of fluid and electrolytes (DiBartola, 1992). If dehydration is not corrected, the volume of fluid should be increased, provided cardiopulmonary and renal function are adequate. As a general rule, the daily fluid volume may be increased by an amount equivalent to 5% of body weight if the initial infusion fails to restore hydration. Remember, the hydration deficit is an estimate based on history and physical examination findings. Therefore, fluid therapy should be tailored to physical examination findings (body weight, moistness of mucous membranes, clearness of urine) over the first 12 hr to few days of fluid therapy.

## COMPLICATIONS OF FLUID THERAPY

Signs of overhydration occur when fluid is administered too rapidly. These include serous nasal discharge, chemosis, restlessness, tachycardia, cough, altered breathing pattern, pulmonary crackles, ascites, polyuria, exophthalmos, diarrhea, and vomiting (Cornelius, Finco, and Culver, 1978). When intravenous or intraosseous routes are used, aseptic catheter placement and proper maintenance are mandatory. The catheter site should be checked periodically for cleanliness, local pain, and swelling. The patient should also be monitored for fever. If any of these signs occur, the catheter should be removed and a new catheter placed in another vein. When the catheter is not in use, it should be flushed frequently with a small volume (<1 ml) of a solution containing 5 U of heparin per milliliter of 0.9% saline ("heparinized saline") solution.

## DISCONTINUATION OF FLUID THERAPY

Fluid therapy should be discontinued when hydration is restored and the puppy or kitten can maintain fluid balance by eating and drinking. As the patient recovers, the volume of fluid administered is usually decreased by 25 to 50% a day (DiBartola, 1992). During this time, the route of administration may be changed from the intravenous or intraosseous to subcutaneous route.

## References and Suggested Reading

Boothe DM and Tannert K: Special considerations for drug and fluid therapy in the pediatric patient. Compend Cont Educ Pract Vet 14:313, 1992.

Cornelius LM, Finco DR, and Culver DH: Physiologic effects of rapid in-fusion of Ringer's lactate solution into dogs. Am J Vet Res 39:1185, 1978.

Cullison RF, Menard PD, and Buck WB: Toxicosis in cats from the use of benzyl alcohol in lactated Ringer's solution. J Am Vet Med Assoc 182:61, 1983.

DiBartola SP: Introduction to fluid therapy. In DiBartola SP (ed): Fluid Therapy in Small Animal Practice. Philadelphia WB Saunders Co, 1992, p 321.

Greene RW and Scott RC: Lower urinary tract disease. In Ettinger SJ (ed): Textbook of Veterinary Internal Medicine 3rd edition. Philadelphia WB Saunders Co, 1989, p 1928.

Hosgood G: Surgical and anesthetic management of puppies and kittens. Compend Cont Educ Pract Vet 14:345, 1992.

Kerner JA and Sunshine P: Parenteral alimentation. Semin Perinatol 3:417, 1979.

# NUTRITIONAL AND ENVIRONMENTAL CONSIDERATIONS IN NEONATAL MEDICINE

DENNIS F. LAWLER

*St. Louis, Missouri*

*and* RICHARD H. EVANS

*Laguna Niguel, California*

The nutrition of neonatal and young growing puppies and kittens is best approached in an integrated fashion. Search of printed and data base sources yields numerous reports of studies involving individual nutrients, nutrient classes, and sometimes nutritional supplements or complete products. The veterinary clinician, however, usually is confronted with neonatal nutritional problems of greater complexity. Some clients may request advice about nutrient requirements for gestating or lactating dams to optimize production and performance of litters. Others seek information about individual neonates or litters in varying stages of health and condition. Practical choices for feeding neonatal puppies and kittens are limited by the availability of relatively few products for complete nutritional support, further complicating the situation.

From a nutritional perspective, the neonate is not simply a prospective product of dam's milk or a milk replacer. Rather, the nutritional, clinical, and physiologic states of neonates result from interaction of genetic and gestational (intrauterine) factors, the process of parturition, and the postparturient external environment. Precise evaluation of the nutritional status of the neonate is quite difficult without specialized assays and equipment. In addition, the response of neonates to a wide variety of insults is limited in scope. Their outward clinical appearance often reflects the level of distress, but infrequently suggests the underlying problem. Insight into the cause of the illness may be obtained by reevaluation of events that preceded and followed parturition or occurred during the birth process, along with historic and environmental information that may be available from kennel or cattery records or elicited by interview of pet owners. Anatomic signs noted at gross necropsy likewise may be helpful or nonspecific. Postmortem examination may provide additional information to help refine the process of differential diagnosis on a population basis.

## THE GESTATIONAL ENVIRONMENT

Many studies indicate that birth weight is the single most important determinant of survival for neonatal puppies and kittens. However, birth weight is the collective result of positive or negative interaction of a variety of influences. Prominent among these are the age and health of the dam; genetic factors; nutrition; placentation; presence of infectious or parasitic agents; and the sanitation, quality, and stress imposed by the dam's gestational environment. Each of these should be considered when evaluating neonates with low birth weight.

One approach to diagnosis is to establish an orderly checklist that specifies points of interview, clinical evaluation, and laboratory analyses designed to detect or eliminate common diagnostic possibilities. Likewise, the process of population diagnosis, much like that of individual physical examination, will be enhanced if it is conducted according to a clear written protocol.

Gestational events are likely to be responsible for low birth weight of live or dead neonates. Incomplete development of a variety of physiologic processes, especially pulmonary and cardiovascular functions, is a frequent cause of death in these subjects (Fox, 1965). An empty stomach and small intestine, and a full gallbladder detected by necropsy of immature neonates that have survived up to 48 hr, suggest nutritional starvation resulting from inability or lack of desire to suckle effectively (Lawler, 1991). Nutritional factors may be complicated if the dam deliberately ignores sick offspring.

## PARTURITION

Transition from the intrauterine to the extrauterine environment involves a series of changes in cardiopulmonary function, acid-base balance, and fluid distribution. Death of neonates with normal birth weights, and lacking other clinical or necropsy signs, suggests problems during or immediately surrounding parturition. Interruption of the transition process associated with parturition may lead directly to severe morbidity. If critical functions are affected, death can occur within minutes to hours of birth, even with aggressive support. Hypoxia or anoxia are the most frequent initiating causes of morbidity and mortality of puppies and kittens at the time of birth. Subsequent detection and management of postparturient nutritional problems are often complicated by abnormalities related to the birth process.

## THE EXTERNAL ENVIRONMENT

Causes of neonatal morbidity and mortality include immature physiologic processes, inborn metabolic errors, anatomic birth defects, dystocia, infections, wasting syndromes, inadequate nutrition, trauma (including cannibalism), and environmental factors. Environmental factors, including behavioral adjustment of the dam, should not be overlooked during the process of urgent evaluation and care. These influences may cause or aggravate inadequate neonatal nutrition.

The primary activities of neonatal puppies and kittens are suckling and sleeping. Thus, stress imposed by inadequate sleep may compromise otherwise well-intentioned efforts at nutritional support. Handling must be sufficiently frequent to accomplish the former without precluding the latter. Feeding small amounts at frequent (2- to 3-hr) intervals may be necessary for very small neonates or for those that require intensive support. However, feeding larger quantities at frequent intervals may increase risk of aspiration, especially if gastric emptying is not optimal.

Pneumonia is relatively common during the neonatal period. As with many bacterial infections that affect populations of animals, high ambient temperature and high humidity seem to be accompanied by increased frequency of neonatal mortality from lower respiratory infection. Bacterial mastitis also occurs more frequently in this situation, and may represent an additional source of infectious agents for neonates.

Healthy neonatal puppies in the presence of the dam generally tolerate fluctuating ambient temperatures better than neonatal kittens in the same situation. However, their adaptive ability has limits. Hypothermia, whether disease associated or environmental, suppresses activity and suckling, and depresses gastrointestinal function. Hypothermic neonates that are fed artificially often continue to deteriorate if not given additional support. Necropsy may reveal that milk replacer has remained in the stomach of these subjects and sometimes has refluxed into the esophagus, accompanied by aspiration into the trachea.

Dams that are young and inexperienced, nervous, aged, or perhaps impatient may ignore or traumatize neonates, thereby complicating problems associated with body temperature regulation, feeding, and digestion. Some dams deliberately ignore hypothermic neonates, perhaps as a natural culling process. Stress resulting from high population concentration also may lead to inadequate nutrition because some dams become distracted or simply do not have enough milk. Environmental concerns involving dam attentiveness or health, cleanliness, temperature, humidity, quiet sufficient to allow adequate sleep, and population concentration may compromise response to nutritional support of sick neonates.

## CONTRIBUTING PHYSIOLOGIC PROBLEMS

Anoxic injury, commonly complicated by hypothermia, is the most frequent cause of morbidity and death in neonatal puppies and kittens. However, studies of adaptive responses have shown that the length of the anoxic episode does not necessarily predict outcome. Physiologic responses such as bradycardia reduce myocardial oxygen demand and consumption. There is also considerable individual variation in the degree of complicating acidosis. *Healthy* neonatal puppies maintain circulation at very low blood pressure, and can be resuscitated effectively (Swann, Christian, and Hamilton, 1954). In a study of energy regulation and anoxia, it was shown that *starved* neonates responded paradoxically to hypothermia because their lower metabolic rate allowed some preservation of glycogen reserves (Shelly, 1961). One possible interpretation of the results of these studies is that the combination of anoxia and hypothermia may allow longer survival of some subjects. In practical clinical situations, however, additional complicating factors often include hypoglycemia, dehydration, maternal malnutrition, placental insufficiency or early separation, induced hyperthermia, infection, or other problems that deplete glycogen reserves (Shelly, 1961). Adaptive responses may be compromised by excessively rapid warming of hypothermic neonates, inappropriately timed attempts to stimulate cardiovascular function, or lack of recognition of environmental problems. Fox suggested that irreversibility of neonatal cardiopulmonary failure occurs secondary to a self-reinforcing cycle of circulatory insufficiency, capillary rupture, anoxia, and hypothermia. Pressor responses in neonates are not optimally functional, and therefore anoxia, hypercapnia, and acidosis are not accompanied by vigorous cardiovascular and respiratory responses (Fox, 1965). In light of the subsequent circulatory stasis, the combination of continued hypoxia and induced hyperthermia might be lethal. Thus, attempts at rapid warming followed by early feeding may be correspondingly less effective.

Maintaining hydration is critical to survival of neonates. Total body water of neonates of most species is greater than adults, and maintenance needs for healthy and compromised neonates may be substantially higher, depending on the environment and nature of any illness. If neonates are mildly dehydrated, rehydrating and maintenance fluids may be administered orally or subcutaneously to properly warmed subjects. Oral administration is preferred, recalling that milk replacer solutions will supply some of the fluid requirement of the neonate. More severe dehydration (10 to 12%) usually must be managed intravenously (Evans, 1987) or by intraosseous techniques.

The metabolism of drugs is influenced by the degree of maturity of various organs and systems. Enzymes that metabolize drugs, renal excretory function, serum protein levels and drug binding, and permeability of the blood-brain barrier affect drug metabolism and potential toxicity in neonatal puppies and kittens (Short, 1984). The nutritional state of the subject influences these activities and their rate of maturation. Individuals with slow rates of growth and maturation during the neonatal and early lactation periods, or those affected by wasting syndromes, may remain vulnerable to adverse drug effects for periods that substantially exceed the first month of life.

## NUTRITIONAL CONSIDERATIONS

Milk consists mainly of water that contains various lipids, proteins, sugars, minerals, and minor constituents (Jenness and Sloan, 1970). In an extensive review, it was noted that important analytic differences in milk composition exist in phylogenetically different animal groups (Oftedal, 1984). For example, species that synthesize more lactose, which has osmotic effects, would be expected to produce milk having more water and less dry matter. Milk that is energy dense should be higher in fat, and lower in sugar and water. Species with very small body size logically should produce milk with greater energy density to compensate for small gastric capacity of neonates. Carnivores' milk generally has higher protein and total solids, and lower sugar. However, even considering groups that are defined by phylogeny, expected phenomena do not occur with consistency. The types of amino acids, fatty acids, and carbohydrates, as well as quantities of vitamins and minerals, may vary significantly. Milk also may vary somewhat in composition within species as a function of stage of lactation (Oftedal, 1984), and perhaps other factors. The population selected for study and methodologic decisions may influence results as well (Keen et al., 1982).

Several chemical analyses of milk have been reported. Some authors emphasize the need to consider unavoidable sampling biases when interpreting results of these studies. For example, collection methods should stimulate milk flow that occurs during natural suckling as closely as possible. Stage of lactation, time since last suckling, use of stimulants such as oxytocin, completeness of evacuation of mammary glands, stress, and method of collection may all influence analytic results (Oftedal, 1984).

Presumably, varying concentrations of nutrients in dam's milk that occur during lactation reflect changing nutritional needs of neonatal and suckling puppies and kittens. However, the composition of milk replacers necessarily represents only an average of phylogenetic knowledge; analytic studies with given methodologic biases; time-related lactational changes; and varying amino acid, carbohydrate, and fatty acid content of ingredients. Compared to bitch milk, milk replacers prepared from cow's milk and egg yolks ordinarily would be expected to contain less protein, calories, calcium, and phosphorus, as well as more cholesterol (Chandler et al., 1993). These differences, combined with differences in immunologic and perhaps undefined growth factors, may be part of the reason that healthy hand-reared offspring often do not match expected growth rates of healthy, naturally reared individuals (Chandler et al., 1993). Therefore, reduced growth rates associated with milk replacers should not be regarded as universally abnormal, provided that hydration, health, nutritional status, and weight gain remain acceptable.

The quality of response of neonates to nutritional support also depends partly on ingestion of colostrum. One study demonstrated a direct relationship between suckling and increases in IgG, IgM, and IgA in neonatal serum (Yamada, Nagai, and Matsuda, 1991). Results of this study also suggested that kittens receiving inadequate colostrum may be particularly susceptible to infection after 35 days of life. The clinical significance of these observations relative to nutritional demands is that kittens and puppies in the 3- to 4-week age group undergo important maturational changes, such as visual and sound orientation and development or extinction of some neurologic responses. At this time, intake of solid food also should be initiated, if not already established. If delay of growth and maturation at this critical time is complicated by susceptibility to infection secondary to inadequate colostrum intake, increased morbidity and mortality may occur. Therefore, the timing of weaning should be carefully assessed, including subjects receiving intensive nutritional support. In one study, colostrum ingestion by kittens was accompanied by dramatic increases in serum alkaline phosphatase and gamma-glutamyltransferase. Evaluation of these analytes may provide more rapid and less expensive assessment of colostrum intake than immunoglobulin assay (Center et al., 1991).

Hypoglycemia is a frequent complication of neonatal disorders. In a study of healthy neonatal puppies, the availability of glucose was maintained during a 24-hr fast as a result of glycogenolysis and induced gluconeogenesis. However, fatty acid production declined following 24 hr of fasting, suggesting that less oxidizable substrate was available as a consequence (Kliegman and Morton, 1987). In a related study, puppies developed lower blood glucose concentrations after fasting for 3 to 9 hr if they were also deprived of nutrition as a result of fasting the dam for 72 hr before their birth (Kliegman, 1989). These studies indicate that hypoglycemia may not always be associated with lack of feeding, at least in healthy neonatal puppies. However, neonates that experience multiple insults *in utero*, during parturition, or after birth are more likely to become hypoglycemic. These observations may provide an explanation as to why subjects in need of nutritional support do not always respond to glucose administration. Some individuals may require more thorough diagnostic evaluation and would perhaps benefit from more balanced nutritional therapy.

When evaluating results of studies of commercial or experimental milk replacer products, several factors should be considered. Prominent among these are the vigor, health, or mortality of the animals being evaluated. Reports of weight gains and outcomes equaling or exceeding natural rearing should specify how assignment to treatment groups was made, methods and frequency of artificial feeding compared to allowed natural feeding, and whether growth rates of naturally reared individuals approached normality for the breed and litter size. For example, where litters are split and assigned to different treatment groups, dam-reared offspring should perform better than breed expectation because they are fewer in number and present less demand to the dam. Detailed comparative analysis of dams' milk and experimental products should also be specified. It should be noted whether the authors considered associated clinical events, such as effects of diarrhea, when formulating their conclusions. Finally, knowledge of ages and reproductive histories of dams selected for the study will aid assessment of whether the study population was representative of actual clinical conditions.

## References and Suggested Reading

Center SA, Randolph JF, ManWarren T, et al: Effect of colostrum ingestion on gamma-glutamyltransferase and alkaline phosphatase activities in neonatal pups. Am J Vet Res 52:499, 1991.
*An evaluation of hepatic enzyme activity in neonatal pups before and after colostrum ingestion, demonstrating increases that might be used as an indicator of colostrum intake after birth.*
Chandler ML, Miller E, Olson PN, et al: Serum chemistry and lipid profiles in neonatal beagle puppies fed homemade milk replacer formulas. Cornell Vet 83:107, 1993
*A thorough experimental study comparing bitch-reared pups with siblings given homemade milk replacer containing either of two levels of calcium and phosphorus, and providing extensive physiologic evaluations of the study subjects.*
Evans RH: Rearing orphaned wild mammals. Vet Clin North Am 16:755, 1987.
*A discussion of management and clinical care of orphaned wild mammals, and techniques for rehabilitation and reintroduction to natural habitat.*
Fox MW: The pathophysiology of neonatal mortality in the dog. J Small Anim Pract 6:243, 1965.
*A review of known causes of canine neonatal mortality, with emphasis on associated physiologic considerations.*
Jenness R and Sloan RE: The composition of milks of various species: A review. Dairy Sci Abstr 32:599, 1970.
*An evaluation of quantitative differences in the milk of various animal species.*
Keen CL, Lonnerdal B, Clegg MS, et al: Developmental changes in composition of cat's milk: Trace elements, minerals, protein, carbohydrate, and fat. J Nutr 112:1763, 1982.
*An analytic study comparing the nutrient content of queen's milk at various stages of lactation.*
Kliegman RM and Morton S: The metabolic responses of the canine neonate to twenty-four hours of fasting. Metabolism 36:521, 1987.
*An experimental study examining changes in energy production and utilization in fasted, healthy neonatal pups.*
Kliegman RM: Alterations of fasting glucose and fat metabolism in intrauterine growth-retarded newborn dogs. Am J Physiol 256:E380, 1989.
*An experimental study examining the effect of temporary growth retardation during late gestation on the energy metabolism of neonatal puppies.*
Lawler DF: Wasting syndromes in young cats. *In Small Animal Reproduction and Pediatrics.* St. Louis, Ralston Purina Company, 1990, pp 52–68.
*A discussion of clinical presentation, causes, and management of wasting syndromes in young cats.*
Oftedal OT: Milk composition, milk yield, and energy output at peak lactation: A comparative review. Symp Zool Soc Lond 51:33, 1984.
*An examination of the variation of milk composition in animals by phylogenetic grouping, with a discussion of sampling and analytic problems to be considered when comparing and evaluating related studies.*
Shelly HJ: Glycogen reserves and their changes at birth and in anoxia. Br Med Bull 17:137, 1961.
*An study of glycogen reserves of neonatal animals, and the effects of anoxia.*
Short CR: Drug disposition in neonatal animals. J Am Vet Med Assoc 184:1161, 1984.
*A short review of neonatal physiologic responses that influence drug metabolism and toxicity, with emphasis on practical clinical considerations.*
Swann HG, Christian JJ, and Hamilton C: The process of anoxic death in newborn pups. Surg Gynecol Obstet 99:5, 1984.
*An experimental study of physiologic responses during respiratory and circulatory failure resulting from anoxia in neonatal pups.*
Yamada T, Nagai Y, Matsuda M: Changes in serum immunoglobulin levels in kittens after ingestion of colostrum. Am J Vet Res 52:393, 1991.
*An examination and comparison of feline sera before and after ingestion of colostrum, demonstrating immunoglobulin transfer involving IgG, IgM, and IgA.*

# PRINCIPLES OF DRUG THERAPY FOR THE PRACTICING VETERINARIAN

DAWN MERTON BOOTHE
*College Station, Texas*

## Adverse Drug Reactions

The intent of drug therapy is to induce a desired pharmacologic response for a sufficiently long period while avoiding adverse drug reactions. Two types of adverse drug reactions, referred to as types A and B, can follow drug administration. Type A drug reactions commonly reflect plasma drug concentrations that have exceeded the therapeutic range and entered the toxic range. Thus, these reactions are often manifested as an exaggerated but otherwise normal pharmacologic response to a drug. An example is hypotension caused by the negative inotropic and chronotropic effects of the nonselective β-blocker, propranolol. Type A responses may also reflect a secondary pharmacologic response (e.g., bronchoconstriction induced by propranolol) or cytotoxic effect (e.g., acetaminophen-induced methemoglobinemia). However, each of these reactions is predictable, dose dependent, and usually avoidable. Therapeutic failure due to inappropriately low plasma drug concentrations (i.e., below the effective minimum concentration) might be considered a subcategory of type A adverse reactions. In contrast to type A reactions, type B adverse drug reactions are not related to the expected pharmacologic effect of the drug. They are unpredictable, not dose dependent, and are thus difficult to avoid. An example is a drug hypersensitivity (allergy) or genetic idiosyncrasy. Differences in receptor numbers or receptor sensitivity to a drug may also result in adverse reactions among species. Often, however, the adversities are predictable and reflect use of a dose that does not take into account these receptor differences.

## Dose-Response Relationship

For most drugs, the magnitude of pharmacologic response is proportionately related to the (log of) drug concentration at the tissue (receptor) site. Because tissue samples cannot be collected easily, drug concentration at the tissue site are approximated by measuring plasma drug concentration (PDC). The *therapeutic range* provides a target for the dosing regimen. It consists of a minimum effective PDC ($C_{min}$), below which therapeutic failure is likely; and a maximum effective PDC ($C_{max}$) above which a type A adverse reaction is more likely (Fig. 1). Fixed dosing regimens are comprised of a dose (mg/kg) and interval. The dose of the regimen should result in a PDC that approximates without exceeding $C_{max}$. The relationship between the dose of drug administered and PDC achieved following

**Figure 1.** Determinants of plasma drug concentration following administration of a fixed dosing regimen act in concert. The drug must first be absorbed, most commonly from the gastrointestinal tract. Orally administered drug passes through the liver prior to reaching systemic circulation. Drug must be distributed from circulation into tissues and back again. Only free drug may distribute, thus protein binding may prevent distribution in either direction. Elimination of the drug from the body occurs through either hepatic metabolism and/or renal or biliary secretion of the drug or its metabolites. Once in the bile or urine, drugs can be recirculated either through passive resorption (kidney) or enterohepatic circulation (bile).

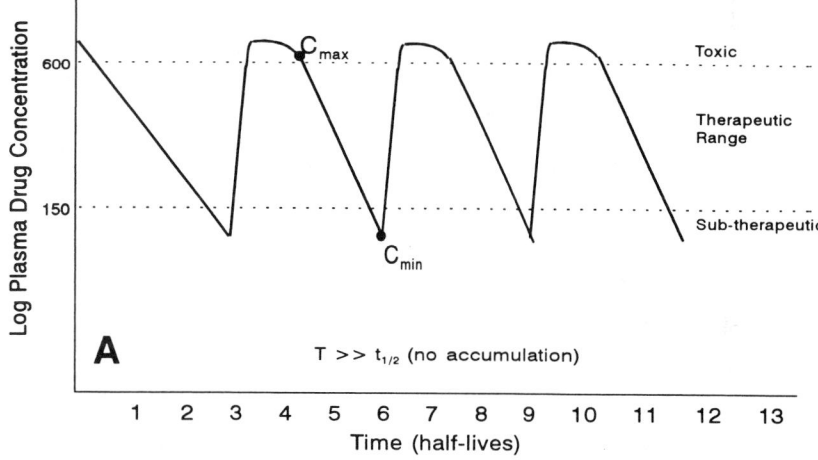

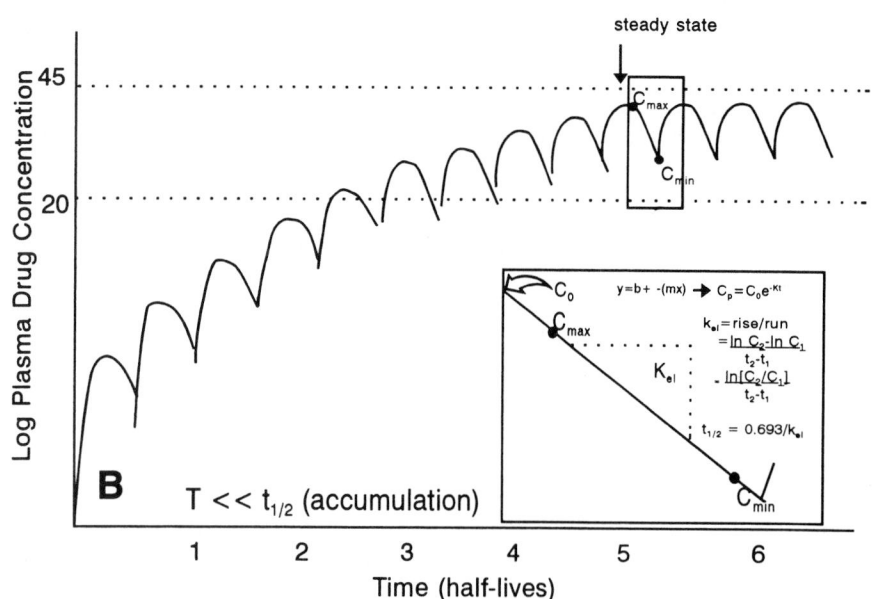

oral administration is complex. Likewise, the determinants of dosing interval or the time that can elapse before PDC drops below $C_{min}$ are also complex.

Type A adverse reactions should be anticipated when using doses that are anecdotal, rather than based on scientific, controlled studies. Yet, drug therapy may fail even if the recommended fixed dosing regimen is based on scientific data, since the populations from which inferences about the patient are based tend to be healthy and small in number. Individualization of drug therapy for the patient that is based on the principles of clinical pharmacology will increase the likelihood of therapeutic success.

## DETERMINANTS OF DRUG DISPOSITION

Following administration of a fixed dose of a drug, several drug movements act in concert to determine PDC (Fig. 2). These movements are largely dependent on passive diffusion and include: (1) absorption from the site of administration to systemic circulation, which includes the major vessels and well-perfused organs; (2) distribution of the drug from systemic circulation to tissues and back again; and (3) elimination of the drug from the body by metabolism and excretion. These movements are dynamic, occurring simultaneously, and their net effects determine PDC at any time during the dosing interval. The movements of drug through the body can be described scientifically by plotting drug concentrations measured following administration of a known dose against time on semilogarithmic paper. The PDC-versus-time curve is linearized on semilogarithmic paper if it follows *first order* kinetics: a constant fraction rather than a constant amount moves from the plasma (absorbed, distributed, or eliminated) per unit time (Fig. 3). The rate of each movement is described by the slope of the line or component comprising the movement. Each drug movement is affected by a num-

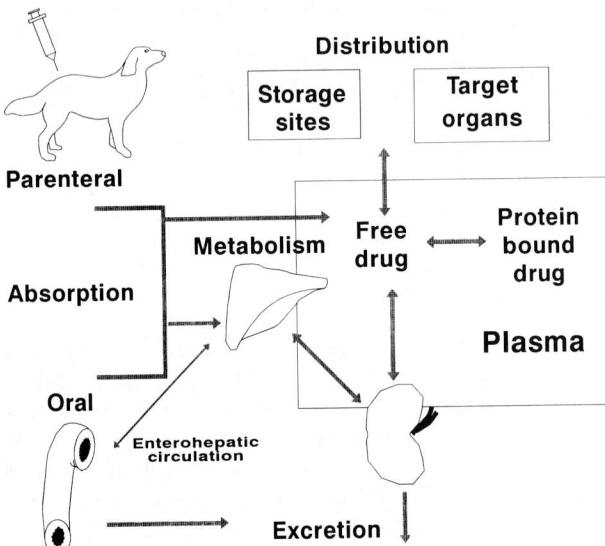

**Figure 2.** Plasma drug concentration (PDC) -versus-time curves. *A*, Following intravenous administration, a drug that fits a one-compartment open model will plot as a straight line on semilogarithmic paper. Such drugs are either very rapidly distributed to peripheral tissues or are bound to plasma proteins to the point that they can not easily leave the plasma. Both situations are lacking a distribution phase. The volume of distribution of both drugs is based on the PDC extrapolated (*dotted line*) back to time zero. *B*, Following intravenous administration, a drug characterized by distribution into peripheral tissues generally results in two components or phases when plotted on semilogarithmic paper. The PDC declines in the first phase due to both distribution into tissues and elimination. Once a distribution equilibrium has been reached, PDC declines only due to elimination. The two phases can be separated by stripping, most effectively accomplished by linear regression. The Vd for such a drug is usually determined by extrapolating (*dotted line*) the terminal or elimination phase of the PDC-versus-time curve. The second PDC-versus-time curve results from oral administration of the dose of drug. The absorption rate constant can be derived from the upswing of the curve, but only after the elimination component of the curve is stripped. Generally, the distribution phase of non-IV doses is masked by the absorptive phase. Bioavailability of the drug would be determined from the ratio of area under the curve measured from the extravascular dose and the IV dose. Note that Vd and thus Cl can only be determined following IV administration.

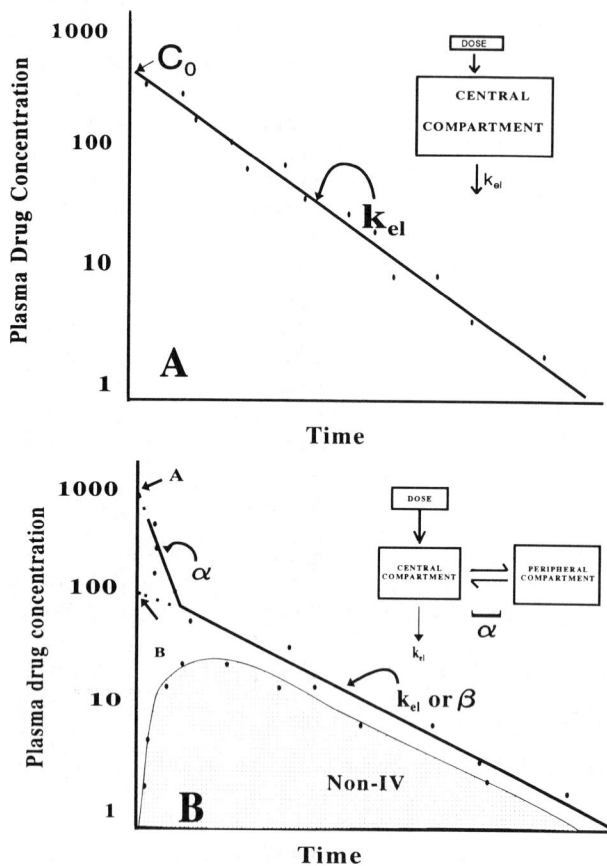

**Figure 3.** The relationship between dosing interval $T$ and drug half-life ($t_{1/2}$) determines the amount of drug accumulation. A drug whose dosing interval is longer than its half-life (*A*) is not likely to accumulate, since most of the drug will be eliminated during a dosing interval. In contrast, a drug administered at an interval shorter than its half-life (*B*) will accumulate, since most of the drug is still in the body by the next interval. Steady state occurs at 5 drug half-lives, when the amount of drug eliminated during a dosing interval equals the amount of the dose reaching systemic circulation. Drug half-life can be determined from peak ($C_{max}$) and trough ($C_{min}$) plasma drug concentrations (inset, *B*).

ber of physiologic factors, the most important being the rate and extent of passive diffusion. Lipid solubility, molecular weight, and drug $pK_a$, which are characteristics of the drug that cannot be easily altered, are important determinants of passive diffusion. The concentration gradient of nonionized drug across the site of drug movement is one of the most important determinants of passive drug diffusion. In its ionized form, a drug cannot traverse lipid membranes and thus becomes "trapped" in the environment. A drug is generally ionized when surrounded by an environmental pH that is more than 2 pH units greater than its $pK_a$ if a weak acid, or 2 pH units less than its $pK_a$ if a weak base. Orally administered aminoglycosides are weak bases ($pK_a$ 9 to 10), and thus become ionized and trapped in the acidic environment of the gastrointestinal tract. They are not absorbed. Other host determinants of passive diffusion include thickness of the membrane to be traversed (i.e., edematous compared to normal tissues); permeability of the membrane; surface area (e.g., small intestine versus stomach); and temperature.

## Absorption

Most orally administered drugs reach systemic circulation following absorption from the small intestine. The rate and extent of drug absorption in the gastrointestinal tract is dependent on a number of host factors, most of which affect passive diffusion. These include gastrointestinal pH, which favors absorption of weak acids; surface area, which favors absorption in the small intestine compared to the stomach; motility, which mixes the drug, thus increasing the concentration of diffusible drug at the site of movement; permeability and thickness of the mucosal epithelium; and intestinal blood flow, which maintains the drug concentration gradient across the mucosal epithelium. This latter factor is important only for drugs capable of rapid transfer across the epithelium.

The percentage of an administered dose that reaches systemic circulation is referred to as *bioavailability* (*F*). Bioavailability is determined by measuring the area under a PDC-versus-time curve (AUC) following non-IV administration (Fig. 3) and comparing this number with the AUC measured following IV administration of the same dose. If the AUC for both curves are equal, bioavailability is 100% (*F*=1). Bioavailability is used to predict drug efficacy following different routes of administration or administration of different formulations of the same drug. The factors that determine absorption of a drug will also determine its bioavailability. In addition, bioavailability of an orally administered drug is decreased if the drug is metabolized by intestinal epithelial cells, intestinal microbes, or the liver. Hepatic metabolism can profoundly affect PDC of an orally administered drug. Following gastrointestinal absorption, drugs enter the portal vein, and then the liver. Thus, an orally administered drug is exposed to hepatocytes prior to entering the systemic circulation. Drugs characterized by a high hepatic extraction (>70%) are al-

most completely removed from the blood by hepatocytes during the first passage of blood through the liver. As a result, the drug may not reach the systemic circulation in concentrations sufficiently high to cause a pharmacologic response. Despite good to excellent oral absorption, such drugs are characterized by poor bioavailability and must either be administered parenterally or at oral doses high enough to compensate for first-pass metabolism by the liver. Examples of drugs that undergo significant first-pass metabolism include some cardiac drugs (propranolol, diltiazem in some species, hydralazine, nitroglycerin), diazepam, and opioid analgesics. The negative effects of first pass metabolism on pharmacologic response may be reduced if the drug metabolites are also pharmacologically active (e.g., propranolol and diazepam).

Obviously, the greater the extent of absorption of a drug, the greater the anticipated pharmacologic response to the drug. However, pharmacologic response may vary even if bioavailabilities are equal. A drug whose rate of absorption is slower may be completely absorbed, but PDC may not reach the same magnitude or peak as another preparation or route. For example, while a drug may be completely absorbed (*F*=1) from slow-release preparations, a therapeutic concentration may never be reached since absorption occurs very slowly. The absorption rate constant, $k_a$, of a drug is derived from the slope of the upswing of the PDC versus time curve following non-IV drug administration (Fig. 3). Absorption half-life, derived from $k_a$, is a clinically useful parameter that indicates the time necessary for 50% of a drug to be absorbed. At 3 drug absorption half-lives, 87.5% of a drug has been absorbed.

## Distribution

Once a drug reaches the systemic circulation, it may be distributed from the central (blood) compartment to peripheral tissues, including the site of drug action. The major factors that determine drug distribution to and from tissues include a drug concentration gradient, the lipid solubility of the drug, and its ability to penetrate cell membranes, the degree to which the drug is bound to plasma or tissue proteins, ionization of the drug, and regional (organ) blood flow.

The amount of tissue to which a drug is distributed, often estimated by the *volume of distribution (Vd)* of the drug, directly influences PDC. This theoretic volume is the volume to which a drug would have to be distributed if it were present throughout the body in the same concentration as that measured in the blood. This parameter can be exemplified by adding 5 gm of dextrose to two beakers, each containing a different but unknown volume of water. Assume that the dextrose is allowed to distribute equally (reach equilibrium) in each beaker. The concentration of dextrose after equilibrium has been reached in beaker A is 5% (50 mg/ml or 5 gm/dl) while the concentration in beaker B is 2.5% (25 mg/ml or 2.5 gm/dl). The volume of water contained in beaker A (its Vd) must be 1 dl, while that in beaker B is 2 dl. The volume of distribution for a drug in an animal is measured in a similar manner: a known amount (dose) is administered intravenously to assure that all drug reaches systemic circulation (i.e., $F=1$). The maximum PDC is determined after (distribution) equilibrium has been reached but before elimination has begun. Because the PDC cannot be measured immediately at time 0, it is often based on extrapolation of the PDC curve back to time 0, and hence is referred to as $C_o$ (Figure 2). The Vd is calculated:

$$Vd = Dose/C_o$$

Note that Vd can only be determined following IV administration, since that is the only route for which 100% of the administered dose reaches systemic circulation (i.e., bioavailability is 100%). Since dose is generally in milligrams per kilogram and $C_o$ is generally milligrams per milliliter (or grams per liter), Vd is generally reported as liters per kilogram.

Plasma drug concentrations following administration of a fixed dose vary inversely with Vd. Volume of distribution differences among species and age (pediatric versus geriatric) can dramatically affect PDC following administration of a known dose. In addition, diseases requiring intensive fluid therapy or those associated with fluid retention or obesity are likely to increase Vd of many drugs (and thus decrease PDC), while dehydration or weight loss is likely to decrease Vd and thus increase PDC.

Drug binding to proteins affects several determinants of drug movement, but particularly distribution and thus Vd. Weakly acidic drugs tend to bind to albumin, while weakly basic drugs tend to bind to $\alpha_1$-glycoproteins. Many drugs are also bound to tissue proteins. Proteins are water soluble and much larger than the drug. Plasma protein-binding renders a drug more water soluble, thus facilitating its movement. However, the protein-bound drug cannot be distributed from plasma into tissues, or from tissues back to plasma. In addition, the protein-bound drugs are not pharmacologically active, cannot be excreted by the kidneys, and for many drugs, are more slowly metabolized by the liver. Drugs that are highly protein bound (>80%) may be more likely to be involved in adverse reactions early in the dosing regimen, since displacement of only a small proportion of drug from the protein (i.e., due to competition with other protein-bound drugs, or hypoalbuminemia) can increase the total amount of free, active drug. For example, displacement of only 1% of a drug that is 99% protein bound (e.g., nonsteroidal anti-inflammatories) can double the availability of pharmacologically active drug. However, clearance of these drugs is often increased (see later discussion). Therefore, PDC eventually returns to normal as a new equilibrium is reached. Displacement from plasma proteins also increases Vd, since the drug is more likely to enter tissues when freed.

Drugs highly protein bound do not distribute into tissues, but remain in systemic circulation. Because the Vd is small, such drugs may distribute to their total volume almost instantaneously. The PDC-versus-time line might appear as a single component or a one-compartment open model (open, since drug leaves the system), since the decline in PDC reflects only elimination from the body (Fig. 3). The volume of distribution of drugs that are highly (>80%) bound to plasma proteins (e.g., albumin or $\alpha$-glycoproteins) tends to be small (i.e., <0.1 L/kg), reflecting the plasma central compartment, which is about 5% of body weight. If a semipermeable membrane divides the beakers used to exemplify Vd into two compartments, distribution of the dextrose throughout each beaker would take longer. Plasma drug concentrations should not be measured until a distribution equilibrium has been reached (i.e., the amount of drug passing through either side of the membrane was equal). The membrane may not allow equal distribution of the drug. Thus both rate and extent of distribution could be altered. The same scenario exists in an animal, but because the semipermeable membrane is complex, multiple compartments may result. For example, drugs that distribute to extracellular fluid (ECF) or intracellular fluid (ICF) (i.e., total body water [TBW]) generally take longer to reach equilibrium compared to drugs that remain in the plasma compartment. The PDC-versus-time line of such drugs may appear as two components or a two-compartment open model (Fig. 2). The first component of the line declines due to both elimination and distribution; the second component declines due to elimination alone, since a distribution equilibrium has been reached (i.e., drug distributing from tissues into circulation equals drug distributing from circulation into tissues). Water-soluble drugs tend to be distributed to extracellular fluid and thus are often characterized by a Vd approximating 0.1 to 0.6 L/kg. Lipid-soluble drugs may cross cell membranes and distribute to total body water; such drugs have a larger volume of distribution ($\geq$0.6 L/kg). Drugs that are bound to tissues may take even longer to reach distribution equilibrium and the PDC-versus-time curves may be comprised of three or more components. The Vd of such drugs (e.g., digoxin in cardiac tissue and aminoglycosides in renal tubular cells) is often greater than 2 L/kg, which is greater than total body water. Although Vd is a useful parameter with which to predict the magnitude of distribution of a drug, and thus dose, it is theoretical only, and does not confirm where (i.e., ECF, ICF, TBW or binding to tissues) the drug has distributed. The ability of a drug to penetrate cell membranes is important when therapeutic success is dependent upon reaching intracellular sites. Many bacterial infections are intracellular, and antibiotic selection might be based on drugs capable of reaching intracellular sites. For example, doxycycline rather than tetracycline may be the preferred treatment for ehrlichiosis.

The rate at which a drug is distributed to tissues can be scientifically represented by the slope of the initial component or phase of the PDC-versus-time line. The elimination component of a two-compartment model must first be mathematically "stripped" or subtracted before the distribution slope or rate constant ($\alpha$) can be determined (Fig. 3). The *distribution half-life*, derived from α, measures the time necessary for 50% of distribution to be completed and offers a means for estimating the time that must elapse before drug distribution to tissues is complete. Clinically, this parameter becomes important because $C_{max}$ will not be achieved in tissues until distribution has reached an equilibrium. If PDC is being monitored in a patient, blood samples for peak drug concentrations should not be collected until distribution has reached an equilibrium. For many drugs, both absorption and distribution are complete within 1 to 2 hr after administration.

## Metabolism

The rate at which a drug is eliminated from the body is the final determinant of plasma drug concentration. Most drugs are eliminated by hepatic metabolism or renal excretion or both. Lipid-soluble drugs require conversion to a water-soluble form before they can be eliminated by the kidney. Such drugs usually are subjected to hepatic metabolism, which occurs in two phases. Phase I metabolism chemically changes the drug so that it is (usually) more water soluble and more susceptible to phase II metabolism. Phase I metabolites are usually inactive. However, they can also be equally, more or less active, or toxic compared to the parent compound. Phase II metabolism, also known as conjugation, occurs when a large water soluble molecule is chemically added to either the parent drug or a phase I metabolite. With rare exceptions, phase II metabolites are inactive. Most drug metabolites are eliminated in the urine. Factors that can affect hepatic drug metabolism include the amount and activity of drug metabolizing enzymes, and, hepatic blood flow if the drug is characterized by a high hepatic extraction (>70%). Changes in protein binding of highly bound drugs can also affect the rate of hepatic metabolism of drugs characterized by a low (<70%) hepatic extraction. The greater the binding, the slower the rate of metabolism. The rate of elimination of such drugs is inversely proportional to their degree of protein binding. Disease, drug interactions, and species differences can have a profound impact on drug metabolism and thus PDC.

## Renal Excretion

Renal excretion is the most important route of drug elimination for both parent drugs and their metabolites. The elimination of water-soluble drugs (e.g., aminoglycosides) is particularly dependent upon renal excretion. Host factors that determine renal excretion include glomerular blood flow, active tubular secretion, tubular resorption, and urinary pH. Except for urinary pH, each of the determinants of renal excretion can be influenced by renal blood flow. The kidney is also capable of metabolizing some drugs (e.g., imipenem), although this capacity is only occasionally of clinical importance.

Glomerular filtration is a passive process. Drugs enter the glomerulus by bulk flow, being excluded if too large (>60,000 daltons) or if bound to large molecules such as albumin. In contrast, active transport is very efficient and rapid, but is susceptible to competition among drugs. Separate transport proteins exist for acidic, basic, and neutral drugs. Probenicid has been used clinically to compete with and thus inhibit the renal excretion of expensive β-lactam antibiotics (e.g., imipenem), thus prolonging their therapeutic PDC. Resorption of drugs from renal tubules into peritubular capillaries slows renal excretion. The extent to which a drug is reabsorbed depends upon its concentration gradient across the tubule, its lipid solubility, and its ionization. Weakly acidic drugs are more likely to be resorbed in acidic urine but will be trapped and excreted in alkaline urine. Urine pH can be therapeutically altered such that the renal excretion rate of a drug can be modified. Note that for drugs renally excreted (e.g., amoxicillin), minimum inhibitory concentrations based on plasma drug concentrations are inappropriate guides to drug therapy of urinary bladder (but not renal) infections, since drug concentrations achievable in the urine are much higher than those in the plasma.

In contrast to renal excretion, biliary excretion is very slow and is much less clinically important. However, drugs excreted by this route are in greater contact with the intestine and its flora compared to other drugs and are thus more likely to cause adverse reactions in the gastrointestinal tract. In addition, drugs excreted by this route may enter the enterohepatic circulation. When excreted into the bile in conjugated form, drugs cannot be reabsorbed from the intestine because of the large molecule weight. However, bacterial degradation can result in free, unconjugated drug that can then be reabsorbed back into systemic circulation. Enterohepatic circulation prolongs drug half-life.

## Elimination

The combined effects of renal and biliary excretion, as well as other routes of elimination (i.e., pulmonary, sweat) irreversibly remove drug from the body. The rate of drug elimination, $k_{el}$, (also β or γ, depending on the number of linear components that comprise the PDC-versus-time curve) describes the fraction of drug in the body irreversibly eliminated per unit time (time$^{-1}$) (Fig. 3). This rate is represented by the slope of the terminal component of a PDC-versus-time curve (the initial components, if present, following IV administration, generally represent both distribution and elimination).

Since $k_{el}$ is a slope, it can be calculated from only two points on the PDC-versus-time curve, such as might be obtained from a peak and trough sample collected as part of therapeutic drug monitoring. The slope, or $k_{el}$, is simply the rise/run or $C_1$-$C_2$-$t_2$-$t_1$, where $C$ = concentration of sample 1 or 2 and $t$ = time that sample 1 and 2 were collected (Fig. 1). Since the PDC is plotted logarithmically, the actual equation becomes:

$$\frac{\ln C_1 C_2}{t_2 - t_1}$$

For example, if gentamicin concentration in blood samples collected at 2 hr and 12 hr following an IV dose were 10.5 and 2.0 µg/dl, the $k_{el}$ for gentamicin in this animal would be 0.17 hr$^{-1}$. The elimination half-life of a drug, derived from $k_{el}$ ($t_{1/2} = 0.693/k_{el}$) (Fig. 1) is one of the most useful parameters for determining an appropriate dosing interval. In the above example, the half-life of gentamicin in this patient is 4.2 hr. At 1 drug elimination half-life, 50% of the dose has been eliminated; by 5 drug half-lives, over 97% of the drug has been eliminated. For gentamicin in this patient, approximately 21 hr must elapse before most of the drug has been eliminated.

Clearance is a parameter often used to assess the elimination capacity and thus physical well being of an organ. Plasma clearance (Cl) is the volume of plasma irreversibly cleared of the drug per unit time and represents the sum total of organ clearance. Note that it differs from elimination because it is a volume per unit time, not a rate. If the drug is cleared exclusively by one organ (e.g., renal clearance of aminoglycosides or hepatic clearance of doxycycline), then plasma clearance also represents clearance of the specific organ. The volume of blood cleared per unit time by an organ is independent of PDC. The same volume of blood will be irreversibly cleared of drug by an organ regardless of how much drug is in the blood. The Cl of a drug represents the fraction ($k_{el}$) of the Vd of a drug that is cleared per unit time. Thus, if the Vd and $k_{el}$ (or half-life) of a drug are known, the Cl of the drug can also be determined:

$$Cl = Vd \cdot k_{el}$$

Note that Cl can only be determined following IV administration of a drug, since Vd can only be measured if bioavailability is known to be 100%.

## FIXED DOSING REGIMENS

A fixed dosing regimen is comprised of a dose and interval (or frequency). The dose necessary to achieve a specified target PDC (e.g., $C_{max}$ for many antimicrobials) depends on the volume of tissue that will dilute the dose administered, estimated by Vd:

$$Dose = C_{max} [Vd]$$

The dose of drug must be increased or decreased proportionately with changes in Vd in order to achieve the same target PDC. Often the dose is not intended to reach $C_{max}$, but rather $C_{min}$ (i.e., phenobarbital) or midway between the two extremes of the therapeutic range. The target concentration depends on the drug efficacy and safety.

The frequency of dosing or the dosing *interval* is determined by the time ($T_{max}$) it takes for maximum plasma drug concentrations ($C_{max}$) to drop to a point below which the desired response no longer occurs, $C_{min}$. Thus, $T_{max}$ depends on the amount of fluctuation in PDC desired during the dosing interval and the elimination rate constant ($k_{el}$). If $C_{min}$ for a drug is close

to half of $C_{max}$, then approximately 1 drug half-life (i.e., $T_{max} = t_{1/2}$) can elapse before the next dose must be administered. A more appropriate interval can be calculated using $k_{el}$ if $C_{min}$ does not approximate half of $C_{max}$:

$$T_{max} = ln \frac{C_{max} \, C_{min}}{k_{el}}$$

The longer the elimination half-life of a drug, the longer can be the interval (or $T_{max}$) between doses.

In order to effect a pharmacologic response or to maintain owner compliance, clinicians are frequently tempted to modify the recommended dosing interval. Yet decreasing a dosing interval is of no benefit for drugs whose half-life is long. For example, an 8-hr dosing interval for phenobarbital (or primidone) (drug half-life 50 to 100 hr) offers no advantage to a 12-hr interval, since very little drug will be eliminated during the 12-hr period between doses. An exception is made if induction of drug-metabolizing enzymes by phenobarbital has decreased drug half-life. In contrast, prolonging a dosing interval for convenience may be dangerous for drugs with a short half-life (e.g., many antibiotics). For drugs with short half-lives, prolonging the dosing interval from every 8 hr to every 12 hr may be accompanied by a dramatic decrease in PDC, probably below $C_{min}$. Note, however, that some drugs are effective even though PDC is essentially nondetectable. Examples include antimicrobials that exhibit a postantibiotic effect (e.g., aminoglycosides); drugs that accumulate in tissues (e.g., omeprazole); drugs whose metabolites are active (some with metabolite half-lives longer than the parent compound), and drugs that inactivate chemicals or receptors that must be resynthesized (e.g., antiprostaglandins). These drugs need not be given every half-life in order to remain effective. Half-life also determines the time that must elapse before a substantial amount of drug has been eliminated in the case of overdose. Although 5 drug half-lives must elapse before 97% of a drug is eliminated, loss of pharmacologic or toxic effect may be evident after only 1 or 2 half-lives have elapsed.

Drug half-lives can be as short as 2 min or less (e.g., epinephrine and dobutamine) or as long as several weeks (e.g., potassium bromide). Drugs with half-lives that are too short for convenient dosing are either given as constant IV infusion (e.g., lidocaine), or may be prepared as slow-release preparations (e.g., benzathine penicillin). Although the elimination half-life of the drug does not vary for these preparations, the absorption of the drug is much slower. The intent, although not always successful, is to maintain constant therapeutic concentrations by assuring continuous addition of drug into plasma. Note, however, that absorption may be so slow that therapeutic concentrations are never reached. Many oral drugs are prepared as slow or continuous-release preparations (e.g., quinidine, or theophylline). However, these preparations have been formulated for humans and the release kinetics may vary substantially in animals.

For drugs with very long half-lives, dosing intervals

are correspondingly prolonged. However, a dosing interval that is too long is also often inconvenient. In addition, for many drugs, the therapeutic range is very narrow and fluctuation of PDC during the dosing interval must be minimized. In both situations, the recommended dosing interval is often shorter than drug elimination half-life. With each subsequent dose of drug administered at an interval (T) that is much shorter than drug half-life, the majority of the previous dose is still in the body and the drug begins to accumulate with multiple doses (Fig. 1). Eventually, a steady state is reached for the drugs such that the amount of drug administered with each dose equals the amount eliminated during the dosing interval. As with drug elimination, approximately 5 drug half-lives must elapse following a fixed dosing regimen before steady state is reached. Steady state is a relevant issue only for drugs administered at a dosing interval that is shorter than the drug elimination half-life (e.g., phenobarbital, potassium bromide, digoxin).

Drugs that accumulate present clinical problems that are not encountered with drugs administered at an interval that precludes accumulation. Maximum therapeutic efficacy will not be realized until steady-state concentrations have been reached, which may be an unacceptable time for some patients (i.e., epileptic dogs receiving potassium bromide). In such situations, a loading dose (i.e., 450 mg/kg potassium bromide) can be administered. This single dose, based on Vd of a drug (0.3 L/kg for KBr) and target concentrations (usually between $C_{max}$ and $C_{min}$) is intended to achieve therapeutic concentrations with the first dose (1.5 mg/ml for KBr). The maintenance dose (e.g., 20 to 40 mg/kg for KBr) is administered after the recommended dosing interval has elapsed. A disadvantage that may preclude administration of a loading dose is that the body is not allowed to gradually adapt to the drug.

For drugs that accumulate, the contribution of a single maintenance dose of drugs to the total amount of drug in the patient's body at steady state can be considerably small, particularly if the dosing interval is much shorter than the drug elimination half-life (e.g., phenobarbital or KBr). If a pet owner fails to administer a dose of such a drug, PDC is not likely to decrease below $C_{min}$ and the patient is not likely to react adversely. A double dose can be given at the next interval. Similarly, if the patient fails to respond to the drug because PDC is inadequate, administration of a single "extra" dose is not likely to be beneficial, since PDC is not likely to change much. Rather, a (smaller) loading dose must be administered or the maintenance dose will need to be increased and a new steady state reached at 5 drug half-lives.

Therapeutic drug monitoring offers a means to guiding the dosing regimen of some drugs. Therapeutic ranges used in veterinary medicine generally have been extrapolated from human medicine (e.g., antibiotics, anticonvulsants, and cardioactive drugs). Note that a range for any particular drug reflects a mean for the population studied, and the range may not accurately

predict outcome in an individual patient. Thus, clinical response remains an important determinant of therapeutic success. Also note that the guidance provided by a therapeutic range varies with the drug. Many dosing regimens are designed such that the highest concentrations during the dosing interval come close to but do not surpass $C_{max}$. Subsequent doses are administered before enough drug has been eliminated to allow plasma drug concentrations to drop below $C_{min}$. However, for some drugs, efficacy or safety depends upon plasma drug concentrations dropping below the minimum concentration during each dosing interval. Efficacy of some antimicrobials is enhanced by the postantibiotic effect, which occurs only after plasma drug concentrations drop below the $C_{min}$. Aminoglycosides represent another variation: PDC must fall below the $C_{min}$ in order to avoid nephrotoxicity. For some drugs, the $C_{max}$ may not be the initial target, but rather represents the point at which therapeutic failure should be considered. For example, the therapeutic range suggested for phenobarbital is 15 to 45 μg/ml. Initial therapy should begin with a dose intended to reach, but not necessarily surpass, the minimum effective dose. However, if the patient continues to seizure unacceptably despite plasma drug concentrations above 15 μg/ml, an appropriate response is to increase the dose proportionately to the desired change in plasma drug concentration:

$$\text{New Dose} = \text{Old Dose} \frac{[\text{Target PDC}]}{\text{Patient PDC}}$$

The dose for this patient can be continually increased if necessary until the maximum target concentration, 45 μg/ml, is reached. Increases beyond the maximum concentration are more likely to lead to hepatotoxicity.

Plasma drug concentrations themselves are susceptible to changes by a number of factors. Factors to be taken into account when modifying recommended doses in a patient include: physiologic factors such as species and age; pathologic factors, particularly cardiac, renal, or hepatic diseases; and pharmacologic factors (i.e., drug interactions) resulting from administration of the drug alone or in combination with other drugs. Each of the factors can alter any drug movement and profoundly alter an animal's response to a drug. Therapeutic success relies on a thorough knowledge of the principles of clinical pharmacology and the drug(s) and individual patient to whom the drug is administered.

## References and Suggested Reading

Beal SL, Benet LZ, Benowitz NL, et al: *Pharmacokinetic Basis for Drug Treatment*. New York, Raven Press, 1985.
Brown SA, Budsberg SC, Calvert CA, et al: *Small Animal Medical Therapeutics*. New York, JB Lippincott Company, 1992.
Ritschel WA: *Handbook of Basic Pharmacokinetics Including Clinical Applications*. Hamilton, Drug Intelligence Publications, 1992.
Rowland M and Tozer TN: *Clinical Pharmacokinetics: Concepts and Applications*. Philadelphia, Lea & Febiger, 1989.

# UNAPPROVED USE OF DRUGS IN SMALL ANIMALS

MARK G. PAPICH
and GIGI DAVIDSON
*Raleigh, North Carolina*

When veterinarians administer Food and Drug Administration (FDA) –approved drugs in an extralabel manner to their small-animal patients, *technically they are in violation of the law*. The Federal Food, Drug, and Cosmetic Act (FFDCA), Sections 501(a)(5) and (6), 512(a)(1)(A) and (B), 512(a)(2), states that any use of a drug in an animal must be according to its approved indication (i.e., according to the dose, route, frequency, indication, and for the species listed on the label) or it is a violation, subject to prosecution and penalty. By contrast, drug labels on human drugs have wide dose ranges and physicians are allowed to administer them for unapproved uses and at unapproved dosages without violation of the law. Veterinarians who treat small animals have not been prosecuted under the FFDCA because the FDA's Center for Veterinary Medicine (FDA-CVM) has used discretion in taking regulatory action. The FFDCA was intended primarily to protect public health by ensuring that foods of animal origin would be safe for human consumption. When it was amended in 1968, the lawmakers did not anticipate, or consider, the tremendous scientific advances that were to occur in companion animal practice. Veterinarians take an oath to do whatever is in their power to ensure animal health and relieve suffering. In order to fulfill the responsibilities of that oath, veterinarians often must administer veterinary drugs or human-labeled drugs to patients in a manner for which the drug is not approved. There is an obvious conflict between the ethics and activities of modern veterinary practice and the law. How can veterinarians responsibly care for the health of their patients and still legally practice veterinary medicine?

## WHAT CONSTITUTES EXTRALABEL DRUG USE?

The FDA-CVM has clearly stated that extralabel drug use is the actual or intended use of a new animal drug in a manner that is not in accordance with the drug labeling. This includes, but is not limited to, use in species or for indications not listed in the labeling, use at dosage levels higher than those stated in the labeling, and (for food-producing animals) failure to observe the stated withdrawal time (*FDA Compliance Guide*, 1992a).

## What is the Extent of Extralabel Drug Use?

Human-labeled drugs are administered for the treatment of many diseases in small animals. At the NCSU Veterinary Teaching Hospital Pharmacy, over 60% of the drugs dispensed for small-animal use are human-labeled drugs. In a survey of three large teaching institutions, 52% of the drug inventory was human-labeled drugs; the rest of the drugs were veterinary drugs that often were used for another species or for another claim on the label (Welser, 1993).

## Why is Extralabel Drug Use Necessary?

Extralabel drug use is common because the labels for approved drugs are so restrictive that one must often prescribe the drug at doses, or for indications, that are not on the label in order to treat the variety of conditions that are encountered in veterinary medicine. Drug labels for veterinary drugs usually list a specific dose, dosage interval, and duration of therapy, but principles of clinical pharmacology (see "Principles of Drug Therapy for the Practicing Veterinarian," this volume, p 40) recognize that each animal should be treated as an individual, unique patient. There is no "average patient" and therefore no single dosage that applies to each patient; dosages often must deviate from what is approved. Human-labeled drugs are used for many conditions in small-animal medicine simply because there are not enough veterinary-labeled drugs available to treat all of the medical conditions that occur in animals. The drug approval process is lengthy and expensive. There is not a sufficient incentive for a drug manufacturer to sponsor drugs to treat all of the specific diseases for which dogs and cats are evaluated by veterinarians.

## The FDA Compliance Policy Guide

The FFDCA was amended in 1968 to restrict the use of animal drugs to the species and usages specified on the label. The FDA-CVM recognized that the practice of veterinary medicine was so diverse that there could not possibly be broad enough dose ranges, or indications on the label, to accommodate all aspects of veterinary practice (The FDA-CVM does not write the laws, Congress does!). Until 1984, the FDA-CVM adopted a policy that veterinarians could use any drug according to their own discretion that they could legally obtain, provided that the veterinarian was responsible for any adverse effects caused by the drug and as long as use of the drug did not cause violative residues in food-producing animals (Crawford, 1993). "Legally obtained" means that the drug could be an FDA-approved animal drug for another species, or it may be a human-labeled FDA-approved drug. A drug is not legally obtained if it is not approved in the United States and is imported (smuggled) from another country.

Because there was widespread use of unapproved drugs in food-producing animals without methods available to detect the drug residues, the FDA-CVM issued a Compliance Policy Guide (CPG) in 1984. The CPG allowed for regulatory discretion in extralabel drug use in animals and guided practitioners administering drugs to food-producing animals. Before the FDA-CVM would pursue regulatory action under this policy, the severity of the disease and whether there were any available drugs labeled for the specific use would be taken into consideration. However, the highest priority was given to investigating cases of extralabel drug use that resulted in residues in food-producing animals.

### REVISIONS TO THE COMPLIANCE POLICY GUIDE

Since 1984 there have been four revisions of the CPG, with the most recent in July, 1992. The current CPG (Table 1) states that veterinarians may consider the extralabel use of drugs in non–food-producing animals without fear of enforcement action. Therefore, as far as companion animals are concerned, the current CPG reaffirms the privilege of veterinarians to use any drug they can legally obtain; however, extralabel drug use in food-producing animals remains more restrictive. The absence of FDA-CVM regulatory action does not imply that veterinarians can recklessly use extralabel drugs in small animals. When prescribing drugs in an extralabel manner, (1) veterinarians are responsible for adverse effects caused by the drug, (2) veterinarians should ensure that a valid veterinarian-client-patient relationship (VCPR) exists (Table 2), (3) there must be scientific evidence that the drug will be safe and effective, and (4) the drug should be properly labeled (Table 3). The American Veterinary Medical Association (AVMA) also has published guidelines for dispensing prescription drugs (AVMA, 1994).

**Table 1.** *FDA Compliance Policy Guide 7125.06: Use of Extralabel Drugs*

"Under usual circumstances veterinary practitioners may consider the extralabel use of drug products in non–food-producing animal practice without being subject to FDA enforcement actions."

**Table 2.** *Valid Veterinarian-Client-Patient Relationship (VCPR)*

1. The veterinarian has assumed the responsibility for making clinical judgments regarding the health of the animal(s) and the need for medical treatment, and the client has agreed to follow the veterinarian's instructions.
2. The veterinarian has sufficient knowledge of the animal(s) to initiate at least a general or preliminary diagnosis of the medical condition of the animal(s). This means that the veterinarian has recently seen and is personally acquainted with the keeping and care of the animal(s) by virtue of an examination of the animal(s) or by medically appropriate and timely visits to the premises where the animal(s) are kept.
3. The veterinarian is readily available for follow-up evaluation in the event of adverse reactions or failure of the treatment regimen.

### The Future of Extralabel Drug Use

#### THE AVMA LEGISLATIVE INITIATIVE

The current FDA-CVM's CPG states that extralabel drug use in companion animal practice will *not* be subject to prosecution. However, the CPG is not law; it is merely a guideline for federal investigators. Technically, extralabel drug use may still constitute a violation of the FFDCA. Veterinarians have felt uneasy about conducting their veterinary practice in a manner that stretches the legal boundaries of drug use, and they are aware that the CPG can be rescinded at any time. This dilemma has prompted the AVMA to support a legislative initiative that would amend the FFDCA. This amendment will allow veterinarians to legally prescribe extralabel drugs and would require the FDA-CVM to issue regulations defining the circumstances under which this use could be allowed. The amendment to the current act would not differ substantially from the current CPG. This legislation will not allow extralabel drug use by nonveterinarians. Opponents of the legislation suggest that it would undermine the drug approval process by removing the incentive to animal drug manufacturers to seek additional drug approvals (Zeller, 1993).

### INTERPRETATION OF FDA-APPROVED DRUG RECOMMENDATIONS

Most of the information currently available on the label of a drug is listed to inform veterinarians and to prevent unapproved use. Drug labels typically contain a list of the active ingredients, the drug vehicle (if the

**Table 3.** *Required Information on a Drug Label*

Name, address, and phone number of veterinarian
Identity of patient
Date
List of active ingredient(s)
Name of drug and quantity of drug dispensed
Directions for use
Dose, frequency, and duration of administration
Precautionary statements

drug is a liquid), and ingredients added as preservatives and buffers. The drug label also lists the name and address of the manufacturer, the expiration date, instructions for use, and withdrawal times for drugs approved for food-producing animals.

## Instructions for Use

The instructions for use and dosages are limited to those that the sponsor of the drug (the manufacturer) has listed on the application and have been approved by the FDA-CVM. The approved indications and dosages are usually narrow and inflexible. Veterinarians often are unsure of the rationale for specific limitations on doses and duration for treatment. For example, a label may state that a drug must be administered at a particular dose (e.g., 2.2 mg/kg) for a duration that is not to exceed a specified time limit (e.g., 10 days). There are many examples of conditions for which veterinarians may wish to exceed the dose or duration of therapy beyond that specified on the label. What then, is the harm in reasonable deviations from the approved labeling requirements? In most cases, very little. The label is specific because of the conditions under which the toxicology tests or clinical trials were conducted for the new-drug application. A drug that lists 10 days as the duration of therapy may be safe if administered for longer than 10 days, but specific trials to establish this safety may not have been conducted or submitted with the new-drug application. A label may list a dose of 2.2 mg/kg, but may be safe if used at a slightly higher dose. However, usually there is no information on the label to guide veterinarians who, in their best judgment, have decided that a higher dose may be necessary in a particular patient. The drug label also may list that the safety of a drug in pregnant animals has not been established. It is possible that the drug is safe during pregnancy, but specific studies may not have been conducted to establish this safety in the target species.

This discussion is not intended to imply that limits on dosages, duration of therapy, and the conditions of therapy listed on a drug label are trivial and can be exceeded without consideration. When there is a question regarding the safety of a drug in a patient, a reputable authority or published data should be consulted before exceeding the label recommendations.

## Expiration Date

Some veterinarians administer drugs to their patients after the drug expiration date, or after the shelf life has been exceeded for a drug reconstituted from its dry form to a solution. The shelf life, or the expiration date, usually is the time for a drug to lose 10% of its potency, after which loss of potency is not necessarily linear. Administering a solution that has exceeded its recommended shelf life can be dangerous. The patient's health is at risk because it may not receive an effective drug, or an expired drug may contain breakdown products or insoluble precipitates in an intravenous solution that are harmful. The stability of drugs under the storage conditions listed on the label are very specific and should be taken seriously. Although it is tempting for veterinarians to continue to administer drugs beyond the expiration date, this practice should be discouraged. Expired drugs are considered "adulterated" by the FFDCA and dispensing such drugs is a misdemeanor. The package insert, or a reliable reference (*USP*, 1994), contains information on the proper storage and shelf life of most drugs. If veterinarians have questions about the safety or potency of particular products beyond their expiration dates, the manufacturer of the drug or a pharmacist should be consulted.

## USE OF HUMAN-LABELED DRUGS IN ANIMALS

The use of human-labeled drugs in companion animals is extremely common. In fact, this group of drugs may comprise the majority of drugs administered to dogs and cats on a regular basis. While this practice can be regarded as extralabel drug use, the CVM covers this use in a separate guideline.

### To What Extent are Human-Labeled Drugs Allowed?

The FDA-CVM recognizes that there are no approved animal drugs for many diseases encountered in small animal practice. Effective therapy of conditions such as cancer, diabetes, cardiovascular disease, poisonings, systemic mycoses, and many bacterial infections require use of human-labeled drugs. Many of the commonly used analgesics and anesthetics are not labeled for animal use. There is a separate CPG (FDA Compliance Guide, CPG 7125.35, 1992) that deals with human-labeled drugs distributed and used in animals (Table 4). It is not the intent of the FDA-CVM to prohibit veterinarians from administering valuable drugs to their patients when there are no available alternatives. The present policy allows regulatory discretion for these uses. The CPG states that the FDA-CVM will refrain in *ordinary circumstances* from enforcement actions when human drugs are used or dispensed by veterinarians in treating non–food-producing animals. In rare circumstances, regulatory action will be considered when the health of the treated animals is harmed.

The primary intent of the current CPG is to elimi-

**Table 4.** *FDA Compliance Policy Guide 7125.35: Use of Human-Labeled Drugs in Small Animals*

"Under usual circumstances, veterinary practitioners may consider the use of human-labeled drug products in non–food-producing animal practice without the threat of FDA enforcement actions. In rare circumstances, for example, when the health of the treated animals is harmed, regulatory attention by FDA would be considered or, preferably, referred to the State veterinary licensing authority for investigation."

nate the promotion of human-labeled drugs for veterinary use by manufacturers, distributors, pharmacies, and veterinarians. The FDA-CVM prohibits the advertising or promotion (either oral or written) of human-labeled drugs for veterinary use because such a practice subverts the drug-approval process by creating disincentives for drug manufacturers to seek approval for animal drugs. A high priority will be placed on taking regulatory action against manufacturers that promote human-labeled drugs when there already is a veterinary-labeled equivalent. To ensure that there is no promotion of these drugs, the FDA-CVM insists that the distribution and dispensing of human-labeled drugs by veterinarians be practitioner driven (Teske, 1993). The FDA-CVM will not interfere with the ordinary distribution of human-labeled drugs by manufacturers directly to veterinarians.

The simple listing of human-labeled drug products in price sheets and catalogues distributed to veterinarians is acceptable. When veterinarians dispense human-labeled drugs to their clients, they must adhere to the same requirements for drug labeling on the container as for extralabel drugs (Table 2). The FDA-CVM does not consider communication about a drug as promotional marketing or advertising when human-labeled drugs are the subject of an article in a veterinary scientific journal. The FDA-CVM recognizes that this is an important source of communication. The FDA-CVM will not take action against the communication of how and when to use various human-labeled drugs in companion animals when such communication occurs in a textbook, review article, or continuing education seminar.

### DISPENSING OF HUMAN-LABELED DRUGS BY RETAIL PHARMACISTS

The FDA-CVM will allow retail pharmacists to dispense human-labeled drugs according to a veterinarian's prescription, provided the dispensing pharmacist labels the drugs with the name, address, and telephone number of the dispenser, name and quantity of the drug, name of the veterinarian, directions for use, and any precautions. The guidelines for prescribing these drugs are listed in the *AVMA Directory* (1994).

### SOURCES OF INFORMATION ON HUMAN-LABELED DRUGS

Since no promotion or advertising of human-labeled drugs is allowed, it is the responsibility of practicing veterinarians to keep informed of the availability of drugs, their potential clinical uses, their pharmacology, and toxicology. This presents a challenge to veterinary practitioners. In human medicine, for most drugs prescribed, there is advertising in popular journals and widespread dissemination of promotional material by the drug distributors. There is usually readily available sources of information regarding the therapeutic uses, appropriate dosages, and possible adverse effects on the package insert, or sources such as the *Physician's Desk Reference (PDR)*. When these drugs are admin-istered to dogs and cats, human prescribing information is not applicable and reliable information is difficult to obtain.

It is the veterinarian's responsibility to keep well informed. The drug manufacturer has no responsibility for informing veterinarians of the therapeutic use and potential toxicoses for a human-labeled drug. Veterinarians should consult well-referenced, or reputable textbooks, or refereed scientific journals for information about the safe and effective use of off-label or human-labeled drugs. The *USP-DI* is an excellent, authoritative source of information on the labeled and extralabel uses of drugs. Veterinary monographs are gradually being added to the *USP-DI* so that by 1995 most of the veterinary and human-labeled drugs used in practice will be included in a veterinary volume of the *USP*.

## NON–FDA-APPROVED DRUGS

The current CPG pertains only to FDA-approved drugs. Veterinarians are prohibited from using drugs that are not approved by the FDA. Therefore, it is technically illegal for veterinarians to purchase bulk drugs from a chemical supply company and formulate their own unapproved drugs. It also is illegal for veterinarians to import drugs from another country without approval by the FDA.

### How Can Non–FDA-Approved Drugs be Used Legally?

If there are conditions for which veterinarians must obtain unapproved drugs from another country or purchase raw chemicals from a domestic supply house, the FDA may allow veterinarians to purchase limited quantities for clinical use. The federal regulations (CFR 511.1) are very specific with respect to the conditions that must be met to obtain an unapproved drug.

### INVESTIGATIONAL NEW ANIMAL DRUG APPLICATION (INADA)

An INADA must be filed with the CVM prior to importing a drug from another country as well as purchasing bulk chemicals domestically. Obtaining an INADA can be a lengthy process. The veterinarian must serve as the sponsor to request an investigational exemption. The CVM requires that veterinarians inform them of the source of the drugs and all intermediaries involved in delivery of an investigational drug. The sponsor must provide the amount and identity of the drug, proposed use, species intended for use, name and address of the foreign or domestic manufacturer, origin and destination of the shipment, and the approximate date of shipment. When the drug is obtained, each container of the drug must be labeled: "Caution. Contains a new animal drug for use only in investigational animals in clinical trials. Not for use in humans. Edible products of investigational animals are not to be used for food unless authorization has been granted by the U.S. Food and Drug Administration or by U.S. Department of Agriculture." Once the investigational drug is obtained, the sponsor must not commercially distribute the drug. The conditions under which the investigational exemption is made limits use of the drug only to the veterinary practice indicated on the sponsor's application. Additional information on obtaining a compassionate investigational exemption may be obtained from the FDA-CVM.

Veterinarians using an investigational drug must keep accurate records for 2 years on each patient in which the drug is used, including: species, sex, age, weight, dose, concomitant therapy, history, diagnosis, treatment results, and adverse effects. All of the drug that has been shipped to the sponsor must be accounted for accurately.

## VETERINARY DRUG COMPOUNDING

There is no precise definition (especially a legal one) of drug compounding. Many veterinarians have regarded compounding as just another form of extralabel drug use and have compounded without regard for their professional responsibility. In a broad definition, drug compounding is any alteration of the drug from its original packaged form. There are many examples of drug compounding in a small-animal veterinary practice. It may be the altering of the dosage form so that it may be administered to a small animal more easily than the original drug formulation (e.g., crushing a tablet and mixing it with a liquid in order to produce an oral solution), admixing two anesthetics in a syringe (e.g., admixing ketamine plus diazepam in a syringe for injection to a cat), or making a solution from a powder (e.g., preparing potassium bromide oral solution to treat an epileptic patient).

### To What Extent is Drug Compounding Allowed by the FDA?

The current regulations do not allow for drug compounding. However, it is recognized that compounding is a small but essential part of veterinary practice because drug formulations are not available for all of the conditions veterinarians treat. The lack of a current CPG by the FDA-CVM has left veterinarians in a dilemma as to what is acceptable. At the time of this writing, the FDA-CVM is in the process of writing a CPG that will outline the responsibilities of veterinarians with regard to drug compounding. It is expected that some drug compounding will be allowed by veterinarians within the confines of their own veterinary practice. A limited amount of compounding may be acceptable: (1) when an FDA-approved drug does not exist; (2) when the available dosage form is inappropriate because of the patient's size, demeanor, physiology, or in a case in which it is necessary to protect the patient or hospital personnel safety; (3) when there

are no clinically effective FDA-approved dosage forms available for specifically diagnosed entities; and (4) when it can minimize side effects or increase efficacy. Veterinarians should be knowledgeable of the compatibilities and stability of compounded formulations. They should keep good records of all compounded formulations. In some instances the complexity of compounding will exceed the veterinarian's knowledge or skills. In these cases veterinarians are advised to seek the advice and assistance of a reputable pharmacist. Veterinarians cannot advertise or promote for distribution drug formulations that they have compounded in their practice. They must only produce enough for short-term anticipated needs. Because of the drug incompatibilities that are possible, admixing more than one active ingredient in the same container or significantly altering the drug's vehicle or inactive ingredients in a solution is risky unless veterinarians have prior knowledge that the admixed ingredients are compatible and one ingredient does not affect the stability of the other drug. The FDA has indicated that regulatory discretion will be used in investigating admixtures of anesthetic agents.

## SUMMARY

### Veterinarian's Responsibilities

Veterinarians will not ordinarily be subject to prosecution when prescribing animal drugs in an extralabel manner, or human-labeled drugs to companion animals. Veterinarians should follow the guidelines listed by the AVMA (AVMA, 1994) when prescribing drugs. Veterinarians should especially ensure that there is a valid VCPR (Table 1), and that drugs that are dispensed to clients contain specific labeling requirements (Table 2).

### Veterinarian's Liabilities

The fact that the FDA-CVM allows veterinarians to prescribe extralabel drugs and human-labeled drugs for use in small animals does not excuse veterinarians from their responsibilities. If adverse reactions occur in a patient, the veterinarian is responsible. If an adverse reaction occurs in a patient in which a veterinarian has used a drug according to his or her best judgment and knowledge, what is the protection to avoid an unfair disciplinary or civil action? The drug manufacturer or the FDA-CVM is not obligated to come to the aid of a veterinarian in these instances. As long as extra-label use and compounding remain illegal, insurance companies can refuse to cover claims that are the result of extralabel drug use. One should justify the unapproved use of drugs with reputable references and documentation. A signed waiver may be recommended for drugs that carry an unusually high risk of adverse effects, but a waiver form is not needed each time a veterinarian administers an unapproved drug to a patient. Whenever possible, veterinarians should discuss use of unapproved drugs with their clients before therapy is instituted.

## References and Suggested Reading

American Veterinary Medical Association: Guidelines for supervising use and distribution of veterinary prescription drugs. *1994 AVMA Directory.* Schaumburg, IL, 1994, pp 90–92.

Crawford LM: History of extra-label use of animal drugs. J Am Vet Med Assoc 202:1618, 1993.

Food and Drug Administration: Compliance Policy Guide 7125.06, Chapter 25—Veterinary Drugs, July 20, 1992.

Food and Drug Administration: Compliance Policy Guide 7125.35, Chapter 25—Veterinary Drugs, July 20, 1992.

Teske RH: Current FDA policy on use of human-labeled drugs in animals. J Am Vet Med Assoc 202:1632, 1993.

United States Pharmacopeial Convention Inc: *Drug Information for the Health Care Provider,* volume I. Rockville, MD, United States Pharmacopeial Convention Inc, 1994.

Welser JR: Extra-label drug use: Pharmaceutical industry view. J Am Vet Med Assoc 202:1635, 1993.

Zeller M: FDA responsibilities in regulation of drugs for use in animals: Congressional perspective. J Am Vet Med Assoc 202:1609, 1993.

# MEDICAL IMPLICATIONS OF FASTING AND STARVATION

TIMOTHY A. ALLEN
*and* PHILIP W. TOLL

*Topeka, Kansas*

## PHYSIOLOGY

### Overview

Fasting is abstinence from food. Although fasting implies self-denial or willful denial of appetite, it is commonly used in veterinary medicine in circumstances where food is withheld from animals. In general usage, starvation is defined as the state of suffering or death resulting from extreme or prolonged lack of food. For the purposes of this review, starvation is fasting of greater than 4 or 5 days' duration.

In clinical practice, animals frequently are anorectic, or are deprived of food for variable periods to facilitate diagnosis or treatment. Sadly, owner neglect and animal abuse can also be causes of fasting and starvation. The purpose of this review is to discuss changes associated with food deprivation at the enzymatic, organ, and whole-animal levels in the postabsorptive, fasted, and starved states. The clinical relevancy of these changes will also be discussed.

The major fuels are carbohydrate, fats, and proteins. Proteins are not primarily fuel reservoirs. Each protein molecule serves a nonfuel function: as an enzyme, or a contractile or structural protein. Fuel components are obtained from the diet and stored in body depots. Whenever there is a shift in the quantity or type of fuel, the body adapts to more efficiently utilize available fuels. Physiologic and biochemical adaptations in fat, carbohydrate, and protein metabolism occur in absorptive, postabsorptive, fasted, and starved states. These adaptations are best understood from the perspective of nutrient balance.

After a meal, ingested fuel is used to satisfy the immediate energy needs of the body and excess fuel is stored in body depots. Animals go through a period of food deprivation each day while they sleep. Concentrations of enzymes rise and fall during the day in response to diurnal variation in food consumption. During fasting, stored fuels are used to provide sufficient energy to survive to the next meal. During starvation, changes occur in fuel utilization that permit survival for prolonged periods.

### Nutrient Balance

All tissues are involved in nutrient balance. All cells consume energy from carbohydrate, fat and, to a small extent, protein. The gastrointestinal tract is responsible for nutrient intake and some excretion. The primary role of the kidney is excretion of minerals, nitrogen, and water. Water loss also occurs in the respiratory tract. The liver processes and stores nutrients. Nervous and endocrine tissues are involved with control of nutrient balance. Blood is the transport medium for both nutrients and hormonal control signals. Muscle is the main consumer of energy.

In the adult animal under homeostatic conditions, nutrient balance is zero; intake equals use and excretion and mass is conserved. Positive nutrient balance occurs immediately following meals and other select circumstances. Growth requires positive balance of all nutrients. Protein synthesis requires positive nitrogen and energy balance. Excess dietary energy results in energy storage in adipose tissue. Excess nitrogen (protein) intake results in increased nitrogen excretion, not storage. Positive water balance results in edema and fluid retention. Negative nutrient balance occurs when intake is less than obligatory use and excretion.

Nutrient intake includes the complex mixture of nutrients that are digested and absorbed in the gastrointestinal tract. The nutrients of primary interest are water, carbohydrate, protein minerals, and vitamins. This discussion will focus on those nutrients contributing to the energy budget. Energy used by the body is stored in chemical bonds of carbon-containing molecules (carbohydrate, fat and, to a small degree, protein). Once these nutrients are absorbed and reach the blood they are transported to specific tissues for use or storage. The energy required to form adenosine triphosphate (ATP), the common fuel for all cells, comes from the energy released during the breakdown of hydrocarbon molecules. The tricarboxylic acid (TCA) cycle is the primary means of producing ATP from hydrocarbons (Fig. 1). Breakdown products of glucose, fatty acids, and amino acids are all substrates for the TCA cycle, where they are oxidized to carbon dioxide and water. Glucose enters this pathway as pyruvate, the product of glycolysis. Fatty acids enter as acetyl-CoA, following $\beta$-oxidation. Both glycolysis and $\beta$-oxidation are energy-yielding processes. Amino acids may enter the TCA cycle at various points following deamination, an energy-using process.

Different tissues have different abilities to utilize these substrates. All cells can utilize glucose, either through the glycolytic and TCA pathways or through glycolysis alone. Many cells lack the ability to use fatty acids (e.g., nervous tissue and red blood cells), and are therefore dependent on glucose as an energy substrate. Dietary energy in excess of that needed for immediate use is stored instead of being excreted. Only very small amounts of hydrocarbons are excreted in the urine as bicarbonate, lactate, pyruvate, or ketones.

## METABOLIC PRIORITIES

Energy metabolism is regulated so that when dietary energy is plentiful, excess energy-containing compounds are directed toward storage. When energy is in short supply, the needs of vital organs, like the brain and kidney, are met first. Maintenance of blood glucose is the next metabolic priority, and provides a readily available supply of an energy substrate that can be used by any tissue. Blood glucose is the substrate pool that is most tightly regulated. Physical activity is a large consumer of energy and is the next highest priority. Maintenance of body condition (i.e., maintenance of protein and fat stores) is the lowest metabolic priority.

## DAILY NUTRIENT BALANCE

ABSORPTIVE PHASE. When food enters the gastrointestinal tract, it is digested by acid in the stomach and a variety of enzymes in the intestine to smaller molecules that can be absorbed and carried to specific organs by the blood stream. Smaller molecules entering the gastrointestinal tract, like water, minerals, and simple sugars, can be absorbed without further processing.

Nutrients in the gastrointestinal tract and in blood cause hormonal responses needed for digestion, transport, use, or storage. Once food enters the stomach, the antral portion of the mucosa secretes gastrin. Food stimulates the gastrin mechanism in two ways. The physical presence of food distends the stomach and causes gastrin release. Certain substances, called secretagogues, such as partially digested proteins, also cause gastrin release. Both food and secretagogues elicit gastrin release by means of a local nerve reflex. Food in the stomach causes local reflexes in the intrinsic nerve plexus of the stomach and vasovagal reflexes. Both local and vasovagal reflexes cause parasympathetic stimulation of the gastric glands and contribute to the secretion produced by the gastrin mechanism. Cholecystokinin is secreted primarily by the jejunal mucosa in response to the presence of acid, fat, and protein breakdown products in the intestines. Cholecystokinin markedly increases the contractility of the gallbladder, thus increasing bile secretion into the small intestine. After chyme enters the small intestine, pancreatic secretion becomes copious, primarily in response to the hormone secretin. Cholecystokinin also greatly increases secretion of pancreatic enzymes. Cholecystokinin is released in response to food in the upper small intestine. Protein breakdown products, proteases and

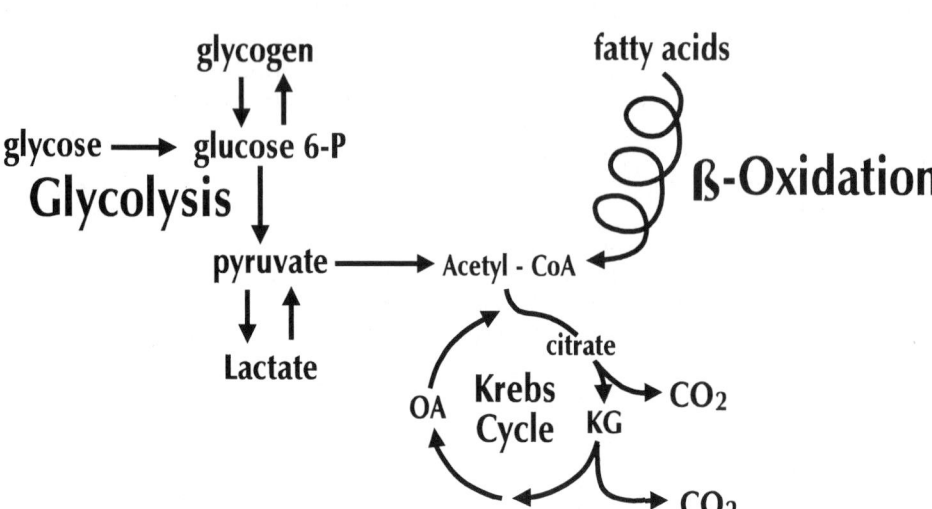

**Figure 1.** The relationship of the three major catabolic pathways. Abbreviations: OA = oxaloacetic acid, KG = α-ketoglutarate.

peptones, fat and, to a lesser degree, acid stimulate cholecystokinin release.

Dietary carbohydrate, fat, and protein provide carbon skeletons to meet immediate energy needs. Excess carbon skeletons are transported to storage sites. Carbohydrates that can be used by monogastric animals are monosaccharides (glucose, fructose, and galactose) and polymers of monosaccharides (disaccharides and starch). Monosaccharides are absorbed intact by the intestinal epithelium. Larger carbohydrate molecules must be cleaved into monosaccharides to be absorbed. Disaccharides are cleaved by specific enzymes. For example, lactase cleaves lactose into glucose and galactose. Starch is broken down into oligo- and disaccharides by salivary and pancreatic amylase. The conversion to monosaccharides is completed by dextrinases, α-glucosidases, and disaccharidases found on the brush border of intestinal epithelial cells. Monosaccharides are transported by the blood to target organs where they are used or stored. Glucose reaching the liver is oxidized to meet the energy needs of the liver, stored as glycogen, or synthesized into fatty acids and glycerol that combine to form triglycerides. Triglycerides are packaged as very-low-density lipoproteins (VLDLs) and exported to adipose cells to be stored for future use. Glucose is used by all cells to meet their immediate energy needs. Most cells produce ATP from glucose through the TCA cycle forming carbon dioxide and water. Red blood cells use glycolysis to produce ATP, resulting in release of pyruvate and lactate to the blood. Under the action of insulin, glucose enters muscle cells, where it is oxidized for energy or as glycogen for future use by muscle. Insulin also stimulates use of glucose by adipose tissue to meet its energy needs or for synthesis of the glycerol moiety of triglyceride.

Dietary fat, in the form of triglycerides, is emulsified by bile salts and digested into glycerol and free fatty acids by pancreatic lipase. These molecules are packaged into micelles and absorbed into the intestinal epithelium, where they are synthesized back into triglycerides and repackaged into chylomicrons. Chylomicrons are transported via the lymph to the blood and on to the target organs for use or storage. Lipoproteins, both chylomicrons from the intestine and VLDLs produced from glucose in the liver, are acted upon by lipoprotein lipase found on the capillary walls of various tissues. The triglycerides in the chylomicrons and VLDLs are converted to fatty acids and glycerol. The fatty acids are taken up by adipose tissue, converted to triglycerides, and stored.

Digestion of protein begins in the stomach with pepsin, and continues with the action of the pancreatic enzymes trypsin, chymotrypsin, elastase, and carboxypeptidases, which are active in the intestine. The process is completed by the action of amino-, di-, and tripeptidases produced by epithelial cells. The resultant amino acids are absorbed by epithelial cells, where some are metabolized but most are released into the blood. Amino acids are used by most cells for protein synthesis. Protein turnover is constant, but balance is zero if adult animals are in nutrient balance. Amino acids are important structural components of cells, especially muscle. Proteins are also crucial building blocks for functional molecules like hormones, enzymes, heme, and deoxyribonucleic acid (DNA). In some tissues, such as muscle, amino acids can be oxidized for energy. In the absorptive state, the energy contribution from oxidation of amino acids is minor.

POSTABSORPTIVE PHASE. The postabsorptive phase is characterized by a shift from storage, and immediate use of nutrients, as they are absorbed to mobilization and use of stores. As blood glucose concentration declines after a meal, insulin decreases. Glucagon increases to mobilize stored energy (Table 1). The liver responds first with glycogenolysis followed by gluconeogenesis. Glycogenolysis begins a few hours after a meal in response to falling blood glucose. Under resting, fasting conditions, liver glycogen is depleted in about 1 day. However, long before liver glycogen is depleted, gluconeogenesis begins and is the main means of maintaining blood glucose. Gluconeogenesis is an energy-consuming process that synthesizes glucose from other carbon sources like lactate from red blood cells and muscle, glycerol from triglyceride metabolism, and amino acids from muscle protein. Fatty acids are mobilized from adipose stores under the influence of glucagon. Fatty acids are used by muscle and liver for energy through β-oxidation. β-Oxidation produces acetyl-CoA which can be used in the TCA cycle for further ATP production. β-Oxidation may produce acetyl-CoA at a rate greater than the TCA cycle can use it, especially if glucose is in short supply. When this happens, acetyl-CoA levels rise. As the concentration of acetyl-CoA increase, the liver produces the ketones,

***Table 1.*** *Hormonal Response to Altered Food Availability/Need*

| Condition | Insulin | Glucagon | Growth hormone | Epinephrine | Cortisol |
|---|---|---|---|---|---|
| Glucose ingestion | Increased | Decreased | Decreased | Unchanged | Unchanged |
| Protein ingestion | Increased | Increased | Increased | Unchanged | Unchanged |
| Mixed-meal ingestion | Increased | Unchanged | Unchanged | Unchanged | Unchanged |
| Starvation | Decreased | Increased | Increased or unchanged | Increased or unchanged | Decreased |
| Exercise | Decreased | Increased | Increased | Increased | Increased |

***Table 2.***  *Enzyme Adaptations to Starvation*

| Metabolic Function | Increased | Decreased |
|---|---|---|
| Pancreatic enzymes | None | All hydrolytic enzymes |
| Fatty acid synthesis (adipose tissue and liver) | None | fatty acid synthase<br>acyl-CoA desaturase (liver)<br>lipoprotein lipase (adipose tissue)<br>NADP-malate dehydrogenase<br>citrate cleavage enzyme<br>acetyl-CoA carboxylase |
| Fatty acid utilization | carnitine palmitoyl transferase (liver) | None |
| Glucose utilization | none | glucokinase (liver) |
| Gluconeogenesis | serine dehyratase<br>alanine aminotransferase (liver)<br>pyruvate carboxylase<br>phospho-*enol*-pyruvate carboxykinase<br>glucose-6-phosphatase | None |

acetoacetate and β-hydroxybuterate. Ketones can be oxidized by muscle and kidney. Glycerol is used for gluconeogenesis by the liver.

FASTING. Fasting occurs when the postabsorptive phase becomes prolonged. The metabolic priority during fasting is to mobilize stores to meet body needs. Hormones involved with mobilization are increased and those involved with absorption and storage are decreased (Table 1). Many of these changes occur daily during the postabsorptive phase, but become extended during fasting. Prolonged disuse of the intestinal tract during fasting results in morphologic changes, such as villus atrophy. Liver glycogen supplies become depleted. Thus, gluconeogenesis becomes the sole means for maintenance of normal blood glucose concentrations and supply of glucose to critical tissues, such as brain and red blood cells, unable to use fatty acids as an energy substrate. Muscle protein is degraded to supply amino acids for gluconeogenesis in the liver. Triglyceride mobilization is increased to meet the needs of tissues able to oxidize fatty acids.

STARVATION. Arbitrarily, fasting for greater than 4 or 5 days is starvation. The metabolic priority during starvation is preservation of structural and functional proteins. During starvation, muscle adapts by using less ketones and more fatty acids. This increases blood ketone concentration. As the blood concentration of ketones increases, the brain begins to use ketones and decrease the use of glucose. As the need for glucose decreases, fewer amino acids are used for gluconeogenesis, thus sparing muscle protein and decreasing urea production. The end result is greater utilization of fat as the primary energy source, conserving functional protein. Starvation reduces the need for digestion in the gastrointestinal tract, fatty acid synthesis in the liver, and fatty acid storage in adipose tissue. Simultaneously, there is an increase in mobilization of fatty acids and gluconeogenesis.

During starvation, synthesis of enzymes specific for fat storage are decreased. These enzymes include acyl-CoA desaturase and lipoprotein lipase. Acyl-CoA desaturase introduces more double bonds into fatty acids, and lipoprotein lipase clears transport lipids from blood for storage. Although liver pyruvate carboxylase is involved in synthesis of fatty acids from glucose, its activity does not decrease because it is also involved in gluconeogenesis. Enzymes specific for gluconeogenesis, such as phosphopyruvate carboxykinase, are produced in increased quantities in starvation. Glucose-6-phosphatase (the enzyme responsible for release of glucose from the liver) activity increases during starvation. Glucokinase, the enzyme that takes up glucose in the liver when blood concentrations of glucose are high, decreases during starvation. Enzyme adaptations to starvation are summarized in Table 2.

## MEDICAL INDICATIONS FOR FASTING

Fasting is frequently utilized in the management of acute gastritis and acute pancreatitis. The presence of food in the stomach stimulates the antral portion of the stomach mucosa to secrete gastrin. Gastrin in turn stimulates gastric acid secretion. Gastric acid can diffuse back across damaged mucosa, preventing healing of eroded or ulcerated mucosa. After chyme enters the small intestine, pancreatic secretion becomes copious, primarily in response to the hormone secretin. Cholecystokinin is released in response to food in the upper small intestine. Cholecystokinin also greatly increases secretion of pancreatic enzymes. Secretion of pancreatic enzymes may exacerbate the inflammatory changes associated with acute pancreatitis.

Fasting is also recommended prior to obtaining blood samples. Physiologic or postprandial lipemia may persist for up to 12 hr after a fat-containing meal is consumed. Hyperlipidemia is detected in blood samples by visualization of lactescence or by finding elevated concentrations of total cholesterol or triglycerides or both.

In the past, starvation has been suggested as a means to treat obesity (Anderson and Lewis, 1980). The use of complete and balanced, reduced-caloric-density diets is more acceptable to pet owners and probably less stressful to the obese pet animal.

## CLINICAL IMPLICATIONS OF FASTING/STARVATION

In human beings, prolonged fasting is accompanied by decreased body weight; decreased body water; increased urinary loss of sodium, calcium, and magnesium; decreased extracellular and plasma volume; postural hypotension; negative nitrogen balance with loss of lean body mass; ketonemia; ketonuria; mild metabolic acidosis; hyperuricemia; hypoglycemia; decreased serum cholesterol; depletion of water-soluble vitamins; and reduction of body fat stores. The extent and rate of weight loss is proportional to initial body weight. The heaviest subjects experience the greatest and most rapid weight loss. Rate of weight loss is hyperbolic, with the rate of weight loss slowing over time. Initial rapid weight loss is primarily due to loss of body water. Hunger is experienced only for the first 2 to 4 days.

### Immunologic

A number of malnutrition-related abnormalities of the immune system have been reported. Most studies have involved prolonged protein calorie malnutrition rather than simple fasting/starvation. However the effect of 72 hr of food deprivation on immune function has been studied in rats (Nohr et al., 1985). In this rodent model, delayed type hypersensitivity and humoral immune responses to 72 hr of fasting followed by a refeeding period of 7 days were evaluated. The 72-hr fast was associated with a 15% decrease in body weight. Both delayed type hypersensitivity and humoral responses were depressed. The mechanisms altering these immunologic tests were unknown. However because the immune responses evaluated were maximally depressed at different times, different mechanisms may have been responsible. Delayed type hypersensitivity was maximally depressed during the refeeding period that followed the 72-hr fast. The adverse effects of the 72-hr fast persisted beyond restoration of body weight.

### Endocrine

In starvation, thyroid function undergoes rapid changes both centrally and at the level of peripheral metabolism of thyroxine. The central effect is characterized by decreased basal serum TSH levels and decreased response to intravenous injection of TRH. Within the first hour of refeeding, serum TSH levels increase rapidly. In eight healthy human beings fasted for 30 hours, serum triiodothyroinine ($T_3$) levels were significantly lower as compared to the fed state. Refeeding did not produce a significant change in $T_3$ levels. Glucocorticoids influence monodeiodination and thyroid-stimulating hormone (TSH) secretion. However, in this study in fasted healthy human volunteers, cortisol levels did not change (Hugues et al., 1984).

The endocrine effects of a longer fast (72-hr) without electrolyte supplementation were studied in 17 normal human subjects (Beer et al., 1989). Immediate effects included a marked increase in plasma cortisol, adrenocorticotrophic hormone, (ACTH), $\beta$-endorphin, adrenaline, noradrenaline, and dopamine. These endocrine changes were present the first day of the fast, although plasma glucose concentrations were unchanged. Presumably these changes were not due to hypoglycemia. Triiodothyronine and TSH levels were decreased, but thyroxine concentrations were unchanged. Possible causes for reduced $T_3$ concentrations were reduction in TSH concentration and increased corticosteroid concentrations. The decrease in TSH concentration might be due to inhibition by increased corticosteroids or dopaminergic activity. As expected for hormones directly influenced by food in the gut, the concentration of gastrin and enteroglucagon decreased during fasting.

Plasma insulin-like growth factor (IGF-1) and growth hormone (GH) were studied in seven normal dogs before and during starvation and during refeeding (Eigenmann, deBruijne, and Froesch, 1985). Mean body weight decreased from 18.3±1.0 kg to 14.5±1.4 kg at day 19 of starvation (21% decrease in body weight). Starvation reduced the level of IGF 1 and increased the level of GH. During refeeding, IGF-1 levels increased. During starvation, GH-secretory capacity measured by central $\alpha$-adrenergic (clonidine) stimulation was enhanced.

Glucagon has pronounced glycogenolytic, gluconeogenic, and lipolytic actions. As these processes are accelerated during fasting, it is reasonable to predict that glucagon concentrations are increased. However, in a study of 11 dogs subjected to a 72-hr fast, immunoreactive glucagon levels were unchanged. Plasma glucose concentrations also were unchanged during the fast, while immunoreactive insulin levels decreased moderately.

Obese men were fasted for 10 days and followed during a 5-day refeeding period. These men lost at least 4.1% of total body weight and were ketonemic and ketonuric. Reproductive function was altered as follows: (1) serum follicle-stimulating hormone (FSH) concentration was decreased, (2) the pituitary responsiveness to luteinizing hormone-releasing hormone (LRH) was blunted, (3) serum testosterone was decreased, and (4) the urinary excretion of LH and FSH increased. The decreased FSH response to LRH suggests a decreased sensitivity of the pituitary gland to hypothalamic stimulation during fasting. Increased gonadotropin excretion without an increase in gonadotropin secretion is consistent with altered renal gonadotropin clearance.

## Renal, Electrolyte, and Acid-Base

During chronic starvation, the kidney may account for a larger proportion of endogenous glucose production. There is net renal extraction of lactate, pyruvate, amino acids, and glycerol. The carbon backbone of these compounds is converted to glucose. With long-term starvation, free fatty acids and $\beta$-hydroxybutyrate are also extracted by the kidney and acetoacetate is released.

In animals with no phosphorus intake because of food deprivation, the phosphate filtered in the kidney is largely reabsorbed to conserve body phosphate stores. Therefore, less phosphate is excreted in the urine and the capacity to excrete acid in the urine is reduced. Consequently, if an acid load is administered, acidemia is more likely to occur.

Starved animals may have reduced urine specific gravities and increased urine volumes. Reduced urine concentrating ability may be due to reduced protein intake and subsequent reduced urea synthesis. Serum urea nitrogen is reduced, and less urea is filtered by the glomerulus and reabsorbed by the renal medulla. This reduces medullary hypertonicity and the tendency for water to move from the distal tubule and collecting duct to the medulla. The ability to form dilute urine should not be influenced by starvation.

Fasting may artifactually increase the serum creatinine concentration when measured by the Jaffe method (Mascioli et al., 1984). So-called noncreatinine chromagens are known to interfere with the Jaffe method. It appears that aceteoacetate produced during fasting in human beings is a noncreatinine chromagen. In five healthy volunteers fasted for 96 hr, mean serum creatinine concentration increased from 1.0±0.08 to 1.7±0.11 mg/dl. Fasting does not appear to influence measurement of serum urea nitrogen and creatinine measured by enzymatic methods.

Plasma and urine electrolytes were measured in healthy, nonobese human beings before, during, and after a 4-day fast (Elia, Crozier, and Neale, 1984). Progressive weight loss of 2.9 kg was observed. During the fasting period the experimental subjects received only distilled water. Plasma sodium, chloride, magnesium, and bicarbonate concentrations decreased, and the sum of hydroxybutyrate and acetoacetate increased, in all subjects. Plasma concentrations of sodium and chloride decreased in all experimental subjects by approximately 4 mmol/l and increased to prefasting levels within 24 hr of refeeding. These changes occurred without detectable alteration in state of hydration or vascular volume. Plasma zinc levels rapidly increased during fasting and returned to normal upon refeeding. Urine zinc levels increased threefold and continued to rise after refeeding. During the period of fasting, no significant changes in the urinary excretion of calcium, magnesium, and phosphate were noted.

Acute starvation may increase catabolism of nucleic acids, purines, and amino acids, and thus can increase uric acid production. Hyperuricemia may result in increased urinary levels of uric acid and predispose to urate urolith formation.

In adult dogs, blood gas profiles obtained 4 and 24 hr after eating were statistically different (Lawler et al., 1992). These data suggested a tendency for fasted adult dogs to develop mild metabolic acidosis with respiratory compensation. By comparison, normal human beings fasted for 18 days develop systemic alkalosis (Stinebaugh and Schloeder, 1972). Metabolic alkalosis persists, to some degree, for as long as 2 weeks. Results of this study indicate that the alkalosis is due to increased renal tubular bicarbonate reabsorptive capacity during fasting that is accentuated upon refeeding carbohydrates. These changes appear to be related to changes in renal sodium handling during fasting and refeeding.

## Cardiac

Starvation in dogs results in gross cardiac edema, myofibrillar atrophy, and interstitial edema. Cellular effects associated with starvation include decreased glycogen content, decreased protein synthesis, activation of proteinases, and mitochondrial swelling. Functional changes associated with starvation include decreased contractile force, decreased cardiac output, and decreased ventricular compliance. Clinical changes associated with starvation in human beings include bradycardia, hypotension, ectopic rhythms, mitral valve prolapse, and decreased exercise capacity.

Cardiac mass is relatively well preserved during short-term starvation and is rapidly restored with refeeding . The mechanism for decreased cardiac protein synthesis in starvation is decreased cardiac microsomal RNA and mRNA synthesis.

Congestive heart failure has been reported during recovery from starvation and anorexia nervosa (Schocken, Holloway, and Powers, 1989). The so-called refeeding syndrome was first described in survivors of concentration and POW camps in World War II. The refeeding syndrome can be seen following oral intake or parenteral perfusion of calorically dense fluids. It has been suggested that the cardiac decompensation observed during refeeding is due to abnormal energy metabolism associated with hypophosphatemia and rapid fluid expansion.

## Hepatic

Energy and protein restriction have been implicated as a cause of feline idiopathic hepatic lipidosis (IHL). With severe energy restriction, triglyceride from adipose tissue is mobilized to the liver. Starvation may be required for the development of IHL, although not all starved cats develop IHL. Two of five previously obese cats subjected to fasting for 4 to 6 weeks developed clinical signs and light microscopic changes in the liver consistent with IHL. In another study, cats fed 25% of their calculated maintenance energy requirement for 2 months developed hepatic lipid accumulation without signs of clinical disease. A third study suggests that the development of IHL is related to the degree of food deprivation in previously obese cats. Hepatic lipidosis was diagnosed in 6 of 25 cats after changing the diet from a dry commercial diet to a purified diet (Biourge et al., 1993). Seven of the 25 cats were judged to be obese at the time of dietary change. Hepatic lipidosis developed in six of the initially obese cats. Clinical signs were first noted 6 to 7 weeks after the diet change. At this time, affected cats lost 30 to 40% of their initial body weight. The cats that did not develop hepatic lipidosis lost 0 to 23% of their initial body weight. The amount of food actually consumed was unknown; however, the rate of weight loss was consistent with little or no food intake.

## Metabolic

During starvation the concentration of plasma ketones increased from 0.06 to 0.28 mmol/L in lean dogs, but remained unchanged in obese dogs. The reduced ketonemia observed in dogs compared with human subjects is due to efficient peripheral utilization, rather than decreased hepatic production (Lewis, Morris, and Hand, 1987). Compared with starved human beings, starved dogs have a mild decrease in blood glucose and serum insulin.

In six obese dogs subjected to 24 to 42 days of starvation, no adverse clinical or biochemical effects were observed (Anderson and Lewis, 1980). Even though, dogs lost 8% of their body weight by the end of week 1, 5% more by the end of week 2, and 3 to 4% per week thereafter, ketoacidosis was not observed. The majority of dogs developed polyuria and polydipsia.

In seven normal dogs starved for 19 days, serum free fatty acids rose continuously and significantly from $0.99 \pm 0.05$ mmol/L at the start to $1.61 \pm 0.12$ mmol/L at the end of starvation (Eigenmann, deBruijne, and Froesch, 1985).

## References and Suggested Reading

Anderson GL and Lewis, LD: Obesity. *In* Kirk RW (ed): *Current Veterinary Therapy VII*. Philadelphia, WB Saunders Co, 1980, p 1034.
*A report of six obese dogs subjected to starvation for periods of 24 to 42 days.*

Beer SF, Bircham PMM, Bloom, SR, et al: The effect of a 72-h fast on plasma levels of pituitary, adrenal, thyroid, pancreatic and gastrointestinal hormones in healthy men and women. J Endocrinol 120:337, 1989.
*The endocrinological effects of a 72-hr fast without electrolyte supplementation were studied in 17 normal human subjects.*

Biourge V, Pion P, Lewis J, et al: Spontaneous occurrence of hepatic lipidosis in a group of laboratory cats. J Vet Intern Med 7:194, 1993.
*In a group of 25 laboratory cats, hepatic lipidosis was diagnosed in six of seven obese cats who had lost 30 to 40% of their initial body weight.*

Eigenmann JE, deBruijne JJ, Froesch ER: Insulin-like growth factor I and growth hormone in canine starvation. Acta Endocrinol 108:161, 1985.
*Plasma insulin-like growth factor (IGF-1) and growth hormone (GH) were studied in seven normal dogs before and during starvation and during refeeding.*

Elia M, Crozier C, and Neale G: Mineral metabolism during short-term starvation in man. Clin Chim Acta 139:37, 1984.
*Plasma and urine electrolytes were measured in healthy, nonobese human beings before, during, and after a 4-day fast.*

Hugues JN, Burger AG, Pekary AE, et al: Rapid adaptations of serum thyrotrophin, triiodothyronine and reverse triiodothyronine levels to short-term starvation and refeeding. Acta Endocrinol 105:194, 1984.
*Thyroid status and cortisol levels were evaluated in this study of eight healthy human beings fasted for 30 hr.*

Lawler DF, Kealy RD, Ballam JM, et al: Influence of fasting on canine arterial and venous blood gas and acid-base measurements. Vet Emergen Crit Care 2:80, 1992.
*In adult dogs, blood gas profiles obtained 4 and 24 hr after eating were statistically different.*

Lewis LD, Morris ML Jr., Hand MS: *Small Animal Clinical Nutrition III*. Topeka, KS, Mark Morris Associates, 1987. pp 6–27.
*This secondary reference describes research on ketone metabolism in fasting dogs.*

Mascioli SR, Bantle JP, Freier EF, et al: Artifactual elevation of serum creatinine level due to fasting. Arch Intern Med 144:1575, 1984.
*In human beings, fasting may artifactually increase the serum creatinine concentration when measured by the Jaffe method.*

Nohr CW, Tchervenkov JI, Meakins JL, et al: Malnutrition and humoral immunity: Short-term acute nutritional deprivation. Surgery 98:769, 1985.
*The effect of short term acute food deprivation (72 hr) on immune function was studied in rats.*

Schocken DD, Holloway JD, and Powers PS: Weight loss and the heart. Arch Intern Med 149:877, 1989.
*In the so-called refeeding syndrome, congestive heart failure has been reported during recovery from starvation and anorexia nervosa.*

Stinebaugh, BJ and Schloeder FX: Glucose-induced alkalosis in fasting subjects. J Clin Invest 51:1326, 1972.
*Normal human beings fasted for 18 days developed systemic alkalosis.*

# DIAGNOSIS AND MANAGEMENT OF ADVERSE FOOD REACTIONS

PHILIP ROUDEBUSH

*Topeka, Kansas*

An *adverse reaction to food* is an abnormal response to an ingested food or food additive. In general, pathogenic mechanisms that lead to adverse food reactions include ingestion of inciting agents followed by interaction of the agents with biologic amplification systems that lead to inflammation and clinical signs.

In view of the number of diverse foods that are routinely ingested by the dog and cat, it is not surprising that there are adverse reactions to dietary substances. The fact that food-related reactions appear relatively infrequently is testimony to the effectiveness of the intestinal mucosal barrier and oral tolerance. Adverse reactions to food have been blamed for a variety of clinical syndromes in dogs and cats, especially those involving the skin and gastrointestinal tracts.

## TERMINOLOGY

Adverse reactions to food are comprised of a variety of subclassifications based on pathomechanisms (Anderson, 1986). The following terms and definitions are those recommended by the American Academy of Allergy and Immunology (Anderson, 1986) (Fig. 1). *Food allergy (food hypersensitivity)* is an adverse reaction to a food or food additive with a proved immunologic basis. *Food anaphylaxis* is an acute food allergy with systemic consequences such as respiratory distress, vascular collapse, and urticaria. *Food intolerance* is a nonimmunologic, abnormal physiologic response to a food or food additive. Food intolerance can be further classified as food idiosyncracy, food poisoning, and pharmacologic reactions to food. *Food idiosyncracy* is an abnormal response that resembles food allergy, but does not involve immune mechanisms. A direct nonimmunologic action due to food or a toxin in food is termed *food poisoning*. Adverse reactions due to a drug-like or pharmacologic effect of a food stubstance are termed *pharmacologic reactions to food*. Adverse reactions resulting from such behaviors as gluttony, pica, or ingestion of indigestible materials are called *dietary indiscretion*. The terms "food hypersensitivity" or "food allergy" have been traditionally used to describe all adverse reactions to food in dogs and cats, including reactions that were truly food intolerance.

## IMMUNOLOGIC REACTIONS TO FOOD

### Food Antigens

Food allergy and food anaphylaxis are two adverse reactions to food with an immunologic basis. Over 6000 food antigens exist; these are almost exclusively proteins or glycoproteins. The most common food allergens in humans are found in egg, peanut, cow's milk, fish, soy, and wheat. Food allergens incriminated in North American dogs include food preservatives and dyes, wheat, beef, egg, corn, poultry, soy, and dairy products. Food allergens incriminated in North American cats include fish, beef, chicken/poultry, dairy products, preservatives, and dyes (Roudebush and Cowell, 1992). Unfortunately, few pet owners and veterinarians complete the extensive feeding trials required to identify offending food allergens. Therefore, very few specific dietary allergens have been documented in food-allergic dogs and cats. Further controlled clinical trials are needed to determine if the current perceptions of offending food allergens are correct.

### Mucosal Barrier and Oral Intolerance

The defense against hypersensitivity to dietary antigens includes an effective mucosal barrier and oral tolerance generated by the cellular immune system of gut-associated lymphoid tissue (GALT). An important adaptation of the gastrointestinal tract is development of a mucosal barrier that prevents the overwhelming uptake of food antigens (Murphy and Walker, 1991). Efficient functioning of the mucosal barrier excludes the majority of ingested antigens, thus minimizing an-

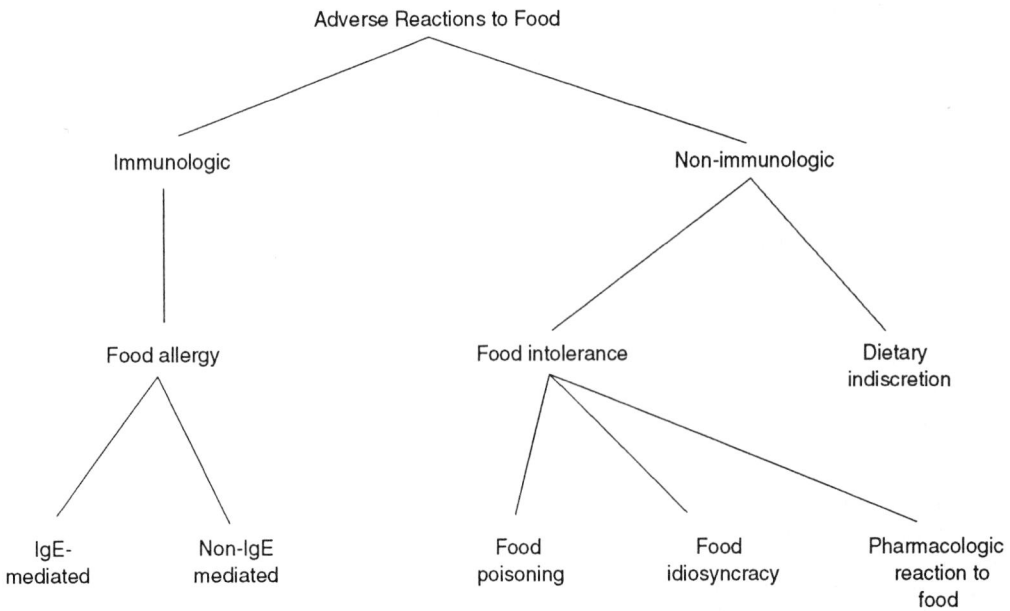

**Figure 1.** Classification of adverse reactions to food.

tigen exposure to GALT. The concept of a mucosal barrier includes effective digestion, the mucous layer, intact and functioning epithelial cells, and immunoglobulin A (IgA).

Complete digestion of food protein results in free amino acids and small peptides that are probably poor antigens. However, an incompletely digested food protein has the potential to incite an allergic response because of residual antigenic proteins and large polypeptides. The thickness and composition of the mucous coat overlying the intestinal surface contributes to the defense against antigen attachment and penetration. Mucus contains carbohydrate moieties that may act as receptor inhibitors, thereby interfering with attachment of antigen to the intestinal microvillus surface (Murphy and Walker, 1991). A direct association between intestinal cell membrane protein/phospholipid ratios and antigen uptake has been demonstrated in some species. Changes in cell membrane composition and function occur early in life, but how these changes effect food antigen uptake is unknown. IgA is the major immunologic component of the mucosal barrier. IgA may prevent the transport of food antigens by complexing with them in the intestinal lumen or within the mucous coat.

Despite these defense mechanisms, the mucosal barrier is not completely impervious to macromolecules. Dietary proteins cross the intact intestinal mucosa in small but significant amounts. Antigens that enter and escape the lamina propria are removed by the mononuclear-macrophage (reticuloendothelial) system of the liver and mesenteric lymph nodes.

The intestine, traditionally viewed as an organ of digestion and absorption of nutrients, maintains an indispensable immunologic function (Murphy and Walker, 1991). The gut is one of the largest immune organs in the body. Absorbed food antigens are presented to the gut-associated lymphoid tissue in such a manner that a potent gut-associated, cell-mediated suppressive response to that antigen develops. This suppressor response is the basis of oral tolerance. Conversely, an allergic response may result if the antigen encounters a defective suppressor arm of GALT or escapes into the systemic circulation. The concept of "immune exclusion" of food antigens is important, since systemic lymphoid tissue does not respond with active immune suppression (tolerance), but active immunoreactivity that could lead to allergic clinical signs.

Abnormalities in gastrointestinal defense mechanisms may predispose patients to food allergies. Predisposing factors for food allergy include mucosal barrier failure (poorly digestible proteins, incomplete protein digestion, increased intestinal mucosal permeability, age-related changes in microvillus cell membrane composition, inflammatory-induced changes in mucous composition) and defective immunoregulation (decreased IgA secretion, deranged cell-mediated responses of GALT, monocyte-macrophage system dysfunction). Which of these pathomechanisms are important predisposing factors in dogs and cats awaits further investigation.

## Clinical Features of Food Allergy in Dogs and Cats

Adverse reactions to food were reported in dogs and cats as early as 1920. Adverse food reactions are usually suspected when a client or veterinarian establishes an historic association between ingestion of certain foods and the appearance of certain clinical signs. No gender predisposition is noted in reported canine or feline cases. Ages of reported cases have ranged from 6 months to 12 years for cats, and 4 months to 14 years for dogs. Up to one third of canine food allergy cases may occur in dogs less than 1 year old. Most of the reported adverse reactions have been termed food allergy, although no specific tests were performed to confirm an immunologic basis for the clinical signs. Two series of cases could not relate the onset of clinical signs with recent changes in the diet. This suggests that dogs and cats may develop food allergy after prolonged exposure to one brand, type, or form of food.

Clinical signs of food allergy in cats are usually confined to the integumentary and/or gastrointestinal systems (Carlotti, Remy, and Prost, 1990; Roudebush, 1994). Dermatologic signs include several different clinical reaction patterns such as severe generalized pruritus without lesions; miliary dermatitis; pruritus with self-trauma centered around the head, neck, and ears; alopecia; and scaling dermatoses. Adverse reactions to food may cause self-inflicted alopecia, eosinophilic plaques, and indolent ulcers of the lip in some cats.

Dermatologic reaction patterns seen in cats with food allergy resemble the patterns seen with other feline skin diseases. Food allergy can mimic idiopathic miliary dermatitis, atopy, flea bite hypersensitivity, psychogenic alopecia, dermatophytosis, and parasitic infestation (cheyletiellosis, pediculosis, scabies, trombiculidiasis). In cats with suspected food allergy, concurrent flea allergy dermatitis or atopy occur in up to 20% of cases.

Gastrointestinal signs of feline food allergy include intermittent vomiting and mild to severe diarrhea. Some cats with vomiting and diarrhea associated with inflammatory bowel disease respond to dietary modification alone. It is not known if the inflammatory bowel disease in these cats is a direct manifestation of an adverse food reaction or if dietary modification is merely palliative.

In dogs, food allergy typically is manifested as nonseasonal pruritic dermatitis that is occasionally accompanied by gastrointestinal signs (Carlotti, Remy, and Prost, 1990; Rosser, 1993). The pruritus is of varying severity. The location of pruritus is often indistinguishable from that seen with inhalant allergies: feet, face, axilla, perineal region, inguinal region, rump, and ears. One-quarter of food-allergic dogs only develop lesions in the ear region. Dogs with chronic or recurrent otitis externa should be closely evaluated for food allergy.

A variety of primary and secondary skin lesions occur in food-allergic dogs (see this volume, p 628). These lesions include papules, erythroderma, excoriations, hyperpigmentation, epidermal collarettes, pododermatitis, seborrhea sicca, and otitis externa. Food allergy often mimics other common canine skin disorders including pyoderma, pruritic seborrheic dermatoses, folliculitis, and ectoparasites. As in cats, 20 to 30% of dogs with suspected food allergy have concurrent allergic disease such as flea allergy dermatitis or atopy or both.

Gastrointestinal signs of canine food allergy include vomiting and diarrhea. Clinical response to dietary modification suggests that hypersensitivity to food antigens plays a role in dogs with chronic idiopathic or plasmacytic-lymphocytic colitis (Nelson et al., 1988). It is not known if the chronic colitis or other forms of inflammatory small-bowel disease are a direct manifestation of an adverse food reaction or if dietary modification is merely palliative in some dogs.

## Diagnosis of Food Allergy

Dietary elimination trials are the main diagnostic method used in dogs and cats with suspected adverse food reactions or food allergy. At the present time, intradermal skin testing, radioallergosorbent (RAST) tests, enzyme-linked immunosorbent assay (ELISA) testing, and endoscopic challenge tests for food hypersensitivity are considered unreliable in animals.

Before an elimination diet is initiated, the client should feed the dog or cat its usual food for 7 to 14 days. During this time the client should record the type and amount of food ingested; any other ingested food items such as table scraps, treats, or snacks; and the occurrence and character of adverse reactions. The patient is then fed a controlled elimination diet for 4 to 12 weeks. The ideal elimination diet should include a novel, highly digestible protein source, avoid protein excesses, be free of additives, and be nutritionally adequate for the animal's life stage and condition. In addition to the dietary change, no other ingested substances such as treats, flavored vitamin supplements, or chew toys should be offered. The client should continue daily documentation of the type and amount of food ingested, and the occurrence and character of adverse reactions. Observation of at least 50% improvement in clinical signs is necessary to make a tentative diagnosis of food allergy. Clinical improvement will usually occur within a few days to weeks.

In a recent survey of veterinarians in the American Academy of Veterinary Dermatology (AAVD), homemade diets were recommended most often as the initial test diets for dogs and cats with suspected food allergy (Roudebush and Cowell, 1992). Homemade test diets usually included a single protein source, or a combination of a single protein source and a single carbohydrate source. Ingredients recommended most often for homemade feline diets include lamb baby food, lamb, rice, and rabbit. Ingredients recommended most often for homemade canine diets include lamb, rice, potato, fish, rabbit, venison, and tofu. Homemade diets contain a novel, highly digestible protein source and

are usually free of additives. However, they are usually high in protein and are often nutritionally inadequate. In the previously mentioned survey, most of the homemade diets recommended for initial management of dogs and cats with suspected food allergy were nutritionally inadequate for adult maintenance. Failure to meet nutritional requirements occurs in most homemade diets because rations are devised to include a minimum of ingredients. In general, homemade diets lack a source of calcium, essential fatty acids, certain vitamins, and other micronutrients.

Nutritionally adequate homemade diet recipes are available and should be used (Codner and Thatcher, 1990; Remillard and Thatcher, 1989; Roudebush, 1994). These recipes include a source of calcium and other essential vitamins and minerals. Additive-free vitamin and mineral supplements that do not contain animal or vegetable proteins are unlikely to be a source of ingested allergens. A source of essential fatty acids, such as vegetable oil, animal fat, or fish oil should also be included.

A smaller percentage of veterinarians in the survey recommended commercial pet food for initial test diets. Commercial diets most often recommended in suspected food-allergic cats are canned Hill's Prescription Diet Feline d/d, dry and canned Hill's Prescription Diet Feline c/d, and Wysong Feline Angergen. Commercial diets most often recommended in suspected food-allergic dogs are dry and canned Hill's Prescription Diet Canine d/d, dry Nature's Recipe Lamb and Rice, and dry Wysong Anergen.

A definitive diagnosis of adverse food reaction is made if the animal's former diet and other ingested substances subsequently offered as a challenge are associated with a return of clinical signs within a few minutes to a week. Reinstituting the elimination diet should resolve the clinical signs induced by the food challenge. Food challenge can be performed in an "open," "single-blind," or "double-blind" manner. In an open food challenge, both the client and veterinarian are aware that a specific food or previous diet is being fed. In a single-blind food challenge, only the client is unaware of what food is being given. In a double-blind food challenge, both the client and veterinarian are unaware of whether a specific food is being given. Double-blind, placebo-controlled food challenges are considered to be most reliable in human beings. Only half the human patients believed to be allergic to a food react to the food when they are challenged in controlled, blinded conditions. Unfortunately, all reports and most recommendations of food challenge in the veterinary literature have been open challenges. Open challenges will continue as the most practical method of establishing a tentative diagnosis of food allergy in dogs and cats, but are subject to false interpretation by both the client and veterinarian.

Provocation involves introducing single dietary ingredients until as many positive reactions as possible can be documented. Clients and veterinarians are often reluctant to pursue challenge and provocation once clinical signs have improved or been eliminated. Provocation may also be difficult in many dogs and cats because commercial pet foods contain such a large number of ingredients and because these ingredients cannot often be duplicated in challenge studies. An example of such an ingredient is poultry by-product meal, which is frequently used as an animal protein source in dry pet foods. Poultry by-product meal is the ground, rendered, clean parts of the carcass such as necks, feet, undeveloped eggs, and viscera, exclusive of feathers. Use of chicken meat in a provocative food challenge may not duplicate the types of antigens found in poultry by-product meal.

Elimination trials will also be difficult to interpret in some dogs and cats because of concurrent allergic skin disease. In several studies of food-allergic dogs and cats, 20 to 30% had concurrent hypersensitivities. Flea-allergic dermatitis and atopy are the most common canine and feline allergies and should be eliminated through other diagnostic testing.

## Treatment of Food Allergy

For most food allergies, avoiding offending foods is the most effective treatment. How selective or meticulous an avoidance diet must be depends upon the individual animal's sensitivity. Some dogs and cats may suffer adverse reactions to even trace quantities of an offending food, while others may have higher tolerance levels. Concurrent allergies will influence the threshold level of clinical signs in some animals. Symptomatic therapy in pruritic animals can also include corticosteroids and antihistamines. Corticosteroids along with dietary change are often used to treat cats with inflammatory bowel disease. One third of humans that have consumed a strict avoidance diet for 1 to 2 years tolerated reintroduction to their diet of food allergens. This suggests that strict avoidance in animals with food allergy may allow some dogs and cats to tolerate exposure to certain food allergens later in life.

Both homemade and commercial diets can be used for long-term maintenance of patients with suspected food allergy. It is very important that any homemade recipe for long-term maintenance should ensure a nutritionally adequate ration. An attempt should always be made to find an acceptable commercial diet that will raise owner compliance with the dietary change and ensure a nutritionally adequate ration.

## NONIMMUNOLOGIC REACTIONS TO FOOD

Nonimmunologic reactions to food include food intolerance and dietary indiscretion (Fig. 1). Dietary indiscretions such as gluttony, pica, and ingestion of garbage usually cause gastrointestinal signs and are easily diagnosed by a thorough environmental and dietary history. Food intolerance may mimic food allergy, except that it can occur on the first exposure to a dietary substance, since nonimmunologic mechanisms are involved. The incidence of food intolerance versus food hypersensitivity or allergy is unknown.

Food additives, preservatives, or dyes are frequently mentioned as causes of adverse food reactions in dogs and cats (Roudebush and Cowell, 1992). Food additives are purposely put into foods to give them some desirable characteristic such as color, flavor, texture, stability, or resistance to spoilage. Many additives enhance the nutritional quality or acceptability of the food, while others are merely added to enhance the consumer appeal of the product. The words preservative and additive are often used synonymously, but they are distinctly different. Preservatives are added to foods to protect or retard decay, discoloration, or spoilage under normal conditions of use or storage. Thus, all preservatives are additives, but not all additives serve a preservative function. The word preservative is often used in a generic sense, but there are several different categories of preservatives such as antioxidants, antimicrobials, and color enhancers.

Additives are found least often in canned pet foods, and most commonly in soft-moist foods, treats, snacks, and dry foods. Many canned commercial pet foods are free of additives. Although individual additives may be harmful, they rarely cause hypersensitivity reactions in humans (Hannuksela and Haahtela, 1987). Very few of the untoward reactions to food additives have a true immunologic basis. Reactions to food additives are best described as food intolerance because they cause clinical signs due to nonimmunologic mechanisms. Azo dyes, nonazo dyes, and antioxidants can all cause histamine release from the leukocytes of normal humans. Benzoates and tartrazine, two of the most frequently incriminated additives in human foods, are rarely found in commercial pet foods. However, other additives documented to cause problems in human beings are found in pet foods, including sodium bisulfite, sodium glutamate, sodium nitrate, BHA, spices, sodium alginate, guar gum, and propylene glycol. Further studies are needed to document the true incidence and mechanisms of food intolerance to pet food additives.

Another cause of food intolerance is pharmacologic reactions to substances found in food. Vasoactive amines, such as histamine, cause clinical signs in human beings when present in excessive levels in food. Scombroid fish (tuna, mackerel, skipjack, and bonito) that undergo bacterial spoilage before consumption are a frequent cause of histamine toxicosis in human beings. Clinical signs usually include diarrhea, flushing, sweating, nausea, vomiting, urticaria, facial swelling, and erythroderma. Recent surveys of histamine in pet foods revealed the highest levels of histamine in canned fish–based cat foods and those cat foods containing fish solubles. Other vasoactive amines (tyramine, spermine, spermidine, phenethylamine, putrescine, and cadaverine) have also been found in pet foods. The role of histamine and other vasoactive amines in food intolerance in animals is unknown. Vasoactive amines may not be present in levels high enough to cause clinical signs, but could lower threshold levels for allergens in individual dogs and cats.

## References and Suggested Reading

Anderson JA: The establishment of common language concerning adverse reactions to foods and food additives: J Allergy Clin Immunol 78:140, 1986.
*A review of the new terminology that is recommended for describing food allergy and food intolerance.*

Carlotti DN, Remy I, and Prost C: Food allergy in dogs and cats. A review and report of 43 cases. Vet Dermatol 1: 55, 1990.
*A review of clinical cases of adverse food reactions in European dogs and cats.*

Codner EC and Thatcher CD: The role of nutrition in the management of dermatoses. Semin Vet Med Surg 5:167–177, 1990.
*Nutritionally complete and balanced homemade diets are summarized.*

Hannuksela M and Haahtela T: Hypersensitivity reactions to food additives. Allergy 42: 561, 1987.
*Review of adverse reactions to food additives in human beings.*

Murphy MS and Walker WA: Antigen absorption. *In* Metcalfe DD, Sampson HA, and Simon RA (eds): *Food Allergy: Adverse Reactions to Foods and Food Additives.* Boston, Blackwell Scientific, 1991, p 52.
*An excellent review of normal antigen absorption and abnormalities that may occur in patients with food allergy.*

Nelson RW, Stookey LJ, and Kazacos E: Nutritional management of idiopathic chronic colitis in the dog. J Vet Intern Med 2:133, 1988.
*Use of low-residue and hypoallergenic diets in dogs with chronic colitis is described.*

Remillard RL and Thatcher CD: Dietary and nutritional management of gastrointestinal diseases. Vet Clin North Am 19: 809, 1989.
*Nutritionally complete and balanced homemade diets are summarized.*

Rosser EJ: Diagnosis of food allergy in dogs. J Am Vet Med Assoc 203: 259, 1993.
*Clinical signs and diagnostic techniques are described for 51 dogs with adverse reactions to food.*

Roudebush P and Cowell CS: Results of a hypoallergenic diet survey of veterinarians in North America with a nutritional evaluation of homemade diet prescriptions. Vet Dermatol 3: 23, 1992.
*Results of a diet survey that outlines the use of both commercial and homemade elimination diets for dogs and cats. Evalution of homemade diet recipes recommended by veterinarians is also given.*

Roudebush P: Nutritional management of the allergic patient. *In* August JR (ed): *Seminars in Feline Internal Medicine,* 2nd edition. 1994, pp 201–208.
*Review of adverse food reactions in cats.*

# OXYGEN FREE RADICALS AND REPERFUSION INJURY

GARY C. LANTZ

*West Lafayette, Indiana*

Evidence continues to emerge implicating oxygen-derived free radicals as major factors in the pathogenesis of many disease processes. These include: oncogenesis, inflammatory diseases, skin burns, lung damage with respiratory distress syndrome, acute renal tubular necrosis, transplant rejection, aging, drug-induced myocardial and hepatic damage, and postischemic "reperfusion injury." Free radicals are also of major importance in the bactericidal mechanisms of leukocytes. In veterinary practice, reperfusion injury may be of major concern for patients in shock. Shock, from any cause, results in underperfusion of tissue; the treatment goal for shock is to improve tissue perfusion. However, this necessary therapy could contribute to further tissue injury.

## REPERFUSION INJURY

Although restoration of oxygen to ischemic tissue is essential for cell survival, a significant portion of tissue damage that occurs is caused from reintroduction of oxygen to the ischemic tissue in addition to that caused by ischemia. This phenomenon is called reperfusion injury or oxygen paradox. The paradoxic oxygen toxicity is initiated by biochemical events occurring during ischemia that result in the generation of partially reduced oxygen species that cause cell injury or death. They include superoxide anions, hydrogen peroxide and other nonradical peroxides, and hydroxyl radicals. In practical terms, patients in shock need restoration of tissue perfusion and tissue oxygen levels. However, in administering the necessary therapy to achieve this goal, the clinician may also contribute to morbidity and mortality associated with reperfusion injury.

Free radicals are unstable, highly reactive molecules because they contain an unpaired electron in their outer orbital or shell. Most molecules exist in orbitals that hold two electrons that spin in opposite directions and make the molecule stable. Oxygen has two unpaired electrons in different orbitals and is, therefore, a naturally occuring free radical. However, the same direction of spin of the two electrons in an oxygen molecule limits the ability of oxygen to abstract electrons from other molecules, thereby preventing spontaneous combustion. If two radicals react, both radicals are eliminated. If a free radical reacts with a nonradical molecule, another free radical must be produced. Therefore, free radicals may participate in chain reactions that can be thousands of events long. Free radicals have half-lives of nanoseconds to milliseconds.

In oxidative phosphorylation, oxygen reduced by four electrons forms water. However, one electron reduction results in the formation of superoxide anion, two-electron reduction results in hydrogen peroxide, and three-electron reduction results in the hydroxyl radical.

Oxygen-derived free radicals induce lipid peroxidation of cell membranes, destruction of intracellular enzymes, and cleavage of deoxyribonucleic acid (DNA) strands. These events result in damaged or disrupted cellular functions. Lipid peroxidation results in formation of lipid radicals that in turn promote further lipid peroxidation and further cell injury. This cascading reaction will stop: (1) when radical meets radical to form a nonreactive molecule, (2) following intervention with radical scavenger drugs, or (3) following death of the patient.

## BIOCHEMISTRY OF FREE-RADICAL GENERATION

During hypoxia, intracellular adenosine triphosphate (ATP) is degraded to hypoxanthine. Hypoxanthine is normally oxidized by xanthine dehydrogenase to xanthine using nicotinamide adenine dinucleotide (NAD). During this reaction, NAD is converted to NADH. Shortly after the onset of ischemia, extracellular calcium concentrations fall, and intracellular calcium concentrations increase secondary to ischemia-mediated breakdown of cell membrane gradient maintenance. Xanthine dehydrogenase is present in large quantities and, in ischemia, is converted to xanthine oxidase secondary to protease stimulation from increased intracellular calcium (Fig. 1). This enzymatic conversion is essential to oxygen radical–mediated reperfusion injury. Excess levels of hypoxanthine accumulate in tissue because xanthine dehydrogenase is no longer present. Xanthine oxidase, which uses oxygen rather than NAD as a substrate, is unable to catalyze the conversion of hypoxanthine to xanthine in absence of oxygen. Increased intracellular calcium also contributes to cell membrane injury by activation of phospholipases, which in turn release free fatty acids from membranes. As a consequence, the arachidonic acid cascade is activated.

At the time of tissue reperfusion, secondary to initiation of shock therapy, molecular oxygen is reintroduced to ischemic tissues. Xanthine oxidase conversion of hypoxanthine to xanthine results in generation of large amounts of superoxide anion. This burst of superoxide formation occurs within 10 to 30 sec after the onset of reperfusion and begins a chain of reactions that produces other radicals. The major site of radical production is the vascular endothelium. Superoxide anion free radicals are very unstable and spontaneously react or dismutate to yield hydrogen peroxide and water. Hydrogen peroxide by itself is not a potent oxidizing agent.

The next key step is reduction of intracellular ferric iron to ferrous iron by superoxide anion. Iron is stored in the protein ferritin found in all cells. Iron released from ferritin during ischemia is readily oxidized at the time of reperfusion. Hydroxyl radicals are formed by the Haber-Weiss reaction in the presence of hydrogen peroxide and iron in an aqueous medium (Fig. 2). The hydroxyl radical is the most destructive and short lived of all the radicals.

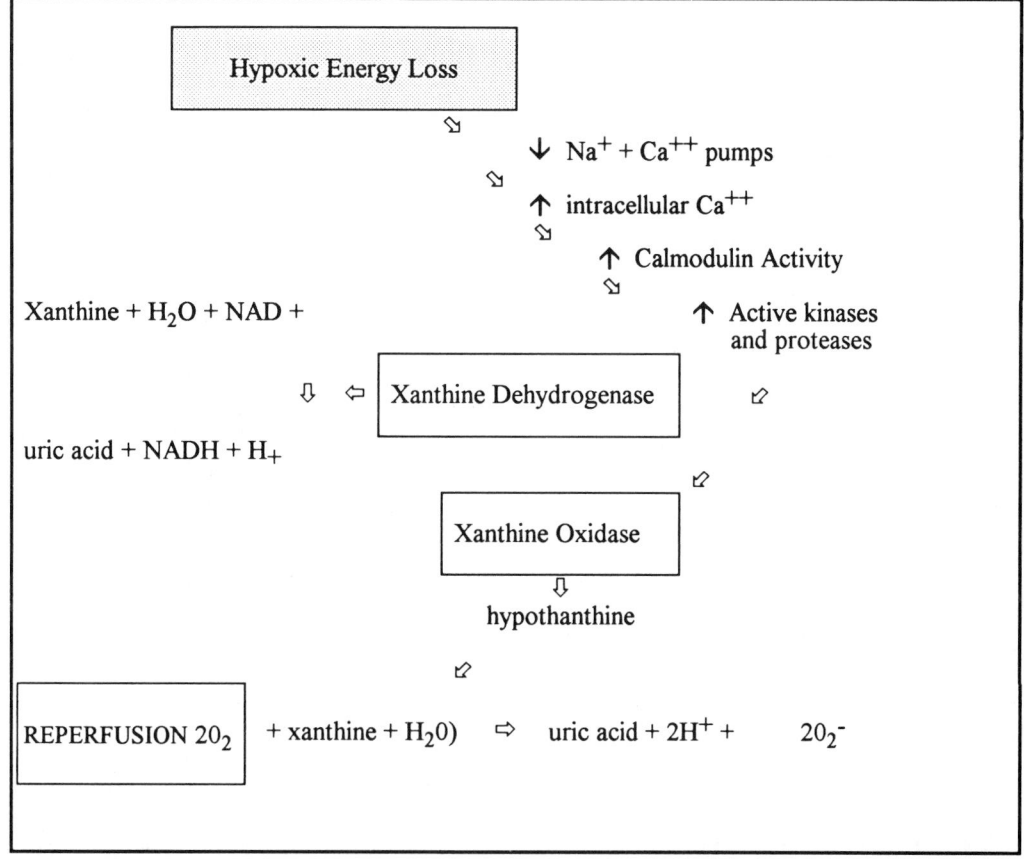

**Figure 1.** An example of enzymatic generation of superoxide radicals $(O_2^-)$ dependent on reperfusion. Conversion of xanthine dehydrogenase to xanthine oxidase is illustrated. (Modified from Hitt ME: Oxygen-derived free radicals: pathophysiology and implications. Compend Cont Educ Pract Vet 10:939, 1988, with permission.)

$$O_2^- + Fe^3 \rightarrow O_2 + Fe^2$$

$$2O_2^- + 2H^+ \rightarrow H_2O_2 + O_2$$

$$H^+ + Fe^2 + H_2O_2 \rightarrow OH^- + Fe^3 + H_2O$$

**Figure 2.** The iron-catalyzed Haber-Weiss reaction. Ferric iron ($Fe^3$) is reduced by superoxide ($O_2^-$). Superoxide readily combines to form hydrogen peroxide ($H_2O_2$). The reduced ferrous iron ($Fe^2$) combines with hydrogen peroxide to produce the hydroxyl radical ($OH^-$).

Accumulated radicals disrupt cellular proteins and membranes by hydrogen ion abstraction. Loss of hydrogen ions results in development of additional radicals in a self-perpetuating process. Lipid radicals generated by lipid peroxidation of cell membranes combine with molecular oxygen and, through biochemical processes in the presence of ferrous iron, produce additional lipid radicals. The effect of these radicals on cells is progressive cellular membrane dysfunction, loss of selective membrane permeability, damage to DNA, and degradation of structural proteins and membrane-bound enzyme activity.

## FREE RADICALS AND CELLULAR DEFENSES

Free radicals are normally generated from a variety of biologic processes. Many cellular enzymes and electron transport processes involve one-electron transfers that produce free-radical intermediates. Oxygen-centered free radicals are often mediators of these reactions because of the ubiquity of molecular oxygen and its ability to readily accept electrons. Intracellular oxygen-derived free radicals are generated by various enzyme reactions, mitochondrial electron transport, and endoplasmic reticulum and nuclear membrane electron transport.

Several cellular defenses protect against the potentially harmful effects of oxygen free radicals normally generated as a physiologic by-product. Superoxide and hydrogen peroxide are decomposed by enzymes to water and molecular oxygen before they contribute to hydroxyl radical formation. The enzymes involved in dismutation are superoxide dismutase, catalase, and glutathione peroxidase. Nonenzymatic lines of defense also scavenge residual free radicals that escape these enzyme systems. This includes vitamin E, which reduces various radical species; and ascorbate, vitamin A, and $\beta$-carotene, which are radical scavengers. During the time of reperfusion and generation of supraphysiologic levels of free radicals, all of the natural defenses are quickly overwhelmed.

## ROLE OF THE NEUTROPHIL

The initial generation of oxygen free radicals occurs primarily in vascular endothelial cells during the re-perfusion period. However, in addition to creating cellular injury these radicals are also responsible for neutrophil chemotaxis and activation. Once adhered to the endothelium, neutrophils mediate damage by secretion of additional oxygen free radicals and proteolytic enzymes. In addition, the increased adhesiveness of neutrophils, cellular swelling from neutrophil injury, and the large number of neutrophils involved may contribute to mechanical obstruction of some capillary beds. This sequence of events is called the "no-reflow" phenomenon. Ischemia continues in these tissue beds and results in necrosis due to the inability to reestablish blood flow.

The steps in chemotaxis related to oxygen radical production are not well understood. However, arachidonic acid, complement, and superoxide anion appear to be key factors. In the presence of superoxide, arachidonic acid products activated by increased intracellular calcium are thought to be primarily responsible for neutrophil chemotaxis, adherence, and activation. The result of neutrophil activation is lysis of structural proteins, lipid peroxidation with perpetuation of reperfusion injury leading to increased microvascular permeability, and cellular injury or death. Reperfusion causes tissue injury that is considerably more severe than injury created by ischemia alone. Neutrophils are the major cause of this additional tissue injury.

The severity of metabolic injury that occurs during the reperfusion period is influenced by the duration and severity of ischemia. Complete ischemia results in death of 100% of the cells in the affected area in a length of time varying from minutes to hours. The time lapse before cells die is influenced by temperature, anaerobic glycolysis, available stored substrate (primarily glycogen), and other factors. Increasing ischemia from 30 to 90 min results in marked intracellular calcium rises and ATP depletion. In general, as the duration of ischemia increases, the severity of ischemic injury increases as measured by percentage of tissue necrosis. Therefore, the longer the period of ischemia, the greater the extent of ischemic injury and reperfusion injury. In the experimental setting, tissue injury can be significantly reduced by filtering blood to reduce the number of neutrophils perfusing the affected area or by the administration of neutrophil monoclonal antibodies to reduce neutrophil adhesiveness. This underscores the importance of neutrophils in the pathogenesis of reperfusion injury.

## TREATMENT FOR REPERFUSION INJURY

Because the duration and severity of ischemia contribute directly to tissue injury and augment reperfusion injury, shock resuscitation therapy to improve tissue perfusion is essential. Many drugs are currently being investigated for their ability to modify or eliminate effects of oxygen-derived free radicals. Experimental studies have revealed that many drugs are effective; however, the laboratory setting can only partially mimic the clinical physiopathogenesis of certain conditions. Unfortunately, specific treatment recommendations with drugs designed to limit oxygen radical production and effects cannot be made at this time due to the lack of clinical experience and well-controlled prospective clinical trials.

Generation of oxygen free radicals occurs very rapidly after the onset of reperfusion. The detrimental effects that radicals cause can best be ameliorated if the drugs are in the tissues at the time of reperfusion. This will allow them to interrupt the cascade of radical development and thus limit cell damage. The drug(s) should be administered intravenously at the start of shock therapy.

Two promising approaches to drug therapy are: (1) chelation of iron and (2) scavenging of radicals. Deferoxamine chelates ferrous iron, which prevents activation of the Haber-Weiss reaction, and therefore inhibits production of the hydroxyl radicals. It effectively attenuates reperfusion injury.

Dimethylsulfoxide (DMSO) is a scavenger of hydroxyl radicals. Its metabolite, dimethyl sulfide, traps other oxygen-derived free radicals. However, the effectiveness of radical scavenging of DMSO in the context of reperfusion injury is controversial (see "Use and Misuse of DMSO," this volume, p 68). Other radical scavengers include mannitol and superoxide dismutase, however these drugs may be more appropriate for chronic inflammatory conditions. Another class of radical scavengers are 21-aminosteroids. These drugs have proven effective in the scavenging of all oxygen and lipid radicals. They are also more effective than deferoxamine in the binding and inactivation of iron.

Allopurinol is a specific inhibitor of xanthine oxidase, thereby preventing the development of superoxide an-

ions at the time of reperfusion. Experimentally, allopurinol has been most effective when administered before the onset of ischemia. Prevention of conversion of xanthine dehydrogenase to xanthine oxidase also has been accomplished experimentally with protease inhibitors and calcium channel blockers.

## References and Suggested Reading

Flaherty JT and Weisfeldt ML: Reperfusion injury. Free Rad Biol Med 5: 409, 1988.
*An in-depth review of experimental studies of reperfusion injury pathophysiology.*

Gutteridge JMC and Halliwell B: Reoxygenation injury and antioxidant protection: A tale of two paradoxes. Arch Biochem Biophys 283:223, 1990.
*A review of the generation and prevention of reperfusion injury.*

Hagland U and Gerdin B: Oxygen-free radicals (OFR) and circulatory shock. Circ Shock 34:405, 1991.
*A review of experimental evidence of reperfusion injury in shock.*

Hitt ME: Oxygen-derived free radicals: Pathophysiology and implications. Compend Cont Educ Pract Vet 10:939, 1988.
*A review of oxygen radical generation and their potential role in various diseases.*

McCord JM: Oxygen-derived free radicals in postischemic tissue injury. N Engl J Med 312:159, 1985.
*A discussion of the theory of reperfusion injury.*

Opie LH and Phil D: Reperfusion injury and its pharmacologic modification. Circulation 80:1049, 1989.
*A review of modulating the tissue effects of oxygen radicals by different types of drugs.*

Vedder NB, Fouth BW, Winn RK, et al: Role of neutrophils in generalized reperfusion injury associated with resuscitation from shock. Surgery 106: 509, 1989.
*A review of neutrophil function in shock.*

Welbourn CRB, Goldman G, Paterson IS, et al: Pathophysiology of ischaemia reperfusion injury: Central role of the neutrophil. Br J Surg 78:651, 1991.
*A review of the neutrophil role in reperfusion injury and potential methods of alternating neutrophil-induced tissue injury.*

Zimmerman JJ: Therapeutic application of oxygen radical scavengers. Chest 100:189S, 1991.
*A review of pharmacologic manipulation of oxygen radicals by radical scavengers in the experimental setting.*

# USE AND MISUSE OF DMSO

CORY F. BRAYTON
*New York, New York*

*and* WAYNE SCHWARK
*Ithaca, New York*

Dimethyl sulfoxide (DMSO) is a powerful organic solvent used widely in industry. In veterinary and human clinical situations it is used primarily as anti-inflammatory and analgesic agent, and as a translocator and potentiator of other therapeutic agents (Brayton, 1986; David, 1972; Jacob, 1986; Kligman, 1965; Knowles, 1967).DMSO's greatest toxic potential probably lies in its intended or unintended combinations with substances that it translocates and potenti-

ates (Brayton, 1986; Rubin, 1983; Schuh, Ross, and Meschter, 1988).

## FDA-APPROVED APPLICATIONS OF DMSO

The only DMSO-containing products approved by the Food and Drug Administration (FDA) for veterinary use are **Domoso** and **Synotic** *(Syntex Animal*

*Health Inc, Des Moines, IA).* **Domoso**, 90% DMSO, in gel or liquid formulations, is approved for use in dogs and horses "as a topical application to reduce acute swelling due to trauma" (package insert). **Synotic**, 60% DMSO and 0.01% fluocinolone acetonide otic solution, is approved for use in dogs "for the relief of pruritus and inflammation associated with acute and chronic otitis" (package insert). **Rimso-50**, 50% w/w aqueous DMSO solution, (Research Industries Corp, Midvale UT) is the only product approved for use in humans and only for intravesical administration to patients with interstitial cystitis. **Cryoserv**, 100% DMSO, (Research Industries Corp, Midvale UT), used in cryopreservation, is not approved for medicinal use. Industrial grade DMSO in concentrations of 90 to 100% may be readily obtained from distributors of chemicals and pharmaceuticals, and may be found in some "health food stores" and drug stores. Although industrial-grade DMSO may contain impurities, it is used widely by veterinary and medical professionals and by the lay population. Some states have laws or statutes that permit physicians to use DMSO for applications other than those specifically approved by the FDA (CBPC).

## PHYSICAL, CHEMICAL, AND BIOLOGIC CHARACTERISTICS

DMSO is a clear, colorless to yellow liquid that freezes at 18.5°C (67°F). Concentrated preparations of DMSO freeze in the refrigerator. A sample that does not solidify is either dilute or impure.

DMSO is extremely hygroscopic. It dilutes rapidly to a concentration of 66 to 67% when exposed to ambient air. Therefore, containers of DMSO should be airtight and closed tightly after use.

DMSO is a bipolar nondissociable solvent. Substances that are not water soluble dissolve readily in DMSO. Some rubber or plastic materials (as in gloves or containers) are penetrated by DMSO (David, 1972).

Hydration of DMSO is exothermic. The heat evolved can be detected when concentrated solutions ($\geq$90%) are mixed with aqueous solutions, or are applied to skin and react with water from air and from underlying tissue.

DMSO acts as an antifreeze at concentrations of 20% (5M) or lower, because its hydrogen bonding with water molecules interferes with their tendency to form a crystalline matrix (ice). DMSO is effective in cryopreservation of cells and tissues (Brayton, 1986; Jacob, 1986).

DMSO is an effective scavenger of hydroxyl radicals (·OH) (Brayton, 1986; Jacob, 1986). In certain experimental systems investigators use DMSO to detect or eliminate hydroxyl radicals.

DMSO inhibits or stimulates various enzymes *in vitro* and *in vivo*, depending on its concentration and other conditions. DMSO is a powerful inhibitor of cholinesterases and of alcohol dehydrogenase (Brayton, 1986; David, 1972; Jacob, 1986).

## PHYSIOLOGIC AND PHARMACOLOGIC EFFECTS, AND TOXICITY

DMSO readily penetrates skin and other membrane barriers. It most effectively penetrates skin in concentrations of 80% or greater. Within minutes of topical or parenteral administration to animals, a characteristic garlic-like or oyster-like halitosis or generalized odor usually is discerned, and may be quite objectionable. The odor is caused by the dimethyl sulfide (DMS) metabolite. Within 20 minutes of topical application, DMSO is found in all organs of the body. Unlike most penetrating solvents, penetration is not associated with irreversible membrane damage. After topical or parenteral administration to animals, most DMSO is excreted unchanged in the urine. Some is metabolized to dimethyl sulfone ($DMSO_2$); small amounts are excreted in feces and metabolized to DMS (Blythe et al., 1986; David, 1972).

DMSO transports or "translocates" many substances across membrane barriers, and influences pharmacologic effects of some substances *in vivo*. It enhances cutaneous and/or mucous membrane penetration of various dyes, local anesthetic agents, salicylates, tetracyclines, antiperspirants, testosterone, phenylbutazone, heparin, sulfadiazine, curare, and other compounds (Brayton, 1986; David, 1972; Jacob, 1986; Kligman, 1965; Knowles, 1967). Because corticosteroids are translocated readily, topical application of DMSO with corticosteroids can produce high tissue levels and systemic effects (Brayton, 1986; David, 1972; Kligman, 1965). Effects of insulin are potentiated when DMSO is administered topically or parenterally (Brayton, 1986). Effective and toxic doses of digitalis compounds are reduced by DMSO (Jacob, 1986; Rubin, 1983). Anesthetic and toxic effects of barbiturates are enhanced when DMSO is administered topically or parenterally (Brayton, 1986; David, 1972). Organophosphate penetration and toxicity is markedly enhanced when administrated with DMSO (Knowles, 1967). DMSO's own anticholinesterase activity likely contributes to this toxic effect. Lethal results in horses are attributed to heavy metal (mercury) poisoning after topical applications of mercury-containing "red" blister with DMSO.

DMSO has anti-inflammatory effects, and can protect against ischemic insult and ionizing radiation (Brayton, 1986; Jacob, 1986). Although other mechanisms may be involved, these effects are mediated largely via scavenging of hydroxyl radicals. Free radicals are released from leukocytes (neutrophils and macrophages predominantly) in inflammatory processes, and from cells injured by ischemia or ionizing radiation. Timely application of an effective radical scavenger can protect adjacent cells from radical-mediated injury.

"Membrane stabilizing" effects of DMSO also are considered to contribute to its anti-inflammatory and protective effects (Jacob, 1986). "Stabilization" of platelet and lysosomal membranes reduces or slows release of inflammatory mediators. "Membrane stabilization" may also contribute significantly to protection against other insults (e.g., radiation, freezing, ischemia).

Paradoxically, however, DMSO causes hemolysis *in vitro* and *in vivo* (Blythe et al., 1986; David, 1972). The hemolytic effect *in vivo* is exacerbated when intravenous administration is rapid and the DMSO concentration is greater than 40%.

DMSO has varied effects on coagulability (Brayton, 1986; Jacob, 1986; Rubin, 1983). Its antithrombotic or antithrombogenic activity possibly contribute to its protective effect against ischemic insult.

DMSO is reported to have an excellent analgesic effect for some types of pain. The primary mechanism of analgesia may be slowed conductance in nerve fibers, especially nonmyelinated, C-type, somatosensory (pain) fibers (Evans, Reid, and Sharp, 1993).

DMSO degranulates mast cells. Local vasodilation and "wheal and flare" after topical application of DMSO is histamine mediated (Kligman, 1965). The potential for massive and morbid histamine release after administration of DMSO to animals with undetected mast cell tumor should be considered.

Toxicity of DMSO is considered to be low (Brayton, 1986; David, 1972; Jacob, 1986; Kligman, 1965; Knowles, 1967; Rubin, 1983). Median lethal doses ($LD_{50}$) of DMSO administered topically, orally, or parenterally to various species are high. Ocular toxicity of DMSO has been reported in laboratory animals; concerns about design and documentation of some human and non-human animal trials precipitated DMSO's withdrawal from Investigational New Drug (IND) status by the FDA (Brayton, 1986; Rubin, 1983).

Teratogenic effects of DMSO have been reported in laboratory animals. Therefore, such effects on a pregnant recipient or administrator of DMSO should be considered (Knowles, 1967; Rubin, 1983).

The greatest toxic potential of DMSO probably lies in its combination with other compounds that it translocates or potentiates, or both (Brayton, 1986; David, 1972; Knowles, 1967; Rubin, 1983; Schuh, Ross, and Meschter, 1988). Such combinations may be: (1) unintended, (2) due to contamination of the source of DMSO, (3) due to contamination of materials with which or in which DMSO is administered, (4) due to skin contamination, or (5) due to concomitant therapies.

## REPORTED AND POTENTIAL CLINICAL APPLICATIONS

Therapeutic applications of DMSO generally take advantage of: (1) penetration, (2) translocation, (3) potentiation of some agents *in vivo*, (4) radical scavenging, and (5) analgesia.

Acute traumatic injury is the condition for which topical application of Domoso is approved. Reported positive effects of DMSO on bruises, strains, and so forth vary from equivocal to remarkable. An anecdotal caution is that DMSO may mask pain and swelling due to fractures.

DMSO is commonly recommended to treat central nervous system (CNS) trauma and consequent cerebral edema. In horses, dogs, cats, and humans, a therapeutic dose of 1.0 gm/kg, in a 10 to 45% solution, administered slowly, IV has been recommended (Blythe et al., 1986).

Free radicals, especially hydroxyl radicals, are believed to be largely responsible for "reperfusion injury." Situations wherein an ischemic area is reperfused (as in surgical correction of intestinal torsions, intestinal volvuli, or canine gastric dilatation-volvulus [GDV], or intraoperative situations where blood supply to an area is abrogated temporarily [e.g., tourniquet]) may benefit from timely application of radical scavengers based on experimental studies. Results with DMSO therapy have been mixed (Arden et al., 1989). Other agents that interfere with the radical cascade, such as the iron chelator deferoxamine, have shown promising results in treatment of GDV (Lantz et al., 1992).

In endotoxemia, where beneficial effects from DMSO radical scavenging might be expected, DMSO may exacerbate hypotensive and hypoglycemic effects of endotoxin (Semrad, 1993).

"Differentiation" of certain immortalized or neoplastic cell lines by DMSO *in vitro* is reported (Kohlhuber, Strobl, and Eick, 1993). Reports vary concerning its efficacy as an antineoplastic or chemotherapeutic agent in different experimental systems.

DMSO dissolves amyloid fibrils and alters precipitability of Bence Jones proteins *in vitro* (Brayton, 1986; Jacob, 1986). Varied clinical responses to treatment of amyloidosis in humans, dogs, and cats are reported.

DMSO is collagenolytic and inhibits fibroblast proliferation *in vitro* (Brayton, 1986; Jacob, 1986). Varied clinical effects of DMSO therapy in connective tissue disorders and in fibrosing conditions such as scarring, peritoneal adhesions, scleroderma (human), and endometrial fibrosis (equine) are reported.

Combinations of DMSO with steroids, nonsteroidal anti-inflammatory drugs (NSAIDs), antiviral agents, antibiotics, antifungal agents, parasiticidal agents, and other compounds have been reported to be beneficial (Stone, 1993). In contrast, minimal and occasionally morbid effects have been reported when DMSO was used to treat a variety of conditions including persistent cutaneous ulcers; "canine lick granulomas"; viral, bacterial, and mycotic dermatitides; and habronemiasis ("summer sores" in horses). Anecdotes and empiric reports are abundant and should be interpreted with caution. The toxic potential of such combinations should be appreciated.

## CONCLUSIONS

DMSO's therapeutic potential has not been investigated thoroughly. Well-controlled, double-blind studies required for FDA approval are difficult to design because of DMSO's characteristic odor, and because often the data involve subjective evaluations (e.g., pain, range of movement, return to function, neurologic assessment). DMSO is relatively inexpensive to produce, and is readily available. Such considerations render

DMSO of little potential profit or interest to the pharmaceutical industry.

The toxicity of DMSO, by itself, is sufficiently low that it does not deter clinicians or members of the lay population from nonapproved applications. Intraperitoneal, intravenous, intra-articular, intrathecal, intrauterine, and intravesical routes for administration of DMSO have been used to treat a variety of conditions. The vast majority of these situations constitute "extra-label" drug use. In today's regulatory environment, clinicians must consider seriously the consequences of such actions (see "Unapproved Use of Drugs in Small Animals," this volume, p 48). Investigators must be judicious when they publish recommendations for such use.

## References and Suggested Reading

Arden W, Stick J, Parks A, Chou C-C, and Slocombe R: Effects of ischemia and dimethyl sulfoxide on equine jejunal vascular resistance, oxygen consumption, intraluminal pressure, and potassium loss. Am J Vet Res 50:380, 1989.

Blythe L, Craig A, Christensen J, Appell L, and Slizeski M: Pharmacokinetic disposition of dimethyl sulfoxide administered intravenously to horses. Am J Vet Res 47:1738, 1986.

Brayton C: Dimethyl sulfoxide (DMSO): A review. Cornell Vet 76:61, 1986.

California Business and Professions Code: California Pharmacy Laws: Section 4212: DMSO.

David N: The pharmacology of DMSO 654. Ann Rev Pharmacol 12:353, 1972.

Evans MS, Reid KH, and Sharp JB Jr: Dimethylsulfoxide (DMSO) blocks conduction in peripheral nerve C fibers: A possible mechanism of analgesia. Neurosci Lett 150:145, 1993.

Jacob S, and Herschler R: Pharmacology of DMSO. Cryobiology 23:4, 1986.

Kligman A: Topical pharmacology and toxicology of dimethyl sulfoxide, part 1. JAMA 193:140, 1965.

Knowles R: Clinical experience with DMSO in small animal practice. Ann NY Acad Sci 141:478, 1967.

Kohlhuber F, Strobl L, and Eick, D: Early down-regulation of c-myc in dimethyl sulfoxide-induced mouse erythroleukemia (MEL) cells is mediated at the p1/p2 promoters. Oncogene 8:1099, 1993.

Lantz G, Badylak S, Hiles M, and Arkin T: Treatment of reperfusion injury in dogs with experimentally induced gastric dilatation-volvulus. Am J Vet Res 53:1594, 1992.

Rubin L: Toxicity of dimethyl sulfoxide, alone and in combination. Ann NY Acad Sci 243:98, 1983.

Schuh J, Ross C, and Meschter C: Concurrent mercuric blister and dimethyl sulfoxide (DMSO) application as a cause of mercury toxicity in two horses. Equine Vet J 20:68, 1988.

Semrad S: Comparison of flunixin, prednisolone, dimethyl sulfoxide, and a lazaroid (U74389F) for treating endotoxemic neonatal calves. Am J Vet Res 54:1517, 1993.

Stone RW: Clinical update on the use of dimethyl sulfoxide. Can Practice 18:16, 1993.

# USES AND MISUSES OF ASPIRIN

MOLLYANN HOLLAND
*and* C. B. CHASTAIN
*Columbia, Missouri*

Aspirin is one of the most-consumed drugs in the United States. It is available in plain, coated, buffered, timed-released, and enteric-coated tablets of various strengths.

For centuries, willow bark was known to have antipyretic effects. This was found to be due to the presence of salicin. In 1829, Leroux isolated sodium salicylate from salicin. Hoffman, a chemist for the Bayer Company, first prepared acetylsalicylic acid, which was also called aspirin. Aspirin began to be marketed around the turn of the century and was shown to have anti-inflammatory and analgesic effects (Fuster et al., 1993).

## CLINICAL PHARMACOLOGY

Aspirin is readily absorbed from the stomach and upper small intestine in both dogs and cats. After absorption, aspirin is hydrolyzed to salicylic acid, which is about 70 to 90% bound to plasma proteins, especially albumin. Salicylate is later conjugated with glucuronate and glycine and excreted in the urine. The rates of elimination vary among species, with the half-life of salicylate ranging from 8 hr in the dog to 38 hr in the cat (Davis, 1980). Cats have a relative deficiency of glucuronate, which accounts for the prolonged elimination time in that species. Aspirin has a relatively long shelf life, but when it ages, aspirin will decompose into acetic acid, which emits a vinegar odor, and salicylic acid.

## MECHANISM OF ACTION

The usefulness of aspirin is dependent upon its anti-inflammatory, analgesic, antithrombotic, and antipyretic properties. Aspirin produces these effects by inhibiting prostaglandin (PG) synthesis through inhibition of the cyclooxygenase enzyme. Prostaglandins' actions include vasoconstriction, vasodilation, and platelet aggregation. They may also cause myalgia and fever.

Prostaglandins are unsaturated fatty acid compounds derived from 20-carbon essential fatty acids, of which the most important is arachidonic acid. Prostaglandins are considered local hormones, as they exert their primary effects at their site of production. Prostaglandins

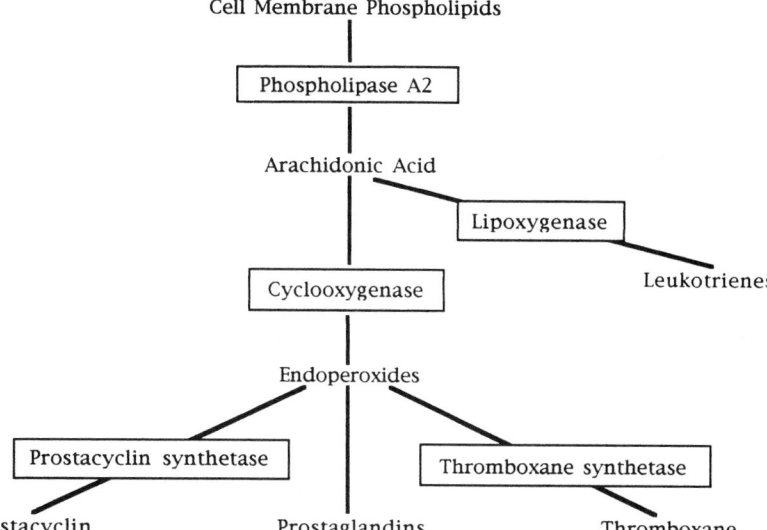

**Figure 1.** Biosynthesis of prostaglandins and related substances from arachidonic acid.

are not stored, and their synthesis occurs immediately before release. Their synthesis is initiated by the release of arachidonic acid from the phospholipid pool of cell membranes. The stimuli for arachidonic acid release is phospholipase $A_2$ or mechanical trauma to the cell membrane (Clive and Stoff, 1984). Arachidonic acid is then converted by cyclooxygenase to the cyclic endoperoxide $PGG_2$, or by lipoxygenase to leukotrienes. The endoperoxide is degraded to $PGH_2$, which is further degraded to prostaglandins of the D, E, or F series (Fig. 1). Aspirin exerts its effects by irreversibly acetylating the cyclooxygenase enzyme. Most cells can synthesize new cyclooxygenase, but platelets do not have this ability. Aspirin does not affect lipoxygenase.

### Anti-Inflammation

Several prostaglandins are responsible for manifestations of the inflammatory response such as vasodilation, increased vascular permeability, edema, leukocyte migration, and local pain (Jenkins, 1987). Aspirin decreases the inflammatory response by inhibiting the cyclooxygenase enzyme and decreasing PG synthesis. Aspirin also suppresses the release of several inflammatory mediators including bradykinin, hista-

mine, and serotonin, and causes an uncoupling of the oxidative phosphorylation of adenosine diphosphate. This latter effect decreases the energy available to sustain an inflammatory response (Davis, 1980). A recommended anti-inflammatory dose of aspirin in the dog is up to 25 mg/kg, every 8 hr and in the cat up to 25 mg/kg, every 24 hr.

### Analgesia

Prostaglandins, especially PGE and $PGI_2$, have a major role in peripheral nociception. They bind to receptors on sensory nerve endings, which facilitate the discharge of impulses and intensify pain (Jenkins, 1987). Aspirin acts peripherally to block the production of inflammatory mediators, which would irritate sensory nerve endings. Therefore, mild to moderate somatic pain resulting from inflammation of joints, tendons, muscles, or superficial wounds responds well to aspirin therapy. Aspirin is not effective in severe somatic or visceral pain (Davis, 1980). A recommended analgesic dose of aspirin in dogs is 10 to 20 mg/kg, every 12 hr, and in cats is 10 mg/kg, every 48 hr.

**Table 1.** *Aspirin Doses for Dogs and Cats*

| Species | Dose° | Time Interval | Route |
|---|---|---|---|
| Dogs | | | |
|   Anti-inflammatory | 25 mg/kg | q8h | PO |
|   Analgesic | 10–20 mg/kg | q12h | PO |
|   Antithrombotic | 0.5 mg/kg | q12h | PO |
| | 10 mg/kg | q24h | PO |
|   Antipyretic | 10 mg/kg | q12h | PO |
| Cats | | | |
|   Anti-inflammatory | 25 mg/kg | q24h | PO |
|   Analgesic | 10 mg/kg | q48h | PO |
|   Antithrombotic | 25 mg/kg | q56–84h | PO |
|   Antipyretic | 10 mg/kg | q48h | PO |

°See precautions in text. Therapeutic doses are frequently associated with gastric irritation, erosion, or ulceration.

## Antithrombotic

When the endothelium of blood vessels is damaged or stretched from hypertension, the subendothelial tissue is exposed, allowing platelet attachment. Arachidonic acid released from both the platelet and from the vessel wall is converted to thromboxanes and prostacyclin. Thromboxanes cause vasoconstriction, which promotes platelet aggregation; and prostacyclin causes vasodilation, which inhibits platelet aggregation. There is, therefore, a delicate balance between maintaining adequate hemostasis and preventing excessive platelet aggregation, which can lead to thromboembolism (Conlon, 1988).

The antithrombotic effects of aspirin were not recognized until the 1960s. By acetylating cyclooxygenase, aspirin prevents the formation of thromboxane, which promotes platelet aggregation. However, aspirin also prevents the formation of prostacyclin, which inhibits platelet aggregation. A dose-related response permits the use of aspirin to inhibit selectively thromboxane formation. Lower doses result in irreversible acetylation of cyclooxygenase in platelets, while allowing nucleated endothelial cells to produce additional cyclooxygenase. Thus, endothelial cells will still produce prostacylin.

In dogs, aspirin's antithrombotic effect has its most important use during the treatment of dirofilariasis. Adult *Dirofilaria immitis* damage the endothelium of pulmonary arteries. This causes platelet adherence and aggregation, which eventually leads to myointimal proliferation. Myointimal proliferation causes an increase in pulmonary vascular resistance pressure, and may lead to right-sided heart failure. By inhibiting platelet adherence, aspirin can decrease pulmonary vascular lesions seen in thiacetarsamide-treated dogs. In heartworm-infected dogs, aspirin has been recommended at doses ranging from 0.5 mg/kg, every 12 hr, to 10 mg/kg, every 24 hr for 4 weeks after adulticide therapy (Keith, Rawlings, and Schaub, 1983; Rackear, Feldman, and Farver, 1988). Use of aspirin for this purpose is controversial, however. The 1992 American Heartworm Society advocated anti-inflammatory doses of corticosteroids rather than aspirin for the treatment of severe thromboembolism, particularly to reduce lung parenchymal injury. Due to the narrow margin of safety of aspirin dosages in cats, it is not recommended during adulticide therapy (Rawlings, 1990).

Aspirin has been used in cats with cardiomyopathy. Atrial enlargement associated with cardiomyopathy results in platelet aggregation and thrombus formation. These thrombi often embolize, occluding systemic arteries such as the distal aorta, external iliac arteries, renal arteries, or mesenteric arteries. Aspirin can be used to minimize formation of thromboemboli in cats with cardiomyopathy; however, there are no studies demonstrating either efficacy or a lack thereof (see "Coumadin," this volume, p 868). The recommended antithrombotic dose of aspirin in cats is 25 mg/kg, every 56 to 84 hr.

## Antipyretic

Aspirin has no effect on normal body temperature, but it does act to normalize body temperature if a fever is present. Aspirin lowers fever in two ways. Centrally, it acts on the hypothalamus, which is normally responsible for maintaining body temperature. Peripherally aspirin causes vasodilation and heat dissipation (Davis, 1980). A recommended antipyretic dose of aspirin in dogs is 10 mg/kg, every 12 hr, and in cats is 10 mg/kg, every 48 hr.

## SIDE EFFECTS

### Gastrointestinal

The most common side effect of aspirin therapy is gastric irritation. Prostaglandin E and $PGI_2$ decrease the volume, acidity, and pepsin content of gastric secretions. Prostaglandins also stimulate secretion of bicarbonate by epithelial cells. In addition, they play a cytoprotective role by producing vasodilation of the gastric mucosa and by increasing gastric and small-intestinal mucus production. Turnover and repair of gastrointestinal epithelial cells are stimulated by prostaglandins. Loss of these protective mechanisms due to cyclooxygenase inhibition by aspirin can lead to mucosal erosions, ulcerations, hemorrhage, anemia, and death.

Local irritation and damage from aspirin hydrolysis to salicylic acid can also contribute to formation of gastroduodenal ulcers.

Several medications are available for treatment of gastrointestinal ulceration caused by aspirin. Cimetidine (Tagamet, SmithKline and French Laboratories), an $H_2$ antagonist, given at a dose of 5 to 10 mg/kg, every 6 to 8 hr, may speed recovery of gastric ulcers induced by aspirin therapy. However, if aspirin therapy is continued during ulcer treatment, cimetidine is ineffective (Jenkins et al., 1991). Omeprazole (Prilosec, Merck, Sharpe & Dohme) is a substituted benzimidazole. It inhibits the hydrogen-potassium ATPase that produces hydrogen ions in parietal cells. Omeprazole is more effective at reducing gastric acidity than cimetidine. Because it is effective for 24 hr, it need be administered only once daily. The recommended dose for omeprazole is 0.7 mg/kg, every 24 hr. (Jenkins et al., 1991). Misoprostol (Cytotec, G. D. Searle & Co) is a $PGE_1$ analogue. Since PGE is one of the prostaglandins normally responsible for gastrointestinal protection, development of a synthetic PGE provides specific drug for prevention and therapy of gastroduodenal ulcers. The dose of misoprostol is 2 to 5 $\mu$g/kg, every 8 hr (Murtaugh et al., 1993).

### Renal

Prostaglandins help regulate renal blood flow. Conditions that cause vasoconstriction, such as dehydration, congestive heart failure, or shock, induce prostaglandin synthesis. Prostaglandin $E_2$ and $PGI_2$ then produce a compensatory vasodilation that increases renal blood flow.

Because prostaglandins are more important in maintaining normal renal perfusion under adverse conditions, patients receiving long-term aspirin therapy are at increased risk of acute renal failure following a renal insult. Long-term, high-dose aspirin therapy may also increase the risk of developing chronic renal failure characterized by renal papillary necrosis. The proposed mechanism is medullary ischemia due to the loss of vasodilation (Clive and Stoff, 1984).

Aspirin use may also lead to sodium retention. In response to vasoconstriction, renal blood flow is redistributed from the cortical nephrons to the juxtamedullary nephrons. These nephrons have an increased ability to absorb sodium. Sodium retention may aggravate hypertension if present (Clive and Stoff, 1984).

## CONTRAINDICATIONS

Aspirin should not be administered to patients with coagulation disorders, and it should be discontinued in any patient 1 week prior to surgery to avoid increased bleeding times. It should be avoided in patients with known gastrointestinal ulceration. Aspirin should be used cautiously in patients with hypoalbuminemia, since the drug will be more metabolically active due to decreased plasma binding.

## FORM OF ASPIRIN

Aspirin is available in many different forms. One of the most commonly recommended is antacid-buffered aspirin. However, the amount of antacid buffering is insufficient to protect the gastrointestinal system. Enteric-coated forms may offer more protection from gastric ulceration; however, the coating may not dissolve, leading to passage of an intact tablet or to erratic drug absorption. Film-coated aspirin manufactured by one of the major drug companies (versus a generic product) is probably more reliable in its stability and absorption. Administering the aspirin with a meal is advisable to decrease the risk of gastric irritation; however, systemic effects of aspirin may still promote gastric ulceration.

## References and Suggested Reading

Clive DM, and Stoff JS: Renal syndromes associated with nonsteroidal anti-inflammatory drug. N Engl J Med 310:563, 1984.
*A review of the physiology and clinical manifestations of the effects of nonsteroidal anti-inflammatory drugs on the renal system.*

Conlon PD: Nonsteroidal drugs used in the treatment of inflammation. Vet Clin North Am [Small Anim Prac] 18:1115, 1988.
*A review of aspirin and other nonsteroidal anti-inflammatory drugs used in the treatment of inflammation.*

Davis LE: Clinical pharmacology of salicylates. J Am Vet Med Assoc 176:65, 1980.
*A review of the pharmacologic effects, dose recommendations, clinical uses, and toxic side effects of aspirin.*

Fuster V, Dyken ML, Vokonas PS, et al: Aspirin as a therapeutic agent in cardiovascular disease. Circulation 87:659, 1993.
*A report on the uses of aspirin in various forms of cardiac disease.*

Jenkins CC, DeNovo RC, Patton CS, et al: Comparison of effects of cimetidine and omeprazole on mechanically created gastric ulceration and on aspirin-induced gastritis in dogs. Am J Vet Res 52:658, 1991.
*A prospective study comparing gastric ulcer healing time in dogs treated with cimetidine or omeprazole.*

Jenkins WL: Pharmacologic aspects of analgesic drugs in animals: An overview. J Am Vet Med Assoc 191:1231, 1987.
*A review of the pharmacologic aspects of opioid and nonopioid analgesics in small animals.*

Keith JC, Rawlings CA, and Schaub RG: Pulmonary thromboembolism during therapy of dirofilariasis with thiacetarsamide: Modification with aspirin or prednisolone. Am J Vet Res 44:1278, 1983.
*A prospective study comparing the pulmonary vascular and perivascular lesions in dogs treated with thiacetarsamide following experimental infection with* Dirofilaria immitis.

Murtaugh RJ, Matz ME, Labato MA, et al: Use of synthetic prostaglandin $E_1$ (misoprostol) for prevention of aspirin-induced gastroduodenal ulceration in arthritic dogs. J Am Vet Med Assoc 202:251, 1993.
*A prospective study evaluating the endoscopic changes associated with aspirin or aspirin/misoprostol therapy in arthritic dogs.*

Rackear D, Feldman B, and Farver T: The effect of three different dosages of acetylsalicylic acid on canine platelet aggregation. J Am Anim Hosp Assoc 24:23, 1988.
*A prospective study evaluating effects of different doses of aspirin on platelet aggregation in normal dogs.*

Rawlings CA: Pulmonary arteriography and hemodynamics during feline heartworm disease. J Vet Intern Med 4:285, 1990.
*A prospective study evaluating effects of aspirin during treatment in cats experimentally infected with* Dirofilaria immitis.

# CYCLOSPORINE

SHELLY L. VADEN
*Raleigh, North Carolina*

Cyclosporine (Cy) was discovered serendipitously while screening fungal products for antibiotic properties. It was later shown to be a potent inhibitor of T-cell activation and is now the drug of choice for preventing allograft rejection. There have been over 15,000 papers published about Cy. This vast list of references reflects the importance of Cy usage, not only as a therapeutic agent, but also as a probe to study immunologic mechanisms. Despite the extensive study of this agent in human medicine and research laboratories, there is a relative paucity of information regarding Cy in the veterinary literature. The purpose of this article is to provide a brief review of the mechanism of action, pharmacokinetics, expected drug interactions and toxicities, and clinical usage of Cy in veterinary medicine.

## MECHANISM OF ACTION

Although Cy has been in clinical use for over a decade, it is only recently that a more thorough understanding of its mechanism of action has been attained. Cyclosporine is functionally related to FK506 (Prograf) and rapamycin. These agents bind specific intracellular receptors, called immunophilins, and inhibit calcium-dependent signal transduction pathways leading to T-cell activation. Cyclosporine becomes active only after binding to its intracellular receptor, cyclophilin. The Cy–cyclophilin complex probably inhibits the activity of calcineurin, a calmodulin-dependent protein phosphatase. Inhibition of this phosphatase activity may prevent translocation across the nuclear membrane of the cytoplasmic subunit of NF-AT (nuclear factor of activated T-cells), a factor that is essential for the transcription of the interleukin 2 (IL-2) gene. Blocking IL-2 transcription leads to impaired proliferation of activated T-helper and T-cytotoxic lymphocytes. Cyclosporine also inhibits transcription of α-interferon, a cytokine that provides amplification signals for macrophage and monocyte activation (Schreiber and Crabtree, 1992).

This early inhibitory effect on T cells leads to many secondary effects on the immune response. The production of other cytokines, including IL-3, IL-4, IL-5, tumor necrosis factor-α, macrophage migration inhibition factor, and γ-interferon, may be impaired. Through inhibition of cytokine production and calcium-dependent pathways, Cy indirectly inhibits mononuclear cell function, antigen presentation, mast cell and eosinophil production, histamine and prostaglandin release from mast cells, neutrophil adherence, natural killer cell activity, and growth and differentiation of B-cells (Thomson, 1992).

## PHARMACOKINETICS

The therapeutic index of Cy is low; high concentrations are toxic and low concentrations are ineffective. The clinical use of Cy is further complicated because blood concentrations achieved following a specific dose vary from patient to patient and within each patient over time. These variabilities are largely determined by differences in absorption, distribution, and metabolism.

Blood Cy concentrations are variable following oral administration. Peak concentrations usually occur between 2 and 4 hr after oral administration, but can be delayed in some animals. In general, the bioavailability following oral administration is low, with approximately 15 to 60% of the dose being absorbed (White et al.,

1986). The bioavailability of Cy may increase with prolonged dosing. The drug is extremely lipophilic, and absorption may be increased when Cy is administered with a fatty meal or decreased with cholestasis. Diarrhea will impair gastrointestinal absorption of Cy.

Highest Cy concentrations are attained in fat and liver, with somewhat lower concentrations found in pancreas, kidneys, skin, and heart. Cyclosporine does not readily penetrate the blood-brain barrier. Blood Cy concentrations may also increase over time due to saturation of tissue binding sites. The drug is largely metabolized by the P-450 microsomal enzyme system. Most metabolites undergo biliary excretion, although a small percentage is eliminated in the urine.

## THERAPEUTIC DRUG MONITORING AND DOSING STRATEGIES

Frequent drug monitoring is needed to maintain blood Cy concentrations in an effective range, while avoiding toxicities. Because blood Cy concentrations can change over time, prolonged usage mandates that drug monitoring continue beyond the initial dosing period. Several assays can be used to measure Cy in biologic fluids. Assays that measure only the parent compound are preferred because the immunosuppressive potency of Cy metabolites is unknown, though probably insignificant. Serum, plasma, or whole blood samples can be used, but the hemolysate of whole blood collected in ethylenediaminetetraacetic acid (EDTA) is the matrix of choice. Only a few studies have addressed therapeutic Cy concentrations in veterinary patients. Table 1 summarizes the assays available and recommended trough concentrations, primarily based on human studies. Concentrations needed to suppress lymphocyte responses appear to be similar across species lines.

In general, initial Cy doses of 10 mg/kg PO, every 24 hr in dogs and every 12 hr in cats, should be used. Many cats find Cy oral solution unpalatable, resulting in ptyalism and head shaking, which can in turn lead to subtherapeutic concentrations. An alternative is to give Cy diluted in olive oil (1 to 4% solution), 5 mg/kg OU every 6 hr (Gregory et al., 1989). Cyclosporine can be given IV (4 to 6 mg/kg/day as a 4-hr infusion) to animals that are unable to receive oral medication. Because the diluent used in the IV solution (cremophor) is extremely irritating, care must be taken to prevent its extravasation. Cremophor may cause acute anaphylactoid reactions in dogs.

During the first months of treatment, Cy concentrations should be measured at regular intervals (two to four times monthly) to ensure that desired blood concentrations are maintained. After this time, drug monitoring can be done at somewhat longer intervals (6 to 12 times per year). It is likely that dosage requirements will actually decrease with chronic administration due to increased intestinal absorption and saturation of binding sites.

***Table 1.*** *Assays Available for Measuring Cyclosporine in Biological Fluids*[*]

| Method | Specific for Parent Compound | Matrix | Recommended Trough Concentration (ng/ml) |
|---|---|---|---|
| HPLC | Yes | Whole blood | 100–300[†] |
| | | Whole blood | 250–600[‡] |
| RIA/MAb | Yes | Serum, plasma | 50–125[†] |
| | | Whole blood | 150–400[‡] |
| RIA/PAb | No | Serum, plasma | 50–300[†] |
| | | Whole blood | 200–800[‡] |
| FPIA | No | Serum, plasma | 150–300[†] |
| | | Whole blood | 250–1000[‡] |
| | | Whole blood | 250–400[§] |

[*]Data derived from Sandimmune (cyclosporine) dosing strategies for long-term maintenance therapy. Sandoz Pharmaceutical Corp, East Hanover, NJ, 1992.
[†]Based on human studies.
[‡]Based on feline studies.
[§]Based on canine studies.
Abbreviations: HPLC = high performance liquid chromatography, RIA = radioimmunoassay, MAb = monoclonal antibody, PAb = polyclonal antibody, FPIA = fluorescence polarization immunoassay, TDx.

## DRUG INTERACTIONS

The potential for polypharmacy leading to detrimental drug interactions is great when Cy is used. Numerous drug interactions have been reported that either potentiate the toxicity of Cy or alter blood Cy concentrations. Table 2 lists well-substantiated Cy drug interactions in people (Lake, 1991). Numerous other drugs are listed as having the potential to interact with Cy. Ketoconazole-induced increases in Cy concentrations have been documented in dogs. The use of ketoconazole, diltiazem, and verapamil to increase Cy concentrations, thereby decreasing dosage requirement and expense, has been suggested. However, this should be done only with

***Table 2.*** *Drugs that May Interact with Cyclosporine*

Drugs that may increase cyclosporine concentrations in the blood
  Bromocriptine
  Danazol
  Diltiazem
  Doxycycline
  Erythromycin
  Fluconazole
  Itraconazole
  Ketoconazole
  Methylprednisolone
  Nicardipine
  Verapamil

Drugs that may decrease cyclosporine concentrations in the blood
  Carbamazepine
  Phenobarbital
  Phenytoin
  Rifampin
  Trimethoprim-sulfamethoxazole (IV only)

Drugs that may potentiate cyclosporine-induced renal dysfunction
  Aminoglycosides
  Amphotericin B
  Cimetidine
  Erythromycin
  Ketoconazole
  Melphalan
  Ranitidine
  Vancomycin

extreme caution because these drugs may also obscure the relationship between drug concentration and effect and alter the ratio of parent drug to metabolite, making dosing of Cy even more complicated.

## TOXICITY

As with use of any immunosuppressive agent, Cy administration is associated with an increased risk of infection and malignancy. Lymphoma and lymphoproliferative disorders have been associated with prolonged Cy usage in people and a cat (Gregory et al., 1991). Cats seem to be relatively tolerant of Cy administration, with soft feces being the primary side effect reported (Gregory et al., 1992). However, Cy has caused anorexia, nausea, vomiting, diarrhea, weight loss, gingival hyperplasia, papillomatosis, hirsutism, and involuntary shaking in dogs (Rosenkrantz, Griffin, and Barr, 1989; White et al., 1986). We have found that many dogs developed these effects when their whole-blood concentrations (by fluorescence polarization immunoassay [FPIA]) exceeded 400 ng/ml. Dosage adjustments with reductions in blood concentrations frequently led to abatement of these clinical signs. Vomiting that occurs shortly after drug administration may be avoided by administering Cy with food. Whereas dogs are somewhat resistant to the nephrotoxic side effects of Cy, high doses have been shown to decrease glomerular filtrating rate. There have been a few reports of nephrotoxicity. High Cy concentrations may also cause defective hepatic protein synthesis, inhibition of insulin release, and peripheral insulin resistance in dogs. Additional adverse effects noted in people are hepatotoxicity, hypertension, and paresthesia.

## CLINICAL USAGE

### Transplantation

Cyclosporine has been used in dogs and cats for clinical and research organ transplantation. Renal allografts can be successfully maintained in cats by the use of cyclosporine (7.5 mg/kg every 12 hr) and prednisolone (0.125 to 0.25 mg/kg every 12 hr). Cyclosporine dosages are adjusted to maintain whole-blood trough concentrations (by high-performance liquid chromatography [HPLC]) of 500 ng/ml or greater prior to and for 30 days after transplantation, but can be reduced to maintain concentrations of 250 ng/ml thereafter (Gregory et al., 1992). Renal transplantation in dogs has been less successful, although combining Cy with antilymphocyte serum, fractionated donor bone marrow, rapamycin and/or FK506 hold promise for the future. Cyclosporine has also been used successfully for bone marrow transplantation in cats, and experimentally for pancreatic islet, lung, and other transplantation procedures in dogs.

## Ophthalmologic Disorders

Cyclosporine has been used extensively for the treatment of keratoconjunctivitis sicca (KCS) in dogs (Morgan and Abrams, 1991; Olivero et al., 1991). Cyclosporine oral solution should be diluted in olive oil (by a licensed pharmacist) to make a 1 to 2% solution. When one drop is applied OU every 12 hr, Cy administration is about 80% successful in decreasing corneal neovascularization, pigmentation, and mucoid ocular discharge, and increasing tear secretion. Drug administration can be decreased in some patients to every 24 or 48 hr. It is uncommon that Cy administration can be completely discontinued. The use of a 1.5% solution has also been shown to be beneficial in the treatment of chronic superficial keratitis (pannus) in dogs (Jackson et al., 1991). Systemic side effects generally do not occur following this protocol because there is no appreciable systemic absorption of Cy.

## Dermatologic Disorders

Cyclosporine has been efficacious in the treatment of psoriasis, pemphigus, bullous pemphigoid, male pattern baldness, and dermatomyositis in human patients. However, in one study, only a limited number of dogs with cutaneous immune-mediated skin diseases and none of the dogs with epitheliotrophic lymphoma showed improvement following Cy administration (Rosenkrantz, Griffen, and Barr, 1989). Unfortunately, therapeutic drug monitoring was not employed in this study. Therefore, treatment failure due to subtherapeutic Cy concentrations cannot be ruled out. There is a single case report of a dog with Cy-responsive granulomatous sebaceous adenitis (Carothers, Kwochka, and Rojka, 1991).

## Glomerulonephritis

Results of many studies have demonstrated reduction in proteinuria associated with Cy administration to people with minimal change glomerulopathy, focal segmental glomerulosclerosis, membranous glomerulonephritis, membranoproliferative glomerulonephritis, and mesangioproliferative glomerulonephritis. However, in a prospective, placebo-controlled clinical trial, there was no proven benefit of Cy in reducing proteinuria associated with glomerulonephritis in dogs (Vaden et al., 1991).

## Miscellaneous Disorders

There have been sporadic reports of people with a variety of refractory immune-mediated disorders responding to Cy administration. These conditions include hemolytic anemia, thrombocytopenia, pure red cell aplasia, systemic lupus erythematosus, rheumatoid arthritis, polymyositis, polyradiculoneuritis, and inflammatory bowel disease. High doses of Cy have been used in people to reverse multidrug resistance during cancer chemotherapy, although dosage regimens have not been published for this use in dogs or cats.

## References and Suggested Reading

Carothers MA, Kwochka KW, and Rojko JL: Cyclosporine-responsive granulomatous sebaceous adenitis in a dog. J Am Vet Med Assoc 198:1645, 1991.
*This is a single case report of a dog with dermatologic disease that was treated with Cy.*

Gregory CR, Hietala SK, Pedersen NC, et al: Cyclosporine pharmacokinetics in cats following topical ocular administration. Transplantation 47:516, 1989.
*This paper describes the ocular administration of Cy.*

Gregory CR, Madewell BR, Griffey SM, et al: Feline leukemia virus-associated lymphosarcoma following renal transplantation in a cat. Transplantation 52:1097, 1991.
*This is a single case report in which a cat developed lymphosarcoma while receiving Cy.*

Gregory CR, Gourley IM, Kochin EJ, et al: Renal transplantation for treatment of end-stage renal failure in cats. J Am Vet Med Assoc 201:285, 1992.
*This paper describes the use of Cy in cats for the purposes of preventing renal allograft rejection.*

Jackson PA, Kaswan RL, Merideth RE, et al: Chronic superficial keratitis in dogs: A placebo controlled trial of topical cyclosporine treatment. Prog Vet Comp Ophthalmol 1:269, 1991.
*This paper describes the use of topically administered Cy for the treatment of chronic superficial keratitis in dogs.*

Lake KD: Management of drug interactions with cyclosporine. Pharmacotherapy 11:110S, 1991.
*This paper details potential cyclosporine drug interactions.*

Morgan RV and Abrams KL: Topical administration of cyclosporine for treatment of keratoconjunctivitis sicca in dogs. J Am Vet Med Assoc 199:1043, 1991.
*This paper describes the use of topically administered Cy for the treatment of keratoconjunctivitis sicca in dogs.*

Olivero DK, Davidson MG, English RV, et al: Clinical evaluation of 1% cyclosporine for topical treatment of keratoconjunctivitis sicca in dogs. J Am Vet Med Assoc 199:1039, 1991.
*This paper describes the use of topically administered Cy for the treatment of keratoconjunctivitis sicca in dogs.*

Rosenkrantz WS, Griffin CE, and Barr RJ: Clinical evaluation of cyclosporine in animal models with cutaneous immune-mediated disease and epitheliotrophic lymphoma. J Am Anim Hosp Assoc 25:377, 1989.
*This paper describes the use of Cy for the treatment of specific dermatologic disorders in dogs.*

Schreiber SL and Crabtree GR: The mechanism of action of cyclosporin A and FK506. Immunol Today 13:136, 1992.
*This paper details the proposed mechanism of action of Cy and the related compound, FK506.*

Thomson AW: The effects of cyclosporin A on non-T cell components of the immune system. J Autoimmun 5(SA):167, 1992.

*This paper details the effects that Cy may have on components of the immune system besides its well-characterized effects on T lymphocytes.*
Vaden SL, Armstrong PJ, Polzin DP, et al: Effects of cyclosporine versus standard care in dogs with idiopathic immune-complex glomerulonephritis: A blinded multicenter prospective clinical trial. J Vet Intern Med 5:129, 1991.

*This abstract describes the results of a prospective, placebo-controlled clinical trial addressing the effects of Cy in glomerulonephritis.*
White JV, Davis WR, Nachreiner R, et al: Cyclosporine pharmacokinetics in normal and pancreatectomized dogs. Transplantation 42:390, 1986.
*The pharmacokinetics of Cy in normal and pancreatectomized dogs are described.*

# PROPOFOL: A NEW SEDATIVE-HYPNOTIC ANESTHETIC AGENT

ELAINE P. ROBINSON,
SHERRY L. SANDERSON,
*and* ROSLYN G. MACHON
*St. Paul, Minnesota*

Propofol (2,6-diisopropylphenol), is an alkylphenol derivative, intravenous anesthetic agent, commonly used in human and veterinary anesthetic practice (Morgan and Legge, 1989; Sebel and Lowdon, 1989). Jokingly referred to as the "milk of amnesia" because of its milky white appearance, propofol is available as an oil-in-water emulsion (Diprivan, Stuart Pharmaceuticals, Wilmington, DE). Propofol has gained wide popularity, particularly in the human field, because of its versatility and unique recovery qualities. Its rapid-onset, ultrashort duration of action and lack of cumulative effects make propofol ideally suited for induction and maintenance of anesthesia. In particular, propofol is associated with quick, smooth and "clear-headed" recoveries. It is superior to all other available anesthetics in these respects. However, propofol is certainly not a "perfect anesthetic." It is costly, contains no preservative, and shares many properties common to other injectable agents, including significant cardiovascular and respiratory depression, and lack of analgesia. When compared to less expensive drugs such as the thiobarbiturates and ketamine, the advantages of propofol may not justify the extra expense for use by veterinarians.

## FORMULATION OF PROPOFOL: PRACTICAL PROBLEMS

Although broadly classified as a sedative-hypnotic, propofol is chemically unrelated to the more familiar members of this group, which include barbiturate and steroidal anesthetic agents (Sebel and Lowdon, 1989). Like many alkylated phenol compounds, propofol exists as an oil at room temperature. Because of its poor water solubility, a solubilizing agent is needed to make propofol suitable for intravenous administration. In 1983, propofol was reformulated to its present composition as a 1% w/v solution in a soybean oil, glycerol, and purified egg phosphatide emulsion, which received Food and Drug Administration (FDA) approval in the United States for human use in 1989 (Zoran et al., 1993). It is available in sealed glass 20- or 50-ml vials, at a concentration of 10 mg/ml. Improved design of the vials in 1993 by the manufacturers promises to reduce the problems of glass splintering when vials are opened. At present, propofol is not approved for use in animals in the United States. An approximate price of propofol is $8.60 for a vial containing 200 mg (equivalent to a single induction dose for a 33-kg dog).

The propofol emulsion is a free-flowing, isotonic solution, with a neutral pH (7.0 to 8.5). Although a very small percentage of dogs and cats may exhibit pain during intravenous administration, accidental, extravascular injection is reported to cause neither irritation nor sloughing. Both the incidence and severity of the pain associated with injection may be reduced by administering propofol through an intravenous catheter in conjunction with free-flowing fluids. Propofol has been shown to be readily compatible with lactated Ringer's solution and 5% dextrose, but should not be allowed to mix with blood products such as plasma. Strict aseptic techniques must always be maintained when handling this agent. Vials of propofol should be protected from light and shaken well before use. Propofol does not contain an antimicrobial preservative, and its soybean oil solubilizing vehicle will readily support the growth of a variety of microorganisms, including *Staphylococcus* and *Candida* species. Fever, bacteremia, sepsis, and endophthalmitis have been documented in human beings receiving contaminated propofol. Propofol should be drawn into sterile, labeled, and dated syringes as soon as the vial has been opened. The manufacturers recommend that unused portions of propofol be discarded within 6 hr; they do not recommend storage or refrigeration. However, many veterinarians have stored propofol at 4°C in sealed sterile syringes or tubes for 24 hr.

## PROPERTIES OF PROPOFOL

### Induction of Anesthesia

Propofol produces rapid induction of anesthesia in a similar time to the ultrashort-acting barbiturates (30 to 60 sec). Induction is generally very smooth and free of excitement, making this an ideal drug to administer without preanesthetics or in high-risk patients in which slow injection is desirable. Occasionally, paddling, myoclonic twitching, or opisthotonus has occurred in dogs at induction of anesthesia. Usually these effects are short lived. However, if they continue into the anesthetic period, the patient can be treated with diazepam (0.1 mg/kg IV, slowly) (Ilkiw, 1992).

### Respiratory Effects

Rapid administration of propofol has been found clinically to produce a high incidence of cyanosis and respiratory arrest. Therefore, we recommend the drug be given more slowly to avoid these respiratory effects. Apnea occurred in 34 of 40 dogs receiving propofol (6 mg/kg IV, given in 5 sec) alone or after acepromazine, diazepam, or acepromazine and butorphanol as preanesthetics in a recent clinical study in dogs (Smith et al., 1993).

### Cardiovascular Effects

Cardiac arrhythmias are extremely rare after propofol injection, which makes it a better choice than thiobarbiturates for animals with cardiac disease or preexisting arrhythmias. However, a recent study in dogs revealed that enhancement of epinephrine-induced arrhythmias is similar during propofol anesthesia to that produced by halothane, and greater than that produced by etomidate. Caution is warranted when administering propofol to excitable animals in which catecholamine levels may be elevated before anesthesia. Other cardiovascular changes produced by propofol administration have come to light after recent clinical and experimental studies in human beings and animals. Propofol may produce significant arteriolar dilatation, negative cardiac inotropy, and arterial hypotension, especially after administration of preanesthetics such as acepromazine or in hypovolemic animals (Ilkiw et al., 1992). Such decreases in arterial blood pressure may not be tolerated by shocked or traumatized patients, or by those with cardiopulmonary diseases. Propofol may also produce decreases in heart rate, although this does not always occur. However, this effect might be accentuated if propofol is given with potent opioid narcotics without concurrent administration of anticholinergics such as atropine. In one experimental study in dogs, the combination of propofol and alfentanil produced cardiac asystole in all dogs evaluated; these effects were reversed by administration of atropine (Flecknell, 1990).

### Quality of Propofol Anesthesia

Low, subanesthetic doses of propofol can be used for sedation alone. Sedation is associated with central nervous system depression, restraint, and lack of awareness of surroundings. Anesthesia is similar to the thiobarbiturates, and is characterized by unconsciousness and sleep. Neither sedation nor anesthesia produced by propofol are associated with complete pain relief. Lack of reflex response may only be complete at deep levels of anesthesia.

### Recovery

Recoveries after propofol anesthesia are characteristically fast, smooth, and excitement free. After single-bolus injections, anesthesia lasts for only 2 to 5 min. Dogs sit up within 10 min and walk within 15 min (Zoran et al., 1993). Return of psychomotor function is fast and complete, and animals return to normal functions, including eating, climbing stairs, and negotiating obstacles within the same day. Some exceptions to this rule exist. The use of premedicants or other anesthetic agents will prolong recovery times, depending on the drugs given. Greyhounds are reported to have slightly prolonged recovery times after single injections or after continuous infusions of propofol; however, recoveries in greyhounds are still more acceptable in both quality and duration than after thiobarbiturate anesthesia (Zoran et al., 1993). Although constant infusions of propofol exceeding 30 or 60 min usually produce longer recovery times, these times are still shorter than any other comparable injectable anesthetic technique.

### Metabolism

Propofol is highly protein bound. It is rapidly conjugated in the liver mainly by glucuronidation to inactive metabolites, which are then excreted by the kidney. Cats with hepatic lipidosis or other hepatic disease may have reduced glucuronidation ability, and therefore may take longer to recover from propofol anesthesia. We have observed cats with hepatopathy take several hours to recover fully. Drugs that inhibit hepatic metabolism may prolong recovery. A recent study in greyhounds showed increased recovery times when dogs were pretreated with chloramphenicol (a P-450 inhibitor) before propofol injection. Plasma levels quickly decline following an intravenous bolus injection, due to both high metabolic clearance and the rapid redistribution of drug into the tissues. The high clearance values, which exceed liver blood flow, suggest that some extrahepatic uptake and metabolism also occurs. Pulmonary uptake (60% of injected dose) has been documented in cats; this uptake was inhibited by fentanyl and by halothane. The significance of this is not yet known in clinical feline patients, but could prolong anesthesia if fentanyl or halothane or other basic lipophilic drugs are given concurrently with propofol. Extrahepatic metabolism may compensate for reduced organ function in the face of liver disease. Preliminary reports in the human literature infer that neither hepatic nor renal disease alter the pharmacokinetics of this agent.

## Anaphylactoid Reactions

Propofol has two potential allergenic molecules: the diisopropyl side chain (which is found in many dermatologic products), and phenol. Both molecules cause histamine release when tested in patients who have experienced an anaphylactoid reaction to propofol. Such reactions have occurred in people both with and without a history of previous exposure to the drug (Laxenaire et al., 1992). However, some patients had previously received the total parenteral nutrition solution, Intralipid, which is almost identical to soybean oil/egg phosphatide solubilizing agent contained in the present formulation of propofol. These reactions occur rarely, and anaphylactoid reactions to propofol have not been reported in animals. However, an anaphylactoid reaction should be suspected in any dog or cat who displays an acute onset of such typical signs as vomition, defecation, profound hypotension, or the sudden development of erythema and/or urticaria, during or immediately after the administration of propofol.

## Anticonvulsant/Convulsant Reactions

Propofol may possess both proconvulsant and anticonvulsant properties. Propofol has been used to control status epilepticus in human patients refractory to standard medical therapy such as benzodiazepines and thiobarbiturates and has been recommended for seizure control in animals (Ilkiw, 1992a). However, propofol has been associated with "seizure" like activity and opisthotonos during recovery from anesthesia, particularly in epileptic human patients. Minor myoclonic twitching and muscle tremors have been observed occasionally in dogs and cats at induction of anesthesia. It is unknown whether these neurologic sequelae represent true seizure activity or merely nonepileptic myoclonia. In our hospital, one 10-year-old Labrador retriever seizured during recovery from propofol anesthesia. Until further investigations are performed, caution should be considered when administering propofol to patients with epilepsy.

## Antiemetic–Appetite Stimulant Properties

Propofol anesthesia has been associated with fewer incidences of postoperative nausea and vomiting than many other anesthetic agents. Propofol, given to human patients receiving chemotherapy, at subhypnotic doses by continuous IV infusion, was associated with significantly lower incidences of nausea and vomiting, even in patients previously refractory to standard anti-

emetic medications, such as metoclopramide. The exact mechanism of the antiemetic effect of propofol is unknown.

In a pilot investigation conducted at our hospital, propofol was used to anesthetize six patients for various diagnostic and therapeutic procedures of short duration. Prior to propofol administration, all patients had been anorexic for varying durations (24 to 96 hr). Three of the patients had been vomiting. Immediately upon recovery from propofol anesthesia, all six patients voluntarily started to eat. Some of the patients were trying to eat even before they were able to stand. We speculated that the patients had some degree of nausea that was minimized by propofol, or that propofol may stimulate appetite.

## Consecutive-Day Administration

Propofol has been recommended for anesthesia that must be repeated daily over a number of consecutive days, due to the lack of cumulative effects of the drug. In dogs this may be a safe protocol. In cats, propofol may produce adverse effects when used repeatedly. In a recent study of healthy cats anesthetized for 30 min daily with propofol, there was significant Heinz-body production in red blood cells after 3 days and cats were recovering more slowly; by the fifth day cats were anorexic, lethargic, and had diarrhea and malaise. By the sixth or seventh day the study was abandoned (Day et al., 1993). The formation of Heinz bodies was attributed to oxidative injury of red blood cells by propofol, a phenomenon produced by other phenolic compounds in cats.

## INDICATIONS

The unusual chemical structure of propofol as an anesthetic may be one reason for the varied reported properties and uses of the drug. These include sedation, outpatient anesthesia, anesthesia (short and long duration), anticonvulsant, antiemetic, appetite stimulant, antioxidant, aphrodisiac, and drug of addiction in human beings. Propofol can only be administered intravenously.

Propofol can be used in single doses for induction of anesthesia. If necessary, anesthesia can be prolonged by frequent repeated bolus injections or by constant infusion. Recommended dose rates for induction of anesthesia in dogs and cats vary between 2 and 8 mg/kg body weight, with an average calculated dose of 6 mg/kg (Table 1) (Ilkiw, 1992; Morgan and Legge, 1989). Lower doses are needed in premedicated or sick animals. To avoid apnea, the drug should be injected slowly intravenously, giving approximately 25% of the calculated dose every 30 sec until the desired effect is achieved. If the anesthesia is to be continued with propofol alone, then incremental doses of propofol at the rate of 1 ml (10 mg) per 12 to 25 kg body weight should be injected each minute, starting approximately 3 min

**Table 1.** *Clinically Accepted Dose Rates of Propofol for Dogs and Cats*

| | |
|---|---|
| Single injection | |
| Healthy, unpremedicated dog or cat | 6 mg/kg IV |
| Healthy premedicated dog or cat | |
| After tranquilizer (e.g., acepromazine) | 4 mg/kg IV |
| After sedative (e.g., xylazine, opioids) | 3 mg/kg IV |
| Constant infusion rate | |
| For sedation only | 0.1 mg/kg/min |
| For minor surgery | 0.6 mg/kg/min, or 1 ml (10 mg)/min/12–25 kg |

**Table 2.** *Adverse Effects of Propofol Associated with Clinical Use in Dogs and Humans*

| | Reported Incidence (%) | |
|---|---|---|
| | **Dog°** **(n = 40)** | **Human†** **(n=25,981)** |
| Respiratory depression, cyanosis, apnea | 85 | <1 |
| Arterial hypotension | NR | 15.7 |
| Bradycardia | NR | 4.8 |
| Premature ventricular contractions | <1 | <1 |
| Excitement on induction | NR | 1.3 |
| Pain on injection | 7.5 | 5.2 |
| Retching/vomiting on recovery | NR | 1.9 |
| Excitement on recovery | 5 | NR |
| Prolonged recovery (>15 min) | NR | 6.8 |

°Data derived from Smith et al., 1993.
†Data derived from McLeskey et al., 1993.
Abbreviation: NR = incidence not reported.

after induction. For periods of anesthesia longer than 15 min, it is more convenient to infuse at the constant rate of 0.4 to 0.8 mg/kg/min, depending on the depth of anesthesia required. Lower infusion rates of 0.115 to 0.3 mg/kg/min have been used in dogs after preanesthetic sedatives. Propofol can be diluted 50:50 with dextrose (5%) or lactated Ringer's to make up a free-flowing infusion solution; the manufacturers recommend that the infusion be discarded after 6 hr exposed to room temperature.

Propofol is particularly useful for induction before endotracheal intubation and inhalation anesthesia. Inhalation anesthesia must be started immediately after intubation or else further doses of propofol will be necessary to keep the patient asleep. Most commonly used preanesthetic tranquilizers and sedatives have been used before propofol inductions; dose rates of propofol must be lowered according to the effect produced by the preanesthetic. Opioid narcotic analgesics should always be given concurrently with an anticholinergic (atropine or glycopyrrolate), to prevent propofol-induced bradycardia. Analgesics should be used if painful surgery is anticipated, as propofol has minimal analgesic properties itself. Painful animals will wake up rapidly with distress if propofol anesthesia is used without analgesics.

Propofol is ideal as an "outpatient" anesthetic for diagnostic or minor procedures, such as radiography, laceration repair, eye examinations, minor dentistry, ultrasound-directed biopsies and other minor biopsies, upper airway examinations, and laryngeal surgery. It is also useful for gastrointestinal endoscopy because it is antiemetic. It apparently does not affect gastrointestinal motility.

The beneficial effects of propofol have also made it a popular choice for greyhound anesthesia and for patients with cardiac arrhythmias. Propofol has also been used as an appetite stimulant, anticonvulsant, and antipruritic drug (the latter in human patients treated with epidural morphine).

## CONTRAINDICATIONS FOR USE OF PROPOFOL

Shocked, stressed, and injured animals may respond adversely to propofol because of the depressant cardi-

ovascular and respiratory effects, especially arterial hypotension. It is imperative to give fluid therapy to such animals before and during propofol anesthesia. Because propofol is highly bound to plasma proteins, hypoproteinemia is a relative contraindication for its use. The drug would have greater activity in hypoproteinemic patients and it is easier to overdose them.

Adequate equipment for respiratory support (endotracheal tubes, oxygen source) are vital when propofol is administered because respiratory arrest may occur in any patient and is a common side effect in dogs (Table 2). Therefore, it would be inadvisable to anesthetize an animal with airway problems, such as a brachycephalic dog, without such equipment available. Likewise, a procedure that demands high levels of analgesia is best not performed with propofol alone.

Patients with histories of hyperlipidemia, anaphylaxis, or seizures might be best anesthetized with another agent, as discussed above.

The major practical contraindications for veterinarians are the expense of the drug and the fact that the drug cannot be preserved once a vial is opened.

## References and Suggested Reading

Day TK, Andress JL, and Day DG: Effects of consecutive day propofol anesthesia on feline red blood cells. *Proc Ann Mtg Am Coll Vet Anesth*, Washington DC, 1993, p 15.
*An abstract of a study of the effects of repeated propofol administration in cats.*
Flecknell PA, Kirk AJ, Fox CE, and Dark JH: Long-term anaesthesia with propofol and alfentanil in the dog and its partial reversal with nalbuphine. J Assoc Vet Anaesth 17:11, 1990.
*An experimental study in dogs in which combinations of propofol and the opioid, alfentanil, produced cardiac asystole.*
Ilkiw JE: Other potentially useful new injectable anesthetic agents. Vet Clin North Am [Small Anim Pract] 22:281, 1992.
*A detailed review of propofol for clinical anesthesia in dogs and cats.*
Ilkiw JE, Pascoe PJ, Haskins SC, and Patz JD: Cardiovascular and respiratory effects of propofol administration in hypovolemic dogs. Am J Vet Res 53:2323, 1992.
*A prospective study of the effects of propofol (6 mg/kg) given to hypovolemic dogs 30 min after significant experimentally induced hemorrhage.*
Laxenaire MC, Mata-Bermejo E, Moneret-Vautrin DA, and Gueant JL: Life-threatening anaphylactoid reactions to propofol (Diprivan). Anesthesiology 77:275, 1992.

*Results of an investigation of 14 human patients who had developed serious anaphylactoid reactions resulting from use of propofol.*

McLeskey CH, Walawander CA, Nahrwold ML, et al: Adverse events in a multicenter phase IV study of propofol: Evaluation by anesthesiologists and postanesthesia care unit nurses. Anesth Analg 77:S3, 1993.
*Results of a large clinical study of surgical patients carried out between 1989 and 1990 in 1722 human hospitals, identifying the incidence of adverse effects of propofol.*

Morgan DW, and Legge K: Clinical evaluation of propofol as an intravenous anaesthetic agent in cats and dogs. Vet Rec 124:31, 1989.
*A clinical study undertaken in the United Kingdom of 290 dogs and 207 cats receiving propofol as a sole anesthetic or as part of an anesthetic regimen.*

Sebel PS, and Lowdon JD: Propofol: A new intravenous anesthetic. Anesthesiology 71:260, 1989.
*A comprehensive and detailed review of propofol in humans patients and in animal studies.*

Smith JA, Gaynor JS, Bednarski RM, and Muir WW: Adverse effects of administration of propofol with various preanesthetic regimens in dogs. J Am Vet Med Assoc 202:1111, 1993.
*A clinical study of the adverse effects of propofol in 40 dogs.*

Zoran DL, Riedesel DH, and Dyer DC: Pharmacokinetics of propofol in mixed-breed dogs and greyhounds. Am J Vet Res 54:755, 1993.
*Results of a study comparing greyhounds and mixed breed dogs in terms of pharmacokinetics of propofol and recovery parameters.*

# PHYSICAL THERAPY AND REHABILITATION

ROBERT A. TAYLOR

*Denver, Colorado*

Current veterinary surgical texts and proceedings of surgical meetings are replete with details of procedures, and discussion of techniques and results. The days of "the sutures were removed at 10 days and the patient made an uneventful recovery" are gone. Veterinarians are more aware of the need for detailed patient follow-up and implementation of a rehabilitation plan for all surgical patients and often are requested by clients to provide such a rehabilitation plan. Human physical therapy has become a "stand-alone" discipline and is one of the most rapidly growing allied health professions (Bureau of Labor Statistics, 1993). It is widely acknowledged that human patients, regardless of age or athletic status, benefit physiologically and psychologically from postsurgical physical therapy.

Physiologic benefits of postsurgical physical therapy include (1) early resolution of inflammation, (2) increased blood flow and lymphatic drainage, (3) increased collagen production, (4) prevention of periarticular contractions, (5) promotion of normal joint hemostasis, (6) prevention or reduction of muscle atrophy, and (7) promotion of normal joint mechanics (Taylor, 1992). Summation of these physiologic events means an earlier and more complete return of function for the injured area.

Physical therapy results in psychologic benefits for the patient and owner. Animals respond positively to "hands on" attention associated with physical therapy. By becoming "part of the solution," owners share in the responsibility for the patients' recovery. Animal owners who have participated in physical therapy often become strong advocates for this discipline.

## PATIENT ASSESSMENT

When the need for physical therapy is anticipated, the nature of the patient's injury and mechanisms involved in repair must be considered. The surgical team and the physical therapist should have a good understanding of the wound healing process, especially how individual tissues (such as bone, nerve, and tendon) temporarily regain strength. With this knowledge, physical therapy plans can be customized to the patient's injuries. For example, patients with fractures immobilized by rigid fixation may be given physical therapy the day of surgery, whereas fractures managed with less rigid stabilization may require a delay before initiating physical therapy.

Following some surgical procedures it is helpful to follow an established physical therapy protocol to allow standardization of therapy.

## DOCUMENTATION

The goal of physical therapy is to hasten functional return. In order to validate the benefits of physical therapy, it is critical to assess findings and chart the patient's response. Evaluation of range of joint motion with a goniometer, limb circumference, and weight-bearing status are recommended for most orthopedic cases. Muscle strength, pain associated with manipulation, and gait analysis may also be determined. Documenting and comparing results of physical therapy facilitates objective assessment of response.

## PHYSICAL THERAPY MODALITIES

Cryotherapy effectively reduces temperature and metabolic rate of injured tissue. Cold therapy reduces destructive enzymatic activity, inflammation, and swelling of damaged tissues. Cold decreases the severity of postsurgical pain by presynaptic inhibition of pain stimuli and reduction of nerve-conduction velocity (Whitney, 1989). In clinical trials, continuous surface cooling of the knee resulted in reduction of analgesic needs in humans. It is reasonable to conclude that the same concept benefits animals (Lemann, 1982). I recommend reusable cold packs to provide safe surface cooling (CP2 Cold Packs, PI Medical) for every surgical patient. These packs can be contoured to the patient's body, wrapped in a clean towel, and applied as the patient recovers from anesthesia. Cold therapy is most effective during the first 7 postoperative days. It is very effective in alleviating pain and swelling during the weeks following the injury, and may be used to reduce discomfort associated with more strenuous forms of physical therapy.

## HEAT APPLICATION

Heat is one of the oldest methods of physical therapy. Beneficial effects of heat include (1) local vasodilation, (2) increased metabolic rate, (3) muscle relaxation, and (4) increased viscosity of collagen (Lemann, 1982). External sources of heat have a narrow therapeutic range (40° to 45°C). Care must be used to avoid thermal burns. This is especially important when external heat is used to treat patients with sensory nerve impairment. Heat application should not be used for at least 2 weeks following surgery, since early use exacerbates vasodilation and swelling of tissue.

## ULTRASOUND

Ultrasonography is a form of acoustic vibration at frequencies greater than or equal to 17,000 Hz. The energy of vibration causes component atoms of the medium to vibrate about their positions of equilibrium, resulting in propagation of energy. The wave propagation and vibration of atoms produces heat in tissue. The depth of penetration is determined by the configuration of the therapeutic unit and treatment head. A 1-MHz treatment head allows for deeper tissue penetration, while a 3-MHz head will work better in smaller areas, where it penetrates superficially. Propagation of ultrasound energy depends on reflections of energy at tissue interfaces and tissue absorption characteristics. Absorption of ultrasound by solids is higher than by liquids. Muscle absorbs twice the energy that fat does; energy absorption for bone is ten times greater than for soft tissues (Esposito, Veal, and Farman, 1984). Bone damage can occur with excessive ultrasound exposure resulting in periosteal burns and bone pain.

Ultrasound increases cell membrane permeability, which promotes nutrient and gas exchange. Ultrasound decreases inflammation, increases vasodilation, accelerates lymph flow, and enhances metabolic events. Ultrasound acts upon fibroblasts and collagen and can hasten wound healing and tensile strength of skin wounds (Drastichova, Samohyl, and Slavetinska, 1973) and may stimulate bone growth (Duarte, 1983).

Ultrasound increases tissue and vascular permeability and can help alleviate edema associated with inflammation (Fyfe and Chahl, 1980). Ultrasound also has been shown to significantly increase tensile strength of the achilles tendon (Enwemeka, 1989; Enwemeka, Rodriguez, and Mendosa, 1990).

### Indications

Ultrasonography can be used postsurgically, and it can be used to treat various musculoskeletal problems. We use it to treat injured muscle, to prevent muscle spasms and fibrosis associated with fractures, and to alleviate pain associated with disk herniation. Contraindications for ultrasonography include direct use over metallic implants and application to malignant tumors. Therapeutic ultrasound should not be used on the eye, heart, or gravid uterus. It should be used with caution over prominent cutaneous nerve, and over extremities with little soft tissue over bone, as periosteal burns may occur.

### Ultrasound Dosimetry

An average power setting of 0.5 to 4 W/sec emitted from the ultrasound head is recommended for therapeutic ultrasound. Coupling media must be used for proper sound-wave propagation. Ultrasonography can be performed in water to treat extremities with little soft tissue covering bone. Ultrasound units may be combined with neuromuscular stimulation capabilities to provide dual treatment modalities.

### MASSAGE

Digital manipulation of soft tissue may enhance circulation, loosen and stretch tendons, and enhance scar remodeling. Results of recent studies indicate that massage enhanced spinal motor neuron excitability (Sullivan et al., 1991). Because massage is physically pleasing, it can help soothe anxious or uncomfortable patients. Massage therapy can often be initiated the day of surgery and continued throughout the physical therapy period.

### HYDROTHERAPY AND SWIMMING

Hydrotherapy is suited for neurologically compromised patients that can be manually supported in a shallow tub of water. Reduction in weight bearing may facilitate early use of the affected limbs. Hydrotherapy can also help prevent urine scalding and decubital ulcers associated with paralysis.

Swimming can provide vigorous joint and muscle action in a reduced weight-bearing and -resistant environment. It should be done in a controlled and supervised environment, ideally in a therapy pool specially designed for animals. Therapy pools should be equipped with an electric pump that creates a current (resistance) against which the animal swims. Patients in deep therapy pools must be closely supervised to prevent injury or drowning. Specially designed flotation vests may be used. Because swimming is a vigorous form of exercise, it should be limited to 3 to 5 min daily.

## NEUROMUSCULAR STIMULATION

Battery-powered transcutaneous neuromuscular stimulators can be used to stimulate muscle with the objective of diminishing atrophy. This modality should be differentiated from transcutaneous electrical nerve stimulators (TENS) used primarily for relief of chronic pain. Electrical stimulation can provide muscle relaxation and muscle reeducation, prevent muscle atrophy, and enhance resolution of edema and inflammation (Windsor, Lester, and Herring, 1993). Significant muscle atrophy, which can occur within the first several days after surgery, may be significantly compounded by use of casts, bandages, or fixator immobilization devices. Electrical stimulation of muscle has been shown to reduce muscle atrophy following anterior cruciate ligament surgery. The device consists of a pulse generator and electrodes that are placed over select muscle groups. It is possible to select pulse amplitude, pulse rate, and cycle length to suite the comfort of the patient. When this device is combined with massage and passive range of motion, muscle fibrosis, such as that which occurs after distal femoral or humeral fractures, can be prevented.

## PASSIVE RANGE OF MOTION

Cycling affected joints through their physiologic range of motion is a simple and easy procedure. Passive range of motion (PROM) can reduce tissue adhesion, promote normal joint dynamics and cartilage nutrition, enhance venous and lymphatic drainage, and minimize contracture of muscles and joints. Ideally, PROM may be initiated the day of surgery and continued for an additional 2 or 3 weeks. The goal of PROM is to maintain or achieve normal range of motion for affected joints. The range of motion of normal contralateral joints can be used for comparison. Because age-related changes in joint range of motion are insignificant, substantial loss of joint mobility should be measured as abnormal and not age related (Roach and Miles, 1991). PROM should not be utilized to manage unstable fracture sites, luxations, hypermotile joints, osteopenic bones, bone tumors, or areas with recent skin grafts.

## EXERCISE

Exercise can play a major role in rehabilitation. Exercise should be graduated to reflect normal tissue repair time, stability of complex fracture repair, and function of the animal on recovery.

Open kinetic chain activity occurs when the extremity is cycled through a normal range of motion without encountering ground contact or pressure. This is difficult to achieve in domestic animals and is therefore rarely done. Closed chain activity such as walking where the distal extremity strikes the ground is a vital rehabilitation tool. It is a safe way to begin active exercise and can include short circles or figure-of-eight patterns to improve muscle strength. Incline walking can be added later during rehabilitation. Walking exercise increases circulation in the limb while improving sensory awareness and muscle strength. Patients with paraparesis or tetraparesis may be exercised while the limb is supported with a body sling.

Several other walking exercise plans also have merit. Syringe caps can be placed over the tarsal and carpal pads of the normal limbs to encourage use of a limb during rehabilitation. Through use of repetitive "sit" and "stay" commands, the quadriceps and biceps femoris as well as the semitendinous and semimembranous muscles can be strengthened. Malleable lead leg weights can also be used to further strengthen atrophied muscles. The weight load is steadily increased over several days to progressively strengthen the limb.

Stair climbing is an excellent form of exercise to strengthen muscles. Stairs should be climbed slowly to ensure limb use during the exercise. When possible, the patient should walk up the steps with the affected limb next to a supporting wall; the patient and therapists should climb the stairs together to prevent skipping of steps.

It is possible to concentrate weight-bearing stresses by "wheelbarrowing" either the front or rear limbs. In this way, the animal is rendered bipedal. This activity can also be useful in proprioceptive training.

## References and Suggested Reading

Draper V and Ballard L: Electrical stimulation versus electromyographic biofeedback in the recovery of quadriceps femoris muscle function following anterior cruciate ligament surgery. Phys Ther 71:455, 1991.

Drastichova V, Samohyl J, and Slavetinska A: Strengthening of sutured skin wound with ultrasound in experiments on animals. Acta Chir Plast 15:2, 1973.

Duarte LR: The stimulation of bone growth by ultrasound. Arch Orthop Trauma Surg 101:153, 1983.

Enwemeka CS: The effects of therapeutic ultrasound on tendon healing. Am J Phys Med Rehabil 68:283, 1989.

Enwemeka CS, Rodriguez O, and Mendosa S: The biomechanical effects of low-intensity ultrasound on healing tendons. Ultrasound Med Biol 16:801, 1990.

Esposito CJ, Veal SJ, and Farman AG: Alleviation of myofascial pain with ultrasonic therapy. J Prosthet Dent 51:106, 1984.

Fyfe MC and Chahl LA: The effect of ultrasound on experimental oedema in rats. Ultrasound Med Biol 6:107, 1980.

Lemann JF (ed): Therapeutic Head and Cold, 3rd edition. Baltimore, Williams & Wilkins, 1982.

Roach KE and Miles TP: Normal hip and knee active range of motion: The relationship to age. Phys Ther 71:656, 1991.

Sullivan SJ, Williams LRT, Seaborne DE, et al: Effects of massage on alpha motoneuron excitability. Phys Ther 71:555, 1991.

Taylor RA: Postsurgical physical therapy: The missing link. Compend Cont Educ 14:1583, 1992.

Whitney SL: Physical agents: Heat and cold modalities. In Scully RM and Barnes MR (eds): Physical Therapy. Philadelphia, JB Lippincott Co, 1989, p 849.

Windsor RE, Lester JP, and Herring SA: Electrical stimulation in clinical practice. Physician Sportsmed 21:85, 1993.

1992–93 U.S. Dept of Labor report from the Bureau of Labor Statistics.

# NONPHARMACOLOGIC MANAGEMENT OF COMMON BEHAVIORAL DISORDERS

BONNIE V. BEAVER

*College Station, Texas*

A number of articles that surveyed owners about their animal's behavior and that reviewed behavioral referrals to veterinarians revealed differences in the ranking of problems between the two groups. Five behavior problems are, however, near or at the top of each list: aggression, housesoiling, excessive barking, destructive chewing, and digging. Given the complexity of determining the proper diagnosis and treatment for the various types of aggression, the reader is referred to a number of other papers on that subject, including Voith and Marder (1988).

## HOUSESOILING

Animals eliminating in the house constitute a large portion of complaints presented to behaviorists. It is the number-one problem cited by cat owners and second only to aggression cited by dog owners. Each species has unique features and will be considered separately.

### Housesoiling by Dogs

The typical description of a dog soiling in the house includes information that the dog had previously been well trained and that it was either urinating or defecating somewhere in the house while the owner was at work. By the time the veterinarian learns about the behavior, the problem has been occurring for several days. The owner often describes the dog showing a "guilty" look or a "he knows" attitude. In response the owner shoves the dog's nose in the mess, and pushes it outside. Coincidentally, these problems often begin during inclement weather, a fact that the veterinarian has to add to all the pieces of the historic puzzle.

Many dogs are reluctant to step outside during rain, snow, or extreme cold. If pushed out, they stand next to the door waiting to come back in. Owners, on the other hand, are busy doing their own things, assuming that if the dog is outdoors it must be "doing its business." The dog comes back in, the owners leave, and 2 or 3 hr later the urge to urinate or defecate is overpowering.

The first step to solving many canine soiling problems is to go back to basic house training. The owner must go out with the dog, regardless of the weather, and stay out until the dog has completed urinating and/or defecating, as appropriate for the individual. While the dog is eliminating, the owner is to lavish it with praise. The schedule for going out should be the same as that successfully used in the past. Occasionally an owner may not be taking a dog out often enough. A dog that eliminates at a specific time, even though the owner is home, may indicate this. Simply add another outing to the dog's schedule.

A second step the owner must take is to discontinue negative feelings for the dog. They must also learn that the submissive behavior they call "the guilty look" is a learned response to a combination of an owner's presence plus an odor of excreta. Since punishment for a behavior must occur at the time of the behavior, the dog quickly learns to associate the return of the owner with punishment for an active approach.

### Housesoiling by Cats

There are two major concerns relative to the complaint of a cat eliminating in the house. The first is to be absolutely sure which cat is causing the problem. A "guilty" look or other trait that can be misinterpreted is not appropriate. Seeing the behavior or hard physical evidence, such as a unique characteristic of the feces, is necessary. The second important piece of information is to determine whether the behavior is that of elimination or marking. If an owner sees the cat squatting to urinate or defecate, most of the time the behavior is that of inappropriate elimination. If the cat is standing, spraying vertical surfaces with streams of urine, the behavior is urine marking.

#### FELINE INAPPROPRIATE ELIMINATION

Housesoiling by urination or defecation is really a normal behavior in an unacceptable location from the owner's perspective. The development of the behavior is often related to an aversion to a location or litter/litter box, or to the preference for a new location or surface (Borchelt, 1991; Voith and Marder, 1988). Probably the most common cause is a litter box that is too dirty, from the cat's perspective. Abrupt changes in litter type, heavy traffic coming into the litter box area, or frequent attempts by an owner to catch the cat while it is in the litter box are other ways an aversion might develop. The absorbing action of carpet may make a new area desirable for urination. In other cases, the litter box may be extremely inconvenient for the cat. The back bedroom on the third floor might just as well be Siberia when the cat spends most of its time in the first floor living room. Instead the cat chooses a spot behind the sofa.

Treatment must address the aversion or preference or both by identifying related factors that play a role. Approaches to solving the problem depend on these factors and may include daily cleaning of the litter box, adding multiple boxes for multiple cats, putting a box on the new location, offering several boxes each with a different type of litter or one at each floor level, preventing access to a new location, or confining the cat in a room without carpeting (Beaver, 1992).

### FELINE SPRAYING

Spraying urine is a marking behavior related to the invasion of the cat's territory or the perception of a stress. This behavior is most commonly associated with the presence of new cats. Even outside cats passing by a window can trigger spraying by an indoor animal. The start of mating season in the spring means more cats are roaming and visible to the resident cat, even though their presence may not be recognized by the owner. The location of the urine mark gives information about the location of the stress. Urine on curtains, by windows or doors, or on objects where the cat views the out-of-doors indicates stress caused by other cats or some other stress outside. Urine on items of a specific person may indicate a strained relationship with that individual (as well as one that has not improved lately either).

Treatment can be multifaceted. By identifying the source of the stress, it may be possible to eliminate or minimize it. The owner could find another home for the new kitten. The roommate could direct energies to feeding the cat instead of yelling at it for spraying dirty clothes. When it is not possible to eliminate the source, it might be possible to change the environment. For the cat stressed by outdoor cats, relief might come by closing the drapes, using window shades, preventing the cat from coming into the room it sprays, or confining the cat to a single room. Most cases can be managed without medication, but in severe cases, appropriate tranquilizers may be needed.

## EXCESSIVE BARKING

Barking dogs are viewed as problems in two primary situations. Nocturnal barking keeps the owner awake and can be a strong motivator to find a solution. Daytime barkers often bother neighbors, especially if the noise lasts most of the day. The motivation to change the daytime behavior may come from a visit by authorities, perhaps to enforce a no-barking ordinance or at least for disrupting the peace.

Dogs tend to be more vocal than their wolf relatives. Barking may have been inadvertently selected at the same time specific physical or other behaviors were chosen for selective breeding. Barking is used as a threat or warning; however, as the tendency to bark

increases so does the disassociation with the distance-increasing message. Domestic dogs bark for attention and in situations when there are no other activities. They also bark in distress, such as with separation anxiety.

### Nocturnal Barking

Dogs barking at night are often rewarded for the behavior by the owner. While the stimulus for the barking may have been a response to another noise, the owner does not care. The voice yelling for quiet or the owner's physical presence are social rewards and increase the likelihood of repeated episodes.

Instead of accidentally rewarding the act, the owner must look for ways to ignore or punish the behavior without the dog perceiving something desirable. The simplest treatment is to totally ignore the barking. Over time the behavior is extinguished because it is no longer rewarded. Since it may not be possible to wait that long, a negative reinforcer can be used. The owner can leave a garden hose with pistol-grip sprayer attached turned on and near the window so that the dog can be blasted with water instead of words. If the dog is kept in a relatively confined area, such as a dog run, a nail above its head will break balloons that are reeled over on a pulley clothesline. The techniques are limited only by the depth of imagination.

### Barking When the Owner is Gone

Because the owner is not particularly bothered by the dog that barks only when no one is home, they may lack the motivation to put much effort into affecting change. If the barking occurs because there is nothing else to do ("boredom barker"), the barking collars may be the most effective. For most boredom barkers, the collar that produces a clicking noise in response to a bark works reasonably well. Shock collars help some problem barkers, but they can be very harsh.

When separation anxiety is expressed by excessive vocalization, extinction of the problem takes time and effort by the owner (Borchelt and Voith, 1982; McCrave, 1991). While the training sessions are ongoing, the owner should use the regular routine for times when they must be gone. The training session activities should be kept distinct from those used daily. The stimulus that starts the anxiety may be detectable with careful observation by the owner. It could be jingling keys, frantic hustling in the kitchen, or the turning off of the radio. That event should be minimized. The owner can divert the dog's attention before giving it a favorite toy, a rawhide chew, or bone coated with a good-tasting smearable food. Then the owner leaves, and quickly returns before the dog even notices. Gradually the owner steps out for longer periods, but always returns before the dog becomes anxious. If a problem with anxiety or barking is noted during these training sessions, shorten the time before the owner returns until it is not stressful. Only after the owner can be gone for several hours in a training session is that routine substituted for the original.

## DESTRUCTIVE CHEWING

Dogs that are mouth oriented will show destructive chewing as a stress-induced behavior. As puppies they can severely try the patience of owners and may need to be controlled by confinement in a crate or use of a muzzle or both. In either case, the puppy should gradually become acquainted with the crate or muzzle and these items should not be used as a punishment, only as a preventative.

As young adults, coping with various types of stress is managed with the most natural, available behavior. If that method is chewing, the problem will be directed toward objects in the environment—furniture, clothes, plants, structural parts of the house, and garden equipment. Stress can result from many areas, particularly not enough exercise. Large breeds, in particular, are genetically designed to be able to work for long periods if in proper condition. The hunting breeds can be in the field all day. Draft breeds can pull heavy loads for many miles. The energy gained from consumption of a good quality diet cannot be expended by a four-block daily walk with the owner. The surplus energy will be used, and if not channeled, it will present itself as a problem such as chewing. Thus, greatly increasing the amount of exercise for a dog that is a destructive chewer can be very useful. The dog can do the majority of work by having it play a game of fetch or Frisbee or road working the animal next to a car or bicycle. If the owners are elderly and unable to accomplish this type of exercise, they may be able to have a grandchild or neighbor child exercise the dog for them.

Destructive chewing can also be an expression of separation anxiety. If the problem is mild and the chewing occurs immediately after the owner leaves or shortly before the owner returns, the type of interactions at that time might be the reason. It is important that the owner not leave or return home in such a way as to excite the dog. Things in the home should be relatively calm for at least 30 min before leaving so that a simple "good bye" is all that is given when the owner leaves. Coming home should also be relatively low key. A "hi" is sufficient when the owner returns, then another specific action, such as changing clothes or starting dinner, becomes the key that positive interactions will soon start. For the long-term problem and the one where the damage is severe and the problem getting worse, a more intense approach will be necessary. If the owner is committed to taking the time and effort to work with this problem, the basic program is the same as that outlined above under the section on barking. First the owner diverts the dog's attention with a favorite item. The owner will gradually leave the house for longer periods of time, always returning before signs of anxiety or chewing begin.

## DIGGING

The location of a dog's digging often tells something about the reason behind it. It is important to realize the owner may make assumptions about the problem that have no bearing on the actual situation, such as the dog is doing the behavior in "spite." Digging is usually considered to be an outdoor problem; however, it can occur indoors as well. Each location will be examined and suggestions made for working with the problem dog.

### Digging Indoors

Dogs that dig indoors are generally one of two types. The first type is the geriatric individual that digs in the carpet during the winter or summer months or both. With the energy-saving consciousness currently in vogue and the decrease in thermoregulatory ability of the older dog, high and low temperatures may trigger problem behaviors. Cold drafts on the floor are chilling, and digging is the instinctive attempt to structure a nest so that lying in that nest will help conserve body heat. The build-up of heat during the hot days of summer may result in digging, especially if the house is built on a concrete slab. Any geriatric dog that is digging should be checked medically for coexisting conditions such as hypothyroidism. In addition to giving appropriate medications, owners can adjust the thermostat to warmer or cooler readings. Another method the owner can use is to wrap the dog up in a blanket to stop the cold draft of winter, or leave a box fan running to help with summer cooling.

Separation anxiety can also cause a dog to dig inside the house, especially near doors. Seldom is digging the sole expression of the problem, however. As described for the barker with separation anxiety, owners committed to changing the behavior can use a gradual program to get the dog used to their absence.

### Digging Outdoors

The majority of problem diggers are outdoor dogs, and most owners with this type of dog try to address the outcome of the problem, forgetting about the cause. Filling a hole with water and stuffing the dog's head under the surface, putting an electric fence along the bottom of the fence, or covering the excavated site with chicken wire may temporarily stop the digging. But because the cause of the problem has not been removed, the behavior will either reoccur or a new behavior will be substituted.

In the hot summer temperatures, an afternoon shady spot may become an area for the dog to cool off. Cool ground, especially if it is a flower bed with moist earth, provides the dog with a spot for conductive cooling to compliment the evaporative cooling of panting. It is not realistic for the owner to think that this type of behavior can be eliminated while the weather is hot. The owners can provide a cool spot for the dog, such as a child's wading pool or an indoor location in the afternoon. Another alternative is to actually encourage the dog to dig in a specific location that meets its needs, but one where the owner can actually landscape. Loose dirt, kept moist and in the shade, can be provided, while the other parts of the flower bed or yard are protected.

Digging near a fence often indicates there is activity on the other side that is attracting the dog's attention. It might be a neighbor child playing, another dog running, or even a cat walking the top of the fence. Digging near a gate should also be viewed relative to activities that are immediately outside. If the dog actually escapes, does it stay in the front yard only to get a better view of the neighborhood activities? Does it run to the closest people for social interaction? Or, does it run off and resist coming when called, indicating an excess of energy to be burned off first? There is a strong human tendency to gradually isolate the backyard dog from human interaction. Eventually mealtime becomes the only time the dog really sees anyone. The addition of another dog will allow most dogs to do well socially, but if left alone, the dog will seek companionship. Interactions with the dog should occur at the same time each day, with 30 min being the minimum any dog would probably need. Several times of interaction, instead of just one, would be preferable.

Dogs that dig in the middle of the yard or in flower beds in the center of the yard may be going after gophers or other small animals, or they may be using up stored energy in their most natural method. Excess energy can also cause a dog to escape from the yard and not return until it is tired. If there are small animals burrowing in the yard, they must be removed as a possible stimulus for the digging. Until that is done, the stimulus for digging after them remains. The veterinarian and owner should evaluate and adjust the energy in the diet and the amount of exercise the dog gets daily as necessary to bring the amount of digging under control.

Housesoiling, barking, chewing, and digging are behaviors of dogs and cats that can be bothersome to their owners. There are many causes of these behaviors, but they are often expressions of environmental stresses to the animal. As pharmacologic agents become more commonly used in veterinary medicine, it is important for the practitioner to remember that drugs do not stop all the various problems. In some conditions they will be useful only when combined with behavior modification. Many situations are best handled through environmental manipulation, using nonpharmacologic therapies.

## References and Suggested Reading

Beaver BV: *Feline Behavior: A Guide for Veterinarians.* Philadelphia, WB Saunders Co, 1992, p 208.
  *A review of normal and abnormal forms of elimination.*
Borchelt PL: Cat elimination behavior problems. Vet Clin North Am [Small Anim Prac] 21:257, 1991.
  *Discusses preferences and aversions.*
Borchelt PL and Voith VL: Diagnosis and treatment of separation-related behavior problems in dogs. Vet Clin North Am [Small Anim Prac] 12:625, 1982.
  *Discusses several approaches to use with separation anxiety.*
McCrave EA: Diagnostic criteria for separation anxiety in the dog. Vet Clin North Am 21:247, 1991.
  *Offers criteria to determine if separation anxiety is part of the problem.*
Voith VL and Marder AR: Canine behavioral disorders. *In* Morgan RV (ed): *Handbook of Small Animal Practice.* New York, Churchill Livingstone, 1988, p 1033.
  *Includes a general comparison between different types of aggression.*
Voith VL and Marder AR: Feline behavioral disorders. *In* Morgan RV (ed): *Handbook of Small Animal Practice.* New York, Churchill Livingstone, 1988, p 1045.

# FACILITATING OWNER-PRESENT EUTHANASIA

CAROLYN BUTLER
*and* LAUREL LAGONI
*Fort Collins, Colorado*

In spite of growing knowledge confirming companion animal loss as a significant life event (Gage and Holcomb, 1991), most veterinarians still receive little or no training in providing grief education and support to pet owners. Lack of training extends to procedures surrounding euthanasia. For example, few veterinarians receive adequate instruction in either the medical or emotional protocols that can be used to effectively facilitate owner-present euthanasia.

More and more frequently, euthanasia is viewed, by veterinary professionals and companion animal owners alike, as a medical privilege and as a gift that can be lovingly bestowed upon dying animals. Thus, today, many euthanasias are conducted like ceremonies, with the process itself treated with the respect and reverence it deserves. To effectively facilitate owner-present euthanasias, veterinarians require expertise in two main areas. First, they must prepare owners to be present (if this is what they choose to do) during the animal's death. Second, they must understand how to facilitate the actual euthanasia procedure with both technical efficiency and emotional sensitivity.

## PREPARING OWNERS FOR COMPANION ANIMAL EUTHANASIA

Once owners have decided to euthanatize their companion animals, veterinarians need to prepare them for what lies ahead. Successful euthanasias begin with thorough preparation. Preparation minimizes the regrets, "what if's," and "if only's" that inevitably follow euthanasias that are not well planned. There are two main components of euthanasia preparation: (1) educating owners about the option to be present during a pet's euthanasia, and (2) facilitating agreements regarding the logistic details of the procedure.

### The Option of Owner Presence

Without question, it is emotionally painful for owners to watch their dearly loved companion animals die. However, clinical experience with owners shows that *not* being present when companion animals die potentially increases their feelings of pain and distress. There are several reasons owners want to be present when their companion animals die. These are:

1. Owners feel their companion animals have always "been there" for them; therefore, owners don't want to feel they abandoned their pets at the time of death.
2. Owners want to know for certain that their companion animals died peacefully, without pain, and that their deaths actually occurred.
3. Owners want the last thing their animals hear and feel to be the owner's soothing words and the owner's loving touches. They also want the chance to say good-bye to their companion animals, not before or after death, but at the moment death occurs.

It is intimidating for some owners to ask to be present with their animals when they die. From the perspective of companion animal owners, veterinarians are authority figures. It is the veterinarian's responsibility, then, to offer companion animal owners the choice to be present.

In order to make educated and informed choices about this option, owners need to know what the procedure entails. Veterinarians might provide this information to pet owners by saying something similar to the following:

"Mary, we know that Pepper is very important to you and to your family. Therefore, we are committed to making the euthanasia experience as meaningful and as positive for you as possible. In order to decide whether or not you want to be with Pepper when he dies, you need accurate information about euthanasia. Would you like me to explain the procedure to you now?"

With the owner's permission, the veterinarian continues:

"The first thing we may do in preparation for euthanatizing Pepper is to take him back to our treatment area, shave a small area of fur, and place an intravenous catheter in a vein, most likely in one of his rear legs. The use of a catheter simply means that we can administer the euthanasia solution more smoothly. It also means that we can accomplish what we need to do without interfering with your desire to pet or to hold Pepper's head.

"After this, Pepper will be brought back to you and you will be given time to spend with him, if you so desire. Then, when all of us agree that it is time to proceed, we will begin the euthanasia process. The method we prefer to use involves three injections. The first is merely a saline solution flush. This ensures that the catheter is working. The second is a barbiturate, usually thiopental, which places Pepper into a soothing state of relaxation. The third injection is the euthanasia solution, usually pentobarbitol sodium. This injection will actually stop Pepper's heart, brain activity, and other bodily functions, and ultimately cause his death. Many people are surprised by how quickly death takes place, as it occurs within a matter of seconds after the last injection is given.

"You should also know that, although humane death by euthanasia is usually peaceful, Pepper may urinate, defecate, twitch, or even let out a few loud sighs. He will not be aware of any of this, though, and he will not feel any pain. In addition, Pepper's eyes may not close. Do you have any questions about any of this?"

If the owner expresses understanding, the veterinarian concludes:

"Mary, after Pepper has died, you can stay with his body as long as possible."

Altogether, this explanation need take only about 10 minutes. It should be emphasized that this information is not delivered in a dry, continuous monologue, as during the veterinarian's explanations, it is not uncommon for owners to cry or to interrupt so they can ask questions. This explanation is greatly enhanced when the conversation is conducted in a private, quiet setting with both owners and veterinarians sitting or standing at the same eye level. It is also enhanced when veterinarians demonstrate their sense of compassion by offering tissues or gentle touches to owners who cry or openly express their feelings.

### Euthanasia Logistics

The second component of euthanasia preparation is planning and agreeing upon the logistic details of the procedure (Table 1). For example, appropriate times and sites for the procedure must be determined (Figs. 1 and 2). Owners must also decide who else, if anyone, they want to accompany them to the euthanasia. For example, with proper preparation, children often choose to be present when their companion animals die. It is a good idea for veterinarians to encourage owners to ask someone to attend their companion animal's euthanasia with them, as even sensitively conducted euthanasias are difficult to bear alone.

Regardless of where and when euthanasia occurs, procedural matters should be dealt with prior to the euthanasia, if possible. For instance, consent forms should be signed and arrangements for payment should be made. If appropriate, the option of necropsy should

**Table 1.** *Checklist for Euthanasia Procedures*\*†

**Before the Procedure, it is Helpful to:**
Inform owners that the time to consider euthanasia has arrived
Educate owners about the methods you use to facilitate the process
Prepare owners for what may happen during the procedure (possible side effects, their own grief manifestations)
Offer owners a choice about being present
Help owners plan the logistic details of euthanasia (where, when, body care, body container, bringing a friend for support)
Offer reading materials, videotapes, tours
Ask owners to sign consent forms and pay their bills ahead of time

**During the Procedure, it is Helpful to:**
Ask another veterinary professional to team the case with you
Prepare the euthanasia site
Place a catheter
Offer owners time alone with their pets
Pronounce the animal dead
Allow clients to clip fur, remove collars, or carry through with any activity that may be symbolic and meaningful to them

**After the Procedure, it is Helpful to:**
Notify other owners who are waiting for appointments if there are unexpected delays
Position/prepare the body for viewing, storage, and/or transport
Escort owners out a side or rear door
Update patient files and records
Send condolence cards or letters
Make follow-up telephone calls
Make referrals to support groups or grief counselors, if appropriate
Plan and carry out debriefing or stress-management strategies

\*Several steps facilitate owner-present euthanasias. The categories used here are somewhat arbitrary, but can be used as a guide to assist pet owners with the process.

†If the veterinarian tends to get nervous during owner-present euthanasias, this checklist can be kept on on a clipboard or inside the patient's file so the veterinarian can discreetly refer to it, if needed.

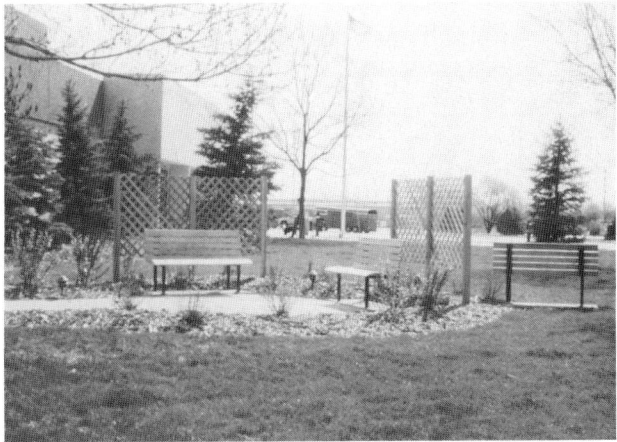

**Figure 2.** Many clients, whose animals have always loved the outdoors (or hated the veterinarian's office), are comforted when they can help their animals die in nonclinical, natural settings.

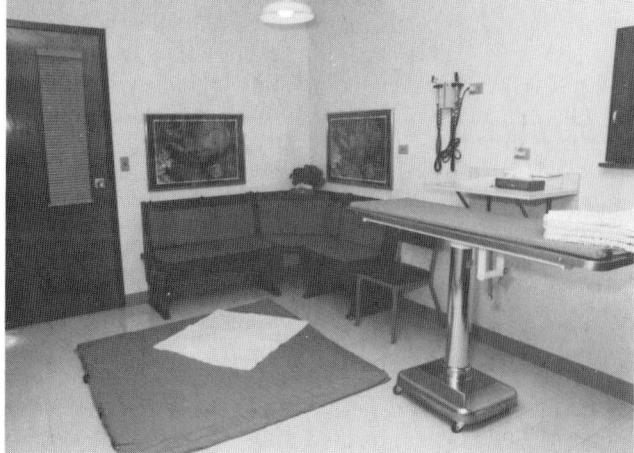

**Figure 1.** This examination room is designed to encourage owner presence during companion animal euthanasia. Special features include comfortable seating (corner bench and floor mat), lowered lighting, window coverings to ensure privacy, and plenty of facial tissues.

be explained. If time allows, suggestions for how to memorialize a pet can also be discussed.

Whenever possible, decisions about body care should be made prior to euthanasia. Owners should be offered all of the options available to them and each should be explained with honesty and sensitivity. It is helpful to use visual aids during this explanation. For example, if veterinarians make caskets or urns available for owners to purchase, samples can be shown (Fig. 3). Body care options can be explained by either veterinarians or technicians. Again, it is important to emphasize that this information is not delivered in the form of a dry, continuous monologue, as owners often respond to it by crying or by asking several questions. When offering body care options, veterinarians and staff might say something like:

"Mary, we can offer you three options for taking care of Pepper's body after he dies. The first option is that you can take him with you and bury him in a pet cemetery or in another appropriate place. If that is your choice, we encourage you to bring something with you to the euthanasia that you feel will be okay for transporting his body. This might be a blanket or a box. We also have caskets available if you would like to purchase one.

"Second, we can cremate Pepper's body and either dispose of the cremains for you or return them to you, if you so desire. If you want them returned to you, you may want to choose an urn or another kind of container for them. Some people like to keep their companion animal's cremains, while others like to spread them in an appropriate location. Since so many people today move quite often, many owners choose cremation so they can take their companion animal's cremains with them.

"Your third option, Mary, is to have us take care of his body for you. If you would like to know specifically how we dispose of animals' bodies, I can discuss this with you. Would you like to have that information?"

If the owner answers "yes," the veterinarian continues with an honest and specific explanation of the disposal method and final location. The veterinarian can soften the explanation by saying something like:

"I wish we had more aesthetically pleasing options to offer you, but the only choice we have is _____."

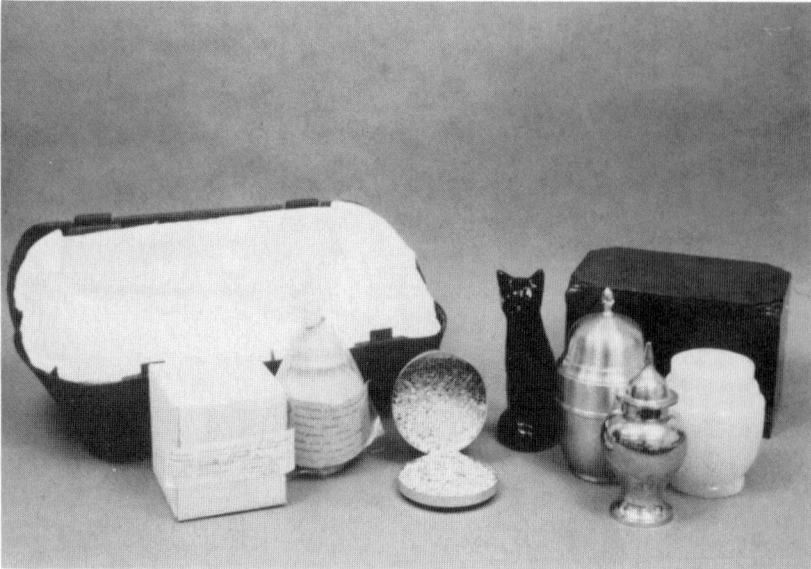

**Figure 3.** Veterinary professionals can use brochures, pictures, and sample items (e.g., caskets, urns, cremains) when helping pet owners make decisions about body care.

Clinical experience has shown that, for some owners, once their companion animals are dead, their bodies no longer have meaning for them. Typically, these owners have no objections to mass burial in a landfill. In fact, when given the option of mass burial at the city landfill, one client quipped, "That's perfect for my dog. His favorite thing to do was to get into the garbage!"

However, because the thought of burying their companion animals at the landfill might be abhorrent for other owners, veterinarians have an ethical responsibility to offer this information to anyone who considers this option. Clinical experience shows that the omission of pertinent details often serves to complicate owner's grief. For example, an elderly woman who decided to have her veterinarian dispose of her dog's body was simply told that her dog would be buried in a mass grave. A month after her dog's death, she contacted her veterinarian and told him she wanted to know where the mass grave was located so she could visit her dog. At that time, the veterinarian reluctantly told the woman that the mass grave was located at the landfill. The woman found this information extremely upsetting and told the veterinarian that, had she known this during her decision-making process, she would have certainly chosen another body care option.

## FACILITATING OWNER-PRESENT EUTHANASIAS

Ideally, owner-present euthanasias are scheduled during times when veterinarians feel most able to meet the demands of the procedure. This may be during the early morning, late afternoon, or even during evening hours. If all involved have agreed that the veterinary facility is the best environment for the euthanasia, owners who arrive for euthanasia appointments should never be kept waiting. Rather, they should be given first priority over everything except medical emergencies. They should also be immediately escorted to the euthanasia site.

It is highly recommended that all owner-present euthanasias be conducted by a team of at least two veterinary professionals. This allows whoever is assisting the veterinarian to focus on the owner's needs and allows the veterinarian to concentrate on the medical aspects of the procedure.

It is also highly recommended that, if an owner has elected to be present, the use of a catheter be carefully evaluated. Catheters are not always necessary and they do not always improve the medical procedures involved with euthanasia. However, they are often an enhancement to the emotional side of euthanasia, as they provide extra insurance that animals die peacefully, without adverse side effects. As previously explained, if the veterinarian decides to use a catheter, it may be best to place it in a rear leg. This allows the owner free access to the face and head of the pet.

After the intravenous catheter has been placed and the animal has been returned to the euthanasia site, owners should be given the opportunity to spend a short time alone with their companion animals, if they so desire. If owners are left alone to say their last goodbyes, the veterinarian should state when he or she will return. For instance, the veterinarian may say, "I will be back in about 10 minutes."

If, after about 10 min, owners are still saying goodbye, the veterinarian can approach them and gently say, "It is time for us to proceed. May we begin?" Most owners will indicate their answer by either nodding or shaking their heads. If their answer is "no," it is appropriate for the veterinarian to give them 5 or 10 min more. Any statement to this effect, though, must be made in a calm, quiet voice with no overtones of impatience or scolding detectable. Owners often report that they felt rushed through the euthanasia process by their veterinarian and feel this negated all of the other positive aspects of their experience.

When owners are ready to proceed, it is normal for the veterinary team members to feel somewhat awkward as they enter the environment in which the eu-

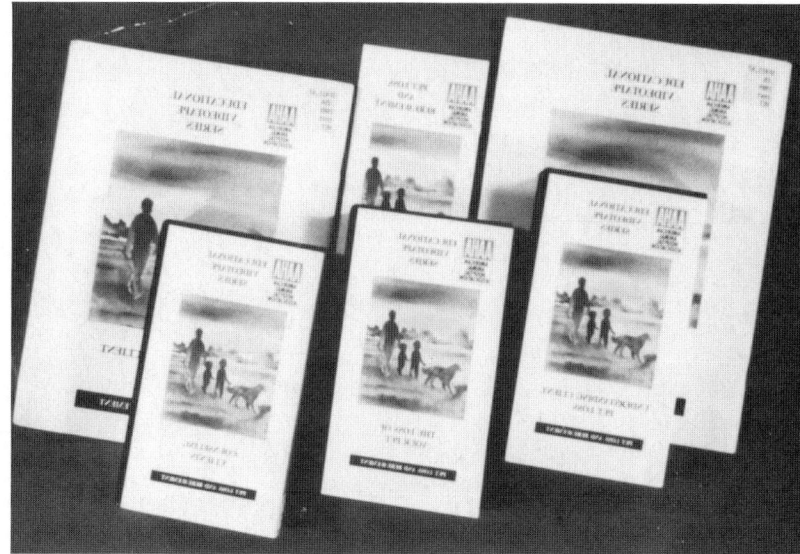

**Figure 4.** Numerous ways to support pet owners during grief are discussed in the American Animal Hospital Association's videotaped educational series on pet loss counseling and client relations.

thanasia is to be performed. Many wonder what they should say or do to comfort their grieving clients. Often, no words are necessary. A touch on an owner's arm or a hug around their shoulders communicates support and understanding quite well.

Before veterinarians begin the lethal injections, they should again tell the owners that they are ready to begin. Whenever possible, syringes should be kept out of sight (e.g., in the pocket of a laboratory coat or a smock) and handled very discreetly, as some people become very alarmed at the sight of syringes and needles. Once the procedure has begun, the drugs should be injected quickly, with little or no lapse of time between them. As they are injected, each may be named so owners are kept abreast of how the procedure is progressing. For example, veterinarians might say:

"Mary, I am injecting the first solution, the saline flush, to make sure the catheter we have inserted is working properly." Once that has been done, the next might be announced by saying, "Now I am giving Pepper a barbiturate that will make him sleepy and help him drift off into a soothing plane of anesthesia." When it is time for the last injection, the veterinarian might say, "Now I am injecting the final drug."

Aside from these statements, it is best for veterinarians to remain silent. Most owners want to focus on saying good-bye to their animals, and find comments, questions, and chatter distracting to their concentration.

With this combination of drugs, adverse side effects rarely occur. Thus, this method of facilitating euthanasia usually goes so smoothly that owners often don't realize their pets have actually died. It is very important, then, for the veterinarian to use a stethoscope to listen for a final heartbeat. When the veterinarian can do so with certainty, the animal should be pronounced dead. Veterinarians should do this with a clear, simple statement such as: "Mary, Pepper is dead." At this time, owners may gasp, cry, sob, or sigh with relief. They may make remarks about how quickly death came and about how peaceful the experience was.

Once death has occurred, owners may review their pets' lives by sharing special or funny stories about the pet. During this time, owners and veterinary professionals alike may feel a need to say good-bye, to comfort one another, and to express their feelings of grief. Creating opportunities to fulfill these needs is important, as support and emotional catharsis are variables known to have positive impact on peoples' overall grief outcomes (Maddison and Walker, 1967; Rando, 1984).

## CONCLUSION

After euthanasia, some people want to leave the euthanasia site quickly, while others need more time alone with their pets. When owners are ready to leave, they should be escorted out a side or back door, if possible, so they don't have to exit through the busy waiting area. Also, if possible, a staff member should stay with the animal's body if the owners are not taking it with them. Almost every owner takes one last look back at their pet before they actually leave. When they see a friendly, familiar face next to their pet, they feel reassured that their companion animal will not be forgotten or treated with disrespect once they leave.

Contacting owners after their companion animals have been euthanatized is a crucial part of retaining their trust. Sending clients personalized condolence cards, letters, or even contacting them by telephone should be standard procedure. When euthanasias are facilitated with compassion and sensitivity, they can soothe and reassure all involved that the decision to end a companion animal's life was the right one (Fig. 4).

### References and Suggested Reading

Gage G and Holcomb R: Couples' perceptions of the stressfulness of the death of the family pet. *Fam Relations* 40:103, 1991.
Maddison D and Walker WL: Factors affecting the outcome of conjugal bereavement. *Brt J Psychiatry*, 113:1057, 1967.
Rando TA: *Grief, Dying, and Death: Clinical Interventions for Caregivers.* Champaign, IL, Research Press Company, 1984.

# Section

# 2

# CRITICAL
# CARE

ROBERT J. MURTAUGH
*Consulting Editor*

***Still Current Information Found in Current Veterinary Therapy XI:***

### Elsewhere in Current Veterinary Therapy XII:

# OUTCOME PREDICTION IN EMERGENCY AND CRITICAL CARE PATIENTS

LESLEY G. KING
*and* RICHARD A. ROCKAR
*Philadelphia, Pennsylvania*

As veterinary critical care has become more sophisticated, we have become adept at maintaining life in very critically ill canine and feline patients. Often, such heroic efforts are associated with considerable investment of time, effort, and money on the part of both the owner and the veterinary hospital staff. Clinicians in veterinary intensive care are therefore becoming increasingly concerned about the economic and social cost of current practices of critical patient management. We routinely face situations where considerable time and energy has already been expended to provide support for a patient, and a subsequent decision to withdraw therapy or to euthanize a patient is fraught with uncertainty. We must therefore look for objective ways to make informed decisions about therapy.

An important consequence of the knowledge explosion in veterinary critical care has been an increased interest in clinical research studies. Research in veterinary patients with naturally occurring illness is an essential part of the development of any new specialty: both to emphasize the similarities between animal and human disease processes, and therefore serve as a model for human disease; and also to elucidate the differences between species, and therefore improve our ability to care for our veterinary patients. As clinical research studies have become an important part of our mission in critical care, we need to find objective ways to quantify the severity of disease in individual patients, regardless of the disease process. This allows us to provide risk stratification; that is, to allow clinical patients to be objectively grouped according to the severity of their disease. Such stratification then allows meaningful comparisons to be made between groups with respect to response to the therapy being studied.

Prognostic indicators have been well established for many specific naturally occurring disease processes. One of the best examples of this is found in the specialty of veterinary oncology, where survival can often be accurately predicted based on extent of neoplasia and metastasis at the initiation of therapy. Prognosis has also been clearly estimated or established in well-controlled, experimentally induced disease processes in research animals. In clinical practice, however, we often do not know the diagnosis, or the severity of the process, at the beginning of hospitalization. Therefore, prognostic estimates based on a specific diagnosis may not be useful. Similarly, predictions of outcome based on experimental studies may be of diminished value clinically. Patients with naturally occurring disorders are often presented for treatment at different or advanced stages of disease. They often receive different therapies from animals in experimental protocols, and they may suffer from complicating factors; for example, age, or concurrent disease such as chronic renal or cardiac insufficiency. Outcome in any individual therefore depends on the type and severity of disease; physiologic reserve and the presence of concurrent disease processes; and the type, amount, and response to therapy.

Thus, we can recognize a need for objective estimates of outcome for veterinary patients with critical illness. Ideally, such estimates should be applicable to any patient, regardless of diagnosis. They should be easily obtained or calculated early in the course of hospitalization, and should be based on objective, measurable parameters that are reproducible from one institution to another. Such parameters should be a routine part of management of critically ill patients, and should be relatively safe, easy, and inexpensive to obtain.

We must recognize the limitations of any estimate of prognosis in individual patients. In using such systems, we hope to identify patients who will benefit from intensive care or specific therapies, and those for whom intensive care will not improve chances of survival. Although outcome prediction is valuable, the confidence level of the prediction varies directly with sample size; that is, the accuracy of the system depends on the number of patients that have been studied. It is statistically impossible to predict survival in an individual based on records of previous patients. The most we can say is that no individual with a given set of characteristics has ever survived.

In human medicine, a variety of prognostic systems have been developed. Although some apply to specific disorders or situations, many frequently used systems are applicable to patients with a wide variety of problems. Investigators in veterinary medicine have begun to modify and apply some of these systems. We can consider the use of systems that apply "scores" to an individual patient, numerically quantifying the severity of disease, or alternatively, we can evaluate the function of one vital organ system as a global indicator of prognosis. Three major types of predictive systems will be considered:

1. Scoring the extent of physiologic derangement (severity-of-disease scoring systems) at admission. This is potentially applicable to any patient admitted.

2. Trauma scoring systems including the Small Animal Coma Score, designed specifically to evaluate trauma patients.

3. Prognostic indicators of severity of disease based on function of one key organ system; for example, pulmonary function or thyroid hormone secretion. This is potentially applicable to any critical patient.

## SEVERITY-OF-DISEASE SCORING SYSTEMS

A severity-of-disease scoring system modeled on the human Acute Physiology and Chronic Health Evaluation (APACHE) system has been developed for use in dogs, and is currently undergoing evaluation. The premise of this scoring system is that any illness can lead to abnormalities in physiologic variables, and the extent of derangement depends on the severity of the disorder. A number of physiologic variables are measured within the first 24 hr after admission to the intensive care unit (ICU). These variables can be divided into three major groups: (1) tests that define the function of the vital organ systems (e.g., heart rate, mean arterial pressure, oxygenation, creatinine, bilirubin, and neurologic status); (2) tests that define the overall metabolic condition of the animal and that are often abnormal in critical patients, including acid-base status, plasma glucose and electrolytes, serum total protein and albumin, packed cell volume, white blood cell count, and body temperature; and (3) parameters that define the expected physiologic reserve (e.g., the age and body weight of the animal or the presence of chronic disease or immunosuppression). All of these parameters are routinely measured in critically ill patients; therefore, collection of data needed for calculation of a severity of disease score should not represent a significant burden to the animal, the owner, or the veterinary staff.

Preliminary data from a pilot study in 200 dogs conducted at the University of Pennsylvania are shown in Figure 1.

Current information suggests that this scoring system will account for at least 75% of the variance in mortality in individual patients. It is important to recognize that this information is very preliminary, and that as we collect more data we hope to improve our ability to objectively predict outcome in the veterinary ICU patient. To date, researchers have studied thousands of human patients—the most recent version, "APACHE III," presented data from over 17,000 human intensive care patients (Knaus et al., 1991). Investigators using the APACHE system in human patients have found that outcome prediction using this system varies with different disease processes (McAnena et al., 1992; Rhee et al., 1990). As we enlarge the data base of veterinary patients, we also hope to establish the limitations of this type of prediction, both within and among various diseases.

## TRAUMA SCORING SYSTEMS

A trauma score is a numerical characterization of injuries sustained from a traumatic incident. Trauma scoring systems can be based on either an anatomic or a physiologic assessment of the patient's condition. The most widely used anatomic scoring system in human trauma medicine is the Injury Severity Score (ISS). The patient's injuries are assigned an Abbreviated Injury Scale (AIS) number value in each of six body regions: external, head/neck, face, chest, abdominal/pelvic contents, and extremities/pelvic girdle. Each region receives an AIS point score for its most serious injury. The ISS is the sum of the squares of the AIS values for the three highest scoring regions. Maximum ISS value is 75 ($5^2 + 5^2 + 5^2$).

Physiologic scoring systems include the Glasgow Coma Scale (GCS) and the Revised Trauma Score (RTS). These scales assess physiologic derangement independent of trauma focus. The GCS was developed specifically for evaluation of neurologic function and assigns a point value for the performance of three functions: eye opening, motor response, and verbal response. The RTS assigns a point value to the patient's GCS and then adds point values for respiratory rate and systolic blood pressure.

Two major forces have driven the implementation of trauma scoring systems in human emergency medicine: the development of specialized regional trauma centers and third party reimbursement. Triage trauma scores, such as the RTS, enable emergency medical technicians to direct the critically injured patient to a high-level trauma center without overburdening the center with the relatively stable victims. Objective assessment of overall injuries with the ISS has allowed the development of formulas for third-party reimbursement appropriate to the level of medical care received by the trauma patient.

Third-party reimbursement for veterinary emergency care and transport to the veterinary emergency

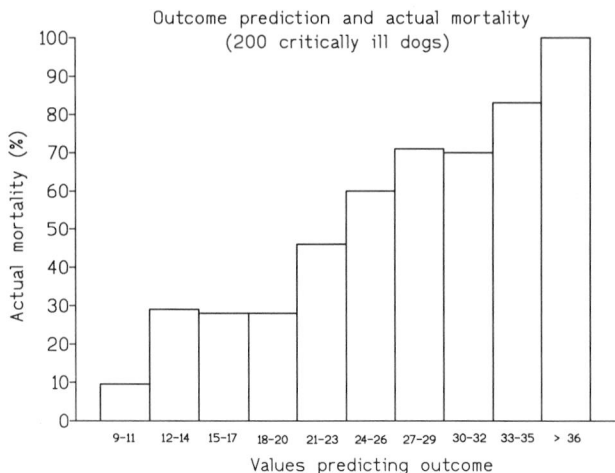

**Figure 1.** Preliminary data from a pilot study of severity-of-disease scoring in 200 dogs at the University of Pennsylvania School of Veterinary Medicine, indicating increased mortality at higher scores.

center by trained veterinary personnel is unlikely to become widespread in the near future. The use of trauma scoring, however, can greatly facilitate the administration of emergency care to the individual veterinary trauma patient. Kirby and Brasmer (Kirby, 1991; Brasmer, 1984) each have emphasized the importance of categorizing traumatic injuries as mild, moderate, severe, or catastrophic. A trauma scoring system provides an objective and organized means of identifying critical injuries and prioritizing emergency care. The trauma scale can also be used to monitor the response to initial therapy. A deteriorating score suggests the need to reevaluate the patient and adjust the therapy. Lastly, a scoring system standardizes the categorization of trauma within an emergency center.

Trauma scoring systems also facilitate the comparison of trauma patient populations. Using the numerical values of the trauma scale, well-defined subpopulations of trauma patients are established. The most obvious use of these groups would be outcome prediction. On its own, a trauma scoring system probably won't show a direct linear relationship to the final bill or chance of survival. However, the trauma score could be used to establish a prognostic scale after evaluation of a large data base with sophisticated statistical treatment. This equips the emergency clinician for a frank and honest discussion of the owner's financial commitment. Developing a prognostic scale also allows for simplified quality assurance evaluation of emergency care. The outcome for a given trauma score could be compared for different time intervals to evaluate an institution, or cases producing unexpected outcomes could be identified for further review.

Developing trauma patient subsets based on trauma scores could also facilitate clinical research. An innovative therapy for shock may significantly improve the outcome of patients with midrange trauma scores, but have no effect on those patients with mild or catastrophic trauma. This beneficial response may not be identified if the analysis only looks at the whole trauma patient population. Furthermore, collaborative research among emergency centers is facilitated with a standard trauma classification system.

Evaluation of veterinary trauma scoring systems has been limited to date. Shores has developed the Small Animal Coma Score (SACS), modeled from the Glasgow Coma Scale (Shores, 1989). The SACS assigns a point score (1 to 6; 6 = normal) to motor activity, brain stem reflexes, and level of consciousness. Initial results seem promising, but statistical evaluations of the importance of total score and the individual components have been limited.

## PROGNOSIS BASED ON FUNCTION OF ONE ORGAN SYSTEM

### Thyroid Function Testing as an Indicator of Outcome

In animals and people with normal thyroid function, severe illness is associated with decreased secretion of hormones from the thyroid gland, and with diminished peripheral conversion of the inactive thyroxine ($T_4$) to active triiodothyronine ($T_3$), a condition known as the "euthyroid sick syndrome." In people, the extent of depression of thyroid hormone secretion is dependent on the severity of illness, and there is a significant correlation between serum concentrations of $T_3$ and mortality rate (Kaptein et al., 1982). Recent retrospective studies in canine intensive care patients at the University of Pennsylvania have shown that a similar correlation exists in veterinary patients. The euthyroid sick syndrome was commonly found in critically ill dogs. There was a significant correlation between the extent of depression of canine baseline $T_3$ and $T_4$, and mortality rate for a given hospitalization in the ICU. Evaluation of thyroid function may therefore be useful for early prediction of a poor outcome, and for identification of dogs that appear to be doing well, but that are suffering from hidden underlying complications that may later affect survival. Further prospective studies are necessary to fully evaluate this type of predictive index.

### Oxygen Tension–Based Indices as Indicators of Survival

In a large retrospective study at Colorado State University, results of arterial blood gas analysis were evaluated for correlation with survival (Van Pelt et al., 1991). Several oxygen tension–based indices were evaluated to determine if they were predictive of severity of disease. Of these, the alveolar-arterial oxygen tension gradient ($P(A\text{-}a)O_2$) (see "Monitoring the Critically Ill Patient," this volume, p 98) was found to be significantly correlated with outcome ($p<.014$). Other factors that contributed to the model predictive of survival included age and base excess. It is important to recognize that the $P(A\text{-}a)O_2$ is an index of overall pulmonary function, and does not distinguish between individual pulmonary disease processes; it is, however, also affected by cardiovascular factors such as cardiac output. Since respiratory function is vital to survival and respiratory dysfunction is very common in critically ill patients, such a simple prognostic indicator might be expected to be of considerable value. Interestingly, the model for survival did not appear to be influenced by the underlying disease. Further prospective studies may confirm the value of this simple and informative way of predicting outcome.

## APPLICATIONS AND LIMITATIONS OF DISEASE SCORING SYSTEMS

Development of a valid severity-of-disease scoring system for animals requires a large data base and rigorous statistical analysis of the data base. In suitable applications, disease scoring systems can create population subsets to highlight the effect of experimental therapeutic protocols. A severity-of-disease score can identify unexpected outcomes or changes in population outcome to focus our internal review of critical care delivery. From an individual standpoint, we can derive statistical prediction of prognosis to assist with client consultations. Therapeutically, a changing numerical score gives us another parameter to evaluate an individual's response to treatment. Properly used, severity of disease scores provide a powerful tool in patient assessment.

Severity of disease scores can lead to dangerous conclusions if the limitations of the system are ignored. First and foremost, predictions are valid only if they come from a patient population similar to that used in validating the disease score. A trauma score developed for blunt motor vehicle injuries may not accurately predict survival of those animals falling from the fifth floor. Secondly, the issue of euthanasia can complicate our statistical assessment of a scoring system. We have all euthanized animals that may have survived had there not been restricted finances or an owner that directed us otherwise. Lastly, we must remember that our patients are individuals within our statistical population. We should neither become lackadaisical in our approach to the trauma patient because a trauma score is near normal, nor should we condemn the dog with pancreatitis based only on the severity of disease score.

## References and Suggested Reading

Brasmer TH: The acutely traumatized small animal patient. *In Major Problems in Veterinary Medicine,* volume 2. Philadelphia, WB Saunders Co, 1984, p 45.
  *A description of the examination of the veterinary trauma patient.*
Kaptein EM, et al: Relationship of altered thyroid hormone indices to survival in nonthyroidal illness. Clin Endocrinol 16:565, 1982.
Kirby R: Approach to the trauma patient. *In* Campfield WW (ed): *The Kal Kan Waltham Symposium for the Treatment of Small Animal Diseases: Emergency Medicine and Critical Care.* Vernon CA, Kal Kan Foods Inc, 1991, p 15.
  *An overview of veterinary trauma patient triage.*
Knaus WA, et al: The APACHE III prognostic system. Risk prediction of hospital mortality for critically ill hospitalized adults. Chest 100:1619, 1991.
  *Results of the most recent evaluation of the APACHE system.*
McAnena OJ, et al: Invalidation of the APACHE II scoring system for patients with acute trauma. J Trauma 33:504, 1992.
Rhee KJ, et al: APACHE II scoring in the injured patient. Crit Care Med 18:827, 1990.
Schuster DP: Predicting outcome after ICU admission—the art and science of assessing risk. Chest 102:1861, 1992.
  *A review of severity of disease scores and their statistical evaluation.*
Shores A: Craniocerebral trauma. *In* Kirk RW (ed): *Current Veterinary Therapy X: Small Animal Practice.* Philadelphia, WB Saunders Co, 1989, pp 847.
  *A review describing the Small Animal Coma Score.*
Van Pelt DR, et al: Oxygen-tension based indices as predictors of survival in critically ill dogs: Clinical observations and review. J Vet Emerg Crit Care 1:19, 1991.
  *An evaluation of blood gas parameters in dogs with regard to outcome.*
Wisner DH: History and current status of trauma scoring systems. Arch Surg 127:11, 1992.
  *A review of trauma scoring systems used in human emergency medicine.*
Yates DW: Scoring systems for trauma. BMJ 301:1090, 1990.
  *A review, with examples, of trauma scoring systems used in human emergency medicine.*

# MONITORING THE CRITICALLY ILL PATIENT

JANET ALDRICH
*and* STEVE C. HASKINS

*Davis, California*

## GENERAL EXAMINATION

There are certain questions that should be asked of every patient, every day (Table 1). Many of these can be addressed by performing a complete physical examination. Monitoring should be sufficiently frequent and extensive to warrant that the animal stays out of harm's way. The problem is that one never is really certain from which direction harm will come. When in doubt as to whether to monitor a given parameter—do so; if it is important enough to ask the question, it is important enough to monitor.

The most important aspect of critical care monitoring is the frequent physical evaluation of the patient by individuals who can properly interpret what they see, hear, and feel. Expensive equipment and extensive technology helps in some situations, but does not replace the frequent "laying on of the hands" by people who care. Following a careful physical examination, additional tests, studies, and procedures should be considered.

## BIOCHEMICAL MEASUREMENTS

### Hemoglobin

Hemoglobin (grams per deciliter) and red blood cells (RBCs) must be structurally normal and in sufficient concentration for adequate oxygen transport. Packed cell volume (PCV) is the relative volume (%) occupied by RBCs in proportion to the amount of total blood

**Table 1.** *A Critical Care Checklist*

1. Cardiovascular
   Electrical, mechanical, arterial blood pressure, tissue perfusion
2. Pulmonary
   Ventilation, oxygenation
3. Central nervous system
   Mentation, behavior, locomotion
4. Other organ systems
   Gastrointestinal, hematology, biochemistries
5. Hydration, fluid and electrolyte status
6. Nutritional status
7. Comfort
   Physical, emotional, pain
8. Asepsis status, including temperature
9. Weight
10. Trends or obvious changes

measured. The hematocrit (Hct) obtained from automated cell counters is calculated from measured parameters of mean corpuscular volume (MCV) and the RBC count. This value can differ from that obtained by the microhematocrit method, and we prefer the more readily available microhematocrit method when comparing serial samples. When using the microhematocrit method, adequate centrifugal force and time must be applied in order to obtain consistent results.

## Colloid Oncotic Pressure

Plasma proteins exert an osmotic pressure because they do not readily diffuse through the capillary membrane. This osmotic pressure is called colloid pressure or colloid oncotic pressure (COP). The COP retains water within the vascular space. Protein molecules account for approximately 60% of the total COP. Since albumin has an average molecular weight about one half that of globulin, albumin exerts the majority (75%) of the COP attributable to plasma proteins. The total COP is greater than that accounted for by plasma proteins because the negatively charged proteins attract cations (mostly Na), thus increasing the number of osmotically active particles. This additional osmotic pressure, called the Donnan effect, accounts for the other 40% of total COP. COP may be calculated from the total plasma proteins; however, in critically ill patients this value may be unreliable because sick animals may have altered albumin/globulin ratios. Malnutrition and increased capillary permeability can enhance the effects of hypoalbuminemia in causing intravascular volume loss. Blood and plasma have the same COP because RBCs exert no osmotic effect. The COP may be measured in a membrane-transducer oncometer in which plasma is placed on one side of a semipermeable membrane and a protein-free solution on the other. Fluid moves through the membrane until the pressures on either side are equal. This pressure is the COP. The COP is approximately 25 mm Hg for ambulatory human patients and 18 to 20 mm Hg in critically ill patients. The correlation, if any, between the refractive index of infused hetastarch or dextran and COP is not

known; therefore, we do not use changes in the refractive index to monitor therapy with these products.

The physical examination should be correlated with the COP (estimated or measured). It is helpful to separate the physical examination findings related to intravascular volume (mucous membrane color, capillary refill time, heart rate, pulse quality) from those related to interstitial volume (skin turgor, mucous membrane moistness). In critically ill patients with decreased COP or increased capillary membrane permeability, the ratio of vascular/interstitial volume is altered; therefore, adequate or even increased interstitial volume cannot be assumed to guarantee adequate intravascular volume.

## Glucose

A deficit in glucose availability to the cells occurs with either hypoglycemia or with an absolute or relative insulin deficiency. Hypoglycemia can occur rapidly and unexpectedly in critically ill patients, and frequent monitoring, especially in the face of changing clinical states, is indicated. Hypoglycemia should be considered in any patient that is septic, hypothermic, seizuring, or exhibiting altered mentation. Marked hyperglycemia can be associated with coma.

## Osmolality

Osmolality is a measure of the total number of solute particles in solution; however, only those solutes whose movement is restricted by a cell membrane will effect the movement of water. The concentration of such solutes is the *effective* osmolality or tonicity of a fluid. Sodium and its associated anions, and glucose are the major contributors to plasma tonicity. Urea contributes to measured osmolality but is not an effective osmol because it is freely diffusible. Measured osmolality is compared to the value calculated from the equation

$$2 \times [Na^+] + BUN/2.8 + glucose/18$$

When measured osmolality minus calculated osmolality exceeds 10 mOsm/kg, an abnormal osmolal gap is present. This finding indicates the accumulation of a solute not represented in the equation such as ethylene glycol, mannitol, or an organic acid (see "Strong Ions and Acid-Base Disorders," this volume, p 121).

## Sodium and Fluid Balance

Serum (or plasma) sodium concentration is a solute/solvent expression. In most cases, changes in serum sodium concentration reflect changes in plasma water. Hypernatremia decreases cell volume, while hyponatremia causes a fluid shift into the intracellular compartment. Neither hypernatremia nor hyponatremia is associated with specific clinical signs (see *CVT XI*, p 301). However, one important clinical consequence of marked changes in serum sodium is altered cerebral function including coma and seizures.

As plasma osmolality increases, vasopressin is released and renal water conservation is enhanced; however, only a portion of the total urine volume is solute-free water available for reabsorption. If plasma osmolality continues to rise, thirst is stimulated, although not all solutes are equally potent in stimulating thirst. Thirst is the major defense against volume contraction and hypernatremia, provided the patient has access to water and is able to drink. The vascular volume is primarily regulated by renal sodium conservation but, if necessary, vascular volume can be defended by renal free-water conservation even at the expense of inducing hypo-osmolality. This is one cause of hyponatremia in volume-depleted patients or in animals with severe congestive heart failure.

The volume of the extracellular space is regulated by total body sodium. Total body sodium depletion contracts the intravascular volume, but total body sodium excess may be associated with increased, normal or decreased intravascular volume.

Volume overload of the extracellular space may be due to renal failure or abnormal renal function—in which case sodium excretion is insufficient—or to decreases in the effective arterial volume, as occurs with congestive heart failure or nephrotic syndrome. The renal response to vascular volume depletion should be retention of sodium so that the urine sodium is less than 10 mEq/L. Urine sodium concentration greater than 20 mEq/L in volume-depleted patients suggests renal sodium wasting or diuretic therapy.

Deficits of total body sodium may be recognized in the patient as decreases in interstitial volume (decreased skin turgor, decreased mucous membrane moistness) or deficits of intravascular volume (blood pressure, mucous membrane color, capillary refill time, heart rate, pulse quality). Most of these assessments are subjective and most useful when serial examinations are made by the same, experienced examiner. Excesses in extracellular volume may be recognized as peripheral edema in dependent areas and periorbital tissues (chemosis), distention of the jugular veins, hydrothorax, or ascites. The volume of the overexpanded extracellular space may be partitioned normally between intravascular and interstitial spaces or maldistributed with the intravascular space smaller than expected. This is most likely to occur when COP is low so that plasma water is not adequately retained within the vascular space.

## Potassium

Disorders of serum (or plasma) potassium are commonly encountered related to fluid therapy, diuretic use, vomiting, acute renal failure, and diabetes mellitus. Of the total body potassium, only 2 to 5% is extracellular. The intracellular/extracellular potassium ratio is a major determinant of resting membrane potential required for proper muscle and nerve function. The distribution of potassium across cell membranes is affected by acid-base balance, tonicity, cell integrity, and

hormones such as insulin and epinephrine. Insulin, for example, increases cellular potassium uptake. Alkalosis may cause a net potassium movement into cells, while acidosis may cause potassium to leave cells. Hypertonicity causes potassium to move out of cells, an effect particularly important in diabetes mellitus. Regulation of the balance between potassium intake and excretion, primarily by the kidney, maintains total body potassium over the long term. Regulation of the ratio between intracellular and extracellular potassium guards against acute changes in serum potassium. Thus, serum potassium can change without any alteration in total body potassium, a condition commonly seen in critically ill patients. In more chronic conditions, changes in serum potassium may reflect changes in total body potassium. This effect is most noticeable when total body potassium is increased, in which case serum potassium rises steeply. Proportionally greater changes in total body potassium are required to cause noticeable changes in serum potassium in cases of total body potassium depletion. Clinical signs of potassium disorders are reviewed elsewhere (see *CVT XI*, p 301). Muscle weakness (hypokalemia) and cardiac arrest (hyperkalemia) are serious consequences.

## Ionized Calcium

The most important physiologically active fraction of extracellular calcium is the ionized fraction, the other fractions being chelated and protein bound. The protein-bound fraction is primarily bound to albumin. Ionized calcium determinations, which measure the physiologically active form, are the most useful in the critically ill patient. This fraction cannot be reliably predicted from total serum calcium concentration because of changes in pH and serum protein concentration that are common in critically ill patients. Acidosis increases ionized calcium because of decreased protein binding, while alkalosis has the opposite effect. Hypoalbuminemia results in decreased ionized calcium in human subjects. In dogs it is helpful to adjust total serum calcium values upward to account for hypoalbuminemia in order to avoid diagnosing abnormalities of calcium homeostasis where none exist. Ionized calcium is measured with ion-selective membrane electrodes. Samples must be handled anaerobically and processed promptly. Clinical manifestations of hypocalcemia are usually manifested as tremors, shaking, or seizures.

## Metabolic Acidosis

Metabolic acidosis is a common condition in critically ill patients and is characterized by a decrease in pH and $[HCO_3^-]$. Calculation of the anion gap ($Na^+ - [Cl^- + Tco_2]$) may help in classifying a metabolic acidosis (see "Strong Ions and Acid-Base Disorders," this volume, p 121). The normal anion gap is 8 to 16 mEq/L. Total $CO_2$ ($Tco_2$) is a measure of both $[HCO_3^-]$ and dissolved carbon dioxide and is usually determined from a venous sample. Therefore $TCO_2$ is usually higher than arterial $[HCO_3^-]$ by 2 to 5 mmol/L. The $TCO_2$ is often used in calculating the anion gap. An increase in production of lactate or ketoacids, excess retention of phosphate or sulfate in renal failure, or generation of organic acids from ethylene glycol poisoning will increase the difference between measured cations and anions, causing an anion-gap acidosis. Decreased $H^+$ excretion by the kidney, or base loss by the kidney or gastrointestinal tract, or acid ingestion will cause a hyperchloremic acidosis without an anion gap. The widening of the anion gap may be obscured by changes in pH and albumin, since the charge of albumin is related to pH, with acidemia decreasing and alkalemia increasing the anion gap. Therefore, patients with lactic acidosis and hypoalbuminemia might not have an anion gap but would nonetheless have metabolic acidosis.

Strict classification of acid-base disturbances, as with the use of a nomogram, can be misleading because critically ill patients often have more than one disorder affecting acid-base status and because incomplete compensation is common in acute disorders. It is most useful to review the entire clinical picture in order to assess the factors that are affecting acid-base balance. While an abnormal laboratory value indicates at least one disturbance, a normal value may result from multiple disturbances acting in opposite directions (see "Strong Ions and Acid-Base Disorders," this volume, p 121).

### Lactate

Adequate tissue perfusion and oxygen delivery to cells is needed for aerobic metabolism. When oxygen demands are not met, lactic acidosis occurs. The severity of the acidosis and the concentration of lactate are rough indicators of the extent of the oxygen debt. Lactate concentrations greater than 2 mEq/L indicate abnormal lactate accumulation and are a common cause of an increased anion gap.

### Evaluation of Primary Hemostasis: Vascular and Platelet

The physical examination provides the first important means of evaluating bleeding disorders. Petechiation indicates a defect in platelet number or function. If vascular integrity is compromised, the effect can be widespread peripheral edema and ecchymoses. Defects in primary hemostasis (platelet/vascular) can cause continuous bleeding from venipuncture sites and bleeding from mucosal surfaces evidenced by melena, epistaxis, hematuria, and hematochezia. These findings are indications for additional studies.

Platelet counts less than 30,000/$\mu$l are often associated with bleeding, although some patients with counts as low as 5000 do not have clinical evidence of bleeding. The bleeding time (BT) test, also called the buccal mucosal bleeding time, measures the ability to form the primary platelet plug *in vivo* and, therefore, tests for the vascular and platelet response. This test is indicated if platelet count is adequate yet signs of a primary hemostatic defect are present. It is not indicated if the platelet count is markedly decreased, since no additional information would be gained. The test is a crude evaluation and subject to a wide range of error. If the platelet count is normal but the BT is prolonged, a defect in platelet function or in vascular integrity is suspected. Additional diagnostic tests include assay of von Willebrand's factor and laboratory evaluations of platelet function, the latter usually undertaken with the consultation of a veterinary hematologist.

### Evaluation of Secondary Hemostasis: Fibrin Formation

Fibrin formation is the result of the secondary hemostatic system. Defects in this system are likely to cause hematomas or bleeding into joints or body cavities. Venipuncture sites that have undergone primary hemostasis may show rebleeding due to failure of the fibrin system to stabilize the primary platelet plug.

Should these signs be observed, an activated clotting time (ACT) should be done. The ACT evaluates the contact phase of coagulation, the intrinsic and common pathways. The ACT is dependent on platelet factor 3 (PF-3), and severe decreases in platelet numbers can prolong this test due to a decreased amount of phospholipid available for activation of clotting factors. Additional evaluation of coagulation factors can be made with the activated partial thromboplastin time (APTT) for the intrinsic system and the one-stage prothrombin time (OSPT) for the extrinsic system. Coagulation factors must be decreased to less than 30% of normal before these tests are prolonged. Fibrinogen is a coagulation factor with the highest concentration of any coagulation factor. Fibrin degradation products (FDPs) are produced when plasmin causes degradation of the fibrin clot.

### Liver Function

Liver dysfunction either as the presenting or secondary problem is common in critically ill patients. The physical examination may show an enlarged, possibly painful liver, especially if the disease is acute. However, chronic hepatitis and portosystemic shunts cause a small, nonpainful liver. Icterus may be noted but is not specific for liver disease. In addition to the liver-related tests in the usual chemistry panel (aminotransferases, alkaline phosphatase, bilirubin, glucose, albumin, blood urea nitrogen [BUN], cholesterol), liver function tests such as ammonia tolerance and bile acids may help identify acute decreases in liver function. Liver dysfunction may result in decreased production of coagulation factors so that OSPT and APTT are prolonged, while the presence of low-grade disseminated intravascular coagulation (DIC) may complicate the evaluation.

Patients with suspected hepatic encephalopathy should be evaluated for secondary causes of encephalopathy including hypoglycemia, hypoxemia, sepsis, electrolyte abnormalities, acid-base disturbances, and cerebral edema.

## Renal

Azotemia is common in critical care patients, often related to decreased renal perfusion or preexistent disease. The physical examination is the first step in evaluation of azotemia. Particular attention should be paid to an assessment of both the interstitial and the vascular volumes, since both volume depletion and edematous disorders can be associated with decreased renal perfusion. One of the most important steps in preventing acute renal failure is a daily review of every therapy and diagnostic procedure in order to avoid those that may compromise renal function. Vascular volume must be adequately maintained and urine output closely monitored. Although there is a risk of infection with indwelling urinary catheters, the benefit of having an accurate measure of urine output may outweigh this risk. Systemic hypertension is common in patients with renal disease and should be controlled to prevent further renal injury. A urinalysis is helpful in monitoring for acute renal disease, such as that caused by aminoglycoside therapy.

## PHYSIOLOGIC MONITORING

Monitoring cardiorespiratory variables can be crucial to the critical care patient (Table 2). However, unless a measurement is extremely low or high, proper interpretation of its clinical importance can only be assessed by correlating the current measurement with previous trends, other findings, and the patient history.

## PULMONARY

### Observation

The breathing rate, per se, is of limited value without some reference to tidal volume and previous trends. A change in breathing rate, however, is often a sensitive indicator of an underlying problem. The rhythm, nature, and effort of breathing should be characterized. Arrhythmic breathing patterns are indicative of a medullary respiratory control problem and central nervous system disorders. Abnormal breathing patterns and exaggerated breathing efforts are indicative of pain, fever, or respiratory disease and require investigation.

### Ventilometry

Ventilation volume can be estimated by visual observation of chest or rebreathing bag excursions, or measured by ventilometry. Normal tidal volume ranges between 10 and 20 ml/kg. A small tidal volume may be acceptable if the rate is sufficient to accomplish normal alveolar minute ventilation. Normal total minute ventilation ranges between 150 and 250 ml/kg/min. Actual alveolar ventilation may be as low as 20% of this total in animals with rapid and shallow ventilation or with increased upper airway dead space; it may be as high as 70% of the total if the patient's breathing is slow and deep and if endotracheally intubated.

## Blood Gases

The analysis of carbon dioxide and oxygen in an arterial blood sample defines pulmonary function. Venous samples interpose a tissue bed between the lungs and the sample site, and provide little information about pulmonary function. An arterial blood sample should be collected anaerobically and analyzed as soon as possible to minimize *in vitro* RBC metabolism. The sam-

**Table 2.** *Approximate Normal Ranges for Commonly Measured Parameters in Dogs and Cats*[*]

|  | Dog | Cat |
|---|---|---|
| Heart rate (bpm) | 60–180 | 140–220 |
| Mean arterial pressure (mm Hg) | 90–120 | 100–150 |
| Cardiac output | | |
| (ml/kg/min) | 100–200 | 167±39 |
| (L/M²/min) | 4.72±1.09 | |
| Systemic resistance | | |
| (mm Hg/ml/kg/min) | 0.64±0.16 | |
| (dynes/sec/cm) | 2162±458 | |
| Mean pulmonary | | |
| arterial pressure (mm Hg) | 14±3 | |
| Central venous | | |
| pressure (cm $H_2O$) | 3±4 | |
| Pulmonary artery | | |
| occlusion pressure (mm Hg) | 5±2 | |
| Oxygen delivery | | |
| (ml/kg/min) | 29±8 | |
| (ml/M²/min) | 815±234 | |
| Oxygen consumption | | |
| (ml/kg/min) | 4–11 | 3–8 |
| (ml/M²/min) | 198±53 | |
| Blood volume (ml/kg) | 75–90 | 47–66 |
| Total plasma proteins | | |
| (gm/dl) | 6.0–8.0 | 6.8–8.3 |
| Albumin (gm/dl) | 2.5–3.5 | 1.9–3.9 |
| Packed cell volume (%) | 37–55 | 29–48 |
| Hemoglobin (gm/dl) | 12–18 | 9–15.1 |
| Breathing rate | | |
| (breaths per min) | 10–30 | 24–42 |
| Minute ventilation | | |
| (ml/kg/min) | 170–350 | 200–350 |
| Arterial $Po_2$ (mm Hg) | 85–105 | 100–115 |
| Arterial $Pco_2$ (mm Hg) | 30–44 | 28–35 |
| Arterial pH | 7.36–7.46 | 7.34–7.43 |
| Bicarbonate (mEq/L) | 20–25 | 17–21 |
| Base deficit (mEq/L) | 0 to −4 | −1 to −8 |
| Sodium (mEq/L) | 145–154 | 151–158 |
| Potassium (mEq/L) | 4.1–5.3 | 3.6–4.9 |
| Chloride (mEq/L) | 105–116 | 113–121 |
| Total $CO_2$ (mEq/L) | 16–26 | 15–21 |

[*]Differences between laboratories are common, especially in serum chemistries.

**Table 3.** *Levels of Concern for PaO₂ and SaO₂*

| PaO₂ | SaO₂ | Importance |
|------|------|------------|
| >80 | >95 | Normal |
| <60 | <89 | Serious hypoxemia |
| <40 | <75 | Lethal hypoxemia |

ple can be kept in ice water for several hours before significant changes occur.

## Carbon Dioxide

The arterial $PCO_2$ ($PaCO_2$) is a measure of the ventilatory status of the patient and normally ranges between 35 and 45 mm Hg. A $PaCO_2$ below 35 mm Hg indicates hyperventilation; a $PaCO_2$ above 45 mm Hg indicates hypoventilation. A $PaCO_2$ in excess of 60 mm Hg may be associated with a severe respiratory acidosis and hypoxemia (when breathing room air), and is sufficient to warrant definitive airway or ventilator therapy. $PaCO_2$ values below 20 mm Hg are associated with severe respiratory alkalosis and decreased cerebral blood flow, which may impair cerebral oxygenation.

Venous $PCO_2$ is usually 3 to 6 mm Hg higher than arterial in stable states. It may be higher in transition states, during anemia, and with carbonic anhydrase inhibitor therapy. Venous $PCO_2$ is a reflection of tissue $PCO_2$, which depends on arterial $PCO_2$ and tissue metabolism. The use of venous $PCO_2$, in general, is a reasonable estimate of arterial $PCO_2$.

The $PaCO_2$ is normally measured with a blood gas analyzer. An economical, portable, reliable, battery-operated blood gas analyzer is available (StatPal, Biomedical Systems Division, Pittsburgh Plate Glass Industries, Pittsburgh, PA). The $PaCO_2$ may also be estimated by measuring the carbon dioxide concentration in a sample of gas taken at the end of an exhalation. Although there is some variability in the correlation between end-tidal carbon dioxide and $PaCO_2$ in patients with rapid breathing rates or with pulmonary disease, the correlation is sufficient for most clinical purposes (see "End-Tidal Carbon Dioxide Monitoring," this volume, p 119).

Hypercapnia may be caused by hypoventilation due to medullary, cervical, or neuromuscular disease; upper or lower airway obstruction; pleural filling disorders; pulmonary parenchymal disease; and abdominal or thoracic restrictive disorders.

## Oxygen

The arterial $PO_2$ ($PaO_2$) is a measure of the oxygenating efficiency of the lungs. The $PaO_2$ measures the tension of oxygen dissolved in physical solution in the plasma, irrespective of the hemoglobin concentration. Hemoglobin saturation measures the percentage saturation of the hemoglobin and is related to the $PaO_2$ by the sigmoidal hemoglobin-oxygen dissociation curve. The clinical information derived from the measurement of hemoglobin saturation is analogous to that obtained from a $PaO_2$ measurement; however, the "numbers of concern" are different (Table 3). Oxygen content is dependent upon both hemoglobin concentration and $PO_2$:

$$O_2 \text{ content} = ([Hb \times 1.34] \times \% \text{ saturation}) + (0.003 \times PO_2)$$

Oxygen partial pressure, saturation, and content are related, but their relationship varies depending upon the underlying disease (Table 4).

The $PaO_2$ is normally measured with a blood gas analyzer. Economical, portable, reliable, battery-operated blood gas analyzers are available (StatPal). *In vitro* oxygen-hemoglobin saturation analyzers are commercially available, economical, and easy to operate. They could be used to evaluate blood oxygenation if the cost of a blood gas analyzer is prohibitive.

Pulse oximeters attach to a patient externally—tongue or lips. These devices are very popular in human medicine and there are many products from which to choose. Performance in dogs and cats may be sporadic with some instruments. A pulse oximeter is an ideal monitor in that it is an automatic, continuous, audible monitor of mechanical cardiopulmonary function (see "End-Tidal Carbon Dioxide Monitoring," this volume, p 119). Pulmonary function and cardiovascular function are tested by this technique. Accuracy should be verified periodically with an arterial blood gas measurement.

The normal $PaO_2$ is between 90 and 100 mm Hg. A $PaO_2$ of 50 to 60 mm Hg is a commonly selected minimum value at which support procedures such as enriching the inspired oxygen concentration or ventilation therapy should be instituted. Venous $PO_2$ reflects tissue $PO_2$ and bears no consistent correlation to arterial $PO_2$. Venous $PO_2$ is usually between 40 and 50 mm Hg. Values below 30 mm Hg may be caused by decreased delivery of oxygen to the tissues (hypoxemia, anemia, low cardiac output, vasoconstriction); values above 60 mm Hg (while breathing room air) suggest reduced

**Table 4.** *Correlation Between PaO₂, SaO₂, and CaO₂ in Different Disease States*

| Disease | PaO₂ | SaO₂ | CaO₂ |
|---------|------|------|------|
| Anemia | Normal | Normal | Reduced |
| Polycythemia | Normal/Reduced | Normal/Reduced | Increased |
| Methemoglobinemia | Normal | Reduced | Reduced |
| Pulmonary disease | Reduced | Reduced | Reduced |
| Hyperoxemia | Increased | Normal | Slightly Increased |

tissue uptake of oxygen (shunting, septic shock, metabolic poisons). Venous blood for such evaluations must be obtained from a central vein such as the jugular vein or cranial vena cava, or from the pulmonary artery.

### Venous Admixture

Venous admixture is the collective term for the multiple mechanisms by which blood can pass from the right side of the circulation to the left side of the circulation without being properly oxygenated: (1) low ventilation/perfusion regions (e.g., bronchoconstriction); (2) no ventilation/perfusion regions (e.g., atelectasis); (3) diffusion impairment (e.g., inhalation toxicities); and (4) anatomic right-to-left shunt. Venous admixture can be estimated by the alveolar air equation:

$$\text{Alveolar } P_{O_2} = \text{Inspired } P_{O_2} - Pa_{CO_2} \; (1.1)$$

where $P_{IO_2}$ = barometric pressure $\times$ 21% and 1.1 = 1/RQ assuming the respiratory quotient (RQ) = 0.9. The normal A-a $P_{O_2}$ = 10 mm Hg when the animal is breathing 21% oxygen and about 100 mm Hg when the animal is breathing 100% oxygen. An above-normal A-a $Pa_{O_2}$ is indicative of a reduced ability of the lung to oxygenate blood (venous admixture). If the animal is breathing 21% oxygen at sea level, and has an approximately normal body temperature, a simplified version of the alveolar air equation is to add the measured $Pa_{O_2}$ and $Pa_{CO_2}$ values. If the added value is less than 120 mm Hg, there is venous admixture; the lower the added value, the greater the magnitude of the venous admixture.

Patients breathing an enriched oxygen mixture should have an elevated $Pa_{O_2}$. A rough estimate of the expected $Pa_{O_2}$ can be obtained by multiplying the inspired oxygen concentration by 5. A $Pa_{O_2}$ measurement below this value indicates venous admixture.

## CARDIOVASCULAR

### Electrical

Abnormal electrical activity includes bradycardia, tachycardia, and arrhythmias. The electrocardiogram does not measure mechanical performance and can appear quite normal in the face of poor myocardial performance. Ectopic pacemaker activity does not necessarily require treatment. It indicates the presence of an underlying abnormality that should be identified, if possible, and treated. Specific ventricular antiarrhythmic treatment is indicated when the rate exceeds the upper limit of normal for the species; when it is multifocal; when the ectopic beat occurs over the preceding T wave; or if there is evidence of impairment of myocardial performance, arterial blood pressure, or tissue perfusion. Total elimination of the arrhythmia is not necessarily the objective of therapy. A simple decrease in the rate or severity of the arrhythmia may be

a suitable end point to the titration of antiarrhythmic drugs, which are not without their own toxic effects.

### Peripheral Perfusion

Perfusion of visceral and other peripheral organs is primarily regulated by vasomotor tone. Vasodilation improves peripheral perfusion but, if excessive, causes hypotension. Vasoconstriction may increase blood pressure but decreases peripheral perfusion. Vasomotor tone is assessed by mucous membrane color, capillary refill time, urine output, and toe-web/core temperature gradient.

### Central Venous Pressure

Central venous pressure (CVP) is the luminal pressure of the intrathoracic vena cava. Peripheral venous pressure is variably higher than CVP, is subject to extraneous influences such as venous compression, and is not a reliable indicator of CVP. Catheters are usually positioned via the jugular vein into the cranial vena cava. Contact with the endocardium of the right atrium or ventricle should be avoided, since this may stimulate ectopic beats. Verification of a well-placed, unobstructed catheter can be ascertained by observing small fluctuations in the fluid meniscus within the manometer synchronous with the heart beat, and larger excursions synchronous with ventilation. Very large fluctuations synchronous with each heart beat may indicate that the catheter is positioned within the right ventricle. Direct observation of the catheter pressure and waveform may help identify proper location of the catheter tip. Measurements should be made between ventilatory excursions, since changes in pleural pressure affect the luminal pressure. A horizontal line drawn between the estimated level of the tip of the catheter (the manubrium or thoracic inlet) and the manometer establishes the "zero" reference level. The vertical difference between the zero level and the meniscus of fluid in the manometer represents the CVP.

The normal CVP in small animals is 0 to 10 cm $H_2O$. Values below 0 cm $H_2O$ indicate relative hypovolemia (or improperly positioned zero reference) and suggest that fluids should be administered. Values above 10 cm $H_2O$ indicate relative hypervolemia and that further fluid therapy should be conservative. The CVP is a measure of the relative ability of the heart to pump the venous return and should be measured when right heart failure is suspected. The CVP does not correlate, however, to pulmonary venous pressure in patients with left-sided heart failure. The CVP is also an estimate of the relationship between blood volume and blood volume capacity; it should be measured as an end point to very large fluid infusions.

The CVP measurement is used to determine whether there is "room" for additional fluid therapy. Subcutaneous edema is not always an indication that fluid therapy has been excessive (only that crystalloid therapy has been excessive) and may not indicate an effective circulating blood volume, because edema may occur in the face of hypovolemia if the patient is hypoproteinemic or if there is increased vascular permeability. Likewise, the CVP measurement cannot "see" what is happening in the interstitial fluid space and edema can occur in the setting of a normal or low CVP.

## Arterial Blood Pressure

Arterial blood pressure is the product of cardiac output, vascular capacity and resistance, and blood volume. Normal systolic, diastolic, and mean blood pressures are approximately 100 to 160, 60 to 100, and 80 to 120 mm Hg, respectively. Adequate mean arterial blood pressure establishes a perfusion pressure for the brain and the heart. It is generally considered to require a mean systemic blood pressure of at least 50 to 60 mm Hg. Arterial blood pressure can be measured in animals by indirect and direct techniques (see "Blood Pressure Measurement," this volume, p 110).

## Cardiac Output

Arterial blood pressure may be normal in the face of low cardiac output and high peripheral vascular resistance. Cardiac output is a flow parameter and is more relevant to systemic perfusion than is pressure. Cardiac output is stroke volume times heart rate. Stroke volume is determined by preload, contractility, and afterload. Cardiac output is usually determined by thermodilution techniques and requires cardiac catheterization and expensive equipment.

Cardiac output may be reduced by insufficient venous return and end-diastolic ventricular filling volume (hypovolemia, positive airway and pleural pressure, or inflow occlusion); by decreased ventricular compliance (hypertrophic cardiomyopathy, pericardial tamponade, or pericardial fibrosis); by decreased contractility; by marked bradycardia or tachycardia or arrhythmias; by insufficient atrioventricular valves; or by outflow tract obstruction (stenosis).

Poor cardiac output should be improved by treating the underlying problem when possible. Preload should be optimized. Sympathomimetic therapy is indicated when fluid therapy alone has failed to restore acceptable arterial blood pressure, cardiac output, and tissue perfusion (see elsewhere in this section). Adequate blood volume restoration may be functionally defined as a CVP of 10 cm $H_2O$ or a pulmonary capillary wedge pressure (PCWP) of 15 mm Hg.

## Oxygen Delivery

Oxygen delivery is the product of cardiac output and blood oxygen content. It is the "bottom line" of cardiopulmonary function. Disease becomes life threat-

ening when, in spite of compensatory mechanisms, oxygen delivery is reduced below the critical level for the patient (the point at which oxygen consumption becomes flow dependent).

When cardiac output is not measured, the adequacy of oxygen delivery must be extrapolated from parameters that are measured, such as pulse quality, capillary refill time, urine output, toe-web/core temperature gradient, base deficit, venous $P_{O_2}$, blood lactate concentration, or tonometric measurements of gastrointestinal mucosal pH (see "Monitoring Gastrointestinal Mucosal pH in Critical Care Patients," this volume, p 133).

## RENAL

The presence of urine output is used as an indirect measure of renal blood flow; renal blood flow is used as an indirect measure of visceral blood flow. Urine output can be assessed by serial palpation of the urinary bladder or by actual measurement following the aseptic placement of a urinary catheter. Normal urine output should be 1 to 2 ml/kg/hr, but this is markedly influenced by infused fluid volumes or diuretic therapy.

## WRITTEN RECORDS

A written record of all observations, treatments, and events is crucial to an effective critical care endeavor. The retrospective display of physiologic trends, therapeutic responses, and thought processes is vital to learning and legal processes.

No particular recording format is any more valid than any other. A person may choose an existing form, but more logically one would tailor records to their own practice situation.

## References and Suggested Reading

Carlson RW and Geheb MA (eds): *Principles and Practice of Medical Intensive Care.* Philadelphia, WB Saunders Co, 1993.
  *A comprehensive, multiauthored text with a strong emphasis on physiology that fulfills its goal of being useful in the clinic and as a general reference.*
DiBartola SP: *Fluid Therapy in Small Animal Practice.* Philadelphia, WB Saunders Co, 1992.
  *An excellent, multiauthored text integrating physiology with the clinical presentation that provides the clinician with a solid basis for formulating therapeutic plans.*
Kaplan PM: Monitoring. *In* Murtaugh RJ and Kaplan PM (eds): *Veterinary Emergency and Critical Care Medicine.* St. Louis, Mosby Year Book, 1992, pp 21–37.
  *A comprehensive review of veterinary emergency and critical care; an essential book for the emergency medicine practitioner.*
Shapiro BA: *Clinical Application of Blood Gases,* 4th edition. Chicago, Year Book Medical Publishers, 1989.
  *A well-written, easy-to-understand discussion of determinants and clinical interpretation of blood gas measurements.*
Shoemaker WC, Ayres S, Grenvik A, Holbrook PR, and Thompson WL (eds): *Textbook of Critical Care.* Philadelphia, WB Saunders Co, 1989.
  *Comprehensive and authoritative reviews of the field by multiple authors, of special interest to the veterinarian wishing to review oxygen delivery and fluid therapy.*
Sprung CL (ed): *The Pulmonary Artery Catheter.* Baltimore, University Park Press, 1983.
  *A good discussion of thermodilution cardiac output catheters, their introduction, and interpretation of measurements.*

# CRITICAL CARE NURSING

MELBA L. McGEE,
CHERYL L. SPENCER,
*and* DEBORAH R. VAN PELT
*Fort Collins, Colorado*

Nursing is defined as the "scientific care of the sick," while critical is defined as "pertaining to crisis" (Grove et al., 1967). "Critical nursing," therefore, becomes "the scientific care of the sick in a crisis." The purpose of this article is to evaluate the scope of this broad definition and describe the scope of critical care nursing. The critical care nurse must have a solid scientific and medical background, as well as expertise in technical skills such as intravenous catheterization. Because of advancing technology, the equipment used in the critical care setting can be complicated and the critical care nurse is expected to operate and troubleshoot this equipment. Critical care nursing is a vital component in the successful treatment of many critically ill patients, and even with the most sophisticated diagnostic testing and advanced monitoring techniques, the critical patient has little chance of recovery without competent nursing care.

Not all patients admitted to the critical care unit are in a "crisis situation," but for some reason, these patients need more intensive monitoring, nursing care, or observation than less ill patients. Murtaugh describes three types of patients admitted to the critical care unit: (1) animals with increased risks of complications admitted for intensive observation/monitoring, such as the postoperative patient with compensated preexisting organ dysfunction; (2) animals that are stable physiologically, but require extensive nursing care, such as the patient requiring ventilator support; and (3) animals requiring constant medical attention, such as the multiple trauma patient with cardiopulmonary dysfunction (Murtaugh, 1992). The critical care nurse must be comfortable with nursing patients in any one of these three categories.

## GENERAL ASSESSMENT

The nursing process may begin even before the patient arrives at the hospital. Owners often telephone ahead with questions concerning their pet, and the nurse should be able to correctly answer basic emergency treatment questions, such as how to transport an injured pet, how to prevent further hemorrhage, or when and if a pet should be induced to vomit.

At certain times in an active practice, the critical care nurse may be called upon to make decisions as regards prioritizing patients for treatment. This is called "triaging." Each animal is evaluated and its injuries classified according to the immediate threat to life. Assessments must be made rapidly and without hesitation. Appropriate treatment is then directed at the patient's most life-threatening injuries. Experience, intuition, and common sense all play important roles in initial patient evaluation, intervention, and treatment.

## EMERGENCY MANAGEMENT AND DAILY NURSING CARE

On hospital admission, a team approach is used to evaluate the patient, with the veterinarian and nurse working together to assess the condition and stability of the patient. The critical care nurse's (or animal health technician's) responsibility is to anticipate the needs of the patient and the veterinarian. In any emergency, time and efficiency are vitally important, and the critical care nurse must always be prepared. In some situations, the critical care nurse may be called upon to initiate appropriate treatment in an effort to stabilize the patient. It is therefore important for the nurse to be familiar with treatment protocols for common emergency situations (see "Cardiopulmonary Resuscitation," this volume, p 167).

In less life-threatening situations, the nurse may be responsible for obtaining the patient's history and performing an initial physical examination. The information gathered by the nurse must be accurate and complete to enable the veterinarian to make informed decisions regarding patient care. A thorough patient history must be obtained, whether the patient is being admitted for postoperative observation or as an emergency. Patient age, sex and breed, onset and duration of the complaint, history of previous problems or medication administration, and environment and vaccination status should all be determined.

A hands-on approach using all five senses is important in patient evaluation and treatment. Baseline data should include temperature, pulse rate, and respiratory rate, as well as packed cell volume, total serum solids, and urine specific gravity. By observation, judge respiratory rate and effort, mucous membrane color, and mentation. From palpation, determine pulse strength and character, capillary refill time, degree of hydration, and the presence of fractures or abdominal injuries. By auscultation, note breath sounds and the presence of heart arrhythmias or murmurs. Smell, seemingly not as important as the other senses, can detect the fruity breath of the ketoacidotic diabetic or detect the aroma of a *Pseudomonas*-infected wound.

Once the patient is stabilized, a more extensive physical examination is performed and further diagnostic tests are usually submitted or ordered. At the same time, a treatment plan or orders are implemented. The order sheet should include the patient's signalment, weight, problems—which may be updated and changed during the course of therapy—and a list of priority monitoring, such as sepsis, dyspnea, or disseminated intravascular coagulation (DIC) alerts. The orders should indicate the type and frequency of monitoring desired and medications to be administered, including the dosage in milligrams, route of administration, and frequency. The orders should also give consideration to the patient's diet and caloric intake. The order sheet should provide space to request laboratory and other diagnostic tests. Finally, special nursing considerations should be noted on the patient's record. Examples include frequently turning the patient, passive range-of-motion exercises, and massaging pressure points to prevent decubital ulcers; nebulization and chest physiotherapy for the patient with pneumonia; or expressing the bladder of patients with neurologic dysfunction. Frequent reevaluation of the patient is necessary to determine appropriate changes in therapy.

In addition to the order sheet, a patient flow sheet should be recorded. The flow sheet provides documentation that the orders have been carried out; information such as the patient's temperature, pulse, and respiration (TPR); and medication and fluid administration. Space should be provided on the flow sheet to note appetite; amount of food consumed; urination/defecation; and presence and character of any pain, vomitus, or diarrhea.

Because the flow sheet covers a 24-hr period, trends in patient status are easily monitored. The nursing chart should record subjective and objective assessments of patient progress, which may aid the veterinarian in prescribing appropriate therapy. Because the nurse is in intimate contact with the patient throughout the day, he or she can denote any subtle changes and relay observations to the veterinarian, as well as make suggestions for improved treatment.

With the change of each nursing shift, rounds should be conducted to inform and update the oncoming nurse about changes in patient status. Relayed information should include the patient's signalment; history of present disease; problem list; treatment schedule; specific problems with handling, treatment, or equipment; and the results of diagnostic tests that were performed during the previous shift. This ensures continuity of treatment and patient care. The oncoming nurse should then review the patient's treatment orders and flow sheet. A baseline physical examination should also be performed by the oncoming nurse. The remainder of this chapter discusses nursing considerations for each of the major organ systems.

## SYSTEMS EVALUATION

### Respiratory

The primary nursing consideration involving the respiratory system is to correct the patient's hypoxia and decrease the work of breathing. Characteristic breathing patterns aid in localizing the source of a patient's respiratory difficulty. For example, an obstructive breathing pattern (slow, deep respirations) suggests upper airway disease (e.g., inspiratory stridor of the dog with laryngeal paralysis), while a restrictive breathing pattern (rapid, shallow respirations) suggests pulmonary parenchymal or pleural space disease (e.g., pneumothorax). Because of the potential risk of respiratory arrest in such patients, frequent observation and monitoring are essential. Of importance are respiratory rate, character of breath sounds, breathing patterns, and mucous membrane color. Mucous membrane color is a fair indicator of oxygenation but should not be relied on exclusively, since arterial partial pressure of oxygen may fall to 50 mm Hg or less before cyanosis is present. Arterial blood gas measurements are the best means of monitoring the ventilation and oxygenation of the dyspneic patient. Recently, pulse oximetry has become popular as a noninvasive means of monitoring oxygen saturation (see "Pulse Oximetry," this volume, p 117).

Care should be taken not to further stress the dyspneic patient by trying to place a mask or nasal catheter for oxygen administration. Cats are especially susceptible to stress-induced dyspnea and respiratory arrest. Often, placing the dyspneic patient in an oxygen-enriched environment such as an oxygen cage will partially alleviate the respiratory distress.

Animals with a tracheostomy are among the most challenging cases entrusted to the veterinary nurse. Tracheostomy care is labor intensive and patients must be monitored constantly (see "Temporary Tracheostomy," this volume, p 179). Because the upper airway is bypassed, the ability to warm, filter, and humidify the lower airway is diminished. Even with supplemental humidification, these patients have increased or thickened respiratory secretions. Tracheostomy tubes can easily be occluded by airway secretions, skin folds, and even bedding, with subsequent respiratory arrest. Small-diameter tracheostomy tubes present a greater hazard of occlusion. Close patient monitoring and sterile suctioning of the tracheostomy are required to prevent airway occlusion. Dogs and cats with tracheostomies lose the ability to thermoregulate because of the decreased air movement across the tongue during panting. This predisposes to hyperthermia. These patients also have increased susceptibility to pneumonia, especially in the critical care unit where resistant nosocomial infections can occur. Strict asepsis and chest physiotherapy will help to decrease the incidence of pneumonia in tracheostomy patients.

### Circulatory

Maintaining adequate tissue perfusion is the nurse's primary concern as regards the circulatory system. There are many causes of circulatory collapse, including shock, heart failure, arrhythmias, and hemorrhage. Multiple causes of circulatory collapse may be present in a single patient. Monitoring pulse rate and quality, rate, blood pressure, capillary refill times, and cardiac auscultation are all methods of evaluating the circulatory system. Again, a hands-on approach is emphasized. Subtle changes in cardiovascular variables may indicate the onset of a clinically significant problem. An increasing heart rate may indicate sepsis, hyperthermia, hypovolemia, pain, or hypoxia, while decreasing heart rate may indicate a problem like hyperkalemia, hypothermia, or increasing intracranial pressure. Thoracic auscultation allows recognition of cardiac murmurs as well as muffled heart or lung sounds which may indicate the presence of pericardial or pleural effusions.

The ideal method of monitoring blood pressure is by direct cannulization of an artery, but the indirect methods, Doppler and oscillometer (Dinamap, Critikon, Tampa, FL), are adequate in larger patients (see "Doppler Assessment of Blood Flow and Pressure in Surgical and Critical Care Patients," this volume, p 113) Acute onset of hypotension in association with tachycardia should be treated with aggressive fluid administration and possibly administration of positive inotropic agents. Capillary refill time (CRT) should not be relied on as the sole indicator of adequate circulation, as normal CRT has been observed even several minutes after cardiac arrest. Venous blood gases, however, often are a good means of evaluating tissue perfusion because poor perfusion leads to greater oxygen extraction with lowering of venous $Po_2$.

Electrocardiograms, performed intermittently or continuously, provide a means of detecting potentially life-threatening cardiac arrhythmias. The critical care nurse must be able to recognize the most common cardiac arrhythmias, such as ventricular premature contractions, asystole, ventricular fibrillation, atrial standstill, and electrical mechanical dissociation or pulseless bradyarrhythmias.

Intravenous catheterization is often a responsibility of the critical care nurse. Long and short catheters of various types are available, but long catheters offer some advantages. First, repeated blood samples can be easily drawn, which means less venipunctures to the patient. Second, when placed in the jugular vein, a long catheter provides access to a central vein allowing measurement of central venous pressure. Site selection is another important consideration in catheter placement, and should be based on the condition of the patient. The jugular vein is optimal in most cases, but other sites that can be used include the lateral saphenous vein in the dog, the medial saphenous vein in the cat, and the cephalic vein in both species. Aseptic technique must be used in catheter site preparation, insertion, and aftercare to prevent contamination and infection. Air emboli must be avoided. If intravenous access cannot be established, an intraosseous catheter can be used (see *CVT XI*, p 107). These are especially helpful in neonates and rodents, when veins are too small for intravenous catheterization, or in severely hypovolemic patients when intravenous catheterization is difficult.

## Neurologic

Important nursing concerns in patients with neurologic disease are the provision of supportive care, min-

imization of complications, and the ability to respond to rapid changes in patient status. Seizing patients require immediate attention aimed at controlling seizures and preventing self-trauma. The nurse should be mindful of safety and should choose a catheter site away from the head, such as the lateral saphenous vein, to decrease the risk of bites. Blood glucose should be evaluated early in the course of treatment, since hypoglycemic seizures can be easily treated with intravenous dextrose administration.

It is important to closely monitor body temperature in seizing patients, as hyperthermia commonly occurs secondary to muscle fasiculations. If body temperature increases above 105°F, the patient can be externally cooled by using fans and by wetting the footpads and thoracic and abdominal areas with cool water.

Supportive care for the neurologic patient requires monitoring for changes in mentation, pupillary light response and ocular movement, posturing, changes in heart rate or respiratory pattern, and signs of hypoxia. Some seizures can be triggered by loud noises and bright lights, making it necessary to place the patient in a quiet, low-light area that is easily accessible for patient monitoring. When intravenous fluids are administered, volume should be controlled by an infusion pump or pediatric infusion set to prevent an inadvertent overdose of fluids that could cause or worsen cerebral edema.

When a patient with neurologic disease recovers from anesthesia or myelography, close monitoring for seizures is in order. Keeping the head elevated will help prevent increased intracranial pressure, as well as decreasing the flow of contrast material into the brain. Patients recovering from spinal surgery are commonly nonambulatory and require supportive care which may include: elevating the extremities with a rolled towel to prevent strain on the spinal column and joints; turning the animal every 4 hr to prevent pulmonary atelectasis and decubital ulcers; and palpation and expression of the bladder at least every 6 hr. It may also be the nurse's responsibility to instruct the owner about physical therapy and exercises that assist the patient's recovery at home. These may consist of passive range-of-motion exercises, massaging pressure points, application of warm or cold packs and, in some instances, hydrotherapy (see "Physical Therapy and Rehabilitation," this volume, p 82).

## Musculoskeletal

Nursing responsibilities often include patients with musculoskeletal disease secondary to trauma, postoperative amputation, or fracture repair. Fractures and associated soft-tissue injury may be complicated by hemorrhage at the fracture site, shock, infection, or DIC.°

---

°The nurse's responsibilities also include assessing patient comfort and reporting to the veterinarian when there is a need for analgesics. Several parameters can be evaluated in making this assessment, including patient vocalization, increased heart or respiratory rate, increased temperature, and dilated pupils (see also *CVT XI*, p 82).

Often, patients with significant musculoskeletal disease are recumbent and require involved nursing care. This includes turning them at least every 4 hr to prevent atelectasis, massaging pressure points and padding with fleeces to prevent decubital ulcers, and thoracic auscultation for signs of atelectasis or pneumonia. The head and limbs can be supported with rolled towels to decrease strain on the joints and spine. Elevating the patient from the cage floor by using racks and mats will prevent urine scalding. The bladder should be palpated at least every 6 hr and expressed as needed to prevent urine retention, which may lead to a urinary tract infection or an atonic bladder.

## Gastrointestinal

In all patients, but especially those with digestive tract disorders, it is important to chart on the flow sheet any changes in appetite; presence, character, or consistency of stools and vomitus; and any change in body weight. Amounts of vomitus and diarrhea should be estimated to calculate contemporary fluid or electrolyte losses. In addition, changes in packed cell volume and total serum solids that may occur as a result of dehydration and fluid loss should be recorded.

Nutritional requirements and feeding orders can vary greatly in critically ill patients and may range from nothing per os (NPO), to nasogastric tube feeding, to enteral feeding with jejunostomy or gastrostomy tubes, or even intravenous hyperalimentation. The nurse should be familiar with these various routes and the specialized diets and fluids available for each technique (see *CVT XI*, pp 32 and 117; *CVT X*, pp 25 and 30).

Careful feeding of the recumbent animal is required to prevent aspiration. If possible, elevate the head or feed small meatballs made from canned food. A gruel made from diluted canned food can be administered in small amounts via a syringe. Water can also be given by syringe. It is important to account for increased caloric requirements, especially if the patient is facing a prolonged recovery period.

Treatment of anorexic patients requires patience and gentle handling. Tempting the animal frequently with palatable foods such as meat baby food, canned commercial pet food, lunch meats, or cheese may be effective. Food left uneaten for more than an hour should be removed and replaced with fresh food each time it is offered. In the partially anorectic animal, administration of diazepam (Valium) may act as an appetite stimulant. A variety of foods should be ready before administering the valium, since the effect is almost immediate. This method should not be substituted for aggressive nutritional support when indicated, as it will not succeed in meeting caloric requirements of the patient.

## Genitourinary

The most important nursing concerns in patients with renal disease are to maintain and monitor the patient's fluid and electrolyte balance. Any changes in frequency or quantity of urination, physical appearance of the urine, or fluctuations in body weight should be recorded. Changes in hydration status or renal function can have a direct impact on fluid requirements. It is important to determine if the patient is voluntarily voiding or whether any urine output observed is secondary to bladder distention and overflow. This is accomplished by palpating the bladder at least four times a day and by noting if the patient is posturing to urinate and actively applying abdominal press.

Daily physical examinations should include bladder palpation, weighing, and checking for vaginal or prepucial discharge. Collecting a free-catch urine sample is an easy way to monitor changes in the physical appearance, urine specific gravity, and chemical components. If unable to obtain serial free-catch samples, samples may be obtained via catheterization or cystocentesis.

Patients in renal failure are often maintained by aggressive intravenous fluid administration to promote diuresis, and should therefore be monitored closely for signs of overhydration. This can be achieved by frequently monitoring body weight (two to four times a day), respiratory rate, measuring central venous pressure through a jugular catheter, auscultating the lungs for crackles, watching for signs of chemosis, and by serial assessment of packed cell volume and total serum solids. Animals with renal failure are often anemic. Vomiting and gastrointestinal ulceration are common complications of renal disease. These gastrointestinal losses can further complicate anemia along with the fluid and electrolyte requirements of the animal.

Patients with renal disease are usually polyuric but can also present with or develop anuria or oliguria. This occurrence necessitates the placement of an indwelling urinary catheter. An aseptic closed urinary collection system should be used to accurately quantitate urine output. Even with a urinary catheter in place, the urinary bladder should be palpated four times a day to ensure that the catheter is patent and the bladder is staying empty. If the bladder is distended, the urinary catheter should be aseptically aspirated or, if necessary, gently flushed with sterile saline. The amount of urine produced should be quantified four times a day, since this will directly affect the volume of fluid therapy. The urethral entry site of urinary catheter should be disinfected and checked daily or as needed for signs of inflammation and discharge. The urine collection system should be changed daily to minimize potential for ascending bacterial infections and to ensure accuracy in measuring the amounts of urine produced.

## SUMMARY

Through patient treatment, monitoring, and assessment, the critical care nurse provides a vital link between the veterinarian and the critically ill patient. A thorough understanding of common emergency conditions and the potential problems association with various underlying diseases is necessary for the critical care nurse to provide optimal treatment in critically ill patients. Use of a hands-on, systematic approach to patient care by the critical care nurse will aid in the successful treatment and recovery of the critically ill patient.

## References and Suggested Reading

Doenges ME, Moorehouse MF, and Geissler AC: *Nursing Care Plans*. Philadelphia, FA Davis Co, 1989.
  *A comprehensive guide to patient care planning.*

Gove et al (ed): *Websters Third New International Dictionary*. Springfield, G & C Merriam Co, 1967.
Murtaugh RJ, Kaplan PM, et al: *Veterinary Emergency and Critical Care Medicine*. St. Louis, Mosby Year Book, 1992.
  *A comprehensive text providing state-of-the-art information regarding emergency and critical care.*
Aanes WA, Allen R, et al: *In* Pratt PW (ed): *Medical Nursing for Animal Health Technicians*. Santa Barbara, American Veterinary Publications, Inc, 1985.
  *A comprehensive text for the animal health technician regarding medical nursing of small and large animals.*
Shaffron N. Critical care nursing. Vet Tech 14:395, 1993.

# BLOOD PRESSURE MEASUREMENT

BERNIE HANSEN

*Raleigh, North Carolina*

Measurement of systemic arterial blood pressure (BP) is a central component of hemodynamic monitoring of critically ill dogs and cats. When combined with careful physical examination and continual electrocardiogram (ECG) monitoring, repeated evaluation of arterial and central venous BP provides adequate surveillance of cardiovascular function in most animals.

Arterial BP can be measured by noninvasive (indirect) techniques that utilize occlusive cuffs encircling a limb or tail or by direct measurement via an indwelling catheter connected to a pressure measuring device.

## BLOOD PRESSURE

The hydraulic pressure within the arterial tree is the dynamic result of the combined forces of the left ventricle of the heart and the arteries to the level of the resistance arterioles. The arterial pressure waveform and the values of systolic, diastolic, and mean pressures vary with location in the arterial tree. Blood pressure monitoring represents an attempt to sample these pressures in a way that provides a clinically useful approximation of actual hemodynamic events. Because many compensatory mechanisms may be invoked to control BP, the presence of normal BP does not guarantee adequate cardiovascular function.

## NONINVASIVE BLOOD PRESSURE MONITORING

Most noninvasive BP monitoring techniques depend on the use of an occlusive cuff and indirectly measure BP by detecting blood flow in an artery distal to the cuff. Detection methods include auscultation, palpation, ultrasonic flow detection, and measurement of cuff inflation pressure oscillations.

Encircling cuffs provide a means to completely occlude a limb or tail artery. A controlled and monitored release of cuff pressure provides means to estimate BP based on detection of return of blood flow. The pressure in the cuff can be measured with an aneroid manometer, mercury manometer, or automated pressure transducer.

Cuff size is an important variable in obtaining indirect pressure measurements. Some pressure applied by the cuff is "lost" to tissue compression, and narrow cuffs are more severely affected by this phenomenon than are wider cuffs. Therefore, pressure measurements obtained from cuffs that are too narrow will be falsely elevated. Cuffs that are too wide may yield BP measurements that are falsely low, although this artifact is less pronounced than that seen with use of narrow cuffs. The optimal width of a cuff bladder is 40 to 60% of the circumference of the extremity to which it is applied, and it should be long enough to encircle at least 60% of the limb. Bladder lengths that exceed limb circumference do not appear to degrade accuracy. The cuff should be applied snugly (not tight) with the bladder centered over the largest artery at that level.

Manual methods of BP determination have been widely used for routine BP measurement in human beings. In spite of evidence that some of these techniques may be useful in normo- and hypertensive dogs (e.g., the auscultatory technique described by Harvey et al., 1983), these techniques have not been routinely employed to monitor companion animals because of the technical difficulties related to the anatomy of dog and cat limbs. The only indirect measurement techniques that have been widely employed in clinical veterinary medicine are and ultrasonic and automated oscillometric determinations.

### Oscillometric Method

As the air in a pressurized cuff is released, oscillations in cuff pressure develop when the pressure in the cuff approaches that of systolic BP. These oscillations increase in amplitude when cuff pressure approximates systolic pressure, increase further at mean arterial pressure, and rapidly decline as diastolic pressure is reached. The manual oscillometric method of BP determination by observation of sphygmomanometer oscillations is a time-honored technique used by physicians; however, this method is often very inaccurate. Accurate detection and interpretation of cuff pressure oscillations became possible only after the development of microprocessor and transducer technology that allowed precise and reproducible automated measurement. One such device (Dinamap Veterinary Blood Pressure Monitor Model 8300, Critikon Inc, Tampa, FL) is marketed for veterinary use. The functions of all automated oscillometric BP measurement devices are based on similar principles and differ mainly in the rules and algorithms used to determine pressures and detect and respond to artifacts or rhythm disturbances (Ramsey, 1991).

The first step in BP measurement is cuff inflation to a suprasystolic value, typically 160 mm Hg. After the cuff is pressurized, the pressure is held constant while the microprocessor samples pressure oscillations. The cuff is gradually deflated in a stepped fashion in increments of 5 to 10 mm Hg. At each step, the microprocessor measures, averages, and records the amplitude of pressure oscillations. Stepped deflation and sampling continues for approximately five steps after oscillation amplitudes peak and begin declining. The shape and size of oscillations are used to determine and reject artifacts. The systolic BP and diastolic BP are estimated by identifying the pressure regions where the oscillation amplitude increases and decreases rapidly, respectively. The mean pressure is generally the lowest cuff pressure with the greatest averaged oscillations, and is a measured, rather than calculated, estimate.

Automated oscillometry has been used in clinical veterinary medicine for over a decade now and provides measurements that closely correlate with direct measurements (Coulter and Keith, 1984; Hamlin et al., 1982; Pettersen et al., 1988). Automated oscillometric devices are relatively expensive; the veterinary model is available for approximately $3000. Successful use of this technique depends on fastidious adherence to recommendations provided by the manufacturers. Five consecutive readings should be obtained, the lowest and highest values discarded, and the remaining three averaged.

## Ultrasonic Method

The ultrasonic BP method depends on the Doppler effect to detect arterial wall or red cell movement underneath an ultrasonic piezoelectric probe (see "Doppler Assessment of Blood Flow and Pressure in Surgical and Critical Care Patients," this volume, p 113). High-frequency energy is transmitted into the tissue underlying the probe and the reflected energy is detected electronically. The frequency of the ultrasound wave

reflected from moving tissue is shifted slightly relative to that which was transmitted, and this difference is converted into an audible signal. Upon cuff deflation, the return of arterial flow or wall motion is detected with the probe placed directly over a superficial artery distal to the cuff. The orientation of the probe relative to the long axis of the artery influences the relative sensitivity of the probe to blood flow or arterial wall motion. Different models are configured to respond optimally to flow (systolic pressure determination) or arterial wall motion (systolic and diastolic pressure determination).

Ultrasonic systolic BP determinations correlate closely with direct measurement in normal and hypertensive dogs (Weiser, Spangler, and Gribble, 1977). Disadvantages include difficulty in obtaining measurements in hypotensive or small animals, interference by body motion, inability to determine mean arterial pressure (MAP), and potential for operator error resulting in overestimation of systolic BP.

Several types of ultrasound probes have been evaluated for veterinary clinical use. Some utilize a probe attached directly to the cuff at an orientation that makes it most sensitive to arterial wall motion. The cuff is placed so that the probe overlies the distal cranial tibial artery. The cuff must be securely taped in place once the optimal placement has been determined. Another design (Parks Medical Electronics Inc, model 811B, Aloha, OR) has a probe not attached to a cuff that is optimized to detect flow. This device may be used on smaller arteries (dorsal metatarsal, common digital), and is available for about $600.

## INVASIVE (DIRECT) BP MONITORING

Indirect methods of BP determination can work well in normal or hypertensive patients, and routine use of these modalities may greatly improve veterinary preventative health care. However, these techniques are most likely to fail in critically ill animals, especially if they are hypotensive or tachycardic. Thus, the very patients most in need of BP monitoring are the least likely to benefit from indirect methods. Use of indwelling catheters for direct BP monitoring in these animals affords more accurate measurement and allows painless removal of multiple blood samples. Disadvantages of this method include the technical difficulty of placing arterial catheters, the expense of equipment, and the risk of hemorrhage or catheter infection.

The usual location for arterial catheterization is the dorsal metatarsal artery. Advantages of using this vessel include its superficial location over the bones of the metatarsus. If hemorrhage results from unsuccessful attempts at catheterization or following catheter removal, the artery is easily compressed to control bleeding. The femoral artery may also be used, but the risk of serious hemorrhage is very high, and constant surveillance of the catheter site is mandatory.

The dorsal metatarsal artery courses parallel with, and medial to, the dorsal extensor tendons of the proximal metatarsus. A pulse is readily palpated in this location in many animals. The hair is widely clipped and the skin is wiped clean with an alcohol swab. The point of cutaneous entry for the catheter is determined and the skin and subcutaneous (periarterial) tissues are blocked with 0.1 to 0.5 ml of 2% lidocaine. Diluting the lidocaine with 1 part 8.4% sodium bicarbonate to 9 parts lidocaine will render the injection nearly painless and hasten onset of complete block. The skin is then prepared aseptically while the block takes effect. The operator dons clean disposable exam gloves and makes a small full-thickness facilitation incision in the skin just distal to the palpable pulsation. A 1- to 2¼-inch, 22- to 18-gauge over-the-needle type catheter that has been primed with heparinized saline is advanced through the incision and into the artery. Specially designed arterial catheters utilizing guidewire techniques increase the success rate (Radial Aterial Catheterization Set, Arrow International Inc, Reading, PA). The catheter is initially oriented at a 30- to 45-degree angle to the long axis of the artery with the bevel facing away from the skin. The advancement of the catheter into the artery is heralded by the (sometimes pulsatile) flow of blood that rapidly purges the saline solution from the needle hub. The catheter-needle assembly is then positioned more parallel to the artery and the needle is advanced another 1 to 3 mm to ensure that the catheter tip has entered its artery. The needle is then held stationary while the catheter is rotated and advanced up the lumen. The catheter is attached to saline-primed, low-compliance arterial pressure tubing with a Luer lock stopcock at the opposite end, and is sutured in place. The stopcock may be attached to the Luer fittings of a disposable, fluid-primed pressure dome, which is in turn fitted to a high-fidelity electronic pressure transducer (such as the Hewlett Packard 1290 C Universal Quartz Pressure Transducer, Andover, MA). The remaining stopcock port(s) is capped with an injection plug. The patency of the catheter may be maintained with periodic flushing with heparinized saline solution via a 25-gauge needle through the injection cap, or by constant infusion of pressurized saline through a unidirectional flushing device (Intraflo Continuous Flush, Abbott Critical Care Systems, Mountain View, CA).

The pressure transducer should be kept at the same level as the heart, or the BP readings must be mathematically corrected for the distance above or below the heart. Accurate systolic, diastolic, and calculated mean pressure measurements may be gathered continuously by an electronic monitor. Ideally, an intensive care BP monitor should include an ECG channel, two pressure ports (one for arterial BP and one for CVP or pulmonary artery pressure), and two temperature ports.

Blood pressure may also be measured with an aneroid manometer. The manometer is connected to three 30-inch intravenous extension tubes (with Luer lock fittings or glued at all connections). The tube closest to the patient is separated from the middle tube by a three-way stopcock. The stopcock, patient extension tube, and middle tube are maintained aseptically and the stopcock and patient tube are primed with saline solution. The end of the saline column in the tubing should be maintained at the level of the heart. To determine BP, sterile saline is injected through the stopcock toward the manometer until the compressed air in the tubing causes the manometer to read higher than the expected mean arterial BP. The stopcock is then turned so that the manometer is open to the patient. The compressed air forces sterile saline into the catheter until the manometer pressure equilibrates with MAP. The highest excursion of the manometer gauge approximates MAP.

## CONCLUSION

Blood pressure monitoring can be life saving if it results in timely and appropriate therapeutic decisions. However, BP measurements must be interpreted in conjunction with other clinical findings and should not be relied on as the sole method of cardiovascular monitoring. Unfortunately, BP values may be easily misinterpreted, resulting in catastrophic treatment errors. For the veterinarian, a fundamental understanding that many critically ill dogs and cats do not become hypotensive until terminal will prevent therapeutic inaction that may result from observing reassuringly normal BP values.

## References and Suggested Reading

Coulter DB and Keith JC Jr: Blood pressures obtained by indirect measurement in conscious dogs. J Am Vet Med Assoc 184:1375, 1984.
*A survey of blood pressure values obtained by automated oscillometry in normal dogs and dogs with cardiac or renal disease.*
Hamlin RL, Kittleson MD, Knowlen G, and Seyffert R: Noninvasive measurement of systemic arterial pressure in dogs by automatic sphygmomanometry. Am J Vet Res 43:1271, 1982.
*Report of a prospective study that compared BP measurements obtained by automated oscillometry with direct measurement in normal dogs and in dogs made hypo- or hypertensive.*
Harvey J, Falsettim H, Cooper P, and Downing D: Auscultatory indirect measurement of blood pressure in dogs. Lab Anim Sci 33:370, 1983.
*A description of a method that successfully adapted the manual auscultatory technique for use on the canine thoracic limb.*
Pettersen JC, Linartz RR, Hamlin RL, and Stoll RE: Noninvasive measurement of systemic arterial blood pressure in the conscious beagle dog. Fund Appl Toxicol 10:89, 1988.
*A report of a prospective study to evaluate the suitability of automated oscillometry for long-term daily monitoring of arterial BP in dogs used in toxicologic studies.*
Ramsey M III: Blood pressure monitoring: Automated oscillometric devices. J Clin Monit 7:56, 1991.
*A review of modern automated sphygmomanometers.*
Weiser MG, Spangler WL, and Gribble DH: Blood pressure measurement in the dog. J Am Vet Med Assoc 171:364, 1977.
*A report of a survey of BP in normal and sick dogs monitored with an ultrasonic Doppler device.*

# DOPPLER ASSESSMENT OF BLOOD FLOW AND PRESSURE IN SURGICAL AND CRITICAL CARE PATIENTS

DENNIS T. CROWE, Jr.
*and* DAVID E. SPRENG

*Milwaukee, Wisconsin*

Doppler ultrasound was introduced in medicine in 1959 for measurement of blood flow velocities. The use of Doppler technique outside the research laboratory began in 1967, when it was used clinically for assessment of arterial blood flow in peripheral vessels, and for the detection of thromboembolism and arteriosclerosis (Hagood, Mozersky, and Tumblin, 1975). Kemmerer et al. reported in 1969 the use of a Doppler device for the indirect measurement of blood pressure (BP) in human beings.

The use of the Doppler effect to measure blood pressure in cats and dogs was first described in the veterinary literature in 1977 (Weiser, Spangler, and Gribble, 1977; McLeish, 1977). In the last 10 years, continuous blood flow monitoring and assessment of arterial blood pressure with Doppler methods has become commonly employed in many veterinary emergency, critical care, and surgical practices.

There are several types of Doppler units available commercially. One unit, manufactured by Parks Medical Electronics, Aloha, OR, Model 811, is relatively low cost ($550 to $650). It detects the flow of blood via an audible sound from a loudspeaker or earphones. Some other models (Parks Medical Electronics, Model 812) have a recorder output designed to work with the DC input of an electrocardiograph that has a high input impedance. A waveform that corresponds to the strength of the electrical signal generated with the Doppler can be charted. These Doppler units are meant for the detection and assessment of blood flow (arterial and venous) and for monitoring arterial blood pressure when used in conjunction with a pneumatic cuff and sphygmomanometer.

We have used both of these Doppler units for over 12 years in clinical and research settings, monitoring several thousand dogs and cats. Species in which we also have had experience with use of the units include humans, rabbits, rats, mice, gerbils, guinea pigs, various birds, horses, deer, cattle, and lions. The Doppler units are easy to use and are able to detect blood flow in even the smallest patient, such as a 50-gm rat or a 25-gm bird with the application of a small plastic probe. It is from both this clinical and research experience, and from others that have performed similar investigations, that we provide strong encouragement and recommendations for the use of Doppler monitoring in clinical practice today.

The purpose of this article is the following:

1.   Introduce essential equipment for the monitoring of blood flow (continuously) and blood pressure (intermittently).
2.   Describe basic mechanisms and principles associated with Doppler flow detection.
3.   Describe practical methods used to monitor blood flow and arterial pressure that are beneficial in patient care decision making.
4.   Describe indications for use of Doppler techniques in clinical practice.

## DOPPLER FLOW DETECTION: BASIC PRINCIPLES AND EQUIPMENT

The Doppler unit consists of an electronic amplifier, speaker, and internal rechargeable battery; and an attached flat flow probe, measuring $9 \times 15 \times 2$ mm (Fig. 1). The probe is a continuous wave Doppler (CW-Doppler) transducer consisting of two piezoelectric quartz crystals. One of the crystals is used to transmit a continuous ultrasonic beam at a set frequency (between 2 and 10 MHz) while the other crystal acts as a continuous receiver. The sound waves traverse the tissue and some echo with a different frequency. The change of frequency that occurs when the reflecting wave has hit a moving object is called Doppler shift.

The Doppler shift principle is a well known phenomenon in everyday life and can be illustrated. When a fire truck approaches and recedes, the sound of the siren (and the waves generated and perceived by the human ear) will change in its intensity and pitch (frequency). Similar changes in intensity and pitch occur with ultrasound waves generated by the Doppler unit, when sending and receiving ultrasound as it becomes influenced by the moving blood flow nearby.

The Doppler and its frequency shifts can be used in various measurements of blood flow in vessels that are sufficiently near a surface for the technique to be effective. The echoes that are detected in the Doppler originate from the red blood cells moving at different velocities in the blood vessels (Hagood, Mozersky, and Tumblin, 1975). If the cells are moving toward the transducer, the frequency of sound waves is increased and the wavelength decreased. If sound waves strike blood flow moving away from the transducer, the frequency of the sound waves that are reflected will decrease and the wavelength will be increased. The difference in sound wave frequencies are converted to equivalent electrical impulses by the receiving piezoelectric crystal. Hence, the swishing sound heard with each pulse wave generated.

The equation, where $F$ is the Doppler shift in Hz, $F_0$ is the transmitted frequency of ultrasound, and V is the velocity of blood flow in m/sec, is shown to demonstrate the direct relationship between the amount of Doppler shift, as represented by strength of the sound generated, and the velocity of the mass of red cells detected:

$$V = \frac{(\Delta F) \times (C)}{(2) \times (F_0) \times \cos \theta}$$

In the equation, the Doppler shift $F$ is directly proportional to V. In the same equation, the angle $\theta$ between the transmitter beam and the direction of blood flow is represented by a cosine function in the Doppler equation. Therefore, the Doppler shift frequency increases as the angle between the ultrasonic beam and the vessels becomes less (Moise, 1988). This is important as regards the position of the flow probe. The probe should be held as flat against the surface of the skin as possible to allow the best detection of blood flow in vessels laying parallel to this surface. Movement of the probe must also be minimized to eliminate "noise" and provide accurate detection of the blood flow velocity.

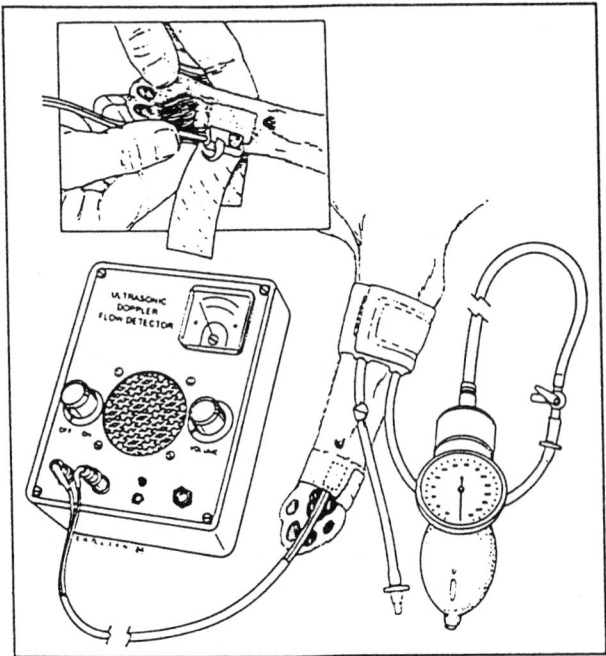

**Figure 1.** Application of the Doppler flow probe and a pneumatic cuff on the forelimb of a cat. (From Grady JL, Dunlop CI, Hodgson DS, Curtis CR, and Chapman PL: Evaluation of the Doppler ultrasonic method of measuring systolic arterial blood pressure in cats. Am J Vet Res 53:1166, 1992, with permission.)

## SENSITIVITY OF PULSE, BLOOD FLOW DETECTION, AND ACCURACY OF BP ESTIMATES WITH DOPPLER COMPARED TO PALPATION, OSCILLOMETRIC, AND DIRECT MEASUREMENTS

It is axiomatic that arterial blood flow and pressure measurements are helpful in the management of anesthetized, ill, or injured patients. Noninvasive methods are preferred in most cases if the procedure used is easy to perform and is accurate and reliable (see "Blood Pressure Measurement," this volume, p 110). The noninvasive methods currently available are palpation, Doppler, and oscillometric.

The oscillometric method involves the use of a microcomputer that senses the oscillations produced in an air-filled cuff encircling the limb that are the result of pulsatile blood flow in the limb. Although systolic and diastolic pressure and pulse rate can be determined by this method, continuous blood flow cannot be monitored. Oscillometric blood pressure detection also requires the patient to be still. Our experience suggests that this method is difficult to use in very hypotensive, cold, or shivering and moving animals.

Palpation alone is not accurate, as exemplified by a research study we performed in anesthetized cats in which direct pressures were being monitored using a catheter placed into the femoral artery and attached to a Statham transducer. As anesthesia was deepened, pulses were palpated and an estimation of strength of femoral pulses and tarsal pulses was made. In some animals we were still able to detect actual pulsations when systolic pressures were below 40 mm Hg, while in others, pulses were undetectable at pressures of 60 to 70 mm Hg. Body confirmation and differences in pulse pressure (systolic pressure minus diastolic pressure) were believed responsible for this variability.

In an unpublished study in dogs in which shock was induced by bleeding, a direct relationship was observed for the strength of the pulse on palpation versus the directly measured arterial blood pressure, but considerable variability existed with respect to detection of blood pressures by palpation. It has been suggested that detection of pulses is dependent on the sensitivity of the individual doing the palpation. A weak femoral pulse without a palpable tarsal pulse has been stated to indicate a systolic pressure under 60 mm Hg. If tarsal pulses are present, the systolic pressure is estimated to be over 80 mm Hg. Nevertheless, adequate femoral pulses were detected in several dogs with systolic pressures well below 60 mm Hg, and pulses were also characterized as "weak and thready" in several dogs that had measured direct arterial pressures well above 100 mm Hg. This latter finding was explained by noting the pulse pressure (systolic-diastolic) was lower than normal due to proportionally greater changes in diastolic pressure as compared to systolic pressure. In the aforementioned dogs, there was good correlation with measured systolic pressure (using a direct arterial catheter) and pressures found with indirect Doppler methods. Diastolic pressures are difficult to determine with Doppler in the cat, but were detected accurately in approximately 70% of the measurements from these dogs. Other investigators also report good clinical correlation between direct and Doppler ultrasonic methods of measuring systolic arterial blood pressure in animals (Grandy et al., 1992). In both studies, Doppler-determined pressure was slightly lower than direct pressures (10±3 mm Hg).

## MONITORING ARTERIAL FLOW AND PRESSURE

The following protocol is recommended for the monitoring of blood pressure and flow with the Parks Medical Electronics Doppler Flow Detector (Model 811, 811-AL, 811-B, and 812):

To begin, the flat flow probe (9 × 15 × 2 mm) is connected to the charged receiver-amplifier-speaker. The receiver-amplifier-speaker unit (15 × 19 × 8 cm) is powered by a rechargeable cadmium battery, which can be used continuously for 4 to 6 hr before it requires recharging. The battery life can often be extended by keeping the loudness of the sound heard through the audio speaker at a minimum. Using earphones rather than speakers to listen to the audio output also increases battery life. It is recommended keeping the flow probe plugged into the receiver-amplifier-speaker to prevent loosening of connections (Parks).

The hair of the patient is clipped just above the palmar metacarpal or plantar metatarsal pad to create a hairless patch at least as big as the probe. Ultrasonic jelly is placed in the concave portion of the flow probe and the probe is taped snugly into position. The ultrasonic jelly is necessary because ultrasound does not travel readily through air. The amplifier is turned on and the probe is manipulated until a clear swishing sound can be heard. This sound is generated by blood flow through the superficial palmar or plantar arterial arch fed by the common digital branches of radial or caudal tibial arteries, respectively.

Monitoring of blood flow can be continued by simply keeping the volume on the amplifier adjusted so that the swishing sound is easily recognized but not so loud that conversations cannot be heard over the sound generated. Each time the heart beats and flow is generated a swishing sound is heard. Therefore, on a continuous basis, a "swish, swish, swish, swish" is heard over the speaker, with the relative intensity of the sound corresponding to strength and amount of blood flow generated.

To measure blood pressure with the Doppler, the method of Korotkoff has been modified, with the Doppler rather than a stethoscope used to "listen" to blood flow. This requires a proper size blood pressure cuff placed proximal to the flow probe and attached to an aneroid sphygmomanometer. The appropriate cuff size is determined by wrapping the cuff around the limb and noting where the "index line" or edge of the cuff falls in relation to the "range" marked on the cuff.

These are small lines marked on the side of the cuff. The "range" lines, if not marked clearly on the cuff, extend from the edge of the air bladder to 30% more of cuff length. The cuff should be of proper fit to allow an accurate estimate of arterial blood pressure (Simpson, Jamieson, and Dickhaus, 1965). The use of an overly large cuff will produce falsely low values (proportional to the oversize of the cuff) and using too small a cuff will produce falsely high values. For the foreleg, the cuff is wrapped around the antebrachium midway between the elbow and the carpus. For the hind limb, apply the cuff in the mid crus or tibial region. The cuff should not be placed over skeletal prominences. The cuff should also be placed so that the main artery (on the medial aspect of the limb in both the front and rear legs) is under the middle of the inflatable bladder.

Two sizes of blood pressure cuffs, "infant" and "newborn" are available from Parks Medical Electronics, and generally are sufficient to monitor pressure accurately in most dogs and cats. The infant cuff is used in dogs weighing more than 15 kg, and the newborn cuff is used on smaller dogs and cats. Cuffs manufactured by Vital Signs or Critikon are available in 1- to 8-cm widths and correspondingly can be used in patients with limbs of similar diameters. After selecting a cuff, it is secured to the limb and taped around to ensure that the Velcro does not loosen. The sphygmomanometer is attached to the cuff and the cuff is inflated to 200 to 250 mm Hg (at least to a pressure 30 mm Hg past when the swishing sound ceased). The valve on the manometer is gradually opened to slowly deflate the cuff. The point at which the swishing sound is first heard again is the systolic pressure. The point where the swishing sound changes from its short pulsatile characteristic sound to a more continuous swishing, longer lasting sound, is the approximate diastolic pressure. This change is heard as "switsh, switsh, switsh" (systolic) to a "swi-ish, swi-ish, swi-ish" (diastolic). If no change in the sound is able to be detected, then diastolic pressure cannot be determined. This is common in small vessels or those that are "stiff" or under high catecholamine influence.

Alternative sites for use with the Doppler flow probe to measure flow and pressure include the cranial aspect of the tarsus, where cranial tibial artery blood flow can be monitored; and the ventral aspect of the tail, where ventral coccygeal artery blood flow can be monitored. Occasionally, the medial aspect of the distal radius can be clipped and radial artery blood flow can be monitored.

Anatomic locations where the Doppler flow probe can be placed to monitor only the presence of arterial blood flow are the following:

1. The ventral aspect of the tongue in unconscious animals to monitor flow through the lingual artery.
2. The surface of the eye (with plenty of ultrasound jelly added) in unconscious animals to monitor blood flow through the ophthalmic arterial plexus behind the eye.

3. The medial aspect of the humerus to monitor blood flow through the brachial artery.

4. The lateral aspect of the neck, flank region, and medial aspect of the thigh to determine blood flow through the common carotid artery, aorta and kidney, and femoral arterial branches, respectively. Because the probe cannot be fixed well to these areas, only periodic rather than continuous monitoring is possible.

## CLINICAL APPLICATIONS OF DOPPLER MONITORING

Continuous Doppler monitoring of blood flow is indicated for any animals believed cardiovascularly unstable or potentially unstable. This includes, in our opinion, all animals undergoing general anesthesia. Not only is pulse rate monitored, but changes in strength of cardiac contraction and stroke volume can be subjectively assessed. This information cannot be assessed with other monitoring methods (e.g., esophageal stethoscope, electrocardiogram (ECG), pulse oximetry, pressure monitored by oscillometrics, and even pressure monitored by direct arterial catheter).

In animals that are unconscious and apparently pulseless, the Doppler probe can be placed on the eye and the presence of blood flow, if any, serially determined. If no flow is evident, cardiac function is nil and cardiopulmonary resuscitation is required. In cases in which resuscitation is elected, it is recommended that the Doppler probe be left in place and used to monitor blood flow generated by the resuscitation.

Indirect blood pressure monitoring has become a very useful tool as compared to palpation of pulses alone. For example, a patient may actually have a high blood pressure with the clinical signs of shock (pale mucous membrane, slow capillary refill time, trembling, anxious level of consciousness and a weak and rapid pulse) caused by severe pain. The weak pulse in this commonly observed example could be caused by a narrow pulse pressure associated with increased diastolic pressure due to high catecholamine release. Without actual blood pressure monitoring, even the expert clinician might have treated this patient with a shock dose of fluids. Knowing the actual pressure is high rather than low allows the animal to be treated much more appropriately with analgesics.

Constant or repeated measurements of blood pressure are a cornerstone in modern anesthesia. It has been our experience that one of the complications (vasodilation) associated with the use of isoflurane and halothane anesthetics would go undetected without arterial blood pressure monitoring. Indirect blood pressure measurement is recommended every 5 to 10 min in stable patients and more often in critical or unstable patients. In emergency settings, some patients will have to be anesthetized even though a very poor physical condition is present. Minimal systolic pressures (60 mm Hg) are required to ensure an adequate major organ blood flow (e.g., kidney, brain, liver). Minimal diastolic pressure (40 mm Hg) is also required to ensure adequate coronary blood flow. Pressures have to be maintained above these critical limits. If monitored, pressures that approach these critical values can be addressed with appropriate therapy to augment the pressures and prevent complications that would otherwise occur. In many cases, simply decreasing the vaporizer setting is all that will be required. In other cases, infusion of crystalloid or colloid solutions will help correct the relative volume depletion responsible for the hypotension. Occasional use of pressor agents such as dopamine, given to effect, will also be required to treat anesthetic-induced hypotension. The assessment of patient response (increasing blood pressures) can be easily monitored with the Doppler and is also of key importance.

## PRACTICAL USE IN CASES OF LIMITED ASSISTANCE

The use of Doppler blood flow monitoring in minor surgical procedures performed by a surgeon, without the help of a technician to monitor anesthesia, is very valuable. The swishing rhythmic sound of the arterial blood flow is a source of information about the anesthetic depth of the patient. Provided probe position and gain settings remain constant, the strength of the sounds is proportional to the amount of blood flow generated with each heartbeat. If the intensity of flow sounds increases substantially, the anesthesia may be too light and the patient may be feeling pain; if the intensity decreases below normal, the anesthetic depth might be too profound. Premature ventricular contractions can be heard as an irregular pulse, indicating the need for ECG monitoring.

## USE OF THE DOPPLER IN CARDIOPULMONARY CEREBRORESUSCITATION

The success of cardiopulmonary cerebroresuscitation (CPCR) is greatly dependent upon generating adequate blood flow to the brain and the heart. Brain perfusion is dependent upon a sufficient systolic pressure gradient (difference between aortic and right atrial systolic pressure) generated by cardiac compression. The difference between aortic diastolic and right atrial diastolic pressure is called coronary perfusion pressure and determines the amount of flow to the cardiac muscle. The measurements of these indices in emergency situations are not possible and external blood flow meters can be used to indicate flow.

For assessment of blood flow to the brain, the Parks Doppler can be used in a very simple application. The 9-mm flat flow probe can be used on the cornea of an animal undergoing CPCR (Crowe, 1992). In preliminary studies, we have found that the presence of swishing sounds was a more reliable indicator of blood flow through the common carotid artery during cardiac massage than are flow measurements using Doppler techniques at peripheral sites (e.g., metacarpus)(Spreng et al., 1994).

## SUMMARY

Transcutaneous Doppler methods of assessing arterial blood pressure and flow are useful for monitoring critical animal patients. Good correlation between direct measured blood pressure and indirect Doppler-assisted pressure monitoring has been shown in dogs and cats. Continuous pressure and blood flow monitoring during anesthesia is recommended in all patients. Monitoring the trends of change in pressures of patients with shock or a low-flow state is important to ensure adequate therapy. Potentially hypotensive patients (pancreatitis, gastric dilation) or potentially hypertensive patients (hyperthyroidism, renal disease) benefit greatly from blood pressure measurements. Doppler blood flow measurements in CPCR appear effective in assessing adequacy of cardiac massage. The ease of use and affordability of Doppler equipment strongly suggests its application be considered by all clinicians performing general anesthesia and when managing seriously injured or ill patients.

## References and Suggested Reading

Crowe DT: Evaluation of a Doppler flow detector and probe on the eye for determining effectiveness of blood flow generation with cardiac massage in dogs (abstr). *Third International Veterinary Emergency and Critical Care Symposium* 3:837, 1992.
*Abstract about the use of the Parks Doppler on the eye in CPR.*

Grady JL, Dunlop CI, Hodgson DS, Curtis CR, and Chapman PL: Evaluation of the Doppler ultrasonic method of measuring systolic arterial blood pressure in cats. Am J Vet Res 53:1166, 1992.
*Indirect systolic blood pressure measurements in 16 cats.*

Hagood CO, Mozersky DJ, and Tumblin RN: Practical office technics for physiologic vascular testing. South Med J 68:17, 1975.
*Overview about noninvasive vascular testing methods with the Doppler in humans.*

Janis KM, Kemmerer WT, and Hagood CO: Doppler blood pressure measurement in infants and small children. J Pediatr Surg 6: 1971.
*Indirect blood pressure measurement in three pediatric patients.*

McLeish I: Doppler ultrasonic arterial pressure measurement in the cat. Vet Rec 100:290, 1977.
*Subjective assessment of Doppler-generated blood pressure in cats.*

Moise NS: Echocardiography. *In* PR Fox (ed): *Canine and Feline Cardiology.* New York, Churchill Livingstone, 1988, p 116.
*Overview of echocardiography in veterinary medicine.*

Simpson JA, Jamieson G, and Dickhaus DW: Effect of size of cuff bladder on accuracy of measurement of indirect blood pressure. Am Heart J 70: 208, 1965.
*Comparison of indirect and direct blood pressures in 24 human subjects using the Korotkoff method.*

Spreng D, Crowe DT, DeBehnke D, and Swarl G: Usefulness of ocular and metacarpal Doppler blood flow sounds in experimental canine cardiopulmonary resuscitation (abstr). Fourth International Veterinary Emergency and Critical Care Symposium, 1994.
*Metacarpal blood flow cannot be used to assess CPR.*

Weiser MG, Spangler WL, and Gribble DH: Blood pressure measurement in the dog. J Am Vet Med Assoc 171:364, 1977.
*Evaluation of Doppler systolic blood pressure measurements in dogs with good correlations.*

# PULSE OXIMETRY

JOAN C. HENDRICKS
*Philadelphia, Pennsylvania*

Pulse oximetry is a technique that allows the instantaneous estimation of arterial oxyhemoglobin saturation by transmitting light through a skin fold. By sensing the difference between light absorption during pulsations (presumed to be arterial) and the background absorption (presumed to be due to venous blood, tissue, and bone), the instruments produce a percentage value for hemoglobin saturation and also a value for pulse rate (Severinghaus and Koh, 1990; Alexander, Teller, and Gross, 1989). Although oxyhemoglobin saturation ($SaO_2$) is not linearly related to arterial $PO_2$, the $SaO_2$ provides information about tissue delivery of oxygen that is clinically important and is complementary to $PO_2$ (Alexander, Teller, and Gross, 1989; Rossing and Cain, 1988).

Despite routine use in human medicine, the application of oximetry to veterinary patients has not become widespread. The potential advantages, in comparison to arterial blood gas analysis, especially in a population of critically ill animals, are readily apparent: a continuous, immediate, noninvasive estimation of oxygenation. However, a number of factors can complicate the interpretation of pulse oximetry, and these factors must also be considered in evaluating its practicality and usefulness (Severinghaus and Koh, 1990; Alexander, Teller, and Gross, 1989; Schnapp and Cohen, 1990; Hannhart et al., 1991). Among the factors that interfere with accurate pulse oximeter saturation ($SpO_2$) measurements in man, variation in skin color, decreased perfusion, hypothermia, increased serum bilirubin concentration, and anemia (Severinghaus and Koh, 1990; Alexander, Teller, and Gross, 1990; Schnapp and Cohen, 1990) might be expected to be present in critically ill small animal patients. Although several models have been calibrated in anesthetized healthy dogs (Hendricks et al., 1987; Hendricks, 1990; Jacobsen et al., 1992) and horses (Whitehair et al., 1990), the validity of oximeter readings in critically ill animals has only recently been established.

## EVALUATION OF PULSE OXIMETRY IN CRITICAL SMALL ANIMAL PATIENTS

A study of continuous monitoring of 21 critical dogs for 2 hr or more (Fairman, 1992) and a study of 51 paired samples of $SaO_2$ and $SpO_2$ in 25 critically ill dogs and eight cats (Hendricks and King, 1993) have recently been reported. In these studies, the measurements were taken from a representative sample of critically ill animals. The major syndromes in these patients were respiratory, cardiovascular, hematologic, gastrointestinal, neurologic, metabolic, and renal. Four animals were in septic shock. Many patients had more than one syndrome. About half of the animals were admitted to the intensive care unit (ICU) immediately after major body cavity surgery performed to correct a life-threatening condition. The patients included several with the clinical features thought to potentially interfere with oximetry. Fifteen readings were taken in anemic animals (packed cell volume, 11 to 33%) and two had elevated serum bilirubin concentration (12 and 21.6 mg/dl). Four were hypothermic (rectal temperatures ranging from 32.2° to 37.4°C). Four of the 33 animals in one study (Hendricks and King, 1993) died within 12 hr of data collection.

Of 51 attempts to obtain both arterial blood and oximetry readings, 12 (23.5%) attempts to obtain arterial blood were unsuccessful, while only three (5.9%) attempts to obtain oximeter readings were unsuccessful (Hendricks and King, 1993). Similarly, during continuous monitoring, all 21 patients tolerated the digital sensor with no or minimal evidence of discomfort (Fairman, 1992). The ease of obtaining readings may have its most significant impact in cats, in whom readings were obtained in eight, while arterial blood gases could be obtained in only three.

The accuracy of the oximeters appears to be acceptable for clinical applications, although the readings are affected by a number of factors, such as the location of the sensor. Hendricks and King (1993), found that 13 of 35 placements on the ear (36%) yielded an ac-ceptable $SpO_2$ reading using the Biox 3740. The next most common placement was the lip, where 62% of 29 placements, were judged to be acceptable. The axilla (25 placements, 64% accepted) and inguinal skin folds (25 placements, 72% accepted) were also used commonly. For continuous monitoring, Fairman found the metacarpals, the gastrocnemius, and the digits to yield acceptable readings with the Nellcor-200 (Fairman, 1992); however, this instrument did not appear to read reliably on densely pigmented skin. Movement (Fairman, 1992) and respiratory artifact (Hendricks and King, 1993) affected the readings in some patients, but these false readings were readily detected and rejected.

When 38 paired $SpO_2$ and $SaO_2$ measures were compared, the mean difference between the $SpO_2$ and the $SaO_2$ was $0.26 \pm 2.2\%$, with the $SpO_2$ being slightly below the $SaO_2$ ($r = .87$; $p < .0001$). The 95% confidence interval was $\pm 4.4\%$, well within the range accepted in humans and claimed by the manufacturers (Alexander, Teller, and Gross, 1989; Gravenstein, 1990). An $SpO_2$ of 90% would thus have a 95% chance of reflecting an $SaO_2$ of 85.6 to 94.4%. However, in two animals with grossly impaired perfusion (one in the midst of CPR efforts after cardiorespiratory arrest, and the other exhibiting generalized thromboembolism), the $SpO_2$-$SaO_2$ difference was much greater (6.3% and 11.4%, respectively).

In using the Nellcor-200 for continuous monitoring, seven hypoxic episodes were detected by the oximeter that were not otherwise noted by observers (Fairman, 1992).

## RECOMMENDATIONS FOR USE OF PULSE OXIMETRY IN CRITICAL PATIENTS

In conclusion, oximetry can be a useful clinical tool in monitoring the oxygenation of critical patients with adequate perfusion, including cats. These instruments can give reasonably accurate readings in a variety of sites, and will provide a reading in over 90% of patients. Presently, we have no basis to suggest limiting the use of the instruments even in cases with anemia, icterus, hypothermia, or primary cardiovascular disease, provided adequate perfusion is present. It is a safe, simple, quick, easy-to-use, and well-tolerated technique. However, in the absence of an arterial blood gas, the limits of the oximeter must be recognized, and severely impaired perfusion may yield grossly inaccurate $SpO_2$ readings.

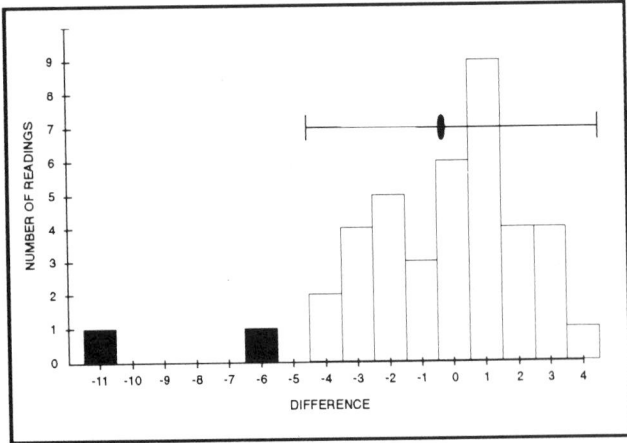

**Figure 1.** A histogram of the number of oximeter readings differing from the actual arterial $SaO_2$ by $-11$ to $+4\%$. The two readings filled in black were in an animal who had suffered a cardiac arrest and a dog who died of diffuse thromboembolic disease. These two outlying values were thus eliminated from further analysis. The mean and 95% confidence interval is displayed above the histogram ($0.26 \pm 4.4\%$). (From Hendricks JC and King LG: Practicality, usefulness, and limits of pulse oximetry in critical small animal patients. J Vet Emerg Crit Care 3:5–12, 1993, with permission.)

### References and Suggested Reading

Alexander CM, Teller LE, and Gross JE: Principles of pulse oximetry: Theoretical and practical considerations. Anesth Analg 68:368, 1989.

Brunel W and Cohen NH: Evaluation of the accuracy of pulse oximetry in critically ill patients. Crit Care Med 16:432, 1988.

Fairman NB: Evaluation of pulse oximetry as a continuous monitoring technique in critically ill dogs in the small animal intensive care unit. J Vet Emerg Crit Care 2:50, 1992.

Gravenstein JS: *Gas Monitoring and Pulse Oximetry*. Boston, Butterworth-Hennemann, 1990, p 148.

Hannhart B, Haberer JP, Saunier C, and Laxemaite MC: Accuracy and precision of fourteen pulse oximeters. Eur Respir J 4:115, 1991.

Hendricks JC, Kline LR, Kovalski RJ, O'Brien JA, and Morrison AR: The English bulldog: A natural model of sleep-disordered breathing. J Appl Physiol 63:1344, 1987.

Hendricks JC: Variable characteristics of two models of ear oximetry in the dog. *Proc Int Vet Emer Crit Care Soc* 1990, p 652.

Hendricks JC and King LG: Practicality, usefulness, and limits of pulse oximetry in critical small animal patients. J Vet Emerg Crit Care 3:5, 1993.

Jacobsen JD, Miller MW, Matthews NS, Hartsfield SM, and Knauer KW: Evaluation of accuracy of pulse oximetry dogs. Am J Vet Res 53:537, 1992.

McGough EK, and Boysen PG: Benefits and limitations of pulse oximetry in the ICU. J Crit Illness 4:23, 1989.

Rossing RG and SM Cain: A nomogram relating pO₂, pH, temperature and hemoglobin saturation in the dog. J Appl Physiol 21:195, 1988.

Schnapp LM and Cohen NH: Pulse oximetry: Uses and abuses. Chest 98:1244, 1990.

Severinghaus JW and Koh SO: Effect of anemia on pulse oximeter accuracy at low saturation. J Clin Monit 6:85, 1990.

Whitehair KJ, Watney GC, Leith DE, and Debowes DM: Pulse oximetry in horses. Vet Surg 19:243, 1990.

# END-TIDAL CARBON DIOXIDE MONITORING

JOAN C. HENDRICKS

*Philadelphia, Pennsylvania*

Carbon dioxide monitors (capnographs) became small and inexpensive enough for clinical use in the early 1980s (Severinghaus and Koh, 1990). These instruments generally use one of two basic types of technology (infrared absorption spectrophotometry or mass spectrometry). They continuously aspirate gas from plastic tubing placed in the patient's airways and analyze the concentration of carbon dioxide (Raemer and Calalang, 1991; Szaflarski and Cohen, 1991). Theoretically, the plateau of the end-tidal carbon dioxide measure for each breath reflects alveolar gas, which in turn equilibrates quickly with arterial carbon dioxide ($Pa_{CO_2}$) in the healthy, normally perfused lung (Szaflarski and Cohen, 1991). Thus, end-tidal carbon dioxide measures have the potential to reflect $Pa_{CO_2}$, and to serve as a noninvasive measure of alveolar ventilation (Szaflarski and Cohen, 1991). If the end-tidal carbon dioxide sample truly reflects alveolar gas, the difference between end-tidal carbon dioxide and $Pa_{CO_2}$ could also be used to calculate the physiologic dead space (Szaflarski and Cohen, 1991), a clinically important parameter.

The use of carbon dioxide monitors in hospital operating rooms to reduce the incidence of ventilatory mishaps (Raemer and Calalang, 1991) has now become routine. This rapid increase in the application of a relatively new technology is due, in part, to the fact that the use of capnography is highly recommended by the American Society of Anesthesiologists (ASA) and also recommended or even required by some medical malpractice insurance carriers (Raemer and Calalang, 1991). Some recent articles advocate the usefulness of the end-tidal carbon dioxide for predicting $Pa_{CO_2}$ in anesthetized equine patients (Cribb, 1988) or waking human adults (Lenz, Heipertz, and Epple, 1991), whereas other reports in human adults and children (Hoffman et al., 1989) and in adult horses (Meyer and Short, 1985) and foals (Geiser and Rohrbach, 1992) have suggested caution in using end-tidal carbon dioxide measures for patient management in at least some clinical situations, as the relationship to $Pa_{CO_2}$, even within an individual patient (Hoffman et al., 1989), may vary greatly.

A study of the usefulness and accuracy of end-tidal carbon dioxide monitoring was conducted in the intensive care unit (ICU) of the Veterinary Hospital of the University of Pennsylvania (Hendricks and King, 1993). Both spontaneously breathing and mechanically ventilated patients were studied.

## END-TIDAL CARBON DIOXIDE MEASURES IN WAKING, SPONTANEOUSLY BREATHING ANIMALS

A method for sampling exhaled gas in waking, spontaneously breathing animals was developed in normal cats and dogs (Hendricks and King, 1993) using a Normocap 100 infrared carbon dioxide monitor (Datex Medical Instrumentation, Tewkesbury, MA). The sample of end-tidal gas was obtained by inserting the plastic tubing 3 to 7 mm into one nostril and closing the alar fold gently around the tubing to minimize aspiration of room air. The mouth was held closed if necessary to ensure nasal breathing. After approximately 30 sec of regular, deep breaths, the respiratory rate and the peak carbon dioxide level were recorded. The procedure lasted 1 to 2 min and was well tolerated by all the normal animals. The range of end-tidal carbon dioxide values obtained in the normal animals was 32 to 35 mm Hg for cats, and 35 to 46 mm Hg in dogs. These values compare well with the published ranges for $Pa_{CO_2}$ in these species (Haskins, 1983). Fifty-four paired end-tidal carbon dioxide and PaCO₂ measures were then obtained in 43 spontaneously breathing ICU patients. The overall range of PaCO₂ in the ICU patients sampled ranged from 20 to 77 mm Hg. The range of respiratory rates was 7 to 90 breaths per minute. The procedure was not tolerated in three additional patients; two were extremely dyspneic and one was vicious.

Overall, the values of the nasal end-tidal carbon dioxide and the PaCO₂ value in nonpanting animals were significantly correlated ($r=.84$; $p<.0001$), and both the $r$ values and the 95% confidence interval ($-1.81$ to $-5.98$) compared well with published values for end-tidal carbon dioxide and PaCO₂ comparisons in humans (Lenz, Heipertz, and Epple, 1991; Hoffman et al., 1989) and animals (Meyer and Short, 1985; Geiser and Rohrbach, 1992). These data are illustrated graphically in Figure 1. However, in animals with respiratory rates above 60, no significant correlation was found ($r=.37$; $p=.27$). Thus, it appears that the nasal sampling technique may be reasonably accurate when used in nonpanting dogs with healthy lungs.

### END-TIDAL CARBON DIOXIDE MEASURES IN MECHANICALLY VENTILATED ANIMALS

Fifty-six patients were mechanically ventilated during the 1-year study period, and the carbon dioxide monitor was used during ventilation in 28 dogs and 6 cats. None of these patients was managed with positive end-expiratory pressures of greater than 5 cm H₂O. The respiratory rates were less than 30 in all patients. Approximately 50% of the patients suffered from primary lung disease; the others were hypoventilating due to metabolic, neural, or muscular conditions.

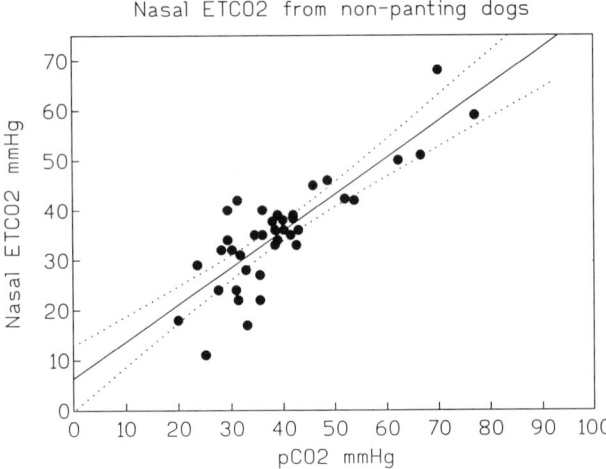

**Figure 1.** Forty-five nasal end-tidal carbon dioxide measures and paired PaCO₂ measures taken from dogs with respiratory rates less than 60 are plotted. The measures are highly correlated ($r=.84$); $p<.0001$). Dotted lines: 95% confidence interval. (From Hendricks JC and King LG: Practicality, usefulness, and limits of end-tidal carbon dioxide monitoring in critical small animal patients. J Vet Emerg Crit Care, 3:5–12, 1993, with permission.)

In eight animals, the end-tidal carbon dioxide values were used to monitor weaning from the ventilator. In an additional two dogs, after removal from the ventilator, the end-tidal carbon dioxide was periodically or continuously monitored at the tracheostomy site to decide when to take arterial blood gas samples or to resume ventilator therapy.

The PaCO₂ values were obtained in 28 of these patients, and ranged from 13 to 96 mm Hg. When the range of end-tidal carbon dioxide values was compared to the range of PaCO₂ values for each patient, the ranges correctly indicated the patient's ventilatory status throughout the duration of ventilation in 26 of the 28 cases. In two measures in 2 of the 28 cases, the end-tidal carbon dioxide failed to detect hypoventilation. In both patients, technical or pulmonary difficulties or both precluded accurate readings (alveolitis, lung collapse, and endotracheal tube occlusion). However, as in a previous similar study in humans (Hoffman et al., 1989), the values for the end-tidal carbon dioxide and the PaCO₂ diverged unpredictably within individual intubated patients. For example, in a cat who was hypoventilating because of cerebral depression, the end-tidal carbon dioxide ranged from 4.4 to 10.3 mm Hg lower than the PaCO₂ with no clinical change in respiratory parameters. Because the end-tidal carbon dioxide and PaCO₂ measures were not always significantly correlated, devising a formula to "correct" the end-tidal carbon dioxide would not improve the ability to predict the PaCO₂ (Hoffman et al., 1989).

### RECOMMENDATIONS FOR USE OF END-TIDAL CARBON DIOXIDE MONITORING IN CRITICAL PATIENTS

In considering the entire patient population, only 1 end-tidal carbon dioxide measure out of 54 from waking patients, and 2 from 28 ventilated patients, incorrectly indicated that the patient was ventilating normally, when hypoventilation was actually present. In the other 53 waking comparison and 26 ventilated cases, the categorization was correct. The sensitivity for diagnosing hypoventilation in the entire patient population was 75%; the specificity was 100%; the positive predictive value was 100%, and the negative predictive value was 97%.

In general, we agree with authors who have suggested that the use of end-tidal carbon dioxide measures alone to predict PaCO₂ and serve as the basis for clinical management cannot generally be supported (Hoffman et al., 1989; Meyer and Short, 1985; Geiser and Rohrbach, 1992). Appropriate uses include: (1) identifying hypoventilation in nonpanting patients; (2) continuous monitoring between arterial blood samples; (3) reducing the frequency of arterial blood samples; (4) verifying continuity of the patient's airway; (5) serving as an apnea monitor, especially during weaning from mechanical ventilation; and (6) providing some information about carbon dioxide in patients in whom arterial samples absolutely cannot be obtained.

## References and Suggested Reading

Cribb PH: Capnographic monitoring during anesthesia with controlled ventilation in the horse. Vet Surg 17:48, 1988.

Dunphy JA: Accuracy of expired carbon dioxide partial pressure sampled from a nasal cannula (Letter to the Editor). Anesthesiology 68:960, 1988.

Geiser DR and Rohrbach BW: Use of end-tidal $CO_2$ tension to predict arterial $CO_2$ values in isoflurane-anesthetized equine neonates. Am J Vet Res 53: 1617, 1992.

Haskins SC: Blood gases and acid-base balance: Clinical interpretation and therapeutic implications. In Kirk RW (ed): Current Veterinary Therapy VIII: Small Animal Practice. WB Saunders Co, Philadelphia, 1983, p. 201.

Hendricks JC and King LG: Practicality, usefulness, and limits of end-tidal carbon dioxide monitoring in critical small animal patients. J Vet Emerg Crit Care, in press.

Hightower CE, Kiorpes AL, Butler HC, et al: End tidal partial pressure of $CO_2$ as an estimate of arterial partial pressure of $CO_2$ during various ventilatory regimens in halothane-anesthetized dogs. Am J Vet Res 41:610, 1980.

Hoffman RA, Krieger BP, Kramer MR, et al: End tidal carbon dioxide in critically ill patients during changes in mechanical ventilation. Am Rev Respir Dis 140:1265, 1989.

Lenz G, Heipertz W, and Epple E: Capnometry for continuous postoperative monitoring of nonintubated, spontaneously breathing patients. J Clin Monit 7:245, 1991.

Meyer RM and Short CE: Arterial to end-tidal $CO_2$ tension and alveolar dead space in halothane or isoflurane-anesthetized ponies. Am J Vet Res 46:597, 1985.

Moens Y and Verstraeten W: Capnographic monitoring in small animal anesthesia. J Am Anim Hosp Assoc 18:659, 1982.

Raemer DB and Calalang BS: Accuracy of end-tidal carbon dioxide tension analyzers. J Clin Monit 7:195, 1991.

Szaflarski NL and Cohen NH: Use of capnography in critically ill adults. Heart Lung 20:363, 1991.

# STRONG IONS AND ACID-BASE DISORDERS

HELIO S. AUTRAN DE MORAIS

*Londrina, Paraná, Brazil*

*and* WILLIAM W. MUIR

*Columbus, Ohio*

Hydrogen ion concentration ($[H^+]$) in arterial plasma is maintained within a narrow range in order to maintain normal metabolic activity. Relatively small changes (mEq/L) from normal $[H^+]$ are not compatible with life. Breathing regulates one end product of tissue metabolism, carbon dioxide (usually measured as carbon dioxide tension $[P_{CO_2}]$), while renal and gastrointestinal mechanisms indirectly regulate the concentration of bicarbonate ($[HCO_3^-]$) and electrolytes. Bicarbonate ion concentration (sometimes used as a measurement of nonrespiratory or metabolic acid-base disorders) is dependent on $P_{CO_2}$, the total concentration of plasma weak nonvolatile acids ($[A_{TOT}]$, composed mostly by albumin and inorganic phosphates), and the difference between the strong cations and the strong anions (the so-called strong ion difference [SID]) (Stewart 1981; Fencl and Leith, 1993). Strong ions are substances that are completely dissociated in plasma at body pH. The most important strong ions in plasma are $Na^+$, $K^+$, $Ca^{2+}$, $Mg^{2+}$, $Cl^-$, lactate, $\beta$-hydroxybutyrate, acetoacetate and $SO_4^{2-}$. The influence of strong ions on pH and $[HCO_3^-]$ can always be expressed in terms of the SID. Changes in SID of a magnitude capable of altering acid-base balance usually occur as a result of increasing concentrations of $Na^+$, $Cl^-$, $SO_4^{2-}$ or organic anions, or decreasing concentrations of $Na^+$ or $Cl^-$. An increase in SID (by decreasing $[Cl^-]$ or increasing $[Na^+]$) will cause nonrespiratory alkalosis, whereas a decrease in SID (by decreasing $[Na^+]$ or increasing $[Cl^-]$, $[SO_4^{2-}]$ or organic anions) will cause nonrespiratory acidosis.

Body homeostatic mechanisms indirectly regulates $[H^+]$ (and pH) and $[HCO_3^-]$ by changing $P_{CO_2}$ (by changes in alveolar ventilation relative to carbon dioxide elimination rate) and SID (by differential reabsorption of $Na^+$ and $Cl^-$ in the kidneys). Although changes in $[A_{TOT}]$ will change $[HCO_3^-]$ and $[H^+]$, control of albumin production and inorganic phosphate concentration is not primarily directed at acid-base homeostasis.

## COMPENSATION

Simple acid-base disturbances occur when abnormalities in one of the principal determinants of $[H^+]$ (e.g., $P_{CO_2}$, SID, or $[A_{TOT}]$) is present. A simple acid-base disturbance includes both the primary process and the compensatory mechanism. That is, if a sustained primary disturbance occurs in $P_{CO_2}$, a compensatory change of regulated magnitude normally occurs in the SID and vice-versa. If the primary disturbance results from a change in $[A_{TOT}]$, however, renal or ventilatory compensation do not occur (Fencl and Leith, 1993). The magnitude of compensation in a given clinical situation cannot be determined with certainty, but the expected degree of compensation based on experimental data from dogs (using $[HCO_3^-]$ instead of SID) has been reviewed (Table 1) (see *CVT XI*, p 26; de Morais and DiBartola, 1991). It is important to remember that compensation does not return pH to normal (with the exception of chronic respiratory alkalosis), overcom-

***Table 1.***   *Compensatory Response to Simple Acid-Base Disturbances in Dogs**

| Disturbance | Clinical Guide for Compensation | |
|---|---|---|
| Metabolic acidosis | For each 1 mEq/L $\Downarrow$ $HCO_3^-$ | $P_{CO_2}$ $\Downarrow$ by 0.7 mm Hg |
| Metabolic alkalosis | For each 1 mEq/L $\Uparrow$ $HCO_3^-$ | $P_{CO_2}$ $\Uparrow$ by 0.7 mm Hg |
| Respiratory acidosis | | |
|   Acute | For each 1 mm Hg $\Uparrow$ $P_{CO_2}$ | $HCO_3^-$ $\Uparrow$ by 0.15 mEq/L |
|   Chronic | For each 1 mm Hg $\Uparrow$ $P_{CO_2}$ | $HCO_3^-$ $\Uparrow$ by 0.35 mEq/L |
| Respiratory alkalosis | | |
|   Acute | For each 1 mm Hg $\Downarrow$ $P_{CO_2}$ | $HCO_3^-$ $\Downarrow$ by 0.25 mEq/L |
|   Chronic | For each 1 mm Hg $\Downarrow$ $P_{CO_2}$ | $HCO_3^-$ $\Downarrow$ by 0.55 mEq/L |

*Adapted from de Morais HSA and DiBartola SP: Ventilatory and metabolic compensation in dogs with acid-base disturbances. J Vet Emerg Crit Care 1:39, 1991, with permission.

pensation does not occur, and sufficient time must elapse for compensation to reach a steady state. Little is known about compensation in cats with simple acid-base disturbances, but there is some suggestion that cats do not compensate as effectively as dogs in the presence of metabolic acidosis. Acid-base balance formulas for dogs or human beings should not be extrapolated to cats.

## CLINICAL DISTURBANCES

Based on the approach proposed by Peter Stewart, a new classification of primary acid-base disorders has been developed (Fencl and Rossing, 1989; Fencl and Leith, 1993). This classification provides a mechanistic view of the causative disturbances, and integrates serum electrolytes and albumin concentration into the interpretation of acid-base status. The clinical implications of the most important diseases affecting $P_{CO_2}$, SID, and $[A_{TOT}]$ will be discussed.

### Disorders of $P_{CO_2}$

Primary respiratory disturbances result from increases (respiratory acidosis) or decreases (respiratory

***Table 2.***   *Principal Causes of Respiratory Acid-Base Disorders*

***Respiratory Alkalosis (Hyperventilation $\Downarrow$ $Pa_{CO_2}$)***
Hypoxia
Low cardiac output
Severe anemia
Pulmonary disease (stimulation of peripheral reflexes, e.g., pneumonia)
CNS-mediated hyperventilation (e.g., drugs, CNS inflammation or tumor, liver disease, fear, pain)
Overzealous mechanical ventilation

***Respiratory Acidosis (Hypoventilation $\Uparrow$ $Pa_{CO_2}$)***
Airway obstruction
Respiratory center depression (e.g., drugs, neurologic disorders)
Cardiopulmonary arrest*
Neuromuscular diseases (e.g., botulism, polyradiculoneuritis)
Severe pulmonary disease
Pleural space disease (e.g., pleural effusion, pneumothorax)
Diaphragmatic hernia
Chest wall trauma
Inadequate mechanical ventilation

*During cardiopulmonary resuscitation $Pa_{CO_2}$ may be below normal.

alkalosis) in $P_{CO_2}$. Carbon dioxide tension can be changed by alveolar ventilation, which has a profound effect on $[HCO_3^-]$ and $[H^+]$. Approximately 50% of daily variability of $[HCO_3^-]$ in normal dogs can be attributed to changes in $P_{CO_2}$ alone. Because arterial $P_{CO_2}$ ($Pa_{CO_2}$) is inversely proportional to the alveolar ventilation, measurement of $Pa_{CO_2}$ provides the clinician with direct information about the adequacy of alveolar ventilation. Respiratory acidosis is therefore caused by and synonymous with hypoventilation, whereas respiratory alkalosis is caused by and synonymous with hyperventilation. The principal disorders associated with primary respiratory acid-base disturbances are listed in Table 2. Therapy of respiratory acidosis should be directed toward the elimination of the underlying cause of alveolar hypoventilation. Airway obstruction should be identified promptly and relieved. Medications that depress ventilation should be discontinued if possible. Pleurocentesis should be performed to remove fluid or air when pleural effusion or pneumothorax is present. Ventilatory assistance, if necessary, must be provided. Respiratory acidosis is not an indication for bicarbonate therapy. Administration of $NaHCO_3$ will decrease $[H^+]$ and decrease ventilatory drive, thus worsening hypoxemia and hypercapnia. It is not usually possible to remove the underlying cause of hypercapnia in patients with chronic pulmonary disease, but appropriate treatment of the underlying disease should be attempted.

Hypocapnia itself is not a major threat to the well-being of patients with respiratory alkalosis. The arterial pH in chronic primary respiratory alkalosis is usually normal or slightly alkalemic due to efficient renal compensation in this setting. The underlying disease responsible for hypocapnia should be the primary focus of therapeutic attention in patients with respiratory alkalosis.

### Disorders of $[A_{TOT}]$

Albumin and inorganic phosphate are nonvolatile weak acids and collectively are the major contributors to $[A_{TOT}]$. Consequently, changes in their concentrations will change $[H^+]$. Hypoalbuminemia will tend to decrease $[A_{TOT}]$ and cause a nonrespiratory alkalosis. Although less common, an increase in albumin concentration causes nonrespiratory acidosis due to an increase in $[A_{TOT}]$. Phosphate is the second most important component of $[A_{TOT}]$ and is normally present in plasma at a low concentration. Hypophosphatemia, therefore, does not cause a nonrespiratory alkalosis. Severe hyperphosphatemia, however, can cause a large change in $[A_{TOT}]$, which can result in nonrespiratory acidosis. The principal causes of nonrespiratory acid-base disturbances resulting from changes in $[A_{TOT}]$ are shown in Table 3. The treatment for hyperphosphatemic acidosis, hyperalbuminemic acidosis, and hypoalbuminemic alkalosis should be directed at the underlying cause.

## Disorders of SID

Changes in SID usually are recognized by changes in $[HCO_3^-]$ or base excess (BE). A decrease in SID produces nonrespiratory acidosis, whereas an increase in SID produces nonrespiratory alkalosis. There are three general mechanisms by which SID can change (Table 4): changing the water content of plasma, changing the $Cl^-$ concentration, and increasing the concentration of unidentified strong anions $(XA^-)$.

### FREE-WATER ABNORMALITIES

Changing the water content of the various body fluid compartments will dilute or concentrate both strong anions and cations. Consequently, SID will change by the same proportion. Changes in free water can be identified by evaluating the $[Na^+]$. An increase in SID due to increases in $[Na^+]$ results in concentration alkalosis, whereas a decrease in SID due to decreases in $[Na^+]$ results in dilution acidosis. It has been suggested that changes in extracellular fluid (ECF) volume alone lead to acid-base disturbances. Changes in ECF volume by themselves do not change SID, $PCO_2$ or $[A_{TOT}]$ and therefore cannot change acid-base status (Fencl and Rossing, 1989). The so-called contraction alkalosis believed to be due to decrease in ECF volume is caused by a decrease in $[Cl^-]$ (see Galla et al., 1991, and de Morais, 1992a for reviews). The principal causes of concentration alkalosis and dilution acidosis are listed in Table 5.

Therapy for dilution acidosis and concentration alkalosis should be directed at treating the underlying cause responsible for changing $[Na^+]$. If necessary, $[Na^+]$ and osmolality should be corrected. Nonrespiratory acidosis should only be treated in patients with severe acidemia (pH <7.2).

### ISONATREMIC CHLORIDE ABNORMALITIES

If there is no change in the water content of plasma, plasma $[Na^+]$ will be normal. Other strong cations (e.g., $K^+$) are regulated for purposes other then acid-base balance and their concentration never changes sufficiently to significantly affect SID (Fencl and Rossing, 1989). Consequently, SID changes only as a result of

**Table 3.** *Principal Causes of $[A_{TOT}]$ Abnormalities*

*Decreased $[A_{TOT}]$*
Hypoalbuminemia
  Protein-losing enteropathy
  Nephrotic syndrome
  Liver disease
  Malnutrition

*Increased $[A_{TOT}]$*
Hyperphosphatemia
  Nutritional hyperparathyroidism
  Renal failure
  Hypertonic sodium phosphate enema toxicity
  Urinary acidifiers containing phosphate toxicity
Hyperalbuminemia
  Dehydration

**Table 4.** *Disorders of SID*

| Abnormality | Disorder |
|---|---|
| Free Water Abnormalities | |
|   Increase in $[Na^+]$ | => Concentration alkalosis |
|   Decrease in $[Na^+]$ | => Dilution acidosis |
| Chloride Abnormalities | |
|   Decrease in $[Cl^-]_{corrected}$ | => Hypochloremic alkalosis |
|   Increase in $[Cl^-]_{corrected}$ | => Hyperchloremic acidosis |
| Unidentified Strong Anions Abnormalities | |
|   Increase in $[XA^-]$ | => Organic acidosis |

**Table 5.** *Principal Causes of Free-Water Abnormalities*

*Concentration Alkalosis ($\Uparrow[Na^+]$)*
Pure water deficit
  Primary hypodipsia
  Diabetes insipidus
  Fever
  Inadequate access to water
  High environmental temperature
Hypotonic fluid loss
  Vomiting
  Peritonitis
  Pancreatitis
  Burns
  Nonoliguric renal failure
  Postobstructive diuresis
Sodium gain
  Salt poisoning
  Hypertonic fluid administration (e.g., hypertonic saline, $NaHCO_3$)
  Hyperaldosteronism
  Hyperadrenocorticism

*Dilution Acidosis ($\Downarrow[Na^+]$)*
Severe liver disease
Nephrotic syndrome
Advanced renal failure
Congestive heart failure
Psychogenic polydipsia
Hypotonic fluid administration (e.g., 0.45% NaCl solution)
Vomiting
Diarrhea
Uroabdomen
Burns
Hypoadrenocorticism
Diuretic administration

changes in strong anions when water content is normal. If [$Na^+$] remains constant, changes in [$Cl^-$] can substantially increase or decrease SID. Evaluation of [$Cl^-$] must be considered in conjunction with measurement of [$Na^+$] because $Cl^-$ can change for reasons other than a change in water balance. Patient $Cl^-$ is therefore "corrected" for changes in [$Na^+$] applying a formula developed for use in human medicine (Leith, 1990) and adapted for use in small animal medicine (de Morais, 1992b) for dogs:

$$[Cl^-]_{corrected} = [Cl^-] \times 146/[Na^+]$$

and for cats:

$$[Cl^-]_{corrected} = [Cl^-] \times 156/[Na^+]$$

where [$Cl^-$] and [$Na^+$] are the patient $Cl^-$ and $Na^+$ concentrations. The values 146 and 156 (in milliequivalents per liter) are the normal [$Na^+$] for dogs and cats, respectively. Normal [$Cl^-$]$_{corrected}$ is approximately 107 to 113 mEq/L for dogs and approximately 117 to 123 mEq/L for cats (de Morais, 1992a). These values may vary for different laboratories and different analyzers. An increase or decrease in [$Cl^-$]$_{corrected}$ indicates that $Cl^-$ is responsible at least in part for the changes in SID. An increase in [$Cl^-$]$_{corrected}$ (i.e., increase in [$Cl^-$] relative to [$Na^+$]) results in a hyperchloremic acidosis, whereas a decrease in [$Cl^-$]$_{corrected}$ (i.e., a decrease in observed [$Cl^-$] relative to [$Na^+$]) results in hypochloremic alkalosis. A normal [$Cl^-$]$_{corrected}$ in presence of an abnormal [$Cl^-$] indicates that SID changes are caused by dilution acidosis or concentration alkalosis.

The principal causes of hyperchloremic acidosis and hypochloremic alkalosis are shown in Table 6. Treatment of hyperchloremic acidosis should be directed at correction of the underlying disease. Administration of $NaHCO_3$, when needed, will tend to correct hyperchloremic acidosis because this solution has an SID greater than plasma.

Hypochloremic alkalosis can be caused by excessive loss of $Cl^-$ relative to $Na^+$ or by administration of substances containing more $Na^+$ than $Cl^-$ compared to ECF. The former can occur following the administration of diuretics that cause $Cl^-$ wasting (e.g., furosemide) or when the fluid lost has a low or negative SID, as in the case of vomiting of stomach content. Treatment in hypochloremic alkalosis should be directed at correction of the SID. Renal $Cl^-$ conservation ordinarily is enhanced in hypochloremic states, but renal $Cl^-$ ion reabsorption does not return to normal until plasma $Cl^-$ concentration is restored to normal or near normal (Galla et al., 1991). In cases where expansion of extracellular volume is desired, intravenous infusion of 0.9% NaCl is the treatment of choice. This solution has an SID of 0 and will decrease plasma SID (Fencl and Rossing, 1989). If hypokalemia is present, KCl should be added to the fluid. When volume expansion is not necessary, $Cl^-$ can be administered using salts without $Na^+$ (e.g., $NH_4Cl$, KCl, $CaCl_2$, $MgCl_2$). These salts will correct the alkalosis because $Cl^-$ is given together with cations that are regulated within narrow limits for pur-

***Table 6.*** *Principal Chloride Disorders*

***Hypochloremic Alkalosis*** [*]   ($\Downarrow$[$Cl^-$]$_{corrected}$)
    Excessive loss of chloride relative to sodium
        Vomiting of stomach contents
        Therapy with thiazides or loop diuretics
        Hyperadrenocorticism
    Excessive gain of sodium relative to chloride
        $NaHCO_3$ therapy

***Hyperchloremic Acidosis*** [†]   ($\Uparrow$[$Cl^-$]$_{corrected}$)
    Excessive loss of sodium relative to chloride
        Diarrhea
    Excessive gain of chloride relative to sodium
        Fluid therapy (e.g., 0.9% NaCl, KCl-supplemented fluids)
        Salt poisoning
        Total parenteral nutrition
        $NH_4Cl$ or KCl therapy
    Chloride Retention
        Renal failure
        Renal tubular acidosis
        Hypoadrenocorticism
        Diabetes mellitus
        Drug induced (e.g., acetazolamide, spironolactone)

[*]Chronic respiratory acidosis will cause a compensatory decrease in [$Cl^-$]$_{corrected}$

[†]Chronic respiratory alkalosis will cause a compensatory increase in [$Cl^-$]$_{corrected}$

poses not related to acid-base balance (Fencl and Rossing, 1989). Acetazolamide can be used orally to decrease SID and correct hypochloremic alkalosis because it causes $Cl^-$ retention by the kidneys. Administration of substances containing more $Na^+$ than $Cl^-$ (e.g., $NaHCO_3$) increases SID, causing nonrespiratory alkalosis.

### ISONATREMIC ORGANIC ACID ABNORMALITIES

Accumulation of metabolically produced organic anions (e.g. lactate, acetoacetate, citrate, $\beta$-hydroxybutyrate) or addition of exogenous organic anions (e.g., salicylate, glycolate from ethylene glycol poisoning, and formate from methanol poisoning) will cause nonrespiratory acidosis because these strong anions decrease SID. Addition of some inorganic strong anions (e.g., $SO_4^{2-}$ during renal failure) will resemble organic acidosis because these substances decrease SID without changing electrolytes. The most frequently encountered causes for organic acidosis in small animal practice are uremic acidosis, diabetic ketoacidosis, lactic acidosis, and ethylene glycol poisoning (Table 7).

***Table 7.*** *Principal Disorders of the Unidentified Strong Anions*

| Organic Acidosis ($\Uparrow$[$XA^-$]) | |
| --- | --- |
| ***Disorder*** | ***Strong Anions Changing SID*** |
| Uremic acidosis | $SO_4^{2-}$ and other anions of renal failure |
| Diabetic ketoacidosis | Acetoacetate, $\beta$-hydroxybutyrate |
| Lactic acidosis | Lactate |
| Salicylate intoxication | Salicylate |
| Ethylene glycol toxicity | Glycolate |
| Methanol toxicity | Formate |

Treatment of organic acidosis should be directed toward the primary disorder and stabilization of the patient. Treatment with $NaHCO_3$ should be done cautiously because metabolism of accumulated organic anions will normalize SID and increase $[HCO_3^-]$. The initial goal in patients with severe organic acidosis is to raise systemic pH to 7.20.

ESTIMATION OF $XA^-$ CONCENTRATION. The anion gap (AG) is a useful clinical tool to distinguish between different forms of metabolic acidosis. Organic acidosis causes an increase in the AG, whereas hyperchloremic acidosis does not. The AG is used clinically to estimate the concentration of "unmeasured anions" $(UA^-)$. Unfortunately, $UA^-$ include the strong $(XA^-)$ and weak (variable charges of albumin and phosphates) unmeasured anions. The AG is therefore heavily influenced by the concentration of plasma proteins, and changes in albumin concentration significantly change AG (Fencl and Rossing, 1989). Hyperphosphatemia may also increase the AG. The major determinant of AG $([HCO_3^-])$ and its major component (variable charges of albumin and phosphates) will change secondarily to changes in $PCO_2$, SID, or $[A_{TOT}]$ (Fencl and Leith, 1993). Thus, changes in AG do not always reflect a stoichiometric change in $UA^-$ even in the presence of organic acidosis. Two mathematical models have been developed for estimation of $XA^-$ in human beings (Leith, 1990; Figge et al., 1992). Unfortunately, these models have not yet been validated in dogs and cats. The history (e.g., ingestion of ethylene glycol), clinical condition (e.g., shock), increases in serum creatinine concentration, blood urea nitrogen (BUN), or serum glucose, and the presence of ketonuria may help in establishing a diagnosis of organic acidosis. Plasma lactate concentration may be measured in patients with suspected lactic acidosis.

## HOW FAR CAN YOU GO WITH A BIOCHEMICAL PROFILE?

From the previous discussion it is apparent that acid-base homeostasis is intertwined and, from a clinical standpoint, principally dependent upon three variables: $PCO_2$, SID, and $[A_{TOT}]$. The biochemical profile can provide useful information about ongoing nonrespiratory acid-base disturbances. Unfortunately, evaluation of the respiratory component of acid-base disturbances requires knowledge of the $PCO_2$. The total carbon dioxide $(TCO_2)$ is a good estimation of the plasma $[HCO_3^-]$ in samples handled aerobically. An increase in $TCO_2$ may result from a nonrespiratory alkalosis (increase in SID or decrease in $[A_{TOT}]$) or from compensation for respiratory acidosis, whereas a decrease in $TCO_2$ may be due to nonrespiratory acidosis (decrease in SID or increase in $[A_{TOT}]$) or compensation for respiratory alkalosis. Increases in $[A_{TOT}]$ can be recognized by an increase in inorganic phosphate or albumin concentration. Hypoalbuminemia is the only potential cause for a decrease in $[A_{TOT}]$. Changes in SID caused by changes in $[Cl^-]$ or $[Na^+]$ also affect $TCO_2$ and can

be identified in the biochemical profile. Dilution acidosis can be detected by the presence of hyponatremia, whereas concentration alkalosis is associated with hypernatremia. Hyperchloremic acidosis and hypochloremic alkalosis are recognized respectively by an increase and decrease in $[Cl^-]_{corrected}$. Compensation for chronic respiratory acid-base disorders, however, is also associated with $[Cl^-]_{corrected}$ changes. Chronic respiratory alkalosis is associated with a compensatory hyperchloremic acidosis and chronic respiratory acidosis is associated with a compensatory hypochloremic alkalosis (de Morais, 1992a).

A high AG in the biochemical profile raises the suspicion of an organic acidosis if albumin and phosphate concentrations are normal. Changes in SID caused by changes in $[Na^+]$ (dilution acidosis and concentration alkalosis) or $[Cl^-]$ (hyperchloremic acidosis or hypochloremic alkalosis) can be assessed as explained above. A quick way to screen for the presence of a $Cl^-$ disorder in the presence of normal $[Na^+]$ is to calculate the difference between $Na^+$ and $Cl^-$ concentration (Na-Cl), which is normally between 32 and 40 mEq/L. Increase in this difference usually implies the presence of a hypochloremic alkalosis, whereas a value below 32 mEq/L is associated with a hyperchloremic acidosis. The use of the biochemical profile in the assessment of nonrespiratory acid-base disorders is summarized in Table 8.

## CLINICAL APPROACH USING STEWART'S SID MODEL

A stepwise approach should be followed in all animals with suspected acid-base disorders. After obtaining the samples, the first step is to determine the pH and the nature of the primary disorder from the blood gas result. The possibility of a mixed respiratory and nonrespiratory acid-base disorder should be assessed by calculating the expected compensation (Table 1). If a nonrespiratory acid-base disorder is present, it should be determined if it is caused by a change in $[A_{TOT}]$ (due to changes in albumin or inorganic phosphate concentration), SID (due to changes in free water, $[Cl^-]$ or $[XA^-]$), or a combination of these factors. Unfortunately, evaluation of changes in SID caused by an increase in $[XA^-]$ is not straightforward. An increase in $[XA^-]$ may be suspected in acidotic patients with diseases known to be associated with organic acidosis (e.g., renal failure, diabetic ketoacidosis). Measurement of lactate concentration permits the quantification of one of the many $XA^-$.

After considering the blood gas results, electrolytes and albumin concentration in conjunction with other laboratory data that may be useful (e.g., serum creatinine concentration, presence of ketonuria, blood glucose concentration), the clinical and laboratory data should be integrated and individual therapy should be planned.

***Table 8.***    *Simple Primary Nonrespiratory Acid-Base Disorders*

| Nonrespiratory Disorder | Na-Cl° | AG[†] | TCO$_2$ | Respiratory Compensation[‡] | Biochemical Profile |
|---|---|---|---|---|---|
| ***Alkaloses*** | | | | | |
| Hypoalbuminemia | N | N,⇓ | ⇑ | No | ⇓ Albumin |
| Hypochloremia | ⇑ | N | ⇑ | Yes | ⇓ [Cl⁻]$_{corrected}$ |
| Concentration | ⇑ | N | ⇑ | Yes | ⇑ [Na+] |
| ***Acidoses*** | | | | | |
| Hyperalbuminemia | N | N,⇑ | ⇓ | No | ⇑ Albumin |
| Hyperphosphatemia | N | N,⇑ | ⇓ | No | ⇑ Inorganic phosphate |
| Hyperchloremia | ⇓ | N | ⇓ | Yes | ⇑ [Cl]$_{corrected}$ |
| Dilution | ⇓ | N | ⇓ | Yes | ⇓ [Na+] |
| Organic | N | ⇑ | ⇓ | Yes | None specific |

°Na-Cl = difference between sodium and chloride concentration.
[†]See text for limitations in using Na-Cl and AG.
[‡]Expected respiratory compensation => for each 1 mEq/L change in the [HCO$_3^-$], Pco$_2$ changes 0.7 mm Hg in the same direction
*Key*: AG = anion gap, Tco$_2$ = total carbon dioxide, ⇑ = increased, N = normal, ⇓ = decreased.

## Evaluation of the Nonrespiratory Component

Two quantitative clinical approaches for assessment of nonrespiratory acid-base disturbances will be discussed, one based on the use of BE and the other based on a mathematical relationship to estimate SID.

Base excess has been used to assess changes in the nonrespiratory component because SID is synonymous with buffer base. Base excess is a measurement of the deviation of buffer base (and therefore SID) from normal values. It should be pointed out, however, that Siggaard-Andersen studied blood, not plasma, and protein was not a variable in that work. The BE has been used clinically for more than a decade to assess the nonrespiratory acid-base status in human patients (Leith, 1991) and has recently been applied to dogs and cats (de Morais, 1992b; DiBartola and de Morais, 1992). Formulas to estimate changes in base excess due to changes in SID and [A$_{TOT}$] are presented in Table 9. A complete description of the derivation of these formulas, as well as their limitations, can be found elsewhere (de Morais, 1992b). These formulas were helpful in understanding complex acid-base disorders in dogs and cats (DiBartola and de Morais, 1992). Unfortunately, no controlled clinical studies have been performed in dogs and cats with acid-base disturbances to assess the accuracy of these formulas.

Figge et al. (1992) developed and successfully tested a new mathematical approach to evaluate nonrespiratory acid-base disorders. The estimation of XA⁻ is calculated by subtracting the "effective SID" (SID$_{eff}$) from the "apparent SID" (SID$_{app}$) (XA⁻ = SID$_{app}$ − SID$_{eff}$). The SID$_{app}$ is calculated using electrolytes measured in the serum (SID$_{app}$ = {[Na⁺] + [K⁺] + [Ca²⁺] + [Mg²⁺]} − [Cl⁻]) and SID$_{eff}$ is a satisfactory approximation of the "real SID." The XA⁻ obtained using this formula is not constrained by the limitations mentioned above for the AG and UA⁻. Despite being a very promising model for assessment of nonrespiratory acid-base disorders, Figge's model, as well the BE model, were de-

veloped using protein behavior based on human albumin. In addition, calculation of SID$_{eff}$ using Figge's model is not simple and may be clinically impractical.° Some of the electrolytes employed to calculate the SID$_{app}$ (magnesium and ionized calcium) are not routinely measured in the biochemical profile and it is not known if approximations (e.g., magnesium = 1.5 mEq/L and ionized calcium = 50% of total calcium) will work clinically in dogs and cats.

## Evaluation of the Respiratory Component

The presence of a respiratory acid-base disorder can be detected by the presence of an abnormal Paco$_2$. When a nonrespiratory acid-base disturbance caused by changes in SID is present, the estimated compensatory change in Pco$_2$ (see Table 1) should be calculated to rule out the possibility of a mixed respiratory and nonrespiratory disorders. Mixed acid-base disturbances are characterized by the presence of two or more separate primary acid-base abnormalities in the same patient (see *CVT XI*, p 24). Mixed acid-base disturbances should be suspected whenever the adaptive compensatory response in Table 1 exceeds or falls short of that expected, the pH is changing in a direction opposite to that predicted by the primary disorder, or Pco$_2$ and [HCO$_3^-$] are changing in the opposite directions.

An example of a mixed respiratory and nonrespiratory acid-base disorder can be found in a dog presented for liver disease and the following data from the blood gas analysis and biochemical profile: albumin and phosphate concentration normal, [Na⁺] = 146 mEq/L, [Cl⁻] = 120 mEq/L, pH = 7.296, [HCO$_3^-$] = 10.4 mEq/L,

---

°SID$_{eff}$ in Figge's Model is estimated as:

$$SID_{eff} = 1000 \times 2.46E\text{-}11 \times Pco_2/(10^{-pH}) + 10 \times [Alb] \times (0.123 \times pH - 0.631) + [Pi] \times (0.309 \times pH - 0.469)$$

where [Alb] is the patient albumin concentration and [Pi] is the patient phosphate concentration.

***Table 9.*** *Estimation of changes in base excess due to changes in SID and [A$_{TOT}$]*

***Changes in [A$_{TOT}$]***

Changes in albumin concentration

$$\Delta \text{ Albumin (mEq/L)} = 3.7 \times ([\text{Alb}]_{normal} - [\text{Alb}]_{patient})$$

Changes in phosphate ([Pi] in mmol/L)

$$([\text{Pi}] = \text{phosphate in mg/dl x } 10/30.97)$$

$$\Delta \text{ phosphate (mEq/L)} = (1.6 \text{ x } [\text{Pi}]_{patient}) + (0.2 : [\text{Pi}]_{patient})$$

***Changes in SID:***

Changes in free water

$$\Delta \text{ Free water (mEq/L)} = 0.25 ([\text{Na}^+]_{patient} - [\text{Na}^+]_{normal})$$

Changes in chloride concentration

$$\Delta \text{ Cl}^- \text{ (mEq/L)} = [\text{Cl}^-]_{normal} - [\text{Cl}^-]_{corrected}$$

Changes in unidentified anions

$$\Delta \text{ XA}^- \text{ (mEq/L)} = \text{BE} - (\Delta \text{ free water} + \Delta \text{ Cl}^- + \Delta \text{ Albumin} + \Delta \text{ phosphate})$$

*Key:*[Alb]$_{normal}$ = normal albumin concentration, [Alb]$_{patient}$ = patient albumin concentration in gm/dl, [Pi]$_{patient}$ = patient phosphate concentration in mmol/L, [Na$^+$]$_{normal}$ = normal [Na$^+$], [Na$^+$]$_{patient}$ = patient sodium concentration in mEq/L, [Cl$^-$]$_{normal}$ = normal [Cl$^-$] concentration, [Cl$^-$]$_{corrected}$ = patient [Cl$^-$] in mEq/L after corrected for changes in free water; XA$^-$ = unidentified strong anions, BE = patient base excess. Normal values for the author's laboratory: [Alb]$_{normal}$ = 3.1 gm/dL, [Na$^+$]$_{normal}$ = 156 mEq/L for cats and 146 mEq/L for dogs, [Cl$^-$]$_{normal}$ = 120 mEq/L for cats and 110 mEq/L for dogs.

PCO$_2$ = 22 mm Hg. This dog is acidemic based on the pH, and the low [HCO$_3^-$] indicates a nonrespiratory acidosis. The normal [A$_{TOT}$] and [Na$^+$] with an increase [Cl$^-$] (and normal AG) indicate a hyperchloremic acidosis. To evaluate the respiratory component in presence of a primary SID abnormality, the expected compensatory change in PCO$_2$ has to be calculated. Using the compensatory rules presented in Table 1, the expected PCO$_2$ for a [HCO$_3^-$] of 10.4 mEq/L is 29.6 mm Hg.[†] The observed PCO$_2$ in this patient is 22 mm Hg, which is more than 2 mm Hg below the expected value. Thus, this patient also has a PCO$_2$ disorder (the PCO$_2$ is lower than it should be for the degree of change in the SID). The final diagnosis in this patient is a mixed respiratory alkalosis and hyperchloremic acidosis.

## CONCLUSIONS

The traditional approach for evaluation of acid-base status using pH, PCO$_2$, and HCO$_3^-$ has several important clinically relevant limitations. It does not give a complete assessment of the sources of pathophysiologic changes in the nonrespiratory component (HCO$_3^-$), it may lead to the conclusion that changes in electrolytes are only secondarily related to acid-base status, and it does not recognize changes in [H$^+$] due to changes in albumin or inorganic phosphate concentration. A thorough evaluation of commonly measured ions (e.g., Na$^+$, Cl$^+$, K$^+$, inorganic phosphate) and serum albumin concentration in addition to history and physical examination provides a basis for a more comprehensive evaluation of acid-base status and greater insights into possible causes and their therapy.

ACKNOWLEDGMENT: The authors thank Dr. Dave E. Leith for his contribution to this manuscript.

## References and Suggested Reading

de Morais HSA: Chloride ion in small animal practice: The forgotten ion. J Vet Emerg Crit Care 2:11, 1992a.
*A review of pathophysiology and treatment of chloride disorders with emphasis on the role of chloride in acid-base disorders.*

de Morais HSA: A non-traditional approach to acid-base disorders. *In* DiBartola SP, (ed): *Fluid Therapy in Small Animal Practice.* Philadelphia, WB Saunders Co, 1992b, p 297.
*A discussion of the applications of the Stewart's SID model to evaluate acid-base disorders in dogs and cats.*

de Morais HSA and DiBartola SP: Ventilatory and metabolic compensation in dogs with acid-base disturbances. J Vet Emerg Crit Care 1:39, 1991.
*A review of the metabolic and respiratory compensation for acid-base disorders in dogs.*

DiBartola HS and de Morais HSA: Case examples. *In* DiBartola, SP, (ed): *Fluid Therapy in Small Animal Practice.* Philadelphia, WB Saunders Co, 1992, p 599.
*Presentation of clinical cases, many of which had complex acid-base disorders. The clinical utility of Stewart's SID approach is exemplified in the assessment of these cases.*

Fencl V and Rossing TH: Acid-base disorders in critical care medicine. Ann Rev Med 40:17, 1989.
*A discussion of the acid-base disorders in critical care medicine with special emphasis on the increasing occurrence of hypochloremic alkalosis and hypoalbuminemic alkalosis.*

Fencl V and Leith, DE: Stewart's quantitative acid-base chemistry: Applications in biology and medicine. Respir Physiol 91:1, 1993.
*A review of the Stewart's quantitative approach to acid-base chemistry. Historic aspects, implications for cellular and membrane processes in acid-base physiology, and clinical implications are reviewed.*

Figge J, Mydosh T, and Fencl, V: Serum proteins and acid-base equilibria: A follow-up. J Lab Clin Med 120:713, 1992.
*A review of the author's mathematical model to assess the acid-base behavior of blood plasma. A new method to estimate the unidentified strong anions was proposed and validated.*

Galla JH, Gifford JD, Luke RG, and Rome L: Adaptations to chloride-depletion alkalosis. Am J Physiol 261:R771, 1991.
*An editorial review of chloride-depletion alkalosis showing the role of chloride in generation and maintenance of hypochloremic alkalosis. The hypothesis that volume depletion is necessary for development of nonrespiratory alkalosis and that volume expansion is necessary for its correction is refuted based on the authors previous experimental work.*

Leith DE: The new acid-base: Power and simplicity. Proc 9th ACVIM Forum, 1991, pp 611–617.
*A very didactic description of the Stewart SID approach.*

Stewart PA: *How to Understand Acid-Base. A Quantitative Acid-Base Primer for Biology and Medicine.* New York, Elsevier, 1981, p 186.
*The original book where most of the Stewart concepts where first explained in detail.*

---

[†]Expected PCO$_2$ = PCO$_{2normal}$ − 0.7 ([HCO$_3^-$]$_{patient}$) where PCO$_{2normal}$ in dogs is usually assumed to be equal to 37 mm Hg, [HCO$_3^-$]$_{normal}$ is equal to 21 mEq/L, and [HCO$_3^-$]$_{patient}$ is the patient's HCO$_3^-$ concentration. Applying the formula for this patient: expected PCO$_2$ = 37 mm Hg − 0.7 (21 mEq/L − 10.4 mEq/L) = 29.6 mm Hg.

# MAGNESIUM AND THE CRITICALLY ILL PATIENT

LINDA G. MARTIN,
DEBORAH R. VAN PELT,
*and* WAYNE E. WINGFIELD

*Fort Collins, Colorado*

Serum magnesium ($Mg^{2+}$) is an infrequently measured electrolyte in veterinary medicine, and until recently, $Mg^{2+}$ therapy was considered unconventional. Several factors make much of the current interest and research in $Mg^{2+}$ especially relevant to veterinary critical care and emergency medicine. First, there appears to be a high incidence of hypomagnesemia in critically ill human patients, and recent evidence suggests that certain populations of critically ill animals are at risk for the development of hypomagnesemia. Second, abnormalities in serum $Mg^{2+}$ may predispose patients to a wide variety of cardiovascular, metabolic, or neuromuscular complications, including cardiac arrhythmias, refractory hypokalemia, and seizures. Finally, the high therapeutic index and low cost of $Mg^{2+}$ may make its empiric use worthwhile in such desperate conditions as cardiopulmonary arrest and shock. The majority of the information presented in this article is derived from research into the role of $Mg^{2+}$ in critically ill human patients, but experimental models using canine subjects also suggest that this forgotten electrolyte may be important in animals as well.

Magnesium is the second most abundant intracellular cation, exceeded only by potassium. The vast majority of $Mg^{2+}$ is found in bone and muscle: 60% of the total body $Mg^{2+}$ content is present in bone, while 20% is located in skeletal muscle and the remainder in other tissues, primarily the heart and liver. Approximately 1% of total body $Mg^{2+}$ is present in the serum. In serum, $Mg^{2+}$ exists in three distinct forms: an ionized fraction, an anion-complexed fraction, and a protein-bound fraction. The ionized fraction is believed to be the physiologically active component.

Magnesium homeostasis is regulated principally by renal and gastrointestinal mechanisms. Absorption of ingested $Mg^{2+}$ occurs primarily in the jejunum and ileum. Under normal circumstances, regulation of serum $Mg^{2+}$ is achieved by renal glomerular filtration and tubular reabsorption. In humans there does not appear to be any tubular secretion of $Mg^{2+}$. Renal excretion of $Mg^{2+}$ varies with dietary changes and, more directly, with the load of $Mg^{2+}$ presented to the kidney. High dietary $Mg^{2+}$ content and high serum $Mg^{2+}$ levels lead to diminished renal tubular reabsorption. Conversely, the kidney conserves $Mg^{2+}$ in response to a deficiency in serum $Mg^{2+}$.

Magnesium is an essential cation required for many metabolic and cellular functions, most notably those involved in the production and use of adenosine triphosphate (ATP). Magnesium is necessary for normal function of the sodium-potassium ($Na^+/K^+$) ATPase pump, which regulates intracellular $K^+$ balance. The calcium ($Ca^{2+}$) ATPase and proton pumps also require $Mg^{2+}$. In addition to transfer, storage, and utilization of energy, $Mg^{2+}$ is required for protein and nucleic acid synthesis, regulation of vascular smooth muscle tone, cellular second messenger systems, and signal transduction.

## HYPOMAGNESEMIA

### Prevalence

Hypomagnesemia appears to be the most clinically significant $Mg^{2+}$ abnormality seen in critically ill patients. Magnesium deficiency appears to be rare in healthy individuals; however, hypomagnesemia is a common electrolyte abnormality in human emergency room patients and in adult and pediatric critically ill patients. Based on available data, hypomagnesemia may be the most underdiagnosed electrolyte disorder in clinical medicine. Incidence rates for hypomagnesemia of greater than 50% have been reported in critically ill human patients (Sachter, 1992). Studies of critically ill patients have also found abnormalities of serum $Mg^{2+}$ to be the most common electrolyte disorder (Sachter, 1992). Several studies have documented concurrent deficiencies in both $Mg^{2+}$ and potassium. Magnesium deficiencies have been reported in 36 to 61% of the hospitalized patients with hypokalemia (Arsenian, 1993; Sachter, 1992). Recent evidence suggests that certain populations of critically ill animals are at risk for the development of hypomagnesemia, including animals on peritoneal dialysis and dogs with congestive heart failure treated with furosemide.

### Etiologies

The causes of $Mg^{2+}$ deficiency are both numerous and complex. In general, they can be divided into: (1) decreased intake, (2) increased losses, and (3) alterations in distribution. Potential causes of hypomagnesemia are listed in Table 1. Decreased dietary intake of

$Mg^{2+}$, if sustained for several weeks, can lead to significant $Mg^{2+}$ depletion. In addition, catabolic illness and prolonged intravenous fluid therapy without $Mg^{2+}$ replacement can contribute to $Mg^{2+}$ depletion.

Increased $Mg^{2+}$ losses may occur through the gastrointestinal tract or the kidneys. Increased gastrointestinal losses of $Mg^{2+}$ may result from extensive small-bowel resection, enteropathies, or cholestatic liver disease. Malabsorption syndromes associated with a decrease in fat absorption also lead to increased intestinal loss of $Mg^{2+}$.

Since the kidney is the primary pathway of $Mg^{2+}$ excretion, it often serves as a focal point for the development of hypomagnesemia through renal loss of $Mg^{2+}$. Acute renal dysfunction as a consequence of glomerulonephritis, interstitial nephritis, or the nonoliguric (diuretic) phase of acute tubular necrosis is often associated with a rise in the fractional excretion of $Mg^{2+}$. A number of endocrinopathies are also associated with an increase in the fractional excretion of $Mg^{2+}$, including diabetic ketoacidosis, hyperthyroidism, and primary hyperparathyroidism.

Numerous drugs administered to critically ill patients may increase renal $Mg^{2+}$ loss. Most of the commonly administered diuretic agents (furosemide, thiazides, mannitol) induce hypomagnesemia by increasing $Mg^{2+}$ excretion. Administration of cardiac glycosides has frequently been associated with hypomagnesemia because these drugs increase urinary magnesium excretion. Other agents that predispose to renal tubular injury and excessive renal $Mg^{2+}$ loss include aminoglycosides, amphotericin, cisplatin, carbenicillin, and cyclosporine.

Disease states or therapeutic modalities may cause the redistribution of circulating $Mg^{2+}$ by producing extracellular to intracellular shifts, chelation, or sequestration. Acute administration of glucose, insulin, or amino acids causes $Mg^{2+}$ to shift intracellularly. Elevation of catecholamines in animals with sepsis, trauma, or hypothermia may cause hypomagnesemia. $\beta$-Adrenergic stimulation of lipolysis appears to generate free fatty acids that chelate $Mg^{2+}$, thereby producing insoluble salts. When administered in large quantities, citrated blood products avidly chelate $Mg^{2+}$ ions. In acute pancreatitis, $Mg^{2+}$ can form insoluble soaps and sequestration of significant amounts of $Mg^{2+}$ may occur in areas of fat necrosis within the pancreas.

### Clinical Manifestations

In the human critical care setting, hypomagnesemia is most often manifested by its effects on the cardiovascular system. The effects of $Mg^{2+}$ on myocardial contraction are linked to its role as a regulator of other ions, primarily $K^+$ and $Ca^{2+}$. This is due to the fact that $Mg^{2+}$ is a coenzyme for the membrane-bound $Na^+/K^+$ ATPase pump. Magnesium deficiency may inhibit pump function and cause intracellular levels of $K^+$ to fall, leading to a decreased intracellular/extracellular $K^+$ ratio. This decreases the resting membrane potential and leads to increased Purkinje fiber excitability, with consequent arrhythmia generation. Magnesium deficiency has been associated with several cardiac arrhythmias including atrial fibrillation, supraventricular tachycardia, ventricular tachycardia, and ventricular fibrillation. Hypomagnesemia also predisposes patients to digitalis-induced arrhythmias. Magnesium deficiency not only enhances digitalis uptake by the myocardium but also inhibits the myocardial $Na^+/K^+$ pump, as does digitalis. This results in disturbances in the resting membrane potential and the repolarization phase of the action potential. Magnesium's $Ca^{2+}$ channel–blocking effect appears to be decreased in states of $Mg^{2+}$ deficiency and subsequently increases intracellular $Ca^{2+}$ content. This results in enhanced sensitivity to the toxic effects of cardiac glycosides and the development of digitalis-mediated arrhythmias. There is also evidence that $Mg^{2+}$ deficiency plays a role in hypertension, coronary artery vasospasm, and platelet aggregation.

Magnesium deficiency can result in various nonspecific neuromuscular signs. Concurrent hypocalcemia and hypokalemia may also contribute to these signs. Magnesium is known to decrease acetylcholine release from nerve terminals and to depress the excitability of nerve and muscle membranes. Magnesium also plays a

***Table 1.*** *Causes of Hypomagnesemia*

**Decreased Intake**
 Inadequate nutritional intake
 Prolonged intravenous fluid therapy without magnesium
  replacement

**Increased Losses**
 Gastrointestinal
  Malabsorption syndromes
  Extensive small-bowel resection
  Chronic diarrhea
  Inflammatory bowel disease
  Cholestatic liver disease
 Renal
  Intrinsic tubular disorders
   Glomerulonephritis
   Acute tubular necrosis
   Postobstructive diuresis
   Drug-induced tubular injury
    Aminoglycosides
    Amphotericin B
    Carbenicillin
    Cisplatin
    Cyclosporine
  Extrarenal factors influencing renal magnesium handling
   Diuretic-induced states
    Furosemide
    Thiazides
    Mannitol
   Digitalis administration
   Diabetic ketoacidosis
   Hyperthyroidism
   Primary hyperparathyroidism

**Alterations in Distribution**
 Acute administration of glucose, insulin, and amino acids
 Cardiopulmonary bypass surgery
 Sepsis
 Trauma
 Hypothermia
 Pancreatitis
 Massive blood transfusion

role in muscle contraction and relaxation by regulating $Ca^{2+}$ channels. Clinical manifestations of $Mg^{2+}$ deficiency can include muscle weakness, which may be manifested by dysphagia or dyspnea if esophageal or respiratory muscles are affected, muscle fasciculations, seizures, ataxia, and coma. Table 2 lists additional clinical manifestations of $Mg^{2+}$ deficiency.

## EVALUATION OF MAGNESIUM STATUS

Magnesium deficiency should be suspected in patients predisposed to its development and exhibiting clinical signs or laboratory features of $Mg^{2+}$ depletion. Unfortunately, the precise clinical diagnosis of $Mg^{2+}$ depletion can be difficult. Since 99% of the total body $Mg^{2+}$ is located in the intracellular compartment, serum $Mg^{2+}$ levels do not always reflect total body $Mg^{2+}$ stores. Therefore, a normal serum $Mg^{2+}$ level can occur in the presence of total body $Mg^{2+}$ deficiency. In addition to utilizing serum $Mg^{2+}$ concentrations, alternative methods of evaluating $Mg^{2+}$ status include determining ultrafilterable $Mg^{2+}$ ($\mu Mg^{2+}$) and ionized $Mg^{2+}$ ($iMg^{2+}$) levels. Until recently, there was no ion-selective electrode commercially available for the determination of $iMg^{2+}$ concentrations. With the advent of a commercially available ion-selective electrode for determining $iMg^{2+}$ levels (NOVA Biomedical, Waltham, MA), the physiologically active fraction of $Mg^{2+}$ can be quantified. Intracellular $iMg^{2+}$ appears to be quite comparable to extracellular $iMg^{2+}$. In addition, $iMg^{2+}$ passes through the cell membrane relatively quickly, suggesting that the intracellular and extracellular $iMg^{2+}$ reservoirs are in dynamic equilibrium. These observations suggest that the measurement of $iMg^{2+}$ in whole blood reflects the dynamic intracellular-extracellular $Mg^{2+}$ homeostasis. This method of measuring $iMg^{2+}$ correlates well with traditional methods of measurement, such as absorption spectroscopy. The ion-selective electrode for $Mg^{2+}$ has proven to be accurate over a wide range of values.

The technique of $uMg^{2+}$ provides an indirect assay for determining the ionized fraction of serum $Mg^{2+}$ (Amicon Corporation, Beverly, MA). This method is based on low-speed centrifugation through a nonabsorptive filter allowing a high degree of protein retention. The ultrafiltrate contains the ionized and anion-complexed fractions of serum $Mg^{2+}$, while the protein-bound fraction remains in the chamber above the filter. Studies have shown that $uMg^{2+}$ is a better predictor of the true physiologically active $Mg^{2+}$ concentration than total serum $Mg^{2+}$ levels.

A practical clinical approach to establishing a diagnosis of $Mg^{2+}$ deficiency involves administering a $Mg^{2+}$ loading dose, and then determining the percentage of $Mg^{2+}$ retained by the body. Since $Mg^{2+}$ is excreted primarily in the urine, retention of an intravenously administered dose of $Mg^{2+}$ can be viewed as evidence of $Mg^{2+}$ depletion. In the human medical population, studies indicate that retention of more than 40 to 50% of the administered $Mg^{2+}$ load indicates $Mg^{2+}$ depletion, while retention of less than 20% indicates that a $Mg^{2+}$ deficiency is less likely. This test is contraindicated in patients with renal insufficiency, disturbances in cardiac conduction, or elevated serum $Mg^{2+}$. These requirements are based on the fact that normal renal function is essential for the reliability of the loading test, that $Mg^{2+}$ administration may further aggravate cardiac conduction disturbances through the AV node, and that $Mg^{2+}$ administration is contraindicated in patients with elevated serum $Mg^{2+}$ levels.

**Table 2.** *Clinical Manifestations of Magnesium Deficiency*

***Cardiovascular***
  Arrhythmias
    Atrial fibrillation
    Supraventricular tachycardia
    Torsades de pointes
    Premature ventricular contractions
    Ventricular tachycardia
    Ventricular fibrillation
    Digitalis-induced arrhythmias
  Electrocardiographic changes
    Prolonged P-R
    Widened QRS
    Depressed ST
    Peaked T
  Coronary artery vasospasm
  Hypertension
  Anemia
  Platelet aggregation

***Metabolic***
  Refractory hypokalemia
  Hypocalcemia

***Neuromuscular***
  Muscle weakness
  Muscle twitching
  Hyperreflexia
  Ataxia
  Seizures
  Coma

## THE USE OF MAGNESIUM IN THE CRITICAL CARE SETTING

Therapeutic investigations in canine subjects indicate that $Mg^{2+}$ supplementation may be beneficial in the treatment of several disorders relevant to critical care and emergency medicine, such as shock, cardiopulmonary arrest, and cardiac arrhythmias. The beneficial effects of $Mg^{2+}$ have been demonstrated in animal models of both hemorrhagic and septic shock. The majority of these studies used magnesium chloride ($MgCl_2$) complexed to ATP, and there is evidence that the beneficial effects require both agents. Improved cellular function, organ function, and survival have been documented when ATP-$MgCl_2$ was infused following a period of shock or ischemia. Studies in canine models of cardiopulmonary arrest have also shown that $Mg^{2+}$ administration prevented cerebral hypoperfusion following resuscitation and raised the ventricular fibrillation threshold (100 mg/kg magnesium sulfate IV over

5 to 15 min) (Billman and Hoskins, 1988; White et al., 1983). These investigations indicate that the use of $Mg^{2+}$ may be efficacious in cardiopulmonary arrest and in the treatment of reperfusion injury. Hypomagnesemia also appears to facilitate digitalis toxicity in dogs, but the digitalis-associated arrhythmias could be promptly terminated with the administration of magnesium sulfate.

Dogs with congestive heart failure being treated with furosemide demonstrate a significant reduction in serum $Mg^{2+}$ levels as compared to healthy controls (Cobb et al., 1992). Another clinical report of dogs with congestive heart failure and concurrent ventricular arrhythmias showed that a small percentage of these animals were responsive to $Mg^{2+}$ antiarrhythmic therapy, regardless of their serum $Mg^{2+}$ level (Edwards, 1991). In addition, hypomagnesemia has been associated with clinical cases of peritoneal dialysis, and routine measurement of serum $Mg^{2+}$ should be performed on patients undergoing peritoneal dialysis for more than 3 to 4 days. These studies indicate that hypomagnesemia may be a clinically significant electrolyte abnormality present in critically ill animals, which warrants further investigation.

## CLINICAL SIGNIFICANCE IN VETERINARY MEDICINE

Unfortunately, to this point, very little research has been performed in clinical veterinary medicine regarding $Mg^{2+}$ status in normal and ill animals. Preliminary research performed by the authors indicates that abnormalities in serum $Mg^{2+}$ may occur commonly in critically ill dogs. To date, of 39 ill dogs studied on admission to the Critical Care Unit at Colorado State University, 21 (54%) were hypomagnesemic, eight (20%) were normomagnesemic, and ten (26%) were found to be hypermagnesemic. Other serum electrolytes were also assessed as part of the initial evaluation of each patient. Several patients had abnormalities of serum electrolytes other than $Mg^{2+}$; however, abnormalities in serum $Mg^{2+}$ occurred with the highest frequency. Several hypomagnesemic critically ill patients in this study population had another electrolyte abnormality present. Thirteen of 39 (33%) critically ill patients had concurrent hypomagnesemia and hypokalemia, and 13 of 39 (33%) were hypomagnesemic and hyponatremic.

The high prevalence of hypomagnesemia observed in this population of critically ill dogs appears to be similar to the rates reported in critically ill humans. Such a high prevalence of hypomagnesemia is not surprising in view of the presence of conditions that can lead to both urinary and gastrointestinal $Mg^{2+}$ wasting in critically ill veterinary patients. Several studies in human patients have also noted a strong association between hypomagnesemia and hypokalemia or hyponatremia. These preliminary values for our population of critically ill dogs appear to be consistent with those reported in medical literature for multiple electrolyte abnormalities. In addition, there appears to be a significant relationship between the concentrations of serum $Mg^{2+}$ and other electrolytes. Since serum $Mg^{2+}$ is not routinely measured in ill animal patients, the detection of either hypokalemia or hyponatremia should alert the clinician to the possibility of coexisting hypomagnesemia.

## CONCLUSION

Despite the provocative research performed in the human medical field, little information is available regarding $Mg^{2+}$ status in hospitalized animals. Before studies can be conducted to determine the role of $Mg^{2+}$ in the pathophysiology and treatment of disease states, studies must be performed to develop accurate methods to assess $Mg^{2+}$ status in normal and critically ill animals.

## References and Suggested Reading

Arsenian MA: Magnesium and cardiovascular disease. Prog Cardiovasc Dis 35: 271, 1993.
*A review of magnesium deficiency as a risk factor for cardiovascular disease and the benefits of magnesium therapy in vascular disease processes.*
Billman GE and Hoskins RS: Prevention of ventricular fibrillation with magnesium sulfate. Eur J Pharmacol 158:167, 1988.
*A prospective study evaluating the effect of magnesium sulfate on ischemically induced ventricular fibrillation.*
Cannon LA, Heiselman DE, Dougherty JM, and Jones J: Magnesium levels in cardiac arrest victims: Relationship between magnesium levels and successful resuscitation. Ann Emerg Med 16:1195, 1987.
*A prospective study evaluating serum magnesium levels with success of resuscitation from cardiac arrest.*
Cobb M and Michell AR: Plasma electrolyte concentrations in dogs receiving diuretic therapy for cardiac failure. J Small Anim Pract 33:526, 1992.
*A prospective study of the effects of diuretic therapy in canine congestive heart failure on serum electrolyte levels.*
Edwards NJ: Magnesium and congestive heart failure. *Proc 9th ACVIM Forum.* New Orleans, LA, 1991, p 679.
*Results of an experimental study evaluating dogs with congestive heart failure while receiving unspecified therapies.*
Sachter JJ: Magnesium in the 1990s: Implications for acute care. Top Emerg Med 14:23, 1992.
*A review of the causes, clinical signs, and therapy of hypomagnesemia and hypermagnesemia.*
Salem M: Hypomagnesemia in critical illness: A common and clinically important problem. Crit Care Clin 7:225, 1991.
*A review of the etiologies, pathophysiology, manifestations, and therapeutic strategies for hypomagnesemia.*
White BC, Winegar CD, Wilson RF, and Krause GS: Calcium blockers in cerebral resuscitation. J Trauma 23:788, 1983.
*A prospective study evaluating the effects of calcium channel–blocking agents on cerebral resuscitation.*

# MAGNESIUM THERAPY

NISHI DHUPA

*Floral Park, New York*

The pathophysiology and clinical conditions associated with hypomagnesemia have been discussed in the previous article by Martin, Van Pelt, and Wingfield. This article provides therapeutic information based on clinical experience with critically ill small animals. Currently magnesium ($Mg^{2+}$) is supplemented on an empiric basis. Although a low serum $Mg^{2+}$ indicates an existing deficit, $Mg^{2+}$ depletion can coexist with a normal serum $Mg^{2+}$. Better evaluation of intracellular $Mg^{2+}$ will allow more accurate dose regimens in the future.

## INDICATIONS

### Susceptible Patients

Factors predisposing critical patients to hypomagnesemia include stress and catabolic illness. Aggressive intravenous (IV) fluid therapy; peritoneal dialysis; nasogastric suction; total parenteral nutrition (TPN); massive blood transfusion; and administration of diuretics, digoxin, and aminoglycosides exacerbate hypomagnesemia. Specific disease processes, such as severe small-intestinal disease, nonoliguric renal dysfunction, postoperative diuresis, diabetic ketoacidosis (with hypophosphatemia), sepsis, pancreatitis, and congestive heart failure (associated with diuretic and digoxin therapy) can result in $Mg^{2+}$ depletion. In small animals, hypomagnesemia is recognized with prolonged hospitalization and often coexists with other electrolyte abnormalities, particularly hypokalemia.

### Clinical Signs

The manifestations of hypomagnesemia are nonspecific and often due to concurrent hypokalemia or hypocalcemia or both. There is no specific serum $Mg^{2+}$ level that results in clinical signs, which include muscle weakness, dyspnea, muscle twitching, seizures, and alterations in mentation. Hypomagnesemia can cause refractory hypokalemia (incomplete response to replacement doses of potassium), and this may be the most important subclinical indicator of magnesium depletion in small animal patients. Refractory hypocalcemia, related to concurrent hypomagnesemia, has also been observed in patients receiving massive blood transfusions. These potassium ($K^+$) and calcium ($Ca^{2+}$) abnormalities can only be corrected if the associated hypomagnesemia is treated. Cardiac arrhythmias have been seen observed in hypomagnesemic patients, particularly in those receiving digitalis and long-term diuretic therapy.

## ADMINISTRATION OF MAGNESIUM

Mild hypomagnesemia may resolve with treatment of underlying disease, modified IV fluid therapy, and correction of hypophosphatemia. Dogs on long-term diuretic and digoxin therapy may benefit from oral supplementation of $Mg^{2+}$ or the use of $K^+$ (and $Mg^{2+}$)-sparing diuretics. Total parenteral nutrition and enteral solutions should be supplemented with $Mg^{2+}$. Supplementation is recommended if serum $Mg^{2+}$ levels are lower than 1.2 mg/dl (normal range=1.7 to 2.4 mg/dl), but may be necessary at higher serum concentrations in the presence of clinical signs, refractory hypokalemia, or hypocalcemia. Renal function, serum $Mg^{2+}$, and serum $Ca^{2+}$ levels must be assessed prior to administration of $Mg^{2+}$. In azotemic patients, the $Mg^{2+}$ dose is reduced by 50 to 75% with frequent monitoring to obviate the risk of hypermagnesemia. Magnesium supplementation is contraindicated in patients with cardiac conduction disturbances.

### Parenteral Supplementation

Both sulfate (8.13 mEq $Mg^{2+}$/gm) and chloride (9.25 mEq $Mg^{2+}$/gm) salts are available in 50% solutions. The IV route is preferred for rapid repletion of $Mg^{2+}$. Intramuscular administration may cause pain. The IV dose is 0.75 to 1 mEq/kg/day, administered by continuous rate infusion (CRI) in 5% dextrose in water (D5W). The $Mg^{2+}$ solution should be diluted to at least 20%. The mixture is incompatible with $Ca^{2+}$ and sodium bicarbonate. A lower dose (0.3 to 0.5 mEq/kg/day), may be used for an additional 3 to 5 days, as complete repletion occurs slowly. For treatment of life-threatening ventricular arrhythmias, a dose of 0.15 to 0.3 mEq/kg of $Mg^{2+}$ is administered over 5 to 15 min.

### Oral Supplementation

Oxide and hydroxide salts of $Mg^{2+}$ are available for oral administration. The suggested dose is 1 to 2 mEq/kg/day. The main side effect is diarrhea.

## OUTCOME

The goal of $Mg^{2+}$ therapy is the resolution of clinical signs. In cases of refractory hypokalemia and hypocalcemia, serum concentrations will increase slowly in response to $Mg^{2+}$ therapy. The observed rate of increase in serum $Mg^{2+}$ concentration will vary with the degree of $Mg^{2+}$ depletion. The $Mg^{2+}$ dose is tailored to individual requirements. Daily monitoring of serum $Mg^{2+}$ levels is required when $Mg^{2+}$ salts are given. Parenteral administration of $Mg^{2+}$ sulfate may result in significant hypocalcemia—especially where predisposing conditions exist—such that $Ca^{2+}$ infusion may be necessary. Other side effects of magnesium therapy include hypotension and atrioventricular and bundle-branch blocks. Adverse effects are usually associated with IV boluses of $Mg^{2+}$ rather than with a CRI. Overdoses of $Mg^{2+}$ may cause respiratory depression and cardiac arrest. Overdoses are treated with $Ca^{2+}$ gluconate at 10 to 50 mg/kg, given as an IV bolus.

# MONITORING GASTROINTESTINAL MUCOSAL pH IN CRITICAL CARE PATIENTS

ROBIN E. WALL
*Mission, Kansas*

## BACTERIAL TRANSLOCATION

### Intestinal Defenses

The intestinal tract, through its numerous metabolic, immune, and barrier functions, serves as a major local defense preventing bacteria and bacterial toxins from entering the systemic circulation. In shock states resulting from sepsis, trauma, and hemorrhage, it has been recognized that the intestinal barrier functions are impaired. The mechanism is not entirely understood, but has been attributed to tissue injury from reactive oxygen metabolites during reperfusion, intracellular hypoxia, inflammatory mediators such as platelet-activating factor and tumor necrosis factor, and impaired utilization of key nutrients (Fink, 1991).

One of three factors must be present for bacterial translocation to occur: disruption of the ecologic balance of the intestinal microflora with overgrowth of certain bacteria, impairment of host immune defenses, or disruption of the intestinal mucosal barrier. The physical barrier may be of primary importance, since limitation of mucosal injury decreases the incidence of bacterial translocation and subsequent sepsis. Ileus, tissue edema, and microvascular thrombosis, which frequently complicate critical illness, may also contribute to intestinal mucosal injury (Fink, 1991). Additionally, critically ill patients are immunosuppressed and often receiving drugs that disrupt the normal gut microflora and promote bacterial overgrowth, such as antibiotics, antacids, $H_2$-receptor antagonists, and narcotics.

### Bacterial Translocation in Critical Illness

Translocation of intestinal bacterial across the intestinal mucosa, with the development of subsequent life-threatening enteric bacteremia, is a major complication of many low blood flow states including hemorrhagic shock and trauma (Fig. 1). It is becoming increasingly clear that gastrointestinal alterations can influence patient outcome in the intensive care unit. Many patients dying of sepsis and multiple organ failure develop bacteremia for which no septic focus can be identified. These infections, often due to enteric bacilli, are postulated to arise from the gastrointestinal tract (Deitch, 1990).

## SPLANCHNIC ISCHEMIA

In low blood flow states, endogenous vasoconstrictors (e.g., angiotensin II, norepinephrine, vasopressin) are released that invariably affect the splanchnic vasculature in an effort to redistribute blood flow and preserve perfusion to essential organs. Subsequently, cellular hypoxia, anaerobic glycolysis, and tissue acidosis result in the gastrointestinal tract secondary to hypoperfusion. Since the mesenteric vasculature is affected frequently, consistently, and early in low blood flow states, detection of gastrointestinal mucosal acidosis may be a sensitive and early indicator of splanchnic ischemia and the risk for bacterial translocation (Grum et al., 1984).

### Pathophysiology of Tissue Acidosis

Ischemia occurs when tissue oxygen requirements are not met and oxygen consumption ($\dot{V}O_2$) becomes dependent upon oxygen delivery ($\dot{D}O_2$). Ischemia occurs when systemic oxygen delivery is decreased as with hypoxemia and anemia or in hypermetabolic states during which tissue demands for oxygen are increased. It is possible for regional ischemia to occur despite apparently adequate systemic oxygen delivery (Fink, 1991). Therefore, the only way to detect localized ischemia before significant injury occurs is to assess the adequacy of regional tissue oxygenation relative to the oxygen demand of the tissue. As tissue oxygen demands are not met, tissue hypoxia and anaerobic glycolysis result, which are reflected by decreased tissue pH, increased carbon dioxide production, and tissue lactic acidosis. In fact, an increase in intestinal intraluminal $PCO_2$ is a very sensitive indicator of intestinal ischemia, occurring before histologic evidence of ischemic injury. The degree of hypercarbia also correlates strongly with the degree of mucosal injury (Bass et al., 1985).

## Gastrointestinal Mucosal pH

A strong correlation has been noted between the change in gastrointestinal mucosal pH ($pH_i$) and $\dot{V}O_2$ as $\dot{D}O_2$ decreases (Grum et al, 1984). Both $pH_i$ and $\dot{V}O_2$ are maintained at normal levels as oxygen delivery de-

creases until a critical point is reached. At that point, $\dot{V}O_2$ becomes dependent on $\dot{D}O_2$, tissue oxygen demand is not met, and $pH_i$ starts to decline. Hemorrhagic, cardiogenic, and traumatic shock cause intestinal mucosal acidosis, the degree of which has been correlated with complications such as bacterial translocation, sepsis, and multiple organ failure (Fink, 1991) and increased mortality of critical care patients (Doglio et al., 1991). Massive bleeding from stress ulceration in human patients has been associated with decreases in $pH_i$. Additionally, a decrease in $pH_i$ was more specific than cardiac index, blood pressure, arterial pH, and urine output for predicting complications following cardiovascular surgery in human patients (Fiddian-Green and Baker, 1987). Normalizing $pH_i$ may improve outcome in select groups of patients by preventing splanchnic organ hypoxia and development of a systemic oxygen debt (Gutierrez et al., 1992).

### MEASURING GASTROINTESTINAL MUCOSAL pH

Gastrointestinal intramucosal pH can be measured directly with microelectrodes or indirectly by measur-

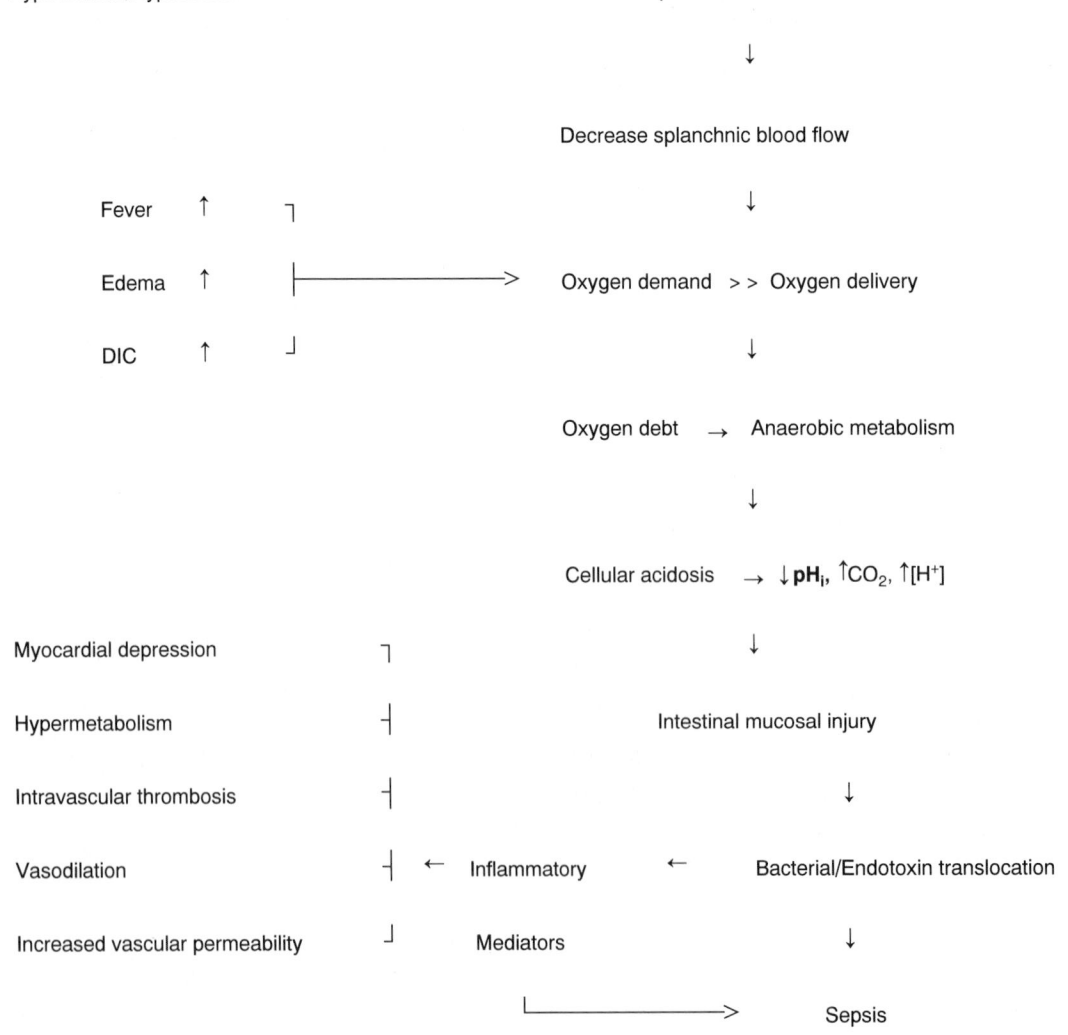

**Figure 1.** Pathogenesis of intestinal ischemia and systemic complications.

ing intraluminal $Pco_2$ (Bass et al., 1985; Fiddian-Green, Pittinger, and Whitehouse, 1982). Measurement of $pH_i$ using microelectrodes tends to be cumbersome, inconvenient for clinical application, and may cause tissue trauma. Conversely, the indirect method (tonometry) has proved useful in both experimental and clinical settings. The validity of indirect tonometry rests on three basic assumptions: (1) carbon dioxide readily diffuses along its concentration gradient and equilibrates between tissues and cavities; (2) tissue and arterial bicarbonate concentrations are similar; and (3) the dissociation constants of $HCO_3^-$ in tissue and plasma are equal (Fiddian-Green, Pittinger, and Whitehouse, 1982). Despite these potential sources of error, primarily in the assumption regarding bicarbonate concentrations, the indirect measurement of $pH_i$ has excellent agreement with direct microelectrode measurements. Indirect tonometry has been validated under limited conditions for dogs and it appears to be a good marker of tissue oxygenation of intact dog intestine (Grum et al., 1984).

A minimally invasive method, using a rectally (preferred) or nasogastrically placed tonometer (Tonomiter, Tonometrics Inc, Worcester, MA), has been developed that permits the measurement of gastrointestinal intramucosal carbon dioxide concentration and subsequent calculation of intramucosal pH (Fig. 2). The device has a distally placed silicone balloon, freely permeable to carbon dioxide, that can be inflated from a sampling port outside of the animal. After inserting the tonometer approximately 10 to 15 cm into the distal large bowel, the balloon is inflated with physiologic saline. Since carbon dioxide freely diffuses along its concentration gradient, saline within the balloon reflects the tissue carbon dioxide ($Ptco_2$) levels following equilibration. The saline is withdrawn following an equilibration period of 30 to 60 min and $Ptco_2$ measured using a blood gas analyzer. An arterial blood sample is obtained simultaneously for measurement of bicarbonate concentration. The $pH_i$ can be calculated using the Henderson-Hasselbalch equation:

$$pH_i = pK_a + \log [HCO_3^-]/\alpha(Pco_2)$$

where $pK_a$ = 6.1, $[HCO_3^-]$ = arterial bicarbonate concentration, $\alpha$ = solubility of carbon dioxide in plasma ($\alpha$ = 0.03), and $Pco_2$ = partial pressure of carbon dioxide in saline from the silicone balloon. In clinical studies involving human patients, $pH_i$ below 7.35 indicated tissue acidosis, ischemia, and increased risk of complications (Doglio et al., 1991; Gutierrez et al., 1992). Dogs appear to be less sensitive to the effects of decreased splanchnic perfusion and can tolerate more severe decreases in oxygen delivery (Papa et al., 1983). The significance of mucosal acidosis in veterinary patients is not yet determined. However, the author's experience suggests that colonic $pH_i$ above 7.35 is strongly associated with a positive outcome, whereas colonic $pH_i$ below 7.15 ($Ptco_2$ >150 mm Hg) is correlated with impending mortality in dogs with otherwise acceptable systemic hemodynamic data, such as mean arterial blood pressure greater than 85 mm Hg and central venous pressure between 3 and 8 cm $H_2O$ ($n=12$).

### CLINICAL APPLICATIONS OF MONITORING $pH_i$

In a veterinary critical care setting, indirect tonometry and monitoring of $pH_i$ can provide a minimally invasive method for monitoring response to therapy, assessing adequacy of oxygenation, and predicting complications in animals with questionable tissue oxygenation (e.g., anemia, hypoxemia, congestive heart failure) or hypermetabolic conditions (sepsis, pancreatitis, trauma). Detection of a low $pH_i$ early in the course of hospitalization permits early intervention to improve tissue oxygenation, potentially minimizing the risk of complications related to an oxygen deficit, such as stress ulceration, sepsis, increased hospitalization time, and death. Tonometric methods may also allow evaluation of the efficacy of various promising therapies for

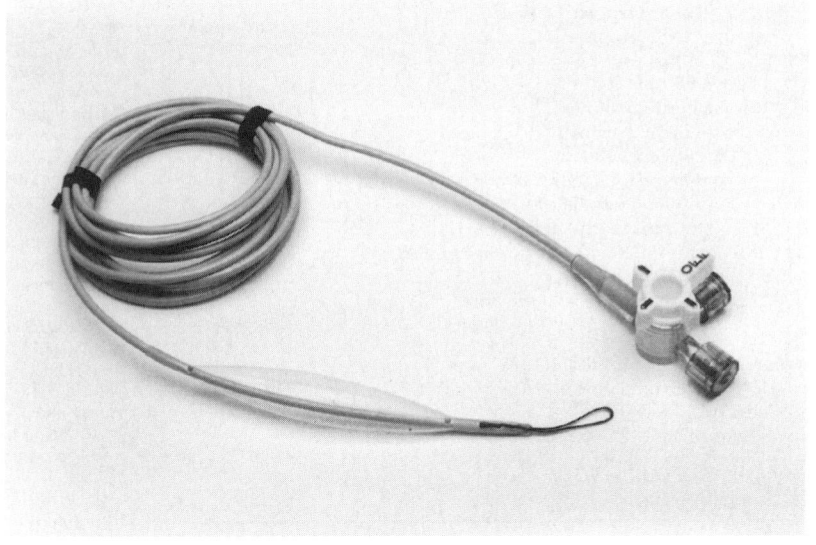

**Figure 2.** Sigmoid tonometer with distally placed Silastic balloon and proximal sampling port.

improving patient outcome following shock, such as hypertonic saline solutions, iron chelators, and oxygen radical scavengers.

### LIMITATIONS OF INDIRECT GASTROINTESTINAL TONOMETRY

Although there is no significant difference in the change in $pH_i$ of the various portions of the gastrointestinal tract in response to ischemia, stomach $pH_i$ is more likely to be influenced by the systemic acid-base status of the patient. The accuracy of gastric tonometry is also influenced by back-diffusion of gastric acid into the mucosa. Therefore, administration of $H_2$-receptor antagonists is recommended if gastric tonometry is performed. Complete occlusion of mesenteric blood flow and intravenous administration of bicarbonate result in underestimation of intramucosal acidity whereas respiratory acidosis–induced tissue hypercarbia may overestimate the degree of injury.

## MINIMIZING TISSUE ISCHEMIA

Intestinal mucosal pH can be optimized and systemic oxygen debt minimized by improving oxygen transport and decreasing tissue oxygen demands (Table 1). Oxygen transport is a function of cardiac output and the oxygen-carrying capacity of blood. To ensure oxygen delivery and minimize tissue ischemia in critical care patients may require intravascular volume loading, vasopressor support (see "Use of Catecholamines in Critical Care Patients," this volume, p 188), oxygen supplementation, and/or ventilatory support. Tissue oxygen demands can be decreased by administration of sedatives or muscle relaxants and by the appropriate use of mechanical ventilation.

**Table 1.** *Minimizing Gastrointestinal Mucosal Ischemia and Related Complications*

**Improve Tissue Oxygen Delivery**
Improve oxygen transport
  $SaO_2$ >90%
  $PaO_2$ >65 mm Hg
  Hematocrit 25–35%
Optimize hemodynamics
  CVP 7–12 cm $H_2O$
    Volume resuscitation
      Isotonic crystalloids
      Dextrans (5–20 ml/kg/24 hr)
  Mean arterial blood pressure >70 mm Hg
    Vasopressor support
      Dopamine (1–10 µg/kg/min)
      Dobutamine (5–20 µg/kg/min)

**Decrease Oxygen Demands**
Mechanical ventilation
Sedation
  Butorphanol (0.2–0.8 mg/kg SC, IV q2–6h)

**Protect Mucosal Barrier**
Enteral feeding

## PROTECTING THE MUCOSAL BARRIER

The best option for promoting villus growth and protecting the intestinal mucosa is enteral feeding. Experimentally, early enteral feeding has been shown to bolster host antibacterial defenses, blunt the hypermetabolic response to injury, maintain intestinal mucosal mass and barrier functions, and prevent disruption of the normal gut microflora (Deitch, 1990).

In the future, therapeutic options to prevent, limit, and speed repair of mucosal injury will become available. Administration of antacids and $H_2$ antagonists may prevent worsening of mucosal injury due to gastric acid secretion. Selective gut decontamination with oral antibiotic administration has been suggested; however, the results of experimental and clinical studies are contradictory and overall patient outcome does not appear to be affected. Preventing reperfusion injury and minimizing the effects of oxygen radicals during the resuscitation phase are other potential options that may become available for preventing gastrointestinal mucosal ischemia and subsequent bacterial translocation.

Presently, the best options for preventing mucosal ischemia and the associated consequences are rapid and adequate resuscitation from shock, maintenance of adequate tissue oxygenation in seriously ill patients, and protection of the intestinal mucosa with early enteral feeding. The use of serial gastrointestinal mucosal pH monitoring in emergency and critical care patients offers a potential benefit in the achievement of these goals.

### References and Suggested Reading

Bass BL, Schweitzer EJ, Harmon JW, and Kraimer J: Intraluminal $pCO_2$: A reliable indicator of intestinal ischemia. J Surg Res 39:351, 1985.
*A study demonstrating the relationship between increased intraluminal $PCO_2$, intestinal blood flow, and mucosal injury in rabbits.*

Deitch EA: Bacterial translocation of the gut flora. J Trauma 30:s184, 1990.
*Discusses evidence supporting the occurrence of bacterial translocation and its role in the critically ill patient.*

Doglio GR, Pusajo JF, Egurrola MA, et al: Gastric mucosal pH as a prognostic index of mortality in critically ill patients. Crit Care Med 19:1037, 1991.
*A prospective study evaluating the prognostic significance of gastric intramucosal pH measured upon admission to the ICU and 12 hr later.*

Fiddian-Green RG and Baker S: Predictive value of the stomach wall pH for complications after cardiac operations: Comparison with other monitoring. Crit Care Med 15:153, 1987.
*Compares the predictive value of gastric intramucosal pH to blood pressure, cardiac index, arterial pH, and urine output on patient outcome.*

Fiddian-Green RG, Pittinger G, and Whitehouse WM: Back diffusion of $CO_2$ and its influence on the intramural pH in gastric mucosa. J Surg Res 33:39, 1982.
*Demonstrates accurate calculation of gastric intramucosal pH from arterial bicarbonate concentration and luminal carbon dioxide.*

Fink MP: Gastrointestinal mucosal injury in experimental models of shock, trauma, and sepsis. Crit Care Med 19:627, 1991.
*A review of etiologies, mediators, and detection of gastrointestinal mucosal ischemia.*

Grum CM, Fiddian-Green RG, Pittenger GL, et al: Adequacy of oxygenation in intact dog intestine. J Appl Physiol 56:R1065, 1984.
*A study demonstrating the relationship between intramural pH, oxygen consumption, and oxygen extraction following decreased oxygen delivery.*

Gutierrez G, Palizas F, Doglio G, et al: A prospective trial of gastric intramucosal pH as a therapeutic index in critically ill patients (abstr). J Trauma 20:65, 1993.
*Clinical study of human patients suggesting that $pH_i$-guided resuscitation may improve outcome from the ICU.*

Papa M, Halperin Z, Rubinstein E, et al: The effect of ischemia of the dog's colon on transmural migration of bacteria and endotoxin. J Surg Res 35:264, 1983.
*Demonstrated translocation of endotoxin from the intestines of dogs following temporary mesenteric ischemia.*

# DIAGNOSIS OF BACTEREMIA IN CRITICALLY ILL DOGS AND CATS

STEVEN W. DOW

*Denver, Colorado*

Bacterial infections remain a major cause of mortality in companion animal patients treated in critical care units. Bacteremia occurs frequently in these patients and is the most serious and life-threatening infection with which critical care clinicians are faced. Animals with serious underlying diseases are at particular risk of developing bacteremia. Illness and intensive medical and surgical treatment disrupt innate host microbiologic defenses, resulting in the progressive colonization and replacement of normal bacterial flora with more pathogenic strains of bacteria, particularly gram-negative bacteria of the Enterobacteriaceae family. In addition, host immune responses are often impaired, due in some cases to effects of the underlying disease (e.g., diabetes mellitus, neoplasia), or to the immunosuppressive effects of certain medications (e.g., high doses of corticosteroids administered to patients with neurologic disease). Invasive procedures and the use of medical devices that bypass cutaneous and mucosal barriers to bacterial invasion (e.g., intravenous or urinary catheters) also promote entry of bacteria into the bloodstream.

## PATHOGENESIS OF BACTEREMIA

Bacteria frequently enter the bloodstream and in healthy individuals rarely cause noticeable effects; the blood-borne bacteria are rapidly removed, primarily by neutrophils and tissue macrophages. Serious bacteremic infections generally only develop when patients either receive an overwhelming challenge dose of bacteria or, more often, when immune defenses are impaired, resulting in delayed bacterial clearance. In these patients, failure to control the infection locally leads to uncontrolled bacterial replication and systemic spread via the bloodstream. Three patterns of bacteremia are possible: transient, intermittent, and continuous. Most critical care patients that develop bacteremia probably exhibit the intermittent pattern, characterized by periodic showering of bacteria into the bloodstream, often from an extravascular source such as urinary tract infection or tissue infection. A fever spike typically follows 1 to 2 hr after bacteria enter the bloodstream. Transient bacteremia occurs frequently, as during routine dentistry, and in healthy patients is of no consequence. Severe bacterial endocarditis is associated with continuous bacteremia and is often fatal.

## CLINICAL FEATURES OF BACTEREMIC INFECTIONS

Bacteremic infections in companion animal critical care patients is a serious problem that until recently has received little attention. We retrospectively evaluated 100 critical care patients that had blood cultures done as part of their medical management in a large veterinary hospital critical care unit, to determine the frequency of bacteremia, characterize the microbiology of the infection (Table 1), and assess the effect of bacteremia on patient morbidity and mortality.

Three clinical abnormalities have often been associated with the occurrence of bacteremic infections in hospitalized patients: fever (or hypothermia), neutropenia or left shift (or both), and shock. When the results of blood culture in our canine and feline patients were correlated with the presence or absence of either of these three signs, each abnormality was significantly more likely to occur in animals with positive blood cultures. The particular type of infecting organism (i.e., gram-positive versus gram-negative) could not, how-

**Table 1.** *Diseases Present in Critically Ill Dogs and Cats with Bacteremia**

| Disease | Number with Disease | Number of Culture-Positive | (%) |
|---|---|---|---|
| Urinary tract infection | 3 | 3 | (100) |
| Leukemia | 2 | 2 | (100) |
| Portosystemic shunt | 2 | 2 | (100) |
| FeLV-positive | 1 | 1 | (100) |
| Diabetes mellitus | 7 | 6 | (86) |
| Pneumonia | 6 | 4 | (67) |
| Postoperative infection | 3 | 2 | (67) |
| Abscess | 3 | 2 | (67) |
| Lymphosarcoma | 5 | 3 | (60) |
| Peritonitis | 7 | 4 | (57) |
| Neutropenia | 6 | 3 | (50) |
| Fever of unknown origin | 4 | 2 | (50) |
| Trauma | 2 | 1 | (50) |
| Endocarditis | 2 | 1 | (50) |
| Discospondylitis | 2 | 1 | (50) |
| Gastroenteritis | 11 | 5 | (45) |
| Tumor | 4 | 1 | (25) |
| Immune-mediated disease | 13 | 3 | (23) |
| Gastric dilatation-volvulus | 5 | 1 | (20) |
| Severe dermal lesions | 6 | 1 | (17) |
| Other | 6 | 1 | (17) |

*From Dow SW, Curtis CR, Jones RL, et al: Bacterial culture of blood from critically-ill dogs and cats: 100 cases (1985–1987). J Am Vet Med Assoc 195:113–117, 1989, with permission.

ever, be distinguished based on the severity of signs or the pattern of abnormalities. Thus, the unexplained development of fever, neutropenia, or shock in a critical care patient is a strong predictor of bacteremia.

Veterinary critical care patients with severe underlying diseases that had positive blood cultures also experienced significantly increased mortality relative to patients with severe underlying diseases who had negative blood cultures. Bacteremia also occurred significantly more often in patients with serious underlying diseases, consistent with studies in human critical care patients indicating that severe illness is itself a strong risk factor for the development of bacteremia. By contrast, bacteremia did not significantly increase mortality in patients without severe underlying disease, presumably because they were better able to control the infection. Thus, efforts to prevent the development of bacteremia should be particularly directed toward the most seriously ill patients, since these are the patients at greatest risk and also those most likely to die after becoming bacteremic.

## MICROBIOLOGY OF BACTEREMIA IN CRITICAL CARE PATIENTS

Clinicians probably underestimate the prevalence of bacteremic infections in critical care patients. In our studies, we found that nearly half (49%) of canine patients and 71% of feline patients that were blood cultured had positive cultures. In dogs, gram-negative bacteria (especially *Escherichia coli*) were most common, followed by gram-positive cocci and obligate anaerobes. Polymicrobial infection was also common, occurring in 17% of canine patients, and was typically comprised of a gram-negative enteric pathogen plus an obligate anaerobe. Notably rare in both dogs and cats were *Pseudomonas* isolates (only three positive cultures over a 3-year period). This is similar to a trend observed in human medicine, where *Pseudomonas* has been replaced by bacteria of the Enterobacteriaceae family and more recently by staphylococci as the most common pathogens in intensive care units.

Bloodstream isolates from cats were either gram-negative bacteria of the Enterobacteriaceae family or obligate anaerobes. *Salmonella* was the most common gram-negative pathogen isolated from cat blood cultures, an indication that salmonellae may be an important but overlooked pathogen in cats. Gram-positive cocci were not recovered from feline blood cultures, although the number of animals studied was small. Most episodes of bacteremia in cats were also polymicrobial.

Despite previous suggestions that certain bacteremic pathogens are associated with higher mortality, we did not find any evidence that infection with any particular type of bacterial pathogen increased mortality, once the severity of the underlying disease was taken into account. In addition, clinical findings alone were not sufficient to discriminate between the type of bacterium (aerobe versus anaerobe; gram-positive versus gram-

negative) with which an animal was infected. Finally, in 18 animals with positive blood cultures, the bacteriologic results led to a treatment change from an ineffective to a more effective antimicrobial drug.

We concluded from these studies that bacteremia was a common complication in veterinary critical care patients and was associated with significantly increased mortality in those patients with severe preexisting disease. Blood culture should therefore become a more routine diagnostic test for the optimal management of veterinary critical care patients. Blood culture is indicated in patients with suspected bacteremia to (1) confirm that infection exists, (2) identify the organism(s) present, and (3) facilitate optimal antimicrobial therapy.

## GUIDELINES FOR BLOOD CULTURE

Blood cultures are indicated in any critical care patient that develops fever, neutropenia or left shift (or both) or other signs of sepsis that cannot be explained by a preexisting infection. Blood cultures are particularly important in the management of severely immunosuppressed patients such as those undergoing cytotoxic chemotherapy for neoplasia, and other patients at risk of developing infection, including those with diabetes mellitus and with urinary tract infection (Table 1).

In all cases, a minimum of two and preferably three blood cultures should be obtained. This not only increases the chances of obtaining a positive culture, but also facilitates accurate interpretation of culture results (Table 2). Timing of cultures is less important, since most bacteremic patients will have intermittent bacteremia and the time of bloodstream showering cannot be predicted. Generally, three cultures taken over a 24-hr period will suffice for patients without severe sepsis. For animals with advanced sepsis, three cultures should immediately be taken over a 2-hr period. Whenever possible, at least 10 ml of blood should be cultured at each time point, since the concentration of blood-borne bacteria is often low.

For most uses, a general purpose blood culture medium such as anaerobic brain heart infusion (BBL, Becton Dickinson Company, Cockeysville, MD) that facilitates growth of both aerobic and anaerobic bacteria is satisfactory. The medium should be warmed to room temperature before inoculation and the blood culture bottles then maintained at room temperature until they are transported to the microbiology laboratory. Typically, preliminary blood culture results will be available within 48 hr, particularly for pathogens likely to be important in critical care patients. We and others have found that prior administration of antimicrobial drugs does not reduce the frequency of positive cultures. Prior or concurrent antimicrobial therapy should therefore not preclude use of blood cultures, particularly in those animals that become septic during antimicrobial therapy, since they are likely to have become infected with an antibiotic-resistant pathogen.

For routine blood culture, blood should be collected

**Table 2.** *Interpretation of Blood Culture Results**

| Organism Isolated | Likely Source | Interpretation |
|---|---|---|
| *Staphylococcus aureus or intermedius* (coagulase-positive) | Skin, intravenous catheter, endocarditis, discospondylitis | Significant |
| *Staphylococcus* (coagulase-negative) | Skin, intravenous catheter | Possible contaminant[†] |
| *Streptococcus* (β-hemolytic) | Skin, endocarditis, discospondylitis | Significant |
| *Streptococcus* (α-hemolytic) | Skin, mouth | Possible contaminant[†] |
| Enterococcus (enteric *Streptococcus*) | Gastrointestinal tract | Significant |
| *Corynebacterium* | Skin, endocarditis | Probably significant |
| *Erysipelothrix* | Skin, endocarditis | Probably significant |
| *Bacillus* | Skin | Possible contaminant[†] |
| Enterobacteriaceae[‡] | Gastrointestinal, urinary, respiratory tract | Significant |
| *Pseudomonas* | Skin, gastrointestinal, urinary tract | Significant |
| *Bacteroides* | Gastrointestinal tract, abscesses | Significant |
| *Clostridium* | Skin, gastrointestinal tract, abscesses | Significance uncertain |

*From Dow SW and Jones RL: Bacteremia. Diagnosis and prognosis. Compend Cont Educ 11:432–441, 1989, with permission.
[†]Unless isolated from multiple cultures.
[‡]The Enterobacteriaceae family includes *Escherichia coli, Salmonella, Klebsiella, Enterobacter, Proteus,* and *Serratia.*

by jugular venipuncture after the neck has been thoroughly disinfected. The same site can be used for all cultures, unless there is evidence of a specific focus of infection such as phlebitis, in which case several different veins should be used. Blood can in some instances also be drawn from indwelling venous catheters, provided they are long enough to provide central venous access, have not been in place for longer than 48 to 72 hr, and have been carefully covered and maintained in a sterile fashion.

## INTERPRETATION OF BLOOD CULTURE RESULTS

Negative blood culture results from two or three successive cultures generally rules out bacteremia caused by common pathogens, although less common, more fastidious bacteria may take days to weeks to grow out. On the other hand, positive blood culture results do not necessarily indicate true bacteremia. The biggest pitfall to interpreting blood culture results is inadvertent contamination of the specimen with normal commensal skin bacteria, particularly coagulase-negative staphylococci, α-hemolytic streptococci, *Micrococcus,* and *Acinetobacter*. The only reliable way to rule out contamination is to culture multiple blood specimens and isolate the same bacterium from at least two. Recovery of potentially pathogenic bacteria that are not normal skin commensals is also taken as presumptive evidence of true bacteremia, although isolation from multiple specimens is very helpful in reaching a diagnosis (Table 2).

## References and Suggested Reading

Abramowicz M: The choice of antibacterial drugs. Med Lett Drugs Ther 34: 49–56, 1992.
Dow SW, Curtis CR, Jones RL, et al: Bacterial culture of blood from critically-ill dogs and cats: 100 cases (1985–1987). J Am Vet Med Assoc 195: 113–117, 1989.
Dow SW and Jones RL. Bacteremia: Diagnosis and prognosis. Compend Cont Educ 11:432–443, 1989.
Weinstein MP, Murphy JR, Reller JB, et al: The clinical significance of positive blood cultures: A comprehensive analysis of 500 episodes of bacteremia and fungemia in adults. II. Clinical observations with special reference to factors influencing prognosis. Rev Infect Dis 5:54–70, 1983.

# SEPTIC SHOCK

REBECCA KIRBY

*Milwaukee, Wisconsin*

There are a group of diseases that share a common pathophysiology: some inciting stimulus causes the production and release of circulating mediators that cause inflammatory changes throughout the body. This results in peripheral vasodilation, increased capillary permea- bility, and depressed cardiac function. The inciting stimulus can be different; however, once the cascade of mediators has been initiated, the clinical progression and complications are the same. Diseases that fall into this category include sepsis and septic shock, pancreatitis, heat stroke, multiple trauma, snake bite, viremia, parasitemia, fungemia, and pansystemic neoplasia. This disease process is called the systemic inflammatory response syndrome (SIRS), and the resultant organ pathology is termed multiple organ dysfunction syndrome (MODS).

Sepsis, and its complications, is becoming a more frequent complication in the small animal patient. Proposed reasons for the increase in incidence include widespread use of catheters and other invasive equipment, administration of corticosteroids and other immunosuppressive agents, and improvement in the ability to manage neoplastic and immunodeficiency disorders.

In the past, the systemic changes that occurred secondary to microorganism invasion into the bloodstream were termed the sepsis syndrome. Recent published definitions from the American College of Chest Physicians and the Society of Critical Care Medicine provide a common ground for discussion and may be adapted to small animals (Table 1).

The presence of microorganisms, their toxins, and the resultant mediators of inflammation separate the pathogenesis of septic shock from other forms of shock. The most toxic and biologically active properties of endotoxin have been attributed to the lipid A portion of the endotoxin molecule. This is released from gram-negative bacteria when their cell walls are disrupted such as during rapid growth and proliferation or death. The cellular effects of endotoxin are mediated by cell surface receptors for endotoxin and by receptors specific for individual mediators.

Although the presence of endotoxin is most frequently recognized as an initiating event, canine models of septic shock demonstrated the same pattern of hemodynamic abnormalities regardless of whether *Escherichia coli* or *Staphylococcus aureus* was used to induce sepsis. Gram-positive bacteria do not contain endotoxin but do possess a variety of cellular constituents, including muramyldipeptides and peptidoglycans that can stimulate the production of tumor necrosis factor (TNF) and interleukin-1 (IL-1).

Mononuclear cells, phagocytes, neutrophils, vascular endothelial cells, and platelets are the primary target cells responding to endotoxin stimulation. Once activated, these elements secrete several substances or mediators, called *cytokines*, that act synergistically to contain the infection. Cytokines are defined as soluble, nonantibody regulatory proteins secreted by the activated immunocytes, mediating both local and systemic responses resulting from infection (see *CVT XI*, p 461). *Lymphokines* are nonantibody regulatory protein secreted by lymphocytes and *monokines* are nonantibody proteins secreted from mononuclear phagocytes. Among these mediators, TNF, platelet-activating factor (PAF), prostaglandins, leukotrienes, lysozymes, interleukins, procoagulant tissue factors, interferon, and toxic oxygen radicals play a dominant role in implementing the containment strategy of inflammation. If bacteria, bacterial products, or inflammatory mediators leak into the bloodstream, the cellular inflammatory response is pansystemic.

## CELLS

The mononuclear phagocyte is considered to be the most critical cell in the host response to endotoxin and in the recruitment of components of the inflammatory response. The binding of endotoxin to mononuclear phagocyte cell surface receptors results in the activation of protein kinases. Protein kinase C has a major role in endotoxin induced production of mediators by macrophages, leading to the release of cytokines such as IL-1, TNF-$\alpha$, PGE$_2$, interferons, and PAF (Fig. 1; Table 2).

The neutrophils play a central role in sepsis. Endotoxin and TNF-$\alpha$ are potent stimulators of neutrophil chemotaxis and expression of neutrophil adherence to endothelium. The adherence to vascular endothelium leads to the spread of endotoxin effects from the blood to multiple organs.

Vascular endothelial cells communicate freely with the circulating cells, mediators, and endotoxin. Exposure of vascular collagen and release of tissue thromboplastin will stimulate the coagulation cascade.

## CYTOKINES

Tumor necrosis factor-$\alpha$, IL-1, and IL-6 have been proven to play a primary role in the pathogenesis of SIRS. Other cytokines and nitric oxide have also been implicated (Table 2).

**Table 1.** *Definitions°*

*Infection:* Microbial phenomenon characterized by an inflammatory response to the presence of microorganisms or to the invasion of normally sterile host tissue by those organisms.

*Systemic inflammatory response (SIR):* The systemic inflammatory response to a variety of severe clinical insults. The response is manifested by two or more of the following criteria:

1. T> 103.5° F or < 100° F
2. Heart rate >160 bpm (dog).
   Heart rate >250 bpm (cat).
3. RR >20 bpm or PaCO$_2$ <32 mm Hg
4. WBC >12,000, <4000, or >10% bands.

*Sepsis:* The systemic response to infection. This systemic response is manifested by two or more of the above criteria.

*Septic shock:* Sepsis with hypotension, despite adequate fluid resuscitation, along with the presence of perfusion abnormalities that may include, but are not limited to lactic acidosis, oliguria, or an acute alteration in mental status. Patients receiving inotropic or vasopressor agents may not be hypotensive at the time that perfusion abnormalities are measured.

*Hypotension:* A systolic BP <90 mm Hg or a reduction of more than 40 mm Hg from baseline in the absence of other causes for hypotension.

*Multiple organ dysfunction syndrome (MODS):* Presence of altered organ function in the acutely ill patient such that homeostasis cannot be maintained without intervention.

°Adapted from American College of Chest Physicians/Society of Critical Care Medicine: American College of Chest Physicians/Society of Critical Care Medicine Consensus Conference: Definitions of sepsis and organ failure and guidelines for the use of innovative therapies in sepsis. Crit Care Med 20:864, 1992, with permission.

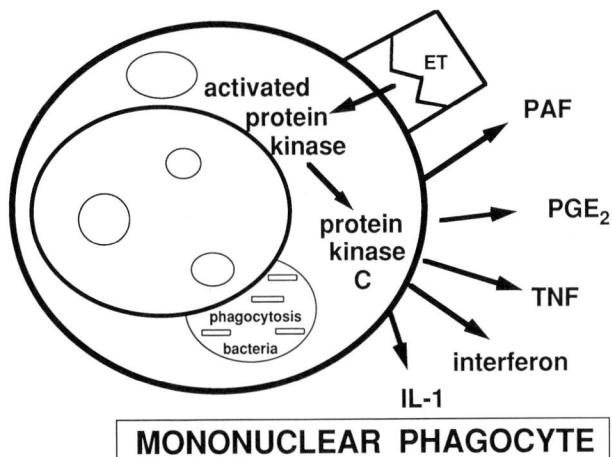

**Figure 1.** Endotoxin binds with cell specific receptors, resulting in the activation of protein kinases. Protein kinase C plays an integral role in the release of septic mediators. The mononuclear cell is believed to be the most critical cell in the initiation of endotoxin-induced inflammatory cellular response. Abbreviations: ET = endotoxin, PAF = platelet-activating factor, $PGE_2$ = prostaglandin E2, TNF = tumor necrosis factor, IL-1 = interleukin-1.

*Tumor necrosis factor* may provide the primary afferent signal initiating many of the metabolic responses of sepsis and endotoxemia. It binds to high affinity receptors in normal tissues and triggers multiple effects, including the release of IL-1, IL-4, and IL-6. Locally, the result is the containment of infection. When TNF enters the circulation, signs of septicemia develop, with

*Table 2.   The Principal Cytokines and Their Actions*

**Tumor necrosis factor**
  T-cell activation
  Pyrogen activity
  Induction of endothelial surface antigen
  Procoagulant activity
  Eicosanoid synthesis
  Granulocyte/monocyte colony-stimulating factor synthesis
  Inhibition of enzymes of lipid metabolism
  Activation of osteoclastic bone resorption
  Triggers production of IL-1, IL-4, and IL-6

**Interleukin-1**
  T-cell release of IL-2
  Release of arachidonic acid metabolites
  Polymorphonuclear cell chemotaxis
  Secretion of inflammatory proteins
  Fibroblast proliferation
  Endothelial cell release of:
    Platelet activating factor, prostacyclin, PMN adherence
      protein, procoagulant activity
  B-cell activation and antibody production

**Interleukin-6**
  T-cell stimulation
  Hepatic acute-phase protein synthesis and release
  B-cell stimulation

**Platelet-activating factor**
  Cardiac: negative inotrope, vasoconstriction
  Pulmonary: vasoconstriction
  Gastrointestinal: ulcers, smooth muscle contraction
  Vasculature: vasodilation, WBC activation, platelet activation,
    protease activation, increased permeability

high TNF concentrations lethal. *Interleukin-1* is produced primarily by stimulated mononuclear phagocytes and has many of the properties of TNF. The principal biologic activity is believed to be the interaction with antigen-stimulated T cells to induce the release of IL-2 by T cells and the synthesis of IL-2 receptors in natural immunity (Green and Adams, 1992). *Interleukin-6* is produced by macrophages, monocytes, fibroblasts, vascular endothelial cells, T lymphocytes, and mast cells. The major stimulus for production is IL-1, with endotoxin, TNF, platelet-derived growth factor, and viral infections providing a lesser stimulus (Green and Adams, 1992). *Platelet-activating factor* is synthesized by leukocytes, endothelial cells and platelets from a phospholipid cell membrane precursor in the presence of calcium.

## NITRIC OXIDE

Nitric oxide is synthesized from L-arginine by the calcium dependent enzyme nitric oxide synthase. A constitutive nitric oxide synthase is present normally in endothelial cells, certain neurons, endocardium, myocardium, and platelets (Vallance et al., 1993). This acts as a physiologic mediator of cell-to-cell communication and intracellular communication. The second type of nitric oxide synthase, an inducible enzyme, is expressed in endothelial cells, vascular smooth muscle cells, macrophages, neutrophils, cardiac myocytes, and endocardial cells after exposure to endotoxin for cytokines such as TNF or IL-1. Actions of this inducible nitric oxide appear to play a key role in the pathophysiology of septic shock and include: inhibition of mitochondrial respiration, reaction with oxygen free radicals to form harmful species, vascular relaxation and poor response to vasoconstrictors, damage to endothelial cells, increase in vascular permeability, inhibition of platelet aggregation and adhesion, neurotransmission, and reduction of duration of cardiac constriction and acceleration of relaxation.

## EICOSANOIDS

Phospholipase $A_2$ is an early mediator, stimulated by TNF-$\alpha$, IL-1, and PAF. It is capable of promoting the release of arachidonic acid from the cell membrane which, when metabolized by cyclooxygenase and lipoxygenase, produce prostaglandins and leukotrienes. Platelet aggregation, neutrophil accumulation, increased vascular permeability, bronchoconstriction, and vasoconstriction of vascular beds in the lungs, heart, intestines, and kidneys are some of the effects of thromboxane $A_2$. Prostaglandin $E_2$ and prostacyclin are vasodilators and increase blood flow. During sepsis, these exert beneficial effects on tissue perfusion and may decrease the severity of tissue damage. Down-regulation of $PGE_2$ can occur by IL-1 and TNF. Leukotrienes have three effects in sepsis: (1) $C_4$, $D_4$, and $D_3$ alter vascular reactivity; (2) $B_4$ promotes PMN accumulation and activation; and (3) all four leukotrienes increase vascular permeability.

## SYSTEMIC EFFECTS

Bacteria entering the bloodstream initiate the response described above. Common sites of invasion are the gastrointestinal tract, respiratory system, and urinary tract. Local inflammatory responses occur due to exposure of immunocytes to endotoxin, exotoxin, or other bacterial substances. Immunocytes are recruited and release cytokines and eicosanoids. There is a systemic inflammatory response when the antigen affects the general circulation. Some of these mediators stimulate immunocytes to produce other mediators, with the cycle eventually perpetuated without regard for the inciting agent.

Septic shock is a combination of three forms of shock: hypovolemic, distributive, and cardiogenic. Uneven vasoconstriction and maldistribution of flow are directly related to tissue hypoxia, tissue oxygen debt, shock, shock-related organ failure, and death. Adaptive responses occur, with some aimed at increasing oxygen delivery, others aimed toward more efficient utilization of oxygen. Alternate sources of energy such as anaerobic glycolysis are activated and energy and oxygen demands are decreased.

Two serious abnormalities in the cardiovascular system occur in septic shock: (1) an increased cardiac output and (2) a decreased systemic vascular resistance (SVR). Arteriolar vasodilation and increased permeability of capillaries leads to a decrease in SVR and loss of intravascular fluid volume, respectively. Hypovolemia occurs, with reduced cardiac preload. There is evidence for a circulating myocardial depressant factor. Cardiac filling and contractility are impaired.

Neutrophils move through the capillaries into the tissues, releasing proteolytic enzymes and superoxide radicals. Platelets adhere to damaged endothelial cells and tissue surfaces, aggregating and releasing their substances. The microvasculature becomes partially occluded by thrombi of white blood cells (WBCs) and platelets, further impairing blood flow.

When death occurs, it is usually the result of physiologic mechanisms and biochemical mediators that lead to multiple vital organ failures. The common denominator is tissue hypoxia from poor tissue perfusion due to unevenly distributed blood flow that occurs *early* in the course of septic shock and prior to organ failure (Shoemaker et al, 1993).

## DIAGNOSIS

Sepsis and septic shock should be suspected in any animal with hypotension, tachycardia, hypovolemia, either fever or hypothermia, high or low WBC count, and signs of multiple organ involvement. Suspicion demands diagnostic studies be done and appropriate monitoring and therapeutic procedures instituted im-

mediately. Noninfectious causes of SIRS, including acute pancreatitis, multiple trauma, snake bite, heat stroke, other causes of ischemia, and diffuse infiltrative neoplastic disease, should be evaluated as inciting causes; however, sepsis also can occur secondary to each of these disorders.

The areas of highest suspicion for harboring the infective focus are: urinary tract, reproductive tract, abdominal cavity, respiratory tract, teeth and gums, and heart valves. *An infection hunt* is initiated. The signalment, history, and physical examination provide a great amount of information for localizing the nidus of infection. Intact male and female patients are suspects for pyometra or prostatic infections. Historic signs of vomiting, diarrhea, and abdominal discomfort directs examination of the abdomen. Increased frequency, straining, blood, or difficulty in urination suggest urinary tract infection. Any history of recurrent infections or recent teeth cleaning are important. Historic questioning should aid in ruling in or out the nonbacterial causes of SIRS.

Physical examination needs to be thorough, with particular attention given to cardiac auscultation and abdominal palpation. A murmur or abnormal rhythm ausculted warrants further diagnostic evaluation of the heart for bacterial endocarditis. Abdominal palpation requires that the clinician examine the four quadrants carefully for fluid, masses, pain, or foreign bodies. The kidneys are palpated for size, contour, and pain, common signs of kidney infections. Careful palpation and close examination of the skin, subcutis, and muscles for areas of myositis, cellulitis, fasciitis, or abscessation is essential.

Blood samples should be obtained for complete blood count (CBC), serum biochemical profile, coagulation profile, pancreatic enzymes, rickettsial or fungal titres as indicated, immune profiles, and blood cultures (see "Diagnosis of Bacteremia in Critically Ill Dogs and Cats," this volume, p 137). Urine should be collected by cystocentesis for urinalysis and culture and sensitivity. Other diagnostic procedures that may be required are directed toward identifying the focus of infection and determining whether emergency surgical or pharmacologic intervention is indicated. Radiographs of the chest and abdomen are obtained looking for mass lesions, pleural fluid, air bronchograms, loss of abdominal detail, dilated gas-filled bowel, or specific organ enlargements or deformities. Ultrasound examination of the abdomen may reveal a mass or abscess, infiltrative changes, or other organ abnormalities. Echocardiography can demonstrate the contractility of the myocardium and assess the heart valves for endocarditis, pericardial effusion, or mass lesions.

Diagnostic peritoneal lavage provides diagnostic assistance in determining if an abdominal abnormality warrants immediate surgical intervention. Fluid retrieved that has the appearance of "prune juice" is often indicative of severe acute pancreatitis. Other indications of pancreatitis from diagnostic lavage are increased inflammatory WBC count with degenerative neutrophils and no bacteria, an elevation in lavage fluid amylase or lipase concentration compared to serum values, and at least temporary pain relief through dilution and drainage of free-abdominal enzymes. Findings that warrant emergency surgical intervention once the animal has hemodynamic stability include WBCs with intracellular bacteria, the presence of meat or vegetable fiber in the sediment, and removal of large quantities of blood from suspected on-going hemorrhage.

## THERAPEUTICS

The key to successful management of animals with septic shock or other forms of SIRS is anticipation— *not* reaction. It takes 24 to 48 hr before the appropriate antibiotics have the desired effects, requiring that the clinician monitor and support organ functions during this period.

*The "wait and see" approach often leads to a worsening condition that requires much more fluids and missed opportunities as patients progress from potentially correctable states to irreversible states.*

WC Shoemaker

Anticipation of multiple organ complications prior to organ failure, and aggressive intervention at the earliest stages are vital to survival. Animals with SIRS are hypermetabolic and have a tissue oxygen debt. This oxygen debt demands supranormal cardiac output, blood volumes, and oxygen delivery to tissues. In a study in human patients, the optimal values (supranormal values) for cardiac performance, oxygen distribution, and oxygen consumption were used as therapeutic goals and attained in 8 to 12 hr, leading to a marked and significant reduction in mortality and morbidity rates (Shoemaker et al., 1993). It is appropriate to then drive the oxygen distribution further in an effort to ensure oxygen consumption is at its maximum.

### Rule of 20

The *Rule of 20* identifies 20 critical clinical parameters that should be assessed at least daily in animals with evidence of SIRS (see "Monitoring the Critically Ill Patient," this volume, p 98). A checklist should be placed into the record with the daily progress notes for easy evaluation and comment. The order of importance will be specific for each patient.

FLUID BALANCE. Animals with septic shock can have massive loss of fluid from the intravascular compartment into third body fluid spaces. This results from the increased capillary permeability and decreased SVR. Perfusion (intravascular volume) must be restored immediately. Replacement of interstitial volume deficits should occur over 1 to 2 hr with balanced electrolyte solutions such as lactated Ringers or Normosol-R (Abbott, North Chicago, IL). Replacement crystalloid volumes can be required that are two to three times the calculated amount, due to continued loss from the abnormal microvasculature as hydrostatic pressure increases. The concurrent use of colloids during resuscitation will reduce the amount of crystalloid required by 40 to 60%, reducing the amount of fluid that extravasates into vital organs such as the lung. Unfortunately, the patient in septic shock can become less responsive to cardiac filling pressures such that preload augmentation may not correct hypotension and will predispose to pulmonary edema in some patients.

When initial resuscitation of catastrophic shock requires peracute restoration of intravascular volume, $7\frac{1}{2}\%$ hypertonic saline (Concentrated Sodium Chloride 23.4%, Am Regent Lab, Shirley, NY) in hydroxyethyl starch (Hetastarch, DuPont Pharmaceuticals, Wilmington, DE) or dextran 70 (6% Gentran 70, Baxter Healthcare Corp, Deerfield, IL) (dogs, 4 to 8 ml/kg; cats, 2 to 6 ml/kg) is administered. The interstitium must be hydrated for hypertonic saline administration. This is followed by 16 ml/kg hydroxyethyl starch or dextran 70 infusion with crystalloids. For acute volume resuscitation, hydroxyethyl starch or dextran 70 is given (dogs, 20 ml/kg; cats, 10 to 15 ml/kg) as an IV bolus followed by crystalloids. These fluids will rapidly restore intravascular fluid volume and decrease the total amount of crystalloid required for resuscitation. Maintenance fluid therapy is then performed utilizing a balanced crystalloid solution.

Successful intravenous fluid resuscitation is suggested when the central venous pressure (CVP) is supranormal (8 to 12 cm $H_2O$), heart rate slows, optimal mean arterial pressures are obtained, and oxygen distribution and oxygen consumption have been driven to supranormal levels. Serum lactate values can be monitored as a reflection of overall tissue oxygen utilization.

ONCOTIC PULL. The presence of large-molecular-weight, negatively charged molecules in the blood vessels has the effect of pulling water from the interstitial space into the vasculature. It holds it there as long as the intravascular oncotic pull is greater than that in the tissues. Serum proteins, especially albumin, provide this pull in the normal animal. However, when anticipating massive extravasation through leaky, vasodilated capillaries, the administration of colloids can prevent peripheral and pulmonary edema and retain intravascular fluid volume.

Choices of colloids that are utilized include whole blood, fresh frozen plasma, dextran, and hydroxyethyl starch. When the albumin is less than 2.0 gm/dl, fresh frozen plasma is administered as the colloid of choice. However, as many as 6 U of plasma can be required in large-sized dogs to achieve the desired oncotic effect. Therefore, plasma is administered until the albumin is above 2.0 gm/dl and then synthetic colloids are infused to add the remaining volume of colloid. Following the initial resuscitation phase, hetastarch (10 to 20 ml/kg IV) is administered by drip over 4 to 6 hr as part of the daily maintenance fluids when MODS is anticipated from SIRS. It is important that the CVP be monitored and that the volume of crystalloids infused be reduced by 40 to 60% of what would be used without the hetastarch. When SIRS is present, the author uses this fluid for at least 3 days.

Another option is dextran 70. This can be administered in a dosage and protocol similar to the hetastarch. The oncotic pull of dextran is not as long lasting as that of hetastarch. In addition, the dextran can decrease platelet adhesion and potentiate bleeding in some animals.

GLUCOSE. The blood glucose should be maintained between 100 and 200 mg/dl. Initial fluid resuscitation should not be done with a glucose-containing solution.

ELECTROLYTES (CALCIUM, SODIUM, CHLORIDE, POTASSIUM) AND ACID-BASE BALANCE. Total calcium (and more importantly, ionized calcium), sodium, potassium, and chloride should be maintained within normal limits. It is usually necessary to supplement potassium in the maintenance fluids. The blood pH and bicarbonate level should be monitored by venous and arterial blood gas. Metabolic acidosis is typically a result of poor perfusion and hypotension and is treated first by improving tissue blood flow.

OXYGENATION AND VENTILATION. Arterial blood gases should be evaluated to show any evidence of hypoxemia, hypercarbia, or hyperventilation. This is important for early detection of pulmonary edema or acute respiratory distress syndrome (ARDS) common to animals with SIRS. Oxygen supplementation is generally needed, and should carbon dioxide accumulate, ventilation therapy is employed (see *CVT XI*, p 98). Prevention and early intervention to improve capillary flow and prevent excessive interstitial fluid accumulation is the key to success. Aspiration pneumonia is anticipated in vomiting patients and gastric suctioning may be warranted if there is gastric distention.

MENTATION. When depression develops, precautions are taken to prevent aspiration and causes of increased intracranial pressure are considered. Serum osmolality should be monitored, especially if the animal is being given parenteral nutrition. Severe elevations or rapid changes in osmolality can cause cerebral edema and alterations in mentation. Glucose levels must be maintained, and appropriate nursing procedures employed (e.g., turning every 4 hr, lubricating the eyes)

BLOOD PRESSURE. Blood pressure should be monitored by either direct or indirect methods (see "Blood Pressure Measurements," this volume, p 110). Systolic pressure must be maintained above 90 mm Hg, and the mean arterial pressure above 60 mm Hg. Should the patient be hypotensive, the following interventions are considered in the following order, unless directed otherwise by specific patient concerns: (1) volume infusion (crystalloids and colloids to drive CVP to 8 to 12 cm $H_2O$, (2) oxygen supplementation, (3) pain control, (4) cardiac support with dobutamine (Dobutrex, Lilly, Indianapolis, IN) (dogs, 5 to 10 µg/kg/min IV constant rate of infusion [CRI]; cats, 2.5 to 5 µg/kg/min IV CRI), and (5) pressor therapy if cardiac support is unsuccessful. Dopamine (Elkins-Sinn, Inc, Cherry Hill, NJ) at low dosage (1 to 3 µg/kg/min IV CRI) will increase renal perfusion. Doses of 5 to 20 µg/kg/min causes peripheral vasoconstriction through α-adrenergic stimulation. Norepinephrine (0.5 to 1 µg/kg/min IV CRI) can provide stronger α-adrenergic stimulation if

dopamine causes tachycardia or is unsuccessful (Vincent and Preiser, 1993); however, the risk of arrhythmias is higher.

HEART RATE, RHYTHM AND CONTRACTILITY. Hypotension, myocardial depressant factor, volume loss, hypoxia, and inflammatory mediators all contribute to development of cardiac arrhythmias and impaired contractility. Tachycardia is most frequently a reflection of hypovolemia, hypotension, or pain. Initial therapy for arrhythmias included oxygen, pain control, and volume replacement. Echocardiography can be helpful in evaluating cardiac function, especially in animals with primary heart diseases, and can guide therapeutics.

ALBUMIN. Serum albumin concentration should be maintained above 2.0 gm/dl. Values persistently below this are associated with increased mortality (Safar, 1982). When albumin is below 2.0 gm/dl, oncotic pull is provided by fresh frozen plasma or whole blood transfusion.

COAGULATION. Disseminated intravascular coagulation (DIC) is expected in patients with SIRS until proven otherwise. Platelet estimate and activated clotting time are in-hospital coagulation monitoring tests and should be done at least daily. Rapid and severe hemodynamic changes can cause sudden and severe coagulation changes, necessitating aggressive monitoring and therapy. Coagulation screening tests for DIC include prothrombin time (PT), activated partial thromboplastin time (APTT), platelet count, fibrinogen, fibrin degradation products, and antithrombin III (AT-III). Antithrombin III decreases early in DIC and the amount in the blood can guide therapy.

Therapy for DIC includes five components. First, oxygenation and tissue perfusion are improved and capillary stasis reduced by aggressive fluid therapy. Second, the underlying disease must be treated. Third, the target organs of DIC—lungs, kidney, heart, brain, and intestines—must be supported. Fourth, if there is active bleeding and consumption of coagulation proteins and AT-III, replacement with fresh frozen plasma is required (Cates et al., 1993). Active hemorrhage necessitates transfusion. Fifth, the interaction of AT-III with thrombin is greatly accelerated when heparin is available as a cofactor. When there is ample AT-III, heparin (Elkins-Sinn, Inc, Cherry Hill, NJ) (50 to 100 U/kg SC every 8 hr) can be administered alone. When AT-III is provided in fresh frozen plasma, one heparin dose is added to the plasma and allowed to incubate for 30 min prior to administration. The next subcutaneous dosage is skipped.

RED BLOOD CELL/HEMOGLOBIN CONCENTRATION. The PCV should be maintained above 20% at minimum, and above 30% ideally. This is accomplished through whole blood or packed red cell transfusion as indicated.

RENAL FUNCTION. Urine output should be assessed on an ongoing basis as a reflection of renal function and fluid balance. The serum creatinine or blood urea nitrogen in the urine sediment (casts) should be assessed daily during the crisis period of SIRS.

Renal failure is managed in the following order: (1) ensure intravascular volume is adequate and that MAP is greater than 60 mm Hg with a fluid challenge, (2) infuse mannitol (Anpro Pharmaceuticals, Arcadia, CA) (0.1 gm/kg IV) when renal insufficiency is diagnosed early, and (3) dose furosemide (Lasix, Ag-Vet Co, Somerville, NJ) (1 mg/kg/hr IV every hr for 4 hr) combined with a dopamine infusion (1 to 3 $\mu$g/kg/min IV CRI) for as long as required.

IMMUNE STATUS, ANTIBIOTIC DOSAGE AND SELECTION, WBC COUNT. The total WBC count and differential cell count are assessed as an indicator of the ability to fight infection. Antibiotic selection, dosage and route of administration are reviewed daily, and backed by appropriate microbiological culture and antibiotic sensitivity data (e.g., blood cultures, see p 138). Persistent fever and high or low left-shift WBC counts found in sick animals on apparently appropriate antibiotics (aerobic microbiologic culture results) suggest anaerobic bacterial, viral, rickettsial, or fungal infections. Anaerobic bacteria must always be considered when the infection is from intestinal, hepatic, or biliary origins.

Antibiotics are initially selected without the benefit of microbiologic culture and antibiotic sensitivity results. Gram stain of urine, sputum, aspirates, or discharges aid in identifying gram-positive or gram-negative cocci or rods and guiding empiric antibacterial therapy. A broad-spectrum bactericidal intravenous antibiotic is selected and given at therapeutic dosages. Bacterial endocarditis is commonly due to gram-positive cocci. Systemic infection from teeth or gums are most frequently due to gram-positive cocci or anaerobes or both. Bacteria from gastrointestinal and reproductive tract origin infections are often gram-negative rods. However, peritonitis can result from gram-negative rods and anaerobic bacteria.

It is better to restrict the empiric use of antibiotics in a critical care unit to a standard few. This helps to reduce the incidence of resistant nosocomial organism infection. Gram-positive cocci can usually be managed with penicillin derivatives such as ampicillin (Totacillin, Beecham Lab) (10 to 50 mg/kg every 6 to 8 hr IV). Gram-negative rods (with or without gram-positive cocci) in a septic animal without shock can be treated with the first generation cephalosporin, cefazolin (Keflin, Lilly, Indianapolis, IN) (40 mg/kg first dose then 20 mg/kg/day every 6 hr IV). When a more aggressive approach is required, gentamicin (Steris Lab, Inc, Phoenix, AZ) (3 to 5 mg/kg/day divided every 8 hr; or 6 mg/kg every 24 hr IV) is administered once the animal is rehydrated and the renal function is adequate. Anaerobic pathogens are treated with metronidizole (Flagyl, Schiapparelli-Searle, Chicago, IL) (20 to 30 mg/kg/day divided every 6 hr IV) by slow infusion.

GASTROINTESTINAL MOTILITY AND MUCOSAL INTEGRITY. The patient should be ausculted at least three times daily for presence of bowel sounds. Ileus predisposes the patient to gastrointestinal ulceration and vomition. Oral glucose and electrolyte solutions help protect against gastric ulceration. The use of $H_2$ antagonists is controversial, as raising the gastric pH can predispose to gastric bacterial translocation and aspiration pneumonia. Gastric ileus associated with refractory vomiting is best treated by nasogastric tube suctioning, removing this peripheral receptor stimulation. In nonpancreatitic patients with SIRS, metoclopromide (Reglan, AH Robbins, Richmond, VA) (1 to 2 mg/kg/day IV CRI) promotes gastric and duodenal motility and blocks the chemoreceptor trigger zone.

Antiemetics are required in the critical vomiting patient that is recumbent, has bradycardia, has compromised breathing, or has a depressed gas reflex. Initially, metoclopromide is used. Alternatively, chlorpromazine (Steris Lab Inc, Phoenix, AZ) (dogs, 0.05 to 0.1 mg/kg IV every 4 to 8 hr; cats, 0.01 to 0.025 mg/kg every 4 to 8 hr IV) can be administered following hemodynamic stabilization.

DRUG DOSAGES AND METABOLISM. It is important to consider the mode of metabolism and excretion of drugs. If liver or renal insufficiency is present, drug selections and dosages may need to be altered. It is always wise to review drug dosages daily in critical animals that are administered "polypharmacy." Errors in calculation can lead to devastating complications.

NUTRITION. Nutrition is important from the moment the animal is admitted to the hospital. Recent data implicate the disuse of the bowel as a predisposing factor in bacterial translocation and secondary sepsis. This factor makes the use of enteral nutrition the preferred route when possible. The immediate goal of nutrient support is to prevent further autodigestion of the body's tissues. It is ideal to maintain body weight.

Animals willing to eat can be started with a small amount of liquid diet (e.g., Clinicare, PetAg, Hampshire, IL). Then a bland diet (e.g., I/D, Hills, Topeka, KS) can be given in small dilute amounts. Animals unwilling to eat are either force fed or tube fed. Force feeding can prove stressful to critical patients and is not to be attempted if there is depressed mentation, difficulty swallowing, or potential of stress-induced complications. Tube feeding can be done by orogastric, nasoesophageal, esophagostomy, gastrostomy, duodenostomy, or jejunostomy tubes.

If it is not possible to immediately initiate enteral feedings, partial parenteral nutrition can be provided with a 3.5% amino acid solution with glycerine in a maintenance electrolyte solution (Procalamine, McGaw, Irvine, CA). Enteral feeding is then initiated by giving small amounts of a glucose and electrolyte solution (0.5 to 2 ml/kg PO) to test how well the animal tolerates oral feeding and to provide microenteral nutrition to the gastric mucosa. If successful, the animal can be weaned onto enteral nutrients.

Enteral nutritional support is first provided by a dilute solution of low volume. Solutions of high osmolality can induce osmotic diarrhea and reflux vomiting. The following protocol has been found to be effective:

1. Calculate the caloric requirements based on the extra energy needs of the disease.
2. Provide one third of the daily caloric requirements utilizing a diluted liquid diet. The diet is diluted

to half strength with water. This is given by small frequent boluses or is placed into an empty IV bag and dripped into the feeding tube over the 12 to 24 hr period.

3. Increase the concentration to two thirds liquid diet and provide two thirds of the daily caloric requirement over 24 hr.

4. Increase the concentration to full strength liquid diet and provide 100% of the calories.

5. Consider lowering the concentration, decreasing the volume, or checking the tube placement should vomiting occur during this weaning process.

6. Administer metoclopromide to promote gastric emptying, reduce esophageal reflux and decrease vomiting if necessary.

7. Wean the animal onto bolus administration of the solution prior to discharge if tube feeding is still required.

In the patient with pancreatitis or gastroduodenal disease, it is best that nutrients do not pass from the stomach into the duodenum. Total parenteral nutrition has been the method of choice in the past; however, enteral feeding is recommended as soon as possible. Should this patient be surgically explored, a jejunostomy tube should be placed.

PAIN CONTROL. Pain can be manifested by tachycardia, restlessness, severe mental depression, or poor attitude. Pain control is important to the cardiovascular function and mental well-being of the animal. Butorphanol (Torbugesic, Aveco, Fort Dodge, IA) (0.2 to 1.2 mg/kg IV every 2 to 4 hr) or buprenorphine (Buprenix, Reckitt & Coleman) (0.01 to 0.02 mg/kg IM every 6 to 8 hr) can be used initially. Preemptive analgesia is recommended for surgical patients. Narcotics and local analgesics have proven effective (see *CVT XI*, p 82).

NURSING CARE AND PATIENT MOBILIZATION. The recumbent patient must be turned every 4 hr. Urine scalding and fecal soiling is to be avoided. Catheter sites must be checked and each catheter labeled appropriately to avoid confusion of lines and misuse of the tubes. When the animal is immobile for an extended time, gentle passive manipulation of the limbs is required. Careful recording of patient status, procedures performed, and drugs administered is essential to accurate patient assessment. Any case-specific procedures, such as peritoneal dialysis or CVP monitoring, requires skilled and informed nurses (see "Critical Care Nursing," this volume, p 106).

WOUND CARE/BANDAGE CHANGE. Many animals with SIRS require wound debridement or surgical correction. The incision site or wound should be examined daily to ensure appropriate healing. Areas of ecchymosis or swelling should be outlined on the skin with a marker pen to monitor progression of size. Bandage changes are required whenever bandages become moist or as dictated on a case-by-case basis.

TENDER LOVING CARE. The mental health of the critically ill animal is very important and most pets are likely to be affected by separation. Visits by the owners are encouraged when it appears to benefit the pet. The veterinarian and nursing staff should speak kindly and softly when working with the animal. The ICU lights are usually on 24 hr/day; when possible, it is a good idea to turn down the lights to promote sleep.

## SURGICAL INTERVENTION

The underlying septic focus must be eliminated as quickly as possible. When abdominal surgery is required for septic peritonitis, open abdominal drainage should be considered. The surgeon should place a gastric or intestinal feeding tube in anticipation of postoperative anorexia. Microenteral nutrition is begun with a glucose and electrolyte solution beginning immediately postoperatively (see *CVT XI*, p 117).

Abscesses should be drained and débrided. Large areas of necrotic skin or fasciitis can require *en bloc* excision and debridement and drainage of underlying tissues. Penetrating wounds should be explored, débrided, and drained.

## References and Suggested Reading

American College of Chest Physician/Society of Critical Care Medicine: American College of Chest Physicians/Society of Critical Care Medicine Consensus Conference: Definitions of sepsis and organ failure and guidelines for the use of innovative therapies in sepsis. Crit Care Med 20:864, 1992.
*A review of the consensus findings on clarification of the sepsis syndrome in man.*
Bottoms GD and Adams RA: Involvement of prostaglandins and leukotrienes in the pathogenesis of endotoxemia and sepsis. J Am Vet Med Assoc 200:1842, 1992.
*A review of the involvement of prostaglandins and leukotrienes in the pathogenesis of endotoxemia and sepsis.*
Cate H, Brandjes DPM, Wolters HJ, et al: Disseminated intravascular coagulation: Pathophysiology, diagnosis, and treatment. New Horizons 1:312, 1993.
*A review of the human and animal studies on DIC in septic shock.*
Green EM and Adams HR: New perspectives in circulatory shock: Pathophysiologic mediators of the mammalian response to endotoxemia and sepsis. J Amn Vet Med Assoc 200:1849, 1992.
*A review of the literature on cytokines and their role in sepsis.*
Safar P: Resuscitation in hemorrhagic shock, coma and cardiac arrest. In Crowley RA and Trump BF, (eds): *Pathophysiology of Shock, Anoxia, and Ischemia.* Baltimore, Williams & Wilkins, 1982, p 428.
*A progressive review of the pathophysiology and aggressive resuscitation of hemorrhagic shock, coma and cardiac arrest.*
Shoemaker WC, Appel PL, Kram HB, et al: Hemodynamic and oxygen transport monitoring to titrate therapy in septic shock. New Horizons 1:145, 1993.
*A review of human and animal studies on hemodynamics and oxygen transport in septic shock.*
Vallance P and Moncada S: Role of endogenous nitric oxide in septic shock. New Horizons 1:77, 1993.
*A review the physiology and role of nitric oxide in septic shock.*
Vincent JL and Preiser JC: Inotropic agents. New Horizons 1:137, 1993.
*A review of human and animal studies on inotropic agents in sepsis.*

# COUNTERPRESSURE USE IN SHOCK AND HEMORRHAGE

DENNIS T. CROWE, Jr.

*Milwaukee, Wisconsin*

This discussion will concentrate on the use of externally applied pressure to the pelvic limbs, pelvis, and abdominal cavity for treatment of shock and control of hemorrhage. Counterpressure is a very practical technique that can be used to control or partially control severe abdominal hemorrhage. This includes hemorrhage caused by injury to the renal artery and vein, abdominal vena cava, and abdominal aorta.

## DEFINITION AND INDICATIONS FOR COUNTERPRESSURE USE

A clinical definition of counterpressure is: external pressure applied to afford an effect on the vascular structures under its influence. The broad indications for counterpressure use include severe hemorrhage from intra-abdominal organs and blood vessels and noncardiogenic shock. Where shock is associated with hemoabdomen, as determined by needle paracentesis or diagnostic peritoneal lavage (DPL) (hematocrit of 5% or greater), external counterpressure should be considered. External counterpressure, when applied to the pelvic limbs and caudal abdomen, can be very effective in slowing or stopping hemorrhage, even that associated with major vessel trauma (e.g., abdominal aorta, vena cava). The use of counterpressure can also be effective in immobilization of pelvic and femoral fractures and limiting associated hemorrhage. Intrathoracic disorders resulting in compromised ventilation first must be excluded by careful examination, as the presence of these conditions represents relative or absolute contraindications to counterpressure application.

Counterpressure may also *temporarily* increase systemic arterial blood pressure and central venous pressure, augmenting cardiac output while directing blood flow to the myocardium and brain (Roth, 1971). The transient rise in central venous pressure facilitates catheterization of peripheral veins. Central vascular replenishment is enhanced by the use of counterpressure, as blood in the capacitance veins and venules is moved toward the central circulation. Although this "autotransfusion" may not be as important as the influence of counterpressure on peripheral vascular resistance, it is the author's opinion that this venous autotransfusion becomes important in patients with loss of vasomotor tone (severe shock). This effect is possibly augmented by movement of interstitial fluid into the vascular system via counterpressure influences on increasing perivascular tissue pressure.

## METHODS OF APPLICATION

Counterpressure is applied using a specially designed, commercially available, small animal "antishock" pneumatic garment or by wrapping towels followed by tape or elastic roller bandage on the pelvic limbs (starting at the toes), pelvis, and caudal abdomen.

### Small Animal Antishock Pneumatic Garment

With the small animal antishock pneumatic garment (SAASPG) (Jobst, Inc, Toledo, OH), the patient is simply wrapped in a garment that contains one or more rubber balloons or bladders. Application should encompass all of the pelvic limbs, pelvis, and abdomen caudal to the rib cage. After the garment is secured, the bladders are inflated, starting with that most caudal or distal until the patient's systemic arterial blood pressure normalizes or all bladders are inflated. As the abdominal bladders or segment of the garment are inflated, ventilation must be monitored and supported as necessary, since abdominal counterpressure reduces thoracic compliance and consequently tidal volume in spontaneously ventilating animals. This approach is particularly important in patients with conditions such as a diaphragmatic hernia or pneumothorax, as the addition of external counterpressure may be fatal, if ventilatory support is not provided (Maull et al., 1986).

### Towel Application

Towels followed by wide elastic rolls or tape are wrapped on the patient starting at the feet and wrapping in a circular "barber pole" fashion. If a blood pressure cuff and sphygmomanometer are available, these can be used to estimate the amount of pressure applied. The bladder of the cuff is partially inflated and laid on the ventral midline of the abdomen. The abdominal towel wrap holds the cuff in place. The sphygmomanometer is brought out from the wrap so the gauge can be read. A second towel is wrapped around the abdomen and pressure applied to raise the pressure in the bladder cuff to approximately 60 mm Hg. If respiratory compromise is observed, then the pressure is lessened. Tape or elastic wrap is used to hold the towel in place at the desired pressure. Abdominal pressures of 40 mm Hg can substantially decrease bleeding from the liver, spleen, and kidney (Crowe, 1982; Cangiano, 1972; Eddy, 1968).

If a blood pressure cuff is not available, ½ to 1 lb of rolled cotton is placed on the ventral abdomen before starting to apply the towels. Correct application allows one to place a finger between the bandage and the skin. The amount of pressure that should be placed on bleeding structures to significantly slow hemorrhage is not as great as one might think; only 2 lb per square inch is enough pressure to stop or drastically reduce blood flow to tissues under the bandage (Crowe and Downs, 1986).

## BENEFITS OF COUNTERPRESSURE

As vessel diameter becomes smaller, due to the influence of counterpressure, the flow through the bleeding vessel reduces by a power of 4. This corrresponds to a reduction in bleeding rate also by a power of 4. Counterpressure for internal hemorrhage control may provide sufficient time to prepare the animal and personnel for surgical intervention. Occasionally, bleeding may be completely controlled with the use of counterpressure. When counterpressure remains in place for several hours, spontaneous hemostasis may occur in some patients. This provides a potential treatment option for owners who cannot afford the costs of surgical treatment (Crowe et al., 1990).

There is experimental support for this treatment. To evaluate the effectiveness of external counterpressure, a circumferential bandage as previously described was applied to the abdomen, pelvis, and pelvic limbs in 6 of 12 anesthetized, *heparinized* dogs instrumented with a device that severed the left renal artery and vein. All dogs were allowed to hemorrhage until significant hypotension occurred (mean arterial pressure [MAP] <60 mm Hg) and clinical signs of shock were apparent. At this time, six of the dogs received external counterpressure. Arterial and central venous pressure significantly increased in all dogs that received the counterpressure, while those pressures continued to fall in the six untreated dogs. All 12 dogs died; however, those receiving the counterpressure had a significantly increased survival time. Mean time of death in the untreated dogs was 12 minutes, while it was 43 minutes in the treated dogs (Crowe and Down, 1986). These results suggest that counterpressure can lengthen "the window" for definitive surgical intervention in patients with catastrophic hemorrhage.

In a series of 30 clinical cases of severe hemorrhagic shock studied by the author, 20 animals responded to external counterpressure as evidenced by increased systemic arterial blood pressure, pulse pressures, and level of awareness. Some of these animals were initially unconscious and regained consciousness following application of counterpressure (Crowe et al., 1990). Similar results have been reported following the use of a similar garment in human patients suffering from catastrophic hypovolemic shock (Ali and Duke, 1991; Shane and Campbell, 1965). In studies involving peo-

ple, the results have been so profound in the resuscitation of certain trauma patients that one author recently stated: "The development of this (external counterpressure) is as important to the circulatory support of the trauma patient as mouth-to-mouth breathing has been to the cardiopulmonary arrest patient" (Safer, 1986).

## FOLLOWING COUNTERPRESSURE APPLICATION

Counterpressure should remain until vascular volume and blood pressure have been restored. If animals demonstrate unstable vital signs or hypotension after volume replacement, this usually indicates catastrophic hemorrhage that will require surgical intervention. In these patients, the counterpressure is continued until just before the surgery is to begin. Counterpressure is then removed quickly, and a rapid skin preparation and aseptic surgical approach performed. The skin preparation should be done while a hand is kept on the abdomen and continues to place pressure on the midabdominal area. In many cases only a few passes are made with the clippers, the skin is quickly sprayed with a surgical preparation solution (such as 2% chlorhexidine or 1% povidone iodine), and the abdomen is opened.

In the majority of animals, treated with counterpressure and the intravenous volume infusion, vital signs stabilize. Following the restitution of vital signs, blood pressure, and pulse pressure to normal or supranormal values, the counterpressure device can be slowly removed while blood pressure and heart rate are continually monitored. With pneumatic devices, small amounts of air are released sequentially every few minutes, provided the patient's systemic arterial blood pressure does not fall more than 5 mm Hg. If a compressive circumferential dressing was used, it is gradually removed by cutting or loosening, starting at the cranial border. As with pneumatic counterpressure devices, if systemic arterial blood pressure decreases more than 5 mm Hg, then removal of the counterpressure should be stopped and more volume replacement instituted until hemodynamic stabilization is reestablished. Rapid removal of counterpressure devices can result in catastrophic hypotension secondary to significant decreases of systemic vascular resistance (Wilson, 1989).

## COMPLICATIONS

### Improper Application

In studies by the author on dogs in which a circumferential pressure bandage ("belly band") was applied without pressure being applied to the pelvic limbs and pelvis, venous distention occurred caudal to the counterpressure application. This resulted in a decrease in cardiac output as measured by thermodilution. Therefore, it is emphasized that when abdominal counterpressure is used, it should be applied first at the most distal aspect of the pelvic limbs, and include the entire circumference of the pelvic limbs and pelvis before involving the abdomen. Bladder necrosis has been observed as a complication of improperly applied wraps; however, this complication has not been observed either experimentally or clinically when counterpressure was evenly distributed from the toes of the pelvic limb through the umbilical region.

## Compartmental Syndrome

This condition results in necrosis of those muscle and nervous tissues in the pelvic limbs under the influence of the counterpressure. The necrosis is a consequence of pressure on blood flow to these structures (Basinger et al., 1987). Fortunately, the prevalence of this syndrome is rare. Compartmental syndrome can result following continuous application of high pressure (>100 mm Hg) for several hours or in the instance of counterpressure applied nonuniformly, which results in venous distention distally (Heppenstall et al., 1979).

## Hemorrhage

When the application of the counterpressure increases systemic arterial blood pressure, there is the potential for increasing hemorrhage at sites cranial to the zone of high pressure. This is a major concern when counterpressure is applied in the trauma patient that is hypotensive secondary to blood loss. If hemorrhage is controlled directly by the counterpressure, the increased systemic arterial blood pressure will have no adverse effect. However, if hemorrhaging sites are not under the influence of counterpressure, as blood pressure rises, hemorrhage will increase (Wilson, 1989).

## Compromised Ventilation

The pressure placed on the abdominal organs consequent to the application of the counterpressure forces the diaphragm cranially and restricts its movement. This complication can be minimized in spontaneously breathing, conscious animals if the counterpressure applied is limited to the caudal one third to one half of the abdomen (Crowe, 1982). If pressure is

applied more cranially, the clinician must be prepared to provide positive-pressure ventilation. If the diaphragm is torn, application of counterpressure is contraindicated in most cases. However, it can be considered in those patients following institution of general anesthesia, tracheal intubation, and positive-pressure ventilation.

## References and Suggested Reading

Ali J and Duke K: Timing and interpretation of the hemodynamic effects of the pneumatic antishock garment. Ann Emerg Med 20:1183, 1991.

Basinger RR, Aron DN, Crowe DT, et al: Osteofascial compartment syndrome in the dog. Vet Surg 16:427, 1987.

Bickell WH, Pepe PE, Bailey ML, et al: Randomized trial of pneumatic antishock garments in the prehospital management of penetrating abdominal injuries. Ann Emerg Med 16:653, 1987.

Burgess AR and Brumback RJ: Early fracture stabilization. In Cowley RA, Conn A, and Dunham MC (eds): Trauma Care, volume I: Surgical Management. Philadelphia, JB Lippincott Co, 1987, pp 184–195.

Cangiano JL and Kest L: Use of G-suit for uncontrollable bleeding after percutaneous renal biopsy. J Trauma 107:360, 1972.

Committee on Trauma, American College of Surgeons: Abdomen. In Early Care of the Injured Patient. Philadelphia, WB Saunders Co, 1985, pp 180–192.

Cowley RA and Dunham CM: Introduction. In Cowley RA and Dunham CM (eds): Shock Trauma/Critical Care Manual: Initial Assessment and Management. Baltimore, University Park Press, 1982, pp xi–xv.

Crowe DT: Diagnostic abdominal paracentesis techniques: Clinical evaluation in 129 dogs and cats: J Am Anim Hosp Assoc 20:223, 1984.

Crowe DT: Internal and external abdominal counterpressure. Abstract Presentations of the Advanced Session of the Vet Crit Care Soc Ann Mtg. Las Vegas, NV, 1982.

Crowe DT: Performing life-saving cardiovascular surgery. Vet Med 84:77, 1989.

Crowe DT and Downs MO: Physiological effects of abdominal binding in normal and intraabdominally bleeding dogs (abstr). Vet Surg 15:24, 1986.

Crowe DT, MacDonald M, Gaston J, Miller G, and Wells M: The use of a pneumatic garment in the management of hemorrhage and hypovolemic shock in dogs and cats: A prospective clinical investigation. Sci Proc 2nd Internat Vet Emerg Crit Care Sympos. 2:650, 1990.

Eddy DM, Wangensteen SL, and Ludewig RM: The kinetics of fluid loss from leaks in arteries tested by an experimental ex vivo preparation and external counterpressure. Surgery 64:541, 1968.

Heppenstall RB, Balderston R, and Goodwin C: Pathophysiologic effects distal to a tourniquet in the dog. J Trauma 19:234, 1979.

Ludweig RM and Wangensteen SL: Aortic bleeding and the effect of external counterpressure. Surg Gynecol Obstet 128:252, 1969.

Maull KI, Krahwinkel DJ, Rozycki GS, and Nelson HS: Cardiopulmonary effects of the pneumatic anti-shock garment on swine with diaphragmatic hernia. Surg Gynecol Obstet 162:17, 1986.

Roth JA and Rutherford RB: Regional blood flow effects of G suit application during hemorrhagic shock. Surg Gynecol Obstet 133:637, 1971.

Safer P: Cardiopulmonary cerebral resuscitation: Basic and advanced life support. In Schwartz GR, Safer P, Stone J, et al (eds): Principles and Practice of Emergency Medicine, 2nd edition. Philadelphia, WB Saunders Co, 1986, pp 194–319.

Shane RA and Campbell GS: Protective effects of external counterpressure in acute hemorrhagic hypotension. Am J Surg 110:355, 1965.

Wilson RF: Accidental and surgical trauma. In Shoemaker WC, Ayres S, Grenvik A, Holbrook PR, and Thompson WL (eds): Textbook of Critical Care. Philadelphia, WB Saunders Co, 1989, pp 1230–1271.

# SYSTEMIC ANAPHYLAXIS

ROBERT D. COHEN

*North Grafton, Massachusetts*

Anaphylaxis is a common clinical entity in small animal practice, and is believed to play a significant role in such diverse clinical syndromes as insect bite, vaccine, and drug reactions; and feline asthma, feline eosinophilic granuloma complex, and lymphocytic-plasmacytic gastroenteritis/colitis. Most of these syndromes are considered forms of localized anaphylaxis and involve chronic intermittent clinical signs or self-limiting clinical signs that are rarely life threatening. Anaphylactic shock, or systemic anaphylaxis, can develop subsequent to localized anaphylactic syndromes or may develop unexpectedly with no prior clinical warning. Although the prevalence of systemic anaphylaxis in small animal practice is unknown, the many localized anaphylactic syndromes that are seen and the potential to develop acute life-threatening systemic anaphylaxis necessitates a thorough understanding of the pathophysiologic mechanisms involved to ensure rapid and comprehensive treatment.

Anaphylactic reactions involve the classic immunologic pathways of the type I or immediate hypersensitivity reaction. This pathway involves an initial exposure to an antigen, induction of immunoglobulin E (IgE) (and rarely IgG) antibody production, and the binding of this cytotropic antibody to tissue mast cells and circulating blood basophils, which renders these cells "sensitized." Subsequent exposure to the same antigen activates mast cells and basophils and leads to release of preformed mediators and to synthesis of additional mediators. These vasoactive and proinflammatory mediators cause the clinical signs associated with an anaphylactic reaction, and it is helpful to think of anaphylaxis as a mast cell–mediated syndrome.

Anaphylactoid reactions are identical to anaphylactic reactions and involve activation and degranulation of mast cells and basophils. These reactions differ in pathogenesis from anaphylactic reactions in that nonimmunologic factors cause the activation of the mast cells. Many chemicals and pharmaceuticals have been found to promote mast cell activation directly and may lead to anaphylactoid reactions. These include nonsteroidal anti-inflammatory drugs (NSAIDs), opiate analgesics, mannitol, iodinated radiographic contrast agents, and dextrans. Any process that activates complement may lead to an anaphylactoid response, in that C3a and C5a are potent initiators of mast cell activation. It should be stressed that distinguishing whether a reaction is anaphylactic or anaphylactoid in nature is of far less importance than recognizing and treating the clinical syndrome.

## PATHOPHYSIOLOGY

The primary preformed mediator released at degranulation of activated mast cells is histamine. Histamine is formed by decarboxylation of the amino acid histidine, and is bound to heparin in mast cell granules. Histamine binds to $H_1$-receptors, leading to an increase in cyclic guanosine monophosphate (cGMP), (which mediates smooth muscle contraction in bronchi and small intestine, pulmonary vasoconstriction, increased vascular permeability, increased leukocyte chemotaxis, and increased production of arachidonic acid metabolites. At $H_2$-receptors, histamine causes an increase in cyclic adenosine monophosphate (cAMP), which results in increased mucus production in airways, decreased leukocyte chemotaxis, and bronchodilation. Although some of the effects at $H_1$- and $H_2$-receptors tend to balance each other, the overall effects of histamine favor the development of peripheral vasodilation, increased capillary permeability, hypotension, bronchial and intestinal smooth muscle spasms, cardiac arrhythmias, and pruritus.

Mast cells also release preformed eosinophilic chemotactic factor of anaphylaxis (ECF-A) and neutrophilic chemotactic factor of anaphylaxis (NCF-A). These mediators serve to recruit eosinophils and neutrophils to the area, and explains the prominence of eosinophils commonly associated with histopathologic evaluation of hypersensitivity reactions. Eosinophils can release leukotriene $C_4$ ($LTC_4$) and platelet-activating factor (PAF), which are proinflammatory, along with the anti-inflammatory compounds histaminase and arylsulfatase B. Neutrophils may adhere to endothelial cells and can, if activated to undergo oxidative burst, damage these cells, causing increased prostaglandin synthesis, which further amplifies the inflammatory process.

Another important group of preformed mediators includes the serine proteases and kallekreins. Serine proteases may serve to activate complement and produce the anaphylatoxins C3a and C5a. These anaphylatoxins promote further release of histamine from mast cells, increased vascular permeability, and C5a is a potent chemoattractant for neutrophils. Kallikreins are proteases that act on kininogens to produce kinins, of which bradykinin is most important. Kinins contribute to increased vascular permeability, smooth muscle contraction, release of prostaglandins and leukotrienes, and stimulation of pain receptors.

At the same time that mast cell activation results in

degranulation and release of preformed mediators, there is induction of additional mediator synthesis. Arachidonic acid metabolites include the prostaglandins and leukotrienes, which are produced by activation of phospholipase $A_2$ during antigen binding to sensitized mast cells. The effects of the arachidonic acid metabolites varies greatly, but in general leads to increased vascular permeability, bronchoconstriction, and leukocyte chemotaxis.

Amplification of the inflammatory reaction associated with anaphylaxis occurs through involvement of the inflammatory cytokines and activation of the complement, coagulation, and fibrinolytic systems. Tumor necrosis factor (TNF), interleukin-1 (IL-1), and interferon promote vasodilation, procoagulant activity, secretion of chemotactic factors, increased cell adherence proteins on endothelial cells, and production of prostaglandins and chemotactic cytokines (see *CVT XI*, p 461). The complement and coagulation systems may also become activated by damage to endothelial cells with possible initiation of disseminated intravascular coagulation (DIC).

## CLINICAL PRESENTATION

The clinical presentation of an animal with anaphylaxis may be variable and will depend on the species involved; the sensitivity of the individual patient; and the type, amount, and route of antigen exposure. The reaction may occur locally or may occur systemically and lead to anaphylactic shock. In systemic involvement, the primary factor leading to shock is hypovolemia from increased vascular permeability and pooling of blood from vasodilation.

In the dog, the splanchnic viscera and liver are the major "shock organs." Dogs suffering from anaphylaxis commonly exhibit restlessness and excitement, followed by vomiting, diarrhea (which may be bloody), collapse, convulsions, coma, and finally death. It should be noted that this entire process may occur in less than an hour.

In cats, the respiratory system is the primary "shock organ." Cats often show facial pruritus initially, followed by ptyalism, vomiting, incoordination, collapse, and death. Cats suffer from severe bronchoconstriction, pulmonary hemorrhage, and laryngeal edema.

## TREATMENT

An animal presented with a history and clinical signs suggestive of systemic anaphylaxis should be considered a medical emergency. Circulatory collapse and the resulting deficits in oxygen delivery to tissues constitute the manifestations of anaphylactic shock, and initial emergent therapy should address these abnormalities. Fluid therapy and epinephrine are the initial therapies of choice for treatment of anaphylactic shock. Endotracheal intubation, oxygen therapy with ventilatory assistance (see *CVT XI*, p 98), and cardiopulmonary

cerebral resuscitation (CPCR; see "Cardiopulmonary Resuscitation," this volume, p 167) may need to be initiated in animals presenting with systemic anaphylaxis.

Epinephrine should be administered at 0.01 to 0.02 mg/kg IV, or the dosage may be doubled and administered through the endotracheal tube into the pulmonary airways if an intravenous line has not yet been established. In less severe cases, epinephrine may be administered IM or SC. The $\alpha$-adrenergic properties of epinephrine cause vasoconstriction, which leads to an increase in systemic vascular resistance, resulting in increased systemic arterial blood pressure, an increase in cardiac output due to increased venous return, and increased coronary blood flow. The $\beta$-adrenergic properties of epinephrine relieve bronchospasm and aid cardiac output through positive inotropic and chronotropic effects. Epinephrine administration also decreases further mediator release from mast cells by causing an increase in intracellular cAMP. Aminophylline (5 to 10 mg/kg IM or slowly IV) may be useful to aid in relief of bronchospasm. Both of these drugs can cause cardiac arrhythmias such that electrocardiographic monitoring is useful.

Fluid therapy should be aggressive in anaphylactic shock. Rapid administration of large volumes of crystalloid solutions are indicated, and a central venous line for central venous pressure (CVP) measurement can be very helpful in monitoring fluid therapy. If available, dextrans (6% Gentran 70, Baxter Healthcare) or hetastarch (Hespan, Dupont Critical Care) may offer significant advantages over crystalloids, providing a more rapid and prolonged hemodynamic response. These colloids can be administered at 5 ml/kg as an intravenous bolus, and can be repeated as needed up to a total daily dosage of 20 ml/kg IV.

After initial volume repletion and epinephrine administration, continued cardiac and respiratory monitoring should be used to help guide further therapy. Serial monitoring of packed cell volume (PCV) and total serum solids (TS), along with measurement of systemic arterial blood pressure and CVP monitoring can be helpful in titrating fluid therapy. If hemoconcentration and a low CVP remain a problem after initial volume loading, additional fluid therapy would be indicated. Lactated Ringer's or 0.9% NaCl can be administered at incremental dosages of 10 to 20 ml/kg IV, or additional boluses of colloids may be administered as recommended above. Optimal fluid therapy should attain a goal of a normal PCV and TS, and a CVP of 3 to 5 cm of $H_2O$. If hypotension remains a problem after adequate volume loading, additional circulatory support in the form of inotropic therapy would be indicated. Dopamine (2 to 10 $\mu$g/kg/min IV constant-rate infusion [CRI]) can be utilized as an inopressor to help maintain splanchnic circulation, cardiac output, and systemic arterial blood pressure.

Important adjunct therapy for systemic anaphylaxis includes the use of corticosteroids and antihistamines. It should be remembered, however, that these drugs may be helpful in controlling ongoing effects if persistent mediator release is occurring, but these agents are of little benefit in acute, life-threatening situations. As these agents can have a permissive effect on vasodilation or negative inotropic effect, these drugs should be used only after adequate treatment of circulatory collapse. Dexamethasone sodium phosphate can be administered at a dosage of 1 to 4 mg/kg IV, or prednisone sodium succinate (Solu-Delta-Cortef, Upjohn Company) may be administered at 10 to 25 mg/kg IV. Corticosteroids have multiple effects, including enhancement of $\beta$-adrenergic–receptor sensitivity, inhibition of histamine synthesis, and limitation of phospholipase $A_2$ activity. Antihistamines bind at histamine receptors and block the effects of histamine via competitive inhibition. Diphenhydramine hydrochloride (Benadryl, Parke-Davis) can be administered at 0.5 to 1.0 mg/kg IV to a total dose of 50 mg.

There are several important guidelines that may help to minimize the chance of precipitating an anaphylactic reaction. Administer all intravenous medications slowly. Always use care when administering medications that are known to cause histamine release or are associated with anaphylaxis, and use care with blood and blood product transfusions. It may be a consideration to pretreat an animal with antihistamines or corticosteroids when that animal has a history of previous reactions. Pretreatment will not prevent the reaction, but may blunt the physiologic response. Like many problems seen in small animal practice, the best treatment is prevention, but unfortunately, this is not always possible. A thorough history is helpful in alerting the clinician to potential situations or medications that might create a problem in an individual patient. Most important of all, it is important to be ready to react. Systemic anaphylaxis may occur extremely rapidly and often unexpectedly, and immediate aggressive therapy is paramount to a successful outcome.

## References and Suggested Reading

Frick OL: Immediate hypersensitivity. In Stites DP, Stobo JD, and Wells JV (eds): Basic and Clinical Immunology, 6th edition. Norwalk, CT, Appleton & Lange, 1987, p 197.
    A comprehensive and detailed text addressing the pathophysiology of type I hypersensitivity reactions. Includes definitions and descriptions of allergens, regulation of IgE antibody production, cell receptor and target cell reactions, mediators, autonomic nervous system involvement, and approach to treatment.
Haupt MT and Carlson RW: Anaphylactic and anaphylactoid reactions. In Shoemaker WC, Ayres SA, Grenvik AG, et al. (eds): Textbook of Critical Care Medicine, 2nd edition. Philadelphia, WB Saunders Co, 1989, p 993.
    The current theory and approach to anaphylaxis in human medicine.
Kapin MA and Ferguson JL: Hemodynamic and regional alterations in dog during anaphylactic challenge. Am J Physiol 249 (Heart Circ Physiol 18): H430, 1985.
    A clinical study of cardiac and circulatory changes associated with anaphylactic shock produced by horse serum sensitization and challenge in the dog.
Mueller DL and Noxon JO: Anaphylaxis: Pathophysiology and treatment. Compend Cont Educ Pract Vet 12:157, 1990.
    A general review of terminology, pathogenesis, and treatment of anaphylaxis in small animal practice.
Tizard I: Veterinary Immunology, An Introduction, 4th edition. Philadelphia, WB Saunders Co, 1992, p 335.
    An excellent comprehensive text on veterinary immunology.
Wilcke JR: Allergic drug reactions. In Kirk RW (ed): Current Veterinary Therapy IX. Philadelphia, WB Saunders Co, 1990, p 444.
    An overview of mechanisms and examples of types of reactions related to drug administration.

# CANINE IMMUNE-MEDIATED HEMOLYTIC ANEMIA

JORG BÜCHELER
and SUSAN M. COTTER
North Grafton, Massachusetts

Immune-mediated hemolytic anemia (IHA) is defined as an increased destruction of erythrocytes by autoantibodies. Affected dogs that have compensated for the increased red cell destruction by increased production may not be anemic, but typically they have overt, sometimes life-threatening hemolytic anemia. One of the most common hematologic disorders in dogs, IHA can be primary (idiopathic, or autoimmune hemolytic anemia), can coexist with another disease (secondary IHA), or can follow administration of certain drugs.

## PATHOGENESIS

All breeds may be affected, but a possible predisposition may exist for old English sheep dogs, cocker spaniels, poodles, Lhasa apsos, Shih Tzus, and several other breeds. Studies in rodents have shown that genetic factors influence the susceptibility to autoimmunization and its clinical manifestations. This is supported by the high occurrence of IHA in certain families of humans and dogs. The disease is more frequently seen in intact or spayed female dogs (sex predominance up to 4:1). A correlation between the female sex and autoimmunity has long been recognized in many species, but the pathogenic mechanisms of female sex hormones are still not clear. The administration of androgens or antiestrogens can, however, prevent or diminish autoimmune reactions in females. Even though IHA occurs at any age, the disease is most commonly observed in middle-aged dogs. Interestingly, IHA has been observed in dogs with increased antibody titers to viral antigens (particularly parvovirus and distemper virus), recent viral infections, or occasionally recent vaccinations, which suggests that viral antigens may be implicated in the cause of some cases of IHA. A recent study in Philadelphia found 40% of all cases of IHA to occur in May and June (Klag, Giger, and Shofer, 1993). This clustering of clinical cases is interesting and opens the discussion of correlations to seasonal exposures or iatrogenic manipulations.

Immune-mediated hemolytic anemia is characterized by a shortened red cell survival time with an immune response that destroys red cells by coating them with immunoglobulin or complement. Two types of IHA, warm and cold reacting, can be identified on the basis of laboratory studies. By far the majority of cases of IHA are mediated by red cell coating with incomplete and warm-type autoantibodies. Warm antibodies react optimally at temperatures between 35°C and 40°C, and incomplete antibodies are so called because they do not agglutinate red cells in saline. Most warm incomplete antibodies detected by the direct antiglobulin test (DAT) are immunoglobulin G (IgG), but may rarely be IgA or IgM. Cold antibodies react optimally at temperatures below 30°C and are virtually always IgM. Those antibodies may cause agglutination or hemolysis of red cells at lower body temperatures in the periphery of the body such as the ear tips, paws, and tail. Cold agglutinin disease in dogs has been observed very rarely and will not be discussed further.

Red cells may be destroyed by intravascular or extravascular hemolysis. Intravascular hemolysis represents a type II immunologic injury mediated by complement bound to IgM or high titers of IgG antibodies. The initiation of events that culminate in the deposition of $C_3b$ on the red cell surface requires at least two IgG molecules bound in close proximity on the membrane. If complement activation continues to completion, the cells may be lysed directly intravascularly. In contrast to IgG antibodies, IgM antibodies bind complement easily and may overwhelm the protective complement-inhibiting mechanisms and lead to intravascular hemolysis. However, the occurrence of IgM autoantibodies is rare, and their titer often is too low to overcome the protective threshold of the complement system. In the usual case of IgG incomplete warm antibodies, adherence to Fc receptors on macrophages and monocytes results in phagocytosis and lysis of the sensitized red cells. This extravascular hemolysis usually takes place in the spleen, since the spleen's unique hemoconcentrating circulatory system allows for a prolonged and intimate contact between sensitized red cells and Fc and complement receptors on the membranes of the abundant splenic macrophages. Complement components on the red cell membrane in addition to IgG molecules rapidly accelerate the rate of destruction by macrophages. Immunoglobulin A incomplete warm antibodies are rarely found on canine red cells, and the mechanism of hemolysis is thought to be similar to that with IgG antibodies.

The severity of hemolysis caused by red cell auto-antibodies depends on its titer, the avidity for the autoantigen, the ability to fix complement (IgG subclass), the antigen density on the membrane, and the state of activation of the macrophage system. Of human patients with warm antibody IHA, 97% have IgG on the red cell membrane. Several studies in dogs with IHA have shown that most have either IgG or IgG and complement-coated red cell membranes, with the latter being more common (Slappendel, 1979). Complement components alone were present on the red cells of over 50% of dogs with mild anemia secondary to other coexisting diseases. It was concluded that the finding of complement components alone on red cells is common in many diseases and rarely associated with significant hemolytic anemia. Complement components can be deposited on the membrane by IgM molecules that subsequently elute from the membrane, or by circulating immune complexes that may adhere nonspecifically to the red cell. The mechanisms that trigger the immune response leading to red cell destruction are poorly understood. At the end of its life, every red cell undergoes changes that trigger an immune response; namely, phagocytosis by a macrophage. The failure of immunologic tolerance that results in premature destruction of red cells in IHA is poorly understood and is probably multifactorial in origin.

## DIAGNOSIS

When a dog is presented with signs of hemolytic anemia, one must rule out other causes of hemolysis or secondary IHA, such as infections (babesiosis, ehrlichiosis, leishmaniasis, hemobartonellosis; dirofilariasis); neoplasms (lymphoma, hemangiosarcoma), granulomatous diseases; splenic torsion; inherited hemolytic disorders such as pyruvate kinase or phosphofructokinase deficiencies; and recent exposure to drugs, toxins, and vaccines. In cases with accompanying signs such as polyarthritis, skin lesions, or glomerulonephritis, lupus erythematosus or other autoimmune disorders should be considered. The autoimmune blood cell destruction will often resolve once an underlying condition or drug has been identified and treated or removed.

The clinical and laboratory features associated with canine IHA have been described in detail (Switzer and Jain, 1981; Cotter, 1992). Dogs with acute IHA usually present with weakness, tachycardia, tachypnea, mucous membrane pallor, and sometimes icterus and splenomegaly. A complete blood count (CBC) often reveals a regenerative anemia with reticulocytosis, spherocytosis, anisocytosis, polychromasia, and a sometimes dramatic reactive leukocytosis with neutrophilia and a left shift. Thrombocytopenia may be present due to antibodies recognizing both red cell and platelet antigens, or due to disseminated intravascular coagulation (DIC). Occasionally schistocytes and nucleated red cells are observed. The serum chemistry profile often shows elevations in serum bilirubin, lactate dehydrogenase (LDH) and alanine aminotransferase (ALT) levels. In cases with intravascular hemolysis, hemoglobinemia and hemoglobinuria may develop. The bone marrow usually shows signs of active regeneration with erythroid hyperplasia, a few plasma cells, and occasionally erythrophagocytosis. The occurrence of spherocytes is highly suggestive of IHA, since other disease conditions causing spherocytosis are rare. Macrophages sometimes ingest opsonized red cells only partially, or proteolytic enzymes on their surface may digest bits of the red cell membranes, producing a spherocyte. Spherocytes are more rigid and fragile, and are prone to removal by splenic macrophages.

The absence of reticulocytosis does not exclude the diagnosis of IHA. In one study, 33% of dogs with IHA initially presented without a reticulocytosis (Klag, Giger, and Shofer, 1993). Reticulocytopenia may indicate a recent onset of hemolysis within the past 3 days, or it may be caused by the destruction of young red cells in the marrow. A persistent reticulocytopenia warrants a bone marrow aspirate to rule out other primary bone marrow diseases. The finding of saline autoagglutination is considered to be diagnostic for IHA and makes the DAT unnecessary. Autoagglutination is secondary to bridging antibodies that overcome the negative membrane zeta-potential that normally separates red cells.

The diagnosis of IHA is established by demonstrating the presence of antibodies on the surface of red cells and by ruling out other causes of anemia. The DAT uses polyvalent pooled serum containing antibodies against all immunoglobulins and complement that bind to coated red cells and lead to bridging, which can be observed. The DAT is positive in approximately 60% of all cases of IHA, depending on the test conditions. A negative DAT in patients with the clinical picture of IHA may be due to a low number of immunoglobulin molecules on the red cell, since the DAT under normal conditions detects only cases with more than 200 to 500 molecules on the red cell membrane. As few as ten IgG molecules on the membrane can cause hemolysis with subsequent anemia (Foerster, 1993). Other causes for a negative DAT include poor test systems, spontaneous antibody elution during washing (low-affinity antibodies), incomplete washing, inadequate dilution of reagents (prozone effects), ongoing immunosuppressive treatment, or incorrect diagnosis.

## THERAPY

### Supportive Care

The clinical course of IHA varies from mild and almost inapparent, to fulminant and fatal hemolysis. In these severe cases it is crucial to avoid secondary complications that may be fatal. Coagulation profiles should be done periodically to detect early signs of DIC from release of thromboplastic substances by hemolyzed red cells. The sudden occurrence of tachypnea or respiratory distress should warrant a work-up for pulmonary thromboembolism (see *CVT XI*, p 139). Klein, Dow, and Rosychuk, (1989) found that 32% of dogs that died

during an episode of IHA had pulmonary thromboemboli on necropsy. The presence of pulmonary thromboembolism seemed to be associated with high serum bilirubin levels, the presence of intravenous catheters, and a high number of transfusions (see *CVT XI*, p 137). Pulmonary thromboembolism may be caused in part by endothelial damage by circulating immune complexes, prednisone therapy, and the release of thromboplastic substances secondary to hemolysis. When pulmonary thromboembolism is present, the blood gas analysis may show hypoxemia and normocapnia. Thoracic radiographs can remain normal or may show an increased interstitial pattern and a small amount of pleural effusion. A ventilation-perfusion scan may aid in the diagnosis, but the equipment is not readily available and the procedure is technically difficult. Dogs with severe hemolysis should be given intravenous fluids at a maintenance dose to ensure adequate renal perfusion, since the by-products of hemolysis such as membrane fragments potentially may cause renal damage thought to be secondary to vasoconstriction and hypoperfusion rather than the direct tubular damage as seen in humans.

### Transfusions

Transfusions may be needed if the anemia is severe or has occurred acutely and before physiologic compensation has occurred. Some clinicians believe that transfusions may accelerate the hemolytic crisis, enhance antibody production; precipitate DIC, pulmonary thromboembolism, or renal failure; and suppress the regenerative response of the bone marrow. However, hypoxia seen in severely anemic dogs may cause serious and potentially fatal multiorgan damage as evidenced by ventricular arrhythmias, centrilobular hepatic necrosis, and renal tubular necrosis. Because of these complications, dogs with signs of hypoxia such as tachypnea, tachycardia, and weakness require red cell support until other treatment modalities reduce the hemolysis. The autoantibody is usually directed against red cell antigens present on most canine red cells, which may make typing and crossmatching difficult or impossible. If the patient cannot be typed, DEA-1–negative blood should be given (see *CVT XI*, p 104). It is likely that the transfused cells will survive or be destroyed at the same rate as the patient's own cells. Packed red cells are preferred, since they minimize circulatory overload in a patient already compromised by a high cardiac output state. It may be more beneficial to give several smaller transfusions than one large volume. The volume of red cells to be transfused should be calculated to raise the hematocrit into a range (usually over 16%) that improves signs of hypoxia.

When signs of DIC are present, fresh frozen plasma should be administered at 10 ml/kg IV or at a volume needed to normalize prothrombin time (PT) and activated partial thromboplastin time (APTT). The use of heparin in dogs already hemorrhaging from DIC is controversial, since it may worsen bleeding, and should not be given unless clotting factors are given as well. Heparin may be most beneficial in severe IHA as a prophylactic measure before bleeding occurs to decrease the potentially harmful effects of thromboplastic substances released from hemolyzed red cells and to minimize the danger of developing pulmonary thromboembolism. Some clinicians routinely recommend this prophylactic use of heparin, although controlled studies are lacking and the practice is not universally accepted.

## Corticosteroids

Corticosteroids usually have a rapid favorable effect on hemolysis, due to a pronounced anti-inflammatory and immunosuppressive action that suppresses both lymphocyte proliferation and interleukin-2 (IL-2) production. T-cell function, natural killer (NK) cell function, monocyte maturation and macrophage antigen handling, chemotaxis, and cytotoxic action are all impaired. The synthesis of many inflammatory mediators is diminished, and microvascular and lysosomal integrity is restored. High doses of corticosteroids eventually suppress IgG production, but this occurs too slowly to account for the rapid improvement often seen clinically. If hemolysis is severe, prednisone at 2 mg/kg/day may be given for 2 weeks, initially IV or IM and later PO. For maintenance, treatment is continued at 1 mg/kg PO every other day as improvement occurs. Treatment may be discontinued 2 to 4 months after the first uncomplicated episode of IHA as indicated by the patient's response, although some dogs will require treatment for a much longer time. The CBC should be periodically rechecked during and after treatment for early signs of relapse. Since corticosteroids may improve red cell survival by interfering with macrophage recognition of antibody and complement-coated red cells, the DAT may remain positive in the face of an improved red cell survival for a period of several weeks. Corticosteroids usually lead to a rapid improvement of the clinical signs of IHA, but reticulocytosis may be delayed, particularly if antibodies are directed against red cell precursors. The objective of initial treatment is to stabilize the patient and the hematocrit, since the rate of increase to normal may be slow. Most dogs can be maintained with supportive care and prednisone until the hematocrit begins to rise.

## Cytotoxic Agents

More aggressive therapy should be initiated in autoagglutinating or nonregenerative forms of IHA considering the high mortality of these conditions. No clinical studies have yet proven a benefit of combination therapy over prednisone alone or demonstrated the most optimal drug combination for specific disease states. The most commonly used cytotoxic agents are azathioprine (Imuran, Burroughs Wellcome Co) and cyclophosphamide (Cytoxan, Bristol Myers Oncology Division). Both cause a generalized suppression of the immune system by inhibiting cell division and cytokine production. The thiopurine azathioprine has its main effect on T-cell function, while the alkylating agents such as cyclophosphamide act on both T and B cells. Cytotoxic agents have sometimes been added to corticosteroids when a rise in hematocrit is not observed after a few days, but probably they should be reserved for dogs with fulminant intravascular hemolysis, autoagglutination, or those that require repeated transfusions or have persistent reticulocytopenia. Azathioprine is used initially at a dose of 2 mg/kg/day PO. This should be reduced to 1 mg/kg/day after the first 7 to 10 days. Adverse effects are usually mild but can include myelosuppression, gastroenteritis, pancreatitis, and elevation of liver enzymes. Cyclophosphamide can be used at a dose of 2 mg/kg/day IV or PO for 4 days, no treatment for 3 days, and the cycle repeated. Adverse effects include myelosuppression and rarely hemorrhagic cystitis. There is no known difference in efficacy or onset of action between azathioprine and cyclophosphamide. Treatment of dogs with azathioprine significantly suppressed the lymphocyte blastogenic response, whereas treatment with cyclophosphamide did not (Ogilvie, Felsburg, and Harris, 1988). The dosage of cytotoxic agents should be individually adjusted. If the neutrophil count drops below $3000/\mu l$, the drug is discontinued until the count returns to normal, and treatment is then reinitiated at a lower dose. Cytotoxic drugs should be tapered slowly over several months in recovering dogs to monitor for early signs of relapse. Their rapid withdrawal may lead to a period of rebound hyperimmune responsiveness.

## Danazol

Danazol (Danocrine, Winthrop Pharmaceuticals) is an attenuated androgen that has been successfully used in human immune-mediated disorders. It acts as an immune modulator by normalizing the suppressor/helper T-cell ratio, activating suppressor T cells, and downregulating Fc receptors on macrophages. The drug is also incorporated into the red cell membrane, stabilizing the membrane and rendering the red cells more resistant to osmotic stress and hemolysis. Preliminary data in human patients with IHA indicate that danazol is effective, and is considered a valuable alternative to prednisone therapy. Moreover, danazol has a sparing effect on the need for corticosteroids, avoiding the adverse effects of long-term corticosteroid use, such as polyuria, weight gain, and increased susceptibility to infections, and may be used by itself to maintain remission. Additionally, some human patients treated with danazol have had more sustained remissions after discontinuation of the drug than patients treated with other drugs. Danazol has been reported rarely to cause weight gain, lethargy, masculinization, and mild elevations of liver enzymes. A few cases described in the veterinary literature support a beneficial role of danazol for the treatment of canine IHA, but controlled clinical trials have not yet been done. Initial treatment should consist of prednisone alone or in combination with danazol (10 mg/kg/day PO), since corticosteroids have a more rapid onset of action. Once the anemia improves, the corticosteroid dose can be gradually tapered and eventually discontinued. When remission has been maintained by danazol alone, the dose can be lowered to 5 mg/kg/day. The dose of danazol may be tapered after 2 to 3 months of normal hemograms, with frequent monitoring for relapse.

## Intravenous Gamma Globulin

Intravenous human gamma globulins (Gamimune, Miles Inc.) are produced by alcohol precipitation of pooled plasma, and are structurally and functionally intact IgG molecules. Several small studies investigating the use of intravenous gamma globulin (IVGG) in human patients with IHA indicate a high response rate to treatment. The mechanism of action of IVGG is unknown, but most responders were hypogammaglobulinemic before treatment. Initially it was believed that most IVGG effects were due to competition for Fc receptors between the IVGG and the autoantibodies, but recent studies indicate that the main benefit is secondary to immune modulation. Intravenous gamma globulin also may enhance functionally defined T-suppressor cells and impair Fc receptor–mediated phagocytosis by macrophages, NK-cell activity, and additionally may lead to a decreased production of inflammatory cytokines such as IL-1 and promote the release of immune-modulatory mediators. Adverse effects in humans may include anaphylactic reactions and an unexplained, reversible increase in serum creatinine concentrations. Scott-Moncrieff et al. (1993) recently administered human IVGG at 0.5 to 1.5 gm/kg as a 12-hr IV infusion to five dogs with nonregenerative IHA that were unresponsive to corticosteroids with or without cyclophosphamide. A marked increase in hematocrit and reticulocyte count occurred in all dogs as well as a normalization of abnormal lymphocyte blastogenic responses and lymphocyte subset distribution. Two dogs showed a long-term complete resolution of IHA, one dog had a long-term partial remission, and two dogs had a transient improvement of anemia and again responded to a repeated infusion of IVGG. No adverse effects were observed in the treated dogs. Whether alloantibody formation would preclude long-term treatment has not been established.

## Cyclosporine

The role of cyclosporine (Sandimmune, Sandoz Pharmaceuticals) has been studied only in a small number of human cases, but some responses have been seen. Cyclosporine selectively inhibits the antigenic activation of T-helper cells by interfering with the production of IL-2, γ-interferon, and the expression of IL-2 receptors by these cells. Cyclosporine suppresses T-helper cell counts, while the number of T-suppressor cells remains normal. Cyclosporine has been given to dogs at a dose of 10 to 20 mg/kg/day IM or PO for 5 days, discontinued for 2 days, and readministered at 5 mg/kg for 5 days. The lower dose is then continued on a 5-days-on, 2-days-off cycle as long as clinically indicated. Adverse effects are usually mild and include gastrointestinal irritation, gingival hypertrophy, papillomatosis, hirsutism, and local irritation after intramuscular injection. Nephrotoxicosis and hepatotoxicosis are rare in the dog. Absorption of the drug from the gastrointestinal tract has been variable, suggesting that at least initially, parenteral administration should be used. If the drug is given orally, monitoring of serum drug levels will ensure adequate treatment.

## Splenectomy

Because the destruction of red cells by IgG incomplete warm autoantibodies takes place mainly in the spleen, splenectomy has been a successful treatment in some recurring or resistant cases. Dogs with evidence of extravascular red cell destruction or splenomegaly are most likely to benefit. Splenectomy may also make it possible to decrease the dose of immunosuppressive drugs in dogs that require continuous treatment to prevent relapse of IHA. Splenectomy may increase the risk of infections with red cell parasites and certain bacteria.

## Experimental Treatments

Plasmapheresis removes autoantibodies and complement components from the plasma. Some human patients unresponsive to other therapy have benefitted from plasmapheresis. A small number of dogs treated with plasmapheresis showed improvement, but they were receiving concurrent immunosuppressive therapy, which makes the interpretation difficult. The reason for inconsistent response to plasmapheresis may be that more than half of the IgG is in the extravascular space and cannot be cleared with a single treatment.

Responses in a few human patients with IHA have been reported following infusion with vincristine-laden platelets, total lymphoid irradiation, antilymphocyte serum, autoantigen-toxin complexes, and dietary therapy (with caloric restriction and supplementation with eicosapentaenoic acids). The benefits of these treatment modalities are unproven.

## PROGNOSIS

Several studies attempting to elicit prognostic factors in IHA reported that a higher mortality was observed in cases that had a low hematocrit on presentation and required a transfusion on the first day in the hospital, and in cases with a serum bilirubin concentration greater than 10 mg/dl (Hohenhaus 1992, Klag et al., 1993). Patients with autoagglutination, intravascular hemolysis, and DIC on presentation also have a poor prognosis (Cotter, 1992). These data most likely reflect the fact that the mortality is directly correlated to the severity and rapidity of hemolysis. There may be also a prognostic correlation between reticulocytosis and improved survival. The overall mortality of IHA has been reported to be between 20 to 40%, but it may be over 80% in fulminant cases. Large controlled studies are needed to compare commonly used immunosuppressive drugs. New treatment regimens including danazol, IVGG, and cyclosporine in corticosteroid-resistant cases may play a promising role in the management of IHA in the future.

## References and Suggested Reading

Cotter SM: Autoimmune hemolytic anemia in dogs. Compend Cont Educ Pract Vet 14:53, 1992.
  *A review of clinical and laboratory features and case management.*
Foerster J: Autoimmune hemolytic anemia. *In* Lee GR, et al (eds): *Wintrobe's* *Clinical Hematology*, 9th edition. Philadelphia, Lea & Febiger, 1993, p 1170.
  *A current review of IHA and its treatment in human medicine.*
Hohenhaus AE: Canine autoimmune hemocytic anemia: Predisposing and prognostic factors. *Proc 10th ACVIM Forum* San Diego, 1992 p 146.
  *A study about predisposing factors and prognostic indicators in IHA.*
Klag AR, Giger U, and Shofer FS: Idiopathic immune-mediated hemolytic anemia in dogs: 42 cases (1986–1990). J Am Vet Med Assoc 202:783, 1993.
  *A case review of IHA.*
Klein MK, Dow SW, and Rosychuk RAW: Pulmonary thromboembolism associated with immune-mediated hemolytic anemia in dogs: 10 cases (1982–1987). J Am Vet Med Assoc 195:246, 1989.
  *A study evaluating the predisposing factors involved in the pathogenesis of pulmonary thromboembolism in IHA.*
Ogilvie GK, Felsburg PJ, and Harris CW: Short-term effects of cyclophosphamide and azathioprine on selected aspects of the canine blastogenic response. Vet Immunol Immunopathol 18:119, 1988.
  *A study comparing the effects of 2 cytotoxic drugs in dogs.*
Scott-Moncrieff JC, Reagan WJ, Glickman LT, et al: Treatment of immune mediated anemia in dogs with intravenous human immunoglobulin (absr). *Proc 11th ACVIM Forum.* Washington, 1993, p 128.
  *A study evaluating the effects of IVGG in five dogs.*
Slappendel RJ: The diagnostic significance of the direct antiglobulin test (DAT) in anemic dogs. Vet Immunol Immunopathol 1:49, 1979.
  *An evaluation of the frequency of different proteins on the red cell surface.*
Switzer JW and Jain NC: Autoimmune hemolytic anemia in dogs and cats. Vet Clin North Am 11:405, 1981.
  *A review of epidemiology, clinical findings, and treatment of IHA.*

# APPROACH TO THE HYPOTHERMIC PATIENT

ALBERT H. AHN
*North Grafton, Massachusetts*

Hypothermia is a pathologic condition that occurs in veterinary patients when core body temperature falls below the physiologically normal range for the species. Maintenance of normal temperature is critical for optimal function of enzyme systems, and this homeostatic process requires a balance between heat production and heat loss by the animal. All organ systems in an animal are affected by this condition and profound hypothermia has been associated with high mortality.

## THERMOREGULATION

The hypothalamus functions as the thermostat for an animal and is responsible for coordinating activities directed at maintaining normal core body temperature (i.e., set point). Responses to cold environmental conditions originate from the posterior hypothalamus, while exposure to excessive heat stimulates responses originating from the anterior hypothalamus. Homeostasis is maintained by complex interactions involving autonomic, somatic, endocrine, and behavioral responses to environmental temperature fluctuations.

The major source of heat production in the body is skeletal muscle activity, with the assimilation of food and the basal metabolic processes of the body representing secondary sources. Excessive heat production without appropriate dissipation can lead to hyperthermia (see *CVT XI*, pp 143–146).

Loss of body heat occurs through several mechanisms. Conduction represents exchange of heat between two objects with different temperatures, with transfer of thermal energy to the object with the lower temperature. Convection, the movement of heated gas or liquid, can amplify the heat loss effects of conduction as warmed air moves away from the animal and is replaced with colder air. Radiation represents another factor involved in heat loss through the transfer of heat by an infrared electromagnetic process between two objects at different temperatures. Evaporation of water from the skin, mucous membranes, and respiratory passages also represents a significant source of heat loss. Panting in dogs and cats takes advantage of this phenomenon, since the rapid, shallow breathing serves to increase evaporation from the mouth and airways while not significantly altering the alveolar gas composition. Minute amounts of heat are lost through urination and defecation.

Animals will attempt to optimize heat production and minimize heat loss to prevent hypothermia in a cold environment. Heat conservation can be mediated behaviorally by seeking shelter from the cold. Reflex responses are key to the heat conservation and production process:

1. Piloerection minimizes loss of heat to the environment by creating a zone of trapped air that acts as an additional layer of insulation.

2. Vasoconstriction in peripheral tissues directs blood away from exposed surfaces (feet, ears, and face).

3. Shivering, an involuntary heat-generating response by the skeletal muscles to cold conditions.

Animals that have acclimated to the cold environment are better able to conserve heat, as thick fur minimizes heat loss due to convection and conduction.

## PATHOPHYSIOLOGY

The degree of organ dysfunction is dependent upon the duration and severity of hypothermia. Increased circulating catecholamine concentrations and vasoconstriction in peripheral tissues initially lead to increases in heart rate, cardiac output, and mean systemic arterial blood pressure in response to mild (1° to 2°C) decreases in body temperature. Subsequently, with progressive duration or severity of hypothermia, heart rate and cardiac output decline. In a study involving dogs, when the core body temperature dropped to 25°C, cardiac output fell by 50% and heart rate decreased 20%.

The electrocardiogram of animals with hypothermia demonstrates abnormalities that are a result of generalized slowing of conduction. Bradycardia resistant to the effects of anticholinergic administration and prolongation of the P-R, Q-T, and QRS intervals and T-wave inversion can be commonly seen in hypothermic animals. An Osborn, or J, wave represents a characteristic and acute elevation of the ST segment, and may be seen commonly in human patients with body temperatures between 32° and 33°C (Elder, 1989). Its presence in dogs has only rarely been documented. Ventricular fibrillation and cardiac arrest are commonly seen in patients with severe hypothermia (temperature <28°C).

Respiratory system changes with hypothermia are typified by tachypnea in the early phases and later, in the presence of progressive cooling of core temperature, there is central and reflex-mediated respiratory depression that leads to decreased respiratory rate and tidal volume. At temperatures below 25°C, decreased vagal activity can lead to a 50% increase in anatomic dead space and a 28% increase in physiologic dead space (Elder, 1989), with a resultant decrease in effective alveolar ventilation.

With hypothermic conditions of 25°C or less, mucociliary activity progressively decreases, while bronchiolar and alveolar epithelial edema develops. These processes further impair respiratory function by promoting bronchiolar mucus plugs and atelectasis as well as decreasing diffusion of oxygen across alveolar surfaces. The resultant conditions put patients surviving a hypothermic crisis at greater risk of developing bronchitis and bronchopneumonia. The aforementioned factors of impaired pulmonary oxygen exchange accompanying shivering and decreased peripheral tissue perfusion contribute to the development of clinically significant lactic acidosis in hypothermic animals.

Compromised oxygen delivery to tissues in hypothermic animals is further exacerbated by a temperature-related shift of the oxygen-hemoglobin dissociation curve to the left. This effect leads to decreased release of bound oxygen from the hemoglobin molecule at various partial pressures of oxygen in tissues.

"Cold diuresis" develops with progressive hypothermia and can result in the development of severe dehydration in these patients. This phenomenon can be seen in animals with a 2° to 3°C drop in core temperature. Cold diuresis results from (1) peripheral vasoconstriction, which transiently increases glomerular filtration rate; (2) the presence of hyperglycemia; and (3) decreased renal tubular cell reabsorptive function, which promotes diuresis through increased excretion of sodium, glucose, and water (Lee-Parritz and Pavletic, 1992).

Abnormalities in hematologic, biochemical, and coagulation parameters occur with hypothermia. Isotonic dehydration from cold diuresis may cause elevation of the hematocrit, hemoglobin concentration, and total serum solids. Leukopenia and thrombocytopenia may be seen with splenic and perivascular sequestration of white blood cells (WBCs) and platelets. Hyperglycemia and ketosis may develop, as hypothermia promotes stress-induced gluconeogenesis, and depresses insulin release and inhibits its action on peripheral receptors. Disseminated intravascular coagulation (DIC) can develop after prolonged hypoperfusion of the extremities as a result of microvascular disruption and activation of clotting cascades.

Intestinal motility decreases with hypothermia, and multiple punctate erosions have been described (Wischnevsky ulcers) in the stomach, ileum, and colon of human patients. These erosions probably result from the effects of the vasoactive amines histamine and serotonin released in response to vascular compromise to the gastrointestinal tract. Gastrointestinal blood loss associated with the development of these erosions is most often minimal.

The liver is relatively resistant to the effects of cold injury; however, glycogen depletion does occur early in hypothermia and there is a generalized decrease in metabolic function that leads to depressed conjugation and detoxification activity. Additionally, the development of mild to severe acute pancreatitis has been associated with hypothermic injury in human patients.

Depending on the degree of hypothermia, the neurologic signs in an animal may be mild (lethargy, increased muscle tone, shivering), moderate (stupor, incoordination, loss of shivering reflex, unconsciousness), or severe (collapse, agonal respirations, fixed and dilated pupils). These clinical signs are attributable to a combination of decreased neuronal enzymatic function, hemoconcentration (increased blood viscosity), decreased oxygen delivery, and vascular changes that can all affect neurologic status.

## DIAGNOSIS

Animals exposed to extreme cold, particularly without an acclimation period, are at risk. In the absence of known exposure to low environmental temperatures, pursuit of predisposing systemic disease along with administration of corrective therapy becomes paramount for the clinician (Table 1).

Hypothyroidism alters thermoregulatory ability by decreasing the hypothalamic set point and thereby decreasing endogenous heat production. Other systemic diseases should be suspected in the absence of exposure, anesthetic and surgical events, or hypothyroidism.

Anesthesia and surgical intervention pose major risks for the development of hypothermia in animals. Elimination of skeletal muscle activity, depression of metabolic processes, impairment of thermoregulation, and loss of heat through breathing of nonhumidified, cold anesthetic gases can result in hypothermia. Preparation of the skin over the surgical site with alcohol increases heat loss by evaporation. Surgical procedures, particularly those involving open body cavities, contribute greatly to the development of hypothermia. Wrapping distal extremities of the animal with insulating materials, using warm water blankets or water bottles, minimizing surgical time, and careful usage of heat lamps during anesthetic recovery will help decrease the likelihood of hypothermia in surgical patients.

## PHYSICAL EXAMINATION

On presentation, the animal may have diminished consciousness. Shivering is often present, although it may be absent in cases of profound hypothermia. Respirations may be shallow and infrequent. Tachycardia or bradycardia may be present in conjunction with poor to absent peripheral arterial pulses and cold extremities. The pupils may be dilated and reflexes diminished or delayed. Confirmation of the hypothermic condition is made through the use of a rectal thermometer. In cases of severe hypothermia, special low temperature thermometers need to be employed to accurately and serially assess the patient's temperature.

**Table 1.** *Causes of Hypothermia*

*Iatrogenic*
 Surgery
 Anesthesia
 Overzealous treatment of hyperthermia

*Systemic Disease*
 Cardiac
 Hypothyroidism
 Sepsis
 Chronic renal failure
 Hypoadrenocorticism
 Malnutrition
 Hypoglycemia
 Neurologic
  Head trauma
  Neoplasia
  Cerebrovascular accident

*Environmental*
 Exposure
 Trauma

## MANAGEMENT

The cornerstone of clinical treatment of hypothermia rests with restoring the core body temperature to the normal range. It has been stated in human medicine that "No one is dead until warm and dead!" (Reuler, 1978). This is in reference to the inaccuracy that may occur with respect to organ function assessment in the hypothermic patient. Rewarming techniques can be divided into two major categories: external and internal.

External rewarming can be performed using passive or active methods. The former is most appropriate for the mildly hypothermic animal and consists of removing the patient from the cold environment and wrapping with blankets or other insulatory materials to allow rewarming of the animal through generation and conservation of its own heat. The use of warm water bottles, circulating warm water blankets, electric heating pads, and immersion in warm water tubs represent active external rewarming techniques that augment the patient's warming capacity.

Internal or core rewarming techniques are generally reserved for use in animals with severe hypothermia. These options may include (1) administration of warm intravenous fluids, (2) peritoneal dialysis using dialysate heated to 43°C, and (3) colonic or gastric lavage or both using warm physiologic saline solutions. Warm peritoneal dialysis is an easy technique to perform and rapidly increases the body core temperature in the patient. Using a diagnostic peritoneal dialysis catheter (Baxter Healthcare Corporation, Deerfield, IL), warmed dialysate (10 to 20 ml/kg) is instilled into the abdomen and exchanged every 30 min. This procedure may be repeated several times until the rectal temperature registers at least 36°C (96°F). With colonic lavage, the inability to procure accurate rectal temperatures subsequent to administration represents a potential disadvantage. The use of infrared otic thermometers (Exergen Corporation, Natick, MA) can circumvent this situation. Care must be exercised in administering warm fluids by gavage, as hypothermic animals are at increased risk for development of aspiration pneumonia from vomition as a result of hypothermia-induced ileus and diminished laryngeal reflex and airway functions.

## COMPLICATIONS

A number of complications may develop during the treatment of hypothermic patients. During the rewarming process, the extremities that have been subjected to increased vasoconstriction to preserve the core temperature begin to vasodilate and sequestered pools of cold blood begin shifting to the central circulation. Furthermore, relatively warm core blood is now perfusing the previously cold peripheral tissues and is cooled in the process. For these two reasons, patients may demonstrate the phenomenon of "afterdrop" (a decrease in body temperature during the rewarming period) even though the cold stress has been removed. The presence of metabolic acidosis should be suspected and measurement of blood gases or total carbon dioxide content, if available, will allow for assessment of the metabolic acid-base status and help determine whether intervention with sodium bicarbonate administration is indicated.

Since the function of hepatic metabolic enzyme systems has been decreased by cold injury, it is important to recognize that metabolism of any administered medications is likely to be prolonged, even after rewarming is complete. This consideration extends to intravenous fluid selection, and it should be recognized that hepatic conversion of lactate to bicarbonate for buffering purposes is likely to be affected.

The neurologic status of hypothermic animals should be closely monitored during rewarming. Deterioration of mentation or development of seizures may indicate increased intracranial pressure from osmotic gradients (fluctuating serum glucose concentrations), ischemic injury, or cold-induced edema. Administration of mannitol (Mannitol injection, USP 25%, American Regent Laboratories, Inc) (0.25 to 2 gm/kg over 15 to 60 min IV; repeat in 6 hr if necessary) and corticosteroids: prednisolone sodium succinate (Solu-Delta-Cortef, The Upjohn Company) 15 to 30 mg/kg IV or dexamethasone sodium phosphate (Dexamethasone Sodium Phosphate, The Butler Company) 4 to 6 mg/kg IV and ventilatory support to decrease $PaCO_2$ may be warranted.

The development of cardiac arrhythmias is a major concern during and after the hypothermic crisis. Continuous electrocardiographic monitoring should be performed and the development of aberrant rhythms should be addressed appropriately (see "Cardiac Arrhythmias in Systemic Disease," this volume, p 161).

Fluid therapy considerations are crucial in the treatment of the hypovolemic, hypothermic patient. Monitoring urine output and central venous pressures (CVP) will allow "fine tuning" of volume support as well as alerting the clinician to the development of any acute renal insufficiency. Serum creatinine and blood urea nitrogen (BUN) concentrations should be assessed serially following rewarming to ensure normal renal function. As most patients will receive aggressive fluid administration rates, it is wise to select warm fluids to amplify the rewarming efforts.

After restoration of normothermia, continued temperature monitoring and supportive treatment are necessary to prevent hyperthermia from overaggressive treatment and to avoid recurrent hypothermia, particularly in the debilitated patient whose thermoregulatory abilities may be compromised. The use of radiant heat lamps, and electric and warm water blankets, is common practice in the latter instance. When using these devices, it is imperative that the patient be vigilantly monitored and turned regularly to avoid the development of cutaneous burns. The placement of heat lamps to provide indirect heat to the animal and the use of a towel or cloth over electric heating pads or warm water blankets diminishes the likelihood of iatrogenic burn injury.

The development of pneumonia is a concern upon recovery from hypothermia in these patients. Clinical signs of coughing, fever, or increased breath sounds warrant survey thoracic radiographs and transtracheal aspiration to obtain samples for cytologic evaluation and microbiologic culture. While pending the results of the diagnostic tests, broad-spectrum antibiotic administration in conjunction with intermittent nebulization and coupage should be instituted.

In cases of exposure, the animal should be closely examined for signs of frostbite injury, particularly to the extremities. The tail, pinnae of the ears, and footpads are commonly affected in cats. External genitalia and footpads are more typically injured in dogs. Upon recovery, return of warmth and sensation to any potentially affected areas is a good prognostic sign. Persistence of anesthesia, pallor, or cold to any of these areas warrants further monitoring for tissue devitalization and sloughing. Within 7 to 10 days of the injury, nonviable tissue can be readily identified and débrided (see *CVT XI*, p 43). In the interim, the patient may require application of an Elizabethan collar to prevent self-mutilation of the frostbitten tissues.

## SUMMARY

Clients must be educated about responsible pet ownership and the importance of providing appropriate shelter for their animals. Neonates, with an increased body surface/body weight ratio as compared to adult animals, and debilitated patients especially must be provided with a warm, draft-free environment. As the vast majority of hypothermic patients encountered have iatrogenically induced hypothermia, veterinary clinicians must be equally diligent. Surgical patients require particular attention and must be closely monitored intraoperatively and during anesthetic recovery to minimize occurrence and severity of this condition. Hypothermia is a life-threatening, complex condition involving multiple organ systems. Prompt treatment and vigilant monitoring are necessary to decrease morbidity and optimize survival.

## References and Suggested Reading

Elder PT: Accidental hypothermia. *In* Shoemaker WC (ed): *Textbook of Critical Care*, 2nd edition. Philadelphia, WB Saunders Co, 1989, pp 101–108. *A review of thermoregulatory physiology, pathophysiology, and management principles of hypothermia in humans.*
Farmer JC: Temperature-related injuries. *In* Civetta JM (ed): *Critical Care*. Philadelphia, JB Lippincott Co, 1988, pp 693–700. *Management of hypothermia in humans.*
Ganong WF: Central regulation of visceral function. *In* Ganong WF (ed): *Review of Medical Physiology*. Norwalk, CT, Appleton & Lange, 1991, pp 231–236. *A review of thermoregulatory physiology in humans and other higher mammals.*
Guyton A: Body temperature, temperature regulation and fever. *In* Guyton

A. (ed): *Textbook of Medical Physiology*, 8th edition. Philadelphia, WB Saunders Co, 1991, pp 797–807.
  *A review of thermoregulatory physiology in humans.*
Haskins SC: Hypothermia and its prevention during general anesthesia in cats. Am J Vet Res 42:856, 1981.
  *A review of general anesthesia employed in veterinary medicine and hypothermia.*
Lee-Parritz DE and Pavletic MM: Physical and chemical injuries: Heatstroke, hypothermia, burns, and frostbite. *In* Murtaugh RJ and Kaplan PM (eds):

*Veterinary Emergency and Critical Care Medicine*. St. Louis, Mosby Year Book, 1992, pp 196–199.
  *A review of pathophysiology, diagnosis, and management of hypothermia in small animal medicine.*
Reuler JB: Hypothermia: Pathophysiology, clinical settings, and management. Ann Intern Med 89:519, 1978.
  *Pathophysiology and clinical management of hypothermia.*
Smith M: Hypothermia. Compend Cont Educ Pract Vet 7:321, 1985.
  *A review article of hypothermia in companion animals.*

# CARDIAC ARRHYTHMIAS IN SYSTEMIC DISEASE

LISA C. RUSSELL
*and* JOHN E. RUSH
*North Grafton, Massachusetts*

Dogs and cats with systemic diseases are often presented with clinical signs of cardiovascular insufficiency. The secondary cardiovascular dysfunction may be the predominant clinical finding or may complicate treatment of the primary disease and thereby contribute to morbidity or mortality. Cardiac arrhythmias are often the first indication that the heart is affected by the underlying disease. Some of these arrhythmias are benign and do not require treatment; others are life threatening and aggressive treatment is indicated. This article provides a review of several pathophysiologic mechanisms that may lead to arrhythmia formation, followed by a specific discussion of the management for several common arrhythmias.

## FACTORS CONTRIBUTING TO ARRHYTHMIA FORMATION

### The Sympathetic Nervous System

Activation of the sympathetic nervous system commonly occurs with systemic disease in response to fever, hypovolemia, hypotension, or shock. Increased sympathetic tone helps to maintain normal blood pressure through increased cardiac output and vasoconstriction. Cardiac output is increased as a result of the positive inotropic and chronotropic effects of catecholamines on the heart. Blood flow is redistributed to "essential" organ systems such as the brain and heart. While these compensatory mechanisms help to maintain perfusion of vital organ systems in the acute setting, detrimental effects, including arrhythmias, also may result.

Catecholamines can potentiate arrhythmia formation, but also can have direct arrhythmogenic effects through the cellular mechanisms of enhanced automaticity, triggered automaticity, and reentry. Automa-

ticity, normally only a property of cardiac pacemaker cells, refers to the slow influx of calcium and sodium ions across the cell membrane during diastole (spontaneous phase-4 diastolic depolarization), which eventually causes the cell to reach threshold. Once threshold is reached, an action potential is generated, the cell depolarizes, and the impulse is propagated to other myocardial cells. Catecholamines increase the slope of phase 4-depolarization by enhancing the influx of sodium and calcium, thereby increasing automaticity and heart rate. This is a compensatory response of the normal heart that results in sinus tachycardia. In some diseases, however, damaged ventricular Purkinje fibers can exhibit enhanced pacemaker activity that may cause ventricular arrhythmias.

Triggered automaticity refers to the low-amplitude oscillations, or afterpotentials, that occur following a cardiac cell action potential. These oscillations are "triggered" by the preceding action potential and, in most instances, are subthreshold and clinically inapparent. Delayed afterpotentials are the result of altered states of repolarization or calcium influx, which is augmented with sympathetic nervous system stimulation or infusion of calcium or digitalis. Catecholamines can increase the amplitude of these oscillations, making it more likely that the impulse will reach threshold and result in arrhythmia.

Reentry occurs when two conduction pathways are joined both proximally and distally, thereby forming a circuit or loop. For reentry to occur, the two pathways of the loop must have different electrophysiologic characteristics such that conduction is blocked in one direction while the impulse is conducted down the other limb of the circuit. If the previously depolarized tissue has repolarized by the time that the impulse has gone full circle and returns, then a reentrant or circus arrhythmia can occur. These conditions are most commonly met when diseased myocardium is present. Sympathetic stimulation, which can alter conduction through the diseased myocardium, can also result in nonuniform repolarization of the myocardium, which is a situation favorable for reentrant arrhythmias. Therefore, by these mechanisms sympathetic stimulation favors the development of reentry and resultant arrhythmia formation.

In addition to the above direct arrhythmogenic effects, catecholamines also can provoke hypokalemia and ischemia, both of which can contribute to arrhythmia formation. Stimulation of $\beta_2$-receptors facilitates the entry of potassium into cells and may provoke hypokalemia-induced arrhythmias. Catecholamines can negate the beneficial electrophysiologic actions of antiarrhythmic drugs through this mechanism (Podrid, Fuchs, and Candinas, 1990). Arrhythmias may be indirectly induced following $\alpha$-adrenergic stimulation and attendant coronary vasoconstriction, which may lead to diminished coronary blood flow and ischemia.

On the basis of the available information, the cautious administration of adrenergic blocking drugs may be useful in the management of some cardiac arrhythmias (see below). In addition to their antiarrhythmic effects, $\beta$-blockers reduce the heart's vulnerability to lethal arrhythmias by increasing the threshold for ventricular fibrillation (Podrid, Fuchs, and Candinas, 1990).

### Reperfusion Injury, Oxygen Free Radicals, and Nitric Oxide

Reperfusion injury has been hypothesized to be a factor in myocardial cell necrosis and arrhythmia development (see "Oxygen Free Radicals and Reperfusion Injury," this volume, p 64). After a period of ischemia, reperfusion of the myocardium leads to generation of superoxide radicals. Xanthine oxidase, produced during ischemia, is a major contributor to the development of oxygen free radicals. Once produced, oxygen free radicals are highly reactive substances that are extremely damaging to cell membranes.

Nitric oxide also may play a significant role in the development of reperfusion injury. Nitric oxide is the compound that was previously identified as endothelium-derived relaxing factor. Nitric oxide is synthesized from the amino acid L-arginine by the enzyme nitric oxide synthase. Production of nitric oxide by endothelial cells causes vasodilation. Vascular relaxation occurs through cyclic guanosine monophosphate (cGMP) and is both calcium and calmodulin dependent. Nitric oxide also is an inhibitor of both platelet aggregation and platelet adhesion, and is known to inhibit leukocyte adherence to the endothelial wall.

In reperfusion injury, elaboration of nitric oxide by the endothelium is markedly diminished, and nitric oxide–mediated vasodilation is lost. The lack of nitric oxide permits neutrophil adherence to the vessel wall and can lead to neutrophil-derived myocardial damage through free radical formation and subsequent necrosis (Cooke and Tsao, 1993). Platelet adhesion and aggregation is enhanced, which may result in microvascular thrombus formation. In addition, reperfusion injury to ischemic myocardium leads to sarcolemmal and sarcoplasmic reticular damage, which can elicit cellular electrophysiologic disturbances of sufficient magnitude to initiate arrhythmias.

The hydroxyl radical is one of the damaging oxygen free radicals produced during reperfusion injury. Iron serves as a vital cofactor in the Haber-Weiss reaction that generates the hydroxyl radical. Deferoxamine, an iron chelator, is known to reduce reperfusion injury. In a canine model of gastric dilation-volvulus (GDV), deferoxamine administration prior to decompression and reperfusion was demonstrated to improve survival and prevent myocardial necrosis or fibrosis (Lantz et al., 1992). While data on cardiac arrhythmia formation were not reported, the authors concluded that the cardiac changes, and therefore perhaps the arrhythmias, may be related to reperfusion injury. Unfortunately, without clinical studies, firm recommendations regarding the routine clinical use of deferoxamine (or other compounds such as dimethylsulfoxide or allopurinol, which mitigate free radical–induced injury) cannot be made at this time.

### Myocardial Necrosis/Contusion

Myocardial necrosis and subendocardial hemorrhage have been reported in dogs in association with many clinical and experimental situations. Experimentally, these lesions can be seen following hemorrhagic shock, isoproterenol or norepinephrine administration, cervical sympathetic ganglion stimulation, thoracic or abdominal trauma, and stimulation of the central nervous system with electricity or certain drugs. In clinical settings, myocardial necrosis has been reported in dogs with GDV (Muir and Weisbrode, 1984), neural lesions, splenic masses (Keyes et al., 1993), and trauma (Macintire and Snider, 1984). Histopathologic findings include multifocal areas of acute degeneration and necrosis of muscle fibers, occasionally with mineralization. Myocardial necrosis can have negative effects on myocardial performance, and these lesions may be directly responsible for or may contribute to the development of ventricular arrhythmias seen in these conditions.

Myocardial contusion has been postulated to play a role in the development of ventricular arrhythmias in dogs after trauma. The significance of myocardial contusion in the development of these arrhythmias, however, has recently been questioned. It is recognized that arrhythmias can occur in dogs with significant trauma—for instance, pelvic fractures—but without evidence of thoracic injury. The occurrence of cardiac arrhythmias in animals with trauma may be related not only to myocardial contusion, but also to shock, reperfusion injury after shock, neurologic injury, or sympathetic stimulation.

### Neurologic Disease and Neurologic Injury

Neurologic disease is another potential cause of cardiac arrhythmias. Arrhythmias may occur in animals with either spinal disorders or intracranial disease processes. Subarachnoid and intracerebral hemorrhage have been shown to cause cardiac arrhythmias and myocardial necrosis in a number of species. In addition, traumatically induced spinal cord lesions in dogs can cause the previously mentioned myocardial lesions of degeneration and myocardial necrosis (Podrid, Fuchs, and Candinas, 1990; Oppenheimer, Cechetto, and Hachinski, 1990).

Experimental studies in a number of species have demonstrated the relationship between stimulation of the central nervous system, especially the hypothalamus, and alterations in cardiac repolarization with the development of cardiac arrhythmias. Arrhythmias reported to occur in association with nervous system injury include ventricular premature beats, ventricular tachycardia, sinus bradycardia, periods of asystole, atrial fibrillation, and atrioventricular (AV) dissociation due to AV nodal rhythms. Of these arrhythmias, sinus bradycardia and ventricular arrhythmias are the most frequently encountered arrhythmias in animals with neurologic disease.

The mechanism underlying ventricular arrhythmias in nervous system injury appears to be activation of the sympathetic nervous system. The threshold for ventricular fibrillation, for example, is lowered following sympathetic stimulation in dogs, and administration of $\beta$-blockers prevents arrhythmia formation in this model (Podrid, Fuchs, and Candinas, 1990). This information provides strong support for consideration of adrenergic-blocking drugs in the management of ventricular arrhythmias in patients with neurologic disease.

Bradycardia also is commonly observed in animals with head trauma or increased intracranial pressure. One mechanism underlying the bradycardia is the Cushing's response, a reflex stimulated by increases in intracranial pressure. Mixed vagal and sympathetic stimulation can occur when the pons is subjected to increased pressure. Systemic hypertension develops in response to increased intracranial pressure to ensure adequate blood flow to the central nervous system. The hypertension in this response is attended by bradycardia, which occurs due to vagal stimulation. Spinal cord injuries also can lead to sinus bradycardia. Sinus bradycardia in spinal injuries is vagally mediated and, when treatment is needed, typically responds to atropine administration (Stauffer et al., 1988).

## Electrolyte Disturbances

### POTASSIUM

Hypokalemia is frequently observed in anorectic animals with severe systemic disease, and is a recognized risk factor for the development of cardiac arrhythmias. The resting membrane potential is determined in part by the concentrations of extracellular and intracellular potassium. When the extracellular serum potassium concentration is lower than normal, the cell becomes hyperpolarized, which enhances cell excitability and automaticity.

Systemic illnesses that commonly result in hypokalemia include diabetic ketoacidosis, hyperadrenocorticism, prolonged vomiting and diarrhea, and hyperaldosteronism. Intensive diuretic therapy also can contribute to the development of hypokalemia, and fluid therapy with potassium-deficient fluids in anorectic patients can precipitate hypokalemia. The incidence of ventricular arrhythmias in people with myocardial infarction is increased if hypokalemia is present. Recent evidence suggests that even mild hypokalemia can contribute to ventricular arrhythmia formation.

Hypokalemia also is very important when antiarrhythmic therapy is being considered. Many of the commonly used antiarrhythmics (i.e., lidocaine, procainamide, quinidine) are less effective in the face of hypokalemia, as low potassium concentrations negate the beneficial electrophysiologic effects of these drugs. Some patients—especially cats—may develop normal sinus rhythm following establishment of normokalemia.

Potassium supplementation is essential in patients with ventricular arrhythmias and hypokalemia. Maintenance of serum potassium levels in excess of 4.0 mEq/L is desirable, and daily evaluation of serum potassium is often appropriate. Potassium supplementation in animals with systemic disease is usually accomplished by addition of potassium chloride (KCl) to intravenous fluids. The degree of supplementation depends on the degree of hypokalemia. The addition of 40 mEq of KCl to 1 L of lactated Ringer's solution is commonly infused in animals with mild hypokalemia receiving maintenance volumes of fluid therapy.

### MAGNESIUM

Magnesium is a metabolic cofactor in hundreds of enzymatic reactions, including a requisite role in the sodium potassium-ATPase pump and several reactions that involve energy production and utilization (see "Magnesium and the Critically Ill Patient," this volume, p 128). Arrhythmia formation in magnesium deficiency can be caused by dysfunction of the sodium potassium-ATPase pump, which can lead to intracellular potassium depletion and arrhythmia formation. The myocardium has high magnesium concentrations, and alterations in magnesium concentrations have been demonstrated to affect cardiac impulse formation, conduction, and myocardial repolarization (Arsenian, 1993).

A number of studies in people have demonstrated an association between hypomagnesemia and ventricular arrhythmias. Magnesium also may be important in the development of atrial fibrillation, especially in dogs given digitalis. Unfortunately, serum magnesium levels do not accurately represent body stores of this electrolyte, which makes documentation of magnesium deficiency syndromes difficult. Circumstantial evidence for the role of hypomagnesemia in arrhythmogenesis is the fact that many arrhythmias are abolished by magnesium administration. Magnesium administration may be helpful in paroxysmal supraventricular tachycardia, multifocal atrial tachycardia, refractory ventricular arrhythmias, and ventricular arrhythmias related to myocardial infarction. In addition, magnesium administration has definite benefits in treating ventricular arrhythmias resulting from digitalis intoxication. Antiarrhythmic therapy with magnesium (see "Magnesium Therapy," this volume, p 132) should be considered to be unconventional at this time, although future studies may clarify the role of magnesium in arrhythmia formation and its potential role in the management of refractory arrhythmias.

### Hypoxemia, Anemia, and Acid-Base Disturbances

Hypoxemia, anemia, and disturbance of acid-base status are common in systemically ill veterinary patients. These factors can all contribute to arrhythmia formation. Metabolic acidosis occurs commonly in patients with diabetes mellitus, renal failure, and in shock patients secondary to anaerobic metabolism and lactic acidosis. Acidosis alters the myocardial cell membrane and favors the development of arrhythmia. Measurement of arterial or venous blood gases in these patients is appropriate. Correction of acidosis with appropriate fluid therapy, rapid resuscitation from shock and, in some instances, sodium bicarbonate administration may be the only measures necessary for arrhythmia control.

Hypoxemia, commonly occurring in patients with chronic respiratory disease, pneumonia, thoracic trauma, and acute respiratory distress syndromes, also contributes to arrhythmia formation. Measurement of arterial blood gas is appropriate when hypoxemia is suspected. If the partial pressure of oxygen ($PaO_2$) is less than 65 mm Hg, then oxygen supplementation is indicated. Interestingly, some animals with cardiac arrhythmias and mild hypoxemia ($PaO_2$ 65 to 80 mm Hg) will experience significant reductions in the number of abnormal beats following oxygen supplementation.

Anemia may also contribute to arrhythmogenesis. Anemic animals may have myocardial tissue hypoxia, owing to diminished oxygen-carrying capacity of the blood and compensatory activation of the sympathetic nervous system. When ventricular arrhythmias occur in anemic patients, the anemia should be corrected with blood transfusion. Maintenance of a packed cell volume (PCV) of at least 25% is desirable.

## MANAGEMENT OF CARDIAC ARRHYTHMIAS

### General Supportive Measures

General measures for the therapy of arrhythmias in animals with systemic disease should include management of the underlying disease, as well as initial treatment of shock, injuries, and acid-base or electrolyte disturbances. Oxygen administration and attempts to improve oxygen delivery are recommended. Maintenance of a PCV of at least 25% is indicated to optimize oxygen delivery. Prompt correction of hypokalemia and other metabolic abnormalities is frequently sufficient to suppress many acute arrhythmias. Analgesics for management of patient pain and discomfort also is recommended, in part to reduce sympathetic tone. Arterial blood pressure should be maintained to ensure myocardial perfusion and to partially mitigate the adverse effects of arrhythmias on hemodynamics.

Cardiac arrhythmias may not be manifested until 12 to 48 hr after initial treatment of GDV, trauma, or hypovolemic shock. Therefore, careful patient and electrocardiographic (ECG) monitoring is essential to detect and adequately manage arrhythmias in these patients. Periodic ECG monitoring is recommended in these patients during the first 48 hr of hospitalization. The goals of therapy are straightforward: to prevent serious hypotension, clinical signs, and sudden cardiac death. Therapy for specific arrhythmias is discussed below.

### Treatment of Specific Arrhythmias

#### SINUS BRADYCARDIA

Sinus bradycardia in animals with intracranial disease often signifies elevated intracranial pressure or a pontine lesion. Treatment of the arrhythmia is rarely required, and efforts should be directed at improving the patient's neurologic status (i.e., oxygen supplementation, mechanical ventilation, corticosteroids, mannitol). The patient's blood pressure and overall cardiovascular status should be assessed. If there is evidence of diminished cardiac output (i.e., weak arterial pulses, poor mucous membrane color, or slow capillary refill time), therapy with atropine (0.02 to 0.04 mg/kg IV or IM) or glycopyrrolate (0.011 mg/kg IV or IM) is indicated. Similarly, treatment is recommended if the animal is thought to be at risk for cardiopulmonary arrest. Bradycardia that is unresponsive to anticholinergic drugs may be managed by cardiac pacing or by dopamine infusion (5 to 20 $\mu$g/kg/min). Caution is advised when using dopamine to avoid increases in blood pressure that might contribute to increases in intracranial pressure.

Sinus bradycardia also may occur in hypothermic or hypoxic animals, in animals with severe vomition, and as a premonitory arrhythmia in critically ill animals prior to cardiopulmonary arrest. Aggressive treatment of shock or sepsis or both in combination with physical efforts to increase body temperature (i.e., hot water bottles, heating blanket, warm fluids) are recommended for hypothermic patients. In addition to blood volume resuscitation, atropine or dopamine infusion (or both) may be used in critically ill animals with bradycardia. Refractory vomiting in some animals can precipitate bradycardia and attendant collapse at the time of vomition; these patients may benefit from anticholinergic drugs.

#### SUPRAVENTRICULAR ARRHYTHMIAS

Sinus tachycardia is the appropriate response of the cardiovascular system to hypovolemia, shock, fever, anxiety, and pain. Specific treatment of sinus tachycardia is usually unwarranted. Therapy should be directed at the cause of sinus tachycardia, with intravenous fluids, colloids, or blood products infused to treat shock or hypovolemia; analgesics administered for pain; and antibiotics or other specific therapy given to patients with fever. Serum potassium also should be measured and corrected if low.

Sinus tachycardia is common and does not require antiarrhythmic therapy. However, it must be differentiated from supraventricular tachyarrhythmias, which do require antiarrhythmic therapy. Supraventricular tachycardia is caused by abnormal depolarization or reentry within the atria or AV junctional tissues. Sometimes, a regularly conducted atrial tachycardia or atrial flutter can be manifested as a regular "supraventricular" tachycardia. With sinus tachycardia a vagal maneuver (e.g., ocular pressure) may result in transient slowing of the heart rate, whereas most supraventricular tachycardias typically manifest a constant, fixed heart rate. Alternatively, abrupt changes in heart rate, blocking of P-waves or flutter waves, or a return to normal sinus rhythm following vagal maneuver is characteristic of some supraventricular tachyarrhythmias. Supraventricular tachycardias often have a P-wave morphology that is different than the sinus conducted beats.

Drug therapy should be considered for patients with supraventricular tachyarrhythmias (rates > 260 bpm in the cat or > 220 bpm in the dog) or for slower supraventricular arrhythmias that persist after hypotension and pain have been effectively treated. When treatment is indicated, therapeutic options for supraventricular tachycardia include calcium channel blockers (diltiazem, verapamil) and β-adrenergic blocking drugs (propranolol, esmolol). Although digoxin may be the drug of choice when supraventricular arrhythmias are accompanied by heart failure, calcium channel blockers and β-blockers are safer, more effective, and result in fewer side effects in animals with systemic disease. Intravenous therapy is preferred for hemodynamically unstable arrhythmias, while oral therapy is recommended for most "stable" patients. Selection of calcium channel blocker or β-blocker is usually empiric and based on personal preference.

For intravenous use of calcium channel blockers, both diltiazem and verapamil are available and effective. The authors' preference is diltiazem (Cardizem, Marion Merrill Dow, Kansas City, MO), which can be administered in an initial 0.25-mg/kg IV bolus over 2 min. Subsequent 0.25-mg/kg boluses can be repeated at 15-min intervals until conversion occurs or until a maximum dose of 0.75 mg/kg has been given. Verapamil is given intravenously in a series of 0.05-mg/kg IV boluses administered slowly to a maximum dose of 0.15 mg/kg. Propranolol can be administered intravenously at a dose of 0.02 to 0.06 mg/kg slowly every 8 hr. Esmolol (Brevibloc, Du Pont Pharmaceuticals, Garden City, NJ) is an ultra-short-acting β-blocker that is given in incremental doses of 0.05- to 0.1-mg/kg boluses every 5 min up to a maximum dose of 0.5 mg/kg or as an infusion of 50 to 200 μg/kg/min. Esmolol is preferred over propranolol, as the effects are short lived,

and if arrhythmia conversion does not occur, then other drugs with negative inotropic properties (i.e., diltiazem or verapamil) can be safely given 30 min after esmolol administration.

It should be stressed that supraventricular tachycardia is uncommon. Most rapid supraventricular rhythms represent sinus tachycardia and are "cured" following analgesic therapy or treatment of hypotension or shock. Drug therapy is rarely required.

Atrial fibrillation is common in large-breed dogs. Although these dogs are predisposed to the development of atrial fibrillation with dilated cardiomyopathy, some dogs with apparently normal hearts develop atrial fibrillation in association with trauma, anesthesia, or systemic disease. Careful auscultation, thoracic radiography, and echocardiography should be performed to determine whether the arrhythmia is associated with congestive heart failure or myocardial disease. If the atrial fibrillation does not result from dilated cardiomyopathy or valvular heart disease, then attempts should be made to convert the arrhythmia back to sinus rhythm. While atrial fibrillation may resolve spontaneously, progressive cardiac enlargement and myocardial failure have been observed to develop in some dogs with chronic atrial fibrillation.

In dogs with atrial fibrillation resulting from systemic disease, the ventricular rate response (after treatment of hypotension) is often 70 to 180 bpm, which is somewhat slower than what is considered "typical" for atrial fibrillation. Conversion of atrial fibrillation to sinus rhythm is initially attempted with quinidine gluconate (6 to 11 mg/kg IM, every 6 hr). Most dogs convert to sinus rhythm within the first 24 hr of therapy. Quinidine has a vagolytic effect, which can dramatically increase AV nodal conduction and lead to a very rapid ventricular response to atrial fibrillation. Digitalis or a β-blocker may be useful to slow the rate of ventricular conduction across the AV node if tachycardia develops. Alternatively, some have reported success with diltiazem (0.5 to 1.5 mg/kg PO every 8 to 12 hr) or verapamil for conversion of atrial fibrillation. Electrocardiographic synchronized cardioversion may be attempted if quinidine and diltiazem are unsuccessful, although this technique has some risk and requires very heavy sedation or anesthesia to be performed safely. If attempts to convert the arrhythmia to sinus rhythm are unsuccessful, the conventional treatment as for animals with atrial enlargement and congestive heart failure is appropriate (i.e., digitalis, diltiazem, or β-blockers, or a combination; see *CVT XI*, p 745).

## Ventricular Arrhythmias

Ventricular arrhythmias are common, and in some cases treatment is necessary. Determination of which cardiac arrhythmias require treatment is often difficult, and specific therapeutic guidelines are lacking. In all cases, the therapies outlined in the section "General Supportive Measures," above, should be employed. Isolated ventricular premature depolarizations usually do not require treatment unless they are initiated on the previous T wave or represent markers for a prior bout of ventricular tachycardia. In animals without pre-existing heart disease, it is recommended that ventricular tachycardia be treated when the rate is rapid, typically when the heart rate during arrhythmias is greater than 160 bpm. In addition, when ventricular arrhythmias are felt to contribute to hypotension, weakness (collapse or difficulty rising or clinical markers of poor perfusion weak pulses, pallor, slowed capillary refill time), therapy should be initiated. Ventricular arrhythmias in animals thought to be at risk for cardiopulmonary arrest also should be treated. When ventricular arrhythmias are at slow heart rates, typically those less than 160 bpm, and the patient does not exhibit any of the aforementioned signs, treatment may be unnecessay.

For ventricular arrhythmias that require treatment, lidocaine infusion (40 to 80 $\mu$g/kg/min) should be given if initial bolus(es) of lidocaine (2 to 4 mg/kg IV slowly) resulted in improvement. If the initial lidocaine boluses fail to improve the arrhythmia, procainamide administered intravenously (2 mg/kg every 5 min up to 20 mg/kg cumulative dose; thereafter a CRI of 20 to 50 $\mu$g/kg/min) or intramuscularly (6 to 20 mg/kg every 4 to 6 hr) also may be attempted.

In many animals, initial therapy with a class I antiarrhythmic drug (lidocaine, procainamide, quinidine) is minimally effective. The addition of a $\beta$-blocker to these drugs should be considered if the patient has responded adequately to treatment for shock (i.e., catecholamine infusions will not likely be required). $\beta$-blockers such as propranolol (0.2 to 0.4 mg/kg PO every 8 to 12 hr), or metoprolol (0.2 to 0.4 mg/kg PO every 12 hr) when added to a class I antiarrhythmic drug, are often effective in controlling the arrhythmia. Care must be exercised in using drugs that reduced liver blood flow (propranolol) in conjunction with lidocaine, which is eliminated by hepatic mechanisms. Similarly, cimetidine should be used cautiously, if at all, in patients receiving lidocaine infusions. Alternatively, many arrhythmias can be successfully managed simply using oxygen administration and analgesics such as butorphanol (0.2 to 0.4 mg/kg SC or IM every 4 to 6 hr) or buprenorphine (0.01 to 0.02 mg/kg IM every 6 to 8 hr).

The end point of antiarrhythmic therapy is not necessarily total alleviation of arrhythmia. Ventricular arrhythmias in animals with systemic disease often are self-limiting and, in most cases, spontaneously resolve within 3 to 10 days. It seems that few animals actually die as a direct result of the arrhythmias, especially when the animal's medical condition is stable or improving. Adequate therapy for ventricular arrhythmias may simply be reduction of the rate of ventricular tachycardia (perhaps <140 bpm) or alleviation of arrhythmias that result in weak arterial pulses, hypotension, patient weakness, or other evidence of diminished cardiac output. In some animals, antiarrhythmic therapy can be discontinued after a few days. Ventricular arrhythmias persist beyond the duration of hospitalization in other patients and oral therapy is required for 7 to 10 days. In this situation, the authors' preference is propranolol or metoprolol, although other clinicians prefer a class I antiarrhythmic or combination. A repeat ECG should be obtained 24 to 48 hr after discontinuation of the antiarrhythmic medications.

## References and Suggested Reading

Arsenian MA: Magnesium and cardiovascular disease. *Progress in Cardiovascular Diseases.* Philadelphia, WB Saunders Co, 1993, p 271.
  *A comprehensive review of the role magnesium plays in cardiac arrhythmias, myocardial function, and maintenance of blood pressure.*
Cooke JP and Tsao PS: Cytoprotective effects of nitric oxide. Circulation 88: 2451, 1993.
  *The interactions between nitric oxide formation, vasodilation, neutrophil adhesion, and their potential for causing reperfusion injury are described.*
Keyes ML, Rush JE, Autran de Morais HS, and Couto CG: Ventricular arrhythmias in dogs with splenic masses. Vet Emerg Crit Care 3:33, 1993.
  *Retrospecive study of dogs with splenic masses indicates a high incidence of ventricular arrhythmias.*
Lantz GC, Badylak SF, Hiles MC, et al: Treatment of reperfusion injury in dogs with experimentally induced gastric dilatation-volvulus. Am J Vet Res 53:1594, 1992.
  *Experimental study evaluating the effects of deferoxamine and DMSO on survival and myocardial injury in dogs with surgically created GDV.*
Macintire DK and Snider TG: Cardiac arrhythmias associated with multiple trauma in dogs. J Am Vet Med Assoc 184:541, 1984.
  *Management of ten dogs with traumatic injuries that subsequently developed cardiac arrhythmias.*
Muir WW and Weisbrode SE: Myocardial ischemia in dogs with gastric dilatation-volvulus. J Am Vet Med Assoc 181:363, 1982.
  *Histopathologic findings indicate myocardial necrosis and ischemia is common in dogs with GDV and ventricular arrhythmias.*
Oppenheimer SM, Cechetto DF, and Hachinski VC: Cerebrogenic cardiac arrhythmias. Cerebral electrocardiographic influences and their role in sudden death. Arch Neurol 47:513, 1990.
  *A review of the evidence that neurologically mediated cardiac injury and arrhythmias may be responsible for sudden death syndromes.*
Podrid PJ, Fuchs T, and Candinas R: Role of the sympathetic nervous system in the genesis of ventricular arrhythmia. Circulation 82(suppl I):I-103, 1990.
  *A comprehensive review of the pathophysiologic mechanisms for causes of sympathetically mediated cardiac arrhythmias, as well as discussion of the evidence supporting use of $\beta$-blockers for ventricular arrhythmias.*
Stauffer J-L, Gleed RD, Short CE, et al: Cardiac dysrhythmias during anesthesia for cervical decompression in the dog. Am J Vet Res 49:1143, 1988.
  *Bradycardia and ventricular arrhythmias are described in dogs undergoing surgical decompression for cervical but not thoracolumbar lesions.*

# CARDIOPULMONARY RESUSCITATION

TIMOTHY B. HACKETT
*and* DEBORAH R. VAN PELT
*Fort Collins, Colorado*

Cardiopulmonary arrest (CPA) is defined as the abrupt and unexpected cessation of spontaneous, effective ventilation and circulation. Cardiopulmonary resuscitation (CPR) provides artificial ventilation and circulation until advanced cardiac life support can be provided and spontaneous cardiopulmonary function is restored.

Biblical and mythological accounts of resuscitation notwithstanding, CPR had its beginnings in the late nineteenth and early twentieth centuries in experiments performed by physicians using animal models. In 1906, a report by Crile described an experimental method of resuscitation in dogs using thoracic compression, artificial ventilation, and parenteral epinephrine. He described both "direct" (i.e., open-chest) and "indirect" cardiac massage, and anticipated the thoracic pump theory of circulation by stating that "pressure upon the thorax alone is capable of producing an artificial circulation. This is by no means accomplished by its action upon the heart solely, but by its action upon all the large vessels—arteries, veins, and capillaries together." In the early 1960s, following a series of animal experiments in which researchers from Johns Hopkins University described artificial ventilation, external cardiac compression, and electrical defibrillation, CPR was gradually adopted as a medical intervention following CPA.

The guidelines for CPR in human beings have evolved through five national conferences starting in 1966. The purpose of these conferences was to review and update published materials concerning CPR in light of scientific advances and clinical experience. Because many of these guidelines have been drawn from experimental animal studies, they are directly relevant to veterinary medicine and are included in these recommendations.

Very little has changed in the actual treatment of cardiac arrest over the last 15 years. With success rates from 0 to 22% reported, the experience in treating CPA is far from encouraging. In a review of 265 nonanesthetized critical care unit cases receiving CPR, only 4.1% of dogs and 9.6% of cats were ultimately discharged from the hospital (Wingfield and Van Pelt, 1993). Many clinicians are understandably skeptical about the usefulness of current treatment protocols, as current recommendations have been implemented and become standard practice without any strong scientific support. Critical evaluation of new and even standard procedures is hampered by a lack of uniformity in reporting clinical treatments and outcomes. The "Utstein style" for uniform reporting of data from human out-of-hospital cardiac arrests has been put forward as the standard method of reporting cardiac arrest and resuscitation data (Cummins, 1993). Outcome measures limited to survival rates are of little value. Outcome measures following CPA must include a measure of duration and quality of survival. By establishing standards like the Utstein reporting scheme, veterinarians will be better able to compare treatments and results.

## READINESS

Cardiopulmonary arrest is the terminal event in most disease processes, and the underlying conditions should always be considered before CPR is attempted. When communicating with the owners of pets in critical condition, clinicians should discuss the possibility of CPA, prognosis, and associated expenses, so that the owners of terminally ill animals can be actively involved in the decision-making process.

By recognizing animals at increased risk of CPA, training of both technical and support staff in early recognition of CPA and use of a team approach in treating the arrest patient, CPR can be initiated in a timely and coordinated manner. When the underlying cause of CPA is reversible, every effort should be made to support vital circulation and oxygenation in a coordinated attempt to save the life. Although patients with primary respiratory arrest are associated with a higher resuscitation rate than those with cardiac arrest, few animals that undergo CPA are resuscitated and even fewer subsequently leave the hospital as normal pets. The major reasons for unsuccessful resuscitation include a delay in the diagnosis of CPA and a subsequent delay in administering appropriate therapy. For the benefit of patients with potentially reversible problems, hospitals should have a fully stocked "crash cart" available and staff should be trained in basic life support (BLS).

Advanced life support (ALS) with electrical defibrillation and emergency drug administration also involves advanced planning. Calculating emergency drug dosages in the environment of an arrest is difficult. The use of computer programs, clinical algorithms, and pre-prepared charts giving intravenous and intratracheal dosages of the commonly used emergency drugs can be invaluable during an arrest (Fig. 1).

All hospital personnel can be trained in some aspect of managing an arrest. For example, nontechnical staff can learn to ventilate patients after intubation, administer abdominal counterpressure, record the drugs administered and time intervals of CPR for later review, and even draw up syringes of drugs and flush. Having regular CPR drills can help emphasize the team approach, not only to CPR, but to health care in general.

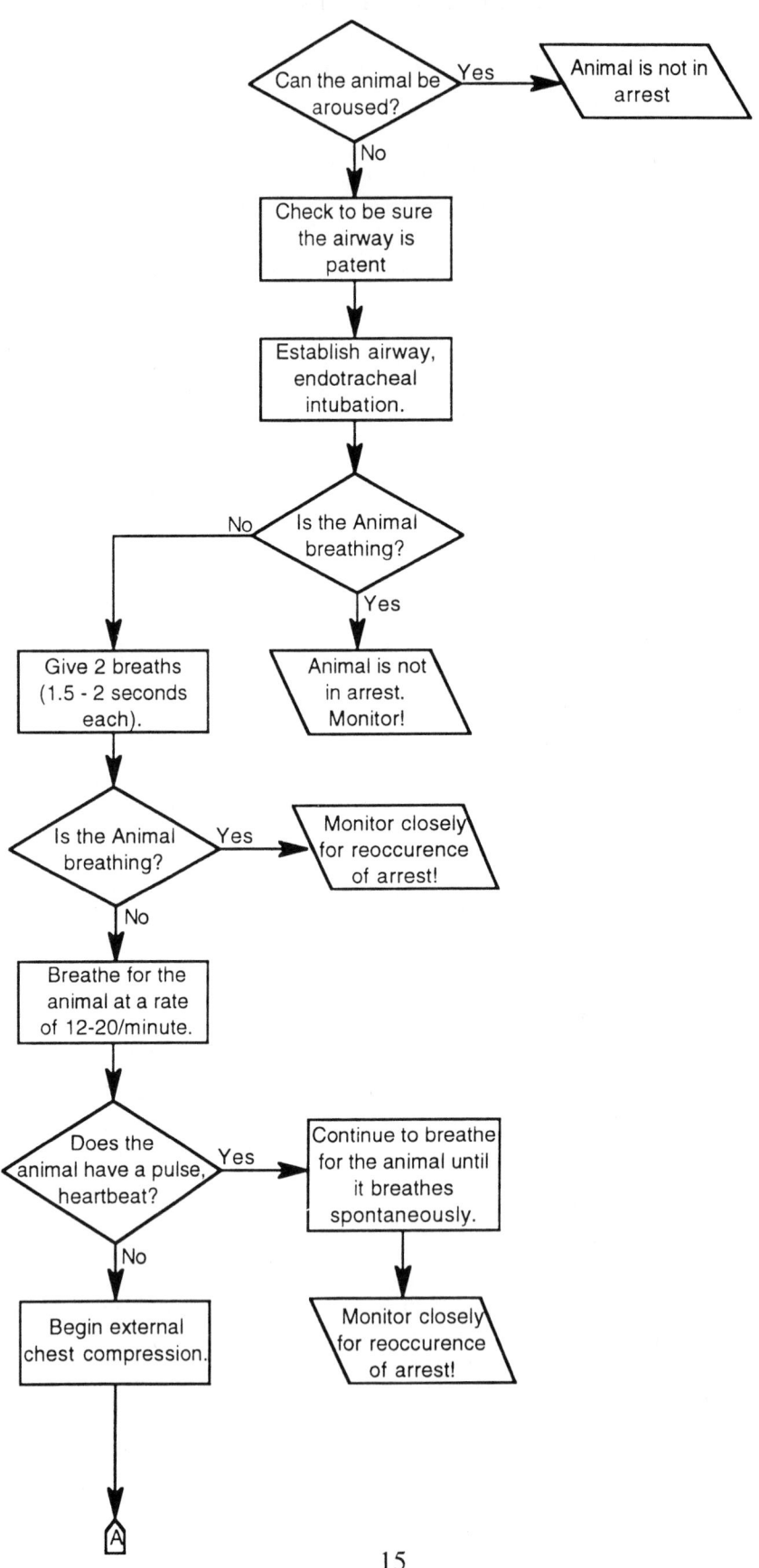

15

**Figure 1.** Cardiopulmonary resuscitation algorithm using recommendations in the text. *Illustration continued on opposite page*

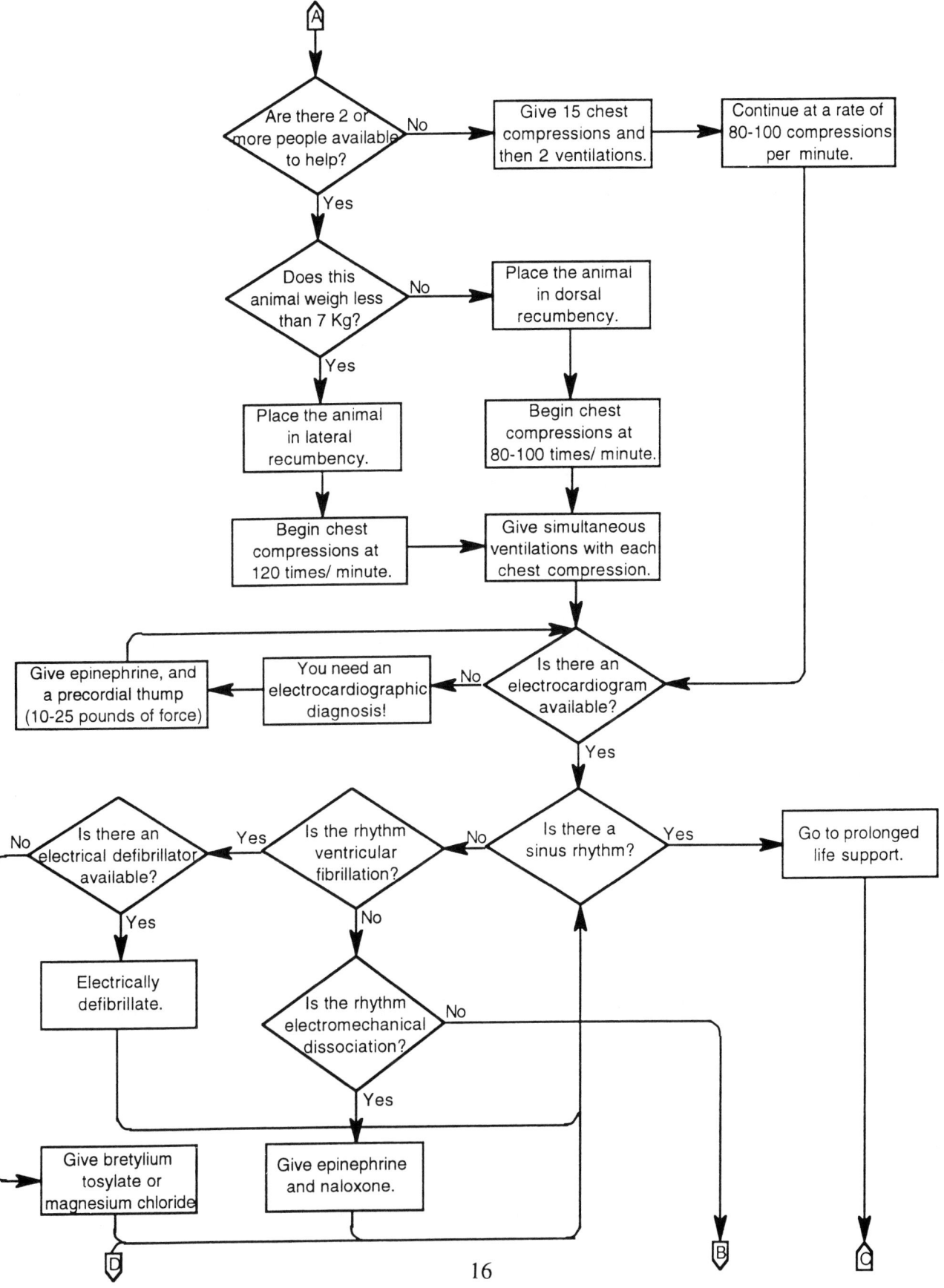

16

**Figure 1.** *Continued*

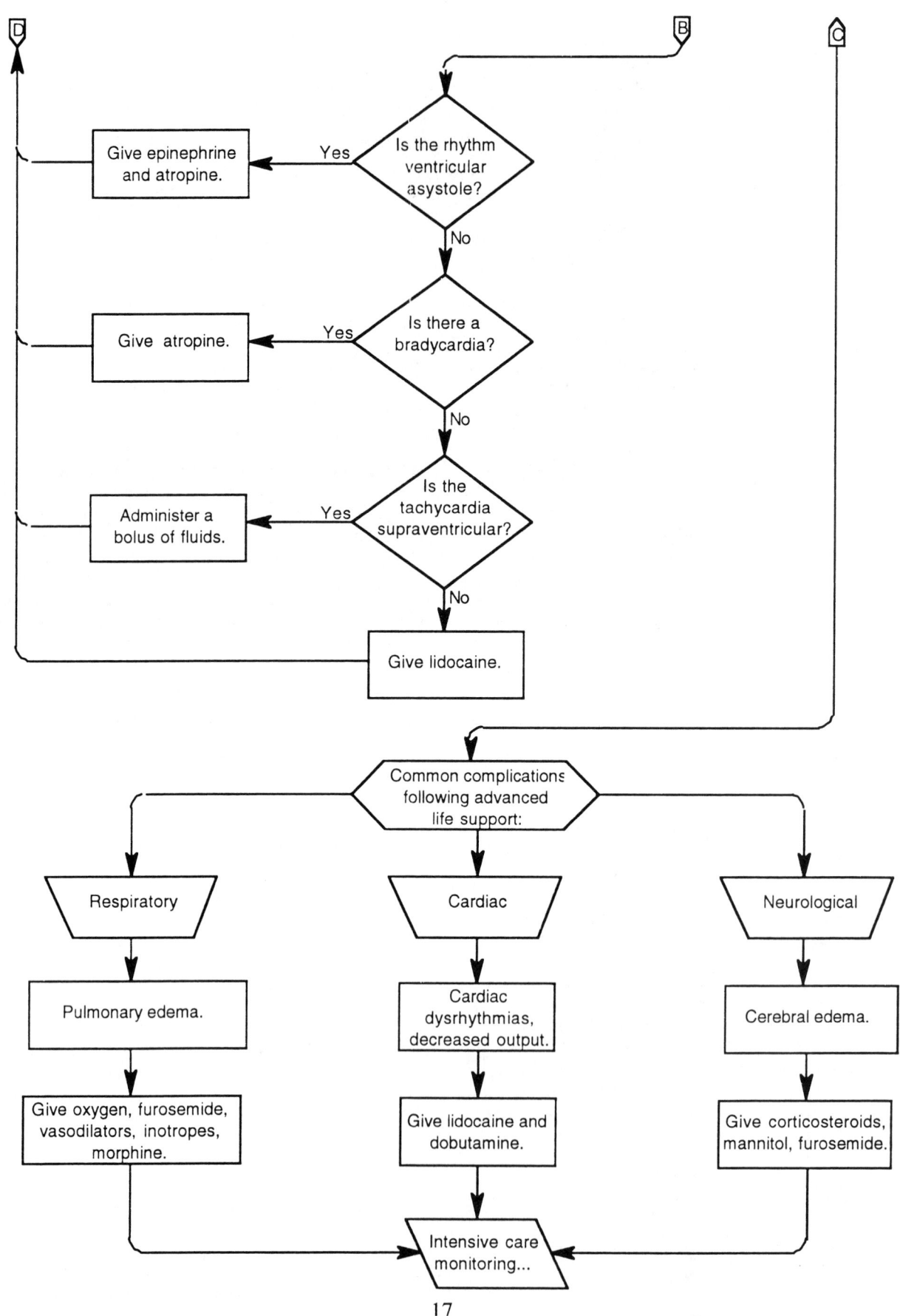

17

**Figure 1.** *Continued*

Staff meetings in which all members of the hospital are present can serve as an ideal time to practice basic life support in a coordinated, low-stress environment.

## CAUSES OF CARDIOPULMONARY ARREST

Cardiopulmonary arrest is usually the result of a cardiac arrhythmia, either a primary cardiac problem or secondary to respiratory arrest. The arrest may be the result of primary cardiac disease or diseases that affect other organs. In animals, arrest most frequently occurs with diseases of the respiratory system (pneumonia, laryngeal paralysis, neoplasia, thoracic effusions, and aspiration pneumonitis), as a result of severe multisystemic disease or trauma, or following cardiac arrhythmias. Recognition of predisposing causes of CPA and diligent monitoring of high-risk patients are necessary to diagnose and treat CPA in a timely manner.

Predisposing causes of cardiopulmonary arrest include the following: (1) cellular hypoxia, (2) vagal stimulation, (3) acid-base and electrolyte abnormalities, and (4) anesthetic agents. Any clinical condition causing cellular hypoxia predisposes the patient to CPA. This can include either primary cardiac disease resulting from inadequate cardiac output and peripheral vasoconstriction, or primary pulmonary pathology leading to arteriolar hypoxia (airway obstruction, hypoventilation, ventilation-perfusion imbalance, shunting or impairment of oxygen diffusion across the blood-air barrier). Anemia and peripheral vasoconstriction secondary to shock can also lead to tissue hypoxia.

In the face of hypoxemia, hypercarbia, or hyperkalemia, vagal stimulation can precipitate ventricular asystole. Procedures associated with increased vagal tone include the following: surgical manipulation of cervical, thoracic, and abdominal tissues; ophthalmic procedures; endotracheal intubation and extubation; tracheal suctioning; and proctoscopic examination.

Acid-base and electrolyte imbalances predispose to CPA. Hypoxia, hypercarbia, and acidemia stimulate the release of catecholamines, which increase cardiac automaticity and metabolic rate. The resultant sinus tachycardia can progress to ventricular tachycardia or fibrillation in the presence of metabolic abnormalities. Acidemia also lowers the myocardial fibrillation threshold. Thus, any patient having a metabolic disorder should be carefully monitored to avert possible CPA.

Many anesthetic agents decrease cardiovascular and respiratory functions and may induce CPA. These agents may depress respirations, sensitize the myocardium to circulating catecholamines resulting in the development of ventricular arrhythmias, or cause hypotension and subsequent tissue hypoxia.

## RECOGNITION OF CARDIOPULMONARY ARREST

Changes in the respiratory rate, depth, or pattern; a weak or irregular pulse; bradycardia; hypotension;

unexplained changes in the depth of anesthesia; cyanosis; and hypothermia are all warning signs of potential impending CPA. Obvious signs of CPA include cyanosis, the absence of effective ventilation, or the absence of a palpable pulse. Animals at risk for CPA should be monitored with this in mind. For busy practices where constant observation is not practical, there are several commercially available apnea monitors that sense the subtle chest-wall movements of ventilation and can alert staff should these cease. More elaborate monitoring includes continuous electrocardiography (ECG) or intermittent automatic blood pressure monitors. Telemetry units are available that provide continuous ECG, respiration, temperature, and blood pressure monitoring, and can be programmed to recognize and alert staff to a variety of life-threatening arrhythmias.

Capillary refill time is a poor indicator of the circulatory status of an animal. Normal refill times may be observed after the heart has stopped. In the dog, a peripheral pulse is absent once the systolic blood pressure falls below 60 mm Hg, while heart sounds are not auscultable below 50 mm Hg systolic pressure. The absence of heart sounds may indicate inadequate cardiac output, although not necessarily cardiopulmonary arrest. Pupillary dilatation begins within 20 sec of circulatory arrest and is maximal by 45 sec. It is important to note that pupillary dilatation is not a reflection of irreversible neurologic damage and should be used as an indicator of effective therapy rather than as an indicator of when to abandon resuscitative efforts. Knowledge of prior drug administration is necessary to accurately evaluate pupil size and reactivity, since previous administration of ganglionic blocking drugs such as epinephrine and atropine will lead to pupillary dilatation.

## BASIC LIFE SUPPORT

The assessment phases of BLS are crucial. No patient should undergo any one of the more intrusive procedures of CPR until the need for it has been established by appropriate assessment. Each of the ABCs of CPR, *airway*, *breathing*, and *circulation*, begins with an assessment phase: "determine the lack of responsiveness," "determine breathlessness," and "determine pulselessness," respectively. Assessment also involves a more subtle, constant process of observing patient responses.

### Airway

Determine the unresponsiveness of the patient and call for help from a coworker. Open the airway to assure its patency. Clean any foreign material or blood from the mouth and pharynx. A simple suction device can help remove fluid or blood from the upper airways. In cases of upper airway obstruction, a tracheostomy can rapidly provide a patent airway.

## Breathing

Determine the breathlessness of the patient. Watch for the chest to rise and fall, listen for air escaping during exhalation, and feel for air flow. The assessment phase should last no longer than 3 to 5 sec. After breathlessness has been confirmed, breathe for the patient. Artificial ventilation should begin with 100% oxygen, if available. Ventilation should be initiated with two large breaths, each 1.5 to 2 sec in duration. If the animal does not begin to breathe within 5 to 7 sec, begin to ventilate at a rate of 12 to 20 times per minute.

The use of acupuncture to stimulate respirations has been reported. Needling the acupuncture point Jen Chung (GV26) may reverse respiratory arrest under clinical conditions. Controlled studies in sheep with induced respiratory arrest have shown increased ventilation in response to acupuncture when compared to other noxious stimuli (Davies, Janse, and Reynolds, 1984). The technique involves using a small (25- to 28-gauge, 1- to 1.5-inch) needle, placing it in the nasal philtrum level at the ventral limit of the nares, to a depth of 10 to 20 mm, twirling it strongly and moving it up and down, while monitoring for improvement in respiration.

## Circulation

Determine the pulselessness of the patient, palpating either the carotid or femoral pulse. This should require no more than 5 to 10 sec. If no pulse is palpated, the diagnosis of cardiac arrest is confirmed and full CPR is begun. Cardiac compression in cats and small dogs (<7 kg) is best accomplished in lateral recumbency. Compression is applied directly over the heart and the chest wall is compressed 25 to 30% of its dimension. Thoracic compression in dogs weighing over 7 kg is performed with the patient in dorsal recumbency. This position maximizes the increase in intrathoracic pressure, due to the larger ventrodorsal dimension of the thorax, resulting in improved blood flow. Chest compression is applied over the distal one third of the sternum, with enough force to compress the thorax 25 to 30% of its dimension. Cardiopulmonary resuscitation in animals requires a rapid rate of compression (80 to 120 compressions per minute). The time of release should equal the time of compression. With one-person CPR, the ratio of chest compression to ventilation is 15:2. Give 15 chest compressions and then two long ventilations. Use a rate of 120 chest compressions per minute when the animal weighs <7 kg and 80 to 100 compressions per minute when the animal weighs more than 7 kg. When two persons are available to do CPR, simultaneous compression and ventilation will maximize intrathoracic pressure. In animals weighing less than 7 kg, the recommended rate of ventilation and compression is 120 times per minute. In animals weighing more than 7 kg, the rate of compression and ventilation is 80 to 100 times each minute. To improve venous return during external thoracic compression, have one person press upon the abdomen between each compression of the chest.

The effectiveness of CPR should be assessed by palpating pulses, or with the use of a flow-detection device such as a Doppler ultrasound transducer (see this volume, p 113). If compressions are not generating adequate blood flow, the resuscitation technique should be altered to increase intrathoracic pressure, or emergency thoracotomy and open-chest cardiac compression considered. A number of studies clearly indicate that open-chest direct cardiac compression produces greater cardiac output and higher cerebral and coronary perfusion gradients than does closed-chest CPR. However, open-chest CPR is of questionable value after prolonged (>10 min) closed-chest CPR, and therefore, if open-chest CPR is to be performed, we believe it should be initiated immediately. Generally, open-chest CPR should be restricted to the operating room and in selected instances of penetrating thoracic injury in cardiac tamponade.

Patients who are resuscitated with basic life support techniques alone are more likely to survive to discharge when compared to those requiring advanced techniques (i.e., drugs and defibrillation). Basic life support skills are essential. Organized, timely implementation of the ABCs will revive more patients than multiple advanced interventions.

## ADVANCED LIFE SUPPORT

Of the many cardioactive drugs available, those used most commonly during CPR include epinephrine, atropine, lidocaine, and naloxone. If a central intravenous (IV) line is available, that is the route of choice for drug administration during CPR. Medication administered intravenously should be followed with large boluses of saline to rapidly carry the agent to the heart. Intratracheal (IT) administration of drugs is advocated in cases without central vascular access. Drugs delivered to the lungs will be absorbed and rapidly carried to the left heart, where these agents can reach the coronary circulation. Severe pulmonary edema and pulmonary disease, which might prevent rapid absorption of the agent, are relative contraindications to intratracheal drug administration. Sodium bicarbonate should never be given via the airways, as it destroys alveolar surfactant and may potentially worsen respiratory distress. A peripheral catheter is the third route of choice for drug delivery. Again, large volumes of saline should be used to "push" these agents toward the coronary circulation. In animals where vascular collapse or small size makes catheterization difficult, an intraosseus catheter provides an excellent means of vascular access. Drugs, crystalloid fluids, whole blood, and other colloids can all be given through an intraosseous catheter. Intracardiac injection has many potential problems, including difficulty injecting into the left ventricle in sustained systole or asystole, the injection of drugs into the myocardium (causing refractory ventricular fibrillation), and possible laceration of coronary vessels. Intracardiac in-

**Table 1.** *Drugs Commonly Employed During and Following Cardiopulmonary Resuscitation*

| Drug | Indications | Dosage | Actions |
|---|---|---|---|
| Atropine sulfate | Sinus bradycardia, AV nodal block, ventricular asystole | 0.04 mg/kg IV<br>0.4 mg/kg IT | Parasympatholytic |
| Bretylium tosylate | Ventricular tachycardia, ventricular fibrillation | 10 mg/kg IV<br>1 to 2 mg/kg CRI | Chemical defibrillator, ventricular antiarrhythmic |
| Calcium chloride 10% solution | Hyperkalemia, hypocalcemia, calcium channel–blocker toxicity, hypermagnesemia | 1 to 2 ml IV to effect; closely observe the ECG | Positive inotrope |
| Deferoxamine mesylate (Desferal) | Postresuscitation, reperfusion injury | 10 mg/kg IV, IM, 2h twice, then t.i.d. for 24 hr | Iron chelator |
| Diltiazem (Cardizem) | Supraventricular tachycardia, hypertrophic cardiomyopathy | D: 0.5–1.5 mg/kg t.i.d. PO<br>C: 1.75–2.4 mg/kg t.i.d. to b.i.d. PO<br>D+C: 0.25 mg/kg IV bolus, to cumulative dose of 0.75 mg/kg | Calcium channel blocker |
| Dobutamine (Dobutrex) | Myocardial failure | 5–20 μg/kg/min CRI | Synthetic catecholamine positive inotrope |
| Dopamine (Intropin) | Low cardiac output, low renal or mesenteric blood flow | 3–5 μg/kg/min CRI for increased renal perfusion; 5–10 μg/kg/min for increased cardiac output | Dopaminergic, $\beta_1$ agonist, norepinephrine precursor |
| Epinephrine | Ventricular fibrillation, ventricular asystole, electromechanical dissociation | 0.02–0.2 mg/kg IV bolus q 5 min<br>0.04–0.4 mg/kg IT<br>1.0 μg/kg/min IV, CRI | $\alpha$- and $\beta$-agonist |
| Furosemide (Lasix) | Pulmonary edema, congestive heart failure, hypertension, anuria, oliguria | D: 2–4 mg/kg q.i.d. to t.i.d. PO, IM, IV<br>C: 1–2 mg/kg o.i.d. to b.i.d. PO, IM, IV | Loop diuretic |
| Lidocaine | Ventricular arrhythmias | D: 2–8 mg/kg IV bolus followed by 50–100 μg/kg/min CRI<br>C: 0.25–0.75 mg/kg IV, slowly | Class IB ventricular antiarrhythmic |
| Magnesium chloride | Unresponsive ventricular dysrhythmias, chemical defibrillator, severe hypotension | 2 gm given slowly over 2 min IV | Electrolyte, chemical defibrillator |
| Mannitol (Osmitrol) | Cerebral edema, anuria, oliguria | 0.5–1 gm/kg IV | Osmotic diuretic |
| Morphine sulfate | Analgesic, vasodilator, pulmonary edema, sedative | 0.04–0.08 mg/kg IM, IV, SC | Narcotic analgesic |
| Naloxone (Narcan) | Electromechanical dissociation, narcotic overdose | 0.03 mg/kg IV or IT | Opiate antagonist |
| Nitroprusside | Congestive heart failure, pulmonary edema | 1 to 5 μg/kg/min CRI | Venous and arterial vasodilator |
| Sodium bicarbonate | Severe metabolic acidosis | 1 to 2 mEq/kg IV | Alkalinizing agent |

Abbreviations: CRI = constant rate infusion, IT = intratracheal, IV = intravenously, IM = intramuscularly, PO = orally, SC = subcutaneously, D = dogs, C = cats, ECG = electrocardiogram.

jection should only be attempted when the heart can be visualized following thoracotomy and pericardiotomy.

## Electrocardiographic Manifestations of CPA

The most commonly encountered arrhythmias during CPA include ventricular asystole, electromechanical dissociation, and ventricular fibrillation. Without an ECG, differentiation is impossible.

Ventricular asystole, with an absence of both mechanical and electrical activity from the ventricles, appears as a straight line on an ECG, or as P waves without QRS complexes. Usually the result of severe myocardial ischemia from prolonged periods of inadequate coronary perfusion, it carries a grave prognosis.

In addition to effective basic CPR, treatment includes administration of atropine and epinephrine (Table 1).

Nonperfusing rhythm (electromechanical dissociation [EMD]) results in electrical activity without sufficient mechanical activity to cause adequate cardiac output or pulses. The failure of contractility is likely due to depletion of myocardial oxygen stores and may be perpetuated by endogenous endorphins. Treatment with the opiate antagonist naloxone may be associated with improved responsiveness of the heart to catecholamines, without significantly affecting blood pressure and aortic blood flow.

Ventricular fibrillation is chaotic, disorganized ventricular electrical activity resulting in sustained ventricular systole. Since the coronary arteries perfuse the myocardium during diastole, no coronary perfusion occurs as long as the animal is in ventricular fibrillation. Should ventricular fibrillation be recognized prior to establishing an airway or intravenous line, defibrillation should be attempted first. The cardiac response to countershock is largely time dependent. After extended ventricular fibrillation (5 to 15 min), countershock rarely results in a spontaneous perfusing rhythm; asystole, EMD, or persistent ventricular fibrillation are the usual results.

## Electrical Defibrillation and Epinephrine

Early electrical DC defribillation is the treatment of choice for ventricular fibrillation. Care must be exercised, as the defibrillator is a very dangerous instrument that can cause injury to the patient and death to the operator if improperly used. Always announce "ALL CLEAR!" and look around to be sure that no one is in contact with the animal, table, or instruments before discharging the defibrillator. The optimal delivered energy to the myocardium for external defibrillation is roughly 2 to 4 J/kg. When delivering this countershock to the myocardium, it is only necessary to "hit" about 28% of the myocardial cells to defibrillate the heart. Thus, paddle position is not as important as once believed. One should make every effort to reduce transthoracic impedance during electrical defibrillation by following these guidelines:

1. Use large surface area paddles.
2. Countershocks applied close together may be most effective.
3. Use an electrode-skin interface material such as electrolyte paste or gel. Do not use alcohol!
4. Apply pressure to the electrodes.
5. Defibrillate during expiration.

If initial countershock(s) fails to convert the ventricular fibrillation or the ECG manifestation of CPA is EMD or asystole, epinephrine should be administered (IV or IT) (Table 1). The beneficial effects of epinephrine depend primarily on its α-adrenergic effects, which include arterial vasoconstriction and selective redistribution of cardiac output. Epinephrine increases the CPR diastolic aortic–to–right atrial myocardial perfusion gradient (coronary perfusion pressure) by increasing aortic diastolic pressure, and improves the cerebral perfusion gradient by increasing carotid arterial pressure.

## Ancillary Therapies

Chemical defibrillators have unproven efficacy in clinical veterinary medicine. Unfortunately, many veterinarians do not have electrical defibrillators and thus chemical defibrillating drugs may be the only option. Drugs that may be used in attempting to convert ventricular fibrillation include bretylium tosylate and magnesium chloride (Table 1). Reports in the literature demonstrate that these drugs have been effective in terminating ventricular fibrillation when electrical countershock has failed. Lidocaine may prevent the re-

currence of malignant ventricular arrhythmias but is of questionable efficacy in the treatment of ventricular fibrillation.

With regard to the use of sodium bicarbonate, therapy aimed at correction of acid-base abnormalities during CPR should be conservative. By lowering blood $PCO_2$, adequate ventilation will provide natural buffering without the risk of overcompensation and adverse effects associated with bicarbonate administration (i.e., hypernatremia, hyperosmolality, hypokalemia, increased dysrhythmias, decreased plasma calcium, and oxyhemoglobin dissociation changes causing decreased tissue oxygen delivery).

Calcium entry into cells has been implicated in a cascade of events involved in reperfusion injury, including vasospasm, membrane degeneration, and production of cytotoxic compounds. Unless indicated by specific disease processes (e.g., hypocalcemia, severe hyperkalemia, hypermagnesemia, or overdose of a calcium channel–blocking agent) calcium should not be routinely used in CPR.

Intravenous fluids should only be administered during CPR when hypovolemia is the cause of the arrest. Fluid loading during CPR may result in decreased cerebral blood flow. Increased right atrial pressures from intravenous fluid loading will also decrease coronary perfusion pressures, causing decreased coronary blood flow.

## PROLONGED LIFE SUPPORT

Reoccurrence of either respiratory or cardiopulmonary arrest is the biggest concern following resuscitation. In most cases, rearrest will occur within 4 hr of the first episode of CPA, necessitating careful monitoring during this time. Postarrest patients should receive oxygen, using either an oxygen cage, nasal insufflation, or a facemask. If cardiopulmonary resuscitation was successful, the myocardium must be supported during the postresuscitation phase. Positive inotropic support with dobutamine or dopamine, preload and afterload reduction using vasodilatory drugs (sodium nitroprusside), and specific antiarrhythmic agents such as lidocaine will be useful in reducing the cardiac arrhythmias and pulmonary edema commonly seen following arrest (Table 1). Furosemide may be administered to further reduce pulmonary edema in normotensive animals.

Following arrest, cerebral resuscitation becomes the next most important concern. Due to the low blood flow to the brain during CPR, ischemia and hypoxia will lead to cerebral edema. Treatment for cerebral edema includes administration of mannitol and corticosteroids (Table 1). Additional drugs that may be used in an attempt to improve cerebral resuscitation include calcium channel–blocking drugs, which may reverse cerebral vasospasm, and barbiturates. Barbiturates have several potentially beneficial effects. They are mild calcium antagonists, which further decrease arachidonic acid and free fatty acid levels in neurons, and they decrease metabolic demands of the brain. However, the sedative effects of barbiturates will mask any changes in patient mentation, making sequential neurologic assessment impossible. To date, there is no conclusive evidence to support the routine postresuscitative use of barbiturates.

For the treatment of post-CPR reperfusion injury, drugs such as iron-chelating agents (deferoxamine) and other free radical scavengers have been proposed (see p 64). Although still experimental, with critical clinical evaluation, these drugs may become useful adjuncts to treatment in the future.

### References and Suggested Reading

Crile GW and Dolley DH: An experimental research into the resuscitation of dogs killed by anesthetics and asphyxia. J Exp Med 8:713, 1906.

Crowe DT: Cardiopulmonary resuscitation in the dog: A review and proposed new guidelines (part I). Semin Vet Med Surg 3:32, 1988.
Crowe DT: Cardiopulmonary resuscitation in the dog: A review and proposed new guidelines (part II). Semin Vet Med Surg 3:328, 1988.
Cummins RO: The Ulstein style for uniform reporting of data from out-of-hospital cardiac arrest. Ann Emerg Med 22:37, 1993.
Davies A, Janse J, and Reynolds GW: Acupuncture in the relief of respiratory arrest. NZ Vet J 32:109, 1984.
Gilroy BA, Dunlop BJ, and Shapiro HM: Outcome from cardiopulmonary resuscitation in cats: Laboratory and clinical experience. J Am Anim Hosp Assoc 23:133, 1987.
Haskins SC: Internal cardiac compression. J Am Vet Med Assoc 200:1945, 1993.
Henik RA: Basic life support and external cardiac compression in dogs and cats. J Am Vet Med Assoc 200:1925, 1993.
Kass PH and Haskins SC: Survival following cardiopulmonary resuscitation in dogs and cats. J Vet Emerg Crit Care 2:57, 1993.
Paraskos JA: History of CPR and the role of the national conference. Ann Emerg Med 22:275, 1993.
Van Pelt DR and Wingfield WE: Controversial issues in drug treatment during cardiopulmonary resuscitation. J Am Vet Med Assoc 200:1938, 1993.
Wingfield WE and Van Pelt DR: Respiratory and cardiopulmonary arrest in dogs and cats: 265 cases (1986–1991). J Am Vet Med Assoc 200:1993, 1993.

# OXYGEN SUPPLEMENTATION

KENNETH J. DROBATZ,
*Philadelphia, Pennsylvania*

SUSAN HACKNER,
*Gaithersburg, Maryland*

*and* SALLY POWELL
*Philadelphia, Pennsylvania*

Maintenance of adequate oxygen delivery to tissues is one of the primary goals in critical care medicine. When tissue oxygen delivery is inadequate, cells must use less efficient, anaerobic means to produce energy and maintain cell metabolism. Lactic acid accumulates and cell energy supply becomes depleted, resulting in cellular as well as organ dysfunction and possibly death. The clinician must understand the major components determining tissue oxygen delivery, which include the amount of oxygen entering the lungs, the adequacy of pulmonary gas exchange, tissue blood flow, and the capacity of the blood to carry oxygen. This article discusses optimizing blood oxygen content through various modes of oxygen supplementation.

## INDICATIONS FOR OXYGEN SUPPLEMENTATION

The amount of oxygen in the blood is determined by the amount of dissolved oxygen, the hemoglobin content, and the oxygen saturation of the hemoglobin. The most common methods of assessing the oxygen content of blood in our practice is arterial blood gas analysis and pulse oximetry. The arterial partial pressure of oxygen ($PaO_2$) measures the amount of dissolved oxygen in the plasma, while pulse oximetry measures the oxygen saturation of hemoglobin ($SaO_2$). The relationship between $PaO_2$ and hemoglobin saturation is depicted in

Figure 1. This relationship will vary under different conditions. For example, the curve shifts to the right with a decrease in pH, or an increase in temperature or 2,3-diphosphoglycerate. Conversely, the curve shifts to the left with an increase in pH, or a decrease in temperature or 2,3-diphosphoglycerate.

Oxygen supplementation is clearly indicated with arterial hypoxemia ($PaO_2$ <80 mm Hg), or a decrease in hemoglobin saturation. Patients with hemoglobin sat-

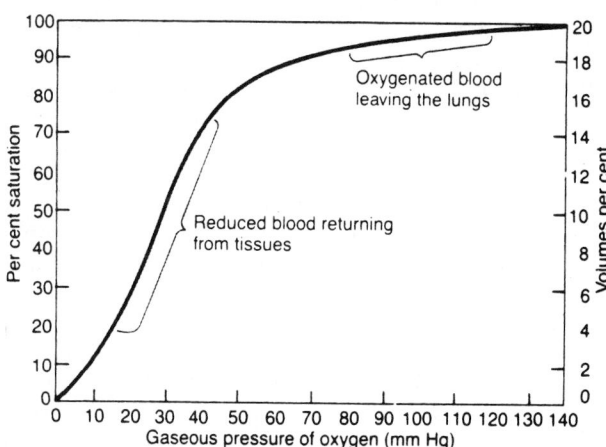

**Figure 1.** Oxygen-hemoglobin dissociation curve. (From Guyton AC: *Textbook of Medical Physiology,* 8th edition. Philadelphia, WB Saunders Co, 1991, p 436, with permission.)

uration close to the steep portion of the curve (Fig. 1) should also receive supplementation. A change in position or a therapeutic procedure on these patients may make only a minor change in $PaO_2$ but a life-threatening decrease in hemoglobin saturation and arterial oxygen content.

Arterial blood gas analysis and pulse oximetery are not routinely available to the practicing veterinarian (see "Pulse Oximetry," this volume, p 117). Therefore, diminished arterial oxygen content is often implied from physical examination findings and the underlying disease process.

There are five pathophysiologic causes of hypoxemia. *Low partial pressure of oxygen in the inspired gas* may result in diminished arterial oxygen content. This most commonly occurs in patients on anesthetic machines or ventilators in which the inspired gas is oxygen poor, or there is excessive rebreathing of dead-space gas. *Hypoventilation* is another cause of hypoxemia and is most commonly detected with airway obstruction, neuromuscular diseases, pleural space or thoracic wall abnormalities, or diaphragm dysfunction. *Diffusion impairment* of oxygen from the alveoli to the pulmonary capillaries is an uncommon cause of hypoxemia in animals, but may occur in lung diseases in which the respiratory membrane is thickenend by proliferation of granular pneumocytes, or accumulation of fibrin deposits or cellular infiltrates or both. We have seen diffusion impairment in patients with diffuse lung injury and histopathologic characteristics of adult respiratory distress syndrome (ARDS). *Ventilation/perfusion mismatch* is the leading cause of arterial hypoxemia in our clinical patients and is seen in diseases that affect the pulmonary interstitium or alveoli such as pulmonary edema, hemorrhage, pneumonia, neoplasia, or embolism. *Right-to-left pulmonary vascular shunt* is the fifth cause of hypoxemia and is an extreme example of ventilation/perfusion mismatch. This cause of hypoxemia does not respond to oxygen supplementation (e.g., lung atelectasis).

The hallmark clinical sign of diminished arterial oxygen content is cyanosis of the mucous membranes. For cyanosis to be detected, there must be greater than 5 gm/dl of unoxygenated hemoglobin in the peripheral capillaries. Therefore, anemic patients may have significant hypoxia without cyanosis. Other clinical signs of hypoxemia that may be noted include an anxious expression; extended head and neck; open-mouth breathing; abducted elbows; and restlessness or agitation, especially during restraint. Respiratory rate is often elevated as well as the heart rate in hypoxemic patients. The brain is one of the most sensitive organs to oxygen deprivation, and hypoxemic patients may be syncopal, obtunded, or even comatose.

Not all patients with respiratory signs are hypoxemic. For example, any disease process that results in diminished perfusion or oxygen delivery to the medulla such as shock, pericardial tamponade, or anemia may result in respiratory stimulation and tachypnea. Tachypnea may also occur with hyperthermia, fear, anxiety, metabolic acidosis, or certain anesthetic drugs

such as narcotics. In the clinical situation, the requirement for oxygen supplementation may not always be clear. If in doubt, oxygen supplementation should be administered.

## MODES OF OXYGEN THERAPY

There are several methods of oxygen delivery available to the small animal practitioner. These include: (1) face mask, (2) nasal catheter, (3) tracheal catheter, (4) oxygen cages and other oxygen-enriched environments, and (5) mechanical ventilation. Selection of the optimal technique depends on the patient's respiratory status and the desired inspired oxygen content ($FIO_2$), the anticipated duration of therapy; the equipment available; and the size, conformation, and temperament of the animal.

### Face Mask

Face masks are used for the short-term delivery of oxygen in emergency situations, for initial therapy, or to evaluate the need for supplemental oxygen in equivocal cases. The advantage of this method is that it may be initiated immediately, with minimal equipment (commercially available oxygen masks and an oxygen source). With a well-fitted mask, high inspired oxygen concentrations can be achieved. As a general guide, flow rates of 8 to 12 L/min achieve an $FIO_2$ of 0.5 to 0.6. To allow elimination of carbon dioxide, an anesthetic machine with a circle system or a nonrebreathing circuit can be used as an oxygen source. The usefulness of this technique is limited in brachycephalic dogs and in many cats, where ill-fitting masks limit the delivered oxygen concentration and create dead space that increases the work of breathing. In addition, masks are generally poorly tolerated, except in moribund animals, necessitating that the patient be continually attended to prevent removal. Many animals will struggle, increasing oxygen consumption and negating the beneficial effects of supplementation. In these patients, an oxygen-enriched environment or immediate placement of a nasal catheter is preferred.

Oxygen may also be administered in acute situations via a plastic bag placed over the animal's head and secured around the neck. Tubing from an oxygen source is passed through a hole punctured in the bag. Oxygen flow rates are similar to those used with a face mask. Like the face mask, this method has the benefit of allowing free access to the patient. The disadvantages, however, are numerous: patients become rapidly hyperthermic; gas leakage invariably occurs, reducing the $FIO_2$; and some patients struggle. While this represents a crude and inefficient method of oxygen supplementation, it may be indicated for short-term therapy in the critically unstable patient that cannot tolerate a mask or catheter.

## Nasal Catheter

The nasal catheter is one of the most efficient, convenient, and cost-effective methods of oxygen administration in small animal patients. It is most commonly indicated for prolonged therapy, but its rapidity and ease of application make it an attractive option for initial therapy in animals that do not tolerate a mask.

The major advantage of this method is that a high $FIO_2$ can be achieved (up to 90%), while allowing free access to the patient. This is particularly important in the critical animal that requires continual monitoring or frequent manipulations. The disadvantages are that the $FIO_2$ cannot be accurately determined, and some patients do not tolerate the catheter and make repeated attempts to dislodge it.

The technique of nasal catheterization is described in Table 1. The catheter should be replaced every 48 hr with a new catheter in the opposite nare.

The flow rate of oxygen is dependent on the size of the animal and the required $FIO_2$, and varies with changes in the respiratory pattern. Table 2 provides guidelines. Animals with tachypnea and reduced tidal volumes may have markedly higher $FIO_2$ at these flow rates. High flow rates may be irritating to the animal, and may be associated with complications such as jet damage to the nasal mucosa or gastric dilation. The

**Table 2.** *Approximate Oxygen Flow Rates for Oxygen Administration Via a Nasal Catheter*[*]

| Weight (kg) | Oxygen Flow Rates (L/min) Required to Deliver an $FIO_2$ of: | | |
| --- | --- | --- | --- |
| | 30–50 % | 50–75 % | 75–100 % |
| 0–10 | 0.5–1 | 1–2 | 3–5 |
| 10–20 | 1–2 | 3–5 | >5 |
| 20–40 | 3–5 | >5 | ? |

*From Court MH: Respiratory support of the critically ill small animal patient. *In* Murtaugh RJ and Kaplan PM (eds): *Veterinary Emergency and Critical Care Medicine.* St. Louis, Mosby Year Book, 1992, p 575, with permission.

minimum flow rate to produce the desired effects should be used. Where high rates are needed, the authors prefer bilateral nasal catheter placement.

Because the catheter bypasses the nasal passages, humidification of the inspired gases is essential to prevent drying of the respiratory mucosa and associated complications. This can be achieved using a commercial in-line bubble humidifier, which attaches to the oxygen wall outlet. This system can be approximated by bubbling the oxygen through an intravenous fluid bottle filled with warm sterile water. With the bottle upright, the oxygen source is connected to the vent port and the tubing to the patient exits from the infusion-line port.

**Table 1.** *Technique of Nasal Catheterization for Oxygen Therapy*

**Equipment:**
  Oxygen source
  In-line bubble humidifier
  Rubber pediatric feeding tube: largest bore possible for patient's nare
  Catheter adaptor
  Syringe barrel without plunger: 5 or 10ml
  Suction tubing (sterile)
  Lidocaine (2%) or proparacaine: 0.5–1.0ml
  Lubricant
  Medical adhesive tape and suture material (nylon), or cyanoacrylate adhesive

**Procedure**
  Infuse lidocaine or proparacaine into the nare, and elevate the muzzle.
  Premeasure the catheter between the medial canthus of the eye and the nare, and mark it at the level of the nare.
  Lubricate the tip of the catheter.
  Insert the catheter into the ventromedial aspect of the nare, and advance it aborally in the ventral meatus to the predetermined length.
  Secure the catheter to the side of the face, as close as possible to the nare, by means of adhesive glue, or by fashioning a tape "butterfly" around the catheter and suturing this to the skin.
  Secure a more proximal portion of the catheter to the skin, either ventral to the ear or on the forehead. (The latter is preferred in cats, who appear to be more tolerant of a catheter if it avoids the whiskers.)
  Attach the syringe barrel to the proximal end of the catheter, using the adaptor.
  Connect the syringe to the humidified oxygen source, by means of the suction tubing.
  Select the appropriate flow rate.

## Tracheal Catheter

A tracheal catheter may be used in patients that do not tolerate a nasal catheter, or where facial conformation or pathology prohibits nasal placement. They are less irritating than nasal catheters, but are more invasive and technically more difficult to place. In the authors' experience, they are difficult to maintain if the animal is able to move its head.

The technique of placement is similar to a transtracheal wash. A large-gauge, long, flexible catheter is used. The end of the catheter should be fenestrated with a sterile blade to prevent jet damage to the tracheal mucosa. In smaller patients, insertion is via the cricothyroid ligament, and in larger dogs between two tracheal rings. The area over the site is clipped and surgically prepared. Local anesthesia of the overlying skin facilitates atraumatic insertion. Aseptic technique should be followed throughout the procedure. The needle of the catheter is introduced percutaneously into the trachea, and the catheter is passed so that the tip lies just cranial to the carina (at approximately the fifth intercostal space). The needle is then withdrawn and the catheter is secured in place with a neck wrap and attached to an oxygen source. Oxygen flow rates and humidification similar to those for nasal catheters are recommended. Complications of this technique include jet damage to the tracheal mucosa and tracheitis.

## Oxygen Cages and Alternative Oxygen-Enriched Environments

An oxygen cage is a sealed compartment with mechanisms to regulate oxygen concentration, eliminate expired carbon dioxide, and control ambient temperature and humidity. Oxygen cages designed for small animal use are available commercially or may be custom built. These systems, however, tend to be expensive, and many of the models currently on the market do not provide the optimal features. Veterinarians should therefore be extremely cautious when purchasing such equipment. The most important aspect to consider is the maximum attainable oxygen concentration. Several commercially available units merely provide a "controlled environment" and do not achieve concentrations above 21% (room air). Most oxygen cages can provide an $FIO_2$ of 0.4 to 0.5. Few machines, however, are able to deliver oxygen concentrations that exceed this (Intensive Care Unit, Plas Labs). The cage door should be made of plexiglass to allow clear visualization of the patient, and it should have portals for entry and exit of fluid lines and monitoring leads. These portals should be designed to minimize oxygen leakage. To this end, we prefer adjustable plastic sleeves to stoppered holes. These also allow some manipulation of the patient without opening the door of the cage. A reliable thermostat and a humidity control device are also essential.

The advantage of an oxygen cage is that it is noninvasive and allows for accurate monitoring and control of the $FIO_2$, temperature, and humidity. It is commonly used for patients that will not tolerate more invasive means of oxygen supplementation. Ambient temperature should be maintained at approximately 22°C (70°F), with a relative humidity of 40 to 50% (Court, 1992). The patient's temperature should be monitored frequently. Large dogs, particularly, tend to become hyperthermic, further compromising their respiratory status. In these patients, nasal catheterization is preferable whenever possible.

The major disadvantage of an oxygen cage, or other oxygen-enriched environment, is that the patient is effectively isolated from the clinician. Evaluation of the animal necessitates opening the cage, thus decreasing the $FIO_2$, with potential decompensation of the patient. Assessment of the animal's respiratory status, by means of a clinical examination or arterial blood gas analysis, does not reflect the status of the animal in the cage. (This deficit can be overcome to some extent, however, with the use of pulse oximetry, which allows remote monitoring of the animal's arterial oxygen saturation within the cage.) An additional disadvantage of the oxygen cage is the large amount of oxygen required to fill the cage, and the enormous gas wastage that occurs with opening. This makes the cage an expensive method of oxygen therapy.

Human neonatal incubators provide an efficient and less expensive option to the oxygen cage for pediatric canine patients and small cats. These systems allow temperature control and, due to their small size, can achieve high oxygen concentrations with relatively small flow rates.

Alternative oxygen-enriched environments have been described for use in small animals. These include a human oxygen tent, and a cage with a "fitted door" into which oxygen is pumped. These systems do not provide a means of carbon dioxide removal or control of ambient temperature and humidity, and may be extremely detrimental to the critical patient. High oxygen flow rates are required to achieve oxygen concentrations of 21 to 50%, and gas leakage invariably occurs. These systems are therefore an inefficient, expensive, and potentially hazardous means of oxygen supplementation.

## Mechanical Ventilation

Mechanical ventilation is indicated in the following situations: (1) hypoventilation, (2) failure of appropriate oxygen supplementation to correct the hypoxemia, (3) high $FIO_2$ requirements for extended periods, (4) clinical signs of respiratory fatigue and impending failure, and (5) intracranial hypertension. A review of ventilator techniques is beyond the scope of this article, and can be found elsewhere (Moon and Concannon, 1992).

## COMPLICATIONS OF OXYGEN THERAPY

Prolonged exposure to high oxygen tensions can result in pulmonary oxygen toxicity. The pathogenesis of this syndrome is likely associated with the production of cytotoxic free oxygen radicals that result in severe pulmonary changes and functional impairment. Evidence suggests that the production of these oxygen radicals is a function of the duration of exposure and the $PaO_2$, rather than the $FIO_2$. There is considerable species and individual variation in susceptibility to toxicity, and diseased lungs do not appear to be more susceptible. Administration of 50% oxygen for longer than 24 hr, or 100% oxygen for longer than 12 hr, should be avoided. Prolonged exposure to less than 50% oxygen, however, does not produce significant lesions in experimental dogs.

Oxygen supplementation can suppress the respiratory drive in patients with severe chronic pulmonary disease. These animals have chronic carbon dioxide retention, and the sensitivity of the central chemoreceptors is lost. Under these conditions, hypoxemia becomes the chief stimulus to ventilation. If such an animal receives oxygen supplementation to relieve the hypoxemia, ventilation may be significantly depressed. These patients require positive-pressure ventilation. Other clinically significant changes that may be associated with oxygen therapy include absorption atelectasis, decreased erythropoiesis, pulmonary vasodilation, and systemic arteriolar vasoconstriction (Fisher, 1980).

In spite of the potential deleterious effects of oxygen supplementation, they remain less significant than the effects of hypoxemia, and the clinician should not hesitate to administer oxygen when indicated. The minimum

F$IO_2$ to relieve the hypoxemia should be used. When the maintenance of adequate oxygenation necessitates prolonged administration of high oxygen concentrations, mechanical ventilation should be considered.

## WEANING FROM OXYGEN THERAPY

In spite of the frequency with which oxygen therapy is used, discontinuation of such therapy has received little attention. It is clear that the administration of high concentrations of oxygen for extended periods is not therapeutic, rational, or safe. Oxygen should be viewed as any other drug and should be given when clinically indicated, only in the amounts required, and reduced and discontinued as soon as feasible. During this period, the causes of hypoxemia should be identified and specific therapy instituted. The duration of oxygen therapy will be dictated by the progress of the patient's primary disease. When this shows evidence of improvement, discontinuation of oxygen therapy can be attempted.

Abrupt cessation of oxygen supplementation can result in rapid respiratory decompensation, even when the patient is receiving a low F$IO_2$. An F$IO_2$ as low as 0.3 can mask the hypoxic effects of lung areas with low ventilation/perfusion ratios. It is prudent to reduce the F$IO_2$ in small decrements over a 24- to 48-hr period, depending on the patient's response. The animal should be closely monitored, and oxygen therapy should be reinstituted if signs of respiratory compromise become apparent. Periodic determination of Pa$O_2$ provides the most objective means of assessing the patient's response to weaning.

### References and Suggested Reading

Court MH: Respiratory support of the critically ill small animal patient. *In* Murtaugh RJ and Kaplan PM (eds): *Veterinary Emergency and Critical Care Medicine.* St. Louis, Mosby Year Book, 1992, p 575.
 *A review of the methods and effects of oxygen supplementation and mechanical ventilation.*
Fisher AB: Oxygen therapy: Side effects and toxicity. Am Rev Respir Dis 122: 61, 1980.
 *A review of oxygen-related complications.*
Moon PF and Concannon KT: Mechanical Ventilation. *In* Kirk RW and Bonagura JD (eds.): *Current Veterinary Therapy XI.* Philadelphia, WB Saunders Co, 1992, p 98.
 *A review of current veterinary techniques of mechanical ventilation.*

# TEMPORARY TRACHEOSTOMY

ROGER B. FINGLAND
*Manhattan, Kansas*

*It is necessary that the tracheostomy serve its purpose well without creating complications of its own."*
Patrick D. Kenan, M.D.

Temporary tracheostomy is indicated to relieve life-threatening upper airway obstruction or prevent its development, to facilitate removal of lower airway secretions (when the cough reflex is abolished), to enable assisted ventilation, to create a vent to reduce pressure effects related to a closed glottis (which undesirably raises cerebrospinal fluid pressure in patients with cerebral edema), and to facilitate inhalation anesthesia during an upper airway or intraoral surgical procedure when per os endotracheal intubation is undesirable. The most common indication for temporary tracheostomy in animals is relief of obstruction from congenital or acquired upper airway disease.

Cuffed and uncuffed metal, plastic, and rubber tubes are available for tracheostomy. Tubes with inner removable cannulae (Shiley, Inc, Irvine, CA) are preferred because the airway is maintained by the outer sheath, while the inner cannula is removed for cleaning. Most tracheostomy tubes designed for use in human patients are disposable but may be sterilized a limited number of times. Ventilatory support via temporary tracheostomy requires a tube with a soft, high-volume, low-pressure cuff. Overinflation of the cuff must be avoided (see "Complications," below). Uncuffed tracheostomy tubes (Shiley, Inc, Irvine, CA) are acceptable; perhaps preferred, for most veterinary applications. The tracheostomy tube diameter should permit movement of normal respiratory volumes through as well as around the tube if it becomes obstructed, approximately two thirds to three quarters the diameter of the trachea. Excessively large tubes predispose to postintubation stenosis.

Suction catheters of appropriate size and texture must be used for tracheal suctioning. Large, stiff, open-ended catheters damage tracheal mucosa. A soft suction catheter with a blunt end, side holes, and a device (side port or T-connector) that allows precise control of suction at the catheter tip may be used. A whistle-tip suction catheter (Argyle, St. Louis, MO) is ideal because the suction control mechanism is built-in and the catheter is soft, pliable, and has side holes.

## TECHNIQUE

Tracheostomy is rarely an emergency procedure. The safest way to establish an emergency airway is by insertion of an endotracheal tube per os. Most obstructive upper airway lesions can be bypassed in this way so that the patient can be maintained until definitive surgical procedures can be performed. Aseptic conditions and precise hemostasis are desirable, although emergency situations require that tracheostomy be performed under less than ideal conditions. The procedure should be performed in the operating room, if only to maintain the most aseptic conditions and impress the operator with the need for meticulous technique.

The patient is positioned in dorsal recumbency with a roll of towels placed under the neck to maintain cervical dorsiflexion. The ventral cervical region is prepared for aseptic surgery in all but emergent circumstances. A ventral cervical midline incision is made from the caudal aspect of the cricoid cartilage to approximately the level of the sixth tracheal cartilage. The paired sternothyroideus and sternohyoideus muscles are bluntly separated on the midline. Various approaches to tracheal incision have been proposed, and there is considerable controversy regarding which incision results in fewer and less-severe postoperative complications.

### Transverse Tracheostoma

Using a No. 10 scalpel blade, a full-thickness stab incision is made through the annular ligament between the third and fourth tracheal cartilages (Fig. 1A). Vital structures are retracted as the tracheostoma is extended laterally from the stab incision (Fig. 1B and 1C). Approximately 65% of the tracheal circumference is incised. A loop of 2-0 silk suture material is placed around the ventral aspect of the tracheal cartilage cranial and caudal to the tracheostoma to facilitate exposure of the stoma during intubation and reintubation (Fig. 2A).

The tracheostoma must be sufficiently large, and the tracheal cartilages must be compliant and flexible to permit atraumatic insertion of the tracheostomy tube through a transverse incision (Fig. 2B). If the tracheostoma is too small or the tracheostomy tube too large, the tracheal cartilage cranial to the tracheostoma is deformed into the tracheal lumen as the tube is inserted. Pressure necrosis of adjacent tracheal cartilage and mucosa can result. Transverse and longitudinal tracheostomas have been evaluated experimentally in animals of different species and age. Although conflicting results exist, many studies have shown no significant difference in the two stomal incisions with regard to immediate and long-term postintubation complications. Most investigators and this author recommend transverse tracheostoma despite the lack of overwhelming experimental evidence to support its superiority.

### Longitudinal Tracheostoma

A ventral midline full-thickness incision is made in the tracheal wall between but not including the second and sixth tracheal cartilages. Although tracheal carti-

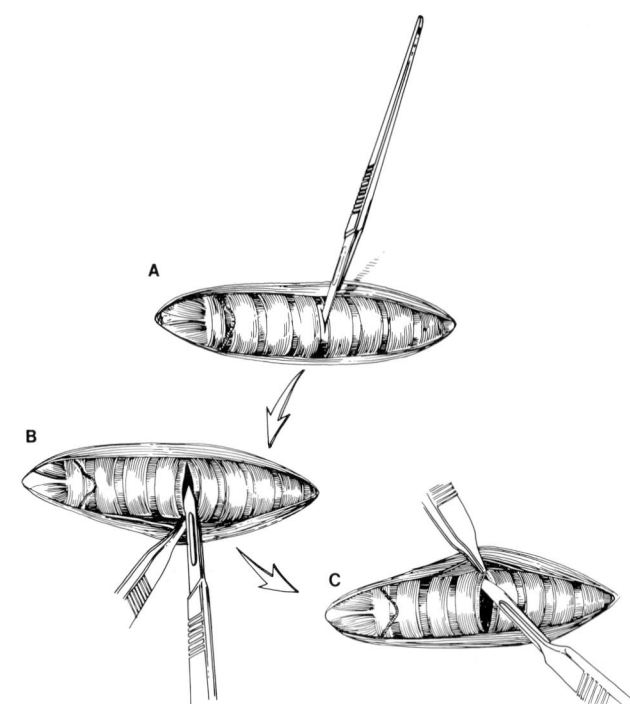

**Figure 1.** Technique for creating a transverse tracheostoma. *A*, A full-thickness stab incision is made on the ventral aspect of the trachea between the third and fourth tracheal cartilages. *B* and *C*, While protecting lateral neurovascular structures with thumb forceps, the tracheal incision is extended laterally on both sides to include approximately 65% of the tracheal circumference.

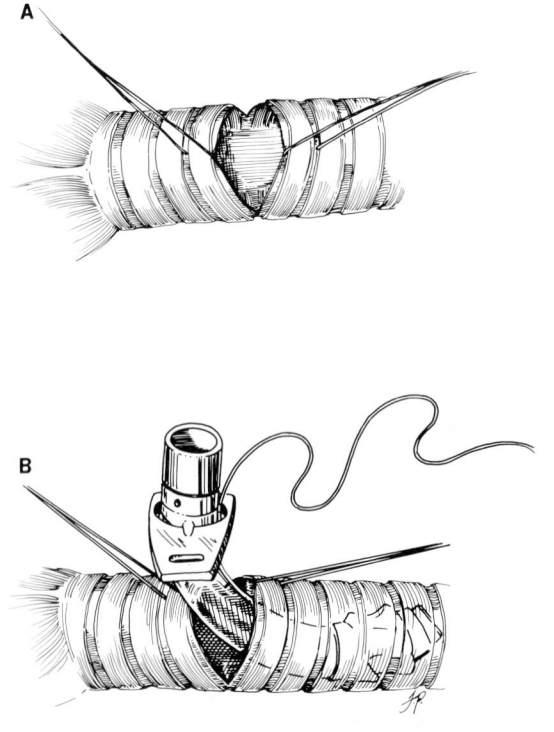

**Figure 2.** *A*, A loop of 2–0 silk suture material is placed around the tracheal cartilage cranial and caudal to the tracheostoma to facilitate exposure during intubation. *B*, The tracheostomy tube is positioned in the trachea, making certain that the tracheal cartilage cranial to the tracheostoma is not distorted.

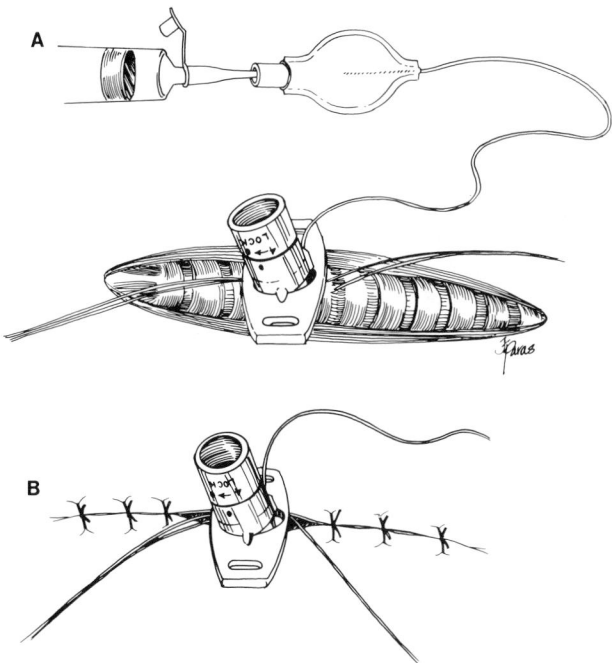

**Figure 3.** *A*, The tracheostomy tube cuff is inflated *only* if ventilatory assistance is required. *B*, The subcutaneous tissue and skin are apposed cranial and caudal to the tracheostoma. The remaining opening must be large enough to accommodate reintubation.

lages are transected, neurovascular structures lateral to the trachea are at less risk for injury. Excessive distraction of the longitudinal tracheostoma during tube insertion can result in tearing of adjacent annular ligaments. The everted ends of the transected cartilages lie against the tracheostomy tube, predisposing the tracheal mucosa to pressure necrosis. Medial collapse of

the transected cartilages may result in postintubation segmental tracheal collapse.

## Tracheal Flap

A U-shaped full-thickness incision, based on the second tracheal cartilage and extending two cartilages caudally, is made on the ventral aspect of the trachea. The flap of ventral tracheal wall is preserved. Creation of a tracheal flap may eliminate excessive pressure on tracheal cartilage and mucosa from a tight-fitting tracheostomy tube. Proponents of this tracheostoma technique emphasize the theoretical advantage of being able to close the stoma by suturing the flap. Unfortunately, anatomic reconstruction frequently is not possible due to destruction or deformation of the flap. The tracheal flap technique has limited usefulness in veterinary medicine and should be reserved for patients that require long-term (weeks to months) tracheostomy.

After the tracheostoma is created, the trachea is gently suctioned to remove blood and mucus and the tracheostomy tube inserted (Fig. 3*A*). The subcutaneous tissue and skin are apposed cranial and caudal to the tube, making certain the incision remains large enough to accommodate reintubation (Fig. 3*B*). The tube is secured by placing a loop of gauze around the patient's neck and through the tieing flange. A cervical bandage is optional.

The tracheostomy tube must be positioned properly within the trachea. If the tube is twisted or inserted too deeply, pressure is exerted on the dorsal tracheal wall by the arch of the tube and on the ventral tracheal wall by the tip of the tube. Prolonged improper positioning can lead to mucosal erosion and cartilage injury (Fig. 4).

**Figure 4.** Complications associated with temporary tracheostomy. *A*, Overinflation of the tracheostomy tube cuff results in distortion of the tracheal wall and excessive pressure on the tracheal mucosa. *B*, Obstructive lesions that may result from temporary tracheostomy. Ventrolateral stricture (*a*) or granuloma (*b*) at the tracheostoma. Granuloma (*c*) at the tip of the tube. Circumferential stricture (*d*) at the level of the cuff.

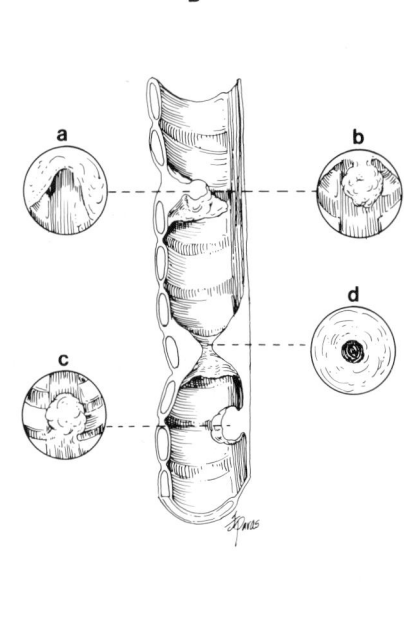

The tracheostomy tube cuff is inflated *only* if positive-pressure ventilation is required. The cuff is inflated so that a slight leak is detected when airway pressures are maximal. If a seal cannot be obtained with an inflation pressure of 25 mm Hg, a larger diameter tube should be used.

## TRACHEOSTOMY TUBE CARE

Tracheostomy tube care requires vigilant patient monitoring and close attention to aseptic technique. Patients with a temporary tracheostomy require 24-hr monitoring, preferably in an intensive care unit. Less frequent observation risks fatal airway obstruction from tube occlusion or dislodgment. Personnel should wash their hands before performing tracheostomy tube care and should wear sterile surgical gloves when handling tubes or suction catheters. Tracheostomy tube care consists of tube (or inner cannula) exchanges, airway suctioning, and humidification or nebulization.

The inner cannula or single-lumen tracheostomy tube should be replaced at least every 24 hr and as needed to maintain a patent airway. Tube exchanges may be needed every 3 or 4 hr for the first 12 hr of intubation. Several inner cannulae can be kept on hand, allowing personnel to simply exchange the soiled cannula with a clean, sterile cannula. Single-lumen tracheostomy tubes should be replaced with a new or resterilized tracheostomy tube of the same diameter. Cold sterilization of tracheostomy tubes or inner cannulae is not recommended. If this sterilization technique must be used, make certain the tube or cannula is rinsed thoroughly with sterile saline solution prior to insertion.

Tracheal suctioning to remove respiratory secretions is necessary because tube tracheostomy prevents coughing. Suctioning frequency varies from 15-min to 8-hr intervals depending on how rapidly the tube becomes occluded with blood, mucus, or exudate. Patients that have conditions commonly associated with copious respiratory secretions such as bronchopneumonia and tracheitis require more frequent suctioning. In many patients, suctioning is required at frequent intervals for the first 24 hr of intubation and then much less frequently. Close attention to the patient's respiratory pattern between scheduled suctioning is critical; suctioning should be performed whenever the need arises.

The patient should be preoxygenated immediately prior to suctioning. One to three hyperventilations (150% of tidal volume) using 100% oxygen will protect the patient from a suction-induced fall in $PaO_2$ for 120 sec after suctioning (Skelley, Deeren, and Powaser, 1980). The suction catheter is inserted without vacuum to the carina or until an obstruction is detected. The catheter is retracted as intermittent, light suction is applied. Rotating the catheter during retrieval minimizes mucosal damage and facilitates removal of secretions. The total time that vacuum is applied to the airway must not exceed 15 sec.

Complications that can result from tracheal suctioning include hypoxemia, gagging, retching, or vomiting from vagal stimulation; cardiac arrhythmias secondary to hypoxia or vagal stimulation; arterial hypotension from vagus-induced bradyarrhythmias; atelectasis from prolonged or excessive suction; and mucosal damage from excessive suction pressure or indiscriminate catheter placement (Wheeler, 1993). Complications related to increased vagal tone can be avoided by atropine administration; however, atropine increases the viscosity of airway secretions, which is of increased consequence in patients with tracheostomy.

Maintenance of airway hydration is essential to prevent dehydration of the mucous layer and subsequent interference with mucociliary flow or damage to respiratory epithelium. The mucous layer is the primary source of water for inspired air when the nasopharynx is bypassed by a tracheostomy tube. Airway hydration can be maintained during tracheostomy by humidification, nebulization, or less efficiently, by instillation of fluid directly into the trachea.

Humidifiers saturate air with water vapor by bubbling air through a liquid reservoir. Nebulizers produce a suspension of very fine particles of liquid in a gas. Humidifiers are helpful in preventing dehydration of airways but are unable to deliver fluid. Pneumatic nebulizers work well for maintaining hydration of airways, although more expensive ultrasonic nebulizers are capable of delivering a larger volume of fluid to the entire respiratory tract. Only sterile solutions (saline or distilled water) should be nebulized because nebulizers are capable of transmitting bacteria from a contaminated reservoir. The patient should be nebulized for 15 min four to six times daily. Pneumatic nebulizers can be attached directly to the tracheostomy tube or placed in-line when a ventilatory circuit is in place.

Hyperventilation, inspiration of dry gases, elevated body temperature, and diuretic therapy (particularly loop diuretics) increase water loss from the respiratory tract and predispose to dehydration of the mucous layer. Patients with elevated body temperature, systemic dehydration, or that require assisted ventilation or diuretic therapy may require systemic fluid administration and more frequent nebulization.

If humidification or nebulization of the airway is not possible, sterile saline solution should be instilled directly into the trachea via a small catheter inserted caudal to the end of the tracheostomy tube. The volume of saline solution to instill is 0.1 ml/kg with a minimum of 1 ml and a maximum of 5 ml regardless of weight. This procedure should be repeated as needed or at 2-hr intervals.

Daily local wound care consists of cleaning the skin adjacent to and beneath the tracheostomy tube flange with sterile cotton-tipped applicators and saline solution. Antiseptic soaps and antibacterial ointments can be irritating to the exposed tracheal mucosa and should be avoided. Prophylactic systemic antibiotic therapy is not indicated and increases the patient risk for infection by antibiotic-resistant bacteria. Tracheostomy is a major risk factor for nosocomial pneumonia by *Pseu-*

*domonas* or gram-negative enteric bacteria that have limited antibiotic susceptibility. Bacterial pneumonia or tracheobronchial infection secondary to tracheostomy should be treated based on culture and susceptibility testing.

## TUBE REMOVAL

The majority of small animal patients require intubation for less than 3 days and about one third for less than 12 hr (Harvey and O'Brien, 1982). Long-term intubation predisposes to postintubation complications, including stenosis. The tracheostomy tube should be removed as soon as the patient is able to move a normal respiratory volume past any obstruction or when assisted ventilation is no longer needed. Extubation consists (in cases of upper airway obstruction diseases) of a series of tube exchanges, each being smaller in diameter, followed by an observation period of at least 15 minutes. If at any time the patient becomes dyspneic, the next larger size tube is inserted and extubation is delayed for at least 12 hr. If ventilation is adequate with a small tube in place, the occlusion cannula (or a cork) is placed in the tracheostomy tube and the patient is observed for 30 min. Extubation is safe if respiratory distress is not observed.

## PATHOLOGIC EFFECTS OF TUBE TRACHEOSTOMY

Tracheostomy, regardless of the orientation of the tracheostoma, results in some degree of luminal stenosis in all patients because the stoma heals by circular cicatrization. Healing of a transverse tracheostoma following short-duration (4 hr) intubation is rapid, with complete reepithelialization occurring by 10 days (Harvey and Goldschmidt, 1982). Tracheostomy does not significantly affect tracheal growth in puppies.

The presence of a tracheostomy tube for 24 hr results in loss of cilia, epithelial ulceration, and submucosal inflammation from the tracheostoma to the carina. Tracheal foreign body (including tracheostomy tubes), assisted ventilation, and high $FIO_2$ predispose to retained respiratory secretions. Retained secretions predispose to mucosal inflammation, atelectasis from obstruction of bronchioles, and bronchopneumonia. The trachea becomes colonized with bacteria from the oropharyngeal flora within 24 hr of intubation.

The trachea at the site of an inflated tracheostomy tube cuff shows a spectrum of changes ranging from superficial inflammation and mucosal ulceration, to necrosis of tracheal cartilages. Cuff inflation pressure has a direct influence on the severity of the tracheal lesion. Severe lesions lead to stenosis due to cicatricial healing.

In human patients on ventilatory support, there is a direct, statistically significant correlation between the potential for tracheal injury and the severity and refractiveness of respiratory failure reflected by elevated oxygen alveolar-arterial difference, need for high $FIO_2$, and need for positive end-expiratory pressure (PEEP) (Kastanos et al., 1983). Respiratory failure may predispose to mucosal injury through the development of increased local hypoxia. Maintenance of local and systemic hydration and close attention to cuff inflation pressure are critically important in intubated patients with severe respiratory disease.

## COMPLICATIONS

Immediate and early complications associated with tube tracheostomy include hemorrhage, damage to peritracheal neurovascular structures, obstruction, dislodgment, and infection. Postintubation complications are observed less frequently and include luminal stenosis and, rarely, tracheocutaneous fistulae. Complications often can be avoided by meticulous surgical technique and disciplined tracheostomy tube care (see "Preventing Complications," below).

Airway obstruction is the most common complication of tracheostomy, both during and after intubation. Tube occlusion can result from kinking, displacement of the deflated cuff over the end of the tube, or impaction with dried secretions. Occlusion of a tracheostomy tube with dried secretions represents the most common and most deadly of all complications associated with temporary tracheostomy. The importance of continuous patient monitoring and meticulous tube care cannot be overemphasized.

### Postintubation Stenosis

Postintubation airway obstruction (stenosis) occurs, to some degree, in all patients that have had a tracheostoma. Patients with less than 75% reduction in tracheal diameter typically are asymptomatic. Clinical signs of luminal stenosis include progressively worsening stridor and dyspnea beginning approximately 4 weeks after extubation. The majority of patients with luminal stenosis following tracheostomy remain asymptomatic for life.

Controversy exists over which tube- or procedure-related factors are most important in the etiology of postintubation stenosis. Infection, movement of the tracheostomy tube within the trachea, pressure on the tracheal wall from the tube or inflated cuff, and surgical technique are known to influence the development of stenosis. Infection, motion, and excessive pressure result in mucosal damage and loss of structural integrity of the tracheal cartilage. Healing of damaged tracheal tissues by cicatrization results in stenosis.

Postintubation stenosis can occur at tracheostoma, cuff site, tip of the tracheostomy tube, or between the stoma and cuff site (Fig. 4). Most patients with stenotic lesions can be managed successfully by resection of the affected segment of trachea followed by precise anastomosis.

Obstruction can result from a polypoid granuloma on the mucosal surface adjacent to the tracheostoma or from collapse or cicatricial healing of damaged tracheal cartilages. Improper surgical technique or tearing of the tracheal wall from traction on the tracheostomy tube may result in an excessively large tracheostoma that is predisposed to complications during healing.

Clinical, pathologic, and experimental data clearly demonstrate the cause-and-effect relationship between excessive cuff pressure and postintubation stenosis at the cuff site. Cuff stenoses typically are circumferential masses of fibrous tissue with small eccentric openings (Fig. 4B).

Tracheal cartilages between the tracheostoma and cuff site can become malacic from chronic inflammation or can be damaged by repeated traumatic intubation. The result usually is dynamic collapse of the affected segment of trachea rather than static luminal stenosis. This condition is rare and may require support from extraluminal prostheses.

The tracheostomy tube tip can cause significant trauma to the tracheal mucosa, especially when the cuff is not inflated. Obstruction results from granulation tissue forming at the point of mucosal erosion (Fig. 4B).

## Preventing Complications

Complications of tracheostomy often can be avoided by thoughtful preparation, meticulous surgical technique, and vigilant tube care. Ideally, tracheostomy should be performed as an elective procedure in a controlled environment. The clinician should consider the likelihood of airway obstruction (e.g., following oral or pharyngeal surgery in brachycephalic breeds), and make certain that personnel and equipment are available for emergency tracheostomy. Alternatively, and often preferably, tracheostomy can be performed elec-

tively prior to performing a procedure that is likely to result in critical airway obstruction.

Patients that require assisted ventilation are at much greater risk for postintubation complications because the tracheostomy tube cuff must be inflated and ventilator hoses must be attached to the tracheostomy tube. A high-volume, low-pressure, thin-wall cuff that does not distort the trachea when inflated minimizes the risk of tracheal injury. The best protection from stenosis lies in utilizing the lowest cuff pressure sufficient to allow adequate mechanical ventilation. Intermittent deflation of the tracheostomy tube cuff does not reduce the risk of mucosal necrosis. The linkage to mechanical respirators should be light and have a swivel adapter to reduce movement of the tracheostomy tube within the trachea.

## References and Suggested Reading

Harvey CE and O'Brien JA: Tracheotomy in the dog and cat: Analysis of 89 episodes in 79 animals. J Am Anim Hosp Assoc 18:563, 1982.
　*A review of the indications and outcomes of temporary tracheostomy in 79 dogs and cats.*
Harvey CE and Goldschmidt MH: Healing following short duration transverse incision tracheostomy in the dog. Vet Surg 11:77, 1982.
　*Clinical and histopathologic evaluation of the effects of transverse tracheostomy (6 hr to 28 days) on the canine trachea.*
Kastanos N, Miro RE, Perez AM, et al: Laryngotracheal injury due to endotracheal intubation: Incidence, evolution, and predisposing factors. A prospective long-term study. Crit Care Med 11:362, 1983.
　*An assessment of the incidence and outcome of laryngotracheal lesions due to intubation and an analysis of correlative factors.*
Skelly BFH, Deeren SM, and Powaser MM: The effectiveness of two preoxygenation methods to prevent endotracheal suction-induced hypoxemia. Heart Lung 9:316, 1980.
　*An evaluation of the effectiveness of two preoxygenation methods in preventing a fall in PaO$_2$ during and after endotracheal suctioning.*
Wheeler SL: Care of respiratory patients. *In* Slatter D (ed): *Textbook of Small Animal Surgery.* Philadelphia, WB Saunders Co, 1993, p 804.
　*A detailed review of normal and abnormal airway physiology in tracheostomy patients and an in-depth description of tracheostomy tube care.*

# THE PRACTICAL USE OF CONSTANT-RATE INFUSIONS

DOUGLASS K. MACINTIRE
*Auburn, Alabama*

The continuous intravenous (IV) delivery of medications through electronic infusion control devices has become commonplace in intensive care units (ICUs) and in referral centers specializing in critical care medicine. Many cardiac and vasoactive drugs have a rapid onset of action and short elimination half-life and must be administered by constant-rate infusion (CRI) to maintain constant serum concentrations and achieve desired pharmacologic effects. With adequate monitoring and accurate delivery systems, these drugs can pro-

vide immediate hemodynamic improvement and the dosage can be titrated to achieve the desired effects.

Despite the many advantages of a CRI, few veterinarians use this technique routinely in their practices. The reasons most practitioners avoid CRI drugs are threefold. First, the proper administration of CRI drugs requires specialized equipment, such as infusion pumps and blood pressure monitors, devices that are lacking in many practices. Second, many of the drugs delivered by CRI are relatively new, and many practitioners have little experience with these drugs. Third, the mathematics used to calculate CRI dosages can be intimidating and unfamiliar, and miscalculations can be fatal. This article will attempt to address these concerns and provide an overview of the drugs and equipment used in CRI therapy, and present some examples of "user-friendly" formulas to make calculations easy.

## EQUIPMENT

Most of the latest models of infusion pumps are volumetric, meaning that they deliver fluids at a constant preset volume in milliliters per hour. Nonvolumetric infusion pumps deliver fluids at a constant drop rate (drops per minute). Nonvolumetric pumps are considered less accurate because the drop size varies with the viscosity of the fluid infused. Thus, flow rates may vary among different fluids.

Infusion pumps generate their own pressure to overcome the resistance of the patient's venous or arterial pressure. Normal venous pressure is 0.8 pounds per square inch (psi), normal diastolic arterial pressure is 1.5 psi, and normal systolic arterial pressure is 2.3 psi (Koch, 1984). Most infusion pumps deliver fluids at an average pressure of 1 to 3 psi, a pressure that is comparable to gravity flow. When the intravenous line becomes occluded, the pressure increases to 4 to 25 psi, depending on the pump manufacturer's specifications. If the flow restriction remains despite the added pressure, an alarm will sound. Low-pressure pumps such as the AVI Guardian (3M AVI, St. Paul, MN), which has a variable occlusion pressure of 4 to 9 psi, may be associated with more frequent episodes of venous occlusion at the low-pressure setting. Although responding to frequent alarms seems bothersome, it may be safer than the alternative. When compared to a high-pressure pump with a venous occlusion pressure of 25 psi (IMED 928, IMED Corporation, San Diego, CA), the low-pressure pump had a significant decrease in the rate of extravascular tissue infiltration (5.1% versus 29.3%) (Engler and Engler, 1986). It appears that high-pressure pumps can potentiate extravasation of infusate at the site of the IV catheter, and they probably should not be used to deliver drugs that have the potential to cause severe perivascular reactions should extravasation occur. Another potential problem with high-pressure pumps is that the alarm will not sound until the maximum occlusion pressure is reached, which can result in a considerable time lapse before an occlusion is detected. If a patient is receiving life-sustaining pharmacologic agents at a low infusion rate, the time delay before the occlusion is detected may be life threatening.

There are three basic types of infusion pumps. A syringe pump is used to deliver small volumes of fluid. The syringe is manually loaded and the pump "pushes in" the plunger. Peristaltic pumps work by compressing and releasing tubing to propel the fluid forward. They are available in linear or rotary models. A third type is the cassette pump, which requires a special administration set. These pumps have a two-cycle delivery system in which first a fluid reservoir fills and then a preset volume is delivered under pressure. Pumps with a membrane filter set cannot be used to deliver suspensions, emulsions, blood, or blood components.

Many pumps require special administration sets that can cost $5 to $10 each. The cost of tubing and administration sets should be considered when purchasing a pump. Some pumps are made specifically to deliver enteral nutrition. In general, these pumps are not as accurate, but administration sets are generally cheaper. Pumps used to deliver critical care medications should have an accuracy rating of ±2% certified by the manufacturer.

Most pumps are equipped with safety alarms that detect air in line, occlusion, completion of infusion, and low battery power. As pumps become more sophisticated, new options become available. One example is the piggyback option, which allows the pump to deliver a secondary infusion at a different flow rate. Another option available on newer pumps is the ability to interface with a hospital computer, which can allow for accurate monitoring of patient responses to vasoactive drugs. As human hospitals upgrade their equipment, infusion pumps should become available to the veterinary market at reasonable cost. The cost of a new pump ranges from $1000 to $3000, but used pumps can be purchased for $200 to $500 (e.g., from Universal Hospital Services, Equipment Resale Program, Bloomington, MN, 1-800-535-1656).

A final consideration in choosing a pump that will be used to deliver cardiovascular drugs, is avoidance of pumps that deliver fluid by a pulsatile (bolus) rather than continuous (flow) method. Adverse pharmacodynamic effects can occur when drugs are delivered by periodic bolus, especially when using very low flow rates and high-concentration infusions. One study showed a variation in blood pressure of 30 mm Hg in dogs receiving epinephrine infusion at 1 ml/hr using a pulsatile diaphragm infusion pump (Abbott, Model II D) (Klem, Farrington, and Leff, 1993). At higher flow rates (5 ml/hr and 10 ml/hr), there was no difference between the different types of pumps tested, and the variability in blood pressure was not observed. The most accurate pump tested for very low flow rates was a linear piston syringe pump (Auto-Syringe, Model 20G, Hooksett, NH).

## DRUGS COMMONLY ADMINISTERED BY CRI

A list of drugs commonly administered by CRI is presented in Table 1. In addition, some of the more common drugs and their indications are discussed here.

### Positive Inotropes

*Dobutamine* is a synthetic catecholemine with selective $\beta_1$ (cardiac) activity, mild $\beta_2$ (vasodilatory) and dose-dependent $\alpha$-adrenergic effects. It is the preferred positive inotrope for the treatment of cardiac

**Table 1.**  *Drugs Commonly Administered by CRI**

| Drug | Actions/Indications | Dosage |
|---|---|---|
| Dopamine (low-dose) | Dilates renal arteries, increases renal blood flow, prevents acute renal failure | 1–3 $\mu$g/kg/min |
| Dopamine (moderate-dose) | Positive inotrope, cardiogenic or septic shock | 4–6 $\mu$g/kg/min |
| Dopamine (high-dose) | Pressor agent, promotes peripheral vasoconstriction, increases BP | 7–20 $\mu$g/kg/min |
| Dobutamine | Positive inotrope, cardiogenic or septic shock | Dogs: 2–20 (rarely as high as 40) $\mu$g/kg/min<br>Cats: 2.5–15 $\mu$g/kg/min |
| Amrinone | Positive inotrope, systemic vasodilator | 0.75 mg/kg IV bolus (slowly over 3–5 min), then 5–10 $\mu$g/kg/min |
| Atacurium | Induction of respiratory paralysis for controlled mechanical ventilation | 0.2 mg/kg IV, then 3–8 $\mu$g/kg/min |
| Epinephrine | Anaphylaxis, cardiac and blood pressure support | 0.1–1.0 $\mu$g/kg/min |
| Fentanyl | Analgesia, sedation, mecahnical ventilation | 10 $\mu$g/kg IV, then 0.3–0.6 $\mu$g/kg/min |
| Norepinephine | Pressor agent, short term blood pressure support | 0.05–1.0 $\mu$g/kg/min |
| Furosemide | Diuretic, promotes diuresis in acute oliguric renal failure | 3–8 $\mu$g/kg/min |
| Nitroprusside | Vasodilator, acute congestive heart failure | 0.5–10 $\mu$g/kg/min |
| Isoproterenol | Vasodilator, positive inotrope, bronchodilator | 0.02–0.10 $\mu$g/kg/min |
| Lidocaine | Ventricular antiarrhythmic | Dog: 2–4 mg/kg IV bolus, then 25–80 $\mu$g/kg/min<br>Cat: 0.25 mg/kg IV bolus, then 10 $\mu$g/kg/min CRI |
| Procainamide | Ventricular antiarrhythmic | Dog: 2 mg/kg bolus, repeated to maximum cumulative dose of 20 mg/kg, then 10–40 $\mu$g/kg/min |
| Verapamil | Supraventricular arrhythmias, tachycardias | 0.05–0.15 mg/kg IV, then 2–10 $\mu$g/kg/min |
| Metoclopramide | Antiemetic | 0.7–1.4 $\mu$g/kg/min |
| Esmolol | Short-acting $\beta$-blocker, decreases tachycardia | 25–200 $\mu$g/kg/min following a 500 $\mu$g/kg loading dose (over 1 min) |

*Certain chemotherapeutic agents, TPN, enteral feedings can also be administered by CRI.

depression associated with septic shock (see "Septic Shock," this volume, p 139) and increases cardiac output while decreasing systemic vascular resistance (at low to moderate doses). In humans, short periods of infusion have been associated with long-term (up to 4 weeks) improvement in cardiac performance (Liang et al., 1984). In veterinary medicine, the drug is used most often in dogs with dilated cardiomyopathy or myocardial failure secondary to sepsis or cardiopulmonary resuscitation. Dobutamine may cause seizures in cats and a lower dosage is recommended for this species.

*Amrinone* is a phosphodiesterase inhibitor with combined positive inotrope and vasodilator effects. It is indicated for the acute treatment of left ventricular failure when blood pressure is adequate. The positive inotropic effects may be less consistent when compared to dobutamine; however, the vasodilation can be potent in dogs. Amrinone cannot be diluted with solutions containing glucose and should not be exposed to light.

*Dopamine* is one of the most versatile hemodynamic drugs available. At low doses (1 to 3 $\mu$g/kg/min), it produces selective vasodilation of renal, splanchnic, and cerebral vasculature through stimulation of dopaminergic receptors. At moderate doses (3 to 10 $\mu$g/kg/min), a strong, predominantly $\beta$ agonist, positive inotropic effect is produced. At higher doses (7 to 10 $\mu$g/kg/min), increasingly prominent $\alpha$ adrenergic effects result in peripheral vasoconstriction. Dopamine is a precursor to norepinephrine, and at very high doses (>20 $\mu$g/kg/min) the $\alpha$ effect produces a strong pressor effect. Dopamine is indicated at low doses to prevent acute oliguric or anuric renal failure following shock, anesthesia, or the administration of nephrotoxic drugs. Concurrent administration of furosemide may be synergistic (Lindner, 1983). At moderate to high doses, dopamine is indicated to support cardiac function and blood pressure in states of shock or after resuscitation. Adverse effects may include tachycardia, arrhythmias, or profound vasoconstriction.

### Pressor Agents

*Epinephrine* is a combined $\alpha$- and $\beta$-adrenergic agonist that is indicated for treatment of anaphylaxis and hypotension resistant to dopamine. Adverse effects include serious arrhythmias, myocardial necrosis, and acute renal failure from excessive vasoconstriction. Like any of the pressor agents, this drug should be dosed with caution, titrated to the lowest dose necessary to maintain adequate blood pressure, and tapered as soon as possible. Pressor agents should not be used until fluid support has been administered to hypovolemic patients.

*Norepinephrine* infusion leads to prominent α-agonist activity. It is also used as a secondary agent to treat hypotension refractory to volume replacement and a CRI of dopamine.

### Vasodilator Drugs

*Nitroprusside* is a balanced vasodilator that dilates systemic arteries and veins. It may also have a prominent effect on pulmonary artery vasodilation and is effective in reducing the preload and afterload in fulminant heart failure with pulmonary edema. An initial CRI of 0.5 to 2 μg/kg/min is used. The base concentration is increased by 1 μg/kg/min every 30 min until there is an improvement in clinical signs (decreased pulmonary crackles and respiratory rate), a decrease in the pulmonary capillary wedge pressure, or identification of systemic hypotension. The effective dose may be as high as 5 to 8 μg/kg/min, but it is usually necessary to start at a lower dose and gradually increase it to prevent hypotension. Since this is a potent vasodilating agent, blood pressure monitoring is essential. When systolic blood pressure decreases to less than 90 to 100 mm Hg, the CRI dose should be decreased. The solution must be shielded from light and should not be continued more than 72 hr in order to prevent cyanide toxicity.

### Antiarrhythmic Drugs

*Lidocaine* is the preferred agent in dogs for acute control of life-threatening ventricular arrhythmias, which may be related to shock, trauma, gastric dilatation-volvulus, electrolyte imblance, myocardial disease, or following resuscitation. The drug is given initially to effect by slow IV bolus (1 to 4 mg/kg). Because lidocaine is rapidly cleared by the liver, steady-state concentrations can be achieved only by CRI. Signs of toxicity include central nervous system depression and seizures. The drug is relatively ineffective in the setting of hypokalemia.

*Procainamide* is often used for the acute suppression of ventricular arrhythmias in dogs when lidocaine is ineffective. Hypotension can occur with rapid IV loading, and either multiple small IV boluses or a CRI should be used to deliver this drug.

*Verapamil* is a calcium channel blocker that is recommended for the acute control of supraventricular tachyarrhythmias. The drug has negative inotropic effects and can produce hypotension secondary to peripheral vasodilation and should be administered in a manner similar to procainamide.

*Esmolol* is a newly introduced ultra-short-acting β-blocker that may be useful in terminating some tachyarrhythmias. Adverse reactions include hypotension, negative inotropic effects, and bronchospasm. Following an initial IV bolus, a CRI is required to maintain effective plasma concentrations.

### Other Drugs

Other drugs commonly administered by CRI include metoclopramide for antiemetic effects, regular insulin for the management of complicated diabetes, certain chemotherapeutic agents (cisplatin, cytosine arabinoside, bleomycin), antifungal agents (amphotericin B), parenteral nutrition, and enteral feedings.

### CALCULATING DOSAGES

There are three formulas that can be used to quickly prepare constant-rate infusions. In general, dosages for most CRI drugs are expressed in *micrograms*, but the drugs themselves are available in concentrations of *milligrams* per milliliter. The following formulas provide "short cuts" that allow the clinician to convert directly from micrograms to milligrams.

This formula allows the veterinarian to formulate an infusion that will last for 6 hr:

$$\text{Drug dosage } (\mu g/kg/min) \times \text{BW (kg)} \times 0.36$$
$$= \text{\# mg required for 6 hr}$$

The veterinarian must choose the total volume of fluid to mix with the drug, and set the drip rate to deliver the total volume in 6 hr. The main benefit of this formula is its simplicity; it requires the veterinarian to remember only one conversion factor—0.36. The calculated amount of drug can be administered by a syringe or infusion pump over 6 hr.

The second formula allows the clinician to convert directly from the drug dosage in micrograms per kilogram per minute to milligrams, *provided a set volume (250 ml) and infusion rate (15 ml/hr) are used*:

$$\text{Drug dosage } (\mu g/kg/min) \times \text{BW (kg)}$$
$$= \text{\# mg to add}$$
$$\text{to 250-ml base solution at a rate of 15 ml/hr}$$

The following formula is versatile, since it is possible to solve for any of the variables.

$$M = \frac{(D)\,(W)\,(V)}{(R)\,(16.67)} \qquad R = \frac{(D)\,(W)\,(V)}{(M)\,(16.67)}$$

where $M$ = number of milligrams of drug to add to base solution, $D$ = dosage of drug in micrograms per kilogram per minute, $W$ = body weight in kilograms, $V$ = volume in milliliters of base solution, $R$ = rate of delivery in milliliters per hour, and 16.67 = conversion factor.

To understand how this formula would be used in a clinical case, consider the following example.

## Example Case

A 6-year-old, 28-kg male Doberman pinscher presents with severe left-sided heart failure and pulmonary edema due to dilated cardiomyopathy. After treatment with furosemide (2 mg/kg IV) and oxygen, pulses remain weak, blood pressure low, and perfusion poor. Dobutamine, at a relatively high dosage of 15 $\mu$g/kg/min, is chosen to provide immediate positive inotropic effects. Since the dog has pulmonary edema, a low fluid rate of 10 ml/hr is chosen to administer the drug.

$$M = \frac{(15\ \mu g)\ (28\ kg)\ (100\ ml)}{(10)\ (16.67)} = 250\ mg$$

Dobutamine is available in 250-mg vials. One vial is added to the base solution to make a total volume of 100 ml and is administered at 10 ml/hr.

To illustrate how the above formula can be used to adjust the dosage based on clinical signs, consider the following problem.

The dog develops tachycardia at a dosage of 15 $\mu$g/kg/min of dobutamine. The dosage can be decreased to 10 $\mu$g/kg/min and we can solve for $R$ to determine the rate adjustment necessary to deliver the drug at the reduced dosage.

$$R = \frac{(D)\ (W)\ (V)}{(M\ (16.67)} = \frac{(10)\ (28)\ (100)}{(250)\ (16.67)} = 7$$

The fluid rate is decreased to 7 ml/hr.

## References and Suggested Readings

Beaumont E: IV infusion pumps. Nursing Management 18:26, 1987.
   *Excellent review of infusion pumps including addresses of manufacturers.*
Engler MM and Engler MB: Comparative evaluation of intravenous therapy regulating devices. Heart Lung 15:262, 1986.
   *Results of an in-hospital study comparing high-pressure and low-pressure infusion pumps.*
Khan MG: *Manual of Cardiac Drug Therapy*, 2nd edition. London, Ballière Tindall/WB Saunders Co, 1988.
   *A reference book for indications, precautions, and mechanism of action of hemodynamic drugs.*
Klem SA, Farrington JM, and Leff RD: Influence of infusion pump operation and flow rate on hemodynamic stability during epinephrine infusion. Crit Care Med 21:1213, 1993.
   *A comparison of four types of infusion pumps at very low flow rates.*
Koch P: What's new in infusion pumps ... and how they provide more effective I.V. therapy. Nurs Life 4:54, 1984.
   *An overview of different types of infusion pumps.*
Koszuta LE: Choosing the right infusion control device for your patient. Nursing 14:55, 1984.
   *A brief review of equipment needed.*
Liang CS, Sherman LG, Loherty JV, et al: Sustained improvement of cardiac function in patients with congestive heart failure after short-term infusion of dobutamine. Circulation 69:113, 1984.
   *A study detailing the effectiveness of dobutamine infusion in human patients with congestive heart failure.*
Lindner A: Synergism of dopamine and furosemide in diuretic-resistant oliguric renal failure. Nephron 33:121, 1983.
   *Low-dose dopamine infusion enhanced the effect of furosemide in human patients with oliguric renal failure.*
Wall RE and Rush JE: Cardiac emergencies. *In* Murtaugh RJ and Kaplan PM, *Veterinary Emergency and Critical Care Medicine*. St. Louis, Mosby Year Book 1992, p 213.
   *An overview of the diagnosis and treatment of cardiac emergencies in veterinary patients.*

# USE OF CATECHOLAMINES IN CRITICAL CARE PATIENTS

JAMES S. WOHL
*and* ROBERT J. MURTAUGH
*North Grafton, Massachusetts*

Catecholamines are endogenous or exogenously administered amines that stimulate receptors of the sympathetic nervous system. These receptors are classified as $\alpha$-adrenergic ($\alpha_1$, $\alpha_2$), $\beta$-adrenergic ($\beta_1$, $\beta_2$), and dopaminergic (DA$_1$,DA$_2$). Endogenous catecholamines include epinephrine (released by the adrenal medulla), norepinephrine (released by postganglionic nerve terminals and the adrenal medulla), and dopamine (secreted from postganglionic nerve terminals). Dobutamine and isoproterenol are synthetic catecholamines.

The biochemical structure of catecholamines consists of a benzene ring and a terminal amino group separated by two carbon atoms. Specific receptor affinity is determined by substitutions on the terminal amino group. The greater the size of an alkyl attachment to the amino group, the greater the $\beta$ effect. Hydroxyl substitutions on the benzene ring and substitutions on the carbon side chain affect potency and duration of action, respectively. Thus, catecholamines that affect both $\alpha$ and $\beta$ receptors usually have individual dose–effect relationships with each receptor. For example, the $\beta$ effects of epinephrine predominate at lower dosages, while $\alpha$-mediated effects predominate at higher dosages. Table 1 lists the catecholamines and their relative adrenergic receptor activities.

The sympathomimetic response is generally thought to result in increases in heart rate, cardiac output, and blood pressure ("fight-or-flight" responses). Hemodynamic changes occur through alterations in the balance of activity between various adrenergic receptors within the sympathetic nervous system (SNS). $\alpha_1$-Receptor activation generally results in constriction of smooth mus-

***Table 1.*** *Adrenergic Receptor Activity of Catecholamines*

| Drug | $\alpha$ | $\beta_1$ | $\beta_2$ | DA$_1$ | DA$_2$ |
|---|---|---|---|---|---|
| Norepinephrine | ++++ | ++++ | O | O | O |
| Epinephrine | ++++ | ++++ | ++ | O | O |
| Dobutamine | + | ++++ | ++ | O | O |
| Dopamine | ++++ | ++++ | ++ | ++++ | ++++ |
| Isoproterenol | O | ++++ | +++ | O | O |

cle (e.g., vascular smooth muscle). Most references to $\alpha$-stimulatory effects of catecholamines refer to $\alpha_1$-mediated vasoconstriction. $\alpha_2$ Activity is more complex and is thought to modify norepinephrine release in the central nervous system and at postganglionic sympathetic nerve terminals. $\alpha_2$-Receptor stimulation may also cause an early transient peripheral vasoconstriction that is overpowered by the $\alpha_2$ central effects that modify norepinephrine release. $\beta_2$-Receptor stimulation results in relaxation of smooth muscle. $\beta_1$ Receptors are cardiostimulatory, providing both inotropic and chronotropic effects. Dopaminergic DA$_1$ receptors are usually postsynaptic and, when activated, relax the smooth muscle of vascular beds. Presynaptic DA$_2$ receptors also relax smooth muscle by inhibiting the release of norepinephrine; DA$_2$ receptors are also located in the emetic center of the brain.

As a consequence of the location and concentration of individual adrenergic receptors, *generalizations* can be made regarding the effects of receptor stimulation in critical care patients. $\alpha_1$-Receptor stimulation results in vasoconstriction of cutaneous, splanchnic, and renal vasculature, causing an increase in peripheral vascular resistance. $\beta_1$ Stimulation results in increases in heart rate (chronotropy), contractile force (inotropy), conduction velocity through the atrioventricular (AV) node, and myocardial irritability. $\beta_2$ Stimulation causes bronchiolar dilation and vasodilation as well as an inotropic and chronotropic cardiac response. Dopaminergic 1 (and possibly DA$_2$)–receptor stimulation will increase renal, splanchnic, cerebral, and coronary blood flow through vasodilatory effects.

Metabolic changes occur as a consequence of adrenergic receptor stimulation. $\alpha_2$ Stimulation results in release of growth hormone from the pituitary gland, while dopaminergic stimulation inhibits the release of prolactin. Lipolysis ($\beta_1$) and glycogenolysis ($\beta_2$) result from $\beta$ stimulation. Therefore, diabetic patients receiving catecholamine infusions should be monitored closely for hyperglycemia, as these animals may have higher insulin requirements.

## USE OF SPECIFIC CATECHOLAMINES

Most indications of catecholamines in critical care patients are directed at manipulating the sympathetic tone of the cardiovascular system (Table 2). Control of cardiovascular responses are mediated by the sympathetic arm of the autonomic nervous system, vagal parasympathetic modulation of heart rate being the major exception. The inherent level of sympathetic activity, particularly vascular resistance, is maintained by the vasomotor center of the lower pons and medulla. Constant slow transmission of impulses through sympathetic nerve fibers maintain vascular tone at approximately 50% constriction. Thus, increases or decreases in vasomotor activity change sympathetic tone in response to physiologic changes in cardiovascular status. Interventions with exogenous catecholamines override

***Table 2.*** *Indications for Catecholamines in the Critical Care Setting*

Cardiac arrest
Epinephrine (0.05–0.2 mg/kg IV or by intrabronchial administration), repeated if necessary every 3 to 5 min. Dopamine (or dobutamine) may be used after stable hemodynamics are established.

Anaphylactic shock
Epinephrine (0.02 mg/kg IV) in conjunction with antihistamines, corticosteroids, and volume-expanding fluids. Epinephrine can be repeated in 15–20 min. Dopamine or dobutamine may be used for further inotropic support.

Cardiogenic shock/acute myocardial failure
Dobutamine (2.5–20 $\mu$g/kg/min) in conjunction with diuretics, vasodilators, and oxygen. Dopamine (5–10 $\mu$g/kg/min) if MAP <65 mm Hg or systolic BP <80–90 mm Hg. Norepinephrine (1–4 $\mu$g/min) can be attempted as a final measure if dopamine fails to correct hypotensive shock.

Septic shock
Dopamine (2–10 $\mu$g/kg/min) or dobutamine (2.5–20 $\mu$g/kg/min). Dopamine is preferred if hypotension or compromise to renal and mesenteric blood flow is a concern.
Norepinephrine (0.05–0.3 $\mu$g/kg/min) can be attempted as a final measure if dopamine and dobutamine fail to correct hypotensive shock.

Oliguric renal failure
Dopamine (0.5–5 $\mu$g/kg/min) in conjunction with diuretics.

Asthma/severe bronchoconstriction
Epinephrine (0.02 mg/kg SC) in conjunction with corticosteroids, bronchodilators, and oxygen.

this control system by directly stimulating adrenergic receptors to increase sympathetic tone. Whether desired effects are achieved with a particular agent is a function of that agent's effects on specific adrenergic receptors and the dosages employed.

### Epinephrine

Epinephrine (EPI) has $\alpha_1$, $\beta_1$, and $\beta_2$ activity, and its potent vasopressor action is blunted by the $\beta_2$-vasodilatory effect. Its positive inotropic and chronotropic effects increase cardiac output but also increase myocardial oxygen consumption. As $\beta$ receptors are more sensitive to EPI than $\alpha$ receptors, increases in heart rate, cardiac output, and stroke volume along with decreased peripheral resistance dominate at low dosages (0.04 to 0.1 $\mu$g/kg/min IV constant-rate infusion [CRI]). Epinephrine administration may be associated with hyperglycemia, hypokalemia, lypolysis, decreased renal perfusion, and increased platelet aggregation. The vasopressor ($\alpha_1$) and bronchodilatory ($\beta_2$) effects of EPI make it the catecholamine of choice in the treatment of cardiopulmonary arrest, systemic anaphylaxis, status asthmaticus, and as a local vasoconstrictor to control hemorrhage.

Epinephrine-induced systemic arteriolar vasoconstriction increases systemic arterial blood pressure and optimally affects the pressure gradients that control myocardial and cerebral blood flow. This effect is more important than the cardiostimulatory effect of EPI during cardiopulmonary resuscitation (CPR) (Lollgen and Drexler, 1990).

The optimal dosage of EPI for use in CPR is controversial. The traditional dosage in CPR has been 0.01 mg/kg. Dosage response studies indicate a dosage range between 0.03 and 0.2 mg/kg IV delivered by a central venous injection may be effective in restoring spontaneous circulation (Koscove and Paradis, 1988). Further complicating this issue is a recent study in humans with cardiac arrest that showed no significant difference in return of spontaneous circulation, neurologic outcome, or survival between low-dosage (0.02 mg/kg) and high-dosage (0.2 mg/kg) EPI administration (Brown et al., 1992).

Dosages of 0.05 to 0.2 mg/kg repeated every 5 min (0.25 to 1 ml 1:1000 EPI per 5 kg BW) by IV bolus or endotracheal route are recommended and seem consistent with available data. As EPI may have a dose–response relationship with the induction of ventricular fibrillation, the higher dosage may be best reserved for facilities with electrical defibrillation capabilities (Moses, 1992). Delivery of EPI through a catheter passed down an endotracheal tube and wedged into a bronchus will allow greater and more rapid plasma absorption than a bolus injected directly down an endotracheal tube (Mazkereth et al., 1992). This intratracheal administration technique is preferred in CPR and other low-flow states when intravenous routes are inaccessible.

The dosage of EPI for the treatment of anaphylactic shock is 0.02 mg/kg IV. Administration can be repeated in 15 to 20 min. Epinephrine should be used as the primary treatment along with administration of intravenous fluid therapy. Corticosteroids, antihistamines, and bronchodilators may be used as adjunctive therapy in systemic anaphylaxis (see "Systemic Anaphylaxis," this volume, p 150). In addition to its cardiostimulatory and bronchodilatory effects, EPI also increases intracellular cyclic adenosine monophosphate (cAMP), thereby decreasing the synthesis and release of mediators of anaphylaxis. Epinephrine administration is generally avoided in animals with nonanaphylactic shock. However, for animals in severe hypotensive shock where irreversible circulatory collapse may occur before fluid therapy has time to restore blood volume and cardiac output, EPI (0.05 to 0.2 $\mu$g/kg IV bolus) will support systemic arterial blood pressure and perfusion to vital organs while fluids are administered.

Epinephrine (0.5 to 0.75 ml 1:10,000 SC or 0.02 mg/kg SC) can be administered to cats with severe bronchoconstriction associated with feline allergic bronchitis. This treatment is used in conjunction with corticosteroids, oxygen therapy, and bronchodilators.

Gauzes soaked in EPI (1:10,000) can be used to control hemorrhage in areas where ligation or application of pressure is impossible (e.g., epistaxis). Epinephrine-soaked gauzes can be packed in the area of hemorrhage in the sedated animal for 5 to 20 min or until bleeding is controlled.

### Dopamine

Dopamine (DA) (Inotropin, American Critical Care; Dopastat, Parke-Davis) is a complex catecholamine that stimulates a variety of adrenergic receptors in a dose-dependent fashion when administered intravenously by CRI. At very low dosages (0.5, perhaps up to 3 $\mu$g/kg/min), DA-mediated coronary, renal, and splanchnic arteriolar vasodilation occurs, resulting in increased blood flow to these vascular beds. At intermediate dosages (3 to 10 $\mu$g/kg/min), predominantly $\beta$-adrenergic effects are evident, resulting in increased heart rate, cardiac output, and stroke volume, with little effect on systemic vascular resistance. Therefore, dopamine can also be considered in the treatment of myocardial failure accompanied by marked hypotension, although close monitoring of heart rate and blood pressure are essential. At high dosages ($\geq$10 $\mu$g/kg/min), $\alpha$-mediated vasoconstriction obliterates the DA and $\beta_2$-vasodilatory effects. This effect results in increases in systemic arterial blood pressure and left ventricular filling pressures and decreases in renal, mesenteric and, possibly, coronary blood flow. For the above reasons, dopamine administration is commonly used to reverse oliguric renal failure, to provide inotropic support in animals with septic or maldistributive shock, and for hemodynamic stabilization following CPR. Dopamine can be diluted in lactated Ringer's solution, normal saline, dextrose 5% in water (D5W), and other common preparations. Dopamine will be inactivated in alkaline solutions and should never be infused with sodium bicarbonate. Once in solution it is stable at room temperature for 24 hr. A

200-mg vial of dopamine added to 1 L of fluids will yield a 200-$\mu$g/ml solution. A pediatric intravenous administration set (60 drops/ml) would then yield 3.3 $\mu$g/drop.

For inopressor support, dopamine can be initiated at 2 to 5 $\mu$g/kg/min by CRI and can be increased by 25 to 50% increments every 30 min to achieve desired results. The onset of action is usually within 5 min of administration. Side effects such as tachyarrhythmias and vasoconstriction to renal, mesentery, and coronary vascular beds are more likely to occur at dosages greater than 10 $\mu$g/kg/min. If tachyarrhythmias occur, dopamine should be discontinued for 20 min and reinitiated at a lower (25 to 50%) dosage. Serial blood pressure measurement and continuous electrocardiographic (ECG) monitoring are desirable during dopamine therapy.

Dopamine, at infusion rates of 0.5 to 5 $\mu$g/kg/min, may benefit patients in oliguric acute renal failure that have not responded to volume expansion, hyperosmotic agents, and diuretic therapy. Low-dose dopamine administration is often used in concert with furosemide (1 mg/kg IV every hour) to increase urinary output. Dopaminergic 1–receptor stimulation causes a decrease in renal vascular resistance, allowing increased renal blood flow. Increased cardiac output and activation of DA$_2$ receptors may also augment renal perfusion. The antiemetic metoclopramide is a DA$_2$-receptor antagonist. Its use may interfere with the potential DA$_2$-mediated increase in renal blood flow and should be discontinued while oliguric patients are receiving dopamine administration. Dopaminergic receptors may be present at renal tubular sites to account for the diuresis and natriuresis observed in dogs. Cats do not appear to express DA receptors in the renal vasculature or tubules and do not experience increased renal blood flow or glomerular filtration rate (GFR) with dopamine administration. Despite this, diuresis and natriuresis do occur with dopamine infusion in cats. This effect is thought to represent a result of $\alpha$-receptor activation, which increases systemic arterial blood pressure and decreases sodium resorption in the distal and collecting tubules (Chew, 1992). It is essential that strict control of infusion rates be maintained, as effects of dopamine at higher dosages can be detrimental in oliguric renal failure. Heart rate and rhythm should also be monitored, although tachyarrhythmias are less common at dosages used to treat oliguria. Although dopamine may increase urine output, effects on GFR are variable and decreases in serum creatinine concentrations may not occur with induced diuresis.

## Dobutamine

As primarily a $\beta_1$ agonist with relatively weak $\alpha$ and $\beta_2$ action, dobutamine (Dobutrex, Eli Lilly and Company) provides positive inotropic effects with little effect on systemic vascular resistance. At lower dosages, its inotropic effects are also greater than its chronotropic effects, and heart rate usually remains unchanged. Increased cardiac output, stroke volume, and the resultant decrease in ventricular filling pres-

sures contribute to improvements in coronary arterial perfusion pressure and ventricular performance. These factors make dobutamine the catecholamine of choice for short-term therapy of low-output congestive heart failure (e.g., dilated cardiomyopathy). Dobutamine can also be used at similar dosages to improve cardiac performance and improve oxygen delivery to poorly perfused tissues in noncardiogenic shock. Due to its extremely short half-life, dobutamine must be administered by continuous IV infusion (dog, 2.5 to 20 $\mu$g/kg/min; cat, 0.5 to 3$\mu$g/kg/min). Dobutamine is compatible with most balanced electrolyte solutions, although it is often administered in D5W to minimize sodium intake in cardiac patients. Effects are seen within 2 min after initiating the infusion and peak at approximately 10 min. Mixing a 20-ml vial (250 mg) in 500 ml of fluid will result in a 500-$\mu$g/ml concentration. Ideally, the use of infusion pumps should be employed to control the rate of delivery. Alternatively, a pediatric IV administration set (60 drops/ml) will deliver 8.3 $\mu$g/drop of the aforementioned concentration of solution. Once in solution, dobutamine should be stable for roughly 24 hr at room temperature.

Dobutamine infusions should be initiated at a low dosage (1 to 3 $\mu$g/kg/min) and the infusion rate can be increased by 25% increments every 10 to 20 min to achieve desired results. At higher dosages (e.g., $\geq$10 $\mu$g/kg/min IV CRI), the chronotropic effect of dobutamine is more likely to be observed. Thus, continuous ECG monitoring is desirable to identify complications such as sinus and ventricular tachycardia or increased ventricular rate response to atrial fibrillation. If tachyarrhythmias or other side effects (vomiting, restlessness, and seizures in cats) are observed, the dobutamine infusion should be discontinued for 15 to 20 min and reinstituted at a lower dosage.

Myocardial $\beta_1$ receptors may become desensitized to dobutamine (and other catecholamines). A lack of response to dobutamine due to this "down-regulation" may be observed 24 to 72 hr after initiation of a CRI (Lollgen and Drexler, 1990). Higher doses may partially overcome this effect.

Dobutamine and other $\beta_1$ agonists will increase AV conduction velocity and may detrimentally increase the ventricular rate in patients with supraventricular tachycardias (e.g., atrial fibrillation, atrial tachycardia). Increasing atrioventricular refractory period helps to control the ventricular rate and maintain cardiac output. Thus, patients may benefit from therapy (digoxin, calcium channel blockers) that slows the ventricular response rate and is initiated prior to catecholamine therapy. Obviously, treatment with a $\beta$-blocker would be inappropriate in this instance.

## Norepinephrine

Norepinephrine (NE) (Levophed, Winthrop) has $\alpha_1$ and $\beta_1$ activity but virtually no effect on $\beta_2$ receptors. Therefore, NE is a potent vasopressor that will significantly increase systemic arterial blood pressure. It is both a positive inotrope and chronotrope, although its chronotropic effects are usually blunted by a vagal reflex–mediated slowing of heart rate induced by the rise in blood pressure. Norepinephrine usually increases myocardial oxygen consumption due to cardiostimulation and increased afterload. The perceived risk of ischemia to coronary and renal vascular beds and exacerbation of peripheral tissue hypoxia have resulted in limited use of NE in veterinary critical care patients. However, recent studies in man (Schreuder et al., 1989) and dogs (Bakker and Vincent, 1993) suggest that the effect on peripheral resistance may be tolerated and that NE administration may improve the delivery and utilization of oxygen in critical patients.

Norepinephrine use is best reserved for cardiogenic or septic shock with severe hypotension that does not respond to intravascular volume expansion with fluid therapy and a dopamine or dobutamine infusion. A dosage rate of 0.05 to 0.3 $\mu$g/kg/min is infused until adequate blood pressure is achieved. Heart rate will usually remain constant, cardiac output may fall due to increased afterload, cardiac arrhythmias may occur, and decreased mesenteric and renal perfusion are limiting potential concerns. The use of gastrointestinal tonometry to assess splanchnic perfusion (see "Monitoring Gastrointestinal Mucosal pH in Critical Care Patients," this volume, p 133) may provide a practical means of monitoring visceral perfusion.

### Isoproterenol

Isoproterenol (Isuprel, Winthrop) is a $\beta_1$ and $\beta_2$ agonist without any $\alpha$-mediated effects. It use, therefore, can induce a profound lowering of peripheral vascular resistance and blood pressure. Isoproterenol can also increase myocardial oxygen consumption while decreasing coronary perfusion pressure. Previously, isoproterenol has been advocated in the treatment of cardiac arrest (usually electromechanical dissociation) and allergic reactions such as asthma. The deleterious effects on blood pressure and myocardial oxygen utilization limit the use of isoproterenol in CPR. Specific $\beta_2$ agonists (e.g., terbutaline, albuterol) have been developed that have supplanted isoproterenol as a bronchodilator. Isoproterenol can still be advocated as a short-term treatment in some cases of complete AV block. In patients where ventricular contractions are infrequent or weak, isoproterenol (0.04 to 0.08 $\mu$g/min) can be used by CRI until a cardiac pacemaker is placed. Isoproterenol should be considered in only those patients requiring short-term continual ventricular stimulation, as the concomitant lowering or peripheral vascular resistance may severely limit perfusion of vital organs in these animals with low cardiac output. Dopamine has been used as an alternative treatment in this setting.

### Use of Catecholamines in Shock

In shock states, the aim of therapy is to increase the delivery and utilization of oxygen to supranormal levels to meet the hypermetabolic demands of critical illness (Shoemaker et al., 1989). Oxygen delivery ($Do_2$) is a function of arterial oxygen content and cardiac output. Mediators of inflammation present in shock may diminish cardiac performance. This decrease in cardiac output and oxygen delivery may occur in the presence of normal or even elevated systemic arterial blood pressure. The utilization of oxygen ($\dot{V}o_2$) by ischemic tissues can be diminished even in high cardiac output states by a maldistribution of blood flow due to uneven vasoconstriction of metarteriolar networks (Shoemaker et al., 1989). While invasive monitoring of cardiac output, $Do_2$ and $\dot{V}o_2$ is impractical in most veterinary clinical settings, comparing arterial and venous $Po_2$ tension may be useful. A low venous partial pressure of oxygen ($Pvo_2$) (ideally obtained from a central venous or pulmonary arterial catheter) in a patient with normal hemoglobin concentration and normal arterial partial pressure of oxygen ($Pao_2$) infers low cardiac output and inadequate oxygen delivery. Conversely, an elevated $Pvo_2$ in a patient with increased cardiac output (septic shock) suggests maldistributive blood flow and impaired oxygen utilization by peripheral tissues.

Volume expansion with intravenous administration of resuscitative dosages of crystalloid (90 ml/kg/hr), colloid (6% dextran or hetastarch; 10 to 20 ml/kg over 2 to 4 hr), or hypertonic (7%) saline (4 to 6 ml/kg) solutions is the most essential treatment of shock. If hemoglobin content is diminished (packed cell volume [PCV] <25%) or hypoproteinemia (total protein <3.5 gm/dl) is present, the appropriate blood product (whole blood, packed red blood cells [RBC], plasma, or colloids) should be administered to enhance oxygen delivery. Parameters indicating restoration of oxygen delivery and utilization include qualitative improvements in the patient's mucous membrane color and warmth, capillary refill time, mentation, heart rate and rhythm, pulse quality, and breathing patterns. Quantitatively measured improvements should include increased urinary output (>2 ml/kg/hr), restoration of adequate systemic arterial blood pressure (mean arterial pressure [MAP] >80 mm Hg), maintenance of central venous pressure (CVP) between 5 and 12 cm $H_2O$, and normalization of gastrointestinal pH, core toe-web temperature differentials and $Pvo_2$ values (to 35 to 45 mm Hg). Central venous pressures less than 5 cm $H_2O$ generally indicate inadequate volume expansion. Central venous pressures above 12 cm $H_2O$ in a patient with low systemic arterial blood pressure (MAP <80 mm Hg) indicate the need for inotropic support.

Dopamine or dobutamine are commonly used in the treatment of septic or maldistributive shock when volume expansion has not restored adequate $Do_2$ and $\dot{V}o_2$. Both dopamine and dobutamine administration will increase cardiac output primarily through $\beta_1$ adrenergic effects. The effects of dopamine and dobutamine at comparable dosages differ; dopamine will generally cause a greater increase in systemic vascular resistance and a greater increase in heart rate. Dobutamine administration provided superior improvement in oxygen transport in critically ill postoperative human patients compared to dopamine administration (Shoemaker et al., 1989). The superiority of dobutamine administration in these patients may have resulted from greater relative $\beta_2$-adrenergic effects that enhanced blood flow to previously vasoconstricted metarteriolocapillary networks (the $\beta_2$ activity of dopamine being counteracted by its greater $\alpha$-mediated effects). This selective lowering of vascular resistance provides improved distribution of blood flow to ischemic tissues. In volume-resuscitated patients (CVP >5 cm $H_2O$) with shock characterized by increased cardiac output (hyperdynamic shock) and elevated $Pvo_2$ values, dobutamine can be instituted at 2.5 to 20 $\mu g/kg/min$ (see previous discussion of dobutamine administration). Dopamine administration is often preferred over dobutamine in the treatment of shock when volume resuscitation has failed to correct systemic arterial hypotension and restore oxygen delivery (Lollgen and Drexler, 1990). Should dopamine administration fail, norepinephrine may be instituted at the previously mentioned dosage range.

## SUMMARY

Although catecholamines provide sympathomimetic effects, differences in receptor activity prohibit interchangeable use. The variability of the dose–effect relationships of some catecholamines mandates strict control of infusion rates, ideally by means of infusion pumps. Monitoring responses both clinically and through measurement of blood pressure (see " Blood Pressure Management" and "Doppler Assessment of Blood Flow and Pressure in Surgical and Critical Care Patients," this volume, p 113) is crucial. Since all catecholamines used in veterinary patients provide some $\beta_1$-stimulatory effect, premature beats and tachyarrhythmias can occur as side effects. Catecholamines with $\alpha$ activity can cause severe tissue necrosis upon extravasation due to local vasoconstriction and ischemia. Although general indication can be made for the use of specific catecholamines in the critical care setting, the individual patient's hemodynamic status should be the primary decision-making consideration when using these powerful agents.

## References and Suggested Reading

Bakker J and Vincent JL: Effects of norepinephrine and dobutamine on oxygen transport and consumption in a dog model of endotoxic shock. Crit Care Med 21:425, 1993.
*An original study investigating the effects of norepinephrine and dobutamine on oxygen delivery, oxygen consumption, and oxygen extraction in a dog model of endotoxic shock.*

Brown CG, Martin DA, Pepe PE, and Steven H: A comparison of standard-dose and high-dose epinephrine in cardiac arrest outside the hospital. N Engl J Med 327:1051, 1992.
*This study demonstrates no significant difference in outcome between use of two different doses of epinephrine in human cardiac arrest patients.*

Chew DJ: Fluid therapy during intrinsic renal failure. *In* DiBartola SP (ed): *Fluid Therapy in Small Animal Practice.* Philadelphia, WB Saunders Co, 1992, p 554.
*A broad discussion of pathophysiology and approach to treatment of intrinsic renal failure.*

Hosgood G: Pharmacologic features and physiologic effects of dopamine. J Am Vet Med Assoc 197:1209, 1990.
*A short review of the clinical pharmacology of dopamine in veterinary therapy.*

Kittleson MD: Dobutamine. J Am Vet Med Assoc 177:642, 1980.
*A short review of the clinical pharmacology of dobutamine in veterinary therapy.*

Koscove EM and Paradis NA: Successful resuscitation from cardiac arrest using high-dose epinephrine therapy. JAMA 259:3031, 1988.
*Case reports and literature review of epinephrine dosing schedules in experimental studies.*

Lollgen H and Drexler H: Use of inotropes in the critical care setting. Crit Care Med 18:556, 1990.
*A brief review of catecholamines and newer inotropic agents and their indications in human critical care patients.*

Mazkereth R, Paret G, Ezra D, and Aviner S: Epinephrine blood concentrations after peripheral bronchial versus endotracheal administration of epinephrine in dogs. Crit Care Med 20:1582, 1992.
*This study compares two different techniques of endotracheal delivery of epinephrine in anesthetized dogs.*

Moses BL: Cardiopulmonary resuscitation. *In* Murtaugh RJ and Kaplan PM (eds): *Veterinary Emergency and Critical Care Medicine.* Boston, Mosby Year Book, 1992, p 508.
*A discussion of pathophysiology and treatment of cardiopulmonary arrest.*

Schreuder WO, Schneider AJ, Groeneveld AB, and Thijis LG: Effect of dopamine vs. norepinephrine on hemodynamics in septic shock. Chest 95:1282, 1989.
*This study compares the effects of dopamine and norepinephrine on hemodynamics, oxygen metabolism and right ventricular performance in human patients with septic shock.*

Shoemaker WC, Appel PC, Kram HB, et al: Comparison of hemodynamic and oxygen transport effects of dopamine and dobutamine in critically ill surgical patients. Chest 92:120, 1989.
*This study suggests the $\beta_2$-mediated effects of dobutamine are responsible for improved microcirculatory flow distribution in human surgical patients during the early postoperative period.*

Stephens KA: Catecholamines and their use in shock. Compend Cont Educ 5:671, 1983.
*A review of the veterinary applications of catecholamines with special emphasis on the shock patient.*

Van Pelt DR and Wingfield WE: Controversial issues in drug treatment during cardiopulmonary resuscitation. J Am Vet Med Assoc 200:2938, 1992.
*A detailed discussion of pathophysiologic and pharmacologic considerations in cardiopulmonary resuscitation.*

# INCOMPATIBLE CRITICAL CARE DRUG COMBINATIONS

MARK G. PAPICH

*Raleigh, North Carolina*

In emergency and critical care situations, potent drugs and drug combinations are administered to very ill patients. These combinations may interact to produce toxicosis, inactivate a drug, or potentiate a pharmacologic effect. There are not very many examples of drug interactions and incompatibilities in the veterinary literature, but interactions are not species dependent, and examples taken from human medicine or experimental studies should predict potential incompatibilities and interactions in veterinary patients. The drugs discussed in this article primarily will be those drugs that can be administered via injection and that have the narrowest therapeutic index. The patients most at risk for an adverse reaction caused by an incompatibility are those that are critically ill, because they may have lost their physiologic reserve in one or more systems and are affected tremendously (either positively or negatively) by the actions of drugs.

## *IN VITRO* VERSUS *IN VIVO* INCOMPATIBILITIES

There are two kinds of interactions possible: those that occur before the drug is administered to the patient (*in vitro*) are pharmaceutical interactions, and those that occur after the drugs have been administered to the patient (*in vivo*) are pharmacologic interactions. Sources of information for these interactions are listed in the reference list at the end of the chapter. In addition, a valuable but frequently overlooked source of information for the practicing veterinarian is a phone call to a local pharmacy.

### Pharmaceutical Interactions

Pharmaceutical interactions occur primarily because of a drug's physical incompatibility with another drug, a fluid solution, or the drug's container. Some drug interactions are acid-base interactions. Other reactions are caused by an affinity of a drug to charged particles in another solution; the affinity of a drug for the container; or degradation of the drug because of pH, temperature, or solubility changes.

#### SIGNS OF INCOMPATIBILITY

Many unstable solutions may not show obvious changes, but the instability of some solutions is obvious because there may be a change in the solution's color, the solution may appear cloudy, or a precipitate may form. For example, outdated thiobarbiturates often contain insoluble precipitates, and when injectable penicillin and cephalosporin solutions decompose, sulfur is released from the molecule and the solution may turn yellow. Never administer an intravenous solution that is cloudy, contains a precipitate, or in which an unexpected color change has occurred.

Consult the manufacturer to determine if a color change in a solution is significant, because for some drug solutions, a color change may not affect potency. Dopamine solutions will form a violet or pink color when stability has been compromised. However, a pink discoloration may occur with dobutamine solutions without affecting potency if they are used within 24 hr. Oxidation may darken the color of some solutions without affecting the drug potency.

#### EFFECTS OF STORAGE ON DRUG STABILITY

Reading the package insert will, in most instances, provide a clinician with information regarding the stability of a drug once a vial is opened or reconstituted with a fluid. Drugs that the manufacturer has packaged in a brown glass vial or container may be sensitive to light. Transferring these solutions to clear containers is risky.

EFFECT OF TEMPERATURE. Many of the antibiotics intended for injection must be reconstituted with water or saline before injection. In general, these drugs are stable only for a few hours at room temperature (Table 1). Usually, the rate of drug degradation is faster at higher temperatures, and cooling or freezing a solution will decrease the number of molecular collisions, causing the drug to remain stable longer (Stella, 1986). For example, injectable cephalosporins such as cefazolin (Ancef, Kefzol), cefoxitin (Mefoxin), ceftiofur (Naxcel), and cefotaxime (Claforan) will decompose within 12 to 48 hr at room temperature, but are stable for 3 to 10 days in the refrigerator, and for several weeks if frozen at −20°C (Table 1). Frozen solutions can be thawed in a microwave oven without losing potency, but once a solution has been thawed it should not be refrozen.

Freezing solutions to increase the shelf life after reconstitution will not always prevent drug degradation, and the manufacturer's package insert should be consulted for precise recommendations. Ampicillin sodium will decompose within 4 hr at room temperature and

**Table 1.** *Table of Stability and Incompatibilities for Common Injectable Critical Care and Emergency Drugs*

| Drug | Stability | *In Vitro* Compatibility With Other Drugs and Containers |
|---|---|---|
| Amikacin | Stable in IV fluids at room temperature for 24 hr; may be pale yellow color without affecting potency | Compatible with all IV fluid solutions; do not mix with heparin, penicillins, or cephalosporins (affected less than other aminoglycosides by interactions with $\beta$-lactams) |
| Aminophylline | Stable at room temperature | Do not mix in a syringe with other drugs; stable with IV fluid solutions |
| Amphotericin B | Stable at room temperature for 24 hr, or in refrigerator for 1 week; do not expose to light for more than 8 hr | Physically incompatible with electrolyte solutions |
| Ampicillin sodium | Unstable; use solutions within 1 hr at room temperature, 4 hr in refrigerator, or 24 hr in freezer | Do not admix with aminoglycosides or heparin; reconstitute with saline or water; stability decreased in dextrose solutions |
| Bicarbonate sodium | Stable at room temperature | Physically incompatible with Ringer's solutions, dobutamine, dopamine, tetracyclines, pentobarbital, vitamin B complex, and insulin |
| Calcium chloride | Stable at room temperature | Compatible with IV fluid solutions; do not mix with sodium bicarbonate, other carbonates, phosphates, sulfates, or tartrates |
| Cefazolin | Stable for 4 days at room temperature, 2 weeks, in refrigerator, 12 weeks in freezer | Stable with all IV fluid solutions, but concentrated solutions in saline (330 mg/ml) may crystalize at room temperature; do not mix with aminoglycosides |
| Cefotaxime | Stable for 24 hr at room temperature, 10 days in refrigerator; 13 weeks in freezer | Compatible with IV fluid solutions; do not mix with alkaline solutions |
| Cefoxitin | Stable for 48 hr at room temperature, 7–30 days in refrigerator, 30 weeks in freezer | Do not mix with aminoglycosides; compatible with other fluids; may be reconstituted with 1% lidocaine for IM use |
| Cephalothin | Stable for 12 hr at room temperature 96 hr in refrigerator, 12 weeks in freezer | Compatible with IV fluids; slight discoloration does not affect potency |
| Ciprofloxacin | Stable | Compatible with IV fluid solutions; compatible with most other drugs, except aminophylline and clindamycin |
| Diazepam | Stable; protect from light | Low solubility in aqueous solutions; significant absorption to plastic infusion system (see text) |
| Dopamine | Stable in fluids for 24–48 hrs | Do not mix with alkalinizing solutions; do not use if the solution is a pink or violet color |
| Dobutamine | Stable for 6 hr at room temperature, and 48 hr in refrigerator; IV solutions should be used within 24 hr; protect from freezing | Do not mix with alkalinizing solutions; pink discoloration indicates slight oxidation, but there is no loss of potency if used within recommended time periods; do not administer through the same IV catheter as heparin, hydrocostisone, and cephalosporins. |
| Flunixin meglumine | Stable at room temperature | Physically incompatible with most fluid solutions |
| Furosemide | Stable (protect from light and from freezing) | Unstable in acidic fluid; do not administer if discolored |
| Gentamicin | Do not store in plastic syringes | Physically incompatible with most penicillins and cephalosporins |

*Table continued on following page*

195

***Table 1.***  *Continued*

| Drug | Stability | *In Vitro* Compatibility With Other Drugs and Containers |
|---|---|---|
| Heparin | Stable at room temperature; protect from freezing | Do not use if discolored; solution is strongly acidic and is incompatible with aminoglycoside antibiotics, erythromycin, penicillin G and many other drugs (see text) |
| Insulin, regular | Refrigerate; protect from freezing | Significant sorption to infusion system, plastic bags, and tubing; loss may be as high as 80%; flush system with insulin prior to IV infusion (see text) |
| Lidocaine | Stable in IV fluids for 24 hr at room temperature | Compatible with IV fluid solutions; stable when stored in plastic syringes |
| Methylprednisolone succinate | Use reconstituted solution within 48 hr | Reconstitute only with special diluent; physically compatible in IV solutions, but may form a haze |
| Metronidazole | Protect from light; protect from freezing | |
| Penicillin G | Stable for 24 hr at room temperature; 7 days in refrigerator, 12 weeks in freezer | Stable in most IV solutions |
| Pentobarbital | Stable | Compatible with most IV fluid solutions, but may precipitate in acid pH; do not mix with alkali-labile drugs |
| Procainamide | Stable in fluids at room temperature for 24 hr; protect from light; protect from freezing | Slight yellow color does not affect potency, but do not use if color is dark yellow; decomposes if admixed with dextrose solutions |
| Propranolol | Stable; protect from light | Stable in all fluids |
| Quinidine | Stable; protect from light; protect from freezing | Compatible with fluid solutions and most other drugs |
| Ticarcillin | Stable in fluids for 48–72 hr at room temperature | Do not mix with aminoglycosides |
| Vitamin B complex | Stable | Compatible with IV fluid and TPN solutions; do not mix with sodium bicarbonate |

Abbreviations: IV = intravenous, IM = intramuscular, TPN = total parenteral nutrition.

in only 24 hr if the solution is frozen at $-20°C$. Freezing of suspensions (e.g., insulin) is not recommended because clumping of the suspended material may occur with thawing, or the drug may crystallize out as larger crystals when it is thawed. Drugs such as procainamide, quinidine, heparin, dobutamine, and furosemide should be protected from freezing because they may crystallize.

### INTERACTIONS WITH FLUID SOLUTIONS

The possibility of drug interactions with the IV fluid solutions should not be overlooked when using an IV fluid delivery system to infuse drugs into patients (Table 1). Only a few drugs have been tested for their compatibility with total parenteral nutrition (TPN) solutions, and unless their compatibility is known, clinicians should avoid admixing drugs with TPN solutions.

ACID-BASE INTERACTIONS. An optimum pH is critical to the stability of drugs that may be admixed with fluid solutions. Saline solutions have a pH of 5 to 6, and 5% dextrose solutions have a pH of approximately 5. Aminophylline and sodium salts of weak acids, such as penicillin and barbiturates, are examples of acid-labile drugs that are subject to degradation when added to an acidic fluid solution. Alternatively, weak bases that are formulated as salts of hydrochloric acid (HCl) are alkali labile and must be kept an acidic state to maintain their stability in an aqueous solution. Therefore, drugs such as epinephrine HCl, isoproterenol HCl, dopamine HCl, and dobutamine HCl are incompatible with alkaline solutions such as sodium bicarbonate.

CALCIUM IN SOLUTIONS. Calcium-containing solutions (e.g., Ringer's) will interact with solutions containing carbonate ions (e.g., sodium bicarbonate), resulting in a precipitation of calcium carbonate salts. Calcium in solutions also will interact with phosphates, sulfates, and tartrates.

HEPARIN IN SOLUTIONS. Sodium heparin often is used as an anticoagulant in IV flush solutions. It is physically incompatible with aminoglycoside antibiotics (gentamicin, amikacin, kanamycin), penicillin G sodium, and erythromycin. If these drugs are added to an IV fluid line in which there is heparin, immediate precipitation will result. This interaction can be avoided by simply using a 0.9% saline solution to flush IV catheters, because saline is as effective as heparin in maintaining patency and preventing phlebitis in intravenous catheters (Goode et al., 1991).

### INTERACTIONS WITH THE DRUG CONTAINER OR IV DELIVERY SYSTEM

Adsorption of drugs to the glass or plastic surface of a container often is overlooked. Adsorption is caused by a physical interaction between functional groups on the molecule and binding sites on the container surface. For example, insulins bind to glassware, polyethylene, and polyvinyl chloride (PVC) plastic (Stella, 1986; D'Arcy, 1983). The amount of insulin bound to an IV infusion system can be highly variable because of the differences in fluid used and length of tubing, but has been reported to be in the range of 5 to 80%. The binding appears to be saturable and most of the sorption occurs in the first 10 to 15 min of the infusion. Therefore, protocols for IV administration of insulin to patients recommend infusing 50 ml of the IV insulin solution through the delivery system before connecting it to the patient.

Highly lipid-soluble drugs such as diazepam (Valium) can be absorbed into the plasticizer used in PVC plastic infusion systems. The manufacturer's insert should be consulted to determine if other lipid-soluble drugs are absorbed into plastic. For diazepam, the amount absorbed can be as high as 80% (D'Arcy, 1983). This absorption is not saturable at the usual concentrations administered, and is dependent upon the temperature, concentration of drug, flow rate (the slower the flow rate, the more time for absorption), length of infusion tubing, and the amount of plasticizer in the plastic. Because of this interaction, the dose of diazepam infused into a patient cannot be calculated with any reliability, and an IV infusion of diazepam is not an approved method of administration (D'Arcy, 1983; Stella, 1986). Lorazepam (Ativan) or midazolam (Versed), which are other benzodiazepines with good anticonvulsant activity, are not absorbed to infusion systems. Plastic syringes do not contain flexible plasticizers and therefore do not absorb diazepam. (Although sorption to rubber syringe plungers will occur if stored for several days.)

### INCOMPATIBLE DRUG ADMIXTURES

Admixing drugs that have different vehicles, preservatives, and buffers compromises the chemical stability that the drug manufacturer has assured. These concoctions constitute bad medical practice. Examples of incompatible combinations are listed in Table 1. For example, do not admix aminoglycosides such as gentamicin with penicillins in the same syringe or vial because there is mutual inactivation. Diazepam (Valium) is unstable when mixed with many drugs, although many veterinarians have admixed diazepam with ketamine in the same syringe without any apparent loss of potency of either drug. Heparin sodium is incompatible with many other drugs because it is a strongly acidic solution.

## Pharmacologic Interactions (*In Vivo* Interactions)

Drug interactions that occur in the patient can be considered *pharmacokinetic interactions* if there is an interference with absorption, distribution, or elimination. They are considered *pharmacodynamic interactions* if there is an interference with the drug's action or an interaction at the drug's binding site.

### PHARMACOKINETIC DRUG INTERACTIONS

INTERACTIONS THAT AFFECT ORAL DRUG ABSORPTION. Antimuscarinic anticholinergic drugs, such as atropine or glycopyrrolate, will decrease stomach emptying, intestinal secretions, and intestinal motility, which can impair absorption of orally administered drugs in a critically ill patient. Many of the antiemetic drugs, including some of the drugs classified as phenothiazine derivatives (e.g., chlorpromazine [Thorazine]), also have antimuscarinic effects.

Oral absorption of a drug can be impaired because it binds or adsorbs to a drug administered simultaneously. For example, activated charcoal, kaolin-pectin combinations (Kaopectate), bismuth subsalicylate (Pepto Bismol), and some antacids will decrease the oral absorption of digoxin and some antibiotics. When critically ill patients are receiving these combinations, it is best to administer the oral drug approximately 30 min prior to the administration of the agent that is acting as an adsorbent. The ability of an adsorbent such as activated charcoal and cholestyramine (Questran) to interfere with intestinal drug absorption is the basis for their use in treating acute poisonings.

*Interactions with Sucralfate.* Sucralfate (Carafate) is commonly administered to critically ill patients to prevent or treat gastrointestinal ulcers. Sucralfate may decrease the oral absorption of orally administered fluoroquinolones (e.g., ciprofloxacin), theophylline, and digoxin. Clinicians have considered the importance of three possible interactions with H₂-receptor blocking drugs and sucralfate: (1) inhibiting the absorption of orally administered cimetidine or ranitidine because of adsorption, (2) preventing the absorption of orally administered cimetidine or ranitidine because of sucralfate coating the intestinal mucosa, and (3) cimetidine or ranitidine decreasing the acidity of the stomach sufficiently to inhibit the activation of sucralfate. The available evidence, including studies performed in dogs, has shown that none of these interactions appear to be significant (Hansten and Horn, 1985; Danesh et al., 1987).

DRUG INTERACTIONS INVOLVING DRUG METABOLISM. Drug interactions may occur because of inhibition or induction of the activity of microsomal hepatic enzymes. Drugs can be metabolized by a number of different pathways, making prediction of the consequences of metabolic interactions difficult.

*Inhibitors of Hepatic Metabolism.* Some hepatic enzymes are inhibited by drugs such as cimetidine (Tagamet), chloramphenicol (Chloromycetin), ketoconazole (Nizoral), metronidazole (Flagyl), erythromycin, and phenothiazines. This interaction can potentially increase the concentration of a coadministered drug by decreasing its clearance. For example, cimetidine inhibits the metabolism of theophylline, and chloramphenicol inhibits the metabolism of barbiturates. Chloramphenicol should be avoided in a critical care patient receiving multiple drugs. If one is administering other drugs with cimetidine, and a drug interaction is suspected, exchange cimetidine for ranitidine (Zantac), which does not affect hepatic enzymes as much as cimetidine. Drug enzyme inhibition may be a favorable interaction. For example, ethanol or 4-methylpyrazole is used to inhibit the enzyme alcohol dehydrogenase, which transforms ethylene glycol (antifreeze) to nephrotoxic metabolites.

*Inducers of Hepatic Metabolism.* Inducers of the hepatic enzymes increase the metabolism of drugs that are administered simultaneously. Well-known inducers of hepatic enzymes are anticonvulsants (phenobarbital and primidone), rifampin, and griseofulvin. Chronic administration of the inducer is necessary, because enzyme induction requires several days. This is important to realize, because enzyme inducers cannot be used to increase the clearance of a toxin. However, if a patient is receiving a drug known to be an enzyme inducer, the effectiveness of other drugs metabolized by similar routes may be diminished.

The metabolism of dexamethasone and prednisolone is enhanced via hepatic microsomal enzyme induction by phenobarbital administration. A decreased therapeutic effect should be considered when corticosteroids are administered to patients receiving anticonvulsant treatment, and an increase in the corticosteroid dosage may be needed in order to maintain the desired therapeutic response (Gambertoglio, 1983).

### PHARMACODYNAMIC DRUG INTERACTIONS

POTENTIATION OF A PHARMACOLOGIC EFFECT. In most instances, the potentiation of another drug can be predicted when there is knowledge that two drugs act at the same receptor, or have a similar pharmacologic effect. For example, more than one drug acting as a central nervous system depressant (e.g., a phenothiazine plus a barbiturate) will result in increased depression. Or, if one administers more than one drug that is a vasodilator, such as nitroglycerin, hydralazine, captopril, or acepromazine, severe hypotension may result.

POTENTIATION OF A TOXICOSIS. One drug can potentiate the toxicosis or side effects of another drug. Coadministration of furosemide (Lasix) with gentamicin may increase drug uptake into the renal tubules and increase the risk of gentamicin nephrotoxicosis. The coadministration of any diuretic with angiotensin-converting enzyme (ACE) inhibitors, such as captopril (Capoten) or enalapril (Enacard, Vasotec), should be done so cautiously because hypotension, decreased renal perfusion, and azotemia may result. Since ACE inhibitors reduce potassium excretion, the administration of an ACE inhibitor with a potassium-sparing diuretic may cause hyperkalemia. The administration of ACE inhibitors concurrently with high doses of potassium penicillin G also may produce hyperkalemia.

INTERACTIONS INVOLVING NSAID. The adverse effects of nonsteroidal anti-inflammatory drugs (NSAIDs) on the gastrointestinal tract may be enhanced by the coadministration of glucocorticoids (Dow et al., 1990). Both drugs decrease the protective effect of mucus in the gastrointestinal tract and decrease normal epithelial cell turnover and repair. Bleeding in the gastrointestinal tract can be complicated by the antiplatelet effects of the NSAID.

Some drugs act via prostaglandin synthesis stimulation or potentiation. Furosemide and ACE inhibitors stimulate prostaglandin synthesis to increase renal blood flow, produce vasodilation, or a natriuresis. Nonsteroidal anti-inflammatory drugs, via their inhibition of prostaglandin synthesis, may decrease the action of ACE inhibitors and furosemide.

## CONCLUSION

Many of the details from this discussion are not easy to recall each time one uses these drugs in clinical practice. Examples used here were intended to illustrate common, potential interactions that may have previously been overlooked. The best advice is to read the package insert that accompanies each drug and become familiar with the fluids and drugs with which it is used. Veterinarians should have access to reliable references such as the *USP-DI*, which describe possible interactions and their appropriate management.

### References and Suggested Reading

Danesh BJZ, Duncan A, and Russell RI: Is an acid pH medium required for the protective effect of sucralfate against mucosal injury? Am J Med 83(suppl 3B):11, 1987.
*This symposium contains several articles entirely devoted to sucralfate and its properties.*
D'Arcy PF: Drug interactions with medical plastics. Drug Intell Clin Pharm 17:726, 1983.
*This article summarizes the possible drug interactions with plastic of infusion systems and the principles of these interactions.*
Dow SW, Rosychuk RAW, McChesney AE, and Curtis CR: Effects of flunixin and flunixin plus prednisone on the gastrointestinal tract of dogs. Am J Vet Res 51:1131, 1990.
*This study demonstrated that the combination of corticosteroids plus an NSAID is more toxic to the gastrointestinal tract than NSAIDs alone.*
Gambertoglio JG: Corticosteroids and anticonvulsants. Drug Interact Newslett 3:55, 1983.
*This article provides several references regarding potential interactions with corticosteroids in patients receiving anticonvulsants.*
Goode CJ, Titler M, Rakel B, et al: A meta-analysis of effects of heparin flush and saline flush: Quality and cost implications. Nurs Res 40:324, 1991.
*This analysis of 15 studies concludes that saline is as effective as heparin for flushing IV catheters.*
Hansten PD and Horn JR: Interactions between antiulcer medications. Drug Interact Newslett 5:11, 1985.

*This reference presents evidence for several possible interactions involving antiulcer medications. Of particular interest are the references to studies in dogs that show that sucralfate does not produce a significant interaction with cimetidine.*

The Medical Letter Inc: *Handbook of Adverse Drug Interactions* 1000 Main St. New Rochelle, NY 10801-7537.

*This is a handy reference listing most in vivo interactions; this handbook is also available for IBM-PC or Macintosh computer.*

Stella VJ: Fundamentals of drug stability and compatibility. *In* Trissel LA (ed): *Handbook on Injectable Drugs*, 4th edition. American Society of Hospital Pharmacists, 1986.

*This is an excellent chapter that provides a scientific explanation for drug*

*decomposition due to storage or temperature, and incompatibilities that occur between drugs and fluids, or drugs and other drugs.*

Trissel LA (ed): *Handbook on Injectable Drugs*, 4th edition. American Society of Hospital Pharmacists, 1986.

*This book is an excellent reference that contains a list of all possible interactions for most injectable drugs.*

USP-DI, 1994, United States Pharmacopeial Convention Inc, Beltsville, MD, 1994.

*This is the most comprehensive reference source available that lists the pharmacology, pharmacokinetics, drug interactions, adverse effects, incompatibilities, and dosages for all drugs available; a veterinary version of the USP-DI is scheduled for 1995.*

# DISASTER MEDICINE: MEETING THE NEEDS OF THE SMALL ANIMAL PATIENT

GARY L. STAMP
*San Antonio, Texas*

Thousands of pets have died, been seriously injured, become separated from their owners, and been left to fend for themselves in the aftermath of recent devastating disasters. Hurricanes Andrew, Iniki, and Hugo; the Oakland fire of 1991; and the great Mississippi River Basin flood of 1993 created animal care and animal control challenges of mammoth proportion. It has become clear from these experiences that animal emergency relief efforts should address the basic issues of animal health care/treatment, veterinary public health/animal control, and revival of the veterinary infrastructure.

The efforts and vast resources applied to animal relief programs often fall short of expectations due to lack of preplanning and poor coordination between participating groups. There are many local, state, and national animal welfare agencies that have tremendous resources and expertise available to apply to a postdisaster relief program. The difficulty is integrating them with the veterinary community into a synergistic effort to meet the unique challenges of animal care and animal control (Norman, 1992). Disaster response plans must be developed to address local, regional, and state animal relief contingencies if the chaos of past efforts (e.g., Oakland, Hugo, Andrew) is to be avoided. Veterinarians must play leading roles in development of such plans to ensure a coordinated and effective response to disasters affecting the animal community (Stamp, 1993).

## POSTDISASTER CHALLENGES

The immediate concerns following any major disaster are to save lives and relieve suffering; the long-term goal is to return the community to its predisaster status.

From the veterinary perspective, the basic issues of emergency animal care, veterinary public health, and animal control must be addressed first. Another challenge, reestablishing the veterinary infrastructure as quickly as possible, will facilitate accomplishment of the basic objectives and help eliminate the well-intended but chaotic distribution of care. The character and complexity of these issues will obviously depend on the type disaster, be it fire, hurricane, earthquake, flood, or oil spill.

## EMERGENCY ANIMAL CARE

Preplanning for disasters will help answer the "what," "who," "how," "where," and "when" questions related to performing disaster relief veterinary medicine. The medical problems encountered will vary with geographic location, time of year, and type of disaster.

### Animal Care Problems

*What* medical emergencies should be anticipated? Traumatic injuries to include minor lacerations, abrasions, and puncture wounds as well as life-threatening blunt trauma, head injuries, and fractures are very common, especially following hurricanes and tornados. Heat exhaustion, dehydration, and respiratory problems were frequently treated by veterinarians in the wake of Hurricane Andrew, due to the prevailing environmental conditions in South Florida. With much of the water and food supplies contaminated by the unsanitary conditions created by most natural disasters, mild to severe gastrointestinal disease can be expected as a common presenting complaint. The increased numbers of loose, roaming domestic and wild animals will result in numerous bite wound cases as they compete for food and territorial rights.

Additionally, the stress of the situation may unmask or exacerbate conditions in the small animal patient such as cardiac disease, renal failure, and endocrinopathies. Internal and external parasitism become more of a concern due to the environmental conditions and the inherent low priority attached to prevention by distraught animal owners. Subsequently, vector-borne diseases may increase. Past experience indicates that routine minor medical problems such as dermatoses progress in significance also, due to lack of proper attention and inadequate husbandry practices.

## Health Care Providers

*Who* is expected to provide the postdisaster animal care and from *where*? Again it will depend greatly upon the type of disaster and the extent of damage to veterinary practices in the immediate area. Generally, veterinary facilities in the disaster area should be considered nonfunctional until an area assessment proves otherwise. This situation mandates that much of the initial animal relief be performed by volunteers from outside the area and by those veterinary personnel indigenous to the disaster area having remained with their practices. This in fact was the case with Hurricane Andrew.

Within a few hours of the passing of Andrew, hundreds of animal care volunteers representing at least 15 organizations (Table 1) started arriving in Dade County, FL. This has been the case with other recent natural disasters as well; multitudes of volunteers come in support of animal relief. The problem is on-site organization of these seemingly similar groups and individuals to avoid conflict, redundancy, and inefficiency of effort. The various organizations and volunteer groups are unified in their intent to aid the animal victims, but individual priorities, parochial interests, and lack of cohesion are frequently detrimental to that end (Dee, 1993; Stamp, 1993). Unfortunately, that was this author's observation in Dade County. Despite this fragmented approach, volunteers are essential to care for the thousands of animals abandoned, lost, and injured following a natural disaster.

The animal disaster relief contingent generally will consist of two factions: veterinary medical and animal welfare personnel. The local and state veterinary medical associations (VMAs) have in the past played the lead role in organizing the veterinary support. This was the case in South Florida. Hundreds of veterinary volunteers were coordinated by the South Florida VMA and the Florida VMA to staff the emergency relief centers located in temporary clinic facilities established in the disaster area. Such assistance provided by volunteers is essential to meet the emergent needs of the animal victims and to make up the shortfall in veterinary services that occur due to closed practices. A coordinated plan is critical, however, to effectively place the available personnel assets where and when they are most needed. Obviously, cooperation and a spirit of teamwork are needed.

Nonveterinary groups and individuals such as animal welfare agencies, kennel clubs, rescue associations, and concerned citizens constitute a resource that should be used to support animal relief efforts. A variety of local and national groups may be involved, but the American Humane Association (AHA), a national animal welfare organization headquartered in Denver, can be expected to take the lead. This national organization is the one designated by the American Red Cross to take responsibility for animal relief efforts when disaster strikes; it has established an Emergency Animal Relief Fund. Volunteers from these many groups can be counted on to transport animals, distribute food and supplies, assist in clinics, and augment animal control efforts. The problem again is usually not in having enough personnel but in *coordinating them* to work together, aside from their individual interests, and to focus them on the entire animal relief effort.

The magnitude of many disasters, with the resulting community infrastructure chaos and overwhelming need for relief, will severely challenge the efforts of the disaster team. In the first few days after the disaster, the animal care needs may well outpace the capability and resources of the relief team. This certainly was the case in Hurricane Andrew but not so in the Mississippi River Basin flood where the gradual progression of events allowed relief teams to adequately handle animal care problems.

Additional manpower may be needed when the regional and state resources are insufficient. National groups such as the American Veterinary Medicine Association (AVMA) and the American Animal Hospital Association (AAHA) can provide assistance in a variety of ways, to include mobilizing more volunteers and assigning trained personnel to organize and perform specific functions. The Army Veterinary Corps (VC) can also be utilized if request for their support is coordi-

***Table 1.*** *List of Organizations Supporting Hurricane Andrew Animal Relief**

American Animal Hospital Association
American Veterinary Medical Association
American Humane Association
American Association of Equine Practitioners
American Veterinary Academy of Disaster Medicine
American Red Cross
Florida Animal Control Association
Florida Veterinary Medical Association
Humane Society of the United States
Humane Society of Broward County
Humane Society of Treasure Coast
International Fund for Animal Welfare
South Florida Veterinary Medical Association
United Animal Nations
U.S. Department of Agriculture
U.S. Public Health Service
U.S. Army Veterinary Corps

*These organizations all participated in the Hurricane Andrew animal relief effort and are typical of those that would respond to most major animal-related disasters.

nated through the Federal Emergency Management Agency (FEMA) and the Department of Defense. The VC can provide veterinarians, technicians, field hospitals, and organizational skills.

## Animal Relief Facilities

Facilities and locations must be identified for veterinary relief teams to function. In the aftermath of Andrew, 28 practices in the immediate area were damaged, ten being totally destroyed and eight severely damaged. Injured animals were brought into these facilities for care regardless of the structural condition, if the veterinarian was present and able to attend them. In these conditions, veterinarians should administer emergency treatment until more suitable facilities can be obtained.

The keys to establishing the most functional and most efficient animal relief centers are centered on a *disaster plan*. First, this plan should have plotted all practices in the area and identified suitable facilities as temporary clinics. Facilities should also be designated for support (e.g., command and control center, supply storage, volunteer housing, animal holding). Second, an area assessment should be performed as soon as possible after the disaster by the predesignated animal relief coordinators. Through integration of the disaster plan with the area assessment, the best locations and facilities from which to provide disaster relief can be determined. These may be in existing clinics or temporary facilities modified for animal care.

Utilization of existing clinics is preferred as much as possible for several reasons. The veterinarian may still have access to basic utilities, equipment, and supplies, and is familiar with the workplace. Clients, old and new, probably know the location of the practice and how to find it, which is important during the postdisaster disruption of the community. The regular veterinarian may be better able to care for the patient and provide comfort to the owner. Volunteer veterinary personnel can be used to staff the relief operation while the incumbent is trying to recover property and tend to personal needs.

Temporary animal relief facilities certainly will be needed in disasters of any magnitude. This was the case in Miami after Hurricane Andrew, where three emergency centers were operated. Several factors should be considered when establishing and operating these centers:

1. The disaster plan should have a predesignated veterinary operations coordinator and alternates to organize and assign volunteers.

2. Responsibility and "ownership" of the clinic operation must rest with the veterinary community (e.g., local VMA, state VMA) versus animal welfare agencies.

3. Objectives of the temporary facility (understood by all staff) should be provision of emergency treatment for disaster victims, distribution of food and husbandry supplies as needed to owners, and referral of follow-up care and nondisaster patients to full-service facilities.

4. Signs must be posted advising of services offered, and location/directions to nearest full-service practices.

5. Temporary animal holding (for lost or stray animals) and food distribution services should be provided if possible.

6. A storage area with security for medical and nonmedical supplies must be planned.

7. Relief centers should transition postdisaster animal care to nearby traditional practices once these have returned to operation.

8. Field hospitals (with staff) can be made available from military units if properly requested through the state emergency management agency and FEMA.

The essential elements for success are preplanning and coordination. Veterinary associations must be proactive in developing disaster plans that integrate the interests and resources of animal welfare agencies. Should this not occur, these groups will establish and operate emergency treatment facilities as they see fit, outside the purview of local and state veterinary associations. Utilizing independent volunteers, autonomous relief groups may conduct "their" clinics in a manner inconsistent with sound veterinary practice.

Table 2 lists the criteria and characteristics of an *ideal* temporary animal relief facility. Preplanning and consideration of these factors will greatly influence the effectiveness of the operation as it is deluged with disaster victims. Postponing critical decisions to the impact period (0 to 48 hr postdisaster) jeopardizes the ultimate success of the operation and certainly compromises patient care. Again, reference is made to author's experience in Hurricane Andrew where no predisaster plan existed (Stamp, 1993) and animal relief efforts were hampered by suboptimal placement and

***Table 2.*** *Criteria for Ideal Temporary Animal Relief Facility**

**Location**
  Near dense concentration of lost animals; near population centers; within the disaster area
  Easy access to the public
  Compatible with the neighborhood
  Known site, identifiable
  Out of way of impending disaster (e.g., flooding, fire)

**Utilities**
  As many services as possible, including water, electricity, telephone, heat, air conditioning

**Area**
  Parking available
  Fenced or able to be fenced for animal holding
  Lighted for security

**Structure**
  Sturdy, good condition; masonry desired
  Multiple rooms for receiving, triage, outpatient/exam, minor surgery and treatment; ICU
  Medical and nonmedical storage (e.g., food, water, cleaning agents, cages)
  Securable

**Security**
  Premises and controlled drugs if necessary

---

*A school with athletic field is an excellent choice, if available. Solid structure, fenced area, and familiar location near population centers are desirable characteristics.

building selection of some of the temporary clinics. Storage, security, and animal holding capabilities are often overlooked factors, but are extremely important features of a well-designed facility.

## Temporary Clinic Operations

How does or should the animal emergency relief clinic operate? First and foremost, it is understood that the facility is meant to serve disaster victims, not replace routine veterinary care. The primary objectives are to save lives and relieve suffering. To best accomplish this, the principles of mass casualty care and triage should be practiced. Elective procedures and routine preventive care should be referred to functional full-service practices so as not to clog the emergency system and consume resources. A clearly posted sign, a brief flyer, or both, advising pet owners of this, with directions to other clinics, can help prevent misunderstandings between the clinic staff and clientele. Care must be taken, however, not to inflame or offend owners who also are victims and are understandably distraught.

The principles of emergency medicine should be applied, including triage of patients (Kirby, 1989). The clinic receiving team must recognize those catastrophic patients needing immediate attention and direct them appropriately. A sign-in log should be used to track patients, document presenting complaints, and prioritize problems. Personnel with experience in emergency clinics are obviously an excellent choice for the receiving team. Severe, moderate, and minor injuries and illnesses should then be sequentially managed considering the limitations posed by the temporary facility. Seriously ill or injured patients generally should be stabilized and referred to the nearest full-service practice where definitive care can be provided. The less serious are treated, released, and advised on any follow-up that may be necessary, also at a full-service, traditional clinic.

In some instances, the relief centers may attempt to function as full-service facilities, performing semielective procedures, hospitalizing patients, vaccinating, heartworm testing, and so forth. This obviously is not the mission of these relief operations and should be discouraged from the outset starting with the disaster plan. A preventative medicine vaccination and parasite control program may be relevant, however, in some scenarios such as the Mississippi floods where vector-borne and infectious diseases constituted significant risks. Liberal distribution of one or two broad-spectrum monthly anthelmintic prevention tablets per dog should provide sufficient coverage for the postdisaster period. Vaccination of high-risk patients may also be indicated. The scope of these prevention programs should be determined by a veterinary operations committee.

Again, the health care needs following disasters will vary; they should be assessed immediately by the disaster relief committee and priorities modified appropriately. Services provided are then matched to the needs and resources, with the temporary treatment facilities and the remaining functional veterinary clinics playing specific roles. The established clinics in the disaster area that are operational are utilized to the fullest extent possible. Patients are referred from the temporary treatment centers to these clinics in the disaster area, or to full-service hospitals outside the disaster as the case dictates.

## Documentation

Are medical records necessary for disaster victims? If so, what and how should information be recorded? From past experience, this author strongly advises that a standardized medical record system be utilized by all the veterinary disaster relief treatment centers. The record system, albeit essential, must be very simplistic and should not impede, but should enhance, the delivery of veterinary care. Adequate numbers of volunteers, if used properly, are normally available for this record-keeping function. Patient documentation is comprised of two components; the *sign-in log* and the medical *treatment* record.

The purpose of the sign-in log is to facilitate a smooth flow of patients through the treatment center. Additionally, it will be useful later in providing data on the numbers and types of cases managed by all the treatment centers. These data will assist development of future disaster plans. The log itself should include the basics of owner and patient's name, species, time of arrival, presenting complaint, and perhaps the name of regular veterinarian. Patients may then be triaged by color coding their log entry and seen by the veterinary staff according to severity of injury and time of arrival. Such a simple system will greatly aid distribution of care.

Once in the treatment room, or earlier if time permits, a permanent record is initiated. This may be done by a volunteer assisting in the reception area using information from the sign-in log, or by a technician in the exam room. A form routinely used by emergency clinics is ideal for this situation. This form (Fig. 1) allows for annotation of the signalment, presenting problem, care provided, medication dispensed, and follow-up instructions. Since it is a multiple carbon form, a copy can be given to the owner as a permanent record of care, for referring to the follow-up instructions, and to aid the next clinician ministering to the patient.

This emergency medical record will also be of benefit to owners in filing insurance claims, in obtaining reimbursements for care, and in completing their animal's permanent medical record. It will greatly assist the veterinary disaster relief committee in documenting the cases managed, and drugs and supplies utilized. It also can serve as a basis for reimbursement from the disaster relief fund to veterinarians for free service provided to disaster victims.

## Funding for Service

How is animal medicine relief funded? What is the source? Who manages the funding? Is service provided free, for cost, and to whom? Are private practitioners supported by a relief fund, and how? These are very real questions and the answers will greatly determine the success or failure of the disaster relief efforts. Plans for funding should be well outlined in state and regional disaster plans.

Animal relief groups can anticipate that there will be a tremendous outpouring of donations in the form of supplies and money. Management and distribution of such donations can become very complex and competitive with the various groups and interests involved. Such was the case in Dade County, FL in 1992, when hundreds of thousands of dollars in cash and supplies were donated, and at least a half-dozen separate organizations were actively soliciting, collecting, and distributing funds and supplies. Fiscal oversight of these funds varied tremendously. Donations of money and supplies must be used for the intended purpose.

Management of donations must be specified in the disaster plan. If possible, funds should be received and processed centrally and should be earmarked for one of two broad categories: emergency animal relief or veterinarian assistance. The latter is vital, considering that many veterinary practices will require support to regain operation, and the sooner they are functional the quicker veterinary care in the area will approach predisaster status. The disaster plan should designate the fund managers (disaster relief committee), who then will determine how funds and supplies will be distributed and used. In light of the major natural disasters of 1992 and 1993, some states and national organizations (e.g., AAHA) have now established trust funds to make support available immediately for veterinary disaster operations. Funds in these trusts are intended to relieve the financial burden on both pet owners and victimized veterinarians as they recover from the disaster.

## REVIVING THE VETERINARY INFRASTRUCTURE

Providing postdisaster veterinary care rests with the practitioners in the private sector. Of course, veterinary practices will have been partially or completely de-

**EMERGENCY PET CLINIC, INC.** - 8503 Broadway Suite 101 San Antonio, Texas 78217

CLIENT #: ______ PVS: ______ Telephone (210) 822-2873

| | | | | |
|---|---|---|---|---|
| Date / / | Time A.M. P.M. | Attending Veterinarian(s) / | Employer | Receipt Number 38567 |
| Owner | Phone: Home | Work | | |
| Address | Zip | Regular Veterinarian | | |
| Pet's Name | Breed C F | M ☐ - F ☐ Neutered Y N | DOB Wt. Color | |
| Vaccinations: Date: | FVRCP FELV DHLP/PV RV Not Current | On Heartworm Prevention Y ☐ N ☐ | | |
| Primary Complaint: | | | | |
| | | T P R | | |
| Therapy | Tentative Diag: | | | |

| | | |
|---|---|---|
| SEND | TOTAL CHARGES - - (1) | ______ |
| ☐ MEDS | DEPOSIT - - - - - - - - (4) | ______ |
| ☐ LAB | BALANCE DUE - - - - (4) | ______ |
| ☐ RADS | TOTAL PAID - - - - - (4) | ______ |

Method of Payment: Cash ☐ Check ☐ M/C ☐ Visa ☐ Other ☐

Contact Your Regular Veterinarian The Next Working Day Regarding This Case. RELEASED BY: ______ TIME: ______

**Figure 1.** Example of an emergency clinic form.

stroyed. There is not a veterinary counterpart to the federal, state, and local health care systems that can accommodate disaster victims or disenfranchised animals and animal owners. No government agency exists to ensure care. Practice owners must (and invariably do) make every effort to quickly restore their hospital operations allowing emergency or routine care to be administered in a more optimal and traditional manner. This benefits both the patient and the veterinarian. Even with rapid reestablishment of full-service veterinary care, some independent groups may advocate that a subsidized (but lower quality) care be provided from the temporary clinics for months following the disaster. This would not seem to be in the best interest of most patients or the local veterinary community.

It is recommended that all animal disaster plans acknowledge the requirement to reestablish the community veterinary infrastructure as soon as possible. Use of grants, trust funds, corporate, and national organizational support should be planned. A "buddy system" matching an unaffected practice with one victimized would greatly assist a damaged practice to become operational. Trust funds can be used to obtain needed supplies or to reimburse private practices for supplies consumed in the treatment of disaster victims. A strong veterinary infrastructure is vitally important to meet immediate and long-term animal health care needs, and cooperation is needed from paraveterinary, animal welfare, and allied health care groups.

## ANIMAL CONTROL AND VETERINARY PUBLIC HEALTH

The animal control problem (with its related veterinary public health issues) is extremely difficult to manage in the postdisaster devastation for several reasons. First, the existing local animal control system likely is already stretched in meeting the needs prior to the disaster. Second, the destruction and community disruption result in excessive numbers of homeless, roaming animals. With homes destroyed, families relocated, and familiar landmarks gone, pets may become disoriented and eventually roam. Dogs tend to pack and aimlessly wander through the neighborhood, potentiating a public health problem.

A sufficient holding facility must be established on short notice, or captured animals will have to be transported to facilities outside the disaster area. It is critically important that a confinement facility be available in close proximity to population centers where pets may have been lost. This will afford owners a much better chance to retrieve their animals. Should animals be transferred to shelters or foster homes outside the immediate area, it is unlikely that they will ever by reunited with their owners. Holding centers near temporary housing for disaster refugees will also serve to keep pets close to their owners for visitation, since most refugee housing does not allow pets. The human-animal bond issue must be recognized and accommodated.

Poor owner compliance with tagging and registering their animals also will significantly contribute to the animal control problem and hamper successful retrieval of lost pets. A tagging ID system must be used on all animals treated in the likelihood that they may become lost again. The microchip ID system may well be the best way to permanently identify these animals.

With the increased number of stray animals, there is great potential for bite incidents. The appropriate county, state, or metropolitan veterinary public health office must work closely with animal control and other health care agencies to monitor animal bites, zoonotic diseases, and veterinary-related community health problems (Moore, 1992).

## DISASTER PLAN AND ORGANIZATION

In disasters the magnitude of Andrew or Hugo, an Emergency Operations Center (EOC) will be established to conduct the overall relief effort. The EOC will be under the authority of FEMA, and the United States Public Health Service (USPHS) will have responsibility for the Health Task Force. The armed forces may be activated to support the relief effort if deemed necessary by FEMA, and appropriately requested through the Department of Defense. The American Red Cross and American Humane Association will be actively involved. There also will be a variety of state and local agencies participating in the effort.

In view of the agencies involved and the volunteer personnel available, a basic consideration is organization and planning. Until recently, disaster preparedness plans for animal emergencies were virtually nonexistent. In 1992 and 1993, several states and the AVMA developed plans to address animal-related disaster relief. The AVMA generated a plan (Anderson and Tennyson, 1993), approved by the Department of Health and Human Services (HHS) and the United States Department of Agriculture (USDA), which is intended to provide care for sick and injured livestock, wildlife, and pets; restraint and control of stray and abandoned animals; proper disposal of dead animals; protection of the animal food supply; and infection control. This is an extremely ambitious and broad-based plan calling for the establishment of a cadre of 100 veterinarians and 200 technicians trained in disaster relief services, to serve as a reserve force capable of deploying whenever and wherever a disaster strikes.

The state disaster preparedness plans vary somewhat but primarily are based on the state VMA as the lead agency integrating and organizing relief efforts within their state (Casper, 1993; Marshall et al., 1993; Dorn, 1993). Maryland has developed a pet-sheltering plan; California has produced a county-oriented, comprehensive resource guide for services available and necessary to manage animal-related disasters; Ohio has aligned their VMA Disaster Medicine Committee with the State Emergency Operations Center and the Department of Health.

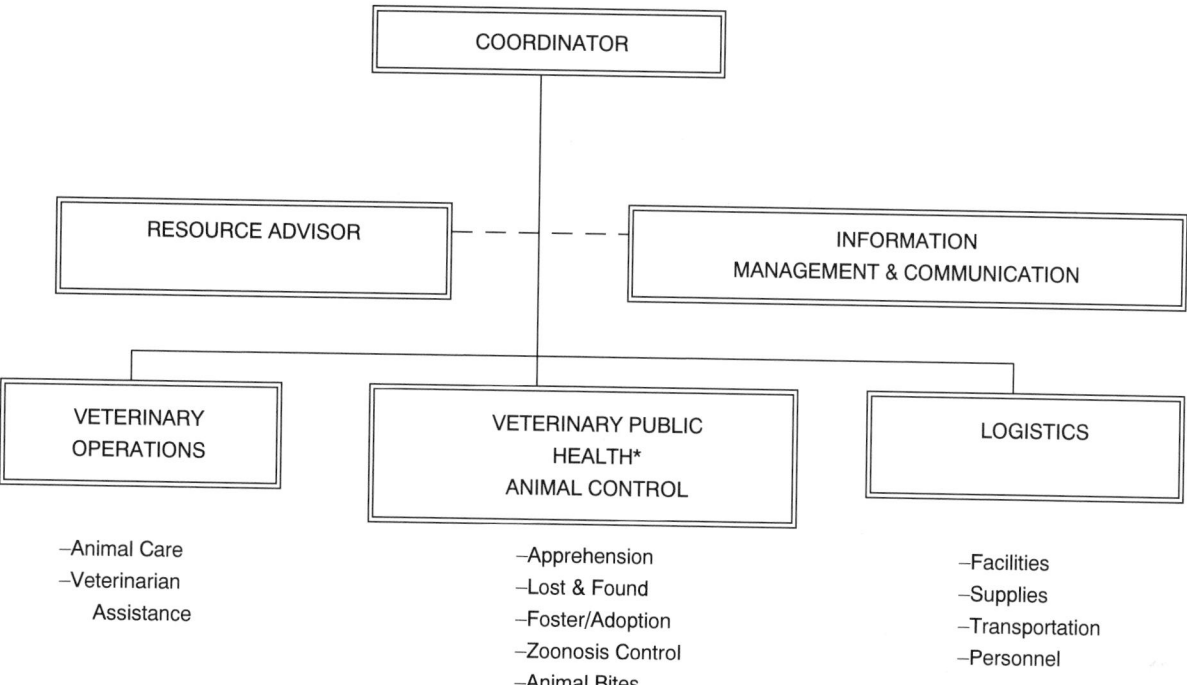

**Figure 2.** Proposed animal emergency disaster relief plan. *May be separated as distinct function.

Major problems to overcome in implementing any plan include an effective and authoritative *command and control center* and coordination of the volunteers. State and local government offices may be overwhelmed immediately and incapable of responding to increased demands for services. Loosely organized groups of volunteers will initiate animal relief operations in a well-meaning but somewhat inefficient manner. It is important that county, regional, and state plans designate organizational structure. An authoritative Disaster Animal Relief Coordinator is needed. Furthermore, the State Veterinarian and state public health representatives must be key players in any major animal relief effort. A few hours of diligent preplanning and coordinating will save countless days of chaos after the disaster.

Based on experience in Hurricane Andrew, this author proposes that to achieve optimum coordination between all the players, the disaster plan should be structured as shown in Figure 2. This plan would designate a governmental officer as the coordinator; one who is unbiased by personal involvement and clearly recognized as an authority figure. The State Veterinarian would be the obvious choice for this position. Another consideration might be the designated representative of the AVMA task force. If the coordinator is from one of the volunteer organizations or associations, command and control authority will be greatly weakened. Whoever is selected, it is *essential* that the coordinator strongly liaison and interact with the EOC.

The proposed plan in Figure 2 would allow for a staff to direct the functions most familiar to them, and to participate in decisions affecting the entire relief effort.

It also considers the importance of managing resources and information while controlling the flow of both. The logistics section is needed to specifically address the enormous task of handling supplies, coordinating and training personnel, and managing the key facilities. Note that the *veterinary operations* branch addresses both animal care and veterinarian assistance, thus acknowledging the importance of supporting the victimized veterinarians so that they can regain their capacity to care for patients. Veterinary public health and animal control are presented under one branch because of the closely related problems, but clearly these could be separated depending on the regional disaster scenario. This plan should provide the appropriate organizational structure to serve most animal emergency relief operations.

## References and Suggested Reading

Anderson DA and Tennyson AV: AVMA preparedness planning. J Am Vet Med Assoc 203:1008, 1993.

Casper J: The Maryland pet-shelter plan. J Am Vet Med Assoc 203:994, 1993.

Dee L: Lessons learned from Hurricane Andrew. J Am Vet Med Assoc 203: 986, 1993.

Dorn CR: Veterinary service and animal care emergency operations plans. J Am Vet Med Assoc 203:1005, 1993.

Kirby R: Critical care-overview. Vet Clin North Am [Small Anim Pract] 19: 1007, 1989.

Marshall K, Norman BB, Schumacher R, et al: Veterinarians as advocates during disasters: The California Veterinary Medical Association's disaster response program. J Am Vet Med Assoc 203:1002, 1993.

Moore RM Jr: The role of the veterinarian in hurricanes and other natural disasters. Ann NY Acad Sci 65:367, 1992.

Norman BB: A different kind of an emergency. Calif Vet 46:23, 1992.

Stamp GL: Hurricane Andrew: The importance of coordinated response. J Am Vet Med Assoc 203:989, 1993.

# Section 3

# TOXICOLOGIC DISORDERS

GARY D. OSWEILER

*Consulting Editor*

*Still Current Information Found in Current Veterinary Therapy XI:*

*Elsewhere in Current Veterinary Therapy XII:*

# INCIDENCE OF SMALL ANIMAL POISON EXPOSURES IN A MAJOR METROPOLITAN AREA

CARL S. HORNFELDT

*Minneapolis, Minnesota*

*and* MICHAEL J. MURPHY

*St. Paul, Minnesota*

This article briefly summarizes the prevalence of small animal poison exposures reported by the Hennepin Regional Poison Control Center. This information is provided to give practitioners and students an indication of the most common toxins encountered by small animals so that rational decisions on preparing for such exposures may be made.

The Hennepin Regional Poison Control Center serves an area comprised of approximately 1.9 million people and has been designated one of 37 regional centers by the American Association of Poison Control Centers. To encourage the veterinary community to utilize the resources available, a special telephone line was designated as the Pet Poison Information Service, and phone stickers bearing this number were distributed throughout the state in 1989. Since that time, the number of animal-related calls to the poison center has grown to 5000 annually. The following data were obtained from calls received through the veterinary line from 1990 through 1992. While this telephone number was distributed to veterinarians for professional use only, veterinarians obviously have referred clients to the poison center, since approximately 50% of calls currently come directly from the public.

It should be noted that data reflect exposure and not toxicosis. A poison exposure is defined as an actual or suspected contact with any substance that when ingested, inhaled, absorbed, applied to, or injected into the body may cause damage to structure or disturbance of function to living tissue (Hornfeldt and Murphy, 1992).

Poison exposures involving dogs made up 69% of cases received during this period, while cats made up 17.7%. The balance was made up of rodents and lagomorphs, birds (e.g., parrots), nondomesticated animals (e.g., squirrels), and exotics (e.g., iguana, ferrets). Large animals made up less than 0.1% of all calls.

The data in Table 1 reveal that pesticides (insecticides and rodenticides) were the largest contaminant group for canine exposures, followed by plants, prescription medications, and over-the-counter medications. The largest contaminant category for exposures in cats were plants, followed by pesticides, household products, and prescription medications.

Insecticides and rodenticides are the most frequently

**Table 1.** *Incidence of Poison Exposures of Small Animals*

| Poison | Dog | Cat | Other/ Unknown | Total | Percentage |
|---|---|---|---|---|---|
| Pesticides | 1911 | 447 | 307 | 2665 | 20.6 |
| Plants | 1401 | 633 | 351 | 2385 | 18.5 |
| Prescription | 1139 | 146 | 163 | 1448 | 11.2 |
| Over-the-counter medications | 1034 | 119 | 187 | 1340 | 10.4 |
| Household products | 776 | 262 | 142 | 1180 | 9.1 |
| Foreign bodies, miscellaneous | 539 | 142 | 107 | 788 | 6.1 |
| Lawn garden products | 361 | 73 | 86 | 520 | 4.0 |
| Cosmetics | 362 | 42 | 68 | 472 | 3.7 |
| Veterinary products | 244 | 114 | 66 | 424 | 3.3 |
| Building supplies | 206 | 101 | 45 | 352 | 2.7 |
| Automotive products | 207 | 87 | 36 | 330 | 2.6 |
| Art/crafts | 207 | 36 | 46 | 289 | 2.2 |
| Food poisoning | 242 | 13 | 31 | 286 | 2.2 |
| Industrial products/ chemicals | 167 | 58 | 53 | 278 | 2.2 |
| Bites, stings, Envenomations | 46 | 7 | 8 | 61 | 0.5 |
| Drugs of abuse | 35 | 0 | 10 | 45 | 0.3 |
| Fumes, gases | 17 | 9 | 6 | 32 | 0.2 |
| Tobacco products | 25 | 3 | 2 | 30 | 0.2 |
| Total | 8919 | 2292 | 1714 | 12,925 | |
| Percentage | 69.0 | 17.7 | 13.3 | | 100.0 |

encountered pesticides. Herbicides and molluscicides are occasionally encountered. The specific insecticides that are commonly reported are cholinesterase inhibitors, pyrethrins, and chlorinated hydrocarbons. Arsenic-containing insecticides are occasionally encountered. Anticoagulant rodenticides, strychnine, zinc phosphide, bromethalin, and cholecalciferol are the most frequently encountered rodenticides. When properly applied, herbicides are rarely responsible for toxicosis in small animals. Metaldehyde used for snail or slug control occasionally causes toxicosis in small animals. These toxins are reviewed elsewhere in this section and *CVT X and XI.*

The plants most frequently associated with toxicosis in small animals are those with cardiac effects (rhododendrons and Japanese yew), nightshades, and members of the Araceae family. Occasionally, onions (*Allium*), sago palms (*Cyas revoluta*), bleeding heart (*Dicentra*), and marijuana (*Cannabis*) cause toxicoses.

Exposures to human prescription medications involve a wide variety of products. Virtually everything in the medicine cabinet has been ingested by a pet. Tricyclic antidepressants, cardiac and blood pressure medications, and cholesterol-lowering products are commonly encountered.

On the other hand, over-the-counter preparations encountered are primarily ibuprofen, naproxen, and acetaminophen.

Household products such as lead, zinc, methylxanthines, detergents, caustic agents, gasoline, ethylene glycol, and alcohol-containing products comprise the fourth most frequently encountered exposure group.

### References and Suggested Reading

Hornfeldt CS and Murphy MJ: 1990 Report of the American Association of Poison Control Centers: Poisonings in animals. J Am Vet Med Assoc 200: 1077, 1992.

# TOP 25 GENERIC AGENTS INVOLVING DOGS AND CATS MANAGED BY THE NATIONAL ANIMAL POISON CONTROL CENTER IN 1992

WILLIAM B. BUCK
*Urbana, Illinois*

During the 12-month period, January 1 through December 31, 1992, the National Animal Poison Control Center assisted in the management of 12,611 cases involving one or more dogs and 5351 cases involving one or more cats. The top 25 generic agents involved are listed in Table 1.

### Table 1.°

| Dogs | Cats |
|---|---|
| **Rodenticides** | **Insecticides** |
| **Anticoagulants** | **Pyrethrins/pyrethroids** |
| Brodifacoum | Allethrin |
| Diphacinone | Permethrin |
| **Cholecalciferol** | Pyrethrins |
| **Insecticides** | Resmethrin |
| **Organophosphates** | Tetramethrin |
| Chlorpyrifos | Tralomethrin |
| Diazinon | **Organophosphates** |
| Phosmet | Chlorpyrifos |
| **Carbamates** | Diazinon |
| Carbaryl | Phosmet |
| Methomyl | Propetamphos |
| Propoxur | Tetrachlorvinfos |
| **Amitraz** | **Carbamates** |
| **Ivermectin** | Carbaryl |

| Dogs | Cats |
|---|---|
| Pyrethrin/pyrethroids | Propoxur |
| Allethrin | **DEET** |
| Pyrethrins | **d-Limonene** |
| Permethrin | **Ivermectin** |
| Tralomethrin | **Rotenone** |
| **DEET** | **Ethylene glycol** |
| **Naphthalene** | **Drugs** |
| **Theobromine/caffeine** | Acetaminophen |
| **Drugs** | Ibuprofen |
| Ibuprofen | Piperazine |
| Pseudoephedrine | **Plants** |
| **Ethylene glycol** | Rhododendron |
| **Metaldehyde** | Lily, Easter and tiger |
| **Mushrooms** | Philodendron |
| **Petroleum distillates** | **Quaternary ammonium chloride** |
| **Zinc/zinc oxide** | |

°The National Animal Poison Control Center (NAPCC) is a nonprofit service of the University of Illinois providing advice to animal owners and consultation with veterinarians about poisoning exposures. The around-the-clock service is supported in part by user fees charged to the caller by credit card (1-800-548-2423) or via a telephone statement (1-900-680-0000). For more information about the center's various services, please contact Dr. Louise M. Cote, NAPCC, University of Illinois College of Veterinary Medicine, 2001 S. Lincoln Ave., Urbana, IL 61801, 217-333-2053.

# EMERGENCY TREATMENT OF TOXICOSES

DAVID C. DORMAN

*Research Triangle Park, North Carolina*

Increasingly, people and their pets live in an environment filled with potentially toxic agents. Unfortunately, the extent of potential poisons far exceeds the number of safe and effective antidotes available to veterinarians for the treatment of toxicoses. Although antidotal treatments are often emphasized in the management of toxicoses, veterinary patients will often benefit as much (if not more) from intensive supportive therapy. Discussion of these supportive therapies will constitute a major part of this article. Different antidotes may serve to counteract the effect of toxicants in various ways. Many "antidotes" are simply directed toward achieving stabilization of vital signs, decreasing exposure, and facilitating toxin removal, while others specifically antagonize the toxicant at a primary or secondary site of action. For specific antidotal regimens, the reader is referred to previous editions of this textbook for listings of antidotes and their indications (Bailey, 1991).

Faced with a seemingly endless number of potential animal-toxicant interactions, veterinarians, must rely upon their general knowledge of how toxicants may affect the animal, and what general means can be employed in order to reduce the extent of an exposure. Critical concepts that should be considered in the treatment of the acutely poisoned animal include:

1. The dose of the toxin determines its effect.
2. Exclusive reliance on antidotal action can be dangerous.
3. Inherent risk is associated with the use of any therapeutic regimen.
4. Determination that a toxicosis has occurred is essential to effective treatment.
5. Goals for the management of acutely poisoned animals include:
   a. Stabilization of vital signs.
   b. Ongoing clinical evaluation.
   c. Prevention of continued exposure to the toxicant.
   d. Administration of an appropriate antidote.
   e. Facilitation of the removal of the absorbed toxicant.
   f. Supportive therapy.
6. *Always* treat the patient and not the toxicant.

All toxicologic therapy is based on two principles. First, the dose of the toxicant determines its effect. Second, there are only three general methods by which a poisoned animal can be treated. These methods include: (1) initiation of life-support measures, (2) modification of the toxic agent's pharmacokinetics (e.g., its absorption, distribution, metabolism, and excretion) in an effort to lower the effective dose reaching receptors, and (3) antagonism of the toxicant's pharmacodynamic effects. The primary goal of this article, therefore, is to discuss initial management of the poisoned animal. Special emphasis will be given to methods that may alter the disposition of a toxicant. Accordingly, the article is subdivided into sections based on the time frame during which these certain treatment modalities would be most effective (e.g., the first few minutes). These time frames should be used only as a general guideline. They may need to be further modified, depending on the individual toxicant, dose ingested, and initial response to therapy.

## THE FIRST FEW MINUTES

### Life Support

The initial management of a poisoned animal is critical. The objective of the first few minutes is to preserve the life of the animal regardless of the toxicant or disease etiology, thereby buying time for detoxification measures to be effective and for specific antidotes to have their pharmacologic action. When multiple animals (e.g., kennels or catteries) are involved, a system of triage may be necessary. During the first few minutes, patient stabilization and toxicant identification should be achieved. Vital treatment considerations for the acutely poisoned animal have been summarized in Tables 1 and 2.

Similar to other aspects of emergency veterinary medicine, it is important to emphasize the need for: (1) a patent airway, (2) adequate ventilation, and (3) prevention of aspiration of vomitus. If the animal is comatose or anesthetized, a patent airway can be provided using a cuffed, inflated, endotracheal tube. Mechanical or manual forced ventilation may be necessary for poisoned animals suffering from paralysis, severe central nervous system (CNS) depression or, rarely, when deep anesthesia is necessary to control convulsions (see *CVT XI*, p 98).

If cardiovascular dysfunction (e.g., arrhythmias) is associated with toxic insult, prompt correction of electrolyte imbalances and acid-base status may result in restoration of normal function. Ideally, blood samples for electrolytes, blood glucose, and serum chemistry determinations should be collected before initiating fluid therapy. There is no single fluid that will fulfill the fluid requirements of all poisoned patients. If shock or hypotension develops, balanced electrolyte solutions (e.g., lactated Ringer's solution) or normal saline are indicated. Daily fluid administration should account for both daily requirements as well as ongoing fluid losses (e.g., vomiting, diarrhea, polyuria). Treatment for cardiac arrhythmias may be required in some toxicoses. In many cases, correcting the underlying or electrolyte disorder may "cure" an arrhythmia without the use of specific antiarrhythmic agents. When used, antiarrhythmic therapy should be tailored for the type of arrhythmia present and the species involved. Before attempting treatment for a cardiac arrhythmia, it is important to establish the possible agent involved and determine whether the animal is already taking medication, especially digoxin. Agents that may potentially result in sinus bradycardia include organophosphate and carbamate insecticides, β-blockers, calcium channel blockers, digitalis glycosides, and phenothiazines (e.g., acepromazine). Parenteral atropine (0.01 to 0.02 mg/kg IV, IM) or glycopyrrolate (0.005 to 0.01 mg/kg IV, IM) are the initial antiarrhythmic agents of choice for symptomatic sinus bradycardia or atrioventricular block.

In the poisoned patient, acid-base homeostasis may also be disrupted by a variety of mechanisms, because: (1) the toxicant or its metabolites have acidic or basic character, (2) the agent causes seizures or other forms of profound muscle exertion, (3) the agent causes circulatory impairment of peripheral tissues (usually secondary to shock), (4) the agent causes respiratory dysfunction, (5) the agent causes prolonged vomiting or diarrhea, and/or (6) the treatment causes electrolyte imbalance (e.g., a diuretic). Acidosis is the most commonly encountered acid-base disturbance. Metabolic acidosis may be observed in toxicoses resulting from ethylene glycol, metaldehyde, and aspirin, among other agents. To correct metabolic acidosis, fluids with added sodium bicarbonate (1 to 3 mEq/kg administered in fluids over 1 to 3 hr: an 8.4% solution sodium bicarbonate = 1 mEq/ml) are used (see "Strong Ions and Acid-Base Disorders," this volume, p 121).

The treatment of status epilepticus must be considered a medical emergency due to potential adverse sequelae (e.g., hypoxia, acidosis) if left untreated. Diazepam (0.5 mg/kg IV or IM, repeated every 10 min for up to three doses) may be used to control seizures from a wide variety of etiologies. Therefore, diazepam is a logical first choice for the management of an animal in convulsions when causation is unclear. When diazepam fails, generally phenobarbital (6 mg/kg IV to effect) is

**Table 1.** *Emergency Treatment to be Considered in the Severely Poisoned Animal*

| Body System Affected | Indications or Goals of Treatment | Methods |
|---|---|---|
| Respiratory | Maintain:<br>1. Patent airway<br>2. Adequate ventilation<br>3. Prevention of aspiration of vomitus | Cuffed, inflated endotracheal tube if the animal is comatose or anesthetized; mechanical or manual forced ventilation may be necessary for poisoned animals with paralysis or severe central nervous system (CNS) depression |
| Cardiovascular | 1. Hypotension | 1. Balanced electrolyte solutions (e.g., lactated Ringer's solution) or normal saline; Catecholamines |
| | 2. Acidosis (e.g., ethylene glycol, metaldehyde, and aspirin) | 2. Acidosis is the most commonly encountered acid-base disturbance. Sodium bicarbonate (1–3 mEq/kg administered in fluids over 1–3 hr) |
| | 3. Cardiac arrhythmias | 3. Correction of underlying disorder may "cure" an arrhythmia without the use of antiarrhythmic drugs; when used antiarrhythmic therapy should be specific for the type of arrhythmia present and the species involved |
| | 4. Bradycardia (e.g., organophosphate or carbamate insecticides) | 4. Atropine (0.01–0.02 mg/kg IV, IM) |
| Nervous System | 1. Seizures (e.g., strychnine, lead) | 1. Diazepam (0.5 mg/kg IV or IM doses may be repeated every 10 min for 3 doses); Phenobarbital (6 mg/kg IV to effect) or pentobarbital (slowly to effect) may be required |
| | 2. CNS excitation (e.g., metaldehyde, lindane, methylxanthines) | 2. Avoid phenothiazine tranquilizers, may be epileptogenic; diazepam (2.5–10 mg IV or PO total dose to effect) could be considered |
| | 3a. CNS depression (e.g., d-limonene, ethylene glycol, marijuana, ivermectin) | 3a. Analeptics generally not recommended, as rebound depression may occur with these agents |
| | 3b. Exogenous opiates (e.g., morphine, codeine) | 3b. Naloxone is administered in dogs at 0.04 mg/kg IV, IM, or SC is repeated as needed; naloxone's duration of action is short (45–90 min) |
| Control body temperature | 1. Hypothermia may occur during anesthesia, heavy sedation, or coma | 1. Blankets and circulating warm water pads may be helpful in maintaining body temperature |
| | 2. Hyperthermia often occurs with persistent seizures | 2. Hyperthermia is controlled with ice or cold baths |

tried next. If seizures still persist, pentobarbital (slowly to effect) is administered to induce light anesthesia. Human beings with CNS stimulation due to ingestion of amphetamines or certain hallucinogens (e.g., lysergic acid diethylamide [LSD] and phencyclidine [PCP]) have been treated with phenothiazine tranquilizers. This therapy, however, has not proven reliable enough to be widely recommended. As a rule, the phenothiazine tranquilizers are best avoided, as they may aggravate CNS depression and in some cases may actually be epileptogenic. If tranquilization is required (e.g., self-trauma), diazepam (2.5 to 10 mg IV or PO total dose to effect) should be considered.

Poisoned animals often present with varying degrees of CNS depression. The use of analeptics (e.g., doxapram) for the treatment of toxicant-induced CNS depression is at best debatable, since it is difficult to stabilize an animal receiving these drugs. In addition, convulsions and rebound depression may follow abrupt discontinuation of these agents. By contrast, naloxone is widely recommended for the treatment of excessive opiate (e.g., morphine, codeine) consumption. Be aware, however, that naloxone's duration of action is fairly short (45 to 90 min), and that when used for the treatment of opiate-induced coma, relatively higher doses may be required. Naloxone is administered to dogs at 0.04 mg/kg IV, IM, or SC, and may be repeated as necessary. Experimental and clinical data in rabbits

and humans indicate that naloxone is also efficacious when administered by the endotracheal route.

Toxicant exposure may also result in abnormal body temperature regulation. Hypothermia may occur in severely depressed or comatose poisoned animals, or it may also occur as a secondary effect owing to prolonged anesthesia. In these cases, blankets and circulating warm water pads may be helpful in maintaining body temperature. Alternatively, hyperthermia is often a problem with toxicosis due to uncouplers of oxidative phosphorylation (e.g., disophenol, pentachlorophenol, and dinitrophenol). When handling patients with potentially toxic exposures to these agents, it is important to keep the animal as calm and cool as possible even prior to the onset of any signs. Hyperthermia may also occur in poisoned animals with persistent seizures. In general, toxicant-induced hyperthermia is controlled with ice or cold water baths, not with antipyretic drugs. Concomitant dehydration may also occur and should be reversed with appropriate replacement fluid therapy.

## Corrosive Exposures (Dilution)

Ingestion of corrosive agents should be managed by rapidly diluting the corrosive with water or milk, along with administration of demulcents and gastrointestinal

**Table 2.** *Treatment (Decontamination) Considerations for the Management of the Poisoned Animal.*[*]

| Decontamination Method | Indications | Contraindications |
|---|---|---|
| Bathing skin[†] | All dermal exposures | None |
| Emetics[‡] | Recent (<2 hr) oral exposures | Rodents and rabbits; corrosive agents; hypoxia, dyspnea, seizures, coma, abnormal pharyngeal reflexes, or other marked neurologic impairments that could lead to aspiration pneumonia; CNS stimulants may precipitate seizures associated with vomiting; petroleum distillates. |
| | Generally more efficient than simple gastric lavage | |
| Activated charcoal[§] | Most recent (<6 hr) ingestions | Caustic agents |
| | | May produce constipation |
| Gastric lavage | Massive ingestions (>LD$_{50}$). Emesis was unproductive or cannot be used (e.g., seizures). Delayed GI emptying is anticipated | Caustic agents |
| | | Seizures (unless anesthetized) |
| Diuresis | Toxicants that are weak acids or weak bases | Renal insufficiency |
| | Alkalinization: 2,4-D, salicylate, phenobarbital | Pulmonary edema (fluid diuresis) |
| | Acidification: strychnine | Heart disease (fluid diuresis) |
| Ion trapping[‖] | Alkalinization: 2,4-D, salicylate phenobarbital | Rhabdomyolysis, myoglobinuria, and hepatic or renal insufficiency |
| | Acidification: strychnine | |

[*]From Dorman DC: Diagnosis and therapy of neurotoxicological syndromes in dogs and cats: general concepts. Part 1. Prog Vet Neurol 4:95–103, 1993, with permission.
[†]Mild handwashing detergent shampoo.
[‡]Includes syrup of ipecac (dog, 1–2 ml/kg; cat, 3.3 ml/kg or 3% hydrogen peroxide (1–5 ml/kg). Apomorphine is generally limited to the dog (0.03 mg/kg, IV; 0.04 mg/kg, IM). Xylazine (cat, 1.1 mg/kg, IM or SC) is somewhat effective as an emetic in cats. These emetics usually initiate vomiting within 5 to 15 min. Apomorphine use may be associated with CNS depression. Xylazine may aggravate respiratory depression and result in vagal-mediated slowing of the heart. Yohimbine (cat/dog, 0.1 mg/kg, IV), has been used effectively to reverse xylazine-induced depression, bradycardia, and hypotension. Salt (sodium chloride) is *not* recommended.
[§]Activated charcoal powder (1–4 gm/kg) combined with a saline (magnesium or sodium sulfate at 250 mg/kg) or osmotic cathartic as a suspension in water (10 × volume) can be administered orally or by gastric tube. Repeated administration of activated charcoal is commonly recommended for many toxicants. Magnesium-based cathartics may be associated with CNS depression.
[‖]Ammonium chloride (100 mg/kg in the dog or 20 mg/kg in the cat, b.i.d.) is used orally to acidify the urine. Ammonia intoxication can also develop and is most often manifested by depression and coma. Forced alkaline diuresis is generally achieved with sodium bicarbonate at 1–2 mEq/kg administered intravenously every 3–4 hr.

protectorants (e.g., sucralfate). The oral administration of water or milk is also frequently recommended in the initial management of other types of poisoning. Several studies, however, demonstrate that administration of large volumes of water actually increases gastrointestinal absorption of toxicants, resulting in a decreased oral $LD_{50}$. Therefore, the routine administration of water or milk to facilitate dilution of a toxicant is controversial.

### Ocular Exposures

Irrigation of chemically injured eyes with water or physiologic saline solutions should never be delayed. A minimum of 20 to 30 min of water irrigation is recommended. The use of neutralizing agents (e.g., boric acid) is generally not recommended. The animal should be examined as soon as possible thereafter. Following adequate irrigation, chemical burns to the eye should be treated with lubricant ointments and lid closure techniques (e.g., third eyelid or conjunctival flap) to protect the damaged ocular surface. Atropine may be considered as a cycloplegic agent. Frequent follow-up examinations or referral to an ophthalmologist is required, since epithelial damage may be delayed (especially with alkali burns), and it is difficult to predict the extent of the ocular damage.

### Diagnostic Efforts

One must maintain a high level of suspicion to toxicoses. The diagnosis of toxicologic diseases on the basis of signs alone is very often difficult, moreover, the animal with signs of illness or poisoning may manifest only one phase of the toxic syndrome. Confirmation of a toxicologic diagnosis often rests upon: (1) a known exposure history, (2) development of appropriate clinical signs and lesions, (3) a time of onset compatible with the toxicant in question, and (4) duration of effects that are consistent with the agent's toxicity. Ideally, the diagnosis will also be supported by the detection of a level of toxicant in the animal sufficient to cause the observed clinical signs.

## THE FIRST FEW HOURS

### Decontamination

The goal of all decontamination procedures is directed toward reducing additional exposure to the toxicant. The five most common routes of exposure to toxicants are: oral, dermal, inhalation, injection (including envenomation), and ocular. It must be recognized that more than one route of exposure (e.g., dermal absorption combined with oral absorption secondary to grooming) may have occurred, and thus several decontamination methods may be beneficial. For example, bathing an animal with a mild handwashing detergent or shampoo is recommended for all cases in which der-

mal exposure may have occurred. Similarly, irrigation (20 to 30 min) of chemically exposed eyes with water or physiologic saline should not be delayed.

### Emetics Versus Gastric Lavage

The use of emetics or gastric lavage in emergency treatment of poisoning is a matter requiring good clinical judgment. Emetics should *not* be given to rodents or rabbits or animals that are hypoxic, dyspneic, extremely weak, comatose, lacking normal pharyngeal reflexes, or suffering other marked neurologic impairments that could lead to aspiration pneumonia. Additionally, if the animal has ingested a CNS stimulant, further stimulation associated with vomiting may precipitate seizures. Emetics and gastric lavage are contraindicated whenever potentially corrosive agents (e.g., petroleum distillates) are ingested and in seizuring animals (unless anesthetized). Salt (sodium chloride) should never be used as an emetic due to its unreliability and the danger of inducing salt toxicosis. Emesis is generally favored over gastric lavage whenever the status of the patient allows for emesis to be produced. In addition, vomiting is generally more effective at removing stomach contents, is easier to induce, and is more effective at removing sizable amounts of particulate matter or tenacious mucus. Gastric lavage is occasionally recommended for cases in which massive ingestions ($>LD_{50}$) occur, emesis is unproductive, or delayed gastrointestinal emptying is anticipated.

In general, emetics are most effective when administered as quickly as possible after toxicant ingestion, and when food is present in the stomach. The response to emetic drugs varies, but gastric emptying is generally effective in removal of 40 to 60% of the gastric chyme when vomiting successfully occurs. Various toxicants are absorbed at different rates and in different parts of the gastrointestinal tract. Small unchanged molecules (e.g., ethylene glycol) or the uncharged fraction of acidic drugs (e.g., aspirin) are typically absorbed relatively rapidly through the gastric mucosa. Basic drugs (e.g., amphetamine) are predominantly charged while in the stomach, and are therefore poorly absorbed in this location. At times, abdominal radiographs may reveal the location of sufficiently radiodense or radiolucent ingesta, which may be of use when deciding whether to employ an emetic. In all cases, to be maximally effective when dealing with compounds absorbed directly from the stomach, emesis must be induced as rapidly as possible following exposure. Some drugs and toxicants actually delay normal gastric emptying. Therefore, no strict rule of thumb applies to how long after ingestion an emetic may be of benefit.

Commonly recommended emetics include syrup of ipecac (dogs, 1 to 2 ml/kg; cats, 3.3 ml/kg) and 3% hydrogen peroxide (1 to 5 ml/kg). These emetics usually induce vomiting within 5 to 15 min. If, however, an animal has not vomited by 15 min, a single repeat administration is recommended. Owners should be warned that prolonged vomiting and depression may occur. Emetic administration by owners is usually indicated for minimal exposures, or cases in which substantial delays in transportation to a veterinarian may occur. Apomorphine and xylazine can be effective emetics for veterinary clinic use. Apomorphine can be given subconjunctivally or by intravenous or intramuscular injection. Apomorphine tablets should be dissolved in sterile water prior to subconjunctival use to limit ocular irritation. As apomorphine solutions are not stable in air or light, they must be freshly prepared before each use. The use of apomorphine may be associated with CNS depression. Apomorphine use is generally limited to the dog (0.03 mg/kg, IV; 0.04 mg/kg, IM). Xylazine (1.1 mg/kg, IM or SC) is somewhat effective as an emetic in cats. Xylazine may aggravate respiratory depression and result in vagal-mediated slowing of the heart rate. The $\alpha_2$-antagonist, yohimbine (cat/dogs, 0.1 mg/kg, IV), has been used effectively to reverse xylazine-induced depression, bradycardia, or hypotension.

To adequately perform gastric lavage when indicated, large-bore gastric lavage tubes and copious amounts of lavage fluid are required. Other factors that influence the efficacy of lavage are: lavage fluid temperature (tepid water preferred, colder water increases gastric emptying time), agent ingested, and frequency of lavage. Minimal pressure should be used, since the stomach wall may be weakened. The procedure is performed on unconscious or lightly anesthetized animals intubated with a cuffed endotracheal tube. A 2- to 4-ft-long clear plastic tube with as large a diameter as possible and having the end fenestrated with one or two oblong holes is used. The tube is inserted to a length equivalent to the distance from the tip of the nose to the xiphoid cartilage. After the stomach tube is in place, the mouth should be kept lower than the chest. A watery activated charcoal suspension is recommended for the lavage fluid after the initial washings have been collected for analysis. Gently creating turbulence by pumping the fluid in under slight pressure, as from a bilge pump, mixes the contents near the end of the tube, allowing gradual removal by gravity flow. Several cycles (perhaps 15 to 20) of 5 to 10 ml/kg each may be required to thoroughly rinse out the stomach. The last few washings should be clean or contain only activated charcoal. The end of the tube should be closed as the tube is removed in order to prevent aspiration. A thick activated charcoal suspension is instilled after either gastric lavage or cessation of vomiting. Small animals generally require the use of a short-acting barbiturate or gas anesthetic before initiating this procedure.

### Activated Charcoal and Cathartics

Medical-grade activated charcoal contains large pore sizes and surface areas that allow for the nonspecific binding of many toxicants. Inactivation of a compound by charcoal is not equivalent to chemical destruction.

The number of drug or toxin molecules that can be adsorbed varies, but sometimes is approximately proportional to molecular size of the xenobiotic and surface area of the activated charcoal. Nonpolar large molecules are most rapidly adsorbed. In addition, ionized solutes are less firmly adsorbed than neutral solutes. Nevertheless, even in the case of a small, uncharged, rapidly adsorbed molecule like ethlylene glycol, the addition of activated charcoal to the treatment regimen is reportedly beneficial even when given as late as 6 hr after oral exposure. Fortunately, animal studies evaluating oral and topical exposure to activated charcoal have shown a lack of toxicity of this adsorbent.

Activated charcoal- administration is indicated for most toxicant ingestions. Activated charcoal powder (1 to 4 gm/kg) combined with a saline (magnesium or sodium sulfate at 250 mg/kg) or osmotic cathartic (e.g., 70% sorbitol) as a suspension in water (10 × volume) can be administered orally or by gastric tube. Repeated administration of activated charcoal is commonly recommended for many toxicants, including those that undergo enterohepatic or enteric recirculation. A variety of activated charcoals are available for veterinary use. One commonly used product (Toxiban) contains 70% activated charcoal, 8% kaolin, and 22% wetting agents. Charcoal tablets or universal antidotes are not as effective. Charcoal tablets are approximately 25% less adsorptive than powders. Coadministration of activated charcoal with vegetable or mineral oil, milk, or other flavorings is generally not recommended. Owners should be forewarned that dark black stools and diarrhea are commonly associated with the administration of activated charcoal.

In evaluating whether a saline cathartic should be administered, several factors should be considered: (1) saline cathartics should not be administered if the ingested agent will have similar cathartic effects (e.g., laxative ingestions; (2) some formulations (e.g., enteric coated, microencapsulated) may have decreased bioavailability if a cathartic is administered; (3) activated charcoal may cause constipation and cathartics may minimize this effect; and (4) magnesium sulfate, if administered repeatedly, could be harmful. Osmotic cathartics are administered per os preferably by stomach tube as a 20% (or more dilute) solution in water.

### THE FIRST DAY

### Facilitating Removal of Absorbed Toxicants

The next concern is the systemic poison that has already been absorbed. Measures to promote the removal of absorbed toxicants include methods to (1) enhance metabolism to less toxic forms, (2) increase excretion rates of the toxicant, or (3) remove the poison from the affected animal directly (e.g., hemoperfusion). Enzyme-inducing drugs such as phenobarbital take at least a couple of days to significantly increase monooxygenase activity. Therefore, they have generally not been recommended for use in reducing residues of persistent xenobiotics in the tissues of small animals. Specific antidotal therapies, such as alcohol dehydrogenase inhibitors with ethylene glycol toxicosis, are occasionally employed to modify the metabolism of a toxicant. Owing to the limitations on our ability to enhance toxicant metabolism, attention must be focused on ways of promoting excretion. The urinary tract and biliary tract represent the two principal routes by which exogenous chemicals are most commonly removed. As discussed above, enterohepatic recirculation may be disrupted with periodic administration of activated charcoal.

## Diuresis

Promotion of renal excretion of toxicants is frequently very beneficial to the patient and is heavily relied upon in the management of many toxicoses. However, diuresis is of benefit only for compounds that are present in significant concentrations in the plasma. In general, organic acids are present in plasma in greater concentrations than organic bases, due to the fact that plasma is slightly more alkaline than is the intracellular environment. This pH gradient results in the partitioning of charged organic acids and bases. Clinical indications for measures to promote renal elimination of absorbed toxicants include: (1) the toxicant is filtered or secreted by the kidney, (2) the presence of serious clinical toxicosis with clinical signs (e.g., hypotension, coma, arrhythmias), (3) a potentially lethal dose has been ingested, (4) normal route(s) of excretion are impaired (e.g., organ injury, concentration-dependent elimination rates), and (5) there is progressive deterioration of an animal's clinical condition in the face of intensive therapy. The effect of excessive water administration (i.e., water diuresis) on the excretion of most substances is minimal. Furthermore, the use of forced diuresis may be associated with the following complications: (1) pulmonary edema, (2) cerebral edema, (3) metabolic acidosis or alkalosis, and (4) electrolyte imbalances (e.g., hyponatremia, hypokalemia). For these reasons, vigorous attempts at forced diuresis should be limited to situations in which benefit can be expected. For toxicoses in which acute renal failure does not respond to osmotic diuresis, the use of furosemide or dopamine or both may be warranted.

## Ion Trapping

The basic premise of ion trapping is that ionized compounds do not readily traverse cell membranes and are therefore not resorbed by the renal tubules. Many chemicals, particularly drugs, are weak acids or weak bases. The ratio of nonionized to ionized drug is calculated from the Henderson-Hasselbalch equation and is pH dependent. For example, at a pH equal to the $pK_a$, an agent will be 50% ionized and 50% nonionized. If the urinary pH favors the ionized form, an agent becomes "trapped" in the tubular fluid and is more likely to be excreted. Acidic compounds such as aspirin remain ionized in alkaline urine. Thus, alkaline drugs such as amphetamines are ionized in acidic urine. Accordingly, alkaline urine generally favors increased excretion of acidic drugs and vice versa. Strong bases ($pK_a > 8.0$) and strong acids tend to be already charged in the glomerular filtrate and are therefore readily excreted by the kidney without further modification of the urine pH. For an agent to respond to pH manipulation of the urine, the following criteria must be met: (1) the toxicant or its toxic metabolite(s) must be significantly eliminated by the kidneys in an unconjugated form, (2) the agent or its toxic metabolite(s) must have a $pK_a$ (acidic or basic) that is near the range of common urinary pHs, and (3) the agent must be neither extensively protein bound nor highly lipophilic.

Administration of ammonium chloride to acidify the urine requires monitoring of metabolic status and is contraindicated if hepatic or renal insufficiency is present. In addition, acidification of the urine is also contraindicated if severe rhabdomyolysis or myoglobinuria is present, since the nephrotoxicity of myoglobin is considered to be enhanced in acid urine. Ammonia intoxication can also develop and is most often manifested by depression and coma. Ammonium chloride (100 mg/kg in the dog or 20 mg/kg in the cat, b.i.d.) is used orally to acidify the urine.

Alkalinization of the urine has been used successfully to treat ethylene glycol, salicylate, phenobarbital, and 2,4-dichlorophenoxyacetic acid (2,4-D) poisoning. Forced alkaline diuresis is generally achieved with sodium bicarbonate at 1 to 2 mEq/kg administered intravenously every 3 to 4 hr. Sodium bicarbonate should be infused intravenously at a very slow rate or, better, may be added to fluids for infusion. Acid-base status must be monitored.

## Gastrotomy

On rare occasion, a gastrotomy or gastric endoscopy may be required in order to remove foreign bodies from the stomachs of small animals. Examples of cases in which gastrotomy should be considered include metal ingestions (e.g., lead weights, pennies, zinc bolts) or, rarely, large quantities of ingested drugs that form coalesced masses (e.g., meprobamate). Although this method is effective, its use should usually be reserved for cases where more conservative methods have failed or are likely to fail. An alternative to gastrotomy would be endoscopic retrieval. Appropriate probes may be used to disrupt masses or remove foreign bodies from the stomach (see *CVT XI*, p 578).

The treatment methods discussed in this article can be used in a number of potential poisonings. Decontamination of the poisoned animal is often the only procedure available for the treatment of many suspected poisonings (e.g., unknown toxicants). Antidotal therapy can be used when the toxicant has been identified and the antidote is available. Specific antidote doses, routes of administration, and indications for use require a complete understanding of the toxicant in question, and are best addressed by other available references. The ultimate outcome in many poisonings depends upon prevention of further toxicant exposure and rational supportive care.

### References and Suggested Reading

Bailey EM: Emergency and general treatment of poisonings. In Kirk RW (ed): Current Veterinary Therapy XI. Philadelphia, WB Saunders Co, 1990, pp 135–144.

*This article provides an overview of the treatment of toxicosis and provides extensive tables of antidotal therapies.*
Beasley VR and Dorman DC: Diagnosis and management of toxicoses. Vet Clin North Am [Small Anim Pract] 20:307, 1990.
*Well-referenced article that reviews treatment considerations of the poisoned animal.*
Cupit GC and Temple AR: Gastrointestinal decontamination in the management of the poisoned patient. Emerg Med Clin North Am 2:15, 1984.
*Review article of decontamination methods available to physicians for reducing human exposures to toxicants.*
Wilcke JR and Turner JC: The use of adsorbents to treat gastrointestinal problems in small animals. Semin Vet Med Surg [Small Anim] 2:266, 1987.
*Review article focusing on the use of activated charcoal and other adsorbents as therapies for the poisoned animal.*

# TOXIC ORNAMENTAL AND GARDEN PLANTS

TAM GARLAND
*and* E. MURL BAILEY
*College Station, Texas*

Often clinicians are confronted with a pet that has a suspected plant intoxication. The purpose of this article is to characterize the effects and treatments of some selected plant intoxications and not to overwhelm the reader with scientific names or toxic principles. Plants, in some form, are found almost everywhere. With the advent of greenhouses and indoor cultivation, plants that previously were encountered only in the tropics or in Europe are now in or around our homes and exposed to our pets. Hybridization has altered many plants in such a way that they are able to withstand climates that heretofore would have killed the plant. Plants are around us in the foodstuffs that we consume, such as rhubarb and onions. Confined birds are still at risk of exposure through the various seeds and vegetables they are fed.

It is obvious that plants are all around us. But what makes a plant toxic? A poisonous plant is one that contains, in its entirety or in any of its parts, substances that even in relatively small quantities can cause varying degrees of disease or death. Various parts of a plant may be toxic: leaves, stems, fruits, seeds, roots, or even the whole plant. There is no uniform or universal test to recognize the degree of toxicity of a plant. Often the plant is attractive and frequently appears to be palatable to the animal. (This is certainly true involving poisonings in human beings.)

Several plant-related factors may play a role in the intoxications of pets. The age of the plant is an important factor. Some plants are more toxic when immature and others when mature. Plants may be more palatable when they have been stressed by such elements as drought or frost. The dry state may be more palatable and possibly more toxic. Likewise, soil, climatic, or other growing conditions affect a plant's toxicity and palatability.

There are also various animal-related factors to consider, such as species and age. Puppies and kittens are much like young children in the sense that many items are taken orally to be tasted or mouthed. Adult animals are less frequently victims of plant intoxications. However, boredom or other behavioral abnormalities are major reasons that adult animals will ingest plants. Caged or penned animals are more apt to experiment with plants within reach than are free-roaming pets or at least yard-contained animals. Changes in a pet's environment can lead to plant intoxications. Feeding of kitchen scraps can be a source of plant toxicants. When both meat and vegetable matter is included in the feeding regimen, gluttonous animals are likely to consume all of it. This provides a source for ingestion of sprouted potato peels, peach, cherry or apricot pits, rhubarb leaf blades, and onions. Animals that are garbage feeders are at risk for plant intoxications. In an analogous fashion, most pet birds prefer the seeds of plants, and some are attracted to the brightly colored blossoms of plants. Psitticine birds are at higher risk with plants that are seed producers since, by nature, these birds are seed consumers. Similarly, birds may become intoxicated by pecking certain plants. Cats that shred a plant with their claws and then clean their claws may become poisoned by the plant if it is highly toxic.

Establishing a diagnosis of plant poisoning is difficult. A thorough and exhaustive history is occasionally enlightening. Establishing this diagnosis is a difficult challenge, since plant intoxications can mimic any disease of bacterial, viral, or parasitic origin, and can affect any organ system or the body as a whole. The signs may be relatively specific or as nonspecific as vomiting or anorexia. The onset of clinical signs will depend upon the kind and part of the plant eaten, the amount consumed, the state of plant growth, the amount and type of other food consumed at the same time, and the individual tolerance of that species to the specific poison. Some toxins are cumulative and require extended periods of ingestion before producing clinical signs. Similarly, some innocuous plants may seem toxic after treatment with an insecticide or herbicide; of course, the insecticide is the problem here. Clinical signs and plant evidence may provide support for a plant intoxication theory.

Evidence of ingestion is important. Some animals will shred a plant without ingesting the plant. Birds and cats are particularly apt to do this. Certain plants, however, do not need to be ingested to cause an effect. These plants produce their effect through local irritation or contact dermatitis or even eliciting allergies in the pet. Some primary conditions, such as nocardiosis, may be secondary to penetration by a foreign body, usually a plant structure of some kind. Therefore, the type of clinical signs and the type of involvement with the plant are important correlating factors.

Perhaps the most confusing issue concerning plants is the use of common names. Common names may refer to a variety of plants depending upon one's regional location. Some scientific names may have the same common name. Table 1 is arranged alphabetically by common names. The use of scientific names can eliminate confusion when consulting with colleagues, but it is rare to find a client versed in scientific names. Thus, it is helpful to be versed in the common names of local plants as well as recognizing some necessary scientific names. Table 2 is a clinical compilation arranged alphabetically by the body system affected showing the plant's common name and principles of therapy.

Some plant intoxications are very specific in their mode of action and therefore necessitate a specific treatment. An example of such a plant would be yellow jessamine (*Gelsemium sempervirens*). This plant seems to contain a chemical substance similar in action to that of strychnine and treatment is the same as for strychnine poisoning. Other plants tend to cause a more generalized syndrome and, consequently, have a more supportive nature of treatment. In most plant intoxications, it is wise to limit continued absorption of the plant toxin. Generally, an emetic followed by activated charcoal and a cathartic will accomplish this task, with the exception of birds (see "Emergency Treatment of Toxicoses," this volume, p 211). Emetics are not recommended in birds. Most birds display intoxication related to digestive disturbances, such as vomiting, anorexia, diarrhea, pasting of the vent space, and a progressively enlarging abdomen. Since plants will pass through the stomach in 2 to 4 hr beyond this time an emetic is not very beneficial to the patient. Once adsorption has been limited, it is advisable to treat the clinical signs.

**Table 1.** *Toxic Ornamental and Garden Plants, Arranged Alphabetically by Common Names*

| Common Name | Scientific Name | Toxic Parts | System Affected |
|---|---|---|---|
| Alpenrose | *Rhododendron ferrugineum* | Flowers, leaves | Gastroenteric |
| American ivy (see Virginia creeper) | *Parthenocissus quinquifolia* | | |
| American mistletoe | *Phoradendron flavescens* | Berries | Gastroenteric |
| Apricot | *Prunus armeniaca* | Pits | Cyanide producers° |
| Azalea | *Azalea* spp. | All parts | Gastroenteric |
| Bitter almond | *Prunus dulcis* var. *amara* | Bark, leaves, especially seeds | Cyanide producers |
| Black locust | *Robinia pseudoacacia* | Bark, green growth, seeds probably, thorns = mechanical hazard | Gastroenteric, cardiac, neurologic |
| Black nightshade | *Solanum nigrum* | All parts especially seeds | Gastroenteric |
| Bluebonnets | *Lupinus* spp. | Seeds | Neurologic |
| Bog bilberry | *Vaccinium uliginosum* | Berries (very susceptible to a fine mold, which may be responsible for any toxicities) | Neurologic, gastroenteric |
| Boxwood or box | *Buxus semervirens* | All parts, especially berries | Mainly cardiac, gastroenteritis, neurologic |
| Bulbous corydalis | *Corydalis cava* | Bulb, usually | Neurologic |
| Buttercup (meadow) | *Ranunculus acris* | All top growth | Gastroenteric, neurologic, renal |
| Buttercup (celery-leafed) | *Ranunculus sceleratus* | All top growth | Mainly gastroenteric, neurologic |
| Caladium (sometimes called elephant's ear) | *Caladium* spp. | Leaf, stem, stalk | Stomatitis-glossitis |
| Castor bean | *Ricinus communis* | All parts, especially seeds | Gastroenteric, neurologic |
| Cherry laurel | *Prunus laurocerasus* | Pits or seeds | Cyanide producer |

*Table continued on opposite page*

**Table 1.** *Continued*

| Common Name | Scientific Name | Toxic Parts | System Affected |
|---|---|---|---|
| Chinaberry | *Melia azedarach* | Fruit | Neurologic |
| Chinese evergreen | *Aglaonema* spp. | Leaves | Stomatitis-glossitis |
| Chinese primrose | *Primula obconica* | Sap | Mainly dermatitis, slightly gastroenteric |
| Chinese wisteria | *Wisteria sinensis* | Seeds | Hepatogenous |
| Christmas cherry | *Solanum pseudocapsicum* | Berries | Gastroenteric |
| Christmas rose | *Helleborus niger* | Leaves, stems | Cardiac, gastroenteric, neurologic |
| Climbing lily | *Gloriosa superba* | All parts | Gastroenteric |
| Common bean | *Phaseolus vulgaris* | Green, uncooked pods and tendrils | Gastroenteric, neurologic |
| Common privet | *Ligustrum vulgare* | All parts, especially berries | Gastroenteric, mild |
| Crocus | *Crocus sativus* *Colchicum autumnale* | Primarily bulbs | Gastroenteric, renal, cardiac |
| Croton (variegated) | *Codiaeum variegatum* | Sap and stems | Dermatitis, mild (sap), stomatitis (stems) |
| Croton | *Croton tiglium* | Especially the seeds | Gastroenteric, neurologic |
| Cycad | *Zamia* spp., *Zamia floridana, Cycas revoluta* | Seed especially, occasionally meal | Hepatic |
| Cyclamen | *Cyclamen purpurascens* | Tuberous rhizomes and sap | Gastroenteric, neurologic, dermatitis |
| Daffodil | *Narcissus pseudonarcissus* | Primarily bulbs, but all of plant | Gastroenteric |
| Deadly nightshade | *Solanum nigrum* or *Atropa belladonna* | All parts | Gastroenteric |
| Dieffenbachia or mother-in-law plant | *Dieffenbachia* spp. | Leaf, stem, stalk | Stomatitis-glossitis |
| Elder | *Sambucus nigra* | All parts, especially berries, roots and sap | Gastroenteric, mild cyanide producer |
| Elephant's ear | *Alocasia* spp., *Colocasia antiquorum, Philodendron* spp. | All parts | Stomatitis-glossitis |
| Euonymus | *Euonymus* spp. | Leaves, berries, stem, sap | Cardiac |
| False acacia (see black locust) | *Robinia pseudoacacia* | | |
| Firethorn | *Pyracantha coccinea* | Berries | Gastroenteric, mild; mild cyanide producer |
| Foxglove | *Digitalis purpurea* | All parts, seeds especially | Cardiac |
| Glory lily | *Gloriosa superba* | Whole plant | Gastroenteric |
| Golden chain | *Laburnum anagyroides* | All parts, especially seeds, sap, and flowers | Gastroenteric, neurologic |
| Golden pothos (potted ivy) | *Epiprenum (Scindapsus)* spp. | All parts, leaves less so than other parts | Stomatitis-glossitis |
| Heavenly blues or Morning Glory | *Ipomoea purpurea* | Seeds especially | Neurologic |
| Henbane | *Hyoscyamus niger* | Whole plant | Neurologic (resembles atropine overdose) |
| Holly | *Ilex aquifolium* | Seeds especially | Gastroenteric, neurologic |
| Hydrangea | *Hydrangea macrophylla, H. quercifolia, H. arborescens* | All parts | Gastroenteric (mild cyanide producer, no clinical signs associated with this), cardiac |
| Ivy (English) | *Hedera helix* | Seeds or fruits | Gastroenteric, neurologic |
| Japanese wisteria | *Wisteria floribunda* | Seeds | Gastroenteric |
| Jerusalem cherry (see Christmas cherry) | *Solanum pseudocapsicum* | | |
| Jessamines (day or night blooming) | *Cestrum diurnum* or *Cestrum nocturnum* | Berries (ripe and unripe) | Gastroenteric, Neurologic: (*C. diurnum* contains vitamin D) |
| Jimson weed, moon trumpet, thornapple | *Datura stramonium* | All parts, especially seeds | Neurologic (resembles atropine overdose) |
| Kafir lily | *Clivia miniata* | Bulbs mostly | Gastroenteric |
| Lantana | *Lantana camara* | Fruit | Gastroenteric, mildly cardiac |

*Table continued on following page*

**Table 1.** *Continued*

| Common Name | Scientific Name | Toxic Parts | System Affected |
|---|---|---|---|
| Larkspur | *Delphinium elatum* | Flowers and seeds | Gastroenteric, cardiac, neurologic, death |
| Lily of the valley | *Convallaria majalis* | Whole plant, especially bulbs | Cardiac, renal |
| Matrimony vine | *Lycium barbarum, L. halimifolium L. carolinianum* | Leaf, stem, stalk | Neurologic, gastroenteric |
| Monkshood | *Aconitum napellus* | All parts, especially seeds | Gastroenteric, neurologic, cardiac, death |
| Moon trumpet (see Jimson weed) | *Datura stramonium* | | |
| Morning glory (see heavenly blues | *Ipomoea purpurea* | | |
| Mother-in-law plant (see dieffenbachia) | *Dieffenbachia* spp. | | |
| Nandina | *Nandina domestica* | Foliage and berries | Cyanide producers |
| Oleander | *Nerium oleander* | All parts | Cardiac |
| Peach | *Prunus persica* | Seeds | Cyanide producers |
| Plum | *Prunus domestica* | Seeds | Cyanide producers |
| Poinsettia | *Euphorbia pulcherrima* | All parts, especially seeds | Gastroenteric |
| Poppy | *Papaver* spp. | Berries, stems, sap | Neurologic, secondary effects on respiratory |
| Potato | *Solanum tuberosum* | Edible tubers, but green growth and sprouts are toxic; most top parts | Gastroenteric, cardiac |
| Purple flag iris | *Iris versicolor* | Bulbs | Gastroenteric |
| Pyracantha (see firethorn) | *Pyracantha coccinea* | | |
| Rhododendron | *Rhododendron ferrugineum* | All parts, especially seeds | Gastroenteric |
| Rhubarb | *Rheum rhaponticum* | Leaves | Stomatitis-glossitis |
| Sowbread (see cyclamen) | *Cyclamen purpurascens* | | |
| Split-leaf philodendron | *Philodendron* spp., *Monstera* spp. | All parts | Stomatitis-glossitis |
| Spurge laurel | *Daphne laureola* | All parts, especially fruits | Cardiac, gastroenteric, neurologic |
| Star-of-bethlehem | *Ornithogalum umbellatum* | Bulbs | Gastroenteric, neurologic |
| Stinking iris | *Iris foetidissima* | Whole plant, all parts | Gastroenteric, severe |
| Sweet pea | *Lathyrus odoratus* | Foliage and seeds | Neurologic |
| Sweetheart vine | *Philodendron* spp. | Leaves, stems, stalk | Stomatitis-glossitis |
| Thornapple (see jimson weed) | *Datura stramonium* | | |
| Tobacco | *Nicotiana tabacum* | Leaves | Neurologic |
| Tulip | *Tulipa* spp. | Bulbs | Gastroenteric, neurologic |
| Virginia creeper, American ivy | *Parthenocissus quinquefolia* | Leaves, stems | Stomatitis-glossitis |
| Wild Rosemary | *Ledum palustre* | Essential oil contained in leaves | Gastroenteric, mild |
| Wolf's bane | *Aconitum vulparis* | All parts, especially seeds | Gastroenteric, neurologic, cardiac, death |
| Wood laurel | *Daphne laureola* | All parts, especially seeds | Cardiac, gastroenteric, neurologic |
| Woolly foxglove | *Digitalis lanata* | Leaves (extremely bitter) | Cardiac |
| Yellow iris | *Iris pseudacorus* | Bulbs | Gastroenteric, neurologic |
| Yellow jessamine | *Gelsemium sempervirens* | Berries and roots | Neurologic |
| Yew | *Taxus* spp. | Foliage, bark, seeds | Cardiac, neurologic |
| Youpon holly | *Ilex vomitoria* | Berries | Gastroenteric |

***Table 2.*** *Body Systems Affected by Toxic Ornamental and Garden Plants*

| System Affected/Plant Name | Clinical Signs | Treatment |
| --- | --- | --- |
| **Cardiac**<br>Black locust, box or boxwood, Christmas rose, crocus, lantana, larkspur, monkshood, potato, spurge laurel, wolf's bane, wood laurel, yew, euonymus, foxglove, hydrangea, lily of the valley, oleander, woolly foxglove, | Cardiac arrhythmias including premature ventricular contractions, ventricular tachycardia, shock, thready pulse; cardiac problems may present with vomition, diarrhea, nausea, even anorexia and cramps; neurological signs are likely to accompany cardiac signs. | Treat clinical signs with sufficiently sustained antiarrhythmia therapy<br>Treat as for digitalis overdose |
| **Cyanide Producers**<br>Apricot, bitter almond, cherry laurel, elder, firethorn, pyracantha, nandina, peach, plum | Resembles signs seen with cyanide intoxication and may include some nausea and vomiting, weakness | Intravenous treatment with sodium nitrite and sodium thiosulfate; supportive and symptomatic care. |
| **Dermatitis**<br>Chinese primrose, croton (*Codiaeum variegatum*), cyclamen | Erythematous skin, possibly pruritis and hair loss; secondary bacterial infection is possible | Wash the animal and apply appropriate ointment; systemic antibiotics may be necessary |
| **Gastroenteric**<br>Alpenrose, American mistletoe, azalea, black locust, black nightshade, bog bilberry, box or boxwood, buttercup (meadow and celery-leafed), castor bean, Chinese primrose, Christmas cherry, Christmas rose, climbing lily, common privet, common bean, crocus, croton (*Croton tiglium*), cyclamen, daffodil, deadly nightshade, elder, firethorn, pyracantha, glory lily, golden chain, hydrangea, holly, ivy, Japanese wisteria, jessamines (day and night blooming), kaffir lily, lantana, larkspur, matrimony vine, monkshood, poinsettia, potato, purple flag iris, rhododendron, spurge laurel, star-of-bethlehem, stinking iris, tulip, wild rosemary, wolf's bane, wood laurel, yellow iris, youpon holly | Nausea, vomition, diarrhea, bloody diarrhea, fever, mydriasis; abdominal pain, glazed eyes; may be accompanied by tremors and/or hypotension; anorexia may be present | Emetic (if no contraindication), lavage with activated charcoal followed by a saline cathartic; intravenous fluids; correct electrolyte imbalances; ventilator therapy may be necessary |
| **Hepatic**<br>Chinese wisteria, cycad | Ascites, icterus, and gastrointestinal signs such as vomiting or anorexia; hemorrhagic gastroenteritis, subcutaneous bruising, thrombocytopenia; possibly a cardiotoxin and a carcinogen | Induce emesis (if no contraindication), lavage with activated charcoal followed by saline cathartic; symptomatic and supportive therapy |
| **Neurological**<br>Black locust, bluebonnets, bog bilberry, box or boxwood, bulbous corydalis, buttercup (meadow and celery-leafed), castor bean, Chinaberry, Christmas rose, common bean, croton, cyclamen, golden chain, heavenly blues, henbane, holly, ivy (english), jessamines (day and night blooming), jimson weed, larkspur, matrimony vine, monkshood, poppy, spurge laurel, star-of-Bethlehem, sweet pea, tobacco, tulip, wolf's bane, wood laurel, yellow iris, yellow jessamine, yew | Excitement or depression, trembling, convulsions that may include cessation of respiration, coma (stiffness in hindquarters, evidence of painful locomotion, may have shifting leg lameness; these clinical signs especially applicable to sweet pea) | Induce emesis (if no contraindication), lavage with activated charcoal followed by saline cathartic; appropriate anticonvulsive therapy; pentobarbital or diazepam (Valium) is recommended; symptomatic and supportive therapy |
| **Renal**<br>Buttercup (meadow), lily of the valley | Polyuria/polydipsia are the earliest signs; Lily of the valley especially affects cats | Induce emesis (if no contraindication), lavage with activated charcoal followed by saline cathartic; symptomatic and supportive care; treat appropriately for the stage of renal failure |
| **Stomatitis-Glossitis**<br>Caladium, Chinese evergreen, croton (variegated), dieffenbachia, elephant's ear, golden pothos, rhubarb, split-leaf philodendron, sweetheart vine, Virginia creeper | Salivation, pawing at the mouth or throat area. Severe cases may show some difficulty swallowing; in severe cases swelling in the pharyngeal region may occlude respiration. | In mild cases, fluid therapy; in more severe cases where respiration is impaired, respiratory and nutrition supportive measures are appropriate. |

An exception to this general recommendation of treating the signs is when the plant contains a specific toxicant, such as cyanide or strychnine. Of course, it is appropriate to treat these specific plant intoxications with specific antidotes.

Various plants, such as the cacti, produce mechanical injuries. Some species of cacti have barbs, much like a fish hook, on the end of the quill or needle. This type of injury is relatively straightforward in its treatment. Local or topical anesthetic may be helpful to remove the offending quill. Antibiotics are generally advisable. Recall that various grass awns, seed heads, and burrs are capable of migrating through ear canals, nasal passages, interdigital spaces, and even in the conjunctiva of the eye. Removal of these may be quite simple or may require surgery, especially if an awn is lodged in the nasal turbinates or deep in an ear canal. Systemic antibiotics effective against anaerobic bacteria may be necessary depending upon the location of the awn and the length of time it was present in the animal.

There is no need to try to remove all plants from an environment where there are pets. Some simple precautions are all that is necessary to let plants and animals live in harmony. Solutions may be as simple as fencing off the garden or moving a potted plant to a higher location until the animal is more mature. Other solutions may include not allowing birds to fly into a room where there is a seed producing plant that would put the pet at risk of intoxication. Finally, remember that intoxications resulting from plants are manageable and treatable for a successful outcome.

## References and Suggested Reading

Bailey, EM, Jr. and Garland, T: Toxicologic emergencies. In Murtaugh RJ and Kaplan PM (eds): Veterinary Emergency and Critical Care Medicine. St. Louis, Mosby Year Book, 1992, p 427.

Case AA: Poisoning and injury by plants. In Kirk RW (ed): Current Veterinary Therapy VII. Philadelphia, WB Saunders Co, 1983, p 145.

Clay BR: Poisoning and injury by plants. In Kirk, R. W. (ed): Current Veterinary Therapy VI. Philadelphia, WB Saunders Co, 1977, p 179.

Fowler ME: Plant poisoning in Small Companion Animals. St. Louis, Ralston Purina Company, 1981.

Frohne D and Pfander HJ: A Colour Atlas of Poisonous Plants. London, Wolfe Publishing Ltd, 1984.

Hall J: Illinois National Animal Poison Control, personal communication, April, 1993.

Kingsbury JM: Poisonous Plants of the United States and Canada. Englewood Cliffs, New Jersey, Prentice-Hall, Inc, 1964.

Oehme FW and Davis JW: Plants poisonous to free-living or caged mammals and birds. In Hoff GL and Davis JW (eds): Noninfectious Diseases of Wildlife. Ames, IA, The Iowa State University Press, 1982 p 8.

Ruhr LP: Ornamental toxic plants. In Kirk RW (ed): Current Veterinary Therapy IX. Philadelphia, WB Saunders Co, 1986, p 216.

Woodward L: Poisonous Plants, A Color Field Guide. New York, Hippocrene Books Inc, 1985.

# RISKS ASSOCIATED WITH HERBAL REMEDIES

ROBERT H. POPPENGA
*Kennett Square, Pennsylvania*

There is an increasing interest in and use of non-traditional therapies by both veterinarians and pet owners. These therapies include naturopathy, herbology, chiropractic, acupuncture, and homeopathy. Often these therapies are part of a holistic approach to preventing and treating disease.

Herbology and homeopathy utilize naturally occurring chemicals, primarily plant derived, in lieu of synthetic chemicals for disease prevention or treatment. Broadly defined, herbs are plants used for medicinal purposes or for their olfactory or flavoring properties. Herbology emphasizes the use of herbal leaves, roots, and flowers to promote healing. Homeopathy is a system of medicine in which the cure of disease is believed to be effected by administering minute doses of chemicals that produce the same signs and symptoms in a healthy person as are present in the disease for which they are administered. The chemicals used in homeopathy, as in herbology, are primarily derived from plants.

Many of these plant-derived chemicals are biologically active and potentially toxic, if exposure is of sufficient magnitude. There are numerous case reports of human poisonings following the ingestion of such naturally occurring chemicals.

The degree to which herbal and homeopathic remedies are used in veterinary medicine is unknown. However, there are many publications written for pet owners that advocate the use of such remedies (de Bairacli Levy, 1986; Pitcairn and Pitcairn, 1982). In addition, the American Association of Holistic Veterinary Medicine advocates the use of alternative therapies for preventing and treating animal diseases. A number of publications describing the use of herbs are available in bookstores (e.g., see Stuart, 1979). The use of herbal and homeopathic remedies in animals is not regulated by the Center for Veterinary Medicine and most of these have not been rigorously tested for safety and efficacy. Although the number of recorded instances of pet intoxication following the use of herbal remedies is small, based upon human poisoning reports, the risks to pets are real.

There are various ways in which poisoning of an animal might occur.

1.   Use of a remedy that contains a known toxin is one possibility. For example, chronic use of herbal remedies containing hepatotoxic pyrrolizidine alkaloids may result in liver failure.

2.   Misidentification of plants or inappropriate use of herbal remedies can result in pet intoxication.

3.   Contamination of commercially prepared herbal remedies with toxic plants has been documented in the human literature (DeSmet, 1991). Seeds of poison hemlock (*Conium maculatum*) have been found in anise seed.

4.   Some herbal remedies may contain inorganic contaminants such as arsenic or intentionally-introduced drug agents such as glucocorticosteroids or phenylbutazone.

5.   Pet intoxication following accidental ingestion of improperly stored remedies may occur. This is particularly true with dogs due to their indiscriminate eating habits.

Many herbal or homeopathic remedies contain numerous bioactive chemicals. When these remedies are used in conjunction with other more traditional drugs, the potential exists for adverse chemical interactions. In addition, several naturally occurring chemicals found in herbal remedies cause liver enzyme induction (DeSmet, 1991). This may result in altered metabolism of other drugs or chemicals, resulting either in enhanced or diminished efficacy or toxicity. The concentrations of biologically active plant constituents may vary depending on the time of year or from one year to the next. Thus, unless specific analyses are conducted on the remedy ingredients, the potency of the final product may vary. There is also the potential for species differences in response to administered, biologically active chemicals. For a given chemical, the route of exposure and age of animal may be important factors in the potential for intoxication. Unfortunately, for most animal species, information on the pharmacokinetics and toxicity of these chemicals is not available.

This article will discuss some of the commonly used herbal remedies and their potential adverse effects. A more in-depth discussion of these topics can be found in several of the references provided. In addition, a more complete compilation of herbal remedies and potential adverse effects following their use is given in Ellenhorn and Barceloux (1988), Lewin, Howland, and Goldfrank (1990), and Spoerke (1990).

## SPECIFIC HERBAL REMEDIES

### Aloe

There are several species of aloe including *Aloe barbadensis*, *A. vera* and *A. officinalis*. Sap from the aloe leaf contains various anthraquinone glycosides collectively called aloin. One of these, barbaloin, is broken down into a sugar and an aglycone called emodin; the latter stimulates large-bowel peristalsis. Aloe has been used topically to treat burns and is found in a wide range of commercial skin products. Due to its irritant action on the colon, emodin has been used as a cathartic.

External application of aloe is unlikely to be associated with adverse effects; minor skin irritation is possible. Vomiting, diarrhea, and abdominal pain may result following oral administration of aloe. Thus, ingestion by grooming animals following dermal application may cause gastrointestinal upsets.

### Camphor

Camphor is an aromatic, volatile, terpene ketone derived from the wood of *Cinnamomum camphora* or synthesized from turpentine oil. Camphor is a component of many over-the-counter products that vary in form and in camphor content. It is used as a topical rubefacient and antipruritic agent.

Camphor is rapidly absorbed from the skin and gastrointenstinal tract, and toxic effects can occur within 15 to 20 min of exposure. In humans, signs of camphor intoxication include vomiting, abdominal distress, excitement, tremors, and seizures, followed by central nervous system (CNS) depression characterized by apnea and coma. Chronic ingestion in children may result in hepatotoxicity and neurotoxicity (DeSmet, 1991). Based upon increased sensitivity of children to the toxic effects of camphor, young animals may be more sensitive than adults.

### Eucalyptus Oil

The genus *Eucalyptus* contains over 500 species of trees indigenous to Australia. Economically, *E. globulus* is the most important species. Notable constituents of *Eucalyptus* are an essential oil and tannins. Medicinal oils distilled from *E. globulus* primarily contain eucalyptol (up to 95%). Tannins occur in both the leaf and bark of the tree. One sample of *E. globulus* leaf powder sold in capsule form had a tannin content of 11%.

Eucalyptus oil is used as an antiseptic and an antispasmodic stimulant agent in bronchitis, asthma and minor respiratory complaints. The dried leaf is sold as a treatment for respiratory tract infections. Eucalyptus oil and eucalyptol have been granted generally recognized as safe (GRAS) status by the Food and Drug Administration (FDA) and both are approved for food use.

Reported $LD_{50}$ values for eucalyptus oil and eucalyptol in rodents are on the order of several grams per kilogram body weight (DeSmet, 1991). Thus, the oil would appear to be relatively safe. However, there are reports of deaths and other acute toxic reactions in humans who have taken the oil orally. In humans, transient coma followed ingestion of as little as 1 ml and fatalities have resulted following consumption of 3.5 ml. The onset of toxic effects is rapid and signs include abdominal pain, vomiting, respiratory distress, bronchospasm, tachypnea, respiratory depression, seizures, depression, and coma. Tannins found in the preparation prepared from leaves can cause mild constipation with repeated use.

Eucalyptus leaves, eucalyptus oil and eucalyptol induce microsomal enzyme activity. Thus, there is the potential for interactions with other drugs or chemicals.

## Garlic

Garlic (*Allium sativum*) is a member of the onion family. Garlic contains 0.1 to 0.3% of a strong-smelling volatile oil containing allyl disulfides such as allicin. Extracts from garlic bulbs or garlic oil have been reported to have bactericidal, insecticidal, antiviral, and fungicidal activities; to decrease serum lipid and cholesterol levels; to prolong bleeding and clotting times; to inhibit collagen-induced platelet aggregation; and to incease fibrinolytic activity (DeSmet, 1990).

Acute toxicity of allicin for dogs and cats is not known; its $LD_{50}$ for mice when administered subcutaneously, or intravenously is 120 mg/kg and 60 mg/kg, respectively. The $LD_{50}$ for garlic extracts given by various routes to rats and mice range from 0.5 ml/kg to greater than 30 ml/kg. In chronic toxicity studies with garlic oil or garlic extracts, anemia has been observed in dogs. Exposure to garlic can evoke allergic reactions such as contact dermatitis and asthmatic attacks. Topical application of garlic oil causes local irritation that can be quite severe.

## Ginger

The ginger plant (*Zingiber officinale*) contains a volatile oil and the fresh or dried rhizome is used as a stimulant, carminative and antiemetic. In general, the toxicity of ginger is low and its use in normally available amounts is not expected to produce toxicity.

## Ginseng

Ginseng is the common name for deciduous perennial plants of the genus *Panax*. The dried root of ginseng has been used in traditional oriental medicine for over 2000 years as a tonic for increasing general strength and removing fatigue.

The active components of ginseng are numerous, although its pharmacologic activity is believed to be due to triterpenoidal saponins called ginsenosides. Metabolic effects of ginseng include decreases in serum glucose and serum and liver cholesterol levels; increases in erythropoiesis, hemoglobin production and iron absorption from the gastrointestinal tract; CNS stimula-

tion; and increases in blood pressure, heart rate and gastrointestinal motility (DeSmet, 1991).

Toxicologic effects of ginseng have been produced in animals only at extremely high doses. Oral administration of an alcoholic extract of ginseng to beagle dogs at 15 mg/kg for a period of 3 months had no apparent adverse effect.

## Nux vomica

Nux vomica is the dried, ripe seeds of *Strychnos nux-vomica*, which contain 1.1 to 1.5% strychnine and about an equal amount of brucine. The tincture is a 10% solution in 70% alcohol (0.12% strychnine). Nux vomica fluid extract is 1.0 to 1.2% strychnine and the dried, powdered extract is 7 to 7.7% strychnine.

Nux vomica has been recommended for administration to cats to treat digestive disturbances resulting from overindulgence and as an initial treatment for feline leukemia. The approximate oral lethal doses of strychnine for dogs and cats are 0.75 and 2.0 mg/kg, respectively. Thus, a lethal dose of a 1.0% fluid extract for a 5-kg cat would be 1 ml.

## Oil of Wintergreen

Oil of wintergreen is derived from *Gaultheria procumbens* and contains a glycoside that when hydrolyzed releases methyl salicylate. The oil is readily absorbed by the skin and is used to treat muscle aches and pains.

While methyl salicylate is potentially toxic, there have been no reports of intoxication in humans from oil of wintergreen. Salicylates are toxic to dogs and cats. Salicylate intoxication of dogs is manifested by nausea, vomiting, and restlessness that progresses to seizures and coma. Hematemesis and gastric ulceration have been reported in dogs given 100 to 300 mg/kg/day orally for 4 weeks. Cats metabolize salicylates much more slowly than dogs and are more likely to be overdosed. Intoxicated cats may present with depression, anorexia, vomiting, gastric hemorrhage, toxic hepatitis, anemia, bone marrow hypoplasia, hyperpnea, and hyperpyrexia.

## Pennyroyal

Pennyroyal oil is a volatile oil derived from *Mentha pulegium* and *Hedeoma pulegioides*. Pennyroyal oil has a long history of use as a flea repellant. Additionally, pennyroyal oil has been used in humans to induce menstruation and as an abortifacient. Health food and pet stores sell products containing pennyroyal oil including flea shampoos and powders.

There are several case reports of pennyroyal toxicosis in the human and veterinary literature. The toxin in pennyroyal oil is a ketone called pulegone, which constitutes 85% of the oil. Pulegone is bioactivated to a hepatotoxic metabolite, menthofuran, by the liver. In the one veterinary case report, a dog was exposed to pennyroyal oil dermally at approximately 2000 mg/kg (Sudekum et al., 1992). Within 1 hr of application, the dog became listless, and within 2 hr began vomiting. Thirty hours after exposure, the dog exhibited diarrhea, hemoptysis and epitaxis. Soon thereafter, the dog developed seizures and died. Histopathologic examination of liver tissue showed extensive hepatocellular necrosis.

### Sassafras

*Sassafras albidum* is an aromatic, decidous tree native to North America. Sassafras oil is approximately 50% safrole, 10% pinene and phennadrene, and 6 to 8% d-camphor. The root wood and root bark have been used as a carminative, stimulant, diaphoretic and diuretic. Also, the root bark has antiseptic properties due to its phenolic content. Sassafras oil is used externally as a rubefacient and insecticide.

The oil should be considered toxic if taken internally. As little as 5 ml of the oil is toxic for an adult human. Based upon toxicity to laboratory animals, a single sassafras tea bag may exceed a human toxic dose. Clinical signs of intoxication include nausea, vomiting, dilated pupils, cardiovascular collapse and CNS depression. Cats may be particularly sensitive to the toxic effects of phenolics in the oil, since they are unable to efficiently metabolize phenolic compounds. Safrole is hepatoxic and hepatocarcinogenic and a potent inhibitor of some liver microsomal enzymes (Ellenhorn and Barceloux, 1988).

Other herbal preparations potentially toxic to pets are given in Table 1.

## DIAGNOSIS

Without a history of exposure to a herbal remedy, the diagnosis of intoxication is difficult. Clinical signs are often nonspecific and the animal may have concurrent signs due to an underlying disease condition. In some instances, a constituent of a herbal remedy may be detected in a biologic specimen. For example, pulegone was found in a liver sample from a dog intoxicated by pennyroyal oil (Sudekum et al., 1992). However, many veterinary diagnostic laboratories do not have such capability, and laboratory confirmation of exposure or intoxication is often impossible. In suspected herbal poisonings, a veterinary toxicologist should be consulted about available laboratory procedures and appropriate tissue samples for submission.

## TREATMENT

Treatment is directed toward undertaking decontamination procedures such as inducing emesis and ad-

***Table 1.*** *Other Herbal Preparations Potentially Toxic to Pets*

| Herb Name | Botanical Source | Pharmacologic Principle | Herbalist's Use | Clinical Effects |
|---|---|---|---|---|
| Cayenne pepper or capsicum | *Capsicum frutescens* | Several volatile oils including capsaicin | External irritant, gastric stimulant | Irritation to mucous membranes, vomiting and diarrhea, exacerbation of preexisting inflammatory bowel disease |
| Camomile | *Anthemis flores* or *A. nobilis* | Volatile oil and aromatic bitter (anthemic acid) | Antispasmodic, digestive aid, treatment of abscesses, poultice | Vomiting, ataxia |
| Cinnamon oil | *Cinnamomum camphora* | Volatile oil containing local mucous membrane irritants such as cinnamaldehyde | Bark of cinnamon is used as an astringent in the treatment of diarrhea and flatulence | Nausea and vomiting, nephro- and neurotoxic in humans |
| Lily of the valley | *Convallaria majalis* | Digitalis-like glycosides, irritant saponins | Cardiotonic and diuretic | Nausea, vomiting, diarrhea, cardiac arrhythmias |
| Mistletoe | *Phoradendron* spp. | Stimulant amines such as tyramine and β-phenylethylamine | Oxytocic, treatment of high blood pressure, sedative | Acute gastrointestinal upset; CNS signs including ataxia, coma or hyperesthesia, opisthotonus, and seizures, cardiovascular collapse |
| Senna | *Cassia angustifolia* | Anthraquinones | Cathartic to relieve constipation | Catharsis, nausea, vomiting, abdominal pain |
| Witch hazel | *Hamamelis virginiana* | Tannins | Mild astringent | Nausea, vomiting, constipation; tannins are hepatotoxic if ingested in sufficient amounts |
| Wormwood | *Artemisia absinthium* | Volatile oil | Sedative, digestive aid, treatment of colic | Gastrointestinal upset, CNS signs including seizures and coma |

ministering activated charcoal with or without a cathartic (see "Emergency Treatment of Toxicoses," this volume, p 211). Indications and contraindications for decontamination procedures should be followed. For example, inducing emesis is contraindicated if ingestion was greater than 2 hr previously or if the animal is seizuring. Cathartics should not be administered to animals exhibiting severe diarrhea. If herbal remedies have been applied dermally, thorough bathing of affected animals is warranted. Ocular exposure to irritating chemicals should be followed by thorough flushing of affected eyes with copious amounts of tepid tap water.

Other treatment is symptomatic and supportive: intravenous fluids are indicated if dehydration is present; acid-base imbalances should be corrected; seizures should be controlled with valium or, if refractory to valium, barbiturates. Electrocardiograms (ECGs) should be monitored in instances of ingestion of cardiotoxins such as cardiac glycosides, and cardiac arrhythmias should be treated appropriately.

### References and Suggested Reading

de Bairacli Levy J: *The Complete Herbal Handbook for the Dog and Cat.* New York, Arco Publishing, 1986.

*Layperson's guide to the use of herbal remedies to treat a variety of dog and cat diseases.*

DeSmet PAGM: *Adverse Effects of Herbal Drugs.* New York, Springer-Verlag, 1991.

*Review of the scientific literature on the toxicity of many bioactive constituents of herbs.*

Ellenhorn MJ and Barceloux DG: *Medical Toxicology: Diagnosis and Treatment of Human Poisoning.* New York, Elsevier, 1988, p 1292.

*In-depth literature review of the toxicity and adverse effects of bioactive constituents of selected herbs.*

Lewin NA, Howland MA, and Goldfrank, LR: Herbal preparations. *In* Goldfrank LR, Flomenbaum NE, Lewin NA, Weisman RS, and Howland MA (eds): *Goldfrank's Toxicologic Emergencies.* Norwalk, CT, Appleton & Lange, 1990, p 587.

*Written and tabulated review of adverse effects in humans of commonly employed herbal remedies.*

Pitcairn RH and Pitcairn SH: *Natural Health for Dogs and Cats.* Emmaus, PA, Rodale Press, 1982.

*Layperson's guide to the use of herbal and homeopathic remedies for treating a variety of dog and cat diseases.*

Spoerke, DG: *Herbal Medications.* Santa Barbara, Woodbridge Press, 1990.

*Concise review of the indications for use and adverse effects of a number of herbal remedies.*

Stuart M: *VNR Color Dictionary of Herbs and Herbalism.* New York, Van Nostrand Reinhold Co, 1979.

*Layperson's guide to descriptions and indications for use of a number of herbs.*

Sudekum M, Poppenga RH, Raju N, and Braselton WE: Pennyroyal oil toxicosis in a dog. J Am Vet Med Assoc 200:817, 1992.

*Case report of death of a dog following dermal application of pennyroyal oil for flea control.*

# MANAGEMENT OF BEE AND OTHER HYMENOPTERA STINGS

ANNETTE K. COWELL
*and* RICK L. COWELL
*Stillwater, Oklahoma*

Each year many pets are stung by insects of the order Hymenoptera. Families responsible for the most severe reactions are: Apidea (bees), Vespidae (yellow jackets, wasps, and hornets), and Formicidae (imported fire ants) (Wright and Lockey, 1990). Most of these insects are social and live in colonies. Worker bees have a barbed, modified ovipositer that sticks in the skin and, along with the entire venom sac, is pulled out of the bee's abdomen. Constriction of muscles associated with the poison gland allow the stinger to continue pumping poison into the animal for 2 to 3 min after it has detached from the bee's abdomen (Wright and Lockey, 1990). Honey bees are herbivorous and tend not to sting unless disturbed. They are frequently found in fields of flowering plants, man-made hives, and trees. Members of the family Vespidae are much more aggressive than bees. Their stingers are not barbed and each individual is capable of inflicting many stings. Generally, yellow jackets are ground nesting, while wasps and hornets live in trees, shrubs, or other aerial structures. Vespids and imported fire ants are predaceous carnivores. Their stings are more likely to become infected. Imported fire ants produce a unique circular pattern of stings. They attach to the pet with their jaws and then pivot in a circle administering multiple stings. Imported fire ant mounds are about a foot tall and are found throughout the southeast United States. Their range is likely to spread, since they have few natural enemies and are very adaptable (deShazo et al., 1990).

Hymenopteran venoms contain a complex mixture of substances that produce toxic and allergic effects. Bee and wasp venom is principally composed of protein. Some of the proteins that have been identified from these venoms are phospholipase $A_1$, phospholipase $A_2$, hyaluronidase, acid phosphatase, antigen 5, melittin, and apamin (Wright and Lockey, 1990). Imported fire ant venom is 95% alkaloid and only 5% protein. The proteins present are similar to those found in other Hymenoptera (deShazo, Butcher, and Banks, 1990).

Dense fur helps protect pets from insect stings. Most stings are found on exposed areas of the head and paws.

Reactions to stings can range from mild to severe and can be divided into four general groups:

Group 1—small local (toxic in origin).

Group 2—large local (allergic in origin).

Group 3—systemic allergic.

Group 4—systemic toxic.

Small local reactions are the most common result of insect stings and are rarely presented to veterinary practitioners. These lesions are characterized by transient redness, swelling, and pain that is the result of the toxicity of the venom to the tissue. Most of these reactions will resolve without treatment in a few hours. If a bee was involved, the stinger should be quickly scraped from the skin and the lesion cleaned. Ice or a topical lidocaine spray may be used to relieve some of the discomfort.

Large local reactions usually have an immunologic basis and involve the whole face or an entire limb. The swelling is contiguous with the sting and can persist for several days (Wright and Lockey, 1990). Experience in humans indicates future stings are not likely to produce systemic reactions in these patients (Schmidt, 1986). Treatment of this type of lesion should include those listed for small local reactions and antihistamines (diphenhydramine 2 to 4 mg/kg b.i.d.), if the lesions are still progressing when presented. If the swelling is particularly severe, prednisolone (1 mg/kg b.i.d.) should be administered with doses tapered over 5 days.

Imported fire ants frequently produce large local reactions. Sterile pustules develop at the site of the sting within 24 hr and may remain for 3 to 10 days. No treatment has been shown to prevent or resolve the pustules (Wright and Lockey, 1990). Treatment is directed at preventing infection, reducing swelling, and controlling severe pruritis. Topical and systemic glucocorticoids as well as antihistamines have been used in people to control the pruritis associated with large local reactions that resulted from imported fire ant stings.

Anaphylaxis is one of the most frightening presentations following a hymenopteran sting. Symptoms usually become apparent within 15 min of the attack. If a severe systemic allergic reaction has not begun within 30 min, it is unlikely to occur (Frazier, 1976). The symptoms of anaphylaxis in dogs include swelling, vomiting, defecation, urination, muscular weakness, depressed respiration, and terminally convulsions. Death may occur within an hour of the first symptoms. Feline anaphylaxis is characterized by pruritis, dyspnea, salivation, incoordination, and collapse (Tizard, 1987). These symptoms result from antigen-induced IgE-mediated release, or formation, of chemical mediators whose target tissues are blood vessels and smooth muscles. In dogs, the shock organ is the liver (hepatic veins). Chemical mediators produce contractions of the hepatic veins and intestinal smooth muscles, and cause local vasodilatation with splanchnic pooling of blood. The shock organ in cats is the lung, and the chemical mediators of anaphylaxis may produce pulmonary hemorrhage and edema of the glottis (Tizard, 1987).

Anaphylaxis associated with insect venom is rarely reported. When it does occur, treatment must be rapid. Epinephrine 1:1000 (0.1 to 0.5 ml) should be given subcutaneously and repeated at 10 to 20 min intervals as needed (Reedy and Miller, 1989). If it becomes necessary to give epinephrine intravenously, it should be diluted to 1:10,000 and 0.5 to 1 ml administered with careful attention to pulse rate, blood pressure and heart rhythm. The value of this drug diminishes as shock progresses. Intravenous fluids are essential to combat the impending vascular collapse, and shock volumes (90 ml/kg in the dog; 60 ml/kg in the cat) of crystalloid solutions should be given rapidly during the first hour of therapy, unless there is pulmonary edema wherein fluid therapy should be judicious. Antihistamines (diphenhydramine hydrochloride, 2 mg/kg, given slowly IV) may be helpful very early in the reaction, and intravenous glucocorticoids (prednisolone sodium succinate, 10 mg/kg) may be helpful. Intubation and oxygen therapy should be included if needed.

Urticaria is a superficial systemic allergic reaction that appears as wheals in the skin. Angioedema can be thought of as deep wheals where deep blood vessels are affected and the edema causes a diffuse swelling in one area. These cutaneous reactions appear suddenly and will spontaneously regress (Reedy and Miller, 1989). The animal frequently rubs its mouth or eyes with its paws or the ground. Signs of vascular collapse are not present. Antihistamines can help stop the progression of the reaction if given early. Patients with urticaria should be observed for an hour after treatment or until the condition improves.

Immunotherapy may be indicated for dogs who have had severe generalized allergic reactions to hymenopteran venom. The products and protocols are adapted from human medicine and have been used with some success (Baker, 1990).

Massive envenomation resulting from large numbers of stings may produce severe systemic reactions as a result of the venom's toxicity rather than an allergic response. Dogs that disturb the nests of hornets, bees, wasps, or fire ants may be attacked by hundreds of insects. The neurotoxic, hepatotoxic, nephrotoxic, and cytotoxic effects of venom have been demonstrated in dogs and cats. The damage produced by the venom may be present immediately or may not be recognized for several days following the initial stings. Variation in type and amount of venom produces several clinical presentations.

Patients suffering from massive envenomation are markedly depressed and frequently febrile. They may not present with the swelling that characterizes allergic responses. Neurologic signs, including ataxia, facial paralysis, and seizures, are common on admission. Red to brown urine, dark brown vomitus, and bloody feces are also part of the clinical picture. Laboratory values reflect the hepatotoxic, cytotoxic, and nephrotoxic properties of the various components of the venom. Alanine amino transferase levels of 16,484 IU/L and total bilirubin levels of 8.5 mg/dl have been reported (Cowell et al., 1991). The hemogram generally reveals an inflammatory leukogram characterized by a leukocytosis with a left shift (Cowell et al., 1991; Wysoke, Van-Den Berg, and Marshall, 1990). In one review of three dogs with bee sting induced reactions, anemia due to intravascular hemolysis with marked spherocytosis was reported (Wysoke, Van-Den Berg, and Marshall, 1990). Also, thrombocytopenia may be present, especially if disseminated intravascular coagulation (DIC) develops (Cowell et al., 1991). Urinalysis may reveal granular casts, which suggest renal tubular damage and may be secondary to the nephrotoxic aspect of the venom. Acute tubular necrosis resulting from hemolysis or from direct renal toxicity may cause acute renal failure.

Victims of multiple hymenopteran stings should be hospitalized and carefully monitored for immediate and delayed systemic toxic reactions. The correction of hypovolemia and prevention of vascular stasis by the rapid administration of fluids and electrolytes is the most important aspect of treatment of severe reactions. Septicemia is a possible complication, and the prophylactic use of broad-spectrum antibiotics is warranted. Corticosteroids are beneficial in the treatment of neurologic symptoms and intravascular hemolysis. Prednisolone sodium succinate (10 mg/kg) should be given intravenously and followed by oral prednisolone (2 mg/kg divided b.i.d.). The prednisolone should be tapered as the signs resolve. Antihistamines and epinephrine are only of value very early in treatment and only if there is a marked allergic component to the reaction (Cowell et al., 1991; Wysoke, Van-Den Berg, and Marshall, 1990).

The natural curiosity of dogs and cats exposes them to aggressive members of the hymenopteran family whose stings can have life-threatening consequences. Most single stings produce a local self-limiting lesion that will respond to the removal of the stinger, gentle cleansing, ice, and possible topical medication for pain. Urticaria and angioedema can be treated with antihistamines and corticosteroids. Anaphylaxis requires prompt intensive therapy with epinephrine and intravenous fluids. Antihistamines, corticosteroids, and oxygen may be of value in selected cases. Acute toxic reactions to multiple hymenopteran stings require vigorous treatment with fluids and corticosteroids and careful monitoring of hepatic, renal, and hematologic parameters for several days.

## References and Suggested Reading

Baker E: *Small Animal Allergy: A Practical Guide.* Philadelphia, Lea & Febiger, 1990, p 123.
  *Discussion of Hymenoptera sting hypersensitivity and immunotherapy in canine patients.*
Cowell AK, Cowell RL, Tyler RD, and Nieves MA: Severe systemic reactions to Hymenoptera stings in three dogs. J Am Vet Med Assoc 198:1014, 1991.
  *Review of three dogs' hematologic, hepatic, renal, and hemostatic abnormalities resulting from Hymenoptera stings.*
deShazo RD, Butcher BT, and Banks WA: Reactions to the stings of the imported fire ant. N Engl J Med 323:462, 1990.
  *Review of the current concepts of imported fire ant sting reactions.*
Frazier CA: Anaphylactic response to insect stings. Compr Ther 2:67, 1976.
  *Epidemiology and treatment of human anaphylactic response to insect stings.*
Reedy LM and Miller WH Jr: *Allergic Skin Diseases of Dogs and Cats.* Philadelphia, WB Saunders Co, 1989, p 28.
  *Discussion of urticaria, angioedema, and anaphylaxis in dogs and cats.*
Schmidt JO: Allergy to Hymenoptera venoms. *In* Piek T (ed): *Venoms of the Hymenoptera: Biochemical, Pharmacological and Behavioural Aspects.* London, Academic Press, 1986, p 509.
  *Comprehensive review of Hymenoptera venom including human reactions and treatment of hypersensitivity.*
Tizard I: *Veterinary Immunology: An Introduction,* 3rd edition. Philadelphia, WB Saunders Co, 1987, p 292.
  *Readable review of mechanisms and clinical presentation of anaphylaxis in domestic animals.*
Wright DN and Lockey RF: Local reactions to stinging insects (Hymenoptera). Allergy Proc 11:23, 1990.
  *Hymenoptera biology and cutaneous reactions in people to stinging insects is reviewed.*
Wysoke JM, Van-Den Berg PB, and Marshall C: Bee sting-induced haemolysis, spherocytosis and neural dysfunction in three dogs. Tvdskr S Afr Vet Ver 61:29, 1990.
  *Review of three dogs diagnosed and treated for hematologic and neurologic dysfunction resulting from massive bee envenomation.*

# *CVT* UPDATE: ANTICOAGULANT RODENTICIDES

LAWRENCE J. FELICE
*and* MICHAEL J. MURPHY
St. Paul, Minnesota

Anticoagulant rodenticide exposure is frequently encountered in companion animal practices. These rodenticides are consistently responsible for exposures, toxicoses, and deaths of dogs and occasionally cats. They accounted for 8.4% of 41,854 calls and 9.2% of 454 deaths reported by 37 poison control centers in 1990. Comparable incidences of exposure, toxicity, and death are also observed in veterinary teaching hospitals and state veterinary diagnostic laboratories. This article focuses on the recognition, diagnosis, and treatment of anticoagulant rodenticide poisoning in small animals, then concludes with comments on three unique clinical situations. The reader is referred to *CVT X* (p 143) for a more expansive discussion of this topic. Since these previous articles were published, advances have primarily been in the development of confirmatory diagnostic tests utilizing serum and liver samples.

carboxylation of these proteins eliminates their ability to bind calcium, which prevents their participation in the clot formation process. Vitamin $K_1$ is given therapeutically to circumvent the need for recycling of vitamin $K_1$ epoxide, thus allowing the synthesis of clotting factors II, VII, IX, and X. For this reason, vitamin $K_1$ therapy *must be continued for as long as toxic concentrations of the anticoagulant rodenticide persist in the liver.*

## RECOGNITION

### Sources and Mechanisms of Action

Recognition of anticoagulant rodenticide toxicity will be discussed in terms of the sources, mechanisms of action, and clinical signs of toxicity. Sources of anticoagulant rodenticides include a wide variety of baits including, but not restricted to, those listed in Table 1. Mechanistically, anticoagulant rodenticides inhibit the "recycling" of vitamin $K_1$ epoxide (see Fig. 1). The resultant depletion of vitamin $K_1$ causes reduced carboxylation of precursors to clotting factors II, VII, IX, and X (i.e., PIVKA proteins II, VII, IX, and X). The lack of

### Clinical Signs

Dogs and cats experiencing anticoagulant rodenticide toxicosis commonly exhibit tachypnea or dyspnea. Anorexia and lethargy may also be reported by owners. Classic signs of hemorrhage, including melena, epistaxis, hematuria, and bleeding from venipuncture sites, may also be observed as the coagulopathy progresses. Animals occasionally die from anticoagulant rodenticide toxicosis without external evidence of bleeding. The most common necropsy findings are

***Table 1.*** *Trade Names and Common Chemical Names of Anticoagulant Rodenticides*

| Trade Name | Chemical Name | Trade Name | Chemical Name |
|---|---|---|---|
| Actosin C | Chlorophacinone | Racumin | Coumatetralyl |
| Boot Hill | Bromadiolone | Racumin 57 | Coumatetralyl |
| Bromone | Bromadiolone | Ramik | Diphacinone |
| Caid | Chlorophacinone | Ramucide | Chlorophacinone |
| Contrax-W | Warfarin | Ratak | Difenacoum |
| Controx-D | Diphacinone | Ratak Plus | Brodifacoum |
| Coumafene | Warfarin | Ratimus | Bromadiolone |
| Co-RAX | Warfarin | Ratomet | Chlorophacinone |
| Diachem | Chlorophacinone | Raviac | Chlorophacinone |
| Diphacin | Diphacinone | RAX | Warfarin |
| Drat | Chlorophacinone | Redentin | Chlorophacinone |
| d-CON | Brodifacoum | Rodentin | Coumatetralyl |
| d-CON Mouse Prufe II | Brodifacoum | Rodex | Warfarin |
| Endox | Coumatetralyl | Rodex Blox | Warfarin |
| Endrocid | Coumatetralyl | Ropax | Brodifacoum |
| Endrocide | Coumatetralyl | Rozol | Chlorophacinone |
| Enforcer Mouse Kill | Brodifacoum | Super Caid | Bromadiolone |
| Havoc | Brodifacoum | Talon | Brodifacoum |
| Just-One-Bite | Bromadiolone | Talon-G | Brodifacoum |
| Kill-Ko Rat Killer | Diphacinone | Tomcat | Diphacinone |
| Klerat | Brodifacoum | Topitox | Chlorophacinone |
| Lapit | Chlorophacinone | Tox-Hid | Warfarin |
| Lim-N8 | Brodifacoum | Tri-ban | Pindone |
| Liphadione | Chlorophacinone | Volid | Brodifacoum |
| LM 91 | Chlorophacinone | Warfarin Plus | Warfarin |
| Maki | Bromadiolone | Weather-Blok | Brodifacoum |
| Matikus | Brodifacoum | Zoocoumarin | Warfarin |
| Microzul | Chlorophacinone | | |
| Mouse Out | Chlorophacinone | | |
| Neosorexa PP580 | Difenacoum | | |
| Parakakes | Diphacinone | | |
| PCQ Rodent Cake | Diphacinone | | |
| Pivacin | Pindone | | |
| Pival | Pindone | | |
| Pival Parakakes | Pindone | | |
| Pivaldione | Pindone | | |
| Pivalyn | Pindone | | |
| PMP Tracking Powder | Valone | | |
| Promar | Diphacinone | | |

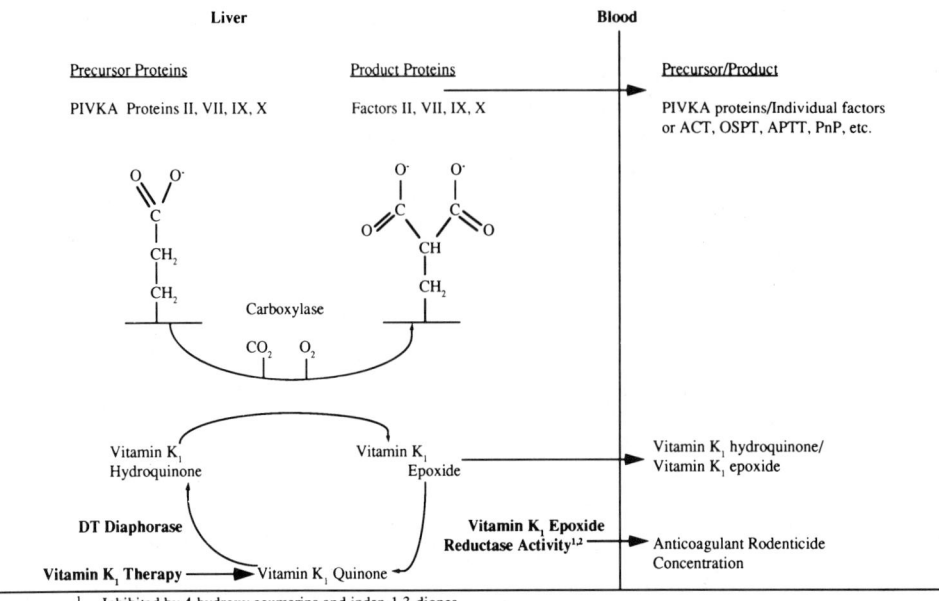

**Figure 1.** Mechanism of action of anticoagulant rodenticides.

intrapulmonary, intrathoracic, or intra-abdominal hemorrhages which are consistent with the dyspnea observed antemortem. Anticoagulant rodenticide toxicosis should be considered as a differential diagnosis for small animals with dyspnea or hemoptysis. Dogs with intrapulmonary hemorrhage associated with anticoagulant rodenticide exposure may develop a secondary bacterial pneumonia. These animals may then develop a productive or nonproductive cough, fever, and further depression.

## DIAGNOSIS

### Clinical Diagnosis

A clinical diagnosis of rodenticide toxicosis is commonly reached following a history of exposure to a potentially toxic dose of an anticoagulant rodenticide (Table 2). Remission of clinical signs and return of coagulation parameters towards normal, 24 to 48 hr after initiating appropriate vitamin $K_1$ therapy, is a commonly used aid for the clinical diagnosis of anticoagulant rodenticide toxicosis. The presence of dye-colored feces may be used as evidence of ingestion of a rodenticide product.

### Supportive Laboratory Tests

Abnormal prolongation of coagulation parameters (activated coagulation time [ACT] > 120 to 150 sec, one-stage prothrombin time [OSPT], activated partial thromboplastin time [APTT]) are commonly used diagnostic aids. Platelet counts can be normal or de-

creased. The ratio of vitamin $K_1$ to vitamin $K_1$ epoxide ($K_1$:$K_1$ epoxide) in serum has been postulated to be a means of determining exposure and duration of action of vitamin $K_1$ epoxide reductase inhibitors. This method is promising for detecting exposure of an animal to a vitamin $K_1$ epoxide reductase inhibitor. It is highly unlikely, however, that it will supplant coagulation parameter testing for this purpose. The $K_1$:$K_1$ epoxide ratio has also been examined as a tool for determining the length of vitamin $K_1$ therapy required in an individual animal. Use of the ratio has been promising in the case of one product (diphacinone), but has proven inappropriate for another (brodifacoum), and is therefore not recommended for this purpose.

### Conclusive Laboratory Tests

A conclusive diagnosis of anticoagulant rodenticide poisoning may be obtained by analytical confirmation of one of the products listed on Table 2 in serum or liver. The presence of these compounds in conjunction with coagulopathy is conclusive evidence of an anticoagulant rodenticide-associated coagulopathy. Experimental studies have shown that animals that have recovered from some long-acting anticoagulant rodenticides still have detectable concentrations of the compound in the serum or liver. Therefore, the detection of an anticoagulant rodenticide in the absence of a coagulopathy may be an incidental finding. The clinician should contact a veterinary diagnostic laboratory or college of veterinary medicine for suggestions on the appropriate sample for confirmatory testing for anticoagulant rodenticides.

## TREATMENT

General, symptomatic, and specific treatment is available for anticoagulant rodenticide toxicosis. Peak serum rodenticide concentrations generally occur 12 hr after experimental exposure; therefore, emetics, adsorbents, and cathartics may be helpful in preventing further absorption prior to this time.

### Symptomatic Therapy

Symptomatic therapy depends on the clinical condition of the animal. Animals with a packed cell volume (PCV) below 15 should be given 9 to 20 ml/kg fresh whole blood to provide both red cells and clotting factors. Animals with a severe coagulopathy (ACT >300 sec, OSPT >20, or APTT >50 sec) should be immediately given clotting factor replacement in the form of either: plasma frozen for less than 1 week; fresh frozen plasma (frozen at −40°C within 6 hr of collection; good for 1 year); or fresh whole blood. Some animals may benefit from fluid therapy.

### Specific Therapy

Vitamin $K_1$ is the specific antidote for anticoagulant rodenticide toxicosis. The recommended dose is 1 to 5 mg/kg/day depending on the compound involved (see Table 2). The majority of products currently on the market contain potent long-lasting compounds, so the 2.5-mg/kg dose is recommended as a starting therapy when the particular rodenticide is not known. Vitamin $K_1$ has the greatest bioavailability after oral administration. So, this route is recommended for animals that are not vomiting. Bioavailability is enhanced by the concurrent feeding of a small fatty meal, so 1 teaspoon of canned dog food is commonly given with the vitamin $K_1$. Once-daily dosing has proven effective in experimental studies. Therapy must be maintained for as long as the anticoagulant rodenticide is inhibiting vitamin $K_1$ epoxide recycling. This time period is commonly 2 to 4 weeks (see Table 2). Previous editions of *CVT* (*IX* and *X*) have detailed recommendations for long-term monitoring of coagulation status. Prothrombin complex status should be checked 2 to 5 days after therapy is discontinued.

Vitamin $K_3$ therapy is not efficacious for treatment of anticoagulant rodenticide poisoning and for that reason is *not recommended*. Vitamin $K_1$ may be given SC if the animal is vomiting or reluctant to take oral therapy. Anaphylactic reactions may occur if vitamin $K_1$ is given IV and extensive hemorrhage has occurred after IM therapy, so neither of these routes is recommended.

## UNIQUE CLINICAL SITUATIONS

### Lactating Bitches

Lactating bitches exposed to anticoagulant rodenticides present a unique dilemma. Although data on the passage of anticoagulant rodenticides in the milk of lactating bitches is not available, warfarin is reported to pass in the milk of lactating women taking the drug. Additionally, pups or kittens are likely to have reduced hepatic drug metabolizing activity and may consequently be more sensitive to toxic effects, especially from long-acting anticoagulant rodenticides. Depending on the amount of product available to the bitch, the most conservative approach may be to wean the pups and provide them with oral vitamin $K_1$ therapy daily for 2 to 3 weeks. The coagulation parameters of the bitch should be used to determine whether she needs therapy. Alternatively, the pups can be left on the bitch and treated immediately with vitamin $K_1$ while the

***Table 2.*** *Toxicity and Therapy of Anticoagulant Rodenticides*

| Chemical Name | Bait Concentration (ppm) | Acute Oral LD$_{50}$ | | | Vitamin K$_1$ Therapy | |
| | | Compound (mg/kg) | | Bait° (oz/#) | Dose (mg/kg) | Length |
| | | Dog | Cat | Dog | | |
| --- | --- | --- | --- | --- | --- | --- |
| Short-Acting: | | | | | | |
| Warfarin | 250 | 20–300 | 5–30 | 1.3 | 1 | 4–6 days |
| Unknown: | | | | | | |
| Bromadiolone | 50 | 11–15 | >25[‡] | 3.5 | 2.5 | ? |
| Fumarin | 250 | ? | ? | ? | 1 | 4–6 days[†] |
| Pindone | 250 | 5–75 | ? | 0.3 | 1 | 4–6 days[†] |
| Valone | 250 | ? | ? | ? | 1 | 4–6 days[†] |
| Long-Acting: | | | | | | |
| Diphacinone | 50 | 0.9–8 | 15 | 0.3 | 2.5–5.0 | 3–4 weeks[§] |
| Chlorophacinone | 50 | ? | ? | ? | 2.5–5.0 | 3–4 weeks[§] |
| Brodifacoum | 50 | 0.2–4 | 25[‡] | 0.06 | 2.5 | 2–3 weeks[§] |

°Ounces of finished bait per pound of body weight required to achieve the lowest LD$_{50}$ value reported in the dog.
[†]Animals should be closely observed/reexamined at the end of therapy.
[‡]Limited data.
[§]Reexamination following therapy is strongly recommended.
?-No data available.

bitch is left untreated. Her coagulation status should be checked 1, 3, and 5 days after suspected exposure. If she does not experience a coagulopathy, vitamin $K_1$ therapy of the pups may be discontinued in 1 week, but the pups should be closely monitored. If she does experience a coagulopathy, the pups should be maintained on vitamin $K_1$ for 1 week after cessation of therapy in the bitch. Vitamin $K_1$ therapy is unlikely to cause toxic problems in pups or kittens. Again, the bioavailability of vitamin $K_1$ is greatest when given orally.

### Pregnant Bitches

At least one anticoagulant rodenticide (diphacinone) has been detected in the amnionic fluid of a bitch at whelping. Since the developing pups or kittens may not be able to eliminate an anticoagulant rodenticide while *in utero*, an anticoagulant rodenticide–exposed pregnant bitch should be maintained on vitamin $K_1$ therapy until she whelps. Vitamin $K_1$ therapy for the offspring should be begun immediately and continued for at least 1 week or until their coagulation status can be monitored.

### Reexposed Animals

Some long-acting anticoagulant rodenticides are present in the liver of dogs weeks after they have clinically recovered from a coagulopathy episode. These animals may consequently be sensitive to much lower doses of anticoagulant rodenticides than listed on Table 2 if reexposed within weeks to months of initial recovery.

# ANTIFREEZE POISONING

MARY ANNA THRALL,
GREGORY F. GRAUER,
*Fort Collins, Colorado*

*and* SHARON M. DIAL
*Phoenix, Arizona*

Antifreeze poisoning is common in small animals and has the highest fatality rate of all common poisons. Widespread availability, pleasant taste, small minimum lethal dose, and lack of public awareness of the toxicity of the compound contribute to the frequency of antifreeze poisoning. Most commercial antifreeze solutions contain 95% ethylene glycol (EG), the toxic agent. Ethylene glycol is rapidly absorbed from the gastrointestinal tract, although absorption may be delayed if food is present in the stomach. The minimum lethal dose of undiluted ethylene glycol is 1.4 ml/kg in the cat, and 4.4 to 6.6 ml/kg in the dog. While the incidence of poisoning is similar in the cat and dog, fatality rates are higher for cats. Antifreeze poisoning occurs most commonly in the fall, winter, and spring, the seasons in which antifreeze is most commonly used.

Ethylene glycol per se is no more toxic than ethanol. Other than causing central nervous system (CNS) depression, ataxia, vomiting, and osmotic diuresis, it has no major toxic effects prior to catabolism. However, EG is metabolized in the liver to glycoaldehyde, glycolic acid, glyoxalic acid, and oxalic acid, substances that result in severe metabolic acidosis and renal epithelial damage. Glycoaldehyde causes CNS dysfunction by inhibition of respiration, glucose metabolism, serotonin metabolism, and alteration of amine concentrations. The other metabolites are directly cytotoxic to renal tubular epithelium. In addition, oxalate combines with calcium in the blood to form a soluble calcium oxalate complex that is filtered by the glomerulus and then crystalizes within the lumina of the tubules. Crystals are light yellow and arranged in rosettes, prisms, and sheaves, and are birefringent when viewed with polarized light (Fig. 1). Although renal tubular epithelium in contact with crystals often appears disrupted, crystal deposition is thought to have a relatively minor role in the pathogenesis of renal tubular damage.

## CLINICAL SIGNS

Clinical signs of ethylene glycol toxicosis are dose dependent and can be divided into those caused by the unmetabolized ethylene glycol, observed from 30 min to 12 hr postingestion, and those caused by the toxic metabolites of EG, which are frequently fatal. In the dog, early clinical signs associated with gastric irritation and high ethylene glycol blood concentrations include nausea and vomiting, mild to severe depression, ataxia and knuckling, muscle fasciculations, decreased withdrawal reflexes and righting ability, and polyuria and polydipsia. As depression increases over time, dogs drink less but polyuria continues, resulting in dehydration. Cats have similar clinical findings, but appear

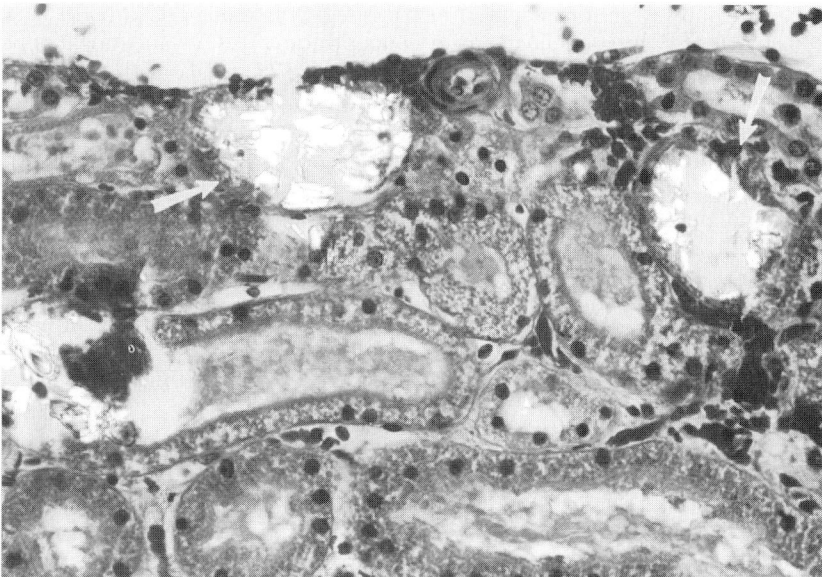

**Figure 1.** Histopathology of dog kidney showing calcium oxalate crystals within the tubular lumen (*arrows*) and tubular epithelial damage (× 400, polarized light).

more depressed, and polydipsia is not observed. Polyuria and polydipsia are caused by EG-induced osmotic diuresis and stimulation of the thirst center by serum hyperosmolality. Central nervous signs are a result of the direct effect of ethylene glycol and glycoaldehyde on the CNS, and are probably attributable in part to metabolic acidosis and increased plasma osmolality. In the dog, CNS signs abate after approximately 12 hr, and patients may appear to have recovered. Cats, however, usually remain markedly depressed. Animals may present severely hypothermic in winter months if depressed and housed outdoors.

Clinical signs associated with oliguric renal failure occur from 48 to 72 hr in the dog, and 12 to 24 hr in the cat following ethylene glycol ingestion. These may include severe depression or coma, seizures, anorexia, vomiting, oral ulcers and salivation, and oliguria with isosthenuria. Anuria often develops by 72 to 96 hr postingestion. Kidneys are often swollen and painful on palpation, particularly in the cat.

## LABORATORY FINDINGS

Laboratory findings may also be divided into those related to ethylene glycol per se, and those related to toxic metabolites.

### Serum Osmolality and Osmolal Gap

Serum osmolality is markedly increased by 1 hr after ingestion, in parallel with serum ethylene glycol concentrations. Hyperosmolality occurs because ethylene glycol is an osmotically active, small-molecular-weight substance (62 daltons), which is why it effectively lowers the freezing point of water. When measured serum osmolality is compared to calculated serum osmolality, the difference is referred to as the osmolal gap. Os-

molality in milliosmoles per kilogram may be calculated using the following formula:

$$1.86 \, (Na^+ + K^+) + glucose/18 + BUN/2.8 + 9$$

The constant, 9, is added to adjust for osmotically active particles such as phosphates and sulfates that are not accounted for in the above formula. Normal serum osmolality for dogs and cats is 280 to 310 mOsm/kg. The normal osmolal gap in dogs and cats is less than 10 mOsm/kg. Dogs that were experimentally poisoned with 10.5 gm ethylene glycol per kilogram body weight (9.5 ml of ethylene glycol or 10 ml of antifreeze per kilogram body weight) had a mean serum osmolality of 440 mOsm/kg and a mean osmolal gap of 134 mOsm/kg at 3 hr postingestion. Both the gap and measured osmolality remained significantly high for approximately 18 hr postingestion. Cats that were experimentally poisoned with 1.6 gm ethylene glycol per kilogram body weight had a mean osmolal gap of 53 mOsm/kg at 3 hr postingestion.

### Serum and Urine Ethylene Glycol Concentrations

In studies in which ethylene glycol was given to evaluate various therapies, EG serum concentrations peaked at 1 hr in cats given EG after a 12-hr fast; in dogs fed a mixture of EG and food, concentrations peaked at 3 to 6 hr postingestion. Approximately 50% of ingested ethylene glycol is excreted unchanged in the urine, while the remainder is rapidly metabolized. Urine concentrations of ethylene glycol peak at approximately 6 hr postingestion in both dogs and cats. Ethylene glycol is usually not detectable in the serum or urine by 72 hr postingestion.

Both serum and urine concentrations are dependent on the quantity of ethylene glycol ingested and absorbed. For example, in dogs given 10.5 gm EG per kilogram body weight, mean serum concentration was 930 mg/dl at 3 hr and mean urine concentration was 3975 mg/dl at 6 hr postingestion; in cats given 1.6 gm EG per kilogram body weight, mean serum concentration was 380 mg/dl at 3 hr and mean urine concentration was 1500 mg/dl at 6 hr postingestion.

Commercial kits (EGT Test Kit, PRN Pharmacal, Inc, 5830 McAllister Ave, Pensacola, FL 32504) are available that appear to accurately measure blood ethylene glycol concentrations at 50 mg/dl or greater. Preliminary studies show that the results appear to correlate with other established methods of measuring ethylene glycol concentrations (Dennis Chew, personal communication). Many hospitals and diagnostic laboratories can also determine concentrations quickly enough to be diagnostically useful. Serum osmolality can also be used to accurately estimate serum ethylene glycol concentrations by multiplying the osmolal gap by 6.2. For example, if the osmolal gap were 100 mOsm/kg, the predicted serum ethylene glycol concentration would be 620 mg/dl.

## Blood Gases, Total Carbon Dioxide and Anion Gap

The metabolites of ethylene glycol, especially glycolic acid, are potent organic acids that cause severe metabolic acidosis. By 3 hr postingestion, total carbon dioxide ($TCO_2$), plasma bicarbonate concentration, and blood pH are decreased. By 12 hr postingestion, they are markedly decreased and remain so throughout the intoxication. The $PCO_2$ often decreases as a result of partial respiratory compensation.

The anion gap is increased by 3 hr postingestion, peaks at 6 hr postingestion, and remains increased for approximately 48 hr. Anion gap is determined by subtracting the measured anions (bicarbonate and chloride) from the measured cations (sodium and potassium). The normal anion gap for dogs and cats is 10 to 15 mEq/L and is comprised of phosphates, sulfates, and negatively charged proteins that are not included in the equation. Metabolites of ethylene glycol significantly increase the pool of unmeasured anions and cause the increased anion gap.

## Urine Analysis

Dogs are isosthenuric (urine specific gravity of 1.012 to 1.014) by 3 hr postingestion of EG due to osmotic diuresis and serum hyperosmolality–induced polydipsia. The urine specific gravity in cats is also markedly decreased by 3 hr postingestion (range = 1.012 to 1.023). Animals remain isosthenuric in the later stages of toxicosis as a result of renal dysfunction and impaired ability to concentrate urine.

Calcium oxalate crystalluria (Fig. 2) is a consistent finding and may be observed as early as 3 and 6 hr postingestion in the cat and dog, respectively, as a result of oxalic acid combining with calcium. Calcium oxalate monohydrate crystals are variable sized, clear, six-sided prisms that are similar in appearance to hippurate crystals and have historically been misidentified as hippurate. In animals poisoned with ethylene glycol, the monohydrate form is observed more frequently than the dihydrate form (Fig. 3), which appears as an envelope or maltese cross. Dumbell or sheaf-shaped crystals (Fig. 4) are observed infrequently. Laboratory personnel should be cognizant of the wide variety of calcium oxalate crystal shapes and the high frequency with which calcium oxalate monohydrate crystalluria occurs following ethylene glycol ingestion.

Urine pH consistently decreases following ethylene glycol ingestion. Inconsistent findings include hematuria, proteinuria, and glucosuria. Granular and cellular casts, white blood cells, red blood cells, and renal epithelial cells may be observed in the sediment of some patients.

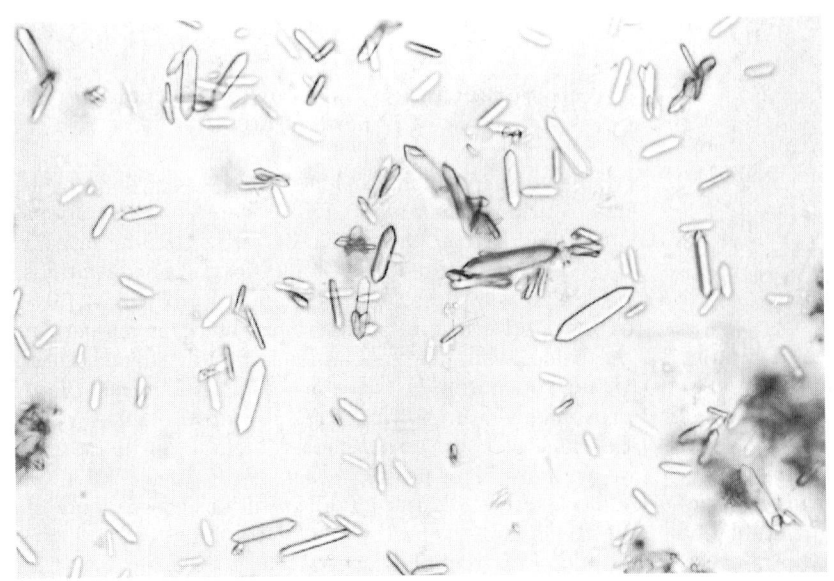

**Figure 2.** Monohydrate calcium oxalate crystals in urine sediment of a dog with ethylene glycol toxicosis ($\times$ 400).

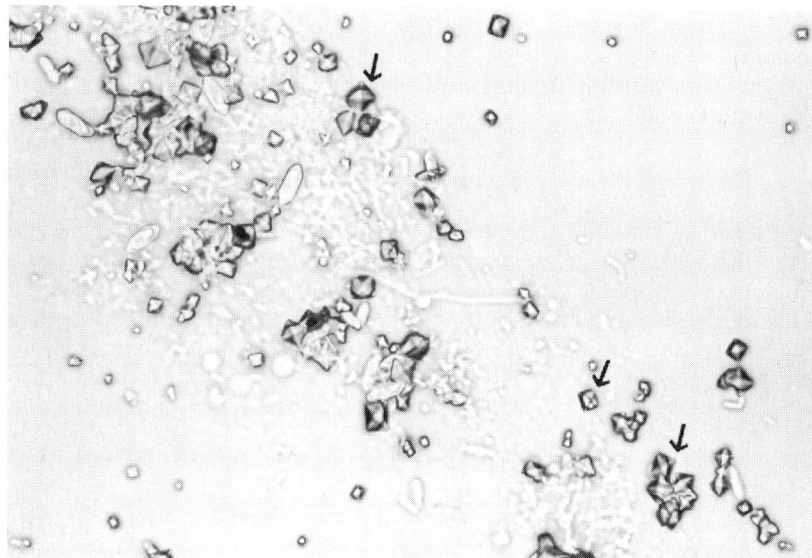

**Figure 3.** Urine sediment containing both dihydrate (envelope shaped) (*arrows*) and monohydrate calcium oxalate crystals from a dog with ethylene glycol toxicosis (x 250).

## Biochemical Profile and Complete Blood Count

### AZOTEMIA

With the onset of renal damage and subsequent decreased glomerular filtration, serum creatinine and urea nitrogen (SUN) concentrations increase. In the dog, these increases begin to occur between 36 and 48 hr following EG ingestion. In the cat, SUN and creatinine begin to increase approximately 12 hr postingestion; however, since cats do not develop polydipsia, this may in part be due to dehydration. Serum phosphorus concentrations increase due to decreased glomerular filtration, but increases as high as 10 mg/dl can also be observed 3 to 6 hr following antifreeze ingestion due to the phosphate rust inhibitors present in the antifreeze solution. In this case, serum phosphorus concentrations return to normal, then increase again with the onset of azotemia. It is important to realize that hyperphosphatemia in the absence of an increased SUN or creatinine is most likely due to increased intake and not an indication of compromised renal function. Hyperkalemia develops with the onset of oliguria and anuria.

### HYPOCALCEMIA

A decrease in serum calcium concentration is observed in approximately half of patients due to chelation of calcium by oxalic acid. Clinical signs of hypocalcemia are infrequently observed because acidosis results in a shift to the ionized, physiologically active form of calcium.

### HYPERGLYCEMIA

Increased serum glucose concentration is observed in approximately half of the patients, and is attributed

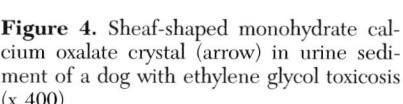

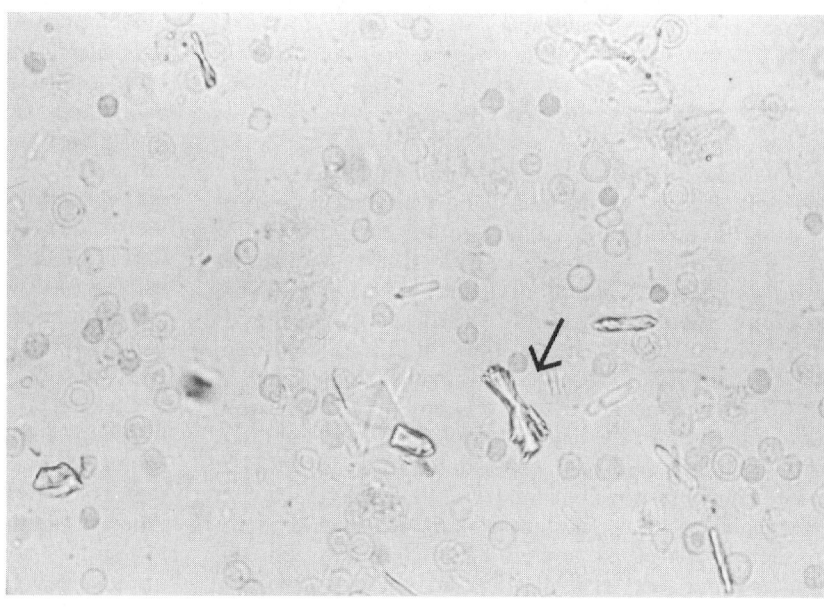

**Figure 4.** Sheaf-shaped monohydrate calcium oxalate crystal (arrow) in urine sediment of a dog with ethylene glycol toxicosis (x 400).

to inhibition of glucose metabolism by aldehydes, increased epinephrine and endogenous corticosteroids, uremia, and possibly inhibition of insulin release due to hypocalcemia.

### COMPLETE BLOOD COUNT

Packed cell volume and total protein are often markedly increased due to dehydration. Stress leukograms (mature neutrophilia, lymphopenia) are commonly observed, presumably as a result of endogenous corticosteroid release secondary to CNS abnormalities, vomiting, metabolic acidosis, and uremia.

## DIAGNOSIS

History, clinical signs, laboratory findings, and histopathology are of diagnostic usefulness. Early diagnosis is critical to successful therapy, since EG is metabolized rapidly; therapy to inhibit EG metabolism should be instituted within at least 8 hr postingestion. Ethylene glycol toxicosis should always be considered when there is history of possible exposure and acute onset of CNS signs and polyuria. Diagnosis can be confirmed by serum or urine EG concentrations or serum osmolality. Urinalysis is also helpful in making an early diagnosis, since calcium oxalate crystalluria is seen in almost all patients by 6 hr postingestion. Marked increases in osmolal gap are almost always due to EG toxicosis. Antifreeze poisoning should also be considered in any animal with acute onset of renal disease. By the time azotemia develops in the dog, most of the EG has been metabolized, and osmolal gap and serum EG concentrations may have returned to near normal, but crystalluria may persist for 2 weeks. Cats, on the other hand, may become azotemic by 12 hr following ingestion, before all of the EG has been metabolized, so that azotemia may occur concurrently with increased EG serum concentrations and increased osmolal gap. If the animal is anuric, a kidney biopsy may be necessary to confirm the diagnosis.

## THERAPY

Therapy for ethylene glycol poisoning is aimed at preventing absorption, increasing excretion, and preventing metabolism of the compound. Supportive care to correct fluid, acid-base, and electrolyte imbalances is also helpful. If ingestion of antifreeze is witnessed, vomiting should be induced. Gastric lavage with activated charcoal is indicated within 1 to 2 hr of ingestion; beyond this time, the procedure is of little benefit.

A critical aspect of therapy is based on preventing the metabolism of ethylene glycol to its toxic metabolites by inhibiting liver alcohol dehydrogenase (ADH), the enzyme responsible for the initial reaction in the metabolic pathway. Inhibition of ADH can be accomplished by giving a compound that combines with the enzyme and renders it inactive, or by giving competitive substrates that have a higher affinity for ADH than does ethylene glycol. The most effective ADH inhibitor in the dog is 4-methylpyrazole (4-MP), a nontoxic pyrazole which, unlike most competitive inhibitors, does not contribute to CNS depression and serum osmolality. When given to dogs as early as 3 hr following EG ingestion, approximately 90% of ethylene glycol is excreted unmetabolized. In dogs, treatment with 4-methylpyrazole has been successful when given as late as 8 hr after ingestion of 10 ml of antifreeze per kilogram body weight. Even if animals are presented as late as 36 hr following EG ingestion, prevention of any remaining unmetabolized EG may be of benefit. The recommended dose of 5% (50 mg/ml) 4-methylpyrazole is 20 mg/kg body weight IV initially, followed by 15 mg/kg IV at 12 and 24 hr, and 5 mg/kg IV at 36 hr. To make a 5% solution of 4-methylpyrazole, 5 gm of 4-MP (Aldrich Chemical Company) is added to 50 ml of polyethylene glycol (400) and 46 ml of bacteriostatic water to make 100 ml. The solution should be filtered with a 0.22-$\mu$m filter before use. The refrigerated solution is stable for at least 2 years. While 4-MP is not approved by the Food and Drug Administration (FDA) for use in animals, veterinarians may obtain 4-MP and use it in their practice without approval from the FDA. If suppliers of 4-MP require evidence of FDA's current regulatory position, a letter may be obtained from the Division of Compliance, Center for Veterinary Medicine, FDA, 5600 Fishers Lane, Rockville, MD 20857; telephone 301-295-8812.

While 4-MP is the recommended therapy in dogs, it is not recommended for use in cats. Although it is nontoxic, it does not effectively inhibit EG metabolism unless given at the same time as EG. Cats died of renal failure even when 4-MP was given as early as 2 hr following EG ingestion. Future investigations using varying doses of 4-MP in the cat may be helpful.

Ethanol and other alkydiols such as propylene glycol and 1,3-butanediol have a higher affinity for ADH than does ethylene glycol, and can be used effectively to inhibit EG metabolism. However, they have numerous disadvantages, including CNS depression and a tendency to further increase serum osmolality. Ethanol became established as treatment of choice for ethylene glycol poisoning because it is a very effective competitive inhibitor for ADH. However, the effective dose of ethanol is high enough to cause CNS depression, and patients often become comatose from the additive effects of EG and ethanol. Also, ethanol is metabolized rapidly, necessitating frequent or constant therapy. The suggested dose for dogs is 5.5 ml of 20% ethanol per kilogram body weight given IV every 4 hr for five treatments, and then every 6 hr for four more treatments. If possible, the same dose can be more safely given as a constant IV infusion, since bolus injections may result in serum concentrations high enough to suppress respiration. Constant serum ethanol concentrations of 100 mg/dl will inhibit most ethylene glycol metabolism. Dogs treated with ethanol at 3 hr following EG ingestion excrete approximately 80% of the EG unmetabolized.

For the present, therapy of choice in the cat is ethanol. The recommended dose is 5 ml of 20% ethanol per kilogram body weight given IV every 6 hr for five treatments and then every 8 hr for four more treatments. In our experience, this results in peak blood ethanol concentrations (BEC) as high as 350 mg/dl, and BEC will drop as low as 40 mg/dl at the end of each treatment interval. The $LD_{50}$ of ethanol in most species is 400 to 500 mg/dl, and respiratory arrest and death have been reported in human patients at 260 mg/dl. We recommend a constant IV infusion of ethanol in fluids to prevent the high BEC observed with bolus infusion. Cats given ethanol often develop severe CNS depression and usually become hypothermic, necessitating an external heat source.

Supportive therapy consists of intravenous fluids to correct dehydration, increase tissue perfusion, and promote diuresis. The fluid volume administered should be based on the maintenance, deficit, and continuing loss needs of the patient. In addition, bicarbonate should be given slowly IV to correct the metabolic acidosis. If possible, dose of sodium bicarbonate should be based on serial plasma bicarbonate concentrations using the following formula:

$$0.3 - 0.5 \times \text{body weight in kg} \times (24 - \text{plasma bicarbonate}) = \text{mEq of sodium bicarbonate needed.}$$

Monitoring the urine pH in response to therapy may also be helpful.

In dogs that present azotemic and in oliguric renal failure, almost all of the EG will have been metabolized, and treatment to inhibit alcohol dehydrogenase is of little benefit. In these patients, the prognosis is poor. Fluid, electrolyte, and acid-base disorders should be corrected, and establishment of diuresis is desirable. Diuretics, particularly mannitol, may be helpful. The tubular damage caused by ethylene glycol may be reversible, but may take weeks to months. Supportive care to maintain the patient during the period of renal tubular regeneration is necessary, and peritoneal dialysis may be useful. Animals may take up to 1 year to regain concentrating ability, and some will always be isosthenuric.

## PROGNOSIS

The prognosis is excellent in dogs that present within 5 hr following ethylene glycol ingestion if 4-MP is given to prevent its metabolism. Most dogs will recover if treatment is initiated as late as 8 hr following ingestion. Quantity of EG ingested, rate of absorption, and time interval prior to institution of therapy are variables that will affect prognosis. The prognosis for cats is also good if treatment with ethanol is instituted within 3 hr following ingestion. Unfortunately, dog and cat owners are frequently unaware of the acute clinical signs, resulting in delayed presentation. Dogs and cats presenting with azotemia have a poor prognosis; in a retrospective study, the only animals presenting with azotemia that recovered were those less than 6 months of age. It is possible that the regenerative capacity of the kidney is greater in young animals.

## PREVENTION

Increasing client awareness of the toxicity of ethylene glycol will aid in preventing exposure and result in earlier presentation of patients. In addition, antifreeze manufacturers should provide more prominent warning labels and additives to make products unpalatable. One of the most promising recent developments for prevention of EG poisoning is the recent introduction of an antifreeze product containing propylene glycol, which is relatively nontoxic.

### References and Suggested Reading

Dial SM, Thrall MA, and Hamar DW: The use of 4-methylpyrazole as treatment for ethylene glycol intoxication in the dog. J Am Vet Med Assoc 195: 73, 1989.
  *An evaluation of the efficacy of 4-methylpyrazole as therapy in dogs with naturally occurring ethylene glycol poisoning.*
Grauer GF, Thrall MA, Henre BA, et al: Early clinicopathologic findings in dogs ingesting ethylene glycol. Am J Vet Res 45:2299, 1984.
  *A report of early clinical and laboratory findings in 15 dogs experimentally poisoned with ethylene glycol.*
Grauer GF, Thrall M, Henre BA, and Hjelle JJ: Comparison of the effects of ethanol and 4-methylpyrazole on the pharmacokinetics and toxicity of ethylene glycol in the dog. Toxicol Lett 35:307, 1987.
  *The efficacy of 4-methylpyrazole and ethanol as therapies for ethylene glycol intoxication in the dog were compared.*
Mueller DH: Epidemiologic considerations of ethylene glycol intoxication in small animals. Vet Hum Toxicol 24:21, 1981.
  *A report of the epidemiology of ethylene glycol poisoning in Minnesota.*
Rowland J: Incidence of ethylene glycol intoxication in dogs and cats seen at Colorado State University Veterinary Teaching Hospital. Vet Hum Toxicol 29:41, 1987.
  *A report of the incidence of and mortality due to ethylene glycol poisoning in dogs and cats presenting to a veterinary teaching hospital in Colorado.*
Thrall MA, Grauer GF, and Mero KN: Clinicopathologic findings in dogs and cats with ethylene glycol intoxication. J Am Vet Med Assoc 184:37, 1984.
  *A retrospective evaluation of clinical and laboratory findings in 26 cats and 24 dogs with ethylene glycol poisoning.*
Thrall MA, Winder D, and Dial SM: Identification of calcium oxalate monohydrate crystals by x-ray diffraction in urine of ethylene glycol intoxicated dogs. Vet Pathol 22:625, 1985.
  *A report of the incidence of monohydrate and dihydrate calcium oxalate crystals in urine of dogs with experimentally induced ethylene glycol poisoning; hippurate-like crystals were shown to be calcium oxalate monohydrate by x-ray diffraction.*

# CVT UPDATE: ZINC TOXICITY

KATHRYN M. MEURS

*College Station, Texas*

*and* EDWARD B. BREITSCHWERDT

*Raleigh, North Carolina*

Toxicity from the ingestion of zinc ointment or zinc-containing objects has become a frequently reported problem in domestic animals. Severe intravascular hemolysis and gastrointestinal irritation are the most commonly reported clinical findings. When therapeutic intervention is delayed, zinc toxicity causes failure of multiple organ systems, and is associated with a high mortality rate (Meurs et al., 1991). Successful therapy is primarily directed at removal of the source of zinc toxicity. Additionally, supportive care may be helpful in decreasing the mortality. The appropriate use of chelating agents, such as calcium ethylenediaminetetraacetic acid (CaEDTA), may be helpful but remains to be validated by further studies.

The most commonly reported sources for zinc toxicity in small animals are zinc nuts from transport cages, zinc plumbing nuts, zinc oxide ointment, zinc game pieces from board games, and pennies minted after 1982 (Allison, Evan, and McDonald, 1989; Breitschwerdt et al., 1986; Meurs et al., 1991; Ogden, 1992; Torrance and Fulton, 1987). These items are all composed of at least 98% elemental zinc. Zinc oxide ointment (Desitin) usually causes gastic irritation (vomiting). Chronic ingestion could possibly result in the hemolytic syndrome.

## TOXICITY

The oral dose of zinc required to induce poisoning appears to be dependent on the degree of intestinal absorption, the form of the zinc salt, and the pH of the gastrointestinal environment (Ogden, 1992). The acidity of the stomach would appear to provide the ideal environment for the gradual release of zinc from objects that have a high zinc content. Following absorption into the blood vascular system, zinc is distributed to various organs preferentially. In humans, the highest concentrations of zinc are found in the uveal tract, prostate, bone, skin, muscle, liver, pancreas, and kidney (Breitschwerdt et al., 1986). Normally, zinc is primarily excreted in the feces, with a small percentage (approximately 25%) excreted in the urine (Basinger and Jones, 1981).

Most heavy metal toxicities deleteriously affect multiple organ systems. The pathogenesis of metal toxicities is often mediated by inhibition of specific biochemical enzymes and/or direct damage to cell membranes or organelles. Cells involved in the transport of metals such as gastrointestinal, hepatic, or renal tubular cells are particularly susceptible to heavy metal toxicity.

## CLINICAL SIGNS

In animals, clinical abnormalities associated with zinc toxicity include gastrointestinal dysfunction (anorexia, vomiting, diarrhea), icterus, and severe intravascular hemolytic anemia accompanied by hemoglobinuria and hematuria. Increased nucleated red blood cells, basophilic stippling, target cells, and polychromasia are frequently observed. Hematologic abnormalities, azotemia, elevations in alkaline phosphatase and alanine aminotransferase activities, and disseminated intravascular coagulation (DIC) are indicators of multiple organ failure (Meurs et al., 1991; Ogden, 1992). Fatalities appear to be secondary to generalized organ failure, severe anemia associated with a hemolytic crisis, or cardiopulmonary arrest (Meurs et al., 1991).

## DIAGNOSIS

The diagnosis of zinc toxicity is frequently dependent on obtaining a history of possible zinc exposure in a dog with clinical abnormalities indicative of gastrointestinal dysfunction or severe hemolytic anemia. Adjunctive diagnostic tests for zinc toxicity include abdominal radiographs indicating the presence of a metallic object in the gastrointestinal tract and a complete blood count (CBC) demonstrating severe intravascular hemolytic anemia. Serum chemistry panel, urinalysis, and coagulation panel should be assessed to establish the severity of organ dysfunction. Serum samples for zinc analysis should be collected carefully to avoid zinc contamination from the syringe or vial. If possible, special tubes for elemental analysis should be used as well as syringes without rubber grommets. Normal canine serum zinc concentrations range from 0.7 to 2.0 $\mu$g/ml (Torrance and Fulton, 1987).

## THERAPY

Treatment of zinc toxicity begins with patient stabilization followed by rapid removal of the zinc object, by endoscopy or laparotomy. Most cases have to be treated for zinc toxicity based on suspicion of the problem; zinc serum concentration levels usually take at least 24 hr for the results. Aggressive supportive therapy as well as removal of the metal object should not be withheld until zinc serum levels are available. Stabilization of the patient requires attention to the many pathologic processes that occur in zinc toxicity. Severe intravascular hemolysis often necessitates a blood transfusion. Thrombocytopenia and evidence of DIC may warrant heparin therapy (initially, we use 150 U/kg SC every 6 hr). Additionally, because the rate of release and absorption of zinc appears to be somewhat dependent on the acidity of the stomach, it may be useful to decrease the gastric acidity of the stomach with an $H_2$-receptor blocker (cimetidine, ranitidine). The risk of acute renal failure, a serious sequela of zinc toxicity, may be lessened by maintaining hydration and avoiding aminoglycoside antibiotics.

Recent studies using rodents have demonstrated a significant decrease in mortality as well as organ damage secondary to zinc toxicity when metal chelators have been given orally or intraperitoneally (Basinger and Jones, 1981; Brownie and Aronson, 1984; Domingo et al., 1988). Although several chelating agents effectively decrease serum and organ zinc concentrations, CaEDTA is the most readily available and effective. In rodents, CaEDTA significantly decreases concentrations of zinc in the serum, heart, bones, and spleen and increases both urine and fecal zinc concentrations (Domingo et al., 1988).

Recent studies provide sufficient support to recommend the use of CaEDTA as a zinc chelator in cases of zinc toxicity (Bassinger and Jones, 1981; Brownie and Aronson, 1984; Domingo et al., 1988). Therapy with CaEDTA should probably be given immediately after the diagnosis of zinc toxicity has been made. CaEDTA can be nephrotoxic, so careful attention should be given to dosing as well as to maintaining the animal's state of hydration. We use 100 mg/kg of CaEDTA divided into four subcutaneous doses per day. CaEDTA should be diluted in 5% dextrose to help decrease local irritation. The most effective dose of CaEDTA for zinc toxicosis in the dog is not known. The dose given here has been adapted from therapeutic regimens for lead toxicity. At this time it is unclear how long chelator therapy should be continued. Serum zinc concentrations appear to decrease very rapidly after removal of the source (48 hr in one case). However, in several cases the serum zinc concentration has remained elevated for at least 3 weeks after removal of the foreign object. If possible, the decision to discontinue chelator therapy should be based on normalization of the serum zinc concentration.

Due to the high mortality associated with zinc toxicosis, these cases should be treated as serious emergencies. The source of zinc toxicity should be eliminated as soon as possible after patient stabilization with fluids or blood transfusions as needed. Hopefully, additional treatment including $H_2$-receptor blockers and CaEDTA may help decrease mortality (Meurs et al., 1991). Further studies are needed to provide additional information in the areas of pathogenesis and effective therapy of zinc toxicity.

## References and Suggested Reading

Allison N, Evan S, and McDonald RK: When pets ingest zinc: How likely is toxicosis? Vet Med 84:777, 1989.
*A case report of zinc toxicosis from ingestion of pennies and a board game piece in a dog.*

Basinger MA and Jones MM: Chelate antidotal efficacy in acute zinc toxicosis. Res Commun Chem Pathol Pharmacol 33:263, 1981.
*Comparative study of the efficacy of different chealtors to decrease mortality in experimental zinc toxicosis in rodents.*

Breitschwerdt EB, Armstrong PJ, Robinette CL, et al: Three cases of acute zinc toxicosis in dogs. Vet Hum Toxicol 28:109, 1986.
*Case reports and review of the pathogenesis of zinc toxicosis in dogs.*

Brownie CF and Aronson AL: Comparative effects of Ca-ethylenediamine-tetraacetic acid (EDTA), ZnEDTA, and ZnCaEDTA in mobilizing lead. Toxicol Appl Pharmacol 75:167, 1984.
*Comparative study of the efficacy of EDTA as a chelating agent.*

Domingo JL, Liobet JM, Paternain JL, and Corbella J: Acute zinc intoxication: Comparison of the antidotal efficacy of several chelating agents. Vet Hum Toxicol 30:224, 1988.
*Comparative study of the effects of different chelating agents to decrease zinc intoxication in rats and mice injected intraperitoneally with zinc compounds.*

Meurs KM, Breitschwerdt EB, Baty CJ, and Young MA: Postsurgical mortality secondary to zinc toxicity in dogs. Vet Hum Toxicol 33:579, 1991.
*Review of the pathogenesis of zinc toxicosis and the causes of mortality associated with zinc intoxication.*

Ogden L: Zinc toxicosis. *In* Kirk RW and Bonagura JD (eds): *Current Veterinary Therapy XI.* Philadelphia, WB Saunders Co, 1992, p 197.
*Review of clinical signs, diagnosis, and therapy of zinc toxicosis.*

Torrance AG and Fulton RB: Zinc-induced hemolytic anemia in a dog. J Am Vet Med Assoc 191:443, 1987.
*Case report of zinc toxicosis in a dog associated with penny ingestion.*

# IRON TOXICOSIS

WILLIAM F. GREENTREE

*Ames, Iowa*

*and* JEFFREY O. HALL

*Urbana, Illinois*

The use of iron in human pregnancy supplements, multivitamins, and general dietary supplements has resulted in it becoming a toxic hazard to pets. High concentrations of iron can also be found in some mineral-fortified fertilizers. Many of these iron-containing products are available over the counter and are therefore accessible in large quantities. Often the dietary products are sugar coated, highly palatable, and not thought of as toxic by pet owners. During 1992, the National Animal Poison Control Center (NAPCC) received 165 calls regarding accidental ingestion of iron-containing products.

## ABSORPTION, DISTRIBUTION, METABOLISM, AND EXCRETION

Iron is the most abundant trace mineral in the body and has a complex metabolism. Unlike many nutrients, the body concentrations of iron are regulated primarily by absorption, not excretion. Ferrous iron is absorbed by the mucosal cells of the duodenum and jejunum utilizing an energy-dependent carrier mechanism. Iron must be in an ionized form for absorption, so metallic iron or its oxide salt are not generally of concern when ingested. Once absorbed, the iron is oxidized to the ferric state and transported across the cell membrane into the plasma where it is rapidly bound to transferrin, a $\beta_1$ glycoprotein. Complexed with transferrin, iron is distributed throughout the body. Of the normal body load of iron, approximately 70% is found in hemoglobin and 10% in myoglobin. The remaining body iron is either utilized in enzymes such as peroxidase, catalase, and cytochrome C, or stored in the liver, spleen, and bones.

The carrier-mediated uptake of iron by the gastrointestinal mucosal cells is generally the rate-limiting factor for its absorption. However, in an acute overdose it appears to be absorbed in a passive, concentration-dependent fashion. This suggests that the carrier-mediated mechanism is either exceeded or not involved in situations of high exposure. There is a possibility that gastric mucosal damage allows increased iron absorption, but it is not required for toxic concentrations of iron to be absorbed. When abnormally large amounts of iron are absorbed, it can surpass the binding capability of transferrin, which results in free iron circulating in the plasma.

A unique feature of iron metabolism is the virtual absence of any means for its active excretion. The small amount of iron that is lost daily in the urine and feces cannot be significantly increased, even in a case of overdose. Iron released by hemoglobin degradation, associated with the removal of senescent erythrocytes, is rapidly adhered to transferrin and transported to the bone marrow for resynthesis of hemoglobin.

## MECHANISM OF ACTION

Acute iron toxicosis exerts its primary effect on the gastrointestinal tract, liver, and cardiovascular system. This is a consequence of both its direct corrosive effect on the gastrointestinal mucosa and the presence of unbound iron in the circulation. Iron salts are corrosive agents and cause a variable degree of hemorrhagic necrosis to the lining of the stomach and small intestine. Pills can adhere to the gastric mucosa and, as they dissolve, can result in extremely high focal concentrations.

Once absorbed into the circulation, iron precipitates a wide variety of metabolic disorders. Free circulating iron penetrates cells of the liver, heart, and brain, resulting in hepatic damage, myocardial failure, and seizures. The degree of hepatic damage can vary from minor swelling of the hepatocytes to widespread necrosis. Iron exerts its most profound effect, however, on the cardiovascular system. Fatty necrosis of the myocardium, postarteriolar dilation, and increased capillary permeability lead to reduced cardiac output, venous pooling, and diminished tissue perfusion. Histamine and serotonin release are stimulated by free iron and can account for some of the cardiovascular effects. Systemic metabolic acidosis subsequently develops from an accumulation of lactic acid, as well as the release of hydrogen ions during the oxidation of ferrous iron to the ferric state. Early pathologic changes are due to free iron's irritant properties, while later changes are linked to mitochondrial poisoning, free radical generation, and the initiation of lipid peroxidation of cellular membranes by free circulating iron. The culmination of these effects is gastrointestinal distress, hepatic necrosis, acute cardiovascular collapse, and potentially death.

## CLINICAL SIGNS

Clinical signs of iron toxicosis reported to the NAPCC include depression, vomiting, hematemesis, diarrhea, bloody stools, tremors, shock, and death. The clinical manifestations of acute iron toxicosis are divided into four stages. The first, 0 to 6 hr postingestion, is characterized predominantly by gastrointestinal effects. Vomiting, diarrhea, and gastrointestinal hemorrhage are a direct consequence of iron's corrosive effect on the mucosa of the stomach and intestines. The second phase, 6 to 24 hr postingestion, is a period of apparent clinical recovery. In cases of severe poisoning, the remission is only transient and soon progresses into the third stage. It is during this third period that the most serious clinical signs of iron toxicosis develop. It is characterized by severe lethargy, a recurrence of the gastrointestinal signs, metabolic acidosis, liver necrosis, cardiovascular collapse, shock, and occasionally death. With severe liver damage, coagulation deficits can also occur. The severe metabolic derangements seen in this stage are primarily due to the effects of free circulating iron. The final phase of iron toxicosis develops several weeks later when the gastrointestinal ulcerations heal, resulting in scarring and stricture formation. Even those animals who did not progress beyond the first stage are at risk for developing strictures.

## EVALUATION

Treatment of acute iron toxicosis varies with each patient and includes stabilization of vital signs, decontamination, chelation, and supportive care. The degree of intervention should be based upon a physical examination of the patient, calculation of the maximum estimated exposure, and the results of diagnostic tests and radiographs. The tablet form of iron supplements is radiodense and can often be seen even when they have been partially chewed.

The relative potential for toxicosis is determined by the amount of elemental iron ingested, regardless of the type of iron salt involved. Human data indicate doses less than 20 mg/kg are considered nontoxic, 20 to 60 mg/kg may cause mild to moderate toxicosis, and ingestions greater than 60 mg/kg are regarded as serious. These ranges appear to be applicable in the dog as well, based on cases at the NAPCC. Dosages greater than 100 to 200 mg/kg are potentially lethal unless prompt treatment is instituted. Table 2 shows the percentage of elemental iron in some of the more common iron salts. For tablet ingestions, an estimated dosage of elemental iron is made by multiplying the amount of the salt form by the percentage of iron in the salt form.

Because it is frequently difficult to accurately estimate the exposure, it is critical that the patient's clinical status be evaluated and monitored. Early clinical signs, particularly vomiting, diarrhea, and abdominal pain, warrant symptomatic and supportive care even if the estimated exposure is low. If signs of shock develop, chelation treatment is indicated regardless of the amount of iron reportedly ingested. Animals who remain asymptomatic for 6 to 8 hr are unlikely to develop clinical signs. These pets can be released and monitored at home by the owner, with instructions to return if any clinical signs occur.

In instances where a pet is symptomatic or the exposure is large, determination of serum iron concentration and iron-binding capacity (available at most human hospitals), complete blood count (CBC), serum chemistry, and abdominal radiographs are recommended. Since both normal serum iron and normal total iron-binding capacity can vary from animal to animal, it is important to measure both. Normal serum iron-binding capacity is only 25 to 35% saturated. When serum iron exceeds the binding capacity, severe systemic effects can be expected. Normal serum iron concentrations in the dog can range from 85 to 240 $\mu$g/dl. Abdominal radiographs may indicate whether a large mass of tablets remains to be absorbed. In humans, the presence of both hyperglycemia and leukocytosis often correlates with a serum iron concentration greater than 30 $\mu$g/dl.

The timing of collection is important when measuring serum iron concentrations. Iron undergoes multicompartmental kinetics, and serum concentrations can change dramatically during the first few hours following ingestion. Additionally, the variable rates at which the tablets may dissolve will also affect the serum iron concentration over time. As a result, it is recommended that serum iron concentrations be measured 4 to 6 hr postingestion for a more accurate clinical evaluation. However, if extremely large ingestions have occurred or the patient is in clinical distress, earlier sample collection may be desired.

**Table 1.** *Stage of Acute Iron Poisoning**

| | Time | Clinical Signs |
|---|---|---|
| Stage I | 0–6 hr | Nausea, vomiting, diarrhea, gastrointestinal hemorrhage |
| Stage II | 6–24 hr | Apparent recovery |
| Stage III | 12–96 hr | Vomiting, diarrhea, gastrointestinal hemorrhage metabolic acidosis, coagulation disorders, hepatic failure, cardiovascular collapse |
| Stage IV | 2–6 wks | Gastrointestinal obstruction |

*These time frames are a guide and some animals vary from these times.

**Table 2.** *Percentage of Elemental Iron in Common Iron Salts*

| Salt | % Elemental Iron |
|---|---|
| Ferric ammonium citrate | 15 |
| Ferric chloride | 34 |
| Ferric hydroxide | 63 |
| Ferric phosphate | 37 |
| Ferric pyrophosphate | 30 |
| Ferroglycine sulfate | 16 |
| Ferrous fumarate | 33 |
| Ferrous carbonate | 48 |
| Ferrous gluconate | 12 |
| Ferrous lactate | 24 |
| Ferrous sulfate (anhydrous) | 37 |
| Ferrous sulfate (hydrate) | 20 |
| Peptonized iron | 16 |

## TREATMENT

Gastrointestinal decontamination is the initial treatment step. If the animal is alert, 3% hydrogen peroxide is the NAPCC's emetic of choice in the home setting. The earlier the material is emptied from the stomach, the better chance the animal will not absorb enough to be of clinical significance. If the quantity of iron ingested is large, if emesis does not result in dislodging of the pills, or if inducing vomiting is contraindicated by the clinical status of the patient, then gastric lavage under anesthesia with a cuffed endotracheal tube in place is indicated. An emergency gastrostomy would be considered if radiographs indicate pills are adhered to the stomach wall or if there is the presence of a drug bezoar. Activated charcoal does not bind iron effectively. It has been recommended that gastric lavage with sodium phosphate or sodium bicarbonate would precipitate the iron into a nonabsorable form, but these treatments have since been shown to have little to no effect.

Restoration of fluid, electrolyte, and acid-base balance is critical for the successful management of iron toxicosis. Intravenous fluids are necessary to support circulatory volume in order to prevent or treat hypovolemic shock. As always, the amount and rate of fluids administered should be determined by calculating the animal's maintenance and replacement needs, and estimating its ongoing losses. When available, blood gas evaluations should be used to guide and assess treatment of metabolic acidosis. If severe gastrointestinal damage has occurred, it is important that the electrolytes be monitored and abnormalities corrected. Other symptomatic measures include the use of gastrointestinal protectants such as sucralfate to treat gastric and intestinal ulcerations.

Chelation therapy is indicated for only those dogs at risk of developing, or already exhibiting, signs of severe toxicosis. Deferoxamine (Desferal) has the highest affinity for iron of any known chelating agent. Treatment should be initiated as soon as possible, or at least within 12 hr of ingestion, to be of any benefit. A continuous intravenous infusion of 15 mg/kg/hr is recommended. More rapid administration has been demonstrated to precipitate cardiac arrhythmias as well as aggravate existing hypotension. If close monitoring of infusions is not possible, deferoxamine may be administered intramuscularly at 40 mg/kg every 4 to 8 hr, depending on the patient's clinical status. Chelation therapy should be continued until serum iron levels decrease below 300 $\mu$l/dl or the total iron-binding capacity, whichever is lower. Chelation of the excess iron may require 2 to 3 days of treatment.

Following recovery from the acute toxicosis, all pets should be monitored for signs of gastrointestinal obstruction, which can develop 4 to 6 weeks postingestion. If this occurs, corrective intervention or supportive management may be required.

### References and Suggested Reading

Adams HR: Drugs acting on the cardiovascular system. *In* Booth and McDonald (eds): *Veterinary Pharmacology and Therapeutics*, 6th edition. Ames, IA, Iowa State University Press, 1988, pp 478–480.

Eisen TF, Lacouture PG, and Lovejoy, FH: Iron. *In* Haddad and Winchester (eds): *Clinical Management of Poisoning and Drug Overdose*, 2nd edition. Philadelphia, WB Saunders Co, 1990, pp 1010–1017.

Gosselin RE, Smith RP, Hodge HC, and Braddock JE: Ferrous salts. *In* Clinical *Toxicology of Commercial Products*, 5th edition. 1984, pp III-179–III-185.

Goyer RA: Toxic effects of metals. *In* Amdul, Doull, and Klassen (eds): *Casarett and Doull's Toxicology. The Basic Science of Poisons*, 4th edition. New York, Pergamon Press, 1991, pp 655–656.

# MANAGEMENT OF ADVERSE REACTIONS TO PYRETHRIN AND PYRETHROID INSECTICIDES

STEVEN R. HANSEN

*Des Plaines, Illinois*

Pyrethrins occur naturally in *Chrysanthemum cinerariaefolium* and related plant species, whereas pyrethroids are synthetic compounds that vary significantly in structure and potency. Pyrethrin and pyrethroid-containing products are marketed by many manufacturers to control flea and tick infestations on dogs and cats. Pyrethroid products used on pets contain allethrin, fenvalerate, permethrin, resmethrin, or sumethrin. Premise products and insect sprays, which are not intended for topical use on dogs or cats, may include pyrethrins, cyfluthrin, cypermethrin, fenvalerate, fluvalinate, permethrin, resmethrin, tetramethrin, tralomethrin, or other pyrethroids as well as organophosphate or carbamate insecticides. Insect growth regulators such as methoprene or fenoxycarb may be included and are very unlikely to cause adverse effects.

Generally, pyrethrin or pyrethroid insecticidal products cause no adverse effects when used according to label directions. Repeated heavy applications, oral ingestions, application on unusually sensitive animals, or direct dermal application of premise products are more likely to result in adverse reactions. In many instances, product reactions are mild and self-limiting or require simple conservative therapies. Overly aggressive treatment is generally not warranted.

## MECHANISM OF ACTION

Pyrethrins and pyrethroids are fat-soluble compounds that undergo rapid metabolism and excretion following oral or dermal exposure. Synthetic pyrethroids have been developed in an attempt to increase product stability and efficacy.

Both pyrethrins and pyrethroids affect nervous tissue by altering the activity of sodium ion channels of nerves. During normal membrane depolarization sodium channels open and permit an influx of sodium ions into the nerve axon. Inactivation of the action potential occurs as the sodium conductance decreases. Potassium channels open in the axonal membrane at the peak of the action potential to permit movement of potassium out of the cell, which returns the membrane potential to the resting state. Energy-dependent sodium and potassium pumps return the membrane to the normal resting state. Pyrethrins and pyrethroids reversibly prolong sodium conductance, producing increased depolarizing afterpotentials that result in repetitive nerve firing. No permanent changes occur in affected nervous tissue. This mechanism is similar to the mechanism of the organochlorine insecticides.

## CLINICAL SIGNS OF ADVERSE REACTIONS

Call data compiled by the National Animal Poison Control Center (NAPCC) provide an overview of adverse reactions as reported by animal owners and veterinarians in dogs, cats, and other species to pyrethrin/pyrethroid insecticidal products (Trammel and Buck, 1990). Clinical signs reported to the NAPCC after using pyrethrin/pyrethroid products may be caused by the active ingredient, carrier, or synergists or may be unrelated and actually result from disease, injury, or exposure to other insecticides or toxicants.

Combined clinical signs in all reported species to the NAPCC from most to least for all routes of pyrethrin exposure (dermal, oral, inhalation) are depression, hypersalivation, muscle tremors, vomiting, ataxia, dyspnea, and anorexia. Less common symptoms from most to least include hyperthermia, hypothermia, weakness, and seizures. Clinical signs reported for fenvalerate from most to least are vomiting, hypersalivation, muscle tremors, depression, seizures, anorexia, ataxia, and diarrhea. Most exposures involving fenvalerate also included the insect repellent diethyltoluamide (DEET). Clinical signs reported following permethrin exposures are muscle tremors, depression, ataxia, vomiting, and seizures/anorexia. Permethrin toxicoses more commonly occur in cats treated with products labeled for use on dogs only. Exposures resulting in death have been reported with both pyrethrins and pyrethroids. In such situations a complete and thorough diagnostic investigation is required to rule out other causes. In many cases, gross product misuse, diseases, or other toxicant exposures can be identified as the actual cause of death.

Salivation is considered a minor side effect in cats and results from oral sensory stimulation by pyrethrins/pyrethroids. To complicate diagnosis, some cats will salivate when stressed or when sprayed with water. Cats also occasionally exhibit ear flicking, paw shaking, and repeated contractions of the superficial cutaneous muscles. These clinical signs may result from agitation or from topical stimulation of peripheral sensory nerves in the skin. Ataxia, especially in kittens and puppies, may result from heavy applications of products containing isopropyl alcohol. Animal owners often confuse paw flicking and hyperesthesia with muscle tremors and seizures and heavy salivation with vomiting.

## TOXICITY

The toxicities of pyrethrins and pyrethroid compounds vary considerably but are much lower than toxicities of organophosphate or carbamate insecticides. Frequently, animal owners will heavily apply pyrethrin/pyrethroid sprays to cats and small dogs, and this gross overuse of products can occasionally result in adverse symptoms. Overapplication of products on cats is more likely to result in adverse reactions because cats have a greater surface area/body weight ratio, making it easier to overdose a small pet but difficult to overdose a large pet. Long-haired cat breeds also have a greater coat surface area than short-haired breeds, and when soaked will retain on their haircoat a much larger dose. Idiosyncratic or allergic hypersensitivity reactions can rarely happen at low dosages.

Appropriate application quantities of pyrethrin-containing sprays are 3.3 to 9.9 ml/kg or 0.5 to 1.5 ounces on a 4.5-kg pet. Many hand-held trigger sprayers deliver approximately 1.5 ml per pump, resulting in a general application rate of one to two squirts per pound of body weight on small pets. The veterinarian is encouraged to consult the manufacturer for specific recommended application rates. Adverse reactions are unlikely when products are applied in this manner.

If a professional pest control operator has treated the house, the operator should be contacted for information on the exact compound, final dilution, amount used, and areas treated. During premise treatment, animals, including birds and reptiles, should be removed and not returned until the areas have dried, and fish tanks should be sealed with plastic wrap with the aerators disconnected.

## DIAGNOSIS

Laboratory analyses to diagnose pyrethrin/pyrethroid exposure or toxicosis are not routinely available. Interpretation of tissue residues, when obtained, is difficult and of little value except to confirm exposure. Metabolites have not yet been identified in dogs or cats for pyrethrins or pyrethroids. Analysis for insect repellents, synergists, or isopropanol (when used as a carrier) may be a more reliable indicator of exposure (Dorman et al., 1990; Mount, Moller, and Cook, 1991).

Marked neurologic symptoms of several days' duration are inconsistent with pyrethrins/pyrethroids, but do occur following accidental or intentional exposure to organophosphate insecticides. Many dips containing organophosphates labeled for dogs only are available through pet stores, feed stores, and veterinary clinics. Because flea control requires the use of products to treat the pet, yard, and house, organophosphate insecticides can be easily misused, resulting in tremors, weakness, and anorexia lasting days to weeks (see "Management of Organophosphate/Carbamate Insecticide Toxicoses," this volume, p 245). Cats inappropriately exposed to the organophosphate chlorpyrifos can remain anorexic for days to weeks and during this period will have reduced whole blood cholinesterase enzyme activity (See *CVT XI*, p 188). Correct use of organophosphate insecticides on pets and in the house and yard will not result in adverse symptoms in cats or dogs if the areas are allowed sufficient time to dry.

Due to the similarity of some clinical signs between organophosphate/carbamate insecticides and pyrethrin/pyrethroid insecticides including hypersalivation, vomiting, diarrhea and muscle tremors, a whole blood cholinesterase is a recommended laboratory test. Whole blood cholinesterase, a sensitive indicator of organophosphate/carbamate exposure, is not depressed by pyrethroid insecticides (Dorman et al., 1990). Samples should be submitted to a diagnostic laboratory that has established normals for cats and dogs to permit a meaningful interpretation.

Even if assay methodology is available, interpretation of pyrethrin/pyrethroid tissue residues is limited to confirming exposure because of a lack of reference values, relating signs, dose, and tissue residue values. A presumptive diagnosis of pyrethrin/pyrethroid toxicosis can only be made if clinical signs, dose, and exposure history are consistent. Exposures to other classes of insecticides or toxicants as well as infectious diseases or trauma must be ruled out. Reduced cholinesterase activity is suggestive of an exposure to an organophosphate or carbamate insecticide.

## TREATMENT

A detailed history is crucial and should include exposure dose, onset, and duration of clinical signs as well as information on the previous use of flea control products on the pet and in the premises. Maintenance of a normal body temperature is important because hypothermia, induced by heavy spray applications, bathing or dipping, can enhance the effects of pyrethrins/pyrethroids on nervous tissue. Sedatives should also be avoided or used with caution in cats prior to dipping, because sedatives may further reduce body temperature. Hyperthermia may occur as a result of muscle fasiculations or seizures and should also be controlled.

Most cats who develop only hypersalivation following topical exposure to a pyrethrin product return to normal without veterinary care. To reduce grooming and therefore hypersalivation, the animal owner can dry the pet with a towel that has been warmed in a clothes dryer and then brush thoroughly with a grooming brush. The affected animal will groom less, feel better, and return to normal quickly. Once the patient is stabilized, a mild detergent bath is recommended to reduce further dermal absorption and ingestion from grooming. Recommended detergents include liquid hand dishwashing products, but not electric dishwasher products.

Oral ingestions of a pyrethrin/pyrethroid can be treated with an emetic such as 3% hydrogen peroxide (2 ml/kg, maximum of 45 ml, PO) given after a moistened meal if treatment is begun within 1 hr and the animal is asymptomatic (Beasley and Dorman, 1990). Activated charcoal (2 gm/kg, PO; see *CVT XI*, p 173) should be given with a cathartic such as magnesium sulfate (Epsom salts, 250 mg/kg, PO) or, preferably, 70% sorbitol (3 ml/kg, PO). Sorbitol is available over the counter in many pharmacies. Because of the grooming habits of cats, and because there is potential enterohepatic recirculation of some pyrethrin/pyrethroid compounds, activated charcoal may be of benefit in cases of dermal exposures showing marked neurologic symptoms (Valentine, 1990).

Seizure activity is uncommon following exposures to pyrethrins but may result from high doses of permethrin or fenvalerate. Clients may interpret an agitated or shivering cat as "seizuring." Diazepam (0.5 to 1.0 mg/kg IV) will usually control muscle tremors resulting from pyrethrin/pyrethroid overdose. Phenobarbital may be used if seizure activity is not adequately controlled by diazepam.

Atropine sulfate is not antidotal when treating pyrethrin/pyrethroid adverse reactions and has been shown to have no effect on increasing survival in laboratory animals. A test dose of atropine sulfate (0.01 to 0.02 mg/kg, IV) can help differentiate organophosphate/carbamate from pyrethrin/pyrethroid toxicosis. A test dose of atropine sulfate will not significantly reverse cholinergic symptoms induced by an organophosphate/carbamate insecticide overdose such as hypersalivation, bradycardia, respiratory depression, or miosis. If necessary, low doses of atropine sulfate (0.02 to 0.04 mg/kg, IM or SC) can be used to control hypersalivation associated with pyrethrin exposures. Excessive use of atropine sulfate should be strictly avoided. Repeated high doses of atropine sulfate (0.2 mg/kg), as would be appropriate for organophosphate or carbamate toxicity, can result in central nervous system (CNS) stimulation and tachycardia.

Most pets recover from adverse reactions to dermal applications of pyrethrin products within 24 hr. Recovery time may be longer for a pyrethroid toxicosis. Increased salivation alone does not warrant aggressive treatment and is usually self-limiting. Some animal owners confuse heavy salivation with vomiting. Atropine sulfate is not antidotal or necessary. If the animal is vomiting, lethargic, having diarrhea or protracted salivation, a detergent bath is warranted. Animals showing muscle tremors must be differentiated from shivering due to hypothermia, ear and paw flicking due to agitation or from dermal sensations induced by direct pyrethrin skin contact and should be managed with diazepam, activated charcoal, and fluid support. Cholinesterase enzyme activity is not reduced by pyrethrin/pyrethroid insecticides and can be used to identify exposure to an organophosphate or carbamate insecticide. Animals not markedly improved within 24 hr should be further evaluated for other causes or predisposing conditions.

Subsequent applications of pyrethrin/pyrethroids to sensitive pets should be reduced (use 1 or 2 squirts of most spray products per pound body weight) or a towel should be sprayed and wrapped around the pet, leaving the head exposed for 15 min. Alternatively, a grooming brush can be sprayed and the product brushed evenly into the haircoat. These application methods can reduce salivation in cats that demonstrate no other symptoms.

## References and Suggested Reading

Beasley VR and Dorman DC: Management of toxicosis. Vet Clin N Am [Small Anim Pract] 20:307, 1990.
  *Detailed chapter on decontamination procedures.*
Dorman DC, Buck WB, Trammel HL, et al: Fenvalerate/N,N-diethyl-m-tolumide (Deet) toxicosis in two cats. J Am Vet Med Assoc 196:100, 1990.
  *Case report of pyrethroid product toxicosis in cats.*
Mount ME, Moller G, and Cook J: Clinical illness associated with a commercial tick and flea product in dogs and cats. Vet Hum Toxicol 33:19, 1991.
  *Summary of research conducted on commercial pyrethroid product demonstrating adverse reactions.*
Trammel HL and Buck WB: *Tenth Annual Report of the Illinois Animal Poison Information Center.* Dubuque, Kendall-Hunt 1990.
  *Summary of call data from 1988 received by the Illinois Animal Poison Information Center, now the National Animal Poison Control Center.*
Valentine WM: Pyrethrin and pyrethroid insecticides. Vet Clin of N Am [Small Anim Pract] 20:375, 1990.
  *Detailed chapter on mechanism of action of pyrethrins and pyrethroids.*

# MANAGEMENT OF ORGANOPHOSPHATE AND CARBAMATE INSECTICIDE TOXICOSES

STEVEN R. HANSEN
*Des Plaines, Illinois*

Organophosphate and carbamate insecticides are commonly formulated for use on dogs and cats and in the house and yard for control of fleas, ticks, and mites. Agricultural and household products may also contain organophosphate or carbamate insecticides and must be considered as possible sources of insecticide exposure. As a result of the wide use of organophosphate- and carbamate-containing products, toxicoses can occur from accidental exposure, intentional misuse, and rarely from idiosyncratic or allergic hypersensitivity reactions in dogs and cats. However, the use of an insecticide product alone is rarely sufficient to support a diagnosis of insecticide toxicosis. Correct interpretation of exposure dose, onset of clinical signs, duration of clinical signs, previous insecticidal use, diagnostic data, and response to therapy is important. A basic understanding of the mechanism of action of organophosphate and carbamate insecticides and adverse reactions in animals will help the clinician diagnose and manage toxicoses. Responsible use of pesticides will help ensure that animal toxicoses are avoided whenever possible. Organophosphate and carbamate compounds differ markedly in structure, but toxicoses will be considered together because of similarities in clinical signs, diagnosis, and treatment.

## MECHANISM OF ACTION

Both organophosphate and carbamate compounds produce effects on nerves through the inhibition of the enzyme acetylcholinesterase. Normal activity of acetylcholinesterase is to hydrolyze the neurotransmitter acetylcholine in the synaptic space, thereby stopping nerve impulses. Carbamate insecticides reversibly inhibit acetylcholinesterase, whereas organophoshate insecticides permanently disable acetylcholinesterase by an irreversible binding known as aging.

Clinical signs of toxicoses are usually correlated with overriding stimulation of parasympathetic pathways, but may also result from sympathetic stimulation. Specifically, acetylcholine stimulates nicotinic receptors of the somatic nervous system, parasympathetic preganglionic nicotinic and muscarinic postganglionic receptors, and sympathetic preganglionic nicotinic receptors. The effector organ of the somatic nervous system is skeletal muscle. Effector organs of the parasympathetic nervous system are the iris, cardiac muscle, blood vessels, smooth muscle of the lung and gastrointestinal tract, and exocrine glands. Effector organs of the sympathetic nervous system can be stimulated through preganglionic cholinergic neuron stimulation of postganglionic adrenergic neurons in the adrenal gland, cardiac muscle, iris, blood vessels, smooth muscle of the lung and gastrointestinal tract, and exocrine glands. The degree to which the parasympathetic or sympathetic nervous pathways are stimulated is a function of many factors and helps to explain the mix of clinical signs that can occur.

## CLINICAL SIGNS OF TOXICOSES

Flea, tick, and other insect control products contain many different active ingredients including organophosphate or carbamate insecticides designed to kill during various life cycle stages, and in the case of fleas and cockroaches, may be combined with insect growth regulators. As a result, rarely does a homeowner, pest control operator (PCO), or veterinarian use a single product or use products exclusive to one manufacturer when designing an integrated pest management plan. Therefore, the clinician must investigate all premise, house, yard, and agricultural products in the vicinity regardless of whether the animal owner feels the pet was exposed.

Toxicoses from organophosphate or carbamate insecticides can occur in dogs and cats when yard or agricultural formulations are ingested or misused, when dips are incorrectly diluted, when cholinesterase-inhibiting compounds are used in conjunction with other topical or systemic organophosphates, when products labeled for dogs only are used on cats, or when unusually sensitive pets are exposed. Commonly, chlorpyrifos formulations are inappropriately used on cats and can result in acute and/or chronic toxicoses (Fikes, 1992; see *CVT XI*, p 188). Dips containing chlorpyrifos or phosmet, which rarely produce toxicoses when used as labeled, are available through veterinary clinics, pet stores, and feed stores and may be applied inappropriately on cats.

Clinical signs of organophosphate or carbamate toxicoses are commonly a result of parasympathetic stimulation. Clinical signs, include vomiting, depression, hypersalivation, muscle tremors, diarrhea, ataxia, anorexia, hyperthermia, dyspnea, seizure, weakness, and death (Trammel and Buck, 1990). Other classic symptoms include miosis and bradycardia. Chronic anorexia, muscle weakness, and twitching can occur in cats with or without episodes of acute toxicoses. Because of potential stimulation of the sympathetic nervous system, as described earlier, the lack of some classic parasympathetic symptoms or evidence of sympathetic stimulation such as tachycardia should not necessarily be considered inconsistent. Agricultural products containing carbamates such as carbofuran and flybaits containing the carbamate methomyl can produce rapid onset of seizures and respiratory failure and should be treated aggressively without delay.

## TOXICITY

Examples of organophosphate compounds used for insect control on or around pets include chlorpyrifos, cythioate, diazinon, dichlorvos, fenthion, phosmet, tetrachlorvinphos, and safrotin. Carbamate insecticides include carbaryl, propoxur, methomyl, and bendiocarb. Individual compound toxicity is variable and is highly dependent on route of exposure and dose.

Premise treatments applied by PCOs often contain chlorpyrifos or safrotin. Commonly, application dilutions are 0.2 to 1.0% active ingredient in water. Flea treatments applied by PCOs are broadcast over the entire area of the house, whereas cockroach applications are limited to baseboards and cabinets. All pets should be strictly removed from the premise when insecticidal products are applied and not returned until the premises are dry. Residues that can be dislodged from properly treated carpets allowed to dry will not induce toxicoses in companion animals. Cats exposed to wet carpeting during or immediately after organophosphate application are at risk and should undergo basic dermal decontamination procedures immediately. Generally, PCOs are cautious around pets and knowledgeable regarding insecticides and should be contacted to obtain exact details regarding pesticide applications.

Agricultural products may also represent risk to rural pets or wandering pets and may include the organophosphates chlorpyrifos, phosmet, coumaphos, diazinon, dichlorvos, fenthion, fonofos, malathion, parathion, naled, ronnel, or carbamates such as carbofuran (Osweiler et al., 1985). Many agricultural organophosphates are no longer available; however, these products may remain in sheds, garages, or barns for years and continue to be a potential hazard.

## DIAGNOSIS

Tentative diagnosis of organophosphate or carbamate toxicosis is made when clinical signs and exposure history are consistent with toxicosis. Reduction to less than 25% of normal in whole blood, retinal, or brain cholinesterase activity is a reliable indicator of organophosphate exposure and may suggest toxicosis. In live animals, whole blood cholinesterase determination is recommended. Consult the diagnostic laboratory prior to sample submission. Cats are especially sensitive to cholinesterase depression without concomitant clinical signs and may remain clinically normal with whole blood cholinesterase values less than 10% of normal. Therefore, whole blood cholinesterase depression alone is not diagnostic for toxicosis unless combined with consistent exposure history and clinical signs.

Whole blood cholinesterase determinations should be part of the diagnostic work-up for cats experiencing anorexia and weakness lasting days to weeks of unknown cause. Whole blood cholinesterase will remain depressed for the duration of the anorectic syndrome. Dogs generally do not experience chronic organophosphate toxicoses similar to cats. Carbamate insecticides will not cause chronic anorexia and weakness in cats. Tissue analysis for organophosphate and carbamate insecticides can provide additional evidence of exposure, but further interpretation of tissue concentrations is not generally meaningful. In live animals, analysis of fur is helpful in identifying compounds applied to pets when accidental use of an organophosphate is suspected as evidenced by whole blood cholinesterase depression.

## TREATMENT

A detailed history including previous pesticide use, active ingredients, clinical signs, onset of clinical signs, duration of clinical signs, and exposure dose are important. Vomitus or gastric lavage washings should be frozen and saved for possible analysis and for legal reasons.

Correct decontamination procedures are important when managing toxicoses (Beasley and Dorman, 1990). If the patient has ingested an organophosphate or carbamate product within the past 2 hr and is asymptomatic, then an emetic such as 3% hydrogen peroxide (2 ml/kg, PO, maximum of 45 ml) should be administered after feeding a moistened meal. Emesis from hydrogen peroxide is reliable if there is adequate ingesta in the stomach. Induction of emesis following ingestion of liquid organophosphate products should be avoided due to potential aspiration and lung damage from petroleum distillate solvents. Induction of emesis following the ingestion of carbamates such as methomyl should be avoided or attempted with caution due to the potential for rapid onset of seizures. Further decontamination from oral ingestions should include activated charcoal (2.0 gm/kg, PO, or stomach tube; see *CVT XI*, p 173) mixed with a cathartic such as 70% sorbitol (3.0 ml/kg) diluted with water and given by dose syringe or preferably stomach tube. Symptomatic patients recently ingesting significant quantities of an insecticidal product should be anesthetized and a gastric lavage performed using a large-bore stomach tube with a cuffed endotracheal tube in place using repeated washings of an activated charcoal slurry 15 to 40 times or until no more ingesta is evident. If the time since ingestion is more than a couple of hours, activated charcoal and sorbitol without induction of emesis or gastric lavage may be superior because the risk of anesthesia may be greater than the benefits of minimal recovery of insecticide from the stomach.

If the pet is presented seizuring, intravenous diazepam (Valium) or phenobarbital and atropine sulfate (0.2 mg/kg, one fourth IV, remaining SC) should be administered immediately. Atropine sulfate is administered as needed to control life-threatening clinical signs such as respiratory depression, bronchoconstriction, and bradycardia. Atropine sulfate should not be used unless clinical signs are present, and the dose and frequency should be titrated to control muscarinic signs. Care should be taken not to overuse atropine sulfate. Atropine sulfate toxicosis can result in tachycardia and CNS stimulation. Oxygen or ventilator therapy (see *CVT XI*, p 98) may be indicated until respirations return to normal.

Clinical signs, such as muscle fasiculations, resulting from nicotinic receptor stimulation by an organophosphate, can be reduced using pralidoxime chloride (Protopam, Wyeth-Ayerst Laboratories, New York, NY) administered at 10 to 15 mg/kg, IM or SC, given two to three times daily and continued until recovery. Pralidoxime chloride is most beneficial when started within 24 hr of exposure. In situations where dermal exposures to organophosphates have occurred for several days involving anorectic, weak cats, pralidoxime chloride may still be of benefit. Pralidoxime chloride should be continued for 36 hr before ceasing administration due to lack of improvement. Chlorpyrifos-exposed chronic, anorectic cats may begin eating after two to three doses of pralidoxime chloride. Reconstituted bottles of pralidoxime chloride kept refrigerated and wrapped in tin foil have been successfully used for up to 2 weeks.

Once the patient is stabilized, a detergent bath using a hand dishwashing detergent is indicated in cases of dermal exposure to organophosphate or carbamate products to reduce further cutaneous absorption or ingestion from grooming. Activated charcoal may be of benefit even in cases of dermal exposure due to biliary excretion and intestinal reabsorption of some organophosphate compounds or metabolites. Repeated doses of activated charcoal should be administered at 1 gm/kg at 6- to 8-hr intervals or until improvement is evident. Sorbitol should continue to be administered with activated charcoal to avoid constipation unless diarrhea develops.

Supportive care such as intravenous fluids, nutritional management, and maintenance of normal body temperature are critical for recovery. The animal owner must understand that adequate nursing care, especially nutritional support, may be needed for 1 to 4 weeks and complete recovery may take longer. Chronic anorectic cats treated in this manner have an excellent chance of recovery without permanent neurologic dysfunction.

Consulting an animal poison control center staffed around-the-clock with veterinarians trained in veterinary toxicology such as the National Animal Poison Control Center at the College of Veterinary Medicine, University of Illinois, Urbana, IL can be crucial for product identification, treatment, and diagnostic information. Insecticide product manufacturers can be a further source of information.

## References and Suggested Reading

Beasley VR and Dorman DC: Management of toxicoses. Vet Clin North Am [Small Anim Pract] 20:307, 1990.
Fikes JD: Feline chlorpyrifos toxicosis. *In* Kirk RW and Bonagura JD (eds): *Current Veterinary Therapy XI: Small Animal Practice.* Philadelphia, WB Saunders Co, 1992, pp 188–191.
    *Clinically oriented material regarding diagnosis and management of chlorpyrifos toxicoses in cats.*
Fikes JD: Organophosphorus and carbamate insecticides. Vet Clin North Am [Small Anim Pract] 20:353, 1990.
    *Detailed chapter on mechanism, diagnosis, and management of organophosphorus and carbamate toxicoses in small animals.*
Munro NB, Shugart LR, Watson AP, et al: Cholinesterase activity in domestic animals as a potential biomonitor for nerve agent and other organophosphate exposure. J Am Vet Med Assoc 199:103, 1991.
    *Review article on cholinesterase determination and normals between species.*
Osweiler GD, Carson T, Buck WW, et al: *Clinical and Diagnostic Veterinary Toxicology,* 3rd edition. Dubuque, Kendall/Hunt Publishing Co, 1985, pp 298–317.
    *Management of organophosphorus and carbamate insecticides with extensive product listings.*
Trammel HL and Buck WB: *Tenth Annual Report of the Illinois Animal Poison Information Center.* Dubuque, Kendall-Hunt, 1990.
    *Summary of call data from 1988 received by the Illinois Animal Poison Information Center, now known as the National Animal Poison Control Center.*

# LAWN CARE PRODUCTS

DIANE F. GERKEN
*Columbus, Ohio*

Health concerns about the use of lawn care products have received considerable media attention in the past 10 years. As a result, public perception is that these products are primarily pesticides and that these products are very toxic or pose a significant health threat to humans and animals. Scientific and forensic animal data do not support the perception that exposure to these products results in a significant number of confirmed intoxications. Information about product use and actual small animal intoxications is not readily available to most veterinarians; therefore, some practitioners may rely on anecdotal reports to form their opinions about the products.

In the experience of this author, veterinarians often pose similar questions about lawn care products. Hence, the "most-often-asked-question" format was chosen for this article. Although questions and answers about specific products have not been included, more specific information about individual products and the actual risk assessment process is available.

## WHAT ARE THE MOST COMMON CHEMICALS USED IN LAWN CARE?

The most commonly used lawn care chemicals are listed in Table 1 under the appropriate use. These chemicals usually are formulated in liquid or granules for application. Liquid formulations are often purchased as a concentrate and must be diluted with water by the homeowner or commercial company before application. Typically, a liquid application for the entire lawn will consist of more than 90% water, approximately 5 to 7% fertilizer, and less than 1% total pesticides. Liquid spot treatment products are usually more concentrated but are used sparingly. Granular applications usually contain 30% or less fertilizer and less than 5% total pesticides. Typical product formulations contain fertilizer only, fertilizer plus one or more pesticides or, infrequently, one or more pesticides only.

## HOW CAN AN ANIMAL BECOME EXPOSED TO LAWN CARE PRODUCTS?

The two most common routes of exposure are oral and dermal. Exposure to liquid concentrates and granules is possible with homeowner storage. Exposure to the diluted liquids is possible during application or before foliar drying. Exposure to applied granular material usually is the result of spills during loading equipment, spreader equipment failure, or spreading granules on nonlawn surfaces such as driveways and sidewalks.

**Table 1.**   *Most Commonly Used Lawn Care Chemicals*

| Fertilizers | Fungicides |
|---|---|
| Polyphosphates | Iprodione |
| Urea/reaction products | Thiophanate methyl |
| Potassium chloride | |
| Ammonium phosphates | |
| Sulfates | |

| Insecticides | Herbicides |
|---|---|
| Diazinon | 2,4-Dichlorphenoxyacetic acid |
| Chlorpyrifos | MCPP |
| Isofenphos | MCPA |
| Carbaryl | Dicamba |
| Cyfluthrin | Pendimethalin |
| | Triclopyr |
| | Glyphosate |

## DOES EXPOSURE RESULT IN TOXICOSIS?

Intoxication from these products is dose related. In most cases, exposure will not result in any adverse effects, but there are some exposures that could. Consumption of liquid concentrates while mixing or granules in storage is more likely to result in toxicosis than any other common exposure. This is because of the higher chemical concentration and total amount of product available to the animal. Consumption to excessive amounts of granules such as in driveways or from spills may result in mild clinical signs.

Oral or dermal exposure to lawns where diluted liquids or granules are properly applied generally are of negligible risk. This statement is made when considering (1) the low chemical concentration of the liquid application, (2) the large area of application, (3) low liquid volumes applied per unit area of lawn, (4) low percentage of dislodgeable chemical residue from foliage, (5) granular deposition in the thatch layer, and (6) less than 100% dermal and oral bioavailability in determining the exposed dose. The exposed dose is then often compared to the no observable effect level (NOEL) determined in chronic experimental studies and other experimental forensic data.

## DO LAWN CARE CHEMICALS CAUSE CANCER IN ANIMALS?

Long-term chronic experimental studies in dogs do not support the conclusion that the chemicals identified in Table 1 are carcinogenic. The only scientific data that are in conflict with that conclusion is the much-publicized work of Hayes et al. (1992). It is the author's opinion that serious flaws in this epidemiologic study have negated the conclusions of this study. Unfortunately, there are no other epidemiologic studies.

## WHAT INFORMATION DO I NEED TO STRONGLY SUSPECT LAWN CARE CHEMICAL TOXICITY?

The clinical signs and clinical history must be compatible with specific chemical exposure. In the case of death, a postmortem examination should reveal the appropriate chemically related target tissues, and gross and histopathologic findings. The amount of chemical in the exposure must be sufficient to cause adverse effects. Any clinical pathologic findings should be compatible also. An example would be an alleged acute organophosphate-related death and depression of brain cholinesterase. Exposure alone is not sufficient evidence to diagnose intoxication. Currently, in most cases, there is not enough information available for these chemicals to determine an expected lethal or toxic concentration in tissues or body fluids. Therefore, the analytical finding of a chemical in animal tissues or body fluids is evidence of exposure but not necessarily intoxication.

## IS THERE A TOXICOLOGIC CONCERN ABOUT INERT INGREDIENTS?

Since the majority of the applied liquid products are soluble in water and are diluted when mixed with water, inert ingredients in the products themselves are of little concern. In general, the inert ingredients in granular products are also not of toxicologic concern.

## IS THERE A CONCERN ABOUT MIXTURES?

There are not many good experimental studies using standard mixtures of these products. Because most of these products have different mechanisms of producing toxicity and based on current experimental work with mixtures, it does not appear that most mixtures result in toxicologic potentiation or synergy.

## WHY DOES POSTING OF LAWN APPLICATIONS OCCUR?

In many states and localities, posting of lawn care product applications is required by law. Posting serves as a notification that lawn care applications occurred. It is part of the community's right to know. Posting is not related to the toxic potential of the materials used.

## WHY IS IT RECOMMENDED THAT ANIMALS AND HUMANS STAY OFF LAWNS UNTIL LIQUID APPLICATIONS DRY?

It is recommended that animals and humans stay off of the lawn until the liquid application is dry to limit exposure. As with any chemical (e.g., lawn care product, detergent), there should be an effort by the public to limit exposure. The amount of chemical that is dislodgeable decreases as the liquid dries. The overall difference between the actual exposure dose and a toxic dose is changed little by foliar drying; therefore, the risk is still negligible without drying.

### References and Suggested Reading

Hayes HM, Tarone RE, Cantor KP, Jessen CR, McCurin DM, and Richardson RC: Case-control study of canine malignant lymphoma: Positive association with dog owner's use of 2,4-dichlorphenoxyacetic acid herbicides. J Natl Cancer Inst 83:1226, 1991.

# ILLICIT DRUG INTOXICATION IN DOGS

GENEVIEVE A. DUMONCEAUX

*Davis, California*

Illicit chemicals are encountered daily in the United States. Due to their curious nature, dogs are the domestic animal at highest risk of exposure. Pets, as well as working police dogs (Dumonceaux and Beasley, 1990), can become victims of toxic or fatal exposures to illicit drugs. The most dangerous aspect of such exposures is the rapid onset of effects from commonly encountered agents. Familiarity with agents commonly abused in the community is helpful, since detailed histories are often difficult to obtain. Owners are usually reluctant to offer information about illegal substances in their homes. Prompt action to minimize the effects of the ingested agents increases the chance of recovery.

## MARIJUANA

Marijuana (*Cannabis sativa*) can be found in households in all socioeconomic areas. The alkaloid tetrahydrocannabinol (THC) is the primary active principle in the *Cannabis* plant (Godbold, Hawkins, and Woodward, 1979). Its effects on dogs are similar to those in humans. Signs may include behavioral changes, ataxia, incoordination, muscle weakness, conjunctival injection, mydriasis, depression, stupor, vomiting, increased pulse rate, decreased blood pressure, hypothermia, hyperthermia, hyperesthesia, hyperactivity, tachypnea, bradycardia, tremors, and seizures (Godbold, Hawkins, and Woodward, 1979; Kisseberth and Trammel, 1990). The therapeutic index of THC is very high; therefore, death from acute intoxication is rare (Kisseberth and Trammel, 1990).

The cannabinoids are rapidly absorbed by oral and inhalation exposure. They are metabolized by the liver and undergo enterohepatic recirculation. As a result, only about 6 to 20% of an oral dose reaches the systemic circulation (Coppock, Mostrom, and Lillie, 1989). First aid for exposed dogs consists of inducing emesis early (within 1 hr of ingestion) before clinical signs of a toxicosis develop. This can be accomplished by crushing one tablet of apomorphine hydrochloride (Lilly) and adding 0.5 ml of sterile water. Administer one to three drops of the suspension into the conjunctival sac. When vomiting is finished, the eye should be rinsed thoroughly with sterile water or sterile saline. Alternative (although less effective) methods of inducing emesis are with 3% hydrogen peroxide at a dose of approximately 1 ml/kg body weight PO (repeated once if necessary), or syrup of ipecac (Roxane) administered at a dose of 2.2 ml/kg body weight PO (do not repeat). If vomiting continues past the desired effect, an antiemetic can be administered to control emesis so that

further therapeutic measures can be instituted. When vomiting has ceased, 1 to 4 gm of activated charcoal per kilogram body weight (Toxiban, Vetamix) and 1.25 ml/5 kg of a 10 to 20% saline cathartic solution, such as sodium sulfate (Glauber's salt) or magnesium sulfate (Epsom salt) in water, should be administered orally or by gastric intubation (Dumonceaux and Beasley, 1990).

Activated charcoal is used to bind the agent in the digestive tract, lessening its systemic absorption. After the onset of clinical signs, emesis may be contraindicated. However, activated charcoal and a cathartic are still highly recommended. Two or three doses of activated charcoal given several hours apart may be necessary to interrupt the enterohepatic recirculation and shorten the syndrome.

Treatment after the initial detoxification procedures is mainly supportive and based on clinical signs. Recovery is usually good with supportive care. Monitoring should continue until signs of toxicosis are resolved. This may take up to 3 days.

## COCAINE

Cocaine is frequently encountered in today's society. It is rapidly absorbed from mucous membranes, including the membranes lining the oral cavity, gastrointestinal tract, and nasal passages. It is rapidly metabolized by the liver and excreted mainly in the urine. Effects are related to central nervous system (CNS) excitation, peripheral vasoconstriction, hyperthermia secondary to the vasoconstriction, and increased muscular activity. Death results from respiratory arrest, cardiac arrest, and often hyperthermia (Catravas and Waters, 1981; Kisseberth and Trammel, 1990).

Detoxification should be instituted quickly prior to clinical signs of toxicosis. Emesis, activated charcoal, and a saline cathartic should be instituted immediately to facilitate removal of the toxicants from the gastrointestinal tract. However, significant absorption may occur rapidly before detoxification can be instituted. Sedation or general anesthesia followed by enterogastric lavage may be safer and more beneficial than emesis because of the highly toxic nature and rapid onset of effects of this drug. When entire bags of the drug are ingested, endoscopy or surgery to remove the plastic bags of the concentrated drugs may be of value (Dumonceaux and Beasley, 1990).

In addition to limiting gastrointestinal uptake, steps should be taken to combat the effects of systemically absorbed cocaine. Experimental pretreatment with chlorpromazine (Elkins-Sinn) has been shown to antagonize many of the systemic effects of the cocaine. It may also decrease the incidence of seizures and help control hyperthermia (Catravas and Waters, 1981). Tracheal intubation and oxygen or a resuscitator bag (AMBU Bag, AMBU Inc) and face mask may be beneficial in cases for which respiratory support is needed. A mechanical respirator may be necessary with severe or prolonged respiratory depression.

If seizure activity is evident, 0.5 to 1 mg of diazepam (Valium, Schein) per kilogram body weight should be administered IV (to effect) to a maximal total dose of 20 mg (Dumonceaux and Beasley, 1990; Kisseberth and Trammel, 1990). Body temperature should be monitored closely for the duration of the dog's hospitalization. If hyperthermia develops as a result of seizure activity or as a primary effect of the cocaine, measures to decrease the core body temperature by external means should be instituted immediately.

The use of propranolol (Inderal, Wyeth-Ayerst) for the treatment of cocaine overdosages has been somewhat controversial (Catravas and Waters, 1981). The cardiovascular effects of cocaine are usually short lived and usually without rhythm disturbances other than tachycardia (Adams, 1988). In human cases, the use of propranolol is reserved for treating life-threatening (tachy)arrhythmias.

## NARCOTICS

There are several types of narcotics used legally and illegally. Heroin is a popular illegal narcotic in this country. It is a morphine derivative and a favorite opiate of morphine addicts (Gosselin, Smith, and Hodge, 1984).

Narcotics exert effects on the gastrointestinal tract, cardiovascular system, and central nervous system. Early clinical signs related to ingestion of narcotics include drowsiness, ataxia, decreased sensory and pain perception, transient excitation, vomiting, defecation, and increased respiratory rate. Later clinical signs may include delirium, convulsions, miosis, coma, respiratory depression, and a marked decrease in blood pressure. Pulmonary edema often occurs in fatal cases. Death is most often attributed to respiratory arrest and can occur within 12 hr (Gosselin, Smith, and Hodge, 1984; Kisseberth and Trammel, 1990).

Treatment should include early induction of emesis (before signs develop), or enterogastric lavage under general anesthesia, followed by oral or gastric administration of activated charcoal and a saline or sorbitol cathartic (see "Marijuana," above). A patent airway should be maintained.

Naloxone (Narcan, DuPont Multisource Products) is the most effective and reliable antagonist for most narcotic agents. This should be given at a dose of 0.01 to 0.02 mg/kg IV, IM, or SC to effect. Because the effects of many narcotics outlast the effects of this antagonist, naloxone should be repeated as needed to antagonize the effects of the narcotic (Easom and Lovejoy, 1983; Dumonceaux and Beasley, 1990). If several doses are

administered with little response, its efficacy is unlikely. Alternatively, the dog may not have been exposed to an opioid (Dumonceaux and Beasley, 1990; Gosselin, Smith, and Hodge, 1984).

Additional measures for treatment of dogs following narcotic ingestion involve: (1) constant monitoring, (2) respiratory support, (3) seizure control with diazepam, and (4) intravenous fluid therapy as dictated by the dog's hydration and cardiovascular status.

## AMPHETAMINES

Amphetamine (d,l-$\alpha$-methylphenethylamine) has some adrenergic properties. It is a noncatechol, sympathomimetic amine that has greater CNS stimulant activity than epinephrine and other catecholamines (Litovitz, 1983). The term "amphetamine" also refers to a whole group of amphetamine derivatives.

Amphetamines are rapidly absorbed from the gastrointestinal tract. High concentrations occur in the brain and cerebrospinal fluid. They are metabolized by the liver. Acute effects of amphetamine overdosage include restlessness, behavioral changes, hyperactivity, mydriasis, polypnea, hyperthermia, tachycardia, tachypnea, tremors, hypertension or hypotension, respiratory depression, cardiac arrythmias, heart block, and circulatory collapse (Kisseberth and Trammel, 1990; Litovitz, 1983). Effects usually persist in humans for 4 to 24 hr. However, some sustained-release formulations are also available and will result in prolonged effects (Kisseberth and Trammel, 1990).

Treatment consists of stabilization of the patient if needed, then detoxification of the digestive tract. Emesis or gastric lavage are recommended if exposure was less than 2 hr before presentation and there are no contraindications (i.e., onset of clinical signs of intoxication). If a sustained-release product is involved, repeated doses of activated charcoal and a saline cathartic may be indicated. Close monitoring is essential along with supportive care and treatment of specific clinical signs. External stimuli should be minimized and sedatives (i.e., short-acting barbiturates) may be administered as needed. Fluids and corticosteroids are indicated if hypovolemia or shock develop. Urinary acidification by oral administration of ammonium chloride or ascorbic acid and increasing urine volume will enhance renal excretion (Litovitz, 1983). This therapy should be used only when the dog is not acidotic and has uncompromised hepatic function.

Phenothiazines and butyrophenones (dopamine antagonists) have also been demonstrated to protect against the lethal effects of amphetamines (Litovitz, 1983). Chlorpromazine at 10 to 18 mg/kg IV (Schein Pharmaceutical, Inc) or haloperidol at 1 mg/kg IV (Haldol, McNeil Pharmaceutical) have been shown to have antidotal effects in experimental dogs that had been administered a lethal IV dose of an amphetamine (Kisseberth and Trammel, 1990; Litovitz, 1983). These agents have been demonstrated to combat the drug-related hyperthermia, convulsions, and hypertension.

Diazepam may also be used to control excessive CNS stimulation. Electrocardiograms should be monitored periodically and severe arrhythmias treated as indicated. Increases in intracranial pressure should be counteracted with measures to decrease cerebral edema, congestion, and hemorrhage (Litovitz, 1983).

## SUMMARY

The key to saving dogs exposed to illicit substances is rapid action. Removal from the gastrointestinal tract, absorption, and catharsis are the first steps.

If bags of the drugs are ingested intact, immediate endoscopy or surgery may be required to remove the bag to prevent obstruction or rapid absorption of a lethal dose. Injectible medications to antagonize the effects of the drugs should be administered based on the agent(s) ingested and apparent clinical signs. Continuous monitoring is critical in any case of known or suspected drug intoxication. Familiarity with possible side effects of the pharmacologic antagonistic agent will aid in monitoring and treatment of the patient.

### References and Suggested Reading

Adams HR: Adrenergic and antiadrenergic drugs. *In* Booth NH and McDonald LE (eds): *Veterinary Pharmacology and Therapeutics*, 6th edition. Ames, IA, Iowa State University Press, 1988, p 91.
*Information on the clinical effects of adrenergic and antiadrenergic agents.*
Catravas JD and Waters IW: Acute cocaine intoxication in the conscious dog: Studies on the mechanism of lethality. J Pharmacol Exp Ther 217:350, 1981.
*A study of acute effects and treatments of cocaine poisoning in dogs.*
Coppock RW, Mostrom MS, and Lillie LE: Ethanol and illicit drugs of abuse. *In* Kirk RW (ed): *Current Veterinary Therapy X: Small Animal Practice.* Philadelphia, WB Saunders Co, 1989, p 171.
*Information on toxicology and management for nonmedically administered agents.*
Dumonceaux GD and Beasley VR: Emergency treatments for police dogs used for illicit drug detection. J Am Vet Med Assoc 197:185, 1990.
*A report on drug intoxications, clinical effects, and emergency treatments in drug detection dogs on the job.*
Easom JM and Lovejoy FH: Opiates. *In* Haddad LM and Winchester JF (eds): *Clinical Management of Poisoning and Drug Overdose.* Philadelphia, WB Saunders Co, 1983, p 424.
*An in-depth description of opiates including history, metabolism, clinical and physiologic effects, and treatments for intoxications.*
Godbold JC, Hawkins BJ, and Woodward MG: Acute oral marijuana poisoning in the dog. J Am Vet Med Assoc 175:1101, 1979.
*A description of* Cannabis sativa *intoxication in dogs.*
Gosselin RE, Smith RP, and Hodge HC: *Clinical Toxicology of Commercial Products,* 5th edition. Baltimore/London, Williams & Wilkins, 1984, p III–284.
*Toxicologic information on many commercially available agents.*
Jaffe JH and Martin WR: Morphine and related opioids. *In* Goodman LS, Gilman AG, Rall TW, et al (eds): *The Pharmacological Basis of Therapeutics,* 7th edition. New York, Macmillan Publishing Co, 1985, p 509.
*Information on toxicology, clinical effects, and treatment for opioid agents.*
Kisseberth WC and Trammel HL: Illicit and abused drugs. Vet Clin North Am 20:405, 1990.
*A review of clinical signs, toxicity, and emergency treatment for intoxication of dogs and cats by illicit agents.*
Litovitz T: Amphetamines. *In* Haddad LM and Winchester JF (eds): *Clinical Management of Poisoning and Drug Overdose.* Philadelphia, WB Saunders Co, 1983, p 469.
*A comprehensive look at amphetamines.*

# A BRIEF GUIDE TO INDOOR AIR POLLUTANTS AND RELEVANCE TO SMALL ANIMALS

JANICE A. DYE
*Chapel Hill, North Carolina*

*and* DANIEL L. COSTA
*Research Triangle Park, North Carolina*

Whether fueled by recent lay press accounts of "sick-building syndromes" or "multiple chemical sensitivity syndromes," or simply part of a general trend toward improved health awareness, concern over indoor residential as well as outdoor environmental air quality has been growing. Accordingly, concerned owners may approach their veterinarians to inquire about the possibility of air pollutants causing disease or cancer in their pets. This article is intended to provide a brief overview of the potential adverse health effects of commonly encountered air pollutants. Since many dogs and cats spend virtually all of their lives within the family domicile, the focus of the review will be on indoor air pollutants and select environmental (i.e., outdoor) air pollutants.

Pet animals have been previously proposed as ideal sentinels for studying chemical-induced carcinogenesis (Glickman and Domanski, 1986). Whereas experimen-

This paper has been reviewed by the Health Effects Research Laboratory, U.S. Environmental Protection Agency, and approved for publication. Approval does not signify that the contents necessarily reflect the views and policies of the Agency nor does mention of trade names or commercial products constitute endorsement or recommendations for use.

tal carcinogenesis testing typically utilizes relatively high-level exposures over relatively short periods of time, pet animals receive low-level exposure to potential environmental carcinogens throughout their entire lives, thereby closely paralleling the natural exposure of their owners. Furthermore, owing to the shorter lifespan of animals compared to human beings, shorter latency periods would allow data acquisition in less time than would be possible using strictly human-based epidemiologic studies. As presented below, reports on pet-based epidemiologic studies regarding exposure to asbestos, pesticides, and secondhand cigarette smoke are currently available. Unfortunately, little epidemiologic information on the health effects of other air pollutants in small pet animals exists. Nevertheless, it would seem reasonable to assume that pets undergo comparable, if not greater, exposure to indoor air pollutants as their owners.

The most common indoor air pollutants and their principal sources are listed in Table 1. Much of the information presented here has been extrapolated from human-based epidemiologic studies or experimentally exposed laboratory animals. It should be understood that the relationships between air pollutant exposure and consequential adverse health effects are complex. Estimates of disease induction must take into account the numerous factors that influence the development of pulmonary injury or respiratory tract disease. Factors include distinct pollutant chemical characteristics (e.g., solubility, reactivity), differing experimental conditions (e.g., resting versus exercising subjects), variable routes of exposure (e.g., nasal versus mouth breathing), and so forth. Detection of pulmonary injury may be influenced by both the pollutant concentration and duration of exposure, whether single or multiple exposures were utilized, and the length of recovery period allowed prior to disease assessment. Additive or synergistic effects of combined pollutant exposures are also possible. Perhaps most importantly, differences in host susceptibility due to age, sex, diet, or unique species sensitivities must be recognized. Disproportionately increased risks may be present in very young or aged individuals, or in subjects with preexisting respiratory disease such as chronic bronchitis, asthma, or respiratory tract infections. Along these lines, a previous study comparing radiographic evidence of pulmonary disease in rural versus urban dogs found no differences in the urban-rural distribution of pulmonary disease in the younger dogs; however, older urban dogs (>7 years) exhibited greater thoracic disease than did older rural dogs (Reif and Cohen, 1970). The following discussion is intended only as a general, necessarily cursory, review of air pollutant health effects.

## POLLUTANTS

### Nitrogen Dioxide

Nitrogen dioxide ($NO_2$), a poisonous, brownish gas, is both a major indoor and outdoor air pollutant. Home concentrations, however, may be as much as five times that found in the external environment (ALA, 1986), well in excess of the level of $NO_2$ that the Environmental Protection Agency has established as the safe level in the outdoor air. Resulting almost entirely from combustion processes, the major household sources are poorly ventilated or maintained gas appliances (e.g., ranges, clothes dryers, water heaters), fireplaces, and coal- or wood-burning stoves. Adverse health effects include alterations in host defense mechanisms such as decreased alveolar macrophage function. Thus, $NO_2$ exposure may result in increased frequency or severity of respiratory tract infections in small animals. Long-term (e.g., near-lifetime) exposures to $NO_2$ are also suspected of causing chronic lung disease (i.e., emphysema).

### Carbon Monoxide

Carbon monoxide (CO) is a colorless, odorless gas. As a product of incomplete fuel combustion, sources of CO are similar to those of $NO_2$. The principal source is motor vehicle exhaust. Classic cases of human poisonings, whether accidental or intentional, arise from car engines left running in attached garages or sheds. Significant exposure may also result during use of charcoal grills or unvented kerosene heaters in relatively closed air spaces, or when chimneys or other venting ducts of central heating systems are obstructed. Birds are especially sensitive to this air toxicant, as evidenced by their classic use as sentinels in coal mine shafts. Carbon monoxide poisoning is also an important cause of the morbidity and mortality in pets managing to es-

***Table 1.*** *Most Common Indoor Air Pollutants and Their Principal Sources*

| Air Pollutants | Potential Source(s) |
|---|---|
| Nitrogen dioxide ($NO_2$) | Gas appliances, water heaters, stoves, coal- and wood-burning stoves |
| Carbon monoxide (CO) | Charcoal burning or auto exhaust in garages, unvented kerosene heaters |
| Ozone ($O_3$) | A tropospheric photochemical by-product of fuel combustion products |
| Sulfur dioxide ($SO_2$) | Industrial burning of sulfur-containing coal and oil, unvented kerosene heaters |
| Secondhand cigarette smoke | Contents include CO, HCHO, acrolein, and various gases and particles |
| Formaldehyde (HCHO) | Foam insulation, wood or fiber products, carpets, upholstery, draperies |
| Asbestos | Flooring or roofing materials, especially older wall and pipe insulation |
| Radon (Rn) | Water or natural gas passing through radon-emitting ground or rock |
| Microbial and fungal agents | Air conditioners, air ducts and filters, humidifiers, airtight buildings |
| Household products | Cleaning agents, personal care products, pesticides, paints, varnishes |

cape from burning homes. Owing to its tremendous affinity for hemoglobin as well as myoglobin, CO prevents cellular oxidation, causing severe cellular anoxia and death. Unlike many of the other air pollutants where problems arise principally due to chronic low-level exposures, single (likely to be encountered) exposures of CO, may prove lethal. Clinical signs range from lethargy and fatigue, to headache and depression, confusion, nausea, and ultimately, unconsciousness and death.

## Ozone

Ozone ($O_3$) is primarily considered an outdoor air pollutant, although lesser concentrations may occur indoors as well. In the environment, $O_3$ is not emitted directly, rather it is produced in the lower atmosphere by the photochemical interaction of sunlight with various combustion products, nitrogen oxides, volatile organic compounds (from gasoline, solvents, or consumer products), and oxygen. Hot temperatures and air inversion patterns serve to increase ambient air concentrations. When significant accumulations of $O_3$ occur near ground level, the commonly recognized phenomenon of "smog" is observed. Indoor $O_3$ arises principally from outdoor $O_3$ that has permeated into the structure with normal air exchange. Typically, indoor $O_3$ concentrations are less than half that measured outdoors, but during smog episodes these indoor levels may be sufficient to affect human health. On occasion, $O_3$ can be emitted directly into the indoor air from electric generators, from certain office equipment (e.g., photocopy and fax machines, laser printers), and ironically, from some "air-purifiers" that actually use $O_3$ to rid tobacco or microbial odors. Under these latter conditions, $O_3$ concentrations in the indoor air can exceed those outdoors, even in smog.

As an oxidant gas, $O_3$ is among the most injurious of the atmospheric pollutants. When inhaled, ozone can penetrate down to the small peripheral airways, potentially oxidizing respiratory tissues along the way. Airway responsiveness is defined as the ease with which the airways constrict in response to nonspecific stimuli. Increased airway responsiveness is considered an important characteristic of asthma. Acute $O_3$ exposure in healthy dogs and humans has been shown to increase airway responsiveness and cause airway epithelial inflammation. Exposure to relatively low $O_3$ concentrations, comparable to that occurring in many urban areas, has been shown to further increase airway responsiveness during allergen challenge in humans with atopic asthma (Molfino et al., 1991). Chronic exposure to low $O_3$ concentrations has been shown to induce bronchiolitis in rhesus monkeys. In humans and rabbits, $O_3$ has been shown to have variable effects on mucociliary clearance, a primary mechanism for clearing inhaled particles or offending microorganisms from the airways, thereby raising concerns regarding host resistance against infection.

## Sulfur Dioxide

Sulfur dioxide ($SO_2$) is also primarily an outdoor air pollutant. The product of metal smelting processes or industrial burning of sulfur-containing coal or oil, it is considered the major precursor to acidic deposition (i.e., acid rain). While pet owners may be familiar with the problems associated with acid rain, with one exception, veterinary interest in $SO_2$ pollution principally involves environmental concerns over aquatic and wildlife health effects. The exception is unvented kerosene space heaters which, when used indoors, emit significant amounts of $SO_2$ and associated acid aerosols. Most of the aerosol is complexed with ammonia, thereby reducing its intrinsic acidity, but total airborne concentrations can be astronomical in closed-space situations. Moreover, when $SO_2$ gas is combined with other organic acid emissions, these heater gases can be quite irritating to the eyes and respiratory tracts of animals as well as humans. Additionally, acid aerosol exposures from ambient $SO_2$ pollution may occur in pets housed outdoors, or pets exercising outdoors for several hours during the day. Laboratory animal studies have shown that acidic aerosols may cause airway constriction, impairment of mucociliary clearance of particles, changes in airway inflammatory responses, and generalized increases in airway responsiveness. Risk appears to accrue in children or adult humans active out-of-doors for several hours a day (ATS Workshop, 1991). Since even brief exposures to acidic atmospheres (which may occur with downdrafts of smokestack plume) may trigger severe bronchoconstriction, people with hyperresponsive airways (e.g., asthmatics) are considered to be at particular risk. Certain cats with chronic bronchopulmonary disease also appear to have increased airway responsiveness, based on anecdotal evidence as well as limited airway challenge testing information. It would seem likely that such pets with preexisting airway hyperresponsiveness would be at similar peril to this irritant gas-particulate complex, and especially indoor kerosene space heater emissions.

## Secondhand Cigarette Smoke

Cigarette smoke contains numerous toxins and ciliotoxins, causing pulmonary connective tissue damage, mucus hypersecretion, and mucus pooling. Firmly established as an important risk factor for human lung cancer, cigarette smoking has also been causally linked to chronic obstructive pulmonary disease, chronic bronchitis, emphysema, increased airway responsiveness, exacerbations of asthma, and impaired immune function; hence, increased frequency of pulmonary infections. Older studies of cigarette smoking by trained tracheostomized dogs confirmed the development of comparable histologic changes and pulmonary neoplasia in veterinary species as well (Hammond et al, 1970; Auerbach et al., 1970).

Secondhand smoke, also known as environmental tobacco smoke (ETS), is simply the smoke from someone else's cigarette. Although its effects are still being debated, secondhand smoke contains carbon monoxide, formaldehyde, acrolein, and various assorted gases and particles. The dwell-time in the air and cooling of ETS alters the chemical composition and gas-particle associations of the smoke, and may well alter its toxicity. There are reports of enhanced bacterial mutagenicity (Ames Assay) of ETS particulate matter when compared to mainstream cigarette smoke.

Secondhand smoke is known to cause ocular and respiratory tract irritation, especially in poorly ventilated air spaces. Associated with reduced resistance to respiratory tract infections, secondhand smoke is especially a problem in young children, leading to increased incidence of bronchiolitis, pneumonia, and middle-ear infections. Pet animals are similarly exposed to the smoke of their owner's cigarettes (see Fig. 1). Predisposition toward analogous disease conditions is likely.

Of even greater concern, recent studies in humans and dogs have associated exposure to secondhand smoke with increased risks of pulmonary neoplasia. Recently, the Environmental Protection Agency declared secondhand smoke, ETS, as a definitive carcinogen in

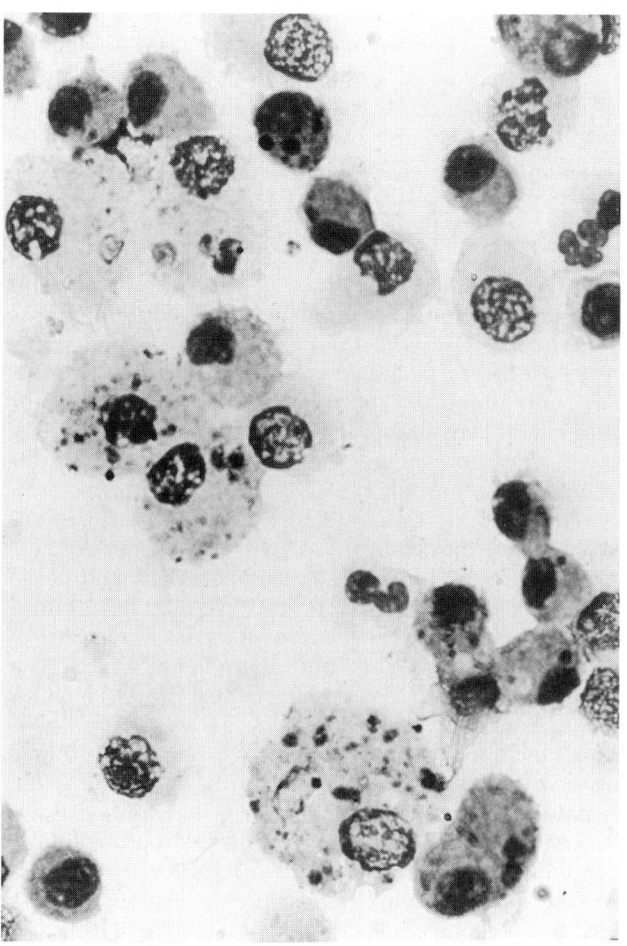

**Figure 1.** A transoral tracheobronchial wash from a cat exposed to secondhand cigarette smoke in the household revealed numerous macrophages containing darkly pigmented intracytoplasmic particles. (Wright-Giemsa, original magnification × 1000.)

humans. In one study, cigarette smoke exposure during childhood and adolescence was found to double the risk of developing lung cancer (Janerich et al., 1990). Studies in pet animals have been limited. In one study, the increased risk for lung cancer in dogs was restricted to brachycephalic and mesocephalic breeds (Rief et al., 1992). Conversely, a previous report of cancer risk in dogs showed that dolichocephalic breeds were at increased risk for developing nasal cancer (Hayes, Wilson, and Fraumeni, 1982). It was postulated that these trends reflect the tendency for carcinogens to be deposited in the nasal regions of dolichocephalic breeds, thereby preventing deposition into the lower respiratory tract. Unfortunately, increased nasal carcinogen deposition may in turn be associated with increased risk of nasal neoplasia. It should be noted, however, that these trends in the dog may reflect chronic exposure to more than just secondhand cigarette smoke.

## Formaldehyde

Formaldehyde is a pungent, highly water-soluble, reactive gas. Indoor exposures may occur during offgassing of formaldehyde from resins present in particleboard, fiberboard, and wood paneling. Other sources may include foam insulation, carpeting, upholstery, and drapery fabrics. Mobile homes, being relatively airtight and constructed from many of these materials, are especially problematic. Formaldehyde gas is an ocular and upper respiratory tract irritant. Exposures may cause headaches, nausea, and dizziness. Recognizing that relative to humans, rodents are obligate nasal breathers with extensive nasal epithelial mucosa, chronic exposure to toxic concentrations of formaldehyde has been shown to induce nasal epithelial injury, increased cell proliferation, and nasal cancer in rats.

## Asbestos

Asbestos constitutes a group of naturally occurring mineral (hydrated silicate) fibers. In the past, asbestos was used extensively as a cheap source of noncombustible insulation for walls and pipes. Asbestos was also used in many types of flooring and roofing materials, cement and spackling compounds, and friction products (e.g., brake shoes and clutch pads). Asbestos fibers are small and when abraded or disturbed, readily become airborne. They are easily inhaled and deposited within the airways; however, pulmonary defense mechanisms have great difficulty removing or destroying these fibers. Asbestos-induced diseases typically have latency periods of up to 30 years in humans, and have been associated with the development of pleural plaques, asbestosis (i.e., interstitial fibrosis), bronchogenic carcinoma, and the otherwise extremely rare neoplasia, malignant mesothelioma. Although production of asbestos-containing pipe wrap and insulations was banned in the late 1970s, many older public and residential buildings still contain considerable amounts of asbestos that is slowly being eroded and released into the air. Asbestos removal and containment remain costly and controversial issues.

A retrospective epidemiologic study associated development of mesothelioma in dogs with exposure of their owners to asbestos (Glickman, Domanski, and Maguire, 1983). Several of the owners were shipyard workers or auto mechanics. Interestingly, the wives and children of asbestos workers (especially of miners) have also been found to be at higher risk of mesothelioma due to asbestos exposure from re-entrained asbestos dust from clothing. Male dogs appeared to be at a higher risk for developing mesothelioma for reasons not readily apparent (Glickman, Domanski, and Maguire, 1983). Mesothelioma has also been found more commonly in human males; however, this predisposition was previously assumed to reflect occupation exposure patterns.

## Radon

Radon is a type of radioactive gas emitted by soil or rock containing trace amounts of radium or uranium. Radon or its progeny (i.e., radon daughters) may enter the home via the underlying soil through cracks in the foundation or holes in the geologic deposits beneath the home. Once inside, radon gas decays with a half-life of 3.8 days. The ionized atoms adsorb to dust particles and may be subsequently inhaled. Alternatively, water or natural gas passing through underground regions containing radon may serve as potential sources of radon exposure. Differing geographic locations vary considerably in the amount of radon present in the soil. As an $\alpha$-emitter, the primary target for radon is the lung. In contrast, the target organs for uranium are the bone and kidneys, and for radium, the bone. Previous health concerns have been largely occupational, involving the increased risk of uranium miners for developing cancer. Despite the prevalence of recent lay press reports on radon risks, and the various home detection kits available in many local department stores, the current scientific evidence for an association between residential radon exposure and lung cancer is weak. More extensive case-control epidemiologic studies are forthcoming.

## Microbial and Fungal Agents

Owing to the tremendous increases in home heating costs during the 1970s, extensive efforts were made to more efficiently insulate residential dwellings. As a result, many homes are currently far more airtight than ever before. Decreased air flow through a dwelling, possibly combined with extensive use of wall-to-wall carpeting, has allowed microbes, bacteria, fungi, and dust (including dust mites and their excreta), to accumulate in the indoor air at higher concentrations than were previously present. This trend has been proposed as one of several explanations for the emerging in-creases in asthma and other atopic disease syndromes, although increased exposure to environmental air pollutants is another potentially confounding factor. While the role of microorganisms or their by-products in the worsening of atopic conditions is uncertain, their potential for inflicting infectious disease is epitomized by "legionnaire's disease," which arose from microbial overgrowth within air conditioning systems. Molds and fungi (or their volatile emission products) have also been implicated in the so-called sick-building syndrome which frequently affects office workers enclosed in "tight" buildings. Unfortunately, the links between microbial-associated pollutants and evident disease in humans (and animals) are more speculative than certain. The potential, however, is real.

Ironically, for the purpose of this review, pets in general and specifically the airborne feline saliva allergen (*Fel d I*) are considered important sources of indoor air pollutants to human beings. Preventative measures can assist in lowering the overall allergen build-up within the home. Frequent washing of the cat was found to markedly reduce the concentration of *Fel d I* allergen in the air (deBlay, Chapman, and Patts-Mills, 1991). This may prove to be a viable alternative to euthanasia of cats whose owners have developed atopic disease. To ensure proper home ventilation, existing air ducts must never be blocked. Instead, air ducts should be maintained by changing air duct and air conditioning filters on a regular basis. Humidifier and dehumidifier filters should also be changed regularly.

## Household Products

The potential for exposure to various and assorted chemical compounds within the home environment is tremendous. Pets and their owners are oft times exposed to fumes from carpeting, paints, varnish, furniture, and draperies after moving into new homes or during extensive remodeling. Additionally, it is estimated that the average home contains at least 45 different aerosol products. These products range from modern cleaning agents (air fresheners, furniture polish) and personal care items (hair sprays, deodorants, static guards, perfumes), to solvents, paints, and pesticides (insect and roach sprays, fumigants, flea control products). In turn, these compounds are composed of a variety of active and inert ingredients including a multitude of volatile organic compounds (VOCs). When used in well-ventilated areas, as per label instructions, most people (and pets) experience minimal adverse effects from use of these products. However, as potential sensory irritants, exposure may be associated with ocular, dermal, or respiratory tract irritation. Dizziness, headache, nausea, and even allergic reactions may arise during excessive or prolonged contact with these agents. Retrospective epidemiologic studies in dogs have associated chronic topical insecticide application, especially in obese dogs, with increased risk of developing transitional cell cancer of the bladder (Glickman, Schofer, and McKeen, 1989).

Perhaps most importantly, many owners fail to read or heed the warning label instructions. They insist on using these products carelessly or excessively. An extreme example of this is the owner that decided to put both the cat and activated flea bomb together in a large plastic bag in order to "kill the fleas once and for all." Sadly, the point of this incident is to stress that home exposure to chemicals, be it through seemingly appropriate but chronic exposure, or acute and inappropriate product usage, is a realistic cause of illness in small animal medicine. It should be considered when formulating a list of differential diagnoses, especially if the signs reflect relatively acute onset of ocular, dermal, or respiratory system disease. Avian veterinarians should be especially attuned to this possibility. As with carbon monoxide, pet birds may be exceedingly sensitive to aerosolized VOCs. Even the fumes from overheated cooking pans lined with polytetrafluoroethylene (Teflon or Silverstone) have been associated with acute and fatal toxicosis (Wells, 1983).

## RECOMMENDED PRECAUTIONS

Simple preventative measures can help to ensure that neither the owner nor the pet are exposed unnecessarily to air pollutants. Gas appliances should be functioning properly. Gas stoves and heaters should be free of cracks and properly vented to the outside of the house. When available, exhaust fans should be used while cooking with gas ranges. If the tip of the gas burner flame appears yellow or orange instead of blue, the range should be inspected or adjusted. Lastly, gas ranges should never be used as heat sources.

Kerosene heaters should be used carefully and only as per the manufacturer's instructions. Heaters should be refueled outdoors and only low-sulfur fuel should be used. The heater should be kept clean and properly adjusted. Kerosene heaters should be used with great caution and should be vented outdoors or used only in spaces with significant air leakage. Cars or lawn mower engines should never be left running inside a garage or shed. This is especially critical if the garage is ever used to house a pet.

Aerosol household products should be used only in well-ventilated areas. If cleaning agents, remodeling materials, new paint or varnish, new or refinished furniture, new carpeting or draperies, and so forth, are associated with an offensive odor or seem to cause headaches and ocular irritation to the owners, the owners should ensure that neither they nor their pet maintain prolonged exposure to the fumes until the odors dissipate. If this is not possible, efforts to improve air ventilation are a must. Along these lines, flea-control dips, shampoos, and spray products should be applied only as directed and in well-ventilated areas.

The above precautions may be especially important for puppies and kittens, geriatric dogs and cats, and pets with known respiratory disease. Analogous to the human situation, it is reasonable to assume that dogs with chronic bronchitis or cats with chronic bronchopulmonary disease are at increased risk of exacerbating their underlying respiratory conditions following prolonged exposure to air pollutants. Perhaps the one precaution that would result in the most benefit to the pet as well as the owner(s), is for the owner to stop cigarette smoking altogether or at least restrict smoking to outside the family domicile.

## References and Suggested Reading

American Lung Association (ALA): Air pollution in your home? Public Information Pamphlet #1001, 1986.

American Thoracic Society (ATS) Workshop: Health effects of atmospheric acids and their precursors. Am Rev Respir Dis 144:464, 1991.

Auerbach O, Hammond EC, Kirman D, and Garfinkel L: Effects of cigarette smoking on dogs. II. Pulmonary neoplasms. Arch Environ Health 21:754, 1970.

deBlay R, Chapman MD, and Patts-Mills TAE: Airborne cat allergen (*Fel d I*) environmental control with the cat *in situ*. Am Rev Respir Dis 143:1334, 1991.

Glickman LT, Domanski LM, Maguire TG, et al: Mesothelioma in pet dogs associated with exposure of their owners to asbestos. Environ Res 32:305, 1983.

Glickman LT and Domanski LM: An alternative to laboratory animal experimentation for human health risk assessment: Epidemiologic studies of pet animals. Altern To Lab Anim 13:267, 1986.

Glickman LT, Schofer FS, and McKeen LJ: Epidemiologic study of insecticide exposures, obesity, and risk of bladder cancer in household dogs. J Tox Environ Health 28:407, 1989.

Hammond EC, Auerbach O, Kirman D, and Garfinkel L: Effects of cigarette smoking on dogs. I. Design of experiment, mortality, and findings in lung parenchyma. Arch Environ Health 21:740, 1970.

Hayes HM, Wilson GP, and Fraumeni JF Jr: Carcinoma of the nasal cavity and paranasal sinuses in dogs: Descriptive epidemiology. Cornell Vet 72:168, 1982.

Janerich DT, Thompson WD, Varela LR, et al: Lung cancer and exposure to tobacco smoke in the household. N Engl J Med 323:632, 1990.

Molfino NA, Wright SC, Katz I, et al: Effect of low concentrations of ozone on inhaled allergen responses in asthmatic subjects. Lancet 338:119, 1991.

Reif JS and Cohen D: Retrospective radiographic analysis of pulmonary disease in rural and urban dogs. Arch Environ Health 20:686, 1970.

Reif JS, Dunn K, Ogilvie GK, and Harris CK: Passive smoking and canine lung cancer risk. Am J Epidemiol 135:234, 1992.

Wells RE: Fatal toxicosis in pet birds caused by an overheated cooking pan lined with polytetrafluoroethylene. J Am Vet Med Assoc 182:1248, 1983.

# Section

# 4

# INFECTIOUS DISEASES

### EDWARD B. BREITSCHWERDT
*Consulting Editor*

*Still Current Information Found in Current Veterinary Therapy XI*

**Elsewhere in Current Veterinary Therapy XII:**

# OPTIMIZING LABORATORY DIAGNOSIS OF INFECTIOUS DISEASES

DWIGHT C. HIRSH

*Davis, California*

A key consideration, usually made early in the diagnostic work-up, is whether or not a patient has an infectious disease. This decision is important, since drugs used to treat conditions with noninfectious etiologies are oftentimes contraindicated for treatment of conditions with an infectious etiology (e.g., corticosteroids versus antibiotics). Although the results of cytologic examination of a sample obtained from an affected site may be useful in the determination of the etiology, frequently this is not the case, particularly if the numbers of microorganisms are not high. Thus, the results of bacteriologic culture of an affected site becomes important.

## CLINICAL SIGNIFICANCE OF AN ISOLATE

The major goal of the microbiology laboratory is to isolate clinically relevant microorganisms from an affected tissue or body cavity, and if more than one type of microorganism is present, to isolate them in approximately the same ratio as *in vivo*. What defines a "clinically relevant" microorganism is an important diagnostic consideration. Whether an isolate is relevant to the patient's disease depends upon the circumstances of isolation. For example, the isolation of large numbers of a particular microorganism from a normally sterile site in the presence of an inflammatory cytology would be interpreted as clinically relevant. The identification of microorganisms and assessment of a "positive culture" are the thrusts of this article. Serologic diagnosis is discussed only briefly, and the reader is directed elsewhere in this section for details of serologic and immunodiagnostic techniques.

Attention must be given to the site cultured as well as the method of obtaining the sample for culture. The determination of relevance is made a great deal easier if the sample is obtained from a normally sterile site. Obtaining a sample from the alimentary canal, and expecting meaningful answers, may be unrealistic, unless one is looking for the presence or absence of a particular microorganism (e.g., *Salmonella* or *Campylobacter*).

## SAMPLE COLLECTION

Care must be given to the way a sample is collected; otherwise, interpretation of results may be difficult. Most infectious processes arise subsequent to the contamination of a compromised surface or site by microorganisms that exist as flora on a contiguous mucosal surface. In other words, microorganisms isolated from an affected site are often similar (if not identical) to those found as part of the normal body flora.

Below is a discussion of sample collection from the perspective of a clinical microbiologist with the responsibility of providing the clinical veterinarian with meaningful information.

### Respiratory Tract

Samples from the upper respiratory tract (proximal to the larynx) are limited in usefulness due to the presence of an abundant normal flora. However, fungal diseases involving the upper tract can be diagnosed by culture techniques. The main fungal diseases are cryptococcoses and aspergillosis. Since neither microorganism is routinely found in the upper tract, their demonstration together with serologic evidence is usually sufficient to make the diagnosis. Cryptococcal disease involving the upper tract and associated structures (sinuses) can be diagnosed by examination of smears (see below) and culture of affected material. Serologic detection of cryptococcal antigen in the bloodstream will help with the interpretation in some cases (e.g., cases in which no microorganisms are seen in the direct smear together with very small numbers grown in culture). A commercial kit (e.g., Crypto-LA Test, Wampole Laboratories) is available for this assay. Diagnosis of *Aspergillus*-mediated disease of the nasal turbinates is made by "traumatic" flush or biopsy of affected tissues. Isolation (on blood agar or other suitable fungal medium) of *Aspergillus* confirms the diagnosis. Serologic examination of the blood for antibodies to *Aspergillus* corroborates the culture results. Commercially available kits (e.g., Aspergillus Agar Gel Immunodiffusion Test, Meridian Diagnostics) are available for serologic testing. These kits only test for presence of antibodies to *A. fumigatus*. Fortunately, *A. fumigatus* is the most common species of *Aspergillus* involved in nasal cavity disease.

Samples from the lower respiratory tract (distal to the larynx) are obtained either by transtracheal aspiration or by broncoalveolar lavage or brush. The lower tract is not entirely sterile in normal animals, but the number of microorganisms ($<10^3$/ml) is usually too small to be of concern (i.e., isolation of microorganisms from a normal animal's lung without enrichment is unusual).

From the microbiologist's perspective, wash (lavage) fluid is superior to brush material. The amount of material that is obtained from brushing the affected site is too small for the manipulations needed for acquisition of meaningful results.

### Feces

Diarrheal disease of bacterial etiology may be caused by a number of different microorganisms. Only two species are easily identified as causative agents, *Salmonella* and *Campylobacter*. Freshly voided fecal material should be sent to the laboratory. Although the amount of feces to send to the laboratory has not been established for small animals, about 1 gm (lima bean size) should be sufficient. A rectal swab is not as useful. Culture techniques (*Salmonella* and *Campylobacter*) together with direct smear analysis (*Campylobacter*) are methods used to make the microbiologic diagnosis.

### Urinary Tract

The diagnosis of bacterial cystitis is made by culturing bacteria from the urinary bladder. Normal bladder urine, though not totally sterile, has too few bacteria to demonstrate bacteriologically. Bladder urine can be obtained to catch (voided urine), catheter, or by cystocentesis. Because urine obtained by catheter or by catch may be contaminated by the normal flora in the distal urethra (those same species that may potentially contaminate the bladder), the numbers of bacteria per milliliter must be determined. If there are greater than or equal to $10^5$ bacteria per milliliter of urine, statistically, the chances are good that they came from the bladder and not the distal urethra. However, if the sample was obtained by percutaneous aspiration, then any cultured bacteria are of clinical relevance, unless there is contamination due to inadvertent bowel penetration. Thus, documentation of the method for urine collection is important in order to correctly process and interpret the results of urine culture.

### Reproductive Tract

The vagina contains a normal bacterial flora. Members of this flora increase in numbers when there is vaginitis, as well as some changes in the relative prevalence of the involved species. However, it is our contention that microbiologic analysis of the vagina (other than determining the presence of *Brucella*) yields very little diagnostic information with respect to the determination of the cause of a vaginitis or as a guide to reproductive health. The uterus is normally sterile. Samples obtained through the cervical os must be obtained through a sterile speculum with a guarded swab. To do otherwise, is to risk contamination of the sample with commensal vaginal flora that will usually contain the same bacteria responsible for contaminating the uterus. Culture results of exudates from the vulvular area of bitches with open pyometra are uninterpretable, since these samples will be contaminated with members of the normal vaginal flora (which also contains the most frequently isolated bacteria from pyometra, *Escherichia coli*).

### Abscesses/Draining Tracts and Other Fluids

Whenever possible, samples of abscesses should be obtained by aspiration. Obtaining samples from draining tracts that will yield meaningful data is somewhat more difficult. Swabs placed into the tract will almost always become contaminated with bacteria growing around the external opening of the tract. Some of these same bacteria may also be deep within the tissue and a part of the etiology of the condition, while others may simply be living around the external opening and have nothing whatsoever to do with the etiology of the condition—from a bacteriologic standpoint, there is no way to tell.

### Skeletal

Samples of the skeletal system are best obtained by biopsy of the affected site. Some sites, however, are not easily sampled. In these cases, the blood culture provides a potentially rewarding alternative (e.g., dogs with discospondylitis).

### Skin

Skin is a normally contaminated surface. Interpretation of the results of bacterial culture of the skin is difficult unless care is taken not to "sample" normal skin microorganisms, which may also contain the suspected bacterial pathogen. Unfortunately, it is impossible to clean the skin prior to sample collection for bacterial culture without removing the etiologic agent as well. Skin biopsy followed by analysis of the normally sterile subcutaneous tissue alleviates this problem. Likewise, culture of the contents of a pustule also reduces the possibility of confusing results.

Culture of the skin for dermatophytes is a different story, since selective media are used. Nevertheless, it is still important to reduce the bacterial "load" on the skin to avoid bacterial overgrowth, which can obscure slower growing dermatophytes. Precleaning the skin with soap and water, followed by swabbing the area to be sampled with alcohol, greatly reduces the number of bacterial contaminants without affecting the isolation of fungi. If precleaning the skin with soap and alcohol is difficult (e.g., painful), cleaning the area with sterile water will help. Since a selective medium will be inoculated (see below), demonstration of the fungus should be possible.

## Blood

Culture of the peripheral blood is relatively expensive and must be done correctly if interpretable results are to be expected. Crucial to generating meaningful results is the realization that placing 1 bacterium or 100 bacteria in the culture bottle, can result in the same result in 24 hr, when the bottle is examined by the laboratory technologist. Therefore, contamination of the needle by a bacterial skin contaminate (just one!) will yield confusing (and erroneous) results. Thus, skin preparation, which includes removing the hair and disinfecting the skin over the vein, is critically important. Disinfection should include application of 70% alcohol (ethyl or isopropyl) followed by application of 1 to 2% tincture of iodine or 10% povidone-iodine solution (1% available iodine). Individually wrapped units prepared for skin disinfection are commercially available (e.g., Frepp/Sepp Kit, Marion Scientific).

It is also important to realize that microorganisms may not circulate in the blood of a septic patient at all times. For this reason, samples should be obtained over several hours (see "Diagnosis of Bacteremia," this volume, p 137). We collect at least three samples, spaced no closer than 1 hr apart, within a 24-hr period. Because there may be fewer than 1 microorganism per milliliter of blood in a septic animal, as much blood as possible should be collected. The maximum amount of blood is dictated by the size and condition of the animal, as well as the size and volume of the blood culture bottle (the blood sample must be diluted at least 1:10 so that the detrimental bacteriologic effects of the complement proteins and phagocytic cells are reduced).

## SAMPLE TRANSPORT (HOLDING)

The sooner the sample is processed in the microbiology laboratory, the better. Realistically, the time between sample collection and processing may range from minutes to the next morning. The main danger in waiting is sample drying (all microorganisms) and exposure to a noxious atmosphere (oxygen for obligate anaerobes). For this reason, it is important that the sample be kept moist (for a syringe full of exudate, this is obviously not an important consideration) and, if conditions warrant (see below), air excluded. Moistness is usually maintained by placing the sample in a transport (holding) medium. Transport (holding medium) is nothing more than a balanced salt solution usually in a gelled matrix. Because this medium does not contain any nutrient material, microorganisms in the sample do not multiply (and thereby the relative number and ratios are preserved), but remain viable for a time, at least for overnight. How long a bacterial species survives in transport media depends upon the microorganism involved; β-hemolytic *Streptococcus*, for example, does not survive as long as *Escherichia coli*. Swabs should always be placed in transport medium, regardless of the interval between processing and collection (e.g., Culturette Systems, BBL). Fluids that

may contain anaerobic bacteria (exudate from draining tracts, peritoneal and pleural effusions, abscess material) should be cultured right after collection. If this material is contained in a syringe, then the air should be expelled and a sterile stopper placed over the needle. If a swab is used to collect the sample, it should be placed in an anaerobic transport medium (e.g., Anaerobic Transport Medium, Anaerobe Systems). If a syringe-full of sample cannot be processed immediately, the syringe should be emptied into an anaerobic transport medium and held at room temperature. Do not refrigerate samples suspected of containing anaerobes, because some species do not tolerate reduced temperatures.

Urine samples should be refrigerated if not processed immediately, especially if the sample was obtained by catch or catheter where the concentration of microorganisms is important. How long a sample of urine can be stored in the refrigerator is not known, but probably no longer than overnight.

Fecal material, if not processed within an hour or two should be placed in transport medium (e.g., Fecal-Enteric Plus Vials, Trend Scientific). Feces held without addition to a holding medium will dry, decreasing the number of *Salmonella* or *Campylobacter* in the sample, thereby reducing the chances they will be detected.

## SAMPLE PROCESSING

Samples of fluid, other than frank pus, should be spun in a desk-top centrifuge (full speed) at room temperature for 15 min. Fluids handled in this fashion are usually cerebrospinal fluid (CSF), material obtained from the lower respiratory tract, and urine obtained by percutaneous aspiration. The supernatant is decanted, and the pellet (which may be invisible) resuspended in the small volume of supernatant that usually remains in the tube.

## Direct Smear

In addition to cytologic characterization of the patient's inflammatory response, information obtained from examination of a stained smear of material is valuable because it may be the first indication (and sometimes the only) that an infectious process is present. Also, what is seen (e.g., shape, gram-staining characteristics) will help guide the choice of therapy 24 hr before culture results are available. However, it must be kept in mind that at least $10^4$ microorganisms per milliliter or gram of material must be present in order to be readily detected microscopically.

As is the case of a sample obtained from a normally sterile site, the presence of bacteria in bladder urine is a significant finding. However, interpretation of the results of analysis of urine samples obtained by catheter or by catch is difficult because of the confounding presence of flora in the distal urethra. Finding bacteria by direct smear in concentrated (the preferred) or unconcentrated urine obtained by percutaneous aspiration is a clinically relevant finding. Demonstration of one bacteria per oil field in a drop of unconcentrated urine (which has been allowed to dry and then stained) represents about $10^5$ to $10^6$ bacteria per milliliter of urine.

Two types of stains are available, the Gram stain and Romanowsky-type stain, such as Wright's (e.g., Diff-Quik, Harleco). Each type of stain has advantages and disadvantages. The Gram stain is useful in that the shape and the gram-staining characteristics of the agent are seen. The disadvantage of the Gram stain is that the cellular content of the sample is not readily discerned. On the other hand, a Romanowsky-type stain gives the observer a feeling for the cellular nature of the sample and whether or not there are bacteria present. The shape of the bacteria is important, and the Gram-staining characteristics of the microorganism can be deduced (i.e., cocci are almost always gram-positive, rods are almost always gram-negative). So the disadvantage of not knowing for sure whether the observed microorganisms are gram-positive or gram-negative is really not much of a disadvantage. We believe that an assessment of the cytology of the sample is very important in assessing the relevance of the microorganism seen and subsequently grown.

Direct examination of hair or squamous epithelium for the presence of dermatophytic fungi is a procedure that takes practice, but the rewards are immense. Diagnosis of dermatophytosis can be made while the patient is still on the premises (rather than waiting for the results of culture, which may take up to 10 days). Hair and affected skin (nail) are scraped from the lesion, and placed in a drop or two of 10% potassium hydroxide. After the preparation is gently heated (no boiling!), it is examined microscopically (low power) under low light intensity. Affected hairs will appear to have a grayish coat, which, if examined under high-dry magnification, are the arthroconidia (spherical structures a little smaller than a red blood cell) of dermatophyte fungi. Sometimes hyphae are seen, especially in areas that are hairless. Fungal structures can more readily be visualized by adding a drop of 0.1% Calcofluor white to the drop of 10% potassium hydroxide and then observing with fluorescent microscopy. Fungal hyphae and arthroconidia will appear green or blue-white.

## Media Inoculation

Before considering the types and kinds of media that have to be inoculated to ascertain the presence or absence of an infectious agent, a discussion of how the media is inoculated is necessary.

Determination of the relative numbers of microorganisms in a sample greatly help interpretation of significance. Colonies of microorganisms growing on all four quadrants of a Petri plate indicate that there are large numbers of microorganisms in the sample. If a sample yielded one or two colonies growing on the plate, significance of these colonies and thus the ques-

tion as to the infectious etiology of the condition would be in doubt. "Enrichment" prior to plating of a sample obtained from a normally sterile site should never be done because one microorganism can grow to numbers equalling many thousands in a very short period of time. Obviously, more credence will be given to a process from which 1000 microorganisms were isolated versus a sample from which one was isolated. The only exception to this "rule" is whether the presence or absence of a particular microorganism is significant (e.g., *Salmonella*). From a clinical perspective, the author believes that the use of enrichment broths, other than for the determination of the presence or absence of a particular species of bacterium, are more trouble than they are worth. Too often, enrichment culture results lead to the unnecessary work-up and treatment of a contaminating microorganism.

Determination of relevance is aided by the cytology of the sample obtained from the affected site. Isolation (demonstration) of numerous microorganisms from a normally sterile site without the presence of inflammatory cells should be viewed with suspension. One exception to this rule is cryptococcal infection wherein the sample may contain a large number of yeast cells but very few inflammatory cells (the cryptococcal capsule is immunosuppressive). Perhaps another is urinary tract infection in dogs with Cushing's disease (or taking glucocorticosteroids). Situations that may explain the isolation or demonstration of a "significant number" of microorganisms from a normally sterile site without evidence of an inflammatory response include: contaminated collection devices; contamination of the collection device from a contiguous, normally nonsterile site; contamination of the medium inoculation device in the microbiology laboratory; or contamination of the medium before inoculation. Collection devices sterilized by liquid disinfectants quite often become contaminated by microorganisms able to live in such fluids (*Pseudomonas* is notorious for this).

Plates may be streaked in any fashion as long as individual colonies are produced after incubation. Assessing relative numbers is very subjective, and every laboratory has their own way of doing this. Relative numbers of microorganisms may be reported by noting how much growth occurs on the surface of the plate. Obviously, growth of one colony (the offspring of one bacterium) versus growth over the whole plate would be viewed differently with respect to clinical importance. Determination of the actual numbers of bacteria present is only important when analyzing urine obtained by catch or catheter (because of the problem of contamination of the sample by bacteria in the distal urethra). In this instance, calibrated loops (we use disposable loops) containing 0.001 or 0.01 ml of urine are used to inoculate appropriate media (blood/MacConkey, for example). We inoculate blood and MacConkey agars with 0.01 ml of urine. If we find 100 colonies or more after overnight incubation, which translates into greater than or equal to $10^5$ bacteria per milliliter, we interpret this as a significant bacteriuria. There are a number of commercially available "kits" designed to rapidly determine if there is a significant bacteriuria. However, these kits are designed for analysis of urine obtained by clean midstream voiding, a collecting method that is most amenable to human patients. Thus, samples containing less than $10^4$ to $10^5$ bacteria per milliliter (as might be the case with bladder urine) might not test positive by one of these commercial kits, which are designed to detect concentrations greater than $10^5$ bacteria per milliliter.

## Aerobic Bacteria

The standard medium inoculated for the isolation of facultative microorganisms is a blood agar plate. Many laboratories include a MacConkey agar plate as well (or as a "split" plate with blood agar on half and MacConkey agar on the other half). MacConkey agar is useful because enteric microorganisms (e.g., *E. coli, Klebsiella, Enterobacter*) grow very well, as does the nonenteric *Pseudomonas*. Most other nonenteric gram-negative rods and all gram-positive microorganisms do not grow well on this medium. *Bordetella* will grow as tiny pinpoint colonies after 24 hr, and after 48 hr of incubation, the colonies will be quite large. Assessing the growth on MacConkey agar will help greatly to detect the presence or absence of enteric organisms, the group of bacteria most difficult to deal with therapeutically.

## Anaerobic Bacteria

Anaerobic bacteria grow on blood agar. However, specially prepared blood agar is used. The blood agar is prepared in such a way as to rid the medium as much as possible of oxygen and its products. The plates come from the manufacturer in specially sealed pouches designed to exclude air. After anaerobic plates are inoculated they should be placed in a container of flowing oxygen-free carbon dioxide or placed directly into an anaerobic environment (note that anaerobic blood plates that have been removed from their pouches should be stored in flowing oxygen-free carbon dioxide or in an anaerobic environment).

When to inoculate media for anaerobic incubation depends upon the source of the sample. Processing samples for anaerobes is time consuming and expensive. The most common sites or conditions that contain anaerobic bacteria are draining tracts (40% will contain anaerobic bacteria); abscesses (36%); pleural, pericardial, and peritoneal effusions (87%); pyometra (23%); osteomyelitis (21%); and lungs (13%). Anaerobic culture of sites that contain a population of anaerobic bacteria as part of the normal flora is wasteful (feces, vagina, distal urethra, oral cavity). An exception would be culture of duodenal aspirates for assessment of bacterial overgrowth. In this instance, the relative numbers found is what is sought (overgrowth is usually considered present when the total numbers of bacteria, anaerobes and aerobes, exceeds $10^8$/ml of contents). An-

aerobic culture of the urinary tract is not routinely performed because the recovery of these microorganisms from this site is extremely rare.

## Blood Culture

There are two types of techniques that are used to determine whether there are bacteria in the bloodstream or not. In one method, a quantity of blood is inoculated into a bottle containing a broth medium. The inoculated medium is then incubated at 37°C and analyzed at various times to determine if there is bacterial growth (see below for examples of various types of blood culture bottles available). In the other type of procedure, the host cells in the sample are lysed and the sample centrifuged (e.g., ISOLATOR, DuPont). The pellet is processed to determine whether there are bacteria present or not.

The advantages of the lysis method are numerous. First, if the pellet is inoculated onto blood and MacConkey agars, then presumptive identification is possible 24 hr after the blood has been drawn from the patient. Second, lysis and centrifugation removes the microorganisms from the fluid phase of the blood, which may contain antibiotics as well as complement proteins and phagocytic cells. And third, some measure of quantification is possible, which helps in the determination of significance of the isolate.

The main advantage of using the blood bottle method is that samples containing significant but very few bacteria per milliliter will test positive, whereas this might not be so in the lysis method. Second, some bacteria do not grow readily when removed from the blood and put onto a solid surface (as would be the case in the lysis method). This may be especially true for those bacteria that have been damaged by an antibiotic drug. There are various devices (e.g., Antibiotic Removal Device, ARD, BBL) that are used to remove antimicrobial drugs from the blood sample. These are usually resins that remove commonly used antibiotics such as ampicillin, aminoglycosides, and tetracyclines. On the other hand, processing of the sample by the blood bottle method is more difficult and time consuming. Although this method is not as labor intensive at the time of receipt of the sample, subsequent sample processing is very time consuming. Consider, at 24-hr after inoculation a portion of the bottle is removed and stained. Another portion is inoculated onto media for anaerobic and aerobic incubation. These tasks are done daily, or every other day for at least 1 week. Various modifications have been devised to save processing time. A technique used quite commonly in laboratories that process samples obtained from human patients is to add a radioactive substrate to the bottle. At various times thereafter, the gas in the bottle is automatically analyzed for radioactivity (e.g., BACTEC, Johnston Labs). Another method utilizes a "paddle" coated with bacteriologic media (e.g., blood agar on one side and MacConkey agar on the other) in direct communication with the broth in the bottle by being built into the top within a clear plastic cylinder (e.g., Septi-Chek, Roche). By tilting the bottle and "flooding" the cylinder, the paddle is inoculated. The paddle is observed daily (and flooded daily) to see if colonies develop.

## Fungi

It is important to realize that virtually all medically important fungi will grow on blood agar incubated aerobically at 37°C. These include *Aspergillus* (as a mold), *Coccidioides* (as a mold), *Cryptococcus* (as a yeast), *Candida* (as a yeast), *Sporothrix* (as a yeast), *Histoplasma* (as a yeast), and *Blastomyces* (as a yeast). The only thing to remember is that they take some time (24 to 48 hr instead of 24 hr) for the colonies to be big enough to be manipulated. A notable exception is *Malassezia* (the yeast involved with otitis externa in dogs) which does not grow at all well on blood agar. This organism is best demonstrated in direct smear.

Most dermatophytes do not grow on blood agar, and most do not grow well at 37°C (the one common exception is *Trichophyton verrucosum*, the cause of ringworm in cattle). Selective media containing inhibitors of saprophytic fungi, as well as antibiotics to inhibit skin bacteria, are inoculated with suspected hair and scabs. One such medium is dermatophyte test medium (DTM). Dermatophyte test medium also contains glucose, proteins, and a pH indicator that turns red if the conditions around the growing colony are alkaline. Saprophytic fungi will utilize the glucose more readily than the dermatophyte fungi, thereby producing an acid environment around a growing colony. Dermatophytes, on the other hand, will choose the protein as an energy source, which results in an alkaline environment around the colony. There are two disadvantages to exclusive use of DTM. One, if the inoculated medium is not examined daily for the appearance of the first color change, erroneous results may occur. This is because saprophytic colonies (almost always fast growers) run out of their preferred substrate (glucose) and start utilizing protein. This results in a color change from yellow (acid) to alkaline (red). The second disadvantage is that the dermatophyte fungi do not sporulate well on DTM. In a microbiology laboratory, asexual structures are used to identify dermatophyte fungi. An alternative method is to use both DTM and rapid sporulating medium (a medium designed to prompt dermatophyte fungi into sporulating) (e.g., Derm Duet, Bacti-Lab, Inc).

## INTERPRETATION OF RESULTS

Results of observation of the direct smear should be available within 24 hr of sample collection. These results should tell the clinician whether there are inflammatory cells present, their nature, and whether bacteria (or fungi) were observed. However, it should be kept in mind that not seeing bacteria does not rule out their presence, since it takes approximately $10^6$/ml or gm of tissue to see at least one bacteria per oil immersion field. Observing cocci (regardless of the stain that is used) almost always means that there are *Staphylococcus*, *Streptococcus*, or *Peptostreptococcus* (anaerobic streptococcus) present in the sample. On the other hand, presence of rods almost always indicates that there are gram-negative microorganisms present. The presence of filaments is sometimes confusing unless a Gram stain is performed. This is so because some filaments are gram-positive (*Actinomyces*, *Nocardia*), and other filaments, albeit shorter, may be gram-negative anaerobic rods such as certain members of the genus *Fusobacterium*. Since treatment of conditions in which filamentous species are found (*Actinomyces/Nocardia* versus anaerobic rods) is so different, it is important to obtain supporting data when confronted with such a situation. Supporting data may include culture results, nature and site of the condition (e.g., pyothorax in the cat almost never contains *Actinomyces*), and history (e.g., recent removal of a plant awn).

In summary, the author believes the most important goals of a microbiology laboratory are to determine whether an infectious agent is present in an affected site, and if present, to characterize the microorganism. When an infectious agent contaminates a normally sterile site, this assessment is made considerably easier. However, it is vitally important that steps taken by the clinician, as well as by the technologist in the laboratory, be consistent with the above-stated goals. To do otherwise makes detection of the infectious agent more difficult, and may confuse the issue by introducing microorganisms uninvolved in the disease process, or eliminating clinically significant microorganisms. In either case, improper treatment can result: an inappropriate antibiotic is administered or antibiotics are not given, when in fact, they should be.

## References and Suggested Reading

Hirsch DC and Ruehl WW: Clinical microbiology as a guide to treatment of infectious bacterial diseases of the dog and the cat. *In* Scott FW (ed): *Contemporary Issues in Small Animal Practice, volume 3, Infectious Diseases*. New York, Churchill Livingstone, 1986, pp 1–28.

Isenberg HD, Schoenknecht FD, and von Graevenitz A: Collection and processing of bacteriological specimens. *In* Rubin SJ (ed): *Cumitech 9*. Washington, DC, American Society for Microbiology, 1979.

Isenberg HD, Washington JA, Doern GV, and Amsterdam D: Specimen collection and handling. *In* Balows A, Hausler WJ, Herrmann KL, Isenberg HD, and Shadomy HJ (eds): *Manual of Clinical Microbiology*, 5th edition. Washington, DC, American Society for Microbiology, 1991, pp 15–28.

# IMMUNOPATHOLOGIC CONSEQUENCES OF INFECTIOUS DISEASE

STEVEN W. DOW

*Denver, Colorado*

*and* MICHAEL R. LAPPIN

*Fort Collins, Colorado*

Development of an immune system capable of mounting both innate and acquired immunologic responses was driven largely by selective pressures imposed by pathogenic microorganisms. These immune responses may either block infection outright or prevent the development of severe disease if infection does occur. However, there are situations where immunologic responses to infection, particularly chronic infections caused by persistent pathogens of relatively low virulence, are actually more detrimental to the host than the consequences of unchecked infection. In this article, we will discuss several examples of clinically important infectious diseases of dogs and cats where abnormal or exaggerated immune responses contribute substantially to the disease pathogenesis, and introduce the concept of superantigen-mediated diseases and their possible clinical relevance to companion animal medicine.

Although immune responses to some pathogens may become so exaggerated that they resemble autoimmune diseases, there is as yet no convincing evidence that any infectious disease of animals can induce a state of true autoimmunity. Nonetheless, it is important clinically to distinguish the immunologic sequelae of infection from diseases of an immune-mediated, noninfectious nature. A prime example is immune-mediated anemia (IMA), which may develop spontaneously due to abnormal immunoregulation or may be triggered by infection with any of several erythrocyte-tropic pathogens. An accurate diagnosis in such situations is critical because the long-term therapeutic options are generally diametrically opposed. Prolonged, potent systemic immunosuppression is indicated for patients with non-infectious IMA, whereas antimicrobial therapy (possibly combined with a short course of corticosteroid therapy) is indicated for patients with an infectious cause of IMA. An erroneous diagnosis may have dire consequences for the patient.

Mechanistically, immune responses can be grouped into four broad categories, although recent developments suggest that for completeness a fifth category will be necessary. In most infections, multiple immunologic mechanisms operate simultaneously, although one mechanism is usually predominant. For example, both T lymphocytes and antigen-presenting cells (either macrophages, B cells, or dendritic cells) are required to develop immunologic responses in diseases that may appear clinically to be mediated only by antibodies and complement, such as IMA.

The best studied immunologic reactions caused by infectious diseases in animals generally involve antibody-mediated responses to exogenous antigens or to altered self-antigens, although it is likely that T-cell–mediated immune responses play the predominant role in these and other immunopathologic processes. Our knowledge of cell-mediated immune responses in companion animals is limited, primarily due to technical difficulties inherent to the study of these processes, although recent advances in molecular immunologic research have begun to answer some questions in this area.

Immediate hypersensitivity reactions occur when the host is reexposed to an antigen that has previously induced formation of cytophilic immunoglobulin E (IgE) antibodies. Only certain antigens, especially oligosaccharide helminth antigens, trigger IgE production. After the first antigenic exposure, secreted IgE binds to the surface of mast cells and basophils. When antigen is encountered a second time, it binds to the specific cytophilic IgE, which in turn triggers sudden and massive release of vasoactive substances (e.g., histamine, heparin, prostaglandins, leukotrienes) from mast cells and basophils, followed by an influx of eosinophils. Depending on the antigen dose and site of exposure and the amount of IgE present, the reaction may trigger either a localized reaction or a systemic anaphylactic response. Helminth parasites are most often associated with this type of immune sequelae, including allergic pneumonitis due to *Dirofilaria immitis* infection.

Antibody-mediated cytotoxicity and immune complex formation are the most common mechanisms by which infectious agents induce immunologic injury. In cytotoxic reactions, antibody binds to the surface of infected cells (or cells that have been rendered antigenic), followed by complement binding. This results in cell destruction, either by direct complement-mediated cell lysis or by phagocytosis and destruction by mononuclear phagocytes in extravascular sites, especially the spleen. Platelets and erythrocytes are common targets for this type of reaction. Infectious disease examples include *Haemobartonella felis* and *Babesia canis* infections.

Immune complex deposition in tissues occurs when soluble antigen-antibody complexes form, usually a consequence of the host response to persistent, low-level infection. Antigen-antibody complexes are most likely to induce injury when they involve very-high-avidity antibodies, or form under conditions where there is slight antigen excess. Soluble immune complexes are most often deposited in organs with an end-arterial circulation, including renal glomeruli, joint capsules, the uveal tract, skin, and meninges. Immune complexes, once deposited in an organ, are able to bind complement, thereby eliciting a perivascular inflammatory reaction characterized by an influx of neutrophils, platelets, and monocytes. Vasoactive substances and inflammatory cytokines released by these cells then destroy parenchymal cells in the immediate vicinity of the reaction, leading over time to progressive, irreversible organ injury. Examples of antigen-antibody complex–mediated diseases include feline infectious peritonitis (FIP), *Toxoplasma gondii*–induced uveitis, feline leukemia virus (FeLV)–associated glomerulonephritis, and corneal edema following canine infectious hepatitis virus infection.

Granulomatous inflammation characterizes chronic, slowly progressing infections caused by pathogens such as systemic fungi (*Blastomyces, Histoplasma*) and mycobacteria that are able to survive within macrophages. Often, the organism is contained but never eradicated and a state of equilibrium between the organism and the host ensues. In some cases, the granulomatous response to the organism induces more tissue destruction and organ pathology than the infectious agent itself.

A fifth type of immunologic response to pathogens has been described recently. The reaction involves widespread, simultaneous activation of many T lymphocytes by a substance (often a toxin) that can be produced by certain bacteria, mycoplasmas, and viruses. These compounds are collectively referred to as superantigens because of their ability to simultaneously activate many T cells by a mechanism distinct from that by which mitogens or conventional antigens activate T cells. When many lymphocytes are activated simultaneously, they release large quantities of cytokines, which in turn trigger systemic sequelae, including fever, vascular collapse, diarrhea, and shock. The toxic shock syndrome (caused by *Staphylococcus aureus*) and scarlet fever (caused by *Streptococcus pyogenes*) are two examples of superantigen-mediated diseases in humans.

Lymphocytes activated by superantigens are usually rendered functionally incompetent and may disappear entirely if the antigen persists for more than several weeks. Thus, the host response to the microorganism causes serious morbidity and occasionally mortality, yet does not lead to eradication of the agent. Evolutionarily, it is unclear why diverse pathogens have developed superantigens, although they may function to transiently inactivate T-cell immunity and thereby provide the pathogen with an opportunity to establish infection.

## RICKETTSIAL AND BACTERIAL INFECTIONS

Acute *Haemobartonella felis* infection is lethal in one third of cats, due to rapid-onset anemia. However, a carrier state develops in nearly all the remaining recovered cats and these animals are at risk of developing chronic or acute immune-mediated anemia. Chronic and repeated parasitemia results in antibody-mediated erythrocyte destruction, due in large part to antibody-dependent cytotoxicity.

The presence of the *Haemobartonella* organism on the erythrocyte surface may expose normally sequestered antigens, induce novel erythrocyte antigens, or induce complement fixation on the erythrocyte surface, with the erythrocyte being indirectly damaged as a result. Many *Haemobartonella*-infected cats will have immunoglobulin or complement bound to erythrocyte membranes, which gives a positive reaction in the Coombs' test. As a consequence of having surface-bound immunoglobulin, erythrocytes will be removed from circulation by splenic macrophages; if the rate of removal exceeds the rate of replacement, regenerative anemia results. A similar condition may also develop in dogs infected with the parasite *Babesia canis*.

Effective treatment for severely affected cats includes antibiotics (usually doxycycline) to eliminate the organism from the erythrocyte surface, plus immunosuppressive therapy to slow erythrocyte destruction. Prednisone (2 to 4 mg/kg daily for 1 to 2 weeks) is indicated in severely anemic cats, cats with autoagglutination of erythrocytes, or cats that have had multiple episodes of anemia. Any infected cat, even after successful treatment, should be presumed a chronic carrier, and retreatment may be periodically necessary.

Rickettsial infections of dogs, especially canine ehrlichiosis (*Ehrlichia canis*) and Rocky Mountain spotted fever (*Rickettsia rickettsii*), are associated with immunologic sequelae that may be more severe than the direct effects of infection. Vasculitis involving small arterioles is a prominent feature of canine rickettsial infections. *Rickettsia rickettsii* infects and replicates in vascular endothelial cells; *E. canis*–infected peripheral blood mononuclear cells settle in small vessel beds. Endothelial cell damage triggers activation of local innate immune responses, which includes complement deposition. Complement deposition and activation induces neutrophil influx and lysis, liberating cytotoxic mediators that cause further vessel damage and induce thrombosis. In the later stages of vasculitis, a perivascular mononuclear cell infiltrate consisting of lymphocytes and macrophages develops.

Persistent *E. canis* infection leads to pronounced activation of humoral immune responses, resulting in hypergammaglobulinemia, bone marrow plasmacytosis, and occasionally monoclonal gammopathies. Although rickettsia within monocytes are virtually impervious to the effects of humoral immune responses, the overabundance of anti-*Ehrlichia* antibodies has adverse consequences for the host. Circulating immune complexes in dogs chronically infected with *E. canis* may bind to the glomerular endothelium, thereby precipitating glomerulonephritis, with resultant polyuria and proteinuria. This condition is potentially reversible after successful antibiotic elimination of the organism. For treatment of *Ehrlichia*-induced glomerulonephritis, doxycycline should be used instead of tetracycline, as tetracycline is potentially nephrotoxic. Circulating immune complexes also commonly lodge in the synovial membranes and uveal tract, inducing nonseptic, suppurative polyarthritis and uveitis.

Chronic rickettsial infection can induce low titers of antinuclear antibodies and positive Coombs' tests. Monoclonal gammopathy (immunoglobulin G) and bone marrow plasmacytosis in dogs with chronic ehrlichiosis makes the differentiation from multiple myeloma and chronic lymphocytic leukemia difficult. In severe chronic ehrlichiosis, bone marrow hypoplasia with resultant anemia, neutropenia, and thrombocytopenia may develop. It is not clear if these hypoproliferative phenomena are immune mediated or are a direct rickettsial effect. Since these clinical and laboratory abnormalities are also common with immune-mediated diseases like systemic lupus erythematosus, the complete diagnostic evaluation of a dog with nonspecific immunologic abnormalities should include rickettsial serology. In severe cases, it may be prudent to initiate treatment by combining glucocorticoid therapy (prednisone, 1 to 2 mg/kg daily) with a tetracycline antibiotic until results of serologic testing are available.

Several bacteria, especially certain strains of both streptococci and staphylococci, can produce toxins (superantigens) that exert profound immunologic effects. Although the original infection may be mild or self-limited, liberation of these toxins results in rapid and severe systemic signs, including shock and serious organ damage, especially to the kidney and heart.

Bacterial superantigens activate large numbers of T lymphocytes by simultaneously binding the T-cell–receptor $\beta$ chain and the class II MHC molecule of an adjacent antigen-presenting cell. This binding provides a potent activating stimulus, capable of activating up to one third of all circulating T cells simultaneously (depending on which T-cell–receptor $\beta$ chains they express), whereas normally fewer than 1 in 10,000 T cells are capable of responding to a foreign antigen. The mechanism by which bacterial superantigens activate T cells differs in two ways from the lymphocyte activation induced by nonspecific T-cell mitogens such as concanavalin A. First, superantigens stimulate only T cells whose T-cell receptors bear certain $\beta$-chain configurations, whereas mitogens nonspecifically trigger all T cells. Secondly, the superantigens must be presented by MHC class II expressing antigen-presenting cells, whereas there is no requirement for class II molecules in mitogen-induced responses.

*Staphylococcus aureus* produces several enterotoxins, which can induce typical symptoms of food poisoning and occasionally shock in humans. Some strains of *S. aureus* also produce toxic shock syndrome toxin-1, which has been associated with most cases of toxic shock syndrome. Group A streptococci (*Streptococcus pyogenes*) also produce toxins with superantigen properties. These are the streptococcal pyrogenic exotoxins, which have also been referred to as erythrogenic toxins or scarlet fever toxins. Toxins that meet the criteria for designation as superantigens have also been isolated from *Clostridium* and *Pseudomonas*. *Mycoplasma ar-*

*thritidis*, which induces chronic, relapsing arthritis in rodents, secretes a small protein with superantigen properties, designated *Mycoplasma arthritidis* mitogen.

Several important viruses may also produce superantigens. A number of superantigens are produced by endogenous and exogenous murine retroviruses, with important effects on development of the T-cell repertoire in mice. There is preliminary, albeit controversial, evidence that HIV may mediate T-cell depletion at least in part via a superantigen-like effect. Two primate herpesviruses, including Epstein-Barr virus, encode proteins with superantigen effects, and the rabies virus nucleocapsid also has superantigen properties.

Circumstantial evidence suggests that bacterial and viral superantigens are also relevant to diseases of dogs and cats. Staphylococcal enterotoxins A and B are potent *in vitro* activators of canine and feline lymphocytes. *In vivo*, staphylococcal enterotoxins are thought to be responsible for some severe, acute gastrointestinal illnesses in dogs. *Mycoplasma* infection can induce a chronic polyarthritis syndrome in cats that resembles *Mycoplasma* arthritis in rodents. An FIV protein has been identified that is a potent inducer of T-cell proliferative responses. Thus, it is likely that there are other as yet unidentified superantigens that may mediate clinically important disease syndromes in dogs and cats. With increased availability of canine and feline immunologic reagents, it may become possible to detect the changes in T-cell subsets and functional status that characterize superantigen-mediated diseases. It may also become possible in the future to utilize specific neutralizing antibodies to block the systemic effects of superantigens early in the disease course.

## VIRAL INFECTIONS

Immunologic abnormalities figure prominently in the pathogenesis of several important viral diseases. During acute infection, the canine infectious hepatitis virus spreads widely and infects many different cell types. If the infected dog mounts an effective immune response and develops high virus neutralizing antibody titers, the infection is controlled. If, on the other hand, the animal cannot mount an effective immune response and develops only low neutralizing antibody titers, then viral infection may persist in organs such as the liver and eventually lead to organ damage via direct viral cytopathic effects. Infectious canine hepatitis virus may occasionally gain access to the eye, where it infects corneal endothelial cells. Antiviral antibodies bind to infected corneal endothelial cells and activate complement, leading eventually to immune complex–mediated corneal injury, which is manifested clinically as corneal edema. Thus, the ocular injury is immunologically mediated, whereas hepatocyte injury is due directly to viral cytopathic effects. Specific treatment for corneal edema is not indicated, as the condition usually resolves spontaneously.

A different immunologic mechanism accounts for

central nervous system (CNS) injury in chronic canine distemper virus–induced encephalitis. If the initial viremic episode is not adequately controlled, the virus spreads to and infects glial cells within the CNS. Here, the virus undergoes slow, noncytopathic replication. Months to years after the initial infection is cleared from peripheral tissues, antiviral immune responses begin to attack virus-infected cells within the CNS. In this disease, cell-mediated immune responses are the major effectors. Virus-specific T cells attack and destroy distemper virus–infected cells, including microglia and astrocytes. In the process, adjacent oligodendrocytes are also damaged, leading eventually to demyelination, the major pathologic lesion in chronic canine distemper virus encephalitis. In this example, it is the immune response to the virus, rather than the virus itself, that triggers CNS injury. Immune suppression with corticosteroids may temporarily slow the tempo of chronic canine distemper encephalitis, but long-term disease remission is rare.

Virulent strains of FIP virus primarily infect tissue macrophages and circulating monocytes, as well as endothelial cells of small veins and venules. Migration of virus-infected monocytes into blood vessel walls and deposition of antiviral immune complexes induces an intense vasculitis, which in turn leads to leakage of fibrin-rich fluids into intercellular spaces. A characteristic protein-rich exudate subsequently develops in most infected cats. Some infected cats, for reasons not clear, develop the dry form of FIP without appreciable fluid accumulation, although vasculitis still occurs.

Feline infectious peritonitis is clearly a disease mediated by humoral antiviral immune responses. The virus itself is relatively nonpathogenic, particularly to the host macrophage. Infected cats, despite developing strong antiviral antibody responses, are unable to clear the virus from infected cells. These same antiviral antibodies are, however, largely responsible for the immune-mediated pathology, especially vasculitis, that develops in cats infected with pathogenic strains of FIP. Vaccination against FIP with a killed vaccine actually significantly worsens disease, probably because antiviral antibodies actually enhance FIP infection of macrophages via Fc receptor–mediated uptake of the opsonized virus.

Since ineffective humoral antiviral responses figure prominently in the pathogenesis of FIP, most treatment attempts have focused on suppressing this response. Immunosuppressive doses of corticosteroids and cytotoxic drugs have been used most often, with evidence of transient effectiveness but not long-term cure. Cell-mediated immune responses are likely to be much more effective at controlling virus replication and spread than humoral immunity. Therefore, more specific immunosuppressants have been sought, along with drugs that work to specifically stimulate cell-mediated immunity. It may soon be possible to utilize recombinant feline cytokines such as interferon-γ and interleukin-12 to boost cell-mediated immunity, while at the same time suppressing humoral immune responses with drugs that block interleukin-4 (one of the primary cytokines required for antibody formation) activity. Use of recombinant feline interferon-α may also prove efficacious in suppressing viral replication in infected cats. Vaccination with an apathogenic temperature-sensitive mutant FIP strain also appears to induce protective immune responses in some cats.

Chronic FeLV infection may also lead to immune-mediated injury in infected cats, through different mechanisms than in FIP infection. Coomb's-positive anemia can develop. Viremic animals have very high levels of circulating FeLV antigens, much of which may be complexed to antiviral antibodies. These immune complexes may be deposited in vascular beds, especially in the kidneys, resulting in progressive glomerulonephritis. One potentially effective treatment is suppression of viral replication, primarily by employing inhibitors of virus replication such as interferon-α (Interferon alpha 2b, Roche; 10,000 U/kg SC b.i.d.) and/or azidothymidine (10 mg/kg, PO b.i.d.). In select cases, a brief course of immunosuppressive therapy to reduce immune complex formation may be indicated. In this particular FeLV-associated disease, as in fatal FIP, it is the immune response to the virus, rather than the virus itself, that causes disease.

## PARASITIC INFECTIONS

In the parasitized host, many of the detrimental immunologic reactions induced by infection are mediated by antiparasite antibodies. *Babesia* spp. infect canine erythrocytes leading to erythrocyte lysis and destruction. In chronic infection, the degree of erythrocyte destruction often exceeds the number of parasitized cells. Therefore, immune-mediated erythrocyte destruction is generally felt to contribute more to the pathogenesis of chronic anemia than *Babesia* infection per se. In babesiosis, as in feline hemobartonellosis, immunoglobulin-coated erythrocytes are destroyed in the spleen or lysed *in situ* by anti-*Babesia* antibodies plus complement. Positive Coomb's tests are common.

*Trypanosoma cruzi* causes American trypanosomiasis. Cardiomyopathy is common in infected dogs. The pathogenesis of cardiomyopathy is unclear but may be due to parasite-derived toxins, overstimulation of the sympathetic nervous system, or immune-mediated reactions.

*Leishmania* spp. are obligate intracellular protozoan parasites. As with ehrlichiosis, the humoral immune responses are dramatic but nonprotective. Antibodies against *Leishmania* spp. lead to opsonization and phagocytosis by macrophages. The organism survives within macrophages and ultimately stimulates histiocytic proliferation in reticuloendothelial organs including the liver, spleen, and lymph nodes. The humoral immune responses can result in autoantibody production or innocent bystander reactions leading to Coomb's-positive anemia or thrombocytopenia. Immune complex production can cause vasculitis, polyarthritis, or glomerulonephritis. Renal failure secondary to glomerulonephritis is a common cause of death in *Leishmania*-infected dogs.

Formation of persistent tissue cysts is a key feature of the immunopathogenesis of *Toxoplasma gondii* infection, because these cysts serve as an antigen depot. Although *T. gondii* bradyzoites are not actively dividing while encysted within tissues, they remain metabolically active and release bradyzoite-specific antigens into their immediate environment, thus ensuring that the host remains sensitized to parasite antigens. One consequence of this persistent immune stimulation is development of immune-mediated sequelae. In humans, circulating immune complexes may trigger fever and muscle pain in *Toxoplasma*-infected patients. Recurrent retinochoroiditis in transplacentally infected people is likely due to cell-mediated immune responses.

Endogenous uveitis, an important ocular disease of cats, has been linked to immunologic consequences of *T. gondii* infection. Intraocular production of *T. gondii*–specific immunoglobulins is common in cats with endogenous uveitis; intraocular production of *T. gondii*–specific IgM has only been documented in cats with endogenous uveitis. Cats with endogenous uveitis are more likely than healthy cats to be positive for serum *T. gondii*–containing immune complexes. In addition, *T. gondii*–specific immune complexes have been detected in aqueous humor, in levels exceeding those found in serum. These results suggest that anti-*Toxoplasma* antibodies and immune complex formation play a role in the pathogenesis of feline toxoplasmosis and especially feline endogenous uveitis. Treatment with clindamycin may lead to clinical improvement or cure in cats with primary *Toxoplasma*-induced uveitis.

Excessive immune complex formation in canine dirofilariasis is most often manifested clinically as glomerulonephritis. This condition is most likely to develop in dogs with longstanding *Dirofilaria immitis* infection and is potentially reversible once the patent infection has been resolved with adulticide therapy.

Pulmonary eosinophilic granulomatosis is another, more serious immune-mediated complication attributed to dirofilariasis. This disorder probably involves a combination of both immediate hypersensitivity and cell-mediated immune reactions to *D. immitis* antigens in some dogs. Histologically, the lesions are comprised of nodular accumulations of eosinophils, plasma cells, and macrophages. Nearly 60% of dogs with these pulmonary lesions, as detected radiographically or surgically, have been found to be *Dirofilaria*-positive by serologic testing. Unfortunately, recurrence is common even after treatment to eradicate the organism. Corticosteroid treatment may induce temporary lesion regression.

## References and Suggested Reading

Appel MJG, Shek WR, and Summers BA: Lymphocyte mediated immune cytotoxicity in dogs infected with virulent canine distemper virus. Infect Immun 37:592, 1982.

Barlough JE and Stoddart CA: Feline coronaviral infections. *In* Greene CE (ed): *Infectious Diseases of the Dog and Cat.* Philadelphia, WB Saunders Co., 1990, pp 299–312.

Calvert CA, Mahaffey MB, Lappin MR, et al: Pulmonary eosinophilic granulomatosis in dogs. J Am Anim Hosp Assoc 24:311, 1989.

Gocke DJ, Morris TQ, and Bradley SE: Chronic hepatitis in the dog: The role of immune factors. J Am Vet Med Assoc 156:1700, 1970.

Greene CE: Host-microbe interactions. *In* Greene CE (ed): *Clinical Microbiology and Infectious Diseases of the Dog and Cat.* Philadelphia, WB Saunders Co., 1984, pp 73–77.

Harvey JW and Gaskin JM: Feline haemobartonellosis: Attempts to reduce relapses in chronically infected cats. J Am Anim Hosp Assoc 14:453, 1978.

Kotzin BL, Leung DYM, Kappler J, and Marrack P: Superantigens and their potential role in human disease. *In* Dixon F (ed): *Advances in Immunology,* vol 54. New York, Academic Press, 1993, pp 99–146.

Lappin MR, Cayatte S, Powell CC, et al: Detection of *Toxoplasma gondii* antigen-containing immune complexes in the serum of cats. Am J Vet Res 54:415, 1993.

Lappin MR, Roberts SM, Davidson MG, et al: Enzyme-linked immunosorbent assays for the detection of *Toxoplasma gondii*-specific antibodies and antigens in the aqueous humor of cats. J Am Vet Med Assoc 201:1010, 1992.

Troy GC and Forrester SD: Canine ehrlichiosis. *In* Greene CE (ed): *Infectious Diseases of the Dog and Cat.* Philadelphia, WB Saunders Co., 1990, pp 404–415.

# PET OWNERSHIP FOR IMMUNOCOMPROMISED PEOPLE

CRAIG E. GREENE

*Athens, Georgia*

## THE PROBLEM

Immunodeficiency occurs in people for a variety of physiologic and pathologic reasons. Age is one determinant, since the fetus, neonates, and young children have underdeveloped immune systems. Similarly, elderly persons, especially those in nursing homes or hospitals, have apparent increased risks of developing infections. Concurrent conditions such as other illnesses, pregnancy, burns, indwelling tubes, catheters, or implants increase the risk of the host by removing natural barriers to infectious agents. Immunodeficiency is also a result of cancer chemotherapy or leukopenic disorders and may be inborn in the case of congenital or hereditary defects in the immune system. The most rapidly advancing cause of immunodeficiency in people is the acquired immunodeficiency syndrome (AIDS) resulting from infection with human immunodeficiency virus (HIV). For this reason, information presented herein will stress documented AIDS-related zoonoses, although all immunodeficient people should apply similar guidelines in handling their pets. Furthermore, because zoonoses can develop in immunocompetent people, many of the principles and practices for sanitation can be applied by anyone with pets.

Zoonoses are defined as infectious diseases shared by people and animals; however, not all zoonoses are transmitted from animals to humans. Those zoonoses that can be contracted from companion animals pose an inherent risk for immunocompromised people with pets. Inhalation or ingestion are the common means by which many zoonotic infections may be transmitted. Transmission can occur by bites or scratches, or by arthropod vectors. Many zoonotic agents are maintained in nature in inanimate conditions such as soil, water, or vegetation. In these zoonoses, animals may contaminate the environment, but in most cases, people and animals acquire these infections simultaneously and independently of each other.

The importance of zoonotic diseases has become more apparent in recent years owing to the AIDS epidemic in the human population. In fact, the appearance of unusual zoonotic infections in people was the way that AIDS was first recognized. The increasing incidence of zoonotic infections in immunosuppressed people makes it imperative that veterinarians keep their knowledge of these diseases current. Most physicians are not as well trained in zoonoses compared to veterinarians. Veterinarians may be in a better position to advise immunocompromised persons about the relative risk of pets and provide them with accurate information on precautionary measures. Surveys have been conducted showing that approximately 50% of patients with AIDS have pets. Although veterinarians are among the best educated concerning animal infections, few have been taking an active role in educating their immunodeficient clients (Spencer, 1992). AIDS patients most frequently consult physicians, nurses, and community health personnel, who give conflicting advice (Gill and Stone, 1992). Surveys have shown that over 90% of HIV-infected people have been advised to give up their pets by human health professionals, while only 5% have followed this advice.

Pets offer important physiologic and psychologic benefits for people, especially the infirmed. Important bonds of friendship exist between people and their pets. While illness and disability often alienate homebound AIDS victims from their family, friends, and acquaintances, pets provide continued companionship and overcome the deleterious effects of loneliness. It may be more detrimental to the well-being of the isolated immunocompromised person to lose their pet companion than to potentially risk acquiring a zoonotic infection.

At a first glance, risk of acquiring animal infections may appear to dominate the medical literature and media reports, but a relatively small fraction of infections in people can actually be attributed to pet contact. People with immunosuppression have an increased risk of acquiring all types of infections including zoonoses. People are more likely to acquire infections from other people than from animals. Furthermore, some of the highly publicized infections in AIDS patients such as toxoplasmosis are due to reactivation of previous infections acquired from meat and do not relate to current pet exposure. Unfortunately, misconceptions about pet-acquired illnesses may cause people to give up their pets unnecessarily. Medical and veterinary health personnel should not automatically recommend that immunodeficient patients give away companion animals when practical precautionary measures exist to reduce the risks of infection. Veterinarians may have to offset the undesirable image that has been projected by unfavorable media coverage of health risk imposed by pets. Not only are many of the pet-associated illnesses of minor consequence, they are much rarer than published reports that document their occurrence suggest. Furthermore, many of the published zoonotic illnesses have occurred in people with intensive animal-related occupations.

Immunoincompetent people may develop emotional and physical limitations that prevent them from adequately caring for their pets. They often need assistance, and numerous organizations are available to help them meet these needs. Veterinarians can advise their clients on the relative risks and care necessary to contain zoonoses and direct them to support groups to help them with home pet care. Pets Are Wonderful Support (PAWS) is a nonprofit organization dedicated to providing information and "at home" support for immunocompromised people that want to keep their pets. PAWS publishes a brochure from their San Francisco office entitled *Safe Pet Guidelines* that gives immunocompromised owners background information on keeping their pets and themselves healthy. A list of the PAWS national network of support organizations and brochures is provided in Table 1. Veterinarians can also assist by channeling donations of money and by offering their professional expertise to these local groups.

## DISEASES

Over 250 organisms are known to cause zoonotic infections. Of these, approximately 30 to 40 involve companion animals. Of these latter infections, a selected few have been reported with greater frequency in people with immunodeficiency and AIDS (Anon, 1990). The appearance of a few of these infections, cryptosporidiosis, *Mycobacterium avium* infection, cryptococcosis, and salmonellosis, has been used to define the onset of AIDS syndrome in HIV-infected people. The AIDS-related zoonoses that are potentially acquired directly from companion animals are cryptosporidiosis, toxoplasmosis, cat scratch disease, campylobacteriosis, salmonellosis, giardiasis, *Rhodococcus equi* infection, *Mycobacterium marinum* infection, psittacosis, dermatophytosis, and bite infections. Other zoonotic infections reported in immunodeficient patients that are probably acquired from environmental exposure rather than pets are pneumocytosis, microsporidiosis, *Mycobacterium avium* complex infection, and cryptococcosis. The zoonoses described below will be restricted to those that have been associated with exposure of immunodeficient people to companion animals.

Toxoplasmosis is the most publicized zoonotic disease acquired from pets, due in part to the emphasis physicians receive in their training in animal diseases. Actually, the overall risk of becoming infected from cats in the household is comparatively low (see "CVT Update: Feline Toxoplasmosis," this volume, p 309). Although it can be acquired by ingestion of oocysts shed by infected cats, infection in people usually occurs by ingestion of undercooked meats, especially goat or pork. Isolated outbreaks of disease have been reported following handling or inhaling soil dust contaminated by cat feces. Toxoplasmosis occurs in 10% of AIDS patients and is thought to be responsible for at least 30% of central nervous system (CNS) complications in this immunodeficient population. Most cases of CNS toxoplasmosis are due to reactivation of quiescent infections rather than recent exposure.

Cryptosporidiosis is an intestinal infection caused by a ubiquitous coccidian parasite that can be acquired from young domestic herbivores (calves, lambs, kids, and piglets) with diarrhea or less commonly pets. Human-to-human transmission occurs without animal reservoirs, and outbreaks have been noted in day-care centers and family groups. The usual source of outbreaks from environmental exposure is drinking of water sources contaminated by animal or human sewage. Water runoff from grazing animals or animal holding facilities or sewage treatment facilities can contaminate surface water supplies. Chlorination of water does not kill these parasites and filtration systems for municipal water must be of high caliber to eliminate these organisms. *Cryptosporidium* oocysts can be found in 90% of untreated municipal water supplies and 30% of treated systems. As a result, most people contact this organism independent of exposure to their pets and approximately 15% of AIDS patients develop this complication (Buckley, Braffman, and Stern, 1990). Immunocompetent people show signs of abdominal pain and a self-limiting diarrhea of 5 to 10 days' duration. Immunodeficient individuals have a severe water debilitating chronic diarrhea that is refractory to therapy. Oocysts in feces are small (2 to 4 $\mu$m) and are difficult to demonstrate without concentration procedures and special staining.

Giardiasis is a disease found in animals and people, although it is not well established whether interspecies transmission is common. As with cryptosporidiosis, outbreaks are usually waterborne or involve young children in day-care centers. Signs of infection in people are a watery, foul-smelling diarrhea with flatus and abdominal distention. The diagnosis in people may be difficult, since finding the parasite on up to three stool examinations is no greater than 50% (Scully, Mark, and McNeely, 1985). For this reason, treatment is often empiric.

Salmonellosis develops in approximately 5% of AIDS patients. Food-borne episodes from contaminated meat account for many exposures, but a few pet-related ex-

**Table 1.** *Resources for Pet Owners with AIDS Compiled by PAWS*

**National Network and Education Resource**
Pets Are Wonderful Support (PAWS), 539 Castro Street, San Francisco, CA 94114, (415) 241-1460

**Local Groups**
Pets Are Wonderful Support (PAWS), 539 Castro Street, San Francisco, CA 94114, (415) 241-1460
PAWS, Chicago, 1153 N. Dearborn, #321, Chicago, IL 60610, (312) 465-3741
PAWS, LA, 8272 Sunset Bl., West Hollywood, CA 90046, (213) 650-7297
PAWS, Orange County, 3111 Via Santo Tomas, San Juan Capistrano, CA 92675, (714) 489-2898
PAWS, St. Louis, 4579 Laclede, St. Louis, MO 63108, (314) 351-8047
PAWS, San Diego, 1278 University Avenue, San Diego, CA 92103, (619) 234-PAWS
Pets Are Loving Support, Inc., 1438 Peachtree Street, Atlanta, GA 30309, (404) 876-7257
Pet Pals, P.O. Box 190712, Dallas, TX 75219, (214) 521-5124
Pals, Pets Are Loving Support, P.O. Box 1539, Guerneville, CA 95446, (707) 869-9473
The Pet Patrol, 1623 Marshall, Houston, TX 77006, (718) 682-5995
Companion Animal Support & Assistance Network (CASAN), P.O. Box 4963, Louisville, KY 40204, (502) 451-2676
Pet Owners with AIDS/ARC Resource Service, Inc. (POWARS), P.O. Box 1116, Madison Square Station, New York, NY 10159, (212) 744-0842
Marin Humane Society, 171 Bel Marin Keys Bl., Novato, CA 94949, (415) 883-4621
Pets Support Network, 1824 12th Avenue, Seattle, WA 98122, (206) 328-8780
Pets, Washington DC, 1747 Connecticut Avenue, NW, Washington, DC 20009, (202) 234-PETS

**General Resources**
The Latham Foundation, 1826 Clement Avenue, Alameda, CA 94501, (510) 521-0920
Center for Animals in Society, University of California, Davis, CA 95616, (916) 752-3602
AAHA, P.O. Box 150899, Denver, CO (303) 986-2800
Delta Society, 321 Burnett Ave., So., 3rd Fl., Renton, WA 98055, (205) 226-7357
California VMA, 5321 Madison Avenue, Sacramento, CA 95841, (916) 344-4988
AVMA, 1931 N. Meacham Road, Ste. 100, Schaumberg, IL 60173, (800) 248-2862

**Recommended Brochures for Clients**
PAWS, Questions you may have about toxoplasmosis and your cat. Pets Are Wonderful Support, San Francisco, CA 94114.
PAWS, Safe Pet Guidelines. Pets Are Wonderful Support, San Francisco, CA 94114.
American Animal Hospital Association, Pet Owner Guidelines for People with Immunocompromised Conditions. For members of AAHA (800) 252-2242 ask for Member Service Center.

posures have involved turtles. Severe recurrent diarrhea and bacteremia are common in AIDS patients.

Cat scratch disease has been recently determined to be caused by *Rochalimaea henselae*. In this disorder, a local papule and regional lymphadenomegaly develop 3 to 10 days after a scratch or puncture wound from a cat. In some cases, cat association without known injury occurs. A similar pathologic process has been seen with injuries produced by dogs, monkeys, and even porcupines and with other disorders such as toxoplasmosis. Many lymphadenopathic illnesses in the past have probably been misdiagnosed as cat scratch disease. Now that this cat-associated organism has been identified, specific characterization of the clinical syndromes it causes can be elucidated. The infection in cats appears to be subclinical and may be transmitted by fleas. *Rochalimaea*-related illnesses are being recognized with increasing frequency in immunosuppressed patients as other forms of the cat scratch syndrome, notably disseminated cat scratch disease and bacillary angiomatosis. In addition, cat-unassociated bacillary angiomatosis has also been shown to be caused by a closely related organism, *R. quintana*.

Campylobacteriosis is caused by a microaerophilic group of gram-negative, curved motile rods that are commensal flora of animals. Although *Campylobacter jejuni* has been the incriminated organism, recent studies have shown a wide variety of related species exist in domestic and wild animals. As regards pets, young dogs and cats with diarrhea have been most commonly associated with household infections. *Campylobacter jejuni* is frequently isolated from dogs or cats recently acquired from pet stores, kennels, animal shelters, or pounds. Uncooked meat, especially poultry, is probably a greater source of infection. Fecal-oral, food-borne, and water-borne transmission are the principal avenues for infection. Contaminated water supply, potentially from migrating waterfowl or herbivores, may be a source of infection for outdoor pets. Children of less than 5 years with a newly acquired puppy have the highest prevalence of infection (Salfield and Pugh, 1987). Signs of infection are intense abdominal discomfort, bloody diarrhea, fever, tenesmus, and fecal leukocytosis. Immunosuppressed individuals with AIDS develop recurrent diarrhea, dehydration, and bacteremia.

*Rhodococcus equi* infections have been reported in AIDS patients that have been exposed to horses or farm animals or from environmental exposure to this soil saprophyte. Clinical signs are related to a pneumonia with pulmonary abscessation.

Dermatophytosis from pet animals is caused by two zoophilic fungi, *Microsporum canis* and *Trichophyton mentagrophytes*. Cats and dogs, respectively, may harbor these fungi asymptomatically. People develop classic lesions with circular alopecia, scaling, crusting, and ulceration. Topical therapy of lesions is often rewarding, but topical and systemic therapy of pets and environmental decontamination is often needed to prevent reoccurrence.

Psittacosis is an endemic infection of birds worldwide caused by *Chlamydia psittacii*. It may be transmitted by direct contact with birds or indirectly by their feces or feathers. Infected birds may remain carriers. Animal care workers have a high risk of becoming exposed. Affected people develop pneumonia with a variety of systemic manifestations including arthralgia and myalgia. The risk of infection has been greatly reduced through the introduction of tetracycline in poultry feeds; however, this has the undesirable consequence of producing antimicrobial–resistant strains and does not reduce the prevalence of infection in pet birds.

Bite infections are a risk to immunosuppressed people with *Pasteurella* and *Capynocytophaga* (DF-2) infections being the most documented. Splenectomy or other immunosuppressive diseases are associated with an increased risk of fatal sepsis from these bacteria. Signs are acute severe cellulitis and bacteremia that may develop within 24 to 48 hr of the bite.

Microsporidiosis has been reported with increasing frequency as a cause of chronic watery diarrhea in AIDS patients. These protozoan parasites are a heterogenous group in the phylum Microspora. Although various microsporidia infect animals, none of the infections in humans have been traced to household pets. A wide variety of environmental exposure exists and a number of species of farm animals, monkeys, rodents, rabbits, and fish have been shown to become infected. The premise that pets are involved has not been well substantiated.

There are a number of other zoonoses that have not been documented with any greater frequency in immunosuppressed individuals as compared to the general population. The references at the end of this article should be consulted for more extensive review of all companion animal–associated zoonoses.

## RECOMMENDATIONS

Handling pets offers no greater danger of acquiring infection for an immunosuppressed person than would contacting other people or the environment. Therefore, simple hygienic measures will greatly reduce the risk of exposure to zoonoses. Factors making animals a potentially greater risk are some of the unique organisms they can harbor and the lack of sanitary behavior that pets often practice. Owners can often institute routines in their own behavior that makes it unlikely they will contract a disease from their companion animal.

In general, precautions should be taken if an immunosuppressed person decides to acquire a pet for companionship or if a pet is being used to provide companionship for people in hospitals or nursing homes. Infectious diseases including zoonoses are more frequently a problem in puppies or kittens. Furthermore, those animals coming from high population densities as exist in humane shelters, pounds, or crowded pet stores may have a greater chance of harboring pathogens. Acquiring a new adult pet from a single-pet household may be the best consideration. Any newly acquired pet should be thoroughly examined by a veterinarian prior to being introduced.

Immunosuppressed people should wash their hands frequently during the course of the day and consistently after handling animals or their excretions. This is especially important before eating, smoking, performing dental hygiene, and putting in corrective lenses. The pet's environment should also be kept clean and free of dirt, uneaten foods, and excrement.

Newly acquired cats should have their vaccinations and routine anthelmintic therapy for roundworms and hookworms. Serologic testing for FeLV, FIV, and toxoplasmosis is recommended. While FeLV and FIV pose no chance of infecting people, cats affected with these immunosuppressive viruses are more likely to develop infectious diseases. Measuring IgG toxoplasmosis titers will help determine prior exposure in cats. Younger kittens are more likely to be seronegative and are of risk in shedding oocysts following their first exposure to *T. gondii*. Immunoglobulin G seropositivity indicates prior exposure and minimal risk, since cats rarely if ever reshed oocysts after initially being infected. Prophylaxis for dirofilariasis should be given to pets in endemic areas. Yearly check-ups and vaccinations are indicated to prevent the possibility of the pet contracting highly infectious illnesses. Illness in any pet should be an important reason to seek veterinary care. In the event of illness, a veterinarian should be consulted without delay.

The animal's hair coat and skin should be kept in good condition by weekly baths, brushing, and trimming of matted fur. Nails of dogs and cats should be trimmed frequently to reduce the chance of scratch injuries. If cats scratch when handled, then declawing should be considered. Fleas should be managed with regular bathing and dipping with insecticides and intensive environmental treatment in the area the animals frequent. This includes indoor floors and carpets, especially where they sleep, their sheltered roaming areas, and other animals in contact. Environment treatment using flea bombs or spraying should include larvicidal growth inhibitors as well as adulticide compounds. Flea collars and powders, sprays, or topical application of concentrated residual insecticides are adjunctive measures, but should be used while observing for toxicity. More effective control of fleas in the environment may require a professional exterminator. To control ticks, routine daily checking of pets is indicated or immediately after leaving tick-infested areas. Prior application of DEET-containing compounds is indicated. Any ticks should be removed with rubber gloves, tweezers, or facial tissues and protected hands should be washed after removal. Ticks should not be removed or crushed with bare exposed hands. Flies, cockroaches, and vermin may also transport infectious organisms. Pets should be restricted from areas where rodents burrow and measures taken to eliminate areas near the home where vermin may nest.

Immunosuppressed individuals should try to avoid direct contact with pet's excretions, and gloves should be worn during handling of fecal material. Diarrheic stools are particularly challenging to remove without becoming exposed. Feline litter boxes should be kept out of eating areas and should be cleaned by a non-immunosuppressed, nonpregnant adult. Litter box dust can be avoided by using bag liners and dust-free litters and by moistening litter before sealing bags. Although the litter box should be emptied outdoors or in well-ventilated areas to avoid inhalation, the litter should not be disposed in the outdoors. Since a minimum of 24 hr is required for *Toxoplasma* oocyst maturation for infectivity, the litter box should be cleaned every 24 to 48 hr where possible. The litter box can be disinfected once monthly by filling it with boiling water from the stove.

In dogs, coprophagia should be discouraged and cat litter boxes should be isolated from other unintended pets. Within communities, animals should be restricted from defecating in playgrounds, parks, and walkways, or provisions should be made for owners to remove the excrement from public places should it occur. Veterinarians should be aware that unrestricted antimicrobial use in pets selects for transferable resistance in enteric pathogens such as *Campylobacter* spp., *Salmonella* spp., and *E. coli* in pets. Improved health education of children should be accomplished. Children should be educated not to practice geophagia or pica and to wash their hands after playing in soil. For those with aquatic or cold-blood pets, rubber gloves should be used for cleaning aquariums or terrariums. Diarrheic pets should not be exposed to the general household and should not contact young children of immunosuppressed members in a household. Animals suffering from diarrhea should be bathed as needed to decontaminate their hair coat. Pet owners should be instructed to wear rubber gloves during cleaning of diarrheic stools and to use sodium hypochlorite at a dilution of 1 ounce per quart of water for disinfection. Similar precautions can be recommended for other body fluids including urine and saliva.

Immunocompromised owners should be advised not to let pets lick them on the mouth and to practice good preventative dental hygiene for themselves and their pets. Routine dental prophylaxis with scaling or brushing is recommended for pets exposed to immunocompromised people. Veterinarians or other household members or assistants should assume these responsibilities. Saliva should be washed from hands or open wounds. Pets should not be kissed on their oral cavity. Rubber gloves should be worn when oral medication is given to pets, or someone else should assume these responsibilities.

Bite wounds are probably the most frequent health risk faced by immunocompromised individuals. Pets that are aggressive in behavior or play should not be kept under these circumstances. People who are inadvertently bitten should wash with soap and water and rinse the wound with dilute organic iodine solutions or quaternary ammonium compounds as an alternative. Pets should not be allowed to lick human wounds. Cats that scratch frequently should be declawed. Children should be taught not to startle feeding or sleeping animals. A physician should be immediately notified of any bites or scratches from pets that do occur. Prophylactic antimicrobial therapy may be considered by physicians knowing the patient's immunocompromised status.

The diet of pets is extremely important in limiting fecal-oral pathogens. Only commercial diets that have been cooked or pelleted should be fed. Raw or unprocessed meat or offal or unpasteurized dairy products should not be used. Pets should be restricted of scavenging and hunting or feeding on carrion. They may have to be confined to meet this end. Water from the tap should always be available to pets. Access to outside surface water or toilet bowl water should be restricted.

### References and Suggested Reading

Anon: Aids patients can acquire some infections from animals. J Am Vet Med Assoc 197:1268, 1990.

Baxter DN and Leck I: Deleterious effects of dogs on human health 2. Canine zoonoses. Community Med 6:185, 1984.

Buckley RM, Braffman MN, and Stern JJ: Opportunistic infections in the acquired immunodeficiency syndrome. Semin Oncol 17:335, 1990.

Current WL, Reese NC, Ernst JV, et al: Human cryptosporidiosis in immunocompetent and immunodeficient persons: Studies of an outbreak and experimental transmission. N Engl J Med 308:1252, 1983.

Gill DM and Stone DM: The veterinarian's role in the AIDS crisis. J Am Vet Med Assoc 201:1683, 1992.

Goldstein EJC: Household pets and human infections. Infect Dis Clin North Am 5:117, 1991.

Greene CE (ed): *Infectious Diseases of the Dog and Cat.* Philadelphia, WB Saunders Co, 1990.

Salfield NJ and Pugh EJ: Campylobacter enteritis in young children living in households with puppies. BMJ 294:21, 1987.

Scully RE, Mark EJ, and McNeely BU: Case records of the Massachusetts General Hospital, case 39-1985. N Engl J Med 313:805, 1985.

Sorvillo FJ, Lieb LE, and Waterman SH: Incidence of campylobacteriosis among patients with AIDS in Los Angeles County. J Aids 4:598, 1991.

Spencer L: Pets prove therapeutic for people with AIDS. J Am Vet Med Assoc 201:1665, 1992.

# EMPIRIC ANTIBIOTIC THERAPY

SHELLY L. VADEN
*and* MARK G. PAPICH
*Raleigh, North Carolina*

Ideally, results of bacterial culture and antimicrobial susceptibility testing should be known so that optimal treatment regimens can be designed. However, this information is frequently not known at the time antibiotic therapy is initiated. Empiric antibiotic therapy is the administration of antibiotics without prior knowledge of the infecting microorganism's identity and antimicrobial susceptibility profile. This article provides an approach to the empiric selection of antibiotics. This approach is based on results of studies that have identified the bacteria most likely to infect specific sites and evaluated tissue distribution and spectrum of activity of specific antibiotics (Papich, 1990). Once the site of infection has been identified, an appropriate antibiotic can be selected (Table 1). Suggested dosage regimens for commonly used antibiotics are listed in Table 2. Although the term "antibiotic" refers to chemical substances produced by microorganisms, usage in this article shall be extended to include synthetic antibacterial agents, such as sulfonamides and quinolones. The reader is encouraged to study other sections of this book for detailed descriptions of ancillary treatment modalities used for infections in specific sites or for the treatment of infections not listed in this article.

There is often a temptation to use antibiotic regimens that are broad spectrum, with activity against gram-negative and -positive, aerobic and anaerobic bacteria. In reality, an extended spectrum of antibacterial activity is often not needed and may in fact be detrimental, leading to the emergence of microbial resistance. Drugs should be selected that have minimal adverse effects on the patient and the patient's normal flora, but that have maximum effect against the suspected bacterial pathogen. Patient factors that should influence the selection of antibiotics include the status of the immune system, the location of the infection, the presence of concurrent diseases (e.g., hepatic or renal failure), and the physiologic status (e.g., pregnant or neonatal animal). An antibiotic regimen with an extended spectrum of activity using bactericidal drugs may be required in an immunocompromised patient while awaiting microbial culture results. Local factors at the site of infection should be considered because they will influence the activity of antibiotics. For example, pus or necrotic debris in an infection will decrease the activity of aminoglycosides and trimethoprim-sulfonamides. An anaerobic environment also will inhibit the antibacterial activity of aminoglycosides. Certain drugs should be used judiciously or not given to animals that are pregnant or growing or have hepatic or renal failure.

## SPECIFIC RECOMMENDATIONS

### Skin

Almost all superficial pyodermas in dogs and cats and most deep pyodermas in dogs are caused by *Staphy-*

**Table 1.** *Partial List of Pathogenic Bacteria Infecting Specific Sites and Reasonable Empiric Antibiotic Choices*°

| Site | Dog Common Pathogen | Cat Common Pathogen | Empiric Antibiotic Choices | |
| --- | --- | --- | --- | --- |
| | | | *Primary* | *Secondary* |
| **Skin** | | | | |
| Superficial pyoderma | *Staphylococcus intermedius* | *Staphylococcus aureus* | Amox/Clav Oxacillin | TMP/Sulfa Chloramphenicol |
| Deep pyoderma/ abscessation | *Staphylococcus* spp. *Proteus* spp. *Escherichia coli* *Pseudomonas aeruginosa* | *Pasteurella multocida* L-form bacteria | Cloxacillin 1Ceph Clindamycin | Enrofloxacin Erythromycin Aminoglycosides Doxycycline |
| **Urinary Tract** | | | | |
| Bladder, kidneys, prostate | *Escherichia coli* *Staphylococcus* spp. *Enterococcus* spp. *Proteus* spp. *Klebsiella* spp. *Pseudomonas* spp. *Enterobacter* spp. | *Staphylococcus* spp. *Escherichia coli* *Proteus* spp. *Enterococcus* spp. *Pasteurella* spp. | Amox or Amp Amox/Clav TMP/Sulfa 1Ceph Enrofloxacin | Aminoglycosides Chloramphenicol Doxycycline |
| **Respiratory Tract** | | | | |
| Trachea | *Bordetella bronchiseptica* *Mycoplasma* spp. | *Bordetella bronchiseptica* *Mycoplasma* spp. | Amox/Clav Doxycycline Chloramphenicol | |
| Bronchi and pulmonary parenchyma | *Escherichia coli* *Klebsiella* spp. *Pasteurella* spp. *Bordetella bronchiseptica* *Pseudomonas* spp. *Staphylococcus* spp. *Streptococcus* spp. | *Pasteurella multocida* *Bordetella bronchiseptica* *Moraxella* spp. *Mycoplasma* spp. | TMP/Sulfa 1Ceph Enrofloxacin Chloramphenicol Amox/Clav Amox or Amp | Doxycycline Aminoglycosides |
| Pleural cavity | *Actinomyces* *Nocardia* Anaerobes | *Pasteurella* spp. Anaerobes | Amp TMP/Sulfa | Clindamycin |
| **Skeletal System** | | | | |
| Joints | *Staphylococcus* spp. *Streptococcus* spp. *Escherichia coli* *Mycoplasma* spp. Anaerobes | *Pasteurella* spp. *Mycoplasma* spp. L-form bacteria | 1Ceph Amox/Clav Doxycycline | Enrofloxacin 1Ceph |
| Apendicular osteomyelitis | *Staphylococcus* spp. *Escherichia coli* *Proteus* spp. *Enterococcus* spp. Anaerobes | *Staphylococcus* spp. *Escherichia coli* *Proteus* spp. *Enterococcus* spp. Anaerobes | 1Ceph Amox/Clav Clindamycin | Aminoglycosides Enrofloxacin Cloxacillin |
| Discospondylitis | *Staphylococcus* spp. *Streptococcus* spp. *Brucella canis* | *Staphylococcus* spp. *Streptococcus* spp. | 1Ceph | Enrofloxacin Cloxacillin |
| **Mastitis** | *Escherichia coli* *Staphylococcus* spp. *Streptococcus* spp. | *Escherichia coli* *Staphylococcus* spp. *Streptococcus* spp. | 1Ceph Amox/Clav | Enrofloxacin |
| **Septicemia** | *Staphylococcus* spp. *Escherichia coli* *Streptococcus* spp. *Salmonella* spp. *Proteus* spp. *Pseudomonas* spp. *Enterococcus* spp. *Enterococcus* spp. Anaerobes | *Escherichia coli* *Klebsiella* spp. *Salmonella* spp. Anaerobes | Aminoglycoside + ampicillin sodium Aminoglycoside, 1Ceph + clindamycin Enrofloxacin + clindamycin Enrofloxacin + ampicillin sodium Imipenem-cilastatin Cefoxitin 3Ceph | |

°Once the site of infection is identified, Table 1 can be used to select an antibiotic. Initially, primary choices should be selected. Secondary choices should be used if a favorable response did not occur after using a primary choice and culture results are not yet available, or if all of the primary choices are contraindicated in a particular patient.

Abbreviations: Amp = ampicillin, Amox = amoxicillin, 1Ceph = first-generation cephalosporin (cephalexin, cefadroxil, cefazolin, cephradine), 3Ceph = third-generation cephalosporin, TMP/Sulfa = trimethoprim-sulfadiazine or trimethoprim-sulfamethoxazole.

***Table 2.*** *Suggested Dosage Regimens for Commonly Used Antibiotics*

| Antibiotic | Species | Dose | Route | Interval | Comments |
|---|---|---|---|---|---|
| Amikacin | Dog, cat | 5–10 mg/kg | IV, IM, SC | q8h | a, b |
| Amoxicillin | Dog, cat | 10–22 mg/kg | PO, SC | q8h | |
| Amoxicillin + clavulanate | Dog | 12.5–25 mg/kg | PO | q8–12h | |
| | Cat | 62.5 mg | PO | q8–12h | |
| Ampicillin sodium | Dog, cat | 10–20 mg/kg | IV, IM, SC | q6–8h | |
| Cephalothin, cephapirin | Dog, cat | 10–30 mg/kg | IV, IM | q6–8h | c |
| Cefazolin | Dog, cat | 20–25 mg/kg | IV, IM | q6–8h | c |
| Cephalexin | Dog, cat | 22 mg/kg | PO | q8h | c, d |
| Cefadroxil | Dog, cat | 22 mg/kg | PO | q8–12h | c, d |
| Cefotaxime | Dog, cat | 25–50 mg/kg | IV, IM, SC | q8h | e |
| Cefoxitin | Dog, cat | 30 mg/kg | IV | q8h | f |
| Ciprofloxacin | Dog, cat | 5–15 mg/kg | PO | q12h | a, g, h |
| Chloramphenicol | Dog | 40–50 mg/kg | IV, IM, SC, PO | q8h | g, h, i |
| | Cat | 50 mg | IV, IM, SC, PO | q12h | |
| Clindamycin | Dog | 5–11 mg/kg | IM, SC, PO | q12h | i |
| | Cat | 5–11 mg/kg | SC, PO | q12h | |
| Cloxacillin | Dog | 20–40 mg/kg | PO | q8h | |
| Doxycycline | Dog, cat | 5 mg/kg | PO, IV | q12h | d, g, i |
| Enrofloxacin | Dog, cat | 2.5–5 mg/kg | PO, IM | q12h | a, g, h |
| Gentamicin | Dog, cat | 2–4 mg/kg | IV, IM, SC | q8h | a, b |
| Imipenem-cilastatin | Dog, cat | 2–5 mg/kg | IV | q6–8h | a |
| Metronidazole | Dog | 10–20 mg/kg | PO | q8–12h | i |
| | Cat | 10–25 mg/kg | PO | q24h | |
| Oxacillin | Dog, cat | 22–40 mg/kg | PO | q8h | |
| Oxytetracycline or tetracycline | Dog, cat | 20 mg/kg | PO | q8h–12h | a, d, g, h, i |
| Ticarcillin + clavulanate | Dog | 40–110 mg/kg | IV, IM | q6h | j |
| Tobramycin | Dog, cat | 2 mg/kg | IV, IM, SC | q8h | a, b |
| Trimethoprim-sulfamethoxazole or trimethoprim-sulfadiazine | Dog, cat | 30 mg/kg | IV, PO | q12h | a, h |

Key: a = avoid or reduce dose in patients with renal failure, b = therapeutic drug monitoring advised, particularly in young animals, c = first-generation cephalosporin, d = administer with food if gastrointestinal upset occurs, e = third-generation cephalosporin, f = second-generation cephalosporin, g = avoid in young animals, h = avoid in breeding or pregnant animals, i = avoid or reduce dose in patients with severe liver failure, j = used primarily for treatment of *Pseudomonas* spp. infections.

lococcus intermedius or *S. aureus* infections. Antibiotic dosages listed in Table 2 will usually produce high drug concentrations in the skin. Whereas 3 weeks of treatment may be sufficient to treat superficial pyoderma, 6 to 8 weeks may be needed for the treatment of deep pyoderma. Although cats frequently get abscesses, deep pyoderma is rare. Cat abscesses can usually be managed by establishing drainage and the administration of amoxicillin, cephalexin, or cefadroxil. If abscesses do not resolve with this treatment, L-form bacteria may be present, and a therapeutic trial with tetracycline should be employed.

## Urinary Tract

Many antibiotics reach very high concentrations in the urine, allowing for the relatively straightforward treatment of uncomplicated urinary tract infections (UTI) by the administration of an antibiotic for 10 to 14 days (Ling, 1984). If after one course of empiric antibiotic therapy, signs of UTI recur, microbial culture and susceptibility testing of the urine is indicated. If after this second course of antibiotics, signs of UTI recur, a more thorough diagnostic evaluation directed toward determining an underlying cause of bacterial infection should be pursued. Prostatitis and py-

elonephritis are two potential causes of recurrent urinary tract infections. Prostatitis should be suspected in any sexually intact male animal presenting with bacterial cystitis. If these conditions are suspected, empiric antibiotic therapy should not be initiated until appropriate samples are submitted for microbial culture and susceptibility testing. Antibiotics that reach effective concentrations in the urine do not necessarily reach effective concentrations in the prostate and kidneys (Klausner, 1983). However, enrofloxacin and trimethoprim-sulfonamides reach high concentrations in these tissues. Antibiotics should be administered for at least 4 weeks to animals with prostatitis and 6 to 8 weeks to animals with pyelonephritis.

## Respiratory Tract

Bacterial rhinitis in the dog and cat almost always occurs secondarily to another disorder. Although antibiotic therapy can lead to clinical improvement, positive results are commonly transient. The nasal passages have abundant normal flora, complicating the interpretation of culture results; however, heavy growth of one or even two pathogenic organisms may suggest infection and aid in antibiotic selection. If a favorable response to the selected antibiotic is noted, treatment should continue for 6 to 8 weeks.

Antibiotic therapy may not be helpful in the treatment of canine infectious tracheobronchitis because most antibiotics do not reach sufficiently high concentrations in the tracheal mucosa and infections are often self-limiting (Bemis and Appel, 1977). However, *Bordetella bronchiseptica* can colonize the lower airways and antibiotic therapy may be warranted. Antibiotic therapy should be administered for at least 10 days, or 5 days beyond resolution of clinical signs.

For lower respiratory tract infections, tracheal or bronchial specimens should be obtained for cytologic examination and microbial culture prior to initiating antibiotic therapy because it is often difficult to predict which bacterial species is responsible for the infections. For most antibiotics, interstitial and alveolar drug concentrations are similar to serum concentrations; however, bronchial concentrations are usually lower and are not influenced by the presence of mucosal inflammation (Pennington and Reynolds, 1973). Because of the impaired diffusion of drugs into bronchial secretions, the high end of the dosage range should be used during antibiotic treatment. In all cases, appropriate supportive care should be provided. The response to therapy should be monitored through repeated physical examination and thoracic radiographs. If drug selection is appropriate, a favorable response should be noted within 48 to 72 hr of initiating appropriate antibiotic therapy. Antibiotic administration should be continued for at least 1 week beyond resolution of clinical signs.

Effective management of pyothorax requires antibiotic therapy, drainage of the pleural cavity, and supportive care. During the initial management, antibiotics should be administered parenterally because these animals are frequently septic. Antibiotic therapy should be continued for 4 to 6 weeks after drainage of the pleural cavity is complete.

## Skeletal System

Septic arthritis requires aggressive management in order to eliminate the infection and salvage the joint. Parenteral antibiotics may be necessary during the initial treatment period. Once inflammation has been reduced, oral antibiotic therapy can be started and should continue for 4 to 6 weeks. The high end of the dose range listed for antibiotics in Table 2 usually will produce adequate drug concentrations in synovial fluid. Arthrotomy and lavage may be required. Likewise, appendicular osteomyelitis requires aggressive management. Most antibiotics reach adequate concentrations in bone tissue when administered at recommended doses (Hall et al., 1980; Wiggins et al., 1978). However, if blood supply is decreased because of a sequestrum, hematoma, or implant, the penetration of antibiotics to the site of infection may be impeded, making the treatment of appendicular osteomyelitis difficult. In contrast, discospondylitis is often readily responsive to antibiotic therapy. Parenteral antibiotics may be needed

if there is evidence of bacteremia or septicemia, but in most cases oral antibiotics administered for 4 to 6 weeks are effective. Tetracyclines should never be administered for bone infections because their antibacterial activity is reduced in bone.

## Mastitis

Bacterial mastitis is uncommon in the dog and quite rare in the cat. Before beginning therapy, a sample of milk or aspirated fluid can be submitted for culture. Antibiotics should continue for 10 to 14 days beyond resolution of inflammation. Hot compresses applied to the affected glands may be useful in promoting drainage. Occasionally, surgical débridement is required.

## Septicemia

In the case of life-threatening septicemia, antibiotics with activity against gram-negative, gram-positive, aerobic, and anaerobic bacteria should be administered intravenously. Because the bacteria responsible for the infection is often difficult to predict, blood culture should be initiated prior to administering antibiotics. This typically includes combination therapy. Once the site of infection is identified and results of microbial culture and susceptibility testing are available, the spectrum can be narrowed to target the known pathogen. Some antibiotics, including cefoxitin, imipenem-cilastatin, third-generation cephalosporins, and ticarcillin-clavulanate, should be reserved for infections with gram-negative bacteria that have proven multiple drug resistance rather than be used for routine broad-spectrum empiric therapy (Dwozack, 1986). Furthermore, third-generation cephalosporins and imipenem-cilastatin may create resistance by inducing $\beta$-lactamase activity (Saunders and Saunders, 1988) and/or altering the microbial microenvironment. Unless ticarcillin-clavulanate is administered at very high doses (approximately 100 mg/kg) it is unlikely to have effective broad-spectrum activity.

## References and Suggested Reading

Bemis DA and Appel MJG: Aerosol, parenteral and oral antibiotic treatment of *Bordetella bronchiseptica* infection in dogs. J Am Vet Med Assoc 170:1082, 1977.
*This study demonstrated that systemic treatment with antibiotics does not produce sufficiently high drug concentrations in bronchial secretions to treat* Bordetella bronchiseptica *infections.*
Dwozack DL: Emergence of resistance in gram-negative bacteria: A risk of broad-spectrum beta-lactam use. Drug Intell Clin Pharm 20:562, 1986.
*A summary of the risks of emergence of resistance associated with the use of broad-spectrum β-lactams.*
Hall BB, Fitzgerald RH, Kelly PJ, and Washington JA: Pharmacokinetics of penicillin in canine osteomyelitic bone. Orthop Trans 4:175, 1980.
*This study demonstrated that antibiotic penetration in osteomyelitic bone does not differ substantially from healthy bone.*
Klausner JS: Management of canine bacterial prostatitis. J Am Vet Med Assoc 182:292, 1983.
*A summary of the principles associated with antibiotic penetration in the prostate gland.*
Ling GV: Therapeutic strategies involving antimicrobial treatment of the canine urinary tract. J Am Vet Med Assoc 185:1162, 1984.

*A summary of the studies by the author in which high concentrations of antibiotics in the urine are demonstrated.*

Papich MG: Tissue concentrations of antimicrobials: The site of action. Prob Vet Med 2:312, 1990.

*This review article with 101 references summarizes the factors that affect the tissue concentrations of drugs and discusses the concentrations of antibiotics in various tissues.*

Pennington JE and Reynolds HY: Concentration of gentamicin and carbenicillin in bronchial secretions. J Infect Dis 128:63, 1973.

*This study demonstrated that antibiotics usually do not reach high concentrations in bronchial secretions.*

Saunders WE and Saunders CC: Inducible β-lactamases: Clinical and epidemiologic implications for use of newer cephalosporins. Rev Infect Dis 10:830, 1988.

*A summary of the studies that have demonstrated inducible β-lactam resistance.*

Wiggins CE, Nelson CL, Clarke R, and Thompson CH: Concentration of antibiotics in normal bone after intravenous injection. J Bone Joint Surg 60A:93, 1978.

*This study demonstrated that β-lactam and aminoglycoside concentrations in bone generally parallel the concentrations in serum following intravenous injection.*

# FELINE IMMUNODEFICIENCY VIRUS

ROBERT V. ENGLISH
*Raleigh, North Carolina*

Feline immunodeficiency virus (FIV) was isolated in 1987 by Pedersen et al. (1987) from a cat with clinical disease strikingly similar to the acquired immunodeficiency syndrome (AIDS) associated with human immunodeficiency virus infection (HIV). The virus was originally termed "feline T-lymphotropic virus," but was renamed FIV in keeping with current lentivirus nomenclature. Because FIV represents a significant health threat to the feline population, as well as an animal model for human AIDS, the biology and pathogenesis of the virus has been intensely studied over the past 6 years. Despite these investigations, the underlying mechanisms responsible for the immune dysfunction and other pathologic changes associated with FIV are unclear. It has become apparent that FIV and HIV share a common immunopathogenesis and that these viruses result in changes in nearly every organ system.

## BIOLOGY OF THE VIRUS

Feline immunodeficiency virus is a member of the lentivirus family of retroviruses and is biologically distinct from feline leukemia virus, an oncornavirus. The virus consists of an outer envelope and a nucleocapsid containing a polymerase, group-specific antigens (*gag* proteins), and two copies of its single-stranded ribonucleic acid (RNA) genome. Similar to other retroviruses, the genome is organized into *gag*, *pol*, and *env* genes flanked by long terminal repeats at the 3' and 5' ends. Replication of FIV is similar to other lentiviruses that include HIV, simian immunodeficiency virus, equine infectious anemia, visna/maedi virus, and bovine immunodeficiency virus. After binding to a cellular receptor, the nucleocapsid is released into the cell and the magnesium-dependent reverse transcriptase activity of the polymerase produces a double-stranded deoxyribonucleic acid (DNA) provirus from the RNA genome. This provirus incorporates into the host cell genome. When provided with the proper molecular signals, the provirus is transcribed by the host cell producing full-length viral genomic RNA, as well as mRNA for the production of viral proteins. Genomic RNA is packaged with nucleocapsid proteins and polymerase, and buds from cell membrane at sites containing the virus encoded envelope glycoproteins.

Nucleotide sequence of the FIV genome suggests regulatory elements similar to those in other lentiviruses are present in FIV. These elements are important in controlling virus expression and infectivity and are therefore potential targets for antiviral therapy (see *CVT XI*, p 211). Some of these regulatory proteins may also contribute to the pathogenesis of clinical syndromes associated with lentivirus infection. It is now clear that the transactivator protein (TAT) of HIV is responsible for stimulation of endothelial cells that leads to the formation of Kaposi's sarcoma in AIDS patients.

## EPIDEMIOLOGY

Feline immunodeficiency virus is endemic in most areas, including the United States, Japan, Australia, and Europe. Retrospective studies have demonstrated antibodies against FIV in sera samples from the late 1960s indicating the virus has been in the cat population for at least several decades (Reid et al., 1992). The prevalence of FIV infection is greatest in outdoor, free-roaming cats. Among all cats, males are 1.5 times more likely to be infected than females, and the mean age at the time of diagnosis is 6 to 8 years. In the United States, the prevalence of FIV is 1 to 4% in healthy pet cats, and 13 to 15% in cats with clinical signs of disease (Yamamoto et al., 1989). In Japan, where a much greater proportion of the cat population is free roaming compared to the United States, the prevalence of FIV is 28.9% in healthy cats and 43.9% in clinically ill cats (Ishida et al., 1989).

There is a higher prevalence of FIV infection in cats with antibodies against feline syncytia forming virus, another retrovirus. The linkage of these two infections is not surprising considering both viruses are probably transmitted by biting and therefore have a higher prevalence in free-roaming cats.

## TRANSMISSION

The high prevalence of FIV in free-roaming male cats suggests fighting is a primary mode of transmission. The virus is present in saliva, and infected cats can transmit the virus by biting (Yamamoto et al., 1989). Parental inoculation of plasma or blood from infected cats also readily transmits the virus. Unlike feline leukemia virus (FeLV), FIV does not produce a high viremia. As a result, transmission from casual contact such as sharing of food bowls and mutual grooming is uncommon. Consequently, within a stable cat household, transmission from an infected cat to uninfected cats is unlikely.

Limited studies have failed to demonstrate sexual transmission. However, transmission from queen to kitten does occur. Approximately 50% of the kittens nursing a queen experiencing acute FIV infection (1 to 2 months after infection) will acquire the virus. Transmission from chronically infected queens is much lower, with only approximately 5% of kittens becoming infected. This suggests the high viremia that occurs 2 to 8 weeks after infection increases the probability of perinatal infection. Current evidence suggests perinatal infection occurs by ingesting FIV present in the milk of infected queens. It is possible that swallowing of maternal blood during parturition may also result in neonatal infection. Interestingly, kittens up to 4 months of age have been infected by oral exposure to high levels of virus. Unlike HIV infection, experimental studies have not documented *in utero* transmission (Wasmoen et al., 1992; Sellon et al., 1993).

## PATHOGENESIS

Because FIV infection in cats represents an animal model for AIDS, research into the pathogenesis of FIV has focused primarily on the immune system. Evidence is mounting that suggests the immunodeficiency associated with lentiviruses is the result of virus-induced disturbance of immune regulatory pathways. Indeed, lentiviruses themselves stimulate strong humoral and cellular immune responses. It may be that this potent immune stimulatory ability is responsible for the immune dysfunction that occurs in infected hosts.

### Cellular Tropism of FIV

The mononuclear cell tropism of FIV is broader than that of HIV or simian immunodeficiency virus. These viruses infect primarily CD4$^+$ lymphocytes and mac-

rophages. Similarly, the primary target of FIV during the first few weeks of infection is the CD4$^+$ lymphocyte, but virus is also detectable in CD8$^+$ cells as well as B cells. As the primary immune response develops and the initial viremia subsides, virus burden among peripheral mononuclear cell switches to the B cell (English et al., 1993). The finding of essentially identical circulating lymphocyte subset changes in FIV-infected cats and HIV-infected patients suggests that despite FIV's broader tropism, these viruses share a similar immunopathogenesis. Tissue macrophages are also a reservoir for FIV, although minimal virus is present in circulating monocytes. The fibroblast adapted Petaluma strain of FIV appears to have a broader tropism compared to other FIV isolates and will infect many cell types including astrocytes in vitro (Dow et al., 1990). There is no evidence that FIV is capable of infecting human cells.

### Lymphocyte Subset Changes Associated with FIV Infection

Most systemic viral infections induce similar lymphocyte changes. Days to weeks after infection a lymphopenia develops, typically associated with peak expression of the infectious agent (Fig. 1A). The decrease in peripheral lymphocytes is probably secondary to corticosteroid-induced redistribution of lymphocytes, and all lymphocyte subsets are affected. This transient lymphopenia is followed by a strong immune response that results in a rebound in lymphocyte numbers to above preinfection levels. As the infectious agent is cleared, the immune response decreases and lymphocyte numbers return to normal.

The hallmark of FIV infection is a decrease in the CD4$^+$:CD8$^+$ cell ratio among peripheral lymphocytes. As with other viral infections, FIV-infected cats develop a panlymphopenia 1 to 3 weeks after inoculation (Fig. 1B). A strong immune anti-FIV response follows, but the nature of the lymphocyte response is different. The major deviation in the immune response to FIV is the lack of an appropriate CD4$^+$ cell response. The CD4$^+$ subset of lymphocytes are helper/inducer cells required for the initiation of immune responses. With FIV infection, the rebound in CD4$^+$ cells after the initial lymphopenia is often incomplete, failing to reach preinfection levels. The CD8$^+$ subset of lymphocytes, or cytotoxic/suppressor cells, do exhibit an appropriate response and rise above preinfection levels. However, instead of returning to baseline values as the FIV viremia decreases, the number of circulating CD8$^+$ cells remains elevated for 12 to 18 months after infection. The result of this dysregulation in the T lymphocyte subsets is an early, persistent decrease in the CD4$^+$:CD8$^+$ ratio. Initially, the decrease in the ratio is predominately due to both an increase in CD8$^+$ cells and a decrease in CD4$^+$ cells. During the subclinical stage of infection that follows, CD8$^+$ cells return to normal levels, while CD4$^+$ cells continue to slowly decline. By the time cats enter the chronic clinical disease stage,

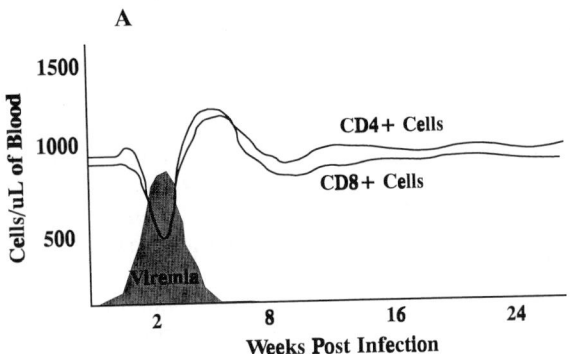

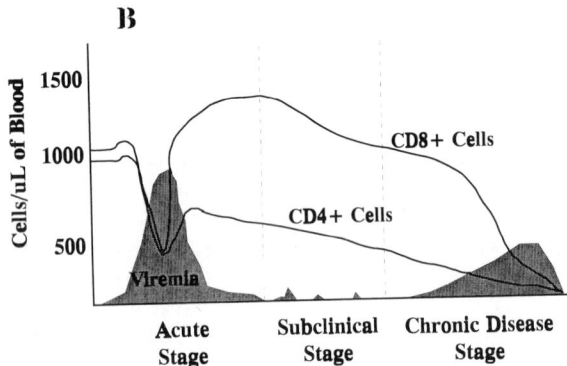

**Figure 1.** *A*, Circulating CD4$^+$ and CD8$^+$ lymphocyte changes during a typical systemic viral infection. *B*, Circulating CD4$^+$ and CD8$^+$ lymphocyte changes during FIV infection. After the initial burst in virus replication (shaded areas), the level of circulating virus is low during the subclinical stage of infection. Virus expression during the chronic clinical disease stage is unknown, but presumed similar to HIV infection. Terminally, virus is often difficult to isolate from infected cats.

the decrease in the CD4$^+$:CD8$^+$ ratio is due to a profound loss of CD4$^+$ cells. Because these changes are occurring in only some subpopulations of lymphocytes, total lymphocyte numbers often remain within normal limits. However, terminally, the number of all lymphocytes is greatly reduced, and total lymphocyte counts below 300 cells per microliter are not uncommon.

The rate at which these lymphocyte changes occur is variable and probably depends on the strain of FIV, the size of the inoculum, and the immunologic background of the host. Furthermore, as in humans, there is great variation among cats in their total lymphocyte numbers. As a result, accurate interpretation of lymphocyte subset changes requires repeated analysis over several months.

Except for the initial burst in virus expression during acute infection, the level of viremia in infected cats is low. Studies of HIV-infected patients have demonstrated transient bursts of virus replication occur during the asymptomatic and early AIDS stages of infection. In late AIDS, overall virus expression increases (Fig. 1*B*). It has also been demonstrated that increased virus expression occurs during periods of immune stimulation, such as after vaccination. These periods of in-

creased expression are associated with further alteration of lymphocyte subsets.

Lehman et al. (1992) recently showed that vaccination of FIV-infected cats with a recombinant feline leukemia vaccine resulted in a decrease in the CD4$^+$: CD8$^+$ ratio, suggesting immune stimulation may also result in increased virus expression in FIV-infected cats.

Transient neutropenias also may occur during acute FIV infection. Neutropenias develop after the lymphopenia, usually 6 to 8 weeks after infection, and may persist for months. The loss of circulating neutrophils can be severe, with levels below 1000 cells per microliter, and secondary septicemias have occurred in acutely infected cats. There is also evidence that neutrophil function is impaired in infected cats (Lafrado et al., 1992).

## Functional Immune Changes Associated with FIV Infection

In addition to quantitative lymphocyte changes, FIV-infected cats have progressive functional immune deficits. Loss of memory responses to soluble antigens occurs early in the infection. Experimental studies have demonstrated that both cellular proliferation and antibody production after stimulation with T-dependent recall antigens (antigens the immune system has previously generated a primary immune response to) are lost by the asymptomatic stage of infection (Torten et al., 1991). Broader immune impairment (as evidenced by loss of proliferative responses to mitogens such as concanavalin A and pokeweed mitogen, and superantigens such as staphylococcus enterotoxins A and B) occurs around the time cats enter the chronic clinical disease stage of infection. Not surprisingly, the ability of peripheral blood lymphocytes from FIV-infected cats to produce interleukin-2, a cytokine produced by CD4$^+$ lymphocytes, is also reduced in FIV-infected cats (Siebelink et al., 1990).

As with HIV, FIV infection also results in chronic B-cell activation. B cells from FIV-infected cats spontaneously produce higher levels of immunoglobulin, especially IgM, *in vitro* than do B cells from uninfected cats. As a result, polyclonal gammopathies with resultant increased serum total protein are common in FIV-infected cats. It is likely that both the direct stimulatory effects of FIV, as well as increased immune stimulation from chronic opportunistic diseases, contributes to the increased B-cell activation in these cats.

How FIV infection brings about these progressive immune alterations is not clear. However, it is likely that alterations in the immune response to acute FIV infection sets the stage for the immunologic deficiencies and clinical diseases that characterize the chronic clinical disease stage of infection.

## DIAGNOSIS

Detection of antibodies against FIV is diagnostic for infection. Antibodies to the virus are present in serum by 3 to 6 weeks after infection, and often reach high titers of 1:2000 or greater by 6 months after infection. Several tests are available for detecting antibodies to FIV. An immunoblot assay, also known as a western blot assay, allows detection of antibody responses to specific viral proteins and is therefore the most specific antibody test. However, it is an expensive and time-consuming assay and not readily available. A membrane bound enzyme-linked immunosorbent assay (ELISA) test (CITE test, Idexx, Portland, ME) as well as a standard 96-well ELISA assay (Idexx, Portland ME; Synbiotics, San Diego, CA) are commercially available. Indirect fluorescent antibody assays are available through veterinary diagnostic laboratories, and require interpretation by experienced personnel.

Reid et al. (1992) recently evaluated the sensitivity and specificity of a commercial plate ELISA test (Petchek FIV antibody test kit, Idexx, Portland, ME), and an IFA assay using infected peripheral blood lymphocytes as targets. Using immunoblotting as the "gold standard," both assays were highly sensitive (ELISA, 100%; IFA, 97.4%) and specific (ELISA, 99.6%; IFA, 100%). It is also our laboratory's experience that the membrane-bound ELISA test (CITE Test, Idexx, Portland, ME) is a sensitive and specific assay as compared to immunoblotting or virus isolation. False-negative results may occur during the first few weeks of infection before seroconversion has occurred. Additionally, cats with end-stage FIV infection will often test negative. These cats are severely lymphopenic with depletion of all lymphoid tissue. It is also difficult to culture virus or detect provirus in these cats. Kittens born to FIV-infected queens may acquire antibodies against FIV through passive transfer. Kittens testing positive for FIV antibodies should therefore be retested after maternal antibodies have declined (4 to 6 months of age) or tested for the presence of virus.

Although the level of viremia is extremely low in FIV-infected cats, virus isolation from peripheral blood lymphocytes is usually possible and must be considered the best standard for infection. Virus isolation can require up to 6 weeks and is therefore of limited clinical value. Assays utilizing the polymerase chain reaction for detection of provirus or viral RNA are routinely used in research laboratories to confirm FIV infection. These assays are rapid and highly sensitive and specific. Although commonly used to clinically diagnose HIV infection, these assays require special equipment and technical support and are not offered by most veterinary diagnostic centers. The recommendations for testing and confirming FIV infection are outlined in Table 1.

**Table 1.** *Recommendations for FIV Testing*

| Signalment | Screening Test | Result | Confirmatory Test | Result | Comments |
|---|---|---|---|---|---|
| Healthy cat with no known exposure | Membrane ELISA | Negative | None | — | High probability the cat is negative |
| | | Positive | Immunoblot or virus detection | Negative | Cat is probably not infected; recommend repeat confirmatory test in 2 months |
| | | | | Positive | Cat is infected |
| Cat with chronic clinical disease | Membrane ELISA | Negative | None unless severely lymphopenic or chronic wasting syndrome present | — | Severely lymphopenic or wasting cats may be at the terminal stages of FIV infection; consider virus isolation assay |
| | | Positive | None | — | High probability the cat is infected |
| Cat with intermittent febrile episodes and/or enlarged lymph nodes | Membrane ELISA | Negative | Repeat ELISA in 2 months | Negative | Cat is probably not infected |
| | | | | Positive | High probability the cat is infected |
| | | Positive | None | — | High probability the cat is infected |
| Cat less than 6 months old | Membrane ELISA | Negative | None | — | Cat is probably not infected |
| | | Positive | Repeat ELISA after 6 months of age | Negative | Cat is probably not infected; initial positive result represented passive transfer of maternal antibodies |
| | | | | Positive | Cat is probably infected; however, virus culture or repeat ELISA at 12 months of age is recommended |

Abbreviation: ELISA = enzyme-linked immunosorbent assay.

# CLINICAL DISEASE ASSOCIATED WITH FIV INFECTION

Clinically and immunologically, FIV infection can be divided into three stages: acute infection, which lasts 3 to 6 months; the subclinical stage, which lasts from months to years; and the AIDS-like or chronic clinical disease stage, which also may last for months to years.

## Acute FIV Infection

Clinical disease associated with acute FIV infection is often mild; consequently, cats are not commonly presented during this stage for veterinary care. Intermittent febrile episodes associated with lethargy and inappetence occur, as well as generalized lymph node enlargement. Lymph node hyperplasia often persists for several months. Nonhealing abscesses and even septicemia may occur in cats with profound neutropenias. Mild to life-threatening neurologic disease (see *CVT XI*, p 1010) has developed 2 to 3 months after inoculation in cats experimentally infected with different strains of FIV and is discussed below.

## Subclinical Stage of FIV Infection

Although cats are healthy during the subclinical stage, it is important to note that a low level of virus expression occurs, clinicopathologic changes are present, and immune function continues to deteriorate. The length of the subclinical stage of infection is variable. Experimental studies with specific pathogen-free cats have demonstrated that cats can remain clinically normal although severely lymphopenic if not exposed to other pathogens. On the other hand, pet cats may develop chronic clinical disease with only minimal lymphocyte changes. This suggests that the progression of FIV-associated disease may be slower in confined cats with minimal pathogen exposure. With HIV infection, the number of CD4$^+$ cells is highly prognostic for risk of disease development, with AIDS usually occurring after CD4$^+$ cell counts are below 200 cells per microliter. A similar statistical association probably exists with FIV, but adequate prospective data on the CD4$^+$ cell counts and prevalence of disease in FIV-infected cats is not currently available.

## Chronic Clinical Disease Stage of FIV Infection

The deterioration of immune function predisposes FIV infected cats to a wide variety of opportunistic diseases (see *CVT XI*, p 223). In addition, it is now clear that some of the clinical disorders that occur in infected cats are directly related to FIV expression.

Chronic stomatitis is one of the most common manifestations of FIV infection. The disease is characterized by gingival hyperplasia and epithelial erosions, especially in the fauces of the oral cavity. Weight loss may develop in severe cases as prehension and mastication become painful. The etiology of the condition is unknown, although calicivirus has been implicated as a possible opportunistic infection. Histopathologic examination reveals predominately a lymphocytic plasmacytic infiltrate.

Other common diseases seen in FIV-infected cats include recurrent upper respiratory infections, chronic enteritis, and persistent dermatomycosis. Small-bowel enteritis can develop during either the acute or chronic stage of FIV infection. The enteritis is often mild but persistent despite symptomatic therapy. With other lentiviruses, virus is present in the lamina propria of the intestinal tract, raising the possibility that enteritis is a primary manifestation of FIV infection. Opportunistic systemic fungal infections have been reported, but appear to be less prevalent in FIV-infected cats than in HIV-infected patients. Polydipsia and polyuria associated with mild elevations in blood urea nitrogen (BUN) and serum creatinine have also been noted in chronically infected cats (Thomas et al., 1991).

Many FIV-infected cats are initially presented for veterinary care because of ocular disease. Routine screening of all FIV-infected cats presented to the North Carolina Veterinary Teaching Hospital revealed 42% had ocular lesions. Retinal abnormalities were the most common finding and included focal areas of retinal degeneration and inner retinal hemorrhages. Cellular infiltrates, predominately plasma cells, into the anterior vitreous were common and appear as "snow banks" behind the lens. These lesions are usually secondary findings, since they do not cause changes observable by the owner. The other major ocular syndrome associated with FIV infection is anterior uveitis. The clinical signs of this potentially blinding disease are the same as for other causes of anterior uveitis and include mild blepharospasms, scleral injection, corneal edema, aqueous flare, hypopyon, and ocular hypotension. The inflammation can be recurrent or persistent, leading to lens luxation or glaucoma. Histopathologic examination of affected globes reveals perivascular lymphocytic plasmacytic infiltrates in the iris, ciliary body, and anterior sclera. Transient conjunctivitis has also been reported in FIV-infected cats and may occur during the acute or chronic stage of infection. Because anterior uveitis is a vision-threatening disorder, it is critical that cats presented with conjunctival inflammation be thoroughly examined for evidence of intraocular inflammation.

The etiology of the ocular changes is unclear. As with HIV, the retinopathy probably represents a primary manifestation of FIV. Anterior uveitis may also be a primary manifestation of FIV or the immune dysregulation it induces, or may be the result of opportunistic *Toxoplasma gondii* infection. Epidemiologic studies have demonstrated a correlation between anterior uveitis in FIV-infected cats and serologic changes consistent with *T. gondii* infection. Unfortunately, the ability of FIV to polyclonally activate B cells raises the possibility that elevated antibody titers to other pathogens may occur without opportunistic disease being present. Nonetheless, it is clear that opportunistic infection does occur, and all FIV-infected cats with intraocular inflammation should be evaluated for *T. gondii* infection.

The development of neurologic disease, lymphomas, and chronic wasting syndromes in specific pathogen-free cats experimentally infected with FIV suggests these disorders are primary manifestations of the virus. The most common neurologic change is altered behavior, which may occur in 30 to 40% of infected cats (Dow et al., 1992). Cats may become aggressive, roam, pace, or become stuporous and out of touch with their environment. In experimentally infected cats, we have observed more severe impairment, including varying levels of paresis and multifocal motor deficits. These changes may develop during the acute (6 to 10 weeks after infection) or terminal stages of infection. In acutely infected cats, neurologic deficits develop suddenly over several days, and slowly improve over 2 to 3 months. Cats with severe motor impairment will often have permanent deficits. Improvement is less likely in chronically infected cats. Clinically apparent peripheral nerve dysfunction has occurred in naturally infected cats, and reduced muscle action potentials after ulnar nerve stimulation has been documented in experimentally infected cats. Cerebrospinal fluid from cats with and without clinical neurologic changes will usually contain antibodies against FIV, increased numbers of mononuclear cells, and mild protein elevations. The virus can be cultured from both the brain parenchyma and the cerebrospinal fluid of infected cats. Electrophysiologic changes occur, including increased retinocortical latency times during visual evoked potential testing, and diffuse high amplitude activity during electroencephalography.

Although FIV is not an oncornavirus like feline leukemia virus, undifferentiated lymphomas and myeloid tumors have been reported in infected cats. These tumors may originate in nonlymphoid organs, including the central nervous system and the eye. The phenotypic characterization of these tumors is unknown. In our laboratory, attempts to isolate virus or detect provirus from lymphomas from three FIV-infected cats were negative. Additionally, flow cytometric analysis of a lymphoma from an FIV-infected cat revealed low levels of surface immunoglobulin and a lack of T-cell–associated proteins such as CD4 or CD8, suggesting the tumor may have been of B-cell origin. These findings suggest FIV-associated lymphomas may be similar to lymphomas in AIDS patients that are typically of B-cell origin and are not infected with HIV.

Terminally, many FIV-infected cats develop a wasting syndrome. Cats may lose 20 to 30% of their body weight over several weeks. Intermittent periods of moderate weight loss and subsequent weight gain are not uncommon, with severe wasting occurring in the last few months of life. The pathogenesis of the cachexia is unclear. Increased tumor necrosis factor expression probably contributes to the weight loss associated with AIDS.

## PATHOLOGIC FINDINGS

The most frequent histopathologic finding in infected cats is bone marrow hyperplasia (Reinacher and Holznagel, 1991). Leukocyte maturation may be dysplastic, with altered ratios of mature and immature cell populations. Megakaryocytosis is also a common finding (Shelton et al., 1990; Reinacher and Holznagel, 1991). Perivascular mononuclear cell infiltrates are often present in most parenchymal organs. In the central nervous system, these infiltrates are accompanied by diffuse gliosis and white matter pallor (Hurtrel et al., 1992). Chronic focal interstitial nephritis and areas of nephrosclerosis may occur. Intestinal changes may include mononuclear cell infiltration of the mucosa and crypt epithelium degeneration. Lymphatic changes present depend on the stage of infection. The lymph node enlargement during acute FIV infection is the result of marked immune stimulation with both B- and T-cell areas hyperplastic with follicular disorganization and dysplasia. As the infection progresses, lymphoid atrophy occurs and reactive lymphocytes are replaced with fibrous tissue (Brown et al., 1991).

## THERAPY

Therapies for lentiviruses have focused on inhibiting reverse transcriptase. Cellular infection is dependent on reverse transcription of the viral RNA into DNA. Nucleoside analogs including azothiouridine (AZT, Retrovir, Burroughs Wellcome, Research Triangle Park, NC), dideoxycytosine, and dideoxyionosine are currently used for the treatment of HIV. While they decrease virus expression, their effectiveness in preventing or slowing the progression of disease is controversial. The use of antiretrovirus drugs early in infection may be required to significantly alter disease progression. Resistance to nucleoside analogs may also diminish their effectiveness. Azothiouridine is highly efficacious against FIV's reverse transcriptase and is well tolerated at 10 mg/kg three times a day. However, treatment of cats with AZT has not prevented experimental FIV infection. Both AZT (5 mg/kg b.i.d. sc) and 9-(2-phosphonylmethoxyethyl) adenine (PMEA) (2.5 mg/kg b.i.d. sc) have been reported to reduce the severity of chronic stomatitis in FIV-infected cats (Hartmann et al., 1991). Because FIV infection is an animal model for AIDS, information on the efficacy and safety of antiretroviral drugs and biologic response modifier therapies in cats should expand rapidly. Institutional drug trials may allow new therapies to be tested in cats with minimal cost to pet owners.

With effective antiretroviral therapy not readily available, the care of FIV-infected cats is primarily supportive. Limiting an infected cat's contact with other cats is important. This decreases exposure to other pathogens that may further compromise immune function and provide a source of opportunistic infection. Infectious diseases should be identified and treated aggressively with appropriate antimicrobial therapy (see elsewhere in this section). Some of the clinical manifestations of FIV infection, such as severe stomatitis and anterior uveitis, require systemic corticosteroid therapy, whereas this treatment is inappropriate in cats with bacterial (e.g., lobar pneumonia) or fungal (e.g., nasal cryptococcal) infections. While intuitively corticosteroids are considered contraindicated in immunodeficiency syndromes, their use early in the chronic disease stage may help control virus expression by decreasing immune activation. Corticosteroid use during the primary viremia is contraindicated and may lead to elevated virus expression by dampening the primary immune response.

Routine vaccination of FIV-infected cats is controversial. During the subclinical and early chronic disease stage of FIV, cats are capable of immunologically responding to vaccines. However, there is evidence that suggests immune stimulation leads to increased virus expression and further compromises immune function. Consequently, vaccination may potentially worsen, not strengthen, a cat's immunity. Until the exact consequences of vaccination are understood, it is recommended that indoor cats with minimal exposure to other cats not be vaccinated except for rabies as required by law (see *CVT XI*, p 202). Furthermore, any vaccines given should be killed preparations, and not modified live vaccines. A vaccine for FIV is not available.

## PROGNOSIS

The average time from diagnosis of FIV infection until death is about 5 years. The progression of disease is much more rapid in cats co-infected with feline leukemia virus. Many of the manifestations of FIV infection require only intermittent supportive care often with antibiotic therapy (see *CVT XI*, p 276). For this reason and the unlikelihood of transmission to other cats within a stable household, euthanasia is not recommended unless a cat has entered the terminal stage of disease. Chronic wasting, the development of tumors, and debilitating neurologic disease are the most common reasons for euthanasia.

## References and Suggested Reading

Brown P, Hopper C, et al: Pathological features of lymphoid tissues in cats with natural feline immunodeficiency virus infection. J Comp Pathol 104: 345, 1991.
*A report on the histopathologic changes in FIV-infected cats.*
Dow S, Drietz M, et al: Feline immunodeficiency virus neurotropism: Evidence that astrocytes and macrophages are the primary target cells. Vet Immunol Immunopathol 35:23, 1992.
*Description of the in vitro tropism of FIV for neurologic tissue.*

Dow SW, Poss ML, et al: Feline immunodeficiency virus: A neurotropic lentivirus. AIDS 3:658, 1990.
*Original report focusing on the neurologic changes in FIV cats and pathologic changes in the nervous system.*
English RV, Johnson CM, et al: In vivo lymphocyte tropism of feline immunodeficiency virus. J Virol 67:5175, 1993.
*Research report identifying the populations of circulating mononuclear cells that are infected with FIV.*
Hartmann K, Donath A, et al: Use of two virustatica (AZT, PMEA) in the treatment of FIV- and of FeLV seropositive cats with clinical symptoms. *First International Conference of Feline Immunodeficiency Researchers*, Davis, CA, 1991.
*Clinical report on the effectiveness of two antiretroviral drugs in reducing the severity of clinical disease in FIV-infected cats.*
Hurtrel M, Ganiere J, et al: Comparison of early and late feline immunodeficiency virus encephalopathies. AIDS 6:399, 1992.
*Pathologic examination of nervous system changes during the first year of FIV infection.*
Ishida T, Washizu T, et al: Feline immunodeficiency virus infection in cats of Japan. J Am Vet Med Assoc 194:221, 1989.
*Seroepidemiologic study on the clinical diseases associated with FIV infection in Japanese cats.*
Lafrado L, Podell M, et al: FIV: A model for retrovirus induced pathogenesis. AIDS Res Rev 2:6, 1992.
*Excellent review of the neurologic and immunologic changes associated with FIV infection.*
Lehmann R, von Buest B, et al: Immunization-induced decrease of the CD4+:CD8+ ratio in cats experimentally infected with feline immunodeficiency virus. Vet Immunol Immunopathol 35:119, 1992.
*Report on lymphocyte subset changes after vaccination of FIV-infected cats for feline leukemia virus.*
Pedersen NC, Ho E, et al: Isolation of a T-lymphotropic virus from domestic cats with an immunodeficiency-like syndrome. Science 235:790, 1987.
*This is an excellent article describing the original isolation of FIV. The article provides information on the range of clinical diseases associated with FIV.*
Reid R, Barr M, et al: Retrospective serologic survey for the presence of feline immunodeficiency virus antibody: A comparison of ELISA and IFA techniques. Cornell Vet 82:359, 1992.
*A large study evaluating the specificity and sensitivity of FIV assays.*
Reinacher M and Holznagel E: Post mortem diagnosis of spontaneous FIV infection. *First International Conference of Feline Immunodeficiency Virus Researchers*, Davis, CA, 1991.
*A conference report on the postmortem findings in 40 FIV-infected cats.*
Sellon R, Jordan H, et al: Feline immunodeficiency virus can be transmitted via milk during acute maternal infection. J Virol 68:380, 1994.
*A report on the vertical transmission of FIV in experimentally infected cats.*
Shelton G, Linenberger M, et al: Hematologic manifestations of feline immunodeficiency virus infection. Blood 76:1104, 1990.
*A report on the hematologic changes in FIV-infected cats, including bone marrow changes.*
Siebelink KH, Chu IH, et al: Feline immunodeficiency virus (FIV) infection in the cat as a model for HIV infection in man: FIV-induced impairment of immune function. AIDS Res Hum Retrovir 6:1373, 1990.
*A report on the immune-function deficits in naturally and experimentally infected cats at different stages of FIV infection.*
Thomas J, Robinson W, et al: Association of renal disease indicators with feline immunodeficiency virus infection. *First International Conference of Feline Immunodeficiency Virus Researchers*, Davis, CA, 1991.
*Conference report on clinicopathologic changes consistent with renal disease in FIV-infected cats.*
Torten M, Franchini M, et al: Progressive immune dysfunction in cats experimentally infected with feline immunodeficiency virus. J Virol 65: 2225, 1991.
*Documentation of early and late immune deficiencies in FIV-infected cats.*
Wasmoen T, Armiger-Luhman S, et al: Transmission of feline immunodeficiency virus from infected queens to kittens. Vet Immunol Immunopathol 35:83, 1992.
*A preliminary report on the vertical transmission of FIV.*
Yamamoto JK, Hansen H, et al: Epidemiologic and clinical aspects of feline immunodeficiency virus infection in cats from the continental United States and Canada and possible mode of transmission. J Am Vet Med Assoc 194: 213, 1989.
*Excellent epidemiologic study of the clinical diseases associated with FIV infection and the seroprevalence of the infection in the United States.*

# FELINE RICKETTSIAL DISEASES

DORSEY L. KORDICK,
*Raleigh, North Carolina*

MICHAEL R. LAPPIN,
*Fort Collins, Colorado*

*and* EDWARD B. BREITSCHWERDT
*Raleigh, North Carolina*

*Rickettsia* are gram-negative bacteria in the order Rickettsiales. This is a diverse order that contains three families: Rickettsiaceae, Bartonellaceae, Anaplasmataceae, and many pathogenic genera that infect a number of vertebrate species.* In this discussion, the term "rickettsial" will be used in reference to organisms currently classified in the order Rickettsiales. Organisms in this order have an obligate intracellular or epicellular existence and are commonly transmitted by arthropod vectors.

*Haemobartonella felis, Coxiella burnetii, Ehrlichia equi, E. risticci,* and *Rochalimaea* spp. are the rickettsial agents known to infect cats. With the exception of haemobartonellosis, clinical disease induced by rickettsial infection is rarely recognized in cats. Because of the historic difficulties in culturing rickettsiae, there is minimal information concerning disease biology for several of these organisms, particularly in animals. Importantly, *Coxiella burnetii,* the *Ehrlichia* spp., and the *Rochalimaea* spp. have zoonotic potential. The following discussion considers the pathogenesis, clinical findings, treatment, prevention, and zoonotic risk of each rickettsia.

## HAEMOBARTONELLOSIS

Haemobartonellosis (feline infectious anemia) is caused by the organism *Haemobartonella felis.* Morphologically, *H. felis* is approximately 0.5 $\mu$m in diameter and is found in an epicellular location on erythrocytes. The organisms appear as short rods or cocci and are occasionally found in chains. It is a non–acid-fast organism and stains deep purple with Wright's and Giemsa stains. Attempts to culture the rickettsiae *in vitro* have been unsuccessful.

Transmission studies have demonstrated infection via oral or parenteral administration of blood from both diseased and apparently healthy cats. Additionally, *in utero* and lactogenic routes of transmission have been proposed as possible routes of infection in kittens. Acute hemolytic disease can be documented in cats of all ages. The frequent observation of cat-bite abscesses prior to clinical haemobartonellosis, coupled with the fact that males (perhaps due to increased fighting behavior) are more often affected with disease signs, has prompted the suggestion that cat bites may be another mode of transmission. Some investigators have observed an increased incidence of haemobartonellosis in flea-infested cats. As yet there is no experimental proof to support this observation, but a common mode of transmission within the order Rickettsiales is through blood-sucking ectoparasites.

Clinical manifestations of haemobartonellosis range from subclinical infection to severe anemia depending upon the immune status of the animal and the stage of disease. Clinical illness is often more severe in cats concurrently infected with the feline leukemia virus; however, *H. felis* can induce disease in immunocompetent cats. Fever, anemia of varying degrees of severity, depression, anorexia, and weight loss are frequent abnormalities. Splenomegaly and icteric mucous membranes may also occur. Rickettsemia is generally cyclical, causing packed cell volume (PCV) values to fluctuate due to sequestration of infected erythrocytes in the spleen. In cats that recover, a chronic carrier state develops during which stressful conditions can reportedly precipitate a relapse in clinical disease. Experimental attempts, however, to induce clinical disease in carrier animals have yet to support this hypothesis. Carrier cats that have recovered from experimental infection were immunosuppressed, splenectomized, and induced with *Pasteurella multocida* abscesses. No relapse into clinical disease was observed in any of the protocols.

Definitive diagnosis of haemobartonellosis can only be accomplished by the observation of *H. felis* in a thin blood smear. Since *H. felis* has not been cultured successfully, serologic confirmation of haemobartonellosis is not possible. Immediate preparation of blood smears following venipuncture may maximize organism visualization. Individual rickettsia are approximately one tenth the size of a red blood cell. Care must be used in differentiating organisms and erythrocyte inclusions such as Howell-Jolly bodies or chromatin remnants in reticulocytes. In view of the episodic nature of the rickettsemia, absence of discernable bacteremia or organisms on erythrocytes does not eliminate *H. felis* infec-

---

*Subsequent to the submission of this article for publication, the order Rickettsiales has been amended to exclude motile organisms and those culturable on bacteriologic media (Brenner et al., 1993). *Rochalimaea* spp. have been reclassified into the genus *Bartonella,* and the family Bartonellaceae has been removed from the order Rickettsiales. This reclassification was based upon the analysis of phenotypic characteristics and extensive phylogenetic studies.

tion. Conversely, when organisms are found in the blood smear of an immunocompetent or immunocompromised cat, *H. felis* may not be the cause of anemia or other disease manifestations. Cats with haemobartonellosis frequently have positive Coombs' tests as a result of antierythrocyte antibodies. Autoagglutination also occurs in some cats. Death due to severe anemia is not uncommon.

If the PCV rapidly declines to below 15%, blood transfusion is usually indicated. Orally administered oxytetracycline at a dosage of 22 mg/kg three times a day for 21 days is the treatment of choice. The authors have also successfully managed some cases with doxycycline administered orally at 5 mg/kg twice daily for 21 days. Another alternative regimen consists of concurrently starting treatment with chlorpromazine orally at 2 to 3 mg/kg once daily for 8 days along with metronidazole orally at 40 to 50 mg/kg once daily for at least 21 days. In the case of severe regenerative anemia accompanied by a positive Coombs' test or autoagglutination, concomitant therapy with orally administered prednisolone at 1 to 2 mg/kg should be employed to inhibit erythrocyte destruction. The dosage should be adjusted as the PCV increases to a normal value. The use of thiacetarsamide sodium or chloramphenicol has been questioned in recent years due to toxicity and frequent lack of efficacy. Their use should be reserved for the treatment of infection unresponsive to tetracyclines.

Cats recovering from haemobartonellosis experience a good long-term prognosis. Tetracycline treatment does not completely clear *H. felis*, and cats that recover from acute haemobartonellosis appear to retain the status of carrier animal. Fleas and ticks should be controlled to prevent potential reinfection. Experimentally, *H. canis* has been transmitted by the brown dog tick. Infection of dogs with *H. felis* has not been demonstrated, although cats have been subclinically infected with *H. canis* experimentally. The organism does not appear to pose a zoonotic threat to humans. Phylogenetic studies may change our ideas regarding the relationship between these two species and other genera.

## COXIELLOSIS

*Coxiella burnetii* is a rod-shaped rickettsia, approximately 0.25 μm in width by 0.5 to 1.25 μm in length, that causes Q fever in humans. The distribution of *Coxiella* is worldwide with reservoir hosts varying with the geographic location. Domestic species of cattle, sheep, goats, swine, camels, several wild mammals, birds, cats, and dogs are known hosts to the organism. Approximately 40 species of ticks and other arthropods have been identified as vectors.

Several routes of natural and experimental transmission have been identified. Rodent ticks and avian mites can successfully transmit the organism through biting. Organisms are shed from carrier animals in the urine, milk, placental tissues, amniotic fluid, and feces. Infectious aerosols during parturition constitute an important mode of transmission. The organism can survive in the environment despite dessication. Feline infection can also result from the ingestion of infected prey species such as meadow mice. Natural transmission between queen and kittens can occur and infection between cats has been produced experimentally.

*Coxiella burnetti* grows in the vacuoles of host cells rather than in the cytoplasm or nucleus, and has an affinity for the urogenital tract of infected animals. A latent period of infection is frequently observed until parturition, when highly infectious fluids are released into the environment. Small blood vessels are the tissue primarily affected by *C. burnetii* in the early phase of infection. During the late phase, damage to the mononuclear phagocyte system, liver, and central nervous system occurs. Both immune-mediated and direct effects of the organism are responsible for late-phase damage.

Naturally occurring coxiellosis is usually subclinical in cats. However, abortion can be a possible consequence of *C. burnetii* infection in animals that are chronic carriers of the organism. Vague and nonspecific clinical abnormalities such as fever, anorexia, and lethargy have been observed within 2 days of subcutaneously infecting cats. These symptoms persisted for 3 days and were not evident in animals receiving orally administered inoculum or cage contact with *C. burnetii*. There have been questions raised regarding a higher risk of human infection associated with stillborn kittens. People experience acute symptoms such as fever, lethargy, muscle tenderness, and severe headache followed by more chronic sequelae such as pneumonitis, hepatomegaly, and endocarditis. Hematologic abnormalities in humans have included lymphocytosis and thrombocytopenia.

Isolation of the rickettsiae from blood inoculated into either embryonated chicken eggs or in L929 mouse fibroblast cell culture is the most definitive method of diagnosis. *Coxiella burnetii* has also been recovered from the urine of cats 2 months following experimental infection. Serologic tests utilizing complement fixation, immunofluorescent antibody, and competitive enzyme immunoassay techniques have been developed, but availability is generally limited to research laboratories.

Effective treatment of chronically infected cats to eliminate carriers and shedding of the organism has not been reported. In cattle, similar attempts to eliminate infection have been unsuccesful. *Coxiella burnetii* has a predilection for the urogenital tract and can persist there asymptomatically. Chemotherapeutic agents used in human infection include tetracycline, chloramphenicol, and some quinolones.

Although other domestic mammals are the primary source of infection for humans, cats are nonetheless an important reservoir that requires consideration. Veterinary health personnel and owners should wear gloves and masks while attending to parturient or aborting cats. All cats not used for breeding should be ovariohysterectomized.

Research into the development of a vaccine against coxiellosis has been ongoing for 55 years. Whole-cell vaccines for humans and animals are considered to be investigational and not licensed in the United States for general administration. The development of a particulate subunit vaccine as an alternative to the whole-cell vaccine is currently being studied.

## ROCHALIMAEA INFECTION

*Rochalimaea* species are short, slightly curved rods approximately 0.5 to 1.0 $\mu$m in length. Four species of the genus have been identified to date. *Rochalimaea henselae* has recently been implicated as the most frequent causative agent of human cat scratch disease (CSD). The rickettsia has been isolated on blood culture from several cats in contact with clinically affected people. *Rochalimaea henselae* has also been associated with vascular proliferative disease, while *R. quintana* and *R. elizabethae* have been reported in two cases of human endocarditis. *Rochalimaea quintana* was the etiologic agent of trench fever during the world wars. *Rochalimaea vinsonii* to date has only been found in voles of Nova Scotia.

The means of transmission of *Rochalimaea* spp. from cats to people and from cat to cat have not been determined. Some investigators have noted an increased rate of cat scratch disease in people contacting flea-infested animals, particularly kittens. Although not definitively established, cats may infect one another via bites, grooming behavior, scratches, and possibly *in utero*.

Investigative efforts are currently being made into the pathogenesis of *Rochalimaea* infection in the cat. Most infected cats appear to be subclinical; however, only limited studies have been reported. Pronounced lymphadenopathy occurs in human patients. Affected lymph nodes reveal granulomatous necrosis with a mixed cell infiltrate and frequently contain argyrophilic (silver) staining rickettsiae. Argyrophilic, intracellular coccobacilli have been observed in some cats with idiopathic peripheral lymphadenopathy. It is likely that *R. henselae* lymphoid hyperplasia occurs in cats.

Demonstration of the bacteremia through blood culture documents infection but does not allow for speciation. Caution should be exercised in attempts to isolate the organism, due to the pathogenicity of *R. quintana*. The rickettsiae are extremely fastidious and require long incubation periods (up to 1 month) on blood agar in an enriched carbon dioxide environment. Preliminary isolation studies of CSD-associated cats suggest that rickettsemia persists for extended periods of time. Alternatively, serologic analysis using an immunofluorescent antibody (IFA) test to detect antibody to *Rochalimaea* is available from the Centers for Disease Control (CDC) for human patients in whom CSD is suspected. Serologic testing of feline serum for antibodies to *R. henselae* is available through our laboratory.[†] *In vitro*, *Rochalimaea* species are susceptible to

gentamicin, rifampin, ciprofloxacin, and trimethoprim-sulfamethoxazole.

Because the pathogenicity for *R. henselae* and potentially other *Rochalimaea* species has not been established, we cannot make definitive treatment recommendations at this time. In those instances where *Rochalimaea* infection is suspected, treatment with an antibiotic with antirickettsial activity would seem prudent. Recently, several *Rochalimaea* species have emerged as important pathogens for humans. Cat scratch disease, peliosis hepatis, bacillary angiomatosis of the skin and spleen, and endocarditis are some of the diseases currently associated with the genus. The rickettsia is able to elicit clinical disease in both immunocompromised and immunocompetent patients; however, clinical manifestations of infection tend to differ depending upon the status of the patient's immune system. Widespread occurrence of human disease within families owning a carrier of *Rochalimaea* is low and supports continued possession of the animal. Immunocompromised individuals, however, should limit exposure to known *Rochalimaea*-infected cats and exercise caution when handling cats of undefined health status.

## EHRLICHIOSIS

The distribution of *Ehrlichia* species is worldwide. *Ehrlichia*-like morulae have been found in cats on three continents. The rickettsiae are pleomorphic, coccoid-ellipsoid, and approximately 0.5 $\mu$m in diameter. The organism lives intracellularly in leukocytes or platelets and occurs as compact inclusions with a mulberry-like appearance, referred to as morulae.

Naturally occurring *Ehrlichia* infection in cats has been documented primarily with *E. risticii*, the cause of Potomac horse fever. The organism is prevalent in the equine population and, given the frequently close association of cats and horses, it is possible that cats may be an important reservoir in the life cycle of the bacterium. Cats can be experimentally infected with *E. risticii* or *E. equi* but not *E. canis*. Cats experimentally inoculated with *E. risticii* or *E. equi* occasionally develop clinical signs of disease including fever, depression, lymphadenopathy, anorexia, and diarrhea. Morulae occur in monocytes following *E. equi* infection but are not associated with *E. risticii* infection.

*Ehrlichia*-like organisms have been identified in leukocytes from a small number of clinically ill cats in Nairobi, Kenya, France, and the United States. Serologic studies were not performed in the Kenya report, but the organism was intermediate in size between *E. canis* and *E. sennetsu*. Clinical signs of disease included fever, anorexia, weight loss, and dyspnea. Normocytic normochromic anemia was common. The cat observed in the United States exhibited intermittent cyclic fever, anorexia, general malaise, and nonlocalizing hyperesthesia. Laboratory abnormalities included normocytic, normochromic, nonregenerative anemia and hyperglobulinemia. Pyogranulomatous lymphadenitis of a mesenteric lymph node was documented histopatho-

---

[†]Tick-borne Disease Laboratory NCSU-CVM, Room C-321 4700 Hillsborough St. Raleigh, NC 27606

logically. Cytologic evaluation of imprints made from the lymph nodes revealed multiple mononuclear cells containing clusters of intracytoplasmic inclusions that resembled *Ehrlichia* morulae. Immunofluorescent antibody testing revealed immunoglobulin G antibody titers to *E. canis* (1:80) and *E. risticii* (1:40). The clinical signs of malaise, hyperesthesia, and fever resolved within 48 hr after initiation of doxycycline administered orally at 5 mg/kg twice daily. The clinical signs combined with pyogranulomatous lymphadenitis, the presence of *Ehrlichia*-like morulae in mononuclear cells, the apparent clinical response to doxycycline, and the exclusion of other common causes of fever suggested that the clinical signs exhibited by this cat were induced by infection by an *Ehrlichia* species.

Serum from multiple cats have been screened at Colorado State University for antibodies against *E. canis* and *E. risticii*. Twelve cats with clinical signs or laboratory evidence of disease consistent with infection by an *Ehrlichia* species including fever, malaise, weight loss, anorexia, lymphadenopathy, nonseptic suppurative polyarthritis, anemia, thrombocytopenia, neutropenia, polyclonal gammopathy, and monoclonal gammopathy have been identified that also had antibodies that reacted with *E. canis* antigens. Each cat had a positive response to doxycycline. Cats with antibodies that reacted with both *E. canis* and *E. risticii* antigens have *E. canis* titers consistently two- to eightfold higher than *E. risticii* titers, suggesting that the *Ehrlichia* species involved is more closely related to *E. canis*. Antibodies against *E. equi* or *E. sennetsu* have not been detected at higher titers in *E. canis*–seropositive cats. Since cats cannot be infected by *E. canis*, it is likely that the *Ehrlichia* species infecting these cats is a separate species.

*Rhipicephalus* spp., *Ixodes* spp., and *Hyalomma* spp. of ticks have been identified as vectors for various species of *Ehrlichia*. The clinically ill cats from Kenya were infested with *Haemophysalis laechi*. No vector has been identified for cases occurring in the United States.

Definitive diagnosis of feline ehrlichiosis is based on demonstration of morulae in leukocytes. A presumptive diagnosis of feline ehrlichiosis can be made by combining appropriate clinical signs of disease with serologic evidence of infection (preferably seroconversion), exclusion of other etiologies, and response to an antirickettsial drug.

Tetracyclines have been traditionally used in both canine ehrlichiosis and Potomac horse fever. Doxycycline given orally at 5 mg/kg twice daily, appears to be effective in feline cases as described previously. Imidocarb dipropionate or tetracycline were used successfully in the three cases diagnosed in Kenya.

At this time, it is unknown whether cats harbor species of *Ehrlichia* transmissible to people. It is also unknown whether cats serve as an intermediate host for infection of horses with *E. risticii*.

## References and Suggested Reading

Bouloy R, et al: Feline ehrlichiosis: Clinical case and serologic survey. J Am Vet Med Assoc 204:1475, 1994.

Brenner DJ, et al: Proposals to unify the genera *Bartonella* and *Rochalimaea*, with descriptions of *Bartonella quintana* comb. nov., *Bartonella vinsonii* comb. nov., *Bartonella henselae* comb. nov., and *Bartonella elizabethae* comb. nov., and to remove the family Bartonellaceae from the order Rickettsiales. Int J Syst Bacteriol 43:777, 1993.

Buoro IBJ, et al: Feline anaemia associated with ehrlichia-like bodies in three domestic short-haired cats. Vet Rec 125:434, 1989.

Charpentier F and Groulade P: Probable case of ehrlichiosis in a cat. Bull Acad Vet Fr 59:287, 1986.

Dawson JE, et al: Susceptibility of cats to infection with *E. risticii*, causative agent of equine monocytic ehrlichiosis. Am J Vet Res 49:2096, 1988.

Gillespie JH and Baker JA: Experimental Q fever in cats. Am J Vet Res 13:91, 1952.

Greene CE and Breitschwerdt EB: Rocky Mountain spotted fever and Q fever. *In* Greene CE (ed): *Infectious Diseases of the Dog and Cat*, 2nd edition. Philadelphia, WB Saunders Co, 1990, pp 430–433.

Harvey JW: Haemobartonellosis. *In* Greene CE (ed): *Infectious Diseases of the Dog and Cat*, 2nd edition. Philadelphia, WB Saunders Co, 1990, pp 434–442.

Pederson NC: *Feline Infectious Diseases*. California, American Veterinary Publications, 1988, pp 221–230.

Regnery RL, et al: Characterization of a novel *Rochalimaea* species, *R. henselae*, sp. nov., isolated from blood or a febrile, human immunodeficiency virus-positive patient. J Clin Microbiol 30:265, 1992.

Williams JC et al: Vaccines against coxiellosis and Q fever. Ann NY Acad Sci 653:88, 1992.

# CANINE EHRLICHIOSIS: CLINICAL IMPLICATIONS FOR HUMORAL FACTORS

RUSSELL T. GREENE

*Phoenix, Arizona*

Canine ehrlichiosis, first recognized in the United States more than 30 years ago, is a disease of worldwide importance. After infection with *Ehrlichia canis*, plasma cell infiltration occurs in many organs, and the resulting humoral response is thought to play an important role in disease pathogenesis. This review emphasizes what is known concerning humoral factors associated with *E. canis* infections, and will discuss these as they relate to information concerning the agent, clinical signs, clinical pathology, and therapeutic alternatives. Excellent reviews detailing many aspects of canine ehrlichiosis have been published (Greene and Harvey, 1984; Troy and Forrester, 1990).

## THE AGENT

For many years, only one pathogenic *Ehrlichia* species, *Ehrlichia canis*, was recognized. More recently, several new species have been characterized, and it is likely that more will be isolated. Currently, the genus *Ehrlichia* can be broadly subdivided into three groups (Brouqui et al., 1992). *Ehrlichia canis*, *E. chaffeensis*, and *E. ewingii* make up one group. *Ehrlichia equi* and *E. phagocytophilia*, which potentially are different strains of the same species, constitute the second group. The third group consists of *E. risticii* and *E. sennetsu*. *Ehrlichia platys* has not been fully categorized in this scheme. An ehrlichial agent is suspected as a cause of feline disease (see "Feline Rickettsial Diseases," this volume, p 287); however, an agent has yet to be isolated. The clinical importance of this genus reclassification is that veterinarians may soon learn of new rickettsial agents and the diseases they cause.

*Ehrlichia canis* is considered to be the type species of the genus. The common features shared by these organisms are their intracellular habitat in leukocytes, and their multiplication within a membrane-lined vacuole of the infected cell. Currently, *Ehrlichia* species are differentiated from each other by their host-animal specificity, their host-cell (either granulocyte or macrophage/monocyte) specificity and, except for *E. canis*, their limited geographic distribution.

## CLINICAL SIGNS

The duration of clinical signs associated with canine ehrlichiosis is quite variable. Classically, the acute phase of the disease occurs 1 to 3 weeks after infection, and clinical signs last only 2 to 4 weeks. Depression, anorexia, lethargy, weight loss, and fever are the most common manifestations of the acute-phase disease.

Despite earlier reports that the subacute phase lasts only weeks, more recent reports have demonstrated that many dogs experience a subacute phase that can last for years (Codner and Faris-Smith, 1986; Perille and Matus, 1991). Oftentimes this subacute stage is subclinical. Therefore, not much is known concerning this stage or the factors that transform subclinical infections into a chronic state. The final stage of ehrlichiosis is the chronic stage, which can be associated with mild or severe manifestations. Nonspecific clinical signs, as observed in the acute condition, can be seen in chronic cases. In addition, bleeding tendencies, lymphadenopathy, splenomegaly, ocular abnormalities, and secondary infections are considered the indicators of chronic ehrlichiosis. Polyarthropathies and neurological signs have also been described.

## CLINICAL PATHOLOGY

Thrombocytopenia, leukopenia, nonregenerative anemia, monocytosis, and lymphocytosis are commonly found in canine ehrlichiosis. These hematologic abnormalities are rarely present simultaneously, and various combinations are more typical.

Thrombocytopathia and Coombs'-positive anemias are infrequently observed and are thought to be, at least in part, mediated by humoral factors. A platelet migration inhibitory factor, distinct from antiplatelet antibody, is produced by lymphocytes of *E. canis*–infected dogs, and contributes to the thrombocytopathia (Kakoma et al., 1977). This factor has been shown to inhibit platelet pseudopod formation, causing the affected platelets to become rounded, clumped, and leaky. In addition, hyperglobulinemia (see below) has an inhibitory effect on migration and adhesiveness of circulating platelets. Coombs'-positive anemias may occur secondary to nonspecific coating of red blood cells by globulins or subsequent to a specific immune response to red blood cell surface antigens.

Canine patients with ehrlichiosis may develop urinary tract infections, septicemia, or opportunistic infections. Decreased leukocyte numbers and function are usually responsible for these infections. Lymphocytes of affected dogs have been shown to secrete a factor that exerts a cytotoxic effect on autologous monocytes (Kakoma et al., 1977). This cytotoxic factor may be the same chemical, mentioned above, that inhibits platelet pseudopod function. In addition, a species-specific leukocyte migration-inhibitory factor has been isolated from *Ehrlichia*-infected dogs. These, as well as other uncharacterized factors, contribute to the potential for concurrent infections.

Mild increases in hepatic enzyme activities (alanine aminotransferase [ALT] and alkaline phosphatase [ALP]) and elevations in blood urea nitrogen (BUN) and creatinine can be detected, although these values are usually normal in ehrlichiosis. Hyperproteinemia, hyperglobulinemia, and hypoalbuminemia are frequently observed (see below). Results of routine coagulation tests (prothrombin time [PT], activated partial thromboplastin time [APTT], and fibrin degradation products [FDPs]) are typically normal, unless a secondary disease process initiated disseminated intravascular coagulation (DIC). However, because of the thrombocytopathia and severe thrombocytopenia, bleeding times and clot retraction times may be prolonged.

Marked abnormalities in serum proteins are routinely found in both experimental and naturally occurring *E. canis* infections. Two weeks after experimental infection, $\alpha_2$ proteins transiently increase, but then gradually decrease during the subsequent month to below normal concentrations. Serum $\gamma$-globulins dramatically increase and serum albumin decreases in chronic experimental infections. $\beta$-Globulins may variably increase.

Dogs in the chronic stage of naturally acquired disease have a similar hypergammaglobulinemia and hypoalbuminemia as is seen in chronic, experimental infections. The magnitude of the increase in γ-globulins typically correlates with the duration of illness. Although polyclonal gammopathies are typical in *E. canis* infections, monoclonal gammopathies are occasionally observed. After therapy, in naturally occurring conditions, the gammopathies usually resolve within 3 to 9 months. However, it may take up to 15 months for globulins to normalize in some cases.

The kidneys are also affected by humoral factors in canine ehrlichiosis (Troy and Vulgamott, 1980; Codner and Maslin, 1992). Glomerular leakage is common in acute infections. Minimal-change glomerulonephropathy accounts for the protein loss. Immunofluorescent staining has revealed mild to moderate depositions of immunoglobulins in glomerular tufts and mesangium. An immune pathogenesis would explain why the glomerulonephritis in chronic cases is occasionally nonresponsive to appropriate antibiotic treatment.

## Serologic Tests

The indirect immunofluorescent antibody (IFA) test for detection of anti–canine *Ehrlichia* antibodies was developed in 1971, and is still routinely utilized for serodiagnostic testing in both animals and humans (Dawson et al., 1991). The relatively recent successful propagation of *E. canis* in a tissue culture cell line has allowed for the production of *Ehrlichia* organisms in large enough quantities for more sophisticated serologic assays, such as enzyme-linked immunosorbent assay (ELISA) and immunoblot methodologies.

There is significant antigenic cross-reactivity between the various ehrlichial species in serologic testing. Using homologous antisera, *E. canis* and *E. sennetsu* cross-react considerably. *Ehrlichia risticii* cross-reacts strongly with *E. sennetsu* and, to a lesser degree, with *E. canis*. *Ehrlichia equi* and *E. sennetsu* have substantial antigenic cross-reactivity, and may actually be very closely related. There is minimal cross-reactivity between *E. equi* and *E. canis* or *E. risticii*. Importantly, there is limited serologic cross-reactivity between *E. canis* and many common nonehrlichial canine pathogens.

Clinicians must remember that all ehrlichial agents induce a specific humoral immune response in their host. This serologic response occurs in every animal exposed to *Ehrlichia* spp., regardless of whether the infection becomes established, or disease is present. This means that detection of an antibody titer does not equate with a diagnosis of disease due to ehrlichiosis. In equine *E. risticii* infections (Potomac horse fever), the higher the patient's titer, the more likely *E. risticii* is associated with the disease process (Rikihisa et al., 1990). A similar situation has been accepted for years with canine *E. canis* infections. Veterinarians should realize that the cut-off titer for positive serology is frequently arbitrarily established and varies among labora-

tories from 1:10 to 1:80. Therefore, the diagnostic significance of a low titer should be interpreted cautiously.

After experimental exposure to *E. canis*, IFA titers can be demonstrated at 1:10 or greater as early as 7 days, and as late as 28 days, after inoculation. Using immunoblot techniques, a 25-kd polypeptide band of *E. canis* is consistently recognized during this early stage of infection. This protein band is found among all members of the genus *Ehrlichia*. Immunofluorescent antibody titers usually remain increased for the duration of an infection. However, it has been documented in at least one instance that, during a terminal chronic infection, antibody titers can drop to less than 1:10 just before death. In chronic infections, typically at least 12 polypeptide bands are recognized on immunoblots. The size ranges for the bands are from 12 to 147 kd and typically there are at least four immunodominant bands (25, 42, 57, and 70 kd) (Nyindo, Kahoma, and Hanson, 1991). Currently, immunoblots are not used on a clinical basis; however, with the classification of many new ehrlichial species, immunoblots may develop into a useful diagnostic tool to differentiate the infecting agent.

A direct correlation cannot be made between the presence of increased antibody titers and cell-mediated immune responses or clearance of the agent. Therefore, the level of antibody titer does not reflect the degree of protection. In addition, clinically normal animals with high titers after treatment are fully susceptible to reinfection with a homologous strain.

The duration of persistence of posttreatment antibody titers appears to be somewhat related to the level of antibody titer at the time of treatment. Dogs with initial low-level antibody titers (1:10–1:160) tend to have their titers return to negative within a few months. However, in dogs with high antibody titers (≥1:1280), persistence of increased antibody titers for over 2 years is common. Although there has been only one report of six dogs with persistence of antibody titers, data from the author's recently completed research involving 100 dogs suggest that this is a common occurrence in naturally exposed patients. It is unclear at this time if this antibody persistence is from continual exposure (since the animals usually are not moved from their place of initial exposure) or persistence from the previous infection.

## TREATMENT

The treatment for canine ehrlichiosis consists of antirickettsial agents and supportive care. Tetracycline (22 mg/kg, every 8 hr for 14–21 days) or doxycycline (5 to 10 mg/kg, every 12 to 24 hr for 7 to 10 days), have generally been considered the drugs of choice (Greene and Harvey, 1984). However, newer literature (Iqbal and Rikihisa, 1994) suggests this length of therapy is inadequate. The author recommends 2 to 3 months of therapy based on preliminary data. Other medications that have been administered successfully include chloramphenicol, imidocarb dipropionate, or amicarbalide.

The quinolones have some antirickettsial effects; however, preliminary evidence suggests that they are not useful in canine ehrlichiosis. In dogs with acute illness, clinical response is usually seen within 24 to 48 hr. Short-term immunosuppressive glucocorticoid therapy may be of value for severe, life-threatening thrombocytopenia during the initial stage of treatment. This is often prescribed out of necessity, because it is often difficult to distinguish between canine ehrlichiosis and immune-mediated thrombocytopenia while awaiting serologic test results.

Some dogs do not respond to the standard antimicrobial therapy. In particular, dogs with chronic ehrlichiosis may have irreversible bone marrow or renal changes. Supportive care, which may include blood transfusions and nutritional supplementation, may be required. Although controversial, bone marrow stimulation with anabolic steroids may also be useful.

If animals live in an endemic area and there is concern of continuous exposure to infected ticks, low levels (6 mg/kg) of once-daily tetracycline can be administered as a preventative. It was demonstrated that this dose of tetracycline will protect dogs from developing disease following a subsequent inoculation.

## SUMMARY

Clearly, humoral factors play an influential role in canine ehrlichiosis. Understanding the significance of serologic titers and humoral factors in clinical cases will help direct clinicians in their diagnostic and therapeutic management. In addition, veterinarians need to be aware that the genus *Ehrlichia* is currently undergoing substantial redefinition. Additional species will likely be identified in the near future, and our understanding of the host response to ehrlichial infections may be further elucidated.

## References and Suggested Reading

Brouqui P, Dumler JS, Raoult D, and Walker DH: Antigenic characterization of ehrlichiae: Protein immunoblotting of *Ehrlichia canis*, *Ehrlichia sennetsu*, and *Ehrlichia risticii*. J Clin Microbiol 30:1062, 1992.

Codner EC and Faris-Smith LL: Characterization of the subclinical phase of ehrlichiosis in dogs. J Am Vet Med Assoc 189:47, 1986.

Codner EC and Maslin WR: Investigation of renal protein loss in dogs with acute experimentally induced *Ehrlichia canis* infection. Am J Vet Res 53:294, 1992.

Dawson JE, Rikihisa Y, Ewing SA, et al: Serologic diagnosis of human ehrlichiosis using two *Ehrlichia canis* isolates. J Infect Dis 163:564, 1991.

Greene CE and Harvey JW: Canine ehrlichiosis. *In* Greene CE (ed): *Clinical Microbiology and Infectious Diseases of the Dog and Cat.* Philadelphia, WB Saunders Co, 1984.

Iqbal Z and Rikihisa Y: Reisolation of *Ehrlichia canis* from blood and tissues of dogs after doxycycline treatment. J Clin Microbiol. 32:1644, 1994.

Kakoma I, Carson CA, Ristic M, et al: Autologous lymphocyte-mediated cytotoxicity against monocytes in canine ehrlichiosis. Am J Vet Res 38:1557, 1977.

Kakoma I, Carson CA, Ristic M, et al: Platelet migration inhibition as an indicator of immunologically mediated target cell injury in canine ehrlichiosis. Infect Immun 20:242, 1977.

Nyindo M, Kakoma I, and Hansen R: Antigenic analysis of four species of the genus *Ehrlichia* by use of protein immunoblot. Am J Vet Res 52:1225, 1991.

Perille AL and Matus RE: Canine ehrlichiosis in six dogs with persistently increased antibody titers. J Vet Intern Med 5:195, 1991.

Rikihisa Y, Reed SM, Sams RA, et al: Serosurvey of horses with evidence of equine monocytic ehrlichiosis (Potomac horse fever). J Am Vet Med Assoc 197:1327, 1990.

Troy GC and Forrester SD: Canine ehrlichiosis. *In* Greene CE (ed): *Infectious Diseases of the Dog and Cat.* Philadelphia, WB Saunders Co, 1990.

Troy GC, Vulgamott JC, and Turnwald GH: Canine ehrlichiosis: A retrospective study of 30 naturally occurring cases. J Am Anim Hosp Assoc 16:181, 1980.

# *CVT* UPDATE: ROCKY MOUNTAIN SPOTTED FEVER

RANCE K. SELLON
*and* EDWARD B. BREITSCHWERDT
*Raleigh, North Carolina*

Rocky Mountain spotted fever (RMSF), the disease caused by *Rickettsia rickettsii*, is but one of a number of diseases caused by infection with organisms of the genus *Rickettsia*. The epidemiology of Rocky Mountain spotted fever and the essential role of ticks in transmission of the disease were first described in detail in the early 1900s by Howard Ricketts, for whom the organism is named. In the United States, RMSF is the most common rickettsial disease in humans and, along with canine ehrlichiosis, one of the most common in dogs. While statistics for the number of canine cases are not available, in 1992, 493 human cases of RMSF were reported to the Centers for Disease Control (CDC). With a mortality rate in humans of approximately 5%, several deaths each year in people (and dogs) are attributed to RMSF, emphasizing the importance of this disease. In addition, dogs may serve as a sentinel species for human RMSF, so an understanding of the epidemiology, transmission, clinical disease, and treatment of canine RMSF may help increase disease awareness in those areas in which the disease is especially prevalent.

## PREVALENCE AND TRANSMISSION

Though originally described in people of the Rocky Mountain states of Montana and Idaho, RMSF is now recognized primarily as a disease of the central and southeastern United States. The states reporting the largest number of human cases of RMSF in 1992 were Oklahoma (90), North Carolina (64), and Tennessee (54). Comparatively fewer cases of RMSF are reported from the western portion of the United States (including Alaska and Hawaii) or New England. Though statistics for the prevalence of canine RMSF are not as comprehensive as for human RMSF, serosurveys of the prevalence in dogs, when reported, generally parallel the human surveys. For example, serosurveys of dogs in Oklahoma and North Carolina indicate that, as is the case for people, there is also a high degree of exposure of dogs in these states to spotted fever group rickettsiae. It is important to understand that extensive serologic cross-reactivity between *R. rickettsii* and other spotted fever group rickettsiae (*R. montana, R. rhipicephali*) may falsely contribute to the apparent seroprevalence of *R. rickettsii* if reactivity to the cross-reacting species is not concurrently determined.

The distribution of RMSF reflects the distribution of the ticks that are the transmitting vector. Two species of ticks, *Dermacentor andersoni* and *D. variabilis*, are the primary ticks transmitting the causative agent, *Rickettsia rickettsii*. The organism is maintained in the tick population through vertical transmission of the rickettsia. Dogs are not a reservoir for the disease, nor are they sources of human infection, because dogs do not develop the degree of rickettsemia necessary to establish infection in ticks. The seasonal activity of *D. andersoni* and *D. variabilis* contributes to the seasonal aspect of RMSF apparent in endemic areas. In North Carolina and other endemic areas, RMSF is primarily a disease of the spring, summer, and fall; winter cases of RMSF are unusual.

## PATHOGENESIS/CLINICAL DISEASE

The pathogenesis of RMSF has been nicely detailed in previous literature (Comer, 1991), so only the prominent features of the disease will be summarized here. RMSF is truly a multisystemic disease that may have a variety of clinical appearances. The clinical signs of RMSF are attributable to invasion of endothelial cells of the small blood vessels, primarily the precapillary arterioles and postcapillary venules, and the vasculitis that follows. The ensuing loss of vascular integrity leads to increased vascular permeability, edema, and coagulopathies that may be manifest as hemorrhage or thrombosis or both. These abnormalities can lead to systemic hypotension, decreased organ perfusion, and organ damage and dysfunction. Clinical signs are thus a reflection of the organs involved. In dogs, the severity of clinical signs reflects the number of organisms at inoculation; fewer numbers result in mild clinical signs and generally self-limiting disease, while inoculation with larger numbers of organisms results in more severe clinical signs or death if untreated. Disease severity may also reflect pathogenic differences between isolates of *R. rickettsii*. There are numerous isolates used in experimental infections that manifest differences in clinical severity within a given species of animal studied. Lastly, disease severity also reflects host factors as well. Some people infected with *R. rickettsii* have antibodies that bind to cultured endothelial cells and to endothelial phospholipids. Though a cause-and-effect relationship has not been firmly established between infection with *R. rickettsii* and the development of antiphospholipid antibodies, it is suspected that antiphospholipid antibodies may diminish the natural antithrombotic properties of the vascular endothelium through an as yet poorly understood mechanism.

Clinical signs associated with canine RMSF have been well characterized, but are not pathognomonic for RMSF. Variations in clinical signs from case to case, and the similarity of clinical signs of RMSF to those of other diseases, contribute to the difficulties in establishing a definitive diagnosis of RMSF during acute infection. Among the most common presenting clinical findings in dogs with RMSF are fever, depression, anorexia, lameness, and neurologic signs. Other common clinical signs associated with RMSF include vomiting and diarrhea, and generalized lymph node enlargement. Clinical signs indicative of disease involvement of other organs may also be present (Table 1). Careful examination of the haired skin and the ocular fundi should not be forgotten, as these organs may reveal evidence of hemorrhage and increase the suspicion of RMSF.

As is the case for clinical signs, laboratory abnormalities associated with RMSF are not pathognomonic for the disease and may be similar to those observed in other diseases. Clinical laboratory abnormalities in-

***Table 1.*** *Common Historical Complaints and Clinical Signs Associated with RMSF in Dogs*

Fever
Anorexia
Depression
Lameness
Lymph node enlargement
Increased bronchovesicular sounds
Scleral injection
Neurologic signs
   Para/tetraparesis
   Vestibular disease
   Seizures
   Hyperesthesia
Gastrointestinal disease
   Vomiting
   Diarrhea
Petechial hemorrhage
Dermal necrosis
Peripheral edema

clude early leukopenia followed later by leukocytosis that is characterized primarily by neutrophilia. Thrombocytopenia is reported as the most common hematologic abnormality observed in RMSF. The thrombocytopenia observed with RMSF is typically mild to moderate in degree (175,000 to 50,000/$\mu$l). Platelet counts greater than 100,000/$\mu$l may be interpreted as normal if their numbers are estimated from an examination of a stained blood smear. Thus, an absolute platelet count is most useful in detecting mild thrombocytopenia and increasing the clinical suspicion of RMSF. Since bleeding due solely to thrombocytopenia is unusual when platelet counts are above 10,000/$\mu$l, animals that have evidence of hemorrhage with platelet counts greater than 10,000/$\mu$l should be suspected of having a vasculitis and RMSF considered as a differential diagnosis. Other abnormalities of the complete blood count (CBC) and biochemical profile may be observed, but there is no one pattern characteristic of RMSF infection (Table 2).

Clinical RMSF may resemble other diseases and can present the clinician with diagnostic and therapeutic dilemmas. Differential diagnoses for RMSF include acute ehrlichiosis, sepsis syndrome, pancreatitis, and some immune-mediated diseases (e.g., immune-mediated thrombocytopenia, immune-mediated polyarthritis). Distinguishing acute RMSF from sepsis syndrome may be particularly difficult because of the similarities of these two diseases in physical examination abnormalities, and abnormal results of hematologic and biochemical profiles (see "Septic Shock," this volume, p 139). In the authors' experience, abnormalities of coagulation tests (prothrombin time [PT], activated partial thromboplastin time [APTT]) are not as pronounced in RMSF as in sepsis syndrome, and RMSF is not as commonly associated with disseminated intravascular coagulation (DIC), though DIC may develop in severe cases of RMSF.

## IMMUNE RESPONSE

Studies of experimental RMSF infection in dogs have characterized the kinetics of antibody responses to *R. rickettsii*. Typically, immunoglobulin M (IgM) titers rise quickly following infection, becoming detectable around day 9 of infection and peaking around day 20, and are undetectable by about day 80. In contrast, IgG titers do not become detectable until days 22 to

28 of infection and reach their peak around day 42 of infection. Immunoglobulin G titers gradually decline over the course of 6 to 9 months after infection. In experimental settings, challenge inoculation of dogs with *R. rickettsii* 3 years after recovery from RMSF has not resulted in clinical disease, suggesting that immunity to *R. rickettsii* may be lifelong.

## DIAGNOSIS

Because the clinical presentation of canine RMSF can be extremely variable, a high index of suspicion must be maintained for dogs presenting with compatible historical complaints and physical examination abnormalities, particularly in areas where the disease is prevalent. A tentative diagnosis of RMSF is supported by appropriate historical, physical, and laboratory findings in endemic areas during the months of April through September, the time of the year when the disease is most prevalent. A history of recent tick exposure or the presence of ticks on the patient adds further support to the presumptive diagnosis, but the absence of such should not lessen the degree of suspicion for this disease. Definitive diagnosis is based on serologic conversion, the demonstration of *R. rickettsii* organisms by immunohistochemical methods in affected tissue, or culture of the organism. The mainstay of diagnosis of RMSF is serologic testing, but there are potential pitfalls in the interpretation of serologic assays. Results of a recently reported comparison of three serologic assays illustrate that no one serologic test currently available will accurately identify all infected dogs if a single acute or convalescent sample is assayed. The most reliable serologic diagnosis (defined as a fourfold increase in titer between acute and convalescent sera) is provided by assays that measure the composite IgM/IgG response. Submission of acute samples greater than a week into infection may potentially result in less pronounced (i.e., less than fourfold) increases in the convalescent titers if assays that detect only IgM antibodies are used.

An additional confounding factor in the use of serology for the diagnosis of RMSF is the observation that dogs exposed to other nonpathogenic spotted fever rickettsiae can develop antibodies that cross-react with *R. rickettsii*. Titers to these other rickettsial organisms can be high enough to create confusion and misinterpretation of acute titers if solely relied upon for diagnosis. Even following early administration of antirickettsial drugs, submission of convalescent sera for testing will usually document a fourfold increase in titer to *R. rickettsii* that will then confirm the diagnosis of RMSF. These findings point out the necessity of (1) obtaining acute and convalescent sera at appropriate times whenever possible for a definitive diagnosis of RMSF, and (2) an understanding of the assay used by any particular laboratory for the diagnosis of RMSF. Failure to appreciate these aspects of serologic testing may result in inaccurate diagnoses.

A last pitfall of serodiagnosis of RMSF is potential

***Table 2.*** *Clinical Pathologic Abnormalities Observed with RMSF*

Hematology
  Thrombocytopenia
  Leukopenia/leukocytosis
  Anemia
Chemistry
  Hypoalbuminemia
  Increased serum alkaline phosphatase activity
  Hyponatremia
  Hypokalemia

variability in reported results of antibody titers that may arise if samples are tested at different laboratories, or are assayed at different times or by different individuals within the same laboratory. To avoid these confounding factors, clinicians are encouraged to freeze a serum sample from blood obtained during the acute presentation, obtain a second serum sample during the convalescent period 4 to 6 weeks later, and submit both samples to one laboratory for simultaneous assay.

In addition to serologic testing, a diagnosis of RMSF may also be made by immunohistochemical demonstration of R. rickettsii organisms in biopsies of lesions induced by the infection. In dogs, this test appears to have limited usefulness due to the unpredictability of finding organisms within a lesion. Experimental studies of the utility of an immunofluorescent assay for detection of RMSF organisms in dogs have demonstrated the necessity of testing several sections of a given biopsy to accurately evaluate the lesion for organisms; examination of few sections from any one biopsy may result in a false-negative test result. It is suspected that prior treatment with antirickettsial antibiotics may further reduce the sensitivity of this particular assay, as antibiotic treatment results in the rapid clearance of the organism from tissues, so samples should ideally be collected before the initiation of therapy for optimal sensitivity. The test is less useful late in the course of disease (beyond 2 weeks) because the organisms will be cleared by specific immune responses at this time. It is important to obtain a biopsy of affected tissue, as normal-appearing tissue is unlikely to contain organisms. Modifications of immunohistochemical detection assays using a two-antibody system and immunoperoxidase conjugates instead of fluorescein have been developed. Compared to immunofluorescent assays for demonstration of rickettsial organisms in tissues, potential advantages of immunoperoxidase assays include increased sensitivity and ease of performing the assay; however, direct comparison of the different tests has not been reported.

Diagnosis of RMSF during the acute phase of the disease continues to be hampered by the lack of a sensitive and specific test. Developments in molecular biology are providing tools that are revolutionizing the study and diagnosis of numerous diseases of people and animals, and may fill this diagnostic void. Use of the polymerase chain reaction (PCR) for the early diagnosis of RMSF has been described. The PCR employs small R. rickettsii–specific sequences of deoxyribonucleic acid (DNA) (primers) and a heat-stable DNA polymerase to amplify larger segments of the R. rickettsii genome from blood or tissue. The amplified DNA products are then visualized by gel electrophoresis or other methods. Detection of specific amplified DNA products confirms the presence of the organism in the tissue of interest, and thus confirms the diagnosis of RMSF. Under proper conditions of amplification, the PCR can be highly sensitive and very specific, but its use is limited at present to research laboratories.

## THERAPY

Definitive treatment of RMSF relies upon antibiotics with antirickettsial activity. Tetracycline and related compounds (oxytetracycline, doxycycline) are the historical standards for therapy and remain as some of the most useful drugs for treatment of RMSF. Tetracycline is administered orally at a dose of 22 mg/kg every 8 hr for 14 to 21 days. Chloramphenicol (15 to 20 mg/kg every 8 hr PO, IM, or IV for 14 to 21 days) has excellent activity against R. rickettsii and has the advantage of parenteral routes of administration for animals with vomiting or other conditions that may preclude the oral route. Chloramphenicol also will not stain the tooth enamel of puppies that must be treated. Response to treatment in most animals is rapid, and improvements in clinical and laboratory abnormalities are often observed within 24 to 48 hr of initiating therapy.

While tetracycline and chloramphenicol are the most commonly used drugs for the treatment of RMSF, other drugs have been evaluated for antirickettsial therapy. A recent experimental study in dogs has shown that enrofloxacin was as effective as tetracycline and chloramphenicol in the treatment of experimental RMSF. When administered at a dose of 3 mg/kg orally every 12 hr, enrofloxacin was very effective in resolving the clinical, hematologic, and vascular abnormalities caused by a sublethal RMSF infection. However, it should be emphasized that the experimentally infected dogs did not have severe disease, and the efficacy of enrofloxacin in the face of severe RMSF infection, or infection with field isolates of R. rickettsii, awaits clarification from properly controlled laboratory and clinical trials.

Supportive therapy (intravenous fluids, analgesics, nutritional maintenance, wound management) will be indicated in some cases of RMSF. Fluid therapy, when indicated, should be closely monitored, as the vasculitis that characterizes RMSF may increase the risk of edema formation if fluid therapy is too aggressive; pulmonary or cerebral edema could have disastrous consequences in susceptible patients. Aspirin or other compounds that interfere with platelet function should not be used as analgesics. Because of the frequent delay from initial presentation to definitive diagnosis, specific antirickettsial therapy should not be withheld pending definitive diagnosis in cases of suspected RMSF. Rapid improvement following therapy may further support a tentative diagnosis of RMSF.

## PREVENTION

Currently, methods of preventing RMSF focus on prevention of contact between ticks and susceptible hosts. Avoiding tick-infested areas is the best, though not always the most practical, means of preventing RMSF. Control of tick populations with yard sprays and dips for pets is an important aspect of disease control. Prompt removal of ticks is another mainstay of prevention. Ticks should be removed with hemostats or tweezers and not fingers, and the tick should not be crushed if at all possible. Vaccinations against *R. rickettsii* have met with some success in protecting laboratory rodents from infection, but the use of vaccines has not yet moved beyond the laboratory into clinical practice.

## SUMMARY

Rocky Mountain spotted fever remains an important tick-transmitted disease of humans and dogs, and is prevalent throughout most of the United States. The clinical disease in dogs is varied, and routine laboratory tests are not pathognomonic, therefore, a high index of suspicion for this disease is critical for submission of appropriate samples for definitive diagnosis and therapy. A presumptive diagnosis of RMSF in animals that are evaluated for compatible historical complaints, and physical examination and laboratory abnormalities during the spring, summer, and fall, justifies initiation of specific antirickettsial therapy. The best prevention is avoiding tick-infested areas and implementation of tick control on the premises and on the pet.

## References and Suggested Reading

Breitschwerdt EB, Levy MG, Davidson MG, et al: Kinetics of IgM and Ig G responses to experimental and naturally acquired *Rickettsia rickettsii* infection in dogs. Am J Vet Res 51:1312, 1990.
*A description of the immunologic response in dogs with RMSF illustrating changes in specific immunoglobulins over time following infection and resistance to clinical disease following challenge exposure.*
Breitschwerdt EB, Davidson MG, Aucoin DP, et al: Efficacy of chloramphenicol, enrofloxacin, and tetracycline for treatment of experimental Rocky Mountain spotted fever in dogs. Antimicrob Agents Chemother 35: 2375, 1991.
*Results of a comparison of these three drugs in the treatment of canine RMSF that showed that all three drugs were equally effective in resolving mild clinical infections.*
Comer KM: Rocky Mountain spotted fever: Vet Clin North Am 21:27, 1991.
*A comprehensive description of the epidemiology, pathogenesis, clinical signs, treatment, and prevention of RMSF.*
Greene CE, Marks MA, Lappin MR, et al: Comparison of latex agglutination, indirect immunofluorescent antibody, and enzyme immunoassay methods for serodiagnosis of Rocky Mountain spotted fever in dogs. Am J Vet Res 54:20, 1993.
*A comparison of three serologic assays for RMSF diagnosis that illustrates that the there is no one perfect test for the serologic diagnosis of RMSF, especially during the acute stage of the disease.*
Ricketts HT: Some aspects of Rocky Mountain spotted fever as shown by recent investigations. Med Rec 76:843, 1909 (reprinted in Rev Infect Dis 13:1227, 1991).
*A fascinating account of the early investigations into RMSF pieced together to form an epidemiologic model of RMSF before the causative agent was known.*
Tzianabos T, Anderson BE, and McDade JE: Detection of *Rickettsia rickettsii* DNA in clinical specimens by using polymerase chain reaction technology. J Clin Microbiol 27:2866, 1989.
*A description of a protocol for the use of the polymerase chain reaction to detect* R. rickettsii *DNA from infected human patients.*

# SALMON POISONING DISEASE

YASUKO RIKIHISA
*Columbus, Ohio*
*and* GARY ZIMMERMAN
*Livingston, Montana*

## GEOGRAPHIC DISTRIBUTION

Salmon poisoning disease (SPD) is not an actual poisoning, but rather an acute and highly fatal rickettsial disease of domestic and wild Canidae. The disease is normally transmitted to dogs upon ingestion of raw fish of the family Salmonidae harboring rickettsia-infected metacercariae of the fluke *Nanophyetus salmincola*. The disease is indigenous around rivers in the Pacific coast region from northwestern California to southwestern Washington. Additionally, several SPD cases were reported in Vancouver Island, Canada (Booth, Stogdale, and Grigor, 1984). Salmon poisoning disease has been reported from outside the indigenous areas when fish migrate through fluke-infested rivers or infected fish are transported.

## SALMON POISONING DISEASE AGENT

The etiologic agent of SPD is *Neorickettsia helminthoeca*, a gram-negative minute coccoid rickettsia in the tribe Ehrlichieae. *Neorickettsia helminthoeca* stains dark blue to purple by Romanowsky stain. *Neorickettsia helminthoeca* infects monocytes/macrophages (but not seen in other types of cells) and can be isolated from liver, spleen, and blood and propagated in tissue culture (Rikihisa, Stills, and Zimmerman, 1991). *Neorickettsia helminthoeca* has not been grown in ordinary bacteriologic media, yolk sac, fibroblasts, or small laboratory rodents. In the past, a small quantity of organism was isolated and cultured in primary canine blood monocyte in a medium containing 20 or 40% canine serum. The organism has been recently efficiently cultured using a dog macrophage cell line, DH82 cells (Rikihisa, Stills, and Zimmerman, 1991), in a medium containing 10% fetal bovine serum, in a sufficient quantity to allow molecular and antigenic studies (Pretzman et al., 1992; Rikihisa, 1991). *Neorickettsia helminthoeca* multiply by binary fission and are found in membrane-lined vacuoles in the cytoplasm. The organisms were individually tightly enveloped by the host membrane or enveloped as a cluster (morulae). The morulae were less compact and smaller in size compared to those of *Ehrlichia canis* in DH82 cells (Rikihisa, Stills, and Zimmerman, 1991). Two layers (outer and inner) of membrane, ribosomes, and fine deoxyribonucleic acid (DNA) strands were evident in the organism by transmission electron microscopy (Rikihisa, Stills, and Zimmerman, 1991). Like the members of the genus *Ehrlichia*, there was no thickening of inner leaflet of the outer membrane or outer leaflet of the inner membrane (Rikihisa, Stills, and Zimmerman, 1991).

*Neorickettsia helminthoeca* is antigenically and genetically most closely related to *Ehrlichia* spp. By Western immunoblot analysis and indirect fluorescent antibody (IFA) labeling, *N. helminthoeca* is reciprocally cross-reactive strongly with *E. risticii* (the agent of Potomac horse fever) and *E. sennetsu* (the agent of human sennetsu fever in Japan), but weakly with *E. canis* (the agent of canine ehrlichiosis) (Rikihisa, 1991). The percentage 16SrRNA gene sequence homology between *N. helminthoeca* is 94.3% with *E. risticii*, 94% with *E. sennetsu*, and 82.3% with *E. canis* (Pretzman et al., 1992). The 16SrRNA gene sequence comparison is currently considered the most reliable means to determine phylogenetic relatedness among bacteria, and the result suggests *N. helminthoeca*, *E. sennetsu*, and *E. risticii* but not *E. canis* belong to the same genus, although they are currently classified under different genera (as it was named "new rickettsia"). The 16SrRNA gene sequence homology between *Rickettsia rickettsii*, the agent of Rocky Mountain spotted fever, is 79.9% (Pretzman et al., 1992).

The Elokomin fluke fever agent was reported to occur along the Elokomin River in the State of Washington. The agent responsible has been cultured in primary canine blood monocytes by continuous passages for up to 2 months, and no morphologic differences between *N. helminthoeca* and Elokomin fluke fever agent were noted at either the light or electron microscopic level (Frank, McGuire, and Gorham, 1974). Infection of one organism does not protect the dog from infection with another (Frank et al., 1974) and were weakly cross-reactive with *N. helminthoeca* by IFA. The agent has a wider host range than *N. helminthoeca* and is reported to infect bear, raccoon, and ferret in addition to the Canidae. Clinical signs of Elokomin fluke fever are milder than those of SPD. With *N. helminthoeca* infections, dogs develop a fever with more of a temperature spike, whereas Elokomin fluke fever produces a longer plateau-type fever (Gorham and Foreyt, 1990). The lymph node pathology is also different between *N. helminthoeca* and Elokomin fluke fever agent. Follicles are active in *N. elokominica* infection, but in *N. helminthoeca* infection, follicles disappear accompanied by histiocytosis (Frank et al., 1974). Metacer-

cariae can harbor both organisms simultaneously. The agent has not been cultured in a continuous cell line and based upon current information is considered as a strain of *N. helminthoeca*.

## EPIZOOTIOLOGY

The vector and reservoir of SPD is a digenetic trematode, *Nanophyetus salmincola*, which harbors the rickettsia throughout its life cycle stage from egg to adult. Three different hosts are required for the completion of the trematode life cycle: the freshwater snail *Oxytrema silicula* in which *N. helminthoeca* asexually multiply, salmonid fish in which the trematode encysts as metacercaria, and carnivorous animals in which the metacercaria develops into adult and produce fertilized eggs (Knapp and Millemann, 1981). Evidence of existence of the rickettsia in all development stages of the trematode was supported by transmission studies. Ingestion of adult flukes, metacercariae, helminth-infected snail livers, and helminth eggs can cause SPD. *Neorickettsia helminthoeca* has never been seen or directly isolated from the fluke. The distribution of SPD roughly corresponds to the distribution of *O. silicula* and thus the distribution of *N. salmincola* in North America. In the enzootic area, essentially 100% of salmonid fish are infested with trematodes. Ocean-caught fish are not free from infection. Thirty-one per cent of 542 ocean-caught king salmon, 53% of 2049 coho salmon, and none of 35 pink salmon were infected with metacercariae of *N. salmincola* (Weiseth, Farrell, and Johnston, 1974). It is, however, unknown what percentage of trematodes harbor *N. helminthoeca* or whether there are strains of *N. helminthoeca* of varying degrees of virulency. Although *O. silicula* and *N. salmincola* are common in certain river basins in the former Soviet Union (Dovgalev, 1988), SPD is limited to the above restricted areas in North America.

*Neorickettsia helminthoeca* is transmitted from the fluke in the intestinal lumen to the dog's macrophages. Although the trematode infects a wide variety of species of animals, SPD was found chiefly in Canidae (dogs, coyotes, foxes) and occasionally seen in other species of immunosuppressed animals. *Neorickettsia helminthoeca* infects neither fish nor snail.

Venereal transmission from infected male to a female was also reported. Rectal and aerosol transmission is also possible (Frank, McGuire, and Gorham, 1974). Blood, feces, and lymph node aspirants are infectious; thus, infected dogs must be isolated and care used so as not to induce iatrogenic transmission.

## PATHOGENESIS/IMMUNE RESPONSE

Ingested metacercaria in salmonid fish mature in 5 to 6 days in the gut, and the adult stage attaches deep in the interior of intestinal mucosa, inducing inflammation (i.e., hyperemia), inflammatory cell migration, and edema around the parasites. By unknown mechanisms, *N. helminthoeca* transfers to monocytes and macrophages that migrate through blood and lymphatic vessels and lodge in somatic and visceral lymph nodes. *Neorickettsia helminthoeca* circulate in the blood of orally infected dogs starting 8 to 12 days after infection as evidenced by successful reisolation of *N. helminthoeca* from the blood from 8 to 11 days after infection until death (Rikihisa, Stills, and Zimmerman, 1991). Before 8 to 11 days after infection, *N. helminthoeca* cannot be reisolated, suggesting that migration or infection of blood monocytes does not occur by that time. Lymph nodes appear to be the primary site of multiplication of neorickettsiae, since *N. helminthoeca* was found primarily in lymph nodes. Like *E. risticii*, *N. helminthoeca* appears to have intestinal tissue trophism, since not only the oral route of infection but also the intravenous inoculation of cell-cultured organisms induced severe hemorrhages throughout the small intestine (Rikihisa, Stills, and Zimmerman, 1991). In contrast to *E. risticii*, *N. helminthoeca* induces severe inflammatory responses in the intestinal wall and hypertrophy of lymph nodes, especially mesenteric lymph nodes with a large number of histiocytes present. Tremendous enlargement of mesenteric lymph nodes is related to the port of entry of *N. helminthoeca*. Intravenous injection of *N. helminthoeca* makes dogs sick faster and more severely, but mesenteric lymph nodes did not become as large as those by oral route of infection. Nonsuppurative meningitis or meningoencephalitis brain lesions have also been noted in both natural and experimental infection of *N. helminthoeca*. Infected blood monocytes appear to cross the blood-brain barrier as suggested by the presence of infected histiocytes in cerebellar meninges (Hadlow, 1957). Severe central nervous system depression seen in SPD is probably related to these brain lesions.

The dogs experimentally infected with *N. helminthoeca* orally developed IgG antibody at 13 to 15 days after infection as detected by IFA test (Rikihisa, Stills, and Zimmerman, 1991). In contrast to *E. canis* infection, persistent or chronic infection with *N. helminthoeca* is uncommon.

## CLINICAL FINDINGS

A typical incubation period for *N. helminthoeca* infection is approximately 5 to 7 days. However, prolonged incubation periods of 19 to 33 days have also been reported. Clinical signs are characterized by anorexia, inactivity, depression, and sudden onset of fever, above 39.8°C or up to 42.7°C, followed by hypothermia over the next 4 to 8 days, resulting in sharp peak-like temporal temperature curve (Rikihisa, Stills, and Zimmerman, 1991). Vomiting may precede the typical watery yellowish diarrhea that is sometimes tinged with blood. Rapid weight loss is evident, and the lack of ingestion of water coupled with fluid loss through vomiting and diarrhea results in severe dehydration with both electrolyte and acid-base imbalances. Serous nasal and ocular discharges are sometimes seen. Lymphad-

enopathy of the major nodes is easily palpable. Many clinicians report a typical odor of the diarrhea of SPD. It is important that the disease not be confused with distemper, hepatitis, or parvovirus infection, since the prognosis for appropriately treated dogs with SPD is generally good.

## DIAGNOSIS

In enzootic areas, SPD should be considered based on clinical signs. To confirm the diagnosis, a cytocentrifuged lymph node aspirate should be examined after Romanowsky staining (we prefer Diff-Quik) for the presence of *N. helminthoeca*, as *N. helminthoeca* are most frequently seen in the lymph node. Although *N. helminthoeca* can be reisolated into the macrophage cell line culture from the spleen, liver, and blood monocyte fractions (Rikihisa, Stills, and Zimmerman, 1991), the organism is less frequently visualized in these tissues, and blood smears are not useful for diagnosis. Tissue culture rickettsial isolation is not routinely used, as it requires special facilities and trained personnel. Infected dogs develop specific antibodies by 2 weeks after infection as determined by IFA and Western immunoblot analysis (Rikihisa, 1991; Rikihisa, Stills, and Zimmerman, 1991). Because of the acute nature of SPD, one cannot wait for serologic test results before treating dogs; thus, serologic tests are not routinely done. Appearance of the light brown trematode eggs, approximately 87 to 97 $\mu$m $\times$ 35 to 55 $\mu$m, in dog feces also supports the diagnosis. As clinical signs develop during the prepatent period, not finding the fluke eggs in feces does not rule out SPD. Hematologic observation is nonspecific, characterized by leukopenia followed by rebound leukocytosis. Like other ehrlichial infections, large monocytoid cells similar to elicited or activated monocytes appear in the blood during the course of infection.

## PATHOLOGIC FINDINGS

Remarkable lymphadenopathy, splenomegaly, hepatomegaly, and edema are seen. Intestinal hemorrhage and inflammation are the characteristic lesions and are more severe than those caused by the fluke alone. Neuropathology was found in our and other's experimentally infected dogs (Hadlow, 1957). Brains appeared swollen, and engorgement of meningeal blood vessels was evident in some experimentally infected dogs.

Microscopically, lesions are generally mild and proliferative in character with very little evidence of degeneration and necrosis in various organs including brain, although extensive necrosis may accompany the proliferative response in lymphoid tissue. Lesions consist of mononuclear cell infiltration instead of granulocytic suppurative infiltration. Intimal proliferation and vascular necrosis or thrombosis seen in rickettsial infection, such as Rocky Mountain spotted fever, are not observed. Generalized lymph node enlargement is due to marked infiltration of macrophages accompanied by severe depletion of small lymphocytes and a loss of germinal centers. Splenic follicular central hemorrhage and necrosis and obliteration of thymic architecture by macrophage infiltration are common. Lesions in the central nervous system are different from those of viral infections of dogs (e.g., rabies, canine distemper, and infectious canine hepatitis or toxoplasmosis).

## THERAPY AND PROGNOSIS

Sulfonamides, chlortetracyclines, oxytetracyclines, and chloramphenicol have been the most common agents used for SPD. Doxycycline, 10 mg/kg, IV given twice a day for at least 7 days, is useful. Because diarrhea and vomiting are usually present, the intravenous route is preferred to oral administration. As with other rickettsial infections, sulfonamides, penicillin, or aminoglycosides are not effective. Keeping the dogs dry, clean, and warm is important. General supportive therapy is required to replace and maintain fluid losses and maintain electrolyte and acid-base balance. Because the intestinal flukes can by themselves cause severe enteritis, anthelmintic therapy such as praziquantel should be used. Nonsteroidal anti-inflammatory drugs may be also used.

Dogs treated early in the course of the infection have a better chance of full recovery than those treated later in the infection. Nearly 90% of untreated dogs will succumb to SPD, due to dehydration, acid-base imbalances, and anemia resulting from the diarrhea. Those dogs that survive initial infection from SPD, either naturally or following therapy, will have a lifelong immunity to the SPD agent but not to either Elokomin fluke fever or repeated infections of *N. salmincola*.

## PREVENTION

The best practical preventive measure is to prevent exposure to raw, infected fish. With known recent ingestion of raw salmonid fish, emetics may be helpful in reducing the potential of SPD from developing. *Neorickettsia helminthoeca* can survive in dead fish without refrigeration for up to 1 month, and at −20° or −80°C for several months. Infected fish should be cooked above 60°C more than 15 min to inactivate *N. helminthoeca* before feeding dogs. With any known exposure to salmonid fish, dogs should be observed for early signs of SPD, followed by appropriate intervention therapy. Because dogs can be infected, not only orally, but also intravenously, intradermally, and by the ocular route, dogs that are confirmed as being infected with SPD should be isolated until they are well. Because of the development of solid immunity in recovered dogs and the development of an effective tissue culture method, a vaccine is theoretically possible, but no vaccine has yet been developed for SPD.

## References and Suggested Reading

Booth AJ, Stogdale L, and Grigor JA: Salmon poisoning disease in dogs on southern Vancouver Island. Can Vet J 25:2, 1984.

Bosman DD, Farrell RK, and Gorham JR: Nonendoparasite transmission of salmon poisoning disease of dogs. J Am Vet Med Assoc 156:1907, 1970.

Dovgalev AS: Distribution and invasion rate of mollusks, the intermediate hosts of trematodes in the middle Amur river region Russian SFSR USSR. Med Parazitol Parazit Bolezai 71, 1988.

Frank DW, McGuire TC, and Gorham JR: Cultivation of two species of *Neorickettsia* in canine monocytes. J Infect Dis 129:257, 1974.

Frank DW, McGuire TC, Gorham JR, and Farrell RK: Lymphoreticular lesions of canine neorickettsiosis. J Infect Dis 129:163, 1974.

Gorham JR and Foreyt WJ: Salmon poisoning disease. *In* Green CE (ed): *Infectious Diseases of the Dog and Cat.* Philadelphia, WB Saunders Co, 1990, pp 397–403.

Hadlow WJ: Neuropathology of experimental salmon poisoning of dogs. Am J Vet Res 18:898, 1957.

Knapp SE and Millemann RE: Salmon poisoning disease. *In* Davis JW (ed): *Infectious Diseases of Wild Mammals.* Ames, IA, Iowa State University Press, 1981, pp 376–387.

Pretzman C, Rikihisa Y, Ralph D, and Fuerst P: 16SrRNA sequence comparison between *Neorickettsia helminthoeca* and *Ehrlichia* spp. (abstr H86). New Orleans, LA, American Society for Microbiology, May 26–30, 1992, p 197.

Rikihisa Y: Cross-reacting antigens between *Neorickettsia helminthoeca* and *Ehrlichia* spp. shown by immunofluorescence and Western immunoblotting. J Clin Microbiol 29:2024, 1991.

Rikihisa Y, Stills H, and Zimmerman G: Isolation and continuous culture of *Neorickettsia helminthoeca* in a macrophage cell line. J Clin Microbiol 29:1928, 1991.

Simms BT and Muth OH: Salmon poisoning. Transmission and immunization studies. *Proc 5th Pacific Science Congress* (Canada, 1933), 4:2949–2960, 1934.

Weiseth PR, Farrell RK, and Johnston SD: Prevalence of *Nanophyetus salmincola* in ocean-caught salmon. J Am Vet Med Assoc 165:849, 1974.

# MYCOPLASMA INFECTIONS OF DOGS AND CATS

SØREN ROSENDAL

*Guelph, Ontario, Canada*

Mycoplasmas are prokaryotic microorganisms enclosed in a cytoplasmic membrane, but without an outer cell wall. Taxonomically, they belong within the class Mollicutes, a name emphasizing the pleomorphism and the contrast to bacteria with distinct morphology bestowed by the rigid peptidoglycan wall. Like most bacteria, they can be cultured in the laboratory on rich cell-free substrates, providing lipids, carbohydrates, and amino acids for metabolism. Mycoplasmas are fastidious and slow growing, and are sensitive to antimicrobials interfering with nucleic acid and protein synthesis, but not those with activity against cell-wall synthesis, such as penicillin. The organisms most frequently associated with domestic animals are classified in the genera *Mycoplasma*, *Ureaplasma*, and *Acholeplasma*; the former two groups require cholesterol for survival and growth, but the latter does not.

Dogs and cats host many species of mycoplasmas, few of which are proven pathogens. Mycoplasmas are part of the mucosal membrane bacterial flora of the respiratory, genital, and intestinal systems. They are generally not significant pathogens in their natural sites, but may incite an inflammatory response if they spread to parts of the systems not normally occupied by a natural microbial flora, or if they spread to the conjunctiva. Mycoplasmas of dogs and cats are not invasive but may cross the mucosal barriers under conditions of general debilitation, such as immunosuppression or malignancies, in which cases they may disseminate to joints and various tissues. At least in the cat, mycoplasmas may establish in subcutaneous tissue of traumatized skin.

The process of isolating and identifying mycoplasmas is slow and only feasible in laboratories with experience and proper typing reagents. Nevertheless, efforts to look for mycoplasmas should be encouraged in conditions of possible infectious nature, where other agents are ruled out.

There are at least 15 species of the genus *Mycoplasma* represented in the dog and cat mycoplasma flora in addition to *Acholeplasma laidlawii* and ureaplasmas. The canine ureaplasmas have not been further classified, whereas those recovered from the cat are speciated into *U. felinum* and *U. cati*.

## DOG

The mycoplasma flora in the larynx, pharynx, and nasal cavity of the dog is rich and varied, but has not been implicated in any disease conditions of these sites.

However, disease conditions in the lower respiratory tract predisposes to invasion of the lung. Of the several different species recovered from lungs of dogs with pneumonia, only *M. cynos* has been shown to cause pathology in experimentally inoculated puppies. A strain of *M. bovigenitalium* has produced equivocal inflammatory changes, whereas *M. spumans*, *M. canis*, or *M. gateae* were innocuous. In an unrelated study of bronchopneumonia in laboratory dogs, Kirchner et al. (1990) found mycoplasmas of unknown identity, but suggested that they had etiologic significance based on the histopathologic changes.

Practitioners should evaluate carefully any positive mycoplasma findings in transtracheal wash samples and attempt to rule out any primary reasons for invasion of the lower airways. If mycoplasmas are suspected of contributing to bronchitis and pneumonia, treatment with antimicrobials, such as those listed below, should be administered over 1 to 2 weeks.

There are undoubtedly cases of reproductive failure in the dog where mycoplasmas have a primary etiologic role, although the evidence is largely circumstantial (see "Canine Genital Mycoplasmas and Ureaplasmas," this volume, p 1090). Mycoplasmas should be ruled in or out by submitting appropriate samples for culture when the following conditions are recognized: poor conception, early embryonic death, embryo or fetal resorption, abortion, stillborn pups, and weak or dying pups.

In the male dog, cases of epididymo-orchitis associated with mycoplasmas have been described. In a large-scale survey of fertile and infertile male and female dogs, the prevalence of mycoplasmas in vagina, prepuce, and semen was highest in infertile animals. The rate of ureaplasma infection in the vagina of infertile dogs was almost twice the rate in fertile dogs and only ureaplasmas were isolated from semen of infertile males with low sperm count, subnormal motility, and morphologic abnormalities.

Since mycoplasmas are normal inhabitants of the vagina and prepuce in dogs, it is not surprising that mycoplasmas also appear to play an opportunistic role in disease conditions of the urinary tract. They have been isolated from clinical samples taken by cystocentesis at a rate of 4%, and in many cases in pure culture and numbers above $10^4$/ml. Increased number of inflammatory cells in urine of dogs with mycoplasma urinary tract infection is further evidence of their etiologic significance.

In both reproductive and urinary tract conditions, *M.*

*canis* seems to be the most frequently isolated type. Inoculation of the vas deferens through experimentally created fistula in male dogs has resulted in orchitis and epididymitis. *Mycoplasma canis* has also been inoculated into the uterus of female dogs, who became cervical shedders and in a few cases developed purulent endometritis.

Mycoplasmas may be sporadically involved in polyarthritis of dogs, but more work is needed to determine if mycoplasma polyarthritis similar to the syndromes occurring in other animal species also occur in the dog and cat.

## CAT

Mycoplasmas are frequently associated with conjunctivitis in the cat. *Mycoplasma felis* appears to be the type most commonly isolated, and it likely contributes significantly to the disease, since experimentally exposed cats have developed inflammation of the conjunctiva.

Like dogs, cats harbor a rich mycoplasma flora in the nasopharyngeal-laryngeal mucosa. The lower airways of healthy cats are free of mycoplasmas, whereas pneumonic cats often have *M. felis* isolated from samples of lung tissue. In general, mycoplasma isolates from the lung are probably rarely of primary significance, except in the case of *M. felis* isolation, since pneumonia has been seen in experimentally exposed kittens. This organism may also disseminate to the joints of animals with immunocompromising disease conditions. Polyarthritis caused by *M. gateae* has been recognized in a cat with reduced γ-globulin and assumed immunoinsufficiency. However, the isolate caused arthritis in both immunosuppressed and normal cats upon intravenous inoculation.

There is no experimental evidence for the role of mycoplasmas in reproductive failure of cats, but this should not discourage practitioners from submitting samples for mycoplasma culture in conditions similar to those listed above for the dog.

Interestingly, mycoplasmas seem occasionally to be causing chronic subcutaneous abscesses in the cat. The abscesses may follow bites inflicted by other cats, with the mycoplasmas originating from the teeth or oral cavity. It is also possible that dog bites can initiate the lesions, since *M. canis* has been isolated from one ab-scess. The mycoplasma wound infections in cats may pose risks to owners and others in contact. A case of wound infection in a cat where the attending veterinarian contracted cellulitis in the hand has been described. The cellulitis required surgery and was unresponsive to penicillin but treatable with vibromycin. Although the mycoplasma was only isolated from the veterinarian, both the cat and the veterinarian had growth-inhibiting antibodies to the mycoplasma. This isolate or most of those recovered from cat abscesses have as yet not been classified as one of the described species.

## TREATMENT

If persuasive evidence speaks for mycoplasmas having a primary role or contributory role in inflammatory conditions of dogs or cats, antimicrobial therapy should constitute prolonged administration of quinolones, chloramphenicol, tetracycline, tylosin, lincomycin, or spiramycin (see Appendix). Minimal inhibitory concentrations (MIC) of macrolide drugs, except for erythromycin and oleandomycin, are relatively low. The MIC values obtained with tetracyclines, aminoglycosides, chloramphenicol, and lincomycin are within the range where they should have clinical efficacy. The newer fluoroquinolone drugs have proven efficacious against other mycoplasmas and would presumably also be useful in mycoplasmoses of dogs and cats.

## References and Suggested Reading

Haesebrouck F, Devriese LA, van Rijssen B, and Cox E: Incidence and significance of isolation of *Mycoplasma felis* from conjunctival swabs of cats. Vet Microbiol 26:95, 1991.

Jang SS, Ling GV, Yamamoto R, and Wolf AM: *Mycoplasma* as a cause of canine urinary tract infection. J Am Vet Med Assoc 185:45, 1984.

Keane DP: Chronic abscesses in cats associated with an organism resembling *Mycoplasma*. Can Vet J 24:289, 1983.

Kirchner BK, Port CD, Magoc TJ, Sidor MA, and Ruben Z: Spontaneous bronchopneumonia in laboratory dogs infected with untyped *Mycoplasma* spp. Lab Anim Sci 40:625, 1990.

Lein DH: Canine mycoplasma, ureaplasma, and bacterial infertility. *In* Kirk RW (ed): *In* Current Veterinary Therapy IX: Small Animal Practice. Philadelphia, WB Saunders Co, 1986.

McCabe SJ, Murray JF, Ruhnke HL, and Rachlis A: Mycoplasma infection of the hand acquired from a cat. J Hand Surg 12A:1085, 1987.

Moise NS, Crissman JW, Fairbrother JF, and Baldwin C: *Mycoplasma gateae* arthritis and tenosynovitis in cats: Case report and experimental reproduction of the disease. Am J Vet Res 44:16, 1983.

Rosendal S: Canine mycoplasmas: Their ecologic niche and role in disease. J Am Vet Med Assoc 180:1212, 1982.

# CVT UPDATE: CANINE LYME DISEASE

MAX J. G. APPEL
*and* R. H. JACOBSON
*Ithaca, New York*

Canine Lyme disease is commonly observed by veterinarians practicing in areas endemic for the Lyme spirochetal agent, *Borrelia burgdorferi*. The spirochetes are transmitted by ticks, including *Ixodes scapularis* (formerly *I. dammini*) in the eastern and north central United States, *I. pacificus* in California and Oregon, and *I. ricinus* in Europe. Many wildlife mammals and birds become subclinically infected with *B. burgdorferi* and serve as reservoirs for tick infection. In contrast, dogs and humans—and apparently to a lesser extent, horses, cattle, and cats—develop clinical disease. Lyme borreliosis has become the most common arthropod-borne disease of humans, and probably of dogs, in the United States. A clear understanding of canine Lyme disease and its management has been thwarted, however, because it mimics other diseases, serotests have tended to lack specificity, and the natural infection has been difficult to reproduce in the laboratory. Lack of information has often led to misinformation about the disease that only now is starting to be clarified through more detailed clinical and experimental observations.

## EPIZOOTIOLOGY

### The Organism

The causative agent of Lyme disease, *Borrelia burgdorferi*, is most closely related to *B. hermsii*, which causes tick-borne relapsing fever in the southwestern United States. Better known but more distantly related spirochetes cause leptospirosis (*Leptospira* spp.) and syphilis (*Treponema* spp.).

All species of *Borrelia* are host-associated spirochetes with alternate arthropod and vertebrate hosts. They do not live in water or soil and are not transmitted by aerosols or fecal contamination. Borrelias are predominantly extracellular pathogens. However, they can invade endothelial or fibrous tissue cells.

Strain differences have been found between isolates from various regions in the United States, Europe, and Asia; these may account for differences observed in clinical syndromes in Europe as compared with the United States.

### Vectors

Deer ticks, hard-shelled ticks of the genus *Ixodes*, transmit *B. burgdorferi* by attaching and feeding on various hosts. Other blood-sucking insects also may be involved, but evidence indicates that they are of minor importance as vectors. The primary way in which an animal or human being becomes infected is by tick bite.

After a tick attaches and begins to feed, spirochetes residing in the midgut of the tick begin to migrate to the salivary glands and from there into the host. The probability of infection increases when infected ticks are allowed to feed for prolonged periods and become engorged. There is little danger of infection during the first 12 to 24 hr of tick feeding.

*Ixodes* ticks require three hosts and four different developmental steps to complete their 2-year life cycle. The female tick lays about 2000 eggs in the spring. If the female was infected with *B. burgdorferi*, the larvae that emerge from the eggs do not carry sufficient bacteria to induce infection in a host upon which they feed. In the northeastern and midwestern United States, the larvae feed primarily on the white-footed mouse *Peromyscus leucopus*. Many infected mice harbor *B. burgdorferi* for their lifetime without developing disease. Larvae become infected by ingesting blood of persistently infected mice, then drop off the host and enter a resting stage for the winter.

The larvae molt into nymphs the following spring. On average, 25% of unfed nymphs in the northeastern United States are infected. During spring and early summer, the nymphs attach and feed on new hosts, again most commonly on the white-footed mouse or any of a wide range of animals including dogs and humans. An infected nymph may transmit *B. burgdorferi* to a new host during its 4-day feeding period. Conversely, an uninfected nymph becomes infected by feeding on a previously infected animal. In our experimental studies on dogs, nymphs are less effective vectors than are adult ticks.

In the fall of the second year, nymphs molt again and enter the adult stage. Up to 80% (average of 50%) of the adult ticks in areas endemic for Lyme disease in the northeastern United States may be carrying *B. burgdorferi*. These ticks are the most important source of infection for dogs. As long as temperatures remain above 2°C (35°F), adult ticks can be found on shrubs where they gain access to white-tailed deer and other larger animals.

Adult ticks mate on the host. Male ticks tend to stay on the host and die, but the females engorge for 5 to 7 days and then drop off and reside under fallen leaves during the winter. The following spring, they lay eggs and complete the 2-year cycle. Adult ticks that do not find a host in the fall may survive over the winter and become active again from early spring until about mid-May in the northern United States.

In the southern United States, *I. scapularis* larvae and nymphs feed primarily on lizards, which do not maintain infection with *B. burgdorferi*. Consequently, nymphal and adult infection rates are low, often less than 1%. Rates of infection with *B. burgdorferi* are also low in *I. pacificus* in California (1 to 5%).

## Transmission to Dogs

Experimental infections have indicated that dogs exposed to *B. burgdorferi*–infected adult ticks in the fall and early spring have a higher probability of acquiring the infection than if exposed to nymphs in late spring. Contact transmission from dog to dog did not occur. There is presently no evidence for transmission by other vectors.

A recent report indicates that when pregnant bitches are repeatedly inoculated with large numbers of *B. burgdorferi*, the fetuses may become infected. However, this route of exposure to *B. burgdorferi* is highly artificial and does not mimic what occurs in nature. Using an experimental model of tick attachment, pregnant bitches did become infected but their fetuses did not. Neither did the pups of an infected bitch acquire the infection from her. Furthermore, there is no epidemiologic or anecdotal evidence from veterinarians that newborn pups are afflicted with Lyme disease.

## Prevalence of Infection

The proportion of dogs in endemic areas that develop clinical disease is relatively small. Serologic studies suggest that while more than 75% of the dog population in hyperendemic areas may be exposed to infected ticks, only about 5% of exposed dogs actually develop clinical signs that may be attributable to Lyme disease. Within endemic areas, foci of tick infestation are intermingled with noninfested areas, resulting in "hot spots" where dogs have a much greater probability of acquiring an infection than in adjacent areas where the habitat is not favorable to the vector tick.

On a national scale, Lyme disease is to a large extent a regional problem. Its distribution is highly correlated with the distribution of the principal tick vectors. Although human Lyme disease cases in 1992 were reported to the Centers for Disease Control and Prevention for patients residing in 45 states, established enzootic foci are known in only 19 states, which account for 94% of the cases reported during 1991 and 1992. Eighty-five per cent of the cases reported were from the northeastern and mid-Atlantic focus (all coastal states from North Carolina to and including Maine plus New York, Pennsylvania, and New Hampshire), 10% were from the midwestern focus (Wisconsin, Minnesota, Michigan, Illinois, Missouri, and Iowa), and 4% were from the western focus (California and Oregon).

Only 1% of the cases were from the remaining states, which represent approximately two thirds of the land mass of the United States. The occurrence of sporadic cases in states without established enzootic foci may be due to infectious exposure in limited foci, exposures during visits to enzootic foci outside the state of residence, or misdiagnosis. The conclusion from the human data is that dogs in areas representing most of the United States are currently at a very minimal risk, if any, of acquiring Lyme disease.

## CLINICAL MANIFESTATIONS

### Onset

Clinical manifestations of disease, particularly lameness, did not appear in experimental dogs subjected to tick-induced infections until 2 to 5 months after exposure, indicating a much longer latent period in dogs than previously thought. It is not known, however, if reported recurrence at 6 months to 1 year after the first episode is due to recrudescence of a persistent primary infection or reexposure to infected ticks.

### Signs

Lyme disease in dogs is primarily an arthritis in either an acute or subacute form; the acute form may be transient and in some cases recurrent. The devastating chronic arthritis and severe central nervous system involvement seen in humans with systemic disease is rarely seen in dogs irrespective of how long they have been in endemic areas or how long they may have been infected.

Dogs may present with sudden lameness and sometimes signs of severe pain. One or more joints may be involved. Joints are often swollen, hot, and painful on manipulation. Fever, anorexia, and lethargy are commonly observed in affected dogs. Some become severely depressed and are reluctant to move. In our experimental studies, dogs that developed lameness in one leg as a result of exposure to infected ticks recovered in 3 to 4 days in the absence of antibiotic therapy. One or two episodes of recurrent lameness occurred in some dogs at intervals of several weeks or months, with apparent full recovery after each episode. Swollen axillary and popliteal lymph nodes were frequently observed in these dogs.

In a series of 91 symptomatic dogs from endemic areas that proved to be infected based on Western blot serology, lameness, joint pain, and/or myalgia was the primary complaint. Depression, lethargy, and/or inappetence was the next most common complaint, while fever was observed in only a few of these dogs. These data confirm clinical observations reported in the literature. Rare instances of other clinical signs, reported among seropositive dogs, have included complete heart block; renal failure; and neurologic changes such as seizures, aggression, and other behavioral changes.

The skin rash representing the first stage of human Lyme disease (erythema chronica migrans) is rarely seen in dogs. In our experience, only 1 of approximately 30 dogs exposed to infected adult or nymphal stages of *I. scapularis* displayed a rash.

## Clinical Pathology

Occasional fever that lasts for 1 or 2 days may be seen in infected dogs. In experimental dogs that developed lameness, total and differential white blood cell (WBC) counts and hematocrits as well as electrolyte and serum enzyme panels remained in the normal range. Creatine kinase was slightly elevated in a few dogs during acute lameness. Antinuclear antibody or rheumatoid factor were not found in any of the dog sera. Total immunoglobulin G (IgG) levels were elevated in some dogs after infection.

Total WBC counts in synovial fluid from affected joints with acute arthritis were between 7000 and 50,000 cells/mm$^3$ (mean = 21,000). Differential counts revealed between 43% and 85% neutrophils (mean = 21%), with macrophages, monocytes, and synovial lining cells constituting the remainder. Approximately 1% of the cells were lymphocytes.

## Duration

Canine Lyme disease, induced experimentally by a single exposure to infected ticks, presents as episodic lameness, with each episode lasting only several days. It is not documented, however, whether disease signs would persist in the absence of antibiotic therapy among dogs in endemic areas where repeated exposure to large numbers of infected ticks occurs over extended periods of time. Anecdotal information from many veterinarians suggest that chronic intractable signs attributable to Lyme disease are exceedingly rare.

Asymptomatic dogs probably remain infected for years even following proper regimens of antibiotic therapy. In one case, a Connecticut dog moved to Wyoming (a nonendemic area) in 1989 was symptomatic for Lyme disease at that time, and following rigorous antibiotic therapy, the signs diminished. The dog has remained seropositive for 4 years, while a seropositive littermate that was asymptomatic but also treated is now seronegative.

Our experimental dogs, infected by one exposure with adult ticks, had infections that persisted for at least 12 months and high antibody titers that remained essentially unchanged for at least 18 months (the longest periods studied). High levels of antibody suggest persistence of the antigen that stimulate its production. If the organisms had been killed by the immune response, the expectation is that antigen would be cleared and

titers would have subsided. For example, waning of vaccine-induced antibody titers is what we have observed in dogs inoculated with the killed commercial bacterin; as the antigen is cleared, titers fall to nearly undetectable levels in about 7 to 10 months. Persistence of infection is apparently the norm for the Lyme agent.

## DIAGNOSIS

### Diagnostic Criteria

We consider four criteria as important to establish the diagnosis of Lyme disease in dogs: (1) history of exposure to *Ixodes* ticks in an endemic area, (2) typical clinical signs, (3) a positive serology using a properly validated test, and (4) a prompt response to antibiotic therapy. One or two of these criteria alone are usually not sufficient to confirm a diagnosis. For example, if a dog has never been in an area known to be infested with *Ixodes* ticks carrying *B. burgdorferi*, it is very unlikely that the dog has Lyme disease. The clinical diagnosis must rule out confounding factors such as rheumatoid, infectious, or immune-mediated arthritis; osteopathies; degenerative joint diseases; or other infectious diseases such as Rocky Mountain spotted fever, ehrlichiosis, and bacterial endocarditis. Hemograms, analysis of synovial fluid, radiographs, and serology for other infectious agents should thus be performed to exclude other common canine diseases (see "Neurologic and Musculoskeletal Disorders," this volume, p 1109 for details about other joint diseases).

### Diagnostic Tests

Following exposure to infected ticks, anti–*B. burgdorferi* antibodies began to appear in dogs within 4 to 6 weeks. Antibody titers increased for several weeks to high levels and then remained constant for at least 18 months. This pattern has been seen repeatedly in our studies. Based on samples submitted by veterinarians to our diagnostic laboratory and anecdotal conversations with veterinarians that do their own in-house testing, when the clinical diagnosis of Lyme disease is highly probable, dogs virtually always have a significant antibody titer to the Lyme agent. False-negative test results are rare. If the tests are properly validated, they may also have a high degree of specificity, thus minimizing false-positive results. Therefore, contrary to some reports, tests for antibody can be useful as one factor in the diagnosis of Lyme disease of dogs.

Vaccination of dogs against the Lyme agent elicits antibodies that react in the Lyme antibody tests. Therefore, routine serology of vaccinated dogs is not useful. A recent development, however, using Western blot technology (as detailed below) distinguishes between antibodies generated in response to infection versus antibodies that develop following vaccination with the Lyme bacterin. This test can thus determine if symptomatic dogs that have been vaccinated also have antibody to tick-induced infection with the Lyme agent.

Detection of IgM antibodies against infectious agents is usually indicative of an early stage of infection preceding the switch to IgG antibodies. In the case of Lyme disease, however, IgM antibodies persist for many months and are not useful as indicators of early infection.

### SEROLOGY

ELISA.     The enzyme-linked immunosorbent assay (ELISA) test for detection of canine antibodies to the Lyme agent is very useful in the differential diagnosis of Lyme disease, if the laboratory has properly validated the test and if the dog has not been vaccinated (vaccinal antibodies interfere in the ELISA test). Suggestions that antibody tests are not very useful are derived in part from observations with human serology, which tends to be equivocal for Lyme disease. Also, early ELISA tests for canine lyme antibodies were not confirmed through experimental infections and had a tendency to be false-positive.

It should be pointed out that seropositivity in an endemic area is not sufficient for a diagnosis of Lyme disease. The higher the rate of seroprevalence, the less useful becomes a positive serum titer.

When human patients experience the erythematous rash, they usually have not yet developed antibody to the organism and thus test negative. If they are then treated with antibiotics, they may never develop antibody to B. burgdorferi. Some human patients with chronic Lyme disease are apparently anergic, resulting in no detectable antibodies to the Lyme agent. Extrapolation of this knowledge to dogs was unfortunate because dogs generally are faithful in producing antibody when infected and are virtually always seropositive by the time they exhibit clinical signs.

It is imperative that ELISA tests are properly validated by the laboratory that is used. Any laboratory can legally offer testing services with no evaluation of the tests by outside regulatory agencies. Thus, inquiries should be made about how a given test was validated and the basis for its interpretation. In our experience with the commonly used Lyme antigen in ELISA tests, uninfected dogs have small amounts of cross-reactive antibodies elicited by other agents such as Leptospira spp., which may be interpreted as anti-Lyme antibody if the test is not corrected for this activity. This observation is based on having validated our ELISA using sera drawn periodically over 18 months from experimental dogs that were exposed to infected ticks and from submissions of samples by veterinarians from dogs in hyperendemic areas in which the clinical diagnosis was Lyme disease.

Dogs vaccinated against Lyme disease with the commercial bacterin will develop strong antibody responses to the bacterin that react in conventional ELISA tests designed to detect infected dogs. Therefore, the ELISA is not useful in determining the infection status of vaccinated dogs.

Several commercial test kits that use ELISA technology are available to veterinarians for detecting canine antibodies to the Lyme agent. However, well-controlled ELISA tests and other tests run in reputable diagnostic laboratories are probably more reliable.

WESTERN BLOT.     The Western blot is a confirmatory test that can distinguish between dogs that have been or are infected with B. burgdorferi versus dogs that have been vaccinated with the Lyme bacterin; it can also detect the dog that has experienced both an infection and a vaccination with the Lyme bacterin. While ELISA is a quantitative determination of all of the antibodies produced against many antigenic moieties of B. burgdorferi, the Western blot determines the unique pattern of antibodies produced against antigens of a tick-induced infection, which is different than the pattern produced following vaccination.

OTHER TESTS.     The indirect fluorescence antibody (IFA) test functions on a similar principle as ELISA except that the antigen used to detect antibody is usually whole bacterial cells of B. burgdorferi fixed on slides. Antibodies primarily directed against surface components of B. burgdorferi are thus detected. The IFA test interpretation is subjective and thus prone to variation between laboratories.

### DETECTION OF ORGANISMS OR THEIR ANTIGENS

The definitive diagnosis for bacterial infections is to isolate the causative organism. In veterinary and human studies, B. burgdorferi has been extremely difficult to culture from body fluids and tissues. The vast majority of isolation attempts have been unsuccessful, apparently because of the lack of organisms in the samples. In our experimental studies, the only locus from which the organism was consistently isolated over a period of several months after tick exposure was near the site of bites by infected ticks. If the site of the tick bite is known, a skin biopsy from that area provides the best chance for successful isolation of the organism. Even if the area of the bite is not known, there is a better chance of isolating the organism from skin, even at sites distant to the bite, than from blood or urine. This approach is not recommended, however, because isolation of B. burgdorferi is time consuming and expensive.

Detection of deoxyribonucleic acid (DNA) of B. burgdorferi in tissues and body fluids is an alternative to bacterial culture but suffers from some of the same limitations in sensitivity as culture because of the apparent lack of organisms or their DNA in urine or blood. In the assay, DNA in the sample is amplified using the polymerase chain reaction (PCR) and then detected using a genetic probe that is unique to B. burgdorferi. The PCR results on skin biopsies from experimental dogs have been comparable with isolation results.

## TREATMENT

Antibiotics are the treatment of choice for Lyme disease in dogs and in humans. Several tetracyclines, such as doxycycline (10 mg/kg every 24 hr PO for 21 to 28 days), or β-lactam antibiotics such as amoxicillin (22 mg/kg every 12 hr PO for 21 to 28 days), have been found empirically to be very effective. Dogs usually respond with complete clinical recovery within 24 to 48 hr. The long duration of therapy is warranted because of the tendency of *B. burgdorferi* to persist in dogs and the very slow multiplication of the organism (the doubling rate is about 12 hr compared with about 15 min for most bacteria). Tetracyclines should not be given to growing dogs. However, considering the fact that Lyme disease in dogs appears to be self-limiting, the need for a long-duration therapy may prove to be questionable.

Dogs with recurrent episodes of Lyme disease, whether acquired from reinfestation of infected ticks or a relapse from an initial infection, are highly responsive to antibiotics given at the same doses as for a primary episode. This is in contrast to humans who do not respond as favorably to antibiotics when they are in the chronic stage of Lyme disease.

It is often debated whether asymptomatic seropositive dogs should be treated with antibiotics. In general, the answer is no. Most infected dogs having antibodies to *B. burgdorferi* never develop Lyme disease. Moreover, dogs are at extremely low risk of developing the chronic arthritis seen in humans. Nevertheless, chronic Lyme disease apparently may occur in isolated instances, so the risk of disease must be weighed against the cost and complications of antibiotic therapy. A further consideration is that most attempts to rid asymptomatic dogs of all organisms seem to be unsuccessful even with repeated regimens of antibiotics. This is based on antibody titers remaining high for long periods of time in dogs that are repeatedly treated. If antibiotics do not clear the infection, why do they ameliorate clinical signs of Lyme disease? It is theorized that antibiotic therapy reduces the bacterial load, with an attendant elimination of clinical signs, but does not totally eliminate the organism. This would explain the persistence of antibodies that could be elicited by a constant trickle of *B. burgdorferi* emerging from their intracellular location and other sites inaccessible to antibiotics.

Should antibiotic treatment be initiated in dogs carrying *Ixodes* ticks? If dogs in endemic areas are exposed frequently to ticks, treatment is impractical. A more practical approach may be removal of ticks from dogs on a daily basis because the ticks must at least partially engorge before the organism is transmitted.

Corticosteroids and other anti-inflammatory drugs are sometimes used to alleviate the arthritic signs associated with Lyme disease in dogs. Although the initial result may be impressive, corticosteroids mask the diagnostic value of antibiotic treatment. Anti-inflammatory drugs seem to ameliorate the clinical problems.

## PROGNOSIS

Dogs respond very well to antibiotic treatment. Even with recurrent disease, dogs again respond as they do in a primary occurrence. Complete recovery can be expected in the vast majority of cases. Chronic disease, which can be devastating in humans, has rarely been seen in dogs. When it has been diagnosed, one must question the possibility of other etiologies. It should be noted that dogs may recover spontaneously in the absence of antibiotic therapy as seen repeatedly in our experimental dogs.

## ZOONOTIC IMPLICATIONS

It has been speculated that *B. burgdorferi* in the saliva or urine of infected dogs might be transmissible to humans. Our experiments to test this hypothesis have failed to provide any evidence of transmission from infected to noninfected dogs kept in close contact and subject to urine contamination. The risk to humans would be even less. Although the antigens of *B. burgdorferi* have been found in canine urine, viable organisms deteriorate quickly in urine and saliva, and are virtually impossible to isolate by culture. Also, the organisms are rarely found in the kidneys of infected dogs. If the organism is readily transmitted from dogs to humans, one would expect dog owners, veterinarians, and kennel caretakers to be at greater risk than people in the general population who do not own dogs. There is no evidence of increased risk among those who own or handle dogs.

It also has been speculated that dogs can transport ticks into the house that could then fall off and become attached to humans, thereby inducing infection. Although this scenario is possible, it is improbable because ticks are thermotropic and once on the dog's hair, will quickly go to the skin and start embedding; no instance of humans becoming infected by ticks transported into the house by dogs has been clearly documented. Once a tick starts feeding on the dog, it will feed to repletion. Ixodid larvae, nymphs, or adults are not intermittent feeders.

## PREVENTION AND CONTROL

### Preventing Tick Bites

Tick engorgement on dogs may be prevented by controlling the tick population in the environment, use of tick repellents, or by grooming dogs daily. Tick collars and dips may be used to control ticks on dogs, and some repellents containing diethyltoluamide (DEET), permethrin, or amtraz ("Preventick") are marketed for veterinary use. Attempts to reduce the deer tick population by radically reducing the deer population, even by as much as 70%, have been only partially successful. Rodents and other wildlife can replace deer as hosts, and efforts to reduce the primary host, the white-footed mouse, are not feasible.

Selective chemical control of ticks appears to be more promising, although only relatively small areas can be controlled. The Boston-based company, Eco

Health, Inc, has developed biodegradable tubes containing permethrin-treated cotton batting (Damminix) that can be placed in infested areas. Mice use the cotton for nesting material. The acaricide-covered nesting material rapidly kills exposed *I. scapularis* larvae and nymphs. Contradictory reports have appeared about the effectiveness of this approach.

## Vaccination

A commercial bacterin consisting of killed *Borrelia burgdorferi* in a proprietary adjuvant is currently the only licensed Lyme disease vaccine for dogs. Several million doses have been sold and, according to the manufacturer, there appear to be no immediate adverse reactions to its use other than transitory fever. Efficacy of the vaccine was originally based on studies in which vaccinated and control dogs were challenged by needle inoculation of large numbers of organisms over 7 consecutive days. Based on Western blot analysis in several laboratories, it is known that challenge infections induced by injection of cultured *B. burgdorferi* elicits a very different antibody response than does a challenge by infected ticks. It is, therefore, important to ascertain efficacy of the vaccine under properly controlled field trials in which challenge is by tick-induced infection. No randomized field trials or cohort studies on vaccinated and control dogs, naturally or experimentally challenged by tick-induced infections, have been reported. A nonrandomized retrospective study conducted at three veterinary practices in the northeastern United States suggests that the bacterin may reduce the rate of clinical Lyme borreliosis in dogs from about 4.4% of all seropositive dogs seen in these clinics to about 1%.

The manufacturer claims, in the insert accompanying their vaccine, that the vaccine may protect even those dogs that already are infected but asymptomatic. This claim seems unwarranted based on queries from veterinarians indicating a clinical diagnosis of Lyme disease in vaccinated dogs, and on evidence from Western blot analysis of samples submitted to us by veterinarians. We evaluated histories and Western blot results for a series of 140 dogs that had developed classic Lyme disease as determined by a conservative case definition: stiffness or lameness with depression and anorexia that responded to antibiotic therapy in an endemic area. This definition excluded cases where Lyme disease was considered an equivocal etiology. Of these dogs, 109 had been vaccinated, often repeatedly over 2 to 3 years. Based on Western blot serology, 37 of the vaccinated dogs (34%) had evidence of antibody to both the vaccine and to a tick-induced infection by *B. burgdorferi*. The vaccine either did not protect these dogs from infection or they became infected prior to vaccination and the vaccine did not induce protection against disease via neutralizing antibody as suggested in the insert accompanying the commercial vaccine. Recommendations of the company to vaccinate seropositive dogs thus seems unwarranted and needs further investigation.

Surprisingly, 49 of 109 symptomatic vaccinated dogs (45%) had antibodies only to the Lyme bacterin. One could postulate that these dogs were infected but never developed antibody to a tick-induced *Borrelia* infection. This is unlikely because antibody responses to tick-induced infections occurred in all of the dogs that developed clinical signs of Lyme disease in our experimental studies. An alternative explanation is that these vaccinated dogs were misdiagnosed. If that were true, one would have expected an equivalent rate of misdiagnoses in nonvaccinated dogs that were seronegative; however, of 37 nonvaccinated symptomatic dogs for which the Western blot was requested, only three dogs (8%) were diagnosed as probable Lyme disease but were serologically negative.

This apparent vaccine-related syndrome may be due to *Borrelia* antigens in the bacterin that may elicit pathology. *Borrelia burgdorferi* contains heat shock proteins and other proteins known to induce inflammatory and pathologic changes that are similar to some of the symptoms seen in human Lyme disease. This concern has precluded development of a whole-cell bacterin from consideration as a human vaccine. It would be desirable to have a single-protein vaccine such as outer surface protein A (Osp A). Studies to develop such a vaccine are in progress in several laboratories.

## Recommendations for Vaccination

It is misleading to suggest that Lyme disease is endemic in 44 of 50 states when the three endemic foci, accounting for 99% of reported human Lyme cases, represent only one third of the land mass in the United States. Vaccination of dogs outside the three foci (mid-Atlantic, northeastern, midwestern, and western) is not needed even if the vaccine were considered unequivocally effective and safe.

We cannot recommend vaccination of dogs in endemic areas with the whole cell bacterin until questions are resolved about clinical Lyme disease developing in dogs that have been properly vaccinated. The risk of not vaccinating is minimal, since the disease in dogs is not fatal, is probably self-limiting in the majority of cases, and is effectively treated with antibiotics even among dogs that have recurrent episodes of Lyme disease. Furthermore, the risk of ever developing clinical disease appears to be relatively low.

The risk of vaccination may be greater than previously thought, based on the observation that dogs having no antibody to tick-induced infection can develop classic signs of Lyme disease. Because the vaccine is reported to reduce cases of Lyme disease from about 4.4% to 1% of dogs at risk, if only 1 to 2% of vaccinated dogs in endemic areas experience this phenomenon, the possible advantages of vaccination would probably be offset by the risk of its use. The basis for the observation that vaccinated dogs develop Lyme disease is not understood and must be investigated further before firm conclusions can be drawn.

bilirubin, alanine aminotransferase activity, alkaline phosphatase, and lipase can develop depending on the organ system involved. Urinalyses were normal in all cats evaluated in one study. None of the clinical laboratory changes are pathognomonic for toxoplasmosis. However, the combination of clinical manifestations of ocular disease, fever, and CNS disease with hyperglobulinemia may lead to some cats being incorrectly diagnosed with feline infectious peritonitis (FIP). Cerebrospinal fluid (CSF) analyses from subclinically ill cats experimentally inoculated with *T. gondii* are generally normal. Protein levels ranging from normal to 149 mg/dl and nucleated cell counts ranging from normal to 28 cells/mm³ were detected in a series of cats with suspected CNS toxoplasmosis. The predominant white blood cells were lymphocytes. Tachyzoites can be found in blood, cerebrospinal fluid, transtracheal wash fluids, peritoneal effusions, and pleural effusions. Documentation of tachyzoites in fluids from an infected cat is unusual and is more likely to occur in acutely infected, clinically ill cats.

## Radiology

Pulmonic toxoplasmosis most commonly causes diffuse interstitial to alveolar patterns. Alveolar coalescence was described in one cat. Pleural effusion may develop in some cases. Abdominal radiographic findings may include homogenous increased density due to peritoneal effusion, organomegaly due to hepatomegaly, lymphadenopathy, intestinal masses, or loss of contrast in the cranial right quadrant of the abdomen due to pancreatitis. An intracranial mass lesion was detected in one cat with suspected CNS toxoplasmosis. Diffuse swelling of the spinal cord was documented by myelography in one cat. It is not known if radiographic abnormalities occur in clinically normal cats or cats undergoing the enteroepithelial cycle.

## Demonstration of *T. gondii* in Tissues

Cytology or mouse inoculation (bioassay) rarely demonstrates tachyzoites in urine, pulmonary aspirates, CSF, and peritoneal or pleural effusions from acute clinical cases. If tachyzoites are found, a definitive diagnosis of active infection and possibly clinical disease can be made. Histologically, demonstration of clones of tachyzoites also can be diagnostic of active infection and possibly clinical disease. Tissue cyst demonstration by bioassay, immunoperoxidase staining, or histologic examination of tissue is suggestive of chronic infection but does not differentiate subclinical infection from clinical disease.

## Serologic Tests

*Toxoplasma gondii*–specific antibodies, antigens, and antigen-containing immune complexes can be detected in the serum of cats following infection (Fig. 2). Immune complexes are one mechanism for the removal of circulating antigens released during the dissemination phase of infection or from encysted bradyzoites. Antibodies are most commonly detected in serum using enzyme-linked immunosorbent assay (ELISA), indirect immunofluorescent antibody (IFA) assay, or agglutination procedures. Assays are available for the detection of immunoglobulin M (IgM) and immunoglobulin G (IgG). Agglutination assays potentially detect all antibody classes against *T. gondii*. Some commercially available agglutination assays fail to accurately detect anti-*Toxoplasma* IgM. Contact your commercial laboratory concerning the classes of antibodies detected in the assay used.

*Toxoplasma gondii*–specific IgM is detectable in serum by ELISA in approximately 80% of subclinically ill cats within 2 to 4 weeks following experimental induction of toxoplasmosis; these titers generally are negative within 16 weeks after infection. Positive IgM titers greater than 1:256 have only been detected within the first 12 weeks following experimental induction of toxoplasmosis. Detectable IgM titers were present in the serum of 93.3% of the cats in a recent paper on clinical toxoplasmosis; IgG titers were detected in 60% (Lappin et al., 1989). Some clinically ill cats will have IgM titers greater than 1:256 that persist for longer than 12 weeks. Persistent IgM titers (>16 weeks) have been documented commonly in cats coinfected with FIV and in cats with ocular toxoplasmosis. It has been hypothesized that FIV-coinfected cats have either long-term activated infection or have immunologic deficits that impede antibody class shift. Following repeat inoculation with *T. gondii*, primary inoculation with the Petaluma isolate of FIV, and administration of glucocorticoids, some cats with chronic toxoplasmosis will have short-term recurrence of detectable IgM titers. Thus, the presence of IgM in serum does not correlate to recent infection or oocyst shedding in all cats.

Following experimental induction of infection in subclinically ill cats, *T. gondii*–specific IgG can be detected by ELISA in serum in the majority of cats within 3 weeks after infection. Positive IgG antibody titers generally last for years after infection. It has been suggested that single, high IgG titers suggest recent or active infection. The author has demonstrated IgG antibody titers greater than 1:16,384 in subclinically ill cats up to 5 years after experimental induction of toxoplasmosis. Thus, the presence of a positive IgG antibody titer in a single serum sample only indicates exposure, not recent or active disease. The demonstration of an increasing IgG titer can document recent or active disease. Unfortunately, in experimentally infected cats, the time span from the first detectable positive IgG titer to the maximal IgG titer is approximately 2 to 3 weeks, leaving a very narrow window for the documentation of an increasing titer. Many cats with clinical toxoplasmosis have chronic low-grade clinical signs and may not be evaluated serologically until their IgG antibody titers have reached their maximal values. In humans with reactivation of chronic toxoplasmosis, IgG

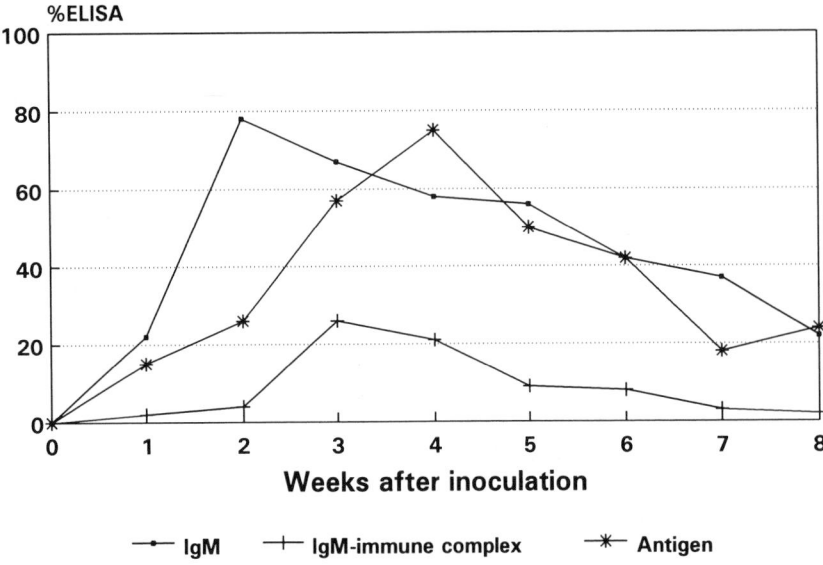

%ELISA

Weeks after inoculation

IgM    IgM-immune complex    Antigen

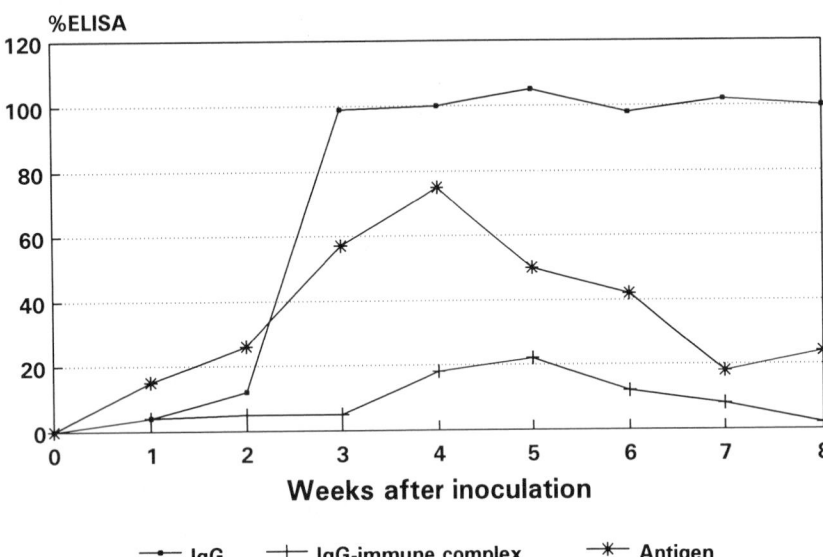

%ELISA

Weeks after inoculation

IgG    IgG-immune complex    Antigen

**Figure 2.** Serum antibody, antigen, and immune complex responses as determined by ELISA sequentially following experimental infection of cats with *T. gondii*.

titers only rarely increase. It appears that this occurs in cats as well.

*Toxoplasma gondii*–specific antigens can be detected in serum from cats using ELISA. Following experimental induction of toxoplasmosis, most subclinically ill cats will develop circulating antigenemia within 4 weeks after inoculation. Circulating antigenemia can be detected intermittently in some cats for months to years after infection. It has been hypothesized that these antigens are intermittently released from tissue cysts.

*Toxoplasma gondii*–containing immune complexes can be detected in the serum of cats using ELISA. Cats experimentally inoculated with *T. gondii* will develop detectable levels of *T. gondii*–specific IgM immune complexes and *T. gondii*–specific IgG immune complexes transiently. Cats with ocular toxoplasmosis are more likely than healthy cats to have *T. gondii*–containing immune complexes in serum and often have higher im-

mune complex concentrations in aqueous humor than serum. These results suggest that *T. gondii*–specific immune complexes may play a role in the pathogenesis of ocular toxoplasmosis. Some naturally infected cats with clinical signs of disease referable to toxoplasmosis and clinical response to anti-*Toxoplasma* drugs have been seronegative for *T. gondii*–specific antibodies but seropositive for *T. gondii*–specific antigens or immune complexes. Formation of *T. gondii*–specific immune complexes in the serum of some cats may lead to negative antigen and antibody assay results.

## Aqueous Humor and Cerebral Spinal Fluid Measurement of Antibodies

Local production of IgM and IgG antibodies can be determined in the aqueous humor and CSF of cats in some laboratories. Documentation of local production of antibodies suggests active infection of that body system. Submission of serum and aqueous humor or serum and CSF is suggested in cats with suspected intraocular or CNS toxoplasmosis.

## CLINICAL DIAGNOSIS

There is currently no one test that can document clinical feline toxoplasmosis. Exposure to *T. gondii* is suggested by the presence of *Toxoplasma*-specific antibodies, antigens, or immune complexes in serum. Recent or active toxoplasmosis is suggested by the presence of an IgM titer greater than 1:64, a fourfold or greater increase in IgG titer over a 2- to 3-week period, antigen without antibodies, immune complexes without antibodies, or local production of antibodies in aqueous humor or CSF. Since *T. gondii*–specific antibodies develop in the serum of subclinically ill cats as well as those with clinical signs of disease, it is impossible to make an antemortem diagnosis of clinical feline toxoplasmosis based on these tests alone. The antemortem diagnosis of clinical feline toxoplasmosis can be tentatively based on the combination of

1. Demonstration of serologic evidence of infection.
2. Clinical signs of disease referrable to toxoplasmosis.
3. Exclusion of other common etiologies.
4. Positive response to appropriate treatment.

## THERAPY

Cats with suspected clinical toxoplasmosis have been administered supportive care as needed. Clindamycin hydrochloride (Antirobe, The Upjohn Company, Kalamazoo, MI) has been used in the management of many cases. Clindamycin hydrochloride is administered at an oral dosage of 25 mg/kg divided two or three times daily for 4 weeks. Clinical signs not involving the eyes or the CNS usually resolve within the first 2 to 3 days of drug administration. Recurrence of clinical signs may be more common in cases treated for less than 4 weeks. There is no evidence to suggest that this drug can totally clear the body of the organism. Ocular and CNS toxoplasmosis respond more slowly to therapy. Clindamycin hydrochloride crosses the blood-brain barrier in cats, and has been used successfully in a limited number of cases with suspected CNS toxoplasmosis. Trimethoprim-sulfa combination therapy at a dosage of 15 mg/kg given orally twice daily has resulted in the resolution of central nervous system disease in some cats. Pyrimethamine combined with sulfa drugs is recommended for the treatment of clinical feline toxoplasmosis but commonly results in toxicity.

Most cases with ocular involvement are treated with clindamycin hydrochloride in combination with topical, oral, or parenteral corticosteroids. Retinochoroiditis often responds rapidly to clindamycin hydrochloride alone. Anterior uveitis should be treated with an anti-*Toxoplasma* drug and corticosteroids initially to avoid secondary damage to the eye induced by inflammation. Occasionally, anterior uveitis will initially worsen following clindamycin hydrochloride administration. It has been hypothesized that this is due to increased release of antigen from tissue cysts, leading to magnification of immune-mediated disease. Cats with concurrent FIV infection are more difficult to manage therapeutically.

## PUBLIC HEALTH RISKS

The role of the cat in the human zoonosis is primarily related to the production of oocysts and perpetuating the disease in the environment and food chain. Individual adult cats generally only shed oocysts once in their life and the oocyst shedding period usually has a duration from days to several weeks. Repeat exposure of adult cats to *T. gondii* generally does not result in oocyst shedding. Oocyst shedding in cats with chronic toxoplasmosis can be induced with extremely high doses of glucocorticoids. Clinical doses of glucocorticoids failed to induce oocyst shedding in recent or chronically infected cats. While oocyst production in the intestines was documented in a cat with clinical signs of hepatitis, most cats with clinical toxoplasmosis are not shedding oocysts. Coinfection with feline leukemia virus (FeLV) or FIV does not lead to prolonged oocyst shedding periods. Primary-phase FIV infection failed to induce oocyst shedding in cats with chronic toxoplasmosis.

Infection from direct contact with oocyst-shedding cats is extremely unlikely. Since oocysts have to sporulate to be infectious, contact with fresh feces cannot cause infection. Cats are very fastidious and usually do not allow feces to remain on their skin for time periods long enough to lead to oocyst sporulation. Due to the short oocyst shedding period and the failure of most cats to repeat oocyst shedding on repeated exposure, it may not be necessary to remove pet cats from the home environment of pregnant or immunosuppressed individuals. Oocysts can live in the environment for months to years. Human contact with sporulated oocysts likely occurs most frequently via geophagia when working with soil or drinking contaminated water. Oocyst induction of infection is rarely confirmed, but has been implicated as the source of at least two outbreaks of clinical toxoplasmosis. Accidental hosts including filth flies, cockroaches, earthworms, and dung beetles have been shown to transport *T. gondii* oocysts and may be a source of infection for cats housed indoors. To avoid oocyst induction of infection, high-risk individuals should:

- Avoid feeding cats undercooked meats.
- Not allow cats to hunt.
- Clean the litterbox daily and incinerate or flush the feces.

- Clean the litterbox daily with scalding water or use a litterbox liner.
- Wear gloves when working with soil.
- Keep childrens' sandboxes covered.
- Boil water for drinking that has been obtained from the general environment.
- Control potential transport hosts.

Some species of *Hammondia* and *Besnoitia*, two non-pathogenic protozoans, lead to the shedding of oocysts in cat feces that are indistinguishable microscopically from those of *T. gondii*. Due to public health risks, if a fecal sample from a cat is shown to contain oocysts measuring 10 X 12 $\mu$m, it should be assumed that the organism is *T. gondii*. The feces should be collected and incinerated daily until the oocyst shedding period is completed. Administration of clindamycin (25 to 50 mg/kg/day PO), sulfonamides (100 mg/kg/day PO), or pyrimethamine (2.0 mg/kg/day PO) can reduce levels of oocyst shedding.

Humans are commonly infected following the ingestion of tissue cysts in undercooked meats. In the United States, pork products have the highest incidence of *Toxoplasma* cysts. Meats should be cooked to at least 65.5°C (150°F) for 20 min. Gloves should be worn when handling raw meats (including field dressing) for cooking or hands should be cleansed thoroughly. Freezing meat at −20°C for several days greatly reduces tissue cyst viability.

Pregnant women, AIDS victims, and other immunosuppressed people commonly question their veterinarian concerning the likelihood of individual cats shedding *T. gondii* oocysts in their environment. Fecal examination is an adequate procedure to determine when cats are actively shedding oocysts but is not helpful in predicting when a cat has shed oocysts in the past. There is no serologic assay that accurately predicts when a cat has shed *T. gondii* oocysts. Some recommendations can be made by assessing the results of fecal examination combined with *T. gondii*–specific serologic test results:

1. If an adult cat is *T. gondii*–seropositive and is negative for oocysts on fecal examination, it is unlikely that the cat will shed oocysts again in the future.

2. If a cat is *T. gondii*–seronegative, it is likely that the cat would shed oocysts if infected by *T. gondii* and appropriate prevention measures should be taken.

If an owner is concerned that they may have toxoplasmosis, they should see their doctor for testing. There is currently no way to determine if an owner acquired toxoplasmosis from contact with individual cats.

## PREVENTION

The key to the prevention of feline toxoplasmosis is to avoid exposure to the organism as previously discussed. A mutant strain of *T. gondii* that fails to lead to oocyst formation has been identified. This strain is being evaluated as a potential vaccine. Following vaccination with *T. gondii* clone T-263, oocyst shedding after challenge with oocyst-forming strains of *T. gondii* is blocked.

## References and Suggested Reading

Beneson MW, Takafuji ET, Lemon SM, et al: Oocyst-transmitted toxoplasmosis associated with ingestion of contaminated water. N Engl J Med 307: 666, 1982.
   *A report of an outbreak of toxoplasmosis in people suspected to have been infected by oocyst ingestion.*
Dubey JP and Beattie CP: *Toxoplasmosis of Animals and Man.* Boca Raton, FL, CRC Press, 1988, pp 1–220.
   *A comprehensive review of the* T. gondii *literature.*
Dubey JP and Carpenter JL: Histologically confirmed clinical toxoplasmosis in cats: 100 cases (1952–1990). J Am Vet Med Assoc 203:1556, 1993.
   *A review describing the clinical and histologic findings in cats with toxoplasmosis.*
Dubey JP, Zajac A, Osofsky SA, et al: Acute primary toxoplasmic hepatitis in an adult cat shedding Toxoplasma gondii oocysts. J Am Vet Med Assoc 197: 1616, 1990.
   *A case report of a cat with hepatitis and active enteroepithelial toxoplasmosis.*
Fishback JL: Prospective vaccines to prevent feline shedding of *Toxoplasma* oocysts. Compend Cont Ed Pract Vet 12:643, 1990.
   *A review article that details the development of a* Toxoplasma *vaccine that blocks oocyst shedding.*
Lappin MR: Immunodiagnosis and management of clinical feline toxoplasmosis. *Proceedings, Waltham Feline Medicine Symposium,* Orlando, FL, 1993, pp 19–26.
   *A review article that describes the immunologic and clinical findings in cats with toxoplasmosis.*
Lappin MR, Greene CE, Winston S, et al: Clinical feline toxoplasmosis: Serologic diagnosis and therapeutic management of 15 cases. J Vet Intern Med 3:139, 1989.
   *Results of diagnostic testing and treatment of 15 cats with clinical toxoplasmosis.*
Lappin MR, Marks A, Greene CE, et al: Effect of feline immunodeficiency virus infection on *Toxoplasma gondii*-specific humoral and cell-mediated immune responses of cats with serologic evidence of toxoplasmosis. J Vet Intern Med 7:95, 1993.
   *Description of the immunologic and clinical findings in cats with FIV and toxoplasmosis.*
Lappin MR, Roberts SM, Davidson MG, et al: Enzyme-linked immunosorbent assays for the detection of *Toxoplasma gondii*-specific antibodies and antigens in the aqueous humor of cats. J Am Vet Med Assoc 201:1010, 1992.
   *Description of the use of aqueous humor antibody and antigen measurement in the diagnosis of clinical toxoplasmosis.*
O'Neil SA, Lappin MR, Reif JS, et al: Clinical and epidemiological aspects of feline immunodeficiency virus and *Toxoplasma gondii* coinfections in cats. J Am Anim Hosp Assoc 27:211, 1991.
   *Description of naturally occurring feline toxoplasmosis in FIV-coinfected cats.*
Patton S, Legendre AM, McGavin MD, et al: Concurrent infection with *Toxoplasma gondii* and feline leukemia virus. J Vet Int Med 5:199, 1991.
   *A study that evaluated the effect of feline leukemia virus and* T. gondii *coinfection on oocyst shedding.*

# CANINE BABESIOSIS

JOSEPH TABOADA

*Baton Rouge, Louisiana*

Babesiosis is a disease of worldwide significance caused by tickborne hematozoan organisms of the genus *Babesia*. *Babesia canis* and *Babesia gibsoni* are the two species capable of infecting the dog. Clinical signs caused by *Babesia* cover a wide spectrum, ranging from asymptomatic carrier states to fulminant hemolytic anemia resulting in death. Ixodid ticks serve as carriers of the parasite; the geographic distribution correlates with the range of the specific tick vector. In the United States, canine babesiosis occurs most commonly along the Gulf Coast and in the south central and southwestern states. Arkansas, Florida, Oklahoma, and Arizona seem to have the highest prevalence. Outbreaks are often localized to a relatively small area and most typically occur in kennels. Veterinarians in one practice may see large numbers of affected dogs, while neighboring practices in the same state may see few if any cases.

## ETIOLOGY

Of the 73 identified species of *Babesia*, only two are known to naturally infect the dog. *Babesia gibsoni* is found primarily in northern Africa and the southern parts of Asia. It has recently been described as endemic in the southwestern United States (Conrad et al., 1991). It is sporadically seen in areas near military bases where military working dogs are housed after being transported back to the United States from overseas. The parasite is a small, pleomorphic (1.0 × 3.2 μm) organism usually found singly within erythrocytes. The primary vector tick of *B. gibsoni* is *Haemaphysalis bispinosa*; but *Rhipicephalus sanguineus* is thought to be the vector tick in the United States. *Babsenis canis* is larger (2.4 × 5.0 μm), piriform shaped, and often paired within erythrocytes (although singly infected erythrocytes are also common). The range of *B. canis* is greater, covering most of southern Europe; Africa; Asia; and North, Central, and South America. Vector ticks include *Rhipicephalus sanguineus*, *Dermacentor reticulatus*, and *Haemaphysalis leachi*. Based on serologic and cross-immunity studies as well as noted differences in pathogenicity and transmitting vectors, a trinomial nomenclature system has been proposed to describe *B. canis* (Uilenberg et al., 1989). *Babesia canis vogeli* is the proposed name for the strain occurring in tropical and subtropical regions of most continents and transmitted by the brown dog tick, *R. sanguineus*. It is the least pathogenic of the three strains and is probably the one found in the United States. *Babesia canis canis* is proposed for the strain occurring in Europe and parts of Asia. It is intermediate in pathogenicity and is transmitted by ticks of the *Dermacentor* genus. Finally, *Babesia canis rossi* is the proposed name given to the highly pathogenic strain transmitted by *H. leachi* and found in southern Africa.

## LIFE CYCLE, TRANSMISSION, AND PATHOGENESIS

Babesias are introduced into the susceptible host by the bite of infected ixodid ticks. All stages of the tick are thought to be infective, but the adult female is most important in parasite transmission. Once in the host, *Babesia* spp. parasitize only erythrocytes. Merozoites of *B. canis* multiply within the erythrocytes by repeated binary fission. As many as 16 merozoites may be seen in a single red cell. Erythrocytes infected with one or two merozoites are most commonly noted on blood smears from affected dogs. The host immune response to the parasite and to altered antigenic determinants on affected erythrocyte membranes are important in determining the extent of clinical signs.

Ticks become infected following ingestion of infected host erythrocytes during feeding. Once in the tick, both trans-stadial and transovarial transmission can occur. The *Babesia* parasite may lie dormant for long periods of time. When the tick feeds on the blood of a susceptible vertebrate host, sporozoites are passed with the tick's saliva into the host circulation. The tick must feed a minimum of 2 to 3 days for transmission of *B. canis* to occur. After infection, there is usually a significant host immune response generated, but the immune system does not appear able to completely clear infections and recovered animals are usually chronic carriers of the parasite.

Parisitemia results in hemolysis (usually of an intravascular nature) and subsequent anemia. However, the severity of anemia is not proportional to the degree of parasitemia. Both direct parasitic damage and secondary immune system–induced damage following formation of antierythrocyte membrane antibodies are important in the pathogenesis of the hemolysis (Adachi et al., 1992). The formation of antierythrocyte antibodies is reflected in the fact that in one study, nearly 85% of dogs with babesiosis were positive on direct antiglobulin (Coombs') tests (Farwell, Legrand, and Cobb, 1982). Thrombocytopenia is common, especially in dogs infected with *B. gibsoni*. Like the hemolytic anemia, the pathogenesis of the thrombocytopenia is probably partially immune mediated. Membranoproliferative glomerulonephritis is seen in some infected dogs and also may have an immune-mediated pathogenesis. Vascular stasis from sludging of parasitized cells within capillary beds also contributes to many of the observed clinical signs. Soluble parasite proteases activate the kallikrein system and induce fibrinogen-like protein (FLP) formation. It has been suggested that FLPs increase erythrocyte "stickiness," leading to sludging of erythrocytes in the capillaries. The most severe sludging appears to occur in the central nervous system and muscles.

## CLINICAL DISEASE

### Prevalence

Reported seroprevalence to *Babesia canis* antigen in the United States has ranged from 3.8 to 59%. The seroprevalence is higher in adult dogs than in dogs less than 1 year of age. The prevalence of *Babesia* antibodies appears to be high in some populations of dogs in the southeastern part of the United States. Few serologic surveys have been reported outside of the south, and in most parts of the United States the prevalence of *Babesia* infection is probably low. In a serologic survey of dogs in Florida, 46% of 393 greyhounds but none of 50 adult nongreyhound pet dogs were seropositive, implicating both environment and breed susceptibility as factors in determining seroprevalence in endemic areas (Taboada et al., 1992).

### Clinical Signs

Dogs younger than 6 months of age are more susceptible to babesial infection than adult dogs. This factor appears to be especially important in the pathogenicity of *B. canis*. Puppies in the 4- to 12-week age range are probably most susceptible. Maternally derived antibodies may be protective in some puppies less than 8 weeks of age. Age may be a less important factor in the pathogenesis of clinical disease caused by *B. gibsoni* and the more virulent strains of *B. canis*.

Two syndromes, one characterized by hypotensive shock (hyperacute disease) and the other by hemolytic anemia (acute disease), account for most of the clinical signs observed in animals with babesiosis. Hyperacute disease is characterized by hypotensive shock, hypothermia, tissue hypoxia, extensive tissue damage, and vascular stasis. A high percentage of dogs with this form of babesiosis die despite therapy. Hyperacute disease has not been documented in adult dogs in the United States but may occasionally occur in infected puppies. Shock, coma, or death following a less than 1-day history of anorexia, lethargy, and hemoglobinuria is usually seen. Shock and metabolic acidosis are thought to result from severe anemia, babesial protease release, and vascular stasis. Activation of kallikrein by babesial proteases results directly in vasodilation and contributes to shock. Vasodilation and vascular stasis also result in erythrocyte sequestration. This sequestration

contributes to the acute drop in packed cell volume (PCV). Dogs with hyperacute babesiosis are usually heavily parasitized with *Babesia* organisms and have a history of heavy tick infestation.

Acute disease is characterized by anorexia, lethargy, hemolytic anemia, thrombocytopenia, lymphadenopathy, and splenomegaly. Fever and vomiting are also commonly observed. Fatalities may occur, especially in puppies of *B. gibsoni*–infected adults, but most animals with acute disease will recover (Abdullahi, 1990). Hemoglobinuria and icterus may be noted, especially in *B. canis*–infected dogs, and periorbital edema can be seen. Immune-mediated hemolytic anemia and systemic lupus erythematosus are the primary diseases that must be differentiated from this form of babesiosis.

Chronic babesiosis is primarily reported in *B. canis*–infected dogs in southern Africa and is characterized by intermittent fever, decreased appetite, and marked loss of body condition. Anemia is not usually seen in chronically infected dogs. The chronic form of the disease may occur in *B. gibsoni*–infected dogs in the United States but has not been well documented following *B. canis* infection.

A wide variety of "atypical signs" have been reported in *Babesia*-infected dogs (Table 1). These signs are less common than those seen with the hyperacute and acute presentation described above. Unfortunately, it is difficult to say whether the atypical signs are induced by *Babesia* alone or are caused by concurrent disease. Mild upper respiratory signs and dyspnea may be seen. Gastrointestinal signs may include vomiting, constipation, diarrhea, and ulcerative stomatitis. Vascular manifestations include edema, ascites, and purpura. Rarely, hemorrhages varying from petechiae to ecchymotic patches occur secondary to thrombocytopenia or disseminated intravascular coagulation (DIC). A *Babesia*-associated masticatory myositis has been described. Other atypical musculoskeletal manifestations have included joint swelling and back pain. Central nervous system manifestations, secondary to so-called cerebral babesiosis, include seizures, weakness, and ataxia. The neurologic manifestations are thought to be caused by sludging of parasitized erythrocytes within capillaries of the central nervous system and occur most often in hyperacutely affected dogs. Many of the other atypical manifestations may have a similar pathogenesis. Duel infections with *Babesia* spp. and *Ehrlichia canis* may contribute to the diversity of clinical signs described.

Subclinical infection is probably more common than is currently being recognized in the United States. Parasites will rarely be found on blood smears from asymptomatic carriers, making identification of this group of dogs difficult without performing serologic screening tests. The importance of this group of dogs may be in their role as potential source of infection to susceptible puppies. Babesiosis can be an important cause of morbidity and mortality in puppies in breeding kennels located in endemic areas. Veterinarians often attribute anemic puppies to ecto- and endoparasitism without thinking about the possibility of babesiosis. The diag-

**Table 1.** *Clinical Findings in Dogs With Babesiosis*

| Nonspecific Clinical Signs | | Atypical Clinical Signs |
| --- | --- | --- |
| Anorexia | Ascites | Ocular and nasal discharge |
| Lethargy | Edema | Respiratory distress |
| Weakness | Constipation | Masticatory myositis |
| Pyrexia | Diarrhea | Temporomandibular joint pain |
| | Ulcerative stomatitis | Back pain |
| | Hemorrhage | Central nervous system signs |
| | | Seizures |
| | | Ataxia |
| | | Paresis |

| Hyperacute Presentation | Acute Presentation | Chronic Presentation |
| --- | --- | --- |
| Hypothermia | Hemolytic anemia | Intermittent pyrexia |
| Shock | Icterus | Partial anorexia |
| Coma | Splenomegaly | Loss of body condition |
| DIC | Lymphadenopathy | Lymphadenopathy |
| Metabolic acidosis | Vomiting | |
| Death | | |

nosis can be difficult to make in affected puppies but adults in affected kennels can serve as serologic markers for the disease. Serologic surveys of adult dogs from kennels where babesiosis is causing anemia in puppies will often reveal a seroprevalence of over 75%. Rarely will any of the adult dogs be showing clinical signs of babesiosis, however.

## Clinical Pathology

The primary hematologic abnormalities in animals with babesiosis include anemia and thrombocytopenia. A mild, normocytic, normochromic anemia is generally

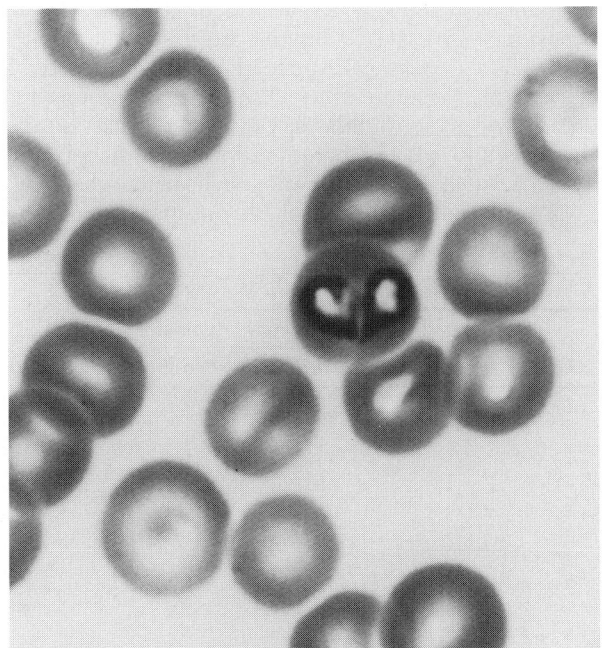

**Figure 1.** A pair of large piriform-shaped merozoites of *Babesia canis* within an erythrocyte from a 3-week-old neopolitan mastiff puppy with acute babesiosis.

noted in the first few days after infection. The anemia becomes macrocytic, hypochromic, and regenerative as the disease progresses, the reticulocytosis being proportional to the severity of the anemia. Leukocyte abnormalities are inconsistently seen and may include leukocytosis, neutrophilia, neutropenia, lymphocytosis, and eosinophilia. Leukocytosis is more likely in hyperacute disease than in the acute presentation. Low-grade thrombocytopenia is common in symptomatic cases, but is rarely low enough for spontaneous bleeding to occur.

Serum chemistry values are usually normal. Hypokalemia may be seen in severely affected animals but is probably a nonspecific finding due to decreased potassium intake. Hyperkalemia, hypoglycemia, and increased alanine aminotransferase (ALT), aspartate aminotransferase (AST), and creatine phosphokinase (CPK) was noted in severely affected puppies in one study (Irwin and Hutchinson, 1991). Azotemia and metabolic acidosis are common, and appear to contribute to morbidity and mortality. Hyperbilirubinemia is a consistent finding during acute disease caused by *B. canis*, but not by *B. gibsoni*. Bilirubinuria, hemoglobinuria, proteinuria, and granular casts may be seen on urinalysis.

## DIAGNOSIS

Diagnosis of babesiosis is made by demonstrating the presence of *Babesia* organisms within infected erythrocytes. Large piriform-shaped organisms, usually present singly or in pairs, is indicative of *B. canis* infection (Fig. 1), while smaller singular intracellular organisms are likely to be *B. gibsoni*. Parasitemias are often low, and thorough examination of thin blood smears is necessary to find the organisms. Blood smears made from the peripheral capillary beds in the ear tip or nail bed may yield higher numbers of parasites. Red blood cells adjacent to the buffy coat are also more likely to be infected. Giemsa-stained blood smears are superior to

Wright's-stained smears for finding organisms. While the organisms are sometimes easy to find in acutely infected animals, they are rarely evident in chronically infected or asymptomatic carriers. Subinoculation of blood into a splenectomized dog will yield more obvious parasitemias, making the diagnosis much easier. After experimental inoculation, a transient parasitemia is noted on days 1 through 5, with a more significant parasitemia occurring around day 14. Logistics, expense, and animal welfare considerations make subinoculation generally unfeasible.

Serology is reliable at detecting patent or occult parasitemias. While many serologic tests for canine babesiosis are available, the indirect fluorescent antibody (IFA) test is the most commonly used. Generally, titers greater than or equal to 1:80 are considered positive. A positive titer on one sample appears to be sufficient for diagnosis. Very young dogs, or dogs early in the disease course, may be serologically negative, however, making convalescing serum necessary in those cases. Cross-reactivity between *B. canis* and *B. gibsoni* make parasite identification necessary to differentiate between the two species.

## THERAPY

Therapy of canine babesiosis involves both supportive and babesiacidal measures. Supportive therapy is important and often all that is required in treating acute disease caused by the strains of *B. canis* found in the United States. Intravenous fluids should be administered to animals that are dehydrated or in shock. Whole blood or packed erythrocytes should be transfused to patients that are severely anemic (see "Practical Guidelines for Transfusion Therapy," in *CVT XI*, p 475). Sodium bicarbonate infusion is recommended in animals that are severely acidemic. Acidosis is a poor prognostic factor if left untreated. Treatment of concurrent stressors, especially gastrointestinal parasitism, is also important.

Many babesiacidal drugs (Table 2) have been used in the treatment of *Babesia* infection. Unfortunately, the most effective of these, diminazene aceturate,

phenamidine isethionate, and imidocarb dipropionate, are not available or approved for use in the United States except on a limited experimental basis. Of these, diminazene aceturate is the most commonly used worldwide. It is effective against both canine babesias at an intramuscular dose of 3.5 mg/kg. Imidocarb is very effective against *B. canis* but not as effective against *B. gibsoni*. At the suggested dose of 5 mg/kg given intramuscularly twice at 14-day intervals, imidocarb eliminates the babesia infection and also eliminates infectivity of ticks engorging on treated animals for up to 4 weeks after treatment. Imidocarb has also proven effective against *Ehrlichia canis* and is therefore the drug of choice in dual infections. *Babesia gibsoni* is less responsive to babesiacidal therapy than *B. canis*. Unfortunately, it is also less likely to respond to symptomatic therapy alone.

Other drugs that have been used include oxytetracycline, which is effective against *Babesia* organisms of cattle but not dogs; and metronidazole, which has been used with limited success in the treatment of *B. gibsoni* infections. There have been numerous anecdotal reports of success in treating canine babesiosis with clindamycin at 25 mg/kg orally divided twice daily. However, it should be noted that many infected dogs will recover completely without specific babesiacidal therapy if adequate supportive measures are taken, making interpretation of uncontrolled treatment observations difficult. This author presently recommends that infected dogs be treated by aggressive supportive care and clindamycin if the unapproved drugs listed above are not available. Controlled trials evaluating the efficacy of clindamycin are needed.

Whether glucocorticoids are indicated is controversial. The immune system is implicated in many of the clinical manifestations of canine babesiosis, especially the hemolytic anemia. Therefore, treatment with immunosuppressive doses of glucocorticoids should be beneficial (see "Clinical Applications of Glucocorticoid Therapy in Nonendocrine Disease," this volume, p 406). However, steroid therapy may predispose to other infections and has the potential to induce babesial relapse (Masuda, 1983). The monocyte-macrophage system is important in control of *Babesia* parasitemia, and

***Table 2.*** *Babesiacidal Compounds Used in the Treatment of Canine Babesiosis*

| | | | Effectiveness Against | |
|---|---|---|---|---|
| **Drug** | **Proprietary Name** | **Dosage** | *Babesia canis* | *Babesia gibsoni* |
| Diminazene aceturate° | Berenil Ganaseg | 3.5 mg/kg IM | +++ | ++ |
| Imidocarb dipropionate° | Imizol | 5 mg/kg IM | +++ | ? |
| Phenamidine isethionate° | Lomadine Phenamidine | 15 mg/kg SC on 2 consecutive days | +++ | ++ |
| Primaquine phosphate | Primaquine | 0.5 mg/kg IM | ? | + |
| Clindamycin | Antirobe Cleocin | 25 mg/kg PO divided b.i.d. | ? | ? |
| Metronidazole | Flagyl Protostat | 25–65 mg/kg PO s.i.d. | — | + |

°Not available or approved for use in the United States without an FDA-approved NAID number.
Effectiveness: +++ = very good, ++ = good, + = fair, — not effective, ? = unknown.

reduction in this system's function will often result in more severe parasitemia shortly after glucocorticoid therapy is initiated. Glucocorticoids are probably indicated in dogs with acute hemolytic anemia or other signs attributable to immune mechanisms. Long-term use is probably not indicated, however. When glucocorticoids are given, the dog should be monitored closely for secondary infections and adverse effects.

## PREVENTION

The lack of approved babesiacidal compounds in the United States makes prevention of paramount importance. Preventative measures alone may be sufficient to control *B. canis* outbreaks in kennels in the southeastern United States. The primary means of prevention is control of the vector tick. Frequent inspection of the skin and hair coat for ticks is important, since it takes a minimum of 2 to 3 days' feeding for transmission of the *Babesia* to occur. The initiation of dipping programs and environmental control measures is also important in endemic areas. Before introducing new animals into a colony, they should be serologically tested, dipped, and quarantined. Flea and tick collars, while not very effective for flea control, are reasonably effective for tick control when used in conjunction with inspection, dips, and environmental management.

A vaccine produced from cell culture–derived exoantigens of *B. canis* is available in Europe. An efficacy of 70 to 100% has been reported, with the disease occasionally seen in the vaccinates generally being mild (Moreau, Martinod, and Fayet, 1988). The beneficial aspects of the vaccine were particularly evident in immunosuppressed dogs, which are recognized as a high-risk group. Other field studies have been less impressive. This conflicting information, together with the high cost of the vaccine, has limited its use. The vaccine does represent the first antiprotozoan vaccine ever produced commercially and is therefore a landmark advancement that may eventually herald a new era in the control of babesiosis and other protozoal diseases.

*Babesia* organisms can be transmitted by blood transfusion, making control in a blood donor especially important. All prospective canine blood donors should be serologically tested for babesiosis. Positive animals should be identified and culled from the program. Splenectomy will increase the likelihood of finding parasites in animals with occult infection and is therefore indicated. Blood smears should be examined for *Babesia* daily for 2 weeks after splenectomy and then periodically thereafter.

## BABESIOSIS IN GREYHOUNDS

The greyhound may be more susceptible to infection than other breeds of dogs (Taboada et al., 1992). Greyhound racing is a rapidly growing, economically important industry in many states. In 1987, the industry value (not including parimutuel betting) was nearly $1 billion in the state of Florida alone. The racing greyhound is a tremendous athlete that must be in top shape to adequately compete. Anything that decreases performance, even slightly, can have a dramatic impact on the animal's competitive and economic standing. The high prevalence of babesiosis in greyhounds and the potential impact the disease has on performance make it an important issue to the industry.

Greyhounds begin training and racing at an early age, and impaired development may keep an animal from reaching athletic potential. Babesiosis primarily affects puppies at an age when they are rapidly maturing, thus potentially disrupting the developmental process and causing economic losses to the breeders and owners of affected dogs. Transplacental transmission magnifies the importance in breeding kennels. Overt clinical signs of babesiosis are rare in adult greyhounds, but the impact that subclinical infections may have on the canine athlete is not known.

An individual greyhound may train and race in many different states. The highly mobile nature of large numbers of potential carriers may have a significant epidemiologic impact on disease prevalence. Additionally, retired greyhounds are often used as blood donors because of their large size, docile nature, and high red blood cell numbers. This is another, although probably epidemiologically insignificant, source of *Babesia* spread.

## References and Suggested Reading

Abdullahi SU, Mohammed AA, Trimnell AR, et al: Clinical and haematological findings in 70 naturally occurring cases of canine babesiosis. J Small Anim Pract 31:145, 1990.

Breitschwerdt E: Babesiosis. *In* Greene CE (ed): *Clinical Microbiology and Infectious Diseases of the Dog and Cat.* Philadelphia, WB Saunders Co, 1984, pp 796–805.

Breitschwerdt EB, Malone JB, MacWilliams P, et al: Babesiosis in the greyhound. J Am Vet Med Assoc 182:978, 1983.

Conrad P, Thomford J, Yamane I, et al: Hemolytic anemia caused by *Babesia gibsoni* infection in dogs. J Am Vet Med Assoc 199:601, 1991.

Farwell GE, LeGrand EK, and Cobb CC: Clinical observations on *Babesia gibsoni* and *Babesia canis* infections in dogs. J Am Vet Med Assoc 180:507, 1982.

Harvey JW, Taboada J, and Lewis JC: Babesiosis in a litter of pups. J Am Vet Med Assoc 192:1715, 1988.

Irwin PJ and Hutchinson GW: Clinical and pathological findings of *Babesia* infection in dogs. Aust Vet J 68:204, 1991.

Kuttler KL: Chemotherapy of babesiosis. *In* Ristic M (ed): *Babesiosis of Domestic Animals and Man.* Boca Raton, FL, CRC Press, 1988, pp 227–242.

Levy MG, Breitschwerdt EB, and Moncol DJ: Antibody activity to *Babesia canis* in dogs in North Carolina. Am J Vet Res 48:339, 1987.

Masuda T, Baba E, and Arakawa A: Relapse of canine babesiosis after prednisolone treatment. Mod Vet Pract 64:931, 1983.

Moreau Y, Martinod S, and Fayet G: Epidemiologic and immunoprophylactic aspects of canine babesiosis in France. *In* Ristic M (ed): *Babesiosis of Domestic Animals and Man.* Boca Raton, FL, CRC Press, 1988, pp 191–196.

Schetters TH PM, Kleuskens J, Scholtes N, et al: Vaccination of dogs against *Babesia canis* infection using parasite antigens from in vitro culture. Parasite Immunol 14:295, 1992.

Taboada J and Merchant SR: Babesiosis of companion animals and man. Vet Clin North Am [Small Anim Pract] 21:103, 1991.

Taboada J, Harvey JW, Levy MG, et al: Seroprevalence of babesiosis in greyhounds in Florida. J Am Vet Med Assoc 200:47, 1992.

Uilenberg G, Franssen FFJ, Perie NM, et al: Three groups of *Babesia canis* distinguished and a proposal for nomenclature. Vet Q 11:33, 1989.

# CANINE AND FELINE MYCOBACTERIAL INFECTION

HOLLY L. JORDAN

*Raleigh, North Carolina*

Once regarded as a disease of declining importance, mycobacteriosis has become a growing concern of public health professionals over the past decade. There has been a resurgence of human mycobacteriosis, particularly in individuals with acquired immunodeficiency syndrome (AIDS). Tuberculosis due to *Mycobacterium bovis* or *M. tuberculosis* is uncommon in dogs and cats, but as observed in the human population, there has been an increasing variety of nontubercular, atypical species associated with disease in companion animal patients. Manifestations of mycobacterial infections may mimic a number of chronic diseases. Due to the zoonotic potential of these bacteria, early recognition and diagnosis are essential.

## ETIOLOGY

Mycobacteria are nonmotile, non–spore-forming, acid-fast, aerobic bacilli. Due to a complex lipid-rich cell wall, they are weakly gram-positive. Classification of mycobacteria is based largely on pathogenicity for humans and animals, rate of growth, and biochemical characteristics (Greene, 1990; Inderlied, Kemper, and Bermudez, 1993). *Mycobacterium tuberculosis* and *M. bovis* are considered to be "typical" mycobacteria and are responsible for the classic granulomatous disease, tuberculosis, in mammals. These species are slow-growing (2 to 6 weeks in culture), facultative intracellular organisms with pathogenicity against humans, dogs, and cats. Their natural reservoirs are animal hosts; they survive poorly in the environment. *Mycobacterium lepraemurium* causes the nodular cutaneous disease, feline leprosy, in cats. It is a slow-growing, obligate intracellular bacteria that is difficult to culture. Other mycobacterial species can be subgrouped according to *in vitro* characteristics, but they are generally classified as "atypical" mycobacteria, nontuberculous mycobacteria (NTM) or, more recently, potentially pathogenic environmental mycobacteria (PPEM). Most of these species are saprophytes associated with opportunistic infections. This group includes some slow-growing species (e.g., *M. avium*), and many fast-growing (7 days in culture) species.

## IDENTIFICATION

Preliminary identification of mycobacteria in tissues may be accomplished with the Kinyoun, Ziehl-Neelsen, or Fite-Faraco acid-fast stains, or fluorescent dyes. Kinyoun stain is packaged in kits similar to Gram stains and is easily performed in practice. Mycobacteria bacilli stain variably—they may have a beaded appearance or club shape. Rod-shaped forms may be found within macrophages, multinucleated giant cells, and occasionally in neutrophils. Some cells may be distended with intracytoplasmic stacks or bundles of bacilli. With Romanovsky stains, such as Diff-Quik, the bacilli appear as linear "negative images" or short bars that fail to take up stain. In addition to mycobacteria, *Nocardia*, some bacterial spores, and some *Corynebacterium* spp. are also weakly acid-fast; positive identification necessitates bacterial isolation.

Clinicians should consult a clinical microbiology laboratory or their state health department for advice on appropriate handling of specimens for mycobacterial culture. The National Jewish Center for Immunology and Respiratory Medicine (1400 Jackson Street, Denver, CO 80206) provides clinical mycobacteriology services. Culture and sensitivity may require weeks for slow-growing species. Laboratory animal inoculation is no longer commonly used to speciate these organisms.

## IMMUNOPATHOGENESIS

Mycobacteria enter the host by ingestion or inhalation. The bacilli are phagocytized by macrophages, where they multiply intracellularly. Several factors permit these organisms to survive inside phagocytic cells: a resistant waxy cell wall, antioxidants (e.g., catalase), cytotoxic factors, and the ability to prevent fusion of the phagosome and lysosome or to escape the phagosome and live freely in the cytoplasm. Cell-mediated immunity prevents dissemination of mycobacteria. If the host is unable to clear the intracellular organisms, a chronic immune response ensues, resulting in granulomatous inflammation. Mycobacteria elicit a humoral response, but antibodies appear to play a small role in protection against infection. Conditions that limit cell-mediated immunity, such as human immunodeficiency virus (HIV), may predispose hosts to mycobacterial infection.

## MYCOBACTERIAL DISEASE IN DOGS AND CATS

Mycobacterial infections in companion animals tend to be manifested as either primary cutaneous disease or multisystemic illness. Primary dermatologic manifestations have been described in association with atypical and lepromatous mycobacteria. Though *M. bovis* and *M. tuberculosis* may also cause skin lesions, infections most frequently result in generalized involvement.

## Cutaneous Nontubercular Mycobacterial Disease

Nontubercular mycobacteria comprise a diverse group of species found in a variety of habitats. In the 1950s, Runyon classified NTM into four groups based on growth and pigment production. Recent examination of nucleic acid homology between mycobacteria has essentially corroborated this classification scheme. Organisms implicated in cutaneous atypical mycobacteriosis in pets include *M. avium*, *M. fortuitum*, *M. chelonei*, *M. xenopi*, *M. thermoresistibile*, *M. smegmatis*, *M. phlei*, and *M. ulcerans*. Cats appear to be infected more often than dogs.

The route of entry is unknown, but infections have been associated with fight wounds, trauma, and subcutaneous injections (Künkle et al., 1983). Direct transmission between companion animals or between humans and animals has not been reported. Cats and dogs commonly present with chronic cutaneous nodules, granulomas, abscesses, or ulcers, with or without sinuses and fistulous tracts. Nodules vary in size and number. They are frequently nonpainful and may be freely movable. Typical sites include the cutis and subcutis of the caudal abdomen, groin, lumbar region, and extremities. These pyogranulomatous lesions are often poorly responsive to antibiotics. Animals usually appear relatively healthy. Pyrexia, lymphadenopathy, and splenomegaly have been reported, but systemic illness is uncommon. Some patients develop an inflammatory leukogram; however, many animals have no laboratory abnormalities.

The differential diagnosis for nodular or ulcerative dermatitis includes chronic bacterial infections, nocardiosis, actinomycosis, dermatophytosis, neoplasia (e.g., squamous cell carcinoma, mast cell tumor, mammary tumors, cutaneous lymphoid tumors), mycotic infections (e.g., cryptococcus, blastomycosis), panniculitis, eosinophilic granuloma, foreign body reaction, and other mycobacterial infections (e.g., feline leprosy in cats). Acid-fast stains of cytologic imprints, aspirates, or biopsy material from lesions may provide rapid diagnosis. However, some species (e.g., *M. fortuitum*), may be missed due to small numbers of intralesional organisms. Histologically, the inflammatory infiltrate consists of numerous macrophages, epithelioid cells, and neutrophils. Occasionally clear vacuoles are present that may contain small numbers of acid-fast organisms. Differentiation of NTM from other mycobacterial species is important due to the zoonotic potential of the tubercle bacilli. Definitive diagnosis, therefore, requires culture of tissue lesions; multiple attempts may be necessary if bacterial populations are small.

Routine antibiotic therapy is often unrewarding due to drug resistance in NTM. Quinolones, aminoglycosides, cephalosporins, erythromycin, tetracycline, doxycycline, and amoxicillin trihydrate/clavulanic acid have been used with variable success. Unfortunately, *in vitro* sensitivities do not always correlate with effectiveness in animals. Studdert and Hughes (1992) reported successful treatment of cutaneous *M. fortuitum* and *M. smegmatis* infections in cats with enrofloxacin (Baytril, Haver/Mobay; 5 mg/kg every 24 hr, PO) for 3 to 7 weeks. Ciprofloxacin (Cirpo, Miles; canine dose, 10 to 15 mg/kg every 12 hr, PO) may be more effective against some mycobacteria (Mundell, 1990). Therapy for cutaneous mycobacteriosis may be required for weeks to months. Surgical resection is often unsuccessful due to poor wound healing and the high likelihood of recurrence. Spontaneous remissions have been reported (Muller, Kirk, and Scott, 1989), but the prognosis is usually guarded.

## Feline Leprosy

The etiology of this nodular-ulcerative disease is *M. lepraemurium*. It is associated with a granulomatous skin disease similar to human leprosy (also called Hansen's disease) caused by *M. leprae*. Cats, rats, mice, and guinea pigs may be infected with *M. lepraemurium*. The route of transmission is unclear, but cats may be exposed by contact with rodents. Feline leprosy is reported most frequently in cool, damp climates: northwestern North America, western Europe, New Zealand, and Australia. No breed or sex predilection is known. It is reported more frequently in cats less than 3 years of age.

These very slow-growing bacilli apparently incubate in the feline host for weeks to months, but once formed, the lesions can grow rapidly. One or more freely movable nodules (up to 3 cm in size) develop in the dermis and subcutis on any area of the body, particularly the head and extremities. Nodules are usually nonpainful, soft, and fleshy. Ulceration may occur, but unlike NTM, fistulous tracts and exudate are not typical. Spread to regional lymph nodes and spleen has been reported. Histologic evidence of peripheral nerve involvement is a consistent feature of human leprosy, but it is a variable finding in cats. Systemic disease is uncommon; most cats appear healthy on examination.

The differential diagnosis for feline leprosy is similar to that for skin disease due to NTM. In contrast to other mycobacteria, *M. lepraemurium* are usually present in large numbers in tissue samples, especially within phagocytes. The inflammatory cell infiltrate in NTM dermatitis generally includes more neutrophils. In feline leprosy, the predominant inflammatory cells are foamy macrophages and epithelioid cells interspersed with smaller numbers of neutrophils or lymphocytes. Unlike infections with *M. bovis* and *M. tuberculosis*, caseation necrosis and encapsulation are rare. In addition, other mycobacteria can be cultured more easily; a negative culture may support a diagnosis of *M. lepraemurium*. With diligence, successful growth has been accomplished with Ogawa egg yolk medium.

The treatment of choice is surgical excision. Like NTM lesions, recurrence is not uncommon. Spontaneous regression of small lesions has been observed. The most promising medical therapy is clofazimine (Lamprene, Ciba-Geigy), a human leprosy drug (Mundell, 1990). The dose for feline leprosy is 2 to 3 mg/kg once daily PO for at least 1 month beyond the resolution of lesions. Skin discoloration may occur and cats should be monitored for possible hepatotoxicity. Rifampin, dapsone, and streptomycin have been used in cats with variable success and variable toxicity (Greene, 1990).

## Systemic Nontubercular Mycobacterial Disease

Members of the *M. avium-intracellulare* complex and *M. fortuitum-chelonei* complex are the most frequent atypical mycobacteria associated with systemic infections in companion animals. Healthy cats and dogs are fairly resistant to the avian tubercle bacillus, *M. avium*, but systemic infections have been reported sporadically. Immunosuppression, such as chronic steroid administration, may enhance susceptibility. Interestingly, feline immunodeficiency virus has not been associated with increased susceptibility to these organisms. *Mycobacterium avium* also infects poultry, cattle, and pigs. Transmission to pets may occur by ingestion of infected animal by-products; however, *M. avium* is ubiquitous in the environment and may remain viable for up to 2 years in water, soil, bedding, plant material, and housedust. *Mycobacterium fortuitum* is the most commonly isolated mycobacterium in soil and hospital dust; exposure probably occurs by inhalation.

There is no age or sex predilection; basset hounds and Siamese cats appear to be predisposed. A genetic component is also suggested by reports of *M. avium* infections in related animals (Carpenter et al., 1988). The clinical signs and physical findings of generalized NTM infection are indicative of chronic disease. Nonspecific signs are common: anorexia, weight loss, lethargy, depression, and pyrexia. Vomiting, diarrhea, coughing, dyspnea, lymphadenopathy, splenomegaly, submandibular swelling, icterus, spinal pain, and lameness have been described. Dogs with systemic *M. fortuitum* infection may develop pleural effusion, bronchopneumonia, and hypertrophic osteopathy (Wylie, Lewis, and Pechman, 1993). Common hematologic abnormalities include nonregenerative anemia, leukocytosis, neutrophilia with or without a left shift, and monocytosis. Hypoproteinemia and hypoalbuminemia are typical serum chemistry changes. Elevated liver enzyme activities and total bilirubin concentration are not uncommon.

The differential diagnosis for systemic mycobacteriosis encompasses many chronic conditions, including generalized infection with bacteria, fungi, protozoans, parasites, or rickettsia; neoplasia; and immunosuppression due to drugs, viruses, or congenital immunodeficiencies. The lymphadenopathy of mycobacteriosis may look clinically very similar to lymphosarcoma (Orr, 1980). The periosteal changes and hypertrophic osteopathy observed in dogs with *M. fortuitum* may mimic *Hepatozoon canis* (Wylie, Lewis, and Pechman, 1993).

Presumptive diagnosis of mycobacterial infection may be made by identifying acid-fast organisms in cytologic or histologic specimens of tissues, such as lymph node and bone marrow. Occasionally, organisms may be observed in neutrophils or monocytes in peripheral blood or buffy coat smears. Granulomatous or pyogranulomatous inflammation is the principal histologic change. *Mycobacterium avium* may be present in large numbers, both intracellularly and extracellularly. *Mycobacterium fortuitum* is usually more difficult to find. Discreet granuloma formation, caseation necrosis, and calcification are less common in disseminated NTM infections than in infections due to *M. bovis* or *M. tuberculosis*.

Nontubercular mycobacteria are resistant to standard antituberculosis medications, such as isoniazid and ethambutol. Lung lobectomy and administration of kanamycin or amikacin and amoxicillin-clavulanate potassium resulted in recovery from *M. fortuitum* pneumonia in dogs (Wylie, Lewis, and Pechman, 1993). Clofazimine has been used to treat NTM in cats and dogs at a dose of 8 to 12 mg/kg every 24 hr, PO (Mundell, 1990). *Mycobacterium avium* is particularly difficult to treat due to a lack of effective drugs and the fact that most animals present late in the disease course. *In vitro* sensitivity results for this slow-growing organism may take longer than is practical in many cases. *Mycobacterium avium* is one of the most common causes of bacteremia in patients with HIV and new drugs have been introduced to treat these individuals; however, there have been no studies confirming effectiveness or toxicity in cats and dogs. Current recommendations for treatment of systemic *M. avium* in humans are to administer a combination of medications for months and possibly years (Inderlied, Kemper, and Bermudez, 1993). Two new macrolides, azithromycin (Zithromax, Pfizer) and clarithromycin (Biaxin Filmtabs, Abbott), have shown promise, and according to Inderlied et al. (1993) may be used in combination with ethambutol (Myambutol, Lederle) and a third drug, such as rifampin (Rifadin, Marion Merrell Dow), enrofloxacin, or rifabutin (Mycobutin, Adria). Amikacin, clofazimine, ansamycin, streptomycin, cylcoserine, and ethionamide have also been prescribed. The prognosis for systemic *M. avium* infection is poor.

## Tubercular Mycobacterial Disease

Due to regulatory programs in food animals, tuberculosis in dogs and cats is currently very uncommon. Dogs are moderately susceptible to *M. tuberculosis*. Cats are less susceptible to *M. tuberculosis* than dogs, but are more likely to be infected with *M. bovis*. *Mycobacterium tuberculosis* is most often spread by airborne routes, and infection of pets typically requires long-term close contact with infected people. Transmission of *M. tuberculosis* from animals to humans has not been shown. Pets are a potential source of *M. bovis* for other animals (e.g., cattle) and possibly humans. Exposure to *M. bovis* frequently occurs by ingestion of tainted milk, meat, or offal, allowing colonization of the gastrointestinal tract. Airborne transmission and respiratory tract localization also occur. Organisms are excreted in feces and sputum. Exposure via exudative skin lesions has also been described (Isaac et al., 1983).

Clinical disease is usually nonspecific. Lymphadenopathy and gastrointestinal or respiratory signs are most common. Weight loss, anorexia, and fever are often evident. Respiratory signs include bronchopneumonia, pulmonary nodule formation, and hilar lymphadenopathy. Oropharyngeal lymphadenopathy is associated with dysphagia, retching, and hypersalivation. Vomiting, diarrhea, mesenteric lymphadenopathy, and abdominal effusion are typical gastrointestinal manifestations. Cutaneous ulcers, nodules, abscesses, or plaques similar to lesions caused by NTM or *M. lepraemurium* may be observed, though animals with *M. tuberculosis* or *M. bovis* appear generally sick. Disseminated disease may involve the liver, spleen, heart, or nervous system. Potential laboratory changes include nonregenerative anemia, leukocytosis, hyperglobulinemia, and hypoalbuminemia. Radiographic findings such as lymphadenopathy, interstitial lung infiltration, hepatosplenomegaly, and miliary calcification may resemble neoplastic changes.

A preliminary diagnosis of mycobacteriosis can be made by finding acid-fast organisms associated with granulomatous inflammation in cytologic or histologic samples. Encapsulation may be evident with focal areas of necrosis and possibly calcification. Serologic testing of cats and dogs is generally unreliable. Skin testing in dogs has been used, but it is not accurate in cats. Dogs may be tested by injecting 250 TU (tuberculin units) (0.1 ml) of purified protein derivative (PPD) intradermally on the inner surface of the pinna. Purified protein derivative is a preparation of the soluble proteins found in medium in which mycobacteria have been cultured. The injection site should be examined 48 to 72 hr after injection. Positive reactors will have a raised, indurated, and subsequently necrotic swelling at the site (Greene, 1990). False-positives may occur. Bacterial isolation provides definitive diagnosis.

Consistent, effective treatment of tuberculosis in cats and dogs has not been developed. Current therapy involves combinations of agents, such as isoniazid (available as a generic drug from various sources), rifampin, and ethambutol for 6 to 9 months (Greene, 1990). These drugs can cause toxicity, especially hepatotoxicity. Isoniazid has been used prophylactically in people

exposed to tubercle mycobacteria. Due to the potential public health hazard of these organisms, euthanasia of infected dogs and cats is generally recommended. People exposed to animals with tuberculosis (e.g., owners, veterinary care givers) should consult their physicians or public health departments for examinations and appropriate skin testing. *Mycobacterium tuberculosis* and *M. bovis* are reportable diseases.

## ZOONOTIC POTENTIAL AND CONTROL

*Mycobacterium tuberculosis* and *M. bovis* are human pathogens. Animals infected with these organisms must be considered potential sources of infection for people. *Mycobacterium lepraemurium* has shown no ability to infect humans. Atypical mycobacterial infections occur in people, especially in immunosuppressed individuals; however, pets are an unlikely source of infection, given the wide range of environmental habitats for NTM. Mycobacteria are resistant to many disinfectants. Tuberculous species survive less than 2 weeks in the environment, but other species may survive for years outside animal hosts. Mycobacteria can be killed by dilute (5%) phenol or (5%) bleach, sunlight, or ultraviolet radiation (Greene, 1990).

## References and Suggested Reading

Carpenter JL, Myers AM, Conner MW, et al: Tuberculosis in five basset hounds. J Am Vet Med Assoc 192:1563, 1988.
  *Case reports of systemic* M. avium *infection in related and unrelated basset hounds.*
Greene CE: Mycobacterial infections. *In* Greene CE (ed): *Infectious Diseases of the Dog and Cat.* Philadelphia, WB Saunders Co, 1990, pp 558–572.
  *General review that includes antituberculosis drug dosages.*
Inderlied CB, Kemper CA, and Bermudez LE: The *Mycobacterium avium* complex. Clin Microbiol Rev 6:266, 1993.
  *Comprehensive review of the disease in people.*
Isaac J, Whitehead J, Adams JW, et al: An outbreak of *Mycobacterium bovis* infection in cats in an animal house. Aust Vet J 60:243, 1983.
  *Investigation of a unique outbreak of feline mycobacteriosis in a research setting.*
Künkle BA, Gulbas NK, Fakok V, et al: Rapidly growing mycobacteria as a cause of cutaneous granulomas: Report of five cases. J Am Anim Hosp Assoc 19:513, 1983.
  *Case studies of dogs and cats with nontuberculous mycobacterial skin disease.*
Muller GH, Kirk RW, and Scott DW: *Small Animal Dermatology.* Philadelphia, WB Saunders Co, 1989, pp 272–278.
  *Discussion of cutaneous mycobacteriosis from the dermatologist's perspective.*
Mundell AC: New therapeutic agents in veterinary dermatology. Vet Clin North Am [Sm Anim Pract] 20:1541, 1990.
  *Review of current drugs available for cutaneous mycobacterial infection.*
Orr CM, Kelly DF, and Lucke VM: Tuberculosis in cats: a report of two cases. J Small Anim Pract 216:247, 1980.
  *Case reports of feline tuberculosis.*
Studdert VP and Hughes KL: Treatment of opportunistic mycobacterial infections with enrofloxacin in cats. J Am Vet Med Assoc 201:1388, 1992.
  *Report of successful treatment of cutaneous atypical mycobacteriosis.*
Wylie KB, Lewis DD, and Pechman RD: Hypertrophic osteopathy associated with *Mycobacterium fortuitum* pneumonia in a dog. J Am Vet Med Assoc 202:1986, 1993.
  *Case report of successful therapy for disseminated atypical mycobacterium.*

# OPPORTUNISTIC FUNGAL AND ALGAL INFECTIONS

ALICE M. WOLF

*College Station, Texas*

## OPPORTUNISTIC FUNGAL INFECTIONS

The systemic mycotic fungi (*Blastomyces dermatitidis*, *Coccidioides immitis*, *Cryptococcus neoformans*, and *Histoplasma capsulatum*) are primary pathogens of animals. A number of other fungal organisms occasionally infect dogs and cats as accidental or opportunistic pathogens. These fungal opportunists apparently gain access to the host through disruption of the cutaneous or mucocutaneous barrier. Although immunosuppressive disorders have been identified in association with many opportunistic mycoses in human beings, affected animals have rarely been identified as being immunosuppressed and the majority are otherwise apparently healthy individuals.

## Pythiosis

The causative agent of pythiosis, *Pythium insidiosum* (previously *Hyphomyces destruens*) is an aquatic organism of the order Peronosporales, phylum Oomycota, kingdom Protoctista. The term "phycomycosis" has also been previously used to refer to infections with this as well as some other fungal organisms now classified in the zygomycosis group. *Pythium* produces biflagellate zoospores that apparently are attracted to areas of damaged tissue and hair.

Pythiosis occurs most commonly in tropical and subtropical regions of the world. In the United States, the organism is endemic in states bordering the Gulf of Mexico. Pythiosis is most common in young, large-breed dogs; cats are rarely affected.

### GASTROINTESTINAL PYTHIOSIS

Gastrointestinal infection is the most common form of pythiosis in dogs. Single or multiple granulomatous fungal lesions can occur in any portion of the gastrointestinal tract. Clinical findings may include dysphagia, halitosis, anorexia, regurgitation, vomiting, diarrhea, or tenesmus, depending on the location of the fungal lesions. Physical examination may reveal weight loss, a thickened intestinal segment, or an abdominal mass. Lymph nodes draining the site of the fungal lesions may also be enlarged due to fungal invasion or secondary to inflammation. Routine hematologic and biochemistry studies are often normal; however, eosinophilia and hypoproteinemia with hypoalbuminemia have been found in some patients. Serum bilirubin and liver enzyme values may be elevated in patients with biliary obstruction secondary to granulomatous duodenitis. Ultrasound imaging or barium studies may demonstrate a mass lesion or filling defect.

### CUTANEOUS/SUPERFICIAL PYTHIOSIS

Cutaneous pythiosis occurs occasionally in dogs. Infection may occur in any site but usually involves the extremities, the tail-head, the perineum, or occasionally the face. The cutaneous fungal lesions are edematous, hairless, proliferative, and may be pruritic. They usually contain multiple ulcerations and drain serohemorrhagic exudate. Nasal and retrobulbar pythiosis has been described in one cat.

### DIAGNOSIS

The diagnosis of pythiosis is based on histopathologic identification of the organism and may be challenging because the condition is often overlooked, few organisms may be present, and staining with routine hematoxylin and eosin stains is inconsistent. Cytology specimens can be obtained with either exfoliative or aspiration techniques and stained with Wright's-Giemsa stain. In these, *Pythium* may be seen as wide, poorly septate, and branching "ghost" hyphae that are unstained amid the cellular debris. The presence of an eosinophilic component to the granulomatous infiltration should also raise the suspicion of pythiosis. Fungal stains may be used on both histopathologic and cytologic specimens to enhance detection of the organisms. *Pythium* may not stain well with periodic acid-Schiff (PAS) stain but is usually demonstrable with Gormori's methenamine silver (GMS) stain. Specific identification of the *Pythium* organism can be obtained by isolation in fungal culture or with indirect fluorescent antibody (IFA) techniques performed on tissue specimens at the Centers for Disease Control (Atlanta, GA).

### PROGNOSIS AND TREATMENT

Because the cell wall characteristics of *Pythium* spp. are different from other fungal agents, most attempts at antifungal chemotherapy for pythiosis have been unsuccessful. One cat with nasal and retrobulbar disease apparently responded to treatment with itraconazole. Complete surgical excision is the most effective treatment for pythiosis; unfortunately, involvement may be extensive by the time a diagnosis has been established.

## ZYGOMYCOSIS

Zygomycosis refers to infection with organisms in the class Zygomycetes that includes the genera *Mucor*, *Rhizomucor*, *Rhizopus*, *Absidia*, *Mortierella*, *Conidiobolus*, and *Basidiobolus*. Because specific identification of the infecting organism was not performed in most patients, infections with these organisms also appear in the older literature under the designation of phycomycosis. It is therefore difficult to separate the clinical signs and lesions caused by this group of organisms from those produced by *Pythium*. Most reported cases have had gastrointestinal tract, abdominal organ, or cutaneous involvement with signs and lesions similar to those described for pythiosis. Widely disseminated disease has been reported in some animals. The diagnosis of zygomycosis is based on finding the broad, poorly septate organisms in cytologic or histopathologic specimens and specific identification of the organism in fungal culture or by IFA testing. The prognosis for patients with zygomycosis is guarded unless the lesions can be completely excised. The sensitivity of these organisms to antifungal agents is variable and the selection of an antifungal agent should be based on specific culture and sensitivity testing.

## HYALOHYPHOMYCOSIS

### PAECILOMYCOSIS

*Paecilomyces* spp. are soil saprophytes with a ubiquitous distribution. Infection in both dogs and cats is rare. The fungal lesions begin as cutaneous granulomas and later disseminate to involve a wide variety of internal organs and tissues. The organism can be identified on fungal culture; cytologic and histopathologic specimens demonstrate thick, septate, pseudohyphae with bulbous dilatations. The prognosis for patients with paecilomycosis is grave because surgical management and antifungal chemotherapy have not been effective to date. Treatment with the newer azole antifungal drugs has not been reported; however, these agents may offer more promise in the treatment of this disease in the future.

### GEOTRICHOSIS

*Geotrichum candidum* is a saprophytic fungus found in soil and decaying organic matter. Disseminated geotrichosis has been described in three dogs. Severe granulomatous fungal pneumonia was the primary clinical finding; however, fungal lesions were disseminated in many organs and tissues. Disseminated geotrichosis was rapidly progressive and fatal in all reported patients. Two of these dogs had received corticosteroid therapy before a definitive diagnosis of fungal infection was made and it is not known whether steroid treatment affected the progression of their disease. Nevertheless, the prognosis for dogs with disseminated geotrichosis is grave.

### PSEUDOALLESCHERIOSIS

*Pseudoallescheria boydii* (*Scedosporium* or *Monosporium apiospermum*, *Pteriellidium boydii*, *Allescheria boydii*) is a saprophytic fungus that has been isolated from soil or sewage. Pseudoallescheriosis has only been reported in the dog and clinical findings include fever, orchitis, and abdominal organ involvement associated with diffuse peritonitis and peritoneal effusion. Diffuse fungal pneumonia attributed to *P. boydii* has been described in one dog; however, this diagnosis is in question because the organism can be a cultural contaminant and the organism was identified only on sputum culture in this patient. The prognosis for patients with pseudoallescheriosis is grave. Surgery is the treatment of choice for localized lesions. Successful antifungal chemotherapy of abdominal pseudoallescheriosis has not been reported; however, many isolates of *P. boydii* are reported to be susceptible to miconazole and the newer azole antifungals may be effective if extensive disease is not present.

## PHAEOHYPHOMYCOSIS

Phaeohyphomycosis in dogs and cats is caused by many organisms including those of the genera *Bipolaris* (*Dreshlera*), *Xylohypha* (*Cladosporium*), *Phialophora*, *Curvularia*, *Helminthosporium*, *Alternaria*, *Stemphylium*, *Exophiala* (*Phialophora*), *Fonsecaea*, *Rhinocladiella*, *Moniliella*, and *Phialemonium*. Most of these are ubiquitous fungal saprophytes found in wood and soil.

### SUBCUTANEOUS PHAEOHYPHOMYCOSIS

Subcutaneous infection on the extremities or head is the most common form of disease and probably results from wound contamination. Phaeohyphomycosis lesions begin as cutaneous papules or subcutaneous nodules that may develop fistulous tracts and ulcers exuding purulent material. Osteomyelitis of the underlying bone is present in some patients. The diagnosis of phaeohyphomycosis is made by recognition of the organism on cytologic or histopathologic examination and cultural identification of the causative agent. The prognosis for animals with subcutaneous phaeohyphomycosis is guarded. Complete surgical excision is the treatment of choice and has been effective in early, well-circumscribed lesions. Varying degrees of success have been achieved with antifungal agents including amphotericin B, flucytosine, ketoconazole, and itraconazole (see Legends).

### DISSEMINATED PHAEOHYPHOMYCOSIS

Cerebral or disseminated phaeohyphomycosis has been reported in both dogs and cats. Neurologic signs are acute in onset; rapidly progressive; and include seizures, opisthotonos, nystagmus, gait disturbances, and protrusion of the nictitating membranes. Disseminated infection produces a variety of signs involving organs of the respiratory, gastrointestinal, or urinary tract. Cerebral and disseminated phaeohyphomycosis have not been treated successfully and the diagnosis usually is made by identification and culture of the organism on necropsy examination.

## TRICHOSPORONOSIS

*Trichosporon* spp. are filamentous saprophytic yeasts that are ubiquitous in nature and are occasionally found as part of the normal cutaneous or mucous membrane flora. Trichosporosis has been described in three cats. Clinical findings in these patients included nasal cavity infection with fever; a nasal granuloma with associated nasal discharge; and regional lymphadenopathy in one patient, cutaneous nodules progressing to disseminated disease in another, and cystitis with urinary bladder invasion in the third. Diagnosis is based on the identification of the pleomorphic, septate, branching hyphae; arthroconidia; and budding yeast-like *Trichosporon* fungal elements in tissue sections. Identification can be confirmed by direct immunofluorescence testing. The prognosis for cats with trichosporosis is grave. Although azole antifungal agents may be effective against *Trichosporon* spp., treatment with ketoconazole was unsuccessful in the cat with nasal disease, and death occurred before treatment was initiated in the other two patients.

## CANDIDIASIS

*Candida albicans* is part of the normal flora of the nasal, genital, and gastrointestinal mucosa. Oral candidial overgrowth has been reported secondary to oral and mucocutaneous ulcerative diseases in immunosuppressed animals. Generalized cutaneous or systemic candidiasis has been described in several dogs and cats but is rare. Clinical findings in affected animals include fever, dermatitis, anterior uveitis, pleural effusion, myositis, osteomyelitis with fistulous tracts, diarrhea, and brainstem or cerebellar dysfunction. Diagnosis is based on recognition of budding yeasts, pseudohyphae, or true hyphae in cytologic specimens or tissue sections, and microbiologic isolation of *Candida albicans* in fungal culture. The prognosis for patients with cutaneous or mucocutaneous candidiasis is fair. Superficial candidial lesions can be treated with topical antifungal agents (miconazole, clotrimazole, amphotericin B lotion). Systemic or disseminated candidiasis may respond to treatment with amphotericin B or the azole antifungal agents; however, the prognosis for these animals is grave.

## OPPORTUNISTIC ALGAL INFECTIONS

### Protothecosis

The *Prototheca* spp. are colorless algae with a saprophytic, fungus-like mode of nutrition. They are ubiq-

uitous in the environment and have a worldwide distribution. Two species, *Prototheca wickerhamii* and *P. zopfii*, are pathogenic for mammals. Animals are probably constantly exposed to *Prototheca* in the environment, yet clinical disease is rare, suggesting that *Prototheca* are of low virulence or that animals possess a high level of natural resistance to this organism.

#### CUTANEOUS PROTOTHECOSIS

Cutaneous protothecosis caused by *Prototheca wickerhamii* probably results from percutaneous inoculation of the organism via trauma or wound contamination. Cutaneous disease is most common in the middle-aged or older cat. Lesions include solitary, soft or firm, mass lesions most frequently found on the limbs or head. Cutaneous protothecosis involving the skin or footpads has been reported in a few dogs. These lesions were deeper and more extensive than those reported in cats and affected large areas of skin, subcutaneous tissue, and some regional lymph nodes.

#### DISSEMINATED PROTOTHECOSIS

*Prototheca zopfii* causes disseminated protothecosis, the most common form of disease in the dog. There is no age predilection for this disease. Female dogs slightly outnumber males and the collie dog predominates in reported cases. The gastrointestinal tract is suspected to be the portal of entry for *P. zopfii* because colonic lesions causing chronic, intermittent, bloody diarrhea are present in most affected patients. Ocular lesions are also common and include chorioretinitis, exudative retinitis with retinal detachment, anterior uveitis, and panophthalmitis. Central nervous system (CNS) infection causes paresis, vestibular deficits, seizures, and deafness in some dogs. Kidney involvement may produce signs of renal insufficiency. Myocardial lesions are present in a few dogs, but clinical evidence of cardiac dysrhythmias or failure has not been reported.

Hematologic parameters in patients with protothecosis are often normal; a neutrophilic leukocytosis has been reported in several dogs. Biochemical profiles may be normal or reveal only minimal changes. Moderate increases in serum liver enzymes, blood urea nitrogen (BUN), or creatinine levels have been reported in a few patients. In a dog with CNS involvement, the analysis of cerebrospinal fluid (CSF) revealed an eosinophilic pleocytosis and elevated protein level. Proctoscopic examination may reveal diffuse thickening, reddening, and hemorrhage in the colonic and rectal mucosa. Radiographic examinations have not been performed in most patients but generally reveal only nonspecific enteritis.

#### DIAGNOSIS

The diagnosis of protothecosis is made most readily by identification of the organism on cytologic or histopathologic examination of affected tissues. *Prototheca* appear as round, unicellular organisms, 5 to 15 $\mu$m in diameter, with a definite, slightly refractile capsule. Pathogenic *Prototheca* spp. grow well on blood agar incubated at 37°C, producing small, flat, nonhemolytic, gray-white colonies within 72 hr. On Sabouraud dextrose agar incubated at 25°C, light tan to white, waxy, yeast-like colonies appear within 72 hr. Organisms taken from cultures can be readily identified with Gram stain. *Prototheca* may stain poorly with hematoxylin-eosin but can be more clearly defined by Giemsa, GMS, or PAS techniques. Definitive diagnosis and speciation of *Prototheca* can be obtained with IFA testing performed on formalin-fixed tissues or unstained tissue sections at the Centers for Disease Control.

### PROGNOSIS AND TREATMENT

The prognosis for patients with cutaneous protothecosis is guarded. The treatment of choice is surgical removal of affected tissues. Several cats have apparently responded to excision of well-circumscribed cutaneous lesions; however, long-term follow-up has not been reported. In reports of *in vitro* susceptibility studies of *P. zopfii* isolates from animals, about one third to one half of all pathogenic *Prototheca* strains were susceptible to gentamicin sulfate, amphotericin B, or polymyxin B, and all isolates were susceptible to nystatin. Unfortunately, amphotericin B, ketoconazole, oral nystatin with tetracycline, and simazine (an aquarium algicide) have not been clinically effective in the treatment of disseminated protothecosis in dogs. One dog was apparently successfully treated with liposome-encapsulated amphotericin B; however, long-term follow-up on this patient is not yet available and the prognosis for these patients remains grave.

## References and Suggested Reading

Allison N, McDonald RK, Guist SR, et al: Eumycotic mycetoma caused by *Pseudoallescheria boydii* in a dog. J Am Vet Med Assoc 194:797, 1989.

Beale KM and Pinson D: Phaeohyphomycosis caused by two different species of *Curvularia* in two animals from the same household. J Am Anim Hosp Assoc 26:67, 1990.

Bissonnette KW, Sharp NJH, Dykstra MH, et al: Nasal and retrobulbar mass in a cat caused by *Pythium insidiosum*. J Med Vet Mycol 29:39, 1991.

Connole MD: Review of animal mycoses in Australia. Mycopathologica 111:133, 1990.

Dhein CR, Leathers CW, Padhye AA, et al: Phaeohyphomycosis caused by *Alternaria alternata* in a cat. J Am Vet Med Assoc 193:1101, 1988.

Doster AR, Erickson ED, and Chandler FW: Trichosporonosis in two cats. J Am Vet Med Assoc 190:1184, 1987.

Elad D, Orgad U, Yakobson B, et al: Eumycetoma caused by *Curvularia lunata* in a dog. Mycopathologica 116:113, 1991.

Fiske RA, Choyce PD, Whitford HW, et al: Phaeohyphomycotic encephalitis in two dogs. J Am Anim Hosp Assoc 22:327, 1986.

Foil CS: Miscellaneous fungal infections. In: Greene CE (ed): *Infectious Diseases of the Dog and Cat*. Philadelphia, W.B. Saunders Co, 1990, p 731.

Fulton RB and Walker RD: *Candida albicans* urocystitis in a cat. J Am Vet Med Assoc 200:524, 1992.

Howerth EW, Brown CC, and Crowder C: Subcutaneous pythiosis in a dog. J Vet Diagn Invest 1:81, 1989.

Kettlewell P, McGinnis MR, and Wilkinson GT: Phaeohyphomycosis caused by *Exophiala spinifera* in two cats. J Med Vet Mycol 27:257, 1989.

Littman MP and Goldschmidt MH: Systemic paecilomycosis in a dog. J Am Vet Med Assoc 191:445, 1987.

Mancianti F, Giannelli C, Bendinelli M, et al: Mycological findings in feline immunodeficiency virus-infected cats. J Med Vet Mycol 30:257, 1992.

Migaki G, Casey HW, and Bayles WB: Cerebral phaeohyphomycosis in a dog. J Vet Med Assoc 191:997, 1987.

Miller WW and Albert RA: Ocular and systemic candidiasis in a cat. J Am Anim Hosp Assoc 24:521, 1988.

Pichler ME, Gross TL, and Kroll WR: Cutaneous and mucocutaneous candidiasis in a dog. Compend Cont Educ Pract Vet 7:225, 1985.

Rhyan JC, Stackhouse LL, and Davis EG: Disseminated geotrichosis in two dogs. J Am Vet Med Assoc 197:358, 1990.

Sharkey PK, Graybill JR, Rinaldi MG, et al: Itraconazole treatment of phaeohyphomycosis. J Am Acad Dermatol 23:577, 1990.

Walker RL, Monticello TM, Ford RB, et al: Eumycotic mycetoma caused by *Pseudoallescheria boydii* in the abdominal cavity of a dog. J Am Vet Med Assoc 192:67, 1988.

# ANTIMYCOTIC DRUG THERAPY

ALFRED M. LEGENDRE

*Knoxville, Tennessee*

The treatment of systemic fungal infection has been improved by two new imidazole drugs. Itraconazole and fluconazole are antifungal agents of the triazole group that can be given orally. These agents are effective and produce minimal adverse effects. In this article, the efficacy of these drugs is compared to that of more traditional drugs, amphotericin B and ketoconazole. Recommendations for treating specific fungal infections will be made.

## AMPHOTERICIN B

Amphotericin B remains the "gold standard" of antimycotic drugs. It produces a rapid response in fulminating fungal infections and is effective against many pathogenic fungi. It must be given intravenously and usually produces renal toxicosis. In fulminating life-threatening infections, amphotericin B is an excellent choice for initial treatment. Itraconazole may be an equally effective treatment for fulminant disease, but that is yet to be proven.

The principal toxicity of amphotericin B therapy is renal. Because renal toxicosis is more severe when amphotericin B is given to a dehydrated, sodium-depleted animal, rehydration prior to amphotericin B therapy is mandatory. An effective and safe treatment protocol for the dog is to give 0.5 mg/kg of amphotericin B diluted in 5% dextrose. In dogs with normal renal function, amphotericin B can be diluted in 60 to 120 ml and given by a slow intravenous injection over 15 min. When renal function is compromised, amphotericin B should be diluted in 500 ml to 1 L and given over 3 to 6 hr. The slower infusion rate minimizes the likelihood of renal injury. Amphotericin B should be given every other day if the serum blood urea nitrogen (BUN) concentration remains below 50 mg/dl. The BUN concentration should be measured before each dose to avoid irreversible renal failure. When the BUN concentration increases, intravenous fluid therapy may be beneficial. If the BUN value exceeds 50 mg/dl, discontinue amphotericin B therapy until the BUN concentration decreases to 35 mg/dl or less. A cumulative dose of at least 8 to 10 mg/kg of amphotericin B is necessary for cure of blastomycosis and histoplasmosis. A larger cumulative dose is needed for coccidioidomycosis, aspergillosis, and other fungal infections.

Amphotericin B usually improves the dog's clinical condition in 3 to 4 days. This rapid effect is not seen in dogs treated with ketoconazole, but in dogs with blastomycosis treated with itraconazole, the response time is similar to amphotericin B treatment. Cats are more sensitive than dogs to the nephrotoxicosis of amphotericin B. Cats have been effectively treated with doses of 0.25 mg/kg given slowly over 3 to 6 hr. With the introduction of newer, more effective triazole drugs, the situations that would warrant the use of amphotericin B in cats are extremely rare.

Although amphotericin B remains a mainstay of initial therapy, its use should be restricted to the first few days of a life-threatening systemic infection or in fungal infections that are unresponsive to other treatments. Because of the cost of intravenous administration and frequent laboratory testing, the total cost of amphotericin B therapy is similar to the cost of therapy with new triazoles.

## KETOCONAZOLE

Ketoconazole was the first antifungal drug of the imidazole family that could be given orally for treatment of systemic mycoses. It is effective against a number of the systemic fungi. Clinical response to treatment may take 10 days to 2 weeks. Ketoconazole can produce anorexia, vomiting, and hepatic toxicosis. The incidence of adverse effects is fairly low at the therapeutic dosage (10 mg/kg b.i.d). Ketoconazole interferes with steroid hormone synthesis and will decrease serum concentrations of testosterone and cortisol. Because of this it has been used to treat dogs with hyperadrenocorticism. The hormonal suppression may be harmful to pregnant animals and can produce infertility in male dogs. The triazoles do not affect steroid hormone concentrations.

Ketoconazole has effectively eliminated remaining fungal organisms when given after a short course of amphotericin B. Ketoconazole can be used as the sole therapy in more chronic infections when rapid onset of improvement is unnecessary. For some fungal infections, such as aspergillosis, the ketoconazole minimum inhibitory concentrations (MICs) measured for many of the isolates are high. The MICs may exceed the serum concentrations of ketoconazole that can be achieved without drug-induced toxicosis.

Ketoconazole has been very useful in cats with cryptococcosis but the 10 mg/kg twice-daily dosage can produce anorexia and debility in cats. Hepatic toxicosis is the principal toxicity of the drug in cats. The triazoles, itraconazole and fluconazole, are more effective and better tolerated by cats than is ketoconazole.

The principal advantage of ketoconazole over the newer triazoles is price. In coccidioidomycosis, long-term treatment is required to cure or control the disease. Ketoconazole appears to be as effective in this disease as itraconazole. At a therapeutic dosage for each drug, the cost of ketoconazole is about half that of itraconazole.

## FLUCONAZOLE

Fluconazole is a new triazole that is effective against *Candida* and *Cryptococcus* species. It is a water-soluble drug that attains concentrations in the central nervous system that approximate plasma concentrations. The drug is eliminated in large part by the kidneys, producing high concentrations in the urine. Adverse effects are similar to those produced by the other drugs of the imidazole family including anorexia and hepatic toxicosis. Malik et al. (1992) cured 28 of 29 cats with cryptococcosis involving the nasal passages and skin of the head. The cats were given 50 mg of fluconazole twice a day. The treatment was effective even in cats with concurrent feline immunodeficiency infections. Cure was achieved in 2 to 4 months in most cats but treatment should be continued 1 month beyond resolution of clinical signs. Serum concentrations of fluconazole vary greatly from cat to cat. This suggests that the dose could be increased in unresponsive cryptococcosis if the cat shows no drug toxicosis. The adverse effects noted by Malik et al. were mild anorexia initially in some cats and slight increases in serum alanine aminotransferase (ALT) activity. Fluconazole appears to be an excellent drug for feline cryptococcosis and the prognosis in this disease has been improved markedly. Malik's study did not include cats with ocular and central nervous system disease, but the good penetration of fluconazole into these tissues justifies an attempt at therapy with this drug.

Fluconazole is available from pharmacies in 50, 100- and 200-mg tablets and comes in an injectable form. It will cost about $18 a day to treat a cat with 50 mg twice daily (Diflucan, Roerig Division of Pfizer Inc). There are no drugs, including the triazoles, currently approved for the treatment of veterinary patients with systemic fungal infections.

## ITRACONAZOLE

Itraconazole is the latest triazole to become commercially available. We have been evaluating this drug in dogs and cats since 1987. Itraconazole is a lipid-soluble drug that is best given with food to enhance intestinal absorption. It has a broad spectrum of activity against the pathogenic fungi. It is effective in aspergillosis, blastomycosis, coccidioidomycosis, cryptococcosis, histoplasmosis, as well as some of the Zygomycetes and the pigmented fungi that cause phaeohyphomycosis. We have also seen improvement in dogs with Prototheca infections. Itraconazole appears to have a spectrum of activity that equals or exceeds that of amphotericin B.

The MICs of itraconazole against *Aspergillus* and *Blastomyces* species are about one tenth the MICs of ketoconazole for these organisms. Serum drug concentrations can be attained that are many times the MICs without producing significant toxicosis. Itraconazole is not found in urine or cerebrospinal fluid (CSF) in significant concentrations. In spite of low CSF concentrations, itraconazole was shown by Perfect et al. (1986) to be effective in a rabbit model of cryptococcal meningitis. This suggests that the lipid-soluble itraconazole is tissue bound in the nervous system and not free in the CSF.

About 10% of dogs given a 5-mg/kg dose twice daily of itraconazole developed hepatic toxicosis that was severe enough to temporarily require discontinuation of the therapy. About 5% of dogs given itraconazole at 5 mg/kg/day had hepatic toxicosis that required discontinuation of the drug. The most significant serum biochemical abnormality associated with itraconazole treatment is an increase in ALT activity. Less than 10% of dogs given 5 mg/kg/day and about 15% of dogs given 10 mg/kg/day of itraconazole developed increases in ALT activity greater than 200 IU/L. Increases in ALT activity above 200 IU/L were usually present by the time dogs developed drug-associated anorexia. Anorexia is an excellent way to monitor for itraconazole toxicity. When anorexia occurs, it usually develops during the second month of treatment. This helps to separate anorexia associated with fungal disease from anorexia due to the itraconazole treatment. Appetite usually returns 3 or 4 days after discontinuing itraconazole. Monthly measurements of serum ALT activity is recommended to monitor hepatic effects of treatment.

Hepatic injury tends to occur in dogs with the highest serum concentrations of the drug, though some dogs with modest serum itraconazole concentrations have developed liver toxicosis. The serum drug concentrations may vary up to tenfold in dogs receiving the same dose of the drug. Serum concentrations can be measured (Dr. Mike Rinaldi at the Fungus Testing Lab, University of Texas Health Science Center, 7703 Floyd Curl Drive, San Antonio, TX 78284, (Tel. 512-567-4131). Without a serum concentration to guide dosage adjustments, it is wise to stop treatment until the appetite returns. Itraconazole treatment can be restarted at half the original dosage. Most dogs that develop hepatic toxicosis have high serum drug concentrations and will still benefit from therapy at the reduced dose.

A bizarre adverse effect attributed to itraconazole therapy is ulcerative dermatitis and limb edema. It occurs in less than 10% of the dogs given 10 mg/kg/day of itraconazole. It has not been seen in cats given 10 mg/kg/day or in dogs given 5 mg/kg/day of itraconazole. The affected dogs develop 1- to 2-cm circular areas of necrotic skin that eventually slough and ulcerate. These skin changes are due to a vasculitis. The lesions resolve after discontinuation of the itraconazole treatment. When dogs with ulcerative dermatitis were retreated at half the original dosage the skin lesions did not recur.

Although the incidence of adverse effects in cats has not been quantified, cats tolerate itraconazole better than ketoconazole. A number of cats that were anorexic on ketoconazole tolerated itraconazole at dosages of 5 mg/kg twice daily. Cats may develop hepatic toxicosis and anorexia on itraconazole therapy. The anorexia usually resolves quickly after the drug is discontinued, but there is always concern about inducing anorexia-related hepatic lipidosis.

Itraconazole comes in 100-mg capsules (Sporanox, Janssen Pharmaceutical). The capsules contain small pellets that can be put into food. This is especially useful in treating cats. The cats will readily eat the food containing the itraconazole. Treatment of a 20-kg dog given 10 mg/kg/day costs about $10 a day.

## RECOMMENDATIONS FOR SPECIFIC FUNGAL INFECTIONS

### Nasal Aspergillosis

Most nasal fungal infections are caused by *Aspergillus fumigatus*. Sharp et al. (1993) describe the treatment of 24 dogs with nasal flushes containing 10 mg/kg of enilconazole twice a day for 7 to 14 days. This treatment eliminated the infection in 20 of the 24 dogs. Surgical implantation of tubes into the nasal cavity and the frontal sinus are required because enilconazole must have direct contact with the infected tissues. Animals with deep tissue infections of the nasal area are not suitable for enilconazole therapy. Enilconazole is available from Sterwin Laboratories Inc, Millsboro, DE 19966-0537 (Tel 1-800-633-0462). The brand name is Clinafarm-EC and the drug is distributed as a fungicide to control *Aspergillus* in hatcheries.

Itraconazole and amphotericin B are effective in the treatment of aspergillosis, but resistance may develop to amphotericin B therapy. Itraconazole will cure approximately 60 to 70% of dogs with nasal aspergillosis when given at 5 mg/kg twice daily for at least 60 to 90 days. It is difficult to be specific about the response rate in newly diagnosed cases because many of the dogs treated in our study had received multiple prior treatments.

The considerations to be weighed are cost, convenience, and the concerns about surgery and anesthesia. Enilconazole cures a greater number of dogs than itraconazole but requires surgical implantation of tubes in the nasal passages. Aspergillosis occurs mainly in large dogs, which makes the cost of long-term treatment with itraconazole expensive (see this volume, p 899).

## Systemic Aspergillosis

*Aspergillus tereus* and other species of *Aspergillus* cause infection of long bones, vertebrae, and the kidneys. Before itraconazole became available, systemic aspergillosis had a guarded to hopeless prognosis because prolonged treatment with amphotericin B caused renal toxicosis. Many dogs with systemic aspergillosis can be maintained with 5 mg/kg twice daily of itraconazole, but cure is uncommon. Aspergillosis of the urinary tract makes treatment difficult because itraconazole is not excreted through the kidneys.

## Blastomycosis

*Blastomyces dermatitides* organisms are very sensitive to itraconazole. Treatment with 5 mg/kg/day of itraconazole appears as effective as amphotericin B alone or amphotericin B plus ketoconazole. An initial drug loading with 5-mg/kg twice daily for 4 days is recommended. The 5 mg/kg daily dose in dogs with blastomycosis is as effective as the 10-mg/kg/day dose. This makes the cost of itraconazole therapy more affordable. Cats with blastomycosis are treated with 5 mg/kg twice daily because they don't seem to absorb the drug as well as dogs. We have had good results with itraconazole treatment of cats with blastomycosis.

Treatment in blastomycosis should be continued for at least 60 days or until all clinical signs have been resolved for 30 days. Serum antibody titers are not helpful in monitoring the course of the disease or in the identification of recurrence of disease. Severity of disease at the initial examination can be used to determine the duration of treatment. Dogs with severe lung involvement should be treated for at least 90 days. Relapse will occur in about 20 to 25% of dogs regardless of treatment. Dogs that have recurrence can be retreated with itraconazole because the organisms don't seem to develop drug resistance.

A study done by Brooks et al. (1991) showed that 76% of dogs with ocular blastomycosis of the posterior segment (subretinal granulomas, retinitis, and chorioretinitis) responded to itraconazole. Involvement of the anterior segment responded poorly to itraconazole. This study suggest that itraconazole will penetrate into infected eyes. Blind eyes should be removed to eliminate a possible nidus of disease.

## Coccidiodomycosis

Based on a very limited experience with itraconazole in the treatment of coccidioidomycosis, itraconazole does not seem to be superior to ketoconazole. The general recommendation of initial therapy with amphotericin B at 0.5 mg/kg intravenously every other day to control fulminating disease and ketoconazole at 10 mg/kg twice daily to continue treatment is still valid. Antibody titers are helpful in monitoring the response of coccidioidomycosis to treatment. Long-term treatment is usually required.

## Cryptococcosis

Cryptococcosis is mainly a disease of cats, although dogs are occasionally affected. The response to fluconazole treatment reported by Malik et al. (1992) is superior to our experience with itraconazole therapy, but many of our cats with cryptococcosis had disseminated disease. Fluconazole, 50 mg per cat twice a day, for at least 2 to 4 months is recommended. Fluconazole penetrates well into the CSF and the eye, giving it additional therapeutic advantages. Long-term therapy appears to be necessary to eliminate the infection. The latex agglutination cryptococcal capsular antigen titers of serum are helpful in determining the proper time to discontinue therapy. All signs of infection should be resolved for at least 1 to 2 months and the antigen titers should be negative before therapy is discontinued.

In cryptococcosis refractory to fluconazole, itraconazole at 5 mg/kg twice daily can be used. Cats, like dogs, have very variable plasma concentrations of fluconazole and itraconazole. In unresponsive cats, the dose may be increased if there are no signs of drug-induced toxicosis.

## Histoplasmosis

Histoplasmosis in cats responds well to itraconazole given at a dose of 5 mg/kg twice daily. The cats should be treated for at least 60 to 90 days or until all signs have been resolved for 1 month.

Histoplasmosis in dogs generally responds well to itraconazole given at a dose of 5 mg/kg twice daily. Some dogs that did not respond well were treated with amphotericin B at 0.5 mg/kg intravenously every other day for four or five doses and the treatment was completed with itraconazole. Dogs with intestinal histoplasmosis and malabsorption may require an initial course of amphotericin B therapy before adequate absorption of the itraconazole can be expected. Histoplasmosis usually requires at least 3 months of treatment to resolve the infection or treatment for at least 1 month beyond the resolution of clinical signs. Titers are not helpful in evaluating response to treatment.

## Sporotrichosis

Sporotrichosis in dogs and cats appears to be relatively sensitive to itraconazole therapy. Treatment with 5 mg/kg twice daily is recommended for dogs and cats. Itraconazole is more expensive than the standard sodium iodide therapy but is better tolerated, especially by cats. Therapy should be continued for at least 1 month after clinical signs have resolved. Care should be taken in the treatment of cats with sporotrichosis because infection in people can occur from contact with infected cats.

## Miscellaneous Fungal Infections

A number of the pigmented fungi that are normally saprophytic organisms in the soil can be pathogenic. There are insufficient data to quantitate the number of these infections that will respond to itraconazole, but itraconazole is effective against some of the isolates of these organisms. A trial of itraconazole at 5 mg/kg twice daily for 1 month is worthwhile. Surgery may be helpful to remove mycetomas that cannot be cured with medical therapy.

## References and Suggested Reading

Brooks DE, Legendre AM, Gum GG, et al: The treatment of canine ocular blastomycosis with systemically administered itraconazole. Progress Vet Comp Ophthalmol 1:263,1991.
Grant SM and Clissold SP: Itraconazole—a review of its pharmacodynamic and pharmacokinetic properties, and therapeutic use in superficial and systemic mycoses. Drugs 37:310–344, 1989.
Malik R, Wigney, DI, Muir, DB, et al: Cryptococcosis in cats: Clinical and mycological assessment of 29 cases and evaluation of treatment using orally administered fluconazole. J Med Vet Mycology 30:133, 1992.
Perfect JR, Savani DV, Durack DT: Comparison of itraconazole and fluconazole in treatment of cryptococcal meningitis and candida pyelonephritis in rabbits. Antimicrob Agents Chemother 29:579, 1986.
Sharp NJH, Sullivan M, Harvey CE, et al: Treatment of canine nasal aspergillosis with enilconazole. J Vet Intern Med 7:40, 1993.
Supplement 1. Rev of Infect Dis. 9:S1–152, 1987.

# Section

# 5

# ENDOCRINE AND METABOLIC DISORDERS

MARK E. PETERSON
*Consulting Editor*

# *CVT* UPDATE: SAMPLE COLLECTION AND TESTING PROTOCOLS IN ENDOCRINOLOGY

ROBERT J. KEMPPAINEN
*Auburn, Alabama*

*and* TERRENCE P. CLARK
*De Pere, Wisconsin*

This article is an update to material in *Current Veterinary Therapy X* (p 761) (Kemppainen and Zerbe, 1989). That article described our recommendations for performing routine veterinary endocrine diagnostic tests. Our recommended protocols for several of the tests, listed in Table 1, have not changed and are not covered here. Instead, this article discusses revisions to some of the testing protocols and adds new procedures to the list. In addition, sample collection and submission recommendations followed by the Auburn University Endocrine Diagnostic Laboratory for measurement of specific hormones are included.

## COLLECTION AND SUBMISSION OF SAMPLES FOR HORMONE MEASUREMENT

### General Instructions

Because of the potential loss of hormone immunoreactivity, special consideration should be given to sample collection and handling. Endocrine diagnostic laboratories vary in their protocols recommended for collection, storage, and shipping of samples. It is therefore important for clinicians to adhere to the methods recommended by the reference laboratory they choose.

In general, a plasma or serum sample is recommended for hormone measurement, and under no circumstance should whole or clotted blood be submitted to the laboratory. Samples should not be mailed in glass containers (including serum separator tubes). Samples should be mailed in protected containers and not in envelopes. We recommend that one ship samples early in the week and use a fast, reliable form of delivery service. Before collecting samples, tubes should be prelabeled with the appropriate information including the owner's name, patient's name, and the hormone to be measured. If baseline and one or more post-samples are required for a test procedure, the tubes should be clearly labeled to indicate the time on each sample. If the clinician is interested in obtaining interpretive assistance concerning the results, a brief description of the history and clinical status is helpful. It is best to contact the reference laboratory prior to submitting samples from species that are less commonly seen in veterinary practice.

We recommend that serum samples be collected into plain glass (red-top) tubes. Blood should be allowed to completely clot at room temperature, centrifuged as soon as possible, and the serum collected. For plasma, we recommend collecting the sample into an ethylenediaminetetraacetic acid (EDTA) (purple-top) tube. The sample should be centrifuged within 15 min of collection, and the plasma collected. Samples of serum or plasma should be preferably placed into snap-top plastic (polypropylene) tubes. If the sample is not immediately packaged for shipment to the laboratory, the serum or plasma should be refrigerated or frozen until shipment. One should avoid submission of samples with severe hemolysis or lipemia, although this is sometimes impossible. Specific instructions for each hormone are discussed below.

### CORTISOL

A minimum of 1 ml of serum or plasma is required for cortisol measurement. Given a choice, we prefer plasma aspirated from blood collected into EDTA tubes. The sample should be securely packaged in an insulated container with at least one frozen refrigerant pack. It is ideal to mail the sample using next-day or second-day delivery service (to avoid more than 3 days in transit). Cortisol is sensitive to the effects of temperature, and data from our laboratory suggest that this loss of cortisol is reduced when plasma is obtained using EDTA compared with storage in serum.

### TOTAL THYROXINE AND TRIIODOTHYRONINE

A minimum of 1 ml of plasma or serum is required to measure thyroxine ($T_4$) and triiodothyronine ($T_3$). Unlike cortisol, cold conditions for shipment are not required for thyroid hormones. Therefore, securely packaged samples can be shipped by regular mail service. Although it was reported that hemolysis and lipemia had relatively little effect on measurement of $T_4$ and $T_3$ (Reimers, 1989), we have noticed artifactual elevations in $T_3$ concentrations in occasional highly lipemic samples.

335

**Table 1.**  *List of Endocrine Testing Procedures Described Previously°*

Basal or resting plasma or serum cortisol
ACTH stimulation test
Low-dose dexamethasone suppression test
High-dose dexamethasone suppression test
Combined dexamethasone suppression–ACTH stimulation test
Plasma endogenous ACTH measurement[†]
Metyrapone suppression test
Basal or resting plasma or serum thyroxine ($T_4$) or triiodothyronine ($T_3$)
Thyrotropin (TSH) stimulation test[†]
Fasting serum insulin
Serum or plasma progesterone and other gonadal hormones
Basal and stimulated growth hormone

°Data from Kemppainen RJ and Zerbe CA: Common endocrine diagnostic tests: Normal values and interpretation. *In* Kirk RW (ed): *Current Veterinary Therapy X: Small Animal Practice.* Philadelphia, WB Saunders Co, 1989, p 961, with permission.
[†]Updated in this article.

### GONADAL STEROIDS

A minimum of 1 ml of plasma or serum should be submitted for testosterone or progesterone measurement. These hormones are temperature sensitive; therefore, packaging samples in insulated containers with frozen refrigerant packs and rapid mail delivery are recommended.

### INSULIN

A minimum of 1 ml of plasma or serum should be submitted for insulin measurement. Insulin is temperature sensitive; therefore, packaging in insulated containers with frozen refrigerant packs and shipment using next-day or second-day mail service is recommended. In addition, insulin measurement is affected by hemolysis, so this should be avoided. Because a validated feline insulin assay is not always available in laboratories offering canine insulin measurement, check with your lab before submitting a sample for feline insulin measurement.

### Plasma Endogenous ACTH, Free $T_4$ By Equilibrium Dialysis, Urinary Cortisol/Creatinine Ratio

Recommendations for collection and submission of samples for determination of plasma endogenous adrenocorticotrophic hormone (ACTH), free $T_4$ ($FT_4$), and urinary cortisol/creatinine ratio are discussed below in the sections on endocrine testing protocols.

## UPDATES ON ENDOCRINE TESTING PROTOCOLS PREVIOUSLY DISCUSSED IN *CVT X*

### Thyroid-Stimulating Hormone Stimulation Test

USE.    To diagnose hypothyroidism in dogs.
PRINCIPLE.    In most dogs, hypothyroidism is due to direct destruction of the thyroid gland. Consequently, dogs with complete thyroid loss or with a failing thyroid gland lack a reserve and fail to show a significant increase in plasma or serum $T_4$ levels after thyroid-stimulating hormone (TSH) injection. In contrast, TSH injection in euthyroid dogs results in a clear increase in $T_4$ concentrations in a period of a few (4 to 8) hours.

METHOD.    Thyroid-stimulating hormone is difficult to obtain, and the veterinary product is often unavailable. Another source is TSH supplied for human use (Thyropar, Rhone-Poulenc Rorer Pharmaceuticals, Collegeville, PA). Thyroid-stimulating hormone is stable for several months when diluted and frozen (Kobayashi, Nichols, and Peterson, 1990). The TSH can be diluted and stored frozen in aliquots in syringes. To perform the test, collect a baseline (pre-TSH) blood sample for plasma or serum $T_4$ determination, and inject 0.1 U TSH/per kilogram intravenously. Collect a post-TSH sample for $T_4$ determination 4 to 6 hr later. The response to even lower doses of TSH (1.0 U/dog) has been reported in normal dogs (Beale, Helm, and Keisling, 1990).

NORMAL VALUES.    The magnitude of the increase in plasma or serum $T_4$ after TSH is directly related to the dose of TSH. In healthy dogs, normal pre-TSH $T_4$ concentrations are 20 to 55 nmol/L (1.5 to 4.3 $\mu$g/dl), and normal post-TSH $T_4$ values (after 0.1 U TSH/kg) are greater than 40 nmol/L. If TSH is given at 1 U/dog, normal post-TSH $T_4$ concentrations were reportedly greater than 32 nmol/L (Beale, Helm, and Keisling, 1990).

INTERPRETATION.    In dogs with primary hypothyroidism, pre-TSH $T_4$ values are either below normal or in a borderline low range, and have little to no increase in $T_4$ in response to TSH administration. Dogs with pre-TSH $T_4$ concentrations in the mid-normal range or greater are unlikely to be hypothyroid. Equivocal responses are seen occasionally in response to TSH. When an equivocal response occurs, the veterinarian has the following options: (1) to observe the clinical progression for several weeks to months, (2) to repeat testing with TSH in 2 to 4 months, (3) to perform $FT_4$ measurement using equilibrium dialysis (see below), or (4) to conduct a therapeutic trial using $T_4$ replacement therapy.

### Plasma Endogenous ACTH Measurement

USES.    To differentiate pituitary-dependent hyperadrenocorticism (PDH) from hyperadrenocorticism due to an adrenocortical tumor (AT) in dogs. Plasma ACTH measurement is recommended only in cases where the diagnosis of hyperadrenocorticism has been clearly established. The test is particularly useful when administration of high doses (0.1 to 1.0 mg/kg) of dexamethasone has failed to significantly suppress serum or plasma cortisol concentrations. Plasma ACTH concentrations are also used to differentiate primary from secondary hypoadrenocorticism.

PRINCIPLE. Plasma ACTH concentrations are in mid-normal to above-normal range in dogs with PDH and low to nondetectable in dogs with AT (due to cortisol negative feedback on the "normal" pituitary in this condition). Concentrations of ACTH are elevated in primary, but low in secondary, hypoadrenocortisim.

METHOD. The easiest way to submit a sample for ACTH determination is to obtain a sample collection tube from a veterinary endocrine reference laboratory containing EDTA and the enzyme inhibitor, aprotinin (Sigma Chemical, St. Louis, MO; Trasylol, Miles Inc, FBA Pharmaceutical, West Haven, CT). At our laboratory* we add aprotinin to EDTA-containing vacutainer tubes and mail them upon request to veterinarians. The aprotinin is added to provide 500 kallikrein inactivator units per milliliter of whole blood; it is important to fill these tubes to their total draw capacity.

Once the blood is collected into these tubes, the sample is centrifuged immediately at room temperature, and the plasma collected is placed into plastic tubes and stored at 4°C. The sample should be shipped immediately (within 1 day of collection) in a container with two frozen refrigerant packs using next-day or second-day delivery. The endocrine diagnostic laboratory used should ensure a valid assay for dog ACTH, and they should also indicate that they have tested the effectiveness of aprotinin to preserve ACTH. Because canine ACTH is unstable when collected in the absence of aprotinin, substantial loss of the hormone in plasma will occur within 2 days of collection even when stored at 4°C.

NORMAL VALUES. Normal values for canine ACTH in our laboratory are 10 to 80 pg/ml (2 to 16 pmol/L). In cats, normal values are 5 to 85 pg/ml (1 to 17 pmol/L).

INTERPRETATION. In our laboratory, endogenous ACTH measurement is recommended most commonly in dogs with confirmed hyperadrenocorticism that do not show suppressed plasma cortisol in response to high doses of dexamethasone. This occurs in up to 20% of dogs with subsequently proven PDH. In our experience, about half of dogs with hyperadrenocorticism that fail to have suppressed cortisol concentrations after administration of a high dose of dexamethasone have PDH, whereas the remaining half have AT.

One reason for the limited use of plasma endogenous ACTH measurement is related to the (previous) stringent requirements for sample collection and submission (e.g., centrifugation of blood at 4°C, submission of frozen plasma in dry ice). These restrictions often made the test impractical in clinical situations. Collection of blood into aprotinin-containing tubes preserves accurate estimation of ACTH without the need to maintain frozen plasma and, therefore, packing with several pounds of dry ice for transport to the reference laboratory. It is possible that use of aprotinin as a preservative, or use of other practical methods to preserve the hormone in plasma, will increase the use of measurement of this hormone by veterinarians in practice.

---

*Auburn University Endocrine Diagnostic Laboratory

## ENDOCRINE TESTING PROTOCOLS NOT DISCUSSED IN *CVT X*

### T₃ Suppression Test

USE. To diagnose hyperthyroidism in cats, especially cats with clinical signs of the disease and $T_4$ and $T_3$ concentrations that remain within the normal range (mild hyperthyroidism).

PRINCIPLE. Exogenous $T_3$ will suppress secretion of pituitary TSH and therefore lower $T_4$ (and $T_3$) secretion from the thyroid. In cats with hyperthyroidism, secretion of $T_4$ and $T_3$ is autonomous and TSH is already suppressed. Multiple doses of exogenous $T_3$ will suppress $T_4$ in normal but not hyperthyroid cats.

METHOD. To perform the test, first obtain a blood sample for plasma or serum $T_4$ and $T_3$ measurement. Next administer $T_3$ (liothyronine; Cytobin, SmithKline Beecham Animal Health, Exton, PA) at a dosage of 25 mg per cat every 8 hr PO for 2 days, then give the seventh dose on the morning of the third day. Obtain a blood sample for plasma or serum $T_4$ and $T_3$ measurement 4 hr after the last dosage of liothyronine. Submit both the baseline and postliothyronine plasma or serum samples to a reference laboratory for $T_4$ and $T_3$ assay.

NORMAL VALUES. The $T_4$ concentration after liothyronine administration should be less than 20 nmol/L (1.5 $\mu$g/dl). The $T_3$ concentration after liothyronine administration should be increased relative to the baseline $T_3$ concentration.

INTERPRETATION. A $T_4$ concentration greater than 20 nmol/L after liothyronine administration is consistent with hyperthyroidism. The $T_3$ measurement after liothyronine administration is necessary to ensure that the $T_3$ was properly administered. The $T_3$ concentration after liothyronine administration is usually increased 50 to 100% relative to the baseline concentration (before liothyronine administration). Inadequate $T_3$ pill administration by owners can lead to false-positive test results, since sufficient $T_3$ may not be absorbed to suppress TSH, and therefore $T_4$ concentrations, in euthyroid cats.

### T₄ by Equilibrium Dialysis

USE. To diagnose hypothyroidism in dogs.

PRINCIPLE. Most of the $T_4$ in the circulation is bound to proteins, whereas a small fraction circulates free. Because this free fraction is thought to be biologically active, it is the best indicator of thyroid function at the cellular level. Variations in $T_4$-binding-protein status could have a large effect on total $T_4$ ($TT_4$) concentration, while $FT_4$ concentration would not be affected by such changes.

Equilibrium dialysis provides a more accurate means to estimate $FT_4$ than other procedures (e.g., $FT_4$ analog methods), especially in dogs with nonthyroidal illness or dogs receiving certain drugs (e.g., glucocorticoids). It has been shown, however, that approximately 25%

of dogs with hyperadrenocorticism had low $FT_4$ concentrations, in conjunction with low $TT_4$ (Ferguson and Peterson, 1992). Free $T_4$ by equilibrium dialysis is more time consuming and costly than some other commercially available methods to estimate $FT_4$, but it presently appears to provide the most accurate estimation.

METHOD. Obtain a blood sample under resting conditions and collect approximately 1 ml of *serum*. Ship the sample in an insulated container with frozen refrigerant packs. Preferably, sample should arrive at testing laboratory within 2 days.

NORMAL VALUES. In dogs, normal $FT_4$ by equilibrium dialysis in our laboratory is 8 to 40 pmol/L.

INTERPRETATION. Values less than 8 nmol/L are consistent with hypothyroidism. Although our laboratory offers this test, we have not had extensive experience with it (see "Free Thyroid Hormone Determinations in the Diagnosis of Thyroid Disease," this volume, p 360). We hope that measurement of $FT_4$ by this method (Nichols Institute, San Juan Capistrano, CA) will allow for a more definitive separation of hypothyroidism from euthyroidism, compared with determination of $TT_4$. A test with clear discrimination potential would be of particular value in dogs with borderline low $TT_4$ concentration, or in animals with low $TT_4$ concentration that also have nonthyroidal disease or are receiving drugs that may suppress serum $T_4$ and $T_3$ concentrations. Since TSH is expensive and may be difficult to obtain, alternative testing methods are needed.

## Thyrotropin-Releasing Hormone Stimulation Test

USES. May be used in the diagnosis of hypothyroidism or for the diagnosis of feline hyperthyroidism. This test, like the $T_3$ suppression test, is especially useful in cats with mild hyperthyroidism that have clinical signs of the disease and normal or only mildly elevated basal or resting concentrations of $T_4$ and $T_3$ (Peterson, Broussard, and Gamble, in press).

PRINCIPLE. Thyrotropin-releasing hormone (TRH) is a hypothalamic peptide that stimulates the release of TSH from the pituitary gland. Injection of TRH should increase TSH concentration, followed by an increase in levels of $T_4$. Because assays to accurately measure canine or feline TSH are not yet available, only $T_4$ concentration is determined. The increase in $T_4$ in response to TRH is reduced or absent in dogs with either secondary (i.e., lesion at the pituitary) or primary (i.e., lesion at the thyroid) hypothyroidism. In cats with hyperthyroidism, autonomous secretion of $T_4$ and $T_3$ suppress TSH synthesis and secretion so that cats with the disease have little to no increase in $T_4$ after TRH.

METHOD. For dogs, obtain a baseline (pre-TRH) blood sample for plasma or serum $T_4$ measurement. Inject TRH (protirelin; Thypinone, Abbott Laboratories, North Chicago, IL) at 0.1 mg/kg IV, and collect a post-TRH blood sample 6 hr later. Submit pre-TRH and post-TRH plasma or serum samples for $T_4$ mea-

surement. Higher dosages of TRH are associated with side effects (e.g., salivation, vomiting).

For cats, collect a pre-TRH sample and give 0.1 mg/kg TRH IV, and obtain a post-TRH plasma or serum sample 4 hr later. Side effects (vomiting, tachypnea, salivation) are common in cats immediately following injection of TRH.

NORMAL VALUES. In normal dogs, baseline serum $T_4$ concentrations range from 20 to 55 nmol/L (1.5 to 4.3 $\mu$g/dl). On average, TRH injection results in a 1.5-fold increase in $T_4$ from the pre-TRH concentration (i.e., a 30 nmol/L $T_4$ pre-TRH value should increase to 45 nmol/L post-TRH).

In normal cats, baseline serum $T_4$ concentrations range from 10 to 50 nmol/L; TRH injection results in an increase in $T_4$ by at least 50 to 60% relative to the pre-TRH value (i.e., a 20 nmol/L pre-TRH $T_4$ value should increase to 32 nmol/L or greater).

INTERPRETATION. A normal increase in $T_4$ in response to TRH indicates a functional pituitary-thyroid axis. Triiodothyronine concentrations change little in response to TRH and, therefore, are of limited diagnostic value in the TRH stimulation test.

In our experience, the usefulness of the TRH stimulation test in dogs is somewhat limited by the fact that the response to TRH is quite small and a percentage (about 25%) of even healthy dogs show little to no increase in $T_4$ after injection of TRH. This is in contrast to the increase in $T_4$ in response to even relatively low doses of TSH, which is more consistent. A normal response to TRH tends to rule out hypothyroidism, but a reduced response should not be used as definitive evidence to confirm hypothyroidism. The $T_4$ response to TRH has not been thoroughly evaluated in dogs with nonthyroidal illness or in dogs receiving drugs possibly affecting the thyroid.

In cats with hyperthyroidism, the magnitude of the increase in $T_4$ is reduced compared with the response in euthyroid cats. Whereas euthyroid cats show at least a 60% increase in $T_4$ concentration comparing baseline to post-TRH samples, an increase of 50% or less is consistent with a diagnosis of hyperthyroidism (Peterson, Broussard, and Gamble, in press). Increases between 50 and 60% relative to basal $T_4$ are considered equivocal.

## Urinary Cortisol/Creatinine Ratio

USE. As a screening test for hyperadrenocorticism in dogs.

PRINCIPLE. Cortisol and its metabolites are excreted in the urine, and the amount of this excretion increases in hyperadrenocorticism. Determination of the ratio of urine cortisol to creatinine corrects for variations in urine concentration (of dilution).

METHOD. Collect a urine sample, centrifuge to remove debris, and submit (1 ml) to a reference laboratory in an insulated container containing frozen refrigerant packs.

NORMAL VALUES. Normal urine cortisol/creatinine

ratios in dogs range from 0.5 to $20 \times 10^{-6}$ in our laboratory (there are no units and usually the $10^{-6}$ is omitted).

INTERPRETATION. In dogs with hyperadrenocorticism, urine cortisol/creatinine ratio is almost always increased above the normal range. However, the ratio is also elevated in many dogs with nonadrenal illness (Smiley and Peterson, 1993). Therefore, while this test appears highly sensitive in detecting hyperadrenocorticism, it is nonspecific. The test can be used as a screening procedure, and values in the normal range can be interpreted to mean that hyperadrenocorticism is highly unlikely. As with other screening tests for hyperadrenocorticism (such as the low-dose dexamethasone suppression and ACTH stimulation tests), false-positive results are not uncommon. The best way to avoid this problem is to restrict use of these tests to patients that have clear historical and clinical evidence of hyperadrenocorticism. Results of any of these screening procedures should be interpreted cautiously in patients with evidence of nonadrenal illness.

## References and Suggested Reading

Beale KM, Helm LJ, and Keisling K: Comparison of two doses of aqueous bovine thyrotropin for thyroid function testing in dogs. J Am Vet Med Assoc 197:865, 1990.

Comparison of the increase in serum $T_4$ concentration in healthy dogs in response to either 1 or 5 U of bovine TSH.

Ferguson DC and Peterson ME: Serum free and total iodothyronine concentrations in dogs with hyperadrenocorticism. Am J Vet Res 53:1636, 1992.

Comparison of total $T_4$, $T_3$, reverse $T_3$, and free $T_4$ concentrations in healthy dogs and 42 dogs with hyperadrenocorticism.

Kemppainen RJ and Zerbe CA: Common endocrine diagnostic tests: Normal values and interpretation. In Kirk RW (ed): Current Veterinary Therapy X: Small Animal Practice. Philadelphia, WB Saunders Co, 1989, p 961.

Discussion of methods for and interpretation of endocrine tests commonly used in small animal practice.

Kobayashi DL, Nichols R, and Peterson ME: Serum thyroid hormone concentrations in clinically normal dogs after administration of freshly reconstituted vs previously frozen and stored thyrotropin. J Am Vet Med Assoc 197:597, 1990.

Findings indicate that reconstituted TSH maintained biologic ability for at least 3 months when stored at $-20°C$.

Lothrop CD, Tamas PM, and Fadok VA: Canine and feline thyroid function assessment with the thyrotropin-releasing hormone response test. Am J Vet Res 45:2310, 1984.

Normal thyroidal responses to TRH injection in dogs and cats.

Peterson ME, Broussard J, and Gamble DA: Use of the thyrotropin-releasing (TRH) stimulation test to diagnose mild hyperthyroidism in cats. J Vet Intern Med 8:279.

Evaluation of the thyroidal responses of normal cats, cats with hyperthyroidism, and cats with nonthyroidal illnesses to TRH.

Reimers TJ: Guidelines for collection, storage, and transport of samples for hormone assay. In Kirk RW (ed): Current Veterinary Therapy X: Small Animal Practice. Philadelphia, WB Saunders Co, 1989, p 968.

Discussion of factors affecting accurate measurement of hormones in samples from veterinary species.

Smiley LE and Peterson ME: Evaluation of a urine cortisol:creatinine ratio as a screening test for hyperadrenocorticism in dogs. J Vet Intern Med 7: 163, 1993.

Comparison of urine cortisol/creatinine ratios in normal dogs, dogs with hyperadrenocorticism, dogs with clinical signs resembling those in hyperadrenocorticism, and dogs with nonadrenal illness.

---

# EFFECTS OF DRUGS ON ENDOCRINE TESTS

DAWN MERTON BOOTHE
*College Station, Texas*

Drugs may interfere with an endocrine diagnostic test either by acting directly at the level of the analytical procedure (*in vitro*) or by inducing a physiologic change in the patient (*in vivo*). Of the two types of interference, it is likely that analytical interference will occur regardless of the species from which the sample was collected. Thus, interference affecting analytical procedures are better documented in veterinary medicine, since these effects generally can be extrapolated from analytical testing in human subjects. Mechanisms of *in vitro* interference with endocrine tests vary with the hormone being measured and the procedure being used.

If drug interference is suspected, the laboratory should be contacted and questioned. This is particularly important if the patient is receiving drugs structurally similar to the hormones being measured. Cross-reactivity between the drug and the hormone tested can falsely increase test values. For example, therapeutic corticosteroids cross-react with endogenous corticosteroid hormones, although the percentage of cross-reactivity varies with the assay and drug. Drugs that increase plasma corticosteroid concentrations *in vitro* include aldosterone, corticosterone, cortisone, 11-deoxycortisol, heparin (containing impurities), progesterone, spironolactone, and testosterone. Urine concentrations of corticosteroids are increased *in vitro* by ascorbic acid, colchicine, dexamethasone, potassium iodide, quinidine, spironolactone, and phenothiazines.

The effects of *in vivo* interference of endocrine tests in human patients are numerous and have been well documented. Such interference may result in clinical manifestations of disease (e.g., adrenal gland suppression by glucocorticoids, or the effects of progestins on multiple endocrine organs) (Eigenmann and Venker-Van Haggen, 1981). Compared to analytical interference, identifying the mechanisms of *in vivo* interference is more difficult and frequently is not possible. Mechanisms of drug interference with the thyroid, adrenal, and sex hormone axis have been best documented in human patients.

Hormone concentrations may be decreased because of suppression of hormone release at each level of the endocrine axis (i.e., hypothalamus, pituitary, or target organ), often because hormone synthesis is decreased, as well as because of altered peripheral hormone metabolism. This latter effect is often the result of induction of hepatic drug-metabolizing enzymes. Potent inducers of hepatic drug-metabolizing enzymes include phenobarbital, phenytoin, and rifampin.

Less commonly, hormone concentrations are physiologically increased by drugs; again, changes in hepatic metabolism are a common cause. Potent inhibitors of hepatic drug metabolism include cimetidine, chloramphenicol, and ketoconazole. Drugs can also increase hormone concentrations by competing with and displacing the hormone from carrying proteins. The protein from which hormones are most likely to be displaced is albumin, a nonspecific carrier of many weakly acidic drugs (e.g., nonsteroidal anti-inflammatory drugs). Competition for albumin-binding sites may be less important for those hormones carried by specific carrier proteins, although competition for binding sites has been documented for such proteins as well. Displacement of hormone from a binding protein increases the concentration of free, pharmacologically active hormone. Although total hormone concentrations initially may not change following displacement, as unbound hormone is cleared more rapidly, concentrations of total and unbound hormone are likely to decrease. In some cases, a drug may influence blood hormone concentrations simultaneously at several physiologic sites, complicating interpretation (e.g., the effects of phenytoin on thyroid hormone concentrations). Because animals differ physiologically, extrapolation between species must be done cautiously. Caution is also advised when extrapolating results of studies in normal animals to the animal suffering from disease of an endocrine system. For example, propranolol decreases thyroid hormone concentrations in hyperthyroid humans, but not in euthyroid dogs (Center et al., 1981).

In some instances, the effect of a drug on concentrations of a hormone is well known and is used either diagnostically (e.g., dexamethasone-induced decrease in serum cortisol concentration or xylazine-induced growth hormone secretion) or therapeutically (e.g., antithyroid drug inhibition of thyroxine secretion). More commonly, the effect is undesirable. Several examples of undesired, drug-induced physiologic changes in endocrine function have been documented in small animal patients. The examples most documented in small animals are the effects of drugs, particularly glucocorticoids, on the hypothalamic-pituitary-adrenal axis. Interference with this axis can become clinically detrimental. Suppression of the adrenal axis by glucocorticoids is most marked following administration of depo- (repositol) forms (Spencer et al., 1980). However, interference has also

been documented after administration of a single dose of prednisolone or triamcinoline, multiple doses of methylprednisolone (Spencer et al., 1980), topical administration of triamcinolone (Roberts et al., 1984), and ophthalmic administration of prednisone (Zenoble and Kemppainen, 1987).

Glucocorticoids are not the only drugs that interfere with the hypothalamic-adrenal axis. The imidazole antifungal drug, ketoconazole, inhibits the cytochrome P-450 enzymes responsible for the synthesis of both sex and adrenal steroids (Hostetler et al., 1988). Suppression of testosterone and cortisol has been documented in dogs following oral administration of 10 mg/kg once daily (Willard et al., 1986); hormone concentrations are lowered by day 1 and remain low at day 5. Progesterone concentrations increase as testosterone concentrations decrease. The magnitude of testosterone inhibition by ketoconazole apparently resolves, with testosterone concentrations being less predictable a month after therapy has started. The inhibitory effect of ketoconazole on testosterone and adrenal steroids has been used therapeutically in the treatment of prostatic cancer, benign prostatic hypertrophy, and hyperadrenocorticism. The newer imidazole antifungal drugs do not appear to inhibit steroid synthesis as effectively as ketoconazole.

Drug interference with evaluation of the thyroid axis is also of importance because of the prevalence of thyroid dysfunction in small animals. Several drugs, targeting various sites, interfere with thyroid function testing (see Table 2) (Wenzel, 1981). Thyroid-stimulating hormone (TSH) response to thyrotropin-releasing hormone (TRH) is altered by a number of drugs that modulate neurotransmitter (e.g., serotonin and dopamine) concentrations in the brain. Glucocorticoid suppression of the TSH response to TRH administration has been well documented. Higher doses appear to suppress hypothalamic inhibition of TSH, whereas low doses interfere with the hypothalamic response (Wenzel, 1981). Note however, that interference of the thyroid axis by glucocorticoids does not preclude simultaneous testing of the thyroid and adrenal axes in healthy dogs (Moriello, Halliwell, and Oakes, 1987; Reimers, Concannon, and Cowan, 1992). Antithyroid drugs such as propylthiouracil and methimazole are used therapeutically to block thyroid hormone synthesis. The effects of iodide- and iodine-containing products (including radiographic contrast agents) on thyroid hormone concentrations are well recognized and used therapeutically. Through hypothalamic regulation, iodines cause a rapid increase in TSH response to TRH as thyroxine ($T_4$) and triiodothyronine ($T_3$) concentrations decrease.

The effects of anticonvulsant drugs, especially phenobarbital and phenytoin, on thyroid hormone disposition are less appreciated. Several sites of interference have been identified for anticonvulsant drugs. Displacement of $T_4$ by highly-protein-bound drugs (e.g., phenytoin) from thyroxine-binding globulin will increase the $T_4$ concentrations; induction of hepatic drug-metabolizing enzymes results in increased clearance of both $T_4$ and $T_3$; increased conversion of $T_4$ to $T_3$ by peripheral tissues further decreases serum $T_4$ concentrations. This latter mechanism has been postulated as the reason that $T_3$ concentrations remain normal despite increased $T_3$ clearance in patients receiving phenytoin (Senuty, Baker, and Yuen, 1988). Clinical signs of hypothyroidism may not be apparent in such cases. However, note that both serum $T_4$ and free $T_4$ may be decreased in some patients receiving anticonvulsants. Anticonvulsants (phenytoin) may also have a direct negative effect on TSH response to TRH. Drug-induced changes in thyroxine-binding globulins have also been documented in human patients receiving anticonvulsants. Thyroxine and TSH concentrations should be used to diagnose hypothyroidism in animals receiving anticonvulsants (Senuty, Baker, and Yuen, 1988). Note that thyroid supplementation will suppress response to

TSH and testing should not be performed until supplementation has been discontinued for 4 to 6 weeks.

Tables 1 through 4 list drugs capable of physiologically interfering with tests that measure hormone concentrations in blood and plasma. The information is based primarily on published reports in human medicine as reported by the American Clinical Chemistry Society. Few of these interactions have been documented in veterinary patients. Although it is likely that the mechanisms of interference are similar and the effects the same, extrapolations must be made cautiously. A variety of drugs have been tested for their physiologic effect and were found to have no effect. These results are not included in the tables. Most drug effects listed are either statistically or clinically significant, but not

**Table 1.** *Drug-Induced Physiologic Changes in the Adrenocortical Axis*°

| Hormone Affected | Effect | Drug Administered | Comment |
|---|---|---|---|
| **Corticosteroids** | | | |
| | Increased | Corticotropin | Maximal response at 4 hr |
| | Increased | Insulin | 60 min after IV injection |
| | Increased | Phenytoin | Altered metabolism |
| | Decreased | Albuterol | After IV administration |
| | Decreased | Androgens | May induce cholestasis |
| | Decreased | Dexamethasone† | 24 hr after dosing |
| | Decreased | o,p′-DDD (mitotane)† | Therapeutic intent |
| | Decreased | Rifampin | Hepatic enzyme induction |
| **Corticotropin** | | | |
| | Increased | Etomidate | Mild increase; direct suppression of adrenal |
| | Increased | Insulin | After IV administration |
| | Increased | Metoclopramide | After IV administration |
| | Increased | Vasopressin | After IV administration |
| | Decreased | Clonidine | — |
| | Decreased | Dexamethasone | — |
| | Decreased | Methylprednisolone | — |
| **Cortisol** | | | |
| | Increased | Anticonvulsants | — |
| | Increased | Corticotropin | Diagnostic intent |
| | Increased | Cortisone | For at least 24 hr |
| | Increased | Estrogen | Increases binding globulin concentrations |
| | Increased | Ethanol | High IV doses |
| | Increased | Fluocinolone | Following topical administration |
| | Increased | Hydrocortisone | For at least 24 hr |
| | Increased | Insulin | Marked effect; insulin-induced hypoglycemia |
| | Increased | Lithium | — |
| | Increased | Metoclopramide | Following IV dosing |
| | Increased | Opiates | Usually within 1 hr of IV administration |
| | Increased | o,p′-DDD (mitotane)† | Therapeutic intent |
| | Increased | Prostaglandin $F_2$ | Slight increase |
| | Increased | Vasopressin | Slight increase |
| | Decreased | Barbiturates | Preoperative use |
| | Decreased | Beclomethasone | Following inhalant administration |
| | Decreased | Clonidine | In growth hormone deficiency |
| | Decreased | Danazol | Displacement from binding sites |
| | Decreased | Deoxycorticosterone | Following topical administration |
| | Decreased | Dexamethasone† | Diagnostic intent |
| | Decreased | Ephedrine | Accelerated clearance due to increased hepatic blood flow and enzyme activity |
| | Decreased | Etomidate | Direct suppression of adrenal function |
| | Decreased | Fluocinolone | Following topical administration |

°Table reflects serum or plasma values only and is based on information reported in Young DS: *Effects of Drugs on Clinical Laboratory Tests*, 3rd edition. Washington DC, American Association for Clinical Chemistry Press, 1990.
†Reported in veterinary literature.

***Table 2.*** *Drug-Induced Physiologic Changes in Hormones of the Thyroid Axis**

| Hormone Affected | Effect | Drug Administered | Comment |
|---|---|---|---|
| **Thyroid-Stimulating Hormone (TSH)** | | | |
| | Increased | Furosemide | When drug therapy discontinued |
| | Increased | Iodides | Increased response to TRH |
| | Increased | Metoclopramide | Maximum effect 3–6 hr after administration |
| | Increased | Morphine | In hypothyroid and euthyroid patients |
| | Increased | Potassium iodide | — |
| | Increased | Prednisolone | Twofold increase; response to TRH unchanged |
| | Increased | TRH | Threefold increase in 30 min |
| | Increased | Phenytoin | — |
| | Decreased | Apomorphine | In hypothyroidism |
| | Decreased | Aspirin | — |
| | Decreased | Carbamazepine | Long-term therapy |
| | Decreased | Glucocorticoids | Inhibits TRH at hypophysis |
| | Decreased | Dopamine | Antagonizes TRH at hypophysis |
| | Decreased | Heparin | Interferes with binding to protein |
| | Decreased | Levothyroxine | — |
| | Decreased | Triiodothyronine | In euthyroid and hypothyroid patients |
| **Thyroxine** | | | |
| | Increased | Desiccated thyroid | — |
| | Increased | Estrogens | Increased binding capacity for up to 1 month |
| | Increased | Fluorouracil | Increased binding capacity |
| | Increased | Glucocorticoids | Inhibition of conversion |
| | Increased | Halothane | Increased release from liver |
| | Increased | Insulin | Increased release from liver |
| | Increased | Levothyroxine | Suppression of endogenous hormone; exogenous measured |
| | Increased | Phenytoin | — |
| | Increased | Propranolol | Blockage of iodothyronine deiodination |
| | Increased | Prostaglandins | Direct effect |
| | Increased | Tamoxifen | — |
| | Increased | Thyroid | — |
| | Increased | Thyrotropin | — |
| | Increased | TRH | — |
| | Decreased | Aminosalicylic acid | Prolonged administration may cause hypothyroidism |
| | Decreased | Anabolic steroids | Decreased binding to globulins |
| | Decreased | Androgens | Decreased binding to globulins |
| | Decreased | Anticonvulsants | — |
| | Decreased | Asparaginase | — |
| | Decreased | Aspirin | Displaces thyroxin from binding sites to prealbumin |
| | Decreased | Barbiturates | Competition for binding to prealbumin |
| | Decreased | Bromocriptine | In hypothyroidism (response to TRH unchanged) |
| | Decreased | Carbamazepine | Induction of hepatic enzymes; increased extrathyroidal metabolism |
| | Decreased | Chlorpromazine | Increased metabolism by liver |
| | Decreased | Cholestyramine | Decreased intestinal absorption |
| | Decreased | Glucocorticoids | Up to 1 week posttherapy |
| | Decreased | Diazepam | Competition for transport proteins |
| | Decreased | Furosemide | Displacement from binding sites and enhanced clearance |
| | Decreased | Growth hormone | Inhibition of TSH response to TRH (?) |
| | Decreased | Heparin | Modified binding to transport proteins? |
| | Decreased | Iodides† | Decreased synthesis (therapeutic) |
| | Decreased | Lithium | Reduced thyroidal iodine uptake, iodination of tyrosine, release of $T_4$; hepatic metabolism of $T_4$ to $T_3$ |
| | Decreased | Methimazole† | Therapeutic intent |
| | Decreased | Mitotane | Competes with $T_4$ for binding globulin |
| | Decreased | Penicillin | Competes for binding globulin |
| | Decreased | Phenobarbital | Induction of hepatic enzymes |
| | Decreased | Phenylbutazone | Impaired synthesis; competition for binding to albumin |
| | Decreased | Phenytoin | Displacement from binding proteins; induction of hepatic enzymes |

*Table continued on opposite page*

**Table 2.**  *Continued*

| Hormone Affected | Effect | Drug Administered | Comment |
|---|---|---|---|
| | Decreased | Potassium iodide | |
| | Decreased | Propylthiouracil[1] | Inhibits synthesis (iodination of tyrosine) Therapeutic intent |
| | Decreased | Ranitidine | Slight reduction |
| | Decreased | Salicylate | Competition for transport proteins |
| | Decreased | Somatostatin | Inhibition of TSH release (?) |
| | Decreased | Stanozolol | — |
| | Decreased | Sulfonamides | Acts like thiourea on thyroid gland |
| | Decreased | Terbutaline | Mild decrease |
| | Decreased | Triiodothyronine | — |
| ***Triiodothyronine*** | | | |
| | Increased | Estrogens | Increased binding to proteins |
| | Increased | Fluorouracil | Increased binding to proteins |
| | Increased | Heparin | Interference with binding to protein |
| | Increased | Insulin | Release from liver |
| | Increased | Phenytoin | — |
| | Increased | Prostaglandins | |
| | Increased | Tamoxifen | — |
| | Increased | Terbutaline | — |
| | Increased | TRH | Percentage free $T_3$ unchanged |
| | Increased | Levothyroxine | — |
| | Increased | Triiodothyronine | — |
| | Decreased | Androgens | Decreased binding capacity (diminution of transport proteins) |
| | Decreased | Anticonvulsants | |
| | Decreased | Asparaginase | |
| | Decreased | Aspirin | |
| | Decreased | Carbamazepine | Increased extrathyroidal metabolism |
| | Decreased | Cimetidine | Reduced response to TRH |
| | Decreased | Furosemide | |
| | Decreased | Glucocorticoids | Inhibition of conversion |
| | Decreased | Iodides | Inhibition of conversion |
| | Decreased | Lithium | See thyroxine |
| | Decreased | Phenytoin | See thyroxine |
| | Decreased | Potassium iodide | |
| | Decreased | Propranolol | Membrane stabilization (see thyroxine) |
| | Decreased | Propylthiouracil | |
| | Decreased | Salicylate | See thyroxine |
| | Decreased | Somatostatin | See thyroxine |
| | Decreased | Stanozolol | See thyroxine |
| ***Free Thyroxine*** | | | |
| | Increased | Aspirin | Interference with binding to globulin and prealbumin |
| | Increased | Danazolol | Displacement from protein |
| | Increased | Estrogens | Increased binding to globulin |
| | Increased | Furosemide | — |
| | Increased | Heparin | Modification of thyroxin binding |
| | Increased | Phenytoin | |
| | Increased | Propranolol | Blockade of iodothyronine deiodination and peripherally, due to deiodination of thyroxine and metabolism of binding protein |
| | Increased | Thyroxine | — |
| | Decreased | Anticonvulsants | — |
| | Decreased | Asparaginase | — |
| | Decreased | Furosemide | — |
| | Decreased | Levothyroxine | — |
| | Decreased | Lithium | — |
| | Decreased | Phenylbutazone | Long-term |
| | Decreased | Phenytoin | Increased degradation, including that displaced from binding proteins |
| | Decreased | Ranitidine | — |
| ***Thyroxin-Binding Globulin*** | | | |
| | Increased | Anticonvulsants | Due to increased extrathyroidal metabolism of hormones |
| | Increased | Epinephrine | Increased binding capacity |
| | Increased | Estrogen | Increased binding capacity |
| | Increased | Phenothiazines | Prolonged use |
| | Increased | Tamoxifen | — |

*Table continued on following page*

***Table 2.*** *Continued*

| Hormone Affected | Effect | Drug Administered | Comment |
|---|---|---|---|
| | Decreased | Anabolic steroids | Direct effect |
| | Decreased | Androgens | Direct effect |
| | Decreased | Cortisone | Reduced synthesis |
| | Decreased | Danazolol | — |
| | Decreased | Methyltestosterone | Direct effect |
| | Decreased | Nandrolone | Anabolic effect |
| | Decreased | Oxymethalone | Direct effect |
| | Decreased | Prednisolone | Decreased globulin; increased prealbumin |
| | Decreased | Propranolol | Inhibition of thyroxine deiodination and binding protein metabolism |
| | Decreased | Stanozolol | — |
| | Decreased | Testosterone | Direct effect |

°Table reflects serum or plasma values only and is based on information reported in Young DS: *Effects of Drugs on Clinical Laboratory Tests*, 3rd edition. Washington DC, American Association for Clinical Chemistry Press, 1990.
†Reported in the veterinary literature

***Table 3.*** *Drug-Induced Physiologic Changes in Reproductive Hormones* °

| Hormone Affected | Effect | Drug Administered | Comment |
|---|---|---|---|
| **Testosterone** | | | |
| | Increased | Barbiturates | Decreased metabolic clearance |
| | Increased | Bromocriptine | — |
| | Increased | Cimetidine | Displaced hormone from binding sites at pituitary and hypothalamic level |
| | Increased | Danazol | — |
| | Increased | Estrogens | Increased binding and decreased clearance |
| | Increased | Gonadotropin | — |
| | Increased | Phenytoin | — |
| | Increased | Rifampin | Increased microsomal activity and increased biosynthesis |
| | Increased | Testosterone | In hypogonadal men and following self-steroid administration in athletes |
| | Decreased | Carbamazepine | Induction of hepatic enzyme activity |
| | Decreased | Cyclophosphamide | Testicular atrophy |
| | Decreased | Danazolol | Altered binding and increased free hormone |
| | Decreased | Dexamethasone | Decreased clearance and binding |
| | Decreased | Diethylstilbestrol | — |
| | Decreased | Digoxin | — |
| | Decreased | Halothane | Mechanism unclear; inhibited release of gonadotropin (?) |
| | Decreased | Ketoconazole† | Transient block of testosterone synthesis |
| | Decreased | Methylprednisolone | Suppression of gonadotropin-releasing hormone secretion |
| | Decreased | Prednisolone | See methylprednisolone |
| | Decreased | Spironolactone | Inhibits biosynthesis in testis and displaces testosterone from cytosolic receptors |
| | Decreased | Stanozolol | — |
| | Decreased | Tetracycline | — |
| **Progesterone** | | | |
| | Increased | Ketoconazole† | — |
| | Decreased | Ampicillin | Decreased synthesis (?) |
| | Decreased | Danazol | To nondetectable levels in women |
| | Decreased | Prostaglandin $F_{2\alpha}$ | Marked decrease with successful abortion |
| | Decreased | Testosterone | Self-steroid administration in athletes |
| **Estrogen** | | | |
| | Increased | Digoxin | — |

°Table reflects serum or plasma values only and is based on information reported in Young DS: *Effects of Drugs on Clinical Laboratory Tests*, 3rd edition. Washington DC, American Association for Clinical Chemistry Press, 1990.
†Reported in the veterinary literature

**Table 4.** *Miscellaneous Drug-Induced Physiologic Changes in Hormone Concentrations**

| Hormone Affected | Effect | Drug Administered | Comment |
|---|---|---|---|
| **Angiotensin I** | Increased | Enalapril | As angiotensin II falls |
| | Increased | Nifedipine | — |
| **Angiotensin II** | Increased | Estrogens | — |
| | Increased | Furosemide | — |
| | Increased | Nifedipine | — |
| | Increased | Spironolactone | — |
| | Decreased | Captopril | — |
| | Decreased | Enalapril | — |
| **Antidiuretic Hormone** | Increased | Furosemide | — |
| | Increased | Hydrochlorothiazide | — |
| | Increased | Lithium | — |
| **Erythropoietin** | Increased | Fluoxymesterone | — |
| | Increased | Anabolic steroids | — |
| **Growth Hormone** | Increased | Apomorphine | — |
| | Increased | Clomipramine | |
| | Increased | Clonidine | In children with deficiency |
| | Increased | Corticotropin | |
| | Increased | Dopamine | Stimulates release |
| | Increased | Estrogens | |
| | Increased | Glucagon | Potent stimulant |
| | Increased | Glucose | Diagnostic intent |
| | Increased | Halothane | Response to surgical stress? |
| | Increased | Insulin | With insulin-induced hypoglycemia |
| | Increased | Metoclopramide | After single injection |
| | Increased | Progestins[†] | In dogs |
| | Increased | Propranolol | In hypertensives treated with diuretics |
| | Increased | Vasopressin | — |
| | Increased | Xylazine[†] | Diagnostic intent |
| | Decreased | Chlorpromazine | — |
| | Decreased | Corticosteroids | Suppresses secretion |
| | Decreased | Corticotropin | Reduces maximal secretion during sleep |
| | Decreased | Hydrocortisone | — |
| **Insulin** | Increased | Albuterol | — |
| | Increased | Deoxycorticosterone | — |
| | Increased | Glipizide[†] | Therapeutic intent |
| | Increased | Glucagon | Diagnostic intent |
| | Increased | Glucose | — |
| | Increased | Insulin | — |
| | Increased | Medroxyprogesterone | Metabolic effect |
| | Increased | Prednisolone | — |
| | Increased | Rifampin | — |
| | Increased | Spironolactone | — |
| | Increased | Streptozotocin | — |
| | Increased | Terbutaline | — |
| | Increased | Tolbutamide | — |
| | Increased | Verapamil | — |
| | Decreased | Asparaginase | — |
| | Decreased | Cimetidine | — |
| | Decreased | Furosemide | Intravenous |
| | Decreased | Hydrochlorothiazide | — |
| | Decreased | Morphine | — |
| | Decreased | Phenytoin | — |
| | Decreased | Propranolol | — |
| | Decreased | Tolbutamide | — |
| | Decreased | Xylazine[†] | — |

*Table reflects serum or plasma values only and is based on information reported in Young DS: *Effects of Drugs on Clinical Laboratory Tests*, 3rd edition. Washington, DC, American Association for Clinical Chemistry Press, 1990.
[†]Reported in the veterinary literature.

all listings note the level of significance. Known or suspected mechanisms of the physiologic disturbance have been noted when available. Drugs whose effects on endocrine function are used either diagnostically or therapeutically to treat the endocrine disorders are noted as such.

## References and Suggested Readings

Center SA, Mitchell J, Nachreiner RF, Concannon PW, and Reimers TJ: Effects of propranolol on thyroid function in the dog. J Am Anim Hosp Assoc 17:813, 1981.
*A report of an experimental study focusing on the effects of propranolol on thyroid function in euthyroid dogs.*

Kemppainen RJ and Sartin JL: Effects of single intravenous doses of dexamethasone on baseline plasma cortisol concentrations and responses to synthetic ACTH in healthy dogs. Am J Vet Res 45:742, 1984.
*A report of an experimental study focusing on the effects of dexamethasone on the hypothalamic-pituitary-adrenal axis.*

Moriello KA, Halliwell REW, and Oakes M: Determination of thyroxine, triiodothyronine, and cortisol changes during simultaneous adrenal and thyroid function tests in healthy dogs. Am J Vet Res 48:456, 1987.
*A report of an experimental study that supports performance of simultaneous adrenal and thyroid function tests.*

Reimers TJ, Concannon PW, and Cowan RG: Changes in serum thyroxine and cortisol in dogs after simultaneous injection of TSH and ACTH. J Am Anim Hos Assoc 18:923, 1982.
*A report of an experimental study that supports performance of simultaneous adrenal and thyroid function tests.*

Roberts SM, Lavach JD, Macy DW, and Severin GA: Effect of ophthalmic prednisolone acetate on the canine adrenal gland and hepatic function. Am J Vet Res 45:1711, 1984.
*A report of a study investigating the effects of topically administered glucocorticoids on selected physiologic functions.*

Senuty P, Baker DE, and Yuen GJ: Assessment of thyroid function during phenytoin therapy. DICP: Ann Pharmacother 22:609, 1988.
*A report of a study investigating the effects of anticonvulsants in dogs.*

Spencer KB, Thompson FN, Clekis T, and Lorenz MD: Adrenal gland function in dogs given methylprednisolone. Am J Vet Res 4:1503, 1980.
*A report of a study investigating the effects of a specific glucocorticoid on adrenal function.*

Wenzel KW: Pharmacological interference with in vitro tests of thyroid function. *Metabolism* 30:717, 1981.
*A review article focusing on the effects of drugs on thyroid function.*

Willard MD, Nachreiner R, McDonald R, and Roudebush P: Hormonal and clinical pathologic changes with long-term ketoconazole therapy in the dog and cat. Proc Am Coll of Vet Intern Med 6:13.25, 1986.
*A report of a study that investigates selected physiologic and pathologic effects of long-term ketoconazole administration in dogs and cats.*

Young DS: *Effects of Drugs on Clinical Laboratory Tests*, 3rd edition, Washington DC, American Association for Clinical Chemistry Press, 1990.
*A comprehensive, references review of the effects of drugs on clinical laboratory tests.*

Zenoble RD and Kemppainen RJ: Adrenocortical suppression by topically applied corticosteroids in healthy dogs. J Am Vet Med Assoc 191:685, 1987.
*A report of a study that focuses on the effects of topically administered glucocorticoid on adrenal function.*

---

# PEDIATRIC ENDOCRINOLOGY

### DEBORAH S. GRECO
*Fort Collins, Colorado*

Pediatric endocrine disorders are becoming increasingly recognized as contributing factors to perinatal mortality in puppies and kittens. The purpose of this article is to outline an approach to the diagnosis and treatment of pediatric endocrine disorders in puppies and kittens.

## DIFFERENTIAL DIAGNOSIS OF GROWTH DISORDERS IN CATS AND DOGS

Many pediatric endocrine disorders, including hypothyroidism, hypopituitarism, diabetes mellitus, hyperadrenocorticism, hyperparathyroidism, and hypoadrenocorticism, are manifested as disorders of statural growth. Growth charts for kittens and puppies are readily available in standard veterinary pediatrics texts (Chastain, 1990). Causes of stunted or inadequate growth in small animals may be divided into two broad categories: intrinsic defects of growing tissues (skeletal dysplasias, chromosomal abnormalities, dysmorphic dwarfism), and abnormalities in the environment of growing tissues (nutritional, metabolic, environmental, or endocrine).

Intrinsic defects of growing tissues include most of the genetic and chromosomal abnormalities that result in growth failure. Genetic disorders may be suspected on the basis of clustering of the disease in certain breeds or lines of dogs and cats (i.e., chondrodystrophy of Alaskan malamutes). Diagnosis may require pursuing pedigree analysis or genetic testing or both.

Abnormalities of the environment of growing tissues are the most common and easily identified abnormalities. A thorough dietary history will reveal inadequate quantity or quality of feeding. Metabolic disorders, such as portosystemic shunts, pancreatic insufficiency, chronic renal failure, diabetes mellitus, and congestive heart failure, may be identified by characteristic clinical signs and laboratory data. Endocrine causes of growth retardation include hypothyroidism, hyperadrenocorticism, hypoadrenocorticism, and hypopituitarism.

Endocrine growth abnormalities can be divided into two groups based on the type of dwarfism present. A proportionate dwarf exhibits small stature but precisely the same proportions as the adult animal (Fig. 1); proportionate dwarfism is characteristic of growth hormone deficiency. In contrast, a disproportionate dwarf has a normal size head and trunk but short legs (Fig. 2); disproportionate dwarfism is characteristic of hypothyroid dwarfism. Other endocrine causes of abnormal growth (i.e., diabetes mellitus) result in subnormal stature (not true dwarfism) and a normally proportioned animal.

## JUVENILE HYPOTHYROIDISM

Congenital primary hypothyroidism in puppies may be caused by thyroid dysgenesis; dyshormonogenesis;

**Figure 1.** Illustration of proportionate dwarfism. Note that the length of the leg, size of the head, and size of the trunk are smaller than for the adult.

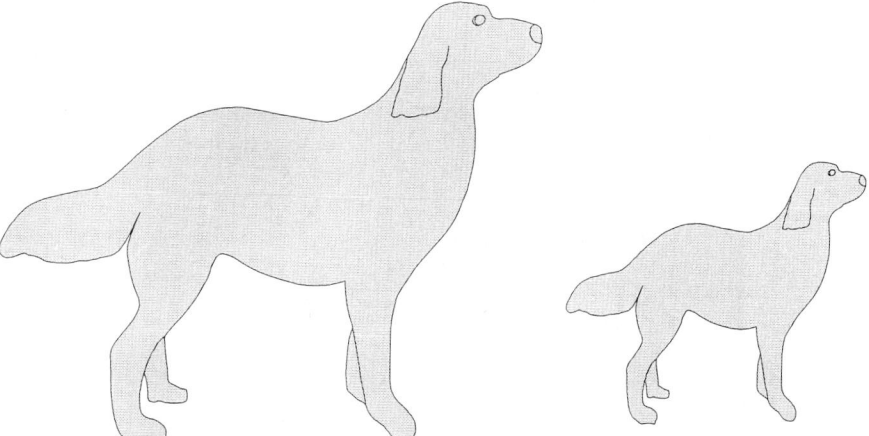

and more rarely, serum transport abnormalities, goitrogens, or severe iodine deficiency (Chastain, 1990). In the dog, thyroid dysgenesis is the most common cause of primary congenital hypothyroidism (Chastain, 1990). Secondary hypothyroidism in dogs may be congenital secondary to thyroid-stimulating hormone (TSH) deficiency (Greco, 1991). Dyshormonogenesis leads to goitrous hypothyroidism, a rare cause of congenital hypothyroidism in kittens (Arnold et al., 1984).

Congenital hypothyroidism is characterized by stunted growth, gait abnormalities, mental dullness, muscular weakness, delayed dental eruption, and constipation (Chastain, 1990; Greco, 1991). Typical physical features of congenital hypothyroidism include disproportionate dwarfism, a broadened skull, macroglossia, hypothermia, lateral strabismus, exophthalmos, bradycardia, alopecia, retention of puppy hair coat, and abdominal distention (Fig. 3). The clinical signs of hypothyroidism in kittens are very similar to those in puppies. In addition, constipation may be a primary feature of congenital hypothyroidism in kittens. The characteristic ragged epiphyses with scattered foci of calcification (epiphyseal dysgenesis) is pathognomonic for congenital hypothyroidism; however, pituitary dwarfs also

exhibit epiphyseal dysgenesis because of TSH deficiency (Fig. 4).

Hypercholesterolemia, mild hypercalcemia, nonregenerative anemia, elevated serum creatine phosphokinase levels, and hypoglycemia are common laboratory findings consistent with congenital hypothyroidism. Diagnosis is based on subnormal total or free thyroxine ($T_4$) concentrations before and after TSH administration. Note that normal total $T_4$ concentrations in young puppies or kittens (15 to 25 $\mu$g/dl) may be 10 to 20 times higher than those of normal adults (Chastain, 1990). Diagnosis of congenital hypothyroidism can also be made on the basis of thyroid scanning with sodium pertechnetate. The perchlorate discharge test using [131]I is helpful in diagnosing organification defects (Chastain, 1990).

Congenital hypothyroidism is treated by levothyroxine supplementation (22 $\mu$g/kg/day, PO). If treatment is started after 3 to 4 weeks of age, mental retardation is likely. Many animals with hypothyroid dwarfism are not diagnosed until relatively late in life. While the mental disturbances caused by congenital hypothyroidism are usually irreversible, the skeletal malformations may be reversible if the hypothyroidism is treated ag-

**Figure 2.** Illustration of disproportionate dwarfism. Note that the head and trunk are similar in size to the adult, but the legs are much shorter.

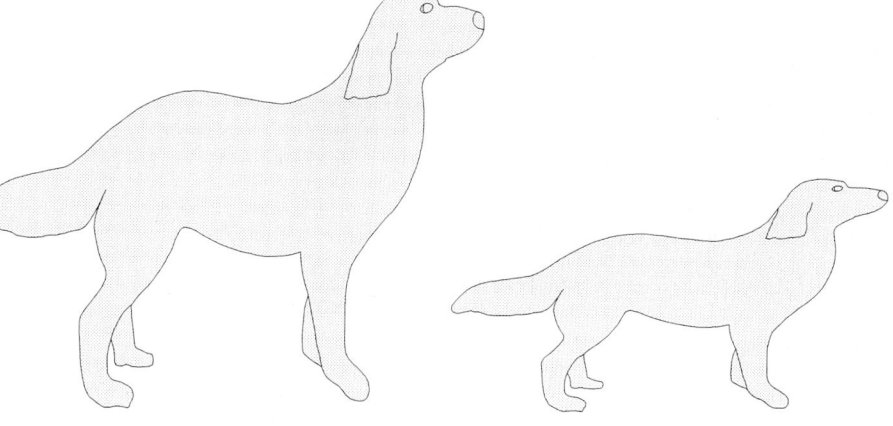

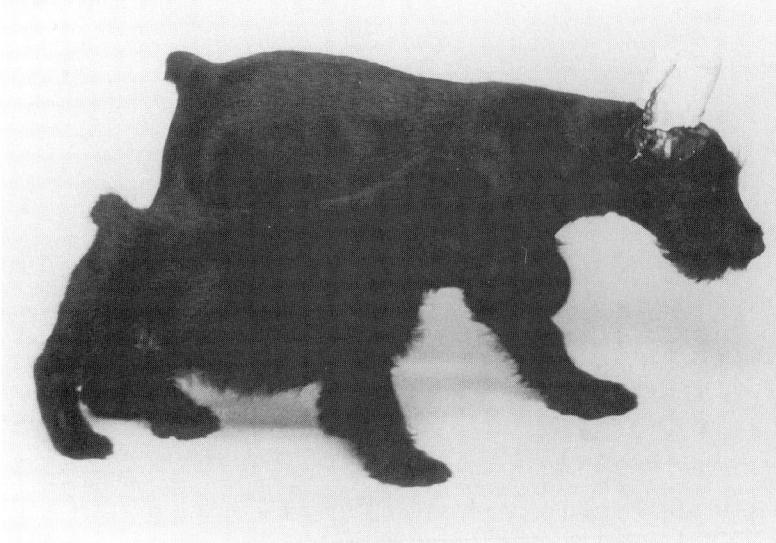

**Figure 3.** Hypothyroid dwarf giant schnauzer puppy (8 weeks) with normal littermate. Note disproportionate dwarfism.

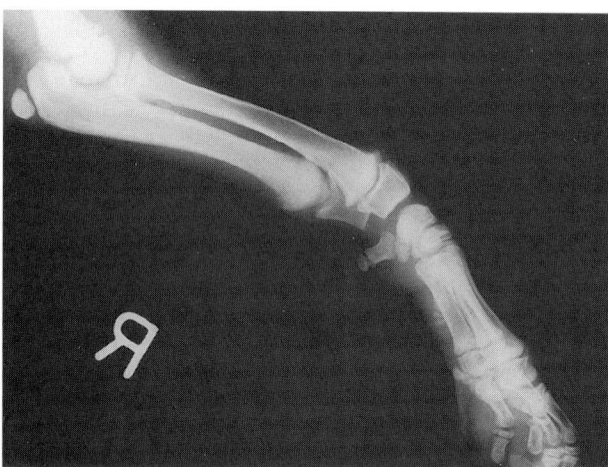

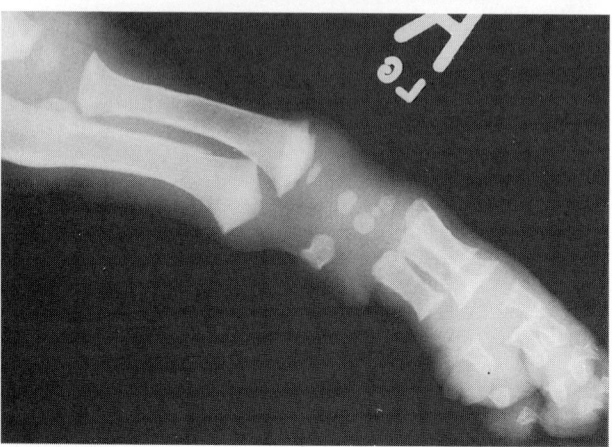

**Figure 4.** Radiographs of the forelimb of a normal puppy (*top*) and a hypothyroid dwarf littermate (*bottom*). Epiphyseal dysgenesis is apparent in the hypothyroid dwarf.

gressively in animals under the age of 8 to 10 months. Treatment is similar to that for canine congenital hypothyroidism except that kittens require a lower dosage of levothyroxine (10 μg/kg/day, PO).

## JUVENILE-ONSET DIABETES MELLITUS

Juvenile-onset diabetes mellitus, defined as insulin-dependent diabetes in dogs less than 1 year of age, is one of the more common endocrine disorders of puppies. However, fewer than 1.5% of diabetic dogs have juvenile-onset diabetes (Chastain, 1990). Diabetes mellitus is thought to be an inherited disorder in several breeds of dogs, most notably keeshond and golden retriever dogs (Table 1). Juvenile-onset diabetes mellitus has not been recognized in the cat. In humans, an association between juvenile diabetes and viral disease is suspected; similarly, viral disease (parvo, distemper) has been suspected in the pathogenesis of canine juvenile diabetes mellitus (Chastain, 1990). Subclinical viral infections may present as juvenile-onset diabetes mellitus and concurrent exocrine pancreatic deficiency (EPI) rather than as isolated β-cell atrophy.

Clinical signs, such as polydipsia, polyuria, and polyphagia, become evident from 2 to 6 months of age; nocturia may be dramatic. Decreased growth rate compared to normal littermates and severe weight loss in the face of polyphagia is another cardinal sign of diabetes mellitus in puppies. Lenticular edema or cataracts and soft stools or small-bowel diarrhea may also be a present. Severe diarrhea or steatorrhea, however, should alert the veterinary clinician to the possibility of concurrent exocrine pancreatic deficiency. Pelvic limb paresis suggestive of polyneuropathy may be observed.

**Table 1.** *Breeds in which Juvenile-Onset Diabetes Mellitus has been Documented*

| | |
|---|---|
| Keeshond° | Old English sheepdog |
| Golden retriever° | English springer spaniel |
| West Highland terrier | Whippet |
| Doberman pinscher | Schipperke |
| Miniature schnauzer | Chow |
| German shepherd | Miniature pinscher |
| Labrador retriever | Finnish spitz |

°Genetic basis suspected.

**Table 2.** *Treatment Outline for Juvenile Diabetes Mellitus*

1. Diet
   a. Energy requirements for growth
   b. High-quality protein
   c. Feeding frequency: t.i.d. to q.i.d.
2. Insulin therapy
   a. Initial dose: 0.5–2 U/kg, SC
   b. Lente or isophane (NPH) insulin
   c. Frequency: at least b.i.d., may need t.i.d.
   d. May administer in combination with regular insulin
3. Monitoring therapy in puppies < 6–8 mo
   a. Assess body weight weekly
   b. Assess glucose curve every 2 wk
   c. Adjust dose based on new weight and glucose curve
4. Exercise
   a. Regularly scheduled, consistent exercise
5. Concurrent exocrine pancreatic insufficiency
   a. Supplement with Viokase (1 tsp/feeding); incubate on food for 1/2 hr
   b. Conservative insulin dosage (1/2 U/kg) until EPI is controlled
   c. Multiple, small meals

Laboratory findings of fasting hyperglycemia (200 mg/dl) in conjunction with glucosuria are diagnostic for juvenile diabetes mellitus. Elevations in serum cholesterol, serum glutamic pyruvic transaminase (SGPT), and alkaline phosphatase (ALP) are not uncommon. Often, ketonemia and ketonuria are observed. If ketoacidosis is present, metabolic acidosis, increased anion gap, hyponatremia, hyperkalemia, and hypochloremia may also be evident. Concurrent EPI may be diagnosed by measuring serum trypsin-like immunoreactivity or by fat absorption tests.

Emergency treatment of juvenile diabetic ketoacidosis is the same as for adult ketoacidosis. Long-term management of juvenile diabetes includes use of intensive insulin therapy using an intermediate-acting insulin (0.5 to 2.0 U/kg, SC) to maintain blood glucose concentrations within a narrow range (80 to 200 mg/dl) (Table 2). Nutritionally balanced diets with protein of high biologic value should be fed. The quantity of food should be calculated using standard age and breed feeding charts, and energy needs should be recalculated every 2 weeks during periods of rapid growth (ages 1 to 6 months). Puppies should be fed at least twice daily; if more frequent feedings are given, supplemental injections of regular insulin may also be administered. Physical activity, water consumption, and urine output should be maintained within normal limits (Table 2).

Management of concurrent EPI may be particularly problematic. The veterinarian should be alerted to the possibility of EPI by the persistence of clinical signs such as diarrhea or steatorrhea, weight loss or lack of weight gain in a growing puppy, or by hypoglycemic episodes after administration of relatively low doses of insulin (<1U/kg). Replacement therapy with exocrine pancreatic enzyme preparations is indicated in puppies with concurrent EPI. Insulin dosage should be increased after pancreatic enzyme replacement to compensate for the increased caloric intake.

## PITUITARY DWARFISM

Pituitary dwarfism, a well-documented syndrome of German shepherd dogs, is inherited as a simple autosomal recessive trait (Campbell, 1988). Pituitary dwarfism has also been observed in other breeds such as the spitz, carnelian bear dog, toy pinscher, and Weimaraner (Campbell, 1988). In German shepherd dogs, failure of oral ectoderm to differentiate into pars distalis results in a cystic Rathke's pouch. Eventually, mucin-filled cysts enlarge and impinge on the remaining pituitary tissue, resulting in diminished production of all anterior pituitary hormones (e.g., TSH, ACTH, GH).

Clinical signs appear in affected German shepherd puppies during the first 2 to 3 months of life. Proportionate dwarfism, shrill barking, and mental retardation manifesting as problems with house training are common signs. Retention of a puppy hair coat with failure to grow primary guard hairs is a characteristic dermatologic sign. Truncal alopecia that spares the head and extremities is common in older pituitary dwarfs; the skin is often thin, hypotonic, scaly, and hyperpigmented (Campbell, 1988). Other clinical signs, such as delayed physeal closure and delayed dental eruption, may be related to secondary thyroid hormone deficiency rather than to growth hormone (GH) deficiency alone. Delayed onset of puberty and infantile external genitalia are probably caused by secondary pituitary luteinizing hormone (LH) and follicle-stimulating hormone (FSH) deficiency.

Clinicopathologic findings may include mild normocytic normochromic anemia (secondary to GH, ACTH, and TSH deficiency), hypoglycemia (secondary to ACTH deficiency), and hypophosphatemia (secondary to GH deficiency).

The characteristic signalment and clinical signs may allow a presumptive diagnosis, but diagnosis should be confirmed by documentation of inadequate growth hormone concentrations or reserve. Canine growth hormone assays are not currently available, at least in the United States; however, serum insulin-like growth factor (IGF) assays are available in some endocrine laboratories. Normal serum IGF-1 concentrations, in German shepherd puppies, are 345±50 ng/ml; higher than that of adult German shepherd dogs. The mean insulin-like growth factor level for dwarf dogs is 11±2 ng/ml (Campbell, 1988).

Growth hormone preparations are expensive and

may be difficult to obtain. If available, recommended therapy includes growth hormone (bovine, porcine, or human) at a dosage of 0.1 U/kg SC three times weekly for 4 to 6 weeks. Growth hormone treatment can be repeated if clinical signs recur (Campbell, 1988). Thyroid hormone supplementation (20 μg/kg/day, PO) will reverse many of the dermatologic and skeletal consequences of TSH deficiency, as many clients cannot afford somatotropin therapy.

## JUVENILE DIABETES INSIPIDUS

Diabetes insipidus (DI) may be central or nephrogenic in origin. Nephrogenic DI is an inherited disorder in dogs that results in resistance to the action of antidiuretic hormone (ADH) in the kidney. Central diabetes insipidus (CDI) may be congenital (ADH deficiency) or acquired (trauma). See *CVT X* for a complete discussion of diabetes insipidus (Nichols, 1989).

The primary clinical signs of idiopathic CDI are excessive thirst and severe polyuria. Urine volume may exceed 50 ml/kg/day and water consumption may be greater than 100 mg/kg/day. Unlike most of the other pediatric endocrine diseases, juvenile DI does not lead to dwarfism. Laboratory abnormalities are limited to hyposthenuria (urine specific gravity <1.006) and elevated plasma osmolality. Diagnosis is made by excluding other differentials for polydipsia and polyuria (e.g., renal disease, diabetes mellitus) after reviewing a minimum data base and by a water deprivation test. Failure to concentrate urine adequately (>1.025 in dogs; >1.030 in cats) during a water deprivation test followed by response to exogenous ADH or desmopressin (DDAVP) (increase in urine specific gravity) is diagnostic for central diabetes insipidus.

Following the discontinuation of production of repositol, vasopressin preparation (Pitressin tannate in Oil, Parke-Davis), desmopressin (DDAVP, Ferring), a synthetic arginine ADH, has become the only viable therapy for CDI. Administration of DDAVP results in complete resolution of polydipsia and polyuria caused by vasopressin deficiency. Although there is considerable variability in the pharmacokinetics of DDAVP in different patients, many animals can be managed by administering DDAVP in the conjunctival sac once or twice daily (Nichols, 1989).

Adjuvant therapy includes the use of diuretics and sulfonylureas; however, some clients are unable to afford medication and may opt for no treatment other than unlimited access to water. Chlorpropamide is a sulfonylurea that stimulates secretion of ADH (for patients with partial DI), and sensitizes the renal tubules to ADH by increasing cyclic adenosine monophosphate (cAMP) within renal tubular cells. The recommended dosage is 10 to 40 mg/kg/day, and common side effects include hypoglycemia (frequent feedings are recommended), nausea, and skin eruptions (Nichols, 1989). Both nephrogenic and central diabetes insipidus patients may benefit from thiazide diuretic therapy. Thiazide diuretics cause extracellular fluid volume contrac-

tion, increased proximal tubular sodium, and water reabsorption, and hence decreased water delivery (reducing urine volume) by inhibition of sodium reabsorption in the ascending loop of Henle (Nichols, 1989). An initial starting dose of chlorothiazide is 20 to 40 mg/kg twice daily.

## JUVENILE HYPERADRENOCORTICISM

Spontaneous juvenile hyperadrenocorticism has been identified in four dogs less than 1 year of age (Feldman, 1987). However, a more common cause of juvenile hyperadrenocorticism in young dogs is iatrogenic Cushing's syndrome. Regardless of the etiology, signs of juvenile hyperadrenocorticism are similar to those of adult-onset hyperadrenocorticism including polydipsia, polyuria, and dermatologic signs (e.g., alopecia, comedones). In addition, dogs with juvenile-onset hyperadrenocorticism usually suffer from stunted growth because of the effects of glucocorticoid excess on epiphyseal growth centers. Diagnosis of juvenile hyperadrenocorticism is achieved through use of the ACTH-stimulation test or low-dose dexamethasone suppression test; etiology (iatrogenic versus endogenous) may be more easily identified via the ACTH-stimulation test. Treatment of juvenile hyperadrenocorticism is similar to that for adult dogs with hyperadrenocorticism.

## JUVENILE HYPOADRENOCORTICISM

Primary hypoadrenocorticism, a deficiency in glucocorticoids or mineralocorticoids or both, is usually caused by immune-mediated destruction of the adrenal glands; however, congenital adrenal hypoplasia has been described in an 8-week-old puppy (Chastain, 1990). Adrenocorticotrophic hormone (ACTH) deficiency resulting in secondary hypoadrenocorticism is relatively common in puppies that suffer from pituitary dysfunction. Hypoadrenocorticism is rare in cats, and never reported in kittens.

Clinicopathologic signs of juvenile hypoadrenocorticism are identical to those in the adult (Chastain, 1990). Unlike most of the other pediatric endocrine diseases, juvenile hypoadrenocorticism does not lead to dwarfism. Primary hypoadrenocorticism is characterized by weight loss, anorexia, and episodes of hypovolemic shock. Weak pulse, bradyarrhythmias, vomiting, diarrhea, and abdominal pain are characteristic clinical signs. Often, constipation, dehydration, and hypothermia are observed. Classic signs include depression, anorexia, weak muscles and a history of waxing and waning episodes of gastrointestinal upset. Typical laboratory findings include hyponatremia, hyperkalemia, and prerenal azotemia. Hypochloremia, hyperphosphatemia, hypercalcemia, and occasionally hypoglycemia may be observed. An electrocardiogram may show peaking and elevation of T waves, small or absent P waves, increased P-R interval, and prolonged Q-T interval.

Emergency treatment of primary juvenile hypoadrenocorticism consists of fluid therapy, glucocorticoid, and mineralocorticoid replacement. Puppies presented in a hypovolemic crisis should be treated with shock doses of fluids (NaCl, 0.9%) and glucocorticoids. Use of dexamethasone phosphate will allow concurrent diagnostic testing via the ACTH-stimulation test.

Chronic treatment of juvenile hypoadrenocorticism is also similar to treatment of adult dogs suffering from hypoadrenocorticism. Maintenance therapy with Florinef (0.1 mg/5 kg) or repositol agents such as deoxycorticosterone pivalate (DOCP; 2.2 mg/kg every 28 days) is recommended. Mineralocorticoid dosages should be adjusted based on clinical signs and serum sodium and potassium concentrations. Glucocorticoid therapy should be used judiciously, as excess glucocorticoids can cause premature closure of the epiphysis in young dogs. Most addisonian puppies do not require glucocorticoid supplementation except during periods of stress. Small, physiologic doses of prednisone (0.2 mg/kg, PO daily) may be used during stressful periods.

## JUVENILE HYPERPARATHYROIDISM

German shepherd dogs may suffer from primary hyperplasia of the parathyroids. The condition is inherited as an autosomal recessive trait. Clinical findings include stunted growth, polyuria, polydipsia, and muscular weakness (Chastain, 1990). Laboratory findings consist of hypophosphatemia with increased fractional clearance of phosphorus, elevated plasma PTH, and hypercalcemia. Radiographs may reveal decreased bone density. Differential diagnoses include hyper- or hypovitaminosis D, bone neoplasia, and osteomyelitis.

## References and Suggested Reading

Arnold U, Opitz M, Grosser I, et al: Goitrous hypothyroidism and dwarfism in a kitten. J Am Anim Hosp Assoc 20:753,1983.
  *Case report of goitrous hypothyroidism in a 14-week-old kitten.*
Campbell KL: Growth hormone-related disorders in dogs. Compend Cont Educ Small Anim Pract 10:477, 1988.
  *Excellent review of growth hormone deficiency syndromes and dermatologic manifestations of growth hormone deficiency.*
Chastain CB: Endocrine and metabolic systems. *In* Hoskins JD (ed): *Veterinary Pediatrics.* Philadelphia, WB Saunders Co, pp 249–269, 1990.
  *Thorough review of current veterinary pediatric endocrinology; excellent reference list.*
Feldman EC: *Canine and Feline Endocrinology and Reproduction.* Philadelphia, WB Saunders Co, 1987.
  *Excellent reference for endocrine disorders of adult animals with specific reference to juvenile endocrinology when appropriate.*
Greco DS: Congenital hypothyroid dwarfism in a family of giant schnauzers. J Vet Intern Med 5:57, 1991.
  *Clinical report of secondary hypothyroid dwarfism in a family of giant schnauzer puppies.*
Nichols CE: Diabetes insipidus. *In* Kirk RW (ed): *Current Veterinary Therapy X.* Philadelphia, WB Saunders Co, 1989, p 973.
  *Current review of diagnosis and treatment of diabetes insipidus in dogs and cats.*

# DIAGNOSIS AND TREATMENT OF MACROTUMORS IN DOGS WITH PITUITARY-DEPENDENT HYPERADRENOCORTICISM

CYNTHIA A. DUESBERG,
ELIZABETH HERST BERTOY,
*and* EDWARD C. FELDMAN
*Davis, California*

Canine pituitary-dependent hyperadrenocorticism (PDH) results from excessive secretion of adrenocorticotrophic hormone (ACTH) from the pars distalis or pars intermedia of the pituitary gland, which in turn induces bilateral adrenocortical hyperplasia and hypercortisolism. Excess secretion of ACTH may arise from hyperplastic or neoplastic pituitary tissue. Adenomas of the pars distalis are the most frequent histologic finding in dogs with PDH. These tumors are usually small and clinically silent, except for their endocrine effects. Less commonly, dogs with PDH develop large tumors that grow to compress or invade adjacent neural structures, resulting in central nervous system (CNS) dysfunction. Based on criteria used for human beings, pituitary tumors are defined as macrotumors if 10 mm or larger in diameter. Although this criterion is also used to define a macrotumor in the dog, it is somewhat arbitrary. Because of variability in the size of the pituitary gland and calvaria among different breeds, an absolute size criterion may not be appropriate for all dogs.

## ANATOMY AND HISTOPATHOLOGY

The effect of macrotumor growth on the structure and function of the canine brain can be best appreciated after reviewing the anatomy of the canine pituitary gland and its relation to adjacent neural structures. The pituitary gland is suspended by a stalk-like projection (the pars tuberalis) from the ventral surface of the hypothalamus. A thin layer of dura mater, the diaphragma sella, covers the dorsal aspect of the pituitary gland, separating it from the overlying hypothalamus. A large foramen, in the center of the diaphragm, loosely encircles the pars tuberalis. The remainder of the gland occupies an oval depression in the basisphenoid bone, which gives rise to a complex of bones, the sella turcica. The sella turcica surrounds the pituitary gland and resists the growth of macrotumors in all but a dorsal direction. Tumor-related destruction of the sella turcica is an uncommon finding in dogs with macrotumors. In contrast, the thin, incomplete diaphragma sella provides minimal resistance to dorsal tumor expansion, which may then compress or invade suprasellar structures, including the hypothalamus, third ventricle, and thalamus, but tends to spare the more rostrally located optic chiasm. Severe compression of the third ventricle can obstruct the flow of cerebrospinal fluid and lead to hydrocephalus.

Information on the histopathology of macrotumors is limited, but the origin and cell type appear to be similar to ACTH-secreting microtumors. The majority of macrotumors evaluated histologically have originated in the pars distalis, and have been classified as adenomas. Adenocarcinomas have been identified infrequently. Even less is known about the biologic behavior of pituitary tumors in dogs with PDH. It is not possible to identify dogs that will develop CNS signs from a large tumor on the basis of patient signalment, endocrine test results, responsiveness of hypercortisolism to $o,p'$-DDD or ketoconazole treatment, or site of tumor origin within the pituitary gland.

## CLINICAL FEATURES

Pituitary-dependent hyperadrenocorticism is most frequently diagnosed in middle-aged and geriatric dogs. Breeds recognized most commonly include dachshunds, miniature poodles, and boxers. A distinct breed or sex predilection has not been identified for dogs with PDH caused by macrotumors. However, in a recent study of 13 dogs with CNS signs caused by macrotumors, large dogs ($\geq$20 kg) predominated.

The clinical signs exhibited by dogs with macrotumors often reflect both the endocrinologic and the space-occupying effects of the tumor. In the majority of dogs with macrotumors, the endocrinologic manifestations of the disorder are limited to excessive ACTH secretion, resulting in the typical clinical signs associated with hyperadrenocorticism (e.g., polyuria, polydipsia, polyphagia, endocrine alopecia, a pendulous abdomen and muscle atrophy). Uncommonly, dogs with macrotumors also develop complete or partial hypopituitarism as a consequence of destruction of the remaining pituitary gland by the expanding tumor. Although the prevalence of hypopituitarism in dogs with macrotumors is unknown, this complication has been recognized in fewer than 10% of those we have evaluated. Injury to the pituitary gland or hypothalamus may disrupt the synthesis and secretion of growth hormone, thyrotropin, gonadotropin (follicle-stimulating hormone, luteinizing hormone), prolactin, oxytocin, and vasopressin (antidiuretic hormone). Insufficient secretion of thyrotropin or vasopressin are the most clinically significant, and are the only manifestations of hypopituitarism recognized in our patients. The diagnosis of hypopituitarism may be difficult because assays for pituitary hormones, other than ACTH, are not routinely available, necessitating indirect assessment of pituitary function by evaluation of target organ function. In dogs with poorly regulated PDH, recognition of hypopituitarism is further complicated by the effects of hypercortisolism on pituitary hormone synthesis and peripheral receptor sensitivity. Hypercortisolism causes feedback inhibition of synthesis and release of thyrotropin, gonadotropin, and growth hormone, resulting in secondary hypothyroidism and gonadal atrophy. In addition, hypercortisolism appears to either reduce pituitary secretion of vasopressin (central diabetes insipidus) or reduce renal sensitivity to vasopressin (nephrogenic diabetes insipidus). Either syndrome may be difficult to evaluate on the basis of water deprivation studies alone.

### Neurologic Abnormalities

Neurologic abnormalities associated with macrotumors are quite variable in their onset and severity. The majority of dogs with PDH are neurologically normal, but the absence of CNS signs does not rule out the presence of a macrotumor. In as many as 50% of dogs with a macrotumor identified at necropsy or with survey CNS imaging, signs of hypercortisolism were the only clinical abnormalities expressed (Nelson, Ihle, and Feldman, 1988; Kipperman et al., 1993). When CNS signs are exhibited by dogs with macrotumors, their onset may precede, coincide with, or follow the recognition of signs of hyperadrenocorticism. The majority of dogs that develop CNS signs in association with a macrotumor are initially evaluated for signs of hyperadrenocorticism, and the CNS signs develop weeks to years after the diagnosis and treatment of PDH. Less commonly, CNS signs are the inciting reason for presentation to a veterinarian, and the clinical suspicion of hyperadrenocorticism arises from additional information obtained from the history and physical examination.

When neurologic abnormalities are first recognized, they may be limited to subtle behavioral changes and specific deficits may not be detected on neurologic examination. Signs commonly reported by the owners of these dogs include anorexia, restlessness, loss of interest in normal household activities, delayed response to stimuli, and brief episodes of disorientation. In addition to a macrotumor, differential diagnoses for these signs include hypocortisolism resulting from *o,p'*-DDD (mitotane) overdosage, *o,p'*-DDD–induced neurotoxicity, and concurrent disease unrelated to PDH or its treatment. Mitotane-induced neurotoxicity is rare and transient, lasting for 24 to 48 hr after drug administration. A diagnosis of hypocortisolism can be established by results of ACTH stimulation test, in combination with response to glucocorticoid supplementation.

When more definitive neurologic signs are exhibited by dogs with macrotumors, those most frequently observed in our patients include altered mentation (i.e., obtundation and stupor), ataxia, symmetric tetraparesis, and pacing. Neurologic deficits observed less frequently include rotary nystagmus, a tendency to circle, and head-pressing. These signs can be attributed to the destruction of portions of the hypothalamus or thalamus. Anisocoria, strabismus, and facial hypothesia or paralysis may result from damage to cranial nerves. Neurologic signs that tend to occur with advanced disease include thermoregulatory dysfunction, behavioral changes (e.g., aggression), blindness, seizures, and coma. However, blindness may be misdiagnosed in dogs with macrotumors because their mental dullness results in inappropriate responses to visual stimuli (e.g., absent menace response).

## DIAGNOSIS

After confirming a diagnosis of hyperadrenocorticism with results of ACTH-stimulation or low-dose dexamethasone suppression tests, PDH may be differentiated from adrenocortical tumor using endocrine discriminatory tests (i.e., high-dose dexamethasone suppression test, plasma endogenous ACTH concentration), and/or evaluation of the size and shape of the adrenal glands using ultrasonography, radiography, or computed tomography (CT) (see *CVT XI*, p 10). Inadequate suppression of cortisol concentration after a high dose of dexamethasone has been advocated as a means of identifying dogs with PDH caused by macrotumors. However, there is no blood or urine test that can always identify dogs that have or will develop macrotumors.

### Advanced Diagnostic Imaging

Advanced imaging of the CNS is the only reliable means of establishing an antemortem diagnosis of a pituitary macrotumor. Three-dimensional imaging, using CT (see *CVT XI*, p. 10) or magnetic resonance imaging (MRI), is a noninvasive method to identify pituitary tumors and assess their effect on adjacent neural structures. Suprasellar extension of macrotumors, and compression of the overlying hypothalamus, thalamus, and third ventricle, can be readily detected using CT or MRI (Figs. 1 and 2). The pituitary gland lacks a complete blood-brain barrier, and macrotumors demonstrate enhancement with iodinated or paramagnetic contrast agents administered during CT or MRI, respectively. Contrast enhancement of the macrotumors may improve their detection. It also allows better delineation of tumor from peritumoral edema and adjacent neural structures, and facilitates the differential diagnosis of the tumor.

Diagnostic imaging of the pituitary gland is recommended for dogs with PDH that develop CNS signs not attributable to a metabolic cause. The information yielded by imaging studies is essential for determining the prognosis and appropriate treatment for dogs with

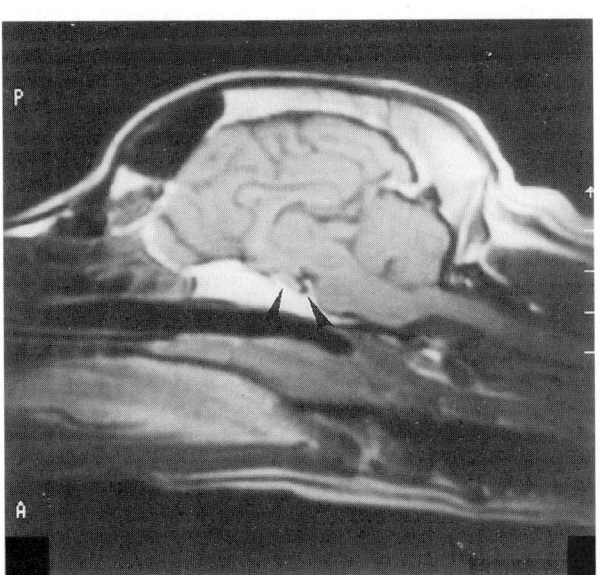 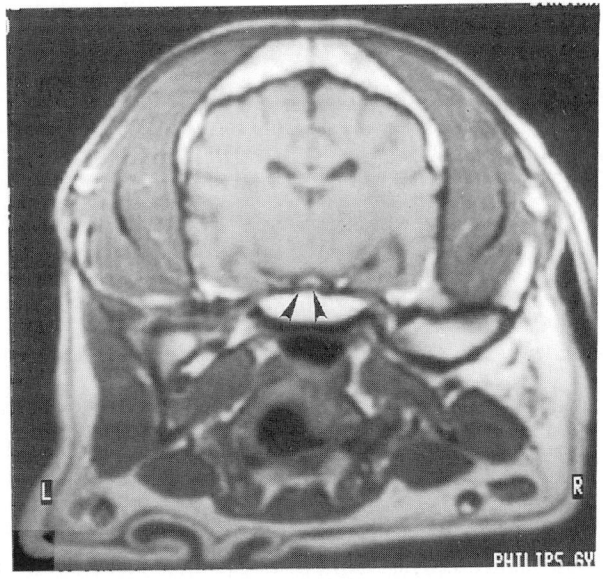

A          B

**Figure 1.** Magnetic resonance image of a 10-year-old cocker spaniel with PDH, and no neurologic signs. *A,* Midline sagittal view. *B,* Transverse view (*arrowheads* demonstrate a normal pituitary gland within the sella turcica).

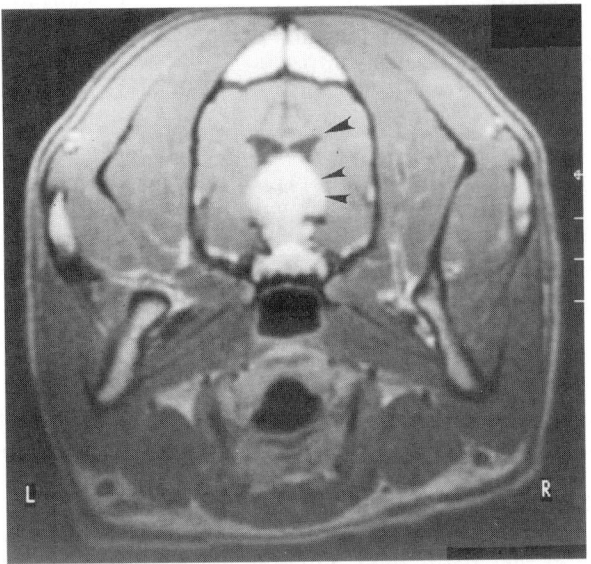

**Figure 2.** Post-gadolinium MRI of a 7-year-old bull terrier with PDH that developed signs of disorientation and ataxia. Transverse view demonstrating a 2.4-cm densely enhancing mass arising from the pituitary fossa (*small arrowheads*). Dilatation of the lateral ventricles indicates obstructive hydrocephalus (*large arrowhead*).

PDH and CNS signs. Treatment is indicated for dogs with mild or moderate CNS signs that have a visible pituitary tumor identified by advanced imaging. If not treated, most dogs develop significant progression of neurologic signs within weeks to months, with a tendency for neurologic deterioration to accelerate as it progresses.

The decision to perform CT or MRI of the pituitary gland in dogs with PDH that lack CNS signs must be tempered by the realization that imaging facilities are not readily available, the procedure is usually quite expensive, and the dog will need to be anesthetized. A degree of risk is associated with general anesthesia of any middle-aged to geriatric patient. The powerful magnet used in MRI further complicates anesthesia because it prohibits the use of common anesthetic machines and monitoring equipment. In dogs undergoing MRI, anesthesia can be safely induced and maintained using injectable agents (i.e., pentobarbital or a combination of ketamine and diazepam). However, minimal monitoring of vital signs is possible during the 8- to 10-min period each scan is performed.

The significance of identifying a pituitary tumor in a dog that lacks CNS signs is uncertain. In a recent study using MRI to evaluate the pituitary gland in dogs with newly diagnosed PDH and no CNS signs, visible tumors (3 to 12 mm) were found in more than half of the dogs (Bertoy et al., in press). It is not clear which, if any, of these dogs will develop CNS signs at some future time. It remains to be determined whether the finding of a relatively large tumor is predictive of future tumor growth and development of CNS signs. However, since at least 50% of dogs with macrotumors do develop CNS signs, treatment appears to be warranted when tumors exceed 10 mm, even if CNS signs are

lacking. Dogs that have compression or invasion of parasellar structures by a pituitary tumor should also be treated, regardless of absolute tumor size or CNS signs. Large-scale studies to evaluate the biologic behavior of pituitary tumors in dogs with PDH are needed before detailed guidelines for preventative treatment can be established.

## TREATMENT AND PROGNOSIS

Objectives for the treatment of macrotumors include the removal or destruction of tumor mass, reversal of neurologic dysfunction, and resolution of hypercortisolism, while sparing remaining pituitary function. Of these objectives, reduction of tumor mass-effect and improvement in neurologic function receive the highest priority. Cytoreduction of canine macrotumors has been attempted using radiation therapy or, rarely, surgical excision. Following advances in microsurgery, partial hypophysectomy became the treatment of choice for PDH caused by microtumors in human beings. Unfortunately, even in the most sophisticated surgical settings, the size and location of most canine macrotumors would contraindicate surgical intervention.

### Radiation Therapy

Radiation therapy has been the primary modality used for the treatment of macrotumors in dogs (see "Radiation Therapy for Pituitary Tumors," this volume, p 356). Reported treatment regimens have consisted of using cobalt-60 teletherapy to administer 40 to 54 Gy, in 10 to 18 equal fractions, over a 4- to 6-week period. Results achieved within any group of dogs reported have been quite variable. In our experience, approximately 70% of dogs with CNS signs caused by a macrotumor show improvement in neurologic function after radiation therapy. The remaining 30% show progression of neurologic signs, despite treatment. Dogs that show progression of CNS signs often die, or are euthanatized, before radiation treatment is completed.

Approximately 50% of the dogs that have a favorable response to radiation treatment demonstrate rapid improvement, with partial or complete resolution of neurologic abnormalities before radiation treatment is completed. In the remaining 50%, progression of CNS signs cease, but improvement is not evident until 1 to 2 months after radiation treatment is completed. Dogs from either group may show continual, gradual improvement in CNS signs for several months after treatment is completed.

Complications resulting from pituitary irradiation have been mild, most frequently including depigmentation of hair in the radiation field, hearing loss, and vestibular signs. Infrequent complications include trigeminal nerve damage and keratoconjunctivitis sicca. Hypopituitarism is a reported complication of pituitary irradiation in human beings, but has not been reported in dogs. However, surveillance for clinical signs of hypothyroidism, hypoadrenocorticism, or diabetes insipidus should be maintained, and endocrine function testing performed, if clinically indicated.

## Concurrent Medical Treatment

The effect of pituitary irradiation on ACTH secretion by canine macrotumors is not predictable. Excessive ACTH secretion may decline weeks to months after radiation treatment, or may persist indefinitely. In one report, ACTH secretion declined in three of six dogs, 5 to 17 months after radiation therapy (Dow et al., 1990). If excessive ACTH secretion persists, resolution of hypercortisolism requires medical treatment to destroy or inhibit adrenocortical function. Medical treatment for PDH has been reviewed elsewhere (see *CVT X, XI*). The decision to initiate or resume medical treatment for hypercortisolism in a dog with a macrotumor must be based on the perceived risks and benefits for the pet and owner. Medical treatment of hypercortisolism has no direct effect on pituitary tumors, but has been postulated to remove negative feedback to ACTH secretion and promote growth of pituitary tumors. Furthermore, medical treatment of PDH requires close observation of the dog's attitude and appetite in order to prevent hypocortisolism and is not recommended for dogs exhibiting CNS signs or anorexia. If CNS signs resolve following radiation therapy, medical treatment of hypercortisolism is recommended only if warranted by clinical or metabolic manifestations of hypercortisolism. These include behavioral problems (e.g., inappropriate urination, food-related aggression), severe muscle weakness, nonhealing wounds, recurrent infections, diabetes mellitus, and pancreatitis. Because dogs undergoing treatment for hypercortisolism may have a delayed decline in ACTH secretion, a complete history, physical examination, and endocrine evaluation (basal endogenous ACTH concentration and ACTH stimulation test) should be performed every 2 to 3 months to assess pituitary adrenocortical function.

## Prognostic Determinants

Recurrence of CNS signs is common, and may occur weeks to years after radiation treatment. When CNS signs relapse, deterioration of neurologic function may be quite rapid. In a group of nine dogs with macrotumors that we treated, CNS signs relapsed 5 to 26 months after radiation treatment, and median survival time was 11 months. This contrasts with median survival times of 2.5 and 25 months after radiation treat-

ment reported by others (Mauldin and Burk, 1990; Dow et al., 1990).

The degree of neurologic impairment appears to be an important determinant of short- and long-term prognosis. Dogs exhibiting mild CNS signs, limited to subtle behavioral abnormalities, tend to have more rapid, complete, and lasting remission of neurologic signs. Dogs exhibiting more advanced CNS signs, such as stupor, seizures, or head-pressing, often show minimal or no response to radiation, and are more likely to die before treatment is completed. The degree of neurologic impairment has been strongly correlated with tumor volume, determined by CT imaging or postmortem examination. However, some dogs with tumors 10 mm or larger show no neurologic abnormalities, whereas others with relatively small tumors may be severely impaired. This disparity between tumor volume and neurologic signs probably reflects the rate of tumor growth. Slow-growing tumors allow compensation for injury to nervous tissue before reaching a critical mass that results in neurologic signs.

## References and Suggested Reading

Bertoy EH, Feldman EC, Nelson RW, et al: Magnetic resonance imaging of the brain in dogs with recently diagnosed but untreated pituitary-dependent hyperadrenocorticism. J Am Vet Med Assoc (in press).
*A prospective study using magnetic resonance imaging to determine the incidence of visible pituitary tumors in dogs with newly diagnosed, untreated pituitary-dependent hyperadrenocorticism.*

Dow SW, LeCouteur RA, Rosychuk AW, et al: Response of dogs with functional pituitary macroadenomas and macrocarcinomas to radiation. J Small Anim Pract 31:287, 1990.
*A prospective study evaluating the effects of pituitary irradiation on the size and endocrinologic function of large pituitary tumors.*

Duesberg CA, Feldman EC, Nelson RW, et al: Brain magnetic resonance imaging for the diagnosis of pituitary macrotumors. J Am Vet Med Assoc (in press).
*A description of magnetic resonance imaging characteristics of pituitary macrotumors in 13 dogs with PDH and neurologic signs.*

Kipperman BS, Feldman EC, Dybdal NO, et al: Pituitary tumor size, neurologic signs, and relation to endocrine test results in dogs with pituitary-dependent hyperadrenocorticism: 43 cases (1980–1990). J Am Vet Med Assoc 201:762, 1992.
*A comparison of endocrine test results in dogs with PDH caused by microtumors versus those with macrotumors or neurologic signs or both.*

Mauldin GN and Burk RL: The use of diagnostic computerized tomography and radiation therapy in canine and feline hyperadrenocorticism. Prob Vet Med 4:557, 1990.
*A description of the clinical course of eight dogs with macrotumors treated with cobalt-60 radiation.*

Nelson RW, Ihle SL, and Feldman EC: Pituitary macroadenomas and macroadenocarcinomas in dogs treated with mitotane for pituitary-dependent hyperadrenocorticism: 13 cases (1981–1986). J Am Vet Med Assoc 194:1612, 1989.
*A review of clinical, laboratory, and tumor characteristics in 13 dogs with pituitary macrotumors.*

Sarafaty D, Carrillo JM, and Peterson ME: Neurologic, endocrinologic, and pathologic findings associated with large pituitary tumors in dogs: Eight cases. J Am Vet Med Assoc 193:854, 1988.
*A description of neurologic signs, endocrine test results, and tumor characteristics for eight dogs with macrotumors.*

# RADIATION THERAPY FOR PITUITARY TUMORS

SUSAN M. LARUE

*Fort Collins, Colorado*

The past decade has been an exciting period in the diagnosis and treatment of dogs and cats with pituitary tumors. Hormonal assays have been developed and normal values established. High-resolution computed tomography (CT) and magnetic resonance imaging (MRI) have been made increasingly available to veterinary patients. Radiation therapy is also more accessible and is becoming an important tool in the management of patients with pituitary tumors.

Pituitary-dependent hyperadrenocorticism (PDH) resulting from excessive secretion of adrenocorticotrophic hormone (ACTH) by the pituitary gland is a common endocrinopathy in dogs and cats. Pituitary-dependent hyperadrenocorticism is associated with the presence of either microscopic or macroscopic tumors, generally adenomas. Although these tumors are benign, the physical presence of a macroadenoma can cause neurologic signs. Macroscopic pituitary tumors cannot be distinguished from microscopic tumors antemortem without the aid of CT or MRI evaluation. Macroscopic tumors, termed "macroadenomas," were defined as tumors visible on CT evaluation. This terminology has become somewhat confusing as CT and MRI technology has evolved, permitting smaller and smaller lesions to be diagnosed.

Originally, it was presumed that the vast majority of patients with PDH had only a microscopic focus of tumor, termed "microadenoma." More recently, it has been observed that some patients with PDH can have macroadenomas without the presence of neurologic abnormalities. These tumors are being recognized because more animals with PDH routinely undergo CT or MRI evaluation and possibly because improved survival in medically treated PDH allows time for tumor progression from microscopic to macroscopic.

Pituitary macroadenomas are also associated with acromegaly syndromes in dogs and cats. Adenocarcinomas of the pituitary have been reported, and while some are nonfunctional, others secrete ACTH and cannot be distinguished from adenomas using laboratory evaluation (Kipperman et al., 1992) or appearance on CT or MRI. Other enhancing tumors such as meningiomas can occur in the pituitary fossa and cannot be distinguished by CT or MRI from tumors of pituitary origin.

In animals with macroadenomas, neurologic signs vary and depend on the size and extent of the lesion. Signs reported have included behavioral abnormalities such as lethargy, pacing, wandering, hiding, circling, head pressing, depression, aggression, and somnolence.

Seizures, cranial nerve deficits, and paresis have also been reported. Patients with neurologic signs secondary to pituitary tumors undergo rapid demise if left untreated (Sarfaty, Carillo, and Peterson, 1988).

Radiation therapy has been reported as a treatment option for dogs with neurologic signs resulting from pituitary macroscopic tumors. In the report by Dow et al. (1990), neurologic signs resolved in six dogs treated with radiotherapy. Signs associated with pituitary ACTH secretion persisted for at least 1 year after treatment despite a reduction in tumor size. Median survival was 24 months, a vast improvement over the mean survival of 4.7 months reported in eight dogs with large pituitary tumors treated with medical management alone (Sarfaty, Carillo, and Peterson, 1988). A later report had a comparable median survival (21 months) if the neurologic status of the animal was good prior to treatment, but there was limited survival in patients that had moderate to severe neurologic signs when radiotherapy was initiated (Mauldin and Burk, 1990). These data imply that early diagnosis and treatment is important in the management of this condition. Therefore, patients with PDH should be closely observed for the presence of any neurologic sign compatible with the presence of a macroscopic tumor. When animals return for reevaluation, owners should be questioned about any subtle changes in behavior. At Colorado State University, anorexia has been an early and consistent finding in patients with PDH that have developed macroadenomas. Computed tomography or MRI is recommended in any patient with PDH having anorexia or other subtle neurologic signs.

The diagnosis of PDH and pituitary macroadenomas has been covered in detail in previous articles. This discussion focuses on performing imaging techniques in patients where radiotherapy is a treatment option, and on the principles of treating and managing a patient with radiotherapy.

## CT EVALUATION

If an animal is undergoing CT or MRI evaluation for a possible pituitary mass, special care should be taken with the diagnostic studies to facilitate radiotherapy. The CT image should include the external contour of the patient. The positioning of the patient for CT scan should duplicate as closely as possible the positioning that will be used for radiotherapy. If the patient is positioned differently for radiotherapy than for the CT scan (on which treatment planning was based), the dose to the tumor may not be accurate. At Colorado State University, patients undergoing CT scan are positioned in sternal recumbency. The head is positioned with no rotational or axial deviation and adjusted until the hard palate is parallel to the couch. If the region of interest is limited to the pituitary, the scan begins caudally at the middle of the bullae and proceeds rostrally to encompass the entire tumor. A slice thickness of 4 mm with a 1-mm overlap is desired. After an initial scan without contrast, 160 mg/kg iodine in the form of triiodinated contrast material should be injected intravenously. Nonionic contrast agents are also acceptable at the same dosage.

Images should be reconstructed on the dorsal and sagittal planes to accurately define the shape and extent of the lesion. The same positioning criteria are applicable to MRI evaluations.

## RADIATION THERAPY

Radiation therapy for pituitary tumors is indicated in the following situations: in animals with a pituitary tumor and associated neurologic signs; in animals with a pituitary tumor but without neurologic signs if the pituitary tumor is greater than or equal to 1 cm diameter; and in animals that have a pituitary tumor that is causing compression or invasion of adjacent normal tissues on CT or MRI. The role of radiotherapy in animals with microadenomas or small, noninvasive tumors (<1 cm) has not been determined.

External beam radiotherapy for pituitary tumors must be administered using megavoltage irradiation, generally available from a Cobalt-60 machine or clinical linear accelerator. Orthovoltage radiotherapy of pituitary tumors is contraindicated for a variety of reasons. The low-energy orthovoltage x-rays attenuate rapidly so the intervening normal tissues receive an inappropriately high dose of irradiation. Dosimetry is further complicated by the disproportionately high dose that is delivered to the skull, and the uncertainly of what dose reaches the tumor.

## Treatment Planning

The goals of treatment planning are to administer the desired dose to the tumor while minimizing the dose to normal tissue structures. The simplest method of treating is to use parallel-opposed portals, calculating the dose to a point in the center of the tumor. However, advances in radiotherapy have allowed for more sophisticated treatment planning. Computerized systems enhance treatment planning by allowing multiple beams from various angles and the use of beam attenuators, known as wedges. Ideally, there should be less than 5% variation between the minimum tumor dose and the maximum dose administered to the patient.

Parallel-opposed portals constituted the first method reported in the veterinary literature for treating pituitary tumors. The advantage of the technique is that it can be easily calculated without the aid of a computerized system, and that it provides an even distribution of dose to the tumor (Fig. 1A). The disadvantage of this approach is that both the inner and external ear canal are in the treatment field and receive a dose comparable to the tumor dose. This can result in important early and late effects to the ear from irradiation. The most profound early effect is ulcerative otitis externa. Late effects include hearing impairment that can vary from mild to complete deafness. By using more sophisticated treatment planning, the dose to the inner and external ear canal can be decreased. Methods include using more than two beams or using wedges or both (Fig. 1B).

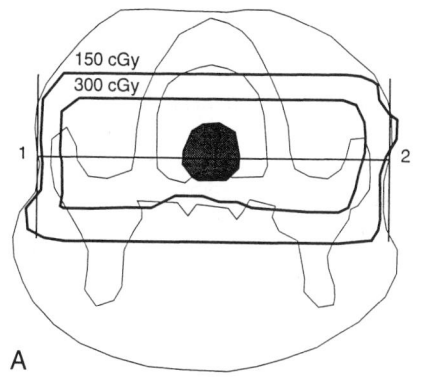 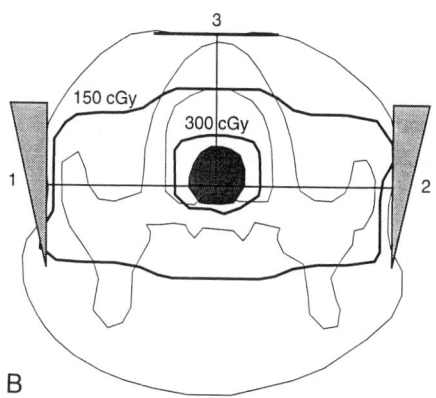

**Figure 1.** *A,* This is a computer-generated treatment plan based on the CT image of a patient with a macroadenoma. The gray hatched region represents the tumor and desired margin. Parallel-opposed portals are used. This plan is similar to what is obtained when dose calculation is performed without a computer. The region of interest receives the minimum tumor dose of 300 cGy per fraction, but a large volume of normal tissue also receives the same dose. *B,* Computer-generated treatment plan on same patient as in *A.* This plan uses wedges and three beams. The overall result is to restrict the 300-cGy isodose line to the region of the tumor and decrease the dose administered to the rest of the brain and other normal tissue structures. The inner ear apparatus and external ear canal cannot be seen from this central axis view; however, the field extends caudally to include those structures. This method reduces the dose to these structures, which should result in a decreased probability of hearing impairment.

In general, if the lesion is believed to be an adenoma, the region being treated should include the tumor and a 1-cm margin. A larger margin is often included by necessity because the megavoltage radiotherapy equipment available in veterinary medicine requires the minimal field sizes that are often much larger than these small tumors! This is particularly true when treating small dogs and cats, where even the smallest field sizes available incorporate almost the entire brain. If there is reason to believe that the tumor may be an adenocarcinoma, the field size should be increased to include at least a 2-cm margin.

## Patient Positioning

After a treatment plan is developed, the animal needs to be positioned to receive therapy. The position of the portals should be determined from the treatment plan, using bony landmarks to assist in alignment. If the animal is to be treated in sternal recumbency, it is recommended that the hard palate be adjusted with a small sponge until parallel with the treatment couch. For dogs being treated in lateral recumbency, foam pads positioned between the legs to keep the extremities parallel may help decrease axial rotation, and a small foam pad placed under the rostral maxilla will maintain axial alignment of the head. Laser positioning lights can be used to aid in positioning, although tattoos are less reliable in animal patients than in human patients, where skin is less mobile. It is best to use the relation between bony landmarks and the positioning lasers in veterinary patients.

The region being treated must be confirmed using port films. Port films are radiographs in which the film is exposed by photons emitted directly from the radiotherapy machine. The film, X-omat TL (Kodak), is made specifically for this purpose. Two brief exposures are made: the first includes only the treatment field, and the second includes a wider area so the location of the field in relation to surrounding structures can be evaluated. At initial observation, port films look like diagnostic radiographs of the poorest quality. However, on closer observation, important bony structures can be identified (Fig. 2). For pituitary tumors, the field should be centered at the pituitary fossa. The ventral aspect of the field should extend into the oral pharynx. For most patients, a 4- × 4-cm or 4- × 5-cm field will adequately encompass the tumor and margins.

## Radiation Protocol and Dose

In general, radiation dose administered to any tumor is limited by the tolerance of late-responding normal tissues in the field. Slow- or nondividing tissues, such as bone and neural tissues, are susceptible to late effects from irradiation, particularly when administered in the large fraction sizes commonly used in veterinary medicine. The radiation dose administered to the region should have a minimal probability of causing a

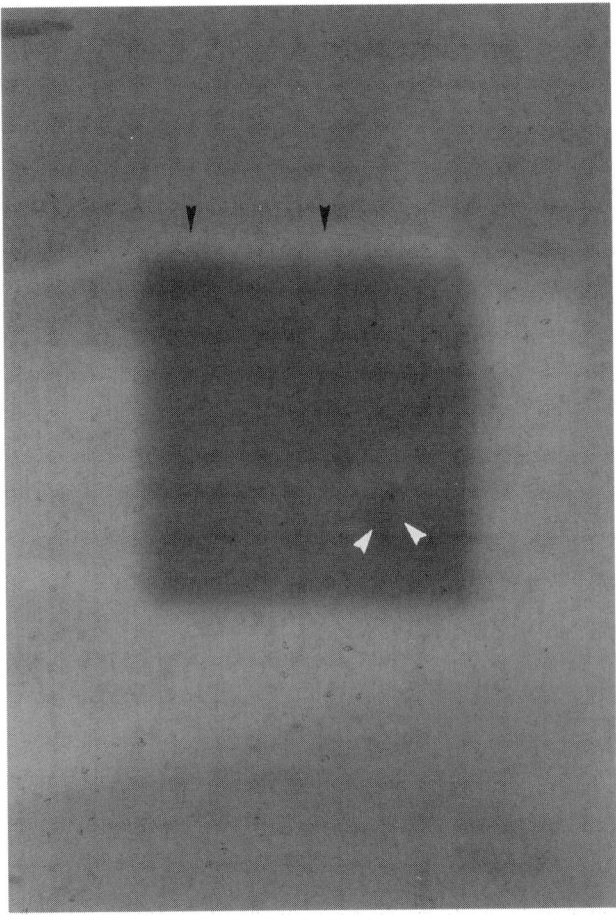

**Figure 2.** Port film indicating the treatment volume in a cat receiving radiotherapy for a pituitary tumor. *Black arrows* show the dorsum of the skull and *white arrows* mark the bullae. On close inspection the ear, frontal sinus, and hard palate can be observed.

significant late effect. Increasing the duration of radiotherapy administration does not reduce to the probability of late effects.

The brain is the dose-limiting tissue when treating pituitary tumors. Histologically, late effects to brain include vascular lesions, vacuolar changes in white matter, gitter cells in areas of malacia and necrosis, and parenchymal atrophy, which can result in hydrocephalus. Necrosis, when it develops, is irreversible, although in human patients surgical excision of the necrotic region is sometimes beneficial. These late effects of irradiation generally occur 6 months or more after radiotherapy. These changes can be manifested by a variety of clinical signs, the most common of which is exacerbation of the original signs. Animals may also experience different neurologic signs, seizures, or generalized depression and somnolence. It is often very difficult to distinguish the clinical signs associated with late effects of irradiation from signs associated with tumor recurrence. Computed tomography and MRI scans can be difficult to interpret because some brain tumors do not completely disappear following irradiation. Therefore, the presence of a mass does not necessarily imply tumor regrowth. Although steroid administration may cause some relief of signs by decreasing associated edema, the signs are generally progressive.

At Colorado State University, animals undergoing radiation therapy for a variety of brain tumors underwent necropsy evaluation at the time of euthanasia. The brains of these patients were closely evaluated for tumor recurrences and brain necrosis associated with irradiation. Based on this information, it is believed that the radiation tolerance for brain is 45 to 48 Gy administered in 3-Gy fractions. If surgery or surgical biopsy has been performed, 45 Gy in 3-Gy fractions should not be exceeded. Fortunately, pituitary adenomas appear to be responsive to modest doses of irradiation; in humans, the radiation dose used for treating adenomas usually does not exceed 45 Gy (Halberg and Sheline, 1987). The current protocol used for most pituitary macroadenomas at Colorado State University is 45 Gy administered in 15 fractions of 3 Gy on a Monday-through-Friday schedule. If the tumor is 2 cm or larger, if there is severe compression of adjacent brain, or if there is clinical evidence that suggests that the tumor may be malignant, the patient should receive 48 Gy in 16 fractions of 3 Gy.

## CLINICAL MANAGEMENT DURING AND AFTER RADIOTHERAPY

Unless the patient is profoundly depressed, general anesthesia is administered to patients prior to treatment. The anesthetic regimen should be based on the individual patient's clinical status and biochemical panel, keeping in mind the principles of neuroanesthesia. Preanesthesia with meperidine, followed by induction with ultra-short-acting barbiturate and maintenance with isoflurane and oxygen has been used successfully in a large number of dogs and cats with brain tumors. The use of a ventilator in animals with brain tumors undergoing radiotherapy is recommended.

While all animals undergoing radiotherapy need close observation and continued evaluation during the course of treatment, this is especially true for patients with brain tumors. In many animals, the neurologic signs will often improve dramatically within the first week of therapy. It is unclear what mechanism is responsible for the clinical improvement, inasmuch as significant reduction in tumor volume would not be expected in such a short time. Although dogs with a better neurologic function may have an improved prognosis, some animals with severely compromised neurologic function will dramatically improve during therapy and have a durable remission. A few patients, however, will experience an initial worsening of signs, perhaps due to brain edema associated with the radiotherapy. Anti-inflammatory doses of dexamethasone or prednisolone have been successful in controlling these signs in some patients. If at all possible, scheduled radiotherapy should be continued during this period. Otitis also may develop in the second or third week of therapy; in these animals, treatment with otic preparations containing a steroid or dimethyl sulfoxide (DMSO) may be helpful. In these animals, there may be a transient period of decreased hearing during this time as the result of the ear canals becoming swollen and filled with cellular debris.

Changes to the skin will be evident by 2 weeks after the end of therapy. Changes vary depending on the dose to the skin and the sensitivity of the patient; however, dry to moist desquamation and regional alopecia are common. In almost all cases, the fur will grow back, but it may return with a different color or texture.

Neural tissue is unique from other tissues because of the development of "early delayed" effects from irradiation. These effects, which usually occur from 2 weeks to 3 months after therapy, are due to transient demyelination. Clinically, this results in an exacerbation of the original signs, or it can result in generalized depression. Computed tomography or MRI studies performed at this time will probably not assist in making the diagnosis. The demyelinization is not profound enough to be discernable and evaluation of the tumor can be misleading. Clinical signs may improve or stabilize with steroidal therapy or resolve with time. Supportive care should be initiated and the owners made aware that signs *may* improve over a period of weeks.

The primary goal of treating pituitary tumors with irradiation is to diminish associated neurologic signs. However, in some patients with PDH, ACTH production decreases and medication (e.g., mitotane) for Cushing's disease can be discontinued; this usually does not occur for at least a year after therapy. It is important that patients be monitored at regular intervals following irradiation for changes in their endocrine status.

Patients should also be evaluated on a regular basis for late effects from radiotherapy. Hearing impairment has been reported, as has transient central vestibular disease. Late effects to the brain have been discussed and are difficult to distinguish from tumor recurrence. If an animal presents with compelling evidence of a tumor recurrence, treatment options are limited. Reirradiation of the brain is not advocated because of the extremely high probability of complications. If the tumor recurs or there are neurologic signs associated with late effects of irradiation, palliative treatment with steroids may improve the quality of life for a brief period. A postmortem examination, including histologic evaluation of the tumor bed, is strongly recommended in any animal with a pituitary tumor treated with radiotherapy. Important information such as the histologic identity of the tumor and the effect of irradiation on the brain relative to dose, fraction size, and treatment volume cannot be determined any other way. This knowledge is necessary for continued advances in the treatment of these tumors.

## References and Suggested Reading

Dow SW, LeCouteur RA, Rosychuk RAW, et al: Response of dogs with functional pituitary macroadenomas and macrocarcinomas to radiation. J Small Anim Pract 31:287, 1990.

*A retrospective study of six dogs with pituitary tumors treated with radiotherapy.*
Halberg FE and Sheline GE: Radiotherapy of pituitary tumors. Endocrinol Metab Clin 16:667, 1987.
    *A review of treatment of pituitary tumors in human patients with radiotherapy.*
Kipperman BS, Feldman EC, Dybdal NO, et al: Pituitary tumor size, neurologic signs, and relation to endocrine test results in dogs with pituitary-dependent hyperadrenocorticism: 43 cases (1980–1990). J Am Vet Med Assoc 201:762, 1992.
    *A retrospective study evaluating pituitary tumor size and endocrine test results in 43 dogs.*

Mauldin GN and Burk RL: The use of diagnostic computerized tomography and radiation therapy in canine and feline hyperadrenocorticism (sic). Prob Vet Med, 2:557, 1990.
    *A review of hyperadrenocorticism in humans and in veterinary patients and retrospective data on diagnosis and treatment in ten patients.*
Safarty D, Carrillo JM, and Peterson ME: Neurologic, endocrinologic and pathologic findings associated with large pituitary tumors in dogs: Eight cases (1997–1984). J Am Vet Med Assoc 193:854, 1988.
    *A retrospective study of eight dogs with large pituitary tumors.*

# FREE THYROID HORMONE MEASUREMENTS IN THE DIAGNOSIS OF THYROID DISEASE

DUNCAN C. FERGUSON

*Athens, Georgia*

Tests for the measurement of free thyroid hormone concentrations are now being offered by veterinary diagnostic laboratories. The following discussion outlines the theoretical value of the measurement of free hormone concentrations in the diagnosis of thyroid disease, and then considers the methodology for measurement of free thyroid hormones. The discussion focuses upon the measurement of free thyroxine ($FT_4$) and free triiodothyronine ($FT_3$) in the diagnosis of canine hypothyroidism and feline hyperthyroidism.

## THE "FREE HORMONE" HYPOTHESIS

The free hormone hypothesis, proposed by Robbins and Rall over 30 years ago, states that it is the unbound fraction of hormone which is available to tissues and therefore proportional to the action, metabolism, and elimination of that hormone. This hypothesis has stood the clinical test of time; direct or indirect measurements of $FT_4$ have become the mainstay in the diagnosis of thyroid disease in human medicine (Mendel, 1989).

## FREE THYROXINE MEASUREMENTS AS APPLIED TO HUMAN PATIENTS

The experience with accurate free hormone measurements in domestic animals is still being developed. Because of its potential for appropriate use in veterinary medicine today, it is worthwhile examining why serum $FT_4$ has such diagnostic value in humans. In humans, the diagnostic accuracy of a single $FT_4$ measurement is approximately 90%. When both endogenous thyrotropin (TSH) and $FT_4$ measurements concur, the diagnostic accuracy approaches 100%. The $FT_4$ concentration correlates highly with thyroid secretory function. An estimate of $FT_4$ is theoretically not subject to the spontaneous or drug-induced changes that may occur in total $T_4$ ($TT_4$) concentration measurements. Furthermore, it is the free hormone fraction that is available to peripheral tissues and converted there to the more biologically active $T_3$ (Fig. 1). In fact, it is the intrapituitary conversion of $T_4$ to $T_3$ that links the $FT_4$ value inversely to the large changes in endogenous TSH concentrations seen as serum $FT_4$ falls. The $FT_4$ concentration is inversely proportional to the logarithm of the serum TSH concentration; that is, an approximately 100-fold increase in serum TSH is seen with a twofold fall of $FT_4$ (Nicoloff, 1991). The relationship between serum $FT_4$ and TSH is therefore a functional one, and since $FT_4$ can currently be measured accurately in the dog, this relationship should be of interest to veterinarians.

## PLASMA THYROID HORMONE BINDING IN THE DOG AND CAT

The circulation of the lipophilic thyroid hormones in plasma is dependent upon binding by plasma proteins like albumin and thyroxine–binding globulin (TBG), which serve to "buffer" hormone delivery into tissue and provide a hormone reservoir, as well as some proteins like thyroid hormone-binding prealbumin (transthyretin [TBPA]), which may serve as intermediary carriers for specific tissue hormone uptake. The dog has approximately 15% of the amount of TBG in plasma compared to humans, while the cat does not appear to

**Figure 1.** *In vivo*, thyroid hormones (T₄, T₃) are in equilibrium with PBP and CTBP in the cytosol. The free (unbound) form of thyroid hormones (FT₄, FT₃) distribute across the plasma membrane and determine hormone action at the mitochondria (oxygen consumption and energy metabolism) and the nucleus (protein synthesis). Furthermore, FT₄ intracellularly serves as the substrate for the 5'-deiodinase enzyme, which converts T₄ to the more active hormone T₃.

*In vitro*, in the dialysis chamber, the free fraction of T₄ can equilibrate across a dialysis membrane where it can be sampled or assayed. Abbreviations: PBP = plasma-binding proteins, T₃ = triiodothyronine, T₄ = thyroxine, FT₄ = free thyroxine, FT₃ = free triiodothyronine, CTBP = cytosolic thyroid hormone-binding proteins, 5'-D = 5'-deiodinase enzyme.

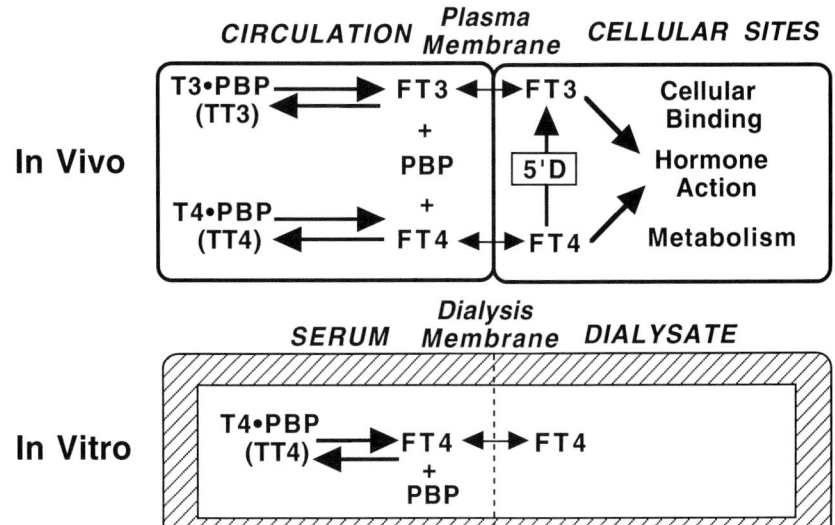

have this high-affinity binder. In the dog, in addition to albumin, TBG, and TBPA, T₄ appears to bind to the plasma lipoprotein high-density lipoprotein 2 (HDL₂) and to very-low-density lipoprotein (VLDL). Serum thyroid hormone–binding proteins in the cat include primarily albumin and prealbumin.

Transthyretin is present in the plasma of species ranging from fish to humans, suggesting its importance in tissue hormone delivery. The overall affinity of the thyroid hormone–binding proteins for T₄ is lower in the dog than in humans. As will be pointed out later, many of the rapid "nondialysis" methods for free hormone measurement are extremely TBG dependent, providing inaccurate results when TBG concentrations are low to undetectable. Partly as a result of this weaker protein binding, TT₄ concentrations are lower and the unbound or free fraction of circulating T₄ is higher in dogs and cats. The proportion of free hormone is a primary determinant of the rate of fractional metabolic and excretory turnover of thyroid hormones. In the healthy euthyroid dog or cat, about 0.1% of total serum T₄ is unbound or free, whereas about 1% of T₃ is free, while the fractional FT₄ in humans is 20 to 30% of these values. In the dog, the plasma half-life of T₄ has been estimated to be between 10 and 16 hr, compared with about 7 days in humans; the plasma half-life of T₃ in the dog is estimated to be 5 to 6 hr (Larsson, Pettersson, and Carlstrom, 1985; Peterson and Ferguson, 1990; Ferguson and Peterson, 1992).

## CLINICAL SITUATIONS THAT MAY ALTER THE FREE THYROID HORMONE FRACTION

In theory, measurement of FT₄ should account for changes in serum binding associated with medical conditions and drug competition. As the FT₄ fraction rises or falls, the negative feedback of the absolute FT₄ concentration on the hypothalamus and pituitary causes a fall or rise in TSH secretion, resulting in alteration of

thyroid secretion and TT₄ concentration. We have been able to demonstrate *in vitro* that the fatty acid, oleic acid, a putative hormone-binding inhibitor in nonthyroidal illness, increases the FT₄ fraction of undiluted serum by over 200%. Furthermore, the commonly used drugs furosemide, flunixin, and diphenylhydantoin increases the FT₄ fraction *in vitro* by 50 to 200%. Any drug that is highly protein bound (> 90%) has the potential of increasing the FT₄ fraction. If this mechanism occurs in the circulation, the absolute FT₄ concentrations would transiently rise, increasing negative feedback on the pituitary TSH secretion, resulting in a fall in thyroid hormone secretion, and eventually lowering TT₄ concentrations but returning FT₄ to normal. The development of thyroid hormone–binding antibodies in autoimmune thyroid disease may decrease the free hormone fraction in selected cases with high titers, although an extensive study has not yet been performed.

## METHODS FOR THE MEASUREMENT OF FREE THYROID HORMONE CONCENTRATIONS

### Serum FT₄ Concentration by Equilibrium Dialysis

The standard reference technique ("gold standard") for the measurement of the FT₄ involves the determination of the FT₄ fraction (% FT₄ when expressed as a percentage) by equilibrium dialysis of a radioactive T₄ tracer and the TT₄ concentration by radioimmunoassay (RIA). The absolute FT₄ concentration is then calculated as follows:

$$FT_4 \text{ (pmol/L)} = \% FT_4 \times TT_4 \text{ (nmol/L)} \times 10$$

Equilibrium dialysis requires special dialysis chambers and attention must be paid to the purity of the radioactive tracer so that iodide contamination does not result in artificially elevated results. Present radioisotopic dialysis methods are tedious, and large numbers of samples cannot be assayed at the same time. It has been observed that the dilution of dog serum by greater than fourfold is likely to result in an underestimate of the $FT_4$ fraction (Ferguson and Peterson, 1992). However, "direct" dialysis methods have recently been developed and are used in at least one commercial assay (Table 1) that include the dialysis of undiluted serum followed by radioimmunoassay of the dialysate with an ultrasensitive radioimmunoassay. Preliminary results using this nonisotopic equilibrium dialysis assay indicate good agreement (high correlation, slope approximating 1) with the isotopic equilibrium dialysis procedure. This assay is now starting to be used by certain veterinary endocrine diagnostic laboratories (see Table 1).

## "Analogue" Immunoassays for Measurement of Free Thyroid Hormones

Commercial "analogue" $FT_4$ assays, which theoretically measure the $FT_4$ concentration directly by radioimmunoassay, are available and are being used by a large number of veterinary diagnostic laboratories. These assays were developed for use on human serum and contain reagents optimal for this application. Some assays use antibodies inside of microcapsule dialysis membranes or thyroid hormone analogues that theoretically do not bind serum proteins. Undoubtedly, these methods are more rapid and practical than equilibrium dialysis. Because most of these assays depend upon the dominance of the high-affinity protein TBG, there is even more reason to question the validity of these assays for veterinary use, as TBG concentrations

**Table 1.**  *Commercial Laboratories Performing Direct Dialysis Free Thyroxine Assays**

1. Auburn University Endocrine Diagnostic Laboratory
   Endocrine Diagnostic Service
   P.O. Box 2148
   Auburn, AL 36831-2148
   Phone: 205-844-5400
   Contact: Dr. Robert Kemppainen

2. Endocrine Laboratory
   Dept. of Clinical Sciences
   College of Veterinary Medicine
   Kansas State University
   Manhattan, KS 66506
   Phone: 913-532-5690
   Contact: Dr. David Bruyette

3. Endocrinology
   Animal Health Diagnostic Laboratory
   P.O. Box 30076
   Lansing, MI 48909
   Phone: 517-353-0621

4. Veterinary Research
   10 Executive Blvd.
   Farmingdale, NY 11735
   Phone: 800-872-1001
   Contact: Dr. Rhett Nichols

*Other laboratories may have developed this capability at the time of publication.

are low in the dog and nonexistent in the cat (Larsson, Pettersson, and Carlstrom, 1985). Those kits that use an analogue method have been seriously questioned, because the labeled analogue of thyroxine binds to serum albumin and results are subject to variation with the serum albumin and nonesterified free fatty acid concentrations (Nelson, Wilcox, and Pandian, 1992).

The commercial analogue $FT_4$ assays have been classified by the American Thyroid Association only as free hormone indices (also thyroid hormone binding ratios) (Larsen, Alexander, and Chopra, 1987). The commercial free thyroid hormone assays have received considerable technical criticism for their use in humans (Kaptein et al., 1981). The American Thyroid Association went as far as stating that the analogue (nondialysis) methods for measuring $FT_4$ did not measure $FT_4$ at all, but likely were detecting something proportional to $TT_4$.

Despite the concern for some of these assays in human medicine, analogue $FT_4$ assays have been rapidly adopted in veterinary endocrine diagnostic laboratories. Unfortunately, very few validation studies have been reported. A recent summary report from the Endocrine Quality Assurance Program service coordinated by the Society for Comparative Endocrinology and Michigan State University revealed that, of the laboratories reporting $FT_4$ values from their commercial assays, the results averaged 50 to 60% of the results as measured by equilibrium dialysis. More disconcerting, the range of values measured on the same pooled sample was anywhere from 10 to 120% of the equilibrium dialysis value. As a result, some of these assays provide a normal range of $FT_4$ concentration as 3 to 5 pmol/L, very low concentrations compared to the relatively species-constant average of approximately 25 pmol/L.

Why are the commercial assays so inaccurate in conditions where greater discrimination is really needed? Methodologic idiosyncrasies (including steps requiring serum dilution) with these kits result in artificially reduced or inaccurate values, particularly in the presence of serum hormone-binding inhibitors (such as with nonthyroidal illness and drugs) (Ferguson, 1992). This dilutional effect can be minimized in dialysis systems; however, it is unavoidable in most commercial $FT_4$ assays. At the present time, the author can report encouraging results with the commercial direct dialysis $FT_4$ assay that utilizes a nonradioactive dialysis step and a very sensitive radioimmunoassay on the dialysate (see Table 1). Direct dialysis $FT_4$ results correlate well with tracer equilibrium dialysis even when animals with other diseases are included.

In summary, the analogue $FT_4$ assays are unlikely to provide much more diagnostic value than measurement of $TT_4$ concentrations, whereas the direct dialysis assay holds promise for improvement of diagnostic accuracy. These assays are not as rapid and are more expensive to purchase and run than the analogue assays (wholesale cost about $20; cost to practitioner between $25 and $40). Analogue $FT_3$ measurements, performed by some diagnostic laboratories, have the same methodologic problems as the commercial $FT_4$ measurements, and have dubious diagnostic value in the diagnosis of hypothyroidism for the same reasons as measurement of $TT_3$ concentrations. There are no commercial direct dialysis assays for $FT_3$, although some are under development.

## CLINICAL ACCURACY OF DIALYSIS METHODS FOR MEASURING $FT_4$

The performance of the dialysis assays should be evaluated over the range of conditions that veterinarians are attempting to distinguish diagnostically. Comparison of analogue $FT_4$ assays to dialysis methods generally results in reasonably high correlations in healthy dogs ($r \sim 0.9$ where 1.0 is perfect correlation). This performance in the healthy dog may be the result of the high correlation between $FT_4$ and $TT_4$ concentrations in the normal dog ($r \sim 0.7$ to 0.8). When samples from dogs with all thyroid and nonthyroid conditions were evaluated, the correlation coefficient falls to between 0 and 0.5.

It is also critical to consider the diagnostic accuracy of the assay methods in comparison to dialysis methods. Accuracy is considered to be the percentage of dogs labeled appropriately as euthyroid with normal $FT_4$ values and hypothyroid with low $FT_4$ values. Using the TSH stimulation test result and therapeutic response as the standard, $FT_4$ by equilibrium dialysis is 90% accurate, while other assays have an accuracy no better than $TT_4$ measurements ($\sim 70\%$). Therefore, early studies appear to indicate that only the dialysis methods for $FT_4$ measurement will provide the additional information needed to distinguish animals with low $TT_4$ concentrations due to nonthyroidal conditions from those with hypothyroidism.

## FREE $T_4$ MEASUREMENT IN THE DIAGNOSIS OF HYPOTHYROIDISM IN DOGS

In the absence of a single superior test for the diagnosis of hypothyroidism, such as an endogenous canine TSH immunoassay, and particularly with the sporadic availability of bovine TSH, greater attention has been paid to the identification of tests that can be performed on a single sample of blood. The results of multiple static tests are then compared by discriminant analysis to more rigorous diagnostic criteria (e.g., histology, response to therapy, TSH stimulation tests). Of the combinations of static tests, the following relation between $FT_4$ (commercial direct RIA) and cholesterol was found to give the highest diagnostic accuracy as a screening test (Larsson, 1988):

$$0.7 * FT_4 \text{ (pmol/L)—cholesterol (mmol/L), or}$$
$$9 * FT_4 \text{ (ng/dl)—0.027 * cholesterol (mg/dl)}$$

Although this algorithm does not employ the results of a dialysis $FT_4$ measurement, and normal ranges must be confirmed independently by each laboratory, it il-

lustrates an important principle in the use of any of the diagnostic tests for thyroid insufficiency: the value of a new test or combination of tests should be judged against independent objective criteria.

Hyperadrenocorticism is often a differential diagnosis for the dermatologic abnormalities seen in hypothyroidism. Total $T_4$, $T_3$, reverse $T_3$ ($rT_3$), and $FT_4$ by equilibrium dialysis were measured in 42 dogs with hyperadrenocorticism, and 38% of the dogs had low $TT_4$ values. However, of these animals, $FT_4$ concentrations were also low in 62%, indicating that roughly 25% of the dogs with hyperadrenocorticism also had low $FT_4$ concentrations (Ferguson and Peterson, 1992). In spontaneous hyperadrenocorticism, as has been shown with exogenous glucocorticoids, glucocorticoid excess likely suppresses TSH secretion and therefore $FT_4$ concentrations, raising the possibility that a secondary hypothyroidism might occur (Moore, Ferguson, Hoenig, 1993). Regardless of the mechanism, the $TT_4$ concentrations return to normal following therapy of the hyperadrenocorticism (Ferguson and Peterson, 1992).

## $FT_4$ MEASUREMENTS IN CATS WITH HYPERTHYROIDISM

In cats suspected for hyperthyroidism, studies have generally showed significant correlations between $TT_4$ and $FT_4$ concentrations determined by equilibrium dialysis, as well as between $FT_4$ itself determined by both equilibrium dialysis and by analogue assays. These data are consistent with an elevation of $FT_4$ in hyperthyroidism leading to increased concentrations of $TT_3$, $rT_3$, and $FT_3$. Therefore, at least for routine use in cats with hyperthyroidism, $FT_4$ measurements do not appear to provide any additional diagnostic information over use of $TT_4$ alone.

## SUMMARY AND COMMENTARY

The goal of this discussion was to summarize the current information available on free thyroid hormone measurements in veterinary diagnostics. One of the problems with this task is that the facts are not entirely collected. It is not sufficient to evaluate the tests in normal animals; rather, the measurements should be made in those situations where the $FT_4$ fraction is likely to be altered (e.g., uremia, drug therapy with furosemide, and hypoalbuminemia). Until proven useful in these situations in the dog and cat, the "analogue" methods for $FT_4$ measurement, which includes most assays now being offered by veterinary diagnostic laboratories, should be interpreted with caution. Despite the theoretical diagnostic advantages of free hormone measurements, it is significant to note that the analogue assays are more appropriately classified as free hormone indices rather than a true measurement. Currently, it appears that valid methodology will stem only from methods that mimic equilibrium dialysis of undiluted serum; that is, the direct dialysis method.

## References and Suggested Reading

Ferguson DC: Can hypothyroidism really be diagnosed? Analysis of tests of thyroid hypofunction in dogs and humans. *Proceedings of the 15th Waltham/OSU Symposium*, 1992, p 13.
*A review comparing thyroid function tests in dog to those used currently in humans.*

Ferguson DC and Peterson ME: Serum free and total iodothyronine concentrations in dogs with spontaneous hyperadrenocorticism. Am J Vet Res 53:1636, 1992.
*A manuscript describing the free $T_4$ assay by equilibrium dialysis applied to euthyroid dogs and dogs with hyperadrenocorticism.*

Kaptein EM, MacIntyre SS, Weiner JM, et al: Free thyroxine estimates in nonthyroidal illness: comparison of eight methods. J Clin Endocrinol Metab 52:1073, 1981.
*A systematic review of the analogue free $T_4$ assays as applied to human serum.*

Larsen PR, Alexander NM, and Chopra IJ: Revised nomenclature of tests of thyroid hormones and thyroid-related proteins in serum (Letter to the Editor). J Clin Endocrinol Metab 64:1089, 1987.
*A statement prepared by members of the American Thyroid Association on free thyroid hormone assays.*

Larsson MG: Determination of free thyroxine and cholesterol as a new screening test for canine hypothyroidism. J Am Anim Hosp Assoc 24:209, 1988.
*A study using the discriminant analysis of an analogue free $T_4$ assay and serum cholesterol to distinguish thyroidal states in dogs.*

Larsson M, Pettersson T, and Carlstrom A: Thyroid hormone binding in serum of 15 vertebrate species: Isolation of thyroxine-binding globulin and prealbumin analogs. Gen Comp Endocrinol 58:360, 1985.
*A description of the serum thyroid hormone–binding proteins in mammals.*

Mendel CM: The free hormone hypothesis: A physiologically based mathematical model. Endocrine Rev 10:232, 1989.
*A recent review of the evidence supporting the free hormone hypothesis.*

Moore GE, Ferguson DC, and Hoenig M: Effects of oral administration of anti-inflammatory doses of prednisone on thyroid hormone response to thyrotropin-releasing hormone and thyrotropin in clinically normal dogs. Am J Vet Res 54:130, 1993.
*A study evaluating the effect of oral glucocorticoids on thyroid function tests.*

Nelson JC, Wilcox RB, and Pandian MR: Dependence of free thyroxine estimates obtained with equilibrium tracer dialysis on the concentration of thyroxine-binding globulin. Clin Chem 38:1294, 1992.
*A study demonstrating the dependence of accurate $FT_4$ estimates with equilibrium dialysis on serum TBG concentrations.*

Nicoloff J: *Guide to Thyroid Function Testing for Laboratorians and Physicians.* Abbott Diagnostics Educational Services, 1991.
*A monograph prepared by Abbott Laboratories describing the current state of thyroid function testing in humans.*

Peterson ME and Ferguson DC: Thyroid diseases. *In* Ettinger SJ (ed): *Textbook of Veterinary Internal Medicine*, volume 2. Philadelphia, WB Saunders Co, 1990, p 1632.
*A textbook review of thyroid physiology, diagnostic testing, and diseases.*

# MONITORING THYROID HORMONE REPLACEMENT THERAPY

KENT R. REFSAL
*and* RAYMOND F. NACHREINER

*East Lansing, Michigan*

Treatment of canine hypothyroidism with oral administration of iodothyronines has been part of veterinary practice for many years. Probably every veterinarian engaged in small animal practice has observed the dramatic reversal of clinical signs of hypothyroidism achieved with thyroid replacement therapy. When compared to topics such as pathophysiology and diagnosis, the subject of thyroid hormone replacement has received very little attention. Veterinarians are presented with a variety of recommendations for dosage and schedule of treatment. A number of thyroid hormone preparations are available and differences in cost are considerable. Questions arise as to differences in potency and bioavailability among these products.

Application of diagnostic tests has provided better insight into the pathophysiology of canine hypothyroidism, but has also provided new questions. In addition to measurement of total concentrations of thyroxine ($T_4$) and triiodothyronine ($T_3$), assays to quantify or estimate free iodothyronines and autoantibodies that bind to thyroglobulin, $T_3$, or $T_4$ are available. There is controversy among internists as regards utility and interpretation of these various tests. A validated assay for thyrotropin (TSH) in the dog is not available. There

has also been documentation and speculation of additional clinical presentations of hypothyroidism. These less typical manifestations include neurologic deficits, lameness, megaesophagus, and changes in behavior. With a wider array of potential clinical signs and possibility of equivocal or false-positive test results, veterinarians may employ a trial course of thyroid treatment as a "bioassay" to help decide whether or not a dog may be hypothyroid. In these circumstances, monitoring the success of treatment is of paramount importance. The purpose of this article is to review physical changes and end points of endocrine testing in assessment of thyroid replacement therapy.

## PHYSICAL RESPONSE TO THYROID SUPPLEMENTATION

The clinical response of the patient is the most important end point in evaluation of thyroid hormone supplementation. This is especially pertinent when treatment is initiated from the perspective of a therapeutic trial. The time-trend sequence of physical improvement has been previously summarized (Rosychuk,

1982; Nelson and Ihle, 1987). The first sign of improvement is often an increase in activity and alertness during the first week of treatment. There is usually some improvement in dermatologic signs within 4 to 6 weeks of treatment as characterized by evidence of regrowth of hair. However it may take several months to shed old hair and accumulation of keratin. Sometimes the first growth of hair is atypical. We have seen an instance where the first hair growth on the dorsum of a hypothyroid Doberman pinscher was long and wavy following treatment. This hair was subsequently replaced with a normal coat. The rate of weight loss in overweight dogs is variable. Subjectively, we associate the most consistent patterns of weight loss in dogs that also show lethargy and dermatologic abnormalities. There may be evidence of some improvement of neurologic signs by 2 weeks of treatment but expectations are not well defined. Lastly, improvement of problems related to infertility is unpredictable.

In human medicine, there is concern for subclinical thyrotoxicosis as a sequel to thyroid supplementation (Helfand and Crapo, 1990). Complications from subclinical hyperthyroidism may be related to decrease in bone density, elevation of liver enzymes, or changes in electrocardiographic findings. This has not been a concern in the dog; however, prospective clinical studies have not been done. Dogs are resistant to development of iatrogenic thyrotoxicosis, presumably related to a rate of thyroid hormone metabolism that is considerably more rapid than in people. In our experience, overt iatrogenic thyrotoxicosis in the dog is rare and is often associated with a dose of $T_4$ that is well above recommended therapeutic regimens. Clinical signs of thyrotoxicosis include increased heart and respiratory rates, restlessness, and weight loss accompanied by an increased appetite. Serum concentrations of $T_4$ and $T_3$ are clearly elevated (see later discussion).

In human medicine, initiation of thyroid hormone replacement may be introduced more gradually in the presence of concomitant nonthyroidal illness or in geriatric patients. The rationale is to increase metabolism more slowly to prevent adverse interactions with other treatments. Recommendations for gradual initiation of thyroid supplementation have been made for dogs with cardiac disease, diabetes mellitus, hypoadrenocorticism, liver disease, and renal failure. This approach has theoretical merit but has not been evaluated in clinical studies.

## MONITORING THYROID REPLACEMENT WITH ENDOCRINE TESTS

### Considerations From Human Medicine

In dogs and people, the most common form of hypothyroidism is primary hypothyroidism. The mainstay of treatment is oral administration of synthetic thyroxine. In a hypothyroid patient, $T_4$ supplementation results in increases in serum concentrations of both $T_4$

and $T_3$, the latter reflective of deiodination of $T_4$ by peripheral tissues. One end point of endocrine testing is to measure serum concentrations of iodothyronines as an assessment of absorption and metabolism of exogenous $T_4$. The availability of sensitive assays for human TSH provides another end point to evaluate thyroid replacement therapy. Baseline serum concentrations of TSH are elevated in primary hypothyroidism as is the increase of TSH with administration of thyrotropin-releasing hormone (TRH). Normalization of these variables with thyroid supplementation would provide an end point of appropriate negative feedback of the pituitary-thyroid axis. In human medicine, sensitive TSH tests or TRH stimulation tests are regarded as sensitive indicators of inappropriate thyroid replacement therapy (Helfand and Crapo, 1990). Use of TSH assays may account in part for the trend of lowering doses of $T_4$ in human medicine over the past 20 years. However, body tissues differ in dependence on intracellular deiodination of $T_4$ versus the circulation as a source of $T_3$. The brain is more dependent on intracellular deiodination. Therefore, there is question whether pituitary suppression as an end point for subclinical thyrotoxicosis reflects the response of other tissues to thyroid supplementation. In their review of monitoring thyroid hormone supplementation, Helfand and Crapo (1990) emphasize consideration of clinical response and laboratory tests.

Can results from therapeutic monitoring studies in people have relevance in veterinary medicine? Normalization of baseline TSH was accomplished when serum $T_3$ was similar to and serum $T_4$ was higher than controls (Fish et al., 1987). This finding raises question over the importance of the role of serum $T_3$ in the negative feedback of TSH. Until demonstrated otherwise, research in therapeutic monitoring of dogs should not overlook measurement of $T_3$.

### Endocrine Monitoring of Thyroid Replacement in the Dog

In the euthyroid dog, the serum concentration of $T_4$ remains fairly constant over a 24-hr period, with minor episodic fluctuations (Kemppainen and Sartin, 1984). Because of the short half-life of $T_4$ in the dog (estimates from 8 to 16 hr), it is not practical to mimic the normal physiologic pattern with oral administration of $T_4$. In the period between treatments, dogs are exposed to absorption curves with peak and nadir concentrations. Recommendations for daily dose of $T_4$ for the dog vary considerably, based either on body weight or metabolic size. On a weight basis, daily doses of 20 to 40 ug/kg, on a once-daily or divided twice-daily schedule are most commonly used (Ferguson, 1986). A daily dose of 0.5 mg/m² based on metabolic size has also been proposed (Chastain, 1982). The dose of $T_4$ given to a dog at a single treatment could thus vary more than twofold, depending on the regimen of treatment selected.

Results from two recent studies provide further insight into relationships between administered dose of

$T_4$ and serum concentrations of iodothyronines. A clinical survey contained data obtained from individual samples submitted to an endocrine laboratory to monitor thyroid hormone supplementation (Nachreiner and Refsal, 1992). Individual data entries contained information about the dose and product given, the time of post-treatment sampling, and the weight of the dog. Although not readily apparent by inspection of means and standard errors of $T_4$ and $T_3$ concentrations, there is tremendous variation of therapeutic concentrations within a given regimen of treatment. Undoubtedly, some may reflect errors in data records. However, we suspect that much of this variation reflects differences among dogs in efficiency of absorption of $T_4$. Some dogs maintain low concentrations of $T_4$ and $T_3$ despite receipt of substantial doses of $T_4$. Some of the factors associated with nonthyroidal illness or drug therapy have the potential to alter therapeutic concentrations of iodothyronines (Ferguson, 1986). However, the large number of samples in the clinical survey still provided an opportunity to examine the effects of dose, time of sampling, and $T_4$ product on serum concentrations of iodothyronines. As might be expected, overall serum concentrations of $T_4$, $T_3$, and estimates of free $T_4$ and free $T_3$ increased with daily dose. Serum $T_4$ and estimates of free iodothyronines were higher at 4 to 6 hours after treatment than other times, but $T_3$ did not differ among sampling intervals. In the statistical analysis of the clinical survey, body weight was entered as a covariate. There was an inverse relationship (negative slope) between body weight and serum $T_3$ and estimates of free $T_4$ and free $T_3$. There was no significant relationship with body weight and $T_4$. This result suggests that therapeutic concentrations of iodothyronines do not predictably get higher in large dogs that are dosed by body weight rather than metabolic weight. It has been our subjective experience that treatment may not be adequate in many large dogs receiving $T_4$ dosed on the basis of metabolic size.

Questions arise as to differences in $T_4$ products. Our clinical survey found that $T_4$ and estimates of free hormones were highest in dogs receiving a brand of levothyroxine marketed to veterinarians (Soloxine, Daniels Pharmaceuticals). Products could differ in potency or bioavailability or both. Potency reflects the quantitative accuracy of the amount of $T_4$ in a tablet. Bioavailability reflects rate of release of $T_4$ with dissolution of the pill. At present, data from prospective studies are very limited that provide direct comparison of $T_4$ products used by veterinarians. One study in dogs did not show a relationship between rate of *in vitro* dissolution of three $T_4$ products and therapeutic concentrations of $T_4$ *in vivo* (Wood et al., 1990). However, the findings of that study may be challenged because treatments were not administered long enough for equilibration of absorption curves and the dose was potentially suboptimal. Recognition of differences among products should be based both on clinical efficacy and analytical comparison of potency and bioavailability.

Are there differences among products? In our interaction with veterinarians, one scenario regularly occurs.

Thyroxine supplementation is initiated in a large dog with a brand-name product, with subsequent clinical improvement. For economic reasons, the veterinarian then changes to a less expensive product of the same dose. A return of clinical signs is noted, with concern of association with the change of products. Clinical improvement is often reinstated with switching back to the brand-name product or increasing the dose of the less expensive product.

The influence of dose and schedule of $T_4$ administration on serum concentrations of $T_4$ and $T_3$ was investigated in detail in a recent study (Nachreiner et al., in press). Surgically thyroidectomized dogs received each of six regimens of treatment in a Latin-square experimental design. The six treatments were daily doses of 44, 22, or 11 $\mu g/kg$ levothyroxine sodium (Soloxine, Daniels Pharmaceuticals) administered orally on a once-daily or divided twice-daily schedule. After 28 days of each treatment regimen, blood samples were collected in a schedule to allow estimations of pharmacokinetics of oral absorption of $T_4$. Results from weekly monitoring during each treatment schedule indicate that absorption curves of $T_4$ and consequent production of $T_3$ have stabilized by 1 week of treatment (Fig. 1). There is evidence for a subtle decline of serum $T_4$ and $T_3$ from 1 to 4 weeks of treatment, which may reflect an increase in rate of metabolism. However, these results indicate that assessment of absorption of exogenous $T_4$ could be made after 1 week of treatment. As expected, there was a positive relationship between daily dose of levothyroxine and serum concentrations of $T_4$ and $T_3$ (Fig. 2). At doses of 44 $ug/kg/day$, especially if given once daily, serum $T_4$ exceeds the reference range but corresponding concentrations of $T_3$ still remain within the normal range. This suggests autoregulation of $T_4$ deiodination and may be a mechanism to prevent thyrotoxicosis. The half-life of $T_4$ was shorter with 44-$ug/kg/day$ doses than 11 $ug/kg/day$, indicating that kinetics of $T_4$ may be dose dependent. Variation of therapeutic concentrations among dogs was also a pronounced feature of this experimental study. Across all treatments the highest and lowest therapeutic concentrations were fairly consistent in the same respective dogs. These differences in serum $T_4$ were of a two- to threefold magnitude. The duration of treatments in this study was not sufficient to assess the clinical response. However, it was our subjective impression that some dogs developed seborrhea, dry hair coats, and were less active with daily doses of 11 $ug/kg$.

## RECOMMENDATIONS

Monitoring thyroid replacement in the dog can involve assessment of both clinical response and therapeutic concentrations of iodothyronines. Results from our data reinforce the recommendation that the daily dose of 20 to 40 $ug/kg$ is adequate for most dogs. It is convenient to initiate treatment with administration of 22 $\mu g/kg$, repeated twice daily (0.1 mg/10 lb b.i.d.). This regimen provides a balance between optimal

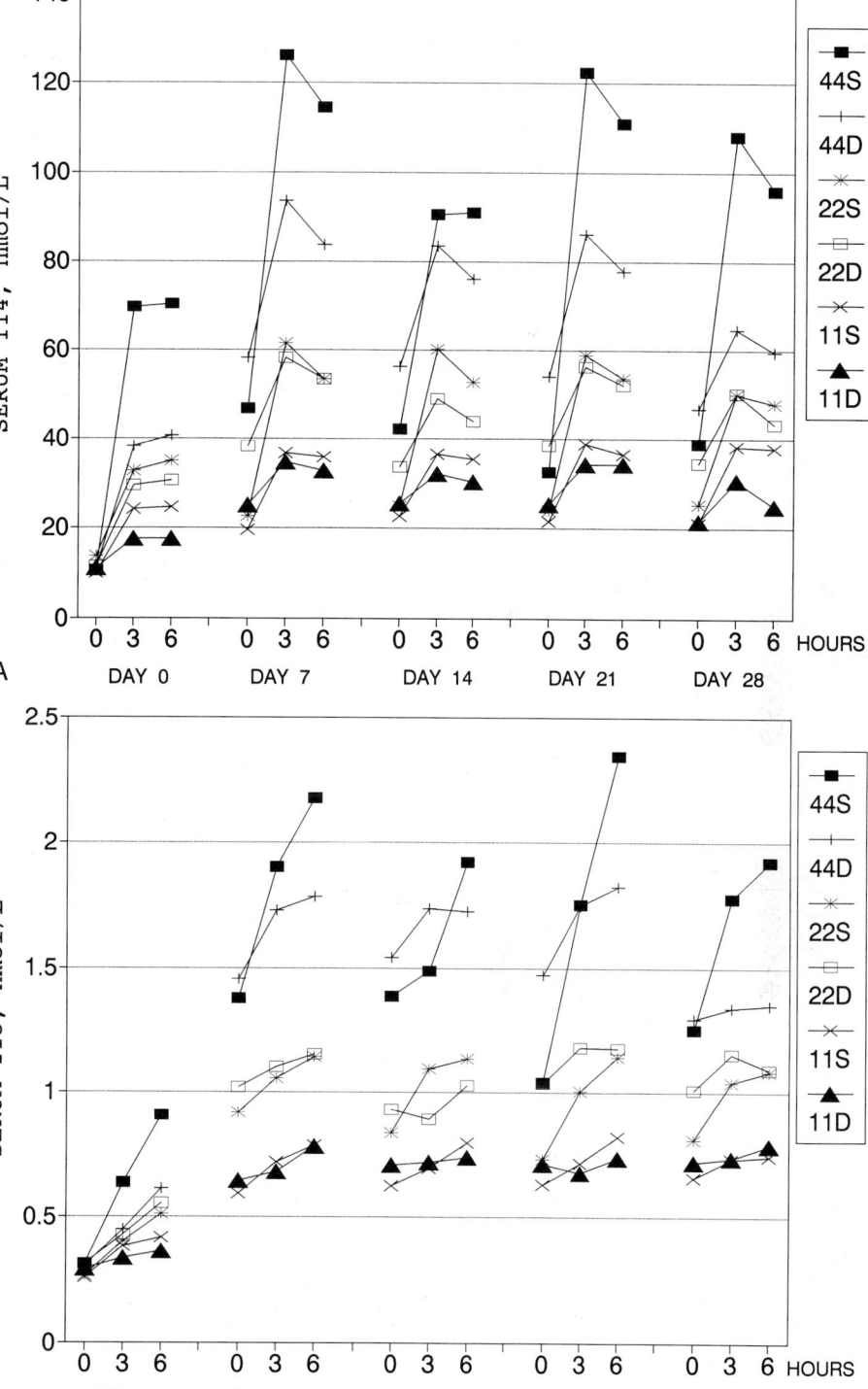

**Figure 1.** Effect of duration of treatment on mean serum concentrations of thyroxine (A) and triiodothyronine (B) in thyroidectomized adult dogs (n=12) receiving different doses of levothyroxine per os. Daily doses were 44, 22, or 11 ug/kg, given on either once-daily (S) or divided twice-daily (D) schedules. All dogs received each treatment regimen in a Latin-square experimental design. The laboratory reference range for thyroxine is 20 to 40 nmol/L and for triiodothyronine is 1.0 to 3.1 nmol/L in normal dogs. (Reprinted with modification from Nachreiner RF, Refsal KR, Ravis WR, et al: Pharmacokinetics of l-thyroxine after its oral administration in dogs. Am J Vet Res, 54: 2091, 1993.)

chances for clinical improvement with the unlikely outcome of iatrogenic thyrotoxicosis. It is still advantageous to wait 4 to 8 weeks to monitor therapeutic concentrations of iodothyronines because the clinician can evaluate the clinical response. Therapeutic monitoring samples should be drawn at 4 to 8 hours after treatment, a time that provides good correlation with the area under the curve for $T_4$ and a good indication of formation of $T_3$. If the clinical response is satisfactory and serum $T_4$ is elevated ($\geq$60 nmol/L, for example), the option is available to decrease the dose to 22 ug/kg once daily. If the clinical response is not satisfactory despite compliance of treatment, the clinician must either reconsider the need for $T_4$ supplementation or increase the dose. In some hypothyroid dogs, thyroid hormone concentrations, as measured by routine radioimmunoassay procedures, are not accurate because of assay interference by antithyroid autoantibodies that

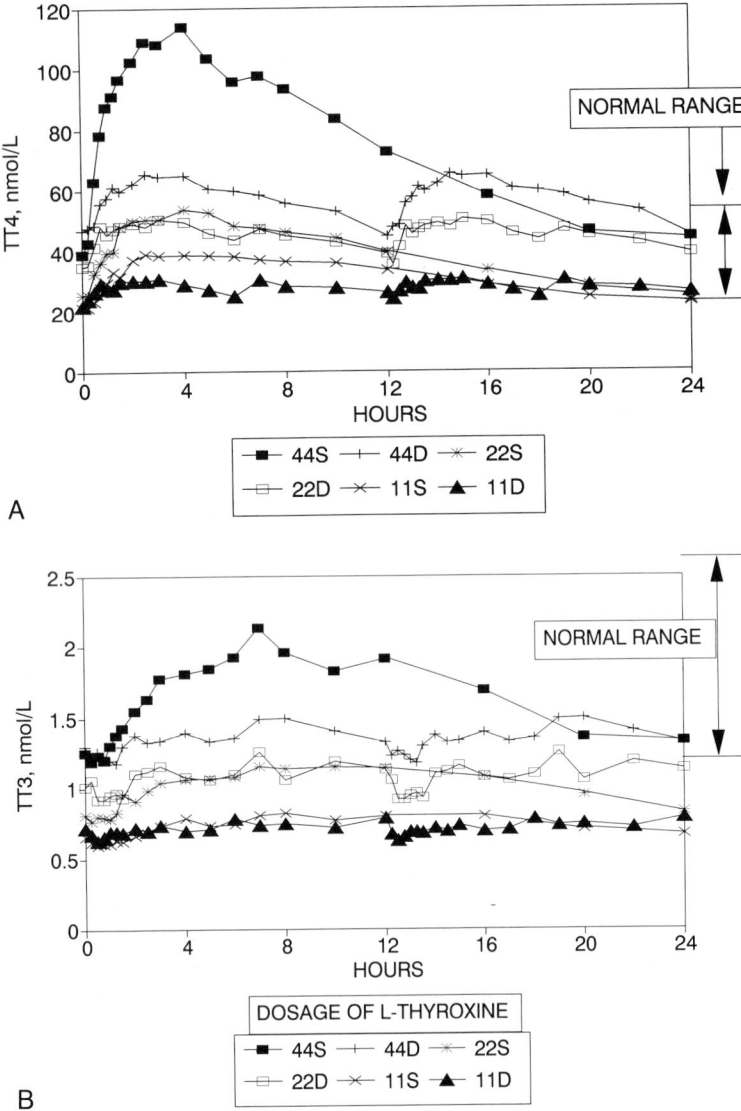

A

B

**Figure 2.** Time trend changes in mean concentrations of thyroxine (*A*) and triiodothyronine (*B*) in sera of thyroidectomized adult dogs (*n*=12) receiving different doses of levothyroxine per os. Daily doses were 44, 22, or 11 *u*g/kg, given on either once-daily (S) or divided twice-daily (D) schedules. Data were collected on day 28 of a treatment schedule. All dogs received each treatment regimen in a Latin-square experimental design. The laboratory reference range for thyroxine is 20 to 40 nmol/L and for triiodothyronine is 1.0 to 3.1 nmol/L in normal dogs. (Reprinted with modification from Nachreiner RF, Refsal KR, Ravis WR, et al: Pharmacokinetics of l-thyroxine after its oral administration in dogs. Am J Vet Res, 54:2091, 1993.)

bind to $T_4$ and $T_3$. In these dogs, the clinician will have to rely on the clinical response to evaluate the success of thyroid replacement therapy. Measurement of free $T_4$ by equilibrium dialysis techniques can provide an assessment of $T_4$ absorption in dogs with these autoantibodies.

## References and Suggested Reading

Chastain CB: Canine hypothyroidism. J Am Vet Med Assoc 181:349, 1982.
*Overview of clinical signs, diagnosis, and treatment of canine hypothyroidism.*
Ferguson DC: Thyroid hormone replacement therapy. *In* Kirk RW (ed).: *Current Veterinary Therapy IX: Small Animal Practice.* Philadelphia, WB Saunders Co, 1986, p 1018.
*Review of thyroid physiology and clinical application of thyroid replacement therapy in the dog and cat.*
Fish LH, Schwartz HL, Cavanaugh J, et al: Replacement dose, metabolism, and bioavailability of levothyroxine in the treatment of hypothyroidism. Role of triiodothyronine in pituitary feedback in humans. N Eng J Med 316:764, 1987.
*Clinical study of bioavailability of levothyroxine and relationships with serum thyroxine, triiodothyronine, and thyrotropin.*
Helfand M and Crapo LM: Monitoring therapy in patients taking levothy-roxine. Ann Intern Med 113:450, 1990.
*Review of the use of thyroid function tests to monitor therapy in people taking levothyroxine.*
Kemppainen RJ and Sartin JL: Evidence for episodic but not circadian activity in plasma concentrations of adrenocorticotropin, cortisol, and thyroxine in dogs. J Endocrinol 103:219, 1984.
*Experiment to characterize daily patterns of secretion of adrenocorticotropin, cortisol, and thyroxine in dogs.*
Nachreiner RF and Refsal KR: Radioimmunoassay monitoring of thyroid hormone concentrations in dogs on thyroid replacement therapy: 2674 cases (1985–1987). J Am Vet Med Assoc 201:623, 1992.
*Clinical survey to evaluate relationships between dose of levothyroxine, schedule of treatment, product, and body weight on therapeutic concentrations of iodothyronines in dogs.*
Nachreiner RF, Refsal KR, Ravis WR, et al: Pharmacokinetics of l-thyroxine after its oral administration in dogs. Am J Vet Res 54:2091, 1993.
*Experiment to quantify effects of dose and schedule of oral levothyroxine treatment on pharmacokinetic variables in thyroidectomized dogs.*
Nelson RW and Ihle SL: Treating hypothyroidism through hormone supplementation. Vet Med 87:153, 1987.
*Overview of clinical considerations of thyroid hormone replacement in dogs.*
Rosychuk RAW: Thyroid hormones and antithyroid drugs. Vet Clin North Am [Small Anim Pract] 12:111, 1982.
*Review and overview of treatment of hypothyroidism and hyperthyroidism.*
Wood RW, Martis L, Gillum AW, et al: In vitro dissolution and in vivo bioavailability of commercial levothyroxine sodium tablets in the hypothyroid model. J Pharm Sci 79:124, 1990.
*Experiment to compare bioavailability of three brands of levothyroxine in dogs with [131]I-induced hypothyroidism.*

# COMPLICATIONS OF TREATMENT AND CONCURRENT ILLNESS ASSOCIATED WITH HYPERTHYROIDISM IN CATS

THOMAS K. GRAVES

*East Lansing, Michigan*

The small animal veterinarian is faced with a variety of treatment options for the cat with hyperthyroidism. Most of the traditional treatments for the disease are effective and relatively safe. However, none are free of the possibility of serious complications. Recent advances in the knowledge of occult hyperthyroidism and studies on the effects of nonthyroidal illness on feline thyroid function have thrown another wrench into the therapeutic decision-making process. The hyperthyroid cat may have a concurrent disease that masks its hyperthyroidism. This can make both the diagnosis of hyperthyroidism and the choice of treatment somewhat difficult. Conversely, recent study has suggested that hyperthyroidism itself can mask serious underlying disease. Complications of treatment of hyperthyroidism are quite common in cats. Some of these complications are relatively trivial. Others are life threatening. If left untreated, feline hyperthyroidism has severe long-term consequences. However, which treatment to use is only one of the dilemmas faced in the clinical management of the disease. In some cases, the most important question may be whether to treat at all.

## RENAL FUNCTION AND HYPERTHYROIDISM

As the number of cats treated for hyperthyroidism increases, many small animal practitioners have noticed what appears to be a relatively high incidence of overt renal failure following treatment of hyperthyroidism. The relationship between hyperthyroidism and renal failure is difficult to sort out epidemiologically, since both diseases are very common in the aging feline population.

Hyperthyroidism in humans and in cats causes tachycardia and increased cardiac output, and hypertension has been documented in cats with hyperthyroidism. Although the normal kidney possesses autoregulatory capabilities that hold glomerular filtration rate (GFR) relatively constant despite changes in blood pressure, the hyperthyroid cat, probably due to either chronic thyrotoxicosis or concurrent intrinsic renal disease, may have limited renal autoregulatory ability. Thyrotoxicosis, therefore, could conceivably elevate GFR and mask underlying renal disease. In human beings, hyperthyroidism causes both increased renal blood flow and in-

creased urinary creatinine excretion. Following treatment of feline hyperthyroidism and return to euthyroidism, cardiac output and, hence, GFR could drop, causing clinical development of overt renal failure in cats with underlying disease.

Studies have recently been conducted to test the hypothesis that renal function in cats often deteriorates following treatment of hyperthyroidism. Using plasma disappearance of $^{99m}$Tc-DTPA to estimate GFR, we demonstrated a significant drop in mean GFR in cats following treatment of hyperthyroidism by surgical thyroidectomy. All of the cats of our study experienced decreases in GFR, some declining as much as 80% of the prethyroidectomy rate. In all cats, serum concentrations of creatinine and urea nitrogen increased following thyroidectomy. Several of the cats became azotemic (with isosthenuria) within a month of treatment of hyperthyroidism; none of the cats we studied were azotemic prior to treatment.

Although further studies are needed, it would seem prudent to consider carefully the renal health of a cat when choosing a treatment option for hyperthyroidism. Meticulous physical examination, complete blood counts and serum chemistry profiles, as well as urinalyses are essential steps in the work-up of feline hyperthyroidism. Cats with obvious renal failure and azotemia would probably not benefit from treatment of hyperthyroidism unless the clinical signs of thyrotoxicosis were so severe as to be unmanageable. For instance, if a cat develops congestive heart failure associated with thyrotoxic heart disease, there may be no choice as to whether or not to treat the hyperthyroidism. In such a case, an antithyroid drug might be the initial treatment of choice. Should azotemia worsen and signs of overt renal failure and uremia develop following the return to euthyroidism, the treatment might be easily reversed by simply stopping antithyroid drug administration. Unfortunately, the owners and veterinarians of many hyperthyroid cats may find themselves in the unenviable position of deciding between the lesser of two evils.

As feline hyperthyroidism can mask underlying renal disease, the converse is also apparently true. A recent report showed that basal serum thyroid hormone concentrations are low or low-normal in a majority of cats with chronic renal failure (Peterson and Gamble, 1990). In that study, nearly 50% of 128 cats with renal failure had serum thyroxine ($T_4$) concentrations below the normal range. Another approximately 30% had serum $T_4$ concentrations in the low-normal range. The same effect of lowering basal serum $T_4$ concentrations was found in a variety of other diseases including diabetes mellitus, hepatic disease, heart failure, neoplasia, inflammatory bowel disease, and inflammatory pulmonary disease. Mean serum $T_4$ concentrations in cats in all of these disease categories were significantly lower than in healthy cats. These results suggest a plausible explanation for occult hyperthyroidism in some cats, and should be taken into consideration when formulating diagnostic and treatment plans for cats with clinical signs of thyrotoxicosis.

## COMPLICATIONS OF SURGICAL THYROIDECTOMY

Surgical thyroidectomy is a commonly used and effective means of treating feline hyperthyroidism. While the aged thyrotoxic cat would seem a poor surgical candidate, it is uncommon for a hyperthyroid cat to die from anesthetic or surgical complications. Fortunately, the surgical complications of thyroidectomy are well documented in the veterinary literature and, once recognized, are manageable.

### Hypocalcemia

The most common complication of surgical thyroidectomy is hypocalcemia. A likely mechanism for the development of post-thyroidectomy hypocalcemia is inadvertent damage to the parathyroid glands or their blood supply resulting in hypoparathyroidism. While this might seem obvious, there is very little solid evidence to support hypoparathyroidism as the sole mechanism for the development of hypocalcemia in cats undergoing thyroidectomy. There appears to be little correlation between the surgeon's clinical impression of the degree of parathyroid gland trauma during surgery and the actual development of hypocalcemia. Hypocalcemia sometimes develops even in cases where very little manipulation of the parathyroid glands has occurred. Conversely, surgeons are sometimes surprised by the lack of development of hypocalcemia in cases where parathyroid glands were poorly visualized or severely traumatized during surgery. Studies in human patients with hypocalcemia following thyroidectomy for thyrotoxicosis suggest mechanisms other than parathyroid gland damage (Michie, Stowers, and Duncan, 1971). Increased osteoclast activity, osteomalacia, and osteoporosis, as well as increased serum calcium and phosphorus concentration, are observed in human thyrotoxic patients. A possible contributory mechanism for post-thyroidectomy hypocalcemia may be the sudden reversal of "thyrotoxic osteodystrophy." Studies of calcium balance perioperatively, bone histology, and parathyroid gland function are lacking in feline thyroidology.

Regardless of the cause, post-thyroidectomy hypo-

calcemia can be severe, necessitating immediate treatment. Early signs of hypocalcemia include anorexia and facial twitching. More diffuse muscle fasciculation can develop. Severe clinical signs of hypocalcemia include tetany and generalized seizures. Serum calcium concentrations should be monitored postoperatively regardless of clinical signs. However, mild hypocalcemia in the absence of clinical signs is quite common and probably does not require treatment. Should overt hypocalcemia develop, immediate treatment is essential. Emergency treatment of hypocalcemia entails intravenous administration of 10% calcium gluconate at a dosage of 0.5 to 1.5 ml/kg (Peterson and Randolph, 1989; Chew, Nagode, and Carothers, 1992). The drug should be delivered over a 10- to 20-min period. Electrocardiographic monitoring during intravenous calcium gluconate infusion is recommended; infusion should be stopped if signs of toxicity (e.g., bradycardia, cardiac arrest, vomiting, shortened Q-T interval) occur. Following acute correction of hypocalcemia, maintenance calcium gluconate therapy should be instituted. Several regimens for intravenous calcium gluconate infusion have been recommended. Most recommend the addition of one or two 10-ml vials of 10% calcium gluconate (depending on severity of hypocalcemia and response to treatment) to a 500-ml bag of 0.9% sodium chloride (fluids containing bicarbonate, lactate, or acetate should be avoided due to the potential for calcium salt precipitation). The mixture is then administered at a standard maintenance rate. Serum calcium concentrations should be monitored two or three times daily. Obviously, care must be taken to ensure that calcium-containing fluids are not administered too rapidly. If careful monitoring is not possible, 10% calcium gluconate can be administered subcutaneously at a dosage of 1 to 2 ml every 8 hr. The 10% calcium gluconate solution should be diluted at least 1:1 with saline prior to administration to help minimize pain and tissue damage caused by the hypertonicity of the solution.

Maintenance treatment of post-thyroidectomy hypocalcemia involves administration of oral calcium supplements as well as vitamin D preparations (Peterson and Randolph, 1989; Chew, Nagode, and Carothers, 1992). Calcium supplementation is recommended at a dosage of 25 to 50 mg/kg/day. The most common and practical approach is to administer Tums Antacid Tablets (SmithKline Beecham, Philadelphia, PA), which are available over the counter and are inexpensive, at a dosage of one or two tablets divided into three or four daily doses. This degree of calcium supplementation is only necessary for the first week or two of treatment, after which time normal dietary calcium content should be sufficient to maintain serum calcium concentrations within the normal range.

Oral vitamin D therapy should be instituted concurrent with the start of calcium administration. The most commonly used vitamin D preparation has been dihydrotachysterol (DHT, Roxane, Columbus, OH), a synthetic form of vitamin $D_3$. The initial dose of DHT is 0.02 to 0.03 mg/kg/day for 3 to 4 days, followed by a reduction of the dose to 0.01 to 0.02 mg/kg given every

24 to 48 hr. The dosage of the drug should be adjusted to maintain serum calcium within the normal range. The ideal vitamin D supplement, however, is probably calcitriol (Chew, Nagode, and Carothers, 1992). Calcitriol (1,25-dihydroxycholecalciferol; Rocaltrol, Roche Laboratories, Nutley, NJ) is the active form of vitamin D and has several advantages over other vitamin D preparations. The time of onset of action and maximal effect is shorter than with DHT. In addition, there is a shorter duration of action with calcitriol than with DHT. This means that toxic effects of hypervitaminosis D are easier to manage with calcitriol. The time for toxicity effects to resolve following excess treatment with calcitriol is 2 to 14 days versus 1 to 3 weeks with DHT. The recommended dosage of calcitriol is 2.5 to 10 ng/kg/day. Rocaltrol is supplied commercially as 0.25- and 0.50-$\mu$g capsules. The author empirically uses one 0.25-$\mu$g capsule every 48 hr for long-term treatment of post-thyroidectomy hypocalcemia. Regardless of the vitamin D and calcium preparations used, treatment is usually not necessary after 2 to 3 weeks and drugs can be discontinued. Serum calcium concentrations should be measured after discontinuation of therapy and owners should be instructed to monitor their cats for signs of recurrence of hypocalcemia.

## Neurologic Complications

Voice change, transient Horner's syndrome, and laryngeal paralysis are infrequent complications of surgical thyroidectomy. Horner's syndrome can occur following damage to the cervical sympathetic trunk. Laryngeal dysfunction (either voice change or paralysis) can occur following damage to the recurrent laryngeal nerves. These complications are rare. In an early retrospective study of thyroidectomy in cats with hyperthyroidism (Birchard, Peterson, and Jacobsen, 1984), voice change and transient Horner's syndrome occurred in 1 each of 85 cases. Neither of these complications required treatment. Bilateral laryngeal paralysis has been observed following thyroidectomy. It is unclear whether this complication is the result of bilateral recurrent laryngeal nerve damage or direct damage to the larynx during intubation. Regardless of the cause, bilateral laryngeal paralysis can result in complete airway obstruction requiring surgical intervention.

## COMPLICATIONS OF ANTITHYROID DRUGS

Complications of antithyroid drugs have been well documented in the veterinary literature. The most commonly used antithyroid drugs in the United States are methimazole (Tapazole, Eli Lilly, Indianapolis, IN) and propylthiouracil (PTU). These drugs are used either as sole treatment for hyperthyroidism, or, in many cases, as a preparatory treatment for surgical thyroidectomy. Adverse side effects occur in approximately 15% of cats treated with methimazole (Peterson,

Kintzer, and Hurvitz, 1988). These effects include such clinical signs as vomiting, anorexia, lethargy, facial pruritis, self-excoriation, and bleeding; as well as laboratory abnormalities such as eosinophilia, lymphocytosis, leukopenia, agranulocytosis, thrombocytopenia, positive antinuclear antibody and Coombs' tests, and increases in liver enzymes. Many of these effects are mild and resolve without cessation of methimazole therapy, while others persist until drug administration is stopped. The more dangerous side effects (e.g., thrombocytopenia, agranulocytosis, and hepatopathy) are uncommon, affecting less than 3% of patients, and necessitate immediate cessation of methimazole therapy. The incidence of adverse effects is reportedly higher in cats treated with PTU, with 20 to 25% of cats experiencing side effects. In one study, 8% of cats treated with PTU developed severe hematologic complications (Peterson et al., 1984). Half of those patients were euthanatized due to severity of adverse effects of PTU.

Carbimazole is a pro-drug that is converted to methimazole in the body. Carbimazole is not available in the United States, but is used widely in Europe. A recent study of the efficacy and safety of carbimazole in the treatment of hyperthyroidism in cats suggests that it may be associated with less adverse effects than either methimazole or PTU (Mooney, Thoday, and Doxey, 1992). In that report, only 4% of cats developed hematologic abnormalities (lymphocytosis and leukopenia). These abnormalities were very mild and cessation of carbimazole therapy was not necessary. Similarly to methimazole, approximately 11% of cats developed clinical side effects due to carbimazole therapy. These effects included vomiting, anorexia, and depression. While results of this study seem promising, the number of cats studied by Mooney et al. was far less than that of Peterson's study of methimazole (45 versus 262 cats), and it would be premature to compare the safety and efficacy of the two drugs based on these studies alone. Further studies comparing carbimazole to the other antithyroid drugs would seem a welcome addition to the veterinary literature.

## Effect of Methimazole on Hemostasis

The relationship between hemostasis and antithyroid drugs is extremely complex and poorly understood. Bleeding disorders have been observed in cats treated with methimazole; these effects have not always been associated with thrombocytopenia (Peterson, Kintzer, and Hurvitz, 1988). Although undocumented in the literature, many veterinarians have observed that cats treated with methimazole, regardless of platelet counts, are prone to bleeding from venipuncture sites and during surgical thyroidectomy. Although rarely, PTU administration to human patients has been shown to cause hypoprothrombinemia that is partially reversible with vitamin K therapy. This factor has not been investigated in cats undergoing thioureylene drug (methimazole, PTU, and carbimazole) treatment. In addition, there may be a functional similarity between the thioureylene drugs and dicoumerol-type drugs. For example, dicoumerol and warfarin, like the thioureylenes, are capable of blocking the peripheral conversion of $T_4$ to $T_3$. At present, platelet aggregometry is being used to investigate the effects of methimazole on platelet function in cats with hyperthyroidism, and preliminary results suggest that methimazole may cause decreased platelet function in some hyperthyroid cats. While these observations warrant careful monitoring of thiourylene-treated cats for signs of hemorrhage, further investigation is needed before firm conclusions can be drawn.

## IATROGENIC HYPOTHYROIDISM

Iatrogenic hypothyroidism is extremely rare regardless of the treatment used for hyperthyroidism in the cat. Most cats are euthyroid following radioiodine treatment. Antithyroid drugs, when used properly, result in low-normal serum thyroid hormone concentrations. Even bilateral surgical thyroidectomy usually results in only slightly low or low-normal circulating concentrations of thyroid hormones. When bilateral thyroidectomy was first being done as a treatment for feline hyperthyroidism, postsurgical thyroid hormone supplementation was a common practice. However, while the need for thyroid hormone supplementation following bilateral thyroidectomy seems obvious, it is almost never needed. Cats in which thyroid hormone is not given following bilateral thyroidectomy rarely develop overt clinical hypothyroidism. In fact, results of thyroid hormone measurement in serum from thyroidectomized cats suggest that complete thyroidectomy is nearly impossible in the cat and that the very small amount of residual thyroid tissue left behind after thyroidectomy is sufficient to produce adequate thyroid hormone in the cat. In rare instances, cats can develop iatrogenic hypothyroidism presenting with clinical signs that include obesity, lethargy, nonpruritic seborrhea sicca, and loss of hair on the pinnae. More diffuse or truncal alopecia is not a feature of iatrogenic hypothyroidism in the cat (Peterson and Randolph, 1989). The clinical signs of hypothyroidism resolve following treatment with thyroxine at a dosage of 10 to 20 $\mu g/kg/day$.

## References and Suggested Reading

Birchard, SJ, Peterson ME, Jacobsen A: Surgical treatment of feline hyperthyroidism: Results of 85 cases. J Am Anim Hosp Assoc 20:705, 1984.
  *An early retrospective of results in hyperthyroid cats.*
Chew DJ, Nagode LA, and Carothers M: Disorders of calcium: Hypercalcemia and hypocalcemia. *In* DiBartola SJ, (ed): *Fluid Therapy in Small Animal Practice.* Philadelphia, WB Saunders Co, 1992, p 168.
  *A comprehensive textbook chapter covering pathophysiology, diagnosis, and treatment of calcium disturbances.*
Graves TK, Kruger JM, Nachreiner RF, et al: Glomerular filtration rate decreases following treatment of feline hyperthyroidism. Personal observations.
  *A prospective study showing decreases in glomerular filtration rate, increases in serum urea nitrogen and creatinine, and development of renal azotemia following treatment of feline hyperthyroidism.*
Michie W, Stowers JM, Duncan T, et al: Mechanism of hypocalcemia after thyroidectomy for thyrotoxicosis. Lancet 1:508, 1971.
  *A study supporting mechanisms other than hypoparathyroidism for development of post-thyroidectomy hypocalcemia in thyrotoxic human patients.*
Mooney CT, Thoday KL, and Doxey DL: Carbimazole therapy of feline hyperthyroidism. J Small Anim Pract 33:228, 1992.
  *A study of the efficacy and safety of carbimazole in 45 cats with hyperthyroidism.*
Peterson ME and Gamble DA: Effect of nonthyroidal illness on serum thyroxine concentrations in cats: 494 cases (1988). J Am Vet Med Assoc 197:1203, 1990.
  *A large retrospective study showing low or low-normal serum thyroxine concentrations in a wide variety of nonthyroidal diseases in cats.*
Peterson ME, Hurvitz AI, Leib MS, et al: Propylthiouracil-associated hemolytic anemia, thrombocytopenia, and antinuclear antibodies in cats with hyperthyroidism. J Am Vet Med Assoc 184:806, 1984.
  *A retrospective study documenting adverse effects of propylthiouracil in cats.*
Peterson ME, Kintzer PP, Hurvitz AI: Methimazole treatment of 262 cats with hyperthyroidism. J Vet Intern Med 2:150, 1988.
  *A comprehensive prospective study of the efficacy and safety of methimazole.*
Peterson ME and Randolph JF: Endocrine diseases. *In* Sherding RG (ed): *The Cat: Diagnosis and Clinical Management.* New York, Churchill Livingstone, 1989, pp 1095–1161.
  *A comprehensive review of endocrine disorders in cats, including hyperthyroidism and hypothyroidism.*

# RADIOACTIVE IODINE (RADIOIODINE) TREATMENT FOR HYPERTHYROIDISM IN CATS

MARK E. PETERSON
*New York, New York*

Hyperthyroidism, the condition resulting from secretion of excess thyroid hormone, is the most common endocrine disorder in the cat. This condition usually results from adenomatous hyperplasia or adenoma of the thyroid gland, with carcinoma being a relatively very rare cause of hyperthyroidism in cats.

Hyperthyroidism can be treated medically, surgically, or with radioiodine. Medical treatment in cats generally consists of daily administration of an antithyroid drug (e.g., methimazole); such treatment is not a cure and must be given for the rest of the cat's life. Surgery, on the other hand, can cure the hyperthyroidism because the adenomatous thyroid tissue responsible for the disorder is removed. Like surgery, radioactive iodine (radioiodine) will also cure the hyperthyroid condition. The procedure for this treatment is relatively simple, usually consisting of administration of a single injection of a solution of radioiodine.

Of the three treatment options, radioiodine is considered by many to be the treatment of choice for most hyperthyroid cats when the treatment is available. The purpose of this article is to give an overview of aspects of radioiodine treatment germane to the practicing veterinarian who is referring hyperthyroid cats for this treatment. A list of the institutions or treatment centers licensed to administer radioiodine to cats in the United States and abroad is given in Tables 1 and 2, respectively.

## ADVANTAGES OF RADIOIODINE THERAPY OVER MEDICAL OR SURGICAL TREATMENT FOR HYPERTHYROIDISM IN CATS

Medical treatment will be effective in controlling hyperthyroidism in most cats, but there can be several reasons it may not be the best choice. First, some cats are difficult or impossible to medicate (antithyroid drugs must be administered orally, generally one to three times daily). Second, mild reactions (e.g., loss of appetite, vomiting) are common, whereas a few cats develop serious untoward reactions to the antithyroid drugs (e.g., thrombocytopenia, leukopenia, hepatopathy). Because of the potential for these side effects, periodic blood tests (including complete blood and platelet counts) are necessary to monitor the cat's condition. Finally, some owners may not want to have to medicate their cat on a daily basis for the rest of the cat's life, especially if the cat is only middle-aged.

Surgery is an effective treatment for hyperthyroidism in most cats but may have disadvantages. Many cats with hyperthyroidism have secondary cardiomyopathy and are higher surgical and anesthetic risks; therefore, preoperative preparation of hyperthyroid cats with antithyroid drugs or a $\beta$-adrenergic–blocking agent (or concurrent administration of both drugs) is generally recommended. There is also a risk that there will be damage to the adjacent parathyroid glands during thyroid surgery, resulting in transient or, less commonly, permanent hypoparathyroidism and hypocalcemia. This complication can be life threatening and results in extra hospitalization and cost. After surgery, cats may occasionally develop hypothyroidism (usually transient), necessitating treatment with thyroid hormone replacement. Finally, there is always the potential that the hyperthyroidism will not be cured with surgical treatment or that the condition will reoccur a few months to years after successful thyroidectomy. The prevalence

that hyperthyroidism will persist or recur is higher among cats that have only one thyroid lobe removed at time of surgery because most cats have adenomatous hyperplasia involving both thyroid lobes. In addition, there is always a chance that the cat may have hyperfunctioning thyroid tissue at ectopic sites, usually in the anterior mediastinal area; such ectopic adenomatous thyroid tissue may be difficult to resect surgically.

Radioiodine therapy has some distinct advantages over use of medical or surgical treatment. Overall, radioiodine provides a simple, effective, and safe treatment for cats with hyperthyroidism. With radioiodine, the need for anesthesia and the risk of hypoparathyroidism (the major disadvantages with surgery) are eliminated. Antithyroid drug treatment is not needed; in fact, most investigators recommend that drug treatment must be discontinued for a short time (usually 1 to 2 weeks) before radioactive iodine is administered to the cats. The administered radioactive iodine concentrates in and destroys hyperactive thyroid tissue within the cat's body, whether in the normal cervical area or in ectopic sites. The major drawback is that after administration of radioiodine, the cat must be kept hospitalized (1 to 3 weeks in most treatment centers).

## MECHANISM OF ACTION OF RADIOIODINE TREATMENT

Thyroid hormones are the only iodinated organic compounds in the body. Therefore, the only function of ingested iodine is for thyroid hormone synthesis. Ingested stable iodine ($^{127}$I) is converted to iodide in the gastrointestinal tract and absorbed into the circulation. In the thyroid gland, iodide is concentrated or trapped by active transport mechanisms of the thyroid follicular cell, resulting in intracellular iodide concentrations that are 10 to 200 times that of serum. Once inside the thyroid cell, iodide is oxidized to iodine, which is incorporated into tyrosine residues of thyroglobulin (organification) to form the thyroid hormones, thyroxine ($T_4$) and 3,5,3'-triiodothyronine ($T_3$).

The radioisotope used to treat hyperthyroidism is radioiodine-131 ($^{131}$I). The basic principle behind treatment of hyperthyroidism with $^{131}$I is that thyroid cells do not differentiate between stable and radioactive iodine; therefore, radioiodine, like stable iodine, is concentrated by the thyroid gland after administration. In cats with hyperthyroidism, radioiodine is concentrated primarily in the hyperplastic or neoplastic thyroid cells, where it irradiates and destroys the hyperfunctioning tissue. Normal thyroid tissue, however, tends to be protected from the effects of radioiodine, since the uninvolved thyroid tissue is suppressed and receives only a small dose of radiation (unless very large doses are administered).

When administered to a cat with hyperthyroidism, a large percentage of radioiodine accumulates in the thyroid gland. The remainder of the $^{131}$I is excreted primarily in the urine and to a lesser degree in the feces.

**Table 1.** *Radioiodine Treatment Centers Licensed to Treat Cats in the United States**

| State | Institution or Center | Phone Number | Doctor to Contact |
|---|---|---|---|
| Alabama | Auburn University<br>College of Veterinary Medicine<br>Auburn University, AL 36849 | (205) 844-4690<br>(205) 844-5045 | Medicine Service<br>or<br>Dr. William R. Brawner |
| Arizona | Southwest Veterinary Oncology<br>141 East Ft. Lowell<br>Tucson, AZ 85705 | (602) 327-8131 | Dr. Mary K. Klein |
| California | University of California-Davis<br>Veterinary Medical Teaching Hospital<br>Davis, CA 95616 | (916) 752-8498 | Dr. Alain Theon |
|  | Veterinary Nuclear Imaging<br>34 Creek Road<br>Suite D<br>Irvine, CA 92714 | (714) 559-7289 | Dr. Michael R. Broome |
|  | Veterinary Tumor Institute<br>2585 Soquel Drive<br>Santa Cruz, CA 95065 | (408) 476-5777 | Dr. Jay L. Stone |
|  | Veterinary Oncology Specialties<br>225 Carmel Avenue<br>Pacifica, CA 94044 | (415) 359-9870 | Dr. Jane M. Turrel |
| Florida | Veterinary Radiology Services of So.<br>Florida<br>University Animal Hospital<br>9410 Stirling Road<br>Cooper City, FL 33024 | (407) 479-0460<br>(305) 432-5611 | Dr. Ronald L. Burk |
| Georgia | University of Georgia<br>College of Veterinary Medicine<br>Athens, GA 30602 | (706) 542-8309<br>(706) 542-3221 | Dr. Royce E. Roberts |
| Illinois | University of Illinois<br>Department of Veterinary Biosciences<br>1008 Hazelwood Drive<br>Urbana, IL 61801 | (217) 333-6507 | Dr. Robert A. Twardock |
| Indiana | Purdue University<br>School of Veterinary Medicine<br>West Lafayette, IN 47907 | (317) 494-1107 | Dr. Catherine Scott-Moncrieff |
| Kansas | Kansas State University<br>College of Veterinary Medicine<br>Manhattan, KS 66506 | (913) 532-5690 | Dr. David S. Bruyette |
| Louisiana | Louisiana State University<br>School of Veterinary Medicine<br>Baton Rouge, LA 70803 | (504) 388-1181 | Dr. Karen J. Wolfsheimer |
| Massachusetts | Angell Memorial Animal Hospital<br>350 South Huntington Avenue<br>Boston, MA 02130 | (617) 522-7282 | Dr. Jean M. Duddy |
| Minnesota | University of Minnesota<br>College of Veterinary Medicine<br>St. Paul, MN 55108 | (612) 625-6722 | Dr. Gary R. Johnston |
| Missouri | University of Missouri<br>College of Veterinary Medicine<br>Columbia, MO 85211 | (314) 882-7821 | Dr. Louis A. Corwin |
| New Mexico | Aardvark Veterinary Clinic<br>217 East Marcy Street<br>Sante Fe, NM 87501 | (505) 989-4343 | Dr. John A. Romero |
| New York | The Animal Medical Center &<br>Cornell University Medical College<br>510 East 62nd Street<br>New York, NY 10021 | (212) 838-8100 | Dr. Mark E. Peterson |
|  | Cornell University<br>College of Veterinary Medicine<br>Ithaca, NY 14853 | (607) 253-3241 | Dr. Nathan L. Dykes |
| Ohio | The Veterinary Referral Clinic<br>5035 Richmond Road<br>Cleveland, OH 44146 | (216) 831-6789 | Dr. Terrance A. Hamilton |
|  | The Ohio State University<br>Columbus, OH 43210 | (614) 253-1040 | Dr. Michael Q. Bailey |

*Table continued on opposite page*

**Table 1.** *Continued*

| State | Institution or Center | Phone Number | Doctor to Contact |
|---|---|---|---|
| Oregon | Feline Thyroid Clinic 1045 F. Gateway Loop Springfield, OR 97477 | (503) 744-2966 | Dr. Douglas M. Evans |
| Tennessee | University of Tennessee College of Veterinary Medicine Knoxville, TN 37901 | (615) 974-5806 | Dr. William H. Adams |
| Texas | Animal Radiology Clinic 2353 Royal Lane Dallas, TX 75229 | (214) 484-5637 | Dr. Catherine S. Lustarten |
| | Texas A & M University College Station, TX 77843 | (409) 845-2351 (409) 845-3408 | Small Animal Clinic or Dr. Sheri R. Keele |
| Washington | Feline Hyperthyroid Treatment Center 22226 Highway 99 Edmonds, WA 98026 | (206) 771-2287 | Dr. Dennis L. Wackerbarth |

°As of date of printing.

**Table 2.** *Radioiodine Treatment Centers Licensed to Treat Cats in Countries Outside of the United States°*

| Country | Institution or Center | Phone Number | Doctor to Contact |
|---|---|---|---|
| Australia | University of Melbourne School of Veterinary Science Veterinary Clinic and Hospital Werribee, Victoria 3030 | (03) 741-3500 | Dr. R. W. Mitten |
| | The University of Sydney Veterinary Teaching Hospital Sydney, NSW 2006 | (02) 692-3437 | Dr. David B. Church |
| | Gladeville Veterinary Hospital 449 Victoria Road Gladesville, NSW 2111 | (02) 817-5758 | Dr. R. M. Zuber |
| Canada | University of Saskatchewan Department of Veterinary Internal Medicine Western College of Veterinary Medicine Saskatoon, Saskatchewan S7B OWO | (306) 966-7126 | Dr. Susan M. Meric |
| England | University of Bristol Department of Veterinary Medicine Langford House, Langford Bristol BS18 7DU | (0934) 852581 | Dr. Tim Gruffydd-Jones Dr. A. Sparkes |
| Scotland | University of Glasgow Veterinary School Department of Veterinary Medicine Bearsden Road Bearsden, Glasgow G61 1QH | (041) 339-8855 (041) 330-5700 | Dr. Carmel T. Mooney |
| South Africa | Department of Medical Physics Medunsa 0204 | (012) 529-4389 | Dr. W. J. Strydom |
| New Zealand | Department of Veterinary Clinical Sciences Massey University Palmerston North | (06) 354-3374 | Dr. Boyd R. Jones |
| | Chartwell Veterinary Clinic P.O. Box 12-014 Hamilton | (07) 855-9072 | Dr. Ian Robertson |
| | Dunedin South Veterinary Clinic 29 McBridge Street Dunedin | (03) 455-5718 | Dr. Alistair Newbould |

°As of date of printing.

Iodine-131 has a half-life of 8 days and emits both $\beta$ particles and $\gamma$ radiation. The $\beta$ particles, which cause 80% of the tissue damage, travel a maximum of 2 mm in tissue and have an average path length of 400 $\mu$m. Therefore, $\beta$ particles are locally destructive but spare adjacent hypoplastic thyroid tissue, parathyroid glands, and other cervical structures.

## AVAILABLE TREATMENT SITES FOR CATS WITH HYPERTHYROIDISM

Although radioactive iodine treatment itself is relatively simple and safe, sites that are licensed to perform the treatment are not widely available (see Tables 1 and 2). The limited availability of the radioiodine treatment sites for cats with hyperthyroidism is a result of the strict radiation safety precautions and procedures that must be followed after treatment. Following administration of the radioiodine, cats must remain hospitalized in the nuclear medicine isolation ward until the amount of radiation within their body has decreased to a level that has been deemed to be safe by the radiation safety office. This time of hospitalization in the nuclear medicine isolation ward will vary depending on the treatment site, but generally ranges from 1 to 4 weeks.

The institutions or treatment centers that are licensed to administer radioiodine to cats with hyperthyroidism are listed in Tables 1 and 2. These lists of referral centers were compiled in the fall of 1993 through a questionnaire sent to members of the Society for Comparative Endocrinology. Therefore, it is possible that other treatment centers might have been inadvertently excluded, or that other institutions have started offering this treatment after the survey was performed. In general, information concerning referral of a hyperthyroid cat to one of these treatment facilities should be made by the practicing veterinarian; Tables 1 and 2 list the appropriate person to contact, along with their address and phone number.

## PATIENT SELECTION FOR RADIOIODINE TREATMENT

Routine diagnostic testing and work-up generally should be performed by the referring veterinarian prior to referral for radioiodine treatment. This is very important, inasmuch as these cats tend to be middle- to old-aged and therefore may have other unrelated geriatric problems. In general, cats should be relatively stable before being considered for radioiodine therapy. Cats that have clinically significant cardiovascular, renal, gastrointestinal, endocrine (e.g., diabetes), or neurologic disease may not be very good candidates for this treatment, especially due to the length of boarding required after the $^{131}$I treatment is administered. Any known concurrent medical problems should be discussed with the veterinarian in charge (see Tables 1 and 2) to determine if the cat is an appropriate candidate for the therapy and required isolation.

In some cats, the veterinarian may choose to stabilize the cat for a few weeks or months before time of referral by administering cardiac medications, $\beta$-blocking agents, or antithyroid drugs. Although concurrent administration of $\beta$-blocking agents does not interfere with radioiodine treatment, one should realize that radioiodine is generally less successful in curing hyperthyroidism in cats receiving antithyroid drugs. Therefore, if antithyroid drugs have been administered, most authorities recommend that they be discontinued for at least 1 to 2 weeks before treatment with radioiodine in order to increase the likelihood of restoring euthyroidism with a single treatment. Any history of antithyroid drug treatment should always be discussed with the veterinarian performing the radioiodine treatment when scheduling the referral (see Tables 1 and 2). In some cats with severe, life-threatening hyperthyroidism, one may decide that it is not wise to stop antithyroid drug treatment; however, that matter should be discussed with the veterinarian performing the radioiodine treatment.

## RADIATION SAFETY PRECAUTIONS AFTER RADIOIODINE TREATMENT IN CATS

After radioiodine has been administered to cats with hyperthyroidism, there are certain radiation safety restrictions and procedures that must be followed. The cats must be confined to a restricted area of the hospital (e.g., nuclear medicine isolation ward) that has minimal traffic. Also, the cats should be housed in appropriate cages so that urine and feces can be collected safely. All personnel handling the cats, cages, food dishes, and excreta are required to wear long laboratory coats, disposable plastic gloves, and film badges. All material removed from the cage must be handled as radioactive waste and disposed of accordingly. The cats are discharged from the hospital when the radiation dose rate has decreased to a safe level as determined by the radiation control office (generally after a 1- to 3-week period in most treatment centers).

Upon discharge, the cats will still be excreting a small amount of radioiodine in their urine and feces. The remaining radioactivity will be gradually eliminated from the cat over the next 2 to 4 weeks through radioactive decay and excretion into the urine and feces. Until this is complete, however, the cat will continue to emit low levels of radiation. Because of this, most authorities recommend avoiding close (i.e., <3 to 6 feet), prolonged contact with the cat for the first 1 to 2 weeks after release. If the owner cannot avoid close, prolonged contact with the cat during this period, it is generally recommend that the cat be boarded with the referral veterinarian during this period. Additional information concerning handling of the cat upon release to the owners and related radiation safety issues should be discussed with the veterinarian in charge of the radioiodine therapy (see Tables 1 and 2).

## ADVERSE EFFECTS ASSOCIATED WITH RADIOIODINE TREATMENT IN CATS

Overall, side effects associated with radioiodine treatment of cats are extremely rare. Because radioiodine is relatively specific in its site of action, there is no hair loss or increase in skin pigmentation, as may be seen with external radiation therapy (cobalt radiation). Some cats appear to develop mild, transient discomfort of the thyroid gland during the first few days after treatment (probably as a result of radiation thyroiditis), but this condition is self-limited and resolves spontaneously. The most serious problem associated with radioiodine treatment in cats is permanent hypothyroidism (see below), which develops a few months after treatment with radioiodine in a small percentage of cats.

## FOLLOW-UP THYROID FUNCTION TESTING AFTER RADIOACTIVE IODINE TREATMENT

The ideal goal of $^{131}$I therapy is to restore euthyroidism with a single dose of radiation without producing hypothyroidism. Indeed, most hyperthyroid cats treated with radioactive iodine are cured by a single dose. Thyroid hormone concentrations in the blood are normal within 2 weeks of therapy in approximately 70 to 80% of cats, and in over 90% of cats by 3 months. Although cats appear to feel better within days after treatment, the owner will notice gradual clinical improvement and resolution of the signs of hyperthyroidism over a 1- to 3-month period.

Approximately 5 to 10% of cats, however, fail to respond completely and remain hyperthyroid after treatment with radioiodine. These cats may show clinical improvement and in some cases have resolution of all signs of hyperthyroidism, but their serum thyroid hormone concentrations remain high. If these cats are not re-treated, their signs of hyperthyroidism will usually return a few months later. Therefore, if the hyperthyroid state persists for longer than 3 months after initial treatment, the referring veterinarian should discuss the possibility of re-treating the cat with radioiodine with the veterinarian in charge of the radioiodine therapy (see Tables 1 and 2). In such cats, re-treatment is generally recommended because virtually all cats that remain hyperthyroid after the first treatment can be cured by a second treatment.

In contrast, a few (generally <5%) cats treated with radioiodine will develop permanent hypothyroidism, which develops a few months after treatment with radioiodine in a small percentage of cats. Clinical signs associated with iatrogenic hypothyroidism in these cats may include lethargy, nonpruritic seborrhea sicca, matting of hair, and marked weight gain; bilateral symmetric alopecia does not develop. If hypothyroidism develops (diagnosis based upon clinical sign, subnormal serum $T_4$ concentration, and response to replacement therapy), lifelong thyroid hormone supplementation is generally needed (i.e., 0.1 mg levothyroxine per day).

After administration of radioiodine to cats, cure of hyperthyroidism is generally permanent, but studies have recently demonstrated that the disorder can reoccur. However, relapse is very uncommon, with a prevalence of less than 5%, and the time between treatment with radioiodine and relapse is generally 3 or more years. Therefore, such relapse might indicate the development of new hyperplastic or neoplastic nodules arising from any remaining normal thyroid tissue, rather than reoccurrence of the first adenomatous thyroid tumor that was treated with radioiodine. Nevertheless, the fact that both hypothyroidism and relapse can occur after treatment of cats with radioiodine indicate that continued, periodic monitoring of thyroid function (e.g., at least once yearly) is advisable once euthyroidism is restored.

## CONCLUSIONS

The choice of treatment of a cat with hyperthyroidism may be influenced by many factors, including the severity of the disease, the presence of concurrent disease, and the availability of treatment, especially radioiodine. Overall, use of radioiodine may be the optimum treatment for cats with hyperthyroidism when an institution or treatment center licensed to administer radioiodine to cats is located nearby.

Radioactive iodine treatment involves a single, nonstressful procedure that is without associated morbidity or mortality. Untoward systemic effects have not been observed. Unlike surgery, anesthesia is not required. A single $^{131}$I treatment will restore euthyroidism in most cats with hyperthyroidism, whereas cats that remain persistently hyperthyroid can be successfully retreated with radioiodine and those that become hypothyroid can be supplemented readily with levothyroxine. At present, the major disadvantage of radioiodine therapy is the limited availability of facilities licensed to handle $^{131}$I and treat cats with hyperthyroidism (see Tables 1 and 2).

### References and Suggested Reading

Jones BR, Cayzer J, Dillon EA, et al:Radio-iodine treatment of hyperthyroidism in cats. NZ Vet J 39:71, 1991.
*Of 32 cats with hyperthyroidism treated with relatively low doses of radioiodine, 28 (88%) responded to treatment, three remained hyperthyroid, and one became hypothyroid.*
Meric SM, Hawkins EC, Washabau RJ, et al:Serum thyroxine concentrations after radioactive iodine therapy in cats with hyperthyroidism. J Am Vet Med Assoc 188:1038, 1986.
*Of 31 hyperthyroid cats treated with radioiodine, 29 (83%) had normal serum $T_4$ concentrations when retested 1 month after treatment, three cats remained hyperthyroid, and two cats had low serum $T_4$ values.*
Meric SM and Rubin SI: Serum thyroxine concentrations following fixed-dose radioactive iodine treatment in hyperthyroid cats: 62 cases (1986–1989). J Am Vet Med Assoc 197:621, 1990.
*Of 60 cats with hyperthyroidism that were treated with a fixed dose of 4 mCi of radioiodine and then reexamined, 50 (84%) had a complete response, five (remained hyperthyroid, and five developed a low serum $T_4$ concentration unassociated with any clinical signs of hypothyroidism.*
Peterson ME: Results of radioactive iodine treatment in cats with hyperthyroidism: 524 cases (1986–1992). J Vet Intern Med 1995 (in press).
*Of a large series of hyperthyroid cats treated with radioiodine, high serum $T_4$ concentrations fell to within normal range in over 90% of cases, whereas*

*less than 5% of cats remained hyperthyroid and less than 5% became hypothyroid.*

Peterson ME, Randolph JF, and Mooney CM: Endocrine diseases. *In* Sherding RG (ed): *The Cat: Diagnosis and Clinical Management*, 2nd edition. New York, Churchill Livingstone, pp 1403–1506, 1994.
*Provides an in-depth review of the treatment methods for cats with hyperthyroidism, and discusses diagnosis and management of hypothyroidism in cats.*

Turrel JM, Feldman EC, Hayes M, et al. Radioactive iodine therapy in cats with hyperthyroidism. J Am Vet Med Assoc 184:554–559, 1984.
*Of 11 hyperthyroid cats treated with radioiodine, seven had a complete response, two had a partial response but remained hyperthyroid, and two became hypothyroid.*

Turrel JM, Feldman EC, Nelson RW, et al: Thyroid carcinoma causing hyperthyroidism in cats: 14 cases (1981–1986). J Am Vet Med Assoc 193: 359–364, 1988.
*Cats with thyroid carcinoma generally require higher doses of radioiodine to cure the hyperthyroid state.*

# UTILITY OF DIAGNOSTIC ASSAYS IN THE EVALUATION OF HYPERCALCEMIA AND HYPOCALCEMIA: PARATHYROID HORMONE, VITAMIN D METABOLITES, PARATHYROID HORMONE–RELATED PEPTIDE, AND IONIZED CALCIUM

DENNIS J. CHEW,
LARRY A. NAGODE,
THOMAS J. ROSOL,
MARCIA A. CAROTHERS,
*and* PATRICIA SCHENCK

*Columbus, Ohio*

Hypercalcemia and hypocalcemia are each associated with many underlying disease processes. The magnitude of either hypercalcemia or hypocalcemia is not sufficient by itself to provide a diagnosis. Information from the history and physical examination, hematology, serum biochemistry, imaging of the body cavities and skeleton, and cytology or biopsies commonly provide important direction as to the likely cause for hypocalcemia or hypercalcemia. A more definitive diagnosis for the causes of hypercalcemia and hypocalcemia is now possible in most cases due to the recent development and availability of serum hormone assays related to calcium metabolism that have been validated in animals. Table 1 provides an overview of the anticipated changes in routine laboratory results and serum hormone assays related to calcium metabolism in different disease states associated with hyper- and hypocalcemia.

## PARATHYROID HORMONE

Measurement of serum parathyroid hormone (PTH) concentrations is the most commonly employed clinical assay related to calcium metabolism. Its greatest use is to identify hypercalcemic patients in which parathyroid hormone plays a major role in the development of hypercalcemia. This assay may also provide convincing evidence for the diagnosis of primary hypoparathyroidism in patients with hypocalcemia.

## Assays for PTH

The clinical validity and usefulness of serum PTH measurement to evaluate parathyroid gland function in dogs and cats is greatly influenced by the type of assay selected (i.e., amino-terminus, carboxy-terminus, mid-molecule fragments, or intact molecule). Sensitive and validated immunoreactive PTH (i-PTH) assays for use in dogs are now available. The most popular commercial assay employs a two-site immunoradiometric (IRMA) method that recognizes both the amino- and carboxy-terminal end of the intact PTH (1-84) molecule (Fig. 1). Proper storage and handling of the serum sample is necessary to ensure that degradation of intact PTH does not occur prior to analysis. Serum should be separated, immediately frozen, and the sample sent on ice to an appropriate laboratory. Sera from cats have

***Table 1*** *Overview of the Anticipated Changes in Routine Laboratory Results and Serum Hormone Assays Related to Calcium Metabolism in Disease States Associated with Hyper- and Hypocalcemia*

| Disorder | Total Calcium | Ion-Calcium | Phosphorus | Creatinine | PTH | Calcitrol | 25(OH)-D | PTHrP |
|---|---|---|---|---|---|---|---|---|
| Primary hyperparathyroidism | ↑ | ↑ | –, ↓ | –, ↑ | ↑ | –, ↑ | – | – |
| Secondary hyperparathyroidism | | | | | | | | |
|   Nutritional | ↓, – | ↓, – | ↑, – | | ↑ | ↓, – | – | – |
|   Renal-chronic | – | –, ↓ | ↑, – | ↑ | ↑ | ↓, – | – | – |
|   Renal-chronic | ↓ | ↓ | ↑, – | ↑ | ↑ | ↓, – | – | – |
|   Renal-chronic | ↑ | ↓, –, ↑ | ↑, – | ↑ | ↑ | ↓, – | – | – |
|   Renal-acute | ↓, – | ↓, – | ↑, – | ↑ | ↑ | ↓, – | – | – |
| Malignancy-associated hypercalcemia | | | | | | | | |
|   Humoral | ↑ | ↑ | –, ↓ | – | ↓, – | ↓, –, ↑ | – | ↑ |
|   Local osteolytic | ↑ | ↑ | ↑, – | – | ↓ | ↓ | – | – |
| Elevations in vitamin D metabolites | | | | | | | | |
|   Cholecalciferol toxicity | ↑ | ↑ | ↑, – | –, ↑ | ↓ | –, ↑ | ↑↑ | – |
|   Lymphosarcoma | ↑ | ↑ | –, ↓ | – | ↓ | ↑ | – | ↑ |
|   Granulomatous inflammation | ↑ | ↑ | –, ↑ | – | ↓ | ↑ | – | – |
| Addison's disease | ↑ | –, ↑ | –, ↑ | ↑, – | ↓ | – | – | – |
| Dehydration | ↑ | ↑, – | – | –, ↑ | – | – | – | – |
| Primary hypoparathyroidism | ↓ | ↓ | ↑, – | – | ↓ | –, ↓ | – | – |
| Hypoalbuminemia | ↓ | –, ↓ | – | – | – | – | ↓ | – |
| Hypovitaminosis D | ↓ | ↓ | – | – | –, ↑ | ↓ | ↓ | – |
| Eclampsia | ↓ | ↓ | –, ↓ | – | ↑ | ↑ | – | – |

Key: ↑ = high concentration, ↓ = low concentration, – = normal or no change.

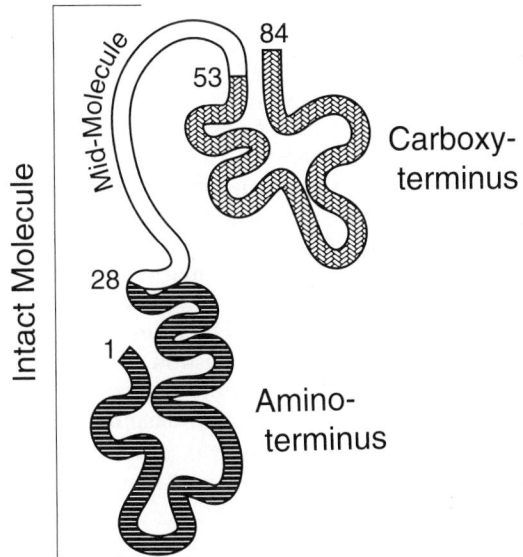

**Figure 1.** Regions of the PTH molecule potentially recognized by immunoreactive assays. The amino-terminus (amino acids 1-28) is highly stable and is the bioactive part of the molecule that associates with the PTH receptor. The carboxy-terminus (amino acids 53-84) has a role in facilitating secretion of PTH from the parathyroid gland but apparently has no additional role (no bioactivity). Single antigenic site assays have been developed against the amino-terminus, carboxy-terminus, and mid-molecule areas. The intact molecule (amino acids 1-84) is assayed with dual antibodies directed against both the amino- and carboxy-terminus. Most recently, a dual antibody assay has become available with both antigenic sites on the amino-terminus.

recently been validated using this methodology. In our laboratory, this method is not as sensitive as the amino-terminal assay for the detection of i-PTH in cats.

Some laboratories measure amino-terminal PTH using a single-site assay. Degradation of intact PTH to fragments during storage or shipment of serum does not substantially reduce the PTH as measured in this assay. The amino-terminal part of PTH is stable in serum. No amino-terminal fragments circulate in blood; therefore, amino-terminal PTH measured in a serum sample was originally part of circulating intact PTH (Fig. 1). This method measures PTH from dogs or cats with good sensitivity, but the methodology is cumbersome and slow (6 days). The availability of reagents for this measurement has recently been restricted; it is likely that this assay will not be generally available in the near future, although it will continue to be performed in a few research laboratories.

A new method that shows potential for PTH measurement in our laboratory detects the stable amino-terminus by the two-site IRMA methodology (Nichols Institute, San Juan Capistrano, CA 92675). This convenient method is rapid (24 hr) and detects a wide range of PTH concentrations without the need for sample dilution. Preliminary results suggest that this assay is effective for dog and horse PTH; cat PTH is also under investigation.

Carboxy-terminal and mid-molecule PTH assays suffer from the serious limitation that biologically inactive fragments of PTH are detected by these methods. Carboxy-terminal and mid-molecule PTH fragments are excreted by the kidney and therefore accumulate in the serum of dogs and cats with renal failure (Fig. 1). We do not recommend the assay of serum PTH using these methods, since overinterpretations may be made in animals with decreased renal function. In renal failure, impaired clearance of PTH fragments possessing no biologic activity results in large increases in measured PTH that is not proportional to biologically active PTH.

## Interpretation of PTH Determinations

Serum ionized calcium is the major physiologic stimulus to either increase or inhibit the secretion of PTH. Consequently, it is necessary to interpret PTH concentrations simultaneously with the corresponding serum calcium concentration. In most instances, the serum total calcium and serum ionized calcium concentrations change proportionally.

If the parathyroid glands are healthy, PTH will be suppressed or within the normal range in animals with functional hypercalcemia. High PTH at the time of hypercalcemia strongly suggests the diagnosis of primary hyperparathyroidism, although PTH values within the normal range are occasionally encountered in patients with primary hyperparathyroidism (Table 1). Patients with renal failure usually have high PTH concentrations (secondary hyperparathyroidism) regardless of serum calcium concentration (Table 1). This can create confusion for the small population of renal failure patients that also present with hypercalcemia (see "Ionized Calcium" below for further discussion).

Normal parathyroid glands will be stimulated to secrete high concentrations of PTH during times of functional hypocalcemia. Parathyroid hormone levels that are either low or normal during times of hypocalcemia support a diagnosis of primary hypoparathyroidism (Table 1).

## VITAMIN D METABOLITES

Cholecalciferol from the skin, diet, or exogenous sources is rapidly converted by enzymatic hydroxylation in the liver to 25(OH)–vitamin $D_3$ (calcidiol). The 25(OH)–vitamin $D_3$ is subsequently further hydroxylated in a highly regulated manner within the kidney to the physiologically active vitamin D metabolite 1,25(OH)$_2$–vitamin $D_3$ (calcitriol).

Measurement of serum 25(OH)-vitamin $D_3$ is a clinically useful vitamin D metabolite determination. It is commercially available at an affordable price and provides information useful in the evaluation of animals with hypercalcemia suspected of vitamin D intoxication. Determination of serum 1,25(OH)$_2$–vitamin $D_3$ concentrations is occasionally helpful in the evaluation of hypercalcemia, but this measurement is not readily available and is expensive.

## Assays for 25(OH)–Vitamin $D_3$

A variety of assays have been developed for 25(OH)–vitamin D (calcidiol) including both radioimmunoassay (RIA) and competitive protein binding assays. The later are simple, work well in our laboratory, and are the type most commonly used. A preliminary chromatographic purification step is used to separate calcidiol from calcitriol and other vitamin D metabolites. The purified calcidiol competes with tritium-labeled calcidiol for binding to the naturally occurring serum protein that binds all circulating vitamin D metabolites. This vitamin D–binding protein is an inexpensive reagent compared to antibodies required for RIA tests. Commercial kits are available from a number of vendors (e.g., Amersham Inc). Because vitamin D is a steroid and is identical in all species, these assays require no specific validation for individual species. It is very stable in serum stored frozen but, like all vitamin D metabolites, is photosensitive and should be stored protected from light. The Michigan State University Endocrinology Laboratory offers this assay.

## Interpretation of 25(OH)–Vitamin $D_3$ Determinations

Normal serum concentrations of 25(OH)–vitamin $D_3$ indicate an adequate nutritional supply of vitamin D, whereas animals with nutritional rickets have low serum concentrations of 25(OH)–vitamin $D_3$. High serum concentrations of 25(OH)–vitamin $D_3$ provide definitive evidence for overexposure to cholecalciferol (vitamin $D_3$) (Table 1). Cholecalciferol is rapidly converted to 25(OH)–vitamin $D_3$ in the liver, largely as a function of the amount of cholecalciferol substrate presented for metabolism. Rodenticides containing cholecalciferol are the main cause of hypercalcemia associated with high serum 25(OH)–vitamin $D_3$ concentrations, although overtreatment with vitamin D as replacement therapy during primary hypoparathyroidism occasionally may have the same result. High serum concentrations of serum 25(OH)–vitamin $D_3$ persist for weeks to months following ingestion of enough cholecalciferol to cause hypercalcemia. The concentration of 25(OH)–vitamin $D_3$ remains high despite the return of serum calcium to normal concentrations during this period of treatment.

## Assays for 1,25(OH)$_2$–Vitamin $D_3$

This seco-steroid hormone, produced in significant amounts only by mitochondria in cells of the renal proximal convoluted tubule, is important in some disorders of calcium metabolism. It circulates in very low concentrations compared to calcidiol and other steroid hormones (i.e., picograms per milliliter rather than nanograms per milliliter). As in calcidiol assays, a preliminary purification of calcitriol is required. The naturally occurring receptor for calcitriol is used in this assay in which tritium-labeled calcitriol competes with calcitriol purified from the sample. It is properly termed a "radioreceptor" assay.

Calcitriol is extremely stable in frozen serum but, like calcidiol, must be protected from light. As a steroid hormone, it is equally detectable regardless of animal species. Both vitamin $D_3$ and vitamin $D_2$ produce calcitriol, which are detectable identically with the calf thymus gland receptor now most commonly used in this radioreceptor assay.

Although a kit from Amersham Inc is available for this assay, it is best performed in laboratories with considerable experience with calcitriol measurement. It is performed commercially by Nichols Institute Reference Laboratories, Roche Biomedical Laboratories, and Continental Assays; Continental requires a 20-sample minimum but is the least expensive at $100 per assay.

### Interpretation of 1,25(OH)₂–Vitamin D₃ Determinations

Serum calcitriol concentrations are usually low or normal in patients with any form of functional hypercalcemia. Some dogs with lymphosarcoma and hypercalcemia comprise a distinct subset of patients with humoral hypercalcemia of malignancy (HHM), in which serum calcitriol concentrations are high. In these instances, the high serum concentration of calcitriol is possibly due to synthesis of calcitriol by the malignant neoplasm. Alternatively, the high serum calcitriol concentration may be due to increased renal synthesis of the hormone, which is produced in response to another hormone elaborated by the malignant neoplasm; that is, parathyroid hormone–related polypeptide (see below).

Although the renal 1α-hydroxylation of 25(OH)–vitamin $D_3$ to 1,25(OH)₂–vitamin $D_3$ is tightly regulated, evidence from our laboratory suggests that pharmacologic concentrations of 25(OH)–vitamin $D_3$ may overload this system. We have documented high serum concentrations of 1,25(OH)₂–vitamin $D_3$ in some dogs with cholecalciferol intoxication. High serum concentrations of calcitriol may be expected in patients with hypercalcemia associated with severe granulomatous inflammation (e.g., blastomycosis), but this has yet to be documented in dogs.

Some patients with primary hyperparathyroidism may have high serum calcitriol concentrations due to activation of the renal 1α-hydroxylase system by PTH. High serum calcitriol may be transient or intermittent, however, as elevated blood calcium can exert direct inhibition of renal 1α-hydroxylase.

Measurement of serum calcitriol is not necessary in the evaluation of most hypocalcemic patients, since the cause of the low calcium is usually apparent by other means. High or normal serum concentrations of calcitriol are expected in those dogs and cats with functional hypocalcemia and a normal renal capability to produce calcitriol (Table 1). Low serum concentrations of cal-citriol during hypocalcemia may be encountered in patients with renal failure or sustained hyperphosphatemia or both. Serum calcitriol concentrations are often apparently normal during the early phases of renal failure due to the stimulatory effects of high circulating PTH, which increases the synthesis of calcitriol in the remaining renal tubules via the 1α-hydroxylase system. In more advanced renal failure, the absolute serum concentrations of calcitriol are low (Table 1). Serum calcitriol measurement may be useful in the evaluation of obscure hypocalcemia, especially in young animals that may have metabolic defects in vitamin D metabolism.

### PARATHYROID HORMONE–RELATED PROTEIN

Parathyroid hormone-related protein (PTHrP) is a recently identified hormone that was isolated from malignant neoplasms in patients with hypercalcemia. Some malignant tumors develop the ability to secrete high levels of biologically active PTHrP, leading to high circulating concentrations of the hormone. PTHrP is capable of binding to PTH receptors in bone and kidneys, resulting in a syndrome that mimics primary hyperparathyroidism (i.e., HHM).

In contrast to PTH, which is made only by the parathyroid glands, PTHrP is normally produced by many tissues in the adult animal, such as epidermis, endocrine glands, muscle, uterus, mammary gland, and brain. PTHrP functions as a local (paracrine) hormone in adult tissues and is not secreted into the circulation in significant or measurable quantities. The function in most adult tissues is unknown, but PTHrP may be important in regulation of differentiation and local calcium metabolism.

Circulating levels of PTHrP in normal animals are undetectable in most assays and are below 1 picomole ($10^{-9}$ mol/L). PTHrP is similar to PTH in that the biologically active region is the amino-terminus. The carboxyl-terminal region has little or no effect on calcium regulation. The carboxyl-terminal region is rapidly cleaved from the amino-terminal region in blood and is excreted by the kidneys. Therefore, animals with renal failure will have high concentrations of biologically inactive, carboxyl-terminal PTHrP in the blood.

### Assays for PTHrP

Two types of assays have been developed for measuring circulating, biologically active PTHrP concentrations. The first is an N-terminal RIA specific for human PTHrP (Incstar Corp, Stillwater, MN). The sensitivity of the assay is 1.8 pmol/L. This assay has been useful in measuring circulating concentrations of PTHrP in dogs because the amino-terminal region of canine PTHrP is identical to human PTHrP. The assay requires special handling of samples to ensure reliable results. A blood sample should be collected in a tube with ethylenediaminetetraacetic acid (EDTA) (7.2 mg/ml). A protease inhibitor (aprotinin, 400 KIU/ml) should be added immediately to prevent degradation of PTHrP. The plasma is removed after centrifugation and may be stored at −20°C. Serum samples from dogs with high PTHrP concentrations often result in lower values than plasma samples collected with aprotinin.

The second assay that has been developed is a two-site IRMA for human PTHrP (Nichols Institute, San Juan Capistrano, CA). Two-site assays are more sensitive than one-site assays for PTHrP; this is important in detecting the low concentrations present in normal individuals. The sensitivity of the two-site IRMA is 0.3 pmol/L. This assay also requires proper sample handling with the use of protease inhibitors to prevent proteolysis of PTHrP. The manufacturer of the assay supplies tubes that contain protease inhibitor for blood collection. The two-site IRMA has not been validated for use in animals. It is possible that the carboxyl-terminal region of animal forms of PTHrP will differ from human PTHrP, which would make the assay less useful in veterinary medicine. Nichols Institute will perform the IRMA on samples for $145 if the sample has been collected in one of their special tubes containing protease inhibitors.

### Interpretation of PTHrP Determinations

Measurement of PTHrP can be clinically useful during the evaluation of patients with hypercalcemia, but has no role in evaluation of those with hypocalcemia. A variety of hypercalcemia-inducing substances can be secreted by malignant tumors that are not secreted in appreciable quantities by normal tissues; of these, PTHrP appears to be the most important. Additionally, it is the only mediator of HHM for which there is a commercially available kit for measurement. PTHrP is not detectable in the sera from normal dogs or from those without malignancy.

High concentrations of PTHrP have been associated with a variety of tumors (Table 1), most notably lymphosarcoma and anal sac adenocarcinoma; miscellaneous other carcinomas comprise most of the remaining tumors that elaborate PTHrP. For some tumors, it appears that PTHrP is necessary and sufficient to create hypercalcemia (i.e., anal sac adenocarcinoma). For other tumors (i.e., lymphosarcoma), it is likely that PTHrP is not sufficient by itself to result in hypercalcemia. In either case, detectable concentrations of PTHrP may serve as a marker of underlying neoplasia as well as the cause of the hypercalcemia. Following effective ablative treatment of the tumor (surgery, chemotherapy, or radiation therapy), PTHrP concentrations rapidly decline. Persistently high PTHrP concentrations following treatment may serve as a marker of tumor burden that has not been sufficiently decreased.

For example, using the Incstar amino-terminal RIA to measure PTHrP in dogs with HHM, dogs with apocrine gland adenocarcinomas of the anal sac and hypercalcemia have plasma concentrations ranging from 10 to 100 pmol/L; apocrine gland adenocarcinoma of the anal sac and normocalcemia, undetectable to 10 pmol/L; miscellaneous carcinomas, 4 to 50 pmol/L; lymphoma and hypercalcemia, undetectable to 15 pmol/L; lymphoma and normocalcemia, usually undetectable; and normal dogs, usually undetectable. Small numbers of cats with HHM have been evaluated. Preliminary data suggest that the assay will detect high circulating concentrations of PTHrP in cats.

Low or nondetectable concentrations of PTHrP during episodes of hypercalcemia indicate that HHM is not likely. Neoplasms that induce hypercalcemia secondary to bone metastasis and local bone osteolysis (uncommon in veterinary medicine) would be associated with undetectable levels of PTHrP. PTHrP has not been detectable in a variety of other conditions known to result in hypercalcemia, including primary hyperparathyroidism and cholecalciferol intoxication.

### IONIZED CALCIUM

Serum total calcium consists of three fractions: ionized (free), protein-bound, and complexed fractions. Ionized calcium measurements are superior to total serum calcium measurements, since it is ionized calcium that is physiologically important. Serum ionized calcium concentration usually parallels serum total calcium concentration during hypercalcemia. In normal animals and in most animals with hypercalcemia, ionized calcium approximates 55% of total calcium values for dogs and 60% for cats. The most important exception is encountered in patients with renal failure, in which the ionized calcium is frequently below that expected, based on the total calcium. The relationship of ionized calcium to total serum calcium has been less well studied during hypocalcemia, but the same relationship appears to exist when patients with hypoalbuminemia are excluded.

Some commercial laboratories report values for serum ionized calcium that are calculated from total calcium, albumin, and other serum biochemical parameters, rather than by actual determination of the ionized calcium concentration. These formulas are based on human criteria that are not accurate in animals and should not be used.

Measurement of serum ionized calcium is useful to confirm that hyper- or hypocalcemia based on assay of total calcium is associated with actual changes in ionized calcium. Measurement of ionized calcium is most useful in patients with renal failure and hypercalcemia.

### Assay for Ionized Calcium

Ionized calcium is determined by the use of potassium chloride–saturated ion-specific electrodes. A variety of machines are available to measure ionized calcium, but not all commercial laboratories are equipped to offer this measurement. Additionally, special handling of blood samples is necessary in order to allow clinically relevant interpretation of results.

Blood should be collected from a free-flowing vein in order to minimize any chances for local pH decreases during venous occlusion. Jugular venous blood is preferred over peripheral limb veins for this reason. We recommend the determination of ionized calcium from serum rather than from plasma samples. If plasma measurement is desired, the use of titrated heparin tubes is recommended; silicone separator tubes are not recommended for serum collection, since variable binding of calcium to silicone can occur.

Exposure of the serum sample to air results in loss of carbon dioxide, which increases the pH and decreases the ionized calcium (shifting of free to bound calcium). Consequently, minimizing exposure to air following collection, separation, storage, and measurement is mandatory. Ideally, the serum sample should be analyzed immediately following clot formation and centrifugation with the tube cap in place. After centrifugation, the cap is removed and the instrument probe inserted directly into the serum.

If transport to a lab is necessary, serum must be anaerobically aspirated through the tube cap into a small syringe, taking care to ensure there are no air bubbles in the syringe. The syringe should be capped (B-D Luer-Lok) and then secured with parafilm. Pilot studies in our laboratory indicate that serum samples carefully collected from dogs in this manner yield very similar results compared with those analyzed immediately for up to 72 hr of storage at 4°C (standard refrigerator temperature). This should provide enough time for anaerobic serum samples to be transported to a laboratory on ice. Heparinized canine plasma samples yield similar results for up to 9 hr of 4°C storage. Formulas designed to "correct" the ionized calcium concentration to a serum pH of 7.4 have not been critically evaluated as to their accuracy or clinical usefulness, and are not presently recommended.

## Interpretation of Ionized Calcium Determinations

Evaluation of ionized calcium concentrations serves to confirm that hyper- or hypocalcemia based on total serum calcium concentration may have functional consequences. Patients with renal failure often exhibit low ionized calcium concentrations in the face of low, normal, or high concentrations of serum total calcium (Table 1). The primary renal failure patient with hypercalcemia will also have a high i-PTH measurement (renal secondary hyperparathyroidism). Typically, animals with primary hyperparathyroidism have high serum ionized calcium and i-PTH concentrations. In contrast, renal failure patients that subsequently develop hypercalcemia usually have a normal or low ionized calcium in association with a high i-PTH concentration. This is presumed to result as a consequence of increased calcium complexes with phosphate, citrate, or sulfate that can occur in uremia. Some dogs with severe renal secondary hyperparathyroidism develop ionized hypercalcemia that is indistinguishable from that encountered in primary hyperparathyroidism. In such instances, exploration of the parathyroid glands may be inevitable to exclude a focal parathyroid gland tumor (primary hyperparathyroidism) or to confirm diffuse parathyroid gland hyperplasia (secondary renal hyperparathyroidism).

Total serum calcium and ionized calcium decrease proportionately during functional hypocalcemia. Serum total calcium concentration below 6.5 mg/dl in dogs cannot occur without some decrease in ionized calcium concentration. Patients with hypoalbuminemia and low total serum calcium concentration usually are assumed to have normal ionized calcium concentrations, based largely on formulas that "correct" the total calcium to the normal range when serum albumin or total protein concentrations are factored into an equation. Such equations are useful only to remind us that the total calcium measurement depends in part on a protein-bound fraction of calcium. Correction of total calcium to the normal range does not guarantee that the ionized calcium is normal. Ionized calcium is disproportionately low in some patients with hypoalbuminemia.

## References and Suggested Reading

Barber PJ, Elliott J, Torrance AJ: Measurement of feline parathyroid hormone: Assay validation and sample handling studies. J Small Anim Pract 34:614, 1993.
*This paper demonstrates the validity of feline serum and plasma PTH measurements using a two-site intact molecule immunoradiometric assay.*

Chew DJ, Nagode LA, Carothers M: Disorders of calcium: Hypercalcemia and hypocalcemia. In Dibartola SP (ed): *Fluid Therapy in Small Animal Practice.* Philadelphia, WB Saunders Co, 1992, pp 116–176.
*This chapter provides further detail on calcium-related hormone assays and normal values, as well as a review of normal calcium homeostasis.*

Rosol TJ and Capen CC: Biology of disease, mechanisms of cancer-induced hypercalcemia. Lab Invest 67:680, 1992.
*This review paper provides more detailed insight into the mechanisms for humoral hypercalcemia of malignancy.*

Rosol TJ, Nagode LA, Couto CG, et al: Parathyroid hormone (PTH)-related protein, PTH, and 1,25-dihydroxyvitamin D in dogs with cancer-associated hypercalcemia. Endocrinology 131:1157, 1992.
*This paper provides detailed hormone data related to abnormal calcium metabolism in dogs with clinical disease, with special emphasis on PTHrP.*

Szenci O, Brydl E, and Bajcsy CA: Effect of storage on measurement of ionized calcium and acid-base variables in equine, bovine, ovine, and canine venous blood. J Am Vet Med Assoc 199:1167, 1991.
*This paper reviews factors that can alter ionized calcium during storage and provides data from heparinized blood samples collected from dogs and then stored.*

# COMPLICATIONS AND CONCURRENT DISEASE ASSOCIATED WITH DIABETIC KETOACIDOSIS AND OTHER SEVERE FORMS OF DIABETES MELLITUS

RHETT NICHOLS
*Farmingdale, New York*

*and* KATHY L. CRENSHAW
*New York, New York*

Many animals with diabetes mellitus are severely ill on clinical presentation. The spectrum of disease is quite variable and includes diabetic ketoacidosis, ketosis without acidosis, hyperosmolar nonketotic syndrome, and other nonketotic variants (negative urine ketones, serum osmolality <340 mOsm/kg with or without acidosis). These more severe forms of diabetes are often precipitated by concurrent diseases such as pyelonephritis, pancreatitis, pyometra, hyperadrenocorticism, renal failure, and heart failure. To make matters worse, in-hospital treatment of diabetic dogs and cats is commonly associated with serious complications, including hypoglycemia, hypokalemia, and hypophosphatemia.

## CONCURRENT DISEASE ASSOCIATED WITH DIABETES MELLITUS

In human diabetics, the major factors that precipitate diabetic ketoacidosis, hyperosmolar nonketotic syndrome, and other nonketotic variants are too little insulin, infection, severe stress, hypokalemia, renal failure, drugs that decrease insulin secretion or cause insulin resistance, and inadequate fluid intake for any reason. Many of these precipitating factors also play an important role in veterinary medicine. For example, diabetic dogs and cats frequently suffer from concurrent urinary tract infections, pyometra, pancreatitis, prostatitis, pneumonia, renal failure, or congestive heart failure. In a recent study of 60 diabetic cats at the Animal Medical Center (the AMC study) 43% were azotemic on admission. Although the majority of cats had mild renal insufficiency (serum creatinine <2.5 mg/dl), the degree of renal impairment was assessed as moderate to severe (serum creatinine >3.0 mg/dl) in 20% of the cases. Other concurrent diseases or drug therapy included inflammatory bowel disease, asthma, urinary tract infection, pancreatitis, hyperthyroidism, heart disease, neoplasia, and corticosteroid administration.

In a previous study of 59 diabetic dogs at the University of California Teaching Hospital, Davis, CA (the Davis study), concurrent diseases and complications recognized during the initial management were as follows: ketosis, heart disease, urinary tract infection, pancreatitis, Cushing's syndrome, renal impairment, skin infection, neoplasia, pancreatic insufficiency, and several miscellaneous disorders (Ling et al., 1987). The most frequent causes of death in these patients were severe ketoacidosis accompanied by renal shutdown and acute necrotizing pancreatitis. Since a wide variety of disorders can be associated with diabetes mellitus, a careful search should always be made, both at the time of physical examination and during therapy, for underlying problems that may have precipitated an episode of decompensated diabetes. A complete data base should include a complete blood count, serum biochemical profile with amylase and lipase, urinalysis with culture and sensitivity, chest and abdominal radiographs and, in select cases, abdominal ultrasonography.

## COMPLICATIONS ASSOCIATED WITH INITIAL PRESENTATION AND THERAPY

### Dehydration, Acidosis, and Hyperosmolarity

Most diabetic patients with diabetic ketoacidosis, hyperosmolar nonketotic syndrome, and other nonketotic variants are moderately to severely dehydrated (7 to 12%) on initial presentation. In addition, many patients are acidotic ($TcO_2$ <15 mEq/L) and markedly hyperosmolar (>330 mOsm/kg). In the Davis study, medium serum bicarbonate concentrations were below normal. In the AMC study, nearly 50% of diabetic cats were ketoacidotic and over 40% were hyperosmolar. Several diabetic cats with ketosis were not acidotic. The majority of the cases of acidosis ($TcO_2$ range: 7 to 14 mEq/L) were successfully treated with replacement fluids and insulin therapy; only rarely was sodium bicarbonate administered.

While there is no question that severe acidosis is a dangerous consequence of diabetic ketoacidosis and may result in decreased cardiac contractility and direct peripheral vasodilatation, certain disadvantages of bicarbonate therapy outweigh its advantages in many clinical settings. Major disadvantages of bicarbonate therapy include acceleration of the development of hypokalemia and hypophosphatemia, cerebral edema, increased hemoglobin affinity with resulting peripheral tissue hypoxia and fluid overload, and paradoxical cerebrospinal fluid acidosis. Moreover, in human studies, the clinical course of diabetic ketoacidosis was not significantly altered in patients given bicarbonate versus patients not given bicarbonate. Therefore, it is generally recommended not giving bicarbonate unless the pH approaches 7.

The effective serum osmolality in the significantly hyperosmolar diabetics in the AMC study ranged from 331 to 350 mOsm/kg. Effective serum osmolality (tonicity) is calculated based on the following formula:

$$2(Na + K) + glucose\ (mg/dl)/20$$

This formula accounts for only those substances that are biologically active in pulling water from the cellular and interstitial space into the vascular compartment and, therefore, can be used to more accurately estimate the degree of dehydration. Without exception, an effective serum osmolality greater than 330 mOsm/kg is associated with severe water deficits.

In terms of clinical frequency, the nonketotic hyperosmolar variants (serum osmolality between 330 and 340 mOsm/kg, with or without acidosis, negative urine ketones) were the most common clinical presentation, followed by hyperosmolar ketoacidosis and true or pure hyperosmolar nonketotic syndrome (>340 mOsm/kg, $TCO_2$ >15 mEq/L, negative or minimal urine ketones). Clinically, diabetic ketoacidosis and hyperosmolar nonketotic syndrome appear to represent a continuum of disease. At one extreme, pure diabetic ketoacidosis without significant hyperosmolality typically indicates the total absence of insulin. And at the other extreme, pure hyperosmolar nonketotic syndrome without ketoacidosis typically occurs in the non–insulin-dependent diabetic.

Treatment of the hyperosmolar-ketoacidotic patient is aimed at restoring intravascular volume such that optimal tissue perfusion is present to ensure delivery of administered insulin to the peripheral tissues. The type of fluid chosen is usually based on the serum sodium concentration. Serum sodium may be low, normal, or elevated; however, total body sodium is always low. If the serum sodium concentration is below 140 mEq/L, then 0.9% saline is administered. If the sodium levels are 140 to 160 mEq/L, then 0.9% saline or lactated Ringer's solution is used for fluid replacement. If the serum sodium concentration is above 160 mEq/L, 0.45% saline is recommended. Generally, half of the calculated water deficit is given intravenously over 4 to 6 hr, followed by maintenance requirements over the next 18 to 20 hr. Fluid therapy must be adequate prior to insulin administration, as insulin will cause glucose and water to shift from the vascular space into the cells. The result is an acute loss of vascular volume and worsening hypernatremia. Past fears of cerebral edema secondary to rapid fluid administration appear unwarranted. A number of recent studies have documented that cerebral edema in diabetic ketoacidosis or hyperosmolar nonketotic syndrome is unrelated to the rate of fluid replacement or rate of correction of the hyperglycemia or hypernatremia (Rosenbloom, 1986).

## Hypoglycemia

The major "toxic" reaction associated with insulin therapy is hypoglycemia. It has been estimated that people with insulin-dependent diabetes mellitus (IDDM) experience one to two episodes of mild to moderate symptomatic hypoglycemia per week, while the incidence of hypoglycemia in patients hospitalized for diabetic ketoacidosis is 30 to 37% (Fischer et al., 1986; Siperstein, 1992). Risk factors identified for hypoglycemia (other than high doses of insulin) include "tight" diabetic control, hepatic and renal disease, fever, and "nothing orally" status.

In the AMC study, the incidence of hypoglycemia during hospitalization was 13%, although 70% of the hospitalized patients required dextrose supplementation to maintain a blood glucose greater than 200 mg/dl (>11 mmol/L). In most cases, a low dose of regular beef-pork insulin (1/2 to 1 U) was being given subcutaneously four times daily prior to the hypoglycemic event. The majority of the hypoglycemic episodes in hospitalized animals were noted to be asymptomatic; however, symptomatic hypoglycemia was occasionally observed. Avoidance of hypoglycemia in the hospitalized patient is best achieved by periodic monitoring of blood glucose levels (e.g., every 6 hr), initially using low doses of insulin (0.25 U/kg in the dog; 0.1 U/kg in the cat), and supplementation of dextrose into maintenance or replacement fluids when the blood glucose falls below 200 mg/dl (<11 mmol/L).

Some cats with diabetic ketoacidosis regain their ability to produce normal amounts of insulin weeks to months after exogenous insulin therapy has been initiated (this rarely occurs in the dog). These patients are referred to as transient diabetics and are commonly presented for clinical signs related to episodes of hypoglycemia. Long-term monitoring of the diabetic state with periodic blood sugar and urine glucose determinations (if possible) is recommended to avoid this problem. Transient diabetes mellitus in cats is believed to be related to a phenomenon referred to as "glucose toxicity," whereby hyperglycemia per se causes downregulation of the glucose transport mechanism and the ability of pancreatic B cells to produce insulin. Control of hyperglycemia with oral hypoglycemics or exogenous insulin administration may allow repair of this defect and the discontinuation of these modes of therapy.

## Hypokalemia

In the 1930s, even after the discovery of insulin, the average mortality rate for human patients with diabetic ketoacidosis was 29% (Siperstein, 1992). One of the major reasons for the high mortality rate was the general unawareness of hypokalemia-induced cardiac arrhythmias. Because of osmotic diuresis, metabolic acidosis, vomiting, diarrhea, and anorexia, a deficit in total body potassium (up to 5 to 10 mEq/kg) is present in diabetic ketoacidosis. Nevertheless, serum potassium levels are often normal or even elevated despite severe total body potassium depletion. Acidosis causes a shift of potassium from the intracellular to extracellular compartments. Hyperglycemia, likewise, promotes intracellular potassium depletion and contributes to a falsely high estimation of total body potassium.

Clinically, most dogs and cats with untreated diabetic ketoacidosis have normal or decreased serum potassium. The normal serum potassium levels are misleading because, as mentioned above, there is a universal depletion of total body potassium stores. In the AMC study, two thirds of the diabetic cats had normal potassium concentrations on admission, while one third were hypokalemic. Most hypokalemic cats had mild (3.0 to 3.5 mEq/L) to moderate (2.5 to 3.0 mEq/L) hypokalemia prior to therapy. In the Davis study, pretreatment medium serum potassium concentrations were below normal in over 75% of the diabetic dogs.

During therapy for diabetic ketoacidosis, the serum potassium concentration declines in virtually all patients because of rehydration (dilution), correction of acidosis (shift of hydrogen out of the cells in exchange for potassium), insulin-mediated cellular uptake of potassium, and continued urinary losses. If potassium concentration is low or normal on admission in the face of severe metabolic acidosis, immediate institution of intravenous potassium is required. If the potassium concentration is above the normal range, potassium therapy should be withheld for 2 to 4 hr until it is certain that the patient is not anuric or oliguric. Potassium supplementation is best provided by potassium chloride solution, which is added to parenteral fluids. Intravenous potassium supplementation can be given based on the guidelines shown in Table 1.

If an accurate measurement of serum potassium is not available, potassium should be added at the rate of 10 mEq/250 ml (40 mEq/L) of intravenous fluids. It is very important to monitor potassium supplementation and serum potassium levels, given that there is a steep decline in potassium concentration immediately after the institution of therapy, with the lowest levels reported during the first few hours of therapy. Hypokalemia carries the risk of cardiac arrhythmias, respiratory failure, and lesser complications of generalized muscle weakness, gastrointestinal stasis, and poor renal water

conservation. Daily serum electrolyte determinations and necessary treatment adjustments are made until normal values are obtained. In the AMC study, despite low-dose insulin therapy, appropriate volumes of intravenous fluids, and potassium supplementation, mild or moderate hypokalemia or worsening hypokalemia occurred after initiation of therapy in 40% of the diabetic cats. The majority of these cats had ketosis without acidosis of diabetic ketoacidosis. These results suggest that the published general guidelines for potassium supplementation in intravenous fluids, especially for patients with diabetic ketoacidosis, may be too low.

## Hypophosphatemia

Phosphorus is an important component of adenosine triphosphate (ATP) and is therefore critical in certain energy-dependent physiologic processes. If serum phosphorus levels drop below 1 mg/dl, a crisis may develop in body cells that are high energy users, including red blood cells, skeletal muscle cells, and brain cells. Signs of acute hypophosphatemia include rapid hemolysis; muscle weakness and rhabdomyolysis; and decreased cerebral function leading to seizures, stupor, and coma. Phosphate depletion is common in diabetic ketoacidosis and, like hypokalemia, is caused by decreased intake from anorexia and vomiting, increased urinary losses from osmotic diuresis and replacement fluid therapy, and translocation following insulin or alkali administration.

In veterinary medicine, despite sporadic cases of hemolytic anemia associated with hypophosphatemia and diabetes mellitus, phosphate depletion is considered by many clinicians as a clinically silent abnormality that is only apparent in laboratory measurements. However, results from the AMC study would suggest that hypophosphatemia is a major contributor to patient morbidity. While only 5% of the diabetic cats were hypophosphatemic (<2.0 mg/dl) prior to therapy, 25% developed hypophosphatemia or worsening hypophosphatemia following treatment. Most of the cats with pretreatment- or treatment-induced hypophosphatemia presented with ketosis or diabetic ketoacidosis. In several cats, the hypophosphatemia was associated with intravascular hemolysis and severe anemia that required transfusion or aggressive phosphate supplementation or both. In all cases, phosphate was supplemented as potassium phosphate at a dose of 0.03 to 0.12 mmol/kg/hr followed by repeated phosphate determinations every 12 to 24 hr until the serum phosphate level was greater than 2.5 mg/dl. The dose of phosphate used for treating severe hypophosphatemia was much higher than previously recommended (0.01 to 0.03 mmol/kg/hr) in the veterinary literature (Willard et al., 1987). Experience from the AMC study indicates that the published dose of phosphate for correction of severe hypophosphatemia is often inadequate. In most cases, two to four treatments of potassium phosphate at 6-hr intervals was necessary to raise the phosphate concentration above 2.5 mg/dl. In general, patients with dia-

***Table 1.***

| Serum Potassium (mEq/L) | Potassium Supplement/250 ml (mEq) |
|---|---|
| >3.5 | 5 |
| 3.0–3.5 | 7 |
| 2.5–3.0 | 10 |
| 2.0–2.5 | 15 |
| <2.0 | 20 |

betic ketoacidosis and pretreatment phosphate levels below 3.0 mg/dl appear at risk for worsening hypophosphatemia and hemolysis. The biggest concern over phosphate therapy is that intravenous phosphate will lower serum calcium and cause deposition of calcium phosphate in soft tissues. If phosphate replacement is attempted, serum calcium and phosphate levels must therefore be carefully monitored.

### References and Suggested Reading

Fischer KF, Lees JA, and Newman JH: Hypoglycemia in hospitalized patients, causes and outcomes. N Engl J Med 315:1245, 1986.
*A large retrospective human study.*

Ling GV, Lowenstein LJ, Pulley LT, and Kaneko JJ: Diabetes mellitus in dogs: A review of initial evaluation, immediate and long-term management, and outcome. J Am Vet Med Assoc 170:521, 1977.
*The largest retrospective study of diabetes mellitus in dogs.*

Rosenbloom AL: Intracerebral crisis during treatment of diabetic ketoacidosis. Diabetes Care 13:22, 1990.
*A retrospective study of the causes of changing neurologic status in treated diabetic ketoacidotic patients.*

Siperstein MD: Diabetic ketoacidosis and hyperosmolar coma. Endocrinol Metab Clin North Am 21:415, 1992.
*An in-depth discussion of precipitating causes and treatment of diabetic ketoacidosis and hyperosmolar coma.*

Willard MD, Zerbe CA, Schall WD, et al: Severe hypophosphatemia associated with diabetes mellitus in six dogs and one cat. J Am Vet Med Assoc 190:1007, 1987.
*A retrospective review of the clinical presentation, clinical course, and treatment of severe hypophosphatemia secondary to diabetes mellitus in small animals.*

---

# *CVT* UPDATE:
# INSULIN AND INSULIN SYRINGES

MARK E. PETERSON
*New York, New York*

*and* GARY R. SAMPSON
*Indianapolis, Indiana*

Insulin was discovered in 1921, and the pharmaceutical industry has since made great strides in improving its purity and stability, modifying its duration of action, and producing it from different sources. Until recently, all insulin came from beef or pork pancreata, and its purity and strength were not always reliable. Today there are more than 30 insulin preparations available in the United States, including human insulin, which is genetically engineered by recombinant deoxyribonucleic acid (DNA) technology. Today's insulins are extremely pure, with human insulin being the purest and purified pork insulin a close second. However, even the beef and beef/pork insulins are purer today than they were a decade or two ago.

Changes in the available sources and formulations of insulin products for use in humans are having a great impact on treatment in veterinary medicine. There has been a trend among the manufacturers of insulin toward production of an increasing number of human insulin preparations, which offers several advantages to human patients over previously used animal products. Because of the declining use of animal-source insulins in human patients, both Eli Lilly and Novo Nordisk, the two largest manufacturers of insulin in the United States, recently discontinued some of their animal-source (e.g., beef/pork) insulin preparations. Protamine zinc insulin (PZI), a long-acting insulin favored for use in cats, has not been manufactured for use in humans since 1991, but this beef/pork PZI preparation is sched-

uled to be reintroduced for use in dogs and cats by the Anpro Pharm Company (Table 1). These changes in the species source of available insulin (i.e., human versus animal), plus the fact that there are so many new insulin preparations available, may make selecting the correct insulin for use in the diabetic dog or cat difficult. In addition, an increasing number of improved insulin syringes (low-dose syringes, ultrafine needles) have become available, confusing the issue further (Table 2). Therefore, our purpose in this article is to clarify some of these issues concerning the selection and use of insulin and insulin syringes in the treatment of dogs and cats with diabetes mellitus.

All mammalian insulin is structurally similar, containing 51 amino acids in two polypeptide chains, the 21–amino acid A chain and the 30–amino acid B chain (Smith, 1972). Until recently, most commercial insulins produced in the United States were beef/pork combinations composed largely of beef insulin, since beef pancreata far outnumber pork pancreata as a byproduct of the meat-packing industry. Beef/pork insulin preparations contain a mixture of approximately 90% beef and 10% pork insulin. Pork insulin is close to human insulin in structure, differing only by one amino acid in the B chain, and beef insulin differs by three amino acids. Pork insulin is identical to the insulin of dogs in its amino acid structure. Cat insulin, which differs from pork and dog insulin by four amino acids, is most similar to beef insulin, differing in only one po-

***Table 1.*** *Insulin Preparations*

| Product | Manufacturer | Kind | Species | Strength |
|---------|--------------|------|---------|----------|
| ***Short-Acting*** | | | | |
| Humulin R | Lilly | Regular | Human | U-100 |
| Ilentin I Regular | Lilly | Regular | Beef/Pork | U-100 |
| Iletin II Regular | Lilly | Regular | Pork | U-100, U-500 |
| Novolin R | Novo Nordisk | Regular | Human | U-100 |
| Novolin R Penfill | Novo Nordisk | Regular | Human | U-100 |
| Purified Pork R | Novo Nordisk | Regular | Pork | U-100 |
| Velosulin Human | Novo Nordisk | Regular | Human | U-100 |
| ***Intermediate-Acting*** | | | | |
| NPH Anilin | Anpro Pharm | NPH | Beef/Pork | U-40 |
| Humulin L | Lilly | Lente | Human | U-100 |
| Humulin N | Lilly | NPH | Human | U-100 |
| Iletin I Lente | Lilly | Lente | Beef/Pork | U-100 |
| Iletin I NPH | Lilly | NPH | Beef/Pork | U-100 |
| Iletin II Lente | Lilly | Lente | Pork | U-100 |
| Iletin II NPH | Lilly | NPH | Pork | U-100 |
| Novolin L | Novo Nordisk | Lente | Human | U-100 |
| Novolin N | Novo Nordisk | NPH | Human | U-100 |
| Novolin N Penfill | Novo Nordisk | NPH | Human | U-100 |
| Purified Pork L | Novo Nordisk | Lente | Pork | U-100 |
| Purified Pork N | Novo Nordisk | NPH | Pork | U-100 |
| ***Long-Acting*** | | | | |
| Humulin U | Lilly | Ultralente | Human | U-100 |
| Protamine Zinc & Anilin | Anpro Pharm | PZI | Beef/Pork | U-40 |
| ***Mixtures*** | | | | |
| Humulin 50/50 | Lilly | 50% NPH, 50% Regular | Human | U-100 |
| Humulin 70/30 | Lilly | 70% NPH, 30% Regular | Human | U-100 |
| Novolin 70/30 | Novo Nordisk | 70% NPH, 30% Regular | Human | U-100 |
| Novolin 70/30 Penfill | Novo Nordisk | 70% NPH, 30% Regular | Human | U-100 |
| Novolin 70/30 Prefilled | Novo Nordisk | 70% NPH, 30% Regular | Human | U-100 |

sition, amino acid 18 of the A chain (Hallden et al., 1986).

In human diabetic patients, human insulin is generally preferred, especially in individuals that develop allergies or immune resistance to animal-derived insulin preparations. In dogs and cats, human insulin will usually be effective in controlling the diabetic state. However, most diabetic cats and dogs can be successfully treated with beef/pork insulin, which is the least expensive preparations available. Although insulin antibodies do develop in some dogs and cats treated with beef/pork combinations, the development of insulin resistance secondary to these antibodies appears to be rare. If insulin resistance secondary to the development of insulin antibodies is suspected in a diabetic dog or cat, however, a change in insulin type may be warranted. Because dog and pork insulin are identical in structure, pork insulin is the most appropriate for use in dogs with insulin resistance. Since human insulin differs from dog insulin in only one position, human preparations might also be used in dogs with insulin resistance and, since they are so widely available, may be easiest to obtain. However, since cat insulin differs considerably from human and pork, these insulins may or may not be helpful in the treatment of cats with insulin

resistance. Although the sole use of beef insulin has not been reported in cats with insulin resistance, beef or beef/pork insulin may be the preparation of choice because of their similarity.

If a change in insulin is contemplated, it is important to realize that different types and brands of insulin have different pharmacologic properties. For example, pork insulin has a shorter duration of action than does beef/pork insulin in dogs, as does human insulin in humans. A similar short duration of action has been seen in some dogs treated with human neutral protamine Hagedorn (NPH) or Lente insulin. Thus, choosing pork or human over beef/pork insulin may necessitate more frequent injections in some dogs.

Insulin is available in short-, intermediate-, and long-acting preparations that are usually injected separately but may be mixed together in the same syringe (Table 1). At present, all short-acting preparations include human and animal source regular insulins. Intermediate-acting preparations include NPH and Lente insulins. Long-acting preparations include Ultalente insulins and PZI. Although not commonly used in animals, insulin preparations with a predetermined proportion of NPH mixed with regular insulin (e.g., 70% NPH to 30% regular) are also commercially avail-

***Table 2.*** *Insulin Syringes*

| Product | Manufacturer | Insulin Strength | Needle Gauge | Needle Size | Packaging |
|---|---|---|---|---|---|
| ***1-cc Syringes*** | | | | | |
| HSW Soft-Jet (Anilin) | Anpro Pharm | U-40 | 26-gauge | 1/2″ | 150 (individually wrapped) |
| HSW Soft-Jet (Anilin) | Anpro Pharm | U-40 | 27-gauge | 1/2″ | 150 (individually wrapped) |
| B-D Micro-Fine IV | Becton Dickinson | U-100 | 28-gauge | 1/2″ | 100 (10 packs of 10) |
| B-D Ultra-Fine | Becton Dickinson | U-100 | 29-gauge | 1/2″ | 100 (10 packs of 10) |
| Can-Am-E-Z Ject | Can-Am Care | U-100 | 27-gauge | 1/2″ | 100 (individually wrapped) |
| Can-Am E-Z-Ject | Can-Am Care | U-100 | 28-gauge | 1/2″ | 100 (individually wrapped) |
| Monoject Ultra Comfort 28 | Kendall-Futuro | U-100 | 28-gauge | 1/2″ | 100 (individually wrapped) |
| Monoject Ultra Comfort 29 | Kendall-Futuro | U-100 | 29-gauge | 1/2″ | 100 (individually wrapped) |
| Pharma-Plast | Pharma-Plast USA | U-100 | 28-gauge | 1/2″ | 100 (10 packs of 10) |
| Pharma-Plast | Pharma-Plast USA | U-100 | 29-gauge | 1/2″ | 100 (10 packs of 10) |
| Terumo | Terumo Medical | U-100 | 27-gauge | 1/2″ | 100 (individually wrapped) |
| Terumo | Terumo Medical | U-100 | 29-gauge | 1/2″ | 100 (individually wrapped) |
| ***1/4-cc Syringes*** | | | | | |
| Terumo | Terumo Medical | U-100 | 29-gauge | 1/2″ | 100 (individually wrapped) |
| ***1/2-cc Syringes*** | | | | | |
| B-D Micro-Fine IV | Becton Dickinson | U-100 | 28-gauge | 1/2″ | 100 (10 packs of 10) |
| B-D Ultra-Fine | Becton Dickinson | U-100 | 29-gauge | 1/2″ | 100 (10 packs of 10) |
| Can-Am E-Z-Ject | Can-Am Care | U-50 | 28-gauge | 1/2″ | 100 (individually wrapped) |
| Monoject Ultra Comfort 28 | Kendall-Futuro | U-100 | 28-gauge | 1/2″ | 100 (individually wrapped) |
| Monoject Ultra Comfort 29 | Kendall-Futuro | U-100 | 29-gauge | 1/2″ | 100 (individually wrapped) |
| Pharma-Plast | Pharma-Plast USA | U-100 | 28-gauge | 1/2″ | 100 (10 packs of 10) |
| Pharma-Plast | Pharma-Plast USA | U-100 | 29-gauge | 1/2″ | 100 (10 packs of 10) |
| Terumo | Terumo Medical | U-100 | 27-gauge | 1/2″ | 100 (individually wrapped) |
| Terumo | Terumo Medical | U-100 | 29-gauge | 1/2″ | 100 (individually wrapped) |
| ***3/10-cc Syringes*** | | | | | |
| B-D Micro-Fine IV | Becton Dickinson | U-100 | 28-gauge | 1/2″ | 100 (10 packs of 10) |
| B-D Ultra-Fine | Becton Dickinson | U-100 | 29-gauge | 1/2″ | 100 (10 packs of 10) |
| Monoject Ultra Comfort 29 | Kendall-Futuro | U-100 | 29-gauge | 1/2″ | 30/100 (individually wrapped) |

able. Confusion can result if one does not realize that different companies have adopted different names for the same short-, intermediate-, and long-acting forms of insulin or their mixture (Table 1).

Insulin is commercially available in concentrations of 40, 100, and 500 U/ml (designated U-40, U-100, and U-500). One unit of insulin equals approximately 36 $\mu$g of insulin. U-40 insulin is favored by some veterinarians for use in diabetic dogs and cats, because a small dose can be more easily measured than with U-100 insulin. However, in the United States, U-100 insulin has replaced U-40 insulin as the most commonly used in human patients. In the United States, the only U-40 insulins available are NPH and PZI, manufactured by Anpro Pharm (Table 1). In addition, U-40 insulin is still widely available in other parts of the world, including Europe and Latin America. The U-500 concentration, the only insulin that requires a prescription, is indicated only in rare cases of insulin resistance when an insulin dosage of hundreds of units per day is required.

Whatever insulin preparation is used, it is critical that owners purchase the correct syringe to match the concentration of insulin to be administered. In other words, one must use U-40 syringes with U-40 insulin, and U-100 syringes with U-100 insulin. If U-100 insulin is inadvertently drawn with a U-40 syringe, the dose would be more than twice what it should be. Until recently, this was not a major problem in the United States because only U-100 insulin was available; how-ever, because of the recent availability of U-40 NPH and PZI insulins, U-40 insulin syringes must again be used for those insulins.

Over the past few years, a variety of improvements in insulin syringe and needle technology have been made. For example, insulin syringes have become smaller, and the needles have sharper points (i.e., ultrafine needles) and special coatings that work to make injections less painful. As before, the syringes are marked in insulin units, but there may be some differences in the way units are indicated, depending on the size of the syringe and the manufacturer. Hard-to-read syringes may be a problem for visually impaired owners; syringe attachments that magnify the number and unit markers are also available for these owners.

In general, there are four different insulin syringes available (Table 2). U-100 insulin syringes are manufactured with a 0.3-, 0.5-, and 1-ml capacity, whereas only one U-40 insulin syringe is available with a 1-ml capacity and a 26- or 27-gauge needle (Anpro Pharm; Table 2). The smaller sized U-100 syringes are designed for patients that require a smaller dosage of U-100 insulin. For example, the 0.3-ml syringes are designed for patients that require less than 30 U of insulin per injection. These syringes make it easy to accurately draw up a small dosage of U-100 insulin without the need for dilution of the insulin preparation. In dogs and cats that require very small dosages of insulin, the U-100 insulin preparations can be diluted with the appropriate pH-adjusted diluent specific for the individual insulin obtained from the manufacturer (free of charge).° A recent study reported that administration of less than 2.0 U of undiluted U-100 insulin to children with diabetes commonly resulted in marked overdosage (up to 95%); therefore, these investigators recommended that U-100 insulin be diluted if the prescribed dose is less than 2.0 U (Casella et al., 1993). Special care must be taken to ensure that the correct dose of the diluted insulin is administered with an ordinary insulin syringe. For example, if a 1:10 dilution of insulin is prepared, a full 1-ml, U-100 insulin syringe will hold only 10 U, a full 0.5-ml syringe will hold only 5 U, and a full 0.3-ml syringe will hold only 3 U.

Of the more recently developed insulin injection devices, pen injectors and jet injectors have achieved some popularity, especially in Europe. The pen injectors have been used with some success in dogs. These pen-sized syringes house a cartridge containing 1 to 2 ml of insulin. After setting the dose by a dial, the needle is inserted in the skin, and a plunger delivers the dose. Insulin cartridges come in limited total capacities of regular (Novolin R Penfill), NPH (Novolin N Penfill), and premixed 70/30 insulins (Novolin 70/30 Penfill, Table 1). Theoretically, pen injectors should increase both accuracy and convenience, but one major disadvantage of these pen injectors is that dose adjustments can only be made in 1- and 2-U dose modifications.

Jet injectors deliver insulin transcutaneously by an air-jet mechanism rather than by a needle. These devices release a tiny jet stream of insulin, forcing the insulin through the skin with pressure. Although these jet injectors may work satisfactorily for some pet owners, a major disadvantage of these devices is their expense (>$1000). In addition, these devices are somewhat cumbersome and often traumatize the skin; therefore, many human diabetic patients find use of jet injectors to be no less uncomfortable than standard injections.

---

°To obtain approprate diluent for Lilly insulins, the veterinarian should call the manufacturer directly at (317) 276-1610. To obtain appropriate diluent for Novo Nordisk insulins, call the manufacturer directly at (609) 987-5837.

## References and Suggested Reading

Casella, SJ, Mongilio MK, Plotnick LP, et al: Accuracy and precision of low-dose insulin administration. Pediatrics 91:1155, 1993.
*Insulin injections of less than 2.0 U of U-100 insulin have an unacceptable large dosing error, and insulin should be diluted if the prescribed dose is less than 2.9 U.*
Hallden G, Gafvelin G, Mutt V, et al: Characterization of cat insulin. Arch Biochem Biophysics 247:20, 1986.
*Description of the isolation and characterization of the insulin amino acid structure in cats.*
Neubauer H and Schone H: The immunogenicity of different insulins in several animal species. Diabetes 27:8, 1978.
*Because the insulins of dogs and pigs have identical amino acid sequences, no antigenicity of porcine insulin in dogs could be observed.*
Position Statement of the American Diabetes Association. Insulin administration. Diabetes Care 16:31, 1993.
*Reviews the current recommendations of the American Diabetes Association concerning use of insulin and insulin syringes.*
Saudek CD: Future developments in insulin delivery systems. Diabetes Care 16 (suppl 3):122, 1993.
*A review of the insulin injection devises, including pen injectors and jet injectors, in human patients.*
Schernthaner G: Immunogenicity and allergenic potential of animal and human insulins. Diabetes Care 16 (suppl 3):155, 1993.
*A review of the immunologic complications of insulin therapy in human patients.*
Smith L: Amino acid sequences of insulins. Diabetes 21 (suppl 2):457, 1972.
*A review of the amino acid sequence of insulin in a variety of species, including the human, pig, cattle, and dog.*

---

# INSULIN RESISTANCE IN DIABETIC DOGS AND CATS

RICHARD W. NELSON

*Davis, California*

## DEFINITION AND ETIOLOGY

Insulin resistance is a condition in which a normal amount of insulin produces a subnormal biologic response. There is no insulin dose that clearly defines insulin resistance. When assessing insulin effectiveness in a diabetic dog or cat, the insulin dose relative to body weight and adequacy of glycemic control should be evaluated simultaneously. For most diabetic dogs, good glycemic control (i.e., blood glucose concentra-tion between 100 and 250 mg/dl) can be achieved with less than 1.0 U of intermediate- or long-acting insulin per kilogram of body weight given once or twice daily. For most diabetic cats, adequate glycemic control can be achieved with 5 U or less of long-acting insulin per cat given once or twice daily. Insulin resistance is suspected if the insulin dosage is above 1.5 U/kg per injection (dog) or more than 6 U per injection (cat) and all blood glucose concentrations are greater than 300 mg/dl. Insulin resistance is also suspected when excessive amounts of insulin (i.e., insulin dosage >2.2 U/kg) are necessary to maintain the blood glucose concentration below 300 mg/dl.

Insulin resistance may result from problems occurring before the interaction of insulin with its receptor (i.e., prereceptor), at the receptor, or at steps distal to the interaction of insulin and its receptor (i.e., postreceptor) (Ihle and Nelson, 1991). Prereceptor problems reduce free metabolically active insulin concentration and include increased insulin degradation and insulin-binding antibodies. Receptor problems include alterations in insulin-receptor–binding affinity and concentration and insulin-receptor antibodies. Postreceptor problems are difficult to differentiate clinically from receptor problems and both often coexist. In dogs and cats, receptor and postreceptor abnormalities are usually attributable to obesity or a disorder causing excessive secretion of a diabetogenic hormone; that is, cortisol, glucagon, epinephrine, and growth hormone. An excess or deficiency of thyroid hormone may also result in resistance (Ford et al., 1993).

## DIAGNOSTIC EVALUATION

Whenever insulin resistance is suspected, problems with insulin activity or administration technique should be ruled out before a diagnostic evaluation for insulin resistance is undertaken. Failure to administer an appropriate dosage of biologically active insulin can mimic insulin resistance because of unrecognized insulin underdosage. Insulin underdosage can result from administration of biologically inactive insulin (e.g., outdated, overheated, mixed by shaking), administration of diluted insulin, use of inappropriate insulin syringes for the concentration of insulin (e.g., U-100 syringe with U-40 insulin), or problems with insulin administration technique (e.g., misunderstanding on how to read the insulin syringe, inappropriate injection technique). The easiest way to identify these types of problems is to administer new, undiluted insulin by the clinician and measure several blood glucose concentrations throughout the day. If an insulin-resistant type of serial blood glucose curve persists, a diagnostic evaluation to identify the cause of insulin resistance may be warranted.

There are two avenues to pursue during the diagnostic evaluation of insulin resistance. Both can be pursued at the same time, if necessary. One avenue is designed to rule out problems created by insulin therapy itself, and the other avenue is designed to rule out concurrent diseases that are interfering with insulin action (Table 1). Obtaining a complete history and performing a thorough physical examination is the first and perhaps most important step in determining which avenue to pursue.

## Changes in Insulin Therapy

There are several changes in insulin therapy that can be tried to improve insulin effectiveness. Diluted insulin should be replaced with full-strength insulin. In some dogs and cats, insufficient amounts of insulin may be administered when diluted insulin is used, despite appropriate dilution and insulin administration techniques; inadequacies which are corrected when full-strength insulin is used. Small insulin syringes (U-100, 0.3-ml) can be used with full-strength U-100 insulin for cats and small dogs receiving small amounts of insulin (see elsewhere in this section).

Secretion of diabetogenic hormones during the Somogyi phenomenon may induce insulin resistance, which we believe can last 24 to 72 hr following the hypoglycemic episode (Feldman and Nelson, 1982). If serial blood glucose concentrations are evaluated on the day of the hypoglycemia, the Somogyi phenomenon will be identified and the insulin dosage lowered accordingly. However, if the blood glucose is monitored after secretion of the diabetogenic hormones, insulin resistance will be diagnosed and the insulin dosage may be increased, further exacerbating the Somogyi phe-

**Table 1.** *Recognized Causes of Insulin Ineffectiveness or Insulin Resistance in the Diabetic Dog and Cat*

| Caused by Insulin Therapy | Caused by Concurrent Disorder |
| --- | --- |
| Inactive insulin | Diabetogenic drugs |
| Diluted insulin | Hyperadrenocorticism |
| Improper administration technique | Diestrus (bitch) |
| Inadequate dose | Acromegaly (cat) |
| Somogyi phenomenon | Infection, especially oral cavity and urinary tract |
| Inadequate frequency of insulin administration | Hypothyroidism (dog) |
| Impaired insulin absorption, especially Ultralente insulin | Hyperthyroidism (cat) |
| Anti-insulin antibody excess | Renal insufficiency |
| | Liver insufficiency |
| | Cardiac insufficiency |
| | Chronic pancreatitis |
| | Exocrine pancreatic insufficiency |
| | Glucagonoma (dog) |
| | Hyperlipidemia (?) |
| | Pheochromocytoma (?) |

nomenon. Reducing the insulin dose and evaluating the patient's response over the ensuing 2 to 5 days can be done to rule out insulin resistance associated with the Somogyi phenomenon. If clinical signs of diabetes worsen following a reduction in the insulin dose, another cause for the insulin resistance should be pursued. However, if the owner reports no change or improvement, continued gradual reduction of the insulin dosage should be pursued.

Administration of insulin under the skin does not necessarily guarantee that the insulin will be absorbed into the circulation for subsequent interaction with insulin receptors. Slow or impaired absorption of subcutaneously deposited insulin is most commonly observed in diabetic cats receiving Ultralente insulin. Changing the type of insulin may be beneficial in the patient with poor subcutaneous absorption of insulin. When changing type of insulin, a more potent insulin should be substituted for the previous insulin. Market insulins, listed in order of increasing potency, are Ultralente, Lente, neutral protamine Hagedorn (NPH), 70% NPH/30% regular and then regular crystalline insulin. Inadequate insulin potency is particularly common in cats on Ultralente insulin. We have had success in these cats by switching from Ultralente to Lente or NPH insulin given twice a day (Bertoy, Nelson, and Feldman, in press).

Excessive insulin-binding antibodies may develop in some diabetic dogs and cats receiving beef/pork insulin. Dog insulin is similar to human and pig insulin, while cat insulin is similar to cow insulin (Hallden et al., 1986). Purified pork insulin and presumably recombinant human insulin are relatively nonantigenic following chronic administration in the dog, while beef/pork insulin is antigenic because of the beef component (Feldman, Nelson, and Karam, 1983). Similar studies have not been reported in the cat. Presumably, purified beef insulin is relatively nonantigenic in the cat, while purified pork insulin and recombinant human insulin are antigenic.

Changing species of insulin may be beneficial when excessive insulin-binding antibodies are suspected. Unfortunately, a commercial assay for measurement of insulin-binding antibodies is not available for the dog and cat. However, circulating insulin antibodies may interfere with some radioimmunoassay (RIA) techniques used to measure serum insulin concentration in a manner similar to the effects of thyroid hormone antibodies on RIA techniques for serum thyroid hormone concentrations. This interference can be used to raise the clinician's index of suspicion for insulin-binding antibodies as a cause for insulin resistance in a diabetic dog or cat. A single-phase separation system utilizing antibody-coated tubes is used in our laboratory to measure serum insulin concentration. The presence of insulin antibodies in the serum sample will cause spuriously high insulin values using this RIA. Serum insulin concentration is less than 50 µU/ml (<360 pmol/L) 24 hr after the previous insulin injection in the diabetic dog and cat without antibodies causing interference with the RIA. In contrast, serum insulin concentration is typically greater than 400 µU/ml (>2800 pmol/L) and may be greater than 1000 µU/ml (>7000 pmol/L) 24 hr after the previous insulin administration when insulin antibodies that interfere with the RIA are present in the serum sample. When insulin resistance due to insulin-binding antibodies is suspected, a switch to recombinant human insulin (i.e., Humulin, Eli Lilly) should be tried for the dog and either human insulin or beef insulin (Novo Nordisk) should be tried for the cat. In our experience, glycemic control is usually improved within 2 weeks of changing the species of insulin when insulin-binding antibodies are the cause of the insulin resistance.

## Pursuing Concurrent Disorders

There are many disorders that can interfere with insulin therapy (Table 1). Obtaining a complete history and performing a thorough physical examination is the most important step in identifying these concurrent disorders. Is the patient taking any medications that may have insulin-antagonistic properties? Has the female diabetic dog been spayed, and if not, when was the last estrus observed? Has the owner noticed any clinical signs that may suggest concurrent infection (e.g., hematuria, vaginal discharge)? Abnormalities identified on a thorough physical examination may suggest a concurrent insulin-antagonistic disorder or infectious process, which will give the clinician direction in the diagnostic evaluation of the patient.

If the history and physical examination are unremarkable, a complete blood count (CBC), serum biochemical analysis, serum thyroxine concentration, adrenocorticotrophic hormone (ACTH) stimulation test, and urinalysis with bacterial culture should be done to further screen for concurrent illness. If insulin resistance is identified in an intact bitch, diestrus should always be suspected regardless of the history. A serum progesterone concentration can be obtained to document the presence of functional corpora lutea. For most commercial endocrine laboratories, a serum progesterone concentration greater than 2 ng/ml (>6 nmol/L) is consistent with diestrus.

Hyperadrenocorticism should always be considered in the diabetic dog with insulin resistance. Many of these dogs have mild or no dermatologic alterations consistent with hyperadrenocorticism. In addition, the polyuria, polydipsia, hepatomegaly, and hepatic enzyme alterations are often ascribed to the poorly controlled diabetic state. Because of the high incidence of iatrogenic hyperadrenocorticism, the ACTH stimulation test is perhaps the best initial diagnostic test for hyperadrenocorticism in the diabetic dog and cat. When interpreting the ACTH stimulation test, the influence of poorly regulated diabetes mellitus on adrenocortical function and subsequent results of the test should be considered. A mildly exaggerated adrenocortical response to ACTH may be seen in some diabetic dogs and cats with insulin resistance, yet the pituitary and adrenal glands are histologically normal. Presumably, the chronic "stress" related to poorly regulated diabetes mellitus is responsible for these results. For these patients, the diagnosis of hyperadrenocorticism should also be based on clinical pathologic abnormalities, results of additional pituitary-adrenal function tests, abdominal ultrasonography, and clinical suspicion for the disorder.

Abdominal and thoracic radiographs, abdominal ultrasonography, an electrocardiogram, and serum trypsin-like immunoreactivity should be evaluated if prior diagnostics have failed to identify a cause for insulin resistance. Special attention should be paid to the pancreas and adrenal glands when performing abdominal ultrasonography. Diabetic dogs and cats with exocrine pancreatic insufficiency are difficult to regulate with insulin; have persistent weight loss despite polyphagia, ultimately becoming emaciated; and typically have large quantities of stools that may be normal or soft, not the voluminous, rancid stools considered classic for exocrine pancreatic insufficiency.

Acromegaly is still possible in the cat when diagnostic tests and alterations in insulin therapy have failed to identify a cause for insulin resistance. Acromegaly in the cat is characterized by insulin-resistant diabetes mellitus and slowly progressive organomegaly (Peterson et al., 1990). Acromegaly should be considered in the cat with poorly controlled diabetes mellitus and weight gain rather than weight loss. Historically, the diagnosis was established by documenting increased baseline plasma growth hormone concentration. Unfortunately, measurement of growth hormone concentration in the cat is no longer commercially available. An alternative approach is to identify a pituitary mass using contrast-enhanced computed tomography or magnetic resonance imaging. This finding would support acromegaly in the cat with normal pituitary-adrenocortical axis test results.

The role of insulin receptor and postreceptor defects has yet to be documented in dogs and cats. Problems in this area should be suspected when all other causes of insulin resistance have been ruled out, insulin absorption following subcutaneous administration has been documented, and there has been minimal improvement in glycemic control with the use of less antigenic insulin preparations. Therapy is frustrating and usually involves the progressive increase in the insulin dosage to obtain some semblance of glycemic control.

## References and Suggested Reading

Bertoy EH, Nelson RW, and Feldman EC: Effect of Lente insulin for treatment of diabetes mellitus in cats. J Am Vet Med Assoc (in press).
*Study that evaluated the effectiveness of Lente insulin in a group of diabetic cats.*

Feldman EC and Nelson RW: Insulin-induced hyperglycemia in diabetic dogs. J Am Vet Med Assoc 180:1432, 1982.
*Retrospective study describing the Somogyi phenomenon in a group of diabetic dogs.*

Feldman EC, Nelson RW, and Karam JH: Reduced immunogenicity of pork insulin in dogs with spontaneous insulin-dependent diabetes mellitus. Diabetes 32:153A, 1983.
*Synopsis of prospective study evaluating antigenicity of beef and pork insulin in diabetic dogs.*

Ford SL, Nelson RW, Feldman EC, et al: Insulin resistance in three dogs with hypothyroidism and diabetes mellitus. J Am Vet Med Assoc 202:1478, 1993.
*Retrospective study describing insulin resistance in three diabetic dogs with hypothyroidism and resolution of resistance after initiation of thyroid hormone supplementation.*

Hallden G, Gafvelin G, Mutt V, et al: Characterization of cat insulin. Arch Biochem Biophys 247:20, 1986.
*Study describing the amino acid sequence of the insulin molecule in the cat.*

Ihle SL and Nelson RW: Insulin resistance and diabetes mellitus. Compend Cont Educ 13:197, 1991.
*Review of causes and diagnostic approach to insulin resistance in the diabetic dog and cat.*

Peterson ME, Taylor RS, Greco DS, et al: Acromegaly in 14 cats. J Vet Intern Med 4:192, 1990.
*Retrospective study describing the clinical aspects of acromegaly in 14 cats.*

# INSULIN TREATMENT OF DIABETES MELLITUS IN THE DOG AND CAT

JOHN D. BROUSSARD

*Columbus, Ohio*

*and* MELISSA S. WALLACE

*New York, New York*

Diabetes mellitus is a heterogeneous group of disorders in which insulin production is deficient or the action of insulin on peripheral tissues is impaired. Depending on the metabolic manifestations of the disease process, diabetes mellitus may be mild and chronic, or acutely life threatening.

In order to better understand and treat the different forms of this disease in dogs and cats, diabetes mellitus may be roughly classified into two main categories similar to those used in human medicine. Insulin-dependent diabetes mellitus (IDDM), or type I, is the most common clinically recognized form in dogs and cats. It is characterized by low to absent endogenous serum insulin concentrations and by lack of β-cell response to the administration of insulin secretogogues. The pathogenesis of IDDM, which ultimately leads to β-cell injury and death, is poorly understood and is undoubtedly multifactorial. Genetic susceptibility plus acquired environmental factors such as infection, autoimmune disease, or pancreatitis appear necessary. In cases of IDDM, loss of β-cell function is irreversible, and lifelong insulin therapy is usually necessary to maintain glycemic control and prevent ketoacidosis.

Non–insulin-dependent diabetes mellitus (NIDDM), or type II diabetes, is characterized by hyperglycemia despite the ability to secrete insulin. The patient suffers from a relative deficiency of insulin, usually due to a combination of insufficient or delayed secretion and peripheral resistance to the action of insulin. In people and animals, factors that are known to promote insulin resistance include obesity, diseases such as infections or endocrinopathies, and certain drugs (see "Insulin Resistance in Dogs and Cats," this volume, p 390). Animals with NIDDM sometimes require less insulin than IDDM patients, and some may be managed successfully without insulin, using dietary therapy or oral hypoglycemic agents (see "Treatment of Feline Diabetes Mellitus with the Oral Sulfonyurea, Glipizide," this volume, p 401).

While two distinct disease processes seem to exist in human medicine, differentiation of IDDM and NIDDM in dogs and cats is sometimes difficult. Measurement of basal and stimulated serum insulin concentrations will usually help classify the type, but are not reliable in all cases (Kirk, Feldman, and Nelson, 1993). In cats, NIDDM and IDDM appear to be part of a continuum of disease in which insulin resistance ultimately can lead to loss of β-cell function. Compared with dogs, cats have a much higher incidence of NIDDM and transient diabetes. They also more commonly respond to treatment without the use of exogenous insulin. In general, animals who develop ketoacidosis have moderate to severe deficiency of insulin and can, for practical purposes, be classified as having IDDM. Conversely, lack of development of ketoacidosis in a chronic diabetic dog or cat that is not treated with exogenous insulin implies some level of β-cell function and a diagnosis of NIDDM (Peterson, Randolph, and Mooney, 1994).

For the clinical management of dogs and cats with diabetes mellitus, it is helpful to distinguish the uncomplicated (i.e., simple) from the complicated diabetic patient. Animals with uncomplicated diabetes mellitus can be managed as outpatients or nonintensive-care inpatients. Pets with complicated diabetes mellitus require hospitalization with an intensive-care level of management. For the purposes of this discussion, the uncomplicated diabetic is defined as an animal that has early symptoms of insulin deficiency manifested as polyuria, polydipsia, polyphagia, and weight loss, but is otherwise normal. In other words, this is a diabetic who is still compensating for the disease. The complicated diabetic is defined as the animal that has developed serious sequelae of insulin deficiency, such as dehydration, ketoacidosis, mental depression, anorexia, and vomiting. If critical care is not available, it may be best for the veterinarian to refer these cases, if possible. Ketoacidotic diabetes mellitus is responsible for the majority of complicated cases, but nonketoacidotic hyperosmolar diabetes mellitus is occasionally recognized. Other illnesses that complicate a diabetic case include hepatic lipidosis, cholangiohepatitis, pancreatitis, pyelonephritis, and hyperadrenocorticism (see "Complications and Concurrent Disease Associated with Diabetic Ketoacidosis and Other Severe Forms of Diabetes Mellitus," this volume, p 384).

## INSULIN THERAPY OF COMPLICATED DIABETES MELLITUS

Therapy of complicated diabetes mellitus requires management of fluid balance, electrolyte balance, acid-base disturbances, and control of blood glucose. The control of hyperglycemia is the least important aspect of initial therapy. Prior to the administration of insulin, fluid deficits and electrolyte abnormalities must be addressed. A thorough review of these aspects of treatment are beyond the scope of this article, but may be found elsewhere (see *CVT XI*, p 359). The focus of this section will be protocols for insulin therapy in the sick diabetic patient.

Diabetic dogs and cats suffering from dehydration, anorexia, ketoacidosis, vomiting, or other complications should be treated with a short-acting insulin such as regular crystalline insulin. Regular insulin may be given by any parenteral route. The advantages of short-acting insulin are rapid onset, and short, reliable duration, allowing frequent dosage adjustments based on the blood glucose concentration of the animal. Blood glucose measurements can be performed with glucose reagent strips or a glucose meter. There are three general protocols for the initial therapy of the complicated diabetic dog or cat: low-dose constant-rate intravenous infusion, hourly intramuscular injections, and subcutaneous injections every 6 hr. There are inherent advantages and disadvantages of each approach.

The most common protocol used for humans with diabetic ketoacidosis is a low-dose constant-rate intravenous insulin infusion. This provides a steady-state concentration of insulin to inhibit ketogenesis and glycogenolysis. The result is a gradual lowering of blood glucose and reduction of ketones as they are metabolized. The major disadvantages are that this protocol requires frequent monitoring of blood glucose and will occasionally result in hypoglycemia. Whether hypophosphatemia and hypokalemia are more common with this protocol is unknown, but is a potential concern. In dogs, a safe and reliable protocol is to administer 2.2 U/kg/day of regular insulin diluted in 0.9% saline or lactated Ringer's solution and given via infusion pump at a constant rate (Macintire, 1993). A suggested dose for cats is 1.1 U/kg/day (Diehl and Wheeler, 1991). Because insulin adheres to glass and plastics, 50 ml of an insulin-saline mixture should be flushed through the infusion set prior to administering it to the pet. The blood glucose should be monitored hourly or every 2 hr. When the blood glucose reaches 250 mg/dl (13.9 mmol/L), the insulin infusion may be reduced by 25 to 50%, and enough 50% dextrose is added to the intravenous fluids to make a 2.5 to 5% solution to prevent hypoglycemia (Macintire, 1993). Serum electrolytes and acid-base balance should be monitored every 6 hr, if possible, until the patient is stable. Once ketosis is resolved and the animal is eating, a longer acting subcutaneous insulin protocol may be initiated.

Another popular initial protocol for complicated diabetic animals is hourly intramuscular injections of regular insulin. Similar to the intravenous infusion, the goal is to provide insulin in the circulation at all times to reverse ketogenesis and hyperglycemia. This protocol requires hourly injections and blood glucose measurements. The dose is 0.2 U/kg initially, followed by 0.1 U/kg hourly until the blood glucose is 250 mg/dl (13.9 mmol/L). The insulin injections are then reduced to every 4 to 6 hr, given subcutaneously if the animal is hydrated or intramuscularly if dehydration is still present. At this time dextrose (50%) is added to the intravenous fluids to make a 5% solution to maintain the blood glucose in the 200- to 300-mg/dl range. Once the pet is nonketoacidotic, eating, and maintaining normal hydration, a longer acting insulin can be initiated, as for an uncomplicated diabetic animal.

A protocol that is practical, safe, and reliable is the use of regular insulin subcutaneously every 4 to 6 hr. Regular insulin is normally rapidly absorbed and has a duration of 4 to 6 hr after subcutaneous administration. Because dehydration may delay insulin absorption, the initial two or three dosages may be administered intramuscularly to avoid accumulation of subcutaneous insulin with later absorption and overdosage. The starting dose is 0.25 U/kg, and the initial dose is considered a test dose. The blood glucose is reassessed 4 to 6 hr later, and the next dose is selected based on both the absolute value and the incremental decrease in blood glucose obtained since the prior dose. The goal is to provide enough insulin to gradually lower the blood glucose by approximately 50 to 70 mg/dl/hr (2.8 to 3.9 mmol/L/hr). For example, if the initial insulin dose and fluid therapy lowered the patient's blood glucose from 800 to 500 mg/dl (44.4 to 27.8 mmol/L), the second dose should be the same as the first to continue lowering the blood glucose at a reasonable rate. However, if the second blood glucose concentration was 300 mg/dl (16.7 mmol/L), the next insulin dose should be lowered by at least half, so as not to cause hypoglycemia. If the second blood glucose concentration was 700 mg/dl (38.9 mmol/L), then the insulin dose could be safely increased by 50 to 100%. Once the patient's general response to insulin and fluid therapy is known, a chart for that patient can be provided for the veterinary technician to establish subsequent insulin dosages based on blood glucose levels. The chart specifies decreasing insulin dosages with decreasing blood glucose measurements (Table 1). The chart will be different for each

**Table 1.** Dose Adjustment Chart for Subcutaneous Regular Insulin Administration in the Ketoacidotic Diabetic Dog or Cat*

| Blood Glucose (μg/dl) | Dose of Regular Insulin | | Fluids to Administer |
|---|---|---|---|
| | 5-kg B.W. | 20-kg B.W. | |
| >800 | 1.5 U | 7 U. | LRS |
| 401–800 | 1 U | 5 U | LRS |
| 241–400 | 0.5 U | 3 U | LRS |
| 181–240 | 0.5 U | 3 U | LRS/2.5% dextrose |
| 121–180 | 0.5 U | 2 U | LRS/2.5% dextrose |
| 81–120 | 0 U | 1 U | LRS/2.5% dextrose |

*Example of a chart for the veterinary technician prescribing the type of fluid therapy and dosage of subcutaneous regular insulin to be administered every 6 hr to a 5-kg or 20-kg cat or dog. Adjustment are made to the chart if the patient does not have a gradual lowering of blood glucose followed by a steady maintenance of blood glucose concentration between 180 and 300 mg/dl.
Abbreviations; LRS = lactated Ringer's solution, B.W. = body weight.

pet, based on body size and sensitivity to insulin. Similar to the other protocols, 50% dextrose is added to the intravenous fluids to make a 2.5 to 5% solution once the glucose reaches 180 to 250 mg/dl (10 to 13.9 mmol/L). This allows insulin therapy to be continued so as to reverse ketogenesis. When the patient is eating and drinking well and is no longer ketoacidotic, a longer acting insulin may be instituted. This protocol rarely induces hypoglycemia in our experience and is effective at lowering blood glucose and reversing ketogenesis. Because infusion pumps are not strictly required and because monitoring can be less intense, this protocol is less expensive for the veterinarian and the client.

All three protocols described above are effective. The correct protocol will vary with the practice type, level of veterinary technician care available, the practitioner, and perhaps the patient. Regardless of the insulin protocol used, good clinical judgment, strict attention to detail, and careful patient monitoring are required to successfully manage the complicated diabetic patient.

## INSULIN THERAPY IN THE UNCOMPLICATED DIABETIC

The uncomplicated diabetic patient generally shows the classic signs of polyuria, polydipsia, polyphagia, and poor condition without concurrent electrolyte imbalances, ketoacidosis, renal failure, or gastrointestinal compromise. These patients generally require little or no supportive care and may safely begin insulin therapy at home. As maintenance insulin requirements are greatly effected by diet, activity level, and stress, home is the ideal environment to establish a therapeutic regime.

## Diet Therapy

Nutritional management is an important factor in the treatment of all diabetic patients. In some cases, particularly obese cats, it may be the most important part of therapy. Several factors must be considered when formulating a diet plan. The timing and caloric content of meals should be formulated to maintain consistency and avoid postprandial hyperglycemia. In terms of timing, caloric intake should occur when insulin is still present in the circulation and capable of promoting glucose metabolism. For animals on twice-daily therapy, this often means that two meals a day are optimal. Animals on once-daily therapy may benefit by being allowed to eat multiple meals throughout the day. In terms of dietary content, diets high in complex carbohydrates and soluble fiber tend to slow glucose absorption. Semimoist foods should be avoided because they contain disaccharides and propylene glycol and promote hyperglycemia.

Abnormalities of body condition should be addressed when formulating a diet plan. Thin patients should gain weight and obese patients should reduce. Weight reduction in obese patients requires careful reduction of caloric intake. In general, reduction of intake to 60 to 70% of caloric requirements for ideal body weight will facilitate weight reduction. Weight loss in excess of 3% of body weight per week is considered dangerous, particularly in cats. Diets high in fiber are particularly useful in obese diabetic patients, as they promote weight loss and slow glucose absorption. However, high-fiber diets are contraindicated in thin diabetic patients, because they cannot supply adequate nutrition for weight gain. In thin patients, high-calorie, dense, low-fiber diets are fed until optimum body weight is achieved (see CVT X, p 1008).

## Maintenance Insulin Therapy

Several insulin formulations are available for maintenance therapy in dogs and cats. In these preparations, substances such as protamine and zinc are bound to insulin molecules to slow the subcutaneous absorption and prolong the duration of effect. In general, these augmented insulin preparations are classified as intermediate acting (e.g., neutral protamine Hagedorn [NPH], Lente), or long acting (e.g., protamine zinc insulin [PZI], Ultralente), based on human pharmacokinetic properties. The species of origin of insulin used in these preparations may be beef, pork, a combination of both, or synthetically produced human insulin (see "CVT Update: Insulin and Insulin Syringes," this volume, p 387).

Several factors must be considered when choosing the insulin regimen for maintenance therapy. One must designate the frequency of administration, insulin preparation, species of origin, and a starting dose. Ideal therapy for each animal will be different based on the special needs of the patient and the owner.

The frequency of administration is often a compromise between the needs of the patient and the limitations of the owner's schedule. Intermediate-acting insulins are generally administered twice daily in cats and dogs. Long-acting insulins are initially given once daily, but twice-daily administration may sometimes be needed. As there can be marked variability between the response to long-acting insulins, the ultimate frequency of administration must be based on the individual animal's response.

The goal for frequency of administration will help determine the insulin preparation used. We recommend the use of intermediate-acting insulins administered twice daily for initial therapy when possible (especially in dogs). In our clinical experience and based on pharmacokinetic studies in dogs and cats, the response of patients to intermediate-acting insulins is more predictable than that of long-acting insulins. The inconvenience of twice-daily therapy is often justified by the considerable decrease in incidence of treatment failure.

The choice of species of origin for insulin therapy is primarily based on commercial availability, and in some cases based on antigenicity and bioavailability (i.e., the percentage absorbed). The commercial availability of insulin products is ultimately controlled by trends in human diabetes therapy. Some insulin formulations, such as those containing insulin of beef/pork or pork origin, are currently unavailable in the United States (see "CVT Update: Insulin and Insulin Syringes," this volume, p 387). Therefore, we generally use insulins of human recombinant or beef origin at this time. The antigenicity and absorption of these insulins is known to differ (Broussard and Peterson, 1994). However, in most diabetic patients, these differences are not clinically significant. In general, the insulin species of origin used in a given patient should remain constant, and one should proceed with caution when changing the species of origin.

The initial dose of insulin used for maintenance therapy should attempt only to supply insulin at physiologic levels without risking hypoglycemia. The dose may then be increased as needed based on the individual patient's response. In the cat, we begin with a dose of 0.2 to 0.5 U/kg. Our initial insulin dose in dogs is 0.4 to 0.7 U/kg. Large dogs tend to be dosed at the low end of the range. As intermediate-acting insulins tend to be more bioavailable and clinically more potent, they are dosed at the low end of the range. Starting doses for long-acting insulins tend to be higher (Wallace, Peterson, and Nichols, 1990; Wallace and Kirk, 1990).

In cases that have been stabilized on subcutaneously administered short-acting insulin, the initial insulin requirements may help determine the initial maintenance insulin dose. On a per-unit basis, intermediate- and long-acting insulins tend to be less bioavailable and, therefore, less potent. Generally, one may safely begin maintenance insulin therapy at a dose that is comparable to the established short-acting insulin requirements. In most cases, this will provide a smooth transition to maintenance therapy without risking insulin overdose (Wallace and Kirk, 1990).

## Monitoring and Initial Dose Adjustments

Client education is the most important step in preparing a diabetic patient for maintenance insulin therapy. Initial instructions must go beyond technical training in subcutaneous injection. The client should understand the terminology used to describe the preparation, concentration, and species of origin of the insulin used. The handling of insulin to include proper storage and mixing should be explained. The relationship between syringe calibration and insulin concentration, as well as the technique for measuring doses, must be understood. Also, the client should be taught how to use and interpret reagent strips for urine monitoring. Finally, the signs of hypoglycemia should be discussed with the owner and recommendations given for emergency treatment. As this large amount of information may be difficult for the owner to assimilate in a short time, it is often helpful to prepare written instructions to reinforce the major points.

Initial home monitoring of the diabetic patient will involve assessment of clinical response (lessening of polyuria, polydipsia, and changes in body condition) and evaluation of urinary glucose and ketone levels. The owner should measure urinary glucose and ketone levels once or twice daily, preferably prior to insulin administration. Ideally, low levels of glucosuria, 100 to 250 mg/dl (5.5 to 13.9 mmol/L), and no ketones should be detected. Consistently high urine glucose readings (>500 mg/dl or >28 mmol/L) indicate that the insulin dose may be inadequate. Consistently negative readings indicate that insulin doses are adequate or excessive. The insulin dose should be adjusted by 0.5- to 1-U increments every 3 to 4 days based on recurring effects. The initial dose adjustments are usually made based on consultation with the veterinarian over the phone.

Although monitoring urine for glucosuria and ketonuria is helpful in the initial regulation of the diabetic patients, the clinician and owner must not lose sight of the inherent limitations of these test results. This technique is sometimes misleading, as there are many reasons other than insulin underdosing that can cause marked morning glucosuria, such as rapid metabolism of insulin, or insulin overdose with rebound hyperglycemia. Also, urine glucose measurements cannot differentiate euglycemia from hypoglycemia, as both conditions are characterized by negative urine glucose readings (Wallace and Kirk, 1990).

## Serial Blood Glucose Determinations

After 1 to 2 weeks of treatment, the animal should return to the hospital for an evaluation of serial blood glucose concentrations. To adequately evaluate diabetic control, the onset, peak, and duration of current insulin therapy should be determined. This requires multiple blood glucose measurements over at least one dosing interval. The following protocol is recommended on the day of a serial blood glucose curve. In the morning, the owner should feed the patient and administer insulin as usual. As soon as possible, the patient is brought to the hospital for the first blood glucose determination (using blood glucose test reagent strips). Additional samples for blood glucose measurement should be collected at 2- to 3-hr intervals for at least 12 hr with twice-daily therapy and 24 hr with once-daily therapy. During the day, the patient's normal feeding schedule should be simulated if possible. Based on the results of these glucose determinations, adjustments in insulin dosage, frequency of administration, or formulation are made as necessary.

Interpretation of the serial blood glucose curve involves assessment of insulin effectiveness, the glucose nadir, and the duration of insulin effect. The ability of insulin to lower blood glucose concentrations determines its effectiveness. If the insulin is not effective in lowering the blood glucose concentration, inappropriate insulin administration technique, insulin underdosage, poor insulin absorption, or insulin resistance should be considered (see "Insulin Resistance in Dogs and Cats," this volume, p 390). The next parameter to assess is the lowest blood glucose level (i.e., the glucose nadir). The glucose nadir aids in the evaluation of the insulin dose. The glucose nadir should ideally fall between 80 and 125 mg/dl (4.4 and 7.0 mmol/L). If it falls below the ideal range, the insulin dosage should be decreased. This often requires beginning regulation again at a very conservative insulin dose. If the glucose nadir remains above the ideal range, an increased insulin dose is usually necessary. The duration of insulin effect is used to evaluate the frequency of administration and the insulin preparation. The duration of effect is essentially the part of the dosing interval during which the patient's blood glucose remains between 80 and 250 mg/dl (4.4 and 13.9 mmol/L). Ideally, glucose levels should remain within this range during 80 to 90% of the dosing interval. If the duration of effect is too short, increasing the frequency of insulin administration or changing to a longer acting insulin preparation may be necessary. Serial blood glucose curves should be repeated at 2- to 3-week intervals until satisfactory glycemic control is achieved.

The results of serial blood glucose curves can be adversely affected by stress and inappetence. The insulin antagonistic effects of stress hormones may give the false impression of insulin resistance. Decreased appetite in the hospital may cause underestimation of the insulin needs of a patient. These inherent problems with the test may be partially overcome by carefully managing the patient's in-hospital environment. When the results of serial glucose curves are inconsistent with one's clinical impression of regulation, these problems should be considered.

## Long-Term Monitoring

Once the animal is reasonably well controlled, subsequent rechecks every few months are recommended. These rechecks should consist of a history, physical examination, review of the urine glucose measurements and, in some cases, serial blood glucose evaluations. During long-term insulin treatment, owners should continue to monitor for recurrence of clinical signs, as well as monitor urine for glucose concentration and ketones at least once or twice a week. If the patient consistently has high levels of glucosuria, or if ketonuria is detected on more than 2 or 3 consecutive days, the patient should be brought to the hospital for reevaluation. If regulation of the patient's diabetic control is ever in question, evaluation of a serial blood glucose curve is recommended.

Other means of monitoring long-term glycemic control, commonly used in human patients with diabetes, include glycosylated hemoglobin and fructosamine determinations. The value of these assays is their ability to accurately reflect the average blood glucose concentration over the preceding few weeks. Results of these measurements would not replace the need for occasional serial blood glucose determinations, as they indicate failure of regulation without defining the problem. Both glycated hemoglobin and fructosamine have been measured in cats and dogs with diabetes, but with conflicting results. Additional studies need to be done before these determinations can be routinely recommended for use in cats and dogs (Peterson, Randolph, and Mooney, 1994) (see "Monitoring Long-Term Control in the Diabetic Patient," this volume, p 403).

## References and Suggested Reading

Broussard JD and Peterson ME: Comparison of two ultralente insulin preparations with protamine zinc insulin in clinically normal cats. Am J Vet Res 55:127, 1994.
*A comparison of the subcutaneous absorption of PZI and Ultralente insulins of beef/pork and human origin.*

Diehl KJ and Wheeler SL: Pathogenesis and management of diabetic ketoacidosis. *In* Kirk RW and Bonagura JD (eds): *Current Veterinary Therapy XI.* Philadelphia, WB Saunders Co, 1991, p 359.
*A review of the pathogenesis, diagnosis, and clinical management of diabetic ketoacidosis in dogs and cats.*

Kirk CA, Feldman EC, and Nelson RW: Diagnosis of naturally acquired type-I and type-II diabetes mellitus in cats. Am J Vet Res 54:463, 1993.
*A prospective study of serum insulin and glucose concentrations before and following stimulation with glucagon in obese, lean, and diabetic cats.*

Macintire DK: Treatment of diabetic ketoacidosis in dogs by continuous low dose intravenous infusion of insulin. J Am Vet Med Assoc 202:1266, 1993.
*Results of a prospective clinical trial using continuous low-dose intravenous insulin infusion protocol in 21 diabetic dogs.*

Nelson RW: Dietary therapy for canine diabetes mellitus. *In* Kirk RW (ed): *Current Veterinary Therapy X.* Philadelphia, WB Saunders Co, 1989, p 1008.
*A discussion of diet therapy as an adjunct to insulin therapy in the chronic management of diabetes mellitus in the dog.*

Peterson ME, Randolph JF, and Mooney CM: Endocrine diseases *In* Sherding RG (ed): *The Cat: Diagnosis and Clinical Management,* 2nd edition. New York, Churchill Livingstone, pp 1403–1506, 1994.
*Provides an in-depth review of the treatment methods for cats with complicated and uncomplicated diabetes.*

Wallace MS and Kirk CA: The diagnosis and treatment of insulin dependent and noninsulin-dependent diabetes mellitus is the dog and the cat. Probl Vet Med 2:573, 1990.
*A review of the maintenance therapy of diabetes mellitus in dogs and cats.*

Wallace MS, Peterson ME, and Nichols CE: Absorption kinetics of regular, isophane and protamine zinc insulin in normal cats. Domes Anim Endocrinol 7:509–515, 1990.
*Comparison of the absorption kinetics of short-, intermediate-, and long-acting insulins in cats.*

# TRANSPLANTATION AS A MEANS OF TREATING DIABETES MELLITUS

EDWARD C. FELDMAN,
RICHARD W. NELSON,
*Davis, California*

*and* PATRICK SOON-SHIONG
*Los Angeles, California*

Diabetes mellitus is an extremely common endocrine disorder in human beings, dogs, and cats. It is estimated that each year approximately 800,000 Americans are diagnosed as having diabetes mellitus. Millions of Americans have diabetes mellitus. A small percentage of these people (approximately 10%) have a form of diabetes that has been labeled variously: juvenile type, insulin-dependent type, or type I. Put simply, these individuals have pancreatic islets that have completely lost the ability to synthesize insulin. These human beings require exogenous insulin, by injection on a daily basis, to survive. However, even with these injections, insulin-dependent diabetics are susceptible to ketoacidosis, their blood glucose fluctuations may be both wide and difficult to control (they are "brittle"), and they are prone to a variety of potentially catastrophic long-term complications. These short- and long-term complications of diabetes mellitus are the impetus to investigators who continue their search for better methods of treating or even curing diabetes mellitus. While this work is directed at helping human beings, veterinary patients always have the potential of benefiting from this broadening base of knowledge and care.

## WHOLE PANCREAS TRANSPLANTATION

Interest in pancreas transplantation continues, in part because of the difficulties in achieving optimal metabolic control with subcutaneous insulin injections in most patients with diabetes mellitus and in part because of the increasing utilization of organ transplantation in the management of people with a variety of disorders. The first human pancreatic transplantation was performed by Kelly and Lillehei in 1966 and only a few others were performed over the next 14 to 15 years. Since 1980, there has been a dramatic and steady increase in the number of these procedures. The International Pancreas Transplant Registry reports approximately 300 transplants per year for 1986 and 1987, the most recent years for which data are published. One of the most common techniques utilizes a duodenal segment of pancreas anastomosed to the urinary bladder. The University of Minnesota has performed 285 of these procedures between July 1986 and November 1992. The bladder-drained-pancreatic-transplant provides a mechanism for eliminating pancreatic exocrine secretions. Urinary amylase concentrations can then be monitored, and a decrease has been found to be a sensitive and early marker of graft rejection.

A total of 1394 transplants were performed from 1966 to 1988 and, in 1988, 514 were still functioning, with the longest functioning for 9.8 years. Graft survival (and function) has continued to improve and, for the period 1983 to 1988, the 1-year survival rate for technically successful grafts worldwide was 61%. Individual centers have reported even higher success rates. The University of Minnesota has obtained a 77% 1-year survival for simultaneous pancreas and kidney grafts, identical to the data from Stockholm, and the University of Wisconsin has reported an 83% graft survival at 2 years. Improvements in surgical techniques, donor and recipient selection, and immunotherapy have probably all contributed to this improved outcome.

The reason that transplantation holds a tremendous amount of interest are the catastrophic long-term complications of diabetes mellitus in people, which typically occur following decades of being afflicted with this disorder. Diabetes mellitus remains one of the most common causes of heart disease, kidney failure, blindness, and stroke in the United States. Diabetes mellitus is the most common cause of limb amputation and kidney transplantation in the United States. Notwithstanding the apparent transplant successes, it is important to emphasize that pancreas transplantation is major surgery with all the attendant risks. Furthermore, these people must be significantly immunosuppressed to prevent rejection of the transplant. Therefore, whether a successful pancreas transplant will prevent the end-organ complications of diabetes becomes the determining factor in deciding if, and in whom, pancreas transplants should be recommended. Pancreas transplantation, for example, does appear to stop the progression of diabetic nephropathy but not retinopathy. Whether retinopathy would respond if the transplantation were performed earlier is unknown. Successful pancreas transplantation also appears to halt the progression of diabetic neuropathy. It should not be understated that the quality of life in these people is definitely improved following successful transplantation. These and other data strongly suggest that pancreas transplantation, when successful, may be a major benefit to some patients with diabetes.

Because of the short-term operative risks, the long-term risks of immunosuppressive therapy, and the inability to accurately predict the 30 to 40% of diabetic patients in whom severe end-organ complications will develop, most physicians restrict pancreas transplantation to patients with end-stage diabetic nephropathy. More recently, especially with the emerging data that at least nephropathy and neuropathy can be halted by successful pancreas transplantation, there has been increasing interest in performing pancreas transplants before end-stage renal failure. In most centers this remains a research procedure, but at the University of Michigan, criteria for performing pancreas transplants prior to development of end-stage diabetic nephropathy have been established and debated. These criteria include established but not severe nephropathy defined as proteinuria greater than 150 mg but less than 3 gm in 24 hr; a creatinine clearance greater than or equal to 60 ml/min; autonomic neuropathy defined as gastroparesis, orthostatic hypotension, or abnormal cardiac vascular reflexes; or labile diabetes, defined as prolonged hospitalization for glycemic control, repeated severe episodes of hypoglycemia, or repeated episodes of ketoacidosis. If other institutions adopt similar criteria, the desire for pancreas transplants will soon exceed the available supply.

Since the major goal of transplantation is prevention or reduction of long-term complications, the value of transplantation in pets must be questioned. Diabetic dogs and cats do not live long enough, even surviving past normal life expectancy, to develop the long-term complications known to occur in people with insulin-dependent diabetes. The reasons for transplantation in pets are, therefore, far less critical in terms of need when compared with people. However, as the technology improves, application to pets remains a possibility. Whole pancreas transplantation has been successfully performed in dogs with graft survival of more than 1 year. This procedure has been utilized exclusively in research, with the pancreatic ducts either surgically drained into the urinary bladder or the exocrine secretions allowed to flow free into the peritoneal cavity.

Due to a lack of demand by the public, insufficient expertise within the veterinary profession, ethical questions regarding suitable donors, and the significant expense for these procedures (currently approximately $70,000 per transplant in humans), this method of treatment has not been utilized in clinical veterinary medicine. Furthermore, without considerable coordination throughout the profession to harvest pancreata from dogs with terminal problems but a healthy pancreas, one donor dog would have to be killed to transplant one recipient. Additionally, the negative side effects of immunosuppression would or could be of greater concern to diabetic dogs or their owners than the problems inherent to insulin administration.

Criteria regarding potential candidates for pancreas transplantation are becoming less rigorous (but the number of available pancreata available for transplantation is limited). The surgery is both difficult and expensive, and the need for host immunosuppression cannot be eliminated. The cost for each procedure is great and the number of potential recipients is huge. These are among the factors that have prompted continued research into pancreatic *islet* transplantation rather than whole organ transplantation (i.e., potential for a much larger population who could be treated with lower morbidity and mortality rates and at a significantly reduced cost).

## PANCREATIC ISLET TRANSPLANTATION

Transplantation of pure islets of Langerhans is an attractive alternative to whole pancreas transplantation for the reversal of diabetes: islets can be transplanted with little risk to the recipient, the immunogenicity of donor tissue might be altered to reduce immunosuppression requirements, cost can be moderated, and a greater number of individuals can be treated. In the past decade, methods of islet separation from whole pancreas have been described that have improved the yield from each donor pancreas. Islet transplantation to resolve diabetes has been successful in several small laboratory animal species, in dogs, and in a limited number of humans.

### Autograft

If a pancreas is surgically removed from a dog and the islets harvested, one can transplant those cells back into that same individual (autotransplantation) and prevent diabetes mellitus from occurring in the short term. This can be achieved without immunosuppression, since the recipient receives no foreign tissue. However, in the past, diabetes eventually occurred because the number of islets transplanted were probably insufficient (due to losses in the isolation procedures), those remaining become "exhausted" resulting in further cell loss, and because it is not possible to locate the graft in a "normal" anatomic site. These and other factors decrease long-term survival of transplanted cells.

### Allograft

The next logical step in islet research was transplantation from one individual to another within the same species (allograft). This allows utilization of more than one donor per recipient, thus allowing more islets to be transplanted. It was hoped that the need for immunosuppression to prevent graft rejection, as in whole pancreas transplantation, would be circumvented with islet allografting. However, it was quickly demonstrated that the pancreatic islets are potent antigenic stimuli and that without recipient immunosuppression, rejection of this tissue typically was complete within 5 to 12 days of transplantation. Furthermore, the amount of immunosuppression required to prevent rejection correlated directly with the number of donors contributing to the graft. In other words, if cells from one donor are implanted, that recipient requires less immunosuppression to prevent rejection than a recipient receiving tissue from three donors. To complicate matters, numerous studies demonstrated that duration of graft survival could be correlated with the number of islets transplanted. The more islets transplanted, the better the control of the blood glucose concentrations in both the short and long term. Transplanting an "ideal" number of islets, however, often required transplantation of islets collected from at least three to five donors.

The dilemma now begins to become more clear: tissue from several donors allows better control of diabetes mellitus. Utilization of several donors increases the need for levels of immunosuppression that might harm the recipient. Also, the need for multiple donors creates the ethical question of multiple dog lives being sacrificed in order to treat one dog that could already be treated with exogenous insulin. Adding to the confusion: immunosuppression with drugs like cyclosporine is not benign. Dogs receiving long-term cyclosporine develop a number of problems directly due to the effects of the drug: weight loss, papillomatosis, anemia, hypoalbuminemia, and polyclonal gammopathies. To further complicate a complicated situation, blood concentrations of cyclosporine required to prevent pancreatic islet rejection are actually harmful to those very islets being "protected."

### Immunoprotected Islet Transplantation

#### MICROENCAPSULATION

Many techniques have been used to circumvent the problems of immune rejection and to avoid the need for immunosuppression. One approach to this problem has been to utilize a technology called microencapsulation. The first report on microencapsulation appeared in *Science* in 1980. This novel approach to the previously mentioned rejection problems completely encloses each viable islet within a semipermeable membrane. The microcapsular membrane, composed of cross-linked alginate, a nontoxic polysaccharide, is permeable to small molecules such as glucose or insulin but totally impermeable to large molecules such as immunoglobulins. Tissue transplanted within such membranes are essentially invisible to a recipient's immune system. Preliminary results in a group of naturally occurring type I diabetic dogs have reinforced the potential value of microencapsulation. To date, transplantation has involved allografts (within species). A group of 12 pet dogs with naturally occurring diabetes mellitus received microencapsulated canine islets, transplanted free into the peritoneal cavity. Blood glucose concentrations fell to or below normal levels within 8 to 12 hr. These dogs remained euglycemic for 1 to 6 months, with a mean of 3.5 months. Five of these dogs received second transplants following recurrence of insulin dependence. Success following the second transplant was equivalent to that observed after the first.

### ARTIFICIAL PANCREAS

Several additional technologies are being actively pursued in an attempt to immunoprotect transplanted islets. One publicized approach is to place the islets into a sealed, surgically implantable chamber. The chamber is then anastomosed to the recipient's vasculature, but islets are separated from the recipient by unique semipermeable membranes. This methodology also has great potential.

### SUMMARY

Transplantation of microencapsulated islets has been valuable in gathering information, but each donor must undergo extremely sophisticated surgery or be killed in order to harvest the pancreas. Allografting of islets, therefore, has limited potential in people and would not be utilized in dogs. However, if such technology can be developed to a situation where pig pancreas (currently used in the production of insulin) is utilized in harvesting islets of Langerhans, one can visualize a large resource for this novel treatment of diabetes mellitus. If such a tool is developed for humans, it will likely become available for veterinary medicine as well.

## References and Suggested Reading

Alejandro R, Feldman EC, Shienvold FL, et al: Advances in canine diabetes mellitus research: Etiopathology and results of islet transplantation. J Am Vet Med Assoc 193:1050, 1988.
*This manuscript reviews the results of intrahepatic islet transplantation in immunosuppressed canine recipients.*

Dafae DA and Uinik AI: Is pancreas transplantation for insulin-dependent diabetes mellitus worthwhile? N Engl J Med 322:1608, 1990.
*The controversies regarding transplantation are reviewed.*

Kennedy WR, Xavier N, Goetz FC, et al: Effects of pancreatic transplantation on diabetic neuropathy. N Engl J Med 322:1031, 1990.
*This is one of many manuscripts regarding the potential benefit of transplantation to long-term complications of diabetes mellitus in human beings.*

Palmer JP: Current management of type I diabetes: Insulin, transplantation and immunotherapy. 42nd Postgraduate Assembly, The Endocrine Society 1, 1990.
*This is an excellent review of transplantation technology and immunosuppression in diabetic patients.*

Soon-Shiong P, Feldman EC, Nelson RW, et al: Successful reversal of spontaneous diabetes in dogs by intraperitoneal microencapsulated islets. Transplantation 54:769, 1992.
*Review of our results of treating diabetic pet dogs with microencapsulated islets.*

Soon-Shiong P, Feldman EC, Nelson RW, et al: Long-term reversal of diabetes by the injection of immunoprotected islet cells. *Proceedings of the National Academy of Sciences* 90:5843, 1993.
*Long-term results are reported regarding dogs with naturally occurring diabetes, transplanted with microencapsulated islets.*

Sutherland DER, Moudry KC, and Fryd DS: Results of pancreas-transplant registry. Diabetes 38(suppl 1): 46, 1989.
*A review of pancreatic transplantations since 1966.*

Tattersall R: Is pancreas transplantation for insulin-dependent diabetics worthwhile? N Engl J Med 321:112, 1989.
*The controversies regarding pancreas transplantation are reviewed.*

University of Michigan Pancreas Transplant Evaluation Committee: Pancreatic transplantation as treatment for IDDM. Diabetes Care 11:669, 1988.
*This manuscript reviews some of the new concepts regarding criteria for potential whole pancreas transplantation candidates.*

---

# TREATMENT OF FELINE DIABETES MELLITUS WITH THE ORAL SULFONYLUREA, GLIPIZIDE

RICHARD W. NELSON
*and* EDWARD C. FELDMAN

*Davis, California*

Two classes of oral antihyperglycemic drugs are used for the treatment of non–insulin-dependent diabetes mellitus (NIDDM) in human beings, the biguanides (phenformin and metformin) and the sulfonylureas. Metformin is available in Canada and Europe, but is not currently available in the United States. Sulfonylureas are the only orally administered antihyperglycemic drugs approved for use in human beings in the United States. The second-generation sulfonylureas, glipizide and glyburide, are commonly used for the treatment of NIDDM (Table 1).

## MECHANISM OF ACTION

The mechanism of action by which sulfonylurea drugs exert their hypoglycemic effects is debated. Pancreatic and extrapancreatic effects have been identified. The primary effect of sulfonylureas is the direct stimulation of insulin secretion by the $\beta$ cells of the pancreas (Gerich, 1989). Extrapancreatic effects include improvement of tissue sensitivity to circulating insulin, either through increased insulin receptor binding or improved postbinding action, inhibition of hepatic glycogenolysis, increased hepatic glucose utilization, and decreased hepatic insulin extraction. These extrapancreatic effects may be a direct action of the drug itself or secondary to the resultant stimulation of insulin secretion.

## INDICATIONS FOR USE

Some endogenous pancreatic insulin secretory capacity must exist for sulfonylureas to be effective in improving glycemic control. As such, sulfonylurea treatment is ineffective as the sole form of treatment for human beings with an absolute deficiency of insulin, (i.e., insulin-dependent diabetes mellitus [IDDM]), but is a valuable therapeutic aid for people with NIDDM. Sulfonylurea treatment has not been effective in most diabetic dogs, presumably because of the high incidence of IDDM in this species.

Type-II or NIDDM has been reported in cats (Kirk et al., 1993) and accounts for as many as 30 to 50% of diabetic cats seen at our hospital. The etiogenesis of NIDDM in cats may be analogous to NIDDM in human beings (Johnson et al., 1989); therefore, sulfonylureas may be effective in some cats with NIDDM. The oral administration of the second-generation sulfonylurea, glipizide (Glucotrol, Pfizer), stimulates insulin secretion in healthy cats (Miller et al., 1992). In a recent study, glipizide treatment was shown to be effective in improving glycemic control in some cats with diabetes mellitus (Nelson et al., 1993). Clinical response was variable, ranging from excellent (i.e., blood glucose concentrations decreasing to <200 mg/dl) to partial response (i.e., clinical improvement but failure to resolve hyperglycemia) to no response. Presumably, the population of functioning $\beta$ cells varied from none (severe IDDM) to near normal (mild NIDDM) in the cats studied, resulting in a response range from none to excellent. Cats with a partial response to glipizide have some functioning $\beta$ cells but not enough to decrease blood glucose concentration to less than 200 mg/dl. These cats may have severe NIDDM or the early stages of IDDM.

Ideal candidates for sulfonylurea treatment are NIDDM cats who still have adequate $\beta$-cell function.

**Table 1.** *Some of the Oral Sulfonylurea Drugs Available in the United States.*

| Generic Name | Trade Name | Relative Potency |
| --- | --- | --- |
| First generation: | | |
|   Tolbutamide | Orinase | 1 |
|   Acetohexamide | Dymelor | 2.5 |
|   Tolazamide | Tolinase | 5 |
|   Chlorpropamide | Diabinase | 6 |
| Second generation: | | |
|   Glipizide | Glucotrol | 100 |
|   Glyburide | Micronase | 150 |
| | Diabeta | 150 |

Unfortunately, no consistent clinical parameters (e.g., obesity) have been identified that allow the clinician to prospectively determine which cats will respond to glipizide therapy. Insulin secretagogue tests (e.g., intravenous glucose tolerance test, glucagon tolerance test) are used in human beings to assess $\beta$-cell function and differentiate IDDM from NIDDM. Unfortunately, measurement of baseline serum insulin concentration or serum insulin concentration following administration of an insulin secretagogue has not been a consistent aid in differentiating IDDM from NIDDM in the cat (Kirk et al., 1993; Nelson et al., 1993). A fasting serum insulin concentration greater than the normal mean concentration (>12 $\mu$U/ml in our laboratory) or any postsecretagogue insulin concentration greater than one standard deviation above the reference mean (>18 $\mu$U/ml in our laboratory) would suggest the existence of functional $\beta$ cells and the possibility for a beneficial response to glipizide treatment. Unfortunately, cats subsequently identified as having IDDM and many of those with NIDDM have a low baseline serum insulin concentration and do not respond to a glucose or glucagon challenge. This apparent insulin deficiency in cats subsequently identified with NIDDM is presumably because of concurrent "glucose toxicity." Because of the inability to prospectively identify those cats that will respond to glipizide treatment, selection of diabetic cats for treatment with glipizide must rely heavily on the veterinarian's assessment of the cat's health, severity of clinical signs, presence or absence of ketoacidosis, other diabetic complications (e.g., neuropathy), and owner desires.

## ADVERSE REACTIONS

Adverse reactions of glipizide treatment in cats include hypoglycemia, vomiting shortly after administration of the drug, hepatic enzyme alterations, and icterus. The incidence of adverse reactions is less than 15%. Hypoglycemia, hepatic enzyme alterations, and icterus resolve after discontinuing glipizide. It is not known whether the hepatic enzyme alterations are a result of hepatocellular damage and leakage or cellular death. In cats with gastric or hepatic reactions, glipizide treatment can be reinstituted using a lower dosage, once clinical signs and/or hepatic enzyme abnormalities or icterus have resolved. In some cats, the side effects do not recur; however, in others, reactions recur regardless of the glipizide dosage.

## CURRENT TREATMENT RECOMMENDATIONS

Currently, we administer glipizide, 2.5 mg per os two times a day in conjunction with food (preferably containing increased amounts of fiber), to those diabetic cats that are nonketotic and relatively healthy on physical examination, and to those cats whose owners refuse to administer insulin to their pet. Glipizide treatment is not recommended in lieu of insulin in those cats previously well regulated with insulin treatment, unless hypoglycemia is a persistent problem despite small amounts of insulin. Glipizide treatment has been ineffective in improving glycemic control in cats with insulin resistance and is not recommended in this circumstance.

Each cat is examined weekly during the first month of glipizide therapy. A history, complete physical examination, body weight and urine glucose/ketone measurement, and several blood glucose concentrations are evaluated at each examination. If vomiting, icterus, and euglycemia have not occurred after 2 weeks of treatment, the glipizide dosage is increased to 5.0 mg two times per day. Therapy is continued as long as the cat is stable. An effect on blood glucose concentrations may not be apparent for 4 to 8 weeks after initiating treatment. If euglycemia or hypoglycemia develop, glipizide dosage may be tapered down or discontinued and blood glucose concentrations reevaluated 1 week later to assess the need for the drug. If hyperglycemia recurs, the dosage is increased or glipizide is reinitiated, with a reduction in dosage in those cats previously developing hypoglycemia. Glipizide is discontinued and insulin therapy initiated if clinical signs continue to worsen, the cat becomes ill or develops ketoacidosis, blood glucose concentrations remain greater than 300 mg/dl after 1 or 2 months of therapy, or the owner becomes dissatisfied with the treatment.

There are several possible outcomes utilizing this therapeutic approach. The most common is failure to control hyperglycemia and the clinical signs of diabetes mellitus. For these cats, glipizide therapy is discontinued and insulin is used to control the blood glucose concentration. In a small percentage of these cats, insulin therapy may be discontinued in the future. Less commonly, the blood glucose concentration and clinical signs are controlled without the use of exogenous insulin. Glipizide can be discontinued in some of these cats, while others require glipizide to maintain control of the diabetic state. For some of these cats, glipizide becomes ineffective and exogenous insulin is ultimately required to control the diabetic state. For these cats, the time from initiation of glipizide therapy to initiation of insulin therapy is unpredictable and quite variable, ranging from a few weeks to greater than a year. Most cats remain on insulin for life once a requirement for insulin is established. Rarely, insulin requirements will continue to wax and wane. Presumably, the transition from NIDDM to IDDM is due to progression of the underlying pathophysiologic mechanisms (e.g., islet-specific amyloid deposition) responsible for the development of diabetes in the cat. The more rapid the rate of progression, the shorter the beneficial response to glipizide.

### References and Suggested Reading

Gerich JE: Oral hypoglycemic agents. N Engl J Med 321:1231, 1989.
  *A review of the oral hypoglycemic drugs used to treat non–insulin-dependent diabetes mellitus in humans.*
Johnson KH, O'Brien TD, Betsholtz C, et al: Islet amyloid, islet-amyloid polypeptide, and diabetes mellitus. N Engl J Med 321: 513, 1989.
  *A comparative review of the association between islet amyloid and diabetes mellitus in several species, including the cat.*
Kirk CA, Feldman EC, and Nelson RW: Diagnosis of naturally acquired type-I and type-II diabetes mellitus in cats. Am J Vet Res 54:463, 1993.
  *A study documenting the existence of type-I and type-II diabetes mellitus in cats using the glucagon tolerance test.*
Miller AB, Nelson RW, Kirk CA, et al: Effect of glipizide on serum insulin and glucose concentrations in healthy cats. Res Vet Sci 52:177, 1992.
  *A study evaluating the effects of different dosages of glipizide on serum insulin and glucose concentrations in healthy cats.*
Nelson RW, Feldman EC, Ford SL, et al: Effect of an orally administered sulfonylurea, glipizide, for treatment of diabetes mellitus in cats. J Am Vet Med Assoc 203:821, 1993.
  *A prospective study evaluating the efficacy of glipizide for the treatment of diabetes mellitus in 20 cats.*

# MONITORING LONG-TERM CONTROL IN THE DIABETIC PATIENT

C. B. CHASTAIN

*Columbia, Missouri*

Assessment of the long-term control of diabetes mellitus is best evaluated by the average highest daily value of blood glucose level and by the average daily range of the blood glucose level. Ideal control of diabetes in dogs and cats is often arbitrarily defined as confinement of the blood glucose level within a range of 100 to 150 mg/dl throughout the day and night. Multiple daily home blood glucose determinations are not practical for routine home care of diabetic dogs and cats.

## PROBLEMS WITH URINE GLUCOSE TESTS

Urine samples are more easily collected than blood samples by owners of diabetic pets. Testing of random daily urine samples for glucose has often been recommended to monitor the control of diabetes in dogs and cats. But for owners, the collection and testing of urine for glucose is an inconvenience, an added expense, and often misleading.

Measurement of urine glucose cannot be assumed to reflect blood glucose values unless the renal threshold is established on an individual basis. An individual animal's renal glucose threshold varies widely. In dogs, the usual renal threshold for glucose is 175 to 220 mg/dl; in cats, it may be higher. Urine glucose levels are therefore not detectable until blood glucose levels exceed the desired upper range. Conversely, if urine glucose is undetectable, the blood glucose may be undesirably low.

Also, urine with high glucose concentration formed in the morning may not be voided and tested until the afternoon, when the blood glucose has become normal or subnormal. Increasing the dose of insulin based on a random urine glucose concentration can be dangerous. Urine voiding should be monitored closely enough to know the interval during which the urine tested was collected in the bladder. This is difficult and generally undesirable.

False-negative and false-positive results may occur with conventional tests for urine glucose. Glucose oxidase–impregnated strips may give false-negative results from inhibitory substances such as salicylates. Testing for urine glucose by the copper reduction technique may give false-positive results in the presence of other reducing substances such as ascorbic acid.

The measurement of urine glucose levels is only an indication of the circumstances involving the last insulin injection, the last meal, recent exercise, and other recent unknown factors. An abnormally high urine glucose measurement may be atypical of the average results using the same treatment protocol on another day. Concern and changes in insulin dosage should be based on repeated abnormal findings involving more than one insulin injection, meal, period of exercise, and other events that affect blood glucose concentrations.

## HOME PARAMETERS OF DIABETES CONTROL

Control of diabetes should be assessed at home by a variety of practical, inexpensive means. The owner should keep a log of the parameters (Table 1) to be reviewed by the veterinarian during office reexaminations. Diabetic dogs or cats should be examined by a veterinarian if abnormalities are detected by monitoring at home for 2 or more days in a row or whenever ketones are detected in the urine. Routine office reex-

***Table 1.***   *Home Parameters of Monitoring Diabetic Control*

| Evaluation | Frequency |
| --- | --- |
| Attitude | Daily |
| Appetite | Daily |
| Physical activity | Daily |
| Water consumption* | Daily |
| Urinary continence | Daily |
| Body weight | Weekly |
| Urine ketones | As necessary† |

*Daily water consumption should not exceed 60 ml/kg (1 oz/lb) body weight.
†Measurement of urine ketones is indicated if there is concern if any of the routine assessments are repeated abnormal.

aminations on diabetics should be recommended every 3 months regardless of home monitoring results.

Single daily "spot checks" of blood glucose represent only a single point in a dynamic event that is also influenced by many variables such as patient struggle and stress, sedation with xylazine, exercise, and food intake. Blood glucose curves determined by multiple samples taken throughout a day are stressful and not necessarily representative of home control.

Two semiquantitative laboratory markers of diabetic control, glycohemoglobin (GHb) and fructosamine, provide a convenient means of determining the mean blood glucose concentration during the preceding 5 days to 12 weeks. Samples required are a single whole blood sample for GHb determination, or a serum sample for fructosamine determination.

## SEMIQUANTITATIVE LABORATORY MARKERS OF LONG-TERM CONTROL

### Glycohemoglobin

Small amounts of glucose nonenzymatically and irreversibly bind with a portion of hemoglobin (Hb). The binding is a ketoamine formation of glucose with N-terminal valine of the $\beta$-chain, lysine of the $\alpha$-chain, and internal lysines of the $\alpha$- and $\beta$-chain of Hb. This irreversible binding occurs slowly throughout the life of the red blood cell. Normally less than 10% of Hb is affected.

The major form of GHb is $HbA_{1c}$. The remaining GHb is phosphorylated glucose or fructose called $HbA_{1a}$ and $HbA_{1b}$, respectively. Most assays measure all forms of GHb. By measuring the combination, an indirect assessment of the mean blood glucose can be determined for the preceding several weeks, depending on the half-life of circulating red blood cells (RBCs).

Glycohemoglobin is a tissue (RBC) glucose rather than a serum or plasma glucose. The binding of glucose with Hb interferes with its binding to 2,3-diphosphoglycerate. There also is a greater Hb affinity to oxygen, impeding its release. The resulting decreased delivery of oxygen to the tissues may cause some of the complications of diabetes.

Blood is a collection of new, middle-aged, and aged RBCs. The rate of decline of elevated GHb is related to the removal of old RBCs. A rise in blood glucose levels must result in an elevated mean blood glucose for at least 1 to 3 weeks before the GHb level is abnormally elevated. Recent anemia will result in low GHb concentrations because of the shortened duration of glucose exposure to the newly generated RBCs.

Glycohemoglobin can be measured by chromatographic, electrophoretic, and colorimetric methods. Glycohemoglobin assays lack universal reference standards. Normal ranges vary among laboratories and erroneous results occasionally occur.

The most common problem leading to false results involves chromatographic methods and is the detection of reversible aldimine, called preHb$_{1c}$. The first step in glycosylation of Hb is binding of glucose to HbA to form preHbA$_{1c}$, a labile intermediate compound. This step occurs readily and is reversible. A second step in which preHbA$_{1c}$ undergoes a rearrangement to a stable compound, HbA$_{1c}$, is irreversible and occurs slowly. Red blood cells allowed to be in contact with high plasma glucose concentrations will rapidly form high concentrations of preHb$_{1c}$. Some chromatographic procedures measure preHbA$_{1c}$ and yield falsely elevated GHb level results.

Other conditions that may cause falsely elevated GHb levels as measured by column chromatography are lipemia, acetylated Hb from high-dose aspirin therapy, carbamylated Hb from uremia, and fetal hemoglobin. The most reliable methods of measuring GHb are high-performance liquid chromatography (HPLC) or gel electrophoresis, which separate HbA$_{1c}$ from other Hb. Colorimetric procedures are based on Hb interacting with certain organic phosphates.

Normal GHb values in dogs are about 4 to 8%, depending on the laboratory and method of determination. Poorly controlled diabetic dogs have values of greater than 10%. Dog RBC have a circulation life of about 120 days. The GHb concentration indirectly reflects the mean blood glucose level over the preceding 8 to 12 weeks.

Cats have less than 5% GHb and less HbA$_{1c}$ than dogs or humans (Hasegawa et al., 1992). Yet, with some chromatographic methods, GHb concentration may be falsely reported as more than 80%. Column cation exchange chromatography on RBC hemolysates has resulted in falsely elevated GHb levels from normal cats. This may be due to a lower HbA isoelectric pH in cats than in dogs and humans. More rapid elution from the columns then results. Valid GHb levels in normal cats should be less than 12%.

Affinity chromatography that measures all GHb have been reported to be normally less than 12% in normal cats (Akol, Waddle, and Wilding, 1992). Cat RBC turnover (66 to 78 days) is only slightly more than half as long as the RBC turnover in dogs. Therefore, GHb in cats represents the mean glucose over the preceding 5 to 6 weeks, a shorter evaluation period than in dogs.

## Fructosamine

In addition to Hb, other blood proteins are also irreversibly glycosylated. By determining these proteins' glycosylated concentration and considering their half-life, an estimate of the duration of hyperglycemia can be made. Fructosamine is a ketoamine product containing fructose and albumin formed by nonenzymatic glycosylation of the amino group on lysine in albumin (Reusch et al., 1993).

Since albumin has a shorter life (12-day turnover) than hemoglobin (120-day turnover in dogs; 70 days in cats), serum albumin fructosamine levels assess the mean blood levels over a shorter preceding time (5 to 8 days) than does GHb levels (8 to 12 weeks) (Kawamoto et al., 1992). Serum fructosamine levels will become normal faster than GHb in a newly controlled diabetic. Rising serum fructosamine concentrations may signal deteriorating control of diabetes earlier than GHb concentrations.

Fructosamine is usually measured by a nitroblue tetrazolium reduction in alkaline conditions method (Roche Diagnostic Systems). The upper normal limit in dogs is about 3.38 mmol/L in dogs (Kawamoto et al., 1992) and 3.47 mmol/L in cats (Kaneko et al., 1992). Levels above 3.5 mmol/L are therefore abnormal. Fructosamine is stable in serum refrigerated at 4°C for 7 days or frozen at −20°C for 28 days (Jensen, 1992; Kaneko et al., 1992).

## RECOMMENDED IN-OFFICE REEXAMINATION OF DIABETICS

Glycohemoglobin or fructosamine determinations in diabetic dogs and cats are probably not as sensitive in detecting poor diabetic control as careful daily home-monitoring of the appetite, attitude, water consumption, physical activity, urinary continence, and weekly monitoring of the body weight. The sensitivity of these home-monitoring parameters is owner dependent. Glycohemoglobin or fructosamine measurements are valuable whenever owner monitoring is not completely reliable.

Diabetics should be physically reexamined, their home-monitoring log reviewed, and blood examinations repeated every 3 months. Recommended components of an outpatient recheck examination are listed in Table 2.

Compared to GHb determinations by chromatography, serum fructosamine levels by colorimetry are less susceptible to false elevations, particularly in cats. The selection of a reference laboratory to measure GHb should be limited only to those that have established normal levels in dogs or cats and whose normal ranges are less than 10%. Reference laboratories for fructosamine determinations also should have normals established for dogs or cats, and the normal ranges should be less than 3.5 mmol/L.

Glycohemoglobin levels may be preferable for routine 3-month reevaluations of diabetic dogs. However,

**Table 2.**   *Recommended Routine Diabetic Outpatient Examinations*

1. Review owner's observations and home monitoring results
2. Perform and record routine physical examination
3. Collect urine for urinalysis
4. Collect blood for a hemogram and serum chemistry panel
5. Collect serum for a fructosamine determination or whole blood for a glycohemoglobin determination

serum fructosamine levels may be more useful in diabetics that have had recent hemolysis, since hemolysis will decrease GHb concentration in uncontrolled diabetics. Fructosamine determinations will also indicate satisfactory home control of diabetes earlier than GHb levels.

Serum fructosamine levels may be misleadingly low in cases with hypoalbuminemia. Fructosamine levels can be adjusted to a normal albumin level of 2.5 gm/dl in hypoalbuminemic dogs by the following formula:

2.5/albumin level in gm/dl X fructosamine level

= adjusted fructosamine level

However, a recent study's results indicated that calculations of adjusted fructosamine levels may not be necessary in dogs (Jensen, 1993). Glycohemoglobin levels are not affected by hypoalbuminemia.

### References and Suggested Reading

Akol KG, Waddle JR, and Wilding P: Glycated hemoglobin and fructosamine in diabetic and nondiabetic cats. J Am Anim Hosp Assoc 28:227, 1992.

*Poorly controlled or untreated diabetic cats have glycohemoglobin concentrations above 12%.*

Hasegawa S, Sako T, Takemura N, et al: Glycated hemoglobin fractions in normal and diabetic cats measured by high performance liquid chromatography. J Vet Med Sci 54:789, 1992.

*Cats have lower concentration of HbA$_{1c}$ than dogs or humans.*

Jensen AL: Serum fructosamine in canine diabetes mellitus. An initial study. Vet Res Commun 16:1, 1992.

*Fructosamine is stable in canine serum refrigerated for 5 days or frozen for 28 days.*

Jensen AL: Various protein and albumin corrections of the serum fructosamine concentration in the diagnosis of canine diabetes mellitus. Vet Res Commun 17:13, 1993.

*Correcting the fructosamine concentration for altered total plasma protein or serum albumin concentrations in dogs may not be necessary.*

Kaneko JJ, Kawamoto M, Heusner AA, et al: Evaluation of serum fructosamine concentration as an index of blood glucose control in cats with diabetes mellitus. Am J Vet Res 53:1797, 1992.

*Serum fructosamine concentration is a valid evaluation of glycemic control in diabetic cats.*

Kawamoto M, Kaneko JJ, Heusner AA, et al: Relation of fructosamine to serum protein, albumin, and glucose concentrations in healthy and diabetic dogs. Am J Vet Res 53:851, 1992.

*Fructosamine concentration in canine blood is correlated with serum albumin concentration.*

Reusch CE, Liehs MR, Hoyer M, et al: Fructosamine: A new parameter for diagnosis and metabolic control in diabetic dogs and cats. Vet Intern Med 7:177, 1993.

*Serum concentration of fructosamine is a valuable parameter of assessing the control of diabetes in dogs and cats.*

# CLINICAL APPLICATIONS OF GLUCOCORTICOID THERAPY IN NONENDOCRINE DISEASE

ELLEN N. BEHREND
*and* DEBORAH S. GRECO
*Fort Collins, Colorado*

Glucocorticoids are one of the most commonly prescribed classes of medication in veterinary medicine. As such, the potential for misuse of glucocorticoids is quite great. Corticosteroids should be used to achieve strict therapeutic goals while minimizing the potentially life-threatening side effects of these compounds (see "Rational Use of Glucocorticoids in Dermatology," this volume, p 573).

## PHYSIOLOGY OF GLUCOCORTICOIDS

The term "corticosteroid" refers to a set of hormones synthesized and secreted by the adrenal cortex. Glucocorticoids account for 95% of the corticosteroids released from the adrenal glands. The cells within the adrenal cortex that synthesize the glucocorticoids function as part of the hypothalamic-pituitary-adrenal (HPA) axis. The hypothalamus produces corticotrophin-releasing hormone (CRH) which, in turn, stimulates cells of the pars distalis of the pituitary to secrete adrenocorticotrophic hormone (ACTH). Adrenocorticotrophic hormone is the only direct stimulus of glucocorticoid release. The secretion of CRH, ACTH, and glucocorticoids in the canine and feline occurs in an episodic, rather than circadian, rhythm. Glucocorticoids act directly on the hypothalamus to decrease the release, synthesis, and storage of CRH and on the pituitary to inhibit the secretion of ACTH. Prolonged use of exogenous glucocorticoids that maintains serum glucocorticoid concentrations at supraphysiologic levels will suppress basal and ACTH-stimulated secretion of glucocorticoids.

## TISSUE EFFECTS

### Anti-inflammatory

The anti-inflammatory and immunosuppressive properties of glucocorticoids can be utilized to decrease or prevent tissue destruction and fibrosis. In general, glucocorticoids act to maintain the integrity of the microcirculation, decrease capillary blood flow, protect cell membranes, and diminish the response of inflammatory cells either by slowing their migration to an inflammatory site or curtailing their phagocytic and bactericidal capacities. Other anti-inflammatory actions include inhibition of histamine production by mast cells, reduced clearance of antigens by the reticuloendothelial system and, possibly, stabilization of lysosomal membranes.

### Immunosuppressive

Glucocorticoids have additional actions that specifically affect the immune system, although these effects are minimal in dogs and cats. Production of new antibodies is decreased by glucocorticoids. Lymphopenia occurs secondary to increased concentrations of glucocorticoids for two reasons. Initially, a reduction in lymphocyte numbers occurs due to a sequestration of the cells into the bone marrow, where they will not be activated. Secondly, prolonged glucocorticoid use slows the rate of division of immature lymphocytes. Glucocorticoids also affect nonspecific immunity by decreasing cell migration and cytokine production; in fact, these actions are more profound than the effects on the specific immune responses.

### Other

The principal biochemical actions of glucocorticoids include stimulation of gluconeogenesis, inhibition of peripheral tissue protein synthesis, and stimulation and induction of protein synthesis in the liver and of lipogenesis. Other general effects of glucocorticoids include maintenance of cardiac and skeletal muscle strength, brain activity, and normal water distribution. Glucocorticoids exert a permissive effect on the pressor and bronchodilatory effects of catecholamines and also enhance diuresis, glomerular filtration rate, and free water clearance. With respect to calcium homeostasis, intestinal absorption is decreased, renal excretion is increased, and body stores are redistributed, resulting in a decrease in serum calcium. Lastly, other endocrine organs can be influenced by glucocorticoids. The thyroid gland, testes, and ovaries can be inhibited directly by glucocorticoids and the conversion of thyroxine ($T_4$) to the active triiodothyronine ($T_3$) is reduced. The release of multiple anterior pituitary hormones, such as prolactin, thyroid-stimulating hormone, luteinizing hormone, and follicle-stimulating hormone, is suppressed by glucocorticoids.

## CLINICAL PHARMACOLOGY OF GLUCOCORTICOIDS

At the current time, ten synthetic glucocorticoids are licensed for use in the United States and are available in a myriad of topical and systemic preparations (Table 1). All glucocorticoids are absorbed well from any administration site and can be administered via the topical, enteral, subcutaneous, intramuscular, intralesional, or intravenous routes; intravenous therapy is reserved for emergency situations.

In general, when compared to cortisol, the synthetic glucocorticoids have greater glucocorticoid activity and less mineralocorticoid activity; the only synthetics that possess mineralocorticoid activity are hydrocortisone, prednisone, and prednisolone. Synthetic glucocorticoids bind less avidly to serum protein and, as a result, diffuse more readily into the tissues. Furthermore, the synthetic glucocorticoids have a higher affinity for the steroid receptor, slower degradation and, hence, a longer duration of action (Chastain, 1989).

The potency of the synthetic glucocorticoids is assessed by their anti-inflammatory activity and rated relative to hydrocortisone that is given an arbitrary value of 1.0 (Table 2). No difference exists between the synthetic glucocorticoids with respect to the quality or mechanism of action of the anti-inflammatory activity. Prednisone and cortisone must be activated in the liver to prednisolone and cortisol, respectively; therefore, topical use of these glucocorticoids is inappropriate. The hepatic conversion of prednisone to prednisolone is curtailed only in the face of severe end-stage liver failure.

Duration of action is a property inherent to each synthetic glucocorticoid. The synthetic glucocorticoids are divided into three categories depending upon their duration of action. Cortisone and hydrocortisone are short acting, while prednisone, methylprednisolone, and triamcinolone are intermediate acting. Paramethasone, flumethasone, dexamethasone, and betamethasone are all long acting (Table 2).

Tissue penetration and the intrinsic duration of action is further influenced by the chemical form of the

**Table 1.** *Commonly Used Veterinary Products Containing Glucocorticoids*

| Compound | Systemic Preparation | Manufacturer | Topical Preparation | Manufacturer |
|---|---|---|---|---|
| Betamethasone | Betasone | Schering | Topagen | Schering |
| | | | Gentocin Topical | Schering |
| | | | Gentocin Otic | Schering |
| Dexamethasone | Azium | Schering | | |
| | Voren | Bio-ceutic | | |
| Flumethasone | Flucort | Syntex | | |
| Hydrocortisone | Cortef° | Upjohn | | |
| | Hydrocortone° | Merck | | |
| | A-hydrocort° | Abbott | | |
| Methylprednisolone | Medrol | Upjohn | | |
| | Solu-medrol° | Upjohn | | |
| | Depo-medrol° | Upjohn | | |
| | A-methaPred | Abbott | | |
| Prednisone | Delta-cortef | Upjohn | | |
| | Prelone | Muro | | |
| | Solu-delta-cortef | Upjohn | | |
| | Deltasone | Upjohn | | |
| | Meticorten | Schering | | |
| | Orasone | Reid-Powell | | |
| Triamcinolone | Vetalog | Solvay | Panalog | Solvay |

°Approved for human use only.

glucocorticoid in the preparation. The synthetic glucocorticoids are synthesized as esters, and the nonglucocorticoid moiety of the compound has a profound effect on bioavailability. The less soluble the ester, the slower the rate of absorption, the less the daily glucocorticoid activity supplied, and the longer the inherent duration of action will be prolonged. Highly soluble esters that release the glucocorticoid moiety for absorption and receptor binding within minutes include succinate, hemisuccinate, and phosphate (e.g., Solu-delta Cortef, Upjohn; Azium-SP, Schering). Glucocorticoids bound to polyethylene glycol will be available within minutes to hours (e.g., Azium, Schering; Meticorten, Schering). The moderately insoluble esters, which include acetate, diacetate, isonicotinate, and tebutate, remain bound to the glucocorticoid for days to weeks (e.g., Depo-Medrol, Upjohn), while the acetonide, hexacetate, pivalate, and diproprionate esters are poorly soluble and release the glucocorticoids over a period of weeks to months (e.g., Vetalog, Solvay).

## INDICATIONS FOR USE OF GLUCOCORTICOIDS

In general, there are six nonendocrine disease states for which the use of glucocorticoids are indicated: inflammatory, immune-mediated, and neoplastic disorders; cerebral edema; shock; and hypercalcemia (Tables 3 and 4). Dosage of medication varies in accordance with the desired effect and the compound utilized; less potent glucocorticoids require relatively higher doses (Tables 2 and 3). Which glucocorticoid is preferred also varies with the condition being treated. Methylprednisolone acetate (Depo-Medrol, Upjohn), for example, is recommended for the treatment of feline gingivitis-stomatitis. In contrast, this glucocorticoid is not recommended for therapy of inflammatory bowel disease. Furthermore, a more potent glucocorticoid may succeed in obtaining remission of a given disease in an individual patient where a less potent glucocorticoid has failed. For example, oral triamcinolone or dexa-

**Table 2.** *Comparison of the Synthetic Glucocorticoids*

| Compound | Duration of Action° | Anti-inflammatory Potency (per mg) | Equivalent Dose (mg) | Appropriate for Alternate-Day Use |
|---|---|---|---|---|
| Cortisone | Short | 0.8 | 5.0 | No |
| Hydrocortisone | Short | 1.0 | 4.0 | No |
| Prednisone[†] | Intermediate | 4.0 | 1.0 | Yes |
| Methylprednisolone | Intermediate | 5.0 | 0.8 | Yes |
| Triamcinolone | Intermediate[‡] | 5.0 | 0.8 | No |
| Paramethasone | Long | 10.0 | 0.4 | No |
| Flumethasone | Long | 15.0 | 0.3 | No |
| Dexamethasone | Long | 30.0 | 0.15 | No |
| Betamethasone | Long | 35.0 | 0.12 | No |

°Short = <12 hr, intermediate = 12–36 hr, long = >48 hr.
[†]Prednisone or prednisolone.
[‡]May be up to 48 hr.

**Table 3.**  *Examples of Recommended Initial Doses and Treatment Regimens*[*][†]

| Disease | Preferred Glucocorticoid | Initial Dose[‡] | Treatment Protocol |
|---|---|---|---|
| Inflammatory disease | Prednisone | 0.25–0.5 mg/kg q12h | Taper in 5- to 7-day intervals |
| Chronic/allergic bronchitis | Prednisone | 0.25–0.5 mg/kg q12h | Taper in 5- to 7-day intervals. May require lifelong q.o.d. therapy |
| Pulmonary heartworm hypersensitivity | Prednisone | 0.5–1.0 mg/kg q12h | Taper over 7–14 days; use before adulticide therapy |
| Chronic active hepatitis | Prednisone | 0.5 mg/kg q12h | Taper after 14 days if improving; if not, use adjunct therapy |
| Eosinophilic enteritis/colitis (canine) | Prednisone | 0.5–1.0 mg/kg q12h | Taper in intervals of 7 to 14 days |
| Eosinophilic enteritis/colitis (feline) | Prednisone | 2.0–4.0 mg/kg q12h | Do not taper |
| Plasmacytic/lymphocytic enteritis | Prednisone | 1.1 mg/kg q12h | Decrease by 50% after 5 to 10 days, then taper in 14-day intervals |
| Lymphangiectasia | Prednisone | 1.0–1.5 mg/kg q12h | Taper after remission |
| Feline gingivitis/stomatitis | Methylprednisolone acetate | 2.0–5.0 mg/kg IM | Give every 2 wk until response, then PRN (≥q6–8 wk) |
|  | Prednisone | 1.0–2.0 mg/kg b.i.d. | Taper slowly after remission |
|  | Triamcinolone | 4 mg/cat q24h | After remission, taper to q.o.d. then lowest effective q.o.d. dose |
| Granulomatous meningoencephalitis | Prednisone | 0.5–1.0 mg/kg q12h | Taper after 14 days; therapy required for life |
| Atopy/flea allergy dermatitis | Prednisone | 0.5 mg/kg q12h (dog) 1.0 mg/kg q12h (cat) | Taper in 5- to 7-day intervals |
| Immune-mediated disease | Prednisone | 1.0–2.0 mg/kg q12h | Taper in 10- to 28-day intervals |
| Immune-mediated anemia/thrombocytopenia | Prednisone | 1.0–2.0 mg/kg q12h | Taper in 10- to 28-day intervals |
| Immune-mediated skin disease | Prednisone | 2.2 mg/kg q12h | Treat until remission, then taper slowly to lowest effective dose |
| Neoplasia | Prednisone | 1.0–2.0 mg/kg q12h | Consult chemotherapy protocols |
| Cerebral edema | Dexamethasone | 2.0 mg/kg q6h IV | Use for 24 hr then taper; switch to prednisone PO after 2 to 3 days if needed |
| Hypercalcemia | Prednisone | 1.0–2.0 mg/kg q12h | Taper in 2- to 3-day intervals |
| Shock | Prednisolone sodium succinate | 15.0 mg/kg IV | Give once |
|  | Dexamethasone | 5.0 mg/kg IV | Give once |
| Insulinoma | Prednisone | 0.25 mg/kg q12h | Use 3 to 5 days; increase or decrease as needed to maintain blood glucose |
| Intervertebral disk disease | Prednisone | 0.25–0.5 mg/kg q12h | Use for 2 to 3 days, then daily for 3 to 5 days |
| Spinal cord trauma | Methylprednisolone sodium succinate | 30 mg/kg q6h IV | Use up to 24 hr, then discontinue |
| Glomerulonephritis | Prednisone | 1.0–2.0 mg/kg q12h | Controversial; may not affect course of disease |

*Consult other texts for alternate protocols and for treatment of other disorders (e.g., Plumb, 1991; Serra, 1991).
†Glucocorticoids may be required in combination with other medications in some disorders.
‡Glucocorticoid administered PO unless otherwise stated.

methasone may be beneficial in treatment of certain cases of feline gingivitis-stomatitis that are refractory to prednisone. In cases where a sustained high level of potent steroid for a short period is desirable, such as in cerebral edema or shock, dexamethasone is recommended.

Glucocorticoids are most commonly used for their anti-inflammatory or immunosuppressive effects due to their properties discussed above. In the treatment of neoplastic conditions, glucocorticoids are used as chemotherapy for tumors such as lymphosarcoma, multiple myeloma, or mast cell tumor where the glucocorticoids may affect the tumor cells themselves. Glucocorticoids,

utilized at anti-inflammatory doses, can alleviate the inflammation and concomitant pain associated with many neoplasms. The effects of glucocorticoids on calcium homeostasis allow for their utilization in the treatment of hypercalcemia. This effect of glucocorticoids is transient and only occurs at high dosages (Table 3). Utilization of glucocorticoids in this manner should be initiated only after the cause for the hypercalcemia has been determined. Glucocorticoid use can alter the cytologic properties of lymphocytes and/or can initiate remission of lymphosarcoma, therefore obscuring the diagnosis. Glucocorticoids can be utilized to treat cerebral edema associated with various disorders.

**Table 4.** *Partial List of Other Indications for Glucocorticoid Use*

| System/Disease | Condition | System/Disease | Condition |
|---|---|---|---|
| Allergic disease | Angioneurotic edema | Neoplasia | Central nervous system tumors |
| | Contact or parasite dermatitis | | Leukemia |
| | Drug reactions | | Lymphosarcoma |
| Dermatologic | Feline eosinophilic/granuloma complex | | Mast cell tumor |
| | | | Multiple myeloma |
| | Pyotraumatic dermatitis | Neurologic | Acute trauma |
| Gastrointestinal | Inflammatory bowel disease | | Vestibular disorders |
| | Ulcerative colitis | Ophthalmic | Acute uveitis |
| Multisystemic | Heat stroke | | Choroiditis |
| Musculoskeletal | Polymyositis | | Optic neuritis |
| | Immune-mediated arthritis | Pulmonary | Bronchial asthma |
| | | | Eosinophilic/lymphoid granuloma |
| | | | Inhalation injury |
| | | | Pulmonary eosinophilic infiltrates |

Short-term glucocorticoid therapy can be efficacious for interstitial edema associated with conditions such as neoplasia and hydrocephalus. The efficacy of glucocorticoids in the treatment of trauma or cytotoxic edema is questionable.

The use of glucocorticoids for the treatment of shock has long been advocated but remains controversial. The strongest indication for glucocorticoid use occurs in the setting of septic shock. Glucocorticoids are never recommended as a substitute for fluid therapy and can cause hypotension, so they must be used in combination with volume replacement.

## SELECTION OF A GLUCOCORTICOID AND INDUCTION OF THERAPY

### Short-Term Therapy

Intensive short-term glucocorticoid use can decrease the morbidity and mortality of potentially fatal conditions such as allergic emergencies, shock, severe asthma, central nervous system trauma, and heat stroke in which alleviation of the inflammatory response is of primary concern. Long-acting and potent glucocorticoids, such as dexamethasone, are indicated, because a single dose is commonly all that is required.

### Chronic Glucocorticoid Therapy

As a rule when considering chronic use of glucocorticoids (e.g., for the treatment of immune-mediated or inflammatory diseases), the smallest possible dose that is effective should be administered in the least toxic interval over the shortest time period sufficient to control the disease activity. In order to obtain a remission at the initiation of therapy, anti-inflammatory or immunosuppressive therapy should be instituted at a 12-hr dosing interval (i.e., twice daily) and then the dosing interval lengthened. A given dose of relatively short-acting agents like prednisone is more potent in its anti-inflammatory activity when administered twice daily when compared to once daily. Inflammatory conditions usually require induction doses for 5 to 7 days, whereas 10 to 28 days are required for induction of immunosuppression.

### Tapering the Dose

If an animal has been treated with intensive glucocorticoid therapy for greater than 24 hr, the dose needs to be tapered over several days in order to avoid signs of hypoadrenocorticism upon withdrawal of therapy. In general, the longer an animal remains on the induction dose or the greater the induction dose, the more stepwise and longer the period between dose reduction (Table 5). Tapering schedules vary with the disease being treated. Alternate-day therapy should be instituted when the daily steroid dose is 0.125 to 0.25 mg/kg. Tapering should be performed cautiously and only when the disease is confirmed to be in remission (i.e., stable or rising packed cell volume in immune-mediated anemia, normal joint fluid cytology in immune-mediated polyarthritis, or absence of gastrointestinal

**Table 5.** *Examples of Schedules for Dose Tapering*

| Protocol | Inflammatory Disease | Immune-Mediated Disease |
|---|---|---|
| Induction | 0.25–0.5 mg/kg q12h for 5 to 7 days | 1.0 mg/kg q12h for 10 to 28 days |
| Maintenance | 0.25–0.5 mg/kg q24h for 5 to 7 days | 0.75 mg/kg q12h for 10 to 28 days |
| | | 0.5 mg/kg q12h for 10 to 28 days |
| | | 0.25 mg/kg q12h for 10 to 28 days |
| | | 0.25 mg/kg q24h for 10 to 28 days |
| Withdrawal | 0.5–1.0 mg/kg q.o.d. | 0.25 mg/kg q.o.d. OR 0.5 mg/kg q.o.d for ≥ 21 days |

signs in inflammatory bowel disease). If an immune-mediated disease recrudesces, remission is much more difficult to obtain than previously. If recrudescence occurs, the glucocorticoid dose should be increased immediately to a dose equivalent to or higher than the initial dose utilized, particularly if the disease is life threatening or the clinical signs are severe (e.g., immune-mediated anemia). If remission is lost on an inflammatory disease and continued therapy is indicated or mild clinical signs associated with immune-mediated disease recur, the dose should be increased to the last regimen that kept the animal disease free.

## Alternate-Day Therapy

Every-other-day treatments are used to maintain remission without the side effects of daily or twice-daily treatments such as HPA axis suppression. Instituting therapy with an alternate-day protocol to avoid side effects, however, is inappropriate due to lack of efficacy. When changing to alternate-day therapy, the same daily dose is given every other day (e.g., change from 5 mg every day to 5 mg every other day), which results in a 50% dose reduction, or the total dose is maintained by doubling the daily dose (e.g., change from 5 mg every day to 10 mg every other day) (Table 5). When using glucocorticoids for immunosuppressive therapy, it is best to utilize the latter tapering scheme when moving from daily to alternate-day therapy. Depending upon the individual patient and the disease being treated (e.g., immune-mediated anemia), glucocorticoid therapy may be required for life. If alternate-day therapy is successful in maintaining disease remission, dosing every third day can be attempted.

Alternate-day use of glucocorticoids is only appropriate with the short-acting and certain intermediate-acting forms (Table 2). The duration of adrenal suppression is as long or longer than the half-life of the medication. Even with administration of certain glucocorticoids (e.g., dexamethasone) every 48 hr, the effects of a given dose will overlap with that of subsequent dose and no benefit will be derived from alternate-day administration. If dexamethasone or betamethasone are to be used long term, they should be given at most every 4 days. Methylprednisolone acetate should be reserved for the cat and not given more often than every 14 days.

## Pulse Therapy

An alternative protocol for systemic glucocorticoid use suggested to achieve early remission with minimal side effects is that of pulse therapy. Pulse therapy is the parenteral administration of suprapharmacologic doses of a short-acting glucocorticoid, usually methylprednisolone sodium succinate, for short periods of time (e.g., 3 days) and has been utilized in humans and dogs for the treatment of immune-mediated skin disease (White, Stewart, and Bernstein, 1987). Theoretical

advantages of pulse therapy include immediate symptomatic relief, the avoidance of side effects associated with high-dose oral administration of glucocorticoids, efficacy in patients unresponsive to high-dose oral administration, and the ability to decrease or discontinue glucocorticoid maintenance therapy after pulse therapy is completed. The long-term efficacy of pulse therapy to sustain control of the immune-mediated skin disease on alternate-day maintenance therapy has been questioned. In one study, pulse therapy (methylprednisolone sodium succinate, 11 mg/kg IV once daily for 3 days) was utilized in five dogs with autoimmune skin disease. All five had rapid improvement of their skin lesions but then relapsed on standard maintenance therapy. In spite of their relapses, treatment was ultimately successful in four of the dogs; combination immunosuppressive therapy was required, but the dogs were eventually well controlled without institution of the common immunosuppressive dose (2.2 mg/kg) of prednisone (White, Stewart, and Bernstein, 1987).

While pulse therapy can avoid the more common adverse effects associated with prolonged high-dose oral glucocorticoid use, this regimen is associated with numerous other side effects in humans. The complication rate has been reported to range from "low" to as high as 56% and includes arthralgia, facial swelling, nausea, and osteopenia, among others. Other severe adverse reactions such as sepsis, seizures, pulmonary thromboembolism, and sudden death have also been documented. In the canine, one dog may have experienced arthralgia secondary to this treatment (White, Stewart, and Bernstein, 1987) and, in another case, a permanent diabetes mellitus has been induced (Jeffers, Shanley, and Schick, 1991). In the latter patient, a prediabetic state may have existed prior to glucocorticoid use. Thus, pulse therapy can be used to obtain remission of an immune-mediated skin disease, but it should be reserved for cases that are intolerant to the standard induction protocol (Table 3) and the owners must be advised of the potential adverse effects.

## Repository Therapy

The repository glucocorticoids methylprednisolone acetate and triamcinolone acetonide (Vetalog) can be used for short-term intensive therapy of inflammatory disease in the cat when administration of oral medication is not possible. The repository form is not recommended in the canine. Methylprednisolone acetate should never be given more frequently than every 2 weeks. Use of the repository does not maintain constant blood levels of glucocorticoid, but chronic suppression of the HPA axis will occur. Furthermore, the medication cannot be discontinued if an adverse reaction occurs.

## Topical and Intralesional Therapy

Topical and intralesional therapy can provide high concentrations of a potent glucocorticoid at the disease site while minimizing the systemic effects. Glucocorticoids applied via any route will be absorbed, however, and can lead to adverse results; the more glucocorticoid absorbed, the greater the effects. Absorption from topical sites is increased in human pediatric patients, in the presence of inflammation, and with the use of occlusive wraps. Other factors include the preparation vehicle, concentration of the glucocorticoid, anatomic site, frequency, and size of the area treated. Delivery rate to the tissues increases in the order: ointment, cream, lotion, foam, gel, solution. Fluorinated products should be used short term only, due to their potent effects. Acetonide and valerate esters bind to affected tissue enhancing the glucocorticoid effect, acetate esters are lipid soluble and quickly absorbed, and the succinate and phosphate esters are absorbed less readily.

## POTENTIAL ADVERSE EFFECTS

A multitude of undesirable effects have been associated with glucocorticoid use, although a cause-and-effect relationship has not been proven in all cases (Table 6). These effects can be divided into the alteration of the HPA axis versus nonspecific tissue effects (Plumb, 1991).

All the synthetic glucocorticoids suppress CRH and ACTH secretion, but their effects are not equivalent. In general, the greater the anti-inflammatory capability of the glucocorticoid, the greater the capacity to suppress the HPA axis. If ACTH concentrations remain diminished over time, the adrenal cells that synthesize glucocorticoids atrophy and the responsiveness of the HPA axis is progressively diminished. In most species, adrenal atrophy is generally apparent within 10 days of initiating high-dose glucocorticoid therapy (Melby, 1977). However, cats are more resistant to the nonadrenal effects but not to the adrenosuppressive effects of exogenous glucocorticoids than are dogs.

With loss of adrenal cells, suppression of the HPA axis will persist after treatment is withdrawn. Adrenal atrophy secondary to glucocorticoid administration is reversible. However, adrenocortical insufficiency can become a clinical problem either with sudden withdrawal of glucocorticoid supplementation or if the patient encounters a stressful situation and no longer possesses sufficient adrenocortical reserve to meet physiologic demands. The length of time required for recovery ultimately depends upon the duration and dosage of exogenous steroid use as well as the degree of adrenal atrophy. Return to full function is best assessed by use of the ACTH-stimulation test. Abrupt discontinuation of medication can result in steroid withdrawal syndrome (see "Corticosteroid Withdrawal Syndrome," this volume, p 413).

The rapidity of onset and duration of adrenal suppression secondary to glucocorticoid use should not be underestimated. In dogs, a single intravenous dose of dexamethasone at a dose of 0.01 mg/kg suppressed the HPA axis for 16 hr and 0.1 mg/kg caused decreased adrenal activity for 32 hr (Kemppainen and Sartin, 1984). Systemic effects of glucocorticoids have also been reported with cutaneous, ophthalmic, or otic administration in dogs and with intranasal administration in humans. Administration of 1% prednisolone acetate in both eyes four times daily for 4 weeks in dogs suppressed the HPA axis through 2 weeks beyond discontinuation of treatment (Eichenbaum et al., 1988); cutaneous administration of compounds such as betamethasone can significantly decrease basal levels of cortisol within 7 hr and repeated treatments suppress the HPA axis further (Zenoble and Kemppainen, 1987). Suppression of the HPA axis will be minimal with short-duration use.

Pharmacologic doses of glucocorticoids also affect cells outside the HPA axis. Use of glucocorticoids for greater than 2 weeks can cause adverse results ranging from polyuria/polydipsia and polyphagia to steroid he-

**Table 6.**  *Adverse Effects Associated with the Use of Glucocorticoids*

| System | Effect | System | Effect |
|---|---|---|---|
| Cardiovascular | Hypertension | Host defenses | Immunosuppression |
| | Sodium/water retention° | Metabolic | Hyperlipidemia |
| | Peripheral edema | | Glucose intolerance |
| Cutaneous | Acne/comedones | | Hepatomegaly° |
| | Atrophy of dermis/subcutis° | | Obesity° |
| | Excess bruising | | Polyuria/polydipsia° |
| | Alopecia | | Polyphagia° |
| Endocrine/reproductive | Infertility | Musculoskeletal | Osteoporosis |
| | Iatrogenic hyperadrenocorticism | | Myopathy/muscle weakness |
| | Hypoadrenocorticism (adrenal atrophy) | Nervous system | Behavior changes |
| | | | Peripheral neuropathies |
| | Growth failure | | Seizures |
| | Birth defects | Ocular | Cataracts |
| | Abortion | | Glaucoma |
| Gastrointestinal | Gastric ulceration° | | |
| | Gastric hemorrhage | | |
| | Intestinal perforation | | |
| | Pancreatitis | | |

°Most common.

patopathy and iatrogenic Cushing's syndrome. Glucocorticoids cause insulin resistance and can precipitate diabetes mellitus if a prediabetic state exists. Use of glucocorticoids can facilitate the formation of gastric ulcers. Risk of ulceration is increased in animals with neurologic disease. Due to their effect on sodium retention, use of glucocorticoids can result in hypertension; animals with heart disease may decompensate due to the extra workload on the heart and failure ensues. Potential adverse effects of intensive short-term glucocorticoid use include rare multifocal preventricular contractions, precipitation of ketoacidosis in a diabetic, gastric ulceration, and burning or itching at a muscular injection site.

Glucocorticoids have a definite place in the treatment of numerous diseases. However, their adverse effects must not be discounted. In emergency situations, the more potent long-acting steroids like dexamethasone are desirable. For chronic use, the short-acting and certain intermediate-acting glucocorticoids are preferable. The dose should be tapered and changed to alternate-day therapy as soon as possible, but caution should be taken not to allow recrudescence of a disease.

## References and Suggested Reading

Chastain CB: Use of corticosteroids. *In* Ettinger SJ (ed.): *Textbook of Veterinary Internal Medicine.* Philadelphia, WB Saunders Co, 1989, pp 413–428.
*An excellent and thorough review of the physiology of the HPA axis and the use of glucocorticoids.*

Eichenbaum JD, Macy DW, Severin GA, et al: Effect in large dogs of ophthalmic prednisolone acetate on adrenal gland and hepatic function. J Am Anim Hosp Assoc 24:705, 1988.
*Five adult dogs were treated in both eyes four times a day for 1 month with 1% prednisolone acetate; suppression of the HPA axis was demonstrated during treatment and 2 weeks beyond and abnormal carbohydrate metabolism was exhibited during treatment.*

Jeffers JG, Shanley KJ, and Schick RO: Diabetes mellitus induced in a dog after administration of corticosteroids and methylprednisolone pulse therapy. J Am Vet Med Assoc 199:77, 1991.
*Report of a single dog that developed permanent diabetes mellitus subsequent to glucocorticoid pulse therapy.*

Kemppainen RJ and Sartin JL: Effects of single intravenous doses of dexamethasone on baseline plasma cortisol concentrations and responses to synthetic ACTH in healthy dogs. Am J Vet Res 45:742, 1984.
*Duration of adrenocortical suppression subsequent to a single intravenous injection of different concentrations of dexamethasone was determined in dogs.*

Melby JC: Clinical pharmacology of systemic corticosteroids. Ann Rev Pharmacol Toxicol 17:511, 1977.
*An excellent review of the physiology and effect of glucocorticoids with recommendations on their therapeutic uses.*

Plumb DC: *Veterinary Drug Handbook.* White Bear Lake, PharmaVet Publishing, 1991, pp 324–348.
*An excellent review of the pharmacology of synthetic glucocorticoids including treatment protocols for many disorders for which glucocorticoids are utilized as therapy.*

Serra DA: Glucocorticoid therapy. *In* August JR (ed): *Consultations in Feline Internal Medicine.* Philadelphia, WB Saunders Co, 1991, pp 271–277.
*A thorough discussion of the use of glucocorticoids in cat including recommended doses for certain feline diseases and general recommendations for glucocorticoid use.*

White SD, Stewart LJ, Bernstein M: Corticosteroid (methylprednisolone sodium succinate) pulse therapy in five dogs with autoimmune skin disease. J Am Vet Med Assoc 191:1121, 1987.
*Report on five dogs that received glucocorticoid pulse therapy for autoimmune skin disease.*

Zenoble RD and Kemppainen RJ: Adrenocortical suppression by topically applied corticosteroids in healthy dogs. J Am Vet Med Assoc 191:685, 1987.
*Marked HPA axis suppression of rapid onset but prolonged duration was demonstrated after administration of three topical corticosteroid preparations.*

---

# CORTICOSTEROID WITHDRAWAL SYNDROME

DEBORAH S. GRECO
*and* ELLEN N. BEHREND
*Fort Collins, Colorado*

Corticosteroid withdrawal syndrome is a poorly understood phenomenon that results from acute withdrawal of glucocorticoids. The disorder has been variously termed "steroid pseudorheumatism," "steroid-induced panmesenchymal reaction," or the "steroid withdrawal syndrome" (Fauci, 1985). Both subjective and objective manifestations of adrenal suppression may be observed in steroid withdrawal syndrome. The syndrome was first described in patients suffering from rheumatoid arthritis whose steroid dosage was erratic or who were initially treated with high doses of steroids then rapidly tapered off steroids (Slocumb, 1953). The initial clinical description of the syndrome included fever, musculoskeletal aching, malaise, lupus-like syndromes, hypertension, debility, and emotional lability. Because of the highly emotional and subjective nature of this disorder, corticosteroid withdrawal syndrome is rarely recognized in veterinary patients.

## ETIOLOGY

The etiology of corticosteroid withdrawal syndrome is poorly understood. However, the hallmark of this disorder is the presence of clinical signs attributable to corticosteroid deficiency (hypoglycemia, hypotension) and/or hypothalamic-pituitary-adrenal (HPA) suppression. Some human patients may appear to have psychologic dependence on glucocorticoids based on clinical signs (e.g., depression, weakness) in the absence of any objective evidence of adrenal suppression. Nevertheless, physical dependence may exist in the face of normal HPA function. Tissues may become accustomed to high levels of glucocorticosteroids for such a period of time that the glucocorticoid receptors are "down-regulated." The body perceives rapid glucocorticoid withdrawal as a "relative" deficiency and the patient experiences signs of steroid deprivation. Although most cases of corticosteroid withdrawal syndrome are described in human patients receiving exogenous glucocorticoids, corticosteroid withdrawal syndrome can occur following treatment for hyperadrenocorticism or following endogenous glucocorticoid stimulation by exogenous adrenocorticotrophic hormone (ACTH) (Synacthen) (Rippere, 1989).

Four subgroups of human patients with this syndrome have been recognized: type-I patients are symptomatic and have biochemical evidence of HPA suppression; type-II patients have recrudescence of the disease for which steroids were originally prescribed; type-III patients show dependence upon corticosteroids, either physical or psychologic, normal HPA axis function, and no recrudescence of underlying disease; type-IV patients have biochemical evidence of HPA suppression without symptoms and without recrudescence of underlying disease (Dixon and Christy, 1980).

## CLINICAL FEATURES

Clinical signs of corticosteroid withdrawal syndrome are usually observed immediately after acute withdrawal of corticosteroids or following treatment for hyperadrenocorticism. Clinical features of corticosteroid withdrawal syndrome may include vague or subjective symptoms such as weakness, malaise, and lethargy. In humans, psychologic disturbances, such as depression, are common. Nausea, anorexia, and weight loss are common gastrointestinal signs of corticosteroid withdrawal syndrome. Cardiovascular conditions, such as hypertension or orthostatic hypotension with syncope, may also be observed. The most well-recognized symptoms, however, are those related to "pseudorheumatism" or lupus-like syndromes. Fever, malaise, arthralgia, musculoskeletal aching, fever, and desquamation of the skin are the most common clinical signs of corticosteroid withdrawal syndrome (Slocumb, 1953). Unfortunately, exacerbation of underlying disease (i.e., systemic lupus) may manifest with similar symptoms making it difficult to distinguish from corticosteroid withdrawal syndrome. Type-IV corticosteroid withdrawal syndrome is characterized by the absence of clinical signs attributable to corticosteroid withdrawal.

## DIAGNOSIS

In type-I and -IV corticosteroid withdrawal syndrome, the ACTH-stimulation test can be used to diagnose the disorder; suppression of the HPA axis is demonstrated by a lack of response to exogenous ACTH administration. Type-I patients exhibit signs of corticosteroid dependence and suffer from withdrawal of the drug; in contrast, type-IV patients exhibit no clinical signs of disease and their diagnosis is usually serendipitous. In humans and probably in veterinary patients, type-II and -III corticosteroid withdrawal syndrome will be more difficult to document. Normal HPA axis function is observed as evidenced by adequate stimulation and response to exogenous ACTH administration; however, the patient experiences recrudescence of the disease for which steroids were originally prescribed or exhibits physiologic or psychologic dependence on pharmacologic doses of glucocorticoids.

Many patients with steroid withdrawal syndrome have positive serologic tests for lupus erythematosus including positive antinuclear antibody tests and positive lupus erythematosus cell preparations. This feature can make differentiation of steroid withdrawal syndrome from autoimmune disorder relapse extremely difficult (Hardin, 1973).

Diagnosis is based on characteristic clinical signs, compatible diagnostic tests, and response to treatment with reinstitution of glucocorticoid therapy or an increased dosage of corticosteroids (Dixon and Christy, 1980). Compatible diagnostic tests may vary depending on the type of corticosteroid withdrawal syndrome present. In veterinary patients, type-III steroid withdrawal syndrome would be difficult to diagnose, since animals are not capable of articulating "psychologic" dependence on corticosteroids. Type-I and type-IV corticosteroid withdrawal syndrome can be diagnosed based on subnormal response to ACTH coupled with compatible clinical signs (type I) (Dixon and Christy, 1980). Type-II corticosteroid withdrawal syndrome may be diagnosed in an animal with recrudescence of clinical signs after withdrawal or reduction in steroid dosage and a normal adrenal response to ACTH stimulation.

## TREATMENT

The entire symptom complex may relate to tissue acclimation to high doses of corticosteroids; therefore, replacement therapy with glucocorticoids is indicated in all forms of corticosteroid withdrawal syndrome except type IV. Corticosteroid withdrawal syndrome can be avoided by judicious glucocorticoid therapy; avoidance of high doses and rapid withdrawal is the best prevention. Depending on the type of steroid withdrawal syndrome (types I, II, and III are treated), treatment usually consists of increasing the dosage of glucocorticoids until remission occurs. The increased dosage should be continued for 1 to 2 weeks, at which time the dose may be decreased slowly (25% every 2 weeks) until the desired maintenance dose is achieved. Eventually, alternate-day glucocorticoid therapy is desirable, but in patients with corticosteroid withdrawal syndrome this may not be possible. Some human patients with corticosteroid withdrawal syndrome (particularly type III) require daily doses of corticosteroids, albeit small doses, indefinitely to remain symptom-free (Dixon and Christy, 1980)

## CASE ILLUSTRATIONS

The following case illustrations are included to provide the veterinary clinician with clinical situations that may be suspicious for corticosteroid withdrawal syndrome.

*Type I:* A 4-year-old male castrated golden retriever presents for evaluation of skin disease (flea-allergy dermatitis), lethargy, vomiting, weakness, and stiff gait. The dog has received daily corticosteroids for treatment of the dermatitis since the age of 2 years. The owner discontinued the prednisone (40 mg/day) this morning. Physical examination reveals classic signs of iatrogenic hyperadrenocorticism including calcinosis cutis. An ACTH response test reveals undetectable baseline cortisol and no response to ACTH. This dog shows classic signs of type-I corticosteroid withdrawal syndrome including stiff gait, weakness, lethargy, and gastrointestinal signs. Objective evidence of adrenal suppression is observed. Treatment would consist of reinstitution of glucocorticoid therapy at the same dose that was discontinued (40 mg/day) followed by a slow taper (25% reduction every 2 weeks, every-other-day therapy when dose is <1 mg/kg) until adrenal function becomes normal.

*Type II:* A 5-year-old male collie with systemic lupus erythematosus (SLE) presents with a history of treatment with prednisolone (1 mg/lb every 24 hr) for the last 3 weeks. Clinical signs resolved with the initial dose of steroids; however, when the dose was decreased to 0.5 mg/lb every 24 hr, the dog began to show clinical signs (desquamation of the skin, arthralgia, proteinuria). An ACTH stimulation test reveals a normal response; repeat antinuclear antibody (ANA) titer is positive. Addition of Imuran (1 mg/kg, PO daily) for 4 weeks resulted in no improvement. Improvement was noted only when the prednisolone dosage was increased to 2 mg/lb twice daily. Is this a relapse of SLE or corticosteroid withdrawal syndrome? Probably not a relapse of SLE because of the lack of response to other immunosuppressive agents (e.g., Imuran). The normal adrenal response to ACTH and clinical remission only after increasing the dose of corticosteroids would suggest type-II corticosteroid withdrawal syndrome.

*Type III:* An 11-year-old female spayed cocker spaniel is presented for evaluation of Lysodren therapy of 3 days, duration for pituitary-dependent hyperadrenocorticism. The dog was started on Lysodren at 50 mg/kg divided once daily; however, after only 3 days of therapy, she began to exhibit a stiff gait, anorexia, weakness, and fever. Laboratory parameters were consistent with Cushing's syndrome (increased SAP, hypercholesterolemia) and an ACTH response test revealed a high baseline cortisol (7 μg/dl) and a normal response to ACTH (14 μg/dl). Is this corticosteroid withdrawal syndrome or true Lysodren-induced hypoadrenocorticism? In this case, the normal response to ACTH and the history

of short duration of treatment with Lysodren suggests that this dog is suffering from corticosteroid withdrawal syndrome. Concurrent treatment with Lysodren and prednisone followed by slow tapering of the dose of prednisone should resolve the clinical signs in this dog.

*Type IV:* A 3-year-old female spayed Tibetan terrier is being evaluated for therapy of autoimmune thrombocytopenia. The dog has remained symptom-free since remission following treatment with corticosteroids at immunosuppressive doses. The dog is now receiving 0.25 mg/kg prednisolone once every day. An ACTH response test shows undetectable levels of cortisol and no response to ACTH stimulation. The lack of clinical signs and objective evidence of adrenal suppression is suggestive of type-IV corticosteroid withdrawal syndrome. One might argue that treatment is not necessary because of the lack of clinical signs, but if this dog were to undergo stress (e.g., boarding), an addisonian crisis might ensue. Treatment might consist of reducing the steroid dose further to stimulate endogenous ACTH secretion to stimulate an adrenal response or providing additional steroid therapy during periods of stress.

Although corticosteroid withdrawal syndrome is an unusual syndrome in animals, veterinarians should be aware of clinical situations in which corticosteroid withdrawal syndrome may occur. In particular, animals receiving high doses of glucocorticoids and those with iatrogenic or naturally occurring hyperadrenocorticism are at highest risk of developing corticosteroid withdrawal syndrome. In human patients, corticosteroid withdrawal syndrome is prevented by judicious use of glucocorticoids and by avoiding "self-medication." In veterinary patients, the clinician should prescribe glucocorticoid therapy according to strict therapeutic guidelines. The client must be made aware of the potential side-effects of glucocorticoids, including corticosteroid withdrawal syndrome, and instructed to avoid the indiscriminate administration of glucocorticoids.

## References and Suggested Reading

Dixon RB and Christy NP: On the various forms of corticosteroid withdrawal syndrome. Am J Med 68:224, 1980.
   *Excellent review of corticosteroid withdrawal syndromes in five human patients and discussion of diagnosis and treatment strategies.*
Fauci AS: Glucocorticosteroid therapy. *In* Wygaarden JB, Smith LH (eds): *Cecil Textbook of Medicine.* Philadelphia, WB Saunders Co, 1985, p 111.
   *Concise review of the uses of glucocorticosteroids in humans with guidelines for their utilization.*
Hardin JG: Steroid-induced morbidity mimicking active systemic lupus erythematosus. Ann Intern Med 78:558, 1973.
   *Two clinical examples of steroid pseudorheumatism mimicking SLE in human patients; illustrates the similarity of corticosteroid withdrawal syndrome to SLE.*
Rippere V: Possible steroid withdrawal syndrome following short Synacthen test—a personal report. Med Hypotheses 28:187, 1989.
   *Single case report of corticosteroid withdrawal syndrome following a diagnostic ACTH-stimulation test in a human patient.*
Slocumb CH: Rheumatic complaints during chronic hypercortisonism and syndromes during withdrawal of cortisone in rheumatic patients. Mayo Clin 28:655, 1953.
   *Original description of the clinical syndrome of corticosteroid withdrawal syndrome in human patients.*

# MITOTANE (o,p'-DDD) TREATMENT OF HYPERADRENOCORTICISM IN DOGS

PETER P. KINTZER

*North Grafton, Massachusetts*

*and* MARK E. PETERSON

*New York, New York*

Mitotane (o,p'-DDD; Lysodren, Bristol-Myers Oncology Division) is the drug most commonly used for the treatment of hyperadrenocorticism in dogs. Management of canine pituitary-dependent hyperadrenocorticism with mitotane was first described over 20 years ago (Schecter et al., 1973). Furthermore, protocols to treat canine hyperadrenocorticism resulting from cortisol-secreting adrenocortical neoplasia have recently been reported (Kintzer and Peterson, 1993). The use of mitotane as an adrenocorticolytic agent evolved from the work of Nelson and Woodard who, in the late 1940s, observed that dogs given the insecticide DDD developed severe adrenal cortical necrosis and atrophy. Further investigation (Cuerto and Brown, 1958) demonstrated that the o,p' isomer was primarily responsible for the adrenocorticolytic effect.

## MECHANISM OF ACTION AND PHARMACOLOGY

Mitotane exerts a direct cytotoxic effect on the adrenal cortex, resulting in a selective, progressive necrosis and atrophy of the zonae fasciculata and reticularis. Because the zona glomerulosa is relatively resistant to the cytotoxic effects of mitotane, normal secretion of aldosterone is usually maintained. After conversion to an active metabolite by the P-450 system, mitotane binds to critical mitochondrial macromolecules. This causes destruction of the mitochondria, resulting in cell death and necrosis (Schteingart, 1989). In addition, mitotane interferes with steroid biosynthesis, primarily through inhibition of the 11-$\beta$-hydroxylase and cholesterol side-cleavage enzymes. The exact mechanism by which mitotane impedes steroid hormone synthesis is not known but may be related to inhibition of the glucose-6-phosphate dehydrogenase enzyme or decreased production of reduced triphosphopyridine in the adrenal cortical cells (Gutierrez and Crooke, 1980).

The systemic availability of mitotane administered as intact tablets to fasting dogs is poor. One study demonstrated that the availability of mitotane was improved with an emulsion of the drug in oil, better with intact tablets given in food, and best with ground tablets mixed in oil given in food (Watson, Rijnberk, and Moolenaar, 1987). Furthermore, the availability of intact tablets given with food was significantly greater in dogs with pituitary-dependent hyperadrenocorticism than in normal dogs. Poor absorption of mitotane could contribute to the apparent resistance to the effects of the drug that develops in some dogs with hyperadrenocorticism. Therefore, based on these studies, it is recommended that mitotane be administered with meals; however, crushing the tablets cannot be recommended due to the cytotoxic nature of the drug and the risk of human exposure. Intestinal fat absorption is above normal in dogs with hyperadrenocorticism and decreases after treatment with mitotane (Simpson and Van Der Broek, 1990). Therefore, even if mitotane is given with food, such a decrease in intestinal fat absorption might decrease the availability of mitotane as treatment proceeds.

In dogs, the exact metabolic fate of mitotane is not known. In humans, however, it is well known that mitotane undergoes oxidative biotransformation by the hepatic microsomal enzyme system. It is likely that the disposition of mitotane is similar in dogs, since microsomal oxidation is the most prominent metabolic pathway for lipid-soluble drugs (such as mitotane) in most mammalian species. If this is the case, any drug that stimulates the hepatic microsomal enzyme system would enhance the metabolism of mitotane, resulting in decreased mitotane concentrations and a diminished adrenocorticolytic effect. In accord with that, concurrent administration of phenobarbital, a potent inducer of hepatic microsomal enzymes, can dramatically increase mitotane dosage requirements in dogs being treated for hyperadrenocorticism. Furthermore, mitotane itself may accelerate its own biotransformation through induction of the hepatic microsomal enzyme system; this may partly account for the finding that many dogs will require higher maintenance dosages of mitotane over time.

In human patients, the elimination of mitotane becomes more prolonged after chronic administration (Moolenaar et al., 1981). This results from the gradual liberation of mitotane from adipose tissue where the drug is concentrated. Watson, Rijnberk, and Moolenaar (1987) found a gradual, progressive increase in plasma mitotane concentrations in dogs with pituitary-dependent hyperadrenocorticism given loading doses of mitotane for approximately 14 days. Whether this results from adipose tissue storage of mitotane in the dog has not been determined, but a correlation between mitotane concentrations in plasma and adipose tissue has been documented in human patients treated with the drug (van Slooten et al., 1982).

## TREATMENT OF PITUITARY-DEPENDENT HYPERADRENOCORTICISM

Since the first protocol was described by Schecter et al. in 1973, mitotane has become the drug most frequently used for the treatment of dogs with pituitary-dependent hyperadrenocorticism. We recently evaluated long-term mitotane treatment of pituitary-dependent hyperadrenocorticism in 200 dogs (Kintzer and Peterson, 1991). The results of that study indicated that mitotane is effective and relatively safe for the treatment of pituitary-dependent hyperadrenocorticism in dogs.

The initial induction dosage of mitotane is 40 to 50 mg/kg/day for 7 to 10 days, administered with food. Induction dosages of greater than 50 mg/kg/day are rarely required and will result in a higher incidence of hypoadrenocorticism. Concurrent glucocorticoid supplementation with prednisone or prednisolone (0.2 mg/kg/day) is recommended to mitigate the adverse effects associated with serum cortisol concentrations rapidly falling into the normal or subnormal range during this initial treatment period. In dogs with concomitant insulin-resistant diabetes mellitus (daily insulin requirements >2.2 U/day), a lower initial daily dose of mitotane (25 mg/kg) and a higher daily maintenance dose of prednisone or prednisolone (0.4 mg/kg) are recommended to prevent rapid alterations in daily insulin requirements during the induction period. Most dogs are stronger, less lethargic, and will show at least some resolution of polyuria and polydipsia during the initial induction period.

The efficacy of the initial 7- to 10-day induction period is determined by an adrenocorticotrophic hormone (ACTH) stimulation test. Since prednisone and prednisolone both cross-react in most cortisol assays to falsely elevate serum cortisol concentrations, daily glucocorticoid administration must be discontinued on the morning of ACTH stimulation testing. To ensure adequate control of hyperadrenocorticism, both the basal and post-ACTH serum cortisol concentrations must be lowered into the normal resting range (1 to 4 $\mu$g/dl or 25 to 125 nmol/L). In most dogs with pituitary-dependent hyperadrenocorticism, initial daily mitotane treatment succeeds in decreasing both basal and post-ACTH serum cortisol concentrations into the normal resting range. In about one third of dogs, however, both basal and post-ACTH cortisol concentrations fall to subnormal values (<25 nmol/L) after the initial treatment period. In this situation, mitotane is stopped and glucocorticoid administration continued until serum cortisol concentrations normalize. These low serum cortisol concentrations typically increase spontaneously into the normal resting range within 2 to 6 weeks; however, in a few dogs, levels will remain low for 6 to 18

months without further mitotane. Conversely, about 10 to 15% of dogs still respond to exogenous ACTH with serum cortisol concentrations above the normal resting range (>125 nmol/L) after initial daily mitotane treatment. In these dogs, daily mitotane administration should be continued and ACTH stimulation tests repeated at 7- to 10-day intervals until circulating cortisol concentrations fall into the normal resting range. There is individual sensitivity to mitotane among dogs during the induction period, and the length of daily therapy needed to adequately reduce adrenal reserve can range from 5 days to 2 months.

Once adrenal reserve has been appropriately reduced, mitotane should be continued at a maintenance dosage of 50 mg/kg/week in two to three divided doses. Daily glucocorticoid supplementation is rarely necessary during maintenance mitotane therapy. During periods of stress, however, appropriate dosages of glucocorticoids should be administered. Complete resolution of all clinical signs of hyperadrenocorticism may require up to 6 months in some dogs.

Despite initial control of hyperadrenocorticism, relapses are common during maintenance mitotane therapy, developing in about one half of dogs during the first year of treatment. Several factors may contribute to relapse in these dogs:

1. An initial weekly maintenance dosage of less than 50 mg/kg. Less than a quarter of the dogs in our study could be controlled on a long-term basis on less than 50 mg/kg/week, and very few could be controlled with a weekly dose less than 40 mg/kg (Kintzer and Peterson, 1991).

2. The development of progressively higher circulating ACTH concentrations, which may overwhelm the adrenocorticolytic effect of mitotane and stimulate regeneration of the adrenal cortex. Increased pituitary ACTH secretion occurs as the result of diminished negative feedback due to the decrease in circulating cortisol concentrations.

3. Poor absorption of mitotane may lessen the effects of the drug. As previously mentioned, absorption of mitotane is enhanced when given with a fatty meal. Furthermore, dogs with pituitary-dependent hyperadrenocorticism demonstrate higher-than-normal intestinal fat absorption that normalizes after mitotane therapy; mitotane absorption, therefore, may fall as treatment proceeds.

4. Increased clearance of mitotane leading to lower serum mitotane concentration may contribute to apparent resistance to the drug. Drugs (e.g., phenobarbital) that induce the hepatic microsomal enzyme system may accelerate the biotransformation of mitotane. In addition, mitotane itself may induce the hepatic microsomal enzymes responsible for its degradation. Overall, the resulting fall in mitotane concentrations would decrease the adrenocorticolytic effects of the drug.

The effectiveness of maintenance mitotane therapy should be monitored with an ACTH-stimulation test at

1, 3, and 6 months of therapy and every 6 months thereafter. Should the basal or post-ACTH serum cortisol concentrations increase above the normal resting range, daily mitotane should be reinstituted at 40 to 50 mg/kg for 5 days. Once circulating cortisol values have been appropriately reduced to within normal resting range, the weekly maintenance dosage should be increased by approximately 50%. As a result of repeated relapse, maintenance dosages as high as 300 mg/kg/wk may be necessary to control signs of hyperadrenocorticism in some dogs (Kintzer and Peterson, 1991).

Side effects are relatively common and should be expected when mitotane is administered. The adverse effects most commonly observed include lethargy, weakness, anorexia, vomiting, diarrhea, and ataxia. About one quarter of dogs develop one or more of these problems during the initial period of daily mitotane administration, but they are relatively mild in most dogs. These adverse effects develop as serum cortisol concentrations fall rapidly to normal or subnormal levels (glucocorticoid withdrawal) and typically resolve rapidly when mitotane is discontinued and glucocorticoid supplementation increased. When side effects develop during the initial induction period, mitotane should be discontinued and the glucocorticoid dosage doubled until the dog can be evaluated. Persistence of problems longer than a few hours after increasing the glucocorticoid dosage usually signifies another medical problem.

Likewise, mild adverse reactions occur in almost one third of dogs during maintenance mitotane therapy, and usually develop shortly after beginning maintenance therapy or during relapses when daily therapy is reinstituted. Again, the development of side effects is associated with subnormal circulating cortisol concentrations in most cases. If side effects occur during maintenance therapy, mitotane should be discontinued and glucocorticoid supplementation administered. Should adverse signs persist for longer than a few hours after administration of glucocorticoid, the dog should be evaluated as soon as possible to exclude other disorders, including mineralocorticoid insufficiency. In most cases, it will be necessary to resume maintenance mitotane therapy in 2 to 8 weeks as determined by ACTH-stimulation test results and clinical signs.

The most serious side effect associated with mitotane administration is complete glucocorticoid and mineralocorticoid insufficiency (Addison's disease), developing in about 5% of dogs during maintenance therapy. Although it can occur at anytime during maintenance therapy, iatrogenic Addison's disease is most likely to develop during the first year of treatment. Unfortunately, it does not seem to be possible to predict which dogs will develop Addison's disease; in our study, we found no difference in the maintenance dosages of mitotane between those dogs that developed complete adrenocortical insufficiency and those that did not (Kintzer and Peterson, 1991). In general, Addison's disease should be suspected if a dog developing side effects during mitotane therapy does not promptly respond to glucocorticoid supplementation. Iatrogenic

Addison's disease is confirmed in these dogs by ACTH-stimulation testing (i.e., undetectable serum cortisol concentrations) and serum electrolyte determinations (i.e., hyperkalemia and hyponatremia). If Addison's disease does develop, mitotane is discontinued and appropriate supplementation with glucocorticoid and fludrocortisone acetate instituted immediately. In our experience, dogs developing iatrogenic adrenal insufficiency require glucocorticoid and mineralocorticoid replacement therapy for the remainder of their lives; therefore, further mitotane administration is usually unnecessary.

## TREATMENT OF ADRENAL-DEPENDENT HYPERADRENOCORTICISM

Surgical excision is the treatment of choice of a unilateral adrenocortical tumor, since a complete cure is attainable. Surgical adrenalectomy, however, is a difficult procedure associated with a high rate of intraoperative and postoperative complications, including death. Furthermore, approximately half of these tumors are malignant, and many are not completely resectable. In addition, gross metastatic disease may be evident by radiography, computed tomography, ultrasonography, or at exploratory laparotomy. Finally, the dog may be an unacceptable anesthetic or surgical risk, or the owner may refuse surgery.

Mitotane is considered the treatment of choice for nonresectable or recurrent adrenocortical carcinoma, at least in human beings. Mitotane is of limited effectiveness in most dogs with cortisol-secreting adrenal tumors when administered at dosages used to treat dogs with pituitary-dependent hyperadrenocorticism (Feldman et al., 1992). We recently reported the results of a study of the effectiveness and safety of higher doses of mitotane administered for long periods in 32 dogs with adrenal tumors (Kintzer and Peterson, 1993). Overall, that study demonstrates that medical adrenalectomy with mitotane is an effective and relatively safe therapeutic alternative for most dogs with cortisol-secreting adrenocortical tumors.

When treating dogs with adrenocortical neoplasia, mitotane should be employed as a true chemotherapeutic agent, with the goal being the destruction of all tumor tissue (as indicated by undetectable basal and post-ACTH serum cortisol concentrations). Although complete destruction of neoplastic adrenocortical tissue is unnecessary in the treatment of adrenal adenomas, most dogs will either have known adrenal carcinoma or have not been surgically explored (and therefore have a 50% chance of having adrenal carcinoma). Thus, the induction of overt hypoadrenocorticism is not discouraged in these dogs and may well improve long-term prognosis. Unfortunately, the development of direct mitotane toxicity limits the induction of complete adrenocortical insufficiency and precludes use of this approach in many dogs.

Initially, mitotane should be given at a dosage of 50

to 75 mg/kg day for 10 to 14 days. Concurrent prednisone supplementation at 0.2 mg/kg/day is indicated throughout the period of mitotane administration. At the completion of this initial period of daily therapy, an ACTH-response test is performed. Glucocorticoid supplementation must be withheld on the morning of the test to avoid interference with the cortisol assay. Although not correlated with tumor response in all dogs, serum cortisol determinations are a practical and relatively reliable means of assessing response to therapy, with the therapeutic objective being undetectable to low concentrations of both basal and post-ACTH serum cortisol values (<25 nmol/L). Should serum cortisol concentrations decrease but remain within or above the normal resting range, daily mitotane is continued (50 to 75 mg/kg/day) and ACTH-response testing repeated every 10 to 14 days until serum cortisol concentrations fall below normal.

If this initial daily dose is essentially ineffective and the serum cortisol response to ACTH remains unchanged from pretreatment values, the daily dosage of mitotane should be increased by 50-mg/kg/day increments every 10 to 14 days until serum cortisol concentrations decrease or drug intolerance develops. In these dogs, daily mitotane is continued at the dosage at which some response was seen or at the highest tolerated dosage, and ACTH-stimulation testing is continued at 10- to 14-day intervals until circulating cortisol concentrations fall below the normal resting range. Dogs with adrenal tumors require higher daily induction dosages of mitotane than those generally needed by dogs with pituitary-dependent hyperadrenocorticism (Table 1). More importantly, a longer period of induction (>2 weeks) will be necessary in about half of the dogs to satisfactorily decrease serum cortisol concentrations. In dogs with pituitary-dependent hyperadrenocorticism, the cumulative induction dose of mitotane is usually 400 to 500 mg/kg (e.g., 50 mg/kg/day for 10 days equals a cumulative dose of 500 mg/kg), whereas we found that dogs with adrenal tumors often require a cumulative induction dose up to ten times higher (Kintzer and Peterson, 1993).

Once undetectable to low-normal serum cortisol concentrations are documented, an initial maintenance mitotane dose of 75 to 100 mg/kg/week in divided doses together with daily maintenance glucocorticoid supplementation are recommended. To ensure that serum cortisol concentrations remain suppressed to desired levels, an ACTH-stimulation test should be repeated 1 to 2 months after initiation of maintenance therapy. If basal and post-ACTH serum cortisol concentrations remain at low to undetectable levels, the original maintenance mitotane dose should be continued. If serum cortisol concentrations rise into the normal resting range (25 to 125 nmol/L), however, the weekly maintenance dose should be increased by 50%. If basal or post-ACTH serum cortisol concentrations rise above normal resting range (>125 nmol/L), daily mitotane treatment is reinstituted at 50 to 100 mg/kg/day until cortisol concentrations fall to low or undetectable values; the weekly maintenance dose is then increased by 50%. Such dosage adjustments are followed by repeat ACTH-stimulation testing in 1 month to ensure an adequate response to the new maintenance dose.

Subsequent dosage adjustments are based on periodic ACTH stimulation tests at 3- to 6-month intervals, as well as the dog's tolerance of the medication itself. Relapses are not uncommon and can be expected in 50 to 70% of dogs during maintenance mitotane therapy. Although a too-low initial mitotane dosage is an obvious reason, continued adrenal tumor growth or metastasis or both will contribute to relapse in some dogs. For the most part, dogs with known metastatic disease will not be as well controlled on a long-term basis as dogs without evidence of metastasis, presumably because of progression of disease.

In general, dogs with adrenal tumors require higher maintenance dosages of mitotane than those needed by dogs with pituitary-dependent hyperadrenocorticism (Table 1). We have found the mean final maintenance dosage of dogs with adrenal tumors to be almost double the final maintenance dosage required in dogs with pituitary-dependent hyperadrenocorticism (Kintzer and Peterson, 1991; Kintzer and Peterson, 1993). About 25% of dogs with adrenal tumors can be expected to need a maintenance dose of over 150 mg/kg, a dose necessary in only about 5% of dogs with pituitary-dependent hyperadrenocorticism. Moreover, some dogs would be given even higher doses of mitotane in an attempt to control clinical signs or tumor growth except that adverse reactions became a limiting factor. Some dogs will, however, respond to mitotane dosages used to treat pituitary-dependent hyperadrenocorticism. Of the 32 dogs we studied, six (18.8%) were treated successfully with the protocol most commonly recom-

***Table 1.*** *Guidelines for Use of Mitotane in the Treatment of Hyperadrenocorticism in Dogs**

| Cause of Hyperadrenocorticism | Initial Daily Dose | Initial Maintenance Dose |
|---|---|---|
| Pituitary dependent | 40–50 mg/kg/day until serum cortisol concentrations in normal resting range (generally 7–10 days) | 50 mg/kg/wk (in divided doses) |
| Adrenal dependent | 50–75 mg/kg/day until cortisols low to undetectable; dosage increased until effective or to highest tolerated (may take 3–6 weeks or longer) | 75–100 mg/kg/wk (in divided doses) |

*See text for specific details regarding dosage adjustments and monitoring of therapy.

mended for pituitary-dependent hyperadrenocorticism (i.e., induction dosage of 40 to 50 mg/kg/day for 7 to 10 days, followed by maintenance dosage of 50 mg/kg/wk). Most dogs that respond to these comparatively low dosages of mitotane probably have either an adenoma or small carcinoma without widespread metastasis. Although a decrease of serum cortisol concentrations into or below the normal resting range indicates successful control of disease, we have seen some dogs nevertheless still succumb to tumor progression. Such progression is presumably due to drug-resistant nonfunctional neoplastic cells.

Adverse effects, including anorexia, lethargy, weakness, and diarrhea, develop in about 60% of dogs with adrenal tumors treated with mitotane. In some cases, adverse reactions result from the development of subnormal serum cortisol concentrations, as has been reported in dogs with pituitary-dependent hyperadrenocorticism overtreated with mitotane. In about half of the dogs, however, these adverse reactions result from a direct drug toxicity independent of mitotane's effect on cortisol secretion. In such cases, side effects do not appear to be related to low circulating cortisol concentrations for the following reasons: (1) the dogs are receiving at least maintenance daily glucocorticoid supplementation, (2) no resolution in adverse signs occurs when the glucocorticoid dose is increased, and (3) post-ACTH cortisol concentrations are not low when adverse effects develop. Moreover, a similar drug reaction develops in up to 80% of human patients with adrenal carcinoma treated with large dosages of mitotane.

If severe side effects occur, mitotane should be stopped, glucocorticoid supplementation continued, and the dog reevaluated as soon as possible to exclude glucocorticoid and mineralocorticoid deficiency (i.e., one should perform an ACTH-stimulation test and serum electrolyte determinations). In dogs with normal serum electrolyte concentrations and subnormal serum cortisol concentrations, the daily glucocorticoid supplementation is increased (to 0.4 mg/kg/day) to exclude cortisol deficiency as the cause of the adverse side effects. If the adverse side effects recur when maintenance mitotane is reinstituted despite such an increase in daily glucocorticoid dosage, a direct drug toxicity is likely. In dogs suspected of suffering such direct drug toxicity, maintenance mitotane is reinstituted at a 25 to 50% lower dose after signs of toxicity have resolved. As a result, cortisol concentrations will usually rise to within or above the normal resting range on repeat ACTH-stimulation testing. The resting and post-ACTH cortisol concentrations must, however, be kept in the normal resting range to prevent recurrence of signs of hyperadrenocorticism. Reinstitution of the higher weekly maintenance dosage can be attempted at a later date; unfortunately, recurrence of adverse signs is likely.

Complete glucocorticoid and mineralocorticoid deficiency (Addison's disease), although rare, can develop in some dogs with adrenal tumors given high doses of mitotane. If iatrogenic Addison's disease does develop, one should discontinue mitotane and institute appropriate supplementation with glucocorticoid and mineralocorticoid (e.g., fludrocortisone acetate or desoxy-corticosterone pivalate) therapy. Additional mitotane is not necessary unless hypoadrenocorticism resolves and cortisol concentrations again increase into or above normal resting range. Unfortunately, one cannot predict in which dogs Addison's disease will occur. A high maintenance mitotane dosage and, likewise, whether the tumor is benign or malignant are not unequivocal portents of the development of Addison's disease. We have treated one dog with adrenal carcinoma that had pulmonary metastases that resolved after administration of mitotane and subsequent development of adrenal insufficiency. Iatrogenic Addison's disease is not undesirable and, in fact, may enhance the dog's long-term prognosis, since all functional neoplastic adrenocortical tissue (as well as any remaining normal adrenal tissue) has probably been destroyed.

## References and Suggested Reading

Cuerto C and Brown JH: Biological studies on an adrenocorticolytic agent and the isolation of the active components. Endocrinology. 62:334, 1958.
*Describes isolation of o,p'-DDD as the active agent responsible for the adrenocorticolytic effect of DDD in dogs.*

Feldman EC, Nelson RW, Feldman MS, et al: Comparison of mitotane treatment for adrenal tumor versus pituitary-dependent hyperadrenocorticism in dogs. J Am Vet Med Assoc 200:1642, 1992.
*Study demonstrates that dogs with adrenocortical tumors are typically more resistant to adrenocorticolytic effects of mitotane.*

Gutierrez ML and Crooke ST: Mitotane (o,p'-DDD). Cancer Treat Rev 7: 49, 1980.
*Good review of mitotane therapy of adrenocortical tumors in human patients.*

Kintzer PP and Peterson ME: Mitotane (o,p'-DDD) treatment of 200 dogs with pituitary-dependent hyperadrenocorticism. J Vet Intern Med 15:182, 1991.
*Evaluation of mitotane therapy in a large series of dogs with pituitary-dependent hyperadrenocorticism.*

Kintzer PP and Peterson ME: Mitotane (o,p'-DDD) treatment of togs with cortisol-secreting adrenocortical neoplasia: 32 cases (1980–1992). J Am Vet Med Assoc 205:54, 1994.
*Study that demonstrates that mitotane is fairly successful in controlling hyperadrenocorticism in dogs with adrenocortical tumor if high dosages are employed.*

Moolenaar AJ, van Slooten H, van Seters AP and Smeenk D: Blood levels of o,p'-DDD following administration in various vehicles after a single dose and during long-term treatment. Cancer Chemother Pharmacol 7:51, 1981.
*Good study of pharmacokinetics of mitotane in human patients.*

Nelson AA and Woodard G: Severe adrenal cortical atrophy (cytotoxic) and hepatic damage produced in dogs by feeding 2,2 bis (parachlorophenyl)-1,1-dichloroethane (DDD or TDE). Arch Pathol 48:387, 1949.
*First study that demonstrates the adrenocorticolytic effect of DDD in dogs.*

Schecter RD, Stabenfeldt GH, Gribble DH, et al: Treatment of Cushing's syndrome in the dog with an adrenocorticolytic agent (o.p'-DDD). J Am Vet Med Assoc 162:629, 1973.
*First report of use of mitotane treatment in dogs with hyperadrenocorticism.*

Schteingart DE: Cushings syndrome. Endocrinol Metab Clin North Am 18: 311, 1989.
*Good review paper concerning the diagnosis and management of adrenocortical tumors in human patients.*

Simpson JW and Van Den Broek AHM: Assessment of fat absorption in normal dogs and in dogs with hyperadrenocorticism. Res Vet Sci 48:38, 1990.
*Study demonstrates that fat absorption is increased in dogs with hyperadrenocorticism.*

van Slooten H, van Seters AP, Smeenk D, and Moolenaar AJ: o,p'-DDD (mitotane) levels in plasma and tissues during chemotherapy and at autopsy. Cancer Chemother and Pharmacol 9:85, 1982.
*Measurement of drug concentrations of mitotane in various tissue in human patients.*

Watson ADJ, Rijnberk A and Moolenaar AJ: Systemic availability of o,p'-DDD in normal dogs, fasted and fed, and in dogs with hyperadrenocorticism. Res Vet Sci 43:160, 1987.
*Study demonstrates that administration of mitotane with food enhances absorption of the drug in dogs.*

# ALTERNATIVES IN THE TREATMENT OF HYPERADRENOCORTICISM IN DOGS AND CATS

DAVID S. BRUYETTE

*Manhattan, Kansas*

While o,p'-DDD (mitotane [Lysodren]) and keto-conazole (Nizoral) are the most commonly used med-ications in the medical management of hyperadreno-corticism, a number of other treatment options exist or are on the horizon. These treatments are directed at a number of different sites involved in the regulation of the hypothalamic-pituitary-adrenal (HPA) axis. Poten-tial sites for medical intervention include drugs that affect the hypothalamus or pituitary, adrenal gland, or peripheral glucocorticoid receptors. To date, there is only limited clinical experience with most of the med-ications to be discussed. With some drugs, clinical trials are currently underway. Prior to using any of these al-ternative therapies, consultation with a veterinary en-docrinologist is recommended.

## DRUGS THAT ACT ON THE HYPOTHALAMIC-PITUITARY-ADRENAL AXIS

Pituitary-dependent hyperadrenocorticism (PDH) is by the far the most common cause of hyperadrenocor-ticism, and accounts for approximately 90% of all cases in dogs. Although the underlying pathophysiology of hyperadrenocorticism is unknown, a number of poten-tial etiologies exist. Alterations in hypothalamic neuro-transmitter concentration (e.g., dopamine depletion), decreased glucocorticoid receptor concentration, and the occurrence of somatic mutations leading to the de-velopment of pituitary adenomas may either singly or in combination result in pituitary hypersecretion of ad-renocorticotrophic hormone (ACTH). Little is known regarding the etiology of functional adrenal neoplasia leading to ACTH-independent hyperadrenocorticism. Adrenal neoplasia accounts for approximately 10% of cases of spontaneous hyperadrenocorticism in dogs and cats.

Several drugs may result in amelioration of the clin-ical signs and laboratory abnormalities associated with PDH by attempting to modulate the HPA axis. They include bromocriptine, cyproheptadine, and l-deprenyl.

## Bromocriptine

Bromocriptine (Parlodel) is a dopamine agonist used in the treatment of human patients with prolactin-se-creting and growth hormone–secreting pituitary tu-mors, as well as Parkinson's disease. Several lines of evidence point to the possibility of hypothalamic do-pamine depletion resulting in ACTH hypersecretion and the development of PDH (see discussion below, l-deprenyl). Dopamine concentrations are decreased in some dogs and human patients with PDH, and treat-ment with oral dopamine agonists (in humans and dogs) and dopamine infusion (in horses) has been ben-eficial in some patients with PDH.

The utility of bromocriptine therapy has been dem-onstrated in some human patients with PDH. In one study, treatment with bromocriptine resulted in a fall in ACTH and cortisol concentrations and remission of clinical signs in over 80% of patients with PDH or Nel-son's syndrome (Lamberts et al., 1980). Response to treatment may occur as the result of either dopami-nergic influences or a direct effect of bromocriptine on the pituitary. Other studies, however, have shown treat-ment with bromocriptine to be of only minimal efficacy, even when bromocriptine response tests were utilized before treatment to identify those patients most likely to respond.

Bromocriptine has been evaluated in normal dogs and dogs with PDH with doses ranging from 0.01 to 0.1 mg/kg either as a single daily treatment or in di-vided doses (Peterson and Drucker, 1981; Rijnberk et al., 1988). The overall efficacy has been low, partly due to unwanted side effects including vomiting, anorexia, and behavioral changes. However, an occasional dog with PDH will respond to the drug with remission of clinical signs and normalization of low-dose dexame-thasone suppression tests. The use of bromocriptine seems to be of limited value in the dog because of the development of side effects. No experience with the use of this agent in cats has been reported.

## Cyproheptadine

Cyproheptadine (Periactin) is an antiserotonin drug with antihistamine and anticholinergic effects. Seroto-nin has been speculated to play a role in the regulation of corticotropin-releasing hormone (CRH) or ACTH release, and may be effective in patients with PDH secondary to an abnormality in serotonin metabolism or turnover. Currently, it is not possible to identify this subset of patients prior to treatment with cyproheptadine, and the number of patients with PDH as the result of a serotonin abnormality is probably fairly small.

Cyproheptadine has been effective, however, in the management of some humans and dogs with PDH. In humans, successful treatment is accompanied by a return of cortisol secretion to normal and restoration of normal cortisol suppression by dexamethasone; relapse of the disease occurs soon after withdrawal of cyproheptadine treatment in such patients. In humans, a few months may be required in order to obtain maximal benefit, so its use may not be acceptable in patients requiring more rapid correction of their hypercortisolemia.

In dogs, cyproheptadine doses ranging from 0.3 to 3.0 mg/kg day have resulted in complete and partial clinical and biochemical responses in less than 10% of cases with PDH (Peterson and Drucker, 1978; Peterson and Drucker, 1981). The major side-effect of cyproheptadine in dogs is polyphagia. The use of cyproheptadine appears to warrant further investigation. No information exists regarding its use in cats with PDH.

### l-Deprenyl

l-Deprenyl (Eldepryl) is a selective monoamine oxidase type B (MAO-B) inhibitor that is currently approved for the treatment of Parkinson's disease in humans. In addition, l-deprenyl may also affect presynaptic reuptake of dopamine and have a neuroprotective effect. Inhibition of MAO-B leads to increased concentrations of dopamine in the nigrostriatal area and partial to complete amelioration of the symptoms of Parkinson's disease.

There are several reasons why dopamine depletion and monoamine oxidase inhibitors may play a role in the pathogenesis and treatment of PDH. First, dopamine concentrations are decreased in some dogs and human patients with PDH. Second, PDH is a geriatric disease, and it is known that the concentration of MAO-B increases with age. Together, these events lead to further functional dopamine depletion. Lastly, as described in the section on bromocriptine, treatment with oral dopamine agonists or dopamine infusion has been beneficial in some patients with PDH.

Dopamine affects the HPA axis primarily through tonic inhibition of ACTH release from the pars intermedia, as well as indirectly affecting ACTH secretion from the pars distalis. Based on previous studies, approximately 30% of dogs with PDH have adenomas or adenomatous hyperplasia that arise in the pars intermedia; therefore, monoamine oxidase inhibitors might be effective in restoring the role of dopamine to inhibit the oversecretion of ACTH in these dogs. In addition, it appears that dopamine depletion also plays a role in enhancing CRH-mediated ACTH release from the pars distalis. This suggests that central nervous system (CNS) dopamine depletion can increase ACTH secretion from either the pituitary pars intermedia or pars distalis, and that dopamine depletion may play a role

in the pathogenesis of at least some cases of PDH in dogs.

In normal dogs, chronic daily oral administration of l-deprenyl has been shown to effectively and irreversibly inhibit MAO-B activity without the development of adverse side effects. Treatment with l-deprenyl at the dosage of 2 mg/kg/day has recently been reported to be effective in a preliminary study of dogs with PDH (Bruyette, Ruehl, and Smidberg, 1993). In that study, five of seven dogs with PDH showed improvement of clinical signs and normalization of low-dose dexamethasone suppression tests. Of the seven dogs, two have remained normal while receiving treatment for longer than 18 months. In addition, recent dose-titration studies have indicated that 1 mg/kg/day may be equally effective in the treatment of canine PDH. No adverse side effects have been noted in any of the dogs with PDH treated with l-deprenyl. A large multicenter clinical trial is currently underway in Canada and the United States. Currently, no data are available on the efficacy or safety of l-deprenyl therapy in cats.

### DRUGS THAT ACT ON THE ADRENAL GLAND

Several medications are currently available that interfere with adrenal steroid synthesis, either through transient enzyme inhibition or a direct adrenolytic effect. These drugs include metyrapone, aminoglutethimide, trilostane, etomidate, and suramin. Most of these drugs have been evaluated in normal dogs and humans, as well as in patients with PDH and functional adrenal neoplasia. Experience in dogs or cats with hyperadrenocorticism has been limited.

### Metyrapone

Metyrapone (Metopirone) reduces cortisol concentrations by inhibiting the action of the adrenocortical enzyme $11\beta$-hydroxylase, thus blocking the conversion of 11-deoxycortisol to cortisol. A reciprocal rise in plasma ACTH concentrations occurs as circulating cortisol concentrations are lowered.

Metyrapone has been effectively used in humans to treat hyperadrenocorticism secondary to functional adrenal neoplasia, ectopic ACTH syndrome, and PDH (Verhelst et al., 1991). Efficacy rates of 70 to 80% have been reported in both the short and long term, especially with respect to amelioration of the clinical signs of hypercortisolemia. Use of the drug can improve the quality of life of patients with adrenal carcinoma or the ectopic ACTH syndrome, conditions where the long-term prognosis is generally very poor. The effectiveness of metyrapone for long-term management in humans is reduced by the rise in plasma ACTH concentrations that occurs after administration of metyrapone, which eventually overrides the enzymatic block and results in the return of clinical signs of hyperadrenocorticism. Successful long-term management of patients with

PDH has been obtained in conjunction with pituitary irradiation.

To date no information exists on the use of metyrapone in the management of hyperadrenocorticism in dogs, although limited information is available for the cat. In a recent report describing the successful use of metyrapone in a diabetic cat with severe cutaneous lesions (Daley et al., 1993), signs of glucocorticoid insufficiency developed after treatment with metyrapone (65 mg/kg PO every 8 hr) for 2 days, and the cat was treated with injectable glucocorticoids. The cat improved rapidly, and the dose of metyrapone was reduced (65 mg/kg PO every 12 hr). Serum cortisol response to exogenous ACTH administration was greatly reduced after 5 days of metyrapone treatment. During drug treatment, the skin lesions had markedly improved, and the cat subsequently underwent successful bilateral adrenalectomy.

Two of three other cats reported in the literature also showed clinical improvement during metyrapone treatment, although the follow-up periods were short. The use of metyrapone in the cat at doses of 65 mg/kg every 8 to 12 hr appears to be effective, at least in some cases. It remains to be seen whether long-term therapy will be successful in controlling hyperadrenocorticism, or if loss of adrenal blockade secondary to rising circulating ACTH concentrations will prevent its long-term effectiveness, as occurs in humans. Use of metyrapone in the short term may allow for rapid correction of hyperadrenocorticism and its complications prior to considering adrenalectomy.

## Aminoglutethimide

Aminoglutethimide (Cytadren) reduces cortisol concentrations by inhibiting the cholesterol side-chain cleavage enzyme, which is the first step in the synthesis of adrenal steroids from cholesterol. In human patients, its use has been reported in both the management of PDH and adrenal carcinoma. Like metyrapone, it does not produce a sustained decrease in cortisol secretion because of the compensatory increase in circulating ACTH concentrations. The combination of aminoglutethimide and metyrapone may be more effective in some patients, presumably through enhanced adrenal blockade. As with metyrapone, combination treatment with aminoglutethimide in combination with pituitary irradiation may increase its long-term effectiveness.

Aminoglutethimide has not been evaluated in the management of hyperadrenocorticism in dogs or cats. Administration of aminoglutethimide to normal dogs, however, does result in suppression of both adrenal and testicular steroid hormones, and no side effects have been reported (LaCoste et al., 1989). The blockade of androgen synthesis is incomplete, however, and the combination of ketoconazole and aminoglutethimide is more effective in lowering sex steroid concentrations. The use of aminoglutethimide in dogs with hyperadrenocorticism requires further investigation. No information is available regarding its use in cats.

## Trilostane

Trilostane (Modrastane) has been shown to inhibit adrenal, ovarian, and placental steroid synthesis in a number of species. It appears to act by competitive inhibition of 3β-hydroxysteroid dehydrogenase, leading ultimately to decreased synthesis of cortisol. The drug has been used in the management of PDH and functional adrenal neoplasia in humans. Results have been inconsistent, with some patients exhibiting only partial enzyme inhibition and little or no improvement in clinical signs (Dewis et al., 1983). Like the other drugs that act to block adrenal steroid synthesis, plasma ACTH concentrations increase following successful treatment with trilostane, so adjunct therapy with pituitary irradiation may be necessary to obtain complete remission. The use of trilostane appears to be well tolerated with few side-effects. Currently, no information is available regarding its efficacy in dogs or cats with hyperadrenocorticism.

## Etomidate

Etomidate (Amidate), an imidazole derivative, is an ultra-short-acting hypnotic agent used to induce general anesthesia and to maintain sedation in critical care patients. Etomidate also inhibits the normal increase in plasma cortisol and aldosterone that occurs during surgical stress. Adrenal suppression occurs for 1 to 6 hr following a bolus injection of etomidate, with maximal suppression 3 to 4 hr after induction of general anesthesia. In vitro, etomidate directly inhibits adrenal steroidogenesis by inhibiting the cholesterol side-chain cleavage enzyme and 11β-hydroxylase. Several reports have highlighted the potential role of adrenal suppression that may develop after etomidate administration, thereby contributing to patient morbidity and mortality. Constant low-dose infusions have been used in the short-term successful management of human patients with severe psychologic manifestations of hyperadrenocorticism, but long-term administration has not been reported.

In the dog, etomidate given as an intravenous bolus (2 mg/kg) for the induction of general anesthesia results in marked adrenal suppression for 2 to 6 hr. When compared with barbiturates for induction of general anesthesia, etomidate causes a greater decrease in basal cortisol concentrations and also results in a blunted cortisol response to exogenous ACTH administration within 2 hr of induction of anesthesia. However, despite the suppressive effects of etomidate on cortisol secretion, serum cortisol concentrations (basal and post-ACTH administration) increased after induction of anesthesia and no adverse cardiovascular changes were noted, indicating that etomidate is generally a safe agent for induction of general anesthesia (Dodam et al., 1990).

Because of the suppressive effects of etomidate on adrenal steroidogenesis, etomidate may be beneficial in the short-term management of the dog with hyperadrenocorticism, especially if administered in doses that do not induce general anesthesia. The effects of etomidate need to be evaluated both in normal dogs and dogs with hyperadrenocorticism. The effects of etomidate on cortisol secretion have not been evaluated in either normal cats or cats with hyperadrenocorticism.

### Suramin

Suramin (Germanin) has been used as an antitrypanosomal drug in humans since the 1920's. Recent studies have shown that suramin is an inhibitor if reverse transcriptase, and several investigators have evaluated the efficacy of the drug in patients infected with human immunodeficiency virus (HIV). In addition, suramin appears to inhibit a variety of growth factors, suggesting that it might be an effective chemotherapeutic agent for certain types of cancer. Reports of adrenal insufficiency have been reported in human patients undergoing treatment with high doses (550 to 830 mg/m$^2$) of suramin. Its mechanism of action with respect to adrenal dysfunction is unknown.

In one study, cynomolgus monkeys were treated with high doses of suramin for 5 weeks. Treated animals had a progressive decrease in adrenal reserve, with an increase in circulating ACTH concentrations. Serum electrolyte values remained within the reference range. Histopathologic examination of the adrenal glands revealed a diffuse inflammatory cell infiltrate and thinning of the zona glomerulosa and zona fasciculata (Feuillan et al., 1987).

In humans, use of suramin for patients with adrenocortical carcinoma and Cushing's disease is currently undergoing clinical trials. A few reports of complete or partial responses to suramin have been reported in patients with metastatic adrenocortical carcinoma (La-Rocca et al., 1990).

Suramin has been used in both dogs and cats with nonadrenal disease (i.e., trypanosomiasis, benign prostatic hyperplasia, feline leukemia virus [FeLV]-related disease), and minimal toxicity has been observed at the doses employed. The effects of suramin on adrenal function in dogs and cats has not been studied. Further work on dose titration, toxicity, and effects on adrenal steroid synthesis are needed before suramin can be recommended for the management of hyperadrenocorticism in dogs and cats.

## DRUGS THAT ACT ON THE PERIPHERAL GLUCOCORTICOID RECEPTOR

Mifepristone (RU 486) is a synthetic antiprogestin that binds to both glucocorticoid and progesterone receptors; therefore, it has both antiprogesterone and antiglucocorticoid properties. The mechanism of action of mifepristone is complex (Spitz and Bardin, 1993).

Because of the drug's antiprogesterone properties, mifepristone is an effective abortifacient in humans, dogs, and cats. In both dogs and cats, doses of 20 to 30 mg/kg as a single subcutaneous injection or 2.5 mg/kg every 12 hr for 4.5 days results in effective pregnancy termination after day 32 of gestation (Sankai et al., 1991). Few side effects have been reported.

The dose of mifepristone required to induce an antiglucocorticoid effect is higher than that required to antagonize progesterone. The antiglucocorticoid properties have been examined in normal subjects and in human patients with hyperadrenocorticism secondary to PDH, ectopic ACTH syndrome, and adrenal neoplasia. In normal subjects, mifepristone blocks the feedback effect of cortisol on ACTH secretion in a dose-dependent fashion. Long-term administration results in persistently elevated plasma ACTH and cortisol concentrations. The response to CRH is unchanged and the diurnal rhythm of ACTH and cortisol is maintained.

In humans, signs of glucocorticoid deficiency have been observed at doses of 4 to 10 mg/kg/day, and the symptoms resolved following treatment with dexamethasone. Unfortunately, since measurement of serum cortisol cannot be used to evaluate functional hypocortisolism during receptor blockade, hypocortisolemia is evaluated with indirect parameters such as remission of clinical signs of hyperadrenocorticism, and the appearance of eosinophilia, hypoglycemia, and decreased free water clearance.

Mifepristone has been effective in eliminating the clinical signs of hypercortisolemia in 60 to 70% of patients with hyperadrenocorticism secondary to ectopic ACTH secretion and functional adrenocortical neoplasia. Patients with PDH may not sustain long-term remissions, as the glucocorticoid receptor blockade may be overcome by rising cortisol and ACTH concentrations.

In normal dogs, administration of mifepristone (20 to 50 mg/kg/day PO) for 10 days resulted in a three- to fourfold rise in plasma ACTH and cortisol concentrations. These elevations persisted for several days after discontinuation of the drug. Plasma aldosterone concentrations rose in the dogs treated with 50 mg/kg/day, possibly secondary to the increase in ACTH concentrations. No difference in serum sodium or potassium concentrations or osmolality was observed between dogs treated with any dose of mifepristone and those treated with placebo. No side effects were observed throughout the treatment period (Wade et al., 1988).

No studies have been performed to evaluate the efficacy of mifepristone in the treatment of hyperadrenocorticism in the dog, and the effects of the drug on adrenal function in dogs and cats has not been studied. Further work is warranted, although the difficulty in assessing the response to therapy and the potential lack of a long-term effect in management of PDH may limit its widespread use. Mifepristone may be useful in the management of patients with adrenal-dependent disease either as single-agent therapy or as short-term preparation of patients for adrenalectomy. Currently, mifepristone is not available in the United States; however, the political and ethical issues surrounding its importation may soon be resolved.

## References and Suggested Reading

Bruyette DS, Ruehl WW, and Smidberg TL: l-Deprenyl therapy of canine pituitary-dependent hyperadrenocorticism. J Vet Intern Med 7:114, 1993.
*This abstract describes the beneficial effects of l-deprenyl therapy in the management of dogs with PDH.*

Daley CA, Zerbe CA, Schick RO, et al: Use of metyrapone to treat pituitary-dependent hyperadrenocorticism in a cat with large cutaneous wounds. J Am Vet Med Assoc 202:956, 1993.
*This paper describes the use of metyrapone in a cat with hyperadrenocorticism and reviews the rationale for metyrapone in the management of PDH.*

Dewis P, Anderson DC, Bullock DE, et al: Experience with trilostane in the treatment of Cushing's syndrome. Clin Endocrinol 18:533, 1983.
*A review of the mechanism of action of trilostane and its efficacy in Cushing's syndrome in humans.*

Dodam JR, Kruse-Elliott KT, Aucoin DP, et al: Duration of etomidate-induced adrenocortical suppression during surgery in dogs. Am J Vet Res 51:786, 1990.
*This article outlines the effects of etomidate on adrenal function in dogs.*

Feuillan P, Raffeld M, Stein CA, et al: Effects of suramin on the function and structure of the adrenal cortex in the cynomolgus monkey. J Clin Endocrinol Metab 65:153, 1987.
*This paper characterizes the biochemical and histologic effects of suramin on adrenal function in normal monkeys.*

LaCoste D, Caron S, Belanger A, et al: Effect of three week treatment with [D-trp6, des-GLY- NH10(2)] LHRH ethylamide, aminoglutethimide, ketoconazole, or flutamide alone or in combination on testicular, serum, adrenal, and prostatic steroid levels in the dog. J Steroid Biochem 33:233, 1989.
*This article describes the effects of aminoglutethimide on adrenal steroid production in normal dogs.*

Lamberts SW, Klijn JG, DeQuijada M, et al: The mechanism of the suppressive action of bromocriptine on adrenocorticotropin secretion in patients with Cushing's disease and Nelson's syndrome. J Clin Endocrinol Metab 51:307, 1980.
*This paper outlines the efficacy of bromocriptine administration in human patients with Cushing's syndrome.*

LaRocca RV, Stein CA, Danesi R, et al: Suramin in adrenal cancer: Modulation of steroid hormone production, cytotoxicity in vitro, and clinical antitumor effect. J Clin Endocrinol Metab 71:497, 1990.
*A review of the utility of suramin in the medical management of adrenal carcinoma in humans.*

Peterson ME and Drucker WD: Cyproheptadine treatment of spontaneous pituitary ACTH-dependent canine Cushing's disease. Clin Res 26:703, 1978.
*This abstract presents information on the use of cyproheptadine in the management of dogs with pituitary-dependent Cushing's disease.*

Peterson ME and Drucker WD: Advances in the diagnosis and treatment of canine Cushing's syndrome. *Proceedings of the 31st Gaines Veterinary Symposium*, pp 17–24, 1981.
*Reviews the effects of bromocriptine and cyproheptadine in the treatment of dogs with pituitary-dependent Cushing's disease.*

Rijnberk A, Mol JA, Kwant MM, et al: Effects of bromocriptine on corticotropin, melanotropin, and corticosteroid secretion in dogs with pituitary-dependent hyperadrenocorticism. J Endocrinol 118:271, 1988.
*Reviews the effects of bromocriptine administration in dogs with PDH.*

Sankai T, Endo T, Kanayama K, et al: Antiprogesterone compound, RU 486 administration to terminate preganancy in dogs and cats. J Vet Med Sci 53:1069, 1991.
*Describes the efficacy of mifepristone as an abortifacient in dogs and cats.*

Spitz IM and Bardin CW: Mifepristone (RU 486)—a modulator of progestin and glucocorticoid action. N Engl J Med 329:404, 1993.
*A review of the physiology of mifepristone and its use in conditions where progestin or glucocorticoid blockade is desirable.*

Verhelst JA, Trainer PJ, Howlett TA, et al: Short and long-term responses to metyrapone in the medical management of 91 patients with Cushing's syndrome. Clin Endocrinol 35:169, 1991.
*Describes the efficacy of metyrapone in the short- and long-term management of human patients with Cushing's syndrome.*

Wade CE, Spitz IM, Lahteenmaki P, et al: Effects of the antiglucocorticoid RU 486 on adrenal function in dogs. J Clin Endocrinol Metab 66:473, 1988.
*Describes the effects of daily RU 486 administration on cortisol and ACTH concentrations in normal dogs.*

# HYPOADRENOCORTICISM IN DOGS

PETER P. KINTZER
*North Grafton, Massachusetts*
*and* MARK E. PETERSON
*New York, New York*

Hypoadrenocorticism is an uncommon endocrinopathy that typically develops in young to middle-aged female dogs and is most commonly characterized by deficient secretion of both mineralocorticoids and glucocorticoids. In dogs, spontaneous hypoadrenocorticism results from atrophy or destruction of the adrenal cortices (primary hypoadrenocorticism or Addison's disease) or, in rare instances, deficient pituitary adrenocorticotrophic hormone (ACTH) production (secondary hypoadrenocorticism). Primary hypoadrenocorticism usually results in inadequate glucocorticoid and mineralocorticoid secretion and, in the vast majority of cases, is thought to be the end result of an immune-mediated process. Primary adrenocortical insufficiency can also develop secondary to the administration of the adrenocorticolytic drug mitotane (*o,p'*-DDD). In secondary adrenal insufficiency, deficient pituitary ACTH secretion results in inadequate glucocorticoid production, whereas mineralocorticoid secretion is usually preserved because ACTH has little trophic effect on mineralocorticoid production.

Occasionally, dogs with untreated primary hypoadrenocorticism may have normal serum electrolyte concentrations (i.e., serum sodium and potassium). In some, it is likely that previous therapeutic intervention obscured any alterations in serum electrolyte concentrations. Multiple blood sampling over a period of weeks is necessary in some dogs with primary hypoadrenocorticism to demonstrate hyperkalemia and hyponatremia. These cases have been termed "atypical" hypoadrenocorticism and can be explained by the fact that the progression of the disorder is a gradual process in which glucocorticoid secretion becomes subnormal before mineralocorticoid secretion is substantially affected.

## HISTORICAL AND CLINICAL FINDINGS IN HYPOADRENOCORTICISM

Common historical and clinical findings seen in dogs with hypoadrenocorticism are listed in Table 1. Unfortunately, no set of clinical signs is pathognomonic for hypoadrenocorticism, and the signs listed are common to a wide variety of more prevalent diseases. The severity and duration of these clinical findings vary greatly among dogs. The majority of dogs are examined because of chronic progressive problems that have been present a variable period of time, ranging up to 1 year in duration. Conversely, those dogs in an acute adrenal crisis may present as a true medical emergency. Careful questioning, however, often elicits a history consistent with hypoadrenocorticism preceding the onset of acute adrenocortical crisis by days to months. An important diagnostic clue is a waxing-waning course of illness that is exacerbated by stress and responds to nonspecific treatment and supportive care (e.g., parenteral fluid administration or cage rest).

Given that the historical and clinical findings associated with hypoadrenocorticism in dogs are vague, nonspecific, often intermittent, and similar to those seen in a variety of more common disorders, it follows that the key to the diagnosis of hypoadrenocorticism is a high index of suspicion.

## ROUTINE LABORATORY FINDINGS IN HYPOADRENOCORTICISM

Common clinicopathologic abnormalities found in dogs with hypoadrenocorticism are listed in Table 2. Classic findings on the serum biochemical profile are hyperkalemia, hyponatremia, azotemia, and mild to moderate metabolic acidosis (total carbon dioxide [$TCO_2$] <15 mEq/L). In addition, hypercalcemia may be seen in up to 30% of cases. Serum electrolyte disturbances alone cannot be relied upon for the definitive diagnosis of primary hypoadrenocorticism, however. Hyperkalemia may occur in a variety of other diseases, particularly renal failure, gastrointestinal disorders, and acidosis. Azotemia is typically prerenal in origin and resolves with adequate fluid replacement. In the unusual instance that serum concentrations of creatinine and urea nitrogen do not quickly return to normal, inadequate fluid therapy or ischemic renal damage resulting in at least a degree of renal azotemia should be considered. Serum biochemical evaluation in dogs with secondary adrenocortical insufficiency are usually unremarkable, although hyponatremia and azotemia may be seen.

Hematologic evaluation may reveal a mild to moderate nonregenerative normocytic normochromic anemia and the absence of a stress leukogram. Urinalysis frequently reveals a dilute urine specific gravity, especially when the specific gravity is considered in the context of prerenal azotemia. In our experience, over 50% of dogs have an impaired ability to concentrate their urine (specific gravity <1.030) in the presence of high serum concentrations of creatinine and urea nitrogen. This decreased renal concentrating ability has been attributed to medullary washout and decreased medullary blood flow.

## ELECTROCARDIOGRAPHIC FINDINGS IN HYPOADRENOCORTICISM

An electrocardiogram (ECG) should be performed in all dogs with marked hyperkalemia (>6.5 mEq/L), especially if bradycardia is present. Abnormalities of cardiac conduction may have grave consequences for dogs with hypoadrenocorticism. In our experience, electrocardiographic abnormalities are found in over 50% of dogs with untreated hypoadrenocorticism in which an ECG is performed. Sinoatrial standstill is by far the most common arrhythmia recorded, whereas ventricular premature contractions and atrial fibrillation occur occasionally.

There are a number of classic electrocardiographic findings that are reported with hyperkalemia (i.e., prolonged QRS duration, decreased R-wave amplitude, increased T-wave amplitude, prolonged P-R interval, and absence of P waves). However, these ECG changes often correlate poorly with serum potassium levels in dogs with hypoadrenocorticism. The reason for this poor relationship is unclear, but appears to result from the interaction of other concurrent electrolyte abnormalities, metabolic acidosis, azotemia, and decreased tissue perfusion on the cardiac conduction system. Therefore, the ECG cannot be used to closely estimate the serum potassium concentration, at least in dogs with hypoadrenocorticism.

## RADIOGRAPHIC FINDINGS IN HYPOADRENOCORTICISM

Radiographs, typically taken in dogs in an acute adrenal crisis or in those with severe clinical signs associated with hypoadrenocorticism, may demonstrate abnormalities associated with volume depletion and decreased tissue perfusion. These findings include microcardia, a narrowed vena cava or descending aorta, and hypoperfused lung fields. Megaesophagus may also be demonstrated on thoracic radiography, but this finding is very rare (<1% of dogs); with successful treatment of hypoadrenocorticism, megaesophagus should resolve completely.

## DIAGNOSIS OF HYPOADRENOCORTICISM

Definitive diagnosis of hypoadrenocorticism requires demonstration of inadequate adrenal reserve. A low resting serum cortisol concentration coupled with a subnormal or negligible cortisol response to exogenous ACTH administration is diagnostic for hypoadrenocorticism. The ACTH-response test can be performed using either ACTH gel or synthetic ACTH (cosyntropin). When using ACTH gel, serum cortisol concentrations are determined before and 2 hr after intramuscular injection of 20 U. If cosyntropin is used, samples are drawn before and 1 hr after intravenous or intramuscular administration of 0.25 mg.

In dogs with presumed acute adrenocortical insufficiency, the ACTH-response test can be done immediately. Alternatively, it can be performed following several hours of stabilization with parenteral fluid and glucocorticoid administration. Prednisone, prednisolone, hydrocortisone, and cortisone all cross-react with serum cortisol assays and should be withheld until completion of ACTH-response testing. On the other hand, dexamethasone does not interfere with cortisol determination and can be used in the initial treatment of acute adrenocortical insufficiency without interfering with ACTH-response testing. In those dogs that have received prednisone, prednisolone, hydrocortisone, or cortisone treatment, glucocorticoid therapy must be switched to dexamethasone for at least 24 hr before an ACTH-response test can be performed. In dogs with hypovolemia or marked dehydration, it is advisable to delay ACTH-response testing until initial fluid replacement has been administered. In such cases, decreased tissue perfusion may impede absorption of the ACTH preparation, particularly if ACTH gel is administered intravenously, resulting in inaccurate and misleading data. If these dogs are tested when still markedly dehydrated, ACTH should be administered intravenously as cosyntropin.

The presence of serum electrolyte abnormalities (e.g., hyperkalemia and hyponatremia) along with a subnormal cortisol response to ACTH is indicative of primary hypoadrenocorticism. It must be remembered, however, that some dogs with secondary hypoadrenocorticism also develop hyponatremia. Determination of plasma endogenous ACTH should be used to differentiate primary from secondary adrenal insufficiency in dogs with normal serum electrolyte levels and in dogs with hyponatremia alone. Plasma ACTH concentrations are very high in dogs with primary hypoadrenocorticism as a consequence of the loss of negative feedback of cortisol on the pituitary gland. In contrast, plasma ACTH concentrations are low to undetectable in dogs with secondary hypoadrenocorticism. Plasma samples for endogenous ACTH determination must be drawn before corticosteroids are administered or after a long period of withdrawal, because glucocorticoid treatment will rapidly lower high plasma ACTH values to normal or low concentrations. In addition, samples for ACTH determination must be appropriately handled to ensure accurate results (see "*CVT* Update: Sample Collection and Testing Protocols in Endocrinology," this volume, p 335).

## TREATMENT OF HYPOADRENOCORTICISM

### Acute Adrenocortical Insufficiency

Acute adrenocortical insufficiency (addisonian crisis) is a life-threatening emergency requiring immediate intervention. If the history and presentation are compatible with acute hypoadrenocorticism, appropriate therapy should be instituted without delay, and the definitive diagnostic work-up begun while the initial

**Table 1.** *Historical and Clinical Findings in Spontaneous Canine Hypoadrenocorticism*

| Sign | Approximate Percentage of Cases |
|---|---|
| Lethargy/depression | 95 |
| Anorexia | 90 |
| Vomiting | 75 |
| Weakness | 75 |
| Weight loss | 50 |
| Dehydration | 45 |
| Diarrhea | 40 |
| Waxing/waning course | 40 |
| Collapse | 35 |
| Previous response to therapy | 35 |
| Hypothermia | 35 |
| Slow CRT | 30 |
| Shaking | 27 |
| Polyuria/polydipsia | 25 |
| Weak pulse | 20 |
| Bradycardia (<60 bpm) | 18 |
| Melena | 15 |
| Painful abdomen | 8 |
| Hair loss | 5 |

Abbreviations: CRT = capillary refill time, bpm = beats per minute.

**Table 2.** *Common Clinicopathologic Abnormalities in Canine Hypoadrenocorticism*

| Finding | Approximate Percentage of Cases |
|---|---|
| Hyperkalemia | 95 |
| Hyponatremia | 80 |
| Na/K ratio <27 | 95 |
| Hypochloremia | 40 |
| Hypercalcemia | 30 |
| Azotemia | 85 |
| Decreased $TCO_2$ | 40 |
| Elevated ALT/AST | 30 |
| Hyperbilirubinemia | 20 |
| Hypoglycemia | 17 |
| Anemia | 25 |
| Eosinophilia | 20 |
| Lymphocytosis | 10 |
| Urine specific gravity <1.030 | 75 |

Abbreviations: Na = sodium, K = potassium, $TCO_2$ = total carbon dioxide, ALT = alanine aminotransferase, AST = aspartate aminotransferase.

treatment is in progress. Before initiating therapy, however, one must collect blood for determination of complete blood count (CBC) and serum chemistry profile (including electrolyte levels), as well as urine for complete urinalysis therapy.

Of primary importance in the treatment of acute adrenocortical insufficiency is the rapid administration of large volumes of intravenous fluids, preferably 0.9% NaCl. In our experience, use of lactated Ringer's solution in the initial therapy of adrenal crisis is not inappropriate; the small amount of potassium in lactated Ringer's solution does not appear to be detrimental and is far outweighed by the benefit of rapid correction of hypovolemia. Fluid therapy is initiated at a rate of 60 to 80 ml/kg/hr for 1 to 2 hr to ensure prompt correction of hypovolemia, and the infusion rate is then decreased. Such rapid fluid administration is also a dependable means of quickly decreasing the serum potassium concentration as the result of its dilutional effect, as well as by improving renal perfusion and increasing potassium excretion. Urine output should be monitored to assess the adequacy of urine production and to help guide fluid therapy. Fluids are tapered to a maintenance rate and eventually discontinued over a few days based on the dog's clinical status, response to therapy, urine output, and laboratory parameters.

Also of great importance in the treatment of acute adrenocortical insufficiency is the intravenous administration of a glucocorticoid. A rapid-acting formulation such as dexamethasone sodium phosphate (2 to 4 mg/kg) or prednisolone sodium succinate (15 to 20 mg/kg) is preferred, and dexamethasone must be used if the ACTH-response test is in progress (in order to avoid cross reaction with the cortisol assay). The initial dose of rapid-acting glucocorticoid can be repeated in 2 to 6 hr if necessary. Glucocorticoid supplementation is gradually tapered to a maintenance dosage of prednisone or prednisolone (0.2 mg/kg daily) as the dog's condition improves. Supplementation should be administered parenterally until vomiting has ceased.

A rapid-acting parenteral mineralocorticoid formulation is no longer available for use in the treatment of acute adrenocortical insufficiency. However, this does not appear to be of much clinical importance, because rapid correction of hypovolemia, amelioration of shock, and restoration of vascular integrity with glucocorticoids are sufficient to stabilize the dog with hypoadrenocorticism. Nevertheless, oral mineralocorticoid supplementation with fludrocortisone acetate (Florinef, Squibb, Princeton, NJ) can be instituted immediately; this will not do any harm and may help correct serum electrolyte disturbances.

Other clinicopathologic derangements, such as metabolic acidosis or hypoglycemia, may require attention. In most cases, metabolic acidosis is corrected by fluid and glucocorticoid therapy; administration of sodium bicarbonate is rarely necessary. Severe acidosis (pH <7.2), however, should be treated. The total dose of bicarbonate is calculated using the following formula:

$$\text{deficit in mEq} = (\text{body weight in kg}) \times (0.5) \times (\text{base deficit})$$

Of the calculated deficit, 25% is given in the intravenous fluids over the initial 6 to 8 hr, and the acid-base status is then reevaluated. It is unusual for a dog to require additional sodium bicarbonate administration. Hypoglycemia, if present, should also be addressed. If the animal is not dehydrated, glucose can be added to the intravenous fluids at a concentration of 2.5%. Symptomatic hypoglycemia should be treated with a slow intravenous bolus of 0.5 to 1 ml/kg of a 50% dextrose solution.

Cardiac conduction abnormalities associated with severe hyperkalemia can progress to ventricular fibrillation or asystole. Rapid fluid infusion alone will lower serum potassium concentrations and dramatically improve ECG abnormalities within 30 to 60 min in most dogs. Should severe hyperkalemia persist despite such fluid administration, or if death from hyperkalemic myocardial toxicity appears to be at hand, sodium bicarbonate followed by intravenous insulin and glucose can be given. Regular insulin is given at a dosage of 0.5 U/kg; 2 to 3 gm of glucose per unit of insulin is administered, half as an intravenous bolus and half in the intravenous fluids over the next 6 to 8 hr. Such dogs must be closely monitored for signs of hypoglycemia, as dogs with adrenocortical insufficiency are very sensitive to the hypoglycemic action of insulin. Intravenous glucocorticoid supplementation, as described above, will help minimize the occurrence of severe hypoglycemia, especially if given before the administration of insulin. An alternative therapy, slow intravenous administration of 10% calcium chloride solution (0.1 ml/kg), may antagonize the effects of potassium on myocytes.

## Chronic Adrenocortical Insufficiency

Most dogs with hypoadrenocorticism do not present in acute adrenocortical insufficiency but have a more chronic form of hypoadrenocorticism, with clinical signs of varying severity and duration. These dogs generally do not require the aggressive treatment needed in dogs with acute hypoadrenocorticism. However, fluid therapy and parenteral glucocorticoid replacement may be indicated in dogs with chronic hypoadrenocorticism, especially if azotemia, dehydration, or vomiting is present; such parenteral therapy should be continued until these abnormalities have resolved and maintenance corticosteroid therapy can be initiated. Similarly, in dogs recovering from an adrenal crisis, maintenance therapy is instituted once the dog is stable and oral medication can be tolerated. In dogs, maintenance corticosteroid treatment of hypoadrenocorticism consists of lifelong mineralocorticoid supplementation, usually together with glucocorticoid replacement therapy. Either fludrocortisone acetate (Florinef, Squibb, Princeton, NJ) or deoxycorticosterone pivilate (DOCP; Percorten-V, CIBA-GEIGY Animal Health, Greensboro, NC) can be administered for chronic mineralocorticoid replacement.

Fludrocortisone acetate should be instituted at an initial oral dosage of 10 to 20 μg/day, with the daily dosage adjusted by 0.05- to 0.1-mg increments on the basis of serial serum electrolyte determinations (i.e., sodium and potassium). After initiation of fludrocortisone administration, serum concentrations of electrolytes, urea nitrogen, and creatinine should be monitored weekly until stabilized within the normal range. Once this is achieved, the dogs should be reevaluated monthly for the first 3 to 6 months of treatment, then every 3 to 6 months thereafter. In many dogs in which fludrocortisone is used as long-term mineralocorticoid replacement, the daily dose required to control the disorder gradually increases; such an increasing dosage requirement is usually most evident during the first 6 to 24 months of treatment. In most dogs, the final fludrocortisone dosage needed to control hypoadrenocorticism is 20 to 30 μg/kg/day. Very few dogs can be controlled on a dosage of 10 μg/kg/day or less. Adverse effects (usually polydipsia and polyuria), development of a relative resistance to the effects of the fludrocortisone, or financial considerations (especially when treating large or giant breed dogs) may necessitate a change to DOCP therapy in some dogs.

In those dogs in which DOCP is used as long-term mineralocorticoid replacement, the drug should be initiated at a dosage of 2.2 mg/kg given by deep intramuscular injection every 4 weeks. After the first two to three injections of DOCP, serum concentrations of electrolytes, urea nitrogen, and creatinine should be monitored at 2, 3, and 4 weeks after DOCP administration in order to determine the drug's duration of action and to help make dosage adjustments, if needed. The duration of action of DOCP varies between dogs, with most requiring the drug at 3- to 4-week intervals, but with a few dogs requiring treatment with DOCP every 2 weeks. Once stabilized, the serum concentrations of electrolytes, urea nitrogen, and creatinine should be monitored at 3- to 6-month intervals, at time of DOCP administration. Although many dogs could be controlled on a maintenance DOCP dosage somewhat lower than 2.2 mg/kg, this dosage is still recommended, at least for initial treatment. Almost all dogs with hypoadrenocorticism will be well controlled with this dosage, and use of this dose obviates the need for the practitioner to incrementally increase the dosage of DOCP over the first 6 to 12 months of therapy, which occurs in many dogs in which DOCP is initiated at a lower dose. Furthermore, no adverse effects such as hypertension or sodium retention have been seen in dogs treated with this recommended dose of 2.2 mg/kg. Nevertheless, one can attempt to gradually lower the monthly maintenance dosage of DOCP in order to determine a minimally effective dose, particularly if cost is a factor.

Daily glucocorticoid replacement with prednisone or prednisolone (0.2 mg/kg, PO) is necessary in only about half of dogs with hypoadrenocorticism. In general, all dogs are initially treated with both mineralocorticoid and glucocorticoid replacement. If warranted because of the development of side effects, the glucocorticoid dosage can be tapered to alternate days and then discontinued in order to evaluate if glucocorticoids are needed as part of maintenance therapy. The fact that glucocorticoids can be discontinued without development of severe adverse effects in many dogs with hypoadrenocorticism is especially important in those dogs that have developed signs of iatrogenic hyperadrenocorticism (e.g., polyuria and polydipsia) after treatment. In many of those dogs, cessation of glucocorticoids will reverse signs of iatrogenic hyperadrenocorticism, and mineralocorticoid replacement alone will control signs of hypoadrenocorticism. Nevertheless, additional glucocorticoid supplementation (two to ten times normal recommended dosage) may be necessary during periods of stress such as illness, trauma, or surgery; therefore, the owner should always have some glucocorticoid on hand and be informed of the situations when the dog might require glucocorticoid supplementation.

Dogs with documented secondary adrenal insufficiency require only glucocorticoid replacement. Daily administration of oral prednisone or prednisolone (0.2 mg/kg) is usually sufficient, except during periods of stress when higher dosages are required. If primary pituitary ACTH deficiency has not been confirmed by demonstrating undetectable to low plasma ACTH concentrations, however, one must continue to monitor serum electrolyte concentrations on a regular basis. Many dogs with "atypical" primary hypoadrenocorticism, originally presenting with normal serum electrolyte concentrations and suspected of having secondary hypoadrenocorticism, will subsequently develop the classic electrolyte abnormalities (i.e., hyperkalemia and hyponatremia) of primary hypoadrenocorticism and require mineralocorticoid replacement.

## References and Suggested Reading

Feldman EC and Peterson ME: Hypoadrenocorticism. Vet Clin North Am [Small Anim Pract] 14:751, 1984.
  *An overview of hypoadrenocorticism in dogs.*
Kintzer PP and Peterson ME: Mineralocorticoid treatment of 176 dogs with spontaneous hypoadrenocorticism. J Vet Intern Med 6:112, 1992.
  *Report of large series of dogs in which the maintenance dosages of fludrocortisone acetate and desoxycorticosterone pivilate needed to treat hypoadrenocorticism were determined.*
Rogers W, Straus J, and Chew D: Atypical hypoadrenocorticism in three dogs. J Am Vet Med Assoc 179:155, 1981.
  *A description of atypical hypoadrenocorticism.*
Schrader LA: Hypoadrenocorticism. *In* Kirk RW (ed): *Current Veterinary Therapy IX.* Philadelphia, WB Saunders Co, 1986, pp 972–977.
  *Another excellent review of hypoadrenocorticism.*
Willard MD, Schall WD, McCaw DE, et al: Canine hypoadrenocorticism: Report of 37 cases and review of 39 previously reported cases. J Am Vet Med Assoc 192:1091, 1988.
  *Clinical report of a large series of dogs with adrenocortical insufficiency.*

# HYPERLIPIDEMIA

JOAN BARRIE

*Wetherby, West Yorkshire, United Kingdom*

*and* TIMOTHY D.G. WATSON

*Glasgow, United Kingdom*

Hyperlipidemia is defined as an increase in plasma concentrations of cholesterol or triglyceride or both. The condition may arise as the result of a primary, often inherited, defect in lipoprotein metabolism or as a consequence of an underlying systemic disease. In humans, plasma lipid and lipoprotein concentrations may be influenced by medical status, hormonal factors, dietary composition, and genetic determinants. The current understanding of these interactions in the dog and cat is based mainly on observations made during experimental studies and a small but rapidly expanding number of clinical reports. The following is a review of the current information regarding the etiology, investigation, and management of hyperlipidemia in the dog and cat.

## LIPOPROTEIN STRUCTURE AND FUNCTION

Lipids are water-insoluble biomolecules that are essential for normal physiologic function. Triglycerides are the most abundant dietary lipids and are a source of chemical energy that may be stored in adipocytes or mobilized according to tissue demand. Cholesterol is a major component of cellular membranes and is an essential precursor of steroid hormones, vitamins, and bile acids.

The transport of these insoluble lipids through the aqueous phase of plasma to their sites of utilization or storage is achieved by the formation of lipid-protein complexes that act as vehicles for the transport of cholesterol, cholesteryl esters, and triglycerides. Lipoproteins are composed of a surface coat made up of phospholipid, cholesterol, and apolipoproteins surrounding a hydrophobic lipid center of triglycerides and cholesteryl esters. The apolipoproteins are specific proteins that direct the lipoproteins to their site of metabolism by acting as ligands for cell surface receptors and as cofactors in the enzymatic hydrolysis of triglyceride and the esterification of cholesterol. There are a number of discrete populations of lipoproteins that may be classed on the basis of their size, hydrated density, lipid, and apolipoprotein composition and electrophoretic mobility. The classes recognized in the dog are chylomicrons, very-low-density lipoproteins (VLDL), low-density lipoproteins (LDL), and high-density lipoproteins (HDL). The chylomicrons and VLDL are triglyceride-rich lipoproteins, in contrast to HDL and LDL, which act predominantly as vehicles for cholesterol and cholesteryl esters. Each lipoprotein species has a specific function, and the coordinated interactions between lipoprotein populations and tissues ensure the efficient transport of lipid in response to physiologic demand (Watson and Barrie, 1993). Chylomicrons are responsible for the delivery of dietary triglycerides to body tissues and cholesterol to the liver. These lipoproteins are formed in intestinal lacteals following a fat-containing meal and enter the circulation via the lymphatic duct. Very-low-density lipoproteins, the major plasma vehicle of endogenous triglyceride, are structurally similar to chylomicrons and are synthesized continuously by the liver. In the circulation, the core triglycerides of chylomicrons and VLDL are hydrolyzed by the enzyme lipoprotein lipase, which is bound to the endothelial lining, predominantly of skeletal and cardiac muscle and adipose tissue. The action of this enzyme liberates fatty acids from the lipoprotein core for storage or utilization by those tissues. The cholesteryl ester–dense chylomicron remnants formed by this mechanism are removed from the circulation by the liver, while VLDL remnants are further modified to LDL. In humans, LDL are quantitatively the most important plasma cholesterol carrier, whereas the HDL plays the major role in the dog and cat. High-density lipoproteins are synthesized by the liver and intestines and interact with peripheral tissues, resulting in an accumulation of cholesterol within the lipoprotein core. The particles are then transported to the liver where the cholesterol may be utilized or excreted. Progressive cycles of cholesterol accumulation and esterification within the core of HDL particles results in a cholesteryl ester–enriched lipoprotein called $HDL_1$, which is found in the plasma of hypercholesterolemic dogs.

Other lipoprotein species have been isolated from the plasma of hyperlipidemic dogs including $\beta$-very-low-density lipoprotein ($\beta$-VLDL), a cholesteryl ester–enriched lipoprotein believed to have a major atherogenic potential. This lipoprotein has been isolated from the plasma of dogs with hypothyroidism and may play a role in the development of vascular lesions in some dogs with thyroid dysfunction.

## ETIOLOGY OF HYPERLIPIDEMIA

Hyperlipidemia may arise as a consequence of disturbances of lipoprotein formation or metabolism. The presence of hypercholesterolemia or hypertriglyceridemia or both depends on which of the lipoprotein classes are affected. Lipid abnormalities arising as a consequence of systemic disease processes (secondary hyperlipidemia) are common in dogs and have been recognized in cats. Hyperlipidemias resulting as the sequelae of inherited defects of lipoprotein metabolism are termed primary or familial, while cases in which neither a heritable basis nor an underlying metabolic disease can be documented are termed idiopathic. The most common cause of hyperlipidemia in the dog and cat is postprandial hyperlipidemia, a physiologic phenomenon resulting from the appearance of chylomicrons in the circulation between 2 and 6 hr after fat ingestion. The triglyceride concentration at this time may be sufficient to impart an opaque or milky appearance to the plasma (lipemia) as a result of the refractive properties of the large triglyceride-rich lipoproteins. Lipemia is not recognized in association with hypercholesterolemia. Clearance of chylomicrons from the circulation allows a return to fasting triglyceride concentrations between 8 and 16 hr after a meal. Plasma cholesterol concentrations show a small postprandial rise that does not usually exceed the upper limit of species-specific reference ranges.

## HYPERTRIGLYCERIDEMIA

Fasting hypertriglyceridemia may result from impaired clearance of chylomicrons and VLDL from the circulation (e.g., a deficiency of lipoprotein lipase) or from overproduction of VLDL. This hyperlipidemia phenotype is most commonly seen in association with diabetes mellitus in both the dog and cat, and in hypothyroidism, hyperadrenocorticism, and protein-losing nephropathy in the dog (Barrie et al., 1993). Obesity in the dog has not been associated with overt fasting hyperlipidemia, but it appears that a relationship between adiposity and impaired plasma triglyceride clearance does exist. This may result in a more severe or prolonged postprandial hyperlipidemia and thus predisposes obese dogs to the clinical consequences of hypertriglyceridemia. An association also exists between acute pancreatitis in the dog and hypertriglyceridemia, and it is believed that the lipid abnormalities may initiate or contribute to the pathologic process. An accumulation of triglyceride-rich lipoproteins in the circulation may therefore predispose dogs to the development of pancreatic disease.

Familial hypertriglyceridemia is rare in the dog. However, a heritable defect, the exact nature of which has not yet been elucidated, is believed to be the cause of hypertriglyceridemia in the miniature schnauzer (Ford, 1993). This disorder is characterized by an increase in the plasma triglyceride concentration secondary to an excessive accumulation of chylomicrons and VLDL in the plasma. A moderate increase in the plasma cholesterol concentration may also be noted. The majority of affected animals are middle-aged and older, but no sex predilection has been identified. In addition to hyperlipidemia in miniature schnauzers, idiopathic hypertriglyceridemia and hyperchylomicronemia has been reported in pedigree and cross-bred dogs (Watson and Barrie, 1993).

An inherited deficiency of lipoprotein lipase has been identified as the cause of inherited hyperchylomicronemia of cats, a well-recognized entity that has been described worldwide (Jones, 1993). The defect is inherited as an autosomal recessive trait and the hyperlipidemia is characterized by the accumulation of chylomicrons and VLDL in the plasma of fasted cats. The age of onset of the clinical disease and the nature of the clinical signs associated with the hyperlipidemia are variable.

## HYPERCHOLESTEROLEMIA

Hypercholesterolemia is most commonly recognized secondary to systemic diseases; in particular, hypothyroidism, diabetes mellitus, hyperadrenocorticism, protein-losing nephropathies, and obstructive jaundice. It is possible to induce hypercholesterolemia in the dog by dietary manipulation, but the fat content of conventional dog food is insufficient to achieve this in animals with normal lipid metabolism.

Primary hypercholesterolemia has not been confirmed in the dog and cat, but increased plasma concentrations of $HDL_1$ have been reported in briards in the United Kingdom.

## THE CONSEQUENCES OF HYPERLIPIDEMIA

Hypertriglyceridemia is associated with a number of clinical consequences in the dog and cat; therefore, the presence of excessive fasting triglyceride concentrations (>500 mg/dl or >5.5 mmol/L) should be considered a possible health risk. The severity of the clinical signs may not correlate with the degree of hypertriglyceridemia.

Most commonly, hypertriglyceridemia in the dog is associated with gastrointestinal signs including intermittent episodes of nonlocalizing abdominal pain, anorexia, and vomiting. In some individuals, the results of laboratory investigations are supportive of a diagnosis of acute pancreatitis; however, in many cases the plasma amylase and lipase activities and the appearance of abdominal radiographs are considered within normal limits. Alimentary signs may be recognized in any hypertriglyceridemic dog but are most frequently seen in miniature schnauzers over 4 years of age. As the affected dog ages, the severity and frequency of the episodes of abdominal pain may increase. The gastrointestinal disease may be self-limiting, since anorexia, resulting in a prolonged fast, allows clearance of the triglyceride-rich lipoproteins from the circulation. Alimentary signs of this type have not been documented in cats with hyperchylomicronemia.

Primary and secondary hyperlipidemias may produce ocular abnormalities, but many lesions are the result of interaction between local and systemic factors (Crispin, 1993). Ocular manifestations of hyperlipidemia therefore display a variable incidence. Just as lipemia may be detected in whole blood collected from kittens with marked hyperlipidemia, so may the milky appearance of the retinal vessels in nontapetal areas be detected on funduscopic examination. This finding is referred to as lipemia retinalis and may be recognized in animals with a triglyceride concentration greater than 2500 mg/dL (28 mmol/L), or at concentrations lower than this in anemic individuals (Crispin, 1993). Lipemia retinalis is one of the most common clinical manifestations of inherited hyperchylomicronemia in the cat. The lactescence of the retinal vessels does not impair visual function, but should alert the clinician to the presence of hyperlipidemia. Lipid-laden aqueous humor has also been reported in a hypertriglyceridemic dog and a cat.

Xanthomata are the result of lipid accumulation in the skin or other tissues. Cutaneous xanthomata have been described rarely in animals, but are recognized in association with feline hyperchylomicronemia and diabetes mellitus in the dog and cat. Peripheral neuropathies resulting from the formation of xanthomata over bony tuberosities are a common clinical entity in cats with inherited hyperchylomicronemia. The affected cats most frequently present with Horner's syndrome, tibial nerve paralysis, or radial nerve paralysis.

Other clinical signs associated with hypertriglyceridemia include generalized seizures, which have been described as the initial presenting sign in some miniature schnauzers with hyperlipidemia. The relationship between the disturbances of lipid metabolism and those of the central nervous system is not understood. Moderate to severe anemia has been reported in a number of young kittens (<4 weeks of age) with inherited hyperchylomicronemia, but the relationship between hyperlipidemia and anemia has not been fully elucidated.

Hypercholesterolemia is associated with few clinical signs in the dog and cat. Ocular abnormalities include arcus lipoides corneae, which is an annular lipid infiltration of the peripheral cornea and perilimbal zone of the sclera. The condition has been recognized as an infiltration of cholesterol, fatty acids, and phospholipids in German shepherd dogs with hypothyroidism and hyperlipidemia. Lipid keratopathy, a rare condition of the dog, is a corneal lipid deposition (unilateral or bilateral) with associated vascularization. The plasma cholesterol concentration in affected dogs is often increased.

Atherosclerosis is a relatively rare consequence of hyperlipidemia in the dog and is most commonly seen in association with hypothyroidism. The vascular lesions may be the result of deposition of cholesteryl esters from LDL or β-VLDL. The clinical presentation of affected individuals depends upon the location of the diseased vessels, but may include iliac thrombosis, behavioral signs, and generalized seizures.

## INVESTIGATION

Hyperlipidemia is often noted during routine laboratory investigations. The recognition of lipemia is of considerable importance, since the plasma turbidity may result in the production of spurious laboratory results. Where blood parameters are measured by spectrophotometric methods, the presence of lipemia may give rise to false-negative or false-positive results. It is worthy to note that amylase and lipase assays are affected by lipemia; therefore, the confirmation of pancreatic disease in hypertriglyceridemia patients often provides a diagnostic challenge. It is preferable that plasma should be separated from the red cells as soon as possible after sample collection, since lipemia may predispose a sample to in vitro hemolysis, further compounding the interference with laboratory procedures.

When presented with a case of hyperlipidemia, it is first necessary to confirm the presence of fasting hyperlipidemia by ensuring that the sample was drawn after a prolonged period of food withdrawal (12 to 16 hr). In kittens with suspected idiopathic hyperchylomicronemia where this fasting period is unacceptable, the clinician must interpret the lipid concentrations in the light of the postprandial triglyceride peak, which is expected in normal animals between 2 and 6 hr after food ingestion. The investigation of hyperlipidemia requires the measurement of both plasma cholesterol and triglyceride concentrations. After confirmation of hyperlipidemia, the clinician's diagnostic efforts should be directed at excluding the presence of an underlying metabolic or endocrine disease. In cases of secondary hyperlipidemia, it is often unnecessary to proceed further than this, but in dogs with secondary lipid abnormalities that have not normalized after the treatment of the underlying disease, and in dogs with primary or idiopathic hyperlipidemia, it may be necessary to further categorize the lipid disturbances.

The chylomicron test is a simple means of confirming the presence of chylomicrons and VLDL. When plasma or serum is left at 4°C overnight (12 hr), the chylomicrons float to the top of the sample, forming a "cream layer." The presence of chylomicrons in the plasma of fasted animals is a pathologic finding. An increase in the VLDL concentration is characterized by an overall opalescence of the plasma infranatant.

Lipoprotein electrophoresis has been used in a number of laboratories to qualitatively study the plasma lipoprotein concentrations of the dog and cat (Whitney, 1992). Ideally, the analysis should be performed within 72 hr of collection, and the plasma maintained at 4°C until that time. Ethylenediaminetetraacetic acid (EDTA) is generally considered the anticoagulant of choice, but individual laboratories should be approached regarding the details of sample collection and transportation. Lipoprotein electrophoresis allows the rapid identification of the lipoprotein classes present in the plasma and, in particular, facilitates the recognition of β-VLDL and $HDL_1$.

Recent advances in the development of combined ultracentrifugation and precipitation techniques have provided methods for the quantification of canine and feline lipoproteins. Currently these methods are restricted to use in research establishments, but their employment may allow the accurate characterization of primary and idiopathic hyperlipidemias, allowing rational therapeutic approaches in individual cases.

In animals with primary or idiopathic hypertriglyceridemia, it is helpful to differentiate a deficiency of lipoprotein lipase from an overproduction of triglyceride-rich lipoproteins. The plasma activity of lipoprotein lipase may be measured in a blood sample collected 10 min after the intravenous administration of heparin (70 to 100 IU/kg). The total lipase activity of a sample collected in this fashion is the sum of the individual activities of lipoprotein lipase and hepatic lipase. Clinicians should therefore ensure that the selected assay provides a means of measuring specific lipoprotein lipase activity. Such assays are currently only performed in a small number of research laboratories.

## MANAGEMENT

The plasma lipid concentrations in dogs and cats with secondary hyperlipidemia generally return to normal, or near normal, after successful stabilization or treatment of the underlying disease process. The plasma lipid concentrations may decline rapidly, as is the case with canine hypothyroidism, or remain abnormal for a more prolonged period, as frequently seen in dogs with diabetes mellitus. If specific treatment for any underlying disease process does not cause resolution of the hyperlipidemia, then introduction of lipid-lowering strategies should be considered. The following guidelines may be used for the management of unresolved as well as idiopathic hyperlipidemias.

Dogs with a fasting plasma triglyceride concentration greater than 500 mg/dl (5.5 mmol/L) are considered at risk of the development of pancreatitis, and lipid-lowering intervention should be instituted. Miniature schnauzers with triglyceride concentrations higher than this on consecutive samples (2- to 4-week intervals) are candidates for dietary intervention, irrespective of the presence or absence of clinical signs at the time of investigation. Hypertriglyceridemic dogs presenting with signs typical of acute pancreatitis should be treated symptomatically, including the maintenance of fluid and electrolyte balance and the withdrawal of food where necessary. The primary approach in the management of hypertriglyceridemia is the reduction of the dietary fat intake. A number of proprietary low-fat, high-fiber diets are available in canned and dry preparations: these include Veterinarian Canine Low Fat (WALTHAM), Prescription Diets Canine r/d and w/d (Hills Pet Products), CNM OM-Formula Canine Veterinary Diet (Ralston Purina Company), and Eukanuba Lite (The Iams Company). The diets should be fed according to the manufacturer's guidelines for maintenance, except in the case of obese animals, where a weight-reduction program should be instituted. The selected diet must be the only food source for the affected pet, and the plasma lipid concentrations should be monitored at 1 month after its introduction. In many dogs with idiopathic hyperlipidemia, it may be difficult to maintain lipid concentrations within laboratory reference ranges; therefore, the goal of therapy is to maintain a triglyceride concentration less than 500 mg/dl (5.5 mmol/L). If, after 1 month of dietary management, the triglyceride concentration has not decreased significantly it is important to exclude a failure of owner compliance as the cause of the ineffective response, particularly since low-fat, high-fiber diets may have poor palatability. A diet with a moderately restricted fat content (between 8 and 12%, on a dry-matter basis) is often sufficient to control the hypertriglyceridemia of miniature schnauzers with familial hyperlipidemia, but as these dogs grow older, the episodes of alimentary signs increase in severity or frequency and may require further dietary fat restriction for the control of the clinical manifestations. In cases of hypertriglyceridemia that are not adequately controlled by a proprietary diet, it is possible to formulate a homemade diet (Lewis, Morris, and Hand, 1987) in which the fat is replaced by medium-chain triglycerides (MCT Oil, Mead Johnson Nutritional Division; 0.5 ml/kg PO every 24 hr), which are absorbed directly into the portal circulation and oxidized by the liver. Since medium-chain triglycerides do not provide all the essential fatty acids for the dog, it is also necessary to provide a source of these (e.g., corn oil).

Dietary fat restriction is also the primary means of managing feline hyperchylomicronemia. Low-fat, high-fiber preparations include Prescription Diets Feline r/d and w/d (Hills Pet Products), CNM OM-Formula Feline Veterinary Diet (Ralston Purina Company), and Iams Lite (The Iams Company). Affected kittens should be weaned and maintained on a selected product. Cats presenting with peripheral neuropathies generally show resolution of clinical signs over 4 to 12 weeks. Additional methods of lowering plasma lipid concentrations in the cat have rarely proved necessary.

In order to maintain low plasma triglyceride concentrations in some dogs, it may be necessary to use medical therapy in addition to dietary fat restriction. A number of lipid-lowering therapies are used in human medicine, where the selection of a specific agent is determined predominantly by the nature of the underlying abnormality of lipid metabolism. None of these products are licensed for use in the dog and cat. Until controlled therapeutic trials have been conducted in these species, lipid-lowering drugs should be used with caution and the animals monitored at frequent intervals.

The authors have found that marine oils (10 to 30 mg/kg PO every 24 hr) reduce both fasting triglyceride concentrations and the postprandial peak in dogs with hypertriglyceridemia. The supplements are well tolerated and no side effects of their use have been observed. Other lipid-lowering drugs may prove beneficial. The authors have used gemfibrizol (Lopid, Parke Davis; 150 to 300 mg PO every 12 hr) in a small number of dogs with hypertriglyceridemia. The drug has been shown to be well tolerated in both short- and long-term studies at dosages greater than 15 times in excess of those used for lipid-lowering effect. Although no side effects have been noted in dogs treated with gemfibrizol, it is advisable to monitor hematologic and biochemical parameters at regular intervals. Gemfibrizol therapy has produced variable reductions in plasma triglyceride concentrations, but it may be a useful adjunct to dietary therapy in cases in which alternative methods have failed to control triglyceride concentrations. The administration of the drug should be discontinued if no response has been noted within 3 months of the initiation of therapy.

Hypercholesterolemia in the dog is currently considered a useful indicator of underlying endocrine or metabolic disease, rather than an immediate health risk to the animal. However, prolonged marked increases in the plasma cholesterol concentration (>750 mg/dl or >20 mmol/L) have been associated with the development of atherosclerosis. It is therefore important to consider dietary fat restriction in cases of marked idiopathic hypercholesterolemia. Cholestyramine, a bile acid–binding resin (Questran, Bristol Laboratories; 1 to 2 gm PO every 12 hr) may be used in cases of persistent idiopathic hypercholesterolemia, but its use may increase hepatic VLDL synthesis; therefore, the plasma triglyceride concentrations should be monitored closely.

In summary, the successful management of the clinical manifestations of hyperlipidemia in the dog and cat depends upon the reduction of the plasma lipid concentrations followed by regular clinical and laboratory evaluation.

## References and Suggested Reading

Barrie J, Watson TDG, Stear MJ and Nash AS: Plasma cholesterol and lipoprotein concentrations in the dog: The effects of age, breed, gender and endocrine disease. J Small Anim Pract 34: 507, 1993.
*A study of the plasma lipid and lipoprotein cholesterol concentrations associated with secondary hyperlipidemia in the dog.*
Crispin SM: Ocular manifestations of hyperlipoproteinaemia. J Small Anim Pract 34:500, 1993.
*A review of the ophthalmic abnormalities associated with local and systemic disturbances of lipid metabolism.*
Ford RB: Idiopathic hyperchylomicronaemia in miniature schnauzers. J Small Anim Pract 34:488, 1993.
*A review of the clinical signs and management of canine familial hypertriglyceridemia.*
Jones BR: Inherited hyperchylomicronaemia in the cat. J Small Anim Pract 34:493, 1993.
*A review of the lipid abnormalities and clinical features of feline lipoprotein lipase deficiency.*
Lewis LD, Morris ML, and Hand MS. Index of dietary management. *In* Lewis LD, Morris ML, and Hand MS (eds): *Small Animal Clinical Nutrition III*, 3rd edition. Topeka, KS, Mark Morris Associates, 1987, p 13.
*The formulation of homemade low-fat diets.*
Watson TDG and Barrie J: Lipoprotein metabolism in the dog and cat: A review. J Small Anim Pract 34: 479, 1993.
*A detailed review of the structure, function, and metabolism of plasma lipoproteins in the dog and cat.*
Whitney MS: Evaluation of hyperlipidemias in dogs and cats. Semin Vet Med Surg Small Anim 7: 292, 1992.
*A guide to the investigation of hyperlipidemia, including the interpretation of lipoprotein electrophoresis profiles.*

# Section

# 6

# HEMATOLOGY, ONCOLOGY, AND IMMUNOLOGY

BRUCE R. MADEWELL
*Consulting Editor*

435

# HEMATOLOGIC TECHNOLOGY FOR DIAGNOSING ANEMIAS

GLADE WEISER

*Fort Collins, Colorado*

This article is intended to provide the practicing veterinarian with (1) an appreciation for the technologic capabilities emerging in veterinary hematology, and (2) the knowledge for using hematologic information to characterize the common clinical problem of anemia.

The availability of automation in human hematology has been extrapolated with success to veterinary hematology. Initially, this required invention of instrument modification and calibration protocols. Over the past 10 to 15 years, the objectives of utilizing this technology in centralized laboratories have been to maintain low relative cost, provide more sensitive analyses, and improve reliability of data. We now have an experience base that greatly enhances the ability to perform hemograms in commercial veterinary laboratories.

Currently, the cost of technology is decreasing dramatically enough that sophisticated analyzers are feasible in most veterinary practice facilities. Hematology systems are now produced and supported specifically for veterinary applications, eliminating much of the need for complex knowledge necessary for use of human instrument systems. Species-specific cell analysis requirements are engineered into the systems. These incorporate the advantages of individual cell analysis that provide sophisticated information about erythrocytes (e.g., Mascot Multispecies Hematology Analyzer, CDC Technologies, Inc, Oxford, CT). This development places technology in the veterinarian's hands that was only present in large commercial laboratory facilities a few years ago. However, with this capability comes a responsibility. For on-site hematology to be successful, this responsibility involves a commitment to attention to detail and a knowledge of when to utilize the consultative expertise of a hemopathologist. One danger is that analyzers will be used to generate numbers while neglecting other important parts of the hemogram. Another pitfall is laxity in rigorous assurance of accurate instrument performance as specified by the manufacturer. If this commitment to expertise cannot be assured, it is recommended that laboratory work be delegated to the reference laboratory. Central facilities still provide the advantage of expertise in all components of the complete blood count (CBC). One of the most important of these components is examination of the blood film to link important morphologic abnormalities with data findings. Whether the veterinarian uses the central laboratory facility or attempts to develop on-site capabilities in hematology, interpretation of results depends on an up-to-date knowledge of erythrocyte analysis.

## DETERMINATION OF HEMATOLOGIC DATA BY AUTOMATED INSTRUMENTATION

The preferred technology for blood analysis incorporates varying degrees of procedural automation and rapid individual cell analysis. Instrumentation provides the ability to count cells and also measure individual cell volume. On more sophisticated systems, a histogram or volume distribution curve of the erythrocyte population may be displayed. Representative histograms are shown in Figure 1. The histogram is a visual display of the distribution of individual erythrocyte volume. It is generated by analysis of several thousand erythrocytes in a few seconds. The shape characteristics of normal histograms are similar across species.

Complete blood analysis for the hemogram is depicted in a flow diagram in Figure 2. The instrument will divide blood analysis into two independent pathways. One pathway involves an isotonic dilution of blood in which erythrocytes and platelets may be analyzed. The blood erythrocyte and platelet concentrations are determined by cell counting. The mean corpuscular volume (MCV) value may be determined from analysis of the volume distribution. The hematocrit is computed by multiplying the MCV by the erythrocyte concentration. An additional value, the red cell distribution width (RDW), is provided by mathematical analysis of the histogram. It is an approximation of the coefficient of variation of the erythrocyte volumes. This is an index of volume heterogeneity or volume anisocytosis; it is not strictly related to diameter anisocytosis traditionally observed on stained blood films. The second pathway involves making a dilution of blood in which a lytic agent is added to obliterate erythrocytes. This agent lyses cell membranes, liberating hemoglobin which is measured by spectrophotometry. Naked leukocyte nuclei are remnant particles that can be counted to determine blood leukocyte concentration. The hemoglobin concentration and hematocrit values are used to calculate the mean corpuscular hemoglobin concentration (MCHC). Because of the constant nature of this value across most species, this value may be used as a cross-validation of the two separate analysis pathways. A major analytical error in one or both of the pathways is likely to be reflected in a major error in the MCHC.

Similar counting and sizing functions exist for evaluation of platelets. Instruments have an analytical routine to separate platelets and erythrocytes. This routine works with varying success when using human instru-

437

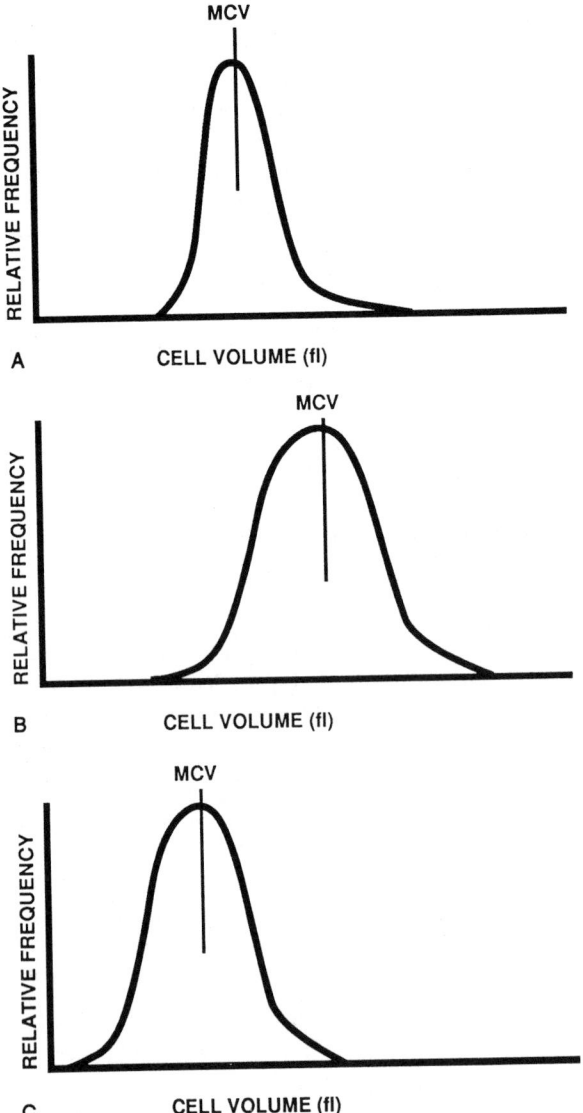

**Figure 1.** Representative histogram curves showing distribution of canine erythrocyte volume. *A,* Normal histogram. *B,* Example of macrocytosis. *C,* Example of microcytosis. Note the increased volume heterogeneity seen as increased histogram width in *B* and *C.* From the data in the curve, the mean corpuscular volume can be determined; in these examples it is indicated by the vertical line marked "MCV."

mentation. On most instruments, the separation is reliable for canine blood. Feline platelets are at least twice as large as platelets of other species. This results in variable degrees of overlap between erythrocyte and platelet populations. Most human analyzers do not separate feline platelets and erythrocytes well.

## Limitations Encountered in Contemporary Hematology

Some veterinarians utilize the services of a human hospital laboratory. When interfacing with a human laboratory, it will generally be the responsibility of the vet-

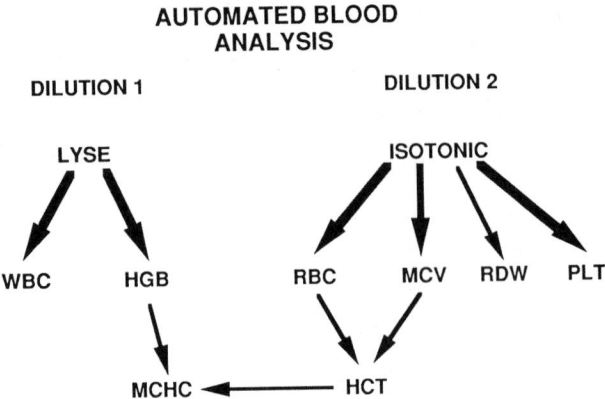

**Figure 2.** Diagram depicting sample processing and data generation in automated blood analysis. In dilution 1, the cells are treated with lyse, and in dilution 2, the cells are suspended in an isotonic medium. Heavy arrows indicate direct measurements and thin arrows indicate data derived by calculations.

erinarian to provide some technical information to the laboratorians. The instrumentation used will be configured for analysis of human blood. With these systems, automated erythrocyte analysis is reliable for canine blood. However, erythrocytes of cats and other common domestic species are too small to be properly analyzed. The erythrocyte counting and sizing measurements are not accurate. Therefore, human medical laboratories should use microhematocrit centrifugation for measuring hematocrit values in cats and other species with small erythrocytes. Alternatively, the laboratory may choose to maintain an animal-specific instrument.

Some veterinary hospital facilities performing in-house hematology still utilize manual procedures. In these cases, analysis should be limited to determination of hematocrit by microhematocrit centrifugation. Most cases of anemia established by the hematocrit should be referred to a veterinary reference laboratory for further characterization. It is recommended that hemoglobin measurement and manual microscopy erythrocyte counts not be done. These were done historically for purposes of calculating erythrocytic indices. Mean corpuscular volume values calculated by this method have poor reproducibility. The effort/benefit ratio in performing manual erythrocyte procedures is not favorable.

## INTERPRETATION OF ERYTHROCYTIC INDICES

The following tools are obtained from hematology instrument systems described above.

## Red Cell Distribution Width and Histogram Characteristics

The RDW value is an expression of volume anisocytosis or heterogeneity. It is of use to the laboratorian as an adjunct to evaluation of erythrocyte pathology on blood films. Reference ranges for RDW should be supplied for each instrument. Target values are up to 15 for dogs and up to 20 for cats. An increase in the RDW value indicates that there is a disturbance in the normal degree of heterogeneity of cell volume. This is usually due to a change in the size of erythrocytes produced in bone marrow in response to the underlying disease. Abnormal subpopulations are either large or small, and are due to the causes of macrocytosis or microcytosis, respectively (Fig. 1). One advantage of the histogram and RDW is that they allow detection of cell volume disturbances much earlier than examination of MCV alone. For example, there are cases of iron deficiency anemia with development of a microcytic subpopulation, yet the MCV value is still in the low-normal range. With experience, examination of these factors prompts the laboratorian to suspect specific morphologic abnormalities that may be confirmed by examination of the blood film. When separated from blood film examination, the RDW and histogram has little value to the clinician.

## Mean Corpuscular Volume

Target reference ranges for MCV are 60 to 72 fl for dogs and 37 to 49 fl for cats. When there is considerable progressive disturbance of cell volume in the direction of microcytosis or macrocytosis, the MCV value may become abnormal. Microcytosis is a feature of advanced iron deficiency anemia. The presence of this anemia is a clue that the animal has had chronic external blood loss sufficient to deplete body iron stores. The Akita breed of dog has microcytic erythrocytes compared with dogs of other breeds. Mean corpuscular volume values for Akitas are usually between 54 and 60 fl. Macrocytosis accompanies prominent erythrocyte regeneration in most species. Under conditions of maximal erythroid marrow stimulation in severe regenerative anemia, cells with about twice normal volume may be produced in all species except the dog. Interestingly, under conditions of maximal regeneration, dogs produce cells that are only slightly to 1.5× increased in volume. Poodle dogs frequently have a phenomenon known as poodle macrocytosis. The erythron is normal, but macrocytic cells are present. Mean corpuscular volume values in poodle macrocytosis may range from 75 to 100 fl.

## Mean Corpuscular Hemoglobin Concentration

The MCHC consistently falls in a range of approximately 32 to 37 gm/dl in dogs and cats. Traditionally, this value was useful in classifying anemia. Using manual techniques, this value would decrease in the range of 25 to 32 gm/dl in cases of iron deficency anemia. This was regarded as a useful artifact that was likely related to incomplete packing of abnormal erythrocytes

when using the microhematocrit technique. Using analyzer-based erythrocyte sizing and counting, the MCHC is usually normal to only slightly decreased in iron deficiency anemia. The MCHC may decrease slightly in extremely regenerative anemia when there is a very high percentage of polychromatophilic erythrocytes. These slightly immature cells have not yet reached their full hemoglobin concentration.

The MCHC has taken on a different role in the age of automated hematology. It has relatively little value to the clinician for interpretation of anemias. It is more important as a quality-control tool in the laboratory and is therefore of value to astute laboratorians using automated instrumentation. As mentioned above, the two values used to calculate the MCHC (PCV and hemoglobin) are measured in two separate pathways in the instrument. Major changes in MCHC indicate the presence of a problem with either the sample or the instrument analysis. Gross errors indicate the presence of an instrument malfunction or individual sample misanalysis that needs reconciliation. Increases in MCHC are not related to erythrocyte disease. They are due to turbidity that can falsely increase the spectrophotometric determination of hemoglobin. Common examples include gross *lipemia* and *sample hemolysis* in all species and high concentrations of Heinz bodies in cats. Mean corpuscular hemoglobin concentration values of 38 to 80 gm/dl may occur with these problems. It is also possible for extreme leukocytosis (>200,000/μl) to increase the MCHC. A high MCHC should prompt the examination of the sample for these causes. If these causes are eliminated, then a high MCHC indicates the presence of an instrument analytical problem. Decreases below 25 to 27 gm/dl indicate the presence of an instrument analytical problem.

## MORPHOLOGY ON STAINED BLOOD FILMS

As described above, the various erythrocytic indices serve to sensitize the hemopathologist to important morphologic abnormalities likely to be present. This sensitization increases the chances of recognizing abnormalities. The information provided by automated instrumentation has limited diagnostic value without skilled examination of blood films. The morphologic assessment of abnormalities is essential to diagnosis of most hematologic disease. The recognition of morphologic abnormalities is central to confirming a process or disease. For example, the determination of most causes of hemolysis requires identification of erythrocytic defects on the stained blood film. Readers are referred to reference texts for encyclopedic treatment of erythrocyte morphology in disease (Jain, 1986; Jain, 1993; Meyer, Coles, and Rich, 1992; Weiser, 1981, 1988, 1989, 1994a, 1994b).

## Reticulocyte Count

This manual technique is essential to diagnosis of anemia. Because it is labor intensive, it is unfortunately not routinely done. A reticulocyte count should be performed by laboratories as part of the hemogram on *all* anemic patients, for this count is the preferred method of quantifying the bone marrow response to anemia. Reticulocytes are visualized by staining blood with a vital stain such as new methylene blue or brilliant cresyl blue. The count is performed by differentiating 1000 consecutive erythrocytes as either reticulocytes or nonreticulocytes. The resultant percentage of reticulocytes may be multiplied by the erythrocyte count to yield reticulocytes per microliter of blood. The absolute reticulocyte count eliminates the need to interpret a reticulocyte percentage corrected relative to the hematocrit or erythrocyte concentration. Interpretive guidelines are as follows: counts of 0 to 60,000/$\mu$l indicate nonregenerative anemia, and counts of 60,000 to 500,000/$\mu$l encompass the range of mild to marked responses in regenerative anemias. Automation of the reticulocyte count will likely occur in the near future. This will improve the frequency of use and reproducibility of this measurement.

## APPROACH TO ANEMIA

Anemia is a very common clinical problem that is secondary to many primary disease processes. Characterization is important in managing the problem of anemia, but it is more important to provide clues to the underlying process or disease. Recognition of a hematologic process or disease depends on accurate, integrated interpretation of numerical data and morphologic findings on the hemogram. The clinician must develop a mental technique to rapidly analyze the hematologic data into meaningful interpretations. This is facilitated if the clinician follows an order for examination of information and has knowledge of the priority different pieces of information have in making an interpretation. In-depth discussion of specific diseases in relationship to this approach scheme is beyond the scope of this article. The reader is referred to the reference list for more in-depth details of anemias in dogs and cats (Jain, 1986; Jain 1992; Weiser, 1988, 1989, 1994a, 1994b; also see "Approach to the Anemic Patient," this volume, p 447).

When considering anemia, the clinician should develop an order that works from the least specific to the most specific interpretations. A flow chart (Fig. 3) will help the clinician develop a clear order to categorizing anemia.

### Regeneration or Nonregeneration

The first interpretative consideration is to determine if the anemia is regenerative or nonregenerative. This assessment will immediately eliminate about half of the potential causes of anemia. The most important piece of information for this interpretation is the reticulocyte count, using the guidelines given above. Other pieces of information that are supportive of regeneration, but

of lesser priority, include the subjective assessment of increased polychromasia on the Wright's-stained blood film, an increase in erythrocyte volume histogram width in the direction of larger cell volume with associated increase in the RDW value, an increased MCV, and metarubricytosis. These latter findings do not conclusively support regeneration unless there is accompanying reticulocytosis. The MCV is the last value to increase out of the reference range. As macrocytes accumulate during the regenerative response, there is a progressive widening of the histogram to the right. This is associated with an increase in the RDW. A large fraction of the circulating cells must be produced under these conditions before the MCV finally becomes macrocytic. Because cells produced during regeneration in dogs are not as increased in volume as in other species, macrocytosis is less frequently observed in canine regenerative anemia.

### REGENERATIVE ANEMIA

A regenerative pattern indicates that the animal has either blood loss (hemorrhage) or hemolysis and that the bone marrow is responding at an accelerated rate to replace lost cells. The next pieces of information to assess are the plasma protein concentration and erythrocyte morphology. Both hemolysis and internal hemorrhage may cause hyperbilirubinemia if the rate of hemoglobin catabolism is sufficient to exceed hepatic processing of heme pigment. Because this rate is usually greater with hemolytic disease, hemolysis is more frequently associated with hyperbilirubinemia. Bone marrow examination is not useful in regenerative anemia. If there is reticulocytosis, it can be predicted that the marrow will reflect erythroid hyperplasia.

HEMORRHAGE. When blood is lost from the vascular space, fluid replacement will occur over a period of hours in the body's attempt to restore circulating volume. This process will dilute plasma proteins such that hypoproteinemia will develop when there has been moderate to severe hemorrhage. External hemorrhage results in more severe hypoproteinemia than internal hemorrhage. In adult animals, protein concentrations of less than 6.5 gm/dl in the face of regenerative anemia suggests that the problem is hemorrhage. Protein values in the 4.0- to 5.5-gm/dl range may occur when there has been moderate to marked external hemorrhage. Erythrocyte morphology is usually normal aside from the features associated with regeneration. One exception is that hemorrhage associated with splenic hemangiosarcomas is frequently accompanied by acanthocytes and fragmented erythrocytes.

Recognition of the hemorrhage pattern should prompt a diligent search for the physical site of blood loss if it is not obvious on the initial presentation. Hemorrhage at a single site should be approached as a local problem, whereas hemorrhage at multiple sites should be approached as a coagulation disorder.

HEMOLYSIS. Because hemolytic disease results in selective loss of erythrocytes from blood, the plasma protein concentration remains normal. In adult animals

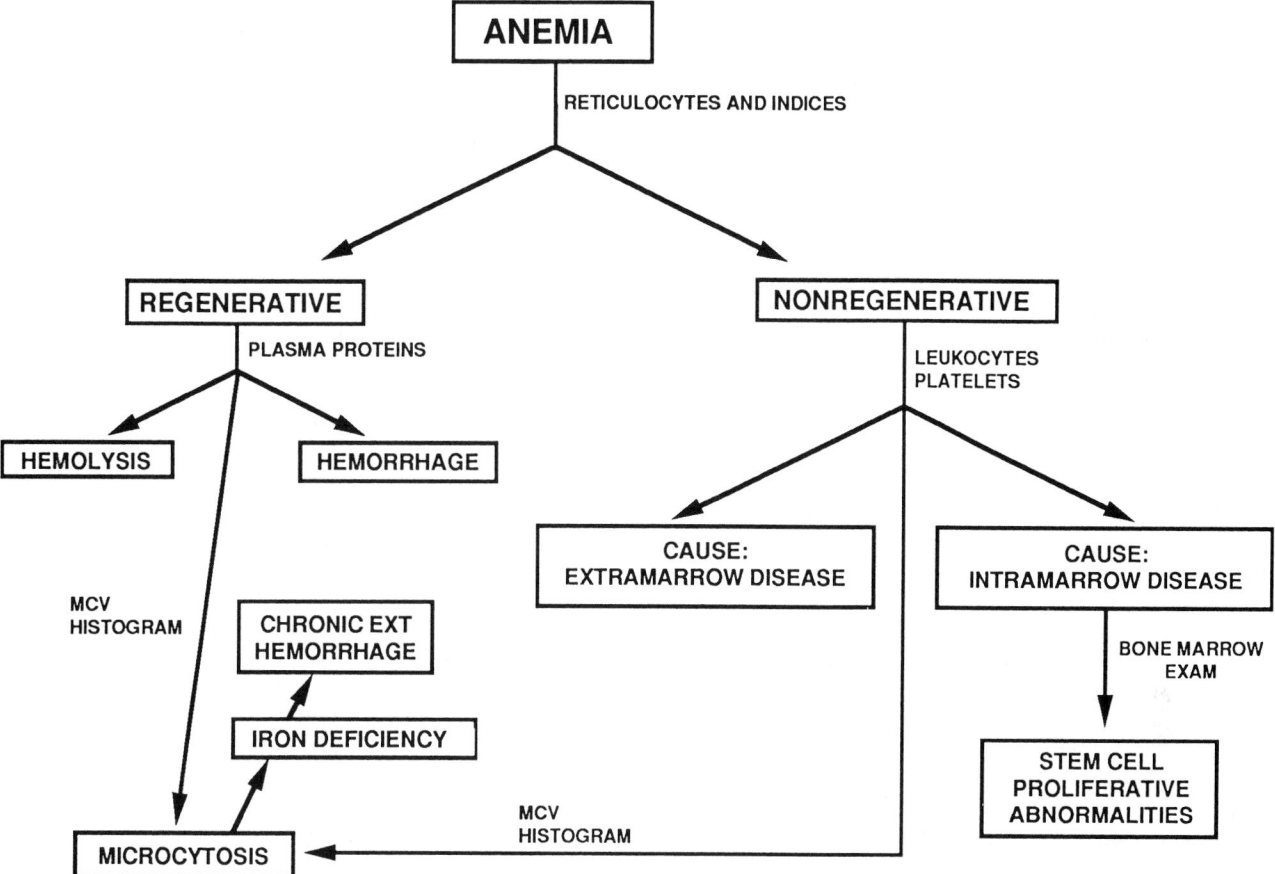

**Figure 3.** Flow chart diagram for approach to anemia. Items enclosed in rectangles represent interpretations. Text items not enclosed in rectangles indicate pieces of data that should be examined to lead to various interpretations. Please refer to text and references for in-depth discussion.

it is usually above 7.0 gm/dl when measured by refractometry. When a hemolysis pattern is present, the diagnosis usually depends on identifying a specific erythrocyte defect on the Wright's-stained blood film. Because an accurate morphologic assessment of these problems requires considerable experience, blood films should be referred to the clinical pathologist for consultation. Morphologic RBC defects commonly associated with specific diseases include spherocytes, Heinz bodies, and the hemotropic parasites known to cause shortened erythrocyte survival. Relatively rare causes of hemolysis include erythrocyte enzyme deficiencies that result in shortened erythrocyte survival. These usually occur in purebred dogs and are elucidated by a process of elimination and specialized testing recommended by the reference laboratory.

### NONREGENERATIVE ANEMIA

A nonregenerative pattern indicates that the anemia has developed as a result of bone marrow failure to produce erythrocytes at an adequate rate. The next pieces of information to assess are the erythrocyte morphology, the leukogram, and platelets. Following consideration of these cell lines, it may become appropriate to examine bone marrow.

NON-REGENERATIVE ANEMIA CAUSED BY EXTRA-MARROW DISEASE. In this category, selective depression of erythropoiesis is associated with normal production of platelets and leukocytes. Platelet concentration should be normal. Leukocyte concentration will be normal or will reflect a pattern of responsiveness to processes such as steroid release or inflammation. This type of anemia may be caused by a variety of chronic, extramarrow, medical disorders. Examples include hypothyroidism, hypoadrenocorticism, chronic renal disease, and chronic inflammatory diseases. The bone marrow shows nonspecific erythroid hypoplasia in these disorders and therefore examination of bone marrow does not provide a definitive diagnosis. Once the above categories of systemic disease are ruled out, it is then appropriate to examine marrow. It is also possible for primary marrow disorders to be manifested as selective nonregenerative anemia early in the course of disease.

NONREGENERATIVE ANEMIA CAUSED BY INTRA-MARROW DISEASE. Diseases in this category may be regarded as a variety of stem cell abnormalities that result in disturbances to production of multiple hematopoietic cell lines. This category is recognized when *nonregenerative* anemia is accompanied by any one or combination of the following findings: thrombocytopenia, neutropenia, or abnormal leukocytes in the blood. Abnormal leukocytes are those that may be associated with a hematopoietic cell neoplasm; this may be blasts of any cell lineage.

Stem cell disorders may manifest in at least three different categories that should be regarded as a morphologic and behavioral continuum. These categories include myeloaplasia, myelodysplasia, and myeloproliferative disease. A stem cell disorder resulting in myeloaplasia will eventually result in cytopenias of all cell lines in blood (see *CVT XI*, pp 479 and 478, respectively). Myelodysplasia is a stem cell disturbance that results in less severe cytopenias and subtle morphologic abnormalities. This is recognized most frequently in cats. The most frequent cytopenias are nonregenerative anemia and recurring neutropenia. Altered synchrony of cell maturation events result in morphologic abnormalities such as platelet and erythrocyte macrocytosis. Erythrocyte volume heterogeneity may be increased; this is associated with a widened histogram, increased RDW, and macrocytosis that is not associated with a regenerative response. Myeloproliferative disease is a stem cell disorder that may be regarded as a hematopoietic cell neoplasm of marrow cell origin. The prominent features include hyperproliferation of an abnormal cell line and marked reduction of normal cell lines. The proliferating cell line loses the normal orderliness of maturation or the ability to eventuate in mature cells. Abnormal cells often enter the blood as a leukemia. Lymphoproliferative disorders may also involve marrow and result in lymphocytic leukemia. What all these proliferative diseases have in common is failure to deliver adequate concentrations of various normal cell types to blood.

### IRON DEFICIENCY ANEMIA

It is important to recognize iron deficiency anemia because it usually indicates that a specialized form of hemorrhage is present. In juvenile animals of most species except the dog, iron deficiency may result during rapid growth while on an all-milk diet. However, in adult animals, iron deficiency almost always develops secondary to *chronic external blood loss*. This form of anemia may be either regenerative or nonregenerative. In the author's experience, chronic blood loss associated with gastrointestinal neoplasms usually is associated with bone marrow responsiveness evidenced by reticulocytosis, and blood loss due to hookworm infestation in puppies is frequently nonregenerative. Overused blood donors may develop marked features of iron deficiency but retain the ability to regenerate erythrocytes.

Iron deficiency is recognized by examination of the MCV, histogram, RDW, and blood film in concert as decribed below. The most important hematologic feature of iron deficiency anemia is microcytosis. When iron becomes limiting to erythropoiesis, the rate of hemoglobin synthesis may become reduced. Associated with this reduction are additional cell divisions that result in smaller cells. The newly produced cells released from marrow have smaller volume than normal. As this process continues over time, the erythrocyte volume heterogeneity increases. This is recognized as a widening of the histogram to the left, an increase in the RDW, and a decreasing MCV. In early iron deficiency, the increased RDW and widened histogram will occur before the MCV decreases into the microcytic range. With very-long-standing iron deficiency, all the normal cells may be replaced with a homogeneous population of microcytic cells. When this occurs, the histogram may appear normal in width, but the MCV is very low (35 to 50 fl in dogs). On the blood film, erythrocyte hypochromia may be observed as increased central pallor in dogs. Hypochromia is not observed in the cat. Another morphologic feature is a fragmentation process. This is likely due to oxidative injury to erythrocyte membranes.

### References and Suggested Reading

Jain NC: *Schalm's Veterinary Hematology*, 4th edition. Philadelphia, Lea & Febiger, 1986.
 *Comprehensive veterinary hematology reference text.*
Jain NC: *Essentials of Veterinary Hematology.* Philadelphia, Lea & Febiger, 1993.
 *Applied veterinary hematology text.*
Meyer DJ, Coles EH, and Rich L: *Veterinary Laboratory Medicine—Interpretation and Diagnosis.* Philadelphia, WB Saunders Co, 1992.
 *Comprehensive clinical pathology text.*
Weiser MG: Correlative approach to anemia in dogs and cats. J Am Anim Hosp Assoc 17:286, 1981.
 Weiser MG: Erythrocyte disorders. *In* Ettinger SJ (ed): *Ettinger's Textbook of Veterinary Internal Medicine*, 3rd edition. Philadelphia, WB Saunders Co, 1989, p 2145.
 *Review of erythrocyte pathophysiology and anemias in dogs and cats.*
Weiser MG: Erythrocyte responses and disorders. *In* Ettinger SJ (ed): *Ettinger's Textbook of Veterinary Internal Medicine*, 4th edition. Philadelphia, WB Saunders Co, 1994a, pp 1864–1891.
 *Review of erythrocyte pathophysiology and anemias in dogs and cats.*
Weiser MG: Erythrocytes and associated disorders. *In* Sherding RG (ed): *Diseases of the Cat.* New York, Churchill-Livingstone, 1988, p 529.
 *Review of erythrocyte pathophysiology and anemias in cats.*
Weiser MG: Disorders of erythrocytes and erythropoiesis. *In* Sherding RG (ed): *Diseases of the Cat.* 2nd edition. New York, Churchill-Livingstone, 1994b, p 691.
 *Review of erythrocyte pathophysiology and anemias in cats.*

# METHEMOGLOBINEMIA AND HEINZ-BODY HEMOLYTIC ANEMIA

JOHN W. HARVEY

*Gainesville, Florida*

Hemoglobin is a protein consisting of four polypeptide globin chains, each of which contains a heme prosthetic group within a hydrophobic pocket. Heme is composed of a tetrapyrrole that contains a central iron molecule that must be maintained in the ferrous ($+2$) state to reversibly bind oxygen.

Methemoglobin differs from hemoglobin only in that the iron moiety of heme groups has been oxidized to the ferric ($+3$) state. About 3% of hemoglobin is oxidized to methemoglobin each day in normal animals as a result of autoxidation of hemoglobin and/or secondarily to oxidants produced in normal metabolic reactions. Methemoglobin usually accounts for less than 1% of total hemoglobin, however, because it is constantly reduced back to hemoglobin by an enzyme reaction within erythrocytes (Harvey, 1989).

Heinz bodies are large aggregates of precipitated hemoglobin that are attached to the internal surfaces of erythrocyte membranes. In contrast to dogs and other species, normal cats may have 5 to 10% Heinz bodies within their erythrocytes. Not only is cat hemoglobin more susceptible to denaturation by endogenous oxidants, but when compared to other species, the cat spleen is less efficient in the removal ("pitting") of Heinz bodies from erythrocytes.

## METHEMOGLOBINEMIA

Methemoglobinemia results from either increased production of methemoglobin by oxidants or decreased reduction of methemoglobin associated with a deficiency in the erythrocyte methemoglobin reductase enzyme. Experimental studies and clinical reports indicate that many drugs can produce methemoglobinemia in dogs and cats. Significant methemoglobinemia has been associated with clinical cases of benzocaine, acetaminophen, and phenazopyridine toxicities in cats and dogs (Harvey, 1989). These drugs can also produce Heinz-body hemolytic anemias (discussed later in this article).

### Clinical Signs

Mucous membranes of animals with significant methemoglobinemia have a cyanotic appearance that may be difficult to recognize in heavily pigmented animals. Lethargy, ataxia, and stupor, resulting from hypoxia, do not become apparent until methemoglobin content reaches 50%, with a coma-like state and death ensuing when it reaches 80% (Harvey, 1989).

### Laboratory Findings

Methemoglobinemia may not be apparent in normally dark venous blood samples, but a spot test can be used to determine if clinically significant levels of methemoglobin are present. One drop of blood from the patient is placed on a piece of absorbent white paper and a drop of normal control blood is placed next to it. If the methemoglobin content is 10% or greater, the patient's blood should have a noticeably brown coloration, compared to a bright red color of the control blood. Accurate determination of methemoglobin content requires that blood samples be placed in ice and rapidly submitted to a laboratory that has this test available (Christopher and Harvey, 1992).

### Therapy

Mild to moderate methemoglobinemia does not require specific treatment to reduce the methemoglobin content, but elimination of oxidant exposure, intravenous fluids, and N-acetylcysteine (see below) may be indicated to combat other forms of tissue injury caused by oxidants. If the oxidant exposure is eliminated, erythrocytes can convert much of the methemoglobin back to hemoglobin within 24 hr. Oxygen therapy is of limited value, because methemoglobin cannot bind oxygen, and only a small increase in blood oxygen content can be obtained from an increase in dissolved oxygen.

Methylene blue, given slowly over several minutes as a 1% solution (1 mg/kg) IV, may be administered in cases with severe methemoglobinemia. A dramatic response should occur during the first 30 min after treatment. While this dose can be repeated if necessary, methylene blue should be used cautiously in cats and dogs, because it can cause Heinz-body hemolytic anemia in these species. In the case of drugs that cause substantial Heinz-body formation as well as methemoglobinemia, methylene blue treatment can potentiate the formation of Heinz bodies and anemia. Consequently, it is prudent to measure the hematocrit for 3 days after methylene blue treatment to ensure that a significant anemia does not develop.

Ascorbate has been recommended for the treatment

of methemoglobinemia associated with acetaminophen toxicity in dogs and cats (Cullison, 1984); however, ascorbate is not effective in reducing methemoglobin in dogs (Harvey et al., 1991), and has not been evaluated in cats.

## Methemoglobin Reductase Deficiency

Methemoglobin is reduced to hemoglobin, primarily by the NADH-dependent methemoglobin reductase (cytochrome $b_5$ reductase) enzyme. Persistent methemoglobinemia associated with methemoglobin reductase deficiency has been recognized in Chihuahua, borzoi, English setter, terrier-mix, cockapoo, poodle, corgi, Pomeranian and toy Eskimo dogs (Harvey et al., 1991), and recently in a domestic shorthair cat. The deficiency is presumed to be an inherited disorder, as it is in humans, but family studies have not been reported.

Affected animals have cyanotic-appearing mucous membranes, and may exhibit lethargy or exercise intolerance at times, but frequently have no clinical signs of disease. In several cases, the methemoglobinemia was recognized for the first time during surgery when mucous membranes and blood remained dark even though animals were given supplemental oxygen.

Venous blood samples remain dark with a brownish tinge, rather than turning bright red, when exposed to air (see methemoglobin spot test above). When assayed spectrophotometrically, methemoglobin concentrations in deficient dogs vary from 13 to 41%. The methemoglobin content in the deficient cat was 50%. Hematocrits in deficient dogs are usually normal, but the hematocrit in the reported cat was increased. A definitive diagnosis is made be measuring erythrocyte methemoglobin reductase enzyme activity. This assay is done in a few research laboratories and requires that prior arrangements be made before blood samples are submitted (Harvey et al., 1991).

Treatment is unnecessary because the methemoglobinemia is not life threatening. Affected dogs appear to have normal life spans.

## HEINZ-BODY HEMOLYTIC ANEMIA

The oxidation of globin sulfhydryl groups causes conformational changes in hemoglobin molecules, making them unstable. Heinz bodies form following the coalescence of many denatured hemoglobin molecules, and generally increase in size for 1 or 2 days after exposure to the oxidant.

In addition to Heinz-body attachment, oxidants can injure erythrocyte membranes by the peroxidation of unsaturated fatty acids and oxidation of membrane sulfhydryl groups, resulting in the polymerization of membrane phospholipids and proteins. While methemoglobinemia is reversible, Heinz-body formation and membrane damage are not. Oxidatively damaged erythrocytes have increased membrane rigidity and decreased deformability, which make them more likely to be removed from the circulation.

## Clinical Signs

Clinical signs vary depending on the nature of the oxidant involved and the time elapsed since administration or consumption. Mucous membranes may appear cyanotic if there is methemoglobinemia, pale if there is moderate to severe anemia, or icteric if there is hyperbilirubinemia. Weakness, depression, rapid heart rate, and rapid respiratory rate may be observed as a result of hypoxia from methemoglobinemia or severe anemia. Vomiting, anorexia, and diarrhea may also occur. Hemoglobinuria may be evident in some cases secondary to severe intravascular hemolysis. Subcutaneous edema, especially involving the face, and excessive salivation have been reported in cats with acetaminophen toxicity.

## Laboratory Findings

Heinz bodies are often unrecognized on routinely stained blood films, because they either do not stain, or stain similarly to the remaining intact hemoglobin. They can be especially difficult to recognize in dogs, because multiple small Heinz bodies tend to develop in dog erythrocytes, in contrast to the large single inclusions typical of cat erythrocytes. If large, Heinz bodies may appear as pale inclusions within erythrocytes or as bulges from the surface of erythrocytes. If intravascular hemolysis has occurred, Heinz bodies may be visualized as red inclusions within an erythrocyte "ghost." Heinz bodies are readily visualized as dark, refractile inclusions in new methylene blue "wet" preparations (Fig. 1) and as light-blue inclusions with reticulocyte stains (Christopher and Harvey, 1992).

Another erythrocyte abnormality that suggests oxidant injury to erythrocytes is the presence of eccentrocytes, erythrocytes with the hemoglobin concentrated to one side of the cell (Fig. 2). Eccentrocytes are formed by the adhesion of opposing areas of the cytoplasmic face of the erythrocyte membrane.

Except for splenectomized dogs that may have occasional small Heinz bodies, normal dogs do not have detectable Heinz bodies in their erythrocytes; consequently, their presence in dogs is usually indicative of Heinz-body hemolytic anemia. Careful history-taking usually reveals the source of oxidant responsible for the erythrocyte damage.

In contrast to dogs, a high percentage of Heinz bodies does not necessarily correspond to development of significant hemolytic anemia in cats. Increased numbers of Heinz bodies occur in some cats with other diseases, such as diabetes mellitus, hyperthyroidism, and lymphoma, but are associated with only mild anemia (Christopher, 1989). Conversely, a cat that has ingested an oxidant may develop severe, life-threatening anemia in conjunction with Heinz-body formation.

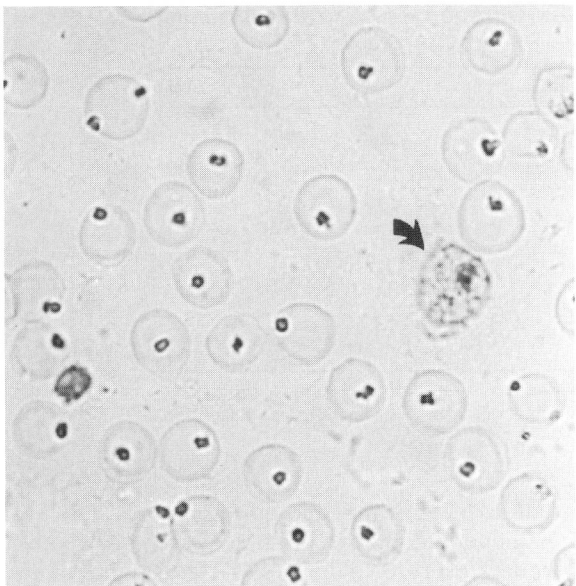

**Figure 1.** Erythrocytes from a cat containing darkly staining Heinz bodies as visualized using a new methylene blue wet mount preparation. The arrow indicates an aggregate reticulocyte.

Thus, it is very important to interpret the number of Heinz bodies in conjunction with the history, clinical setting, and severity of anemia.

Heinz-body hemolytic anemias are usually regenerative, as evidenced by increased reticulocyte counts and increased polychromasia on routinely stained blood smears (see "Hematologic Technology for Diagnosing Anemias," this volume, p 437). However, if an animal is examined within one or two days of oxidant exposure, the regenerative response may be minimal, because several days are required for increased production of reticulocytes.

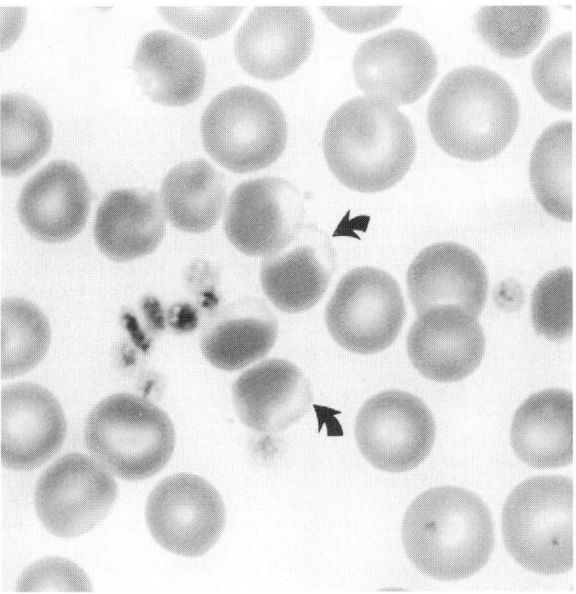

**Figure 2.** Eccentrocytes (*arrows*) in blood from a dog with acetaminophen toxicity as visualized using a Wright-Giemsa stain.

The mean corpuscular volume (MCV) may be increased if substantial numbers of large reticulocytes are present. The mean corpuscular hemoglobin concentration (MCHC) may be above normal because the presence of Heinz bodies makes the hemolysate turbid, when analyzed in a spectrophotometer, thereby artifactually raising the hemoglobin value used to calculate this index (see "Hematologic Technology for Diagnosing Anemias," this volume, p 437).

In most cases of Heinz-body hemolytic anemia, erythrocyte destruction results primarily from increased phagocytosis of injured erythrocytes by macrophages. Erythrocytes may lyse within the circulation following extreme oxidant injury, however, resulting in hemoglobinemia and hemoglobinuria. Significant intravascular hemolysis causes a number of abnormal clinical chemistry tests. Hyperbilirubinemia or hyperbilirubinuria may be present following rapid decline in hematocrit or when concomitant liver injury is present.

## Substances Causing Heinz-Body Formation

Experimental studies indicate that many drugs can produce Heinz-body formation in dogs and cats. Only those substances that have caused Heinz-body formation in clinical practice (Harvey, 1989; Houston and Myers, 1993) are listed in Table 1.

Cats are particularly susceptible to acetaminophen toxicity, with as little as one half of a tablet causing clinical disease in small cats. Toxicity usually results when clients give their animals acetaminophen-containing analgesics. Methemoglobin values are elevated within 2 to 4 hr after acetaminophen administration, followed by Heinz-body formation and anemia over subsequent days. While dogs can also develop methemoglobinemia and anemia, hepatic necrosis may be a more important sequelae to excess acetaminophen administration than the hematologic abnormalities.

Fresh, cooked, and dehydrated onions can cause Heinz-body hemolytic anemias. Most clinical cases have occurred in small dogs. One report describes Heinz-body hemolytic anemia in two cats fed onion soup.

Zinc toxicity has primarily resulted from the consumption and retention of zinc-containing objects within the stomach of dogs. Sources of zinc include U.S. pennies minted after 1982, metallic hardware, and ointment containing zinc oxide. The mechanism(s) by which zinc produces hemolytic anemia is unclear, but Heinz bodies have been recognized in some clinical cases (see "*CVT Update: Zinc Toxicity*," this volume, p 238).

Benzocaine toxicity has resulted from the application of over-the-counter antipruritic products to the skin of dogs and cats. Clinical signs result primarily from the resultant methemoglobinemia. Experimental studies have demonstrated substantial methemoglobinemia following administration of a benzocaine-containing spray to the larynx of cats. Heinz-body formation and anemia

***Table 1.*** *Oxidants Reported to Cause Clinical Cases of Methemoglobinemia or Heinz-Body Hemolytic Anemias in Cats or Dogs*°

| Oxidant | Methemoglobinemia | Anemia |
|---|---|---|
| Acetaminophen | +++ | +++ |
| Onions | NCS | +++ |
| Zinc | ? | +++ |
| Benzocaine | +++ | ± |
| Methylene blue | NCS | +++ |
| Phenazopyri-dine | +++ | ++ |
| Vitamin K | ? | + |
| Methionine | NCS | ++ |
| Propylene glycol | − | ± |

°The plus and minus signs indicate propensity of a drug to produce methemoglobin and/or Heinz bodies. NCS = not clinically significant and ? = unknown, but probably not clinically significant. See text for more information about these substances.

may occur, but hemolytic anemia, if present, appears to be mild.

Heinz-body hemolytic anemia has occurred following the oral administration of methylene blue–containing urinary tract antiseptics in cats and following the intravenous injection of methylene blue to outline pancreatic islet-cell and parathyroid gland tumors in dogs. Urinary tract products containing methylene blue are no longer approved for use in cats or dogs.

The administration of phenazopyridine, a urinary tract analgesic, can cause marked methemoglobinemia and Heinz-body hemolytic anemia in cats.

Excess vitamin K administration can cause Heinz-body hemolytic anemia in dogs. Vitamin $K_3$ (menadione) is more likely to cause a hemolytic anemia than is vitamin $K_1$. (Menadione should not be used in dogs, because it is not efficacious in the treatment of coumarin rodenticide poisonings.)

High doses of DL-methionine, given as a urinary acidifier in the treatment of feline urologic syndrome, have produced Heinz-body hemolytic anemia in cats.

Propylene glycol has been used as a humectant in soft-moist cat and dog food in the past. At the levels included in these foods, it caused prominent Heinz-body formation and shortened erythrocyte life spans, but minimal anemia, in cats. Propylene glycol is no longer added to cat food in the United States.

## Therapy

When possible, the oxidant source should be removed (e.g., endoscopic or surgical removal of zinc objects from the stomach). If less than 2 hr have elapsed since ingestion of an oxidant, vomition should be induced, and activated charcoal may be given at a dosage of 2 gm/kg body weight as a 20% saline slurry (Cullison, 1984) (see "*CVT* Update: Zinc Toxicity," this volume, p 238).

*N*-Acetylcysteine (Mucomyst, Mucosil) is efficacious in the treatment of acetaminophen toxicity if given within a few hours following drug administration. Since acetaminophen is slowly eliminated by cats, *N*-acetylcysteine should be given if clinical signs are present,

regardless of the time since drug administration. The recommended dosage is 140 mg/kg PO, followed by 70 mg/kg PO every 6 hr for seven treatments (Cullison, 1984). The absorption of *N*-acetylcysteine from the intestinal tract will be impaired by concurrent activated charcoal administration. The potential usefulness of this drug in treating other oxidant-induced hemolytic anemias has not been evaluated.

Once Heinz bodies are recognized, the hematocrit should be monitored closely, because the hematocrit usually does not reach the nadir until several days after oxidant exposure. Whole blood transfusions should be given when marked anemia is present, or when the hematocrit is decreasing rapidly and clinical signs suggest the condition is deteriorating (see *CVT XI*, p 475). If severe intravascular hemolysis is present, intravenous fluid therapy is recommended to minimize the chance of a hemoglobin nephrosis. Fluid therapy and correction of electrolyte and acid-base disturbances may also be indicated if severe vomiting or diarrhea occurs, renal injury develops, or shock occurs.

## References and Suggested Reading

Christopher MM: Relation of endogenous Heinz bodies to disease and anemia in cats: 120 cases (1978–1987). J Am Vet Med Assoc 194:1089, 1989.
   *A clinical study that determines what diseases in cats are associated with increased percentages of Heinz bodies.*
Christopher MM and Harvey JW: Specialized hematology tests. Semin Vet Med Surg Small Anim 7:301, 1992.
   *A review of hematology tests including preparation and examination of Heinz-body stains and determination of methemoglobin content of blood.*
Cullison RF: Acetaminophen toxicosis in small animals: Clinical signs, mode of action, and treatment. Compend Cont Educ Pract Vet 6:315, 1984.
   *A review of the diagnosis and treatment of acetaminophen toxicity in dogs and cats.*
Harvey JW: Erythrocyte metabolism. In Kaneko JJ (ed): Clinical Biochemistry of Domestic Animals, 4th edition. San Diego Academic Press, 1989, p 185.
   *A review of erythrocyte metabolism including methemoglobin formation and reduction, Heinz-body formation, and oxidants associated with methemoglobin and/or Heinz-body formation.*
Harvey JW, King RR, Berry CR, and Blue JT: Methaemoglobin reductase deficiency in dogs. Comp Haematol Int 1:55, 1991.
   *A report of three cases of methemoglobin reductase deficiency in dogs and review of previously reported cases.*
Houston DM and Myers SL: A review of Heinz-body anemia in the dog induced by toxins. Vet Hum Toxicol 35:158, 1993.
   *A review of toxins producing Heinz-body hemolytic anemia in dogs.*

# APPROACH TO THE ANEMIC PATIENT

ALBERT H. AHN
*and* SUSAN M. COTTER
*North Grafton, Massachusetts*

Anemia is a clinical finding characterized by a decrease in total red blood cell mass with a resultant insufficiency of oxygen delivery to peripheral tissues. It is a commonly recognized clinical sign in dogs and cats and often indicates a serious underlying disorder requiring prompt diagnostic and therapeutic intervention.

Anemia can be classified as regenerative, with increased red blood cell production; or non-regenerative, with insufficient bone marrow response (see this volume, p 440). Furthermore, anemia can be characterized based on red cell morphology, mean corpuscular volume (MCV), and mean corpuscular hemoglobin concentration (MCHC). These classification schemes are used to direct diagnostic testing and therapy. The approach to the anemic animal should be with the initial objective of determining whether the cause is blood loss, hemolysis, or decreased production (Table 1). The most appropriate diagnostic and therapeutic procedures can then be instituted.

## HISTORY AND PHYSICAL EXAMINATION

The signalment and history are important in narrowing the list of rule-outs. Young animals may be affected with a congenital disease or iron deficiency secondary to blood loss from gastrointestinal or dermatologic parasitism. Middle-aged animals are more likely to have immune-mediated disease such as hemolytic anemia. Older patients are at greater risk of developing malignancies such as leukemia and hemangiosarcoma. Recent drug therapy or vaccination may predispose to hemolysis, marrow suppression, thrombocytopenia, or abnormal platelet function. Travel to certain locations might alert the clinician to test for ehrlichiosis, babesiosis, or other red cell parasites. Since the majority of anemic cats are infected with feline leukemia virus (FeLV), questions should be asked about FeLV testing or contact with other cats. Dietary indiscretion (onions, pennies, nuts, and bolts) can lead to hemolytic anemia.

Clinical signs of anemia include tachycardia, tachypnea, pale mucous membranes, and pronounced peripheral pulses. Animals with acute hemorrhage or hemolysis will develop clinical signs at a higher hematocrit than will an animal with a gradual onset of anemia from decreased production of red cells. Fever is a nonspecific sign, but may accompany acute hemolysis or an underlying infectious disease. While icterus may be observed in the patient with hemolytic anemia, hepatic or biliary disease also must be ruled out. Petechiation may be noted with thrombocytopenia from immune-mediated disease, marrow failure, or disseminated intravascular coagulopation (DIC). Halitosis or oral ulcers could indicate renal failure with anemia from decreased erythropoietin. Lymphadenopathy may be present in lymphoma or secondary to a systemic infection such as ehrlichiosis. The abdomen should be carefully palpated for organomegaly, masses, or fluid. Splenomegaly can occur in hemolytic or nonregenerative anemia and hematopoietic or splenic neoplasia. Abdominal, pleural, or pericardial effusion can be the result of bleeding from trauma, tumors such as hemangiosarcoma, or from clotting factor deficiencies. Sertoli cell tumors or rarely ovarian tumors can cause marrow aplasia from hyperestrogenism.

## DIAGNOSTIC TESTING

A hemogram (complete blood count [CBC]), including red cell indices and reticulocyte count, should be performed on every anemic animal. The presence or absence of reticulocytes is the basis by which anemia is classified as regenerative or nonregenerative. Nucleated red cells in the absence of reticulocytosis are not evidence of regeneration.

The onset and duration of anemia are important, as the diagnostic and therapeutic approach may vary. A hematocrit (Hct) taken in an acute hemorrhagic episode may be misleading, as fluid shifts from extravascular to intravascular compartments can take up to 24 hr to occur. Therefore, one may underestimate the severity of a hemorrhagic crisis by relying on a single measurement of the Hct.

A drop of blood placed on a microscope slide can be observed for evidence of autoagglutination. If present, true agglutination, which occurs in some cases of immune-mediated hemolytic anemia, must be differentiated from rouleaux, which may occur if concentration of fibrinogen or globulin is increased. Rouleaux are common in cats, and even normal feline blood may sometimes appear to agglutinate on a slide. Adding a drop or two of saline will disperse rouleaux, but true agglutination remains. Gross evaluation of a blood sample may provide immediate additional information. Chocolate brown discoloration indicates methemoglobinemia from oxidant injury to the red blood cells. The presence of icteric plasma suggests hemolysis or hepatobiliary disease. The buffy coat layer can be smeared and stained to look for *Ehrlichia* inclusions in

***Table 1.*** *Causes of Anemia*

**Hemorrhage**
  Surgery/trauma
  Coagulopathy
    von Willebrand's disease/thrombopathia
    Thrombocytopenia
    Hemophilia A, B/decreases in other factors
    Disseminated intravascular coagulopation (DIC)
  Ectoparasiticism (fleas, ticks, lice)
  Gastrointestinal (hookworms, neoplasia, ulceration)
  Neoplasia (hemangiosarcoma)

**Hemolysis**
  Antibody-mediated
    Warm-reactive IgG AIHA
    Cold-reactive IgM AIHA
    Transfusion reaction
  Congenital
    Phosphofructokinase deficiency (English springer spaniels,
      American cocker spaniel)
    Familial nonspherocytic, hemolytic anemia (poodles)
    Elliptocytosis (one cross-bred dog)
    NADH methemoglobin reductase deficiency (several breeds
      of dogs)
    Hemolytic anemia secondary to RBC membrane defect
      (beagles)
    Pyruvate kinase deficiency (beagles, Basenjis, West Highland
      white terriers, giant schnauzers, Abyssinian cats)
    Vitamin $B_{12}$ deficiency (giant schnauzers)
    Predisposition to oxidant injury, high erythrocyte potassium,
      and low glutathione levels (Akitas, Shebas)
  Toxin/drug-induced
    Propylthiouracil
    Lead
    DL-methionine
    Cephalosporins
    Fenbendazole
    Dapsone
    Gold salts
    Modified live virus vaccines
    Oxidants
    Onions
    Acetaminophen
    Methylene blue
    Phenacetin

Propylene glycol
    Phenol compounds (mothballs)
    Benzocaine
    Hydroxyurea
    Vitamin $K_3$
  Parasites
    Hemobartonellosis (*Haemobartonella canis, Haemobartonella
      felis*)
    *Cytauxzoon felis*
    Babesiosis (*Babesia canis, Babesia gibsoni*)
    Ehrlichiosis (*Ehrlichia canis*)
  Microangiopathic
    Splenic torsion
    Vena cava syndrome
    Hemangiosarcoma

**Decreased Production**
  Bone marrow disorder
    Hematopoietic malignancy
    Myelofibrosis
    Idiopathic aplastic anemia
    Irradiation
    Myelodysplasia
  Systemic disease
    Anemia of chronic disease/inflammation
    Feline leukemia virus
    Parvovirus
    Renal failure
    Liver disease
    Endocrine disease (hypothyroidism, hypoadrenocorticism)
    Neoplasia
  Toxin/drug
    Estrogen
    Chemotherapy
    Phenylbutazone
    Trimethoprim-sulfadiazine
    Griseofulvin
    Quinidine
    Thiacetarsamide
    Non-steroidal anti-inflammatory agents
  Nutritional
    Mineral deficiency (iron)
    Vitamin deficiency (B complex)
    Inadequate protein intake

white blood cells, although these are rarely found. Serologic testing is the method of choice for diagnosis of ehrlichiosis.

A blood smear can be examined to estimate white blood cell and platelet counts, and to look for morphologic or color changes in red cells, abnormal cells, or parasites such as *Haemobartonella* or *Babesia*. Presence of spherocytes indicates immune-mediated hemolysis. Schistocytes or helmet cells may be observed in microangiopathic hemolysis or DIC. Heinz bodies composed of denatured hemoglobin indicate oxidant injury. A few Heinz bodies are normal in cats.

The feces should be examined for change in color, which could indicate blood loss or hemolysis. Certain medications such as bismuth can darken the feces and be mistaken for melena. A fecal occult blood (guaiac) test may detect gastrointestinal blood loss, though the specificity of this test in animals eating meat diets is uncertain. A urinalysis is warranted to detect blood loss, increases in bilirubin or urobilinogen indicative of hemolysis or hepatobiliary disease, decreased specific gravity, proteinuria, or sediment changes suggestive of

renal disease. Significant changes in the chemistry profile of an anemic patient include increases in bilirubin (hemolysis or liver disease), alanine aminotransferase (ALT), alkaline phosphatase (ALP) (liver disease or hypoxic damage from severe anemia), blood urea nitrogen (BUN), creatinine (renal failure), calcium (lymphoproliferative disease), and globulin (myeloma, ehrlichiosis). Hypoproteinemia may be a sign of hemorrhage, although disorders of the liver, kidneys, intestine, and skin may also be associated with hypoproteinemia.

A positive direct antiglobulin (Coombs') test in an anemic patient indicates the presence of immune-mediated hemolysis, which may be primary or secondary to infections or previous transfusion. A coagulation profile (fibrinogen, fibrin degradation products [FDPs], platelet count, prothrombin time [PT], activated partial thromboplastin time [APTT]) may be performed if a coagulopathy is suspected. A buccal mucosal bleeding time may be measured to test for a platelet function defect. Radiographic and ultrasonographic imaging are used to rule out gastric foreign bodies or thoracic or abdominal abnormalities such as neoplasia. A bone marrow aspirate and core biopsy will provide diagnostic and prognostic information in nonregenerative anemia or if abnormal circulating cells are present. Evaluation of the marrow is particularly useful in cats in which marrow suppression or neoplasia may be caused by retroviruses. Anemic cats should be tested for FeLV and feline immunodeficiency virus (FIV). Red cell enzyme concentrations should be measured in young animals with unexplained Coombs'-negative hemolytic anemia, especially in breeds predisposed to these disorders.

In summary, blood loss anemia is primarily diagnosed on physical examination, and aided by finding microcytic hypochromic anemia with hypoproteinemia and guaiac-positive stools. Hemolysis is usually associated with macrocytic anemia with reticulocytosis, sometimes icterus and spherocytosis, or other changes in red cell morphology. Nonregenerative anemia most typically is associated with reticulocytopenia, and normocytic, normochromic red cells, sometimes with leukocytopenia and/or thrombocytopenia, or signs of other systemic disease.

## MANAGEMENT OF SPECIFIC DISEASES

Acute hemorrhage is rarely a diagnostic problem, and is treated by removing the cause and restoring circulatory blood volume. The Hct may be normal and red cells are required only after loss of greater than 30 to 40% of the blood volume. Diagnosis and treatment of chronic blood loss requires a different approach, since anemia does not develop until iron stores are depleted. Since younger animals have smaller stores of iron, they will become iron deficient sooner with ongoing blood loss than will adult animals. The anemia is variably regenerative, and usually microcytic and hypochromic. Thrombocytosis may be present. The red cell distribution width (RDW) may show a bimodal peak, reflecting microcytic cells and some macrocytic reticulocytes. Since iron deficiency is not likely to result from nutritional deficiency, every case requires a search for the source of blood loss, which is usually from the gastrointestinal tract. In puppies and kittens, treatment of endo- and ectoparasites may be all that is needed. In adult animals, however, tremendous numbers of blood-sucking parasites would be needed to cause anemia, so even if such parasites are present, additional diagnostic testing (e.g., endoscopy, ultrasonography, barium study) is indicated to rule out any underlying cause. Treatment with ferrous sulfate (50 to 300 mg/day), or in severe cases, red cell transfusion is indicated while the cause of the blood loss is investigated and treated.

Thrombocytopenia or abnormal platelet function as seen with von Willebrand's disease, is usually characterized by petechiae or bleeding from mucosal surfaces. In most coagulopathies, signs of hemorrhage overshadow the signs of anemia.

Hemolytic anemia can result from many causes in dogs and cats (Table 1). Immune-mediated hemolytic anemia (IHA) is the most common cause of hemolysis in dogs, and is discussed in detail elsewhere in this volume (p 152). Treatment consists of immunosuppression and supportive care with transfusions. High doses of corticosteroids (prednisone 2 mg/kg/day) are often successful. However, refractory or fulminating disease requires more aggressive treatment with drugs such as azathioprine or cyclophosphamide. Although IHA is usually a typical hemolytic anemia, some dogs will have a nonregenerative anemia. The bone marrow may show evidence of erythrophagocytosis and increased proliferation of early red cell precursors that are destroyed before they reach the reticulocyte stage, or may have an overall decrease in red cell production. These dogs are usually Coombs'-negative but may have spherocytosis. Diagnosis often is made by ruling out other causes of nonregenerative anemia and by therapeutic trial with immunosuppressive drugs. Thrombocytopenia can be seen in IHA either from concurrent immune-mediated thrombocytopenia (Evans' syndrome) or DIC.

Hemolytic anemia caused by congenital red cell defects usually becomes evident in young dogs with clinical signs that may mimic IHA. Phosphofructokinase (PFK) deficiency, seen in English springer spaniels and American cocker spaniels, is most likely to be confused with IHA for several reasons (Giger and Harvey, 1987). Cocker spaniels are predisposed to IHA, and the signs of hemolysis in PFK deficiency occur acutely when the blood pH rises at times of excitement. These dogs present with acute intravascular hemolysis and a rapid drop in the Hct, followed by spontaneous recovery. If immunosuppressive drugs are given at that time, the improvement may be erroneously attributed to the drug, reinforcing the misconception that the dog has IHA. Excessive exercise and excitement should be avoided in animals with PFK deficiency. The prognosis is better than for pyruvate kinase deficiency, where terminal development of osteosclerosis is common. Specific treatment is not available for most congenital anemias, but confirmation of the diagnosis is important so that genetic counseling may be offered and ineffective treatments avoided.

Red cell parasites may cause hemolysis in dogs and cats. Primary infection with *Haemobartonella felis* should be an acute regenerative anemia. More commonly it acts as an opportunist in cats with an underlying abnormality such as FeLV or FIV infection. The current treatment of choice for haemobartonellosis is a tetracycline such as doxycycline (Vibramycin, Pfizer) at 5 mg/kg every 12 hr. A recent anecdotal report claimed success in ten cats with anemia secondary to haemobartonellosis treated with enrofloxacin (Baytril, Miles Inc) 22.7 mg/day for 10 to 14 days (Winter, 1993). If this is verified by others, it would be an improvement over current treatment.

Canine babesiosis has been known to cause hemolytic anemia in certain geographic areas, but it may be more common and widespread that previously believed. Almost half of approximately 400 racing greyhounds in Florida were found to be seropositive and presumed infected (Taboada et al., 1992). Since retired greyhounds are often used as blood donors, testing of these dogs is indicated before their blood is used. *Babesia gibsoni*, endemic in Asia, was unknown in this country prior to 1979, but recently caused hemolytic anemia in 11 dogs from southern California (Conrad et al., 1991). Most recovered dogs become chronic carriers, so the prevalence of infection may continue to increase. Treatment with the babesiacidal agents diminazene aceturate or imidocarb dipropionate require special authorization from the Food and Drug Administration (FDA) prior to use (see "Canine Babesiosis," this volume, p 315).

The list of drugs and toxins reported to cause hemolytic anemia in dogs and cats continues to increase. The majority fall into the category of oxidant toxins, to which feline hemoglobin is especially sensitive. Cats with oxidant injury to their red cells develop methemoglobinemia and Heinz-body anemia. Acetaminophen has been the drug most commonly reported to cause hemolysis and hepatic necrosis in cats, but others are listed in Table 1. Propylene glycol, a common additive to semimoist cat foods, has been reported to shorten red cell life span in cats (Christopher, Permon, and Eaton, 1989). Normal cats can increase the rate of red cell production and maintain a normal Hct, but cats whose marrow is less able to compensate, such as those with chronic diseases, renal failure, or FeLV infection, may become anemic. Foods containing propylene glycol should not be fed to these cats. Recently, two cats with polycythemia vera developed acute methemoglobinemia while being treated with hydroxyurea (Hydrea, Squibb; 500 mg/wk PO), a drug with oxidant properties. Although this dose has safely been given to other cats, careful monitoring or a lower dose is indicated. Treatment of anemia from oxidant toxins, discussed in detail elsewhere in this section, consists of acetylcysteine to replenish glutathione stores. Treatment should be started within the first 12 hr after toxin ingestion before irreversible damage has occurred. Additional treatment for acetaminophen toxicity includes cimetidine, an inhibitor of the P-450 cytochrome oxidase system that is responsible for producing the toxic metabolites. Vitamin C has also been advocated for its antioxidant properties. Red cells of Japanese breeds of dogs such as Akitas and Shebas have increased potassium and decreased glutathione concentrations compared to other dogs. Since glutathione protects against oxidant damage, these breeds are at greater risk for hemolysis when exposed to oxidants. This may explain why hemolysis secondary to onion ingestion is prevalent in Japan, where these breeds are common. If a drug or toxin is suspected as a cause of hemolysis, removal of the offending agent and supportive care may be all that is required for treatment. Endoscopy is less stressful than gastrostomy for removal of pennies or other toxic foreign bodies from the stomach of young dogs with hemolysis secondary to zinc toxicity (see *CVT* Update "Zinc Toxicity," this volume, p 238).

Microangiopathic hemolysis is usually associated with a serious underlying disease, often with coexisting DIC. Characteristic findings are schistocytes, sometimes in association with hemoglobinemia. Treatment must be directed toward the underlying cause.

The most common cause of nonregenerative anemia is probably chronic disease or inflammation. The anemia is usually mild, with the Hct in the range of 25 to 35%, and the clinical signs of the underlying disease usually predominate. Anemia of chronic disease does not require specific treatment and will resolve if the underlying disease is treated successfully. Although serum iron concentration is usually low, the problem is decreased utilization rather than decreased stores, so iron supplements should not be given.

Cats are most likely to present with nonregenerative anemia most commonly secondary to FeLV, but sometimes is associated with FIV (Cotter, 1990). The anemia in FeLV-positive cats is characteristically macrocytic but nonregenerative and may require blood transfusion for supportive care. To date, no therapy has been found to reverse or mitigate the effects of FeLV, although the anemia will improve in some cats if a coexisting infection or other reversible problem is treated successfully. The work-up of an anemic FeLV-positive cat should proceed in the same manner as for an FeLV-negative cat. Potentially treatable causes such as haemobartonellosis or hemolytic toxins must not be overlooked.

Aplastic anemias are relatively uncommon but very serious causes of anemia or pancytopenia. Causes and management of these conditions are described in *CVT XI*, p 479.

The anemia of end-stage renal failure is a result of decreased production of erythropoietin. Recombinant human erythropoietin (Epogen, Amgen Inc) has been effective in increasing the Hct and improving the quality of life in dogs and cats with renal failure (see *CVT XI*, p 486). Dogs with Hct's below 30% and cats with Hct's below 25% are good candidates for therapy. Prior to treatment, animals are evaluated for evidence of iron deficiency, underlying infections, or other problems that might inhibit optimal erythropoiesis. The dose is 100 U/kg SC three times weekly for 12 weeks or until the Hct reaches 37 to 45% in dogs and 30 to 40% in cats. Then the dose schedule is decreased to once or twice weekly. Monitoring the Hct on a weekly basis during the induction period will prevent overdosing, which will result in polycythemia. Prolonged use of erythropoietin has been associated with the development of antibodies that cause refractory anemia in 20 to 50% of patients (Cowgill, 1992).

The bone marrow should be examined in both dogs and cats with unexplained persistent nonregenerative anemia, especially if neutropenia or thrombocytopenia is present, or if abnormal cells are present in the circulation (see *CVT XI*, p 488). A biopsy can be examined for degree of cellularity or fibrosis, and an aspirate for evidence of dysplastic or neoplastic changes. Not all animals with hematopoietic malignancy have large numbers of abnormal circulating cells; some present with pancytopenia. Myelodysplasia is a relatively common cause of anemia and other cytopenias in FeLV-positive cats and rarely in dogs. The marrow is cellular with ineffective maturation and release of all hematopoietic cell lines. Megaloblastic changes have sometimes been confused with those seen in folate or vitamin $B_{12}$ deficiency; however, concentrations of those nutrients have been normal in cats with myelodysplasia, so supplementation with hematinics is not likely to be of value.

With toxin, drug-induced, or idiopathic nonregenerative anemia, the goals are to remove any offending agent and to support the patient with transfusions until the marrow can regenerate. Erythropoietin is not useful in these patients, since endogenous erythropoietin production is adequate. Patients with pancytopenia from aplastic anemia are at risk for sepsis or hemorrhage. Recombinant granulocyte colony-stimulating factor (Neupogen, Amgen Inc) has been used with some success to stimulate neutrophil production (see *CVT XI*, p 466).

## TRANSFUSIONS

The mainstay of supportive care for the anemic patient is red blood cell transfusion. In acute blood loss, however, it is critical that the hypovolemic state be reversed first with crystalloid or colloid solutions. Packed red cells are the treatment of choice for patients with hemorrhagic shock and anemia of any cause. If both red cells and clotting factors are needed, fresh whole blood or recombined packed red cells and fresh frozen plasma would be needed. Components can be prepared if one has access to separation equipment or a cooperative local human blood center. Alternatively, an increasing number of veterinary blood centers offer blood components for sale. The use of specific blood components has been described in more detail elsewhere (Cotter, 1991; Stone and Cotter, 1992; *CVT XI*, p 475).

Canine blood donors should be tested for at least DEA-1 blood group antigens. Unless recipients can be typed prior to transfusion, only DEA-1–negative donors should be used. Several other erythrocyte antigens are variably reactive; thus, if a dog has received a transfusion previously, a major crossmatch should be performed. Most cats are type A, but the prevalence of type B varies depending on the breed. If the donor cat is known to be type A, a major crossmatch is all that is needed prior to transfusion. This is necessary for even the first transfusion, since type-B cats have strong anti-A antibodies and a type-B donor must be found (Giger, 1992).

The prognosis for recovery of an anemic patient varies with the cause. As a general rule, regenerative anemia has a better prognosis than does nonregenerative anemia. Since exceptions to this rule exist, a systematic approach to each patient will allow for the most accurate diagnosis, prognosis, and for the most appropriate treatment.

## References and Suggested Reading

Christopher MM, Perman V, and Eaton JW: Contribution of propylene glycol-induced Heinz body formation anemia in cats. J Am Vet Med Assoc 194:1045, 1989.
*A study of the effect of various concentrations of propylene glycol on Hct and red cell life span.*

Conrad P, Thomford J, Yamane I, et al: Hemolytic anemia caused by *Babesia gibsoni* infection in dogs. J Am Vet Med Assoc 199:601, 1991.
*A retrospective study of 11 dogs with hemolytic anemia induced by infection with* Babesia gibsoni *in southern California.*

Cotter SM: Feline retroviral infections. In Greene C (ed): *Infectious Diseases of the Dog and Cat.* Philadelphia, WB Saunders Co, 1990, p 316.
*An overview of feline retroviral infection and discussion of associated clinical disorders.*

Cotter SM: *Comparative Transfusion Medicine.* Orlando, FL, Academic Press, 1991.
*A textbook on all aspects of transfusion medicine, with emphasis on canine and feline issues.*

Cowgill LD: Applications of recombinant human erythropoietin in dogs and cats. In Kirk RW and Bonagura JD (eds): *Current Veterinary Therapy XI.* Philadelphia, WB Saunders Co, 1992, p 486.
*A review article describing clinical uses of recombinant human erythropoietin in dogs and cats.*

Giger U and Harvey JW: Hemolysis caused by phosphofructokinase deficiency in English springer spaniels: Seven cases (1983–1986). J Am Vet Med Assoc 191:453, 1987.
*A description of a hereditary acute hemolysis associated with alkaline fragility of red cells.*

Giger U: The feline AB blood group system and incompatibility reactions. In Kirk RW and Bonagura JD (eds): *Current Veterinary Therapy XI.* Philadelphia, WB Saunders Co, 1992, p 472.
*A review of clinical transfusion medicine in the cat.*

Stone MS and Cotter SM: Practical guidelines for transfusion therapy. In Kirk RW and Bonagura JD (eds): *Current Veterinary Therapy XI.* Philadelphia, WB Saunders Co, 1992, p 475.
*A review of clinical transfusion medicine in the dog.*

Taboada J, Harvey JW, Levy MG, et al: Seroprevalence of babesiosis in greyhounds in Florida. J Am Vet Med Assoc 200:47, 1992.
*A survey demonstrating high prevalence of* Babesia canis *antibodies in racing greyhounds.*

Winter RB: Using quinolones to treat haemobartonellosis. (Letter to the Editor). Vet Med April:306, 1993.
*Letter describing use of enrofloxacin for treatment of ten cats with haemobartonellosis.*

# LEUKOCYTE DISORDERS AND THEIR TREATMENT

DOUGLAS J. WEISS

*St. Paul, Minnesota*

The continuous migration of neutrophils into tissues that interface with body surfaces provides the primary defense against bacterial invasion. In health, egress of neutrophils into the tissues is balanced by production, keeping the number in blood relatively constant. However, because of the short circulation time and the presence of large marginated and storage pools, the numbers of neutrophils in the blood can change rapidly.

Six hematopoietic growth factors are primarily involved in the regulation of granulopoiesis. Stem cell factor, interleukin-1 (IL-1), interleukin 3 (IL-3), interleukin 6 (IL-6), and granulocyte/macrophage colony-stimulating factor (GM-CSF) stimulate the proliferation of multipotential stem cells. Stem cell factor is a glycoprotein produced by marrow stromal cells. Interleukin-1 and IL-6 are inflammatory cytokines which, in addition to their effects on hematopoiesis, mediate many of the systemic manifestations of acute inflammation (see "Cytokines and Biologic Response Modifiers in Small Animal Practice," this volume, p 547). When administered to humans, IL-3 increased both granulocyte and platelet production. GM-CSF and granulocyte colony-stimulating factor (GCSF) are produced by a variety of tissues in the body in response to IL-1, IL-3, tumor necrosis factor, and endotoxin. GM-CSF, administered by itself, stimulates production of granulocytes and monocytes. When given together with IL-3 and erythropoietin, GM-CSF stimulates erythropoiesis and, when given together with IL-3, stimulates thrombopoiesis. G-CSF specifically stimulates neutrophil production and function.

Granulocyte disorders encountered in dogs and cats include neutropenia and neutrophil function disorders. The causes and treatment of each of these conditions will be discussed. Although broad-spectrum antibiotic treatment remains the primary treatment regimen for neutrophil disorders, new therapeutic modalities such a hematopoietic growth factor treatment, bone marrow transplantation, and granulocyte transfusion have greatly expanded the clinician's capacity to treat animals with neutrophil disorders. Specific treatments to stimulate granulopoiesis include administration of G-CSF, GM-CSF, stem cell factor, and IL-3. Bone marrow transplantation techniques have been successfully applied to dogs and cats in treatment of diseases such as pyruvate kinase deficiency, cyclic hematopoiesis, mucopolysaccharidosis, Chédiak-Higashi syndrome, lymphosarcoma, and feline retrovirus infections (Gasper, Fulton, and Thrall, 1992).

## NEUTROPENIA

Neutropenia (i.e., <3000 neutrophils per microliter in dogs and less than 2500 neutrophils per microliter in cats) indicates an imbalance in the production, distribution, and/or utilization of neutrophils. Dogs and cats with less than 500 segmented neutrophils per microliter should be considered highly susceptible to infection; however, some animals are not highly susceptible until neutrophil numbers drop below 200/μl. Immature and toxic neutrophils should not be considered when assessing susceptibility to infection because they are likely to be less functional. Irrespective of the cause, dogs and cats with less than 500 segmented neutrophils per microliter should be treated with antibiotics and appropriate supportive care.

### Neutrophil Consumption/Destruction

Neutropenia, due to demand for neutrophils in body tissues, is usually associated with septicemia, endotoxemia, or bacterial sepsis involving the lungs or body cavities (Table 1). The presence of a marked left shift and toxic changes in the hemogram indicate the need

***Table 1.*** *Causes of Neutropenia in Dogs and Cats*

| | |
|---|---|
| Neutrophil consumption/destruction | |
|   Bacterial septicemia | Dog, cat |
|   Endotoxemia | Dog, cat |
|   Immune-mediated neutropenia | Dog |
| Decreased neutrophil production | |
|   Therapeutic drugs | |
|     Chemotherapeutic drugs | Dog, cat |
|     Estrogen | Dog |
|     Phenylbutazone | Dog |
|     Sulfonamides | Dog |
|     Cephalosporins | Dog |
|     Chloramphenicol | Cat |
|     Propylthiouracil | Cat |
|     Methamizole | Cat |
|     Griseofulvin | Cat |
|   Infectious disease | |
|     Ehrlichosis | Dog |
|     Feline leukemia virus | Cat |
|     Feline lentivirus | Cat |
|     Parvovirus | Dog, cat |
|     Cyclic hematopoiesis | Dog |
| Marrow stromal disorders | |
|   Marrow necrosis | Dog, cat |
|   Myelofibrosis | Dog, cat |
|   Inflammation | Dog, cat |
| Myelodysplastic syndrome/leukemia | Dog, cat |

for intensive antibiotic therapy and supportive care. Administration of a broad-spectrum bactericidal antibiotic is essential to control infection. As a general rule, expect the first antibiotic to be effective for 5 to 7 days in controlling fever and infection. Administration of a second antibiotic usually controls infection for up to 5 days, while subsequent antibiotics may control infection for only 1 or 2 days. Choice of antibiotic should be based on bacterial culture and sensitivity whenever possible. In the absence of culture and sensitivity results, broad-spectrum antibiotics such as cephalosporins or a combination of antibiotics should be used. A combination of gentamicin (1 mg/lb IV t.i.d.) and cephalothin (20 mg/lb IV t.i.d.) or gentamicin and ticarcillin (20 mg/lb IM q.i.d.) has been recommended to treat neutropenic animals that are febrile. Since mediators of inflammation stimulate production of hematopoietic cytokines, administration of exogenous hematopoietic cytokines would likely not be beneficial. Granulocyte transfusions are technically difficult to perform and are of questionable value to the neutropenic patient (Weiss, 1991).

Immune-mediated destruction of neutrophils have not been well documented in dogs or cats likely due to the lack of tests to detect antineutrophil antibodies. Steroid-responsive neutropenias have been reported for dogs.

## Decreased Neutrophil Production

Decreased neutrophil production can result from destruction of hematopoietic stem cells or granulocytic progenitor cells, damage to the marrow microenvironment (i.e., stroma), or hematopoietic myelodysplasia/neoplasia. Hematopoietic stem cell destruction causes suppression of all hemic cell lines, bone marrow hypoplasia, and pancytopenia in the blood. The term "aplastic anemia" has been used to describe this condition. In acute aplastic anemia, severe destruction of stem cells results in marked neutropenia and thrombocytopenia within 10 days. Affected dogs and cats usually have clinical signs referable to bacterial sepsis or hemorrhage. In chronic aplastic anemia, less severe suppression of hematopoiesis enables the animal to maintain neutrophil and platelet numbers at levels that prevent sepsis and hemorrhage, but prolonged suppression of erythropoiesis for weeks to months results in severe nonregenerative anemia. Causes of stem cell destruction include irradiation; drug toxicities; and viral, fungal, and rickettsial infections. Idiopathic aplastic anemia, that is commonly seen in humans, is rarely observed in dogs or cats.

### CHEMOTHERAPEUTIC DRUGS

Bone marrow is a target for most chemotherapeutic drugs because of their predilection for actively proliferating tissues. Rapidly proliferating cells include progenitor cells and the lineage-specific precursor cells. Stem cells tend to be spared, since they are not rapidly proliferating cells. Because of their short half-life in the blood, neutropenia is the first change noted in the hemogram. The nadir of the neutropenia usually occurs within 4 to 7 days. Depression and fever are clinical signs of note. Hematologic recovery predictably occurs within 2 to 4 weeks. Hematopoietic growth factor therapy is highly effective in reducing the duration of chemotherapy-induced neutropenia in dogs (see *CVT XI* p 466). Recombinant canine G-CSF (5 $\mu$g/kg every 24 hr SC), administered to dogs with mitoxantrone-induced myelosuppression, reduced the severity and duration of neutropenia. Broad spectrum antibiotic therapy should be given to all animals with total segmented neutrophils less that 500/$\mu$l.

### ESTROGEN TOXICITY

Dogs are highly susceptible to bone marrow suppression associated with estrogen administration or estrogen-secreting tumors (Weiss and Klausner, 1990). A single large dose of estrogen results in a predictable hematologic response in blood and bone marrow. Early suppression of erythropoiesis and thrombopoiesis results in thrombocytopenia within 9 to 14 days and a mild decrease in the packed cell volume (PCV). Granulopoiesis is initially stimulated, resulting in myeloid hyperplasia in the bone marrow and neutrophilia in the blood that peaks between days 17 and 23. Thereafter, myeloid hypoplasia and neutropenia develop. Hematopoietic recovery commonly occurs beginning at 25 to 30 days. Some dogs develop severe, chronic aplastic anemia when given two or more doses of estrogen at or near the recommended dosage. Many of these dogs have been euthanatized shortly after diagnosis; however, prolonged treatment may result in recovery after 2 to 3 months. Therapy consists of administration of platelet-rich plasma to prevent bleeding and broad-spectrum antibiotics to prevent bacterial sepsis. The utility of hematopoietic growth factors in treatment of estrogen toxicity has not been extensively investigated. G-CSF and GM-CSF would be expected to enhance residual granulopoiesis in affected dogs. Treatment with IL-3 or stem cell factor may stimulate thrombopoiesis as well as granulopoiesis.

### NONSTEROIDAL ANTI-INFLAMMATORY DRUGS

Although the incidence appears to be low, phenylbutazone and meclofenamic acid have been associated with hematologic dyscrasias in dogs (Weiss and Klausner, 1990). Syndromes include severe aplastic anemia, agranulocytosis, and agranulocytosis with thrombocytopenia. Agranulocytosis with or without thrombocytopenia may be an immune-mediated disorder and is usually reversible when the drug is discontinued. Aplastic anemia associated with nonsteroidal anti-inflammatory drugs is associated with severe stem cell destruction. Hematologic recovery has not been documented. Response to treatment with hematopoietic cytokines has not been evaluated.

### SULFONAMIDES

Both aplastic anemia and immune-mediated cytopenias have been reported in dogs treated with sulfonamides. A probable immune-mediated anemia, neutropenia, and/or thrombocytopenia has been reported for Doberman pinschers treated with trimethoprim-sulfadiazine. The dogs recovered promptly when the drug was discontinued. Aplastic anemia, characterized by pancytopenia and acellular bone marrows, has been seen in several dogs treated with trimethoprim-sulfadiazine. In the author's experience, affected dogs recover rapidly when treatment is discontinued.

### CEPHALOSPORINS

Administration of large doses of cefazedone to beagle dogs resulted in pancytopenia, neutropenia, thrombocytopenia, or nonregenerative anemia in most animals. Bone marrow specimens were cellular, but ultrastructural changes, including mitochrondrial damage and arrested maturation, suggested that erythroid and granulocytic precursor cells were being destroyed in the marrow. Neutropenia has been observed in both dogs and cats treated with therapeutic doses of cephalosporins. In all cases, the hematologic dyscrasia resolved rapidly after the drug was discontinued.

### CHLORAMPHENICOL

Chloramphenicol, administered to cats for 2 to 3 weeks, may induce leukopenia and hypocellular bone marrows with dysplastic features in the granulocytic series. A dog given chloramphenicol for 8 days had mild anemia and thrombocytopenia associated with marked increases in erythroid cells containing iron deposits (i.e., sideroblasts and siderocytes); however, most dogs do not show hematologic changes. Both cats and dogs recovered promptly after chloramphenicol treatment was discontinued.

### ANTITHYROID DRUGS

Leukopenia has been reported in 8% of cats receiving propylthiouracil and 3.8% of cats treated with methamizole (see "Complications of Treatment and Concurrent Illness Associated with Hyperthyroidism in Cats," this volume, p 369). Positive direct Coombs' test results in some cats suggested an immune-mediated cause of the disorder. Cats recovered rapidly after withdrawal of the drugs.

### EHRLICHOSIS

Pancytopenia, leukopenia, or thrombocytopenia commonly accompany acute monocytic and granulocytic ehrlichiosis. Although leukopenia frequently resolves, thrombocytopenia tends to persist. Since bone marrow hypoplasia is present, destruction of marrow precursor cells is the likely cause. In chronic forms of ehrlichiosis, cytopenias occur less frequently (see "Canine Ehrlichiosis: Clinical Implications for Humoral Factors," this volume, p 290). Antibiotic therapy and supportive care are often curative in acute cases but chronic cases may be refractory to treatment. Platelet-rich plasma transfusions may be beneficial for dogs that are actively bleeding.

### FELINE LEUKEMIA VIRUS

Anemia and neutropenia are commonly seen in cats infected with feline leukemia virus (FeLV). Toxic neutrophils and thrombocytopenia may also be seen. Bone marrow may appear normal, hypoplastic, or hyperplastic. Hyperplastic bone marrows, associated with nonregenerative anemias or neutropenia, have been classified as myelodysplastic or preleukemic syndromes. Clinical studies indicate that the neutropenia associated with FeLV-induced myelodysplasia responds to treatment with canine recombinant G-CSF. Allogeneic bone marrow transplantation has been performed in FeLV-infected cats in an attempt to resolve cytopenias and eliminate the viral infection. Although bone marrow transplants are approximately 80% successful, most cats remain infected with the virus (Gasper, Fulton, and Thrall, 1992).

### FELINE LENTIVIRUS INFECTION

Anemia, lymphopenia, and neutropenia commonly accompany lentivirus infection in cats. Dysplastic features observed in bone marrow samples from affected cats suggest a myelodysplastic syndrome.

### PARVOVIRUS INFECTION

Parvoviruses in both dogs and cats invade and destroy rapidly proliferating tissues such as crypt epithelium in the intestine, bone marrow progenitor cells and committed proliferating cells, and lymphoid tissue. Severe leukopenia, with left shifts and toxic changes, commonly develop in both dogs and cats 5 to 8 days after infection. Since infection is transient and stem cells are spared, hematologic recovery usually occurs within a week. Because of concurrent destruction of intestinal epithelium and leukopenia, both dogs and cats are highly susceptible to bacterial infection and endotoxemia. Broad-spectrum antibiotic therapy and supportive care are essential to recovery. Since the leukopenia is severe but of short duration and the threat of infection is high, affected animals may benefit from granulocyte transfusions. Therapeutic granulocyte transfusions are technically difficult to perform and, because of the short half-life of circulating neutrophil, a minimum of 4 daily transfusions has been recommended (Weiss, 1991).

### CANINE CYCLIC HEMATOPOIESIS

Cyclic hematopoiesis is a hereditary disorder of hematopoietic stem cells seen in gray collie dogs. The disorder begins within the first weeks of life and is characterized by cyclic fluctuations in leukocyte, reticulocyte, and platelet numbers every 10 to 13 days. Neutropenia is marked and persists for 2 to 4 days. Subsequently, neutrophilia and monocytosis occur. Antibiotic therapy and supportive care prolongs life, but dogs usually die by 3 years of age. Treatment with G-CSF, endotoxin, or lithium carbonate reduces or eliminates the cyclic neutropenia. Endotoxin and lithium carbonate have adverse side effects. Recombinant canine G-CSF (1 to 2.5 µg/kg, every 12 hr SC) prevented the neutropenia but did not completely eliminate the cyclic hematopoiesis. Bone marrow transplantation is curative.

## Bone Marrow Stromal Disorders

Bone marrow stromal disorders include necrosis, myelofibrosis, and inflammation. Bone marrow necrosis has been associated with leukemia, lymphoma, sepsis, endotoxemia, and drug toxicities. Unless severe, cytopenias in the blood are not seen. Myelofibrosis is commonly the end result of marrow injury and should not be viewed as a primary neoplastic process. Inflammatory disorders of bone marrow include purulent, fibrinous, and granulomatous inflammations. Purulent inflammation is associated with sepsis and endotoxemia. Fibrinous inflammation has been seen in dogs with disseminated intravascular coagulation (DIC). Granulomatous inflammation is common in dogs and cats with blastomycosis and histoplasmosis and has been seen in one dog with a systemic fungal infection. The approach to treatment involves antibiotic administration to prevent secondary injection, supportive care, and treatment of the underlying disease process.

## Myelodysplastic Syndrome/Neoplasia

Myelodysplastic syndrome (MDS) and hemic neoplasia are suspected by the paradoxical finding of cytopenias due to decreased marrow production in the face of a hypercellular bone marrow. Generally, hemic neoplasia is differentiated from MDS by the presence of greater than 30% blast cells in the marrow. Cytopenias associated with hemic neoplasia have been ascribed to crowding out of normal hemic cells (i.e., myelophthisis). Myelodysplastic syndrome is confirmed by the presence of dysplastic features in one or more of the hemic cells and variable increases in blast cells up to 30%. Myelodysplastic syndrome has been described in association with FeLV infection, drug toxicities (i.e., cephalosporin and chloramphenicol), and as a rapidly fatal preleukemic disorder. Treatment of human MDS patients with GM-CSF and G-CSF has resulted in some improvement in neutrophil counts in the blood. An additional benefit of GM-CSF and G-CSF treatment is enhancement of the impaired neutrophil function frequently associated with MDS.

# NEUTROPHIL FUNCTION DEFECTS

To protect the body from invading microorganisms, neutrophils must be able to adhere to endothelial cells at a site of infection; move through the endothelium toward an increasing concentration of a chemotactic agent; and attach, ingest, and destroy the organism. Both congenital and acquired defects in each of these functions have been documented for dogs, but few have been reported for cats (Table 2). Neutrophil function defects should be suspected in animals that have multiple episodes of bacterial sepsis. Detection of the neutrophil function defects is dependent on the application of sensitive tests that evaluate all aspects of neutrophil function.

## Acquired Neutrophil Function Defects

In dogs, acquired neutrophil function defects have been associated with poorly controlled diabetes mellitus, bacterial pyoderma, lead intoxication, protothecosis, hyperalimentation, and treatment with corticosteroids. The only disorder in cats associated with acquired neutrophil function defects is FeLV infection. Treatment of affected animals should be directed toward resolving the causative disease if possible and administration of broad-spectrum antibiotics to prevent and/or control bacterial sepsis. Administration of GM-CSF or G-CSF may enhance neutrophil function as well as stimulate granulopoiesis.

## Congenital Neutrophil Function Defects

### CHÉDIAK-HIGASHI SYNDROME

Chédiak-Higashi syndrome is seen in smoke-blue Persian cats with yellow eyes. Affected cats have increased susceptibility to bacterial infections because of defective chemotaxis, degranulation, and bacterial killing as well as episodes of neutropenia. Neutrophils,

**Table 2.** *Disorders of Neutrophil Function in Dogs and Cats*

| | |
|---|---|
| Adherence | |
| Leukocyte adhesion deficiency | Dog |
| Diabetes mellitus | Dog |
| Chemotaxis | |
| Chédiak-Higashi syndrome | Cat |
| Leukocyte adhesion deficiency | Dog |
| Complement (C3) deficiency | Dog |
| Staphylococcal pyoderma | Dog |
| Feline leukemia virus | Cat |
| Phagocytosis | |
| Leukocyte adhesion deficiency | Dog |
| Complement (C3) deficiency | Dog |
| Bacterial killing | |
| Doberman pinscher syndrome | Dog |
| Weimaraner syndrome | Dog |
| Leukocyte adhesion deficiency | Dog |
| Feline leukemia virus | Cat |
| Lead intoxication | Dog |

eosinophils, and monocytes have large cytoplasmic granules that result from fusion of primary and secondary granules. Despite the neutrophil dysfunction, affected cats can survive for many years with only infrequent episodes of bacterial sepsis. Bone marrow transplantation and treatment with canine recombinant G-CSF have been used successfully in cats with Chediak-Higashi syndrome. Bone marrow transplantation was found to restore both the defective neutrophil and platelet function (Colgan et al., 1992). Administration of recombinant canine G-CSF (10 μg/kg every 24 hr SC) for 10 days resulted in normalization of neutrophil counts within 3 days and enhanced chemotactic responses and bacterial phagocytosis.

### PELGER-HUËT ANOMALY

Pelger-Huët anomaly occurs in both dogs and cats and is characterized by failure of granulocyte nuclei to lobe. Nuclei of mature neutrophils and eosinophils appear round, oval, or dumbbell shaped. In cats, monocytes and megakaryocytes are also affected. No increase in susceptibility to infection has been reported and neutrophil function has generally been found to be normal.

### CANINE LEUKOCYTE ADHESION DEFICIENCY

A defect in the CD11/CD18 family of adhesive glycoproteins has been documented in Irish setter dogs as well as in mixed-breed dogs. The CD11/CD18 cell membrane glycoprotein is a member of the integrin family of intercellular adhesive proteins and is involved in adhesion of neutrophils to endothelial cells, complement-mediated chemotaxis, and complement-mediated phagocytosis. All affected puppies have evidence of bacterial sepsis within the first 12 weeks of life. Neutrophils from affected dogs have severely impaired capacity to ingest particles opsonized with immunoglobulin G (IgG) and complement as well as diminished adherence to nylon wool. Impaired adherence to endothelium reduced the number of neutrophils reaching sites of infection. Therefore, affected puppies fail to form pus at sites of infection. Affected puppies die within the first 6 months of life despite antibiotic therapy .

### CHRONIC INFLAMMATION IN DOBERMAN PINSCHERS

A defect in neutrophil bactericidal activity has been described in eight Doberman pinschers. Affected dogs

had chronic rhinitis and pneumonia but survived for years with intermittent antibiotic therapy to control infection. The bactericidal defect was associated with reduced production of superoxide.

### RECURRENT INFECTIONS IN WEIMARANERS

Recurrent and persistent bacterial infection have been reported in Weimaraner dogs (Couto et al., 1989). Neutrophil chemiluminescense for affected dogs is reduced, indicating reduced capacity to generate oxygen radicals, which are necessary for bacterial killing.

## References and Suggested Reading

Colgan SP, Gasper PW, Thrall MA, and Boone TC: Neutrophil function in normal and Chediak-Higashi syndrome cats following administration of recombinant canine granulocyte colony-stimulating factor. Exp Hematol 20: 1229, 1992.
*A study of the use of G-CSF in attenuating the neutrophil function defects as well as the neutropenia associated with Chediak-Higashi syndrome.*

Couto CG, Krakowka S, Johnson G, et al: In vitro immunologic features of Weimaraner dogs with neutrophil abnormalities and recurrent infections. Vet Immunol Immunopath 23:103, 1989.

Gasper PW, Fulton R, and Thrall MA: Bone marrow transplantation: Update and current considerations. *In* Kirk RW (ed): *Current Veterinary Therapy XI.* Philadelphia, WB Saunders Co, 1992, p 493.
*A review of progress in bone marrow transplantation for treatment of cats infected with feline leukemia virus.*

Obradovich JE, Ogilvie GK, Stadler-Morris S, et al: Effect of recombinant canine granulocyte colony-stimulating factor on peripheral blood neutrophil counts in normal cats. J Vet Intern Med 7:65, 1993.
*Discusses the dosage and route of administration of G-CSF to cats.*

Ogilvie GK, Obradovich JE, Cooper MF, et al: Use of recombinant canine granulocyte colony-stimulating factor to decrease myelosuppression associated with the administration of mitoxantrone in the dog. J Vet Intern Med 6:44, 1992.
*Discusses the beneficial effects of G-CSF in treating chemotherapy-induced neutropenia.*

Mishu L, Callahan G, Allebban Z, et al: Effects of recombinant canine granulocyte colony-stimulating factor on white blood cell production in clinically normal and neutropenic dogs. J Am Vet Med Assoc 200:1957, 1992.
*A study of the response of healthy and neutropenic dogs to administration of G-CSF.*

Schuening FG, Appelbaum FR, Deeg HJ, et al: Effects of recombinant canine stem cell factor on hematopoietic recovery after otherwise lethal total body irradiation. Blood 81:20, 1993.
*A study of the response of healthy and irradiated dogs to the administration of canine stem cell factor.*

Trowald-Wigh G, Hakansson L, Johannisson A, et al: Leukocyte adhesion protein deficiency in Irish setter dogs. Vet Immunol Immunopathol 32:261, 1992.
*A study of neutrophil functions in dogs affected with leukocyte adhesion deficiency.*

Weiss DJ: White cells. Vet Sci 36:57, 1991.
*A review of neutrophil disorders and therapeutic granulocyte transfusion in animals.*

Weiss DJ, and Klausner JS: Drug-associated aplastic anemia in the dog. J Am Vet Med Assoc 196:472, 1990.
*A review of adverse hematologic disorders associated with the administration of therapeutic drugs.*

# SPONTANEOUS BLEEDING DISORDERS

C. GUILLERMO COUTO

*Columbus, Ohio*

The components of hemostasis constitute a finely tuned system in charge of maintaining the fluidity of the blood, and of preventing blood from escaping outside blood vessels when injury occurs. When one recognizes the profusion of operative procoagulant and anticoagulant systems, it is remarkable that the prevalence of clinically relevant, spontaneous hemostatic disorders is relatively low. Despite this, patients are oftentimes presented for evaluation of spontaneous bleeding, or they are further evaluated when an otherwise healthy dog or cat experiences marked intraoperative or postoperative bleeding. This article briefly discusses the physiology of hemostasis from a clinician's standpoint, and emphasizes clinical recognition and interpretation of abnormalities in hemostasis screens.

## PHYSIOLOGY OF HEMOSTASIS FOR THE CLINICIAN

The hemostatic system interacts intimately with the vessel wall. In general, it is best to think about the intact endothelial surface of normal blood vessels as possessing anticoagulating properties, whereas the hemostatic system is mainly thought to possess procoagulating properties. Although this is a fairly accurate generalization, multiple exceptions to the rule exist (see below).

Traditionally, the hemostatic system is thought to be composed of three main arms: *primary hemostasis, secondary hemostasis,* and *fibrinolysis.* Primary hemostasis describes the interaction between platelets and vessel wall; secondary hemostasis describes the formation of fibrin through activation of the coagulation cascade; and fibrinolysis refers to the lysis of a clot or thrombus through activation of plasminogen into plasmin. The secondary hemostatic system is traditionally referred to as the "coagulation cascade," which is composed of intrinsic, extrinsic, and common pathways (Fig. 1). This concept has recently been disputed, and it now appears that the pathway of fibrin generation is a common one, since the three traditional pathways are closely interrelated. Clotting factors are designed by using Roman numerals; the addition of "a" to the designation of a clotting factor indicates an activated factor.

### Primary Hemostasis

Upon injury to the endothelial surface of a blood vessel and exposure of the flowing blood to the subendothelium, platelets adhere to the injured area by a variety of mechanisms. In most mammalian species, one of the many mediators of platelet adhesion to the subendothelial collagen is von Willebrand's factor (VWF). This adhesive protein, which circulates in blood in the form of large multimers and is a carrier for factor VIII, the antihemophilic factor, binds to subendothelial receptors and to glycoprotein receptors on the platelet surface, initiating adhesion. The platelets thus adhere to the underlying tissues and undergo aggregation, forming the temporary primary hemostatic plug, which is short lived (i.e., seconds to minutes). In addition to adhering to the subendothelial tissue, platelets also contain a large number of procoagulants and clotting factors, so that they provide an optimum milieu for activation of the clotting cascade.

### Secondary Hemostasis

In concert with the activation of the primary hemostatic system, fibrin formation is initiated in the milieu of the platelet plug. This occurs through activation of both the intrinsic, extrinsic, and common pathways of blood coagulation (Fig. 1). Most clotting factors, with the exception of factors VIII and VWF, are produced in the hepatocytes. Factors II, VII, IX, and X are vitamin K dependent (i.e., vitamin K is required in order to attach calcium-binding sites postribosomally to these proteins).

Traditionally, an irregular vascular surface is the contact stimulus necessary for activation of factor XII into factor XIIa, initiating the *intrinsic pathway;* activation of factor X initiates the *common pathway* of coagulation, resulting in fibrin formation. In the *extrinsic pathway,* tissue factor (TF), a transmembrane glycoprotein

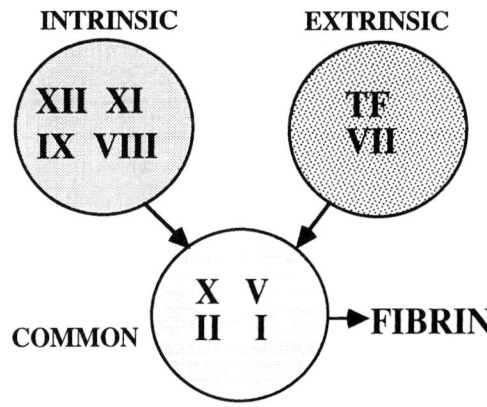

**Figure 1.** The traditional coagulation cascade.

present in most nonendothelial cell membranes, complexes with factor VII, resulting in activation of factor IX and factor X. Once factor X is activated, the common pathway of coagulation is initiated, and insoluble fibrin is generated (Fig. 1). This system results in the formation of a long-lasting secondary hemostatic plug, which is eventually reshaped to allow normal blood flow through the affected area.

### Fibrinolysis

The main role of the fibrinolytic system is to destroy or lyse fibrin clots or thrombi. In addition to lysing fibrin and fibrinogen, plasmin may biodegrade factors V, VIII, IX, and XI, as well as some other plasma proteins such as insulin, adrenocorticotrophic hormone (ACTH), and growth hormone. The fibrinolytic system is prohemorrhagic; enhanced fibrinolysis typically results in spontaneous bleeding.

Plasminogen, a proenzyme, is activated by either factor XIIa or by a variety of poorly defined tissue activators. Several tissue activators of plasminogen have been recognized, including streptokinase, urokinase, and tissue-type plasminogen activator (t-PA); these are used therapeutically in human patients and small animals with thromboembolic disorders. The fibrinolytic system also has built-in inhibitory mechanisms that have a net procoagulant effect. Inhibitors of fibrinolysis include $\alpha$-2-antiplasmin, $\alpha$-2-macroglobulin, and tissue-type plasminogen activator inhibitors 1 and 2 (t-PAI–1 and –2).

Plasmin biodegrades fibrinogen and fibrin, generating fibrin-degradation products (FDPs), which can be detected in plasma of dogs and cats by using diagnostic kits (see "Laboratory Evaluation"); FDPs also exert a profound inhibitory effect on platelet function, contributing to the petechiae and ecchymosis in patients with disseminated intravascular coagulation (DIC).

### Physiologic Anticoagulants

In order to maintain the delicate balance between clotting and bleeding, the hemostatic system also possesses several inhibitory mechanisms. In addition to the fibrinolytic system, the most important physiologic anticoagulants are antithrombin III (AT-III), a cofactor for heparin, and proteins C and S, two vitamin K–dependent factors that inhibit mainly factors V and VIII.

## CLINICAL RECOGNITION OF HEMOSTATIC DISORDERS IN DOGS AND CATS

Dogs frequently present for evaluation of spontaneous bleeding tendencies detected by the owner. A tendency towards excessive bleeding may also be discovered while performing invasive procedures, such as venipuncture, catheterization, or surgery. In contrast to dogs, cats with bleeding disorders may not bleed spontaneously, but they tend to bleed excessively while any of these procedures are being performed.

When evaluating a dog or cat with a spontaneous bleeding disorder, the information obtained during history taking and physical examination usually allows the clinician to differentiate between disorders of primary and secondary hemostasis (see below). These disorders can then be confirmed in the majority of the patients by performing simple tests.

As discussed above, the formation of the primary hemostatic plug (i.e., vascular-platelet interaction) is rapid, but short lived. Therefore, the following occurs in a dog or cat with thrombocytopenia or platelet dysfunction (or less frequently, with a vasculopathy): millions (or billions) of endothelial cells die daily in normal individuals, thus exposing the subendothelium to the circulating blood; in a normal animal, multiple primary hemostatic plugs will be formed, preventing noticeable bleeding. In a dog or cat with a nonfunctional primary hemostatic plug, blood starts exiting the superficial (and deep) blood vessels, and it does so during a few seconds to minutes, until a permanent secondary hemostatic plug is formed. This is analogous to what happens when one opens a faucet attached to an irrigator hose (one with multiple perforations), which allows the water to flow for a few seconds to minutes, and then closes it. Upon examining the ground, the "blood vessel" (in this case the irrigator hose) is surrounded by small "hemorrhages" (i.e., puddles) along its course. These superficial hemorrhages along the course of a blood vessel represent petechiae (pinpoint hemorrhages) and ecchymoses (hemorrhages approximately 1 cm in diameter) in a patient with thrombocytopenia or platelet dysfunction. Therefore, in animals with primary hemostatic disorders, the typical clinical findings include petechiae, ecchymoses, and bleeding from mucous membranes (e.g., epistaxis, hematuria, melena); in other words, *superficial bleeding* (Table 1). These animals also tend to bleed immediately after venipuncture (i.e., upon removing the needle).

In a dog or cat unable to form fibrin (i.e., a defect in secondary hemostatic plug formation), stretching or damage to a vessel wall results in minimal immediate bleeding. For example, upon performing venipuncture, there is almost no immediate bleeding, but the affected animal starts bleeding profusely after a few minutes. This delayed onset of bleeding occurs because the defect (hole) in the blood vessel is temporarily sealed by the platelet plug. However, because this patient cannot generate fibrin, once the primary hemostatic plug is no longer functional, blood starts to flow through the defect, and it continues to do so unimpaired, resulting in a large deep hemorrhage. This is analogous to opening up a faucet connected to a regular garden hose and allowing the water to run for several minutes to hours. Upon closing the faucet, rather than having multiple small puddles (i.e., petechiae and ecchymoses), there is a very large puddle at the end of the hose (analogous to a hematoma around the defect in the blood vessel). In a patient with a *secondary hemostatic defect*, this

**Table 1.** *Clinical Manifestations of Primary and Secondary Hemostatic Defects**

| Primary Hemostatic Defect | Secondary Hemostatic Defect |
|---|---|
| Petechiae common | Petechiae rare |
| Hematomas rare | Hematomas common |
| Bleeding at mucosal membranes | Bleeding into muscles, joints, and body cavities |
| Bleeding from multiple sites | |
| Bleeding immediately after venipuncture | Delayed bleeding after venipuncture |

*Adapted from Couto CG: Disorders of hemostasis. *In* Nelson RW and Couto CG (eds): *Essentials of Small Animal Internal Medicine.* St. Louis, Mosby Year Book, 1992, p 927, with permission.

translates into deep bleeding (i.e., formation of large hematomas or bleeding into body cavities) (Table 1). Dogs and cats with congenital secondary hemostatic defects may also have a high frequency of abortions or stillbirths, and high perinatal mortality. For reasons unknown thus far, the prevalence and severity of spontaneous secondary hemostatic bleeding are considerably lower in cats than in dogs with equivalent clotting factor levels.

Dogs and cats with mixed hemostatic defects (primary plus secondary) develop a combination of petechiae, ecchymoses, mucosal bleeding, hematomas, and intracavitary bleeding. Mixed hemostatic defects are almost exclusively associated with DIC, and are common in dogs and cats.

## LABORATORY EVALUATION OF THE BLEEDING PATIENT

Several laboratory tests are available to confirm a presumptive diagnosis in a dog or cat with spontaneous or excessive bleeding. The screening (or cage-side) tests will be discussed in some detail, since they are frequently performed by the clinician. The routine laboratory tests for hemostatic evaluation as well as the specialized hemostatic tests used to confirm specific defects will be briefly summarized, since they are always performed by referral laboratories, and thus, the methodology is not important for the clinician.

### Screening (Cage-Side) Tests

Four rapid semiquantitative tests are available. These tests allow for a rapid characterization of the defect as either a primary, secondary, or mixed hemo-static defect; or as enhanced fibrinolysis. The four tests are: examination of the blood smear, activated coagulation time (ACT), buccal mucosa bleeding time (BMBT), and determination of FDPs (Table 2).

### EXAMINATION OF THE BLOOD SMEAR

The first step in evaluating a dog or cat with a bleeding tendency, particularly if the clinical signs are suggestive of a primary hemostatic defect, is to examine a good-quality blood smear. The average number of platelets per monolayer field under oil immersion should be obtained. In normal dogs and cats, there are 11 to 25 platelets per field; each platelet in a monolayer field under oil immersion is equivalent to approximately 15,000 platelets per microliter. It is important to screen the smear at low power to search for platelet clumps that may result in pseudothrombocytopenia prior to evaluating the counting area.

If a dog or cat with evidence of primary hemostatic bleeding has more than four to five platelets per field, in all likelihood the bleeding is not due strictly to thrombocytopenia, and a platelet dysfunction syndrome may be present. Most patients with spontaneous bleeding due to thrombocytopenia have less than two platelets per oil immersion field.

### ACTIVATED COAGULATION TIME

The ACT evaluates the ability of whole blood to clot when diatomaceous earth, a contact activator, is added to the sample in a test tube. The test is performed by drawing 3 ml of blood in a syringe (without anticoagulant) by atraumatic venipuncture; 1 ml of blood is discarded, and the remaining 2 ml are placed in a tube containing diatomaceous earth (ACT tubes, Beckton Dickenson). The sample is mixed with the contact

**Table 2.** *Simple Cage-Side Tests for the Rapid Classification of Hemostatic Disorders**

| Test | Most Likely Disorder(s) if Prolonged (or Positive) |
|---|---|
| Platelet estimation in blood smear | Thrombocytopenia |
| Activated coagulation time | Intrinsic system defect |
| Fibrin degradation products | Enhanced fibrinolysis, DIC |
| Buccal mucosa bleeding time | Thrombocytopenia, thrombocytopathia |

*Adapted from Couto CG: Disorders of hemostasis. *In* Nelson RW and Couto CG (eds): *Essentials of Small Animal Internal Medicine.* St. Louis, Mosby Year Book, 1992, p 929, with permission.

agent by gently rocking the tube four or five times, and it is then placed in a warm plate or water bath at 37°C. The stopwatch is started when the blood is placed in the tube. After the first minute, the tube is removed every 5 to 10 sec, gently tilted, and then replaced in the plate or bath. At the first indication of gel formation, the stopwatch is stopped and the time read. The ACT in normal dogs ranges from 60 to 90 sec, and in cats is usually under 65 sec.

Because the ACT results in activation of factor XII, it evaluates primarily the *intrinsic* (factors XII, XI, IX, and VIII) and *common* (factors X, V, II, IIa, and fibrinogen) pathways. Since isolated defects in the extrinsic system are extremely rare, the ACT can be used as a reliable screening test for evaluation of secondary hemostasis. Platelet factor 3 (PF-3), a phospholipid, is a cofactor for clotting factors *in vitro*; thus, in theory, thrombocytopenia can result in prolongation of the ACT. However, this is extremely rare in practice. In general, prolongation of the ACT parallels prolongation in the activated partial thromboplastin time (APTT) (see below). The following disorders are usually associated with prolongation of the ACT: liver disease, congenital coagulopathies, vitamin K–responsive coagulopathies, and DIC, among others.

### BUCCAL MUCOSA BLEEDING TIME

This test evaluates the interaction between platelets and endothelium (or subendothelium) that leads to formation of the primary hemostatic plug. The BMBT is performed using a template (Simplate II, American Diagnostics) that is used to make a small incision of standard width and depth in the inner surface of the upper lip (i.e., buccal mucosa). Upon performing this incision using manual restraint in dogs and chemical restraint with ketamine and acepromazine (15 to 20 mg/kg of ketamine and 0.2 mg/kg of acepromazine IM) in cats, the time it takes for the blood to clot is determined. A gauze tourniquet is placed around the buccal mucosa to increase the venous hydrostatic pressure. Excessive blood flowing from the incision is blotted using a gauze pad or filter paper, exerting care not to dislodge the forming clot. Reference values for normal dogs and cats range from 1 to 3 min.

Prolonged BMBT occurs mainly in dogs and cats with thrombocytopenia and platelet dysfunction syndromes. In a patient with evidence of primary hemostatic bleeding and a normal platelet count, a prolonged bleeding time is usually an indication of a platelet dysfunction syndrome. Although in theory the BMBT should be prolonged in dogs and cats with vascular disorders, this rarely occurs in practice.

### FIBRIN DEGRADATION PRODUCTS

Fibrin (fibrinogen) degradation products are formed when plasmin biodegrades one or both of these coagulation proteins. Four fragments are generated upon the action of plasmin on fibrin (fibrinogen): fragments X, Y, D, and E. Only fragments D and E are detected by most commercially available assays. The ThromboWellcoTest is the most widely used assay for FDPs in dogs and cats, and being rather simple, it can be easily performed in-house by most practitioners. Two ml of whole blood are collected in a plastic syringe by direct atraumatic venipuncture. The sample is then transferred to a tube containing thrombin and a trypsin inhibitor (ThromboWellcoTest tubes), where in normal dogs and cats, it clots almost instantly. Two dilutions of serum (1:5 and 1:20) are then incubated with polystyrene latex particles coated with sheep anti-FDP antibodies, and at 2 min the presence or absence of agglutination at each dilution is recorded.

In most normal dogs and cats described in the literature and evaluated in our hospital, the test is negative; however, positive FDPs at a dilution of 1:5 and 1:20 were reported in normal cats (O'Rourke, Feldman, and Ito, 1982) (the significance of these results is unknown). The presence of positive results in the ThromboWellcoTest should be considered abnormal and regarded as an indication of active fibrinolysis; in our hospital, the most common syndrome associated with positive FDPs is DIC. Positive FDPs can also occur in dogs and cats with venous or arterial thrombosis and in dogs with anticoagulant rodenticide toxicity.

Based on the combination of the clinical signs and physical examination findings, and on the results of these simple tests of hemostatic function, the clinician can rapidly characterize the majority of the bleeding syndromes in dogs and cats (Tables 2 and 3).

## Routine Laboratory Tests

Several routine tests of hemostatic function are available in most university and commercial diagnostic laboratories. In general, a hemostasis screen (coagulation screen or coagulogram) is composed of five tests: a platelet count; the APTT, which evaluates the intrinsic and common coagulation pathways; the one-stage prothrombin time (OSPT), which evaluates the extrinsic and common pathways; fibrinogen concentration; and determination of FDPs. Some referral laboratories also perform AT-III determinations.

In most laboratories, coagulation tests are performed using a concurrent control sample of pooled canine or feline plasma. When interpreting the results of the APTT and OSPT, it is best to compare them to the controls. Prolongation (or shortening) of more than 25% above (or below) the control is considered clinically meaningful. In general, more than a 70% decrease in the activity of an individual clotting factor is necessary to result in prolongation of these assays. Interpretation of hemostasis screens is given in Table 3.

Decreased fibrinogen concentration is usually an indication of abnormal production (i.e., liver disease), or increased consumption (i.e., DIC), whereas increased fibrinogen concentrations are common in dogs and cats with inflammatory disorders or renal disease. Decreased AT-III activity is observed mainly in patients

**Table 3.** *Clinical and Hemostatic Abnormalities in Dogs and Cats with Spontaneous Bleeding Disorders*

| Disorder | Type | Species° | Clinical Signs† | Laboratory Abnormalities | Treatment |
|----------|------|----------|-----------------|--------------------------|-----------|
| IMT | Primary | D>C | P, E, MB | TP, ↑ BT | Immunosuppression |
| VWD | Primary | D>C | P, E, MB, PM | ↑BT, ↓ VWF | WFB, FP, FFP, DDAVP, thyroxine |
| Hemophilias | Secondary | D>C | H, BBC, PM | ↑APTT‡, ↑ ACT | WFB, FP, FFP |
| Rodenticide poisoning | Secondary | D>C | H, BBC | ↑APTT, ↑ ACT, ↑OSPT | WFB, FP, FFP, vitamin K |
| Liver disease | Secondary or mixed | D, C | H, P, E, BBC | As above plus TP | WFB, vitamin K |
| DIC | Mixed | D, C | P, E, MB, H, BBC | ↑APTT, ↑ ACT, ↑OSPT? TP, ↓ fibrinogen, + FDPs | Remove cause, heparin, WFB, FFP, fluids |

°Clinically more prevalent than.
†Prolonged intraoperative bleeding occurs in all these disorders.
‡See text.
Abbreviations: IMT = immune-mediated thrombocytopenia, P = petechiae, E = ecchymosis, MB = mucosal bleeding, TP = thrombocytopenia, ↑ = prolonged, BT = bleeding time, VWD = von Willebrand's disease, PM = perinatal mortality, VWF = von Willebrand's factor activity, WFB = whole fresh blood, FP = fresh plasma, FFP = fresh frozen plasma, ? = unproven efficacy, H = hematomas, BBC = bleeding into body cavities, DIC = disseminated intravascular coagulation, D = dog, C = cat, APTT = activated partial thromboplastin time, ACT = activated clotting time, OSPT = one-stage prothrombin time, FDP, = fibrin-degradation products, DDAUP = desmopressin.

with liver disease, protein-losing nephropathy or enteropathy, and DIC.

## Specialized Laboratory Tests

Some diagnostic laboratories specialized in hemostasis can perform specific assays, such as individual clotting factor determination. Properly collected samples should be mailed overnight (frozen or refrigerated) to the laboratory for evaluation. The laboratory should be contacted first.

## MANAGEMENT OF THE BLEEDING PATIENT

Basic principles in the management of dogs and cats with bleeding tendencies include mainly halting the bleeding by addressing its primary cause, and minimizing trauma while handling and treating these patients. It is important to minimize trauma by prescribing absolute cage rest in patients with bleeding disorders. It is also important to perform venipunctures with small-gauge needles to prevent excessive bleeding, keeping pressure in the area with a gauze pad for several minutes; injectable medication should be administered only by the intravenous route (and preferably, through an indwelling intravenous catheter) to prevent development of subcutaneous or intramuscular bruising and hematomas; and unnecessary surgical or medical procedures that could exacerbate bleeding should be avoided.

There are few nonspecific therapeutic measures that can be implemented in dogs and cats with spontaneous bleeding, including administration of whole fresh blood or plasma to patients with secondary or mixed bleeding defects to replenish clotting factors and fibrinolytic components, and administering immunosuppressive doses of corticosteroids (equivalent to 2 to 4 mg/lb of prednisone s.i.d.); the latter appears to decrease the frequency and severity of bleeding in dogs and cats with primary (and possibly secondary) bleeding disorders by decreasing vascular permeability, even if the thrombocytopenia causing bleeding is not due to immune mechanisms.

## COMMON HEMOSTATIC DISORDERS IN DOGS AND CATS

The clinical and hemostatic features of selected spontaneous bleeding disorders in dogs and cats are depicted in Table 3.

## References and Suggested Reading

Couto CG: Disorders of homostasis. *In* Nelson RW and Couto CG (eds): *Essentials of Small Animal Internal Medicine*, St. Louis, Mosby Year Book, 1992, p 926.
Couto CG and Hammer AS: Disorders of hemostasis. *In* Sherding RG (ed): *The Cat: Diseases and Management*, 2nd edition. New York, Churchill Livingstone, 1994, p 739.
Dodds JW: Hereditary and acquired hemorrhagic disorders in animals. Prog Hemost Thromb 2:215, 1974
Feldman BF: Coagulopathies in small animals. J Am Vet Med Assoc 179:559, 1981.
O'Rourke L, Feldman BF, and Ito RK: Coagulation, fibrinolysis, and kinin generation in adult cats. Am J Vet Res 43:1478, 1982.

# DEFINITIVE SURGICAL TREATMENT FOR CANCER

STEPHEN J. BIRCHARD

*Columbus, Ohio*

Surgical oncology in veterinary medicine has improved significantly in recent years. Surgery for neoplasia remains one of the most important methods of treatment for the cancer patient. Although surgery alone rarely effects a cure of malignant neoplasia, *en bloc* excision of tumors can significantly prolong the patient's life without causing untoward effects.

Many surgeons have developed more liberal attitudes toward cancer. What was once thought to be unresectable, such as certain oral tumors, may now be routinely excised via radical surgery. When surgical therapy is combined with other modalities, such as chemotherapy or radiation therapy, the surgeon becomes part of a multidisciplinary team. Therefore, the oncologic surgeon finds it necessary to become familiar with the principles not only of oncologic surgery, but also of chemotherapy, radiation therapy, tumor biology, and other aspects of cancer medicine.

Veterinary oncologic surgeons are also being asked to operate on animals with advanced malignant disease. It is no longer automatically assumed that a patient with metastatic cancer is not a surgical candidate. Cytoreductive surgery, combined with other modalities, may make sense in certain patients with advanced disease. The more willing we are to take some aggressive surgical steps in animals with diffuse disease, the more we will learn about tumor behavior, life spans, and so forth. Although anecdotal, the author has had experiences with certain tumors that were excised even though the animal had diffuse metastatic disease and had the animal live a good quality of life for several months to a year.

One of the most important concepts for the oncologic surgeon is to not lose sight of the big picture. Before performing radical procedures, several basic questions should be asked: what is the extent of the disease? What other diseases are present? How feasible is resection and reconstruction? Can the whole tumor be removed? And what are the owner's and the clinician's expectations? These factors will be considered later in this article. A thoughtful approach to the patient combined with a positive relationship with the owner increases the likelihood of a successful outcome.

Experience with oncologic surgery teaches the veterinarian many important lessons. One of the most important of these lessons is that the most success will be attained if one treats a "small lesion with a big operation." In other words, discover the malignancy early and treat it with a radical procedure. This gives the patient the best chance for a reasonably good outcome.

## DEFINITIONS

Incisional biopsy is the procurement of tissue from a lesion without removing it in its entirety. It is strictly a diagnostic procedure. Incisional biopsies are indicated to define the type of tumor present, helping the surgeon to plan the type of operation necessary. Some normal tissue should be included in the biopsy specimen in order for the histopathologist to better characterize the lesion. Incisional biopsy is ideal for peripheral lymph nodes that are draining a tumor to determine the stage of disease. Excisional biopsy also allows for procurement of tissue, but involves removal of the entire tumor. Removal of a tumor by this method does not imply wide or radical excision, however.

Wide excision of a tumor means removal of sufficient normal tissue with the tumor so that there is an increased chance of removal of all macroscopic and microscopic tumor. The amount of normal tissue removed depends upon tumor type and location. In general, for most malignancies, a 1- to 2-cm margin of normal tissue should be excised with the tumor to be considered a wide excision. However, for mast cell tumors, a 3-cm margin is recommended. This recommendation applies not only to the lateral and medial margin, but also to the deep margin. A common error is to disregard the deep margin and resect an inadequate amount of tissue.

*En bloc* removal of a tumor is defined as removal of a tumor as a "whole." In other words, the tumor is excised with a section of all surrounding tissues being removed as well. For example, to remove a tumor in the subcutaneous space by *en bloc* excision, the surgeon excises the overlying skin, surrounding subcutaneous tissues, and underlying muscle and fascia. The tissues are removed as a "block" of tissue with the tumor in the center.

Radical excision of a tumor is the most aggressive oncologic surgery performed. Radical excision involves extensive dissection and removal of tissues some distance from the primary tumor. For example, radical mastectomy is the removal of an entire chain of mammary glands along with lymph nodes, all underlying subcutaneous tissues and possibly some muscle, and regional lymph nodes, even if there was only one tumor in the chain. Another example of radical excision would be removal of a large section of thoracic or abdominal body wall in order to completely excise a tumor attached to the muscle.

## OVERVIEW OF CLINICAL APPROACH TO SURGICAL NEOPLASTIC LESIONS

Many factors should be considered before embarking on an oncologic surgical procedure. Define and stage the disease. Is it benign or malignant, invasive or localized, and metastatic or confined to a single lesion? What organ's systems are involved and can resection be safely performed? Is a radical surgical procedure feasible considering tumor location and tissue involvement? What other options are available for the disease and how does nonsurgical treatment compare to surgical treatment in terms of results, complications, and cost? Will surgery be part of an integrated treatment plan including chemotherapy or radiation therapy or both? How will these adjunctive treatments affect tissue healing? What is the overall condition of the animal? Is it a good risk for anesthesia and surgery? Obtain sufficient information from the patient to help gauge this risk, such as complete blood count (CBC), serum chemistry profile, urinalysis, thoracic radiographs, and so forth. Last but definitely not least: What are the expectations and attitude of the owner? How far is the owner willing to go, and are they realistic about the outcome? The veterinarian should not only inform the client about the disease and its treatment, he or she should develop a working relationship with the owner, especially if extensive and costly treatments are planned. The owner needs to feel as comfortable and confident as possible about the doctors and their plan, and the veterinarian needs to feel that the owner supports the decisions that are being made.

## PRINCIPLES OF ONCOLOGIC SURGERY

"Early, wide, and deep" is frequently quoted as one of the most important aspects of oncologic surgery. Detect the tumor early and treat it with an aggressive surgery. The first goal is to completely remove the tumor, the second goal is to close the wound. The surgeon must not compromise the aggressiveness of the resection because of anxiety over how to close the wound. Large skin wounds can be closed with rotating flaps or grafts or left open to heal by second intention. Large wounds of the oral cavity or nose can also be left open if necessary and the animal fed via a gastrostomy tube. Delayed closure can then be performed if necessary. If the tumor is attached to bone, it is not helpful to scrape the tumor tissue off the bone; the bone must also be removed.

Tumors should be removed *en bloc* whenever possible. Handling of the tumor should be minimized, and invasion of its capsule avoided. The surrounding tissues should be frequently lavaged with sterile saline and closure performed with clean gloves and instruments.

Resected tissues should always be biopsied, no matter how obvious the tumor appears to be. Give the histopathologist an adequate history, and orient the pathologist by marking tumor margins with sutures or India ink. Biopsies should also be obtained from surrounding tissues, lymph nodes, or other organs that could have metastatic lesions in order to stage the tumor.

If postoperative radiation or chemotherapy is anticipated, adjustments may be needed in the use of sutures or other implants in the wound. Nonabsorbable sutures may be indicated if postoperative chemotherapy will impair wound healing, especially in dangerous situations such as with intestinal anastomosis.

## EXAMPLES OF SURGICAL TREATMENT OF SPECIFIC NEOPLASMS

### Mammary Neoplasia

Considerable evolution has occurred in the surgical approach to mammary tumors. Several years ago, radical mastectomy (removal of all glands along with regional lymph nodes and underlying tissues) was recommended for virtually all mammary tumors of dogs and cats. Clinical studies have now clearly shown that radical surgery is not necessary for most mammary tumors (MacEwen and Withrow, 1989). Long-term survival is not enhanced by aggressive surgical removal of all glands compared to simple mastectomy (removal of one gland only) or lumpectomy. However, the principle of removal of sufficient tissue to achieve complete resection should not be compromised. Strategies for mastectomy are now dependent not so much on tumor type, but on location and extent of neoplasia, directions of lymphatic drainage, and how to achieve complete resection. Glands 1 and 2 drain cranially to the axillary lymph node, glands 4 and 5 drain caudally to the inguinal lymph node, and gland 3 can drain either cranially or caudally. Lymphatic drainage can occur to the other mammary chain and can also be altered by the neoplastic invasion.

Masses located between glands 4 and 5 are usually best removed by removing both glands 4 and 5 (regional mastectomy), especially if they are large. It is simply easier and less traumatic to the tissues to remove both glands than to try to separate them. If gland 5 is removed, the inguinal lymph node is usually also removed and should be examined histologically. Masses on glands 1, 2, or 3 can be removed by lumpectomy, simple mastectomy, or regional mastectomy. The axillary lymph node is usually removed only if it is palpably enlarged or has cytologic evidence of neoplastic cells present in it.

Removal of all mammary glands is still recommended for those animals that have tumors in all glands. Bilateral mastectomy has been described for selected patients, but the author prefers to stage the resection and do one side at a time (see "Mammary Tumors in the Dog," this volume, pp 508 and 1098).

Surgical complications consist of seroma, wound infection, dehiscence, and blood loss. These complications are minimized by adhering to sound principles of tissue handling, closure of dead space, and hemostasis. In mastectomy closure, the subcutaneous suture layer is of utmost importance to wound healing. The subcutaneous sutures are used to close dead space and relieve skin tension, allowing skin sutures to be placed loosely and decreasing the need for drains or postoperative bandages.

Like many other situations in oncologic surgery, knowing when not to recommend surgery is important to the animal with mammary neoplasia. Inflammatory mammary carcinoma, characterized by rapidly growing, invasive, and diffusely inflamed tumors, is not amenable to resection. These tumors cannot be completely resected and surgery can induce severe complications such as disseminated intravascular coagulation (DIC).

## Oral Neoplasia

Aggressive surgical resection of oral neoplasms has become the treatment of choice for most patients. Before reports of successful removal of oral tumors by mandibulectomy and maxillectomy, tumors were removed by scraping off bone, electrocautery, or just removing the soft tissue component. These conservative procedures were largely unsuccessful; rapid recurrence or metastasis or both usually occurred. It is now well established that early and aggressive resection of oral tumors by mandibulectomy or maxillectomy can result in long periods of disease-free life or even cure in some cases (Salisbury and Lantz, 1988; Schwarz et al., 1991a). Benign oral masses such as fibrous or ossifying epulis may require mandibulectomy or maxillectomy if bone is involved, and results are usually excellent. Of the common malignant oral tumors, the most encouraging results of surgery tend to be on the squamous cell carcinoma (SCC) in dogs. The most common malignant oral tumor in cats is SCC; however, it is a more difficult tumor to manage than in dogs. Squamous cell carcinoma in cats grows rapidly and is very locally invasive. Oral malignant melanoma tends to rapidly metastasize, and fibrosarcoma tends to recur. However, even with these tumors, very early recognition and *en bloc* excision can be successful. One recent study suggested that tumors located rostrally in the mouth have a better prognosis than those located caudally (Schwarz et al., 1991b).

Surgical strategy for the patient with an oral tumor depends upon tumor type, location, and extent of tissue involvement. Preoperative radiographs are imperative to determine if bone is involved and to what extent. Even if the bone appears normal on radiographs, if the tumor is thought to be malignant, *en bloc* excision of the tumor with the underlying bone is recommended. Extensive removal of bone and associated soft tissue can be performed without untoward effects on the animal. For example, for tumors located at mid-mandible or maxilla, complete unilateral hemimandibulectomy or maxillectomy can be done followed by standard soft tissue reconstruction. For tumors located at the rostral mandible, bilateral partial mandibulectomy can be performed back to and including the second or third premolar tooth. Extending the excision more caudally than

this can result in difficulty eating. The author has also performed bilateral maxillectomy in a dog with an osteosarcoma of the hard palate (Figs. 1 through 4). Multiple surgeries were required to achieve soft tissue closure of the defect, but complete resection was accomplished.

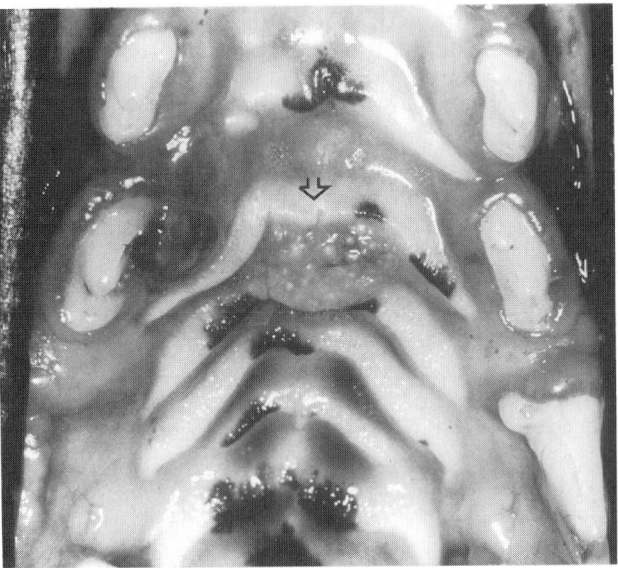

**Figure 1.** Intraoral view (nose is to the top of the photograph) of an osteosarcoma involving the hard palate in a collie.

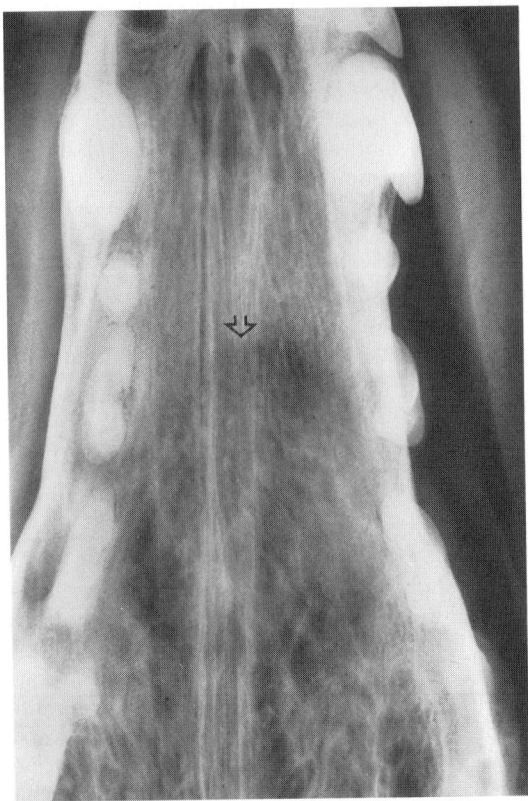

**Figure 2.** Ventrodorsal radiograph of the hard palate in same dog as in Figure 1.

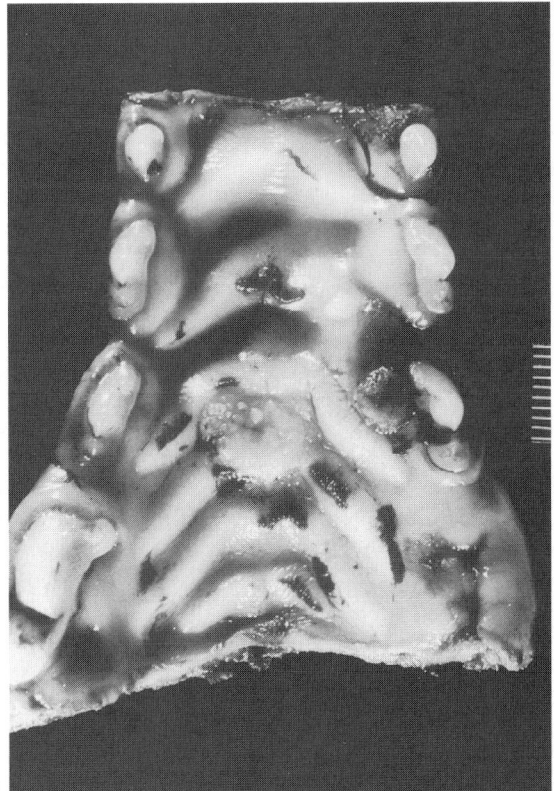

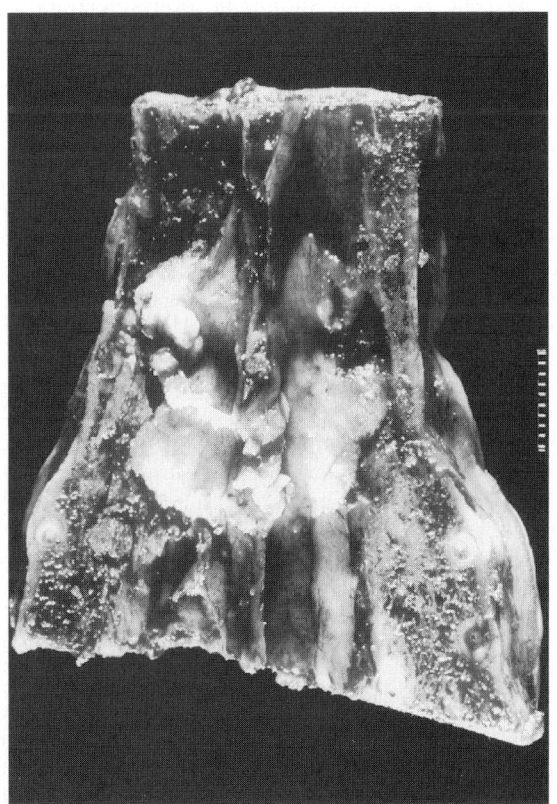

**Figure 3.** Postoperative tissue specimen from collie in Figure 1 showing ventral (*A*) and dorsal (*B*) aspect of the involved portion of hard palate and maxilla.

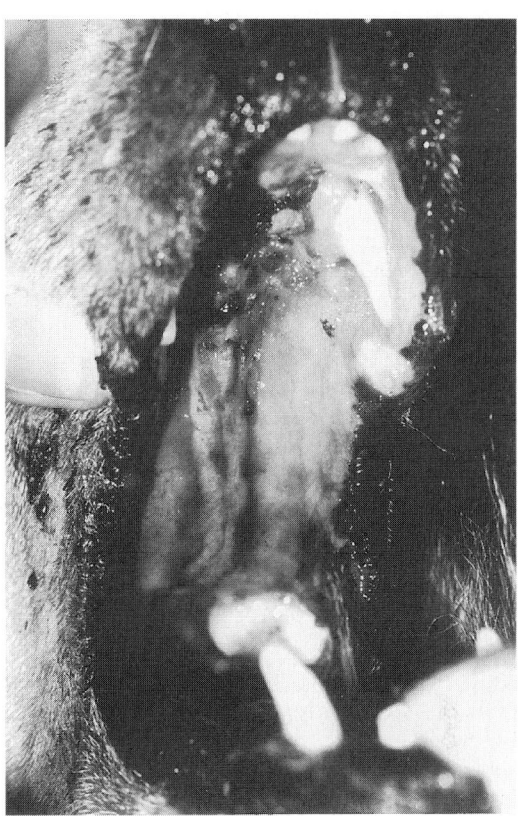

**Figure 4.** Postoperative intraoral view of collie shown in Figure 1 showing results of reconstruction of the soft tissues after removing the neoplasm.

Cats are not quite as resilient as dogs in their response to extensive oral surgery. Hemimandibulectomy and hemimaxillectomy are frequently performed and are well tolerated by cats, but more intensive nutritional support may be necessary. Percutaneous gastrostomy tubes are frequently used by us to supply nutrition during the first several weeks postoperatively.

## Cutaneous Neoplasia

Tumors of the skin are some of the most common seen in veterinary practice. A wide variety of tumors occur, both benign and malignant. One of the most important principles of surgical management of these tumors is to establish a diagnosis before planning the operation. A very practical and accurate biopsy method of skin masses is fine-needle aspiration. This information allows the clinician to plan an appropriate treatment. A benign skin tumor, such as an epidermal inclusion cyst, requires only a marginal excision and routine skin closure. Malignant skin tumors, such as mast cell tumor (MCT), require extensive tissue resection (e.g., 3-cm margin exision for MCT) followed by more complicated reconstruction. As mentioned previously, a 3-cm margin means the deep tissue margin as well as the lateral and medial margins. Many times it is impossible to achieve adequate deep tissue resection because of adverse effects on the patient, but the deep margin should at least be carefully considered when removing any skin mass.

It is very important to be sure that a complete resection has been peformed before performing an extensive skin reconstruction or graft. If doubt exists concerning the skin margins, the wound may be left open and covered with appropriate dressings until the biopsy results are available. If histopathology reveals inadequate excision, the patient can be reoperated to remove more tissue, or other options such as radiation therapy can be considered.

Massive skin defects that result from extensive resection can be closed using a variety of reconstruction methods. Random or axial pattern skin flaps are used to close large skin wounds when appropriate tissues are available. Free skin grafts, such as mesh grafts, are used if local skin is not sufficient to close the wound. However, free skin grafts must be preceded by a period of open wound management to establish a bed of healthy granulation tissue. Our experience with mesh grafts has been very good in cats and fair in dogs.

## Gastrointestinal Neoplasia

The gastrointestinal tract is another system where surgery can be a definitive treatment for tumors. Benign tumors of the stomach, such as fibroma and leiomyoma, can be completely excised with surgery. Gastric leiomyoma is frequently found at the cardia of the stomach, making removal difficult. However, the tumor can be approached via a greater curvature gastrotomy and removed by submucosal resection within the stomach lumen. Even malignant tumors of the stomach, such as lymphosarcoma and adenocarcinoma, are sometimes resectable. We have operated on several cats with early lymphoma of the stomach that were resectable and resulted in reasonable disease-free intervals. Adenocarcinoma of the stomach in dogs, unfortunately, is frequently located at the lesser curvature and may extend from cardia to pylorus. However, the author has seen some tumors that were not so extensive and were removable by partial gastrectomy.

Resectability of intestinal tumors varies according to location and tumor type. Adenocarcinoma in dogs is frequently seen in the duodenum and colon. Duodenal resection is complicated by its relationship to the pancreas and gallbladder, but tumors can be removed via resection and anastomosis, especially if present in the distal duodenum and not involving the major duodenal papilla. Surgical removal of an intestinal tumor may be only palliative if metastasis has already occurred. However, significant prolongation of life can occur after removal of the primary tumor. The author has experience with one dog with a duodenal carcinoma and diffuse metastasis to the omentum and lymph nodes that lived for 1 year after duodenal resection and no adjunctive therapy.

Intestinal tumors are amenable to wide resection, since animals can function well after removal of a significant portion of the tract. Important surgical consid-erations are: maintain adequate blood supply to the tissues, be sure that the anastomosis is tension free, use nonabsorbable sutures (e.g., 4-0 or 5-0 polypropylene) for anastomosis if postoperative chemotherapy is anticipated, and be sure to perform biopsy of other affected organs and tissues such as regional lymph nodes and liver.

## Lung Neoplasia

Primary lung tumors are frequently amenable to surgical removal, especially if they are solitary and not adhered to surrounding structures. Although lung tumors are usually malignant (e.g., adenocarcinoma, squamous cell carcinoma), significant postoperative survival times are possible after complete resection. If the tumor is resected before metastasis has occurred, postoperative life span up to 1 year is possible (Withrow, 1989). If the neoplasm has metastasized to mediastinal lymph nodes, postoperative survival is shorter.

There are some principles of lung tumor removal that should be considered. These tumors are frequently located near the hilus. The tumor may be adhered to the left or right atrium, or the pericardium. Careful dissection is required to free the tumor from these structures. In some cases, a section of pericardium is removed with the lung lobe to be sure that all of the tumor is removed. When a complete lobectomy is performed, the bronchus should be doubly clamped and severed between the clamps, leaving one clamp attached to the resected lobe. This is to prevent drainage of bronchiolar fluid into the surgical site. Also, the surgeon should warn the anesthetist that some bronchial fluid may drain into the trachea during manipulation of the affected lung lobe. This can complicate ventilation by plugging the endotracheal tube. Periodic suction of the tube may be necessary during the procedure. Surgical stapling devices are very useful for partial or complete lung lobectomy. The device is used to close the bronchus or lung parenchyma by delivering two rows of B-shaped stainless steel staples into the tissue.

After resection of the lung, check the bronchial stump for air leakage by flooding the site with warm saline and asking the anesthetist to give a positive-pressure inspiration. If leakage occurs, additional staples or sutures may be required. Also, check the remaining lung lobes and mediastinal lymph nodes for evidence of disease.

## PRINCIPLES OF POSTOPERATIVE CARE

The postoperative cancer patient has several needs that should be addressed. First, postoperative analgesia should be provided, especially after extensive resection of tissue such as with mandibulectomy or maxillectomy. Opiates such as morphine, bupremorphine, or butorphenol can be used. Fluid support of the patient is also very important. Intravenous fluids should be administered until the animal appears able to maintain hydration with oral intake.

Nutritional support is also critical. Cancer patients tend to be in a poor plane of nutrition to begin with, and major surgery can delay return to an adequate level of food intake. If the surgeon anticipates a prolonged period of anorexia or inability to eat adequately, some kind of nutritional access device should be planned preoperatively and placed during the procedure (e.g., a gastrostomy tube).

Long-term follow-up is very important to monitor the patient for evidence of tumor recurrence or metastasis. The frequency of reevaluations will depend upon the type of tumor. Maintaining good follow-up with the patient and owner also helps oncologists to collect data concerning disease-free intervals and long-term prognosis. Future trends in cancer treatment will be influenced by objective analysis of large patient populations and results of therapy.

### References and Suggested Reading

MacEwen EG and Withrow SJ: Tumors of the mammary gland. *In* Withrow SJ and MacEwen EG (eds.): *Clinical Veterinary Oncology.* Philadelphia, JB Lippincott Co, 1989, p 292.

Salisbury SK and Lantz GC: Long-term results of partial mandibulectomy for treatment of oral tumors in 30 dogs. J Am Anim Hosp Assoc 24:285, 1988.

Schwarz PD, Withrow SJ, Curtis CR, et al: Mandibular resection for oral cancer. J Am Anim Hosp Assoc 27:601, 1991a.

Schwarz PD, Withrow SJ, Curtis CR, et al: Partial maxillary resection for oral tumors. J Am Anim Hosp Assoc 27:617, 1991b.

Withrow SJ: Tumors of the respiratory system. *In* Withrow SJ and MacEwen EG (eds.): *Clinical Veterinary Oncology.* Philadelphia, JB Lippincott Co, 1989, p 215.

---

# INDICATIONS AND APPLICATIONS OF RADIATION THERAPY

ALAIN P. THÉON

*Davis, California*

Veterinary radiation oncology has benefitted from the progress made in medical radiation oncology. Many advancements have been made possible through better understanding of the biologic processes that underlie radiation responses. Technologic advances have resulted in increasingly sophisticated treatment units and treatment planning. These improvements have led to a greater role for radiation therapy in both local and regional treatments.

Radiation therapy is the most important nonsurgical treatment for animals with solid tumors. Numerous reports have documented the efficacy of radiation therapy for the treatment of selected tumor types, with cure now being a realistic goal. The small number of radiation therapy facilities and the cost of treatment have limited the impact of radiation therapy in overall animal cancer management.

## CLINICAL PRINCIPLES OF RADIATION THERAPY

### Methods of Irradiation

Methods of irradiation include teletherapy, brachytherapy, and systemic therapy. In teletherapy, irradiation is delivered at some distance from the tumor. Three teletherapy techniques are available in small animal practice: external-beam, intraoperative, and endocavitary. Usually, radiation therapy is carried out by external-beam irradiation, also called transcutaneous irradiation. This is the only method of irradiation that will be covered in this article. Treatment may be done with a variety of radiation sources including low-energy orthovoltage x-rays, high-energy megavoltage x-ray or γ-ray photon beams, and electron beams. The treatment plan is based on the size, depth, and anatomic location of the tumor.

### Treatment Prescription

During a course of external-beam radiotherapy, the total radiation dose is given as a series of small equal-sized doses called dose fractions. Each dose fraction is given to the animal while under general anesthesia to ensure adequate immobilization and positioning. A radiation therapy course is prescribed in terms of overall treatment duration (time), total radiation dose (dose), and dose fractionation pattern (fractionation) which includes the dose per fraction and the frequency of administration: daily (Monday through Friday), alternate-day (Monday/Wednesday/Friday), or twice-weekly (Monday, Friday) schedules.

A typical treatment prescription for a person includes a dose of 60 to 70 Gy (1 Gy=100 rad) given over

6 to 7 weeks with daily dose fractions of 1.8 to 2 Gy. Time dose-fractionation schemes used for animals are referred to as coarse because fewer dose fractions using larger doses per fraction (>2 Gy/fraction) are prescribed for essentially logistic reasons. Treatment prescriptions typically use lower total doses in a shorter overall time, with 6 to 16 fractions of 3 to 6 Gy over a period of 3 to 4 weeks.

There is biologic and clinical evidence that such coarse fractionation protocols may be suboptimal for selected tumors. The use of large doses per fraction places the animal at risk for serious radiation complications, thus limiting the total dose that can be delivered. In addition, the use of fewer dose fractions given on an alternate-day or twice-weekly schedule allows tumor cell repopulation during the interfraction time interval. Several clinical trials are in progress to evaluate the benefit of reducing the dose per fraction and using daily fractionation in selected tumors, such as intranasal and brain tumors in dogs and oral tumors in cats.

The cardinal principle of radiation therapy is the delivery of a dose that sterilizes all viable tumor cells and allows survival of critical organs and tissues in the irradiated (target) volume.

The radiation oncologist's objective is to determine individual radiation prescriptions that are a compromise between the dose required for tumor sterilization and the dose that is tolerated by surrounding normal tissue.

## The Role of Radiation Therapy in Cancer Management

Radiation therapy can be used alone or in combination with other treatment modalities. The goals of a combined approach are to improve the efficacy and reduce the morbidity of the treatment. The indications for radiation therapy have been expanded by the development of multimodality treatments.

The combined treatment protocol may be aimed at a single target, the local-regional tumor. This is called "local cooperation," and the goal is to increase the local efficacy. It is used for tumors where treatment failure results from the inability of a single treatment to control the primary tumor. Combinations of surgery, chemotherapy, or hyperthermia with irradiation can be used for local cooperation.

Combined treatment modalities may also be aimed at several targets. Each treatment modality is aimed at a target (macroscopic or microscopic) missed by the other modality; this is called "spatial cooperation." Combinations of definitive radiation (with or without surgery) for treatment of local disease and adjuvant systemic chemotherapy for treatment of subclinical metastatic disease are used for spatial cooperation. Localized lymphoma in the cat is a good example of a tumor that could benefit from such a combination. The indications and applications of spatial cooperation will not be discussed further in this article.

## RADIATION THERAPY AS A SINGLE TREATMENT MODALITY

Radiation therapy is primarily used for the treatment of localized and invasive solid tumors. The single most important factor affecting the probability of local control is tumor volume. The T symbol of the TNM system for staging cancer (Owen, 1980) followed by a number is conventionally used to express the volume and extension of the primary tumor. An inverse relationship between the probability of local control and the tumor volume has been shown for several tumor types: mast cell tumor (Turrel et al., 1988), oral tumors (Théon, Rodriguez, and Madewell, 1993), carcinomas of the nasal planum in cats (Théon, Madewell, Shearn, et al., 1993b), intranasal tumors (Théon, Madewell, Harb, et al., 1993a; Théon, Peaston, Madewell, et al., 1994a) and soft tissue sarcomas (McChesney, Withrow, Gillette, et al., 1989). Other factors such as histologic type, histologic grade, tumor proliferative activity, tumor location, species, and history of previous treatment have been shown to affect local control.

The goal of radiation therapy is to eradicate the cancer and thereby cure the patient. Although cure is possible in many cases, tumor recurrence or development of metastasis will occur in others. In the limited number of long-term animal studies available for review, the 3-year relapse-free survival rate appears to be a reliable estimate of the statistical cure rate, because if the patient is alive and free of disease after that period, the probability for tumor recurrence and metastasis is very small. Because the yearly recurrence rate appears constant over the first 3 years following treatment, the local control rate (%) at $\alpha$ years ($\alpha<3$) after treatment can be estimated by 100 x (3-year local control rate/ 100)$^{\alpha/3}$.

Depending on the characteristics of the primary tumor, the goals of treatment can be either cure or palliation. The treatment objective should be defined at the time of development of the therapeutic strategy. Animals are treated with curative intent when it is projected that the animal has a finite probability of surviving after treatment, even if that chance is low. Palliation is defined as noncurative treatment and can be subdivided into growth restraint/local control and symptom control.

### Curative Radiation Therapy

Radiation therapy plays an important role in the curative treatment of most common solid tumors and localized lymphomas. It is also used in the management of benign adenomas of the pituitary and perianal glands. Tumors irradiated with curative intent should have a good to high probability of local control, with no evidence of metastasis at the time of treatment. Depending on the efficacy and morbidity of radiation therapy compared to other treatment modalities, the indications of curative radiation therapy are either absolute or relative.

## ABSOLUTE INDICATIONS FOR RADIATION THERAPY

These include tumors that are very sensitive to radiation or tumors for which irradiation may be of unique advantage (Table 1). Transmissible venereal tumors at all sites are usually highly curable with moderate (20 to 30 Gy) doses of radiation. For extranodal solitary lymphomas (stage I), in dogs and cats, radiation therapy alone is standard management. When the minimum tumor dose is in excess of 36 Gy (4 Gy/fraction, alternate-day schedule), there is virtually no local recurrence rate. Dogs with localized mycosis fungoides of the oral mucosa require more aggressive treatment with doses in excess of 40 Gy because of the high rate of locoregional failure when lower doses are used.

Radiation therapy is the mainstay of treatment for central nervous system (CNS) tumors, since most lesions are inoperable. The overall median survival times reported for dogs with intracranial tumors ranges from 5 to 15 months. At the University of California–Davis Veterinary Medical Teaching Hospital (UCD-VMTH) the median survival of dogs ($n$=50) with gliomas and inoperable meningiomas treated with an aggressive protocol using focal irradiation (48 Gy, 4 Gy/fraction, alternate-day schedule) was 11.9 months. Gillette et al. (at Colorado State University) have reported an overall median survival time of 13.5 months after radiation therapy (with or without surgery). Radiation therapy is curative for small pituitary macroadenomas associated with minimal or no neurologic signs. In 17 dogs with pituitary macrotumors treated at the UCD-VMTH with focal radiation therapy (48 Gy, 4 Gy/fraction, alternate-day schedule), nine dogs with minimal neurologic signs had long-term remissions with a mean and median relapse-free survival of 18 and 24 months, but eight dogs with severe neurologic signs that did not improve during treatment had short survival times (median=2 weeks post-treatment). Six cats and 11 dogs with spinal lymphoma were treated at UCD-VMTH with craniospinal axis irradiation with a radiation boost to the primary tumor; all had local control, but a high rate of distant relapse was observed.

Nonlymphoproliferative intranasal tumors in both dogs and cats are difficult to control. Most studies in dogs have reported a 1-year survival rate of 60% and a 2-year survival rate of 25 to 50%. Analysis of the results of dogs ($n$=77) and cats ($n$=16) with carcinomas and sarcomas (chondrosarcomas and fibrosarcomas) of the nasal cavity and paranasal sinuses treated similarly with 48 Gy indicate similar results in both species (Théon, Madewell, Harb, et al., 1993a; Théon, Peaston, Madewell, et al., 1994a). The mean and median times to tumor progression are 16 and 10 months after treatment.

## RELATIVE INDICATIONS FOR RADIATION THERAPY

These include operable lesions where curative surgery may cause anatomically or physiologically undesirable sequelae. In small lesions where documented local control rates by both surgery and irradiation are similar, the choice should be based on relative morbidity for the site. Poor general health of the animal precluding multiple anesthetic episodes as well as logistics and cost may be factors in favor of surgery. Superficial cutaneous lesions covering large areas or multiple synchronous lesions, and patients with involvement of the regional lymph nodes, are best treated by radiation therapy. Additional consideration is given to radiation therapy when the probability of local control by either modality is less than 50%, since surgical salvage of recurrent or persistent tumor after irradiation is more likely than radiation salvage after surgery. A recurrence after irradiation is likely to be at the epicenter of the original lesion rather than at the periphery. Therefore, a surgical procedure is more likely to encompass the recurrence with a reasonable margin.

In tumors of the head, radiation therapy is preferred to surgery when the surgical procedure leads to suboptimal function or cosmesis. Radiation therapy is particularly well suited for early lesions of the facial skin including carcinomas of the nose, eyelids, or pinnae and certain more extensive lesions of the forehead and cheeks. In cats with early (1- to 2-cm diameter) squamous cell carcinomas of the nasal planum, 1-year local control rates of 85% have been reported (Théon, Madewell, Shearn, et al., 1993b). In dogs, however, squamous cell carcinomas of the nasal planum are usually large at presentation and the results are not as good. In a study of 15 dogs at UCD-VMTH, the local control rate 12 months after treatment was 20%. When adjustments are made for tumor size, local control rates in dogs and cats are similar.

Ceruminous gland carcinomas of the ear canal are radiocurable in both dogs and cats (Théon, Barthez, Madewell, et al., 1994b). T1 (<2-cm diameter lesion) tumors of the external ear canal and middle ear are

***Table 1.*** *Tumors for Which Radiation Therapy is Indicated*

| Highly Indicated and/or of Unique Advantage | Often Indicated and Equivalent to Surgery | Indicated Mainly in Combination Therapy | Rarely Indicated |
|---|---|---|---|
| Oral mycosis fungoides | Squamous cell carcinoma (facial skin and oral cavity) | Fibrosarcoma (oral and cutaneous) | Prostate carcinoma |
| Extranodal localized lymphoma | | Hemangiopericytoma | Mammary carcinoma |
| Pituitary macroadenoma | | Liposarcoma | Bladder carcinoma |
| Nasal tumors | Mast cell tumors | Osteosarcoma | |
| Transmissible venereal tumor | Epulis (acanthomatous, fibromatous) | Adenocarcinoma (perianal, thyroid, salivary) | |
| Brain tumors | Adamantinoma | | |
| | Perianal adenoma | | |

successfully treated with radiation therapy. Perianal gland adenomas in dogs are also radiocurable; one study indicated a 60% 1-year local control rate (Gillette, 1976). At UCD-VMTH, a low response rate was observed in ten dogs with sweat gland carcinomas and in four cats with meibomian gland carcinomas.

For oral tumors, radiation therapy is preferred when a high risk of oral incompetence is anticipated following radical excision. In dogs, good to excellent local control (Table 2) is achieved with irradiation for T1 to T2 (2- to 4-cm diameter) tumors of most sites in the oral cavity (Théon, Rodriguez, and Madewell, 1993). For more advanced tumors (with the exception of squamous cell carcinoma of the tonsil, tongue tumors, and melanomas), a local combined treatment modality is the treatment of choice for cure.

Radiation therapy may be preferred at specific sites on the trunk or extremities for small lesions where wide excision would be technically difficult. Local control for early-stage mast cell tumors as well as soft tissue sarcomas in dogs is very good. The 3-year local control rate for localized (stage I and II) mast cell tumors, irrespective of histologic grade, has been reported as 84% (Turrel, Kitchell, Miller, et al., 1988). A 67% 1-year local control rate for T1 to T2 (2- to 5-cm diameter) hemangiopericytomas and fibrosarcomas was obtained in dogs receiving radiation doses of 45 to 50 Gy (McChesney, Withrow, Gillette, et al., 1989).

## Palliative Radiation Therapy

In some cancers, local control of the disease and increased survival time can be expected, but cure is unlikely. Palliation should not be viewed as an unworthy goal, since many animals may live for long periods in comfort with residual tumor or metastasis. This approach should be used for tumors with a low probability of local control and no evidence of metastasis at the time of diagnosis, or tumors with a good probability of local control and a high likelihood of developing metastasis.

Cats with oral squamous cell carcinoma (gingiva, tongue, and sublingual structures) have a poor prognosis with conventional radiation therapy. Tumors are radioresponsive but predictably recur, often with regional and distant metastasis. The survival time of dogs with oral melanoma and tonsillar squamous cell carcinoma is substantially increased and quality of life is improved when the primary tumor is controlled, but the development of metastasis usually causes death.

Monostotic plasmacytomas can be treated with radiation therapy. At UCD-VMTH, six dogs irradiated with 40 Gy had local control greater than 1 year, but all ultimately developed systemic disease.

Surgical resection of a tumor that persists after irradiation may be used to attempt salvage. Surgery is recommended as additional treatment for selected tumors that have regressed in size but persist 3 to 6 months after irradiation. For example, dogs with large T3 (>5-cm diameter lesion) inoperable thyroid carcinomas are treated with palliative intent, but with curative doses of radiation. If substantial tumor regression is observed, these dogs are reevaluated for surgery and elective surgical salvage is attempted. Indeed, this approach is entirely different from postoperative irradiation, which is a planned combined modality using surgery and radiation. Reirradiation of a recurrent tumor after radiation failure may be used in selected cases to significantly prolong survival (Turrel and Théon, 1988).

Finally, radiation therapy can be used for tumors for which no other treatment modality is currently available. Although local control of large inoperable soft tissue sarcomas is modest (40% 1-year local control) (McChesney, Withrow, Gillette, et al., 1989), treatment should not be withheld. In dogs with large tumors (gliomas, pituitary adenomas, meningiomas) requiring whole-brain irradiation, treatment is palliative in nature.

Radiation may also be used to relieve distressing symptoms and improve the quality of life. Radiation therapy plays a limited role in the treatment of small animals with metastatic neoplasms in a terminal stage. Dogs with appendicular osteosarcoma that are not candidates for amputation may benefit from palliative radiation therapy. The recommended treatment includes 4 to 6 weekly dose fractions using large doses per fraction (7.5 to 10 Gy). Prompt pain relief was observed in 11 dogs treated at UCD-VMTH, with duration of relief up to 8 months. Most dogs died of metastatic disease prior to return of pain.

## RADIATION THERAPY USED IN COMBINATION WITH SURGERY

Radiation therapy and surgery may be equally beneficial in the treatment of small lesions, but they are

**Table 2.**    *Oral Tumors in 140 Dogs Treated at UCD-VMTH with Telecobalt: 3-Year Local Control Rates*[*]

| T stage (WHO) | T1 (<2-cm diameter) | T2 (2–4-cm diameter) | T3 (>4-cm diameter) |
|---|---|---|---|
| Acanthomatous epulis (n=37) | 87% | 81% | 55% |
| Fibromatous epulis (n=7) | 100% | 75% | — |
| Adamantinoma (n=15) | 100% | 71% | 33% |
| Squamous cell carcinoma (n=31) | 64% | 31% | 28% |
| Fibrosarcoma (n=17) | 64% | 34% | 16% |
| Malignant melanoma (n=33) | 40% | 28% | — |

[*]Lesions of hard palate, gingivae, or buccal mucosa.

mutually beneficial for treatment of large lesions. Local cooperation of the two modalities is more likely to eliminate the locoregional neoplasm and results in reduced morbidity. The general indications for tumors for which improved local control may be obtained include tumors with low cure rates by either surgery or radiation therapy alone. As a rule, large tumors should not be treated with radiation alone if the gross tumor can be resected simply (i.e., when there is a good probability that all of the gross tumor can be removed). Similarly, large tumors should not be treated with surgery alone if total extirpation of all neoplastic tissue is not anticipated.

The biologic rationale for combining these two techniques is well established. Radiation therapy efficiently sterilizes microscopic foci of tumor cells present at the periphery of the tumor, and surgery is efficient in removing the gross tumor mass. The central idea in combining the two modalities is that conservative surgical resection and irradiation is as effective as radical excision. This combination reduces the cosmetic or functional deficit of radical surgery.

The main combinations of radiation therapy and surgery revolve around preoperative and postoperative radiation therapy. There is uncertainty as to which combination is more effective. Treatment combinations are contingent on (1) anatomical structures involved, (2) extent of anticipated surgical resection, and (3) dose of radiation and volume to be irradiated. As a rule, preoperative radiation leads to a slight increase in surgical complications, and postoperative radiation leads to a slight increase in radiation complications.

### Postoperative Irradiation

By convention, postoperative irradiation has been the usual treatment method in veterinary medicine. The main advantage of postoperative radiation therapy is that the treatment is directed at known residual tumor in the operative field that has been assessed by direct visualization and pathologic examination of the surgical specimen. Good communication between the radiation oncologist and the surgeon is imperative. Information regarding the total extent of tissue involvement, the estimated volume of residual tumor, and the quality of the surgical margins is required for radiation treatment planning. A cutaneous surgical scar, in most cases, is inadequate to accurately predicate a treatment. Radiopaque markers (clips, wires) may be used by the surgeon to mark the limits of the surgical field.

The potential disadvantage of postoperative irradia-

tion is that radiation therapy must be postponed until wound healing is complete, which may allow tumor repopulation. A delay of 2 to 4 weeks is satisfactory in most cases. If the surgeon anticipates that wound healing or surgical reconstruction will delay the start of irradiation by more than 6 weeks, preoperative irradiation is preferred.

Selective postoperative irradiation should be used after surgical (visible residual disease) or histologic evidence of incomplete excision of a primary tumor. The status of the surgical margin has a direct impact on the likelihood of achieving local control at the primary site. For optimal results, surgery must reduce tumor burden to microscopic levels. Debulking (cut-through) and marginal excision give very little therapeutic advantage. For example, a surgical excision that removes 99% of a tumor containing $10^{10}$ cells (~10 gm of tissue) leaves $10^8$ cells. In a study of 144 dogs with T2 to T3 (>2-cm diameter lesion) tumors of the skin and subcutaneous tissues treated at the UCD-VMTH, the presence of histologically positive margins or macroscopic residual disease after resection of mast cell tumors, cutaneous fibrosarcomas, and hemangiopericytomas significantly affected the efficacy of postoperative irradiation (Table 3). After macroscopically incomplete excision, the results of postoperative irradiation are similar to irradiation alone.

In dogs, large operable intraoral tumors and tumors of the salivary, perianal, ceruminous, and thyroid glands are best treated with conservative surgery and postoperative irradiation. At UCD-VMTH, the 3-year local control rates in dogs with perianal gland tumors (n=19) and thyroid adenocarcinomas (n=18, T2a and T2b tumors) treated with postoperative irradiation were 65% and 89%, respectively. Osteosarcomas of the mandible and maxilla may also benefit from postoperative irradiation, because treatment failures are usually due to inability to control the primary tumor rather than from metastastic disease.

In dogs, postoperative irradiation of accessible intracranial and spinal meningiomas offers the highest probability of tumor control. In cats, complete surgical excision alone seems to be adequate treatment in most cases. Spinal soft tissue sarcomas can be treated successfully, after surgical decompression, with irradiation. Three spinal neuroblastomas in young dogs (<2 years of age) have been irradiated postoperatively at UCD-VMTH; two dogs with local control developed distant metastasis within 6 months after treatment, one dog is still alive with no evidence of disease 2 years after treatment.

Elective postoperative irradiation should be done for

***Table 3.*** *Postoperative Irradiation of Cutaneous and Subcutaneous Tumors in Dogs Treated at UCD-VMTH: 3-Year Progression-Free Survival Rate Estimates*

| Postoperative Residual Disease | Mast Cell Tumors (n=80) | Fibrosarcoma (n=39) | Hemangiopericytoma (n=25) |
|---|---|---|---|
| Macroscopic | 58% | 30% | 51% |
| Microscopic | 90% | 76% | 100% |

tumors with documented high rates of recurrence after surgery. The failure rate for some tumors with histologically negative margins may be substantial. Clean surgical margins are not a guarantee that all tumor cells have been removed, as cell aggregates greater than $10^6/cm^3$ or higher are required for histopathologic detection. Fibrosarcomas, hemangiopericytomas, cutaneous hemangiosarcomas, infiltrative lipomas and liposarcomas, and lymphangiomas and lymphangiosarcomas conservatively resected with clean surgical margin may benefit from postoperative irradiation.

Irradiation of a surgical failure when gross disease is present is not considered postoperative irradiation and is unlikely to succeed. Recurrence at the primary site after surgery most likely occurs at the periphery of the original tumor, in the margin of resection. The difficulty in discerning recurrent tumor in scarred, distorted tissue and the presence of radioresistant tumor cells in this relatively avascular tissue may account for the lack of efficacy of radiation therapy in this setting.

## Preoperative Irradiation

Preoperative irradiation presents several advantages. In contrast to postoperative irradiation, preoperative treatment can be given to a smaller treatment volume with lower radiation doses for comparable tumor control. Treatment fields are limited to encompass the gross disease and expected patterns of local extensions and do not need to incorporate areas that have been contaminated by surgical dissection. By disturbing the vascular supply to the tissues, surgery may result in the formation of a relatively radioresistant population of residual tumor cells in the hypoxic environment of the surgical scar. As a result, the microscopic disease surrounding the gross tumor mass requires higher doses of radiation in the postoperative setting than in the preoperative setting. Preoperative irradiation may also decrease shedding of viable tumor cells at the time of resection.

The principal disadvantage of preoperative irradiation is the risk of increased surgical complications. The risk is difficult to assess, since most lesions treated with preoperative irradiation are inoperable and would be associated with a high risk of complications with surgery alone. The current experience with people is that despite a higher risk, the surgical wounds do heal in virtually all patients. Surgery should be performed 3 to 4 weeks after radiotherapy completion when the acute radiation reactions have resolved.

Frequently, irradiation results in partial tumor regression, improving the resectability of the tumor. Animals with large tumors in which resection would require a major ablative procedure should be treated with preoperative irradiation. We treat dogs with large unresectable carcinomas or soft tissue sarcomas of the face (lip and chin), oral cavity, and trunk with preoperative irradiation with doses of 32 to 40 Gy. Large T3 to T4 (>5-cm diameter) fibrosarcomas, hemangiopericytomas, and mast cell tumors of the extremities are also treated with preoperative irradiation in an effort to avoid amputation. If the surgical margins are grossly positive, a radiation boost (16 to 20 Gy) is given after complete healing. Preoperative irradiation is also recommended for cats with large (T4) facial carcinomas (Théon and Peaston, 1992).

Operable and relatively localized lesions for which surgical manipulation may contribute to dissemination of viable tumor cells may be best treated with preoperative irradiation. Large subcutaneous soft tissue sarcomas with anticipated regional microextensions are also candidates for preoperative irradiation. Truncal fibrosarcoma in the cat is a good example of a tumor that could be better treated by preoperative irradiation. In a study conducted at UCD-VMTH, 13 cats with truncal subcutaneous fibrosarcomas treated postoperatively with large-field (100 to 120 $cm^2$) irradiation (40 Gy, 4 Gy/fraction) had tumor recurrence either on the surgical scar or at the periphery of the irradiated field. These results indicate that the radiation dose was too low and that the radiation fields were not large enough. Unfortunately, the risks of severe complications associated with large irradiation fields and high radiation doses prevent further improvement in the postoperative setting. There is a good biologic rationale for the use of preoperative irradiation for these tumors, because lower doses are required to sterilize microscopic extensions, and the preoperative field of irradiation can be reduced. For instance, a cat with a 3- to 4-cm diameter tumor would be treated adequately preoperatively with a 35- to 50-$cm^2$ radiation field at the skin. Seen after surgery, the same cat with a scar 6 to 8 cm long will require a radiation field at the skin of 65 to 80 $cm^2$ or more depending on the oncologic technique of the surgeon and the complexity of the skin scar.

# RADIATION THERAPY USED IN COMBINATION WITH RADIATION ENHANCERS

Several strategies have been developed for treatment of animals with locally advanced tumors to overcome radioresistance as a cause of local treatment failure. Local cooperation between radiation (with or without surgery) and radiation enhancers have shown great promise. Many agents, chemical and physical, have been shown to enhance the cytotoxic effects of radiation. The interaction of irradiation with antineoplastic agents or hyperthermia has received special consideration in veterinary medicine.

## Radiation Therapy and Chemotherapy

As a general principle, a combination of radiation therapy and cytotoxic chemotherapy is successful when the drug employed is active against the tumor. Radiation therapy and chemotherapy are administered concurrently in order to take advantage of a direct interaction. An improvement in the therapeutic index results from concurrent administration only if the combination produces a proportionally greater increase in antitumor efficacy than in normal tissue toxicity. Many classes of drugs have been found to interact with radiation by enhancement of cytotoxicity and inhibition of cellular radiation repair. In veterinary medicine, the platinum-coordination complexes (cisplatin, carboplatin) have been most studied.

Traditionally, chemotherapy is given intravenously (systemically). However, the radiation-enhancing effects of a drug are limited by low drug concentrations in the tumor and the systemic toxicity associated with the drug. New routes of administration, including intra-arterial and intratumoral, have been investigated for use with irradiation. These techniques are designed to maximize the drug concentration in tumors and minimize systemic exposure. Intra-arterial drug administration has been developed essentially for use in the treatment of canine appendicular osteosarcoma. Intra-arterial administration of cisplatin results in significantly greater tumor necrosis than intravenous administration. A therapeutic gain has been reported for needle-directed intralesional administration of several antineoplastic agents including cisplatin, carboplatin, 5-fluorouracil, and bleomycin. Further pharmacologic improvement may be achieved by using slow-release formulations such as proteinaceous or oily emulsions of drugs. In cats, the extreme toxicity of 5-fluorouracil and cisplatin preclude their safe use for intratumoral chemotherapy alone or in combination with irradiation. Because of limited diffusion of the drugs in tissues, a carefully planned pattern of intratumoral injections is required to allow adequate dose distribution; for example, cisplatin does not diffuse in tissue more than 5 mm from the site of injection.

Enhancement of tumor response by concurrent irradiation and chemotherapy can be achieved with either a concomitant or simultaneous schedule of administration. Concomitant treatments involve the administration of one or several chemotherapy cycles using full or nearly full-intensity dosages during the course of radiation therapy. As a result, the drug may have a direct cytotoxic effect in addition to enhancing the effect of radiation. Concomitant irradiation and intra-arterial cisplatin chemotherapy provides excellent palliation in dogs with appendicular osteosarcoma that are ineligible for amputation or limb-sparing surgical procedures (Heidner, Page, McEntee, et al., 1991). A cisplatin chemotherapy regimen of two doses of 70 mg/m$^2$ is given at a 3-week interval during the radiation therapy course prior to the first and last dose of radiation. Furthermore, in selected dogs with appendicular osteosarcoma, a trimodality approach including concomitant intra-arterial cisplatin and irradiation (32 to 40 Gy) followed by limb-sparing surgery results in a 92% 1-year local control rate (Withrow, Thrall, Straw, et al., 1993). Because of local and systemic toxicities, concomitant irradiation and administration of doxorubicin (30 mg/m$^2$; UCD-VMTH data) or mitoxantrone (5 mg/m$^2$; Larue, Gillette, McChesney Gillette, 1990) is not recommended. At the UCD-VMTH, concomitant irradi-

ation and intratumoral chemotherapy using cisplatin in dogs and carboplatin in cats has shown very encouraging results for treatment of advanced carcinomas and sarcomas. Lesions suitable for this combined modality treatment include T2 to T3 (>2-cm diameter) oral soft tissue tumors with minimal bony involvement. Bone-producing tumors, such as some epulides, are not suitable because intratumoral injection would not be possible. The technique may be used successfully for conservative treatment of T2 to T3 (>2-cm diameter) soft tissue sarcomas of the extremities when preoperative irradiation alone would not make the lesion operable. Complete response was observed in 83% ($n=12$) of dogs with T2 to T3 soft tissue sarcomas of the head and extremities, treated with concomitant irradiation (48 Gy) and four weekly intratumoral cisplatin injections (0.5 mg/cm$^3$ of tissue treated) (Théon, Madewell, Ryu, et al., 1994c). The good initial tumor response and the lack of enhanced radiation complications indicate that a therapeutic gain is achievable using this combined modality.

Simultaneous irradiation and chemotherapy treatment consists of drug administration at low dosage prior to each radiation fraction during the course of irradiation. As a result, the drug has minimal cytotoxic effect and functions essentially as a radiosensitizer in the target volume. We have used simultaneous treatment with cisplatin (10 mg/m$^2$, IV) and irradiation (40 Gy) has been used successfully for palliation of dogs with appendicular osteosarcoma and advanced carcinomas of the head, neck, and urinary bladder. The role of carboplatin as a radiation enhancer is currently under investigation. It may prove to be more effective than cisplatin as a sensitizing agent, since higher dosages can be achieved safely. Intravenous carboplatin chemotherapy given at doses of 30 to 45 mg/m$^2$ concurrently with irradiation (40 Gy, 4 Gy/fraction, 3½ weeks) is being evaluated for treatment of canine intranasal carcinomas. Signs of systemic toxicity have not been observed in the eight dogs treated.

## Radiation Therapy and Hyperthermia

Clinical hyperthermia is the use of heat at supranormal temperature for cancer treatment. Hyperthermia is cytotoxic when used alone, but it is most useful when combined with radiation therapy for local cooperation. In selected human tumors, the rates of complete response obtained with radiation alone may be doubled by the combined use of hyperthermia and radiation therapy.

The biologic effect of a combination of heat and radiation is due to complementary cytotoxicity and heat-induced radiosensitization. Important factors affecting the efficacy of this combination are the timing and sequence of the two modalities; radiation time-dose fractionation; and hyperthermic parameters including thermal dose, number of heat treatments, and tumor volume.

In clinical practice, protocols using radiation doses

of 25 to 55 Gy with two to four hyperthermia treatments at 42° to 44°C for 30 to 60 min prior to or following a radiation dose fraction have been used. We use four weekly hyperthermia sessions (43.5°C, 30 min), given immediately after a radiation dose fraction during the course of irradiation (48 Gy, 4 Gy/fraction, 4 weeks). The optimal duration, frequency, and total number of hyperthermia sessions are still under investigation. In a series of 24 dogs with T2 to T3 (>2-cm diameter) oral fibrosarcomas treated at UCD-VMTH with two or four hyperthermia treatments, no significant difference in response duration was seen.

Several prospective randomized veterinary studies have been published that compare rates of tumor response and response durations with irradiation alone and irradiation plus hyperthermia. Improved complete response rates and preliminary evidence of therapeutic gain have been observed for almost all tumor types and locations in dogs and cats (Gillette, McChesney, Dewhirst, et al., 1987; Dewhirst and Sims, 1984; McChesney Gillette, Dewhirst, Gillette, et al., 1992).

Tumor volume significantly affects the efficacy of the combination. For small tumor volumes ($<10$ cm$^3$), response duration in animals treated with the combined modality is superior to that in animals treated with radiation alone (Dewhirst and Sim, 1984). For larger tumors, however, analysis of response duration has not shown a significant difference in long-term local control. This may be explained by the low doses of radiation used and the inability to adequately heat large tumors.

An absolute requirement for cure of a solid tumor is the eradication of the primary and regional disease. There is no doubt that for some tumors, including oral malignant melanomas, tonsillar carcinomas, and appendicular osteosarcomas, the principal cause of failure is early development of metastasis, and improvement in local control has not resulted in increased survival. For some tumors, including soft tissue sarcomas, nasal tumors, perianal adenocarcinomas, and localized lymphomas, the introduction of more effective locoregional therapy has resulted in prolonged survival after treatment, but a higher frequency of distant metastasis has been observed. Prior to effective locoregional treatment, animals died from local recurrence before metastasis became clinically apparent. The identification of subgroups of animals at risk and development of

effective adjuvant systemic chemotherapy will have a direct impact on cure rates. For most large tumors, however, local tumor recurrence is the major cause of treatment failure leading to death (natural or iatrogenic). This provides powerful incentive for aggressive investigation of new locoregional treatments.

## References and Suggested Reading

Dewhirst MW and Sim DA: The utility of thermal dose as a predictor of tumor and normal tissue responses to combined radiation and hyperthermia. Cancer Res 44:4772, 1984.

Gillette EL: Radiation therapy of canine and feline tumors. J Am Anim Hosp Assoc 12:359, 1976.

Gillette EL, McChesney SL, Dewhirst MW, and Scott RJ: Response of canine oral carcinomas to heat and radiation. Int J Radiat Oncol Biol Phys 13:1861, 1987.

Heidner GL, Page RL, McEntee MC, et al: Treatment of canine appendicular osteosarcoma using cobalt 60 radiation and intraarterial cisplatin. J Vet Intern Med 5:313, 1991.

Larue SM, Gillette EL, and McChesney Gillette SL: Irradiation plus mitoxantrone for treatment of canine nasal tumors. Proc ACVR, 1990, p 38.

McChesney SL, Withrow SJ, Gillette EL, et al: Radiotherapy of soft tissue sarcomas in dogs. J Am Vet Med Assoc 194:60, 1989.

McChesney Gillette SL, Dewhirst MW, Gillette EL, et al: Response of canine soft tissue sarcomas to radiation or radiation plus hyperthermia: A randomized phase II study. Int J Hyperthermia 8:309, 1992.

Owen LN: TNM Classification of Tumours in Domestic Animals, 1st edition. Geneva, World Health Organization, 1980.

Théon AP, Madewell BR, Harb MF, and Dungworth DL: Megavoltage irradiation of neoplasms of the nasal and paranasal cavities in 77 dogs. J Am Vet Med Assoc 202:1469, 1993a.

Théon AP, Peaston AE, Madewell BR, and Dungworth DL: Irradiation of nonlymphoproliferative neoplasms of the nasal and paranasal cavities in 16 cats. J Am Vet Med Assoc 204:78, 1994a.

Théon AP, Barthez PY, Madewell BR, and Griffey S: Radiation therapy of ceruminous gland carcinomas in dogs and cats. J Am Vet Med Assoc (in press), 1994b.

Théon AP and Peaston AE: Preoperative irradiation of facial tumors in cats. Proc ACVIM, 1992, p 805.

Théon AP, Madewell BR, Shearn V, and Moulton JE: Prognostic factors for squamous cell carcinomas of the nasal planum: A study of ninety cats treated with radiotherapy. J Am Vet Med Assoc (Submitted, 1993b).

Théon AP, Rodriguez JR, and Madewell BR: Prognostic factors for canine oral tumors treated with megavoltage irradiation: A study of 140 dogs. J Am Vet Med Assoc (Submitted).

Théon AP, Madewell BR, Ryu J, and Castro J: Concurrent irradiation and intratumoral chemotherapy with cisplatin: A pilot study in dogs with spontaneous tumors. Int J Radiat Oncol Biol Phys (in press), 1994c.

Turrel JM, Kitchell BE, Miller LM, and Théon AP: Prognostic factors for radiation treatment of mast cell tumors in 85 dogs. J Am Vet Med Assoc 193:936, 1988.

Turrel JM and Théon AP: Reirradiation of tumors in cats and dogs. J Am Vet Med Assoc 193:465, 1988.

Withrow SJ, Thrall DE, Straw RC, et al: Intra-arterial cisplatin with or without radiation in limb-sparing for canine osteosarcoma. Cancer 71:2484, 1993.

# SAFE HANDLING AND ADMINISTRATION OF CHEMOTHERAPEUTIC AGENTS IN VETERINARY MEDICINE

KRISTA L. DICKINSON
and GREGORY K. OGILVIE

*Fort Collins, Colorado*

The use of and potential exposure to chemotherapeutic agents is rapidly expanding as the benefits of these anticancer agents become more apparent. Antineoplastic drugs at therapeutic dosages have the potential to be teratogenic, mutagenic, and carcinogenic in animals and humans (ASHP Technical Assistance Bulletin, 1990; Cancer Chemotherapy Guidelines, 1988; OSHA Work Practice Guidelines, 1993; Ringlein, 1987). The actual risk to health care workers is not known. Until that risk is clearly defined, care should be taken to minimize exposure to owners, veterinarians, and allied veterinary health care professionals who handle these drugs and the animals that are treated with these pharmacologic agents.

The purpose of this article is to review the advisory or regulatory organizations that are involved in establishing guidelines for handling these drugs, ways in which veterinary health care workers can be exposed to chemotherapeutic agents, methods of handling these important therapeutic agents, and finally, methods of disposing materials used for mixing and administering chemotherapeutic agents. In addition, a brief summary of how cytotoxic agents can be safely administered is also discussed.

## REGULATORY AND ADVISORY ORGANIZATIONS

One of the Occupational Safety and Health Administration's (OSHA) prime responsibilities is to help publicize "known hazards" that specific professions have already identified as areas of risk, such as handling chemotherapeutic agents. The Occupational Safety and Health Administration publishes guidelines for health care professionals regarding the handling of cytotoxic agents (ASHP Technical Assistance Bulletin, 1990). These guidelines are straightforward and generally applicable to veterinary medicine. Current copies of these guidelines may be obtained from OSHA, Director of Technical Support, Room H-3651, Washington, DC 20210. The OSHA guidelines have been designed to assist all health care professionals who may be exposed to hazardous drugs, specifically antineoplastic agents.

These guidelines have been compiled from information, publications, and personnel in medical and pharmaceutical communities (OSHA Work Practice Guidelines, 1993). These are not mandatory standards; they are only recommendations. However, under the Occupational Safety and Health Act of 1970, public law 91-596, section V(a)(1) has been deemed the "general duty clause." This clause mandates that it is the general duty of all employers to provide a safe and healthful work place for all employees. It is this section that allows for lawful intervention of OSHA in some cases to mandate specific standards. Considering the lack of data on the risks of long-term low-dose exposure to chemotherapeutic agents and the need to protect employees from all occupational health hazards, the veterinary community must recognize, promote, and institute procedures that facilitate the safe handling and disposal of anticancer drugs. Remaining current on new information is imperative for veterinarians and staff who are working with chemotherapeutic agents. One nationwide nursing organization, the Oncology Nursing Society, has published a series of cancer chemotherapy guidelines (Ringlein, 1987). The recommendations are current, concise, easy to obtain, relatively inexpensive, and generally applicable to veterinary medicine. The address for these documents from the Oncology Nursing Society is 501 Holiday Drive, Pittsburgh, PA 15220-2749. Another resource created specifically for the veterinary community is a videotaped series provided by the American Animal Hospital Association (AAHA). The address for AAHA is PO Box 150899, Denver, CO 80215-0899. Additional resources will undoubtedly become available for the health care professional in the years to come.

## METHODS OF EXPOSURE

The means of exposure to cytotoxic agents can occur in three ways: (1) inhalation during mixing and/or administration due to aerosolization of the drug; (2) absorption of the drug through the skin; and (3) ingestion through contact with contaminants such as food or cigarettes (ASHP Technical Assistance Bulletin, 1990;

Cancer Chemotherapy Guidelines, 1988; OSHA Work Practice Guidelines, 1993; Ringlein, 1987). Common clinical examples of situations where exposure may occur include: (1) withdrawal of a needle from a pressurized drug vial; (2) drug transfers between various equipment; (3) opening of glass ampules; (4) expulsion of air from drug-filled syringes; (5) failure of equipment or improperly set-up equipment; (6) exposure to excretia from patients who have received certain cytotoxic drugs; and (7) crushing or breaking tablets of cytotoxic drugs. In the last situation, cytotoxic powder has been documented for up to 12 inches away from where the tablets are crushed. Therefore, *drugs should be dispensed only when whole tablets are used.* For ease of dosing, veterinarians should prescribe tablets by rounding down to the next whole tablet. In any case, individuals should document any acute exposure to antineoplastic agents. All veterinary health care workers should have routine health examinations. Finally, women of childbearing age should exercise extreme caution when handling cytotoxic agents.

## DRUG HANDLING EDUCATION

The Occupational Safety and Health Administration has determined that specific educational procedures are essential to minimize the risk for employees that handle cytotoxic agents (ASHP Technical Assistance Bulletin, 1990; Cancer Chemotherapy Guidelines, 1988; OSHA Work Practice Guidelines, 1993; Ringlein, 1987). Personnel with any exposure risks should be made aware of the potential hazards and what precautions may be taken to minimize their exposure. This can be accomplished by providing pertinent written information from the sources listed previously, by initiating "in-house" training, and by exposure to formal education sessions available within the community. In this way, veterinary personnel can work safely with cytotoxic drugs. Each veterinary clinic that handles chemotherapeutic agents should establish a procedures manual to help identify those cytotoxic agents and the risks and benefits of each drug. The manual should contain a material safety data sheet (MSDS) for each hazardous drug used. This drug data sheet obtained from the drug manufacturer lists pertinent information regarding the drug, such as what protective precautions should be taken in the case of a spill or other emergencies, and what first aid information should be utilized in the case of drug exposure. A drug insert should also be in this manual. This drug insert is provided by the manufacturer with each container of cytotoxic agent. The insert includes recommendations on dosage and administration information for human use. Other important items to be included in the cytotoxic drug procedures manual should be standard protocols for various drug administrations, extravasations, anaphylaxis antidotes, and information on appropriate spill cleanup. Another section should pertain to hospital policy on disposal and waste management. Again, all of the aforementioned information that is provided by the manufacturer such as the drug insert deals almost exclusively with human patients; therefore, items such as dosages for animal use should be obtained from veterinary resources. Veterinary health care workers can acquire information from local hospitals that have ongoing cytotoxic drug-handling seminars or from regional university veterinary teaching hospitals with an active oncology unit.

## EQUIPMENT FOR MIXING DRUGS

Ideally, OSHA has recommended a biologic safety cabinet (BSC) to mix chemotherapeutic agents safely. If installation of a class-II vertical flow-containment hood or BSC is beyond the scope of the practice, there are other pieces of equipment that can aid in providing a safe environment in which to mix drugs. The respirator with a high-efficiency filter, preferably a powered air-purifying respirator (PAPR), provides the best protection against aerosolized cytotoxic particles. Surgical masks do not protect the handler from breathing aerosolized materials. Latex, surgical quality, nonpowdered gloves should be used when handling cytotoxic agents. All gloves are permeable to some extent to most agents, so gloves should be changed often. Double gloving increases protection from absorption. Nonsterile, heavyweight latex gloves are commercially available and specifically designed for use when handling cytotoxic agents. A large-animal OB glove may be used under the latex glove to protect the fore and upper arms from aerosolization. A protective, nonporous gown that is lint free and closed in the front with long sleeves and knit cuffs to be covered by latex gloves should also be utilized in ideal situations. In preparing drugs outside of a BSC, goggles should also be worn. Other equipment needed for some mixing and handling of antineoplastic agents should be disposable, plastic-backed, absorbable paper "diapers" to be used on the mixing surface to help contain spills. Syringes and IV sets should have Luer-Lok fittings to prevent separation of needle and/or IV line during the administration. All IV lines should be primed with a noncytotoxic agent. Chemotherapy hazardous drug labels should be placed on all cytotoxic medications prepared. Ziploc-style bags to store or transport these agents assist in containing a spill in the event of an accident. Whenever possible, do not use glass containers. Chemotherapy spill kits should be located in areas where drugs are mixed and administered. These kits are available commercially. They can also be assembled to contain two pairs of disposable latex gloves, disposable protective gowns, shoe covers, safety goggles, respirator, absorbent plastic back pads, two reusable hazardous waste bags, and a container for sharps. In any case, the area where drugs are prepared should be a low-traffic, well-ventilated area. Direct exposure to heat and cooling vents should be avoided. Storage for hazardous drugs should be secure and separate from all other drugs. No eating, drinking, smoking, chewing gum, applying makeup, or storing food should be allowed in the area to prevent contamination through ingestion. Frequent hand washing is encouraged before and after any procedure that involves a chemotherapeutic agent.

## DISPOSAL PROCEDURES

All equipment used for compounding and administration of chemotherapeutic agents should be placed in a leakproof, puncture-proof container labeled "hazardous waste." Housekeeping personnel should receive instructions on safe handling procedures and should wear surgical latex gloves and gowns with cuffs and back closure when handling these containers. If any chemotherapeutic agent is administered by an owner at home, a leakproof container should be dispensed with instructions for disposal. Specific arrangements should be made with a certified disposal company for the destruction or disposal of antineoplastic agents. Two major methods exist. One is incineration at temperatures of 1000°C (1800°F); or disposal in a landfill. Both methods should be done with approval of the Environmental Protection Agency and all state, local, and national regulations.

## DRUG ADMINISTRATION

Proper administration of chemotherapeutic agents is essential for the veterinary health care professional to ensure a safe environment for patient, owner, and caregiver. Adequately prepared personnel who are specifically trained and technically skilled in administering cytotoxic drugs should assume this responsibility. Knowledge about each specific agent utilized as regards reconstitution, stability, storage, dosage, mode of administration, various toxicities, and known antidotes should be readily available. Oncologic emergencies that may occur at the time of administration, such as extravasation, anaphylaxis, or a cytotoxic drug spill, may be handled effectively if appropriate guidelines for treatment are in place. Be prepared. The ability to access pertinent laboratory values for those administering chemotherapy is important due to possible bone marrow toxicity or potential organ damage caused by some antineoplastic agents. The following information is a chemotherapy administration checklist modified from the Cancer Chemotherapy Guidelines issued by the Oncology Nursing Society (Ringlein, 1987).

1. Check patient's prior chemotherapy administration history and review appropriate laboratory data prior to reconstituting drug.
2. Measure and record all masses or lymph nodes.
3. Verify and calculate veterinarian's written order for specific drug, dosage, and route of administration.
4. Reconfirm calculated dose.

5. Wash hands before and after handling all chemotherapeutics.
6. Reconstitute drugs under aseptic conditions, utilizing appropriate safety precautions while handling cytotoxic drugs (gloves, gown, goggles, respirator, if not under BSC).
7. Label drug with patient's name, date, drug dose, amount and type of diluent used, and place a cytotoxic drug label and place in ziplock bag, store appropriately until use.
8. Prepare administration area.
   Have written protocols for oncologic emergencies easily available.
   Have a chemotherapy spill kit available.
   Assemble all items for venipuncture.
9. Personnel administering chemotherapy and patient restrainer put on protective equipment necessary (minimum—gloves).
10. Confirm patient identity.
11. Reconfirm drug dosage.
12. Select venipuncture site based on:
    No other venipuncture same day if using a vesicant chemotherapy.
    Ease of restraint of patient.
13. Perform standard aseptic venipuncture utilizing one clean stick into the vein.
14. After securing catheter, do a "vein challenge" by flushing a bolus of $\geq$ 12 ml normal saline into catheter in vein.
15. Monitor patient during administration for any local or systemic reaction.
16. Upon completion of chemotherapy, again flush catheter with a bolus of normal saline and pull catheter, placing bandage.
17. Place all equipment utilized in the drug administration into a Ziplock bag and dispose of in a proper container according to practice policies.
18. Document procedure in medical record.

## CONCLUSIONS

In summary, antineoplastic agents are being utilized more and more in private practice. These agents are of tremendous benefit for the treatment of a wide variety of neoplastic disorders in veterinary patients. The drugs utilized for the treatment of these patients will almost certainly contain some risk for veterinary health care professionals. The degree of risk for these professionals is not known. Care should be taken when handling chemotherapeutic agents or animals that are treated with these drugs.

### References and Suggested Reading

*ASHP Technical Assistance Bulletin on Handling Cytotoxic and Hazardous Drugs.* Am J Hosp Pharm 47:1033, 1990.
*This bulletin reviews safe handling procedures for the professional dealing with anticancer drugs.*

*Cancer Chemotherapy Guidelines: Module 1—Recommendations for Cancer Chemotherapy.* Oncology Nursing Society, 1988, p 1.
  *This succinct monograph discusses the handling of antineoplastic agents.*
*OSHA Work Practice Guidelines for Personnel: Dealing with Cytotoxic Drugs.* OSHA Instructional Publication, Washington, DC, Office of Occupational Medicine, 1993.

*This monograph reviews the guidelines for handling chemotherapeutic agents.*
Ringlein JW: Principles of oncology nursing and safe handling of chemotherapeutic agents. *In* Skeel RT (ed): *Handbook of Cancer Chemotherapy.* Boston, Little, Brown & Co, 1987, p 493.
  *The chapter in this book describes the salient principles of handling cytotoxic drugs.*

# ANTICANCER DRUGS: DOSE SCHEDULE AND GUIDELINES

MARY KAY KLEIN

*Tucson, Arizona*

## CONVENTIONAL CHEMOTHERAPY

The narrow therapeutic index and potentially life-threatening side effects of antineoplastic agents make their careful dosage calculation imperative. Individual pharmacokinetic profiles would be the most desirable method; however, the technological expertise and financial support required are prohibitive. A complete and accurate chemotherapy listing can be found in the formulary near the end of this volume. Several chemotherapeutic regimens are also outlined in subsequent articles (also see this volume, p 1446). The doses recorded in these references have been widely used and will be safe for most animals; however, careful monitoring and support are always indicated. Before using any chemotherapeutic regimen, the clinician should be completely familiar with the handling and pharmacology of the agents used (including their mechanism of action and metabolism; predicted effects on normal tissues, especially the bone marrow; and pharmacokinetic alterations associated with renal, gastrointestinal, and hepatic dysfunction), the spectrum of drug effectiveness as determined through clinical trials, the biologic characteristics of the neoplastic disease, and the clinical condition of the patient. Each patient presents a unique set of circumstances. The following article is designed to provide rationale for the use of chemotherapy; logical treatment plans have evolved through our understanding of tumor biology.

### Dose Intensity

The response to chemotherapy has classically been described according to first-order kinetics; that is, assuming a constant growth rate and relative sensitivity, the number of cells killed by chemotherapy is directly proportional to one variable—the dose administered. However most tumors do not grow at a constant exponential rate, but rather by a gompertzian model, whereby the growth fraction decreases exponentially with time. An alternative model explains clinical tumor regressions by the relative growth fraction present at the time of treatment (DeVita, 1993): very small and very large tumors should be less responsive than those of intermediate size where the growth fraction is maximal. Undoubtedly, each mechanism influences the outcome observed clinically.

Changes in dose intensity can be made in the dose administered or the administration schedule. Whenever consideration is given to decreasing the dose intensity, perhaps to prevent toxicity, it is important to remember that a marked decrease in cure rate occurs before a significant reduction in response rate is apparent. Although the complete response rate is the most important indicator of efficacy and a prerequisite for cure, *in vitro* modeling indicates that a dose reduction of only 20% may lead to the loss of 50% of the cure rate **without** affecting the complete response rate seen (DeVita, 1993).

Combination drug protocols are often required to optimize response and survival rates. Logical combination chemotherapeutic regimens provide for maximal cell kill within a toxicity range that is acceptable to the patient and allow for broad range of coverage of the resistant cells present in a heterogenous tumor population. In order to successfully be incorporated into a combination regimen, the chosen chemotherapeutic agent must meet four criteria:

1. Each drug must have some efficacy as a single agent.
2. Toxicities of each drug must not overlap and activities should be enhanced or synergistically affected.
3. Each agent must be used at its optimal dose.
4. Each drug must be scheduled at the shortest possible interval required to allow for recovery of the most sensitive target tissue, usually the bone marrow (DeVita, 1993).

## Dose and Schedule Calculation

The therapeutic and toxic effects of chemotherapy are related to the amount of time cells are exposed to an effective concentration of drug. The majority of published drug dosages are described on the basis of body surface area (BSA). Body surface area is thought to be the most accurate means of calculating dose and predicting toxicity, as it is found to be more predictive of basal metabolic rate than body weight. Organs with high metabolic rates, such as the kidney, are responsible for metabolism and excretion of many chemotherapeutic agents, and the function of the kidneys is found to correlate better with BSA than body weight. Small animals generate more heat and use more oxygen than large animals, and the basal metabolic rate of the animal increases as the body size of the animal decreases. Small patients have a greater BSA/body weight ratio compared to larger patients; therefore, they receive a comparatively higher milligrams-per-kilogram dose.

Two drugs are notable exceptions to the accuracy of BSA: melphalan (Page et al., 1988) and doxorubicin (Arrington et al., 1993). Melphalan-induced toxicity in dogs is more accurately predicted when it is dosed on the basis of body weight rather than BSA. Two explanations are proposed: (1) metabolism or excretion of melphalan occurs independent of metabolic rate (therefore, small dogs are inadvertently overdosed), or (2) basal metabolic rate does not adequately predict hematopoietic sensitivity. Pharmacokinetic studies will be required to address the first hypothesis. The second warrants further consideration in that BSA has never been positively correlated with hematopoietic stem cell activity and in at least one study was found to correlate better with body weight than BSA (Vreiesendorp and Von Bekkom, 1980).

Regarding doxorubicin, pharmacokinetic profiles have now been completed in the dog to indicate that drug metabolism and excretion occur at the same rate regardless of the size of the dog. Whereas a 5-kg dog will receive doxorubicin at a dose of 1.74 mg/kg when calculated on BSA basis, a 40-kg dog will receive only 0.88 mg/kg, a difference of almost twofold. Small dogs dosed according to their body surface areas achieved greater peak plasma concentration and plasma drug concentration versus time curves (AUC), and longer drug elimination half-lives. In the smaller dogs, clinical signs of toxicosis were more pronounced, as was myelosuppression. Dosing doxorubicin on a milligrams-per-kilogram body weight basis produced more consistent plasma concentration and excretion rates in dogs with widely variable body weights and BSAs. The doxorubicin toxicity was found to directly relate to plasma concentration. A previous study indicates that smaller dogs dosed according to their body surface area can be expected to show increased morbidity (Ogilvie et al., 1989), and another study demonstrated an increase in survival times for small dogs compared to large dogs (MacEwen et al., 1981), which would make sense in light of the increased dose intensity in the small dogs. Although the pharmacokinetics indicate that the milli-grams-per-kilogram dosing method delivers the same therapeutic dose to all dogs, the optimal dose to achieve the longest survival time with tolerable toxicity has not yet been identified. Until that optimal dose is identified, clinicians may want to warn the owners of small dogs that their risk for side effects may be higher and consider using decreased doses when unacceptable toxicity is predicted or seen. Furthermore, because doxorubicin undergoes significant metabolism in the body and is eliminated via the biliary system, dosage adjustments are also considered prudent in any animal with elevations in total bilirubin concentrations.

Other situations require some caution when dosing animals on the basis of BSA. The disposition of both doxorubicin (Rodvold, Rushing, and Teuksbury, 1988) and cyclophosphamide (Powis et al., 1987) has been shown to be altered in the obese human patient. Whether the decreases in clearance are secondary to fatty infiltration of the liver or changes in enzyme activity is not known. At the very least some caution should be used in the obese, small dog. The very immature animal could also be expected to metabolize agents at a different rate. Whenever treatment modalities are combined, pharmacokinetic changes may also occur. The addition of whole body hyperthermia to cisplatin regimens significantly altered the pharmacokinetics of that compound (Page et al., 1992). The possible interactions with concurrently administered antibiotics, analgesics, and antiemetics should also be considered. In addition, there is significant variation among species as indicated by the contraindication for cisplatin in cats.

Dose scheduling should be based on two factors: (1) the potential doubling time of the tumor, and (2) time required for sensitive host tissues to recover. Doses must be given at intervals less than the tumor doubling time, otherwise, even if drug resistance does not develop, the tumor will be able to repopulate and expand despite an otherwise effective treatment. Fortunately, repair by normal tissues generally occurs more rapidly than that for tumors. Drugs are often scheduled on a weekly basis; when drugs are given on days 1 and 8, bone marrow suppression is unchanged when compared to drug administration on day 1 alone, probably because the marrow stem cell compartment is still in a quiescent state (DeVita, 1993). When doses are repeated during the phase of early recovery of the marrow (days 16 to 21), severe neutropenias can result. The interval that is of greatest importance in monitoring chemotherapy patients is the duration of the nadir of leukocytes and platelets; durations of less than 4 to 7 days are tolerated by most patients.

## Predicting Toxicity

Conventional cytotoxic agents typically interfere with cell replication, and their therapeutic index arises from the slower growth rates of most normal tissues in comparison to those having undergone malignant transformation. It is this difference between dose–response curves of normal and tumor tissue that must be exploited. The dose-limiting toxicity remains related to the effects of cytotoxic agents on normal tissues. Those toxicities can be predicted by reviewing the cell kinetics of normal tissues. Hair loss is expected in those breeds of dogs with continuous hair growth. The potential for anorexia, vomiting, and/or diarrhea exists, as the lining of the gastrointestinal tract is replaced every 3 to 5 days. Myelosuppression is the dose-limiting toxicity for most drugs, as segmented neutrophils are replaced twice in every 24-hr period. The exceptionally high turnover rate in this tissue explains why myelosuppression is often the dose-limiting toxicity associated with the administration of many chemotherapeutic agents. It must be remembered, however, that each chemotherapeutic agent tends to have its own unique set of attendant precautions.

As a general rule, the potential for toxicity of an anticancer drug correlates with the specificity of the drug for a specific phase of the cell cycle. Those drugs that are active throughout the cell cycle and also affect resting cells can be expected to be associated with the greatest potential for morbidity. The nitrosoureas fit into this category. On the other hand, those drugs that are active only in dividing cells and in a select portion of the cell cycle, such as vincristine, can be expected to have less of an effect on normally renewing tissues. Hormonal agents, whose effects are thought to be mediated via receptor mechanisms, and compounds that take advantage of unique biochemical differences such as L-asparaginase, are truly selective in their activities. A high therapeutic index is generally associated with their use.

## Drug Resistance

Some tumors are intrinsically drug resistant by virtue of compromised drug delivery to areas of poor vascularization and/or pharmacologic barriers such as the blood-brain barrier. In others, lengthy remissions are induced in newly diagnosed patients, but the development of acquired drug resistance ultimately results in death for patients with many hematologic and solid tumors. The Goldie-Coldman hypothesis holds that cells survive by expanding clones that have spontaneously mutated to resistant forms. This hypothesis predicts that resistance should be a problem even with small tumor burdens, and that the maximal chance for cure will occur when all available drugs are given simultaneously.

There are four major cellular mechanisms responsible for the development of acquired drug resistance: decreased drug accumulation, altered drug metabolism, altered drug targets, and enhanced deoxyribonucleic acid (DNA) repair capacity (DeVita, 1993). Examples of each are given in Table 1. One of the most widely studied mechanisms is the overexpression of P-glycoprotein and its association with multidrug resistance (MDR), the phenomenon of resistance to multiple drugs with little similarity in chemical structure and mechanism of action. P-glycoprotein appears to function as an energy-dependent efflux pump that rapidly decreases the intracellular concentration of many natural products such as doxorubicin and the vinca alkaloids. Multidrug resistance has been effectively manipulated in human lymphoma, myeloma, and myelogenous leukemia patients (Dalton, 1993). Numerous studies are currently underway in veterinary medicine to identify the presence of MDR-associated P-glycoprotein. Preliminary clinical trials in our laboratory indicated no improvement in first disease-free interval following the addition of verapamil, the most widely studied resistance reversal agent, to canine lymphoma patients given doxorubicin as a single agent. There was, however, a trend toward increased length of second remission intervals following treatment with doxorubicin and verapamil at the time of relapse. A combination of chemosensitizers, verapamil, and quinine was found to have unacceptable morbidity in canine lymphoma patients. The number of patients in these studies was small, however, and larger studies with concurrent evaluations of MDR expression are needed before conclusions or treatment recommendations can be made.

## Limitations of Chemotherapy

Limitations to chemotherapy in clinical settings are attributed to:

1. The inability to precisely identify metastatic disease at the time of diagnosis and detect minimal residual disease following a clinical complete response.

*Table 1.* *General Mechanisms of Cellular Resistance to Antineoplastic Agents*

| Mechanism | Example |
|---|---|
| Decreased drug accumulation | Overexpression of P-glycoprotein |
| | Altered methotrexate transport components |
| Altered drug metabolism | Changes in activation (cyclophosphamide) |
| | Changes in inactivation (increased deamination of antimetabolites) |
| Altered drug targets | Quantitative and qualitative changes in topoisomerase II, dihydrofolate reductase |
| | Development of alternative pathways |
| Enhanced DNA repair | Demonstrated best for cisplatin and alkylating agents, not yet fully understood |

2. The inability to use doses of effective drugs at levels found at the high end of dose–response curves.

3. The expression of multidrug resistance.

4. The inability to measure the moment-to-moment impact of therapy (DeVita, 1993).

Prognostic factors allowing prediction of metastasis for most tumors have not been determined. This problem is now being addressed at the molecular level by probing for expression of genes that normally control cell migration or metastasis. The development of techniques, such as the polymerase chain reaction, that allow detection of one malignant cell in 1 million normal cells should help with the detection of minimal residual disease following treatment. The availability of colony-stimulating factors may well allow dose escalations, especially if feline or canine recombinant products become available. Multidrug resistance is now manipulated in the clinical setting. Perhaps someday, techniques such as positron emission tomography and magnetic resonance spectroscopy will allow measurements of the impact of the treatment simultaneous with its application, allowing schedule alterations of drug administration so that whatever is required to kill the cancer cells and no more is administered.

## ALTERNATIVE APPROACHES

The development of differentiating agents, and compounds effective in the prevention of carcinogenesis, are attractive alternatives to further refinements in cytotoxic drug therapy. These compounds may prove to be exceptions to the rule that the maximal tolerated dose must be administered to achieve the maximal response.

### Chemoprevention

The retinoids (vitamin A and its natural and synthetic derivatives) are promising pharmaceuticals for cancer chemoprevention. Because these compounds have only recently been introduced, a brief review of their proposed mechanism of action is included, as well as dose schedules and toxicity notes (see "The Use of Synthetic Retinoids in Veterinary Medicine," this volume, p 585). The important role of retinoids in maintaining the integrity of epithelial tissues first sparked an interest in their ability to pharmacologically modify carcinogenic pathways. The multistep character of epithelial carcinogenesis makes it amenable to chemopreventive interventions and 13-cis-retinoic acid, at high doses, has been shown to suppress oral premalignancy and prevent second primary head and neck tumors in human patients (Tallman and Weirnik, 1992). Recommended doses remain somewhat empirical; canine patients treated with etretinate at 1 mg/kg every 12 hr for a minimum of 90 days showed objective responses in some cases of preneoplastic and preinvasive squamous cell carcinoma (Marks et al., 1992). Those authors concluded that although surgery remains the treatment of choice for invasive squamous cell carcinomas, the progression of preneoplastic lesions may be reversed or prevented by use of etretinate.

### Differentiating Agents

Malignant cells maintain their ability to differentiate along mature pathways when exposed to favorable conditions. Phenomenal results have been achieved in the treatment of human acute promyelocytic leukemia (APL) patients with the differentiating agent, all-trans retinoic acid (Huang et al., 1988). The discovery that the gene coding for the production of a nuclear retinoic acid receptor coincides with the breakpoint on chromosome 17 that is translocated in all cases of APL gave new insight into the mechanisms of retinoic acid–induced differentiation (Tallman and Wiernik, 1992). Three nuclear retinoic acid receptors have been identified. The exact function of each has not been identified, but it may someday be possible to design retinoic acid derivatives that interact with a specific receptor, thus separating toxic from beneficial effects.

Cutaneous lymphomas in both human and canine patients have been shown to be responsive to retinoids, and forced differentiation of malignant cells is the proposed mechanism. Six of 14 dogs with cutaneous lymphoma achieved remission following the administration of isotretinoin, with survival times ranging from 5 to 17.5 months (White et al., 1993). The isotretinoin dose used was 3 to 4 mg/kg, every 24 hr. A variety of benign canine tumors were also found to be responsive to retinoids. Responses were seen in five of seven dogs with intracutaneous cornifying epitheliomas, as well as one dog with an inverted papilloma and one with an epidermal cyst. Both isotretinoin and etretinate were found to be effective. Adverse effects included keratoconjunctivitis sicca, polydipsia, pruritus, hyperlipidemia, joint pain, swelling of the tongue, and teratogenesis. Side effects were seen in 29% of cases but did not appear to be dose dependent. Doses administered were 1 to 2 mg/kg every 24 hr of isotretinoin, and 1 mg/kg every 24 hr of etretinate.

Retinoid-induced cellular differentiation is enhanced by a variety of cytokines including the interferons, tumor necrosis factor, and granulocyte colony-stimulating factor. Low-dose cytosine arabinoside also appears to be synergistic with the retinoids. Improved tumor response rates have been seen with combination therapy in human patients with advanced squamous cell carcinoma of the skin and cervix, and etretinate in combination with interferon-α has resulted in improved response rates in human mycosis fungoides patients when compared to results with interferon-α alone (Altomare et al., 1993). This author has seen complete, albeit short-lived, responses to human interferon-α in canine cutaneous lymphomas. Whether or not it holds a place in therapy, or if a canine recombinant interferon would increase efficacy, is an issue for further study.

## References and Suggested Reading

Altomare GF, Cappella GL, Pigatto PD, et al: Intramuscular low dose alpha-2b interferon and etretinate for treatment of mycosis fungoides. Int J Dermatol 32:138, 1993.
*Etretinate potentiated the effectiveness of interferon-α in human cutaneous T-cell lymphoma.*

Arrington KA, Legendre AM, Tabeling GS, et al: Doxorubicin administration in dogs comparing two dosage protocols, body surface area (30 mg/m²) and body weight (mg/kg). Am J Vet Res (in press), 1994.
*Metabolism and excretion of doxorubicin was not different in the smaller patient and doses based on BSA consistently resulted in increased pharmacokinetic values and clinical toxicoses in smaller dogs.*

Dalton WS: Overcoming the multi-drug resistant phenotype. In DeVita VT, Hellman S, and Rosenberg SA (ed): Cancer: Principles and Practice of Oncology. Philadelphia, JB Lippincott Co, 1993, pp 2655–2666.
*A comprehensive review of clinical approaches to manipulating drug resistance.*

DeVita VT Jr: Principles of chemotherapy. In DeVita VT, Hellman S, and Rosenberg SA (eds): Cancer: Principles and Practice of Oncology. Philadelphia, JB Lippincott Co, 1993, pp 276–292.
*A review of the theories behind the application of chemotherapy.*

Huang M, Ye Y, Chen S, et al: Use of all-trans retinoic acid in the treatment of acute promyelocytic leukemia. Blood 72:567, 1988.
*Twenty-three of 24 patients achieved a complete response with all-trans retinoic acid, the last patient achieved a complete response following the addition of cytosine arabinoside.*

MacEwen EG, Brown NO, Patnaik AK, et al: Cyclic combination chemotherapy of canine lymphosarcoma. J Am Vet Med Assoc 178:1178, 1981.
*Response rates, survival times and prognostic factors are identified.*

Marks SL, Song MD, Stannard AA, et al: Clinical evaluation of etretinate for the treatment of canine solar-induced squamous cell carcinoma and preneoplastic lesions. J Am Acad Dermatol 27:11, 1992.
*Therapeutic efficacy for the treatment of preneoplastic lesions in the dog is presented.*

Ogilvie GK, Richardson RC, Curtis CR, et al: Acute and short-term toxicoses associated with the administration of doxorubicin to dogs with malignant tumors. J Am Vet Med Assoc 195:1584, 1989.
*Smaller dogs consistently demonstrated more clinical toxicoses and only body weight was predictive of such.*

Page RL, Macy DW, Thrall DE, et al: Unexpected toxicity associated with use of body surface area for dosing melphalan in the dog. Cancer Res 48: 288, 1988.
*Melphalan-induced toxicity in dogs can be more accurately estimated by body weight than by surface area.*

Page RL, Thrall DE, George SL, et al: Quantitative estimation of the thermal dose-modifying factor for cis-diamminedichloroplatinum (CDDP) in tumour-bearing dogs. Int J Hyperthermia 8:761, 1992.
*Dose must be modified to avoid unacceptable toxicity when cisplatin is combined with hyperthermia.*

Powis G, Reece P, Ahmann DL, et al: Effect of body weight on the pharmacokinetics of cyclophosphamide in breast cancer patients. Cancer Chemother Pharmacol 20:219, 1987.
*Cyclophosphamide disposition is altered in patients with increased body weight.*

Rodvold KA, Rushing DA, and Tewksbury DA: Doxorubicin clearance in the obese. J Clin Oncol 6:1321, 1988.
*Body weight was found to be significantly related to doxorubicin clearance.*

Tallman MS and Wiernik PH: Retinoids in cancer treatment. J Clin Pharmacol 32:868, 1992.
*An excellent review of retinoid therapy and its oncological applications.*

Vreiesendorp HM and Von Bekkum DW: Role of total body irradiation in conditioning for bone marrow transplantation. In Therfelder S, Rodt H, and Kilg HJ (eds): Immunology of Bone Marrow Transplantation. Berlin, Springer-Verlag, 1980, p 269.
*The hematopoietic stem cell activity necessary to rescue 50% of mice, rats, monkeys, and dogs following lethal, total-body irradiation correlated better with body weight than with BSA.*

White SD, Rosychuk RAW, Scott KV, et al: Use of isotretinoin and etretinate for the treatment of benign cutaneous neoplasia and cutaneous lymphoma in dogs. J Am Vet Med Assoc 202:387, 1993.
*Clinical responses are documented and toxicities noted.*

# DRUG INTERACTIONS WITH ANTINEOPLASTIC AGENTS

CAROLYN J. HENRY
*Pullman, Washington*

*and* WILLIAM G. BREWER, JR.
*Auburn, Alabama*

Chemotherapy is defined as the treatment of disease by chemical agents. The treatment of neoplastic disease by chemical agents (i.e., cancer chemotherapy) has become the mainstay of oncologic therapy for systemic neoplasia. Effective chemotherapy requires knowledge of tumor sensitivity; pharmacology, pharmacokinetics, and pharmacodynamics of antineoplastic agents; and drug–drug interactions. Awareness of drug interactions is important not only in determining combination chemotherapy protocols, but also in anticipating complications of treating concurrent neoplastic and other systemic disease or medical conditions. In addition, information regarding *in vitro* drug interactions is obviously crucial to the safe and efficacious preparation and administration of chemotherapeutic agents.

Antineoplastic agents interact with pharmacologic agents, both *in vitro* and *in vivo* through several different mechanisms. This is not surprising, since the action of most chemotherapeutic agents depends on their extremely reactive nature. *In vitro* reactions may occur when two or more drugs are added to the same intravenous fluids, resulting in decreased drug activity due to drug precipitation and inactivation. A classic example of precipitation is the interaction of doxorubicin and heparin when a 1000-U/ml heparin flush is used.

*In vivo* reactions may enhance or decrease drug activity and toxicity depending on factors such as route of administration, mechanisms of activation and degradation, competition for protein binding and/or drug receptor sites, effects on intracellular targets, timing of administration, routes of excretion, and unexplained mechanisms. Examples of each of these mechanisms follow.

Oral cyclophosphamide has been shown to decrease

the absorption of orally administered digoxin, thereby decreasing peak serum concentrations and efficacy of the digoxin. This effect does not occur when digoxin elixirs are utilized. Intravenous administration of cyclophosphamide may be preferable for animals receiving digoxin tablets.

Cyclophosphamide is an example of an antineoplastic agent that requires metabolism to its active form. Chloramphenicol inhibits hepatic activation of cyclophosphamide, and therefore decreases its antitumor effect. Conversely, barbiturates increase activation of cyclophosphamide and may enhance its toxicity.

Inhibition of drug degradation can also enhance toxicity. This occurs with the concurrent administration of azathioprine and allopurinol, since allopurinol inhibits xanthine oxidase, the enzyme that degrades azathioprine.

Competitive protein binding can increase the concentration of free active drug, leading to enhanced toxicity. An example is concurrent administration of aspirin compounds and methotrexate. Bound methotrexate is displaced from albumin by aspirin.

Folates and methotrexate enter the cell by binding the same membrane receptor. Consequently, concurrent administration will inhibit entry of methotrexate into the cell and decrease the intracellular concentration and activity of methotrexate.

The importance of timing of drug administration and effects on cellular targets are seen with the concurrent use of methotrexate and fluorouracil. The antitumor effect of methotrexate occurs through the inhibition of dihydrofolate reductase, an enzyme required for the synthesis of tetrahydrofolate. Tetrahydrofolate is required for nucleic acid synthesis, specifically thymidine. When methotrexate administration precedes fluorouracil by 1 hr, there is a synergistic effect; however, when fluorouracil precedes methotrexate, the fluorouracil inhibits thymidylate synthetase, thus maintaining intracellular pools of tetrahydrofolate. Therefore, the methotrexate-induced inhibition of dihydrofolate reductase is of no consequence.

Competitive inhibition for routes of excretion can enhance toxicity, as exemplified by the increased nephrotoxicity that occurs with the concurrent use of cisplatin and methotrexate, which are both excreted by the kidney.

For unknown reasons, the concurrent administration of actinomycin D and fluorouracil has been associated with an increased frequency of neurotoxicity.

This article tabulates reported drug interactions with various antineoplastic agents used in veterinary clinical oncology. The information is limited to agents applicable to veterinary medicine, but does not exhaust all possible interactions. Many studies reviewed did not list the degree of interaction. Such information was included in this review, if available. Antineoplastic agents with no known incompatibilities are not discussed. The chemotherapeutic agents reviewed are listed according to class of antineoplastic agent in Table 1. Table 2 summarizes the reported physical incompatibilities of antineoplastic agents with other drugs.

**Table 1.** *Interactions with Antineoplastic Agents Used in Veterinary Medicine*

| Antineoplastic Agent | Interacting Drug | Comments |
|---|---|---|
| **Alkylating Agents** | | |
| BCNU | Amphotericin B | Increases antitumor effect secondary to increased cellular uptake |
| | Cimetidine | Potentiates neutropenia and thrombocytopenia due to decreased hepatic degradation |
| | Digoxin | Serum concentrations decreased by agent |
| | Phenobarbital | Decreases efficacy of agent due to increased hepatic clearance |
| | Vitamin A | Increases antitumor effect |
| Chlorambucil | Phenobarbital | Increases cytotoxocity |
| | Prednisone | Synergistic in lymphoid neoplasia |
| Cyclophosphamide | Allopurinol | Enhances bone marrow suppression |
| | Barbiturates | Increases toxicity of agent due to increased rate of conversion to metabolites |
| | Chloramphenicol | Decreases efficacy of agent by interfering with metabolism to active form |
| | Cisplatin | Synergistic |
| | Corticosteroids | Decreases efficacy of agent initially due to interference with metabolism to active form |
| | Digoxin | Decreased oral absorption of digoxin |
| | Diuretics | Increases risk of syndrome of inappropriate ADH secretion |
| | Doxorubicin | Increases risk of cardiotoxicity |
| | Halothane and/or nitrous oxide | Increased anesthetic mortality in humans |

*Table continued on following page*

***Table 1.*** *Continued*

| Antineoplastic Agent | Interacting Drug | Comments |
|---|---|---|
| | Imipramine | Decreases efficacy of agent |
| | Insulin | May alter insulin requirements in diabetes |
| | Phenothiazine | Decreases efficacy of agent |
| | Thiazide diuretics | Prolong leukopenia |
| | Vinblastine | Increases risk of syndrome of inappropriate ADH secretion |
| | Vincristine | Increases toxicity and may induce syndrome of inappropriate ADH secretion |
| | Vitamin A | Decreases efficacy of agent by interfering with metabolism to active form |
| Dacarbazine (DTIC) | Allopurinol | Synergistic inhibition of xanthine oxidase activity |
| | Azathioprine/mercaptopurine | Toxicity enhanced by agent due to inhibition of xanthine oxidase activity |
| | Phenobarbital | Increases metabolic activation of DTIC |
| Melphalan | Cyclosporine | Increases risk of nephrotoxicity |
| ***Antitumor Antibiotics*** | | |
| Actinomycin D | Amphotericin B | Increases cellular uptake of agent |
| | Fluorouracil | May increase risk of neurotoxicity and decreases efficacy of agent |
| | Methotrexate | Decreases efficacy of agent |
| | Vincristine | Decreases efficacy of agent |
| Bleomycin | Amphotericin B | Synergistic |
| | Cisplatin | Decreases excretion and increases risk of cisplatin-induced nephrotoxicity |
| | Digoxin | Decreased serum levels of digoxin |
| | Vinblastine | Raynaud's phenomenon in humans |
| | Vincristine | Synergistic |
| Doxorubicin | Acetominophen | Decreases glutathione pool and sensitizes liver to free radical damage |
| | Amphotericin B | Increases cellular uptake of agent |
| | Barbiturates | Increases total plasma clearance of agent |
| | BCNU | Decreases glutathione pool and sensitizes liver to free radical damage |
| | Cyclophosphamide | Increases cardiotoxicity risk and risk of cyclophosphamide-induced cystitis |
| | Daunorubicin | Increases cardiotoxicity risk |
| | Digoxin | Decreased serum levels of digoxin |
| | Heparin | Precipitates |
| | Mercaptopurine | Increases risk of mercaptopurine-induced hepatotoxicity |
| Mitoxantrone | Cytarabine | Nausea, alopecia, vomiting, stomatitis, mucositis, myelosuppression |
| ***Antimetabolites*** | | |
| Azathioprine | ACE-inhibitors | Severe leukopenia |
| | Allopurinol | Blocks primary pathway for detoxification; should decrease azathioprine dose to 1/3–1/4 dose |
| Cytarabine | Digoxin | Oral absorption of digoxin decreased |
| | Flucytosine | Agent antagonizes the anti-infective activity of flucytosine |
| | Gentamicin | Decreases efficacy against *Klebsiella pneumoniae* |
| | L-Asparaginase | Synergistic |
| | Methotrexate | Simultaneous administration enhances the therapeutic effect of agent |
| Fluorouracil | Actinomycin D | Decreases efficacy of agent and may increase risk of neurotoxicity |
| | Amphotericin B | Increases efficacy of agent and increases risk of nephrotoxicity |

*Table continued on opposite page*

**Table 1.** *Continued*

| Antineoplastic Agent | Interacting Drug | Comments |
|---|---|---|
| | Cimetidine | Increases systemic exposure to agent and increases bioavailability of oral fluorouracil |
| | Cisplatin | Synergistic; neurotoxicity of agent potentiated |
| | Methotrexate | Synergistic if given before agent, antagonistic if given after and incompatible |
| Mercaptopurine | Vincristine | Increases cytotoxicity |
| | Allopurinol | Increases risk of myelosuppression; should decrease dose of agent to 25 to 33% (or by 75%) |
| | Doxorubicin | Increased risk of hepatotoxicity with combination |
| | Methotrexate | Decreases efficacy of agent |
| Methotrexate | Trimethoprim-sulfamethoxazole | Increases bone marrow suppression |
| | Kanamycin | Cellular uptake decreased by agent |
| | Amphotericin B | Increases cellular uptake and cytotoxicity of agent |
| | Bleomycin | Decreases cellular uptake of agent |
| | Cephalothin | Decreases cellular uptake of agent |
| | Chloramphenicol | Displaces from protein binding and increases toxicity |
| | Cytarabine | Agent may potentiate cytotoxocity if given before cytarabine |
| | Etretinate | Increased risk of hepatotoxicity with combination |
| | Fluorouracil | Increases cell kill with concurrent administration and decreases cytotoxicity if given before agent |
| | Folic acid preparations (including vitamins) | May decrease efficacy of agent |
| | Hydrocortisone sodium succinate | Decreases cellular uptake of agent |
| | Hydroxyurea | Decreases cellular uptake of agent |
| | L-Asparaginase | Agent toxicity and cytotoxicity is decreased if given prior to L-asparaginase; decreases cellular uptake of agent |
| | Methylprednisolone | Decrease cellular uptake of agent |
| | Nonsteroidal anti-inflammatory agents | Increase hematologic, renal, and gastrointestinal toxicity |
| | Penicillins | Decrease cellular uptake of agent |
| | Phenylbutazone | Displaces from protein binding and increases toxicity |
| | Probenicid | Delays disappearance of agent from serum due to competition for renal tubular secretion |
| | Procarbazine | Increased risk of nephrotoxicity with combination |
| | Pyrimethamine | Increases toxicity of agent |
| | Salicylates (including Pepto Bismol) | Displace from protein binding and increase toxicity |
| | Sulfonamides | Displace from protein binding and increase toxicity |
| | Tetracyclines | Displace from protein binding and increase toxicity |
| | Vincristine | Increases cellular uptake of agent when vincristine given 0–1 hr prior |
| ***Plant Alkaloids*** | | |
| Vinblastine | Methotrexate | Cytotoxic effects enhanced by agent due to increased cellular uptake |
| | Mitomycin C | Acute pulmonary reactions (shortness of breath and severe bronchospasm) have occurred with this combination in human patients |
| Vincristine | Actinomycin D | Efficacy decreased by agent |
| | Bleomycin | Synergistic, especially when administered 6–12 hr after agent |

*Table continued on following page*

**Table 1.** *Continued*

| Antineoplastic Agent | Interacting Drug | Comments |
|---|---|---|
| | Calcium channel blockers | Increase intracellular concentration of agent by inhibiting outflow from cells |
| | Cyclophosphamide | Agent enhances cytotoxicity |
| | Digoxin | Serum levels decreased by agent |
| | Fluorouracil | Cytotoxicity enhanced by agent |
| | L-Asparaginase | Decreases hepatic clearance when administered before agent; should give vincristine 12 to 24 hr prior to L-asparaginase |
| | Methotrexate | Agent enhances cellular uptake |
| | Mitomycin C | Acute pulmonary reactions (shortness of breath and severe bronchospasm) have occurred with this combination in human patients; agent enhances cytotoxicity |
| ***Miscellaneous Agents*** | | |
| Cisplatin | Interferon-$\alpha$ | Synergistic |
| | Aminoglycosides | Renal damage and ototoxicity with combination |
| | Amphotericin B | Increases risk of nephrotoxicity if given concurrently or within 2 weeks of administration of agent |
| | Anticonvulsant agents | Plasma concentrations are decreased by agent |
| | Bleomycin | Delayed excretion secondary to cisplatin-induced renal damage may lead to increased toxicity of bleomycin |
| | Combination cephalothin/ gentamicin | Increases risk of cisplatin-induced nephrotoxicity |
| | Cyclophosphamide | Synergistic |
| | Fluorouracil | Synergistic |
| | Loop diuretics | Increase risk of ototoxicity of agent |
| | Methotrexate | Renal elimination altered by agent |
| L-Asparaginase | Cyclophosphamide | Agent interferes with activation due to effects on hepatic function |
| | Cytarabine | Synergistic |
| | Mercaptopurine | Detoxification is decreased and hepatotoxicity in enhanced by agent |
| | Methotrexate | Hepatotoxicity is increased by agent; if L-asparaginase is administered 9–10 days prior to or shortly after methotrexate, antitumor effects of methotrexate are enhanced and gastrointestinal and hematologic toxicities of methotrexate are decreased |
| | Prednisone | Hyperglycemia |
| | Vincristine | Agent interferes with detoxification; cumulative neuropathy and disturbances of erythropoiesis; administration of L-asparaginase after rather than before or with vincristine may decrease potential for toxicity |
| Mitotane ($o,p'$-DDD) | Barbiturates | Hepatic metabolism increased by agent |
| | CNS depressants | Enhanced CNS depression with combination |
| | Corticosteroids | Hepatic metabolism increased by agent |
| | Spironolactone | Blocks action of agent |

***Table 2.*** *Physical Incompatibilities of Antineoplastic Agents\**

| | VCR | VBL | 6-MP | MITO | DOX | MTX | DTIC | BLEO | CIS | VP-16 | CYC | 5FU | ARA |
|---|---|---|---|---|---|---|---|---|---|---|---|---|---|
| Furosemide | + | + | − | − | + | − | − | + | − | − | − | − | |
| Heparin sodium | − | +† | − | + | +‡ | − | − | − | − | − | − | − | +§ |
| Dexamethasone SP | − | − | − | − | + | − | − | + | − | − | − | − | − |
| Sulfhydryl groups | − | − | − | − | − | − | − | + | − | − | − | − | − |
| Amino acids | − | − | − | − | − | − | − | + | − | − | − | + | − |
| Riboflavin | − | − | − | − | − | − | − | + | − | − | − | − | − |
| Diazepam | − | − | − | − | + | − | − | + | − | − | − | + | − |
| Hydrocortisone Na succinate | − | − | − | − | + | − | + | + | − | − | − | − | + |
| Divalent & trivalent cations (esp Cu) | − | − | − | − | − | − | − | + | − | − | − | − | − |
| Aminophylline | − | − | − | − | + | − | − | + | − | − | − | − | − |
| 5FU | − | − | + | + | + | + | − | − | − | − | − | − | + |
| Cephalothin | − | − | − | − | + | − | − | + | − | − | − | − | +‖ |
| Benzyl alcohol solutions | − | − | − | − | − | − | − | − | − | − | + | − | − |
| Methotrexate | − | − | − | − | − | − | − | + | − | − | − | + | + |
| Penicillins | − | − | − | − | − | − | − | + | − | − | − | + | + |
| Tetracyclines | − | − | − | − | − | − | − | + | − | − | − | + | − |
| Ascorbic acid | − | − | − | − | − | − | − | + | − | − | − | − | − |
| Insulin | − | − | − | − | − | − | − | − | − | − | − | + | + |
| Multivitamins | − | − | − | − | − | − | − | − | − | − | − | + | − |
| Mannitol | − | − | − | − | − | − | − | − | + | − | − | − | − |
| Na bisulfite | − | − | − | − | − | − | − | − | + | − | − | − | − |
| Dextrose solutions | − | − | − | − | − | − | − | − | +¶ | + | − | +# | − |
| Metoclopramide | − | − | − | − | − | + | − | − | + | − | − | − | − |
| Prednisolone Na succinate and D5W | − | − | + | − | − | − | − | − | − | − | − | − | − |
| Allopurinol Na in D5W | − | − | + | − | − | − | − | − | − | − | − | − | − |
| Prednisolone Na phosphate | − | − | − | − | − | + | − | − | − | − | − | − | − |
| Normal saline | − | − | − | − | − | − | − | − | − | + | − | − | − |
| Mitomycin | − | − | − | − | − | − | − | + | − | − | − | − | − |
| Terbutaline sulfate | − | − | − | − | − | − | − | + | − | − | − | − | − |
| Droperidol | − | − | − | − | − | + | · | + | − | − | − | + | − |
| Na bicarbonate 5% | − | − | − | − | − | − | − | − | + | − | − | − | − |
| Methylprednisolone Na succinate | − | − | − | − | − | − | − | − | − | − | − | − | + |
| Gentamicin | − | − | − | − | − | − | − | − | − | − | − | − | + |
| Ranitidine HCl | − | − | − | − | − | + | − | − | − | − | − | − | − |
| Cefazolin | − | − | − | − | − | − | − | + | − | − | − | − | − |

\*, physical incompatibility has been reported; −, no physical incompatibility has been reported.

†200 U/ml heparin sodium.

‡1000 U/ml heparin sodium and 2 mg/ml doxorubicin injected into Y-site with no flush between.

§Haze formation at 10,000 U/L.

‖2 gm/L cephalothin.

¶Breakdown after 2 hr in solution.

#10% loss of fluorouracil in 7 hr at room temperature.

Abbreviations: VCR = vincristine, VBL = vinblastine, 6-MP = mercaptopurine, MITO = mitoxantrone, DOX = doxorubicin, MTX = methotrexate, DTIC = dacarbazine, BLEO = bleomycin, CIS = cisplatin, VP-16 = etoposide, CYC = cyclophosphamide, 5FU = fluorouracil, ARA = cytosine arabinoside.

## References and Suggested Reading

Chabner BA and Collins JM (eds): *Cancer Chemotherapy: Principles and Practice.* Philadelphia, JB Lippincott Co, 1990, pp 110–490.
*A textbook presenting principles of chemotherapy, standard protocols in human patients, and individual chemotherapeutic agent information.*

Cohen MH, Johnston-Early A, and Hood MA: Drug precipitation within IV tubing: A potential hazard of chemotherapy administration. Cancer Treat Rep 69:1325, 1985.
*A review of in vitro incompatibilities with antineoplastic agents.*

Door RT: Incompatibilities with parenteral anticancer drugs. Am J Intraven Ther Feb/Mar:42, 1979.
*A review of incompatibilities with commonly used antineoplastic agents.*

Dorr RT and Fritz WL: *Cancer Chemotherapy Handbook.* New York, Elsevier, 1980, pp 75–97, 201–711.
*A manual of chemotherapy principles, common protocols used in human patients, individual antineoplastic agent information, and drug interactions.*

Griffin JP, D'Arcy PF, and Speirs CJ: *A Manual of Adverse Drug Interactions,* 4th edition. Boston, Butterworth's, 1988.
*A textbook outlining drug interactions for all classes of pharmaceuticals.*

McEvoy GK: Antineoplastics agents. In *AHFS Drug Information.* Bethesda, MD, American Society of Hospital Pharmacists, Inc, 1993, pp 521–671.
*A pharmaceutical manual providing detailed drug information comparable to that found on drug inserts.*

Olin BR: Antineoplastics. In *Drug Facts and Comparisons.* Philadelphia, JP Lippincott Co, 1992, pp 642–649.
*An updatable manual of complete and current pharmacologic information listed by drug class.*

Perry MC: *The Chemotherapy Sourcebook.* Baltimore, Williams & Wilkins, 1982. *A comprehensive textbook discussing chemotherapy principles, drug interactions, and individual antineoplastic agents.*

Trissel LA: *ASHP Handbook on Injectable Drugs,* 5th edition. Bethesda, MD, ASHP, 1988.
*A textbook that provides information regarding drug stability, drug interactions, and incompatibilities.*

Wittes RE, Leyland-Jones B, Fortner C, et al: Chemotherapy: The properties and uses of single agents. In Wittes RE (ed): *Manual of Oncologic Therapeutics 1989/1990.* St. Louis, JB Lippincott Co, 1989, pp 91–169.
*A handbook of human chemotherapy that provides information regarding mechanisms of action, common uses, toxicity, and drug interactions for antineoplastic agents.*

# TUMOR IMMUNOLOGY AND TUMOR IMMUNOTHERAPY

NEIL T. GORMAN

*Melton Mowbray, Leceistershire, United Kingdom*

There is little doubt that there are antigenic differences between normal and neoplastic cells that are reflected in the composition of antigens within the cell membrane. In the clinical situation, there is a continuing debate as to whether or not an immune response is truly mounted to these antigens and, if so, whether or not the response is of benefit to the patient. If this is so, one of the major goals of cancer medicine must be to devise therapeutic regimens that act specifically against neoplastic cells while leaving normal tissue unimpaired.

Tumor antigens can be defined as antigens that are expressed on the surface of neoplastic cells but not usually expressed on the surface of normal differentiated cells or at low density on the normal cell. The definition of tumor antigens has been expanded to include proteins expressed on tumor cells even though there is no evidence of a host response to these antigens. The origins of these antigens are diverse and arise from viral gene expression, expression of differentiation antigens usually present only on stem cells, or from alterations in glycosylation of glycoproteins and glycolipids that alter the antigenic determinants of the cell surface proteins. The expression of these antigens may be induced by viruses or other exogenous carcinogens such as ultraviolet irradiation and a whole variety of chemicals. These proteins are not usually specific to the tumor cells, often being found at low density on stem cells. Tumor antigens are arbitrarily classified as either tumor-specific transplantation antigens (TSTA) or tumor-associated antigens (TAA).

## TUMOR-SPECIFIC TRANSPLANTATION ANTIGENS

Transplantation of carcinogen-induced tumors from one syngeneic animal to another previously immunized with lethally irradiated cells of the same tumor type is followed by rejection, and lifelong protection is conferred against further transplants of that tumor. This system indicated the presence of tumor-specific transplantation antigens (TSTAs) on the surface of the cell. Cross-protection experiments between different chemically induced tumors, even those of the same histologic type, showed that the TSTAs were unique to an individual tumor. Some transplanted tumors were highly immunogenic and some were weakly immunogenic.

The biochemical characterization of the majority of the TSTAs on experimentally induced tumors remains to be determined. The expression of endogenous retroviral antigens by neoplastic cells causes much of the confusion in this area, but at least one TSTA (gp70) has been reported. Aberrant glycosylation patterns of this glycoprotein may produce the unique and novel cell surface antigenic structures.

## TUMOR-ASSOCIATED ANTIGENS

The strong TSTAs associated with the chemically induced rodent tumors have not been demonstrated in humans or animals. Tumor-associated antigens expressed on nonviral tumors have been defined largely by monoclonal antibodies and can be divided into differentiation antigens and embryonic antigens.

Differentiation antigens represent those that are normally expressed during differentiation and may be turned on and off during differentiation. If a cell becomes neoplastic at a particular stage of differentiation, the clones of cells will simply reflect that stage of differentiation. The classic example of these is the expression of CD antigens on lymphoid cells and the common leukocyte antigen. In contrast, differentiation antigens can be expressed aberrantly on cells when there is de-repression of "normal" differentiation antigens or expression of antigens that are not normally expressed on that cell type and include endocrine receptors and some oncogene products. It is the latter that continue to attract most attention scientifically, but it should be borne in mind that many of the oncogene products act as DNA-binding proteins and are not expressed on the cell surface. Equally, it is important to emphasize that although the protein products associated with oncogenes are often mutated, there is no evidence to suggest that these are a target for the immune response, even when their structures are associated with cell surface expression. The detection of abnormal amounts of the products of an oncogene is a fundamental indicator of neoplastic change within the cell demonstrating that the cellular proto-oncogene has been activated and transformed the cell. Proto-oncogenes are a set of normal cellular genes involved in cell regulation. Their products range from growth factors to growth-factor receptors and signaling proteins associated with the cell membrane down to the DNA-binding proteins.

Embryonic antigens are antigens normally expressed on fetal and embryonic cells and are usually found at very low levels on normal stem cells. It has been recognized for some time that some malignant cells revert to produce a fetal equivalent of an adult protein or cell surface antigen. These have largely been used as indicators for the identification and monitoring of disease states rather than in a serious investigation of the immune response to tumors. As such antigens are usually expressed at low levels on normal stem cells, one might expect them to be nonimmunogenic in their natural hosts. The best examples of embryonic antigens are the carcinoembryonic antigen (CEA) and $\alpha$-fetoprotein expressed by intestinal neoplasia in humans.

A number of the monoclonal antibody-defined tumor antigens appear to be related to glycosylation determinants rather than the polypeptide structure per se. Alterations in glycosylation can produce novel antigenic structures as evidenced by the generation of the Thomson-Friedenreich antigens (or T antigens) expressed on human carcinomas. Similar alterations in the glycosylation of glycolipids can also produce novel antigenic determinants. For example, a monoganglioside has been defined both on colonic carcinoma cells and on adenocarcinomas of stomach, pancreas, and colon, but not on normal adult tissue. Furthermore, this carbohydrate structure is found in the serum of 50 to 60% of colorectal, 80 to 90% of pancreatic, and 70 to 80% of patients with gastric adenocarcinomas. Recently, it has been found that certain glycolipids not normally expressed on human cells are found on some tumor cells.

## ANTIGENS ON VIRUS-INDUCED TUMORS

While several groups of DNA viruses are known to be oncogenic, only one group of RNA viruses, the retroviruses, have been shown to have this property. The mechanisms of transformation by retroviruses and DNA viruses are different and they display distinct relationships with their host cells. In the case of the DNA viruses, productive replication does not occur in the transformed cell, but expression of one or more regions of the virus genome is necessary to initiate transformation. In addition, glycosylated viral proteins that are expressed at the cell surface may also be present on the transformed cell and these can act as targets for the immune response.

Retroviruses have been shown to activate protooncogenes primarily by insertional mutagenesis. Examination of the structure of a feline leukemia provirus indicates that it has three coding regions: *gag*, which codes for the internal proteins; *pol*, which codes for the enzyme reverse transcriptase and endonuclease; and *env*, which codes for the envelope proteins. In addition, at each end of the virus are two directly repeated sequences known as long terminal repeats (LTRs). These sequences contain promoters, which are the site of initiation of transcription; and enhancers, which serve to regulate the level of transcription in a tissue-specific and orientation-independent way. Activation of the *myc*

oncogene, a DNA-binding protein, is associated with the insertion of the provirus adjacent to the first exon of the *myc* gene but is in the opposite transcriptional orientation. The LTR-associated enhancer "takes over" the regulation of the mRNA transcription from the normal *myc* gene promoter. This process often results in increased levels of transcription of *myc* mRNA. The promoter also disrupts upstream regulation of the *myc* gene; for instance, by inserting a de-enhancer region. In companion animal veterinary medicine the most intensively studied retroviruses have been feline leukemia virus (FeLV).

## FELINE LEUKEMIA VIRAL ANTIGENS AND THE ANTIVIRUS RESPONSE

Lymphoid malignancies are common in the cat, and most are associated with a feline leukemia virus infection acquired from a carrier cat either transplacentally or through contaminated body secretions, particularly saliva. After a latent period of months or years, during which time the cat has a persistent infection and associated viremia, lymphoma or less commonly leukemia may develop. The virus replicates in many cell types including those in hemopoietic and epithelial tissues. All of these infected cells will express on their cell surface the envelope viral glycoproteins or gp70s. In addition, glycosylated variants of internal virion structural proteins are also found at the cell surface. Polymorphism in the envelope glycoprotein determines the three subgroups of FeLV known as A, B, and C. These subgroups are defined on the basis of viral interference (i.e., when a cell is infected by one subgroup, it cannot be superinfected by the same subgroups but is open to infection by a different subgroup). This phenomenon is believed to result from blocking of the cell virus receptors by viral glycoprotein expressed on the cell surface.

Following infection, the cat may mount an antiviral response characterized by the production of neutralizing antibody directed at the envelope glycoproteins. Concomitantly, there is an elimination of virus, or modulation of expression in infected cells. Recently, it has been shown that a high proportion of cats that appear to have eliminated the virus have in fact a latent infection in myelomonocytic and lymphoid cells. Furthermore, it has been demonstrated that this latent state is maintained by the presence of neutralizing antibody. When bone marrow from latently infected cats is cultured *in vitro*, spontaneous reactivation of virus production occurs, but this can be suppressed by neutralizing but not non-neutralizing monoclonal antibodies to FeLV.

There is an overwhelming body of evidence demonstrating that when a cat is infected by FeLV, a successful antibody response can be mounted to the virus with the production of virus-neutralizing antibody. Where the challenge is heavy or under circumstances where the cat cannot generate an effective immune response, FeLV-related diseases will occur. FeLV-induced lymphomas have been associated with the production of the tumor-associated antigen, feline oncornavirus-associated cell membrane antigen (FOCMA). FeLV-infected cats with lymphosarcoma demonstrate low titers of anti-FOCMA antibody, while those that resist tumor development maintain high levels. The definition of FOCMA antigens has essentially been a functional one in that either indirect immunofluorescence or complement-dependent cytotoxicity has been used to detect antigens on the reference T-cell lymphosarcoma cell line FL74. Since in early studies anti-FOCMA antibody was found in viremic cats with detectable neutralizing antibody and since this antibody could not be absorbed with viral structural antigens, it was suggested that FOCMA was a transformation-specific, nonstructural antigen of the virus. Later it was concluded that the same or a closely related antigen was expressed on feline sarcoma virus (FeSV) –transformed cells and this might represent the product of a common transforming protein. Data leading to these conclusions were the apparent concordance of antibody titers assayed on FL74 cells and non-virus-producing mink cells. A correlation between FOCMA titers and neutralizing antibody titers to FeLV-C, but not to FeLV-A and B, has been known for some time. There is no correlation between neutralizing antibody titers to subgroups A and B of FeLV and FOCMA, but a positive correlation exists with neutralizing titers to subgroup C. Furthermore, the predominant viral glycoprotein expressed on FL74 cells was found to be that of the subgroup-C virus. A common feature of FOCMA-positive sera is their reactivity with FeLV-C gp70. A particularly interesting observation was that a T-cell lymphosarcoma line releasing only subgroup-A virus, known as F422, reacted with FOCMA antiserum and with certain monoclonal antibodies to FeLV-C gp70. The epitope detected by the monoclonal antibody was present on budding virus particles but was not observed in the mature virion and may account for the failure in earlier studies to absorb FOCMA reactivity with virus preparations. The origin of these FeLV-C epitopes on transformed lymphoma cells is unresolved. It still remains attractive to speculate that they may arise from endogenous envelope gene sequences expressed either directly or after recombination with exogenous feline leukemia viruses. One of the intriguing early observations of FOCMA distribution was that it was detected on lymphosarcoma cells from virus-positive and virus-negative cats, the definition of virus-negative being the absence of virus antigen-positive cells in the blood. Recent molecular analysis has shown that a small percentage of cats with lymphosarcoma that are virus-negative by these criteria contain FeLV genomes in the tumor cells. However, by far, the majority of virus-negative cats with lymphosarcoma do not possess evidence of integrated FeLV proviruses, and it is likely that the cause of these tumors is unrelated to FeLV infection. The reported ubiquity of FOCMA reactivity on lymphosarcoma cells therefore becomes a paradox, but may be resolved if endogenous FeLV genomes are expressed in these tumors. Such a phenom-enon could be independent of FeLV infection. This explanation also raises the wider issue of whether endogenous retroviral genomes in other species could function as tumor-associated antigens even in tumors of nonviral origin.

## IMMUNE RESPONSE

The molecular and cellular basis of the immune response is now quite clear as compared to 5 and 10 years ago. The complete sequence of events in the immune response is beyond the scope of this article, but it is important to understand that there is antigen processing, antigen recognition by antigen receptors, cell cooperation between cells of the immune system, and finally the initiation of effector functions. The key event is antigen recognition by T cells. T cells recognize antigen in association with either class I or class II major histocompatibility (MHC) antigens. $CD8^+$ cytotoxic T cells (Tc) recognize antigen on the surface of cells in association with class I MHC antigens, whereas $CD4^+$ helper T cells (Th) recognize antigen in association with class II MHC antigen on the surface of antigen-presenting cells and some B cells. This system ensures that antigen receptors on the surface of T cells do not become saturated with native antigen, thus preventing the initiation of an appropriate response. Exogenous antigen is taken up initially by antigen-presenting cells. These are usually fixed and circulating macrophages, but other specialized cells such as Langerhans cells in the skin and interdigitating dendritic cells in lymphoid tissue serve in this function. Other cells that act as antigen-presenting cells include: B cells, astrocytes, follicular cells in the thyroid, endothelia, and fibroblasts. Once antigen is internalized, it is degraded into peptide fragments within phagolysosomes, where it becomes associated with a class II MHC antigen. The resultant class II–peptide complex is transported to the cell surface. Endogenous antigen produced within the cell is transported into the rough endoplasmic reticulum (RER) using a series of transporting molecules. Once in the RER, some of the peptides become associated with and stabilize class I MHC molecules. These stabilized molecules are then transported directly to the cell surface. Infection of cells by viruses and parasites are excellent examples of this type of system. It should, however, be noted that cellular antigens of any type could be affected this way, which does have implication as regards self versus nonself and the development of autoimmune disease.

It is comparatively easy to envisage how tumor antigens associated with viral and chemically induced tumors can be processed and presented to the immune system, as in both cases new or modified antigens are produced. Tumor antigens shed from the cell surface can be taken up and processed by antigen-processing cells. In some cases, such as lymphoid tumors and those of the macrophage series, the transformed cell could act as the antigen-presenting cell. The difficulty comes in relation to spontaneous tumors where the tumor antigens are simply differentiation antigens to which there is tolerance. Confusion still reigns as to the mechanism whereby the response is generated and in most spontaneous tumors, the nature of specific immune response has yet to be defined.

## EFFECTOR MECHANISMS IN TUMOR IMMUNITY

The previous section has covered briefly the possible expression of tumor antigens by viral- and non-viral-induced tumors. The belief is that there is an immune response to some of these antigens that culminates with the generation of effector mechanisms that contribute to the removal of tumor cells from the host. There are a number of effector mechanisms that can operate, the most important of which are considered below.

### Antibody

Antibody can act as an effector mechanism either through complement activation or through antibody-dependent cell-mediated cytotoxicity (ADCC). In feline lymphoma there is good evidence that antibody is important not only in the antiviral but also in the antitumor response. A good correlation has been shown between the antitumor antibodies (anti-FOCMA) as determined by complement-dependent lysis of tumor cells in vitro and protection against tumor development. The role of complement is reinforced by the report that hypocomplementemic FeLV viremic cats appear to be predisposed to tumor development despite the presence of anti-FOCMA antibodies. These observations are surprising, as it has been previously found that antibody-dependent complement-mediated lysis of nucleated cells is a very ineffective method of cell lysis. It would also be of great value to know if ADCC is important in the immune response to both FeLV infections and FeLV-induced tumors.

### Antibody-Dependent Cell-Mediated Cytotoxicity

Populations of cells that express a surface Fc receptor can bind and kill cells coated with antibody. The specificity of ADCC is conferred by the immunoglobulin, which binds to the target and then via its Fc portion binds to an Fc receptor–bearing cell. An Fc receptor is essential for a cell to function as an effector cell in ADCC, but not all cells with Fc receptors are effector cells (e.g., B lymphocytes do not mediate ADCC). Certain Tc and natural killer (NK) cells possess an Fc receptor and thus fulfill the requirement for ADCC, but it is clear that other leukocytes mediate damage to the target through secretory processes. Monocytes, neutrophils, and eosinophils can also function as effector cells in ADCC, and their relative importance in the immunopathogenesis of disease is de-

pendent upon the pathogen and the antibody response to that pathogen.

### Natural Killer Cells

The NK cell is derived from the large granular lymphocyte and are $CD3^-$, $CD16^+$, and $CD56^+$, and do not show successful rearrangement of the T-cell receptor. Natural killer cells can be both recruited and enhanced by interleukin-2 (IL-2) and interferon-$\alpha$ and -$\gamma$ (IFN-$\alpha$). The determinants recognized by NK cells in vivo are more prevalent on certain malignant, undifferentiated, infectious, and nonautologous cells, but there is no evidence of any molecular change that converts an NK-resistant cell to an NK-susceptible cell. Natural killer cells bind to many potential targets, but the signal for cytolysis comes from within the target cell itself.

### Cytotoxic T Lymphocytes

Cytotoxic T cells express CD8 and damage viral infected cells and, as mentioned previously, the T-cell receptors recognize this viral antigen only in association with class I MHC antigens. The expansion of Tc cell clones is directly related to the release of cytokines, particularly IL-2, from Th cells.

### Tumor-Isolated Lymphocytes and Lymphocyte Activated Killer Cells

Tumor-isolated lymphocytes (TILs) have been shown to have an in vitro sensitivity to IL-2 and experimentally have shown reactivity to fresh tumor cells. This has been taken as evidence for a tumor response, but the nature of the antigens involved has not been described. As these lymphocytes are isolated from the tumor itself, it is fair to consider this evidence of a cellular antitumor response. TILs have been used in the therapy of neoplastic disease as will be discussed later.

Lymphocyte activated killer (LAK) cells are very different from the TILs in that they are populations of lymphocytes isolated from blood or lymphoid structures and cultured in vitro with IL-2. The resultant population has been shown to have in vitro activity against a wide range of tumor cells.

## MECHANISM OF LYMPHOCYTE-MEDIATED CYTOTOXICITY

The lytic event requires physical contact between the effector cell and the target. The lytic event is in three stages: binding, release of killing substances, and the actual cell lysis. The first stage involves the T-cell receptor–antigen–MHC complex as already discussed. The final stage involves changes in the membrane permeability of the target cell, which leads to swelling and disruption. There are a number of ways that cytotoxic cells can kill nucleated cells. Vesicles in the Tc have been shown to contain a C9-like molecule termed "perforin" that polymerizes to form a transmembrane channel in a $Ca2^+$-dependent manner. These are the ring-shaped structures 10 to 15 nm in diameter that traverse the membrane, but the detail is not as complete as that available for complement. True lysis, as with an erythrocyte, does not occur, as apoptosis is seen with a programmed cell death. It has been proposed that cytoxins are also contained within the vesicles and these are released and pass through the perforin channel to promote DNA fragmentation. Finally, it is well recognized that the vesicles can contain IFN-$\gamma$ and tumor necrosis factors−$\alpha$ and −$\beta$ (TNF-$\alpha$ and -$\beta$), all of which can combine with surface receptors on the target cell.

### Macrophages

Macrophages are found in association with many solid tumors. These cells are attracted and maintained at the tumor cytokines and interferons. *In vitro*, these cells can be activated to exhibit tumoricidal activity by a number of agents including IFN-$\alpha$; -$\beta$; -$\gamma$; IL-2; and TNF-$\alpha$. Activated macrophages can distinguish between normal and neoplastic cells. The true role of macrophages *in vivo* as an antitumor mechanism is by no means clear. There is, however, experimental evidence to show that inhibiting macrophage function *in vivo* (e.g., with silica) impairs the animal's ability to resist tumor challenge and increases the sensitivity of the animal to the tumor challenge.

### Cytokines

The cytokine network has become increasingly important in our understanding of the normal immune response. The predominant cytokines are the ILs, IFNs, and TNFs. All these contribute to the orchestration of the immune response. Tumor necrosis factor was originally investigated for its association with the development of cachexia and the direct destruction of tumor cells, but it soon became clear that it has many roles to play in lymphocyte and macrophage activation. Detailed consideration of cytokines is given elsewhere in this section (see "Cytokines and Biologic Response Modifiers in Small Animal Practice," this volume, p 547).

## MANIPULATION OF THE ANTITUMOR RESPONSE IN THE THERAPY OF TUMORS

The possibility that the immune system could recognize and eventually eliminate tumor cells from the body has always been an attractive possibility for the clinician. The potential of this approach for the clinical management of tumors was first indicated in work that demonstrated an immune response to virus-induced or chemically induced tumors. It is not surprising that the level of success of immunotherapy in experimental animals is not mirrored in human and veterinary patients, as it is quite clear that the same level of antigenicity is not expressed by spontaneously arising tumors of nonviral origin. In immunotherapy, there has been a move away from the insistence that target molecules be truly tumor antigens. It is better to consider the aim of immunotherapy as one of damaging and removing tumor cells while inflicting limited damage upon the normal cell population.

## ANTIBODY THERAPY

This is a form of passive immunotherapy where specific antitumor antibodies are administered and no active participation of the immune response is required. The initial successful application of this approach has used monoclonal antibodies directed at tumor antigens to target drugs such as adriamycin, isotypes such as [131]I, ricin A-chain toxin, or other antineoplastic agents to the sites of the tumor deposits. This selectivity avoids the toxicity to normal tissue so often associated with such agents. There is the potential bonus that the dose of a drug delivered to the tumor cell could be greatly increased compared to conventional methods, but this potential has yet to be realized. Some remarkable successes in the treatment of some B-cell lymphomas using monoclonal antibodies alone directed against the idiotypic determinants of the surface immunoglobulin have been reported. This is even more remarkable when it is considered that the idiotype of the neoplastic B cell can change due to somatic mutation. It would appear that the anti-idiotype–idiotype interaction serves to control the proliferation of the neoplastic B cells. This example is the exception, as other monoclonal antibodies alone have been unsuccessful due to the inability of the isotype to interact with effector mechanisms. Recent work in the dog has been reported demonstrating that a monoclonal antibody against canine lymphocytes can moderate the progression of certain forms of canine lymphoma.

The efficacy of the mouse and rat monoclonal antibodies against human tumor antigens has been limited by host response to the heterologous immunoglobulin. To overcome this problem, chimeric antibodies have been constructed whereby mouse myeloma cells producing antitumor antibodies are transfected with human immunoglobulin heavy chain constant genes. The result is that the myeloma clones produce an antibody that has the heavy chain human constant regions and the variable regions of mouse origin. The resultant chimera is technically less likely to engender an immune response against itself once injected into a patient. There are further imaginative ways in which the antibody can be manipulated to target immune responses. One of these is redirected cytotoxicity, where bispecific antibody is created. One specificity is directed against the tumor cell surface and the other against one of the markers expressed on effector cells, particularly Tc cells. This duality results in the drawing together of target and effector and potentially can increase the kill rate of the tumor cell.

The potential for monoclonal antibody therapy lies most likely in the treatment of nonsolid tumors (e.g., lymphomas) and in the treatment of micrometastatic disease, particularly when it is located in the bone marrow.

## CYTOKINE THERAPY

The potential for the use of cytokines is twofold. First, cytokines can be administered to the patient directly. Second, cytokines can be used to manipulate cells *in vitro* for reinfusion into the patient.

The predominant cytokines in the former category are the interleukins and the interferons. There is theoretical sense in infusing a patient with the major T-cell-activating cytokine in the hope that the appropriate cytotoxic T cells are activated and destroy tumor cells. Implicit in this approach is that many T-cell clones will be activated in an indiscriminate way. The systemic effect on patients has been dramatic in that the morbidity has been very high and a number of deaths have been reported. In the recent past, it is IL-2 that has attracted most attention, having been used on terminally sick melanoma and renal carcinoma patients, and some encouraging reports have emerged. Enthusiasm for using IL-2 to activate T cells *in vitro* and reinfusing them into the patient has been voiced. This process generates the so-called LAK cell but has met with no success.

It is fair to say at this time that the potential for cytokine therapy alone in the management of neoplastic disease is minimal. As all the clinical trials are undertaken on terminally ill patients, it is difficult to see how proper assessment of their efficacy can ever be made. In the veterinary arena, feline and canine interferons have been cloned and sequenced and no doubt will be used in the clinical setting in the near future. In relation to studies undertaken thus far in humans, the potential would seem to be greater than the reality, but time will tell.

*Active immunotherapy* is the attempt to generate a specific immune response against the tumor cell surface antigens. A number of clinical trials have used immunization with either tumor cells or extracts of tumor cell membranes (usually KCl-lysed cells) in combination with chemotherapy to stimulate an appropriate response, but they have had limited success.

An innovative approach to the use of tumor cells as an immunogen has been heterogenization of weak tumor cell surface antigens. Heterogenization of a tumor antigen is when a highly antigenic determinant is inserted or coupled to the tumor cell surface and the resultant heterogenized cells are used as the immunogen. The incorporation of such highly antigenic structures into the cell surface appears to generate an immune response not only to itself but also to the weak cell surface antigen. This acts via Th lymphocytes that expand clones that have antitumor activity. Two basic techniques have been used: insertion of viral antigens into tumor cells, and coupling of haptens, in particular purified protein derivative of tuberculin (PPD), to the cell surface. In the former, a number of viruses have been used experimentally, but vesicular stomatitis virus and influenza show the most promise. In the latter, PPD is covalently coupled to the cell surface and the heterogenized cells injected into the patient previously primed with bacillus Calmette-Guérin (BCG). In both these examples, an antitumor response can be detected *in vivo* and *in vitro* and the experimental results have been encouraging. These approaches have been used in clinical trials in the treatment of neoplastic diseases in humans and dogs, but the results are not as good as in the experimental model. An alternative approach is to combine the tumor cell surface antigens with foreign MHC determinants. This is achieved by fusing the tumor cell with a cell that expresses a different MHC haplotype. This provides an antigenic structure in the cell membrane that acts as a helper determinant in a similar manner to either the viral antigen or the hapten.

It has been possible to isolate the lymphocytes that infiltrate tumors and culture them *in vitro* using IL-2. The basis behind this approach is that the infiltrating lymphocytes are likely to have some antitumor activity. Manipulation of these cells thus has the potential to generate a potent antitumor response. This approach is far more sensible than the LAK cell, which remains far too indiscriminate.

## NONSPECIFIC IMMUNOSTIMULANT THERAPY

There are a number of biologic products that have been shown to nonspecifically stimulate the immune system. Of these products, the most consistent has been the use of bacteria as immunostimulants. The two most common bacterial agents that have been used are BCG and Proprionibacteria. It is fair to say that the results with Proprionibacteria have been most disappointing in both veterinary and human medicine and it is no longer being used. The work with BCG has provided slightly more encouragement in the treatment of neoplasia in humans and animals.

Bacille Calmette-Guérin has been shown to activate and mobilize macrophage populations so that they can kill cells. This is mediated by the lymphocyte's release of macrophage-activating factors, including ILs, IFNs, and TNF-α and -β. There is compelling evidence in experimental systems that attests to the ability of BCG to induce regression of tumors following intralesional and systemic injection. Probably the best application of this in veterinary medicine is the treatment of equine sarcoids with intralesional BCG or extracts of the BCG cell walls (e.g., methanol extractable residue [MER] and cell wall skeleton [CWS]). There are now a number of published series that show complete regression of sarcoids following intralesional BCG, particularly in treatment of periocular sarcoid. This site specificity raises the question of whether or not sarcoids express varying antigenicity according to the site. In addition, there are reports of successful treatment of canine mammary carcinoma using cell wall extracts from mycobacteria, although this does not seem to have much influence on either survival time or metastasis.

Bacille Calmette-Guérin has also been used in the treatment of tumors in the dog including melanomas, mammary tumors, lymphomas, and metastatic disease from osteosarcomas and mammary tumors. There is little convincing evidence that intralesional BCG injection of mammary tumors has any significant effect on the progress and eventual outcome of this disease. Due to the very heterogeneous nature of these tumors, a carefully controlled trial relating both to histologic type and to the clinical stage is required. In the control of metastatic disease, intravenous BCG has been shown to delay the onset of pulmonary metastasis in both osteosarcomas and mammary tumors but failed to produce cures. This has been attributed to the nonspecific activation of pulmonary macrophages. In contrast, treatment with MER had no effect on the outcome of canine osteosarcoma.

Techniques now exist that allow an investigation of the nature of cell surface antigens and the immune response generated against them to a level and detail and understanding that did not seem possible 5 years ago. The future of the science of tumor immunology is therefore clearly very strong, and the data now emerging about the structure of tumor antigens, their coding sequences, and the genetic control processes are at the forefront of knowledge. Eventually, these advances will be translated into the clinical setting, but this will take time in both the veterinary and the human medical fields to have the impact that we believe is possible.

# TREATMENT AND PROGNOSIS OF CANINE MALIGNANT LYMPHOMA

DAVID M. VAIL
*Madison, Wisconsin*

Malignant lymphoma (lymphosarcoma) is the most common hematopoietic tumor encountered in the dog, and as such, is one of the most frequent neoplastic disorders treated by the veterinary clinician. While lymphoma can present in many forms, this article will restrict itself to a discussion of only those dogs with regional or generalized lymphadenopathy, which represent 85% or more of those cases presented to the veterinary practitioner. A discussion of the diagnosis and staging of canine lymphoma and attention to the solitary and extranodal forms of the disease is beyond the scope of this article and the reader is directed to recent textbook coverage of these aspects (Helfand and Vail, 1993).

Without therapy, most dogs with lymphoma succumb to their disease within 4 to 6 weeks following diagnosis. While the achievement of cures is still quite rare in the dog, lymphoma remains a very gratifying disease to treat, as durable (i.e., >6 months) remission rates through the use of chemotherapy approach 90%. Three primary challenges exist for the practitioner for improving the outcomes of dogs presenting with lymphoma: first and foremost, the discovery and employment of new, potentially safer, and innovative treatment protocols to increase the durability of initial remissions; second, the application of more successful and durable rescue protocols in dogs who have lost their initial remission and again show evidence of gross disease; and finally, the ability to prognosticate more accurately to a client as to the likelihood of achieving and maintaining long-term remission in their companion animal in order for them to make informed treatment decisions.

As the vast majority of dogs with lymphoma present with the generalized form of the disease, therapy naturally must be aimed systemically rather than locally. This usually involves systemic chemotherapy, generally applied in two distinct phases. First, induction and maintenance therapy are administered, so that the disease is initially managed with the goal of attaining a durable, complete remission (i.e., clinical absence of neoplastic disease). The second phase is termed "rescue" therapy, defined as an attempt to reestablish a complete remission upon the return of the tumor, or alternative therapy in those dogs that do not respond adequately to initial induction and maintenance therapy.

## INDUCTION AND MAINTENANCE THERAPY

Over the years, many successful chemotherapeutic protocols have been developed and presented in the veterinary literature; a review of the more successful protocols has recently been undertaken (Vail, 1993). Most protocols involve the use of multiple drugs used in alternating combinations and result in response rates of 80 to 90% for periods of 6 months or more. During the induction period, more aggressive drugs and shorter intervals between drug delivery are utilized to ensure a quick and complete attainment of remission. This induction period is typically followed by varying periods of "maintenance," where the intervals between drug treatments are slowly increased in length until they are ultimately discontinued after a period of time. The theoretical goal of maintenance therapy is to maintain the length (i.e., durability) of the complete remission. Some protocols utilize an initial induction period without subsequent maintenance, while in others, maintenance periods vary from 6 months to 3 years. Only one veterinary study (Hahn et al., 1992) attempted to answer the question of whether maintenance therapy is of benefit. Unfortunately, the reported first remission lengths in this study were unusually short and occurred prior to the maintenance phase of the protocol, thereby making conclusions about the efficacy of maintenance difficult. While controversy continues regarding the ideal length and aggressiveness of the maintenance period, extension of therapy beyond 2 years in a dog enjoying a complete remission probably has little if any justification in the author's opinion. Prospective randomized clinical trials will ultimately be necessary to confirm or refute the benefit of maintenance.

The induction and maintenance protocol used at the author's hospital is presented in Table 1. This regimen (UW-M protocol) has resulted in the longest remission durations and survival times reported to date for the chemotherapeutic management of lymphoma (Keller et al., 1993). Remission rates of 91% are achieved, with overall median remission duration and survival times of 36 and 51 weeks, respectively. If the patient presents with a World Health Organization clinical substage "a" (i.e., without systemic signs), as the majority of patients do, the overall median remission duration and survival times improve to 44 and 69 weeks, respectively. Therapy under this protocol was initially developed to continue for 3 years; however, the author now discontinues therapy after 2 years of uninterrupted complete remission.

Alternative protocols are made available if financial constraints or the short treatment intervals will affect the client's willingness to treat. Prednisone alone (1 to 2 mg/kg/ day PO) can inexpensively produce responses that may improve the quality of the animal's life for a short (i.e., 30-day) period. However, the client should be cautioned that, based on a number of reports, it may be more difficult to achieve durable future remission with aggressive chemotherapy in dogs with lymphoma initially treated with just prednisone. This probably reflects the development of multidrug resistance (MDR). Therefore, the initial, protracted use of prednisone alone is probably unwise and should be reserved only for those cases where clients object strongly to the use of more conventional aggressive induction. The addition of oral cyclophosphamide (50 mg/m$^2$ PO for 4 consecutive days each week) to the prednisone is also relatively inexpensive and may produce short (i.e., 1- to 2-month) periods of remission.

An alternate protocol that may fit a particular client's time constraints more effectively is that of single-agent doxorubicin (30 mg/m$^2$ IV every 3 weeks for five total treatments). Reported median remission lengths of 18 to 29 weeks (Postorino et al., 1989; Carter et al., 1987), while shorter than for the UW-M protocol, are still fairly durable. Advantages of this single-agent protocol make it attractive to the practitioner. Only one agent is given; therefore, if adverse effects occur they can easily be attributed to a single drug. Also, treatments are performed in-hospital, ensuring better compliance and

**Table 1.** UW-M Induction and Maintenance Protocol for Canine Lymphoma

| Induction Phase | | | | | | | | | |
|---|---|---|---|---|---|---|---|---|---|
| Drug | Week 1 | Week 2 | Week 3 | Week 4 | Week 5 | Week 6 | Week 7 | Week 8 | Week 9 |
| Vincristine 0.7 mg/m$^2$ IV | X | | X | | | X | | X | |
| L-Asparaginase 400 IU/kg IM | X | | | | | | | | |
| Prednisone° PO daily | X | X | X | X | | | | | |
| Cyclophosphamide 200 mg/m$^2$ IV | | X | | | | | X | | |
| Doxorubicin 30 mg/m$^2$ IV | | | | X | | | | | X |

| Maintenance Phase | |
|---|---|
| Drug | Frequency |
| Vincristine 0.7 mg/m$^2$ IV<br>Chlorambucil 1.4 mg/kg PO<br>Methotrexate[1] 0.8 mg/kg IV or doxorubicin 30 mg/m$^2$ IV | Beginning on week 11, alternate these three treatments every 2 weeks. After week 25, alternate these three treatments every 3 weeks. After week 49, alternate these three treatments every 4 weeks. All drugs are discontinued after 2 years if the dog is in complete remission. |

°Prednisone is used at a dosage of 2 mg/kg/day for week 1, then 1.5 mg/kg/day for week 2, then 1 mg/kg/day for week 3, then 0.5 mg/kg/day for week 4, then discontinued.
[1]Methotrexate and doxorubicin are alternated until the total cumulative dose of doxorubicin reaches 180 mg/m$^2$. At that point, only methotrexate is used.

eliminating the need to send potentially dangerous drugs home with the client. All treatment stops after 15 weeks, minimizing the possibility of drug-induced toxicities from long-term maintenance protocols. Finally, the protocol may be less costly in the long run, as shorter treatment and monitoring intervals are necessary.

## Alternatives or Adjuncts to Chemotherapy

### MONOCLONAL ANTIBODY THERAPY

A monoclonal antibody (Mab 231) has recently been marketed that recognizes some canine lymphoma cell lines (Rosales et al., 1988). Preliminary studies suggest this antibody prolongs remission duration in some dogs with lymphoma when used after attainment of a chemotherapy-induced complete remission. Such therapy would have the distinct advantage of eliminating the need for long-term maintenance chemotherapy. The results of these studies, while encouraging, warrant further controlled clinical trials to evaluate efficacy.

### RADIATION THERAPY WITH OR WITHOUT BONE MARROW TRANSPLANTATION

Staged whole-body radiation therapy alone for multicentric lymphoma holds little promise. Alternatively, total-body irradiation with bone marrow transplant has been used successfully for years in human medicine and has shown promise in the research setting for dogs with lymphoma.

## RESCUE THERAPY

Regardless of the induction protocol used, most dogs eventually relapse. At this point, further client education is in order. In general, reinduction can be achieved in the majority of relapsed dogs; however, the length of subsequent remissions tends to be short lived. In those cases induced and maintained on the UW-M protocol, the author initially attempts rescue by returning to the weekly induction phase as outlined in Table 1. If this fails, alternative rescue protocols are chosen.

A summary of rescue protocols advanced in the literature and at recent gatherings of veterinary oncologists is presented in Table 2 and have been recently reviewed (Vail, 1993). Actinomycin D is an inexpensive rescue agent that initially showed a great deal of promise. It has been used safely at dosages of 0.9 to 1.1 mg/m$^2$ intravenously once every 2 to 3 weeks; however, it has not lived up to expectations in the author's experience. No responses were noted in any of 25 dogs with relapsed lymphoma treated with actinomycin D in a study conducted at three institutions (Moore, Ogilvie, and Vail, 1993). Mitoxantrone (5.0 to 6.0 mg/m$^2$ IV, every 3 weeks) is more costly than actinomycin D; however, if a complete remission is achieved, the durability appears to be superior. Second remissions have also been achieved using a doxorubicin-dacarbazine combination (doxorubicin [30 mg/m$^2$] IV on day 1 and dacarbazine [200 mg/m$^2$] IV on days 1 through 5, cycled every 21 days), and with doxorubicin alone (30 mg/m$^2$ IV every 3 weeks). The latter is only utilized if doxorubicin was not part of the previous induction protocol. The MOPP protocol (methclorethamine, Oncovin [vincristine, Ely Lilly Co], procarbazine, and prednisone) has recently been evaluated as a rescue protocol in the dog. Each cycle of MOPP is 28 days, with dosage and timing as follows. On day 1, methclorethamine (6 mg/m$^2$) and vincristine (0.7 mg/m$^2$) are given intravenously. Procarbazine (100 mg/m$^2$) and prednisone (30 mg/m$^2$) are given orally on a daily basis from days 1 through 14. Significant myelosuppression can result from this protocol; nearly two thirds of dogs developed leukopenia, one third developed thrombocytopenia, and a significant number of deaths attributable to myelosuppression were reported.

Regardless of the rescue agent chosen, nearly 70% of dogs will respond, with approximately one third achieving a complete remission. However, the durability of the new remission is generally poor, with median lengths ranging from 2 to 5 months. Our inability to produce more durable second and third remissions is likely due to the emergence of drug-resistant clones of tumor cells. Significant gains in rescue therapy will probably have to await the development of techniques to overcome multiple drug resistance, a topic discussed in *CVT XI*, p 406.

***Table 2.*** *Summary of Responses for Canine Rescue Protocols*°

| Rescue Protocol | Number of Animals Treated | Overall Response (%) | Complete Response (%) | Median Response Duration (days) | Median Duration of Complete Response (days) |
|---|---|---|---|---|---|
| Actinomycin D | 12 | 83 | 42 | 42 | 63 |
| Actinomycin D | 25 | 0 | 0 | 0 | 0 |
| Mitoxantrone | 44 | 41 | 30 | Not reported | 127 |
| Doxorubicin[†] | 12 | 42 | 33 | 145 | 152 |
| Doxorubicin-dacarbazine | 15 | 53 | 33 | <42 | Not reported |
| MOPP | 17 | 88 | 35 | 28 | Not reported |

°Modified from Vail DM: Recent advances in chemotherapy for lymphoma of dogs and cats. Compend Cont Educ Pract Vet (Small Anim) 15:1034, 1993, with permission.
[†]No dogs in this protocol had previous exposure to doxorubicin.

**Table 3.** *Prognostic Factors Associated with Canine Lymphoma*

| Factor | Strongly Associated | Possibly Associated | Comments |
|---|---|---|---|
| WHO clinical stage | | X | Controversial; probably only stage V dogs with significant bone marrow involvement resulting in cytopenias have a poorer prognosis |
| WHO clinical substage | X | | WHO substage "b" (i.e., with systemic signs of illness) have significantly shorter remission and survival durations |
| Sex | | X | Some larger studies suggest females may enjoy a longer survival duration than male dogs |
| Immunophenotype | X | | T-cell phenotype carries a poorer prognosis than the B-cell phenotype |
| Hypercalcemia | | X | May not be an independent prognostic factor; probably confounded by negative prognosis associated with T-cell phenotype and WHO substage "b" |
| Histologic morphology | | X | NCI working formulation has been found in some studies to be prognostic |

Abbreviations: WHO = World Health Organization, NCI = National Cancer Institute.

## FACTORS AFFECTING PROGNOSIS FOR DOGS WITH LYMPHOMA

One of our most important goals involves education of our clients with respect to prognosis. In the case of lymphoma, the ability to comfortably predict success and durability of remissions in a given situation would be of benefit in helping our clients make informed treatment decisions. The literature on this subject is extensive and in many cases contradictory (Keller et al., 1993; Greenlee et al., 1990; MacEwen et al., 1987). In general, age, breed, and body weight appear to have little or no bearing on outcome. Table 3 lists factors that have been identified in the veterinary literature as having potential for predicting outcome for dogs with lymphoma.

On the horizon, less qualitative and more quantitative prognostic indices for lymphoma may shed light on this topic. We and others are presently determining the potential doubling time ($T_{pot}$) on tumor tissue from dogs with lymphoma prior to treatment. $T_{pot}$, simply put, is a mathematically derived measure of cell cycle proliferation that takes into account the fraction of tumor cells actively proliferating, and the speed with which the proliferation is progressing. It is hoped that information gained from this and other tumor cell kinetic parameters will be prognostic. The quantification of MDR may also result in prognostic information, and a number of laboratories are actively pursuing this end. Quantitative assays such as these may offer several potential benefits to the clinical oncologist of the future. They may prove to have clinical significance independent of that provided by most qualitative prognostic variables (i.e., tumor histology, clinical stage, or patient signalment characteristics), allowing a more accurate prediction of treatment response and long-term survival. They may also allow more individual tailoring of treatment protocols.

## References and Suggested Reading

Carter RF, Jarris CK, Withrow SJ, et al: Chemotherapy of canine lymphoma with histopathological correlation: Doxorubicin alone compared to COP as first treatment regimen. Am Anim Hosp Assoc 23:587, 1987.
*Results of a prospective trial of doxorubicin single agent chemotherapy for induction in dogs with lymphoma.*

Greenlee PG, Filippa DA, Quimby FW, et al: Lymphoma in dogs. Cancer 66:480, 1990.
*A morphologic, immunologic, and clinical study of 176 cases of canine lymphoma in an attempt to determine factors with prognostic significance.*

Hahn KA, Richardson RC, Teclaw RF, et al: Is maintenance chemotherapy appropriate for the management of canine malignant lymphoma? J Vet Intern Med 6:3, 1992.
*A retrospective study comparing two treatment protocols with an attempt to determine the appropriateness of maintenance therapy in managing dogs with lymphoma.*

Helfand SC and Vail DM: Hematopoietic system. In Slatter D (ed): *Textbook of Small Animal Surgery.* Philadelphia, WB Saunders Co, 1993, p 2111.
*A comprehensive review of the epidemiology, diagnosis, and staging of lymphoma in dogs and cats.*

Keller ET, MacEwen EG, Rosenthal RC, et al: Evaluation of prognostic factors and sequential combination chemotherapy with doxorubicin for canine lymphoma. J Vet Intern Med 7:289, 1993.
*Presentation of the UW-M chemotherapy protocol and results of multivariate analysis to determine prognostic factors for dogs with lymphoma.*

MacEwen EG, Hayes AA, Matus RE, and Kurzman I: Evaluation of some prognostic factors for advanced multicentric lymphosarcoma in the dog: 147 cases (1987–1981). J Am Vet Med Assoc 190:564, 1987.
*A retrospective study of a large number of cases of canine lymphoma in an attempt to determine factors with prognostic significance.*

Moore AS, Ogilvie GK, and Vail DM: Actinomycin D for reinduction of remission in resistant canine lymphoma. J Vet Intern Med (in press) 1995.
*A multi-institutional study of 25 dogs with relapsed lymphoma who failed reinduction of remission with actinomycin D.*

Postorino NC, Susaneck SJ, Withrow SJ, et al: Single agent therapy with adriamycin for canine lymphosarcoma. J Am Anim Hosp Assoc 25:221, 1989.
*Results of a prospective trial of doxorubicin single-agent chemotherapy for induction in dogs with lymphoma.*

Rosales C, Jeglum AK, Obrocka M, and Steplewski Z: Cytolytic activity of murine anti-dog lymphoma monoclonal antibodies with canine effector cells and complement. Cell Immunol 115:420, 1988.
*A study indicating that a monoclonal antibody has been developed that recognizes certain canine lymphoma cell lines and can result in their in vitro destruction.*

Vail DM: Recent advances in chemotherapy for lymphoma of dogs and cats. Compend Cont Educ Pract Vet (Small Anim) 15:1031, 1993.
*A referenced review of both induction and rescue protocols advanced in the veterinary literature for dogs and cats with lymphoma.*

# TREATMENT OF FELINE MALIGNANT LYMPHOMA

ANTONY S. MOORE
*and* ORLA M. MAHONY
*North Grafton, Massachusetts*

Cats have a higher incidence of lymphoma than do dogs or humans, and lymphoma accounts for 90% of all feline hematopoietic tumors. However, when compared with the veterinary literature regarding treatment of canine lymphoma, there is very little information about the therapy of feline lymphoma. This article reviews the current literature regarding staging and prognostic factors for feline lymphoma and compares established chemotherapeutic protocols with newer anticancer drugs and different treatment modalities.

The occurrence of feline lymphoma has been strongly associated with feline leukemia virus (FeLV) infection. The majority of cats with lymphoma are FeLV-positive (about 70%); however, both FeLV-positive and -negative lymphoma cells have tumor-specific feline oncornavirus-associated cell membrane antigen (FOCMA) on their membranes, indicating that FeLV may cause both types of feline lymphoma. The average age of occurrence is 3 years for FeLV-positive cats and 7 years for cats that are FeLV-negative. In addition, the occurrence of FeLV in cats with lymphoma varies with the form of the disease. For example, while approximately 80% of cats with multicentric or mediastinal disease test positive for FeLV, fewer than 25% of cats with alimentary lymphoma test positive. FeLV test status has been shown to have some prognostic significance for survival of cats with lymphoma. FeLV status does not, however, appear to influence response to therapy, and survival data may actually be influenced by other concurrent FeLV-related diseases such as anemia and immunosuppression rather than by the cancer itself.

Feline lymphoma has been classified according to two different schemes. The first relates to the primary anatomic site of the lymphoma, and the other relies on the extent of disease (Mooney et al., 1987) (Table 1). Both schemes are complimentary (i.e., an alimentary lymphoma can be further classified as stage 1 to 5, which may have some prognostic significance).

## PROGNOSTIC FACTORS FOR FELINE LYMPHOMA TREATED WITH CHEMOTHERAPY

### Age, Breed, and Sex

These factors have not been shown to affect response to therapy, remission duration, or survival time for cats with malignant lymphoma.

***Table 1.*** *Staging System*°

**Stage 1**
   A single tumor (extranodal) or single anatomic area (nodal)
   Includes primary intrathoracic tumors

**Stage 2**
   A single tumor (extranodal) with regional lymph node involvement
   Two or more nodal areas on the same side of the diaphragm
   Two single (extranodal) tumors with or without regional lymph node involvement on the same
      side of the diaphragm
   A resectable primary gastrointestinal tract tumor, usually in the ileocecal area, with or without
      involvement of associated mesenteric nodes only

**Stage 3**
   Two single tumors (extranodal) on opposite side of the diaphragm
   Two or more nodal areas above and below the diaphragm
   All extensive primary unresectable intra-abdominal disease
   All paraspinal or epidural tumors, regardless of other tumor site or sites

**Stage 4**
   Stage 1–3 with involvement of liver or spleen or both

**Stage 5**
   Stage 1–4 with initial involvement of CNS or bone marrow or both

°From Mooney S, Hayes A, Matus R, et al: Renal lymphoma in cats: 28 cases (1977–1984). J Am Vet Med Assoc 191:1473–1477, 1987, with permission.

## Anatomic Site

Cats with peripheral lymphadenopathy without other system involvement appear to have a good prognosis and have a median survival of 2 years with chemotherapy. To confuse the issue, it is possible that some of these cats reported in earlier studies may have had "atypical" feline lymphoid hyperplasia rather than lymphoma, thereby accounting for the high response rate. Cats with mediastinal lymphoma had the highest rate of complete remission (CR) in one study (89%), with median remission duration of 24 weeks (Cotter, 1983). By contrast, in another study, only 45% of 31 cats with mediastinal lymphoma attained CR, for a median remission of 8 weeks (Jeglum, Whereat, and Young, 1989).

## FeLV Status

As previously stated, FeLV status does not appear to influence response to therapy or remission duration; however, FeLV status has been related to median survival: 9.1 months for FeLV-negative compared to 4.2 months for FeLV-positive (Mooney et al., 1987).

## Stage of Disease

Stage of disease (see Table 1) was significantly related to response to therapy in one study. Complete response rates were as follows: stage 1 (93%), stage 2 (83%), stage 3 (48%), stage 4 (42%), and stage 5 (58%). Stage of disease also related to survival, with less advanced disease (stages 1 and 2) having median survival of 7.6 months, compared with 3.2 months for stage 3 and 2.6 months for stages 4 and 5 (Mooney et al., 1989).

## Stage and FeLV

In the same study reported above, there was no difference in survival times for cats in stages 3, 4, and 5 regardless of FeLV status; however, cats in stages 1 and 2 with a positive FeLV test had a median survival of 4 months compared to 17.5 months for FeLV-negative cats with stage 1 or 2 lymphoma. Similarly, for 28 cats with renal lymphoma, prognosis was best for cats with stage 2 lymphoma that were FeLV-negative.

## INFLUENCE OF CHEMOTHERAPY ON REMISSION AND SURVIVAL

### Response to Therapy

While cats that achieve CR live a median of 5 months (range = 2 to 42 months), those showing a partial remission (PR) seldom maintain this response for more than 4 to 6 weeks. In another study, cats responding to therapy with a CR had median survival of 7 months, compared with cats having a PR (2.5 months) or no response (1.5 months).

## Maintenance Therapy

Twenty-three cats with mediastinal lymphoma were treated with vincristine, cyclophosphamide, and prednisone. A CR was attained in 70% and these were randomized to receive no further treatment or anti-FOCMA serum. The median remission duration for untreated cats was 40 days and all cats relapsed by 84 days compared with a median of 150 days for cats that received maintenance chemotherapy (Cotter et al., 1980). Thus, maintenance therapy beyond the induction phase appears important for durable remissions and survival.

## FELINE LYMPHOMA OF SPECIFIC SITES

In one study, the multicentric form of feline lymphoma was the most commonly observed, with 43.6% of 454 cats having this form of disease (Hardy, 1978). Mediastinal (38.3%) and alimentary (15.2%) were the next most commonly seen sites for lymphoma. In another study of 150 cats with lymphoma, the alimentary form was more common (46.7% of cases) than were the mediastinal (25.4%) or multicentric (18.6%) forms (Meincke et al., 1972). However, the definition of the type of lymphoma varied between the two studies.

In a recent review of biopsy and cytology samples diagnosed as feline lymphoma at Tufts University Diagnostic Laboratory, alimentary lymphoma was the most commonly diagnosed, accounting for more than 30% of the samples. Another 15% of the diagnoses were made from the abdominal cavity; however, the primary site was not specified. Cats with lymphoma of miscellaneous sites was the second most common group.

The clinical features and response to therapy for feline lymphoma of various sites are reviewed below. While alimentary and renal lymphoma are reasonably commonly encountered, spinal lymphoma is relatively uncommon; however, spinal lymphoma is the most common spinal cord tumor in cats.

## Alimentary Lymphoma

This form of lymphoma is defined as involving the gastrointestinal tract itself or the mesenteric lymph nodes. It appears to be rarely associated with FeLV antigenemia, and affects older cats. Definitive diagnosis is often difficult, and some authors recommend laparotomy to obtain tissue samples. This approach results in a delay in instituting chemotherapy while wound healing takes place; however, surgery may permit resection of localized tumor masses, thereby reducing tumor burden or relieving obstructive disease. By contrast, ultrasonography was used to obtain a definitive diagnosis in 22 cats either by fine-needle aspiration or Tru-cut biopsy. This method was found to be safe and reliable, was less invasive, and allowed evaluation of other intra-abdominal structures (Penninck et al., 1994). The low morbidity associated with ultrasonography makes it the method of choice in many cats for obtaining a diagnosis of alimentary lymphoma.

The increased use of endoscopy to examine the upper gastrointestinal tract and the colon allows biopsies to be taken with very low morbidity. Disadvantages of this approach include the inability to examine abdominal organs and lymph nodes for accurate staging, and the possibility of obtaining superficial, nondiagnostic samples that reflect secondary inflammatory processes surrounding the primary lymphoma.

The clinical responses to chemotherapy in 29 cats with alimentary lymphoma were recently reviewed at our hospital. FeLV antigenemia was present in four of these cats, which represented an older population with no gender predilection. Presenting signs included vomiting (15 cats) and diarrhea (five cats); but interestingly, 13 cats showed only anorexia or weight loss as an indication of gastrointestinal disease. Most of the 29 cats had a palpable abdominal mass, and gastrointestinal or mesenteric lymph node involvement was confirmed by ultrasound endoscopy or exploratory surgery or both. Twenty-eight cats were treated with COP protocol (see later section), and one cat received prednisone and chlorambucil. Dependent on clinical response and owner compliance, additional drugs administered included doxorubicin, L-asparaginase, chlorambucil, idarubicin, and mitoxantrone. Response to therapy was determined by improvement in clinical signs, reduction in the size of a palpable mass, or by ultrasonography. The lymphoma primarily involved the intestinal tract (rather than stomach) in approximately 70% of the cats. Due to the difficulty in objectively assessing response, we evaluated survival times in these cats. Median survival with chemotherapy was 50 days, with a mean survival of 230 days (range = 2 to 2120). While most cats responded poorly to chemotherapy, a subpopulation of cats had long survival times, with five cats living longer than 1 year. Survival did not seem to be influenced by the extent of the lymphoma within the gastrointestinal tract, nor by the location or clinical stage. However, those cats that were treated with surgical resection and chemotherapy appeared to live longer than those treated with chemotherapy alone (Mahony et al., 1994).

Nutritional support seems to be extremely important in cats with alimentary lymphoma, as anorexia and vomiting are two of the major clinical signs associated with this form of the disease. It may be necessary to place a nasogastric tube, a pharyngostomy tube, or a gastrostomy or jejunostomy tube in order to maintain alimentation, and hence body weight, in a cat undergoing treatment for gastrointestinal lymphoma.

## Renal Lymphoma

Stage of disease appears to be an important prognostic variable in renal lymphoma. Cats with stage 2 disease (localized to the kidneys alone) have the best prognosis. Cats that are FeLV-positive have shorter survival times, as do cats that are severely azotemic. However, azotemia itself was not an absolute prognostic criterion in one study. Eleven of 28 cats died due to central nervous system (CNS) lymphoma, and cats with renal lymphoma were felt to have a high rate of relapse in the site. Seventeen cats (61%) had a CR with median remission duration of 127 days (range = 20 to 2542+). Treatment with cytosine arabinoside was thought to reduce the risk of CNS relapse (Mooney et al., 1987).

## Spinal Lymphoma

Twenty-one cats were diagnosed with spinal lymphoma, with the majority (81%) presented for hindlimb paresis. Ancillary tests that were considered helpful in making the diagnosis of lymphoma were: FeLV test that was positive in 16 of 19 cats, and bone marrow aspirates that contained lymphoblasts in 11 of 16 cats. Nine cats were treated with chemotherapy, and one with surgical decompression and chemotherapy. For six cats receiving vincristine, cyclophosphamide, and prednisone, three attained a CR, with a median duration of 14 weeks (range = 5 to 28). Three additional cats attained a PR (median = 6 weeks; range = 4 to 10). Three cats were given prednisone. Of those cats, one cat had no response, and two had a PR for 4 and 10 weeks, respectively. The cat treated with surgery and chemotherapy had a CR for 62 weeks, and on relapse, treatment with doxorubicin (30 mg/m$^2$ IV) resulted in a further CR (Spodnick et al., 1992).

## COMBINATION CHEMOTHERAPY PROTOCOLS

As with dogs treated for lymphoma, a combination protocol using vincristine, cyclophosphamide, and prednisone (COP protocol) still provides the basis of most chemotherapy protocols for feline lymphoma.

Thirty-eight cats with lymphoma were treated with vincristine (0.75 mg/m$^2$ IV weekly for 4 weeks, then every 3 weeks), cyclophosphamide (300 mg/m$^2$ PO every 3 weeks), and prednisone (2 mg/kg/day). Complete remission was attained in 79% of cats, with remission durations of 42 days to more than 42 months (median = 150 days). Remission rates varied with anatomic site, with the best being for mediastinal disease or peripheral lymphadenopathy. Cats had a lower complete response rate than did dogs treated with the same chemotherapy protocol, and were more likely to relapse early in therapy than dogs, but a higher percentage of cats remained in CR after 12 months (Cotter, 1983).

In another protocol, lymphoma was treated in 75 cats

with vincristine 0.025 mg/kg IV for weeks 1 and 3, cyclophosphamide 10 mg/kg IV for week 2, and methotrexate 0.8 mg/kg PO (IV if gastrointestinal lymphoma) for week 4. This 4-week cycle was continued. Of 62 cats with follow-up, 32 (52%) attained CR for a median of 112 days. Forty-four cats also received prednisone, and 36 also received L-asparaginase. Cats with mediastinal lymphoma did not fare as well in this study, with only 45% achieving CR for a median of 8 weeks (Jeglum, Whereat, and Young, 1989).

The same protocol as above (with the addition of L-asparaginase 400 IU/kg IP on week 1 of cycle 1) was given to 103 cats with lymphoma. Responses were classified as CR if there was a 75% or greater reduction in tumor volume. Sixty-four cats (62%) had a CR with median survival of 210 days (response durations not given). Thirty per cent of cats showing CR were alive at 1 year. Stage of disease was related to response and survival, while FeLV status was related to survival (but not response) (Mooney et al., 1989).

## Idarubicin

Idarubicin (4-demethoxydaunorubicin) is an anthracycline derivative that is more active *in vitro* than its parent compound, daunorubicin, and yet it is less cardiotoxic *in vivo*. In addition, the drug is active by both parenteral and oral routes of administration. In human cancer trials, orally administered idarubicin has been shown to have antileukemic activity as well as activity in non-Hodgkin's lymphoma. In human patients, gastrointestinal toxicity is more severe after oral administration, but myelosuppression is comparable to that following intravenous administration. Most cats will tolerate oral idarubicin at a dose of 2 mg/day for 2 consecutive days every 21 days. The dose-limiting toxicities are leukopenia and anorexia, as reported with other anthracycline derivatives such as doxorubicin.

Oral idarubicin treatment caused two cats with lymphoma to achieve clinical remission. In a study to further explore the utility of idarubicin for treatment of feline lymphoma, 18 cats that achieved remission following COP therapy were treated from week 4 with single-agent idarubicin. The median remission duration for these 18 cats was 162 days (range = 9 to 804 days), with two cats still alive and off treatment at 330 and 804 days. One cat died in remission at 220 days of unknown causes. Remission time was calculated from the first day of idarubicin therapy. With the addition of COP induction period of 21 days, the median remission duration was 183 days, which compares favorably with other protocols (Moore et al., 1994).

The ease and noninvasive nature of administration makes this drug an attractive option for the client; however, idarubicin still has limited availability. The remissions seen imply that other anthracyclines such as doxorubicin may be useful in the treatment of feline lymphoma. Unfortunately, there is little reported information as to the efficacy of doxorubicin in this disease.

## Current Recommendations

The COP protocol (Cotter, 1983) remains an effective, relatively nontoxic, and inexpensive method of treating feline lymphoma. The most commonly observed toxicities that follow vincristine administration are anorexia and vomiting, resulting in weight loss, during the first 4 weeks of therapy. If severe, these signs warrant a short delay in the next therapy (7 days or fewer) and a reduction in dose (to 0.65 mg/m² is usually sufficient). Supportive measures such as subcutaneous fluid administration and appetite stimulants such as cyproheptadine (4 to 8 mg b.i.d. to t.i.d. PO) assist in rapid recovery. Hemorrhagic cystitis following cyclophosphamide administration is rare in cats; however, myelosuppression often occurs 7 days after administration. A complete blood count should be performed 1 week after each cyclophosphamide dose and the dosage reduced by 25% if the segmental neutrophil count is below 1000 cells per microliter.

If the lymphoma proves resistant to COP, doxorubicin at a dose of 25 mg/m² IV every 3 weeks may be used as a "rescue" agent. Anorexia appears to be the most common toxicity to doxorubicin in cats, and myelosuppression results in a neutrophil nadir at 7 to 10 days. Supportive therapy should be provided as for vincristine toxicity, and a dose reduction to 20 mg/m² in the case of neutropenia is usually sufficient to prevent reoccurrence of doxorubicin toxicity. Doxorubicin-induced cardiomyopathy appears to be less common in cats than in dogs; however, some investigators consider doxorubicin to produce a cumulative renal toxicity. It is probably prudent to monitor renal function in cats receiving long-term doxorubicin therapy until this toxicity is further evaluated.

Other chemotherapeutic agents such as L-asparaginase and chlorambucil are rarely effective in treating feline lymphoma; however, toxicities are uncommon with these drugs, and their use may be warranted in refractory cases. L-Asparaginase, 10,000 IU/m² IM; and chlorambucil, 2 mg/cat every alternate day appear to be safe dosages in the cat.

At present, we are investigating the use of doxorubicin in feline lymphoma by randomizing cats that achieve remission with COP chemotherapy to receive either COP or doxorubicin maintenance chemotherapy for 6 months. Preliminary results show that median remission for cats that continue to receive COP maintenance is 9 weeks, while more than half the cats that received doxorubicin maintenance are alive more than 30 weeks after starting chemotherapy. While most protocols suggest that chemotherapy should continue for at least 12 months, there have not been any investigations of shorter term chemotherapy for maintaining long-term clinical remission.

## Radiation Therapy

While radiation therapy is usually not considered as a primary treatment modality for feline lymphoma due to the systemic nature of the disease, the high level of radiation sensitivity of malignant lymphocytes makes palliative therapy for localized or extranodal lymphoma an attractive option either alone or in combination with systemic chemotherapy.

Ten cats with localized lymphoma that involved the nasal cavity (three cats); retrobulbar area (three cats); and mediastinum, subcutaneous tissue, maxilla, and mandible (one each) were treated with radiation therapy. Four cats also received chemotherapy. Overall median remission time for the eight cats that achieved CR was 114 weeks (range = 4 to 227 weeks). Total radiation dose varied from 6 to 40 Gy and did not appear to predict duration of response. Three cats had recurrence of lymphoma at sites other than the irradiated area, indicating that a combination of radiation and chemotherapy may be useful in delaying or preventing progression of localized lymphoma (Elmslie et al., 1991).

Radiation therapy causes a rapid reduction in tumor burden, and may also be considered for cats that have life-threatening obstructive or space-occupying lymphoma; for example, large mediastinal masses, spinal lymphoma, or pharyngeal/laryngeal disease. The relatively low doses needed to achieve a response mean that toxicities due to radiation therapy are unlikely. The contribution to remission duration is uncertain, however, and studies defining the role of palliative adjunctive radiation therapy have yet to be published.

Major advances have been made in the treatment of canine lymphoma in the last 10 years, with the evaluation of newer agents such as doxorubicin and L-asparaginase and the creation of multidrug chemotherapy protocols. In contrast, the treatment of feline lymphoma has received scant attention; however, it remains a relatively responsive tumor type. As newer drugs and protocols are evaluated, improved remission and survival times for cats with lymphoma can be expected.

## References and Suggested Reading

Cotter S: Treatment of lymphoma and leukemia with cyclophosphamide, vincristine and prednisone: II. Treatment of cats. J Am Anim Hosp Assoc 19: 166, 1983.
*Results of treatment with COP in 38 cats with lymphoma of various anatomic sites.*
Cotter S, Essex M, McLane M, et al: Chemotherapy and passive immunotherapy in naturally occurring feline mediastinal lymphoma. In Feline Leukemia Virus. Elsevier North Holland Inc, 1980, p 219.
*Results of a randomized trial comparing anti-FOCMA antibody immunotherapy with no maintenance therapy in cats with mediastinal lymphoma.*
Elmslie R, Ogilvie G, Gillette E, et al: Radiotherapy with and without chemotherapy for localized lymphoma in 10 cats. Vet Radiol 32:277, 1991.
Hardy W, Jr: Epidemiology of primary neoplasms of lymphoid tissues in animals. In: The Immunopathology of Lymphoreticular Neoplasms. Plenus Publishing, 1978, p 129.
Jeglum K, Whereat A, and Young K: Chemotherapy of lymphoma in 75 cats. J Am Vet Med Assoc 190:696, 1989.
*Results of combination chemotherapy for feline lymphoma.*
Mahony O, Moore A, Cotter S, et al: Chemotherapy for alimentary lymphoma in cats. J Am Vet Med Assoc (in press) 1995.
*Results of combination chemotherapy for feline alimentary lymphoma.*
Meincke J, Hobbie W, Jr, Hardy W, Jr: Lymphoreticular malignancies in the cat: clinical findings. J Am Vet Med Assoc 160:1093, 1972.
Mooney S, Hayes A, MacEwen E, et al: Treatment and prognostic factors in lymphoma in cats: 103 cases (1977–1981). J Am Vet Med Assoc 194:696, 1989.
*Results in combination chemotherapy for feline lymphoma and prognostic significance of a staging protocol.*
Mooney S, Hayes A, Matus R, et al: Renal lymphoma in cats: 28 cases (1977–1984). J Am Vet Med Assoc 191: 1473–1477, 1987.
*Results of combination chemotherapy for feline renal lymphoma.*
Moore A, Ruslander D, L'Heureux D, et al: Toxicity and efficacy of oral idarubicin administration to cats with neoplasia. J Am Vet Med Assoc (in press).
*Evaluation of idarubicin for treatment of various feline tumors, and for utility in the maintenance therapy of feline lymphoma.*
Penninck D, Moore A, Tidwell A, et al: Ultrasonography of alimentary lymphosarcoma in the cat. Vet Radiol (in press).
*Evaluation of ultrasonographic features of feline gastrointestinal lymphoma and of the utility of ultrasound in obtaining a definitive diagnosis.*
Spodnick G, Berg J Moore F, et al: Spinal lymphoma in cats: 21 cases (1976–1989). J Am Vet Med Assoc 200:373, 1992.
*A review of clinical features of feline spinal lymphoma and the clinical response to therapy.*

# NONSURGICAL MANAGEMENT OF SOFT TISSUE SARCOMAS

ALAN S. HAMMER
*Louisville, Kentucky*

*and* C. GUILLERMO COUTO
*Columbus, Ohio*

Soft tissue sarcomas are common in small animals, where they comprise 7 to 16% of all tumors. The incidence of soft tissue sarcomas is 36/100,000 in the dog and 17/100,000 in the cat; boxer dogs are at high risk for developing soft tissue sarcomas (Dorn, 1976). The most common soft tissue sarcomas in dogs are fibrosarcoma, hemangiosarcoma, and hemangiopericytoma; fibrosarcomas are the most common soft tissue sarcomas in cats.

While surgery remains the mainstay of therapy in animals with soft tissue sarcomas (see "Definitive Surgical Treatment for Cancer," this volume, p 462), there are four main indications for adjuvant therapy, including: (1) patients with nonresectable tumors or with incompletely resected tumors in which further surgery cannot be performed; (2) patients with metastatic disease; (3) patients with highly metastatic tumors but no clinical evidence of metastases; and (4) as neoadjuvant treatment in an attempt to decrease the surgical morbidity or to increase the probability of successful surgical excision. Local recurrence of soft tissue sarcomas may result in death or lead to euthanasia. In other patients, although local control may be easily accomplished (e.g., splenectomy for splenic hemangiosarcoma), early metastases may lead to death or euthanasia shortly after diagnosis.

When approaching a patient with a soft tissue sarcoma, it is important to assess several things. First, the patient should be evaluated to ascertain the location of the tumor and whether nearby critical structures are involved; this will determine if the tumor is resectable or not, and whether there is clinical evidence of metastases. In addition to physical examination, various imaging techniques such as radiographs, ultrasound, computed tomography (CT), or magnetic resonance imaging (MRI) of the affected area may be necessary to determine the extent of local invasiveness and to dictate the most appropriate surgical approach. Thoracic radiographs and abdominal ultrasound, CT, or MRI should also be used as deemed appropriate to adequately evaluate the patient for metastatic disease.

Second, the histopathologic characteristics of the tumor should be assessed. This may be predictive of the metastatic rate, and may aid in deciding whether adjuvant therapy is needed. The degree of differentiation, lymphatic or vascular invasion, and mitotic index are some of the histopathologic features that should be evaluated in every biopsy specimen. For example, soft tissue sarcomas with a low mitotic index are less aggressive and the survival times with surgery alone are usually greater than 1 year (Bostock and Dye, 1980; Bostock and Dye, 1979). Table 1 divides the common soft tissue sarcomas into low- and high-metastatic potential categories. Tumors with a metastatic rate of 10% or less on initial presentation are considered to have a low metastatic potential, whereas tumors with a metastatic rate greater than 25% are considered to be highly

**Table 1.** *Metastatic Potential of Soft Tissue Sarcomas in Dogs and Cats*

**Low Metastatic Potential**
Fibrosarcoma
Hemangiopericytoma
Myxosarcoma
Nerve sheath tumors

**High Metastatic Potential**
Hemangiosarcoma
Leiomyosarcoma
Liposarcoma
Lymphangiosarcoma
Malignant fibrous histiocytoma
Malignant mesenchymoma
Rhabdomyosarcoma
Synovial cell sarcoma
Undifferentiated sarcoma

metastatic. It is the authors' opinion that those tumors composed of well-differentiated spindle cells (e.g., fibrosarcoma, nerve sheath tumors, hemangiopericytoma, and leiomyosarcoma) have a different biologic behavior and response to chemotherapy. Consequently, these tumor types are treated with different chemotherapy protocols than undifferentiated sarcomas and hemangiosarcomas. In addition to resectability and biologic behavior, other factors that may influence whether adjuvant therapy is used include financial concerns, the owner's concerns about side effects of treatment, and concurrent illnesses.

Therapeutic modalities available for dogs and cats with soft tissue sarcomas include radiotherapy, hyperthermia, chemotherapy, photodynamic therapy, immunotherapy, and combinations thereof. While chemotherapy and immunotherapy may be used to aid in local control, they are more frequently used in patients with clinical or subclinical metastatic disease. Surgery, radiotherapy, hyperthermia, and photodynamic therapy are typically used to provide local tumor control. If a tumor has not disseminated beyond a local region, a cure may be possible with appropriate local therapy. However, a cure is not likely to be achieved in a patient with a highly metastatic tumor, or when metastases have already occurred. In these instances, chemotherapy or immunotherapy may palliate the disease and provide good quality, long-term remissions.

Surgery, discussed in the article "Definitive Surgical Treatment of Cancer" (this volume, p 462), is the modality most likely to effect a cure, and is the most effective method to cytoreduce a tumor prior to employing other treatment means. Surgical cytoreduction results in an increase in the growth fraction, which may improve the efficacy of adjuvant chemotherapy or radiotherapy. Additionally, surgical cytoreduction improves the blood supply and, consequently, the delivery of oxygen and antineoplastic agents to the tumor; the ratio of immune effector cells to target cancer cells also increases after surgery. Therefore, tumor cells may be more susceptible, after surgical cytoreduction, to the effects of chemotherapy, radiotherapy, or immunotherapy.

Traditionally, soft tissue sarcomas have been considered relatively resistant to radiation therapy; however, recent evidence suggests that this modality may be beneficial in some patients. The local control rate in dogs with hemangiopericytoma was 50%, and in dogs with fibrosarcomas it was 21% (McChesney et al., 1989). In contrast, when radiotherapy was used postoperatively in dogs with incompletely resected soft tissue sarcomas (i.e., fibrosarcoma, hemangiopericytoma, nerve sheath tumor, and myxofibrosarcoma), the local control rate at 3 years was greater than 80% (Mauldin, Meleo, and Burk, 1993).

The combination of radiotherapy and hyperthermia appears to be synergistic, with reported response rates of 63 to 90% (Gillette, 1986; Prescott and Dewhirst, 1992). However, hyperthermia alone does not appear to provide adequate local tumor control. Further discussion of hyperthermia can be found in *CVT XI*, p 418.

Radiotherapy can also be combined with chemotherapy. The drugs most commonly used are doxorubicin and cisplatin, since they have both direct antineoplastic effects and radiosensitizing properties. While these combinations are promising, only anecdotal information is available at this time.

Photodynamic therapy is another form of local tumor control. (For a review of the principles of photodynamic therapy, see "Lasers in Veterinary Oncology" in *CVT XI*, p 414.) This therapy is limited by the depth of penetration of the light, the uniformity of distribution of the photosensitizing compound, and the damage to the surrounding tissues. Large tumors are difficult to treat, though preliminary reports suggest that marked tumor kill is possible, particularly if interstitial fibers are used. Prolonged complete remissions have been reported in 10 of 14 dogs with soft tissue sarcomas using this treatment modality (Beck, 1992). Postoperative photodynamic therapy should increase the response rate due to decreased tumor burden and improved light penetration.

Chemotherapeutic agents considered to have activity against soft tissue sarcomas in dogs and cats include doxorubicin, cyclophosphamide, dacarbazine, vincristine, methotrexate, cisplatin, actinomycin D, and mitoxantrone. Overall, doxorubicin is considered to have the broadest spectrum of activity. In a trial of single-agent doxorubicin, the overall response rate for dogs with soft tissue sarcomas was 22% (Ogilvie et al., 1989). Responding tumor types included fibrosarcoma, hemangiosarcoma, synovial cell sarcoma, undifferentiated sarcoma, liposarcoma, and neurofibrosarcoma. It should be noted that the response rate in tumors considered to have low metastatic potential (e.g., fibrosarcoma, hemangiopericytoma, myxosarcoma, and neurofibrosarcoma) was only 10%. It has been reported that aggressive, poorly differentiated sarcomas in people have a better response rate to doxorubicin chemotherapy than well-differentiated sarcomas (van Haelst-Pisani et al., 1991).

The efficacy of single-agent mitoxantrone in dogs with soft tissue sarcomas is similar to that of doxorubicin (i.e., 21% response) (Ogilvie et al., 1991). In contrast to doxorubicin, the response rate in dogs with tumors of low metastatic potential was 36%; there were no responses to mitoxantrone in dogs with hemangiosarcoma or undifferentiated sarcomas. In a trial of mitoxantrone in seven cats with soft tissue sarcomas, responses were observed in a cat with fibrosarcoma and a cat with rhabdomyosarcoma (Ogilvie et al., 1993).

Combination chemotherapy has several advantages over single agent chemotherapy, and probably represents a better approach to the patient with a soft tissue sarcoma. The advantages include "attacking" the tumor cells from several different biochemical approaches, possible synergistic activity between the agents, and decreasing toxicity by choosing agents that lack overlapping toxicities. A combination of vincristine, methotrexate, cyclophosphamide (VMC), and immuno-

therapy resulted in complete or partial responses in five of six cats with fibrosarcoma (Brown et al., 1978). However, the same protocol did not significantly prolong survival times in dogs with hemangiosarcoma (Brown, Patnaik, and MacEwen, 1985). A second protocol reported in cats with sarcomas is a combination of doxorubicin and cyclophosphamide (AC) (Mauldin et al., 1988). Although the number and type of soft tissue sarcomas in this study was limited, two of three cats with fibrosarcoma had complete or partial responses.

A combination of vincristine, doxorubicin, and cyclophosphamide (VAC) has resulted in a 73% response rate in dogs with soft tissue sarcomas (Couto and Helfand, 1986). Similar to the single-agent doxorubicin trial, the response rate in tumors with low metastatic potential was lower than in those with high metastatic potential.

Another chemotherapy protocol used to treat dogs with soft tissue sarcomas is a combination of doxorubicin and dacarbazine (ADIC). This protocol is efficacious in dogs with canine lymphoma, and we consider it effective in dogs with tumors composed of spindle cells (e.g., fibrosarcoma, nerve sheath tumors, hemangiopericytoma, and leiomyosarcoma). Table 2 lists the doses and schedules for the chemotherapeutic protocols discussed above.

Immunotherapy for soft tissue sarcomas has received little attention. A mixed bacterial vaccine (*Streptococcus pyogenes* and *Serratia spp.*) was used in cats with fibrosarcoma and in dogs with hemangiosarcoma, in combination with surgery and VMC chemotherapy (Brown et al., 1978; Brown, Patnaik, and MacEwen, 1985). The mechanism of action of the mixed bacterial vaccine may be macrophage activation or induction of release of various cytokines such as interleukin-1, interleukin-6, interferon, or tumor necrosis factor. A more defined compound is liposome-encapsulated muramyl tripeptide phosphotidylethanol (L-MTP-PE), a macrophage-activating agent. This compound has had efficacy in dogs with osteosarcoma and is currently being evaluated in dogs with hemangiosarcoma receiving doxorubicin and cyclophosphamide chemotherapy (MacEwen et al., 1989). Finally, another purported macrophage activator, acemannan, is commercially available, but randomized clinical trials to confirm its efficacy have not been performed.

Table 3 lists the current recommendations for traditional adjuvant therapy of soft tissue sarcomas in dogs and cats. Photodynamic therapy and immunotherapy should be considered in dogs and cats that have failed traditional modalities, or in those for which traditional therapies are deemed inappropriate. Adjuvant chemotherapy is particularly indicated for aggressive or undifferentiated sarcomas or for hemangiosarcomas, and should consist of a doxorubicin-containing protocol such as VAC. Tumors that are less responsive to chemotherapy (e.g., hemangiopericytoma and nerve sheath tumors) should be treated with adjuvant radiotherapy with or without hyperthermia. Future treatment for soft tissue sarcoma may involve combinations of surgery, radiotherapy, hyperthermia, chemotherapy, and

***Table 2.*** *Chemotherapy Protocols for Dogs and Cats with Soft Tissue Sarcomas*

| Protocol | Dose | Route | Schedule |
|----------|------|-------|----------|
| Doxorubicin | 30 mg/m$^2$ (dogs) | IV | Every 3 wk |
| | 20–25 mg/m$^2$ (cats) | IV | Every 3–4 wk |
| | Pretreat dogs with diphenhydramine 2.2 mg/kg; administer doxorubicin over 30 min | | |
| Mitoxantrone | 5 mg/m$^2$ (dogs) | IV | Every 3 wk |
| | 3–6 mg/m$^2$ (cats) | IV | Every 3 wk |
| | May be more efficacious if given as a 4-hr infusion | | |
| Cisplatin | 50–70 mg/m$^2$ | IV | Every 3–4 wk |
| | DO NOT USE IN CATS! | | |
| | Administer with saline diuresis as described in Ogilvie[18] | | |
| VMC | Vincristine 0.0125 mg/kg | IV | Weekly |
| | Methotrexate 0.3–0.5 mg/kg | IV | Weekly |
| | Cyclophosphamide 1 mg/kg | PO | Daily to every other day |
| VAC (dogs) | Vincristine 0.75 mg/m$^2$ | IV | Days 8 and 15 |
| | Doxorubicin 30 mg/m$^2$ | IV | Day 1 |
| | Cyclophosphamide 100 mg/m$^2$ | IV | Day 1 |
| | Administer doxorubicin as described above | | |
| | Repeat cycle on day 22 and give 3–5 cycles | | |
| | Administer trimethoprim-sulfadiazine 15 mg/kg PO b.i.d. while on chemotherapy | | |
| AC (cats) | Doxorubicin 20–25 mg/m$^2$ | IV | Day 1 |
| | Cyclophosphamide 50 mg/m$^2$ | PO | Days 3, 4, 5, 6 |
| | Repeat cycle every 21 days | | |
| | Give a total of 3–5 cycles | | |
| ADIC | Doxorubicin 30 mg/m$^2$ | IV | Day 1 |
| | Dacarbazine 800–1000 mg/m$^2$ | IV | Day 1 |
| | DO NOT USE IN CATS! | | |
| | Give dacarbazine over 8 hr in D5W | | |
| | Administer doxorubicin as described above | | |
| | Repeat cycle every 3 wk | | |
| | Give a total of 3–5 cycles | | |
| | Administer trimethoprim-sulfadiazine 15 mg/kg PO b.i.d. while on chemotherapy | | |

***Table 3.*** *Current Adjuvant Treatment Recommendations for Dogs and Cats with Soft Tissue Sarcomas*

| Tumor Type | Treatment Options |
|------------|-------------------|
| Fibrosarcoma | XRT+/-HT; ADIC; VMC; AC |
| Hemangiopericytoma | XRT+/-HT |
| Leiomyosarcoma | ADIC |
| Neurofibrosarcoma | XRT+/-HT; ADIC |
| Hemangiosarcoma | VAC |
| Liposarcoma | VAC |
| Malignant fibrous histiocytoma | VAC |
| Synovial cell sarcoma | VAC, AC |
| Undifferentiated sarcoma | VAC; ADIC |

Abbreviations: XRT = radiotherapy; HT = hyperthermia; ADIC = doxorubicin, dacarbazine; VAC = vincristine, doxorubicin, cyclophosphamide; VMC = vincristine, methotrexate, cyclophosphamide; AC = doxorubicin, cyclophosphamide.

immunotherapy and, it is hoped, will result in prolonged survival times.

### References and Suggested Reading

Beck ER. Lasers in veterinary oncology. *In* Kirk RW and Bonagura JD (eds): *Current Veterinary Therapy XI.* Philadelphia, WB Saunders Co, 1992, p 414.

Bostock DE and Dye MT: Prognosis after surgical excision of canine fibrous connective tissue sarcomas. Vet Pathol 17:581, 1980.
Bostock DE and Dye MT: Prognosis after surgical excision of fibrosarcomas in cats. J Am Vet Med Assoc 175:727, 1979.
Brown NO, Patnaik AK, and MacEwen EG: Canine hemangiosarcoma: Retrospective analysis of 104 cases. J Am Vet Med Assoc 186:56, 1985.
Brown NO, Patnaik AK, Mooney S, Hayes A, Harvey HJ, and MacEwen EG: Soft tissue sarcomas in the cat. J Am Vet Med Assoc 173:744, 1978.
Couto CG and Helfand SC: VAC chemotherapy for metastatic and nonresectable soft tissue tumors in the dog (abstr). *Proc 6th Ann Conf Vet Cancer Society*, West Lafayette, 1986.

Dorn CR: Epidemiology of canine and feline tumors. J Am Anim Hosp Assoc 12:307, 1976.

Gillette EL: Cancer therapy: Radiation and hyperthermia. Semin Vet Med Surg 1:21, 1986.

MacEwen EG, Kurzman ID, Rosenthal RC, et al: Therapy for osteosarcoma in dogs with intravenous injection of liposome-encapsulated muramyl tripeptide. J Natl Cancer Inst 81:935, 1989.

Mauldin GN, Matus RE, Patnaik AK, Bond BR, and Mooney SC: Efficacy and toxicity of doxorubicin and cyclophosphamide used in the treatment of selected malignant tumors in 23 cats. J Vet Intern Med 2:60, 1988.

Mauldin GN, Meleo KA, and Burk RL: Radiation therapy for the treatment of incompletely resected soft tissue sarcomas in dogs: 21 cases. *Proc 13th Ann Conf Vet Cancer Society*, Columbus, OH, 1993, p 111.

McChesney SL, Withrow SJ, Gillette EL, Powers BE, and Dewhirst MW: Radiotherapy of soft tissue sarcomas in dogs. J Am Vet Med Assoc 194:60, 1989.

Ogilvie GK, Krawiec DR, Gelberg HB, et al: Evaluation of a short-term saline diuresis protocol for the administration of cisplatin. Am J Vet Res 49:1076, 1988.

Ogilvie GK, Moore AS, Obradovich JE, et al: Toxicoses and efficacy associated with administration of mitoxantrone to cats with malignant tumors. J Am Vet Med Assoc 202:1839, 1993.

Ogilvie GK, Obradovich JE, Elmslie RE, et al: Efficacy of mitoxantrone against various neoplasms in dogs. J Am Vet Med Assoc 198:1618, 1991.

Ogilvie GK, Reynolds HA, Richardson RC, et al: Phase II evaluation of doxorubicin for treatment of various canine neoplasms. J Am Vet Med Assoc 195:1580, 1989.

Prescott DM and Dewhirst MW: Hyperthermia: Update and current indications. *In* Kirk RW and Bonagura JD (eds): *Current Veterinary Therapy XI.* Philadelphia, WB Saunders Co, 1992, pp 418–423.

van Haelst-Pisani C, Buckner JC, Reiman HM, Schaid DJ, Edmonson JH, and Hahn RG. Does histologic grade in soft tissue sarcoma influence response rate to systemic chemotherapy? Cancer 68:2354, 1991.

# TREATMENT OF CANINE OSTEOSARCOMA

RODNEY C. STRAW
*and* STEPHEN J. WITHROW
*Fort Collins, Colorado*

The most common primary bone tumor of dogs is osteosarcoma, which is also called osteogenic sarcoma. Osteosarcoma is a high-grade malignancy that develops most commonly in the medullary canal, usually in the metaphyses of long bones. Primary tumors that arise in the skull and axial skeleton account for about 25% of cases of osteosarcoma and very rarely these tumors occur primarily in soft tissue sites such as the mammary tissue, spleen, liver, and bowel. There are forms of osteosarcoma that develop from cortical or periosteal surfaces of bone (periosteal, parosteal, or juxtacortical osteosarcoma), but these forms are also rare. The purpose of this article is to share our clinical and research experience with traditional high-grade osteosarcoma. We currently have detailed records of over 500 treated dogs with this tumor. We have drawn from this resource and the literature to produce this overview of the management of canine osteosarcoma.

## DIAGNOSIS

### Signalment and History

Osteosarcoma is most common in giant and large breeds, with males affected slightly more frequently than females; the average age is 7 years (range = 6 months to old age). The most common site is the metaphysis of the distal radius followed by the proximal metaphysis of the humerus and either metaphyses of the femur and tibia. The bones adjacent to the elbow are almost never primary sites for osteosarcoma. Dogs present because of a gradually worsening lameness and the development of a mass at the primary site. However, acute lameness due to a pathologic fracture is not unusual.

### Radiography

High-detail radiographs of craniocaudal and lateral projections usually demonstrate loss of cortical continuity, since the tumor causes lysis and destruction of bone, leading to disruption of periosteum, and evoking pain and lameness. The tumors are therefore outside the medullary canal by the time the dog presents to a veterinarian. Classic radiographic hallmarks for neoplastic disease of bone include loss of trabecular pattern of the metaphysis, cortical lysis, periosteal new bone (Codman's triangle), palisading new bone in the soft tissue (sunburst), soft tissue swelling and indistinct transitional zone (no well-defined sclerotic margin), and pathologic fracture and lesions that do not extend directly across joints. Thoracic radiographs are important for staging, and both lateral projections as well as a dorsoventral or ventrodorsal view should be carefully evaluated for signs of metastasis. For dogs with osteosarcoma, the probability of detecting pulmonary metastasis at presentation is less than 10%. Radiographically detectable nodules need to be 0.5 to 1.0 cm in diameter before they become noticeable by standard thoracic radiography. Radiography is also useful for identifying metastasis in other sites such as bone. Less than 10% of dogs will present with detectable bone metastases or synchronous primary tumors. Nuclear scintigraphy with $^{99m}$Tc methylene diphosphate (MDP) is a more sensitive test for detecting lesions in bone where there is lysis or active bone turnover. Even with this more sensitive technique, less than 10% of dogs will have areas of increased isotope uptake consistent with neoplasia in areas of bone other than the primary site at presentation.

## DIFFERENTIAL DIAGNOSIS

Dogs do not always present with lesions of "textbook" appearance and there are other diseases that must be considered. The major rule-outs include other primary bone tumors, metastatic tumors to bone, bacterial osteomyelitis, and systemic mycoses. Multiple myeloma is a malignant disease of plasma cells, and purely lytic bone lesions can occur with this systemic disease. The lesions, however, are usually multiple and appear as "punched-out" areas of lysis with very little or no proliferative bone component. Similarly, lymphoma of bone causes a purely lytic pattern, but this is a very rare disorder. Other less likely possibilities include benign bone tumors, bone cysts, and degenerative or reparative lesions.

Other primary bone tumors such as chondrosarcoma, hemangiosarcoma, and fibrosarcoma account for 5 to 10% of all primary bone tumor diagnoses. These lesions may occur in smaller dogs as well, and may arise in unusual sites such as the distal humeral metaphysis. These tumors can only be definitively differentiated from osteosarcoma by evaluation of large tissue specimens. Beware of making a definitive diagnosis of chondrosarcoma from small volumes of biopsy tissue. Many osteosarcomas are heterogeneous in their histologic appearance, and tissue taken from one location of the tumor may contain largely a chondroid matrix (chondrosarcoma), whereas another area contains tumor osteoid. Osteosarcomas have been subclassified histologically as osteoblastic, chondroblastic, fibroblastic, osteoclastic, poorly differentiated, and telangiectatic. Subgroups do not seem to have any prognostic significance; however, they are significant from a diagnostic standpoint because chondroblastic, fibroblastic, and telangiectatic subgroups of osteosarcoma may easily be confused with chondrosarcoma, fibrosarcoma, and hemangiosarcoma, respectively. The key to histologic diagnosis of osteosarcoma is the presence of tumor osteoid.

Cancer metastasis to bone should be suspected where the lesion occurs in a diaphyseal location. Metastasis to bone requires hematogenous spread, and lesions often establish adjacent to nutrient foramina at the ends of the diaphyses or in bodies of vertebrae, especially caudal lumbar sites. There is usually a primary tumor detectable elsewhere such as in the mammary glands, prostate, bladder, or other intra-abdominal organ, or there is a history of a malignant tumor removed from such sites within the past year or so.

Osteomyelitis of bacterial etiology in mature dogs requires pathogenic bacteria to gain access directly to the bone and, except in puppies, is usually not a sequel to septicemia or bacteremia. Therefore, there is usually a history of recent surgery or penetrating wound such as gunshot injury, surgery, or a bite. These lesions often drain purulent material, and sequestra are frequently seen radiographically. Fever or changes in the leukogram consistent with infection do not always accompany this diagnosis.

Coccidioidomycosis and blastomycosis are systemic mycoses where bone lesions can occur. Proliferative new bone is the predominant radiographic appearance; however, lysis does occur and many of these lesions look indistinguishable from osteosarcoma. Dogs residing in endemic areas or those with a history of travel to such areas should be considered as candidates for these fungal diseases. There may be intrathoracic lesions (hilar lymphadenopathy or peribronchial lesions), and multiple bone sites may be affected. However, synchronous primary osteosarcoma or metastatic osteosarcoma to bone are also rule-outs for dogs with more than one osteolytic, osteoproliferative lesion. Serology and cytology of draining lesions can be useful to help diagnose fungal osteomyelitis, but the definitive diagnosis relies on histologic interpretation of biopsy tissue.

### Bone Biopsy

A definitive diagnosis lies in correct procurement and interpretation of tissue for histopathology. There are several techniques for obtaining tissue from bone for histopathology; however, there are some pitfalls. Correct interpretation of histopathology requires an experienced pathologist with a good working knowledge of bone pathology. This is especially true where small tissue samples are to be examined. The clinician must be aware that the histologic diagnosis must fit the clinical picture. If the pathologist's report concludes the presence of reactive bone, this must not be accepted as the diagnosis, and does not rule out the presence of a pathologic process. Such a report merely indicates that more tissue must be examined. A lytic and proliferative bone lesion with the above-stated differential diagnoses cannot be merely "reactive." The problem often does not lie in the interpretation of the slide but rather in the sampling. With this in mind, the clinician should consider whether preoperative biopsy is indicated. This is best decided by asking if the result of such a biopsy would alter the treatment given or the owner's willingness to treat. In a middle-aged, giant-breed dog with a lytic and proliferative lesion of the proximal metaphysis of the humerus; with the radiographic characteristics of osteosarcoma where there is no history of travel to an area endemic for coccidioidomycosis or blastomycosis, no history of recent surgery or penetrating wound to the area; and where there are no known primary neoplastic lesions either currently or in the recent past, then it would be possible to consider excision of the bone lesion (either by amputation or limb sparing) without a preoperative biopsy. In other circumstances, where there is considerable doubt about the diagnosis and the owner has unwillingness to treat given certain diagnostic outcomes, then preoperative biopsy becomes important. Bone biopsy may be performed by an open incision with curettage or trephine biopsy, or a closed needle or trephine biopsy. The advantage of the open techniques is that a large sample of tissue is obtained. Unfortunately, these techniques require a fairly involved operative procedure and risks postoperative complications such as hematoma formation, wound breakdown, infection, local seeding of tumor, increased local pain, and pathologic fracture. Although a closed biopsy with a Michel trephine has a high diagnostic accuracy, there is a high risk of evoking pathologic fracture by creating a large stress riser in the already weakened bone. Our preference for bone biopsy in most circumstances is a closed biopsy with a Jamshidi bone marrow biopsy needle (American Pharmaceal Company, Valencia, CA). The surgeon who does the definitive surgery should be the one to perform the preoperative biopsy, particularly if limb-sparing surgery is considered as the possible treatment option for the patient. Limb radiographs are carefully evaluated to select the site of biopsy. The center and the transition bone of the lesion are chosen for biopsy and a small skin incision is made with consideration to subsequent surgery so the biopsy tract can be removed *en bloc* with definitive tumor resection. At our institution, Jamshidi needle biopsy has an accuracy rate of greater than 90% for detecting tumor versus nontumor and the technique has been well described (Powers et al., 1988).

## BIOLOGIC BEHAVIOR

Osteosarcoma is locally destructive, invasive, and has a very high metastatic rate. Virtually all forms of osteosarcoma are high grade histologically, and by the time the dog is presented, the primary tumor has eroded through the cortical bone to escape the medullary canal within which it arose. By convention, such tumors are called stage II-B if there is no evidence of metastatic disease (stage III if metastases are detected). The exceptions to this biologic behavior are surface osteosarcomas, which are lower grade and do not have a high metastatic rate, and osteosarcoma of the mandible. Canine mandibular osteosarcoma has a lower metastatic rate than classic osteosarcoma of appendicular sites. We found that dogs treated with mandibulectomy alone had a 1-year survival rate of 70%. The reason for this is unclear. Rarely, we encounter dogs with osteosarcoma that has been longstanding (several months) and the histology will be interpreted as low grade. It is our experience, however, that dogs with these tumors have the same survival probability as dogs with classic osteosarcoma once treatment is initiated.

## TREATMENT

### Consultation With Owners

Owners are confronted with difficult decisions once their dog is diagnosed with osteosarcoma. Because of the highly malignant nature of this disease, veterinarians have not previously been enthusiastic about treatment and early euthanasia was usually the outcome. If no treatment is given, dogs usually live a median of 1 to 2 months, but because of worsening pain from the primary site or pathologic fracture at that site, euthanasia is usually performed. Amputation alone is a palliative treatment. Dogs treated by amputation alone have a median survival of 162 days, with approximately 10% surviving 1 year. Although amputation alone does not significantly improve survival, quality of life is improved because the pain from the primary disease is resolved. We have performed hundreds of amputations, and results in terms of function, cosmetics, and owner acceptance have been excellent in almost every case. Even very large dogs can do well with three legs. However, dogs treated with amputation alone usually die from lung metastases. Metastatic disease to lungs is usually clinically silent in terms of signs until there is a large tumor burden. Eventually, nonspecific signs such as malaise, weight loss to the point of cachexia, inappetence, and weakness become prominent. Dyspnea, hemoptysis, hypertrophic osteopathy, and other severe signs of respiratory disease occur very late in the course and most owners elect euthanasia before these serious problems develop.

### Multimodal Therapy

Osteosarcoma, by nature of its high metastatic rate, is considered a systemic disease at initial presentation. Therefore, treatment should be directed systemically as well as locally. Amputation is an effective way of completely removing the primary cancer, and stump recurrences are rare. Many chemotherapeutic agents and biologic response modifiers have been used in trials to address the occult metastatic disease that is present in virtually all dogs with osteosarcoma. The drug that has become the "gold standard" adjuvant agent for canine osteosarcoma is cisplatin (Platinol, Bristol Myers Company, Syracuse, NY; also see *CVT XI*, p 395). We recommend administering cisplatin as soon as possible after amputation for at least two cycles. Survival improvement is significant, and approximately 50% 1 year survival rates can be obtained. Survival probability improves with increasing number of cisplatin doses (up to six); however, the major dose-limiting factor in dogs is nephrotoxicity.

## Cisplatin Side Effects

Prior to administration of cisplatin, dogs must have greater than 3000 neutrophils per deciliter, greater than 75,000 platelets per deciliter, the blood urea nitrogen (BUN) and creatinine should be normal, and urine specific gravity should ideally exceed 1.035 without an abnormal sediment. In these circumstances, the rate of serious complications where hospitalization is necessary is less than 5%. Dogs with preexisting renal disease are likely to become worse, to the point of developing decompensated renal failure, following cisplatin treatment. Dogs may vomit while the drug is administered, but protracted vomiting is rare. Many dogs will have a subdued attitude or decreased appetite 3 to 4 days after receiving cisplatin. Bone marrow suppression will occur and usually manifests as neutropenia alone. Occasionally, thrombocytopenia is also seen. The lowest cell counts usually occur 6 and 16 days after administration. We do not perform CBC or platelet counts unless clinical signs occur. At our recommended dose schedule, severe neutropenia with septicemia is very rare. Small-body-weight dogs and perhaps sighthounds appear to be at greatest risk and should be monitored particularly closely. Alopecia may only be a feature in dogs with continuous hair growth. Other breeds may experience delayed hair growth at clipped areas, such as the amputation site. Other uncommon toxicities include hearing loss and peripheral neuropathy. Because cisplatin is a potent tubular toxin, we advocate the use of large volumes of a 0.9% NaCl solution to be given prior to and after each dose to help protect the kidneys.

## Cisplatin Administration Techniques

We generally administer the first dose of cisplatin on the day of amputation and our recommended dose is 70 mg/m$^2$. This dose can be safely given every 21 days for up to six treatments or until clinicopathologic tests indicate early signs of decreasing renal function. It is extremely important to note that this dosage is *not* safe for use in cats. Safe dosage has not been determined in cats. We currently use a short-term saline diuresis protocol for the administration of cisplatin. Following placement of an indwelling large-bore intravenous catheter, a 0.9% NaCl solution is administered intravenously for 3 hours at 25 ml/kg/hr. This usually requires an infusion pump to safely deliver fluids at this high rate. At the end of the third hour, cisplatin (70 mg/m$^2$) is diluted in 6 ml/kg of 0.9% NaCl and administered over 20 min. After cisplatin injection, saline diuresis is continued at 25 ml/kg/hr for 1 more hr. We place dogs on racks above drains during cisplatin administration and subsequent diuresis. Urine should be treated as if contaminated with cisplatin. Hospital staff should wear latex gloves when handling or cleaning up urine. We ensure dogs are washed or hosed off and

allowed to void urine prior to discharge to their owner's care. The dog is released the day after cisplatin administration.

## Other Chemotherapeutic Agents

Doxorubicin (Adriamycin, Adria Labs, Columbus, OH) has some efficacy and can improve survival in dogs with osteosarcoma after amputation; however, it does not appear to be as potent as cisplatin for this cancer. Doxorubicin has been used in conjunction with cisplatin, but in the studies reported so far, there does not appear to be any real advantage over cisplatin as a single agent.

Carboplatin (Paraplatin, Bristol-Myers, Evansville, IN) is closely related to cisplatin, and in a national trial with this drug as a sole adjuvant agent after amputation for dogs with osteosarcoma, survival results were very encouraging (Bergman et al., 1992). This agent may be as active against osteosarcoma as cisplatin. Carboplatin's major dose-limiting toxicity is myelosuppression. It does not have the same high level of nephrotoxicity, so presumably can be used in dogs excluded from cisplatin regimens because of decreased renal function. The drug is given intravenously without saluresis at 300 mg/m$^2$ on 21-day cycles. Unexplained deaths, thought to be drug related, have sporadically occurred and this drug is currently quite expensive.

## SURGERY

### Amputation

The classic guideline for amputation for osteosarcoma is to remove the limb by sectioning proximal to the bone within which the tumor arises. There is no strong evidence, however, that cutting through unaffected medullary canal of the tumor-bearing bone leads to stump recurrence in dogs. However, there is also no real need to leave as much stump as possible as there is in people, because dogs do not need to be fitted with limb prostheses. Hind limbs can be removed by amputation through the proximal one third of the femur, by disarticulation at the coxofemoral joint, or partial hemipelvectomy (Straw et al., 1992). It is our preference to perform disarticulation at the hip joint unless the tumor is in the proximal metaphysis of the femur. For tumors of this site that have soft tissue extension toward the joint capsule and acetabulum, partial hemipelvectomy with removal of the acetabulum is preferred. For lesions involving the front leg, forequarter amputation is the preferred technique except for selected lesions of the scapula, which are treated by partial scapulectomy.

### Scapulectomy

We have successfully removed bone tumors involving proximal locations of the scapula. Dogs can function extremely well with partial scapulectomy; however, pronounced gait abnormalities can be expected after scapulectomy by disarticulation through the scapulohumeral joint (Kirpensteijn et al., 1994).

## Other Ablative Surgery

Mandibulectomy and maxillectomy (Schwarz and Withrow, 1990) are appropriate surgeries for tumors of oral sites. Tumors of periorbital sites can be removed by orbitectomy (Withrow, 1993a). Rib tumors can be removed by chest wall resection and reconstruction with polypropylene mesh (Marlex mesh, CR Bard Inc, Billerica, MD), with plastic plates (Lubra Plates, Fort Collins, CO) for large lesions, or by diaphragmatic advancement for caudally located rib primaries. Selected lesions of the ulna can be removed by partial ulnectomy, and reconstruction with a bone substitute is not always necessary because the radius can provide adequate support for weight bearing in most instances. Selected tumors of the pelvis can be removed by techniques of hemipelvectomy (Straw et al., 1992) and, although these are difficult surgeries, function and cosmetic outcomes have been excellent.

## Limb Sparing

Although most dogs function well with amputation, there are some dogs in which limb sparing may be indicated, such as dogs with intercurrent orthopedic or neurologic disease, very large dogs, or dogs with owners who refuse amputation for their pet. We have performed approximately 200 limb-sparing operations on dogs and have learned a great deal from this experience. Our limb sparing trials are continuing and the development of new technology is ongoing. Suitable candidates for limb-sparing are dogs with osteosarcoma clinically confined to the leg where the primary tumor affects less than 50% of the bone as determined radiographically. The primary tumor site is intensively treated, either before surgery with intra-arterial cisplatin chemotherapy, radiation therapy (Withrow et al., 1993b), or both; or after surgery with intra-operative chemotherapy (see "New Developments," below). In very small tumors or stage I disease where the primary tumor is completely confined within the medullary canal, limb sparing may be possible without this perioperative treatment to the primary. The most suitable cases for limb sparing are dogs with tumors in the distal metaphysis of the radius or ulna. We have performed limb sparing in dogs with tumors located in many other sites, but the surgery for tumors of the distal end of the radius is technically expedient, attended by fewer complications than for other sites, and the functional outcome is predictably good to excellent. Surgery involves tumor removal with close margins. The bone is removed with an osteotomy approximately 5 cm proximal to the proximal radiographically determined limit of the lesion and by an incision, usually through the

radiocarpal joint. Partial ulnectomy is often performed for primary tumors of the radius and it may be necessary to remove the entire ulnar segment adjacent to tumors with abundant lateral soft tissue extension. The defect is reconstructed with a segment of size-matched frozen sterile cortical allograft. The medullary canal of the allograft provides a reservoir for antibiotic-impregnated methyl methacrylate bone cement, which also provides the allograft with support during revascularization, preventing screw backout and fracture (Straw et al., 1992). The entire construct is stabilized with a dynamic compression plate and screws, and a pancarpal arthrodesis is performed (Straw, Withrow, and Powers, 1990). Approximately 90% of dogs have good to excellent limb function with only a slight gait abnormality associated with the arthrodesis. A major complication is infection. Most infected allografts are adequately managed by long-term systemic antibiotics; however, allograft removal or amputation has been necessary for a few uncontrollable allograft infections. Local tumor control rates have ranged from approximately 80 to 90%. When survival rates for dogs treated with limb sparing and cisplatin are compared to the survival rates for dogs treated with amputation and cisplatin, there is no statistically significant difference. Therefore, limb sparing is a viable option to amputation for selected cases; however, it is technically demanding and is part of a multimodal therapy plan with chemotherapy and possibly radiation therapy. This demands a team approach and is not a trivial treatment.

## NEW DEVELOPMENTS

Over the past few years, we have been working to develop a local drug release system for the administration of a high dose of cisplatin to the wound after resection of the tumor-bearing bone, mainly for use in limb sparing. Control rates at the primary site have improved since using this new chemotherapy delivery system. There has also been an unexpected survival advantage seen in dogs receiving this treatment. This form of chemotherapy is not yet commercially available and trials are underway to define the limitations and indications for local drug delivery in cancer therapy.

## RADIATION THERAPY

Another form of local cancer therapy is high-energy external beam radiation therapy. Although we have used fractionated external beam photons delivered by linear accelerator to treat primary sites of osteosarcoma prior to limb sparing, the major role of radiation therapy in this disease currently is to palliatively treat bone metastasis or primaries that cannot be completely resected. Primary osteosarcoma of the vertebrae generally cannot be resected en bloc. We have found that intralesional resection with decompression of the spinal cord, coupled with fractionated external beam radiation therapy and local-release cisplatin in the drug delivery system previously described can produce reasonably good survival rates with good functional results. The premise is that the cisplatin released from the drug delivery system, which is placed distant from the primary site, establishes a low level of systemic cisplatin that can act as a radiation sensitizer during the course of the 15 fractions of radiation administered daily. Bone metastasis with osteosarcoma is an emerging problem and it appears we are seeing more dogs with late bone metastases. These secondary tumors are usually multiple and painful. Radiation therapy given by coarse fractionation (5 Gy x 5 daily fractions) appears to be useful in most cases by decreasing the pain associated with these lesions. Dogs can be pain free for about 6 months or longer, but usually the tumors will ultimately progress and become painful within 2 to 3 months.

## TREATING METASTATIC DISEASE

Pulmonary metastases are the classic cause of treatment failure in osteosarcoma, despite bone metastasis becoming a more frequent problem. Pulmonary metastasectomy has been reported to be a useful technique in selected cases (O'Brien et al., 1993). The guidelines for case selection are that the tumor at the primary site is controlled, preferably for a long relapse-free interval (>300 days) and that fewer than three nodules are detected on thoracic radiography. Dogs that fall into this category have the highest probability of surviving disease-free after thoracotomy and lung lobectomy for pulmonary metastasis. Further chemotherapy with cisplatin, doxorubicin, or other agents has not been effective for the treatment of measurable metastatic osteosarcoma in dogs.

## FUTURE STUDIES

Work continues in many centers to devise better ways to treat osteosarcoma in people and dogs. Osteosarcoma is a solid tumor with a devastatingly high metastatic rate. The key to understanding how to treat this disease is underscored by an understanding of the cellular and molecular abnormalities producing these malignant cells. The goal of future research is to determine prognostically significant variables that can direct "tailor-made" therapeutic protocols with predictable success.

## References and Suggested Reading

Bergman PB, MacEwen EG, Kurzman IL, et al: Amputation and carboplatin for the treatment of dogs with osteosarcoma: 34 cases (1991–1992) (abstr). *Proc Vet Cancer Soc*, Pacific Grove, CA, Oct 18–21, 1992, p 53.
*Results of study using carboplatin to treat dogs with osteosarcoma.*
Kirpensteijn J, Straw RC, Pardo AD, et al: Partial and total scapulectomy in the dog. J Am Anim Hosp Assoc 30:313, 1994.
*A technique for removing part or all of the scapula.*
O'Brien MG, Straw RC, Wilkins SJ, et al: Resection of pulmonary metastasis in canine osteosarcoma: 36 cases (1983–1992). Vet Surg 22:105, 1993.
*The outcome of dogs after pulmonary metastasis removal and prognostic indicators*
Powers BE, LaRue SM, Withrow SJ, et al: Jamshidi needle biopsy for diagnosis of bone lesions in small animals. J Am Vet Med Assoc 193:205, 1988.
*A technique for bone biopsy.*
Schwarz PD and Withrow SJ: Mandibulectomy, maxillectomy and premaxillectomy. *In* Bojrab MJ (ed): *Current Techniques in Small Animal Surgery*, 3rd edition. Lea & Febiger, 1990, p 850.
Straw RC, Withrow SJ, and Powers BE: Management of canine appendicular osteosarcoma. Vet Clin North Am [Small Anim Pract] 20:1141, 1990.
*Techniques for limb sparing are discussed in this paper.*
Straw RC, Powers BE, Withrow SJ, et al: The effect of intramedullary polymethylmethacrylate in healing of intercalary cortical allografts in a canine model. J Orthop Res 10:434, 1992.
*A study of healing of allografts where bone cement filled the medullary canal.*
Straw RC, Withrow SJ, and Powers BE: Partial or total hemipelvectomy in the management of sarcomas in nine dogs and two cats. Vet Surg 21:183, 1992.
*Techniques for amputation of hind legs where there are proximally located osteosarcoma primaries and for removing pelvic bones for tumors of these sites.*
Withrow SJ, O'Brien MG, Straw RC, et al: Orbitectomy in the dog and cat: 21 cases (abstr). *Proc Vet Cancer Soc*, Columbus, OH, Oct 3–5, 1993a, p 128.
Withrow SJ, Thrall DE, Straw RC, et al: Intra-arterial cisplatin with or without radiation in limb sparing for canine osteosarcoma. Cancer 71:2484, 1993b.
*Results of limb sparing in dogs treated preoperatively with chemotherapy or chemotherapy and radiation therapy.*

# TREATMENT OF SKIN CANCER

BRUCE R. MADEWELL
*Davis, California*

Tumors of the skin and subcutaneous tissues are best handled by the surgeon; surgical excision is rapid and cost effective. The recovery time following uncomplicated excision is quick, and the procedure is frequently curative. With these tenets in mind, it is surprising to realize that tumors of the skin and subcutaneous tissues pose so many problems for the clinical veterinarian. Difficulties encountered in effective management of tumors of skin and subcutaneous tissues are related to the late stage of diagnosis of many tumors; the location of a neoplasm near a complex anatomic site that may preclude a wide-margin excision; and poor understanding of the biology of many of these tumors. Furthermore, for most tumors of the skin and subcutaneous tissues, prognostic variables, such as those based on histomorphologic criteria, have not been devised.

The purpose of this article is to offer treatment perspectives for tumors of the skin and subcutaneous tissues. Comments are offered for tumors that are not amenable to surgical excision, and for those that have reoccurred following incomplete surgical excision. Also included are methods of treatment alternative to surgical excision, if available, for particular tumors at anatomic sites that are difficult to access surgically. For simplicity, the tumors are categorized into those derived from epithelium, tumors derived from the supportive structures of the mesenchyme, and the round cell tumors of the skin.

## TUMORS DERIVED FROM EPITHELIUM

### Squamous Cell Carcinoma

Squamous cell carcinomas derived from skin surfaces are unique with respect to their biology and their potential responsiveness to new and innovative treatment methods. From a biologic perspective, the sunlight-associated skin tumors of the facial skin in white cats and ventral abdomen in dogs provide good examples of the evolution of a neoplasm through preneoplastic stages of erythema, actinic keratosis, solar elastosis, carcinoma *in situ*, and invasive squamous cell carcinoma. Although it is assumed that the stages of initiation, promotion, and progression of evolving carcinomas are influenced by one or more genetic or epigenetic events, the influences of factors other than ultraviolet light exposure on a nonpigmented skin surface have not been elucidated in small animal patients. Furthermore, when similar tumors occur in animals with pigmented skin and hair coats, no risk factors have been identified.

Despite the high incidence rate for sunlight-associated squamous cell carcinomas in animals living in the arid and semiarid regions of the western United States, treatment methods have not been optimized. There are descriptions in the veterinary literature on the use of a variety of treatment methods for management of cutaneous squamous cell carcinomas, although for some methods, the results have been derived from small compilations of clinical cases. The treatment methods include surgical excision, radiation therapy, focal hyperthermia or cryosurgery, chemotherapy, and the more recently described photodynamic therapy. Surgical excision is curative for localized tumors; sunlight-associated lesions are slow to metastasize, and thus are amenable to local treatment methods at least during the early stages of their development. Tumors of the external surfaces of the ears, facial skin, and periocular structures are usually managed by the surgeon. Squamous cell carcinomas affecting the skin of the flanks are also associated with low metastatic potential, and are therefore good surgical candidates. Subungual squamous cell carcinomas, despite the high probability

for invasion of underlying bone, are favorably managed by amputation. In one study of 21 dogs with subungual carcinomas treated surgically, local recurrences were not observed, and only one dog developed metastasis (O'Brien et al., 1992).

### RADIATION THERAPY

For the most commonly applied treatment methods, surgery and radiation therapy, end results of treatment for tumors at most sites have not been precisely described. In one study describing the results of radiation therapy for squamous cell carcinomas of the facial skin in cats, cure was most likely to be achieved with small, T1 stage (<2.0-cm maximum diameter and minimally invasive) lesions (Théon et al., 1993a). In that study, the overall progression-free survival rates at 1 and 5 years following therapy for all stages were 60% and 10%, respectively. Histologic criteria were not identified that would allow prediction of response to therapy, but the proliferative fraction was found to be a significant prognostic determinant of response to irradiation; tumors with low proliferating fractions were more likely to respond favorably to irradiation than tumors with high proliferating fractions. Radiation therapy is an attractive treatment option for sunlight-associated tumors compared to focal surgical excision because it provides the opportunity for treatment of a wide field. This is a rational approach for management of tumors that develop by field carcinogenesis (i.e., where a diffuse carcinogenic exposure [ultraviolet light] results in the development of multiple premalignant and malignant lesions within the exposed tissue region).

### PHOTODYNAMIC THERAPY

Photodynamic therapy (PDT) is a relatively new method in veterinary medicine that is undergoing investigation for control of superficial tumors of the skin. The principles of application of PDT were described in *CVT XI*, p 416. Photodynamic therapy offers the theoretical advantage of allowing selective destruction of tumor cells within the irradiated field because of preferential uptake or retention of the photodynamic agent by tumor cells. Another advantage when compared to radiation therapy is that generally, only one or a few treatment sessions are required. As noted with radiation therapy, best results have been obtained following photodynamic therapy for focal, minimally invasive tumors (Peaston, Leach, and Higgins, 1993). Although the results of preliminary studies are promising, whether PDT will provide tumor control as efficiently or consistently as surgical excision or radiation therapy has not been determined. Photodynamic therapy is currently limited in veterinary practice to a few university settings on an experimental basis. Another limitation is that the photodynamic agents in clinical use or under investigation have only been preliminarily tested in dogs and cat (Roberts et al., 1991). Porfimer sodium (Photofrin, American Cyanamid, Pearl River, NY) is the single product currently approved for human clinical use; it is activated at 625 to 635 nm, allowing only superficial (1 to 3 mm) light penetration. Another limitation to the use of Photofrin is that it is cleared slowly from tissues, requiring that the patient remain in subdued light for 4 to 6 weeks following treatment. Other investigational agents are activated by longer wavelengths of light, thus allowing better penetration of light into tissue and the theoretical advantage of allowing deeper volumes of tumor to be irradiated effectively. These agents also cause less cutaneous photosensitization. Several of the compounds being studied appear to interact more efficiently with light, have more selective localization in tumors, and have faster clearance than Photofrin. These agents include chloroaluminum sulfonated phthalocyanine and pyropheophorbide hexyl alpha ether (HPPH-23).

### RETINOIDS

Another therapeutic innovation in human medicine that has seen preliminary application in veterinary medicine for control of squamous cell carcinomas of the skin is the use of retinoids (see "The Use of Synthetic Retinoids in Veterinary Medicine," this volume, p 585). The naturally occurring compounds with vitamin A activity and their synthetic analogs are referred to as retinoids; some retinoid derivatives are capable of inhibiting cell growth and inducing cell differentiation. They are potent modulators of squamous differentiation in normal and malignant keratinocytes. These compounds are used in human patients to reverse the clinical appearance of actinic keratosis, and may be useful in prevention of invasive cancer. The synthetic retinoids isotretinoin (Accutane, Hoffman-La Roche, Nutley, NJ) and etretinate (Tegison, Hoffman-La Roche) have been preliminarily tested in veterinary patients. Those data suggest that some dogs with sunlight-associated skin lesions, including preneoplastic and minimally invasive carcinomas, may benefit from the oral administration of etretinate (1 mg/kg b.i.d. for a minimum of 90 days) (Marks et al., 1992).

### CHEMOTHERAPY

The anticancer drugs 5-fluorouracil, cisplatin, or methotrexate, administered intralesionally as therapeutic implants in a repositol formulation, have been reported for management of some superficial tumors of the skin (Kitchell et al., 1992). Although the results of those studies are encouraging, these proprietary therapeutic implant formulations are not yet available for routine clinical practice. Alternatively, cisplatin may be prepared in a controlled-release formulation using sesame oil; these therapeutic implants have been used favorably in the horse for the control of squamous cell carcinomas (Théon et al., 1993b) but await additional verification in small animal patients.

In human patients, topical 5-fluorouracil (Effudex, Roche Dermatologics, Nutley, NJ) is an effective agent for treating multiple actinic keratoses and Bowen's disease. Topical application of 5-fluorouracil may be useful as part of the overall management for dogs with multiple actinic keratoses on the skin of the ventral abdomen, although a precise schedule of administration has not been described in the dog for this purpose. Topical application of 5-fluorouracil results in skin inflammation and irritant dermatitis in some patients. We have also seen systemic 5-fluorouracil toxicity following topical application of the drug to the skin of the ventral abdomen of dogs. Because optimal use of topical 5-fluorouracil has not been described in dogs, caution is advised when using this product for control of precancerous skin lesions, and discontinuation of treatment is advised if serious adverse reactions develop. 5-Fluorouracil (5% concentration) is applied topically, using latex gloves, to focal lesions once daily for 5 days, and then once weekly for 4 to 6 weeks. An Elizabethan collar is used to prevent the dog from licking the medication. Because of the risk of systemic toxicity, 5-fluorouracil is *not* recommended for use in cats either by topical application or systemic administration.

## Other Epithelial Tumors

Basal cell tumors and tumors derived from more differentiated adnexal structures of the skin are generally benign in dogs and cats. For benign tumors, recurrence following adequate surgical excision is unlikely. For tumors affecting skin adnexae, those derived from sweat glands have the greatest likelihood for malignancy. Sweat gland adenocarcinomas are locally infiltrative, commonly inciting a desmoplastic response. Local and regional metastases may ensue. Aggressive surgical treatment, radiation therapy, and the use of anticancer drugs such as doxorubicin are treatment considerations, but end results following treatment have not been reported.

## MESENCHYMAL TUMORS

The supportive somatic structures of the skin include fibrous and adipose connective tissues, blood vessels, lymphatic structures, nerves, smooth and striated muscle, and fascia. Most of the malignant tumors of the soft tissues are sarcomas, and despite the wide tissue heterogeneity of these neoplasms, they share some common features. Notable is the ability of soft tissue sarcomas to invade tissues locally and to metastasize primarily to the lungs.

### SURGICAL TREATMENT

The curative intent of surgical treatment for soft tissue sarcomas is based on the probability that the neoplasm is localized to the point of origin, and has not yet spread to involve adjacent structures, blood vessels, or regional lymph nodes. Surgical techniques that ensure tumor-free margins markedly improve local control rates for soft tissue sarcomas (see "Definitive Surgical Treatment for Cancer," this volume, p 462).

An *intralesional* incision is made deliberately by the surgeon to procure a biopsy specimen, thus allowing definitive treatment planning once the diagnosis is established. The subsequent wide excision includes the biopsy tract. An intralesional incision might also be done inadvertently by the surgeon if a resection is confined because of anatomic constraints. As a consequence, micro- or macroscopic tumor deposits remain following surgery. A marginal excision is used to remove a tumor in one piece, and is made through the surrounding reactive tissue or pseudocapsule or both. Although a marginal excision might be satisfactory for treatment of some benign tumors, residual tumor may remain in a large number of cases. A marginal excision is used for diagnostic purposes, as a palliative procedure, or as a procedure adjuvant to additional therapy such as irradiation. If a marginal excision is done before radiation therapy, it is important for the surgeon to mark the lateral and deep margins of the tumor using radiopaque material such as stainless steel sutures or staples. These markers may then be used by the radiation therapist to adequately and optimally design a treatment field. A marginal excision constitutes unsatisfactory treatment for most of the commonly encountered soft tissue sarcomas in small animal practice. A *wide-margin* excision is a definitive procedure that involves resection of the tumor and a surrounding margin of normal tissue; all resections are done through normal tissue, but within the involved compartment of that tissue. Although a wide-margin excision may be curative, residual tumor may remain if "skip" lesions had been present; such skip lesions are commonly encountered at the lateral margins of poorly differentiated mast cell sarcomas. The most definitive procedure is a *radical* excision, whereby the entire lesion, pseudocapsule, underlying reactive bone, and muscles associated with that compartment are resected, thus leaving no residual tumor following surgery. Although radical excisions are theoretically appropriate for malignant soft tissue tumors, for some tumors such as malignant melanoma, less aggressive surgical procedure might be adequate because treatment failures occur outside the surgical field, implying that metastases had been present at the time of operation.

### MALIGNANT MELANOMA

The prognosis for dogs with malignant melanoma arising from dermal sites is generally considered more favorable than for dogs with melanomas arising from mucosal sites. Melanomas arising from the dermis that are characterized histologically as benign are associated with good survival times following surgery, whereas in one study, more than 65% of dogs with malignant melanomas arising from the dermis were euthanatized because of local reoccurrence or distant metastasis within 2 years of treatment (Frese, 1978). In that study, the importance of tumor volume was determined by the extremely poor prognosis for dogs with large-diameter (>4-cm) neoplasms; the median postoperative survival time for dogs with large tumors was 4 months with a 100% 2-year death rate, whereas it was 12 months with a 54% 2-year death rate for dogs with small-diameter (<2-cm) tumors. Although malignant melanoma affecting cutaneous sites is uncommon in the cat, the prognosis for cats following surgical excision of cutaneous malignant melanomas is better than that associated with tumors affecting ocular or oral sites.

### HEMANGIOMA AND HEMANGIOSARCOMA

Hemangiomas and hemangiosarcomas may be derived from endothelial structures of the skin. There are several studies suggesting that solar irradiation increases risk in the dog for hemangiomas and hemangiosarcomas of the dermis, but does not influence risk for tumors affecting the subcutaneous tissues. Surgical excision is generally curative for cutaneous hemangiomas. For hemangiosarcoma of the skin, dogs with tumors derived from the dermis have a better prognosis following surgery than dogs with tumors derived from the subcutaneous tissues, especially if the dermal tumor was associated with sunlight-associated solar dermatosis (Hargis et al., 1992). Furthermore, there is considerably greater likelihood for dogs with subcutaneous hemangiosarcomas to have primary tumors elsewhere, in other solid organs—the skin site therefore representing a metastatic focus of a tumor that is unlikely to be favorably managed surgically.

### HEMANGIOPERICYTOMA

Hemangiopericytoma is a cutaneous neoplasm affecting dogs that is often difficult to remove surgically. Local recurrence rates ranging from 7.5 to 56% have been reported in the literature. Local recurrence appears to reflect several factors, including tumor volume and location, but also surgical technique. Because of the highly infiltrative growth pattern but inherently low probability for metastasis of cutaneous hemangiopericytoma, wide-margin or radical excision with appropriate reconstruction is of great importance for good patient management.

### FIBROSARCOMA

Fibroma and its malignant counterpart, fibrosarcoma, occur in both dogs and cats. Wide-margin or radical excisional methods are required to effectively manage fibrosarcomas. Because of the importance of primary surgical excision for effective management of fibrosarcoma, consultation or referral of the patient to a skilled surgeon is advised to optimize treatment. Fibrosarcomas have generally been considered poorly responsive to radiation therapy, and there are few descriptions of response of fibrosarcomas to chemotherapy. More recent results suggest, however, that radiation therapy does provide good local control for many of the soft tissue sarcomas; these methods and results are described elsewhere in this book by Théon (see "Indications and Applications of Radiation Therapy," this volume, p 467).

There appear to be two special circumstances in cats with regard to fibrosarcomas. First, the association of multicentric fibrosarcomas in young cats with feline sarcoma viruses, first described in 1969, is well known to clinical veterinarians. These cats test positively for the feline leukemia virus and respond poorly to treatment. An apparent new syndrome has recently been described in cats—fibrosarcomas that develop at the site of subcutaneous administration of vaccines (Hendrick et al., 1992), including feline leukemia virus and rabies virus vaccinations. Because this is a newly recognized syndrome, optimum treatment has not been devised. It has been our experience that tumor recurrence frequently complicates apparently inadequate primary excision. Recurrent tumors are highly infiltrative, making subsequent excisional surgeries difficult or impossible. Vaccine-induced fibrosarcomas can also metastasize.

For cats with fibrosarcomas, data published before the descriptions of vaccine-associated tumors revealed that tumors affecting the pinna or flank were effectively treated surgically, but tumors derived from the skin of the head, neck, or limbs were associated with poor postoperative survival times. Nearly three fourths of these cats either died or were euthanatized as a consequence of their tumor within 9 months of surgery (Bostock and Dye, 1979). It was further demonstrated that the mitotic index of feline fibrosarcomas was a useful prognostic determinant; cats with fibrosarcomas with less than 6 mitotic figures per high-power field (400X) had median survival times of 128 weeks, compared to only 16 weeks for those cats with more than 6 mitotic figures per high-power field.

## MALIGNANT FIBROUS HISTIOCYTOMA

Although malignant fibrous histiocytoma is one of the most frequently described soft tissue sarcomas in human patients, it occurs infrequently in small animal patients, but occasionally in the cat. These tumors contain an admixture of morphologic cell types, including fibroblast-like cells, histiocytic-appearing cells, and giant cells. Aggressive surgical methods with careful examination of the surgical margins of the specimen are required to effectively manage these neoplasms.

## LIPOMA, INFILTRATIVE LIPOMA, AND LIPOSARCOMA

There are three histologically distinct tumors derived from fat tissues in the dog. Lipomas are excised for cosmetic purposes or if they interfere with function. Infiltrative lipomas pose surgical problems; 50% or more of these tumors will recur because wide-margin excisions are difficult to accomplish. Liposarcomas, very uncommon tumors in the dog, have some probability for metastasis in the dog. I am not aware of treatment options for liposarcomas in the dog beyond primary excision.

## RADIATION THERAPY

Management of soft tissue sarcomas in veterinary medicine has relied upon surgical resection, including amputations for tumors of the extremities. Innovations in treatment, derived from experiences with human patients, are now beginning to be applied to veterinary patients. These methods include chemotherapy and radiotherapy applied prior to surgery or perioperatively, in conjunction with function-sparing ablative and reconstructive surgery.

There is considerable rationale for combining surgery and radiotherapy for management of soft tissue sarcomas. Concurrent radiation therapy should allow less mutilative surgical resections for local tumor control. If radiotherapy is given first, regression of the tumor after irradiation may make surgical resection easier. Preoperative radiotherapy should allow the use of lower total doses and smaller treatment ports because the margins resulting from large surgically manipulated postoperative fields do not have to be included. In addition, shedding of viable tumor cells during the surgical resection may at least theoretically be minimized, decreasing the likelihood of local tumor recurrence or distant spread.

Preliminary results for dogs with hemangiopericytomas treated with radiation therapy (orthovoltage) have been described (Evans, 1987). In that study, 41% of dogs had local tumor control 2 years following treatment. Small tumor size (treatment portal <50 cm$^2$) and hind limb location were identified as factors correlating positively with treatment response. These results suggest that radiation therapy should be considered for those tumors that, because of location, cannot be excised with adequate margins.

## CHEMOTHERAPY

Adjuvant therapy for soft tissue sarcomas following excision remains controversial in both human and veterinary practice. Most systemic chemotherapy regimens for treatment of soft tissue sarcoma in human patients include doxorubicin, which is the most effective single agent. There are few data in the veterinary literature demonstrating significant responses of inoperable soft tissue sarcomas to chemotherapy; however, preliminary data suggest that adjuvant chemotherapy, using the combination of vincristine, doxorubicin, and cyclophosphamide, may provide palliation for dogs with established hemangiosarcomas and delay the onset of metastasis following surgical excision (Helfand, 1989). There are also preliminary data to suggest that some dogs with inoperable malignant melanoma might benefit from treatment with carboplatin.

## NEW THERAPIES

Little progress has been made in veterinary medicine for management of dogs or cats with soft tissue sarcomas that are not surgical candidates. There are few data to show that adjuvant therapy reduces the risk for local reoccurrence of incompletely resected tumors, and the data are similarly scant to suggest that objective responses can be attained in small animals with established metastases. It is hoped that new therapies with biologicals (cytokines with or without peripheral-blood or tumor-associated lymphocytes), multiagent chemotherapeutic regimens, and combinations of chemotherapy and cytokines will produce substantial tumor responses.

## ROUND CELL TUMORS OF THE SKIN

### Mycosis Fungoides and Cutaneous Lymphoma

Theoretically, there are a range of treatment methods that could be used for management of mycosis fungoides (epitheliotropic lymphoma) and cutaneous lymphoma in the dog. Psoralen with ultraviolet light irradiation (PUVA) and electron beam radiotherapy are methods not generally available for veterinary patients, and personnel hazards associated with drug handling generally preclude the use of topically applied nitrogen mustard or nitrosoureas. Biologic response modifiers such as interferon, monoclonal antibodies, and interleukin-2, which are valuable in some human patients with mycosis fungoides, are not yet available for use in animals. In veterinary medicine, for focal lesions, radiation therapy is effective treatment. For multiple or widespread lesions, systemically applied antineoplastic agents (see "Treatment and Prognosis of Canine Malignant Lymphoma," and "Treatment of Feline Malignant Lymphoma," this volume, pp 494 and 498, respectively) may provide palliative responses in some animals, and survival times of 6 months for cutaneous lymphoma and 11 months for epitheliotropic lymphoma have been described. There are new data to suggest that these patients may also benefit from treatment with retinoids. In a preliminary study, objective responses were achieved in more than one third of dogs treated with the retinoid etretinate at 3 to 4 mg/kg every 24 hr (White et al., 1993). It was suggested that concurrent treatment with corticosteroid may decrease patient discomfort associated with scaling and pruritic skin.

### Mast Cell Sarcoma

Mast cell tumors account for as high as one fifth of the cutaneous canine neoplasms in some surveys. Small, confined, and well-differentiated tumors are generally managed effectively surgically, but local recurrence and regional and systemic dissemination preclude effective treatment for many mast cell tumors, particularly those that are graded histologically as poorly differentiated (grade III). Years ago, Bostock described short survival times following surgical excision (median = 18 weeks) for dogs with poorly differentiated mast cell tumors when compared to those with well-differentiated tumors (median = 51 weeks) (Bostock, 1973). Poor survival times following surgical excision for undifferentiated mast cell tumors were confirmed in a later report (Patnaik, Ehler, and MacEwen, 1984). Bostock later reported that quantitation of silver-nucleolar organizer regions ($AgNO_3$) also offered prognostic information that correlated well with histologic grading (Bostock et al., 1989). In that study, 73% of dogs with a high mean $AgNO_3$ count (>4.9/cell) were destroyed as a consequence of tumor-related disease, whereas survival times following treatment of dogs with lower counts were significantly better, and no dog with a low $AgNO_3$ count (<1.7/cell) was destroyed as a consequence of the mast cell tumor (Bostock et al., 1989).

Cutaneous mast cell tumors in cats are generally not associated with visceral lesions. Although a variety of histologic variants of feline cutaneous mast cell tumors have been described, in general, the tumors are benign biologically and are not likely to reoccur following adequate surgical excision.

Radiation therapy has been recommended for management of dogs with incompletely excised mast cell tumors. In one study of 95 mast cell tumors affecting 85 dogs, the survival rates following irradiation at 1 and 2 years were 78.8% and 77%, respectively (Turrel et al., 1988). Ideal responses resulted from irradiation of small, well-differentiated lesions that had a long clinical course, and the prognosis following irradiation was better for dogs with tumors affecting the skin or subcutaneous tissues of the extremities than for those with tumors involving the trunk, especially the inguinal and perineal regions.

There has been recent description of the use of local injection of deionized water at the site of incompletely excised mast cell tumors (Grier et al., 1990). The rationale for that study was based on the apparent sensitivity of mast cells, in vitro, to exposure to deionized water resulting in cell death due to hypotonic shock. Preliminary data were presented in the same study to suggest that dogs and cats with incompletely excised mast cell tumors had less likelihood of local tumor reoccurrence than for those animals treated with surgery alone. For treatment, at the time of surgery or commencing 2 weeks following surgical excision, deionized water was infused into the surgical tumor bed using a 26-gauge needle; the injection was carried through the surgical wound and into the subcutaneous tissues and muscular fascia. For treatment at the time of surgery, a volume of water was used to create a gelatinous appearance of the subcutaneous tissues, whereas for dogs treated initially 2 weeks following surgery, a volume of water was injected along both edges of the excision to create a swollen appearance. Three subsequent treatments with water were given at 10- to 21-day intervals. The efficacy of this seemingly simple method for control of localized or inadequately excised mast cell tumors awaits additional verification.

## PLASMACYTOMA

Solitary plasmacytomas, independent of the syndrome multiple myeloma, have occasionally been described on the skin of dogs, although this tumor is more frequently encountered in the oral cavity. There appears to be some risk for progression of plasmacytoma to multiple myeloma in the dog, and surgical excision is advised.

## HISTIOCYTOMA

Although histiocytomas may regress spontaneously, surgical excision with pathologic confirmation is advised to be certain that the cytologic impression of histiocytoma was correct and not a misinterpretation of a poorly pigmented mast cell tumor.

## CANINE TRANSMISSIBLE VENEREAL TUMOR

The canine transmissible venereal tumor is located primarily on the external genitalia of male and female dogs. Extragenital forms affect the skin and subcutaneous tissues, lymph nodes, and visceral sites. Although tumor control for localized neoplasms may be achieved with surgical excision or cryosurgical treatment, recurrence is common. The canine transmissible venereal tumor is uniquely radiation responsive, and indeed, a single radiation dose of 10 Gy may be curative (Thrall, 1982). Several regimens for tumor control have been described using anticancer drugs, used either as single agents or as combinations of agents. Vincristine sulfate (0.025 mg/kg IV once weekly, for up to seven treatments) appears to be the most active anticancer agent that has been critically tested in the dog, and several studies suggest that the results of treatment using vincristine alone are as good as the results achieved using combination chemotherapy (Calvert, Leifer, and MacEwen, 1982). Although antitumor immune responses have been demonstrated in dogs with naturally occurring and experimentally transmitted venereal tumors, and there are some data to support the use of specific and nonspecific immune stimulants as therapeutic agents, an optimal immunotherapeutic regimen has not yet been described.

## SUMMARY

Surgical treatment is the most widely used and most effective treatment for cutaneous neoplasms in the dog and cat. New treatment methods are now being introduced into veterinary practice for control of cutaneous neoplasms, either adjunctive to surgical treatment, or as alternative treatment. Radiation therapy used prior to surgical excision is a rational treatment approach for large or infiltrative soft tissue sarcomas. Photodynamic therapy is an alternative method for treatment of superficial tumors of the skin that may prove very efficacious for tumor control as new photodynamic agents are developed and tested. The use of anticancer drugs, administered systemically or intralesionally, is now being tested in dogs and cats for selected cutaneous neoplasms. The newly developed biologic response modifiers are certain to have value for management of some cutaneous neoplasms in animals, as precedent information in human patients indicate. The retinoids may provide a means for prevention of cancer in high-risk patients.

## References and Suggested Reading

Bostock DE: The prognosis following surgical removal of mastocytomas in dogs. J Small Anim Pract 14:27, 1973.
*The first clinical description of the differential responses of dogs with cutaneous mast cell tumors to surgical excision based on a tumor grading system.*

Bostock DE, Crocker J, Harris K, et al: Nucleolar organiser regions as indicators of postsurgical prognosis in canine spontaneous mast cell tumors. Br J Cancer 59:915, 1989.
*A description of the use of nucleolar organizer regions to predict response to surgical treatment for dogs with mast cells tumors.*

Bostock DE and Dye MT: Prognosis after surgical excision of fibrosarcomas in cats. J Am Vet Med Assoc 175:727, 1979.
*A description of the end results following surgical excision of fibrosarcoma in the cat.*

Calvert CA, Leifer CE, and MacEwen EG: Vincristine for treatment of transmissible venereal tumor in the dog. J Am Vet Med Assoc 181:163, 1982.
*The responses of 41 dogs with canine transmissible veneral tumors to vincrisitine chemotherapy are described.*

Evans SM: Canine hemangiopericytoma—a retrospective analysis of response to surgery and orthovoltage radiation. Vet Radiol 28:13, 1987.
*The results of treatment of 22 dogs with hemangiopericytoma with orthovoltage irradiation.*

Frese K: Verlaufsuntersuchungen bei Melanomen der Haut und der Mundschleimhaut des Hundes. Vet Pathol 15:461, 1978.
*The responses of dogs with melanomas of the skin to surgical excision.*

Grier RL, DiGuardo G, Schaffer CB, et al: Mast cell tumor destruction by deionized water. Am J Vet Res 51:1116, 1990.
*Description of a novel method for control of mast cell tumors in the dog and cat.*

Hargis AM, Ihrke PJ, Spangler WL, and Stannard AA: A retrospective study of 212 dogs with cutaneous hemangiomas and hemangiosarcomas. Vet Pathol 29:316, 1992.
*A clinical and pathologic study of benign and malignant cutaneous vascular tumors in the dog.*

Helfand SC: Chemotherapy of solid tumors. In Kirk RW (ed): Current Veterinary Therapy X: Small Animal Practice. Philadelphia, WB Saunders Co, 1989, pp 489–493.
*A compilation of chemotherapeutic agents and protocols for treatment of soft tissue sarcomas.*

Hendrick MJ, Goldschmidt MH, Shofer FS, et al: Postvaccinal sarcomas in the cat: Epidemiology and electron probe microanalytical identification of aluminum. Cancer Res 52:5391, 1992.
*A description of the association of fibrosarcomas in the cats with subcutaneous vaccination.*

Kitchell BE, Luck EE, Orenberg EK, et al: Treatment of canine squamous cell carcinoma with intralesional therapeutic implants. In Proc 11th Ann Meet Vet Cancer Soc 1992, p 79.
*The use of intralesional chemotherapy using a repositol formulation is described in dogs with squamous cell carcinoma.*

Marks SL, Song MD, Stannard AA, and Power HT: Clinical evaluation of etretinate for the treatment of canine solar-induced squamous cell carcinoma and preneoplastic lesions. J Am Acad Dermatol 27:11, 1992.
*A clinical report using a synthetic retinoid for the management of squamous cell carcinoma and precursor lesions in dogs.*

O'Brien MG, Berg J, and Engler SJ: Treatment by digital amputation of subungual squamous cell carcinoma in dogs: 21 cases (1987–1988). J Am Vet Med Assoc 201:759, 1992.
*Report on the favorable responses to surgery of dogs with tumors derived from the nail-bed epithelium.*

Patnaik AK, Ehler WJ, and MacEwen EG: Canine cutaneous mast cell tumor: Morphologic grading and survival time in 83 dogs. Vet Pathol 21:469, 1984.
*The responses of dogs with mast cell tumors to surgical excision based on tumor grade.*

Peaston AE, Leach MW, and Higgins RJ: Photodynamic therapy for nasal and aural squamous cell carcinoma in cats. J Am Vet Med Assoc 202:1261, 1993.
*The responses of cats with squamous cell carcinoma to photodynamic therapy.*

Roberts WG, Klein MK, Loomis M, et al: Photodynamic therapy of spontaneous cancers in felines, canines, and snakes with chloro-aluminum sulfonated phthalocyanine. J Natl Cancer Inst 83:18, 1991.
*A description of the application of photodynamic therapy to small animal patients.*

Théon AP, Madewell BR, Shearn V, and Moulton JE: Prognostic factors for squamous cell carcinomas of the nasal planum: A study of ninety cats treated with radiotherapy. Personal observations. 1993a.
*The responses of cats with facial squamous cell carcinomas to megavoltage irradiation.*

Théon AP, Pascoe JR, Carlson GP, and Krag DN: Intratumoral chemotherapy with cisplatin in oily emulsion in horses. J Am Vet Med Assoc 202:261, 1993b.
*The clinical application, with end results, of intratumoral cisplatin chemotherapy in the horse.*

Thrall DE: Orthovoltage radiotherapy of canine transmissible venereal tumor. Vet Radiol 23:217, 1982.
*The responsiveness of the canine transmissible venereal tumor to orthovoltage irradiation is described.*

Turrel JM, Kitchell BE, Miller LM, et al: Prognostic factors for radiation treatment of mast cell tumor in 85 dogs. J Am Vet Med Assoc 193:936, 1988.
*A description of the responses of dogs with mast cell tumors to radiation therapy.*

White SD, Rosychuk RAW, Scott KV, et al: Use of isotretinoin and etretinate for the treatment of benign cutaneous neoplasia and cutaneous lymphoma in dogs. J Am Vet Med Assoc 202:387, 1993.
*A clinical description on the use of synthetic retinoids for treatment of cutaneous neoplasms in the dog.*

# MAMMARY TUMORS IN THE DOG

### G.R. RUTTEMAN
*Utrecht, The Netherlands*

Mammary tumors are important in small animal veterinary practice. In the female dog, the incidence of malignant mammary tumors is higher than that of any other cancer. In California, the annual incidence rate in intact female dogs was estimated to be approximately 260/100,000 dogs (Dorn et al., 1968). About 20 to 40% of dogs with mammary tumors or dysplasias develop malignant neoplasms. It is often difficult to discriminate between benign and malignant mammary nodules by means of clinical criteria. Since some dogs with benign mammary tumors are at higher risk to develop malignant mammary tumors as well (Gilbertson et al., 1983), the proper management of both types of disease is important.

Mammary tumors are rare before the age of 2 years, although fibroadenomatous lesions occasionally occur in dogs as young as 1 year. The incidence increases slowly after the age of 4 years, rises steeply between 6 and 10 years, and then the increase appears to lessen.

There is ample evidence that both endogenous ovarian hormones and synthetic derivatives used in many countries to prevent estrus may stimulate mammary tumor development. In male dogs, the incidence of mammary tumors is only about 1% of that in females.

Much is still unknown about the pathogenesis of mammary tumors and the factors that determine their biologic behavior. However, some important discoveries will be mentioned briefly in this article.

## PATHOGENESIS

### Endocrine Factors

Mammary tumor development in the dog is inhibited by ovariectomy performed before 2½ years of age (Schneider, Dorn, and Taylor, 1969). If carried out later, it may still reduce the risk of benign tumors, but will probably have little or no effect on the risk of malignant tumors. Furthermore, it has been demonstrated that administration of long-acting progestogens to prevent estrus causes a moderate increase in the risk of developing benign mammary tumors but not of malignant tumors. For prevention of estrus in dogs, ovariectomy before 2½ years of age is to be preferred over progestogen treatment with respect to the mammary tumor risk. The role of endogenous hypophyseal hormones in mammary tumorigenesis in the bitch is still controversial. In bitches with mammary tumors, neither growth hormone nor prolactin basal plasma levels were elevated when compared to age-matched controls in the same phase of the estrous cycle (Rutteman and Misdorp, 1993). On the other hand, both endogenous luteal phase progesterone and injected progestin induce growth hormone production in mammary epithelium in the dog (Selman et al., 1994). Differences in the length of time of exposure to progestins and consequently in exposure to growth hormone may be of importance in canine mammary tumorigenesis.

There is no convincing evidence that either pregnancy or lactation significantly alters the mammary tumor risk, although the risk in female dogs used extensively for breeding from an early age onward may be somewhat lower.

Steroid and peptide hormones exert many of their actions in target cells by binding to specific high-affinity binding sites (receptors). Receptors for estrogens, progestins, and prolactin have been found in nearly all specimens of histologically normal mammary tissue of female dogs as well as in a high proportion of benign mammary tumors. They were present in only about half of the primary cancers and at lower concentrations than in nonmalignant mammary tissues (Rutteman and Misdorp, 1993), indicating a loss of function of genes encoding for these receptors. This is consistent with the concept that deviations from normal control mechanisms develop progressively in malignant tumors.

It is still uncertain whether steroid hormones cause mutations, or whether they only enhance tumorigenesis by their growth-promoting effect. The available evidence indicates that steroid hormones act at an early stage in the development of tumors by increasing the number of susceptible cells. Growth may also be stimulated in cells that have undergone partial malignant transformation, but possibly to a lesser extent in fully malignant cells at a late stage of tumor development. Steroid receptor presence is infrequent in metastases of mammary cancers, which may indicate a more autonomous pattern of growth (Rutteman and Misdorp, 1993).

### Genetic Alterations

In experimental animals as well as in humans there is much evidence that genetic alterations are of major importance in the development and progression of tumors. Two types of alterations appear involved. The first includes an alteration of cellular proto-oncogenes in such a way that these become activated oncogenes. One example is that of a mutation of a gene coding for a hormone receptor that leads to the production of a truncated receptor, no longer able to bind its hormonal ligand. These truncated receptors may be constitutively active. Another example is that of a gene amplification leading to overexpression of, for example, a nuclear transcription factor such as c-*myc*.

The second type of alteration involves the loss or inactivation of a tumor-suppressor gene. Under normal circumstances, such a gene may code for control of cell division or cellular senescence. Abrogation of this function may enhance tumorigenesis. It appears that several of the genetic alterations described above are necessary before a cell turns into a tumor cell. Future research may reveal the extent to which the development and behavior of canine mammary tumors are influenced by such genetic alterations.

Gross changes in nuclear deoxyribonucleic acid (DNA) content can be determined by flow cytometry. An abnormal DNA content, or aneuploidy, has been observed in 50 to 60% of primary malignant mammary tumors and found to be related to an adverse prognosis. Some benign proliferative lesions have also been found to contain aneuploid tumor cells. Perhaps this is related to the progression towards a malignant state occasionally observed in such histologically benign lesions. DNA flow cytometry also can be used to determine the number of proliferating cells. The fraction of cells in the S phase of the cell cycle (SPF) has generally been found to be higher in malignant tumors than in benign lesions. In one study, a high SPF was found to be associated with an unfavorable outcome after surgery of mammary tumors in dogs (Hellmén et al., 1993).

## CLINICAL PRESENTATION AND DIAGNOSIS

Mammary tumors may present as a solitary mass or as multiple swellings. The caudal glands are more often affected than the cranial ones, probably because of their greater mass. Multiple lesions occur in more than half of the cases, and in the majority of dogs they represent different primary lesions (Brodey, Goldschmidt, and Roszel, 1983). Sometimes, attentive owners will present a dog with multiple small nodules of only a few millimeters in size during metestrus or after a progestin injection. Once the steroid levels decrease, such lesions may completely disappear. Purely cystic lesions also appear to be dependent upon hormonal stimulation.

Many other dogs are presented with firm nodules larger than just a few millimeters. Clinical signs of malignancy include rapid growth, noncircumscribed growth, fixation to skin and/or underlying tissues, and ulceration. The presence of more than one of these signs signifies a high risk for the presence of a malignant tumor, but their absence does not exclude malignancy. Large size may be either the result of rapid growth or merely the result of long delay before veterinary examination. Seemingly rapid growth can also occur in cystic lesions without necessarily being a grave sign. Although less common in the dog than in the cat, single or multiple soft circumscribed swellings may develop in young animals during metestrus or pregnancy or after treatment with progestogens. These are benign fibroadenomatous lesions that sometimes involve all mammary glands. They usually, but not always, disappear rapidly upon cessation of exposure to exogenous and endogenous sex steroids.

It is often impossible to differentiate between benign and malignant mammary tumors in the dog by physical examination. In some cases, cytology of fine-needle aspiration biopsies (preferably of a solid mass, not cystic fluids or secretions) may provide the diagnosis. The finding of several criteria of cellular malignancy by an experienced cytologist will result in a diagnosis of malignancy with a high predictive value. However, many histologically and clinically malignant tumors lack clear cytologic signs of malignancy and thus a conclusive cytologic diagnosis cannot be made (Allen, Prasse, and Mahaffey, 1986).

Lesions that remained indolent for a long time may suddenly change, and the delay in treatment may turn an operable condition into an inoperable one due to local invasion or metastasis. If a tumor appears to be operable, possible sites of distant metastasis should be examined. These include distant lymph nodes, including the prescapular, sternal, and deep inguinal nodes, and the lungs and other internal organs. Since metastases to other internal organs are infrequent without previous development of lung metastases, attempts to visualize these will rarely be productive if radiographic examination of the thorax does not reveal metastases in the lungs. Enlargement of deep inguinal nodes revealed by radiographic or ultrasound examination of the pelvic area may indicate the presence of metastasis. Such examinations, or lymphatic scintigraphy at highly specialized clinics, are particularly indicated in tumors with involvement of superficial inguinal nodes. In the author's experience, detectable distant metastases are unlikely with circumscribed loose-lying local tumors less than 1 cm in size, and radiographic examination is usually negative. In all other cases and also in dogs that have had previous surgery for a tumor, radiography is an essential preoperative diagnostic procedure.

Mammary tumors may be found in a lactating mammary gland that sometimes also has signs of mastitis. These circumstances may hinder the definition of the extent of the tumor. Cytologic examination of fine-needle aspiration biopsies may help to exclude the differential diagnosis of inflammatory carcinoma (see below) and sometimes will reveal bacterial infection. Systemic antibiotic therapy is indicated for the latter, and the lactation may be suppressed by bromocriptine, which inhibits prolactin secretion, in a dose of 10 $\mu$g/kg two times daily for 2 to 3 weeks. After this treatment, it is usually easier to define whether the tumor can be excised.

### Inflammatory Carcinoma

The most aggressive neoplasm in the dog is the inflammatory type of carcinoma. This tumor often involves several adjacent mammary glands and sometimes the whole mammary chain or even both chains. At physical examination, the mass is warm, erythematous, and painful. These signs are associated with the inflammatory reaction caused by massive invasive growth of tumor cells. Often the nipples are retracted in the edematous tissue. Edema may even involve the limbs at the side of the tumor. At the university clinic in Utrecht, nearly all cases of this type have been presented within 1 to 2 months after estrus or a progestin injection. Perhaps substances produced by the normal mammary epithelium have a growth-stimulatory effect on the tumor cells. Sometimes, the cytologic finding of highly anaplastic tumor cells in fine-needle aspirates may help the clinician to differentiate inflammatory carcinoma from hyperplastic/inflammatory conditions. In our experience and that of many others (Madewell and Theilen, 1987), systemic metastases are present in virtually all dogs presented with inflammatory carcinoma. Due to the rapid infiltrative and invasive nature of this type of tumor, however, nodular-type lung metastases are observed radiographically in only a minority of cases. Surgery cannot be expected to be beneficial. Responsiveness to systemic therapy, to be discussed later in this article, is very poor. Sometimes, hemorrhagic diathesis develops due to disseminated intravascular coagulation (DIC). More frequently, the presence of DIC is recognized by the finding of abnormal clotting times, fibrin split products, and thrombocytopenia. However, DIC may also develop in dogs with or without previous surgery for mammary tumors other than inflammatory carcinoma. Careful examination in such cases will often reveal metastatis to regional lymph nodes if they are still *in situ* or to distant nodes. Lung metastases may be miliary or, if larger, sometimes cannot clearly be recognized radiographically because of the obscuring effects of concurrent hemorrhage in the lungs.

### Clinical Staging

In order to provide a basis for predicting the prognosis of mammary cancers, a clinical staging system has been proposed by the World Health Organization (WHO): The TNM classification. Tumors are staged in different categories. "T" stands for tumor size and fixation, "N" for involvement of regional lymph nodes, and "M" for the presence or absence of distant metastasis, based upon, among other things, radiographic examination of the thorax. The TNM information leads to a division to four clinical stages, with local/locoregional tumor extension progressing from stages I to III and distant metastasis being categorized as stage IV (for further information, see Misdorp, 1987). The advanced stage III was found to be associated with a worse prognosis than earlier stages in one study using some modification of this staging system (see *CVT IX*, p 480). A refinement of this staging system can probably be achieved by using results of cytologic examination of needle biopsies of clinically abnormal lymph nodes, rather than by only using the finding of enlarged nodes. A firm consistency of lymph nodes may be as suggestive of metastasis as nodal enlargement, while the latter may also be caused by reactive lymphadenopathy.

In several studies, the presence of regional lymph node metastasis has been found to be associated with an adverse prognosis, either when studying survival time or time until tumor recurrence (Madewell and Theilen, 1987). In a multivariate analysis, however, Misdorp (1987) found no additional prognostic value of nodal involvement after taking into account the strongly related factor of severe infiltrative growth. Since univariate analysis unequivocally indicates a prognostic effect of nodal involvement, it is a factor that easily can and should be determined by the clinician in order to present the owner with a more accurate assessment of the prognosis. This does not mean that surgery may not be of benefit in node-positive cancer. In many dogs, removal of the tumor *en bloc* with the tumorous node will result in at least local control and sometimes even in a complete cure.

## PATHOLOGY

Histopathologic examination may provide the clinician with information on the type of tumor and the type of growth. In addition, the completeness of removal may be assessed if the entire excised specimen is submitted for examination. For a more extensive description the reader is referred to Moulton (1990) (also see *CVT IX*, p 480).

Benign proliferative lesions, including benign tumors and dysplasias, can be separated into those with and those without cellular atypia. In keeping with observations in humans, the finding in a dog of proliferative lesions with moderate cellular atypia was found to be associated with an elevated risk for development of infiltrative carcinoma in remaining mammary tissue (Gilbertson et al., 1983). The authors used the term "precancerous mastopathy" for such atypic proliferative lesions.

If severe histologic or nuclear atypia is found in a tumor without signs of infiltration through basal membranes in multiple sections, it is termed carcinoma *in situ*. Assuming that no tumor infiltration has occurred in other parts of the tumor that were not examined, this implies that the tumor cells had not yet acquired the capacity to infiltrate and metastasize.

Infiltrative adenocarcinomas can be divided into simple type (tumorous epithelium only) or complex type (tumorous epithelium and myoepithelium). A highly undifferentiated structural and cellular phenotype in which every sign of glandular organization is lost leads to the diagnosis of anaplastic carcinoma. Malignant mesenchymal tumors include fibrosarcoma, osteosarcoma, osteochondrosarcoma, or sarcoma of unspecified type. Sometimes, tumors consist of both carcinomatous and sarcomatous components. Most sarcomas only spread by a hematogenous route, in contrast to carcinomas, which rarely develop hematogenous metastasis without lymphogenous spread. The risk of tumor recurrence ranks as follows: (carcino)sarcomas and anaplastic carcinomas > simple adenocarcinomas > complex adenocarcinomas (Misdorp, 1987). The type of growth (intraductal/infiltrative/invasion of vessels) is highly correlated with completeness of excision. The type of growth further is also important with regard to risk of distant metastasis and, together with completeness of excision, is important with regard to the risk of local recurrence.

## TREATMENT

### Surgery

As stated earlier, millimeter-sized nodules in dogs detected during a period of progestin exposure may sometimes disappear once this exposure ceases. Surgical excision of affected glands or, alternatively, removal of hormonal stimulation by ovariohysterectomy is unnecessary in many cases but may prevent full neoplastic development in others.

Solid tumors or dysplasias larger than 0.5 cm are unlikely to be reversible upon cessation of hormonal stimulation. Surgery should be considered in dogs that are in good general condition (see "Definitive Surgical Treatment of Cancer," this volume, p 462). The tumors should not be fixed to underlying tissues and detectable distant metastases should be absent. Complete local excision must be deemed feasible at a safe distance from the tumor margins. A preoperative biopsy in such cases is redundant and adds unnecessary expense. In other cases, a conclusive cytologic diagnosis or a histologic diagnosis by examination of an incisional biopsy is needed before a decision can be made regarding the type of treatment.

Nodulectomy should be considered to be a diagnostic procedure rather than a possible cure. It is contraindicated in dogs with multiple lesions or a single lesion larger than 1 cm, or if any clinical sign of malignancy can be detected (also see "Mammary Tumors," this volume, p 1098).

Based on the results from diagnostic procedures described above, the clinician should decide whether it is reasonable to aim for a complete cure by surgery; that is, in lesions without signs of malignancy, or in lesions of limited extension if malignancy is likely or certain. In early-stage cancers or benign disease, radical surgery may be curative. In animals in which a long life expectancy is probable, tumor recurrence or the appearance of new primary tumors is best prevented with total chain resection. If the other chain is free of detectable nodules, it is advised to include ovariohysterectomy prior to the chain resection in the same operation. This may reduce the growth of microscopic benign lesions and also will result in atrophy of remaining mammary tissue, facilitating early detection of new tumors.

If a less radical approach is followed, there is a higher likelihood of development of new primary tumors, a risk that may be less important in older animals. In addition, nodulectomy or simple mastectomy has an increased risk of a local recurrence as compared to chain resection or block dissection if the tumor is malignant and invades lymph vessels. If a malignant tumor is present in either one of the two thoracic glands or in the caudal abdominal or inguinal gland, a block dissection does not completely eliminate the risk of a tumor recurrence in the remaining mammary glands or distant regional lymph nodes. In about 10% of dogs, lymph drainage occurs from the two cranial glands to the caudal abdominal gland or vice versa. During resection of caudal mammary glands, the superficial inguinal node is removed because of its intimate anatomic association with the mammary tissue. The axillary nodes are removed only if tumor involvement is likely or certain.

If lesions are poorly circumscribed or fixed to underlying tissues or if there is regional metastasis, the question to be weighed is whether surgery may achieve at least local control. If cytologic or histologic examination demonstrates that the tumor is malignant, local control, by performing chain resection or at least block dissection, is probably the best that can be achieved, in view of the high probability of distant metastasis. Thus, in a dog with a large ulcerating mass with lymph node involvement in one mammary chain and small circumscribed lesions in the other mammary chain, removal of the latter often may be omitted. Extreme extension in width or major fixation of the tumor to underlying tissues may make complete removal impossible, resulting in the diagnosis of locally advanced, inoperable cancer. Follow-up is advised at 1 month after surgery and then at 3-month intervals for the first year.

Apart from tumor-related features, the type of surgery may be limited by advanced age and other factors that influence life expectancy, but also the owner's expectation of the result of the surgery. Malignant tumors without overt distant metastases will have developed micrometastases in 50 to 70% of cases at the time of presentation. Tumor-related death after surgery reportedly occurs in 40 to 60% of dogs and in the majority of cases during the first 2 years.

## Adjuvant Treatment

In only 20 to 30% of human breast cancer patients, protocols using either hormonal or chemotherapy after surgery of primary disease delay recurrent disease, resulting in a significant improvement of the prognosis. Current investigations are concerned with whether very aggressive chemotherapy is more effective, but the related toxicity may preclude the use of such high-dose regimens in canine mammary cancer treatment. In veterinary practice, major improvement in the management of mammary tumors in dogs instead should come from efforts at earlier treatment. Treatment delay at present is found to average from 6 months to over a year.

If pathologic examination of malignant tumors indicates incomplete excision, the first consideration should be whether rapid reoperation may offer a beneficial perspective. If this is unlikely, radiotherapy using equipment that delivers radiation of sufficient energy may achieve or prolong local control.

If examination reveals extensive intravascular invasion by the tumor, there is not only a very high risk of local recurrence but also of distant metastasis. There is also a high risk of distant metastasis if there is regional lymph node involvement or if the tumor is of an aggressive histologic type. In these cases, systemic therapy may interfere with the development of distant metastasis, provided the treatment is effective against the tumor.

Ovariectomy and the administration of antiestrogens have been found to be effective in preventing or delaying metastatic disease in about 50% of human patients with estrogen receptor–positive breast cancer. In the few studies of the effect of ovariectomy in the dog, the development of distant metastasis was not found to be reduced. This is not surprising in view of the frequent absence of steroid receptors in mammary carcinoma metastases in the dog. Yet, adjuvant ovariectomy might reduce the subsequent development of tumors, in particular of benign tumors, in the remaining mammary tissue. The author has used an antiestrogen (tamoxifen, 0.7 mg/kg every 24 hr) for 4 to 8 weeks in ten dogs with advanced mammary cancer, but observed no measurable effect in any of these dogs (for another view, see "Mammary Tumors," this volume, p 1098).

The value of chemotherapy as an adjuvant to surgery is uncertain in canine mammary cancer, in preventing either local recurrence or distant metastasis (see *CVT X*, p 489). The efficacy in aggressive diseases such as anaplastic carcinomas with severe infiltration or vascular invasion appears to be low. Perhaps some benefit can be gained in dogs undergoing surgery for simple carcinomas of clinical stages II to III. There have been isolated reports that drugs such as Adriamycin administered as single agent or in combination with other drugs may improve disease-free survival in such animals. Carefully conducted clinical trials are needed.

Many attempts have been made to augment the activity of the immune system against cancer cells, in particular after removal of the primary tumor. An important condition is that the residual tumor mass is as small as possible. Reported benefits of systemic administration of the nonspecific immunostimulants *Corynebacterium parvum* or bacille Calmette-Guérin (BCG) were not confirmed in a large multicenter trial. Also, intratumoral injection of these vaccines did not improve postsurgical survival (Rutten et al., 1990). Activation of the tumoricidal activity of macrophages can also be produced by muramyl tripeptide phosphatidyl-ethanolamine (MTP-PE), a derivative of a fragment of the cell wall of *Mycobacterium*. Systemic administration of MTP-PE, encapsulated in liposomes in order to enhance its half-life, is presently being investigated for its efficacy as adjuvant therapy in preventing metastatic disease in canine mammary carcinoma.

## Management of Inoperable Disease

The major impediment to surgery is extensive fixation to underlying tissues. In such locally advanced mammary cancers, some dogs may benefit from radiotherapy. If there is sufficient response, surgical excision of remaining tumor may be considered. It should be recognized, however, that many such patients also have systemic dissemination of tumor that leads to symptoms in a short time.

In the author's opinion, no major improvement is to be expected from present chemotherapeutic treatment in dogs with established distant metastases. In isolated cases, there may be tumor remission during chemotherapy (see *CVT XI*, p 427).

A particularly life-threatening condition is pleural effusion due to metastatic carcinoma. Since this effusion is often partly enhanced by the inflammatory response to the cancer cells, basic supportive therapy may achieve short-term palliation. After drainage of as much as possible of the fluid, prednisolone (2 mg/kg/day for 3 days, followed by 0.5 to 1 mg/kg) may be given. There are anecdotal data on the use of chemotherapy in pleural effusion (see *CVT XI*, p 427).

## References and Suggested Reading

Allen SW, Prasse KW, and Mahaffey EA: Cytologic differentiation of benign from malignant canine mammary tumors. Vet Pathol 23:649, 1986
  *A study demonstrating the difficulty in discriminating between benign and malignant mammary tumors.*
Brodey RS, Goldschmidt MH, and Roszel JR: Canine mammary gland neoplasms. J Am Anim Hosp Assoc 19:61, 1983.
  *A review of the background, presentation, and treatment of mammary tumors.*
Dorn CR, Taylor DON, Schneider R, et al: Survey of animal neoplasms in Alameda and Contra Costa Counties, California. II. Cancer morbidity in dogs and cats from Alameda County. J Natl Cancer Inst 40:307, 1968.
  *A epidemiologic study on the cancer incidence in dogs and cats in a California area.*
Gilbertson SR, Kurzman ID, Zachrau RE, et al: Canine mammary epithelial neoplasm: Biologic implications of morphologic characteristics assessed in

232 dogs. Vet Pathol 20:127, 1983.
*A retrospective study on the relation of pathologic features in canine mammary tumors and their biological behavior after surgery.*

Hellmén E, Bergström R, Holmberg L, et al: Prognostic factors in canine mammary tumours: A multivariate study of 202 consecutive cases. Vet Pathol 30:20, 1993.
*A prospective study on the relation of clinicopathologic features, DNA-ploidy, and cell kinetics in mammary tumors and prognosis after surgery.*

Madewell BR and Theilen GH: Tumors of the mammary gland. *In* Theilen GH and Madewell BR (eds): *Veterinary Cancer Medicine*, 2nd edition. Philadelphia, Lea & Febiger, 1987, p 327.Misdorp W: The impact of pathology on the study and treatment of cancer. *In* Theilen GH and Madewell BR (eds): *Veterinary Cancer Medicine*, 2nd edition. Philadelphia, Lea & Febiger, 1987, p 53.

Moulton JE: Tumors of the mammary gland. *In* Moulton JE (ed): *Tumors in Domestic Animals*, 3rd edition. Berkeley, CA, University of California Press, 1990, p 518.

Rutteman GR and Misdorp W: Hormonal background of canine and feline mammary tumours. J Reprod Fertil. 47(suppl):483, 1993.
*A short review on the pathogenetic role of hormones and hormone receptors in canine mammary tumorigenesis.*

Rutten VPMG, Misdorp W, Gauthier A, et al: Immunological aspects of mammary tumors in dogs and cats: A survey including own studies and pertinent literature. Vet Immunol Immunopathol 26:211, 1990.
*A review on immunologic aspects of mammary tumors, with emphasis on possible treatment.*

Schneider R, Dorn CR, and Taylor DON: Factors influencing canine mammary cancer development and post-surgical survival. J Natl Cancer Inst 43: 1249, 1969.
*A retrospective case-control study on the relation of endocrine status and cause and prognosis of canine mammary tumors.*

Selman PJ, Mol JA, Rutteman GR, et al: Progestin-induced growth hormone excess in the dog originates in the mammary gland. Endocrinology (in press) 1995.
*An experimental study revealing some of the mechanisms of progestin-induced growth hormone overproduction in the female dog.*

# SYNDROMES OF HYPERGLOBULINEMIA: DIAGNOSIS AND THERAPY

ANN E. HOHENHAUS
*New York, New York*

Serum protein levels are routinely evaluated in veterinary medicine. In the normal cat or dog, albumin and globulin are present in approximately a 1:1 ratio. Pathologic states resulting in an increase in globulin concentration relative to the albumin concentration warrant further evaluation of serum proteins by cellulose acetate electrophoresis (Table 1). This article focuses on diagnosis and therapy of hyperglobulinemic states.

## INDICATIONS FOR SERUM PROTEIN ELECTROPHORESIS

Serum protein electrophoresis should be considered when there is hyperglobulinemia, or an abnormal albumin/globulin ratio (outside the laboratory's normal range of approximately 0.7 to 1.3). The albumin/globulin ratio can be abnormal if either the albumin or globulin are decreased or the globulin is elevated. Hyperalbuminemia does not occur except in states of hemoconcentration. Infrequently, a serum protein electrophoresis should be performed when the albumin/globulin ratio is normal. Examples might include pathologic fractures, osteoporosis, multifocal osteolytic lesions, malabsorption, thrombocytopenia, or hypercalcemia of unknown etiology. Discovery of a monoclonal globulin in the serum protein electrophoretic pattern dictates a differential diagnosis of numerous disorders known to be associated with a monoclonal gammopathy (Table 2).

## THE NORMAL ELECTROPHORETIC PATTERN

Serum is applied to a cellulose acetate strip, which is then placed in an electrical field. The cellulose acetate strip is stained for protein. A densitometer scans the stained areas and produces a curve consisting of four fractions: $\alpha_1$-globulin, $\alpha_2$-globulin, $\beta$-globulin, and $\gamma$-globulin (Fig. 1A). $\gamma$-Globulins, more commonly called immunoglobulins (Ig), can migrate in the $\alpha_2$-globulin, $\beta$-globulin, and $\gamma$-globulin regions. When evaluating an electrophoretic pattern, the clinician should be aware of other proteins that will migrate in the same regions as the globulins and produce an abnormal electrophoretic pattern (Kyle and Greipp, 1978).

## INTERPRETATION OF THE ABNORMAL ELECTROPHORETIC PATTERN

Abnormalities of the globulin fraction can be either polyclonal or monoclonal in origin (Fig. 1B, C, and D) The electrophoretic pattern of a polyclonal gammopathy is a broad-based peak observed in the $\beta$ or $\gamma$ region in both locations. A polyclonal gammopathy is a nonspecific finding and can occur in chronic infection, inflammation, and neoplasia.

A monoclonal gammopathy is produced by a single plasma cell line and has been associated with only a very small number of disease states in the cat and dog (Table 2). The electrophoretic pattern of a monoclonal

***Table 1.*** *Definition of Terms*

***Immunoglobulin (Antibody)***
Serum protein composed of heavy and light chains
Four classes are described in the dog and cat: IgG, IgA, IgM, and IgE
Produced by plasma cell in response to antigenic stimulation
Migrates in the $\alpha$, $\beta$, or $\gamma$ region

***Electrophoresis***
Electrical separation of charged particles based on differential migration in an electrical field

***Serum Electrophoresis***
Separates protein into albumin, $\alpha$, $\beta$, and $\gamma$ globulins
Commonly performed on cellulose acetate strips
Allows accurate measurements of serum protein fractions

***Urine Electrophoresis***
Used to confirm the presence of a light-chain proteinuria
Requires a 24-hr urine collection and concentration of urine 80–200X

***Immunoelectrophoresis***
Allows identification of monoclonal immunoglobulin as to class, IgG, IgA, IgM, IgE
Used to confirm the existence of a monoclonal gammopathy

***Gammopathy***
Abnormality of immunoglobulins

***Monoclonal gammopathy***
Excessively produced immunoglobulin with a single heavy-chain class and light-chain type
Appears in the $\alpha$, $\beta$, or $\gamma$ region
Most commonly associated with neoplasia
Can be associated with chronic infection

***Polyclonal gammopathy***
Excessively produced immunoglobulins with multiple heavy-chain class and light-chain type
Appears in the gamma region
Associated with chronic infection, inflammation
Most common gammopathy

gammopathy is recognized as a narrow spike occurring in the $\alpha_2$-, $\beta$-, or $\gamma$-globulin region. A spike is considered monoclonal if the width of the spike is less than or equal to the albumin spike.

Hemolysis results in a broad band in the $\alpha_2$-globulin region due to the migration of the haptoglobin–hemoglobin complex. The $\alpha_2$ region may contain acute-phase reactant proteins and be increased in acute inflammation. If plasma is inadvertently used for electrophoresis, a discrete band, representing fibrinogen, appears in the $\beta$ and $\gamma$ regions and in the patient with iron deficiency anemia, transferrin migrates as a band in the $\beta$ region. Bands in these regions should prompt a reevaluation of the patient and the sample.

## CLASSIFICATION OF MONOCLONAL GAMMOPATHIES

### Multiple Myeloma

In dogs, the disease most commonly associated with a monoclonal gammopathy is multiple myeloma. Multiple myeloma occurs rarely in the cat. The diagnosis of multiple myeloma requires fulfillment of two of the four following criteria:

1. Radiographic evidence of osteolytic bone lesions.
2. >10% neoplastic plasma cells in the bone marrow.

3. IgA or IgG monoclonal gammopathy.
4. Bence Jones proteinuria.

Dogs with multiple myeloma have an equal distribution of IgA and IgG monoclonal gammopathies (Matus et al., 1986). A predominance of IgG gammopathies occurs in cats. IgA gammopathy is more likely to result in hyperviscosity syndrome than IgG gammopathy, due to the propensity of IgA molecules to form dimers. Bence Jones proteinuria has a prevalence of about 30% in the cat and 40% in the dog. Osteolytic lesions or diffuse osteoporosis are uncommon in the cat, but occur in about 50% of dogs.

### Waldenström's Macroglobulinemia

Waldenström's macroglobulinemia results from the proliferation of abnormally differentiated B cells. These lymphoplasmacytoid cells represent forms intermediate between B lymphocytes and plasma cells in their level of differentiation. Excessive amounts of IgM are manufactured by the cells, frequently leading to the development of hyperviscosity syndrome.

### Plasma Cell Leukemia

Plasma cell leukemia occurs when neoplastic plasma cells escape from the bone marrow into the peripheral circulation. It is rare.

**Table 2.** *Conditions Associated With a Monoclonal Gammopathy in Veterinary Medicine*

Multiple myeloma
Waldenström's macroglobulinemia
Plasma cell leukemia
Nonsecretory myeloma
Extramedullary plasmacytoma
Monoclonal gammopathy of undetermined significance
Chronic lymphocytic leukemia
Lymphoma
Feline infectious peritonitis
Ehrlichiosis
Amyloidosis
Lymphocytic enteritis

## Nonsecretory Myeloma

Nonsecretory myeloma is a variant of multiple myeloma that does not produce a monoclonal immunoglobulin and, consequently, lacks a monoclonal gammopathy and Bence Jones proteinuria. Cases of nonsecretory myeloma demonstrate all other features of multiple myeloma.

## Extramedullary Plasmacytoma

An extramedullary plasmacytoma is a tumor mass composed of plasma cells located distant from the bone marrow. Mucocutaneous plasmacytomas have been reported in the mouth, on the feet and trunk, or in the ears of dogs (Rakich et al., 1989). Occasionally, mucocutaneous plasmacytomas occur in association with lymphoma or multiple myeloma. Extramedullary plasmacytoma of the intestinal tract can occur in both secretory and nonsecretory forms.

## Monoclonal Gammopathy of Undetermined Significance

Monoclonal gammopathy of undetermined significance is rarely reported in dogs. It is found in 3% of persons over the age of 70. In 11% of these people, the disease progresses to a monoclonal gammopathy associated with malignancy. To make this diagnosis, all other causes of monoclonal gammopathy must be excluded.

## Lymphoma

Lymphoma is a proliferation of neoplastic B or T cells within an organ; these abnormal cells form a mass lesion or replace normal tissue. Monoclonal gammopathies in this disease occur if the phenotype of the neoplastic cell is a B cell capable of secreting immu-

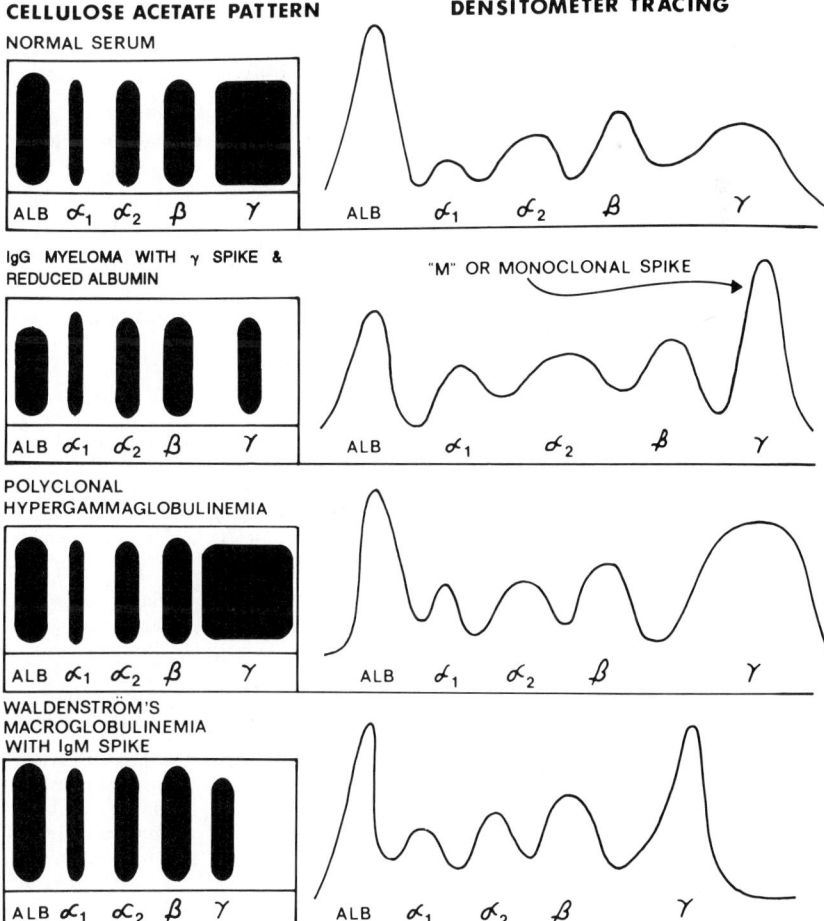

**Figure 1.** Normal and common abnormal electrophoretic patterns. (Modified from Harmenining PD: *Clinical Hematology and Fundamentals of Hemostasis.* Philadelphia, FA Davis Co, 1988, p 272, with permission.)

noglobulin. The percentage of lymphoma cases with a monoclonal gammopathy is unknown. A monoclonal gammopathy has been reported in two cats with lymphoma, one cat with feline immunodeficiency virus (FIV), and one with feline leukemia virus (FeLV).

## Chronic Lymphocytic Leukemia

Chronic lymphocytic leukemia is a tumor of well-differentiated B lymphocytes. Monoclonal gammopathies have been found in 68% of dogs with chronic lymphocytic leukemia. Bence Jones proteins have been identified in 40% of the same dogs. This disease is rarely reported in the cat (Leifer and Matus, 1986).

## Feline Infectious Peritonitis

Feline infectious peritonitis (FIP) is a fatal disease of cats caused by a coronavirus. It is frequently associated with hyperglobulinemia and occasionally associated with monoclonal gammopathies.

## Amyloidosis

This includes a heterogeneous group of disorders that may involve multiple organ systems. Immunoglobulin-associated amyloidosis has been reported in a dog with cutaneous amyloidosis and a cat with an extramedullary plasmacytoma. Both had a monoclonal gammopathy of IgG.

## Ehrlichiosis

Chronic *Ehrlichia canis* infection has been associated with a monoclonal gammopathy and hyperviscosity syndrome (Breitschwerdt et al., 1987). All cases have been reported to have a monoclonal IgG protein, and a plasmacytosis is often found in the bone marrow. Bence Jones proteins can also be identified in the urine.

## Plasmacytic Enterocolitis

One case report of a dog with plasmacytic enterocolitis and a monoclonal gammopathy has been reported. The monoclonal IgG resolved following treatment of the enteritis.

## DIAGNOSTIC EVALUATION OF PATIENTS WITH MONOCLONAL GAMMOPATHIES

The exact diagnostic plan for a patient with a monoclonal gammopathy depends on the clinical signs expressed in that particular patient. The plan can be divided into three components: (1) confirmation of the presence of a monoclonal gammopathy, (2) identification of the causative disease, and (3) establishment of the degree of organ involvement (Table 3).

## Confirmation of the Monoclonal Gammopathy

Confirmation of serum and urine monoclonal gammopathy should be done using immunoelectrophoresis. Immunoelectrophoresis identifies the class of immunoglobulin—either IgG, IgA, or IgM—which comprises the monoclonal protein. This test is essential to differentiate multiple myeloma of the IgG and IgA class from Waldenström's macroglobulinemia, which is of the IgM class. Urine immunoelectrophoresis is cumbersome in clinical practice, since it requires a 24-hr collection of urine that then must be concentrated 80 to 200 times.

Urine should be analyzed for the presence of Bence Jones proteins. Bence Jones proteins are the light chains of the immunoglobulin molecule, which are produced in excess by the plasma cell and filtered by the kidney. Urine dipsticks are sensitive to the presence of albuminuria, but insensitive to the presence of Bence Jones proteins. A special heat precipitation test must be performed to detect these proteins in the urine. Heat precipitation of Bence Jones protein is useful as a screening test, but fails to detect light chains in some cases. It may also give false-positive results in cases of renal insufficiency, connective tissue diseases, or malignancy.

Serum viscosity should be measured in patients with monoclonal gammopathies, especially those with coagulopathies, retinal hemorrhage, or neurologic signs. Hyperviscosity is usually associated with monoclonal IgM due to its large molecular weight or IgA due to the formation of dimers. Serum viscosity is measured using an Ostwald viscosimeter and usually

**Table 3.** *Evaluation of a Patient With a Monoclonal Gammopathy*

*Confirm the Presence of a Monoclonal Gammopathy*
  Immunoelectrophoresis
  Bence Jones proteins
  Urine electrophoresis
  Serum viscosity

*Define Causative Disease Process*
  Bone marrow aspiration or biopsy
  Histology
  Fluid cytology
  *Ehrlichia* titer
  Fluid electrophoresis

*Establish Degree of Organ Involvement*
  Routine thoracic and abdominal radiographs
  Survey skeletal radiographs
  Nuclear bone scan
  Serum chemistry profile
  Complete blood count
  Urinalysis

requires 5 ml of serum. Normal serum viscosity has been reported to be less than 1.8 sec in the dog. Normal relative serum viscosity values for the cat have not been published, but have been reported in two separate studies to be less than 2.5 (Hribernik et al., 1982) and less than 1.7 (Wiedenkeller and Rosenberg, 1994).

### Identification of the Causative Disease Process

Bone marrow aspiration or biopsy is indicated in all patients with monoclonal gammopathy. Bone marrow infiltration is diagnostic in many cases of multiple myeloma, macroglobulinemia, chronic lymphocytic leukemia, or lymphoma. Cases of chronic ehrlichiosis may have plasma cell hyperplasia in the bone marrow and should not be mistaken for cases of multiple myeloma. An *E. canis* titer should be obtained from dogs with a history of residing in areas where *E. canis* is endemic.

Other diagnostic tests that should be considered in patients with chronic diarrhea and monoclonal gammopathy are a barium contrast gastrointestinal study, fiberoptic endoscopy or laparotomy with multiple intestinal biopsies. Incisional or excisional biopsy of any mass or enlarged lymph node should be performed. Suspect cases of FIP may require a biopsy of the liver, omemtum, or kidney for definitive diagnosis, because of the poor correlation of elevated FIP titers with clinical disease. Correlation of pleural or peritoneal effusion levels of albumin and globulin have been suggested for use in the diagnosis of feline infectious peritonitis (Shelly, Scarlet-Kranz, and Blue, 1988). Albumin and γ-globulin percentage of total protein as determined by electrophoresis of the effusion were correlated with a diagnosis of FIP. If the γ-globulin percentage was greater than 32% and the albumin percentage less than 48%, the diagnosis was highly likely to be FIP. Albumin/γ-globulin ratios greater than 0.81 were highly predictive for ruling out a diagnosis of FIP.

### Establishment of the Degree of Organ Involvement

Patients with a monoclonal gammopathy should have a complete blood count (CBC), a differential count, and serum biochemical analysis performed. Particular attention should be directed to the serum calcium level because hypercalcemia can cause significant renal injury. It is essential that serum calcium concentration be corrected for hypoalbuminemia, since many hypergammaglobulinemic patients are also hypoalbuminemic. One formula potentially useful for correction of the calcium in dogs is:

$$\text{corrected calcium (mg/dl)} = \text{serum calcium (mg/dl)}$$
$$- \text{albumin (mg/dl)} + 3.5$$

If the corrected calcium is greater than 12.0 mg/dl, hypercalcemia is strongly suspected and an ionized calcium should be obtained. This formula is not appro-priate for use in the cat. Hypercalcemic patients may also develop azotemia due to prerenal causes (e.g., dehydration from vomiting) or to direct tubular damage.

Routine urinalysis should be obtained and include both a dipstick and sediment analysis. Hyposthenuria is expected in patients with hypercalcemia due to a calcium-induced nephrogenic diabetes insipidus. Renal tubular damage from hypercalcemia can cause cellular casts. White blood cells in the urine sediment may indicate infection and a urine culture should be submitted.

Routine thoracic and abdominal radiographs should be obtained and evaluated critically for the presence of osteoporosis or osteolytic lesions. Spinal radiographs and long-bone radiographs may be necessary to demonstrate a lytic lesion in regions associated with bone pain or neurologic deficits. Bone scintigraphy with [99m]Tc methylene diphosphonate (MDP) may also be useful to localize regions of osteolysis. Radiography or ultrasound examination should also be conducted to identify internal lymphadenopathy, hepatosplenomegaly, or an anterior mediastinal mass.

## TREATMENT AND PROGNOSIS OF DISEASES ASSOCIATED WITH MONOCLONAL GAMMOPATHIES

In addition to the standard methods for monitoring response to therapy, the presence of a monoclonal gammopathy provides the veterinary clinician with a readily obtainable method for monitoring treatment success and failure via repeated serum protein electrophoresis. Electrophoresis is a sensitive indicator of treatment success, because the size of the monoclonal spike is proportional to tumor burden. Sequential analysis of serum or urine immunoelectrophoresis should be performed approximately every 2 to 3 months. A decrease in both the total protein in the 24-hr urine collection as well as resolution of the Bence Jones proteinuria is also a good indication of treatment success.

### Multiple Myeloma/Waldenström's Macroglobulinemia

There does not appear to be any benefit in treating these diseases as separate entities. Melphalan (Alkeran, Burroughs Wellcome) and prednisone are most commonly used to treat myeloma and macroglobulinemia (Table 4). There appears to be no advantage to treating macroglobulinemia with chlorambucil over melphelan. In dogs with heavy tumor burden, cyclophosphamide (Cytoxan, Mead Johnson) can be added to the regimen on a weekly basis during the initial induction period. Doxorubicin (Adriamycin, Adria Labs) can also be used in dogs with a heavy tumor burden during induction therapy, but caution must be exercised when using cyclophosphamide or doxorubicin to avoid total marrow necrosis. Both of these agents should be considered in myeloma or macroglobulinemia resistant to prednisone

**Table 4.**  *Treatment of Canine Multiple Myeloma and Waldenström's Macroglobulinemia*

| | | | |
|---|---|---|---|
| Day 1–10 | Melphalan | 0.1 mg/kg PO | q24h |
| Day >11 | Melphalan | 0.5 mg/kg PO | q24h |
| Day 1, 8 | Cyclophosphamide | 200 mg/m² PO or IV | q24h |
| Day 1–10 | Prednisone | 15 mg/m² PO | q24h |
| Day 11–60 | Prednisone | 15 mg/m² PO | q48h |

and melphalan. The prognosis with chemotherapy alone for myeloma and macroglobulinemia is fair. Median survival is approximately 18 months, and most dogs die or are euthanized due to tumor progression or tumor-related complications. Radiation therapy can be used to treat localized myeloma lesions causing spinal cord compression and neurologic deficits. Such therapy should always be given in conjunction with chemotherapy.

Multiple myeloma and Waldenström's macroglobulinemia carry a much graver prognosis in the cat than in the dog (Wiedenkeller and Rosenberg, 1994). Cats do not respond well to the therapeutic protocol listed for the dog and survival is only 2 to 3 months in treated cats. Feline retroviral infections do not appear to be associated with multiple myeloma and macroglobulinemia and cannot be blamed for the poor survival times.

### Plasma Cell Leukemia and Nonsecretory Myeloma

These diseases can be considered a variant of multiple myeloma and should be treated as such. Because they are so uncommon, optimal therapy and prognosis are unknown.

### Extramedullary Plasmacytoma

Surgical excision appears to be curative in most cases of extramedullary plasmacytoma; however, patients should be evaluated for systemic disease as discussed above and those patients with systemic disease should be treated with chemotherapy (Table 4). In patients with a nonresectable plasmacytoma, radiation therapy is useful. The optimal therapy protocol has not been defined, but as the sole therapy, a 6-week course of 4200 to 5200 rad (42 to 52 Gy) is recommended.

### Monoclonal Gammopathy of Undetermined Significance

By definition, monoclonal gammopathy of undetermined significance requires no treatment. The patient must be monitored routinely for the development of a disease associated with monoclonal gammopathy. Periodic physical examination, CBC and differential count, serum biochemistry, and serum electrophoresis are indicated every 4 to 6 months.

### Chronic Lymphocytic Leukemia

Chronic lymphocytic leukemia is often an incidental finding observed in geriatric dogs under evaluation for unrelated problems. Not every dog with chronic lymphocytic leukemia needs treatment with antineoplastic agents. Dogs who are anemic, thrombocytopenic, or leukopenic should be treated, as well as any dog with a monoclonal gammopathy or clinical signs related to cancer. Vincristine sulfate (Oncovin, Eli Lilly), chlorambucil (Leukeran, Burroughs Wellcome), and prednisone are the drugs most commonly used in the treatment of chronic lymphocytic leukemia (Table 5). A CBC, differential cell count, and platelet count should be monitored weekly for the first month of therapy and thereafter on a monthly basis. Serum electrophoresis should be evaluated every 3 months. Median survival time of dogs treated with this protocol is 348 days (range = 30 to 1000 days).

If one of the rare cats with chronic lymphocytic leukemia is encountered, prednisone should be administered 5 mg twice daily. Prednisone may be tapered to 2.5 mg every other day if the cat develops glucocorticoid toxicity such as recurrent infections or hyperglycemia. As a rule, most cats tolerate 5 mg of prednisone twice daily extremely well. Additionally, chlorambucil should be given at 0.2 mg/kg/day. Practically speaking, cats should get one chlorambucil tablet every 2 to 4 days depending on their body weight. Dividing chlorambucil tablets is inappropriate due to the potential for exposure of owners to the antineoplastic agent.

### Lymphoma

Chemotherapy is the mainstay of lymphoma treatment. The reader is referred to other articles in this section for lymphoma chemotherapy protocols.

### Feline Infectious Peritonitis

Treatment of feline infectious peritonitis is invariably discouraging. No specific antiviral compounds are avail-

**Table 5.**  *Treatment of Canine Chronic Lymphocytic Leukemia*

| | | |
|---|---|---|
| Day 1, 8 | Vincristine | 0.7 mg/m² IV q24h |
| Day 1–7 | Chlorambucil | 0.2 mg/kg PO q24h |
| Day 8–> | Chlorambucil | 0.1 mg/kg PO q24h |
| Day 1–7 | Prednisone | 30 mg/m² PO q24h |
| Day 8–14 | Prednisone | 20 mg/m² PO q24h |
| Day 15–21 | Prednisone | 10 mg/m² PO q24h |

able and therapy consists predominantly of nursing care. The prognosis is grave.

### Ehrlichiosis

Tetracycline (22 mg/kg PO every 8 hr for 14 days) is the treatment of choice for ehrlichiosis (see "Canine Ehrlichiosis," this volume, p 290). Response is variable, especially in chronic infection with pancytopenia.

### Plasma Cell Gastroenteritis

Gastroenteritis is typically treated with prednisone and cytotoxic agents such as azathioprine and chlorambucil. Dietary management may also be beneficial. The reader is referred elsewhere in this volume for treatment protocols.

## COMPLICATIONS OF MONOCLONAL GAMMOPATHIES

### Hyperviscosity Syndrome

The major complication of monoclonal gammopathies is the hyperviscosity syndrome. Serum hyperviscosity produces signs due to increased blood viscosity resulting in coagulopathy, ocular changes, congestive heart failure, and mentation changes (Patterson, Caldwell, and Doll, 1990).

#### COAGULOPATHY

Hyperviscosity syndrome most commonly presents as a bleeding diathesis. Patients typically have ecchymoses, epistaxis, and mucosal hemorrhages. The abnormalities result from a platelet function defect due to coating of platelets with antibody. Patients may also be thrombocytopenic due to myelopthesis. Monoclonal proteins also interact with coagulation factors and act as inhibitors to coagulation.

#### OCULAR CHANGES

Retinal hemorrhage may be a result of thrombocytopenia or other coagulation defects. Congestion of retinal blood vessel contributes to the development of subretinal hemorrhage and retinal detachment. Hyperviscosity can result in papilledema and increased vascular tortuosity, which also contribute to visual disturbances.

#### CONGESTIVE HEART FAILURE

The presence of monoclonal proteins in the serum exerts an osmotic force that draws fluid into the vascular space and results in hypervolemia. Congestive heart failure may ensue.

### Treatment of Hyperviscosity Syndrome

The symptoms of hyperviscosity syndrome can be alleviated by reducing serum viscosity. To achieve a lasting effect, the underlying disease must be treated appropriately, but in cases of severe hemorrhage, altered mentation, or congestive heart failure, plasma exchange must be done. Automated plasmapheresis has been performed in cases of multiple myeloma and ehrlichiosis but is available only in referral centers. Therapeutic phlebotomy can achieve the same effect without special equipment. Blood is withdrawn from the dog at a rate of 20 ml/kg while volume is replaced at a rate of 30 ml/kg IV of crystalloid solution. The patient must be monitored for anemia and red blood cells replaced as necessary. The red blood cells can be either homologous cells from a donor dog or autologous cells obtained by centrifugation of phlebotomized whole blood (2000g for 3 min). The plasma is expressed into a satellite bag and discarded. The red blood cells are resuspended in 250 ml of 1° to 6°C 0.9% NaCl and recentrifuged (5000g for 5 min). The saline is expressed into a satellite bag and discarded. This process is repeated two additional cycles to remove the residual protein. The red cells are resuspended in enough chilled saline, approximately 100 ml, to allow easy transfusion. Phlebotomy may need to be repeated on two consecutive days to significantly decrease serum viscosity. Serum total protein levels should be measured prior to each phlebotomy.

### Azotemia

Renal failure associated with monoclonal gammopathies is a multifactorial problem, involving both the renal tubules and the glomeruli. Bence Jones proteins and hypercalcemia are principally responsible for renal tubular damage; concurrent amyloidosis of the kidney causes glomerulonephritis and albuminuria. Immunodeficiency may predispose to pyelonephritis. Renal hypoxia, due to increased serum viscosity and decreased renal perfusion, has been implicated in the pathogenesis of azotemia in cases of monoclonal gammopathies. Therapy should be directed at the underlying cause and fluids given to diurese the patient. Hypercalcemia is discussed in *CVT XI*, p 301.

### Pathologic Fractures

Severe, localized osteolysis results in pathologic fractures. When fractures occur in weight-bearing bones, the fracture must be stabilized, but will require control of the local tumor for healing to occur. Local tumor control can be accomplished using emergency "bolus" radiation therapy. Doses of 1000 rad (10 Gy) given on days 1, 8, and 15 may control localized myeloma lesions when pathologic fractures result from osteolysis. This protocol can also be used in cases of spinal cord compression from vertebral fracture or tumor mass.

## Hypercalcemia

Several mechanisms for hypercalcemia in cases of monoclonal gammopathies have been proposed. Direct osteolysis and release of calcium from bone or increased levels of humoral substances mediating calcium release such as osteoclast activating factor, tumor necrosis factor, or interleukins have been proposed as causative factors. The fluid requirements of hypercalcemic patients first should be provided using intravenous 0.9% NaCl, which also causes a calciuresis. Although furosemide can induce calciuresis, its use in the dehydrated, vomiting patient may worsen the azotemia. The use of prednisone in the undiagnosed hypercalcemic patient is likely to decrease the serum calcium concentration, but it will also make the diagnosis of lymphoproliferative disorders difficult, if not impossible, and its use in undiagnosed patients cannot be recommended. Successful diagnosis and treatment of the underlying disease will result in resolution of the hypercalcemia (also see *CVT XI*, p 301).

## Immunosuppression

Patients with a monoclonal gammopathy have defects in both cellular and humoral immunity. Any infection in these patients should be treated appropriately and aggressively based on culture results. Bactericidal antibiotics such as ampicillin, aminoglycosides, fluoroquinolones, and trimethoprim-sulfa are appropriate choices.

## References and Suggested Reading

Breitschwerdt EB, Woody BJ, Zerbe CA, et al: Monoclonal gammopathy associated with naturally occurring canine ehrlichiosis. J Vet Intern Med 1:2, 1987.
*A discussion of clinical and immunologic findings in 14 dogs with monoclonal gammopathy secondary to natural infection with* Ehrlichia canis.
Hribernik TN, Barta O, Gaunt SD, and Boudreaux MK: Serum hyperviscosity syndrome associated with IgG myeloma in a cat. J Am Vet Med Assoc 181:169, 1982.
*A case report of a feline IgG multiple myeloma.*
Kyle RA and Greipp PR: The laboratory investigation of monoclonal gammopathies. Mayo Clin Proc 53:719, 1978.
*An excellent discussion of laboratory testing of monoclonal gammopathies.*
Leifer CE and Matus RM: Chronic lymphocytic leukemia in the dog: 22 cases (1974–1984). J Am Vet Med Assoc 189:214, 1986.
*A description of clinical course, laboratory testing, and treatment in 22 dogs with chronic lymphocytic leukemia.*
Matus RE, Leifer CE, MacEwen GE, and Hurvitz AI: Prognostic factor for multiple myeloma in the dog. J Am Vet Med Assoc 188:1288, 1986.
*A description of clinical pathology, treatment, and outcome for 60 cases of canine multiple myeloma.*
Patterson WP, Caldwell CW, and Doll DC: Hyperviscosity syndromes and coagulopathies. Semin Oncol 17:210, 1990.
*A description of the usual presentations and management of the hyperviscosity syndrome.*
Rakich PM, Latimer KS, Weiss P, and Steffens WL: Mucocutaneous plasmacytomas in dogs: 75 cases (1980–1987). J Am Vet Med Assoc 194:803, 1989.
*A characterization of the histologic, clinical, and biologic features of mucocutaneous extramedullary plasmacytomas in the dog.*
Shelly SM, Scarlet-Kranz J, and Blue JT: Protein electrophoresis on effusions from cats as a diagnostic test for feline infectious peritonitis. J Am Anim Hosp Assoc 24:495, 1988.
*A statistical analysis of usage of fluid electrophoresis as a diagnostic aid in feline infectious peritonitis.*
Wiedenkeller DE and Rosenberg MP: Dysproteinemias. In August J (ed): Consultations in Feline Medicine 2. WB Saunders Co, Philadelphia, 1994, p 573.
*An extensive description of the causes and management of feline monoclonal gammopathies.*

# THE PARANEOPLASTIC DISORDERS

LESLIE E. FOX
*Gainesville, Florida*

Paraneoplastic disorders (PND) are the clinical manifestations or "remote effects" produced by a tumor at a site distant from the tumor or its metastases. The frequency of PND is undetermined. Cancer-induced alterations in host energy metabolism or cancer cachexia are probably the most common PND in veterinary and human medicine. Additionally, it is estimated that 15 to 20% of treated human cancer patients will develop a PND, exclusive of cancer cachexia, sometime during their illness, while up to 75% of patients with untreatable neoplasms will experience a PND (Bunn and Ridgway, 1993).

In human patients and small animals, PND are most frequently associated with tumors of the endocrine and hematologic systems. The best characterized of these result from the effects of uncontrolled production of a biologically active hormone normally made by the tumor's tissue of origin. For example, bilateral alopecia, polyuria/polydipsia, and polyphagia are "remote" effects of cortisol production by an adrenal gland adenoma. However, PND are more often caused by ectopic production of a biologically active hormone from a tissue not normally producing that hormone, such as antidiuretic hormone (ADH) from a lung tumor or parathormone-related proteins (PTHrP) from an anal sac apocrine gland adenocarcinoma. Even more common and less well understood are the PND caused by the elaboration of nonendocrine substances produced by the tumor or the host response to that tumor such as antibodies and growth factors, and cytokines such as prostaglandins, interleukins, and tumor necrosis factor (TNF).

The manifestations of neoplasms other than those ascribed to the tumor itself are important aids to determining diagnosis, prognosis, and effectiveness of therapy. The PND may be the only indication of the presence of a neoplasm and may be more detrimental to the patient than the neoplasm itself. For example, the PND of hypoglycemia may be more harmful and is certainly more easily detected than the presence of an insulin-secreting β-cell tumor of the pancreas. Paraneoplastic disorders may be the first sign of a neoplasm's presence, allowing early detection as well as serving as a tumor marker to assess treatment. There is little information regarding the response of paraneoplastic disorders to specific antineoplastic therapies; however, resolution of clinical signs most often parallels successful tumor eradication. Persistence of PND after

**Table 1.** *Paraneoplastic Disorders in Companion Animals*

| Paraneoplastic Disorders | Clinical Features | Associated Neoplasms in Companion Animals |
|---|---|---|
| Malignancy-associated hypercalcemia | Dehydration, depression, muscular weakness, anorexia, polydipsia/polyuria, vomiting, arrhythmias | Lymphoma (thymic, multicentric, extranodal leukemia), carcinomas (nasal, pulmonary, mammary, squamous cell, thyroid, apocrine gland of anal sac, gastric, pancreatic, testicular, parathyroid gland), thymomas, multiple myeloma, epidermoid carcinoma of the lung |
| Extrapancreatic hypoglycemia | Weakness, seizures | Hepatocellular carcinoma, hepatoma, hemangiosarcoma, leiomyosarcoma, splenic hemangiosarcoma, salivary gland adenocarcinoma, metastatic oral melanoma, mammary carcinoma, pulmonary carcinoma, plasma cell tumor, lymphocytic leukemia, renal carcinoma |
| Hyperhistaminemia, mast cell degranulation | Gastrointestinal ulceration with melena and hematemesis, urticaria, erythema, pruritus, poor wound healing, anaphylactoid reaction, hypotension/arrhythmias, altered coagulation | Mast cell tumor |
| Cancer anorexia/cachexia syndrome | Weight loss >5–10% BW kg, anorexia >2–3 days' duration, early satiety | Any tumors |
| Syndrome of inappropriate antidiuretic hormone secretion | Hyponatremia, polydipsia/polyuria, edema | Pulmonary carcinoma (dog) |
| Fever | Persistent pyrexia >39.7°C (103°F) without infection | Lympho- and myeloproliferative, neoplasms, mast cell, hepatic, and brain tumors |
| Polycythemia | Exercise intolerance, seizures, red mucous membranes, PCV >60 | Renal tumors, lymphoma, polycythemia vera, hepatic tumors |
| Hypertrophic osteopathy | Hypertrophic osteopathy, painful swollen limbs, reluctance to walk | Primary lung tumors, rhabdomyosarcoma (bladder), esophageal sarcomas, pulmonary metastatis, carcinoma, renal carcinomas, hepatic adenocarcinoma, pulmonary carcinoma, and renal papillary adenoma (cat) |
| Dermatologic disorders | Nodular, dermatofibrosis, erythema, flushing, necrolytic migratory erythema | Renal cystadenocarcinoma, mast cell tumor, pheochromocytoma, pancreatic adenocarcinoma |
| Renal disorders | Amyloid deposition, glomerulonephritis, concentrating defects, proteinuria, nephrotic syndrome | Many tumors, lymphoma, plasma cell tumors, mast cell tumors |
| Nervous system disorders | | |
| Central nervous system | Hyperviscosity syndrome (seizures, dementia) | Lymphoma, plasma cell tumors |
| Peripheral nervous system Neuromuscular junction | Myasthenia gravis (weakness with exercise that improves with rest) | Thymoma, hepatocellular carcinoma, osteosarcoma, mammary adenocarcinoma, pheochromocytoma, pulmonary adenocarcinoma |
| Neuropathy | Weakness, cranial nerve abnormalities | Lymphoma, bronchogenic carcinoma, insulinoma, leiomyosarcoma, hemangiosarcoma, and undifferentiated sarcomas |
| Neuromyopathy | Weakness, muscle pain, proprioception deficits | Pulmonary carcinoma |
| Myopathy | Myositis | Thymoma |

clinical remission may indicate that metastatic disease persists. Likewise, recrudescence of a paraneoplastic disorder often parallels tumor recurrence even before direct visualization of that tumor is possible.

The PND associated with the unregulated production of polypeptide hormones includes endocrine tumors of the pituitary, adrenal, pancreas, gastrointestinal tract, testicles, and ovaries. These have been reviewed and will not be discussed (Wheeler, 1989).

## ECTOPIC HORMONE/CYTOKINE PRODUCTION

### Hypercalcemia

Malignancy-associated hypercalcemia (MAHC) is defined as a persistent pathologic increase in serum total calcium concentration greater than 12 mg/dl. Up to 40% of human cancer patients will experience hypercalcemia at some time during the course of their disease (Rosol and Capen, 1992). Malignancy-associated hypercalcemia in humans is most commonly observed with tumors of the urinary tract, multiple myeloma, and small cell lung carcinomas. Although uncommon in the cat, as many as 25% of dogs with lymphoma (usually multicentric or mediastinal), 33 to 100% of dogs with anal sac apocrine gland adenocarcinoma, and 17% of dogs with multiple myeloma have MAHC (Chew, Nagoda, and Carothers, 1992). In human patients with lymphoma, hypercalcemia is associated with decreased survival; however, in dogs with lymphoma hypercalcemia has not been associated with shortened survival in most studies.

Common clinical signs of hypercalcemia in the dog include anorexia, weight loss, polyuria with compensatory polydipsia, dehydration with central nervous system (CNS) depression, and generalized weakness. Bradycardia, arrhythmias, vomiting, and constipation are observed less frequently. Cats show anorexia, vomiting, weight loss, and dehydration with or without polyuria/polydipsia.

Osteoclastic bone resorption is usually the source of increased serum calcium, although increased renal tubular reabsorption and intestinal absorption contribute. The primary stimulus for MAHC osteoclastic bone resorption in humans, and probably in dogs, appears to be humoral; however, local release of bone reabsorption stimuli from metastatic cancer cells also contributes. Locally released and blood-borne factors include parathyroid hormone, parathyroid hormone-related protein (PTHrP), cytokines (interleukin-1 [IL-1], interleukin-4 [IL-4], interleukin-6 [IL-6], TNF-$\alpha$, TNF-$\beta$, osteoclast activating factor, D-factor, tumor necrosis factors $\alpha$ and $\beta$, or leukemia inhibitory factor), transforming growth factors (TGF-$\alpha$, TGF-$\beta$), calcitriol, 1,25-dihydroxyvitamin D, granulocyte monocyte colony-stimulating factor (GM-CSF), and prostaglandins such as prostaglandin $E_{2M}$ ($PGE_{2M}$). Tumor-produced PTHrP and other humoral factors bind to receptors on osteoblasts, which in turn stimulate bone resorption by osteoclasts at lo-

cations other than the tumor's location. PTHrP also increases renal reabsorption and promotes intestinal absorption of calcium.

Humoral factors have been determined in dogs with MAHC. Serum PTHrP concentration in dogs with anal sac apocrine gland adenocarcinoma, lymphoma, and various carcinomas was increased when compared to non–tumor-bearing dogs, whereas serum 1,25-$(OH)_2$D levels were usually normal to decreased, and PTH was normal (Peterson et al., 1992). The magnitude of hypercalcemia was linearly correlated to PTHrP activity in dogs with anal sac apocrine gland adenocarcinoma, but not in dogs with lymphoma, suggesting additional mechanisms for MAHC.

Although often compounded by a humorally directed increase in serum calcium, MAHC is observed in association with neoplasms that have locally mediated osteolysis. In dogs, such tumors include bone metastasis (mammary and prostate carcinomas) and plasma cell tumors. Additionally, in dogs with lymphoma and bone marrow involvement, hypercalcemia results from tumor-directed bone reabsorption secondary to local elaboration of $PGE_{2M}$.

Ablation of the tumor is the best way to ameliorate MAHC. Because dehydration stimulates renal reabsorption of calcium with sodium, rehydration with 0.9% NaCl and repeat measurement of serum calcium should be performed before diagnosing hypercalcemia. Death from hypercalcemia is uncommon in companion animals; thus, expansion of the extracellular volume with normal saline infused over 12 to 24 hr and replacement of other electrolytes is recommended before administering other therapy. After rehydration, normal saline diuresis and loop diuretics will enhance renal excretion of calcium. Glucocorticoid are frequently recommended as treatment for MAHC in veterinary patients. Despite cytotoxicity for lymphoid and monocytoid cells, glucocorticoids have been generally ineffective for MAHC in human patients with solid tumors, including primary parathyroid tumors. Malignancy-associated hypercalcemia from hypervitaminosis D will diminish in response to glucocorticoid therapy, because they are most effective as inhibitors of the action of vitamin D. Unfortunately, serum 1,25-$(OH)_2$D levels have been shown to be low in most human and some canine malignancies.

The routine treatment of MAHC involves resolving the primary disease and the use of additional serum calcium-lowering agents such as biphosphonates, plicamycin, gallium nitrate, and calcitonin. These are discussed in *CVT X*, p 988 and *CVT XI*, p 301.

### Hypoglycemia

Hypoglycemia is defined as a fasting blood glucose concentration of less than 70 mg/dl. Paraneoplastic hypoglycemia is usually observed with pancreatic islet cell tumors and some extrapancreatic tumors. The most common cause of cancer-associated hypoglycemia in humans, dogs, and probably cats is hyperinsulinemia from a pancreatic β-cell tumor. The diagnosis and treatment of insulinomas are discussed in *CVT XI*, p 386. Extrapancreatic tumor hypoglycemia (EPHG) is uncommon. In human patients, 60% of extrapancreatic tumors producing hypoglycemia are mesenchymal in origin, whereas in dogs, hepatic tumors (hepatocellular carcinoma and lymphoma) are more common.

Animals with EPHG usually show a constellation of clinical signs referable to the nervous system, because 60% of blood glucose is used by that system. These signs include generalized or hind limb weakness, seizures, behavior changes, focal neurologic abnormalities, collapse, and coma. Tachycardia, hunger, vomiting, and nervousness are signs attributed to compensatory adrenergic effects associated with increased concentrations of plasma catecholamines. Clinical signs are usually observed at blood glucose concentrations of less than 40 to 45 mg/dl, but rapid decline is associated with the more severe clinical abnormalities.

Proposed mechanisms for EPHG in human patients include the following:

1. Tumor production of "big" insulin-like growth factor II ("big" IGF-II) resulting in increased peripheral glucose consumption. Insulin-like growth factors I and II (formerly called somatomedin C) are produced by a variety of tissues. They share extensive amino acid homology with proinsulin and similar activities with insulin. "Big" IGF-II is an abnormally large, tumor-produced form of IGF-II (approximately 12 to 15 kd) (Macauley, 1992).

2. Excessive consumption of glucose by the tumor, particularly hepatic tumors.

3. Increased peripheral glucose utilization as a result of ectopic insulin production, increase in number of insulin receptors, altered binding of insulin, stimulation of insulin release by unknown protein, or binding of insulin by paraproteins.

4. Tumor production of a suppressive factor that either inhibits glucagon release or inhibits glycogenolysis or gluconeogenesis.

5. Destruction of sufficient liver by tumor or metastasis to result in a decrease in glucose.

The most common cause of EPHG is production of an IGF by the tumor. Normally, growth factors IGF-I and -II bind to cell surface IGF receptors, stimulating cell growth and also cross-reacting with the human insulin receptor, resulting in anabolic effects on muscle, adipose tissue, and liver. In human patients, most non–islet cell tumors have elevated levels of abnormal IGF-II mRNA, resulting in high circulating blood levels of immunoreactive "big" IGF-II and normal to low IGF-II levels and decreased growth hormone, insulin, and IGF-I. It has been postulated that "big" IGF-II stimulates glucose uptake by muscle and fat and suppresses hepatic response to hypoglycemia via a negative feedback effect on growth hormone secretion. The degree of hypoglycemia does not always correlate with the concentration of circulating "big" IGF-II, because altered carrier protein binding allows better tissue penetration and enhanced activity (Macauley, 1992).

Complete tumor resection results in resolution of paraneoplastic clinical signs and normalization of blood glucose concentrations. However, large size, unusual tumor location, or presence of metastasis frequently prevent surgical removal, and medical management is required to control hypoglycemia. Extrapancreatic hypoglycemia is rare in humans and animals; therefore, treatment beyond surgical resection is seldom reported. Frequent feedings alone may control clinical signs for many of the patients with EPHG. Oral Karo syrup (0.5 to 1.0 ml/kg PO) or 50% dextrose (1.0 ml/kg IV) is recommended for emergency hypoglycemic crises to be maintained with a 5% dextrose solution infusion. However, to ensure a more consistent blood glucose concentration, the patient should be frequently fed a diet high in complex carbohydrates. Normoglycemia can be achieved by increasing hepatic gluconeogenesis and diminishing peripheral tissue glucose utilization with low-dose glucocorticoids. Drugs traditionally used to increase blood glucose by lowering blood insulin activity, such as diazoxide, are unlikely to be of much value in the treatment of EPHG. In a few case reports, growth hormone or continuous intravenous glucagon infusion led to improvement in human patients with "big" IGF-II EPHG.

## Hyperhistaminemia

Paraneoplastic disease associated with mast cell tumors (MCT) is more common in dogs than other species. Most clinical signs are referable to the elaboration of mast cell granule constituents, particularly histamine, heparin, and proteolytic enzymes. Histamine binds to $H_1$ and $H_2$ receptors, which are ubiquitous in the body. Binding of histamine to gastric mucosal parietal $H_2$ receptors results in hyperacidity; increased mucosal blood flow; edema; and subsequent ulceration, melena, hematemesis, and abdominal pain. In one study, more than 80% of necropsied dogs with MCT had gastric ulceration (Howard, Sawa, and Nielsen, 1969). Spontaneous local release of granule contents leads to edema, erythema, hemorrhage, and pruritus with and without physical manipulation of the tumor. Massive systemic release of histamine, associated with rapid cell kill after hyperthermia or cryosurgery, may induce life-threatening cardiopulmonary effects including hypotension ($H_1$- and $H_2$-receptor binding), arrhythmias ($H_1$- and $H_2$-receptor binding), and bronchospasm ($H_1$-receptor binding). Both histamine binding to macrophage $H_1$ and $H_2$ receptors causing the production of fibroblast suppressor factor (which delays fibroplasia), and proteolytic enzymes released from cells that remain in surgical margins, impair wound healing. Tumor-associated systemic heparin release results in prolonged coagulation times, whereas local heparin release can cause prolonged postoperative bleeding, particularly with larger tumors (3 to 10 cm).

Wide surgical excision is the treatment of choice for resolution of clinical effects of hyperhistaminemia. Pretreatment with an $H_1$ blocker (diphenhydramine; Benadryl, Parke-Davis; 1.0 mg/kg IM) and H₂ blockers cimetidine (Tagamet, SmithKline Beecham; 5 mg/kg every 8 hr) or ranitidine (Zantac, Glaxo; 2 mg/kg every 12 hr) before surgical excision can prevent hypotension and adverse cardiopulmonary effects. Histamine 1 and H₂ blockers may be administered until suture removal to aid in wound healing. Specific therapy for gastro-duodenal ulceration is discussed in detail in *CVT X*, p 911 (also see "Gastrointestinal Ulcer Therapy," this volume, p 706).

## Cancer Cachexia

Cancer results in profound host energy imbalances. Malnutrition associated with neoplasia produces the PND called cancer cachexia. Clinical abnormalities include hypophagia/anorexia, involuntary weight loss, muscle weakness, skeletal muscle and organ atrophy, anemia, glucose intolerance, hypoglycemia, hyperinsulinemia, hyperlactic acidemia, hypoproteinemia, hypertriglyceridemia, and hyperlipemia. No consistent relationship in humans has been observed between cancer cachexia and the duration of clinical illness, clinical stage, tumor location, or histology. However, weight loss is more severe in patients with gastrointestinal malignancies.

The overall prevalence of clinically observable cancer cachexia is difficult to determine in human and veterinary patients, but it is estimated that progressive, relentless tissue wasting results in death of two thirds of human cancer patients. Regardless of treatment type, patients with greater than 6% body weight loss have shorter survival times (Sigal and Daly, 1992). Most tumor-bearing veterinary patients show chronic wasting illness terminally, and evidence of detrimental cancer-associated metabolic alterations have been demonstrated in both dogs and cats.

Major factors contributing to the development of chronic wasting include decreased nutritional intake, inappropriate energy expenditure, and abnormal substrate metabolism. Cancer-associated hypophagia progressing to anorexia may be a result of altered taste perception, early satiety, chronic nausea, feeding-associated hyperthermia, and direct interference with prehension and swallowing. An excellent discussion of anorexia is found in *CVT X*, p 18.

Although inappetence probably contributes most significantly to malignant cachexia, abnormal substrate metabolism precedes tumor detection and measurable weight loss. Human and experimental animal studies have shown that tumors compete with the host for necessary nutrients, at first imperceptibly, and then with obvious tissue wasting. The preferred substrate for tumor cell metabolism is glucose. Inefficient metabolism of glucose to lactate via anaerobic glycolysis meets tumor cell energy needs at a cost of 20% of the host's energy requirements. By altering the metabolic efficiency of the host cells, tumors direct host fat and muscle depletion. Alterations in host glucose metabolism include increased gluconeogenesis from lactate, amino

acids and recycling of glucose, uncoupling of respiration and oxidative phosphorylation, and insulin resistance. Host protein metabolism is deranged, resulting in increased skeletal muscle protein degradation, reduced skeletal muscle synthesis, increased total body protein turnover, and increased liver protein synthesis. Alterations in lipid mobilization include increased serum free fatty acids and glycerol turnover, decreased lipogenesis, and decreased endothelial lipoprotein lipase activity. Most of these alterations have been reported in cancer-bearing dogs (Ogilvie, 1993).

Resting energy expenditure (REE) is altered and nonadaptive in human patients and dogs. Hypermetabolism, eumetabolism, and hypometabolism have been reported with similar frequency in tumor-bearing patients both with and without weight loss. In humans, hypermetabolism is associated with gastric tumors and soft tissue sarcomas. Alteration in REE resolves with successful extirpation of the tumor. Dogs with lymphoma have normal REE but decreased REE after remission with chemotherapy, suggesting that normal REE may actually represent maladaption to malignancy-induced alterations in carbohydrate, lipid, and protein metabolism (Ogilvie et al., 1993). See *CVT XI*, p 433 for a more detailed discussion of metabolic alterations in dogs with cancer cachexia. See *CVT XI*, p 438 for a discussion of cancer cachexia in cats.

The cause of malignancy-associated cachexia is multifactorial, involving both tumor-produced products and tumor-orchestrated host responses. Hormones and cytokines produced by the host and the tumor such as TNF-α, IL-1, IL-6, interferon-γ, and D-factor have been implicated (Sigal and Daly, 1992).

Anorexia and cachexia have numerous effects on the cancer-bearing animal. Limited immunologic antitumor response, decreased cell-mediated immunity, delayed wound healing, decreased responses to therapy, and increased antineoplastic therapy toxicity are frequently observed. Although in animal tumor models, oral and parenteral nutrition can significantly stimulate tumor cell proliferation and distant metastasis, clinically, increased antitumor response and decreased toxicity have been demonstrated with improved nutrition in human studies.

Nutritional support is often delayed until dogs and cats have been inappetent for weeks and/or weight loss is severe. Because tumor-directed metabolic derangements are present prior to visualization of the tumor and may persist during clinical remission, nutritional support of the cancer patient is important. Determining when a patient needs improved nutrition may be difficult. An animal that is unable to consume 75 to 80% of its daily caloric requirements needs additional nutritional support in the form of enteral, or possibly parenteral, feeding. Force-feeding, intermittent orogastric tube feeding, pharyngostomy, nasogastric or enterostomy tube feeding, and total parenteral nutrition are valuable techniques for providing short-term (a few days) nutrition if antineoplastic therapy is forthcoming. However, for supplemental nutrition lasting longer than a few days or for the animal that is unable to meet nutritional requirements at home, percutaneous gastrostomy tube placement is the simplest, safest, most practical approach. See *CVT X*, p 30 for a discussion of enteral nutrition. See *CVT X*, p 25 for management of parenteral feeding. See *CVT XI*, p 32 for a discussion of the use of nasogastric tubes. See *CVT XI*, p 117 and this volume, p 669, for a discussion of nutritional management of the critical care patient, including gastrostomy tube placement.

Anorexia for more than 72 hr is an indication for exogenous appetite stimulation in cats and dogs. Treatment of hypophagia/anorexia is difficult and requires increasing food palatability and administration of pharmacologic agents that consistently promote appetite. Short-term appetite stimulants such as the benzodiazepams or cyproheptadine (cats only) are unlikely to result in adequate food intake by the cancer patient. Use of human recombinant interferon-α improves appetite and quality of life in feline leukemia virus (FeLV) –positive cats with lymphoma. A more detailed discussion of anorexia may be found in *CVT X*, p 19 (Weiss, Cummins, and Richards, 1991).

Weight loss of greater than 5 to 10% of body weight indicates inadequate nutritional intake. Glucocorticoids and the anabolic steroids nandrolone decanoate (DecaDurabolin, Organon Pharmaceuticals, up to 1–5 mg/kg weekly to maximum of 200 mg total dose for dogs) and stanozolol (Winstrol, Winthrop-Breon, 1–2 mg orally q12h or 25–50 mg IM, weekly per dogs) have been recommended to stimulate appetite and weight gain in human and veterinary patients. In humans, corticosteroids and cyproheptadine improve quality of life and appetite without weight gain or improvement in survival. Megestrol acetate will improve appetite and food intake, increase body weight from fat, and decrease nausea and vomiting for patients with advanced cancer (Bruera, 1991). Effects of megestrol acetate on long-term survival have not been evaluated. Adverse effects in cats such as diabetes mellitus, adrenal suppression, and mammary neoplasia may limit long-term use of megestrol acetate for weight gain.

Energy requirements are difficult to determine for the tumor-bearing veterinary patient, because they may be increased, decreased, or comparable to normal animals. Late in the progression of neoplasia when weight loss is severe or during aggressive antineoplastic therapy, energy requirements are probably higher than non–tumor-bearing animals. In contrast, energy requirements early in the course of the disease may be less than that of normal animals. A guideline for maintaining an animal nutritionally is to estimate the resting energy needs at 1500 kcal/m$^2$/day or 132 × BW$_{kg}^{0.75}$ kcal/day for dogs and 200 to 300 kcal/cat/day for the cat (Hill, 1993). If severely catabolic, the resting energy needs should be multiplied by a factor of 1.5.

Specific therapeutic implications from studies of metabolism in canine lymphoma patients suggest that use of lactate- or dextrose-containing fluids should be avoided. Additionally, diets high in simple carbohydrates may exacerbate lactate to glucose conversion at great expense to the dogs with cancer cachexia. High-biologic-value protein should be fed to animals with lymphoma. Because most weight loss in cancer cachexia is due to loss of body fat and fat is a poor substrate for tumor energy, diets containing 30 to 50% nonprotein calories as fat have been associated with improvement in body weight (Ogilvie, 1993).

## Fever

Pyrogens are frequently released directly from tumors and by stimulated macrophages and lymphocytes. Sepsis is a far more common cause of fever in humans and animals with neoplasms than true paraneoplastic fever, thus a thorough search for septicemia is required prior to use of antipyretics (see "Septic Shock", this volume, p 137). Among other mediators, IL-6 and IL-1 have been implicated as factors in malignancy-associated fever.

## Other Ectopic Hormone Syndromes

Ectopic ADH secretion is usually associated with small cell lung cancers in human patients, but has been infrequently reported in the dog. A PND in dogs called the syndrome of inappropriate ADH secretions (SIADH) has been associated with undifferentiated carcinoma and meningeal sarcomas. Clinical abnormalities include urine hyperosmolality relative to plasma hypo-osmolality, normal renal and adrenal function, and natriuresis despite plasma hypo-osmolality and hyponatremia. In people, neurologic signs predominate and include dementia, seizures, and coma. Effective management includes eradication of the tumor and correction of electrolyte and water imbalances.

## HEMATOLOGIC/HEMOSTATIC PARANEOPLASTIC DISORDERS (SEE TABLE 2)

### Anemia

#### ANEMIA OF CHRONIC DISEASE

Anemia is the most common hematologic abnormality associated with cancer in humans and animals. Sometime during the course of their disease, over one half of human patients become anemic. Anemia of chronic disease (ACD) or malignancy-associated anemia is related to decreased red cell survival and is neither due to crowding out of bone marrow precursors with tumor cells nor related to tumor size or the presence of metastasis. It is characterized by a mild to moderate normocytic, normochromic, nonregenerative anemia with normal bone marrow cellularity. Red blood cell survival is usually decreased from 120 days to 60 to 90 days in humans. The cause of increased red cell destruction is unknown; erythrocyte injury resulting from abnormal tumor vasculature, inflammation, or immune-complex or immunoglobulin adherence results in

**Table 2.** *Hematologic/Hemostatic Manifestations of Malignancy*

| Abnormality | Associated Tumor in Small Animals |
|---|---|
| **Thrombocytopenia** | |
|   Decreased production by bone marrow | Lymphoproliferative, myeloproliferative, metastatic tumor, disseminated mast cell tumor, granulosa cell tumors, Sertoli cell tumors |
|   Increased sequestration by spleen and liver | Mast cell tumor, lymphoma, hemangioma/hemangiosarcoma |
|   Increased utilization in tumor-associated hemorrhage or DIC | Large tumors, hemangiosarcomas |
|   Increased destruction by immune-mediated mechanisms | Lympho- and myeloproliferative, mast cell tumor, mammary and nasal adenocarcinomas, fibrosarcoma, other solid tumors |
| **Thrombopathies** | |
|   Defects of adhesion | Plasma cell tumors, lymphoma, polycythemia vera |
|   Acquired von Willebrand's disease | Myeloproliferative neoplasms, plasma cell tumors, and lymphoid leukemias for both |
|   Defects of aggregation and release | |
| **Anemia** | |
|   Anemia of chronic disease | Many tumors |
|   Microangiopathic hemolytic anemia | Hemangiosarcoma, metastatic neoplasms, hepatic tumors |
|   Immune-mediated hemolytic anemia | Hemolymphatic tumors and others |
| **Polycythemia** | Renal and hepatic tumors |
| **Thrombocytosis** | Osteogenic sarcoma, metastatic squamous cell carcinoma, gingival carcinoma, lymphoma |
| **Leukocyte abnormalities** | |
|   Neutrophilia/leukemoid reaction | Lympho- and myeloproliferative |
|   Neutropenia | Not reported in dog or cat |
|   Eosinophilia | Lymphoproliferative, mast cell tumors, carcinomas |
| **Pancytopenia** | |
|   Myelophthisis | Acute myeloproliferative disease, myeloma, lymphoma, many tumors |
|   Hyperestrogenism | Sertoli cell tumor, granulosa cell tumors |
| **Coagulation factor abnormalities** | |
|   Dysfunction, heparinemia | Mast cell tumors |
|   Deficiency V, prekallikrein | Carcinomas |
|   Inhibition | Not reported in small animals |
|   Abnormal structure | Not reported in small animals |
|   Hyperproteinemia | Plasma cell tumor, lymphoma, lymphocytic leukemia, nonmyelomatous tumors |
|   Disseminated intravascular coagulation | Hemangiosarcoma, thyroid carcinoma, inflammatory carcinoma, many tumors, myeloproliferative disease |
| **Vessel abnormalities** | |
|   Vasculitis | Any tumor, lymphoproliferative |
|   Incomplete endothelialization | Large tumors, hemangiosarcoma |

rapid clearing of red blood cells by the reticuloendothelial system in ACD.

Decreased red cell survival time coupled with inadequate bone marrow response result in ACD (Johnson and Roodman, 1989). Sufficient erythropoietin and usable iron are required for an appropriate response to a demand for increased red cell production. Erythropoietin levels are usually normal when assessed by radioimmunoassay, but it is possible that the endogenous erythropoietin response is inadequate for the degree of anemia. The red cell regenerative response is also affected by inflammation-activated macrophages that elaborate cytokines including interferons-$\alpha$, -$\beta$ and -$\gamma$, and TNF-$\alpha$ which are involved in the suppression of erythroid colony formation. Thus, decreased erythroid progenitor cells are available to respond to erythropoietin even if levels are adequate or increased.

Another contribution to poor bone marrow response in ACD is abnormal iron metabolism including decreased serum iron, transferrin, and intestinal iron absorption, and increased serum ferritin and iron storage. During inflammation, lactoferrin, released by neutrophils, complexes to iron, is phagocytized by macrophages, and prevents erythroid precursors from obtaining iron. Additionally, activated macrophages produce IL-1 and TNF, which result in the production of the acute-phase protein, apoferritin. Apoferritin decreases serum iron and increases macrophage sequestered iron. Administration of TNF also causes reduction in red cell count and serum iron, increased storage iron, and impaired reticulocyte production with increased erythropoietin.

Specific treatment is seldom required because animals with ACD are usually asymptomatic; however, erythropoietin supplementation may be valuable in the treatment of symptomatic cancer-associated ACD (see *CVT XI*, p 484).

### RED CELL APLASIA

A severe nonregenerative anemia without erythroid bone marrow precursors is called pure red cell aplasia. It is uncommon and, in human patients, is usually seen in association with thymomas. It has not yet been reported in dogs with thymomas. In humans, most aplastic anemias are caused by autoantibody to early red cell progenitors. However, antierythropoietin antibodies and T-cell suppression have also been reported. Approximately 25% of malignancy-associated aplastic anemias respond to resection of the tumor, suggesting persistence of immune dysfunction (Johnson and Roodman, 1989).

### MYELOPHTHISIS

Myelophthisis, or bone marrow infiltration by tumor cells, is usually a late complication of cancer. In human cancer patients, it is observed most frequently with advanced gastric, prostate, and breast carcinomas. Myelophthisis can result in pancytopenia, leukoerythroblastosis, myelofibrosis, or leukemoid reaction. These effects are not due to tumor cells crowding the bone marrow, but are more likely due to the local production of myelosuppressive cytokines and competition for nutrients. Leukoerythroblastosis has been reported in dogs and cats with stage V lymphoma and acute myelogeneous leukemia. Treatment is aimed at controlling the primary disease. The use of recombinant human erythropoietin in the treatment of anemia associated with multiple myeloma-induced myelophthisis has brought promising results in human patients.

### IMMUNE-MEDIATED HEMOLYTIC ANEMIA

Immune-mediated hemolytic anemia (IMHA) is observed in up to 45% of human patients with selected hematologic malignancies and solid tumors (Johnson and Roodman, 1989). In the dog and the cat, IMHA is usually associated with lymphoid neoplasms, generally those with bone marrow involvement, and may be the only indication of malignant disease. It is also associated with solid tumors and can be observed with thrombocytopenia (Evans' syndrome).

Clinical signs of IMHA include anorexia and lethargy, pale mucous membranes, icterus, hepatosplenomegaly, and hemoglobinuria. Anemia is usually mild to moderate and regenerative with reticulocytosis. Warm reacting IgG is the involved antibody and the direct antiglobulin (Coombs') test is usually positive.

A postulated mechanism of IMHA is a tumor-directed alteration in host immunoregulation. Eradi-

cation of the primary tumor is the key to management of tumor-associated AIHA. Short-term control with a corticosteroid and cyclophosphamide may be achieved, but response is temporary until the inciting cause has been removed. Splenectomy has been used in some humans if primary treatment fails (see "Approach to the Anemic Patient," this volume, p 447).

### MICROANGIOPATHIC HEMOLYTIC ANEMIA

Microangiopathic hemolytic anemia (MAHA) is uncommon in animals and people and is associated with diseases of small blood vessels. Red cell fragmentation, particularly schistocytosis, is observed with or without anemia or thrombocytopenia. Abnormal red cell shape, hemolysis, and fragmented platelets result from intravascular shearing due to fibrin strands from low-grade disseminated intravascular coagulation (DIC), abnormal tumor vasculature with fibrin deposition, or intimal proliferation in the pulmonary vasculature in response to tumor emboli. In human patients, carcinomas most frequently cause MAHA, with gastric (>50%), breast, and prostate tumors being common (Antman et al., 1979). In the dog, hemangiosarcoma is the neoplasm most commonly associated with MAHA. In one study, 50% of dogs with visceral hemangiosarcoma had microangiopathic hemolysis and 12% had MAHA without evidence of DIC (Hammer et al., 1991). Approximately 15% of dogs with other neoplasms including lymphoma, carcinomas, soft tissue sarcomas, and osteosarcomas had evidence of red blood cell fragmentation (Madewell, Feldman, and O'Neill, 1980). Excision of the primary tumor is the recommended treatment.

## Polycythemia

Polycythemia is rarely diagnosed in human and canine cancer patients. In people, renal tumors account for greater than 50% of tumor-associated polycythemia, whereas hepatocellular carcinomas account for 25% (Hammond and Winnick, 1974). In the dog, primary and secondary renal tumors account for most of the reported cases. Ectopic erythropoietin production by the tumor has been documented in both humans and dogs, although increased production of erythropoietin by compression-induced hypoxic renal and hepatic tissues may also be possible. Clinical signs are a result of hyperviscosity, vessel dilation and impaired blood flow, tissue hypoxia, hemorrhage, and thrombosis. In humans, most cases of tumor-associated polycythemia have resolved after resection of the neoplasm. If complete tumor removal is not possible, reduction of the hematocrit to less than 55% by periodic phlebotomy and fluid volume replacement should alleviate clinical signs.

## Pancytopenia

Pancytopenia is observed most often with estrogen-secreting tumors. Bone marrow aplasia that is often irreversible is common with Sertoli cell tumors of the canine testes and granulosa tumors of the ovary of the bitch and queen. Recent evidence suggests that estrogen-induced production of a myelopoiesis-inhibitory factor (MIF) by canine thymic stromal cells inhibits granulocyte-macrophage progenitor cell growth and may therefore lead to pancytopenia (Farris and Benjamin, 1993). Bone marrow recovery is often impossible. (See *CVT IX*, p 495, *CVT X*, p 479, and "Leukocyte Disorders and Their Treatment," this volume, p 452 for discussions of management of pancytopenia.)

## PLATELET DISORDERS

### Thrombocytopenia

Thrombocytopenia is the most common hemostatic abnormality associated with tumors in both dog and human cancer patients. In humans, lymphoma and chronic lymphocytic leukemia are most frequently associated with decreased platelet counts. Thrombocytopenia has been reported in up to 40% of dogs with a variety of tumors (Madewell, Feldman, and O'Neill, 1980). It has been reported most often in dogs with extensive tumor burden such as metastatic adenocarcinomas or stage IV and V lymphoma, but also in association with localized neoplasms, particularly carcinomas and sarcomas (Helfand, 1988). In dogs with hemangiosarcoma, 75 to 90% of these patients have thrombocytopenia some time during the course of their disease (Hammer et al., 1991). Extensive tumor-burden and histology-dependent decreases in platelet survival times and high fibrinogen turnover have been observed in both humans and dogs with solid tumors, particularly carcinomas and lymphomas (Helfand, 1988). Proposed mechanisms for shortened survival times are adherence to incompletely endothelialized tumor vasculature and premature removal from the circulation after tumor-stimulated microaggregation or coating of platelets by tumor-derived proteins.

In human cancer patients, immune-mediated thrombocytopenia (IMT) may be a warning that precedes a diagnosis of lymphoma by months to years. This is in contrast to the development of IMHA, which is usually detected only in the presence of overt malignancy. In a recent study of over 1 million dogs with immune-mediated diseases and lymphoma, dogs with immune-mediated thrombocytopenia had a greater occurrence of lymphoma when compared with dogs without immune-mediated thrombocytopenia (Keller, 1992).

It is often difficult to differentiate IMT from subclinical or overt DIC. Malignancy-associated IMT is usually caused by increased platelet destruction. Postulated mechanisms for increased platelet destruction include antiplatelet antibody production by the tumor, autoantibody production to antigens common to both tumor and platelet, and adherence of tumor antigen–autoantibody immune complexes to platelets causing accelerated destruction. In a recent study, antiplatelet antibodies were found in 21% of dogs with lymphoma.

Mean platelet count was 75,000/$\mu$l, which normalized with chemotherapy-induced remission (Kristensen et al., 1991).

### Thrombocytosis

Thrombocytosis of greater than 500,000/$\mu$l is found in up to 60% of human patients with malignancy (Johnson and Roodman, 1989). It is usually a reflection of a reactive marrow or, sometimes, iron deficiency. Carcinomas of the stomach, lung, and colon, and lymphoid malignancies are most commonly associated with thrombocytosis in these patients. The increased risk for thrombosis seen in humans has not been observed in dogs.

## LEUKOCYTE ABNORMALITIES

Granulocytosis of greater than 20,000/$\mu$l in the absence of overt infection or leukemia has been observed in 20% of human cancer patients, most frequently with carcinomas of the lung (Bunn and Ridgway, 1993). The frequency of this abnormality is unknown in companion animals. Cancer-associated granulocytosis of greater than 75,000/$\mu$l is called a leukemoid reaction and is infrequently observed. Documented cases include renal tubular carcinoma, rectal adenomatous polyp, and metastatic fibrosarcoma in the dog and salivary gland and sweat gland carcinomas in the cat. Clinical signs referrable to leukocytosis were absent. Postulated mechanisms include colony-stimulating factor production by the tumor, local bone marrow stimulation by tumor metastasis, and stimulation of the bone marrow by necrotic tumor by-products. All of the reported canine cases of granulocytosis have resolved within a week of surgical resection.

Neutropenia in the cancer patient is usually caused by antineoplastic therapy or the effects of metastasis to the bone marrow. Paraneoplastic neutropenia has been observed with squamous cell carcinoma in the cat and mammary and thyroid adenocarcinomas in dogs. Immune-mediated mechanisms for leukocyte destruction have been proposed. Both antineutrophil antibody production with subsequent destruction of granulocytes and tumor-produced bone marrow "blocking" factors have been suggested. In both cats and dogs with solid tumors, resolution of neutropenia parallels effective antineoplastic therapy.

Tumor-associated eosinophilia of greater than 5000/$\mu$l is uncommon in canine, feline, and human cancer patients. In people, eosinophilia is observed with lymphomas, solid epithelial tumors, and undifferentiated mesenchymal tumors. It is most often associated with metastatic disease and, if greater than 6% of the total white blood cell count, warrants a poor prognosis in spite of only 20% incidence of tumor cells in the bone marrow. In a few patients, eosinophilia is the first sign of disease. Relationships between eosinophilia and neoplasms in the dog have not been adequately evaluated.

Severe eosinophilia of greater than 10,000/$\mu$l has been reported in dogs with mammary adenocarcinoma, mast cell tumor, and oral fibrosarcoma. Greater than 5000/$\mu$l eosinophils have been observed in cats with lymphomas, mast cell tumors, myeloproliferative diseases, and various carcinomas. Direct tumor production or tumor-induced production of cytokines with eosinophilopoietic or eosinophilotactic abilities by lymphocytes, macrophages, or mast cells, and neoplastic or immune-complex stimulation of histamine release have been implicated as causes of eosinophilia. Tumor-associated eosinophilia usually resolves with eradication of the tumor.

## HEMOSTATIC SYSTEM DISORDERS

Greater than 90% of people with hematologic and solid neoplasms and 83% of dogs with advanced malignancies have abnormal coagulation tests (Madewell, Feldman, and O'Neill, 1980). All measurable coagulation parameters have been reported to be abnormal in human cancer patients; however, the most common abnormalities are increased fibrin/fibrin split products and thrombocytosis. These aberrations are consistent with an overcompensated intravascular coagulation with fibrinolysis. When 53 tumor-bearing dogs were evaluated, decreased platelet survival times, thrombocytopenia (if bone marrow or spleen/liver were involved), prolongation of the activated thromboplastin time, and increased or decreased plasma fibrinogen concentration were observed (O'Donnell et al., 1981).

Although the overall risk for cancer-associated hemorrhosis/thrombosis in veterinary patients is undetermined, it appears to be much lower than in human cancer patients. It is estimated that in untreated cancer-bearing humans, up to 20% experience venous thrombosis and up to 10% overt hemorrhage. Disseminated intravascular coagulation is the most frequently reported hemostatic disorder in dogs and cats with cancer. A single underlying mechanism is unlikely, as the cause of altered coagulation in cancer patients probably involves interaction between tumor-produced products, mononuclear cells and cytokines, and aberrant endothelium. Inappropriate coagulation may be stimulated by the production of procoagulant proteins by tumor cells (tissue factor and non–tissue-factor-dependent cysteine protease) and monocytes. Additionally, tumors elaborate platelet proaggregating substances that promote initial clot formation. The elaboration of TNF produced by inflammation-activated macrophages alters endothelial cell surfaces, and exposure of subendothelial collagen from damaged vessels found within the tumor itself promotes inappropriate coagulation. Decreased factor clearance, factor neutralization, decreased fibrinolysis, and bacterial sepsis also contribute to hypercoagulability. The hemorrhagic diathesis that results from the anticoagulant effect of fibrin split products, thrombocytopenia, and hypofibrinogenemia is associated with an 80% mortality rate in dogs, but is

fortunately infrequent in most cancer-bearing animals. Subclinical DIC is far more common.

Clinical signs of bleeding, bruising, petechiae, and ecchymoses suggest abnormalities of vessels or platelet numbers or function. Overt hemorrhage has been reported in association with monoclonal gammopathies in 60% of dogs and 30% of cats with multiple myeloma and also with canine macroglobulinemia and isolated cases of lymphoma/leukemia in both species. A variety of tumors have been reported to cause DIC-related bleeding diathesis in canine patients, but hemorrhagic DIC is most often associated with hemangiosarcoma, inflammatory mammary carcinoma, and thyroid adenocarcinoma. Even small cutaneous tumors can induce DIC. Hemostatic defects such as persistent hemorrhage from the tumor, thrombocytopenia, decreased fibrinogen, and hemostatic test alterations characteristic of subclinical DIC were present in association with small cutaneous hemangiomas and hemangiosarcomas (Hargis and Feldman, 1991).

Primary antitumor therapy is the best management for altered coagulation and DIC. Individualized therapy is necessary for the management of the patient with DIC. Blood component replacement has not been shown to exacerbate DIC and is indicated in patients with active hemorrhage. Heparinization of human and veterinary patients with DIC is controversial. In human medicine, heparinization is reserved for those patients with either acute uncontrolled bleeding or chronic debilitating DIC. In a recent review of the effect of heparinization in human cancer patients with chronic DIC, approximately 60% showed clinical improvement when antitumor therapy was combined with heparinization. However, long-term control was maintained in only 10 to 20% of these patients if the tumor was not controlled (Bunn and Ridgway, 1993). Treatment of DIC has been reviewed in *CVT X*, p 451, and elsewhere in this section (see "Spontaneous Bleeding Disorder," this volume, p 457).

Monitoring the response to heparinization therapy of malignancy-associated hemostatic abnormalities is often problematic. In human and probably veterinary patients, the rapid turnover of fibrinogen by consumption in DIC and replacement by hepatic synthesis makes plasma fibrinogen determination the most useful measure of resolving DIC. Plasma fibrinogen measurements every 8 to 12 hr during heparinization should indicate response to therapy, whereas the platelet count and fibrin split products may take 2 to 3 days to show significant changes (Colman and Rubin, 1990).

### Hyperviscosity Syndrome

The flow characteristics of blood may be affected by both cellular and soluble components. Hyperviscosity caused by multiple myeloma and other dysproteinemias, polycythemia, hyperleukocytic acute or chronic leukemias results in clinical signs referable to almost any system, but especially the renal and cardiovascular systems, and the blood coagulation cascade in veterinary patients.

Bleeding diathesis manifested by ecchymoses, petechiae, epistaxes, gingival bleeding, melena, and retinal hemorrhages is the most common sign of hyperviscosity syndrome in human and canine patients. The cause of bleeding is multifactorial. Monoclonal protein-coated platelets function abnormally in hemostasis. Paraproteins act as coagulation factor inhibitors and bind coagulation proteins causing actual deficiencies. Additionally, tests show coagulation test times to be abnormally prolonged. Hyperviscosity secondary to paraproteinemia has been reported in a few cats where the physical evidence of bleeding was retinal hemorrhage. A more detailed discussion of dysproteinemia and hyperviscosity syndrome is included in this section (see "Syndromes of Hyperglobulinemia: Diagnosis and Therapy," this volume, p 523).

## NEUROMUSCULAR SYSTEM DISORDERS

In humans, cancer-associated neurologic complications are most often due to the direct effects of the tumor or its metastasis. Less commonly, cancer-associated metabolic encephalopathy affects up to 20% of hospitalized human patients. The presenting clinical signs may be exclusively neurologic, consisting of depression, weakness, dementia, and/or seizures. Organ failures, particularly liver and kidney, electrolyte abnormalities, hypoglycemia, altered drug metabolism, hemorrhage from thrombocytopenia or hypercoagulability, and nutritional deficiencies occur with greatest frequency.

True paraneoplastic neurologic disorders affect only 1% of human cancer patients and precede a diagnosis of cancer in approximately two thirds of these patients. Although considered infrequent in veterinary patients, paraneoplastic neurologic disorders are probably underestimated because diagnosis is difficult. For example, the association between "weakness," a common clinical sign in animals with neoplasms, and confirmation of electrophysiologic evidence of an associated polyneuropathy is difficult to establish.

In human and canine patients, paraneoplastic disorders affect the peripheral nervous system more frequently than the central nervous system. Like the "silent" metabolic alterations preceding the discovery of a tumor in the syndrome of cancer cachexia, abnormalities in the peripheral and central nervous systems have been detected in human cancer patients in the absence of clinical signs, often months to years prior to detection of the tumor itself. Although not symptomatic, it is estimated that up to one third of human cancer patients have electrophysiologic alterations. In one study, 76% of dogs with malignant solid tumors and normal neurologic examinations had marked histologic abnormalities including a mixture of demyelination/remyelination and axonal degeneration similar to sensorimotor polyneuropathy found in tumor-bearing human patients (Braund, 1990). Examples of local or generalized paraneoplastic peripheral neuropathies in the dog have been found with lymphoma, myelomonocytic leukemia, insulinoma, and prostate and pancreatic adenocarcinomas; whereas paraneoplastic neuromyopathies have been observed with thymoma, bronchogenic carcinoma, lymphoma, bile duct carcinoma, intestinal adenocarcinoma, and simultaneous seminoma and perianal gland adenoma.

Proposed mediators of paraneoplastic neurologic disease include biologically active molecules such as hormones, as in the peripheral neuropathies associated with insulinomas, neurotoxins, cytokines, and nutrient deficiencies. A known cause of paraneoplastic neurologic disease in humans, and probably the most common cause in veterinary patients, is autoimmunity. Autoantibodies are formed that cross-react between peripheral or central nervous system cellular antigens and tumor antigens. The presence of a disease-specific autoantibody has been demonstrated in at least ten different paraneoplastic syndromes in people. For example, in myasthenia gravis, an autoimmune response that is directed at the acetylcholine receptor resulting in generalized exertional weakness that improves with rest has been observed in humans and dogs with thymoma. Localized weakness of facial muscles, esophagus, larynx, or pharynx has been seen in both species with this impairment in postsynaptic transmission. Additionally, a presumptively immune-mediated polymyositis has been reported in some dogs and cats with thymomas.

## SKELETAL SYSTEM DISORDERS

Hypertrophic osteopathy (HO) is characterized by painful, nonedematous, warm periosteal soft tissue swelling of the limbs with a radiographic appearance of new periosteal bone formation starting distally in the metacarpals and metatarsals and progressing proximally. Hypertrophic osteopathy is most commonly found in association with mass lesions usually of the peripheral lung field. Although HO is seen most commonly with primary lung tumors in humans, metastatic lung lesions induce HO more commonly in dogs. Abdominal tumors such as rhabdomyosarcomas and a carcinoma of the urinary bladder and nephroblastoma have also been associated with HO. In the cat, pulmonary adenocarcinoma, renal papillary adenoma, thymoma, and bronchogenic carcinoma resulted in HO.

The exact cause of fibrovascular soft tissue proliferation and new bone formation is unknown. Humoral vasoactive substances or neurologic stimulation leading to increased blood flow to the extremities is the proposed mechanism of bone and connective tissue proliferation. Paraneoplastic HO has been reversed following vagotomy and intercostal neurectomy, supporting the theory that stimulation of afferent vagal fibers of the hilum, mediastinum, or parietal pleura result in efferent stimulation of vasculature, connective tissue, and bone.

Optimal treatment for HO is surgical resection of the mass or chemotherapy-induced remission. Resolution of clinical signs is often complete in 2 to 4 weeks. Medical management consists of anti-inflammatory doses of glucocorticoid or nonsteroidal anti-inflammatory agents.

## MISCELLANEOUS PARANEOPLASTIC DISORDERS

### Dermatologic Disorders

Indirect dermatologic consequences of malignancy are underestimated. In human patients, dermatologic PND may antedate the discovery of the tumor, signal its recurrence, or appear simultaneously with recognition of the neoplasm. Purpura, flushing, erythema, urticarial and bullous states, hyperpigmentation, pruritus, erythema nodosum, hypertrichosis, and acanthosis nigricans are just a few of the dermatologic lesions associated with neoplasms in people. In the dog, dermatologic abnormalities have been frequently reported in association with endocrine tumors such as bilateral endocrine alopecia and hyperpigmentation in hyperadrenocorticism. Reports of paroxysmal flushing and generalized erythroderma induced by cellular products from pheochromocytomas, carcinoids, and intrathoracic and cutaneous mast cell tumors are infrequent. The appearance of millimeter to centimeter hyperplastic dermal collagenous nodules up to 1 year prior to the detection of renomegaly or renal insufficiency is an important premonitory dermatologic sign of internal malignancy in German shepherd dogs with nodular dermatofibrosis and renal cystadenocarcinoma.

### Gastrointestinal System Disorders

The most common PND affecting the gastrointestinal system is probably the anorexia/cachexia syndrome discussed previously. Although the frequency in veterinary patients is unknown, hypoalbuminemia of undetermined cause occurs in almost all human cancer patients. The effects of hormone-producing endocrine tumors such as gastrinomas are the best characterized PND with gastrointestinal manifestations. In one study of humans with tumors of the lung, prostate, pancreas, colon, and lymphoid tissue without histologic evidence of small intestine involvement, various degrees of villous atrophy of the small intestinal mucosa were reported in more than half of the cases. Malabsorption was a problem for some of these patients.

In human patients, abnormal liver function, hepatomegaly, hepatic enzymopathy, acute cholestatic jaundice, and alterations in liver-produced plasma proteins that commonly resolve with excision of the primary tumor have been frequently reported without evidence of actual tumor in the liver (Bunn and Ridgway, 1993). The remote effects of neoplasia on the liver, which resolve following surgical resection in some patients, have been reported in patients with renal cell carcinoma (Stauffer's syndrome). The mediator of hepatic dysfunction is unknown; however, renal cell carcinomas produce a hepatotoxic cytokine, IL-6, *in vitro*. Renal transitional cell carcinoma and renal cell carcinoma have been reported in dogs with unexplained increases in serum alkaline phosphatase and alanine aminotransferase activities.

### Renal Disorders

Paraneoplastic renal diseases are most often due to amyloid deposition, paraproteins, hypercalcemia, and tumor-associated immune complex deposition. For example, the effects of multiple myeloma on renal function include renal failure secondary to myeloma protein deposition in collecting ducts, amyloid deposition, Fanconi syndrome with proximal renal tubular acidosis, nephrogenic diabetes insipidus, and nephrotic syndrome. In human patients, protein loss markedly decreases with resolution of the plasma cell tumor. In dogs, glomerulonephritis is common in dogs with neoplasms. It has been reported in 33 to 40% with localized mast cell tumors and 69% with systemic mastocytosis (O'Keefe and Couto, 1988). Resolution of the neoplasm results in improvement in paraneoplastic renal disorders, provided that renal damage is reversible.

### Cardiovascular System Disorders

Cardiovascular system–related manifestations of malignancy in humans and the dog are numerous. In human patients, carcinoid plaque formation and cardiac amyloid deposition, dysrhythmias due to dehydration and electrolyte imbalances, and cardiovascular consequences of inappropriate antidiuretic hormone-secretion are commonly observed in association with neoplasms. A high-output state caused by anemia, blood hyperviscosity, hyperthyroidism, hyperaldosteronism, and shunting of blood through the tumor mass are less common. Cardiovascular system–related PND in the dog and cat occur most commonly as a result of hormone secretion by the tumor, as in, for example, thyroid adenomas in cats and pheochromocytomas and chemodectomas in dogs. Resolution of clinical signs parallels tumor removal.

### References and Suggested Reading

Antman KH, Skarin AT, Mayer RJ, Hargreaves HK, and Canellos GP: Microangiopathic hemolytic anemia and cancer: A review. Medicine 58:377, 1979.
  *Six cases of MAHA in human cancer patients and a review of the literature.*
Bick RL: Coagulation abnormalities in malignancy: A review. Semin Thromb Hemost 18:353, 1992.
  *In-depth review of cancer-associated coagulation abnormalities, correlation with tumors, in humans.*
Braund KG: Remote effects of cancer on the nervous system. Semin Vet Med Surg 5:262, 1990.
  *Discussion of neurologic complications of cancer in dogs.*
Bruera E: Clinical management of anorexia and cachexia in patients with advanced cancer. Oncology 49:35, 1992.
  *Summary of effects of a variety of appetite stimulants and their effect on weight gain in human patients with cancer cachexia.*

Bunn PA and Ridgway EC: Paraneoplastic syndromes. *In* DeVita VT, Hellman S, and Rosenberg SA (eds:) *Cancer: Principles and Practice of Oncology.* Philadelphia, JB Lippincott Co, 1993, p 2026.
*An excellent review of paraneoplastic syndromes in human cancer patients.*

Chew DJ, Nagode LA, and Carothers M: Disorders of calcium: Hypercalcemia and hypocalcemia. *In* DiBartola SP (ed): *Fluid Therapy in Small Animal Practice.* Philadelphia, WB Saunders Co, 1992, pp 116–176.
*Recent review of calcium metabolism with emphasis on hypercalcemia and treatment.*

Colman RW and Rubin RN: Disseminated intravascular coagulation due to malignancy. Semin Oncol 17:172, 1990.
*Review of defects of hemostasis and treatment of DIC in human medicine.*

Farris GM and Benjamin SA: Inhibition of myelopoiesis by serum from dogs exposed to estrogen. Am J Vet Res 54:1374, 1993.
*Part II of a study that demonstrates a myelopoiesis inhibitory factor in canine serum.*

Hammer AS, Couto CG, Swardsen C, and Getzy D: Hemostatic abnormalities in dogs with hemangiosarcoma. J Vet Intern Med 5:11, 1991.
*Evaluation of hemostatic abnormalities in dogs with hemangiosarcoma.*

Hammond D and Winnick S: Paraneoplastic erythrocytosis and ectopic erythropoietins. Ann N Y Acad Sci 230:219, 1974.
*A review of cancer-associated polycythemia.*

Hargis AM and Feldman BP: Evaluation of hemostatic defects secondary to vascular tumors in dogs: 11 cases (1983–1988). J Am Vet Med Assoc 198:891, 1991.
*Cutaneous vascular tumors associated with abnormal coagulation tests and thrombocytopenia.*

Helfand SC: Platelets and neoplasia. Vet Clin North Am 18:131, 1988.
*In-depth review of platelet abnormalities and associated tumors in humans, cats, and dogs.*

Hill RC: A rapid method of estimating maintenance energy requirement from body surface area in inactive adult dogs and in cats. J Am Vet Med Assoc 202:1814, 1993.
*Review of equations commonly used to calculate dietary energy needs in dogs and cats.*

Howard EB, Sawa TE, and Nielsen SW: Mastocytoma and gastroduodenal ulceration. Vet Pathol 6:146, 1969.
*Retrospective report of the association between mast cell tumors and gastroduodenal ulceration.*

Johnson RA and Roodman GD: *In* Bone RC (ed): *Hematologic Manifestations of Malignancy.* Disease-a-Month. Chicago, Year Book Medical Publishers, Inc., 1989, p 725.
*An excellent review of cancer-associated hematologic/hemostatic paraneoplastic disorders.*

Keller ET: Immune-mediated disease as a risk factor for canine lymphoma. Cancer 70:2334, 1992.
*Retrospective investigation involving over 1 million dogs of a variety of immune-mediated diseases and their association with canine lymphoma.*

Kristensen AT, Klausner JS, Weiss DJ, Christie DJ, Liebenstein B, and Laber J: Prevalence of antiplatelet antibody in dogs with lymphosarcoma—a pilot study. *Vet Cancer Soc Proc, 11th Ann Meet,* 1991, p 49.
*A report of the finding of antiplatelet antibodies in dogs with lymphoma.*

Macauley VM: Insulin-like growth factors and cancer. Br J Cancer 65:311, 1992.
*Review of role of insulin-like growth factors in growth of tumors and development of extrapancreatic tumor hypoglycemia.*

Madewell BR, Feldman BF, and O'Neill S: Coagulation abnormalities in dogs with neoplastic disease. Thromb Diath Haemost 44:35, 1980.
*Evaluation of hemostatic disorders associated with neoplasms in the dog.*

O'Donnell MR, Slichter SJ, Weidon PL, and Storb R: Platelet and fibrinogen kinetics in canine tumors. Cancer Res 41:1379, 1981.
*Determination of hemostatic defects associated with a variety of neoplasms in dogs.*

Ogilvie GK: Alterations in metabolism and nutritional support for veterinary cancer patients: Recent advances. Compend Cont Educ 15:925, 1993.
*Up-to-date review of cancer cachexia with particular reference to canine studies with therapy recommendations.*

Ogilvie GK, Walters LM, Fettman MJ, Hand MS, Salman MD, and Wheeler SL: Energy expenditure in dogs with lymphoma fed two specialized diets. Cancer 71:3146, 1993.
*Prospective evaluation of REE in dogs fed a specialized diet.*

O'Keefe DA and Couto CG: Coagulation abnormalities associated with neoplasia. Vet Clin North Am 18:157, 1988.
*Excellent review of malignancy-associated coagulation abnormalities with reference to human, feline, and canine tumors.*

Peterson JL, Couto CG, Hammer AS, Chew DJ, Ayl RD, Nagode LA, Capen CC, and Rosol TJ: Humoral hypercalcemia of malignancy in dogs: Serum parathyroid hormone-related protein. *Vet Cancer So, Proc 12th Ann Conference,* 1992, p 34.
*Recent report of PTHrP measurement in dogs with hypercalcemia.*

Rosol TJ and Capen CC: Biology of disease—mechanisms of cancer-induced hypercalcemia. Lab Invest 67:690, 1992.
*Most up-to-date review of mechanisms and tumor associations of hypercalcemia of malignancy that includes many species including humans, cats, dogs, and laboratory animals.*

Sigal RK and Daly JM: Enteral nutrition in the cancer patient. *In* Rombeau JL and Caldwell MD (eds:) *Clinical Nutrition: Parenteral Nutrition.* Philadelphia, WB Saunders Co, 1992, p 263.
*Excellent review of cancer-associated malnutrition and the consequences of nutritional support of the cancer patient.*

Wallach PM, Flannery MT, and Stewart JM: Paraneoplastic syndromes for the primary care physician. Prim Care 4:727, 1992.
*A basic review of paraneoplastic syndromes in human cancer patients.*

Weiss FC, Cummins JM, and Richards AB: Low-dose orally administered alpha interferon treatment for feline leukemia virus infection. J Am Vet Med Assoc 199:1477, 1991.
*Evaluation of an inexpensive interferon for stimulation of appetite and well-being.*

Wheeler SL: Endocrine tumors. *In* Withrow SJ and MacEwen EG (eds.) *Clinical Veterinary Oncology.* Philadelphia, JB Lippincott Co, 1989, p 253.
*Review of history, clinical signs, diagnosis, and treatment of hormone-secreting endocrine tumors of the dog and cat.*

# MONOCLONAL ANTIBODIES: APPLICATIONS IN DIAGNOSIS AND TREATMENT

LAUREL J. GERSHWIN
*Davis, California*

Medicine has relied on antisera for diagnostics and therapeutics for many years. In 1975, an innovation in the production of antisera was made that created dramatic changes in diagnostics and therapeutics: hybridoma technology was discovered. Hybridomas are cells created *in vitro* by the fusion of a parent myeloma cell with an immune spleen cell. These hybrid cells retain the malignant characteristic of the myeloma parent and the antigen specific immunoglobulin-producing ability of the parent spleen cell. The original hybridomas were made from mouse myeloma parent cell lines and spleen cells, but as the technology has advanced, ad-tional types of hybrids have been created, such as human hybridomas, bovine heterohybridomas (bovine X murine), and porcine heterohybridomas (porcine X murine). The latter cell lines produce bovine and porcine antibodies, respectively.

The process of making "standard" murine hybridomas involves a complex process of cell fusion, selection for those fused cells that have a myeloma and a lymphocyte partner by using a selection medium for their growth, and cloning of the hybridoma cells. The cells are cloned so as to have only a single hybrid cell in a well of a tissue culture plate. This is so that the cell will divide and its progeny will all be identical with regard to the specificity of antibody that they produce. The production of antibody is tested for by analysis of the supernatant from the cloned cells. Once the desired antibody-producing clones are identified, they are grown in large volume and their antibody product is harvested for use in diagnostics or therapeutics or both.

This article summarizes the current and future uses that veterinary medicine has for monoclonal antibodies (see Table 1).

## MONOCLONAL ANTIBODY PRODUCTION: WHY AND HOW

When an animal encounters antigen, the usual antibody response is polyclonal; that is, there are many different antibodies produced against a variety of determinant groups or epitopes on any one antigen. The normal serum electrophoresis pattern that we observe shows a broad peak in the $\gamma$ region, where the antibodies migrate. This broad peak is characteristic of the heterogeneous nature of the normal immune response (Fig. 1). The serum from a patient with multiple myeloma shows a different pattern of electrophoretic mobility: a narrow tall peak (Fig. 1). This is because a myeloma tumor is derived from a single clone of malignant plasma cells and as such it produces a homogeneous antibody population, monoclonal antibodies. In the myeloma patient, we usually neither choose nor know the specificity of the antibodies produced. When hybridomas are produced, however, the specificity of the antibody is chosen, thereby creating a large concentration of antibodies specific to one single antigenic epitope.

### Table 1. Diagnostic and Therapeutic Uses for Monoclonal Antibodies

**Diagnostic**
ELISA test kits (e.g., FeLV, parvovirus, distemper, *Dirofilaria immitis*)
Erythrocyte antigen typing
Lymphocyte subpopulation determination
MHC class-I and class-II testing
Tumor-specific antigen detection

**Therapeutic**
Radioactive imaging
Immunotherapy with cytotoxins
Anti-idiotype vaccines

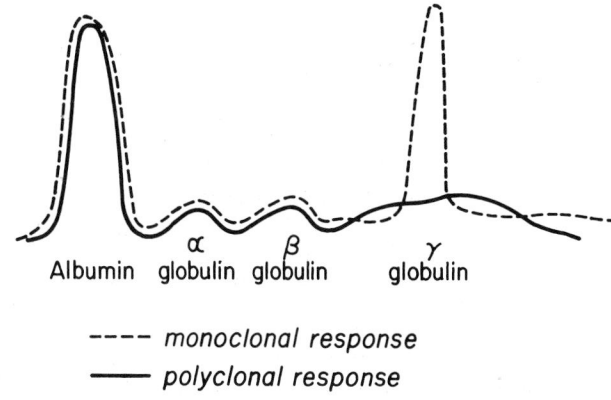

**Figure 1.** Densitometry from serum electrophoresis of normal serum versus serum containing monoclonal antibodies.

To create monoclonal antibodies, first an antigen is chosen. For example, the outer membrane protein from feline leukemia virus (VP21). Then mice are immunized with the virus, and after a time the mouse is killed and the spleen removed. The spleen cells are harvested and mixed with the myeloma fusion partners. While these cells can grow forever in culture, they lack an enzyme (hypoxanthine phosphoribosyl transferase) that allows them to use hypoxanthine supplied in the media. When grown in media (HAT media) that contains aminopterin, they are prevented from *de novo* synthesis of purines and will die. Thus, single myeloma cells or fused myeloma:myeloma cells will die, but myeloma:lymphocyte fusion products will live because the lymphocyte provides the needed enzyme for purine metabolism. The fusion is accomplished with a chemical, polyethylene glycol, and then the cells are dispensed in a tissue culture plate and are allowed to grow in the HAT medium.

After several weeks the supernatants of the fused cells are tested for the production of specific antibodies; those producing antibodies are chosen for continued growth and cloning. Final production of the antibody reagents can be done either in tissue culture or in mice, where the cells will grow as ascites tumors dispensing monoclonal antibodies into the ascites fluid. The process of monoclonal antibody production is summarized in Figure 2.

Why go to all the trouble of creating hybridomas when one can simply immunize and bleed a rabbit and obtain antiserum appropriate for many diagnostic uses? The answer is that the specificity of being able to bind a single epitope creates a variety of possibilities for diagnosis and therapy that would never be possible with polyclonal reagents. For example, one can immunize a mouse with dog lymphocytes and by creating and screening hybridomas, develop a whole panel of antibodies recognizing different surface determinants. Thus we can have reagents to recognize CD4 (helper T cells), CD8 (suppressor/cytotoxic T cells), complement receptors, antibody receptors, and so forth. A rabbit serum would not be able to distinguish these cell populations without extensive purification of the cells prior to immunization. In one recent study, subtle differences in IgG fractions from dog serum were found using monoclonal antibodies. These reagents will assist in better definition of IgG subclasses in the dog (Mazza et al., 1993).

## MONOCLONAL ANTIBODIES AS DIAGNOSTIC TOOLS

### Monoclonal Antibodies Against Canine and Feline Pathogenic Agents

Monoclonal antibodies developed against pathogenic agents of veterinary importance have uses in *in vitro* assays and in studies on pathogenesis and epidemiology of strain variation. For example, neutralizing and nonneutralizing monoclonal antibodies have been produced against a single capsid protein of feline calicivirus. Antigenic variation was noted and was attributed to restricted immunity in populations due to the modified virus vaccine currently in use (Milton et al., 1992). The ability to recognize virus variants is important in tracing virus spread among the population. In another study, a virus receptor on feline cells that appears to be distinct from CD4 was identified using monoclonal antibodies against a feline immunodeficiency virus (FIV)-glycoprotein. The interesting difference between virus neutralization and enhancement of feline infectious peritonitis (FIP) virus was studied with a panel of monoclonal antibodies specific for antigenic epitopes on the spike protein of FIP virus. Monoclonal antibodies are used to detect antigenic differences between rabies virus strains in a variety of species; street virus can be differentiated from challenge virus.

### *In Vitro* Assay Systems

#### ENZYME-LINKED IMMUNOSORBENT ASSAY

Enzyme-linked immunosorbent assay (ELISA) is a technique that has become popular during the past 20 years. The availability of monoclonal antibody reagents specific for antigenic epitopes on a variety of infectious agents has facilitated the development of quick, accurate diagnostic kits for such diseases as feline leukemia, feline immunodeficiency, feline infectious peritonitis, *Dirofilaria immitis*, and parvovirus infection. Monoclonal antibodies specific for canine distemper virus (no cross-reactivity with other paramyxoviruses) were used to develop both antigen and antibody detection ELISA (Potgieter and Ajidagba, 1989). Samples can be derived from serum, cerebrospinal fluid, or tissue, and the assays can be read visually.

There are a variety of test kits available for the diagnosis of FeLV infection. Most kits are antigen detection assays, and they use a monoclonal antibody specific for the VP27 of FeLV to coat the ELISA well. The sample, usually blood or serum, containing the virus is incubated with the well, binding to the monoclonal antibodies and remaining despite the subsequent wash steps. Detection is brought about by the use of another antibody conjugated with an enzyme such as horseradish peroxidase, which catalyzes a color change in the substrate added as the last step.

#### RADIOIMMUNOASSAY

Although less applicable for in-hospital use, the radioimmunoassay (RIA) is used frequently in the diagnostic laboratory. Measurement of levels of hormones and other small molecules, such as prostaglandins and leukotrienes, is performed most commonly by RIA.

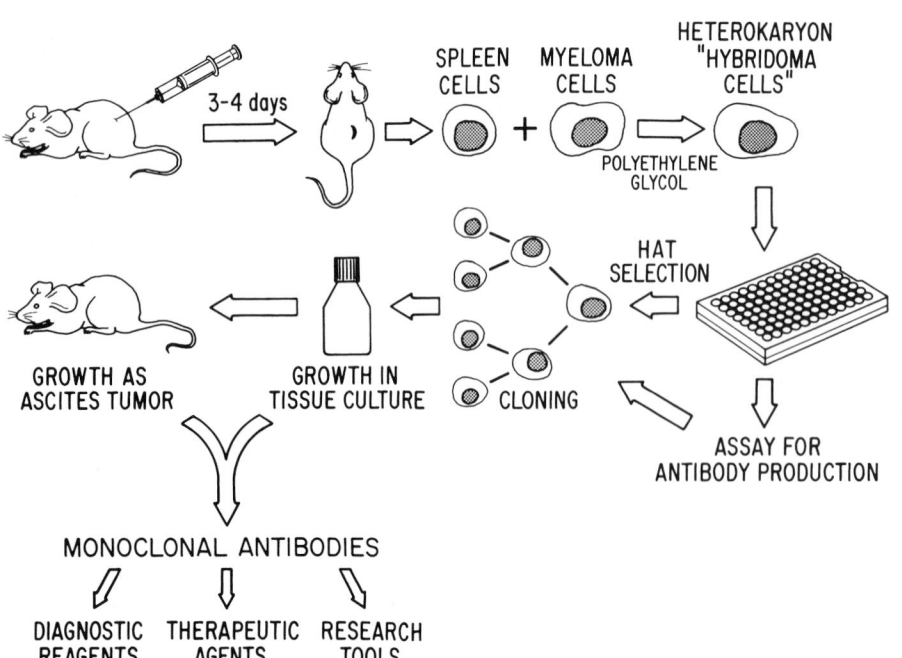

**Figure 2.** Schematic showing the process of monoclonal antibody production.

Competitive RIA can be used to measure progesterone levels, for example. Such an assay utilizes a monoclonal antibody to bind to the hormone. In the competitive format, the patient's sample provides a source of hormone that competes with the standard labeled hormone in the assay.

### TUMOR CELL IDENTIFICATION (*IN VITRO*)

Immunohistochemistry is the staining of tissue sections with antibodies tagged with an indicator, such as an enzyme, for the purpose of staining the particular cell(s) to which the antibodies bind. After binding with the cell-associated antigen, the labeled antibody is reacted with a substrate that produces insoluble color in the area of antibody binding. This technique has been used to identify specific types of tumor cells. Monoclonal antibodies provide a tool for distinguishing between tumor antigens and antigens normally present on the tissue of origin. They can be used to detect antigen and to localize it *in situ*. In human medicine, monoclonal antibodies have been developed that recognize colorectal carcinoma by detection of the carcinoembryonic antigen.

A monoclonal antibody developed to react with canine melanoma tissue detects 82% of melanomas. It distinguishes amelanotic melanoma from spindle cell mesenchymal tumors and differentiates between benign and malignant melanocytic lesions in dogs (Oliver and Wolfe, 1992).

## Recognition of Cell Surface Molecules

### LYMPHOCYTE SUBPOPULATIONS

Immunoregulatory status of a patient can be reflected in the ratio of $CD4^+$ to $CD8^+$ T lymphocytes. In humans where monoclonal antibody reagents capable of binding specifically with either of these T-cell subsets have been available for some time, ratio changes show some interesting patterns in certain diseases. Immunofluorescent labeling of the appropriate monoclonal antibody reagents and the use of a fluorescence-activated cell sorter or scanner are required for such diagnostic applications. In such cases, the ratio of $CD4^+$ to $CD8^+$ T lymphocytes is useful information in prediction of disease prognosis. Examples have been cited for infectious as well as autoimmune and allergic disease. For example, $CD4^+/CD8^+$ ratios were decreased in patients with histoplasmosis. The $CD4^+/CD8^+$ ratios reverted to normal in patients that recovered within 6 to 10 weeks, whereas those patients that developed hypersensitivity showed increased $CD4^+/CD8^+$ ratios. Changes have been documented in several viral diseases, such as hepatitis B virus infection in which a decreased ratio is present during acute infection, due to increased $CD8^+$ cells. Upon viral clearance and appearance of neutralizing antibody, the ratio becomes normal again. An increased $CD4^+/CD8^+$ ratio was seen in patients with active rheumatoid arthritis (RA), but not inactive RA. The ratio was also increased in patients with another autoimmune disease, myasthenia gravis.

Studies similar to those described above have not been performed in small animal medicine, because development of the appropriate monoclonal antibodies has been slow in coming for dogs and cats. With the reported development of such reagents and the development of a machine called the FACSCAN, which analyzes cells for the presence or absence of fluorescent markers (i.e., monoclonal antibodies conjugated to fluorescein), application of T-lymphocyte subset determination is or will be readily available in most clinical veterinary immunology laboratories. Application to diseases such as allergic (atopic) dermatitis, systemic lupus erythematosus, viral disease (distemper, parvovirus, FIV), and a myriad of other diseases will yield useful information for prediction of prognosis and understanding pathogenesis better. One recent study describes the production of monoclonal antibodies against the $\alpha$ subunit of the feline Il-2 receptor. Such reagents will be useful in studying T-cell activation in cat diseases.

### DOG ERYTHROCYTE ANTIGENS

Monoclonal antibodies were produced against dog erythrocyte antigens (DEA) DEA-1.1 (Andrews, Chavey, and Smith, 1992). This is an important allele in the blood group A system. Incompatibility of DEA-1.1 causes hemolytic transfusion reactions (after sensitization has occurred by previous incompatible transfusion). This antigen system may also be implicated in neonatal isoerythrolysis. The antibody was used to develop a card agglutination test, which uses only 50 $\mu$l of blood and can be read macroscopically. Other monoclonal antibodies are available that detect DEA-3.

### MAJOR HISTOCOMPATIBILITY ANTIGENS

The importance of major histocompatibility (MHC) antigens in transplantation and the use of dogs in transplantation studies has initiated production of monoclonal antibodies against these determinants. In one study, antibodies were produced that recognize MHC class-II antigens on canine cells (Lin, Chang, and Chang, 1992). Using these antibodies, it was demonstrated that class-II expression is induced on transplanted lung cells (bronchial epithelium and vascular endothelium) but not on normal lung cells.

## MONOCLONAL ANTIBODIES AS THERAPEUTIC TOOLS

## Radioactive Imaging

The production of monoclonal antibodies specific for tumor-associated antigens has made it possible to develop techniques whereby an antibody can be coupled to a radioactive compound and injected into a patient.

The antibody will home to the tissue containing the tumor antigens for which it is specific. Radiography can then be used to visualize the antibody, thereby localizing the tumor. The technique can be used to access the extent of organ involvement in the neoplastic process. Cytotoxic drugs such as methotrexate and chlorambucil have been used in this type of delivery system.

## Delivery of Cytotoxic Drugs

The same concept as described for imaging can be used for the delivery of cytotoxic drugs to a tumor site. The concept of a "magic bullet" was conceived by Ehrlich in the early 1900s. The modern technology of monoclonal antibodies has brought the concept to fruition. A tumor-specific antibody is coupled to a cytotoxic drug and is injected into the patient. The antibody–drug complex homes to the tumor and a high dose is administered to the affected tissue. Adverse systemic side affects frequently associated with cytotoxic antitumor drugs are thus diminished by this type of delivery system.

A variety of cytotoxic compounds have potential for this type of therapy. Among those that have been tried are: diphtheria toxin; the plant toxin, ricin; and the *Pseudomonas aeruginosa* exotoxin A. Penetration of one molecule of the ricin toxin into a cell has been deemed sufficient for killing. Success with this procedure depends upon the ability to selectively target the toxin to the tumor cells with minimum nonspecific binding to other cells.

## MONOCLONAL ANTIBODIES AS VACCINES

### Anti-idiotype Vaccines

The concept of anti-idiotype vaccines has been popular for the past decade, although the technique has not yielded many finished products marketable as vaccines. Reviewing terminology: the idiotype of an antibody is that part of it which includes the hypervariable regions of the heavy and light chains. It dictates the specificity of the antibody (i.e., the antigen with which the antibody will bind). An anti-idiotype is formed when there is an immune response against the idiotype of the antibody, creating anti-idiotypes, which are actually mirror images of the antigenic determinant for which the first antibody was specific (Fig. 3). This second antibody, the anti-idiotype, can be used as a vaccine to elicit an antibody response to the antigenic determinant that it mimics. Thus, an animal can be immunized with an antigen without ever having been exposed to it.

The greatest application for this technology is in the infectious disease area, particularly when it is difficult to purify the antigens from an organism and it is unwise to use the entire organism as a vaccine, because of adverse side effects. With the anti-idiotype technique,

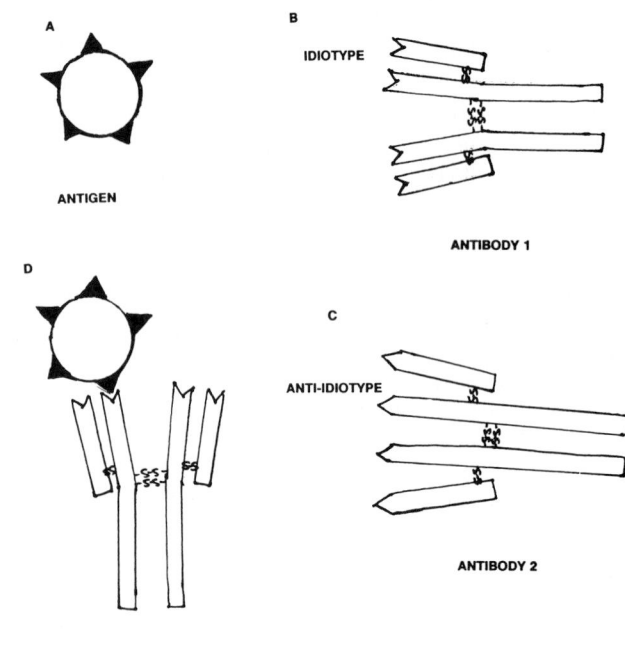

**Figure 3.** Anti-idiotype vaccine production: a mouse is immunized with the antigen and monoclonal antibody 1 is produced; a second mouse is immunized with antibody 1 and produces antibody 2 against the idiotype of antibody 1. This anti-idiotype resembles the original antigen. Immunization of a patient with antibody 2 will elicit a polyclonal antibody response with some antibodies recognizing the anti-idiotype and also antigen. Antibody 3 can bind to and neutralize the antigen.

one can eliminate the need to purify large amounts of bacterial, viral, or parasitic antigens for use in subunit vaccines, yet still retain the advantage of not having to use the whole organism, which might contain toxins or other inflammation-inducing substances. In human medicine, this methodology has been applied to development of candidate human immunodeficiency virus (HIV) vaccines.

## References and Suggested Reading

Andrews GA, Chavey PS, and Smith JE: Production, characterization, and applications of a murine monoclonal antibody to dog erythrocyte antigen 1.1. J Am Vet Med Assoc 201:1549, 1992.
*A card agglutination test that uses only 50 µl microliters of blood developed with the monoclonal antibodies to dog erythrocyte antigen 1.1 is described.*

Corapi WV, Olsen CW, and Scott FW: Monoclonal antibody analysis of neutralization and antibody-dependent enhancement of feline infectious peritonitis virus. J Virol 66:6695, 1992.
*A panel of monoclonal antibodies was developed to study and identify the viral protein neutralization and enhancement epitopes on feline infectious peritonitis virus.*

Fevereiro M, Ronecker C, Laufs A, Tavares L, et al: Characterization of two monoclonal antibodies against feline immunodeficiency virus *gag* gene products and their application in an assay to evaluate neutralizing antibody activity. J Gen Virol 72:617, 1991.
*Monoclonal antibodies against gag gene products of FIV were used in a simple assay for detection and quantification of infectious virus and neutralizing antibody.*

Hara Y, Ejima H, Aoki S, and Tagawa M: Preparation of monoclonal antibodies against dog erythrocyte antigen D1(DEA-3). J Vet Med Sci 53:1105, 1991.
*Monoclonal antibodies that react with D1 antigen from the DEA-3 system*

*were prepared for application to antigen characterization and erythrocyte typing.*

Hosu MJ, Willett BJ, Dunsford TH, Jarrett O, et al: A monoclonal antibody which blocks infection with feline immunodeficiency virus identifies a possible non-CD4 receptor. J Virol 67:1667, 1993.

*A monoclonal antibody was produced that detects a feline cell surface protein that may be an FIV receptor distinct from CD4.*

Lin CY, Chang ZN, Chang SC: The establishment of two monoclonal antibodies that recognize canine MHC class II antigens. Transplant Proc 24: 1304, 1992.

*Monoclonal antibodies that recognize MHC class-II antigens on canine cells were produced and used to show that class-II expression occurs on transplanted but not normal bronchial epithelial cells.*

Mazza G, Duffus WPH, Elson CJ, et al: The separation and identification by monoclonal antibodies of dog IgG fractions. J Immunol Methods 161:193, 1993.

*IgG subclasses were recognized by monoclonal antibodies.*

McMichael AJ and Fabre JW: *Monoclonal Antibodies in Clinical Medicine.* London, Academic Press, 1982.

*This is a good overview of clinical applications of monoclonal antibodies.*

Milton ID, Turner J, Teelan A, et al: Location of monoclonal antibody binding sites in the capsid protein of feline calicivirus. J Gen Virol 73:2435, 1992.

*Three monoclonal antibodies were developed against the capsid protein of feline calicivirus for use in studying the antigenic variation that gives rise to restricted immunity in host populations.*

Oliver JL and Wolfe LG: Antigen expression in canine tissues, recognized by a monoclonal antibody generated against canine melanoma cells. Am J Vet Res 53:123, 1992.

*Monoclonal antibodies were developed against canine melanoma cells and were found to distinguish between amelanotic melanoma and spindle cell mesenchymal tumors, as well as between benign and malignant melanocytic lesions in dogs.*

Potgieter LND and Ajidagba PA: Quantitation of canine distemper virus and antibodies by ELISA using protein A and monoclonal antibody capture. J Vet Diag Invest 1:110, 1989.

*Monoclonal antibodies developed against canine distemper virus were used to detect antigen and antibody in serum, CSF fluid, and tissue, without cross-reactivity with other paramyxoviruses.*

Stern NJ and Gamble HR (eds): *Hybridoma Technology in Agricultural and Veterinary Research.* Totowa, NJ, Rowman & Allanheld, 1984.

*This book contains papers presented at a symposium and demonstrates the variety of applications of monoclonal antibodies to veterinary research.*

# CYTOKINES AND BIOLOGIC RESPONSE MODIFIERS IN SMALL ANIMAL PRACTICE

STEPHEN A. KRUTH

*Guelph, Ontario, Canada*

Therapy directed towards correcting alterations in either immune function or myelosuppression associated with neoplastic, infectious, or autoimmune disease would be useful in small animal practice. Agents that enhance immune responses during immunization are also of interest. *Immunopotentiation* is a general term that implies optimization or augmentation of the immune response, while the term *immunotherapy* is used when defined antigens are targeted (e.g., treating lymphoma with monoclonal antibodies). *Immunoadjuvant therapy* refers to the nonspecific activation of one or more cell populations within the immune system (e.g., the use of bacterial cell wall preparations or cytokines that activate various cell lines). Preparations employed to enhance immune responses are called *biologic response modifiers*, and range from relatively crude cell extracts to molecularly cloned cytokines to highly defined synthetic chemicals.

Small animal veterinarians have been reluctant to use biologic response modifiers largely because specific indications and efficacy have not been clearly defined. As well, the mechanisms by which many of these preparations function remain poorly understood. The preparations are often relatively crude extracts of bacteria or tissue, adding to the impression that these approaches border on the edge of acceptable therapy. Their use has also been limited by potential side effects and lack of availability.

Relatively recent advances in immunology and molecular biology were needed to explain the actions of biologic response modifiers. It now appears that these preparations affect the production and secretion of a number of cellular messengers, termed *cytokines*. Purified cytokines are now being used as therapeutic agents.

Extensive efforts to evaluate the use of biologic response modifiers (including specific cytokines) in the management of cancer and retroviral infections in humans are underway. Unfortunately, the results have usually been disappointing (although there are exceptions, such as the use of interferon-$\alpha$ for the management of human hairy cell leukemia). The information available on cytokines for dogs and cats is derived primarily from investigations using these species as models for human diseases. Most veterinary species-specific cytokine research has been in the prevention and management of infectious diseases in food-producing animals (e.g., mastitis and respiratory infections). As canine and feline cytokines are cloned and biologic response modifiers become better defined, immunopotentiation procedures will probably play roles both in immunization and in the management of diseases of the dog and cat.

The goal of this update is to present immunopotentiation therapy in the context of cytokine physiology. A brief introduction to cytokines is presented, followed by examples of cytokine-based therapy. Finally, examples of biologic response modifiers licensed for use in dogs and cats are given. Examples of nonspecific techniques of immunopotentiation are given in Table 1 (specific means of immunopotentiation, such as vaccination and the administration of hyperimmune globulin or sensitized lymphocytes, are beyond the scope of this article). An excellent general review of biologic response modifiers has been prepared by MacEwen (MacEwen, 1985).

## CYTOKINES

Cytokines are low-molecular-weight protein or glycoprotein mediators involved in the regulation of cell growth and differentiation. They are produced by a wide variety of cells, including lymphocytes, monocytes, granulocytes, endothelial cells, keratinocytes, and fibroblasts. Cytokines mediate and regulate the initial immune response, inflammation, tissue repair, and hematopoiesis. Some are cytolytic for virus-infected and neoplastic cells (Tompkins and Tompkins, 1990). *Cytokine* is the preferred terminology; the terms *lymphokine* and *monokine* suggest that a substance is produced by either lymphocytes or monocytes, when in fact there is considerable overlap. Cytokine nomenclature is confusing, as many of these substances are produced by or act upon cells other than the name implies, and a given cytokine has probably been known historically by a variety of names.

Recombinant molecular biology technology has allowed investigators to define many human and murine cytokines at the DNA level, and assays for cytokine activities are widely available for research purposes. Some cytokines are now available in amounts that can be used in clinical trials. Recombinant cytokines are designated by "r" and the species of origin (e.g., rHuIL-2 for recombinant human interleukin-2). Although cytokines from different species tend to have similar structures, a given cytokine from one species may induce antibodies against itself when administered to another species, potentially limiting the use of some recombinant human cytokines in dogs and cats. Unfortunately, few canine or feline cytokines have been cloned.

Cytokine systems consist of the cytokine and a specific target cell receptor, designated by "R" (e.g., IL-2R), which serve to activate the target cell. Although some cytokines have systemic effects, most function in autocrine and paracrine manners, and are effective in extremely small amounts. Most cytokines are secreted following the activation of cells by appropriate stimuli. Cytokine secretion is closely regulated to avoid pathogenic effects of overproduction. In addition to the short expression of cytokines, circulating natural and specific inhibitors can prevent small amounts of cytokine from having prolonged or diffuse effects. Abnormal cytokine or receptor expression has been associated with some neoplastic disorders; for example, the continuous expression of IL-2 and/or IL-2R has been associated with T-cell leukemia, and the autonomous growth of acute myeloblastic leukemia cells is related to autocrine stimulation by GM-CSF, G-CSF, and IL-6. The hypoproduction of cytokines has also been documented, such as the hypoproduction of IL-2 in systemic lupus ery-

---

**Table 1.**  *Examples of Nonspecific Induction of Immunopotentiation*

**Active (Requires Host Response)**
  Cytokines (e.g., IL-1, IL-2, IFN-γ; activation of cells involved in immunity, inflammation, and
    hematopoiesis)
  Thymosins and other hormone-like thymic extracts (accelerate maturation of T-cells)
  Agents of biologic origin (induction of IL-1, IL-2, TNF, and IFN secretion from macrophages)
    Bacterial preparations
      Bacillus Calmette-Guérin (BCG)
      *Propionibacterium acnes* (previously called
        *Corynebacterium parvum*; Immunoregulin, ImunoVet°)
    Extracts of bacteria
      Methanol extractable residue (MER) of BCG
      Mycobacterial cell wall extract (Regressin-V,
        Vetrepharm, Inc°)
      *Serratia marcescens* extract
    Chemically identified bacterial extracts
      Muramyl peptides (from BCG)
      Lipopolysaccharide
    Complex carbohydrates
      Acemannan (Acemannan Immunostimulant, Carrington Laboratories°)
    Synthetic chemicals
      Levamisol, isoprinosine (inducers of thymic hormone secretion)
      PolyI:C (inducer of interferon secretion)

**Passive (Does Not Require Host Response)**
  Immunoglobulin therapy
  Plasmapheresis (removal of "blocking antibodies")

**Adoptive (Transfer of Activated Cells)**
  Cytokine-activated killer cells

°Licensed for use in dogs and cats.

**Table 2.** *Interleukin-1 Sources, Activities, and Potential Therapeutic Applications*

*Sources*

Antigen-presenting cells, natural killer (NK) cells, B cells, neutrophils, endothelial cells, fibroblasts, others. Two forms have been described in several species: IL-1α, and IL-1β. These represent the products of two distinct genes, but recognize the same receptors.

*Functions*

Activation of T cells in the presence of antigen, induction of IL-2 and IL-2R
Costimulation of thymocyte proliferation
Augmentation of NK-mediated cytotoxicity
Stimulation of B-cell differentiation, proliferation, and Ig secretion
Induction of hematopoietic growth factor synthesis
Induction of insulin secretion; cytolytic to islet cells
Induction of acute-phase protein synthesis
Induction of adhesion molecule expression by endothelial cells
Induction of steoridogenesis
Induction of fever and sleep
Osteoblast and endothelial cell activation
Enhancement of collagen production by epidermal cells

*Potential Therapeutic Applications*

Radioprotective effect (stimulator of hematopoiesis)
Acceleration of wound healing
Antagonists may have utility in the treatment of chronic inflammatory diseases
Vaccine adjuvant

thematosus, advanced malignancies, and primary immunodeficiency syndromes.

Cytokine receptors are subject to transient up- or down-regulation, further controlling cytokine activity. An understanding of receptor physiology is clinically relevant, as cytokine analogues are being developed that have desired biologic activity without dose-limiting side effects. For example, an IL-2 analogue that binds to the intermediate affinity form of IL-2R, but not to the high-affinity form of IL-2R, has recently been described. This analogue induces T-cell cytotoxicity, but should not cause toxic systemic signs associated with activation of the high-affinity form of the receptor. Receptor antagonists may also have therapeutic potential, such as a recently described IL-1R antagonist, which may be useful in the management of chronic arthritis. Additionally, the measurement of circulating levels of soluble receptors may be useful for diagnosis and as a prognostic indicator (e.g., serum IL-2R levels correlate with clinical stage and histopathologic grade of non-Hodgkin's lymphoma in humans).

The production of cytokines and cytokine receptors is normally limited to a few days, and the circulation half-life is short, suggesting that recirculation is not part of normal cytokine physiology. The pharmacologic use of cytokines will thus require the development of novel delivery systems (e.g., liposomes, continuous regional hepatic arterial infusion), as dose-limiting toxicity may be associated with systemic administration.

*Interleukins* (ILs) are defined as messengers acting between leukocytes (Elmslie, Dow, and Ogilvie, 1991). This terminology is also inaccurate in that these substances may be produced by and act upon cells other than blood cells. There are currently 13 interleukins described, designated IL-1 through IL-13. IL-1 and IL-2 are probably the most clinically relevant interleukins; their known activities are presented in Tables 2 and 3. None of the canine interleukins have been

**Table 3.** *Interleukin-2 Sources, Activities, and Potential Therapeutic Applications*

*Source*

Activated T$_H$ cells

*Activities*

Autocrine and paracrine stimulation of T cells
Stimulation of B cells and Ig synthesis
Induction of tumoricidal activity and growth of NK cells and LAK cells
Augments IFN-γ and IL-6 production
Modulation of histamine release from basophils

*Potential Therapeutic Uses*

Induction of LAK and TIL cells
Treatment of immunodeficiency
Vaccine adjuvant
Measurement of serum IL-2 receptor levels for diagnosis and prognosis of various autoimmune disorders, malignancies, transplant rejection, and infectious diseases

Abbreviations: NK = natural killer (cells), LAK = lymphokine activated killer (cells), IFN-γ = interferon-γ, IL-6 = interleukin-6, TIL = tumor-infiltrating lymphocytes, Ig = immunoglobulin.

cloned. Cloning of feline IL-2, IL-6, and IL-10 has recently been reported.

*Interferons* (IFNs) are recognized for their nonspecific antiviral activity. They also have significant immunoregulatory and cytostatic functions. Interferon-$\alpha$ is a mix of glycoproteins referred to as leukocyte or lymphoblastoid IFN (depending upon the cell of origin). Interferon-$\beta$ is produced by fibroblasts; IFN-$\alpha$ and IFN-$\beta$ are structurally and functionally related, and are produced in response to viral infections. Interferon-$\gamma$ is secreted by T cells, natural killer (NK) cells, and other immune effector cells in response to a specific antigenic stimulus. It is one of the most potent immunoregulatory mediators known, influencing the production of immunoglobulin isotypes, up-regulating class I and II MHC complex antigens, and increasing the efficiency of macrophage-mediated killing of intracellular parasites. Canine IFN-$\gamma$ and feline IFN-$\alpha$ have been cloned. Their biologic activities are listed in Tables 4 and 5.

*Growth factors* stimulate the growth of a variety of cell lines. All are cytokines, and some are designated as interleukins. Hematopoietic growth factors are termed *colony-stimulating factors* (CSFs); however, they may have other activities. They include stem-cell factor, IL-3, granulocyte macrophage colony-stimulating factor (GM-CSF), granulocyte colony-stimulating factor (G-CSF), and macrophage colony-stimulating factor (M-CSF). Canine G-CSF has been cloned.

Another clinically important pair of cytokines are the *tumor necrosis factors* (TNFs). TNF-$\alpha$ and TNF-$\beta$ are closely related cytokines that bind to the same cell surface receptors and which play a critical role in normal host resistance to infections and in the destruction of neoplastic cells. TNF-$\alpha$ has also been called *cachectin* due to its role in inducing a cachectic state via inhibition of lipoprotein lipase and fatty acid synthetase, and by stimulating catabolic pathways in myocytes and hepatocytes. The primary sources of TNF-$\alpha$ are activated monocytes and macrophages. TNF-$\beta$ is also called *lymphotoxin*, the primary source being activated T cells. Due to the ubiquity of their receptors, their ability to stimulate several different cell activation pathways, and their ability to induce or suppress the expression of

**Table 4.**   *Interferon-$\alpha$/$\beta$ Sources, Activities, and Potential Therapeutic Applications*

**Sources**
    IFN-$\alpha$: monocytes/macrophages or lymphoid cells stimulated by viruses, bacterial products, or nucleic acids; a family of molecules derived from several genes
    IFN-$\beta$: fibroblasts/epithelial cells; more than one molecular species may be present, depending upon species

**Activities**
    Nonspecific antiviral activity via effects on RNA and protein synthesis, as well as induced extracellular antiviral proteins
    Antiproliferative effects on both normal and malignant cells
    Enhanced natural killer cell activity against tumor cells

**Potential Therapeutic Uses**
    Cross-species activity is often present
    Prophylactic and therapeutic activity against a variety of acute and chronic viral infections
    Adjunctive therapy for hematologic, lymphoid, and limited other malignancies

**Table 5.**   *Interferon-$\gamma$ Sources, Activities, and Potential Therapeutic Applications*

**Sources**
    Activated $T_H$ cells
    NK cells

**Activities**
    Immunoregulatory effects
        Principle macrophage activating factor: up-regulation of type-I and -II MHC antigens, increased antimicrobial activity, increased antitumor activity, increased TNF-$\alpha$ synthesis, inhibition of migration
        Enhancement of IL-2 synthesis, enhancement of cytotoxic T-cell and NK-cell activity
        Induction of antibody-dependent cytotoxicity via induction of Fc receptors on neutrophils and monocyte-macrophages
        Stimulation of B-cell activity
    Inhibition of growth of normal and neoplastic cells
    Nonspecific antiviral activity (<IFN-$\alpha$/$\beta$)

**Potential Therapeutic Uses**
    Adjuvant therapy for cancer patients undergoing immunosuppressive therapy
    Treatment of systemic intracellular infections
    Clinical trials in cancer patients have generally been disappointing

Abbreviations: NK = natural killer (cell), TNF = tumor necrosis factor, MHC = major histocompatibility complex, IL = interleukin, IFN = interferon.

many genes, the two TNFs are capable of producing a wide variety of effects. TNF actions are listed in Table 6.

## Cytokines as Biologic Response Modifiers

Clinical trials designed to investigate the therapeutic utility of cytokines are becoming common in human medicine. For example, IL-2 administered as a single agent to humans with advanced renal cell cancer or melanoma has been associated with partial or complete responses in approximately 20% of cases. Adoptive immunotherapy with lymphokine activated killer (LAK) cells (lymphocytes isolated from peripheral blood and incubated with IL-2) has been associated with partial or complete responses in up to 35% of humans with renal cell cancer, 21% with melanoma, 13% with colorectal cancer, and 57% with non-Hodgkin's lymphoma. Tumor-infiltrating lymphocytes (TIL) (lymphocytes recovered from growing tumors and incubated with IL-2) have induced significant clinical responses in humans where other forms of IL-2 based therapy have failed. Normal canine peripheral blood mononuclear cells stimulated *in vitro* with rHuIL-2 manifest cytotoxicity against a variety of malignant cells, and cells with LAK characteristics have been induced with rHuIL-2 in cats.

There have been few cytokine-based clinical trials in dogs or cats, most of which have evaluated the efficacy of recombinant hematopoietic growth factors (see below). Recombinant HuIL-2 and rHuIFN-α have been evaluated in cats with feline leukemia virus (FeLV) infections, and rHuTNF-α and rHuIL-2 in combination with chemotherapy or surgery was evaluated in dogs with a variety of spontaneous neoplasms. Overall, the results of these trials have been disappointing.

## Cytokines as Vaccine Adjuvants

Classic vaccine adjuvants induce IL-1 secretion, which in turn initiates a cascade of events leading to an enhanced protective response via the induction of receptors for IL-2 and CSFs, and the secretion of IL-2, IL-4, IL-6, and IL-8. Unfortunately, the side effects associated with the proinflammatory actions of IL-1 have prohibited its use as an adjuvant. A synthetic peptide consisting of amino acid residues 163–171 of human IL-1β was described recently. This analogue is devoid of proinflammatory activities but maintains the immunostimulating activity of entire IL-1β, making it a possible adjuvant candidate.

Interleukin-2 has been shown to have utility as an adjuvant in a porcine *Haemophilus pleuropneumoniae* bacterin and in an inactivated rabies virus vaccine in mice. Cytokines, cytokine analogues, or cytokine inducers will be important in the future development of canine and feline vaccines.

## HEMATOPOIETIC GROWTH FACTORS

### Recombinant Canine G-CSF

Recombinant growth factors have potential clinical utility in the management of myelosuppressive disorders (e.g., FeLV-induced neutropenias) or myelosuppression secondary to chemotherapy or radiation therapy. Canine G-CSF has been cloned, but is not commercially available at this time. In a pilot study, five healthy dogs were given 5 μg recombinant canine G-CSF (rcG-CSF)/kg/day SC for 4 weeks. The mean neutrophil counts ± standard deviation increased from 6537/ml ± 1726 to 26,330/ml ± 7066 within 24 hr after the first injection of rcG-CSF. A maximum of 72,125/ml ± 15,073 was reached by day 19. Significant mono-

**Table 6.** *Tumor Necrosis Factor Sources, Activities, and Potential Therapeutic Applications*

---

**Sources**
   TNF-α: activated monocytes or macrophages, also neutrophils, lymphocytes, endothelial cells, other cells
   TNF-β: activated T cell

**Actions**
   Cytolytic or cytostatic activities towards tumor cells
   Induction of MHC antigens
   PMN activation
   Osteoclast activation
   Antiviral activity
   TNF-α can induce hematopoietic growth factor activity
   TNF-α is a major mediator in toxic shock and sepsis

**Potential Therapeutic Applications**
   Adjunct therapy of malignancies
   Antibodies to TNF may be used to treat septic shock
   Monitoring TNF-αR may be useful in chronic inflammatory diseases

---

Abbreviations: TNF = tumor necrosis factor, MHC = major histocompatibility complex, PMN = polymorphonuclear neutrophil.

cytosis also developed. Blood counts returned to normal within 5 days after discontinuing rcG-CSF, and clinically significant toxicoses were not associated with rcG-CSF administration.

In another study using normal dogs, a significant dose-dependent increase in functional neutrophils and monocytes was again demonstrated. These investigators also found that rcG-CSF prevented neutropenia and associated clinical signs (but did not completely eliminate the cycling of neutrophils) in cyclic-hematopoietic dogs when administered at rates of up to 2.5 $\mu$g/kg every 12 hr. The time to bone marrow reconstitution was not decreased in dogs treated with rcG-CSF following autologous bone marrow transplantation, emphasizing that rcG-CSF action is dependant upon the presence of progenitor cells in the bone marrow (Mishu et al., 1992).

To evaluate the utility of rcG-CSF in the management of chemotherapy-induced neutropenia, myelosuppression was induced with mitoxantrone in otherwise normal dogs and then treated with daily rcG-CSF for 20 days. None of those receiving rcG-CSF developed serious neutropenia, while four of five dogs not treated with rcG-CSF did. These findings demonstrate that rcG-CSF is capable of reducing the duration and severity of mitoxantrone-induced myelosuppression (Ogilvie et al., 1992a).

Recombinant canine G-CSF has also been studied in normal cats: 5 $\mu$g rcG-CSF/kg/day SC was administered to healthy cats for 42 days. Mean neutrophil counts increased from 10,966/ml $\pm$ 2324 to 30,688/ml $\pm$ 5296 within 24 hr after the first dose. Neutrophil counts increased and remained elevated until cytokine administration was discontinued. There were no adverse effects associated with the administration of rcG-CSF to healthy cats (Obradovich et al., 1993).

The use of cytokines in the treatment of myelosuppression in cancer patients may involve risks. Receptors for these growth factors have been identified on various tumor cell lines, and varying degrees of *in vitro* tumor proliferation responses to exogenous cytokines have been documented, raising the concern that in some situations cytokines may actually stimulate tumor growth.

## Extract of *Serratia marcescens*

Recombinant colony-stimulating factors are not yet commercially available for use in dogs and cats, and they are likely to be expensive if they are licensed. An alternative approach is to administer a preparation that induces the synthesis and release of cytokines of interest. An extract of *Serratia marcescens* is a potent activator of macrophages, inducing the release of IFN-$\alpha$, IFN-$\gamma$, TNF-$\alpha$, IL-1, IL-6, and GM-CSF. This preparation induces myeloproliferation, either directly by stimulating CSF-producing cells, or indirectly through the actions of other released cytokines. In a study of doxorubicin-induced myelosuppression in normal dogs, increasing the dosage and schedule of administration of extract reduced the duration and severity of induced myelosuppression. There was also an increase in endogenous G-CSF activity 4 to 6 hr after the extract was administered. These findings demonstrate that *S. marcescens* extract reduces the duration and severity of doxorubicin-induced myelosuppression, and that this may be at least partially mediated by G-CSF (Ogilvie et al., 1992b).

## EXAMPLES OF BIOLOGIC RESPONSE MODIFIERS LICENSED FOR USE IN DOGS AND CATS

A large number of preparations, ranging in degree of purity from entire bacterial cells to specific cell components, have been used as biologic response modifiers. Until recently, little was known about the specific mechanisms by which these compounds exert their effects. Most evidence now suggests an interaction with macrophages, resulting in increased antigen uptake, enhanced phagocytosis, cytotoxicity, and the release of cytokines. Activated macrophages can be microbicidal and tumoricidal. Examples of two products licensed for veterinary use in North America follow. One is a mycobacterial cell wall extract, while the other is a complex carbohydrate. It should be emphasized that these preparations have not undergone controlled, prospective, randomized clinical trials, and that the clinical benefits to be derived from the use of these compounds is unknown.

### Mycobacterial Cell Wall Fraction

An emulsion of mycobacterial cell wall fractions (Regressin-V, Vetrepharm, Inc) is licensed for the treatment of mixed mammary tumors and mammary adenocarcinoma in dogs and sarcoid in horses. The following information was supplied by the manufacturer. Regressin-V induces IL-1 and TNF-$\alpha$ secretion from monocytes and macrophages. In a study of seven dogs with mammary adenocarcinoma, five of seven underwent complete remission, with tumor-free survival times of 3 to 19 months; dogs were then lost to followup. There are no data suggesting that Regressin-V had any effect on metastatic disease.

Canine mammary tumors should be treated once 2 to 4 weeks prior to surgery. Low-grade fever and malaise may occur 1 or 2 days after injections, and may last for up to 1 week. Surgical removal of the tumor creates a cosmetic improvement (necrosis and draining of the tumor may be present for weeks following injection); however, survival is not significantly improved. If surgery is not performed, therapy can be repeated every 1 to 3 weeks, up to four treatments. This mycobacterial cell wall extract is also included as an adjuvant in several veterinary vaccines.

## Acemannan

Acemannan (Acemannan Immunostimulant, Carrington Laboratories) is a chemically defined $\beta$-(1,4)–linked mannan-based polysaccharide derived from the *Aloe barbadensis miller* plant. It stimulates the release of IL-1$\alpha$, IL-6, TNF-$\alpha$, and prostaglandin $E_2$ from macrophages, resulting in tumor apoptosis and necrosis. Other actions include enhancement of macrophage phagocytosis and nonspecific cytotoxicity, and interference with glucosidase I activity (leading to the production of abnormal glycoproteins by neoplastic cells, which appears to be associated with tumor cell death). Direct antiviral activity has also been described. This effect is associated with modified glycosylation of both viral infected cells and glycoprotein coats of viruses, leading to inhibition of virus replication and infectivity.

Acemannan is licensed for the treatment of fibrosarcoma in dogs and cats. Intratumoral injection is followed by tumor encapsulation, necrosis, and death, facilitating surgical excision. The dosage regimen is 2 mg injected into the tumor mass and 1 mg/kg IP weekly for 6 weeks. Rapid expansion of the tumor due to cystic fluid accumulation should be expected, and surgical removal of the mass is recommended when tumor delineation or necrosis occurs. No adverse effects of acemannan have been reported at the recommended dosage. Other responding tumors include squamous cell carcinoma, cutaneous histiocytoma, myxosarcoma, adenocarcinoma, lymphoma, mast cell tumor, and infiltrating lipoma (Harris et al., 1991).

Acemannan has been used to treat cats with FeLV and feline immunodeficiency virus (FIV) infections. Clinically affected cats with FeLV or FIV infections treated with acemannan had improved quality of life and longer survival times compared to historical controls (Sheets et al., 1991; Yates et al., 1992); however, a placebo-controlled prospective study has not been published. Interestingly, oral administration of acemannan appeared to have the same efficacy as did parenteral administration; similar findings have been reported in FeLV-infected cats given oral rHuIFN-$\alpha$.

## LOW-DOSE ORALLY ADMINISTERED ALPHA INTERFERON TREATMENT FOR RETROVIRAL INFECTIONS IN CATS

Although not licensed for use in cats, rHuIFN-$\alpha$ may have some efficacy in the management of FeLV (and possibly FIV) infections. Several reports have claimed that FeLV infected cats treated with rHuIFN-$\alpha$ showed one or more of the following: increased activity and appetite, resolution of hematologic abnormalities, clearance of viremia, and prolonged survival times. It was suggested that small but optimal amounts of rHuIFN-$\alpha$ may bind to mucosal macrophages, lymphocytes, or other cells which in turn initiate cytokine cascades, inducing a systemic anti-viral response. The reader is referred to the paper by Weiss et al. for formulation, dosage, and treatment schedules.

## SUMMARY

Although the therapeutic potential of some recombinant cytokines has been studied in dogs and cats, species-specific preparations are not commercially available at this time. Human recombinant preparations are expensive, and may have limited effects. Alternatively, biologic response modifiers in the form of bacterial cell wall extracts and complex carbohydrates are currently licensed for use in dogs and cats. These preparations theoretically have the advantage of inducing a more coordinated cytokine response than do single recombinant cytokines. They should be further evaluated for their efficacy in the treatment of cancer, retroviral infections, and use as vaccine adjuvants with prospective, randomized controlled clinical trials before specific recommendations for their use can be made. However, when alternative therapies have low efficacy and significant adverse effects, these preparations may play a role in the management of malignancies such as fibrosarcoma and mammary adenocarcinoma. Immunopotentiation therapy in small animal practice is in an early developmental stage; however, it raises expectations for the development of more effective therapies for many malignancies, retroviral infections, and myelosuppression.

## References and Suggested Reading

Barta O: Immunoadjuvant therapy. *In* Kirk RW and Bonagura JD (ed): *Current Veterinary Therapy XI: Small Animal Practice.* Philadelphia, WB Saunders Co, 1992, p 217.
  *A review of biologic response modifiers that have been tested in dogs or cats.*
Elmslie RE, Dow SW, and Ogilvie GK: Interleukins: Biological properties and therapeutic potential. J Vet Intern Med 5:283, 1991.
  *A catalogue approach to IL-1 though IL-10.*
Harris C, Pierce K, King G, Yates KM, Hall J, and Tizard I: Efficacy of Acemannan in treatment of canine and feline spontaneous neoplasms. Mol Biother 3:207, 1991.
  *Acemannan induced clinical responses in 12 of 43 animals with a variety of solid tumors.*
MacEwen EG: Approaches to cancer therapy using biological response modifiers. Vet Clin North Am [Small Anim Pract] 15:667, 1985.
  *A general review, including bacterial agents, interferons, monoclonal antibodies, cytokines, and immunoregulatory peptides.*
Mishu L, Callahan G, Allebban Z, Maddux JM, Boone TC, Souza LM, and Lothrop CD: Effects of recombinant canine granulocyte colony-stimulating factor on white blood cell production in clinically normal and neutropenic dogs. J Am Vet Med Assoc 200:1957, 1992.
  *Recombinant canine G-CSF induces myelopoiesis in normal and cyclic-hematopoietic dogs, but not dogs receiving total body irradiation.*
Obradovich JE, Ogilvie GK, Stadler-Morris S, Schmidt BR, Cooper MF, and Boone TC: Effect of recombinant canine granulocyte colony-stimulating factor on peripheral blood neutrophil counts in normal cats. J Vet Intern Med 7:65, 1993.
  *Recombinant canine G-CSF induces neutrophilia in normal cats.*
Ogilvie GK and Obradovich JE: Hematopoietic growth factors: Clinical use and implications. *In* Kirk RW and Bonagura JD (eds): *Current Veterinary Therapy XI: Small Animal Practice.* Philadelphia, WB Saunders Co, 1992, p 466.
Ogilvie GK, Obradovich JE, Cooper MF, Walters LM, Salman MD, and Boone TC: Use of recombinant canine granulocyte colony-stimulating factor to decrease myelosuppression associated with the administration of mitoxantrone in the dog. J Vet Intern Med 6:44, 1992a.
  *Recombinant cG-CSF prevents serious neutropenia in chemotherapy-induced myelosuppression.*
Ogilvie GK, Elmslie RE, Cecchini M, Walters LM, and Pearson FC: Use of a biological extract of *Serratia marcescens* to decrease doxorubicin-induced myelosuppression in dogs. Am J Vet Res 53:1787, 1992b.
  *This extract induces cytokine secretion and myelopoiesis in dogs.*

Sheets MA, Unger BA, Giggleman GF, and Tizard IR: Studies of the effect of acemannan on retrovirus infections: Clinical stabilization of feline leukemia virus-infected cats. Mol Biother 3:41, 1991.
*Administration of acemannan for 6 weeks intraperitoneally to cats with clinical signs improved the quality of life and survival times.*

Tompkins MB and Tompkins WAF: Cytokines in the immunoregulatory network: Potential for therapy in the canine and feline species. *In* Barta O (ed): *MHC, Differentiation Antigens, and Cytokines in Animals and Birds.* Blacksburg, BAR-LAB, 1990, p 81.
*A review of cytokine physiology and their use as immunotherapeutic agents in cats and dogs.*

Tompkins MB and Tompkins WAF: Immunoregulatory cytokines and their potential in therapy. *In* Kirk RW and Bonagura JD (eds): *Current Veterinary Therapy XI: Small Animal Practice.* Philadelphia, WB Saunders Co, 1992, p 461.

Weiss RC, Cummins JM, and Richards AB: Low-dose orally administered alpha interferon treatment for feline leukemia virus infection. J Am Vet Med Assoc 199:1477, 1991.
*A review of the clinical experience with orally administered alpha interferon in HIV and FeLV infections, with practical guidelines for using low-dose orally administered rHuIFN-α in cats infected with FeLV.*

Yates KM, Rosenberg LJ, Harris CK, Bronstad DC, King GK, Biehle GA, Walker B, Ford CR, Hall JE, and Tizard IR: Pilot study of the effect of acemannan in cats infected with feline immunodeficiency virus. Vet Immunol Immunopathol 35:177, 1992.
*Acemannan therapy may induce increased survival times in FIV-infected cats exhibiting clinical signs of disease.*

# AUTOIMMUNITY

CINDY J. BRUNNER
*Auburn, Alabama*

Autoimmunity occurs as a consequence of the immune system's failure to eliminate high-affinity self-reactive lymphocytes in primary lymphoid organs, or its failure to regulate the activity of low-affinity self-reactive lymphocytes that become immunocompetent and are released into the body.

When autoimmune disease results from spontaneous loss of self-tolerance, the disorder is considered to be primary. Autoimmune disease that follows a bout of infection, neoplasia, or severe inflammation is regarded as secondary. In secondary autoimmune disease, the loss of self-tolerance is provoked by the initial appearance of microbial antigens or tumor-associated antigens in close proximity with autoantigens on the cell surface. Then, despite successful elimination of the microorganism or neoplastic cells, tissue damage continues because of activation of self-reactive lymphocytes.

The frequency of occurrence of autoimmune disease in the pet population is low. Most immune-mediated tissue damage in animals can be attributed to an exuberant immune response to exogenous antigen, rather than mistaken recognition of autoantigens as foreign.

It is often difficult to establish with certainty the autoimmune nature of an inflammatory process. Even healthy animals produce antibodies that bind to autoantigens, especially with increasing age. Also, once an inflammatory process begins, one can frequently detect antibodies that are reactive to tissue antigens. The following criteria have been proposed as "Koch's postulates" of autoimmune disease: (1) the autoantibodies should be detectable in all cases of the disease, (2) the disease should be experimentally reproducible by some form of immunization with the antigen, (3) the experimental disease must show immunopathologic lesions that parallel those seen in the natural disease, and (4)

the disease should be transferable from an affected animal to a normal animal by means of either serum or living lymphoid cells.

## CLASSIFICATION OF AUTOIMMUNE DISEASES

As an aid to understanding the pathogenesis and clinical management of autoimmune diseases, it is useful to categorize them according to the extent of organ involvement. Such categorization is relevant because those diseases that are organ-specific can sometimes be managed simply by replacing a missing hormone, whereas successful management of generalized autoimmune disease usually requires aggressive immunosuppressive therapy.

Organ-specific autoimmune disease is one in which illness is referable to dysfunction of a single organ or tissue. The pathologic features of organ-specific autoimmune disease characteristically include a mononuclear cell infiltrate in the affected organ or tissue, with or without deposition of tissue-specific autoantibodies.

Generalized autoimmune disease results from loss of immunologic tolerance to an autoantigen that is widespread throughout the body, either by virtue of its appearance on cells of a wide variety of tissues, or by its dissemination through the circulation. The pathogenesis of generalized autoimmune disease usually includes deposition of antigen–antibody complexes. Systemic signs, including fever, inappetence, and malaise, usually accompany generalized autoimmune disease, and lesions are found in multiple organs.

## ETIOLOGY OF AUTOIMMUNE DISEASE

No single mechanism can account for all forms of autoimmune disease; different mechanisms probably contribute in different organs and tissues. Environmental factors are presumably involved, including infectious agents, allergic reactions, and inflammation. Evidence for the contribution of genetic factors to autoimmune disease is inescapable.

In humans, autoimmune disorders often occur in familial patterns, and sometimes exhibit distinct gender predisposition (females being at greater risk than males). Autoimmune diseases also appear to be more common in certain breeds of dogs, notably the German shepherd and old English sheepdog. The likelihood of developing specific autoimmune diseases, including type-1 diabetes mellitus, rheumatoid arthritis, and multiple sclerosis, is linked in humans to particular antigens of the major histocompatibility complex (MHC). Genetic association of autoimmunity with MHC in the pet population is under investigation, but strong linkage has already been demonstrated in laboratory animals. Inbred rodents, particularly transgenic mice, are of particular value in defining the role of lymphocyte receptors and antigen presentation in establishing immunologic tolerance and in triggering autoimmunity.

Central to an understanding of the etiology of autoimmune disease is recognition of the processes that control induction and maintenance of immunologic tolerance to autoantigens.

### Mechanisms of Central Tolerance

The most widely accepted model of central tolerance is the intrathymic elimination of autoreactive T cells through clonal deletion. Developing T lymphocytes interact with MHC determinants on thymic epithelium, and probably on bone marrow-derived cells, in an environment that is free of exogenous antigens. The selective pressure on these thymocytes is initially positive, favoring survival of those cells able to recognize empty MHC structures that will eventually serve as antigen carriers on antigen-presenting cells. Subsequently, however, thymocytes that react too vigorously with self-peptides in those MHC carriers will be killed via apoptosis. Clonal deletion in the thymus depends on autoantigen concentration as well as on receptor affinity: autoantigens present at high concentration in the thymus readily trigger elimination of autoreactive clones, while autoantigens present at low concentration will only trigger elimination of clones that have receptors with high affinity. Low-affinity autoreactive thymocytes will be allowed to mature and depart the thymus. Because a normal immune response is highly dependent on T lymphocytes, the absence or silencing of autoreactive T lymphocytes effectively prevents most autoimmune reactions from occurring.

Presentation of antigen to immature B lymphocytes with high-affinity receptors also results in the elimination of those cells if the encounter occurs during a critical stage of their development. Immature B lymphocytes that combine with autoantigens cap and shed their receptors. Some self-reactive B cells will die, although most are simply rendered unreactive and must be governed further through peripheral mechanisms.

Appearance of high-affinity autoreactive lymphocytes in the periphery is thought to be due to: (1) escape from clonal deletion, (2) mutation that increases receptor affinity (a normal occurrence in B lymphocytes), (3) development from ectopic sites, or (4) reaction with previously sequestered autoantigens.

### Mechanisms of Peripheral Tolerance

Clonal deletion in primary lymphoid organs can only occur in response to autoantigens that are prevalent enough or superficial enough to appear on thymic epithelium or on antigen-presenting cells in the thymus. Some autoantigens are so well sequestered within distant tissues that they are not available for presentation to developing thymocytes. Immunologic tolerance to sequestered autoantigens is thought to occur through peripheral mechanisms affecting immunocompetent T and B lymphocytes.

Mature autoreactive lymphocytes undergo varying degrees of peripheral tolerization, possibly including deletion. The extent to which tolerance can be maintained is dependent on the antigen receptors on lymphocytes and the antigen density in tissues. Immunocompetent lymphocytes that exist in a state of relatively "soft" tolerance pose a threat because they can be activated during a normal immune response or other process that promotes increased expression of antigens or antigen receptors.

Exogenous antigens (bacteria, viruses, fungi, toxins) are normally processed and presented in combination with class II MHC on macrophages, dendritic cells, B lymphocytes, and other specialized antigen-presenting cells. The $CD4^+$ (helper) T cell only recognizes linear antigen fragments that are displayed with class II MHC on these antigen-presenting cells. By limiting the number of cells with authority to present exogenous antigens, the immune system can prevent haphazard activation of $CD4^+$ T cells. Cells that do not normally express class II MHC may do so if exposed to cytokines or other products of an inflammatory reaction (interferon-$\gamma$ is an especially powerful stimulus of class II MHC expression). Thus, epithelial, endothelial, and glial cells that normally do not present antigens are able to trigger helper T-cell autoreactivity. These autoreactive T cells can then release the cytokines necessary to facilitate differentiation of autoreactive $CD8^+$ (cytotoxic) T cells, as well as autoreactive B cells.

Down-regulation of antigen receptors or their accessory molecules (e.g., CD4 and CD8 on T lymphocytes; B7/BB1 on B lymphocytes) represents one mechanism whereby mature autoreactive lymphocytes can be made refractory to stimulation. Cytokine signals released from nearby inflammatory cells can trigger the tolerant cells to express receptors and initiate autoimmunity.

In addition to causing release of stimulatory cytokines, inflammation and infection can expose tissue antigens that are normally sequestered. This phenomenon explains why animals with underlying deficiencies in T-cell function sometimes develop autoimmune disease. Poorly contained infections lead to tissue damage and release of sequestered antigens.

Suppressor T lymphocytes have long been hypothesized as participants in the maintenance of peripheral tolerance. Unfortunately, the existence of suppressor T lymphocytes has not been verified conclusively. Nevertheless, some experimental evidence suggests that defects in antigen-specific suppressor T-cell function contribute to autoimmune disease.

Alteration of reactivity within the idiotype/anti-idiotype network may contribute to defective immunologic control and subsequent autoimmunity. Anti-idiotype antibodies are generated against the unique amino acid configuration of an antigen-combining site on another antibody or on an antigen receptor of a lymphocyte. Anti-idiotype antibodies have been found at low concentration in healthy animals, where they might contribute to peripheral tolerance or even help to dampen a normal immune response once the antigen has been eliminated. Lack of a balanced idiotype/anti-idiotype reaction could result in expansion of a clone of autoreactive lymphocytes.

Microbial proteins that act as superantigens and do not require antigen processing have been implicated in autoimmunity. Superantigens bind to the lateral surface of the T-cell receptor at a site unrelated to the antigen-binding site, and can activate a large percentage of CD4$^+$ as well as CD8$^+$ T cells by crosslinking the T-cell receptor with an antigen-presenting cell.

Recent research has revealed that mature, autoreactive lymphocytes exist in the body in far greater numbers than had ever been envisioned. Immunologic tolerance may be a precarious state that depends less on the absence of a clone of lymphocytes than it does on the absence of a co-stimulatory signal essential to lymphocyte activation. Rather than searching for immunologic accidents that result in the rare "horror autotoxicus," perhaps we should ask why autoimmune diseases are not more common.

## CLINICAL MANAGEMENT OF AUTOIMMUNITY IN VETERINARY PATIENTS

Many of the laboratory procedures used to diagnose autoimmune disease, as well as the specimens required, are discussed in *CVT XI*, pp 445, 503.

### Autoimmune Endocrinopathies

#### HYPOTHYROIDISM

The most common endocrinopathy in the dog, hypothyroidism is usually attributed to lymphocytic thyroiditis or idiopathic thyroid atrophy. The immunologic mechanism of tissue damage is presumably cell mediated, although the prevalence of antibodies reactive with thyroglobulin, thyroid peroxidase, or the receptor for thyroid-stimulating hormone, suggests a more complex immunopathogenesis. Autoimmune hypothyroidism, like other autoimmune endocrinopathies, is identified through clinical examination, endocrinologic testing, and histopathologic examination of affected tissue. Some diagnostic laboratories offer serologic testing to detect antibodies reactive with thyroglobulin or direct immunofluorescence testing to identify antibodies deposited in the affected tissue. Autoimmune hypothyroidism is treated with thyroid hormone replacement (sodium levothyroxine; 0.1 mg/4.5 kg b.i.d. or s.i.d. PO) (also see "Monitoring Thyroid Hormone Replacement Therapy," in this volume, p 364).

#### AUTOIMMUNE POLYGLANDULAR SYNDROME

Simultaneous immune-mediated destruction of two or more endocrine tissues can result in autoimmune polyglandular syndrome. The most frequent combination of such endocrine dysfunctions in dogs is hypothyroidism with hypoadrenocorticism, although any combination of the following can be seen: primary hypothyroidism, primary hypoadrenocorticism (Addison's disease), insulin-dependent diabetes mellitus (clearly documented as autoimmune in humans but not yet in animals), hypoparathyroidism, and hypogonadism. Diagnosis of autoimmune polyglandular syndrome is inferred from appropriate clinical signs and endocrinologic testing, plus histopathologic evidence of lymphocytic invasion. Like hypothyroidism, autoimmune polyglandular syndrome often can be managed by replacement of the necessary hormones. Autoimmune polyglandular syndrome is described in detail in *CVT XI*, p 383.

### Autoimmune Diseases of Muscle and Nervous Tissue

#### POLYMYOSITIS

Polymyositis is a relatively common myopathic disorder that occurs most often in large-breed adult dogs of either sex. Clinical signs vary but usually consist of weakness, fatigue, stiffness, muscle pain, and swelling. In some affected animals, abnormal clinicopathologic findings include hypergammaglobulinemia, a positive antinuclear antibody (ANA) test, and circulating immunoglobulin G (IgG) antibodies reactive with sarcolemmal membrane. Polymyositis occurs as a manifestation of systemic lupus erythematosus in dogs, and also is associated with primary lymphocytic thyroiditis. Polymyositis is responsive to prednisone (0.5 to 1.0 mg/kg b.i.d.) and the prognosis is favorable.

#### EOSINOPHILIC MYOSITIS

Eosinophilic myositis most often affects the muscles of mastication (masseteric, temporalis, pterygoid) and is especially prevalent among adult German shepherd dogs. The recurrent pain and swelling of this disorder are accompanied by peripheral eosinophilia and eosinophils in the muscle lesions. Diagnosis is made from signalment, clinical signs, and histopathologic examination of a muscle biopsy. Autoantibodies reactive with myofibers of the temporal muscle can be found in the circulation of some patients, but immunofluorescence testing of muscle tissue is not performed routinely. Eosinophilic myositis is responsive to prednisone (0.5 to 1.0 mg/kg b.i.d.) but may recur, so the prognosis is usually considered to be guarded.

### ACQUIRED MYASTHENIA GRAVIS

Acquired myasthenia gravis is an uncommon condition that results from an autoimmune reaction against acetylcholine receptors at neuromuscular junctions (discussed in more detail in *CVT XI*, p 1039). At highest risk are large-breed adult dogs, especially the German shepherd; the mean age of onset is 5 years, and both sexes are affected. Acquired myasthenia gravis has also been reported in cats. Myasthenic patients exhibit progressive muscle weakness with exercise, especially in the thoracic limbs and head, and dysphagia and regurgitation are common because of intrathoracic megaesophagus. Diagnosis of acquired myasthenia gravis in dogs is generally made by clinical examination and by the rapid reversal of clinical signs upon administration of edrophonium chloride (Tensilon, Roche Laboratories; 0.1 to 0.2 mg/kg IV). Some reference laboratories offer radioimmunoassay to detect serum antibodies specific for the acetylcholine receptor. Such testing has demonstrated that 90% of dogs with acquired myasthenia gravis have antibodies against neuromuscular junction. Direct immunofluorescence testing of a muscle biopsy may reveal immune complexes at the neuromuscular junction. Acquired myasthenia gravis is managed by chronic administration of cholinesterase inhibitors such as pyridostigmine bromide (Mestinon, Roche Laboratories; 1 to 3 mg/kg b.i.d. or t.i.d. PO). The prognosis is guarded, in part because great care must be taken to prevent aspiration pneumonia. Also, even though a patient responds initially to a long-acting cholinesterase inhibitor, the condition can become refractory. In animals as well as humans, acquired myasthenia gravis is sometimes associated with a mediastinal tumor, particularly thymoma, and clinical improvement follows removal of the mass.

### ACUTE POLYRADICULONEURITIS (COONHOUND PARALYSIS)

Acute polyradiculoneuritis is a rare peripheral neurologic disorder that affects any breed and both sexes of adult dogs. Traditionally associated with a raccoon bite, the condition is also seen in dogs that have never encountered a raccoon. Ventral roots and spinal nerves are affected symmetrically (motoneurons more than sensory neurons), producing clinical signs of posterior weakness and hyporeflexia. The weakness ascends rapidly until all four limbs are affected with flaccid tetraplegia in an otherwise alert and afebrile patient. Lesions of acute polyradiculoneuritis consist of segmental demyelination with axonal preservation or degeneration, and an accompanying accumulation of leukocytes (mostly macrophages, with scattered aggregates of lymphocytes and plasma cells). The condition in dogs appears to be clinically and pathologically identical to Guillain-Barré syndrome in humans. Recovery is spontaneous if the patient is provided adequate supportive care, although neurologic dysfunction persists in some patients. Additional information about acute polyradiculoneuritis can be found in *CVT XI*, p 1034.

## Autoimmune Hematologic Diseases

### AUTOIMMUNE HEMOLYTIC ANEMIA

Immune-mediated destruction of erythrocytes appears in a variety of clinical forms, depending on the antibody isotype and the degree of participation by the complement cascade. The most common form in dogs involves IgG, which may or may not activate complement sufficiently to trigger intravascular hemolysis. Less often the erythrocytes are coated with IgM, and agglutination or intravascular hemolysis can result, depending again on complement fixation. Rarely, cold-agglutinin disease occurs, in which IgM autoantibodies bind to erythrocytes only at reduced temperature (such as is encountered in body extremities), causing ischemic necrosis.

A minority of patients with autoimmune hemolytic anemia exhibit true autoagglutination that must be distinguished from rouleaux. A few drops of isotonic saline will disperse cells aggregated by rouleaux; persistent agglutination in saline is pathognomonic for immune-mediated hemolytic anemia. A negative "saline test" should not rule out immune-mediated hemolytic anemia, however, because IgG often cannot overcome the zeta potential to bridge adjacent erythrocytes. In patients whose erythrocytes do not autoagglutinate, a direct Coombs' test is done to confirm the presence of antibodies on the erythrocytes. Indirect Coombs' testing is rarely used in veterinary patients because of the complexity of animal blood group systems and the customary absence of circulating autoantibodies.

Coombs' reagent with strong reactivity against IgG will produce a marked prozone effect in the direct Coombs' test. To avoid erroneous interpretation of the prozone as a negative test result, the reagent should be diluted to its optimal concentration. Many laboratories use polyvalent Coombs' reagent, which contains a mixture of antibodies against IgG, IgM, and C3. Because the optimal concentration will differ for each component, it is advisable to conduct the Coombs' test with serial dilutions of reagent.

A presumptive diagnosis of immune-mediated hemolytic anemia can be made in the dog even without a positive Coombs' test. Clinical and laboratory findings consistent with immune-mediated hemolytic anemia include moderate to severe anemia, marked reticulocytosis, polychromasia, significant spherocytosis, and, occasionally, autoagglutination (see "Approach to the Anemic Patient," this volume, p 447).

Autoimmune hemolytic anemia is usually treated with prednisone, although controversy exists regarding the value of high-dose versus low-dose glucocorticoid therapy. Some clinicians recommend prednisone at 1 mg/kg/day, claiming that clinical evidence fails to support the use of higher doses. Other clinicians recommend the usual immunosuppressive dose (2 mg/kg b.i.d. PO).

Patients failing to respond to glucocorticoid therapy alone can often be managed with prednisone combined with azathioprine (Imuran, Burroughs Wellcome; 2 mg/kg s.i.d. PO). If remission is not seen after several weeks with this combination, then prednisone should be replaced with cyclophosphamide (Cytoxan, Bristol-Myers; 2 mg/kg 4 days per week or alternate days), in combination with azathioprine (see "Canine Immune-Mediated Hemolytic Anemia," this volume, p 152).

Blood transfusion in Coombs'-positive patients is usually contraindicated. It is often difficult to find a crossmatch-negative donor for a Coombs'-positive patient because the patient's autoantibodies recognize a common antigen found on the erythrocytes of many donor animals regardless of blood type. If transfusion is absolutely necessary, the prospective donor should be negative for DEA-1.1, DEA-1.2, and DEA-7 blood group antigens; major and minor crossmatches should be negative; and only washed erythrocytes should be administered.

Some patients that suffer repeated bouts of anemia despite chemotherapy will respond favorably to splenectomy. Surgical removal of the spleen impedes the elimination of antibody-coated erythrocytes, many of which can continue to transport oxygen. In addition, the spleen is the source of plasma cells that produce antibodies against antigens in the circulation, so splenectomy removes the major source of autoantibodies.

### IMMUNE-MEDIATED THROMBOCYTOPENIA

Idiopathic thrombocytopenia is relatively common in companion animals, and often is immune-mediated. Unfortunately, laboratory confirmation of suspected autoimmune etiology in thrombocytopenic patients is difficult to obtain. The two laboratory tests used historically are the platelet factor-3 (PF3) test to detect antibodies against platelets, and immunofluorescence testing to detect antibodies against megakaryocytes. The PF3 test is subject to frequent false-positive and false-negative results, and its usefulness is controversial. Direct or indirect immunofluorescence on smears of bone marrow aspirates can detect antimegakaryocyte antibodies, but the results are often difficult to interpret because of high background fluorescence. Most cases of immune-mediated thrombocytopenia are diagnosed clinically (with clinicopathologic support) and respond to prednisone (1 to 2 mg/kg s.i.d.), although some require cyclophosphamide or vincristine (On-covin, Lilly; 0.02 mg/kg once a week IV). Some clinicians have prescribed danazol (5 mg/kg every 12 hr PO) with prednisolone for this condition. Some patients, whose platelet concentrations cannot be maintained with chemotherapy, will enter long-term remission following splenectomy.

## Autoimmune Skin Diseases

### PEMPHIGUS

Autoantibodies against epidermal cell surface glycoproteins initiate an immunopathologic process that results in blister formation characteristic of the various forms of pemphigus. Recent evidence implicates plasminogen activator from epidermal cells in the pathogenesis of pemphigus. Plasminogen activator is released into intercellular spaces, where it cleaves plasminogen into plasmin. Plasmin then destroys intercellular substance and decreases cell adhesion, causing acantholysis. Pemphigus appears in several clinical forms, depending on the location of the lesions and the probable target autoantigen; two forms are of importance in veterinary patients.

Pemphigus foliaceus is the most common form in both the dog and the cat. In pemphigus foliaceus, the skin contains erythematous macules that progress to pustules and then break to form crusts. Lesions are distributed throughout the body, but are most common on the bridge of the nose; on the nasal planum; around the eyes; and on the pinna, foot pads, and nailbeds (see also *CVT X*, p 616, and "Medical Treatment of Canine Pemphigus-Pemphigoid," this volume, p 636). The pathogenesis of pemphigus foliaceus consists of an autoimmune attack in the superficial epidermis, resulting in formation of a fissure between the stratum granulosum and stratum corneum. The fissure fills with fluid plus neutrophils and loose epithelial cells (acanthocytes).

Pemphigus vulgaris is a rare but severe form of bullous autoimmune skin disease. Lesions consist of well-defined ulcers with scalloped edges and are found most often on the oral mucosa, external nares, lips, eyelid margins, ears, anus, and prepuce or vulva. The target antigen is apparently located in the suprabasilar epidermis.

Presumptive diagnosis of pemphigus can be made from clinical signs and examination of an impression smear of a pustule. If the crust from a lesion is carefully peeled back and a slide is touched to the fresh ulcer, the fluid will be found to contain neutrophils and acanthocytes, with few bacteria.

Confirmation of the diagnosis requires histologic examination of a biopsy specimen, with or without immunohistologic testing. Unlike most skin biopsies, specimens collected for diagnosis of pemphigus should contain a margin of apparently normal tissue. A 6-mm biopsy punch should be used, and for direct immunofluorescence testing, the tissue should be divided longitudinally with a scalpel blade to produce a specimen no thicker than 3 mm. Immunofluorescence testing of biopsies from the footpad or nose are of limited diagnostic value because of the high frequency of false-positive reactions in those tissues. Secondary bacteria often invade traumatized pemphigus lesions, necessitating a "pustule watch" to identify fresh bullae suitable for biopsy. The patient can be admitted early in the day and examined hourly for the appearance of new pustules, which are then biopsied. In addition, the most difficult rule-out in pemphigus is canine pyoderma (bacterial folliculitis). A conservative diagnostic approach is to assume the skin condition is caused by pyoderma, and treat with appropriate antibiotics for 2 to 3 weeks. After secondary bacterial infections have resolved, the skin can be examined for new pemphigus lesions.

Biopsy specimens should always be submitted in 10% buffered formalin for routine histopathologic examination, even if immunologic testing is also done. If multiple specimens are collected, replicates should be placed in Michel's fixative and can be stored until histopathologic findings are reported. The specimens in Michel's fixative can then be submitted for confirmation of a positive diagnosis. Michel's fixative is available from histologic supply houses (e.g., Newcomer Supply, Middleton, WI). Technical limitations of immunofluorescence testing are discussed in *CVT XI*, p 503.

Immunoperoxidase staining is a highly sensitive method that has threatened to replace immunofluorescence testing in the diagnosis of autoimmune diseases. Immunoperoxidase offers several advantages over immunofluorescence: (1) formalin-fixed tissue can be used, although some reactivity is lost if the tissue is in formalin longer than 24 hr; (2) paraffin embedding preserves structural details and provides familiar morphologic features; and (3) sections stained with immunoperoxidase provide a reasonably permanent record. However, a high rate of false-positive reactions occurs with immunoperoxidase staining of inflammatory skin lesions that are not autoimmune, especially when bacteria are present.

Management of pemphigus requires aggressive immunosuppressive therapy, often with combinations such as prednisone (2 mg/kg b.i.d. PO) plus azathioprine (2 mg/kg s.i.d. PO); or prednisone plus aurothioglucose (Solganal, Schering; 1 mg/kg weekly IM) (see "Medical Management of Canine Pemphigus-Pemphigoid, this volume, p 636).

## Autoimmune Arthritides

### SYSTEMIC LUPUS ERYTHEMATOSUS

Systemic lupus erythematosus (SLE) is a generalized autoimmune disease manifested as immune complex–mediated inflammation. The most common presenting sign in the dog is lameness due to symmetric, nonerosive polyarthritis. Other organ systems are also affected, resulting in glomerulonephritis, dermatitis, hemolytic anemia, thrombocytopenia, and a variety of less common conditions. Autoantibodies are produced against an assortment of autoantigens (or perhaps against a common epitope found in an assortment of tissues). The most popular diagnostic tests detect antinuclear antibodies, which participate in immune complex formation but are by no means the only contributors to the pathogenesis.

Because of its sensitivity, the ANA test is used as a screening tool to aid in the diagnosis of SLE. Patient's serum is applied to a slide containing fixed cells that have prominent nuclei (e.g., mouse liver sections, HeLa cells, Vero cells). Antinuclear antibodies in the serum bind to the exposed nuclear antigens and are revealed with fluorescein-conjugated species-specific antiglobulin. Most diagnostic laboratories screen sera at a standard dilution (e.g., 1:10) that will allow discrimination between positive and nonspecific reactions; they then retest positive sera after serial dilution to obtain an end-point titer. A high ANA titer is said to correlate with progressive disease, whereas a decrease in titer signifies remission. The clinical significance of a particular titer depends on laboratory methodology, especially the type of cells used to trap the antibodies. Laboratory personnel should be consulted to help interpret the results of this and other immunologic testing.

The LE cell test detects antinuclear antibodies by their opsonizing activity. Some laboratories request that blood for LE cell testing be collected in a tube containing glass beads that will be shaken to disrupt the cells, while others prefer clotted blood that will be forced through a mesh screen. The damaged cells extrude nuclei that are opsonized by antinuclear antibodies in the sample. These opsonized nuclei are then phagocytized by viable neutrophils remaining in the specimen, to generate LE cells. Results of the LE cell test are subject to bias, but a clearly positive test result is considered specific for SLE.

Like polyarthritis, the skin and renal lesions associated with SLE are initiated by immune complex deposition. The immunoglobulin component of the immune complexes can be detected by immunofluorescence microscopy of specimens collected in Michel's fixative.

Immunosuppressive therapy for SLE usually involves prednisone (2 mg/kg b.i.d. PO), often in combination with azathioprine or cyclophosphamide.

### RHEUMATOID ARTHRITIS

Like SLE, rheumatoid arthritis begins as a synovitis and progresses to a symmetric polyarthritis, but the lesions of rheumatoid arthritis are much more aggressive. Characteristic radiographic changes in affected joints include erosion of cartilage and subchondral bone with eventual collapse of the joint space. Immune complexes in the synovium and synovial fluid probably initiate the inflammatory reaction. Serum and synovial fluid from patients with rheumatoid arthritis usually contain autoantibody reactive with IgG. This autoantibody, or rheumatoid factor, can be detected by passive agglutination with the Rose-Waaler test or with a commercially available latex agglutination test (see "The Use of the Laboratory in the Diagnosis of Joint Disorders of Dogs and Cats," this volume, p 1166).

Anti-inflammatory effects of aspirin may provide some comfort in canine patients with rheumatoid arthritis, but the immunopathologic process will not be arrested. Adequate control requires immunosuppressive therapy with prednisone, sometimes in combination with azathioprine; aurothioglucose has also proven effective in dogs with rheumatoid arthritis (see "Treatment of the Immune-Based Inflammatory Arthropathies of the Dog and Cat," this volume, p 1188).

## FUTURE APPROACHES TO TREATMENT OF AUTOIMMUNE DISEASE

Treatment of autoimmune disease is directed toward: (1) reducing the inflammatory process, (2) restoring normal immune regulation (inhibiting further expansion of the clone of autoreactive cells and silencing those already present), and (3) replacing the missing hormone or factor.

Ideally, immunosuppressive therapy should eliminate or control only the autoreactive cells, and have minimal impact on other components of the immune system necessary to the patient's survival. In practice, however, such targeted immunosuppression is not yet available, so management of autoimmune disease entails a balance between achieving remission and creating potentially lethal bone marrow suppression. Cyclosporine, which is widely used in transplantation medicine, may have application in autoimmune disease as well because it offers more precise control of lymphocyte activation than can be obtained with cytotoxic agents.

Anti-idiotype antibodies directed against the antigen receptors of autoreactive lymphocytes are undergoing clinical testing in human patients. By crosslinking and capping lymphocyte receptors, anti-idiotype antibodies inhibit further autoreactivity. Similarly, monoclonal antibodies and recombinant peptides are being used to block MHC determinants on antigen-presenting cells and accessory molecules on autoreactive lymphocytes.

Human trials are also underway to test whether oral tolerization can be used to control autoimmune disease. Laboratory experiments have indicated that animals given autoantigens orally resist subsequent induction of autoimmunity. The mechanism through which oral immunization results in tolerance is not known.

Adjuvants are being tested for their ability to modify inflammatory cytokine release. This approach is consistent with the hypothesis that immunologic tolerance is maintained through the withholding of an essential costimulatory signal. The objective is to shift production of cytokines from those that mediate tissue damage (e.g., interferon-γ) to those that are less destructive (e.g., interleukin-4).

Obviously, advances in the diagnosis and treatment of autoimmune disease in veterinary and human patients will soon rely on breakthroughs in molecular medicine.

## References and Suggested Reading

Halliwell REW and Gorman NT: *Veterinary Clinical Immunology.* Philadelphia, WB Saunders Co, 1989.
 *A comprehensive veterinary immunology textbook that offers excellent diagrams and illustrations depicting a variety of immunologic disorders in animals.*
Jans HE, Armstrong PJ, and Price GS: Therapy of immune mediated thrombocytopenia: A retrospective study of 15 dogs. J Vet Intern Med 4:4, 1990.
 *A retrospective analysis of the management of thrombocytopenia in dogs, including discussion of the value of splenectomy.*
Lewis RM and Picut CA: Veterinary Clinical Immunology—From Classroom to Clinics. Philadelphia, Lea & Febiger, 1989.
 *An inexpensive veterinary immunology textbook that provides descriptions and case studies of immunologic disorders in animals.*
Webb SR: Self/nonself discrimination: The role of T cell tolerance. *Proc 10th ACVIM Forum,* San Diego CA, May 1992, p 149.
 *A review of tolerance mechanisms that involve T lymphocytes.*
Zipfel W, Hewicker-Trautwein M, and Trautwein G: Demonstration of immunoglobulins and complement in canine and feline autoimmune and non-autoimmune skin diseases with the direct immunofluorescence and indirect immunoperoxidase method. J Am Vet Med Assoc 39:494, 1992.
 *A critical comparison of immunoperoxidase staining and conventional immunofluorescence for identification of immunoglobulins in skin lesions of small animals.*

# IMMUNOSUPPRESSION AND IMMUNODEFICIENCY

JAMES A. ROTH

*Ames, Iowa*

The immune system is remarkably efficient at protecting normal young adult animals from infectious disease. The normal immune system is able to prevent clinical signs from developing after low-level exposure to many infectious agents and is able to limit the clinical signs and cause clinical recovery from infection after exposure to the majority of pathogens in most animals. The efficiency of the normal immune system may be most clearly appreciated when one is confronted with infections in an immunocompromised animal. Infections with unusual pathogens may occur, infections with common pathogens may be unusually severe or persistent, and infectious diseases may not respond to therapy as well as expected. These signs should lead the clinician to suspect that the patient has a primary or secondary immunodeficiency. The purpose of this article is to provide an overview of the broad topic of primary immunodeficiency syndromes and the factors associated with secondary immunodeficiencies and to direct the reader to sources where these subjects are covered in more detail.

Primary immunodeficiencies are congenital and due to genetic defects (also see *CVT XI*, p 448). Secondary immunodeficiencies (or immunosuppression) are due to secondary factors that suppress what would otherwise be normal immune function (also see *CVT XI*, p 453). There are also age-related considerations. For example, very young animals and old animals have decreased immune function as compared to normal young adults.

Defects in either native or acquired immune defense mechanisms may lead to increased susceptibility to infection. Native defense mechanisms do not require previous exposure or vaccination to be effective. These include barriers to entry and colonization (e.g., intact skin and mucous membranes, normal flora, mucociliary transport), the complement system, phagocytic cells, antibiotic peptides, and interferons. Acquired immunity develops a few days after exposure or vaccination and is specific for the disease agent with which it was induced. Acquired immunity can be attributed to circulating antibody, cell-mediated immunity, and/or mucosal antibody (IgA).

## PRIMARY IMMUNODEFICIENCIES

Relatively few primary immunodeficiencies have been described in dogs and cats. Many additional primary immunodeficiencies have been described in children. It is likely that many of these same genetic defects in immune function occur in dogs and cats as well, on rare occasions, but have not been detected and characterized. These would manifest as severe, recurrent, and perhaps fatal infections in the first few weeks of life. Diagnosis of a primary immunodeficiency requires tests that are typically only available in research laboratories (see *CVT XI*, p 441). Therefore, an underlying primary immunodeficiency is likely to go undiagnosed in a young puppy or kitten with a serious infectious disease. The primary immunodeficiencies that have been detected in puppies and kittens were reviewed in the previous edition of this text (Felsburg, 1992 in *CVT XI*, p 448).

Establishing the presence of a primary immunodeficiency and characterizing the defect present would be helpful. It would establish that the animal has a poor prognosis and that therapy is not likely to be successful in the long term. In addition, if the mode of inheritance

of the genetic defect is known, the veterinarian can make recommendations regarding the future use of the sire and dam in breeding programs.

## SECONDARY IMMUNODEFICIENCIES

The immune system is a complex system influenced by other systems in the body (notably the neuroendocrine system) and by external factors such as infectious agents, stressors, toxins, drugs, and diet. These factors may cause mild to severe immunosuppression resulting in increased susceptibility to infection, neoplasia, autoimmune disease, and allergy. Many of the causes of secondary immunodeficiency have recently been reviewed (Chandra and Sarchielli, 1993; Greene, 1990; Halliwell and Gorman, 1989; Krakowka, 1992 in *CVT XI*, p 453) and will be summarized here. The patterns of infection associated with immunodeficiency and methods for assessment of immune function in small animal patients were reviewed in the previous volume of this text (Couto, 1992 in *CVT XI*, p 223; Gershwin, 1992 in *CVT XI*, p 441).

### Failure of Passive Transfer

Puppies and kittens receive a small amount of immunoglobulin G (IgG) across the placenta (approximately 10% of the maternal level) before they are born. If they receive adequate amounts of colostrum during the first 24 hr of life, they will attain serum IgG levels similar to those of the dam. This passive transfer is most efficient within the first 6 hr of birth. Failure to receive colostrum apparently does not put puppies at a serious disadvantage if they are well managed under hygienic conditions. Receiving adequate colostrum may be more important in kittens. If puppies and kittens do not receive colostrum, their maternal antibody titers will soon wane, and they will be susceptible to infections at an earlier age (see "Fluid Therapy in the Puppy and Kitten," and "Nutritional and Management Considerations in Neonatal Medicine," this volume, pp 34 and 37, respectively). However, they are also able to respond to vaccines at an earlier age without the interference of maternal antibodies.

### Acquired Immune Deficiency From Infectious Agents

Some viral (e.g., feline leukemia virus, feline immunodeficiency virus, feline panleukopenia virus, canine parvovirus, canine distemper virus) and parasitic (e.g., demodicosis, toxoplasmosis, trypanosomiasis) infections can induce mild to severe immunosuppression. The immune system defects may be responsible for many of the clinical signs observed. Secondary bacterial, fungal, and viral infections may be the reason that the animals are brought to the attention of a veterinarian. If the underlying immunosuppressive infection can be resolved, then the secondary infections should respond better to therapy. The immunosuppressive viral conditions can best be managed by avoidance of exposure and vaccination to prevent infection or reduce the severity of clinical signs.

## Physical and Psychological Distress

There is ample evidence that both physical and psychological distress can suppress immune function in humans and animals. Most of the research demonstrating this in domestic animals has been done on food-producing animals on a population basis, but companion animals are also likely to be affected. The immunosuppression that has been observed is typically mild but may influence the incidence, severity, and outcome of infectious disease. Distress-induced alterations in immune function are mediated by interactions between the neuroendocrine and immune systems. Studies of the effects of distress on the immune system initially focused on the influence of glucocorticoids released by the adrenal cortex in response to stress; these hormones are known to suppress several aspects of immune function. It is now recognized that there are many mechanisms by which the neuroendocrine system can alter immune function in response to distress, including catecholamines produced by the adrenal medulla; endogenous opiates (endorphins and enkephalins) produced by the pituitary, adrenal medulla, and sympathetic terminals; and by direct sympathetic innervation to the parenchyma of the thymus, spleen, and bone marrow. Some psychologically distressing events that may be expected to be mildly immunosuppressive are weaning, a change in environments, hospitalization, and introduction of a new pet into the household.

## Dietary Influences on the Immune System

Both nutritional deficiencies and nutritional excesses may result in impairment of immune function and increased susceptibility to disease (Chandra and Sarchielli, 1993; also see "Nutritional and Management Considerations in Neonatal Medicine," this volume, p. 37). Malnourishment and the potential for immune dysfunction is especially likely in hospitalized patients, small-for-gestational-age neonates, and in advanced age. Obesity has also been associated with immune dysfunction.

Key vitamins and minerals for optimal immune function include vitamins A, C, and E; the B complex vitamins; and copper, zinc, magnesium, manganese, iron, and selenium. The balance of these constituents is especially important, since an excess or deficiency in one component may influence the availability or requirement for another.

Obese dogs have been shown to have a poorer response to challenge with *Salmonella typhimurium* or distemper virus, resulting in higher morbidity and mortality than nonobese controls. Excessive intake of poly-unsaturated fatty acids, iron, and vitamin E have been shown to be immunosuppressive. Obesity, excessive intake of nutrients, and over-supplementation with vitamins and minerals may be the most frequent type of malnutrition in companion animals. There is growing evidence in both humans and animals that overnutrition may impair immune responses and increase the risk of several diseases, including infection and cancer.

## Immunosuppression Associated With Neoplasia

Animals with neoplastic disease often have measurable immune dysfunction and an increased susceptibility to secondary infections. There are many possible mechanisms for the neoplasia-associated immunosuppression. The animal may have had preexisting immune dysfunction which led to the neoplastic disease, the immune dysfunction may be neoplasia induced, it may be due to therapy for the neoplasia (e.g., surgery, irradiation therapy, or cytotoxic drugs), or it may be a combination of these factors. The immunosuppression associated with neoplasia may be mild to profound. Tumors may directly suppress the immune system by secreting immunosuppressive factors, or they may indirectly suppress the immune system by causing the host to release immunosuppressive factors. This tumor-induced immunosuppression may aid in the dissemination of the tumor.

Surgical stress has been shown to suppress natural killer (NK) cell function for several days. Natural killer cells are an important cytotoxic cell in the first line of defense against neoplasia and for controlling circulating tumor emboli. Cytotoxic drugs and irradiation used in tumor therapy may be profoundly immunosuppressive by damaging the rapidly dividing cells of the immune system. An appreciation for the degree of immunosuppression present is important in managing patients with neoplastic disease. Immunosuppression complicates the clinical management of the case because the affected animals will be more susceptible to secondary infection, and the neoplasia will be more difficult to control. The topic of tumor immunology and immunotherapy is covered in "Tumor Immunology and Tumor Immunotherapy," this volume, p 488.

## Immunosuppression Associated With Endocrine Dysfunction

Nearly all hormones have been shown to influence immune function, including glucocorticoids, catecholamines, progesterone, estrogen, insulin, somatotropin, prolactin, thyroxine, and thymic hormones. A deficiency or excess of hormone levels may result in mild to severe immune dysfunction. The normal hormonal fluctuations associated with the estrous cycle and pregnancy have been shown to be associated with minor alterations in immune function and increased susceptibility to infection in other species. Animals with diabetes mellitus or Cushing's disease have fairly severe immune dysfunction. Clinicians should be aware, when dealing with animals with endocrine dysfunction or on hormonal therapy, that there may be an associated immunosuppression and secondary complications.

## Alterations in Immune Function With Age

The immune system begins to develop in the last trimester of pregnancy. Neonatal animals are able to mount an immune response against infectious agents or vaccines, but the magnitude of the response is generally reduced and the onset delayed as compared to young adult animals. The relative immaturity of the immune system, plus the fact that they must mount a primary immune response against all of the pathogens that they encounter, are in large part responsible for the increased susceptibility of young animals to infectious disease. The presence of passively transferred maternal antibody is important for decreasing the susceptibility to infection until the immune system matures and the animal can mount its own immune response. The presence of the maternal antibody also interferes with the response to vaccination. If a young puppy or kitten does not receive maternal antibody against a particular pathogen, they may respond to vaccination at a very young age. However, modified live vaccines should not be used in puppies and kittens less than 5 to 6 weeks of age because there is a risk that the immaturity of the immune system may allow the modified live organism to cause disease.

It is generally believed that immune responsiveness and some native defense mechanisms continue to improve in the early neonatal period and reach a maximum at about puberty. Immune function then begins to decrease in old age, resulting in an increase in the incidence of infectious diseases, neoplasia, and autoimmune phenomenon. These changes have not been thoroughly documented in the dog and cat, but have been shown in rodents and humans.

## MANAGEMENT AND THERAPY OF THE IMMUNODEFICIENT PATIENT

Animals that are suspected of having suboptimal immune function should be isolated from other animals to reduce exposure to infectious agents. If infections do develop, they must be treated aggressively if they are to be controlled (see *CVT XI*, p 223; and "Empirical Antibiotic Therapy" in this volume, p 276). Animals with immunodeficiencies will probably not respond to

therapy as well as a normal animal and, depending on the severity of the immune defect, the prognosis may be poor.

If a primary immunodeficiency is suspected, it is important to attempt to confirm the diagnosis so that an accurate prognosis can be made and the case managed accordingly. If a secondary immunodeficiency is suspected, it is important to identify and remove the cause of the immunodeficiency if possible. Depending on the nature of the immunodeficiency, it may be beneficial to treat the animal with an immunomodulator to attempt to improve immune function. The use of cytokines and other biologic response modifiers as immunomodulators in cats and dogs was reviewed in the last edition of this text (Barta, 1992 in *CVT XI*, p 217; Tompkins and Tompkins, 1992 in *CVT XI*, p 461) and is updated in this volume (see "Cytokines and Biologic Response Modifiers in Small Animal Practice," p 547).

## References and Suggested Reading

Barta O: Immunoadjuvant therapy. *In* Kirk RW and Bonagura JD (eds): *Current Veterinary Therapy XI.* Philadelphia, WB Saunders Co, 1992, p 217.
*A review of immunomodulators used in dogs and cats with dosages and references to the primary literature.*
Chandra RK and Sarchielli P: Nutritional status and immune responses. Clin Lab Med 13:455, 1993.
*A review of nutritional influences on the immune system.*
Couto CG: Patterns of infection associated with immunodeficiency. *In* Kirk RW and Bonagura JD (eds): *Current Veterinary Therapy XI.* Philadelphia, WB Saunders Co, 1992, p 223.
*Classifies the immunodeficiency syndromes in dogs and cats and characteristics of associated infectious complications.*
Felsburg PJ: Primary immunodeficiencies. *In* Kirk RW and Bonagura JD (eds): *Current Veterinary Therapy XI.* Philadelphia, WB Saunders Co, 1992, p 448.
*A review of selected primary immunodeficiencies in the dog and cat including information on diagnosis and clinical management of these syndromes.*
Gershwin LJ: Immunologic assessment of the small animal patient. *In* Kirk RW and Bonagura JD (eds): *Current Veterinary Therapy XI.* Philadelphia, WB Saunders Co, 1992, p 441.
*A review of methods for assessment of immune dysfunction.*
Greene CE: Immunodeficiency and infectious disease. *In* Greene DE (ed): *Infectious Diseases of the Dog and Cat.* Philadelphia, WB Saunders Co, 1990, p 55.
*A review of immunodeficiency as a predisposing factor to infectious diseases with references to the primary literature.*
Halliwell REW and Gorman NT: Diseases associated with immunodeficiency. *In* Halliwell REW and Gorman NT (eds): *Veterinary Clinical Immunology.* Philadelphia, WB Saunders Co, 1989, p 449.
*A review of specific immunodeficiency diseases with extensive references to the primary literature.*
Krakowka S: Acquired immunodeficiency diseases. *In* Kirk RW and Bonagura JD (eds): *Current Veterinary Therapy XI.* Philadelphia, WB Saunders Co, 1992, p 453.
*A review of various causes of secondary immunodeficiency.*
Tompkins MB and Tompkins WAF: Immunoregulatory cytokines and their potential in therapy. *In* Kirk RW and Bonagura JD (eds): *Current Veterinary Therapy XI.* Philadelphia, WB Saunders Co, 1992, p 461.
*A review of the biologic activities of cytokines and their potential as therapeutic agents.*

# TRANSPLANTATION IMMUNOLOGY

CLARE R. GREGORY

*Davis, California*

In the late 1800s and early 1900s, surgeons gained the technical ability to transplant organs and tissues from one animal to another. It soon became evident that, following transplantation, most organs would rapidly become ischemic and necrotic. In 1923, Dr. Carl Williamson, at the Mayo Clinic, demonstrated that cells of the immune system were responsible for the death of transplanted tissues and organs. This discovery set the stage for the study of immune-mediated rejection and the development of effective immunosuppressive strategies.

Transplantation of organs and tissues in veterinary medicine is becoming more common. Corneal transplantation is performed to replace diseased or scarred corneas. Corneoscleral transplantation is performed for the treatment of canine epibulbar melanomas. Allogeneic bone marrow transplantation has been performed in cats to aid in the treatment of lymphohematopoietic neoplasias, aplastic anemias, and feline retrovirus infections (see *CVT XI*, p 493). Renal transplantation for acute and chronic renal failure in the dog and cat is performed at university hospitals and in private veterinary practices (see *CVT XI*, p 870). Feline renal transplant patients have now survived over 4 years with normal renal function.

## NOMENCLATURE

A *graft* is tissue or an organ used in a transplant procedure. An *autograft* is tissue or an organ that is removed from and then transplanted into the same individual. A common example is a cancellous bone graft used to speed fracture healing. Autografts do not incite an immune response. An *isograft* is tissue or an organ transplanted between two genetically identical individuals—identical twins or closely inbred individuals. An *allograft* is tissue or an organ transplanted between genetically nonidentical members of the same species. Virtually all renal transplants performed in clinical veterinary medicine are allografts. A *xenograft* is tissue or an organ transplanted between members of different species.

## MECHANISM OF THE IMMUNE RESPONSE

Rejection of the transplanted tissue or organ is determined by T-cell (lymphocyte) recognition of differences in the composition of cell surface glycoproteins between graft and host tissues. These glycoproteins are termed histocompatibility antigens or histocompatibility molecules. The histocompatibility antigens that incite the most vigorous rejection response are encoded by genes of the major histocompatibility complex (MHC).

## Genetics

An MHC is found in all vertebrates. In dogs, this cluster of genes on a single chromosome is termed the dog leukocyte antigen (DLA), in cats it is termed the feline leukocyte antigen (FLA), and so on. Polymorphism, or the presence of many different variations of the same gene (alleles) at a single location, or locus, is characteristic of the MHC. Each individual will have two, one on each paired chromosome, of many possible alleles at each locus in his or her MHC. This variation in the genetic makeup of the MHC results in the production of a tremendous variety of cell surface histocompatibility antigens. This variety ensures that the host T cells will recognize virtually all tissue and organ allografts as foreign, resulting in a rejection response.

The genes of the MHC are closely linked, and the genetic information inherited from each parent on a single chromosome is transferred as a block. This group of genes is termed the MHC *haplotype*; each offspring receives one haplotype from each parent. The genes of each haplotype are expressed codominantly; therefore, cell surface histocompatibility antigens derived from each parent will be present in the offspring (Fig. 1).

This basic understanding of the genetics of the MHC is important clinically, particularly in a species like the dog, in which it is difficult to immunosuppress or control the rejection response. Since each offspring inherits one haplotype from each parent and each haplotype is expressed codominantly, 25% of littermates have the possibility of being MHC identical, 50% might share one haplotype, and 25% might not share a haplotype. Without the administration of immunosuppressive agents, renal allografts from MHC-nonmatched dogs survive approximately 10 days, renal allografts from dogs matched for one haplotype survive approximately 24 days, and MHC-matched allografts survive for 150 days or more. In the latter group, the rejection response can be controlled using immunosuppressive agents; therefore, selection of MHC-identical littermates as donor/recipient pairs can greatly enhance the chance of long-term graft survival.

The fact that allograft survival is not indefinite when a dog receives a kidney from an MHC-identical donor demonstrates that the MHC is not the only genetic region coding for histocompatibility antigens. Minor histocompatibility genes have been isolated in mice and human beings and probably code for changes in peptide structure in endogenous proteins that allow recognition by host T cells, but do not affect their physiologic function. Fortunately, the rejection response produced by minor histocompatibility differences is relatively easy to prevent using immunosuppressive drugs.

## Transplantation Antigens

It is important to understand that the MHC-encoded cell surface glycoproteins, or transplantation antigens, did not evolve to prevent the transplantation of genetically dissimilar tissue and organs, but rather, to protect the host from invasion by viruses, fungi, nematodes, and other parasites. To do so effectively, the immune system must distinguish between antigens against which an immune response would be beneficial (pathogenic or allogeneic) or harmful (host or self). In the thymus, during fetal development, T cells are propagated or destroyed based on their ability to recognize MHC glycoproteins as "self" or "nonself." The interaction between MHC glycoproteins and T cells, in the presence of antigen, results in a series of transmembrane and cytosolic chemical reactions that result in T-cell cytotoxic activity and the production and/or release of cytokines. Cytokines (interleukins [ILs], tumor necrosis factor [TNF], and others) result in the further activation of T cells, B cells, macrophages, and other immunoreactive cells (see "Cytokines and Biologic Response Modifiers in Small Animal Practice," this volume, p 547).

The cell surface glycoproteins encoded by the genes

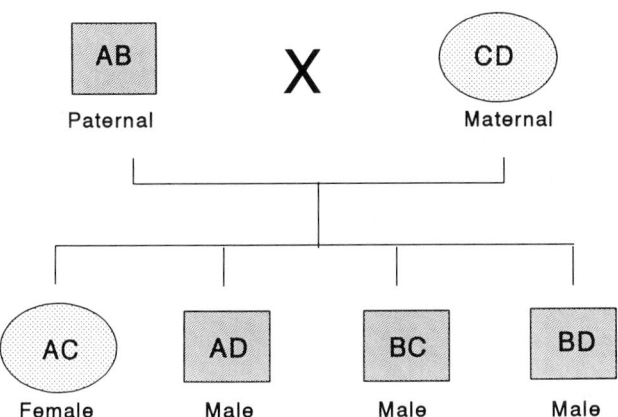

**Figure 1.** Inheritance of MHC haplotypes. A haplotype is the combination of alleles at each locus on a single chromosome and is almost always inherited as a unit. Haplotype designations are given by A, B, C, and D. Paternal haplotypes are A and B, and maternal haplotypes are C and D. Offspring of this mating inherit one haplotype from each parent and will have one of four possible combinations of haplotypes. Statistically, 25% of the offspring will be MHC identical (i.e., AC and AC), 25% will be totally MHC nonidentical (i.e., AC and BD), and 50% will be MHC haploidentical (i.e., AC and AD). (Modified from Schwartz BD: The HLA complex and disease susceptibility. *In* Schwartz BD (ed): *Immunology.* Kalamazoo, Upjohn, 1991, p 22, with permission.)

of the MHC are divided into two major classifications: 1 and 2. Class 1 glycoproteins or molecules are expressed on all nucleated cells. Class 1 molecules have a folded region that holds and presents antigens from virus-infected, tumor, and allogeneic cells to antigen-responsive cytotoxic (CD8$^+$) T cells. The linkage of the T cell receptor–CD8 complex on the surface of cytotoxic T cells with the class I molecule–antigen complex of allograft or antigen-presenting cells (monocytes, macrophages, Langerhans cells of the epidermis, and dendritic cells of lymphoid organs) results in the proliferation and differentiation of a clone of cytotoxic T cells specific for that class 1–antigen combination. Thus, the cytotoxic activity of T cells is both antigen-specific and class 1–restricted.

Class II molecules are only constitutively expressed on the surface of cells that are essential for immune responses. These include B cells (lymphocytes), thymic epithelial cells, and the cells listed above that present antigen to T cells. T cells, vascular endothelial cells, smooth muscle cells, and others can express class II antigens when activated by cytokines such as interferon-$\gamma$ (IFN-$\gamma$). The function of class II molecules is similar to that of class I. Antigen-sensitive T helper cells (CD4$^+$) recognize the class II–antigen complex on allogeneic or antigen-presenting cells. The linkage of the CD4–T-cell receptor complex with the class II–antigen complex results in the proliferation and differentiation of a clone of T helper cells specific for that class II–antigen complex. Activated T helper cells begin the cascade of events responsible for acute allograft rejection by the release of cytokines (IL-2, IL-3, IL-4, IL-5, IL-6, interferon-$\gamma$, TNFs, granulocyte macrophage colony-stimulating factor [GM-CSF], and others) that propagate an inflammatory response, activate cytotoxic cells, and promote antibody formation.

In addition to their role as antigen-presenting molecules, it is believed that class I and class II molecules, alone, may stimulate alloreactive T cells and serve as the stimuli for rejection reactions. Also, rejection may be initiated following T-cell recognition of class I or II–minor histocompatibility antigen complexes.

## Accessory Cell Surface Molecules

T-cell activation by allogeneic or antigen-presenting cells requires cell contact and cell surface molecule interaction. Cell surface molecules that interact are termed "ligand-receptor pairs." A ligand is any molecule that forms a complex with another molecule. In addition to the class 1/antigen-CD8/T-cell receptor ligand-receptor pair and the class 2/antigen-CD4/T-cell receptor ligand-receptor pair, there are a number of additional cell surface ligand-receptor interactions that serve to augment the binding of the cells and enhance the stimulation of the T cell (Fig. 2). The accessory molecular interactions are not antigen specific. Two examples of these T cell–antigen-presenting cell accessory binding pairs are CD2 and LFA-3; and LFA-1 and ICAM-1.

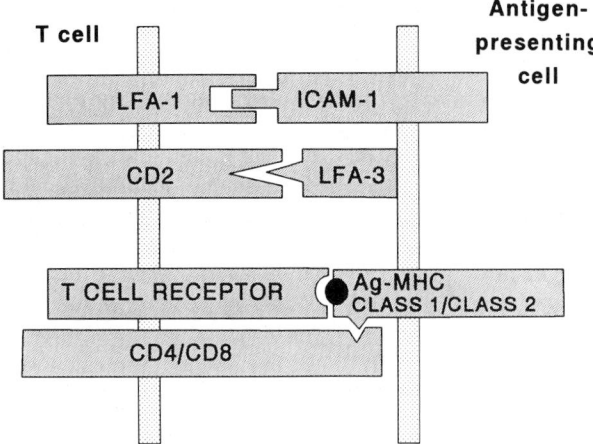

**Figure 2.** Different cell surface receptor-ligand interactions during antigen recognition by T cells. In addition to the critical binding of the T-cell receptor to antigen in association with an MHC molecule, receptor-ligand interactions occur that are not specific for a particular antigen. The interactions shown here enhance the avidity of the binding of the T cell to the antigen-presenting cell. CD2, CD4, and CD8 also influence the generation of intracellular signals that result from antigen recognition. (Modified from Imboden JB: T-cell activation. *In* Schwartz BD (ed): *Immunology.* Kalamazoo, Upjohn, 1991, p 54, with permission)

## REJECTION

The primary mechanism of the destruction of an allograft is generation of T lymphocytes that are cytotoxic for the cells of the graft. Graft cell lysis is accomplished through the direct action of T cytotoxic cells and by the activation of cascading enzyme systems, including the complement, clotting, and probably the kinin pathways. Other cellular mediators such as B cells, plasma cells, macrophages, platelets, and polymorphonuclear leukocytes have both a direct and indirect role in allograft rejection. Xenograft rejection is similar to allograft rejection, but the immune response is generally more severe and the organ is lost more quickly. In addition, many species appear to have naturally occurring antibodies to the cell surface antigens of xenogeneic cells. These naturally occurring antibodies attach to the endothelial cells of the xenograft blood vessels and fix complement. This results in cell lysis, platelet fixation, and thrombosis of the blood vessels followed by necrosis of the organ.

Three overlapping types of organ rejection are recognized clinically. *Hyperacute rejection* is an accelerated form of rejection that is associated with naturally occurring (xenograft) or preformed circulating antibody in the serum of the recipient that reacts with donor cells, particularly the endothelium of blood vessel walls as described above. In hyperacute allograft rejection, the recipient has been sensitized to the allograft MHC antigens by previous blood transfusions, pregnancy, or transplantation. Preexisting antibody can be identified before transplantation by testing leukocytes of the potential donor with the serum of the recipient in the presence of complement. If preexisting antibody is present in the serum, the host leukocytes will be lysed.

*Acute* allograft rejection typically occurs 7 to 21 days after transplantation or when effective immunosuppression is terminated (Fig. 3). Pathologic studies of the rejected organ reveal a predominant pattern of mononuclear leukocyte infiltration in the tissue.

*Chronic* rejection is characterized by gradual loss of organ function over months to years, often without any clinically recognized rejection episode. Chronic rejection is a major cause of death for all human organ transplant recipients and the primary cause of death for heart transplant recipients. Kidneys undergoing chronic rejection show severe narrowing of numerous arteries and thickening of the glomerular capillary basement membrane. Heart transplants show progressive thickening of the coronary arteries caused mainly by smooth muscle cell proliferation and migration. Occlusion of coronary artery blood flow results in diminished function of the cardiac muscle and, eventually, in myocardial infarction. The factors causing chronic rejection have not been defined. Some investigators feel that it is a slow or latent cellular effect, others attribute the lesions to the effects of anti-MHC antibody. In the author's opinion, chronic rejection may not be a primary rejection response, but rather, an inappropriate response of affected tissues to chronic injury. Many growth factors, including transforming growth factor–$\beta$, platelet-derived growth factor, and fibroblast growth factor have been shown to be up-regulated in chronically rejecting organs. Growth factors have been shown *in vitro* and *in vivo* to promote fibroplasia, collagen synthesis, and smooth muscle cell proliferation and migration. Currently, growth factor inhibitors are being investigated for the treatment of chronic rejection.

## MODIFICATION OF THE REJECTION RESPONSE

As the response of the immune system to foreign antigens has been better understood, many schemes or therapies have evolved that attempt to block or reduce the rejection response and protect the transplanted organ or tissue from destruction.

### Antigen Reduction

The most direct form of immunomodulation is to reduce the exposure of the host immune system to the alloantigens. In organ transplantation, this is accomplished by matching the donor and recipient for MHC antigens. Transplantation antigens can also be hidden from allosensitive T cells. Prior to implantation into the peritoneal cavity, pancreatic islet cells can be encapsulated in fenestrated plastic spheres that prohibit T cells from coming into contact with the islet cells.

### Depletion of Immune Cells and Products

Lymphocyte populations can be depleted by the administration of cytotoxic drugs, antilymphocyte serum,

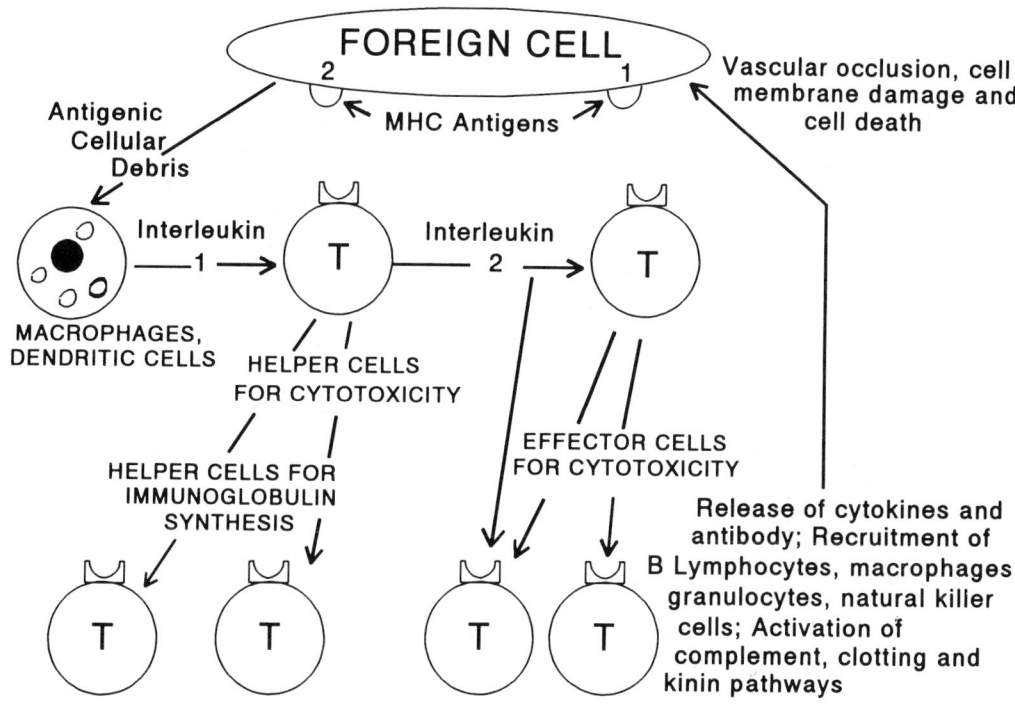

**Figure 3.** Acute allograft rejection produced by activation of T-lymphocytes by alloantigens. (Modified from Gregory CR and Gourley IM: Organ transplantation in clinical veterinary practice. *In* Slatter D (ed): *Textbook of Small Animal Surgery*, 2nd edition. Philadelphia, WB Saunders Co, 1993, p 95, with permission.)

lymphocytapheresis, or by irradiation of lymphoid organs. Organs of the immune system—in particular, the spleen and thymus—can be surgically removed. Splenectomy results in impairment of phagocytic functions and a reduced production of antibodies.

Antibody formation may be suppressed by cytotoxic drugs or lymphoid irradiation of B cells and plasma cells. Destruction of T cells indirectly decreases antibody production by decreasing the effects of T-cell–derived cytokines on B cells. Antibodies and cytokines can be directly eliminated from the host by plasmapheresis.

## Functional Alteration of Immunocompetent Cells

Alteration of cellular function, directly or indirectly, without generalized cytotoxicity has been in the forefront of immunologic research for the past decade. Cyclosporine was the first antirejection agent that specifically altered T-cell function. Other drugs are now in development that inhibit essential metabolic pathways necessary for T-cell activation and/or T-cell–mediated cytotoxicity. OKT3 is a murine monoclonal antibody directed against the human CD3–T-cell receptor complex on the cell surface of T cells. Within minutes of administration, there is a marked decrease in the number of circulating T cells. Gradually, these cells reappear but have internalized the CD3–T-cell receptor complex from the cell surface. Without this receptor complex, T cells cannot respond to the class 1 or class

2–antigen complex on the surface of allogeneic or antigen-presenting cells. OKT3 has been proven to be a valuable treatment for acute rejection in human allograft recipients. Other antibodies have been directed against cytokines and cytokine receptors. Anti–IL-2 receptor, anti-tumor necrosis factor, anti-IFN-γ antibodies, and others have been shown to increase allograft survival in animal models.

Antibodies have also been directed against the accessory cell-adhesion molecules, resulting in reduction of T-cell binding and activation. Interference with the binding of LFA-1 on T cells with ICAM-1 on allogeneic or antigen-presenting cells has prolonged allograft survival in rodent and primate models.

The antibodies used against T-cell receptors, cytokines, and adhesion molecules are usually murine in origin. Mice are challenged with the foreign glycoproteins and produce antibody that is collected and administered to another animal or human being facing a rejection reaction. In most cases, the organ recipient will form antibodies against the murine antibody that eventually neutralize its effect. To reduce this problem in human transplantation, the active portion of the mouse antibody (antigen binding or Fab portion) has been combined to human antibody (Fc and variable regions) to produce antibodies of lower antigenicity. This technology is still experimental.

Other schemes of specific immunosuppression are under investigation; for example, the generation of T-cell–specific antibody–toxin complexes. As T-cell activation and the factors involved in signal transduction are better understood, agents are being directed against the molecular events that occur in the cell membrane and in the cytosol following T-cell antigen recognition.

## IMMUNOSUPPRESSIVE AGENTS USED IN TRANSPLANTATION

For the foreseeable future, in clinical veterinary medicine, immunosuppression of MHC-nonmatched allograft rejection will have to be accomplished using chemotherapies, with the possible short-term administration of antithymocyte antibody. Specific immunosuppression using genetically engineered antibodies, soluble receptor fragments, and other biologic methods is still experimental and not available for clinical application.

### Glucocorticoids

Glucocorticoids, and in particular, prednisolone, have been used to control allograft rejection in human transplant patients for many years, and have both direct and indirect effects on the immune response. Glucocorticoids stabilize the cell membranes of vascular endothelial cells and inhibit the production of local chemotactic factors, thus decreasing infiltration of neutrophils, monocytes, and lymphocytes. In allogeneic tissue, the secretion of destructive proteolytic enzymes, such as collagenase, elastase, and plasminogen activator is inhibited (see "Clinical Applications of Glucocorticoid Therapy in Nonendocrine Disease," this volume, p 406). Glucocorticoids also inhibit the release of arachidonic acid from membrane phospholipids. This prevents the synthesis of prostaglandins, thromboxanes,

and leukotrienes, which are major mediators of inflammation.

Glucocorticoids also redistribute monocytes and lymphocytes from the peripheral circulation to the lymphatics and bone marrow. This affects primarily T cells. T-cell activation and cytotoxicity are also reduced. Glucocorticoids also suppress cytokine activity (interleukins) and alter macrophage function. Prednisolone has been used in both dogs and cats to slow allograft rejection. However, administered as a single agent, prednisolone is not capable of preventing allograft rejection.

### Cyclophosphamide

The major effect of cyclophosphamide results from alkylation of deoxyribonucleic acid (DNA) during the S phase of the cell cycle. The alterations in DNA structure can be lethal to the cell or may produce miscoding errors that inhibit cell replication or DNA transcription. Cyclophosphamide produces T- and B-cell lymphopenia and suppresses both T-cell activity and antibody production (Fig. 4). Following transplantation of baboon livers to human recipients, cyclophosphamide has been administered to aid in the prevention of the production of xenoantibodies.

### Azathioprine

Azathioprine is a purine analog that is metabolized to ribonucleotide monophosphates. Poor conversion to diphosphates and triphosphates leads to an intracellular accumulation of monophosphates that produces a feedback inhibition of enzymes required for the biosynthesis of purine nucleotides. The triphosphates analogs

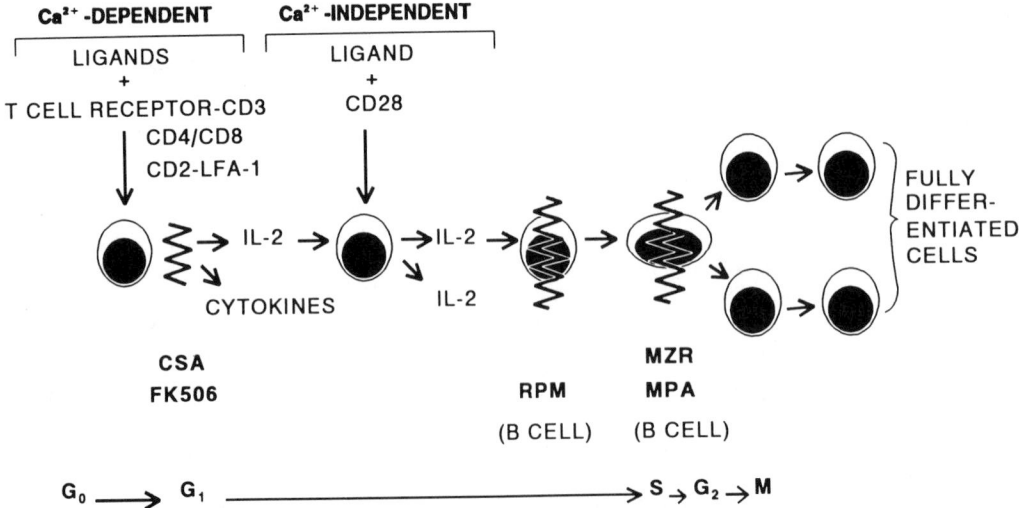

**Figure 4.** Representation of the possible sites of action of immunosuppressive agents on activated T cells. Cyclosporine (CSA) and FK506 prevent the transcription of early-phase cytokine genes, rapamycin (RPM) inhibits the signal transduction of IL-2 bound to its receptor and may have other antiproliferative effects unrelated to lymphokine signals, and mizoribine (MZR) and mycophenolic acid (MPA) inhibit purine nucleotide synthesis. RPM, MZR, and MPA also act on activated B cells at the sites shown. (Modified from Morris RE: Rapamycins: Antifungal, antitumor, antiproliferative, and immunosuppressive macrolides. Transplant Rev 6:39, 1992, with permission.)

that do form become incorporated into DNA and result in ribonucleic acid (RNA) miscoding and faulty transcription. Azathioprine has a greater effect on humoral than on cell-mediated immunity. Azathioprine and prednisolone, when administered at maximally tolerated levels, do not effectively suppress the rejection response against canine MHC-nonmatched renal allografts.

## Cyclosporine

Cyclosporine (CSA) inhibits early T-cell gene activation ($G_0$ phase of the cell cycle) and prevents synthesis of several cytokines, in particular IL-2 (also see "Cyclosporine," this volume, p 74). Without stimulation by IL-2, further T-cell proliferation is inhibited, and T-cell cytotoxic activity is reduced. Unlike the situation in human beings, in cats and dogs, cyclosporine is not hepatotoxic or nephrotoxic when administered at effective immunosuppressive doses. Very high blood levels (trough levels of >750 ng/ml) have been associated with systemic fungal infections in cats. Combination cyclosporine and prednisolone immunosuppression has maintained normal function in MHC-nonmatched feline renal allografts for over 4 years. Unfortunately, the same combination in MHC-nonmatched canine renal allografts only delays immune-mediated destruction of the graft for a few months.

## FK506

FK506 is a macrolide immunosuppressive agent with the same mechanism of action as cyclosporine. However, on an equimolar basis, FK506 is many times more potent. In experimental trials in human beings, FK506 has been used to successfully reverse ongoing rejection of liver transplants. Because of its potency, successful immunosuppression can be achieved, in some situations, without the addition of corticosteroids. This "steroid-sparing" effect is especially beneficial for pediatric transplant patients. Initially, it was hoped that FK506 would be free of the nephrotoxicity associated with cyclosporine. Unfortunately, FK506 has a similar spectrum of toxicities as cyclosporine.

## Rapamycin

Rapamycin (RPM) is another macrolide compound with a molecular structure similar to FK506. However, RPM acts much later in the cell cycle ($G_1$ to S) and blocks multiple effects of cytokines on immune cells, including IL-2–stimulated T-cell proliferation. The antiproliferative effects of RPM are not limited only to T and B cells. Rapamycin also selectively inhibits the proliferation of growth factor–dependent and growth factor–independent nonimmune cells. For this reason, RPM is being assessed for its ability to inhibit the fi-

broplasia and smooth muscle cell proliferation associated with chronic allograft rejection.

## Mizoribine and Mycophenolic Acid (RS 61443)

Both compounds suppress DNA synthesis by inhibiting inosine monophosphate dehydrogenase, an enzyme in the *de novo* pathway leading to the synthesis of guanosine. At relatively low plasma concentrations, these drugs selectively inhibit T- and B-cell proliferation, since these cells lack a salvage pathway necessary for purine biosynthesis. At higher concentrations, they inhibit the proliferation of nonimmune cells as well. Both compounds have been used as experimental immunosuppressants in dogs. When used as solo agents, renal rejection was prevented or delayed, but the dogs died of severe gastrointestinal toxicity and/or central nervous system-induced anorexia.

## Combination Therapy

Cyclosporine can be used as a single agent to effectively suppress allograft rejection in the cat. Effective immunosuppression, in a clinical sense, is defined as patient survival with a normal quality of life for 1 or more years. In human beings, cyclosporine and FK506 have been used effectively as solo agents, but in many situations, the toxicity of each agent precludes the maintenance of dosages that are effective. Most of the currently used and experimental immunosuppressive agents have differing mechanisms of action and affect immune cells at different stages of activation, differentiation, and proliferation. Combining agents often results in more effective immunosuppression with fewer drug-induced side effects (Fig. 4). In human transplant patients, azathioprine, cyclosporine, and prednisolone are often used in combination. Based on work in animal models, future patients will likely receive the combination of either cyclosporine or FK506 with rapamycin or mycophenolic acid.

Early studies suggest that some canine recipients of MHC-nonmatched renal allografts can be effectively immunosuppressed with a combination of antithymocyte serum, cyclosporine, azathioprine, and prednisolone (Mathews KA, personal communication, University of Guelph). However, rejection episodes still remain a problem and the graft can be lost. In veterinary medicine, the search continues for an effective and nontoxic agent for the control of canine allograft rejection.

## References and Suggested Reading

Chandler C and Passaro E: Transplant rejection. Mechanisms and treatment. Arch Surg 128:279, 1993.
Imboden JB: T-cell activation. *In* Schwartz BD (ed): *Immunology*. Kalamazoo, Upjohn, 1991, p 54.

Gregory CR and Gourley IM: Organ transplantation in clinical veterinary practice. *In* Slatter D (ed): *Textbook of Small Animal Surgery*, 2nd edition. Philadelphia, WB Saunders Co, 1993, p 95.

Gregory CR: Cyclosporine. *In* Kirk RW and Bonagura JD (eds): *Current Veterinary Therapy X: Small Animal Practice*. Philadelphia, WB Saunders Co, 1989, p 513.

Kirkpatrick CH and Rowlands DT: Transplantation immunology. JAMA 268: 2952, 1992.

Klippel JH: Immune-modulating therapies. *In* Schwartz BD (ed): *Immunology*. Kalamazoo, Upjohn, 1991, p 207.

Mandel TE: Basic immunology of transplantation. Med J Aust 157:126, 1992.

Morris RE: Rapamycins: Antifungal, antitumor, antiproliferative, and immunosuppressive macrolides. Transplant Rev 6:39, 1992.

Schwartz BD: The human major histocompatibility human leukocyte antigen (HLA) complex. *In* Sites DP and Terr AI (eds): *Basic and Clinical Immunology*, 7th edition. San Mateo, Appleton & Lange, 1991, p 45.

Schwartz BD: The HLA complex and disease susceptibility. *In* Schwartz BD (ed): *Immunology*. Kalamazoo, Upjohn, 1991, p 22.

Stevenson S and Schwartz A: Transplantation immunology. *In* Slatter DH (ed): *Textbook of Small Animal Surgery*. Philadelphia, WB Saunders Co, 1985, p 199.

Tilney NL and Kupiec-Weglinski JW: The biology of acute transplant rejection. Ann Surg 214:98, 1991.

# Section

# 7

# DERMATOLOGIC DISEASES

WILLIAM H. MILLER, JR.
*Consulting Editor*

### Elsewhere in Current Veterinary Therapy XII:

# RATIONAL USE OF GLUCOCORTICOIDS IN DERMATOLOGY

DANNY W. SCOTT

*Ithaca, New York*

The modern era of dermatologic therapy had its origin in 1949 with the commercial unveiling of hydrocortisone. The birth of hydrocortisone drew a line between two eras, felicitously termed "BC" (before corticosteroids) and "AC" (after corticosteroids). Although their worth in treating inflammatory dermatoses is unquestionable, glucocorticoids are decidedly the most used and abused medicaments in veterinary medicine. Their frequent usage is wholly tenable, as there are numerous dermatoses that are greatly benefitted by glucocorticoid therapy. Less tenable, however, is the continued abuse of glucocorticoids, which generally stems from carelessness, lack of close and frequent client communication and patient reevaluation, and occasionally ignorance.

Being a veterinary dermatologist, I am certainly aware of the problems—acute and chronic—that glucocorticoids can create. Indeed, over 50% of the referral cases we see have been complicated and confounded—clinically and diagnostically—by the excessive use of these drugs. The clinical, hematologic, biochemical, immunologic, endocrinologic, and histopathologic abnormalities and masking effects induced by glucocorticoids are legion, well-known, and will not be considered here (Calvert and Cornelius, 1990a; Calvert and Cornelius, 1990b; Ferguson, 1993; Noxon, 1992).

By the same token, I am frequently in the position of having to use glucocorticoids acutely and chronically—for all sorts of clinical, therapeutic, economic, and client compliance considerations. This can usually be done with minimal harm to the patient if the clinician practices the science *and* the art of glucocorticoid therapy in dermatology. If this were done with care and close patient follow-up and client communication, glucocorticoids would not have the dreadful reputation they have among pet owners, the lay public, and some veterinarians.

## INDICATIONS

Without a doubt, the skin absorbs more glucocorticoid pummeling than any other organ system. This is not surprising, as skin disorders may comprise 25 to 75% of all disease-related office calls. Table 1 displays a wide array of canine and feline dermatoses for which glucocorticoids are often used in the therapeutic regimen.

The major indications for glucocorticoid therapy are hypersensitivity (allergic) dermatoses (atopy, flea bite hypersensitivity, other insect- and arachnid-related hypersensitivities, food hypersensitivity), pyotraumatic dermatitis ("hot spot"), acral lick dermatitis, contact dermatitis (irritant or allergic), eosinophilic granuloma, eosinophilic plaque, indolent ulcer, autoimmune diseases (pemphigus, pemphigoid, lupus erythematosus), and immune-mediated disorders (vasculitis, drug eruptions). Glucocorticoids are usually only *part* of the management employed for most dermatoses, and the clinician must control or eliminate other predisposing, precipitating, and complicating factors so as to keep the glucocorticoids in their proper perspective: (1) used as infrequently as possible, (2) used at as low a dose as possible, (3) used in alternate-day regimens when chronic administration is required, and (4) used only when other less hazardous forms of therapy have failed or could not be employed.

## ROUTE OF ADMINISTRATION

Glucocorticoids can be administered orally, by injection (intramuscular, subcutaneous), topically, or in some combination thereof. The decision as to which route(s) to employ depends on several considerations: the nature of the dermatosis, the personality of the patient, the personality and capabilities of the owner, cost, other patient-disease considerations, and patient-drug idiosyncracies.

### Oral

Oral administration is preferred, especially in dogs, because: (1) it is simple, (2) it is inexpensive, (3) it can be more closely regulated (daily dose more precise than with repositol injections: drug can be rapidly withdrawn if undesirable side effects occur), and (4) it is the *only* safe, therapeutic, physiologic way to administer glucocorticoids chronically, especially in dogs.

### Subcutaneous, Intramuscular

Injectable glucocorticoids are usually administered subcutaneously or intramuscularly. Although injectable glucocorticoids are often only licensed for intramuscular use, most clinicians (including the author) administer these drugs subcutaneously. The reasons for choosing the subcutaneous route are: (1) there are

573

**Table 1.** *Canine and Feline Dermatoses Amenable to Anti-inflammatory and Immunosuppressive Doses of Glucocorticoids*

| Anti-inflammatory | Immunosuppressive |
|---|---|
| Atopy | Pemphigus |
| Flea bite hypersensitivity | Pemphigoid |
| Other insect- arachnid-related hypersensitivities | Lupus erythematosus (discoid, systemic) |
| Food hypersensitivities | Cold hemagglutinin disease |
| Contact dermatitis (irritant or allergic) | Vasculitis |
|  | Drug eruption |
|  | Linear IgA dermatosis |
| Urticaria and angioedema | Vogt-Koyanagi-Harada–like syndrome |
| Pyotraumatic dermatitis | Dermatomyositis |
| Acral lick dermatitis | Plasma cell pododermatitis |
| Seborrheic dermatitis | Relapsing polychondritis |
| Solar dermatitis | Sterile panniculitis |
| Acanthosis nigricans | Eosinophilic granuloma, eosinophilic plaque, indolent ulcer |
| Idiopathic mucinosis of Shar-Pei | Sterile granuloma/pyogranuloma syndrome |
|  | Foreign body granuloma |
|  | Sterile eosinophilic pustulosis |
|  | Juvenile cellulitis |
|  | Psoriasiform-lichenoid dermatosis of springer spaniel |
|  | Benign fibrous histiocytoma |
|  | Lymphosarcoma (epitheliotropic and nonepitheliotropic) |
|  | Mast cell tumor |

fewer objections (and pet-owner crises!), especially in cats; and (2) it is clinically just as effective as intramuscular administration. The exception would be in the obese patient, where subcutaneous injections can be sequestered.

## Topical

Owing to the bothersome hairiness of dogs and cats, their tendency to lick and rub anything put on their skin, the widespread nature of most dermatoses, and the fortitude required in applying topical medicaments to a pet, glucocorticoids are usually given parenterally. Because of these considerations, topical glucocorticoids are rarely used as the sole form of therapy. However, there are instances in which topical glucocorticoids are used as the sole therapy, and even more instances in which they are combined with other medicaments to achieve optimal results.

## CHOICE OF GLUCOCORTICOID

One cannot establish a single rule that will apply to all patients with any given glucocorticoid-responsive dermatosis. One must consider the expected duration of therapy; the personality of the patient; the personality, reliability, capabilities, and lifestyle of the owner; the response of the *patient* to the drug; the response of the patient's *disease* to the drug; and other patient-disease considerations.

## Parenteral

If the anticipated duration of systemic glucocorticoid therapy is short term (<1 month), the clinician can generally use whichever glucocorticoid he or she likes. However, for long-term therapy, oral glucocorticoids are indicated, especially in dogs.

At times, the personality of the patient significantly influences the choice of glucocorticoid (e.g., the animal who cannot be medicated orally). Likewise, the capabilities/reliability of the owner can be the deciding factor (e.g., owners who cannot, or will not give oral medicaments).

The clinician will learn by history or personal experience that some glucocorticoids do not seem to work as well as others in certain patients. This probably reflects dosage, absorptive, or metabolic differences in patients. Whatever the explanation(s), the concept of "Not all glucocorticoids are created equal" is an important one to remember. If a disease does not respond well to a particular glucocorticoid, but glucocorticoids are still the preferred treatment, try a different one (or two!).

Occasionally, a glucocorticoid that has been working well for a patient seems to lose its effectiveness, so the clinician begins administering larger doses of the drug. This well-recognized but poorly understood phenomenon is called *steroid tachyphylaxis*. In this instance, the animal will respond well to equipotent doses of a different glucocorticoid and, after a variable length of time, the clinician can usually return to successfully managing the patient with the original glucocorticoid. Steroid tachyphylaxis should *never* be considered until the animal is carefully examined and the owner carefully questioned about possible complicating factors (e.g., bacterial infection, contact dermatitis, fleas) that have caused the pruritus to come out of control.

Some animals may respond better to injectable glucocorticoids than to those administered orally. In our experience, this always reflects a failure to given equipotent doses of the oral glucocorticoid, or failure of the clinician to establish an effective maintenance regimen.

Another approach to glucocorticoid therapy is to give an initial injection, followed by oral tablets. The justification is that "the injection works faster." Pharmacologically, this is untenable, as oral glucocorticoids establish effective plasma levels just as rapidly as subcutaneous or intramuscular injections. Clinically, this fallacy is perpetuated because equipotent doses of oral glucocorticoids are not used.

Finally, the clinician sometimes discovers that a patient can receive some but not other glucocorticoids without significant adverse effects. For instance, extreme polydipsia, polyuria, polyphagia, urinary incontinence, panting (the "locomotive effect"), or personality changes produced by prednisone or prednisolone may be avoided by changing to another corticosteroid such as methylprednisolone, triamcinolone, or dexamethasone. The concept of "Not all glucocorticoids are created equal" applies. If one glucocorticoid disagrees with a patient, but glucocorticoids are still desirable, try others.

## Topical

The choice of topical glucocorticoid is based on the nature of the dermatosis, the stage of the dermatosis, and preference of the veterinarian and the owner. The most important criterion is the stage of the dermatosis. In general, *acute* and *subacute* dermatoses are characterized by varying combinations of papules, vesicles, erosions, ulcers, exudation, edema, and heat, and are best managed with nonocclusive, nonheating glucocorticoids in aqueous or lotion form. *Chronic* dermatoses are characterized by varying degrees of scaling, crusting, lichenification, erythema, and pigmentary disturbances, and are best managed with penetrating, lubricating drugs in cream or ointment form. Studies have shown that many generic topical glucocorticoids are less potent and not equivalent to brand names (Jackson et al., 1989).

Topical glucocorticoids are grouped according to relative anti-inflammatory activity (Table 2), but the activity may vary markedly depending upon the vehicle, site of application, disease, and individual patient. As with systemic glucocorticoids, some patients respond better to one topical glucocorticoid than another. In general, potency is an accurate predictor of efficacy, and the more potent the glucocorticoid the less frequently it need be applied. Nonprescription (over-the-counter)

***Table 2.*** *Relative Anti-inflammatory Potencies of Selected Topical Glucocorticoids*°

| Agent | Brand Name | Company |
|---|---|---|
| **Group I** | | |
| Betamethasone dipropionate, 0.05% cream, ointment | Diprolene | Schering |
| Clobetasol propionate, 0.05% cream, ointment | Temovate | Glaxo Derm |
| Diflorasone diacetate, 0.05% ointment | Psorcon | Dermik |
| **Group II** | | |
| Betamethasone dipropionate, 0.05% ointment | Diprosone | Schering |
| Desoximetasone, 0.25% cream, ointment | Topicort | Hoechst-Roussel |
| Fluocinonide, 0.05% cream, ointment | Lidex | Dermik |
| **Group III** | | |
| Betamethasone valerate, 0.1% ointment | Valisone | Schering |
| Triamcinolone acetonide, 0.5% cream | Kenalog | Westwood-Squibb |
| **Group IV** | | |
| Fluocinolone acetonide, 0.025% ointment | Synalar | Syntex |
| Fluocinolone acetonide, 0.1% solution | Synotic[†] | Syntex |
| Triamcinolone acetonide, 0.1% cream | Vetalog[†] | Solvay |
| **Group V** | | |
| Betamethasone valerate, 0.1% cream, lotion | Valisone | Schering |
| Fluocinolone acetonide, 0.025% cream | Synalar[†] | Syntex |
| Triamcinolone acetonide, 0.1% cream, lotion | Kenalog | Westwood-Squibb |
| **Group VI** | | |
| Desonide, 0.05% cream | Tridesilon | Miles |
| Fluocinolone acetonide, 0.01% shampoo | F/S Shampoo | Hill Dermaceuticals |
| **Group VII** | | |
| Dexamethasone, 0.1% cream | Decaderm | MSD |
| Dexamethasone, 0.04% spray | Decaspray | MSD |
| Hydrocortisone, 1 and 2.5% cream, ointment | Hytone | Dermik |
| Hydrocortisone, 1% spray | Cortispray[†] | DVM |
| Hydrocortisone, 1% spray | Dermacool-HC[†] | Allerderm/Virbac |
| Hydrocortisone, 1% solution | HB 101[†] | Butler |
| Hydrocortisone, 1% spray | Hydro-Plus[†] | Phoenix |
| Hydrocortisone, 1% spray | Hydro-10 Mist[†] | Butler |
| Hydrocortisone, 1% spray | PTD-HC[†] | VRx |

°Group I is most potent, group VII is least potent.
[†] Veterinary label.

products containing 0.5% hydrocortisone are not rated, and are rarely useful in dogs and cats. It is usually necessary to begin topical therapy with a potent fluorinated glucocorticoid in order to bring an active dermatitis under control. We have never used anything more potent than betamethasone valerate or fluocinolone acetonide. In instances where topical glucocorticoids are going to be used chronically, every attempt should be made to use less potent agents, such as 1% hydrocortisone.

Unless there is a specific indication for the inclusion of an antibacterial or antimycotic agent with a glucocorticoid, one should avoid the use of combination ("polypharmaceutical") topical products. If additional antibacterial, antimycotic, keratolytic, ceruminolytic, and local anesthetic agents are not needed, it is best not to expose the patient to unnecessary medications and increase the risk of contact irritant or hypersensitivity reactions. Regrettably, there are few topical products approved for use in dogs and cats that contain only glucocorticoid (Table 2).

## DOSAGE

It is important to remember that every patient is an individual and that *glucocorticoid therapy must be individualized.* Recommended glucocorticoid doses are guidelines and nothing more. Clinicians typically talk in terms of "anti-inflammatory" versus "immunosuppressive" doses, and "induction" versus "maintenance" doses in discussing regimens of glucocorticoids. The two most commonly used oral glucocorticoids are prednisone and prednisolone. We have never managed any animal, nor have we read about or heard of one, that had such severe liver disease that hepatic transformation of prednisone to active prednisolone was compromised. We believe prednisone and prednisolone are completely interchangeable in the clinical situation. Dosage recommendations in this article will be based on prednisone (prednisolone) equivalents. Table 3 contains information on approximately equipotent dosages of other oral glucocorticoids. However, although triamcinolone is traditionally listed as being only 20%

more potent than prednisone or prednisolone, our experience would suggest that it is closer to five to ten times more potent, and this is indicated in Table 3. Thus, our anti-inflammatory induction dose of triamcinolone for a dog would be 0.22 mg/kg/day.

The *anti-inflammatory induction dose* (as most commonly used in allergic dermatoses) of oral glucocorticoid in dogs is 1.1 mg prednisone per kilogram given every 24 hr, in the morning. The *immunosuppressive induction dose* for dogs is 2.2 to 6.6 mg/kg every 24 hr in the morning. Some clinicians will divide these inductions in half and administer them every 12 hr. In our experience, once-a-day administration is equally effective, and usually produces fewer side effects. The *maintenance dose* for dogs should, if at all possible, be no greater than 0.55 mg/kg *every other morning.*

In general, as compared to dogs, cats require about twice the dose of glucocorticoid orally for induction and maintenance therapy. A recent study revealed that normal cats had approximately one half the number of dexamethasone-binding receptors in skin and liver as normal dogs, and that the feline receptors had a lower affinity for dexamethasone (van den Broek and Stafford, 1992). This finding may contribute to the well-known relative glucocorticoid resistance observed in cats compared to dogs.

The most commonly used injectable glucocorticoid in dermatology is methylprednisolone acetate (Table 4). It is well tolerated and is the glucocorticoid of choice in cats dosed at 20 mg/cat subcutaneously. We almost never use injectable glucocorticoids in dogs because of this species' increased susceptibility to acute and chronic glucocorticoid side effects. However, the administration of most repositol glucocorticoids two or three times a year is unlikely to produce serious side effects in most dogs.

## REGIMENS

Glucocorticoid regimens vary with the nature of the dermatosis, the glucocorticoid used, induction versus

***Table 3.*** *Relative Potency and Activity of Oral Glucocorticoids*

| Drug | Glucocorticoid Potency | Equivalent Dose (mg) | Duration of Effect (hr) | Preferred for Alternate-Day Therapy |
|---|---|---|---|---|
| **Short-Acting** | | | | |
| Cortisone | 0.8 | 25 | 8–12 | |
| Hydrocortisone | 1.0 | 20 | 8–12 | |
| **Intermediate-Acting** | | | | |
| Prednisone | 4.0 | 5 | 24–36 | + |
| Prednisolone | 4.0 | 5 | 24–36 | + |
| Methylprednisolone | 5.0 | 4 | 24–36 | + |
| **Long-Acting** | | | | |
| Flumethasone | 15.0 | 1.3 | 36–48 | |
| Triamcinolone | 40.0 | 0.5 | 36–48 | |
| Dexamethasone | 40.0 | 0.5 | 36–54 | |
| Betamethasone | 50.0 | 0.4 | 36–54 | |

***Table 4.*** *Injectable Glucocorticoids for Use in Pruritic Dogs and Cats*

| Agent | Brand Name | Company | Manufacturer's Regimen | |
|---|---|---|---|---|
| | | | Dose | Route |
| Betamethasone | Betasone | Schering | 0.2–0.4 mg/kg in dog | IM |
| Dexamethasone | Azium | Schering | 0.25–1 mg/dog | IM |
| | | | 0.125–0.5 mg/cat | IM |
| Dexamethasone | Voren | Bio-Ceutic | 0.25–1 mg/dog | IM |
| | | | 0.125–0.5 mg/cat | IM |
| Flumethasone | Flucort | Syntex | 0.06–0.25 mg/dog | IM or SC |
| | | | 0.03–0.125 mg/cat | IM or SC |
| Methylprednisolone | Depo-Medrol | Upjohn | 2–40 mg/dog | IM |
| | | | 10–20 mg/cat | IM |
| Triamcinolone | Vetalog | Solvay | 0.1–0.2 mg/kg/dog | IM or SC |
| | | | 0.1–0.2 mg/kg/cat | IM or SC |

maintenance therapy, special patient considerations, and special owner considerations.

## Oral

In generally, dermatoses requiring anti-inflammatory doses of oral glucocorticoid require smaller doses and a shorter period of induction therapy to bring about remission, as compared with dermatoses requiring immunosuppressive doses. Anti-inflammatory induction doses are usually given for 3 to 7 days, and immunosuppressive induction doses are usually given for 10 to 14 days. The key is to continue daily induction doses until disease activity is completely suppressed.

Maintenance therapy with oral glucocorticoid is best accomplished with prednisone, prednisolone, or methylprednisolone on an alternate-day basis. With alternate-day therapy, the daily dose of glucocorticoid used for successful induction therapy is given every 48 hr: in the morning for dogs and in the evening for cats. This alternate-day dose is usually reduced by 50%, every 1 or 2 weeks, until the lowest satisfactory maintenance dose is achieved. In general, if alternate-day prednisone doses must be maintained at greater than 0.55 mg/kg in dogs and greater than 1.1 mg/kg in cats, chronic glucocorticoid side effects will be seen within 1 to 2 years.

It is important here to discuss the concept of "tolerable itchiness" or "tolerable disease" with the pet owner. For instance, when managing allergic pets with chronic glucocorticoid therapy, we tell the owners that we do *not* want to stop all itch. If we give enough glucocorticoid to stop all scratching, rubbing, licking, and chewing, we are probably giving too much and side effects are likely. It is wiser to allow the pet to manifest some evidence of pruritus, as long as dermatitis, alopecia, self-mutilation, and personality abnormalities are not present. By the same token, it is better to tolerate occasional pustules and crusts in an animal with pemphigus foliaceus than to cause much worse disease with excessive doses of glucocorticoid.

If alternate-day therapy with prednisone, prednisolone, or methylprednisolone is successful, one should attempt to give the medication every third day. Occasionally, pets can be satisfactorily controlled with every-third-day or every-fourth-day medication.

If alternate-day therapy with prednisone, prednisolone, and methylprednisolone is ineffective (too much pruritus/dermatitis on the day without medication) or if there are unacceptable glucocorticoid side effects (uncommon), try one of the long-acting glucocorticoids (e.g., triamcinolone or dexamethasone). Unfortunately, the longer duration of effect of these glucocorticoids make them much less effective for long-term alternate-day therapy in dogs. Every-third-day therapy would be preferable, but usually does not control clinical signs on the second day of no therapy. If alternate-day therapy with long-acting oral glucocorticoids is chosen, the owner must realize that regardless of the dose, chronic glucocorticoid side effects are almost guaranteed within 1 to 2 years.

The situation is quite different for the cat. Many cats can be effectively and safely maintained on alternate-day triamcinolone or dexamethasone. Again, some cats can be controlled with dexamethasone given orally once or twice a week, so the veterinarian should always be trying to extend the interval between glucocorticoid treatments.

Finally, most dermatoses *cannot be brought under control* initially with alternate-day glucocorticoid therapy. *Daily* treatment is usually needed for successful induction therapy.

## Injectable

Subcutaneous or intramuscular injections of glucocorticoids are usually fine for induction therapy, but they are usually unsatisfactory and often dangerous for chronic maintenance therapy in dogs. Even single injections of glucocorticoids can have prolonged adrenocortical suppressive effects in dogs (Table 5).

In cats, the situation is very different. Due to the simplicity and cost-effectiveness of giving subcutaneous injections, the difficulty of frequent pilling, and the relative resistance of cats to the side effects of glucocorticoids, repositol methylprednisolone acetate is usually the glucocorticoid of choice in cats. Cats are given 20 mg subcutaneously, every 2 weeks until the dermatosis

**Table 5.** *Effects of Glucocorticoids on Adrenocortical Function in Dogs*

| Drug | Protocol | Route of Administration | Duration of Suppression After Treatment Stopped |
|------|----------|------------------------|------------------------------------------------|
| ***Parental Administration*** | | | |
| Dexamethasone | 0.1 mg/kg once | IV | 32 hr |
| Dexamethasone sodium phosphate | 0.1 mg/kg once | IV | <24 hr |
| Dexamethasone alcohol | 1 mg/kg once | IM | 48 hr |
| Dexamethasone 21-isonicotinate | 0.1 mg/kg once | IM | 10 days |
| Dexamethasone 21-isonicotinate | 1 mg/kg once | IM | 4 weeks |
| Methylprednisolone acetate | 2.5 mg/kg once | IM | 5 wk |
| Methylprednisolone acetate | 4 mg/kg once | IM | 9 wk |
| Methylprednisolone acetate | 0.56 mg/kg once | SC | 3 wk |
| Triamcinolone acetonide | 0.22 mg/kg once | IM | 4 wk |
| Triamcinolone acetonide | 0.22 mg/kg/day for 8 days | PO | 2 wk |
| ***Topical Administration*** | | | |
| Betamethasone valerate | 1.36 mg/kg/day for 5 days | Skin ointment | 4 wk |
| Dexamethasone | 0.03 mg/kg/day for 8 wk | Ophthalmic drops | 2 wk |
| Dexamethasone | 0.31 mg/kg/day for 3 wk | Otic drops | 3 wk |
| Fluocinonide | 0.68 mg/kg/day for 5 days | Skin ointment | 4 wk |
| Prednisolone acetate | 0.75 mg/kg/day for 4 wk | Ophthalmic drops | 2 wk |
| Triamcinolone acetonide | 1.36 mg/kg/day for 5 days | Skin ointment | 4 wk |
| Triamcinolone acetate | 0.31 mg/kg/day for 3 wk | Otic drops | 3 wk |

Abbreviations: IV = intravenously, IM = intramuscular, SC = subcutaneously, PO = orally.

is in remission (rarely are more than two or three induction injections required). Maintenance injections are administered as needed thereafter. If maintenance injections are given no more frequently than every 8 weeks, most cats will experience no side effects.

## Topical

Topical glucocorticoids are most commonly used for the treatment of pyotraumatic dermatitis, allergic otitis externa, acral lick dermatitis, sterile granulomas (eosinophilic, foreign body, or idiopathic), eosinophilic plaque, discoid lupus erythematosus, acanthosis nigricans, localized seborrheic dermatitis, solar dermatitis, and histiocytoma. In addition, topical glucocorticoids may be used as spot treatments in animals receiving systemic glucocorticoids.

Due to the "reservoir effect," topical glucocorticoids need be applied only once or twice daily. Sprays, solutions, or lotions can be used in acute or subacute dermatoses, on superficial dermatoses, and where clipping the hair coat is undesirable. Creams and ointments are used in chronic dermatoses and on thickened lesions where penetration is necessary (Table 2).

Many clinicians treat topical glucocorticoids as if they were totally innocuous agents. This is totally erroneous and potentially disastrous. Several recent studies have shown that topical glucocorticoids—whether applied as ophthalmic, otic, or cutaneous medicaments—produce significant systemic effects that may include iatrogenic Cushing's syndrome and iatrogenic secondary adrenocortical insufficiency (Table 5). If more potent topical glucocorticoids are used, if excessive amounts are used, if large areas of the body are treated, if the epidermal barrier is abnormal or absent, if treatment is administered chronically, and/or if the patient also ingests the product (grooming behavior in

cats, licking behavior in dogs), systemic effects will be more likely. We have seen a number of cases of iatrogenic Cushing's syndrome in dogs caused by excessive use of topical glucocorticoids, most commonly with Panalog, Tresaderm, and Synotic. When applying glucocorticoids to their pets so as to minimize their own exposure, owners must be instructed to take proper precautions (wear plastic or rubber gloves or finger cots; use applicator sticks).

Once the daily induction therapy has brought the dermatosis under control, topical glucocorticoids should be used in the same manner as oral glucocorticoids: no more frequently than every other morning (dog) or evening (cat), and even less frequently, if possible.

## WHEN SYSTEMIC GLUCOCORTICOIDS ALONE ARE UNSATISFACTORY

Alternate-day glucocorticoid therapy is not a panacea. There are some patients that cannot be successfully managed, either because side effects are unacceptable, or disease control on the "off" day is inadequate. This is most often encountered in chronic allergic dermatitis or autoimmune and immune-mediated dermatoses.

A common situation is a patient with chronic allergic skin disease that has been managed for some period of time with a relatively stable oral or injectable glucocorticoid regimen, and suddenly becomes more pruritic. There is a tendency to say that "this animal's allergy has gotten worse," and to immediately increase the dose of systemic glucocorticoid. Certainly, allergies can become worse with time, and can have periods when clinical signs are worse because of an increase in allergen (pollen and mold spore count surges in spring, summer, and fall; increased house dust quantity and dispersion as heating systems kick-in during winter). As previously mentioned, steroid tachyphylaxis is also a possible consideration. In these situations, a short-term increase in glucocorticoid dose or switching to a different glucocorticoid may be indicated. However, in the majority of cases, the sudden worsening of clinical signs is due to the arrival of a complicating factor: bacterial infection, *Malassezia* dermatitis, flea infestation, other insect- or arachnid-related dermatoses, dry skin, and reactions to recently instituted or ongoing topical treatments (shampoos, dips, sprays, and so forth). The clinician must *always* suspect and reevaluate the pet for the development of additional dermatoses. Failure to do this results in the continued "ascension of the steroid mountain," using increasing doses and frequencies. Adverse patient side effects and owner-veterinarian frustration escalate. In summary, never forget the principles of "threshold phenomenon" and "summation of effects" when dealing with pruritic and/or dermatitic dogs and cats (Griffin et al., 1993; Scott and Miller, 1993a; Scott and Miller, 1993b).

The clinician must look for ways to reduce glucocorticoid doses and frequencies when: (1) required systemic glucocorticoid regimens involve doses and frequencies that are too great or produce intolerable side effects, (2) a previously well-controlled pet begins to have problems again (and the exacerbation is known to *not* be the result of some complicating factor[s]), or (3) a patient continues to have focal areas of disease activity.

Some patients with allergic and autoimmune dermatoses will be notably worse when exposed to ultraviolet light (sunshine). Sun avoidance may be useful.

Animals who have occasional or constant problem areas of pruritus, inflammation, and excoriation often benefit from topical applications. Nonsteroidal topicals should be tried first (Table 6). If these are ineffective, topical glucocorticoids can be used (Table 2).

Animals who have multifocal or generalized pruritus will usually require total body topical therapy. The simplest of these are shampoos (Table 6). Shampoos remove surface debris, bacterial by-products, and allergens; cool the skin; and can rehydrate the stratum corneum. As allergic pets tend to have easily irritated,

"sensitive" skin, shampoos used on them should be hypoallergenic, moisturizing, and nonirritating. The clinician should begin with simple products, such as Allergroom and HyLyt°efa, and move up to more potent shampoos as needed. We have been impressed with the antipruritic activity of Epi-Soothe and Histacalm. Shampoos are typically given one or twice a week (remember to allow 10 to 15 min contact time before rinsing!), or as needed. When a more potent humectant and moisturizing effect is needed, rinses may be preferred (Table 6). We have been very pleased with the weekly or biweekly use of MicroPearls Cream Rinse.

More severe degrees of pruritus or pruritus unresponsive to shampoos and rinses may necessitate the use of soaks (Table 6). In this respect, cool water is the simplest, cheapest, least irritating soak solution available! Increased antipruritic activity can be achieved by adding colloidal oatmeal to the water. Soaks should be administered once or twice a day, with a 20- to 30-min contact time. Antipruritic effects may last several hours or 1 to 3 days. Obviously, this type of therapy is time and labor intensive but it can be administered by the owner. *Never* use warm, hot, or cold water for soaks, as in the long run these situations tend to exacerbate pruritus.

If nonsteroidal topical therapy has been unsuccessful in treating generalized forms of pruritus, one can try a glucocorticoid-containing shampoo. F/S Shampoo (Table 2) can be used daily for 5 to 7 days, or once or twice a week for at least 6 months with no adverse clinical, hematologic, biochemical, or adrenocortical suppressive effects (Beale et al., 1993).

If all topical efforts fail, the clinician can try systemic "steroid-sparing" drugs. For the pruritic animal, try antihistamines and/or ω-3/ω-6 fatty acid–containing products (Table 7). They will frequently reduce required doses and frequencies of glucocorticoids (Scott and Miller, 1993a; Scott and Miller, 1993b). For animals with autoimmune or immune-mediated dermatoses, steroid reduction can often be achieved with concurrent use of DVM Derm Caps, azathioprine (dogs only!), chlorambucil, dapsone (dogs only!), or chrysotherapy (gold salts) (Griffin, Kwochka, and MacDonald, 1993).

**Table 6.** *Useful Nonsteroidal Topical Agents for Pruritic Dogs and Cats*

| Product | Active Ingredient(s) | Form | Manufacturer |
|---|---|---|---|
| **Spot Application** | | | |
| Caladryl | 1% diphenhydramine, 8% calamine, camphor | Lotion | Parke-Davis |
| Dermacool | Hamamelis extract, menthol | Spray | Allerderm/Virbac |
| Histacalm | 2% diphenhydramine | Spray | Allerderm/Virbac |
| **Total Body Application** | | | |
| Allergroom | Moisturizing, hypoallergenic | Shampoo | Allerderm/Virbac |
| HyLyt°efa | Moisturizing, hypoallergenic | Shampoo | DVM |
| Epi-Soothe | Colloidal ointment | Shampoo | Allerderm/Virbac |
| Histacalm | 2% diphenhydramine | Shampoo | Allerderm/Virbac |
| MicroPearls Cream Rinse | Humectant, hypoallergenic | Rinse | EVSCO |
| HyLyt°efa | Moisturizing, hypoallergenic | Rinse | DVM |
| Water | Water | Soak | Nature! |
| Aveeno | Colloidal oatmeal | Soak | Rydelle Labs |
| Epi-Soothe | Colloidal oatmeal | Soak | Allerderm/Virbac |

**Table 7.** *Useful Nonsteroidal Systemic Agents for Pruritic Dogs and Cats°*

| Drug | Class | Regimen |
|------|-------|---------|
| **Dog** | | |
| Amitriptyline | Antihistamine | 1 mg/kg q12h |
| Chlorpheniramine | Antihistamine | 0.4 mg/kg 8h |
| Clemastine | Antihistamine | 0.05–0.1 mg/kg q12h |
| Diphenhydramine | Antihistamine | 2 mg/kg q8h |
| Hydroxyzine | Antihistamine | 2 mg/kg q8h |
| DVM Derm Caps® | ω-3/ω-6 fatty acids | 1 capsule/9.1 kg q24h |
| **Cat** | | |
| Chlorpheniramine | Antihistamine | 0.4–0.8 mg/kg q12h |
| Clemastine | Antihistamine | 0.15 mg/kg q12h |
| DVM Derm Caps® Liquid | ω-3/ω-6 fatty acids | 0.5 ml/4.5 kg q24h |

°These agents can be used individually to reduce required glucocorticoid doses in dogs and cats. In addition, an antihistamine can be combined with an ω-3/ω-6 fatty-acid product to achieve nonsteroidal synergism.

## UNCONVENTIONAL USES OF GLUCOCORTICOIDS

Glucocorticoids may be useful in situations where their employment would generally be considered contraindicated. We have seen dogs with severe deep bacterial infection (furunculosis, cellulitis), sometimes in association with demodicosis, where the paws were swollen, painful, and a pitting edema extended proximally, even to the level of the carpi and/or hocks. Appropriate systemic antibiotic and topical therapy for 10 to 14 days had not helped these dogs and some were getting worse. Two to 3 days of oral prednisone (2.2 mg/kg every 24 hr) resulted in rapid resolution of swelling, edema, and pain, and the infection then responded nicely to antibiotics. We assume the massive edema resulted in unsatisfactory delivery of antibiotic to the tissues.

We also have employed glucocorticoids in the treatment of canine histiocytomas. These benign neoplasms usually undergo spontaneous regression. However, at times they are pruritic, ulcerated, bleeding, and cosmetically unacceptable. Usually veterinarians simply excise them. When surgical intervention is impossible (e.g., site of neoplasm, owner refusal to allow anesthesia and surgery), we have had excellent results with the twice-daily topical application of fluocinolone in DMSO (Synotic), until remission is achieved (2 to 4 weeks).

## MONITORING THERAPY

There are no hard and fast scientific data or rules to present here. The individuality of patients, their diseases, and their owners must be considered. Animals on chronic glucocorticoid therapy, whether systemic and/or topical, should be examined every 6 months before more medication is dispensed. Although many authors recommend doing laboratory work (hemogram, urinalysis, serum biochemistry panel, even adrenocorticotrophic hormone [ACTH] response tests), we usually find these to be of limited help and not cost effective. Most animals on chronic glucocorticoid therapy will have one or more hematologic and/or biochemical abnormalities, and variable suppression of adrenocortical responsiveness to ACTH. A urinalysis and bacterial culture of urine may be more worthwhile. Even though one study indicated that about 35% of the dogs on chronic glucocorticoid therapy had bacteriuria, without clinical signs or abnormal urinalysis, the clinical significance of this bacteriuria usually is unclear (Griffin, Kwochka, and MacDonald, 1993). We rarely recognize urinary tract disease coincident with glucocorticoid therapy.

In our experience, the most useful examinations are historical and physical. Are drinking, urinating, and eating habits normal? Is the animal's weight steady? Are personality and activity normal? Do the skin, hair coat, and musculature look and palpate normally? Is the liver palpably enlarged or the abdomen soft and pendulous? If body fat being redistributed? We believe a clinician's skills at history-taking and physical examination are by far the most useful "tests" in monitoring patients receiving chronic glucocorticoid therapy.

## COMMENTS

Clearly, we do not fear glucocorticoids or avoid them at all cost. We *do* respect glucocorticoids—both their benefits and their potential harmful effects. We *do*, for various patient, disease, and owner reasons, use glucocorticoids frequently, both acutely and chronically. We *do* try to insure that owners have a solid understanding of the potential risk and benefits of glucocorticoids. We *do* encourage frequent reassessment, whether over the telephone or in person. If the clinician is committed to these "do's," and can share his or her knowledge of dermatologic science and art with a cooperative patient and owner, then significant side effects attributable to chronic glucocorticoid therapy should be a problem in only about 10% of the cases.

### References and Suggested Reading

Beale KM, Kunkle G, and Keisling K: A study of long-term administration of F/S Shampoo in dogs. Proc Am Acad Vet Dermatol/Am Coll Vet Dermatol 9:36, 1993.

*This 6-month study shows that F/S Shampoo can be used once or twice weekly without producing adverse clinical, hematologic, biochemical, or adrenocortical suppressive effects.*

Calvert CA and Cornelius LM: Avoiding the undesirable effects of glucocorticoid hormone therapy. Vet Med 85:846, 1990a.
*Good review of glucocorticoid side effects and how to minimize their occurrence.*

Calvert CA and Cornelius LM: Corticosteroid hormones: Endogenous regulation and the effects of exogenous administration. Vet Med 85:810, 1990b.
*Good review of the physiology and pathophysiology of glucocorticoids.*

Ferguson EA: Glucocorticoids—use and abuse. *In* Locke PH, Harvey RG, and Mason IS (eds): *Manual of Small Animal Dermatology.* Gloucestershire, British Small Animal Veterinary Association, 1993, pp 233–243.
*Good review of the pathophysiology, side effects, and proper use of glucocorticoids.*

Griffin CE, Kwochka KW, and MacDonald JM: *Current Veterinary Dermatology. The Science and Art of Therapy.* St. Louis, Mosby-Year Book, 1993.
*Good review of the symptomatic therapy of pruritus in dogs and cats.*

Jackson DB, Thompson C, McCormack JK, and Guin JD: Bioequivalence (bioavailability) of generic topical corticosteroids. J Am Acad Dermatol 20:791, 1989.
*Study documents the frequent inferior status of generic topical glucocorticoids when compared to brand names.*

Merchant SR and Caprile KA: Pharmacological management of allergic disease. Semin Vet Med Surg 6:256, 1991.
*Good review of the topical and systemic management of pruritus in dogs and cats.*

Noxon JO: The effect of glucocorticoid therapy on diagnostic procedures in dermatology. *In* Kirk RW and Bonagura JD (eds): *Current Veterinary Therapy XI.* Philadelphia, WB Saunders Co, 1992, pp 498–502.
*Good review of the various hematologic, biochemical, and pathologic "abnormalities" produced by glucocorticoids.*

Scott DW and Miller WH Jr: Nonsteroidal anti-inflammatory agents in the management of canine allergic pruritus. J S Afr Vet Assoc 64:52, 1993a.
*Good review of the pathophysiology and nonsteroidal management of allergic pruritus in dogs.*

Scott DW and Miller WH Jr: Medical management of allergic pruritus in the cat with emphasis on atopy. J S Afr Vet Assoc 64:103, 1993b.
*Good review of the pathophysiology and steroidal/nonsteroidal management of allergic pruritus in cats.*

van den Broek AHM and Stafford WL: Epidermal and hepatic glucocorticoid receptors in cats and dogs. Res Vet Sci 52:312, 1992.
*Study shows that cats have approximately one half the number of dexamethasone-binding receptors in skin and liver as compared to dogs.*

# FELINE IMMUNOMODULATORS

KAREN HELTON RHODES
*New York, New York*

Medications that have the capacity to alter the immune system in either a suppressive or stimulatory fashion can be termed "immunomodulators." The veterinary literature has a limited amount of data regarding the use of feline immunomodulators. Many of the reports are anecdotal or involve a limited number of cases. Evaluation of the immune system in the cat and the response of individual cell types is extremely difficult and therefore leaves clinical response to therapy as the most reliable diagnostic tool in understanding the immunologic response to various drugs. Some therapeutic agents can be clearly categorized as immunosuppressant or immunostimulatory, while others cannot be categorized so precisely. The following discussion is not a comprehensive review of all available immunomodulators, but includes a select group of medications currently being used in cats.

## GLUCOCORTICOIDS

Glucocorticoids are potent anti-inflammatory agents that have a wide variety of immunosuppressive activities. Margination and adherance of white blood cells is decreased as is chemotaxis of cells. Function is also decreased with a reduction in phagocytic activity of inflammatory cells. Steroids inhibit complement activity; suppress the antibody response to antigenic stimulation; increase gamma globulin metabolism, inhibit the release of arachidonic acid from phospholipid, thereby altering the inflammatory response; and are considered

T-cell lympholytic. Glucocorticoids are involved in a number of other immunologic pathways as well.

Anti-inflammatory dosages of glucocorticoid in cats range from 0.5 to 2.2 mg/kg/day and immunosuppressive dosages range from 2.2 to 8.8 mg/kg/day. Methylprednisolone acetate (Depo-Medrol, Upjohn), prednisone, and dexamethosone are the most efficacious forms of glucocorticoid in the cat. Depo-Medrol at 20 mg/cat subcutaneously every 2 weeks for a total of three injections is a standard *initial* protocol for idiopathic eosinophilic granuloma complex (EGC) lesions. Maintenance injections should not exceed a frequency of once every 6 to 8 weeks. Prednisone and dexamethasone are usually ineffective in controlling EGC. Prednisone can be used as a sole immunosuppressive agent or in conjunction with other cytotoxic drugs to control immune-mediated diseases. Dexamethasone has been found to be effective in controlling symptoms of allergic dermatitis when other medications have failed. Diabetes mellitus is a common side effect of corticosteroid therapy; therefore, owners should be instructed to monitor the cat's urine at home for glucose on a weekly basis.

## AUROTHIOGLUCOSE

Aurothioglucose, an injectable gold salt, is used primarily in the management of pemphigus foliaceus and recurrent, resistant EGC lesions. This compound can modulate many phases of the immune system and inflammatory response including neutrophil migration and function, lymphocyte function and immunoglobulin production, and monocyte/macrophage function (Bloom et al., 1988).

Aurothioglucose (Solganal, Schering) is supplied in 10-ml vials at a concentration of 50 mg/ml. Most protocols require weekly intramuscular injections of 1 mg/kg. The induction phase of the drug may take 6 weeks or longer, after which injections are decreased to monthly intervals. During the induction phase a complete blood count, serum biochemistry, and urinalysis should be taken every other week to monitor side effects of the drug. Toxicity is limited in cats but may include glomerulonephritis with proteinuria, bone marrow suppression, thrombocytopenia, aplastic anemia, cutaneous eruptions, toxic epidermal necrolysis, and hepatotoxicosis. Impending toxicities may be heralded by eosinophilia.

## AZATHIOPRINE*

Azathioprine is an imidazole derivative of 6-mercaptopurine and is commonly used in dogs as an immunosuppressive agent. This drug is classified as a purine antimetabolite and, therefore, interferes with deoxyribonucleic acid (DNA) and ribonucleic acid (RNA) metabolism. Azathioprine also modulates cell-mediated immunity and T-lymphocyte–dependent antibody synthesis.

Azathioprine (Imuran, Burroughs Wellcome) is supplied in 50-mg tablets. The dose recommended for the cat is 1.0 mg/kg/day or every other day, which necessitates that the drug be divided into small alliquots of one tenth of a tablet to ensure an accurate dose. This procedure dramatically increases the cost of the medication. More importantly, cats exhibit an idiosyncratic adverse reaction to azathioprine by developing a severe, nonresponsive, fatal leukopenia and thrombocytopenia. Two reported studies (Caciolo, 1984; Beale, 1989) showed myelotoxicity with prominent granulocyte hypoplasia in 9 of 13 cats given azathioprine at a dose range of 1.1 to 2.2 mg/kg every other day. Hematologic abnormalities appeared after a mean of 8.25 doses in one study and 15.4 doses in the other. Cats frequently *do not recover even if the drug is withdrawn.* Four additional cases of fatal azathioprine toxicity have been diagnosed by the author. Other reported side effects include hepatotoxicosis, vomiting, panniculitis, hypersensitivities, alopecia, and cutaneous eruptions. Any cat receiving this medication should be vigorously monitored. Because of the problem in accurate dosing and the potential for fatal toxicity, *this drug is not recommended for use in the cat.*

## CHLORAMBUCIL

Chlorambucil (Leukeran, Burroughs Wellcome) is an alkylating agent similar to cyclophosphamide and

mechlorethamine. These drugs alter DNA synthesis and inhibit rapidly proliferating cells. Chlorambucil is administered orally at a dosage of 0.1 to 0.2 mg/kg/day in conjunction with prednisone at a dosage of 2.2 mg/kg/day. The small pill size of chlorambucil (2.0 mg) allows easy dosing of small animals. Most cats require one half tablet (1.0 mg) per day. Toxicities are uncommon in the cat but may include mild, gradual, and rapidly reversible bone marrow suppression. Anorexia, vomiting, and diarrhea have been reported in the cat but resolve when the drug is changed from a daily to an alternate-day schedule. Rarely reported toxicosis associated with chronic use in humans includes pulmonary fibrosis, hepatotoxicity, drug fever, skin hypersensitivities, peripheral neuropathies, interstitial pneumonia, sterile cystitis, infertility, leukemia, and secondary malignancies.

Chlorambucil is being used by the author (Helton-Rhodes and Shoulberg, 1992) as a routine treatment for feline pemphigus foliaceus and for severe recalcitrant cases of feline eosinophilic granuloma complex. Daily treatment (0.1 to 0.2 mg/kg/day) is maintained until marked resolution of clinical signs has been achieved, or approximately 75% improvement is seen. This degree of improvement may require 4 to 8 weeks of treatment. Alternate-day chlorambucil is then initiated and maintained for several weeks, provided there is no exacerbation of clinical signs. Following this, prednisone (if being used concurrently) and chlorambucil are decreased alternately and gradually until the lowest possible maintenance dose is determined. Most cats do not require continued chlorambucil and may be maintained on low alternate-day doses of prednisone. However, each cat is unique and successful protocols vary. Animals should be monitored by complete blood and platelet counts every 2 weeks while on chlorambucil therapy.

In a 1992 report (Helton-Rhodes and Shoulberg, 1992), The Animal Medical Center had used chlorambucil to successfully treat 26 domestic cats with pemphigus foliaceus and three cats with recalcitrant eosinophilic granuloma complex lesions. Of 26 cats with pemphigus foliaceus, 10 (38%) showed a 75% improvement in clinical symptoms within 4 weeks of combination (chlorambucil and prednisone) therapy; 7 of 26 (27%) at 6 weeks, 8 of 26 (31%) at 8 weeks; and 1 (4%) required 12 weeks of therapy. Six of the 26 cats remained free of disease for a mean of 4 years (range-2 to 6 years) with no medication required. Two have since died of unrelated causes and four are currently alive and free of disease. Of 26, 9 have been maintained on on alternate-day prednisone therapy (2.5 to 5.0 mg) for a mean of 3 years (range-1.5 to 4.0 years) and have remained free of disease. Five of the 26 cats were maintained with alternate-day prednisone and remained free of lesions for a mean of 15 months (range-6 to 22 months), yet each of these cats relapsed while on maintenance therapy and required subsequent treatment with chlorambucil. Four of these cats responded to chlorambucil in a similar or shorter time frame as during induction therapy. The remaining cat

---

*Not recommended for cats.

failed to respond within 8 weeks and the owner elected to euthanize the cat. Five of the 26 cats were lost to follow-up yet were free of disease at a 6- to 12-month visit. Two of the 26 cats died of unrelated causes and the status of their disease at the time of death was unknown.

Two cats, in addition to the 26 cats discussed, failed to respond to chlorambucil after 8 weeks of therapy and both were subsequently treated with azathioprine. One of these cats developed severe myelosuppression within 4 weeks of therapy and was euthanized at the owner's request. The other cat responded to azathioprine within 5 weeks of therapy and showed no adverse effects. Both owners declined the option to use aurothioglucose due to the weekly injection schedule.

In the same report (Helton-Rhodes and Shoulberg, 1992), three cats with severe persistent EGC lesions were treated successfully with chlorambucil. One cat had clinical and histologic eosinophilic plaque lesions that covered approximately two thirds of the body surface; one cat had a linear granuloma of the soft palate and footpads of two digits as well as a 10- × 20-cm truncal eosinophilic plaque; and the third cat had severe indolent ulcers of the maxillary lip margins. Diagnostic procedures to identify a specific underlying etiology for each of these cases were negative. Unsuccessful therapeutic trials prior to chlorambucil included injectable, oral, and topical corticosteroids; antihistamines; allergy testing and hyposensitization; external parasite control; injectable gold salts; and megestrol actetate. Each of these cats responded to chlorambucil therapy within 6 weeks. The first cat with severe eosinophilic plaque showed the most rapid response at 3 weeks, while the other two required 5 to 6 weeks to show an approximate 75% improvement. Once this level of improvement was achieved, a slow taper was initiated. Two cats were maintained on a slow 12-week taper and are currently off of all medication with no recurrence of lesions. The third cat with the severe indolent ulcers remained free of active lesions (residual 3- × 4-mm scarred lesion) for approximately 8 months, at which time the lesions flared and were nonresponsive to chlorambucil. This cat is currently being maintained on interferon therapy with marginal, although acceptable to the client, success.

Chlorambucil is currently the author's drug of choice in the treatment of feline immune-mediated dermatoses because of the drug's efficacy, small tablet size, and lack of severe toxicity. Other severe immunologic disorders that are nonresponsive to conventional therapy also may be considered as candidates for chlorambucil therapy.

## MEGESTROL ACETATE

Megestrol acetate (Ovaban, Schering) is an oral drug that is widely abused in veterinary medicine. The drug is not approved for use in feline dermatoses in the United States but is commonly used anyway to treat a variety of conditions including allergic dermatitis, be-

havioral problems, and EGC lesions. Megestrol acetate has more potent and longer lasting anti-inflammatory and adrenal suppressive effects than corticosteroids. Side effects of the drug (mammary gland fibroadenomatous hyperplasia/neoplasia, diabetes mellitus, behavioral abnormalities, adrenocortical suppression) necessitate serious consideration prior to use. Once owners are warned of the problems associated with the drug[1] and all other options are exhausted, then therapy may be attempted at a dosage of 2.5 to 5.0 mg/cat every other day, declining to 2.5 mg every 7 to 14 days for maintenance. Owners should be instructed to monitor the cat's urine for glucose as an early warning of toxicity.

## LEVAMISOLE

Levamisole (Levasole, Pitman-Moore) is an anthelmintic drug that is also capable of modulating the immune system. It alters the metabolism and function of T lymphocytes, monocytes, and neutrophils. The enhancement of activity occurs in those cells whose function is suppressed or inefficient. There is no enhancement of activity in normally functioning cells. Levamisole stimulates cell-mediated immune reactivity by potentiating the rate of T-lymphocyte differentiation, the responsiveness to antigens and mitogens, and the activity of effector lymphocytes. By altering monocyte and neutrophil function, levamisole may speed antigen localization and clearance. There is no known direct effect on B-cell activity. Levamisole has been used with limited success in canine medicine and is even more rarely utilized in feline medicine. Feline EGC is a common and often frustrating clinical entity. The pathomechanism of the condition is poorly understood but is currently felt to be a manifestation of a severe hypersensitivity reaction. Levamisole, among numerous other medications, has been tried in a limited number of cases. Inflammatory disorders and autoimmunity are often characterized by chronic antigenic stimulation. Levamisole may enhance antigen clearance or increase the activity of suppressor lymphocytes, which are important in the regulation of the immune system.

Side effects of levamisole in general include gingivitis, agranulocytosis due to leukocyte agglutinating antibodies, thrombocytopenia, vasculitis, nausea, vomiting, fever, arthralgias, muscle pain, and cutaneous eruptions. Patients should be closely monitored during therapy for potentially severe side effects. Although this drug has been used in a few cases, exact therapeutic protocols and expected efficacy for levamisole are unknown in the cat and *extreme caution* must be exercised when choosing this drug for therapy.

## ACEMANNAN

Acemannan (Acemannan Immunostimulant, Carrington Laboratories) is a polydispersed complex poly-

---

[1]Informed consent forms should be obtained from owners.

saccharide of high molecular weight. Acemannan has been theorized to stimulate interleukin-1, interleukin-6, tumor necrosis factor-$\alpha$, and prostaglandin $E_2$ production by macrophages and has also demonstrated *in vitro* antiviral activity. The product is packaged as a kit containing a 10-mg vial of acemannan and a 10-ml vial of sterile diluent for injection. The approved mode of administration is intraperitoneal (1 mg/kg) or intralesional (2 mg/tumor) injections. Intravenous, subcutaneous, and oral administrations have also been described (Yates, Raboud, and Tizard, 1992). Acemannan has been used primarily in cases of FIV-infected cats. Efficacy data regarding the use of this medication in feline medicine is still largely anecdotal. Reported side effects include fever, anorexia, depression, diarrhea, syncope, transient bradycardia and disorientation, tachypnea or tachycardia or both, collapse, and pain on injection.

## COLONY-STIMULATING FACTORS

Colony-stimulating factors are hematopoietic growth factors with biologic specificity defined by their ability to support the proliferation and differentiation of blood cells of different lineages. These factors are currently being studied for their use in chemotherapy-induced neutropenias, myelodysplastic syndromes, and bone marrow failure syndromes. Griseofulvin toxicity in the cat with severe neutropenia and bone marrow suppression as well as the frequent use of chemotherapeutic agents are instances of potential use of these factors. Granulocyte colony-stimulating factor (G-CSF) and granulocyte macrophage colony-stimulating factor (GM-CSF) have been used in the cat to accelerate recovery from bone marrow suppression (Ogilvie and Obradovich, 1990; Obradovich, 1993). G-CSF accelerates the recovery of neutrophils and marrow progenitors, while GM-CSF is less restricted in its effects on marrow progenitor cells, including eosinophils, monocytic, erythroid and, sometimes, megakaryocytic lines. GM-CSF also induces mature neutrophils and monocytes to increase phagocytosis, superoxide generation, antibody-dependent cellular cytotoxicity, tumoricidal killing, and cytokine production. The author has limited yet promising experience with colony-stimulating factors in the recovery of cases of griseofulvin-induced bone marrow suppression.

## INTERFERON-$\alpha$-2b

Originally described as an antiviral protein, interferon-$\alpha$-2b has been shown to suppress cell proliferation, induce tumoricidal activity in macrophages, enhance phagocytic activity of macrophages, and augment the specific cytotoxicity of lymphocytes for target cells (Cummins et al., 1988).

Interferon-$\alpha$-2b has been reported as a potentially beneficial component of combination (interferon-$\alpha$-2b, interleukin-2, and zidovudine [AZT]) immunotherapy in the treatment of FeLV-FAIDS complex (Zeidner, 1990) and as a solitary treatment in feline leukemia. It has also been used in combination with tumor necrosis factor-$\alpha$ to treat solid tumors, as a single agent in the treatment of T-cell lymphoma as well as in combination with etretinate, and in combination with chlorambucil to treat non-Hodgkin's lymphoma in humans. In a pilot study at The Animal Medical Center, the author has treated cases of eosinophilic granuloma complex and cutaneous T-cell lymphoma with interferon-$\alpha$-2b. The exact treatment protocol and efficacy is currently under investigation. Preliminary results are limited yet promising.

Feline immunomodulators are becoming more important in the management of severe recalcitrant disease that cannot be controlled by more conventional therapy. Exact treatment protocols and efficacy data are currently under investigation by several institutions.

## References and Suggested Reading

Bloom JC, Thiem PA, Halper LK, et al: The effect of longterm treatment with auranofin and gold sodium thiomalate on immune function in the dog. J Rheumatol 15:409, 1988.
*A review of the proposed immunomodulatory effects of the various forms of gold immunotherapy.*
Brunner CJ and Muscoplat CC: Immunomodulatory effects of Levamisole. J Am Vet Med Assoc 176:1159, 1980.
*A review of the pharmacologic and immunomodulatory activity of levamisole.*
Cummins JM, Tompkins MB, Olsen RG, et al: Oral use of human alpha interferon in cats. J Biol Response Mod 7:513, 1988.
*An introductory paper to the use of interferon in the cat, with an excellent reference list.*
Helton-Rhodes KA and Shoulberg N: Chlorambucil: Effective therapeutic options for the treatment of feline immune-mediated dermatoses. Feline Pract 20:5, 1992.
*A review of previous reported treatments for feline immune-mediated disorders and an introduction of chlorambucil as an excellent treatment option.*
Lieschke GJ and Burgess AW: Granulocyte colony-stimulating factor and granulocyte-macrophage colony-stimulating factor. N Engl J Med 327:28, 1992.
*An excellent review article on G-CSF and GM-CSF—first of a two-part series.*
Lieschke GJ and Burgess AW: Granulocyte colony-stimulating factor and granulocyte-macrophage colony-stimulating factor. N Engl J Med 327:99, 1992.
*The second of a two-part series.*
Obradovich JE, Ogilivie GK, Stadler-Morris S, et al: Effect of recombinant canine granulocyte colony-stimulating factor on peripheral neutrophil counts in normal cats. J Vet Intern Med 7:65, 1993.
*An initial source dealing with factor use specifically in the cat.*
Ogilvie GK and Obradovich JE: Use of colony-stimulating factors in human and veterinary medicine. Proc 8th ACVIM Forum, Washington, DC, 1990.
*An introductory source of possible dosages and protocols, with a good reference list after the abstract.*
Yates KM, Raboud J, and Tizard IR: Pilot study of the effect of acemannan in cats infected with feline immunodeficiency virus. Proc 2nd Ann Nat Conference HIV/AIDS Res, Vancouver, BC, 1992.
Zeidner NS, Myles MH, Mathiason-DuBard CK, et al: Alpha interferon (2b) in combination with zidovudine for the treatment of presymptomatic feline leukemia virus-induced immunodeficiency syndrome. Antimicrob Agents Chemother 34:1749, 1990.

# THE USE OF SYNTHETIC RETINOIDS IN VETERINARY MEDICINE

HELEN T. POWER,
*Los Gatos, California*

*and* PETER J. IHRKE
*Davis, California*

The synthetic retinoid drugs are derivatives of vitamin A. Introduced in the early 1980s, they have increased therapeutic benefit but are less toxic than vitamin A. Vitamin A is required for normal growth, vision, reproduction, and maintenance and differentiation of epithelial tissues. Vitamin A has been used as a therapeutic agent, based on the histopathologic similarities between keratinization disorders and vitamin A deficiency. Interest in vitamin A for cancer prevention and therapy has been based on the association between vitamin A deficiency and the subsequent development of certain cancers.

Currently, there are three synthetic retinoid drugs available. Tretinoin (Retin-A, Ortho), a topical medication, is available as an ointment, gel, or liquid. The two parental synthetic retinoids are: 13-*cis*-retinoic acid, or isotretinoin (Accutane, Roche), available in 10-, 20-, and 40-mg capsules; and etretinate (Tegison, Roche), available in 10- or 25-mg capsules. Acitretin (Soriatane, Roche), the active metabolite of etretinate, with similar therapeutic indications, is available in Europe, and is anticipated to be released in the United States in 1995. Isotretinoin and etretinate, although chemically related, have different spectrums of action and are not therapeutically interchangeable. In human medicine, topical tretinoin is used for the treatment of acne, photoaging, and preneoplastic disease secondary to solar damage. The primary indication for isotretinoin is severe cystic acne, and etretinate is used in treatment of psoriasis and disorders of keratinization.

The mechanisms of action of the synthetic retinoids are not entirely understood. Their effects are mediated through multiple nuclear receptors of the steroid-thyroid hormone superfamily resulting in qualitative, quantitative, and temporal changes in transcription of messenger ribonucleic acid (mRNA), thus altering cellular protein products. Clinically, the retinoids promote desquamation of hyperkeratotic skin and a normalization of deregulated proliferative activity. They are also anti-inflammatory due to a direct but poorly understood effect on the immune system and a suppressive effect on chemotaxsis. In essence, the effect of the retinoids is to normalize abnormal epidermal differentiation.

## CLINICAL APPLICATIONS

The synthetic retinoids have been used in veterinary medicine for approximately 10 years. As these drugs were developed for human use, available research information pertained to human diseases and appropriate applicability to veterinary medicine had to be developed. In human medicine, although the synthetic retinoids have provided remarkable therapeutic benefit, most patients have side effects. Veterinary clinical experience indicates that there are far fewer clinical and clinicopathologic side effects in cats and dogs than in humans. The use of the synthetic retinoids in veterinary medicine for the treatment of disorders of keratinization has been established; their evaluation as adjunctive therapies in the management of cutaneous neoplasia and in the treatment of follicular dysplasias is currently being explored. In the following discussion of the clinical use of the synthetic retinoids, recommendations for some diseases are based on demonstrated efficacy in clinical trials, whereas for other rare disorders the recommendations are based on the treatment of only a few individuals (Table 1). Discussion with a veterinary dermatologist prior to utilizing retinoid therapy will provide the practitioner with the most current information.

## Keratinization Disorders of Cocker Spaniels (Primary Seborrhea)

A primary keratinization disorder (primary seborrhea) has been documented in the cocker spaniel. Affected cocker spaniels have either generalized excessive scaling or multifocal lesions of tightly adherent crusts (seborrheic plaques), with concurrent dull greasy hair coat, odor, pruritus, and often secondary bacterial and/or *Malassezia* infection. Conventional therapy includes frequent bathing using keratolytic/keratoplastic shampoos, antibiotics and/or antifungals for secondary infections, and the judicious use of corticosteroids to decrease inflammation and sebaceous gland secretion.

Etretinate (1 mg/kg every 24 hr or divided every 12 hr PO) is an alternative therapy for affected cocker spaniels (Power et al., 1992). Candidates for therapy should have the clinical diagnosis of primary seborrhea confirmed by histopathology. Response to therapy is usually recognized within 60 days and includes a decrease in scale and keratin adherent to hair shafts, a softening and thinning of seborrheic plaques, less odor, and a decrease in pruritus. More severely affected

**Table 1.** *Indications for Synthetic Retinoid Therapy in Dogs*

| Disease | Retinoid | Dose |
| --- | --- | --- |
| Primary seborrhea in cocker spaniels | Etretinate | 1 mg/kg q24h or divided q12h PO |
| Primary keratinization disorders/ichthyosis | Etreinate | 1 mg/kg q24h or divided q12h PO |
| Schnauzer comedo syndrome | Isotretinoin or etretinate | 1 mg/kg q24h PO or divided q12h PO |
| Sebaceous adenitis in poodles | Isotretinoin | 1–2 mg/kg q24h or divided q12h PO |
| Sebaceous adenitis in Akitas or Samoyeds | Etretinate | 1–2 mg/kg q24h or divided q12h PO |
| Granulomatous sebaceous adenitis in viszlas | Isotretinoin | 1–2 mg/kg q24h or divided q12h PO |
| Hair follicle dysplasias | Etretinate | 1 mg/kg q24h or divided q12h PO |
| Actinic keratosis/solar-induced squamous cell carcinoma | Etretinate | 2 mg/kg q24h or divided q12h PO |
| Epitheliotrophic lymphoma Cutaneous lymphoma | Isotretinoin or etretinate | 2 mg/kg q24h or divided q12h PO |
| Multiple infundibular keratinizing acanthomas | Etretinate | 1–2 mg/kg q24h or divided q12h PO |

cocker spaniels may not show maximum benefit for 4 to 6 months. If significant secondary pyoderma or *Malassezia* dermatitis is present, these disorders should be treated specifically. Etretinate therapy has minimal to no beneficial effect on the coexistent hyperplastic or ceruminous otitis present in some cocker spaniels. Continued therapy is required to maintain clinical benefit. However, less frequent treatment such as 5 days out of 7; 1 week on, 1 week off; or 1 month on, 1 month off may be effective. Alternate-day therapy generally has not been successful. Since dogs require lifelong therapy, the clinician and owner should establish a protocol to monitor for possible side effects (see "Side Effects of Systemic Retinoids and their Management," below). Isotretinoin is ineffective in the treatment of primary seborrhea.

### Keratinization Disorders and Similar Syndromes in Other Dog Breeds

Many canine skin diseases are proposed to be disorders of keratinization (based on clinical and histopathologic features); however, the actual pathomechanism has not been proven. Sporadically, apparent primary keratinization disorders occur in individual dogs of any breed. Until the pathogenesis of these disorders is elucidated, it is difficult to predict if the synthetic retinoids would be useful therapies. However, the response or lack thereof in certain syndromes may in itself be informative as to the underlying pathomechanism. The use of synthetic retinoid therapy should be based on histopathologic findings consistent with a keratinization disorder and the systematic elimination of other causes of scaling and crusting (allergy, ectoparasitism, infection, endocrinopathy).

*Schnauzer comedo syndrome* is a localized keratinization disorder, occurring along the dorsum. Lesions are often better palpated than visualized. Both isotretinoin (1 mg/kg every 24 hr PO) and etretinate (1 mg/kg every 24 hr PO) have been used successfully to manage

this syndrome (Power and Ihrke, 1990; Kwochka, 1993).

*Seborrheic dermatitis of springer spaniels, golden retrievers, and Irish setters* has responded to etretinate (1 mg/kg every 24 hr or divided every 12 hr PO) in a manner similar to cocker spaniels (Power and Ihrke, 1990; Kwochka, 1993). However, West Highland white terriers and basset hounds have not responded (Power and Ihrke, 1990). The use of etretinate for seborrhea sicca in Irish setters, German shepherds, dachshunds, and Doberman pinschers has not been reported but could be considered if secondary causes of scaling (allergy, ectoparasitism, infection, endocrinopathy) are ruled out.

*Canine ichthyosis* is a rare, congenital disorder of keratinization that may occur in any breed. It is characterized clinically by severe adherent verrucous scales, and histologically by extreme hyperkeratosis. Both isotretinoin (1 mg/kg every 24 hr or divided every 12 hr) and etretinate (1 mg/kg every 24 hr or divided every 12 hr) have been used successfully in the management of canine ichthyosis (Power and Ihrke, 1990; Kwochka, 1993). Based on experience in human medicine, etretinate is the preferred retinoid for ichthyosis.

### Sebaceous Adenitis

Sebaceous adenitis is a mature-onset disorder of unknown etiology resulting in destruction of the sebaceous glands. Diagnosis is based on histopathology. The most common variant, seen in standard poodles, Akitas, and Samoyeds, is characterized by severe hyperkeratosis, minimal lymphohistiocytic inflammation, but complete destruction of the sebaceous glands. Clinical features include fine but adherent scaling, keratin collaring of hair shafts, and severe hair loss. Treatment-resistant bacterial folliculitis/furunculosis may be present in Akitas. In standard poodles, sebaceous adenitis has been documented to be an autosomal recessive trait, with variable expression. A less common form of sebaceous adenitis occurs primarily in vizslas but can affect other short-coated breeds. Histologically, this form is characterized by a granulomatous inflammation of sebaceous glands. Granulomatous sebaceous adenitis is characterized clinically by focal to coalescing alopecic plaques or nodular lesions, primarily affecting the trunk. Sebaceous adenitis has been recognized as a sporadic occurrence in other breeds and crossbred dogs.

Response to retinoid therapy has been variable in both forms of sebaceous adenitis. Some dogs have improved remarkably, while others have improved only minimally, seemingly without correlation to duration of disease or severity of signs. Approximately 60 to 70% of dogs will respond to retinoid therapy with 60 to 70% improvement. Some dogs respond better to isotretinoin, while others improve more dramatically while receiving etretinate. Long-term treatment is needed to maintain clinical benefit, although less frequent maintenance therapy may be effective (see comments for cocker spaniels).

In standard poodles, the current recommendation is to begin therapy with isotretinoin (1 to 2 mg/kg every 24 hr or divided every 12 hr PO). If response is poor after 90 days, switch to etretinate (1 to 2 mg/kg every 24 hr or divided every 12 hr PO). Akitas or Samoyeds should be treated initially with etretinate. If response is poor, then switch to isotretinoin (Rosychuk R and Rosenkrantz W, 1993, personal communications). Isotretinoin (1 mg/kg every 24 hr PO) is recommended for the treatment of dogs with the granulomatous form of sebaceous adenitis (Stewart, White, and Carpenter, 1991). The Genodermatosis Research Foundation (1635 Grange Hall Road, Dayton, OH 45432), a nonprofit organization focusing on canine genetic skin diseases, can be contacted for the most current recommendations on shampoo and other adjunctive therapies for dogs with sebaceous adenitis.

## Hair Follicle Dysplasias

The newest application of etretinate is in the treatment of hair follicle dysplasia. This poorly understood group of syndromes is characterized by abnormal growth and development of hair follicles, thus noninflammatory alopecia is the primary clinical feature. Definite breed predispositions strongly suggest a heritable basis. Color dilution alopecia, the most common hair follicle dysplasia, occurs in color-dilute Doberman pinschers, Irish setters, dachshunds, chow chows, Great Danes, Italian greyhounds, and whippets. Affected dogs exhibit partial, patchy alopecia; a dry, lusterless hair coat; scaliness; and papules. Etretinate treatment (1 mg/kg every 24 hr or divided every 12 hr PO) in a limited number of cases has resulted in marked hair growth and elimination of excessive scaling and papules (Rosychuk R and Rosenkrantz W, personal communications, 1993). Beneficial changes are seen within 30 days. Information on long-term therapy necessary to maintain clinical benefit is not available. Early results suggests flank alopecia as seen in boxers, bulldogs,

Airedale terriers, and miniature schnauzers will respond to etretinate treatment, as outlined for color dilution alopecia.

## Neoplastic Diseases

The potential interaction between vitamin A and cancer prevention and therapy has been recognized for decades, from both laboratory research and epidemiologic studies documenting increased incidence of cancer in vitamin A–deficient populations. Early research interest leading to the development of synthetic retinoids was actually directed at their potential as cancer therapies. The antitumor activity of the retinoids is based on their effects on cell differentiation and proliferation, and their action to "normalize" tissues, forcing neoplastic cells back into physiologic equilibrium.

To date, the use of the synthetic retinoids in veterinary cancer medicine has been primarily as sole therapies (Table 1). Although related, isotretinoin and etretinate have different spectrums of action; lack of response of a tumor to one of the retinoids does not preclude response to the other. Thus, there may be indications to switch to another retinoid if there has been poor response to the initial drug after 2 to 3 months. Retinoid therapy can be used in conjunction with other anticancer therapies.

## Actinic Keratosis and Solar-Induced Squamous Cell Carcinoma

Solar-induced disease occurs in the poorly haired regions of lightly pigmented dogs such as Dalmatians, American Staffordshire terriers, pit bull terriers, beagles, and whippets. Affected dogs, generally known as "sun bathers," have large areas of erythema, with finely adherent scale, dorsoventrally oriented linear patterns of induration, multiple comedones, and treatment-resistant secondary bacterial furunculosis. This syndrome can be recognized by the combination of these distinctive features and the lack of lesions in pigmented regions. Diagnosis is confirmed by histopathology. Actinic keratoses are generally multiple, plaque-like, alopecic or hyperkeratotic papillated lesions. Solar-induced squamous cell carcinoma can range from single lesions to multiple lesions too numerous to count; and from small (<1 cm) nonhealing erosions to plaque-like, crateriform, nodular, invasive lesions. Etretinate (2 mg/kg every 24 hr or divided every 12 hr PO) is an appropriate therapy for actinic/preneoplastic disease, minimizing the likelihood of further tumor development, and is partially effective in the management of solar-induced squamous cell carcinoma (Marks et al., 1992). Therapy should be continued for a minimum of 6 months. Further solar exposure should be prevented. Obvious squamous cell carcinoma lesions should be treated specifically with surgery, cryosurgery, and/or radiation. Although synthetic retinoids are useful in the management of solar-induced disease, prevention by appropriate education of owners of high-risk breeds in areas of high sun exposure is more appropriate.

### Epitheliotrophic T-Cell Lymphoma (Mycosis Fungoides) and Cutaneous Lymphoma

Epitheliotrophic T-cell lymphoma is a multifocal to generalized cutaneous neoplastic disease of older dogs. Clinical signs are variable; affected dogs may have plaques, nodules, diffuse erythroderma, or exfoliative dermatitis. Mucosal lesions, particularly of the oral cavity, are common and considered a poor prognostic sign. Cutaneous lymphoma is less common, generally has lymph node involvement, and exhibits patchy to generalized erythema with plaques and scaling. In both diseases, diagnosis is based on histopathology. Untreated dogs with either disease have a short life expectancy. Neither disease responds well to conventional chemotherapy. High-dose etretinate (3 to 4 mg/kg every 24 hr or divided every 12 hr) or isotretinoin (3 to 4 mg/kg every 24 hr or divided every 12 hr) are beneficial, palliative therapies, extending life expectancy. Prednisone or other antineoplastic agents can be used concurrently, if deemed appropriate.

### Miscellaneous Benign Cutaneous Neoplasias

A variety of benign, cutaneous neoplasms occasionally develop in multiple sites and, although not life threatening, may severely compromise the owner-pet relationship and overall quality of life. Examples include multiple sebaceous adenomas, epidermal cysts, infundibular keratinizing acanthomas, and inverted papillomas. Affected dogs have responded to isotretinoin (1 to 2 mg/kg every 24 hr or divided every 12 hr) or etretinate (1 to 2 mg/kg every 24 hr or divided every 12 hr). Response is gradual, but benefit should be seen within 45 days.

Multiple infundibular keratinizing acanthomas (keratoacanthoma, intracutaneous cornifying epithelioma) occur in the Norwegian elkhound, keeshond, German shepherd dog, and old English sheepdog. Current therapy is repeated surgical excision. Affected dogs have responded to both isotretinoin (1 to 2 mg/kg every 24 hr or divided every 12 hr) and etretinate (1 to 2 mg/kg every 24 hr or divided every 12 hr) (White et al., 1993). The most predictable result of retinoid therapy is that new tumors do not develop. Existing tumors may in-

volute with reduction of keratinous exudate. Etretinate is the appropriate retinoid for long-term therapy.

## SYNTHETIC RETINOID THERAPY IN CATS

There is less experience with synthetic retinoid therapy in cats, due to fewer apparent indicated uses (Table 2) and early reports of lack of efficacy of isotretinoin for the treatment of solar-induced squamous cell carcinoma. Cats tolerate the synthetic retinoids well; clinical or laboratory side effects have been minimal. However, anorexia occurs more commonly than in dogs and may be because cats receive a relatively higher dose (approximately 2 to 2.5 mg/kg) due to their size and the available forms of isotretinoin or etretinate. If necessary, less frequent treatment (e.g., every other day, every other week) can be used to minimize this problem. Clinical and laboratory monitoring should be as in dogs (see "Side Effects of the Synthetic Retinoids and their Management," below).

### Solar-Induced Squamous Cell Carcinoma

Isotretinoin was evaluated for the treatment of squamous cell carcinoma in cats at 3 mg/kg/day and found to be ineffective (Evans, Madwell, and Stannard, 1985). Since that study, there has been increasing interest in the synthetic retinoids in human medicine as treatment for photo-aged skin and preneoplastic actinic changes. This has renewed veterinary clinicians' interest in the use of these drugs in cats with solar-induced actinic disease. Etretinate (10 mg/cat every 24 hr PO) appears to be beneficial in cats with preneoplastic actinic disease. It can be used as an adjunctive therapy in addition to specific treatment of established tumors and eliminating further sun exposure. Etretinate has been used as a beneficial but palliative therapy in cats with inoperable solar-induced squamous cell carcinoma (Kitchell B, 1990; Rosychuk R, 1993, personal communications).

### Bowen's Disease

One case of this rare, non–solar-induced multicentric form of squamous cell carcinoma in situ has been treated successfully with etretinate (10 mg/cat every 24

**Table 2.** *Indications for Synthetic Retinoid Therapy in Cats*

| Disease | Retinoid | Dose |
| --- | --- | --- |
| Actinic keratosis/solar-induced squamous cell carcinoma | Etretinate | 10 mg/cat q24h PO |
| Bowen's disease | Etretinate | 10 mg/cat q24h PO |
| Epitheliotrophic lymphoma cutaneous lymphoma | Isotretinoin | 10 mg/cat q24h PO |
| Feline acne | Trentinoin | 0.025% topically q24–48h |
| | Isotretinoin | 10 mg/cat q24h PO |

hr PO) (Olivery T, 1993, personal communication). The response was gradual (60 to 90 days) but complete.

### Cutaneous T-Cell Lymphoma (Mycosis Fungoides)

Both isotretinoin (10 mg/cat every 24 hr PO) and etretinate (10 mg/cat every 24 hr PO) have been used with good but only palliative effect in cats with cutaneous T-cell lymphoma. There is a reduction in lesional erythema and scaling, but when re-biopsied, the neoplastic cellular infiltrate was still present. Isotretinoin is the preferred retinoid (Rosenkrantz W, 1993, personal communication).

### Feline Acne

Topical tretinoin (Retin-A, 0.025% cream) has been reported to be effective therapy for feline acne (Bender W, 1993, personal communication). It must be used *extremely sparely* or cats will exhibit a severe, irritant reaction. Isotretinoin (10 mg/cat) may be effective for cats with recalcitrant feline acne (Rosenkrantz W, 1993, personal communication).

## SIDE EFFECTS OF SYNTHETIC RETINOIDS AND THEIR MANAGEMENT

Current recommendations for clinical monitoring of the synthetic retinoids are based on their use in human medicine. However, the incidence of side effects in companion animals is less than in humans. Side effects of the synthetic retinoids are due to their vitamin A activity and are similar to those seen with hypervitaminosis A.

Two types of side effects occur: pharmacologic and toxic. Pharmacologic side effects, although undesirable, are due to the same mechanisms that produce therapeutic benefit. They occur in most human patients, but are predictable. Their intensity is determined by dose, and is reversible on discontinuation. Examples are mucocutaneous dryness and xerosis, chelitis, conjunctivitis, palmoplantar desquamation, epistaxis, and generalized pruritus. These pharmacologic effects are so consistent in humans that they are used to monitor therapy compliance. Side effects reported in dogs include inappetence, vomiting, diarrhea, increased thirst, pruritus, conjunctivitis, chelitis, stiffness, and behavioral changes (hyperactivity). The most common side effect seen in cats is anorexia with subsequent weight loss. As in human patients, these side effects resolve when the dosage is lowered or discontinued. The incidence of clinical side effects in dogs and cats has been low. Most animals exhibit none.

The one side effect that appears to occur with more frequency in dogs than in humans is keratoconjunctivitis sicca (KCS). Keratoconjunctivitis sicca has not been observed in cats. The synthetic retinoids alter tear composition, resulting in increased tear evaporation. Tear function should be monitored by direct measurement (Schrimer tear test strips) before treatment and on a monthly basis for the first 6 months of treatment. Client education of the clinical signs of KCS is important. Many clients can perform the Schrimer tear test at home and report values to the clinician. Dogs that have developed KCS while receiving retinoid therapy have responded to topical cyclosporine. Dogs may regain tear function if retinoid therapy is discontinued.

Toxic side effects may involve organ systems in which no therapeutic benefit is expected. They are rare, possibly idiosyncratic, and the intensity is believed to be a function of cumulative dose. Such effects include increased liver enzymes, increased triglyceride and cholesterol levels, hepatotoxicity, bone pain and hyperostoses, muscle pain, headache, intracranial hypertension, or visual disturbances. In human medicine, there is appropriate concern over cholesterol and triglyceride elevations, especially in patients needing long-term retinoid therapy. Isotretinoin is more likely to cause these chemistry changes and thus is not recommended for long-term use. Most alterations occur early in therapy and are transitory. Thus, in human patients, liver enzymes, cholesterol, and triglyceride values are monitored initially, and continued if abnormalities develop. If no significant changes occur, further monitoring is repeated only as deemed necessary.

To date, dogs receiving synthetic retinoid therapy have had minor to moderate alterations in serum chemistry values (abnormal transaminases, triglycerides, and cholesterol); however, these have not been associated with clinical signs. Pretreatment and 30-day serum chemistry evaluation should be performed, with subsequent testing if indicated. Individual dogs have had marked increases in fasting serum triglycerides while receiving synthetic retinoid therapy. These dogs did not have any associated clinical signs and responded rapidly to dietary fat restriction ("lite" foods). The risk/benefit of synthetic retinoid therapy must be carefully assessed in any patient with a history of pancreatitis, hepatitis, diabetes-mellitus, or any other metabolic disease that could alter or be exacerbated by increases in cholesterol or serum lipids.

The most serious side effect of the synthetic retinoids is teratogenicity. This is particularly a problem with etretinate, as it is stored in body fat and may result in teratogenicity for as long as 2 years after therapy is discontinued. The synthetic retinoids may also interfere with spermatogenesis. The synthetic retinoids *must not* be used in unspayed females or breeding males. Potential for tetratogenicity must be explained to the owners to minimize the possibility of human ingestion. *Pharmacies should be requested to label prescriptions "Not for Human Use" as a further precaution.*

In summary, any healthy, even geriatric dog or cat can be treated with synthetic retinoids with minimal likelihood of side effects (Table 3). However, close clinical monitoring (monthly) including assessment of tear function is essential. Laboratory evaluation after the initial phase of treatment should be repeated as deemed

**Table 3.** *Guidelines for Synthetic Retinoid Therapy*

Diagnosis confirmed by histopathology
Owner compliance with necessary monitoring (monthly)
No concurrent systemic disorders that could be exacerbated by
  synthetic retinoid therapy
Client education regarding gradual benefit and likelihood of long-
  term therapy
Client education regarding potential side effects (KCS,
  teratogenicity, hepatic enzymes, lipid metabolism, skeletal)

necessary. Owners of animals receiving synthetic retinoid therapy should be instructed to discontinue treatment and present their pet for evaluation if they observe any changes that concern them. Most side effects will be of the pharmacologic type, and with the possible exception of KCS, will resolve with discontinuation of therapy. As these side effects are dose dependent, treatment generally can be reinitiated at a lower dose. It is essential that the clinician be aware of the rare but possible toxic side effects. In these cases, therapy should be discontinued.

Most cases involving synthetic retinoid therapy require long-term or lifelong therapy. There are no data in companion animals on the effects of long-term retinoid therapy. In human medicine, some patients have received therapy for 15 years; and only a few have developed any signs of chronic vitamin A toxicity. It is recommended that monitoring be continued with particular attention to observation for liver, skeletal, or cardiovascular problems. Less skeletal and ocular side effects occur with etretinate than with isotretinoin. Thus etretinate is recommended for diseases requiring long-

term therapy. To date, no specific adverse effects due to chronic retinoid therapy have been reported in companion animals, although follow-up has been limited to approximately 4 years.

## References and Suggested Reading

Evans AG, Madwell BR, and Stannard AA: A trial of 13-*cis*-retinoic acid for treatment of squamous cell carcinoma and preneoplastic lesions of the head in cats. Am J Vet Res 46: 2553, 1985.
  *First report of the use of synthetic retinoids in cats.*
Kwochka KW: Retinoids and vitamin A therapy. *In* Griffin CE, Kwochka KW, and MacDonald JM: *Current Veterinary Dermatology*. St. Louis, Mosby Year Book, 1993, p 203.
  *A detailed discussion of the pharmacology and clinical applications of vitamin A and the synthetic retinoids.*
Marks SL, Song MD, Stannard AA, and Power HT: Clinical evaluation of etretinate for the treatment of canine solar-induced squamous cell carcinoma and preneoplastic lesions. J Am Acad Dermatol 27:11, 1992.
  *Discusses the therapeutic benefit in ten dogs with solar-induced disease treated with etretinate.*
Power HT and Ihrke PJ: Synthetic retinoids in veterinary dermatology. *In* DeBoer DJ (ed): *Advances in Clinical Dermatology*. Vet Clin North Am [Small Anim Pract] Philadelphia, WB Saunders Co, 1990, p 1525.
  *A detailed and complete discussion of the synthetic retinoids and their use in veterinary medicine.*
Power HT, Ihrke PJ, Stannard AA, and Backus KQ: The use of etretinate for the treatment of primary keratinization disorders (idiopathic seborrhea) in cocker spaniels, West Highland white terriers, and basset hounds. J Am Vet Med Assoc 201:419, 1992.
  *Report of first clinical trial evaluating etretinate for the treatment of primary keratinization diseases in dogs.*
Stewart LJ, White SD, and Carpenter JL: Isotretinoin in the treatment of sebaceous adenitis in two vizslas. J Am Anim Hosp Assoc 27:65, 1991.
  *Report of the efficacy of isotretinoin for treatment of granulomatous sebaceous adenitis.*
White SD, Rosychuk RAW, Scott KV, et al: Use of isotretinoin and etretinate of the treatment of benign cutaneous neoplasia and cutaneous lymphoma in dogs. J Am Vet Med Assoc 202:387, 1993.
  *The clinical experience of utilizing the synthetic retinoids for a variety of neoplasms of the skin.*

# SHAMPOOS AND MOISTURIZING RINSES IN VETERINARY DERMATOLOGY

KENNETH W. KWOCHKA
*Columbus, Ohio*

The use of topical therapy programs to help control the many dermatoses seen in small animals has become an important part of everyday practice. The broad range of shampoos and moisturizing rinses has provided the practitioner a real chance to individualize topical therapy for each animal.

It is the veterinarian's responsibility to inform clients of the rationale for and expectations of topical therapy. First, topical therapy rarely works when used alone for most dermatoses. However, it is usually very effective

adjunctive therapy to get more rapid resolution of the dermatoses, quicker comfort for the patient, lower doses of concurrent systemic drugs, and better control of recurrence of the problem.

Second, the proper products must be prescribed based on known activity of the active ingredients and vehicle against the dermatoses being treated, time to and duration of effects, and potential side effects.

Third, it must be understood that long-term topical therapy is no substitute for managing the dermatosis by establishing a definitive diagnosis as soon as possible and prescribing specific treatment based on that diagnosis.

Finally, and most important, the owner must be compliant with the recommended topical treatment program. Proper compliance requires excellent client communication including proper instructions for bathing, using handouts, videotapes, or actual demonstrations.

The purpose of this article is to provide an update for practitioners on current recommendations and recent advances for treating four common and important clinical dermatologic problems with shampoos and rinses. More detailed discussions on general principles of topical therapy and additional indications for its use are available in other references (Kwochka, 1993a; Kwochka, 1993b).

## STAPHYLOCOCCAL PYODERMA

One of the most common clinical presentations to the veterinary practitioner is a dog with pyoderma due to *Staphylococcus intermedius*. This cutaneous infection is usually secondary to an underlying dermatosis. Common precipitating diseases include allergies (atopy, food allergy, flea allergy), endocrinopathies (hypothyroidism, hyperadrenocorticism), demodicosis, and primary seborrhea. The key to successful management is to diagnose and treat the primary disease (Kwochka, 1993c). However, antibiotics and topical therapy are needed to control infection until this can be accomplished.

Topical therapy is an important adjunct in the treatment of recurrent superficial and deep pyodermas. It is also helpful when used prophylactically to decrease the severity and frequency of recurrence of the infection. However, rarely can dogs with idiopathic recurrent pyoderma be completely controlled with topical therapy alone without immunostimulants, periodic administration of full dosages of systemic antibiotics, or subminimal dosage maintenance systemic antibiotics (Kwochka, 1993c). In order to achieve this, antibacterial shampoos would be needed at least every 48 hr, which is too labor intensive and impractical for most clients.

The most effective shampoos are those with benzoyl peroxide or chlorhexidine. They should be administered at least one or two times per week, with a 10-min contact time before rinsing. After bathing, a chlorhexidine rinse (ChlorhexiDerm disinfectant, DVM Pharmaceuticals; Nolvasan solution, Fort Dodge) may result in greater residual antibacterial activity. These 2.0% solutions are diluted with water to result in a final concentration of 0.5%. The rinses are especially helpful in dogs with deep pyoderma.

### Benzoyl Peroxide

Benzoyl peroxide shampoos (OxyDex shampoo and Sulf OxyDex shampoo, DVM Pharmaceuticals; Pyoben

shampoo, Allerderm/Virbac) are especially effective because of their excellent antimicrobial activity, follicular flushing action, and residual effects for 48 hr. Benzoyl peroxide was shown in a controlled quantitative study (Kwochka and Kowalski, 1991) to have superior prophylactic activity against *S. intermedius* when compared to chlorhexidine, complexed iodine, and triclosan. The benzoyl peroxide concentration should not exceed 5%, since the higher percentage products are irritating to dog skin. Owners must be warned about the potential for bleaching of fabrics.

Benzoyl peroxide is also keratolytic and degreasing. Whereas these actions will be beneficial in many cases, they can inhibit long-term usage in others because of excessive drying of the skin. In these cases a bath oil (HyLyt°efa bath oil coat conditioner, DVM Pharmaceuticals; Alpha-Sesame Oil dry skin rinse, Veterinary Prescription) or humectant (Humilac dry skin spray and rinse, Allerderm/Virbac) rinse should be used after each bathing to rehydrate the skin and hair coat. A switch to a nondrying chlorhexidine-containing product should also be considered.

### Chlorhexidine

Chlorhexidine is a synthetic biguanide with broad-spectrum antibacterial and antifungal activity, rapid kill, and good residual activity. It is nonirritating, nontoxic, and works in organic debris. Chlorhexidine ranked second after benzoyl peroxide and ahead of complexed iodine and triclosan in prophylactic activity against *S. intermedius* on dog skin (Kwochka and Kowalski, 1991). It is found in shampoo formulations at concentrations of 1% (ChlorhexiDerm shampoo, DVM Pharmaceuticals) and 0.5% (Nolvasan shampoo, Fort Dodge). Although it does not have the follicular flushing activity of benzoyl peroxide, it has the advantage of being in emollient formulations for long-term use on dry skin and coat.

### Lauricidin

Lauricidin glyceryl monolaurate (2%) is a fatty acid monoester potentiated by 1.5% lactic acid in a new shampoo (Lauricare Medicated Pet Shampoo, 3M). Lauricidin is a broad-spectrum antimicrobial agent in a moisturizing vehicle that has demonstrated excellent *in vitro* activity against gram-positive bacteria, gram-negative bacteria, and *Malassezia pachydermatis*. Studies are currently being conducted at several clinical centers to determine *in vivo* activity against these organisms. This product is scheduled to be marketed in 1995.

## MALASSEZIA DERMATITIS

*Malassezia pachydermatis* is being increasingly recognized as a cause of skin infections secondary to underlying dermatoses in dogs (Mason, 1993). It seems especially prevalent in cases with severe greasy scale, inflammation, and pruritus associated with allergies, superficial pyoderma, and primary seborrhea. The infection must be controlled with appropriate systemic and topical antifungal agents to give the patient relief while a definitive diagnosis of the underlying dermatosis is being pursued.

The best response is seen with systemic ketoconazole (Nizoral, Janssen) at 5 to 10 mg/kg every 12 hr PO or itraconazole (Sporanox, Janssen) at 5 mg/kg every 24 hr PO, for 30 days. The degree of clinical improvement over this time period is the best way to determine how many of the signs are due to the infection versus the primary underlying disease. Since the yeast inhabits only the most superficial layers of the epidermis, it is curious that systemic therapy is so far superior to topical therapy for this condition. Systemic ketoconazole may work by additional mechanisms to improve the skin condition than simply killing the yeast. It may favorably modulate epidermal cell physiology, cutaneous inflammation, and hormonal activity in the skin and hair follicles.

Topical therapy is indicated for initial adjunctive therapy with the systemic ketoconazole and in recurrent cases when a cause for the yeast infection cannot be found. As with recurrent pyoderma, topical therapy should be used at least once or twice per week.

The three most important considerations in topical therapy of *Malassezia* dermatitis are to use products with degreasing activity, specific antifungal activity, and residual activity. Unfortunately, there is not a single product that meets all of these criteria. Combinations of degreasing agents followed by specific antifungal agents are most often employed.

## Degreasing Agents

Degreasing agents are helpful to remove the oily scales and exudate commonly seen associated with *M. pachydermatis* infections. The greasy exudate may have a permissive effect on the growth of the yeast and impede antifungal agents from adequate penetration to kill the organisms. Good degreasing agents include benzoyl peroxide shampoos (OxyDex shampoo, Pyoben shampoo) a sulfur with benzoyl peroxide shampoo (Sulf OxyDex shampoo), and 1% selenium sulfide (Selsun Blue dandruff shampoo, Ross).

## Antifungal Agents

### KETOCONAZOLE

One of the most effective topical therapy combinations for *Malassezia* dermatitis to date has been with a once- or twice-weekly degreasing shampoo followed by a 2% ketoconazole shampoo (Nizoral shampoo, Janssen). The ketoconazole shampoo should be left in contact with the skin for 10 to 15 min before rinsing. Ke-

toconazole shampoo has not been associated with topical or systemic side effects in dogs. This shampoo is expensive, which may limit its use on a continual basis in some patients.

### MICONAZOLE

Miconazole is another imidazole with good activity against *M. pachydermatis* when used topically. Miconazole lotion (Conofite lotion, Pitman-Moore) or cream (Conofite cream, Pitman-Moore) is valuable for locally severe lesions such as pododermatitis, cheilitis, and otitis externa.

Recently, a 2% miconazole and 0.5% chlorhexidine shampoo (Dermazole shampoo, Allerderm/Virbac) has been marketed in the United States. An *in vitro* evaluation (product advertisement) claimed a 99.6% and 99.9% kill rate against *M. pachydermatis* after 5 and 15 min, respectively. However, no clinical studies have been reported using this product for *Malassezia* dermatitis or other fungal infections. I have found this shampoo to be less effective then either 2% ketoconazole or 1 to 2.5% selenium sulfide shampoos. Cost is comparable to that of ketoconazole shampoo.

### SELENIUM SULFIDE

At the 1% concentration, selenium sulfide is effective in *Malassezia* dermatitis because of its degreasing and antifungal activity. At 2.5% (Selsun Rx 2.5% selenium sulfide lotion, Ross), it has superior degreasing and antifungal activity but may cause cutaneous irritation in some patients, especially those with inflamed skin.

### CHLORHEXIDINE

Shampoos containing 0.5% and 1.0% chlorhexidine have been used for *Malassezia* dermatitis. They have no demonstrated *in vitro* or *in vivo* efficacy at these low concentrations; 4% chlorhexidine surgical scrubs are effective alternatives.

### LAURICIDIN

As described above, this novel broad-spectrum antimicrobial agent has excellent *in vitro* activity against *M. pachydermatis* and is currently being evaluated in a shampoo formulation (Lauricare Medicated Pet Shampoo) in clinical trials.

## Agents With Residual Activity

Residual activity with shampoos is predictably short, since they are rinsed off after a 10- to 15-min contact time. The most effective topical formulations would be those with good antifungal activity in a more residual vehicle such as aqueous rinses applied to the total body and left on to dry.

### ENILCONAZOLE

Enilconazole (Imaverol, Janssen) appears to be the most effective topical rinse formulation for *Malassezia* dermatitis. Bathing with a 1% selenium sulfide shampoo to remove scale and sebum followed by application of an enilconazole rinse has been advocated as an effective approach to control the infection (Mason, 1993). Enilconazole is not yet available in the United States.

### ACETIC ACID

Acetic acid is effective against *M. pachydermatis* and is inexpensive. A useful topical rinse formulation with residual activity is made by mixing equal parts of white vinegar and water and applying to the body once or twice weekly after a degreasing shampoo (Selsun Blue dandruff shampoo, Ross).

### CHLORHEXIDINE

The use of topical chlorhexidine rinses diluted with water for a final concentration of 0.5% has been advocated for residual antifungal activity. This low concentration has no demonstrated activity against *M. pachydermatis*.

## ALLERGIC AND IDIOPATHIC PRURITUS

Although by no means appropriate as sole therapy in pruritic skin diseases, topical therapy may be helpful in symptomatic relief of pruritus. The requirements for high levels of systemic steroids and other anti-inflammatory agents will surely be decreased if owners are willing to expend the time and effort needed for administration of topical therapy.

The initial approach in dogs with allergic skin disease, especially atopy, is to treat with systemic antihistamines and fatty acids, try to avoid the offending allergens, and use topical hypoallergenic or antipruritic shampoos followed by a moisturizing or antipruritic rinse once or twice per week. The expectation is that 30 to 40% of atopic dogs can be managed without systemic steroids by using this approach. I find that this number is essentially cut in half if topical therapy is not part of the program. Additionally, when steroids are needed, lower doses can be utilized if a good topical therapy program is in place.

### Hypoallergenic Shampoos

Bathing contributes to relief of pruritus by removing organic and inorganic debris from the skin surface (including surface allergens and bacteria), by cooling the skin surface, and by hydrating the stratum corneum. The hypoallergenic, cleansing-moisturizing shampoos (HyLyt*efa hypoallergenic moisturizing shampoo, DVM Pharmaceuticals; Allergroom hypoallergenic emollient shampoo, Allerderm/Virbac) are excellent for this purpose, since they have less potential to irritate already inflamed pruritic skin. Mild antibacterial shampoos containing chlorhexidine (ChlorhexiDerm shampoo, Nolvasan shampoo) may be preferred when a secondary pyoderma is present.

### Antipruritic Shampoos

Specific antipruritic agents have been incorporated into hypoallergenic shampoos. These agents include colloidal oatmeal (Epi-Soothe shampoo, Allerderm/Virbac), colloidal oatmeal with the antihistamine diphenhydramine hydrochloride (Histacalm shampoo, Allerderm/Virbac), and colloidal oatmeal with the anesthetic agent pramoxine hydrochloride (Relief shampoo, DVM Pharmaceuticals). Colloidal oatmeal has also been added to flea-control shampoos with synergized pyrethrins (Ecto-Soothe shampoo, Allerderm/Virbac) and with synergized pyrethrins and permethrin (SynerKyl shampoo, DVM Pharmaceuticals).

Antipruritic shampoos do offer some enhanced activity over simple hypoallergenic moisturizing shampoos. However, this activity is fairly minimal because the oatmeal concentration is very low. Additionally, if an antipruritic shampoo is used alone without other topical treatment, the residual activity is minimal because it is rinsed off. Therefore, the recommendation is to always follow an antipruritic shampoo with an antipruritic rinse.

### Antipruritic Rinses

#### CREAM RINSES

Two antipruritic cream rinses have been marketed. One contains 20% colloidal oatmeal (Epi-Soothe cream rinse, Allerderm/Virbac) and another has 20% colloidal oatmeal with 1% pramoxine hydrochloride (Relief creme rinse, DVM Pharmaceuticals). I have found the latter product to be more effective, probably because of the addition of pramoxine hydrochloride. Pramoxine hydrochloride is a topical anesthetic agent effective for symptomatic relief of pruritus. Unlike other topical anesthetics, there is an extremely low incidence of dermal irritation or sensitization.

Some clinicians have realized better residual activity with cream rinses by only lightly rinsing off the formulations so that some remains to dry in contact with the skin surface. This only works in short-coated dogs, as those with long coats become greasy. These cream rinses have also been used as "lotions" applied to nonhaired or sparsely haired portions of the body without rinsing. An actual lotion vehicle (Relief Lotion, DVM Pharmaceuticals) has recently been marketed for this purpose.

#### AQUEOUS RINSES

Colloidal oatmeal (Epi-Soothe bath treatment, Allerderm/Virbac; Aveeno colloidal oatmeal, Rydelle) cool water rinses or soaks also provide short-term relief of pruritus. These are very effective topical therapeutics for antipruritic activity because they are applied without rinsing and are 100% colloidal oatmeal. Oilated oatmeal with 43% colloidal oatmeal and mineral oil (Aveeno oilated oatmeal, Rydelle) is available for animals with very dry skin and hair coat. These products may be used as pour-on rinses or total body soaking solutions in a tub. A mixture of 2 tablespoons of powder per gallon of water is usually sufficient as a rinse. For soaking, a packet of the powder should be placed in cheesecloth or nylon stockings which is then placed in the soaking water. Soaks should last for at least 10 to 15 min.

Moisturizing bath oil (HyLyt°efa bath oil coat conditioner, Alpha-Sesame Oil dry skin rinse) or humectant (Humilac dry skin spray and rinse) rinses and sprays can also help control pruritus by rehydrating dry skin by increasing the water content of the stratum corneum. These agents are especially effective when very dry skin and hair coat are contributing to the overall pruritus. Additionally, these may help restore stratum corneum barrier function and thus improve control of the development of bacterial and yeast infections in the skin of pruritic patients.

## DRY AND GREASY SCALING DERMATOSES

Most dogs presented to a practitioner for cutaneous scale formation have secondary scaling not associated with a primary keratinization defect (Kwochka, 1993d). The dermatoses that may result in secondary scaling include ectoparasitism, pyoderma, dermatophytosis, endocrinopathies, autoimmune dermatoses, allergic dermatoses, and environmental dermatoses. Topical therapy is important in these diseases to help control the scaling and keep the animal comfortable until the primary disease is diagnosed and treated.

Symptomatic topical therapy, especially with antiscaling agents in shampoo formulations, is the major form of therapy used to manage most of the primary keratinization defects (Kwochka, 1993a).

In a dog with a scaling dermatosis and long hair coat, it may be beneficial to clip the hair and keep it fairly short during treatment. If there is a large amount of scale formation, bathing with a detergent shampoo (D-BASIC shampoo, DVM Pharmaceuticals) prior to the use of an antiscaling shampoo will allow use of less of the medicated formulation, better contact with the skin surface, and thus enhanced efficacy.

Bathing is instituted two to three times per week until good control of the scale and odor is achieved and then as infrequently as needed for maintenance. A dog with mild dry scale and no odor may be controlled after only 2 or 3 weeks and then maintained with a bath every month. A dog with severe greasy scale and odor may take several weeks before the owners are satisfied with the response and then still need baths every 7 to 10 days for control. The maintenance program may

vary depending on the season, since extremes of heat and humidity may affect the amount of dryness or greasiness, scaling, and secondary bacterial infection.

Antiscaling compounds are keratolytic or keratoplastic or both. A keratolytic agent causes cellular damage of corneocytes, resulting in ballooning of the cells and subsequent cell shedding. Thus, the stratum corneum is softened and removed, resulting in better control of scale formation. A keratoplastic agent results in "normalization" of epidermal cell kinetics and keratinization, usually by cytostatic effects on the basal cell layer. Common antiscaling agents include sulfur, salicylic acid, benzoyl peroxide, tar, and selenium sulfide. Complete details on each of these active ingredients are found in other references (Kwochka, 1993a; Kwochka, 1993b).

### Dry Scaling Dermatoses

Dermatoses generally characterized by dry scale include primary idiopathic seborrhea in certain breeds (e.g., Irish setters, Doberman pinschers), sebaceous adenitis, ichthyosis, ear margin dermatosis, zinc-responsive dermatosis, parasitism (cheyletiellosis, canine scabies, notoedric mange, and endoparasites), pyoderma (usually dry scaling associated with older resolving lesions), allergies, environmental factors (dry heat), and autoimmune dermatoses (pemphigus foliaceus). Patients treated with topical flea-control products, tar, and benzoyl peroxide may also develop severe dry scale formation.

Mild dry scaling may simply respond to a moisturizing, hypoallergenic shampoo (HyLyt°efa hypoallergenic moisturizing shampoo, Allergroom hypoallergenic emollient shampoo). If the dry scaling is more severe and does not respond to a moisturizing shampoo, then a sulfur and salicylic acid combination (Sebolux shampoo, Allerderm/Virbac; SebaLyt antiseborrheic shampoo, DVM Pharmaceuticals; Sebbafon dermatologic shampoo, Upjohn) should next be considered. Sulfur and salicylic acid have synergistic keratolytic activity when formulated in equal concentrations. The combination is ideal for dry scaling conditions because the agents do not have degreasing activity. Bath oil (Alpha-Sesame Oil dry skin rinse), humectant (Humilac dry skin spray and rinse), or oil/humectant combination (HyLyt°efa bath oil coat conditioner) rinses should be applied after the skin has been hydrated by bathing. These moisturizers may also be effectively applied between shampoos using a plant mister bottle.

If the dry scaling is severe and still nonresponsive, then the low-potency tar products (Clear Tar shampoo, Veterinary Prescription; NuSal-T shampoo, DVM Pharmaceuticals; T-Lux shampoo, Allerderm/Virbac) may be necessary. However, since tars are degreasing, further drying may result even though scale formation from the epidermis is being better controlled. After-bath moisturizing rinses are mandatory in these dogs. Additionally, the tar shampoo may need to be alternated with a cleansing and moisturizing shampoo to prevent excess drying.

## Greasy Scaling Dermatoses

Common greasy scaling conditions include primary seborrhea in spaniels, terriers, basset hounds, and German shepherd dogs; epidermal dysplasia of West Highland white terriers, vitamin A–responsive dermatosis, canine acne, greasy ear margin dermatosis, and some pyodermas.

For cases of oily or greasy scaling, benzoyl peroxide (OxyDex shampoo, Pyoben shampoo), benzoyl peroxide with sulfur (Sulf OxyDex shampoo), tars (Clear Tar shampoo; NuSal-T shampoo; T-Lux shampoo; LyTar shampoo, DVM Pharmaceuticals; Allerseb-T shampoo, Allerderm/Virbac), and selenium sulfide (Selsun Blue dandruff shampoo) are useful alone or alternating in combination. High concentrations of these products may be irritating and very drying. Thus, after the severe problem is controlled, switching to the most innocuous agent to control the condition is indicated. For greasy scale complicated by pyoderma, alternating a tar and a benzoyl peroxide product is useful. An emollient antibacterial shampoo with 0.5% (Nolvasan shampoo) or 1.0% (ChlorhexiDerm shampoo) chlorhexidine would be preferred to benzoyl peroxide in the case of dry scaling with pyoderma.

## References and Suggested Reading

Kwochka KW: Symptomatic topical therapy of scaling disorders. *In* Griffin CE, Kwochka KW, and MacDonald JM (eds): *Current Veterinary Dermatology: The Science and Art of Therapy.* St. Louis, Mosby Year Book, 1993a, p 191.
*A review of the specific active ingredients and commercial shampoos and rinses used for primary and secondary scaling disorders of dogs.*
Kwochka KW: Topical therapeutics. *In* Locke PH, Harvey RG, and Mason IS (eds): *Manual of Small Animal Dermatology.* Gloucestershire, United Kingdom, British Small Animal Veterinary Association, 1993b, p 220.
*A review of general principles of topical therapy and all of the specific indications for topical therapy in veterinary dermatology.*
Kwochka KW: Recurrent pyoderma. *In* Griffin CE, Kwochka KW, and MacDonald JM (eds): *Current Veterinary Dermatology: The Science and Art of Therapy.* St. Louis, Mosby Year Book, 1993c, p 3.
*A review of the clinical signs, diagnostic evaluation, and treatment of dogs with chronic recurrent superficial and deep pyoderma.*
Kwochka KW: Overview of normal keratinization and cutaneous scaling disorders of dogs. *In* Griffin CE, Kwochka KW, and MacDonald JM (eds): *Current Veterinary Dermatology: The Science and Art of Therapy.* St. Louis, Mosby Year Book, 1993d, p 167.
*An introduction to primary and secondary scaling disorders of dogs, concentrating on the diagnostic approach to these cases.*
Kwochka KW and Kowalski JJ: Prophylactic efficacy of four antibacterial shampoos against *Staphylococcus intermedius* in dogs. Am J Vet Res 52: 115, 1991.
*A comparison of the prophylactic activity of four commercial veterinary antibacterial shampoos against* Staphylococcus intermedius *in dogs using a quantitative* in vivo *technique.*
Mason KV: Cutaneous *Malassezia. In* Griffin CE, Kwochka KW, and MacDonald JM (eds): *Current Veterinary Dermatology: The Science and Art of Therapy.* St. Louis, Mosby Year Book, 1993, p 44.
*A review of the pathogenesis, clinical signs, diagnostic evaluation, and treatment of* Malassezia *dermatitis in dogs and cats.*

# THE EFFECT OF POTENTIATED SULFONAMIDES ON CANINE THYROID FUNCTION

JAN A. HALL
*Fort Collins, Colorado*

*and* KAREN L. CAMPBELL
*Urbana, Illinois*

Hypothyroidism is the most commonly diagnosed endocrine disorder in dogs. Diagnosis is usually based on evaluation of history, physical examination, and thyroid hormone levels. Thyroid hormone is needed for normal cellular metabolic functions throughout the body. A deficiency in circulating thyroid hormone affects the metabolic function of all organ systems. As a result, the clinical signs of hypothyroidism are often vague and may resemble many other disorders, making diagnosis very difficult.

The measurement of basal tetraiodothyronine ($T_4$) and triiodothyronine ($T_3$) levels are used widely by veterinary practitioners as an indicator of thyroid function. Low levels of basal $T_4$ and $T_3$ are found in animals with primary hypothyroidism (thyroid gland destruction or dysfunction), secondary hypothyroidism (deficiency of thyroid-stimulating hormone [TSH]), tertiary hypothyroidism (deficiency of thyrotropin-releasing hormone [TRH]), "compensatory hypothyroidism" (euthyroid-sick syndrome), and as a result of altered binding of thyroid hormones to serum proteins. In addition, many drugs and diagnostic agents have been shown to alter basal thyroid hormone concentrations in humans. The thyrotropin (TSH) stimulation test is regarded as being the most accurate method of diagnosing primary hypothyroidism.

Because of the wide range of signs associated with impaired thyroid hormone secretion, hypothyroidism is included in the differential diagnosis of almost all dogs with skin disease, lethargy, and reproductive disorders. Many dogs with hypothyroidism present with dermatologic abnormalities and many develop a secondary staphylococcal pyoderma due to the underlying immunosuppression associated with the hypothyroidism.

Potentiated sulfonamides are commonly used antimicrobial drugs in veterinary medicine. There are two veterinary products approved for use in the dog, trimethoprim-sulfadiazine (Tribrissen, Coopers) and ormetoprim-sulfamethoxine (Primor, Roche). A human generic formulation, trimethoprim-sulfamethoxazole (Bactrim, Roche; Septra, Coopers; many generics), is also extensively used in dogs, as it is relatively inexpensive.

Potentiated sulfonamides are often used as a first-line treatment for canine staphylococcal pyoderma. Substantial clinical use has shown that high doses and long treatment periods may be required to control many infections. Most dermatologists recommend using a dose of 30 mg/kg of trimethoprim-sulfadiazine or trimethoprim-sulfamethoxazole twice daily in the treatment of staphylococcal pyoderma and advise that the medication be continued for a minimum of 4 to 6 weeks or a week after the pyoderma clears. This is twice the veterinary manufacturer's dose rate of 15 mg/kg, and two to three times longer than the manufacturer's recommended maximum length of therapy (14 days).

Most veterinarians are aware of the wide range of potential toxic reactions associated with sulfonamide use in the dog including bone marrow suppression, polyarthritis, keratoconjunctivitis sicca, hepatopathy, and drug eruption. However, few veterinarians are aware that long-term use of sulfonamides may also lead to hypothyroidism and interfere with thyroid diagnostic testing.

The potential for thyroid-related side effects from sulfonamides is not widely publicized. Of the two potentiated sulfonamides approved for use in dogs, trimethoprim-sulfadiazine (Tribrissen) and ormetoprim-sulfamethoxine, package inserts do not include hypothyroidism in the list of reported side effects. The package insert for Primor states: "following oral administration of Primor to dogs at 27.5 mg/kg/day for eight weeks, no changes were noted . . . except for elevated serum cholesterol, increased thyroid and liver weights, enlarged basophilic cells in the pituitary and mild follicular hyperplasia. These changes are known to be associated with prolonged administration of sulfonamides to dogs and have been shown to be reversible." The Freedom of Information Act summary for Primor states that the principal treatment-related effect of extended sulfonamide use is hypothyroidism. Under miscellaneous reactions, the package insert for a trade name trimethoprim-sulfamethoxazole combination (Bactrim) states: "Goiter production, diuresis and hypoglycemia have occurred rarely in (human) patients receiving sulfonamides. . . . Rats appear to be especially susceptible to the goitrogenic effects of sulfonamides, and long term administration has produced thyroid malignancies in the species."

## CLINICAL STUDIES

In a recently published study, 20 dogs with recurrent pyoderma and normal thyroid function were treated with a generic potentiated sulfonamide, trimethoprim-sulfamethoxazole at 30 mg/kg twice daily for 6 weeks. $T_3$ and $T_4$ concentrations were measured before and after the treatment period. $T_4$ levels were dramatically depressed in 16 of the 20 dogs at the end of the treatment period. Thyrotropin response tests after therapy were significantly suppressed. In two of these three dogs, response to TSH remained subnormal and within the hypothyroid range for 8 to 12 weeks following therapy.

Another study looked at thyroid function in six healthy beagle dogs treated with trimethoprim-sulfadiazine (Tribrissen) at the manufacturer's recommended dose of 15 mg/kg once daily for 4 weeks. TSH response tests were performed before and after 4 weeks of treatment, and then 3 weeks after the treatment were stopped. No significant differences in thyroid function were noted over the course of the study period. The results of this study strongly suggest that the toxic effects of sulfonamides depend very much on dose and duration of treatment.

## MECHANISM OF ACTION

A variety of compounds are known to inhibit thyroid hormone synthesis and secretion without having major effects on other organ systems. Administration of these compounds leads to decreased levels of circulating thyroid hormones, resulting in increased secretion of TSH and eventual thyroid enlargement or goiter. When inhibition of thyroid hormone synthesis is incomplete, the secretion of thyroid hormones may be sufficient to maintain eumetabolism. When the inhibition is more severe, there will be inadequate secretion of $T_4$ and $T_3$ and the goiter is accompanied by clinical hypothyroidism.

Sulfonamides are aniline derivatives with a parasubstituted aminobenzene ring. The *para*-amino group is believed to be the important structure in conferring antithyroid activity. If the amino group is replaced by a methyl group, the antithyroid activity is markedly reduced. Sulfonamides are believed to inhibit peroxidase activity in the thyroid gland, interfering with thyroglobulin iodination and coupling of the iodotyrosines. This is the same mechanism used to treat feline hyperthyroidism. However, sulfonamides have markedly less activity than propylthiouracil and methimazole.

The antithyroid effect of sulfonamides appears to be vary among species. Rats appear to be especially susceptible to the goitrogenic effects of sulfonamides, and long-term administration has led to thyroid neoplasia. In human studies, although the sulfonamides have antithyroid activity, only mild effects have been reported. At normal suggested doses and duration, they do not appear to cause significant thyroid suppression. The potential goitrogenic effects of sulfonamides have not been adequately evaluated in dogs.

## DIAGNOSIS

Radionuclide thyroid imaging is a sensitive, noninvasive, and clinically useful technique for evaluating thyroid function and for differentiating between hypothyroidism and drug-induced thyroid suppression. A 1:1 ratio normally exists between the uptake in the parotid salivary gland and the uptake in the normal thyroid gland. Dogs with hypothyroidism typically have low or nondetectable pertechnetate accumulation. In contrast, dogs with drug-induced lowering of basal serum thyroid hormone concentrations have normal accumulation concentrations. Two dogs scintigraphically imaged after trimethoprim-sulfamethoxazole treatment at 30 mg/kg for 6 weeks had increased uptake of $^{99m}TcO^{4-}$, indicating increased physiologic iodide trapping. Unfortunately, this technique is limited to veterinary schools and hospitals because of the expensive equipment required.

Because sulfonamides can suppress thyroid function, potentiated sulfonamide use is inappropriate in any dermatologic case when hypothyroidism is considered a possible primary diagnosis. Potentiated sulfonamides may suppress baseline thyroid hormone levels and the effect of TSH stimulation, leading to misinterpretation of results. Potentiated sulfonamides should not be used until after thyroid function has been evaluated. Although it is unclear how long thyroid suppression will last, the limited studies that have been performed suggest that it may take 8 to 12 weeks for thyroid function to return to normal following discontinuation of sulfonamide therapy.

## SUMMARY

Use of potentiated sulfonamides may be responsible for a significant amount of iatrogenic hypothyroidism in the dog, resulting in the misdiagnosis of inadequate thyroid function in animals treated with them. Veterinarians prescribing potentiated sulfonamides need to be aware of the potential adverse effects of these antimicrobials on thyroid function.

### References and Suggested Reading

Ferguson DC: The effect of non-thyroidal factors on thyroid function in dogs. Compend Cont Educ Pract Vet 10:1365, 1988.
*Review of the effects of nonthyroidal illness and drug therapy on thyroid function in the dog.*
Green WL: Antithyroid compounds. *In* Ingbar SH and Braverman LE (eds): *Werner's The Thyroid.* Philadelphia, JB Lippincott Co, 1986, pp 339–411.
*Review of the effects of extrinsic and intrinsic factors, including antithyroid drugs and nonthyroid illness on normal thyroid function in humans and laboratory animals.*
Hall IA, Campbell KL, Chambers MD, et al: Effect of trimethoprim-sulfamethoxazole on thyroid function in dogs with recurrent pyoderma. J Am Vet Med Assoc 202:1959, 1993.
*Twenty dogs with recurrent pyoderma and normal thyroid function were treated with a generic potentiated sulfonamide, trimethoprim-sulfamethoxazole at 30 mg/kg twice daily for 6 weeks. Significant suppression of $T_4$ was noted at the end of the study.*
Panciera DL and Post K: Effect of administration of sulfadiazine and trimethoprim in combination on thyroid function in dogs. Can J Vet Res 56: 349, 1992.
*Six healthy dogs were treated with trimethoprim-sulfadiazine at the manufacturer's recommended dose of 15 mg/kg once daily for 4 weeks. No significant differences in thyroid function were noted.*

# EPIDERMAL DYSPLASTIC DISORDERS OF DOGS AND CATS

WILLIAM H. MILLER, Jr.
*Ithaca, New York*

Under normal conditions, epidermal cell replication and maturation progresses in an orderly fashion such that four cell layers with characteristic cell morphology are easily recognized. In dysplastic disorders, the orderly progression is lost. Cell layers become indistinct, cells mature in a haphazard fashion, and cellular atypia is commonplace. This dysregulated growth could lead to neoplastic transformation and the dysplastic disorders should be considered potentially preneoplastic conditions.

## ACTINIC KERATOSES

Actinic keratoses are uncommon to rare preneoplastic skin lesions of middle-aged to old dogs or cats. They are caused by prolonged exposure to ultraviolet light. For an actinic keratosis to develop, the involved area must be lightly pigmented and sparsely haired. Previously damaged skin (e.g., scars) may be more susceptible to the development of these lesions.

Actinic keratoses can occur in any breed of dog, but

Dalmatians, whippets, Staffordshire terriers, bull terriers, white boxers, beagles, and German shorthaired pointers have an increased risk (Rosenkrantz, 1993). The location of the lesions depends on how the dog sunbathes. Dogs who stay in full sternal recumbency develop lesions on the face and ears. Since most dogs favor a lateral recumbency, the flanks, ventrolateral abdomen, and lateral or medial hock area are commonly involved. Dogs who sleep on their back or who are caged on wire above white concrete can have their entire ventrum involved. Early solar damage is heralded by erythema and scaling. With time, the areas thicken and develop a rough but glistening surface. Papules, plaques, comedones, and nodules also may be seen. In very chronic cases, the lesions ulcerate and this usually is due to progression to an invasive squamous cell carcinoma.

Lesions in the cat are almost exclusively seen on the head, especially on the ears, eyelids, and planum nasale. As in the dog, erythema and scaling is the first sign of solar sensitivity. With time, the area thickens and is lightly crusted. Ulceration and heavy crusting unless induced by self-trauma signifies progression to an invasive squamous cell carcinoma.

The diagnosis of a photodermatitis usually is straightforward. When the signs are recognized and treated early, progression to actinic keratoses or squamous cell carcinoma can be prevented. Treatment involves intense photoprotection (Rosenkrantz, 1993). If such measures are not used or are ineffective, actinic keratoses will develop. If strict photoisolation is instituted at this point, new lesions should not develop but existing ones will persist.

In both dogs and cats, surgical removal of actinic keratoses is the treatment of choice. When this is impossible, treatment options are greatly reduced. For dogs, the topical application of 5-fluorouracil can be beneficial (Gross and Brimacomb, 1986). This drug is neurotoxic to cats.

One veterinary oncologist reports excellent results in cats with $^{90}$Sr plesiotherapy (Turrell JM, 1992, personal communication). Plesiotherapy is basically very superficial radiation therapy but utilizes a relatively inexpensive probe, does not require multiple fractionated treatments, causes little radiation damage, and costs far less than conventional radiotherapy. Approximately 150 Gy are delivered to each lesion. Since the strontium probe used releases $\beta$ rays which only penetrate 2 to 4 mm, multiple separate lesions can be treated at one time with little concern for the development of radiation sickness. Because of the limited penetration, lesions should be treated early. Supposedly, one treatment can eliminate the dysplastic cells and return the skin to near normal. More details on this treatment are eagerly awaited.

## EPIDERMAL DYSPLASIA OF WEST HIGHLAND WHITE TERRIERS

Epidermal dysplasia of West Highland white terriers (EDW) is a genetically determined disorder of keratinization complicated by a secondary *Malassezia* dermatitis (Scott and Miller, 1989). The epidermal dysplasia itself causes mild to moderate greasiness of the skin and hair, while the secondary yeast dermatitis accelerates the seborrheic changes and causes moderate to severe pruritus. Unlike other dogs where the *Malassezia* dermatitis usually is a one-time event (Mason, 1992), dogs with EDW develop recurrent or near constant yeast infections.

Most dogs with EDW present within the first year of their life for a generalized pruritic disorder. Either sex can be affected and the severity of the pruritus and visible skin lesions depends on the timing of the first examination. Early on, the coat tends to be mildly to moderately greasy and needs constant brushing to keep the hairs from clumping together. Some greasy scale may be visible on the skin surface. Pruritus is mild to moderate and tends to involve the face, ears, feet, and intertriginous areas. At this point, the pruritus may lessen or stop with the administration of anti-inflammatory dosages of prednisolone (1.1 mg/kg/day). With advancing time, despite the administration of prednisolone, the pruritus increases in intensity and distribution. Advanced cases have widespread hair loss, erythema and lichenification of the skin, and large seborrheic plaques where the greasy scale adheres to the skin surface. In chronic cases, the traumatized areas, intertriginous areas, and interdigital spaces may be hyperpigmented.

As a breed, the West Highland white terrier is prone to allergy, primary seborrhea, ichthyosis, generalized demodicosis, and EDW, and all these disorders must be included in the differential diagnosis. Demodicosis is eliminated by skin scrapings, while ichthyosis and primary seborrhea usually can be dismissed by the timing at onset and nature of the lesions. Allergy, especially food hypersensitivity, and sarcoptic mange must be considered and are eliminated by the feeding of a home-cooked hypoallergenic diet for 3 to 10 weeks and appropriate scabicidal treatments. Before allergy tests for atopy are performed, skin biopsies should be taken. In some dogs, numerous *Malassezia* yeast can be seen in the cytologic preparation of the seborrheic debris. Since the presence or absence of yeast on cytology does not confirm or negate, respectively, the diagnosis of EDW, the biopsy is necessary. Multiple samples should be taken from seborrheic areas. The keratin layer must not be disturbed by close clipping of the hair or by the application of any cleaning or disinfecting solutions. The biopsies will show the dysplastic change but may or may not demonstrate the yeast.

The major symptoms of EDW are associated with the secondary *Malassezia* infection and must be resolved. Topical treatment may or may not be effective as the sole means of treatment but will be beneficial in all cases. Shampoos containing antifungal agents (Dermazole, Allerderm; Chlorhexiderm, DVM Pharmaceutical) have received wide usage, but no studies on their true efficacy are available. These products are used two to three times weekly for the first 2 weeks and then at least weekly for an additional 2 to 4 weeks. Some investigators use antiseborrheic products containing sulfur or benzyl peroxide, but these shampoos are likely to be too drying or irritating if used as the sole means of treatment.

When shampoos are insufficient, oral treatment with ketoconazole (Nizoral, Janssen Pharmaceuticals) is indicated. The drug is administered orally at 10 mg/kg one to two times daily for 30 to 45 days. Topical treatments may decrease the course of therapy to 21 days. Topical treatment with enilconazole dips (Imaverol, Janssen Animal Health) every third to fourth day for four treatments also is effective, but this product is not currently available in the United States.

When the yeast dermatitis is resolved, the animal's pruritus should be virtually eliminated. If the remaining pruritus is significant, the animal may have an intercurrent atopic condition. Assuming that EDW is the dog's only problem, the yeast dermatitis will recur because the underlying epidermal dysplasia remains. No studies have been published that have suggested effective methods of control for the EDW, and the author's experience with frequent antiseborrheic baths or isotretinoin (Accutane, Roche Laboratories) have been disappointing. Antifungal shampoos may be of some benefit, but probably would not prevent all relapses. The only method of control that has been consistently successful involves the episodic or constant use of ketoconazole.

If the interval between infections is long, each episode is treated for 30 to 45 days and then the drug is stopped. If the interinfection interval is short, as it is in most cases, the ketoconazole is administered on a constant basis. Most dogs in this latter category are euthanized because of the poor prognosis for cure and expense of maintenance therapy. Several dogs have been maintained in a near normal state for several years when they took the ketoconazole every second to third day. Similar control should be achievable with maintenance use of the enilconazole, but that remains unproven.

Since dogs with EDW have severe skin disease, they are not entered into breeding programs. Because of the inherited basis of the disorder, the parents and littermates also should not be used for breeding until the specific mode of inheritance is determined.

## PAPILLOMAVIRUS INFECTION

Until recently, papillomavirus infections were unknown in cats and typically only caused oral papillomatosis in dogs. Papillomavirus infections now have been documented in cats and cause either fibropapillomas (Carpenter et al., 1992) or multiple dysplastic plaque on the skin (Carney et al., 1990). Dysplastic plaques have also been associated with papillomavirus infection in one dog by the author. The virus in cats is a newly recognized one, but it is unclear whether there is a new strain of canine papillomavirus or whether the classic strain can induce differing types of lesions.

Dogs or cats with dysplastic plaques develop multiple lesions of varying size anywhere on the body. The plaques usually are 1 cm or larger in diameter, are haired initially, and are covered by scale or heavy crust.

The lesions in cats tend to be crusted and this crusting can induce pruritus.

Depending on the number and nature of the lesions, the list of differentials can be short or long. Since the lesions do not respond to any conventional treatments, biopsies should be performed. The diagnosis of a dysplastic plaque is easily made, but the confirmation of the viral etiology will require immunohistochemical straining or electron microscopy or both.

Individual lesions can be removed surgically, but new lesions are likely to occur. No data are available on other successful modes of treatment. Patients should be monitored carefully, since the papillomavirus infection probably predisposes these patients to the development of multiple squamous cell carcinomas *in situ* (Bowen's disease).

## BOWEN'S DISEASE

Bowen's disease is the name used in human dermatology to describe patients with one or more squamous cell carcinomas *in situ*. The keratinocytes in the area have become dysplastic and precancerous but remain above the basement membrane of the skin for long periods. Solar induction is the most common cause, but viral induction, especially by papillomaviruses, also is important. The condition has been reported in one dog and multiple cats.

The reported dog was 5 years old and had multiple variably crusted and pigmented papules, plaques, nodules, and verrucous lesions on its ventrum and feet (Gross and Brimacomb, 1986). The dog had a history of frequent sunbathing, so solar induction was suspected. However, the dog developed multiple lesions in its haired skin, so some other cause, perhaps viral, may have been contributory. The dog developed invasive squamous cell carcinoma.

Multiple cats have been recognized with Bowen's disease (Miller et al., 1992). Affected cats are old, do not have lightly pigmented skin or coats, and have long histories of skin disease only. The cats have multiple, variably pigmented hyperkeratotic plaques, especially on the head, neck, shoulder region, and forelimbs. Heavily crusted lesions can be pruritic, but most lesions are asymptomatic. Treatment with antibiotics, glucocorticoids, and various topical agents causes no improvement.

The lesions in the dog and cats have striking clinical and histologic similarity to actinic keratoses and the papillomavirus lesions. Solar induction probably was at least partially causal in the dog and the author has identified papillomavirus antigen in the lesions from one cat.

Insufficient clinical data have been published to define the biologic behavior of this condition in animals. Progression to invasive squamous cell carcinoma has been recognized, but it is very uncommon and occurs late in the course of the disease.

The dog was treated with topical 5-fluorouracil and lesion regression was noted. Plesiotherapy has been used in the cat with very encouraging results. Early lesions can disappear entirely, while old thick lesions respond poorly. Although treated lesions resolve, new ones tend to appear in untreated areas.

## SUMMARY

Aside from epidermal dysplasia of West Highland white terriers, the dysplastic disorders of dogs and cats appear to be due to solar exposure, papillomavirus infection, or combinations thereof. New solar lesions can be prevented by strict photoprotection, but new viral lesions cannot be prevented and should be expected. Progression from dysplasia to frank neoplasia appears to be very slow but can be expected, especially if ultraviolet light exposure continues. Plesiotherapy appears to be the treatment of choice for these preneoplastic conditions.

## References and Suggested Reading

Carney HC, England JJ, Hodgin EC, et al: Papillomavirus infection of aged Persian cats. J Vet Diagn Invest 2:294, 1990.
  *Discussion on two cats with multiple viral plaques.*
Carpenter JL, Kreider JW, Alroy J, et al: Cutaneous xanthogranuloma and viral papilloma on an eyelid of a cat. Vet Dermatol 3:187, 1992.
  *Report on proven viral papilloma.*
Gross TL and Brimacomb BH: Multifocal intraepidermal carcinoma in a dog histologically resembling Bowen's disease. Am J Dermatopathol 8:509, 1986.
  *The original case report of Bowen's disease in the dog.*
Mason KV: *Malassezia* dermatitis and otitis. *In* Bonagura JW and Kirk RW (eds): *Kirk's Current Veterinary Therapy XI.* Philadelphia, WB Saunders Co, 1992, 544.
  *General discussion on* Malassezia *infections.*
Miller WH Jr, Affolter V, Scott DW, et al: Multiple squamous cell carcinomas in-situ resembling Bowen's disease in five cats. Vet Dermatol 3:177, 1992.
  *Report on five cats with multiple squamous cell carcinomas in situ.*
Rosenkrantz WS: Solar dermatitis. *In* Griffin CE, Kwochka KW, and MacDonald JM (eds): *Current Veterinary Dermatology.* St. Louis, Mosby Year Book, 1993, p 309.
  *An excellent review of photodermatitis.*
Scott DW and Miller WH Jr: Epidermal dysplasia and *Malassezia pachydermatis* infection in West Highland white terriers. Vet Dermatol 1:25, 1989.
  *Report on eight dogs with epidermal dysplasia.*

# CONGENITAL ADRENAL HYPERPLASIA-LIKE SYNDROME

LYNN P. SCHMEITZEL,
*Knoxville, Tennessee*

CLINTON D. LOTHROP, Jr.,
*Auburn, Alabama*

*and* WAYNE S. ROSENKRANTZ
*Garden Grove, California*

Adult dogs presented with bilaterally symmetric endocrine alopecia initially involving the rump, perineum, flanks, caudal thighs, and neck without signs of systemic illness, and with normal thyroid and adrenal function tests, are tentatively diagnosed to have either a sex hormone imbalance or growth hormone–responsive alopecia. Congenital adrenal hyperplasia-like syndrome is a newly described disorder caused by an adrenocortical sex hormone imbalance that occurs in dogs with a clinical presentation similar, if not identical, to that of growth hormone–responsive alopecia.

## CLINICAL SIGNS

Dogs with congenital adrenal hyperplasia-like syndrome have similar clinical signs to those with growth hormone–responsive alopecia. Age of onset is usually between 1 and 2 years of age, but the alopecia can develop at any age. Certain breeds are predisposed,

including Pomeranians and chow chows. Males and females, both intact and neutered, are affected.

Symmetric alopecia and hyperpigmentation develops on the rump, perineum, caudal thighs, neck, tail, and trunk while sparing the head and distal extremities. Initially, the guard (primary) hairs are lost with retention of the undercoat (secondary) hairs. Later, complete alopecia develops in these areas. Some dogs may develop alopecia after clipping. Comedones are often present in the alopecic areas. Secondary superficial pyoderma and mild seborrhea sicca may be found concurrently. These dogs have clinically normal (intact or neutered) reproductive structures.

## PATHOGENESIS

The pathogenesis has not been completely elucidated. However, abnormal adrenal steroidogenesis resulting in adrenocortical hyperprogestinism and hyperandrogenism is the suspected cause of the alopecia. A partial deficiency of one of the adrenal enzymes, 11-hydroxylase, 21-hydroxylase, or 3-hydroxysteroid dehydrogenase, may be causing a partial deficiency of aldosterone or cortisol in the affected dogs (Fig. 1). The decreased cortisol and aldosterone concentrations stimulate the anterior pituitary gland to increase adrenocorticotrophic hormone (ACTH) secretion that subsequently causes adrenocortical hyperplasia and increased adrenal sex hormone production.

This syndrome in dogs may be similar to one in people called congenital adrenal hyperplasia. Three forms of congenital adrenal hyperplasia caused by an adrenocortical enzyme deficiency occur: (1) individuals with a total deficiency have a complete lack of aldosterone and cortisol (salt wasting); (2) individuals with a partial deficiency develop hyperandrogenism (short stature, hirsutism, and male patterned baldness), of which two subsets exist (affected individuals develop signs of androgen excess during childhood or at puberty [nonclassic "late-onset"]; and (3) individuals with a cryptic (hidden) partial deficiency (usually relatives of clinically affected individuals) do not have clinical signs of disease, but have the same biochemical abnormalities and may develop signs later.

An alternative hypothesis for the hair loss in some dogs may be an inherent increased production of the adrenocortical sex hormones that causes the abnormal hair coats. The authors believe that the elevated adrenocortical sex hormones bind to the hormone receptors in the skin, causing the hair coat changes observed in this syndrome.

Normal Pomeranians and Pomeranians with growth hormone–responsive alopecia were previously shown to have both decreased growth hormone response tests and increased concentrations of progesterone, 17-hydroxyprogesterone, androstenedione, and dehydroepiandrosterone sulfate before and/or after ACTH stimulation (Schmeitzel and Lothrop, 1990). Plasma endogenous ACTH was also elevated in the dogs tested. Hyposomatotropism (low growth hormone concentration) may be contributing to the alopecia or may be falsely decreased due to the adrenal sex hormone imbalance similar to the decreased growth hormone responsiveness to xylazine observed in hyperadrenocorticism (Cushing's syndrome) and hypothyroidism.

The authors suspect that the breeds at risk for congenital adrenal hyperplasia-like syndrome are being bred for this defect to grow a thick hair coat (e.g., hirsutism). A form of male pattern baldness may be occurring in the alopecic dogs with the elevated adrenocortical sex hormone concentrations.

## DIAGNOSIS

Tentative diagnosis is made by history and clinical signs of an otherwise healthy dog with an apparent endocrine alopecia. Definitive diagnosis is made by ruling out other causes of bilateral symmetric alopecia in dogs

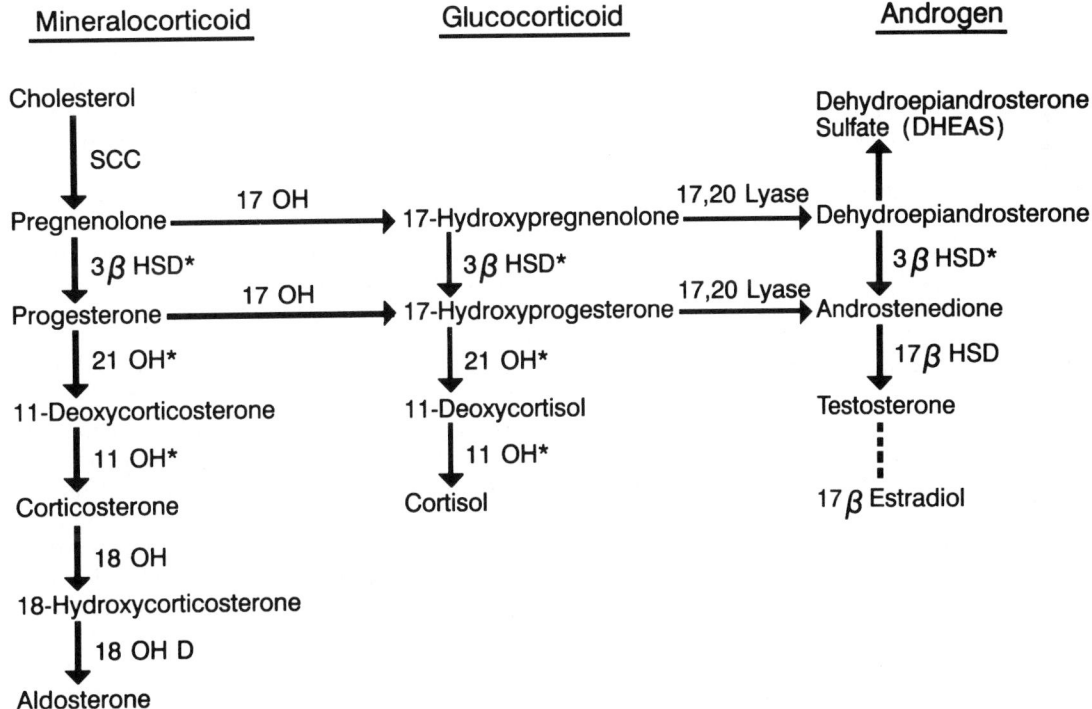

**Figure 1.** Main pathways of adrenocortical steroidogenesis. Abbreviations: SCC = cholesterol side-chain cleavage, HSD = hydroxysteroid dehydrogenase, OH = hydroxylase, OHD = hydroxydehydrogenase, ° = sites of adrenocortical enzyme deficiencies, resulting in excessive adrenocortical androgen production in people. (From Schmeitzel LP and Lothrop CD Jr: Hormonal abnormalities in Pomeranians with normal coat and in Pomeranians with growth hormone-responsive dermatosis. J Am Vet Med Assoc 197:1333, 1990, with permission.)

and by demonstrating elevated concentrations of adrenocortical sex hormones and their precursors with an ACTH response test. Differential diagnoses include other endocrinopathies (hypothyroidism; hyperadrenocorticism [Cushing's syndrome], sex hormone imbalances); anagen or telogen defluxion; postclipping alopecia of sled dogs and other breeds; cyclic flank alopecia; and follicular dysplasias affecting Siberian huskies, Irish water spaniels, Portuguese water dogs, curly coated retrievers, and adult black and red Doberman pinschers (Gross, Ihrke, and Walder, 1992; Miller, 1990).

A complete blood count and serum chemistry panel should be within normal limits. Abnormal laboratory results consistent with hypothyroidism (normocytic, normochromic nonregenerative anemia, elevated cholesterol) or hypercortisolism (stress leukogram, elevated serum alkaline phosphatase) should not be present.

A skin biopsy should demonstrate histologic changes consistent with an endocrinopathy (surface and follicular hyperkeratosis, epidermal atrophy and melanosis, and follicular and sebaceous gland atrophy). Hair follicles may be predominantly in telogen (resting phase of the hair follicle growth cycle) phase arrest, or in catagen (intermediate phase of the hair follicle growth cycle) phase arrest. In some cases, hair follicles may exhibit hypereosinophilic tricholemmal keratinization ("flame follicles").

Ideally, a thyrotropin response test (TSH response test) or a thyrotropin-releasing hormone (TRH) response test and a low-dose dexamethasone suppression test should be performed and found to be normal. If TSH or TRH are not available, baseline serum thyrosine $(T_4)$ and triiodothyronine $(T_3)$ concentrations should be within the middle to high normal range. If baseline serum $T_4$ and $T_3$ concentrations are below normal or within low normal range, a 6-week trial course of L-thyroxine at 0.02 mg/kg PO given every 12 hr is suggested.

If no significant hair regrowth is observed after 6 weeks of L-thyroxine therapy and serum $T_4$ concentration determined 4 to 6 hr after the morning medication was administered is within high normal range, a low-dose dexamethasone suppression test should be performed to determine if hypercortisolism consistent with Cushing's syndrome is present. A low-dose dexamethasone suppression test is considered to be a more sensitive screening test for Cushing's syndrome compared to an ACTH stimulation test. If the results of a TSH and TRH response test and a low-dose dexamethasone suppression test are normal, an ACTH stimulation test should be performed and concentrations of the adrenocortical steroid hormones and their precursors before and after ACTH should be determined.

### ACTH Stimulation Test

Collect blood in both an ethylenediaminetetraacetic acid (EDTA) (2.0-ml) and clot (5.0-ml) tube. Centrifuge and remove the plasma and serum from the tubes and freeze immediately. Administer synthetic ACTH (cosyntropin, Cortrosyn, Organon Inc, West Orange, NJ) 0.5 IU/kg IV or porcine aqueous gelatin ACTH (repository corticotropin injection, USP, H.P. Acthar Gel—40 IU/ml, Rhône-Poulenc Rorer Pharmaceuticals Inc, Collegeville, PA) 2.2 mg/kg IM. Collect post-ACTH stimulation blood samples (2-ml EDTA tube and 5-ml clot tube) 1 hr after synthetic ACTH or 1 and 2 hr after gelatin ACTH. Centrifuge and remove the plasma and serum from the tubes and freeze immediately.

The samples should be kept frozen (preferably on dry ice) and sent to the laboratory by overnight mail. Many laboratories will perform assays for cortisol, progesterone, testosterone, and estradiol. However, the Endocrinology Laboratory at the University of Tennessee College of Veterinary Medicine can determine 17-hydroxyprogesterone, androstenedione, and dehydroepiandrosterone sulfate serum concentrations in addition to the previously mentioned hormones (Schmeitzel and Lothrop, 1990).

If concentrations of adrenocortical sex hormones and their precursors are elevated before and/or after ACTH administration compared to normal dogs, a diagnosis of congenital adrenal hyperplasia-like syndrome is made. Results of the adrenocortical sex hormones and their precursors before and after ACTH in normal intact and neutered dogs are listed in Tables 1 and 2.

Some dogs with congenital adrenal hyperplasia-like syndrome have elevated plasma cortisol concentrations after ACTH stimulation. These dogs do not have the polyuria, polydipsia, polyphagia, or elevated serum alkaline phosphatase that usually occur in dogs with hypercortisolemia due to Cushing's syndrome. The authors believe that the elevated plasma cortisol concentrations after ACTH stimulation in the absence of other clinical signs or biochemical alterations consistent with hypercortisolemia due to Cushing's syndrome are other indications of the abnormal steroidogenesis that causes this disorder, and are not due to Cushing's syndrome.

### TREATMENT

Congenital adrenal hyperplasia like-syndrome may respond to several modes of therapy including castration, methyltestosterone, growth hormone, and o,p'-DDD. Castration is generally recommended, since many of the male dogs will regrow hair for varying periods of time after castration. Castration most likely reduces the overall concentration of the sex hormones, the reduction of which stimulates hair regrowth.

Some dogs do not respond to castration, only partially or temporarily respond to castration, or were neutered before clinical signs developed. A trial course of methyltestosterone may be tried in these dogs. Methyltestosterone is a controlled substance (schedule III), so a Drug Enforcement Administration (DEA) number will be needed to obtain the drug. The dose is 1 mg/kg

**Table 1.** *Range of Sex Hormones in Normal Intact Dogs Before and After ACTH Stimulation (ng/ml Unless Noted Otherwise)*

| Hormone | Mean° | | Range | |
|---|---|---|---|---|
| | *Before* | *After* | *Before* | *After* |
| **Males** | | | | |
| Progesterone (n = 10) | 0.41 (± 0.53) | 1.10 (± 1.23) | 0.00–1.79 | 0.10–3.74 |
| 17-hydroxyprogesterone (n = 10) | 0.30 (± 0.35) | 1.37 (± 0.88) | 0.00–1.09 | 0.48–2.95 |
| DHEAS (n = 10) | 18.52 (± 11.49) | 20.83 (± 10.95) | 6.60–43.38 | 5.76–44.14 |
| Androstenedione (n = 10) | 13.28 (± 10.07) | 12.24 (± 6.74) | 4.08–33.76 | 3.92–23.68 |
| Testosterone (n = 10) | 3.07 (± 4.23) | 2.56 (± 4.14) | 0.37–11.10 | 0.39–14.2 |
| Estradiol 17 β (pg/ml, n = 10) | 18.69 (± 14.58) | 15.63 (± 8.63) | 0.00–44.24 | 5.7–31.84 |
| **Females** | | | | |
| Progesterone (n = 5) | 0.28 (± 0.05) | 0.77 (± 0.31) | 0.20–0.33 | 0.55–1.30 |
| 17-hydroxyprogesterone (n = 5) | 0.22 (± 0.13) | 1.50 (± 0.44) | 0.10–0.43 | 1.11–2.09 |
| DHEAS (n = 5) | 5.67 (± 1.67) | 7.77 (± 1.68) | 3.86–8.32 | 5.66–10.18 |
| Androstenedione (n = 5) | 6.51 (± 8.04) | 2.00 (± 0.86) | 1.12–20.40 | 1.28–3.44 |
| Testosterone (n = 5) | 0.10 (± 0.00) | 0.10 (± 0.00) | 0.10–0.10 | 0.10–0.10 |
| Estradiol 17 β (pg/ml, n = 5) | 24.75 (± 9.36) | 21.99 (± 8.07) | 14.01–39.59 | 15.93–34.21 |

°Data are expressed as mean (± SD).

(maximum dose-30 mg/dog) PO every other day for up to 3 months. Once the hair has regrown, a maintenance dose of 1 mg/kg (maximum-30 mg/dog) should be given one to two times weekly. Potential adverse reactions of methyltestosterone therapy include cholangiohepatitis, seborrhea oleosa, and behavioral changes. The authors know of at least one intact male dog and several neutered dogs affected with congenital adrenal hyperplasia-like syndrome that responded to methyltestosterone supplementation.

Some dogs respond to growth hormone supplementation. The dose is 0.015 IU/kg SC two times a week for 6 weeks. A complete response may be seen in 3 months. Growth hormone is diabetogenic; therefore, it is important to measure a fasting blood glucose before therapy is initiated and at least once a week during the 6-week therapy. If hyperglycemia develops during therapy, the injections should be discontinued immediately. Permanent diabetes mellitus may develop if therapy is continued in the presence of persistent hyperglycemia.

Growth hormone is available at reasonable cost from Dr. A. F. Parlow, Harbor-UCLA Medical Center, 1000 West Carson Street, Torrance, CA 90509.

The most effective therapy for congenital adrenal hyperplasia-like syndrome is o,p'-DDD. o,p'-DDD causes necrosis and atrophy of the zona fasciculata and the zone reticularis of the adrenal cortex. The zona reticularis is the portion of the adrenal cortex that predominantly produces the sex hormones.

o,p-DDD therapy consists of loading and maintenance phases. During the loading phase, the o,p'-DDD is given at 15 to 25 mg/kg PO once daily for up to 7 days. At the end of the 7-day loading period, or earlier if any clinical signs compatible with hypocortisolemia develop, an ACTH stimulation test should be performed to determine the response of cortisol concentrations before and after ACTH. The goal of therapy during the loading phase is to suppress the dog's baseline cortisol concentration to a low normal range and to suppress cortisol concentration after ACTH stimu-

**Table 2.** *Range of Sex Hormones in Normal Neutered Dogs Before and After ACTH Stimulation (ng/ml Unless Noted Otherwise)*

| Hormone | Mean° | | Range | |
|---|---|---|---|---|
| | *Before* | *After* | *Before* | *After* |
| **Males** | | | | |
| Progesterone (n = 9) | 0.05 (± 0.03) | 0.37 (± 0.37) | 0.008–0.09 | 0.05–1.19 |
| 17-hydroxyprogesterone (n = 9) | 0.05 (± 0.03) | 0.58 (± 0.26) | 0.00–0.08 | 0.40–1.22 |
| DHEAS (n = 9) | 2.11 (± 3.33) | 2.93 (± 4.30) | 0.09–10.49 | 0.27–13.78 |
| Androstenedione (n = 9) | 4.79 (± 1.54) | 5.36 (± 2.02) | 2.71–7.97 | 2.97–9.67 |
| Testosterone (n = 9) | 0.01 (± 0.00) | 0.02 (± 0.00) | 0.01–0.02 | 0.01–0.03 |
| Estradiol 17 β (pg/ml, n = 9) | 43.13 (± 9.99) | 41.29 (± 13.45) | 28.40–63.30 | 29.90–69.00 |
| **Females** | | | | |
| Progesterone (n = 8) | 0.07 (± 0.06) | 0.71 (± 0.25) | 0.02–0.19 | 0.35–1.11 |
| 17-hydroxyprogesterone (n = 8) | 0.12 (± 0.13) | 0.91 (± 0.32) | 0.00–0.42 | 0.45–1.45 |
| DHEAS (n = 8) | 3.84 (± 4.48) | 5.00 (± 4.65) | 0.26–12.18 | 0.94–14.30 |
| Androstenedione (n = 8) | 6.50 (± 3.70) | 4.94 (± 0.41) | 2.77–14.28 | 4.44–5.51 |
| Testosterone (n = 8) | 0.02 (± 0.00) | 0.02 (± 0.00) | 0.01–0.02 | 0.01–0.02 |
| Estradiol 17 β (pg/ml, n = 8) | 40.26 (± 8.16) | 40.56 (± 8.08) | 27.70–53.20 | 26.10–51.40 |

°Data are expressed as mean (± SD).

lation to a range of 30 to 50 ng/ml (3.0 to 5.0 $\mu$g/dl). If the cortisol concentrations are suppressed, the adrenocortical sex hormones and their precursor concentrations are also suppressed.

If the cortisol concentrations after ACTH stimulation are too low (<30 ng/ml), o,p'-DDD therapy should be discontinued. The dog should be thoroughly evaluated for clinical evidence of hypocortisolemia, and assays for serum electrolyte concentrations should be performed to determine if hyperkalemia or hyponatremia are present. Prednisolone at a dose of 2.5 to 10 mg/dog PO once daily or every other day should be given if clinical signs of hypocortisolemia are present. If hyponatremia or hyperkalemia are documented, fludrocortisone acetate 0.005 mg/kg PO should be administered every 12 hr. Severe electrolyte imbalances may require fluid therapy and salt supplementation. Desoxycorticosterone pivalate administered at a dose of 12.5 to 100 mg/dog IM every 25 days may be necessary for dogs with persistent electrolyte abnormalities. Since o,p'-DDD generally spares the zona glomerulosa, the aldosterone-producing portion of the adrenal gland, aldosterone deficiency with electrolyte changes are rare (Feldman and Nelson, 1987). A majority of the dogs affected with congenital adrenal hyperplasia-like syndrome treated with o,p'-DDD have no adverse reactions to the therapy.

The goal of the maintenance phase of o,p'-DDD therapy is to maintain suppression of cortisol and the adrenocortical sex hormones and their precursors. When the cortisol concentration after ACTH stimulation is 30 to 50 ng/ml (3.0 to 5.0 $\mu$g/dl), o,p'-DDD should be given at a dose of 25 mg/kg PO once every 5 to 14 days.

Three weeks after starting o,p'-DDD therapy, an ACTH stimulation test should be performed again to determine the response of cortisol concentrations before and after ACTH administration. A complete physical examination and serum chemistries with electrolytes should be determined to document any direct adverse effects from o,p'-DDD, or from hypocortisolemia or hypoaldosteronemia secondary to the o,p'-DDD therapy.

Favorable clinical response is usually observed within 4 to 12 weeks. At first, hair loss may be increased, probably due to loss of the telogen hairs when the anagen phase (growth phase) of the hair follicle cycle is initiated. Hair regrowth is usually observed shortly thereafter.

An ACTH response test should be repeated 10 weeks after the initiation of o,p'-DDD therapy to determine levels of cortisol and adrenocortical sex hormones and their precursors before and after ACTH. The hormone concentrations after ACTH stimulation should be maintained in the low normal ranges for best results.

A number of dogs with this syndrome have been treated with ketoconazole without significant improvement. Two dogs have partially responded to high doses.

## PROGNOSIS

The prognosis of dogs with congenital adrenal hyperplasia-like syndrome is good. Without therapy, these dogs eventually develop complete alopecia and hyperpigmentation of the neck, trunk, perineum, and caudal thighs, with the head and distal extremities spared. Mild seborrhea sicca and recurrent superficial pyodermas will need to be treated. Neutering intact dogs or administering methyltestosterone supplementation to neutered dogs may be efficacious in some cases. To date, the most effective therapy for congenital adrenal hyperplasia-like syndrome is o,p'-DDD therapy.

The authors suspect that many cases of growth hormone–responsive alopecia actually have congenital adrenal hyperplasia-like syndrome. Additional research is needed to determine the actual pathogenesis and the ideal therapy for this disorder.

### References and Suggested Reading

Feldman EC and Nelson RW: Canine and feline endocrinology and reproduction. Philadelphia, WB Saunders Co, 1987, p 55, 137, 195.
    *Reviews of diagnosis and treatment of hypothyroidism, hyperadrenocorticism, and hypoadrenocorticism.*
Gross TL, Ihrke PJ, and Walder EJ: Veterinary dermatopathology. St. Louis, Mosby Year Book, 1992, pp 273, 298.
    *A correlation of clinical and microscopic features of skin disease.*
Miller WH Jr: Follicular dysplasia in adult black and red Doberman pinschers. Vet Dermatol 1:181, 1990.
    *A study of clinical and histologic features of an adult-onset follicular dysplasia affecting adult Doberman pinschers.*
Schmeitzel LP and Lothrop CD Jr: Hormonal abnormalities in Pomeranians with normal coat and in Pomeranians with growth hormone-responsive dermatosis. J Am Vet Med Assoc 197:1333, 1990.
    *A prospective study of hormonal abnormalities, including adrenal sex hormones, in Pomeranians with normal coats and with growth hormone–responsive dermatosis.*

# HEREDITARY LUPOID DERMATOSIS OF THE GERMAN SHORTHAIRED POINTER

STEPHEN D. WHITE

*Fort Collins, Colorado*

*and* THELMA LEE GROSS

*West Sacramento, California*

Hereditary lupoid dermatosis of the German short-haired pointer is a newly described skin disease noted thus far only in this breed. Age of onset is typically by 8 months. No sex predilection has yet been noted in the small number of cases of which the authors are aware. The disease has been recognized in the United States, the Netherlands, and the United Kingdom. Its hereditary nature is suggested by its occurrence in siblings and half siblings, and the shared ancestry in some of the affected dogs.

## CLINICAL SIGNS

The most pronounced clinical signs are scaling and crusting. Fronds of keratin may surround the hair shaft. Initial lesions may occur on the face, ears, and back, but the condition often becomes generalized, and the hocks and scrotum may be severely affected. Pruritus and pain are variable. Peripheral lymphadenopathy and, less often, pyrexia, may be observed. The authors are aware of one dog with a positive antinuclear antibody (ANA) test, and another with a persistent proteinuria.

## HISTOPATHOLOGY

Histologically, as typified by nine affected dogs, the clinical scaling is manifested microscopically by hyperkeratosis and parakeratosis, and there is mild to moderate acanthosis. Basal cell degeneration is characterized by vacuolar change, as well as by individual cell necrosis. This individual cell necrosis also occurs frequently to occasionally throughout the stratum spinosum, and in one dog necrosis became confluent in the superficial epidermis. Basal cell degeneration may lead to dermal/epidermal separation, and even ulceration. These degenerative changes extend to the keratinocytes of the hair follicles to the level of the isthmus.

The dermis is characterized by mild to moderate interface inflammation (often obscuring the dermal/epidermal junction), consisting of lymphocytes, macrophages, and plasma cells. Exocytosis of lymphocytes into the overlying epidermis and follicular epithelium is mild to moderate. Occasional satellitosis is evident around individually necrotic keratinocytes. Neutrophils occur in the areas of severe epidermal degeneration and ulceration. Eosinophilic infiltration and dermal fibrosis are uncommon findings.

Of interest is the fact that sebaceous glands may be completely absent in some to all skin specimens obtained for biopsy. Alternatively, they may be small or normal. In one dog, nodular accumulations of lymphocytes, macrophages, plasma cells, and occasional neutrophils were seen surrounding the isthmus of the hair follicles.

The microscopic appearance of lupoid dermatosis of the German shorthaired pointer bears some resemblance to lupus erythematosus, erythema multiforme, and sebaceous adenitis. Transepidermal keratinocyte necrosis and lymphocyte satellitosis are features of erythema multiforme. Basal cell vacuolation and necrosis, and dermal/epidermal separation, may be features of either lupus erythematosus or erythema multiforme. These features strongly suggest an immunologic basis for this disorder. Sebaceous gland loss may be striking and resemble late-stage sebaceous adenitis (Hargis AM, personal communication, 1993). Sebaceous gland atrophy may be secondary to extension of keratinocyte degeneration and inflammation to the outer hair follicle; other diseases (such as cutaneous leishmaniasis) may involve similar "sweeping up" of sebaceous glands by a perifollicular/periadnexal inflammatory process. As seen in sebaceous adenitis, the loss of sebaceous glands may have resulted in the fine scaling observed clinically in these dogs. Hyperkeratosis is present histopathologically, but generally is not as severe as observed in sebaceous adenitis.

Histopathology of the lymph nodes shows reactive hyperplasia. In at least one case, there was histiocytosis with prominent hemosiderosis.

## THERAPY

Therapy has, at this point, been frustrating. The authors know of several dogs that showed initial improvement to fatty acid supplementation (EFAVet, Efamol; DermCaps, DVM Pharmaceuticals [in one case, this was combined with niacinamide and tetracycline, 500 mg of each drug every 8 hr]), only to eventually relapse. Because of the excessive scaling and involvement of the sebaceous glands, retinoids may prove to be of some therapeutic benefit to these dogs. Antiseborrheic shampoos and corticosteroids have usually been of disappointing efficacy.

## DISCUSSION

The etiology of this disease is uncertain. If this is truly lupus erythematosus (LE), it represents a distinct subset of this disease in dogs. The early age of onset is unusual in either discoid LE or systemic LE, yet the onset is too late to have a convincing similarity to neonatal LE in human beings (in which the mother has evidence of LE as well). Discoid LE in human beings does rarely occur in childhood, often with eventual progression to systemic LE; such a similarity is attractive to the age of onset, but the clinical features of these dogs are not like those described in canine discoid LE.

Alternatively, this condition may be a form of erythema multiforme, a disease that is often seen in response to drug administration, particularly in young dogs. While there has been no convincing drug history in any of the dogs that the authors are aware of, the onset of signs at 5 to 6 months of age has a temporal relationship to the completion of immunizations of most young dogs; and hereditary predisposition to an adverse immunologic reaction to vaccination is therefore possible.

Until more cases are studied, our understanding of this disease must be considered to be in the initial stages. It is hoped that through cooperation of dermatologists and practitioners, our knowledge of this condition and its potential therapies will be expanded.

### References and Suggested Readings

Gross TL, Ihrke PJ, and Walder EJ: Veterinary Dermatopathology. St. Louis, Mosby Year Book, 1992, pp 26–28.

Theaker AJ and Rest JR: Lupoid dermatosis in a German shorthaired pointer (letter). Vet Rec 131:495, 1992.

# ACQUIRED, NONENDOCRINE ALOPECIAS OF THE DOG AND CAT

KEVIN J. SHANLEY

*Valley Forge, Pennsylvania*

The causes of alopecia are numerous and varied. They are often classified as congenital (ectodermal defect in miniature poodles, congenital alopecia, feline alopecia universalis, feline hypotrichosis), inherited (black hair follicular dysplasia, color dilution alopecia, dermatomyositis), psychogenic (feline or canine psychogenic alopecia, acral lick dermatitis), endocrine (hypothyroidism, hyperadrenocorticism, sex hormone imbalances, growth hormone-responsive alopecia, castration-responsive alopecia), folliculitis (bacterial, dermatophytosis, demodicosis), infectious (parasitic, fungal), nutritional (protein deficiency, vitamin A deficiency, fatty acid deficiency, zinc-responsive dermatosis), autoimmune (discoid or systemic lupus erythematosus, the pemphigus group, bullous pemphigoid), neoplastic (cutaneous lymphosarcoma, cutaneous mast cell tumor), or secondary to pruritus as with the allergic diseases or scabies. Alopecia can be further classified into scarring (cicatricial) and nonscarring (noncicatricial) types. Cicatricial alopecias result in scar tissue formation and cause permanent alopecia due to the replacement of the hair follicles in the dermis with fibrotic tracts. Without scar tissue formation, the alopecia is not permanent. Some disorders may be scarring or nonscarring, depending on the severity, extent, and chronicity of the disease (Table 1).

Acquired nonendocrine alopecia is a term given to the remaining diseases that cause alopecia. These "leftover" diseases are an unrelated group of uncommon to rare skin diseases that present with alopecia as the most significant clinical sign. This article will include discussions of anagen defluxion, telogen defluxion, trichorrhexis nodosa, alopecia areata, traction alopecia, and postvaccination reactions. Sebaceous adenitis can be included in this group and is covered in this edition (p 619) and in *CVT XI* (p 534).

## CLINICAL CONSIDERATIONS

There are important considerations and questions common to the clinical approach of any patient with alopecia. Is the alopecia bilaterally symmetric or asymmetric? Is the distribution trunkal or generalized? Is the alopecia focal or multifocal and does the location of the alopecia predispose the site to physical insults or trauma? Is the alopecia complete, where the entire length of the hair shaft is absent or is it traumatic ("stubble") alopecia, where the hairs look as if they have been broken or clipped just above the level of the skin? What other accompanying skin lesions are pres-

**Table 1.** *Causes of Complete Temporary, Complete Permanent, and Traumatic Temporary Alopecia*

| Disease | Complete Temporary | Complete Permanent | Traumatic Temporary |
|---|:---:|:---:|:---:|
| Endocinopathies | X | | |
| Folliculitides | X | X | |
| Allergies | | | X |
| Anagen defluxion | X | | |
| Telogen defluxion | X | | |
| Trichorrhexis nodosa | X | | X |
| Alopecia areata | X | X | |
| Traction alopecia | | X | X |
| Thermal burn | | X | |
| Vaccine/injection reactions | | X | |

ent, such as follicular or nonfollicular papules or pustules, crusts, epidermal collarettes, comedones, or hair follicular casts? It is beyond the scope of this article to discuss a detailed approach to alopecia, and the reader is referred to other sources (Rosenkrantz, 1984).

Alopecia is defined as a loss of hair, or the absence of hair. Defluxion is defined as "a sudden disappearance or falling out" of the hair, whereas effluvium is defined as "an outflowing or shedding" of the hair. Defluxion and effluvium are often used interchangeably. In addition to the common pathomechanisms of alopecia, it is important to be aware of diseases that cause constriction of the hair shaft or a structural defect in hair formation. This will cause weakening and breakage of the hairs and result in clinical alopecia. If the breakage occurs below the level of the follicular orifice, it will appear as complete alopecia even though histopathologic examination of the affected follicles will show an intact hair bulb and proximal hair shaft. If the breakage occurs above the skin, it will appear as traumatic alopecia.

## ANAGEN DEFLUXION

Anagen defluxion (anagen effluvium) is an abnormal loss of hair during the anagen (growing) phase of the hair growth cycle. Normally, hairs should epilate easily only after they have entered the telogen (resting) phase of the hair cycle. Anagen defluxion is a nonscarring alopecia and is a rare disease in dogs and cats. There are no age, breed, or sex predilections and the animal presents with multifocal areas of alopecia in a random pattern. It often affects the majority of the trunk, and will occasionally affect the head and proximal extremities. It is due to an acute, severe synchronous insult to numerous anagen hairs and results in premature loss of the affected hairs, usually several days to 2 weeks after the insult. The alopecia is complete. The most common causes of anagen defluxion are severe systemic diseases or the administration of cytotoxic chemotherapeutic medications. In humans, it has been associated with the administration of anticoagulants, antimetabolites, cytotoxic agents, alkylating agents, and mercury and thallium poisoning. Methotrexate and cyclophosphamide are especially toxic to the hair follicles and may result

in anagen defluvium. Helpful diagnostic clues include the physical examination findings and a history of recent illness or drug administration. Affected hairs epilate easily and show anagen hair bulbs under microscopic examination. Normal anagen hair bulbs can be identified by their blunted expanded root, frequently marked pigmentation, and an intact root sheath. When anagen defluxion is present, there may be acute narrowing of the hair shafts, affecting the portion of the hair within the follicle distal to the hair bulb. Biopsies for dermatopathology show an increased number of empty hair follicles, dystrophic changes of the hair follicle epithelium, and occasional "exclamation point hairs" due to the constriction of the hairs distal to the hair bulb. The exact reason for the alopecia is unknown. There is no treatment for this type of hair loss and the condition will spontaneously resolve. Normal hair growth will occur 2 to 3 months after removal of the stress, medications, or other inciting factors.

## TELOGEN DEFLUXION

Telogen defluxion (telogen effluvium) is an uncommon disease of cats and dogs that results in marked asymmetric, patchy alopecia, similar to anagen defluxion. It usually involves the trunkal hairs, but can involve extensive areas of the body. It is due to a significant insult that causes numerous hairs to prematurely progress from the anagen phase through catagen to telogen. Once these hairs are in telogen, they can be epilated easily, resulting in excessive shedding and alopecia. One to 3 months later, new anagen hairs begin to grow and dislodge the remaining telogen hairs. Stressful insults that can cause telogen defluxion include pregnancy, parturition, lactation, severe systemic illnesses, marked febrile episodes, shock, surgery, and various medications, particularly cytotoxic chemotherapeutics. The trichogram is helpful in identifying numerous telogen hairs. They are identified by a gently tapered "club-shaped" hair bulb with minimal to no pigmentation present and the absence of a root sheath. Histopathology will show an increased number of telogen follicles, including many devoid of hairs. As with anagen defluxion, there is no inflammation in the dermis, and other pathologic changes are not present. A diagnosis can be rendered with a history of stress, excessive epilation of hairs, and an increased number of telogen hairs on microscopic examination (trichogram). Biopsy is useful to confirm an increased number of telogen follicles, an increased telogen/anagen follicular ratio, and to rule out other noninflammatory causes of alopecia. No treatment is necessary. The hair will regrow completely several months after the inciting cause has been identified and removed (Scott, 1989).

## TRICHORRHEXIS NODOSA

Trichorrhexis nodosa is a rare trichodystrophy of dogs and cats. Translated literally, it means "hair fracture nodes." Affected hairs have small, white node-like swellings of the hair shaft. Transverse fracture of the hair cortex occurs, causing the nodal swellings which weaken the hair shaft. Affected hairs break easily, leading to alopecia or dull, lusterless hair that does not achieve significant length. On microscopic examination, the nodes resemble the ends of two brushes pushed into one another, forcing them to interdigitate.

In humans, trichorrhexis nodosa is the most common hair shaft anomaly. Mild traction on the hair will result in its separation at the site of the fracture node. It is classified as either congenital or acquired, although further research may allow more specific classification. Currently it is felt that hair cortical deficiencies and cuticular defects may be the primary factors, leading to trichorrhexis nodosa. Suggested cortical deficiencies include a breakdown of the intercellular cement substance that holds the hair cortex cells together, much in the same way that pemphigus results from a breakdown in the intercellular cement substance that holds epidermal cells together. If the cuticle is damaged or destroyed, the cortex is exposed to more physical trauma and detergents that have a solubilizing effect on the intercellular cement substance. Whether the structural defect is due to a cuticular weakness, cortical defect, or both, the characteristic node shows fragmented and whole spindle cells splayed out at irregular angles to the normal hair shaft (Price, 1990). These changes are not always visible with the naked eye or light microscopy. Acquired trichorrhexis nodosa is usually seen in patients secondary to chemical or thermal straightening, aggressive use of a stiff brush or sharp metal comb, harsh chemical treatments, or tight-fitting apparel. Occasionally, there is no history of excessive trauma or chemical application.

The rarity of this condition in animals is probably twofold: (1) the infrequent use of harsh chemicals on the hair, and (2) the lack of examination of hairs with high-power light microscopy or scanning electron microscopy. The author has seen trichorrhexis nodosa in a cat with flea allergy dermatitis. It is likely that this condition will be recognized more frequently when trichograms are used more routinely. Acquired distal trichorrhexis nodosa should be seen in heavily groomed animals, pets with long hair where the total accumulative trauma due to grooming is greatest, and in pruritic patients. The diagnosis of trichorrhexis nodosa is made with recognition of the transverse fractures of the hair under light microscopy. Absolute confirmation may require scanning electron microscopy. The treatment of trichorrhexis nodosa initially involves the discontinuation of any topical chemical applications (e.g., shampoos, dips), aggressive grooming, or any other damaging or traumatic process to the hair. Secondly, diagnose and treat any underlying cause of pruritus. The condition may require 2 to 4 years to resolve in humans, and an extended period of time may also be needed in veterinary patients.

## ALOPECIA AREATA

Alopecia areata has been recognized in cats, dogs, horses, cattle, and humans. It presents with random, usually asymmetric, sharply demarcated, annular to oval areas of complete alopecia with smooth, normally pigmented skin with no macroscopic evidence of inflammation. It usually involves the head, neck, and trunk and has minimal or no associated pruritus. There is no age, breed, or sex predilection recognized. The exact pathomechanism is unclear. In humans, alopecia areata is a relatively common disorder, affecting 1 to 2% of the population. It may present with a mild tingling sensation or localized pain, with mild palpable dermal edema. It is thought to have an immune-mediated basis, although neurologic, psychosomatic, and local foci of inflammation of the oral cavity have also been proposed as associated factors. A genetic influence is likely, as a familial incidence is present in approximately 25% of human patients. Alopecia areata is often associated with atopy and numerous autoimmune disorders, and is considered one of the manifestations of the polyglandular autoimmune syndrome. It is more common in females and is often associated with other autoimmune dermatoses, particularly vitiligo and Vogt-Koyanagi-Harada syndrome. Since C3 and occasionally IgM and IgG deposits are identified along the basement membrane zone and around the follicles, an autoimmune pathogenesis was suspected, but further studies showed these changes do not correspond to complement-mediated tissue reactions. The presence of C3, IgM, and IgG is generally thought to be a secondary event. In the acute stages of alopecia areata, early changes of the melanocytes in the hair bulb suggest that they may be the initial target of the immune reaction. Alopecia areata is also associated with pitted, dystrophic nails and ophthalmologic disorders including ptosis-miosis, enophthalmos, pigmentary abnormalities, and lens opacities (Gollnick and Orfanos, 1990).

Trichogram examination will show decreased numbers of anagen hairs, many of which are dystrophic, and increased numbers of telogen hairs. Confirmation of the diagnosis is based on biopsy results that show a normal epidermis with a marked inflammatory infiltrate composed of lymphocytes, macrophages, and occasional neutrophils located around the lower portions of the hair follicles. There are increased numbers of catagen and telogen hairs. Later stages show minimal inflammation with few normal follicles, since most have undergone marked atrophy. The progressive margins of alopecia areata lesions may show "exclamation mark hairs" as can be seen in other anagen-destructive diseases such as anagen defluxion (Scott, 1989). In humans, there is a marked peribulbar lymphocytic infiltrate commonly referred to as a "swarm of bees." The infiltrate is composed of small lymphocytes, large granular lymphocytes, and macrophages. The majority of lymphocytes are helper-inducer T cells. Melanophages are present at the original sites of the hair papillae and increased numbers of mast cells are found around fibrous tracts of the telogen hairs.

Little information is available on the treatment of alopecia areata. Dogs may spontaneously recover after 6 months to 2 years. The initial hair regrowth is often thin, in the center of lesions, and new hairs are usually unpigmented or lighter in color than normal. In humans, systemic steroid treatment leads to immediate repigmentaion of regrowing hairs. In humans, there is a good prognosis, as 30 to 50% of patients experience regrowth or complete restitution of their hair within the first 6 to 12 months after onset. There is a high relapse rate if treatment is discontinued (Gollnick and Orfanos, 1990). Treatment with systemic corticosteroids is frequently effective in inducing hair regrowth. Good to excellent results occur with intralesional steroid injections for circumscribed lesions. Psoralens with UVA light (PUVA) exposure and topical minoxidil have had moderate to excellent results and an investigational immunostimulant, inosiplex, has had excellent results. Most treatments are only temporarily successful (Mitchell and Krull, 1984).

## TRACTION ALOPECIA

Traction alopecia is a client- or groomer-induced condition caused by chronic, steady, excessive tension on numerous hairs in a specific area due to various hairstyling procedures including braiding, barrettes or rubber bands. It is seen in humans, and has been reported in four dogs (Rosenkrantz, Griffin, and Walder, 1989). In humans, it is usually a transitory alopecia unless marked follicular damage occurs. None of the affected dogs regrew hair. The clinical signs are complete alopecia involving a well-circumscribed area with otherwise normal looking skin. The patterns vary from circular, if a rubber band was used, to linear, if a barrette was used. The breeds involved were poodle, Maltese, Shih Tzu and Yorkshire terrier. Too few cases have been reported to ascertain any age or sex predilections. As is expected, the lesions are found on the head where hair retaining devices are used. The pathomechanism is unclear, although the current theory suggests that the continual tension on the hairs results in decreased blood supply to the hair bulb. The primary difference between the disease in dogs and humans is that the hair loss is usually temporary in humans. Rosenkrantz theorized that dogs may have anatomic vascular hair

bulb differences, may have the retaining devices left in place longer than in humans, and may not be able to communicate that the devices are too tight and painful, resulting in more significant damage.

Diagnosis is based on the findings of complete alopecia at an appropriate site with no evidence of inflammation with the history of use of a hair retaining device for prolonged periods. Confirmation of the diagnosis is by biopsy. The epidermis is normal and there is minimal dermal inflammation. Hair follicles are few in number, small, and are usually in telogen. They are devoid of hairs and may be filled with keratin. Fibrous tracts may be the only evidence of damaged hair follicles. Melanophages may inhabit the site of dermal papillae. A mild inflammatory infiltrate of macrophages, lymphocytes, and neutrophils may be present in more chronic lesions. There is no treatment to replace fibrotic follicles. It is critical to remove any hair retaining devices immediately, and to avoid their tight placement in the future. Surgery to remove the affected area should give good cosmetic results.

## POSTVACCINATION ALOPECIA AND PANNICULITIS

Recognition of postvaccination alopecia and panniculitis in dogs and cats has increased dramatically over the past 7 years, when it was first reported (Schmeitzel, Loeffler, and Bass, 1986). Several factors are likely to account for this. In 1985, the first rabies vaccine for subcutaneous administration was approved in the United States. In the late 1980s, Pennsylvania and other states enacted laws requiring the vaccination of all cats for rabies. Although rabies vaccine is implicated most often, other vaccines will produce identical reactions, and it is likely that any vaccine can cause this reaction. Clinically, a focal area of complete alopecia develops 4 to 12 weeks after vaccination. Initially the skin is thickened with variable erythema and scaling. Hyperpigmentation occurs at a later stage in some cases. Most lesions are 2 to 6 cm in diameter, although they have been reported to be as large as 10 cm. Sites include the dorsal neck and scapular area, the dorsal lumbar area, the flank, and the dorsolateral thorax. The lesions are usually neither pruritic nor painful. End-stage lesions have marked complete alopecia, with minimal to no increased thickness and no evidence of inflammation. In addition to the common causes of focal complete alopecia such as folliculitis, the differential diagnosis should include alopecia areata, anagen or telogen defluvium, and traction alopecia. In a recent search of biopsy samples received at the Surgical Pathology Laboratory at the University of Pennsylvania between 1988 and 1993, at least 51 dogs and 14 cats were identified with postvaccine alopecia or panniculitis. Fifteen were seen in miniature poodles, a breed previously identified at risk. Fourteen were identified in other small breeds and seven cases were seen in large-breed dogs. Fifteen cases occurred in mongrels. An additional four cases were seen with lesions compatible with, but not diagnostic of, postvaccine alopecia and panniculitis. The ages ranged from 5 months to 12 years and no sex predilections were evident. No age, breed, or sex predilections were noted in cats. Regional lymph nodes showed marked lymphoid hyperplasia in the few cases where they were biopsied. The pathomechanism of this reaction is unclear, although the histopathologic findings suggest an idiosyncratic hypersensitivity or immune-mediated process. The marked predisposition of miniature poodles suggests that genetic factors may play a role as well. The diagnosis is based on the dermatologic findings, historical evidence of a recent vaccination, and skin biopsy. Excisional biopsies are preferable to punch biopsies, since much of the reaction can be missed if superficial punch biopsies are taken. Typical findings include an alopecic, nodular, lymphocytic dermatitis with necrotizing panniculitis. The epidermis may be normal, although mild hyperkeratosis and acanthosis may be present. There may be basal cell vacuolation and lymphocytic infiltration into the epidermis. Hair follicles may be in telogen, severely atrophic, or destroyed. Melanin is engulfed by macrophages in the superficial dermis and in the deep dermis at the sites of previous hair bulbs and dermal papillae. The dermis may be mildly to severely myxomatous. The major reaction occurs in the deep dermis and the panniculus, with a marked, nodular lymphoplasmacytic infiltrate. The lymphoid infiltrate can be so marked as to form lymphoid follicles. Macrophages and neutrophils vary in number, but large numbers can be present. As the lesion progresses, multiple foci of necrosis and extensive fibroplasia develop. The panniculus is eventually replaced with a fine fibrillar connective tissue stroma. Deep muscle may undergo degenerative changes. Macrophages and giant cells may be present and may contain a gray-brown granular or crystalline material. It is likely that this material is aluminum from the adjuvant fraction of vaccines (see discussion below). Immunofluorescent testing with antibodies to rabies antigen shows positive deposits in dermal blood vessel walls and hair follicle epithelium of affected sites.

In addition to the primarily cosmetic problem of alopecia and panniculitis, there is a serious problem of increased risk of developing sarcomas at previous vaccine site reactions in cats. This association is not clear in the dog. Most patients present with fibrosarcomas, although myxofibrosarcomas, osteosarcomas, and giant cell sarcomas are also seen. Hendrick and others have presented convincing evidence supporting this association. They reported 437 feline fibrosarcomas at sites commonly used for vaccinations between 1987 and 1991. This included several cases that were "transitional," with granulomatous inflammation compatible with a postvaccinal reaction existing concomitantly with foci of sarcoma cells. There were also several cases of sarcomas that had arisen from sites of previous postvaccine alopecia and panniculitis, which had been confirmed on biopsies. In this same review, 101 of 198 (51%) of these fibrosarcomas had inflammatory cells composed of lymphocytes and macrophages surrounding and partially infiltrating the tumors. A "gray-brown granular to crystalline foreign material was found within macrophages in the inflammatory foci" in 42 out of these 198 biopsies. (Hendrick et al., 1992). This material was identified as aluminum, which is often used as an adjuvant in many vaccines. Aluminum may have an oncogenic effect to induce sarcomas, or it may only be a marker linking the fibrosarcoma to a previous vaccination site. Recently, vaccines that do not contain aluminum have been incriminated in causing postvaccinal sarcomas, implying that aluminum may not be a factor, or not the sole factor required to induce the sarcoma. Postvaccinal sarcomas frequently recur, so wide surgical excision is necessary. Metastasis is rare, but the lungs are the likely target if metastasis does occur. This situation brings up a host of questions concerning the administration of any vaccine. At this time, no one is advocating a change in vaccine protocols, pending further definition of the cause. However, it is advisable to keep accurate records of the vaccine type, lot number, manufacturer, and the specific location and depth (SC or IM) of administration of the vaccine. When administering more than one vaccine at a time, different locations should be used for each vaccine. Ideally, the same general site of the cat or dog should be used repeatedly for only one given vaccine in that patient. One suggestion is to use the right lumbar area for rabies, or the left lumbar area for DHLP-P or FVRCP each time these vaccines are administered over the patient's life. In this way, further information may show which vaccines are most likely to induce sarcomas. Otherwise, if rabies is given in one area one year and FVRCP in the same area the following year, it will be difficult to prove which vaccine was associated with a sarcoma arising at that site.

The treatment alternatives for postvaccination alopecia and panniculitis include waiting and watching versus surgical excision of the affected area. Because of the marked association of postvaccine alopecia/panniculitis in the cat and later development of fibrosarcomas, the author advises wide surgical excision of the affected area after the inflammation has subsided. Since this association is not clear in the dog, individual veterinarian and client preferences will dictate whether surgery or the wait-and-see approach is best. As further studies clarify the underlying etiology and incidence of occurrence of the alopecia, panniculitis, and sarcomas, more specific recommendations can be made.

## References and Suggested Reading

Gollnick H and Orfanos CE: Alopecia areata: Pathogenesis and clinical picture. *In* Orfanos CE and Happle R (eds.): *Hair and Hair Diseases.* New York, Springer-Verlag, 1990, p 529.
  *This chapter presents a detailed account of the history, epidemiology, associated diseases, pathomechanism, clinical presentation, and prognosis of human patients with alopecia areata.*
Hendrick MJ, Goldschmidt MH, Shofer FS, et al: Postvaccinal sarcomas in the cat: Epidemiology and electron probe microanalytical identification of aluminum. Cancer Res 52:5391, 1992.
  *This article presents statistical evidence supporting the association of feline sarcomas with prior vaccinations, by identifying aluminum from vaccine adjuvants in the tumors.*

Mitchell AJ and Krull EA: Alopecia areata: pathogenesis and treatment. J Am Acad Dermatol 11:763, 1984.
*This review article discusses the pathogenesis of alopecia areata and details a variety of treatment options in humans.*

Price VH: Structural anomalies of the hair shaft. In Orfanos CE and Happle R (eds): Hair and Hair Diseases. New York, Springer-Verlag, 1990, p 363.
*This chapter details trichodystrophies of humans including trichorrhexis invaginata, congenital and acquired trichorrhexis nodosa, and pili torti, with excellent electron photomicrographs.*

Rosenkrantz WS, Griffin CE, and Walder EF: Traction alopecia in the canine: Four case reports. Proc Am Acad Vet Dermatol/Am Coll Vet Dermatol 5:63, 1989.
*This is the original report of traction alopecia in veterinary medicine.*

Rosenkrantz WS: Alopecia in dogs and cats. Dermatol Rep 3:1, Squibb Animal Health Division, 1984.

*A practical approach to alopecia in dogs and cats, based on a diagnostic algorithm.*

Scott DW: The biology of hair growth and its disturbances. In Von Tscharner C and Halliwell REW (eds): Advances in Veterinary Dermatology, London, Bailliere Tindall, 1989, p 3.
*This is a comprehensive review of the ontogeny, histoanatomy, and biochemistry of hair, the hair cycle, and hair diseases in veterinary medicine.*

Schmeitzel LP, Loeffler D, and Bass MC: Focal cutaneous reactions at vaccination sites in a cat and four dogs. Proc Am Acad Vet Dermatol/Am Coll Vet Dermatol 2:39,1986.
*This report identifies postvaccination reactions in veterinary medicine and describes the clinical and histopathologic findings.*

# MANAGEMENT OF CHRONIC AND RECURRENT PYODERMA IN THE DOG

DOUGLAS J. DeBOER

*Madison, Wisconsin*

Staphylococcal skin infection (bacterial pyoderma) is an extremely common skin disorder of dogs. Such infections usually are easy to treat and respond readily to antibiotic administration. In a notable number of patients, the infection can become a chronic or recurrent problem. This article presents a guide to diagnostic tests and treatments particularly useful for managing dogs with recurring or chronic staphylococcal skin infection.

Essentially all staphylococcal skin infections in dogs are caused by *Staphylococcus intermedius*, a coagulase-positive species formerly classified as *S. aureus*. True *S. aureus*, though it is the principal pathogen of human skin, is almost never a cause of canine infections. Owners often inquire about the transmissibility of their pet's infection to human beings in the household. Because the bacterial species involved are distinct, pathogenic staphylococci do not easily pass between humans and dogs; human beings do not serve as a "reservoir" of staphylococci for canine infections and vice versa.

*Staphylococcus intermedius* is a common transient bacterium on the hair coat of dogs. Thus, potentially pathogenic staphylococci are usually present on all dogs' skin; these organisms merely await some trigger or additional cutaneous insult that will allow them to initiate an infection. The key to management of recurrent pyoderma is to identify this underlying insult and correct it.

## CLINICAL PRESENTATIONS OF CHRONIC AND RECURRENT PYODERMA

### Initial Classification

Several defined syndromes of recurrent pyoderma exist. Initially, it is useful to classify a dog with recurrent pyoderma by two criteria: whether the infection is primary or secondary, and the depth of involvement in the skin. *Primary recurrent pyodermas* occur in otherwise healthy skin with no apparent or definable underlying disease. *Secondary recurrent pyodermas*, which are much more common, occur secondary to another skin disease or secondary to an underlying internal medical problem.

The depth of involvement of pyoderma is classified as surface, superficial, or deep. *Surface pyodermas* consist of very superficial erosions of the skin, with *S. intermedius* principally colonizing the surface and not invading into the skin. The most familiar examples are mild versions of intertriginous (fold) pyodermas or early pyotraumatic dermatitis ("hot spot"). With *superficial pyoderma*, there is invasion of bacteria into the hair follicle (folliculitis) and/or microabscessation in the superficial epidermis (impetigo). This form appears grossly as papules, pustules, focal crusting, and epidermal collarettes, and represents the most common canine pyoderma seen in veterinary practice. If the bacterial infection extends to involve structures beyond and beneath the hair follicle, the disease is termed *deep pyoderma*. Deep pyoderma is recognized by the formation of ruptured hair follicles (furuncles), which appear as deep pustular to small nodular lesions that rupture and drain purulent or blood-tinged exudate. Deep infections require longer treatment and are more difficult to manage.

### Common Clinical Presentations of Recurrent Pyoderma

#### RECURRENT SURFACE PYODERMA

Certain breeds with prominent skin folds on the face, lips, base of the tail, vulvar area, or body (e.g., Pekinese, pug, English bulldog, springer spaniel, Chinese Shar-Pei) are predisposed to development of chronic or recurrent intertriginous dermatitis that is frequently secondarily infected with *S. intermedius*. In such cases, the underlying problem is clearly anatomic, and surgical correction to ablate the fold is the only hope of permanent cure. However, many such patients can be managed adequately with lifelong topical treatments.

### RECURRENT SUPERFICIAL PYODERMA

This most common form of recurrent pyoderma can occur in any age, breed, or sex of dog, and is characterized by recurrent episodes of papular to pustular eruption, with formation of multifocal crusts or epidermal collarettes as the lesions heal. Pruritus is usually present, and is often moderate to severe—thus leading some authors to postulate the role of "bacterial hypersensitivity" in this disease. Most recurrent superficial pyoderma is seen secondary to another underlying skin disease or internal medical problem. Some dogs with recurrent superficial pyoderma defy diagnosis, and are grouped under the term "idiopathic recurrent superficial pyoderma."

### RECURRENT DEEP PYODERMA

Less commonly, a dog will be presented with a complaint of recurring deep pyoderma. Nodules, furuncles, or draining tracts can be present at any location on the body, and can drain a purulent to bloody exudate in which staphylococci can be found on cytologic examination. Pruritus is often mild or absent. Some cases can be traced to an underlying disease. In the author's experience, recurrent deep pyoderma is the most common form of pyoderma associated with a documented defect in cell-mediated immunity.

### INTERDIGITAL FURUNCULOSIS

This disease is sometimes called "interdigital cysts," which is a misnomer because histologically the lesions are never actually cystic, but rather are large nodular areas of pyogranulomatous inflammation. Many cases of interdigital cysts are nothing more than deep staphylococcal pyoderma and will respond to vigorous antibiotic treatment. In some dogs the disease is incompletely responsive to antibiotics, and recurrences are frequent. The reasons for this are unclear. Some dermatologists believe that breeds with shorter, bristly hairs between the digits and/or prominent interdigital webs (such as the Labrador retriever or Chinese Shar-Pei) are predisposed to this disease because the short hair shafts are easily forced backwards into the follicles with locomotion (traumatic implantation), leading to a foreign-body reaction to the implanted hair and secondary deep pyoderma. Management as a recurrent deep pyoderma along with the use of antimicrobial foot soaks is appropriate initially. For severe cases, radical surgical correction via fusion podoplasty has been proposed.

### PRESSURE-POINT PYODERMA

Continuous trauma over a pressure point, most often the lateral elbow or hock joint, can create a callus that becomes secondarily involved with deep pyoderma. Traumatic implantation of hair shafts is also common in this area. The result is a chronic, low-grade infection of this thickened, traumatized skin. This condition often becomes a chronic management problem, because the underlying cause (i.e., physical trauma to the area) invariably persists.

### GERMAN SHEPHERD DOG PYODERMA

This syndrome is recognized in German shepherd dogs, and seems more common in dogs bred from European lines. Severe, chronic deep draining lesions are seen over the dorsal lumbosacral area and hind limbs. The often incomplete response of this disease to antibiotic treatment has led to speculation that it is more than merely a staphylococcal infection. One recent study suggested a T-lymphocyte dysfunction in affected dogs. This disease should be considered a clinical syndrome with multifactorial underlying etiologies, rather than a specific diagnosis. It can be caused by a variety of definable underlying diseases ranging from hypothyroidism to food allergy; some cases are truly idiopathic. European studies demonstrated that at least some form of the disease is familial, thus affected individuals should not be used for breeding stock. Initial management should be as a recurrent deep pyoderma, with an especially vigorous search for underlying causes. If antibiotics fail to provide adequate control of an idiopathic case, as an alternative to euthanasia, palliative treatment with corticosteroids can be considered along with lifelong administration of antibiotics.

### JUVENILE CELLULITIS

Mentioned here because of its frequent confusion with deep pyoderma, this condition of young puppies is not a bacterial infection. Typically, the disease occurs in a dog less than 16 weeks of age, and is manifested by an acute onset of severe swelling and deep draining lesions around the face, muzzle, and/or pinnae. The submandibular lymph nodes are enlarged, abscessed, and may rupture to the surface. The etiology is unknown, but the disease is not staphylococcal infection and is thus poorly (if at all) responsive to antibiotics. Because of the severe exudation, it is sometimes erroneously diagnosed as a chronic, unresponsive deep pyoderma. This disease is treated with corticosteroids at relatively high doses (e.g., prednisolone, 2 mg/kg/day

PO until the lesions resolve [10 to 14 days], then tapering the dose over an additional 2 to 4 weeks).

## UNDERLYING CAUSES OF CHRONIC AND RECURRENT PYODERMA IN DOGS

### Persisting Underlying or Coexisting Skin Disease

The most common cause of chronic or recurrent pyoderma in dogs is the persistence of an unidentified or untreated underlying disease condition. *This point cannot be overemphasized, and the clinician must be extremely diligent in pursuing any and all differential diagnoses of underlying diseases appropriate to the individual patient.* It seems that nearly any major or minor insult to a dog's skin can result in a secondary staphylococcal pyoderma. Some possible underlying diseases to consider in evaluating a dog with recurrent pyoderma are listed in Table 1.

### Bacterial Hypersensitivity

Many dogs with recurrent superficial pyoderma have erythematous, inflammatory, rapidly spreading, pruritic lesions that suggest an allergic reaction. Results of research studies incorporating histopathology, intradermal skin testing with staphylococcal antigens, and antistaphylococcal immunoglobulin E (IgE) quantitation suggest a hypersensitivity reaction to *Staphylococcus* bacteria in some dogs. Conclusive cause-and-effect evidence is lacking, and the role of "bacterial hypersensitivity" in the pathogenesis of recurrent superficial pyoderma remains controversial. Intradermal skin testing

**Table 1.** *Underlying or Concurrent Skin and Systemic Diseases Associated With Recurrent Pyoderma in Dogs*

| Category | Examples |
| --- | --- |
| Physical trauma | Maceration of skin by water (swimming) |
| | Trauma over a pressure point |
| External Parasitism | Fleas° |
| | Scabies |
| | Demodicosis |
| | Cheyletiellosis |
| Allergy | Flea allergy dermatitis° |
| | Atopy (allergic inhalant dermatitis)° |
| | Food allergy |
| Seborrheic disease | Primary seborrhea° |
| | Secondary seborrhea (e.g., with hypothyroidism) |
| Infections | Concurrent dermatophyte infection or deep mycosis |
| Endocrinopathy | Hypothyroidism |
| | Hyperadrenocorticism |
| Internal disorders | Early or subclinical major organ dysfunction |
| | Occult neoplasia |

°Especially common causes.

with staphylococcal antigens, or *in vitro* determinations of antistaphylococcal IgE by enzyme-linked immunosorbent assay (ELISA) or radioallergosorbent (RAST) methods are of little practical value in diagnostic evaluation of recurrent pyoderma.

### Immunodeficiency

Only rarely do dogs with recurrent pyoderma have histories of multiple infections in other organs. This suggests that a primary, general state of immunodeficiency is exceptionally rare as a cause of recurrent pyoderma. The author has encountered a few dogs with apparent cellular immune dysfunction that could be documented via a lymphocyte blastogenesis test. These dogs have usually presented with recurrent deep pyoderma. There are a few reports of dogs with severe circulating IgA deficiency, resulting in recurrent respiratory and skin infections. The relationship between serum IgA and recurrent staphylococcal infection is currently an area of controversy. Available evidence suggests that serum IgA may be below normal reference ranges in a variety of canine dermatoses, including parasitic infestation, allergy, and pyoderma, and thus low serum IgA is a nonspecific finding. Thus, the value of serum IgA determination in diagnostic evaluation of canine pyoderma is questionable at present.

### Resistant *Staphylococcus* Strain

The *least* common cause of chronic, recurring pyoderma is a staphylococcal organism that is resistant to all commonly used antibiotics. It is the author's opinion and experience that bacterial resistance is greatly overdiagnosed as a cause of recurrent pyoderma. Certainly, staphylococci regularly and easily acquire resistance to many antibiotics with repeated treatment. However, even with prolonged treatment, *S. intermedius* strains from canine skin have shown a remarkable lack of propensity to develop resistance to antibiotics such as the cephalosporins (e.g., cephalexin) and penicillinase-resistant penicillins (e.g., oxacillin).

### Nonstaphylococcal Pyoderma

Occasionally, a nonstaphylococcal organism will be cultured from a canine pyoderma lesion, usually along with *S. intermedius*. In most cases, this organism represents inconsequential secondary infection or contamination from the environment during sampling, especially if the organism is cultured in low numbers. In these cases, treating with an antibiotic based only on the sensitivity pattern of the *S. intermedius* is generally successful. Very rarely, primary recurrent pyoderma caused by *Pseudomonas* or *Proteus* is seen, and the response to antibiotics used for treating staphylococcal pyoderma is poor. It is helpful to perform cytologic examination of stained smears of the purulent material—the finding of numerous rod-like organisms is highly unusual and should prompt the clinician to consider a primary pathogen other than *Staphylococcus*.

## Nonbacterial Pustular Dermatoses

There are a few uncommon to rare diseases that produce pustular lesions that are not staphylococcal pyoderma. The following such diseases should be considered as differential diagnoses in a chronic or recurrent case: pemphigus foliaceus, sterile eosinophilic pustulosis, subcorneal pustular dermatosis, and pustular drug eruptions. Occasionally, dermatophytosis can present with pustular lesions as well.

## MANAGEMENT OF CHRONIC OR RECURRENT PYODERMA

### Aggressive Evaluation for Underlying Causes

Initial management of a dog with recurrent pyoderma consists of an aggressive search for definable underlying causes (Table 1). If exhaustive evaluation fails to reveal a cause, then a diagnosis of "idiopathic recurrent pyoderma" can be made. A key question in the evaluation is, "*What is the dog's response to vigorous treatment with antibiotics alone?*" This single question is extremely helpful in planning a logical series of diagnostic tests for the individual patient. If the veterinarian has not observed the answer to this question firsthand, the first and most valuable "diagnostic test" to perform is to treat the dog with an appropriate antibiotic for a long enough period of time, excluding all corticosteroid medication, and observe the results. Based on the response to antibiotic treatment, make a list of the most likely underlying differential diagnoses, then formulate a testing plan based on this list. The response patterns of recurrent pyoderma to antibiotics tend to fall into four categories:

1. *Complete clinical response* to antibiotics (neither lesions nor pruritus remaining as long as the dog receives antibiotics) suggests the pyoderma may be secondary to an underlying cause that is not pruritic. Underlying systemic diseases that interfere with immune function, such as hypothyroidism, hyperadrenocorticism, subclinical organ dysfunction, or occult neoplasia should be considered especially in older animals. In younger animals, this response may be seen in early atopic dogs.

2. *Partial clinical response* to antibiotics, with disappearance of all lesions but pruritus remaining suggests that the recurrent pyoderma is secondary to a pruritic disease that produces no lesions by itself. Here, allergic diseases such as atopy or food allergy should be given first consideration in the testing plan.

3. *Partial clinical response* to antibiotics, with some

lesions and pruritus remaining, suggests that recurrence may be related to an underlying, pruritic, lesion-producing disease such as external parasitism, dermatophytosis, or primary seborrhea. Allergy is a possible but less likely cause.

4. *Little or no response* to antibiotics suggests failure of the client to administer medications properly, an antibiotic-resistant bacterium, or a nonbacterial pustular disease. In such cases, bacterial culture and sensitivity and skin biopsy are most valuable.

### Indications for Immunologic Tests

Dogs with recurrent pyoderma frequently are referred to a university practice for evaluation of the immune system. With our current state of knowledge, *the advisability or cost-effectiveness of an "immunologic work-up" is questionable* on a number of grounds. First, documentable immunodeficiency is an uncommon cause of recurrent pyoderma. Second, there are dozens—perhaps hundreds—of individual components that together constitute the entire immune response, and only a very few of these can be measured. Thus, our ability to assess a dog's immunocompetence with laboratory tests is extremely limited, even in university practices with extensive laboratory facilities. Third, these tests are often unavailable to veterinarians in general practice, and even if available are rather expensive. Fourth, even if we are able to document a specific immunodeficiency in a dog, we have only a very few, poorly researched specific treatments to correct these defects. Nevertheless, if a veterinarian does desire to pursue immune dysfunction as a cause of recurrent pyoderma, the following tests could be considered.

#### SERUM IMMUNOGLOBULIN QUANTITATION

These tests are quantitative evaluations of total serum concentrations of IgG, IgA, and IgM, and usually are performed using a radial immunodiffusion method. The results of these tests can vary significantly from laboratory to laboratory, depending on the technique and the manufacturer of the assay plate. Thus, it is critical that any values obtained be compared only to reference ranges from the same laboratory.

#### COMPLETE BLOOD COUNT

Though not specifically a measure of immune function, some authors have found value in examination of the total lymphocyte count. If the total count is below $1000/mm^3$, repeat the test. If this lymphopenia is repeatable, and there is no other explanation for it (e.g., hyperadrenocorticism, stress, viral infection), this may be an indication of lymphocyte dysfunction.

#### LYMPHOCYTE BLASTOGENESIS TEST

Here, the patient's lymphocytes are isolated and cultured for several days in the presence of mitogenic substances such as phytohemagglutinin (PHA). In healthy animals, PHA will stimulate lymphocytes to undergo blast transformation and begin synthesis of deoxyribonucleic acid (DNA). As DNA synthesis proceeds, radioactive DNA precursors added to the culture medium are incorporated into the cells and measured. Despite the relatively complicated reagents and equipment necessary to perform this test, it is at best a crude measure of lymphocyte function and is subject to numerous technical difficulties. Because of equipment requirements and the fact that the blood sample must be processed within hours of collection, it is generally offered only by university laboratories.

### NEUTROPHIL FUNCTION TESTS

Standard immunologic tests such as phagocytosis assays or bactericidal assays (e.g., nitroblue tetrazolium reduction test) are occasionally offered by university laboratories, but have received extremely little study as far as their usefulness in diagnosis of canine pyoderma.

### OTHER "IMMUNE PANEL" TESTS

Other immunologic tests relating primarily to autoimmune disease (e.g., antinuclear antibody, rheumatoid factor, Coombs' test) are of no value in diagnosis of recurrent pyoderma.

## Initial Treatment of Recurrent Pyoderma

### ANTIBIOTIC CHOICES

The cornerstone of initial treatment of an episode of recurrent pyoderma is administration of a systemic antibiotic for a sufficient length of time. Antibiotics ideally should be chosen for each patient based on culture and sensitivity testing. However, potential adverse drug effects, likelihood of development of bacterial resistance, and cost are also considerations. For convenience, the practitioner can consider antibiotics for treatment of pyoderma to fall into four categories:

1. *Useless antibiotics* are those with little or no activity against most strains of *S. intermedius*. This group includes penicillin, ampicillin, amoxicillin, hetacillin, nonpotentiated sulfa drugs, and the tetracyclines.

2. *"First-line" antibiotics* are good choices for initial treatment of many cases of pyoderma; however, from 10 to 30% of staphylococcal strains are resistant. Moreover, resistance commonly develops to these antibiotics with prolonged or multiple-course use; thus, they are often unsuitable for chronic cases. Examples (all given orally) include trimethoprim-sulfadiazine (Tribrissen, Coopers), 30 mg/kg every 12 hr; erythromycin, 10 to 15 mg/kg every 8 hr; lincomycin (Lincocin, Upjohn), 20 mg/kg every 12 hr; chloramphenicol, 25 mg/kg every 8 hr; clindamycin (Antirobe, Upjohn), 5

mg/kg every 12 hr; and ormetoprim-sulfadimethoxine (Primor, Roche), 27 mg/kg/day.*

3. *Excellent antibiotics* are efficacious against all or nearly all strains of *S. intermedius* and have relatively infrequent adverse effects. Resistance does not commonly develop to this group, even with prolonged use, making them more useful in chronic cases. All are more expensive than most other choices. Examples (all given orally) include oxacillin, 20 mg/kg every 8 hr; cephalexin, 20 mg/kg every 8 to 12 hr; and amoxicillin-clavulanic acid (Clavamox, SmithKline Beecham), 20 mg/kg every 8 hr. Note that the dose of the latter drug is higher than that recommended by the manufacturer. In the author's experience, a significant number of dogs with pyoderma fail to resolve completely using the label-specified dose.

4. *Effective but usually unnecessary antibiotics* are generally efficacious against *S. intermedius* pyoderma. However, they have some drawback that makes their use less desirable for chronic pyoderma. For example, most *S. intermedius* strains are susceptible to aminoglycoside antibiotics (gentamicin or amikacin), but their parenteral route of administration and nephrotoxicity make such antibiotics unsuitable for treating pyoderma. Fluoroquinolones such as enrofloxacin (Baytril, Miles) or ciprofloxacin (Cipro, Miles) are also efficacious in canine pyoderma. However, they cannot be used in immature dogs because of potential toxicity, and bacterial resistance develops with prolonged use. Fluoroquinolones are extremely valuable for treatment of serious infections with aggressive pathogens such as *Pseudomonas* and should be reserved for such use; there is currently abundant concern in human medicine regarding overuse of these drugs leading to emergence of resistant strains.

### LENGTH OF INITIAL TREATMENT

An episode of recurring pyoderma initially should be treated for 2 weeks past the point of clinical normalcy. For most recurrent superficial pyodermas, a 3- to 4-week course should suffice. Deep pyoderma often requires antibiotic treatment for 6 to 10 weeks. Failure to treat pyoderma with antibiotics for a long enough period of time is a common mistake.

### DO NOT USE CORTICOSTEROIDS

Concurrent corticosteroid treatment should be avoided in all cases of recurrent staphylococcal pyoderma. There is no physiologic rationale for use of glucocorticoids in a recurrent bacterial infection, and such use may lead to interference with normal immunologic clearance of the organism and persistence of the infection. If glucocorticoids become "necessary" to keep a patient with recurrent staphylococcal pyoderma under control, this is a very strong indication that an uniden-

---

*See page 595 for cautions on long-time, high-dose use of sulfonamides, which may produce iatrogenic hypothyroidism.

tified underlying cause for the recurrence is present and should prompt renewed diagnostic investigation.

### ADJUNCT TOPICAL TREATMENT

SHAMPOOS. Topical treatment with antibacterial shampoos helps with initial resolution of an episode of recurrent pyoderma. Such treatment also aids in prevention of relapse by limiting the bacterial counts on the skin surface. Because the residual action of available shampoos is less than 1 week, frequent shampooing is necessary—twice weekly until the infection is clear, then once weekly thereafter as a maintenance treatment. It is wisest to choose a product with good residual action, yet with minimal drying or irritating effects. Useful products include 0.5% chlorhexidine (Nolvasan, Fort Dodge; ChlorHexiderm, DVM) or 2% benzoyl peroxide with a moisturizing additive (MicroPearls, Evsco; OxyDex, DVM). Iodine-based products are less satisfactory.

CREAMS OR OINTMENTS. Most topical antibiotic products have poor efficacy against *S. intermedius* and often contain a corticosteroid, which may be undesirable. A useful topical antibiotic is 2% mupirocin ointment (Bactoderm, Beecham). This product is just as effective as systemic antibiotics in resolving localized staphylococcal pyoderma in humans. The author has found this product very valuable and well tolerated for long-term management of localized surface or superficial pyodermas, such as fold pyodermas. The cream is applied twice daily until resolution of the infection, then once every 1 or 2 days as needed to prevent relapse.

## Long-Term Management of Recurrent Pyoderma

### CLIENT COUNSELING

Recurrent pyoderma is usually a lifelong disease, and it is necessary to devise a long-term control program acceptable to the owner. To facilitate compliance and minimize client frustration, owners should be informed of the following facts about recurrent pyoderma: (1) permanent cure is rarely achieved; (2) lifelong treatment will likely be necessary; (3) if the disease begins in an immature dog, an occasional patient will appear to outgrow the tendency for recurrence at maturity (1 to 1.5 years of age); and (4) if the disease begins in an older dog, an underlying systemic cause (e.g., occult neoplasia) may eventually manifest itself so the owner must watch for any change that points to emergence of a definable cause.

### IMMUNOMODULATORY DRUGS

The evidence for efficacy of immunomodulatory drugs such as levamisole or cimetidine in canine recurrent pyoderma is very thin, and entirely anecdotal. Controlled trials documenting the efficacy of such drugs in dogs—even *in vitro*—have not been done,

and most veterinary dermatologists have been unimpressed by their usefulness. In some individuals and species, *levamisole* will restore defective T-lymphocyte function and numbers, but will not stimulate normally functioning lymphocytes beyond their normal function. Thus, a trial of levamisole should be contemplated only in documented instances of lymphocyte dysfunction (e.g., an abnormal lymphocyte blastogenesis test or a persistently low lymphocyte count). The most commonly listed dose is 2.2 mg/kg PO, three times weekly. Doses above or below this amount may be immunosuppressive. The available food animal deworming tablet (182 mg) is too large for many dogs; the injectable liquid (13 to 14% = 130 to 140 mg/ml) may be used orally for smaller animals. Adverse effects of ataxia, gastrointestinal disturbances, and cutaneous drug eruptions have been reported. *Cimetidine* theoretically blocks $H_2$ receptors on suppressor T lymphocytes, reducing their suppressive activities. Its effectiveness in dogs has not been documented; however, isolated case reports and clinical reviews advocate a dose of 3 to 4 mg/kg, every 12 hr, PO, for at least 10 weeks past remission of the pyoderma.

### IMMUNOMODULATORY BACTERINS

Immunomodulatory bacterins are an aid in long-term management of recurrent pyoderma, and their efficacy in dogs has been documented in a number of studies. Their major effect is *not* to cure an existing, active episode of relapse, but rather to prevent or delay additional relapses once the active episode has been cured with antibiotics. These bacterins have multiple modes of action under experimental conditions; the actions responsible for efficacy in canine pyoderma are not known. Overall, the author's experience is that about 30 to 50% of dogs with recurrent pyoderma will ultimately benefit from bacterin treatment. Although immunomodulatory bacterins often must be administered as lifelong maintenance treatments, their cost and potential adverse effects are less than with continuous antibiotic administration.

STAPHYLOCOCCUS PHAGE LYSATE (SPL, DELMONT LABORATORIES). SPL is a bacterin prepared by bacteriophage lysis of human-origin *Staphylococcus aureus* bacteria. It is the only commercially available staphylococcal bacterin licensed for use in dogs, and is the author's preferred product. SPL treatment is effective in up to 70% of dogs with idiopathic recurrent superficial pyoderma; it has not been critically evaluated in deep pyoderma. A suggested protocol is given in Table 2. Reported adverse effects are rare.

PROPIONIBACTERIUM ACNES BACTERIN (IMMUNOREGULIN, IMMUNOVET). Prepared from killed *P. acnes* organisms, this bacterin is licensed for use in canine pyoderma, and evidence suggests it may be of benefit as an adjunct treatment in chronic cases. It is administered once to twice weekly, at a dosage of 0.25 to 2 ml, IV, depending on body weight. Anecdotal evidence suggests that if response occurs, it will be seen within 3 months.

**Table 2.** *Protocol for Treatment of Recurrent Pyoderma with SPL*

1. Treat with an effective oral antibiotic for 6 weeks.
2. Concurrently, begin treatment with 0.5 ml SPL, SC twice weekly. Owners are quite capable of administering SPL at home after proper instruction. SPL must be kept refrigerated.
3. After the 6-week course of antibiotics, continue SPL alone.
4. Allow a trial period of 10 to 14 weeks of SPL administration. Patients who do not respond in this time are unlikely to improve with continued SPL treatment.
5. Favorable responses to SPL will be manifested by lack of recurrence of the pyoderma, a substantial lengthening of intervals between relapses, or much milder relapses that are controlled by continued SPL injection or by briefer (2 to 3 weeks) courses of antibiotic treatment.

BOVINE MASTITIS BACTERINS. These products (Staphoid AB, Wellcome; Lysigin, BioCeutic) have been advocated for treatment of recurrent pyoderma in dogs. Their relatively common adverse effects (local swelling at injection site, malaise), lack of documented efficacy, and the availability of alternative efficacious products licensed for dogs should preclude their use for canine pyoderma.

AUTOGENOUS VACCINES. Autogenous vaccines are bacterins "custom-made" from bacteria isolated from an individual patient. No critical evaluation of their usefulness in canine pyoderma has been undertaken. In the author's experience, autogenous bacterins do appear to help some dogs, but adverse reactions (as for bovine mastitis products) are common. Practically, it is difficult to find a commercial laboratory willing to prepare an autogenous vaccine for administration to canine patients.

STAPHYLOCOCCUS INTERMEDIUS LYSATE. A product similar to SPL but prepared from strains of *S. intermedius* isolated from dogs is under development at the time of this writing. Theoretically, such a product would have the advantage of containing bacterial antigens that are more similar to canine pathogens than other, *S. aureus*–based products.

### LONG-TERM USE OF ANTIBIOTICS

Extended administration of antibiotics will maintain remission in many dogs with recurrent pyoderma. This treatment has several important drawbacks, including increased risk of adverse drug effects, induction of antibiotic resistance in the patient, promotion and dissemination of antibiotic-resistant staphylococci, and generally high cost. Long-term antibiotic use thus should be considered only after all other treatment modalities have failed, as an alternative to euthanasia.

Prolonged antibiotic treatment carries an increased risk of adverse drug effects ranging from annoying to life threatening. Inadvertent changes in the normal gastrointestinal flora or direct gastrointestinal irritation from the drug can lead to vomiting or diarrhea. Anaphylactic reactions to an orally administered antibiotic are possible but rare. There is also the possibility of an antibiotic-related cutaneous drug eruption, which can be as mild as a papular or pustular eruption or as severe as the often-fatal syndromes of erythema multiforme and toxic epidermal necrolysis.

Extended use of antibiotics, especially at subtherapeutic doses, exerts selection pressure on bacterial populations and promotes emergence of antibiotic-resistant strains. There is abundant concern on this topic in the medical literature, as similar experience in humans has led to appearance of infections with highly resistant pathogens that can be difficult or impossible to treat. Veterinarians have an ethical responsibility to help avoid a worsening of this phenomenon by prudent antibiotic use.

If long-term antibiotic use becomes necessary for recurrent pyoderma, two treatment regimens are possible. *Pulse therapy* is the best protocol to try initially, because in theory it will minimize the chances of the bacterium becoming antibiotic resistant. In this protocol, once the recurrent episode is clear, antibiotics are given at the full therapeutic dose, but only every other week. If remission is maintained for 2 months, extend the antibiotic-free period to 2 weeks ("1 week on, 2 weeks off"). Thereafter, as long as the dog remains in remission, the antibiotic free period can be gradually increased until control is no longer satisfactory. Most dogs with recurrent pyoderma cannot remain antibiotic free for more than 3 weeks without losing control of the disease. If pulse therapy proves unsatisfactory, *continuous low-dose therapy* can be attempted. With this protocol, a single dose of oral antibiotic is administered once daily, indefinitely, at approximately one half to one third of the usual *total* daily therapeutic dose.

Antibiotic selection is critical if extended antibiotic regimens are used. *S. intermedius* usually becomes resistant to the "first-line" antibiotics (see above) within several months of their use. The possibility of adverse effects such as keratoconjunctivitis sicca with sulfa-based drugs makes these drugs unsuitable for chronic use. Penicillinase-resistant penicillins (e.g., oxacillin) or cephalosporins are good choices, because both development of resistance and adverse effects are uncommon.

# CANINE MUCOCUTANEOUS PYODERMA

PETER J. IHRKE

*Davis, California*

*and* THELMA LEE GROSS

*West Sacramento, California*

Canine mucocutaneous pyoderma is an uncommon to rare syndrome characterized by erythema, swelling, and crusting of the mucocutaneous junctions. The syndrome most frequently involves the lips and perioral skin but occasionally affects other mucocutaneous junctions such as the vulva, prepuce, and anus. Although response to antibacterial therapy supports a bacterial role in the disorder, predisposing or initiating factors are not known. Relapses are common after initially successful therapy.

## CLINICAL FEATURES

Historically, the syndrome is gradual in onset. Erythema and swelling precede crusting. Bilateral symmetry is common in lip and perioral lesions. Affected lips are markedly erythematous and uniformly swollen. The lateral commissures usually are affected. Crusting is especially evident entrapping hairs at mucocutaneous junctions. Depigmentation of the lips is uncommon in early cases but may be noted with chronicity. Fissuring and erosions with adherent crusting may occur in more severe cases. Salivary staining is present ventral to the lip lesions, and exudate may mat the hair surrounding the lesions. The mucocutaneous junction of one naris or both nares may be affected. Bilateral symmetry is not seen in lesions involving the nares. Similar lesions less commonly affect the vulva, prepuce, or anus.

Rubbing is reported frequently by owners, inferring pruritus or pain. Afflicted dogs resent palpation and examination of the lips. Lesions may be mildly malodorous but odor is not as striking as that of lip-fold intertrigo. Regional lymphadenopathy may be present.

The lesions of mucocutaneous pyoderma do not originate in folded skin. The syndrome is distinct clinically from lip-fold pyoderma or other intertrigo. However, perioral mucocutaneous pyoderma may precede or coexist with lip-fold pyoderma.

Age or sex signalment predilections have not been noted. German shepherd dogs and their related crossbreeds may be affected more frequently.

## DIAGNOSIS

Canine mucocutaneous pyoderma involving the lips and perioral skin is visually distinctive. Possible differential diagnoses include discoid lupus erythematosus, lip-fold pyoderma, demodicosis, zinc-responsive dermatosis, and canine acne.

Clinically, mucocutaneous pyoderma primarily affecting the lips or the nares may most closely mimic discoid lupus erythematosus. However, partially symmetric lesions involving the dorsal muzzle and the planum nasale usually are present in discoid lupus erythematosus. Although erythema, crusting, and depigmentation may be similar in these two diseases, the distinctive swelling of the lips seen with mucocutaneous pyoderma is not a clinical feature of canine discoid lupus erythematosus.

In contrast to mucocutaneous pyoderma, lip-fold pyoderma develops in and usually is confined to the deep triangular fold on either side of the lower lip. Spaniels are at markedly increased risk for the development of lip-fold pyoderma.

Perioral, localized demodicosis may appear casually similar to mucocutaneous pyoderma, but the lips are not involved. Demodicosis is seen predominately in young dogs and usually has a relatively rapid onset. Demodicosis should be ruled out by multiple, deep skin scrapings.

Zinc-responsive dermatosis is characterized clinically by scaling, crusting, and alopecia of the perioral skin, vulva, and the perianal area, as seen in mucocutaneous pyoderma. However, periorbital lesions are common in zinc-responsive dermatosis and absent in mucocutaneous pyoderma. Zinc-responsive dermatosis is seen predominantly in Siberian huskies and Alaskan malamutes.

Canine acne is a common skin disease of young dogs characterized by the formation of comedones; crusted papules; and pustules on the chin, lips, and adjacent skin. Although the distribution can be similar to mucocutaneous pyoderma, pustules usually are obvious in canine acne. Canine acne is seen most frequently in short-coated breeds. The onset of canine acne coincides with puberty and commonly resolves spontaneously after puberty.

Skin biopsy may be necessary to achieve a definitive diagnosis. In addition to routine histopathology, direct immunofluorescent or immunohistochemical testing may be useful in differentiating mucocutaneous pyoderma from histologically similar discoid lupus erythematosus.

Histopathologically, mucocutaneous pyoderma is characterized by a hyperplastic epidermis with superficial pustulation and crusting. Erosion or ulceration may be present. A dense, lichenoid band of superficial inflammation composed predominantly of plasma cells with admixtures of lymphocytes, neutrophils, and macrophages is present in the dermis. Although the inflammatory infiltrate closely approximates the overlying epidermis, the dermal-epidermal interface is not obscured. Similar but milder inflammation may surround subjacent adnexal appendages in specimens taken from haired skin at mucocutaneous junctions.

## CLINICAL MANAGEMENT

Canine mucocutaneous pyoderma responds readily to topical or systemic antibacterial therapy, but long-term clinical management may be problematic, since recrudescence is common.

Gently clipping the hair away from the lips prevents the retention of secretions matting the surrounding hair. Topical antibacterial shampoos containing benzoyl peroxide (OxyDex, DVM Pharmaceuticals; Pyoben, Allerderm) or benzoyl peroxide and sulfur (Sulf OxyDex, DVM Pharmaceuticals) are beneficial. The affected area is cleansed gently daily for the initial 2 weeks. After the lesions are patted dry, a 2% mupirocin ointment (Bactoderm, SmithKline Beecham) is applied sparingly to the lesions. This hydrating, ointment-based product has been more successful therapeutically than either antibiotic creams or benzoyl peroxide gels. After 2 weeks of daily therapy, the cleansing and application of topical antibiotics can be decreased to twice weekly and sometimes weekly therapy. More severe cases benefit from systemic antibiotics administered during the first 3 to 4 weeks of topical therapy. Antibiotics useful in the management of canine pyoderma such as erythromycin, lincomycin (Lincocin, Upjohn), ormetoprim-sulfadimethoxine (Primor, Roche), trimethoprim-potentiated sulfonamides, or cephalexin may be used.

When all lesions have resolved (usually 3 or 4 weeks), therapy may be discontinued. Recrudescence is common; some dogs require long-term maintenance therapy with benzoyl peroxide shampoos and mupirocin ointment. Occasionally, systemic antibiotics may be indicated for severe reoccurrences.

## Reference and Suggested Reading

Gross TL, Ihrke PJ, and Walder EJ: *Veterinary Dermatopathology: A Macroscopic and Microscopic Evaluation of Canine and Feline Skin Disease.* St. Louis, Mosby Year Book, 1992, pp 141–143.

# THE DIAGNOSIS OF SEBACEOUS ADENITIS IN STANDARD POODLE DOGS

ROBERT W. DUNSTAN

*East Lansing, Michigan*

*and* ANN M. HARGIS

*Edmonds, Washington*

The term "sebaceous adenitis" is applied to a presumptive group of diseases with the cardinal histologic feature of an inflammatory reaction directed primarily against sebaceous glands. Although sebaceous adenitis has been recognized in many breeds of dogs (Table 1) and in cats and humans in North America, the disease is most frequently diagnosed in standard poodles. Recently, there has been a major effort on the part of breeders and veterinarians to better understand and decrease the prevalence of standard poodle sebaceous adenitis. Although the hope is that knowledge gained from standard poodles will be applicable to sebaceous

**Table 1.** *Canine Breeds in Which Sebaceous Adenitis Has Been Identified*

| | | |
|---|---|---|
| Airedale | Hovawart | Samoyed |
| Akita | Irish setter | Scottish terrier |
| American Eskimo | Labrador retriever | Shih Tzu |
| Cocker spaniel | Lhasa apso | Springer spaniel |
| Collie | Maltese | Saint Bernard |
| Dachshund | Miniature pinscher | Standard poodle |
| Dalmation | Miniature poodle | Toy poodle |
| Doberman pinscher | Mixed breeds | Vizsla |
| German shepherd | Old English sheepdog | Weimeraner |
| Golden retriever | Pomeranian | |

adenitis in other breeds, because of interbreed variability in the histologic features as well as the severity and distribution of clinical lesions, it is premature to utilize standard poodle sebaceous adenitis as a template for this disease.

The purpose of this report is fourfold: (1) to characterize the clinical and histologic features of standard poodle sebaceous adenitis, (2) to define the heritable nature of the disease, (3) to discuss what is known about its pathogenesis, and (4) to describe the Sebaceous Adenitis Registry for standard poodles.

## CLINICAL AND HISTOLOGIC FEATURES

### Clinical Features

Sebaceous adenitis in standard poodles is a disease of marked variability in its clinical severity. In the most typical presentation of the disease there is dry, scaly skin with patchy zones of alopecia of mild to moderate severity involving the dorsal trunk and neck, top of the head, and ear pinna. A characteristic feature is that scales are tightly adhered to hair shafts. Hairs may be dull and brittle and often have a brown to red tint. Infrequently, a secondary staphylococcal pyoderma may develop. In more severely affected dogs, lesions can be much more extensive (i.e., the hair loss may be so diffuse and symmetric that an endocrinopathy is suggested and/or there may be hyperkeratotic plaques). Dogs with severe hyperkeratosis often have a "seborrheic" odor. In contrast, mildly affected dogs can have such subtle lesions that the disease is extremely difficult to detect clinically. In our experience, the mildest forms of standard poodle sebaceous adenitis can only be recognized by microscopic evaluation of a skin biopsy sample. We define such dogs as subclinically affected. Standard poodle sebaceous adenitis has no sex or coat color predilection. In approximately 90% of standard poodles, clinical lesions are first recognized between 1.5 and 5 years.

### Histologic Characteristics

As with all inflammatory diseases, standard poodle sebaceous adenitis goes through early, fully developed, and late phases. The early phase consists of a mild perifolliculitis centered at the follicular isthmus (the midregion of the hair follicle) with involvement of the sebaceous duct. In the fully developed phase, the inflammation intensifies and is associated with a nodular granulomatous inflammatory reaction at the level of the sebaceous gland. The disease progresses into the late stage after the sebaceous gland is destroyed. Once this occurs, the inflammation diminishes and there is a region of perifollicular fibrosis (i.e., a scar), which is most prominent at the level of the follicular isthmus. Late lesions are often accompanied by keratin plugging of follicular infundibula. Hyperkeratosis is a variable feature. Based on sequential biopsies of dogs bred to

develop the disease, progression from early to late stages takes several months.

In standard poodles with clinically recognizable lesions, there is good correlation with the histologic changes. Dogs with more severe scales have more pronounced hyperkeratosis and those with more severe hair loss have a more intense and diffuse inflammatory reaction that resolves with more prominent scarring. However, histologic evaluation of skin biopsy specimens from clinically normal standard poodles, mainly from kennels in which the disease has occurred, defines a population of subclinically affected dogs in which only an occasional sebaceous gland in a 6-mm punch biopsy may have the histologic changes characteristic of sebaceous adenitis. Over 25% of standard poodles diagnosed with sebaceous adenitis may have this subclinical form. Follow-up of these dogs has indicated that a small number will develop an overt form of the disease but most remain clinically normal. Thus, microscopic examination of haired skin is extremely accurate in diagnosing dogs with clinical disease; however, in standard poodles with a normal hair coat, histologic lesions that would allow for the diagnosis of subclinical sebaceous adenitis can be so infrequent that they may not be identified in a given skin biopsy specimen. For this reason, it is very difficult to ever state a standard poodle is "normal" by microscopic examination of skin biopsies.

## HERITABILITY OF STANDARD POODLE SEBACEOUS ADENITIS

Based on pedigree analysis, there is no doubt that sebaceous adenitis in standard poodles is a genetic disease. This same analysis suggests the disease is autosomal recessive; however, because of the variability of clinical signs and the difficulty in calling a dog "normal," breeding studies (now in progress) need to be analyzed for confirmation of the mode of inheritance. What is known is that breeding subclinically affected standard poodles offers the same risk of producing offspring with the disease as breeding dogs with overt sebaceous adenitis, indicating that subclinically affected standard poodles are not carriers but actually have a mild form of the disease. That subclinical dogs apparently have the same genotype as overtly affected standard poodles explains why sebaceous adenitis has become such a frequently recognized disease in this breed.

## PATHOGENESIS

The triggering events responsible for the development of sebaceous adenitis in standard poodles are unknown. Theories concerning etiology include an autoimmune reaction to sebaceous gland antigens or a primary structural defect in sebaceous glands or ducts that results in leakage of sebum and subsequent development of a foreign body inflammatory response that destroys the sebaceous glands. The two major clinical characteristics of sebaceous adenitis in this breed, scaly skin and hair loss, appear to be sequela to the loss of sebaceous gland lipids and perifollicular fibrosis, respectively. Sebaceous secretions are believed to be important in preventing excessive water loss through the skin. Presumably, a decrease in sebaceous secretions results in drying of the stratum corneum, especially in the follicular infundibulum, resulting in the keratin aggregating around hair shafts. Sebaceous adenitis is not the only disease in which an inability to produce sebum is associated with scaly skin. Similar lesions are identified in asebia, a mouse mutation in which sebaceous glands fail to develop. That alopecia is a feature of sebaceous adenitis in standard poodles can be attributed in part to the perifollicular fibrosis that may cause decreased function of stem cells located in the region of the fibrotic reaction. Alopecia of standard poodle sebaceous adenitis is often transient if the hyperkeratosis can be controlled, indicating the hair loss is not due to destruction of hair follicles.

## THE REGISTRY FOR SEBACEOUS ADENITIS

Because sebaceous adenitis in standard poodles is a genetic disease, its prevalence can be decreased by identifying and not breeding standard poodles who are carriers or affected with the disease. To this end, a registry was established in 1992. The Sebaceous Adenitis Registry for Standard Poodles is an "open" registry, meaning its main goal is to identify dogs affected with sebaceous adenitis and to make this information available to any breeder who might request it. Not only is an open registry the most effective means to eliminate a targeted genotype from a genetic pool, but considering our concerns about recognizing "normal," it is the only type of registry that could be established for the disease in standard poodles.

Because the Sebaceous Adenitis Registry for Standard Poodles has only recently been established, there is understandably considerable confusion and controversy concerning the process of registration and what registration means.

### The Process of Registration

Registration is through the Institute for Genetic Disease Control in Animals (GDC),* which will provide a list of participating pathologists, registration forms, and instructions on request. Registration requires evaluation of two 6-mm skin biopsy specimens by a participating pathologist who sends the results of the histologic evaluation to submitting veterinarians and to GDC for addition to their computer files.

Clinically normal standard poodles, 18 months or older, that have been used or are intended to be used

for breeding purposes should be registered as should any dog with a diagnosis of sebaceous adenitis, regardless of the breeding status. There is a charge for registration, but this fee is waived for affected dogs. To maintain active registration, dogs should be biopsied annually.

For clinically normal dogs, two 6-mm punch biopsies should be submitted from the dorsal cervical area. For dogs with skin lesions suggesting sebaceous adenitis, the biopsies should be obtained from clinically affected areas. Breeders often ask that dogs in show coat not be shaved for the biopsy procedure. Although honoring this request will not affect the ability of the pathologist to evaluate the sample, it does increase the risk of infection and subsequent scarring at the biopsy site. Biopsy specimens should be placed in a leak-proof, crush-resistant container containing 10% neutral buffered formalin.

Samples should be sent directly to a GDC-participating pathologist. In addition to the name of the owner/breeder, the following information should be sent regarding the standard poodle on which biopsy was performed: age, sex, coat color, American Kennel Club/Canadian Kennel Club registration number, registered name, a pedigree covering at least four generations, any prior history of sebaceous adenitis in the lineage, and a signed statement from the submitting veterinarian regarding the condition of the coat.

### The Meaning of a Histologic Diagnosis of "Normal"

The pathologist evaluating the biopsy sample will submit to GDC one of three diagnoses based on established criteria: "affected," "questionable," or "normal." All diagnoses of "subclinically affected" or "questionable" will be confirmed by another participating pathologist. The diagnosis of "affected" should be self-explanatory. The diagnosis of "questionable" is applied to samples in which the biopsy is not normal, yet a definitive diagnosis of sebaceous adenitis cannot be established. This can occur when lesions are early in their development or when another skin disease is present that obscures or mimics the disease (e.g., an allergic dermatitis, a folliculitis or demodicosis). When there is a diagnosis of "questionable," a subsequent biopsy is requested to confirm or deny the presence of sebaceous adenitis.

The most important and yet the most confusing diagnosis is "normal." To avoid misconceptions, it is extremely important that veterinarians educate standard poodle owners concerning this diagnosis. To reiterate, evaluation of a skin biopsy specimen is of great value in confirming the diagnosis of clinically evident standard poodle sebaceous adenitis, of moderate value in diagnosing the subclinical form of the disease, and of minimal value in establishing that a dog is free of sebaceous adenitis. Thus, the diagnosis of "normal" should not be interpreted as meaning the animal cannot be a carrier, nor does it imply that a standard poo-

---

*Institute for Genetic Disease Control, P.O. Box 222, Davis, CA 95617 (916)-756-6773.

dle will never develop sebaceous adenitis. What a histologic diagnosis of "normal" means is that based on our current knowledge of standard poodle sebaceous adenitis using the limited technology now available, the owner has done all that is possible to ensure that the dog examined is suitable for breeding. In addition, by having their animal biopsied and registered, information has been contributed that will prove of lasting value to decrease the incidence of the disease in standard poodles.

Over the past 4 years, considerable progress has been made in our understanding of sebaceous adenitis, especially in standard poodles. Defining that standard poodle sebaceous adenitis is heritable and the existance of a subclinical form of the disease has helped explain why the disease in this breed has become so prevalent. Establishing a registry is currently helping breeders select dogs to use in their breeding programs that have the least chance of carrying a genotype which could lead to affected offspring. Still, more work needs to be done. Better methods of diagnosing "normal" standard poodles are needed. Determining whether sebaceous adenitis represents the same disease in all canine breeds also needs to be defined. Hopefully, by the time the next edition of this text is published, further advances will be made to help with our understanding and ability to diagnose sebaceous adenitis not only in standard poodles, but in all breeds and species prone to develop the disease.

## Authors' Note

Since 1990, the Genodermatosis Research Foundation, Inc, a not-for-profit organization founded to facilitate research and knowledge of genetic skin diseases in animals, has been collecting information on sebaceous adenitis and presenting it in a newsletter: *Progress in SA Research*. Future editions can be obtained through: Genodermatosis Research Foundation, 1635 Grange Road, Dayton, OH 45432

## References and Suggested Reading

Brown WR and Hardy MH: A hypothesis on the cause of chronic epidermal hyperproliferation in *asebia* mice. Clin Exp Dermatol 13:74, 1988.

Brucker L and Brucker R: What breeds have been diagnosed with SA? Prog SA Res Winter/Spring, 1993, p 2.

Brucker L and Brucker R: Basic facts about SA. Prog SA Res Summer, 1992, p 1.

Jenkinson DM: Sweat and sebaceous glands and their function in domestic animals. *In* von Tscharner C and Halliwell REW (eds): *Advances in Veterinary Dermatology*, Vol 1. London, Bailliere Tindall, 1990, p 446.

Nicholas FW: *Veterinary Genetics*. Oxford, Clarendon Press, 1987, p 217.

Renfro L, Kopf AW, Gutterman A, et al: Neutrophilic sebaceous adenitis. (Letter to the Editor). Arch Dermatol 129:910, 1993.

Rosser EJ, Dunstan RW, Breen PT, et al: Sebaceous adenitis with hyperkeratosis in the standard poodle: A discussion of ten cases. J Am Anim Hosp Assoc 23:341, 1987.

Rosser EJ: Sebaceous adenitis. *In* Kirk RW and Bonagura JD (eds): *Current Veterinary Therapy XI: Small Animal Practice*. Philadelphia, WB Saunders Co, 1992, p 534.

Scott DW: Granulomatous sebaceous adenitis in dogs. J Am Anim Hosp Assoc 22:631, 1986.

Scott DW: Adenite sebacee pyogranulomateuse sterile chez un chat. Point Vet 21:107, 1989.

# MYCOBACTERIAL SKIN DISEASES IN SMALL ANIMALS

ALAN C. MUNDELL
*Seattle, Washington*

Cutaneous mycobacteriosis refers to a class of skin infections caused by bacteria belonging to the genus *Mycobacterium*. All members of this genus are aerobic, nonmotile, non–spore forming, and have lipid-rich (mycolic acid) cell walls. Mycobacteria are called "acid-fast" bacteria because the high lipid content of the cell wall retains carbolfuchsin stains after acid and alcohol decolorization. In addition, these cell walls inhibit host defense mechanisms and impart greater resistance to common disinfectants. Mycobacterial diseases are rarely observed in small animals; atypical mycobacteriosis and feline leprosy are the principal mycobacterial skin disorders.

## ATYPICAL MYCOBACTERIOSIS

Mycobacteria that are nontuberculous and nonlepromatous have been called "atypical" or "opportunistic" mycobacteria. These organisms are saprophytic and are usually isolated from water and moist soil. Cutaneous infections are rare and typically occur after contamination of traumatized skin. Atypical mycobacteria have been divided into four categories depending on culture characteristics. Most dog and cat infections belong to the group IV category. Group IV atypical mycobacteria are deemed rapid growers, as bacterial growth usually starts within 1 week of inoculation instead of weeks to months. *Mycobacterium fortuitum*, *M. chelonei*, *M.*

*phlei, M. smegmatis, M. xenopi,* and *M. thermoresistible* have been isolated from skin lesions of dogs and cats (Muller, Kirk, and Scott, 1989). In the United States, *M. fortuitum* and *M. chelonei* are the most common isolates. Although there is no apparent age, breed, or sex predilection, cats seem more predisposed than dogs to cutaneous atypical mycobacteriosis (Kunkle, 1990b).

Lesions may be single or multiple and are frequently located in the flank and groin (especially cats). Soft to firm, dermal to subcutaneous nodules will normally ulcerate and fistulate. A seropurulent exudate that does not contain tissue grains is a consistent finding. Even with extensive cutaneous lesions, most dogs and cats display minimal constitutional signs. The differential diagnosis for cutaneous atypical mycobacteriosis is vast and includes feline leprosy (cats only), tuberculosis, foreign body dermatitis, deep mycotic infections, mycetomas, dermatophyte pseudomycetomas, chronic bacterial infections, generalized demodicosis (dogs primarily), sterile nodular panniculitis, pansteatitis, eosinophilic granuloma complex, and neoplasia.

Bacterial cultures and histopathology are the most reliable methods of diagnosis. The exudate or lesional tissue should be inoculated onto both blood agar and special mycobacterial media (Löwenstein-Jensen or Stonebrink). Since most laboratories do not routinely perform mycobacterial cultures when aerobic cultures are submitted, it is best to inform the laboratory that an atypical mycobacterial organism is suspected. Atypical mycobacteria will usually start to grow on blood agar within 1 week of inoculation; however, the medium may become overgrown with more rapidly dividing secondary organisms that were present in the draining fluid (Kunkle, 1990b). In addition, many laboratories discard their blood agar cultures if there has been no growth within 72 to 96 hr. Species identification can be difficult and typically the local laboratory must submit the culture to a select national laboratory.

Histologic examination of lesional tissue often requires special techniques in order to demonstrate the mycobacterial organism. Special techniques such as snap freezing the formalin-fixed tissue or rapid Ziehl-Neelsen staining may be necessary to reveal the organism (White, 1986). Characteristically, fewer acid-fast bacilli are observed in atypical mycobacteriosis than in feline leprosy. Nodular pyogranulomatous dermatitis/panniculitis is the common histologic pattern (Muller,

Kirk, and Scott, 1989). If organisms are found, they are usually located within extracellular lipid vacuoles that are ringed by neutrophils. Besides the paucity of bacteria, atypical mycobacteriosis also differs from feline leprosy by the extracellular location of the organisms.

Laboratory animal inoculation is seldom performed. If cultures fail to identify the mycobacterial organism and the possibility of tuberculosis exists, guinea pig inoculation may be performed.

Treatment options vary greatly, since there are too few reported cases to establish a preferred therapeutic protocol. Most reports of successful disease management are either anecdotal or involve low case numbers. It appears that clinical remission may be more easily achieved in dogs than in cats (Kunkle, 1990b). Because the condition naturally waxes and wanes with occasional prolonged periods of remission, the success of all treatment options must be carefully assessed. Thus, no therapy may be used if the disease involves a reasonably small area and the condition does not bother the animal or owner. Additionally, when owners are unwilling to commit to a prolonged course of therapy, allowing the disease to naturally cycle may be a viable alternative. In time, the skin lesions usually become more extensive, but the disease rarely becomes systemic.

Surgical excision is most successful with small, easily excised lesions. Wide surgical margins must be used. Unfortunately, surgical site dehiscence is common. Surgically debulking lesions while treating the animal with a prolonged course of an appropriate antibiotic may provide a prolonged remission. Surgical excision may be more effective with canine lesions.

Medical management has been attempted using a variety of drugs. Table 1 contains the dosages of the more effective agents (Kunkle, 1990a; Mundell, 1990; White, 1991). Most of these drugs are not Food and Drug Administration (FDA) approved for use in dogs and/or cats. *In vitro* sensitivity testing *may* be helpful when selecting a therapeutic agent. Unfortunately, the clinical response is often less than the sensitivity test would suggest. In general, medication should be administered for 2 to 6 months past clinical cure. If the drug is effective in achieving clinical remission, but lesions return after discontinuing medication, then prolonged or indefinite drug therapy should be used. It is imperative that all therapy be closely monitored for development of adverse side effects. This typically re-

***Table 1.***    *Select Drug Dosages for Treatment of Cutaneous Atypical Mycobacteriosis*

| Treatment | Product (Manufacturer) | Dosage |
|---|---|---|
| Clofazimine | Lamprene (Ciba-Geigy) | 8–12 mg/kg q24h, PO |
| Enrofloxacin° | Baytril (Mobay) | 2.5–5 mg/kg q12h, PO |
| Doxycycline | Vibramycin (Pfizer) | 5 mg/kg q12h, PO |
| Amikacin | Amiglyde-V (Fort Dodge) | 5–7 mg/kg q12h, SC, IM |
| Kanamycin | Kantrim (Fort Dodge) | 5–7 mg/kg q12h, SC, IM |
| Gentamicin | Gentocin (Schering-Plough) | 2 mg/kg q12h, SC, IM |

°An adjunctive transdermal route of drug delivery has also been used by mixing a 1:1 solution of 2.27% enrofloxacin in 90% dimethyl sulfoxide. A dose of 1 ml is applied to affected areas.

quires periodic blood and urine laboratory evaluation, especially when using drugs with known potential toxicities (e.g., aminoglycosides and nephrotoxicity, ototoxicity).

Because of the rare and sporadic nature of the disease, preventative measures that would decrease the likelihood of skin and subcutaneous trauma (e.g., not allowing pets to roam freely) are considered unnecessary. Once atypical mycobacteriosis is present, avoidance of immunosuppressive drugs may help prevent exacerbation or recurrence of the disease.

## FELINE LEPROSY

Feline leprosy is a mycobacterial disease of cats that was first recognized in Australia during the early 1960s. The condition has since been identified in New Zealand, Great Britain, France, the Netherlands, and the west coast of the United States and Canada. The disease is usually confined to cats living in port cities and coastal areas. Feline leprosy has no breed or sex predilection. Age of disease onset is usually 2 to 5 years. The condition occurs most frequently in cats allowed to roam freely.

The etiologic agent of feline leprosy is *Mycobacterium lepraemurium*, the rat leprosy organism. Although the rat leprosy organism had been suspected for many years, only recently have sophisticated culture techniques and biochemical analysis allowed identification of *M. lepraemurium* as the etiologic agent (Mori and Kohsaka, 1986). Mode of transmission is unknown; however, rat bites, insect vectors, and aerosolization of contaminated nasal secretions are proposed methods of transmission. In experimental infections, the incubation period is 2 to 18 months.

Clinical signs consist of skin lesions that may be solitary or multiple, intradermal or subcutaneous, nodular or plaque-like, and haired or ulcerated. Fistulation and exudation are uncommon.

Although skin lesions may occur anywhere on the body, head and limbs are frequently affected. Additionally, lesions may occur on the lips, gums, tongue, and nasal mucosa. Regional lymph nodes may be enlarged with lymphoid hyperplasia and infiltration of epithelioid cells and macrophages. The feline leprosy organism is occasionally isolated from these lymph nodes. The condition rarely disseminates to spleen, bone marrow, liver, kidney, lung, and/or adjacent muscle. Unlike cats with localized cutaneous feline leprosy, cats with disseminated leprosy are usually ill and should be evaluated for underlying immunosuppressive diseases including feline leukemia and feline immunodeficiency viruses.

Diagnosis is achieved primarily through histologic evaluation in conjunction with compatible history, physical examination, cytology, culture, and possibly laboratory animal inoculation. The differential diagnosis for feline leprosy includes atypical mycobacteriosis, tuberculosis, foreign body dermatitis, deep mycotic infections, mycetomas, dermatophyte pseudomycetomas, chronic bacterial infections, eosinophilic granuloma complex, and neoplasia.

Cytology from lesional impression smears consists of mixed inflammatory cells with macrophages and histiocytes containing variable numbers of acid-fast bacilli. Ziehl-Neelsen and a modified Fite's stain are the acid-fast stains most commonly used for these smears.

Biopsies of lesions should be fixed in 10% buffered formalin and evaluated histologically using both hematoxylin-eosin and acid-fast stains (Ziehl-Neelsen and modified Fite's). The histology is somewhat analogous to human leprosy with the presence of both tuberculoid and lepromatous forms (Muller, Kirk, and Scott, 1989). The tuberculoid form consists primarily of nonencapsulated epithelioid granulomas that are interspersed with neutrophils and surrounded by a zone of lymphocytes. Low numbers of organisms are associated with this tuberculoid pattern. The lepromatous form is composed of sheets of large foamy macrophages that contain large numbers of acid-fast bacilli. In humans, the lepromatous form indicates a more immunocompromised host and thus a poorer prognosis. In cats, this correlation has not been demonstrated satisfactorily. One major histologic difference between human and feline leprosy is the lack of consistent cutaneous nerve infiltration by the feline leprosy organism.

Culture of the feline leprosy mycobacterium is difficult, since the organism fails to grow on blood agar and standard mycobacterial media (Löwenstein-Jensen and Stonebrink). A 1% Ogawa egg-yolk medium can grow the organism when incubated under precise temperature and carbon dioxide conditions. Most commercial laboratories do not perform Ogawa egg-yolk cultures. However, tissue maceration cultures (obtained via sterile biopsies) incubated on blood agar and routine mycobacterial media can help differentiate the feline leprosy organism from atypical or tuberculosis-causing mycobacteria that grow on these media.

Laboratory animal inoculation is used primarily in research to propagate and investigate the feline leprosy organism. This procedure is of greatest value when differentiating feline leprosy from tuberculosis. Only the tuberculosis-producing mycobacteria will routinely kill guinea pigs within 6 to 8 weeks after inoculation (Muller, Kirk, and Scott, 1989).

There are a variety of therapeutic options for the treatment of feline leprosy. When lesions are small and unobtrusive, one option is no treatment. However, this strategy is seldom effective and is recommended only for lesions that appear to be spontaneously resolving at the time of diagnosis.

Surgical excision is the treatment of choice when lesions are limited in number and wide surgical margins can be used. However, disease recurrence is common and may require additional surgical intervention and/or medical management.

Medical management has been attempted using drugs that have shown efficacy in treating human leprosy, since the feline leprosy organism is unaffected by common antibiotics. Dapsone and rifampin were the first human antileprosy drugs investigated. Unfortunately, in the cat, toxicity to these drugs is common while efficacy is variable (Kunkle, 1990a; White, 1986). A recent evaluation of another common human anti-leprosy drug, clofazimine (Lamprene, Ciba-Geigy), was more encouraging. Clofazimine is an iminophenazine dye that is suspended in olive oil and packaged in 50- and 100-mg capsules. The antimycobacterial mode of action is not completely understood but is believed to be due to an increase in phagocyte synthesis of lyso-somal enzymes and release of reactive oxidants ($O_2$, $H_2O_2$, and $OH^-$). Although the pharmacokinetics of clofazimine in the cat are unknown, a dosage of 2 to 3 mg/kg/day for 6 to 12 weeks past complete clinical res-olution appears to be effective. At this dosage minimal side effects were noted. Higher dosages may produce transient elevations in liver enzymes. In order to obtain the proper feline dose, the capsule is punctured and the contents proportioned. Latex gloves are worn to prevent staining of the hands. Clofazimine is not ap-proved by the FDA for animal use (Mundell, 1990).

## References and Suggested Reading

Kunkle GA: Feline leprosy. *In* Greene CE (ed): *Infectious Diseases of the Dog and Cat.* Philadelphia, WB Saunders Co, 1990a, p 567.
Kunkle GA: Atypical mycobacterial infections. *In* Greene CE (ed): *Infectious Diseases of the Dog and Cat.* Philadelphia, WB Saunders Co, 1990b, p 569.
Mori T and Kohsaka K: Identification of cat leprosy bacillus grown in mice. Int J Lepr 54:584, 1986.
Muller GH, Kirk RW, and Scott DW: Mycobacterial granulomas. *Small Animal Dermatology.* Philadelphia, WB Saunders Co, 1989, p 272.
Mundell AC: New therapeutic agents in veterinary dermatology. *In* DeBoer DJ (ed): *The Veterinary Clinics of North America: Small Animal Practice.* Philadelphia, WB Saunders Co, 1990, p 1544.
White PD: Enrofloxacin-responsive cutaneous atypical mycobacterial infec-tion in two cats. *Proc 7th Ann Meet Am Assoc Vet Dermatol*, 1991, p 95.
White SD: Cutaneous mycobacteriosis. *In* Kirk RW (ed): *Current Veterinary Therapy IX: Small Animal Practice.* Philadelphia, WB Saunders Co, 1986, p 529.

# TREATMENT OF GENERALIZED DEMODICOSIS IN DOGS

### WILLIAM H. MILLER, Jr.
*Ithaca, New York*

Despite its recognition for years, generalized de-modicosis in the dog is still not completely character-ized. The higher incidence of disease in purebred dogs, the proven predisposition of certain breeds to develop the disease, the repeated occurrence of the disease in different litters produced by the same parents, and the elimination of the disease in certain kennels by a re-strictive breeding program indicate some heritable in-fluence. Various immunologic studies have shown ab-normalities in the cell-mediated immune system of these dogs. The degree of immunosuppression appears to be related to the number of mites present but can be significantly worsened by any intercurrent pyoderma or systemic illness. Elimination of the mites, pyoderma, or systemic illness can return the dog's immune system to normal as far as can be detected by currently avail-able tests. The widely held theory on the pathogenesis of the disease is that affected dogs have an inherited, mite-specific, cell-mediated immunodeficiency which by itself or in conjunction with another immunode-pressive condition results in disease.

## CLINICAL MANIFESTATIONS

A complete description of demodicosis is beyond the scope of this article and the reader is referred to stan-dard textbooks for detailed descriptions. Germane to this discussion are the age at onset and the extent of the clinical lesions. Most cases of demodicosis start dur-ing puppyhood but may not be diagnosed until the dog is a young adult if the owners do not seek veterinary attention or if skin scrapings are not performed. At the other end of the spectrum is the adult dog (>4 years of age) who has never had a skin disease and suddenly develops generalized demodicosis. Dogs with adult-onset disease have some immunodepressive disorder like hyperadrenocorticism, hypothyroidism, diabetes mellitus, or lymphoreticular neoplasia which triggers the demodicosis. Depending on the dog's genetic sus-ceptibility to demodicosis, standard hematologic, bio-chemical, endocrine, or immunologic tests may or may not be able to define the underlying problem at the onset of the demodicosis. The underlying condition will reach some level where it can be diagnosed but can be 12 to 18 months later, so medical evaluations should continue in dogs with seemingly idiopathic adult-onset demodicosis.

Most cases of generalized demodicosis are easy to differentiate from localized demodicosis because large areas of the dog's body are involved. Some dogs at the onset of their disease or during its entire course have more localized lesions. Common examples include dogs with five or more fairly discrete, small areas of disease; involvement of most of the face; or pododemodicosis of two or more feet. Although these dogs have localized lesions, they have generalized demodicosis with all of its prognostic and therapeutic considerations. When acaricidal agents are necessary, the entire body must be treated and not just the involved areas.

## THERAPEUTIC MONITORING

The diagnosis and response to therapy is determined by skin scrapings. Monitoring the patient by its physical appearance is completely unreliable, since all dogs with generalized demodicosis always approach clinical normalcy weeks to months before negative skin scrapings are obtained.

For the most consistent patient monitoring, the same sites should be scraped at each visit and the results should be recorded in tabular form in the record. The number of mites and the percentage that are alive or dead should be noted. The number of sites scraped varies from case to case, but four to six would be considered a minimum. The facial region and at least two feet should be included. Squeezing the skin prior to scraping, and scraping until capillary bleeding occurs is critical, especially as treatment comes to a close. Without these steps, some mites will be missed.

All dogs respond at their own rate and, as long as the skin scrapings at each visit show less mites, the current therapy should be continued for an additional 30 days. If the mite counts start to increase, the odds are that the treatment protocol is not being followed. A more common problem is that the mite counts become stable and cannot be reduced any further. When such a plateau is reached, a modification in treatment will be necessary.

When the scrapings at all sites are negative, treatment should be continued for an additional grace period. Thirty days is the minimum for all dogs. For very chronic cases, 60 to 90 days may be more appropriate. After the grace period, all treatments are discontinued and the patient is watched carefully for the next 12 months. Any skin lesions that occur should be scraped immediately. If no lesions occur, the dog is declared cured and should never develop demodicosis again.

## TREATMENT PROTOCOL

Treatment must be focused on the whole dog and not just the mites. Inadequate nutrition, heavy parasite loads, stressful management situations, intercurrent systemic disorders, and pyodermas all can contribute to the dog's immunosuppression and make it more difficult to resolve the demodicosis. All dogs with generalized demodicosis should have all management problems, systemic illnesses, and pyodermas resolved before specific treatment is instituted.

Upwards of 50% of dogs less than 12 months of age will self-cure their generalized demodicosis with the correction of management problems and the transition from puppyhood to adulthood. No detailed sociologic data are available to characterize these dogs, but they appear to come from litters where not all puppies are affected. Some dogs with adult-onset disease also will self-cure once their underlying systemic disease is identified and resolved. Accordingly, acaricidal treatments may not be necessary in all dogs. All pyodermas should be treated with an appropriate antibiotic, and regular bathing with an antiseborrheic shampoo should be instituted. Shampoo selection depends on the nature of the dog's condition. (See "Shampoos and Moisturizing Rinses in Veterinary Dermatology," this volume, p 590, for a complete discussion of the available products.) The animal's progress or lack thereof is monitored by scrapings. If no response is seen or the animal worsens with this symptomatic treatment, acaricides will be necessary. Some veterinarians will dip these dogs occasionally with amitraz to kill some mites and assist the dog in its self-cure. Since the measurable immunosuppression in these dogs seems to be influenced by mite numbers, this assisted self-cure approach may have some merit.

### Acaricidal Treatments

The literature is replete with studies on the treatment of demodicosis, and some studies show very different results with the same drug. For example, one investigator reported an 86% recovery rate with 4 to 8 amitraz dips (Muller, Kirk, and Scott, 1989), while another study reported a 0% cure rate (Scott and Walton, 1985) with the same product. These contradictory results can be explained in many ways but demonstrate that dogs with generalized demodicosis behave in a very individualized fashion. Any one drug, regardless of how it is used, will not be uniformly successful and some dogs, perhaps as many as 10%, cannot be cured with current methods. With this variability, the prognosis for cure always must remain guarded and treatments must be individualized for each patient.

The only product licensed by the U.S. Food and Drug Administration (FDA) for the treatment of generalized demodicosis is a 19.9% amitraz solution (Mitaban, Upjohn). Another amitraz solution is available (Taktic, Hoechst-Roussel) but this is an Environmental Protection Agency (EPA) -registered external parasiticide for cattle and swine. The reader is reminded that it is a violation of federal law to use a registered pesticide in a manner inconsistent with its labeling.

Mitaban is licensed for application every 14 days at a final diluted strength of 250 ppm (10.6 ml in 7.6 L of water). Product information dictates that dogs with medium to long hair coats be clipped prior to treatment and that all dogs be bathed before the first, if not all dips. Side effects are uncommon but include sedation and an increase in pruritus. Hyperglycemia can occur in some dogs, so diabetic dogs should be monitored carefully.

The product information indicates that the dipping should be continued for two treatments past negative scrapings or until six treatments have been performed. The latter recommendation should be ignored. The dipping should be continued past negative scrapings even if that requires 12 to 18 or more dips. If a plateau is reached with the biweekly dipping, an alternative protocol must be developed. Most investigators will continue with the amitraz solution but apply it on a weekly basis. Concentrations used include 250, 500, 750, and 1000 ppm and success has been reported at each strength. Rate of cure appears to be better with stronger solutions, but these are more expensive and may be more likely to cause side effects. Accordingly, it is best to start at 250 ppm and use this concentration until cure or the next plateau is reached. Most investigators in the United States do not exceed 500 ppm of Mitaban. In Europe, the stronger solutions are routinely used, but their amitraz concentrate appears to be different than Mitaban.

If weekly amitraz dips do not resolve the demodicosis, the owner currently has the option of daily amitraz therapy or the oral administration of either ivermectin (Ivomec, MSD Ag Vet) or milbemycin (Interceptor, Ceiba-Geigy). The new amitraz protocol involves the application of a 0.125% (approximately 1000 ppm) solution to one half of the body on a rotating basis each day. If the feet are involved, they are treated each day by soaking them in small cups of solution. The study with this technique used the large-animal amitraz (Taktic) and reported cure in 56 of 71 (79%) dogs with no serious side effects (Medleau and Willemse, 1991). The mean course of treatment was 3.7 months.

The original work with ivermectin administered at 0.4 mg/kg once weekly showed minimal efficacy (Scott and Walton, 1985). Recent work with milbemycin and ivermectin shows more promising results. Milbemycin has been studied most extensively and, at daily dosages between 1 and 2 mg/kg, 85% of the dogs achieved negative scrapings (Miller et al., 1993). When the drug was administered at 2 mg/kg, 90% of the dogs achieved negative scrapings. With the first dosage, cure rates of between 54 and 71% have been obtained. The study at 2 mg/kg is not yet complete. In either study, the course of treatment varied considerably with ranges from 90 to 300 days. At dosages below 2.5 mg/kg, no side effects were noted. When two dogs received 3.3 mg/kg, they developed mild neurologic signs (ataxia, trembling, stupor) within 24 hr of dosing. The signs disappeared within 24 hr of drug withdrawal with no residual deficits.

The expense of milbemycin has led investigators to reevaluate the efficacy of ivermectin. When ivermectin is given orally at 0.6 mg/kg/day, negative scrapings can be achieved (Paradis and Laperriere, 1992). Courses of treatment vary to as long as 210 days. These studies are still underway, so cure rates are not yet available but should be as high if not higher than those seen with milbemycin. This protocol *cannot be used safely* in collies and probably Shetland sheepdogs, old English sheepdogs, other herding dogs, and their crosses. Side effects to ivermectin are also neurologic, but they tend to be severe and long lasting when 0.2 to 0.6 mg/kg is administered. Some investigators test all dogs for ivermectin sensitivity by administering 0.125 mg/kg/day for

up to 7 days. If a dog is sensitive to high-dose ivermectin, mild neurologic signs should be seen during this period. Drug withdrawal should prevent progression and the signs should disappear within 48 hr.

No studies have been conducted to determine if the topical application of amitraz will shorten the course of milbemycin or ivermectin treatment. The pharmacology of the drugs are different so drug interactions should not occur. Simultaneous topical and systemic treatments should be more effective, but it remains to be seen if the added effort and expense increases the cure rate or significantly shortens the overall course.

If cure cannot be achieved with any of the above treatments, the owner is left with the options of euthanasia, resorting to one of the old topical organophosphate protocols, or long-term control with topical dips. Most dedicated owners elect control, typically with amitraz dips every second to third week. Oral administration of ivermectin or milbemycin could be used, but maintenance protocols have not been developed, and the safety of these products under chronic high-dose usage is unknown.

## RECURRENCE OF DISEASE

The goal of treatment is to kill every *Demodex* mite on the dog's body. Since transfer of *Demodex* mites from one adult dog to another is highly unlikely, eradication of the dog's indigenous population should guarantee lifelong cure regardless of the status of the dog's immunoincompetence towards *Demodex* mites. The question remains as to whether this goal is achieved or if the mite population is just reduced to a level that the dog can tolerate.

Relapses occur commonly and can be attributed to either inadequate treatment or the dog's intolerance level. If the relapse occurs within the first 3 months after treatment, therapy was inadequate. With the mite's approximately 30-day life cycle, it would be difficult for a few mites to replicate to a sufficient number to cause clinical disease within 90 days. If many mites persist, disease-producing levels can occur easily. These treatment failures are usually caused by inadequate scrapings (too few, poor technique, or failure to scrape the face and feet) so treatment was terminated too close to the status of true negative scrapings. These animals could be cured with the same protocol that produced the original remission, but treatment should be longer and monitoring should be more intense.

When relapses occur late, especially during the 7th through 12th month, cure would be unlikely with a repetition of the same protocol. Here, mite numbers are reduced to near zero, but the dog's intolerance to the mites is so great that even a few mites are too many. If mite eradication is to be achieved in this type of case, some other protocol must be followed.

To the author's knowledge, none of the dogs aggressively and successfully treated for demodicosis have relapsed if they remained lesion free for a full 12 months after treatment. This is not true for puppies or adults who self-cured their disease or were assisted in their self-cure by casual acaricidal therapy. These dogs harbor some mites but can tolerate them as long as their underlying immunoincompetence is not worsened by some superimposed immunodepressive condition. If the dog is treated with immunodepressive drugs (corticosteroids, cytotoxic agents) or develops a system illness, the demodicosis is likely to recur. In some dogs, the demodicosis recurs years later for no apparent reason. Since a dog's cell-mediated immunoresponsiveness decreases with advancing age, the relapse in these predisposed dogs may be due to immune exhaustion.

Since there is no way to determine if a dog's mite population is eliminated, all dogs recovered from generalized demodicosis should be kept in the best health possible and they should not be treated with immunodepressive drugs during their entire life (but especially not during the first 12 months after treatment).

## SUMMARY

With current treatments, most dogs can be cured of demodicosis, and those that cannot can be controlled. The ultimate elimination of this disease will be prevention by breeding restrictions. All dogs who have recovered from demodicosis, even if they self-cured their disease, *must not be used for breeding.* Until the genetics of the disorder is established or a reliable screening test is developed to detect susceptible dogs, *the parents of an affected dog and all its littermates must not be used for breeding.* These recommendations will be difficult for most breeders to accept.

## References and Suggested Reading

Medleau LM and Willemse A: Efficacy of daily amitraz therapy for generalized demodicosis in dogs: Two independent studies. *Proc AAVD/ACVD,* Scottsdale, AZ, 1991, p 41.
  *Report on the treatment of 71 dogs with a daily amitraz protocol.*
Miller WH Jr, Scott DW, Wellington JR, et al: Clinical trial on the efficacy of milbemycin oxine in the treatment of generalized demodicosis in adult dogs. J Am Vet Med Assoc 203:1426, 1993.
  *Report on the results of treatment of 30 dogs with chronic generalized demodicosis.*
Muller GH, Kirk, RW, and Scott DW: *Small Animal Dermatology,* 4th edition. Philadelphia, WB Saunders Co, 1989, p 376.
  *General discussion on demodicosis.*
Paradis M and Laperriere E: Efficacy of daily ivermectin treatment in a dog with amitraz-resistant, generalized demodicosis. Vet Dermatol 3:85, 1992.
  *Case report on the efficacy of daily ivermectin treatment.*
Scott DW and Walton DK: Experiences with the use of amitraz and ivermectin for the treatment of generalized demodicosis in dogs. J Am Anim Hosp Assoc 21:535, 1985.
  *Report on the poor efficacy of biweekly amitraz or weekly ivermectin treatment.*

# THE CURRENT IMMUNOLOGY OF ALLERGY

KEVIN T. SCHULTZ

*Madison, Wisconsin*

The function of the immune system is to recognize self and respond to nonself. In general, this response is a protective mechanism against both microbial and environmental agents. However, the immune response can result in disease. This abnormal immune response is typically classified into one of four hypersensitivities. (Also see "Rational Use of Glucocorticoids in Dermatology" and "Insect and Arachnid Hypersensitivity Disorders of Dogs and Cats," this volume, pp 573 and 631, respectively; and *CVT XI,* pp 505, 509, and 513). The following brief review will summarize the pathophysiology of type I immunoglobulin E (IgE) –mediated hypersensitivity.

Type I hypersensitivities are immune-mediated disorders that can involve a variety of organs in afflicted dogs or cats. There are two different types of immediate hypersensitivities in animals. One is a systemic reaction known as anaphylaxis and the second reaction involves a more local and less severe disease. Most noticeable clinical signs in dogs are associated with reactions in the skin and gastrointestinal tract. Organs for IgE-mediated reactives in cats include the skin and gastrointestinal tract but also the respiratory tract and perhaps the urogenital tract. The clinical signs are the result of allergen exposure followed by mast cell/basophil degranulation and mediator release.

There are a number of factors that are required for an animal to develop IgE antibody to a given allergen. The factors can be grouped into those associated with the environment and those associated with the host.

## ENVIRONMENTAL FACTORS

Allergens are antigens that have the unique property of inducing an IgE antibody response. Important allergens in dogs and cats include pollens, parasitic products, certain foods, microorganisms, and, uncommonly, drugs and biologics such as vaccines.

Pollens encompass a very large group of airborne

proteinaceous substances, and pollen exposure is typically seasonal. Parasitic products include excretory/secretory products of internal and external parasites, including injected substances such as saliva or venom. Microbes include sporulation products of certain microbes such as fungi and a variety of infectious agents. In dogs, *Staphylococcus intermedius* or a substance produced by this microbe can act as an allergen. Food products can include almost any material eaten by an animal. Drugs and vaccines can also induce IgE antibodies in some animals. Almost any drug is capable of eliciting such a response; however, certain biologics are more likely to induce an IgE antibody response than are others (bacterial bacterins versus modified live virus vaccines).

In general, the route of exposure will determine the types of clinical signs associated with the allergen reaction. Pollens can be absorbed across mucosal surfaces as well as transdermally. The former route of exposure has been the presumed route of pollen-related allergen reactions in dogs and cats. It is generally believed that inhaled allergens must circulate to the skin from the respiratory tract to cause cutaneous reactions. However, cutaneous absorption may play a more important role in exposure of dogs and perhaps cats than previously thought. For example, the acute cutaneous reaction seen in some dogs that involves the feet, ventral portion of the body, and face after exposure to grass may be the result of cutaneous absorption of the offending allergen. This has yet to be scientifically proven, however, as it may be cutaneous irritation.

Certain infectious processes can result in immunologic changes such that an animal will more likely produce an allergic response to a potential allergen. There have been a number of reports of allergic respiratory disease in children following viral infections. Based on these observations, it has been hypothesized that the viral infection alters immune regulatory pathways. This change in immune regulation will result in IgE antibody response more easily following allergen exposure. There has been at least one study that demonstrated that dogs infected with distemper virus and challenged with an allergen developed IgE antibody to the allergen as compared to dogs only exposed to allergens.

Infections may result in clinical manifestations of allergic reactions. It has recently been shown that dogs with recurrent superficial pyodermas caused by *S. intermedius* have high levels of anti-*Staphylococcus* IgE antibody. The assumption based on this finding is that part of the reason for recurrences of pyoderma in some dogs is because of an allergic cutaneous inflammation that can result in continued staphylococcal skin infection. Parasites are particularly efficient at inducing an IgE response in animals. The mechanisms by which parasites or their products illicit an IgE response are not well understood. However, a number of veterinarians have observed that parasitic infections in dogs and cats can initiate changes in immunity that results in the development of allergies to a broad range of allergens. For example, clinically normal dogs or cats that become flea infested may subsequently develop classic signs of inhalant allergy even after there is no ectoparasite infection. It is presumed that the flea infestation changes some immune-regulating function that activates IgE production to a number of allergens.

## HOST FACTORS

This hypersensitivity reaction is mediated by IgE and in some situations IgG antibody. There is a genetic predisposition to develop IgE antibody; however, the genetic basis for this response is poorly understood. Much more is known about the cellular events responsible for IgE synthesis. When an animal is exposed to an antigen, an antigen-presenting cell (commonly a macrophage) will ingest, process, and then present the antigen to two types of lymphocytes called B cells and T cells. B cells are the lymphocytes that differentiate into antibody-producing plasma cells. T cells function by elaborating a variety of factors and these factors can act directly on the antigen or more commonly will activate host defense mechanisms such as enhancement of phagocytosis by macrophages. Alternately, T lymphocytes may function by producing factors that stimulate B cells to produce antibody or augment other T-cell functions. These T lymphocytes are called T-helper cells. Recent research in human beings and rodents indicates that the development of either an IgE response or an IgM/IgG and delayed-type hypersensitivity is under control of subpopulations of T-helper cells. The two populations are called $T_{H1}$ and $T_{H2}$. It appears that part of the basis for an animal to produce an IgE response or an IgM/IgG response resides with these cells.

$T_{H1}$ cells elaborate two cytokines, interferon-$\gamma$ and interleukin-2, when stimulated with antigen. These two cytokines work together to drive B cells into production of IgG. In contrast, $T_{H2}$ cells elaborate a different cytokine called interleukin-4, which will result in B cells maturing into IgE-producing cells. These cytokines can act locally (i.e., within a very short distance) or systemically (at a distant site in the body). This is the means by which one cell "communicates" to another cell. One of the first steps in the communication pathway between two cells is a binding of one cell to the other cell. The ability to interfere with cell communication such as modifying cytokine production or altering cell–cell binding will undoubtedly prove to be future therapies for IgE-mediated diseases. For example, one such "communication" molecule, CD23, is on the surface of lymphocytes. A recent study has shown that if antibody that binds CD23 is given to a rabbit and then the rabbit is immunized in such a way as would typically induce an IgE response, the rabbit fails to produce IgE. There are a number of ongoing studies aimed at identifying ways to prevent IgE production or dampen an ongoing IgE response.

The IgE antibody system functions as a local immune response in a way analogous to the IgA immune system. Both are antibodies that are concentrated at mucosal and skin surfaces and function as protective

**Table 1.** *Mast Cell Inflammatory Mediators*

| Mediator | Effects |
|---|---|
| **Preformed** | |
| Histamine | Vasoactive, increase in vascular permeability, mucus production, and prostaglandin release |
| Serotonin | Smooth muscle contraction and increase in vascular permeability |
| Eosinophilic chemotactic factor | Influx and activation of eosinophils |
| Heparin | Anticoagulant |
| Chondroitin sulfate | Anticoagulant |
| Neutrophil chemotactic factor | Activation and influx of neutrophils |
| **Synthesized** | |
| Kinin-generating proteases | Activation of the kinin system, induction of pain and itch |
| Leukotrienes | Increased vascular tension, vasoactivation |
| Platelet-activating factor | Platelet and neutrophil activation |
| Prostaglandins/thromboxanes | Vasoactivation-platelet aggregation |

responses against surface pathogens. Moreover, it appears that both the IgE and IgA systems function synergistically. This is especially noticeable when there is a deficiency of IgA production. When such a deficiency is present, there is a substantially elevated incidence of IgE-mediated diseases. This has been described in IgA-deficient people and has been observed in IgA-deficient dogs. Certain breeds, such as shar pei, can have IgA deficiency and, in association with the deficiency, will develop severe food allergies and inhalant allergies. It has been suggested the IgA determination may be useful for predicting atopic dogs that respond poorly to hyposensitization.

When an animal produces IgE to an allergen, the animal is said to be sensitized. The allergen-specific IgE is released from plasma cells and binds to the surface of mast cells and basophils. Degranulation of the mast cell or basophil can occur if the animal is reexposed to the allergen. The allergen must bind to two adjacent IgE molecules on the cell surface for degranulation to occur. The bridging of two molecules results in a cascade effect such that a variety of inflammatory mediators are released into the cells' local environment. The mediators are either preformed substances or are formed after degranulation has occurred. These mediators and their effects are listed in Table 1. It is the action of the mast cell and basophil products that result in the clinical signs of type I hypersensitivities.

In summary, IgE-mediated reactions occur in dogs and cats and affect a number of different organ systems. The IgE immune response is becoming more defined, and this knowledge should be very useful in the near future for control of these immunologic hypersensitivities.

## References and Suggested Reading

Baker E: *Small Animal Allergy: A Practical Guide*. Philadelphia, Lea & Febiger, 1990, p 4.
  *A good, practical guide to allergic disorders of dogs and cats.*
DeBoer DJ, Saban R, Schultz KT, et al: Feline immunoglobulin E: Preliminary evidence of its existence and cross reactivity with canine IgE. *In* White S, Ihrke PJ, and Mason I (eds): *Advances in Veterinary Dermatology* Oxford, Pergamon Press, 1993.
  *The first physicochemical evidence for feline IgE.*
Mueller DL and Noxon JO: Anaphylaxis: Pathophysiology and treatment. Compend Cont Educ 12:157, 1990.
  *A good review of the mechanisms of and treatments for anaphylaxis.*
Thompsen JP: Basic immunologic principles of allergic diseases. Semin Vet Med Surg 6:247, 1991.
  *A good review of the four types of immune hypersensitivities.*

# INSECT AND ARACHNID HYPERSENSITIVITY DISORDERS OF DOGS AND CATS

ROBERT G. BUERGER

*Baltimore, Maryland*

The term "insect and arachnid hypersensitivity" generally brings to mind localized or systemic reactions to stinging (venomous) insects. This is especially true in humans where hypersensitivities to stinging insects are encountered much more frequently than hypersensitivities to biting (feeding) insects. In small animal practice, however, hypersensitivities to biting insects are encountered more frequently. Flea bite hypersensitivity, for example, accounts for as much as 35% of the case load in some veterinary hospitals in the southern United States. Flea bite hypersensitivity will not, however, be the focus of this discussion. Other biting insects have been incriminated in hypersensitivity reactions in small animals including mosquitoes, black flies, tabanids (horse flies and deer flies), midges, and ants. Mosquito allergy may be the most important biting insect hypersensitivity.

Another means of exposure to insect and arachnid allergens is via the air as aeroallergens, and these allergens are derived largely from nonbiting insects. Dust mites, cockroaches, houseflies, moths, ants, crickets, and beetles have been incriminated as important sources of indoor and/or outdoor aeroallergens in humans. Dust mite hypersensitivity is common in atopic dogs and cats, but the importance of other insect aeroallergens is only now becoming clear.

## BITING (FEEDING) INSECT HYPERSENSITIVITY

Reports of severe mosquito hypersensitivity have appeared in the human and veterinary literature. Mosquitoes have been shown to cause a unique type of eosinophilic dermatitis in cats that has been linked clinically and histopathologically to the eosinophilic granuloma complex. In 1984, Wilkinson and Bate first described a corticosteroid-responsive syndrome characterized by seasonal (warm weather), papular, erosive, crusting, and depigmenting dermatitis on the bridge of the nose; papules on the pinnae; granulomatous skin lesions; hyperkeratotic and sometimes hyperpigmented footpads occasionally accompanied by swelling, tenderness, fissures, and depigmentation; peripheral lymphadenopathy; and occasionally fever. There were histologic similarities to the eosinophilic granuloma complex. Several causes were speculated, but it was not

until Mason and Evans (1991) described eight additional cats with similar histories and lesions that a convincing etiology could be established. In that report, the lesions were found to occur at sites where mosquitoes were seen feeding and were found to resolve when the cats were kept behind screening in the same environment. Positive intradermal skin test reactions to a crude mosquito extract were demonstrated in two of four cats. This suggested that a type-I (immediate) hypersensitivity reaction to mosquito allergens is involved in the pathogenesis of the lesions, but in some cases, other immunologic mechanisms (type-IV hypersensitivity, cutaneous basophil hypersensitivity) may be at work as well.

The most impressive lesions of feline mosquito bite hypersensitivity are usually found on the bridge of the nose and on the planum nasale and consist of papules, edema, erosions, crusts, alopecia, and depigmentation. Rule-outs include eosinophilic granuloma, infectious dermatitis (i.e., dermatophytosis, bacterial pyoderma), pemphigus foliaceus, pemphigus erythematosus, lupus erythematosus, and neoplasia. If the clinical history and physical findings are suggestive of feline mosquito bite hypersensitivity, and particularly if skin scrapings and dermatophyte culture are negative, a definitive diagnosis should be pursued. Complete blood count (CBC) in affected cats usually reveals a peripheral eosinophilia. Skin biopsies reveal spongiosis; infiltrates of eosinophils into the epidermis (occasionally with micropustule formation); focal epidermal necrosis; erosions; serocellular crusts; and eosinophilic dermatitis (perivascular [superficial and deep] to diffuse) with variable numbers of neutrophils, lymphocytes, and mast cells. There may also be foci of eosinophilic (collagenolytic) granuloma formation. Intradermal skin testing with mosquito allergen (available commercially as a whole body extract) at a concentration of 500 or 1000 PNU/ml may be helpful in establishing the diagnosis. The author has not yet utilized mosquito allergen in the diagnosis of mosquito bite hypersensitivity; however, two of seven atopic cats tested with insect allergens in the author's clinic developed 3+ or 4+ reactions in response to intradermally injected mosquito allergen at both of the above concentrations. Neither of the two cats had histories or clinical findings that were typical of mosquito bite hypersensitivity. One cat (an indoor cat) had nonseasonal otitis externa and the other (an indoor-outdoor cat) had pruritus of the face, neck, and ears that persisted during the cold winter months and during long periods of indoor confinement. Both cats had other (more significant) reactions on intradermal skin testing for which they have received hyposensitization injections. One might speculate that the reactions in these cats reflect inhalant hypersensitivities to airborne mosquito allergens or represent a cross-reactivity with other (insect or noninsect, biting or non-biting) allergens.

Mosquito hypersensitivity has also been speculated to be a contributing or causative factor in the development of eosinophilic muzzle (nasal) folliculitis in dogs. It is possible that it is a cause of pinnal eosinophilic folliculitis or pinnal insect-bite granulomas as well. Hypersensitivities to other biting or feeding insects may also be important. Given that the dorsal muzzle is sparsely haired or covered only in short hairs in most dogs, feeding or biting insects may have an opportunity for a blood meal at this site. Other sparsely or short-haired areas such as the ears, muzzle, groin, and legs may be other prime targets. The role of insect hypersensitivity in the pathogenesis of muzzle eosinophilic folliculitis is possibly overemphasized given that the planum nasale is almost never affected (it should be a prime location for insect bites given the lack of protective hair) and that the vast majority of dogs go back into the same environment and do not have recurrent disease. Muzzle eosinophilic folliculitis may represent a cutaneous reaction pattern for which there are several causes.

Nasal eosinophilic folliculitis often results in an acute onset of severe pruritus, follicular papules, pustules, furuncles, crusts (sometimes thick, hemopurulent crusts), excoriations, and alopecia on the dorsal muzzle of particularly long-nosed dogs; however, the planum nasale is not usually affected. Lesions may heal with scarring. Rule-outs include bacterial folliculitis, dermatophytosis, demodicosis, contact dermatitis (irritant or allergic), lupus erythematosus, pemphigus foliaceus, pemphigus erythematosus, and drug reactions. In the author's practice, bacteria (*Staphylococcus intermedius*) is the most common cause of eosinophilic folliculitis, and the dermatitis resolves with appropriate antimicrobial treatment. Mosquito hypersensitivity should be suspected, however, if the folliculitis is acute in onset, recurrent, and seasonal; if there is no response to appropriate antimicrobial treatments; if skin scrapings, dermatophyte culture, and bacterial culture are negative; if there is a positive correlation with mosquito exposure; if biopsy reveals eosinophilic folliculitis without microorganisms; if other hypersensitivities (atopy and food allergy) have been ruled out; and if there is a positive reaction to intradermal mosquito allergen.

As with any hypersensitivity, avoidance is the best treatment. Indoor confinement (behind screening) at night is preferred and usually curative. When indoor confinement is not possible, dog- and cat-approved, pyrethrin-containing sprays may provide sufficient repellent activity. However, since sprays are not practical for face and ear applications, the solutions may be dabbed on with cotton, a sponge, or a cloth, being care-ful not to get the solution in the eyes. There are additional comments on reducing environmental insect exposure in the aeroallergen portion of this article. Severely affected cats and dogs will require corticosteroid therapy. Prednisone or prednisolone at a dose of 1 to 2 mg/kg/day (cats) or 0.5 to 1.0 mg/kg/day (dogs) is effective. For cats, a single injection of DepoMedrol 20 mg IM may be effective as well. If maintenance corticosteroid therapy is necessary, the lowest effective dose of prednisone or prednisolone given on alternate days should be sought. Antihistamines may be efficacious, but their use has not been investigated in the treatment of biting insect hypersensitivities.

Hyposensitization is an interesting speculation for the cat or dog whose mosquito bite hypersensitivity cannot be controlled by any other means. However, there are no reports of efficacy. As the pathogenesis of the hypersensitivity appears to involve exposure to mosquito salivary antigens and/or haptens at the feeding site (similar to the pathogenesis of flea bite hypersensitivity), and given that the commercial mosquito allergen is a whole body extract, hyposensitization may prove to be as ineffective for mosquito bite hypersensitivity as it is for flea bite hypersensitivity.

## INSECT AND ARACHNID AEROALLERGENS

Studies have shown that allergens derived from many nonbiting insects and arachnids are capable of inducing allergic reactions in humans and that these allergens are present in outdoor air in quantities comparable to known allergens (Lierl, Riordan, and Fischer, 1986). In outdoor air, insect allergens had seasonal fluctuations with the highest levels being present during warm weather. Peak ant activity was found to occur in July and August (Lierl, Riordan, and Fischer, 1986). Cricket, moth, and housefly activity rose in April and persisted until September (Lierl, Riordan, and Fischer, 1986; Wynn et al., 1988). Other insects are suspected or known to have the ability to induce hypersensitivity reactions including butterflies and honeybees (Kino and Oshima, 1978). Insects and arachnids are also important sources of indoor/nonseasonal aeroallergens, and housedust mites, cockroaches, carpet beetles, spiders, and silverfish (among others) have proven or suspected roles in respiratory allergies in humans (Baldo and Panzani, 1988). In humans, hypersensitivities to these allergens manifest primarily as respiratory disease (i.e., asthma, rhinitis).

In veterinary medicine, hypersensitivities most commonly manifest as pruritus, and the diagnostic approach involves the exclusion of parasitic and infectious causes, elimination diets to rule out food allergy or intolerance, and intradermal skin testing. The cause of the pruritus in approximately 10% of cases cannot be found (Griffin, 1993), and 20 to 50% of canine atopics that undergo hyposensitization do not respond (Muller, Kirk, and Scott, 1989). Some of these diagnostic and hyposensitization failures may be due to allergens that are not currently being considered, including insect allergens. Griffin (1993) reported the results of insect allergy testing in Southern California and Las Vegas, NV, and in these locations, 4.5%, and 6.3% (respectively) of dogs were found to be intradermal skin test–negative to all conventional allergens (including fleas and housedust mites), but were positive to one or more insect allergens. In the author's clinic, 7 of 45 atopic dogs (15.6%) had either very weak 1 to 2+ reactions or were skin test–negative to all conventional allergens including fleas and housedust mite. One of the seven, 14.3% had 3 or 4+ positive reactions to insect allergens. The pursuit of insect allergies is clearly relevant.

Insect aeroallergies should be considered one of the many causes of atopic dermatitis in the dog and so the pathogenesis of insect allergy should involve some of the same mechanisms that are involved in development of pollen, dust, and mold allergies. Dogs inhale, ingest, or absorb percutaneously insect allergens that ultimately lead to a type-I hypersensitivity reaction, although it is possible that other allergic mechanisms are involved (i.e., type-IV hypersensitivity, cutaneous basophil hypersensitivity).

Dogs with atopy tend to have an onset of symptoms early in life, often between 1 and 3 years of age, and those developing insect aeroallergies probably begin with symptoms during this same period of time. There is no known breed or sex predilection for insect allergies, although it would not be surprising if the same breeds that are predisposed to atopy will be predisposed to insect aeroallergies. Pruritus and erythema are the primary presenting complaints and although the pruritus may be generalized, it is usually more severe on the feet, ventral neck and trunk, axillae, face, and ears (Griffin, 1993; Muller, Kirk, and Scott, 1989). The pruritus may ultimately lead to saliva stained hair, self-induced alopecia, excoriations, lichenification, secondary pyoderma, or secondary seborrheic dermatitis. In most patients with outdoor insect aeroallergens, the symptoms are seasonal. However, hypersensitivities to indoor insect/arachnid aeroallergens may result in symptoms that are year-round. Given that most dogs with insect/arachnid hypersensitivities have other hypersensitivities as well (e.g., to fleas, pollens, dust mites, molds), the seasonality of the dermatitis may not be helpful diagnostically (Griffin, 1993).

The diagnosis of atopy is based on the signalment, history, physical examination; on the exclusion of parasitic and infectious dermatoses; on the exclusion of food allergies (via the feeding of an elimination diet); and on positive intradermal skin test results. The diagnosis of insect/arachnid aeroallergies is no different. The author has performed intradermal allergy skin testing with whole insect allergens (Greer Laboratories) in a small number (45) of suspect atopic dogs in Baltimore during the period from February to May. The results are shown in Table 1. Griffin (1993) reported that 15 normal beagles were injected with insect allergens at 500 and 1000 PNU/ml concentrations and were found not to react at these concentrations, but housefly and cockroach allergens were not tested and it is not clear

**Table 1.** *The Results of Intradermal Allergy Skin Testing With Insect and Arachnid Allergens in 45 Atopic Dogs*

| Insect/Arachnid | Antigen (PNU/ml) | % Positive of Dogs (3 or 4+) |
|---|---|---|
| Black ant | (500) | 7 |
| Black ant | (1000) | 11 |
| Cockroach | (500) | 0 |
| Cockroach | (1000) | 0 |
| House fly | (500) | 7 |
| House fly | (1000) | 9 |
| Mosquito | (500) | 11 |
| Mosquito | (1000) | 16 |
| Moth | (500) | 29 |
| Moth | (1000) | 31 |
| Black fly | (500) | 15 |
| Black fly | (1000) | 22 |
| Deer fly | (500) | 25 |
| Deer fly | (1000) | 28 |
| Horse fly | (500) | 13 |
| Horse fly | (1000) | 18 |
| Housedust mite | (25) (mix of *Dermatophagoides Farinae* and *D. Ptheronyssinus*) | 51 |
| Flea (1/1000, w/v) | | 42 |

if a moth allergen was tested. In the author's study, allergens for housedust mite, blackfly, deer fly, and moth clearly had a high degree of reactivity in atopic dogs. Twenty-two (49%) of the 45 atopic dogs tested did not react to any of the insect allergens or had weak 1 or 2+ reactions (housedust mite and flea allergens excluded). If housedust mite and flea are included, then the percentage of insect/arachnid nonreactors drops to 29% (13 of 45 atopic dogs). The reactions to moth are interesting given that the wings and fine scales are readily rubbed off or dislodged in flight, forming a fine dust, and given how readily moths are attracted to homes (Kino et al., 1978). Aeroallergens derived from outdoor insects were found to be present in outdoor air in quantities comparable to those of known allergens (Lierl, Riordan, and Fischer, 1986). In May 1993, Greer Laboratories began offering a serologic test for canine insect allergies (on a research basis). Included on the panel are allergens for housefly, horsefly, deerfly, caddisfly, blackfly, black ant, fire ant, moth, mosquito, cockroach, and flea. Studies are needed to determine if these serologic tests have diagnostic value.

As with all hypersensitivities, a cause-and-effect relationship should be sought when making a diagnosis of insect/arachnid hypersensitivity. This may not be possible considering that other hypersensitivities are often present. Improvement when the dog is put into an insect/arachnid–free environment, and exacerbation when the dog is exposed to insects/arachnids is supportive evidence.

While the therapy of biting insect hypersensitivity is directed at preventing the insect's contact with the host, the treatment of insect aeroallergies must be directed at the dog's environment because exclusive use of topical treatments (repellants) will still allow significant aeroallergen exposure. In the case of housedust mites, a reduction in the mite's habitat by removing carpets; laundering bedding frequently at 130°F; removing or providing impermeable (i.e., vinyl) covers for upholstered furniture, mattresses, and pillows; vacuuming frequently; removing stuffed animals and clutter; treating carpets with benzyl benzoate or tannic acid; and keeping humidity below 50% may lead to a significant reduction in mite numbers and hence improvement in dust mite allergies (Platts-Mills, 1993). Additionally, the flea control programs that veterinarians commonly recommend for flea-allergic patients should benefit the insect/arachnid–allergic patient as well. The author recommends treatment of the home with a permethrin and fenoxycarb–containing spray every 3 weeks for three treatments and then monthly. If employed properly, these regular insecticidal treatments should also reduce the number of housedust mites and other potentially allergenic insects and arachnids indoors. Additionally, the careful treatment of the outdoor environment (i.e., yard, kennel, and dog house) with chlorpyrifos, malathion, or carbaryl as per the manufacturers' instructions every 3 weeks for three treatments and then monthly should greatly reduce insect exposure and help control fleas as well. Screens in place when windows are open will prevent most flying insects from entering the home. Dead insects should be removed regularly from the home and garage (e.g., window sills, corners, light fixtures) and from kennels. Removing the habitat of insects (i.e., ant hills, standing or running water in the case of mosquitoes and black flies, and decaying organic material or uncovered garbage in the case of house flies) will also help reduce exposure to insects.

The effectiveness of hyposensitization for most insect aeroallergens has not been studied in dogs. Of the insect/arachnid allergens tested, the author has used only housedust mite in hyposensitization programs. Benefit to hyposensitization has been seen, and Griffin (1993) too has reported hyposensitization success. However, a double-blind study (Charach, 1993) with housedust mite immunotherapy over a 16-week period of time was unable to demonstrate any efficacy. The study may not have continued long enough. It has been suggested, but not proven, that hyposensitization to other insect/arachnids may work best with black ant allergen.

Symptomatic treatment of the pruritus associated with insect aeroallergies is often necessary, and therapy is similar to that provided for conventional aeroaller-

gens. Antihistamines (e.g., hydroxyzine, diphenhydramine, chlorpheniramine, clemastine) and/or fatty acid supplements help some dogs. The reader is referred to *CVT XI*, p 563 for a complete discussion of nonsteroidal therapy for pruritus (Paradis and Scott, 1992). If the cause(s) of a dog's hypersensitivity cannot be controlled and if nonsteroidal therapy is not effective, alternate-day administration of short-acting corticosteroids such as prednisone or prednisolone at a dose of up to 1.1 mg/kg may be necessary.

## References and Suggested Reading

Baldo BA and Panzani RC: Detection of IgE antibodies to a wide range of insect species in subjects with suspected inhalent allergies to insects. Int Arch Allergy Appl Immunol 85:278, 1988.

Charach M: Specific immunotherapy in dogs with house dust mite allergy: A double blind placebo study. *Proc Ann Member's Meeting AAVD/ACVD* 9:50, 1993.

Griffin CE: Insect and arachnid hypersensitivity. *In* Griffin CE, Kwochka KW, and MacDonald JM (eds): *Current Veterinary Dermatology, The Science and Art of Therapy.* St. Louis, Mosby Year Book, 1993, p 133.

Gross TL, Ihrke PJ, and Walder EJ: *Veterinary Dermatopathology.* St. Louis, Mosby Year Book, 1992, p 210.
*A dermatopathologic discussion of feline mosquito-bite hypersensitivity.*

Kang BC, Johnson J, Morgan C, et al: The role of immunotherapy in cockroach asthma. J Asthma 25:205, 1988.

Kino T, Chihara J, Fukuda K, et al: Allergy to insects in Japan. High frequency of IgE antibody responses to insects (moth, butterfly, caddis fly, and chironomid) in patients with bronchial asthma and immunochemical quantitation of the insect-related airborne particles smaller than 10 μm in diameter. J Allergy Clin Immunol 79:857, 1987.

Kino T and Oshima S: Allergy to insects in Japan. The reaginic sensitivity to moth and butterfly in patients with bronchial asthma. J Allergy Clin Immunol 61:10, 1978.

Lierl MB, Riordan BS, and Fischer TJ: Concentration of airborne insect-derived particles in outdoor air (abstr 412). J Allergy Clin Immunol 85:246, 1986.

Mason KV and Evans AG: Mosquito bite-caused eosinophilic dermatitis in cats. J Am Vet Med Assoc 198:2086, 1991.

Muller GH, Kirk RW, and Scott DW: *Small Animal Dermatology,* 4th edition. Philadelphia, WB Saunders Co, 1989, pp 419 (fly dermatitis), 450 (atopy).

Paradis M and Scott DW: Nonsteroidal therapy for canine and feline pruritus. *In* Kirk RW and Bonagura JD (eds): *Current Veterinary Therapy XI.* Philadelphia, WB Saunders Co, 1992, p 563.

Platts-Mills TAE: Indoor allergens. *In* Middleton EM, Reed CE, Ellis EF, et al (eds): *Allergy Principles and Practice,* 4th edition. St. Louis, Mosby Year Book, 1993, p 514.

Tee RD, Gordon DJ, Lacey J, et al: Occupational allergy to the common house fly (*Musca domestica*): Use of immunologic response to identify atmospheric allergen. J Allergy Clin Immunol 76:826, 1985.

Wilkinson GT and Bate MJ: A possible further clinical manifestation of the feline eosinophilic granuloma complex. J Am Anim Hosp Assoc 20:325, 1984.

Wynn SR, Swanson BA, Reed CE, et al: Immunochemical quantitation, size distribution, and cross-reactivity of Lepidoptera (moth) aeroallergens in southeastern Minnesota. J Allergy Clin Immunol 82:47, 1988.

Yunginger JW: Insect allergy. *In* Middleton EM, Reed CE, Ellis EF, et al (eds): *Allergy Principles and Practice,* 4th edition. St. Louis, Mosby Year Book, 1993, p 1511.

# FIBROPRURITIC NODULES IN THE DOG

EMILY J. WALDER

*Venice, California*

## CLINICAL FEATURES

Fibropruritic nodules are uncommon lesions occurring on the dorsal lumbosacral region of dogs. They appear to be directly associated with chronic flea allergy dermatitis and are rarely observed in conjunction with any other type of cutaneous hypersensitivity. They are most likely nodular scars developing in foci of chronic self-trauma and secondary pyoderma. According to Ihrke, this condition may be more prevalent in purebred or crossbred German shepherd dogs. Most of the affected animals are middle-aged or older. There is no known sex predilection.

The lesions may be solitary but are more often multiple. As many as 50 nodules have been observed on one patient. They appear as dome-shaped, fungiform, or occasionally polypoid masses that range in size from 0.5 to 2 cm. The surface frequently has a papillated configuration. The nodules may be hyperpigmented or hypopigmented. The surrounding skin is frequently alopecic, hyperpigmented, and lichenified, as would be expected in chronic flea allergy. Erosion or ulceration may be present, particularly in larger masses.

Clinical differential diagnoses are limited, since the presentation is usually characteristic. Solitary lesions may be more readily confused with neoplasia. Differential diagnoses include fibroma, nodular sebaceous hyperplasia, papilloma, and fibromatous polyp.

## THERAPY

There is no specific treatment for fibropruritic nodules. Antibiotic therapy may aid in the resolution of ulceration or deep pyoderma within the masses. Surgical excision may be indicated for larger or ulcerated lesions. Without surgical intervention, the nodules are likely to be permanent due to the presence of fibrous scar tissue. Appropriate treatment of the underlying etiology, flea allergy dermatitis, may inhibit development of additional fibropruritic nodules in patients that are predisposed to this condition.

## HISTOLOGIC FEATURES

Fibropruritic nodule is a low or high dome-shaped mass that is not well demarcated from the surrounding skin. The epidermis has moderate to marked, irregular acanthosis. The rete pegs frequently have an angular configuration. Papillation of the epidermis is usually present and may be dramatic. Pseudocarcinomatous hyperplasia may be present. There is variable erosion or ulceration accompanied by serocellular crusting.

The dermis has moderate to marked fibrosis with proportionate effacement of adnexa. The collagen bundles are thicker than in adjacent dermis, but hyalinization is not observed. Vertical "streaming" of collagen in the superficial dermis is a common finding; this is actually a manifestation of vertical orientation of small blood vessels and surrounding pericytes. This phenomenon is also a diagnostic feature of acral lick dermatitis. Earlier lesions have hyperplasia and mild dysplasia of the residual, entrapped hair follicles. Suppurative or pyogranulomatous folliculitis is often evident. Small trichogranulomas may be present in the deep dermis. Later lesions are totally devoid of adnexa.

The superficial dermis within the nodule has mild, perivascular cuffing by variable mixtures of plasma cells, pigmented macrophages, lymphocytes, and neutrophils. The superficial dermis in the skin adjacent to the nodule exhibits perivascular infiltration by mast cells, eosinophils, lymphocytes and, in some cases, pigmented macrophages. The overlying epidermis often shows acanthosis and hyperpigmentation, corresponding to the lichenification and pigmentary alterations observed clinically.

Histologic differential diagnoses are limited. Nodular scar is a reasonable alternative nomenclature; fibropruritic nodule is a type of nodular scar arising in an environment of chronic flea allergy dermatitis. Trichogranuloma is also an appropriate diagnosis when the phase of development is characterized by focal furunculosis. Fibropapilloma provides an adequate description of both the dermal and epidermal features of fibropruritic nodule, but this nomenclature implies a neoplastic process and probably should be reserved for the papillomavirus-induced masses on the penis of bulls. Fibropruritic nodule may resemble focal adnexal dysplasia (folliculosebaceous hamartoma), particularly when residual adnexa have become hyperplastic and distorted. However, abnormal hair follicles and sebaceous lobules are the predominant component of focal adnexal dysplasia; this situation is not observed in fibropruritic nodule. Fibropruritic nodule is not likely to be confused with fibroma, which has a uniform, repetitive pattern of bundles and swirls of small fibrocytes in a collagenous stroma. Additionally, neither focal adnexal dysplasia nor fibroma generally has a component of florid epidermal hyperplasia.

## Reference and Suggested Reading

Gross TL, Ihrke PJ, and Walder EJ: *Veterinary Dermatopathology: A Macroscopic and Microscopic Evaluation of Canine and Feline Skin Disease.* St. Louis, Mosby Year Book, 1992, pp 70–71.

# MEDICAL TREATMENT OF CANINE PEMPHIGUS-PEMPHIGOID

BARBARA A. KUMMEL

*Gaithersburg, Maryland*

## PEMPHIGUS FOLIACEUS

Pemphigus foliaceus (PF) is the *most* common autoimmune skin disease in the dog. It accounts for 1.5% of the cases seen in the author's specialty dermatology practice. This disease in the dog has a great variety of clinical presentations as well as marked variation in the severity of the disease and, therefore, significant variation in the level of patient discomfort. The aggressiveness with which a pemphigus foliaceus patient is treated must depend upon the severity of the disease in that particular patient.

Mild cases of canine pemphigus foliaceus are considered to be those in which the disease does not result in pain or pruritus, the patient appears to "feel well," and the lesions are limited to one or two areas of the body (i.e., face and ears, face and feet, or mild truncal lesions). Treatment of these cases consists of administration of slow intravenous dexamethasone at a dosage of 0.25 mg/kg of body weight and an intramuscular injection of prednisone at a dosage of 2 mg/kg. Oral corticosteroids (prednisone, prednisolone, or methylprednisolone) are prescribed at an initial dose of 0.5 mg/kg administered with food twice daily until clinical signs show significant improvement. This is usually noted within 14 to 21 days, and the dosage of oral corticosteroid is reduced to once daily for 2 to 4 weeks, and then, hopefully, to alternate-day administration at a dosage of 0.5 mg/kg. If the disease remains in "remission" at this dose, the author does not attempt to further decrease the dose, as PF flare-ups often are more difficult to control than the initial disease. The potential adverse side effects of long-term corticosteroid therapy are monitored by reevaluations every 6 months. These evaluations consist of skin scrapings for demodicosis, fungal cultures for dermatophytes, a urinalysis, a complete blood count (CBC) with platelet count, and a chemistry profile. A complete physical examination is performed, with the major concerns being obesity, which may lead to serious joint disease (when coupled with constant corticosteroid use); and cardiac disease, which may be exacerbated by corticosteroid use.

If the patient is showing signs of excessive polydipsia, polyuria, polyphagia, panting, personality changes, and/or weight gain, the type of oral corticosteroid is always changed to methylprednisolone (Medrol) which usually minimizes these discomforting side effects. The disadvantage of methylprednisolone is its excessive expense compared to prednisone or prednisolone.

Severe cases of canine pemphigus foliaceus must be treated more aggressively. These patients often have significant pain and/or pruritus associated with their disease. Many are febrile, anorectic, or lethargic. Secondary bacterial skin infection, due to the extensiveness of the epidermal erosion, is often present. The initial treatment is the same as for mild cases of pemphigus foliaceus, except that azathioprine (Imuran) is added to the initial treatment protocol at a dosage of 1 mg/kg/day. Skin cytologies are also performed to check for evidence of secondary bacterial infection. This is necessary, since PF itself is often a "pustular" disease, making "clinical" evaluation for secondary bacterial infection inaccurate. If numerous cocci and/or rods are evident on cytology, a broad-spectrum bactericidal antibiotic is prescribed for 3 to 6 weeks. Patients receiving azathioprine therapy are evaluated every month. The evaluation consists of a complete physical examination as well as a CBC (with a platelet count) to check for thrombocytopenia, anemia, and leukopenia that may be associated with the azathioprine therapy. If after 3 months, the patient is not showing any CBC abnormalities (associated with the azathioprine therapy), and if clinical signs are significantly improved, the corticosteroid level is reduced to 0.5 mg/kg every *other* day, but the azathioprine dosage is unchanged. At this stage, reevaluations, with a CBC (including platelet count), a chemistry profile, and a urinalysis are performed every 3 months. If the patient is *not* improving at the 3-month reevaluation, the azathioprine is increased to 2 mg/kg/day, and the patient reevaluated every 2 to 4 weeks. If after 3 months of the increased azathioprine therapy either the patient is not responding *or* if the azathioprine is causing bone marrow suppression, the azathioprine is discontinued for 1 month, the corticosteroid is increased to 1.0 mg/kg given twice daily, and the patient is reevaluated in 1 month. At this stage, parenteral gold salt therapy (Solganal) is initiated at a dosage of 1 mg/5 kg IM weekly for 10 weeks, then monthly. Although an oral form of gold salt therapy, auranofin, is available, I believe the parenteral gold salt therapy is far more effective. Several canine PF patients who had not responded to the oral form did respond well to parenteral dosage. I always wait at least 4 weeks between discontinuation of the azathioprine and initiation of injectable gold salt therapy because four of our canine PF patients developed fatal toxic epidermal necrolysis (TEN) when gold salt therapy was initiated immediately upon cessation of azathioprine therapy.

The author has treated over 100 canine pemphigus

patients with parenteral gold salt therapy. Many exhibit pain at the injection site. Two cases of thrombocytopenia with petechia and ecchymoses were observed. Both cases resolved with cessation of therapy. No other adverse side effects have been noted, unless the gold salt therapy was initiated immediately after cessation of azathioprine therapy.

Cyclophosphamide (Cytoxan) is occasionally suggested for treatment of canine pemphigus foliaceus. However, I choose *not* to use this drug because of the extremely common adverse side effects, the most common of which is hemorrhagic cystitis.

## PEMPHIGUS ERYTHEMATOSUS

Pemphigus erythematosus (PE) is the third most common autoimmune skin disease in the dog. (Pemphigus foliaceus and discoid lupus erythematosus are more common.) Some writers feel that it is related to both pemphigus foliaceus and lupus erythematosus. However, I feel that PE is a benign variant of pemphigus foliaceus because the disease is limited to the face and ears, and patients have no systemic signs of disease. In some cases, the facial lesions are mildly pruritic and may be painful.

Treatment of PE also must be based upon severity of the lesions and the level of patient discomfort. Initial treatment consists of injecting the planum nasale with triamcinolone acetonide (Kenalog) at a dosage of 0.4 mg/kg. The human drug Kenalog is less irritating than the veterinary drug Vetalog, perhaps because Kenalog requires dilution with sterile saline, since it is supplied only in vials of 40 mg/ml. The vehicle in Vetalog may be the irritating factor. This initial injection is followed by oral administration of corticosteroids, as discussed under "Pemphigus Foliaceus." In most canine PE patients, the corticosteroid dosage can be reduced to 0.5 mg/kg every other day. Sun avoidance is helpful in preventing further facial (especially nasal) damage due to UV-B radiation. Sunscreens are of little benefit in canine patients due to poor patient tolerance. Most dogs will attempt to rub the material off their faces. This causes further trauma to existing lesions and gets the irritating material in their eyes. Canine PE patients *rarely* require other immunosuppressive drugs or antibiotics. The most frustrating aspect of treatment is the unwillingness of many owners to accept the permanent minor facial lesions, which are only cosmetic. In some patients, unsafe levels of medications are needed to have them "look normal." On the other hand, if left untreated, erosive nasal lesions may result in severe nosebleeds, nose erosion and, in rare cases, secondary squamous cell carcinoma of the nose secondary to the constant "trauma."

## PEMPHIGUS VULGARIS

Pemphigus vulgaris (PV) is an uncommon to rare autoimmune skin disease of the dog. The depth of the lesions (entire epidermis) as well as the location of the lesions (mucocutaneous junctions and virtually any skinned area) make the disease painful. Most patients are presented febrile, anorectic, depressed, and dehydrated. Supportive care is as important as treatment of the disease itself.

Treatment of pemphigus vulgaris is quite involved. Most patients require intravenous fluid therapy. If possible, the lesions should be cleansed and the hair gently trimmed. We never use sedation to facilitate local therapy, as the overall health status of these patients is often compromised, so sedative drugs are contraindicated. Whirlpool baths are helpful, since the lesions are similar to third-degree burns. The potential stress created by using whirlpool baths must be considered, as stress exacerbates most autoimmune skin diseases. Intravenous dexamethasone, intramuscular prednisolone (Meticorten), and oral corticosteroids are initiated as described under pemphigus foliaceus. However, in pemphigus vulgaris cases, we also initiate azathioprine (1 mg/kg) and antibiotic therapy immediately. The patient is best managed at home because the stress of hospitalization may exacerbate the disease. The patient should be encouraged to eat, but those with good appetites should not be allowed to gain excessive weight.

Patients should be reevaluated every 10 to 14 days and a CBC with platelet count performed. A chemistry profile and urinalysis is recommended every 4 to 6 weeks. As the disease responds, the first drug to be tapered off is the corticosteroid. If the disease is *not* responding, the corticosteroid and the azathioprine doses should be doubled, and the patient reevaluated every 5 to 7 days. This treatment regimen is best continued as long as the patient is improving. After 2 to 3 months of high-level corticosteroid and azathioprine therapy if the patient is still not improving, the azathioprine is discontinued for 1 month and gold salt therapy initiated (as described under pemphigus foliaceus). Pemphigus vulgaris is a most difficult disease to treat and manage. Patients do not feel well, the lesions are painful, and the lesions are unsightly and difficult for many owners to manage.

## PEMPHIGUS VEGETANS

Pemphigus vegetans is an extremely *rare* autoimmune skin disease of the dog. It is considered to be a benign variant of pemphigus vulgaris. The author has treated only three cases of canine pemphigus vegetans, but all responded to tapering dosages of corticosteroid therapy. None required other immunosuppressive drugs or antibiotics. In all three cases, the patients were neither painful nor pruritic. They also appeared to be unaware of their cutaneous disease and felt quite well.

## CANINE (BULLOUS) PEMPHIGOID

Canine pemphigoid is an uncommon autoimmune skin disease of the dog. Sixty-five per cent of our 28 cases were collies or Shetland sheepdogs. (It is possible that these were actually ulcerative dermatoses of the collie and Shetland sheepdog; see next chapter in this section.) A few cases of toxic epidermal necrolysis were originally misdiagnosed as canine pemphigoid.

As with pemphigus vulgaris, canine pemphigoid is difficult to treat due to the depth of the lesions, and the areas of involvement (the inguinal areas and axillae), which result in significant pain. Since all patients appear to be in pain upon presentation, and many are febrile, anorectic and/or dehydrated, supportive care is essential. (See pemphigus vulgaris.) Initial therapy consists of intravenous dexamethasone, intramuscular prednisolone, and oral corticosteroids. I also begin azathioprine therapy at once in all patients. Unless skin cytology shows significant evidence of a secondary bacterial infection, antibiotics are *not* prescribed because cases of toxic epidermal necrolysis secondary to drug administration may be initially misdiagnosed as canine pemphigoid, and antibiotic therapy may exacerbate that disease.

## IMPORTANT POINTS IN THE TREATMENT OF CANINE PEMPHIGUS AND PEMPHIGOID

1. Always question: Does the severity of the disease warrant the potential adverse side effects of the medication?

2. Always use as low a dose of *alternate*-day corticosteroid therapy as possible.

3. Obesity is *the* most common adverse side effect of corticosteroid therapy. This may be devastating, as the combination of obesity and corticosteroids leads to joint laxity, osteoporosis, and a marked increase in severe joint injuries. The most common injury is ruptured cruciate ligaments. Obese patients receiving corticosteroids are poor surgical candidates!

4. Azathioprine (Imuran) treatment is best monitored by CBCs with a platelet count and a urinalysis, every month for 3 months, then every 3 months. Most patients who are going to have bone marrow suppression will have it appear during the first 3 months of therapy.

5. Parenteral gold salt therapy (Solganal) is far more effective than oral gold salt therapy (auranofin).

6. Use antibiotics *only* if secondary bacterial skin infection has been documented via skin cytology, bacterial culture, and/or skin biopsies.

## PROGNOSIS FOR PATIENTS WITH CANINE PEMPHIGUS OR PEMPHIGOID

### Pemphigus Foliaceus

Approximately 75% of my patients responded well to therapy and did not have serious side effects resulting from medications. Approximately 15% of patients suffered significant side effects of therapy (including corticosteroid-induced diabetes mellitus; azathioprine-induced bone marrow suppression; and unacceptable, uncomfortable corticosteroid side effects such as personality changes, obesity, joint disease, and excessive polyuria). Approximately 10% of my patients were lost to follow-up, or euthanized due to cost, apparent patient suffering, or poor owner compliance.

### Pemphigus Erythematosus

In almost 90% of my patients, the disease was "controlled" (cosmetically acceptable) on relatively safe levels of medications. Approximately 10% of my patients were lost to follow-up, suffered unacceptable disease complications such as constant nosebleeds or extensive nasal erosion, or were euthanized due to lack of owner compliance/acceptance.

### Pemphigus Vulgaris

Over 50% of my pemphigus vulgaris patients were euthanized within the first 6 months of diagnosis due to lack of response to therapy, side effects of medication, cost of treatment and monitoring, and/or an unacceptable quality of life.

### Pemphigus Vegetans

All three of my patients are leading normal lives on low-dose, alternate-day corticosteroid therapy (2 to 7 years).

### Canine (Bullous) Pemphigoid

Of 28 cases of canine pemphigoid, nine were lost to follow-up, six were euthanized within the first 3 months of therapy, another five were euthanized within the first year of therapy, and one died accidently. The remaining seven dogs are living comfortable lives, relatively lesion free, and with no significant side effects of therapy.

# ULCERATIVE DERMATOSIS OF SHETLAND SHEEPDOGS AND COLLIES

PETER J. IHRKE

*Davis, California*

*and* THELMA LEE GROSS

*West Sacramento, California*

Ulcerative dermatosis of Shetland sheepdogs and collies is a rare, poorly understood syndrome of adult onset. The syndrome is characterized by vesicobullae and ulcerations that predominantly affect the intertriginous regions of the groin and axillae. Lesions may vary markedly in both extent and severity. This dermatosis may represent a variant of canine familial dermatomyositis, since certain cutaneous histopathologic changes are qualitatively similar, coexistent myositis has been noted, and breed predilections are identical.

## CLINICAL FEATURES

Transient vesicobullous eruptions eventuate in coalescing erosions and ulcerations with distinct, serpiginous arcuate borders. The transition from affected areas to adjacent normal skin is often strikingly abrupt. The lesions usually begin in the comparatively glabrous regions of the groin, and frequently spread subsequently to the axillae. Other less common sites of involvement include the eyelids, pinnae, oral mucosa, genitals, anus, and footpads. The localization of lesions may be partially bilaterally symmetric. Larger, serpiginous ulcers may be painful, especially in the flexure surfaces of the groin. Secondary bacterial colonization of the ulcers may lead to suppuration and additional pain. Concerted, frequent grooming of the ulcers by the dog commonly removes any suppurative debris, making the diagnosis of secondary bacterial infection more difficult. Mild to moderate scarring is a feature of severe, chronic lesions. As in canine familial dermatomyositis, estrus may trigger relapse.

Muscle involvement has been asymptomatic in the cases studied to date. Electromyography, performed because skin biopsy findings and affected breeds mirrored canine familial dermatomyositis, revealed concomitant myositis, characterized by fibrillation potentials, positive sharp waves, and unusual high-frequency discharges.

To our knowledge, this syndrome has been seen only in the adult Shetland sheepdog and collie. The syndrome appears to be more common in the Shetland sheepdog. Sex predilection has not been noted. None of the dogs seen by the authors have had a previous history suggestive of juvenile-onset canine familial dermatomyositis.

## DIAGNOSIS

Ulcerative dermatosis of Shetland sheepdogs and collies is a visually distinctive skin disease. Some Shetland sheepdogs and collies previously diagnosed as having bullous pemphigoid (or formerly, hidradenitis suppurativa) may have had this syndrome. Other clinical differential diagnoses include erythema multiforme major, systemic lupus erythematosus, and pemphigus vulgaris.

Canine bullous pemphigoid is a very rare autoimmune disease affecting both skin and mucous membranes. The oral mucosa and pinnae are more commonly affected in canine bullous pemphigoid than in ulcerative dermatosis. Ulceration and scarring generally are considerably more severe in canine bullous pemphigoid. Direct immunofluorescent or immunohistochemical testing should reveal a linear band of immunoglobulin deposition at the basement membrane zone, in contrast to ulcerative dermatosis.

Erythema multiforme major usually presents as a rapidly fulminating, ulcerative syndrome affecting the oral mucosa as well as the skin of the trunk. Early lesions are annular target lesions that quickly coalesce, rather than vesicobullae that slowly eventuate in arcuate ulcerations with distinct serpiginous borders. Most cases of erythema multiforme are drug induced; drug histories have been consistently negative in the case of ulcerative dermatosis seen by the authors.

Systemic lupus erythematosus produces pleomorphic skin lesions in conjunction with evidence of other organ system involvement. Ventral body ulcers may resemble those of ulcerative dermatosis of Shetland sheepdogs and collies. Antinuclear antibody testing is positive in systemic lupus erythematosus and has been negative consistently in ulcerative dermatosis.

Canine pemphigus vulgaris is a very rare autoimmune skin disease usually characterized by severe, expanding ulcerative lesions of the oral mucosa, other mucous membranes, and the skin. The severity and rapidly expanding nature of the skin lesions are substantially more dramatic than ulcerative dermatosis of the Shetland sheepdog and collie. Direct immunofluorescent or immunohistochemical testing should reveal intercellular deposition of immunoglobulin in the epidermis.

Skin biopsy is required for the diagnosis of ulcerative dermatosis of the Shetland sheepdog and collie. The erythematous, crusted margins of the ulcers are most likely to yield diagnostic histopathologic lesions. Wedge technique is preferred due to the fragility of the dermoepidermal junction in this disease, since punch technique can shear weak epidermal attachments, resulting in loss of epidermis from the specimens. Electromyographic and histopathologic evidence of muscle inflammation, if present, also support the diagnosis.

Histopathologically, ulcerative dermatosis of the Shetland sheepdog and collie is characterized by severe basal cell damage, generally characterized by brightly eosinophilic individual cell necrosis, as well as basal cell vacuolation. Basal cell degeneration is most prominent in the epidermis but is also present in the outer wall of superficial hair follicles. Individual cell necrosis may extend more mildly to the stratum spinosum. True vesiculation or Stannard's "usable artifact" (dermoepidermal separation at the margins of a structurally weakened specimen) both may be seen as a result of the basal cell damage. Ulceration and exudation are common. The dermal inflammatory infiltrate is superficial, perivascular to partially lichenoid, and composed of mixed mononuclear inflammatory cells, including lymphocytes and macrophages. Ulcers are subtended by a prominent neutrophilic infiltrate.

The epidermal lesions are qualitatively similar to but more severe than most cases of canine familial dermatomyositis. Follicular atrophy, a prominent feature of canine familial dermatomyositis, is absent in ulcerative dermatosis, possibly reflecting the more fulminating and severe nature of the lesions in ulcerative dermatosis. Individual cell necrosis of keratinocytes of the upper layers of the epidermis in ulcerative dermatosis is very similar to erythema multiforme, but is generally not as severe. Direct immunofluorescent testing for immunoglobulin or complement has been consistently negative in ulcerative dermatosis of the Shetland sheepdog and collie, unlike in canine autoimmune skin diseases.

## CLINICAL MANAGEMENT

Therapeutic management mimics that used for canine familial dermatomyositis. Evaluating therapeutic efficacy is difficult, since symptoms may be quite cyclical. Since fragility at the dermoepidermal junction presumably is responsible for the ulceration, minimization of the potential for trauma and self-trauma is beneficial. Forbidding rough playing with another dog was surprisingly beneficial in one case seen by the first author. All coexistent pruritic skin diseases (especially those affecting the groin and axillae such as flea allergy dermatitis) must be diagnosed and treated appropriately to prevent or reduce potential for self-trauma due to pruritus. Hypoallergenic shampoos may be beneficial.

Clinical or histologic evidence of secondary pyoderma warrants the use of systemic antibiotics. Cephalexin (22 mg/kg PO every 12 hr) for 4 weeks has been beneficial in reducing both the amount of inflammation and the size of the lesions (Mundell AC, personal communication, 1993). This partial response to antibiotics may have led to erroneous diagnoses of hidradenitis suppurativa.

Immunosuppressive dosages of corticosteroids may be beneficial in the management of early cases and in more chronic cases during periods of recrudescence when more severe ulceration is a feature. Initial dosages of prednisone or prednisolone (1 to 2 mg/kg PO every 12 hr) are utilized followed by tapering to lowest efficacious alternate-day therapy.

Pentoxifylline (Trental, Hoechst-Roussel), utilizing 400-mg controlled release tablets either daily or every other day, has been helpful in diminishing inflammation and encouraging healing. Daily medication has been more beneficial, but some dogs vomit with daily therapy. In human medicine, pentoxifylline is administered three times daily. This dosing schedule can be accomplished in veterinary medication if reformulation into smaller dose capsules is performed by a pharmacist. Pentoxifylline increases microvascular blood flow, which presumably leads to enhanced tissue oxygenation. In addition, pentoxifylline inhibits tumor necrosis factor α. Affected dogs also have seemed to benefit from vitamin E administered orally at 200 to 400 mg PO every 12 hours.

Long-term clinical management of ulcerative dermatosis of the Shetland sheepdog and collie can be problematic. While mild cases may be merely troublesome, more severely affected dogs may exhibit lifelong debilitating disease with cyclical recrudescence. The marked breed predilection of ulcerative dermatosis of the Shetland sheepdog and collie, coupled with an apparent link with canine familial dermatomyositis, suggests genetic predilection. The authors recommend that affected dogs should not be used for breeding and should be neutered.

## References and Suggested Reading

Ely H: Pentoxifylline therapy in dermatology: A review of localized hyperviscosity and its effects on the skin. Dermatol Clin 6:585, 1988.

Giroir BP: Mediators of septic shock: New approaches for interrupting the endogenous inflammatory cascade. Crit Care Med 212:780, 1993.

Gross TL, Ihrke PJ, and Walder EJ: Veterinary Dermatopathology: A Macroscopic and Microscopic Evaluation of Canine and Feline Skin Disease. St. Louis, Mosby Year Book, 1992, pp 36–38.

Hargis AM and Mundell AC: Familial canine dermatomyositis. Compend Con Educ 14:855, 1992.

Samlaska CP and Winfield EA: Pentoxifylline. J Am Acad Dermatol 30:603, 1994.

# DISEASES OF THE CLAW AND CLAW FOLD

ROD A.W. ROSYCHUK

*Fort Collins, Colorado*

Diseases restricted to the claw and/or claw fold appear to be uncommonly encountered in clinical practice. Dogs presenting with claw (or claw fold) disorders as the only dermatologic manifestation of disease constituted 1.3% of cases seen by a referral clinic (Scott and Miller, 1992b). In cats, the reported incidence was 2.2% (Scott and Miller, 1992a).

## NORMAL ANATOMY

The claw fold is that fold of skin which covers the proximal dorsal and lateral portion of the claw. The claw is a modified extension of the skin (both epidermis and dermis) covering phalanx 3 (P3). The dermis (corium) covers P3. It contains blood vessels and nerves and is often referred to as the quick. The dermis is continuous with the periosteum of P3 on its inner surface, and supports the epidermis on its outer surface. The epidermis over the dorsal, lateral, and medial surfaces of the claw is modified to become the claw plate (wall), and ventrally, the claw sole. The basal cell layer of the epidermis produces several layers of noncornified keratinocytes that subsequently flatten, cornify, and fuse to become the claw plate and sole. The proximal base of the claw is often referred to as the coronary (crown-like) band region. Basal cells are most active in their production of keratinocytes in the dorsal ridge and coronary band regions. In dogs, claws have been reported to grow by 0.8 to 1.6 mm/wk or by an average of 1.9 mm/wk (Scott and Miller, 1992b).

Histologically, the basal cell layer and adjacent keratinocytes (keratogenous zone) at the very proximal portion of the claw are referred to as the claw matrix. It is this region that is most active in the production of keratinocytes. Damage to the claw matrix generally results in the production of an abnormal claw plate. It is important to note that in normal claws, it is quite common to see intranuclear vacuoles within the basal cell layer and artifactual clefting of the dermoepidermal junction due to decalcification and sectioning, respectively. These changes must be differentiated from those seen with certain autoimmune/immune–mediated diseases.

## DISEASES OF THE CLAW

When disease is restricted to one or two claws, most likely underlying etiologies include trauma, bacterial or fungal infections, or neoplasia. When multiple claws are involved on all feet (often in a symmetric fashion), major consideration is given to autoimmune/immune–mediated, genetic, endocrine, nutritional, or immunosuppressive diseases (Scott and Miller, 1992a,b).

### Terminology

The terms used to describe pathologic changes of the claw are summarized in Table 1.

### General Diagnostic Approach

The work-up of any disease of the claw must begin with a thorough dermatologic history and examination. Asymmetric involvement of only one or two claws warrants fungal culture, Wood's lamp examination, KOH preparation (see "Fungal Infection," below), cytologic examination of exudates, bacterial culture and sensitivity testing or trial systemic antibiotic therapy (see "Bacterial Infection," below), radiographs, and/or P3 amputation for histologic examination. In cases of generalized/symmetric onychodystrophy or onychomadesis, all of the above are generally performed. In addition, the patient is screened for systemic disease (e.g., complete blood count [CBC], serum chemistry panel, urinalysis, antinuclear antibody [ANA] titer, cold agglutinin evaluation, thyroid/adrenal evaluation).

Diseases of the claw produce their most significant changes in the dermoepidermal junction area and dermis overlying P3. Even when claw fold involvement is concurrently noted, biopsies from the claw fold alone often fail to delineate the pathologic process. Histologic examination of P3 and the entire associated claw unit is necessary for these purposes. Routine declawing procedures are adequate for obtaining a sample. Care should be taken to retrieve the entire claw and a small portion of the nail fold. In those diseases where claw plate loosening/sloughing is encountered, secondary changes (e.g., bacterial infection) occur quickly. For diagnostic purposes, emphasis should be placed on amputating P3 when the claw is early in the course of its disease (ideally before extensive claw plate separation has occurred). Early changes are often heralded by serous, serosanguineous, or purulent exudation around the base of the claw plate. In the dog, emphasis should be placed on harvesting an involved dewclaw or the P3 of digits 2 or 5. The claws of digits 3 and 4 are generally

**Table 1.**  *Terminology for Claw/Claw Fold Disorders*°

| Term | Definition |
| --- | --- |
| Paronychia | Inflammation of claw fold |
| Anonychia | Absence of claws (usually congenital) |
| Leukonychia | Whitening of claws |
| Macronychia | Unusually large claws |
| Micronychia | Unusually small claws, often shorter or narrower than normal |
| Onychalgia | Claw pain |
| Onychauxis | Hypertrophy of claws |
| Onychia (onychitis) | Inflammation in the claw unit; usually in the matrix |
| Onychoclasis | Breaking of claws |
| Onychocryptosis | Ingrown claw |
| Onychodystrophy | Abnormal claw formation |
| Onychogryphosis | Hypertrophy and abnormal curvature of claws |
| Onychomadesis | Sloughing of claws |
| Onychomalacia | Softening of claws |
| Onychomycosis | Fungal infection of claws |
| Onychorrhexis | Longitudinal striations associated with brittleness and breaking of claws |
| Onychopathy (onychosis) | Disease or deformity of claw(s) |
| Onychoschizia | Splitting and/or lamination of claws, usually in the horizontal plane at the free edge |

°Modified from Scott DW and Miller WH: Disorders of the claw and clawbed in dogs. Compend Cont Educ 14:1448, 1992b, with permission.

weight bearing and would be last choices. The claw is placed in routine 10% neutral buffered formalin for submission. In order to obtain appropriate sections for histopathologic examination, the pathologist will ideally section the claw sagittally (along the long axis).

### General Principles of Therapy

In most disorders of the claw, emphasis is placed on frequent nail clipping and/or filing to keep the claws short and less likely to catch on material. In claw loosening and sloughing syndromes, claw plates that begin to separate from the claw bed will invariably be lost, in spite of therapy. These loosened claw plates frequently catch on material and are a constant source of discomfort/pain. In such cases, it is appropriate to avulse the entire claw plate. This is best done by firmly grasping and pulling the claw plate with heavy forceps (e.g., needle drivers). All remnant claw plate should be removed. Hemorrhage is variable but transient. Every effort should be made to leave the entire underlying dermis (quick) intact. If this is stripped away, claw regrowth may be poor or absent and there is significant concern for osteomyelitis or avascular necrosis of P3. Claw plates that have not yet begun to separate should not be avulsed. Multiple claw plates may be removed at the same time under general anesthesia. Avulsed claws are covered with a germicidal ointment (e.g., 10% povidone-iodine ointment) and the foot is bandaged for 1 to 2 days. Even with multiple avulsions, discomfort is transient. Following bandage removal, every effort must be made to keep the feet free of debris. Exercise should be minimized and limited to clean, smooth surfaces. Routine cleansing with a germicidal shampoo

may be of benefit. For exudative lesions, soaks with an astringent/germicidal solution such as one packet aluminum acetate (Domeboro, Miles Inc) and 25 ml of 2% chlorhexidine in 1 pint of water may be of benefit. Soaks are repeated every 8 or 12 hr.

When attempts at medical management have failed to benefit a claw disorder, consideration should be given to P3 amputation. 20-nail P3 amputations (all nails on all toes) are routinely performed in the cat. They can also be performed in the dog. Although generally well tolerated in dogs, multiple P3 amputations may result in some lameness following exercise (e.g., working dogs).

### Trauma

Trauma is the most common disorder affecting claws of both dogs and cats. Tearing, crushing, or bite wounds for example, result in fracture and/or avulsion of part of the claw plate and occasionally P3. Affected claws are often painful and variably pruritic. Secondary paronychia due to self-trauma (licking, biting) and secondary bacterial infections are common. Therapy involves clipping, cleansing, removal of the fractured portion of the affected claw, and topical astringent/germicidal soaks every 8 or 12 hr (see "General Principles of Therapy," above). If secondary bacterial infections are suspected, oral antibiotics are indicated (see "Bacterial Infection," below). The prognosis for claw regrowth is good. If the claw matrix is significantly damaged, any new claw plate formation may be abnormal (aberrant curl, ridged, abnormal consistency of claw plate).

## Bacterial Infection

Bacterial infections of the claw are almost invariably secondary to some underlying local or systemic disease. Trauma (e.g., fracture, excessively short nail clipping) affecting only one or a few claws is most common. There is often significant paronychia, toe swelling, pain, lymphadenopathy and, with multiple claw involvement, variable fever and depression. Claw sloughing (onychomadesis) is variable. Osteomyelitis may develop in chronically affected claws.

*Staphylococcus intermedius* is most commonly isolated in dogs, although mixed bacterial infections frequently occur. Samples for bacterial culture are best taken from the proximal portion of a loosened claw plate. Preparation for culture includes clipping, surgical scrubbing, and drying the base of the claw. The claw plate is then avulsed. The proximal portion of the avulsed claw plate is cut away and placed in sterile transport media for submission to a microbiology laboratory.

Therapy for bacterial claw infections secondary to trauma begins with avulsion of fractured portions of the claw. If the entire claw plate is loosened, it should be totally avulsed. Systemic antibiotic therapy is ideally based on culture and sensitivity testing. Empiric choices include standard doses of cephalexin, enrofloxacin, amoxicillin trihydrate/clavulanate potassium, or potentiated sulfonamides. Topical germicidal soaks (e.g., 2% chlorhexidine diluted 1:40 in water) may be of benefit. The prognosis for recovery and claw regrowth is good. Refractory, recurrent disease may be associated with osteomyelitis of P3. In such cases, P3 amputation may be necessary to effect a cure.

Widespread, symmetric onychomadesis due to bacterial infection has been noted in dogs with hypothyroidism or hyperadrenocorticism (Scott and Miller, 1992b). Improvement is noted with systemic antibiotic therapy but is recurrent when antibiotics are discontinued. Therapy includes systemic antibiotics, possible claw plate avulsions, and control of the underlying disease.

It is common to see secondary *Staphylococcus intermedius* infections in canine autoimmune/immune–mediated and idiopathic onychomadesis/onychorrhexis. Systemic antibiotic therapy may lessen inflammation, exudation, pain and pruritus, and slow progression of claw plate fragmentation/loss.

## Fungal Infection

Onychomycosis due to dermatophytosis is a rare cause of claw disease in the dog and cat. When present, *Trichophyton mentagrophytes* is most commonly isolated. There is usually asymmetric involvement of only one or two claws. Attendant paronychia is common. The affected claw plate is often friable and misshapen. *Trichophyton mentagrophytes* may also produce a symmetric, 20-nail onychodystrophy in the dog. In these cases, paronychia or more generalized skin disease may be present. A diagnosis of onychomycosis is made by fungal culture. Samples are best taken from the more proximal portion of the claw plate (coronary band region). Multiple samples should be obtained. They may be washed with alcohol to reduce contaminants. Claw samples are submitted to a microbiology laboratory for culture or are fragmented (mortar and pestle or shave claw with a blade) and placed on a routine dermatophyte culture media. Caution must be employed in interpreting results. It is possible to have transient contamination of the feet with *Trichophyton* spp. and *Microsporum gypseum* (Foil, 1987). Consideration should also be given to the possibility of false-negative cultures. These are noted in 10 to 20% of onychomycosis cases in humans (Zaias, 1990). Arthrospores and/or mycelia may be visualized by clearing claw shavings in 10 to 20% KOH over 24 hr (Foil, 1987) or with special stains of P3 amputations prepared for histologic examination. Claws infected with *Microsporum canis* occasionally may fluoresce under a Wood's lamp.

Therapy for onychomycosis should generally be aggressive. Onychomycosis is well known for its tendency to be refractory or recurrent in humans. This appears to be the case in the dog and cat. Systemic therapy is initiated with higher dosages of microsized griseofulvin (50 to 75 mg/kg every 12 hr). Alternatives favored by some include ketoconazole (5 to 10 mg/kg every 12 hr) or itraconazole (5 to 10 mg/kg every 24 hr). Systemic therapy should be continued for 1 to 3 months beyond complete claw regrowth and negative culture (usually a total of 6 months or more of treatment). Adjunctive topical therapy includes germicidal soaks (2% chlorhexidine diluted 1:30 to 1:40 in water or 10% povidone-iodine diluted 1:10 in water) for 5 to 10 min every 12 hr or one drop of Tresaderm (MSD Ag Vet) per claw every 12 hr. In humans, avulsion of the nail plate has been noted to improve the response to systemic treatment (Zaias, 1990). In the dog, this procedure should be performed only if the nails are loosened/sloughing. Even with aggressive therapy, complete recovery may not be achieved. In such instances, consideration may be given to indefinite low-dose daily systemic therapy (e.g., ketoconazole) or P3 amputations.

Other fungal infections of the claw are only rarely encountered in the dog and cat. Candidiasis secondary to diabetes mellitus produced a symmetric onychomadesis in one dog; a geotrichum infection and cryptococcosis have also been reported to affect the claw of the dog (Scott and Miller, 1992b).

## Autoimmune/Immune–Mediated Disease

In the dog, pemphigus vulgaris, pemphigus foliaceus, bullous pemphigoid, systemic lupus erythematosus, a lupus-like syndrome, cold agglutinin disease, drug eruption, and vasculitis have all been noted to cause symmetric onychomadesis and onychodystrophy, without attendant paronychia. However, it is more common to see concurrent paronychia and/or more generalized cutaneous manifestations. In the cat, these diseases have been noted to cause paronychia, but significant claw plate involvement is exceedingly rare. The author has seen cold agglutinin disease, drug eruption, and vasculitis produce widespread, symmetric onychomadesis in the cat. Diagnosis is supported by CBC, serum chemistry screening, urinalysis, ANA titer, determination of cold agglutinins, and P3 biopsy. Therapy is with immunosuppressive drugs and is discussed elsewhere. If the immunologic phenomenon can be put into remission, normal claw regrowth may be noted.

Perhaps the most common cause of 20-nail onychomadesis in the dog has been referred to as a lupus-like (Scott and Miller, 1992b) or lupoid syndrome. It has been recognized in many breeds, including the miniature schnauzer, golden retriever, Labrador retriever, Rottweiler, and mixed breeds. The age of onset is variable, but tends to be in younger dogs (1 to 6 years of age). Both sexes are affected. Onset of nail loss is usually acute. Affected claws are often painful, pruritic, and result in lameness. Progression to 20-nail loss may be rapid (over 2 to 4 weeks) or protracted over 4 to 6 months. Onychorrhexis is variable. In some cases, it may be the only presenting sign. Paronychia is generally absent, as is a proximal reactive lymphadenopathy or systemic involvement. If present, these signs usually suggest a secondary bacterial infection. Left untreated, the tendency is to have partial regrowth of abnormal, friable nail that continues to be sloughed/pulled off. There is generally no history of other related skin disease. Diagnosis is based on rule-out and histologic evaluation of P3. There is usually widespread hydropic degeneration of the basal cell layer of the epidermis, a mononuclear interface dermatitis, and marked pigmentary incontinence. Dermoepidermal separation may be noted. The author is not aware of direct immunofluorescence (DIF) testing or immunoperoxidase staining performed on affected tissues. Secondary bacterial infections (especially *Staphylococcus intermedius*) are common.

In spite of therapies listed below, loosened claw plates usually will be lost. So they should be removed at the time of anesthesia when diagnostic P3 amputation is performed. Systemic antibiotic therapy is indicated for secondary bacterial infection. Support for the theory of an immune-mediated nature for this disease is provided by the fact that it does respond to immunosuppressive dosages of glucocorticoids (oral prednisone, 2 to 4 mg/kg/day for 2 to 4 weeks, then half this dose for 2 to 4 weeks, then gradually reduce to the lowest every-other-day dose required for maintenance). After several months of successful therapy, one should attempt to discontinue medication. Spontaneous resolutions may occur. An alternative therapy that has been successful in three of four cases treated by the author involves the use of tetracycline and niacinamide as described for discoid lupus erythematosus (White et al., 1991). Doses of 500 mg of tetracycline and 500 mg of niacinamide are given every 8 hr (250 mg of each for patients less than 10 kg) until the claws are significantly regrown (3 to 6 months). The frequency of administration of both drugs is then decreased to every 12 hr for 2 months, then both are given once per day. If the claws remain intact after 4 to 6 months of once-per-day therapy, treatment is stopped. Recurrence of signs warrants indefinite maintenance therapy. The trial treatment period for this drug combination is 3 months. Significant nail regrowth is generally noted within 1 to 2 months; complete regrowth often takes 4 to 8 months. Affected claws will usually regrow normally, although some claws may be deformed or friable. Alternatively, fatty acid therapy (Derm Caps, DVM) at routine dosages may be of benefit in some cases (Scott and Miller, 1992b).

## Neoplasia of the Claw

Squamous cell carcinoma, melanoma, mast cell tumor, keratoacanthoma, inverted papilloma, lymphosarcoma, eccrine adenocarcinoma, neurofibrosarcoma, hemangiopericytoma, fibrosarcoma, osteosarcoma, myxosarcoma, and undifferentiated sarcoma have all been reported to involve the distal digit/claw and/or claw fold in the dog (O'Brien, Berg, and Engler, 1992). The vast majority of cases involve only a single toe. Patients are usually presented for digit swelling, pain, and pruritus. At presentation, there is often toe swelling, paronychia, and variable degrees of erosion/ulceration. The claw may be dystrophic or absent.

Squamous cell carcinoma (SCC) arising from germinal claw epithelium is the most common digital tumor in the dog. Large-breed dogs with black coats, particularly Labrador retrievers and standard poodles, are predisposed. In these breeds, multiple digits may be involved over a course of 2 to 4 years. The tumors appear to be slow growing. Radiographic and histologic evidence of P3 invasion is common. Metastasis is rare, so SCC should be treated by amputation of the involved digit. Prognosis for a cure or prolonged disease-free survival is good. In dogs with regional lymph node metastasis, lymph node excision or limb amputation should be considered (O'Brien, Berg, and Engler, 1992).

Melanomas of the canine digit are highly malignant.

In the cat, a similar spectrum of tumors has been noted. Primary squamous cell carcinomas (originating from claw epithelium) and eccrine carcinomas are aggressively malignant neoplasms. Pulmonary adenocarcinomas and visceral squamous cell carcinoma may metastasize to multiple distal digits in the cat. Digit swelling is the predominant presenting sign. At the time of presentation, there may be no significant evidence of internal involvement. Toe amputation is only palliative (Scott and Miller, 1992a).

## Miscellaneous Causes of Onychomadesis (Claw Sloughing)

Superficial necrolytic dermatitis (hepatocutaneous syndrome) may cause symmetric onychomadesis. Other skin changes are almost always concurrently present (e.g., paronychia, pad hyperkeratosis, alopecia, inflammation, crusting around mouth and eyes). Affected patients usually have concurrent liver disease. Diagnosis is by history, physical examination, and skin biopsy. Response to therapy is generally poor.

An idiopathic, symmetric onychomadesis has been noted in German shepherd dogs in Sweden, whippets in Finland, and English springer spaniels in Norway. No histologic changes were reported (Scott and Miller, 1992b). The author has seen similar presentations. German shepherd dogs appear overrepresented. Claw loss is generally acute. In the very early stages of development, histologic inflammatory changes are minimal. With chronicity, there is a nonspecific diffuse dermal accumulation of neutrophils, macrophages, and lymphocytes. Some degree of improvement is achieved with systemic therapy for secondary infections. This disease must be differentiated from drug eruptions and autoimmune/immune–mediated diseases. In some patients, there is permanent regrowth of normal claw plates; in others, permanent regrowth is noted, but some or all nails are dystrophic. Patients may have recurrent bouts of onychomadesis. There is no apparent therapy for this syndrome, although some have suggested benefit from drug therapy noted to improve peripheral circulation (pentoxifylline, Trental, Hoechst; 400 mg/day) as used in the treatment of canine familial dermatomyositis.

## Miscellaneous Causes of Onychodystrophy (Deformed and/or Friable Claws)

Patients presented with onychodystrophy characterized by variable degrees of onychorrhexis and onychomalacia should have the following differential diagnoses considered:

1. Canine primary seborrhea; dogs have other skin changes consistent with this diagnosis; reported in four cocker spaniels whose skin disease was under control with therapy, but claw abnormalities persisted (Scott and Miller, 1992b).
2. Senile change in old dogs (symmetric); old cats (symmetric, long, curly, dystrophic claws; nutritional imbalance?).
3. Idiopathic symmetric disease in younger dogs (2 to 6 years) with some breeds overrepresented (e.g., dachshund, Siberian husky, Rhodesian ridgeback, German shepherd dog); may be some genetic predisposition.
4. Idiopathic asymmetric (usually one claw) dystrophy in cats, possibly due to previous trauma (also abnormally thick, curved).
5. Canine lupus-like syndrome (see previous discussion).
6. Acrodermatitis in bull terriers.
7. Severe nutritional deficiencies in dogs.
8. Sequela to any of the inflammatory dermatoses noted previously.

9. Hyperthyroidism in cats is noted to produce excessively long and curved claws, due to rapid claw growth.

In the above idiopathic and seborrheic onychodystrophies, therapy is often restricted to frequent nail clipping and filing. The tendency of abnormal claws to catch on material can be minimized with frequent painting of the nails with nail glue (made to attach human artificial nails) or the use of nail caps (Soft Paws, SmartPractice). In one report, three dachshunds responded well to the continuous administration of gelatin (10 grains orally every 12 hr) (Scott and Miller, 1992b). Similar therapy with Knox gelatin (1 packet/15 lb/day) may also be useful. Because biotin-responsive hoof dystrophies have been noted in both horses and pigs (Comben, Clark, and Sutherland, 1984), similar therapy may be of benefit in dogs. Consideration should also be given to retinoid therapy. In refractory cases associated with significant patient discomfort, P3 amputations may be of significant benefit (see "General Principles of Therapy," above).

## DISEASES OF THE CLAW FOLD

Most diseases of the claw fold are inflammatory (paronychia) and involve variable degrees of swelling, alopecia, exudation, crusting, erosion, ulceration, pain, or pruritus. On occasion, changes may be limited to the accumulation of oily/waxy debris. Especially in cats, a caseous, white or yellow exudate can often be expressed from the nail fold area with bacterial, fungal, or autoimmune disease (especially pemphigus foliaceus). Differential diagnoses for paronychia are listed in Table 2.

In general, the work-up of claw fold disease should involve skin scrapings for mites, fungal evaluation (Wood's lamp; KOH-cleared preparations; culture of hairs, crust, and scale), and cytologic examination of exudates. The predominance of degenerative neutrophils, macrophages, and intracellular organisms suggests bacterial or fungal infection. Large numbers of nondegenerative neutrophils and eosinophils with large numbers of acantholytic keratinocytes suggest the pemphigus complex. Large numbers of eosinophils may suggest eosinophilic plaques or eosinophilic granuloma in the cat. Atypical cells suggest neoplasia (Scott and Miller, 1992a). Samples taken for bacterial culture and sensitivity must be interpreted with caution. If debris from the fold is cultured, contaminants and colonizers are usually grown. Results should be interpreted in light of cytologic findings (intracellular bacterial most significant). More reliable results may be achieved by submitting a skin biopsy for culture and sensitivity testing (requires prior surgical cleansing/drying). Multiple samples from multiple sites can often be obtained with a 2-mm biopsy punch. Tissue biopsy (wedge-shaped section) for purposes of histologic and immunologic studies are best taken without surgical cleansing. When

**Table 2.** *Diseases of the Claw Fold*

**Asymmetric (One or More Affected Claw Folds on the Same Paw)**

| | |
|---|---|
| Trauma | |
| Bacterial infection | Most common cause of paronychia in dogs and cats; usually secondary to broken claw; predominantly *Escherichia coli* in cat,[*] *Staphylococcus intermedius* in the dog. |
| Fungal infection | *Cat*: dermatophytosis most common (usually *Microsporum canis*; claw involvement rare); candidiasis (vesiculopustular eruption); blastomycosis, sporotrichosis (abcessation, drainage)[†], cryptococcosis |
| | *Dog*: dermatophytosis most common (*Trichophyton mentagrophytes*); blastomycosis[†] |
| Arteriovenous fistula | More common in cat; toe/foot swelling; generally secondary to trauma |
| Neoplasia | See "Neoplasia of the Claw" |

**Symmetric (One or More Affected Claw Folds on Two or More Paws)**

| | |
|---|---|
| Bacterial infection | Secondary to immunocompromising disease: FeLV and FIV, diabetes mellitus, and iatrogenic hyperadrenocorticism in the cat[*]; hypothyroidism, hyperadrenocorticism,[†] and idiopathic immunoinsufficiencies in the dog |
| Fungal infection | Candidiasis secondary to diabetes mellitus in the dog[†]; geotrichosis and cryptococcosis with onychodystrophy in the dog[†] |
| Demodicosis | *Dog* and *Cat*; expect more extensive involvement (i.e., pododermatitis) |
| Hookworm dermatitis | *Dog*: "Fleshy ring" encircling claw |
| Autoimmune/immune | *Cat*: pemphigus foliaceus most common (initial site of involvement in the majority of cases; claw involvement rare); pemphigus vulgaris, systemic lupus erythematosus, cold agglutinin disease, drug eruption, vasculitis[*] |
| | *Dog*: As for cat; bullous pemphigoid; claw involvement more common than in cat[†] |
| Idiopathic seborrhea | *Dog*: oily/waxy accumulation; generally more extensive skin disease; cocker spaniel, basset hound predisposed |
| Neoplasia | Metastatic pulmonary adenocarcinoma, metastatic squamous cell carcinoma in the cat[*] |
| Miscellaneous | Superficial necrolytic dermatitis in the dog, eosinophilic plaque in the cat,[*] disseminated intravascular coagulation, nutritional deficiencies, thallotoxicosis, ergotism |

[*]Data derived from Scott and Miller, 1992a.
[†]Data derived from Scott and Miller, 1992b.
[‡]Data derived from Foil, 1987.

claw abnormalities are noted, superior diagnostic samples can usually be obtained by P3 amputation.

Therapy for bacterial paronychia includes specific treatment for underlying disease (where present), clipping, cleansing (benzoyl peroxide shampoo, germicidal or astringent/germicidal soaks; see claw diseases), and systemic antibiotics (cephalexin, enrofloxacin, amoxicillin trihydrate/clavulonate potassium) pending culture and sensitivity data. Therapy should extend 1 to 2 weeks beyond apparent clinical remission. Declawing should be considered for recurrent bacterial paronychia in cats. Canine idiopathic recurrent bacterial paronychia may be managed with long-term, low-dose antibiotic therapy (cephalexin) or bacterin therapy (e.g., Staphage lysate).

Therapy for dermatophytosis involves clipping, cleansing with antifungal shampoos such as 1% miconazole (Dermazole, Allerderm/Virbac) or 1% chlorhexi-dine (Chlorhexiderm, DVM), twice-weekly total body dips with 25 to 50 ml/L 2% chlorhexidine or 2% lime sulfur, and focal therapy with an imidazole solution (e.g., miconazole, Conofite, Pitman-Moore). Extensive, severe disease may warrant systemic antifungal therapy with microsized griseofulvin (25 to 30 mg/kg/day), ketoconazole, or itraconazole (see "Claw Diseases," above, for dosages). In the presence of concurrent claw disease, systemic therapy is mandatory. Therapy for fungal paronychia is maintained for 2 weeks beyond remission.

Immune-mediated diseases are generally treated with immunosuppressive dosages of glucocorticoids (to initiate therapy) with or without chlorambucil, or gold salts in the cat; azathioprine, chlorambucil, or gold salts in the dog.

The management and prognosis for neoplasia involving the claw fold are discussed under "Neoplasia of the Claw," above.

## References and Suggested Reading

Comben N, Clark D, and Sutherland JB: Clinical observations on the response of equine hoof defects to dietary supplementation with biotin. Vet Rec 115:642, 1984.
*Case histories of horses with hoof horn abnormalities and their response to biotin therapy.*
Foil CS: Disorders of the feet and claws. Proc Annu Kal Kan Symp 11:23, 1987.
*A review of the clinical presentations, methods of diagnosis, and therapy of diseases of the claw and pododermatitis in dogs and cats.*
O'Brien MG, Berg J, and Engler SJ: Treatment by digital amputation of subungual cell carcinoma in dogs: 21 cases (1987–1988). J Am Vet Med Assoc 201:759, 1992.
*A retrospective study of the neoplasias affecting the digit of the dog with emphasis on the clinical, histopathologic, and long-term follow-up of dogs with subungual SCC treated by digital amputation.*

Scott DW and Miller WH: Disorders of the claw and claw bed in cats. Compend Cont Educ 14:449, 1992a.
*A retrospective study of 65 cases and a review of claw and claw fold diseases in the cat.*
Scott DW and Miller WH: Disorders of the claw and clawbed in dogs. Compend Cont Educ 14:1448, 1992b.
*A retrospective study of 196 cases and a review of normal anatomy, terminology, diseases, and diagnostic aids for claw and claw fold diseases in the dog.*
White SD, Rosychuk RAW, Reinke SI, and Paradis M: Use of tetracycline and niacinamide for treating autoimmune skin disease in 31 dogs. J Am Vet Med Assoc 200:1497, 1992.
*A retrospective study of the use of a combination of tetracycline and niacinamide in the treatment of discoid lupus erythematosus and other autoimmune skin diseases in the dog.*
Zaias N: The nail in health and disease. Norwalk, CT, Appleton & Lange, 1990, p 87.
*A review of onychomycosis presentations, diagnostic aids, and therapy in persons.*

# CANINE OTITIS EXTERNA

PATRICK J. MCKEEVER
*and* HELEN GLOBUS
*St. Paul, Minnesota*

Otitis externa is an inflammation of the epithelial lining of the external auditory canal, which is that portion of the external ear located between the pinna and the tympanic membrane. Depending on the etiology, the inflammation may spread from the auditory canal to the pinna or it may spread from the pinna to the auditory canal.

Incidence of otitis externa in the dog has been estimated to be as high as 20% of the general canine population. It has been reported to account for 4 to 16% of canine hospital admissions. Incidence of otitis in cats has been reported to be from 2 to 6.6%. Variance of reported incidence may be due to such factors as time of year when the surveys were taken, breed popularity in a given area, and the differences in criteria for a diagnosis.

Diagnosis and clinical management of otitis externa is often frustrating because there are numerous factors and diseases that predispose to otitis and numerous secondary pathogens that perpetuate the process. In addition, the tissue and inflammatory response to various pathogenic mechanisms can differ significantly among patients.

## ANATOMY OF THE EXTERNAL EAR

The pinna is funnel shaped and is formed from the distal flaring of the auricular cartilage. It serves to receive air vibrations and to transmit them via the ear canal to the tympanic membrane. The pinnae can be controlled independently and are highly mobile. The shape of the pinna is breed specific and they are covered on both sides with skin that is tightly attached to the perichondrium. The skin that lines the inner surface of the pinnae generally contains fewer hairs.

The majority of the proximal, or deep, portion of the ear canal is formed by the annular cartilage, which is rolled into a narrow band and located between the auricular cartilage and the osseous external acoustic process, to which it is attached by means of ligamentous tissue. The diameter of the ear canal is 5 to 10 mm, depending on the age, breed, and size of the dog. It is approximately 2 cm in length and ends proximally with the tympanic membrane, or ear drum (Getty et al., 1956).

The tympanic membrane is elliptical in outline, and varies markedly in size among individual animals, but averages about 15 × 10 mm (Getty et al., 1956). It is semitransparent, and thinner in the center than peripherally, where it is attached to a circular fibrocartilagenous pad. The pad is fastened to a definite collar of bone in the external acoustic meatus. The manubrium of the malleus can be seen as a white finger-like projection extending into the tympanic membrane.

The skin lining the ear canal is thinnest in the proximal portion of the canal, and becomes progressively thicker as it extends outward to the concave surface of the pinna. The number of hair follicles present in the skin of the ear canal is breed dependent. In short-coated breeds, few hair follicles are found close to the tympanic membrane. However, in long-haired dogs, very fine hairs are often present.

Sebaceous glands form the superficial glandular bed in the dermis of the ear canal and are especially prominent in the more distal or superficial areas of the canal.

The apocrine glands are located below the sebaceous glands in the deeper dermis. The number of sebaceous and apocrine glands present is also breed dependent. Long-haired and fine-haired breeds, such as spaniels and Irish setters, have increased numbers of better developed glands, relative to short-haired breeds.

## PATHOPHYSIOLOGY

Regardless of the inciting factor, inflammation of the ear canal leads to hyperplasia of epidermis and sebaceous glands, resulting in narrowing of the canal. Chronic inflammation will result in severe epidermal hyperplasia (five to six times normal thickness), as well as a persistence of the sebaceous gland hyperplasia. In addition, chronic inflammation results in hyperplasia and dilatation of the apocrine glands and their ducts, further reducing the diameter of the ear canal lumen. If rupture of these cystic apocrine glands occurs, they become surrounded by a dense infiltrate of histiocytes, polymorphonuclear leukocytes, mast cells, giant cells, and fibroblasts. Also, focal accumulations of histiocytes, lymphocytes, and plasma cells may be present within the superficial and deep dermis. All of these factors contribute to a narrowing of the lumen of the ear canal, and in some cases the lumen may become completely stenotic, making otoscopic examination of the deep portion of the canal impossible. In severe, longstanding cases of chronic otitis externa, ossification of the external ear canal and associated cartilage may occur.

## PREDISPOSING CONDITIONS

### Environmental Factors

It has generally been assumed that otitis externa is a primary condition with microorganisms being the etiologic agents. However, further study has shown that otitis is, in fact, secondary to many predisposing factors and other disease states. These other conditions create an environment in the ear that will support the proliferation of bacteria and yeast, which further contributes to the inflammatory process.

Factors predisposing to otitis include foreign bodies (plant awns, seeds, dried ear secretions, excessive hair), parasites (ticks, mites, chiggers, biting flies), trauma, excessive moisture in the ear (from frequent swimming), anatomic abnormalities such as small or restrictive ear canals, and pendulous pinnae (which prevent the circulation of air and results in a high relative humidity in the ear canal).

### Hypersensitivity Diseases

#### ATOPY

The disease most likely to predispose an animal to otitis externa is atopic dermatitis. Approximately 55%

of atopic dogs develop a concurrent otitis, and in 3% of the cases, otitis is the only manifestation of disease (Scott, 1981). Initially, lesions appear as erythema and/or edema with minimal exudation. Chronic inflammation caused by atopy leads to hyperplasia of the epidermis, sebaceous glands, and apocrine glands of the pinna and distal (or most superficial) part of the ear canal. The increased secretions and decreased ventilation resulting from a narrowing of the ear canal create an ideal environment for the proliferation of bacteria and yeast. Changes in the ear associated with atopy are often absent in the proximal (or deep) ear canal. Generally, ear lesions associated with atopy are bilateral, but occasionally they are unilateral. This may be due to localization of secondary bacterial infection to one side.

#### FOOD INTOLERANCE

Approximately 50% of dogs affected by food intolerance will have bilateral inflammation of the ears (Griffin, 1993). Ear lesions associated with food intolerance tend to develop quicker and be more progressive than those of atopy. Severe ceruminous otitis with or without bacterial infection is a common sequela that must be addressed therapeutically. A limited diet is also needed to obtain the best response.

#### CONTACT ALLERGIC OTITIS EXTERNA

Contact allergies of the ears are usually iatrogenically induced in dogs and cats when they become sensitized to certain ingredients in topical otic preparations. Neomycin is most often incriminated, as are, less commonly, propylene glycol and dimethyl sulfoxide. Compared with atopy and food intolerance, otitis due to contact hypersensitivity is rare. However, it should be suspected any time lesions become exacerbated after therapy with a topical agent is instituted.

### Immune-Mediated Diseases

Systemic or discoid lupus erythematosus, as well as diseases of the pemphigus complex, may cause vesicular, pustular, ulcerative, or crusting lesions of the pinna and ear canal, predisposing to otitis externa.

Of the diseases that make up the pemphigus complex, pemphigus foliaceus and pemphigus erythematosus are the ones most likely to be associated with ear lesions and otitis. Although rare, cases involving only the ear have been reported.

The clinical signs of systemic lupus are variable, but when ear lesions are observed, they are associated with one or more of the following: concomitant skin lesions, polyarthritis, fever, proteinuria, anemia, and thrombocytopenia.

Drug eruptions that result in ear lesions are uncommon but can occur as the result of either topical or systemic medications, especially systemic sulfonamide-containing antibacterial agents. Skin lesions may be found on other body regions, as well as the mucocutaneous junctions. The diagnosis is dependent upon an appropriate history of recent drug use and response to drug withdrawal.

## Parasites

### OTODECTES

*Otodectes cynotis* (ear mites) are large, white, free-moving psoroptid mites that causes otoacariasis. These are highly transmissible mites that live on the surface of the epithelial lining of the ear canal, or less frequently on the skin surface. Otodectic mites lack specificity among carnivore host species and are responsible for approximately 10% of otitis in dogs and 50% in cats (Griffin, 1993). The incidence may actually be higher than this because otitis may be produced by low numbers of mites that could go undetected on examination. In addition, mites will often leave the ear canal if severe inflammation or a purulent bacterial or yeast infection develops.

The life cycle is completed in 3 weeks and is initiated with the laying of an egg, which is cemented to a substrate. After 4 days, the egg hatches into a six-legged larva that develops into an eight-legged protonymph in 3 to 10 days. After 3 to 5 days, the protonymph molts into the deutonymph. After an additional 3 to 5 days, the deutonymph becomes attached, end to end, with an adult male. If a male adult is produced from the deutonymph, the attachment has no significance. However, if a female is produced, she must be fertilized at the moment of ecydysis or she will not be able to produce eggs (Muller, Kirk, and Scott, 1989).

Mites feed on lymph and blood, thereby exposing the host to mite antigens. This may allow the host to become sensitized to mites with the production of immunoglubulin E (IgE) reaginic antibodies. This sensitization can be demonstrated in 87% of random source cats, which will have immediate wheal and flare response to mite antigens (Powell et al., 1980). Probably, almost all cats are exposed to small numbers of mites early in life, with the majority developing immune responses that create an aural environment that is not suitable for mite colonization and clinical disease. Other cats may have ineffective immune responses that allow mites to colonize and produce clinical disease.

### DEMODEX

Demodectic mites have been found associated with otitis in both dogs and cats. It is the author's opinion that these mites can be the primary cause of otitis. In other cases, they are secondary invaders taking advantage of a favorable aural environment produced by some other disease. Mites are generally found in mildly inflamed ears that contain excessive wax. Occasionally, they may be an incidental finding in asymptomatic ears.

## Endocrinopathies

Hypothyroidism, male feminizing syndrome, Sertoli cell tumor, and ovarian abnormalities are often associated with chronic otitis externa. Of these, hypothyroidism is most common. The exact pathogenesis associated with the development of endocrine-related otitis is unknown. Most likely, it involves changes in glandular activity and the keratinization process. Most dogs with otitis externa due to endocrinopathies have evidence of a keratinization disorder elsewhere on their bodies.

## Foreign Bodies

Foreign bodies, especially plant awns (foxtail awns) are frequently responsible for otitis externa. In some locales, grass awns are one of the most common causes of otitis. Most cases are acute and unilateral, but in areas with a high density of grass awns, many dogs will have chronic bilateral disease. Grass awns may penetrate the tympanic membrane.

## Tumors

Tumors of the ear should be considered in any chronic case of otitis externa that does not respond to appropriate therapy. They can develop either from the skin or its adnexal structures. Squamous cell carcinoma, histiocytomas, sebaceous gland adenomas and adenocarcinomas, basal cell carcinomas, mast cell tumors, chondromas, chondrosarcomas, trichoepitheliomas, apocrine gland adenomas and adenocarcinomas, fibromas, fibrosarcomas, and papillomas have all been reported. In general, ear tumors in the dog are more common but less malignant than those in the cat.

Squamous cell carcinomas are more common in cats than in dogs and are generally located on the pinnal margins of white-haired cats.

Inflammatory polyps are unique but common ear tumors of cats. They tend to occur in younger animals, as 45% of the cases are found in cats less than 2 years of age. However, inflammatory polyps have been diagnosed in cats ranging in age from 3 months to 5 years. No sex or breed predisposition has been noted. The tumor may tranverse the eustachian tube ventrally, develop in the nasopharynx, and interfere with respiration or swallowing (Harvey and Goldschmidt, 1978).

The stroma of inflammatory polyps consists of either a myxomatous or dense fibrous connective tissue. Inflammatory cells and dilated capillaries are found scattered throughout this tissue. The body of the tumor is covered by either a ciliated or nonciliated columnar epithelium, or by stratified squamous, nonkeratinizing epithelium.

## BACTERIA AND YEAST ASSOCIATED WITH OTITIS

The demonstration of bacteria or yeast in the ear canal does not necessarily mean that these organisms are primary pathogens totally responsible for the development of otitis. Many normal dogs have low numbers of commensal and potentially pathogenic bacteria and yeast present in the ear canal. These organisms can quickly colonize the ear canal if its lining or microclimate becomes altered in a favorable manner. This colonization then exacerbates and perpetuates the inflammatory response within the ear.

In dogs, coagulase-positive *Staphylococcus* spp. have been cultured from 10 to 20% of normal or clean ears, 14% of waxy ears, and from 22 to 40% of otitic ears. Exudates from ears populated with *Staphylococcus* spp. are generally light yellow to light brown in color. Exudates produced due to co-population with *Streptococcus* spp. tend to be light yellow to white.

In dogs, *Streptococcus* spp. can be isolated from approximately 16% of normal ears and 10% of otitic ears. This may indicate that the environment of otitis is less favorable for the growth of *Streptococcus* spp. than the environment of the normal ear. If present, the exudate associated with *Streptococcus* spp. tends to be light brown to yellow in color.

In dogs, *Pseudomonas aeruginosa* can be cultured from approximately 0.4% of normal ears and 20% of otitic ears. It is found frequently in chronic recurrent cases of otitis and in those cases that have had long-term treatment with topical antibacterial drugs. Exudates from ears populated with *Pseudomonas* spp. are yellow in color and generally present in copious amounts. Otitic ears populated with *Pseudomonas* spp. are generally quite painful and often have extensive ulceration of the epithelium lining the ear canal.

*Proteus* spp. have not been cultured from normal ears of dogs. They have been cultured from 11% of otitic ears and are generally associated with dogs that have chronic, ulcerated otitis with light yellow secretions.

*Malessezia pachydermatis* (formerly called *Pityrosporon canis*) is also an oval or peanut-shaped, budding, gram-positive, nonmycelial yeast. In dogs, it has been isolated frequently from both normal and otitic ears so the role it plays in otitis externa is controversial. There is no general agreement as to its incidence in normal (15 to 49%) or otitic (2 to 80%) ears. In our experience, the incidence of *Malessezia* spp. in otitic ear canals of dogs is about 50%. *Malessezia* spp. tend to be found more frequently and present in higher numbers in ear canals with excessive wax.

Because the incidence of *Malessezia* is similar for both normal and otitic ears, it has been suggested that it is a nonpathogenic, normal commensal. However, other evidence, such as otitis cases involving *Malessezia* in monoculture which resolve with appropriate therapy, as well as the production of otitis by the inoculation of *Malessezia* into normal ear canals, suggest that it is pathogenic (Gedek et al., 1979). It is the author's opinion that although *Malessezia* is usually a commensal, it may become pathogenic and contribute to or produce lesions in the ear if the microclimate becomes favorable. Otitic ears with a large population of *Malessezia* spp. will generally have large amounts of chocolate-brown waxy discharge.

## HISTORY

A complete history with questions focused towards dermatology, as well as a complete physical examination, are the initial steps to obtain information necessary for the development of a differential diagnosis.

A complete history is often crucial in providing clues to the cause of the otitis. However, the history is often dealt with in a superficial manner. This difficulty can be overcome by asking the client to complete a dermatology history form before the animal is examined. This form can then be evaluated so that only clarifying questions or questions specific to the ears need be addressed.

The environment often will provide clues towards a diagnosis. If the animal frequents fields, a foreign body in the ear should be considered. If the animal swims frequently, the persistence of moisture in the ear may lead to maceration of the epithelium of the ear canal predisposing to infection. The presence of other animals, especially strays in the environment, or confinement in a dog pound would raise the possibility of parasitic disease.

Information concerning the presence or absence of pruritus and its temporal relationship to the otitis may also be helpful. Bilateral pruritus that proceeds to exudation may indicate hypersensitivity or parasitic diseases.

Determining the chronicity of the condition may also be helpful. Acute, unilateral otitis would raise concerns about the possible presence of a foreign body, and neoplasia should be suspected when unilateral otitis is chronic or nonresponsive to medical therapy. Chronic bilateral otitis is frequently associated with parasites, or as a problem secondary to another disease.

It is also important to ascertain if the animal has had any previous treatment, what specific medications were used, and the response to these medications.

## OTITIC EXAMINATION

The ears, like any other body system, should be examined in a thorough and systematic fashion and the findings recorded. To ensure this, and to minimize the time necessary for the recording of findings, it is very helpful to have an ear examination form. Initially, the pinna and outer ear should be examined visually, noting any inflammation, hyperplasia, exudate, and excessive wax. This should be followed by otoscopic examination of the canal.

### Equipment

An operating head otoscope (Operating Otoscope, Welch-Allyn; Otoscope Set, Medical Diagnostic Services) is preferred because it allows for observations while removing foreign material from the ear via alligator forceps, ear loops, or aspirating the ear with suction. Otoscope cones designed for veterinary medicine are needed to accommodate the various sizes and shapes of canine and feline ears. Because the lumina of the ear canals are often narrowed by hyperplastic tissue, the authors routinely use a cone that is 4 mm in diameter and 5.5 cm in length (Veterinary Speculum, Welch-Allyn or Medical Diagnostic Services). The otoscope of Medical Diagnostic Services offers an advantage in that the specula can be securely fastened to the otoscope head and do not become dislodged as easily as those of the Welch-Allyn unit.

### Restraint

Physical restraint may suffice for otoscopic examination of mild-mannered dogs with minimal problems, and for cursory examination of others. However, to perform a complete and thorough examination of the horizontal canal and tympanic membrane, many animals will require chemical restraint. Chemical restraint also aids in a thorough cleaning of the ear, which is often necessary for visualization of the tympanic membrane. In dogs, ketamine (1.36 to 2.2 mg/kg) in combination with diazapam (0.045 mg/kg) and acepromazine (0.023 mg/kg) given IV has been used satisfactorily by the authors for both examination and cleaning of ears. The higher dose of ketamine (2.2 mg/kg) is preferred, and provides ample restraint for about 20 min.

### Technique

Visualization of the vertical and horizontal ear canal, as well as the tympanic membrane, is best accomplished by pulling the pinna up and out from the head so that the canal is straight. While looking into the otoscope, its cone is slowly inserted to the necessary depth. The otoscope cone may have to be rotated slightly in order to visualize the entire tympanic membrane.

A small amount of pale yellow or yellow-brown wax may be present in the normal ear canal. Hair may have to be removed from the ear canals of some breeds of dogs (poodle, schnauzer, Airedale, wirehair and fox terriers) with an alligator forceps in order to examine the tympanic membrane.

The normal tympanic membrane is translucent, glistening, pearly gray in color, and slightly concave. Cloudiness, opacity, color change, or bulging are signs that generally indicate pathologic changes in the middle ear. Rupture of the tympanic membrane may appear as a small tear in its surface, or it may be so complete that it is difficult to determine where the horizontal canal ends and the middle ear begins. Tympanometry (subjecting the external acoustic meatus to positive, normal, and negative air pressure and monitoring the resultant sound energy flow) has been shown to be superior to otoscopic examination for assessment of the integrity of the tympanic membrane (Little and Lane, 1989).

## DIAGNOSTIC PROCEDURES

From the differential diagnosis, appropriate diagnostic and laboratory procedures may be performed to rule in or out the various primary diseases that could potentially be responsible for, or predispose an animal to, otitis.

Cytologic evaluation of otic exudates or debris is warranted whenever a case of otitis is examined. These examinations can provide immediate diagnostic information about the types of microorganisms and ectoparasites, as well as the type of inflammatory response present. Smears stained with either a modified Wright's stain (Diff-Quick, American Scientific Products) or Gram's stain should be examined for numbers and morphology of bacteria, yeast, leukocytes, and neoplastic cells. Generally, the presence of cocci on smears indicates that either *Staphylococcus* spp. or *Streptococcus* spp. are present. The presence of gram-negative rods may indicate either *Pseudomonas* or *Proteus* spp. Yeast are almost always *Malessezia* spp., but *Candida* spp. are also a possibility. In addition to stained smears, debris from the ear canal can be mixed with mineral oil and examined for ectoparasites and their eggs or larvae.

The decision to submit a sample of ear exudate for culture and sensitivity can be based on the results of cytology. The majority of cases of otitis due to gram-positive cocci or yeast will respond to empiric treatment, and culture and sensitivity are not necessary. However, culture and sensitivity are appropriate for those cases that have not responded to initial therapy. The presence of gram-negative rods is an indication for culture and sensitivity, because they could be *Pseudomonas* spp., which are resistant to the majority of antibacterials.

To diagnose a tumor or differentiate neoplasia from proliferative tissue in the ear canal, a small pinch biopsy may be obtained with an endoscopic biopsy forceps passed through the otoscope cone.

## MANAGEMENT OF OTITIS EXTERNA

Four fundamental steps must be followed to successfully manage otitis externa.

1. Diagnosis and treatment or correction of any primary disease or environmental factor that is predisposing to otitis.
2. Specific identification of bacteria, yeast, parasites, or foreign bodies.
3. Complete cleaning of all hair debris, exudate, and wax from the pinna and vertical and horizontal ear canals.

4. Thorough client education concerning: the etiology of otitis; the anatomy of the ear; instruction in the proper technique of cleaning the ears at home; and proper use of appropriate topical or systemic medications.

## Ear Cleaning

### RATIONALE

Complete removal of all hair, wax, debris, exudate, and foreign material from the horizontal and vertical ear canals is necessary so that: (1) a complete examination of the ear canal and tympanic membrane can be made; (2) exudate and debris do not inactivate medications; (3) topical medications can contact the affected tissues; (4) there is no debris left to serve as a focus for reinfection; and (5) bacterial toxins, degenerating cells, and free fatty acids do not stimulate further inflammation.

### IN-HOSPITAL CLEANING

EQUIPMENT. Routine equipment that is needed includes an operating-head otoscope as previously discussed; a bulb syringe for flushing clean water into the ears; a mosquito and 6-inch alligator forceps for plucking hair and foreign objects from the ears; and ear loops for the dislodgement of wax, crusts, and other debris (Table 1).

Special equipment needed for a thorough ear cleaning is a suction apparatus. If the hospital has such an apparatus for surgery, that is ideal. If not, a suction apparatus can be made very easily and inexpensively from supplies found at home and in hardware stores. From the lamp supply area, purchase three 1/4-inch-diameter brass nipples (two that are 1-inch long and one that is 2-inches long) and six 1/4-inch locknuts. First, place the 2-inch nipple through a hole drilled in a No. 6 rubber stopper and secure it with a locknut on each side of the stopper. Then, take a plastic container or a quart-size Tupperware container with a snap-on lid, and make 1/4-inch diameter holes on opposite sides of the lid. Thread the 1-inch nipples halfway through the lid and put a locknut on either side of the lid. Reattach the lid to the container and place a 2- to 3-m piece of appropriate sized plastic tubing over each of the nipples. To one free end of plastic tubing attach a No. 8-Fr. urinary catheter that has been cut to a length of 12 cm. Attach the other free end of plastic tubing to the nipple protruding from the outer side of the rubber stopper. The stopper can be placed into a hose of any household vacuum cleaner. Adjust the suction control device on the vacuum cleaner hose to achieve the desired level of suction.

TECHNIQUE. With the animal sedated and in lateral recumbency, the ear is evaluated to determine if the tympanic membrane is intact. If it is, the ear is filled with a solution containing dioctyl sodium sulfosuccinate, carbamide peroxide, and tetracaine (Clear-X

Ear Cleansing Solution, DVM Pharmaceuticals). The solution is moved back and forth within the canal by massaging it for 1 to 2 min. If the pinna has exudate or wax on its surface, the cleaning solution should be applied to it also. The pinna can be folded on itself and massaged to loosen the debris. The carbamide peroxide has a foaming action that helps break down larger clumps of debris and float it to the opening of the canal. The dioctyl sodium sulfosuccinate is a ceruminalytic agent that emulsifies the wax so it can be flushed from the ear. After massaging the canal, excess cleaning solution and any exudate and debris that has floated to the surface should be wiped away with a cotton ball. The ear canal is then flushed twice with lukewarm water using a bulb syringe. Failure to thoroughly rinse this solution from the ear may result in irritation to the epithelium lining the ear canal. Next, while observing through an operating-head otoscope, the No. 8-Fr. urinary catheter, attached to a suction apparatus, is used to remove loosened debris, exudate, and any water that is still present. The ear is then examined to verify that it is completely clean. If not, the process should be repeated. The procedure should then be repeated for the other ear. When proficient with this technique, it should be possible to completely clean both ears in less than 20 min. The (Clear-X) solution is not used if the tympanum is ruptured because it may cause vestibular signs.

If the status of the tympanic membrane cannot be determined because the ear canal is filled with exudate or debris or if it is known that the tympanic membrane is ruptured, saline can be used as described above to rinse the ear. If the debris in the ear cannot be rinsed away with the saline, a solution containing propylene glycol, malic acid, benzoic acid, and salicylic acid (Oti-Clens, Beecham) may be considered as an alternative cleaning agent. This product has been used by us and others in ears that have a ruptured tympanum, without any apparent signs of ototoxicity (Neer and Howard, 1982). Its use is always followed by a thorough lavage of the middle ear with saline. One should realize that there is no completely safe solution for cleaning the middle ear. Even water may cause a loss of cochlear and/or vestibular function. After partial cleaning, if it is determined that the tympanum is intact, the (Clear-X) solution can be used to clean the ear more thoroughly. If an animal swallows, gags, or coughs when a solution is placed in the ear, it is a good indication that the tympanic membrane is ruptured. (The liquid has flowed through the ruptured tympanum, to the middle ear, and through the eustachian tube into the pharynx.) A small tear in the tympanum is not a serious defect in a clean ear, as it will usually heal in 5 to 10 days. If the tear is large or if the tympanum has been obliterated, it may never return to the intact state. Transient head tilt or ataxia has been observed in about 1% of the cases that have received flushing and suctioning of the *middle ear*. Although it is extremely rare, permanent deafness or vestibular dysfunction may occur after cleaning the middle ear.

The use of a dental water-propulsion device (such as

***Table 1.*** *List of Drugs and Special Equipment*

| Drugs/Equipment | Uses |
| --- | --- |
| **Drugs** | |
| Ketamine (1.36 to 2.2 mg/kg) Ketaset (Aveco, Fort Dodge) | In dogs IV in combination with diazapam and acepromazine |
| Diazepam (0.045 mg/kg) Valium (Roche) | In dogs IV in combination with ketamine and acepromazine |
| Acepromazine (0.023 mg/kg) Promace (Fort Dodge) | In dogs IV in combination with ketamine and diazepam |
| Dioctyl sodium sulfosuccinate, carbamide peroxide, and tetracaine (Clear-X Ear Cleansing Solution, DVM Pharmaceuticals) | Used topically to clean ears |
| Ivermectin (300 μg/kg SC) (Ivomec, MSD AgVet) | Used to treat ear mites in cats, dose should be repeated in 2 weeks |
| Propylene glycol, malic acid, benzoic acid, salicylic acid (Oti-Clens, Beecham) | Used topically to clean ears |
| Docusate sodium (dioctyl sodium sulfosuccinate [DSS]), (Epi-Otic, Allerderm/Verbac; Otic Blue, Chesterfield) | Used topically to clean wax from ears |
| Hexamethyletracosane (Wax-O-Sol, Life Science Products; Seb-O-Sol, Butler) | Used topically to clean wax from ears |
| Squalene (Cerumene, Evsco) | Used topically to clean wax from ears |
| Lactic acid, salicytic acid, propylene glycol, docusate sodium (Epi-Otic, Allerderm/Verbac) | Used topically to clean exudate and wax from ears |
| Chlorhexidine gluconate (Chlorhexaderm Flush, DVM Pharmaceuticals) | Used topically to clean exudate and wax from ears |
| Neomycin, polymyxin B, pencillin, hydrocortisone acetate, hydrocortisone sodium succinate (Forte-Topical, Upjohn) | Used topically to treat bacterial infection of the ear canal |
| Neomycin, nystatin, thiostrepton, triamcinolone acetonide (Panalog Ointment, Solvay) | Used topically to treat bacterial infection of the ear canal |
| Neomycin, thiabendazole, dexemethasone (Tresaderm, MSD-AgVet) | Used topically to treat bacterial infection or earmite infestation of the ear canal |
| Gentamicin, betamethasone valerate (Gentocin Otic Solution, Schering) | Used topically to treat bacterial infection of the ear canal |
| Chloramphenicol squalane, prednisolone, tetracaine HCl (Liquichlor, Evsco) | Used topically to treat bacterial infection of the ear canal |
| Amikacin (Amiglyde-V Injection, Fort Dodge) | Used topically to treat *Pseudomonas* infection of the ear canal |
| Enrofloxacin (Baytril Injectable, Haver/Diamond Scientific) | Used topically to treat *Pseudomonas* infection of the ear canal |
| Silver sulfadiazine (Spectrum Labs) | Used topically to treat *Pseudomonas* infection of the ear canal |
| Ticarcillin (SmithKline Beecham) | Used topically to treat bacterial *Pseudomonas* of the ear canal |
| Acetic acid hydrocortisone acetate (Clear-X Ear Drying Solution, DVM Pharmaceuticals) | Used topically to treat bacterial infection of the ear canal |
| Acetic acid (Ear/Skin Cleanser, Derma Pet) | Used topically to treat bacterial infection of the ear canal |
| Clotrimazole (Veltrim, Miles) | Used topically to treat yeast infection of the ear canal |
| Miconazole (Conofite Lotion, Pitman-Moore) | Used topically to treat yeast infection of the ear canal |
| Amphotercin B (Fungizone, Squibb) | Used topically to treat yeast infection of the ear canal |
| Rotenone (Ear Mitecide, Vedco or Phoenix) | Used topically to earmite infestations |
| Pyrethrin, squalane, piperonyl butoxide (Cerumite, Evesco) | Used topically to earmite infestations |
| Carbaryl, mineral oil, neomycin, sulfacetamid, tetracaine HCl (Mitox, SmithKline Beecham) | Used topically to earmite infestations |
| Flucinolone acetonid, dimethylsulfoxide (Synotic, Syntex Animal Health) | Used topically in the ear canal as an anti-inflammatory |
| **Equipment** | |
| Operating head otoscope (Operating Otoscope, Welch-Allyn; or Otoscope Set, Medical Diagnostic Services) | |

Water Pik, Teledyne) to flush the ears has been advocated. However, in the author's experience, this technique creates a greater mess, takes longer, and does not clean the ears as well as the technique described above.

Although useful for cleaning the folds of the pinna and outer ear, the longstanding practice of using cotton swabs (Q-tips) to clean the ear canal should be abandoned. Even when done carefully, this technique packs exudate and debris further down the canal closer to the tympanum. If the tympanic membrane is diseased, pressure of the debris may cause it to rupture. If this occurs, or if the tympanum is already ruptured, the debris can be pushed into the middle ear, where it may contribute to the development of otitis media. The physical action of the swab in the canal tends to traumatize and ulcerate the epithelium lining the canal.

### MAINTENANCE CLEANING

Routine, maintenance ear cleaning by the patient's owner is often necessary to resolve longstanding infections. It also may be necessary to control secretions associated with continual inflammation or infection of the ear. The interval for maintenance cleaning may vary from daily to weekly or longer, depending on the rate of formation of exudate or wax in the ear.

PRODUCTS. If the removal of ear wax is the primary concern, a ceruminolytic containing an emulsifying agent such as docusate sodium (dioctyl sodium sulfosuccinate [DSS]), (Epi-Otic, Allerderm/Verbac; Otic Blue, Chesterfield), or hexamethyletracosane (Wax-O-Sol, Life Science Products; Seb-O-Sol, Butler) or squalane (Cerumene, Evsco) is used. All of these agents should be avoided if the tympanum is not intact.

Removal of exudate from the ear can be accomplished by cleaning with one of the following: Oti-Clens; lactic acid, salicylic acid, propylene glycol, docusate sodium (Epi-Otic, Allerderm/Verbac); or chlorhexidine gluconate (Chlorhexiderm Flush, DVM Pharmaceuticals). Routine maintenance cleaning by a patient's owner is not recommended in cases where the tympanum is ruptured.

Either Epi-Otic or Chlorhexiderm Flush can be used to clean an ear if both wax and exudate are present. Neither of these should be used if the tympanum is ruptured.

TECHNIQUE. The client is instructed to grasp the pinna and hold it in a vertical position while the ear canal is filled with the appropriate cleansing solution. The pinna is then folded lengthwise on itself and the ear canal is massaged for 20 to 40 sec to distribute the cleansing solution and allow it to dislodge any exudate or debris and emulsify wax. The cleansing solution, along with any exudate, debris, and wax, is then wiped from the pinna and distal portion of the ear canal. The procedure is repeated until the ear is clean, as evidenced by uncontaminated cleansing solution.

## Topical Treatment

### ANTIBACTERIALS

Initial treatment should be based on stained smears of the ear exudate. If cocci (most likely to be *Staphylococci*) are present, products containing neomycin (Forte-Topical, Upjohn; Panalog, Solvay; Tresaderm, MSD-AgVet), gentamicin (Gentocin Otic Solution, Schering), or chloramphenicol (Liquichlor, Evsco) would be appropriate.

If gram-negative rods are present (often likely to be *Pseudomonas*), gentamicin or polymyxin B (Forte-Topical, Upjohn) would be the products of choice. Chloramphenicol may also be effective against gram-negative rods, but it is less likely to be effective against *Pseudomonas*. Antibacterials that have a high likelihood of being effective against *Pseudomonas* would include injectable amikacin (Amiglyde-V Injection, Fort Dodge) or enrofloxacin (Baytril, Haver/Diamond Scientific) *applied topically*. Silver sulfadiazine (Spectrum Labs) and ticarcillin (SmithKline Beecham) are two additional antibacterials that are often effective for the treatment of *Pseudomonas* spp. A 1% solution of silver sulfadiazine is made by adding 1 gm of silver sulfadiazine powder to 100 ml of water and shaking well. Ticarcillin is an injectable antibacterial that comes lyophilized in a 6 gm bottle. Sterile water (12 ml) is added to the bottle to reconstitute the ticarcillin; 2 ml of this is then added to 40 ml of Oti-Clens, and this is used to both clean and treat the ears twice daily. The length of the activity of ticarcillin in this formulation is not pre-

cisely known, but there is reason to believe that it may not be much longer than 3 days. The remaining reconstituted ticarcillin can be frozen for use at a later date.

Neomycin, gentamicin, chloramphenicol, polymyxin B, and amikacin are known to be ototoxic and *should not be used if the tympanum is ruptured*. The ototoxicity of topical silver sulfadiazine and enrofloxacin are not known. However, the authors have used them in a limited number of cases where the tympanum is ruptured with no apparent side effects. The author's treatment of choice for an ear with a rupture of the tympanic membrane is the ticarcillin–Oti-Clens combination.

Another approach to decrease the bacterial population in the ear is the use of 2 to 6% solution of acetic acid (Clear-X, DVM Pharmaceuticals; Ear/Skin Cleanser, Derma Pet) to lower the pH within the ear canal. *Staphylococcus* and *Streptococcus* can be killed by 5 min of contact with 5% acetic acid and *Pseudomonas* by 1 min of contact with a 2% solution. This form of treatment is especially beneficial for the treatment of infections with *Pseudomonas* spp. when the organism is resistant to other antibacterials. Inflammation, which can be severe, is an occasional side effect of otic treatment with acetic acid. It is more likely to occur when a 5% solution is used.

### ANTIFUNGALS

If *Malassezia* or *Candida* are present, topicals such as clotrimazole (Veltrim, Miles) or miconazole (Conofite Lotion, Pitman-Moore) should be used in the ear. Other drugs effective against yeast would include cuprimyxin (Unitop, Hoffman-La Roche), nystatin (Panolog, Solvay), or amphotercin B (Fungizone, Squibb).

### ANTI-INFLAMMATORY

The anti-inflammatory effects of topical glucocorticoids will benefit most cases of otitis externa by decreasing pruritis, swelling, exudation, and tissue proliferation. Flucinolone acetonide in 60% dimethylsulfoxide (Synotic, Syntex Animal Health) is especially beneficial, as the dimethylsulfoxide serves as a vehicle to allow flucinolone penetration into the tissues. Its use will often result in reduction of the hyperplastic tissue associated with chronic otitis externa. Owners are instructed to fill the affected ear canal with the solution and massage the canal for 20 to 40 sec, two to three times daily. It also decreases wax build-up in the ear that otherwise could result in a concomitant *Malassezia* infection. Long-term topical use of glucocorticoids in the ears may result in systemic absorption, causing elevated liver enzymes and suppressed adrenal response to adrenocorticotrophic hormone (ACTH) stimulation.

### ANTIPARASITICAL

When *Otodectes cyanotes* infestation is diagnosed, the ears should first be cleaned of excess wax and then treated for 20 days with an appropriate miticidal agent. The author prefers a mixture containing 1 ml of rotenone (Ear Mitecide, Vedco or Phoenix) and 10 ml of a solution containing procaine penicillin, neomycin sulfate, polymyxin B, and hydrocortisone (Forte-Topical, Upjohn). Preparations containing pyrethrin (Cerumite, Evesco), carbaryl (Mitox, SmithKline Beecham), and thiabendazole (Tresaderm, MSD AgVet) are also appropriate. All contact animals, both dogs and cats, should be treated as asymptomatic carriers that may be sources of reinfection. In addition, *Otodectes* may be found on other body areas, so use whole-body treatments with pyrethrin sprays weekly for 3 weeks.

### APPLICATION

If there is minimal hyperplasia of the ear canal, the topical medication can be dropped into the ear canal, followed by massage to evenly distribute the formulation. The presence of extensive hyperplasia may prevent drops from penetrating to the deeper portion of the ear canal. This can be overcome by having the client draw the medication into a 1-cc syringe without a needle on it, placing the tip of the syringe in the canal, and then injecting the medication between the folds of hyperplastic tissue. Alternatively, a flexible tom-cat catheter can be cut off (so that it cannot reach the tympanic membrane) and threaded into the ear canal to deliver the medication.

## SYSTEMIC TREATMENT

Most cases of a bacterial infection in the ear can be controlled with topical antibacterials. Systemic antibacterials are indicated if the tympanum is ruptured or the response to topicals is poor. The choice of systemic antibacterials should be based on the results of culture and sensitivity and should be given for 3 to 4 weeks.

Systemic steroids may occasionally be necessary to reduce severe inflammation and swelling of otitis associated with hypersensitivity diseases as well as inflammation and swelling associated with rupture of cystic apocrine glands. Anti-inflammatory doses of a short-acting glucocorticoid such as prednisolone or methyl-prednisolone may be given for 10 to 14 days.

Although no claim is made by the manufacturer, extralabel use of ivermectin (Ivomec, MSD AgVet) is effective for the treatment of *Otodectes cynotes*. It is given subcutaneously at a dose of 300 $\mu$g/kg and repeated in 2 weeks. Collies and collie crosses *should not be treated* with ivermectin because of potential life-threatening neurologic side effects. As with topical treatment for *Otodectes*, all contact animals should be treated.

## INDICATIONS FOR SURGERY

Surgical intervention rarely provides a cure for otitis externa, but rather is a means to make control and treatment easier. It is indicated when the hyperplasia of the ear canal is so great that the resulting stenosis precludes appropriate cleaning and application of medication. Surgical techniques will vary depending on the location and pathology of the lesions and are discussed in other texts (Krahwinkel, 1993).

Surgery is also indicated for otitis resulting from a tumor or polyp of the ear canal. The exact procedure will depend on the size and location of the lesion.

## CLIENT EDUCATION

No matter how thorough a veterinarian has been in diagnosing the patient, cleaning the ears, and dispensing medications, the efforts will be in vain unless the owner properly cleans and treats the ears at home. Therefore, all instructions pertaining to the cleaning or treatment of ears should be typed or clearly printed for the owner. To help ensure client compliance, the veterinarian or an experienced veterinary technician should carefully explain the cleaning and treatment instructions, demonstrate how cleaning and treatment are supposed to be performed, and then watch as the owner repeats the process. Finally, reexaminations should be scheduled at appropriate intervals so that progress can be monitored and any problems with cleaning or treatment can be addressed.

## References and Suggested Reading

Gedek B, Brutzel K, Gerlach R, et al: The role of *Pityrosporum pachydermatitis* in otitis externa of dogs: Evaluation of a treatment with miconazole. Vet Rec 104:138, 1979.
*A study of* Pityrosporum pachydermatitis *and its ability to produce otitis as well as the treatment of this otitis with miconazole.*
Getty R, Foust HL, Prestely ET, et al: Macroscopic anatomy of the ear of the dog. Am J Vet Res 17:364, 1956.
*A study on the anatomy of the canine ear.*
Griffin CE: Otitis externa and otitis media. In Griffin CE, Kwochka KW, and McDonald JM (eds): *Current Veterinary Dermatology*. St. Louis: Mosby Year Book, 1993, p 245.
Harvey CE and Goldschmidt MH: Inflammatory polypoid growths in the ear canal of cats. J Small Anim Pract 19:669, 1978.
*A clinical and histologic description of inflammatory polyps in the ears of cats.*
Little CJL and Lane JG: An evaluation of tympanometry, otoscopy, and palpation for assessment of the canine tympanic membrane. Vet Rec 124:5, 1989.
*A study comparing various methods for determining if the tympanic membrane was intact.*
Krahwinkel DJ: External ear canal. In Slatter D (ed): *Textbook of Small Animal Surgery*. Philadelphia, WB Saunders Co, 1993, p 1560.
*A review of various surgical procedures used for the managment of otitis externa.*
McKeever PJ: Otitis externa. In Locke HP (ed): *Manual of Small Animal Dermatology*. Gloucestershire, British Small Animal Veterinary Association, 1993, p 131.
Muller GH, Kirk RW, and Scott DW: *Small Animal Dermatology*. Philadelphia, WB Saunders Co, 1989, p 367.
*Description of the appearance and life cycle of* Otodectes cynotis.
Neer MT and Howard PE: Otitis media. Compend Cont Educ Pract Vet 4: 410, 1982.
*A review of clinical features, diagnosis, and treatment of otitis media in the dog.*
Powell MB, Weisbroth SH, Roth L, et al: Reaginic hypersensitivity in *Otodectes cynotis* infestation of cats and mode of mite feeding. Am J Vet Res 41:877, 1980.
*A study to determine the pathogenesis of the hypersensitivity that cats develop to ear mites.*
Scott DW: Observations on canine atopy. J Am Anim Hosp Assoc 17:91, 1981.
*Clinical and diagnostic findings in 100 dogs with atopic dermatitis.*

# Section

# 8

# GASTROINTESTINAL DISORDERS

DAVID C. TWEDT

*Consulting Editor*

***Still Current Information Found in Current Veterinary Therapy XI:***

Shelton GD: Megaesophagus Secondary to Acquired Myasthenia Gravis, p 580.
Leib MS: Acute Vomiting: A Diagnostic and Symptomatic Management, p 583.
Guilford WG: Adverse Reactions to Food, p 587.
Dimski DS: Dietary Fiber in the Management of Gastrointestinal Disease, p 592.
Couto CG: Gastrointestinal Neoplasia in Dogs and Cats, p 595.
Twedt DC: *Clostridium Perfringens* Associated Enterotoxicosis in Dogs, p 602.
Tams TR: Irritable Bowel Syndrome, p 604.
Sherding RG and Johnson SE: Intestinal Histoplasmosis, p 609.
Richter KP: Diseases of the Rectum and Anus, p 613.
DeNovo, Jr. and Bright RM: Chronic Feline Constipation/Obstipation, p 619.
Reinmeyer CR: Feline Gastrointestinal Parasites, p 626.
Williams DA: Acute Pancreatitis, p 631.
Hardy RM: Hepatic Encephalopathy, p 639.

# GASTROINTESTINAL DIAGNOSTIC IMAGING

JERRY M. OWENS

*Berkeley, California*

In the assessment of the gastrointestinal (GI) system, the clinician is faced with many imaging choices including survey radiography, contrast studies, fluoroscopy, ultrasound, computed tomography (CT), magnetic resonance imaging (MRI), and nuclear medicine. The selection of imaging studies is dependent on the clinical history, physical examination, suspected clinical problems, and diagnostic rule-outs; the experience, knowledge, and enthusiasm of the clinician; the availability of specialized equipment; and the financial constraints of the owner.

In the imaging work-up of the gastrointestinal tract, the clinician is faced with a number of problems that require solution, including: how to choose the most appropriate examination for the patient's particular problem, how to perform the examination, and how to interpret the finished study. The clinician needs to acknowledge the expected yield of the study and its limitations, the clinician also needs an understanding of pseudolesion, relative to both intrinsic and extrinsic factors.

Since the advent of ultrasound and endoscopy, the need for barium upper GI studies has diminished substantially. Focal gastric diseases, gastric foreign bodies, inflammatory bowel disease, and some malabsorptive diseases can be diagnosed by endoscopy. Abdominal ultrasound readily evaluates the abdomen for masses, lymph node enlargement and some bowel and gastric lesions. In a practice without endoscopy or ultrasound, the GI contrast study can still be used effectively, especially to identify bowel obstruction and large masses.

The clinician's goal should be to obtain an accurate assessment and diagnosis using procedures that are minimally invasive, sensitive, specific, financially justifiable, and performed in a timely manner. The order and extent in which diagnostic tests and imaging procedures are performed should be logical, resulting in a conclusion in which the diagnosis, prognosis, and appropriate therapy can be determined. Routine laboratory studies, including fecal examination, complete blood count (CBC), and serum biochemistries, are usually indicated prior to endoscopy or specialized imaging studies.

readily identified. Esophageal dilation with gas can be identified and the effect of abnormal masses in the cervical region can be assessed by noting displacement of normal structures. Survey thoracic radiographs allow visualization of the esophagus if distended with gas, fluid, or opaque foreign body, and permits the detection of masses in the mediastinum. In addition, the patient can be assessed for concurrent abnormalities affecting the heart, pleural cavity, lung, chest wall, and diaphragm. Survey abdominal radiographs are used for evaluation of the abdominal viscera relative to organ location, size, contour, and density; the presence of free abdominal fluid; the presence of masses; and assessment of the fluid and gas patterns in the bowel.

After interpretation of these radiographs, a diagnosis may be apparent, or perhaps the need for additional studies warranted. The clinician may decide to obtain supplemental projections of the abdomen such as the opposite lateral, a dorsoventral, or a standing lateral with a horizontal x-ray beam to assess the gravitational effects of fluid and gas. Another option would be to proceed to abdominal ultrasound or to obtain a contrast study. Or, it may be appropriate to obtain follow-up films after a few hours or after an enema to see if a suspected gastric foreign body has passed or whether there is a change in the amount of bowel gas or in the appearance of the bowel pattern.

Following the evaluation of the initial data base including survey radiographs and laboratory findings, the clinician needs to make a decision. A *specific diagnosis* (e.g., bowel obstruction) with a recommendation for surgery may be one option. A second option would be a *tentative diagnosis* (e.g., gastritis) with empiric therapy prescribed. A third option would be an *open diagnosis* and the need for either follow-up assessment; other laboratory testing; additional radiographs; or perhaps the application of another diagnostic modality such as ultrasound, endoscopy, or a contrast study. A fourth option is the clinical determination that the primary problem is not a GI problem, but perhaps some other system abnormality such as lumbar disk disease or urinary tract infection, in which other diagnostic studies are needed to complete the work-up.

## SURVEY RADIOGRAPHY

Survey radiographs of the cervical soft tissues aid in assessing a patient with a swallowing disorder or the presence of regurgitation. The pharynx and larynx are

## ULTRASOUND

Ultrasound is gaining popularity in small animal practice for assessing the GI tract as well as other abdominal organs. Many small animal practitioners have their own ultrasound machine, are served by a mobile ultrasound service, or have referral specialists in their geographic area.

Ultrasound is a noninvasive, safe, and reliable technology that has been found to be very effective in recognizing many clinical problems, and has significantly reduced the need for contrast radiography in the small animal practice. Its main value has been in the assessment of solid organs, such as the liver, spleen, kidneys and prostate, but is also helpful in the evaluation of the stomach, small bowel, pancreas, mesenteric lymph nodes, and adrenal gland. Pancreatic and intestinal masses, hypertrophic gastropathy, gastric tumors and foreign bodies, bowel obstruction, and a variety of hepatic and biliary tract lesions have been recognized by ultrasound studies. Ultrasound provides information relative to the internal architecture of many organs, providing an assessment as to the presence of masses, areas of bowel wall thickening, or fluid collections. It also provides the opportunity for guided aspirates or biopsies of lesions.

The diagnostic success depends in part on patient preparation including clipping the hair from the area of examination, and a liberal use of alcohol and acoustic gel to enhance transducer-patient contact and appropriate imaging windows. Image quality is adversely affected by the presence of bowel gas and ingesta within the gastrointestinal tract. In many instances, varying the position of the patient or imaging through additional windows is necessary for complete abdominal evaluation.

The indications for ultrasound are many; however, the limitations of ultrasound are equally significant. Artifacts are very common, and it is important for the sonographer to distinguish real lesions from artifactual ones. Ultrasound is a high-tech, operator-dependent modality in which the quality of the real-time image and the video recording depends on the input of the technician in adjusting the machine for transducer selection, focus, power, gain, and contrast, as well as window selections. This technical input makes significant differences in the overall obtained image and the ultimate conclusion or diagnosis following performance of the examination.

## OTHER IMAGING STUDIES

Computed tomography and MRI are useful procedures in humans and are becoming somewhat more available to veterinary medicine. Both modalities have many applications to the internal imaging of the thorax and abdomen and are complementary to other studies. Overall availability of these studies in small animal practice is low at this time; however, the benefits of these procedures are currently under evaulation at veterinary teaching hospitals and referral practices.

Nuclear imaging is potentially useful in the assessment of many conditions of the abdomen. Scintigraphic studies can be used to obtain morphologic and functional information of the liver, kidneys, and spleen and can assess gastric emptying and pyloric outflow abnormalities. Portal scintigraphy is used to identify the presence of acquired or congenital portosystemic shunts (see "Feline Portosystemic Vascular Shunts," this volume, p 743). It is a valuable modality; however, like many new or expensive technologies, availability is limited.

## Contrast Radiography

Contrast radiography uses a negative or positive contrast medium that is placed within the lumen of the alimentary tract. Positive contrast media include barium sulfate preparations, organic iodinated water-soluable compounds such as Gastrografin or Oral Hypaque and non-ionic iodinated low osmolar preparations, such as iohexol (Omnipaque, Winthrop Pharmaceuticals, NY) and iopamidol (Isovue, ER Squibb, Princeton, NJ). For most esophageal, gastric, and intestinal studies, barium sulfate preparations are preferred over iodinated contrast media, as the barium provides good mucosal coating and high radiographic contrast. The mucosal detail obtained with the water-soluble contrast is inferior to barium media, especially the organic iodinated hyperosmolar products due to the rapid dilution from the mixing of normal luminal fluid as well as the increased fluid drawn into the lumen due to its hyperosmotic effect. In addition, this hyperosmolar effect attracts water, which can be detrimental in a patient that is already dehydrated. One potential use of iodinated contrast is in suspected perforations of the esophagus or stomach, as the extravasated contrast is readily absorbable from the pleural or peritoneal cavities, while barium is not absorbable and causes a local granulomatous reaction.

A potential side effect of an esophageal or upper GI study is the aspiration of contrast medium into the trachea and lung. The low osmolar, non-ionic preparations are safe as they are rapidly absorbed from the alveolar capillary network. The hyperosmolar organic iodides, fluid is drawn towards it and, if aspirated into the lung, a chemical edema will result, which can be fatal. Barium is inert in the lung and when aspirated in small quantities is either expectorated or ultimately phagocytized in the peripheral airspaces. However, if a large volume of barium is aspirated, asphyxiation may result.

Non-ionic contrast media, such as Omnipaque and Isovue, and have been shown to be a safe alternative to the tri-iodinated contrast media as an upper GI contrast medium in assessing the bowel's position and location, the presence of obstruction, or for the detection of intraluminal foreign bodies. A dose of 2 to 3 ml/kg is given per os or via gastric intubation. Radiographs of the abdomen are made immediately and at 15 to 30 minute intervals until either a diagnosis is made or the contrast is detected in the large bowel. As it is nonionic, the side effects of dehydration and excessive contrast dilution are avoided. The only disadvantage is its cost, approximately $1.00 to $1.50 per ml.

Barium sulfate is available in many different preparations. The barium is packaged as a specific particle size with additives to control the charge and absorptive capacity, thus keeping the particles in suspension. Carboxymethyl cellulose is commonly employed as a suspending agent. Overall, the density of the preparation (% w/v) determines its viscosity; the higher the viscosity, the slower the flow. The major bane of barium is the tendency to flocculate, in which there is clumping of the barium, resulting in poor mucosal coating and pseudolesions. This occurs when the barium liquid is not properly mixed prior to its use, if the barium is diluted by increased bowel fluid, or if the patient is dehydrated causing precipitation of the barium particles due to water absorption from the barium mixture. The overall radiographic density varies as well with the different barium concentrations; the more viscous preparations are more opaque and more difficult to "see through." In general, esophageal and gastric mucosal lesions are best evaluated with thicker, more viscous preparations (85 to 100% w/v), the upper GI tract is best assessed with thinner less viscous material (25 to 30% w/v), while the large bowel is best assessed with more dilute compounds (10% w/v).

Negative contrast examinations include pneumogastrography, and pneumocolonography. These are safe procedures, using room air as the contrast agent, and are useful in evaluating the location and position of the stomach and colon, as well as aiding in determining whether a gastric foreign body is present.

A new product called "BIPS" (barium impregnated polyethyene spheres) shows promise in the radiographic diagnosis of bowel obstruction and motility disorders. Small 1.5 mm and 5.0 mm radiopaque markers are administered orally, followed by radiographs exposed at variable intervals. A delay or failure of the spheres to be seen in the large bowel signifies an abnormality. The use of this product is limited in that mucosal assessment is not provided nor can partial bowel obstructions be accurately diagnosed; however, this product does provide an alternative for a barium or iodinated contrast study to document the presence or absence of a complete bowel obstruction.

## Upper GI Series

Barium sulfate mixtures are the preferred contrast media for radiographic examination of the GI tract. Thin barium, 25 to 30% w/v, at a dose of 10 to 15 ml/kg is needed to provide adequate gastric distention. Lower doses of barium will not adequately distend the stomach. The barium can be given via nasogastric or orogastric tube, or given in smaller doses and swallowed. Tubing is preferred as it is faster and easier on the patient. For chemical restraint, dogs can be given acetylpromazine at a dose of 1 mg/10 kg IV (to a maximum of 3 mg) without affecting gastric emptying or small bowel transit times. In the cat, 10 mg of ketamine can be given intravenously; however, a more rapid transit of contrast through the GI tract is frequently a result.

If desired, water soluble iodinated preparations can

be used. These media pass quickly through the GI tract and enable rapid identification of the location (e.g., diaphragmatic hernia) and patency (e.g., bowel obstruction) of the bowel. The major disadvantage is that of poor mucosal coating. In the past, the hyperosmolar iodinated contrast media (e.g., Gastrografin) was most commonly used; however, recent studies have shown that the non-ionic low osmolar contrast media (e.g., Omnipaque) are superior. The lower osmolar agents provide the same rapid transit through the GI tract but do not cause fluid to be withdrawn into the lumen, nor do they cause dehydration. Conversely, the hypertonic, hyperosmolar contrast media draw fluid into the lumen, diluting the contrast media, reducing radiographic contrast, and potentially dehydrating the patient. If used, the recommended doses for the water soluble contrast media are as follows: Gastrografin: 0.5 to 2.0 ml/kg body weight. Omnipaque 240: 2 to 4 ml/kg body weight.

The number and frequency of radiographs needed for a study varies in part with the suspected area of GI disease, the relative rate of gastric emptying, and the bowel transit time. The normal time for barium to reach the colon varies. In the dog, "normal" varies between 90 and 240 min. In the cat, "normal" is 30 to 60 min. There is no fixed standard as to the number of films or views for the optimum GI study. Usually films are made at time zero, with additional films made at 15- to 30-min intervals, until the large bowel is seen. The minimum views per time interval is two (lateral and ventrodorsal); however, opposite lateral, dorsoventral, and oblique projections are sometimes beneficial. The entire GI tract should be visualized during the study for the study to be complete. A suspected lesion should be evident on repeated films. The GI study effectively evaluates for gross anatomic change but is a poor evaluator of physiologic function.

## Double-Contrast Gastrogram

The double-contrast gastrogram is optimum in evaluating the gastric mucosa for subtle mucosal irregularities and for the presence of small gastric foreign bodies. The patient should be heavily sedated or anesthetized. To temporarily paralyze the stomach, intravenous glucagon can be given (0.1 mg for small dogs to 0.35 mg for large dogs). Thick barium (85%) is then administered at a dose of 0.5 to 1 ml/kg. The stomach is then intubated and distended with air to make the stomach tympanic (dose-approximately 5 ml/kg) and four views are taken including right and left lateral, ventrodorsal, and dorsoventral. While potentially useful, this procedure has been largely supplanted by endoscopy.

## Negative Contrast Studies

Negative contrast examinations of the stomach and large bowel are easily performed in the small animal practice and are useful for a rapid assessment of gastric location and position, a subjective assessment of gastric wall thickness, and identification of some large mural masses and ulcers. Determination of the presence or absence of a gastric foreign body can be obtained after insufflating the stomach with room air via a gastric or nasograstric tube at a dose of 2 to 5 ml/kg body weight and obtaining lateral and DV and/or VD projections. For a rapid assessment of colonic location and position, distensibility, ileo-colic or ceco-colic intussusception and evaluating for colonic foreign bodies, room air is injected into the colon via a rubber catheter at a dose of 2 to 5 ml/kg followed by the acquisition of right and left lateral as well as a ventrodorsal or dorsoventral projection of the abdomen.

## PHARYNX AND ESOPHAGUS

Most pharyngeal and esophageal disorders can be evaluated using direct visualization, endoscopy, or barium. Pharyngeal motility is very rapid, and fluoroscopy is best used for barium evaluations. Without fluoroscopy, however, a reasonable swallow can be obtained by using thick barium (85 to 100% w/v), with multiple radiographs obtained. The major abnormal findings include the presence of barium in the nasopharynx, larynx, or trachea indicative of abnormal motility. If no aspiration or reflux occurs, the cricopharyngeal muscle should be readily identified as well as the smooth mucosal folds of the esophagus. Abnormal filling defects in the pharynx due to tumor, polyp, cyst, or foreign body are seen in relief.

For evaluation of esophageal mucosal disease (e.g., esophagitis, neoplasia) or anatomic position (e.g., in patients with a mediastinal mass), thick barium (85 to 100% w/v) works well. Multiple 2- to 10-ml swallows are administered with radiographs obtained after swallowing including lateral, ventrodorsal, and right ventrodorsal oblique projections. For patients with suspected stricture, thick barium mixed with food aids in locating the site and extent of stricture. For the patients with suspected megaesophagus, or vascular ring anomaly, thin barium is preferred (25 to 30% w/v), as the barium water mixture will fill and partially coat the esophagus. Thicker barium tends to drop into the dependent esophagus, and poorly coats the mucosa. Barium studies are ill-advised when megasophagus is obvious from survey films, due to the risk of aspiration.

## THE STOMACH

For suspected gastric disease, additional imaging can include an upper GI study, pneumogastrography, a double-contrast gastrogram, endoscopy, or ultrasound. For many gastric diseases, endoscopy has evolved as an effective diagnostic study, as it allows a visual mucosal assessment, the opportunity to selectively biopsy lesions, and permits retrieval of some foreign bodies.

As the availability of endoscopy is limited, the standard imaging procedure for most small animal clinicians remains the barium upper GI study. This procedure is effective in assessing the distensibility of the stomach, gastric wall thickness, the presence of most gastric foreign bodies, the presence of gastric mucosal masses or large areas of ulceration, and the presence of pyloric outflow obstruction such as pyloric stenosis. A double-contrast gastrogram is better at visualizing minor anatomic lesions such as small areas of gastric ulceration and for identifying small gastric foreign bodies.

Ultrasound can provide important information relative to gastric function and the presence of localized or diffuse thickening of the gastric wall. Gastric contractions are readily seen and the overall wall thickness of the stomach can be determined. In the dog, the thickness of the gastric wall, when measured during physiologic relaxation (noncontracted) and measured from the inner hyperechoic mucosal surface to the outer hyperechoic serosal surface is 3 to 5 mm. If the gastric wall is greater than 7 mm in thickness, it is considered abnormal. Localized areas of gastric wall thickening due to ulceration or neoplasia can be identified. In pyloric stenosis or hypertrophy, the increased thickness of the layers of the pyloric canal can be measured.

Gastric dilation and volvulus is best assessed from survey radiographs alone. The most common form of volvulus is 180 degrees, recognized by identifying the pylorus as displaced dorsally and to the left. If the radiographs are inconclusive for pyloric location, a gastrogram using thin barium (25 to 30% w/v) at a dose of 5 to 10 ml/kg can be done. Obtaining four views of the abdomen (ventrodorsal, dorsoventral, right lateral, and left lateral) will allow gravitational effects of the barium and gas to occur and the ability to confirm the volvulus if present.

## THE SMALL BOWEL

The small bowel loops are assessed by noting their position within the abdomen, the gas pattern of the bowel, intraluminal contents, contour of the bowel wall, and diameter of the bowel. The intraluminal contents normally contain variable amounts of fluid and gas. The density of the fluid normally is homogeneous, but varies depending on diet, amount of food intake, and intestinal motility. Subjective increases in the amount of gas and fluid within the bowel can be seen. Increased gas and fluid without bowel dilation is commonly seen in aerophagia, gastroenteritis, and debilitation. Findings in a partial bowel obstruction, or early in the course of total bowel obstruction can be confusing, and follow-up films may be needed to determine whether persistent, abnormal dilation is present or not.

Dilation of the bowel is termed "ileus," and is recognized by the abnormal accumulation of gas, fluid, or ingesta within the bowel lumen, secondary to luminal obstruction or impaired motor function. The type of ileus can be further classified as mechanical or functional. In mechanical or dynamic ileus, the cause of the bowel dilation is usually a luminal obstruction, caused by a foreign body, intussusception, mural mass (e.g., tumor or granuloma), or extraluminal forces (e.g., adhesions, pressure from a mesenteric mass, or enlarged lymph node). The degree of ileus depends on the etiology of the obstruction, location within the bowel, and duration of obstructive disease. The bowel dilates with fluid and gas proximal to the site of obstruction and is usually empty or normal in size distal to the obstructive site. In functional or adynamic ileus, also referred to as paralytic ileus, gas and fluid accumulates within the bowel due to abnormal bowel motility. This may be from a defect in innervation, of muscular dysfunction, peritonitis, or the result of sympathetic stimulation or parasympathetic inhibition. The ileus may be localized or generalized, depending on the cause. Common causes include severe gastroenteritis, peritonitis, abdominal trauma, vascular compromise (e.g., bowel volvulus or infarction), or severe debilitation. Other potential causes include: hypothyroidism, spinal cord injury, the effect of anesthesia, and amyloidosis. In localized ileus, a single segment of bowel dilates and persists. In generalized ileus, the entire bowel is dilated.

## Bowel Obstruction

Bowel obstruction has a variable clinical presentation depending on the type, location, duration, and associated abnormalities. Multiple causes of obstruction include intraluminal lesions (e.g., foreign body, bezoar, or enterolith) and intrinsic lesions (e.g., neoplasm, granuloma, diverticulum, intussusception, or localized enteritis), or are the result of peri-intestinal disease (e.g., adhesions, hernias, or masses). The survey radiographs may identify the obstructing lesion if it is radiopaque, of abnormal soft tissue density, or surrounded by gas. Abnormal displacement of the small bowel may be seen, as would occur in a linear foreign body with plication or bowel adhesions. Depending on the location of obstruction and whether the obstruction is complete or incomplete, a variable degree of gas or fluid ileus will result. Other potential findings include the loss of peritoneal detail, suggesting free peritoneal fluid or peritonitis and the presence of free abdominal gas indicative of perforation of a hollow viscus.

For confirmation of a suspected diagnosis of bowel obstruction, a barium upper GI study can be done. Alternatively, ultrasound can also be used for this assessment. Ultrasound can show gas- and fluid-dilated bowel loops, a subjective assessment of motility, and in some instances the site of obstruction. Characteristics of the obstructing lesion may differentiate tumors from some foreign bodies, as well as to detect associated lymph node enlargement. Some foreign bodies such as balls or rocks may be identifiable because of their characteristic shape, increased echogenicity, or acoustic shadowing. Linear foreign bodies can often be seen and, when causing plication, cause a pattern that has been described as a "ribbon candy" appearance. Intussusception usually results in a sonographic finding of a multilayered series of concentric rings, representing wall layers of the intussusceptum and intussuscipiens.

## Infiltrative Disease

Infiltrative disease of the small bowel presents a challenge for the clinician. Survey radiographs may appear normal, or may show increased intestinal gas and fluid with the subjective appearance of bowel wall thickening. If a diffuse disease is suspected, endoscopy with gastric and sufficiently deep duodenal biopsies may be effective in establishing the diagnosis of inflammatory bowel disease or GI lymphoma.

The barium UGI series in inflammatory bowel disease usually shows nonspecific changes of mucosal irregularity, prominent peristalsis, prominent villous patterns, and sometimes focal mucosal irregularity (e.g., thumb printing defects). Even an equivocal study, however, is useful in ruling out other lesions such as foreign bodies or bowel tumors. Abdominal ultrasound can evaluate bowel wall thickness and bowel wall irregularity, as well as changes within the architecture of the intestine. Coexistent abnormalities, including lymphadenopathy and peritoneal effusion, can be documented.

Ultrasound can identify diffuse or localized thickening of the bowel wall. The small bowel wall averages 2 to 3 mm in thickness, varying to some degree due to peristalsis; however, the intestine is considered abnormal if the wall is greater than 5 to 6 mm in thickness. The individual layers of the bowel wall, including the mucosa, submucosa, and muscularis portions, can be seen in the normal bowel. As a general rule, symmetric wall thickening without disruption of the layered wall appearance is usually associated with inflammatory disease. Localized asymmetric wall thickening with loss of wall layers is usually due to neoplastic infiltration. Two exceptions exist. In intestinal lymphosarcoma, the neoplastic infiltrate can involve circumferentially long segments of the bowel and in some inflammatory diseases, such as duodenitis associated with pancreatitis, disruption of the wall layers may be recognized.

## Bowel Displacement

Displacement of the bowel can occur with a number of conditions. As the bowel is mobile, changes in bowel position are usually a passive response to changes in the size, shape, or position of other abdominal organs. The most common condition is that of peritoneal herniation involving the diaphragm or abdominal wall with displacement of the bowel and other viscera into the hernia. Peritoneal adhesions can result in fixation of the bowel to the ventral abdominal wall when related to a previous laparotomy, or bowel can adhere to itself secondary to chronic peritonitis, carcinomatosis, or in some cases of linear foreign body in which the bowel is plicated as a mass. Internal hernias, as can occur with mesenteric tears and strangulation of a bowel loop, may result in an abnormal appearance of the small bowel and dilation of the bowel loops depending on the degree of luminal occlusion and vascular compromise. To document the location of the bowel, a barium or iodine upper GI study is usually the most direct approach.

With a diaphragmatic hernia not containing the stomach or bowel, a celiogram (positive-contrast peritoneogram) may confirm the presence of the hernia.

## THE LARGE BOWEL

Diseases of the cecum, colon, and rectum can be assessed by abdominal palpation, digital rectal examination, stool examination, external imaging (radiography and ultrasound), and endoscopy. The clinical presentation of patients with disease of the lower bowel vary depending on the disease (e.g., colitis, neoplasia), degree of obstruction or ileus, and other complications (e.g., perforation, adhesions).

Imaging of the large bowel usually is initiated with survey abdominal films that include the entire colon and pelvic canal. Radiographic signs of disease include marked distention of the cecum, colon, or rectum with gas, fluid, or soft tissue dense material, displacement of the bowel by an enlarged urinary bladder, prostate gland, or other abdominal mass, abnormal density of the bowel wall (e.g., emphysematous colitis), or thickening of the bowel wall. Enlarged lymph nodes in the canal or mesenteric region can displace the bowel or appear to originate from the bowel itself.

Following assessment of the survey radiographs, it may be advisable to perform an enema and obtain follow-up films. Suspected lesions seen on the initial films may subside on the follow-up films, resulting in no further study. If abnormal findings are still present, additional imaging or other diagnostic procedures may be indicated such as:

1. Opposite lateral view (gravitational movement of gas and fluid).

2. Pneumocolon (to differentiate large bowel from small bowel).
3. Barium enema.
4. Double-contrast barium enema.
5. Ultrasound.
6. Endoscopy.

The purpose of an additional procedure would be to evaluate the position and patency of the bowel, the thickness of the bowel wall, and the presence of ulcers or masses involving the mucosa. Intussusception and cecal inversion are other considerations. In patients with suspected colitis or mucosal neoplasia, endoscopy is the preferred diagnostic procedure, as it provides the opportunity to obtain biopsies of abnormal lesions.

## References and Suggested Reading

Agut A, Sánchez-Velverde MA, Lasaosa JM, et al: Use of iohexol as a gastrointestinal contrast medium in the dog. Vet Radiol Ultrasound 34:171, 1993.

Agut A, Sánchez-Velverde MA, Torrecillos FE, et al: Iohexol as a gastrointestinal contrast medium in the cat. Vet Radiol Ultrasound 35:164, 1994.

Allan FJ, Guilford WG: Radiopaque markers: Preliminary clinical observations. Proceedings of 12th Annual Acvim Veterinary Medical Forum, San Francisco, CA, 1994, 982.

Arson E, Carrig CR, and Lattimer JC: Radiology of the gastrointestinal system. In Jones BD (ed): Canine and Feline Gastroenterology. Philadelphia, WB Saunders Co, 1986.

Brawner WR and Daniel GB: Nuclear Imaging. Vet Clin North Am [Small Anim Prac] 23(2): 1993.

Burk RL and Ackerman N: Small Animal Radiology. New York, Churchill Livingstone, 1986.

O'Brien TR: Radiographic Diagnosis of Abdominal Disorders in the Dog and Cat. Philadelphia, WB Saunders Co, 1978.

Strombeck DR: Small Animal Gastroenterology, 2nd edition. Davis, CA, Stonegate Publishing, 1990.

Suter PF: Thoracic Radiography. Wettswil, Switzerland, Peter F. Suter, 1984.

Thrall DE: Textbook of Veterinary Diagnostic Radiology. Philadelphia, WB Saunders Co, 1986.

# SELECTING A GASTROINTESTINAL ENDOSCOPE

ROBERT C. DENOVO
*Knoxville, Tennessee*

Endoscopy has become a valuable diagnostic and therapeutic tool for the small animal clinician. Endoscopy allows direct inspection of the gastrointestinal, respiratory, and lower urogenital tracts and provides a noninvasive method to obtain cytology, biopsy, and culture samples. Therapeutically, endoscopy provides a nonsurgical method to remove foreign bodies from the airways, esophagus, and stomach and is routinely used for percutaneous endoscopic gastrostomy (PEG) tube placement. Gastrointestinal endoscopy comprises over 85% of the endoscopic procedures done in our practice; diagnostic and therapeutic indications for upper and lower gastrointestinal endoscopy are listed in Tables 1 and 2, respectively.

Selection of a gastrointestinal endoscopic system requires knowledge of the types and sizes of endoscopes available as well as an understanding of the functional components of the endoscope. The ideal endoscope for the small animal clinician is an instrument that can be used for a variety of procedures such as retroflexed nasopharyngoscopy, esophagogastroduodenoscopy, and colonoscopy in animals ranging in size from cats to

**Table 1.** *Indications for Upper Gastrointestinal Endoscopy*

| Diagnostic | Therapeutic |
|---|---|
| Dysphagia | Remove esophageal foreign body |
| Regurgitation | Remove gastric foreign body |
| Chronic vomiting | Balloon dilatation or bougienage of esophageal strictures |
| Hematemesis | |
| Chronic small bowel diarrhea | Percutaneous endoscopic gastrostomy or gastroduodenostomy |
| Melena | Gastroduodenal polypectomy |
| Protein-losing enteropathy | |

giant-breed dogs. Although no single endoscope can meet all of these needs, pediatric gastrointestinal endoscopes and the newer veterinary endoscopes are most versatile and provide the best range of application. These endoscopes can also be used for bronchoscopy and vaginoscopy in most medium to large dogs.

## FIBEROPTIC AND VIDEO ENDOSCOPES

There are two basic types of flexible gastrointestinal endoscopes available: fiberoptic endoscopes and video endoscopes. The major parts of a fiberoptic endoscope are the handpiece, the insertion tube, and the universal cord. The handpiece includes the eyepiece, the angulation control knobs, the air/water suction valves, and the opening to the operating channel. The flexible insertion tube contains fiberoptic glass bundles that transmit light from the light source to the distal tip of the endoscope, and fiberoptic glass bundles that transmit the image from the distal tip to the eyepiece. In addition, the insertion tube contains a biopsy/suction channel, an air and water channel, and angulation control wires. The distal part of the insertion tube is the bending section, which produces controlled deflection of the distal tip of the endoscope. The universal cord transmits light from the light source via fiberoptic glass bundles to the endoscope. It also has connections for a water container and suction pump.

Fiberoptic glass bundles are very fragile and can be easily damaged. Broken fibers in the image transmission fiberoptic bundle will cause black spots to appear in the image. For this reason, fiberoptic endoscopes must be handled very carefully to ensure longevity and high-quality images. If purchase of a used or refur-

**Table 2.** *Indications for Lower Gastrointestinal Endoscopy*

| Diagnostic | Therapeutic |
|---|---|
| Chronic diarrhea | Rectal-colonic polypectomy |
| Chronic hematochezia | Balloon dilatation of rectal or colonic strictures |
| Chronic mucoid stools | |
| Chronic tenesmus/dyschezia | |
| Fecal incontinence | |
| Recurrent constipation | |

bished endoscope is being considered, one should avoid endoscopes with many broken fibers.

Video endoscopes are considerably different from fiberoptic endoscopes, although both types of instruments look almost identical. Video endoscope systems have three basic components: the endoscope, a computerized video processor, and a television monitor. A small microelectric video-chip is located on the distal tip of the endoscope and receives the image, which is then transmitted electronically through the endoscope to the video processor. The image is integrated and computer enhanced by the processor and projected to the television monitor where the image is viewed.

This design eliminates the use of fragile fiberoptic bundles and produces a large, high-resolution image that can be viewed by many at one time. This feature improves coordination between endoscopist and assistant during therapeutic procedures, and greatly enhances teaching. Video endoscopes have freeze-frame and video-taping features that facilitate close inspection of specific lesions, photodocumentation, and second opinions. Cost and size are the primary disadvantages of the video endoscopic systems. The smallest video endoscope presently recommended has a 9.5-mm outer diameter insertion tube, which limits its use in small dogs and cats. Video endoscope systems cost approximately twice as much fiberoptic systems.

## SPECIFICATIONS AND COMPONENTS

The primary objective of endoscopy is visualization; therefore, size, brightness, and resolution of the image are important factors to consider when choosing an endoscope. Additionally, endoscopes with slim insertion tubes and large working channels are desirable to maximize versatility, improve ease of insertion into the duodenum, and enhance therapeutic capabilities. A high-quality flexible gastrointestinal endoscope with the following dimensions and features is recommended to meet these objectives.

### Length

A working length of at least 100 cm is necessary for gastrointestinal endoscopic procedures in most small animal patients. This length is sufficient to reach the proximal duodenum in most dogs; however, examination of the duodenum and of the entire colon in giant-breed dogs may require a length of 130 cm or greater.

### Diameter of the Insertion Tube

The diameter of the insertion tube of the endoscope is one of the most important factors to consider when selecting a gastrointestinal endoscope for small animal practice. In general, the insertion tube should be less than 10 mm in diameter. Endoscopes with an insertion tube diameter greater than 10 mm are too large to traverse the pyloric canal and enter the duodenum of cats and small dogs and are generally limited to use in medium and large dogs.

Pediatric gastrointestinal endoscopes range in diameter from 7.8 to 10 mm. Veterinary endoscopes are available with an insertion tube diameter of 8.0 to 9.9 mm. Endoscopes at the smaller end of this range are recommended because they can more easily be inserted into the duodenum of small dogs and cats than endoscopes greater than 9 mm in diameter. This is an important consideration if much feline endoscopy is anticipated. At our practice, however, duodenoscopy is successfully done in most canine and feline patients using a 9.6-mm diameter gastroscope.

There are some trade-offs with smaller diameter endoscopes. The image is usually smaller and not as bright as that obtained with a larger endoscope. The primary difference, however, is a smaller size of the operating channel in pediatric endoscopes. This channel is used for biopsy instruments as well as for suction. Suction through a small channel is not as effective as it is through a larger channel, especially when a biopsy instrument is being used simultaneously. Smaller channels also cannot accommodate some instruments, particularly large grasping forceps. These are minor limitations, however, when compared to the improved ability to do a complete endoscopic examination on a broad range of patients when a smaller diameter endoscope is used.

## Operating Channel

The operating channel of the endoscope is necessary for the passage of biopsy and grasping forceps, cytology brushes, balloon dilators, polypectomy snares, and other instruments for therapeutic procedures. This channel is also used for suction. Large channels are desirable because they allow use of larger instruments and provide better suction. The diameter of the channel is directly proportional to the diameter of the endoscope, ranging from 2 to 3 mm in the pediatric and veterinary gastrointestinal endoscopes, which is adequate for veterinary use. Video endoscopes do not have a fiberoptic bundle for image transmission and can therefore provide a larger operating channel than fiberoptic endoscopes of the same diameter. Therapeutic endoscopes have two operating channels to facilitate operative procedures such as polypectomy; however, the increased diameter of two-channel endoscopes limits their use in veterinary endoscopy.

## Distal Tip Deflection

Gastrointestinal endoscopes should have four-way tip deflection and a small bending radius to allow optimal maneuverability and a wide view for complete endoscopic examination. The maximum bending angle in each direction varies with endoscope diameter and manufacturer. One bending angle should have at least 180-degree deflection to allow retroflexed examination of the nasopharynx, stomach, and rectum. The other three bending angles should have at least 90-degree deflection. Endoscopes with two-way tip deflection do not provide adequate maneuverability for thorough and efficient examination, especially of the stomach and duodenum, and are not recommended for gastrointestinal endoscopy.

The angulation controls for tip deflection are located on the handpiece of the endoscope. The compactness and position of these controls vary from one type of endoscope to another, which can affect the endoscopist's ability to control position with one hand. Ease of handling, comfort, and maneuverability should be determined when testing an endoscope prior to purchase.

## Field of View

Endoscopes with a 90- to 120-degree field of view facilitate orientation and decrease the need to continually reposition the endoscope. Forward-viewing endoscopes are recommended, as side-viewing endoscopes have no routine use in veterinary patients.

## Light Source

High-intensity halogen or xenon light sources of 150 to 300 watts are used for flexible endoscopes. Higher wattage provides greater illumination and image brightness, which is of particular importance when examining a large viscus such as the stomach. Adapters to light sources are available that will allow a light source from one manufacturer to be used with an endoscope from another manufacturer.

## Insufflation and Irrigation

An air pump is necessary for insufflation of the gastrointestinal lumen during endoscopy and is usually built-in to the same unit as the light source. Water flushing is needed to keep the distal lens clean and is also housed in the same unit as the light source.

## Vacuum Source

A vacuum source is a necessary component of the gastrointestinal endoscopy system. Suction provides the ability to aspirate fluid and mucus from the gut lumen to improve visualization of the mucosa, and it facilitates cleansing of the distal lens. A vacuum source is necessary to decompress the gastrointestinal tract at the end of the endoscopic procedure; failure to do so can result in gastric distention, respiratory compromise, and postendoscopic gastroesophageal reflux. Many types of vacuum pumps are available that easily attach to the endoscope; however, these are not sold as a part of the endoscopic system.

**Table 3.** *Manufacturers and Specifications of Fiberoptic Gastrointestinal Veterinary Endoscopes*[*]

| Model | Gastro-Duodeno-Fiberscope | VSF-5 Endoscope |
|---|---|---|
| Manufacturer | Karl Stortz Veterinary Endoscopy—America[†] | Schott Fiber Optics[‡] |
| Working length | 150 cm | 125 cm |
| Insertion tube outer diameter | 8.0 mm | 9.9 mm |
| Working channel diameter | 2.5 mm | 2.8 mm |
| Bending capability (degrees) | | |
| Up | 200 | 180 |
| Down | 120 | 180 |
| Left | 90 | 170 |
| Right | 90 | 170 |
| Field of view (degrees) | 100 | 100 |
| Depth of field of view | | 10–70 mm |
| Immersible | Yes | Yes |

[*]This listing includes examples of current model (August, 1993) endoscopes from major manufacturers. Some specifications for older models vary.
[†]Karl Stortz Veterinary Endoscopy—America, Inc, 175 Cremona Drive, Goleta, CA 93117; Telephone (800) 955-7832.
[‡]Schott Fiber Optics, Inc, 122 Charlton Street, Southbridge, MA 01550; Telephone (508) 765-9744.

## Optional Features

Several optional features are available that improve the use and longevity of an endoscope but which also add to the cost. Independent locks on the deflection controls provide the endoscopist better ability to maintain desired position of the endoscope tip using one hand while the other hand is being used to pass biopsy forceps or for other manipulation. Newer model endoscopes have this as a standard feature. Newer endoscopes are also fluid-tight and can be totally immersed in strong disinfectants for cold sterilization. This feature makes thorough cleaning easier and prevents costly damage caused by water leakage.

Tables 3 and 4 give specifications on fiberoptic gastrointestinal endoscopes currently produced by major manufacturers of veterinary and human endoscopes, respectively, that meet the above recommendations. Specifications on older model equipment may vary.

High-quality used and refurbished endoscopes can be obtained at significantly lower cost from some manufacturers, hospitals, and endoscopy supply retailers.

## ENDOSCOPIC ACCESSORIES

A wide variety of endoscopic accessories are available; however, only a few are essential to perform routine endoscopic procedures such as cytology, biopsy, foreign body removal, and PEG tube placement.

### Biopsy Forceps

These are flexible instruments that can be passed through the working channel of the endoscope and visually directed to specific lesions to obtain 2- to 3-mm pinch biopsies. Several types are available including

**Table 4.** *Manufacturers and Specifications of Fiberoptic Gastrointestinal Human Endoscopes*[*]

| Model | UGI-PE7 Pediatric | UGI-FP7 | GIF TYPE XP20 Pediatric | GIF TYPE PQ20 | FG-24X Pediatric | FG-27X |
|---|---|---|---|---|---|---|
| Manufacturer | Fujinon[†] | Fujinon[†] | Olympus[‡] | Olympus[‡] | Pentax[§] | Pentax[§] |
| Working length | 102 cm | 102 cm | 102.5 cm | 102.5 cm | 105 cm | 105 cm |
| Insertion tube outer diameter | 7.8 mm | 9.8 mm | 7.9 mm | 9.0 mm | 7.9 mm | 9.0 mm |
| Working channel diameter | 2.2 mm | 2.8 mm | 2.0 mm | 2.8 mm | 2.4 mm | 2.8 mm |
| Bending capability (degrees) | | | | | | |
| Up | 210 | 210 | 210 | 210 | 210 | 210 |
| Down | 90 | 90 | 90 | 90 | 120 | 120 |
| Left | 100 | 100 | 100 | 100 | 120 | 120 |
| Right | 100 | 100 | 100 | 100 | 120 | 120 |
| Field of view (degrees) | 105 | 105 | 100 | 100 | 105 | 105 |
| Depth of field of view | 5–100 mm | 5–100 mm | 3–100 mm | 3–100 mm | 3–100 mm | 3–100 mm |
| Immersible | Yes | Yes | Yes | Yes | Yes | Yes |

[*]This listing includes examples of current model (August, 1993) endoscopes from major manufacturers. Some specifications for older models vary.
[†]Fujinon, Inc, 10 High Point Drive, Wayne, NJ 0747-7434; Telephone (800) 872-0196
[‡]Olympus Corporation, 4 Nevada Drive, Lake Success, NY 11042-1179; Telephone (800) 342-1673.
[§]Pentax Precision Instrument Corporation, 30 Ramland Road, Orangeburg, NY 10962-2699; Telephone (800) 431-5880.

standard oval cup, fenestrated oval cup, and long-jaw alligator forceps. Fenestrated forceps do not cause as much crush artifact as nonfenestrated forceps and tend to give larger samples. Alligator-type forceps with long jaws also provide larger samples. Both types are available with a central needle that anchors the forceps to the mucosa. This feature is useful when obtaining biopsies from more elastic tissues such as the esophageal or gastric mucosa or from firm tumors. The central needle prevents the forceps from slipping off the tissue. Preferably, the endoscopist should have at least one fenestrated oval-shaped, one alligator-type, and one alligator-needle biopsy forceps. Disposable forceps intended for single use are available. Although these can be reused, they are not as sturdy or reliable as standard multiuse forceps and are not recommended.

### Grasping Forceps and Retrieval Baskets

Several types of grasping forceps and retrieval baskets are available for foreign body removal and for use in PEG tube placement. Three basic grasping forceps are available; a three- or four-pronged wire forceps, a V-type or "rat-tooth" forceps, and a flattened "duckbill" forceps. The three- and four-pronged forceps have partial hooks on the tips of the prongs. They are particularly useful to grasp coins and irregularly shaped or large objects such as bones, sticks, or trichobezoars. Rat-tooth forceps are most useful for grasping fabric or packaging material or other foreign material that is deformable. Duck-bill forceps are used to grasp coins and other flattened objects in addition to small, smooth-surfaced objects.

Wire basket retrievers are primarily used for removal of rounded or smooth-surfaced objects such as rocks or peach pits. They are also useful to grasp suture that has been passed percutaneously into the stomach during PEG tube placement. At the minimum, the endoscopist should have a rat-tooth forceps and a three- or four-wire retrieval basket.

### Cytology Brushes and Catheters

Sheathed cytology brushes are useful to obtain cytology specimens from specific lesions. Catheters are used to aspirate fluid samples such as duodenal aspirates for *Giardia* testing or culture.

### Balloon Dilators

Balloon dilators are most useful for dilatation of esophageal and rectal strictures. Smaller dilators have an inflated outer diameter of 12 to 20 mm and can be passed through the channel of the endoscope; these are best for strictures in cats and small to medium-sized dogs. Large dilators that range from 30 to 40 mm inflated outer diameter are passed around the endoscope; these are often needed to successfully dilate strictures in large dogs.

## GENERAL GUIDELINES

Here are some suggestions to consider when selecting a flexible gastrointestinal endoscopic system:

1. If you have not had instruction in basic endoscopic technique, get some. Many excellent courses offering a range of basic to advanced endoscopic techniques are available that provide "hands-on" instruction and the opportunity to compare different endoscopic systems. Having practical experience and some degree of aptitude will improve your ability to critically evaluate an endoscope before purchase.

2. Evaluate more than one company's endoscopic system. Schedule a time for a demonstration at your practice, preferably using a patient. This will allow you to evaluate image quality, ease of use, and versatility.

3. Include technical staff in demonstrations, as they will play a central role in development of an efficient endoscopic practice and in proper maintenance of equipment.

4. Determine the terms of equipment warranty; differences exist in length of warranty and in what costs are covered.

5. Determine the availability of service and whether the company will provide an endoscope on loan if your endoscope needs repair. Ask for names of individuals who have recently purchased endoscopes for reference.

# ENDOSCOPIC AND NONENDOSCOPIC PERCUTANEOUS GASTROSTOMY TUBE PLACEMENT

JOHN V. MAUTERER, Jr.

*Columbus, Ohio*

Endoscopic placement of gastrostomy tubes for enteral nutritional support is a relatively safe and effective technique (Kirby et al., 1986; Armstrong and Hardie, 1990). From the time this technique was first introduced to veterinary medicine in 1986 (Mathews and Binnington, 1986), it has rapidly gained acceptance and is now a standard of practice for animals requiring long-term nutritional support. Modifications of this technique, which eliminate the need for an endoscope for percutaneous gastrostomy tube placement, have recently been described (Fulton and Jeffrey, 1992; Mauterer et al., 1994). The purpose of this article is to provide guidelines for decision making concerning enteral nutritional support, gastrostomy tubes, and endoscopic versus nonendoscopic placement techniques.

## INDICATIONS FOR NUTRITIONAL SUPPORT

One should first consider the circumstances that suggest nutritional support is appropriate for a patient. Studies have shown that up to 50% of critical human patients receive inadequate nutritional support (Remillard and Martin, 1990). In veterinary medicine, these percentages are not known, but one would expect the findings to be at least comparable. Clinicians must carefully plan in advance and anticipate when patients will require nutritional support. The indications for enteral nutritional support include: (1) recent weight loss of more than 10%, (2) inappetence for more than 5 to 7 days, (3) anticipated anorexia or inability to eat for more than 5 to 7 days, (4) increased nutrient losses (i.e., open abdominal drainage, large open wounds, burns), (5) increased nutritional needs (i.e., polytrauma, sepsis), (6) serum albumin less than 2.5 gm/dl, (7) hepatic lipidosis in cats, and (8) history of chronic disease. The presence of even one of these criteria warrants serious consideration of nutritional support.

## SELECTING THE ROUTE OF ENTERAL TUBE FEEDING

Once a patient is identified as one requiring nutritional support, the route of administration must be determined. One should always remember the nutritionists' golden rule: "If the gut works, use it!" In line with this thought, numerous methods of enteral feeding have been described that include nasogastric (Crowe, 1986; Abood and Buffington, 1991), pharyngostomy (Bohnign et al., 1970), jejunal (Orton, 1986), esophageal (Rawlings, 1993), and gastric tubes (Bright and Burrows, 1988; Armstrong and Hardie, 1989). Each method has advantages and disadvantages.

Nasogastric intubation is an effective noninvasive method for short-term management, but has the disadvantages of being limited to liquid diets and posing technical difficulties for long-term feeding situations. In addition, access is not always possible as in cases of craniofacial surgery or injury or in some feline breeds with stenotic nares (Mauterer et al., 1994).

Pharyngostomy tubes have been used successfully in the hands of many practitioners; however, technical problems in long-term management and esophageal and respiratory complications have occurred (Crowe, 1986). Recently, a midcervical approach for esophagostomy has been described for use in clinical patients (Rawlings, 1993). The midcervical approach is advocated to decrease respiratory and gastroesophageal complications associated with pharyngostomy. Esophagostomy allows esophageal or gastric feedings without requiring the availability of an endoscope and requires only a minor skin incision, but does require general anesthesia and creation of a small esophageal defect. No ill effects were observed; however, the number of clinical cases reported to date is limited.

Jejunostomy can be useful in cases where gastric pathology or vomiting are part of the clinical disease, but mixed results have been reported in humans and only limited information is available in the veterinary literature concerning the efficacy of jejunostomy tube feeding (Orton, 1986; DiSario et al., 1990).

Gastrostomy tubes can be placed surgically, percutaneously with an endoscope (Mathews and Binnington, 1986; Bright and Burrows, 1988), or percutaneously without an endoscope (Fulton and Jeffrey, 1992; Mauterer et al., 1994). Surgical placement of gastrostomy tubes has the advantages of: direct visualization of the site of placement, suturing of the stomach to body wall, and suturing of the omentum around the tube site to ensure a good adhesion between stomach and body wall. Disadvantages of surgical placement include: the expense of the surgical procedure, morbidity association with celiotomy in a compromised patient, and required general anesthesia. Percutaneously placed gastrostomy tubes offer the advantages of being a quick and relatively noninvasive method, as well as providing a dependable and easily managed route of long-term nutritional support (Armstrong and Hardie, 1990). This technique has the disadvantages of not allowing one to suture the stomach to body wall or omentum to the tube site, and providing only limited control over the exact site of tube placement.

## INDICATIONS FOR GASTROSTOMY TUBE PLACEMENT

Ideally, gastrostomy tube placement is chosen when the patient has a functional gastrointestinal tract from the stomach distally. General indications for use of gastrostomy tubes are: (1) anticipated anorexia or inability to eat for more than 7 to 10 days, (2) inability to use more proximal access to the gastrointestinal tract, and (3) a patient to be maintained at home by the owner for extended time. Specific indications for gastrostomy tube feeding include, but are not limited to: trauma to head and neck, surgery of the head and neck, dysphagia, esophageal disease, hepatic lipidosis, support of neurologically impaired patients, polytrauma, sepsis, chronic renal failure, and unexplained anorexia.

## CONTRAINDICATIONS FOR GASTROSTOMY TUBE PLACEMENT

Contraindications for gastrostomy tube placement include: (1) the ability of the animal to eat its required caloric intake, (2) presence or suspicion of a gastric outflow obstruction, and (3) frequent vomiting as a significant part of the clinical disease process. There are several contraindications that apply specifically for the nonendoscopic technique. First is the animal that requires endoscopy as part of the clinical evaluation. If the patient is to undergo endoscopy for gastric or duodenal examination or biopsy, the gastrostomy tube should be placed with the endoscope. Next is the patient that exhibits signs or is diagnosed with esophageal stricture or obstruction. Attempting to pass a tube placement device blindly could lead to esophageal bleeding, perforation, or further stricture. Similarly, megaesophagus should be considered a potential contraindication for nonendoscopic methods. Though the use of a nonoendoscopic method has been described and safely performed in this situation, extreme caution is advised due to the thin and potentially fragile nature of a chronically distended esophagus (Mauterer et al., 1994).

## INDICATIONS: ENDOSCOPIC VERSUS NONENDOSCOPIC

Endoscopic placement of gastrostomy tubes should be selected for patients with suspected disease of the esophagus, stomach, or duodenum. Endoscopic placement allows visualization and documentation of the size, location, and nature of mucosal lesions and permits mucosal pinch biopsies to be obtained via the endoscope. An additional advantage is that one can visualize the location of tube placement relative to the pylorus.

Nonendoscopic placement of gastrostomy tubes should be reserved for animals that require nutritional support for longer than 7 to 10 days but otherwise do not require endoscopy as part of the diagnostic workup. There are several advantages to the nonendoscopic method. The greatest advantage is the technique does not require an endoscope. The materials required are inexpensive and readily available to most veterinary practices. The technique can consistently be performed in less than 10 min in cats and dogs less than 15 kg. Placement position has been shown to be comparable to that of endoscopy in this group of patients and the technique is not difficult to learn. Short-acting injectable anesthesia is adequate for the nonendoscopic placement technique. Extreme caution is advised when using this technique in dogs that weigh more than 20 kg. Consistent proper tube placement in larger dogs requires experience. Inexperience can result in placement of the tube in the cardia of the stomach, through the gastrosplenic ligament very close to the splenic artery, and/or entrapment of the spleen cranial to the tube. Practice on cadavers is essential until proper placement is consistently achieved.

## TECHNIQUES

Three techniques of percutaneous gastrostomy tube placement are described below: two nonendoscopic (techniques 1 and 2) and one endoscopic (technique 3). All of the materials necessary to perform the techniques except the tube placement devices or endoscope, respectively, are listed in Table 1.

The tube placement device used in technique 1 can be easily made by a local machine shop using 1/4 inch stainless steel tubing or 1/4 inch brake line. The specifications are as follows: 40 cm length, double-lapped flared tip, and a 45 degree bend to the distal 1 cm of the tube. Straight 1/2 inch PVC tubing has also been used successfully in a similar technique (Fulton and Jeffrey, 1992). Technique 2 utilizes a commercially available nonendoscopic placement device.

The landmarks for feeding tube placement are the point 2 cm caudal to the last rib, and one third the distance from the epaxial musculature to the ventral midline on the left lateral body wall. The patient is placed in *right lateral recumbency*, and an 8- × 8-cm area of skin is clipped and prepared with chlorhexidine scrub° followed by 70% isopropyl alcohol. A mouth gag can be placed to simplify passage of the tube placement devices and to protect the endoscope.

---

°Nolvasan surgical scrub, Aveco Co Inc, Fort Dodge, IA, 50501.

**Table 1.** *Materials Required for Percutaneous Nonendoscopic Gastrostomy Tube Placement*

1. Bard Urologic Pezzar catheter° (20-Fr. for <15 kg, 22-Fr. for >15 kg)
2. Sovereign indwelling catheter[†] with accompanying needle: 14- or 16-gauge
3. 3 pieces of No. 1 Braunamid[‡] (two 80-cm and one the length of the prepared Bard catheter)
4. Scissors
5. Hemostat
6. Marks-a-Lot[§] or other permanent marker
7. Catheter adapter″
8. PRN injection port[¶]
9. Mouth gag
10. Chlorhexidine scrub[#] and 70% isopropyl alcohol
11. No. 11 scalpel blade°°
12. Waterproof tape
13. 18-gauge needle[††]
14. Water-soluble lubricant[‡‡]

---

°Pezzar urinary catheter, Bard Inc, Covington, GA, 30209.
[†]Sovereign indwelling catheter, Monoject, St. Louis, MO, 63103.
[‡]Braunamid, B. Braun Melsungen, Melsungen, Germany.
[§]Marks-a-Lot, Carter's Ink Co, Cambridge, MA, 02142.
″Catheter adapter, Becton-Dickinson, Rutherford, NJ, 07070.
[¶]PRN adapter, Deseret, Sandy, UT, 84070.
[#]Nolvasan surgical scrub, Aveco Co Inc, Fort Dodge, IA, 50501.
°°Surgical scalpel blade, Miltex Co, Lake Success, NY, 11042.
[††]Monoject, St. Louis, MO, 63103.
[‡‡]K-Y jelly, Johnson and Johnson Inc, Arlington, TX, 76004.

## Nonendoscopic

The feeding tube[†] is prepared as described as in Figure 1. The dilated proximal end is cut off and discarded. A 2-cm length of the tube is then cut and set aside to be used as the external flange, and the proximal end of the remaining tube is cut at a sharp angle. A strand of suture is cut to the length of the prepared feeding tube and set aside. A circumferential mark is made with a permanent marker[‡] 3 cm from proximal to the mushroom tip.

The length of the tube placement device to be in-

---

[†]Pezzar urinary catheter, Bard Inc, Covington, GA, 30209.
[‡]Marks-a-Lot, Carter's Ink Co, Cambridge, MA, 02142.

serted is estimated by measuring from the tip of the nose, laterally to the last rib. The tube placement device is held with the distal bend oriented to the animal's left side, introduced into the oral cavity, and gently advanced down the esophagus. At the level of the heart, the tube placement device is rotated counterclockwise to follow the path of least resistance. The tube is advanced past the lower esophageal sphincter into the stomach. Once in the stomach, the tube placement device is rotated to bring the distal tip against the left body wall. The proximal end of the tube placement device is lowered to raise the distal end laterally, against the body wall, while a second person palpates the flared end of the tube through the skin. Palpation of the tip is aided by extending the animal's head over the edge of the table.

At this point, the two nonendoscopic techniques differ. In technique 1, the catheter needle[§] is introduced through the skin into the flared tip of the tube placement device″ (Fig. 2A). The 80-cm premeasured suture[¶] (Table 1) is then threaded into the needle and advanced through the tube placement device, exiting at the proximal end where the suture is grasped. Once the suture is passed, the needle and tube placement device are removed. The result is a suture strand that exits the mouth at one end and the left lateral body wall at the other end.

In technique 2, once the tip of the tube placement device[#] is palpable through the body wall, the eyed stylet is forced through the skin (Fig. 2B). The suture is then threaded through the eye of the stylet and the stylet is withdrawn. The tube placement device is then withdrawn from the mouth, pulling one end of the suture with it. The result is a suture strand that exits the

---

[§]Sovereign indwelling catheter, Monoject, St. Louis, MO, 63103.
″Percutaneous non-endoscopic gastrostomy (PNG) placement device, Dr. John Mauterer, MedVet Inc., Columbus, OH 43231.
[¶]Braunamid, B. Braun Melsungen, Melsungen, Germany.
[#]Elb gastrostomy tube applicator, Jorgensen Laboratories Inc, Loveland, CO, 80538 (patent pending).

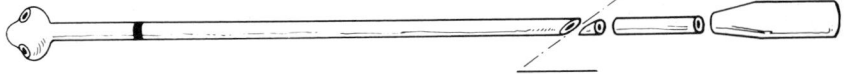

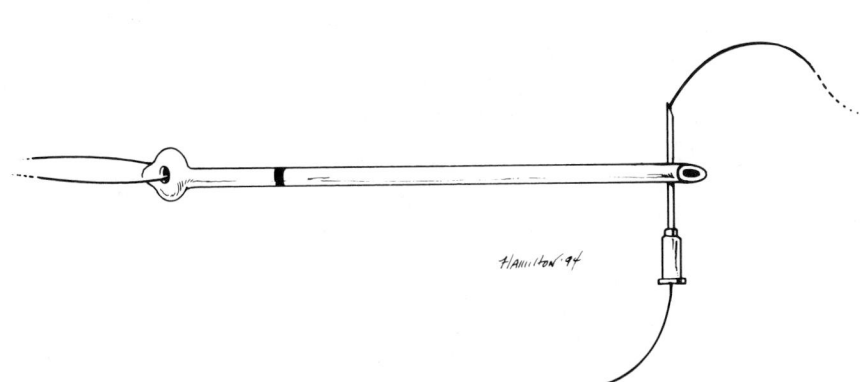

**Figure 1.** Diagrammatic representation of preparation of Bard urologic catheter for percutaneous endoscopic or nonendoscopic placement.

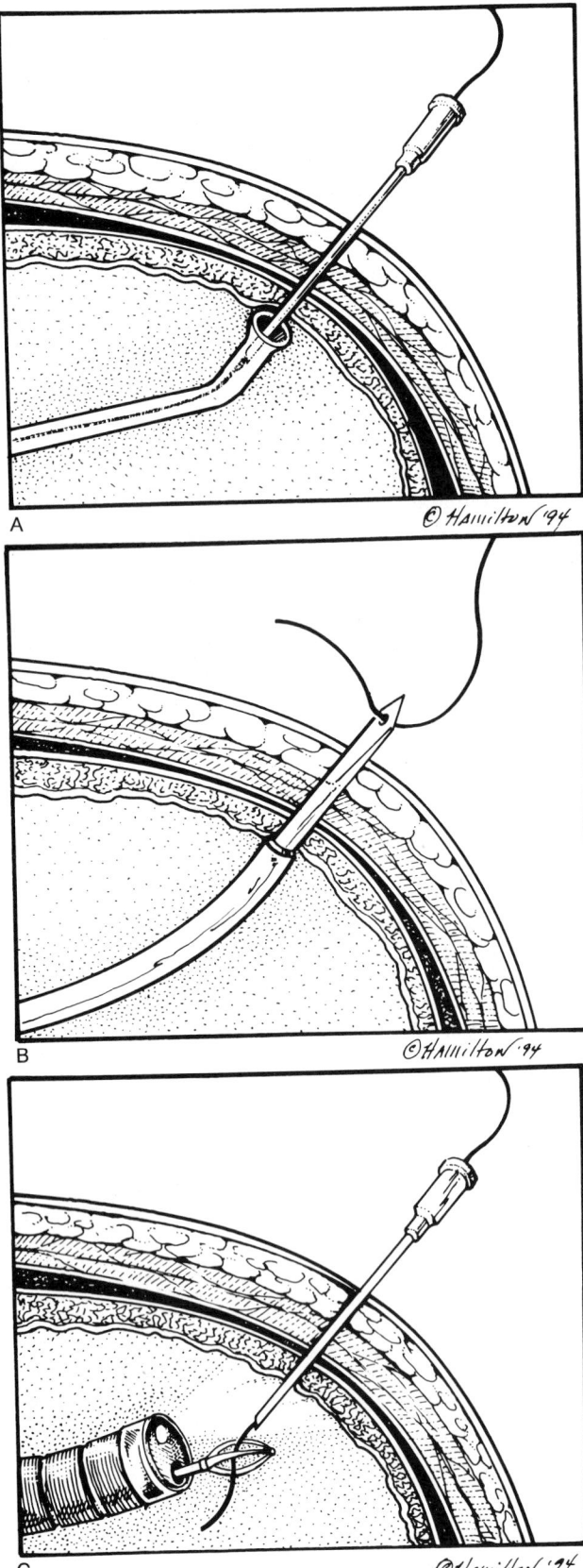

mouth at one end and the left lateral body wall at the other end.

From this point forward, all three techniques can be performed identically. The plastic catheter[§] is threaded, tapered tip first, onto the end of the suture exiting the animal's mouth. An 18-gauge needle[**] is passed through the feeding tube perpendicular to its long axis, 0.5 cm from its tip. The suture then is threaded through the pointed end of the 18-gauge needle (Fig. 1), the needle is removed from the tube, and the suture is tied securely. The cut end of the feeding tube is then seated firmly into the tapered end of the catheter, which acts as a dilator for passage of the tube through the stomach and body wall along the path of the suture. A second 80-cm premeasured suture is passed through the holes in the distal end of the feeding tube and doubled over to permit removal if placement is unsuccessful. A circumferential marking is made with a permanent marker 3 cm from the distal end of the feeding tube to indicate adequate feeding tube passage (Fig. 1).

A water-soluble lubricant[††] is applied to the catheter to aid in passage of the tube. The suture exiting the body wall is grasped and pulled with slow, steady pressure until the catheter tip exits the skin. A 3- to 4-mm skin incision is made with a No. 11 blade[‡‡] at the tube exit site. The suture and catheter are held 90 degrees to the body wall, while the skin is stabilized with two fingers. The suture in the distal end of the feeding tube is held loosely as the tube is pulled through the skin. The suture premeasured to the exact length of the prepared feeding tube is used to determine the length of the tube exiting the stomach. Visualization of the circumferential marking also aids in assessing proper placement. After confirmation of proper tube placement, the safety suture in the distal end of the tube is removed. The external flange is fitted over the feeding tube to the level of the skin and held in place by a butterfly tape-tab.

### Endoscopic

In technique 3 (endoscopic gastrostomy tube placement), the endoscope is advanced into the stomach. The stomach is then insufflated with enough air to visualize the antral region and the area of external digital palpation of the stomach. Landmarks for placement are as previously mentioned; however, minor modifications are made based on what is visualized endoscopically, in order to bring the tube placement site farthest away from the pylorus. Once the placement site is selected, the catheter needle is inserted into the insufflated stomach. The 80-cm strand of suture is threaded through the needle and grasped with the endoscopic foreign body retrieval or basket forceps (Fig. 2C). The endoscope and suture are withdrawn from the mouth.

**Figure 2.** *A*, Needle insertion nonendoscopic technique for gastrostomy tube placement. *B*, Eyed stylet-spear nonendoscopic technique for gastrostomy tube placement. *C*, Endoscopic technique for gastrostomy tube placement.

**Monoject, St. Louis, MO, 63103.
††K-Y jelly, Johnson and Johnson Inc, Arlington, TX, 76004.
‡‡Surgical scalpel blade, Miltex Co, Lake Success, NY, 11042.

***Table 2***  *Bard Urologic Pezzar Catheter Sizes and Flange Recommendations*

| Tube Size (French) | Mushroom Tip (mm) | Shank (mm) | Internal Flange | Food Requires Straining | Body Weight kg |
|---|---|---|---|---|---|
| 14 | 13.0 | 4.8 | Yes | Yes | <15 |
| 16 | 13.5 | 5.6 | Yes | Yes | <15 |
| 18 | 15.0 | 6.2 | Optional | ± | <15 |
| 20 | 15.8 | 6.5 | Optional | No | <15 |
| 22 | 19.0 | 8.0 | Optional | No | >15 |

The result is a suture strand that exits the mouth at one end and the left lateral body wall at the other end. The remainder of the procedure can be performed identically to that described above (Mathews and Binnington, 1986; Bright and Burrows, 1988; Armstrong and Hardie, 1989).

## FEEDING TUBE SELECTION

Feeding tube selection will be limited to a description of the size differences in Bard urologic catheters. Though several other brands of feeding tubes are commercially available, most are either not sturdy, are much more expensive than Bard catheters, or require materials not readily available in most veterinary practices. The author's preference is No. 20-Fr.-tube size for animals less than 35 lb and 22-Fr. for those more than 35 lb. These large sizes allow the feeding of unstrained blenderized food, making owner compliance better, and decreases the incidence of clogged tubes. The size of the mushroom tips are significantly larger, allowing for placement without an internal flange (Table 2). Although I am not aware of any reported cases, there are anecdotal reports of internal flanges not passing out of the stomach of smaller animals following external traction removal of the feeding tube. This prompted the examination of the use of larger size tubes without internal flanges. The larger sizes and lack of internal flanges have not been found to result in increased complication rates relative to previous reports (Mauterer et al., 1994).

## TUBE CARE

After placement, the tube should be flushed with a small amount of water and capped with a catheter adapter[§§] and a PRN injection port.[‖‖]

The tube exit site should be observed daily for signs of redness, pain, swelling, discharge, and migration. If seen, the site should be inspected for possible subcutaneous abscess formation. Treatment of peristomial infections is to establish drainage and institute appropriate antibiotic therapy. The tube does not need to be removed in most cases.

The tube site can be cleaned daily with cotton balls soaked in warm water or hydrogen peroxide. Triple an-

tibiotic ointment[¶¶] applied to the tube site helps to keep daily cleaning and removal of any dried crusts.

Every tube should be secured in some way to prevent inadvertent removal of the tube by chewing or catching the tube on furniture, fences, and so forth. A stockinette[##] "sweater" is very useful for protecting the tube in most patients; however, there are those animals who will not tolerate it. For these patients, the tube can be secured via a Chinese finger-trap suture or a butterfly tape-tab around the tube that is sutured to the skin. Elizabethan collars can also be useful.

There should be no bulky caps or stopcocks placed on the tubes. These items tend to get caught on furniture and in cage grates, resulting in premature removal of the tube.

Cage or crate rest is highly recommended for 10 to 14 days to allow good adhesion of stomach to body wall. After this time, if premature extraction occurs, it is much less likely to result in peritonitis or to require emergency surgery.

## TUBE REMOVAL

The patient should be fasted overnight. Most patients tolerate external traction removal without sedation. The feeding tube is cut to leave 3 cm exiting the skin. The wooden end of a cotton-tipped applicator[°°°] is inserted into the feeding tube. The feeding tube is pulled firmly over the applicator and held tightly to anchor the applicator into the mushroom tip of the feeding tube. While stabilizing the skin at the tube site, firm, steady traction is applied to pull the feeding tube through the body wall. Povidone-iodine ointment[†††] is applied to the tube exit site and a light bandage is maintained for 12 hr. Feeding can resume 12 hr after removal.

## COMPLICATIONS

Complications can be classified as placement related, management related, or miscellaneous. Placement-

---

[§§]Catheter adapter, Becton-Dickinson, Rutherford, NJ, 07070.
[‖‖]PRN adapter, Deseret, Sandy, UT, 84070.

[¶¶]Triple antibiotic ointment, Schein Pharmaceutical Inc, Port Washington, NY, 11050.
[##]Synthetic tubular stockinette, Anago Inc, Fort Worth, TX, 76118.
[°°°]Puritan cotton-tipped applicator, Hardwood Products, Co, Guilford, ME, 04443.
[†††]Povidone-iodine ointment, Rugby Co, Rockville Centre, NY, 11570.

related problems include: placement in abnormal position, pneumoperitoneum, splenic laceration, gastric volume limitation, and delayed gastric emptying (Kirby et al., 1986; Mathews and Binnington, 1986; Armstrong and Hardie, 1990; Fulton and Jeffrey, 1992; Mauterer et al., 1994). The incidence of abnormal placement position can best be reduced by practicing on cadavers to become proficient at the techniques and familiar with the pertinent anatomy. Pneumoperitoneum has been largely a benign radiographic finding. Splenic laceration, though rare, can be a life-threatening complication. In one reported case, inadequate insufflation of the stomach while performing an endoscopic placement was thought to be a significant contributing factor (Armstrong and Hardie, 1990). A similar finding was observed in an ongoing trial using cadavers. Gastric volume limitation and delayed gastric emptying have both been common problems but are easily solved by altering feeding amounts or times, respectively (Armstrong and Hardie, 1990; Mauterer et al., 1994).

Management-related problems include: premature pull-out or chew-out, peritonitis, vomiting secondary to feeding too quickly or administering cold or excessive volume of liquid; and ulceration at the tube site (Mathews and Binnington, 1986; Bright and Burrows, 1988; Armstrong and Hardie, 1990; Mauterer et al., 1994). Premature removal can best be prevented by following the tube care guidelines mentioned above. Client education and compliance is critical in this regard. Vomiting due to a poor feeding protocol can be solved by feeding a room-temperature diet over 5 min at a maximum volume of 17 to 22 ml/kg. Ulceration at the tube exit site can be prevented by being careful to not tighten the external flange against the body wall.

Miscellaneous problems include: abscess or excessive granulation tissue at the tube site. Infection at the tube site is an infrequent problem, but tends to occur within 48 to 72 hr of tube placement. As previously mentioned, it is easily managed with antibiotics and drainage. Excessive granulation tissue at the tube site is a benign problem, primarily a cosmetic concern to clients and no treatment is generally required.

Percutaneous endoscopic and nonendoscopic gastrostomy tubes are useful tools for long-term nutritional support of patients with a wide variety of problems. Care must be taken in the proper selection of each patient and the route of enteral support. Gaining experience using cadavers is of great importance, especially for large-breed dogs. Also, following every detail of described procedures will help reduce procedure-related complications. Aftercare focusing on client education about feeding and tube management will always play a large part in determining the ultimate success of the nutritional support provided and should not be neglected.

## References and Suggested Reading

Abood SK and Buffington CA: Improved nasogastric intubation technique for administration of nutritional support in dogs. J Am Vet Med Assoc 199: 577, 1991.

Armstrong PJ and Hardie EM: Percutaneous endoscopic gastrostomy. Vet Med Rep 1:404, 1989.

Armstrong PJ and Hardie EM: Percutaneous endoscopic gastrostomy: A retrospective study of 54 clinical cases in dogs and cats. J Vet Intern Med 4: 202, 1990.

Bohnign RH, DeHoff WD, et al: Pharyngostomy for maintenance of the anorexic animal. J Am Vet Med Assoc 186:611, 1970.

Bright RM and Burrows CF: Percutaneous endoscopic tube gastrostomy in dogs. Am J Vet Res 49:629, 1988.

Crowe DT: Pharyngostomy complications in dogs and cats and recommended technical modifications: Experimental and clinical investigations. J Am Anim Hosp Assoc 22:493, 1986.

DiSario J, Foutch P, et al: Poor results with percutaneous endoscopic jejunostomy. Gastrointest Endosc 36(3):257, 1990.

Fulton RB and Jeffrey DS: Blind percutaneous placement of a gastrostomy tube for nutritional support in dogs and cats. J Am Vet Med Assoc 201: 697, 1992.

Kirby DF, Craig RM, et al: Percutaneous endoscopic gastrostomies: A prospective evaluation and review of the literature. JPEN 10:155, 1986.

Mathews KA and Binnington AG: Percutaneous incisionless placement of a gastrostomy tube utilizing a gastroscope: Preliminary observations. J Am Anim Hosp Assoc 22:601, 1986.

Mauterer JV, Abood SK, et al: New technique and management guidelines for percutaneous nonendoscopic tube gastrostomy. JAVMA 205:574, 1994.

Orton EC: Enteral hyperalimentation administered via needle catheter-jejunostomy as an adjunct to cranial abdominal surgery in dogs and cats. J Am Vet Med Assoc 188:1406, 1986.

Rawlings CA: Percutaneous placement of a midcervical esophagostomy tube: New technique and representative cases. J Am Anim Hosp Assoc 29:526, 1993.

Remillard R and Martin RA: Nutritional support in the surgical patient. Semin Vet Med Surg 5:197, 1990.

# BIOPSY OF THE GASTROINTESTINAL TRACT

MARK E. HITT

*Annapolis, Maryland*

The most common methods of obtaining biopsy specimens from the gastrointestinal tract (GIT) of dogs and cats include surgical, endoscopic, and "blind" approaches. This article will concentrate on the discussion of endoscopy-assisted biopsy. However, factors involved in the decision as to which method to use will be mentioned. The description of blind biopsy techniques will not be provided but can be found elsewhere (Strombeck, 1990).

## PRACTICAL CONSIDERATIONS FOR BIOPSY

It is important for the reader to be aware of the limitations of gastrointestinal biopsy techniques, both endoscopic and surgical. The author cautions against overlooking other ancillary tests including contrast radiography, fluoroscopic evaluation of motility, and serum biochemical and fecal examinations. Patient status, *time*, and costs must be considered. A common example is the unstable patient with a client who can afford endoscopy *or* surgery. In this situation, endoscopy is less invasive and taxing on the patient than surgery; however, the procedure may be almost as expensive, and surgery may still be required. So which does the veterinarian choose? In such cases, the "big picture" must be considered and all relevant and practical factors assessed.

### Surgical Biopsies

The comparative concerns entailed with a surgical approach to GIT biopsy include increased anesthetic time, and perioperative and postoperative complications (e.g., longer hospitalization, biopsy site and wound healing, risk of sepsis, low serum proteins). These are of increased concern in a debilitated animal. The advantages of surgery include access to all regions of the GIT, "full"-thickness biopsies, and therapeutic options not available to the endoscopist.

If a surgical approach is chosen, then biopsies should routinely be taken. In cases of less than clear localization, it is not uncommon for the author to request a surgeon to biopsy stomach, duodenum, jejunum, ileum, mesenteric lymph node, colon, and the liver. Unfortunately, exploratory surgeries are still performed without biopsies because the GIT "visually appeared" normal to the surgeon. This also serves as a warning to endoscopists. Visual assessment of mucosal detail is helpful, and may on occasion be pathognomonic; however, biopsies should always be taken.

Surgical protocol for suspected GIT disorders should always include careful and gentle palpation of the GIT from the cardia of the stomach to the distal rectum as it enters the pelvic canal. Visual examination of serosal surfaces should be routine. The surgeon looks for evidence of hypoxia, tumor, nonviable tissue, inflammation, and dilation of lymphatics (e.g., lymphangiectasia). The regional lymph nodes (mesenteric, sublumbar or iliac, gastric) should be examined and excisional biopsy considered if they are abnormal in size, color, or texture. Incision into suspect organs for visual examination of the lumen and full-thickness biopsy is the great comparative advantage of exploratory surgery. Wedge biopsies are normally obtained on the antimesenteric side and may only be 1 mm wide. Exception to this is when evaluation of the lymphatic vessels is desired. The organs should be exteriorized and kept moist with lap sponges. Current recommendations are for a simple interrupted pattern using monofilament, absorbable suture material. Prior to replacing the biopsied organ into the abdominal cavity, it should be lavaged with saline. Routine biopsy of the colon, when there is no suspicion of colonic involvement, is discouraged by some surgeons as an unnecessary risk to the patient due to concern for the high bacterial content of the colon and the potential development of bacterial peritonitis. The risk–benefit assessment of obtaining colonic biopsies must be discussed prior to surgery so that the opportunity is not lost. This emphasizes the need for explicit communication of the goals and expectations for the surgery. Presurgical use of oral electrolyte lavage solutions or enemas is at the discretion of the surgeon, but the use of antibiotics to "sterilize the gut" is not generally recommended.

Often overlooked at the time of surgery is the technique of fine-needle aspiration of nonbiopsied regions of the intestinal wall, tumors, and lymph nodes. The diagnosis of infiltrative neoplasia, infection, and inflammation can be made or supported by the cytologic evaluation of specimens obtained from aspiration or impression of cut surfaces of resected tissues. A 12-cc syringe and 22- to 25-gauge needle are used for this technique. Slides may be evaluated immediately following surgery and may influence therapeutic plans prior to return of the histopathology report.

The patient considerations that favor surgical as opposed to endoscopic biopsies include: suspicion of a lesion limited to a specific segment of the GIT not reachable by the endoscope, the client can only afford "one" procedure and surgical treatment is likely to be necessary, and when multiple organ systems need to be examined or biopsied.

## Endoscopic Biopsy

In comparison to surgery, endoscopy is relatively noninvasive. Endoscopy of the GIT provides a means of visually assessing the mucosal (to the lamina propria) characteristics of the target organs but not the deeper submucosal, muscular, or serosal layers. The most commonly performed procedures are esophagogastroduodenoscopy (EGD) and colonoscopy.

A veterinarian needs to think carefully about the motivation for providing endoscopy in a small practice (see "Selecting a Gastrointestinal Endoscope," this volume, p 664). Reasons for obtaining an endoscope include increased choices for patient management, an adequate caseload, enjoyment of using advanced technology, and enhanced knowledge of disease presentation. Advantages of endoscopy for debilitated patients include: the probability of reduced anesthetic time, lessened concern for hypoalbuminemia, reduced incidence of postprocedural complications, reduced patient discomfort, and the elimination of incision management. Percutaneous endoscopically guided feeding tubes can be placed accurately. Complications of pinch biopsies and endoscopy are rare. However, perforation of a diseased organ is possible. Following the procedure, the insufflated organs must be relieved by endoscopic suction and gentle external pressure on the abdomen.

Endoscopy is unable to evaluate the entire length of the intestines. In addition, the technique is limited by the experience of the operator, the luminal conditions present (tumors, GIT contents, bleeding, hypertrophy), and the size of the animal in comparison to the dimensions of the endoscope (e.g., length of the scope versus length of the patient's GIT). Another major consideration is the concept of local (or regional) versus diffuse disease. It is possible for a disorder (i.e., cancer, foreign body, inflammation) to be distant to the area that is visualized. Commonly associated costs include intravenous catheterization, preprocedure enemas and laxatives, preanesthetic evaluation, operator time, anesthesia, and laboratory fees (culture, biopsy, and cytology). Additional costs to the veterinarian include depreciation on the equipment and skilled technical time involved with the preparation and postprocedural care of the endoscope.

### ANESTHETIC CONSIDERATIONS

Veterinarians are familiar with monitoring a patient during surgical anesthesia, and the same considerations need to be given to the endoscopic patient. General anesthesia is highly preferred for endoscopy of the GIT. This is for the patient's comfort and protection of the endoscope. An oral speculum is *always* used with the

endoscope for upper GI procedures and a digital rectal examination is performed prior to each colonoscopy. This prevents accidental damage to the endoscope from teeth or unforeseen rectal debris, respectively. Because endoscopy is often viewed as "high-tech" and novel, attention of staff and operator may be diverted from monitoring of the patient.

The effect of endoscopic insufflation on the anesthetized patient is thought to be a minor concern. However, extrapolation of information from studies of canine gastric dilation and laparoscopic insufflation of the abdomen can be useful. This information reports that intragastric and intra-abdominal pressures above 30 cm $H_2O$ begin to compromise respiration and return of venous blood flow from the abdomen to the heart. With reasonable care, these pressures are not attained with endoscopy.

Problems of abdominal discomfort are commonly reported by humans during insufflation and endoscopic maneuvering. Insufflation should be relieved by suction at the completion of the procedure. An overinsufflated organ results in more difficult maneuvering (especially the pylorus) and evaluation of mucosal detail. Recent information and the author's experience do not support any specific preanesthetic protocol (atropine, glycopyrrolate, diazepam) as superior for endoscopy of the GIT. Therefore preanesthetic and anesthetic protocols should be based upon the patient status.

### PATIENT PREPARATION

The preparation of the patient for esophagoscopy, gastroscopy, and duodenoscopy is simple. No food is offered for 12 to 24 hr and no water is allowed for 6 to 12 hr prior to the procedure. For colonoscopy, the preparation is more involved and varies among endoscopists. If consistent with patient status, no food should be offered for 36 to 48 hr prior to the procedure. Rectocolic enemas using copious amounts of warm water, or saline (0.9%), are essential. These must be done gently, without irritating substances, in order to prevent artifactual lesions. The author's preference is to perform enemas 24, 6, and 2 hr before the colonoscopy. However, two enemas are usually satisfactory. Oral electrolyte lavage solutions (Golytely, Braintree Laboratories), used twice the day before, are helpful if enough volume is administered. The dosage for these is approximately 22 ml/kg of body weight administered per os or by stomach tube. Bisacodyl and magnesium citrate are of questionable benefit, in the opinion of the author.

The patient is positioned in left lateral recumbency for EGD and colonoscopy. This is advantageous because the entry from the pylorus to the duodenum and descending to transverse colon will be upward deflections of the scope. Upward is the greatest deflection of most GI endoscopes. The residual fluids in the lumens also flow away from the target areas by gravity. If difficulty is encountered, then adjusting the patient to sternal or right lateral positions may be helpful. A well-prepared patient normally may not require the use of the endoscope's suction capability. If fluids remain, then suction is very helpful, but clogging of the suction channels is common with colonoscopy and may require removal of the endoscope from the patient for cleansing. It is best to spend more time on preparation of the patient than on cleaning the endoscope during a procedure.

The first purchase that an interested veterinarian should make is a current textbook on endoscopy (Tamms, 1990). The novice endoscopist should expect a learning curve of several months, dependent upon the frequency with which procedures are performed. Despite the desires of most veterinary associates, one or two should be selected to be the "endoscopists." This increases the level of expertise more rapidly and reduces accidental damage to the endoscopic equipment. A short course on endoscopy is advised. It is the author's experience that no matter what your experience level, some cases will be difficult and some cases will be easy, but few will be predictable.

## Specimen Collection and Diagnosis

There are many accessories which are useful for endoscopy of the GIT (see "Selecting a Gastrointestinal Endoscope," this volume, p 664). Specimens for histopathology, cytology, culture, and immunodiagnostic testing (e.g., *Giardia* enzyme-linked immunosorbent assay [ELISA] test, canine parvovirus HA test) can be obtained. Specimens should be collected from all relevant areas of the GIT that are reached. The combinations of these procedures are left to the endoscopist's decision.

### PATHOLOGIST'S ROLE

A detailed clinical history should be provided to the selected pathologist or cytologist. Close communication concerning the clinician's concerns and differential diagnosis does make a difference. The endoscopist should be more concerned with the cytologic description and microscopic diagnosis than with the pathologist's comments. Their comments are based upon the signalment, your clinical history, their biases, and their findings. Inadequate microscopic description in a report can lead the clinician towards over- and underinterpretation and misdiagnosis. An excellent example is the discussions surrounding normal and abnormal numbers of lymphocytes in lymphocytic-plasmacytic inflammatory bowel disease (Jergens, 1992). A histopathologic interpretation of a biopsy specimen may not yield a diagnosis; however, it is rare that it does not provide useful information to the clinician for formulation of further diagnostic and therapeutic plans. The comments useful in a report are: quality of specimen, presence of artifacts, depth (mucosa, lamina propria, submucosa), microvillus height or crypt depth, presence of cellular infiltrates, increases or decreases (hyperplasia, hypoplasia, atrophy) in normal cell populations, inflammation and fibrosis, presence of organisms,

appearance of lymphatic and vascular components, and overall assessment.

### GIT MUCOSAL ASSESSMENT

Endoscopists should complete an endoscopy report for each procedure as part of the medical record. This should include the appearance of all organs traversed as well as the anatomic site and size of any abnormalities. The normal mucosal appearance varies with the organ being evaluated. The esophageal mucosa is pale white to pink, with a moist glistening appearance. Gastric mucosa has slightly more texture and a pink appearance. The fundic area is highlighted by rugal folds, which are distensible. With normal insufflation and mucosal thickness, the submucosal blood vessels can be seen. The antrum often is slightly paler and the rugal folds disappear as the pylorus is approached. The mucosa of the duodenum has a distinctive velvety to "sugar" granular surface due to the microvilli. It is pale pink to reddish normally, but the presence of bile can add a yellowish hue. The Peyer's patches (lymphoid aggregates) may be seen as oval depressions. They should not be biopsied unless they appear abnormal because of confusion with lymphoid inflammatory conditions. The duodenal papillae can be identified on occasion and should not be biopsied routinely. Colonic mucosa is pale pink and moist. Mucus is present in variable amounts dependent upon the irritation due to the procedure or preparation as well as preexisting pathology. In the colon, the presence of submucosal blood vessels is noted with moderate insufflation. The rectum may be more red or be similar to the colon except for the presence of folds of mucosa. The ability of the organs to be distended by insufflation should also be noted, since this can be a clue to intramural or extraluminal disorders.

There is no standardized terminology for abnormal appearances of the mucosa of the GIT. However, some terms are commonly used. The presence of intraluminal mass lesions are noted as sessile or pedunculated. The terms proposed to describe abnormalities of the mucosal surface (Jergens, 1993) are *erythema* (redness), *friability* (ease of damage or tearing), *granularity* (surface texture), *ulcer* (focal, deep crateriform), and *erosion* (irregular surface irritations). If the mucosa appears normal to the endoscopist, then this should be stated. The microscopic description should also include normal patterns and cellular descriptions. Abnormal pathologic results are reviewed concisely in the references (Wilcox, 1992).

### BRUSH CYTOLOGY

Cytologic brushes are used to collect cells from a relatively large surface area of visualized mucosa. The technique should be vigorous. The slides are then prepared by rolling or rubbing the brush on precleaned microscope slides and air drying. These can be examined for evidence of inflammation, neoplasia, and infectious agents. Brush cytology has the disadvantage of being only from the surface of the mucosa. However, its advantages are rapid availability of results and ability to cover a larger surface area than pinch biopsies. Brush cytology should be used in conjunction with pinch biopsies.

### ENDOSCOPIC LAVAGE

Lavage of the organ's lumen, usually the duodenum, with normal saline can be useful for qualitatively identifying bacterial pathogens and overgrowths, and occasionally for diagnosis of *Giardia* by direct microscopic and ELISA tests. This should be performed through a sterilized endoscopic catheter or adapted Silastic tubing. Since the accessory channel does not remain sterile, the clinician's judgment of the relevance of culture results is subjective. The author usually performs the lavage after brushing the duodenal mucosa in order to enhance the collection of debris.

### ENDOSCOPIC PINCH BIOPSY

Pinch biopsy forceps provide the most consistent means of obtaining representative specimens via the endoscope. Specimens of the mucosal epithelium and lamina propria are obtainable. Biopsy forceps can be serrated or smooth, standard or fenestrated, and with or without a needle. The author commonly uses smooth standard forceps for friable proliferative lesions and for the normal duodenal and colonic mucosa. Esophageal and gastric biopsies are somewhat more difficult because of the greater tendency of the instrument to slide along their lumens and the tougher nature of the mucosa in these locations. Here the author uses the serrated (or alligator) with needle style of forceps. Decreasing the level of insufflation and approaching the mucosa from 90 degrees helps improve the quality of the specimens. Whether anticipating a foreign body removal or gastric carcinoma, the endoscopist should always be prepared to perform biopsies at the time of endoscopy. It is recommended to biopsy each organ no matter what its visual appearance. However, this caveat excludes the esophagus unless gross lesions or clinical signs are suggestive of esophageal disease. Correlation between visual reported lesions and histopathologic descriptions is approximately 50 to 80% as reported in

veterinary and human medicine. This covers all levels of endoscopic expertise. The author routinely obtains four to six biopsies from each of the stomach and duodenum, or colon. These are gathered from several locations. If there is a specific visual lesion, then additional biopsies are taken. The standard recommendation is to biopsy the center, margin, and normal surrounding areas of a lesion. The desire to gather specimens from below the surface in the lesion is often frustrated. The repetitive biopsy of one site (hole-in-hole) with the goal of "digging" into the lesion is not proven effective, though it is commonly attempted, for suspected deep neoplastic lesions with superficial inflammation. Experimentally, the use of an endoscopic diathermy (hot electrocautery) snare, to shave off the surface of the lesion and then pinch biopsy the deeper area, has been successful at reaching the submucosal layers. This would enhance the ability to diagnose submucosal or intramural lesions of the GIT. The biopsies are gently teased from the biopsy forceps and placed on foam pads and then enclosed in plastic tissue cassettes (histopathology supplies). These are labeled and placed in 10% buffered formalin. Specimens from proliferative or inflamed lesions can be used to make touch imprints for cytologic evaluation, but these specimens are then sacrificed, since artifactual distortion may occur.

## References and Suggested Reading

Jergens AE, Moore FM, Haynes JS, and Miles KG: Idiopathic inflammatory bowel disease in dogs and cats: 84 cases (1987–1990). J Am Vet Med Assoc 201:1603, 1992.
  *A current update on the microscopic description and histopathologic appearance of the most common diagnosis from endoscopic biopsies.*
Jergens AE: Endoscopic examination of the gastrointestinal tract. *Proc 11th ACVIM Forum*, 1993, p 896.
  *A concise description of terminology describing the appearance of the mucosa.*
Strombeck DR and Guilford WG: *Small Animal Gastroenterology.* Davis, CA; Stonegate Publishing Company, 1990, p 113.
  *Chapter 6 provides a concise overview of blind biopsy techniques, equipment, and ancillary tests of the GIT.*
Tams TR: *Small Animal Endoscopy.* Philadelphia; CV Mosby, 1990.
  *This book is an excellent source of information on all aspects of endoscopic equipment, procedures, and biopsy of the GIT.*
Wilcox B: Endoscopic biopsy interpretation in canine or feline enterocolitis. Semin Vet Med Surg 7:162, 1992.
  *A review of histopathologic terminology and interpretation from the perspective of the pathologist.*

# ANTIEMETIC THERAPY

ROBERT J. WASHABAU
*and* MARC S. ELIE
*Philadelphia, Pennsylvania*

Emesis, or vomiting, is a complex reflex pathway that has evolved in some animal species, particularly the dog and cat, to protect the animal from ingested toxins. While undoubtedly protective, emesis is medically important because of the large number of conditions that may cause or be associated with it. Emesis may occur with such diverse conditions as motion sickness, intestinal obstruction, gastroenteritis, diabetic ketoacidosis, pregnancy, thyrotoxicosis, adrenocortical insufficiency, and uremia. Aspiration pneumonia, fluid and electrolyte depletion, and acid-base disturbances are all potentially serious consequences of vomiting. Under ideal circumstances, definitive diagnosis of a vomiting disorder is established (e.g., gastritis) and specific therapy is initiated. This may not be possible in all circumstances, however. Knowledge of the neuroanatomic pathways as well as the neurotransmitter-receptor systems will facilitate a rational approach to the therapy of emesis in these cases.

## PHYSIOLOGY OF EMESIS

The essential components of the emetic reflex are visceral receptors; vagal and sympathetic afferent neurons; a chemoreceptor trigger zone (CRTZ) located within the area postrema that is sensitive to blood-borne substances; and an emetic center within the re- ticular formation of the medulla oblongata receiving input from vagal and sympathetic neurons, CRTZ, vestibular apparatus, and cerebral cortex (Fig. 1). The current textbook understanding of the physiology of emesis is dominated by concepts elaborated in the early 1950s (Borison and Wang, 1953). A particularly important concept in this model is that vomiting occurs either through activation of the CRTZ by blood-borne substances (*humoral pathway*), or through activation of the emetic center by vagosympathetic, CRTZ, vestibular, or cerebrocortical neurons (*neural pathway*). Thus, activation of the CRTZ by a variety of humoral emetogenic substances (e.g., uremic toxins, cardiac glycosides, endotoxins, and apomorphine) is abolished by surgical ablation of the area postrema, but not by vagotomy or sympathectomy. In contrast, neural activation of the emetic center by gastric disease (e.g., gastritis, intragastric copper sulfate) is abolished by vagotomy or sympathectomy, but not by ablation of the area postrema. Many experimental data have been readily explained by this two-component model.

The model is not without challenge, however, and it has been suggested that there are parallel mechanisms for the initiation of emesis in response to any stimulus, and it is the sum of these inputs that drives the emetic response (Harding, 1990). In other words, emesis need not be simply an either/or response. The concept of a discrete emetic center has also been seriously chal-

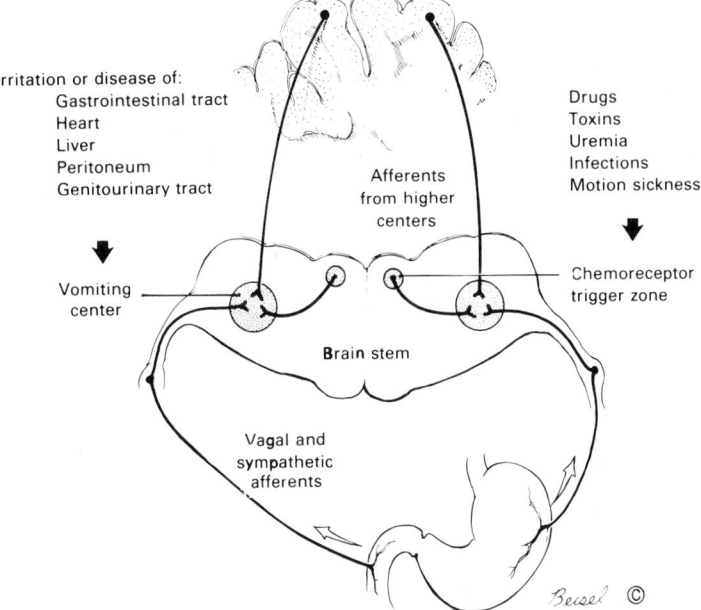

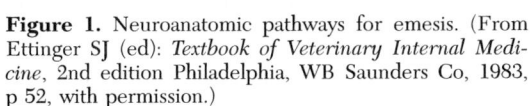

**Figure 1.** Neuroanatomic pathways for emesis. (From Ettinger SJ (ed): *Textbook of Veterinary Internal Medicine*, 2nd edition Philadelphia, WB Saunders Co, 1983, p 52, with permission.)

lenged. Based on more recent electrophysiologic studies, a model of sequential activation of a series of effector nuclei has been proposed that doesn't require a discrete emetic center (Harding, 1990). Despite contemporary reexamination, there still is good agreement on two general patterns of emesis, one humoral and the other neural. Current antiemetic therapy is largely based on these assumptions.

## PHARMACOLOGY OF EMESIS

Most pharmacologic approaches to antiemetic therapy have been based on neurotransmitter-receptor interactions at the CRTZ, emphasizing the humoral pathway of emesis. The neural pathway has received much less emphasis (Table 1).

### Chemoreceptor Trigger Zone

Neurochemical studies in dogs and cats have demonstrated the presence of several neurotransmitters: dopamine, norepinephrine, 5-hydroxytryptamine (5-HT, serotonin), acetylcholine, histamine, and enkephalins; their respective receptors or binding sites: $D_2$-dopaminergic, $\alpha_2$-adrenergic, $5\text{-HT}_3$–serotonergic, $M_1$-cholinergic, $H_1$- and $H_2$-histaminergic, and $ENK_\mu$- and $ENK_\delta$-enkephalinergic; and their respective synthetic or degradative enzymes: DOPA decarboxylase, dopamine $\beta$-hydroxylase, 5-hydroxytryptophan decarboxylase, choline acetyltransferase, histidine decarboxylase, and enkephalinase (Beleslin, 1992). Some neurotransmitter-receptor systems are probably more important than others. For example, apomorphine, a $D_2$-dopamine receptor agonist, is a potent emetic agent in the dog but not the cat (King, 1990) (Fig. 2). This finding has two important implications: (1) that CRTZ $D_2$-dopamine receptors are not so important in mediating humoral emesis in the cat, and (2) that $D_2$-dopamine receptor antagonists (e.g., metoclopramide)

might not be as useful as other antiemetic agents in the cat. On the other hand, xylazine, an $\alpha_2$-adrenergic agonist, is a more potent emetic agent in the cat than in the dog (King, 1990; Lang and Sarna, 1992). The latter finding suggests that $\alpha_2$-adrenergic antagonists might be more useful antiemetic agents than $D_2$-dopamine antagonists in the cat. Cancer chemotherapy (e.g., cisplatinum) –induced-emesis is mediated by activation of $5\text{-HT}_3$ receptors in the CRTZ of the cat (Beleslin, 1992) while visceral and vagal afferent $5\text{-HT}_3$ receptors are activated in the dog (Fukui, Yamamoto, and Sato, 1992). Antagonists of the $5\text{-HT}_3$ receptor are efficacious in the prevention of emesis associated with cisplatinum chemotherapy in dogs (Tucker et al., 1989). Similar information is not yet available in the cat. Finally, histamine and $H_1$- and $H_2$-histaminergic receptors have been demonstrated in the CRTZ of the dog, but not the cat. Histamine is a potent emetic agent in the dog but cats seem resistant to its emetic effects (King, 1990; Beleslin, 1992).

### Emetic Center

At the present time, the $5\text{-HT}_{1A}$ and $\alpha_2$-adrenergic receptors are the only documented receptors involved in the regulation of emesis at the level of the emetic center. It has recently been shown that agonists of the $5\text{-HT}_{1A}$ receptor (e.g., flesinoxan, 8-OH-DPAT, buspirone) suppress emesis associated with motion sickness in cats (Lucot, 1992). These drugs have not been approved for use in the cat, however. The $\alpha_2$-adrenergic receptor, on the other hand, may be antagonized with currently available antiemetic drugs. The emetic center $\alpha_2$-receptor, as well as the CRTZ $\alpha_2$-receptor, may be antagonized by a pure $\alpha_2$-antagonist (e.g., yohimbine) or by mixed $\alpha_1/\alpha_2$-antagonists (e.g. prochlorperazine and chlorpromazine) (Lang and Sarna, 1992). It is likely, however, that most of the antiemetic effect of the $\alpha$-receptor antagonists results from antagonism of the CRTZ $\alpha_2$-adrenergic receptor.

**Table 1.** *Receptors and Neurotransmitters Subserving Emesis in the Dog and/or Cat Only*

| | Neurotransmitter | Receptor |
|---|---|---|
| Emetic center | Norepinephrine | $\alpha_2$-Adrenergic |
| | 5-Hydroxytryptamine | $5\text{-HT}_{1A}$–Serotonergic |
| CRTZ | Dopamine | $D_2$-Dopaminergic |
| | 5-Hydroxytryptamine | $5\text{-HT}_3$–Serotonergic |
| | Acetylcholine | $M_1$-Cholinergic |
| | Histamine | $H_1$- and $H_2$-Histaminergic |
| | Norepinephrine | $\alpha_2$-Adrenergic |
| | *met*-, *leu*-enkephalin | $ENK_{\mu,\delta}$-Enkephalinergic |
| Vestibular apparatus | Acetylcholine | $M_1$-Muscarinic |
| Cerebrum | Enkephalin, endorphin | $ENK_\mu$-Enkephalinergic |
| | Endogenous benzodiazepine? | $\omega_2$/$GABA_A$/chloride channel complex |
| Gut afferents | 5-Hydroxytryptamine | $5\text{-HT}_3$–Serotonergic |
| Gut efferents | Dopamine | $D_2$-Dopaminergic |
| | Acetylcholine | $M_2$-Cholinergic |
| | 5-Hydroxytryptamine | $5\text{-HT}_4$–Serotonergic |
| | Motilin (GI hormone) | Motilin |

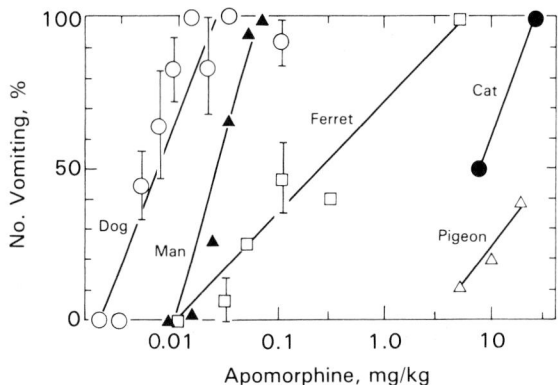

**Figure 2.** Species differences in emetic sensitivity to intravenous apomorphine. (From King GL: Can J Physiol Pharmacol 68: 262, 1990. National Research Council of Canada, Ottawa, Ontario, with permission.)

## Vestibular Apparatus

Muscarinic $M_1$-receptors and acetylcholine have been demonstrated in the vestibular apparatus of the dog and cat. Mixed $M_1/M_2$-antagonists (e.g. atropine and scopolamine) and pure $M_1$-antagonists (e.g., pirenzepine) inhibit motion sickness in both the dog and cat. It is not clear, however, whether the antiemetic effect of these drugs is due solely to $M_1$-receptor antagonism at the vestibular apparatus. Other sites (e.g., cerebral cortex, reticular formation, area postrema) of antagonism are possible (Beleslin, 1992).

## Cerebral Cortex

Opioids (e.g., cannabinoids and nabilone) and benzodiazepines (e.g., diazepam, lorazepam) have been used to reduce anticipatory nausea and vomiting in humans undergoing cytotoxic drug therapy. Cerebrocortical opioid and benzodiazepine receptors have been implicated but have not been very well characterized pharmacologically. These receptors will likely be of minor significance in the pathogenesis of most vomiting disorders in the dog and cat.

## Gut Afferents

There are a number of different mechanisms by which stimuli arising from the gastrointestinal tract cause emesis. For example, ingested toxins, cell degeneration or necrosis, inflammation, luminal distention, chemotherapy, and radiation therapy all induce emesis. Of the many receptors found in the gastrointestinal tract, 5-$HT_3$ receptors likely play an important role in the initiation of emesis (Beleslin, 1992). It is now well established that cytotoxic drugs cause 5-HT release from enterochromaffin cells in the gastrointestinal tract which then activates 5-$HT_3$ receptors on afferent vagal fibers (Fukui, Yamamoto, and Sato, 1992). The vomiting induced by 5-HT release and 5-$HT_3$–receptor ac-

tivation is completely abolished by pretreatment with 5-$HT_3$ antagonists (e.g., ondansetron, granisetron, and tropisetron) (Tucker et al., 1989). Metoclopramide is an antagonist of 5-$HT_3$ receptors also but does not seem to be very effective in preventing chemotherapy-induced emesis. It remains to be determined whether other gastrointestinal tract pathologies are associated with 5-HT release and 5-$HT_3$–receptor activation.

## Gut Efferents

Vagal efferent and myenteric neurons initiate the complex excitation and inhibition of visceral smooth muscle that culminates in emesis. A number of receptors have been identified on myenteric neurons and gastrointestinal smooth muscle cells that regulate gastric emptying and/or intestinal transit. These include $D_2$-dopaminergic, 5-$HT_4$–serotonergic, $M_2$-cholinergic, and motilin receptors. The ability of metoclopramide to facilitate gastric emptying in dogs and cats is thought to involve antagonism at peripheral $D_2$-dopamine receptors, although enhanced cholinergic activity may also be involved. 5-$HT_3$ antagonists also facilitate gastric emptying, but this probably occurs through activation of a neuronal 5-$HT_4$ receptor, instead of antagonism of a 5-$HT_3$ receptor. Cisapride, a substituted benzamide like metoclopramide, facilitates gastric emptying in the dog by this mechanism (Gullikson, Loeffler, and Viriña, 1992). Gastric emptying is also regulated by motilin, a hormone that is released episodically from gastrointestinal endocrine cells. Motilin initiates phase III of the migrating myoelectric complex and facilitates gastric emptying during the fasting state. Low doses of erythromycin (0.5 to 1.0 mg/kg every 8 hr PO, IV) have been shown to stimulate motilin release and facilitate gastric emptying in the dog (Itoh, 1984).

## ANTIEMETIC CLASSIFICATIONS

A number of antiemetic drugs have been formulated based on the aforementioned neurotransmitter-receptor systems. These drugs may be classified as: $\alpha_2$-adrenergic antagonists, $D_2$-dopaminergic antagonists, $H_1$- and $H_2$-histaminergic antagonists, $M_1$-muscarinic cholinergic antagonists, 5-$HT_3$-serotonergic antagonists, 5-$HT_4$-serotonergic agonists, and motilin agonists (see Table 2). Several important points should be made about these classifications.

1. *Some drugs have several mechanisms of antiemesis.* Metoclopramide antagonizes $D_2$-dopaminergic and 5-$HT_3$-serotonergic receptors, and has a peripheral cholinergic effect. The antiemetic properties of metoclopramide may be related to 5-$HT_3$-receptor antagonism, instead of $D_2$-receptor antagonism (King, 1990; Gullikson, Loeffler, and Viriña, 1992). The phenothiazines (e.g., chlorpromazine and prochlorperazine) are antagonists of $\alpha_1$- and $\alpha_2$-adrenergic, $D_2$-dopaminergic, $H_1$- and $H_2$-histaminergic, and muscarinic cholinergic

***Table 2.*** *Antiemetic Classifications*

| Classification | Examples | Anatomic Site(s) of Actions | Dosage | Side Effects |
|---|---|---|---|---|
| $\alpha_2$-Adrenergic antagonists | Prochlorperazine° (Compazine, SmithKline) | CRTZ, emetic center | 0.5 mg/kg q8h SC, IM | Hypotension, sedation |
| | Chlorpromazine° (Thorazine, SmithKline) | CRTZ, emetic center | 0.2–0.4 mg/kg q8h SC | Hypotension, sedation |
| | Yohimbine (Yobine, Lloyd Labs) | CRTZ, emetic center | 0.25–0.5 mg/kg q12h SC, IM | Hypotension, sedation |
| $D_2$-Dopaminergic antagonists | Metoclopramide°″ (Reglan, Robins) | CRTZ, GI smooth muscle | 0.2–0.4 mg/kg q6h PO, SC, IM; or 1–2 mg/kg/day continuous IV infusion | Extrapyramidal signs |
| | Trimethobenzamide°§ (Tigan, Beecham) | CRTZ | 3 mg/kg q8–12h IM | Allergic reactions |
| | Domperidone°† Motilium, Janssen) | GI smooth muscle | 0.1–0.3 mg/kg q12h IM, IV | None reported |
| | Haloperidol° (Haldol, McNeil) | CRTZ | 0.02 mg/kg q12h PO | Sedation |
| | Chlorpromazine° Prochlorperazine° | | | |
| $H_1$-Histaminergic antagonists | Diphenhydramine° (Benadryl, ParkeDavis) | CRTZ | 2–4 mg/kg q8h PO, IM | Sedation |
| | Dimenhydrinate° (Dramamine, Searle) | CRTZ | 4–8 mg/kg q8h PO | Sedation |
| | Chlorpromazine° Prochlorperazine° | | | |
| $M_1$-Cholinergic antagonists | Scopolamine°§ (Hyoscine, Fujisawa) | Vestibular apparatus, CRTZ, other sites? | 0.03 mg/kg q6h SC, IM | Sedation, xerostomia, ileus |
| | Pirenzepine°§† | Vestibular apparatus, CRTZ, other sites? | | |
| | Chlorpromazine° Prochlorperazine° | | | |
| 5-HT₃–Serotonergic antagonists | Ondansetron°† (Zofran, Glaxo) | CRTZ, vagal afferent neurons | 0.5–1.0 mg/kg q12–24h PO, or 0.5–1.0 mg/kg PO 30 min before chemotherapy | Sedation, lip licking, head shaking |
| | Metoclopramide°″ | | | |
| 5-HT₄–Serotonergic agonists | Cisapride°† (Propulsid, Janssen) | Myenteric neurons | 0.1–0.5 mg/kg q8h PO | None reported |
| Motilin agonists | Erythromycin° (Erythrocin, Abbott) | GI smooth muscle | 0.5–1.0 mg/kg q8h PO, IV | Vomiting at microbially effective doses (15 mg/kg q8h) |

°Not approved for use in the dog or cat.
†No dosage information available for the cat.
‡Not available in the United States.
§To be used in dogs only.
″To be used in the cat with caution.
Abbreviations: CRTZ = chemoreceptor trigger zone, GI = gastrointestinal.

receptors (King, 1990). Thus, it may be difficult to discern the exact locus of a drugs antiemetic effect.

2. *Some drugs are nonselective with regard to receptor subtype.* Scopolamine, for example, is a useful antiemetic in the therapy of motion sickness because it crosses the blood-brain barrier and antagonizes $M_1$-cholinergic receptors involved in the pathogenesis of motion sickness. However, scopolamine is a mixed cholinergic receptor antagonist that also binds $M_2$- and $M_3$-cholinergic receptors. Antagonism of gastrointestinal smooth muscle $M_2$-cholinergic receptors may result in delayed gastric emptying and ileus. This is especially true of atropine, aminopentamide (Centrine, Fort Dodge), and isopropamide (Darbid, SmithKline), which is the reason that these drugs are usually contraindicated in the therapy of vomiting disorders. Pirenzepine, a highly selective $M_1$-cholinergic antagonist, is not yet available in the United States.

3. *The mechanism of action of some antiemetics is not even known.* Trimethobenzamide is a substituted benzamide, like metoclopramide, with $D_2$-dopaminergic antagonistic properties. Yet, the antiemetic ef-

fects of trimethobenzamide are not easily explained by $D_2$-dopaminergic antagonism. The antiemetic mechanism(s) of high doses of corticosteroids is also unknown, although inhibition of prostaglandin metabolism is suspected.

4. *Most of these drugs have not been approved for use in the dog or cat.* Of the 14 antiemetic drugs listed in Table 2, only yohimbine (an $\alpha_2$-adrenergic antagonist) has been approved for use in the dog and cat (see "Unapproved Use of Drugs in Small Animals," this volume, p 48).

## RATIONAL CLINICAL USE OF ANTIEMETICS

### Antiemetic Strategies for the Diagnosed Patient

#### MOTION SICKNESS

The neuronal pathways for motion sickness are still incompletely characterized, but motion sickness is believed to arise from stimulation of labyrinthine structures in the inner ear. The chemoreceptor trigger zone is involved in this pathway in the dog, but it is not involved in the cat (Borison and Borison, 1986). $M_1$-cholinergic and $H_1$-histaminergic receptors apparently mediate the emetic response associated with motion sickness because antagonists of these receptors are very effective antiemetic agents. $\alpha_2$-adrenergic, $D_2$-dopaminergic, and $5-HT_3$-serotonergic receptors are not involved in the mediation of this emetic response. Motion sickness in the dog may be treated with $H_1$-histaminergic antagonists (e.g., diphenhydramine, dimenhydrinate) or $M_1$-cholinergic antagonists (e.g., scopolamine, pirenzepine). Motion sickness in the cat, on the other hand, is probably best treated with chlorpromazine instead of a pure $H_1$-histaminergic antagonist. Histamine receptors have not been demonstrated in the CRTZ of the cat, nor is the cat very sensitive to the emetic effects of histamine (King, 1990; Beleslin, 1992).

#### UREMIA

Vomiting associated with uremia has both central and peripheral components. The central component of uremic vomiting is associated with activation of CRTZ $D_2$-dopaminergic receptors by circulating uremic toxins. Other CRTZ receptors (e.g., $\alpha_2$, $5-HT_3$, $M_1$, $H_1$) are apparently not involved in this emetic response. The central component is best treated with a $D_2$-dopaminergic antagonist (e.g., metoclopramide). The peripheral component of uremic vomiting is associated with uremic gastritis and is best treated with $H_2$-histaminergic antagonists (e.g., cimetidine 5 to 10 mg/kg every 8 hr IV) to diminish gastric parietal cell $H^+$ ion secretion, and with sucralfate (0.5 to 1.0 gm every 8 hr

PO for dogs, 0.25 to 0.5 gm every 8 to 12 hr PO for cats) to provide a barrier to $H^+$ ion back-diffusion.

#### CANCER CHEMOTHERAPY

Certain cancer chemotherapies (e.g., cisplatinum, cyclophosphamide) are associated with a high incidence of vomiting. Chemotherapy-induced emesis is mediated by $5-HT_3$-serotonergic receptors, either in the CRTZ (cat) or in vagal afferent neurons (dog). Other receptors are apparently not involved in this response. Antagonists of the $5-HT_3$-serotonergic receptor (e.g., ondansetron, granisetron, tropisetron) abolish the vomiting associated with cisplatinum administration in the dog (Tucker et al., 1989). We currently medicate our canine cancer patients with ondansetron, 0.5 to 1.0 mg/kg PO 30 min before and 90 min after commencing cisplatinum chemotherapy. Although metoclopramide has some $5-HT_3$ antagonistic properties, it has not proved very useful in chemotherapy-induced emesis.

#### DELAYED GASTRIC EMPTYING

Disorders of delayed gastric emptying (e.g., gastritis, metabolic derangements, postoperative gastric dilatation, and volvulus) may cause an animal to experience nausea and vomiting. Treatment of these disorders with cholinomimetic agents in the past was associated with untoward side effects. Contemporary therapy consists of $5-HT_4$ serotonergic agonists, $D_2$-dopaminergic antagonists and motilin agonists. Cisapride, a $5-HT_4$-prokinetic agent facilitates gastric emptying in dogs and cats affected with disorders of delayed gastric emptying (Gullikson, Loeffler, and Viriña, 1992). Metoclopramide facilitates gastric emptying in the dog and cat either through peripheral $D_2$-dopaminergic antagonism or through cholinergic sensitization. Dogs may subsequently be treated with low doses of erythromycin (0.5 to 1.0 mg/kg every 8 hr PO or IV) if they fail to respond to metoclopramide. Erythromycin stimulates motilin release in the dog, which then initiates phase III of the migrating myoelectric complex (Itoh, 1984). It is not known whether erythromycin has similar beneficial effects in the cat.

### Antiemetic Strategies for the Undiagnosed Patient

Antiemetic therapy in an undiagnosed patient may be appropriate when one or more of the following criteria has been satisfied: (1) the vomiting is frequent or severe enough to make the animal feel uncomfortable, (2) persistent vomiting places the animal at risk for aspiration pneumonia or acid-base and electrolyte disturbances, (3) the animal is not suffering from gastrointestinal obstruction or toxicity, or (4) the client does not desire a definitive diagnosis. When these criteria have been met, a systematic approach to antiemesis should be followed (Fig. 3). It should be emphasized that the mechanisms of emesis involved in gastrointes-

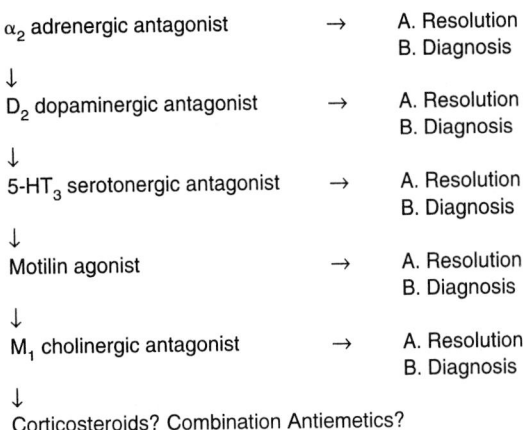

α₂ adrenergic antagonist → A. Resolution
B. Diagnosis

↓

$D_2$ dopaminergic antagonist → A. Resolution
B. Diagnosis

↓

5-HT₃ serotonergic antagonist → A. Resolution
B. Diagnosis

↓

Motilin agonist → A. Resolution
B. Diagnosis

↓

M₁ cholinergic antagonist → A. Resolution
B. Diagnosis

↓

Corticosteroids? Combination Antiemetics?

**Figure 3.** Antiemetic strategies for the undiagnosed vomiting patient.

tinal tract pathologies are poorly understood. The mechanisms likely involve a neural pathway instead of a humoral pathway, and perhaps the participation of a vagal 5-HT₃ receptor. Little else is known. The algorithm proposed in Figure 3 is based on antiemetic efficacies determined from experimental studies in dogs and cats. α₂-adrenergic antagonists are used first because of their established efficacy as potent antiemetic agents, followed sequentially by D₂-dopaminergic antagonists, 5-HT₃-serotonergic antagonists, motilin agonists, and M₁-cholinergic antagonists, depending upon the animals response. Corticosteroids and combination antiemetic therapy could be considered if the animal fails to respond to any of the other antiemetic therapies.

## IRRATIONAL USE OF ANTIEMETICS

Antiemetics may be inappropriate in any or all of the following situations:

1. *Gastrointestinal infection*: antiemetics may prolong gastrointestinal infections, particularly bacterial infections.

2. *Gastrointestinal obstruction*: some antiemetics have peripheral gastric prokinetic effects which, if used, could cause perforation.

3. *Gastrointestinal toxicity*: antiemetics used in this circumstance could prevent the animal from eliminating the toxin.

4. *Systemic hypotension*: the phenothiazines and other α₂-antagonists could worsen hypotension.

5. *Epilepsy*: phenothiazines tend to lower the threshold for seizure activity.

## References and Suggested Reading

Beleslin DB: Neurotransmitter receptor subtypes related to vomiting. *In* Bianchi AL (ed): *Mechanisms and Control of Emesis.* Paris, Inserm, 1992, p 11.
*A review of the neurotransmitters and receptor subtypes involved in emesis.*
Borison HL and Wang SC: Physiology and pharmacology of vomiting. Pharmacol Rev 5:193, 1953.
*A review of pivotal work done in the early 1950s to determine the general mechanisms of emesis in the dog and cat.*
Borison HL and Borison R: Motion sickness reflex arc bypasses the area postrema in cats. Exp Neurol 92:723, 1986.
*Evidence that the neural pathways of motion sickness are different between dogs and cats.*
Fukui H, Yamamoto M, and Sato S: Vagal afferent fibers and peripheral 5-HT₃ receptors mediate cisplatin-induced emesis in dogs. Jpn J Pharmacol 59:221, 1992.
*Evidence that chemotherapy-induced emesis is mediated by vagal 5-HT₃ receptors in the dog.*
Gullikson GW, Loeffler RF, and Viriña AM: Relationship of serotonin-3 receptor antagonist activity to gastric emptying and motor-stimulating actions of prokinetic drugs in dogs. J Pharmacol Exp Ther 258:103, 1991.
*Identification of gastric neuronal 5-HT₄ receptors and their role in the regulation of gastric emptying in the dog.*
Harding RK: Concepts and conflicts in the mechanism of emesis. Can J Physiol Pharmacol 68:218, 1990.
*A review of humoral and neural emesis.*
Itoh Z: Erythromycin mimics exogenous motilin in gastrointestinal contractile activity in the dog. Am J Physiol 247:G688, 1984.
*First evidence that erythromycin at microbially ineffective doses is a potent gastric pro-kinetic agent in the dog.*
King GL: Animal models in the study of vomiting. Can J Physiol Pharmacol 68:260, 1990.
*Excellent review of information derived from emetic studies in several different species.*
Lang IM and Sarna SK: The role of adrenergic receptors in the initiation of vomiting and its gastrointestinal motor correlates in the dog. J Pharmacol Exp Therap 263:395, 1992.
*Experiments that identified a role for CRTZ α₂-receptors in vomiting.*
Lucot JB: Prevention of motion sickness by 5-HT₁ₐ agonists in cats. In Bianchi AL (ed): *Mechanisms and Control of Emesis.* Paris, Inserm, 1992, p 195.
*Experiments that provide first evidence for 5-HT₁ₐ receptors in regulation of emesis in the cat.*
Tucker ML, Jackson MR, Scales MDC, et al: Ondansetron: Pre-clinical safety evaluation. Eur J Cancer Clin Oncol 25:S79, 1989.
*Toxicity studies of ondansetron in the dog.*

# CURRENT CONCEPTS IN CANINE AND FELINE DENTISTRY

SANDRA MANFRA MARRETTA

*Urbana, Illinois*

Dental diseases occur frequently in the dog and cat. A thorough history, complete oral examination, evaluation of clinical pathologic and histopathologic findings, and dental radiography can be instrumental in obtaining an accurate diagnosis.

Dental disease can be subdivided into several basic categories, including: inappropriate number of teeth and developmental anomalies, gingivitis and periodontal disease, and structural injuries with secondary endodontic disease. Depending on the severity of the disease, the age and medical status of the patient, and the financial constraints of the client, various treatment options are available, including: exodontia, periodontal therapy, endodontic therapy, and restorative therapy.

## HISTORICAL AND CLINICAL SIGNS OF DENTAL DISEASE

Eating habits of dogs and cats with dental disease may vary. Owners may report a change in preference from hard food to soft food, dropping food, and chewing on one side of the mouth with the head tilted to one side. Some animals may approach their food dish, attempt to eat, and then run away because of the oral pain associated with eating. Generalized behavioral changes include reclusive behavior, trembling, and changes in temperament.

Clinical signs that may be indicative of a dental problem include: halitosis; bloody, purulent, or excessive salivation; sneezing; nasal discharge; and pawing or rubbing the mouth.

## ORAL EXAMINATION

A complete examination of the oral cavity should be performed whenever an animal is presented for a routine physical examination. A thorough oral examination is essential when a dental problem is anticipated. Uncooperative or painful patients may require tranquilization. Physical findings associated with dental disease may include facial hypersensitivity; swelling or asymmetry; hemorrhagic, purulent, or mucoid nasal discharge; or enlargement of the submandibular lymph nodes. The oral cavity should be systematically examined for missing teeth, supernumerary teeth, overly retained deciduous teeth, and malformed teeth. Changes associated with periodontal disease including gingivitis, gingival recession with root exposure, dental plaque

and calculus, loose teeth, oronasal fistulas, and oroantral fistulas should be evaluated. The dentition should be thoroughly evaluated for structural injuries including dental attrition, dental caries, external root resorptive lesions, and fractures. The teeth should also be examined for proper occlusion.

## CONGENITAL AND DEVELOPMENTAL ANOMALIES

Abnormalities in number of teeth include: supernumerary teeth, retained deciduous teeth, hypodontia, oligodontia, and anodontia. The deciduous and permanent dental formulae for the dog are $2(I_{\frac{3}{3}}, C_{\frac{1}{1}}, P_{\frac{3}{3}}) = 28$ and $2(I_{\frac{3}{3}}, C_{\frac{1}{1}}, P_{\frac{4}{4}}, M_{\frac{2}{3}}) = 42$, respectively. The deciduous and permanent dental formulae for the cat are $2(I_{\frac{3}{3}}, C_{\frac{1}{1}}, P_{\frac{2}{2}}) = 26$ and $2(I_{\frac{3}{3}}, C_{\frac{1}{1}}, P_{\frac{3}{2}}, M_{\frac{1}{1}}) = 30$, respectively. Abnormalities in the formation of teeth include enamel hypoplasia and dilaceration.

### Supernumerary Teeth

Supernumerary teeth are common in the dog. Approximately 10% of dogs have one or more extra teeth. There is some evidence that this condition may be inheritable in some dogs. If the supernumerary teeth are crowding other teeth, causing a malocclusion problem, or contributing to the development of premature periodontitis, then they should be extracted.

### Retained Deciduous Teeth

Retained deciduous teeth occur most frequently in toy-breed dogs and have been reported in cats. A deciduous tooth that is overly retained for as little as 2 weeks following the eruption of the permanent tooth can produce occlusal defects in the permanent dentition. Abnormally retained deciduous teeth should be extracted as soon as possible to minimize malocclusion problems.

### Hypodontia

Hypodontia is the congenital absence of only a few teeth. Absence of teeth in both dogs and cats can be an inherited abnormality or may be the result of a disturbance during the initial stages of tooth formation. Hypodontia is most common in small-breed dogs but does occur in larger breeds. It occurs infrequently in the cat. The teeth that are most frequently missing are the premolar teeth. The canine and carnassial teeth are rarely missing.

## Oligodontia and Anodontia

Oligodontia is the congenital absence of many but not all of the teeth, and anodontia is the total absence of teeth. Both these conditions are rare in the dog and cat. Prior to a definitive diagnosis of anodontia or oligodontia, a dental radiograph must be taken to rule out the possibility of delayed eruption. A familial delayed eruption of up to 2 years has been reported in Tibetan and wheaten terriers and probably occurs in other breeds.

## Malformed Teeth

Abnormalities in the formation of teeth include enamel hypoplasia, gemination, and dilaceration. Enamel hypoplasia can occur secondary to local or systemic factors and is more prevalent in dogs than in cats. Local factors that can result in enamel hypoplasia include periapical inflammation or traumatic injury to a deciduous tooth. Febrile disorders that occur during the development of enamel can interrupt normal enamel deposition on multiple teeth. Gemination is the division of a single tooth bud that results in a single root with two crowns. Dilaceration is any distortion of the crown relative to the root and is usually caused by trauma to the primary tooth with concurrent disruption of the permanent tooth bud.

## GINGIVITIS AND PERIODONTITIS

Periodontal disease is caused by the accumulation of bacterial plaque in the gingival sulcus and between the teeth. Gingivitis, a reversible inflammatory response, is an early form of periodontal disease. Removal of plaque will return the gingiva to a healthy state. Left untreated, gingivitis will progress to periodontitis, causing a deeper inflammatory response that results in permanent damage to the periodontal tissues and loss of supporting tooth structures. Several factors affect the progression of gingivitis to periodontitis, including: amount of plaque, composition of plaque, plaque-retentive areas, and the ability of the animal to respond to the bacterial challenge.

Periodontal disease occurs when the predominant bacterial flora in the gingival sulcus changes from non-motile, gram-positive aerobic coccoid bacteria to more motile, gram-negative anaerobic rod-shaped bacteria. Mixed aerobic-anaerobic flora are commonly found in animals with periodontal disease. An important factor in the progression of periodontal disease is the consumption of large quantities of oxygen by aerobic bacteria. As the number of bacteria increases, the oxygen concentration becomes low, especially in deep periodontal pockets, creating an environment favorable for the growth of anaerobic bacteria.

Chronic periodontal disease can have serious local and systemic effects on an animal's health. The common clinical presentations of periodontal disease in the dog and cat include mobile teeth, periodontal and periapical abscesses with secondary facial swelling, gingival recession, mild to moderate gingival hemorrhage, and deep periodontal pockets with secondary oronasal or oroantral fistulas resulting in a secondary chronic rhinitis. Less frequently, severe gingival sulcus hemorrhage, pathologic mandibular fractures, painful contact buccal mucosal ulcers, intranasal tooth migration, and osteomyelitis occur in animals with severe periodontal disease (Manfra Marretta, 1987).

Dogs and cats with advanced periodontal disease may have difficulty eating and may experience pain when attempting to chew dry food. These animals may become completely anorectic, resulting in malnutrition and weight loss. In cats, inappetence secondary to dental pain may potentially be a contributing factor in the development of hepatic lipidosis. Infected periodontal pockets may serve as a nidus of infection for other organs including the lung, kidney, or heart.

## Periodontal Therapy

The treatment of periodontal disease is based on one principle: a clean periodontium results in a healthy periodontium. Various techniques utilized in the treatment of periodontal disease include: supragingival and subgingival scaling, root planing, subgingival curettage, polishing, gingivectomy, open-flap curettage, extraction, oronasal fistula repair, and home care (Grove, 1990).

### SUPRAGINGIVAL SCALING

Supragingival scaling refers to the removal of dental calculus localized above the gingival margin. Ultrasonic instrumentation with a "universal tip" is an efficient method for removal of supragingival calculus.

A thorough periodontal examination should be performed following supragingival scaling. A periodontal probe is utilized to access the attachment level. Attachment loss or pocket depth is recorded on the patient's dental chart.

### SUBGINGIVAL SCALING, ROOT PLANING, AND SUBGINGIVAL CURETTAGE

Following the removal of supragingival calculus and accessment of periodontal attachment loss, subgingival scaling, root planing, and curettage are performed utilizing a sharp curette such as a Columbia 13/14 or Gracey curette. Subgingival scaling is the removal of dental calculus and debris below the gingival margin. Root planing is the smoothing of the root surface. It is not a distinct entity from subgingival scaling or cleaning of the root surfaces but rather a continuation of the process. Subgingival curettage is performed by directing the edge of the curette toward the pocket wall and scraping the soft tissue wall of the pocket, removing the epithelium and granulation tissue.

Following the removal of all calculus, the teeth are polished with a rubber cup placed on a prophylaxis angle attached to a slow-speed handpiece. Prophylaxis paste is applied directly on the teeth and the cup is gently rotated over all surfaces of the teeth. The teeth are then flushed with forced water and air to remove any residual debris and polish.

### GINGIVECTOMY

A gingivectomy may be necessary in some animals with periodontal disease. A gingivectomy can be utilized to eliminate shallow supraboney pockets. This procedure can also be used in the treatment of gingival hypertrophy or hyperplasia and for obtaining excisional or incisional gingival biopsies.

The performance of a gingivectomy to eliminate a supraboney pocket is initiated by marking the depth of the pocket on the gingiva with the tip of a periodontal probe. An incision is made with a scalpel blade starting slightly apical to the depth of the pocket so that the gingiva postoperatively will have a smooth, beveled, anatomic contour. A minimum of 1 to 2 mm of attached gingiva must be retained when performing a gingivectomy to prevent dehiscence of the alveolar mucosa and painful exposure of alveolar bone.

### OPEN-FLAP CURETTAGE

Open-flap curettage is indicated in cases in which periodontal pockets are greater than 5 to 6 mm deep and do not respond to conservative management. The purpose of open-flap curettage is to reflect the gingiva, gain access to the deeper periodontal structures, and thoroughly treat the affected tissues with the benefit of direct visualization and without loss of attached gingiva. The exposed surface of the tooth is scaled, root planed, and polished. Following liberal irrigation of the surgical site with sterile saline, the flaps are repositioned and held in place with 4-0 chromic, simple interrupted sutures placed interdentally.

### EXTRACTION

Extraction should be performed on teeth that are severely affected with periodontal disease. Severely mobile teeth and teeth with less than 20% residual bone support rarely can be salvaged. These teeth have minimal periodontal support, which results in pain when stress is applied to these teeth. Teeth in which the periodontal pockets extend to the apex of one or more roots should be extracted.

### ORONASAL AND OROANTRAL FISTULAS

Oronasal and oroantral fistulas may be caused by advanced periodontal disease of the maxillary teeth. The most frequent location of oronasal fistulas in the dog is the palatal aspect of the maxillary canine tooth. Any tooth mesial to the maxillary fourth premolar molars including the incisors, canines, and premolars can potentially be associated with an oronasal fistula. Teeth distal to the maxillary third premolar, which can potentially be associated with an oroantral fistula, include the fourth premolars and first molars. Teeth affected with end-stage periodontal disease with a secondary oronasal or oroantral fistula should be extracted and the fistula should be repaired. Oronasal fistulas can be repaired with a single layer or a double-layer flap. Oroantral fistulas are repaired with a single-layer flap (Kapatkin, Manfra Marretta, and Schloss, 1990).

### HOME CARE

Home care is an important part of the treatment and prevention of periodontal disease. Plaque is a combination of food, saliva, and bacteria that accumulate on the teeth. Failure to remove plaque from the teeth will result in the mineralization of the accumulated plaque, which becomes calculus, which is more difficult to remove. Home care should ideally be provided daily and minimally on a weekly basis. There are several home care options, including antibiotic therapy, tooth brushing, dentifrices, chemical plaque control, and dietary/chew toys to reduce plaque and calculus formation.

Antibiotic therapy for animals with mild periodontal disease may include amoxicillin (Amoxil, SmithKline Beecham; 11 to 22 mg/kg PO every 12 hr) perioperatively. A preparation comprised of the broad-spectrum antibiotic amoxicillin and the β-lactamase inhibitor clavulanate potassium (Clavamox, SmithKline Beecham; 12.5 to 25 mg/kg PO every 12 hr) can be utilized in moderate cases for 10 days. In severe cases, amoxicillin can be combined with metronidazole (Flagyl, Searle; 15 mg/kg PO every 12 hr). In a dog with chronic recurrent periodontitis, tetracycline is often beneficial. Tetracycline is secreted in the gingival sulcus, and it has an anti-inflammatory action. The recommended dose of tetracycline (Achromycin, Lederle; 15 to 20 mg/kg PO every 8 hr for 2 weeks, then b.i.d. for 2 weeks, and finally s.i.d. for 2 weeks) can be tapered over a 6-week period.

Tooth brushing can be accomplished utilizing a tooth brush with soft bristles. The tooth brush should be placed in the gingival sulcus at a 45-degree angle and gently rotated to remove plaque from the sulcus.

There are many dentifrices available for cleaning and polishing the tooth surface. An ideal pet dentifrice is an enzymatic toothpaste such as CET (VRx Products) or Enzydent (Schein) toothpaste. These cleansing agents exert their effect by the content of the product, including: (1) abrasives such as calcium phosphate, calcium carbonate, and silicate; and (2) enzymatic hypothiocyanate, which produces a "hydrogen peroxide" reaction that kills the bacteria in plaque.

Chemical plaque control can assist in the reduction of bacterial plaque and gingival inflammation. Chlorhexidine is available on the veterinary market as Ginga-Dent (VRx Products). Two daily rinses with 10 ml of a 0.2% aqueous solution of chlorhexidine will help inhibit plaque and calculus accumulation. Recent evidence has shown that chlorhexidine gluconate (CHx Gel, VRx Products) is the superior form of chlorhexidine. Zinc ascorbate/sulfur amino acid (Maxiguard, Addison Biological Laboratory) has shown some promising results. This type of product stimulates collagen production, assisting in the repair of gingival tissue. Chemical plaque control is not a substitute for proper dental prophylaxis and brushing.

Chewing hard food, rawhide treats, and chew toys has been shown to decrease calculus formation in pets. A new prescription diet (Hill's Canine t/d) has been proven efficacious in slowing the accumulation of plaque, stain, and dental calculus. Hard chew toys should be avoided to prevent trauma to the dentition such as crown fractures. Animals that eat primarily soft food and avoid chew toys tend to require more home care by the owner and often more frequent care by a veterinarian.

## STRUCTURAL INJURIES

Structural injuries of the teeth include dental attrition, dental caries, external odontoclastic resorption, and fractures. The appropriate therapy for structural injuries of teeth is based on the severity of the lesion, the age and medical status of the patient, and the financial constraints of the client. Severe structural injuries of the teeth can affect the pulp, resulting in secondary endodontic disease, necessitating endodontic therapy.

### Dental Attrition

Dental attrition is the abnormal process of teeth wearing down rapidly. Persistent grinding of the teeth on any surface can cause wearing away of the enamel and dentin. Attrition stimulates the odontoblastic processes in the dentinal tubules to produce new dentin on the coronal aspect of the pulpal tissue. This new dentin is called "reparative" or "tertiary" dentin and is darker than primary dentin and appears as a dark solid brown spot on the affected tooth. If attrition is slow enough to permit the pulpal tissues to recede without pulpal exposure, no treatment is necessary. If the attrition rate exceeds the rate of pulpal recession, then the pulp becomes exposed. Pulpal exposure is confirmed if the tip of a dental explorer can enter the pulp canal of the affected tooth. Endodontic therapy is necessary to salvage a tooth that has undergone rapid dental attrition with pulpal exposure.

### Dental Caries

Dental caries is a destructive process that causes decalcification of the tooth enamel and leads to continued destruction of enamel and dentin and cavitation of the tooth. Dental decay or true carious lesions are uncommon in carnivores. In the dog, the teeth most commonly affected are the maxillary first and second molars and the mandibular first molar. Although dental caries occur infrequently in the dog, when they do occur there are often multiple advanced lesions affecting several teeth. Primary dental caries in cats is rare.

Dental caries that are detected early can be managed with restorative procedures. Caries that extend into the pulp require endodontic and restorative therapy or extraction (Harvey and Emily, 1993a).

### External Odontoclastic Resorption

External odontoclastic resorption, also known as external root resorption or cervical line lesions, is common in cats. These lesions are rarely found in other species. They are the result of destructive activity of odontoclasts in the periodontal ligament. The etiology of external root resorption is unknown. They often start as cavitations of the tooth at the cementoenamel junction or neck of the tooth. They can be obscured by normal gingiva in early stages, and then are revealed only by subgingival examination with a dental explorer. Granulation tissue may fill the cavitation located in the crown or neck of the tooth. This tissue must be removed to reveal the defect. These lesions often progress, resulting in painful pulpal exposure, and eventually the crown breaks off, leaving root tips in the alveolar bone. These retained root tips can cause a secondary osteomyelitis with painful mandibular swelling. Dental radiography is essential in the accessment of the full extent of these lesions.

External root resorptive lesions in cats have been categorized into five groups. Class I lesions are cavitations that extend less than 0.5 mm into the tooth's surface. Class II lesions have significant erosions that do not invade into the endodontic system. Class III lesions are deep erosions that invade into the pulp or endodontic system. Class IV lesions are so deep that there is severe loss of tooth structure as well as endodontic involvement. Class V lesions are chronic lesions in which there is complete coronal loss and subsequent granulation tissue covering the retained root.

Treatment of external root resorptive lesions depends on the severity of the lesion (Harvey and Emily, 1993a). Application of a fluoride varnish has been advocated for very early lesions. The most appropriate restorative materials for external root resorptive lesions are glass ionomers. Prior to restoration of feline cervical line lesions, radiographs should be taken to evaluate the root structure of the affected tooth. Frequently, cervical line lesions are extensive and nonrestorable because of extensive loss of tooth structure that may not be evident without a radiograph. It must be remembered that if the pulp is exposed, endodontic therapy is required prior to restoration. Endodontic therapy may not be practical in many of these teeth because of their small size. Additionally, long-term results show that destructive changes continue adjacent to the restoration. Extraction is the treatment of choice for class IV lesions. Class V lesions are treated by extraction of the retained roots. Prevention of external root resorptive lesions is difficult because the cause of the resorptive lesions is not known. Reduction of the gingival inflammatory response and plaque control is recommended to help control the secondary bacterial infections associated with stomatitis.

## Fractured Teeth and Endodontic Disease

Dental fractures should be classified on presentation into two groups: fractures with pulpal exposure and fractures without pulpal exposure. A fracture of the enamel surface without exposure of the pulp requires only that the sharp edges of the fracture site be smoothed off as necessary to avoid any further oral trauma. A fractured tooth with exposed pulp requires endodontic therapy.

Fractured teeth are often noted as an incidental finding on physical examination. However, a series of events may occur in some fractured teeth with exposed pulp that can result in significant clinical presentations. This series of events includes the following conditions: (1) exposed pulp, (2) bacterial pulpitis, (3) pulp necrosis, (4) apical granuloma, (5) periapical abscess, (6) acute alveolar periodontitis, (7) osteomyelitis, and (8) sepsis. The time required for this progression varies from months to years. When a tooth is fractured and the pulp is exposed, the pulp will bleed. Pulpal exposure is extremely painful, and animals with an acutely fractured tooth with pulpal exposure will hypersalivate, be reluctant to eat, and exhibit abnormal behavior. Over several months the pulp becomes necrotic and the animal is no longer painful, until an inflammatory reaction occurs around the apex of the tooth, at which time the animal becomes painful again. An endodontically diseased tooth is not only painful but also is a potential source of infection for other parts of the body.

Clinical signs associated with endodontic disease include: (1) changes in eating habits, (2) pawing at the mouth, (3) abnormal salivation, (4) oral hypersensitivity, (5) facial swelling, (6) oral hemorrhage, (7) sneezing and nasal discharge, and (8) abnormal behavior. Physical examination may reveal fractured teeth, severely worn teeth, discolored teeth, soft tissue fistulas that may be located at or apical to the mucogingival line, teeth that are painful on percussion, external root resorptive lesions in cats, deep dental caries, and pulpal exposure that can be confirmed with a dental explorer.

Radiographic changes associated with endodontic disease include: (1) periapical lysis, (2) apical lysis, (3) large endodontic systems secondary to failure in normal development or endodontic resorption, (4) radiographic loss of tooth structure to the pulp canal such

as in severe external root resorptive lesions or deep dental caries, and (5) secondary destruction of periodontal structures (Eisner, 1990).

## Endodontic Therapy

Numerous treatment options are available for the management of endodontic disease. The various forms of endodontic therapy include: (1) vital pulpotomy with direct pulp capping, (2) conventional or nonsurgical endodontic therapy, (3) nonconventional or surgical endodontic therapy, (4) apexogenesis, and (5) apexification (Harvey and Emily, 1993b). The type of endodontic therapy administered depends on the status of the endodontic system. Factors affecting the type of endodontic therapy administered include: (1) vital pulp versus nonvital pulp, (2) mature versus immature tooth, (3) closed versus opened apex, and (4) exposure time. The endodontic therapy recommended for various types of endodontic problems is defined in Table 1.

Whenever pulp disease is present, it is important to decide which type of endodontic therapy is most appropriate based on the patient's age, time of exposure, and the gross anatomic features and vitality of the tooth. The most frequently performed endodontic therapy is nonsurgical or conventional root canal therapy, followed by vital pulpotomy with direct pulp capping. Infrequently, there are times in which apexogenesis, apexification, and surgical or nonconventional root canal therapy is indicated.

### VITAL PULPOTOMY WITH DIRECT PULP CAPPING

A vital pulpotomy with direct pulp capping is indicated in vital teeth with traumatic pulpal exposure of less than 8 hr. This permissible exposure time may be extended to up to 2 weeks in very young animals with immature teeth. It is also indicated in disarming procedures. Ideally, vital techniques such as vital pulpotomy with direct pulp capping should be limited to use in incompletely developed permanent teeth with pulpal exposure. A vital pulpotomy with direct pulp capping

***Table 1.*** *Various Treatment Modalities for Endodontic Disease*

| | |
|---|---|
| Vital pulpotomy with direct pulp capping | Vital tooth with traumatic pulpal exposure of less than 8 hr; also indicated in disarming procedures |
| Nonsurgical or conventional endodontic therapy | Nonvital mature tooth with closed apex or vital mature tooth with pulpal exposure greater than 8 hr |
| Surgical or nonconventional endodontic therapy | Nonvital mature tooth with apical lysis and immature nonvital tooth with open apex |
| Apexogenesis | Vital, immature tooth with open apex with traumatic pulpal exposure of less than 2 weeks |
| Apexification | Immature, nonvital tooth with open apex |

in an animal less than 18 months of age will permit the tooth to remain vital at least temporarily so that additional dentin can be formed, resulting in an increase in strength of the tooth that has been fractured. Additionally, it can allow the formation of the apex of a very immature tooth.

A pulpotomy with direct pulp capping should never be performed in nonvital teeth, when the pulpal exposure is prolonged, and in teeth in which the pulp is severely traumatized or grossly contaminated.

The objective of a vital pulpotomy with direct pulp capping is to protect the pulp following pulpal exposure by stimulating formation of secondary dentin over the exposed pulp by placing a calcium hydroxide preparation directly over the pulpal tissue and covering over the access site with a restorative material. The owner should be informed that conventional endodontic therapy may be necessary if pulpitis and pulpal necrosis develop.

### CONVENTIONAL ENDODONTIC THERAPY

Conventional endodontic therapy or nonsurgical endodontic therapy is performed through the crown of the tooth. It is the most frequently performed endodontic therapy. This procedure is indicated whenever there is pulpal death of a tooth secondary to inflammation, infection, or trauma. The purpose of endodontic therapy is to preserve the function of the tooth while preventing it from causing adverse effects because of its presence. This is achieved by removing the necrotic or infected pulp and filling the pulp canal with an inert material. Properly performed endodontic therapy will prevent infection or inflammatory products from extending from the tooth into the tissues that surround the apex of the tooth. There are several basic steps involved in performing conventional endodontic therapy. These steps include: (1) making an access to the pulp, (2) débridement of the canal, (3) drying the canal, (4) filling the canal, and (5) restoration of the access site. The owner should be informed that failure of conventional endodontic therapy may necessitate conventional endodontic retreatment or surgical endodontic therapy of the failed root canal. Clinical signs associated with endodontic therapy failure include soft tissue fistulas, teeth that are painful on percussion, periapical swelling, and lost restorations. Dental radiographs should be taken at 6- and 12-month intervals postoperatively and then annually during regular dental appointments to detect potential endodontic failure that would be evident as increased apical or periapical lysis and endodontic resorption.

### SURGICAL ENDODONTIC THERAPY AND CONVENTIONAL ENDODONTIC THERAPY FAILURE

Surgical endodontic therapy refers to the application of endodontic therapy with an approach through soft tissue and bone rather than through the crown of the tooth. Surgical endodontic therapy is always performed in conjunction with nonsurgical or conventional endodontic therapy. There are several indications for surgical endo-

dontic therapy including: (1) apical root resorption, (2) incomplete root development, (3) complication during conventional root canal therapy (broken files), (4) recurrent apical abscessation, (5) horizontal fracture of root tip, and (6) fractured teeth in exotic species.

The major reason for failure of conventional (nonsurgical root canal therapy is an inadequate apical seal. This complication is usually manifested 2 to 3 months postoperatively but can occur 2 to 3 years following conventional root canal therapy, and is usually caused by one of the following: (1) an iatrogenically inadequate apical seal, (2) iatrogenic perforation of the apex, or (3) apical lysis that was undetected because of failure to perform radiography prior to conventional root canal therapy. When conventional endodontic therapy has failed, a radiograph should be taken to determine the extent of pathology of the root involved. Only the affected root needs to be treated either surgically or with conventional retreatment. In most cases, the affected root canal can be managed successfully with nonsurgical endodontic procedures. Conventional retreatment is performed by removing the old gutta-percha with chloroform (a solvent for gutta-percha). The canal is then properly reprepared, and filled with zinc oxide and eugenol and gutta-percha. Approximately 80% of reinfected canals can be successfully managed by retreating the involved root canal with conventional endodontic therapy. If conventional endodontic therapy is likely to fail or if true failure occurs following retreatment, surgical endodontic therapy is indicated.

The teeth most commonly requiring surgical endodontic therapy are the upper 4th premolar, the upper canine, the lower canine and the lower 1st molar in that order of frequency. The mesiobuccal root of the maxillary 4th premolar is the canal that most frequently becomes reinfected. The restricted size of this canal and its slight curvature makes the complete filling of this canal more difficult.

Surgical endodontic therapy is not a substitute for good nonsurgical endodontic therapy. The long-term success rate with surgical endodontics has not been shown to be superior to nonsurgical endodontic therapy. A properly prepared and obturated root canal can be adequately sealed with conventional endodontic therapy in most cases.

### APEXOGENESIS AND APEXIFICATION

Animals that sustain traumatic dental injuries when their teeth are immature present significant problems for the veterinarian. Dental traumatic injuries in young dogs usually present with a crown fracture with secondary pulpal exposure. These problems include: incomplete root formation, structurally weak teeth, large pulp chambers and root canals, and open apices.

The appropriate therapy for fractured immature teeth with pulpal exposure depends on the severity and time of exposure. Animals presented with vital pulpal tissues should be treated with apexogenesis, while animals presented with nonvital pulpal tissue should be treated with apexification. When treating a tooth in which the apex has not completely closed but the pulp is not irreversibly damaged, an "apical development pulpotomy" or apexogenesis procedure is recommended. The injured pulpal tissue is removed while the remaining pulpal tissue is retained to permit further tooth development. Apexification is the treatment of choice for immature teeth with nonvital pulpal tissue. Apexification does not usually result in further development of root length but does result in apical closure by the formation of cementum. This procedure is performed by removing all the pulpal tissue and filling the canal with calcium hydroxide paste. Once apical closure has been achieved following apexogenesis and apexification procedures, conventional endodontic therapy is performed.

## References and Suggested Reading

Eisner ER: Problems associated with veterinary dental radiography. *In* Manfra Marretta S (ed): *Problems in Veterinary Medicine (Dentistry).* Philadelphia, JB Lippincott Co, 1990, p 46.
*A review of intraoral radiographic equipment, positioning, and techniques for use in the dog and cat.*
Grove TK: Problems associated with the management of periodontal disease in clinical practice. *In* Manfra Marretta S (ed): *Problems in Veterinary Medicine (Dentistry).* Philadelphia, JB Lippincott Co, 1990, p 110.
*A review of the origin, clinical presentation, and treatment of periodontal disease in a format that is directly applicable to clinical practice.*
Harvey CE and Emily PP: Restorative dentistry. *In* Harvey CE and Emily PP (eds): *Small Animal Dentistry.* St Louis, Mosby Year Book, 1993, p 213.
*A review of the indications, proper techniques, and materials for restorative dentistry in dogs and cats.*
Harvey CE and Emily PP: Endodontics. *In* Harvey CE and Emily PP (eds): *Small Animal Dentistry.* St Louis, Mosby Year Book, 1993, p 156.
*A review of the signs, radiographic appearance, indications, and appropriate treatment modalities for endodontic disease.*
Kapatkin AS, Manfra Marretta S, and Schloss AJ: Problems associated with basic oral surgical techniques. *In* Manfra Marretta S (ed): *Problems in Veterinary Medicine (Dentistry).* Philadelphia, JB Lippincott Co, 1990, p 248.
*A review of various extraction techniques and management of their associated complications including the management of oronasal and oroantral fistulas.*
Manfra Marretta S: The common and uncommon clinical presentations and treatment of periodontal disease. Semin Vet Med Surg 2:230, 1987.
*A report describing the various clinical presentations of periodontal disease in the dog and cat over a 3-year period at The Animal Medical Center.*

---

# CANINE AND FELINE OROPHARYNGEAL NEOPLASMS

## GARY J. SPODNICK
### *and* RODNEY L. PAGE
*Raleigh, North Carolina*

Oropharyngeal neoplasms are common and account for approximately 6% and 3% of all tumors in dogs and cats, respectively. Tumors can arise from the gingiva, buccal mucosa, tongue, bone, dental structures, and the tonsils. Etiologic factors associated with oropharyngeal neoplasms in dogs and cats have not been identified. In some species such as the rabbit, papillomaviruses have been associated with squamous cell carcinoma. In dogs, oral and ocular papillomas have been reported to progress to carcinoma *in situ* or to squamous cell carcinomas, particularly in young dogs. The incidence of tonsillar squamous cell carcinomas has been reported to be greater in urban dogs, implying environmental carcinogens may be involved in the cause and pathogenesis of this tumor. Currently, however, no other risk factors for oropharyngeal neoplasms have been determined in the dog or cat.

## CLINICAL SIGNS

Oral tumors are most often recognized by the pet owner at a relatively advanced stage when the animal develops clinical signs of increased salivation, halitosis, bloody saliva, anorexia, weight loss, or dysphagia. Occasionally, large tumors may actually interfere with respiration, especially tonsillar tumors or tumors involving the base of the tongue. The oral cavity should be thoroughly inspected for neoplasms during oral examinations and when performing dental prophylaxis. Localized tooth loosening or ulcerated lesions in the oral cavity of a patient with otherwise good dentition detected during routine dental examination or dental prophylaxis should raise the possibility of neoplastic bone lysis. Suspicious lesions should be radiographed and biopsied.

## DIAGNOSTIC EVALUATION

Complete diagnostic evaluation of a patient with an oral neoplasm should be performed to stage the disease, to establish a prognosis, and to determine a course of treatment. Thoracic radiographs should be performed any time an oral malignancy is suspected. Certain neoplasms such as melanomas and tonsillar carcinomas may have pulmonary metastases present at the time of initial diagnosis. Regional radiographs of the primary tumor should be made under anesthesia to accurately determine bony involvement. Radiographic evidence of bony invasion includes cortical bone lysis and loss of normal anatomic detail and symmetry. Radiographic assessment is critical for accurately staging the disease as well as planning the extent of the surgical resection or radiation.

Preoperative biopsy of the tumor should always be performed so an appropriate method of treatment can be planned. Biopsy can be accomplished during the same anesthetic procedure for radiography. A large wedge biopsy that includes a portion of normal tissue is desirable. Oral tumors are often ulcerated, infected, inflamed, or necrotic, changes which can interfere with the histologic diagnosis. A large biopsy specimen may decrease the likelihood of an inaccurate diagnosis and provides additional tissue for any necessary special diagnostic stains. For example, acanthomatous epulides can resemble squamous cell carcinomas, and amelanotic melanomas can often be misdiagnosed as undifferentiated sarcomas or round cell tumors. Biopsy sites should be planned so they may be easily included in the resection or radiation field. Occasionally, excisional biopsy may be performed for small lesions; however, in most cases, incisional biopsy should be performed so that further treatment can be planned with the knowledge of tumor type.

Regional lymph nodes should routinely be evaluated for size, consistency, and symmetry. All abnormal lymph nodes should be aspirated with a fine needle and cytologically examined for the presence of neoplasia. Absence of neoplastic cells from a lymph node aspirate does not guarantee the node is free of tumor; however, presence of neoplastic cells in the lymph node is significant and has importance in staging the disease and treatment planning.

Computed tomography (CT) evaluation of primary oral neoplasms is generally not indicated for surgical planning or radiation therapy. However, if concern exists regarding the extent of nasal cavity invasion or retropharyngeal involvement, a CT evaluation will be necessary.

## TREATMENT OPTIONS

Surgery can be used to effectively manage oropharyngeal neoplasms and has long been the cornerstone of treatment for these tumors (see "Definitive Surgical Treatment for Cancer," this volume, p 462). Maxillectomy and mandibulectomy techniques have been well described (Salisbury, Richardson, and Lantz, 1986; Salisbury and Lantz, 1988; Withrow and Holmberg, 1983). In dogs with all types of cancer involving the mandible, mandibulectomy alone resulted in 1- and 2-year survival rates of 45% and 33%, respectively, and overall median survival time for dogs with malignancies was 11 months (Schwartz et al., 1991a). Similarly, maxillectomy alone resulted in 1- and 2-year survival rates of 46% and 24%, respectively, and an overall median survival time of 8 months in dogs with cancer involving the

upper jaw (Schwarz et al., 1991b). Ideally, margins including at least 2 cm of normal tissue around the neoplasm are necessary when surgically excising oral malignancies such as malignant melanomas, fibrosarcomas, and osteosarcomas in the dog and squamous cell carcinomas in the cat; however, this may not always be possible due to surgical limitations or more extensive involvement than suspected on radiographs. Margins of excised tissue should be histologically examined for neoplasia. Operative sites in which the neoplasm extends to the margin or in which residual tumor remains should be irradiated. Prognostically, dogs survive longer when surgical margins are free of tumor.

Oncologic surgery can result in considerable loss of function and cosmetic alterations. Wound dihiscence is the most common complication following mandibulectomy and maxillectomy. This problem is usually more severe in the maxilla with the formation of oronasal fistula. Dogs and cats are capable of adapting to total hemimandibulectomy; however, prehension is difficult when bilateral mandibulectomy is performed caudal to the second premolars or when total hemimandibulectomy is combined with a partial mandibulectomy on the opposite side. If extensive surgery is planned such that a delay in recovery of oral alimentation is anticipated, a gastric feeding tube should be considered at the time of surgery.

Radiation therapy is indicated when the tumor type is known to be radiation responsive and when potential surgical damage to vital structures in the head and neck region is expected (see "Indications and Applications of Radiation Therapy," this volume, p 467). Radiation is also less likely to result in functional or cosmetic alterations that are associated with wide surgical excision. Radiation therapy may be delivered in a palliative manner when the tumor is considered incurable and when surgical debulking may cause major loss of function or disfigurement. Radiation can be combined with surgery in several ways. Radiation can be used preoperatively to sterilize tumor margins; the tumor can then be surgically excised with less likelihood of recurrence. The incidence of wound healing complications significantly increases when operating in previously irradiated tissues. In one report, dehiscence of maxillectomy sites occurred in 55% of patients receiving radiation (Schwarz et al., 1991b). This emphasizes the need to plan the combination of radiation and surgery with regard for potential complications in order to reduce their frequency. Radiation may also be combined with surgery to treat postoperative residual disease.

Chemotherapy in combination with surgery or radiation may play a useful role in treatment of some oropharyngeal neoplasms, but prolonged survival from adjuvant chemotherapy has not been confirmed in large clinical studies. Canine squamous cell carcinoma is moderately responsive to cisplatin or carboplatin. Doxorubicin-based protocols have demonstrated a 30 to 50% response rate in sarcomas, including those involving the oral cavity. For a more extensive discussion of the use of chemotherapy, the reader is referred to section 6 in this volume.

## References and Suggested Reading

Beck ER, Withrow SJ, McChesney AE, et al: Canine tongue tumors: A retrospective review of 57 cases. J Am Anim Hosp Assoc 22:525, 1986.
*A multi-institutional retrospective study of lingual tumors in the dog.*

Bradley RL, MacEwen EG, and Loar AS: Mandibular resection for removal of oral tumors in 30 dogs and 6 cats. J Am Vet Med Assoc 184:460, 1984
*Results of mandibular surgery performed to resect oral tumors in dogs and cats.*

MacMillan R, Withrow SJ, and Gillette EL: Surgery and regional irradiation for treatment of canine tonsillar squamous cell carcinoma: Retrospective review of eight cases. J Am Anim Hosp Assoc 18:311, 1982
*A retrospective study of eight dogs with tonsillar squamous cell carcinoma treated with a combination of surgery and radiation.*

McChesney SL, Withrow SJ, and Gillette EL, et al: Radiotherapy of soft tissue sarcomas in dogs. J Am Vet Med Assoc 194:60, 1989.
*A report of radiation dose–response relationships for local tumor control and late complications after radiotherapy of dogs with soft tissue sarcomas.*

Salisbury KS, Richardson DC, and Lantz GC: Partial maxillectomy and premaxillectomy in the treatment of oral neoplasia in the dog and cat. Vet Surg 15:16, 1986.
*A description of a technique for and results of partial maxillectomy as treatment for oral neoplasms in 17 dogs and three cats.*

Salisbury KS and Lantz GC: Long-term results of partial mandibulectomy for treatment of oral tumors in 30 dogs. J Am Anim Hosp Assoc 24:285, 1988.
*A retrospective study and review of long-term results of partial mandibulectomy as treatment for oral tumors in 30 dogs.*

Schwarz PD, Withrow SJ, Curtis CR, et al: Mandibular resection as a treatment for oral cancer in 81 dogs. J Am Anim Hosp Assoc 27:601, 1991a.
*Results of long-term follow-up of 81 cases of oral neoplasia in dogs that were treated by mandibular resection.*

Schwarz PD, Withrow SJ, Curtis CR, et al: Partial maxillary resection as a treatment for oral cancer in 61 dogs. J Am Anim Hosp Assoc 27:617, 1991b.
*Results of long-term follow-up of 61 cases of oral neoplasia in the dog that were treated by partial maxillary resection.*

White RAS and Gorman NT: Wide local excision of acanthomatous epulides in the dog. Vet Surg 18:12, 1989.
*Results of wide surgical excision for the treatment of acanthomatous epulides in 25 dogs.*

Withrow SJ and Holmberg DL: Mandibulectomy in the treatment of oral cancer. J Am Anim Hosp Assoc 19:273, 1983.
*A description of various techniques for and clinical results of partial mandibulectomy as treatment for oral neoplasms in 21 dogs.*

# BREED-ASSOCIATED GASTROINTESTINAL DISEASE

W. GRANT GUILFORD
*Palmerston North, New Zealand*

Breed predispositions to many gastrointestinal diseases are suspected in the dog and cat (Table 1). Only on a few occasions have suspected breed predispositions for a disease received sufficient scientific scrutiny to definitively establish the prevalence of the disease in a particular breed. Breeding toward homozygosity by line-breeding from small numbers of imported dogs or cats can establish quite different breed characteristics and disease predispositions in different countries and regions. Therefore, investigations of disease prevalence in popular breeds must be worldwide in scope to be truly representative of a breed. For instance, the prevalence of eosinophilic gastroenteritis in Rottweilers and Samoyeds examined by the author at Massey University, New Zealand, is very much higher than the prevalence I observed in these breeds at the University of California, Davis. The breed predispositions listed in Table 1 are likely to be biased toward North America because they were cited predominantly in North American journals.

## MODES OF HERITANCE

The heritance characteristics of gastrointestinal diseases has received only sporadic attention. Copper-induced hepatopathy of Bedlington terriers is inherited in an autosomal recessive fashion. Idiopathic megaesophagus in wirehaired fox terriers is thought to be inherited in a simple autosomal recessive mode, whereas the same disease in miniature schnauzers has characteristics of an autosomal dominant pattern. These differing heritance patterns of megaesophagus serve to illustrate that the same disease (or syndrome) may be inherited in dissimilar manners in different breeds.

## Importance to the Clinician

To the practicing clinician, breed predispositions are important for a number of reasons. First, they provide the clinician with a high degree of suspicion for certain diseases known to be prevalent in a particular breed. This suspicion affects the ranking of diagnostic possibilities and guides the direction of the work-up. Second, a knowledge of breed predispositions assists veterinarians when advising dog or cat breeders and breed societies concerning future breeding programs. Unfortunately, the lack of information about worldwide prevalence, modes of heritance, diagnostic characteristics, and tests for the carrier state of many diseases limits the depth and value of this advice. Until such information is available, obtaining animals genetically free of the disease for cross-breeding purposes and assisting breed societies in the development and implementation of breeding programs that select against deleterious genes is difficult.

***Table 1.*** *Suspected or Confirmed Breed Predispositions to Gastrointestinal Diseases**

| Breed | Disease |
|---|---|
| Abyssinian | Megaesophagus due to myasthenia gravis |
| Airedale terrier | Pancreatic carcinoma |
| Basenji | Lymphocytic/plasmacytic enteritis, hypertrophic gastritis, lymphangiectasia |
| Beagle | Chronic hepatitis, IgA deficiency |
| Bedlington terrier | Copper-induced hepatopathy |
| Belgian shepherd | Gastric carcinoma |
| Boston terrier | Vascular compression of the esophagus, constipation |
| Boxers | Gingival and circumanal neoplasia, mastocytoma, histiocytic colitis, idiopathic colitis |
| Brachycephalic breeds | Pyloric stenosis |
| Cairn terrier | Microscopic portovascular dysplasia, portosystemic shunts |
| Cocker spaniel | Gingival, oropharyngeal, and circumanal neoplasia; chronic hepatitis, portosystemic shunts |
| Dachshund | Colonic perforation |
| Doberman pinscher | Parvovirus, chronic hepatitis |
| English bulldog | Vascular compression of the esophagus, cleft palate, constipation, fecal incontinence |
| English springer spaniel | Fucosidosis |
| Fox terrier | Circumanal neoplasia |
| German shepherd | Oropharyngeal neoplasia, exocrine pancreatic insufficiency, inflammatory bowel disease, stress-induced diarrhea, megaesophagus, vascular anomaly with compression of the esophagus, sialocele, hepatic angiosarcoma, perianal fistula, bacterial overgrowth |
| German shorthaired pointer | Oropharyngeal neoplasia |
| Golden retriever | Oropharyngeal neoplasia |
| Great Dane | Gastric dilatation-volvulus, megaesophagus |
| Greyhound | Megaesophagus |
| Irish setter | Wheat-sensitive enteropathy, megaesophagus, vascular anomaly with compression of the esophagus, esophageal sarcoma, gastric dilatation-volvulus, perianal fistula |
| Irish wolfhound | Intrahepatic portosystemic shunts |
| Jack Russell terrier | Salivary gland necrosis |
| Labradors | Chronic hepatitis |
| Lundenhund | Protein-losing enteropathy |
| Manx cat | Constipation, fecal incontinence |
| Miniature schnauzer | Hyperlipidemia, pancreatitis, megaesophagus, portosystemic shunts, hemorrhagic gastroenteritis |
| Newfoundland | Megaesophagus |
| Pointer | Hepatic angiosarcoma, esophageal sarcoma, cleft palate |
| Poodle | Sialocele, hemorrhagic gastroenteritis |
| Rottweiler | Parvovirus, gastric eosinophilic granuloma |
| Scottish terrier | Chronic hepatitis |
| Shar-Pei | IgA deficiency, food sensitivity, inflammatory bowel disease, hiatal hernias |
| Siamese cat | Megaesophagus, gastric retention, intestinal adenocarcinoma |
| Siberian husky | Oral eosinophilic granuloma |
| Skye terrier | Copper-associated hepatopathy |
| Standard poodle | Lobular dissecting hepatitis |
| Weimaraner | Oropharyngeal neoplasia |
| West Highland white terrier | Copper-associated hepatopathy, chronic hepatitis |
| Wirehaired fox terrier | Megaesophagus |
| Yorkshire terriers | Portosystemic shunts, lymphangiectasia |

*Abridged from Strombeck DR and Guilford WG: Small Animal Gastroenterology, 2nd edition. Davis, CA, Stonegate Publishing, 1990, p 57, with permission.

## EXAMPLES OF BREED PREDISPOSITIONS

In the author's practice, a vomiting miniature schnauzer with anterior abdominal pain is considered "guilty" of acute pancreatitis unless proven "innocent." Similarly, the diagnostic work-up of a runt Yorkshire terrier puppy begins with the supposition that the dog has a portosystemic shunt. A German shepherd dog with chronic diarrhea has a strong likelihood of affliction with exocrine pancreatic insufficiency, inflammatory bowel disease, or bacterial overgrowth. Ileal adenocarcinoma has a higher degree of probability in a Siamese cat with chronic vomiting than in a domestic shorthair with the same complaint. A middle-aged female Doberman pinscher with depression, anorexia, and vomiting is immediately investigated for chronic hepatitis. Young Rottweilers and Doberman pinschers are predisposed to parvoviral enteritis for unknown reasons. Shar-Peis seem susceptible to food sensitivity, and inflammatory bowel disease, perhaps due to this, breeds predisposition to IgA deficiency. They also develop hiatal hernias frequently.

## CONCLUSION

The clinical acumen of an experienced clinician is in no small part due to a detailed knowledge of the breed predispositions in his or her particular region. The suspected breed predispositions listed in Table 1 serve as a guide, but it is important to reiterate that variations in the genetic make-up of the foundation stock of breeds in different geographic regions may markedly affect the validity and completeness of this list for an individual veterinarian's practice.

## References and Suggested Reading

Andersson M and Sevelius E: Breed, sex and age distribution in dogs with chronic liver disease. J Small Anim Pract 32:1, 1991.
Cox VS, Wallace LJ, Anderson VE, and Rushmer RA: Hereditary esophageal dysfunction in the miniature schnauzer dog. Am J Vet Res 41:326, 1980.
Osborne CA, Clifford DH, and Jessen C: Hereditary esophageal achalasia in dogs. J Am Vet Med Assoc 151:572, 1967.
Patterson DE, Haskins ME, Jezyk PF, et al: Research on genetic diseases: Reciprocal benefits to animals and man. J Am Vet Med Assoc 193:1131, 1988.
Strating A and Clifford DH: Canine achalasia with special reference to hereditary. Southwest Vet 19:135, 1966.
Strombeck DR and Guilford WG: Small Animal Gastroenterology, 2nd edition Davis, CA, Stonegate Publishing, 1990.

# LABORATORY DIAGNOSIS OF CANINE VIRAL ENTERITIS

SANJAY KAPIL
*Manhattan, Kansas*

Enteritis is a common problem in dogs and can be caused by a variety of agents—viruses, bacteria, fungi, protozoa, parasites, and toxicants. Viral enteritis generally has a high morbidity rate and is often difficult to control in kennels. Since there is no specific treatment for enteric viruses, prevention and control of the spread of viral enteritis depends on vaccination and proper disinfection of kennels. Therapy of acute viral enteritis is discussed elsewhere in this section.

Several viruses have been detected in dogs with enteritis, including: canine parvovirus, canine coronavirus, canine rotavirus, canine astrovirus, canine calicivirus, canine herpesvirus, and canine distemper virus. While detection of a virus in normal or diarrheic feces does not qualify it as a cause of enteritis, it should provoke the practitioner's concern regarding the pathogenic potential of that virus and resistance in the kennel environment. It is common to find one or more viral agents in a case of enteritis. The practitioner may find consultation with a diagnostic virologist useful when considering the clinical significance of these observations, especially when a kennel is involved.

Correct identification and characterization of the viral agent is useful in establishing a cause and prognosis for cases of viral enteritis; moreover, proper disinfection of the infected area and determining a probable source of infection often depends on the knowledge of the viral agent involved. In general, enveloped viruses are relatively labile, while nonenveloped viruses are relatively resistant to disinfectants. Also, ribonucleic acid (RNA) and single-stranded deoxyribonucleic acid (DNA) viruses mutate at a higher frequency than double-stranded DNA viruses. Viral mutants can potentially start an outbreak of the disease.

## SPECIMEN SUBMISSION

The diagnosis of enteric viruses in a live dog requires about 10 gm of fresh fecal material placed in a Whirl-Pak (Nasco, Fort Atkinson, WI) and submission to a diagnostic laboratory. Fecal samples should be shipped refrigerated over ice packs. If prolonged transit time is expected, the specimen should be shipped frozen over dry ice. A complete history including the age of dog(s) involved, clinical signs, morbidity, mortality, vaccination, and response to treatment should be provided with the specimen. Due to the zoonotic potential (*Campylobacter*, *Salmonella*, and parasites) of some canine enteropathogens, the specimens should be handled and shipped with care.

The diagnosis of enteric viruses in a dead dog requires submission of three intestinal samples (about 2 cm each) from different regions. Special submission requirements for some enteric viruses will be discussed later. Loss of viruses can occur during sample transit to a diagnostic laboratory and leads to false-negative results.

## LABORATORY TECHNIQUES

Awareness not only of the merits of diagnostic tests available (Table 1) but also of their potential limitations is crucial to effective veterinary practice.

### Electron Microscopy

Electron microscopy is the most valuable technique for diagnosis of viral enteritis. Electron microscopy has the potential for a rapid diagnosis (turnaround time of about 24 hr), permits detection of novel enteric viruses, and permits simultaneous detection of multiple viral agents. In the last 20 years, more than a dozen novel enteric viruses have been detected by negative contrast electron microscopy. Electron microscopy also has some limitations: it requires sophisticated equipment, a trained technician, is an expensive procedure, and can give false-negative and false-positive results.

Electron microscopy suffers from a lack of sensitivity. To diagnose a virus by direct electron microscopy, approximately 1 million viral particles per gram of fecal material should be present (Flewett, 1978). If specimens are improperly shipped, viruses may undergo partial or complete degradation. Partially degraded virus particles cannot be identified or classified and are generally ignored by most electron microscopists. A false-positive result can occur due to the presence of particles that can be confused with viruses. A nonpathogenic virus, such as canine parvovirus 1, is morphologically similar to canine parvovirus 2, the cause of canine enteritis. Similarly, corona-like viruses (Fig. 1) can be confused with coronaviruses on electron microscopy. Moreover, small round viruses, such as enterovirus, parvovirus, calicivirus, and astrovirus, are not

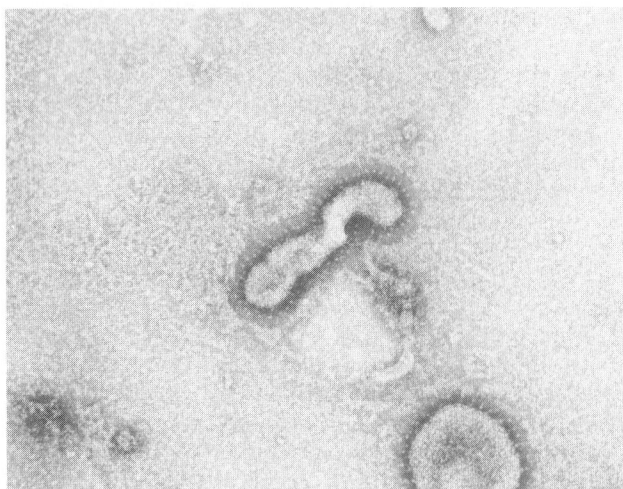

**Figure 1.** Bovine° corona-like virus particles. Surface projections have a thin stalk and a knob at the end.

easy to distinguish on electron microscopy. Often, enteric viruses are clumped by intestinal antibodies and these clumps sometimes contain two or more different viruses. Virus particles in the center of the clump are hard to visualize by electron microscopy. Feces can contain a variety of nonviral particles and bacteriophages that can also be confused with other viruses.

### Immunoelectron Microscopy

Immunoelectron microscopy (IEM) is far more sensitive and has better specificity than direct electron microscopy for diagnosis of canine enteric viruses. Immunoelectron microscopy is more expensive, more time consuming, and more laborious than direct electron microscopy. For diagnosis by IEM, the virus present in a fecal sample is clumped with a standard antiserum. Turnaround time for IEM is about 48 to 72 hr. Immunoelectron microscopy services are not commonly offered by veterinary diagnostic laboratories at this time.

### Enzyme-Linked Immunosorbent Assay

Enzyme-linked immunosorbent assay (ELISA) is commonly used for the detection of canine parvovirus. It offers good sensitivity, good specificity, and rapid diagnosis (turnaround time of about 30 min) of canine parvovirus. Since negative and positive controls are built into each kit, chances of an inaccurate diagnosis are minimized. Because of the simplicity of the procedure and the need for rapid diagnosis, canine parvovirus diagnosis by ELISA (CITE canine parvovirus

**Table 1.** Tests for the Diagnosis of Canine Viral Enteritis

| Virus | Tests Recommended |
|---|---|
| Canine parvovirus | ELISA |
| | HA |
| | EM |
| | FAT |
| Canine coronavirus | EM |
| | VI |
| | FAT |
| Canine rotavirus | EM |
| | ELISA |
| | FAT |
| Canine astrovirus | EM |
| Canine calicivirus | EM |
| Canine herpesvirus | VI |
| | EM |
| Canine distemper virus | FAT |
| | EM |

Abbreviations: EM = electron microscopy, HA = hemagglutination test, VI = virus isolation, FAT = fluorescent antibody test, ELISA = enzyme-linked immunosorbent assay.

°Since viruses in a virus family, even from different animal species, are morphologically similar, electron micrographs from dogs and other species have been used to illustrate the structural difference between viruses.

test kit, IDEXX, Portland, ME) can be performed in veterinary clinics. If additional viral agents are suspected, the specimen should also be submitted to a diagnostic laboratory for direct electron microscopy. ELISA kits for the diagnosis of other canine enteric viruses are not yet available.

## Fluorescent Antibody Test

Fluorescent antibody test (FAT) is a rapid diagnostic technique with a turnaround time of about 2 hr. Unfixed intestinal sections obtained at necropsy can be submitted over ice packs for the diagnosis of canine parvovirus, canine coronavirus, and canine rotavirus. In canine distemper, the viral antigen can be demonstrated in lungs, bladder, and intestine. In the live dog, conjunctival scrapings can be examined for canine distemper virus. For specific fluorescent antibody test(s), the laboratory must know the viral agent(s) suspected. Unlike direct electron microscopy, FAT is used as a confirmatory test, not as a broad-spectrum diagnostic tool.

## Virus Isolation

Virus isolation (VI) in cell culture is not recommended for the diagnosis of most canine enteric viruses. Fecal samples are frequently toxic to cell cultures, as they are loaded with normal intestinal bacteria and fungi. However, canine parvovirus, coronavirus, and rotavirus can replicate if suitable cell culture conditions are provided. Canine herpesvirus is cytopathic and canine distemper virus replicates to low titers in cell culture.

## Polymerase Chain Reaction

Polymerase chain reaction (PCR) is an emerging technology for diagnosis of viral diseases. In PCR, a specific segment of viral genome is amplified. The size of the amplified segment is determined by electrophoresis on agarose gel and diagnosis confirmed by nucleic acid hybridization. Applications of PCR for the rapid diagnosis of novel enteric viruses will no doubt increase in the future. PCR can also differentiate between mutants of a virus. It is a rapid and extremely sensitive diagnostic technique. Presently, most veterinary diagnostic laboratories lack the resources to perform PCR.

## Serologic Techniques

Serologic techniques are not recommended for the diagnosis of enteric viruses. Most adult dogs and pups carry antibodies to enteric viruses due to previous exposure, or from passive antibody immunization transfer from the dam. ELISA and indirect immunofluores-

cence tests that quantitate virus-specific IgM titers do indicate recent exposure to the virus. These IgM-based tests are not available in veterinary diagnostic laboratories at this time. For serology (serum neutralization) to be diagnostic, acute and convalescent serum samples collected 2 to 3 weeks apart should be submitted. It is important to demonstrate a fourfold difference in acute and convalescent viral titers. Hemagglutination followed by hemagglutination inhibition is used for canine parvovirus.

## Histopathology

Histopathology will support the diagnosis of canine viral enteritis syndrome. For example, a veterinary pathologist may be able to detect typical parvovirus lesions in a parvovirus ELISA-negative case. However, for the routine diagnosis of canine enteritis, electron microscopic examination of intestinal contents should be used in conjunction with histopathology on formalin-fixed intestines.

## CANINE ENTERIC VIRUSES

A brief description about some salient and clinically relevant features of canine enteric viruses follows.

## Canine Parvovirus

Canine parvovirus is the most important cause of canine viral enteritis. At the Wisconsin Animal Health laboratory, Madison, (WAHL-M), of 127 samples examined by parvovirus ELISA, 58 tested positive. Also, of 107 samples examined by electron microscopy, 24 were positive for canine parvovirus (Fig. 2). The parvovirus ELISA can distinguish between canine parvovirus 1 (minute virus of canines), a nonpathogenic parvovirus; and canine parvovirus 2, a common cause of

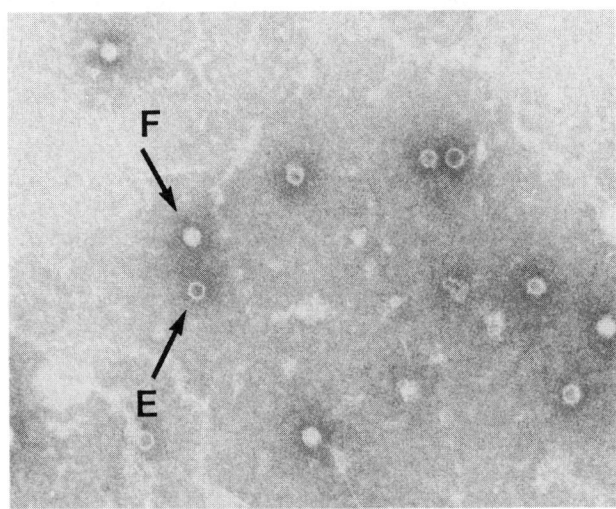

**Figure 2.** Canine parvovirus. Both full (F) and empty (E) virus particles are commonly found.

canine enteritis. Enteric viruses affect a specific anatomic location in the intestine. Using FAT, canine parvovirus viral antigen is present in replicating cells of the intestinal crypts.

Canine parvovirus is a single-stranded DNA virus and, thus, mutates easily. Since its initial identification in 1978, some mutant strains of canine parvovirus have been reported (Parrish et al., 1985). Since canine parvovirus is a nonenveloped virus, it is relatively resistant to mild disinfectants, sunlight, and pH. However, a 1: 10 solution of hypochlorite readily inactivates canine parvovirus. Canine parvovirus survives well in normal kennel conditions. Kenneled dogs may experience repeated outbreaks of canine parvoviral diarrhea. Moreover, immunosuppression is commonly associated with canine parvoviral infection. Dogs affected with canine parvovirus may succumb to adenoviral pneumonia and bacterial endotoxemia.

### Canine Coronavirus

Canine coronavirus is a pleomorphic and an enveloped RNA virus with an average size of 100 nm. On electron microscopy, coronaviruses are easily recognized by the club-shaped projections (peplomers) on their surface (Fig. 3). If canine coronavirus is suspected, the specimen should be shipped refrigerated but not frozen. With repeated freezing and thawing, virus particles lose their peplomers, compromising the ability of an electron microscopist to recognize them. At WAHL-M, canine coronavirus was detected in 4 of 107 fecal samples from dogs with a history of diarrhea. Viral antigens can also be detected in villus enterocytes by FAT. In some clinical cases of enteritis, canine parvovirus and canine coronavirus are simultaneously detected.

### Canine Rotavirus

Canine rotavirus is a nonenveloped RNA virus about 70 nm in size, with a double-stranded, segmented genome (Fig. 4). The virus is relatively resistant to lipid solvents and acidic conditions. Due to its segmented genome, the virus can mutate by genetic recombination.

Unlike other species, rotavirus is not a common cause of canine enteritis. Due to the presence of common group-specific internal capsid antigens, canine rotavirus can be detected in fecal samples by ELISA systems used to diagnose human rotavirus (Rotazyme, Abbott Laboratories, Chicago, IL).

### Canine Astrovirus

Canine astrovirus is an nonenveloped, relatively resistant RNA virus 28 nm in size. It is star shaped with five to six points (Fig. 5). It is occasionally detected in canine enteritis. Canine astrovirus was diagnosed at

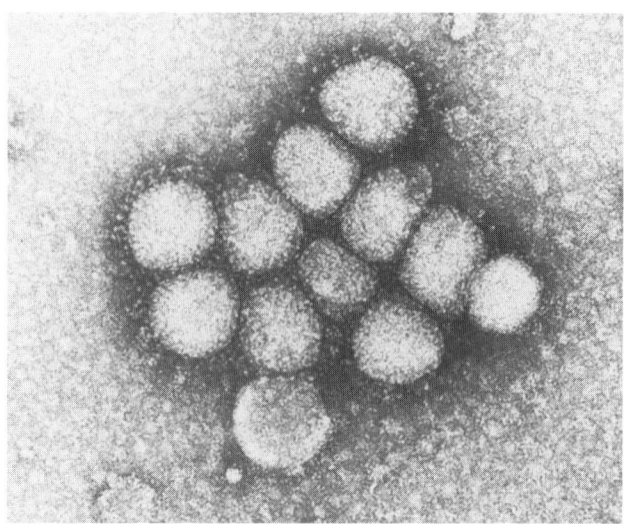

**Figure 3.** Bovine coronavirus. Virus has club-shaped projections.

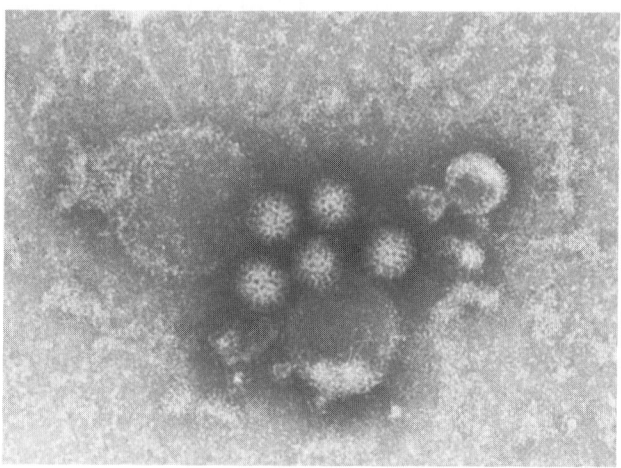

**Figure 4.** Bovine rotavirus. Virus particles have a rimmed cartwheel appearance.

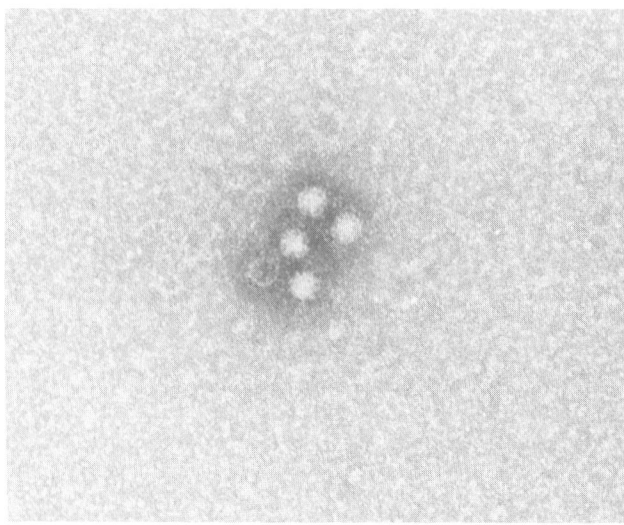

**Figure 5.** Canine astrovirus. Virus particles are star shaped.

WAHL-M in a dog with hemorrhagic enteritis. The dog was negative for parvovirus by ELISA and no significant bacterial pathogen was detected. After 3 days, the dog recovered.

### Canine Calicivirus

Canine calicivirus is an nonenveloped RNA virus about 35 nm in size, with cup-shaped depressions on the surface (Fig. 6). At WAHL-M, canine calicivirus was detected in 1 of 107 samples examined.

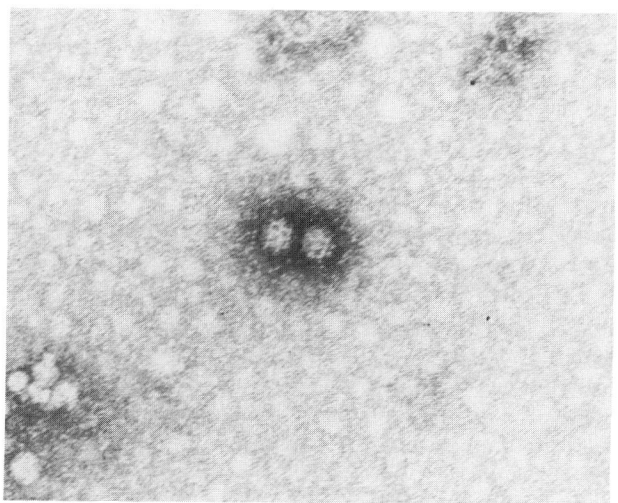

**Figure 6.** Feline calicivirus. Virus particles have cup-shaped depressions on their surface.

### Canine Herpesvirus

Canine herpesvirus has been detected in the feces of dogs with diarrhea (Evermann et al., 1982). However, presence of the virus in feces may be part of a generalized herpes viral infection. It is an enveloped, double-stranded DNA virus.

### Canine Distemper Virus

Canine distemper virus can cause diarrhea and the presence of virus in feces is part of the generalized canine distemper virus infection. It is an enveloped RNA virus.

Our knowledge about canine viral enteritis is limited compared to the information available about human viral enteritis or to the viral enteritis of farm animals. It is believed that other novel enteric viruses will no doubt be detected by direct electron microscopy and PCR techniques in future. Further research needs to be done to determine the presence of enteric viruses in clinically normal dogs.

### References and Suggested Reading

Evermann JF, McKeirnan AJ, Ott RL, et al: Diarrheal condition in dogs associated with viruses antigenically related to feline herpesvirus. Cornell Vet 72:285, 1982.
Flewett TH: Electron microscopy in the diagnosis of infectious diarrhea. J Am Vet Med Assoc 173:538, 1978.
Parrish CR, O'Connell PH, Evermann JF, et al: Natural variation of canine parvovirus. Science 230:1046, 1985.

# ACUTE DIARRHEA

ALBERT E. JERGENS
*Ames, Iowa*

Acute diarrhea is one of the most common clinical problems in veterinary practice, and is a consistent manifestation of intestinal disease in dogs and cats. It is characterized by an abrupt onset of watery or watery-mucoid diarrhea that tends to be self-limiting and of short duration. Mild acute diarrhea with or without vomiting may be caused by a variety of dietary, parasitic, or toxic factors. Other disorders, such as parvoviral enteritis and hemorrhagic gastroenteritis, are more fulminant and potentially life threatening. Although the specific cause for acute diarrhea in most animals is seldom identified, rational symptomatic therapy will reduce morbidity and, potentially, mortality in affected patients.

## PATHOGENESIS OF DIARRHEAS

Acute diarrhea may result from a variety of pathophysiologic processes (Moon, 1978). *Osmotic diarrhea* occurs when increased unabsorbed solutes remain in the intestinal lumen and hold water with them. Dietary overload caused by overeating or abrupt changes in diet are particularly common in young animals. *Secretory diarrheas* occur when abnormal amounts of ions and fluid are secreted into the intestinal lumen. A variety of secretory agents exist, with most generating their physiologic responses through activation of intracellular second messengers such as cyclic adenosine monophosphate (cAMP) and cyclic guanosine monophosphate (cGMP). These second messengers stimulate active chloride secretion and inhibit sodium absorption. The secretory diarrhea caused by *Campylobacter jejuni* infection is largely mediated by cAMP. *Increased intestinal permeability* results from diseases that produce mucosal inflammation, ulceration, or necrosis. Mild lesions alter tight junctions between epithelial cells, allowing the back-leakage of fluid and ions into the bowel lumen. Severe lesions, as seen with hemorrhagic gastroenteritis, cause increased permeability and the loss of large macromolecules such as albumin, globulins, and red blood cells. *Alterations in intestinal motility* can cause diarrhea as a consequence of either increased or decreased intestinal transit. Most diseases that alter motility, such as acute colitis, produce clinical signs because of decreased segmental contractions causing less intestinal resistance to the flow of ingesta.

Identification of the mechanism(s) causing acute diarrhea will assist the clinician in choosing the most appropriate therapeutic regimen. The prevalent causes of acute diarrhea in the dog and cat are listed in Table 1.

## DIAGNOSTIC STRATEGY

A tentative diagnosis of the cause for acute diarrhea is often obtained from history and physical examination. The history should include the patient's signalment; vaccination status; diet; current medications; and environmental exposure to toxins, parasites, or infectious disease. Young animals are prone to dietary, infectious, and parasitic causes for diarrhea. The risks for diarrhea are enhanced with environmental changes, following exposure to infectious agents, and in patients improperly immunized. Animals that roam freely may also develop parasitic, toxic, and infectious disorders. Dietary problems, such as ingestion of spoiled foods or indigestible material and adverse reactions to food, are

prominent causes of acute diarrhea. History should reveal recent dietary changes and identify responsible nutrients. The clinician should note current drug therapy (anti-inflammatory agents, antibiotics, digitalis) that may precipitate diarrhea. Evidence of multisystemic illness is seen with acute metabolic disturbances, toxicities, and certain infectious agents.

The clinical examination provides valuable information concerning the origin of diarrhea and the severity of the patient's present illness (Table 2). The clinician should complete an examination of all body sysytems, with particular emphasis on mentation, cardiovascular status, abdominal palpation, degree of hydration, and rectal examination. Warning signs of serious disease (fever, hypothermia, severe dehydration, abdominal pain, and bloody diarrhea) should be recognized to expedite diagnostic and therapeutic strategies appropriate for the patient.

## LABORATORY FINDINGS

Extensive diagnostic evaluation is seldom required, since most animals with acute diarrhea have mild signs that resolve easily. Visual inspection of feces for fecal consistency, evidence of melena or fresh blood, and the presence of foreign material should be performed. Fecal studies (fecal flotations for parasitic ova and direct fecal smears for protozoa) may detect intestinal parasites. Multiple fecal examinations should be performed to rule out parasitism. Fecal cytology has proven especially useful in the author's practice in identifying etiologic agents (*Clostridium* spores; see *CVT XI*, p 602) or inflammatory disease (fecal leukocytes) as causes for acute large bowel diarrhea. In patients suspected of having infectious diarrhea, perform fecal serology (enzyme-linked immunosorbent assay [ELISA]) for parvovirus or fecal cultures for enteropathogenic bacteria such as *Campylobacter jejuni* and *Salmonella* spp.

Additional laboratory studies (complete blood count [CBC], serum biochemistries, urinalysis, and survey/contrast abdominal radiography) are reserved for animals whose diarrhea is severe, bloody, or who have systemic signs of illness.

**Table 1.** *Possible Causes of Acute Diarrhea*

Dietary
　Abrupt dietary change
　Overeating
　Indiscretion ("garbage," foreign material)
　Food intolerance/allergy
Gastrointestinal inflammation
　Parasitism (helminths, protozoa)
　Bacterial enteritis (*Salmonella* spp.,° *Campylobacter jejuni,*
　　*Clostridium* spp.)
　Viral enteritis (parvovirus,° coronavirus)
　Salmon poisoning disease°
　Hemorrhagic gastroenteritis°
Drugs and toxins
　Anti-inflammatory agents
　Antimicrobials
　Antineoplastic drugs
　Heavy metals/organophosphates°
Functional/mechanical ileus°
Extraintestinal disorders
　Acute pancreatitis°
　Liver disease°
　Kidney disease°
　Hypoadrenocorticism°

°Potentially life threatening.

**Table 2.** *Differentiation of Small and Large Bowel Diarrhea*

| Sign | Small Bowel | Large Bowel |
|---|---|---|
| Quality of feces | Loose to watery | Loose to semisolid |
| Fecal volume | Usually increased | Normal to decreased |
| Frequency of defecation | Mildly increased | Greatly increased |
| Tenesmus | Absent | Present |
| Fecal blood | Melena | Hematochezia |
| Excess mucus | Absent | Present |
| Weight loss | Common | Uncommon |
| Vomiting | May be seen | May be seen |

# SYMPTOMATIC THERAPY OF ACUTE DIARRHEA

Most cases of acute diarrhea in dogs and cats are easily resolved. Symptomatic therapy remains largely empiric, since the causes for diarrheal disorders are often undetermined. The principal goals of symptomatic therapy are restoration and maintenance of fluid and electrolyte balance and bowel rest. Other concerns might include the use of drugs that alter gut motility and antimicrobial therapy for septicemia.

## Fluid Therapy

Fluid therapy in patients with acute diarrhea is directed toward correction of dehydration and acid-base derangements, replacement of electrolyte deficits, and provision for maintenance requirements and ongoing losses (Twedt and Grauer, 1982). Predictable alterations occurring in most patients include variable depletions of sodium, potassium, bicarbonate, and water due to loss of intestinal secretions. The loss of intestinal bicarbonate, the development of hypovolemia, and lactic acidosis from poor capillary perfusion cause metabolic acidosis. Decisions concerning which fluid to use, the route of administration, and the rate of delivery will be largely dictated by the clinical evaluation. Estimation of hydration status is an inexact science, but increased skin turgor, dry mucous membranes, prolonged capillary refill, and weak and rapid pulses are often associated with significant dehydration. Laboratory findings suggestive of dehydration include increased hematocrit, increased total protein concentration, and prerenal elevations of serum urea nitrogen (SUN) and creatinine.

The first-choice rehydration fluid should be a balanced electrolyte solution such as lactated Ringer's solution (LRS). This solution provides small amounts of potassium and large amounts of sodium chloride, and LRS is usually adequate in controlling mild to moderate metabolic acidosis (see "Strong Ions and Acid-Base Disorders," this volume p 121). Potassium chloride (KCl) supplementation to LRS is usually required and should be guided by measurement of serum potassium concentration. In the event that electrolyte analysis is unavailable, a safe dosage used by this author is 10 to 15 mEq of KCl per liter LRS. The volume of rehydration fluid to correct initial fluid deficits should be accurately calculated and given over a 4- to 6-hr period (Table 3). Mildly dehydrated animals may be managed with subcutaneous administration of fluids. The intravenous route is preferred for the rapid replacement of significant fluid deficits. Once replacement fluid losses have been corrected, additional fluid is required to supplant the patient's maintenance requirements (40 to 60 ml/kg/day) and ongoing losses from diarrhea. The adequacy of fluid therapy in correcting fluid deficits is assessed by repeated physical examination, measures of body weight, evaluation of hematocrit and total protein, and estimation of urine output.

***Table 3.*** *Calculation of Fluid Replacement Requirements*

1. Replacement requirement
   (a) Body weight (lb) × % dehydration × 500 = fluid deficit in milliliters
   (b) Body weight (kg) × % dehydration = fluid deficit in liters
2. Maintenance requirement
   40–60 ml/kg/day
3. Contemporary (ongoing) losses
   (a) Secondary to diarrhea
   (b) Secondary to vomiting

The sum of 1, 2, and 3 equals 24-hr fluid requirements

Oral rehydration therapy using isotonic glucose-electrolyte solutions has proven beneficial in animals that can ingest oral fluids. Oral fluid therapy is based on the observation that glucose stimulates small intestinal sodium absorption, creating a concomitant osmotic gradient for water absorption. Use of these solutions is principally indicated in patients having secretory diarrheas in which gut mucosal integrity is preserved (Zenger and Willard, 1989). A veterinary product (Enterolyte, Beecham Laboratories, Bristol, TN) of apparent clinical utility is presently available.

## Dietary Management

The initial dietary goal is to rest the gastrointestinal tract by withholding food for at least 24 hr. The potential benefits of dietary restriction include (1) decreased loss of mucosal epithelia due to the abrasive action of ingesta, (2) reduced risks of dietary hypersensitivity developing from dietary antigens that are absorbed intact, (3) minimizing colonization of the enteric flora by foreign bacteria, and (4) restoration of intestinal brush border disaccharidase activity. Controlled diets that are easily assimilated are recommended when feeding resumes. The ideal controlled diet is highly digestible, is relatively hypoallergenic but contains adequate protein of high biologic value; is reasonably palatable; and contains a minimum of fat, lactose, and additives.

Rice is the preferred carbohydrate in dogs, since it is more completely digested as compared to corn or wheat flours found in most commercial pet foods. This higher digestibility decreases the amount of nutrients remaining in the intestinal tract, a situation which is harmful. Excess nutrients contribute to bacterial overgrowth, which may alter gut motility and cause secretory diarrhea. In contrast, cats tend to be poorly tolerant of starch and should be fed a diet based instead on poultry protein. Acceptable sources of protein in dogs and cats include meat (lamb, lean beef, chicken) or dairy products (cooked eggs, low-fat cottage cheese). Dietary fat should be moderately restricted in dogs, since bacterial metabolites contribute to water secretion by the colon, which exacerbates diarrhea. Feeding the diarrheic cat a low-fat diet often worsens the diarrhea, whereas a diet relatively high in highly digestible fat will often lessen the diarrhea. Avoid feeding high-lactose diets because brush border lactase activities might be insufficient for digestion, and unabsorbed dietary lactose contributes to osmotic diarrhea. High-fiber diets may improve clinical signs of large bowel diarrhea in dogs caused by *Clostridium perfringen* enterotoxicosis (Twedt, 1992).

Examples of appropriate commercial foods used by this author include Prescription Diets canine i/d and feline c/d (Hill's Pet Products). Alternatively, home-prepared diets using a protein/carbohydrate ratio of 1 part protein (lean meats, low-fat cottage cheese) to 3 parts carbohydrate (white rice, pasta, potatoes) may be substituted in dogs. Homemade diets palatable to most cats include baby foods and sliced chicken. The diet is initially fed four to six times daily with one third the amount needed to meet caloric needs. Gradually increase the caloric intake over the next several days. Most acute diarrheas require 5 to 7 days of feeding the controlled diet until the character of the bowel movements normalize. At this time, the patient is weaned back to the normal diet.

### Antimicrobial Therapy

Routine administration of antibiotics for the treatment of acute diarrhea is uncommonly required. Antibiotic use is justified in animals having severe mucosal injury and a high risk for septicemia, as seen with parvoviral enteritis, hemorrhagic gastroenteritis, and salmon poisoning disease (see Section 4) (Dillon, 1984). Evidence of mucosal invasion by bacteria includes hemorrhagic diarrhea; increased fecal leukocytes; severe leukopenia; leukocytosis with a left shift; positive blood cultures; or clinical evidence of sepsis such as fever, depression hypoglycemia, or shock. Antibiotics

are also indicated when specific bacterial pathogens such as *Salmonella* spp., *Campylobacter jejuni*, and *Clostridium* spp. are suspected.

The choice of an appropriate antibacterial drug is dictated by several factors including the suspected etiologic organism, the antimicrobial spectrum of activity, host immunocompetence, and the potential disruptive effects of the antibiotic on the host microflora. Bactericidal drugs are preferred to bacteriostatic drugs in the management of animals with severe hemorrhagic diarrhea or those with compromised immune status. When possible, bacterial culture and antibiotic susceptibility testing should be obtained before antimicrobial therapy is initiated. Animals having positive fecal cultures for specific bacterial enteropathogens should be treated according to the susceptibility pattern of the isolated bacteria (Table 4). Empiric use of antibiotics in uncomplicated acute diarrhea is not recommended because of suppressive effects on the normal host microflora and the risk of promoting resistant status of bacteria.

### Motility Modifying Drugs

Narcotic analgesics (opioids) are probably the most effective motility modifying drugs for the symptomatic treatment of acute diarrhea in dogs (DeNovo, 1986). These drugs include paregoric, loperamide (Imodium, Janssen), and diphenoxylate (Lomotil, Searle). The antidiarrheal effects of these agents are attributed to their pharmacologic actions on intestinal motility and on fluid and electrolyte transport. Opioids directly increase rhythmic segmentation and decrease propulsive contractions of the intestinal smooth muscle. The net ef-

***Table 4.***  *Potential Pharmacotherapy for Acute Diarrhea*

| Drug | Trade Name (Manufacturer) | Dosage | Comment |
|---|---|---|---|
| **Narcotic Analgesics** | | | Contraindicated with infectious diarrhea |
| Paregoric (w/kaolin-pectin) | Parapectolin (Rorer) | .25–.05 mg/kg q8h PO | Do not use opioids in cats |
| Diphenoxylate | Lomotil (Searle) | 0.1–0.2 mg/kg q8h PO | |
| Loperamide | Imodium (Janssen) | 0.1–0.2 mg/kg q8h PO | |
| **Combination CNS Depressants and Anticholinergics** | | | The use of these drugs is uncommonly required; may cause ileus due to anticholinergic |
| Prochlorperazine and isopropamide | Darbazine (Norden) | <10 kg; No. 1 capsule q8h PO <br> >10 kg; No. 3 capsule q8h PO | |
| Chlordiazepoxide and clidinium | Librax (Roche) | 0.1–0.25 mg/kg (clidinium) q8–12h PO | |
| **Antimicrobial Agents** | | | |
| Erythromycin | *Many* | 10 mg/kg q8h PO | Treatment for *Campylobacter jejuni* |
| Enrofloxacin | Baytril (Miles) | 2.5–5 mg/kg q12h PO | Treatment for invasive *Salmonella* spp. |
| Trimethoprim-sulfonamide | Tribrissen (Cooper) | 15 mg/kg q12h PO | |
| Metronidazole | *Many* | 10–20 mg/kg q8–12h PO | Treatment for *Clostridium* spp. |
| **Antisecretory/Protectant** | | | |
| Bismuth subsalicylate | Pepto-Bismol (Proctor & Gamble) | 1.0 ml/kg initially PO, then decrease dosage | Use cautiously in cats, due to salicylate fraction |

fect of narcotic analgesics is to inhibit the flow of intestinal contents. Some opioids are also potent inhibitors of intestinal secretion and they increase mucosal absorption of fluids, electrolytes, and glucose. These drugs are reserved for short-term use, probably no more than 5 to 7 days, and are most appropriate in treating secretory diarrheas (Willard, 1985). Paregoric is most conveniently used in small dogs (<10 kg), since it is available as a liquid. Loperamide reportedly has a faster onset of action and greater antisecretory effects as compared to diphenoxylate.

Narcotic analgesics are not innocuous drugs. Since opioids are narcotics, they may produce central nervous system (CNS) depression in dogs if used inappropriately. Opioids are not recommended for use in cats and are contraindicated in animals having diarrhea resulting from infection with invasive bacteria. In these cases, drug-induced decreases in intestinal transit facilitate microbial proliferation, mucosal invasion, and absorption of bacterial toxins.

Pure anticholinergic drugs serve no useful role in the symptomatic therapy of acute diarrhea. They function to reduce both peristaltic and segmental contractions within the intestinal tract, resulting in less resistance to the flow of ingesta. Due to their generalized suppression of bowel motility, anticholinergics can precipitate ileus and subsequently promote bacterial overgrowth of the small intestine.

Combination CNS depressants with anticholinergics have been successfully used by this author to treat a handful of stress-related gastrointestinal disturbances in dogs. Two drugs that have proven effective include Darbazine (Norden) and Librax (Roche). These drugs should be reserved for use in dogs having large bowel diarrhea refractory to more conventional therapies (also see *CVT XI*, p 604).

## Miscellaneous Therapeutics

A variety of intestinal protectants and absorbents including kaolin, pectin, activated charcoal, and barium sulfate are reported to act locally in the gut by coating the intestinal wall and absorbing various bacteria and toxins. Clinical studies confirming the efficacy of these agents is lacking and their use is not recommended. However, bismuth subsalicylate, the active ingredient in Pepto-Bismol, is an effective agent for the treatment of acute non-specific diarrhea (Dupont et al., 1980). This drug has antienterotoxin, antisecretory, and anti-inflammatory actions that are probably mediated through antiprostaglandin mechanisms. Use this drug cautiously in cats due to their low tolerance for salicylates. Lastly, consider a therapeutic trial with an appropriate anthelmintic (Cornelius and Roberson, 1986) in dogs and cats suspicious for parasitic causes of acute diarrhea.

The prognosis for cure of self-limiting diarrhea is excellent. These animals may be successfully managed with dietary restriction, replacement of mild fluid deficits, and correction of the predisposing cause if identified. Life-threatening causes of acute diarrhea will require in-depth diagnostic evaluation and vigorous intravenous fluid therapy.

## References and Suggested Reading

Cornelius LM and Roberson EL: Treatment of gastrointestinal parasitism. *In* Kirk RW (ed): *Current Veterinary Therapy IX*. Philadelphia, WB Saunders Co, 1986, p 921.
*A listing of clinically useful drugs for treating common canine and feline gastrointestinal parasites.*
DeNovo RC: Therapeutics of gastrointestinal diseases. *In* Kirk RW, (ed): *Current Veterinary Therapy IX*. Philadelphia, WB Saunders Co, 1986, p 862.
*A review of drugs and their dosages commonly employed in the treatment of small animal gastrointestinal diseases.*
Dillon R: Therapeutic strategies involving antimicrobial treatment of the gastrointestinal tract in small animals. J Am Vet Med Assoc 185:1169, 1984.
*The use of antimicrobials in the treatment of gastroenteritis is justified only in specific clinical situations.*
Dupont HL, Sullivan P, Evans DG, et al: Prevention of traveler's diarrhea (emporiatric enteritis) prophylactic administration of subsalicylate bismuth. JAMA 243:237, 1980.
*A human clinical study showing the beneficial effects of bismuth subsalicylate in treating secretory diarrheas.*
Moon HW: Mechanisms in the pathogenesis of diarrhea: A review. J Am Vet Med Assoc 172:443, 1978.
*A review article on the pathophysiologic mechanisms causing diarrhea.*
Twedt DC: *Clostridium perfringens*–associated enterotoxicosis in dogs. *In* Kirk RW and Bonagura JD (eds): *Current Veterinary Therapy XI*. Philadelphia, WB Saunders Co, 1992, p 602.
*A description of the clinical signs, diagnosis, and treatment of* Clostridium perfringens *enterotoxicosis in dogs.*
Twedt DC and Grauer GF: Fluid therapy for gastrointestinal, pancreatic, and hepatic disorders. Vet Clin North Am 12:463, 1982.
*General principles pertaining to fluid therapy in animals with gastrointestinal disorders are discussed.*
Willard MD: Newer concepts in treatment of secretory diarrheas. J Am Vet Med Assoc 186:86, 1985.
*A concise review on the pharmacologic management of secretory diarrhea in the dog and cat.*
Zenger E and Willard MD: Oral rehydration therapy in companion animals. Companion Anim Pract 19:6, 1989.
*This article discusses the indications, pathophysiology, and clinical use of oral rehydration therapy.*

# GASTROINTESTINAL ULCER THERAPY

MICHAEL E. MATZ

*Tucson, Arizona*

The increased use of endoscopy and increased understanding of ulcer pathogenesis have enhanced the awareness of veterinary clinicians to the presence of gastrointestinal (GI) ulcer disease in small animals. The true incidence of GI ulcers in small animals is unknown, but is probably more prevalent than is recognized clinically. Clinical signs in patients with GI ulceration may be inapparent or may be attributed to the more recognizable predisposing cause. Until recently, treatment for GI ulcers centered on neutralizing or reducing gastric acid secretion; however, advancements in the understanding of GI ulceration pathophysiology have resulted in increased therapeutic options. Treatment can be aimed not only to heal, but in certain cases to prevent the development of GI ulcers. Presently, the therapeutic focus has broadened to include agents that enhance mucosal defense mechanisms. These cytoprotective agents exert beneficial effects without changing the concentration of acid in the gastric lumen. The purpose of this article is to review recent information regarding antiulcer drugs and to discuss the use of these drugs in the medical management of GI ulcers in small animals. Due to the limited number of clinical trials evaluating the use of antiulcer drugs in small animals, much of the information presented is based on studies in human patients and on clinical experience in dogs and cats.

## OVERVIEW OF ULCER PATHOPHYSIOLOGY AND MUCOSAL DEFENSE

Gastrointestinal mucosal integrity is maintained through mucosal defense mechanisms which balance the ulcerogenic effects of acid and pepsin. When excessive acid production, impaired mucosal defense, or both situations develop, ulceration may occur. Previously, the presence of excessive gastric acid was emphasized as the primary cause of this imbalance. Although there is clear evidence for the importance of acid in the development of GI ulcers, in most cases the primary pathogenic mechanism appears to be disruption of mucosal defense. Gastrointestinal mucosal defense is the result of many separate and interacting components including mucus and bicarbonate secretion, mucosal hydrophobicity, epithelial cell turnover and restitution, mucosal blood flow, and mucosal prostaglandins.

Mucus and bicarbonate secreted by surface epithelial cells in the stomach and Brunner's glands located in the submucosa of the duodenum are the first level of mucosal defense. Mucus is composed of glycoproteins that adhere to the luminal surface and protect the underlying epithelium by entrapping bicarbonate. These entrapped anions in turn buffer the influxing luminal protons and establish a pH gradient across the thickness of the mucous layer, ranging from a pH of 2 to 3 at the luminal surface to a pH of 7 near the epithelium.

Mucosal hydrophobicity excludes or retards the absorption of potentially damaging water-soluble luminal contents by gastric mucosa. Surface-active phospholipids appear to be the major contributor to this hydrophobicity, although mucus glycoproteins also may play a role. The precise location of this barrier has not been established, but may in whole or part reside in the mucous layer or within the plasmalemma of epithelial cells.

The GI epithelium resists injury through continual rapid cell turnover (2 to 4 days). When damaged, the epithelium may be replaced by migration of surviving cells from the edge of the defect (restitution) or by division of the surviving cells. Cell restitution is the most rapid means of repair. Healthy epithelial cells adjacent to a defect respond by expanding pseudopodia and migrating to cover the epithelial defect. Within 15 to 30 min, minor damage to the epithelial surface can be repaired.

Protection against gastrointestinal mucosal injury is provided by a dense network of capillaries that lie beneath the surface epithelium. In addition to supplying oxygen and nutrients to the epithelium, the high rate of mucosal blood flow allows for the rapid removal of substances that have penetrated the epithelial barrier. Maintenance of gastric mucosal blood flow is essential for the maintenance of mucosal defense, and the extent of damage to this component is central to whether ongoing mucosal damage or restoration will ensue following an insult.

Mucosal defense mechanisms are at least partially dependent on the production of mucosal prostaglandins. These mediators stimulate secretion of mucus and bicarbonate, maintain mucosal hydrophobicity, stimulate cell division and restitution, and sustain mucosal blood flow. In addition, endogenous prostaglandins may inhibit gastric secretion. Mucosal prostaglandins arise from the arachidonic acid pathway as a result of stimulation or perturbation of the GI mucosa. Arachidonic acid is converted to prostaglandins by the actions of the enzymes phospholipase and cyclooxygenase. Prostaglandins of the E type appear to play the most significant in mucosal defense in the gastrointestinal tract.

The consequence of a breach in any superficial component of mucosal defense appears to be minimal so long as the other components remain intact. Disruption of the mucous layer and superficial epithelium (erosion) stimulates the production of mediators (e.g., prostaglandins), which increase blood flow and stimulate cell restitution and replication leading to rapid healing. Failure of these compensatory components of mucosal defense to overcome ulcerogenic factors leads to extension of the injury through the muscularis mucosae into the submucosa (i.e., ulceration).

## PREDISPOSING FACTORS AND CONDITIONS

In general, GI ulceration in small animals is associated with drug administration or clinical conditions that cause mucosal damage. A list of drugs and conditions that have been recognized to be associated with GI ulceration are found in Table 1. The specific pathophysiologic mechanisms by which these drugs and conditions cause or may cause mucosal injury have been well described elsewhere (Moreland, 1988). The majority of these factors predispose to ulcer formation by damaging mucosal defenses. In the author's experience, the use of nonsteroidal anti-inflammatory drugs is the most common cause of GI ulceration in small animals. Gastrinoma and mastocytosis are the only conditions in which hyperacidity is considered to be a primary underlying mechanism for ulcer formation. While liver disease and renal failure do elevate gastrin levels, a corresponding increase in gastric acid secretion has not been demonstrated in human patients or animals.

*Helicobacter pylori* is now known to be a major predisposing factor for the development of gastrointestinal ulcers in human beings. *Helicobacter felis* has been cultured from cats, and other spiral-shaped organisms (possibly *Helicobacter heilmanii*, formerly *Gastrosporillium hominis*) have been found on gastric biopsies from dogs and cats (see "Helicobacter-Associated Gastric Disease in Ferrets, Dogs, and Cats," this volume, p 720). The clinical significance of these organisms in small animals is uncertain and the value of treatment for these organisms is undetermined.

## ANTIULCER DRUGS

### Drugs that Reduce Gastric Acidity

The approach to suppression of gastric acid secretion is based upon evidence that acid reduction heals ulcers in most patients. This evidence supports the opinion that hydrochloric acid is a major factor that interferes with ulcer healing despite considerations that hyperacidity is most often not a contributing factor. By suppressing gastric acid secretion, the balance is tipped toward the mucosal defenses, which allows healing of ulcers. Additionally, a reduction is gastric acidity may significantly decrease the inhibitory effect of pepsin on ulcer healing.

An appreciation of the basic physiology of gastric acid secretion is clinically useful. Gastric acid secretion occurs in the oxyntic (parietal) cell and is stimulated by gastrin, histamine, and acetylcholine. Each of these secretagogues stimulate acid secretion independently, with histamine being the most potent stimulator of gastric acid secretion. However, simultaneous occupation of receptors for gastrin, histamine ($H_2$), and acetylcholine on the basolateral membrane is necessary for maximal stimulation of gastric acid secretion. Receptor stimulation triggers intracellular events involving cyclic adenosine monophosphate (cAMP) histamine, and calcium (gastrin, acetylcholine). This stimulation causes acid secretion to occur at the luminal border through the activation of a hydrogen-potassium ATPase (proton) pump.

#### HISTAMINE $H_2$-RECEPTOR ANTAGONISTS

The histamine $H_2$-receptor antagonists are histamine analogs that selectively and reversibly bind $H_2$-receptors on the oxyntic cell, inhibiting the potent acid secretagogue effect of histamine. $H_2$-Receptor antagonists commonly used in small animals include cimetidine (Tagamet, SmithKline Beecham), ranitidine (Zantac, Glaxo), and famotidine (Pepcid, Merck). These drugs differ in relative potencies, with ranitidine four to ten times more potent and famotidine 20 to 40 times more potent than cimetidine. Despite differences in potency, these drugs have been shown to be equally effective at promoting ulcer healing. Choice of $H_2$-receptor antagonists should be based on considerations of cost, client convenience, and concurrent drug therapy. The longer elimination half-life of ranitidine and

**Table 1.** *Conditions and Drugs Associated with Gastrointestinal Ulceration in Small Animals*

| Impaired Mucosal Defense | Hyperacidity |
|---|---|
| Drugs | Gastrinoma |
|   NSAIDs° | Mastocytosis |
|   Corticosteroids | |
| Stress | |
|   Shock | |
|   Sepsis | |
|   Trauma | |
|   Major surgery | |
| Neurologic disease | |
|   Head trauma | |
|   Intervertebral disk disease† | |
| Metabolic disorders | |
|   Liver disease | |
|   Renal disease | |
|   Pancreatitis | |
| Inflammatory bowel disease | |
| Gastrointestinal neoplasia | |
| Mastocytosis | |
| Gastric motility disorders | |

°NSAIDs that have been associated with GI ulcers in small animals include: aspirin, indomethacin, phenylbutazone, flunixin, ibuprofen, naproxen, and piroxicam.
†Treated with corticosteroids.
Abbreviations: NSAIDs = nonsteroidal anti-inflammatory drugs, GI = gastrointestinal.

famotidine may allow these drugs to be administered less often than cimetidine.

The $H_2$-receptor antagonists are remarkably safe. Cimetidine and, to a lesser extent, ranitidine reversibly bind to the hepatic cytochrome P-450 enzyme system and can interfere with the clearance of drugs metabolized by this route. In most cases this interaction is not of clinical significance. Careful monitoring should be undertaken when administering cimetidine with theophylline, warfarin, or coumadin. The increased intragastric pH associated with the effect of $H_2$-receptor antagonists may decrease the absorption of drugs that require an acid medium for dissolution and absorption such as ketoconazole. Finally, since $H_2$-receptor antagonists undergo 50 to 70% renal excretion, dosages should be reduced by 50% in patients with impaired renal function.

### PROTON PUMP INHIBITORS

Exchange of cellular $H^+$ for luminal $K^+$ by the proton pump on the apical border of the oxyntic cell is the final step in acid secretion. Inhibition of the proton pump ($H^+/K^+$ ATPase) prevents gastric acid secretion by any secretagogue. Omeprazole is currently the only available proton pump inhibitor. Omeprazole as a prodrug requires protonation to become activated. This weak base enters the oxyntic cell from plasma, where it becomes protonated and thereby trapped. The drug, now in its active form, binds irreversibly to the proton pump, producing prolonged acid inhibition. New ATPase must be synthesized before acid production can resume. A single daily dose exerts an effect for up to 24 hr.

Similar to some of the $H_2$-receptor antagonists, omeprazole inhibits the activity of the hepatic cytochrome P-450 system and may influence the disposition of drugs metabolized through this pathway (see "Effects of Hepatic Disease on Drug Disposition," this volume, p 758). Whether this pharmacokinetic effect is of clinical consequence remains to be determined, but no consequential drug interactions have been reported thus far. Like all agents that raise the gastric pH, omeprazole diminishes the absorption of drugs that require acid for absorption such as ketoconazole, ampicillin, and iron.

Unlike the $H_2$-receptor antagonists, omeprazole causes a marked increase in serum gastrin. Prolonged hypergastrinemia has been associated with the development of gastric carcinoids in rats administered high dosages of omeprazole for extended periods. Profound and prolonged acid suppression could predispose to bacterial colonization of the stomach and enteric infections. Despite these concerns, clinically significant side effects of this nature have not been reported in human patients even after long-term administration.

Healing rates of GI ulcers in human beings treated with omeprazole appear to be modestly superior compared to those associated with $H_2$-receptor antagonists. However, these findings are of little clinical significance and do not justify the greater expense of omeprazole

in routine antiulcer medication regimens. Omeprazole is best used for the treatment of ulcers refractory to treatment or ulcers associated with gastrinomas and mastocytosis.

## Cytoprotective Agents

### ANTACIDS

Liquid antacids are as effective as other antiulcer drugs. The use of these drugs in veterinary medicine, however, had been largely abandoned in favor of $H_2$-receptor antagonists and sucralfate, as frequent administration (6 to 12 times daily) of large dosages (0.5 to 1.0 ml/kg) of antacids is required to ensure continuous acid neutralization and promote ulcer healing. Recently, the administration of one antacid tablet containing aluminum hydroxide four times daily has been shown to be as effective as higher dosages of liquid antacids and cimetidine in healing gastric and duodenal ulcers in human patients. This effect appears to occur independent of the acid neutralizing ability of the antacid. Evidence suggests ulcer healing may reside in the ability of aluminum-containing antacids to stimulate mucosal defense mechanisms. In addition, aluminum-containing antacids effectively bind pepsin. This makes aluminum-containing antacid tablets a potential alternative for treatment of GI ulcers in small animals. Such treatment could be useful due to the low cost of these drugs and the ease of administering antacid tablets as compared to antacid liquids in small animals. Clinical studies are needed to evaluate this form of therapy.

The most common side effect of aluminum-containing antacids is constipation. This side effect is minimized on the low-dose regimen and by combining aluminum with magnesium hydroxide. Since aluminum-containing antacids may interfere with the absorption of a number of drugs, it is advisable to separate the oral administration of antacids from other drugs. Aluminum-containing antacids bind phosphate and may result in hypophosphatemia.

### SUCRALFATE

Sucralfate (Carafate, Marion) is a complex salt of sucrose sulfate and aluminum hydroxide. Originally, this drug was thought to promote ulcer healing solely by binding to the surface of the ulcer and providing a physical barrier between luminal contents and the mucosal surface, thereby impairing the diffusion of acid and pepsin. However, the major drug actions of sucralfate that contribute to ulcer healing are related to stimulation of mucosal defense and reparative mechanisms and antipeptic effects. Those mechanisms are induced by both prostaglandin-dependent and prostaglandin-independent pathways. Although sucralfate requires the presence of acid to bind to the ulcer bed, it has been shown to be effective therapeutically even at neutral intragastric pH. Sucralfate has been shown to be as effective as $H_2$-receptor antagonist for healing of GI ulcers in human patients.

As a consequence of its poor solubility, only small amounts of sucralfate are absorbed systemically, and no systemic toxicities have been reported. Sucralfate does not affect the metabolism or elimination of other drugs, but it can affect drug absorption from the GI tract. Drugs that interact with sucralfate include: fluoroquinolones, tetracycline, theophylline, aminophylline, and digoxin. If given 2 hr before sucralfate administration, the bioavailability of tetracycline and digoxin is not reduced. As an aluminum-containing drug, sucralfate can cause constipation and hypophosphatemia.

## THERAPEUTIC CHOICES

### Ulcer Healing

Therapy for GI ulceration is first directed at the initiating cause (e.g., discontinuation of ulcerogenic drugs, tumor removal) and providing supportive care (e.g., fluids, blood transfusion, nutritional support). Antiulcer drug therapy (Table 2) should be based on the confirmed or suspected underlying mechanism(s) involved in ulcer formation.

Ulcers caused by the interference of mucosal defense mechanisms can be effectively treated with either $H_2$-receptor antagonists or sucralfate. Although it is tempting to treat GI ulcers with two drugs such as an $H_2$-receptor blocker and sucralfate, there is no evidence that such a combination is beneficial. Recent evidence regarding low-dose aluminum-coating antacid tablet administration is promising. However, additional clinical experience is needed before this approach can be confidently recommended and the necessity of four-time-daily administration may still be a limiting factor for its use. Based on studies in human patients, routine antiulcer therapy should be continued for a minimum of 4 weeks and preferentially for 6 to 8 weeks. Opti-

mally, ulcer healing should be determined by endoscopic evaluation.

With gastrinoma and mastocytosis, where gastric hyperacidity represents the primary contribution to ulcer formation, omeprazole is the drug of choice. $H_2$-Receptor antagonists, in the author's experience, have been less effective for the treatment of these conditions. Therapy is continued indefinitely unless complete surgical resection of the tumor is possible.

Refractory ulcers are those that do not heal following recommended treatment or that recur promptly after treatment. Owner compliance should be investigated. Poor compliance may be due to cost of medication. It may be better to prescribe a less expensive alternative drug treatment that the owner will administer rather than have the optimal but more expensive drug not administered. Persistent administration of a nonsteroidal anti-inflammatory drug (NSAID) may also cause failure of ulcers to heal or precipitate ulcer reformation. Refractory ulcers should also prompt a search for a gastrin-producing tumor by obtaining a fasting serum gastrin level. A thorough search for evidence of localized or systemic mast cell neoplasia should also be performed. Endoscopic or surgical biopsy of refractory ulcers, unassociated with the aforementioned causes should be done, as the possibility of malignancy, rather than an unhealed benign ulcer, must be considered. If these causes are eliminated, consider continuing treatment with $H_2$-antagonists or sucralfate for a longer period of time or switching to omeprazole.

Severe gastric blood loss resulting from ulceration can be controlled in most cases with aggressive fluid therapy and blood transfusion, along with administration of an $H_2$-receptor antagonist or sucralfate. Surgical intervention is required for patients in which acute bleeding fails to respond to conservative management or when GI perforation is suspected or has occurred. The use of iced gastric lavages, with or without epinephrine, to control gastric bleeding is ineffective, and may worsen the bleeding. In human patients, severe bleeding from GI ulcers may be controlled by endoscopically administered hemostatic therapy and this treatment may also prove effective in small animals.

**Table 2.** *Approximate Dosages for Antiulcer Drugs Used in Small Animals**

| Drug | Dose |
| --- | --- |
| Cimetidine | 10 mg/kg q8h, PO, IM, IV |
| | 12 mg/kg/day continuous IV infusion[†] |
| Ranitidine | *Dog*: 2 mg/kg q8h, PO, IV |
| | *Cat*: 2.5 mg/kg, q12h, IV |
| | 3.5 mg/kg q12h, PO |
| | 2 mg/kg/day continuous IV infusion[†] |
| Famotidine | 0.5 mg/kg q12–24h, PO, SC, IM, IV |
| Omeprazole | *Dog*: 0.7 mg/kg q24h, PO |
| | (>20 kg, 20 mg/dog; <20 kg, 10 mg/dog) |
| | *Cats*: not recommended |
| Aluminum hydroxide tablets | *Dog*: 0.5–1 tablet q6h |
| | *Cat*: 0.25 tablet q6h |
| Sucralfate | *Dog*: 0.5–1 gm, q8–12h, PO |
| | *Cat*: 0.25 gm q8–12h, PO |
| Misoprostol | *Dog*: 2–5 µg/kg q8h, PO[†] |
| | *Cat*: dose not established |

*Modified from Papich MG: Antiulcer therapy. Vet Clin North Am [Small Anim Pract] 234:497–512, 1993, with permission.
[†]Ulcer prophylaxis.

### Ulcer Prophylaxis

#### NSAID-INDUCED ULCERS

Misoprostol (Cytotec, Searle) is a synthetic prostaglandin $E_1$ analog that both inhibits gastric acid secretion and stimulates gastric mucosal defense mechanisms (Table 2). It is as effective as other ulcer-healing agents in treating GI ulcers based on results of studies in human patients. However, the lack of a demonstrated advantage over $H_2$-receptor antagonists and side effects have precluded misoprostol's use as a first-line antiulcer therapy in human patients. The primary therapeutic indication in human patients has been prophylaxis against gastric mucosal injury caused by NSAIDs. Similar therapeutic findings have been demonstrated in a limited number of dogs. Since $H_2$-receptor antagonists have not been shown to be of prophylactic benefit against NSAID-induced gastric ulceration, it is unlikely that the efficacy of misoprostol is the result of its inhibition of gastric acid secretion. Development of gastric mucosal hemorrhage, erosion, and ulceration associated with administration of NSAIDs is largely attributed to reduction of prostaglandin synthesis in the gastric mucosa.

Misoprostol administration is generally well tolerated. A consistent adverse effect associated with misoprostol administration in human beings has been the development of a self-limiting, secretory diarrhea shortly after initiation of treatment. Misoprostol may increase uterine contractility, which could provoke abortion. Therefore, it should not be used in pregnant animals.

The apparently low prevalence of clinically evident NSAID-induced gastric ulcer suggests misoprostol use may be best reserved for patients with a previous history of ulcer requiring chronic NSAID therapy or in older debilitated patients in whom an NSAID-induced ulcer and attendant complications would be life threatening.

### STRESS-RELATED ULCERS

In human beings, stress-related mucosal disease (SRMD) is characteristic of severely ill patients, especially those with burns, central nervous system trauma, sepsis, shock, multiple organ failure, or following a major surgical procedure. The pathophysiologic mechanisms involved in SRMD are not completely understood, but it is known that acid and pepsin play a significant role. Stress-related mucosal disease results in bleeding in a significant number of human patients and can be severe enough in some cases to require aggressive hemodynamic support. Although not well documented, a similar scenario probably exists in small animals. The best approach to SRMD may be prevention. Antacid (high doses), $H_2$-receptor antagonist (cimetidine, ranitidine), and sucralfate administration are equally effective in reducing the incidence of SRMD in human patients. The use of antacids is discouraged due to the need to administer high doses at frequent intervals to maintain intragastric pH above 4, a pH below 4 is required to activate pepsinogen to its proteolytic form, pepsin. Continuous intravenous infusions of $H_2$-receptor antagonists (Table 2) are superior to intermittent bolus administration in maintaining intragastric pH above 4. It is emphasized that the random use of prophylactic therapy is not justified and that therapy should be limited to those cases in which clinical findings support the likelihood of mucosal damage and ulceration.

## References and Suggested Reading

Hurwitz AK: Clinical pharmacology of agents for the treatment of acid related disorders. *In* Lakin D and Dhinnenberg AJ (eds): *Peptic Ulcer Disease and Other Acid Related Disorders.* New York, Academic Research Associates, 1991, p 339.
*Complete review of antiulcer drugs used to treat gastric and duodenal ulcers in humans.*

Jenkins CC, DeNovo RC, Patton CS, et al: Comparison of the effects of cimetidine and omeprazole on mechanically created gastric ulceration and on aspirin induced gastritis in dogs. Am J Vet Res 52:658, 1991.
*A prospective study comparing the ability of cimetidine and omeprazole to heal mechanically induced gastric ulcers and prevent aspirin-induced gastric mucosal injury.*

Moreland KJ: Ulcer disease of the upper gastrintestinal tract in small animals: Pathophysiology, diagnosis and management. Compend Cont Educ Pract Vet 10:1265, 1988.
*A review of pathophysiology, causes, diagnosis, and treatment of gastric and duodenal ulceration in the dog and cat.*

Murtaugh RJ, Matz ME, Labato MA, et al: Use of a synthetic prostaglandin $E_1$ (misoprostol) for prevention of aspirin-induced gastroduodenal ulceration in arthritic dogs. J Am Vet Med Assoc 202:251, 1993.
*A prospective study comparing misoprostol to placebo in the ability to prevent gastric or duodenal ulcers in arthritic dogs administered therapeutic dosages of unbuffered aspirin.*

Nompleggi DJ and Wolfe MM: Peptic ulcer disease, pathogenesis and treatment. *In* Lakin D and Dhinnenberg AJ (eds): *Peptic Ulcer Disease and Other Acid Related Disorders.* New York, Academic Research Associates, 1991, p 33.
*Complete review of pathogenesis, treatment, and prevention of gastric and duodenal ulcers in humans.*

Papich MG: Antiulcer therapy. Vet Clin North Am [Small Anim Pract] 23: 513, 1993.
*A thorough review of the clinical pharmacology of antiulcer drugs used in small animals.*

Stanton ME and Bright RM: Gastroduodenal ulceration in dogs. A retrospective study of 43 cases and literature review. J Vet Intern Med 3:238, 1989.
*Evaluates the causes, clinical findings, treatment, and outcome of 43 dogs with gastric or duodenal ulcers and summarizes previously reported cases of dogs with gastroduodenal ulceration.*

Wallace MS, Zawie DA, and Garvey MS: Gastric ulceration in the dog secondary to the use of nonsteroidal anti-inflammatory drugs. J Am Anim Hosp Assoc 26:467, 1990.
*A retrospective study reviewing the clinical findings and treatment of seven dogs with nonsteroidal anti-inflammatory drug–induced gastric ulceration.*

Wallace JL: Mucosal defense. New avenues for treatment of ulcer disease. Gastroenterol Clin North Am 19:87, 1990.
*Review of current knowledge regarding mucosal defense and its response to injury.*

Weberg R, Aubert E. Dahlberg O, et al: Low dose antacids or cimetidine for duodenal ulcer. Gastroenterology 95:1465, 1988.
*A prospective study comparing low dose of an aluminum-containing antacid to cimetidine in the ability to heal duodenal ulcers in human patients.*

# CANINE GASTROINTESTINAL PARASITES

CRAIG R. REINEMEYER

*Knoxville, Tennessee*

Gastrointestinal parasitism is commonly observed in dogs of all ages, but the prevalence of infection is particularly high in pups because certain routes of transmission are unique to neonates and because young dogs have less acquired immunity to parasitism. In mature dogs, infection usually results from exposure to a contaminated environment or from predation on intermediate or paratenic hosts. The indiscriminate defecatory habits of dogs ensure environmental contamination and perpetuate the risk of parasitic infection for dogs and other hosts, including humans.

Gastrointestinal parasitisms of dogs are diagnosed by demonstration of the parasitic organisms or their reproductive products in feces. The most common diagnostic procedure is fecal flotation, a concentration technique that is adequately described in other sources (Georgi and Georgi, 1990; Sloss, Kemp, and Zajac, 1994). A fecal smear is an inferior substitute, but may be necessary when only a small sample is available. A few canine parasitisms are diagnosed more readily by techniques other than flotation, and those exceptions are noted herein. For additional information about the identification of parasitic products in feces, readers should consult textbooks and diagnostic manuals containing photomicrographs of parasitologic specimens (Georgi and Georgi, 1990; Sloss, Kemp, and Zajac, 1994). Feline gastrointestinal parasites were reviewed in *CVT XI*, p 626.

A great variety of safe and effective drugs are approved for the management of canine gastrointestinal parasitism. With many similar options, drug choices may be affected by issues such as economics, convenience of administration, and an appropriate spectrum of activity to treat multiple parasitisms. Many cases of canine gastrointestinal parasitism are not accompanied by obvious clinical signs, and the benefits of treatment are equivocal. Nevertheless, the aesthetic concerns of dog owners virtually dictate parasite removal. In addition, some parasites of dogs cause important zoonotic conditions, and control is desirable from a public health standpoint.

The major gastrointestinal parasites of dogs are classified in three taxonomic groups: nematodes, cestodes, and protozoa.

## NEMATODE PARASITES OF DOGS

### Ascarids or Roundworms

The canine ascarids *Toxocara canis* and *Toxascaris leonina* are relatively large worms (7 to 8 cm) that reside in the small intestine as adults.

#### TOXOCARA CANIS

*Toxocara canis* is the most prevalent canine ascarid, occurring in up to 90% of all pups by some estimates. The major route of transmission is prenatal infection, in which quiescent (i.e., arrested) *Toxocara* larvae in the tissues of a bitch are stimulated by factors associated with pregnancy to migrate to the uterus and invade the developing fetuses. *Toxocara* eggs appear in the feces of prenatally infected pups within 3 weeks after birth. Alternate routes of infection for *T. canis* include ingestion of embryonated ova or paratenic hosts, and larvae must undergo systemic migration before reaching maturity in the gut.

*Toxocara canis* infections remain patent for a few months, but as early as 5 weeks of age dogs can develop acquired immunity to oral routes of reinfection. Repeated exposure after the development of immunity does not result in patent infections, but rather in the accumulation of arrested larvae in somatic tissues (Parsons, 1987). Arrested larvae constitute a dead-end stage in males and neutered females, however, and can only be transmitted vertically by pregnant bitches.

The ingestion of embryonated *T. canis* eggs by humans results in the liberation and systemic migration of ascarid larvae, with potential damage to the eyes and other organs. These zoonotic syndromes, known respectively as ocular and visceral larva migrans, are distressingly common in North American children.

#### TOXASCARIS LEONINA

*Toxascaris leonina* infects domestic and exotic canids and felids, and is less common than *Toxocara canis*. Infection occurs only through the ingestion of embryonated eggs or intermediate hosts such as small mammals. *Toxascaris leonina* does not migrate systemically and has no zoonotic potential.

CLINICAL SIGNS AND DIAGNOSIS. Ascarid infections are often asymptomatic, but reported clinical signs include poor growth or weight loss, dry hair coat, abdominal enlargement, restlessness, lethargy and weakness, diarrhea, and vomiting. *Toxocara canis* and *T. leonina* infections are diagnosed by demonstration of the typical eggs with fecal flotation, or by direct observation of adult and juvenile worms in vomitus or feces.

TREATMENT. Numerous anthelmintics are approved for treatment of ascarid infections in dogs (Table 1). With similar safety and efficacy profiles, drug choices are based on economic factors, preferences for

**Table 1.** *Anthelmintics for the Removal of Major Gastrointestinal Nematodes of Dogs*

| Drug | Nematode Spectrum | Regimen |
|---|---|---|
| Dichlorvos (Task Tabs, Fermenta) | *Ancylostoma caninum, Toxocara canis, Toxascaris leonina, Uncinaria stenocephala* | 11 mg/kg, PO |
| (Task Granules and Capsules, Fermenta) | *Ancylostoma caninum, Toxocara canis, Toxascaris leonina, Trichuris vulpis, Uncinaria stenocephala* | 33 mg/kg, PO |
| Febantel (Rintal, Miles) | *Ancylostoma caninum, Toxocara canis, Toxascaris leonina, Trichuris vulpis, Uncinaria stenocephala* | 10 mg/kg q24h 3 days, PO |
| Febantel plus Praziquantel (Vercom, Miles) | *Ancylostoma caninum, Toxocara canis, Toxascaris leonina, Trichuris vulpis, Uncinaria stenocephala* | 10 mg/kg FEB and 1 mg/kg PRZ q24h 3 days, PO; increase dosage by 50% for pups <6 months old |
| Fenbendazole (Panacur, Hoechst-Roussel) | *Ancylostoma caninum, Toxocara canis, Toxascaris leonina, Trichuris vulpis, Uncinaria stenocephala* | 50 mg/kg q24h 3 days, PO |
| Mebendazole (Telmintic, Mallinckrodt) | *Ancylostoma caninum, Toxocara canis, Trichuris vulpis, Uncinaria stenocephala* | 22 mg/kg q24h 3 days, PO |
| Milbemycin oxime (Interceptor, Ciba Geigy) | *Toxocara canis, Trichuris vulpis* | 0.5 mg/kg, PO |
| Piperazine base | *Toxocara canis, Toxoscaris leonina* | 44–66 mg/kg, PO |
| Pyrantel pamoate (Nemex, Pfizer) | *Ancylostoma caninum, Physaloptera* spp., *Toxocara canis, Toxoscaris leonina, Vacinaria stenocephala* | 5 mg/kg, PO |
| Thiabendazole° (MSD AgVet) | *Strongyloides stercoralis* | 50–75 mg/kg q24h 3 days, PO |

°Extralabel application.
Abbreviations: FEB = febantel, PRZ = praziquantel.

single treatments versus multiple-day regimens, or a suitable spectrum of activity for simultaneous treatment of coexisting hookworm, whipworm, and/or tapeworm infections (Tables 1 and 3). Because none of the approved compounds is effective against migrating ascarid larvae, it is common practice to repeat treatment in 2 to 3 weeks.

PREVENTION. Because the zoonotic importance of *T. canis* outweighs its impact on the health of dogs, the major objective of ascarid control is prevention of environmental contamination with the highly persistent eggs. To this end, newborn pups can be blocked from developing patent *T. canis* infections by repeated anthelmintic treatment at 2, 4, 6, and 8 weeks of age. The bitch should be dewormed concurrently. A rigorous and expensive alternative is to prevent prenatal transmission from dam to offspring by treating the bitch daily with 50 mg/kg fenbendazole (Panacur, Hoechst-Roussel) from the 40th day of gestation until 5 weeks postpartum (Table 2) (Burke and Roberson, 1983).

**Table 2.** *Anthelmintics for the Prevention or Control of Major Gastrointestinal Nematodes of Dogs*

| Drug | Nematode Spectrum | Regimen |
|---|---|---|
| Diethylcarbamazine citrate | *Toxocara canis* | 6.6 mg/kg q24h, PO |
| Diethylcarbamazine plus Oxibendazole (Filaribits Plus, Smith-Kline Beecham) | *Ancylostoma caninum, Toxocara canis, Trichuris vulpis* | 6.6 mg/kg DEC and 5 mg/kg OXB q24h, PO |
| Fenbendazole (Panacur, Hoechst-Roussel) | *Ancylostoma caninum, Toxocara canis* | 50 mg/kg q24h pregnant bitches from day 40 of gestation to 35 days after whelping, PO |
| Ivermectin plus Pyrantel Pamoate (Heartgard 30 Plus, MSD AgVet) | *Ancylostoma caninum, Toxocara canis, Toxascaris leonina, Uncinaria stenocephala* | 0.006 mg/kg IVM and 5 mg/kg PP once monthly, PO |
| Milbemycin oxime (Interceptor, Ciba Geigy) | *Ancylostoma caninum, Toxocara canis, Trichuris vulpis* | 0.5 mg/kg once monthly, PO |

Abbreviations: DEC = diethylcarbamazine, OXB = oxibendazole, IVM = ivermectin, PP = pyrantel pamoate.

Several compounds are approved for the prevention or control of ascarid infections in dogs (Table 2). Options include daily administration of diethylcarbamazine (DEC) or DEC plus oxibendazole (Filaribits Plus, SmithKline Beecham), and monthly administration of milbemycin (Interceptor, Ciba-Geigy) or ivermectin plus pyrantel pamoate (Heartgard 30 Plus, Merck Sharp & Dohme).

General recommendations for prevention of ascarid infections include twice-weekly removal of feces from the environment and curtailment of predation or scavenging on potential paratenic hosts.

## Hookworms

### Ancylostoma caninum

*Ancylostoma caninum* is the most prevalent gastrointestinal parasite of dogs in all age groups, and is endemic throughout most of the United States. Hookworm eggs are passed in feces and develop to infective third-stage larvae (L3) in about 1 week under favorable conditions. Dogs acquire *Ancylostoma* infections by skin penetration or by ingestion of infective larvae or paratenic hosts; extensive systemic migration occurs before mature worms develop in the gut. One route of transmission unique to neonatal pups is lactogenic infection, in which arrested *A. caninum* larvae in the tissues of a whelping bitch are stimulated to migrate to the mammary glands. These larvae are ingested by nursing pups, and patent infections develop in as little as 2 or 3 weeks.

### Uncinaria stenocephala

*Uncinaria stenocephala* is another fairly common hookworm of dogs in North America. The usual routes of infection involve skin penetration or ingestion of infective larvae. The larvae of all canine hookworm species are able to penetrate intact human skin, causing a pruritic condition known as cutaneous larva migrans.

CLINICAL SIGNS AND DIAGNOSIS. *Ancylostoma caninum* is an avid blood sucker and causes anemia, hypoproteinemia, melena, and stunted growth in pups. Various syndromes of infection, some of which result in peracute or acute fatalities, have been described (Georgi and Georgi, 1990). The clinical signs of hookworm infection in mature dogs are often inapparent, but may include mild to severe blood loss or iron deficiency anemia or hypoproteinemia, weight loss, and a thin hair coat. Mature dogs that are immunosuppressed or malnourished may develop severe clinical signs of hookworm disease.

Hookworm infection is detected by demonstrating the typical ova via fecal flotation techniques. The eggs of *U. stenocephala* are similar to those of *A. caninum*, but are approximately 20% larger.

TREATMENT. Numerous anthelmintics are available for the treatment of hookworm infections in dogs (Table 1). With one important exception, the criteria affecting drug selection for hookworms are similar to those discussed previously for ascarids. The exception is severe hookworm anemia in pups, which requires immediate removal of parasites. Pyrantel pamoate (Nemex, Pfizer) is preferred for this specific application because it acts very rapidly and is comparatively safe in debilitated animals. The other therapeutic compounds for hookworm treatment either have multiple-day regimens, delayed parasiticidal effects, or narrow therapeutic indices. Blood transfusions may be indicated for severe cases of hookworm anemia, and supportive and nutritional care are important for complete management of clinical ancylostomiasis. The relative lack of efficacy of most compounds against migrating larvae supports the common practice of repeating hookworm treatment in 2 to 3 weeks.

PREVENTION. Hookworm disease and patent infections can be prevented in nursing pups by treating the pups at 2, 4, 6, and 8 weeks of age. The bitch should be dewormed concurrently. This same regimen is recommended for ascarid prevention, so the use of an anthelmintic with a suitable spectrum of activity can provide comprehensive nematode control for nursing pups. Transmission of hookworms from the bitch to the pups also can be prevented by the daily fenbendazole regimen proposed previously for ascarids (Table 2) (Burke and Roberson, 1983).

Mature dogs often harbor patent hookworm infections, and it is routine for practitioners to treat the same dog repeatedly throughout the year. To address recurrent infections, several pharmaceutical manufacturers have encouraged comprehensive parasite control by combining compounds for heartworm prophylaxis with other drugs to create products with a broader antiparasitic spectrum. Thus, heartworms and hookworms now can be controlled simultaneously with daily diethylcarbamazine plus oxibendazole, ivermectin plus pyrantel pamoate given monthly, or milbemycin oxime administered monthly (Table 2). These compounds prevent the establishment of adult worms in the intestinal tract or remove them at monthly intervals. In either case, patency is precluded or the duration is shortened, which reduces environmental contamination and the risk of future infection.

General measures for hookworm prevention include disposal of feces every 3 days and placing runs in areas with good drainage and maximum exposure to sunlight. Sodium borate, applied at 4.5 kg/9.3 m², kills hookworm larvae in soil, and 1% bleach solutions are fairly effective on manufactured surfaces.

## Whipworms

### Trichuris vulpis

In most regions of North America, *T. vulpis* is a common parasite of mature dogs and pups older than 4 months. Adult whipworms reside in the ileum, cecum, and colon, and produce eggs that must embryonate to become infective, but can then persist in the environment for several years. Infection results from ingestion of embryonated eggs, and the prepatent period is 7 to 14 weeks.

CLINICAL SIGNS AND DIAGNOSIS.    The lesions of trichuriasis are typhlitis and colitis, with associated diarrhea possibly containing fresh blood and mucus; tenesmus; vomiting; and possibly weight loss, hypoproteinemia, and mild anemia.

Whipworm infection is diagnosed by demonstrating the typical eggs with fecal flotation, or occasionally by retrieving an intact worm with a fecal loop or thermometer. In some dogs with clinical whipworm disease, *Trichuris* eggs cannot be detected in the feces. This condition is attributed to the presence of larval whipworms that are not yet capable of reproducing, so no eggs are passed. Whipworms also can be detected by colonoscopy, but suspected cases of trichuriasis should be treated empirically with anthelmintics before resorting to invasive or expensive diagnostic procedures (Hendrix, Blagburn, and Lindsay, 1987).

TREATMENT.    Several compounds are available for treating whipworm infections, but the majority require a 3-day regimen of therapy (Table 1). All approved compounds must be given orally, which complicates successful management in vomiting dogs.

PREVENTION.    Reinfection with *T. vulpis* is highly probable because the eggs are very persistent in the environment and dogs apparently develop limited immunity to reinfection. General recommendations for whipworm control include weekly collection and disposal of feces. Because of the prolonged egg persistence, dirt runs should be relocated to an area of clean soil, or preferably replaced with concrete or new gravel.

The daily administration of diethylcarbamazine plus oxibendazole or a monthly regimen of milbemycin oxime prevents or controls patent whipworm infections and associated clinical disease (Table 2).

### Miscellaneous Nematodes

Among the nematodes that are encountered infrequently in the canine gastrointestinal tract are *Physaloptera* spp., which normally occur in the stomachs of cats, opossums, raccoons, and other insectivores that ingest arthropod intermediate hosts. In dogs, *Physaloptera* usually appear in vomitus and are mistaken for ascarids based on superficial similarities. The misidentification is recognized when the worms are examined microscopically or when repeated treatment for the mysteriously nonpatent ascarid infections proves unsuccessful.

*Physaloptera* eggs are distinctive, but are rarely detected with routine fecal examination. Successful treatment of *Physaloptera* infection with pyrantel pamoate has been reported (Clark, 1990) (Table 1).

*Strongyloides stercoralis* is encountered infrequently in young pups, and is acquired through skin penetration or ingestion of third-stage larvae. A cycle of autoinfection has been reported in immunosuppressed dogs, re-

sulting in massive worm burdens and disseminated infection. Humans are susceptible to infection with *S. stercoralis*, and transmission between dogs and humans has been documented.

The clinical signs of strongyloidiasis in pups include diarrhea possibly containing blood and mucus, anorexia, coughing, and pruritic dermatitis. Canine *Strongyloides* infection is diagnosed by demonstrating the motile first-stage larvae in smears of fresh feces.

Thiabendazole (Merck Sharp & Dohme) is reportedly effective against canine strongyloidiasis, but emesis is a common side effect (Hendrix, Blagburn, and Lindsay, 1987) (Table 1). Ivermectin demonstrated good efficacy against *Strongyloides stercoralis* in mice, but has not been evaluated in the dog. Preventive actions are similar to the general measures recommended previously for hookworm infections.

## CESTODE PARASITES OF DOGS

The most common cestodes of dogs in North America are *Dipylidium caninum* and *Taenia pisiformis*. Concern about another taeniid cestode, *Echinococcus multilocularis*, is growing in some areas, although its actual prevalence in dogs is quite low. *Echinococcus multilocularis* causes a potentially fatal zoonosis in humans who inadvertently ingest the eggs. The current interest in *E. multilocularis* is based on an apparent expansion of its geographic range and an adaptation from sylvatic to domestic cycles of transmission.

All cestode infections of dogs are transmitted by ingestion of intermediate hosts. The usual intermediate host of *Dipylidium caninum* is the flea. *Taenia* and *Echinococcus* are transmitted by the ingestion of the tissues of rabbits and rodents, respectively (Georgi, 1987).

CLINICAL SIGNS AND DIAGNOSIS.    Despite common opinion to the contrary, adult cestodes in dogs are usually quite harmless. Nevertheless, tapeworm infections have been blamed for various concurrent conditions, ranging from gastrointestinal disturbances to seizures. Cestode infections are usually diagnosed by the detection of fresh proglottids crawling on the feces or the host, or desiccated segments attached to the hair coat. The owner's history regarding observation of proglottids may prove invaluable in the diagnosis of inapparent tapeworm infections.

The detection of cestode infections by fecal flotation is inconsistent because eggs are not always released prior to the time proglottids exit the host. If intact proglottids are recovered, they can be rehydrated and crushed between two microscope slides to release the distinctive eggs. Specific characterization of a cestode infection identifies potential intermediate hosts and assists in efforts to prevent reinfection.

TREATMENT.    Therapy for cestode infections is based more on the aesthetic concerns of the client than the perceived or actual health threat to the dog. Several compounds are approved for treatment of canine cestode infections (Table 3). Broad spectrum cestocides,

**Table 3.** *Anthelmintics for the Removal of Cestode Parasites of Dogs*

| Drug | Cestode Spectrum | Regimen |
|---|---|---|
| Epsiprantel (Cestex, SmithKline Beecham) | *Dipylidium caninum, Taenia pisiformis* | 5.5 mg/kg, PO |
| Febantel plus praziquantel (Vercom, Miles) | *Dipylidium caninum, Taenia pisiformis* | 10 mg/kg FEB and 1 mg/kg PRZ q24h 3 days, PO; increase dosage 50% for pups <6 months old |
| Fenbendazole (Pana-cur, Hoechst-Roussel) | *Taenia pisiformis* | 50 mg/kg q24h 3 days, PO |
| Mebendazole (Tel-mintic, Mallinckrodt) | *Taenia pisiformis* | 22 mg/kg q24h 3 days, PO |
| Praziquantel (Droncit, Miles) | *Dipylidium caninum, Echinococcus granulosus, Taenia pisiformis* | 5–12.5 mg/kg, IM, PO, SC |

Abbreviations: FEB = febantel, PRZ = praziquantel.

such as praziquantel (Droncit, Miles) or epsiprantel (Cestex, SmithKline Beecham), are preferred when the infection has not been characterized. Alternatively, 3-day regimens of benzimidazoles or probenzimidazoles are appropriate when only *Taenia* is present, or when concurrent nematode infection dictates the use of a broad-spectrum anthelmintic.

PREVENTION. Prevention of *D. caninum* infections requires a comprehensive flea-control program, which most practitioners would agree is no simple matter. To avoid infections with *Taenia* and *Echinococcus*, predatory or scavenging dogs should be confined to preclude access to mammalian intermediate hosts, and domestic rodent problems should be alleviated.

## PROTOZOAN PARASITES OF DOGS

### Coccidia

The coccidia are single-celled organisms that reproduce asexually for one or more generations in various tissues, and then undergo a single cycle of sexual reproduction in the gastrointestinal tract. Some species have direct life cycles, others use intermediate hosts, and a few are able to utilize either route of transmission.

The coccidians observed most frequently in young dogs are *Isospora canis* and *I. ohioensis*. Infection with either species is acquired through the ingestion of sporulated oocysts or by predation on rodent, paratenic hosts. The entire life cycle in dogs takes place within the gut. Infection culminates in the passage of unsporulated oocysts in the feces within 1 to 2 weeks of infection. Oocysts sporulate in 2 or 3 days, and may persist in the environment for several months.

CLINICAL SIGNS AND DIAGNOSIS. Most *Isospora* infections, especially those in mature dogs, are asymptomatic. Although the passage of oocysts may be accompanied by diarrhea and hematochezia, some authorities believe that severe clinical signs are more likely due to other enteric pathogens (Kirkpatrick and Dubey, 1987). The pathogenicity of canine coccidiosis remains controversial. The usual method of diagnosis of *Isospora* infection is demonstration of unsporulated oocysts by fecal flotation.

TREATMENT. Many antiprotozoal compounds are "static" rather than "cidal" and are incapable of eradicating protozoal infections independently. Coccidial infections ultimately are eliminated by host defense mechanisms. Sulfadimethoxine (Albon, Roche; Bactrovet, Pitman-Moore) and trimethoprim-sulfadiazine (Tribrissen, Pitman-Moore) reduce the multiplication of coccidia in the gut, decrease oocyst production, and alleviate clinical signs (Table 4). Some consider the clinical improvements following anticoccidial therapy to be attributable to the activity of these drugs against concurrent bacterial enteritis. Treatment of mature dogs with asymptomatic *Isospora* infections is unnecessary unless they represent a potential source of contamination for susceptible pups.

PREVENTION. Daily disposal of feces reduces the number of oocysts in the environment, and cleaning cages with steam or with strong sodium hydroxide so-

**Table 4.** *Compounds for Treatment of Canine Coccidiosis*

| Drug | Spectrum | Regimen |
|---|---|---|
| **Therapy** | | |
| Sulfadimethoxine (Albon, Roche; (Bactrovet, Mallinckrodt) | *Isospora* | 55 mg/kg day 1, PO; followed by 27.5 mg/kg q24h 9 days, PO |
| Trimethoprim-Sulfadiazine° (Tribrissen, Mallinckrodt) | *Isospora* | 30 mg/kg q24h 10 days, PO |
| **Prevention** | | |
| Amprolium° (Corid, MSD AgVet) | *Isospora* | 0.075% solution as drinking water |
| Decoquinate° (Deccox, SmithKline Beecham) | *Isospora* | 50 mg/kg q24h, PO |

°Extralabel applications.

lutions kills oocysts (Kirkpatrick and Dubey, 1987). Predation and scavenging should be discouraged to prevent infections acquired through ingestion of intermediate hosts. Chemoprophylactic measures include the addition of 15 to 30 ml of amprolium (Corid, Merck Sharp & Dohme) to 3.8 L of drinking water for pregnant bitches beginning 10 days prior to whelping, and for weaned pups until 5 months of age (Table 4). Decoquinate (Deccox, Rhône-Poulenc) can be fed to pups from 3 weeks of age until weaning to prevent patent infections and clinical disease (Table 4).

## Miscellaneous Protozoa

*Giardia canis*, a major gastrointestinal protozoan parasite of dogs, is discussed in a separate chapter of this volume.

Practices with superior microscopic skills may occasionally detect the reproductive products of the coccidian parasites *Cryptosporidium*, *Hammondia*, and *Sarcocystis*. Although *Sarcocystis* appears frequently, the other two genera are quite uncommon. None of these protozoa is a significant pathogen in dogs, and effective, chemical treatments have not been identified.

## References and Suggested Reading

Burke TM and Roberson EL: Fenbendazole treatment of pregnant bitches to reduce prenatal and lactogenic infections of *Toxocara canis* and *Ancylostoma caninum* in pups. J Am Vet Med Assoc 183:987, 1983.
   *A report of successful chemoprophylaxis of ascarid and hookworm infections in neonatal pups.*
Clark JA: *Physaloptera* stomach worms associated with chronic vomition in a dog in western Canada. Can Vet J 31:840, 1990.
   *A case report, including presentation and management of* Physaloptera *infection in a dog.*
Georgi JR: Tapeworms. Vet Clin North Am [Small Anim Pract] 17:1285, 1987.
   *A review of the biology and management of cestode infections of small animals.*
Georgi JR and Georgi ME: *Parasitology for Veterinarians*, 5th edition. Philadelphia, WB Saunders Co, 1990, p 412.
   *A textbook presenting fairly complete information on the biology, diagnosis, and management of parasitic infections of domestic animals.*
Hendrix CM, Blagburn BL, and Lindsay DS: Whipworms and intestinal threadworms. Vet Clin North Am [Small Anim Pract] 17:1355, 1987.
   *A review of the biology, pathogenesis, and management of* Trichuris *and* Strongyloides *infections in small animals.*
Kirkpatrick CE and Dubey JP: Enteric coccidial infections. Vet Clin North Am [Small Anim Pract] 17:1405, 1987.
   *A review of the biology, pathogenesis, and management of infections with* Isospora *and other coccidia of the gastrointestinal tract.*
Parsons JC: Ascarid infections of cats and dogs. Vet Clin North Am [Small Anim Pract] 17:1307, 1987.
   *A review of the biology, pathogenesis, and management of* Toxocara *and* Toxascaris *infections in small animals.*
Sloss MW, Kemp RL, and Zajac AM: *Veterinary Clinical Parasitology*, 6th edition. Ames, IA, Iowa State University Press, 1994.
   *A manual of parasitologic diagnostic techniques with numerous photomicrographs for identification of common parasitisms of domestic animals.*

# *GIARDIA:* DIAGNOSIS AND TREATMENT

MICHAEL S. LEIB
*and* ANNE M. ZAJAC
*Blacksburg, Virginia*

*Giardia* is a flagellate protozoan parasite commonly encountered in small animal veterinary practice. *Giardia* isolates from many mammalian hosts are morphologically identical and are currently grouped into a single species, *Giardia intestinalis*. The most common clinical syndrome associated with *Giardia* is acute small bowel diarrhea, but in some cases acute large bowel diarrhea, chronic small or large bowel diarrhea, or rarely acute or chronic vomiting may occur. Clinical signs may be self-limiting in some patients. Surveys throughout the world have found infection rates ranging from 1 to 39% in dogs and cats. In these studies, many animals infected with *Giardia* did not have diarrhea. In most surveys, younger animals have a higher rate of infection.

Severe disease may occur in puppies or kittens, animals with other gastrointestinal parasites or diseases, or debilitated animals, but can occur in otherwise healthy patients. Some of the differences in pathogenicity of *Giardia* may be associated with parasite strain variation. *Giardia* cysts are not routinely identified by commonly used fecal flotation solutions because cysts become shriveled and cannot be readily identified. In addition, the number of cysts shed in the feces fluctuates over time. Common anthelmintics are not effective against *Giardia*. Although the issue is unresolved, *Giardia* may be a zoonotic threat.

## BIOLOGY

The life cycle of *Giardia* is direct. Cysts (9 to 13 $\mu$m) may be ingested from contaminated water, but direct animal-to-animal transmission also occurs, especially where animals are in close contact (e.g., catteries or kennels) (Kirkpatrick, 1987). Cysts are oval and contain two or four nuclei. Excystation occurs in the small intestine and each cyst releases two trophozoites. Maturation and division of the motile trophozoite (12 to 17 $\mu$m long and 7 to 10 $\mu$m wide) occur in the small bowel

(Kirkpatrick, 1987). However, it has been demonstrated that the distribution of trophozoites within the small intestine varies a great deal among individual animals. Trophozoites are teardrop shaped, have four pairs of flagella, a pair of dark median bodies, and are binucleated. Trophozoites attach to the brush border by a ventral disk, where they absorb nutrients. The prepatent period in dogs and cats varies from 5 to 16 days. Little is known about what signals encystation, but it probably occurs in the ileum or colon and may be related to intraluminal bile acids or fatty acids. Although cysts are susceptible to desiccation, they are hardy and can survive for months in a cool, moist environment.

## PATHOPHYSIOLOGY

The specifics regarding the pathogenesis of *Giardia* infection in dogs and cats remain unclear. Studies in laboratory animals and humans have demonstrated malabsorption of nutrients, decreased brush border disaccharidases, defective active transport mechanisms, increased enterocyte turnover, plasma cell and lymphocyte infiltration, villus atrophy, and production of an enterotoxin (Lewis and Freedman, 1992). Some of these changes appear to be associated with the host's immune response. The wide variation in pathogenicity may be related to the host's immune response or nutritional status, presence of other parasites or gastrointestinal diseases, or parasite strain variation. Markers for strain virulence have not been identified.

Both immunoglobulin A and T lymphocytes are involved in the immune response to *Giardia*. Since younger animals are more commonly affected, it is probable that some degree of protective immunity develops. Immunity may protect animals more from the development of clinical signs than from infection, since the authors have observed repeated shedding of cysts in some animals despite treatment.

## CLINICAL SIGNS

Most dogs and cats infected with *Giardia* remain asymptomatic. When clinical signs occur, acute small bowel diarrhea is most common, with the following characteristics: liquid to semiformed feces, moderately increased frequency of defecation, and normal to increased quantity of feces per defecation. Melena (digested blood) is uncommon in cases of giardiasis. Diarrhea may be self-limiting in some patients. Severe diarrhea may be accompanied by dehydration, lethargy, and anorexia. However, most patients remain bright and alert, afebrile, and maintain a normal appetite. Occasionally, acute vomiting may accompany diarrhea. In some cases, the authors have endoscopically observed severe erosion of the duodenum that resolved following successful treatment for *Giardia*. A mild eosinophilia and increased fecal split and unsplit fats have been observed. Chronic small bowel diarrhea with weight loss, poor body condition, and intermittent vomiting may

also occur. *Giardia* may be found in dogs and cats that have other gastrointestinal diseases, especially inflammatory bowel disease. In these cases, the clinical signs and laboratory findings reflect the underlying disease. In humans, *Giardia* infection may mimic inflammatory bowel disease.

Acute or chronic large bowel diarrhea with hematochezia, excess fecal mucus, and tenesmus may occur on occasion. In cases of large bowel diarrhea, frequency of defecation is moderately to greatly increased and quantity of feces per defecation is reduced. Excess fecal mucus is often seen in infected cats (Kirkpatrick, 1987).

## DIAGNOSIS

Diagnosis of *Giardia* can often be made by appropriate fecal examination techniques. If giardiasis is suspected, but cannot be confirmed, a therapeutic trial may be indicated. However, cessation of diarrhea after treatment does not confirm a definitive diagnosis of giardiasis.

Examinations of a fresh fecal saline smear of diarrheic feces may allow identification of motile trophozoites. Trophozoites can be identified by their rapid "falling leaf" motion and concave ventral surface. Trophozoites may be associated with mucus, and the only motility visible may be the flagella. Trichomonads are the only other motile protozoan similar in size to *Giardia* and may be differentiated by an undulating membrane, rolling form of motility, and lack of a concave surface. Trophozoites are not often found in semiformed or firm feces. One study in dogs showed that examination of saline smears of fresh feces on three separate days identified only approximately 40% of dogs infected with *Giardia* (Zimmer and Burrington, 1986b). In that study, approximately 90% of infected dogs were identified after three zinc sulfate fecal examinations.

Examination of feces by zinc sulfate flotation is considered to be the most accurate and practical diagnostic test available (Zimmer and Burrington, 1986b) (Fig. 1). In addition to identifying *Giardia* cysts, eggs of common parasites can also be recognized. Approximately 2 gm of feces are mixed with 15 ml of a 33% solution of zinc sulfate (specific gravity 1.18) and strained into a 15-ml centrifuge tube. The tube is filled with additional zinc sulfate and centrifuged for 3 to 5 min at 1500 rpm. In a free-swinging head centrifuge, additional zinc sulfate is added to create a reverse meniscus and a coverslip placed on the top of the tube. After centrifugation, the coverslip can be transferred to a microscope slide for examination. If a fixed-head centrifuge is used, the surface layer of fluid can be transferred to a microscope slide with a pipette, the bottom of a small glass tube, or bacteriologic loop. A coverslip is added and the slide is examined for cysts. Iodine may be added to the centrifuge tube to stain cysts and make identification easier. Barium sulfate, several proprietary

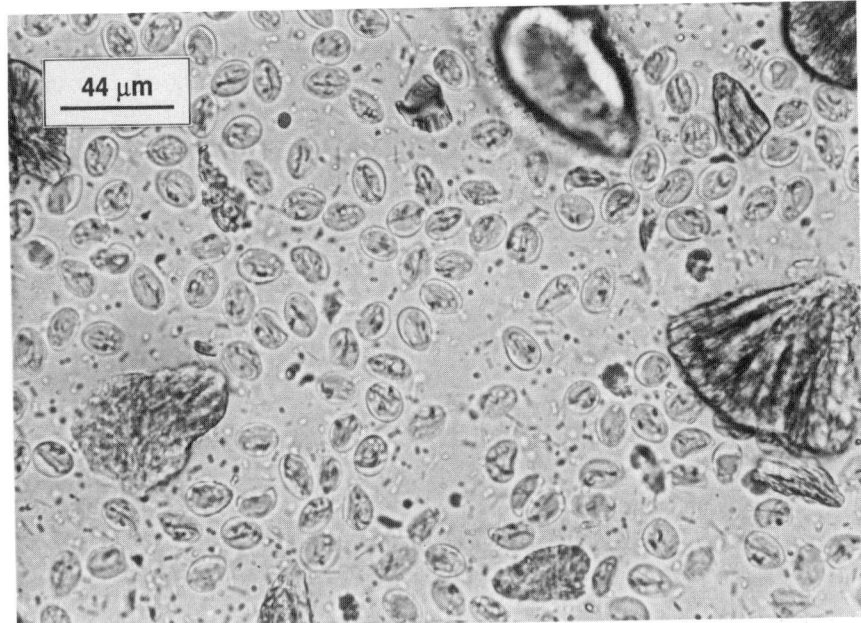

**Figure 1.** *Giardia* cysts cover the microscopic field in this sample prepared by zinc sulfate fecal flotation.

antidiarrheals, and enemas administered prior to collection of feces may interfere with *Giardia* detection.

Duodenal aspiration of fluid with examination of the sediment for motile trophozoites was considered the "gold standard" for diagnosis of *Giardia* in dogs (Pitts, Twedt, and Mallie, 1983). Unfortunately, this requires either endoscopy or exploratory laparotomy. Ten milliliters of saline can be infused into the duodenum through a polyethylene tube passed through the biopsy channel of an endoscope or with a needle during exploratory laparotomy. The fluid should be aspirated, centrifuged, and immediately examined microscopically for motile trophozoites. A study comparing duodenal aspiration with zinc sulfate flotation found that duodenal aspiration was positive in 89% of cases, while a single zinc sulfate flotation was positive in only 39% of cases (Pitts, Twedt, and Mallie, 1983). Two recent studies by the authors have contradicted these findings. In a group of research dogs carefully monitored for parasites during a 17-month period, a single zinc sulfate examination identified infection in 77% of samples, while a duodenal aspirate identified the parasite in 67% of samples (Zajac, Leib, and Burkholder, 1992). More recent investigation in the authors' laboratory found that three zinc sulfate examinations identified approximately 95% of infected dogs versus 88% with duodenal aspiration.

Recently, several fecal enzyme-linked immunosorbent assay (ELISA) tests have been marketed for human use that detect *Giardia*-specific antigens. Preliminary use of one of these tests in the authors' laboratory (Prospect T/Giardia, Alexon Inc, Mountain View, CA) yielded similar results to zinc sulfate flotation in 84% of samples from experimental dogs. However, in 15% of examinations, the ELISA was positive when a single zinc sulfate examination was negative. *Giardia* was identified in half of these cases by examining two additional zinc sulfate flotations. In 1% of fecal samples,

the ELISA was negative while the fecal examination was positive. A recent report using the same ELISA test found that it was falsely negative in 14% of zinc sulfate–positive samples from dogs (Barr et al., 1992). This study also found a positive ELISA in 10% of zinc sulfate–negative samples. These preliminary studies point out that a negative ELISA does not eliminate the possibility of *Giardia* infection. In addition, it is possible that the ELISA may be a more sensitive test and may identify some cases missed with zinc sulfate examination. Further investigation of ELISA testing in dogs and cats is necessary before the authors can recommend the routine use of these tests.

## TREATMENT

The authors' drug of choice in treating giardiasis in dogs and cats is metronidazole 50 mg/kg/day for 5 days. It has also been suggested that the dosage be split and administered twice daily. In one study, metronidazole was effective in clearing 67% of infected dogs at 22 mg/kg twice daily for 5 days (Zimmer and Burrington, 1986a). Tablets should not be divided, as the medication is bitter and unpalatable. Some authors have found that a lower dosage, 10 mg/kg twice daily, is effective in cats (Kirkpatrick, 1987). Severe neurologic side effects, including seizures and coma, have been reported in dogs receiving higher dosages or prolonged treatment (Dow et al., 1989). Mild neurologic signs can occur with recommended dosages but are usually reversible if the drug is discontinued. Metronidazole is a potential mutagen and carcinogen, so treatment of pregnant animals should be avoided.

Metronidazole enters the parasite by passive diffusion. Under anaerobic conditions, the compound is reduced, forming toxic derivatives that bind to deoxyribonucleic acid (DNA), ribonucleic acid (RNA), and other proteins, leading to denaturation and strand breakage. In humans, metronidazole is metabolized in the liver; 60 to 80% of the metabolites and parent compound is eliminated by the kidney. Approximately 15% is eliminated in the feces. Drug interactions are uncommon, but phenobarbital and prednisone may increase hepatic metabolism, while cimetidine may decrease it.

Decreased reductive capability has been demonstrated in several metronidazole-resistant *Giardia* strains isolated from human beings. In addition, trophozoites grown *in vitro* in sublethal concentrations of metronidazole have developed resistance (Upcroft, Upcroft, and Boreham, 1990). This finding could have clinical significance in animals because dosages used to treat inflammatory bowel disease are lower than those used to treat *Giardia*. To prevent the potential development of resistance, the authors recommend eliminating the possibility of a *Giardia* infection by performing three zinc sulfate flotations and treating for an occult infection prior to initiating low-dose (10 mg/kg b.i.d.) long-term metronidazole treatment.

Quinacrine has been shown to be 100% effective in dogs at 6.6 mg/kg twice daily for 5 days (Zimmer and Burrington, 1986a). Approximately half of the dogs treated in this study developed mild and reversible anorexia, fever, or lethargy. Quinacrine has been shown to improve clinical signs in cats, but not to eliminate infection. Unfortunately, quinacrine is not currently available in the United States.

Furazolidone (Furoxone Suspension, SmithKline Beecham) is available as a suspension and is convenient to administer to cats and small dogs (4 mg/kg b.i.d. for 7 days). It has been shown to be effective in cats (Kirkpatrick, 1987). Resistance to furazolidone has recently been demonstrated in *Giardia* isolated from human beings (Upcroft, Upcroft, and Boreham, 1990).

Recently, preliminary investigation has found the anthelmintic albendazole (Valbazen Suspension, SmithKline Beecham) to be a safe and effective treatment in dogs at 25 mg/kg twice daily for 2 days (Barr et al., 1993). Albendazole's mechanism of action is believed to be inhibition of microtubule assembly. It is poorly absorbed from the gastrointestinal tract and has not resulted in toxicity in experimental dogs treated for 13 weeks. However, treatment with higher dosages or for 26 weeks resulted in blood dyscrasias, decreased body weight, and reduced bone marrow cellularity. Effective treatment of cats may require prolonged therapy. Use of albendazole at high dosages has been associated with teratogenicity in some species. Consequently, it should not be used in pregnant animals until additional studies are completed. If further research with albendazole continues to demonstrate safety and efficacy, it may prove to be the preferred treatment for *Giardia*.

Persistent clinical signs after treatment may suggest treatment failure, lack of client compliance, reinfection, underlying gastrointestinal disease, immunologic deficiency, or inaccurate identification of the parasite. Prolonged treatment, use of a different agent, performing

alternative identification procedures (submitting samples to an outside laboratory or using an ELISA test), or instituting further diagnostic testing to identify a primary gastrointestinal disorder is indicated.

## ZOONOSIS

*Giardia* should be considered potentially zoonotic and adequate precautions taken when handling feces. Dog and cat feces should be disposed of promptly and hands washed immediately after contact. Children and immunocompromised adults should avoid contact with feces. Attempts to infect dogs and cats with cysts isolated from humans have yielded contradictory results (Kirkpatrick, 1987). In addition, laboratory properties of canine and human source cysts differ. Some human and cat strains have similar genetic and biochemical properties, while others do not. Some strains may have a wider host specificity than others, and animal strains may be more infective for humans than human strains are for animals.

Cysts are susceptible to drying and many common disinfectants. Quaternary ammonium compounds effectively inactivate cysts. Phenolic disinfectants require longer application times than quaternary ammonium compounds (Zimmer, Miller, and Lindmark, 1988).

### References and Suggested Reading

Barr SC, Bowman DD, and Erb HN: Evaluation of two test procedures for diagnosis of giardiasis in dogs. Am J Vet Res 53:2028, 1992.
  *A fecal ELISA test and a peroral string test were compared with zinc sulfate fecal flotation for the detection of* Giardia *in dogs.*
Barr SC, Bowman DD, Heller RL, et al: Efficacy of albendazole against giardiasis in dogs. Am J Vet Res 54:926, 1993.
  *The efficacy of albendazole for treating three groups of experimental dogs for* Giardia *is described.*
Dow SW, LeCouteur RA, Poss ML, et al: Central nervous system toxicosis associated with metronidazole treatment of dogs: Five cases (1984–1987). J Am Vet Med Assoc 195:365, 1989.
  *Central nervous system toxicity in five dogs treated with metronidazole for* Giardia *or pyothorax is described.*
Kirkpatrick CE: Giardiasis. Vet Clin North Am [Small Anim Pract] 17:1377, 1987.
  *A comprehensive review article on giardiasis in dogs and cats.*
Lewis DJM and Freedman AR: Giardia lamblia *as an intestinal pathogen. Dig Dis 10:102, 1992.
  *A comprehensive review article on giardiasis in human beings.*
Pitts RP, Twedt DC, and Mallie KA: Comparison of duodenal aspiration with fecal flotation for diagnosis of giardiasis in dogs. J Am Vet Med Assoc 182:1210, 1983.
  *The diagnosis of* Giardia *with duodenal aspiration and zinc sulfate fecal flotation was compared in a group of experimental dogs.*
Upcroft JA, Upcroft P, and Boreham PFL: Drug resistance in Giardia intestinalis. Int J Parasitol 20:489, 1990.
  *Resistance to metronidazole and furazolidone in strains of* Giardia *isolated from human beings was detected.*
Zajac AM, Leib MS, and Burkholder WJ: Giardia *infection in a group of experimental dogs. J Small Anim Pract 33:257, 1992.
  *A group of experimental dogs was monitored for* Giardia *by duodenal aspiration and zinc sulfate fecal flotation during a 17-month period.*
Zimmer JF and Burrington DB: Comparison of four protocols for the treatment of canine giardiasis. J Am Anim Hosp Assoc 22:168, 1986a.

*The efficacy of treatment for* Giardia *in a group of dogs with quinacrine, metronidazole, tinidazole, and quinacrine and metronidazole was studied.*
Zimmer JF and Burrington DB: Comparison of four techniques of fecal examination for detecting canine giardiasis. J Am Anim Hosp Assoc 22:161, 1986b.
*Detection of* Giardia *in the feces from an infected dog kennel with a modified zinc sulfate fecal flotation, merthiolate-iodine-formaldehyde concentra-*tion, Wheatley's trichrome stain, and direct fresh fecal smears were compared.
Zimmer JF, Miller JJ, and Lindmark DG: Evaluation of the efficacy of selected commercial disinfectants in inactivating Giardia muris cysts. J Am Anim Hosp Assoc 24:379, 1988.
*Fourteen commercially available disinfectants were evaluated for their efficacy in inactivating* Giardia *cysts in vitro.*

# HELICOBACTER-ASSOCIATED GASTRIC DISEASE IN FERRETS, DOGS, AND CATS

JAMES G. FOX

*Cambridge, Massachusetts*

During the last decade, microaerophilic curved to spiral-shaped, gram-negative bacteria isolated from gastric mucosa of humans and animals have created a great deal of clinical and basic research because of their causal role in gastric disease. The dogma that the euchlorhydric stomach is a predominantly sterile organ, protected from microbial colonization by low gastric pH, has been unequivocally disproven in the last several years. These gastric bacteria belong to the newly named genus *Helicobacter*, and the type species *H. pylori* present in 20 to 90% of adult populations worldwide causes a persistent, active, chronic gastritis and peptic ulcer disease in humans. The organism also has been linked to the development of gastric adenocarcinoma and most recently to gastric mucosal associated lymphoma.

Since the isolation and characterization of *H. pylori*, several additional species of gastric *Helicobacter* have been isolated from stomachs of various mammalian hosts, including dogs, cats, ferrets, cheetahs, and nonhuman primates. Historically, in dogs and cats, these bacteria were described, on a histologic basis, as gastric "spirilla."

The second species of *Helicobacter* isolated from gastric mucosa was *H. mustelae* from ferrets, followed by *H. felis* from cat and dog stomachs. *H. pylori* also has been recently isolated from cat gastric tissue. Another large spiral organism, initially called *"Gastrospirillum hominis,"* is noted frequently in gastric mucosa of dogs, cats, nonhuman primates, and occasionally humans, but thus far has eluded cultivation on artificial media. By using molecular microbial techniques, polymerase chain reaction (PCR) and 16s rRNA ribosomal sequencing, this spiral bacteria has been also classified as a *Helicobacter*, and given the provisional name *"H. heilmannii."*

## PATHOLOGY

To date, chronic or chronic active gastritis due to oral inoculation of *Helicobacter* spp. has been experimentally produced in humans, germ-free pigs, germ-free dogs, and nonhuman primates with *H. pylori*; in the ferret with *H. mustelae*; in germ-free dogs with *H. felis*; and in specific pathogen-free kittens with *H. acinonyx* and *H. heilmannii*.

The *H. pylori*–associated gastritis in humans consisted of an active component (i.e., polymorphonuclear cells) as well as mononuclear cell infiltrates, which depicts a chronic inflammatory response. The persistent *H. pylori* infection in humans, non-human primates, and the domestic cat, like the persistent *H. mustelae* infection in ferrets, also is often characterized by lymphoid aggregates and gastric lymphoid follicles. The presence of these lymphoid elements in dogs and cats historically were considered a normal histologic finding, but experimental evidence suggests that these lymphoid elements are the result of host responses to *Helicobacter* antigens. Also, the presence of eosinophils in gastric mucosa of animals can be a major component of the inflammation, particularly in the acute phase of the infection.

The data presented that causally link duodenal and gastric ulcers with *H. pylori* are now extremely convincing, and peptic ulcer disease in humans is being treated by many gastroenterologists with antimicrobial agents. Although gastric and duodenal ulcer disease in ferrets is strongly associated with chronic *H. mustelae* infection, additional studies are required to ascertain whether duodenal and gastric ulcers have an infections component in dogs and cats.

## EPIDEMIOLOGY

Although infected animals and humans mount a significant systemic IgG response to gastric organisms, the immunoglobulins are not protective and the organism persists in the mucus layer or closely adhered to the gastric epithelium, protected from the gastric acidic milieu. The mechanisms of how the gastric helicobacters are transmitted from host to host are poorly understood. It is known that the gastric helicobacters have specific tissue tropism and colonize only gastric epithelium and not intestinal tissue. Fecal-oral transmission has been suggested, but gastric helicobacters have rarely been isolated from feces of animals or humans. However, *H. mustelae* has been isolated from feces of ferrets, particularly when ferrets have drug-induced hypochlorhydria. This may provide a clue to natural transmission, since gastric *Helicobacter* infection, especially during the early acute phase, can induce transient hypochlorhydria. Also, H. pylori has been isolated from feces of children from a third-world population.

Oral-oral transmission is also possible and is supported by clinical observations of humans infected by exposure to gastric secretions, isolation of *H. pylori* from dental plaque and tissue, and by nosocomial infection due to improper disinfection of gastric pH probes and endoscopic equipment. Similar transmission routes are also probable for gastric helicobacters in animals. Vomitus containing gastric helicobacters is another likely mode of transmission in animals. Irrespective of route of transmission, prevalence of gastric *Helicobacter* infections in colony-raised animals routinely approaches 100%, indicating the organisms' unique ability to selectively and efficiently colonize the stomach of numerous hosts. The domestic cat may also prove to be a reservoir of infection and transmission of *H. pylori* to humans.

## CLINICAL FINDINGS

### Humans

Dyspepsia described as abdominal pain or discomfort centered in the central abdomen is very common, and 40 to 60% of patients with this syndrome have *H. pylori* infection. However, there is no compelling evidence to date to suggest that *H. pylori* is less frequent in infected asymptomatic patients with gastritis. Classic peptic ulcer symptoms also include epigastric pain in addition to pain relieved by food, antacids, or antisecretory medications; hunger or night pain; or episodic pain. Unfortunately, many clinical conditions cause dyspepsia, such as nonulcer dyspepsia, esophagitis, gastric or esophageal cancer, Zollinger-Ellison syndrome, pancreatic disease, and irritable bowel syndrome. Thus, a definitive diagnosis of gastritis and peptic ulcer disease is achieved by endoscopy and often gastric biopsy. The additional benefit of gastric tissue analysis is the ability to culture *H. pylori* and/or visualize the bacteria in the inflamed gastric tissue.

### Animals

In the late 1950s, gastric spiral organisms were mentioned as a possible etiology in cases of clinically apparent gastritis; however, these organisms, like observations of spiral organisms in human gastric tissue during that era, were ignored as modern gastroenterology focused on the theory of acid-induced ulcer disease. The successful incorporation of $H_2$ blockers and other antisecretory drugs in resolution of ulcers in both humans and animals also supported this clinical approach to treatment of peptic ulcer disease. Although the pathogenic potential of gastric *Helicobacter* to produce gastritis in humans and animals is now clearly documented, *Helicobacter* spp. usually cause an asymptomatic infection in the hosts. However, clinical signs in pet animals attributable to *Helicobacter*-associated gastritis are beginning to be recognized. For example, several Persian cats with chronic gastroenterocolitis had large gastric spiral organisms located in areas of stomach with necrosis and proliferation of glandular epithelium. Similarly, an epizootic gastritis associated with gastric spiral bacilli in zoo-maintained cheetahs was clinically recognized by chronic vomiting, weight loss, and in some cases, severe emaciation. Chronic vomiting in dogs linked to gastritis has been classified histologically, but the etiology of the gastritis and the role of gastric bacteria have not been adequately addressed. Clinicians have defined vomiting seen in dogs with chronic superficial gastritis (which may be due to gastric spiral organisms) as intermittent, consistent of mucus or gastric secretions, and sometimes containing bile. Pica, belching, anorexia, and weight loss also are occasionally noted.

*Helicobacter mustelae*–associated gastric and duodenal ulcers in ferrets are well documented. In our experience, ulcers in this species can sometimes be recognized clinically with the presence of blood-tinged vomiting, melena, and chronic weight loss. Acute episodes of massive gastric and/or duodenal bleeding from active ulcers have also been noted infrequently.

## DIAGNOSIS

A diagnosis of chronic gastritis in animals, as in humans, cannot be made by visual examination of the gastric mucosa at endoscopy. A histologic evaluation of gastric biopsies is therefore required; also, the use of a special silver stain or modified Giemsa stain on the gastric tissue reveals the presence of gastric *Helicobacter*-like organisms. A definitive diagnosis requires culture and isolation of the specific species of *Helicobacter*. Unfortunately, the most common spiral organism in dogs and cats is *H. heilmannii*, which to date has been unculturable on artificial media. *Helicobacter felis* is culturable but difficult to isolate, in part because it probably colonizes animal stomachs in smaller numbers than *H. heilmannii*. In practical terms, a histologic diagnosis is therefore required with the presence of gastric spiral organisms on the gastric mucosa or in the gastric mucous layer. Unless the laboratory undertakes electron microscopy on the gastric biopsy tissue, *H. felis* cannot be distinguished from *H. heilmannii*. *Helicobacter mustelae*, like *H. pylori*, however, can be isolated routinely from gastric biopsies by use of antibiotic-impregnated media and growth of the culture under microaerophilic conditions at 37°C.

A provisional diagnosis of gastric helicobacters takes advantage of a unique feature of these organisms—the ability to produce large quantities of urease. Gastric biopsies containing the gastric bacteria can be placed in a urea broth containing a pH indicator (phenol red) and a preservative (sodium azide) to help prevent false-positive reactions due to growth of urease-positive bacterial contaminants during incubation. The broth assay is then visually monitored for the first 8 hr of incubation and then intermittently for the next 16 hours. A positive reaction is indicated by development of a color change in the pH indicator to a deep pink via production of ammonia due to the breakdown of urea. Also, a semiquantitative determination of the number of helicobacters can be achieved by the rapidity of the color change in the assay. A "CLO" test is available commercially, or a microtiter tray with a measured amount of urea test solution delivered to each well can be used very effectively and economically. Other urease tests used in humans, but not perfected in animals except in ferrets under experimental conditions, are the urea breath test, which measures expired radiolabeled carbon dioxide, a by-product of a carbon-labeled urea test meal that is ingested by the patient. An alternative, but less accurate, measure would be direct measurement of ammonia in gastric juice by using a colorimetric assay. Serologic assays are being used to diagnose *H. pylori* in humans and *H. mustelae* infection in ferrets. However, these serologic assays are currently not available to provide a reliable, noninvasive diagnostic test for gastric *Helicobacter* infection in dogs and cats.

## TREATMENT

Various clinical trials using different antimicrobial treatments were initially conducted to assess their ability to eradicate *H. pylori*. A triple-therapy regimen consisting of amoxicillin and metronidazole, or tetracycline and metronidazole, in combination with bismuth subsalicylate given for 2 to 3 weeks has proven to be the most efficient in eradication of *H. pylori*. Indeed, this antimicrobial regimen, plus ranitidine, has proven successful in treating patients with ulcer disease. In studies comparing this treatment to those patients receiving ranitidine alone, ulcers not only healed faster, but the recurrence of ulcers was significantly less in the antibiotic-treated group where *H. pylori* has been eradicated. Recently, therapy regimens using proton pump inhibitors (e.g., omeprazole) in combination with amoxicillin also have shown considerable efficacy in eradicating *H. pylori*. Whether antimicrobial therapy should be instituted in domestic pets with gastritis or ulcer disease is at present unknown. However, studies in ferrets indicate that the triple therapy consisting of amoxicillin (20 mg/kg), metronidazole (20 mg/kg), and bismuth subsalicylate (17.5 mg/kg) (Pepto-Bismol original formula, Proctor & Gamble) three times a day for 3 to 4 weeks has successfully eradicated *H. mustelae* from ferrets.

With eradication, the gastritis diminishes and the IgG *H. mustelae* antibody decreases; these results are consistent with findings in humans after *H. pylori* is eradicated. Omeprazole in ferrets at an oral dose of 0.7 mg/kg once daily effectively induces hypochlorhydria and may be used in conjunction with antibiotics to treat *H. mustelae*–associated duodenal or gastric ulcers. Acute bleeding ulcers must be treated as emergencies, and fluid and blood transfusions are essential.

In preliminary studies, the use of similar treatment regimens has reduced colonization of gastric spiral bacteria in cat stomachs. In addition, it is known that treatment using metronidazole plus bismuth compounds has been used empirically with success to treat undiagnosed gastrointestinal syndromes in cats and dogs. Further controlled studies are warranted to explore the therapeutic benefit of antimicrobial therapies for gastric or duodenal ulcers and chronic gastritis in the dog and cat.

## ZOONOTIC IMPLICATIONS

Because *H. heilmannii* (and to a lesser extent *H. felis*) colonize a small percentage of humans with gastritis, and no environmental source for these bacteria has been recognized, pets have been implicated in zoonotic transmission of the organisms. For example, in one series of *H. heilmannii* infection in humans, two patients had close contact with pets, one lived with 14 cats, and the other owned two Irish setters. In another pediatric case of *H. heilmannii* infection, the household had two cats; a gastric biopsy from one cat indicated it was infected with gastric spiral organisms with similar morphology to that depicted in the child's stomach. Because *H. heilmannii* is not amenable to culture on artificial media, it is difficult to compare the organisms' molecular markers and thereby confirm the identity of their origin. Nevertheless, it is probable that zoonotic transmission does occur with gastric spiral organisms. If, for example, curved to spiral-shaped organisms smaller in size than *H. heilmannii* or *H. felis* sometimes observed in gastric mucosa of pets are *H. pylori* as recently demonstrated in cats, some people suspect, the zoonotic potential would obviously increase substantially. Several laboratories are actively investigating this possibility.

### References and Suggested Reading

Eaton KA, Radin MJ, Kramer L, et al: Epizootic gastritis in cheetahs associated with gastric spiral bacilli. Vet Pathol 30:55, 1993.
  *Provides strong correlation of severe Helicobacter-associated gastric disease in cheetahs associated with significant clinical signs.*
Feinstein RE and Olsson E: Chronic gastroenterocolitis in nine cats. J Vet Diagn Invest 4:293, 1992.
  *This paper notes the possible causal relationship of gastric spiral organisms and presence of gastric disease in cats.*
Fox JG, Correa P, Taylor NS, et al: Helicobacter mustelae associated gastritis in ferrets: An animal model of Helicobacter pylori gastritis in humans. Gastroenterology 99:352, 1990.
  *Describes similarities of gastritis in ferrets to that of* H. pylori *gastritis in humans including histologic features underlying ulcer disease and gastric cancer.*

Fox JG, Otto G, Taylor NS, Rosenblad W, and Murphy JC: *Helicobacter mustelae*–induced gastritis and elevated gastric pH in the ferret (*Mustela putorius furo*). Infect Immun 59:1875, 1991.
*Paper proves Koch's postulate that H. mustelae produces a chronic persistent gastritis in ferrets. Also demonstrates that acute infection with H. mustelae causes transient hypochlorhydria.*

Fox JG, Paster BJ, Dewhirst FE, et al: *Helicobacter mustelae* isolation from feces of ferrets: Evidence to support fecal-oral transmission of gastric *Helicobacter* spp. Infect Immun 60:606, 1992.
*Documents first isolation of a gastric Helicobacter from feces and helps explain likelihood of fecal oral transmission of H. mustelae.*

Fox JG, Blanco M, Polidoro D, et al: Role of gastric pH in isolation of *Helicobacter mustelae* from the feces of ferrets. Gastroenterology 104:86, 1993.
*Demonstrates that drug-induced hypochlorhydria enhances fecal recovery of H. mustelae in ferrets.*

Fox JG and Lee A: Gastric *Helicobacter* infection in animals: Natural and experimental infections. *In* Goodwin S and Worsley BW (eds): *Helicobacter pylori: Biology and Clinical Practice.* Boca Raton FL, CRC Press, 1993, pp 407–430.
*Provides overview on natural and experimental infections with gastric helicobacters in animals.*

Handt LK, Fox JG, Dewhirst FE, et al: *Helicobacter pylori* isolated from the domestic cat: Public health implications. Infect Immun 62:2367, 1994.
*Documents the first isolation of the human pathogen, H. pylori from a domestic reservoir host, the cat.*

Heilmann KL and Borchard F: Gastritis due to spiral shaped bacteria other than *Helicobacter pylori*: Clinical, histological, and ultrastructural findings. Gut 32:137, 1991.
*Provides detailed histological findings of "H. heilmannii"–associated gastritis in a series of human cases.*

Hentschel E, Brandstatter G, Dragosics B, et al: Effect of ranitidine and amoxicillin plus metronidazole on the eradication of *Helicobacter pylori* and the recurrence of duodenal ulcer. N Engl J Med 328:308, 1993.
*Controlled study using antimicrobial regimen plus H₂ blocker in eradication of H. pylori and ulcer regression, and lack of ulcer relapse after H. pylori eradication.*

Labenz J, Gyenes E, Rühl GH, and Börsch G: Amoxicillin plus omeprazole versus triple therapy for eradication of *Helicobacter pylori* in duodenal ulcer disease: A prospective, randomized, and controlled study. Gut 34: 1167, 1993.
*Controlled study demonstrating efficacy of antibiotic treatment and proton pump inhibitor in eradicating H. pylori and regression of duodenal ulcer disease.*

Lee A, Krakowka S, Fox JG, et al: Role of *Helicobacter felis* in chronic canine gastritis. Vet Pathol 29:487, 1992.
*Fulfills Koch's postulate that H. felis can cause lymphofollicular gastritis in dogs.*

Lee A, Fox JG, and Hazell S: The pathogenicity of *Helicobacter pylori*: A perspective. Infect Immun 61:1601, 1993.
*Provides overview of current views on pathogenic mechanisms of gastric helicobacters in both humans and animals.*

Otto G, Fox JG, Wu P-Y, and Taylor NS: Eradication of *Helicobacter mustelae* from the ferret stomach: An animal model of *Helicobacter (Campylobacter) pylori* chemotherapy. Antimicrob Agents Chemother 34:1232, 1990.
*Describes successful eradication of H. mustelae in ferrets with antibiotics and bismuth.*

Otto G, Hazell SH, Fox JG, et al: Animal and public health implications of gastric colonization of cats by *Helicobacter*-like organisms. J Clin Microbiol 32:1043, 1994.
*Provides urease test results and morphologic evidence that gastric helicobacters colonize and are associated with gastric pathology in cats.*

Twedt DC and Magne ML: Chronic gastritis. *In* Kirk RW (ed): *Current veterinary therapy* IX. Philadelphia, WB Saunders, 1986, pp 852.
*Classification of gastritis by histologic criteria; treatment and clinical findings of subsets of gastritis also included.*

# THERAPY OF INFLAMMATORY BOWEL DISEASE

DONNA S. DIMSKI

*Baton Rouge, Louisiana*

Inflammatory bowel disease (IBD) in dogs and cats encompasses a spectrum of diseases that result in the accumulation of inflammatory cells within the mucosa and submucosa of the stomach, small intestine, and/or large intestine. Several types of IBD occur and are classified based on the inflammatory cell infiltrate (Table 1). The cause of IBD is unknown, although certain infections may serve as a predisposing factor. In general, the treatment of IBD is aimed at removing any antigenic source of the inflammation, followed by suppression of the cell-mediated inflammatory response in the gastrointestinal tract.

Inflammatory bowel disease most commonly affects young adult and middle-aged dogs and cats of either sex. Although some forms of IBD have no breed predisposition, certain types occur more frequently in some breeds (Table 1). The clinical signs associated with IBD vary in accordance with the severity and location of cellular infiltration. Animals with IBD of the gastric and small intestinal mucosa usually are afflicted with chronic vomiting, weight loss, and diarrhea, while those suffering from IBD of the large intestine usually experience chronic evidence of tenesmus, frequent defecation, hematochezia, and mucus in the stool. In most cases, physical examination of the dog or cat with IBD will be normal, although some animals will have palpably thickened intestinal loops or evidence of weight loss.

The initial step in the diagnosis of IBD is to rule out metabolic or infectious causes of vomiting and diarrhea. A complete blood count (CBC), serum biochemistry panel, and urinalysis are useful in identifying metabolic abnormalities (such as azotemia or evidence of liver disease) that may cause vomiting or diarrhea. Neutrophilia is occasionally seen in animals with IBD, and a marked eosinophilia (>1500 cells/mm³, often >10,000 cells/mm³) may be seen with eosinophilic gastroenteritis in cats. Animals with severe IBD may manifest a protein-losing enteropathy, with decreases in serum albumin and globulin concentrations. Occasionally, hyperglobulinemia will be seen in dogs with IBD, particularly Basenjis with immunoproliferative enteropathy.

Since the primary treatment for IBD is immunosuppression, ruling out infectious causes of gastrointestinal

**Table 1.**   *Common Types of Inflammatory Bowel Diseases in Dogs and Cats*

| Type | Breed Associations | Comments |
|---|---|---|
| Lymphocytic-plasmacytic | Shar Pei<br>German shepherd dog<br>Other dogs and cats | Most common IBD |
| Immunoproliferative | Basenji | Treat aggressively; poor prognosis |
| Eosinophilic | Dogs | May respond to diet change alone |
| Eosinophilic | Cats | More severe; treat aggressively |
| Hypereosinophilic syndrome | Cats | Severe disease, affecting multiple organs; treat aggressively; poor prognosis |
| Granulomatous | No breed predispositions | Uncommon primary IBD |
| Histiocytic ulcerative colitis | Boxer | Treat aggressively; poor prognosis |
| Wheat-sensitive enteropathy | Irish setter | Feed wheat- and gluten-free diet |

signs and inflammation is imperative (Table 2). *Giardia* may be ruled out by assessment of several zinc sulfate centrifugation tests (see "*Giardia*: Diagnosis and Treatment," this volume, p 716) or by a diagnostic and therapeutic trial with metronidazole (60 mg/kg every 12 hr for 5 days). Fecal cultures, fecal examinations for helminths, and evaluation of intestinal mucosal histopathology may be required to definitively rule out other infectious diseases. Testing for feline leukemia and feline immunodeficiency virus infections in cats is advisable. Although intestinal bacterial overgrowth is difficult to diagnose, identification of low serum cobalamin and elevated serum folate concentrations may support this diagnosis.

The definitive diagnosis of IBD is made by histopathologic evaluation of the gastrointestinal mucosa. Endoscopic evaluation of the stomach and small intestine or colon (depending on the clinical signs exhibited) may reveal visual evidence of disease, although many cases of IBD exhibit normal-appearing mucosa; therefore, biopsy is indicated regardless of appearance (see "Biopsy of the Gastrointestinal Tract," this volume, p 675). Endoscopy is less invasive than surgical biopsy, but endoscopic biopsies are limited in size (approximately 2.8 mm diameter), depth (usually mucosa only), and area (jejunum and ileum are seldom reached). Occasionally, IBD lesions will be missed on endoscopic biopsy, necessitating surgical biopsy. If endoscopy is unavailable, exploratory laparotomy and surgical biopsy can be performed in lieu of endoscopy. Visual inspection of the gastrointestinal serosal surfaces and manual assessment of intestinal wall thickness should be performed. Full-thickness biopsies of the gastrointestinal tract should be collected, even if no gross lesions are detected.

The histologic evaluation of the gastrointestinal biopsy will be confirmatory of IBD, and will specify the type of IBD present based on the cellular infiltrate. Additionally, diagnosis of infectious diseases (such as histoplasmosis) may be noted on histopathology.

**Table 2.**   *Infectious Rule-Outs for Inflammatory Bowel Disease*

| Disease | Method of Ruling Out |
|---|---|
| *Giardia* | Fecal saline smear<br>Zinc sulfate centrifugation<br>Fecal ELISA (?) |
| Intestinal parasites | Fecal flotation |
| *Campylobacter* | Fecal culture<br>Fecal cytology |
| *Salmonella* | Fecal culture |
| Intestinal bacterial overgrowth | Intestinal fluid culture<br>Serum cobalamin and folate |
| Histoplasmosis | Rectal scraping<br>Intestinal biopsy |
| Oomycosis (Pythium) | Intestinal biopsy |

## RATIONALE FOR THERAPY

The pathogenesis of IBD in humans and in animals is poorly understood. In general, IBD is an inflammatory process thought to be initiated by dietary or microbial antigens in the gastrointestinal lumen. These antigens stimulate T lymphocytes, which promote cell-mediated immunity in the gut by modulating the activity of helper, suppressor, killer (K), and natural killer (NK) lymphocytes. In turn, these lymphocytes may cause direct cytotoxicity, attract other inflammatory cells, activate the complement cascade, and lead to local tissue destruction. Therefore, it is the immune response itself that leads to tissue destruction and associated impairment of intestinal digestive and absorptive capabilities.

Because the presumed pathogenesis of IBD involves

antigenic stimulation and an inflammatory response mediated by the mucosal immune system, therapy is aimed at removing the offending antigen and decreasing the immune response. Often, a primary antigen (such as *Giardia* or intestinal bacterial overgrowth) cannot be identified, and a dietary antigen is implicated as the inciting factor. However, it is very difficult in the clinical situation to confirm or disprove the possibility that a certain dietary antigen is the causal factor, and dietary manipulation may or may not be helpful.

## DIETARY MANAGEMENT

The goal of dietary management of IBD is to reduce antigenic stimulation of the intestinal immune system. Proteins, food colorings, and preservatives may all cause adverse gastrointestinal signs, but many of these reactions are direct, not mediated through the immune system. In general, antigenic determinants on proteins are incriminated as the causative factor in many cases of IBD. Therefore, it is advisable to feed a "hypoallergenic" diet to dogs and cats with IBD.

Unfortunately, the term "hypoallergenic diet" is clouded with misconceptions. The primary attributes of a diet formulated for the dog or cat with IBD are that it is free of additives and preservatives, contains an adequate (but not excessive) amount of highly digestable protein, and contains a single, novel protein source. In some cases, additional dietary fiber may have an added benefit.

### Additives and Preservatives

Some pet food companies advertise a product as hypoallergenic if it is free of color additives and preservatives. Foods that contain no additives or preservatives are less likely to induce direct adverse food reactions, and therefore may be beneficial in many animals with IBD; however, they are not necessarily hypoallergenic (see *CVT XI*, p 587).

### Protein Digestibility

The ideal diet for animals with IBD should contain an adequate amount of a highly digestible protein. Excess protein in the diet can lead to increased formation of antigen-antibody complexes in the intestinal wall, which promotes inflammation. The protein fed should be highly digestible, since it is the intact protein, not the polypeptides and amino acids that result from digestion of the protein, that is antigenic. A poorly digestible protein provides increased quantities of antigenic determinants to the intestinal immune system and therefore promotes IBD.

### Protein Source

There are no protein sources that are inherently hypoallergenic, including lamb (which is incorrectly perceived to be the ideal protein source to prevent or treat food allergies manifesting as gastrointestinal or dermatologic diseases). In general, dogs and cats develop immunologic sensitivities to foods that contain antigenic determinants, promote an immune response, and which the animal has eaten with some frequency. Wheat, beef, milk, eggs, horsemeat, fish, and pork can all be allergens promoting IBD in dogs and cats. The practical approach to choosing a protein source, then, is to feed diets that contain only one source of protein that the animal has not eaten before.

In dogs, an ideal approach is to feed a homemade diet based on rice. A single novel protein source such as tofu, cottage cheese, or lamb is added. In cats, homemade diets can include either lamb or chicken, with less rice. If the animal's clinical signs improve on the homemade diet, then switching to a commercial diet with that protein source is advised, unless the homemade diet is made complete by the addition of vitamins, minerals, essential fatty acids, appropriate calcium:phosphorus ratio, and so forth.

Commercial diets are available that meet the criteria of a single, novel protein source. Currently, canned foods containing rabbit, lamb, chicken, fish, venison, or duck as the only protein sources are being used successfully. It is important that the ingredients list of a potentially hypoallergenic diet be thoroughly evaluated, since diets with several protein sources (such as lamb, beef, rice, and wheat) are marketed with a claim to hypoallergenicity. As novel protein sources such as lamb are used in maintenance diets, their potential for use in therapeutic diets is greatly diminished.

### Dietary Fiber

Addition of dietary fiber can be beneficial in some animals with chronic large bowel diarrhea. The diet itself can contain increased quantities of cellulose, an insoluble fiber, or soluble fiber products (such as psyllium) can be added to a diet. Fiber can help in the management of diarrhea by absorbing excess fluid and neutralizing some toxins (see *CVT XI*, p 592). However, it is unlikely that dietary fiber directly affects the intestinal immune system in IBD.

## DRUG THERAPY

While some animals with IBD can be controlled with dietary manipulation alone, many require adjunctive pharmacologic treatment to induce remission of clinical signs. The goal of drug therapy in IBD is to modulate the immune response of the gastrointestinal tract, primarily by suppressing the gut's inflammatory response. To achieve this goal, immunosuppressive agents are chosen as the initial medication. Drug dosages used in the management of IBD are listed in Table 3.

***Table 3.***    *Drugs Used in the Management of Inflammatory Bowel Disease*

| Drug | Dose | Comments |
|---|---|---|
| Prednisone | 0.5–1.0 mg/kg q24h PO | Starting immunosuppressive dose; taper to 0.5 mg/kg q48h when improved |
| Azathioprine (Imuran, Burroughs Wellcome) | 2 mg/kg q24h PO for 1 week, then q48h | Canine dosage; add to prednisone; monitor for bone marrow suppression |
| | 0.3 mg/kg q48h PO | Feline dosage |
| Cyclophosphamide (Cytoxan, Bristol Myers) | 50 mg/m² PO q48h | Add to prednisone; monitor for bone marrow suppression |
| Metronidazole (Flagyl, Searle) | 60 mg/kg PO q24h × 5 days | Dose to treat *Giardia* |
| | 10 mg/kg PO q8–24h | Antibacterial, anti-inflammatory dose |
| Sulfasalazine (Azulfidine, Pharmacia) | 25–50 mg/kg PO q8–12h | Canine dosage |
| | 10–20 mg/kg PO q8–12h | Feline dosage; maximum 10 days |

## Corticosteroids

Prednisone is the primary drug therapy for dogs and cats with IBD. Corticosteroids suppress the immune response and decrease the local inflammation present in the gastrointestinal tract (see "Clinical Applications of Glucocorticoid Therapy in Nonendocrine Disease," this volume, p 406). Additionally, corticosteroids may enhance fluid and electrolyte absorption in the small intestine.

Immunosuppressive doses of prednisone are used initially (1 to 2 mg/kg body weight every 12 hr). Oral preparations are adequate, unless vomiting would preclude their use. Most dogs and cats will show improvement in gastrointestinal signs within 1 to 2 weeks after initiation of prednisone. In most cases, immunosuppressive doses of prednisone should be continued for 1 to 2 months. If clinical signs are in remission at that time, then a slow tapering of the prednisone dose can be attempted, with maintenance of anti-inflammatory doses for 6 to 12 months. In many cases, alternate-day therapy with prednisone must be continued for the remainder of the animal's life, since withdrawal of the drug causes recurrence of clinical signs.

The primary side effects of prednisone therapy in dogs are polyuria, polydipsia, polyphagia, weight gain, and other clinical signs of iatrogenic hyperadrenocorticism (see "Corticosteroid Withdrawal Syndrome," this volume, p 413). These side effects are dose related, and therefore tapering the dose to the least amount of prednisone that will improve the clinical signs is important. Often combination therapy with other immunosuppressive drugs (such as azathioprine) is undertaken with the goal of reducing the corticosteroid dose. Since cats infrequently exhibit clinical signs attributable to corticosteroid usage, addition of azathioprine is seldom warranted in cats.

In humans, other steroid preparations are often used. Corticosteroid enemas are useful in the management of ulcerative colitis, and administration of corticotropin (ACTH) is occasionally substituted for exogenous corticosteroids. However, these methods of corticosteroid administration have not been commonly used in veterinary medicine.

## Other Immunosuppressive Drugs

Azathioprine and cyclophosphamide are immunosuppressive agents that can be used in combination with corticosteroids in the management of IBD. Azathioprine is a synthetic purine analog that is incorporated into DNA. This incorporation inhibits the normal DNA replication process, leading to interference of cellular function. Azathioprine should be considered in the patient with IBD that is not fully responsive to corticosteroids, or when the patient requires a high dose of corticosteroids and experiences unacceptable, corticosteroid-associated side effects. Azathioprine takes 1 to 3 weeks to become fully effective, so corticosteroid doses should not be tapered until the patient has been receiving azathioprine for at least 1 week. The goal of combination therapy is to taper the prednisone until the dose is 0.5 to 1.0 mg/kg on an alternate-day schedule with azathioprine. The major side effect of azathioprine is bone marrow suppression, and complete blood counts should be evaluated every 2 weeks for the initial 2 months of therapy, then every month thereafter. The combination of corticosteroids and azathioprine occasionally can cause pancreatitis, and bouts of vomiting and diarrhea should be evaluated accordingly. The pill size of azathioprine (50 mg) is unwieldy in small animals, but many pharmacists will formulate a suspension of the drug in a palatable syrup when needed.

Cyclophosphamide is an alkylating agent used occasionally in IBD. Like azathioprine, it inhibits cell function. Because of its potency and tendency to induce side effects, this drug should be reserved for patients with severe IBD. Side effects of cyclophosphamide include bone marrow suppression and hemorrhagic cystitis. Complete blood counts should be monitored frequently to assess for thrombocytopenia, leukopenia, or anemia associated with treatment.

## Metronidazole

Metronidazole has many uses in the treatment of IBD. At high doses, it is antiprotozoal, and is the current treatment of choice for *Giardia* infections in dogs and cats. It is antibacterial, and can be used in the management of intestinal bacterial overgrowth. It also inhibits cell-mediated immunity, and thus is a useful drug in the management of IBD. Metronidazole is used as an adjunctive treatment with corticosteroids, and it should be considered if prednisone is unable to control clinical signs without inducing unacceptable side effects. The major side effect of metronidazole is vomiting, although neurologic signs have been seen with overdosage in dogs.

## Salicylates

Salicylates are anti-inflammatory drugs that are useful in the treatment of colonic (but not small intestinal) IBD. The drug most commonly used in veterinary medicine is sulfasalazine, which incorporates sulfa and 5-aminosalicyclic acid (5-ASA) moieties with an azo bond. The drug is not metabolized in the small intestine, but as it reaches the large intestine, colonic bacteria break the azo bond and release the 5-ASA for a local anti-inflammatory effect. Both the sulfa and 5-ASA components are absorbed to some extent across the colonic mucosa. The primary effect of the salicylates is inhibition of the lipoxygenase pathway, which synthesizes leukotrienes. Additionally, salicylates may scavenge oxygen-derived free radicals and may inhibit antibodies directed at colonic antigens.

Sulfasalazine is useful in the management of inflammatory colitis in dogs and cats. The major side effects of sulfasalazine are keratoconjunctivitis sicca (KCS) and salicylate toxicity. The KCS is caused by both components of the drug, although the sulfa component has traditionally been blamed for this side effect. Salicylate toxicity is seen primarily in cats with an excessive dosage or prolonged administration; therefore, a lower dosage should be used in cats, and the recommended duration of therapy is 10 days (Table 3).

Sulfasalazine may be used continuously if needed in canine inflammatory colitis. This drug may also be effective when administered intermittently, as needed when clinical signs recur. Intermittent administration may alleviate some of the expected side effects.

Newer salicylate preparations are currently available for use in humans with colonic diseases. Olsalazine and balsalazide are similar to sulfasalazine, except that the azo bond links two 5-ASA molecules (olsalazine) or a 5-ASA molecule to an inert vehicle (balsalazide). A delayed release form of 5-ASA, mesalamine, is also available that coats the distal ileum and colon with the salicylate. Different 5-ASA preparations are also available as retention enemas. There is currently minimal experience with these newer formulations of salicylates in animals. Caution must be advised in their use in dogs and cats, since these species may have increased risk of toxicity with these drugs. However, it is likely that in the near future a safe and effective dose for animals may be established.

## Newer Drugs

Since IBD, ulcerative colitis, and Crohn's disease are common and severe diseases in humans, current research is focusing on new drugs that will aid in the treatment of inflammatory gastrointestinal diseases. Drugs under investigation include cyclosporine, sodium cromoglycate, clonidine, and eicosapentanoic acid (found in fish oil).

Cyclosporine suppresses cell-mediated immunity, and has been used with moderate success in clinical trials on people with Crohn's disease. The side effects and cost of this drug make it an unlikely candidate for routine use in small animals with IBD.

Sodium cromoglycate decreases inflammation associated with IgE-mediated hypersensitivity, as seen with eosinophilic IBD. Sodium cromoglycate enemas were equal to prednisone enemas in the management of ulcerative colitis in people. This drug has not yet been evaluated in animals.

Clonidine is a centrally acting $\alpha_2$ agonist used primarily for management of hypertension in people. Oral clonidine has been found to equal prednisone in the reduction of inflammation associated with ulcerative colitis in people. There are no reports of its use in IBD in animals.

Eicosapentanoic acid is found in high concentrations in fish oil. This drug inhibits the lipoxygenase pathway, which leads to the formation of leukotrienes; this pathway is thought to be the primary route of arachidonic acid metabolism in the mucosal inflammation of IBD. People with ulcerative colitis showed moderate improvement histologically and clinically when treated with eicosapentanoic acid. This drug is currently available for use in small animal dermatologic diseases (Dermcaps, DVM Inc, Miami, FL), but it has not been evaluated in canine or feline IBD. The dosage of eicosapentanoic acid available in the small animal formulation is much less than that used for treatment of IBD in people.

As more research is performed aiming at a better understanding of the pathogenesis of IBD in small animals, it is likely that more specific therapies will be identified. Until that time, judicious use of accepted dietary and drug regimens offers the best hope for induction of long-term clinical remission of IBD in small animals. Treatment "failures" with standard drug regimens most likely represent an incorrect diagnosis or improper use of currently available drugs.

## References and Suggested Reading

Burrows CF: Canine colitis. Compend Cont Educ Pract Vet 14:1347, 1992.
  *A review of pathophysiology and treatment of colitis in dogs.*
Dennis JS, Kruger KM, and Mullaney TP: Lymphocytic/plasmacytic gastroenteritis in cats: 14 cases (1985–1990). J Am Vet Med Assoc 200:1712, 1992.
  *A retrospective study of lymphocytic-plasmacytic inflammatory bowel disease in cats.*
Dennis JS, Kruger KM, and Mullaney TP: Lymphocytic/plasmacytic colitis in cats: 14 cats (1985–1990). J Am Vet Med Assoc 202:313, 1993.
  *A retrospective study of lymphocytic-plasmacytic colitis in cats.*
Jacobs G, Collins-Kelly L, Lappin M, and Tyler D: Lymphocytic-plasmacytic enteritis in 24 dogs. J Vet Intern Med 4:45, 1990.
  *A retrospective study of lymphocytic-plasmacytic enteritis in dogs.*

Nelson RW, Stookey LJ, and Kazacos E: Nutritional management of idiopathic chronic colitis in the dog. J Vet Intern Med 2:133, 1988.
  *A retrospective study of nutritional management of 13 dogs with lymphocytic-plasmacytic colitis*
Peppercorn MA: Advances in drug therapy for inflammatory bowel disease. Ann Intern Med 112:50, 1990.

  *A review of current and investigational treatment for inflammatory bowel diseases in people.*
Willard MD: Inflammatory bowel disease: Perspectives on therapy. J Am Anim Hosp Assoc 28:27, 1992.
  *A review of currently available therapies for inflammatory bowel disease in dogs and cats.*

# CRYPTOSPORIDIOSIS IN THE DOG AND CAT

STEVEN L. HILL
*and* MICHAEL R. LAPPIN
*Fort Collins, Colorado*

## ETIOLOGIC AGENT

The cause of cryptosporidiosis, *Cryptosporidium* spp. are coccidian parasites in the phylum Apicomplexa, suborder Eimeriina, family Cryptosporiidae. The organisms inhabit the respiratory and intestinal epithelium of many vertebrates including birds, mammals, reptiles, and fish. *Cryptosporidium* spp. are prevalent intestinal parasites of importance to both veterinary and human medicine. Once thought to be a commensal, *Cryptosporidium* spp. are now known to cause gastrointestinal tract disease in a number of species including rodents, dogs, cats, calves, and people. This genus is ubiquitous in nature; some species are pathogenic and can cross-infect between mammalian species. Generally, isolates of *Cryptosporidium* infecting mammals have been infective for other mammals. Transmission of mammalian isolates of *Cryptosporidium* spp. to other vertebrate classes has not been demonstrated. Whether there are multiple species of *Cryptosporidium* that infect mammals is controversial. It is probable that among mammals, *Cryptosporidium parvum* is the only species transmitted in all studies (Dubey, Spreer, and Fayer, 1990).

## LIFE CYCLE

*Cryptosporidium* spp. have an enteric life cycle similar to other coccidian parasites. Immunocompetent mammals develop intestinal tract infection almost exclusively. Immunocompromised mammals can have infections of any section of the gastrointestinal tract including the pancreas, liver, and gallbladder, as well as infection of the respiratory tract. Enteroepithelial development is limited to the luminal enterocytes; extraintestinal tissue cysts do not develop. The enteroepithelial life cycle (Fig. 1) begins with ingestion of sporulated oocysts by a suitable host. Following ingestion of oocysts, four sporozoites are released from each oocyst that penetrate intestinal epithelial cells. Asexual reproduction at the microvillus surface occurs with the production of first- and then second-generation merozoites that are released and penetrate other cells. Gametogony and sporogony occur, resulting in the production of thin-walled and thick-walled oocysts. Sporulated thick-walled oocysts are shed in the feces of an infected host and are immediately infective to a susceptible host. Thin-walled oocysts passed into the intestinal lumen rupture, releasing the sporozoites, which penetrate additional host cells and reinitiate the developmental cycle. *Cryptosporidium* spp. oocysts are spherical to ovoid. *Cryptosporidium parvum* oocysts are the smallest coccidian oocysts, ranging in size from 4.0 to 5.0 $\mu$m in diameter.

## CLINICAL MANIFESTATIONS

### Feline Cryptosporidiosis

*Cryptosporidium* infection in the domestic cat was first reported in 1979 (Iseki, 1979). While *C. parvum* is generally accepted as the cause of feline cryptosporidiosis, at least one murine strain is capable of infecting cats. The prepatent and patent periods in experimentally infected cats were 5 to 6 days and 7 to 10 days, respectively (Dubey, Speer, and Fayer, 1990). Infection of cats by *Cryptosporidium* spp. is generally thought to be subclinical (Asahi, Koyama, and Arai, 1991). It has now been established that *Cryptosporidium* infection in cats can result in clinical disease manifested as diarrhea (Bennett, Baxby, and Blundell, 1985). Two cats with diarrhea were co-infected with feline leukemia virus and *Cryptosporidium* spp. (Goodwin and Barsanti, 1990; Monticello et al., 1987). One cat with chronic diarrhea had intestinal lymphosarcoma and cryptosporidiosis (Lent, Burdhardt, and Bolka, 1993). One cat with chronic diarrhea had detectable oocysts in approximately 20 fecal samples assessed over a 6-week period.

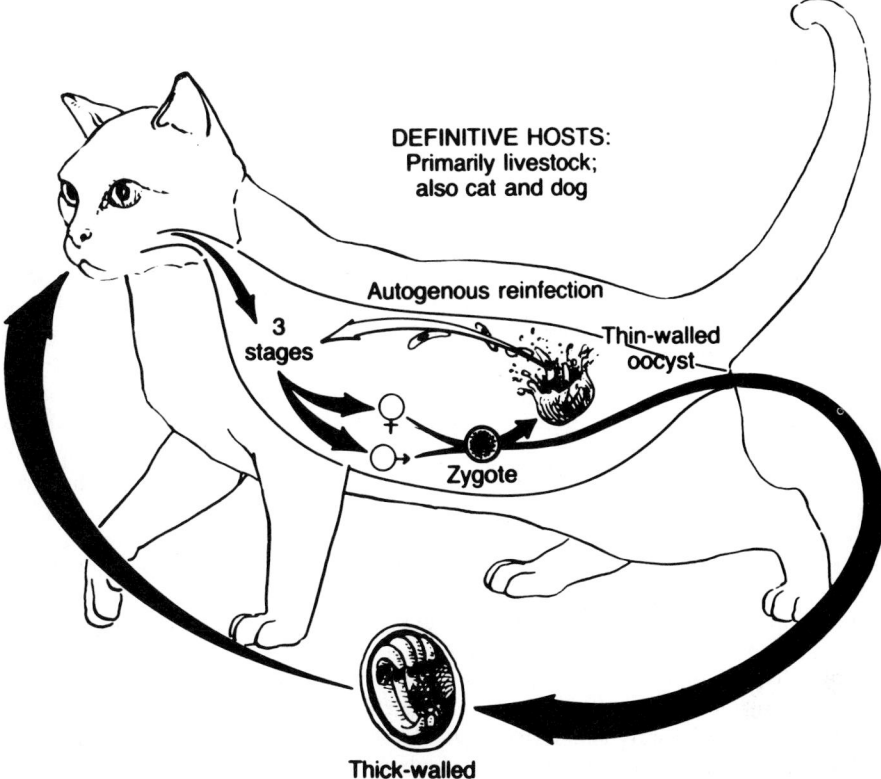

**Figure 1.** Illustrated life cycle of *Cryptosporidium* spp. (From Prestwood AK: Cryptosporidiosis. *In* Greene CE [ed]: *Infectious Diseases of The Dog and Cat.* Philadelphia, WB Saunders Co, 1990, p 848, with permission.)

Laboratory testing of the cat revealed no evidence of immunosuppression. The cat had concurrent lymphocytic/plasmacytic enteritis and duodenal bacterial overgrowth. Antibodies against *Cryptosporidium* spp. were detected in serum (Lappin et al., 1994).

## Canine Cryptosporidiosis

*Cryptosporidium* infection in the domestic dog was first reported in 1983 (Wilson, Holscher, and Lyle, 1983). *Cryptosporidium parvum* appears to be the infecting species. Most reported cases of *Cryptosporidium* oocyst shedding in dogs have been subclinical. Oocyst shedding most commonly has been detected in young dogs. Oocyst shedding can occur in subclinically infected dogs. As in cats, diarrhea is the most common manifestation of intestinal cryptosporidiosis in dogs. With the exception of a 2-year-old dog with intestinal malabsorption resulting in intermittent diarrhea and weight loss (Greene, Jacobs, and Prickett, 1990), clinical cases of intestinal cryptosporidiosis have been in juvenile dogs 6 months of age or less. Co-infection with canine distemper virus was documented in two cases (Fukushima and Helman, 1984; Turnwald et al., 1988).

## DIAGNOSIS

Diagnosis of cryptosporidiosis is based on demonstration of the organism. Histopathologic documenta-

tion of the organism in intestinal biopsies is diagnostic, but is not practical and can be falsely negative. Oocysts are most commonly demonstrated in feces using concentration techniques, staining of fecal smears, and immunofluorescent antibody assays. Enzyme-linked immunosorbent assays (ELISA) for detection of *Cryptosporidium* antigen in feces are available but have not been evaluated extensively using dog or cat feces.[*][†]

The small size of *Cryptosporidium* oocysts makes identification difficult following routine salt solution flotation. The combination of concentration and staining techniques increases the likelihood of oocyst demonstration. Sugar solution centrifugation and zinc sulfate centrifugation using solutions with a specific gravity of 1.18 to 1.20 are effective and can be performed in the veterinary clinic (see *CVT* Update: Feline Toxoplasmosis, this volume, p 309). Fecal sedimentation using formalin-ether or formalin-ethyl acetate is also an effective technique. Fluorescent antibody techniques are thought by some to be optimal for the demonstration of *Cryptosporidium* oocysts, but require special equipment and are only available in some laboratories. We currently perform modified acid-fast staining[‡] of a direct fecal smear and sugar solution centrifugation on

---

[*]ProSpecT Cryptosporidium Microtiter Assay, Alexon Inc, 1190 Borregas Ave., Sunnyvale, CA 94089.

[†]Color-Vue Cryptosporidium, Seradyn, Inc. P.O. Box 1210, Indianapolis, IN 46206.

[‡]Volu-Sol AFB Stain (Carbol Fuchsin), Volu-Sol 700 Sunset Road, Henderson, NV 89015.

samples from animals with suspected cryptosporidiosis. Microscopic examination should be performed at 1000X due to the small size of the oocysts. Phase contrast microscopy is superior to bright-field microscopy for demonstration of unstained oocysts and should be used if available. Identification of oocysts depends on the experience of the individual performing the examination. Many human laboratories have experience with most of the techniques discussed here. Samples submitted to the laboratory should be fresh, mixed one part 100% formalin with nine parts feces to inactivate the oocysts, and clearly marked as suspected cryptosporidiosis to decrease human health risk.

## TREATMENT

A number of therapeutic modalities have been tested for efficacy against cryptosporidiosis in humans and animals. Treatment is required most commonly in immunocompromised patients and includes supportive care, chemotherapeutics, and immunomodulation. Supportive care usually consists of oral or intravenous administration of fluids. Nonspecific antidiarrheal therapy sometimes lessens the volume of diarrheic feces but does not clear the body of the organism. Over 90 drugs have been assessed for anti-*Cryptosporidium* activity; no uniformly successful therapy has been found. Discontinuation of immunosuppressive chemotherapy or administration of immunotherapeutics to improve the immune response has been attempted in some human cases.

Clinical cryptosporidiosis in dogs has generally resulted in death or euthanasia due to the severity of diarrhea. Cryptosporidiosis may not have been the primary problem in most cases, as concurrent diseases such as distemper virus infection were identified. One dog treated with clindamycin hydrochloride continued to shed oocysts in feces (Greene, Jacobs, and Prickett, 1990).

Therapy has been implemented more often for cryptosporidiosis in cats but, overall, response rates have been low. This may be related to concurrent diseases, drug resistance, or incorrect drug dosage. Short-term therapy with sulfadimethoxine and amoxicillin in a cat with intestinal cryptosporidiosis and feline leukemia virus (FeLV) infection was ineffective in controlling diarrhea. This cat was euthanized after only 5 days of therapy, making it difficult to draw conclusions regarding drug efficacy (Goodwin and Barsanti, 1990). One immunocompetent cat with chronic diarrhea, fecal oocyst shedding, and lymphocytic plasmacytic enteritis became normal following the administration of tylosin at 11 mg/kg PO, twice daily for 21 days (Lappin et al., 1994). Oocyst shedding was not documented following treatment for 1 year and the lymphocytic-plasmacytic enteritis resolved. It is unknown whether *Cryptosporidium* induced lymphocytic-plasmacytic enteritis or whether lymphocytic-plasmacytic enteritis predisposed to chronic *Cryptosporidium* oocyst shedding.

## ZOONOTIC ASPECTS

### Canine and Feline Prevalence

The prevalence of *Cryptosporidium* oocysts in cat feces was 8.1% and 3.9%, respectively, in studies performed in Scotland (Mtambo et al., 1991) and Japan (Dubey, Speer, and Fayer, 1990). Seroprevalence has been reported in two studies. Antibodies to *Cryptosporidium* spp. were detected in 20 of 23 (87%) serum samples tested by indirect fluorescent antibody assay in Scotland (Tzipori and Campbell, 1981). ELISA for the detection of anti-*Cryptosporidium* IgG in the serum of cats was developed and validated using serum from experimentally infected and naturally infected cats. The regional seroprevalence of *Cryptosporidium* spp. in cats within the United States is approximately 35% (unpublished data).

The prevalence of *Cryptosporidium* oocysts in dog feces was 2.0% and 1.4%, respectively, in studies performed in California (El-Ahraf et al., 1991) and Japan (Dubey, Speer, and Fayer, 1990). Serum samples from 16 of 21 (80%) dogs in Scotland were positive for antibodies against *Cryptosporidium* spp. using an indirect fluorescent antibody assay (Dubey, Speer, and Fayer, 1990).

Seroprevalence results suggest that dogs and cats are commonly exposed to *Cryptosporidium* spp. Whether seropositive animals are currently harboring the organism is unknown.

Detectable *Cryptosporidium* oocyst shedding can be induced in experimentally infected cats previously negative for oocysts on fecal examination by administering prednisone at a dosage of 10 mg/kg/day (Asahi et al., 1991). Whether clinical doses of glucocorticoids or immunodeficiency-inducing co-infections result in repeated oocyst shedding in *Cryptosporidium* antibody–positive, oocyst–negative cats or dogs is unknown.

### Human Cryptosporidiosis

*Cryptosporidium* spp. are transmitted by fecal-oral spread of the oocyst stage. Ingestion of oocysts by person-to-person contact, person-to-animal contact, or environmental sources (i.e., ingesting contaminated water and possibly fomites, food, or milk products) are the most likely routes of exposure. *Cryptosporidium* infection of people following exposure to calves has been recognized for years. *Cryptosporidiosis* has been reported in veterinary students. Many cases of human cryptosporidiosis in veterinary students go unreported. Human *Cryptosporidium* spp. infection after exposure to an infected dog (Greene, Jacobs, and Prickett, 1990) and infected cats has been reported (Dubey, Speer, and Fayer, 1990; Egger et al., 1990).

The duration and severity of intestinal cryptosporidiosis is determined by the immunocompetence of the patient. Self-limiting diarrhea occurs most commonly in immunocompetent people; immunosuppressed individuals can develop fulminant life-threatening diarrhea. Asymptomatic infections have been reported in immunocompetent persons, and have been described primarily during evaluation of day-care outbreaks and less commonly in geographic surveys. Cryptosporidiosis is of greatest clinical impact in patients with acquired immunodeficiency syndrome (AIDS). Intestinal cryptosporidiosis is implicated as one of the most common causes of chronic diarrhea in AIDS patients. At the time of initial diagnosis, 4% of AIDS patients are infected with *Cryptosporidium* spp. and 10% to 20% will be infected at some time during the course of their disease. *Cryptosporidium* infection is also common in patients undergoing immunosuppressive chemotherapy, patients with hypogammaglobulinemia or agammaglobulinemia, malnourished children, and patients with concurrent viral infections such as measles, chicken pox, or cytomegalovirus (also see, "Pet Ownership for Immunocompromised People," this volume, p 271).

## PREVENTION AND CONTROL

Control and prevention of cryptosporidiosis is primarily directed at elimination or reduction of the exogenous oocyst stage from the environment and avoidance of contact with known sources. With conditions of moisture and moderate temperature, oocysts can remain viable and infectious for extended periods of time. Oocysts of *Cryptosporidium* spp. stored in aqueous suspensions at 4°C can remain infective for 6 to 9 months. Temperature extremes affect oocyst viability. Drying, freeze-thawing, and steam cleaning can inactivate the organism. Water collected in the field should be boiled. As for other coccidian oocysts, few commercial disinfectants have been found effective in killing oocysts of *Cryptosporidium* spp. Immunoprophylaxis is under investigation. Recently, a *Cryptosporidium* autogenous biologic commercial vaccine has become available for use in cattle, but efficacy studies are lacking.

## References and Suggested Reading

Asahi H, Koyama T, Arai H, et al: Biological nature of *Cryptosporidium* sp. isolated from a cat. Parasitol Res 77:237, 1991.
*A report of experimental* Cryptosporidium *infection in cats with recurrence*

*of proliferation of the parasite and subsequently oocyst shedding occurring after prednisolone administration.*
Bennett M, Baxby K, Blundell N, et al: Cryptosporidiosis in the domestic cat. Vet Rec 116:73, 1985.
*A series of three cats with clinical enteric cryptosporidiosis and concurrent cryptosporidiosis in one owner.*
Dubey JP, Speer CA, and Fayer R: *Cryptosporidiosis of Man and Animals.* Boca Raton, FL, CRC Press, 1990.
*A comprehensive, extensively referenced text detailing all aspects of* Cryptosporidium.
Egger M, Nguyen M, Schaad UB, et al: Intestinal cryptosporidiosis acquired from a cat. Infection 18:177, 1990.
*A case of intestinal cryptosporidiosis in an 8-year-old boy after contact with a* Cryptosporidium-*infected cat.*
El-Ahraf A, Tacal JV, Sobih M, et al: Prevalence of cryptosporidiosis in dogs and human beings in San Bernardino County, California. J Am Vet Med Assoc 198:631, 1991.
*A report of* Cryptosporidium *fecal oocyst prevalence in a human and canine population in San Bernardino County.*
Fukushima K and Helman RG: Cryptosporidiosis in a pup with distemper. Vet Pathol 21:247, 1984.
*The first reported case of cryptosporidiosis in a dog.*
Goodwin MA and Barsanti JA: Intractable diarrhea associated with intestinal cryptosporidiosis in a domestic cat also infected with feline leukemia virus. J Am Anim Hosp Assoc 26:365, 1990.
*A case report of a cat with diarrhea co-infected with FeLV and cryptosporidiosis.*
Greene CE, Jacobs GJ, and Prickett D: Intestinal malabsorption and cryptosporidiosis in an adult dog. J Am Vet Med Assoc 197:365, 1990.
*A case report of chronic cryptosporidiosis resulting in intestinal malabsorption in a mature dog.*
Iseki M: *Cryptosporidium felis* sp.n.(Protozoa:Eimeriorina) from the domestic cat. Jpn J Parasitol 28:285, 1979.
*The first description of* Cryptosporidium *in the cat.*
Lappin MR, et al: Tylosin-responsive chronic cryptosporidiosis in a cat. J Am Vet Med Assoc (submitted) 1995.
*A case report of a cat with clinical intestinal cryptosporidiosis that responded to tylosin therapy.*
Lent SF, Burkhardt JE, and Bolka D: Coincident enteric cryptosporidiosis and lymphosarcoma in a cat with diarrhea. Am Anim Hosp Assoc 29:429, 1993.
*Case report of a cat with chronic diarrhea having intestinal lymphosarcoma and persistent cryptosporidiosis.*
Monticello TM, Levy MG, Bunch SE, et al: Cryptosporidiosis in a feline leukemia virus–positive cat. J Am Vet Med Assoc 191:705, 1987.
*A case report of intestinal cryptosporidiosis in a cat with inflammatory bowel disease and toxocariasis.*
Mtambo MMA, Nash AS, Blewett DA, et al: *Cryptosporidium* infection in cats: Prevalence of infection in domestic and feral cats in the Glasgow area. Vet Rec 129:502, 1991.
*Clinical and postmortem survey of domestic and feral cats in the Glasgow area.*
Turnwald GH, Barta O, Taylor HW, et al: Cryptosporidiosis associated with immunosuppression attributable to distemper in a pup. J Am Vet Med Assoc 192:79, 1988.
*Case report of a puppy with distemper virus infection that was co-infected with* Cryptosporidium *spp.*
Tzipori S and Campbell I: Prevalence of *Cryptosporidium* antibodies in 10 animal species, J Clin Microbiol 14:455, 1981.
*Description of an indirect immunofluorescence (IF) procedure for detection of antibodies to* Cryptosporidium *and report of the prevalence of antibody in a number of host species.*
Wilson RB, Holscher MA, and Lyle SJ: Cryptosporidiosis in a pup. J Am Vet Med Assoc 183:1005, 1983.
*A case report of intestinal cryptosporidiosis in a juvenile dog with enteritis.*

# FELINE EXOCRINE PANCREATIC INSUFFICIENCY

DAVID A. WILLIAMS
*West Lafayette, Indiana*

## ETIOLOGY

The most common cause of exocrine pancreatic insufficiency (EPI) in the cat is probably end-stage chronic pancreatitis. In chronic pancreatitis, both endocrine and exocrine pancreatic cells are progressively destroyed, thus exocrine pancreatic insufficiency may be accompanied by diabetes mellitus in some cases.

Pancreatic acinar atrophy (PAA) is by far the most common cause of EPI in dogs, and while there are no well-documented reports of this in cats, the author is aware of at least three cases of feline EPI that at necropsy were shown to have pathologic findings identical to those seen in canine pancreatic acinar atrophy. The etiology of the atrophy is unknown.

Exocrine insufficiency may also develop as a result of obstruction to the flow of pancreatic juice secondary to pancreatic adenocarcinoma or other tumors, although as in dogs this is uncommon. In cats, unlike in dogs, EPI can occur as a complication of proximal duodenal resection and cholecystoduodenostomy, since in cats dual pancreatic ducts are usually absent and therefore damage to the major duodenal papilla blocks pancreatic secretion.

Afflictions of the pancreas that are peculiar to the cat include pancreatic fluke (*Eurytrema procyonis*) infection, aberrant liver fluke (*Amphimerus pseudofelineus*) infection, pancreatitis associated with cholangiohepatitis or hepatic lipidosis, and insular amyloidosis. Of these, only pancreatic fluke infection has been associated with signs suggestive of EPI.

Finally, extremely rare causes of EPI in children include congenital deficiencies of individual pancreatic digestive enzymes or of intestinal enteropeptidase, none of which has been reported in cats.

## PATHOPHYSIOLOGY

Nutrient malabsorption in EPI does not arise simply as a consequence of failure of intraluminal digestion. While there are no reports of experimental studies in cats, observations of both naturally occurring and experimental EPI in several other species have revealed abnormal activities of intestinal mucosal enzymes, and impaired function as indicated by abnormal transport of sugars, amino acids, and fatty acids. Morphologic changes in the jejunal mucosa are seen in some cases, but often functional abnormalities occur in animals with no histologic evidence of mucosal damage. The cause of this mucosal pathology is unknown, but the absence of the trophic influence of pancreatic secretions, concurrent overgrowth of bacteria in the small intestine, and endocrine and nutritional factors may all be contributory.

It has recently been reported that the pancreas is the major source of intrinsic factor in the cat (Fyfe, 1993). This probably accounts for the author's observation that serum concentrations are subnormal, and often undetectable, much more frequently in cats with EPI than is the case in dogs.

## CLINICAL SIGNS

Cats with EPI most commonly present with polyphagia, weight loss, and diarrhea. Although weight loss is often dramatic by the time a final diagnosis is made, the rate of weight loss may be slow initially, and not all animals are obviously polyphagic, so uncharacteristically mild signs may be all that are reported for weeks or months before a more classic clinical picture appears. Greasy soiling of the perineal area and sometimes of the entire hair coat may arise secondary to severe steatorrhea. In many cases, large amounts of semiformed feces are passed, but intermittent severe watery diarrhea may also occur. These signs are all nonspecific and may occur with malabsorption due to any cause.

## DIAGNOSIS

Routine laboratory test results are generally not helpful in establishing the diagnosis of EPI. Serum alanine aminotransferase and alkaline phosphatase activity may be mildly increased, while triglyceride and cholesterol concentrations may be reduced, presumably secondary to malnutrition, but normal serum albumin and globulin concentrations are usually maintained even when patients become severely malnourished. Lymphopenia, lymphocytosis, neutrophilia, and eosinophilia may all be seen, but complete blood count results are often normal and major abnormalities should be pursued as evidence of additional or alternative underlying disorders.

Serum cobalamin concentrations are subnormal in most cats with EPI, and in many cases the vitamin is undetectable. However, it must be remembered that cobalamin malabsorption is not solely a feature of feline

EPI but can also occur with small intestinal diseases. Malabsorption of fat-soluble vitamins is also likely when there is severe steatorrhea, and vitamin K–responsive coagulopathy has been reported in association with feline EPI.

Several laboratory tests for the diagnosis of EPI have been described. Assay of fecal proteolytic activity using a reproducible quantitative method (such as radial enzyme diffusion or azoprotein digestion) will identify most affected patients, but will give false-positive results in a small proportion of cases that have small intestinal disease. Assay of feline serum trypsin-like immunoreactivity (TLI) is a promising new approach, but this method presently has limited availability.

While there are some limited control data in healthy cats, the reliability of other tests for diagnosis of EPI (bentiromide absorption; fat absorption or plasma turbidity; microscopic examination of feces for evidence of undigested food such as fat droplets, starch grains, or muscle fibers) has not been widely evaluated in this species. However, the limited evidence that is available suggests that these latter tests may give misleading results in cats, and that, as has been shown in other species, they often give relatively unreliable results. In any case, they are often not practical for use in cats, so their use is not recommended and will not be discussed further in this article.

## Fecal Proteolytic Activity

Fecal proteolytic activity (often inaccurately referred to as fecal "trypsin") has been used as an index of pancreatic enzyme activity for many years. Unfortunately, the x-ray film gelatin digestion test as widely used is an unreliable assay of fecal proteolytic activity and gives many false-negative and false-positive results. Fecal proteolytic activity assayed using substrates such as azocasein or azoalbumin, or casein in a radial enzyme diffusion assay (Fig. 1) is more reliable. As in dogs, proteolytic activity is present in all normal cats, but results are consistently low in most cats with exocrine pancreatic insufficiency (Fig. 1). At least three fecal specimens should be assayed because normal cats occasionally pass feces with low protease activity. Furthermore, since proteolytic activity in feces is relatively labile, if samples are to be shipped to an outside laboratory for analysis, they should be stored frozen prior to mailing and preferably sent by express delivery service. This type of test is probably the most widely available approach to diagnosis in cats, and can also be applied to other species.

## Serum Trypsin-like Immunoreactivity

Serum TLI refers to the concentration of proteins recognized by antibodies raised against the pancreatic digestive enzyme trypsin. In healthy animals, serum TLI results from the presence of trypsinogen, the inactive zymogen form of the enzyme, which leaks out of the pancreas in trace amounts. Serum TLI can be detected in all normal mammals, provided that a species-specific assay is used. Unfortunately, commercially available immunoassay kits for human or canine TLI do not detect feline TLI. However, a sensitive and specific radioimmunoassay for feline TLI has recently been developed in the author's laboratory.[*] In 28 normal cats from which food had been withheld for 12 to 15 hr, serum TLI concentrations ranged from 31 to 115

[*]Dr. David A. Williams, GI Lab—1248 Lynn Hall, Purdue University, West Lafayette, IN 47907. Telephone (913) 494-0339, Fax (913) 494-8640.

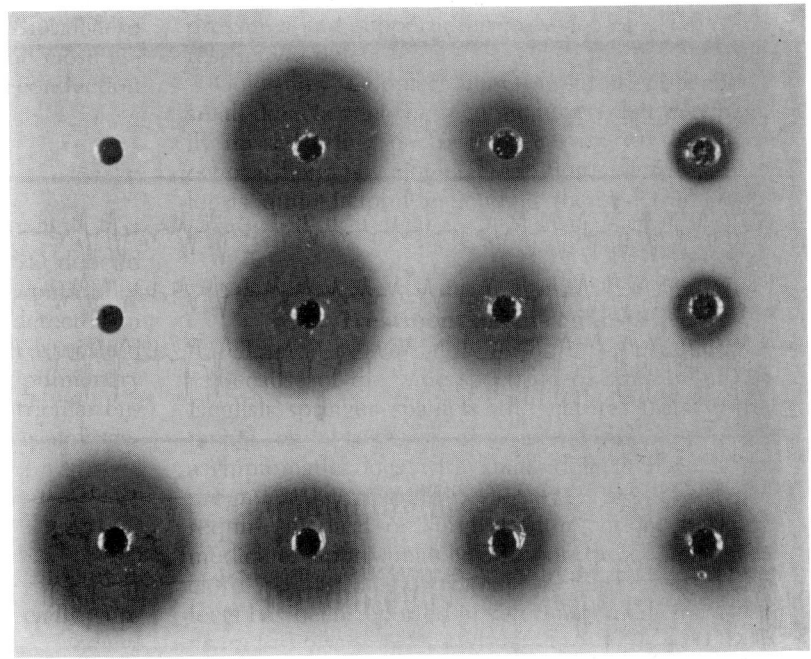

**Figure 1.** Radial enzyme diffusion plate showing proteolytic activity in cat feces. The lower four wells (left to right) are results of serial 50% dilutions of a sample with high activity. The upper four pair of wells are results (duplicate determinations) using feces from a cat with EPI, and clinically normal cats with high, medium, and low normal proteolytic activities, respectively. (From Williams DA, Reed SD, and Perry LA: Fecal proteolytic activity in clinically normal cats and in a cat with exocrine pancreatic insufficiency. J Am Vet Med Assoc 197:210, 1990, with permission.)

μg/L (Medinger, Burchfield, and Williams, 1993). This range of values in normal cats is much greater than the corresponding range observed in dogs using a canine TLI assay.

Trypsin-like immunoreactivity is a pancreas-specific marker, since trypsinogen is synthesized and stored only in pancreatic acinar cells. It is likely that, as in dogs and human beings, loss of acinar tissue must be extensive (>90 to 95%) before signs of EPI become apparent, so serum TLI concentrations will be subnormal in affected cats. Indeed, initial results using this assay showed serum TLI to be subnormal (5 to 27 μg/L) in a group of cats with EPI that had been diagnosed based on observation of consistently negligible fecal proteolytic activity as determined by radial enzyme diffusion (Medinger, Burchfield, and Williams, 1993).

Serum TLI concentrations are likely not to be quite as subnormal in cats with EPI as in affected dogs, since canine PAA is associated with essentially total loss of acinar tissue, whereas inflammation of residual acinar tissue in cats with chronic pancreatitis may lead to greater TLI concentrations than would otherwise be expected. Nonetheless, as in human patients with chronic pancreatitis, subnormal serum TLI concentrations are anticipated in cats with loss of sufficient acinar tissue to cause steatorrhea. In contrast, as in dogs and human patients with small intestinal disease, serum TLI concentrations in cats with small intestinal disease are not likely to be significantly different from those in healthy controls because intestinal disease does not affect serum TLI; pancreatic zymogens and enzymes enter blood directly from the pancreas and are not absorbed intact from the intestinal lumen.

## TREATMENT

Most cats with EPI can be managed successfully by simply supplementing each meal with pancreatic enzyme extracts. If weight gain or control of diarrhea is suboptimal, then antibiotic therapy for potential associated bacterial overgrowth in the lumen of the small intestine, dietary modification, vitamin supplementation, glucocorticoid therapy for potential associated small intestinal mucosal disease, and inhibition of gastric acid output may all be helpful.

### Enzyme Replacement

Enzyme replacement using an initial dose of 1 teaspoonful of powdered nonenteric-coated pancreatic extract (Pancrezyme Powder, Daniels; Viokase-V Powder, Fort Dodge/AH Robins) with each meal is generally effective. Animals that do not show an optimum response to this dose are unlikely to benefit from an increase in the amount of extract fed. Other dietary modifications may benefit such animals. There is no reason to believe that tablets, capsules, and enteric-coated preparations are likely to be more effective than powdered extracts, and indeed, as in dogs, they may be less

effective than powdered extract. The extract should be mixed with a maintenance food immediately prior to feeding, as when treating in dogs. Diarrhea generally improves within 2 to 3 days. As soon as clinical improvement is apparent, owners can determine a minimum effective dose of enzyme supplement that prevents return of clinical signs. This will vary slightly between different enzyme preparations, and also from cat to cat. Affected cats will require addition of enzymes to every meal.

Chopped healthy ox or pig pancreas (1 to 3 ounces per meal) is sometimes an economical alternative to feeding of relatively expensive dried pancreatic extracts. Pancreas can be stored frozen at −20°C for at least 3 months and enzyme activity will be adequately maintained.

Addition of bile salts or antacids and preincubation of enzymes with the food prior to feeding do not increase the effectiveness of enzyme supplements fed to dogs with experimental EPI, and are unlikely to do so in cats. Inhibition of gastric acid secretion by an $H_2$-receptor blocker such as cimetidine probably reduces intragastric destruction of lipase, but is expensive and is unlikely to improve the clinical response in patients that do not respond to enzyme replacement alone.

### Dietary Modification

Fat absorption does not return to normal despite appropriate enzyme replacement therapy in dogs or human patients with EPI. Patients usually compensate by eating slightly more than usual, so up to approximately 20% more than calculated maintenance requirements should initially be fed. This amount of food should be adjusted later to maintain an ideal body weight.

Experimental studies indicate that dietary fiber impairs pancreatic enzyme activity, and high-fiber diets should therefore probably be avoided. There is no evidence that reduced fat content diets are of value in patients with EPI, and their use may exacerbate calorie malnutrition. However, some affected cats may not tolerate diets with high fat contents. Those individuals with poor weight gain that do not tolerate diets with normal or increased fat contents may benefit from supplementation with readily digested and absorbed medium-chain triglyceride oil (MCT Oil, Mead Johnson).

### Vitamin Supplementation

Serum concentrations of cobalamin (vitamin $B_{12}$) and of fat-soluble vitamins are often severely subnormal in cats with EPI. In dogs, serum concentrations do not usually increase in response to treatment with enzymes, even though the clinical response (weight gain and resolution of diarrhea) may otherwise be excellent. Clinical deficiency states are rarely recognized, but vitamin K–responsive coagulopathy has been documented in feline EPI. While appropriate doses are not established, it is reasonable to give oral supplements containing fat-soluble vitamins as well as parenteral cobalamin. Parenteral vitamin $K_1$ (5 to 20 mg every 12 hr SC) should be given when there is clinical or laboratory evidence of a coagulopathy. Tocopherol (30 to 100 IU/day PO with food) and cobalamin (100 $\mu$g every 7 days SC or IM) for 1 month will normalize serum concentrations of these vitamins in most cases.

## Antibiotic Therapy

There are no reports of numbers of duodenal microflora in cats with EPI as compared to normal cats, but duodenal bacterial overgrowth is a common, usually subclinical, complication of EPI in dogs. Antibiotic therapy should not be given routinely to affected cats, but since bacterial overgrowth may contribute to malabsorption and diarrhea in some patients that do not respond completely to routine enzyme supplementation, a course of antibiotic therapy is warranted in such individuals.

Oral oxytetracycline (50 to 100 mg every 12 hr PO for 14 days) is a reasonable initial antibiotic of choice. Metronidazole (25 to 100 mg every 12 hr PO for 14 days) may be more effective if obligate anaerobes are present, as has recently been reported frequently to be the case in normal cats.

## Glucocorticoid Therapy

Concurrent inflammatory bowel disease can complicate feline EPI as in canine patients. If patients do not respond to the above treatments, then a biopsy of the small intestine should ideally be obtained to confirm this possibility. A trial of concurrent oral prednisolone (initial dose 5 mg every 12 hr for 4 to 6 weeks) is probably indicated even if morphologically apparent disease is not confirmed. It is not likely that long-term glucocorticoid administration will be required.

The underlying cause for development of EPI is generally irreversible, and lifelong treatment is likely to be necessary. Provided owners are willing to accept the cost of enzyme replacement, the prognosis is generally good. A few cats may fail to regain normal body weight in spite of all therapeutic measures, but there is usually complete remission of diarrhea and polyphagia, and a generally favorable response to treatment is expected.

## References and Suggested Reading

Anderson WI, Georgi ME, and Car BD: Pancreatic atrophy and fibrosis associated with eurytrema procyonis in a domestic cat. Vet Rec 120:235, 1987.
*A case report of a rare cause of feline EPI.*
Fyfe JC: Feline intrinsic factor (IF) is pancreatic in origin and mediates ileal cobalamin (CBL) absorption. J Vet Intern Med 7:133, 1993.
*New observations on the mechanism of cobalamin absorption in the cat.*
Hawkins EC, Meric SM, Washabau RJ, et al: Digestion of bentiromide and absorption of xylose in healthy cats and absorption of xylose in cats with infiltrative intestinal disease. Am J Vet Res 47:567, 1986.
*A protocol and control values for the bentiromide test in the cat.*
Johnston K, Lamport A, and Batt RM: An unexpected bacterial flora in the proximal small intestine of normal cats. Vet Rec 132:362, 1993.
*Bacterial counts in duodenal juice from cats were much greater than in dogs and included large numbers of obligate anaerobic species.*
Medinger TM, Burchfield T, and Williams DA: Assay of trypsin-like immunoreactivity (TLI) in feline serum. J Vet Intern Med 7:133, 1993.
*New observations on feline serum TLI.*
Nicholson A, Watson ADJ, and Mercer JR: Fat malassimilation in three cats. Aust Vet J 66:110, 1989.
*An account of the difficulties and limitations associated with traditional tests used to investigate suspected fat malabsorption and to diagnose EPI, illustrated by reference to three feline patients with steatorrhea.*
Perry LA, Williams DA, Pidgeon GL, et al: Exocrine pancreatic insufficiency with associated coagulopathy in a cat. J Am Anim Hosp Assoc 27:109, 1991.
*A report of a cat with EPI in which associated vitamin K deficiency and cobalamin malabsorption were documented.*
Sherding RG, Stradley RP, Rogers WA and Johnson SE: Bentiromide:xylose test in healthy cats. Am J Vet Res 43:2272, 1982.
*A protocol and control values for the bentiromide test in the cat.*
Watson ADJ, Church DB, Middleton DJ, and Rothwell TLW: Weight loss in cats which eat well. J Small Anim Prac 22:473, 1981.
*An account of the differential diagnosis for EPI in cats illustrated by reference to four case reports.*
Williams DA and Reed SD: Comparison of methods for assay of fecal proteolytic activity. Vet Clin Pathol 19:20, 1990.
*A revue of methods used for analysis of fecal proteolytic activity, and of precautions that must be taken to obtain reliable results.*
Williams DA, Reed SD, and Perry LA: Fecal proteolytic activity in clinically normal cats and in a cat with exocrine pancreatic insufficiency. J Am Vet Med Assoc 197:210, 1990.
*Control values for fecal proteolytic activity in healthy pet cats and in patient with EPI.*

# BILIRUBIN AND BILE ACIDS IN THE DIAGNOSIS OF HEPATOBILIARY DISEASE

DAVID R. BOSTWICK
*and* D.J. MEYER
*Fort Collins, Colorado*

The objectives of this article are to discuss the pathophysiologic mechanisms responsible for hyperbilirubinemia and an increased serum total bile acid concentration, and the current concepts pertaining to these laboratory tests.

## BILIRUBIN

### Metabolism

Unconjugated bilirubin in healthy dogs and cats is a metabolic waste product derived from three main sources. In dogs, 67% is produced from erythrocyte hemoglobin breakdown, 5.3% from ineffective erythropoiesis, and the remaining 27.7% from the catabolism of other nonerythrocytic heme proteins (myoglobin, catalase, peroxidase, and hepatic cytochrome P-450 enzymes). Aged erythrocytes are removed by the reticuloendothelial system and the majority of unconjugated bilirubin is bound (noncovalently) to albumin for transport to the liver. The albumin–bilirubin complex is carried within the blood to the hepatic sinusoids in close proximity to the sinusoidal hepatocyte membrane. This close association is critical for facilitating the release of bilirubin from albumin. Bilirubin is then transported intracellularly via a nonspecific, bidirectional, carrier-mediated, membrane transport system that is also responsible for the intracellular transport of other organic anions such as sulfobromophthalein (BSP), indocyanine green (ICG), and some xenobiotics. The uptake capacity of the hepatocyte greatly exceeds the excretory transport capacity and thus is not considered to be a rate limiting step in bilirubin metabolism. Within the hepatocyte, bilirubin is bound to cytosolic carrier proteins (ligandins) for transport to the rough endoplasmic reticulum. It is enzymatically conjugated with glucuronic acid forming monoester and diester conjugates, rendering it water soluble. The hepatic uptake, intracellular transport, enzymatic conjugation, and excretion of bilirubin, BSP, and ICG all appear to be similar. In the dog, but not known for the cat, extrahepatic conjugation of bilirubin can occur in the epithelial cells of the jejunum and proximal convoluted tubule in the kidney. The urinary excretion of bilirubin appears to be sex linked; a greater magnitude in males than in females.

Conjugated bilirubin is excreted into the bile via a carrier-mediated active transport system across the canalicular membrane against a concentration gradient. In health, there is evidence to suggest that the conjugation of bilirubin is the rate-limiting step in bilirubin metabolism, but in pathologic conditions, the excretory transport mechanism may be the rate-limiting step. This dichotomy is still the subject of debate concerning bilirubin metabolism. Excreted bilirubin glucuronides are deconjugated and reduced by ileal and colonic bacteria to urobilinogen. Eighty to 90% of the urobilinogen is excreted in the feces as stercobilin, while only a small amount (10 to 20%) of the urobilinogen is reabsorbed to undergo enterohepatic recycling. Most of the recycled urobilinogen is removed through the liver, with only a minute portion being filtered by the kidney for urinary excretion. Urinary urobilinogen is not considered a useful marker of the enterohepatic circulation and lacks diagnostic utility in the differential diagnosis of liver disease.

### Causes of Hyperbilirubinemia

In the healthy dog and cat, there is little circulating bilirubin. Icteric serum and bilirubinuria are first noted when the bilirubin concentration is between 0.6 and 1.0 mg/dl. Icterus is not clinically apparent until the plasma bilirubin concentration exceeds 2.5 to 3.0 mg/dl.

Hyperbilirubinemia can be caused by prehepatic, hepatic, and posthepatic pathophysiologic events. A fourth cause of an increased bilirubin value on the biochemical profile is lipemia. The lactescence of the serum artifactually increases the reported value when determined with most spectrophotometric methods; usually in the range of 1.0 to 2.0 mg/dl. Moderate bilirubinuria is detected in the urinalysis at serum bilirubin concentrations greater than 1.0 mg/dl. If there is no attendant bilirubinuria associated with a reported serum value greater than 1.0 mg/dl, artifact should be considered. Hyperviscosity causes an artifactually increased bilirubin value by "dry reagent" methodology. Moderate to severe hemolysis causes unreliable bilirubin values when determined spectrophotometrically.

The serum bilirubin concentration represents a balance between production and hepatobiliary removal and excretion. Therefore, hyperbilirubinemia is the result of overproduction (hemolysis), impaired uptake or conjugation (hepatic disease), or impaired excretion (cholestasis). Cholestasis is a generic term that defines reduced bile flow, either physiologic or anatomic. Intrahepatic cholestasis involves parenchymal pathology of the hepatocyte and the intrahepatic bile ductules that impair bile flow. Extrahepatic cholestasis is usually secondary to an obstruction of the common bile duct between the gallbladder and the duodenal papilla.

The determination of the packed cell volume (PCV) should be the initial test in the differentiation of hyperbilirubinemia. Erythrocyte destruction sufficiently rapid to cause hyperbilirubinemia usually is associated with a PCV less than 25%. The plasma protein remains within the reference range or is increased. Findings that are supportive of a process causing increased erythrocyte turnover include: autoagglutination, a positive Coombs' test, hemoglobinemia or hemoglobinuria, spherocytosis, reticulocytosis, increased Heinz bodies, or the presence of infectious agents (hemobartonellosis, babesiosis). The reticulocytosis may be only mildly increased in the icteric patient because the maximal hematopoietic response takes 2 to 4 days following the initial hemolytic event. A questionable regenerative response should be evaluated by serial reticulocyte counts. Although hemolysis results in increased circulating concentrations of lipid-soluble, unconjugated bilirubin, which cannot pass through the glomerular membrane, bilirubinuria is a common finding in dogs with hemolytic disease. Two explanations for this phenomenon in the dog include the development of a conjugated hyperbilirubinemia subsequent to decreased canalicular excretion and the unique ability of the renal tubule to metabolize hemoglobin to conjugated bilirubin. Measurement of a marked increase of urine urobilinogen is supportive of a hemolytic process. The colorless urobilinogen is rapidly oxidized to urobilin, imparting a greenish color to urine left standing at room temperature or after prolonged exposure to fluorescent lighting. Thus, a negative or weak positive result should be interpreted judiciously.

The serum total bilirubin concentration is not a sensitive indicator of hepatocellular dysfunction. The presence of hyperbilirubinemia suggests that moderate to marked pathology has altered one or more of the metabolic steps involved in the excretion of bilirubin. Hepatobiliary disease and extrahepatic infections (the cholestasis of sepsis) can cause icterus (Franson et al., 1985). Once increased erythrocyte destruction and an extrahepatic infectious process has been eliminated, the differential diagnosis of icterus becomes problematic.

Acute, diffuse hepatocellular injury is often characterized by marked increases in serum aminotransferase (ALT, AST) activities and mild increases in serum alkaline phosphatase (ALP) activity. Extrahepatic biliary obstruction is characterized by a marked increase in serum ALP activity and lesser increases in serum ALT and AST activities. These biochemical guidelines are fraught with inconsistencies, and additional diagnostic procedures are required. Ultrasonographic and radiographic examination of the icteric patient is useful when there are biochemical findings suggestive of extrahepatic obstruction of the biliary system.

The common causes of feline hyperbilirubinemia include: idiopathic hepatic lipidosis, lymphosarcoma and myeloproliferative diseases, feline infectious peritonitis virus infection, pancreatitis, toxoplasmosis, and cholangiohepatitis. The initial approach to an icteric cat involves the determination of the PCV and examination of a blood smear for *Haemobartonella*. A blood smear made immediately from the ethylenediaminetetraacetic acid (EDTA)-blood is preferable because the organism rapidly "falls off" the erythrocyte. Geographic diseases such as the feline pancreatic fluke infection comprise a considerable proportion of the cases of feline icterus in the southeastern United States and Hawaii. Our mobile society dictates that a travel history should be obtained routinely. All icteric cats do not have idiopathic hepatic lipidosis and a step-wise approach to hyperbilirubinemia is essential. Hyperbilirubinemia in dogs may be associated with chronic liver diseases, cirrhosis, neoplasia, copper storage hepatitis, hepatic toxins or infections, drug reactions, pancreatic carcinoma, and other disorders.

## Bilirubin and Ratios—Is There Diagnostic Utility?

It has been a common misconception that the fractionation or ratio of unconjugated (indirect) and conjugated (direct) bilirubin is beneficial in the differentiation of hemolytic anemia, intrahepatic cholestasis, and extrahepatic cholestasis. Unfortunately, alteration of bilirubin physiology in dogs and cats does not result in the expected changes that are observed in humans. Studies using sophisticated methodology to determine the bilirubin fractions in dogs with immune-mediated hemolysis, intrahepatic disease, and extrahepatic bile duct obstruction have been reported (Rothuizen and van de Brom, 1987). Surprisingly, there were no clinically useful differences in either the magnitude or the ratio of unconjugated-conjugated bilirubin among the groups. The $^3$H-bilirubin clearance parameters indicated that there was increased erythrocyte degradation (decreased survival time) and decreased bilirubin clearance in all three groups. The decreased erythrocyte survival time in hepatobiliary disease may be due to hypersplenism secondary to portal hypertension or direct cytolysis by retained bile acids. Clearance of this supranormal amount of unconjugated bilirubin is further decreased by the hepatocellular dysfunction, resulting in an unconjugated hyperbilirubinemia similar to the magnitude associated with a Coombs'-positive hemolytic anemia. Increased concentrations of conjugated bilirubin found in those dogs with hemolytic anemia were presumably due to cholestasis secondary to pathology induced by centrilobular (zone 3) hepatocellular degeneration caused by hypoxia. These results indicate that there is no diagnostic value in determining the conjugated and unconjugated concentrations of bilirubin in the dog. Our experience in the cat indicates a similar lack of diagnostic utility.

## Delta-Bilirubin—A Future Test

The existence of a novel form of bilirubin was first suspected in 1980, when it was noticed that the total bilirubin concentration in people with cholestatic disease did not equal the sum of the unconjugated and conjugated bilirubin when the assays were performed by an alkaline methanolysis high-performance liquid chromatography (AMHPLC) method. The discrepancy was due to the presence of conjugated bilirubin *covalently* bound to albumin. In the separation process, this bilirubin is not released from albumin and migrates with albumin on the AMHPLC. The new bilirubin (termed biliprotein or delta-bilirubin) was only present in cholestatic disease. Delta-bilirubin formation is dependent upon an intact conjugation mechanism (functional hepatocytes) and impaired biliary excretion (cholestasis). Delta-bilirubin is formed by a relatively slow, nonspecific, nonenzymatic reaction involving the esterified carboxyethyl side chain of the conjugating sugar. The life span is dependent on the half-life of albumin (12 to 14 days).

The strong covalent bond to albumin both prevents the appearance of delta-bilirubin in the urine (even though it is water soluble) and impairs uptake by hepatocytes. Because it requires conjugation to be present, delta-bilirubin does not increase significantly even with prolonged unconjugated hyperbilirubinemia of hemolytic origin. The prolonged life span and lack of renal excretion has implications in the diagnosis and therapeutic monitoring of cholestatic diseases. After the resolution of cholestasis, the unconjugated and the "conventional" conjugated bilirubin are removed from the circulation within several days. The delta-bilirubin remains in the circulation and contributes to the bilirubin concentration. Therefore, even after successful resolution of the cholestatic process, the patient may remain hyperbilirubinemic and even clinically icteric for weeks after liver function has returned to normal. Since delta-bilirubin is not excreted into the urine, it is possible to have hyperbilirubinemia without marked bilirubinuria. In fact, resolution of bilirubinuria may serve as a useful marker of improved hepatic function.* Delta-bilirubin has been documented in the serum of dogs with hepatobiliary disease accounting for 2 to 94% of the total bilirubin concentration. This remarkable

---

*Bilirubin (imparts a yellow to yellow-brown color) is sensitive to fluorescent lighting and is rapidly oxidized to biliverdin (imparts green color). Biliverdin is not detected by the tests for bilirubin; consequently a false-negative test results. Our recommendation is to determine the bilirubin concentration within 30 min or refrigerate the specimen until examined. The sensitivity for detecting bilirubin can be improved by the use of the Ictotest (Ames Company, P.O. Box 70, Elkhart, IN 46515). The dark color of urine does not affect interpretation of the tablet test as it can for the reagent stick.

variability of delta-bilirubin formation probably explains why resolution of icterus appears rapid in some patients and protracted in others. It also emphasizes the value of understanding the kinetics of bilirubin, especially the delta-bilirubin fraction. The simplified determination of delta-bilirubin by dry chemistry methodology will enhance the efforts to evaluate its clinical usefulness.

## BILE ACIDS

### Metabolism

Primary bile acids are synthesized from cholesterol in hepatocytes by the hydroxylation of cholesterol by 7 α-hydroxylase. This enzymatic step is rate limiting and receives negative feedback from bile acids (primarily chenodeoxycholic acid) in the portal venous blood and a positive influence from glucocorticoids and thyroxine. The primary bile acids, cholic acid (CA) and chenodeoxycholic acid (CDCA), are conjugated in the hepatocyte with either glycine or taurine (primarily taurine in the dog and cat). The conjugated CA and CDCA are secreted into the canaliculus by a carrier-mediated, active transport system distinct from the transporter responsible for bilirubin excretion. Canalicular transport is the rate-limiting step in the transport process. Excretion of bile acids provides the primary driving force for bile flow (bile acid-dependent flow).

Most of the bile acids are stored in the gallbladder prior to secretion into the duodenum. Ten to 20% of the bile is continuously secreted into the duodenum, providing the basis for continuous bile acid cycling; this represents the fasting serum total bile acid concentration (FSBA). Within the intestinal lumen, the primary bile acids are deconjugated by bacteria to deoxycholic acid (DCA) and lithocholic acid (LCA). Bile acids are efficiently absorbed by the terminal ileum through a sodium-potassium ATPase active transport system. Ninety-five per cent of the excreted bile acids are absorbed prior to their entry into the colon, allowing only 5% to be excreted with the feces. This efficiency decreases the daily amount of bile acids that need to be replenished by the liver. After absorption, the portal circulation returns the bile acids to the liver. They are efficiently extracted primarily by the periportal (zone 1) hepatocytes by a carrier-mediated, active transport system distinct from the bilirubin transport system. The hepatocellular "recycling" of bile acids is very efficient and little "escapes" to the systemic circulation following a meal; hence, the postprandial serum total bile acid concentration (PPBA) is only slightly greater than the FSBA.

### Indications for Measuring Serum Total Bile Acids

The measurement of serum total bile acid concentrations is helpful in the documentation of occult liver insufficiency, detection of congenital portosystemic shunts, and following the progression or resolution of hepatic disease with therapy. There is no apparent value in determining a FSBA or PPBA when hyperbilirubinemia is present. The most common indications for FSBA and PPBA analysis include: (1) increased serum hepatic enzymes in a patient with clinical signs that are consistent with hepatobiliary disease, (2) persistent chronic increases in serum hepatic enzymes (primarily the aminotransferases) in a breed with a known predisposition for hepatic disease (Doberman pinscher, Bedlington and West Highland white terriers, and the cocker spaniel), (3) as an aid in juvenile animals with signs consistent with hepatic encephalopathy (congenital portosystemic shunting), and (4) in the therapeutic monitoring of hepatobiliary diseases.

## Methods and Normal Values

The FSBA sample is obtained after a 12-hr fast and the PPBA is obtained approximately 2 hr after feeding 2 to 4 tablespoons of canned food (Prescription Diet P/D [dogs] or C/D [cats], Hills Pet Products, Inc). A larger quantity of food is not necessary and may increase postprandial lipemia. If the patient already has signs referable to hepatic encephalopathy, it may be wise to only obtain an FSBA and wait for results prior to provocative stimulation. If the FSBA is markedly increased, a PPBA adds no additional diagnostic information. If the FSBA is normal, however, a PPBA may be increased and of considerable diagnostic aid.

Serum bile acids are stable when refrigerated or frozen. There are two validated laboratory methods for the quantification of serum bile acids; radioimmunoassay (RIA) and an enzymatic method. The RIA method measures conjugated CA and CDCA with a higher specificity for the taurine conjugate, while the enzymatic method measures all nonsulfated conjugated and unconjugated 3 $\alpha$-hydroxy bile acids. Therefore, slightly different values are obtained, but the magnitude is generally not clinically important. Normal values for preprandial and postprandial bile acid concentrations vary with the method used and thus reference ranges are dependent upon each laboratory. In general, most laboratories report 0 to 5 $\mu$mol/L and less than 15 $\mu$mol/L to be normal for the FSBA and PPBA concentrations, respectively. However, it should be recognized that the 95% confidence interval for the PPBA is as high as 24.2 $\mu$mol/L and 29.8 $\mu$mol/L for the enzymatic method and RIA, respectively. Therefore, an interpretive "gray zone" exists within this range. Increased serum bile acid concentrations can be characterized as being in this gray zone or significantly elevated. The "gray zone" is the range between the upper end of normal for the laboratory reference range and about 20 $\mu$mol/L for the dog and cat. When the FSBA is in this range, we suggest one of the following approaches: (1) evaluating the patient for extrahepatic diseases; (2) repeat the FSBA followed by a PPBA looking for at least a twofold increase; (3) repeat the

FSBA in 2 to 4 weeks ensuring an overnight fast; or (4) if combined clinicopathologic findings support chronic hepatitis/cirrhosis or congenital portosystemic shunting, pursue confirmation of the diagnosis. When an FSBA is greater than 20 $\mu$mol/L for the dog and cat, there is a high probability that the histologic findings will define a lesion.

As with any diagnostic test, however, laboratory error must be included in the differential diagnosis of abnormal concentrations. Moderate to marked lipemia artifactually increases the serum bile acid value determined enzymatically but artifactually decreases it when determined by the RIA method. Moderate to marked hemolysis artifactually decreases the serum bile acid value determined enzymatically and probably does not affect the RIA-measured value. Bilirubin has little effect on the recovery of bile acids in canine serum except at bilirubin concentrations greater than 5 mg/dl where there develops a small (<20%) decrease in recovery at low bile acid concentrations.

We have occasionally observed the measurement of an FSBA value greater than the PPBA value. The reason for this disparity is unclear but probably multifactorial. It has been shown that (1) the peak PPBA for individual dogs is variable, (2) fasted dogs store about 40% of the newly produced bile in the gallbladder, (3) a meal stimulates the release of only 5 to 65% of the bile in the gallbladder, and (4) hemolysis can cause the measurement of the bile acid value to be falsely decreased. Postprandial lipemia can predispose to hemolysis. Undoubtedly these physiologic variables in addition to physiologic variation in the intestinal transit time and concurrent underlying intestinal disease contribute to the dichotomy.

## Causes of Altered Bile Acid Concentrations

Bile acid concentrations are a very sensitive but nonspecific indicator of hepatobiliary dysfunction. The FSBA is a reflection of the efficiency and integrity of the enterohepatic circulation. Pathology of the hepatobiliary system (hepatocellular dysfunction or cholestasis) or the portal circulation (portosystemic shunting) results in an increased FSBA prior to the development of hyperbilirubinemia. Low to unmeasurable FSBA is not considered significant in the evaluation of hepatobiliary disease. Even with end-stage cirrhosis, the liver is able to replenish the circulating bile acid pool, since the efficiency of the enterohepatic circulation results in little loss in the feces. Low serum bile acid concentrations are usually a normal variation.

The diagnostic value of determining a PPBA is controversial in the medical literature. The only study evaluating its use in the dog indicated similar test efficiency for FSBA and PPBA measurements, although it increased the sensitivity for the detection of cirrhosis and congenital portosystemic shunting. A PPBA value greater than 25 $\mu$mol/L in the dog and 20 $\mu$mol/L in the cat provided the best sensitivity.

Although bile acids are specific for the liver, increases do not necessarily reflect *primary* hepatic or cholestatic liver disease. Mild to moderate increases can be found with inflammatory bowel disease, hyperadrenocorticism, pancreatitis, and other extrahepatic diseases. The magnitude of increase does not correlate with the severity of the disease process. For example, a dog with extrahepatic bile duct obstruction due to pancreatitis may have an FSBA of greater than 400 $\mu$mol/L and a disease process that can resolve in contrast to a dog with cirrhosis and an FSBA of 70 $\mu$mol/L. Likewise, values between animals with the same disease cannot be compared to determine which is more severely affected. Values can be compared from the same animal, however, to monitor progression or response to therapy.

## References and Suggested Reading

Center S, ManWarren T, Slater M, and Wilentz E: Evaluation of twelve-hour preprandial and two-hour postprandial serum bile acids concentrations for diagnosis of hepatobiliary disease in dogs. J Am Vet Med Assoc 199:217, 1991.
*A retrospective analysis documenting the sensitivity and positive predictive value of serum bile acid concentrations in dogs with hepatobiliary disease.*
Engelking L: Disorders of bilirubin metabolism in small animal species. Compend Cont Educ 10:712, 1988.
*A review of the congenital and acquired disorders that affect bilirubin metabolism.*
Franson T, Hierholzer W, and La Brecque D: Frequency and characteristics of hyperbilirubinemia associated with bacteremia. Rev Infect Dis 7:1, 1985.
*One of several references documenting and discussing the hyperbilirubinemia associated with extrahepatic infections.*
Meyer D and Williams D: Diagnosis of hepatic and exocrine pancreatic disorders. Semin Vet Med Surg [Small Anim] 7:275, 1992.
*A concise review describing the diagnostic utility and interpretation of serum hepatic enzyme alterations and tests of hepatic function.*
Rothuizen J and van de Brom W: Bilirubin metabolism in canine hepatobiliary and haemolytic disease. Vet Quarterly 9:235, 1987.
*Provides evidence that the fractionation of bilirubin into conjugated and unconjugated forms has no diagnostic utility in the discrimination of canine hepatobiliary disease from hemolytic disorders.*
Rothuizen J and van den Ingh T: Covalently protein-bound bilirubin conjugates in cholestatic disease of dogs. Am J Vet Res 49:702, 1988.
*Documentation of delta-bilirubin in dogs with cholestatic and hemolytic disease.*
Rothuizen J, van den Brom W, and Fevery J: The origins and kinetics of bilirubin in healthy dogs, in comparison with man. J Hepatol 15:25, 1992.
*A review article contrasting and comparing bilirubin metabolism in dogs and humans.*

# PATHOGENIC ASPECTS OF CHRONIC LIVER DISEASE IN THE DOG

EWA SEVELIUS
*Helsingborg, Sweden*

*and* LENNART H. JÖNSSON
*Uppsala, Sweden*

Chronic hepatitis with subsequent fibrosis and cirrhosis in dogs has been recognized with increased frequency over the past years. The histopathologic changes of canine liver disease often correspond to those found in humans, but little is yet known about the etiology in dogs. Toxic agents and drugs are known causes of chronic liver disease in the dog. Copper storage hepatitis in the Bedlington terrier is well known. Whether true copper storage hepatitis exists in other breeds is still debated; however, a metabolic copper defect is described in West Highland white terriers in the United States. In human patients, viruses and autoimmunity are common causes of liver disease. For example, Hepatitis B virus and autoimmunity are well known etiologic factors in human chronic active hepatitis. A genetic deficiency of the serum protease inhibitor $\alpha_1$-antitrypsin is another cause of chronic hepatitis and cirrhosis in humans. Recent investigations show that there are distinct differences in the etiology of chronic liver diseases, but also many similarities between dogs and people.

## CLASSIFICATION

Based on histopathologic findings, chronic liver disease has been classified as: chronic active hepatitis, chronic progressive hepatitis, chronic nonspecific hepatitis, cholangiohepatitis, cirrhosis, and copper storage hepatitis. In most dogs affected with a progressive form of hepatocellular disease, the hepatic lesions most closely resemble chronic active hepatitis in humans with mixed inflammatory reaction, piecemeal necrosis, and disruption of the lobular parenchyma by reticulin and fine collagen fibers. In contrast, canine biopsies do not show the prominent portal and periportal mononuclear inflammation characteristic of the condition in people. Nor do they display the bridging necrosis seen in the more severe human cases of chronic active hepatitis. Thus, while the canine lesions are undoubtedly chronic and progressive, because of the morphologic dissimilarities to the human condition, the disorder should rather be labeled chronic progressive hepatitis. The importance of correlating the macroscopic appearance of the liver to the biopsy report should be stressed because a correct histopathologic interpretation of cirrhotic and precirrhotic livers can be difficult and the result misleading.

## BREED, SEX AND AGE INCIDENCE

American and English cocker spaniels, West Highland white terriers, and Labrador retrievers have a significantly high prevalence of chronic liver disease in Sweden (Table 1). Statistically, we also find a high incidence in the Scottish terrier, but there are too few cases to draw any conclusions. The incidence of copper storage hepatitis in the Bedlington terrier is also high, but as this is a well-documented disease all over the world it will not be discussed here (see elsewhere in this section). The breed incidence mentioned above is the result of a demographic study based on histopathologically verified cases of chronic liver disease from all parts of the country. The breed distribution was then compared to dog registration numbers of the Swedish Kennel Club, where about 70% of all Swedish dogs are registered. The frequency of chronic liver disease in the American cocker spaniel and West Highland white terrier is about ten times as high as expected. In English cocker spaniels, the frequency is three times the expected. A recent study, however, shows that the incidence of chronic liver disease in the Labrador retriever is decreasing.

The mean age of West Highland white terriers and cocker spaniels diagnosed with chronic liver disease is 5 years. Male and female West Highland white terriers are equally affected. Male cocker spaniels are more often affected than females. The significantly high incidence of chronic liver disease in both American and English cocker spaniels is consistent with clinical experience in Sweden as well as in the United States.

The most common diagnoses in the cocker spaniel and in the West Highland white terrier are chronic progressive hepatitis or liver cirrhosis. Copper granules are seldom detected in the liver specimens, but when present, the copper is secondary to the chronic inflammatory reaction. Copper accumulation is never as extensive as in the copper-associated hepatitis of Bedlington terriers or in the metabolic copper defect reported in West Highland white terriers in the United States. These differences indicate that there are genetic differences within breeds in different countries. The high incidence of chronic hepatitis and liver cirrhosis in certain breeds indicates that hereditary factors may be of importance in the development of these diseases.

## CLINICAL FEATURES

Many dogs are presented with clinical signs of acute-onset disease, although liver biopsy reveals a chronic liver disease or end-stage liver cirrhosis. Most dogs are lethargic and depressed. Anorexia and weight loss, as well as polydipsia and polyuria, are often reported. Ascites is a much more common clinical finding than icterus. When these signs are present in dogs with chronic progressive hepatitis, the prognosis is more favorable, but when liver cirrhosis has developed, the prognosis is poor. For further information on clinical features and management of liver, the reader is referred to the articles that follow.

## AUTOIMMUNITY

Circulating autoantibodies are important diagnostic markers in humans and are used to discriminate between different forms of chronic liver disease. Cell antinuclear antibody (ANA), smooth muscle antibodies (SMA), and liver membrane antibodies (LMA) are characteristic of human autoimmune, chronic active hepatitis, with ANA occurring in almost 100% of patients. Antimitochondrial antibodies (AMA) are most frequently found in human primary biliary cirrhosis.

In our experience, many dogs with primary as well as secondary acute and chronic hepatitis are ANA positive, at titres of 1:10 to 1:40. Positive ANA is also found in dogs with other liver disorders. The frequent occurrence of ANA in the serum of dogs with different types

**Table 1.** *Most Frequent Breeds Found Among 250 Dogs With Chronic Liver Disease Histopathologically Diagnosed in Sweden 1987–1989.*

| Breed | Males | Females | Mean Age | Total Frequency | Expected Frequency | Significance |
|---|---|---|---|---|---|---|
| Labrador retriever | 5 | 21 | 6.9 | 28 | 12.4 | °°° |
| American cocker spaniel | 19 | 7 | 4.6 | 27 | 2.6 | °°° |
| English cocker spaniel | 15 | 8 | 5.4 | 23 | 6.4 | °°° |
| Golden retriever | 7 | 12 | 5.0 | 20 | 13.3 | |
| West Highland white terrier | 9 | 9 | 4.8 | 18 | 2.1 | °°° |
| German shepherd dog | 7 | 7 | 4.8 | 14 | 20.5 | |
| Dachshund (all types) | 7 | 5 | 6.5 | 12 | 22.9 | |
| Doberman pinscher | 3 | 2 | 7.4 | 6 | 2.2 | ° |
| Scottish terrier | 3 | 3 | 7.7 | 6 | 0.6 | °°° |
| Yorkshire terrier | 3 | 2 | 6.0 | 5 | 3.6 | |

The following diagnoses are included in the material: chronic hepatitis, chronic progressive hepatitis, cirrhosis, and chronic nonspecific cholangiohepatitis. Twenty-one Bedlington terriers with copper toxicosis are not included in the table. Expected frequencies are based on registration records of the Swedish Kennel Club. Significance tested by $\chi^2$ when $n \geq 5$. °°°$p \leq .001$, °°$.001 \leq p \leq .01$, °$.01 < p \leq .05$

of primary chronic hepatitis and cirrhosis as well as in secondary hepatitis indicates a low specificity. Cell nuclear antibodies in dogs are a very heterogenous group of antibodies and are neither organ nor species specific. The fluorescence pattern is granular or speckled and even nucleolar, indicating that the antigen might be ribonucleoproteins or RNA. This is in contrast to the pattern seen in human chronic active hepatitis and in systemic lupus erythematosus, where the fluorescence is homogenous, indicating antibodies recognizing DNA.

Liver membrane antibodies are also present in sera from dogs with chronic liver disease, acute hepatitis, and with other liver disorders including tumors with a smooth and linear fluorescence pattern, again indicating a low specificity of true autoimmunity. Neither AMA nor SMA has been found in dogs and do not seem to be of diagnostic importance in canine liver disease.

Circulating autoantibodies seem to be of minor importance in the etiology and pathogenesis of canine chronic liver disease and when present they might be secondary to the liver damage. The high frequency of autoantibodies, even if secondary, provide a rational reason for treating with corticosteroids. The frequent occurrence of ANA in dogs with different types of chronic hepatitis and cirrhosis can also be of prognostic importance for evaluating therapy because a favorable response to steroids is manifested by decreased titres. The absence of true autoimmunity, however, also supports our view that true chronic, active hepatitis is a rare disease in the dog.

## $\alpha_1$-ANTITRYPSIN

$\alpha_1$-Antitrypsin (AAT) deficiency in humans is an autosomally transmitted disorder associated with a major reduction in serum AAT levels. $\alpha_1$-Antitrypsin is an acute-phase protein that functions as a protease inhibitor, is synthesized in the liver, and increases in inflammatory reactions. Elevated serum levels of AAT are commonly found in humans with chronic active hepatitis and liver cirrhosis. In hereditary AAT deficiency, however, the serum concentration is subnormal in healthy individuals and may increase very little during inflammation. More than 75 human alleles have been identified so far by phenotyping with isoelectric focusing. One of these, the Z-allele, codes for an aberrant protein, PiZ (protease inhibitor Z), which accumulates in the hepatocytes. Severe deficiency of this protease inhibitor in serum is associated with chronic obstructive lung disease, and chronic liver disease in neonates, children, and adults.

In many cocker spaniels with either chronic progressive hepatitis or cirrhosis, periodic acid Schiff–positive, diastase-resistant granules or globules are present in the liver, indicating the presence of a glucoprotein. Immunohistochemistry, using peroxidase/antiperoxidase staining, shows these granules or globules to be AAT. $\alpha_1$-Antitrypsin can be quantified by rocket immunoelectrophoresis. In contrast to what is found in humans, serum AAT levels are within normal ranges instead of decreased in the majority of dogs with AAT-related chronic liver disease. $\alpha_1$-Antitrypsin–related liver disease is also found in breeds other than the cocker spaniel but is less common.

So far three different AAT types have been identified with isoelectric focusing, F (fast), I (intermediate), and S (slow) and these types can appear in either homozygous forms, FF, II, and SS, or as heterozygotes FI, FS, or SI. The F type is most frequently found and the S type is rather unusual. The I type is overrepresented in the cocker spaniel. It either appears as II, FI, or SI. The AAT inclusions are predominantly seen in the liver of dogs having either the homozygous or heterozygous type I of AAT. Rarely, AAT inclusions are observed with the other phenotypes. Individual dogs of other breeds with the type I phenotype also have been recognized with AAT accumulated in the liver and a diagnosis of either chronic progressive hepatitis or cirrhosis. $\alpha_1$-Antitrypsin plays a role in the etiology of canine chronic liver disease, with the I type of AAT in homozygous or heterozygous form predominating. The accumulated AAT might be aberrant in some way resulting in a secretory block, due to aggregation in the endoplasmatic reticulum, especially during acute-phase stimulation. There may also be an increased synthesis or a decreased turnover of AAT due to an elevated inflammatory response. Another explanation might be different secretion rates due to different AAT phenotypes having different affinities for the enzymes necessary for their processing.

## References and Suggested Reading

Andersson M and Sevelius E: Breed, sex and age distribution in dogs with chronic liver disease: A demographic study. J Small Anim Pract 32:1, 1991.

Andersson M and Sevelius E: Circulating autoantibodies in dogs with chronic liver disease. J Small Anim Pract 33:389, 1992.

Lomas DA, Evans DLI, Finch JT, and Carrell RW: The mechanism of Z alpha-1-antitrypsin accumulation in the liver. Nature 357:605, 1992.

Meyer zum Büschenfelde K-H, Lohse AW, Manns M, and Poralla T: Autoimmunity in liver disease. Hepatology 12:354, 1990.

Sharp HL, Bridges RA, Krivit W, and Freier EF: Cirrhosis associated with alpha-1-antitrypsin deficiency: A previously unrecognized inherited disorder. J Lab Clin Med 73:934, 1969.

Sevelius E, Andersson M, and Jönsson L: Hepatic accumulation of alpha-1-antitrypsin in chronic liver disease in the dog. J Comp Pathol (in press) 1995.

Thornburg LP, Shaw D, Dolan M, Raisbeck M, Crawford S, Dennis GL, and Olwin DB: Hereditary copper toxicosis in West Highland white terriers. Vet Pathol 23:148, 1986.

# FELINE PORTOSYSTEMIC VASCULAR SHUNTS

JULIE K. LEVY,
SUSAN E. BUNCH,
*Raleigh, North Carolina*

*and* JAN KOMTEBEDDE
*Cordelia, California*

Portosystemic vascular shunts are diagnosed rarely in cats, occurring at a rate of 2.5 per 10,000 cats examined at North American veterinary schools.[*] The rarity of the disorder and the episodic nature of clinical signs exhibited by affected cats makes this diagnosis a challenge for practitioners.

Portosystemic shunts (PSS) are abnormal vascular connections between the portal and systemic venous circulations. Congenital shunts generally are single anomalous vessels in extrahepatic locations, while acquired shunts are observed most commonly as multiple extrahepatic smaller vessels that become functional as a consequence of portal hypertension. The consequences of the abnormal portal circulation are twofold. First, portal blood containing toxins absorbed from the intestines is delivered directly to the systemic circulation without benefit of hepatic detoxification, leading to hepatic encephalopathy (HE). Second, hepatotrophic factors in the splanchnic circulation draining the gastrointestinal tract and pancreas do not reach the liver, causing inadequate liver development and decreased functional hepatic mass.

On the basis of a search of the hospital accessions at North American veterinary teaching hospitals,[*] records of 78 previously unreported cats with confirmed single congenital shunts were reviewed for this report. Whenever possible, owners were contacted for follow-up. The findings from these cases form the foundation for the observations and recommendations found in this article.

## SIGNALMENT AND TYPICAL CLINICAL SIGNS

Most cases of PSS occurred in mixed-breed cats, but two related breeds, Himalayan and Persian, were at increased risk. Himalayans were diagnosed at nine times their representation in the reference population and Persians at three times their portion of the reference population. Males were diagnosed slightly more frequently than females in our patient series.

Clinical signs were observed by 6 months of age in 75% of cats (Table 1). Many owners reported that their cats exhibited clinical signs from the time they were obtained as 6- to 8-week-old kittens. This was especially apparent when an unaffected littermate also shared the household.

The most common observations were ptyalism, seizures, ataxia, tremors, and depression. Intermittent or permanent blindness and mydriasis were also commonly observed and were believed to be of cerebral cortical origin in most cases, as ocular lesions were rarely observed. Behavior changes such as episodic excessive vocalization, aggression, unusual docility, and hiding were also reported.

Signs related to organ systems other than the central nervous system (CNS) were also observed, although these too may have been manifestations of HE. Vomiting, diarrhea, and anorexia reflected gastrointestinal

**Table 1.** *Clinical Signs and Laboratory Findings in Cats With PSS in Decreasing Order of Frequency*

| Clinical Signs | Laboratory Findings |
|---|---|
| **Common (>50% of cases)** | |
| Ptyalism | Hyperammonemia |
| Seizures | Increased serum bile acid concentration |
| Ataxia | Increased BSP retention |
| **Somewhat Common (25–50% of cases)** | |
| Blindness | Decreased serum creatinine concentration |
| Tremors | Decreased BUN content |
| Depression | Increased ALT or ALP activity |
| Mydriasis | Microcytosis |
| Dyspnea/ tachypnea | Decreased urine concentration |
| **Uncommon (10–25% of cases)** | |
| Head pressing | Hypoalbuminemia |
| Vocalization | Ammonium biurate crystalluria |
| Aggression | Hypoglobulinemia |
| Hiding | Hyperkalemia |
| Diarrhea | Lymphopenia |
| Anorexia | Lymphocytosis |
| Dysuria | Hypokalemia |
| Vomiting | |
| Polyuria/ polydipsia | |
| Anesthetic complications | |

[*]Veterinary Medical Data Bank, Purdue University, 1982–1992. The authors thank Alan Warble for performing the data base searches.

effects. Respiratory system signs included tachypnea, dyspnea, and nasal discharge, despite the fact that specific respiratory lesions were not identified radiographically. Polyuria and polydipsia were observed infrequently. Dysuria was most commonly observed in cats with ammonium biurate cystic calculi and were often the only complaints reported for these cats.

Because by-products of intestinal protein and lipid metabolism are potent contributors to signs of HE, it is not surprising that neurologic signs were precipitated or exacerbated by meals in about half of the cats. In the remainder of cats, however, there was no noticeable pattern to encephalopathic episodes. Decreased functional hepatic mass is presumed to be the cause of anesthetic complications reported in 10% of cats. These complications included prolonged recovery time, postoperative blindness or seizures, and cardiac arrest. Other drugs that may have contributed to encephalopathy included dichlorvos applied topically and methionine administered orally. Both drugs are hepatically inactivated, and methionine is converted to mercaptans, which are potent contributors to HE.

## PHYSICAL EXAMINATION FINDINGS

More than two thirds of cats had stunted body stature on physical examination, and many were thin and unkempt as well. Evidence of other congenital defects was observed during examination of the cardiovascular and reproductive systems. Heart murmurs were detected in nine cats, although few cats had additional tests to characterize the cause of the murmur. Of 43 male cats, 15 were noted to be cryptorchid. One third of cats were exhibiting neurologic signs ranging from depression to coma at the time of examination at the referral center.

## DIAGNOSTIC TESTS

### Laboratory Analysis

Definitive diagnosis is not possible by routine clinicopathologic evaluation, but complete blood count (CBC), serum chemistry analysis, and urinalysis may rule out other causes of reported clinical signs such as renal failure, electrolyte derangements, hypoglycemia, and urinary tract infection.

In our series, about one third of cats exhibited red blood cell (RBC) microcytosis without anemia. Iron deficiency, the most common cause of microcytosis, does not appear to be a factor in PSS. In the authors' experience, clinically stressed cats frequently have lymphopenia. In this series of cases, however, the median lymphocyte count was $3475/\mu l$, and overt lymphocytosis ($>7000/\mu l$) was present in nine cats. Lymphopenia ($<1500/\mu l$) was present in ten cats.

The most common serum biochemical abnormalities occurred in tests of renal function and hepatic enzyme activity. Low creatinine concentration may occur be-

cause cats with PSS have decreased muscle mass and because cats less than 1 year old normally have lower serum creatinine content than do adults. Low blood urea nitrogen (BUN) content may reflect decreased food intake, consumption of low-protein diets, or decreased hepatic production of urea from ammonia. Some authors have theorized that renal function increases in PSS to compensate for decreased hepatic function. Alternatively, HE may be associated with a solute diuresis, which would lower BUN and creatinine concentrations. Modestly increased alanine transaminase and alkaline phosphatase activities were also observed, perhaps associated with decreased hepatic blood flow and bone growth in young cats. Other uncommon serum biochemical abnormalities included mild hypoalbuminemia, hypoglobulinemia, and increases or decreases in potassium content (Table 1).

Hepatic insufficiency leads to the excretion of ammonia and uric acid in the urine, which then form crystals or calculi. Ammonium biurate crystalluria was documented uncommonly in this series and was not correlated with the presence of urinary ammonium biurate calculi. Of nine cats in which calculi were identified, only two cats had urate crystalluria. Urine specific gravity was less than 1.020 in 29% of cats.

Liver function testing is indicated for cats in which a PSS is considered. Delayed sulfobromophthalein (BSP) excretion was present in 85% of the cats tested, making this a sensitive and convenient screening test for PSS. Recently, however, availability of BSP has become restricted, and other tests of liver function have been substituted. High plasma ammonia concentration in the fasting state and after ammonium chloride challenge or consumption of a meal was a very sensitive test. However, plasma samples must be separated immediately and transported on ice to a reference laboratory for accurate analysis, making this test inconvenient for many practitioners. In addition, administration of ammonium chloride may precipitate an encephalopathic crisis, which occurred in several of our cats. Measurement of serum bile acids has gained popularity in the past few years because of its sensitivity, reliability, and convenience. Serum bile acid concentrations were elevated in most fasted samples and 100% of postprandial samples, making this the screening test of choice for feline PSS.

### Radiographic and Ultrasonographic Evaluation

Survey abdominal radiographs support the diagnosis of PSS when microhepatia is identified. This finding is inconsistent and nonspecific, and was present in only half of our cases. Ultrasonographic examination of the abdomen may be used to identify the anomalous vessel and hepatic hypovascularity of PSS patients. The advantage of this technique is the ability to confirm the diagnosis and provide the surgeon with anatomic detail of the PSS without using an invasive procedure. However, the experience of the ultrasonographer is a major factor in the ability to detect a PSS with this modality. The anomalous vessel was located in half of our cases that were examined by ultrasonography. Portal scintigraphy is a reasonably sensitive, noninvasive screening test for PSS, but is available only at selected referral centers. With this technique, radiolabeled technetium pertechnetate is administered by enema, and its distribution is monitored with a gamma camera. In a normal animal, the radiopharmaceutical is absorbed into the portal circulation and subsequently enters the liver before reaching the systemic circulation. In the case of a cat with a PSS, the majority of radiopharmaceutical enters the systemic circulation and radioactivity appears in the heart before it appears in the liver. This study identified 9 of 11 cats with PSS in which it was used. Scintigraphy does not provide anatomic detail about the shunt, however.

Operative portography confirms the diagnosis of PSS and provides the most anatomic detail of all the diagnostic imaging modalities. Anatomic information from the portogram may be helpful in accurately locating the shunt, especially for intrahepatic PSS. Portography is performed by exposing a loop of jejunum during laparotomy. A jejunal vein is catheterized with a 22- or 24-gauge catheter, which is secured in place by ligatures. An extension set is attached to the catheter and flushed with heparinized saline. The intestinal loop is returned to the abdomen, which is closed, temporarily leaving the extension set exposed for administration of contrast medium. With the cat in lateral recumbency, water-soluble contrast medium (1 to 2 ml/kg) is injected as a bolus, and a radiograph is made as the final milliliter is injected. If necessary, a second injection can be made with the cat in dorsal recumbency. The mesenteric catheter is left in place for portal pressure measurements during shunt attenuation. It is not possible to diagnose portal atresia (absence of a portal vein entering the liver) from only the portogram. Hepatic portal flow may appear diminished or absent before shunt ligation, but there is likely to be adequate hepatic vascularity to allow attenuation of the shunt. Repeat portography after shunt occlusion would document adequate intrahepatic portal circulation (Fig. 1).

While the portogram provides excellent imaging of the PSS, the procedure adds considerably to operative time and expense, and is occasionally associated with hemorrhage from the catheter site or anaphylactic reaction to contrast medium. In most cases, an experienced surgeon can locate the PSS without the added information from the portogram.

## TREATMENT

The best clinical outcome for cats with PSS is associated with early diagnosis, followed by medical stabilization and surgery to completely ligate the PSS. Ligation of the anomalous vessel forces portal blood through the liver, where it can be detoxified before entering the systemic circulation. In cats in which excessive portal hypertension occurs allowing only partial shunt ligation, there is a higher risk of continued or recurrent clinical signs. Long-term medical management without surgical correction is usually unsatisfactory.

### Medical Therapy

The cornerstone of medical management is amelioration of the signs of HE. The cause of HE is not precisely understood and is likely multifactorial (see "Medical Management or Chronic Hepatic Encephalopathy," this volume, p 1153). Encephalopathy in PSS occurs when toxic by-products of intestinal metabolism reach the cerebral circulation, either because of shunting from the portal circulation or because of insufficient function of the atrophied liver. Gut-derived am-

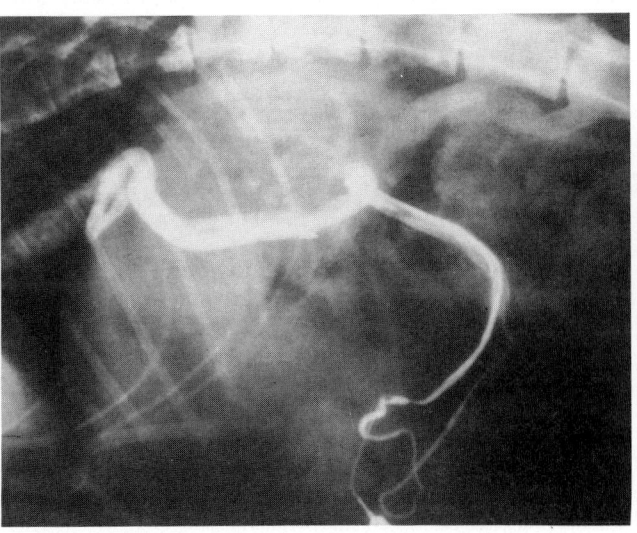
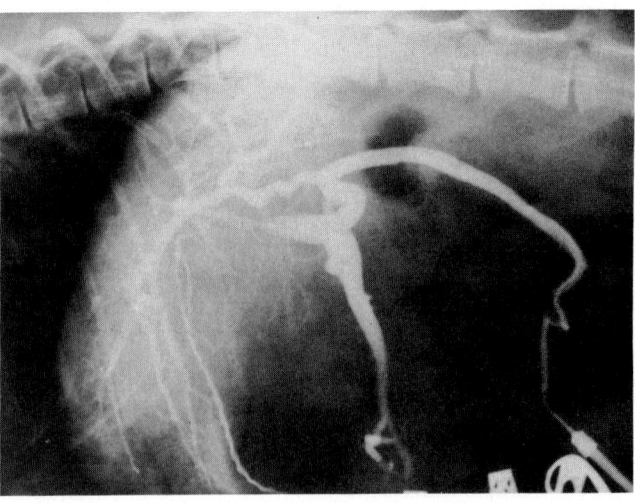

A                    B

**Figure 1.** Mesenteric portogram in a 2.5-year-old neutered male domestic shorthair cat before (A) and after (B) partial ligation of a left gastric–postcaval portosystemic shunt.

monia, imbalanced amino acids and neurotransmitters, fatty acids, mercaptans, and endogenous benzodiazepines have all been implicated in the pathogenesis of HE.

Concurrent conditions that precipitate or potentiate HE include azotemia, hypokalemia, alkalosis, gastrointestinal hemorrhage, infection, dehydration, drug administration, and high-protein diet. While these conditions do not result in HE in normal animals, they may be additive in PSS patients and must be addressed as well.

Abnormal liver function tests in the setting of neurologic clinical signs are suggestive of HE. In a practice situation, however, results of liver function tests may not be available on an emergency basis. Therefore, treatment must often be started empirically if HE is suspected. The first step is to stop intake of food, the fuel for HE, until neurologic signs have resolved. Concurrently, measures are undertaken to decrease the production and absorption of gut toxins, especially ammonia, which are produced by enterocytes and urea-splitting intestinal bacteria. Lactulose is a synthetic disaccharide that is hydrolyzed by colonic bacteria to produce an acid environment and an osmotic catharsis. This traps ammonia in the colon and decreases transit time of ingesta, minimizing the opportunity for bacteria to act on urea that has diffused back into the intestine. The usual starting dosage of lactulose for cats is 1 ml PO every 8 hr. The dosage is titrated to produce stools slightly softer than normal without causing diarrhea. Certain antibiotics are often added to reduce bacterial populations that generate ammonia. Neomycin sulfate (20 mg/kg PO every 8 hr) is a nonabsorbable oral antibiotic that is active against urea-splitting bacteria. It may be used alone or in combination with lactulose. Metronidazole is also effective against ammonia-forming bacteria, and may be administered at 10 mg/kg PO every 12 hr. Antibiotics are usually discontinued after stabilizing the patient because they are usually unnecessary for long-term management and are occasionally associated with side effects of ototoxicity, nephrotoxicity (neomycin sulfate), and neurotoxicity (metronidazole). However, a few patients appear to require antibiotics continuously or intermittently to control signs of HE. Lactulose is most often prescribed when long-term medical therapy is required.

Cats exhibiting severe neurologic signs will benefit from retention enemas to evacuate the colon contents and associated toxins. Dilute lactulose (30% lactulose, 70% warm water) is the most effective enema solution. It is administered at approximately 25 ml/kg and is left in place for 20 to 30 min. Neomycin sulfate (20 mg/kg) or 10% povidone-iodine may also be added to the enema solution to decrease colonic bacteria. The enemas may be repeated until the colon is palpably empty and the pH of the evacuated fluid is less than 6.0 (Hardy, 1992). The benzodiazepine inhibitor flumazenil has shown promise in treating HE in experimental animals and in human patients, but has had little effect at a total dosage of 0.5 mg IV or PO in cats with PSS in the authors' practice.

The ideal anticonvulsant for cats with seizures associated with PSS is controversial. Diazepam is not always effective in controlling cluster seizures, and the possible contribution of endogenous benzodiazepines to the pathogenesis of HE puts the use of this drug further into question. We currently recommend phenobarbital for seizures that fail to respond to standard treatment for HE. Although many reports recommend reducing the dosage of phenobarbital in patients with PSS, it is the authors' experience that normal dosages (2.2 mg/kg IV or PO every 12 hr) are required to achieve therapeutic blood levels in cats. Regardless of the starting dosage selected, phenobarbital blood level monitoring is very important to avoid under- or overdosing PSS patients.

Patients in coma or that exhibit signs of increased intracranial pressure (abnormal pupil responses, hyperventilation, stiff extremities, decerebrate posture) and that fail to respond promptly to treatment with enemas, lactulose, antibiotics, and supportive care, should be treated empirically for cerebral edema. Brain edema is difficult to diagnose in veterinary patients, but nonetheless may cause permanent brain injury or death if not controlled. For this reason, it is safer to treat early for suspected brain edema rather than to wait. Treatment is with mannitol 20% 1 gm/kg IV over 30 min every 4 hr (up to four doses) until improvement occurs. Furosemide may be administered concurrently at 1 to 2 mg/kg IV every 8 hr up to three times. Edema associated with HE is vasogenic in origin and thus is unresponsive to corticosteroids.

When the patient is stable and can eat again, a high-quality, low-protein diet should be offered. For most cats, a commercial diet (Prescription Diet feline k/d, Hill's Pet Nutrition) is adequate. Some cats, however, will become encephalopathic even with this restricted level of protein, and a homemade diet with lower protein content may be substituted (Table 2). Careful attention should be given to assure that adequate amounts of taurine, an essential amino acid in cats, and arginine, which is required to convert ammonia to urea, are present in any commercial or homemade diet for

**Table 2.** *Restricted-Protein Diet for Cats with Portosystemic Shunts**

1/4 lb (115 gm) liver
2 large eggs (100 gm), hard cooked
2 cups (350 gm) cooked rice without added salt
1 T (15 gm) vegetable oil
1 t (5 gm) calcium carbonate
1/4 t (1 gm) potassium chloride (salt substitute)
Balanced supplement that fulfills the feline minimum daily requirement for all vitamins and trace minerals.
Source of taurine (20 mg/day) is needed.

Dice and braise the liver, retaining fat. Combine all ingredients and mix well. This mixture is somewhat dry, and the palatability may be improved by adding water (not milk). Yield 1 1/4 lb (585 gm), 635 kcal/lb, 24.3% protein dry matter basis.

*From Lewis LD, Morris ML, and Hand MS: *Small Animal Clinical Nutrition III.* Topeka, Mark Morris Associates, 1987, pp A3–3, with permission.

cats with PSS. Hyperammonemia and HE has occurred within hours after feeding a commercial casein-based feline diet with low arginine content to normal cats (Diehl and Wheeler, 1992).

## Surgical Correction

Surgical attenuation of the shunt vessel offers the best chance for long-term control of clinical signs. Careful planning and preparation are required, as many cats are in poor condition and are especially sensitive to anesthetics. The authors routinely try to stabilize cats using medical therapy including low-protein diet, lactulose, and anticonvulsants, if indicated, for 1 or more weeks prior to anesthesia and surgery. Hypoglycemia and electrolyte abnormalities should be corrected before anesthesia. If a transfusion is required, only fresh blood should be administered, since ammonia accumulates during storage of whole blood or packed red blood cells. Anesthetic agents with a wide safety margin should be selected. The authors prefer mask or chamber induction, followed by intubation and maintenance with isofluorane. Profound hypothermia develops rapidly in cats undergoing PSS attenuation surgery, and careful usage of heating blankets and warmed fluids should be employed to maintain normal body temperature.

A ventral midline approach is used, and the splanchnic vasculature is carefully evaluated for an anomalous vessel. Detailed knowledge of the splanchnic circulation is essential to reduce the surgery time. If the vessel is not apparent, a portogram may be performed. In this series of cases, the shunt vessel originated from the portal vein, the left gastric vein, and the splenic vein most commonly. In more than half the cases, the anomalous vessel joined the abdominal vena cava, and in another quarter of the cases, it traversed the diaphragm to join a thoracic vein. A large variety of other portosystemic anomalies were noted, including shunts originating from the mesenteric, colic, and right gastric veins and emptying into the renal and phrenicoabdominal veins. Less than 10% of the PSS in this group of cats were intrahepatic.

When the shunt vessel is isolated, it is encircled close to the systemic circulation with a nonabsorbable ligature (3-0 or 2-0 silk) and tied loosely. Portal pressure can be measured with a water manometer or pressure transducer connected to a catheter placed via a purse-string suture in the portal vein, mesenteric vein, splenic vein, or in the anomalous vessel itself. Pressure should be measured as soon as the catheter is placed to minimize the effects of prolonged anesthesia. In dogs, it is speculated that shunt attenuation resulting in postligation portal pressure greater than 20 cm $H_2O$ or an increase of 10 cm $H_2O$ from the resting pressure increases the risk of postoperative splanchnic venous hypertension and death. Acceptable upper limits of portal pressure in cats is unknown, but most surgeons use the same guidelines as for dogs. The small size of feline mesenteric vessels makes their catheterization a technical challenge, and placement in the portal vein could result in portal hypertension if the lumen is reduced excessively as a result of scar contraction. Simple manipulation of the abdominal viscera and extended anesthesia may result in marked variation of pressure measurements without changing the position of the ligature, making pressure interpretation unreliable. In addition, splanchnic venous pressure is correlated with systemic blood pressure. Thus, systemic hypotension may artificially lower splanchnic pressure.

The ligature is gradually attenuated until the shunt is completely occluded, or until portal pressure has reached the accepted upper limits. Excessive congestion, hypermotility, or cyanosis of the intestines or the pancreas indicates overattenuation of the shunt as does a drop in systemic blood pressure. The splanchnic viscera are observed for 10 to 15 min after shunt attenuation for signs of congestion. If these signs are noted, the ligature is removed and reapplied with less vessel attenuation. The catheter used for pressure measurement is removed and hemostasis is carefully established. A liver biopsy is obtained prior to routine abdominal closure (Whiting and Peterson, 1993).

## Cystic Calculi

Of the nine cats in which ammonium biurate cystic calculi were diagnosed, six were greater than 2 years old at the time of diagnosis. Dysuria and hematuria were the only clinical signs exhibited by four of the cats. All nine cats had at least one abnormal liver function test (ammonia, BSP retention, or bile acids), but several had normal or borderline fasting bile acid or ammonia concentration. Ammonium biurate calculi are usually radiolucent, requiring contrast cystography or ultrasonography for identification. Dietary management to dissolve ammonium biurate calculi has not been reported in cats with PSS, and the calculi are routinely removed by cystotomy. Ligation of a PSS responsible for formation of such calculi is indicated to prevent recurrence of calculus formation following cystotomy, even in cats without signs of HE. Because of the high association with PSS, liver function tests are indicated in any cat from which ammonium biurate calculi are removed.

## Postoperative Care

Severe splanchnic venous congestion is the most dreaded complication after shunt attenuation and may occur even if the recommended guidelines are followed. This complication is manifested by severe abdominal pain and abdominal distention, explosive hemorrhagic diarrhea, respiratory distress, and signs of hypovolemic or endotoxic shock within 36 hr after surgery. The only possible treatment is emergency laparotomy to release the shunt ligature, but most animals do not survive. Ascites in the absence of other signs of splanchnic venous congestion is not a reason to remove the ligature and usually resolves within a few days of surgery as portal hypertension becomes less severe.

Because of their small size and the often prolonged anesthetic time, most cats recover from surgery profoundly hypothermic and should be warmed carefully with water blankets or heat lamps. Intraoperative and postoperative hypoglycemia occurs frequently in canine PSS patients, but is uncommon in cats. Nevertheless, it is wise to monitor blood glucose levels until the patient is alert and eating well. Cats exhibiting borderline hypoglycemia preoperatively should be supplemented with dextrose infusion (2.5 to 5%) during and after surgery.

Convulsions in cats without a previous seizure history may occur in the first few days after surgery. The reason for this is unknown and does not appear to be related to blood ammonia or glucose levels. Seizures developed postoperatively in four cats in this series, and in three of these cases they persisted for months to years, requiring long-term treatment with phenobarbital. Because of the severity of the postoperative seizure disorder, some surgeons have elected to routinely administer phenobarbital for 1 week before and a few weeks after surgery for all feline PSS patients. The efficacy of this approach is unknown.

Low-protein diet and lactulose are recommended for 1 month postoperatively to allow time for hepatic regeneration and improved blood flow. A normal diet is then gradually introduced. Results of liver function testing such as measurement of serum bile acids should indicate marked improvement from preoperative values 1 month after surgery. If clinical signs are not adequately controlled or liver function test results remain markedly abnormal, a second work-up should be considered to evaluate for the presence of persistent shunting through a partially ligated vessel or for the presence of functional multiple PSS that developed subsequent to chronically elevated portal pressure. If significant shunting through the original vessel is present, reoperation should be considered to further attenuate the shunt. Several cats in this series suffered recurrence of clinical signs with abnormal liver function tests up to several years after successful shunt attenuation. For this reason, liver function should be monitored once or twice a year to detect deterioration before it is severe enough to cause clinical signs. Cats that fail to return to normal following surgery or for whom surgery is not an option may be managed medically with low-protein diet and lactulose for life, although the long-term outcome is not expected to be as favorable in such patients.

## PROGNOSIS

Of the cats in this series, 73 underwent surgery with the aim of shunt attenuation. The PSS was located and successfully attenuated in 62 cats, of which 55 (89%) were discharged from the hospital. Seven cats died postoperatively with signs of portal hypertension or worsening neurologic status. Several reasons accounted for why the shunt was not ligated in 11 surgical cases. The most common reason was inability to locate the vessel or the (inaccurate) impression that portal atresia was present. Others were not ligated because of the presence of an intrahepatic shunt or because of elevated portal pressure measurements. Most of these 11 cats were euthanatized or died shortly after surgery, but several were successfully managed medically for several years.

Not surprisingly, the 23 cats that were discharged with complete shunt ligation were reported by their owners to be normal or improved more often than were the 32 cats with shunts that were only partially attenuated. Although they did not fare as well as a group, most cats with partial shunt ligation appeared to be normal or improved, while a few showed no change. Importantly, seizures persisted in more cats with partially ligated PSS than in cats with completely ligated PSS. Persistent blindness, although less common than seizures, was also more frequent in the cats with partial shunt ligation. Three cats with partial PSS ligation were euthanatized within 6 months of surgery because of uncontrollable seizures or recurrence of dysuria. One quarter of the cats with partially ligated PSS underwent a second surgery in an attempt to improve their status. In most of these reoperated cases, portal pressure had decreased enough to allow complete PSS ligation, and the cats became normal postoperatively.

## SUMMARY

As a group, cats do not appear to respond as well to corrective surgery for PSS as do dogs (Birchard and Sherding, 1992). This may be in part due to delay in the diagnosis and treatment of this uncommon condition. Many of the cats in this series suffered clinical signs for months to years before a diagnosis was made, perhaps suffering permanent neurologic and hepatic injury or missing a "window" during which a full recovery following surgery is possible. Recognizing PSS as the most likely cause of intermittent ptyalism and neurologic dysfunction in juvenile cats should enable early diagnosis in most cases. In addition, the pathogenesis of HE is complex and incompletely understood, and cats may be particularly susceptible to its effects. Many cats return to normal after surgical intervention, and this remains the best option for owners who desire long-term health for their cats with PSS.

### References and Suggested Reading

Birchard SJ and Sherding RG: Feline portosystemic shunts. Compend Cont Educ Pract Vet 14:1295, 1992.
   *Literature review summarizing the clinical, laboratory, and surgical findings in 40 cats with PSS and comparing surgical outcome of 22 cats with 16 dogs.*
Diehl KJ and Wheeler SL: Evaluation of three enteral feeding formulas in cats (abstr). Proc Am Coll Vet Intern Med, 1992, p 813.

*Report of hyperammonemia and HE associated with the feeding of an arginine-deficient diet.*
Hardy RM: Hepatic encephalopathy. *In* Kirk RW and Bonagura J (eds): *Current Veterinary Therapy XI.* Philadelphia, WB Saunders Co, 1992, p 639.
*A review of the pathogenesis and treatment of hepatic encephalopathy and coma.*

Lewis LD, Morris ML, and Hand MS: Small Animal Clinical Nutrition III. Topeka, Mark Morris Associates, 1990, p A3–3.
*Recipes for patients with PSS and other medical conditions.*
Whiting PG and Peterson SL: Portosystemic shunts, *In* Slatter D (ed): Textbook of Small Animal Surgery, 2nd edition. Philadelphia, WB Saunders Co, 1993, p 660.
*Description of surgical techniques for correcting PSS in cats and dogs.*

# CHRONIC HEPATITIS: THERAPEUTIC CONSIDERATIONS

CYNTHIA R. LEVEILLE-WEBSTER
*North Grafton, Massachusetts*
and SHARON A. CENTER
*Ithaca, New York*

The etiopathogenic mechanisms involved in the development and progression of chronic hepatobiliary disease (CHD) in the dog and cat are poorly understood. As a result, selection of appropriate clinical management is often symptomatic or based on histopathologic changes observed on hepatic biopsy. Therapeutics are further complicated by a lack of information on the clinical efficacy of treatment protocols and on pharmacokinetic data for drugs commonly used to treat animals with CHD (see "Effects of Hepatic Disease on Drug Disposition," this volume, p 758). Veterinary science, therefore, has borrowed heavily from information derived from clinical trials in human patients with CHD.

Definitive treatment of CHD should not be initiated until diagnosis is confirmed with hepatic biopsy. Histopathologic features indicative of CHD include the presence of mononuclear inflammatory cells and/or the presence of fibrosis. Clinicopathologic features that may be seen in CHD include hypoalbuminemia, consistent elevations in serum liver enzymes (alanine aminotransferase [ALT], alkaline phosphatase [ALP] and γ-glutamyl transferase [GGT]), hyperbilirubinemia, and increased serum bile acids.

## AIMS OF THERAPY

Therapeutic goals in the treatment of CHD include the elimination of etiologic factors; suppression of nonspecific mechanisms that contribute to disease progression; provision of an optimum environment for hepatic regeneration; and control of secondary complications including hepatic encephalopathy (HE), ascites, fluid and electrolyte imbalances, coagulopathies, gastrointestinal ulceration, and infections. Therapy for each patient is individualized based on etiology, stage of disease, nutritional status, and the presence of complicating conditions.

## SPECIFIC THERAPY

Specific therapy for CHD is limited to disorders with a known case. Suspected hepatotoxic reactions are treated by discontinuation of drug therapy or removal of the toxic agent. In some cases, with early recognition of toxic effects, discontinuation of the drug may result in complete resolution of hepatic pathology. In many animals, toxicity is recognized after irreversible lesions have developed and symptomatic and supportive care for CHD is necessary.

Copper hepatotoxicity has been well characterized in the Bedlington terrier. In this breed, an inherited defect in biliary copper excretion leads to progressive accumulation of copper in hepatocytes that eventually results in hepatic necrosis, inflammation, and fibrosis. A less well-characterized syndrome associated with aberrant copper storage may occur in the West Highland white terrier. Copper toxicity is treated by chelation therapy with D-penicillamine (Cuprimine, Merck), 2,2,2-tetramine (Syprine, Merck) or 2,3,2-tetramine (not commercially available) at 10 to 15 mg/kg every 12 hr PO (Twedt and Whitney, 1989). Anorexia and vomiting frequently accompany therapy with D-penicillamine in the dog. Other side effects reported in humans include cutaneous eruptions, leukopenia, glomerulopathy, aplastic anemia, and bronchoalveolitis. Adverse reactions with the tetramines have not been noted. Copper chelators work slowly, and it may take many months before reductions in hepatic copper are detectable. Zinc inhibits the intestinal absorption of copper and has been used successfully to treat copper associated hepatic disease (see "Use of Zinc Acetate for the Treatment and Prevention of Canine Copper Hepatotoxicosis," this volume, p 757).

Although increased hepatic copper concentration may develop in cholestatic liver disease in **other** breeds of dogs, copper accumulation is most likely a consequence of reduced biliary copper excretion and not a cause of the disease. The mere recognition of copper-positive staining in a hepatic biopsy or the quantitative determination of a modestly increased hepatic copper concentration does not warrant chelation therapy.

Infectious agents are rare causes of CHD in dogs and cats. Hepatobiliary trematode infestation is well characterized in cats and, if left untreated, can progress to fibrosing cholangiohepatitis. Treatment for 2 days with praziquantel (Droncit, Haver) at 5 mg/kg every 12 hr PO or a single dose of nitroscanate (Lopatol, Ciba-Giegy) at 100 mg/kg have been efficacious. Leptosporosis can cause CHD in dogs. During acute infection, leptosporosis is treated with penicillin (40,000 U/kg every 12 hr for 14 days IM, SC, or PO) to curtail shedding of viable organisms. Doxycycline (2.5 mg/kg/day for 14 days PO) is used to eliminate the chronic carrier state. Elimination of the infectious organism may not prevent progression of CHD. Chronic hepatitis associated with canine adenovirus I has become an uncommon entity since the introduction of highly effective vaccines. For the rare case identified, no specific therapy is recommended. In humans with CHD due to viral infection with hepatitis B or C, $\alpha$-interferon is used to manage the disease.

## SUPPORTIVE THERAPY

### Modulation of Inflammation

When inflammatory changes are present on hepatic biopsy, it is likely that inflammatory cells, their mediators, and local cytokine release are contributing to hepatic necrosis and fibrogenesis. In this circumstance, suppression of the inflammatory response is one way to control disease progression. Glucocorticoids have anti-inflammatory and immune-modulating effects. They inhibit phospholipase A, thereby decreasing production of the proinflammatory mediators, prostaglandins, and leukotrienes. Glucocorticoids also inhibit the movement of leukocytes into sites of inflammation, depress monocyte phagocyte function, and suppress the response of mononuclear cells to cytokines involved in the propagation of the inflammatory response. Some forms of CHD in humans are remarkably responsive to glucocorticoid therapy: patients survive longer, biochemical tests improve, and the histologic progression of the disease slows (Tygstrop, 1989). Similar forms of liver disease in the dog are suspected, but have not been carefully characterized. In one study, dogs surviving more than 1 week beyond initial diagnosis that were treated with prednisone had a significantly increased survival compared to dogs that were not treated (Strombeck, Miller, and Harrold, 1988). Treatment bias in that study and the spectrum of hepatic disorders

included as chronic hepatitis limit definitive conclusions on the treatment efficacy of glucocorticoids in canine CHD. Controlled prospective trials of glucocorticoid therapy in veterinary patients with CHD will be necessary to delineate those patients who might benefit from such therapy.

Presently, glucocorticoid therapy may be considered in patients with CHD when the following criteria are met: (1) infectious causes have been ruled out, (2) active disease exists as evidenced by the presence of significant inflammatory infiltrates on hepatic biopsy or the demonstration of sequential increases in hepatic enzyme concentrations, or (3) evidence of aberrant immune function such as the presence of serum hypergammaglobulemia or antinuclear antibodies or the presence of extrahepatic autoimmune disease exists. In dogs with CHD, a prednisone dose of 1 to 2 mg/kg/day tapered gradually to 0.5 mg/kg/day then to every other day has been recommended (Magne and Chiapella, 1986). In cats, prednisolone has been used at an initial dose of 2.2 mg/kg/day, tapered gradually to 1.0 mg/kg every other day. In humans, tapering prednisone therapy to alternate days is not effective in maintaining histologic remission of steroid-responsive hepatitis. Glucocorticoid therapy in humans must be continued at least 6 months beyond clinical remission to prevent relapse. No information on the efficacy of alternate-day dosing or the length of treatment necessary to sustain remission is available for veterinary patients.

Glucocorticoid therapy may be detrimental when ascites or HE complicate CHD. Residual mineralocorticoid activity in some glucocorticoid preparations may promote sodium and water retention, which can potentiate ascitic fluid accumulation. The catabolic effects of glucocorticoids may precipitate HE. In patients with ascites, use of a glucocorticoid, such as dexamethasone, with little mineralocorticoid activity may be prudent.

The major side effect of glucocorticoid therapy is suppression of the pituitary-adrenal axis, which can result in adrenal atrophy and iatrogenic Cushing's syndrome. Alternate-day therapy with short-acting glucocorticoids, such as prednisone, minimizes axis suppression. Use of longer acting preparations, such as dexamethasone, may require longer intervals between dosing to achieve a similar axis-sparing effect. Other adverse reaction to glucocorticoids include gastrointestinal ulceration, pancreatitis, glucose intolerance, and secondary infections.

Azathioprine (Imuran, Burroughs Wellcome) is an antimetabolite with anti-inflammatory and immune-modulating effects. It is metabolized primarily within the liver and red blood cells to its active form, 6-mercaptopurine. Mercaptopurine disrupts nucleic acid synthesis, thereby inhibiting the proliferation of rapidly dividing cells. It modifies T lymphocyte function, resulting in suppression of cell-mediated immunity and T cell–dependent antibody production. Azathioprine is a valuable adjunct to glucocorticoid therapy in humans. Combination therapy permits prednisone doses to be lowered so that side effects are minimized while clinical efficacy is maintained. Combination therapy with azathioprine (1 mg/kg/day PO) and prednisone (0.5 to 1.0 mg/kg/day) has been recommended for use in the dog (Magne and Chiapella, 1986). If clinical response seems optimal, alternate-day dosing is advised to minimize drug toxicity. Since the major adverse reaction to azathioprine is bone marrow suppression, the hemogram should be monitored initially at 7-day intervals for 2 weeks. A white cell nadir of less than 5000/$\mu$l warrants temporary drug withdrawal. When the white blood cell count returns to normal, azathioprine is reinstituted at 75% of the original dose. Gastrointestinal toxicity and pancreatitis may occur with azathioprine. Hepatotoxicity has been reported in humans, but has not been identified in veterinary patients. Azathioprine is poorly tolerated by cats at doses greater than 0.3 mg/kg every other day PO. Even at this dose, individual tolerance is variable and some cats develop anorexia, vomiting, diarrhea, and serious leukopenia.

Both prednisone and azathioprine require hepatic conversion to active forms. Prednisone is biotransformed to prednisolone in the liver. Studies in humans with CHD comparing the pharmacokinetics of these drugs have shown that reduced formation of prednisolone from prednisone occurs with severe liver disease, but is offset by altered drug binding and biodistribution and delayed elimination. We assume similar factors are operational in veterinary patients. There are no studies on the metabolism of azathioprine in humans or animals with hepatic insufficiency.

## Modulation of Fibrosis

Hepatic fibrosis is an important feature of CHD (for review, see Leveille and Arias, 1993). Fibrosis is characterized by an increase in the hepatic extracellular matrix (ECM). The ECM, composed of collagen, proteoglycans, and glycoproteins, provides the structural framework for the liver. The deposition of ECM in the liver disrupts functional relationships between hepatocytes and impairs sinusoidal perfusion of the liver. If left unchecked, fibrogenesis leads to hepatic cirrhosis. Fibrogenesis is a dynamic and potentially reversible process. An important event in hepatic fibrogenesis is the transformation of the hepatic lipocyte or Ito cell into a fibroblast-like cell. When transformed, these lipocytes synthesize and secrete large amounts of ECM including collagen, the major ECM component in the fibrotic liver.

Therapeutic strategies to modulate fibrogenesis are aimed at inhibiting lipocyte transformation and ECM production. Cytokines released from inflammatory cells have an important role in both processes. The anti-inflammatory actions of glucocorticoids and azathioprine may be effective antifibrotics in this regard. Glucocorticoids also decrease collagen production by inhibiting prolyl hydroxylase, an enzyme specific for collagen formation, and by decreasing the transcription of collagen messenger ribonucleic acid (mRNA).

Colchicine is an inhibitor of microtubular assembly. Collagen secretion from lipocytes requires microtubules and is inhibited by colchicine. Colchicine increases collagenase activity and thus may promote the degradation of existing collagen. Colchicine also inhibits leukocyte migration and this anti-inflammatory action may suppress fibrogenesis. In human clinical trials, colchicine is effective in arresting fibrogenesis associated with cirrhosis (Kerschenobich, Vargas, and Garcia-Tsag, 1988). Three dogs with different types of fibrotic hepatopathies treated with colchicine have been reported in the veterinary literature. Although all dogs responded to combination therapy that included colchicine, a histologic response to therapy was verified in only one dog. The dose used in dogs has been extrapolated from human medicine, 0.03 mg/kg/day PO. Further clinical experience is necessary before the potential benefits of colchicine therapy in canine CHD are defined. There are no reports, to the authors' knowledge, of colchicine use in the cat.

Colchicine therapy in the dog can be associated with nausea, vomiting, and hemorrhagic diarrhea. In humans, rare toxic reactions include agranulocytosis, aplastic anemia, myopathy, and peripheral neuropathies. Colchicine is marketed in two forms, as pure colchicine and as combination product with probenecid. Since probenecid can cause nausea, vomiting, and lethargy in some dogs, the combination product should be avoided.

D-Penicillamine has been touted as an antifibrotic drug. It inhibits lysyl oxidase, an enzyme necessary for collagen synthesis, and also directly binds to collagen fibrils, preventing them from being cross-linked into stable collagen fibers. The use of D-penicillamine as an antifibrotic agent in humans with CHD has been disappointing. This drug has received limited attention as an antifibrotic agent in veterinary medicine. Its use in Bedlington terriers for its copper chelating ability has not provided convincing evidence that it has antifibrotic properties in that disorder.

Human patients with CHD have low serum and hepatic zinc concentrations (McClain et al., 1991). Zinc deficiency is associated with insufficient dietary intake, increased urinary excretion, reduced gastrointestinal absorption, and altered hepatic metabolism. Zinc deficiency may have a role in the immune dysfunction, abnormal protein metabolism, and anorexia that develop in human patients with CHD. Zinc supplementation attenuates the development of pathology in rodent models of induced acute and chronic liver disease. This hepatoprotection may be associated with inhibition of lipid peroxidation and stabilization of lysosomal membranes. Zinc inhibits enzymes involved in collagen synthesis and is necessary for collagenase activity and thus may have antifibrotic properties. Zinc has been given to dogs with CHD as zinc acetate at 200 mg elemental zinc every 24 hr PO. Vomiting limits the administration of zinc as the sulfate or gluconate salt. Plasma zinc levels are monitored every 2 weeks during therapy. The goal is to maintain plasma zinc at 200 to 300 $\mu$g/dl. If concentrations reach 100 $\mu$g/dl, zinc therapy is discontinued to avoid serious hemolytic reactions associated with toxicity. Although zinc can interfere with intestinal iron and copper absorption, the authors have not seen deficiency of these minerals develop in dogs on chronic zinc therapy.

## Choleretics

Serum, bile, and hepatic concentrations of hydrophobic bile acids increase in patients with cholestatic liver disease. Studies show that hydrophobic bile acids interact with hepatobiliary cell membranes and disrupt cellular function. The administration of ursodeoxycholate (Actigall, Ciba-Geigy), a relatively hydrophilic bile acid, to human patients with CHD results in clinical, biochemical, and in some cases, histologic improvement (Poupon and Poupon, 1993). Ursodeoxycholate's cytoprotective effect is related to its ability to displace hydrophobic bile acids from the whole body pool. Other potential benefits of ursodeoxycholate therapy in CHD include stimulation of bile flow and immune modulation related to a decrease in the aberrant expression of major histocompatibility class I antigens on hepatobiliary cells. Expression of these antigens plays a key role in the initiation and propagation of hepatic inflammation in many chronic liver disorders.

Ursodeoxycholate (10 to 15 mg/kg/day PO) has been used as adjunctive treatment by the authors in over 50 dogs with CHD. Vomiting requiring drug withdrawal was seen in one dog. In rabbits and certain nonhuman primates, an inability to sulfate a metabolic derivative of ursodeoxycholate results in serious hepatotoxicity. Toxicity studies conducted for approval of the drug in humans were completed in healthy dogs given considerably higher doses without adverse effects. A preliminary placebo-controlled study of urosodeoxycholate has been conducted in healthy cats. At 15 mg/kg/day PO, no adverse clinical reactions or changes in hepatic histopathology were found. Further work of the safety and efficacy of this bile acid in veterinary patients is needed before its use can be routinely recommended.

Dehydrocholic acid (Decholin, Miles Laboratory) has been recommended as a choleretic agent in veterinary patients, but little data are available on toxicity or clinical efficacy. The availability of ursodeoxycholate has made the use of dehydrocholic acid obsolete. Choleretics are contraindicated when biliary obstruction is present.

## Dietary Management

Dietary therapy is a central issue in the medical management of CHD. In humans, the protein intake required to avoid tissue catabolism and that amount which can be tolerated by the individual differs with various types of CHD. Some patients require protein restriction, while others benefit from supplementation. In light of the relationship between gastrointestinal protein digestion/metabolism and HE, dietary protein restriction has been recommended in veterinary patients with CHD. It is generally believed that an optimal dietary protein amino acid balance in patients with CHD is achieved when branched-chain amino acids exceed aromatic amino acids. This is because increases in aromatic amino acids have been implicated in the pathogenesis of HE. A recent study in dogs with surgically created portosytemic shunts has shown that 12 weeks of severe protein restriction (11% crude protein) results in low serum albumin and total protein concentrations (LaFlamme, Allen, and Huber, 1993). These findings are consistent with inadequate protein intake. Dogs on a 24% crude protein diet maintained normal serum protein concentration but developed signs of HE more frequently than those dogs on the restricted-protein diet. All dogs that developed HE were on a diet in which the amino acid composition was primarily comprised of branched-chain amino acids. This finding is unexpected and contradicts previous studies in human CHD in which encephalopathic patients show improvement on diets high in branched-chain amino acids. In patients with CHD, a delicate balance exists between maintenance of adequate protein intake, provision of protein of optimal quality, and the precipitation of HE.

Until nutritional studies on dietary requirements of veterinary patients with CHD are conducted, the following dietary recommendations are advised. First, dietary protein should at least meet minimal requirements, which are 22% crude protein in the dog and 30% crude protein in the cat. If signs of HE develop, either additional medical therapy can be initiated or the protein content of the diet can be decreased. If additional dietary restriction is undertaken, sequential evaluation of serum albumin and total protein concentrations should be monitored to ensure adequate protein intake. Protein sources with high digestibility and biologic value such as egg or cottage cheese have previously been recommended in veterinary patients with CHD. Eggs, however, contain sulfated amino acids that may contribute to the development of HE. Dairy (cottage cheese) or vegetable (soymeal, cornmeal) protein may be more appropriate than animal (meat, blood) protein. These protein sources are less ammonigenic and contain large amounts of branched-chain amino acids. If nonanimal protein is used in cats with CHD, supplementation with the essential amino acids, taurine and arginine, is recommended. Arginine is essential for optimal function of the Krebs-Henseleit urea cycle, and taurine is required for the obligate taurine conjugation of bile acids in the cat.

It is vital that animals with CHD receive adequate caloric intake. Standard formulas for the calculation of energy requirements in sick or stressed animals may not be accurate in patients with CHD. These formulas, however, should still be used as a guideline until nutritional studies are completed that verify energy needs in spontaneously diseased animals. Carbohydrates should provide the major portion of the energy requirement. In debilitated patients, highly digestible carbohydrate sources, such as rice or pasta, are used because they have optimal intestinal absorption. High-fiber diets have proven beneficial in the dietary therapy of CHD in humans. Previously, these diets have not been recommended in veterinary patients with CHD, since it was felt that colonic fermentation of residues generated by these diets resulted in the formation of toxigenic substances implicated in the pathogenesis of HE. It is now believed that generation of volatile fatty acids by this fermentation acidifies the colon and encourages the proliferation of nitrogen-fixing bacteria, both of which substantially decrease ammonia production and absorption. An additional advantage gained by the use of high-fiber diets is their ability to bind hydrophobic bile acids in the intestinal lumen, resulting in the fecal elimination of noxious bile acids. It is the fiber content of vegetable proteins that likely accounts for the therapeutic benefits of these proteins in patients with CHD. Since it may be difficult to meet daily caloric requirements with high-fiber diets due to their increased bulk and decreased digestibility, they should not be used in animals with poor nutritional status.

Severe fat restriction is not necessary in CHD unless steatorrhea secondary to bile acid malassimilation exists. Dietary fats provide essential fatty acids and fat-soluble vitamins and are important in maintaining palatability of diets, especially in cats. In dogs and cats, fat requirements are met with diets containing 7 to 9% fat on a dry weight basis. Most diets suggested for use in animals with CHD have a high fat content, but in general, are well tolerated.

Humans with CHD develop vitamin deficiencies as a result of reduced dietary intake, decreased hepatic storage and activation, increased intestinal losses, and greater physiologic demand. Vitamin K deficiency is common when the enterohepatic circulation of bile acids is impaired as occurs with bile duct obstruction. The resultant fat malabsorption impairs the intestinal absorption of vitamin K. Severe hepatic insufficiency may also decrease hepatic activation of vitamin K and result in defective carboxylation of vitamin K–dependent coagulation factors. Patients with cholestatic disease or severe hepatic disease may require vitamin K supplementation to avoid bleeding diatheses. Acute therapy to prevent biopsy-associated bleeding requires two to three doses of vitamin $K_1$ (AquaMEPHYTON, Merck) at 0.5 mg/kg every 12 hr IM or SC. Chronic treatment may require administration at 7- to 20-day intervals, determined on the basis of coagulation tests. Deficiencies of B vitamins are common in humans with CHD. Supplementation in veterinary patients may be in order, especially in cats who have very high B vitamin requirements. Use of a balanced multiple vitamin supplement is recommended.

Although benzodiazepines such as valium and oxazepam have been widely used as appetite stimulants in cats, they are contraindicated in all veterinary patients with CHD. Benzodiazepines are encephalopathic toxins capable of precipitating HE. Anorectic cats with CHD are at risk for the development of hepatic lipidosis if they are moderately to severely overweight. Parenteral or enteral nutrition may be necessary to maintain adequate dietary caloric and protein intake in these cats to prevent lipidosis.

## SYMPTOMATIC THERAPY

### Hepatic Encephalopathy

Hepatic encephalopathy, a frequent complication in CHD, is associated with impaired hepatic extraction or metabolism of neuroactive metabolites from the intestinal tract (see "Medical Management of Chronic Hepatic Encephalopathy," this volume, p 1153). Therapeutic measures to minimize interactions between enteric bacteria and nitrogenous substrates are known to ameliorate clinical signs of HE. The cornerstone of therapy for chronic, recurrent HE is dietary management, primarily by dietary protein restriction, as discussed above. When dietary therapy alone is ineffective, the next step is the administration of a nonabsorbable disaccharide. These sugars favorably interact with the alimentary miroflora to decrease the production of encephalopathic toxins. They escape small intestinal absorption and pass to the colon, where they are fermented to organic acids. These acids lower colonic pH and trap ammonia in the ionized form, facilitating fecal excretion. They also optimize bacterial nitrogen fixation and decrease the number of ammonia-generating organisms. Their action as osmotic cathartics purges the intestinal tract of noxious substances and ammonia-generating bacteria. Lactulose (Cephulac, Chronulac, Marrion/Merrill Dow) is the most commonly used disaccharide. It is given initially at 0.1 to 0.5 ml/kg every 6 to 8 hr PO. The dose is adjusted so that clinical signs of HE are controlled and the animal has no more than two to three soft pudding-like stools per day. Excessive lactulose administration can result in diarrhea and metabolic acidosis. Alternatives that may be as effective as lactulose include a more palatable synthetic disaccharide called lactitol or the use of lactose in lactase-deficient patients.

Further modification of the alimentary environment can be accomplished by the combination of disaccharide therapy with an antibiotic. Neomycin (10 to 22 mg/kg every 12 hr PO), a poorly absorbed aminoglycoside, has been shown to be synergistic with lactulose in the treatment of HE. Metronidazole (7.5 mg/kg every 12 hr PO) may also be used. Metronidazole undergoes hepatic metabolism and excretion, and causes neurotoxicity when toxic levels accumulate. The reduced dosage recommended above is based on the dosing of the antibiotic in humans and the authors' clinical experience in veterinary patients. Amoxicillin has been used along with dietary management to successfully allay HE in cats with portosystemic shunts (see "Feline Portosystemic Vascular Shunts," this volume, p 743).

In addition to the dietary and drug therapy, numerous variables known to precipitate HE in patients with CHD must be controlled or avoided. These variables include: (1) gastrointestinal nitrogen loading from excessive protein intake, gastrointestinal bleeding, or administration of ammonium salts; (2) increased systemic mobilization of protein as occurs in catabolic conditions such as infection, neoplasia, and glucocorticoid excess; (3) increased generation of HE toxins in the colon due to constipation; (4) increased circulating concentrations of urea associated with azotemia, which leads to increased alimentary ammonia generation; (5) precipitation of metabolic alkalosis and hypokalemia, which facilitates renal ammonia production and ammonia transfer across the blood-brain barrier; and (6) syner-

**Table 1.**  *Drugs Used to Treat Chronic Hepatic Disease*

| Drug | Dose | Action | Side Effects |
|---|---|---|---|
| Prednisone | *Dog*: 1–2 mg/kg q24h PO tapered to 0.5 mg/kg EOD<br>*Cat*: 2.2 mg/kg q24h tapered to 1.0 mg/kg EOD | Anti-inflammatory<br>Antifibrotic<br>Immune modulation | Iatrogenic Cushing's<br>Increases susceptibility to infection<br>Pancreatitis<br>Glucose intolerance |
| Azathioprine | *Dog*: 1 mg/kg q24h PO combined with prednisone 0.5–1.0 mg/kg EOD<br>*Cat*: 0.3 mg/kg EOD PO | Anti-inflammatory<br>Immune modulation | Neutropenia<br>Vomiting/diarrhea<br>Anorexia<br>Pancreatitis |
| Colchicine | *Dog*: 0.03 mg/kg q24h PO | Antifibrotic<br>Anti-inflammatory | Hemorrhagic diarrhea<br>Vomiting |
| Ursodeoxycholic acid | *Dog/Cat*: 10–15 mg/kg q24h PO | Choleretic<br>Immune modulatoin<br>Hepatoprotective | Vomiting (rare) |
| Zinc acetate | *Dog*: 200 mg elemental zinc q24h PO for 10–25 kg dog: titrate dose with plasma zinc | Decreases intestinal copper absorption<br>Antifibrotic<br>Hepatoprotective | Hemolysis if plasma zinc >1000 $\mu$g/dl |
| 2,2,2-Tetramine | *Dog*: 10–15 mg/kg q24h PO | Copper chelator | None |
| D-Penicillamine | *Dog*: 10–15 mg/kg q24h PO | Copper chelator<br>Antifibrotic<br>Immune modulation | Anorexia<br>Vomiting |
| Lactulose | *Dog/Cat*: 0.1–0.5 ml/kg q8h PO; titrate dose on basis of 2–3 soft stools per day | Modifies intestinal ammonia production and absorption | Diarrhea, cramping<br>Metabolic acidosis with severe overdosage |
| Metronidazole | *Dog/Cat*: 7.5 mg/kg q12–24h PO | Decreases intestinal bacterial ammonia production | Neurotoxicity |
| Neomycin | *Dog/Cat*: 10–22 mg/kg q12h PO | Decreases intestinal bacterial ammonia production | Ototoxicity (rare) |
| Spironolactone | *Dog/Cat*: 1–2 mg/kg q12hr PO; taper to lowest effective dose | Aldosterone inhibitor used to induce diuresis with ascites | Dehydration |
| Furosemide | *Dog/Cat*: 0.25–.05 mg/kg q12–24h PO; taper to lowest effective dose: may use in combination with spironolactone | Loop diuretic used with ascites | Dehydration<br>Hypokalemia<br>Metabolic alkalosis |
| Vitamin K₁ | *Dog/Cat*: 0.5 mg/kg q12h SC, IM × 3 days with bile duct obstruction;<br>*Dog/Cat*: 0.5 mg/kg q7–20 days SC, IM for chronic therapy | Correct coagulation abnormalities associated with vitamin K deficiency | Heinz-body anemia in cat with overdosage |
| Famotidine | *Dog/Cat*: 0.5–1.0 mg/kg q24h PO; q12h IV, SC | H₂-Receptor antagonist | None |
| Cimetidine | *Dog/Cat*: 5 mg/kg q8hr IV, SC, PO | H₂-Receptor antagonist | Inhibits hepatic drug-metabolizing enzymes |
| Ranitidine | *Dog/Cat*: 1–2 mg/kg q8h IV, PO | H₂-Receptor antagonist | Inhibits hepatic drug-metabolizing enzymes |
| Sucralfate | *Dog/Cat*: 0.25–1.0 gm q8–12h PO | Gastric cytoprotection | Constipation<br>Chelates fluoroquinilones |

gistic neural inhibition produced by exposure to anesthetics or sedatives such as barbiturates or benzodiazepines. Acute exacerbations of HE are managed with appropriate fluid therapy to correct dehydration and electrolyte and acid-base abnormalities. Cleansing enemas with warmed polyionic fluids are initially used to remove colonic debris. Retention enemas with Povidone-iodine (Betadine)(1:10 dilution in water, retained for 15 min) or lactulose (5 to 15 ml diluted 1:3 in water, retained for 30 min) are administered to suppress bacterial growth and production of encephalopathic toxins.

## Ascites

The pathogenesis of ascites formation in CHD is complex. Simplistically, ascitic fluid accumulates when Starling forces are disrupted and a new homeostatic balance is established. This occurs in association with portal hypertension, hypoalbuminemia, and avid renal retention of sodium and water due in part to the activation of the renin-angiotensin-aldosterone system. Treatment for ascites includes cage rest, dietary sodium restriction, diuretics, and abdominal paracentesis.

Initial treatment involves strict cage confinement, as this serves to improve renal perfusion and thus promote water and electrolyte excretion. This is usually coupled with dietary sodium restriction. Most commercial pet foods contain excess sodium in the range of 0.5 to 1.0% of dry weight and are not appropriate for patients with ascites. These patients should have their dietary sodium content restricted to 0.1 to 0.3%. Appropriate sodium-restricted commercial diets include canine and feline k/d and h/d (Hill's Pet Products).

Diuretics are used only when ascites is refractory to conservative measures. The goal of diuretic therapy is slow mobilization of fluid so as to minimize the development of complications such as dehydration, hypokalemia, hyponatremia, or metabolic alkalosis.

Theoretically, spironolactone (1 to 2 mg/kg every 12 hr PO), a diuretic with moderate efficacy, would seem the best diuretic to use. Since it is potassium sparing, problems with diuretic-induced hypokalemia are avoided. Spironolactone's action as an aldosterone antagonist directly opposes one of the hormonal excesses associated with the development of ascites. Unfortunately, it is seldom effective when used alone. The potent loop diuretic, furosemide, is more often effective used alone or in combination with spironolactone. A dose of 0.25 to 0.5 mg/kg every 12 hr PO or SC is initially recommended. This dose is increased if the patient fails to respond. Diuretic therapy should be adjusted to the lowest diuretic dose that controls ascitic fluid accumulation. Electrolyte and hydration status, body weight, and abdominal girth are monitored to assess patient condition and treatment efficacy.

Rapid removal of ascitic fluid by abdominal paracentesis is seldom necessary. It is recommended only when fluid accumulation is severe enough to impair respiratory or renal function or to complicate diagnostic or surgical procedures. Complications of large-volume abdominal paracentesis include dehydration, hyponatremia, exacerbation of hypoproteinemia, and peritonitis. The development of hypotension is cautioned in the literature, but has not been recognized as a complication by the authors.

Administration of plasma or whole blood to rectify hypoalbuminemia is used only for crisis intervention such as may occur during surgical procedures or massive gastrointestinal hemorrhage. Extraordinary efforts to control ascites include surgical placement of a LeVeen peritoneovenous shunt to connect the peritoneal cavity with the central venous system, and surgical creation of a portosystemic shunt aimed at palliating portal hypertension. These procedures are associated with many complications including sepsis, catheter occlusion, and worsening of HE. Neither procedure is routinely recommended.

## Bacterial Infections

Bacterial infections may complicate CHD. An increased susceptibility to infection, primarily a consequence of the depressed hepatic reticuloendothelial cell function, accompanies all forms of CHD. The tendency to develop infection is aggravated by the increased translocation of intestinal bacteria into the portal circulation that occurs secondary to portal hypertension. If fever, leukocytosis with a left shift, or significant suppurative inflammation on hepatic biopsy are part of the clinical spectrum, complicating hepatobiliary infections should be suspected. Anaerobic and aerobic cultures of liver tissue and, if possible, bile should be obtained. Empiric antibiotic therapy is often used if cultures have not been submitted or while awaiting culture results. Such therapy is guided by two major considerations: (1) enteric bacteria are the most common isolates in hepatobiliary infection; and (2) drugs that rely on hepatic clearance, metabolism, and excretion are avoided. Amoxicillin, clavulinate-potentiated amoxicillin, certain cephalosporins (cefazolin, but not cephalexin), enrofloxacin, and aminoglycosides are good choices in both dogs and cats with CHD. Drugs to avoid include chloramphenicol (extensive enterohepatic circulation, requires hepatic conjugation and biliary excretion, inhibits drug metabolizing enzymes), tetracyclines (inhibit protein synthesis, may promote hepatic lipidosis), sulfonamides (associated with idiosyncratic hepatotoxicity), and macrolides (undergo biliary excretion).

## Coagulopathy

Many different coagulation abnormalities may accompany CHD. Most of the coagulation factors, coagulation inhibitors (such as antithrombin III), fibrinolytic substances (such as plasmin), and their activators and inhibitors are synthesized, activated, or regulated by the liver. Coagulopathies in CHD may develop as a result of hepatic synthetic failure, vitamin K deficiency from cholestasis, or from quantitative or qualitative platelet defects. Low-grade disseminated intravascular coagulation, which is common in patients with hepatic insufficiency, may also contribute to bleeding tendencies. The tests commonly used to evaluate coagulation status (prothrombin time, partial thromboplastin time, and activated clotting time) reflect inadequacy only after a particular factor is deficient by more than 70%. Overall, there is poor correlation between bleeding tendencies and coagulation test results. Evaluation of mucosal bleeding time is recommended in patients undergoing hepatic biopsy, since this test is more relevant to the patient's clinical response to tissue injury. Candidates for hepatic biopsy with abnormal coagulation tests should be treated as if they had clinical bleeding tendencies. They should receive fresh whole blood transfusions prior to biopsy and be monitored closely for 24 hr after biopsy. If transfusion fails to correct mucosal bleeding time in these patients, biopsy should not be performed. Even patients with normal coagulation tests should remain suspects for bleeding during or after hepatic biopsy, since the tenuous balance of the coagulation system may be upset by even a small amount of hemorrhage during biopsy. All jaundiced patients should receive parenteral vitamin K prior to biopsy.

## Gastrointestinal Ulceration

A recent study has reported a high incidence of duodenal ulcers in dogs with CHD (Stanton and Bright, 1989). The etiopathogenesis of this predisposition includes decreased mucosal blood flow secondary to portal hypertension, reduced mucosal cell turnover, and gastrointestinal hyperacidity from hypergastrinemia associated with reduced hepatic clearance of gastrin and histamine, and bile acid–stimulated gastrin secretion. Evidence of gastrointestinal ulceration in patients with CHD (chronic vomiting, hematemesis, or melena) is managed with $H_2$-receptor antagonists or local cytoprotective agents. The preferred $H_2$ antagonist in patients with CHD is famotidine (Pepcid, Merck, 0.5–1.0 mg/kg/day PO, every 12 hr SC or IV). Famotidine is more potent than cimetidine or ranitidine, requires only once-daily oral administration, and does not inhibit hepatic drug-metabolizing enzymes. The cytoprotective agent sulcralfate (Carafate, Marion/Merrill Dow) is used every 8 to 12 hr PO at a dose of 0.25 gm in animals less than 5 kg and at 0.5 to 1.0 gm in larger animals.

## MONITORING RESPONSE TO THERAPY

Several guidelines are useful in monitoring response to therapy in CHD. Resolution of clinical signs, increased appetite and activity level, weight gain, and reduced ascitic accumulation are subjective indications of successful therapy. Biochemical assessment of response involves monitoring for decreases in serum liver enzyme activity or bilirubin concentration, increases in serum albumin, or a return to normal values on hepatic function tests. Evaluation of serum enzyme activity is invalid in dogs on glucocorticoid or phenobarbital therapy, since these drugs induce elevation in ALT, GGT, and ALP. In human patients with CHD, normalization of bilirubin and albumin values are considered the most significant clinicopathologic indicators of a successful response. Histologic improvement on serial liver biopsies is the "gold standard" in assessing response to therapy.

## References and Suggested Reading

Kershenobich D, Vargas F, and Garcia-Tsag G: Colchicine in the treatment of cirrhosis of the liver. N Engl J Med 318:1709, 1988.
  *A double-blind, randomized, placebo-controlled clinical trial of colchicine therapy in cirrhosis.*
LaFlamme DP, Allen W, and Huber TL: Apparent dietary protein requirements of dogs with portosystemic shunts. Am J Vet Res 54:719, 1993.
  *A study investigating the effect of diets containing either 11% or 24% crude protein on nitrogen balance in dogs with surgically created portosystemic shunts.*
Leveille CR and Arias IM: Pathophysiology and pharmacologic modulation of hepatic fibrosis. J Vet Intern Med 7;73, 1993.
  *A comprehensive review on hepatic fibrogenesis and antifibrotic drug therapy.*
Magne ML and Chiapella AM: Medical management of canine chronic hepatitis. Compend Cont Educ Pract Vet 8:915, 1986.
  *A well-referenced, although somewhat dated, review on medical therapy of CHD included in a symposium on hepatic disease.*
McClain CJ, Marsano L, Burk RF, et al: Trace minerals in liver disease. Semin Liver Dis 11:321, 1991.
  *A review of trace mineral metabolism in human hepatic disease included in a volume dedicated to nutritional therapy of liver disease.*
Poupon RE and Poupon R: Ursodeoxycholic acid for the treatment of cholestatic disease. In Boyer J and Ockner RK (eds): Progress in Liver Disease. Philadelphia, WB Saunders Co, 1993, p 219.
  *An up-to-date review article on the mechanism of action and clinical indications for the use of ursodeoxycholate in human patients.*
Stanton ME and Bright RM: Gastroduodenal ulceration in dogs: Retrospective study of 43 cases and literature review. J Vet Intern Med 3:238, 1989.
  *Description of clinical cases of duodenal ulceration in canine patients with CHD.*
Strombeck DR, Miller LM, and Harrold D: Effects of corticosteroid treatment on survival time in dogs with chronic hepatitis (1977–1985). J Am Vet Med Assoc 193:1109, 1988.
  *A retrospective study of prednisone therapy in dogs with various forms of chronic hepatitis which suggests that glucocorticoid may be beneficial.*
Tygstrop N: Use of corticosteroids in liver disease. In Testa B (ed): Liver Drugs: Pharmacology to Therapeutic Application. Boca Raton, FL, CRC Press, 1989, p 162.
  *A comprehensive review of human clinical trials of prednisone therapy for CHD with a discussion of beneficial pharmacologic properties of glucocorticoids in liver disease.*
Twedt DC and Whitney EL: Management of hepatic copper toxicosis in dogs. In Kirk R (ed): Current Veterinary Therapy X. Philadelphia, WB Saunders Co, 1989, p 891.
  *A discussion of treatment of copper toxicosis in the dog.*

# USE OF ZINC ACETATE FOR THE TREATMENT AND PREVENTION OF CANINE COPPER HEPATOTOXICOSIS

WILLIAM D. SCHALL

*East Lansing, Michigan*

Metallothionein, a low-molecular-weight protein, is found in many mammalian cells, including hepatocytes and intestinal epithelial cells. Metallothionein binds several heavy metals, notably copper and zinc. The production, and hence the intracellular concentration of metallothionein, can be induced by increased intake of heavy metals. Zinc is an excellent inducer of metallothionein, but metallothionein induced by feeding zinc has greater affinity for copper. It is this difference that accounts for the therapeutic efficacy of zinc salts in the treatment and prevention of canine copper hepatotoxicosis. The oral administration of zinc acetate induces increased concentration of metallothionein in intestinal epithelial cells, which then bind dietary copper. Because the copper is nearly irreversibly bound, and because intestinal epithelial cells are sloughed every 3 to 4 days, much of the dietary copper is not absorbed beyond this cell layer. The oral administration of zinc also induces metallothionein in hepatocytes. This, too, is of therapeutic benefit because copper in hepatocytes that is bound to metallothionein is less toxic than copper free in the cytosol. Lastly, the oral administration of zinc acetate promotes the excretion of copper stored in hepatocytes. The mechanism of enhanced excretion is not fully understood and the rate of reduction in copper concentration is relatively slow; hepatic copper concentration is approximately halved over 2 years of therapeutic oral zinc administration.

The therapeutic effects of oral zinc acetate for treating copper hepatotoxicosis are not achieved until the zinc has been administered for several weeks. For this reason, candidates for zinc therapy are any biopsy-proven cases of primary hepatic copper accumulation, including those with minimally to moderately severe hepatitis. Dogs with severe or fulminant hepatitis secondary to copper accumulation are not candidates for zinc therapy alone, although zinc can be used for long-term treatment if copper is successfully chelated (also see "Chronic Hepatitis: Therapeutic Considerations," this volume, p 749) with an agent such as trientine. Zinc treatment can also be started simultaneously with chelation.

The advantages of zinc for treatment of canine copper hepatotoxicosis are efficacy, low cost, and a paucity of side effects. Some dogs vomit orally administered zinc acetate capsules; gastric irritation usually can be prevented by opening the capsules and mixing the zinc acetate in a tablespoon of tuna in oil.

Our current recommendation for treating canine copper hepatotoxicosis is to administer 100 mg of elemental zinc as zinc acetate twice daily for 3 to 6 months. The goal is to achieve plasma zinc concentration of 200 to 600 $\mu$g/dl. After the 3- to 6-month loading period, the dose is decreased to 50 mg twice a day. Plasma zinc concentration and alanine aminotransferase (ALT) activity are determined every 4 to 6 months. If the plasma concentration decreases to less than 150 $\mu$g/dl or if persistent increase in ALT activity occurs, the zinc dose is increased to 100 mg twice daily.

It is important that the zinc be administered separate from food by at least 1 hr because some food constituents such as phytates can bind zinc and diminish its efficacy. If a dog has a tendency to vomit the zinc capsules, however, the contents may be mixed in a tablespoon of tuna fish and fed.

Using this treatment protocol, we have seen no evidence of zinc toxicity. Our experience is limited to treating Bedlington terriers and West Highland white terriers, breeds in which it is clear that hepatitis occurs secondary to copper accumulation.

## Reference and Suggested Reading

Brewer GJ, Dick RD, Schall WD, et al: Use of zinc acetate to treat copper toxicosis in dogs. J Am Vet Med Assoc 201:564, 1992.

# EFFECTS OF HEPATIC DISEASE ON DRUG DISPOSITION

DAWN MERTON BOOTHE

*College Station, Texas*

## THE ROLE OF THE LIVER IN DRUG DISPOSITION

The liver is responsible for over 600 diverse metabolic functions. Among them are the metabolism and elimination of compounds foreign to the body. Although renal excretion is the ultimate mechanism of elimination for most drugs or metabolites, many of these drugs are dependent on hepatic clearance prior to elimination from the body. In addition to the direct role of the liver in drug disposition, the sequelae of liver disease on body fluid compartments, acid-base and electrolyte balance, and renal function can contribute to changes in drug disposition. These changes, in turn, can result in the generation of toxic drug concentrations and adverse effects.

### Hepatic Clearance

The volume of blood-cleared drug by the liver is determined by several factors: the degree to which the drug is protein bound, drug delivery to hepatocytes (blood flow), and the rate and extent of hepatic drug metabolism. Once cleared by the liver, a drug or its metabolite is then eliminated from the body by either biliary or renal excretion.

#### PROTEIN BINDING

Many lipid-soluble drugs are able to circulate in plasma only when bound to plasma proteins. Weakly acidic drugs have the greatest affinity for albumin, the protein to which drugs are most commonly bound. Weak bases more commonly bind to $\alpha_1$-acid glycoproteins such as acute-phase proteins. The extent to which a drug is bound to plasma protein is usually expressed as the fraction of drug free or unbound ($f_{ub}$) to plasma proteins. Binding has several important sequelae on drug activity. Protein essentially acts as a resevoir for the bound drug. The bound drug has limited access to tissues and is not pharmacologically active. Binding of drugs to proteins impairs hepatic clearance of some drugs. Binding is generally reversible and rapidly reaches an equilibrium. Since binding tends to be nonselective, a number of compounds can compete for binding sites, resulting in displacement and an increase in the concentration of unbound, pharmacologically active drug. Decreases in protein concentration will similarly affect the concentration of unbound drug. These sequelae are only likely to occur for a drug that is highly (>80%) protein bound, since only then can the concentration of unbound drug be effectively increased by displacement.

#### HEPATIC DRUG METABOLISM

Those drugs that require hepatic metabolism in order to be eliminated from the body tend to be lipid soluble. Without metabolism, such drugs would remain in the body and eventually accumulate to toxic concentrations. Metabolism renders the drugs more water soluble, and thus more easily excreted in urine. Hepatic metabolism is generally accomplished in the smooth endoplasmic reticulum of the hepatocyte in two phases. Phase I metabolism results in a chemical change (oxidation, reduction, or hydrolysis) in the drug molecule, thus making it more susceptible to phase II metabolism. Phase I reactions are mediated primarily by cytochrome P-450 (microsomal or mixed function oxidase) enzymes. These enzymes have several metabolic requirements in order to react at their maximum capacity. Included are a lipid membrane, several cofactors, oxygen, and iron. The result of phase I drug metabolism varies. Although commonly inactivated, a drug also can be activated to a metabolite of lesser, equal, or greater activity (the parent compound is referred to as a prodrug if it is inactive and its metabolite is active); or the drug can be converted to a toxic metabolite. If toxic metabolites are produced, the liver is a likely target for cytotoxicity. Phase I metabolism is susceptible to changes induced by other drugs or disease.

Phase II metabolism is a synthetic reaction in which a large, water-soluble molecule is conjugated to a drug or its phase I metabolite, thus rendering the drug water soluble. Generally, the phase II metabolite is excreted in urine. Glucuronide, glutathione, and sulfate are examples of molecules to which drugs and phase I metabolites are conjugated. Compared to phase I metabolism, phase II metabolism is less susceptible to the effects of disease and drugs. Both phases vary dramatically among species, affecting both the rate and extent of drug metabolism. The location of the various drug-metabolizing enzymes varies in the liver. Hepatocytes of zone 1 (comparable to the periportal zone of the classic hexagonal lobule) contain a large amount of glucuronidases responsible for phase II metabolism. In contast, hepatocytes of zone 3 (comparable to the centrilobular zone of the hexagonal lobule) contain a larger proportion of cytochrome P-450 enzymes. Zone 2 represents a transition between zones 1 and 3.

### HEPATIC BLOOD FLOW

The portal vein provides 75% of blood flow to the liver, with the remaining 25% provided by the hepatic artery. Because the portal vein drains the small intestine and a large portion of the large intestine in the normal animal, most orally administered drugs are circulated to the liver prior to reaching the systemic circulation. Initial exposure of drugs to hepatocytes can profoundly impact the amount of drug reaching target tissues. The impact depends on the rate at which hepatocytes remove, or extract, the drug from the portal blood. Drugs can be categorized as flow or capacity limited, depending on the rate of hepatic extraction. Identifying the appropriate category is of clinical benefit, because a potential reaction to a medication becomes more predictable in the patient with hepatic disease.

*Flow-limited* drugs are characterized by a very high rate of extraction: greater than 70% of the drug is removed by hepatocytes during a single passage through the liver. In normal animals, the rate of hepatic clearance of flow-limited drugs is determined solely by the rate of hepatic blood flow. Hepatic clearance of flow-limited drugs is generally not altered by changes in the metabolic capacity of the liver unless the changes are profound. In contrast, as liver disease progresses, changes in the relationship between the hepatic parenchyma and perfusion via the hepatic artery and portal vein can dramatically alter the rate of drug delivery to hepatocytes. Clearance of flow-limited drugs decreases in concert with hepatic blood flow. Conversely, because hepatocytes are very efficient at extracting flow-limited drugs from the blood, protein-binding does not generally interfere with hepatic clearance. Hence, flow-limited drugs are also referred to as "binding insensitive." Extraction is not impaired, and in fact may be enhanced (due to better alignment of the bound drug) by protein binding. Examples of flow-limited, binding-insensitive drugs include lidocaine, propranolol, bile salts, and selected anionic dyes such as sulfobromopthalein (BSP) and, in human beings, indocyanine green (ICG).

The term "first-pass metabolism" is used to characterize the disposition of flow-limited drugs because most of the drug is removed the first time it passes through the liver. First-pass metabolism of flow-limited drugs can markedly decrease the systemic bioavailability of orally administered drugs. Drugs that are completely absorbed from the gastrointestinal tract enter the portal circulation and are exposed to the liver prior to reaching the systemic circulation. The amount of drug removed during this first passage through the liver is determined by the amount extracted by hepatocytes; only the portion remaining is available to systemic circulation. Thus, a flow-limited drug with a 70% first-pass extraction is characterized by a less than 30% bioavailability following oral administration. The per-

centage of a dose reaching systemic circulation is further reduced if the drug is less than 100% absorbed from the gastrointestinal tract. Such drugs must either be administered parenterally or at oral doses sufficiently high to compensate for the first-pass effect.

In contrast to flow-limited drugs, *capacity-limited* drugs are characterized by a very inefficient rate of extraction; less than 30% of the drug is removed with each circulation through the liver. Hepatic clearance proceeds at a maximum rate for such drugs regardless of the rate of drug delivery. Changes in hepatic blood flow minimally influence clearance of such drugs. Unlike flow-limited drugs, the hepatic clearance of capacity-limited drugs is hindered by binding to plasma proteins. Capacity-limited drugs characterized by a low concentration (<20%) of unbound drug undergo *restrictive* elimination and are referred to as *binding sensitive*. Since only the free, unbound portion of drug can be cleared by the liver, hepatic clearance of such drugs parallels the fraction of drug unbound to plasma proteins ($f_{ub}$). Examples of capacity-limited, binding-sensitive drugs include nonsteroidal anti-inflammatory drugs, diazepam, and theophylline. Capacity-limited drugs not bound to plasma proteins are *binding insensitive*; hepatic clearance of such drugs approximates the rate of metabolism. Examples of capacity-limited, binding-insensitive drugs include ampicillin, $H_2$-receptor antagonists such as cimetidine, antipyrine, and caffeine. Because serum protein binding and the rate of metabolism of a specific drug varies among species, the classifications for a particular drug also vary among species. In contrast to flow-limited drugs, almost 100% of a capacity-limited drug that is absorbed from the gastrointestinal tract reaches systemic circulation.

The categorization of drugs that depend entirely upon the liver for elimination can be used clinically to quantify different functions of the liver using pharmacokinetic studies. For example, plasma elimination of flow-limited drugs (e.g., ICG, BSP, and bile acids) have been used to estimate hepatic blood flow, while plasma elimination of capacity-limited, binding-insensitive drugs (e.g., antipyrine and caffeine) have been used to evaluate the metabolic capacity of the liver.

### Biliary Excretion

Many of the drugs metabolized by the liver are excreted to some degree in the bile. As with renal secretion, active carrier proteins serve to transport drugs into bile. Transport systems are specific for organic anions, including glucuronides, bile acids, and dyes such as ICG and BSP; organic cations; and neutral compounds such as digoxin. Since the carrier proteins are nonselective, drugs can compete with one another for transport. A separate carrier system is responsible for the transport of steroids and related substances into bile. Molecular weight is an important, although not exclusive, determinant of the role of biliary excretion in the elimination of a drug. In most species there is a threshold molecular weight (e.g., 600) above which compounds are more likely to be eliminated through the bile. The kinetics of biliary excretion are very complex. Compared to renal excretion, biliary excretion is very slow. Drugs can be concentrated up to 10,000-fold in bile compared to plasma. Following biliary excretion, drugs can be eliminated with feces. More commonly, however, they undergo enterohepatic circulation. Biliary elimination of glucuronidated drugs is particularly susceptible to recirculation due to intestinal microbial production of glucuronidases that hydrolize the drug from its conjugate. Once unconjugated from glucuronide, freed drug is more likely to be reabsorbed. The half-life of such drugs can be very long due to constant enterohepatic recirculation.

## EFFECTS OF LIVER DISEASE ON DRUG DISPOSITION

### Measurements of Drug Disposition

The effects of liver disease on drug disposition have been documented through the use of pharmacokinetic studies that have mathematically modeled the behavior of a drug in the body. Such studies depend on measurements of parameters used to estimate drug movement throughout the body. Although estimates, these parameters can be used to predict changes in disposition that will necessitate modifications in a dosing regimen in the patient with liver disease. Parameters that are most useful include volume of distribution, (body) clearance, and elimination half-life. The relationship between these parameters and a dosing regimen are more closely addressed in Section 1 (see "Principles of Drug Therapy for the Practicing Veterinarian," this volume, p 41).

The volume of distribution (Vd) is a theoretical volume of tissue to which a known amount of drug would have to be distributed in order to generate the plasma drug concentration measured after distribution is complete. The Vd of a drug serves as an indicator of how much of the dose of a drug administered to a patient will be diluted by blood and body tissues. The greater the dilution, the smaller the drug concentration in the plasma and target tissue. Volume of distribution should be based on the unbound ($f_{ub}$) fraction of a drug, since binding limits distribution. The volume to which a drug is distributed can be increased in patients with liver disease as sodium and water retention increase. Dehydration and increased protein-binding will decrease the volume to which a drug is distributed. Changes in Vd should necessitate parallel changes in the dose of drug administered: the higher the volume, the greater the dose necessary to achieve a target concentration. Volume of distribution also affects drug half-life. Because a drug is removed from systemic circulation as its volume increases, the drug is no longer available to the organs of clearance. While the volume of blood that is cleared of drug does not decrease, the rate of elimination will since less drug is in that volume. Thus, as the volume increases, drug elimination half-life also increases.

Clearance is the volume of blood irreversibly cleared of drug per unit time. Clearance reflects the capacity of the liver to remove the drug from blood. Thus, this parameter is independent of the Vd of a drug, although mathematically it is calculated from Vd (see this volume, p 41). As with Vd, drug clearance affects drug half-life. The smaller the volume of drug cleared by the liver per unit time, the longer the drug remains in the body and thus the longer the elimination half-life.

The elimination half-life of a drug is the time necessary for 50% of the drug to be eliminated from the body. It is a hybrid parameter determined by both hepatic clearance (if the drug is cleared by the liver) and Vd. Drug elimination half-life changes proportionately with Vd and inversely with clearance.

### Changes in Drug Disposition Induced by Liver Disease

Liver disease is heterogenous in nature. Likewise, its effects on drug disposition are complex and varied. Not only is each determinant of clearance (protein-binding, blood-flow, and metabolism) likely to be affected, but subsequent changes in fluid compartments, acid/base and electrolyte imbalances, and effects on renal function can alter drug disposition.

#### PROTEIN BINDING

Changes in $f_{ub}$ parallel changes in plasma-protein concentrations. Albumin changes both quantitatively (usually decreased) and qualitatively, due to changes in molecular conformation. In addition, drugs must compete with endogenous substrates (i.e., bilirubin and bile acids) that can accumulate in liver disease for the same protein-binding sites. Increased $f_{ub}$ of a drug has several effects. The concentration of pharmacologically active drug in the blood increases as the drug becomes unbound. Minimal changes in the binding of a highly protein-bound drug can result in marked increases in the concentration of active drug. For example, nonsteroidal anti-inflammatory drugs are 99% protein bound. A decrease in protein binding to 98% will double the concentration of free, pharmacologically active drug. Because the drug is free, it will distribute into tissues where it may result in an exaggerated response to the drug. This sequela may, however, be minimized if the drug is capacity limited and binding sensitive. For these drugs, hepatic clearance increases if disease is not sufficiently severe to impair metabolism. Eventually, the concentration $f_{ub}$ of the drug will tend to normalize. Note that clearance will not increase for flow-limited drugs as they become less bound, since the clearance of these drugs is dependent on flow rate and is not influenced by protein binding. Adverse reactions are thus more likely to persist for flow-limited drugs. Note, however, severe hepatic disease may decrease extraction of flow-limited drugs to less than 0.70%, thus causing the drug to act more like a capacity-limited drug. Albumin is not the only drug binding protein affected by liver disease. In acute liver disease, increased plasma concentrations of acute-phase proteins, which often carry basic drugs, may further decrease clearance of capacity-limited, binding-sensitive drugs.

Changes in protein binding that accompany hepatic disease exemplify why half-life often may not reflect changes in drug movement (Table 1). The Vd of a highly protein-bound drug ($f_{ub}$ <20%) will increase as protein-binding decreases and free drug leaves the circulation to be distributed to tissues. Plasma drug concentrations consequently decrease and the drug cannot reach the liver. Note that clearance does not necessarily change in this scenario, however, since the capacity of the liver to metabolize the drug has not necessarily changed. Drug half-life will be prolonged despite normal clearance simply because the Vd has increased. If clearance increases as protein binding decreases (e.g., as with capacity-limited, binding-sensitive drugs), then the volume of drug cleared per unit time increases and drug half-life may be normal, despite changes in the parameters of disposition. The effects of increases in body fluid compartments in patients with liver disease (i.e., ascites, edema) can have the same effect as decreased protein binding, since drugs are likely to be distributed to a larger extracellular volume.

## INTRINSIC METABOLISM

In both cirrhotic and noncirrhotic liver disease, decreased cytochrome P-450 content and hepatocyte mass reduces clearance of capacity-limited drugs. Replacement of hepatocytes with fibrous tissue may further contribute to decreased metabolism in cirrhotic patients. Experimentally induced cholestasis also decreases hepatocyte cytochrome P-450 content. Clearance of capacity-limited drugs declines with changes in cytochrome P-450 enzyme activity. Less commonly, drugs normally characterized by a high extraction may also be affected by profound changes in intrinsic clearance and thus may behave more like capacity-limited drugs.

The effects of liver disease on hepatic metabolism and thus drug clearance may vary with the location of the histologic lesion and the microcirculatory pattern of the liver.

## HEPATIC BLOOD FLOW

Changes in hepatic blood flow in the patient with liver disease can be profound. The progressive nature of hepatic disease is accompanied by progressive decreases in hepatic blood flow. Inflammation accompanies some hepatic diseases and is followed by proliferation of new blood vessels and collagen deposition by activated fibroblasts. With progression to chronic disease, collagen matures, and organized fibrous tissue within sinusoidal spaces contracts around functioning hepatocytes. Collagen and fibrous tissue serve as mechanical barriers to blood able to reach hepatocytes ("capillarization"), so that substrate delivery to metabolic sites is delayed. Regeneration of damaged liver further contributes to delayed substrate delivery. Viable hepatocytes regenerate but the new hepatic parenchyma is nodular. The marked alteration of normal hepatic architecture that accompanies most progressive liver disease alters the intricate relationship between blood supply and hepatocytes. Blood supply from the portal vein and hepatic artery is disturbed, as is passage of blood from hepatic sinusoids to hepatic veins. The portal veins become grossly distorted, and tributaries to functional hepatocytes are lost. Regenerating hepatocyte nodules may be perfused only by branches of the hepatic artery, and fistulae between the portal and hepatic veins may bypass the hepatocytes. Thus, only a portion of total hepatic blood flow ("true hepatic blood flow") may reach hepatocytes. In addition to intrahepatic fistulae, extra hepatic shunts may develop. Distortion of vascular beds increases hepatic vascular resistance and portal pressure. Collateral veins may divert up to 60% of blood away from the liver. These changes in the architecture of the liver profoundly alter the clearance of many drugs. Changes in the clearance of flow-limited drugs are particularly affected because

**Table 1.** *Drugs for Which the Disposition is Affected in Human Patients With Hepatic Disease.*[*][†]

| Category | Drug | CL | Vd | Oral Bioavailability | $t^{1/2}$ |
|---|---|---|---|---|---|
| Flow-Limited Drugs | Lidocaine | −45% | nd | — | +200% |
| | Pentazocine | −45% | nd | +280% | +40% |
| | Propranolol | nd | +130% | +42% | +33% |
| | Verapamil | −35% | +160% | +140% | +380% |
| Capacity-Limited Drugs | Ampicillin | nd | 300% | — | +45% |
| | Chloramphenicol | −65% | −25% | — | +125% |
| | Hexobarbital | −43% | nd | — | +150% |
| | Theophylline | −70% | nd | — | +500% |

[*]Adapted from Williams RL: Drugs and the liver: clinical applications. *In* Benet LZ, Massoud N, Gambertoglio JC (eds): Pharmacokinetic Basis for Drug Treatment. New York, Raven Press, 1984, pp 63–76, with permission.
[†]Percentage changes are approximate. Only differences that were significant were reported.
Abbreviations: Cl = clearance, Vd = volume of distribution, F = bioavailability, $t^{1/2}$ = drug half life, nd = no difference.

they parallel changes in hepatic blood flow. However, clearance of capacity-limited drugs may also decrease in cirrhotic liver disease because substrate delivery is decreased due to capillarization of the vasculature.

### FIRST-PASS METABOLISM

Gastrointestinal absorption and plasma drug concentrations may decline for some drugs in the presence of portal hypertension or profound ascites due to congestion and decreased mucosal blood flow. However, oral bioavailability is likely to be greater for drugs absorbed from the gastrointestinal tract but characterized by first-pass metabolism in the liver (Table 1). Increased bioavailability may reflect both a decline in the metabolic capacity of the liver as well as shunts that allow portal blood to bypass the liver. This effect can be profound even if there is only a modest decrease in the extraction of the drug, since increased bioavailability parallels the fraction of portal blood shunted around the liver. If the drug is normally 90% extracted but decreases to 80% with liver disease, the amount of drug reaching systemic circulation doubles from 10% to 20% of the administered dose. Plasma drug concentrations may also double, which increases the likelihood of an adverse reaction to the drug. Changes in systemic bioavailability of an orally administered drug normally characterized by first-pass metabolism can be used to evaluate the fraction of portal blood shunted past the liver in human patients with liver disease.

### BILIARY EXCRETION

Changes in hepatic clearance induced by diseases afflicting biliary secretion are difficult to characterize and predict. The pharmacokinetics of such drugs are complex because the drugs may undergo enterohepatic circulation, intestinal metabolism, or fecal elimination. Cholestasis is particularly likely to alter biliary elimination of drugs. Extrahepatic cholestasis is likely to interrupt biliary excretion much the same as ureteral obstruction interrupts urinary elimination of renally excreted drugs. This effect can be used diagnostically to document extrahepatic cholestasis using selected radiolabeled pharmaceuticals. The effects of intrahepatic cholestasis on drug metabolism are much harder to describe. Studies addressing these effects depend upon invasive procedures and the collection of blood, biliary, and possibly fecal samples. A few studies have shown that certain causes of cholestasis can result in changes in the function of specific but different intracellular transport mechanisms, depending upon the drug. Cholestasis can reduce cytochrome P-450 activity.

## CLINICAL IMPLICATIONS

The disposition of many drugs is altered in the patient with liver disease. Although drugs metabolized by the liver are most likely to be affected, hepatic disease can affect the disposition of drugs not cleared by the liver due to effects on Vd and protein binding. Table 1 lists examples of flow-limited and capacity-limited drugs used in animals but characterized by significantly smaller clearance in human patients with liver disease. The oral bioavailability of many flow-limited drugs is also increased in these patients.

Although changes in drug Vd in patients with liver disease are less predictable, most often they reflect an increase. Increased Vd results from both water and salt retention (increased extracellular fluid and total body water) and, for protein-bound drugs, decreased plasma proteins. This latter effect has been documented in people with liver disease. The fraction of unbound drug increases for propranolol (40% increase), diazepam (60 to 200% increase), phenylbutazone (up to 500% increase), and quinidine (300% increase). Increased concentration of free drug renders these patients more susceptible to exaggerated pharmacologic effects, particularly for flow-limited drugs, since clearance does not increase. The effect of hepatic disease on protein binding of drugs in dogs has not been studied in depth. In dogs with experimentally induced liver disease, protein binding of ICG did not decrease despite a decrease in serum albumin concentrations to a mean of 2.05 gm/dl. The presence of ascites further complicates drug therapy in the patient with liver disease. The effect on drug response depends in part on whether or not the drug is distributed to the ascitic compartment. Dosing on a milligram-per-kilogram basis will minimize underdosing a patient if the drug is distributed to the ascitic compartment (e.g., many lipid-soluble drugs), but will overdose a patient if the drug is not distributed to the ascitic compartment (e.g., many water-soluble drugs). In dogs with experimentally induced liver disease, the ascitic compartment represents up to 30% of total body weight, yet mean Vd of some drugs does not affect plasma drug concentrations if animals are dosed on a milligram-per-kilogram basis. Thus, it is difficult to predict the effects of ascites on many drugs.

The effect of liver disease on drug elimination half-life is dependent on changes in both Vd and clearance (Table 1). If clearance decreases and Vd increases, then drug elimination half-life will be prolonged. If both Vd decreases or Vd and clearance decrease, changes in drug elimination are less predictable.

Studies that have characterized the disposition of drugs in the small animal patient with liver disease are limited. The elimination of flow-limited drugs such as BSP and lidocaine are decreased up to 50% or more in dogs, depending upon the severity of disease. Indocyanine green elimination has been studied in dogs with experimentally induced liver disease. Although a flow-limited drug in humans, the drug is characterized by a very low (<25%) extraction in dogs, and thus behaves like a capacity-limited drug. Its clearance is decreased up to 80% in experimental models of canine hepatic disease. The clearance of lidocaine that does behave as a flow-limited drug in dogs was decreased up to 50% in dogs with experimental disease. The elimination of capacity-limited drugs such as antipyrine and caffeine (both binding insensitive) also progressively decreases as severity of experimentally induced hepatic disease increases. Again in dogs with severe experimentally induced disease, clearance of antipyrine decreased to less than 75% of control animals.

Recommendations regarding dosing regimens in the patient with liver disease are difficult to make, since the sequelae on disposition are as varied as the diseases and the drugs administered. The magnitude of changes in hepatic function cannot be quantitated as easily as changes in renal function. Although several drugs have been studied in both spontaneous (humans) and experimental disease (animals), none has been used for a basis of drug modification in patients with liver disease. However, the traditional tests of hepatic function can be used to estimate the severity of liver disease. These tests include the static tests such as albumin and blood urea nitrogen (BUN) and dynamic tests such as serum bile acid and bilirubin concentration. Changes in the static tests indicate profound changes in hepatic function including metabolism. It is likely that the elimination of capacity-limited (and possibly flow-limited) drugs cleared by the liver will be similarly affected. Profound changes in serum bile acid concentrations indicate changes in hepatic blood flow, and thus changes in the clearance of flow-limited drugs.

Since drug elimination half-life is the major determinant of dosing interval, the frequency of drug administration should decline as drug half-life increases. Thus, either an increase in the volume to which a drug is distributed (Vd) or and a decrease in the volume cleared per unit time (clearance) should necessitate an increase in the dosing interval of a drug. A decrease in dose may not be necessary if the interval is sufficiently prolonged to avoid drug accumulation (see "Principles of Drug Therapy for the Practicing Veterinarian," this volume, p 41). For drugs administered at an interval that is shorter than drug half-life, the drug will accumulate. The amount of accumulation depends upon the relationship between interval and half-life. The smaller the ratio between the two, the greater the amount of accumulation. For such drugs, maximum drug concentrations and thus maximal response to therapy will not be achieved for 3 to 5 half-lives. The dose of such drugs may need to be reduced along with increasing the drug interval.

In general, drug doses should be reduced for drugs characterized by extraction greater than 70%. In humans, doses are generally reduced by 50%, particularly for orally administered drugs. In patients with severe disease, prolonging the dosing interval of both flow-limited and capacity-limited drugs up to 50% or longer is probably indicated, although this method of compensation has not been documented in clinical patients with spontaneous disease. If the drug is a prodrug (e.g., enalapril, cytoxan, primidone), therapeutic failure due to inadequate metabolism of the prodrug to its active form should be anticipated, and increased dosing may be indicated.

## Renal Effects of Liver Disease

Changes in renal function have been recognized for many years in human patients suffering from cirrhosis. Progressive oliguric renal failure is a common complication of advanced liver disease in humans. Renal failure may occur in up to 75% of human patients dying of cirrhosis. The most dramatic and best studied changes are in renal sodium handling. Sodium chloride retention can be profound, resulting in excessive accumulation of extracellular fluid, which eventually becomes evident as edema and ascites. Spontaneous diuresis can be followed by avid salt retention, underlying the sporadic nature of this renal dysfunction. Salt retention is not necessarily accompanied by water retention. Glomerular filtration frequently is decreased in patients with advanced liver disease, and redistribution of renal blood flow has been documented in patients. The hepatorenal syndrome is a unique form of acute renal failure that frequently occurs as a preterminal event in some human patients with liver disease. These patients eliminate a concentrated urine that is sodium free. Detecting early changes in renal function is difficult in these patients. Blood urea nitrogen concentrations are usually below normal due to imparied hepatic functions. Serum creatinine is subject to interference by exogenous and endogenous (including bilirubin) substances. There are no reports that have focused on changes in renal function in animal patients with liver disease. Yet, it is likely that renal function is impaired in patients with advanced disease. These changes will cause parallel changes in the elimination of most drugs or drug metabolites. Thus, additional care must be given to clinically evaluate response to all drugs administered to patients with advanced or end-stage liver disease, regardless of the route of elimination.

## References and Suggested Reading

Arias IM, Jakoby WB, Popper HP, et al. (eds): *The Liver. Biopsy and Pathology*, 2nd edition. New York, Raven Press, 1988.

Blaschke TF: Protein binding and kinetics of drugs in liver diseases. *In* Gibaldi M and Prescott L (eds): *Handbook of Clinical Pharmacokinetics*. New York, ADIS Health Science Press, 1989, pp 126–139.
  *A review of the effect of changes in protein-binding on drug disposition.*

Blaschke TF and Rubin PC: Hepatic first-pass metabolism in liver disease. *In* Gibaldi M and Prescott L (eds): *Handbook of Clinical Pharmacokinetics*. New York, ADIS Health Science Press, 1989, pp 140–149.
  *A review of the determinants of oral bioavailability and elimination of flow-limited drugs.*

Cornelius CE: A review of new approaches to assessing hepatic function in animals. Vet Res Commun 11:423, 1987.

Epstein M: Hepatorenal syndrome. *In* Epstein M (ed): *The Kidney in Liver Disease*, 3rd edition. Baltimore, Williams & Wilkins, 1988, pp 89–118.
  *A discussion of the factors contributing to and treatment of the hepatorenal syndrome.*

Morgan DJ and Smallwood RA: Hepatic drug clearance in chronic liver disease: Can we expect to find a universal, quantitative marker of hepatic function? Hepatology 10:893, 1989.
  *This review points out the need for a standard marker of hepatic function by delineating the various functions current diagnostic tests assess.*

Poulsen HE and Loft S: Antipyrine as a model drug to study hepatic drug-metabolizing capacity. J Hepatol 6:374, 1988.
  *A review of the use of the capacity-limited drug, antipyrine, as a standard marker of hepatic function.*

Wilkinson GR and Branch RA: Effects of hepatic disease on clinical pharmacokinetics. *In* Benet LZ, et al (eds): *Pharmacokinetic Basis for Drug Treatment*. New York, Raven Press, 1984, pp 49–70.

*An in-depth reveiw of changes in drug disposition which accompany hepatic disease.*

Wilkinson GR and Shand DG: A physiological approach to hepatic drug clearance. Clin Pharmacol Ther 18:377, 1975.
*A scientific summary of the physiological model of hepatic clearance.*

Williams RL: Drugs and the liver: Clinical applications. *In* Benet LZ (ed): *Pharmacokinetic Basis for Drug Treatment.* New York, Raven Press, 1984, pp 53–75.
*A clinically applicable summary of the effects of liver disease on drug disposition and modifications in dosing regimens.*

# MANAGEMENT OF PERITONITIS

## HOWARD B. SEIM III
### *Fort Collins, Colorado*

Generalized peritonitis is a serious and frequently fatal condition in small animals. The mortality rate has been suggested to be as high as 68% (Hosgood and Salisbury, 1988). Successful treatment requires a basic understanding of pathophysiology, knowledge of useful diagnostic techniques, early diagnosis, appropriate medical therapy, and careful surgical planning.

## GENERAL CONSIDERATIONS

The peritoneum is the serous membrane that lines the abdominal cavity (parietal peritoneum) and, by numerous foldings, covers the surfaces of the abdominal viscera (visceral peritoneum). Physiologically, the peritoneum functions by its abilities of absorption, transudation, and exudation, and by the ability to form adhesions in the presence of an inflammatory process. The small amount of free peritoneal fluid normally present provides lubrication for abdominal viscera as they slide over one another. The surface area of the peritoneum is roughly equivalent to the total cutaneous area of the body (Hau et al., 1979).

## PATHOPHYSIOLOGY

### Localized Peritonitis

Localized insult to the peritoneal surface causes a localized inflammatory response characterized by local vasodilatation, cellular infiltration, stimulation of efferent pain fibers, fibrin production, and adhesion of adjacent peritoneal surfaces. Clinically, these changes may appear as a mild pyrexia, increased heart rate, slight hemoconcentration, mild neutrophilia, and occasionally localized pain on palpation. Once the immune system has removed the irritant stimulus, no more fibrin is formed, fibrinolysis effects dissolution of the adhesions, and normal visceral motility returns. If fibrin clots have been present long enough for fibroblast invasion to occur and clot organization begins, permanent adhesions may result. Permanent adhesions are more common in human, bovine, and equine species than in feline and canine species. This localized type of response is seen following minor abdominal soilage as occurs from surgery, intraperitoneal injections, trauma, mild pancreatitis, or surgically induced local peritonitis (i.e., gastropexy, gastrostomy, enterostomy).

### Generalized Peritonitis

Generalized peritonitis is a diffuse inflammation of the peritoneal surfaces and generally represents a more serious threat to the patient than localized inflammation. The near total involvement of an organ capable of large and rapid fluid and ion exchange produces profound alterations in all body systems.

After irritation, the peritoneum responds with an increased vascular permeability (permitting fluid and protein influx into the peritoneal cavity), cellular infiltration with leukocytes and macrophages (in response to the irritant and necrotic debris), and fibrin deposition (increasing the adhesiveness of visceral surfaces). The results of this inflammatory response include neutrophilia progressing to neutropenia, hypovolemia and dehydration, severe hemoconcentration, septicemia, and metabolic alterations (Withrow and Black, 1979). Clinically these changes may manifest as profound septic shock.

#### HYPOVOLEMIA AND DEHYDRATION

Hypovolemia and dehydration are a direct result of an absolute or functional unavailability of body fluid volume. Absolute loss occurs from vomiting, diarrhea, fever, and respiratory and urinary losses. Functional loss can occur through peritoneal effusion (fluid and red blood cells), edema in irritated tissues, and splanchnic pooling secondary to bacterial toxins. The amount of fluid lost is substantial, and clinical signs of hypovolemic shock are usually apparent early.

#### BACTERIA AND LETHAL FACTORS

Presence of bacteria and lethal factors (substrates such as hemoglobin or other proteins) in the peritoneal cavity result in the most rapidly developing and lethal form of peritonitis (Hau et al., 1979). Bacteria may stem from the initial injury site (i.e., ruptured pyometra or perforated bowel) or be acquired later as the adynamic, dilated, irritated, and possibly ischemic intestinal tract loses its ability to isolate bacteria within its lumen, resulting in translocation of bacteria across the intestinal wall. Bacteria cultured from cases of generalized peritonitis are usually a mixed population, but most commonly contain gram-negative bacteria such as *Escherichia coli* and *Streptococcus faecalis*. The most potent lethal factors that contribute to the mortality of patients with generalized peritonitis include presence of hemoglobin, gastric mucin, bile salts, and other bacteria. The presence of bacteria and lethal factors in the peritoneal cavity perpetuate the formation of bacteremia and endotoxemia, resulting in shock or death of the animal. This evidence demonstrates a rationale for meticulous hemostasis and complete lavage of the peritoneal cavity to remove adjuvant substances during contaminated and septic operations.

### METABOLIC ALTERATIONS

Metabolic acidosis occurs rapidly; often secondary to hypovolemia or the primary disease. Acidosis may be compounded by the decreased respiratory minute volume and hypoxia secondary to abdominal pain. Inappropriate renal excretion of hydrogen ions may also lead to acidosis.

Electrolyte abnormalities will vary depending on the etiology and duration of disease. Hyperkalemia secondary to acidosis, shock, poor renal perfusion, and tissue necrosis is a fairly consistent finding. Hyponatremia may develop, but this and other electrolyte changes are generally unpredictable. Serum electrolyte measurements are essential to patient management.

Hypoglycemia may occur early in septic patients due to the presumed "insulin-like" effect of endotoxin. Monitoring blood glucose levels in patients with peritonitis may help predict the development of sepsis and facilitate the clinicians' therapeutic plan.

The endocrine and metabolic effects of generalized peritonitis are similar to those of a thermal burn. The resting metabolic rate may rise 40% above the expected values; subsequent weight loss and muscle wasting is profound. Nutritional support is an important consideration in the management of these severely catabolic patients.

Decreased renal blood flow is part of the initial compensatory change to maintain blood pressure in hypovolemic patients. The decreased glomerular filtration rate that follows does not allow adequate renal excretion of bacterial toxins, acid metabolites, nitrogenous wastes, or excess serum ion concentrations. As a result, accumulation of urea nitrogens, toxins, potassium ions, and hydrogen ions begins. Volume expanding the patient will increase cardiac output and blood pressure and improve renal function.

Hemoconcentration and lowered blood flow allows mixing of the central stream of red cells with the outer flow of platelets and white cells, resulting in a "sludging" effect. This, combined with platelets sensitized by cellular debris, may precipitate disseminated intravascular coagulation and microembolization of organs such as lungs, liver, kidneys, and pancreas.

## ETIOLOGY

The etiology of peritonitis in small animals can be primary or secondary (Hosgood and Salisbury, 1988). Primary generalized peritonitis results from direct infection of the peritoneum, generally through hematogenous spread. This occurs rarely in small animals, with the exception of coronavirus infection associated feline infectious peritonitis. Secondary generalized peritonitis is the predominant form of peritonitis in small animals, and results from septic or chemical contamination of the peritoneal cavity. Chemical contaminants include gastric fluid, bile, pancreatic enzymes, and urine. It is important to emphasize that patients beginning with a chemical irritant in the peritoneal cavity will frequently acquire a secondary bacterial component as normal defense mechanisms are overwhelmed.

The most common cause of peritonitis in small animals is leakage of gastrointestinal contents (Greenfield and Walshaw, 1987). This may occur secondary to gastrointestinal foreign bodies, perforating gastric or duodenal ulcers, breakdown of an intestinal surgical site, or gastric rupture secondary to gastric dilatation-volvulus. Other reported causes include penetrating abdominal wounds, blunt abdominal trauma, ruptured hepatic or prostatic abscess, ruptured pyometra, severe pancreatitis, ruptured gallbladder or bile duct, and ruptured urinary bladder.

## DIAGNOSIS

### Clinical Presentation

There is no age, sex, or breed predilection in patients with peritonitis (Hosgood and Salisbury, 1988). Presenting signs may be extremely varied depending upon the etiology, duration of peritonitis, and severity of disease (localized versus generalized). Patients may present with signs of septic shock including muddy and dry mucous membranes, delayed capillary refill time, cool extremities, and a distended painful abdomen; or be so moribund that it is difficult to elicit responses to external stimuli. Alternatively, patients may present with mild signs of depression only. The history is often noncontributory and may reflect nonspecific signs such as fever, vomiting, anorexia, and depression.

### Physical Examination Findings

A complete physical examination is essential. Areas of attention include: (1) careful examination of the skin for signs of penetrating foreign bodies or bruising secondary to blunt abdominal trauma; (2) careful abdominal palpation for fluid (ballottement), abdominal tenderness, intestinal plication, abdominal mass, enlarged prostate, enlarged uterus, or vomiting during abdominal manipulations; (3) body temperature may be elevated during the acute presentation, normal or subnormal terminally; and (4) mucous membranes may be muddy and dry (suggesting hemoconcentration and sepsis), pale and dry (suggesting hypovolemia), or capillary refill time may be prolonged (suggesting hypovolemia, decreased peripheral perfusion, or shock). As with clinical presentation, the physical examination will vary with duration, severity, and etiology of peritonitis.

## Imaging

Radiographic findings in patients with generalized peritonitis will vary depending upon etiology. Careful examination of survey abdominal radiographs is indicated. Loss of normal detail or presence of a "ground glass" appearance to the abdominal cavity is suggestive of fluid in the abdominal cavity. The clinician should remember, however, that a very young, thin, or dehydrated animal may also have a loss of detail, mimicking the presence of abdominal fluid. A fluid line may be visible on a standing lateral view. Free gas in the abdomen often indicates a rupture of the gastrointestinal tract, a penetrating wound, or recent abdominal surgery. Small quantities of free gas can best be seen on the lateral projection in the sublumbar area or along the diaphragm and appear as wispy, linear air densities. A left lateral recumbent position with a horizontal beam may reveal free gas. Generalized intestinal ileus in combination with findings described above may suggest generalized peritonitis. Generalized ileus alone may be caused by an intestinal disorder unassociated with peritonitis. Careful examination for areas of localized involvement such as loss of detail in the upper right abdominal quadrant (pancreas), cranial one third of the abdominal cavity (liver), middle one third (kidney, spleen), and caudal one third (prostate, uterus, urinary bladder) should be performed.

The use of contrast radiography specifically for the diagnosis of generalized peritonitis is not warranted. It is the opinion of the author that if any one or a combination of the radiographic findings mentioned above are found, further diagnostics, such as abdominocentesis, should be performed.

Ultrasonography has been shown to be useful in the diagnosis of pancreatitis, pancreatic pseudocyst, liver abscess, prostatic abscess, and ruptured gallbladder. Abdominal ultrasonography is recommended in patients suspected of having peritonitis.

## Laboratory Findings

Patients suspected of having peritonitis should have a minimum data base that includes: complete blood count (CBC), serum biochemical profile (including blood urea nitrogen [BUN], total protein, and glucose), electrolytes (sodium, potassium, and chloride), urinalysis, and blood gas analysis, if available. This data base will allow assessment of the patient at the time of presentation and serve as a baseline to evaluate response to treatment. Other tests (e.g., amylase, lipase, liver function) may be indicated depending on the patient's condition and the suspected etiology of peritonitis. Changes in baseline data are monitored as the patient responds to therapy.

## Paracentesis and Diagnostic Peritoneal Lavage

Paracentesis and diagnostic peritoneal lavage have been shown to be safe, reliable means of evaluating various acute conditions of the abdomen (Crowe, 1984). In the majority of cases of generalized peritonitis, the definitive preoperative diagnosis is based on results of paracentesis or diagnostic peritoneal lavage.

The author's preferred technique for abdominal paracentesis is as follows.

1. The patient is placed in lateral recumbency and the abdomen clipped and aseptically prepared.
2. The urinary bladder is catheterized and emptied.
3. A 22- or 20-gauge hypodermic needle is used for the puncture.
4. The needle is placed through the skin, subcutaneous tissue, and into the peritoneal cavity; abdominal fluid is allowed to drip into a collection tube. Gentle abdominal palpation may encourage fluid production.
5. If this technique is unsuccessful, a 3-cc syringe is used to apply gentle negative pressure. First, the syringe plunger is retracted 1/4 cc to break the seal between the syringe barrel and plunger. Then, the syringe is attached to the needle and gentle traction is placed on the syringe plunger, causing slight negative pressure, encouraging aspiration of even the smallest amount of fluid.
6. No matter which technique is used, it is customary to perform a four-quadrant tap; that is, four separate needle punctures.

Generally, punctures are made cranial and caudal to the umbilicus and lateral to the midline on each side; however, needle placement may also be dictated by radiographic presence of an abdominal mass or the presence of a scar on the abdominal skin (could be an old penetrating wound with visceral adhesions). In the event of a negative tap, patient positional changes (standing, rolling to the other side) and a second series of punctures may be necessary, particularly if the index of suspicion for generalized peritonitis is high. It has also been shown that use of an outside-the-needle catheter or a peritoneal dialysis catheter can improve the effectiveness of the tap. It is the author's opinion that a properly performed four-quadrant needle paracentesis will give adequate information in the majority of patients with generalized peritonitis.

Diagnostic peritoneal lavage can be used in patients

suspected of having generalized peritonitis but which have a negative four-quadrant paracentesis. Patient preparation is as described for needle paracentesis. Twenty-two ml/kg body weight of warm sterile saline is gravity infused into the abdominal cavity using an intravenous administration set. The animal is carefully rolled from side to side to distribute and mix the fluid. A sample or fluid is recovered for visual and laboratory examination. No attempt is made to remove all of the fluid (see CVT XI, p 125).

## Cytologic Evaluation of Fluid

Fluid samples should be collected in either an ethylenediaminetetraacetic acid (EDTA) tube, clot tube, or both. If the sample size is of sufficient quantity (>5 ml), it is divided between an EDTA tube and a clot tube. If the sample obtained is small (several drops), an immediate smear should be performed, or the sample collected in EDTA. If culture and susceptibility testing is to be performed, the sample cultured should be collected in a sterile clot tube.

Color, packed cell volume (PCV), white blood cell count, white blood cell morphology (i.e., normal, toxic, or degenerate neutrophils), and the presence or absence of free or phagocytized bacteria, plant fibers, or neoplastic cells should be determined. If the sample is less than 0.5 ml, analysis is generally limited to white cell morphology and presence or absence of bacteria, plant fibers, or neoplastic cells. The diagnosis of bacterial peritonitis, based on the presence of toxic degenerate neutrophils and intracellular bacteria, is associated with 100% accuracy and indicates that surgery is necessary (Botte and Rosin, 1983). Patients suspected of having a chemical peritonitis should have abdominal fluid creatinine and BUN (to detect free abdominal urine), amylase activity (for pancreatitis), alkaline phosphatase (for intestinal trauma), or bilirubin (for leakage of bile) performed to help pinpoint the etiology.

## Treatment

### PREOPERATIVE MANAGEMENT

FLUID THERAPY. When a diagnosis of generalized peritonitis has been established, an indwelling jugular catheter is placed as a means for fluid administration. In order to correct the hypovolemia characteristic of all patients with peritonitis, as well as the metabolic changes discussed earlier (acidosis, electrolyte abnormalities, hypoglycemia, decreased renal blood flow, and decreased cardiac output), volume replacement fluids at a rate up to 90 ml/kg (based on the animal's condition) are started. The use of polyionic isotonic fluid is recommended unless contraindicated by laboratory findings. Acid-base and electrolyte alterations will generally return to normal when the patient is adequately volume expanded. If the patient is septic and hypo-

glycemic, the use of 5% dextrose in Normosol with potassium supplementation based on laboratory values is recommended. It is ideal to base fluid therapy on measurement of central venous pressure (CVP) and urinary output to avoid pulmonary edema, especially in septic animals. The CVP should remain between 0 and 5 and urine output should approach 1 to 2 ml/kg/hr.

ANTIBIOTICS. Antibiotic therapy should be started as soon as the diagnosis of peritonitis is made. Aerobic and anaerobic culture and susceptibility determinations should be performed from the fluid received from the needle paracentesis. A smear and Gram's stain of the sediment from the peritoneal fluid may suggest the nature of the infection. Although initial antibiotic therapy is empirical, the choice can be rational. The antibiotic should be broad spectrum (against gram-positive, gram-negative, aerobic, and anaerobic) and should achieve inhibitory concentrations in the intraperitoneal fluid. Intraperitoneal fluid levels of aminoglycosides, ampicillin, and the cephalosporins are equivalent to serum levels. Ampicillin sodium (Omnipen, Wyeth) at 22 mg/kg IV every 8 hr in combination with an aminoglycoside such as gentamicin (Gentocin, Schering) at 2 to 3 mg/kg every 8 hr is effective against the bacteria commonly found in generalized peritonitis. Care should be taken to evaluate renal function and ensure adequate renal perfusion in patients treated with aminoglycosides, and the dosage should be adjusted accordingly. A third-generation cephalosporin such as cefoxitin sodium (Mefoxin, Merck Sharp & Dohme) at 15 to 30 mg/kg IV every 6 to 8 hr can also be effective, and is commonly used by the author. It is important to remember that patients with chemical peritonitis will likely develop a bacterial component and should be treated with antibiotics.

CORTICOSTEROIDS. Controversy persists regarding the beneficial effects of corticosteroids in sepsis. It is the author's opinion that corticosteroids should be given for the following reasons: (1) they stabilize lysosomal membranes, (2) they decrease capillary permeability, (3) they protect against endotoxin, (4) they have a positive ionotropic effect on the heart, and (5) they help restore normal permeability to the intestinal wall. Appropriate regimens include prednisolone sodium succinate (Solu-Delta-Cortef, Upjohn) at a dose of 15 to 30 mg/kg IV once or dexamethasone sodium phosphate (Dexamethasone sodium phosphate, VEDCO) at 4 to 6 mg/kg IV once. Corticosteroids should be given IV slowly and *after* the patient has been volume expanded.

NONSTEROIDAL ANTI-INFLAMMATORY AGENTS. Studies have documented the beneficial effects of nonsteroidal anti-inflammatory agents (NSAIDS) in the treatment of acute lethal peritonitis in dogs; for example, 100% of dogs in an acute lethal peritonitis model treated with fluids, gentamicin, and flunixin meglumine survived (Hardie et al., 1985). Flunixin meglumine (Banamine, Schering) is given at a dose of 1.1 mg/kg IV once. No evidence of renal or gastrointestinal toxicity was noted in the NSAID group. It has also been shown that the combination of steroids and flunixin meglumine can precipitate the formation of gastric ulcers in normal dogs. It is the author's opinion that either flunixin meglumine or corticosteroids be used in the treatment of sepsis, but not both. Flunixin meglumine should not be used in patients that have a history of renal disease.

ANESTHESIA. Prior to anesthesia, patients should have a shock dose of fluids and the appropriate adjunctive medications discussed above for proper "preoperative stabilization." Patients are given low doses of preanesthetic medications (if any) such as oxymorphone (Numophran, Dupont) prior to mask induction with isoflurane (Aerrane, Anaquest). Isoflurane is the anesthetic maintenance gas of choice for these critical patients. Nitrous oxide should be avoided, especially if patients have developed an adynamic intestinal ileus.

### OPERATIVE MANAGEMENT

SURGICAL AIMS. The surgical aims in patients with generalized peritonitis include: (1) identification and correction of the underlying cause, (2) removal of any foreign material from the peritoneal cavity, (3) provision of adequate drainage and lavage of the peritoneal cavity, and (4) provision of an avenue to ensure nutritional support postoperatively (gastrostomy or enterostomy feeding tube).

Exploratory laparotomy is performed through a ventral midline celiotomy from xyphoid to pubis. A sample of abdominal fluid is obtained for culture and susceptibility testing. Wide and complete exploration to find the source of contamination is important to ensure ultimate success of surgical therapy. Once found, the source is corrected or removed from the peritoneal cavity. Suture material used in an infected area such as this should be monofilament absorbable (polydioxanone or polyglycolic acid) or monofilament nonabsorbable (nylon, polypropylene, or polybutester). Multifilament nonabsorbable (Dacron, braided nylon) and catgut sutures are contraindicated in infected sites. Adhesions are carefully broken down to open all intraabdominal pockets of purulent material. Careful inspection of the peritoneal cavity for multiple sources of contamination (e.g., multiple intestinal perforations from a gunshot wound) is performed. The abdominal cavity is thoroughly lavaged with several liters (200 to 300 ml/kg) of body-temperature, sterile, physiologic saline solution (PSS). The principal effects of copious peritoneal lavage is mechanical removal of debris and dilution of bacteria, endotoxin, and lethal factors. This

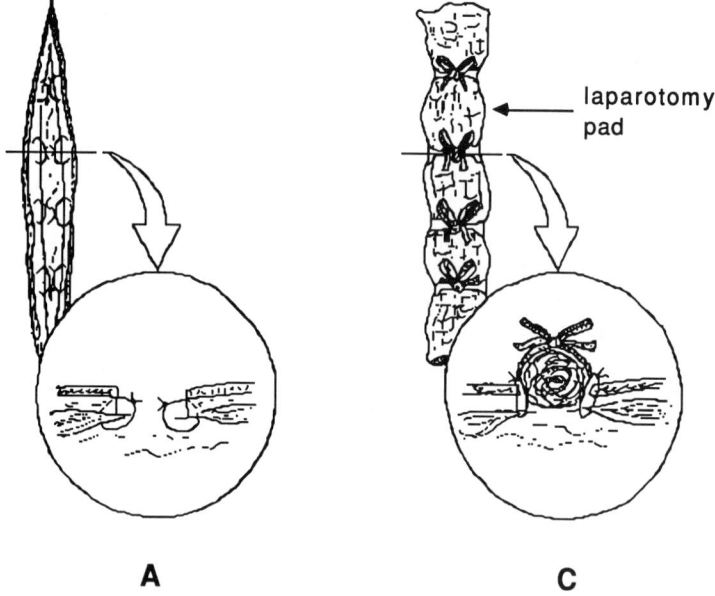

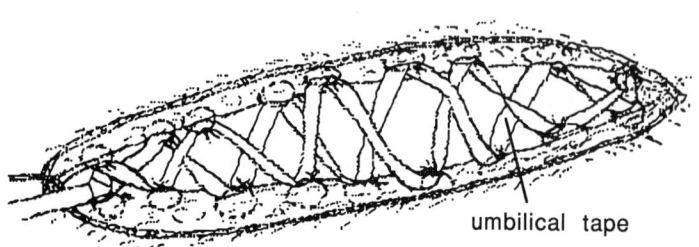

**Figure 1.** *A,* Loops of polypropylene suture are tied in the ventral rectus sheath along both sides of the abdominal incision. Cross-section shows tied loops of suture. *B,* ¼-inch umbilical tape is passed through the loops to loosely "lace-up" the abdominal incision much like lacing a shoe. *C,* A sterile laparotomy pad is placed over the incision to encourage absorption of peritoneal fluid. Umbilical tape is threaded through the loops of polyproplyene and tied over the laparotomy pad to secure it in place.

author recommends the use of PSS without the addition of antiseptics (Betadine, chlorhexidine) or antibiotics. It has been shown experimentally that antiseptics can be detrimental to normal metabolism (causing metabolic acidosis) and intraperitoneal administration of antibiotics is less effective than antibiotics administered systemically.

Nutritional management should be considered in patients with generalized peritonitis. As these patients are in a severe catabolic state, caloric intake immediately after surgery is ideal. Intraoperative placement of a gastrostomy or enterostomy feeding tube is recommended for delivery of appropriate caloric needs postoperatively.

At this point, a decision must be made whether or not to perform open peritoneal lavage and drainage or close the abdominal cavity primarily. Open peritoneal lavage and drainage is defined as a technique that provides postoperative peritoneal drainage through an open or partially open abdominal incision (Woolfson and Dulisch, 1986; Orsher and Rosin, 1984). This decision is based on several factors: (1) an assessment of the degree of peritoneal contamination, (2) ability to surgically remove all remaining debris from the peritoneal cavity, (3) severity of the patient's illness (patients with a more severe illness tend to be treated open), and (4) when continued septic inflammatory processes are anticipated.

If the decision is made to close the abdominal cavity, closure is routine. If the decision is made to "leave the abdomen open," partial closure is performed as follows: (1) loops of polypropylene suture are tied in the ventral rectus sheath (Fig. 1A); (2) 1/4-inch umbilical tape is passed through the loops to loosely "lace-up" the abdominal incision (this acts as a net to support the abdominal viscera when the patient is awake) (Fig. 1B); (3) a sterile laparotomy pad is tied over the incision to encourage absorption of peritoneal fluid (Fig. 1C); (4) a sterile cotton surgical towel is placed over the laparotomy pad as a secondary absorptive bandage; and (5) a cotton roll and gauze covering or commercially available disposable diaper is used to provide further absorption and protection of the abdominal incision.

## POSTOPERATIVE MANAGEMENT

Postoperative therapy includes intravenous fluids, antibiotics, periodic blood glucose analysis (as a monitor for sepsis), high-protein alimentation, and bandage management. Fluid and protein losses can be significant, with hypoproteinemia and hypovolemia reported most frequently (Woolfson and Dulisch, 1986). If hypoproteinemia becomes severe (serum albumin <2.0 mg/dl), plasma transfusions should be considered. Replacement of peritoneal fluid loss is important; quantitating losses is performed by weighing the bandage at each bandage change. High-protein alimentation is provided by the use of commercially available liquid diets given through the gastrostomy or enterostomy tube. Feeding can begin immediately after enterostomy

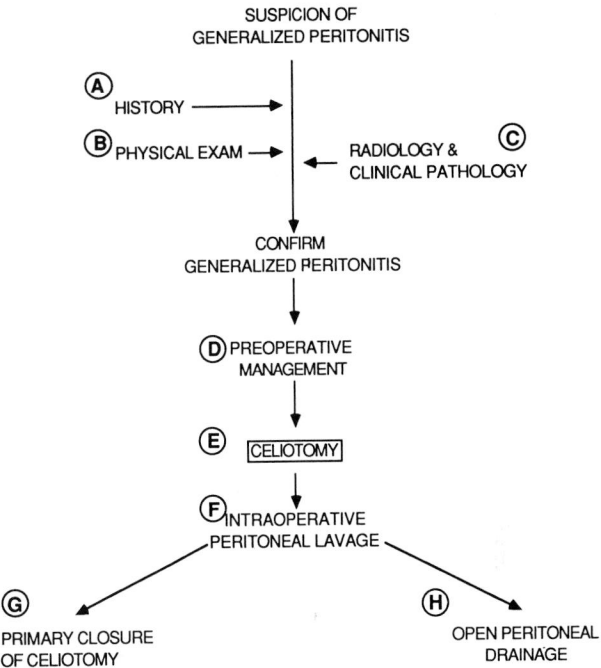

**Figure 2.** Approach to the patient with suspected peritonitis. A. Patients presenting with acute, severe abdominal pain (acute abdomen), vomiting, depression, anorexia, and particularly those patients with a recent history of intestinal surgery or a penetrating abdominal wound should be considered as having generalized peritonitis. B. Physical findings are often nonspecific and may include abdominal tenderness, abdominal distention, fever, severe depression, and purple or muddy-colored mucous membranes. The laboratory data base may reveal early signs of sepsis. C. Confirmation of generalized peritonitis may be accomplished by a combination of radiography and paracentesis. Plain abdominal radiographs may reveal an obstructive pattern or free gas in the peritoneal cavity. Cytology evaluated from a four-quadrant peritoneal tap may reveal characteristic findings associated with generalized peritonitis including: degenerate neutrophils, phagocytized bacteria, free bacteria, and/or free particles of ingesta. A degenerative left shift and decreased glucose level may imply sepsis. D. Preoperative management includes a shock dose of polyionic, isotonic fluids (90 ml/kg), corticosteroids (2 to 4 mg/kg), broad-spectrum antibiotics (aerobic and anaerobic spectrum), and glucose. During the administration of fluids, paracentesis and removal of abdominal fluid is performed. E. An exploratory celiotomy is performed. Fluid that has accumulated in the peritoneal cavity is evacuated by suction to facilitate visualization of abdominal structures. A systematic approach is used when evaluating abdominal viscera in order to locate the source of pertonitis. Once located, the source of peritonitis is corrected or removed. F. After isolation and correction of the source of peritonitis, the peritoneal cavity is irrigated with copious amounts (200 to 300 ml/kg) of sterile PSS. The lavage helps float away debris, dilute organism numbers, and dilute endotoxin load. G. Minor contamination of the peritoneal cavity can be managed by intraoperative peritoneal lavage and primary closure. No postoperative lavage management is needed in these cases. H. Patients with severe intra-abdominal sepsis may be treated by open peritoneal drainage and lavage. The abdominal incision is left open and packed with sterile nonadhering pads, then covered with gauze sponges and held in place with an abdominal bandage. The bandage is changed daily until the cytology of the drainage fluid appears healthy (generally 3 to 5 days). The abdomen is then closed routinely.

tube placement or 24 hr after gastrostomy tube placement.

Bandage changes and continued peritoneal lavage are crucial in successful management of patients treated with open peritoneal drainage. At 24-hr intervals, the patient is taken to the operating room, anesthetized, and the secondary and tertiary bandages removed. The abdomen is prepared for aseptic surgery. The laparotomy pad and umbilical tape are removed and a sample of peritoneal fluid is taken for cytologic evaluation. The abdominal cavity is reexplored (specifically areas of repair: enterotomy, intestinal anastomosis, and so forth) and lavaged (200 to 300 ml/kg PSS). Primary closure of the abdominal incision is dictated by results of the cytologic evaluation at each lavage. As neutrophil morphology becomes normal and bacterial numbers decrease (approaching a serosanguinous exudate), routine abdominal closure is performed.

## Prognosis

The reported mortality for patients with generalized peritonitis is reported to be as high as 68%; however, the type of therapy for each case was not described (Hosgood and Salisbury, 1988). In two series of patients with generalized peritonitis specifically treated using open peritoneal lavage, the mortality rate ranged from 33 to 48% (Woolfson and Dulisch, 1986; Greenfield and Walshaw, 1987). The patients in these series represented the most severe cases of generalized peritonitis. In an experimental study, there was a 100% survival rate in animals treated with open peritoneal drainage, whereas the mortality was 33% in those animals whose peritoneal cavities were closed (Orsher and Rosin, 1984). It is apparent from this information that open peritoneal lavage improves the prognosis of patients with severe generalized peritonitis (Hosgood et al., 1989).

In general, if a positive response to therapy occurs, it is seen by the third or fourth lavage session. In the author's experience, patients requiring open peritoneal lavage beyond 5 or 6 days often develop severe complications such as anemia, electrolyte abnormalities, hypoproteinemia, and the occurrence of nosocomial contamination or infection of the peritoneal cavity. These complications coupled with unresponsive generalized peritonitis often result in an unfavorable to grave prognosis.

## References and Suggested Reading

Botte RJ and Rosin E: Cytology of peritoneal effusion following intestinal anastomosis and experimental peritonitis. Vet Surg 12:20, 1983
*Cytologic evaluation of peritoneal fluid from patients with secondary peritonitis is diagnostic in the majority of cases.*
Crowe DT: Diagnostic abdominal paracentesis techniques: Clinical evaluation in 129 dogs and cats. J Am Anim Hosp Assoc 20:223, 1984.
*The accuracy of diagnostic abdominal lavage in predicting the cause of intra-abdominal injury or disease reaches 95% in dogs and cats.*
Greenfield CL and Walshaw R: Open peritoneal drainage for treatment of contaminated peritoneal cavity and septic peritonitis in dogs and cats: 24 cases (1980–1986). J Am Vet Med Assoc 191:100, 1987.
*Open peritoneal lavage was tolerated well by all patients; the mortality attributable to peritonitis or its complications was 21%.*
Hardie EM, Rawlings CA, and Collins LG: Canine *Escherichia coli* peritonitis: Long-term survival with fluid, gentamicin sulfate, and flunixin meglumine treatment. J Am Anim Hosp Assoc 21:691, 1985.
*One hundred per cent of dogs in an acute lethal peritonitis model treated with fluids, gentamicin, and flunixin meglumine survived.*
Hau T, Ahrenholz DH, and Simmons RL: Secondary bacterial peritonitis: The biologic basis of treatment. Curr Probl Surg 16:1, 1979.
*The biology and principles of therapy in secondary peritonitis is emphasized.*
Hosgood G and Salisbury SK: Generalized peritonitis in dogs: 50 cases (1975–1986). J Am Vet Med Assoc 193:1488, 1988.
*The most common source of peritoneal cavity contamination in dogs with generalized peritonitis was the gastrointestinal tract. Overall mortality was 68%.*
Hosgood G, Salisbury SK, Cantwell HD, and DeNicola DB: Intraperitoneal circulation and drainage in the dog. Vet Surg 18:261, 1989.
*Open peritoneal drainage allows more rapid and complete drainage than sump-Penrose drainage. The use of open peritoneal drainage may therefore be preferable to sump-Penrose drainage in the treatment of peritonitis.*
Orsher RJ and Rosin E: Open peritoneal drainage in experimental peritonitis in dogs. Vet Surg 13:222, 1984.
*Dogs with experimentally induced peritonitis tolerated open peritoneal lavage therapy, and did better clinically than dogs treated with primary closure.*
Withrow SJ and Black AP: Generalized peritonitis in small animals. Vet Clin North Am 9:363, 1979.
*A working knowledge of the anatomy, pathophysiology, diagnostic techniques, and therapeutic modalities is necessary to adequately treat patients with generalized peritonitis.*
Woofson JM and Dulisch ML: Open abdominal drainage in the treatment of generalized peritonitis in 25 dogs and cats. Vet Surg 15:27, 1986.
*Patients with severe generalized peritonitis treated by open peritoneal drainage had a mortality rate of 48%. Complications were hypoproteinemia and nosocomial contamination.*

# Section

# 9

# CARDIOPULMONARY DISEASES

BRUCE W. KEENE
*Consulting Editor*

771

***Still Current Information Found in Current Veterinary Therapy XI:***

Buchanan JW: Causes and Prevalence of Cardiovascular Disease, p 647.
Hellyer PW: Anesthesia in Patients with Cardiopulmonary Disease, p 655.
McKiernan BC: Current Uses and Hazards of Bronchodilator Therapy, p 660.
Fox PR: Current Uses and Hazards of Diuretic Therapy, p 668.
Ware WA: Current Uses and Hazards of Beta-Blockers, p 676.
Pion PD: Current Uses and Hazards of Calcium Channel Blocking Agents, p 684.
Snyder PS and Atkins CE: Current Usage and Hazards of the Digitalis Glycosides, p 689.
Hamlin RL: Current Uses and Hazards of Ventricular Antiarrhythmic Therapy, p 694.
DeLessis LA and Kittelson MD: Current Uses and Hazards of Vasodilator Therapy in Heart Failure, p 700.
Darke PGG: Update: Transvenous Cardiac Pacing, p 708.
Rush JE: Emergency Therapy and Monitoring of Heart Failure, p 713.
Atkins CE: Heartworm Caval Syndrome, p 721.
Miller MW and Fossum TW: Pericardial Disease, p 725.
Harpster NK: Feline Arrhythmias: Diagnosis and Management, p 732.
Hamlin RL: Therapy of Supraventricular Tachycardia and Atrial Fibrillation, p 745.
Moise NS and Gilmour RF, Jr: Inherited Sudden Cardiac Death in German Shepherds, p 749.
Thomas WP: Update: Infective Endocarditis, p 752.
Jacobs G and Panciera D: Cardiovascular Complications of Feline Hyperthyroidism, p 756.
Sisson D: Fixed and Dynamic Subvalvular Aortic Stenosis in Dogs, p 760.
McIntosh Bright J: Update: Diltiazem Therapy of Feline Hypertrophic Cardiomyopathy, p 766.
Calvert CA: Update: Canine Dilated Cardiomyopathy, p 773.
Keene BW: L-Carnitine Deficiency in Canine Dilated Cardiomyopathy, p 780.
Page RL and Keene BW: Doxorubicin Cardiomyopathy, p 783.
Miller MS, Tilley LP, and Atkins CE: Persistent Atrial Standstill (Atrioventricular Muscular Dystrophy), p 786.
Liu S-K and Fox PR: Myocardial Ischemia and Infarction, p 791.
Hawkins EC: Tracheal Wash and Bronchoalveolar Lavage in the Management of Respiratory Disease, p 795.
Mitten RW: Acquired Nasopharyngeal Stenosis in Cats, p 801.
Dye JA and Moise NS: Feline Bronchial Disease, p 803.
Morrison WB: Primary Ciliary Dyskinesia, p 811.
Calvert CA: Eosinophilic Pulmonary Granulomatosis, p 813.

***Elsewhere in Current Veterinary Therapy XII:***

Principles of Drug Therapy for the Practicing Veterinarian, p 41.
Uses and Misuses of Aspirin, p 71.
Blood Pressure Measurement, p 110.
Doppler Assessment of Blood Flow and Pressure in Surgical and Critical Care Patients, p 113.
Pulse Oximetry, p 117.
End-tidal Carbon Dioxide Monitoring, p 119.
Magnesium and the Critically Ill Patient, p 128.
Magnesium Therapy, p 132.
Diagnosis of Bacteremia in Critically Ill Dogs and Cats, p 137.
Septic Shock, p 139.
Counterpressure Use in Shock and Hemorrhage, p 147.
Cardiac Arrhythmias in Systemic Disease, p 161.
Cardiopulmonary Resuscitation, p 167.
Oxygen Supplementation, p 175.
Temporary Tracheostomy, p 179.
The Practical Use of Constant-rate Infusions, p 184.
Use of Catecholamines in Critical Care Patients, p 188.
Incompatible Critical Care Drug Combinations, p 194.
A Brief Guide to Indoor Air Pollutants, p 252.
Empiric Antibiotic Therapy, p 276.
Antimycotic Drug Therapy, p 327.
Clinical Applications of Glucocorticoid Therapy in Nonendocrine Disease, p 406.
Laryngeal Paralysis-Polyneuropathy Complex in Young Dalmatian Dogs, p 1136.
Reference Values for Blood Gases, Bronchoalveolar Lavage, Electrocardiography, Appendices, p 1393.

# SEDATION FOR CARDIOVASCULAR PROCEDURES

REBECCA L. STEPIEN

*Madison, Wisconsin*

The presence of cardiac disease or dysfunction does not obviate the need for sedation in veterinary patients. Sedation facilitates some types of examination (e.g., radiography, echocardiography), and is required for safe and humane performance of certain diagnostic or therapeutic procedures. In addition, unstable states of congestive heart failure (CHF) may be rapidly worsened by patient stress and struggling; sedation of the anxious patient may be life saving. The ideal drug(s) chosen for sedation should provide adequate tranquilization and immobilization. It is desirable that sedatives provide analgesia if required, and have minimal adverse hemodynamic effects. Finally, they should be simple to administer and cost-effective. Methods of general anesthesia of the cardiac patient are discussed in *CVT XI*, p 655.

## SPECIAL CONSIDERATIONS

The fragile hemodynamic balance of many patients with cardiovascular (CV) abnormalities requires careful consideration when choosing a sedative regimen. Hemodynamic effects of individual drugs that are inconsequential in normal patients may be magnified in cardiac patients by their limited ability to compensate for sudden hemodynamic changes. In addition, emergency therapies to rectify adverse reactions to sedative drugs (especially hypotension) are more difficult in animals in whom fluid balance is precarious. Special considerations for sedation in CV patients are summarized in Table 1.

The special needs of the CV patient make a short-acting or reversible sedative regimen preferable. Drugs that cause respiratory depression or increase susceptibility to arrhythmias should be avoided, and vigilant monitoring of ventilation, hemodynamic stability, and vital signs is mandatory. The decision to use local or regional anesthesia for individual procedures in order to avoid systemic hemodynamic effects must be balanced against the precipitation of stress and anxiety to a locally anesthetized but conscious animal (also see *CVT XI*, pp 88 and 95).

In some cases, modification of sedative dose (using the lower end of dosage ranges) or route of administration (intramuscular [IM] rather than intravenous [IV] administration) may help to avoid deleterious effects. Consideration of hemodynamic abnormalities associated with an individual pathologic condition, presedation patient stress level, and concurrent medications allows logical selection of safe and effective sedatives. Sedation of patients with unstable arrhythmias or in overt CHF should be avoided until clinical status is stable. Treatable conditions underlying arrhythmias (e.g., electrolyte or acid-base imbalances) should be addressed prior to sedation. If the patient is on chronic cardiac therapy, cardiac medications should continue as usual up to the time of sedation. For elective procedures, food may be withheld prior to sedation, but animals receiving diuretics or vasodilators should be allowed free access to water. Catheter placement prior to sedation allows rapid emergency drug administration if necessary, and close patient monitoring is essential throughout the period of sedation. Measurement of arterial blood pressure (see Section 2) and pulse oximetry (see "Pulse Oximetry," this volume, p 117) are quite useful in monitoring cardiac patients.

In emergency situations, complete presedation evaluations of the CV patient are neither practical nor possible, but a thorough physical examination is necessary. Severe cavitary fluid accumulations (pleural effusion, ascites), which may limit that patient's ability to ventilate when sedated, should be partially drained. The patient should be evaluated for signs of hypotension and presence of arrhythmias. Blood pressure should be measured. Hypotension may be treated with careful fluid administration and infusion of dobutamine or dopamine when necessary (see "Use of Catecholamines in Critical Care Patients," this volume, p 188); animals with life-threatening atrial or ventricular tachycardias should be treated with appropriate antiarrhythmic medications. If pulmonary edema is severe, administration of diuretics or vasodilators may be used to stabilize the patient prior to sedation. Oxygen may be administered via an oxygen cage, nasal tube, ventilated plastic bag, or mask prior to and during sedation, but care should be taken to avoid additional patient stress due to enthusiastic oxygen masking. If time permits, measurement of packed cell volume (PCV), total protein, blood urea nitrogen (BUN) or creatinine, and serum electrolytes (Na, K, Cl, Mg, Ca) is helpful to detect systemic abnormalities.

## MEDICATIONS INDICATED FOR USE IN CARDIOVASCULAR PATIENTS

Opioids and benzodiazepine-derivative drugs are considered to have the least adverse hemodynamic effects of drugs commonly used for sedation. Alterna-

**Table 1.** *Cardiovascular Conditions Affecting Sedation*

| Cardiovascular Condition | Patient Clinical Consequences |
| --- | --- |
| Chronic myocardial hypoxia | Intolerant of increases in myocardial oxygen consumption, susceptible to arrhythmias |
| Poor cardiac contractile function | Intolerant of myocardial depression, hypotension |
| Decreased myocardial compliance (e.g., HCM), limitations on ventricular filling (e.g., pericardial effusion, MS), outflow obstructions (e.g., AS) | Intolerant of hypotension or decreased filling pressures |
| Decreased cardiac output/increased circulation time | Prolonged effects of sedation, difficulty in assessment of continuous infusions |
| Presence of arrhythmias or administration of arrhythmogenic cardiovascular medications | Susceptible to arrhythmias, intolerant of hypotension |
| Heart rate–dependent cardiac output | Intolerant of bradycardias |
| Catecholamine-dependent cardiac output | Intolerant of reductions in sympathetic tone |
| Hypertension | Intolerant of vasoconstriction |
| Cyanosis due to right-to-left shunting | Intolerant of hypoxia, tachycardias, or bradycardias and decreases in systemic vascular resistance; minimal response to supplemental oxygen |
| Hypotension and/or chronic vasodilator administration | Intolerant of further decreases in blood pressure |
| Pulmonary edema | Intolerant of respiratory depression, adjuvant fluid administration |
| Chronic $\beta$-blocker administration | Limited ability to respond to hypotension and bradycardias, altered response to emergency catecholamine administration possible |
| **Systemic problem related to cardiovascular or systemic therapy** | |
| Hypothermia | Intolerant of further decreases in body temperature |
| Limited hepatic/renal function | Limited or prolonged metabolism and/or excretion of medications |
| Chronic hypoxia | Intolerant of additional respiratory depression, increased risk of arrhythmias |
| Electrolyte imbalances | Susceptible to arrhythmias |
| Unstable systemic fluid balance | Intolerant of hypotension and/or adjuvant fluid administration |

Abbreviations: HCM = hypertrophic cardiomyopathy, MS = mitral stenosis, AS = aortic stenosis.

tively, medications that provide more profound sedation but have more obvious hemodynamic effects (e.g., acepromazine, propofol) may be safely used if dose and effects are carefully monitored. Ketamine and tiletamine/zolazepam are useful sedative agents in both cats and dogs, but the advantage of blood pressure support may be offset by detrimental drug-induced tachycardia in some circumstances.

Morphine and other opioids have long been used for sedation in cardiac patients. Morphine is the prototypical opioid; advantages when used in CV patients include sedation, analgesia, and mild venodilation. Disadvantages include occasional dysphoria, bradycardia, and respiratory depression at high doses. Morphine alone is useful in the initial management of dogs with severe heart failure in whom anxiety and stress appear to be contributing to worsening of signs. Other commonly used opioids include the agonists oxymorphone and meperidine and the partial agonist/antagonists buprenorphine and butorphanol. These drugs vary in potency and reversibility. Oxymorphone is a potent analgesic and sedative (IV or IM), especially combined with a benzodiazepine or acepromazine, but its use may precipitate bradycardia. Meperidine can also be combined with acepromazine or a benzodiazepine but, like morphine, may cause histamine release and hypotension if given IV; this administration route should be avoided. The agonist/antagonists (e.g., buprenorphine, butorphanol) are generally less potent sedatives and analgesics (Cornick and Hartsfield, 1992), but are less res-

piratory depressant than more potent opioids. In the author's practice, various opioid/benzodiazepine combinations are used for sedation of hemodynamically unstable patients, and acepromazine/buprenorphine is used for compensated CV patients when greater levels of sedation are required. Reversal agents should be used with care when longer acting nonreversible agents (e.g., acepromazine) are combined with opioids, or when the reversal agent has a shorter duration of action than the agonist. Reversal agents are less effective when used to reverse agonist/antagonist opioids.

Benzodiazepines are commonly used for sedation, muscle relaxation, and as anticonvulsants. Although benzodiazepines have minimal detrimental hemodynamic and respiratory side effects, administration as a sole sedative agent may not provide adequate sedation for many procedures. In addition, IV benzodiazepine administration may paradoxically cause anxiety and increased excitability in some animals. Benzodiazepines for sedative purposes are most often combined with another agent such as an opioid or ketamine; combining these medications may allow reduction in dosage of the second sedative (see *CVT XI*, p 27). The benzodiazepines in common veterinary use include diazepam and midazolam (Versed, Hoffmann-La Roche, Nutley, NJ) but zolazepam is available in combination with tiletamine (Telazol, AH Robins, Richmond, VA). When used in combination with acepromazine or opioids in CV patients, diazepam is administered as a slow IV bolus 10 to 20 min after IM or subcutaneous (SC) administration of the accompanying drug. Intravenous diazepam is also useful to treat the neurologic manifestations of lidocaine toxicity. Midazolam is water soluble and may be given IV or IM with little adverse hemodynamic effect. The ability to effectively administer midazolam IM (often combined with another agent in a single syringe) is an advantage when venous access is unavailable.

Acepromazine maleate is probably the most commonly used veterinary tranquilizer, either alone or in combination with other drugs. Advantages of use of acepromazine in sedative combinations include low cost, production of more profound sedation than some less hemodynamically active drugs, compatability with other anesthetics, and antiarrhythmic properties. The hemodynamic effects of acepromazine include decreased peripheral vascular resistance, bradycardia (after an initial tachycardia), and direct myocardial depression. In CV patients, adverse effects may include hypotension and worsening of CHF. Although the dose dependency of hemodynamic side effects is controversial, use of acepromazine in CV patients is probably best reserved for those animals who are well compensated and show no evidence of active or impending heart failure. In cases when acepromazine is required, the dose of the drug can be decreased by combining it with opioids or benzodiazepines. In the author's practice, the combination of low doses of acepromazine/buprenorphine (IM) has been safely and effectively used on many compensated canine and feline CV patients.

Ketamine is unique among anesthetic agents used in veterinary medicine in that its overall effects may be cardiostimulatory. Ketamine has been variably shown to increase, decrease, or cause no change in contractile function in isolated myocardial tissue, but in normal animals, myocardial effects may be obscured by sympathetic nervous system–mediated increases in contractility, heart rate, and systemic blood pressure. Adverse effects include increased myocardial oxygen consumption, poor muscle relaxation, and exacerbation of any preexisting systemic or pulmonary hypertension. There are minimal respiratory effects but hypersalivation may occur; atropine administration to control hypersalivation may result in unacceptable tachycardias. Ketamine is contraindicated in hypertensive animals or animals with overt CHF, but may be used in low doses in cats with compensated cardiac disease. Ketamine is commonly administered in conjunction with benzodiazepines given IV (e.g., diazepam), or IM (e.g., midazolam), but may also be combined with acepromazine or opioids (e.g., buprenorphine) to minimize adverse emergence phenomena and aid in muscle relaxation. Tiletamine/zolazepam may be used as an alternative to ketamine, and does not need to be combined with additional sedatives. Occasionally patients in whom compensation is present but precarious will decompensate during or after periods of tachycardia associated with ketamine sedation. When ketamine must be administered IV to patients with CV disease, low doses are preferred. Intramuscular ketamine or tiletamine/zol-

azepam administration may cause local pain and irritation.*

Propofol (Diprivan, Stuart Pharmaceuticals, Wilmington, DE) is a relatively new phenol drug used intravenously for both sedation and anesthesia in veterinary patients (see "Propofol: A New Sedative-Hypnotic Anesthetic Agent," this volume, p 77). Propofol is rapid acting and recovery is prompt and usually excitement free, an advantage for CV patients. Controlled clinical trials of propofol for sedation of cardiac patients have not been reported, but continuous infusion of low doses of propofol has been used for sedation (e.g., for radiography) with few adverse side effects in the author's practice. Administration is facilitated by use of a variable-rate syringe infusion pump, and degree of sedation may be titrated by varying infusion rates (initially, 100 $\mu$g/kg/min). Propofol is reported to cause arterial hypotension via simultaneous direct myocardial depression and vasodilation and transient apnea when given in bolus induction doses; these effects do not appear to be a clinical problem at sedative infusion doses. Rapid recovery upon cessation of infusion is a distinct advantage of propofol, but recovery may take longer in cats due to their reduced capacity for conjugation of phenols. Onset of sedation after initiation of continuous infusion is variable, but may take 10 to 15 min or more unless a "loading" bolus dose is given. For this reason, propofol sedation is best suited for patients with compensated cardiac disease undergoing elective procedures.

Atropine and glycopyrrolate are the anticholinergic medications most commonly used in veterinary medicine. Glycopyrrolate crosses the blood-brain barrier slowly; this quality may help avoid transient bradycardias seen after IV atropine administration. Atropine has a shorter duration of action than glycopyrrolate and is less expensive. Anticholinergic administration has been associated with tachyarrhythmias and bradyarrhythmias in dogs without CV disease; these effects may be due to abolition of vagally mediated protection of the ventricle (tachycardias) or centrally mediated effects (bradycardia). Tachycardia and related increases in myocardial oxygen consumption are generally undesirable in CV patients, but anticholinergics are useful in cases of sedative-induced bradycardia. It has been suggested that anticholinergic medications be administered if the patient's heart rate falls below presedative rate (Bednarski, 1992), but sedative-related vasodilation may render presedation heart rates insufficient to maintain blood pressure. Pulse strength, mucous membrane color, and capillary refill time and blood pressure measurements will aid evaluation of "appropriateness" of the sedated patient's heart rate.

## CONTRAINDICATED MEDICATIONS

Sedatives that are contraindicated for use in CV patients include xylazine and medetomidine. These $\alpha_2$-

*Pain associated with IM ketamine injection may be minimized by changing to a fresh 25-gauge needle and injecting the drug at a slow rate.

agonists produce marked CV depression, characterized by decreased cardiac output and bradycardia coupled with increased systemic vascular resistance, and may cause or complicate arrhythmias (Muir, 1975; Wright et al., 1987). These detrimental effects are dependent on dose, rate, route of administration, and species, but the general cardiodepressant activities of these medications make them contraindicated for CV procedures.

## SEDATION OF PATIENTS WITH SPECIFIC CARDIOVASCULAR CONDITIONS

Individual circumstances always influence the ultimate choice of sedative agents in a given patient, but some general recommendations can be made with regard to specific problems observed in common CV diseases. There have been few specific sedative studies reported in animals with naturally occurring CV disease; most recommendations are based on extrapolations of studies performed on healthy animals com-

bined with clinical experience in patients with CV disease. Rationale for drug selection is outlined below and specific recommendations are summarized in Tables 2 and 3.

### Dilated Cardiomyopathy

Dilated cardiomyopathy (DCM) is a common clinical condition of dogs and still occurs, though infrequently, in cats. Underlying myocardial pathology leads to decreased contractile function, and DCM is commonly complicated by CHF and supraventricular (most commonly atrial fibrillation) or ventricular arrhythmias. For animals in overt CHF when stabilization is not possible, or patients with atrial fibrillation with fast ventricular response but no overt CHF, low-dose opioid/benzodiazepine combinations provide effective and relatively safe sedation. For aggressive dogs, droperidol/fentanyl combinations (Innovar-Vet, Pitman-Moore) may be used, but the dog must be closely monitored for bradycardia and anticholinergics administered as necessary.

**Table 2.** *Recommended and Contraindicated Sedatives in Compensated CV Patients*[*]

| Cardiovascular Conditions | Canine | Feline | Contraindicated |
|---|---|---|---|
| DCM | Innovar-Vet[†] ACP/OPD or BDP PFL | ACP/OPD[‡] or BDP KTM/OPD or BDP | KTM, TLZ if tachyarrhythmic, high-dose ACP |
| HCM | NA | ACP/OPD or BDP KTM/OPD OR BDP TLZ | KTM, TLZ if hypertensive or tachyarrhythmic |
| Thyrotoxicosis | NA | ACP/OPD or BDP | KTM, TLZ |
| Valvular heart disease | ACP/OPD or BDP PFL | ACP/OPD or BDP | KTM, TLZ |
| Pericardial disease | ACP/OPD or BDP ± ANCh, KTM/diaz | ACP/OPD or BDP ± ANCh, KTM/diaz | High-dose ACP, PFL |
| Tachyarrhythmias | ACP/OPD or BDP | ACP/OPD or BDP | KTM, TLZ |
| Bradyarrhythmias[§] | OPD/BDP ± ANCh KTM/diaz | OPD/BDP ± ANCh KTM/OPD or BDP TLZ | ACP, PFL, high-dose OPDs, Innovar-Vet |
| Left-to-right shunts | ACP/OPD or BDP PFL | ACP/OPD or BDP | KTM, TLZ, high-dose OPDs |
| Right-to-left shunts | OPD/BDP | OPD/BDP KTM/OPD or BDP TLZ | ACP, PFL |
| Aortic stenosis | ACP/OPD or BDP | ACP/OPD or BDP KTM/OPD OR BDP TLZ | High-dose ACP, PFL |
| Pulmonic stenosis | ACP/OPD or BDP | NA | High-dose ACP, PFL |
| Heartworm disease[‖] | ACP/OPD or BDP | ACP/OPD or BDP | High-dose ACP, PFL if pulmonary hypertension, KTM, TLZ if tachyarrhythmia |
| Hypertension | ACP/OPD or BDP PFL | ACP/OPD or BDP | KTM, TLZ, high-dose OPDs |

[*]OPD/BDP combinations are recommended for use in debilitated animals or those in overt congestive heart failure; this combination may be used in most patients with compensated heart disease.
[†]Fentanyl/droperidol recommended for more aggressive dogs and may be used in most dogs with compensated cardiac disease if bradyarrhythmias are not present.
[‡]Buprenorphine, butorphanol, oxymorphone, or meperidine are the recommended OPDs for use in cats.
[§]Nonanticholinergic-responsive bradyarrhythmias, temporary or permanent pacing may be required.
[‖]When caval syndrome is not present.
Abbreviations: DCM = dilated cardiomyopathy, HCM = hypertrophic cardiomyopathy, ACP = acepromazine, KTM = ketamine, TLZ = Telazol, PFL = propofol, NA = not applicable, ANCh = anticholinergic, diaz = diazepam.

***Table 3.*** *Recommended Dosages for Sedation of Animals with CV Disease*\**

| Drug | Canine (mg/kg) | Feline (mg/kg) |
|---|---|---|
| Diazepam | 0.05–0.2 IV up to maximum of 5 mg total | 0.05–0.2 IV up to maximum of 5 mg total |
| Midazolam | 0.05–0.2 IV, IM up to maximum of 5 mg total | 0.05–0.2 IV, IM up to maximum of 5 mg total |
| Oxymorphone | 0.05–0.2 IM, IV | 0.05–0.2 IM, IV |
| Morphine | 0.2—0.5 IM | NR |
| Meperidine | 1–5 IM, SC | 1–3 IM, SC |
| Buprenorphine | 0.005–0.01 IV, IM, SC | 0.005–0.01 IV, IM, SC |
| Butorphanol | 0.1–0.5 IV, IM, SC | 0.1–0.5 IV, IM, SC |
| Innovar-Vet† | 0.03–0.1 ml/kg IV, IM, SC | NR |
| Ketamine | NR as sole agent | 2–6 IV, 4–10 IM |
| Telazol | 1–2 IV, 4–8 IM, SC | 0.1–2.5 IV, 2.5–5 IM, SC |
| Acepromazine | 0.02–0.05 IV, IM, SC | 0.02–0.05 IM, SC |
| Propofol | 100–600 μg/kg/min (continuous infusion) | NR |
| Atropine | 0.02–0.06 IV, IM | 0.02–0.06 IV, IM |
| Glycopyrrolate | 0.005–0.01 IV, IM | 0.005–0.01 IV, IM |
| **Combinations** | | |
| Midazolam/oxymorphone | 0.1–0.2/0.05 IM | 0.1/0.05 IM |
| Midazolam/merperidine | 0.1–0.2/1–5 IM | 0.1–0.2/1–3 IM |
| Midazolam/buprenorphine | 0.1–0.2/0.005 IM | 0.1/0.005 IM |
| Midazolam/butorphanol | 0.1–0.2/0.2 IM | 0.1/0.2 IM |
| Diazepam/ketamine | 0.25/2–4 IV | 0.25/2–4 IV |
| ACP/oxymorphone | 0.02–0.05/0.02–0.05 IM | 0.02–0.05/0.02–0.05 IM |
| ACP/meperidine | 0.02–0.05/1–5 IM | 0.02–0.05/1–3 IM |
| ACP/buprenorphine | 0.02–0.05/0.005 IM, SC 0.03/0.008 IV | 0.02–0.05/0.005 IM, SC |
| ACP/butorphanol | 0.02–0.05/0.2 IM, SC | 0.02–0.05/0.2 IM, SC |

\*Animals in overt congestive heart failure or debilitated animals should generally be dosed at the lowest end of the given range.
†Fentanyl/droperidol, dosed as combination in milliliters per kilogram.
Abbreviations: IV = intravenously, IM = intramuscularly, SC = subcutaneously, NR = not recommended, ACP = acepromazine.

For patients with compensated DCM, opioid/benzodiazepine combinations, low doses of acepromazine/opioid, or a low-dose propofol infusion may be used for sedative purposes. Inotropic support (e.g., dobutamine) may be necessary when higher doses of sedative are used.

## Hypertrophic Cardiomyopathy/ Thyrotoxicosis

Hypertrophic myocardial diseases are the most common forms of acquired cardiac disease in cats and are characterized by diastolic dysfunction which may lead to CHF. Reduced ventricular compliance or relaxation abnormalities caused by ventricular hypertrophy may be complicated by dynamic left ventricular outflow tract obstruction in some cats. Sinus tachycardia is deleterious to myocardial oxygen balance and atrial or ventricular arrhythmias also may occur. Hypertrophic heart disease may be idiopathic (hypertrophic cardiomyopathy [HCM]) or secondary to hypertension, thyrotoxicosis, or growth hormone excess. When possible, control of underlying disease should be attempted in cases of secondary hypertrophic heart disease prior to sedation, especially if CHF signs are present. Cats with idiopathic HCM are frequently presented with pulmonary edema or pleural effusion when in CHF; thoracocentesis or diuretic therapy prior to sedation is desirable, but efforts must be limited by patient stress level. Low-dose buprenorphine or butorphanol/benzo-

diazepine combinations are often effective sedatives for cats in CHF, but opioid or acepromazine/benzodiazepine or acepromazine/opioid combinations may be used for compensated patients. Intramuscular ketamine combined with buprenorphine, butorphanol, or benzodiazepines may be used, but should be avoided in cases in which tachyarrhythmias or hypertension are known to be present. Acepromazine when combined with butorphanol is a useful sedative for cats with acute arterial thromboembolism, but hypotensive agents should be avoided in cats with known left ventricular outflow tract obstruction because decreases in systemic blood pressure may increase the left ventricular outflow pressure gradient. Thyrotoxic cats present a unique clinical problem in that systemic hypertension may be present in conjunction with CHF and tachyarrhythmias. Many of the clinical manifestations of thyrotoxicosis are related to increased sympathetic nervous system activity and increased sensitivity to catecholamines. For this reason, if a euthyroid state cannot be achieved prior to sedation, attempts should be made to choose a sedative regimen that will induce minimal sympathetic activity in order to avoid exacerbation of arrhythmias. In overt CHF, opioid/benzodiazepine combinations are recommended. If CHF is not present, opioid/benzodiazepine or acepromazine/opioid combinations may be used. Ketamine and tiletamine are contraindicated for sedation of thyrotoxic cats. If an anticholinergic is necessary to control hypersalivation, glycopyrrolate is preferable to atropine, which may predispose patients to arrhythmias (Muir, 1978).

## Valvular Heart Disease

Valvular heart disease is common in dogs and cats. In cats, mitral dysplasia or mitral insufficiency in conjunction with cardiomyopathies are most common, but in dogs, acquired disease of any of the heart valves may be seen. In cases of uncomplicated mitral or tricuspid insufficiency due to valve dysplasia or endocardiosis, commonly measured indices of myocardial function are usually normal until late in the disease process. For animals with atrioventricular valvular disease and no evidence of CHF, the primary concern is avoidance of extreme variations in heart rate and vascular resistance (Evans, 1992). Use of opioid or acepromazine/benzodiazepine or opioid combination with close heart rate and blood pressure monitoring is recommended. In the case of aortic insufficiency, sedative choice is based on cardiac function. If CHF is present, an opioid/benzodiazepine combination is preferred, but if no CHF is present, acepromazine/benzodiazepine or opioid combinations or propofol may be used. Ketamine is avoided in cases of aortic insufficiency to avoid increasing afterload.

## Pericardial Effusion, Cardiac Tamponade, or Restrictive Pericardial Disease

Pericardial effusion in the dog or cat may be clinically silent or result in signs of right-sided or biventricular congestive heart failure. In cases of constrictive pericardial disease, a noncompliant, thickened pericardium, rather than the presence of large amounts of fluid, limits ventricular filling. When CHF is present, cardiac output is limited and sudden decreases in systemic blood pressure and/or heart rate are poorly tolerated; sedative regimens involving hypotensive agents (e.g., acepromazine, propofol) should be avoided in all patients with clinical pericardial disease and anticholinergics may be needed if bradycardia develops after sedation. In cases where a pericardial effusion results in signs of low cardiac output, an immediate improvement is usually seen after pericardiocentesis. Many dogs may undergo this procedure with local anesthesia only. In those dogs requiring sedation, an opioid/benzodiazepine combination with or without an anticholinergic is recommended. A ketamine/benzodiazepine combination (IV) may be used if more profound sedation is required. Partial drainage of ascites and/or pleural effusion may also ease respiration and decrease patient distress.

## Arrhythmias

The presence of life-threatening tachyarrhythmias or bradyarrhythmias may require administration of atrial or ventricular antiarrhythmics prior to sedation. Sedation choice is based on underlying CV abnormalities after stabilization of cardiac rhythm. Ketamine is contraindicated in patients with tachyarrhythmias, while acepromazine has antiarrhythmogenic effects. In the case of sinus bradycardia, anticholinergic administration may normalize heart rate prior to sedation. If the bradycardia is nonresponsive to atropine and underlying causes cannot be found and corrected (e.g., hyperkalemia), or in cases of third-degree atrioventricular block, a temporary or permanent pacemaker may be required. Permanent transvenous pacemaker implantation is commonly achieved under sedation with use of local anesthesia. The combination of acepromazine/opioid (most often buprenorphine in the author's practice) has proven effective for this procedure, as has the IV combination of ketamine and diazepam. If patient movement is a problem, intermittent IV diazepam administration during the procedure is helpful. Concurrent local anesthetic infiltration at the site of implantation is essential. Once pacing has commenced, inhalation anesthetics can be used for anesthesia during placement of the pulse generator.

## Left-to-Right Shunts

Left-to-right intracardiac (atrial or ventricular septal defect) or extracardiac (patent ductus arteriosus, arteriovenous fistula) shunts result in overload of the cardiac chamber that receives the extra volume from the shunt. Increases in systemic vascular resistance (e.g., as a result of ketamine administration) may increase the shunt volume; sedatives causing decreased vascular resistance are preferred. If no CHF is present, most sedation regimens are well tolerated, but extreme bradycardias or tachycardias should be avoided (avoid high-dose opioids and ketamine). If CHF if present, opioid/benzodiazepine, low-dose acepromazine/opioid combinations, or propofol administration is usually safe and effective.

## Right-to-Left Shunts

Cyanotic heart disease in cats and dogs as a result of right-to-left intracardiac ("reversed" atrial or ventricular septal defect, tetralogy of Fallot) or extracardiac ("reversed" patent ductus arteriosus) shunting leads to chronically reduced oxygen content of systemic arterial blood and eventually to polycythemia. Prolonged polycythemia and hypoxemia, in turn, lead to hyperviscosity syndromes with metabolic acidosis and hypercoagulability. Supplemental oxygen administration is of little assistance in these cyanotic animals because of the anatomic shunt and subsequent venous admixture of systemic arterial blood. The volume of desaturated venous blood that shunts into systemic arterial blood depends on the relative pressures between the right and left side. When systemic vascular resistance decreases due to drug administration, exercise, or therapeutic phlebotomy, the amount of desaturated blood shunted increases, increasing cyanosis. Chronic hypoxemia, polycythemia, and the detrimental effects of hypotension make animals with cyanotic heart disease intolerant of tachycardia, bradycardia, hypotension, and respiratory depression. When sedation cannot be avoided, an opioid/benzodiazepine combination is preferred with an anticholinergic administered as necessary to treat bradycardia. Sedation with IM ketamine/midazolam is useful to maintain systemic blood pressure, but may result in undesirable tachycardia. Indiscriminate use of anticholinergic medications and use of hypotensive sedatives (e.g., acepromazine, propofol) should be avoided.

## Aortic Stenosis/Pulmonic Stenosis

Animals with mild forms of aortic and pulmonic stenosis may be sedated as normal animals of the same age if no concurrent disease exists. In cases where stenosis is accompanied by other defects, clinical signs of low output exist, or when concurrent CHF or arrhythmias are present, sedation regimens must be modified. Animals with aortic or subaortic stenosis are heart rate dependent and somewhat intolerant of systemic hypotension because their ability to increase cardiac output is limited by a fixed obstruction. Aortic and pulmonic stenosis may result in ventricular hypertrophy and patient intolerance of hypoxia and tachycardia-related increases in myocardial oxygen consumption. In animals with severe obstruction and/or several hypertrophied ventricles, an opioid/benzodiazepine combination is most successful; low-dose acepromazine/benzodiazepine or opioid may be useful in animals with less severe obstruction.

## Heartworm Disease/Caval Syndrome

The severity of heartworm disease varies among patients. Complications of severe heartworm disease affecting choice of sedative include pyrexia (with associated systemic vasodilation), pulmonary hypertension/high pulmonary vascular resistance, exaggerated pulmonary hypertensive responses to hypoxia, hypercoagulability, right-sided CHF, disseminated intravascular coagulation (DIC), and the presence of inflammatory pulmonary infiltrates. Filling pressures for the left side are limited by poor right-sided function. Low-stress handling and supplemental oxygen are invaluable in dealing with patients with severe pulmonary parenchymal disease.

Heartworm caval syndrome is a severe complication of heartworm infection that typically occurs in animals with high worm burdens and is associated with high mortality. Affected animals may be presented with acute collapse and signs of low cardiac output, severe pulmonary hypertension with signs of right-sided CHF, hemolytic anemia, and DIC. Varying degrees of hepatic and renal failure are usually present. Immediate therapy includes careful fluid therapy and treatment for DIC, but immediate surgical removal of heartworms from the vena cava, right atrium, and ventricle is the treatment of choice. Worm removal (performed via right jugular venotomy) can often be accomplished with local anesthesia only; if sedation is required, opioid/benzodiazepine combinations are usually effective. Supplemental oxygen may be supplied via mask or nasal intubation in a lightly sedated patient, or endotracheal intubation when deep sedation is used.

## Hypertension

Although detection of hypertension in veterinary patients is increasing, there are few clinical recommendations recorded to date regarding sedation and anesthesia of these patients. Animals in acute hypertensive crisis may be treated with a variety of diuretics and vasodilators, including acepromazine. For chronically hypertensive patients, agents known to decrease blood pressure (e.g., acepromazine, propofol) will usually be tolerated, but hypertensive agents (e.g., ketamine, tiletamine) and bradycardic agents (e.g., high-dose opioids) should be avoided.

## SUMMARY

Safe and effective sedation of CV patients relies on a combination of accurate patient assessment, vigilant monitoring, patience, and understanding of the systemic and pharmacologic effects of both sedative and CV medications. Use of local anesthetics is advocated when possible and if unstable patient status precludes use of systemic agents. In general, combinations of low-dose opioids and benzodiazepines are recommended for use in unstable and/or debilitated CV patients, and may be used in higher doses for more stable patients requiring more profound sedation. If additional restraint is required, low doses of acepromazine combined with an opioid or benzodiazepine may be tolerated by stable CV patients.

## References and Suggested Reading

Bednarski RM: Anesthetic concerns for patients with cardiomyopathy. Vet Clin North Am 22:460, 1992.
  *Recommendations for anesthesia of cardiomyopathic patients.*
Cornick JL and Hartsfield SM: Cardiopulmonary and behavioral effects of combinations of acepromazine/butorphanol and acepromazine/oxymorphone in dogs. J Am Vet Med Assoc 200:1952, 1992.
  *Analgesic, behavioral, and some cardiorespiratory effects of combinations of acepromazine and butorphanol or oxymorphone in six conscious dogs.*
Coyle JP: Sedation, pain relief, and neuromuscular blockade in the postoperative cardiac surgical patients. Semin Thorac Cardiovasc Surg 3:81, 1991.
  *Suggestions for sedation in human postoperative cardiac patients.*
Evans AT: Anesthesia for severe mitral and tricuspid regurgitation. Vet Clin North Am 22:465, 1992.
  *Recommendations for anesthesia in patients with atrioventricular valvular insufficiency.*
Green SM and Johnson NE: Ketamine sedation for pediatric procedures: Part 2, review and implications. Ann Emerg Med 19:1033, 1990.
  *Summary of clinical use and effects of ketamine in human pediatric patients.*
Haskins SC: Injectable anesthetics. Vet Clin North Am 22:245, 1992.
  *A summary of anesthetic and hemodynamic effects of injectable preanesthetic and anesthetic agents.*
Muir WW: Effects of atropine on cardiac rate and rhythm in dogs. J Am Vet Med Assoc 172:917, 1978.
  *Controlled study of effects of atropine administration in 200 dogs.*

Muir WW, Werner LL, and Hamlin RL: Effects of xylazine and acetylpromazine upon induced ventricular fibrillation in dogs anesthetized with thiamylal and halothane. Am J Vet Res 36:1299, 1975.
*Study of arrhythmogenic effects of xylazine and acepromazine in 38 anes-
thetized dogs.*

Wright M, Heath RB, and Wingfield WE: Effects of xylazine and ketamine on epinephrine induced arrhythmia in the dog. Vet Surg 68:398,
1973.
*Study of arrhythmogenic effects of xylazine, ketamine, and xylazine-ketam-
ine in ten nonanesthetized dogs.*

# THERAPY OF HEART FAILURE

BRUCE W. KEENE
*Raleigh, North Carolina*

*and* JOHN D. BONAGURA
*Columbus, Ohio*

Heart failure is a condition characterized by inadequate cardiac output and insufficient delivery of oxygen and nutrients relative to tissue metabolic needs. Heart failure can be distinguished from simple hypovolemia and from most forms of circulatory shock (except cardiogenic shock) by virtue of the normal to elevated venous pressures measured in cardiac failure. Heart failure is not a specific disease, but a clinical syndrome, caused by a structural or functional disorder of the heart. One of the earliest signs of heart failure is exercise intolerance; however, this finding often goes unappreciated by pet owners. Many cases of heart failure remain unrecognized until significant elevations of pulmonary or systemic venous pressures lead to clinical signs of fluid retention, a condition referred to as *congestive heart failure* (CHF).

A number of stereotypical responses develop in response to reduced cardiac output (Table 1), and our appreciation of these compensations is central to the current ideas regarding the therapy of heart failure. This understanding can be enhanced further by considering the pathogenesis of heart failure from any heart disease in three phases (Bristow et al., 1985). These phases are pathophysiologic in basis and not identical to the clinical classification of the New York Heart Association that has been adapted inconsistently to define heart failure in animals.

## PHASES OF HEART FAILURE

### Phase I

The *first phase* of heart failure, the etiology of the cascade of events that eventually leads to the clinical signs of heart failure, is initiated by some usually unrecognized injury (Bristow et al., 1985). In the most common canine situation, the injury involves the atrioventricular valves (resulting in chronic valvular disease) or the myocardium (causing dilated cardiomyopathy [DCM]). The most common injuries causing feline heart disease incite some form of cardiomyopathy or acquired myocardial disease. The injuries responsible for acquired heart disease in dogs and cats may be a genetically predetermined biochemical error, an infectious agent, a disordered immune response, a toxic injury, a nutritional deficiency, or some combination of these events. The response to an identical injury can differ among species, families, and individuals. A number of recent animal investigations aimed at identifying injuries that initiate acquired heart diseases have been conducted; yet, practical therapies directed at avoiding or preventing these inciting injuries still await a more complete understanding of the molecular structure and physiology of the heart. This phase, for practical purposes, is not identified clinically.

### Phase II

Often the initial injury to the heart alters cardiac function but is not otherwise overwhelming or lethal. In this instance, the *second phase* of heart failure ensues. This phase is characterized by activation of the sympathetic nervous system (SNS) and the renin-angiotensin-aldosterone system (RAAS) in response to limited cardiac output and accompanying changes in blood pressure, organ perfusion, and vascular distention. It seems that these compensatory mechanisms developed to enhance the survival of the animal following acute hemodynamic compromise (e.g., hemorrhage) by maintaining circulation to vital organs and restoring intravascular volume. Activation of these systems may support clinically adequate circulatory function for a variable time, depending on the nature and severity of the initial cardiac injury. Despite these short-term benefits, the chronic activation of the SNS and RAAS damages the myocardium and probably hastens the progression of heart failure. In addition to enhanced neurohormonal activity, obvious structural changes in the heart, such as dilatation or hypertrophy, may be evident.

**Table 1.** *Compensatory Adaptations and Adverse Consequences of Neuroendocrine Responses in Heart Failure*

| Adaptive Mechanism | Physiologic Changes | Initial Compensatory Advantages | Adverse Consequences of "Overcompensation" |
|---|---|---|---|
| Activation of the sympathetic nervous system | Arteriolar and venous constriction; tachycardia; enhanced myocardial contractility | Helps to maintain venous return, cardiac output, and arterial blood pressure | Vasoconstriction increases ventricular afterload and leads to redistribution of blood flow; catecholamines lead to myocardial tissue injury, increased myocardial oxygen demand, down-regulation of $\beta$ receptors, and activation of the renin-angiotensin system |
| Activation of the renin-angiotensin-aldosterone system | Angiotensin is a vasoconstrictor and enhances sympathetic activity; release of aldosterone causes sodium retention and expands the plasma volume, and elevated venous pressure | Angiotensin II and norepinephrine maintain arterial blood pressure; aldosterone increases cardiac filling, ventricular preload, and stroke volume via the Frank-Starling mechanism | Angiotensin may cause adverse myocardial remodeling; increased afterload; fluid retention and edema; loss of potassium |
| Arginine vasopressin (antidiuretic hormone) | Vasoconstriction; increases free water retention by the kidney | As above | Increased vasoconstriction augments sympathetic and renin-angiotensin systems; fluid retention and edema |
| Baroreceptor-mediated response to lowered blood pressure | Sympathetic activation, tachycardia, vasoconstriction | Maintains cardiac output and arterial blood pressure | As above for sympathetic nervous system |

This phase of heart failure is generally associated with physical evidence of cardiac disease such as cardiomegaly, heart murmur, gallop sound, or recurrent cardiac arrhythmia. The clinical diagnosis of "heart disease" becomes evident in most cases, although overt signs of cardiac failure are not observed. Detecting cardiac failure in this phase would require a critical examination of cardiac status—such as a maximal exercise test—but this is rarely done, as these animals appear well-adapted to their heart disease. While overt signs of CHF are not evident, some dogs in this phase of heart disease will cough from *mainstem bronchial compression* caused by an expanding left atrium. This is especially common in dogs with mitral regurgitation (MR) and often occurs *before* pulmonary edema can be detected. Most clinicians would consider animals in this phase of heart failure to be *"compensated"* for their heart disease. If the New York Heart Association classification were applied to this phase of heart failure, patients would be designated as class I (no obvious exercise limitations) or class II (slight exercise limitation or coughing with routine physical activity).

In the past, most animals with phase II heart failure have not been treated. However, important advances in the treatment of heart failure have originated from the premise that modulation of compensatory mechanisms in this phase may benefit patients with chronic heart disease. These concepts seem generally applicable to cases of heart failure from a variety of underlying causes. The angiotensin-converting enzyme (ACE) inhibitors (see "Angiotensin-Converting Enzyme Inhibitors," this volume, p 786), digitalis glycosides (see *CVT XI*, p 689), $\beta$-adrenergic blockers (see *CVT XI*, p 676), and calcium channel blockers (see *CVT XI*, p 684) may all prove useful in mitigating some of the adverse effects of the neurohormonal response to heart failure if used under appropriate circumstances. Evidence is accumulating that early intervention to reduce the activation of these "compensatory" mechanisms or to moderate their effects on the heart may actually delay the onset of clinical signs of heart failure in some settings. Clinical application of these ideas is discussed later in this article.

### Phase III

In the *third phase* of the heart failure, overt clinical signs of inadequate cardiac output (exercise intolerance, lethargy, anorexia, cold extremities, prerenal azotemia) or markedly elevated venous pressures (pulmonary edema, pleural effusion, ascites, exercise intolerance, tachypnea, dyspnea, and cough) become apparent. These patients would be classified as New York Heart Association class III (comfortable at rest but clinical signs develop during minimal physical activity) or class IV (clinical signs of heart failure are evident at rest and any exercise is severely limited). Therapy of heart failure is clearly required for these patients and traditionally has been initiated during this phase—after the onset of clinical signs has clearly signaled the presence of serious heart disease. The goals of therapy at this point are alleviation of clinical signs of CHF, improved quality of life, and prolongation of life. These aims can only be achieved if the clinician can successfully orchestrate the administration of various and potent cardiovascular drugs. Understanding the pathophysiology of heart failure, the clinical pharmacology of cardiac drugs, and the hemodynamic abnormalities associated with the common acquired heart diseases are essential for success. This knowledge, coupled with improved clinical methods of assessing cardiac function, have enhanced our ability to pharmacologically optimize preload, afterload, myocardial contractility, and heart rate and rhythm of the individual patient in this phase.

This balance of this article summarizes the authors' views on how new information regarding the pathophysiology of heart failure can be integrated into practical strategies for managing chronic heart failure secondary to valvular disease or dilated cardiomyopathy in dogs, or hypertrophic cardiomyopathy in cats.

## DRUGS FOR TREATMENT OF HEART FAILURE

### Antiotensin-Converting Enzyme Inhibitors

Asymptomatic animals with *clearly defined heart disease* and conclusive evidence of an ongoing (phase II) response to cardiac injury may benefit from therapy directed at diminishing the activity of the RAAS or SNS. The easiest recognized responses to ongoing cardiac injury are cardiac chamber enlargement, hypertrophy, or altered myocardial systolic or diastolic function. Detection of these responses requires thoracic radiography and echocardiography. While cardiac dilatation is usually obvious from the thoracic radiograph, detection of hypertrophy, assessment of systolic function (e.g., shortening fraction), and estimation of diastolic function requires various echocardiographic or even Doppler techniques. A number of studies have identified the usefulness of ACE inhibitor therapy in heart failure of various stages caused by myocardial failure (i.e., DCM). It is not uncommon clinically to identify dogs with DCM prior to the development of overt CHF. When this diagnosis is verified by echocardiography, our therapeutic approach includes prescribing an ACE inhibitor such as enalapril (Enacard, Vasotec; 0.5 mg/kg once or twice daily), captopril (Capoten, 1 mg/kg every 8 hr), or lisinopril (Prinivil, 0.25–0.5 mg/kg once daily) to attenuate the deleterious effects of the RAAS. In dogs with mitral valvular regurgitation, the value of RAAS inhibition during this phase of heart failure is uncertain; however, in dogs with unequivocal evidence of left ventricular and left atrial dilation, we usually prescribe an ACE inhibitor as described above. The merits of this therapy in cats with hypertrophic or restrictive forms of cardiomyopathy is purely speculative, though local myocardial angiotensin systems may promote hypertrophy and contribute to the progression of these diseases.

The use of ACE inhibitors for the overt CHF that develops in phase III heart failure is strongly advocated. Angiotensin-converting enzyme inhibitors have been shown to improve both functional status and survival of humans and dogs in heart failure (CONSENSUS, 1987; SOLVD, 1992) as described elsewhere in this section (see this volume, p 786). We also prescribe enalapril to cats with CHF caused by restrictive cardiomyopathy (see "Restrictive Cardiomyopathy," this volume, p 863), and in cats with hypertrophic cardiomyopathy with progressive CHF characterized by refractory pulmonary edema or development of pleural effusion.

### Digitalis Glycosides

Digitalis glycosides (digoxin and digitoxin) have been shown to sensitize baroreceptors and to induce sustained inhibition of the sympathetic activation that characterizes moderate to severe heart failure in human patients and dogs (Ferguson, 1992). This inhibition precedes any measurable hemodynamic effects of the drug and appears to be independent of the positive inotropic action. Because of these actions, and due to the known deleterious effects of chronic SNS stimulation, digoxin is prescribed more frequently and earlier in the treatment of heart failure. Thus, digitalis can be considered a modest positive inotrope, useful for slowing ventricular rate response in atrial fibrillation, and beneficial in establishing more normal neurohormonal activity.

The authors prescribe digitalis in the management of CHF secondary to DCM, restrictive cardiomyopathy, and chronic valvular heart disease whenever congestive heart failure is present and serious contraindications to the drug (moderate azotemia or hypokalemia; frequent ventricular arrhythmias) are not. A digitalis glycoside is prescribed to virtually all patients with atrial fibrillation. We do *not* consider the examination room heart rate to be a suitable indicator for the need for digitalization, since there is absolutely no evidence that a single heart rate reliably estimates chronic SNS activity or the clinical response attained from digitalization (and digitalis does not effectively slow heart rate in excited or exercising dogs). We also administer digitalis to patients with "asymptomatic" DCM. The indications for digitalization in dogs with MR and phase II heart failure (i.e., enlarged left atrium and ventricle but without pulmonary edema) are less clear. While some cardiologists prescribe digoxin at this time, the authors prefer to initiate therapy with an ACE inhibitor in these dogs unless another indication for digitalization (e.g., frequent atrial premature beats, low ventricular shortening fraction) is identified.

### Diuretics

Loop diuretics such as furosemide are still widely considered by many veterinarians to be "first-line" therapy in the management of fluid retention secondary to heart failure. Many veterinarians initiate therapy of heart failure by prescribing a diuretic administered at a regular interval. There is no doubt that diuretics are effective or that patients with severe or life-threatening edema or effusions should be initially diuresed. The use of chronic diuretic *monotherapy*, however, should be reconsidered. For example, it has been shown that human patients whose symptoms of congestive heart failure are well controlled on diuretics alone deteriorate more quickly than those treated with either ACE inhibitors or digoxin (Captopril-Digoxin Multicenter Research Group, 1988). Clinical deterioration during diuretic monotherapy is thought to be due to volume contraction and diuretic-induced activation of the renin-angiotensin system.

In light of these findings, the authors rarely prescribe chronic diuretic monotherapy even in the initial management of mild CHF caused by MR or DCM. Following initial diuresis, an ACE inhibitor and digoxin should be prescribed and the diuretic dosage lowered or even discontinued if possible. While veterinary studies are needed to address this issue, the authors believe that chronic furosemide monotherapy is inappropriate and that higher doses of diuretics, or combination diuretic therapy, should be reserved for the dog with advanced CHF that is already receiving both an ACE inhibitor and digoxin. In cats with hypertrophic cardiomyopathy, initial diuresis for pulmonary edema is usually essential; however, long-term diuretic therapy can often be attenuated or discontinued if myocardial function is improved by therapy with diltiazem and/or a β-blocker. Cats with CHF caused by restrictive cardiomyopathy generally require daily diuretic doses, but these should be given in conjunction with digoxin and an ACE inhibitor.

## β-Adrenergic Blockers

Activation of the SNS is useful in severe heart failure, since adrenergic activity increases heart rate, myocardial contractility, and arterial blood pressure. Chronic SNS activation is considered deleterious because catecholamines increase afterload, increase myocardial oxygen demand, activate the RAAS, injure myocytes, and down-regulate myocardial β receptors. Mortality in CHF can be predicted in part by the concentration of norepinephrine in the plasma. β-Blockers, including propranolol, atenolol, and metoprolol, appear to restore or "up-regulate" β-adrenergic receptor numbers and sensitivity and protect the myocardium from the cellular effects of excess catecholamines. This benefit is thought to be greatest in DCM, especially when there is recurrent ischemic injury to the myocardium. β-receptor blockade in patients with myocardial failure requires caution, however, since the failing ventricle may be dependent on adrenergic tone to maintain systolic function. Despite their initial depressant effects on the myocardium, long-term β-blocker therapy improves resting hemodynamic indices, exercise tolerance, and functional classification in humans with heart failure (Engelmeir et al., 1985). Recent experiments in dogs have also demonstrated that chronic β-receptor blockade prevents the development of β-receptor subsensitivity in a model of tricuspid valve regurgitation (Liang, Frantz, and Suematsu, 1991) or progressive MR and myocardial dysfunction in ischemic models of DCM. While these studies support the idea that β-blockade may benefit dogs and cats with heart failure, clinical trials are needed to determine whether β-blockade will prolong survival and enhance the quality of the lives of these animals.

While the authors do not yet recommend routine administration of β-blockers in animals with CHF, these drugs are potentially beneficial for a number of specific cardiac conditions. Provided the clinician is mindful of the negative inotropic effects of these drugs, the long-term benefit to the heart may be considerable. In dogs with atrial fibrillation, the concomitant administration of digoxin and a β-blocker provides far better control of ventricular heart rate than digoxin alone. Provided the patient has been diuresed and cardiogenic shock is not evident, incremental doses of a β-blocker can be used to reduce the resting heart rate to 150 beats per minute or less. Initial low doses (e.g., 0.2 mg/kg propranolol PO) can be increased gradually over 2 to 4 days to achieve the desired effect. In dogs with CHF and malignant ventricular arrhythmias, the judicious addition of a β-blocker to a conventional antiarrhythmic drug may provide better control of the rhythm disturbance. In cats with either asymptomatic or symptomatic hypertrophic cardiomyopathy, particularly in those with echocardiographic demonstration of left ventricular outflow obstruction, chronic β-blockade may be beneficial by preventing stress-induced pulmonary edema (see "CVT Update: Feline Hypertrophic Cardiomyopathy," this volume, p 854).

## Calcium Channel Blockers

The calcium channel blocker diltiazem (Cardizem) has been administered for particular cardiac problems associated with heart failure. In animals with atrial fibrillation, diltiazem can be used in place of a β-blocker to control ventricular rate response. Again, the clinician must consider the negative inotropic effects of the drug and start with a low dose (e.g., 0.25 mg/kg PO) and titrate the dosage to the desired heart rate over a number of days. Diltiazem has also been used frequently in cats with hypertrophic cardiomyopathy with either phase II or phase III heart failure (see *CVT XI*, p 766; and this volume, p 854). The potential for regression of left ventricular hypertrophy subsequent to diltiazem administration is intriguing, though the authors have also observed this phenomenon in cats not receiving this drug.

## GENERAL STRATEGIES FOR MANAGING HEART FAILURE

Contemplation of the three phases of heart failure outlined above suggests a general course of action that can be modified based on the clinician's knowledge of the specific heart disease present. Whenever possible, potential underlying causes of heart disease should be identified and corrected or prevented. With the exceptions of heartworm disease, bacterial endocarditis, and DCM associated with taurine-deficiency or L-carnitine–deficiency, such "phase I" therapy (or prophylaxis) is rarely possible because the etiologies of most heart diseases remain unknown.

Management of the common acquired heart diseases of dogs and cats (chronic valvular heart disease and the various cardiomyopathies) requires selection of appropriate treatments that depend on our understanding of pathophysiology as well as the clinical stage of the disease. Classifying animals by the severity of their clinical signs is most useful when making therapeutic decisions with regard to a homogeneous patient population (same species and breed, same disease, same level of activity, similar concurrent problems). Because clinical signs are not easily quantified, classifications such as the New York Heart Association system are subject to considerable interobserver variability. Furthermore, individual patients with similar clinical signs may suffer from pathophysiologically diverse diseases that need different treatments.

The *exact cardiac diagnosis* is therefore important and can usually be attained by considering the species; age; breed; and the results of cardiac auscultation and physical examination, thoracic radiography, electrocardiography (ECG), arterial blood pressure measurement, relevant laboratory tests (which may include a heartworm test, serum thyroxine, blood or plasma taurine, plasma carnitine, complete blood count [CBC], or biochemical profile), and echocardiography. Dogs with chronic mitral and tricuspid valve regurgitation can be identified by age and breed and the characteristic systolic murmurs, and the diagnosis verified by echocardiography. An echocardiogram is essential to the diagnosis of DCM, though the disease can certainly be suspected in susceptible canine breeds based on physical examination, radiography, and ECG. Sorting out the various causes of feline myocardial diseases requires a full work-up with echocardiography as listed above. Once a diagnosis is secured, drug therapy must always be tailored to the specific diagnosis with consideration of the pharmacodynamic effects of the prescribed agents.

Every effort should be made to synthesize all of the information available when constructing a therapeutic plan. Concurrent diseases should be identified with a thorough physical and laboratory examination. Client education regarding the natural history of disease is important, and handouts that discuss the disease and therapy are helpful to many clients. The results of prospective therapeutic trials should be reviewed. The financial and physiologic risks and benefits of therapy should be discussed with the owner prior to formulating a treatment plan.

After a treatment plan is initiated, *follow-up examinations* should be done. The first step involves a careful interview, considering: quality of life, appetite, exercise tolerance, respiratory rate and effort, coughing, ability to sleep without respiratory difficulty, home heart rate (if taken), low output signs (tiring, sudden collapse, syncope), client medication compliance, and potential medication side effects (anorexia, vomiting, diarrhea, weakness). The patient should be examined with attention to: body weight, hydration, heart rate and rhythm, arterial pulses, jugular venous pressure, respiratory rate and breath sounds, liver size and presence or absence of ascites, membrane color, and capillary refill time. The arterial blood pressure should be measured at every visit (see Section 2) because diuretics and vasodilator drugs can cause hypotension and animals with intercurrent diseases may be hypertensive. Thoracic radiographs are useful if the history and physical examination suggest a recrudescence of pulmonary edema, pleural effusion, or another pulmonary complication. The ECG or Holter ECG is helpful if an arrhythmia is detected by auscultation or suspected from the history. Routine serum biochemistries and electrolytes should be obtained regularly or when there are problems such as vomiting or anorexia. Increasing blood urea nitrogen (BUN) or creatinine may indicate hypotension or plasma volume contraction: a sign that the dose of diuretic, and possibly that of any vasodilator, should be reduced. A serum digoxin should be obtained after the initial 1 to 2 weeks of dosing and periodically thereafter. Follow-up echocardiograms are rarely done in dogs because they seldom impact therapy (exceptions include response to taurine or L-carnitine supplementation). It would be foolish, for example, to discontinue digitalis because one did not observe a change in shortening fraction. Similarly, an observed improvement in shortening fraction may be related as much to changes in afterload as inotropism; moreover, the echocardiographic findings may not correspond at all to the clinical examination or radiographs. Of course, the echocardiogram may be indicated in some cases to follow the *progression* of disease. In cats with hypertrophic cardiomyopathy, changes in wall thickness or systolic myocardial function are occasionally observed. Similarly, when the clinical status of a dog with mitral regurgitation suddenly deteriorates, the echocardiogram may show a flail leaflet from a ruptured chordae tendineae or pericardial effusion from a ruptured left atrium.

## Mitral Regurgitation

No pharmacotherapy is currently recommended for the dog with chronic MR without left atrial and left ventricular enlargement. A modestly salt-restricted diet may be offered, but there is no proof this is useful. If left atrial and left ventricular enlargement are obvious, the authors recommend initiating therapy with an ACE inhibitor (enalapril, 0.5 mg/kg every 12 to 24 hr), with or without a modestly salt-restricted diet. While seemingly reasonable, the merits of this recommendation await further clinical trials.

When clinical signs of heart disease develop gradually, the clinician should ascertain by radiography whether the coughing and exercise intolerance are caused by bronchial compression, pulmonary edema, or both. Therapy with an ACE inhibitor, digitalis (digoxin, 0.005 to 0.01 mg/kg every 12 hr), or a diuretic (furosemide, 2 to 3 mg/kg p.r.n.) may all effectively reduce left atrial size, pulmonary congestion, and bronchial compression; consequently, it is likely that coughing secondary to chronic MR can be treated effectively with any one of these drugs, or with all of them in combination. However, for reasons cited previously, the authors prefer combination therapy to monotherapy. Following any necessary diuresis, an ACE inhibitor, digitalis, and a judicious dosage of a diuretic are prescribed for these patients. If follow-up examination reveals complete absence of pulmonary edema and decrease in cardiac size, the diuretic dosage is reduced or discontinued. As CHF progresses, the diuretic dosage can be increased. For owners unable to make the financial commitment required for ACE inhibitor therapy, digoxin and furosemide are prescribed. When digoxin is contraindicated because of poor owner compliance, renal failure, or frequent ventricular arrhythmias, ACE inhibition, modest dietary sodium restriction, and furosemide are usually sufficient to relieve the clinical signs.

Once advanced CHF has developed, the dog should be receiving an ACE inhibitor, digoxin, and furosemide. If clinical signs of left-sided failure persist or recur despite this therapy, an additional vasodilator is prescribed to reduce mitral regurgitant fraction. Therapy with the arteriolar dilating drug, hydralazine (starting at 0.5 and increasing to 1 to 1.5 mg/kg b.i.d.), can be initiated and is often successful in controlling refractory cough or pulmonary edema. The disadvantage of hydralazine is found in the rebound activation of the RAAS caused by the decline in arterial blood pressure. To blunt this response, the dose of the ACE inhibitor can be continued or decreased by 50% (if hypotension becomes a problem). Blood pressure **must** be measured to guide therapy, and systolic blood pressure should be maintained at greater than 90 mm Hg. The risk of hypotension with combination vasodilator therapy is significant, and the dog should be hospitalized to permit frequent measurements of blood pressure (see Section 2). An alternative treatment for refractory pulmonary edema, pleural effusion, or ascites is the addition of spironolactone (2 mg/kg b.i.d. PO) with or without hydrochlorothiazide (2–4 mg/kg; a combination 25 mg/25 mg product is available). The serum potassium concentrations must be monitored closely (3 and 7 days after initiating the drug, then at some appropriate regular interval based on response to therapy) when spironolactone is administered concurrently with an ACE inhibitor. Other treatments that may be useful for symptomatic relief of coughing include hydrocodone and possibly a bronchodilator (see *CVT XI*, p 660). Antiarrhythmic therapy is instituted as needed. As previously discussed, either a β-blocker or calcium channel blocker can be used in dogs with atrial fibrillation and rapid ventricular rate.

Emergency presentations of pulmonary edema are often related to poor client compliance or ruptured mitral chordae tendineae. Initial management for the first 24 to 48 hr includes intravenous furosemide, topical nitroglycerin ointment (½ to 1½ inches), oxygen, morphine (0.1 mg/kg SC), and oral hydralazine (1 to 2 mg/kg PO every 12 hr).

## Dilated Cardiomyopathy

In asymptomatic animals with an unequivocal diagnosis of DCM, ACE inhibition and digitalization (similar doses as for mitral regurgitation) are prescribed. Owners with no financial constraints are also offered a therapeutic trial of L-carnitine supplementation (2 gm every 8 hour PO for 3 months; see *CVT XI*, p 780). Spaniels and small-breed dogs with documented DCM should have a blood or plasma taurine concentration measured, and if low, supplementation with taurine (500 mg every 8 to 12 hr) should be initiated. The value of introducing a β-blocker into this regimen is unresolved. As described in the earlier section, β-blockade may be cardioprotective. However, most studies of cardioprotection in dogs have been in ischemic cardiomyopathy models, and the authors are uncertain if a β-blocker is beneficial or not in dogs with idiopathic DCM. In dogs with recurrent cardiac arrhythmias, a β-blocker is prescribed as adjunctive antiarrhythmic therapy (see "Diagnosis and Management of Ventricular Tachyarrhythmias in Doberman Pinschers with Cardiomyopathy," this volume, p 799).

Once overt CHF has developed, the dog with DCM is treated in a manner similar to that for advanced MR. Digoxin, an ACE inhibitor, and furosemide are the backbone of therapy. Progressively increasing doses of diuretic or combination diuretic therapy (furosemide plus spironolactone or spironolactone-hydrochlorothiazide) are often needed to treat unresponsive edema or body cavity effusions. Some dogs benefit from the addition of hydralazine as described above for MR. Antiarrhythmic therapy is often very important to dogs with DCM. The use of digoxin plus a β-blocker or diltiazem has been described previously for control of heart rate in atrial fibrillation. Calvert (this volume, p 799) and Hamlin (*CVT XI*, p 694) describe the drugs used for management of ventricular rhythm disturbances associated with this condition.

Dogs with DCM may be presented in cardiogenic shock, which is characterized by pulmonary edema or pleural effusion, elevated venous pressures, hypotension, hypothermia, pallor, and other signs of low cardiac output. Emergency measures that include strict cage rest, supplemental oxygen, morphine, transcutaneous nitroglycerin (or intravenous sodium nitroprusside), intravenous furosemide, and infusion of dobutamine or dopamine (see Section 2) are needed during the initial 48 hr of therapy. Bronchodilators, thoracocentesis, and even mechanical ventilatory assistance may be needed to rescue such patients. Once stable, conventional therapy can be initiated. Invasive monitoring in an emergency or critical care hospital may be beneficial to quantify the effects of various drugs on cardiac output, blood pressure, preload, heart rate, rhythm, and indices of afterload and myocardial oxygen demand. Invasive hemodynamic monitoring is expensive and requires intensive nursing care, but it can provide essential information that allows rapid adjustments in the treatment regimen while providing objective evidence of therapeutic effects.

## Hypertrophic Cardiomyopathy

In asymptomatic cats with a (echocardiographic) diagnosis of hypertrophic cardiomyopathy, clients are offered a choice of either diltiazem (7.5 mg every 8 hr PO) or atenolol (12.5 mg every 12 to 24 hr PO). We prefer diltiazem when there is moderate to severe left ventricular hypertrophy (e.g., septum or ventricular wall measurements >8 or 9 mm). When there is echocardiographic or Doppler evidence of significant left ventricular outflow tract obstruction, β-blockade is preferred, either as monotherapy or in combination with diltiazem. If client medication compliance is an issue, once-daily atenolol is recommended.

When congestive heart failure develops in the cat with hypertrophic cardiomyopathy, initial efforts should be directed to reducing pulmonary edema or pleural effusion. Large effusates should be aspirated. Oxygen, topical nitroglycerine ointment (¼ inch every 8 hr), and parenteral furosemide (1 to 2 mg/kg IM or IV every 8 to 12 hr) should be administered until the cat is no longer dyspneic. Subsequently, the diuretic dose is reduced by at least 50% and the nitrate discontinued. Recommended chronic therapy for cats with hypertrophic cardiomyopathy includes avoidance of stress and administration of diltiazem (7.5 mg, t.i.d. PO), which is supplemented as needed with furosemide (1.0 mg/kg PO, p.r.n.). The requirement for diuretic therapy varies greatly among cats, and some cats will need twice-daily treatment, while in others the diuretic can be discontinued. The diuretic dose can be determined by observation of activity, respiratory rate and effort at rest, and periodic chest radiographs. Atenolol (12.5 mg once daily) is used in these cats only if there is substantial left ventricular outflow obstruction, frequent ventricular arrhythmias, or persistent sinus tachycardia. If the cat has experienced more than one episode of heart failure, or has developed a chronic pleural effusion, an ACE inhibitor is added to the regimen (enalapril, 0.25 to 0.5 mg/kg PO every 12 to 24 hr).

## References and Suggested Reading

Bristow MR, et al: Beta-adrenergic function in heart muscle disease and heart failure. J Mol Cell Cardiol 17:41, 1985.
*A comprehensive review of β-adrenergic receptor function in heart failure, including an original conceptual framework of the pathogenesis of heart failure.*

The CONSENSUS Trial Study Group: Effects of enalapril on mortality in severe congestive heart failure; results of the Cooperative North Scandinavian Enalapril survival Study. N Engl J Med 316:1429, 1987.
*Multicenter clinical trial proving the beneficial effects of enalapril on mortality in severe congestive heart failure in humans.*

The SOLVD investigators: Effect of enalapril on mortality and the development of heart failure in asymptomatic patients with reduced left ventricular ejection fractions. N Engl J Med 327:685, 1992.
*Multicenter clinical trial demonstrating the benefit of enalapril in patients with asymptomatic heart disease.*

Ferguson DW: Digitalis and neurohormonal abnormalities in heart failure and implications for therapy. Am J Cardiol 69:24G, 1992.
*Recent comprehensive review by the investigator who first demonstrated the sympathoinhibitory and baroreceptor reflex normalizing effects of digitalis.*

Engelmeir RS, O'Connell JB, Walsh R, et al: Improvement in symptoms and exercise tolerance by metoprolol in patients with dilated cardiomyopathy: A double blind, randomized, placebo-controlled trial. Circulation 72:536, 1985.
*A well-controlled trial documenting the beneficial effects of metoprolol in human dilated cardiomyopathy.*

Liang C-S, Frantz RP, and Suematsu M: Chronic beta-adrenoceptor blockade prevents the development of beta-adrenergic subsensitivity in experimental right-sided congestive heart failure in dogs. Circulation 84:254, 1991.
*Original report of the effect of β-blockade in a model of canine heart failure.*

The Captopril-Digoxin Multicenter Research Group: Comparative effects of captopril and digoxin in patients with mild to moderate heart failure. JAMA 259:539, 1988.
*Multicenter clinical trial in which the effects of diuretics alone are compared to results with captopril and digoxin in human heart failure patients.*

Yusuf S, et al: Need for a large randomized trial to evaluate the effects of digitalis on morbidity and mortality in congestive heart failure. Am J Cardiol 69:64G, 1992.
*Outline of a large, controlled clinical trial to test the effects of digitalis on morbidity and mortality in human heart failure.*

# ANGIOTENSIN-CONVERTING ENZYME INHIBITORS

PHILIP R. FOX
*New York, New York*

*and* D. DAVID SISSON
*Urbana, Illinois*

Heart failure develops when impaired systolic or diastolic function reduces cardiac output below the level needed to support tissue metabolic requirements. Decreased cardiac performance results in a series of complex neuroendocrine mechanisms such as heightened sympathetic drive, renin-angiotensin-aldosterone system activation, and antidiuretic hormone release. Initially, these serve to preserve systemic blood pressure, maintain circulatory homeostasis, and thereby assist the failing heart. Ultimately, they contribute to deteriorating ventricular function, cause progressive hemodynamic embarrassment, and precipitate characteristic signs comprising the clinical syndrome of congestive heart failure.

While rapid progress has been made during the past decade in diagnosing heart disease, less spectacular accomplishments have occurred in heart failure therapy. The prognosis for dogs with congestive heart failure is generally poor. Many die relatively soon—often within months—after the recognized onset of overt clinical signs, due to either the relentless progression of congestive heart failure or the development of lethal arrhythmias.

Data from human trials indicate that a category of vasodilators—the angiotensin-converting enzyme (ACE) inhibitors—prolong survival and are distinctly useful in management of heart failure. In humans, modulation of neurohormonal derangements associated with heart failure offers the best currently available opportunity to improve the quality and duration of life. Recently, several controlled multicenter trials have evaluated the safety and efficacy of enalapril in dogs with heart failure. Similarly, these studies demonstrate a high degree of safety, clinical improvement, and enhanced survival in dogs treated with an ACE inhibitor (enalapril) compared with those who did not receive this drug.

## REVIEW OF NEUROENDOCRINE DISTURBANCES IN HEART FAILURE

Important neuroendocrine alterations in heart failure include heightened sympathetic tone, activation of the renin-angiotensin-aldosterone system, and antidiuretic hormone release. Other compensatory changes tend to blunt excessive vasoconstriction and sodium retention (e.g., endogenous vasodilating substances [prostaglandins, dopamine], atrial natriuretic peptide). As heart failure progresses, however, mechanisms producing vasoconstriction and sodium retention dominate those which induce vasodilation or natriuresis (Table 1). Ex-

amples of the adverse consequences of neuroendocrine activity include increased sympathetic outflow, increasing afterload, and reducing forward stroke volume; systemic vasoconstriction (effects of norepinephrine, angiotensin II, and arginine vasopressin), which leads to further compromise of stroke volume and cardiac output; and sodium and water retention (via renal adaptations and aldosterone release) causing pulmonary and systemic venous congestion. The sympathetic nervous system and renin-angiotensin mechanisms are also linked by multiple positive feedback loops that favor progressive activation of one system when the other is stimulated (Fig. 1).

## PHYSIOLOGIC ACTIONS AND BENEFITS OF ACE INHIBITORS

Converting enzyme inhibitors are the most important class of neurohormonal antagonists currently available for treating congestive heart failure. Agents that inhibit converting enzyme exert their activity at a strategic physiologic junction by blocking conversion of angiotensin I to the circulating octapeptide, angiotensin II (Fig. 1). The latter is a potent vasoconstrictor that contributes to increased cardiac afterload, and is itself a primary stimulus for aldosterone release by the adrenal cortex. Aldosterone enhances renal retention of sodium and water which increases blood volume and cardiac preload. By inhibiting the angiotensin-converting enzyme, many of the deleterious consequences of vasoconstriction (angiotensin II) and sodium retention (aldosterone) can be avoided in heart failure. Some of the anticipated hemodynamic changes resulting from ACE inhibition include decreased atrial and ventricular filling pressures, decreased peripheral vascular resistance, and increased cardiac output.

Other physiologic effects have been reported with ACE inhibitors. For example, decreased concentrations of circulating angiotensin II reduce the facilitory role of this vasoactive peptide on norepinephrine and antidiuretic hormone release. A relationship between de-

***Table 1.*** *Compensatory Adaptations in Adverse Consequences of Neuroendocrine Responses in Congestive Heart Failure*

| Adaptive Mechanisms | Physiologic Changes | Initial Compensatory Advantages | Adverse Consequences ("Overcompensation") |
|---|---|---|---|
| Activation of renin-angiotensin-aldosterone system; ↑ Adrenergic drive | Arteriolar constriction; Tachycardia | Helps maintain blood pressure and tissue perfusion; ↑ Contractility; ↑ Cardiac output | ↑ Afterload; ↓ Stroke volume; Tissue anoxia; ↑ Myocardial oxygen demand; $\beta_1$ receptor "down-regulation"; Sympathetic activation leads to renin release and angiotensin II formation |
| Aldosterone release | Increases blood volume, venous return and cardiac filling | ↑ Filling volumes and pressures; Helps maintain stroke volume via the Frank-Starling mechanism | Fluid retention; Excess venous filling pressure results in pulmonary and systemic congestion; Potassium loss |
| Antidiuretic hormone secretion | Increases blood volume | As above | Extracellular fluid retention, pulmonary and systemic congestion; ↑ Afterload; Hyponatremia |
| Baroreceptor-mediated response to hypotension | Tachycardia | Helps maintain cardiac output | ↑ Cardiac work; ↓ Myocardial perfusion |

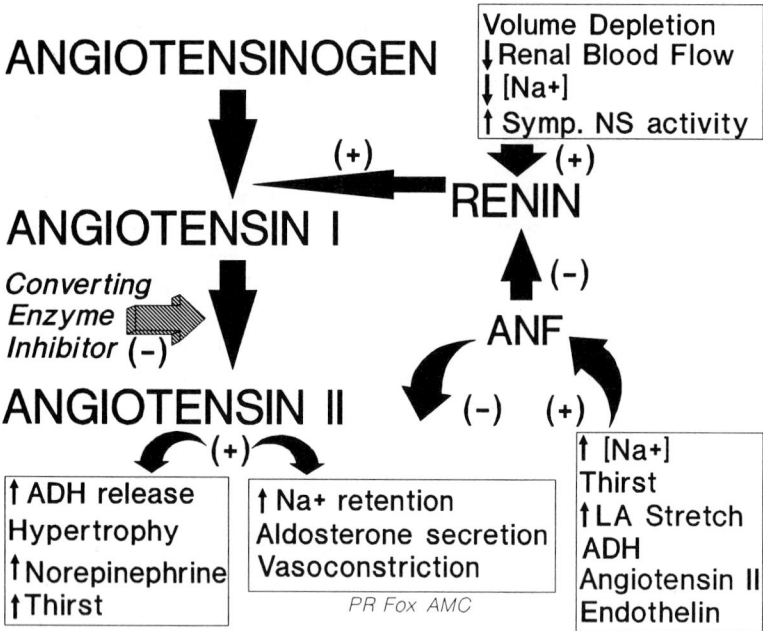

**Figure 1.** Some of the major physiologic alterations activated during heart failure. (+) indicates positive stimulatory feedback; (−) indicates negative or suppressive feedback; ANF, atrial natriuretic factor (peptide); [Na$^+$], sodium concentration; ADH, antidiuretic hormone.

creased ventricular ectopy and sudden death in humans treated with ACE inhibitors, and reduced norepinephrine release, has been suggested. It has also been reported that sulfhydryl-containing ACE inhibitors, such as captopril, can be converted into disulphides, which function as free radical scavengers. The clinical importance of this effect is unclear, but this mechanism might limit some of the adverse consequences of myocardial ischemia. Furthermore, bradykinins, which induce vasodilation by increasing prostaglandin $I_2$ ($PGI_2$) and $PGE_2$ production, are inhibited by converting enzymes. Angiotensin-converting enzyme inhibitors may allow bradykinins to accumulate in tissues and promote favorable hemodynamic effects, although bradykinin levels are not consistently elevated following ACE inhibition. Moreover, local renin-angiotensin systems believed to regulate cellular growth have been demonstrated in cardiac and vascular tissues. Some investigators suggest beneficial effects due to tissue ACE inhibition, mitigating effects on ventricular remodeling, and myocardial fibrosis.

## EVIDENCE TO SUPPORT ACE INHIBITOR USE IN HEART FAILURE THERAPY

In humans with overt congestive heart failure, ACE inhibitors have been shown to improve hemodynamic function, relieve clinical symptoms of heart failure, and reduce overall mortality from cardiovascular disease. As early as 1983, the Captopril Multicenter Research Group reported significant improvement of clinical symptoms in human heart failure patients treated with the ACE inhibitor captopril. In a landmark study published several years later, the Cooperative North Scandinavian Enalapril Survival Study (CONSENSUS) group reported that enalapril treatment significantly re-

duced mortality in humans with severe New York Heart Association ([NYHA] class III/IV) heart failure. The treatment arm of the Studies of Left Ventricular Dysfunction (SOLVD) trial indicated in 1991 that enalapril can reduce morbidity and mortality in patients with less severe heart failure (NYHA class II/III). Moreover, the prevention arm of the SOLVD trial, published in 1992, suggested that onset of heart failure could be delayed by enalapril administration in people with asymptomatic heart diseases caused by dilated cardiomyopathy (DCM) or chronic mitral regurgitation. Studies documenting the clinical efficacy of other ACE inhibitors are in progress.

Recently, large multicenter clinical trials investigated the safety and efficacy of enalapril in the management of canine heart failure caused by DCM or chronic mitral regurgitation. These studies demonstrated substantial benefit to animals managed with enalapril, compared with dogs who did not receive an ACE inhibitor. The Invasive Multicenter Prospective Veterinary Enalapril (IMPROVE) study group reported the primary hemodynamic effect of enalapril (0.5 mg/kg every 12 hr) was a significant decline in pulmonary capillary wedge pressure (PCWP). The clinical consequence of this effect as demonstrated in other trials was improvement of the heart failure state. Not surprisingly, heart rate also declines significantly in dogs treated with enalapril. Interestingly, there was no demonstrable effect of enalapril on systemic vascular resistance or cardiac output in the IMPROVE study. Investigators in the Cooperative Veterinary Enalapril (COVE) study group reported that enalapril, used in combination with conventional therapy (digoxin and furosemide), significantly reduced the clinical signs of heart failure in dogs with DCM or mitral regurgitation. This included reduced severity of pulmonary edema, improvement in the class of heart failure, reduced cough, improved respiratory effort, increased appetite, and improved exercise tolerance. The clinical benefits of ACE inhibitor treatment were most pronounced in those dogs with heart failure caused by DCM. In the enalapril long-term efficacy study, the mean number of days to heart failure or death in the enalapril group for all treated dogs was 169 compared with 90 days in dogs receiving conventional therapy and placebo. The benefits of ACE inhibitor treatment appear to be sustained with chronic therapy.

While other ACE inhibitors might be as effective as enalapril for treating dogs with heart failure, their relative safety and efficacy have not been evaluated in large-scale or long-term clinical trials. The efficacy and safety of ACE-inhibiting drugs in cats has not yet been reported, though these drugs have been used empirically in therapy of CHF.

## PHARMACOLOGY OF ACE-INHIBITOR DRUGS

Currently, there are over 70 different ACE inhibitors under investigation or on the market. Each of these compounds contains either a sulfhydryl-, carboxyl-, or phosphoryl group that acts on the zinc ion-containing active site of angiotensin-converting enzyme. The relative potency of these compounds, as measured by inhibition of circulating ACE, depends on the affinity of the zinc ligand as well as the number of any additional ACE binding sites. Drugs that are more tightly bound to ACE tend to be more potent and more slowly eliminated than drugs that are loosely bound. Thus, enalaprilat and lisinopril are more potent than captopril and they also have a longer duration of action. Differences in potency should not be overemphasized, however, as these are relative differences that generally can be compensated for by adjusting the dosage and/or frequency of administration.

Captopril, lisinopril, and enalapril (after conversion to enalaprilat) are eliminated almost entirely by the kidney via glomerular filtration and tubular secretion. The rate of elimination of these drugs declines with decreased renal function, indicating the potential necessity for dosage adjustment in this circumstance. Captopril and lisinopril are active drugs that are well absorbed orally. Enalapril and the newer ACE inhibitors are prodrugs that must first be converted by the liver to its active compound.

*Captopril*, the first commercially available ACE inhibitor, is a sulfhydryl-containing ACE inhibitor. Its bioavailability is about 75% in fasted dogs, but this is reduced by 30 to 40% when there is food in the gastrointestinal tract. Captopril begins to exert a significant hemodynamic effect within 1 hr after oral administration. Peak effect occurs approximately 1 to 2 hr after administration. Thereafter, the ACE-inhibiting activity of captopril declines rapidly as the compound is excreted. For this reason, captopril must be administered to dogs two to three times daily and is dosed at 0.5 to 2.0 mg/kg PO two to three times a day.

*Lisinopril*, a lysine derivative of enalaprilat, is a carboxyl-containing ACE inhibitor. Its bioavailability is 25

to 50% and is not affected by feeding. Time to peak ACE-inhibiting effect is 6 to 8 hr. The duration of ACE inhibition appears to be much longer for lisinopril than for captopril. Based on limited, and as yet unpublished, clinical studies (Sisson, unpublished data), lisinopril appears to be effective for the treatment of heart failure in dogs with dilated cardiomyopathy when it is administered once daily (0.5 mg/kg/day; blood pressure should be monitored). Trials comparing efficacy of once- versus twice-daily dosing have not been performed.

*Enalapril*, an ester prodrug with very little ACE activity, becomes active when converted (hydrolyzed) in the liver to the diacid enalaprilat, a very potent ACE inhibitor. Enalapril is well absorbed in dogs. Peak absorption of oral enalapril administration occurs at approximately 2 hr and its bioavailability is about 64%. Enalapril must be hydrolyzed to its active diacid form. Peak concentrations of enalaprilat and peak ACE inhibition occur approximately 4 hr after the oral administration of enalapril. At the recommended average starting dose (0.5 mg/kg once daily PO) for enalapril, ACE inhibition is minimal 24 hr after the initial oral dose. For this reason, there is some divergence of opinion regarding the optimal dosing interval. Available evidence suggests that enalapril is effective for the treatment of canine heart failure when given once daily. In some dogs, however, optimal benefit is achieved when the dosing frequency is increased to twice daily.

There are little data concerning the use and efficacy of ACE inhibitors in cats. Sanders and coworkers reported that in healthy cats given oral enalapril (0.25 mg/kg or 0.5 mg/kg) once daily, 95% reduction in ACE was recorded 2 to 4 hr after administration, and ACE levels remained depressed to less than 50% of controls for 2 to 3 days. Clinically efficacious dosages in cardiomyopathic cats have not been documented, and related information is anecdotal. We have safely administered enalapril (0.25 to 0.5 mg/kg s.i.d. to b.i.d. PO) and captopril (0.5 to 1.25 mg/kg s.i.d. to b.i.d. PO) to cats with various forms of cardiomyopathy and heart failure.

## DRUG SAFETY AND POTENTIAL COMPLICATIONS

Overall, ACE inhibitors appear to be safe and well tolerated in dogs with congestive heart failure. This may vary somewhat with the particular type of ACE inhibitor and with concomitant administration of other drugs. Of the ACE inhibitors currently available, the most is known about enalapril based on large multicenter clinical veterinary trials. Accordingly, this drug has become the preferred agent based upon proven safety and efficacy. Captopril, the first available orally active ACE inhibitor, was used extensively in the 1980s. While it was never assessed in large clinical studies, many investigators suggest that captopril is not well tolerated by dogs with congestive heart failure. A high incidence of vomiting, diarrhea, or anorexia often results. Lisinopril has not been as widely used in dogs as enalapril and captopril. Unpublished data (Sisson) suggest that adverse reactions with lisinopril administration are generally mild and similar to those reported with enalapril, although insufficient numbers of dogs have been treated with lisinopril to comment on the prevalence or severity of untoward reactions.

Specific adverse effects of ACE-inhibiting drugs include systemic hypotension, renal dysfunction, gastrointestinal upset (vomiting, diarrhea, anorexia), and hyperkalemia.

*Systemic hypotension* is an infrequently observed complication in dogs when ACE inhibitors are administered in recommended dosages. In the authors' experience, hypotension is most likely to occur in severe heart failure when (1) recommended doses of ACE inhibitor are exceeded; (2) other vasodilating drugs are used in combination with an ACE inhibitor; (3) high doses of potent diuretics such as furosemide are given; and (4) the animal is relatively volume contracted owing to effects of anorexia, fluid third spacing, or overzealous diuresis. In these circumstances, the patient should ideally be hospitalized to initiate therapy and the dog and blood pressure closely monitored. Hypotension is most likely to occur within the first 24 to 48 hr, or if severe volume depletion occurs from heavy diuretic usage. Clinically, affected animals appear depressed, weak, anoretic, and may display an unsteady gait or inability to ambulate. Arterial blood pressure should be measured (see "Doppler Assessment of Blood Flow and Pressure in Surgical and Critical Care Patients," this volume, p 113) to document hypotension and guide therapy. Systolic pressures less than 100 mm Hg should be avoided. Management of symptomatic hypotension or acute renal failure includes reducing the dose of ACE inhibitor, decreasing or eliminating concomitant hypotensive agents (e.g., diuretics, other vasodilators), and judicious intravenous fluid administration.

*Azotemia* may result from functional renal insufficiency in conjunction with ACE-inhibitor therapy. In chronic congestive heart failure, glomerular filtration rate may be preserved despite reduced renal blood flow. This may be due to the effects of angiotensin II effecting relatively greater vasoconstriction on the efferent than afferent renal arteriole. Converting enzyme inhibitors, by blocking conversion of angiotensin I to angiotensin II, may thereby reduce this compensatory mechanism and predispose to renal insufficiency.

In veterinary medicine, evaluations of morbidity are complete only for enalapril. Investigators of the enalapril clinical canine heart failure field studies recorded azotemia (blood urea nitrogen [BUN] >50 mg/dl or creatinine >2.5 mg/dl) in 12% of heart failure dogs (NYHA class II, III, or IV) treated for 2 days with furosemide (mean dose = 4.2 mg/kg/day). After then initiating enalapril or placebo in a double-blind study, 13% receiving placebo were azotemic compared with 22% receiving enalapril ($p$ = .045) at one or more time points (day 2, 14, 21, or 28). It is therefore important to realize that mild to moderate azotemia is common in a substantial percentage of dogs (and most cats) with congestive heart failure, before drug therapy, and especially after furosemide is administered. Azotemia is usually interpreted in these populations as a consequence of decreased renal perfusion (prerenal azotemia) combined with, in older animals, an age-related decline in renal functional capacity.

The magnitude of azotemia may be influenced by factors that further compromise renal blood flow such as volume contraction from diuretics, severe salt restriction, anorexia, vomiting, or fluid third spacing; underlying cardiovascular disease and reduced cardiac output; and development of systemic hypotension. Transient, mild increases in BUN/creatinine may then be related to ACE inhibitors once administration is initiated. It is noteworthy that very mild, nonclinical elevations in BUN or creatinine occurred in the majority of heart failure dogs treated with furosemide plus either enalapril or placebo during the first 3 to 4 weeks of ACE-inhibitor therapy. We therefore believe it prudent to assess a biochemical profile prior to initiating therapy as well as 3 to 7 days after an ACE inhibitor is started. In general, serum creatinine and BUN usually normalize or stabilize at a new steady state with chronic use of ACE enalapril. Since a small percentage of dogs will become azotemic between 1 and 4 weeks after ACE-inhibitor drug therapy, however, the animal's condition should be closely monitored by the owner. A biochemical profile and urinalysis should be promptly reassessed if lethargy, anorexia, or emesis occurs. When mild to moderate azotemia is identified, most dogs respond after diuretic dose reduction. We advocate decreasing the total daily dose of furosemide 50% in this circumstance.

It is important to use the minimal effective diuretic dose when administering ACE inhibitor. In small-breed dogs with first-time congestive heart failure (mild to moderate pulmonary edema) associated with mitral regurgitation, for example, we prefer to administer furosemide starting at 1.1 to 1.6 mg/kg two to three times daily as needed, in combination with ACE inhibitors and digoxin. The lowest effective dose of diuretic should then be utilized when congestion resolves. In cats, we initiate furosemide at 1.1 mg/kg two to three times a day for mild to moderate pulmonary edema. With chronic heart failure, the diuretic dose may rise by gradual, incremental increases according to patient needs, disease progression, and relative drug resistance.

Severe renal failure has been reported with all ACE-inhibitors usually developing shortly after their initiation. Therapy should be altered if serum creatinine concentrations exceed 2.5 to 3.0 mg/dl or BUN concentrations exceed 60 to 70 mg/dl. Most dogs and cats can be adequately managed by skipping one or two doses of diuretic followed by decreasing the diuretic dose by 50%. Occasionally, ACE-inhibitor therapy has to be reduced or abandoned. Judicious administration of fluids is sometimes warranted, especially when animals are anorectic. Subcutaneous administration is often adequate in cats, but intravenous administration may be necessary with severe renal insufficiency.

*Hyperkalemia* is a potential complication with ACE inhibitors. It can result from severely reduced glomerular filtration and diminished release of aldosterone. Practically speaking, however, the degree of observed hyperkalemia in clinical veterinary enalapril trials is negligible. Should severe hyperkalemia occur, discontinuation or reduction in ACE inhibitor dosage is warranted. The use of potassium supplements and potassium-sparing diuretics should probably be avoided in dogs receiving ACE-inhibiting drugs.

## TREATMENT OF CONGESTIVE HEART FAILURE

Therapeutic strategies for heart failure are changing. Traditional management of canine congestive heart failure has relied upon diuretics to reduce intravascular volume and positive inotropes to stimulate myocardial contraction. By the early 1980s, oral vasodilators had become well established for use in acute congestive heart failure to reduce peripheral vascular resistance and ventricular filling pressures. Although employed for chronic therapy as well, no data were available to prove that they prolonged survival. Studies in humans have demonstrated that certain direct-acting vasodilating drugs (hydralazine combined with isosorbide dinitrate), in addition to improving clinical signs, can reduce mortality of congestive heart failure patients. However, these directly acting vasodilator drugs often activate rather than suppress sympathetic nervous system activity and other neurohumoral systems. The potential value of ACE inhibitors over these direct-acting agents results from their beneficial effects of reducing clinical signs and decreasing mortality, while blunting neurohumoral activation.

It is the opinion of the authors that ACE inhibitors should be prescribed, together with appropriate doses of digoxin and furosemide, in most dogs with acquired heart failure caused by dilated cardiomyopathy or mitral regurgitation. In order to afford dogs with acquired heart disease the maximum possible benefit from ACE inhibiting drugs, we advocate their use as soon as conclusive evidence of congestive heart failure is apparent. It is no longer rational to withhold ACE-inhibiting drugs simply because the patient's clinical status improves on conventional therapy (diuretics and digitalis). The use of ACE inhibitors should not be reserved solely for dogs with refractory heart failure. Because of the unique advantages afforded by the physiologic actions of ACE inhibitors, these agents should be used as part of initial and chronic management in most dogs

with acquired heart failure. Since ACE inhibitors provide clinical and hemodynamic benefit in moderate and severe heart failure, the question arises as to whether they are also indicated in animals with left ventricular dysfunction or volume overload but who do not yet have overt heart failure. Currently, recommendations for prophylactic therapy must await outcomes of related studies. While clinical efficacy data are lacking for use of ACE inhibitors with feline cardiomyopathies, our initial impressions are generally positive.

In recognition of the seriousness of congestive heart failure in dogs and cats with acquired heart disease, most patients managed for chronic heart failure should be routinely reevaluated every 2 to 4 months.

## References and Suggested Reading

Captopril Multicenter Research Group: A placebo-controlled trial of captopril in refractory congestive heart failure. J Am Coll Cardiol 2:755, 1983.

Dzau VJ: Renin-angiotensin system and renal circulation in clinical congestive heart failure. Kidney Int 31(suppl 20):S203, 1987.

Fox PR: The effect of drug therapy on clinical characteristics and outcome in dogs with heart failure. *Proc 10th Ann Vet Med Forum*, 1992, pp 592–593.

Francis GS: Neuroendocrine manifestations of congestive heart failure. Am J Cardiol 62:9A, 1988.

Longhofer SL, Ericsson GF, Cifelli S, and Benitz AM: Renal function in heart failure dogs receiving furosemide and enalapril maleate. *Proc 11th Ann Vet Med Forum*, 1993, p 936(A).

Ljungman S, Kjekshus J, and Swedberg K, for the CONSENSUS Trial Group: Renal function in severe congestive heart failure during treatment with enalapril (the Cooperative North Scandinavian Enalapril Survival Study [CONSENSUS] Trial). Am J Cardiol 70:479, 1992.

Packer M, Lee WH, Medina N, et al: Functional renal insufficiency during long term therapy with captopril and enalapril in chronic congestive heart failure. Ann Intern Med 106:346, 1987.

Proceedings of a National Heart, Lung, and Blood Institute Symposium: Mechanisms and management of heart failure: implications of clinical trials for clinical practice. J Am Coll Cardiol 22(suppl A):146A, 1993.

Riegger GA, Liebau G, Holzschuh M, et al: Role of the renin-angiotensin system in the development of congestive heart failure in the dog as assessed by chronic converting-enzyme blockade. Am J Cardiol 53:614, 1984.

Sanders N, Hamlin R, Buffington T, and Blaisdell J: Effects of enalapril on healthy cats. *Proc 10th Ann Vet Med Forum*, 1992, p 822(A).

Salvetti A: Newer ACE inhibitors. A look at the future. Drugs 40:800, 1990.

Sisson DD: Hemodynamic, echocardiographic, radiographic, and clinical effects of enalapril in dogs with chronic heart failure. *Proc 10th ACVIM Forum*, 1992, pp 589–591.

Sisson DD: Evidence for or against the efficacy of afterload reducers for management of heart failure in dots. Vet Clin North Am 21:945, 1991.

Swedberg K, Eneroth P, Kjekshus J, Snapinn S, for the CONSENSUS Trial Study Group: Effects of enalapril and neuroendocrine activation on prognosis in severe congestive heart failure (follow-up of the CONSENSUS trial). Am J Cardiol 66:40D, 1990.

The CONCENSUS Trial Study Group: Effects of enalapril on mortality in severe congestive heart failure: Results of the Cooperative North Scandinavian Enalapril Survival Study (CONSENSUS). N Engl J Med 316:1429, 1987.

The SOLVD Investigators: Studies of left ventricular dysfunction (SOLVD)—rationale, design, and methods: Two trials that evaluate the effect of enalapril in patients with reduced ejection fraction. Am J Cardiol 66:315, 1990.

The SOLVD Investigators: Effect of enalapril on survival in patients with reduced left ventricular ejection fractions and congestive heart failure. N Engl J Med 325:293, 1991.

# TWENTY-FOUR-HOUR AMBULATORY ELECTROCARDIOGRAPHY (HOLTER MONITORING)

N. SYDNEY MOISE
*Ithaca, New York*

*and* TERESA DEFRANCESCO
*Raleigh, North Carolina*

Ambulatory (Holter) electrocardiography (ECG) is a widely used noninvasive modality in human medicine for the evaluation of cardiac rhythm in a variety of disease states. The clinical use of Holter electrocardiography in veterinary medicine is sparse but rapidly increasing despite the technology having been available for over 30 years. A physicist, Normal Jeff Holter, first developed the ambulatory ECG recording after a close friend died of sudden cardiac death. The first Holter recorder weighed over 80 lb; presently, the average recorder (Fig. 1) weighs about 1 lb or less and thus is applicable to the majority of our patients.

The clinical utility of the ambulatory ECG lies in its ability to record the patient's cardiac rhythm over a long period of time (24 to 48 hr) and in the assessment of the ECG during exercise and in a home environment. A typical resting ECG (5 min) only samples 0.3% of a 24-hr period; thus, the Holter recording allows the clinician to make more accurate evaluations of the cardiac rhythm. The purpose of this article is to introduce the veterinary practitioner to Holter technology, its clinical applications, and the interpretation of the 24-hr ECG report.

## EQUIPMENT

### How to Rent a Holter Recorder

A Holter monitor, including an electromagnetic tape with easy-to-follow instructions and hook-up kit, can be acquired by any veterinary practitioner by overnight courier from a Holter monitoring company. Bio-Medical Roche Ambulatory Monitoring Services (RAMS), based in Burlington, NC, is one of these companies that has some experience with veterinary electrocardiography. Their toll-free telephone number is (800) 426-2176. After the recording is completed, the Holter monitoring kit is mailed to the company for data processing. A full report is usually obtained in 5 to 7 days. The current fee for the service is about $130.00. It is advised to check in the veterinarian's local area for other Holter monitoring companies for convenience; however, as detailed below, it is important that the company have experience analyzing canine tapes, preferably with the oversight of a veterinary cardiologist.

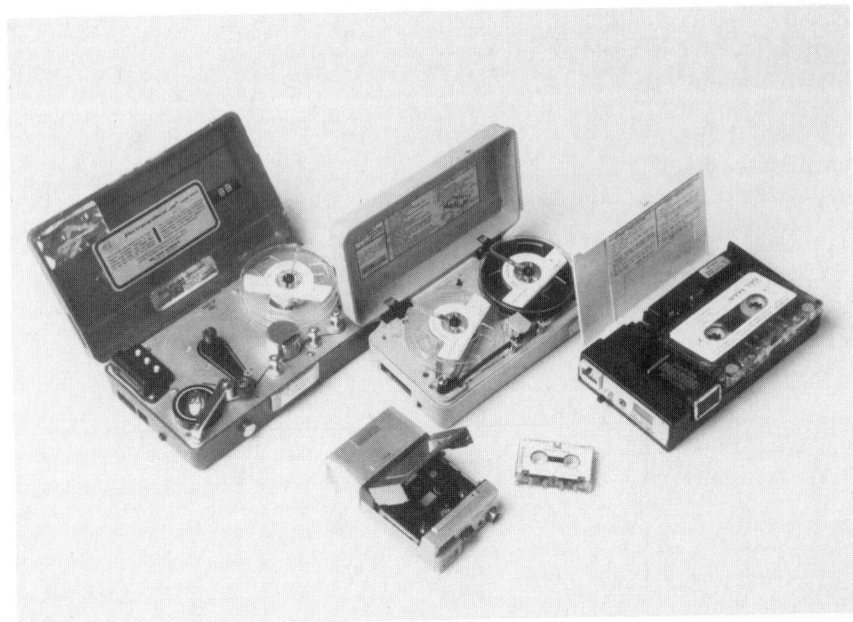

**Figure 1.** Four different Holter recorders. Two are reel-to-reel, two-channel recorders (*left*); one (*right*) is a three-channel cassette recorder; and one is a three-channel microcassette (*center front*) recorder.

## How to Obtain a Holter Recording

A quality recording is essential for accurate rhythm evaluation (Fig. 2). Excessive artifact may result in elimination of important periods of ECG recording. Proper application of the electrodes, careful connection of the leads to the recorder, and proper securing of the recorder to the animal are the first steps to a diagnostic recording (Fig. 3). Two- and three-lead recorders are available, with the three-lead system preferred. Multiple leads are desired because, despite careful application, sometimes one lead may be missing if an error is made in the connections or artifacts result in a lead

that cannot be interpreted. Multiple leads allow for a more accurate interpretation of the ECG (Fig. 4). Depending upon the number of channels, various lead configurations can be used (in Fig. 3, the placement for X, Y, and Z leads and $V_1$, $V_3$, and $V_5$ leads are illustrated). The precordial lead configuration may record larger, more obvious P waves; while the X, Ý, Z lead configuration is preferred for signal averaging.

Some dogs may develop skin irritation from the electrode patches and glue. This problem resolves once the patches are removed. Several applications of a corticosteroid cream can hasten healing. In elderly or weak patients, it is very important not to secure the recorder

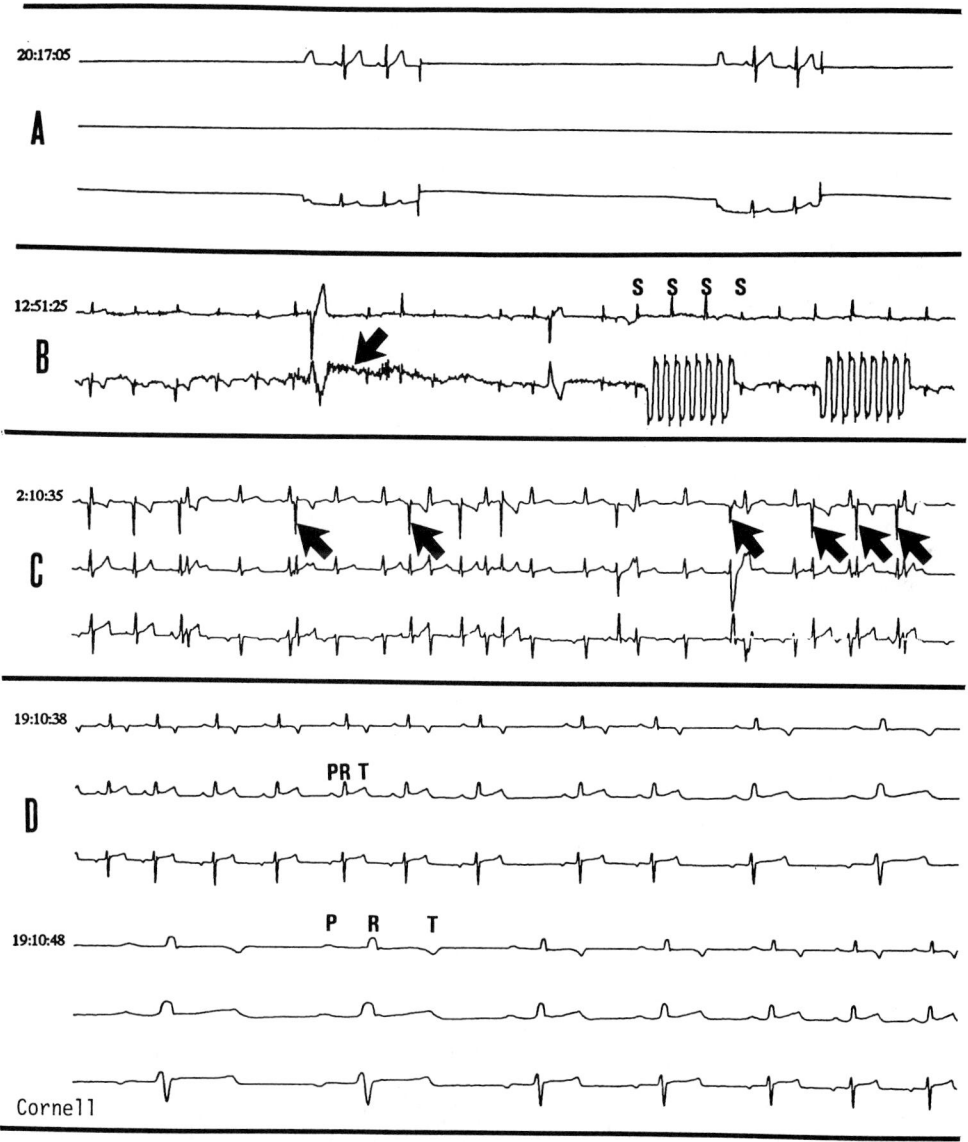

**Figure 2.** *A*, Improper lead connections result in the absence of one lead, and in the other two leads an artifact is seen that could have been mistaken for sinus arrest. *B*, Electrical interference caused an artifact that could have been mistaken for ventricular tachycardia (especially when viewed on the compressed full-disclosure report); however, the value of at least two leads is demonstrated here. In the top lead, a sinus rhythm (S) is seen and alerts the operator to artifact in the other lead. Movement artifact is also seen (*arrow*). *C*, Artifact that mimics an arrhythmia is present here in all three leads. Only careful examination discloses the artifact (arrows indicate some of the artifact). *D*, Improper recording speed caused this artifact, which was mistakenly called "sinus bradycardia." Careful examination reveals the entire P–QRS–T complex to be elongated (two panels shown).

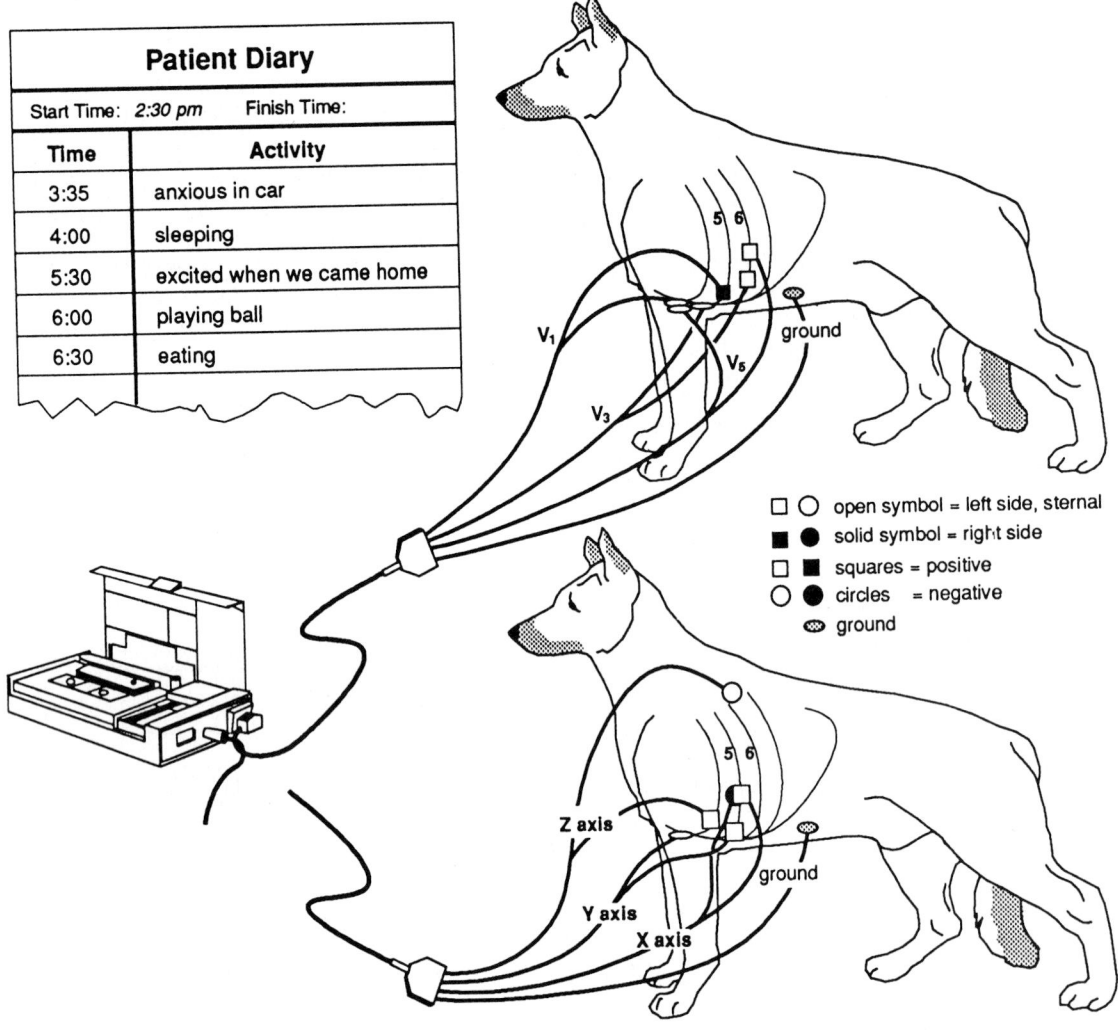

**Patient Diary**

Start Time: *2:30 pm*     Finish Time:

| Time | Activity |
|------|----------|
| 3:35 | anxious in car |
| 4:00 | sleeping |
| 5:30 | excited when we came home |
| 6:00 | playing ball |
| 6:30 | eating |

□ ○ open symbol = left side, sternal
■ ● solid symbol = right side
□ ■ squares = positive
○ ● circles = negative
⊗ ground

1. closely shave hair
2. clean and dry skin
3. apply Vetbond to electrode patches
4. attach leads
5. connect patient cable to recorder input
6. install fresh 9 volt battery
7. connect test cable to ECG machine to check ECG reference strip

8. disconnect test cable
9. unplug patient cable from recorder
10. wrap wires with Kling
11. install cassette tape
12. replace patient cable
13. enter start time
14. place recorder in case, wrap with Elasticon and ideally use vest

**Figure 3.** Steps in the application of the leads for recording a 24-hr ambulatory electrocardiographic recording are shown. The set-ups for recording the precordial leads $V_1$, $V_3$, and $V_5$ and the X, Y, and Z lead system are shown. An Elizabethan collar may be needed in some dogs. We have found that fabric patches provide the best recordings in dogs.

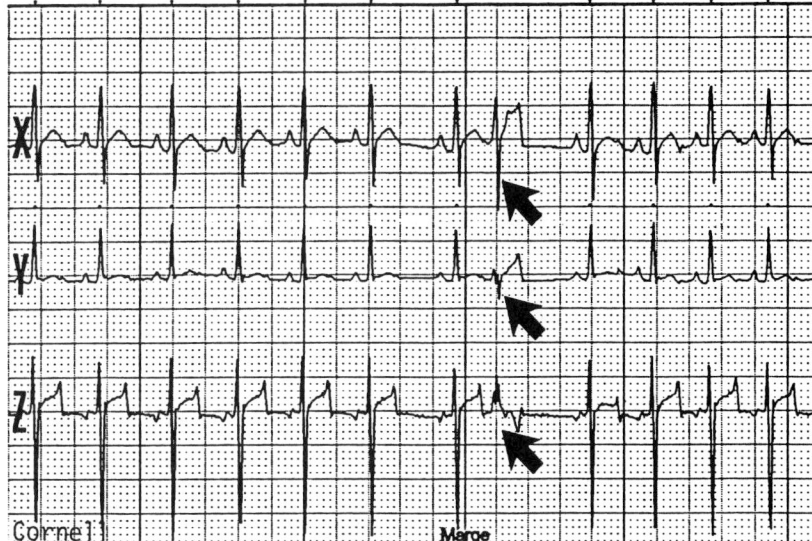

**Figure 4.** X, Y, and Z lead configuration in a dog. If only one lead (X) was being used in the analysis (either because only one lead was recorded or because the operator selected a single lead when performing the analysis), a premature ventricular complex would have been misdiagnosed as a premature supraventricular complex (*arrows*). Although the premature complex is similar to the sinus complexes in lead X, in the Y and Z leads the complex is clearly ventricular in confirmation.

to the dog so snugly that breathing is impaired. Owners should be asked to keep a detailed diary of the activity of the dog. A diary can be helpful when trying to correlate clinical signs with a cardiac arrhythmia, evaluating treatment effects relative to the timing of medication (Fig. 5), evaluating effects of exercise on the ST segment, or when trying to determine the influence of environmental situations on the development of a particular arrhythmia.

## HOLTER ANALYSIS

### How to Evaluate the Holter Report

The completed Holter report provides the details of the patient's arrhythmias, the total number and type of abnormal complexes, and the specific time of day that arrhythmias occurred. These results are graphed and tabulated, and the maximum and minimum heart rates per hour are provided. Special evaluations can be done to assess the ST segment, signal averaging, and heart rate variability. All of these data are helpful in studying the patient if they are accurate. Accurate analysis of canine Holter electrocardiography demands meticulous care and specialized knowledge of the canine ECG.

Because of technical problems in recordings and in the analytic processes, ambulatory electrocardiography has great potential for producing invalid data (Knoebel et al., 1993). Modern Holter analyzing systems are software based and the programs are constantly being updated to improve capability of arrhythmia analysis. However, these systems are not designed for canine electrocardiograms. Even with operator-integrated analysis, substantial numbers of errors in the interpretation of canine electrocardiograms should be expected. Errors are more likely with frequent and complex arrhythmias (Fig. 6) and supraventricular events. Although a beautifully presented report of a dog's 24-hr ECG recording is returned from a service, the vet-

erinarian *must critically examine the raw data* from a full-disclosure printout (24-hr of ECG recording). It is not adequate to assume that the report is accurate based on the service's record of quality control for human ECGs. Also, how the accuracy is determined is important. Correlation coefficients are an insufficient means of evaluation (Salerno, Granrud, and Hodges, 1987). Instead, the most accurate way to ensure a reasonably accurate report is to examine the annotated report (Fig. 7).

The most common error in the analysis of the canine Holter recording is the misinterpretation of sinus arrhythmia as supraventricular ectopic complexes (SVE). Although humans do have sinus arrhythmia, the variation in the RR interval is not as great as in the dog. Frequently, veterinarians simply "ignore" the report of

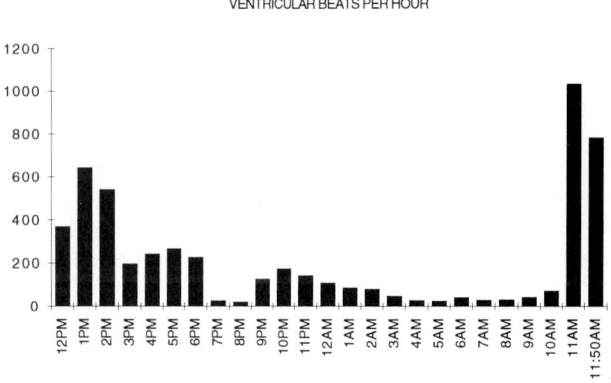

**Figure 5.** A 24-hr histogram of premature ventricular beats from a 9-year-old boxer with cardiomyopathy and syncopal episodes. The Holter was performed to evaluate efficacy of therapy (atenolol, 25 mg PO every 24 hr administered at 5:00 PM). The majority of the ventricular ectopy occurred from 12:00 AM to 6:00 PM, which prompted an increase in the dosing frequency to twice daily. Follow-up 24-hr Holter showed a reduction in the ventricular ectopy from 5461 beats to 80 beats.

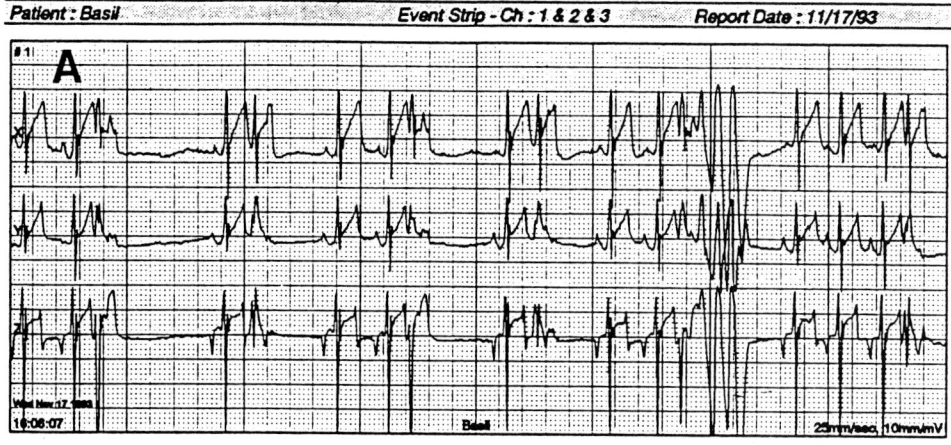

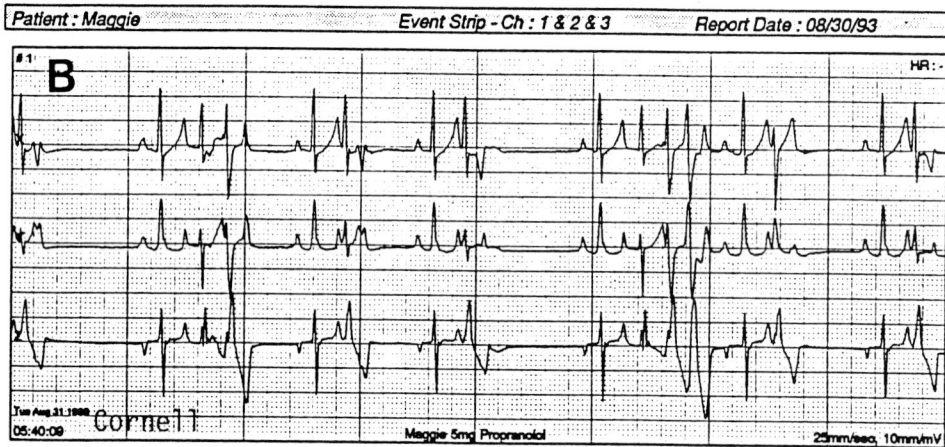

**Figure 6.** Holter recordings from two dogs (*A* and *B*) with complex arrhythmias. Polymorphic ventricular complexes, rapid rates, and short coupling intervals make these Holter recordings very time consuming to annotate for accurate counts of premature beats.

SVEs number. This may be fine as long as there really are no SVEs; however, when this arrhythmia is suspected, a better examination is needed.

While the full-disclosure report is used to check the report, the size of the complexes are too small and the speed too slow to precisely annotate beats. It is not adequate to only examine a few selected strips or "bins" if the actual counts of premature complexes are of importance. In human medicine and perhaps in veterinary medicine, analysis of heart rate variability from Holter recordings is becoming popular; however, unless all sinus beats are annotated correctly, the results are useless. Accurate identification of the QRS complex should be considered in the evaluation of new techniques applied to the canine electrocardiogram. The future for the analysis of the canine recording will depend on improved software developments (i.e., higher frequency digitization, increased logic and learning capability, new methods of arrhythmia identification such as a neural net). Many of the problems faced in the evaluation of the canine ECG also occur in pediatric Holter analysis and in canine research.

Are there so many problems in the analysis of the canine Holter recording that the technique is of little value? No, a 24-hr ECG is valuable. Despite the problems, once a clinician uses the Holter for the evaluation of patients with arrhythmias, the more apparent the inadequacies will be of the typical 1- to 5-min ECG. Therefore, for clinical use in most dogs with arrhythmias, the commercial analysis reports are helpful and adequate as long as the veterinarian checks the full-disclosure report. Dogs with a sinus rate of less than 120 bpm, classic wide monomorphic premature ventricular complexes (PVC), PVC coupling intervals that are not too close to the preceding sinus complex (outside the blanking period), and ventricular tachycardia that is not too fast are more likely to have a more accurate Holter analysis (Fig. 8).

Finally, the interpretation of the Holter report must take into account what is normal for the dog. For instance, the normal sleeping dog may have pauses as long or longer than 3 sec with a heart rate below 40 bpm and periods of low-grade, second-degree heart block. These findings may be misinterpreted as indicating sinus node or atrioventricular nodal disease. Also, older animals appear more likely to have PVCs without cardiac disease. We do not have good documentation of what is normal in dogs at various ages.

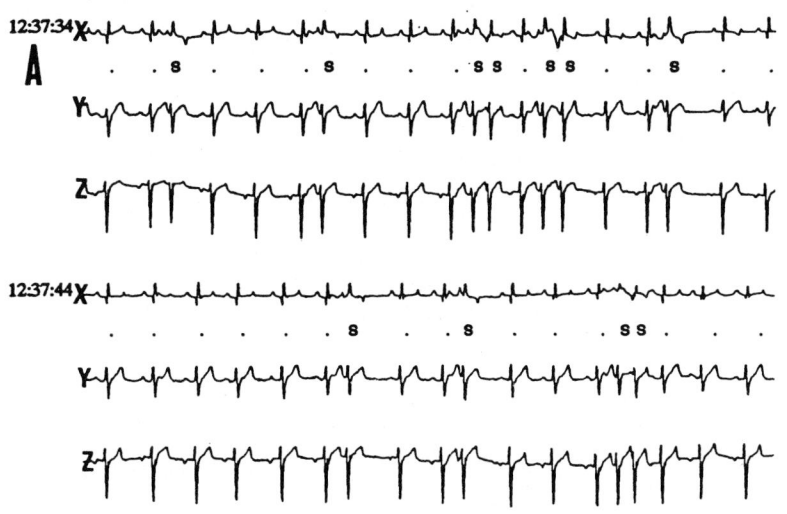

**Figure 7.** *A,* A properly operator annotated Holter report from a dog with premature supraventricular complexes. *B,* An improperly annotated report that may not have been "caught" by the operator during review. Annotation of the premature ventricular complexes (PVCs) is displaced, a T wave of a normal sinus beat is incorrectly labeled as a PVC, and a salvo of four PVCs is identified as only a single PVC. Key: S = supraventricular premature complex, V = premature ventricular complex, ● = normal sinus complex.

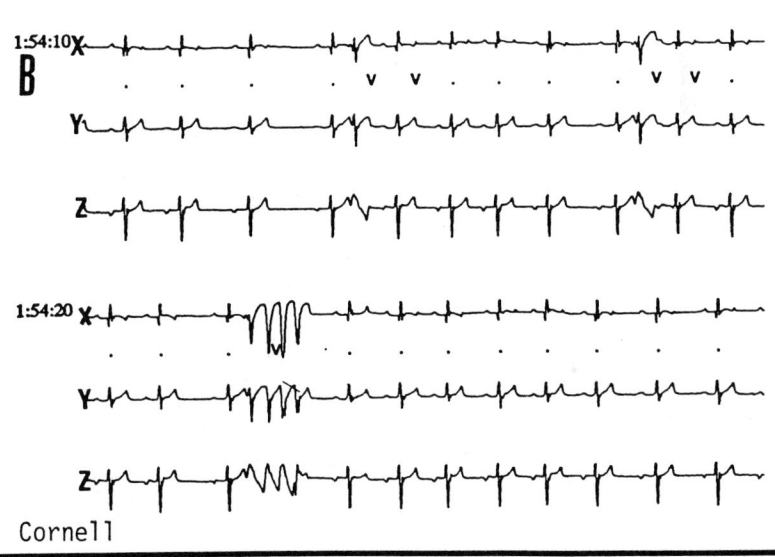

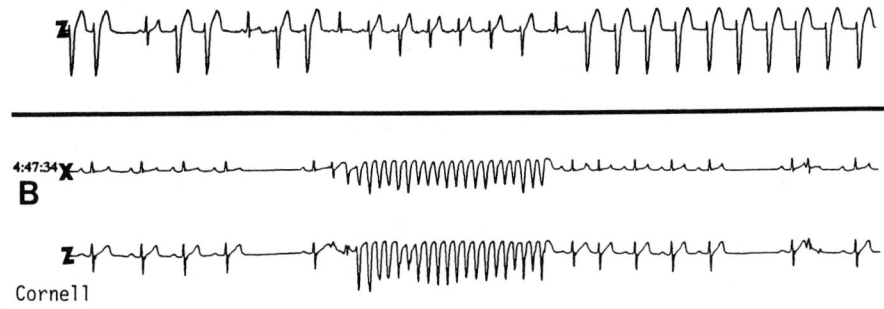

**Figure 8.** *A,* Ventricular complexes from this dog would more likely be correctly identified than those from the dog in *B.*

## CLINICAL APPLICATION

### Diagnosis and Treatment Decisions

Holter monitoring is indicated for the diagnosis of suspect arrhythmias or further assessment of cardiac rhythm disturbances in patients with syncope or near syncope, cardiomyopathy, and ischemic heart disease. The syncopal patient can be a diagnostic challenge because of the episodic nature of the events. When the etiology of the syncopal episodes is not apparent following a complete history and standard cardiovascular evaluation (including thoracic radiographs, blood pressure measurement, echocardiogram, and resting ECG), Holter monitoring increases the likelihood of a diagnosis. Even if a syncopal episode is not recorded, information about the patient's cardiac rhythm may provide important clues as to the cause of the syncope. Causes of syncope related to cardiovascular dysfunction include: (1) bradyarrhythmias; (2) tachyarrhythmias; (3) other cardiac causes of decreased cardiac output (e.g., valvular disease); (4) inappropriate vasodilation (dysautonomia); (5) drug therapy (e.g., vasodilators); (6) volume contraction (e.g., diuretic therapy); and (7) cough-related (tussive) syncope. The ambulatory monitor will clearly define any brady- or tachyarrhythmias, but not other causes.

Holter monitoring is also useful in the assessment of the frequency and malignancy of paroxysmal ventricular arrhythmias in patients with cardiomyopathy, in particular, boxers, Doberman pinschers, and giant breeds. The Holter recording quantitates ventricular ectopy during a 24-hr period, including a breakdown of the type of events (i.e., isolated ventricular premature beat, doublet, triplet, or run of tachycardia). The clinician should inspect disclosure records to verify that Holter interpretation. Ventricular ectopics identified as "couplets" or "runs" may be due to escape or accelerated idioventricular pacemaker activity and not require ther-

apy. So-called R on T ectopics may not actually occur on the prior T wave; instead, they may be classified as such based on an arbitrary cycle-length algorithm. The cardiac rhythm must be correlated to any clinical signs such as exercise intolerance or fatigue. This information is of crucial therapeutic importance. Before deciding to treat a ventricular arrhythmia, one must try to answer the following two questions: (1) Is this arrhythmia causing hemodynamic compromise? (e.g., are clinical signs correlated with the rhythm disturbance), and (2) Is this arrhythmia putting the patient at an increased risk for sudden cardiac death? The first question is answered by correlating clinical signs noted in the diary to the cardiac rhythm. The answer to the second question is a subject of much debate. The frequency, rate, prematurity, and the variability of the arrhythmia determines its malignancy and potential risk of sudden death. However, parameters determining the use of antiarrhythmic therapy are not clearly defined. Despite the lack of precise data, some general recommendations for therapeutic intervention include frequent couplets, triplets, or paroxysms of ventricular tachycardia, especially involving high rates, multiform in morphology, or very premature (e.g., "R-on-T" complexes). Holter monitoring not only provides the clinician with a more accurate assessment of the cardiac rhythm in known cardiomyopathies, but may be useful in the diagnosis of subclinical, borderline cases of dilated or arrhythmogenic cardiomyopathy, which is important for patient follow-up and breeding recommendations.

Ambulatory 24-hr ECG is also useful in patients with potentially ischemic heart disease such as subaortic stenosis or hypertrophic cardiomyopathy. These patients' ischemia can be dynamic and may worsen with exercise. ST segment analysis may be used as a marker of ischemia during exercise (see *"CVT* Update: Canine Subvalvular Aortic Stenosis," this volume, p 822). With a better understanding of the extent of cardiac disease, treatment may be more appropriately implemented.

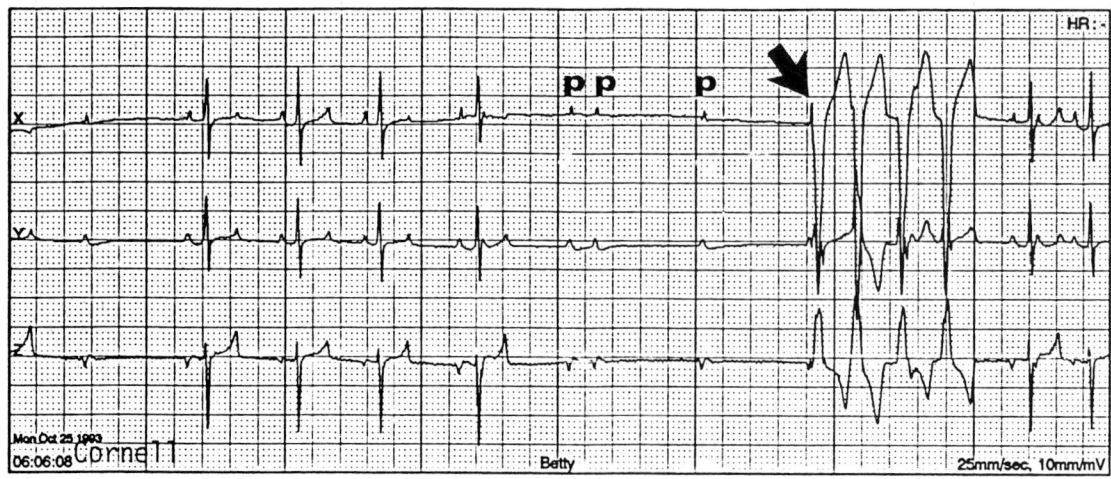

**Figure 9.** Recording from a dog with periods of high-grade, second-degree block. The demand pacemaker interrupts the ventricular pause with a paced beat (*arrow*), but triggers a run of ventricular tachycardia. Paper speed-25 mm/sec.

Another less common clinical application of Holter monitoring is heart rate monitoring in pacemaker patients in whom intermittent failure of the implant is suspected.

## Follow-up Holter Recordings

Once diagnosis has been made and treatment begun, it may be desirable to repeat a Holter recording to assess the safety and efficacy of antiarrhythmic therapy. It must be realized, however, that there can be substantial baseline variation in the frequency of PVCs and SVEs (Raeder et al., 1988). For instance, during a 24-hr monitoring period, a dog has an average of 300 PVCs and three runs of ventricular tachycardia (VT) per hour. Then, during a repeated 24-hr monitoring period, the PVC number drops to an average of 175 PVCs and one run of VT per hour. In this example, the dog had not received any medication. However, had the animal been treated, we may not know if the decrease in number is due to spontaneous variation or antiarrhythmic effect. In humans, it has been found that a decrease of at least 64% for PVCs, 83% for couplets, and 90% for ventricular tachycardia must be seen to say that a true drug effect has occurred (Raeder et al., 1988). Not only can evaluations be made regarding the efficacy of treatment of tachyarrhythmias, but follow-up examinations of patients treated for bradyarrhythmias are helpful as well (Fig. 9).

## References and Suggested Reading

Knoebel SB, et al: Clinical competence in ambulatory electrocardiography. A statement for physicians from the AHA/ACC/ACP task force on clinical privileges in cardiology. Circulation 88:337, 1993.
*A must read for any veterinarian that will be performing 24-hr ambulatory electrocardiography.*
Raeder EA, Hohnloser SH, Graboys TB, et al: Spontaneous variability and circadian distribution of ectopic activity in patients with malignant ventricular arrhythmias. J Am Coll Cardiol 12:656, 1988.
*Discussion of the importance of understanding the spontaneous variability in the frequency of ventricular arrhythmias in humans.*
Salerno DM, Granrud G, and Hodges M: Accuracy of commercial 24-hour electrocardiogram analyzers for quantitation of total and repetitive ventricular arrhythmias. Am J Cardiol 60:1299, 1987.
*Critical analysis of commercial 24-hr ambulatory analyzers and why there are problems with accuracy in rhythm detection.*

# DIAGNOSIS AND MANAGEMENT OF VENTRICULAR TACHYARRHYTHMIAS IN DOBERMAN PINSCHERS WITH CARDIOMYOPATHY

CLAY A. CALVERT

*Athens, Georgia*

## EPIZOOTIOLOGY

Cardiomyopathy is an extremely common disorder in Doberman pinschers. The prevalence of detectable abnormalities increases with age, at least up to 7 to 8 years of age. Approximately 25 to 30% of asymptomatic dogs between 2 and 14 years of age have echocardiographic or arrhythmic evidence of cardiomyopathy (Calvert, 1991a). The overall or cumulative incidence is probably higher. Many Doberman pinschers over 10 years of age have evidence of cardiomyopathy, but these "old" Dobermans often die of intercurrent disease.

Cardiomyopathy in Doberman pinschers may be diagnosed in dogs less than 1 to over 14 years of age. At the time of death, approximately 75% are 5 to 10 years of age. The mean age at the time of onset of congestive heart failure (CHF) is approximately 7.5 years in males and 8.5 to 9.0 years in females. Sudden death occurs at a mean age of approximately 6.5 to 7.0 years. The majority of affected dogs are male (Calvert, Chapman, and Toal, 1982; Calvert, 1986; Calvert, 1991a,b).

## TIME COURSE

Cardiomyopathy in Doberman pinschers is a chronic, insidious, slowly progressive disease that is characterized by two principal abnormalities, cardiac rhythm disturbances and myocardial failure, that eventually lead to one of the two principal clinical manifestations, sudden cardiac death or end-stage congestive heart failure (Fig. 1). The disease evolves over a period of several years in most cases. The time course is accelerated when measurable abnormalities begin in puppies and dogs less than 2 years of age and tends to be prolonged when abnormalities begin after 6 to 7 years of age. Early abnormalities typically begin at 3 to 6 years of age with sudden death or CHF occurring 3 to 4 years later, although some dogs live for 5 to 6 years. There is a long period of subclinical or occult disease during which sudden death occurs in up to 25% of affected dogs (Calvert, Chapman, and Toal, 1982; Calvert, 1986; Calvert, 1991a,b). End-stage CHF is the fate of most of the remaining 75%, associated with a short postonset survival time.

### Arrhythmias and Contractile Dysfunction

Long-term ambulatory electrocardiographic (ECG) (Holter) recordings performed serially beginning at 1 to 2 years of age indicate that ventricular premature contractions (VPCs) are the first detectable abnormalities and appear from months to over 1 year prior to the onset of early, equivocal echocardiographic abnormalities. Ventricular arrhythmias are seldom severe during the first 1 to 2 years, consist of single, isolated, VPC totaling less than 1000 per 24 hr, and are associated with no or equivocal echocardiographic evidence of left ventricular dysfunction. Ventricular arrhythmias usually worsen after the left ventricular shortening fraction decreases below approximately 20%, when the rate of progression of left ventricular dysfunction appears to accelerate and end-stage congestive heart failure typically occurs within a year in those dogs that do not die suddenly (Calvert, 1991a). Progressive left ventricular dysfunction is better monitored by sequential measurements of the left ventricular end-systolic dimension than by the shortening fraction. Approximately 25% of affected dogs will develop life-threatening ventricular arrhythmias at some point after the onset of severe left ventricular dysfunction.

### DIAGNOSIS

Because of the protracted subclinical (occult) disease, the significant incidence of sudden death during the occult phase, and the short survival time after the onset of end-stage congestive heart failure, it is important to diagnose cardiomyopathy early in the course of disease. Not only should a thorough cardiac investigation be conducted in any Doberman pinscher with a complaint of weakness, syncope, exercise intolerance, or a detected arrhythmia or gallop, but also routine annual screening is recommended by the author for adult Doberman pinschers, especially those with a familial history of cardiomyopathy. The two principal means of diagnosis of occult cardiomyopathy are long-term ambulatory ECG (Holter) monitoring and cardiac ultrasound.

### Holter Recording

Holter recording is a practical, easy-to-perform diagnostic technique wherein the heart rhythm is monitored in the home environment for 24 to 48 hr (Fig. 2). Details of this technique were described in the previous chapter (this volume, p 792). Ninety per cent of overtly normal Doberman pinschers less than 4 years of age with no obvious echocardiographic abnormalities have no VPCs, while approximately 10% have less than 50 VPCs/24 hr, usually less than 10. Approximately one third of overtly normal Doberman pinschers between 4 and 6 years of age and 50% over 6 years of age have less than 50 VPCs/24 hr, the rest having none (Calvert, 1991a).

The author's experience and current recommendations for interpretation of Holter recordings in Doberman pinschers are as follows:

1. No VPCs indicates an absence of Holter evidence of cardiomyopathy at that time. Annual examination is recommended in high risk families, since evidence of cardiomyopathy can emerge at virtually any age.

2. Fewer than 50 VPCs/24 hr may be normal, but

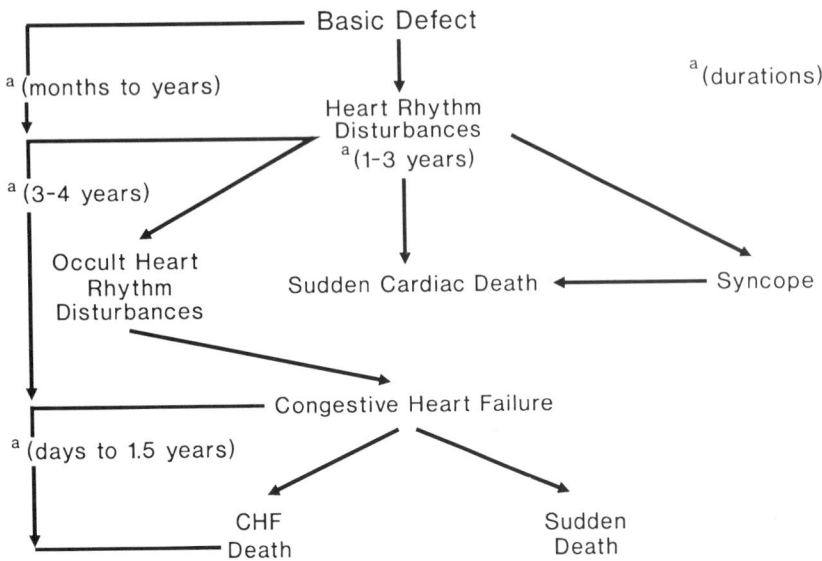

**Figure 1.** Proposed time course of cardiomyopathy in Doberman pinschers. Left ventricular function and heart rhythm disturbances progress slowly, leading to sudden death or CHF.

very early cardiomyopathy cannot be ruled out. Annual examination is recommended.

3.    Between 50 and 100 VPCs/24 hr is probably abnormal. Repeat recordings are recommended at 3- to 6-month intervals.

4.    More than 100 VPCs/24 hr is abnormal. The presence of complex arrhythmias adds weight to the diagnosis. Repeat recordings are recommended at 3- to 6-month intervals.

## Echocardiography

Cardiac ultrasound and Holter recording should be used in combination when evaluating Doberman pinschers for cardiomyopathy. Most overtly normal Doberman pinschers with no Holter-detected arrhythmia have left ventricular wall thicknesses that are at the low end of the normal range for the same sized dogs of breeds not affected by cardiomyopathy, and their papillary muscles do not appear to be highly developed. So-called normal Doberman pinschers, in the author's experience, have a left ventricular shortening fraction of 30 to 36% through a heart rate range of 85 to 110 bpm. Left ventricular end-diastolic and end-systolic wall thicknesses are not less than 7 and 10 mm, respectively, and the left ventricular end-diastolic dimension does not exceed 50 mm in dogs up to 45 kg (Calvert, 1986). Normal test results merely indicate an absence of echocardiographic evidence of cardiomyopathy at that time. Equivocal test results are common in normal dogs (of all breeds) and those with early cardiomyopathy because of inherent limitations of the technique. Left ventricular shortening fractions below 25% are considered unequivocally abnormal. Dogs at risk with normal test results may be examined annually, while those with equivocal or abnormal test results should be examined more frequently.

While the Holter recording and cardiac ultrasound results may be abnormal in randomly tested affected dogs, early in the disease course either test result can be equivocal.* One must always be cautious in declaring a Doberman pinscher as "normal." The older a dog with normal Holter and ultrasound test results, the more likely that the dog is truly normal or at least will not die prematurely of cardiomyopathy. However, it is likely that many Doberman pinschers are affected but that the severity of the cardiac deficiency is sufficiently mild so that overt disease is unlikely until advanced age. Some of these dogs will die of other causes, often without cardiomyopathy having been discovered.

## Identification of Cardiomyopathic Doberman Pinschers at High Risk of Sudden Death

Although virtually all affected Doberman pinschers have ventricular arrhythmias, many do not require antiarrhythmic therapy at the time of diagnosis. A number of general statements can be made based on the author's experience relative to the need for antiarrhythmic therapy in this breed. The arrhythmias are less likely to be life threatening in dogs with left ventricular shortening fractions within approximately 20% of normal. There is a direct relationship among the time course of disease, progressive left ventricular dysfunction, and the likelihood of the emergence of life-

---

*The sensitivity, specificity, and positive predictive value of the author's diagnostic criteria for asymptomatic animals have not yet been reported. Regional breed differences and familial history should be considered in determining the best course of evaluation.

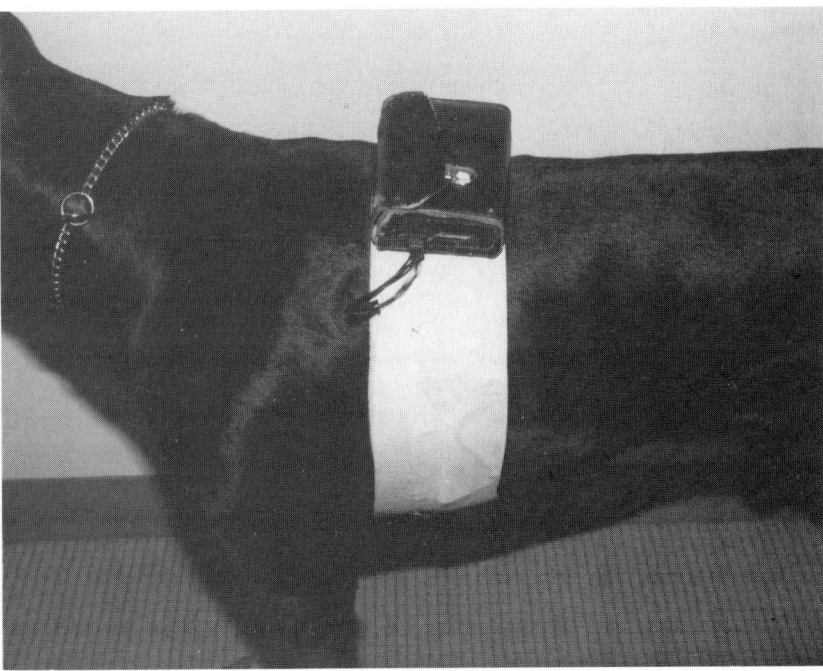

**Figure 2.** A cassette-type, dual-channel Holter recorder (Tracker, Reynolds Medical Ltd, Hertsford, England). The recorder can be easily and compactly attached to allow recording during vigorous activity.

threatening arrhythmias. Approximately 25% of affected dogs will die suddenly, and while "appropriate" antiarrhythmic therapy appears to delay death, current therapy cannot prevent the sudden death of many dogs in the high-risk patient subset. About 20% of affected dogs that reach the end-stage of congestive heart failure are destined to die suddenly of ventricular tachycardia-fibrillation. Many Doberman pinschers that collapse due to ventricular tachycardia die during that episode. Without antiarrhythmic therapy, most dogs surviving the first episode will die during a second episode that usually occurs within 6 weeks and often within 1 to 2 weeks. It is unlikely that an affected dog will survive three syncopal episodes that are initiated by ventricular tachycardia.

Therapy of ventricular arrhythmias is controversial. Adverse affects, including proarrhythmia, lack of efficacy, and the lack of clearly definable indications, are causes for controversy. It is safe to say that many dogs receive antiarrhythmic drugs unnecessarily. However, the high incidence of sudden death in cardiomyopathic Doberman pinschers justifies antiarrhythmic therapy. Once a diagnosis is made, the severity of heart rhythm disturbances must be determined. Arrhythmias may be detected by routine electrocardiography, but temporal fluctuations may result in underestimation of the severity or misinterpretation of therapeutic efficacy. Holter recording is the best method of evaluating heart rhythm disturbances. Syncope, if due to ventricular tachycardia, identifies patients at high risk of sudden death. Signal-averaged electrocardiograms, when abnormal, are associated with severe arrhythmia, the potential to develop severe arrhythmia, and sudden death in Doberman pinschers (Calvert, 1991c). The following criteria are recommended as indications to institute antiarrhythmic therapy.

1. Syncope and documented frequent ventricular premature complexes.
2. Ventricular tachycardia (Fig. 3).
3. Frequent complex ventricular tachyarrhythmias including multiform VPC, triplets, and bigeminy.
4. Signal-averaged ECG evidence suggesting the presence of late potentials (Fig. 4).

The vast majority of dogs fulfilling one or more of the above criteria also have echocardiographic evidence of reduced ejection fraction of 20% or more.

Serial examinations are necessary because the risk of developing life-threatening arrhythmias tends to increase as the disease progresses. It could be argued that it is more practical to initiate therapy for all affected Doberman pinschers with detected arrhythmias. The arguments against such an approach are the high incidence of adverse reactions to antiarrhythmic drugs, including proarrhythmia, the negative inotropic effect of these drugs in those dogs with severely decreased contractility, the potential to suppress escape complexes during bradyarrhythmias, and cost.

Not all Doberman pinschers that experience episodic weakness or syncope do so as a result of ventricular

tachycardia. Cardiomyopathic Doberman pinschers are predisposed to neurocardiogenic syncope that is due to an exertion- or excitement-associated bradycardia (Fig. 5). Doberman pinschers that collapse due to ventricular tachycardia virtually always reveal a severe arrhythmia; although, extended ECG monitoring may be required for accurate assessment. If the arrhythmia is not severe, then neurocardiogenic syncope should be suspected.

## Goals of Antiarrhythmic Therapy

There are a number of aims of antiarrhythmic therapy. A quantitative reduction of ventricular ectopia exceeding 75% is generally recommended and the abolition of ventricular tachycardia is a specific goal. Syncope and exercise intolerance resulting from frequent and severe arrhythmias should be abolished when the first two goals are accomplished. Careful adjustment of drug dosages based on patient response, serial Holter recordings, and serum drug concentrations are important to effective therapy. Surveillance of arrhythmias and response to therapy are indicated (at least every 3 months) and loss of drug efficacy over time is common, requiring treatment alterations.

## Choice of Antiarrhythmic Drug Therapy

### EMERGENCY THERAPY

In the face of immediately life-threatening ventricular tachycardia, intravenous lidocaine is the treatment of choice. Lidocaine (without epinephrine) is administered as a bolus (over 30 sec) of 2 to 2.5 mg/kg IV. The arrhythmia is usually suppressed by one to three boluses. Central nervous system (CNS) toxicity is likely in refractory arrhythmias requiring multiple treatments over a 15- to 30-min period. Diazepam (0.5 mg/kg, IV) is administered to effect for seizures. Arrhythmias refractory to lidocaine are likely to be refractory to the lidocaine cogeners, tocainide and mexiletine.

A constant-rate infusion of lidocaine (40 to 80 $\mu$g/kg/min) is initiated as soon as feasible after bolus conversion. Since approximately five half-lives are required to reach steady state (several hours), small, periodic boluses may be required as the arrhythmia relapses. The infusion rate should not be increased during the first several hours, since toxicity may then be produced. Maintenance antiarrhythmic therapy is initiated as soon as the arrhythmia is stabilized and the lidocaine infusion is gradually withdrawn, with monitoring, after the maintenance drug has reached therapeutic blood levels (16 to 24 hr).

REFRACTORY VENTRICULAR TACHYCARDIA. Lidocaine will be effective in most patients. Occasionally, lidocaine is not effective. Serum electrolyte status, including potassium and magnesium concentrations, should be assessed and corrected if the clinical situation permits this initial therapy. If arrhythmias persist, an alternate drug must be employed. Procainamide can be administered at a dosage of 3 mg/kg IV over a period of 1 to 2 min up to 10 mg/kg over 10 min. If effective, a constant-rate infusion is initiated at a rate of 10 to 30 μg/kg/min. Caution is advised, since procainamide exerts negative inotropic and hypotensive actions and dogs with overt or incipient congestive heart failure may experience a deterioration of cardiovascular function. Consequently, lower dosages are chosen in the cardiac patient. Furthermore, it is useful to know the results of a recent echocardiogram; however, such data may not yet have been obtained. It should also be noted that myocardial function may be transiently depressed following a period of sustained ventricular tachycardia.

### MAINTENANCE THERAPY

Maintenance treatment is required in all dogs receiving emergency treatment and in dogs whose arrhythmia is not immediately life threatening but nonetheless warrants therapy. Examples of the latter include nonsustained (<30 sec) ventricular tachycardia; a history of syncope with subsequently documented frequent VPCs; and frequent VPCs with bigeminy, couplets, or triplets.

Once a determination is made that therapy is indicated, antiarrhythmic drug administration is generally required for the remainder of the patient's life. The severity of arrhythmia and the risk of sudden death tend to increase with time. Class I antiarrhythmic drugs are usually employed first with the choice based on the severity of left ventricular dysfunction: this depends on the severity of cardiomyopathy. Dogs with severely depressed left ventricular ejection fraction are best treated with the lidocaine congeners, mexilitine or to-

cainide, since these drugs exert minimal negative inotropic and hypotensive action and protect against ventricular fibrillation. Impending congestive heart failure is likely when the left ventricular shortening fraction is less than approximately 15%; if there is a gallop heart rhythm; if the R waves are wide and of low voltage; and if there is radiographic evidence of interstitial pulmonary edema, distension of the lobar veins, or severe left atrial enlargement. When left ventricular function is less embarrassed, a number of drugs are appropriate for initial therapy (Table 1). Most available antiarrhythmic drugs have short-term efficacy and arrhythmia control tends to be lost after 3 to 6 months.

TOCAINIDE. Tocainide (Tonocard, Merck Sharp & Dohme) is an effective drug that often reduces ventricular ectopia by greater than 70% and eliminates ventricular tachycardia in approximately 70% of patients. It is often effective when arrhythmias are or have become refractory to procainamide and quinidine. Tocainide produces durable antiarrhythmic control in most dogs. Effective serum concentrations that are maintained for 6 to 8 hr are achieved after three doses. Arrhythmia control can be achieved in 8 hr if two doses are administered at a 2-hr interval and the maintenance schedule is initiated 6 hr later. Loading dosages are not recommended for dogs receiving lidocaine. Low or low normal serum concentrations are often associated with decreased efficacy. In order to maintain a recommended 8-hr trough value of approximately 6 μg/ml, it is often necessary to produce a peak (2-hr) concentration of 12 μg/ml. Values exceeding 12 μg/ml may be associated with neurotoxicity, including unsteady gait, head bobbing or trembling, and excitability or nervousness.

The use of tocainide is severely restricted due to its cost and potential for serious adverse effects during

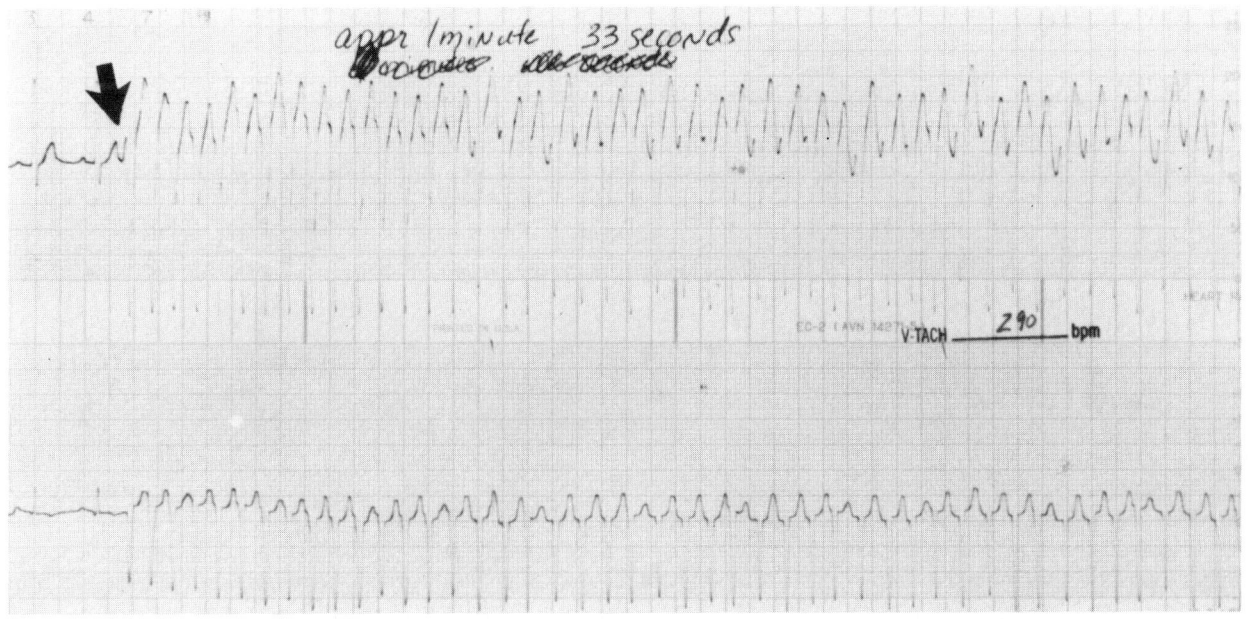

**Figure 3.** Sustained ventricular tachycardia at a high rate (300/min) (25 mm/sec). Antiarrhythmic therapy was prescribed and the dog died suddenly 1 year later.

chronic use. The incidence of anorexia is 20 to 30%, may occur with recommended peak and trough serum concentrations (10 and 6 $\mu$g/L, respectively), and can develop within days of treatment. Progressive corneal endothelial dystrophy has been observed in some Doberman pinschers receiving tocainide for 4 to 14 consecutive months. If corneal edema is not recognized quickly and the drug withdrawn, the condition can progress to blindness. Drug serum concentrations in affected dogs have been similar to those in unaffected dogs.

Acute hyposthenuric, polyuric renal failure has been more commonly associated with chronic therapy. Polydypsia and polyuria with hyposthenuria, usually in association with a degree of anorexia, are consistent signs and have been associated with dosages between 13 and 18 mg/kg three times a day. Acute renal failure can occur if the drug is not withdrawn immediately. Azotemia may or may not resolve; urine specific gravities become isosthenuric, and progression to end-stage renal failure occurs over months to 1 year when azotemia persists. Polydyspsia, polyuria, and hyposthenuria can also develop within 24 hr when loading dosages are administered, but resolve quickly after maintenance therapy is begun.

MEXILETINE. Mexiletine (Mexitil, Boehringer Ingelheim) is another lidocaine congener that the author feels is the best choice for initial maintenance therapy in dogs with overt or impending congestive heart failure and in dogs wherein left ventricular function cannot be immediately determined. Drug cost is a potential limiting factor. Mexitil is less expensive than Tonocard but is more expensive than procainamide and

quinidine. Effective serum concentrations can be achieved after three doses. Mexiletine has been reported to be clinically effective and minimal adverse effects were observed in one report (Lunney and Ettinger, 1991).* In the author's experience, mexiletine has produced few side effects, has produced good efficacy, has occasionally lost efficacy after 3 to 6 months of continuous use, and does not require serum concentrations in the high end of the recommended range for effective use.

PROCAINAMIDE. Sustained-release procainamide (Procan SR, Parke-Davis) is a generally effective, lower cost drug that the author feels is a generally effective initial choice for dogs wherein congestive heart failure is absent and not imminent. Twenty-four hours are usually required to establish sustained, effective blood levels. Long-term efficacy is poor in many dogs and numerous dogs have died suddenly while receiving procainamide. Holter ECG recordings have demonstrated a proarrhythmic effect in some dogs—this is a risk of *all* antiarrhythmic drugs. Some generic sustained-release procainamide products have poor bioavailability and require higher dosages to produce recommended serum concentrations. The Food and Drug Administration (FDA) publishes the Approved Drug Products with Therapeutic Equivalence Evaluations, which compares and rates the efficacy of generic drugs to the original. Generic products rated A are consid-

---

*The safety and efficiency of mexiletine and other antiarrhythmic drugs have not yet been tested in controlled, prospective veterinary clinical trials.

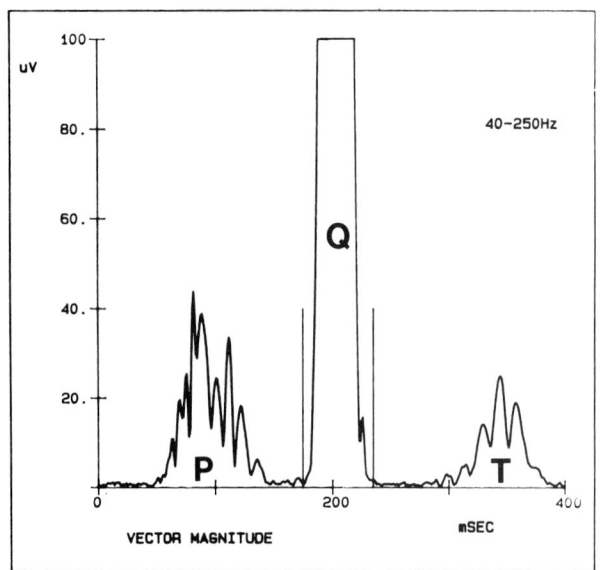

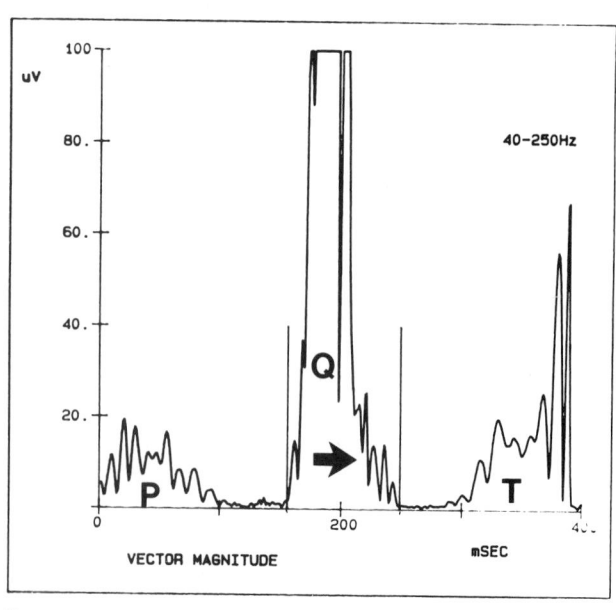

A

B

**Figure 4.** Normal (A) and abnormal (B) signal-averaged ECGs from Doberman pinschers. High-frequency, low-voltage waveforms appear in the terminal QRS complex and early ST segment (*arrow*). These may represent late potentials that have been associated with a high risk of reentrant-type ventricular tachycardias. The abnormal dog (B) had over 78,000 VPCs and over 400 episodes of ventricular tachycardia during a Holter recording performed 3 days previously. Antiarrhythmic therapy was effective and the dog is alive 19 months later. Abbreviations: P = P-wave, T = T-wave, Q = QRS complex.

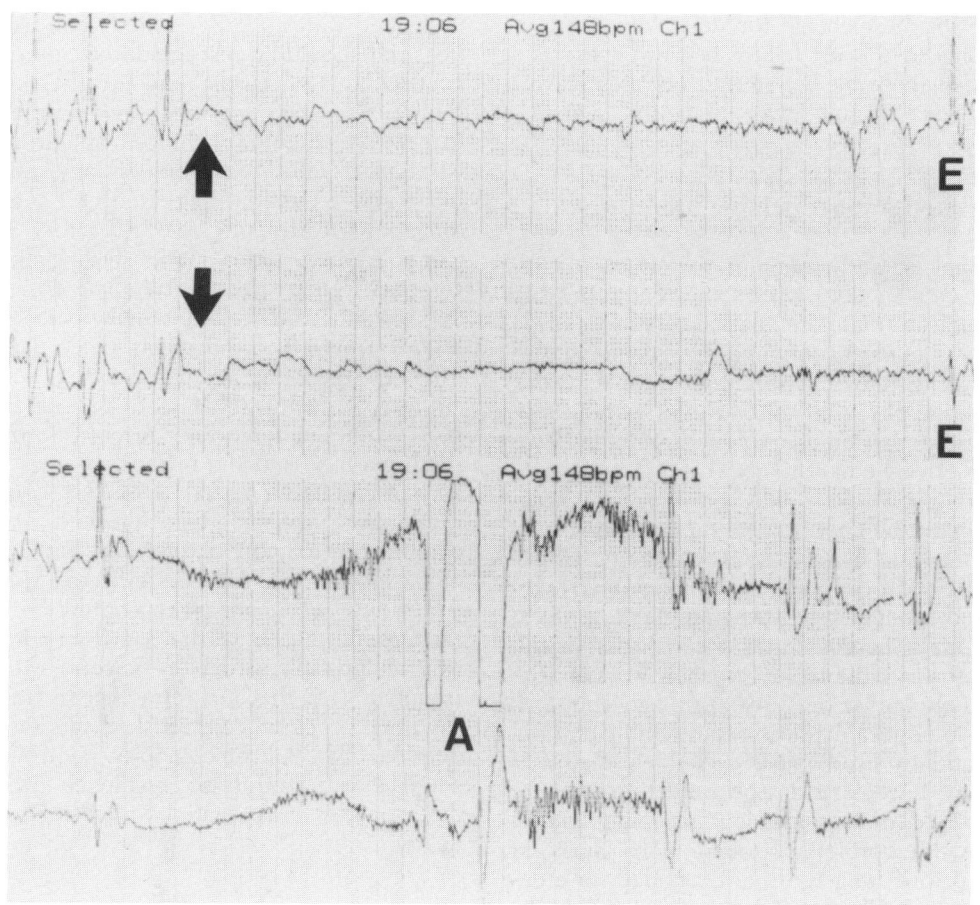

**Figure 5.** Sinoatrial arrest (*arrow*) occurring suddenly within seconds of exertion. Escape beats (E) begin after 7.3 sec. CPR-induced artifact (A) is present.

ered to be equivalent to the original. Those with other ratings are to be avoided.

Adverse effects of procainamide are common but usually not severe. Gastrointestinal disturbances and decreased appetite are the most common side effects. Chronic use is routinely associated with extensive brown hair discoloration in black Doberman pinschers, which partially resolves after the drug is withdrawn. Chronic use also tends to result in subtle, gradual decreased appetite and lethargy that are often not appar-

ent until after the drug is withdrawn. The author feels that procainamide may be less effective in delaying sudden death than the lidocaine congeners.

QUINIDINE. Quinaglute (Berlex) is also a lower cost, sustained-release product that generally demonstrates initial efficacy. Twenty-four hours are usually required to establish sustained, effective blood levels. As with procainamide, efficacy often decreases during chronic use. Anorexia, gastrointestinal disturbances, and weakness are the most common side effects. Qui-

***Table 1.*** *Commonly Recommended, First-Line Antiarrhythmic Drugs*

| Drug | Dosage (mg/kg) | Recommended Serum Concentration (μg/ml) |
|---|---|---|
| Mexilitine (Mexitil) | 5–10 t.i.d. | 0.5–2.0 |
| Tocainide (Tonocard) | 15–20 t.i.d. | Trough (8-hr) 4° Peak (2-hr) 10 |
| Procainamide (Procan SR) | 13–17 t.i.d. | 3–10[†] |
| Quinidine (Quiniglute) | 324 mg t.i.d.[‡] | 2–7[§] |

°Trough value ≥ 6 recommended.
[†]May require up to 13.6 μg/ml for sustained ventricular tachycardia; *N*-acetylprocainamide metabolite not important in dogs.
[‡]One tablet (324 mg) t.i.d. is an appropriate dosage for a 35- to 40-kg dog.
[§]Toxic reactions can occur at levels above 5 μg/ml.

nadine is not the best choice for dogs with overt or impending congestive heart failure because it exerts a modest negative inotropic action and elevates plasma digoxin levels, necessitating lower dosages of digoxin.

## Combined Antiarrhythmic Therapy

Although single agent therapy may be effective, Holter recording data in dogs with somewhat refractory arrhythmias indicate that combination therapy is often more effective. The most commonly used combinations are a class I drug plus a $\beta$-adrenoreceptor–blocking drug or mexiletine plus quinadine, with or without a $\beta$-blocker. Mexiletine in combination with quinidine was reported to be effective in refractory cases (Lunney and Ettinger, 1991). $\beta$-Blockers may prevent ventricular fibrillation. Circumstantial evidence supports the use of sympathetic blockade in Doberman pinschers. Holter recording data typically reveals exacerbation of arrhythmia during and immediately following exertion or excitement and most sudden deaths occur during or following exertion. Arrhythmias are typically worse in the examination room and at the outset of diagnostic studies but improve noticeably during the examination period as the patient's anxiety abates. Sudden death has occurred within 1 week of dosage reduction or withdrawal of a $\beta$-blocker in some dogs receiving combination therapy. Metoprolol (Lopressor, Ciba-Geigy) at a dosage of 0.5 to 1.0 mg/kg three times daily or atenolol (Tenormin, ICI Pharm) at a dosage of 0.5 mg/kg twice daily are effective. $\beta$-Adrenoreceptor–blocking drugs should not be employed as antiarrhythmic therapy at the above dosages in dogs with overt or impending congestive heart failure. Such dogs are heavily dependent on adrenergic drive for maintenance of contractility and blood pressure. The combination of quinidine and procainamide does not appear to be more effective than either alone.

## Amiodarone

Amiodarone (Cordarone, Wyeth-Ayerst) is indicated in humans for life-threatening, recurrent ventricular tachycardia that is not controlled by other drugs (Horowitz and Morganroth, 1987). Amiodarone has been remarkably effective in humans, but its use is associated with numerous adverse effects including dose-dependent gastrointestinal and neurologic effects and non–dose-dependent thyroid dysfunction.

Amiodarone has slow gastrointestinal absorption, delayed onset of action, and a long elimination half-life (Gallagher, Bianchi, and Gessman, 1989; Latini, Con-

nolly, and Kates, 1983). Amiodarone may be useful in dogs but should be restricted to treatment of recurrent ventricular tachycardia uncontrolled by conventional therapy. In dogs, serum concentrations of approximately 1 to 2 $\mu$g/ml achieved by chronic oral administration produce electrophysiologic effects including heart rate reduction, increased Q-T interval, and prolongation of the effective refractory period (Latini, Connolly, and Kates, 1983; Gallagher, Bianchi, and Gessman, 1989; Frame, 1989). A dosage schedule of approximately 10.0 to 15.0 mg/kg twice daily for 7 days followed by 5.0 to 7.5 mg/kg twice daily for 14 days, followed by 7.5 mg/kg once daily has been used by the author. Gastrointestinal disturbances have been the most common adverse effects. Improvement in arrhythmia has occurred in the few dogs treated. Amiodarone causes increased serum levels of other antiarrhythmic drugs, including diltiazem and digoxin. The combination of amiodarone and low-dose $\beta$-blockade or mexiletine may enhance efficacy (Marcus, 1992).

The use of amiodarone should be considered in Doberman pinschers that have rapid, wide-complex ventricular tachycardia or syncope with documented frequent VPC that are refractory to traditional antiarrhythmic drugs, since the risk of sudden death in these dogs is high. Chronic, poorly controlled arrhythmia coupled with ultrasound evidence of advanced cardiomyopathy is associated with a high risk of sudden death.

## References and Suggested Reading

Calvert CA, Chapman WH, and Toal RL: Congestive cardiomyopathy in Doberman pinscher dogs. J Am Vet Med Assoc 181:598, 1982.

Calvert CA: Use of M-mode echocardiography in the diagnosis of cardiomyopathy in Doberman pinschers. J Am Vet Med Assoc 189:293, 1986.

Calvert CA: Long-term ambulatory electrocardiographic monitoring in the diagnosis of occult cardiomyopathy in Doberman pinschers. *Proc ACVIM, New Orleans*, 1991a, p 691.

Calvert CA: Cardiomyopathy in Doberman pinschers. *Proc XVI World Vet Congress, Vienna, Austria*, 1991b, p 27.

Calvert CA: Signal-averaged electrocardiography in Doberman pinschers. *Proc ACVIM, New Orleans*, 1991c, p 693.

Frame LH: The effect of oral and acute intravenous amiodarone administration on ventricular defibrillation threshold using implanted electronodes in dogs. PACE 12:339, 1989.

Gallagher JD, Bianchi J, and Gessman LJ: A comparison of the electrophopiologic effects of acute and chronic amiodarone administration on canine Purkinje fibers. Cardiovasc Pharmacol 13:723, 1989.

Horowitz LN and Morganroth J: Second generation antiarrhythmic agents. J Am Cardiol 9:459, 1987.

James TN and Drake EH: Sudden death in Doberman pinschers. Ann Intern Med 68:819, 1968.

Latini R, Connolly SS, and Kates RE: Myocardial disposition of amiodarone in the dog. J Pharmacol Exp Ther 224:603, 1983.

Lunney J and Ettinger SJ: Mexiletine administration for management of ventricular arrhythmia in 22 dogs. J Am Anim Hosp Assoc 27:597, 1991.

Marcus FI: Drug combinations and interactions with class III agents. J Cardiovasc Pharmacol 20(suppl 2):S70, 1992.

# SUPRAVENTRICULAR TACHYCARDIA ASSOCIATED WITH ACCESSORY ATRIOVENTRICULAR PATHWAYS IN DOGS

CLARKE E. ATKINS

*Raleigh, North Carolina*

*and* KATHY N. WRIGHT

*Knoxville, Tennessee*

Supraventricular tachycardia (SVT) is generally considered a complication of cardiac disease and of heart failure and thought to cause less hemodynamic consequence and lower mortality than ventricular tachycardia. Supraventricular tachycardia, associated with abnormal atrioventricular muscular connections (accessory pathways [AP] or bypass tracts), however, represents a special type of rhythm disturbance, can be recognized in otherwise normal hearts, and may lead to clinical signs that can include apprehension, weakness, syncope, secondary valvular dysfunction, systolic and diastolic cardiac failure, and death. Affected dogs are typically young and otherwise healthy, and SVT associated with AP may be difficult to diagnose and manage. The following is the authors' approach to this increasingly recognized problem in small animal cardiology.

## DEFINITIONS

There is confusion surrounding the nomenclature for accessory pathways and their arrhythmias. For this discussion, the following definitions will be used (Fig. 1). *Accessory pathways* (also termed *bypass tracts* and *Kent bundles*) are abnormal connections between the atria and ventricles, composed of working muscular tissue. These pathways may or may not be of clinical importance in any given animal. The European Study Group for Preexcitation classifies accessory pathways as "tracts" if they insert into specialized conduction tissue and "connections" if the insertion is into working myocardium. These AP may produce *ventricular preexcitation (VPE)* in which the ventricular myocardium is activated earlier than would be expected had the impulse traveled normally through the atrioventricular (AV) node and His-Purkinje system. The electrocardiographic features of preexcitation, which variably include a short P-R interval, wide QRS complex, and slurred onset of QRS complex (*delta wave*), may be termed a "*Wolff-Parkinson-White pattern*" (Fig. 2A). The clinical finding of this electrocardiographic pattern, resultant supraventricular tachycardia, and related clinical signs is termed *Wolff-Parkinson-White (WPW) syndrome* (Figs. 1 and 2). The associated SVT involves a macroreentrant loop composed of the AV node anterogradely and the AP retrogradely (*orthodromic* conduction), or rarely, the AP anterogradely and the AV node retrogradely (*antidromic* conduction), and the electrical abnormality is termed *circus movement* or *atrioventricular reciprocating tachycardia (AVRT)*. Preexcitation may be only sporadically present (so-called *intermittent, latent,* or *nonevident WPW*) or may not be evident at all (*concealed* AP). *Lown-Ganong-Levine (LGL) syndrome* (Fig. 1) exhibits only the shortened P-R interval and is questionably associated with SVT.

## HISTORICAL PERSPECTIVE AND BACKGROUND

Credit for the first description of this syndrome is generally given to Wolff, Parkinson, and White for their 1930 description of SVT associated with bundle-branch block in young people. The first report of ventricular preexcitation in the dog was by Patterson et al. in 1961, while Hill and Tilley described VPE, with and without SVT in seven dogs and nine cats in 1985. There have been a number of other isolated reports of VPE in dogs and cats. We recently reported concealed and latent AP associated with AVRT in Labrador retrievers (Wright, Atkins, and Kanter, 1994).

In people, the incidence of VPE averages 1.5/1000, with males being overrepresented, and a suggested familial predisposition. The age of onset has been reported to range from 0 to 77 years, with the greatest number of diagnoses occurring in the first year of life. The prevalence decreases with age, presumably because of a loss of VPE. Associated cardiac disease, including cardiomyopathy, mitral valve prolapse, and congenital heart disease, is present in less than 20% of cases and often represents only an incidental finding. There does, however, appear to be a clinically important association between WPW and Ebstein's anomaly (see "Tricuspid Valve Dysplasia in the Dog," this volume, p 813).

Ventricular preexcitation is an important cause of SVT in people. In people, the prognosis for asympto-

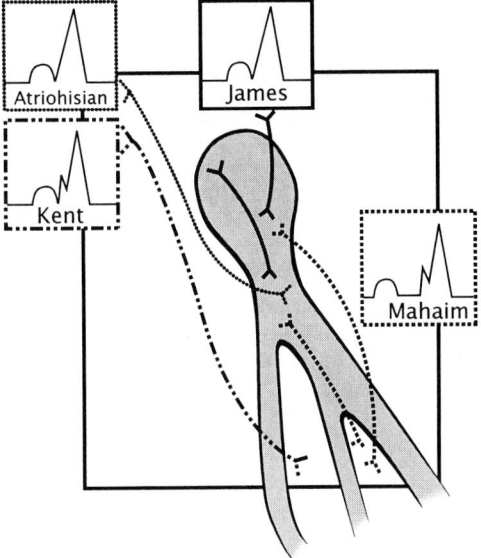

**Figure 1.** Accessory pathways and the expected electrocardiographic morphology during sinus rhythm are depicted schematically. See text for more complete explanation.

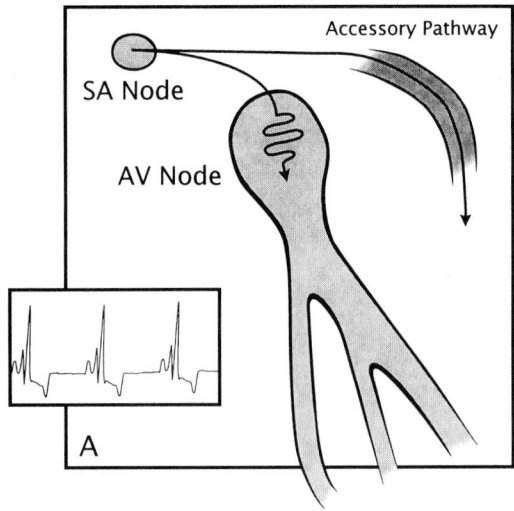

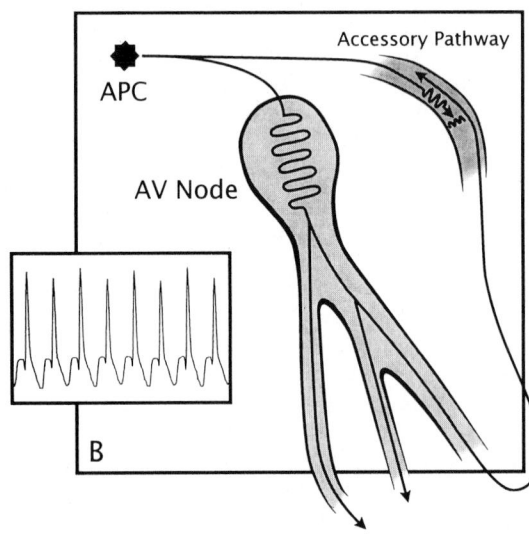

**Figure 2.** Wolff-Parkinson-White syndrome. *A*, Ventricular excitation via a rapidly conducting accessory pathway produces a short P-R interval and delta wave. *B*, An atrial premature complex (APC) finds the accessory pathway refractory and hence conduction occurs anterogradely via the AV node and His-Purkinje system. As the ventricle depolarizes, the accessory pathway is no longer refractory and the impulse can now be conducted retrogradely to the atrium setting up an orthodromic circus movement or atrioventricular reciprocating tachycardia, characterized by retrograde P waves following the QRS complexes and electrical alternans.

matic VPE is excellent and, even if symptomatology develops, the prognosis is generally good with appropriate care. Heart failure is unusual, although more common in those affected with incessant AVRT.

There is little epidemiologic information regarding SVT and AP in dogs (Table 1). Of 3000 total dogs examined, Patterson and colleagues documented 124 abnormal cardiac arrhythmias, one of which was asymptomatic VPE (Patterson et al., 1961). Male dogs do not appear to be predisposed. The average age of our cases and of reported cases is 2.7 years (range-4 months to 11 years), with >70% 3 years of age or less and >35% less than 1 year of age. Hill and Tilley reported SVT in five of seven dogs with demonstrable VPE (Hill and Tilley, 1985). Overall, the reported incidence of SVT in dogs with AP is 82%; atrial fibrillation has not been reported in dogs with VPE. It is quite likely that these reports overestimate the percentage of dogs with VPE that develop SVT, since asymptomatic canine patients are unlikely to undergo electrocardiographic evaluation. Ironically, because latent and concealed AP are not easily recognized, the importance of AP as a cause of SVT is probably underestimated. A variety of concurrent cardiac diseases in dogs and cats with VPE have been reported (Table 1). Systolic and diastolic dysfunction and mitral and tricuspid regurgitation have also been recognized secondary to protracted bouts of AVRT (Table 1). In addition, VPE has been recognized in dogs and cats with mitral or tricuspid valve malformations and in cats with hypertrophic cardiomyopathy.

## ANATOMY AND PATHOPHYSIOLOGY

Early in development, the atrial and ventricular myocardia are continuous. The primitive atrioventricular junction consists of a histologically distinct tissue that eventually evolves into a fibrous barrier separating the atria and ventricles, the only connection normally being via the AV node and His bundle. If the fibrous barrier fails to completely separate the chambers, one or more atrioventricular connections may remain. In humans, these pathways are found in the left lateral (46%), posteroseptal (26%), right free wall (18%), and anteroseptal (10%) locations. These accessory pathways or bypass tracts provide a "preferential" avenue for transmission of an electrical impulse from the atrium to the ventricle because conduction occurs at a more rapid rate than is

**Table 1.**  *Dogs with Reported Accessory Pathways*

| Breed | Sex | Age | Preexcitation | Delta Waves | SVT Documented | CHF | Associated Conditions |
|-------|-----|-----|---------------|-------------|----------------|-----|-----------------------|
| English cocker spaniel | F | 7 yr | Yes | No | No | Yes | DCM |
| Poodle | M | 8 yr | Yes | Yes | Yes | ? | Acquired AV valvular disease |
| Husky | F | 6 mo | Yes | Yes | Yes | ? | ASD |
| German shepherd dog | M | 4 yr | Yes | Yes | Yes | ? | None |
| Boston terrier | M | 5 yr | Yes | Yes | Yes | ? | None |
| Shetland sheepdog | M | 6 mo | Yes | No | No | ? | PDA |
| Not recorded | F | 6 mo | Yes | Yes | Yes | ? | None |
| Great Dane | M | 2 yr | Yes | No | Yes | ? | None |
| Labrador retriever | M | 16 mo | Yes, intermittent | Yes, intermittent | Yes | Yes | None |
| Labrador retriever | F | 2.5 yr | Yes | Yes | Yes | Yes | None |
| Labrador retriever | M | 4 mo | No | No | Yes | Yes | None |
| Labrador retriever | F | 22 mo | No | No | Yes | Yes | Secondary mitral and tricuspid regurgitation |
| Labrador retriever-cross | F | 4 mo | No | No | Yes | Yes | Secondary mitral and tricuspid regurgitation |
| Wirehaired fox terrier | M | 2 yr | Yes | Yes | No | No | None |
| Yorkshire terrier | F | 11 yr | Yes | No | Yes | No | None |
| Great Dane | M | 2 yr | Yes | Yes | Yes | No | None |
| Boxer | F | 1 yr | No | No | Yes | No | None |
| Malamute | M | 11 mo | Yes | Yes | No | Yes | Pulmonic stenosis and tricuspid dysplasia |
| Mongrel | F | 4 mo | Yes, intermittent | Yes, intermittent | Yes | No | None |

Abbreviations: SVT = supraventricular tachycardia, CHF = congestive heart failure, DCM = dilated cardiomyopathy, AV = atrioventricular, ASD = atrial septal defect, PDA = patent ductus arteriosis.

possible via the normal conduction system. Ventricular preexcitation with the potential for "circus movement" tachycardia (AVRT) results.

Kent first described atrioventricular connections (Kent bundles, Fig. 1) which produce preexcitation and AVRT. Mahaim fibers (Fig. 1; normal P-R, delta wave) provide nodoventricular (or nodofascicular) and fasciculoventricular connections, the latter being only questionably associated with AVRT. Intranodal and atrionodal tracts, described by James, and atriohisian tracts, described by Lev et al., are associated with short P-R intervals and no delta wave. These are often found in normal individuals, and their importance in the development of AVRT is unclear (Fig. 1).

Accessory pathways are clinically important *only when SVT results*. The mechanism for the development of the more common type of AVRT (orthodromic; OAVRT) is demonstrated in Figure 2. An atrial premature depolarization typically triggers the event when the electrical impulse finds the "preferred" AP refractory, and hence it follows the normal route through the AV node and His bundle. For the development of OAVRT, the AP must conduct retrogradely when the impulse arrives at its ventricular insertion, allowing the impulse to travel "up" the AP and then "down" (anterogradely) the normal conduction system repetitively. Ventricular premature depolarizations may also trigger OAVRT when the ectopic impulse travels in a retrograde manner "up" the AP and then anterogradely

"down" the normal conduction system to establish the tachyarrhythmia.

Rarely, the cyle direction is reversed, with the ectopic impulse traveling retrogradely "up" the normal conduction system and then from atrium to ventricle (anterograde) "down" the AP. This antidromic AVRT is associated with a more rapid ventricular response, atrial fibrillation, and occasionally, ventricular fibrillation in people. This condition has not been described in veterinary patients and will not be discussed further.

The clinical diagnosis of AVRT is made more difficult when the AP is used only intermittently (intermittent or latent VPE; Fig. 3) or when the AP is capable only of conduction in the retrograde direction (concealed AP; Fig. 4), meaning there is no electrocardiographic evidence of VPE during sinus rhythm. Twenty-three per cent of symptomatic human cases involve a concealed AP. The occurrence of intermittent VPE is determined by the location of the AP and by autonomic balance (e.g., a left lateral AP, with a point of origin some distance from the sinoatrial (SA) node, may be preempted by the normal AV nodal/His bundle route if there is high sympathetic output, enhancing AV nodal conduction). In one large series, 22% of affected people were found negative for VPE on their first electrocardiographic examination. Although the incidence of concealed and latent VPE is unknown in dogs, our experience and that of others (Scherlag et al., 1993) suggests that the problem is more important than previously realized.

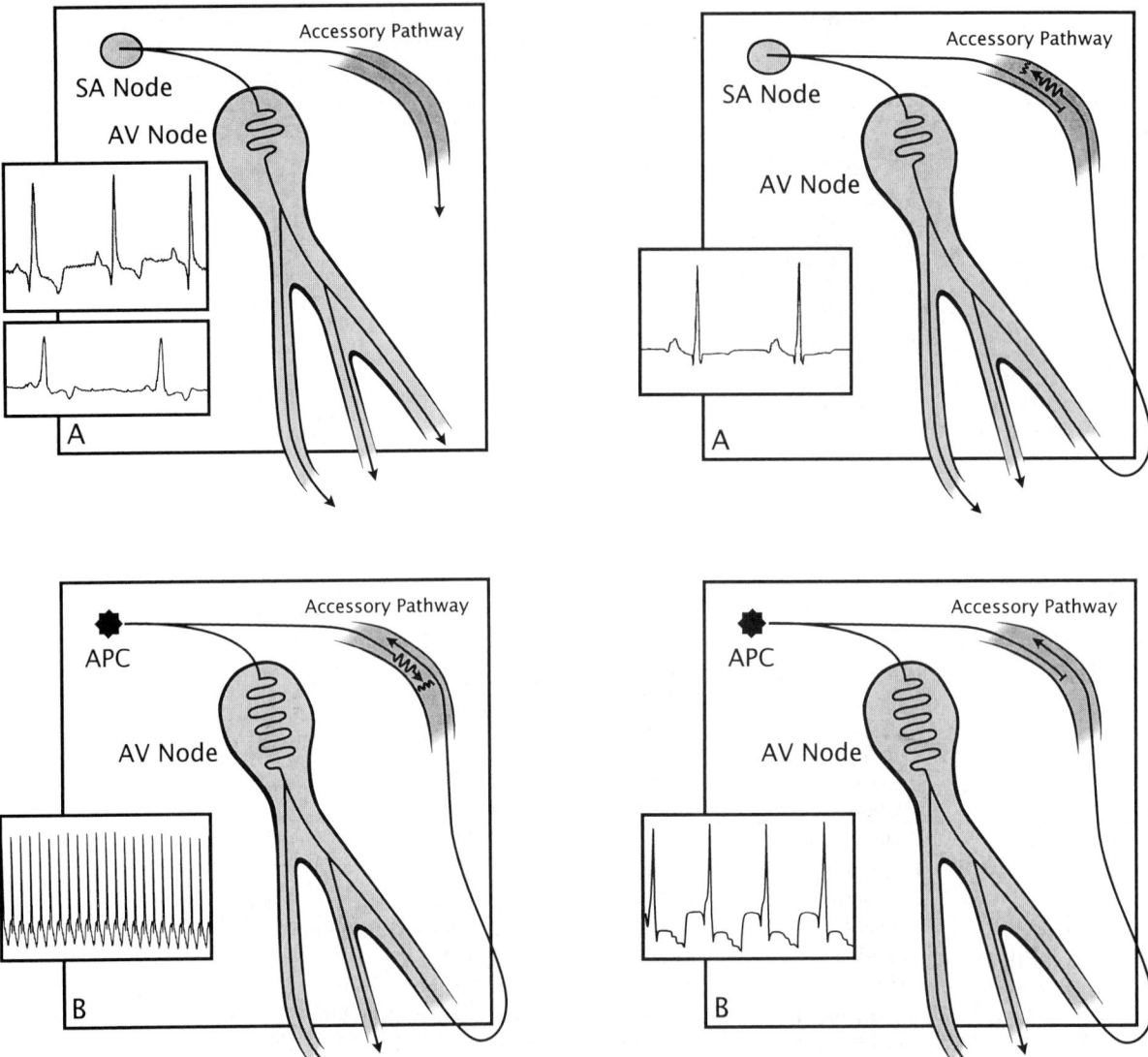

**Figure 3.** Intermittent (latent) Wolff-Parkinson-White syndrome. *A*, Depending on autonomic influences and location of the accessory pathway, sinus beats may be conducted preferentially over the AV node and His-Purkinje system (normal P-R interval and QRS complex) or over the accessory pathway (preexcited complex with short P-R interval and delta wave). *B*, An atrial premature complex (APC) finds the accessory pathway refractory and hence conduction occurs anterogradely via the AV node and His-Purkinje system. As the ventricle depolarizes, the accessory pathway is no longer refractory and the impulse can now be conducted retrogradely to the atrium setting up an orthodromic circus movement or atrioventricular reciprocating tachycardia, characterized by retrograde P waves following the QRS complexes and electrical alternans. This syndrome is more difficult to diagnose because electrocardiographic indicators of preexcitation during sinus rhythm are only intermittently present.

**Figure 4.** Concealed accessory pathway. *A*, Because the accessory pathway can only conduct unidirectionally (retrogradely), all sinus impulses travel through the AV node and His-Purkinje system to activate the ventricles normally (i.e., no preexcitation). The sinus impulse penetrates the accessory pathway such that it is refractory to retrograde conduction and, therefore, no circus movement exists. *B*, An atrial premature complex (APC) arrives at the AV node when it is still partially refractory and conduction time is slowed, giving the accessory pathway time to repolarize and accept the impulse, conducting it to the atrium in a retrograde manner, establishing an orthodromic circus movement or atrioventricular reciprocating tachycardia. This syndrome cannot be diagnosed without specialized studies because there are no electrocardiographic markers (preexcitation) during sinus rhythm.

Clinical signs occur with the abrupt onset of AVRT or the sinus pause (due to overdrive suppression) that follows cessation of the tachycardia. This produces disturbing palpitations in people. Furthermore, with extremely rapid AVRT, the associated decline in both systolic and diastolic ventricular function lowers cardiac output, producing anxiety, weakness, and syncope. This may be aggravated by loss of normal sequential timing

of atrial and ventricular depolarization. Typically, SVT is paroxysmal, but it may also be a sustained, life-threatening arrhythmia. Sustained or frequently recurrent SVT eventually can produce myocardial failure; signs of left, right, or biventricular heart failure; and secondary atrioventricular valvular insufficiency. As discussed above, sudden cardiac death has been described in humans and probably results from antidromic atrial fibrillation over an AP, producing a rapid ventricular response, ultimately deteriorating into ventricular fibrillation.

## DIAGNOSIS

### Clinical Signs

The findings of otherwise unexplained, rapid heart rate (usually >300 bpm) in a young dog without known heart disease is suggestive of the diagnosis. Labrador retrievers are predisposed to SVT, and probably for OAVRT as well. In our experience, accompanying historical and clinical findings have included mucous membrane pallor, weak pulses, apparent apprehension, exercise intolerance, weakness, collapse, syncope, heart murmurs (due to underlying disease or secondary to tachycardia-induced cardiac dilation), pulmonary edema, ascites, and death. We have observed sudden electrical cardiac death in one of these patients.

### Electrocardiography

The electrocardiographic diagnosis of WPW syndrome is relatively straightforward. The diagnostic criteria include rapid SVT and, during sinus rhythm, a short P-R interval (usually ≤50 msec) with QRS prolongation and delta waves in some leads (Figs. 1 and 2). Secondary ST segment and T-wave changes are also noted in people. The accompanying OAVRT is characterized by retrograde P waves following and distinct from the narrow QRS complex, but with a short R-P' interval. Unfortunately, P waves are often difficult to discern, especially with very rapid heart rates. We have observed ST segment depression and QRS alternans with OAVRT. The latter finding is 95% specific and 30% sensitive for OAVRT in humans (Marriott et al., 1989). This tachyarrhythmia tends to begin and end abruptly, typically initiated by an atrial or ventricular premature depolarization. Vagal maneuvers may slow or terminate AVRT by slowing conduction through the AV nodal arm of the reentrant circuit.

Intermittent (latent) VPE with AVRT is more difficult to diagnose, as the electrocardiographic criteria during sinus rhythm are only intermittently present (Fig. 3). The diagnosis may be made in a number of ways: (1) by fortuitously finding electrocardiographic or Holter ECG evidence of VPE; (2) by slowing AV nodal conduction with vagal maneuvers, β-adrenergic blockade, calcium channel blockade, or IV adenosine (these provocative tests favor AP conduction and uncover VPE); or (3) by electrophysiologic testing.

The greatest diagnostic challenge comes from AVRT associated with a concealed AP because there are no electrocardiographic markers of VPE during sinus rhythm (Fig. 4). The diagnosis, therefore, can only be made definitively with electrophysiologic testing. However, in the appropriate clinical setting (young to middle-aged dog lacking underlying cause for arrhythmia, with rapid and characteristic SVT), and characteristic ECG findings during SVT, a tentative diagnosis can be made.

Differential diagnoses for AVRT include sinus tachycardia, SA nodal reentrant SVT, intra-atrial reentrant SVT, automatic atrial or junctional SVT, AV nodal reentrant SVT, and atrial fibrillation and flutter. Tachyarrhythmias such as atrial fibrillation and flutter are usually readily diagnosed electrocardiographically. Irregularity of the ventricular rate response, identification of blocked P waves or flutter waves, and positive P-wave morphology in leads I, II, and AVF argue against OAVRT or AV nodal reentrant SVT. Ventricular tachycardia may also be a differential diagnosis when OAVRT is associated with bundle-branch block or in cases with antidromic AVRT, both of which produce a wide QRS tachycardia. Various authors have provided an approach to the differentiation of these arrhythmias (Bonagura, 1989; Marriott and Conover, 1989; Dreifus, Hessen, and Samuels, 1993).

### Other Tests

Thoracic radiographs should be obtained to determine if cardiomegaly or left heart failure (pulmonary edema) are present. Echocardiography does not provide specific information about AP or the cause of SVT, but can help define systolic and diastolic cardiac function, chamber dimensions, the presence of valvular incompetency, and the presence of underlying cardiac disease (congenital or acquired). It is emphasized that it can be very difficult to distinguish primary from secondary myocardial and valvular dysfunction in the presence of persistently recurrent or sustained tachycardia. Return toward normal function following control of SVT is suggestive of secondary dysfunction ("tachycardia-induced cardiomyopathy"). In young dogs with tachyarrhythmias, serum electrolytes and serologic testing for borrelliosis, Chagas' disease, and toxoplasmosis may also be indicated (see "Myocarditis in the Dog and Cat," this volume, p 842).

## MANAGEMENT AND PROGNOSIS

### General

Management of AP-associated tachycardia is focused on interrupting symptomatic AVRT and preventing its recurrence. In the meantime, therapy for the underlying or resultant cardiac dysfunction must be initiated or continued.

Therapy for AVRT is aimed at impairing conduction or prolonging the refractoriness of one arm of the reentrant circuit (Fig. 5). Vagal maneuvers can be used to enhance vagal tone, thereby slowing AV nodal conduction. Type IA antiarrhythmic agents, such as procainamide, quinidine, or disopyramide, are used to lengthen the refractory period of the accessory pathway. Slowing conduction and prolonging the refractory period of the AV node can be done using a number of drugs: calcium channel blocking agents such as verapamil and diltiazem; adenosine; or β-adrenergic block-

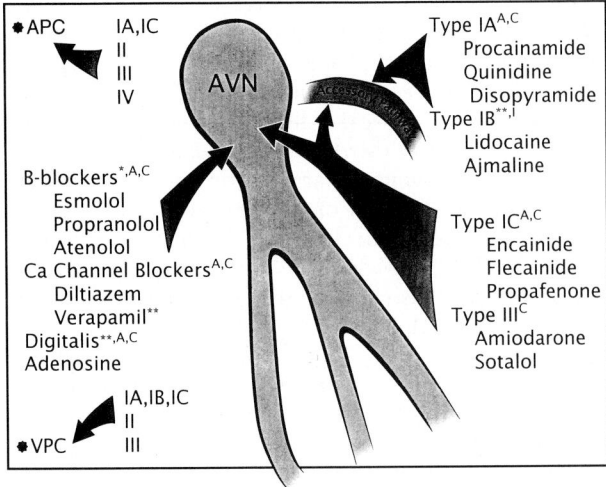

**Figure 5.** The AV node and His-Purkinje system and an accessory pathway are schematized with the site of action of drugs that may be effective in atrioventricular reciprocating supraventricular tachycardia by affecting one or both arms of the macroreentrant loop or the inciting extradepolarizations. Key: ° = may act on both arms of reentrant loop during high sympathetic tone, °° = may enhance conduction over accessory pathway (use cautiously), I = often ineffective; rarely used in this setting.

ing agents, such as atenolol, propranolol, and esmolol. In addition, β-blockers may affect the AP during periods of enhanced sympathetic tone. Though effective, intravenous (IV) verapamil should be used cautiously in the treatment of AVRT, especially in the face of myocardial dysfunction, because of its negative inotropic potential. Verapamil is not administered IV in humans with WPW and atrial fibrillation or flutter, as it may shorten AP refractoriness, leading to ventricular fibrillation. Likewise, digitalis has variable and unpredictable effects on the AP, actually shortening its refractory period in approximately one third of human cases. For this reason, it is generally avoided in AVRT. Type IC agents, such as encainide, flecainide, propafenone, and moricizine (with both IB and IC characteristics) increase both anterograde and retrograde AP and AV nodal conduction time and refractoriness and can be used both acutely and chronically. In humans, the type III antiarrhythmic drug amiodarone is useful chronically because it lengthens the refractory period in all portions of the macroreentrant loop and suppresses triggering extradepolarizations. Sotalol (type III characteristics plus β-blockade) may be similarly effective. Since multiple mechanisms are responsible for atrial and ventricular depolarizations, a number of drugs previously discussed may suppress inciting ectopy (Fig. 4). Because of negative inotropic potential, each of these drugs should be used cautiously in the face of myocardial dysfunction.

## Acute Therapy

Our approach to the tachycardic patient is to first attempt vagal interruption of the circuit, using either bilateral ocular pressure or cautious carotid sinus massage. Though this approach is sometimes effective, the dysrhythmia typically recurs. Likewise, we have experienced short-term response to precordial thumps and induction of emesis. If vagal maneuvers fail, or if AVRT recurs, a calcium channel blocker is administered. Though we have had success with both IV verapamil (0.05 mg/kg over 2 to 3 min; repeated twice, p.r.n.) and diltiazem (0.15 to 0.25 mg/kg over 2 to 3 min), we prefer diltiazem for reasons outlined above. If unsuccessful, other drugs or drug combinations may be employed. Vagal maneuvers, possibly enhanced with morphine (0.2 mg/kg IM) or edrophonium chloride (1 to 4 mg IV), should be again attempted with each drug administration. We have enjoyed success with IV procainamide at recommended (6 to 8 mg/kg) or higher (10 to 25 mg/kg) doses, administered very slowly. With limited experience, adenosine (up to 12 mg IV, very rapidly), propranolol (0.04 mg/kg IV), and esmolol (0.1 to 0.5 mg/kg IV) have been uniformly unsuccessful in our hands. Finally, if all else fails, DC synchronized cardioversion should be employed. Our limited experience with this technique suggests that it should be attempted relatively early in the course of a tachycardic event (first 8 hr), especially in dogs with severe myocardial dysfunction, in an attempt to avoid refractory ventricular arrhythmias and fibrillation that may follow conversion in the severely damaged ventricle.

## Prevention

Prevention and long-term therapy of AVRT can be accomplished by slowing conduction or prolonging refractoriness in either arm of the reentrant circuit, as described above, by preventing inciting atrial (and ventricular) extradepolarizations. Digoxin has not proved to prevent tachycardic events and has eventually been discontinued in all our patients, although it may be useful in the management of heart failure. Combination therapy with procainamide, at conventional doses, and propranolol, with and without digoxin, has proved to be somewhat successful, but relapses have occurred. Diltiazem, while very effective acutely, has not prevented recurrence. Our present approach is to employ sustained-release procainamide at relatively high doses (dosages have ranged from 23 to 42 mg/kg q.i.d.), using target though serum procainamide concentrations established at the time of successful conversion during IV constant-rate infusion (i.e., the serum concentration at time of conversion to sinus rhythm; in our experience between 7 and 20 μg/ml). This method has been successful in a limited number of cases. Therapeutic success (absence of tachycardic episodes) has been maintained even when isolated serum concentrations have fallen below the target levels. If this approach fails, therapeutic options include increasing procainamide doses or adding diltiazem, propranolol, or atenolol at gradually increasing doses, or the substitution of type IC or III antiarrhythmic agents, as described above. The use of digitalis may be considered.

Optimal therapy in human patients now involves special catheters which pinpoint and then ablate the AP using radiofrequency energy. This pinpoint ablation has supplanted surgical procedures. These techniques require electrophysiologic study and special expertise, making them generally impractical for veterinary practice. Scherlag and associates, however, recently reported successful radiofrequency ablation of a concealed AP, thereby curing OAVRT in a dog (Scherlag et al., 1993).*

## Heart Failure

Congestive heart failure is treated with digoxin, furosemide, enalapril, and salt and exercise restriction. Within weeks of control of the AVRT, treatment for cardiac failure can be gradually reduced, and often discontinued. In one case with acute pulmonary edema due to isolated diastolic dysfunction, acute administration of parenteral furosemide and conversion to sinus rhythm were sufficient.

## Prognosis

Without successful management of relentless AVRT, the prognosis is poor. The majority of affected dogs quickly develop congestive heart failure due to diastolic or systolic cardiac dysfunction and secondary atrioventricular valvular incompetence. Without control of

---

*Successful radiofrequency catheter ablation has been performed in other canine cases, as well.

tachycardia, these dogs have died or were euthanatized within 4 to 36 months. With control of the arrhythmia, however, SVT-associated signs, heart failure, and myocardial and valvular dysfunction are potentially reversible.

## References and Suggested Reading

Atkins CE, Kanter R, Wright KN, et al: Orthodromic reciprocating tachycardia and left heart failure associated with a concealed posteroseptal accessory pathway in a young dog. J Vet Intern Med 1995 (in press).

Bonagura JD: Atrial arrhythmias. In Kirk RW (ed): Current Veterinary Therapy X. Philadelphia, WB Saunders Co, 1989, p 271.

Dreifus LS, Hessen S, and Samuels F: Recognition and management of supraventricular tachycardia. Heart Dis Stroke 2:223, 1993.

Hill BL and Tilley LP: Ventricular preexcitation in seven dogs and nine cats. J Am Vet Med Assoc 187:1026, 1985.

Manolis AS and Estes NAM: Supraventricular tachycardia: Mechanisms and therapy. Arch Intern Med 147:1706, 1987.

Marriott HJL and Conover MB: Preexcitation and its arrhythmias. In Advanced Concepts in Arrhythmias, 2nd edition. Philadelphia, CV Mosby Co, 1989, p 141.

Munger TM, Packer DL, Hammill SC, et al: A population study of the natural history of Wolff-Parkinson-White syndrome in Olmstead County, Minnesota, 1953–1989. Circulation 87:866, 1993.

Packer DL and Prytowsky EN: Wolff-Parkinson-White syndrome: Further progress in evaluation and treatment. Prog Cardiol 1:147, 1988.

Patterson DF, Detweiler DK, Hubben K, et al: Spontaneous abnormal cardiac arrhythmias and conduction disturbances in the dog: A clinical and pathologic study of 3000 dogs. Am J Vet Res 22:355, 1961.

Prytowsky EN, Milas WM, Heger JJ, et al: Preexcitation syndromes: Mechanisms and management. Med Clin North Am 68:831, 1984.

Prytowsky EN: Diagnosis and management of preexcitation syndromes. Curr Prob Cardiol 13:225, 1988.

Scherlag BJ, Wang X, Nakagawa H, et al: Radiofrequency catheter ablation of a concealed posteroseptal accessory pathway to treat incessant supraventricular tachycardia in a dog (abstr). J Vet Intern Med 7:116, 1993.

Wright KN, Atkins CE, and Kanter R: Symptomatic supraventricular tachycardia, with and without identified accessory pathways, in Labrador retrievers. Personal observations, 1994.

Zipes DP: Specific arrhythmias: Diagnosis and treatment. In Braunwald E (ed): Heart Disease. Philadelphia, WB Saunders Co, 1992, p 667.

---

# TRICUSPID VALVE DYSPLASIA IN THE DOG

N. SYDNEY MOISE

*Ithaca, New York*

Tricuspid valve dysplasia is a congenital abnormality of the right atrioventricular valve that is characterized by focal or diffuse thickening of the leaflets, underdevelopment of chordae tendineae and papillary muscles, incomplete separation of valve components from the ventricular wall, and focal agenesis of valvular tissue (Fig. 1) (Becker et al., 1971; Liu and Tilley, 1976). As in humans, a pathologic spectrum of dysplasia of the tricuspid valve exists in dogs. Some dogs will have a thick fibrous band of tissue near the tricuspid annulus,

causing tricuspid stenosis. Tricuspid valve dysplasia also may occur with downward (apical) displacement of the valve's basal attachment, a condition called Ebstein's malformation (Liu and Tilley, 1976; Netter, 1978). Because the normal attachment of the septal leaflet of the tricuspid valve is a few millimeters below the annulus and lower than the attachment of the mitral valve, careful examination is required before a diagnosis of Ebstein's malformation is made. Ebstein's malformation may exist with or without dysplasia of the tricuspid valve.

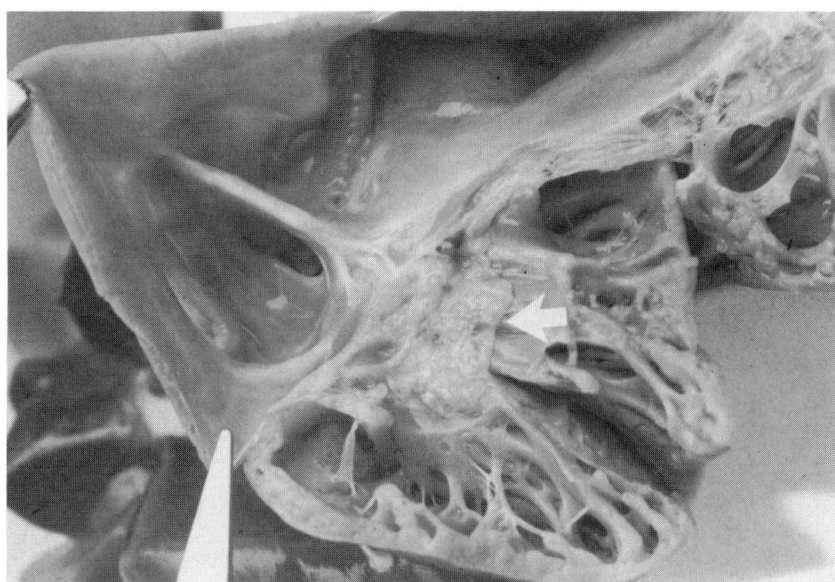

**Figure 1.** Postmortem specimen from a Labrador retriever with severe tricuspid valve dysplasia. The septal leaflet is adhered to the interventricular septum (*arrow*). Right atrial dilatation is evident.

Tricuspid dysplasia may occur in combination with other congenital cardiac defects such as mitral valve dysplasia, atrial septal defect, patent foramen ovale, ventricular septal defects, patent ductus arteriosus, or pulmonic stenosis (Liu and Tilley, 1976), but it most frequently occurs as an isolated defect. The embryonic defect that results in the prominent feature of an adhered septal leaflet involves failure of programmed cell degeneration and consequently inadequate undermining of the valve leaflet (Netter, 1978). The normal loss of these cells permits the valve to be free from the ventricular wall and attached to the papillary muscles via the chordae tendineae.

Tricuspid valve dysplasia results in regurgitation of blood back into the right atrium, such that the right atrium and ventricle become dilated. A prodigious right atrium develops in some dogs, with atrial hypertrophy being especially severe in dogs with coexisting tricuspid stenosis.

## CLINICAL PRESENTATION

Several different breeds (Great Dane, German shepherd dog, Old English sheepdog, Great Pyrenees, borzoi, Irish setter, boxer, Newfoundland, weimaraner, and Shih Tzu) have been reported to be affected with tricuspid dysplasia, most of them large (Liu and Tilley, 1976). At Cornell University, by far the most commonly represented breed is the Labrador retriever (Moise, 1989).* This defect has been identified in black, chocolate, and yellow Labradors (Fig. 1). Several affected puppies within litters have been identified, and preliminary pedigree analysis is suggestive of a familial defect.

Dogs with tricuspid dysplasia usually present as pup-

*Should veterinarians identify affected Labrador retrievers, it is requested that they please send a copy of the pedigree to the College of Veterinary Medicine, Cornell University, Ithaca, New York 14853 (Dr. N. Sydney Moise).

pies without clinical signs and in good body condition. A cardiac murmur is serendipitously found during routine examination. Other affected dogs with soft murmurs may not be identified until later in life or if the dog develops right-sided congestive heart failure. The point of maximum intensity of the murmur is on the right hemithorax at approximately the fourth intercostal space at the costochondral junction. Occasionally, a precordial thrill is palpated in this same location. Femoral pulse quality may be weak or normal depending on the severity and stage of the disease. Jugular distention and jugular pulses may be observed. Mucous membrane color is usually normal unless there is right-to-left shunting across a patent foramen ovale. If congestive heart failure is present, the limbs may be cool to the touch and hepatomegaly and ascites may be palpated. The mucous membrane color of the dogs in severe failure is often gray to pale pink.

## ELECTROCARDIOGRAPHY

Despite the sometimes massive right atrial and ventricular enlargement caused by tricuspid valve dysplasia, the electrocardiogram frequently does not have the classic right heart enlargement features (tall P waves; deep S waves in I, II, III, and aVF; right axis shift). The P waves instead may be normal, or with massive right atrial enlargement they are both wide and tall. The P-wave configuration also may change. Although the standard limb leads may not reveal right heart enlargement, precordial leads recorded on the left hemithorax usually show deep S waves. Deep Q waves and right axis shifts have been reported in some dogs (Liu and Tilley, 1976). Approximately 40% of dogs with tricuspid valve dysplasia display a unique "splintering" of the QRS complex that occurs with an RR, Rr, or rR configuration in leads II, III, and aVF (Fig. 2). This pattern also has been seen in children with Ebstein's malformation (Netter, 1978). The reason for this pattern is not known, but may be due to conduction disturbance in the right bundle branch, conduction through an accessory pathway (atrioventricular [AV] node to ventricular myocardium), or delayed conduction within the atrial myocardium. Accessory pathway tachycardia has been identified in Labrador retrievers with tricuspid valve dysplasia (Dr. Clarke Atkins and Dr. Peter Darke, personal communications). Atrial tachyarrhythmias frequently develop in these dogs because of the enlarged atrium. These arrhythmias include premature complexes, atrial flutter and fibrillation, and probably intra-atrial reentry tachycardias (de Madron et al., 1987). In humans, Wolff-Parkinson-White syndrome is relatively common in Ebstein's anomaly and is usually via the bundle of Kent. Dogs with tricuspid valve dysplasia are sensitive to the development of supraventricular arrhythmias during catheterization procedures. Ventricular arrhythmias seem to develop less frequently.

## RADIOGRAPHY

Right atrial enlargement predominates as a feature of thoracic radiography. Right ventricular enlargement is usually prominent as well. The left heart is dwarfed by the right heart enlargement and there can be marked apex shifting. The pulmonary trunk does not bulge, differentiating tricuspid valve dysplasia from pulmonic stenosis. The pulmonary vasculature may be reduced in size (underperfusion to the lungs). The caudal vena cava may appear enlarged as well as the liver. Selective angiocardiography demonstrates tricuspid valve insufficiency (regurgitation); however, this diagnostic test is not usually needed because the diagnosis is clear from the echocardiogram.

## ECHOCARDIOGRAPHY

Two-dimensional echocardiography is the diagnostic test of choice in evaluating tricuspid valve dysplasia. The septal leaflet of the tricuspid valve appears adhered to the interventricular septum in the right parasternal long and short axis view at the level of the atrioventricular valves and in the four-chamber apical view from the left caudal position (Fig. 3). The lateral free wall leaflet may appear redundant. The leaflets may have varying degrees of thickening. Careful examination is needed to judge the degree, if any, of downward displacement of the leaflets. In dogs with simultaneous tricuspid stenosis, bright fibrous tissue

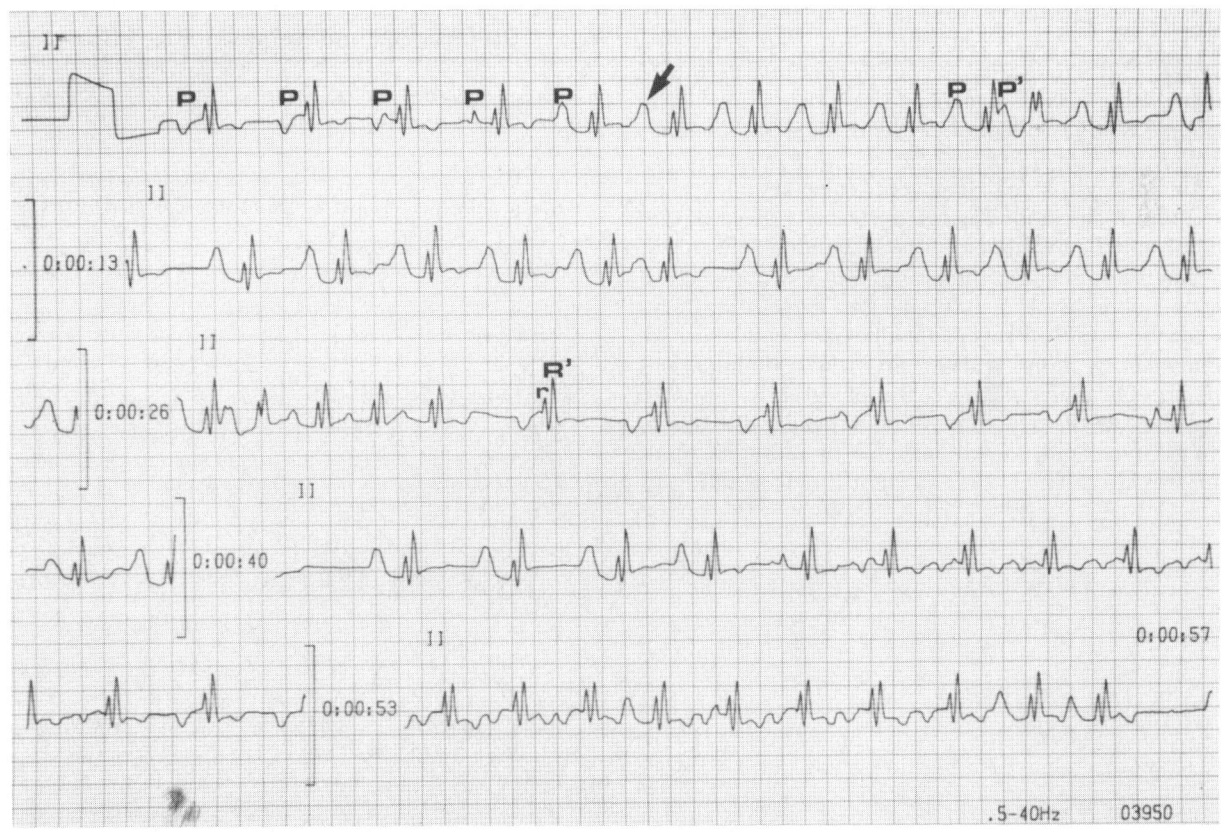

**Figure 2.** Semicontinuous lead II electrocardiogram recorded from a chocolate Labrador retriever with severe tricuspid valve dysplasia. The P-wave morphology changes in polarity and size. At times, the P waves are both wide and tall (*arrow*). The typical splintered QRS complex (rR) is seen. Supraventricular premature complexes and tachycardia are present. This dog eventually developed atrial fibrillation (paper speed = 50 mm/sec, 10 msec = 10 mm).

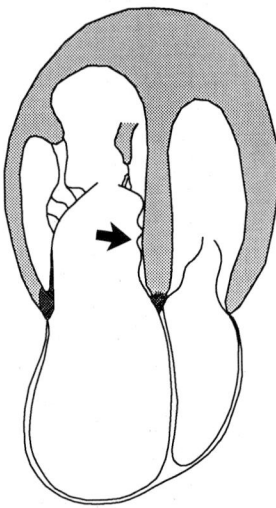

**Figure 3.** Schematic representation of what is seen by two-dimensional echocardiography of a heart with tricuspid valve dysplasia. The four-chamber view shows the septal leaflet to be adhered to the interventricular septum and dilatation of the right atrium and ventricle.

surrounding the tricuspid valve annulus is seen. The right atrium and ventricle will be dilated, although the prominence of the right atrium is most notable. In severe tricuspid stenosis, the right ventricle is normal to small. Frequently, the left ventricle appears too small because of decreased ventricular filling or its relative proportion to the right ventricle is distorted. Diastolic flattening and paradoxical systolic motion of the interventricular septum is present.

Doppler echocardiography reveals tricuspid valve insufficiency; however, the velocity of the regurgitant jet will not be high, since right ventricular systolic pressures are not elevated. The low jet velocity explains the soft murmur heard in some cases. Although the murmur may be subtle and the jet velocity low, these findings do not indicate a mild disease. To the contrary, this can be found in severe insufficiency with marked cardiac deformation of the right heart. Doppler examination of saline contrast echocardiography may also reveal flow across a patent foramen ovale with blood flowing from right to left because of elevated right atrial pressures. The degree of right-to-left shunting is usually insufficient to cause clinical signs of cyanosis unless another defect is present such as pulmonic stenosis.

## PROGNOSIS AND TREATMENT

The prognosis depends on the degree of regurgitation and cardiac enlargement. It is sometimes surprising how long the dogs remain without clinical signs, despite severe disease. However, once the dog develops signs of right-sided heart failure such as ascites, cool extremities, syncope, or exercise intolerance, deterioration is rapid. Specific and clear choices for treating these dogs in right heart failure do not exist. The bottom line is to optimize heart rate and preload and to restrict exercise. Judicious doses of a diuretic (i.e., furosemide 1 to 2 mg/kg, twice daily) can be used to help in the control of the ascites; however, careful monitoring for adequate renal perfusion is mandatory. The angiotensin-converting enzyme inhibitors may be of some value, if not used excessively. Digoxin may be helpful, especially when supraventricular arrhythmias develop. A low-sodium diet can effectively decrease the doses of drugs. Dogs with severe tricuspid valve dysplasia usually die between 1 and 3 years of age, although exceptions occur in either direction.

## References and Suggested Reading

Becker AE, Becker MJ, and Edwards JE: Pathologic spectrum of dysplasia of the tricuspid valve. Arch Pathol 91:167, 1971.
*Complete description of the range of severity of tricuspid valve dysplasia and Ebstein's malformation in children.*
de Madron E, Kadish A, Spear JF, and Knight DH: Incessant atrial tachycardias in a dog with tricuspid dysplasia. J Vet Intern Med 1:163, 1987.
*Description of a boxer with atrial tachycardia and tricuspid valve dysplasia. Electrophysiologic studies are described.*
Liu SK and Tilley LP: Dysplasia of the tricuspid valve in the dog and cat. J Am Vet Med Assoc 169:623, 1976.
*Comparisons of tricuspid valve abnormalities in dogs and cats with electrocardiographic, radiographic, and pathologic characteristics described.*
Moise NS: Uncommon congenital heart defects in large and small animals. Proc Am Coll Vet Intern Med 1989, pp 235–236.
*Selected examples of uncommon congenital heart defects with report of tricuspid valve dysplasia in Labrador retrievers.*
Netter FH: In Yonkman FF (ed). The CIBA Collection of Medical Illustration, volume 5. Rochester, NY, CIBA, Case-Hoyt Corp, 1981, pp 143–144.
*Illustrations and text to describe Ebstein's malformation.*

# THERAPY OF CONGENITAL PULMONIC STENOSIS

WILLIAM P. THOMAS

*Davis, California*

In the last edition of this book, a survey of the records of North American veterinary school teaching hospitals for the years 1987 through 1989 (using the VMDP-Purdue data base) listed congenital pulmonic stenosis (PS) as the third most commonly diagnosed congenital cardiac defect in dogs (18%), behind patent ductus arteriosus (PDA) (32%) and subaortic stenosis (22%) (Buchanan, 1992). By comparison, uncomplicated PS is less common in cats (3%), in which it more often occurs together with other defects. Several specific dog breeds were identified as being predisposed (i.e., at increased risk relative to other breeds, based on odds ratios) to this defect, including the English bulldog, mastiff, Samoyed, miniature schnauzer, cocker spaniel, and West Highland white terrier. In addition, pulmonary valve dysplasia and stenosis has been reported in Boykin spaniels, bull mastiffs, and beagles. A heritable basis for the defect has been proven in beagles (Patterson et al., 1981) and, based on breeding studies of this and other defects, should be suspected in other breeds as well. Both sexes may be affected, although in English bulldogs and bull mastiffs, males have been reported to predominate. Most diagnoses are made within the first year of life. Although it often occurs as an isolated lesion, PS also occurs together with other defects, especially ventricular septal defect, in more complicated deformities (e.g., tetralogy of Fallot).

## ANATOMY AND PHYSIOLOGY

Congenital deformity of the pulmonic valve or the adjacent regions (supravalvular, subvalvular, infundibular) nearly always causes primarily a stenosis with right ventricular (RV) outflow obstruction. Although moderate to severe isolated congenital pulmonic valve insufficiency has been reported in dogs, valvular regurgitation is usually associated with stenosis, is usually mild, and is often inaudible. Several types of deformity may occur, usually singly, but occasionally together. Supravalvular PS is very uncommon. The most common type of PS is valvular dysplasia (88% according to Fingland et al., 1986). The valvular lesion consists of varying degrees of valve leaflet thickening, fusion, or hypoplasia. In some cases, valve fusion results in a dome-shaped valve with a central orifice (Patterson et al., 1981). A fibrous ring may also occur just at the base of the valve (accompanied by valvular deformity) or below the valve in a subvalvular ring. In English bulldogs and boxers, subvalvular stenosis may be caused by an anomalous left coronary artery (Buchanan, 1990). In this anomaly, a single large coronary artery originates from the right aortic sinus of Valsalva and quickly divides into right and left branches. The left coronary branch then encircles and compresses the RV outflow tract just below the pulmonary valve. Occasionally, the obstruction consists of fibromuscular narrowing of the infundibular region of the right ventricle, about 1 to 3 cm below the pulmonic valve. In addition, concentric infundibular hypertrophy may appear to encroach on the RV outflow tract and contribute to the outflow obstruction in some dogs, especially during exercise stress.

In all cases, the obstruction causes increased resistance to RV systolic outflow and a proportional increase in RV systolic pressure. The increase in systolic wall stress (tension) stimulates concentric muscular hypertrophy of the RV wall in proportion to severity of the obstruction and pressure elevation. Beyond the obstructing orifice, blood flow velocity increases, also in proportion to the severity of the obstruction, and flow becomes turbulent, resulting in a poststenotic dilatation of the main pulmonary artery. It is the author's experience that mild, subclinical deformities of the tricuspid valve apparatus often accompany PS in dogs, and more severe tricuspid dysplasia with regurgitation is a major complicating lesion in some dogs. In addition, the foramen ovale remains patent in many dogs with PS, and may allow mild to moderate right-to-left shunting of blood in cases of severe PS with increased right atrial pressure.

## DIAGNOSIS

The clinical diagnosis of pulmonic stenosis uses the standard tests used to evaluate patients for all types of cardiac disease: signalment and history, physical examination, electrocardiography, chest radiography, echocardiography and, occasionally, cardiac catheterization and angiography. Only the last two examinations can definitively diagnose PS and determine or estimate its severity.

Most dogs with PS are asymptomatic during the first year of life, when most initial diagnoses are made, even with moderate to severe obstructions. In very severe cases, exertional fatigue, shortness of breath, or syncope may be reported. Although signs of right heart failure (ascites, pleural effusion, peripheral edema) are possible, they are rare in young dogs unless PS is complicated by another anomaly, particularly tricuspid valve dysplasia and regurgitation.

On *physical examination*, the most important finding

is a systolic murmur of variable quality (from blowing to harsh), originating in the pulmonary artery and heard best at the left heart base (third to fourth intercostal spaces). Often, the murmur radiates loudly dorsally in conjunction with the high velocity jet that is directed into the main pulmonary artery. In some cases, the murmur is heard well just lateral to the sternum on both sides of the cranial thorax. In a minority of dogs (<10%), a diastolic murmur of pulmonic insufficiency may also be heard in the same location or radiating to the right side. The arterial pulse is usually normal. The jugular veins are often judged to be normal, although a mildly exaggerated pulse may be noted in the lower third of the neck. If a marked jugular pulse or jugular venous distention is observed, heart failure or additional defects should be suspected, especially tricuspid dysplasia.

The *electrocardiogram* exhibits one or more of the signs of RV hypertrophy (right axis deviation; S waves in leads I, II, III, and aVF; increased S wave magnitude in the left chest leads $V_3$ and $V_6$) in almost every case. The P waves are usually normal. If P waves are very prominent (increased amplitude and duration), tricuspid dysplasia with marked right atrial dilation should be suspected.

*Radiographs* usually demonstrate mild to moderate cardiomegaly, prominence of the right heart, and poststenotic dilatation of the main pulmonary artery on the dorsoventral view. The pulmonary vasculature appears normal to mildly diminished. If the cardiac silhouette appears markedly enlarged, an additional anomaly such as tricuspid dysplasia should be suspected.

Proof of any vascular obstruction requires demonstration of a pressure differential (gradient) during periods of flow across the obstruction. The characteristic right heart pressure tracings obtained in a dog with PS are shown in Figure 1. The pulmonary artery pressure is normal, but as the catheter is withdrawn into the right ventricle, a sharp increase in systolic pressure occurs, resulting in the systolic pressure gradient between the RV and pulmonary artery. Although the magnitude of the gradient reflects the severity of the obstruction, the recorded gradient varies directly with the flow rate across the fixed obstruction, so that it tends to be significantly lower in anesthetized versus awake patients (Martin et al., 1992). As a result, it is difficult to directly compare gradients and obstruction severity in different patients, or even the same patient, unless the gradients were recorded under similar conditions. Nevertheless, for the purpose of estimating prognosis and making recommendations about intervention, the systolic pressure gradient recorded by catheterization has historically been used to divide patients with PS into mild (<50 mm Hg), moderate (50 to 80 mm Hg), or severe (>80 mm Hg) categories, with allowances for the recording setting (awake, anesthetized).

Right ventricular angiography consistently demonstrates the region(s) of RV outflow narrowing, poststenotic dilatation of the pulmonary artery, and RV hypertrophy. In English bulldogs and boxers with an anomalous left coronary artery, the obstruction is subvalvular, and coronary arteriography demonstrates the abnormal course of the left coronary artery adjacent to the obstruction (Buchanan, 1990). Because of limited resolution and views obtained, it is often difficult to determine the exact configuration of any valvular deformity and whether the obstruction involves the subvalvular region just below the valve.

*Echocardiography* provides the primary means of diagnosis of PS in animals, making confirmation by cardiac catheterization unnecessary in most cases. Examples of two-dimensional images from dogs with PS are shown in Figure 2. Typical findings include: mild to moderate right atrial dilation, concentric RV hypertrophy (Fig. 2A), deformity and narrowing in the region of the pulmonary valve, and poststenotic dilatation of the pulmonary artery (Fig. 2B). Unfortunately, in many cases it is difficult to see enough detail of the pulmonary valve region to clearly define the exact location and anatomy of the deformity (e.g., whether there is valve thickening, valve fusion, fibrosis at the valve base), and to predict the chances of success from valvulotomy. It is generally accepted, however, that fibromuscular subvalvular or infundibular obstructions are more difficult to relieve than valvular obstructions. In dogs with an anomalous left coronary artery, the obstructed region can often be defined as subvalvular, and the enlarged right coronary artery and anomalous left coronary artery may be visualized in some cases.

Doppler echocardiography, which measures blood flow velocity by the shift in sound frequency as the ultrasound beam reflects from moving blood cells, has made it possible to noninvasively identify PS and de-

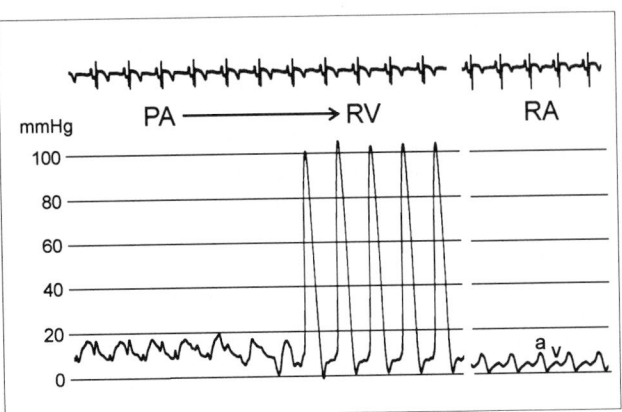

**Figure 1.** Right heart catheterization pressures from a dog with pulmonic stenosis. The pulmonary artery (PA) pressure is normal. As the catheter is withdrawn into the right ventricle (RV), there is an abrupt increase in systolic pressure, resulting in a systolic pressure gradient of 90 mm Hg. The mean right atrial (RA) pressure is normal, but the atrial (A) wave is increased compared to the V wave, indicative of decreased RV compliance from right ventricular hypertrophy.

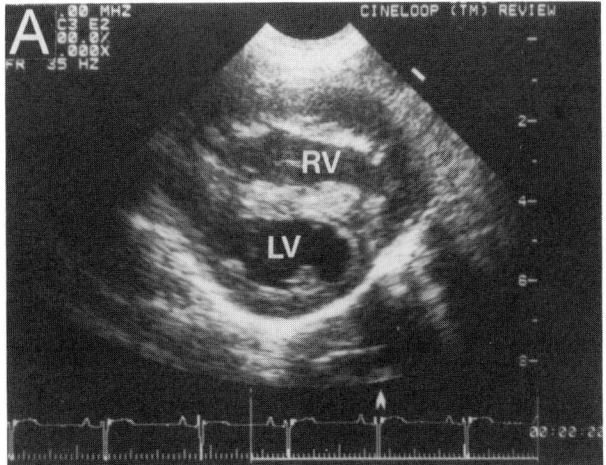

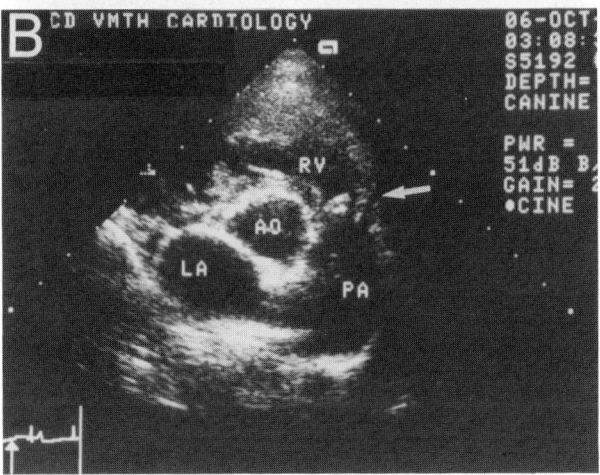

**Figure 2.** Two-dimensional echocardiograms from dogs with pulmonic stenosis. *A,* right parasternal short-axis view, showing concentric hypertrophy of the right ventricle (RV) and ventricular septal flattening, which causes the shape of the left ventricle (LV) to be oval instead of circular. *B,* Right parasternal short-axis view, showing poststenotic dilatation of the pulmonary artery (PA) and a thickened pulmonary valve (*arrow*). Abbreviations: LA = left atrium, AO = aorta.

termine its severity. Two-dimensional, color-coded Doppler produces an image of blood flow velocity superimposed on the familiar gray-scale anatomic image. It readily identifies the turbulent systolic jet distal to the stenosis, and also demonstrates pulmonic valve regurgitation in most cases. It also may help identify the exact location of the obstruction. Using a continuous-wave Doppler beam aligned with flow, the peak velocity of the obstructive systolic jet can be measured. The modified Bernoulli equation, $\Delta P = 4V^2$, relates the pressure gradient across an obstruction ($\Delta P$, in mm Hg) to the peak velocity of the jet distal to the obstruction (V, in m/sec). Peak Doppler jet velocities of 3, 4, and 5 m/sec correspond to peak systolic pressure gradients of 36, 64, and 100 mm Hg, respectively. Doppler estimates of systolic pressure gradients in humans and dogs with PS have shown very good correlation with invasive pressure measurements made under the same conditions. Doppler imaging, which is safe, atraumatic,

and noninvasive, promises to provide the means for accurate evaluation of many more animals with PS (and other defects), whose owners might be reluctant to allow cardiac catheterization.

## THERAPY

### Guidelines for Recommending Therapy

Although firm guidelines for categorizing the severity of PS in dogs and cats for purposes of prognosis and therapy have not been developed, there is general agreement that dogs with resting gradients in the severe category (>80 mm Hg) are at increased risk for syncope, congestive heart failure, or sudden death. Surgical intervention, if available, is usually recommended for these dogs, whether or not they are currently symptomatic. Dogs with resting gradients in the mild category (<50 mm Hg) usually live nearly normal lives and surgery is rarely necessary (Fingland et al., 1986). The exception to this rule is the dog with significant tricuspid regurgitation in addition to mild PS, in which partial relief of the otherwise mild outflow obstruction may be beneficial. Dogs with intermediate resting gradients (50 to 80 mm Hg) often live very comfortably, but the long-term prognosis should be guarded. In these dogs, the decision whether to recommend intervention should include consideration of clinical signs, the activity level and use of the dog, whether the gradient is closer to 50 or 80 mm Hg, and evidence of progressive cardiomegaly and increasing gradient over time.

One possible important exception to these guidelines is dogs with subvalvular stenosis associated with an anomalous left coronary artery. In a recent letter (Kittleson et al., 1992), it was reported that two English bulldogs with this anomaly died acutely during balloon dilation valvulotomy due to rupture of the anomalous vessel. Another dog died during patch-graft surgery due to severing of the artery (Buchanan, 1990). Conduit implantation around the stenosis may be the only option for these dogs.

### Surgery

The options for treatment of pulmonic stenosis are all surgical techniques for relieving or reducing the degree of RV outflow obstruction. Medical therapy is of little benefit unless there are signs of congestion or edema associated with the development of right heart failure. The goal of treatment is to reduce the obstructive pressure gradient from its preoperative level into the mild range postoperatively. Historically, various open surgical techniques have been used to enlarge the right ventricular outflow area. Techniques used in dogs have included (1) right ventriculotomy or pulmonary arteriotomy, and valvulotomy by direct examination; (2) closed valvulotomy, using a valvulotome and dilating instruments inserted through a small incision in the RV wall or pulmonary artery; (3) patch graft application over a previously positioned multifilament wire, which is then used as a saw to perform an arterioventriculotomy under the patch; and (4) implantation of a valved or nonvalved conduit from the RV to the pulmonary artery to create a second route for RV outflow. These techniques are described in detail in other texts (Breznock, 1990). All of these techniques require thoracotomy and knowledge of techniques for handling and incising the heart, and all include significant surgical risk, including operative mortalities of up to 10% or more. Each technique has shown variable success at relieving the RV outflow obstruction and decreasing RV systolic pressure in dogs. However, because of the expense, risk, equipment, and expertise associated with such surgeries, only a small percentage of affected dogs and cats have undergone open chest surgical treatment, and this limited availability is likely to continue. Prior to any surgery, a Doppler-estimated gradient should be measured to provide a means for noninvasive, future follow-up examinations.

## Balloon Dilation Valvulotomy

In the past 10 years, balloon catheter dilation has rapidly become the initial treatment of choice for relieving intracardiac and vascular obstructions in humans. The technique uses a catheter with a strong, cylindrical balloon at its end. When the balloon is positioned across an obstruction and inflated with fluid under pressure, the pressure from the balloon fractures and/or stretches the obstructing tissue, increasing the size of the lumen. Balloon dilation has been particularly successful in both children and adults with congenital valvular PS, resulting in partial reduction of the obstruction in more than 90% of patients (McKay and Grossman, 1988). Because the technique only requires access to a peripheral vein large enough to accept the catheter, it is simpler, less traumatic, safer, and less costly than open chest procedures. Required equipment includes the balloon catheter and fluoroscopy for guidance. The first report of its application in a dog appeared in 1987 (Bright et al., 1987). Since then, it has become the technique preferred by veterinary cardiologists for treatment of PS in dogs (Sisson and MacCoy, 1988; Brownlie et al., 1991; Martin et al., 1992). Successful reduction of the obstructive pressure gradient by 50% or more has been reported in about 75 to 80% of dogs treated. Excluding dogs with an anomalous left coronary artery, major complications (perforation of the heart by the catheter, tricuspid valve damage) are uncommon but potentially life threatening. Minor complications (arrhythmias, right bundlebranch block, entry vein damage requiring ligation, or hemorrhage) are common but not serious.

The procedure is performed as follows: under general anesthesia and using fluoroscopic guidance, right heart catheterization is performed via a jugular or femoral vein approach. Pressures in the pulmonary artery, right ventricle, and right atrium are measured, cardiac output is determined by thermodilution, and right ventricular angiography is performed. The approximate diameter of the pulmonary valve annulus is measured from the angiogram, and a dilation catheter with a balloon diameter of 1.0 to 1.3 times the annular diameter is chosen (McKay and Grossman, 1988). A flexible guidewire is passed through an end-hole catheter and positioned across the obstruction with its tip in a pulmonary artery. The balloon dilation catheter, with the balloon collapsed and wound around its end, is passed over the guidewire and the balloon is positioned across the obstruction by fluoroscopic visualization of the metallic markers at each end of the balloon (Fig. 3). The balloon is then flushed with sterile saline to remove all

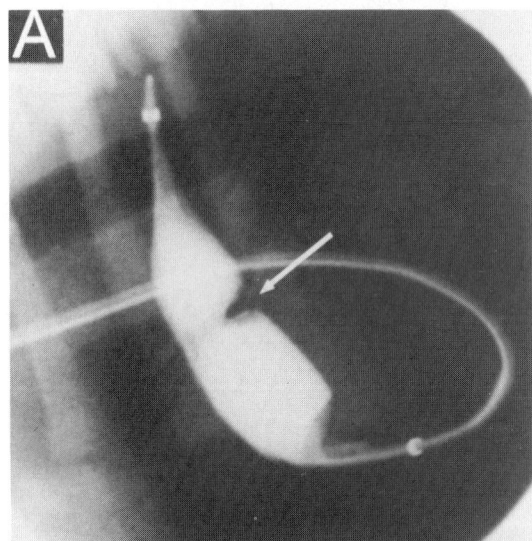

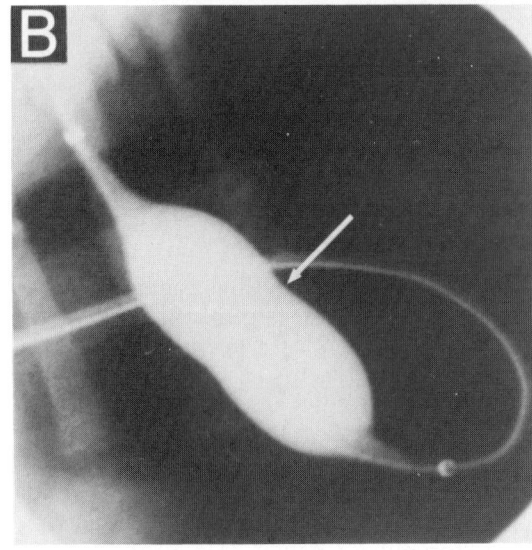

**Figure 3.** Lateral radiographs recorded during inflation of a balloon dilation catheter, from a dog with valvular pulmonic stenosis and a systolic pressure gradient of 84 mm Hg. The balloon has been positioned across the stenotic pulmonary valve. *A*, The balloon is partially inflated and a distinct indentation or waist is seen at the obstruction (*arrow*). *B*, The balloon has been fully pressure inflated and the indentation has been nearly eliminated (*arrow*). The pressure gradient after dilation was 24 mm Hg. (Modified from Sisson DD and MacCoy DM: Treatment of congenital pulmonic stenosis in two dogs by balloon valvuloplasty. J Vet Intern Med 2:92, 1988, with permission.)

air bubbles. Dilation of the obstruction is accomplished by manual inflation of the balloon, using a 5:1 dilution of angiographic contrast solution. During inflation, proper positioning is determined by the appearance of a narrowing or waist in the balloon at the site of the stenosis (Fig. 3A). Pressure is increased in the balloon until it achieves maximal inflation and the narrowing disappears or is reduced (Fig. 3B). After 5 to 10 sec of inflation, the balloon is deflated and the blood pressure and heart rate are allowed to return to normal. The dilation is repeated one to three additional times, depending on how well the obstruction appears to have been relieved. The balloon catheter is then carefully withdrawn over the guidewire, taking care to avoid any resistance at the tricuspid valve. Hemodynamic and angiographic studies are repeated following the procedure to determine the degree of pressure gradient reduction and to make sure that the procedure has not caused a marked increase in tricuspid or pulmonary valve regurgitation. Successful dilation is indicated by a marked reduction in RV systolic pressure (and RV-PA gradient) compared to predilation values (Fig. 4), without a major change in cardiac output. Although any reduction in pressure gradient may be beneficial, the goal should be to reduce the pressure gradient to its lowest possible level. In practice, postoperative gradients of 20 to 50 mm Hg are often achieved and should be considered good results. In some dogs with very severe obstructions and gradients above 150 mm Hg, at least a 50% reduction in gradient is possible, although it may be difficult to achieve postoperative gradients of less than 50 mm Hg. Postoperative care of patients undergoing balloon dilation is minimal, and they can usually be discharged within 12 to 24 hr following the procedure.

Long-term follow-up studies in humans indicate excellent longevity and quality of life for patients whose PS is reduced to a mild level. Although fewer studies are available for dogs, the results appear to be similar. The initial reduction in the pressure gradient persists over succeeding months in most dogs, and the prognosis is probably improved, especially if the gradient can be reduced to less than 50 mm Hg. It is also conceivable that gradients caused by secondary infundibular hypertrophy may regress if the primary valvular or subvalvular obstructive lesion is dilated successfully. Improvements in catheter design, aggressive selection of balloon diameter relative to pulmonary annular diameter, and further experience with the technique should further improve outcomes. Additional work may also indicate whether the technique can be applied to animals with PS as part of more complicated defects.

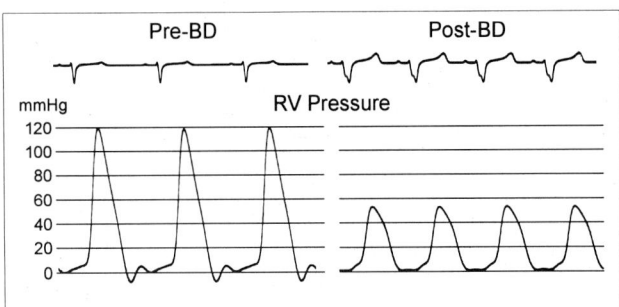

**Figure 4.** Right ventricular pressure from a dog with valvular pulmonic stenosis, recorded before (Pre-BD) and after (Post-BD) balloon dilation valvulotomy. The systolic pressure decreased from 120 mm Hg (gradient = 100 mm Hg, severe) to 55 mm Hg (gradient = 35 mm Hg, mild). Note also the electrocardiographic change above, caused by the development of right bundle-branch block during the dilation.

## References and Suggested Reading

Breznock EM: Surgical relief of pulmonic stenosis. *In* Bojrab MJ (ed): *Current Techniques in Small Animal Surgery*, 3rd edition. Philadelphia, Lea & Febiger, 1990, p 513.

Bright JM, Jennings J, Toal R, and Hood ME: Percutaneous balloon valvuloplasty for treatment of pulmonic stenosis in a dog. J Am Vet Med Assoc 191:995, 1987.

Brownlie JM, Cobb MA, Chambers J, et al: Percutaneous balloon valvuloplasty in four dogs with pulmonic stenosis. J Small Anim Pract 32:165, 1991.

Buchanan JW: Pulmonic stenosis caused by single coronary artery in dogs: Four cases (1965–1984). J Am Vet Med Assoc 196:115, 1990.

Buchanan JW: Causes and prevalence of cardiovascular disease. *In* Kirk RW and Bonagura JD (eds): *Current Veterinary Therapy XI: Small Animal Practice*. Philadelphia, WB Saunders Co, 1992, p 647.

Fingland RB, Bonagura JD, and Myer CW: Pulmonic stenosis in the dog: 29 cases (1975–1984). J Am Vet Med Assoc 189:218, 1986.

Kittleson MD, et al: Letter to the editor. J Vet Intern Med 6:250, 1992.

Martin MWS, Godman M, Fuentes VL, et al: Assessment of balloon pulmonary valvuloplasty in six dogs. J Small Anim Pract 33:443, 1992.

McKay RG and Grossman W: Balloon valvuloplasty for treating pulmonic, mitral, aortic, and prosthetic valve stenoses. *In* Braunwald E (ed): *Heart Disease. A Textbook of Cardiovascular Medicine*, 3rd edition, update 1. Philadelphia, WB Saunders Co, 1988, p 1.

Patterson DF, Haskins ME, and Schnarr WR: Hereditary dysplasia of the pulmonary valve in beagle dogs. Am J Cardiol 47:631, 1981.

Sisson DD and MacCoy DM: Treatment of congenital pulmonic stenosis in two dogs by balloon valvuloplasty. J Vet Intern Med 2:92, 1988.

# CVT UPDATE: CANINE SUBVALVULAR
# AORTIC STENOSIS

LINDA B. LEHMKUHL
*and* JOHN D. BONAGURA
*Columbus, Ohio*

Subvalvular aortic stenosis (SAS) is the second most common canine congenital heart defect, comprising 22% of defects reported to the Veterinary Medical Data Base from 1987 to 1989 (Buchanan, 1992). The left ventricular outflow tract obstruction identified in dogs ranges from an incomplete fibrous ridge to a fibromuscular tunnel (Pyle et al., 1976). Generalized narrowing of the outflow tract and dynamic obstruction have also been described (Sisson, 1992; Buoscio et al., 1994). Current clinical dilemmas in the management of SAS include: (1) preventing transmission of this defect to future generations by identifying mildly affected, asymptomatic dogs; (2) development of effective therapies to decrease or eliminate signs such as exercise intolerance, syncope, and congestive heart failure; and (3) preventing sudden cardiac death in moderate to severely affected dogs.

The pathologic and clinical findings of fixed and dynamic SAS have been thoroughly reviewed in the last edition by Sisson (Sisson, 1992). The focus of this article is to briefly review the recognition of fixed SAS and provide an update on the use of Doppler echocardiography (DE) and Holter monitors in disease assessment, as well as to summarize recent therapeutic advances in the use of balloon catheter dilation (BD).

## CLINICAL FINDINGS

Breeds commonly affected with SAS include Newfoundlands, golden retrievers, Rottweilers, boxers, and German shepherd dogs (Buchanan, 1992). Breeding experiments in Newfoundland dogs have confirmed that SAS is inherited in this breed, but the exact mode of transmission has not been elucidated (Pyle et al., 1976). Of importance is the observation that even mildly affected or clinically normal dogs may transmit the defect to future generations. These studies also revealed development of the lesion in the early postnatal period (perhaps making "congenital" SAS a misnomer) and progression of the lesion with maturity (Pyle et al., 1976).

Clinical features of SAS vary with the severity of the obstruction and the presence of concurrent cardiac lesions. In severely affected dogs, abnormalities are evident on routine cardiac evaluations including physical examination, thoracic radiographs, and the electrocardiogram (ECG). The murmur of severe SAS is a loud, late-peaking systolic ejection murmur heard best over the left subaortic region and the right craniodorsal cardiac base. The murmur often radiates widely—craniodorsally, apically, and even to the head. A soft diastolic murmur of aortic regurgitation is detected in a small percentage of dogs with severe SAS. A holosystolic murmur of mitral regurgitation may be heard over the left apex in some dogs; this murmur can develop from concurrent mitral malformation, envelopment of the mitral valve in the subaortic ring, or from geometric changes in the left ventricle. Additional physical findings include a weak, late-rising arterial pulse and palpable left ventricular heave. In most moderate to severe cases of SAS, radiography demonstrates elongation of the heart, caused by left ventricular hypertrophy, and poststenotic dilation of the ascending aorta. The ECG may demonstrate left ventricular hypertrophy, ST-segment depression, and ventricular extrasystoles.

The dog with mild subaortic obstruction characteristically lacks clinical signs and has a normal thoracic radiograph and electrocardiogram. Physical examination is characterized by normal pulses and precordium, and a soft protomesosystolic murmur heard best immediately caudoventral to the aortic valve area. Exercise can intensify a low-grade murmur; however, post-exercise ventilation and tracheal sounds may prevent detection of these soft murmurs. Exercise may also amplify "physiologic" murmurs. Heavy sedation or anesthesia, probably by decreasing left ventricular contractility, may attenuate the murmur. Distinguishing murmurs caused by mild SAS from "functional" murmurs can be difficult. Generally, functional murmurs are heard best over or craniodorsal to the pulmonary or aortic valve areas. Usually, the electrocardiogram and thoracic radiography are of little or no benefit in evaluation of mildly affected dogs because the obstruction is insufficient to cause detectable changes. Doppler echocardiography is the method used by the authors to screen dogs with soft systolic murmurs for SAS.

## DOPPLER ECHOCARDIOGRAPHY

Diagnosis of SAS in moderately to severely affected dogs (unanesthetized Doppler pressure gradient >75 mmHg) is straightforward inasmuch as a discrete or segmental obstructive lesion, left ventricular hypertrophy, and poststenotic aortic dilation can typically be imaged during two-dimensional echocardiographic studies. In severe cases, hyperechoic segments of the left ventricular myocardium, presumably due to subendocardial fibrosis, may also be appreciated. Doppler studies often demonstrate mitral or aortic regurgitation in these dogs.

Disease severity is quantitated by measurement of the left ventricular–to–aortic systolic pressure gradient. In a normal dog, the aortic valve is open during systole and only a small instantaneous gradient exists between the left ventricle and aorta. In SAS, the left ventricular pressure is elevated to eject blood across the stenosis, and the resultant pressure gradient generally correlates with disease severity. The pressure gradient across a fixed obstruction is a function of not only orifice area but also transvalvular flow; therefore, in states of high or low flow, pressure gradient determination may over- or underestimate lesion severity, respectively.

The pressure gradient can be measured directly by cardiac catheterization or estimated by DE. Although cardiac catheterization has traditionally been the "gold standard" for clinical staging of SAS, there are considerable drawbacks to this invasive and expensive diagnostic study. Doppler echocardiography can provide the same information as catheterization noninvasively. Doppler technology permits measurement of the velocity of red blood cells (RBC) traversing the obstruction. Applying the modified Bernoulli equation to velocity measurements enables pressure gradient determination where:

Pressure gradient = [RBC velocity in m/sec]$^2 \times 4$

Doppler-estimated pressure gradients over 75 mm Hg in lightly sedated dogs are considered to represent a moderate to severe obstruction at the authors' clinic. It should be noted that in some affected dogs the pressure gradient may increase markedly with growth. This is particularly common in giant-breed dogs such as Newfoundlands when they are examined as pups and subsequently as adults. We have not observed large increases in outflow gradients in adult dogs followed for several years.

The relationship between pressure gradients measured by DE and those recorded by cardiac catheterization has been investigated in dogs (Valdes-Cruz et al., 1985; Thomas, 1990). In general, the two methodologies yield very similar gradients over a wide range of values. In comparison studies, it is important that the same gradients are compared under similar physiologic conditions. The possible measured gradients include catheterization and Doppler maximal instantaneous (peak) gradients and mean gradients as well as the traditional peak-to-peak catheterization gradient (Fig. 1). The peak-to-peak gradient is the difference between the peak left ventricular pressure and peak aortic pressure. Note that there is no Doppler correlate to the easily recorded peak-to-peak catheterization gradient because Doppler records instantaneous gradients and the peak aortic pressure occurs later in systole than the peak left ventricular pressure. The peak-to-peak gradient is not "seen" by the left ventricle; the left ventricle works against the more physiologic maximal instantaneous or mean gradient. We compared the mean

and maximal instantaneous gradients recorded by continuous-wave Doppler to gradients measured by dual-tipped micromanometer catheters on a beat-to-beat basis in 15 dogs with SAS. Good agreement between the two techniques was demonstrated (Fig. 2), and high correlation coefficients ($r > .97$) were obtained for both maximal and mean pressure gradients (Fig. 3).

The determined pressure gradient should always be evaluated in light of measurement conditions. We compared the pressure gradients measured in 20 dogs lightly sedated with acepromazine (0.03 mg/kg, IV) and buprenorphine (0.0075 mg/kg, IV) to those gradients obtained in the same dogs under general anesthesia. On average, the peak Doppler gradient decreased under anesthesia by 50%. Errors in severity assessment and diagnosis of SAS may result by neglecting the potential for depression of the myocardium and decreased transvalvular flow decreasing the pressure gradient in dogs under general anesthesia.

Diagnosis of mildly affected dogs is challenging, and it is of critical importance in preventing genetic transmission of SAS and predicting complications such as bacterial endocarditis. Dogs with no murmur are undetectable clinically by any available diagnostic modality. Dogs with a soft murmur and no clinical signs may also go undetected due to lack of owner education or unsuccessful physical examination. Identifying these dogs requires careful auscultation in a quiet room; confirmation of SAS necessitates an echocardiographic evaluation including Doppler. We do not believe that a two-dimensional echocardiogram, without Doppler, is sufficiently sensitive to exclude a diagnosis of mild SAS.

Detection of increased velocity flow across the left ventricular outflow tract and proximal aorta is used to diagnose mild SAS by DE. The normal upper limit for aortic flow velocity is not well established, but the maximal accepted aortic velocity for our laboratory in a dog lightly sedated with either acepromazine (3 mg/m$^2$ subcutaneously) or acepromazine-buprenorphine is 1.7 m/sec. Values between 1.7 and 2.2 m/sec are considered equivocal; however, we believe such values to be compatible with mild SAS when *other* supporting abnormalities are evident. Such abnormalities include sudden velocity acceleration in the left ventricular outflow tract, disturbed flow in the outflow tract or ascending aorta, and aortic regurgitation. Other laboratories use similar but slightly different criteria for diagnosing mild SAS.

When using DE for diagnosis and severity assessment of SAS, multiple transducer placement sites (windows) should be used in order to minimize underestimation of the true velocity caused by poor alignment with flow. We compared the maximal aortic velocity and derived left ventricular to aortic pressure gradient obtained prospectively from 12 dogs with SAS from three transducer windows: subcostal, left apical, and suprasternal notch (Lehmkuhl and Bonagura, 1994). Doppler-estimated pressure gradients calculated from the subcostal velocities were greater than those estimated from the other two windows in most individual dogs and on average for the group. This finding was

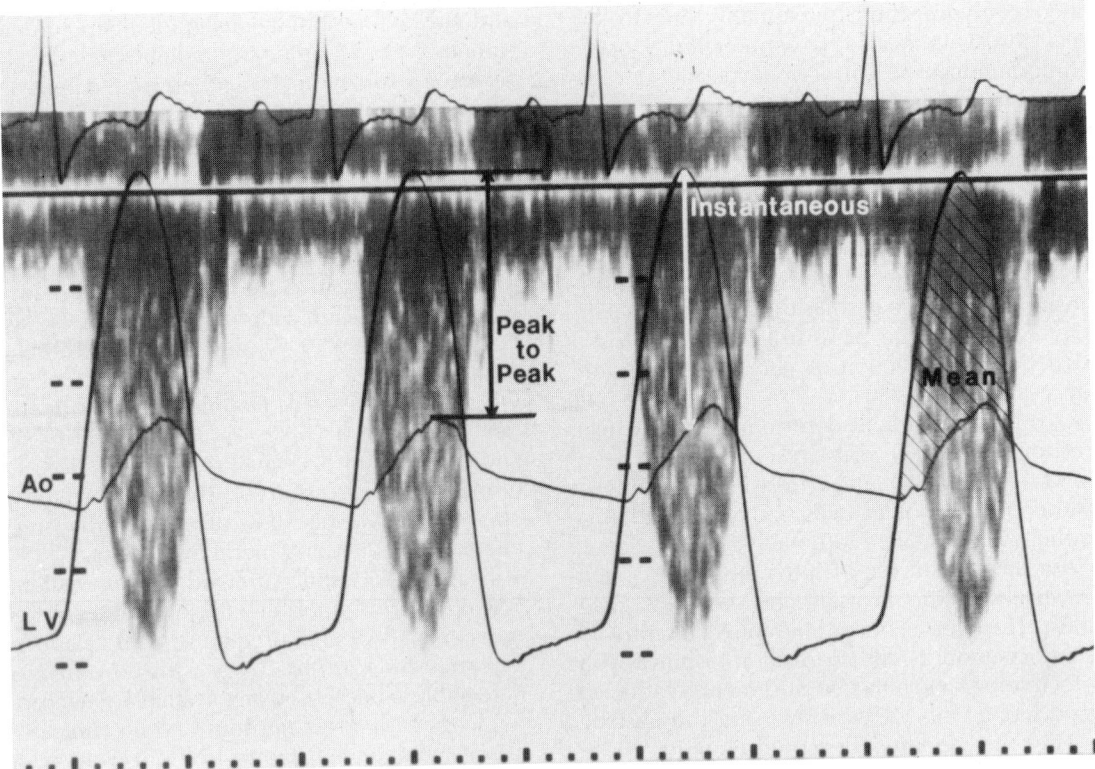

**Figure 1.** Pressure gradient determinations from catheterization and Doppler data. *First curve*: Doppler spectra and left ventricular (LV) and aortic (Ao) pressure traces are shown. The maximal instantaneous Doppler gradient was calculated from the peak aortic velocity and the mean Doppler gradient was calculated by averaging many instantaneous gradients over the ejection period. *Second curve*: The peak-to-peak catheterization gradient is measured by subtracting the peak aortic pressure from the peak left ventricular pressure. *Third curve*: The maximal instantaneous catheterization gradient is the greatest pressure difference at a point in time. *Fourth curve*: Mean catheterization gradient is determined by measuring the area between the left ventricular and aortic pressure curves divided by time. Doppler calibration marks are 1 m/sec. An electrocardiogram is displayed at the top of the figure (paper speed = 100 mm/sec). (Reprinted with permission from the Journal of the American Society of Echocardiography, manuscript #890, 1995.)

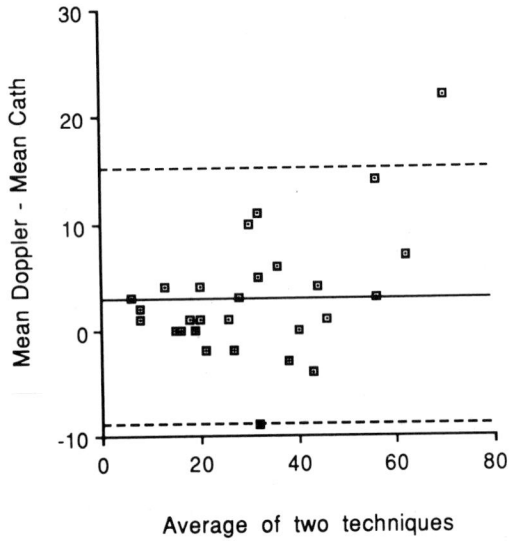

**Figure 2.** The difference between simultaneous Doppler and catheterization mean gradients in relation to the average pressure gradient determined by the two techniques during sinus rhythm. Each data point represents an average of five sinus beats. ————, mean; -----, 2SD. (Reprinted from the Journal of the American Society of Echocardiography, manuscript #890, 1995, in press.)

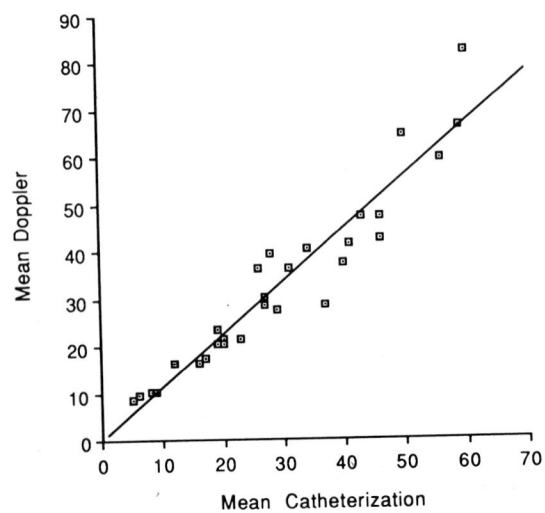

**Figure 3.** Correlation of simultaneous Doppler and catheterization mean gradients measured during sinus rhythm. Each data point represents an average of five sinus beats. (Reprinted from the Journal of the American Society of Echocardiography, manuscript #890, 1995, in press.)

attributed to optimal anatomic alignment with flow from this location. The use of multiple transducer windows decreases the potential for undetection of mildly affected dogs and underestimation of lesion severity.

We consider the use of DE for detection of SAS to be very important. The derived physiologic data are not contaminated by the effects of general anesthesia and can be collected noninvasively. This technique enables us to diagnose SAS and also to establish an accurate prognosis, monitor disease progression, and determine the efficacy of different therapeutic interventions.

## HOLTER MONITORS

Ventricular arrhythmias may account for syncope or sudden death in dogs with moderate to severe SAS. Myocardial ischemia is thought to contribute to the development of lethal arrhythmias. The susceptibility of the hypertrophied left ventricle of affected dogs to development of subendocardial ischemia has been documented experimentally (Borkon et al., 1982), and is evidenced by observed histologic lesions of myocardial necrosis and fibrosis. Myocardial ischemia likely results from a combination of decreased oxygen supply and increased oxygen demands. Abnormal coronary perfusion and intramural coronary artery lesions noted in dogs with SAS contribute to the oxygen debt (Pyle et al., 1973; Muna et al., 1978).

Long-term ambulatory electrocardiographic (Holter) recordings may provide early detection of a cardiac rhythm abnormality and allow us to quantify the frequency and severity of identified arrhythmias. In addition to enabling early institution of antiarrhythmic therapy for serious ventricular arrhythmias, Holter recordings can also be used to assess efficacy of antiarrhythmic therapy. These monitors are available from a number of companies (Roche Ambulatory Monitoring Services) complete with instruction tapes for attachment and removal (see "Twenty-Four-Hour Ambulatory Electrocardiography (Holter Monitoring)," this volume, p 792).

Twenty-four-hour Holter ECGs from dogs with SAS often reveal previously undetected ventricular premature complexes (VPCs) or ventricular tachycardia. In our experience, there is a general trend for dogs with higher pressure gradients to have more frequent VPCs, but considerable variability exists. Holter monitor reports help to characterize the arrhythmia frequency, morphology (uniform or multiform), and timing (single versus couplets or triplets; coupling intervals), as well as identify rhythm disturbances relative to daily activities.

There is a lack of information correlating the characterization of an arrhythmia and the likelihood of syncope or sudden death. However, documentation of sustained ventricular tachycardia or the presence of VPCs on the preceding beats T wave ("R on T"), for example, suggest the need for antiarrhythmic therapy. Institution of antiarrhythmic therapy may be proarrhythmic, expensive, or associated with gastrointestinal and other systemic side effects; therefore, the attending veterinarian must carefully weigh the risks and potential benefits of any antiarrhythmic therapy. Perhaps better characterization of arrhythmias by Holter recordings, combined with long-term patient follow-up, will enable us to develop objective guidelines for the institution of therapy.

Monitoring the effectiveness of antiarrhythmic therapy is initially done by history, physical examination, and routine ECGs. Ideally, a 24-hr Holter monitor is used to verify extended arrhythmia control in the pet's natural environment. Standards previously reported in people suggest that a reduction in VPCs of between 65 and 83% is required to distinguish a therapeutic effect from spontaneous variability (Sami et al., 1980; Morganroth et al., 1978).

In addition to arrhythmia detection, Holter recordings can identify ST-segment deviation. ST-segment depression, probably related to myocardial ischemia, is identified in some dogs with moderate to severe SAS. This change is present more often in dogs with higher pressure gradients and with exercise. As some of the empirically prescribed medications for SAS attempt to reduce myocardial oxygen demand or improve coronary perfusion, Holter monitoring of ST-segment changes (particularly with exercise) may be of benefit in monitoring therapy.

## THERAPY

### Medical Therapy

Therapy of mild SAS is not indicated, with the exception of prophylactic antibiotics for potential bacteremic episodes (dental procedures, surgery, skin wounds) due to the established risk of endocarditis (Muna et al., 1978).

Therapeutic options are frustratingly limited for moderate to severe SAS. Medical therapy with $\beta$-blockers or calcium channel blockers is occasionally utilized to reduce myocardial oxygen demand or increase coronary perfusion, but their benefits have not been documented. We prescribe atenolol (50-mg tablet; $\frac{1}{4}$ to 1 tablet every 12 hr) for dogs with moderate to severe stenosis, in dogs with frequent or malignant ventricular extrasystoles, and when ST deviation is evident on Holter tracings. Resting heart rate and post-therapy Holter ECG are used to monitor treatment. Medical therapy including digitalis, furosemide, and rest have been used in dogs that develop congestive heart failure.

Limited surgical successes have been reported with various techniques; however, the high costs, technical difficulty, restenosis, and high mortality rates associated with surgery have made this option generally disappointing. Recent surgical success has been reported (Orton et al., 1993; Komtebedde et al., 1993) utilizing open resection of the subaortic obstruction during cardiopulmonary bypass, suggesting a possible role for surgery in the future management of this condition. Some dogs develop progressive myocardial failure despite successful surgery (Eyster, 1988).

## Balloon Catheter Dilation

Dilation with a balloon-tipped catheter has been used successfully to relieve the obstruction in children and young adults with discrete subaortic stenosis (De Lezo et al., 1991), and a recent report of BD in nine dogs with SAS by DeLellis and her colleagues was encouraging (DeLellis, Thomas, Pion, 1993). In a third of these dogs, the peak-to-peak pressure gradient decreased by 60% or greater and the remaining six dogs showed a decreased gradient of 25 to 50%. Immediate results at our hospital in 20 consecutive dogs are similar. On average, the gradient decreased by 53%; two thirds of our dogs experienced a drop in pressure gradient by 50% or greater, and excluding one dog with a 19% decrease, the remaining dogs experienced reductions of between 25 and 49%.

Balloon dilation is accomplished under fluoroscopic guidance. To position the balloon dilation catheter, a guidewire is advanced through an end-hole catheter placed in the left ventricle retrograde through the carotid artery. The end-hole catheter is then removed, and a balloon catheter is advanced over the guidewire and centered across the stenosis. The balloon is inflated under pressure (usually multiple times) with dilute contrast agent. Inflation is continued until either the balloon waist disappears, a preselected inflation pressure is reached, or balloon rupture occurs.

Balloon rupture has been reported in humans and dogs (DeLellis, Thomas, Pion, 1993). Manufacturers recommend the use of pressure gauges to guide inflating pressure to a predetermined limit; however, pressure gauges are not always used and higher pressures may be necessary to eliminate the balloon's waist and dilate the stenosis. For economic considerations, we reuse catheters despite the admonition that repeated use, maintenance of high pressure in the balloon, and resterilization increase the risk of balloon rupture. Balloon rupture is problematic if air or catheter emboli result. Fortunately, BD catheters almost always tear in a linear, longitudinal fashion, allowing removal in the event of a rupture, and the risk for air emboli is minimized by proper technique.

The risk for mortality from BD in dogs is low. There were no deaths in our series and only one dog (whose data was excluded) died in the report by DeLellis (DeLellis, Thomas, Pion, 1993). Complications including transient ventricular arrhythmias and conduction disturbances, although potentially life threatening, have not caused any long-term detriment to date. All dogs develop intermittent VPCs or paroxysmal ventricular tachycardia during balloon inflation, but few dogs require antiarrhythmic therapy after recovery. Left bundle-branch block is not infrequent, and third-degree AV block developed in one dog in our experience and one dog in DeLellis' report. In both dogs, the AV block resolved within 30 min.

One concern over the use of BD is the potential for creating or worsening existing aortic regurgitation. In one of our dogs, audible aortic regurgitation developed following BD. However, in children and in the previous veterinary report, there was no significant change detected in the degree of aortic regurgitation following BD (DeLellis, Thomas, Pion, 1993; De Lezo et al., 1991).

Long-term results of BD in dogs are not yet available. The effects of BD on maximal instantaneous pressure gradient (recorded under light sedation) has been evaluated by DE in 18 of our 20 dogs from 2 weeks to 6 months after BD. In some (but not all) dogs, a sustained reduction of the gradient is demonstrable at 6 months after this therapeutic intervention. Six months after BD, one dog had a 65% decrease, 11 dogs had decreases between 26 and 50%, and the rest were decreased by less than 20% (three dogs) or increased (three dogs).

There are still many unanswered questions regarding this technique: Is there an ideal age to perform BD? What is the ideal technique in terms of balloon size and number, or time and pressure of inflation? Are some anatomic forms of SAS more amenable to BD? Importantly, effects of BD on the development of clinical signs or on long-term survival are not yet established. Despite these unknowns, BD merits consideration in dogs with severe SAS (awake or lightly sedated, DE gradients >125 mm Hg) and possibly those with moderate obstruction (awake or lightly sedated, DE gradients >75 mm Hg).

## References and Suggested Readings

Borkon AM, Jones M, Bell JH, and Pierce JE: Regional myocardial blood flow in left ventricular hypertrophy. J Thorac Cardiovasc Surg 84:876, 1982.
*A radioactive microsphere study of regional myocardial blood flow documents a greater susceptibility to development of subendocardial ischemia in dogs with SAS and left ventricular hypertrophy.*

Bouscio DA, Sisson D, Zachary JF, and Luethy M: Clinical and pathological characterization of an unusual form of subvalvular aortic stenosis in four golden retriever puppies. J Am Anim Hosp Assoc 30:100, 1994
*Describes the clinical catheterization and pathologic findings in four puppies with fixed and dynamic SAS.*

Buchanan JW: Causes and prevalence of cardiovascular disease. In Kirk RW and Bonagura JD (eds): Current Veterinary Therapy XI. Philadelphia, WB Saunders Co, 1992, p 647.
*Reviews veterinary literature and summarizes new data from the Veterinary Medical Data Base on the causes and prevalence of cardiovascular diseases in dogs and cats.*

DeLellis LA, Thomas WP, and Pion PD: Balloon dilation of congenital subaortic stenosis in the dog. J Vet Intern Med 7:153, 1993.
*Reports the technique and short-term hemodynamic and clinical results of balloon dilation in nine dogs with subaortic stenosis.*

De Lezo J, Pan M, Medina A, et al: Immediate and follow-up results of transluminal balloon dilation for discrete subaortic stenosis. J Am Coll Cardiol 18:1309, 1991.
*A prospective study detailing the immediate and long-term findings in 33 human patients with discrete subaortic stenosis who were treated by percutaneous balloon dilation.*

Eyster GE: Surgery for aortic stenosis in the dog. Proc 6th ACVIM Forum, 1988, p 594.
*Discusses surgical results of open heart resection of the subvalvular ridge and left ventriculotomy with valve dilation using a valvulotome.*

Follette DM, et al: Resection of subvalvular aortic stenosis. Vet Surg 22:419, 1993.
*This paper focuses on the use of cardiopulmonary bypass, summarizes the results of open heart resection in seven dogs with SAS.*

Lehmkuhl LB and Bonagura JD: Comparison of transducer placement sites

for Doppler echocardiography in dogs with subaortic stenosis. Am J Vet Res 55:192, 1994.
*A prospective comparison of two observers and three transducer placement sites for the determination of maximal aortic velocity and aortic velocity time integral.*

Morganroth J, Michelson EL, Horowitz LN, et al: Limitations of routine long-term electrocardiographic monitoring to assess ventricular ectopic frequency. Circulation 58:408, 1978.
*Prospective Holter study comparing the frequency of VPC on three consecutive 24-hr recordings from 15 human patients with different heart disorders. Spontaneous variation in arrhythmia frequency in individuals was quantified and used to establish a reduction in VPC frequency attributable to therapy rather than spontaneous variation.*

Muna WF, Ferran VJ, Pierce JE, et al: Discrete subaortic stenosis in Newfoundland dogs: Association of infective endocarditis. Am J Cardiol 41:746, 1978.
*A necropsy study of 8 Newfoundlands describes infective endocarditis in four dogs and lesions in the intramural coronary arteries in all eight dogs.*

Orton C, Boon J, Wagner A, et al: Open resection of discrete subvalvular aortic stenosis: Early results. Proc 11th ACVIM Forum, 1993, p 929.
*Abstract summarizes the hemodynamic and clinical results of open resection in nine dogs with subaortic stenosis.*

Pyle RL, Patterson DF, and Chacko S: The genetics and pathology of discrete subaortic stenosis in the Newfoundland dog. Am Heart J 92:324, 1976.
*A detailed genetic and pathologic study involving 139 dogs from 22 test matings.*

Pyle RL, Lowenstein HS, Khouri EM, et al: Left circumflex artery hemodynamics in conscious dogs with congenital subaortic stenosis. Circ Res 33:34, 1973.
*Documents abnormal systolic and diastolic coronary blood flow in dogs with subaortic stenosis.*

Sami M, Kraemer H, Harrison DC, et al: A new method for evaluating antiarrhythmic drug efficacy. Circulation 62:1172, 1980.
*Patients with ischemic heart disease underwent treadmill exercise testing and ambulatory electrocardiography to study spontaneous variability of VPC frequency and establish standards for distinguishing antiarrhythmic effect from spontaneous variability.*

Sisson D: Fixed and dynamic subvalvular aortic stenosis in dogs. In Kirk RW and Bonagura JD (eds): Current Veterinary Therapy XI. Philadelphia, WB Saunders Co, 1992, p 760.
*An excellent review article of the pathology, clinical assessment, and treatment of fixed and dynamic subvalvular aortic stenosis in dogs.*

Thomas W: Doppler echocardiographic estimation of pressure gradients in dogs with congenital pulmonic and subaortic stenosis. Proc 8th ACVIM Forum, 1990, p 867.
*Overviews preliminary comparisons of Doppler-derived and cardiac catheterization–determined pressure gradients in dogs with pulmonic stenosis and subaortic stenosis.*

Valdes-Cruz LM, Jones M, Scagnelli S, et al: Prediction of gradients in fibrous subaortic stenosis by continuous wave two-dimensional Doppler echocardiography: Animal studies. J Am Coll Cardiol 5:1363, 1985.
*Compares pressure gradients determined by Doppler echocardiography and cardiac catheterization in 23 Newfoundlands with subaortic stenosis.*

# VENTRICULAR SEPTAL DEFECTS IN THE ENGLISH SPRINGER SPANIEL

WILLIAM A. BROWN
*Urbana, Illinois*

In recent years, there has been a renewed interest in congenital heart disease in veterinary medicine. This increased interest stems from the more widespread availability and application of echocardiography in diagnosing congenital heart disease and the expanding number of breed-defect relationships that have been described.

Previous epidemiologic studies have reported the overall prevalence of congenital heart disease in the dog as 0.5 to 0.7%. Among the various congenital cardiac defects, ventricular septal defects (VSDs) represent the fifth most common malformation, accounting for approximately 7% of affected dogs. To date, there have been no strong breed predispositions discussed with regard to ventricular septal defects in the dog, although both the keeshond and English bulldog have been reported to be at increased risk.

Recently, however, a group of closely related English springer spaniels that are affected with a disproportionately large number of ventricular septal defects have been identified (Fig. 1). In addition, a review of data contributed to the Veterinary Medical Data Program (Purdue University) between March 1964 and June 1991 confirms that English springer spaniels are at increased risk for developing ventricular septal defects (VSDs) as compared to other breeds. While controlled breeding studies have not been carried out to fully characterize the exact mode of inheritance within this population, it is believed that VSDs in English springer spaniels are inherited as either an autosomal

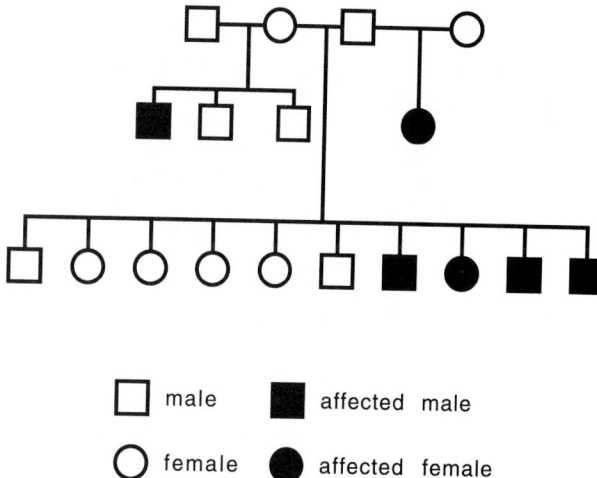

**Figure 1.** Abbreviated pedigree illustrating the familial relationships of English springer spaniels affected with ventricular septal defects.

dominant trait with incomplete penetrance or as a polygenic trait.

## PATHOPHYSIOLOGY

The ventricular septum is made up of four components: the membranous septum, the inlet septum, the trabecular septum, and the outlet or infundibular septum (Fig. 2). Ventricular septal defects are classified according to their location relative to these four regions. While malformations have been described in all four areas in the dog, defects in the membranous septum are the most common.

When viewed from the right ventricle, membranous VSDs are located beneath the septal leaflet of the tricuspid valve. When viewed from the left ventricle, they are located in the left ventricular outflow tract beneath the aortic valve, centered between the right and noncoronary aortic valve cusps. As a result of the location of membranous VSDs high in the interventricular septum, most of the shunted blood goes directly into the

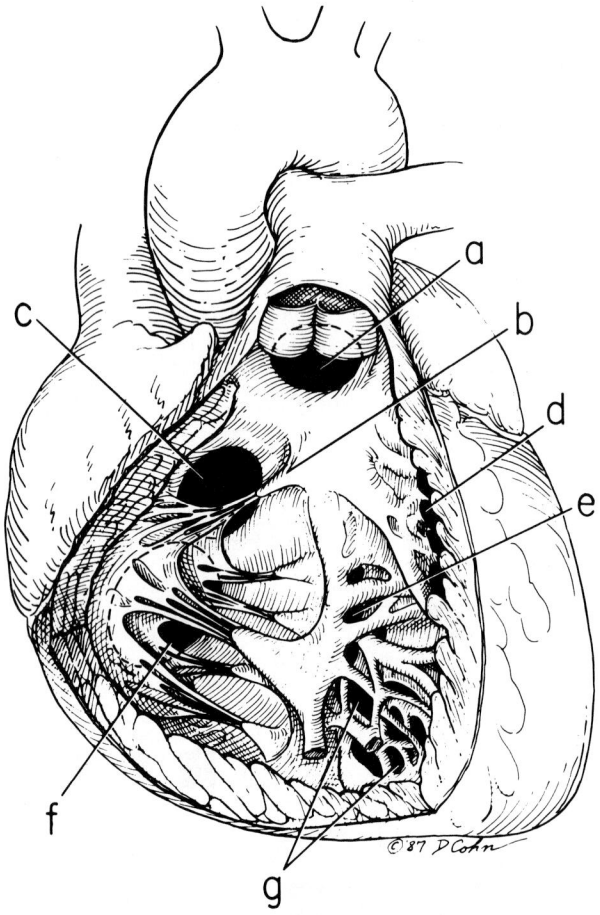

**Figure 2.** Anatomic position of septal defects viewed from the right ventricle: *a*, outlet or infundibular defect; *b*, papillary muscle of tricuspid valve; *c*, membranous septal defect; *d*, *e*, and *g*, muscular septal defects; *f*, inlet defect. (From Adams: Moss' Heart Disease in Infants, 4th edition. Baltimore, Williams & Wilkins, 1990, p 191, with permission.)

right ventricular outflow tract and pulmonary artery. Thus, the hemodynamic burden of the shunt is placed primarily on the left ventricle, which undergoes eccentric hypertrophy. Large shunts and defects located in the lower portions of the interventricular septum often result in volume overload and eccentric hypertrophy of both ventricles.

In some English springer spaniels, the close proximity between the VSD and the aortic valve leads to the development of aortic valvular insufficiency. The pathogenesis of this aortic regurgitation involves the loss of structural support for the aortic valve aparatus as well as the hemodynamic effects of the high-velocity turbulent blood flow through the VSD in systole. Venturi forces generated by the shunting of blood through the VSD draw the poorly supported aortic valve cusps (right coronary cusp and noncoronary cusp) into the defect, causing delayed and abnormal closure of the aortic valve and subsequent aortic regurgitation. Once aortic regurgitation has developed, continuing trauma from the regurgitant jet leads to further damage to the aortic valve leaflets and increased severity of the regurgitation. The additional volume overload that this regurgitation places on the left ventricle often results in progression of left ventricular dilation and development of myocardial failure.

The physiologic consequences of VSDs depend essentially upon two variables, the size of the defect and the pulmonary vascular resistance. In dogs with a small to moderate size VSD, right ventricular and pulmonary artery pressures are maintained at near normal values and the magnitude of the shunt is principally determined by the size and restrictive nature of the defect. In dogs with larger defects (approaching the size of the aorta), the defect does not provide any significant resistance to flow, and the right and left ventricular pressures are allowed to equilibrate. In these cases, the magnitude of the shunt becomes solely dependent upon the difference between pulmonary and systemic vascular resistance. When pulmonary vascular resistance is normal, a large left-to-right shunt will occur. If pulmonary vascular resistance increases, the magnitude of the left-to-right shunt decreases. If the pulmonary vascular resistance exceeds the systemic vascular resistance, the left-to-right shunt is essentially abolished and replaced by a right-to-left shunt. When pulmonary hypertension and right-to-left shunting occur, it is referred to as Eisenmenger's physiology or syndrome. Although this complex defect has been described in the dog, the incidence is quite low. Therefore, the remainder of this discussion will focus on the more typical left-to-right shunting VSD.

## DIAGNOSIS

### History and Physical Examination

Affected dogs are usually detected during auscultation performed as part of a routine physical examination when the dog is presented for vaccination. Most

English springer spaniels are between 2 and 8 months of age and asymptomatic at the time of diagnosis. Occasionally, a dog will be presented with exercise intolerance or respiratory signs due to the development of congestive heart failure. However, these dogs are typically older individuals with longstanding disease or puppies with large defects that cannot tolerate the hemodynamic burden of a large shunt.

The typical murmur of a VSD is a harsh, mixed-frequency holosystolic (regurgitant quality) murmur, heard best over the right precordium, at the third or fourth intercostal spaces. The location can be somewhat variable, however, and in rare instances the murmur may be loudest on the left side. In addition, a left basilar murmur due to relative pulmonic stenosis and a split second heart sound have been reported to occur in some dogs with VSDs. English springer spaniels with VSDs complicated by aortic regurgitation have the typical systolic murmur accompanied by a decrescendo diastolic murmur heard best at the left heart base. The systolic and diastolic murmur must not be confused with the more commonly identified continuous murmur of patent ductus arteriosus (PDA).

The arterial pulse is usually normal except in cases with significant aortic insufficiency, in which the pulses may be bounding.

## Electrocardiography

In most cases observed by the author, the electrocardiogram (ECG) has been unremarkable. The majority of dogs with small to moderate size defects do not experience rhythm disturbances, nor do they have a shift in their frontal plane mean electrical axis. With larger defects, evidence of left atrial and left ventricular enlargement may be present on the ECG. Intraventricular conduction disturbances, including right bundle-branch block and Q-wave abnormalities have also been described in dogs with large membranous VSDs. These conduction abnormalities may be due to the close association between the normal ventricular conduction system and the VSD.

## Thoracic Radiography

The radiographic signs produced by a VSD depend on the size of the septal defect and the magnitude of the shunt. Few radiographic changes are detected in dogs with small VSDs. Larger defects are associated with dilation of the main pulmonary artery, pulmonary hypervascularity, and left atrial and left ventricular enlargement. In some cases, right ventricular enlargement may be observed.

## Echocardiography

Two-dimensional echocardiography, especially supplemented by Doppler examination, is the best diagnostic means of establishing the location and severity of VSDs. Most VSDs can be directly imaged with two-dimensional echocardiography. However, due to limitations in lateral resolution, echocardiography consistently underestimates the size of VSDs, and in smaller dogs actual visualization of the defect can be difficult. A standard two-dimensional echocardiographic evaluation should consist of a thorough examination of the entire interventricular septum using a variety of views. In addition, the left atrial and left ventricular dimensions should be determined, since they both dilate in response to significant left-to-right shunting. The shortening fraction of the left ventricle should also be measured. Ventricular septal defects that cause left ventricular volume overload should result in an increased shortening fraction unless myocardial failure develops.

Doppler echocardiography provides additional information regarding the velocity and direction of blood flow through the VSD and enhances the sensitivity for detecting small lesions not directly visible on the two-dimensional echocardiogram. Methodical interrogation of the right ventricular side of the interventricular septum using color-flow and spectral Doppler is the most effective method for detecting VSDs. Normally, no systolic flow is detected in this region. In dogs with a small to moderate size VSD, a high-velocity (4.0 to 5.0 m/sec) turbulent systolic jet directed toward the right ventricle is detected. In contrast, dogs with a large (unrestrictive) VSD have similar turbulent systolic flow with normal or slightly increased velocity. Application of the modified Bernoulli equation (pressure gradient $= 4 V^2$, where V = maximal velocity in m/s) allows the jet velocity to be converted to the corresponding peak systolic pressure gradient across the VSD. A high pressure gradient (>60 to 70 mm Hg) is consistent with a large difference between right and left ventricular systolic pressures and thus is indicative of a relatively small (restrictive) defect. A small pressure gradient indicates closer equilibration between right and left ventricular pressures and supports the presence of a large (nonrestrictive) defect.

Color-flow Doppler allows rapid identification of small defects or aortic regurgitant jets that may be easily missed using spectral Doppler or two-dimensional echocardiography alone. In addition, color-flow Doppler is quite helpful in guiding the spectral Doppler examination.

## Treatment and Prognosis

Because of the wide spectrum of sizes of VSDs in English springer spaniels, the natural history, treatments, and prognoses are quite variable. Generally, asymptomatic dogs with small defects have a good prognosis. They usually perform well as pets and rarely require medical or surgical intervention. In human medicine, approximately 25% of these small VSDs close spontaneously. Spontaneous closure of small defects has been reported in veterinary medicine but appears to be rare.

Dogs with large defects are frequently symptomatic at presentation or will eventually become so. These patients require surgical treatment to improve their chances for long-term survival. Definitive repair of the VSD or pulmonary artery banding to reduce the magnitude of left-to-right shunting and pulmonary overcirculation are the two surgical options currently available. While primary anatomic repair remains the ideal treatment, it is not frequently attempted because it requires the use of cardiopulmonary bypass and is associated with a much greater risk to the patient and expense to the owner. Pulmonary artery banding has been shown to be an effective palliative alternative for symptomatic dogs when open heart surgery is not available. A cardiologist or surgeon with experience in these procedures should be consulted.

Traditional medical therapy with diuretics, positive inotropes (digoxin), and vasodilators should be considered for those patients in which signs of heart failure develop and surgical correction is not an option. The addition of arterial vasodilators may be especially beneficial in these patients because of their ability to lower the systemic vascular resistance and thus reduce the magnitude of the shunt.

Unfortunately, dogs with VSDs complicated by moderate to severe aortic regurgitation have a poor long-term prognosis. The additional volume overload that aortic insufficiency places on the left ventricle invariably leads to progressive myocardial failure. Definitive therapy for these patients would require surgical closure of the VSD and replacement of the aortic valve.

Evidence from human patients suggests that patients with VSDs are at increased risk for developing bacterial endocarditis. Therefore, it is generally recommended that dogs with VSDs receive prophylactic perioperative antibiotics before undergoing any procedure that may result in a transient bacteremia.

## References and Suggested Reading

Becker AE and Anderson RH: Anomalies of the ventricles. In Becker AE and Anderson RH (eds): Cardiac Pathology: An Integrated Text and Color Atlas. New York, Churchill Livingstone, 1983, p 12.2.
    An excellent pictorial review of the location and pathology of ventricular septal defects.
Buchanan JW: Causes and prevalence of cardiovascular disease. In Kirk RW and Bonagura JD (eds): Current Veterinary Therapy XI. Philadelphia, WB Saunders Co, 1992, p 647.
    A comprehensive review of the recent information regarding breed predispositions to congenital cardiovascular disease.
Feldman EC, Nimmo-Wilkie JS, and Pharr JW: Eisenmenger's syndrome in the dog: Case reports. J Am Anim Hosp Assoc 17:477, 1981.
    A brief review of the clinical findings and diagnosis of several dogs with Eisenmenger's syndrome.
Moise NS: Doppler echocardiographic evaluation of congenital cardiac disease. J Vet Intern Med 3:195, 1989.
    An excellent discussion of the theory and clinical application of Doppler echocardiography in the diagnosis of congenital heart disease.
Olivier NB: Congenital heart disease in dogs. In Fox PR (ed): Canine and Feline Cardiology. New York, Churchill Livingstone, 1988, p 357.
    A brief review of the physiology, diagnosis, and treatment of dogs with ventricular septal defects.
Perloff JK: Ventricular septal defect. In Perloff JK (ed): The Clinical Recognition of Congenital Heart Disease. Philadelphia, WB Saunders Co, 1987, p 365.
    A comprehensive chapter on the pathophysiology, diagnosis, and management of human patients with ventricular septal defects.
Sisson DD, Luethy M, and Thomas WP: Ventricular septal defect accompanied by aortic regurgitation in five dogs. J Am Anim Hosp Assoc 27:441, 1991.
    A report of the clinical findings, diagnosis, and treatment of several dogs with a ventricular septal defect and aortic insufficiency.

# PATENT DUCTUS ARTERIOSUS

SPENCER A. JOHNSTON
Blacksburg, Virginia
and GEORGE E. EYSTER
East Lansing, Michigan

Patent ductus arteriosus (PDA) is a common congenital cardiac abnormality of dogs. Although most frequently diagnosed in the young dog, occasionally it is recognized in the cat as well as in middle age or even older patients. The condition is usually diagnosed due to the characteristic left basilar, continuous, or "machinery" murmur associated with the abnormal blood flow between the aorta and pulmonary artery. Diagnosis can be supported by electrocardiography and thoracic radiograph and confirmed by Doppler echocardiography. Puppies diagnosed with PDA at the time of vaccination are typically asymptomatic, although exercise intolerance, poor growth, and lethargy may be noted. Some puppies and many older dogs are symptomatic at the time of diagnosis, most commonly displaying signs of left-sided congestive heart failure (dyspnea, auscultable pulmonary crackles).

## PATHOPHYSIOLOGY

Once a diagnosis is made, immediate surgical correction is almost always indicated. Beyond the initial pharmacologic management of heart failure, there is no benefit in delaying surgery, since the abnormal physiology associated with this condition will only worsen with time. Briefly, this abnormal physiology consists of a shunt between the aorta and pulmonary artery, such that the left ventricle, aorta, pulmonary artery and vasculature, and left atrium may all be required to carry two to three times the normal volume of blood. This volume overload is manifest as pulmonary overcirculation, left ventricular and left atrial enlargement, and a bulge in the descending aorta in thoracic radiographs. Untreated individuals may develop pulmonary edema, mitral regurgitation, left atrial dilatation, myocardial failure, and atrial fibrillation. They rarely develop pulmonary hypertension or reversed shunting. Due to this progression, untreated PDA is considered to be a potentially fatal disease. Approximately 50% of untreated dogs will die within the first year of life.

Pulmonary edema is present in approximately one half of dogs presenting with PDA (Eyster et al., 1976). These patients will benefit from short-term diuresis immediately prior to surgery. This is done to improve ventilation and oxygenation during anesthesia. Increased compliance of the lungs decreases the force required to maintain adequate ventilation. Furosemide (2 to 4 mg/kg) is administered starting 12 hr preoperatively. This dose may be repeated in 8 hr if clinical signs (harsh lung sounds on thoracic auscultation, coughing) have not resolved. The patient is allowed access to water until 2 hr before surgery. Advanced cases affected by atrial fibrillation or severe congestive heart failure, or aged animals should be managed after consultation with a cardiologist.

## SURGICAL THERAPY

### Thoracotomy

The surgical procedure is done through a left fourth thoracotomy. We find it beneficial to place a small towel roll under the right cranial thoracic wall directly opposite the incision site. This facilitates opening of the intercostal space and improves exposure during surgery. The landmark for the skin incision is the caudal angle of the scapula, which is located at approximately the fourth rib. An incision approximately 1 cm caudal to this landmark will allow access to the fourth intercostal space. The skin incision originates at the angle of the rib and continues distally to near ventral midline.

The cutaneous trunci is incised consistent with the skin incision. The ventral edge of the latissimus dorsi is identified and gently undermined. It is transected dorsally for approximately one half of its width. The insertion of the scalenus is identified on the fifth and sixth ribs. It is transected through its aponeurosis of insertion. The muscle bellies of the serratus ventralis are identified as they insert on each rib, and are bluntly separated between the fourth and fifth ribs. A portion of the origin of the rectus abdominus may require incision to allow adequate exposure ventral to the costochondral junction. The external intercostal muscles are identified and transected as a separate layer, allowing identification of the internal intercostal muscles.

These muscles must be transected to ventral to the costochondral junction to allow adequate exposure. The pleura is penetrated to complete the approach. Once this has been done, a self-retaining rib retractor (Finochietto retractor, Codman & Shurtleff, Inc, Randolph, MA) is placed over moistened pads, and slowly opened to allow adequate visualization.

### Surgical Manipulations

The left cranial lung lobe is reflected caudally to allow uninterrupted viewing of the ductus arteriosus. This can be done by rotating the left cranial lung lobe on its pedicle or by packing it off with a moistened pad. Other than the heart and lungs, the most obvious structures visible will be the phrenic nerve, which courses ventrally over the pericardium; and the vagus nerve, which courses over the brachycephalic artery, aorta, pulmonary artery, and heart base. The ductus arteriosus is located between the aorta and pulmonary artery at the level where the vagus nerve passes over these two structures. The ductus connects the aorta to the pulmonary artery just proximal to the pulmonary artery bifurcation. Patent ductus arteriosus location is confirmed visually and by digitally palpating the thrill ventrally in the pulmonary outflow tract.

### Safety Sutures

Safety sutures are preplaced in patients weighing greater than 7 kg. These are all placed in the Blalock manner, which is to pass the tape around the vessel twice, then grasp the free ends with a hemostat. By pulling up on the free ends, the encircling tape constricts the vessel, stopping blood flow. After gently dissecting the cranial mediastinal pleura away from the aorta and its branches, the aortic safety suture is placed caudal to the ductus. Similar sutures are placed around the brachycephalic and left subclavian arteries. The pericardium is incised longitudinally between the vagus and phrenic nerves. This allows access to the pulmonary and aortic outflow tracts. Should a tear in the ductus occur, the safety sutures are pulled tight, and a single atraumatic clamp, such as a Satinsky clamp (Codman & Shurtleff, Inc, Randolph, MA), is placed cranial and caudal to the pulmonary artery and ascending aorta to effectively occlude all blood flow from the heart. This will allow 2 to 3 min to identify and place a clamp to occlude bleeding from the ductus. Dogs weighing less than 7 kg will bleed to death in the time it takes to tighten all the preplaced sutures, so safety sutures are not placed in these patients.

### Dissection and Ligation

If safety sutures are not required, we do not find it necessary to open the pericardium to ligate the ductus. The first step to ligation is to elevate the vagus nerve and pass a moistened piece of 1/8-inch umbilical tape around the nerve to allow for ventral retraction. Following elevation of the vagus nerve, the natural cleavage plane cranial to the ductus (between the aorta and pulmonary artery) is identified, and dissection proceeds using right-angle forceps, preferably Lahey gall duct forceps with longitudinal serrations (Pilling, Fort Washington, PA). Dissection continues until the cranial mediastinal pleura is penetrated, and can best be described as though the instrument "falls into a hole." Dissection then commences caudal to the ductus in the natural cleavage plane between the aorta and pulmonary artery. Care is taken to avoid the recurrent laryngeal nerve as it passes caudal to the ductus. The majority of the dissection will continue from this direction until the caudal dissection plane communicates with the cranial dissection plane. Care is taken when dissecting so that the instrument always enters the dissection plane closed, is opened within the plane to break down tissue, and is retracted without closing. This is done to avoid trapping tissue between the jaws of the instrument and inadvertently tearing the ductus. Dissection is always done with the tips of the instrument directed towards the relatively thick-walled aorta in order to avoid tearing the fragile ductus.

Once the ductus dissection is complete, two strands of 2-0 silk ligature are passed around the ductus. We recommend these strands be passed individually to avoid twisting of the suture on the back side of the ductus. One strand is gently pulled towards the aorta, while the other is pulled toward the pulmonary artery. With occlusion of the ductus, aortic pressure should increase and the heart rate should drop (Branham reflex). The palpable thrill is eliminated. If the patient tolerates this temporary occlusion, the ligature on the aortic side is tied first. The pulmonic side ligation follows, with an attempt made to have ductal tissue visible between the two ligatures. This may be difficult to accomplish in small dogs.

### Thoracostomy Tube Placement

The preplaced umbilical tapes are removed, the left cranial lung lobe is returned to its normal position, and a thoracostomy tube is placed. We use red rubber catheters (Robinson Red Rubber Catheter, Sherwood Medical, St. Louis, MO), 14- to 18-Fr., placed through a small stab incision over the eighth to tenth rib and entering the thorax at the sixth to seventh intercostal space. The tube is secured with a Chinese finger trap (Crowe, 1983) of 2-0 silk. Silk is used to increase friction between the suture and tube. A commercial trocar catheter (Argyle Trocar Catheter, Sherwood Medical, St. Louis, MO) can be used instead of a red rubber catheter.

### Closure

Prior to closure, an intercostal nerve block is performed using 0.5% bupivicaine (Marcaine, Sterling Drug, New York, NY), injected proximally along the caudal aspect of the fourth rib (Thompson and Johnson, 1991; Berg and Orton, 1986). Thoracic wall closure is with absorbable or nonabsorbable synthetic monofilament suture. It is important to preplace a minimum of four sutures around the ribs, with at least one suture ventral to the costochondral junction. Adjacent sutures are used to bring the ribs together and relieve tension while knots are tied. Once tied, there will frequently be a small step between the fourth and fifth ribs or a slight overlap of the fifth over the fourth rib. Neither the intercostal muscles nor the pleura are sutured directly. The serratus ventralis muscle bellies are reapposed, and the scalenus reattached to its insertion. The latissimus dorsi is closed as a separate layer. Once this layer is closed, the thorax should be airtight, and the thoracic cavity is evacuated using a three-way stopcock and syringe connected to the thoracostomy tube. The cutaneous trunci and subcutaneous tissue are closed as one layer, then skin. The thoracic cavity is evacuated while the patient is placed in the opposite lateral recumbency, as well as dorsal and ventral recumbency. Once the patient seems to be moving an adequate volume of air with each breath, the thoracostomy tube is pulled. We typically preplace a purse-string suture to close the thoracostomy tube incision.

## POSTOPERATIVE CARE

Recovery should be rapid. Patients are usually standing and can be offered food within 4 to 6 hr. Polyuria occurs for 6 to 12 hr due to the need to remove the excess volume associated with physiologic compensation for the PDA. Associated mitral murmurs usually disappear within 24 hr. If a mitral murmur persists beyond 7 days after surgery, it should be addressed as a separate problem. Patients are discharged 24 to 48 hr after surgery. As long as the dog did not have atrial fibrillation prior to surgery, the prognosis for normal life is excellent.

Development of fever and diffuse pulmonary densities up to 3 weeks postoperatively should prompt consideration of suture line infection and hematogenous pneumonia. Interestingly, Doppler studies often demonstrate persistent flow through the ductus; however, no murmur is audible and any residual shunt is clinically insignificant unless there is concurrent infection.

## PROGNOSIS

The overall prognosis for survival of a patient diagnosed with PDA is 89 to 92% (Eyster et al., 1976; Birchard, Bonagura, and Fingland, 1990). The most frequent cause of death associated with surgery is tearing of the ductus. There is no difference in the survival rate of patients treated with the traditional ligation technique, as described here, or with the Jackson-Henderson technique. We prefer the traditional dissection method.

## References and Suggested Reading

Berg RJ and Orton EC: Pulmonary function in dogs after intercostal thoracotomy: Comparison of morphine, oxymorphone, and selective intercostal nerve block. Am J Vet Res 47:471, 1986.
  *An experimental study to evaluate narcotic and local analgesia following thoracostomy.*
Birchard SJ, Bonagura JD, and Fingland RB: Results of ligation of patent ductus arteriosus in dogs: 201 cases (1969–1988). J Am Vet Med Assoc 196:2011, 1990.
  *A clinical retrospective study concentrating on survival statistics and intraoperative complications.*

Crowe DT: Thoracic drainage. *In* Bojrab MJ (ed): *Current Techniques in Small Animal Surgery.* Philadelphia, Lea & Febiger, 1983, p 387.
  *The original description of this method of securing a tube.*
Eyster GE, Eyster JT, Cords GB, and Johnston J: Patent ductus arteriosus in the dog: Characteristics of occurrence and results of surgery in one hundred consecutive cases. J Am Vet Med Assoc 168:435, 1976.
  *One of only two large retrospective studies concerning canine patent ductus arteriosus.*
Thompson SE and Johnson JM: Analgesia in dogs after intercostal thoracotomy. A comparison of morphine, selective intercostal nerve block, and interpleural regional analgesia with bupivicaine. Vet Surg 20:73, 1991.
  *An experimental study to evaluate physiologic parameters associated with analgesia following thoracostomy.*

# RECOGNITION OF CONGENITAL HEART DISEASE IN THE ADULT DOG AND CAT

CLIFFORD R. BERRY

*Raleigh, North Carolina*

The diagnosis of congenital heart disease (CHD) in the adult dog and cat represents a diagnostic challenge. Typically, diagnosis of CHD is made during the early months of life when puppies and kittens are presented for routine vaccination, and a cardiac murmur is auscultated. Complex or severe congenital heart defects that cause significant morbidity (e.g., cyanosis, congestive heart failure, failure to thrive, exercise intolerance, respiratory distress) often result in the death of the animal prior to 2 years of age. Reasons why congenital heart defects remain undetected include: lack of auscultation during routine examination or inadequate time spent on auscultation; soft murmurs that may be misinterpreted as functional or flow murmurs; lack of a murmur or other clinical clue for the presence of congenital heart disease; and the inability to identify a murmur due to the presence of a sinus tachycardia or tachypnea (excited puppies or kittens). For a review of congenital heart diseases in the puppy and kitten, the reader is referred to other articles in this section and to *Current Veterinary Therapy X* (Miller and Bonagura, 1989). Understanding the typical physical examination, auscultation, electrocardiographic, and thoracic radiographic features of each of the common congenital heart defects is helpful.

Dogs and cats 2 years of age or older will be considered adults. This patient population presented for evaluation could include different subsets of dogs and cats, including: asymptomatic or symptomatic animals with undiagnosed congenital heart disease; animals symptomatic for complications of CHD such as endocarditis or atrial fibrillation; asymptomatic or symptomatic patients with residual defects or complications of attempted surgical correction; and the symptomatic patients with congenital heart disease that have received palliative medical therapy.

## OVERVIEW

In a retrospective review of clinical cardiology cases from the Veterinary Teaching Hospitals at North Carolina State University, University of Florida, and University of California, Davis, the most common congenital heart defects that were identified in dogs 2 years of age and older included: left-to-right patent ductus arteriosus (PDA), right-to-left PDA, subaortic stenosis, pulmonic stenosis, and peritoneal pericardial diaphragmatic hernias. Other abnormalities included: atrial septal defect, mitral valve dysplasia, tricuspid valve dysplasia, persistent right aortic arch, combined ventricular septal defect/aortic insufficiency, mitral valve stenosis, and cor triatriatum dexter. In cats, the most common congenital heart defect diagnosed in patients 2 years of age or older included: peritoneal pericardial diaphragmatic hernias, ventricular septal defects, and atrioventricular valve dysplasia.

## DIAGNOSIS

Routine diagnostic testing of adult dogs and cats with congenital heart disease should follow the standard work-up for any animal with a cardiac disorder. Careful auscultation in a quiet environment is the mainstay of the cardiac examination. Murmur evaluation for timing, point of maximal intensity, and areas of radiation should be ascertained. Pulse quality should be evaluated for rapid "run-offs" that may be associated with a PDA, left-to-right shunting, aortiopulmonary window, and aortic insufficiency. In addition, mucous membrane color of the head and tail regions should be evaluated before and after exercise. Cyanosis with polycythemia in the presence of a cardiac murmur are highly suggestive of a congenital heart defect (Table 1). An electrocardiogram (ECG) may demonstrate voltage or axis criteria for cardiomegaly or ventricular conduction delay. The finding of ECG features of right ventricular hypertrophy is particularly noteworthy and should cause the clinician to consider CHD.

## Thoracic Radiographs

Routine evaluation of thoracic radiographs can provide valuable clinical diagnostic clues. High-quality radiographs should include a lateral projection and a perpendicular view (ventrodorsal or dorsoventral). The author's preference is a right lateral and dorsoventral view, as these views provide the most consistent shapes to the cardiac silhouette. On the right lateral radiograph, the heart is an oblong oval shape, with the apex pointing at the diaphragmatic-sternal junction. On the dorsoventral radiograph, the heart has a similar shape, with the apex pointing into the left hemithorax. Rare anomalies may be associated with dextropositioning of the cardiac apex and associated structures (*situs inversus* and other heterotaxic syndromes).

It is critical that both the lateral and dorsoventral radiographs be straight in their positioning. Alignment of the rib heads and costochondrial junctions is a good indicator on the lateral radiograph for accurate positioning. Rotational malpositioning may make interpretation of the cranial and caudal lobar pulmonary vessels, main pulmonary artery, heart base, and apex of the heart inaccurate. Straight positioning of the dorsoventral radiograph can be determined by alignment of the thoracic vertebral bodies and the sternum. This is critical on this radiographic view, as slight obliquity will cause artifactual bulges in the area of the main pulmonary artery or aorta. The dorsoventral view provides the best evaluation of the right and left caudal lobar pulmonary artery and vein for symmetry, size, and distribution. If a dorsoventral radiograph is properly exposed for evaluating the pulmonary parenchyma, underexposure of the central great vessels may result. We routinely take a third exposure (additional dorsoventral view) collimated to the cardiac area, and double the mAs from the original technique. This radiograph can then be used to evaluate the aortic arch, descending aorta, and main pulmonary artery. Careful attention to accurate positioning is again of the utmost importance.

When evaluating thoracic radiographs in dogs and cats for congenital heart defects, the practitioner is encouraged to answer four basic questions regarding the presence or absence of radiographic abnormalities. First, is there cardiomegaly present? If so, is it right sided, left sided, or generalized? Second, is there radiographic evidence of congestive left heart failure (enlarged pulmonary veins, pulmonary edema) or congestive right heart failure (pleural effusion, enlarged caudal vena cava, or ascites)? Third, is there any enlargement of the aortic arch, descending aorta, or main pulmonary artery segment on the dorsoventral cone down view? Finally, is there undercirculation, normal circulation, or overcirculation of the pulmonary vasculature? Once the clinician has answered these questions, the answers should be reviewed for discrepancies. For example, in a dog with right-sided cardiomegaly, bulge in the main pulmonary artery segment, and pulmonary edema, it is not likely that an isolated cardiac anomaly can be diagnosed. These types of discrepancies should be reevaluated and reasonable differential lists established prior to proceeding. Complex or multiple congenital anomalies are often missed until a complete morphologic examination can be done by use of echocardiography, contrast echocardiography, Doppler echocardiography, or selective angiography.

When congenital heart disease is suspected based on the results of physical examination, thoracic radiography, electrocardiography, and laboratory tests (e.g., packed cell volume [PCV] demonstrating polycythemia), the client should be referred to a specialist with experience in the echocardiographic diagnosis of congenital heart disease. Optimal management requires an anatomic diagnosis (two-dimensional echo) and an assessment of hemodynamics using Doppler studies. Contrast echocardiography also can be done to demonstrate right-to-left shunts.

***Table 1.*** *Evaluation of Adult Dogs and Cats With or Without Cyanosis*

| Cyanotic (Secondary Polycythemia) | | Acyanotic (Murmur) | | |
|---|---|---|---|---|
| **Differential Cyanosis** | **Complete Cyanosis** | **Systolic** | **Diastolic** | **Syst/Diast** |
| R-L PDA | R-L VSD | SAS | M Stenosis | L-R PDA (continuous) |
| | R-L ASD ± PS | PS | | VSD/AI |
| | Tetralogy of Fallot | VSD | | SAS/AI |
| | PH ± CHD | M Dys | | AP Window |
| | AP Window | T Dys | | |
| | Complex malformation | AS | | |

Abbreviations: R-L = right-to-left, PDA = patent ductus arteriosus, AP = aorticopulmonary, VSD = ventricular septal defect, ASD = atrial septal defect, PS = pulmonic stenosis, PH = pulmonary hypertension, CHD = congenital heart defect, SAS = subaortic stenosis, AS = valvular aortic stenosis, M Dys = mitral dysplasia, T Dys = tricuspid dysplasia, M Stenosis = mitral valve stenosis, L-R = left-to-right, AI = aortic insufficiency.

## ASYMPTOMATIC ADULT DOGS AND CATS WITH UNDIAGNOSED CHD

Asymptomatic adult dogs and cats with congenital heart defects are usually noted to have a cardiac abnormality based on physical examination (cyanosis, auscultation of a murmur, or muffled heart sounds) or presurgical electrocardiographic or thoracic radiographic screening. Peritoneal pericardial diaphragmatic hernia (PPDH) is one of the most common defects identified in the asymptomatic adult. Physical examination abnormalities may include: muffled heart sounds, borborygmal sounds over the thorax, and absence of expected abdominal contents in the abdominal cavity on palpation. Life-threatening conditions may develop if torsion or vascular compromise of the herniated abdominal viscera occurs as a result of a stricture or strangulation at the hernia site. The most common electrocardiographic abnormality is low-voltage QRS complexes. Variable radiographic abnormalities are seen with dogs and cats with a PPDH including: cardiomegaly, abnormal cardiac contours (not typical of standard chamber enlargement patterns), various roentgen densities within the cardiac silhouette, lack of abdominal viscera within the abdominal cavity, identification of bowel loops (inconsistent) or other discrete abdominal structures within the pericardial space, and contact between the cardiac silhouette and the cranial diaphragm (uncommon in cats). In addition, cats with PPDH may have a mesothelial remnant that can be identified on the lateral thoracic radiograph. This remnant extends between the cardiac silhouette and the diaphragm ventral to the caudal vena cava (Fig. 1).

Other common congenital heart defects that may be recognized in an asymptomatic animal include mild pulmonic or subaortic stenosis, ventricular or atrial septal defect, and atrioventricular valve dysplasia. Patent ductus arteriosus is another relatively common congenital heart defect identified in the adult population. Most defects may be identified based on typical murmur characteristics, but electrocardiographic and thoracic radiographic abnormalities may or may not be present. The use of echocardiography and Doppler echocardiography is diagnostic in experienced hands; angiography is rarely required to determine the nature and extent of the lesion.

## SYMPTOMATIC ADULT DOGS AND CATS WITH UNDIAGNOSED CHD

Symptomatic adult animals with previously undiagnosed congenital heart disease may present to the veterinarian because of congestive heart failure or complications related to the congenital heart defect. Systemic manifestations of congenital heart disease may include: heart failure, ventricular arrhythmias, syncope, exercise intolerance, cyanosis, polycythemia, atrial fibrillation preexcitation syndromes with related tachycardias, and bacterial endocarditis. Any dog or cat with polycythemia that is not corrected after rehydration should be evaluated for congenital heart disease in-

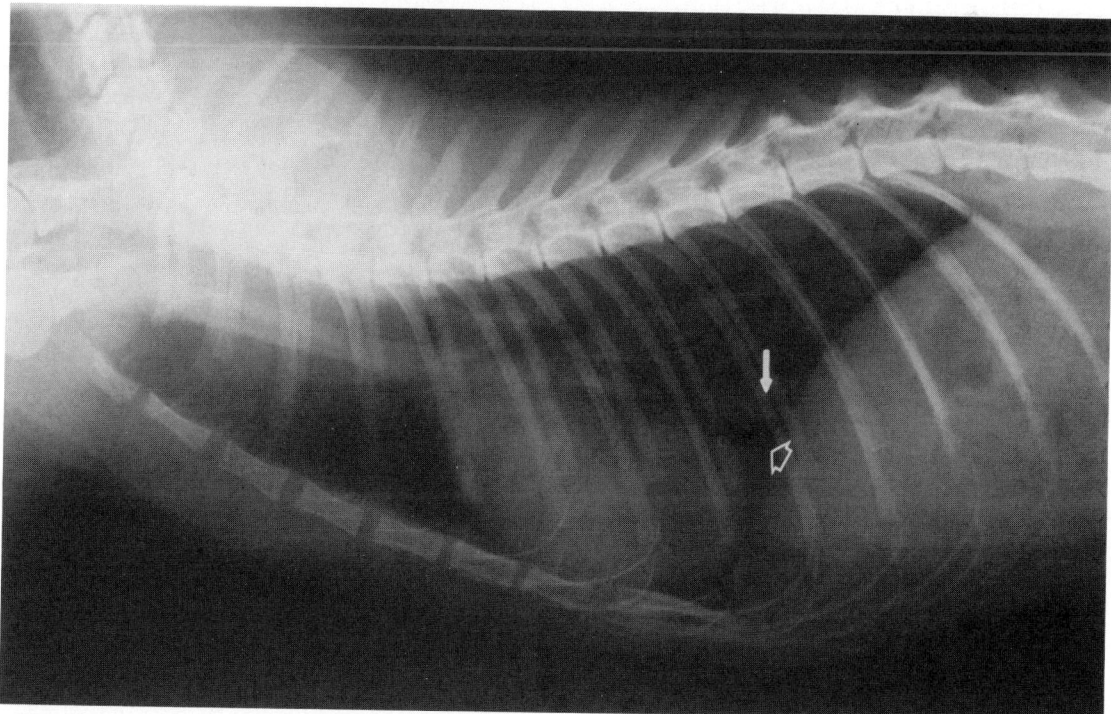

**Figure 1.** Right lateral thoracic radiograph from a 5-year-old domestic shorthair cat that was presented for evaluation of a urinary tract infection. Presurgical evaluation of the thorax documented an enlarged cardiac silhouette with an additional fat/soft tissue opacity noted in the caudal and ventral thorax. On the lateral projection, a dorsal peritoneo-pericardial mesothelial remnant can be seen (*open arrow*) just ventral to the caudal vena cava (*solid arrow*).

cluding right-to-left intra- or extracardiac shunts. A reverse right-to-left PDA is the most common form of Eisenmenger's physiology encountered in veterinary medicine and can lead to polycythemia. Pulmonary hypertension is caused by increased pulmonary vascular resistance, the result of medial hypertrophy and fibrosis along with intimal changes in the pulmonary arteries and arterioles. Enlargement of the main pulmonary artery, right ventricular enlargement, and a bulge in the descending aorta are the characteristic radiographic findings. A heart murmur is frequently absent. Bacterial endocarditis of the aortic valve is a recognized complication in dogs with subaortic stenosis (see *CVT XI*, p 752). Other congenital defects, such as Ebstein's anomaly has been associated with ventricular preexcitation syndromes and supraventricular tachycardias. (For further information, see "Supraventricular Tachycardia Associated With Accessory Atrioventricular Pathways in Dogs," this volume, p 807).

## TREATMENT/MANAGEMENT

Once CHD is recognized in the adult animal, possible treatments should be considered. Management goals include: (1) full identification of the lesion, (2) corrective surgery if needed and if possible, (3) symptomatic treatment of associated complications. Identification of the defect often requires referral for Doppler echocardiography or cardiac catheterization.

The management strategy depends on the lesion, hemodynamics, and severity. Surgical options exist, including ductal ligation, palliative shunt, and reduction of a peritoneal-pericardial hernia. Balloon catheter dilation may be appropriate for some patients with outflow tract obstruction; these options are discussed elsewhere in this section. Medical management of CHF, phlebotomy for polycythemia, and antiarrhythmic drug therapy are indicated in selected cases. Since most practicing veterinarians have little opportunity to manage mature animals with CHD, the best course is to call a cardiologist to discuss the patient and management options.

## SUMMARY

The diagnosis of congenital heart disease in the adult dog and cat requires an awareness of the prevalence of these disorders in this population of patients. Although acquired heart disease is far more common in mature animals, the diagnosis of a congenital lesion should be considered in younger and middle-aged patients (2 to 10 years of age). The use of careful auscultation, identification of characteristic electrocardiographic and thoracic radiographic abnormalities, and the presence of other systemic manifestations of congenital heart disorders should aid the practitioner in identifying cases of congenital heart disease.

## References and Suggested Reading

Berry CR, Koblik PD, and Ticer JW: Identification of dorsal peritoneopericardial mesiothelial remnant as an aid to the diagnosis of congenital peritoneopericardial diaphragmatic hernia in the cat. Vet Radiol 31:239, 1990.
*A retrospective review of cats with congenital pericardial diaphragmatic hernias and a description of a new radiographic finding in some cats with these congenital defects. The clinical utility of this radiographic feature was prospectively evaluated.*

Bonagura J: Congenital heart disease. *In* Bonagura JD (ed): *Contemporary Issues in Small Animal Practice: Cardiology.* New York, Churchill Livingstone, 1987, p 1.
*An excellent review of the work-up with in-depth explanations of the seven most common congenital heart defects in small animals.*

Bonagura JD and Hamlin RL: Treatment of heart disease. *In* Kirk RW (ed): *Current Veterinary Therapy IX.* Philadelphia, WB Saunders Co, 1986, p 319.
*A review of the basics of therapy when treating dogs and cats with congestive heart failure.*

Burrow KM and Braunwald E: Congenital heart disease in the adult. *In* Braunwald E (ed): *Cardiovascular Disease.* Philadelphia, WB Saunders Co, 1991, p 976.
*A review of adult human congenital heart disease.*

Goodwin JK and Lombard CW: Patent ductus arteriosus in adult dogs: Clinical features of 14 cases. J Am Anim Hosp Assoc 28:349, 1991.
*A retrospective review of adult dogs presented for work-up with a cardiac continuous murmur that were diagnosed as having patent ductus arteriosus.*

Miller MW and Bonagura JD: *In* Kirk RW (ed): *Current Veterinary Therapy IX.* Philadelphia, WB Saunders Co, 1989, p 224.
*An excellent review of congenital heart disease in dogs and cats. This should serve as the starting point of all congenital heart work-ups.*

# MITRAL VALVE DISEASE IN CAVALIER KING CHARLES SPANIELS

PETER G. G. DARKE

*Edinburgh, Scotland*

## HISTORICAL BACKGROUND

In 1927, some breeders of King Charles spaniels recognized that modern dogs of their breed no longer resembled those depicted in royal and noble portraits from the 17th century. They therefore undertook to develop a derivative breed, which was larger and less brachycephalic (Fig. 1). Thus the *cavalier* King Charles emerged, from a foundation of only about six dogs. Close interbreeding provided the breed with a very limited gene pool. However, cavalier King Charles spaniels were bred prolifically in the United Kingdom during the 1970s, to become the third most popular pedigree breed, with about 12% of Kennel Club registrations.

Toward the end of the 1970s, it became obvious in Britain that not only was the breed prone to develop mitral regurgitation, as were other small breeds of dog, but that this disease was occurring in young to middle-age dogs. With the cooperation of cavalier King Charles clubs in the United Kingdom, a survey of dogs at shows was made in the 1980s to assess the prevalence of murmurs of mitral regurgitation (MR). The results are presented in Figure 2. Although dogs at shows might not be representative of the breed as a whole, these data confirmed that there was a significant problem, with over 50% of dogs showing MR by 5 years of age, and increased prevalence with age (Darke, 1987). These findings supported a concept of a premature and progressive degeneration of the mitral valve. Furthermore, dogs that had been auscultated several times over a period of years generally demonstrated a progression in the severity of the cardiac murmur.

By this time, numerous dogs with terminal congestive heart failure had been submitted to necropsy. Findings were typical of those reported for other breeds with mitral valve degeneration (MVD): endocardiosis, frequently with ballooning of valve cusps, sometimes ruptured chordae tendineae, and often gross cardiac dilatation that implied severe volume overload or terminal myocardial failure.

A retrospective statistical analysis of the clinical data base at the University of Edinburgh had shown that the prevalence of MR was probably high in cavaliers (Thrusfield, Aitken, and Darke, 1985). They shared this propensity with Chihuahuas, dachshunds, Pekinese, miniature and toy poodles, and whippets. The preponderance of males reported by some other investigators was found in some other breeds (e.g., beagle, cairn, whippet) (Table 1). However, MVD seems to appear equally in both sexes of cavalier. These data were derived mainly from a first-opinion clinic, and might therefore be taken as reasonably representative of the population at large.

## STUDIES IN OTHER COUNTRIES

The breed became popular in other countries, notably Australia and Sweden, and dogs were imported to the United States, gaining fame through President Reagan. Following British reports of the prevalence of MVD, a survey in Australia suggested that the prevalence of MVD in cavaliers might be less (Malik, Hunt, and Allan, 1992). However, investigations in Sweden showed a prevalence similar to that in the United Kingdom.

Dr. Kvart and colleagues at the University of Uppsala then selected cavalier breeders at random in Sweden to evaluate the background prevalence of disease. Their survey would include dogs that might not be brought for auscultation at dog shows. Additionally, these investigators followed the progress of these dogs over 3 years, and demonstrated obvious progression of MVD. Finally, they acquired insurance statistics on cardiac disease in cavaliers, as provided by a large Swedish company. The data provided by this company provided powerful additional evidence of the premature development of cardiac disease in this breed. The frequency of claims for veterinary care related to heart disease was 14 times higher than the mean for all other insured breeds, and claims for death or euthanasia were 13 times higher in dogs 7 to 10 years old (Haggstrom et al., 1992).

A survey of 395 dogs at cavalier shows in Baltimore, MD in 1990 and 1991 revealed a prevalence of murmurs similar to that in the United Kingdom, with more than 50% of dogs aged 4 years and over having murmurs of MR (Beardow and Buchanan, 1993). In 79 dogs reexamined on the second occasion, murmurs were found in 21% of dogs previously found to be murmur free, and of 22 dogs in which murmurs had been detected on the first occasion, the intensity of the murmur had increased in intensity in nine, remained static in nine, and reduced in just four. Investigation of case records in the data base at the University of Pennsylvania also showed that cavaliers were presented prematurely with MVD. Again, both echocardiography and necropsy showed lesions similar to MVD in other breeds, but with prominent mitral valve prolapse and

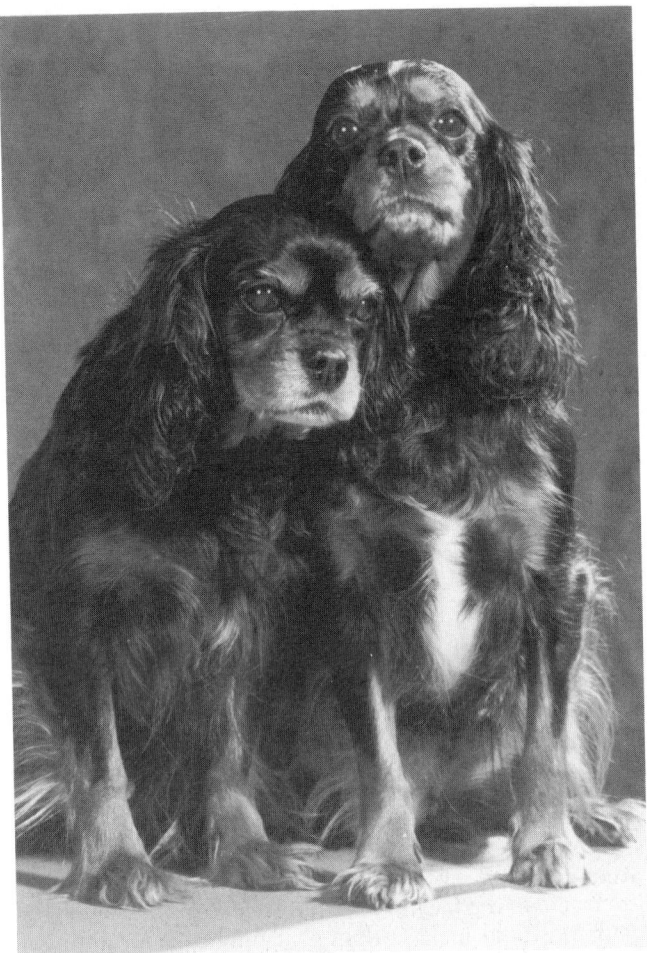

**Figure 1.** Cavalier King Charles spaniel bitches (courtesy of Dr. V. O'Farrell).

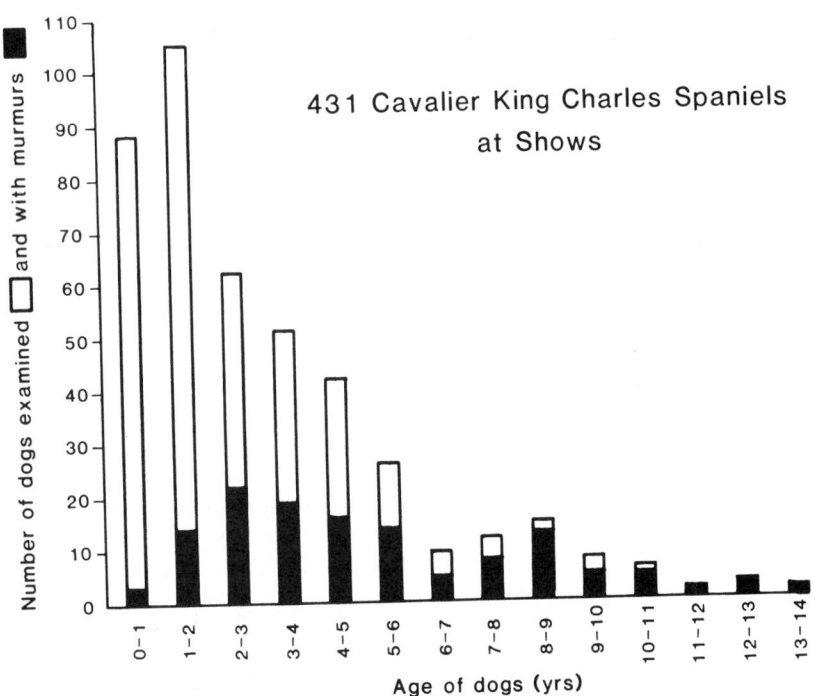

**Figure 2.** Prevalence of murmurs of mitral regurgitation in 431 cavalier King Charles spaniels examined at dogs shows in the U.K. (From Darke, PGG: Valvular incompetence in cavalier King Charles spaniels. Vet Rec 120:365, 1987, courtesy of The Veterinary Record, with permission.)

frequent rupture of chordae tendineae (Beardow and Buchanan, 1993).

## CLINICAL DETAILS

### Presenting Signs

The disease presents in a similar manner to MVD in other breeds, and signs are related to the activity of the dog and the rate and stage of progression of disease, particularly in relation to the size of the left atrium and myocardial function (Reed, 1989). For months or years, the circulation may compensate for MR. Early signs of exercise intolerance may not be noticed by owners, and dogs are often presented with coughing as an early sign of bronchial compression or of heart failure. However, many dogs that compensate well for MR for years may nonetheless develop sudden signs of decompensation. Other dogs show rapid and progressive deterioration in cardiac function over a matter of weeks or months, and signs of inadequate cardiac output (exercise intolerance, weakness, or collapse) may be prominent. Syncope may be associated with cardiac dysrhythmias (particularly paroxysmal tachycardias) or coughing, but the precise etiology is uncertain in most cases. Signs of right-sided cardiac failure (ascites, tachypnea due to hydrothorax, and cardiac cachexia) sometimes develop, due to primary tricuspid valve degeneration, or secondary pulmonary hypertension caused by left-sided failure.

### Cardiac Murmur of MVD

The cardiac murmur in cavaliers is typical of the murmur of MR in many small breeds of dog. The ear-

liest finding by the author in cavaliers with MVD has been a softening and/or prolongation of the first heart sound, followed later by the development of a soft protosystolic murmur, often heard in dogs of only 2 to 4 years of age, and then a murmur increasing in duration and intensity, until it becomes pansystolic, radiating widely. Particularly when rupture of chordae tendineae occurs, a vibrant or musical murmur can be heard, and a flail valve can be demonstrated by echocardiography. In very severe regurgitation, the intensity of the murmur is often reduced, and it usually obliterates the second heart sound, though the intensity of the first heart sound may actually increase. The murmur of MR is typically heard at the fifth intercostal space on the left side of the thorax, most often over the apex, but it usually radiates widely in advanced disease. A systolic murmur in the tricuspid area may represent radiation from the mitral valve, or be a primary murmur of tricuspid regurgitation.

### Other Auscultatory Findings

Diastolic gallop sounds are occasionally heard over the left apex in severe volume overload. However, supraventricular premature beats are frequently found in advanced disease, often heard as a "tripping" in the rhythm. Sinus tachycardia is usually the dominant rhythm in heart failure, but atrial fibrillation has been recorded occasionally in cavaliers.

### Electrocardiography

The electrocardiogram (ECG) typically shows sinus tachycardia in advanced cases, often with supraven-

***Table 1.*** *Odds Ratio and Confidence Intervals for Purebred Dogs With a Statistically Significant Association Between Breed and Heart Valve Incompetence\**

| Breed | Cases | Controls | Odds Ratio | 95% Confidence Intervals | |
|---|---|---|---|---|---|
| **Male Dogs** | | | | | |
| Beagle | 7 | 84 | 2.18 | 1.03 | 4.64 |
| Cairn terrier | 21 | 255 | 2.11 | 1.34 | 3.32 |
| Chihuahua | 10 | 56 | 4.63 | 2.37 | 9.01 |
| Dachshund | 11 | 144 | 1.97 | 1.07 | 3.62 |
| Cavalier King Charles | 22 | 107 | 5.36 | 3.36 | 8.55 |
| Pekinese | 11 | 89 | 3.20 | 1.71 | 5.96 |
| Miniature pinscher | 5 | 15 | 8.75 | 3.29 | 23.28 |
| Miniature poodle | 46 | 338 | 3.68 | 2.66 | 5.10 |
| Standard poodle | 3 | 14 | 5.92 | 1.83 | 19.11 |
| Toy poodle | 9 | 65 | 3.60 | 1.81 | 7.16 |
| Whippet | 10 | 38 | 6.80 | 3.41 | 13.57 |
| **Female Dogs** | | | | | |
| Chihuahua | 7 | 33 | 7.62 | 3.41 | 17.01 |
| Dachshund | 7 | 109 | 2.31 | 1.09 | 4.89 |
| Cavalier King Charles | 23 | 145 | 5.85 | 3.70 | 9.24 |
| Papillon | 4 | 45 | 3.31 | 1.25 | 8.81 |
| Pekinese | 7 | 90 | 2.80 | 1.31 | 5.96 |
| Miniature poodle | 29 | 230 | 4.72 | 3.14 | 7.11 |
| Toy poodle | 5 | 48 | 3.81 | 1.56 | 9.31 |

\*Data modified from Thrusfield MV, Aitken CGG, and Varke PGG: Observations on breed and sex in relation to canine heart valve incompetence. J Small Anim Pract 26:709, 1985, with permission.

tricular ectopy. Ventricular premature beats are less frequently seen. Signs of left-sided cardiac enlargement are usually present (prolongation of P wave and increased duration and amplitude of QRS complex), but these are not sensitive indicators of cardiac enlargement.

### Radiography

Thoracic radiographs are very useful in the evaluation of volume overload in mitral regurgitation. Radiographs reflect left atrial enlargement sensitively and specifically, and progressive enlargement of this chamber can be satisfactorily monitored by this means. Compression of the left mainstem bronchus, probably a significant cause of coughing in many cases, can often be clearly identified. The extent of pulmonary venous congestion and/or edema is easily assessed, and the results of therapy can be monitored. Progressive hepatic

enlargement often accompanies right-sided cardiac enlargement.

### Further Diagnostic Testing

Proof of mitral insufficiency, and evaluation of the severity of regurgitation, requires further investigation, though this is not essential in typical cases. For many years, cardiac catheterization was required to study the hemodynamics of this disease. However, diagnosis can now be verified noninvasively by Doppler echocardiography. Simple echocardiography often suggests valve thickening (Fig. 3A). Abnormal valve motion is often recognized by two-dimensional echocardiography, however, and a prolapsed or flail valve can be seen with stretched or ruptured chordae tendineae, respectively (Fig. 3B). The exact significance and causes of mitral valve prolapse in this disease are unresolved. Echocar-

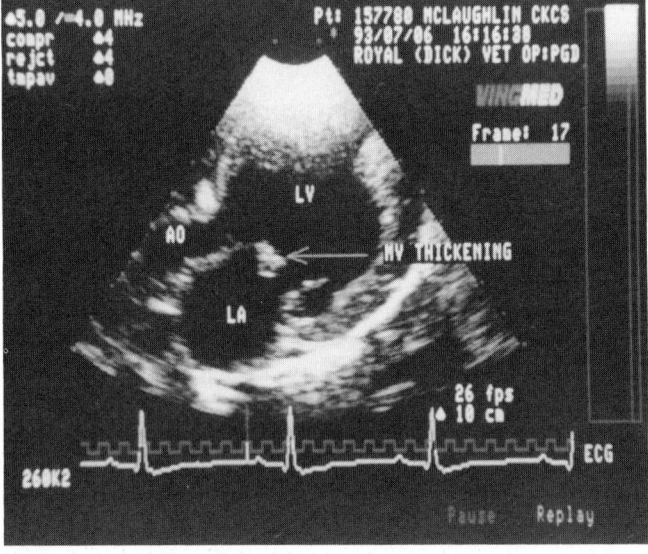

A

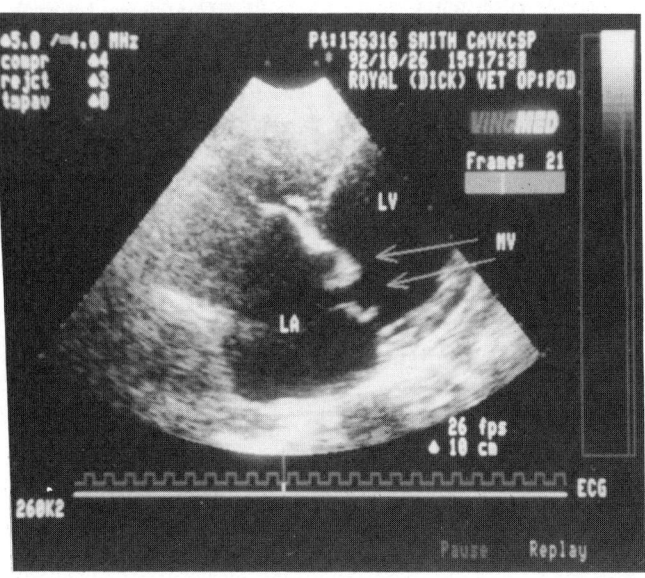

B

**Figure 3.** *A,* Two-dimensional echocardiographic image of a thickened mitral valve. *B,* Two-dimensional echocardiographic image of a flail mitral valve (*arrow*), in cavalier King Charles spaniels. Abbreviations: Ao = aorta, LA = left atrium, LV = left ventricle, MV = mitral valve.

diography suggests hyperkinesis of the ventricle in the early stages of the disease. However, this is misleading: with MR, the ability of the left ventricle to decompress rapidly into the low resistance of the left atrium provides a false impression of enhanced contractility. Color Doppler studies demonstrate the extent (volume) of the regurgitant jet in the left atrium, a semiquantitative indication of severity.

## Definitive Diagnosis of MVD

Definitive diagnosis of MVD depends mainly on finding the typical murmur of MR in this breed. Mitral dysplasia has not so far been reported in cavaliers, and primary cardiomyopathy with secondary MR is almost unknown. However, clinical signs of cardiac failure (e.g., coughing, exercise intolerance, or ascites) can be confused in a dog with compensated MVD that has other concurrent disease (e.g., chronic lower airway disease or hepatic failure). Any dog with chronic coughing and a cardiac murmur should be carefully examined to determine the etiology of the cough. For example, dogs with coughing caused by heart failure (though not necessarily those with just bronchial compression) usually have tachycardia, whereas airway disease is normally associated with a normal heart rate, and often a prominent sinus arrhythmia. Radiography is the most useful arbiter in cases of uncertainty.

## MANAGEMENT

### Case Management

First, the progressive nature of MVD, the inability of clinicians to achieve a cure, and the need for continued therapy must be discussed carefully with the dog's owner. Obese dogs should receive a calorie-restricted diet. The value of low-sodium diets is unproven. However, it can be argued that a reduction in sodium intake at an early stage of the disease may postpone the requirement for diuresis. The author favors such diets less when diuretics or angiotensin-converting enzyme inhibitors are already in use. Because there are no currently available means of stopping or slowing the progression of MVD, therapy is generally limited to general measures to alter the hemodynamic consequences and clinical signs of heart failure (see "Therapy of Heart Failure," this volume, p 780).

## CONTROL OF MVD IN THE BREED

The cavalier King Charles Spaniel Club in the United Kingdom has accepted the need to control

MVD. Although there appears to be no simple pattern of inheritance, the Breed Council has agreed that there is almost certainly a genetic basis for the premature development of MVD. A major problem is that the disease becomes manifest in many dogs after they have started, or even completed, their breeding career. The Club is trying to encourage breeders to select dogs for breeding that are as old as possible while free from murmurs. To this end, a certification scheme has been established whereby breeders have their dogs auscultated annually by a veterinarian; for example, at dog shows or at the time of annual inoculations. The veterinarian then completes a certificate declaring the presence or absence of a cardiac murmur, one copy of which is retained by the breeder; the other copy is sent to the breed club. Breeders are encouraged to ask to see the certificate when selecting a dog for breeding with a bitch, for example.

It is also hoped that the prevalence of MVD in the breed can be monitored from certificates returned to the Breed Club. Furthermore, some aged dogs, especially males, with no evidence of MVD, may provide a foundation for selective breeding. Finally, the history of some of the best known breed lines is being investigated to determine whether any carry a particularly high or low prevalence of disease. It is hoped that these efforts may help to reduce the prevalence of a distressing disorder.

## References and Suggested Reading

Beardow AW and Buchanan JW: Chronic valve disease in Cavalier King Charles Spaniels: 95 cases (1987–1991). J Am Vet Med Assoc 203:1023, 1993.
  *A detailed account of the epidemiology and clinical features of MVD in American cavaliers.*
Darke PGG: Valvular incompetence in cavalier King Charles spaniels. Vet Rec 120:365, 1987.
  *A brief summary of the prevalence of murmurs of mitral regurgitation in cavaliers at UK dog shows.*
DeLellis LA and Kittleson MD: Current uses and hazards of vasodilator therapy in heart failure. In Kirk RW (ed): Current Veterinary Therapy XI. Philadelphia, WB Saunders Co, 1992, p 700.
  *A useful account of the practical aspects of vasodilators in heart failure.*
Fox PR: The effect of drug therapy on clinical characteristics and outcome in dogs with heart failure. In Proc 10th Ann Vet Med Forum. Blacksburg, American College of Veterinary Internal Medicine, 1993, p 592.
  *A brief summary of a multicenter double-blind study with enalapril in congestive failure due to mitral regurgitation or dilated cardiomyopathy.*
Haggstrom J, Hansson K, Kvart C, et al: Chronic valvular disease in the cavalier King Charles spaniel in Sweden. Vet Rec 131:549, 1992.
  *Results of well-structured epidemiologic studies into the prevalence and progression of MVD in cavaliers.*
Malik R, Hunt GB, and Allan GS: Prevalence of mitral valve disease in cavalier King Charles spaniels. Vet Rec 130:302, 1992.
  *A brief account of a survey of mitral insufficiency in cavaliers in Australia.*
Reed JR: Acquired valvular heart disease in the dog. In Kirk RW (ed): Current Veterinary Therapy X. Philadelphia, WB Saunders Co, 1989, p 231.
  *A good resume of the presenting signs, diagnosis, and management of canine heart valve diseases.*
Thrusfield MV, Aitken CGG, and Darke PGG: Observations on breed and sex in relation to canine heart valve incompetence. J Small Anim Pract 26: 709, 1985.
  *A retrospective epidemiologic study of the prevalence of atrioventricular incompetence in a UK veterinary clinic.*

# MYOCARDITIS IN THE DOG AND CAT

SI-KWANG LIU,
*New York, New York*

BRUCE W. KEENE,
*Raleigh, North Carolina*

*and* PHILIP R. FOX
*New York, New York*

Myocarditis is receiving increasing investigative attention by clinicians, pathologists, and molecular biologists interested in the pathogenesis of primary myocardial diseases (cardiomyopathies). This recent interest stems from several important advances, including widespread acceptance of a histologic definition of myocarditis; strong evidence in several mammalian species that cardiotropic viruses play a role in the pathogenesis of myocarditis and cardiomyopathy; and documentation of important links between the host's immune system and genetic make-up and the development, severity, and eventual consequences of myocarditis. The currently accepted criteria for the diagnosis of myocarditis are histologic, requiring the presence of myocardial inflammatory infiltrate and necrosis or degeneration of adjacent myocytes. Because there is no consistently recognizable clinical syndrome or applicable noninvasive diagnostic test, the diagnosis of myocarditis remains problematic and frustrating. Uncertainty may remain even following endomyocardial biopsy because of the often focal nature of the histologic lesions. These problems have prevented an accurate assessment of the true prevalence of myocarditis in dogs and cats, and have blunted the interest of many clinicians and researchers. Increasing numbers of human and animal studies identifying immunologic and genetic links between myocarditis and the eventual development of cardiomyopathy suggest that myocarditis is a more common and important pathophysiologic event with greater epidemiologic significance than previously suspected in both human and veterinary medicine. This article briefly reviews some of the current ideas regarding the occurrence and potential importance of myocarditis in dogs and cats.

## ETIOLOGY AND PATHOGENESIS

It is clear that myocarditis can result from both infectious and noninfectious insults (Table 1). Infectious organisms that have been associated with myocarditis include viruses, bacteria, fungi, protozoa, Rickettsiae, and spirochetes. Infectious organisms may injure the myocardium in many ways, including direct infection, the production of toxic substances, or by inciting immunologically mediated tissue damage. In addition to infectious causes, cardiotoxic drugs and drug hypersen-

sitivity reactions have also been associated with myocarditis. The histopathologic severity of the lesions resulting from any of these agents varies with the severity of the insult, the timing of the histopathologic examination in relation to the insult or infection, and the nature and magnitude of the immune response to the causitive injury or organism. Myocarditis can vary in severity and duration, causing clinical signs acutely in some cases but not for months or possibly even years after the inciting event in others.

## CLINICAL DIAGNOSIS

Classically, the clinical presentation of acute myocarditis is characterized by a rapid onset of heart failure

**Table 1.** *Infectious Pathogens Associated With Canine or Feline Myocarditis*

**Viral**
Parvovirus
Distemper virus
Canine herpesvirus
Feline infectious peritonitis virus
Feline immunodeficiency virus

**Bacterial**
Various

**Rickettsial**
*Rickettsia rickettsii* (Rocky Mountain spotted fever)
*Ehrlichia canis* (Ehrlichiosis)
*Bartonella elizabethae*

**Spirochetal**
*Borrelia burgdorferi* (Lyme disease)

**Fungal**
*Cryptococcus* spp.
*Coccidioides* spp.
*Aspergillus* spp.
*Paecilomyces* spp.
*Blastomyces* spp.
*Histoplasma* spp.
*Actinomyces* spp.

**Algae-like**
*Prototheca* spp.

**Parasitic**
*Toxoplasma gondii* (toxoplasmosis)
*Trypanosoma cruzi* (trypanosomiasis, Chagas' disease)
*Hepatozoon canis*
*Toxocara canis*

or unexplained ventricular arrhythmia associated with a recent history of an infectious disease (upper respiratory infection, gastrointestinal illness, fever) or drug exposure. While many pathogens cause fever during the acute phase of the illness, hypothermia often occurs in critically ill animals with depressed myocardial function, especially puppies and cats. Myocarditis should be suspected in dogs or cats with arrhythmias of unexplained origin (e.g., those without demonstrable structural heart disease or known predisposition for arrhythmia such as gastric dilatation, chest trauma, and so forth), in cases of unexplained systolic myocardial failure in cats and small-breed or other dogs not generally predisposed to dilated cardiomyopathy, and in dogs with echocardiographically demonstrable regional ventricular wall motion abnormalities. Unfortunately, there are no pathognomonic historical, physical, electrocardiographic, radiographic, or echocardiographic findings that allow the clinician to accurately identify myocarditis as an underlying cause of cardiac arrhythmia or failure.

*Physical examination* may be normal. When damage to the myocardium or conduction system is severe, signs of heart failure (dyspnea, exercise intolerance, lethargy, soft cough) or cardiac arrhythmia (episodic weakness, syncope, sudden death) may occur. Thoracic auscultation may disclose evidence of arrhythmia or a murmur of atrioventricular valvular regurgitation (thought to be secondary to papillary muscle dysfunction or concurrent valvular endocarditis) or abnormal lung sounds (e.g., crackles or muffled lung sounds). *Electrocardiography* may reveal a variety of nonspecific abnormalities that have been associated with myocarditis, such as ST- and T-wave alterations, depressed QRS complex voltages, transient or sustained atrial or ventricular arrhythmias, or AV nodal conduction disturbances. *Radiography* may be unremarkable or reflect variable cardiomegaly or venous congestion in cases with congestive heart failure. *Echocardiography* may be enlightening in circumstances where gross cardiac structural changes are present, or where myocardial dysfunction exists. In both humans and dogs, regions of severe ventricular hypokinesis mimicking myocardial infarction have been observed in association with active myocarditis in the absence of biochemical, radionuclide angiographic, or pathologic evidence of ischemia or infarction. Reduced global systolic myocardial performance is also reported in severe cases. On rare occasions, intramyocardial cystic lesions (representing abscesses) or heterogeneous myocardial echogenicity resulting from granulomatous inflammatory infiltrates are imaged. Pericardial effusion is easily detectable if present. In many situations, however, the echocardiographic examination is unremarkable.

When myocarditis is suspected clinically, serologic screening for known infectious causes (including toxoplasmosis, Lyme disease, rickettsial diseases including erlichiosis, Rocky Mountain spotted fever, *Bartonella* spp., and Chagas' disease) may be indicated depending on the clinical laboratory findings and historical or clinical signs of systemic illness present. Unfortunately, lab-

oratory tests (including serum creatine kinase activity) are not consistently altered in myocarditis. In centers with access to *radionuclide angiography*, interesting preliminary experimental data suggest that radionuclides tagged to antimyosin antibodies may eventually become reliable for diagnosis of active myocarditis. *Endomyocardial biopsy* is currently the only means of definitive diagnosis, although limited sampling access, small sample size, and the often multifocal nature of the pathologic lesions combine to limit the sensitivity of this technique. Histologic evaluation of myocyte damage is best appreciated in longitudinal tissue sections by a pathologist experienced in reading through the artifacts common to endomyocardial biopsy specimens. The diagnosis depends on the presence of inflammatory infiltrates as well as myocyte degeneration or necrosis. Fibrosis may be absent or present as perivascular, interstitial endocardial, or replacement type. Recognition of a specific pathogen may be enhanced by the application of molecular techniques to recognize and amplify the genetic material of a specific pathogen in the biopsy specimen. Except for the slim possibility that the etiologic agent will be identified, biopsy-proven diagnosis appears to offer no practical benefit to the patient.

## GENERAL THERAPEUTIC RECOMMENDATIONS

The identification and successful chemotherapeutic elimination of infectious causes (protozoal, bacterial, fungal, and rickettsial) of myocarditis is a top therapeutic priority, since no other effective therapy for myocarditis exists at this time. Whether or not a treatable cause can be identified, therapy must also be directed toward alleviating the clinical signs caused by either cardiac dysfunction or arrhythmia. Because many infectious diseases can cause myocarditis in dogs and cats, and since no well-controlled clinical trials in humans, cats, or dogs provide evidence for any clinical benefit of corticosteroids or other immunosuppressive agents in this setting, their use is not currently advocated in the management of suspected or proven myocarditis. Definitive therapy for or prevention of myocarditis will probably require detailed knowledge of the pathogenesis of viral myocarditis, and the relationship between viral infection, the host immune response and the eventual development of primary myocardial disease.

The prognosis of myocarditis is variable. Many patients no doubt go undiagnosed and recover uneventfully. A conspicuous few die acutely or progress to a form of cardiomyopathy and eventual heart failure.

## FELINE MYOCARDITIS AND RESTRICTIVE CARDIOMYOPATHY

Myocardial disorders constitute an overwhelming majority of acquired feline heart diseases. Idiopathic hypertrophic cardiomyopathy is by far the most common primary myocardial disease of cats. Restrictive cardiomyopathy (RCM) is regularly diagnosed, although opinions vary regarding its clinical characterization (see "Restrictive Cardiomyopathy," this volume, p 863). Restrictive cardiomyopathy (in which the abnormal heart muscle restricts ventricular filling, oftentimes causing contractile dysfunction as well) displays a variety of morphologic and histopathologic features that suggest an inflammatory, possibly immune-mediated, response to some initiating stimulus.

In a series of 461 cats with cardiomyopathy published by Liu in 1977, about 6% were diagnosed with histologic endomyocardial inflammatory lesions and 6% had gross morphologic changes compatible with RCM. Affected cats with endomyocarditis had a mean age of 2.6 years (range = 2.5 months to 8 years); cats with restrictive cardiomyopathy had a mean age of 6.8 years (range = 1 to 11 years). Most (85%) affected with acute myocarditis died unexpectedly. Some cats were dyspneic and depressed and had leukocytosis for 1 to 2 days before death. Of the cats with RCM, all died of cardiac failure (this population was biased toward advanced cases). At necropsy, 45% of RCM cats also had aortic thromboembolism. In a larger series, naturally occurring restrictive cardiomyopathy was diagnosed in 2.4% of 3522 cats that were necropsied from August 1964 to December 1992 at The Animal Medical Center; 73% of the affected cats were male. Ages ranged from 8 months to 15 years (mean = 7.0 years).

The clinical spectrum of endomyocarditis in cats is poorly characterized, and reported cases may be biased toward severe, fulminant infections. The authors most commonly associate a syndrome of acute, severe cardiogenic pulmonary edema in young cats with the necropsy diagnosis of endomyocarditis. It is possible, however, that episodes of nonfatal myocarditis commonly go unrecognized clinically, and eventually result in structural and functional changes that ultimately manifest as cardiomyopathy and congestive heart failure. In practice, it is not uncommon to detect atrial or ventricular arrhythmias (often transient) in cats with hearts that appear either structurally normal or only mildly abnormal by echocardiographic and radiographic examination in absence of recognizable systemic or metabolic disease. The association between these arrhythmias and the presence of chronic or active myocarditis, while suspected, is unknown. Variable degrees of myocardial injury may be detected histologically in affected cats.

The possibility that restrictive cardiomyopathy is a sequela of pathogen-mediated immunologic cardiac injury or to damage related to noninfectious myocarditis is suggested by certain pathologic findings. In cats with acute endomyocarditis, the endomyocardium is focally or diffusely infiltrated by lymphocytes, plasma cells, histiocytes, and a few neutrophils. Adjacent myocytes display abnormal granulation of the sarcoplasmic reticulum, with areas of cell fragmentation and lysis (Fig. 1). Chronic feline endomyocarditis is associated with a minimal inflammatory response, with extensive myocytolysis surrounding areas of granulation and interstitial myocardial fibrosis. Extensive fibrosis, sclerosis and, occasionally, chondroid metaplasia may be present in the left ventricular endocardium (Fig. 2). Massive perivascular and interstitial fibrosis is one of the pathologic hallmarks of restrictive cardiomyopathy. In one study, intramural coronary arterial changes characterized by thickening of the arterial wall and variably decreased lumen size were observed in 71% of the cats with RCM.

Therapy of myocarditis/endomyocarditis in cats is usually supportive and directed at systemic or metabolic derangements caused by the underlying disease, if it can be identified. In cases of congestive heart failure, routine management includes diuretic and vasodilator agents such as nitroglycerin ointment or angiotensin-converting enzyme inhibitors, coupled with

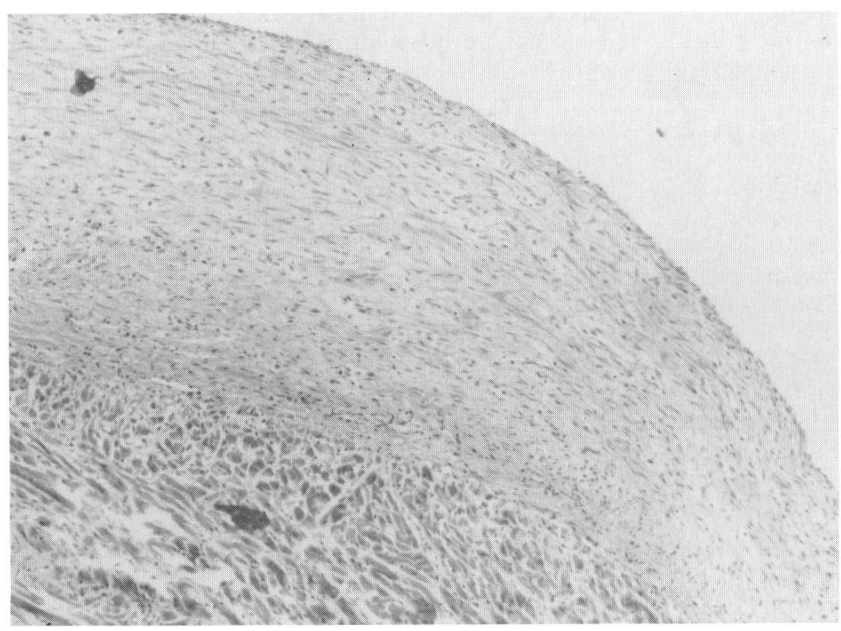

**Figure 1.** Photomicrograph of endocardium from a 4-year-old male domestic shorthair cat that died of cardiac arrest. Extensive proliferation of fibroblasts, fibrous connective tissue, and a few histiocytes are present in the endocardium. Notice infiltration of histiocytes and a few lymphocytes at the junction of fibrous granulation tissue in the myocardium. There was myocytolysis in adjacent myocytes (H & E, ×64).

limitation of activity (see "Restrictive Cardiomyopathy," this volume, p 863). Significant ventricular arrhythmias can be treated with β-adrenergic receptor blockers. These drugs should be avoided in cases with severe systolic myocardial failure, and procainamide may be judiciously substituted (see *CVT XI*, p 732 for a more complete discussion of the diagnosis and management of feline arrhythmias). Supraventricular arrhythmias may be treated with β-blockers, calcium channel blockers, or digoxin.

## MYOCARDITIS AND CARDIOMYOPATHY IN THE DOG

Myocarditis has been reported in the dog in response to a variety of pathogens, with many reports focusing on parvovirus and *Trypanasoma cruzii* (see "Canine Chagas' Myocarditis," this volume, p 850 for more information about trypanosomiasis). Recently, one of the authors (BK) reported a low prevalence (5 to 15%) of biopsy-proven active myocarditis in a sample population of dogs with idiopathic dilated cardiomyopathy, but the role of myocarditis as an initiating event in the pathogenesis of dilated cardiomyopathy remains unknown.

Canine parvovirus was recognized worldwide in 1978 as a cause of peracute, fatal myocarditis in affected puppies. These cases usually involved healthy pups born into parvovirus-contaminated environments with inadequate protective maternal antibody. In 36 affected

dogs from 11 litters, the majority died acutely at about 1 month of age. A number of pups died from 6 to 9 weeks of age with variable signs including cardiomegaly, pulmonary edema, and arrhythmias. The remaining died from about 3½ to 6 months of age, usually unexpectedly, associated with anesthesia or during physical stress.

Histopathologically, the findings of parvoviral myocarditis vary from the finding of large, basophilic, intranuclear inclusion bodies (considered the histopathologic hallmark of the disease) in some of the cardiac myocytes with myocytolysis and minimal or even absent inflammation, to an extensive inflammatory reaction commonly observed in pups dying between 6 and 9 weeks of age. In these pups, lymphocytic and plasmacytic infiltrates surround myocytes showing cytoplasmic coagulation, fragmentation, and lysis. In juvenile dogs, these inflammatory lesions were replaced by histiocytes, fibroblasts, and granulation tissue, with myocytes separated by fibrous connective tissue and foci of myocardium replaced by strands of fibrous connective tissue. The inflammatory, fibrous, and myocytolytic changes are reported to be most severe in the left ventricular free wall and intraventricular septum.

At present, canine parvovirus myocarditis appears to be rare, based on the low incidence of intranuclear inclusions in necropsied hearts. Interestingly, an increasing number of clinical cases of parvovirus infection and subsequent gastrointestinal disease have been observed at many institutions since 1992. Recent evidence using molecular techniques suggests that parvoviral genetic material may be present in the ventricular myocardium of dogs even in the absence of classic intranuclear inclusion bodies. The potential role of persistent viral infections (such as parvovirus) in the pathogenesis of dilated cardiomyopathy is currently under investigation in humans as well as in animals.

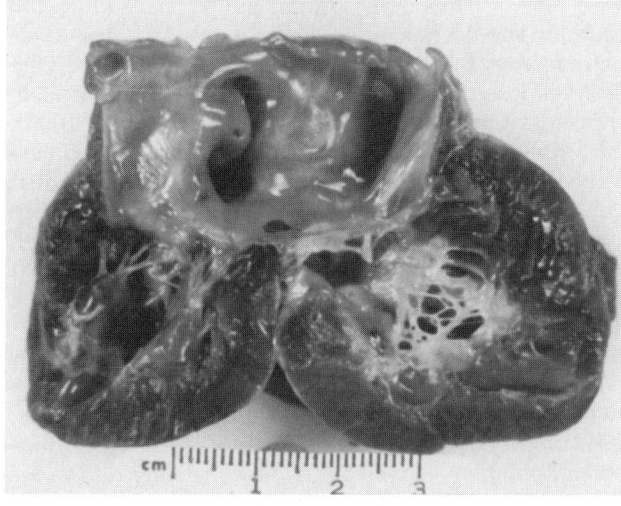

**Figure 2.** Left side of the heart from a 7-year-old male domestic shorthaired cat. Extensive endocardial fibrosis in the outflow tract, and in the midventricular region, with extreme enlargement of the atrium.

## References and Suggested Reading

Fox PR: Feline myocardial disease. *In* Fox PR (ed): *Canine and Feline Cardiology.* New York, Churchill Livingstone, 1988, p 435.
*General review of the pathogenesis, clinical recognition, and treatment of feline myocardial diseases.*
Herskowitz A and Baughman KL: Myocarditis. *In* Gravanis MB (ed): *Cardiovascular Disorders: Pathogenesis and Pathophysiology.* St. Louis, Mosby, 1993, pp 178–209.
*A comprehensive, extensively referenced, current review of myocarditis in humans.*
Liu SK: Myocarditis and cardiomyopathy in the dog and cat. Heart Vessels 1:122, 1985.
*A pathologic description of myocarditis in the dog and cat.*
Meunier PC, Cooper BJ, Appel MJG, and Saluson DO: Experimental viral myocarditis: Parvoviral infection of neonatal pups. Vet Pathol 21:509, 1984.
*Summary of experimental results of parvovirus-induced myocarditis in young puppies.*

# TRAUMATIC MYOCARDITIS

## JONATHAN A. ABBOTT
*Floral Park, New York*

Trauma is an important cause of morbidity and mortality in companion animals. Many animals presented for evaluation of traumatic injury have sustained blunt trauma as the result of road accidents. Complications related to the cardiovascular system are commonly seen in these patients. Most often, these complications are manifest in the form of shock and arrhythmia.

Blunt trauma to the chest may result in a wide array of cardiovascular lesions. Myocardial contusion, pericardial rents, septal perforation, and cardiac rupture may all occur due to nonpenetrating chest trauma. Penetrating trauma to the chest is seen less often in small animal practice. It is important to note however, that trauma to the heart itself is not a prerequisite for the appearance of clinical cardiac abnormalities. Autonomic imbalance, ischemia and reperfusion, electrolyte derangements, and disturbances of acid-base balance may all account for the presence of arrhythmias in traumatized patients. In fact, myocarditis is unlikely to be present at all in these patients; cardiac lesions (if present) are more likely to be necrotic than inflammatory. However, the term "traumatic myocarditis" has become accepted when describing patients who develop arrhythmias following blunt trauma, and will be used in this manner in this article. The syndrome of posttraumatic arrhythmias is observed most frequently in the dog; the following discussion pertains to this species.

The mechanisms by which the heart may be affected in blunt trauma include the following: (1) unidirectional force, (2) bidirectional force (compression), (3) indirect force (e.g., abdominal compression resulting in intravascular pressure changes), (4) decelerative force, and (5) concussive forces. Concussive forces are those that result in alterations of cardiac rhythm but are of insufficient magnitude to cause anatomic lesions (Symbas and Arensberg, 1990). Any of the above, singly or in combination, can occur in road accidents. The general cellular and autonomic causes of cardiac rhythm disturbances are described elsewhere in this volume (see "Cardiac Arrhythmias in Systemic Disease," this volume, p 161).

## DIAGNOSIS

Supraventricular tachyarrhythmias, ventricular arrhythmias, and bradyarrhythmias have all been observed following blunt trauma. However, ventricular arrhythmias such as ventricular premature complexes and ventricular tachycardia are thought to be most common (Alexander, Bolton, and Koslow, 1975). Often, these arrhythmias appear 24 to 48 hr after the occurrence of trauma. Consequently, they may represent an important presurgical consideration in patients who have sustained orthopedic injuries. Surveillance of the cardiac rhythm through careful auscultation or electrocardiography is recommended in patients who have sustained blunt trauma. Accurate electrocardiographic diagnosis of any suspected rhythm disturbance is essential. Remember that sinus or atrial rhythms accompanied by bundle-branch block can mimic ventricular tachycardia!

## Electrocardiographic Features

Dogs that have been struck by automobiles often develop slow ventricular rhythms that are initiated only after a pause in the sinus rhythm (Fig. 1). Unfortunately, the nomenclature of these rhythm disturbances is unclear. Terms such as fast idioventricular rhythm, accelerated idioventricular rhythm, slow ventricular tachycardia, and idioventricular tachycardia have all been employed. Some have applied the term "accelerated idioventricular rhythm" to ventricular rhythms with rates greater than 60 bpm but not exceeding 100 bpm. It should be noted that this premise was likely extrapolated from the human medical literature. That is, rates less than 100 bpm in people do not, as such, represent tachycardias (Marriott and Myerberg, 1990). Experimental data using a canine model of induced atrioventricular block demonstrates that fast idioventricular rhythms generally have rates less than 130 bpm (Ilvento et al., 1982; Vassale et al., 1977). However, there may well be differences between the fast idioventricular rhythms observed in the experimental setting and those observed clinically.

The electrophysiologic basis of these rhythms has not been defined. While abnormal automaticity has been suggested in one experimental model (Ilvneto et al., 1982), others have proposed a form of enhanced normal automaticity in which the idioventricular rate varies (Schamroth, 1980). When the idioventricular rate exceeds the rate of the sinus node, it captures the rhythm and becomes electrocardiographically evident (Fig. 2). When the ventricular rhythm slows, the cardiac rhythm is recaptured by the sinoatrial node and sinus rhythm resumes. This may explain why these rhythms are initiated by late diastolic (escape) beats, and why fusion beats often initiate and terminate the ventricular rhythm (Fig. 3A). Generally, it is reasonable to refer to ventricular rhythms that are initiated after a pause and in which the rate exceeds a prevailing normal sinus rate

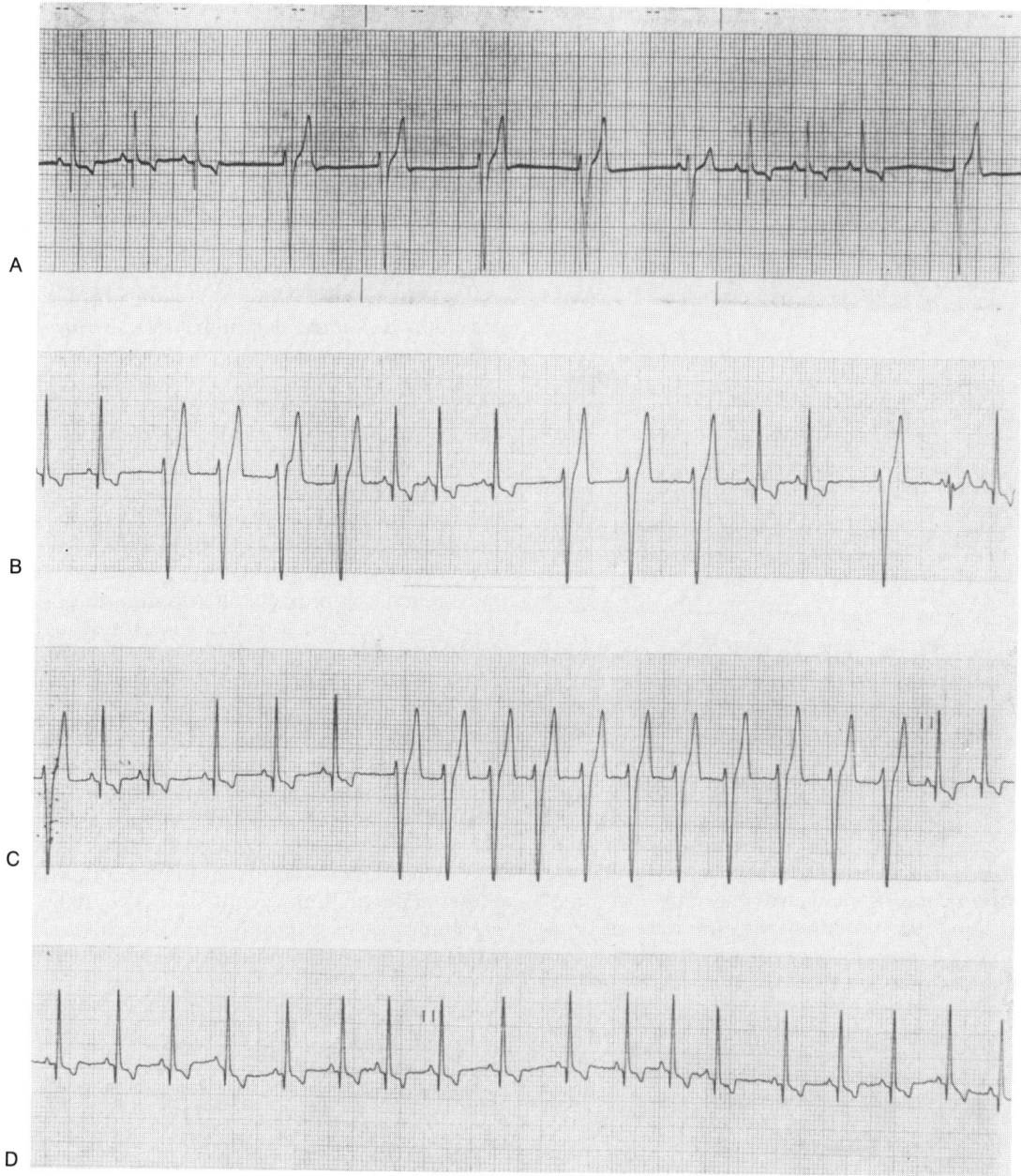

**Figure 1.** Electrocardiograms recorded from a canine patient that had been struck by a car 48 hr previously. *A*, A ventricular rhythm that developed during a pause in the sinus rhythm. The rate of the ventricular rhythm is approximately 70 bpm. The ventricular rhythm is terminated by a fusion complex. *B*, Accelerated idioventricular rhythms with rates of approximately 125 and 107 bpm. Note the second to last complex is a fusion beat. *C*, Accelerated idioventricular rhythm —the rate ranges from 136 to 150 bpm. Note that the rhythm slows before sinus rhythm resumes. *D*, Ventricular rhythms were not noted when the rate of the sinus node increased and the underlying sinus arrhythmia became less pronounced. Interestingly, the morphology of all the ventricular ectopic beats is similar, if not identical. (Electrocardiograms are all lead II and recorded at 25 mm/sec, 0.5 cm = 1 mV.)

by only 5 to 10 bpm as idioventricular tachycardias (Schamroth, 1980) or accelerated idioventricular rhythms. Certainly, ventricular rhythms that are difficult to classify arise in the trauma setting. A labile rate and long, inconsistent pauses preceding the rhythm favor a diagnosis of accelerated idioventricular rhythm. Ventricular tachycardias can be defined arbitrarily as ventricular rhythms that are initiated by early diastolic depolarizations and/or that manifest cycle lengths (R-R intervals) shorter than 375 msec; that is, 160/min (Fig. 3B).

The cause of these accelerated idioventricular rhythms is unknown; a disturbance of autonomic balance or reperfusion of ischemic tissues may explain their presence. The primary importance of identifying these rhythms lies in their clinical significance—they are almost always benign electrically and hemodynamically. As the ventricular rate of these rhythms is

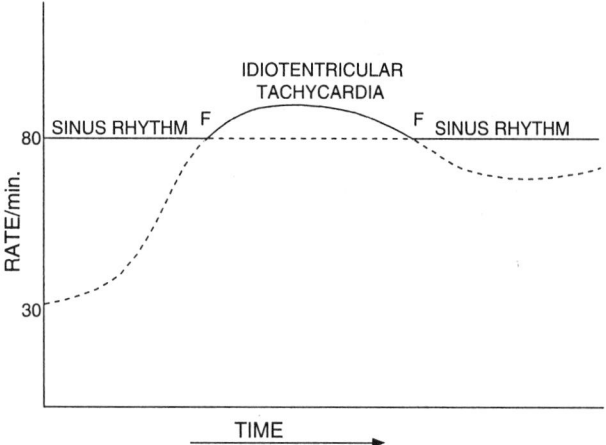

**Figure 2.** A mechanism that may explain the development of idioventricular rhythms in dogs that have sustained blunt trauma in road accidents. F denotes the time when fusion beats occur. (From Schamroth L: Ventricular extrasystoles, ventricular tachycardia, and ventricular fibrillation: Clinical-electrocardiographic considerations. Prog Cardiovasc Dis 23:13, 1980, with permission.)

relatively slow, they are unlikely to have a detrimental effect on blood pressure, though this should be measured. It should be noted, however, that electrocardiographically benign-appearing accelerated idioventricular rhythms are occasionally associated with arterial hypotension and low cardiac output. Preexisting myocardial disease or depressed ventricular function caused by ischemia may predispose the patient to hypotension. Some ventricular arrhythmias are characterized by a progressively increasing or decreasing rate over time. This underscores the importance of accurate electrocardiographic diagnosis and careful attention to the he-

modynamic status (blood pressure, color, refill time, pulse) of the patient.

## THERAPY

Therapeutic decisions in patients with ventricular arrhythmias are based on the clinician's assessment of the risk of lethal arrhythmias, such as ventricular fibrillation, or adverse hemodynamic effects. Very rapid rates reduce ventricular filling time, and the lost atrial contribution to ventricular filling assumes greater importance during tachycardia. Ventricular dyssynergy caused by abnormal ventricular activation can further reduce stroke volume. Sustained ventricular tachycardias can result in myocardial ischemia, increasing ventricular stiffness and further impairing diastolic function and myocardial contraction. Using only the surface electrocardiogram, it is not possible to accurately predict which patients will die suddenly. It is known, however, that the nadir of the ventricular fibrillation threshold occurs at approximately the time the peak of the T wave is inscribed on the electrocardiogram (Katz, 1992). Hence, premature ventricular complexes that occur in early diastole are thought to be more dangerous. This is known as the "R-on-T" phenomenon. It should also be emphasized that late diastolic, ventricular ectopics can precipitate ventricular fibrillation, though this seems far less common.

Another important consideration in the pharmacotherapy of ventricular arrhythmias that has received recent attention is the phenomenon of proarrhythmia. Many antiarrhythmic agents can potentially worsen arrhythmias as well as provide an arrhythmogenic substrate for the development of new arrhythmias (Ham-

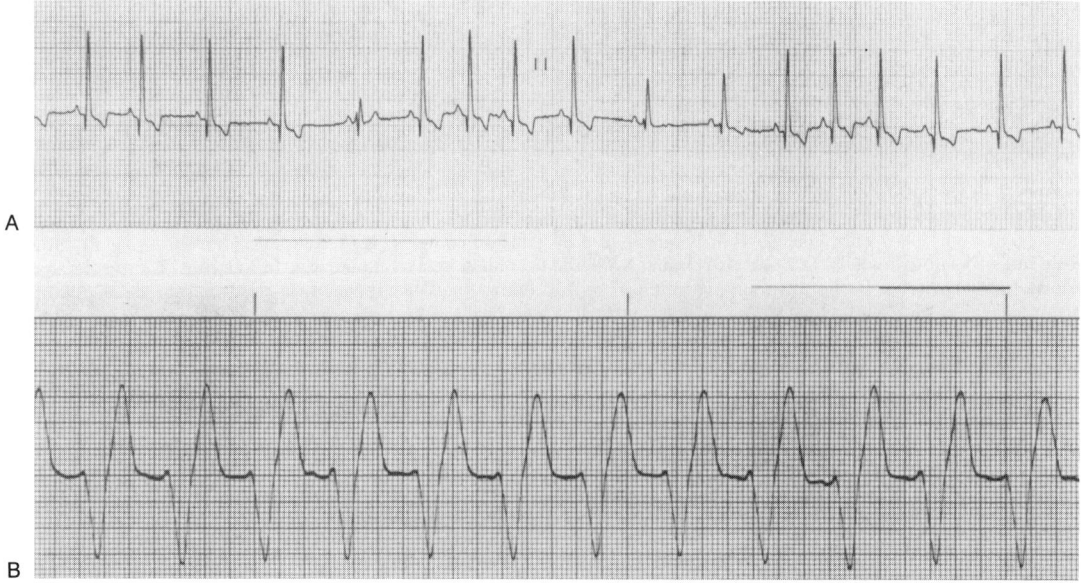

**Figure 3.** *A,* Fusion complexes are noted during pauses in the sinus rhythm. The patient had sustained blunt trauma in a road accident (lead II recorded at 25 mm/sec, 0.5 cm = 1 mV). *B,* Ventricular tachycardia at a rate of 187 bpm in a dog that had been struck by an automobile. Note that the rhythm is regular (lead II recorded at 50 mm/sec, 1 mV = 1 cm).

lin, 1992). In addition to this concern, there is little evidence to support the supposition that a reduction in the frequency of ventricular arrhythmias necessarily reduces mortality. All antiarrhythmic drugs depress myocardial function to some degree; moreover, extracardiac adverse effects can develop. With these factors in mind, it is important to carefully consider each patient before initiating drug therapy.

Ventricular rhythms that begin after a pause and barely exceed the sinus rate do not generally require specific antiarrhythmic therapy. Although these rhythms can usually be suppressed by increasing the sinus rate with atropine, this is generally not recommended, because atropine can also potentiate other, more serious arrhythmias.

Antiarrhythmic therapy is probably indicated if the ventricular rate exceeds an arbitrary limit of 130 to 160 bpm; it is certainly indicated if there is clinical evidence of inadequate cardiac output (poor perfusion, hypotension). The presence of clinical signs may be the single most important and defensible criterion for the initiation of antiarrhythmic therapy. Sustained ventricular rhythms with rates greater than 130 to 160 bpm almost always warrant therapeutic intervention. Therapy of frequent, early diastolic ventricular ectopics may be indicated when there is R-on-T phenomenon; the efficacy of antiarrhythmic therapy for other purposes is unknown.

Prior to the initiation of drug therapy, it is important to consider and, if possible, correct any disorders that may contribute to the genesis of arrhythmias. Hypovolemia should be corrected if present (this alone may decrease the ectopic ventricular rate), and attention must be paid to serum electrolytes (especially serum potassium) and acid-base status. Conditions that may result in hypoxia, such as pneumothorax or anemia, should be identified and remedied if possible. High-quality chest radiographs are essential in patients that sustain blunt trauma regardless of whether or not there is external evidence of injury.

### Antiarrhythmic Strategies

Lidocaine is the drug of choice for the urgent parenteral treatment of hemodynamically significant ventricular arrhythmias in the dog. It is relatively safe and is usually effective, provided the patient's electrolyte are normal. Lidocaine can be administered as a slow intravenous bolus at a dose of 2 mg/kg. If the administration of a single bolus is ineffective in restoring sinus rhythm, repeated bolus injections may be administered. The dose of intravenous lidocaine should not exceed 8 mg/kg over 10 min. If the arrhythmia is responsive to lidocaine, a constant-rate infusion can be initiated (40 to 80 μg/kg/min). Occasionally, it is necessary to administer small, supplemental boluses until a steady-state plasma level is obtained. If lidocaine fails, procainamide can be administered intravenously over 2 to 3 min at a dose of 2 to 3 mg/kg to a total cumulative dose of 6 to 20 mg/kg to normovolemic patients. This drug can be delivered as a constant intravenous infusion at a rate of 25 to 50 μg/kg/min. Some ventricular tachyarrhythmias appear to be adrenergically mediated—the intravenous administration of the short-acting β-blocker esmolol can be used to test this hypothesis in individual patients. This drug can be given as a very slow intravenous bolus at a dose of 0.1 to 0.5 mg/kg. If conversion to sinus rhythm occurs, therapy can be continued with propanolol (0.3 to 1.0 mg/kg PO every 8 hr or, 0.02 to 0.06 mg/kg over 5 to 10 min IV every 8 hr).

Other, less well established, antiarrhythmic strategies that can be contemplated include the use of class 3 antiarrhythmics such as bretylium (5 to 10 mg/kg as a slow intravenous bolus or 5 to 10 mg/kg diluted 1:4 in saline administered over 8 min depending on clinical urgency). Although profound hypomagnesemia is unlikely to accompany an episode of trauma, the intravenous administration of magnesium sulfate appears to have antiarrhythmic properties in some clinical settings. Magnesium sulfate may be administered as a slow intravenous bolus at a dose of 25 to 40 mg/kg (see Section 2 for details of magnesium therapy). If clinical circumstances allow, this dose may be administered diluted in saline over 20 to 60 min. Synchronized, DC cardioversion (½ to 1 J/kg after heavy IV sedation and analgesia) can be considered in hypotensive patients with rapid ventricular rhythms that do not respond to drug therapy. It should be noted that the collective veterinary experience with these interventions is limited.

If it is deemed necessary to attempt conversion with several different agents, it is important to reevaluate the patient and ECG diagnosis at every step. Each time a potentially dangerous drug or therapy is considered, the risk/benefit for the patient should be carefully analyzed. When therapy is deemed necessary it can usually be discontinued after 3 to 4 days. Most of these rhythms require observation rather than drug therapy.

### References and Suggested Reading

Alexander JW, Bolton GR, and Koslow GL: Electrocardiographic changes in nonpenetrating trauma to the chest. J Am Anim Hosp Assoc 11:160, 1975.
  *A case series of patients that developed ventricular arrhythmias following nonpenetrating chest trauma.*
Dangmen KH and Boyden PA: Cellular mechanisms of cardiac arrhythmias. In Fox PR (ed): *Canine and Feline Cardiology.* Philadelphia, WB Saunders Co, 1988, pp 269–289.
  *A textbook chapter that reviews the cellular basis of arrhythmogenesis.*
Hamlin RL: Current uses and hazards of ventricular antiarrhythmic therapy. In Kirk RW and Bonagura JD (eds): *Current Veterinary Therapy XI: Small Animal Practice.* Philadelphia, WB Saunders Co, 1992, pp 694–700.
  *An article that provides a general approach to the therapy of ventricular arrhythmias.*
Ilvento JP, Provet J, Danilo P, and Rosen MR: Fast and slow idioventricular rhythms in the canine heart: Study of their mechanisms using antiarrhythmic drugs and electrophysiologic testing. Am J Cardiol 49:1909, 1982.
  *An experimental investigation of idioventricular rhythms in dogs with induced complete atrioventricular block.*
Katz AM: The arrhythmias III—premature systoles, tachycardias, flutter and fibrillation. In Katz AM (ed): *Physiology of the Heart.* New York, Raven Press, 1992, pp 569–608.
  *A textbook chapter that reviews the electrophysiologic basis of tachyarrhythmias.*

Marriott HJL and Myerburg RJ: Recognition of cardiac arrhythmias and conduction disturbances. *In* Hurst JW (ed): *The Heart, Arteries and Veins.* New York, McGraw-Hill, 1990, pp 489–534.
   *A textbook chapter that reviews principles of electrocardiographic diagnosis in people.*

Schamroth L: Ventricular extrasystoles, ventricular tachycardia, and ventricular fibrillation: Clinical-electrocardiographic considerations. Prog Cardiovasc Dis 23:13, 1980.
   *A review of the electrocardiographic features of ventricular arrhythmias.*

Symbas PN and Arensberg D: Traumatic heart disease. *In* Hurst JW (ed): *The Heart, Arteries and Veins.* New York, McGraw-Hill, 1990, pp 1375–1381.
   *A textbook chapter that reviews the mechanisms and cardiac consequences of trauma.*

Vassale M, Knob RE, Cummins M, et al: An analysis of fast idioventricular rhythm in the dog. Circ Res 41:218, 1977.
   *An experimental investigation of idioventricular rhythms in dogs with induced atrioventricular block and in dogs in which sinoatrial node automaticity was suppressed by vagal stimulation.*

# CANINE CHAGAS' MYOCARDITIS

KATHRYN M. MEURS,
MATTHEW W. MILLER,
*and* R. GAYMEN HELMAN

*College Station, Texas*

Chagas' disease is one of the leading causes of myocarditis in people, and in the dog is associated with a variety of cardiac abnormalities including conduction disturbances, arrhythmias, myocardial dysfunction, and sudden death. The incidence of Chagas' myocarditis in the dog is not known. In the years between 1987 and 1992, 315 canine serum samples were submitted to the Texas Veterinary Medical Diagnostic Laboratory for the indirect fluorescent antibody test for Chagas' disease; 25 were positive. Although the clinical signs of this disease appear to be fairly well documented, the best method for diagnosis and therapy is still controversial.

## EPIDEMIOLOGY

Chagas' myocarditis is caused by the protozoan parasite, *Trypanosoma cruzi.* In the United States, the principal vectors of *T. cruzi* are insects in the family Reduviidae. These insects are usually nocturnal feeders that inhabit animal bedding and housing; they become infected by ingesting the circulating trypomastigote form of the protozoan from the bloodstream of various hosts. Common wild hosts for *T. cruzi* in the southern United States are raccoons, armadillos, and opossums; dogs, cats, and guinea pigs are considered domestic reservoir animals (Barr, 1991).

While in the insect vector, the trypomastigote transforms to the epimastigote form and multiplies by binary fission. The epimastigotes transform back to trypomastigotes in the hind gut of the vector before excretion (Barr, 1991). The classic route of infection in South America is via deposition of the trypomastigote-containing feces by the vector into a fresh bite wound created during the insect's blood meal. Vectors in the United States do not defecate during blood meals and are therefore less efficient transmitters of the disease than their South American counterparts.

Once the trypomastigote has entered the bloodstream of the new host, it enters the cytoplasm of the host's cells (especially macrophages or striated myocytes), where it becomes an amastigote. The amastigotes multiply by binary fission and transform back into trypomastigotes before cell rupture and release of the trypomastigotes into the circulation (Barr, 1991).

## PATHOGENESIS AND CLINICAL SIGNS

There are three phases of Chagas' myocarditis in dogs: acute, latent, and chronic. The acute stage, usually 2 to 4 weeks after infection, may be characterized by lethargy, generalized lymphadenopathy, pale mucous membranes, slow capillary refill time, splenomegaly, and hepatomegaly (Barr, 1991). Experimentally, lymphocytosis is a consistent finding; however, this does not appear to be as common in clinical cases (Barr et al., 1991). Parasitemia can be detected within a few days after infection and peaks within 2 to 3 weeks (Barr, 1991). The electrocardiogram may demonstrate sinus tachycardia, prolonged P-R interval, decreased R-wave amplitude, axis shifts, and conduction disturbances including first-degree atrioventricular (AV) block and right bundle-branch block (Barr, Holmes, and Klei, 1992). The echocardiogram is usually normal (Barr, Holmes, and Klei, 1992).

Sudden death is occasionally seen in the acute state. In experimentally induced canine Chagas' myocarditis, conduction disturbances during the acute stage predicted the occurrence of sudden death. This suggests that abnormalities in the conduction system and perhaps resultant malignant arrhythmias may be the cause of death in these animals (Barr, Holmes, and Klei, 1992).

Clinical findings in the acute stage of Chagas' myocarditis are believed to be a result of damage to the myocardium that occurs as the trypomastigotes rupture from the host's cardiac myocytes. Additional myocardial inflammation may occur as the host's immune system becomes activated against the released trypomastigotes (Barr, 1991). The clinical signs of the acute stage of Chagas' myocarditis are often quite subtle, and are easily overlooked.

Dogs that survive the acute stage may enter a prolonged latent period without clinical signs. In people, the latent period may persist for years before the development of the chronic stage. In the latent period, parasitemia has usually resolved and antibodies to *Trypanosoma cruzi* have developed (Barr, Holmes, and Klei, 1992). The electrocardiogram may be normal or have residual changes similar to those seen in the acute stage. The echocardiogram is usually normal. Sudden death may still occur in this stage (Barr, 1991). It is not clear what percentage of dogs that survive the acute stage will go on to develop the chronic stage, or when they will begin to show clinical signs. Experimentally, dogs that survived the acute stages of Chagas' myocarditis had an average latent period of 77 days (27 to 120 days) (Barr, Gosset, and Klei, 1991).

The chronic stage of Chagas' myocarditis is characterized by progressive, generalized cardiac dilation and ventricular arrhythmias. Clinical signs may be indicative of biventricular failure and include pulse deficits, ascites, pleural effusion, hepatomegaly, and jugular venous distention (Barr, Gosset, and Klei, 1991). It appears that right ventricular failure occurs initially, but is followed rapidly by left ventricular failure (Barr, 1991). Electrocardiographic abnormalities include occasional ventricular premature complexes that frequently progress to paroxysmal and sustained ventricular tachycardia that can be refractory to therapy (Fig. 1). Echocardiographic findings include right ventricular dilation and progressive decreases in left ventricular

function characterized by decreased fractional shortening, reduced ejection fraction, reduced left ventricular free wall thickness, and increases in end-systolic volume (Fig. 2). At this point, heart failure usually progresses to death.

The mechanism for the development of congestive heart failure after the latent period is not well understood. Possible mechanisms that have been suggested include: autonomic nervous system dysfunction, immune-mediated mechanisms, and microvascular disease characterized by irregularities and constrictions of intramyocardial arteriolar vessels and increased platelet adherence and aggregation (Barr, 1991; Tanowitz et al., 1989). An improved understanding of the pathophysiology of this stage of the disease might provide a means for preventing progression of myocardial dysfunction.

## DIAGNOSIS

Historically, the diagnosis of Chagas' disease was made by the isolation of the organism in cell culture or mice. Although this is a fairly sensitive method, it is expensive and very time consuming. Its clinical utility is somewhat limited. Serology has been very useful in the diagnosis of Chagas' disease. Diagnostic methods available include: complement fixation, direct hemagglutination, and indirect fluorescent antibody techniques. False-positive reactions have been reported in humans with leishmaniasis and collagen vascular diseases, so the results of serologic tests should be interpreted with regard to clinical findings (Kirschoff, 1993).

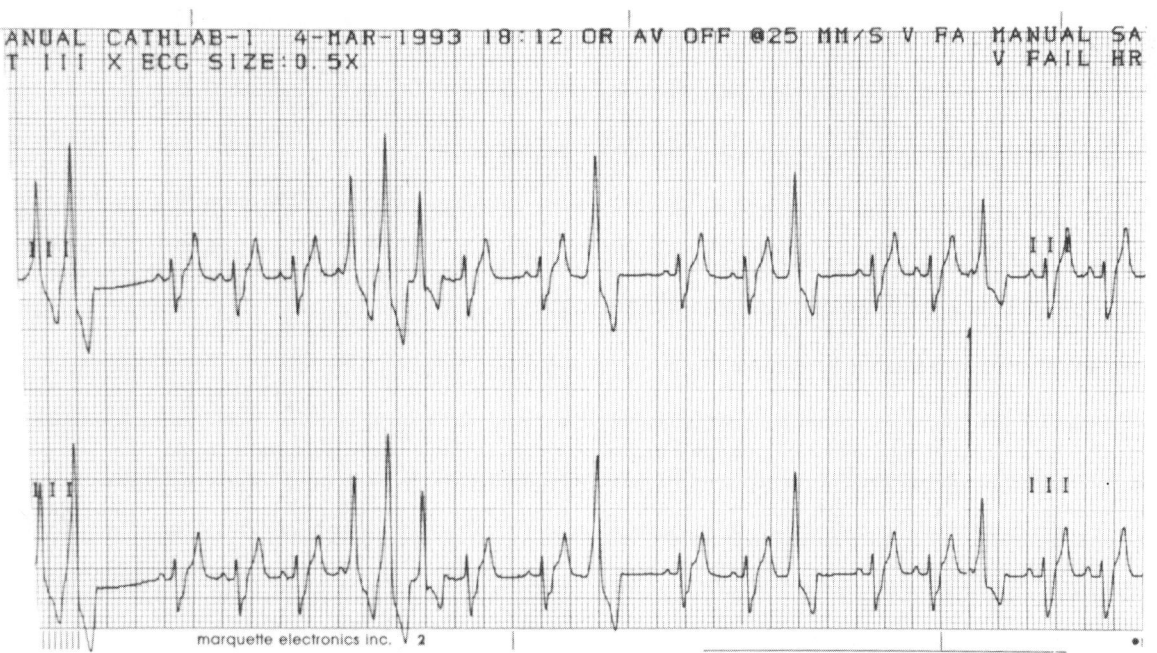

**Figure 1.** Electrocardiogram from a 6-year-old female spayed German shepherd dog with Chagas' myocarditis. Notice that the sinus beats are conducted with a right bundle-branch block pattern (*arrowhead*). Isolated ventricular premature complexes with short runs of paroxysmal ventricular tachycardia are also present (*arrows*). The upright morphology of the ventricular premature complexes in lead II suggest a right ventricular origin (leads II and III, 1 cm = 2 mV, paper speed = 25 mm/sec).

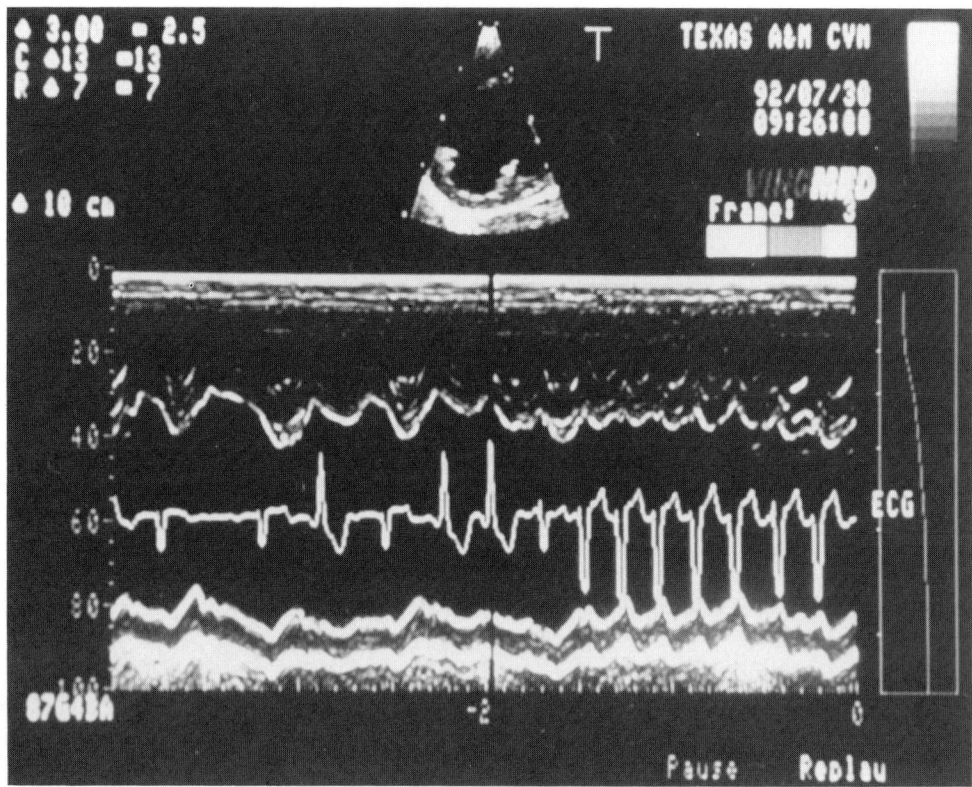

**Figure 2.** M-mode echocardiogram obtained at the chordal level from a dog with chronic Chagas' myocarditis. Notice the multiform ventricular arrhythmia detected during the exam and its effect on myocardial function.

The diagnosis of the acute form of Chagas' myocarditis is made when circulating trypomastigotes are detected on thick blood smears. Trypomastigotes may be identified in peripheral blood within a few days after infection. The level of parasitemia is often low, making detection of trypomastigotes difficult. However, evaluation of a thick blood smear is the best method by which to confirm the acute stage of the disease (Fig. 3). A thick blood smear should be evaluated for the presence of circulating trypomastigotes in dogs with electrocardiographic abnormalities consistent with conduction pathway disease, normal echocardiograms, and that have been in the southern United States or South America. Nonspecific clinical signs coupled with the lack of an easy, accurate diagnostic test make the acute stage of Chagas' disease difficult to diagnose.

The diagnosis of chronic Chagas' myocarditis in our clinic is based on the presence of clinical signs associated with right or biventricular failure, electrocardiographic abnormalities that may include ventricular tachyarrhythmias or conduction disturbances, echocardiographic findings of right ventricular dilation with decreased left ventricular function, and a positive indirect fluorescent antibody test.

## PATHOLOGY

Gross pathology of the myocardium in the acute stage is characterized by mild dilation of the right atrium and ventricle. Multiple yellow, grey to white foci, streaks or pale zones may be present in the subendocardium. Histopathologic evaluation of myocardium from dogs with acute Chagas' myocarditis is characterized by granulomatous myocarditis with pseudocysts containing amastigotes (Fig. 4). Fibrosis is minimal (Barr et al., 1991).

Grossly, chronic Chagas' myocarditis is characterized by biventricular dilation and thinning of the ventricular free walls. Histopathologic evaluation of myocardium from dogs with chronic disease is characterized by multifocal interstitial lymphoplasmacytic and histiocytic infiltrates, perivasculitis, and marked fibrosis (Barr et al., 1991).

## THERAPY

Treatment of dogs with Chagas' myocarditis varies depending on the stage of the disease. Treatment of the acute stage should be directed towards both the peripheral trypomastigote as well as the intracellular amastigote form. Therapy for the chronic stage is usually directed at palliative treatment of congestive heart failure and arrhythmias.

The acute form of Chagas' myocarditis is rarely diagnosed; therefore, therapy directed at elimination of circulating or intracellular parasites is infrequently indicated. Nifurtimox and benzimidazole have reportedly been used to successfully treat acute canine trypano-

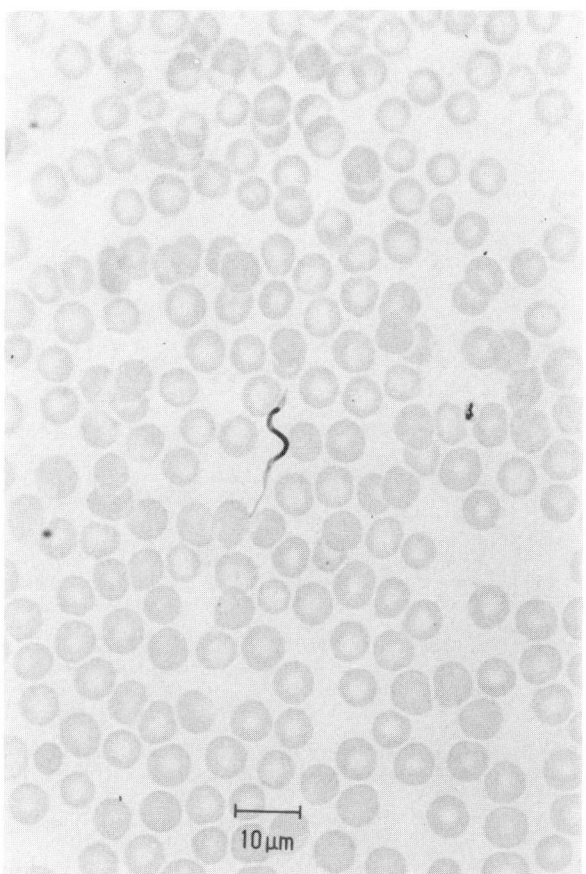

**Figure 3.** Photomicrograph of a blood smear showing a trypomastigote of *T. cruzi* among erythrocytes. (Wright's stain.)

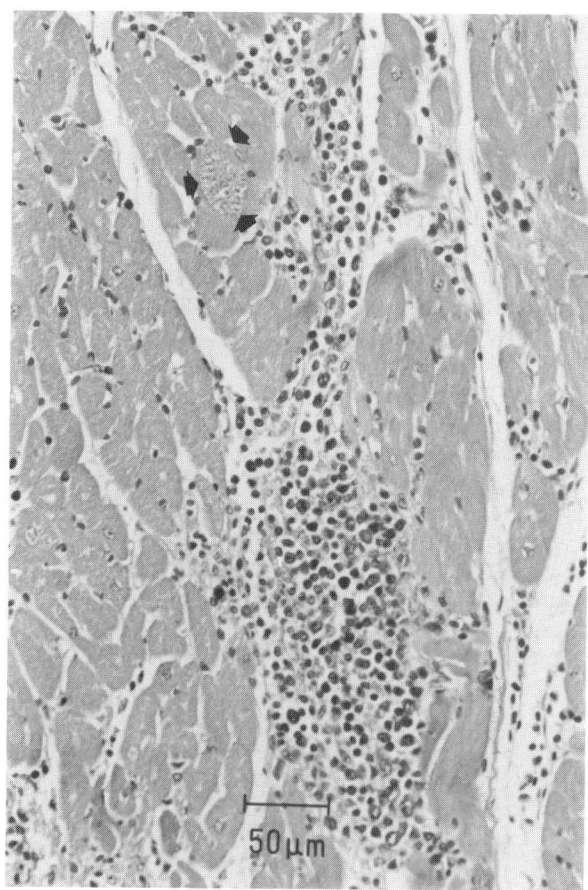

**Figure 4.** Photomicrograph of a section of canine myocardium showing interstitial accumulations of mononuclear leukocytic inflammatory cells consisting of lymphocytes, plasma cells, and mononuclear phagocytes. A myocyte contains intracellular amastigotes of *T. cruzi* (*arrows*). (H&E stain.)

somiasis; however, these drugs do not appear to be highly effective and have been associated with severe side effects (Barr, 1991). The destruction of the intracellular form of *Trypanosoma cruzi* by these drugs is followed by exacerbation of the host inflammatory reaction. Increased severity of myocarditis has been associated with nifurtimox treatment for the acute stage in human beings even though the level of parasitemia decreased (Andrade, Andrade, and Sadigursky, 1980). Additionally, changes that occur in the heart muscle secondary to the intracellular parasite do not resolve, even after the number of intracellular parasites has been decreased. Improved survival has been documented in dogs treated concurrently with anti-inflammatory doses of steroids and nifurtimox (Andrade, Andrade, and Sadigursky, 1980). Treatment for confirmed cases of acute Chagas' myocarditis might include nifurtimox (2 to 7 mg/kg), orally, every 6 hr for 3 to 5 months while simultaneously treating with prednisone (0.5 mg/kg) orally every 12 hr. Nifurtimox is an investigational drug and is only available from the Centers for Disease Control and Prevention in Atlanta, GA.

Unfortunately, the diagnosis of Chagas' myocarditis is usually made after the dog has entered the chronic stage. Therapy directed at destruction of the organism at this stage has not been shown to alter the course of clinical disease. Treatment of this stage is directed to-

wards the clinical signs associated with myocardial failure and the ventricular arrhythmias, which often seem to be refractory to antiarrhythmic therapy. The lack of an effective treatment for Chagas' myocarditis in humans has led to a search for innovative therapy. Two of the most promising areas in therapeutic research include the use of calcium channel blockers (verapamil) and the imidazoles.

## Imidazoles

The imidazoles (ketoconazole, itraconazole) have been recently shown to be useful in the treatment of experimentally induced acute Chagas' disease in mice and in a spontaneous case of Chagas' disease in a person infected with the acquired immunodeficiency syndrome (AIDS) virus (McCabe, Remington, and Araujo, 1984; Solari et al., 1993). The mechanism of action of the imidazoles in this disease is unclear. It has been suggested that they interfere with sterol synthesis and inhibition of the cytochrome P-450 enzyme system. Ketoconazole significantly inhibited the *in vitro* replication of epimastigotes and intracellular amastigotes in experimentally induced Chagas' disease in mice

(McCabe, Remington, and Araujo, 1984). The use of these drugs is currently limited to the acute stage of the disease.

## Calcium Channel Blockers

In rodents, verapamil has been used for both acute and chronic Chagas' infections with some success. Decreased mortality as well as decreased myocardial inflammation and fibrosis were seen in mice with experimentally induced Chagas' disease treated with verapamil. However, verapamil therapy was started at the same time the mice were inoculated. It is theorized that verapamil's direct vasodilatory effects and effect on platelet aggregation may alter the microvascular disease that has been associated with this stage of the disease (Morris et al., 1989; Tanowitz et al., 1989).

The ideal therapy for Chagas' myocarditis is unknown. Therapy of the acute stage is directed at elimination of the organism and reduction of myocardial inflammation. Therapy of the chronic stage consists of palliative therapy for the clinical signs associated with conduction abnormalities and myocardial dysfunction (see elsewhere in this section). Recent research into the use of verapamil and the imidazoles may provide more promising treatment options.

## References and Suggested Reading

Andrade SG, Andrade ZA, and Sadigursky M: Combined treatment with a nitofuranic and a corticoid in experimental Chagas' disease in the dog. Am J Trop Med Hyg 29:766, 1980.

*A comparative study of the survival differences between dogs with experimentally induced Chagas' myocarditis given no treatment, treatment with nifurtimox alone, and treatment with nifurtimox and betamethasone.*

Barr SC: American trypanosomiasis in dogs. Compend Cont Educ 13:745, 1991.

*A general review of clinical findings, diagnosis and treatment of canine Chagas' disease.*

Barr SC, Gosset KA, and Klei TR: Clinical, clinicopathologic and parasitologic observations of trypanosomiasis in dogs infected with North American *Trypanosoma cruzi* isolates. Am J Vet Res 52:954, 1991.

*Clinical findings in dogs experimentally infected with* Trypanosoma cruzi.

Barr SC, Schmidt SP, Brown CC, et al: Pathologic features of dogs inoculated with North American *Trypanosoma cruzi* isolates. Am J Vet Res 52:2033, 1991.

*Pathology findings from dogs experimentally infected with* Trypansoma cruzi.

Barr SC, Holmes RA, and Klei TR: Electrocardiographic features of trypanosomiasis in dogs inoculated with North American *Trypanosoma cruzi* isolates. Am J Vet Res 53:521, 1992.

*Cardiac ultrasound and electrocardiogram findings from dogs experimentally infected with* Trypanosoma cruzi.

Kirchoff LV: American trypanosomiasis (Chagas' disease)—a typical disease now in the United States. N Engl J Med 329:639, 1993.

*A general review of Chagas' disease in the United States.*

McCabe RE, Remington JS, and Araujo FG: Ketoconazole inhibition of intracellular multiplication of *Trypanosoma cruzi* and protection of mice against lethal infection with the organism. J Infect Dis 150:594, 1984.

*Effects of ketoconazole on the development of myocarditis in mice inoculated with* Trypanosoma cruzi.

Morris SA, Weiss LM, Factor S, et al: Verapamil ameliorates clinical, pathologic and biochemical manifestations of experimental chagasic cardiomyopathy in mice. J Am Coll Cardiol 14:782, 1989.

*Results of verapamil treatment in mice with experimentally induced Chagas' myocarditis.*

Solari A, Saavedra H, Sepulveda C, et al: Successful treatment of *Trypanosoma cruzi* encephalitis in a patient with hemophilia and AIDS. Clin Infect Dis 16:255, 1993.

*A case report of an AIDS patient with* Trypanosoma cruzi *encephalitis who responded positively to therapy with itraconazole and fluconazole.*

Tanowitz HB, Morris SA, Weiss LM, et al: Effect of verapamil on the development of chronic experimental Chagas' disease. Am J Trop Med Hyg 41:643, 1989.

*Effect of verapamil on chronic experimentally induced Chagas' myocarditis in mice.*

---

# CVT UPDATE: FELINE HYPERTROPHIC CARDIOMYOPATHY

MARK D. KITTLESON

*Davis, California*

## DEFINITION

Feline hypertrophic cardiomyopathy (HCM) is a disease of the ventricular (primarily left ventricular) myocardium characterized by mild to severe primary concentric hypertrophy. Concentric hypertrophy (thickened wall with normal to small chamber size) of the left ventricle has numerous secondary causes including aortic stenosis, systemic arterial hypertension, hyperthyroidism, and acromegaly. When any of these diseases are present, the diagnosis of hypertrophic cardiomyopathy is excluded and the cardiac abnormality should not be called hypertrophic cardiomyopathy but rather concentric hypertrophy secondary to the primary abnormality (e.g., concentric hypertrophy secondary to hyperthyroidism). In addition to concentric hypertrophy, the myocardium can also thicken due to infiltration, as with lymphoma.

## ETIOLOGY

The etiology of feline HCM is unknown. In humans, it has been known since 1958 that HCM is oftentimes familial. It has been demonstrated that approximately 50% of the human HCM is inherited in an autosomal dominant pattern, with the other cases being sporadic (although oftentimes still genetic in origin). Recently (since 1989), specific genetic abnormalities have been identified in human families that are associated with hypertrophic cardiomyopathy. The first abnormality was a missense mutation identified on the $\beta$-myosin heavy chain gene that resides on chromosome 14q1 (Seidman and Seidman, 1991). Since that time, at least nine missense mutations have been identified on this gene that are associated with hypertrophic cardiomyopathy (Watkins et al., 1992). Most commonly, these mutations have been identified in families, but de novo mutations in individuals with no family history have also been identified. Even more recently, missense mutations in the alpha-tropomyosin gene and missense mutations and a mutation in the splice donor sequence of intron 15 of the cardiac troponin T gene have been identified as causes of familial hypertrophic cardiomyopathy in man (Thierfelder et al., 1994). Since mutations in genes that encode for myosin, for troponin, and for tropomyosin have now been identified, it appears that familial hypertrophic cardiomyopathy in man is a disease of the sarcomere.

Recently, the author and co-investigators have identified the first family of cats (Maine coons) with hypertrophic cardiomyopathy, 35 years after the first identification of a human family (Kittleson, Pion, and Mekhamer, 1993). Because of the close interrelationship in this family of cats, it isn't possible to determine the mode of inheritance of HCM in this family. This is the first clue that HCM in cats may also be genetically linked. Studies are currently in progress to determine if specific gene abnormalities exist in this family of cats.

The author and co-investigators have also identified an increase in serum growth hormone concentration in about 60% of the cats studied in our clinic with HCM. Growth hormone is a known inducer of myocardial hypertrophy. Cats with acromegaly can have quite severe concentric hypertrophy of the left ventricular myocardium. In humans, serum growth hormone concentration is increased in patients with heart failure. In cats with HCM, elevations were identified in cats both with and without heart failure. Whether the increase in serum growth hormone concentration is the cause, is the result, or is unrelated to feline HCM is unknown at this time.

## PATHOLOGY

Cats with severe hypertrophic cardiomyopathy have marked thickening of the left ventricular myocardium (interventricular septum and free wall), with the entire wall commonly being 9 to 11 mm thick. Papillary muscle hypertrophy is oftentimes very prominent. The left ventricular chamber is usually smaller than normal. This is caused by the myocardial thickening encroaching on the left ventricular cavity. In most cats, the left ventricular free wall and the interventricular septum are equally thickened. In some cats, the interventricular septum is significantly thicker than the free wall, while in a few others the free wall is thicker. The left atrium is usually enlarged, oftentimes markedly so. Occasionally, a thrombus is present within the left atrium or the left auricular appendage.

Cats with milder forms of the disease (mild to moderate hypertrophic cardiomyopathy) have lesser wall thickening and a more normal sized left ventricular chamber. The left atrium may be normal in size or mildly to moderately enlarged. It is not unusual to see papillary muscle hypertrophy as the primary manifestation of the disease in these cats.

In humans, myocardial fiber disarray that involves at least 5% of the myocardium in the interventricular septum is found in 90% of patients. This is quite specific for HCM in humans. Other diseases that produce concentric hypertrophy can also cause myocardial fiber disarray, but this almost always involves less than 1% of the myocardium, a level also found in normal human hearts. In cats with HCM, myocardial fiber disarray in the interventricular septum of the same magnitude observed in humans is only identified in approximately 30% of cases (Liu, Roberts, and Maron, 1993).

## PATHOPHYSIOLOGY

In humans, familial hypertrophic cardiomyopathy develops over the first two decades of life. In cats, the disease has been observed in cats as young as 6 months and as old as 16 years. The author has documented one Maine coon cat without evidence of HCM at 3 months of age that died from the disease at 1 year of age and another where the disease progressed from 6 months to 18 months of age. Consequently, the disease may develop in some cats during the first 1 to 2 years of life.

Cats with severe hypertrophic cardiomyopathy are commonly presented because of clinical signs referable to heart failure. Often, cats with lesser forms of HCM never develop overt clinical signs referable to their disease. In severe HCM, left ventricular hypertrophy causes several abnormalities in left ventricular function that can lead to pulmonary edema and decreased cardiac output (heart failure). Cardiac output is stroke volume × heart rate. Stroke volume is determined by end-diastolic volume and end-systolic volume (stroke volume = end-diastolic − end-systolic volume). In cats with severe hypertrophic cardiomyopathy, end-diastolic volume is usually decreased because of the encroachment of the thickened left ventricular myocardium on the left ventricular cavity. Afterload (systolic wall stress = systolic intraventricular pressure × chamber radius/wall thickness) is decreased in hypertrophic cardiomyopathy because of the decrease in chamber size and the increase in wall thickness. Consequently, end-systolic volume is also decreased. However, end-diastolic volume may be decreased relatively more than is end-systolic volume. This would result in a decrease in stroke volume.° Shortening fraction generally is greater in the cat with HCM than in the normal cat (70% versus 50%), yet the stroke volume is reduced because of the decrease in end-diastolic volume. The increased shortening fraction is produced by the decrease in afterload, not an increase in myocyte "contractility."

Edema formation in hypertrophic cardiomyopathy occurs because increased left atrial and pulmonary venous pressures increase pulmonary capillary pressure. These pressure increases can be due to either an increase in left ventricular end-diastolic pressure or mitral regurgitation and are associated with left atrial and pulmonary vein enlargement. Left ventricular end-diastolic pressure can be increased because of abnormalities in diastolic function, because of increased blood volume, and because of mitral regurgitation. Severe concentric hypertrophy, as seen in hypertrophic cardiomyopathy, causes abnormalities in diastolic function. The primary abnormality it causes is an increase in left ventricular chamber stiffness. Chamber stiffness is the ΔPressure/ΔVolume relationship. Because the wall is thickened, it is stiffer than normal, resulting in a greater increase in pressure for any given volume when the ventricle fills in diastole. In addition, cats with hypertrophic cardiomyopathy take a longer time to relax in early diastole, which can cause an increase in diastolic pressure if the heart rate is very fast (if diastole is so short that the ventricle cannot relax to a normal point in the time allotted). Incomplete relaxation of the myocardium may also occur.

Cats with heart failure secondary to hypertrophic cardiomyopathy usually have severe left ventricular thickening, and the most common sign of a cat symptomatic for hypertrophic cardiomyopathy is heart failure. Consequently, veterinarians commonly see cats with heart failure and very thick left ventricles and the common assumption is that the severe hypertrophy must be the only cause of the enlarged left atrium and pulmonary edema. The author has had the opportunity to observe several Maine coon cats with severe thickening but without left atrial enlargement or heart failure over extended periods of time. In addition, people with severe HCM generally often have only a mild to moderate increase in left ventricular end-diastolic pressure.

Consequently, it appears that although severe diastolic dysfunction must result in some increase in end-diastolic pressure, it may not be severe enough to result in severe left atrial enlargement and moderate to severe heart failure in some cats, which suggests that hypertrophy, per se, may not be the only abnormality

---

°As an example, assume that cubing left ventricular chamber diameter predicts chamber volume. If we start with a normal cat that has an end-diastolic diameter of 1.4 cm and an end-systolic diameter of 0.7 cm, this cat's end-diastolic volume would be 2.7 ml and the end-systolic volume would be 0.3 ml. Stroke volume would be 2.4 ml. If we then look at a theoretical case of feline HCM, we can theorize this cat would have an end-diastolic diameter of 1.0 cm and an end-systolic diameter of 0.3 cm. This cat's end-diastolic volume would be 1 ml and end-systolic volume would be 0.02 ml. Stroke volume would essentially be 1 ml.

causing left atrial enlargement, increased left atrial and pulmonary vein pressures, and heart failure.

What else could contribute to edema formation in these cases? We have measured plasma aldosterone concentration in some cats with heart failure secondary to HCM and found it to be elevated. Why might this occur? If cardiac output was reduced in these cats because of a reduction in stroke volume, as explained earlier, renin release would result, ultimately leading to an increase in plasma aldosterone concentration. An increase in plasma aldosterone concentration leads to an increase in blood volume which leads initially to an increase in venous return to the heart which could help lead to the increased diastolic intraventricular pressure, to the increased left atrial size, and to edema formation.

Mitral regurgitation is another consideration. Cats with hypertrophic cardiomyopathy commonly have left apical murmurs and, in the author's experience, cats with hypertrophic cardiomyopathy and left atrial enlargement almost always have evidence of mitral regurgitation on color-flow Doppler examination, whereas cats with hypertrophic cardiomyopathy and normal left atrial size often do not have evidence of mitral regurgitation. Why would mitral regurgitation occur in hypertrophic cardiomyopathy? Most likely because of a phenomenon called systolic anterior motion (SAM) of the mitral valve. Systolic anterior motion is commonly observed in people with hypertrophic cardiomyopathy. It is less commonly documented in cats, probably because the size of the heart and the rapid heart rate make it more difficult to document. However, the author and others have noted that in cats with HCM on color-flow Doppler, one of the most common patterns observed is that of two turbulent jets originating from the same region—one regurgitating back into the left atrium and the other shooting out into the aorta (Fig. 1). This pattern is consistent with SAM. Systolic anterior motion of the mitral valve is the abnormal process of the anterior (septal) mitral valve leaflet being pushed or pulled into the left ventricular outflow tract during ventricular contraction, where it commonly contacts the interventricular septum. Mitral valve SAM can be identified definitively on an M-mode echocardiogram (Fig. 2). Systolic anterior motion produces two abnormalities. First, it obstructs flow out of the left ventricle (dynamic subaortic stenosis). Second, by drawing the anterior leaflet out of its normal position, SAM creates mitral regurgitation. It is the author's belief that mitral regurgitation is the abnormality of primary significance brought about by SAM in cats, since the author believes that mitral regurgitation secondary to SAM of the mitral valve is a significant contributor to the development of heart failure in feline hypertrophic cardiomyopathy. The argument against this is that the color-flow Doppler jet that is present in the left atrium is commonly relatively small when compared to patients that have primary mitral regurgitation and heart failure. It is the author's belief, however, that color-flow Doppler underestimates the amount of regurgitation in cats because of the fast heart rate com-

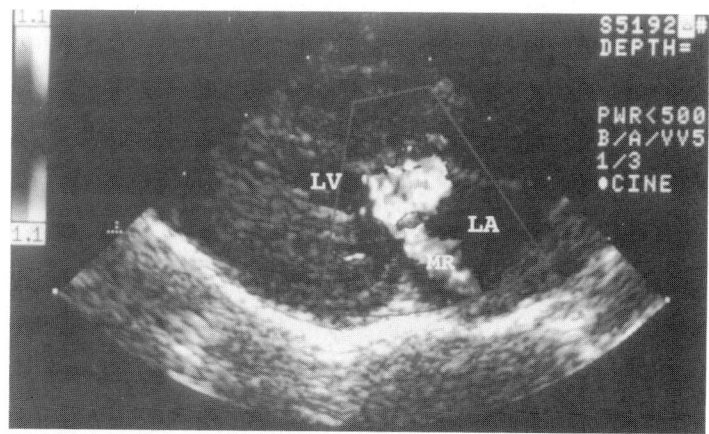

**Figure 1.** A black-and-white rendition of a color-flow Doppler two-dimensional echocardiogram from a Maine coon cat with hypertrophic cardiomyopathy showing two turbulent jets—one of mitral regurgitation going into the left atrium and one of dynamic subaortic stenosis going into the aorta. Abbreviations: LV = left ventricle, LA = left atrium, MR = mitral regurgitation.

pared to a relatively slow frame rate in current machines, so the amount of regurgitation may be greater than perceived. Even if the amount of regurgitation is less than that seen in primary mitral regurgitation, it is probably a combination of increased left ventricular chamber stiffness and mitral regurgitation that creates moderate to severe heart failure in many cats. In this situation, lesser degrees of mitral regurgitation would be required to drive left atrial and pulmonary vein pressures high enough to cause edema formation. This is particularly likely if the dilated and hypertrophied left atrium has a decreased compliance and inability to sufficiently distend and accept the regurgitant and right ventricular stroke volumes.

Cats with severe HCM that present in heart failure most commonly have pulmonary edema. Some cats with HCM, however, have pleural effusion. Usually, this is only a small amount of effusion, but in a few cases the effusion can be considerable. Pleural effusion in cats with heart failure can be a modified transudate, or can be chylous in nature. It is unknown exactly why pleural effusion develops in these cats. There are two likely possibilities. The first is that the elevation in pulmonary vein and pulmonary capillary pressures results in pulmonary vasoconstriction, pulmonary hypertension, and right heart failure. Increased left atrial stiffness may also contribute to pulmonary hypertension. This scenario commonly occurs in humans and horses with left heart failure but does not usually occur in dogs. The overall importance of pulmonary hypertension in the cat is unsolved, although in the author's experience, it is unusual to identify right heart enlargement or other evidence of right heart failure, such as hepatic vein enlargement on an ultrasound exam. The second possibility is that the visceral pleural veins in cats drain into the pulmonary veins such that elevated pulmonary vein pressure (congestive left heart failure) causes the formation of pleural effusion. This is known to occur in humans but has not been proven in the cat.

Thrombi in cats with HCM appear to develop in the left atrium or left auricle. In humans, the presence of echocardiographic "smoke" (an amorphous, swirling, light gray haze) in the left atrium is associated with increased risk of thromboembolic disease. Echocardiographic smoke probably occurs because of red cell aggregation that occurs when blood flow velocity is low. The author and others have also noted echocardiographic smoke in some cats with HCM and an enlarged left atrium, in some cats with HCM and left atrial thrombi, and in some cats with HCM and thromboembolic disease. The presence of moderate to severe left atrial enlargement in a cat with HCM should be considered a risk factor for development of thromboembolic disease. Echocardiographic smoke should be considered an additional risk factor.

## CLINICAL PRESENTATION

Cats with hypertrophic cardiomyopathy may be completely asymptomatic, may have subtle signs of heart failure, may have moderate to severe heart failure, may die suddenly, or may develop thromboembolic disease. Asymptomatic cats can have mild to severe left ventricular thickening. It is likely that many cats with mild to moderate thickening never develop clinical signs referable to their disease and live normal lives. Cats with severe thickening may be completely asymptomatic. More commonly, however, cats with severe disease that appear to be asymptomatic actually show subtle signs of heart failure that can be detected by a very observant owner. Respiratory rate is oftentimes increased in these cats at rest and they may become more tachypneic or even dyspneic if stressed, although they usually recover quickly following stress.

Cats with severe HCM usually have auscultatory abnormalities. A systolic murmur, heard best over the sternum or left apex, is common and probably due either to outflow tract obstruction, mitral regurgitation, or both. A gallop sound is also common. In cats with fast heart rates, rapid ventricular filling and atrial systole (the two times at which gallop sounds are generated) occur very close together so that on an M-mode echocardiogram the mitral valve is observed to only open once. Consequently, it is oftentimes impossible to tell in a cat with tachycardia (typical of heart failure) whether the gallop sound is an audible third or fourth heart sound. This distinction is principally academic, since differentiation of $S_3$ from $S_4$ does not distinguish the form of heart disease.

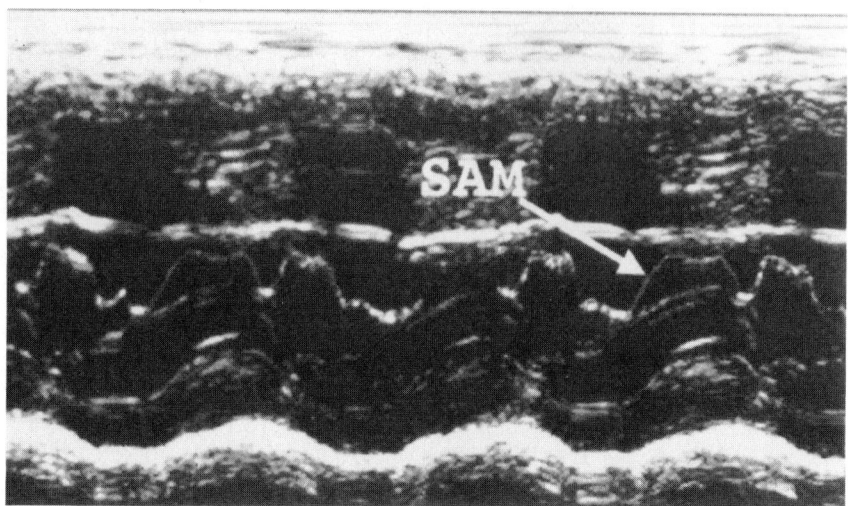

**Figure 2.** An M-mode echocardiogram from a Maine coon cat with severe hypertrophic cardiomyopathy showing systolic anterior motion of the mitral valve. The systolic anterior motion occurs between the diastolic openings of the mitral valve leaflets. The anterior leaflet moves towards the interventricular septum in systole. Abbreviation: SAM = systolic anterior motion.

Cats with severe hypertrophic cardiomyopathy and moderate to severe heart failure are usually brought to a veterinarian because of respiratory abnormalities, usually tachypnea, dyspnea, or infrequently for cough. While coughing is a more common sign of respiratory diseases (infection, asthma, lungworms, heartworms), this sign can develop in cats with heart disease. Coughing in cats can be mistaken for vomiting, so it is not unusual for the owner's chief complaint to be vomiting. To distinguish coughing from vomiting in a cat, the veterinarian should palpate the trachea vigorously enough to produce a cough (one should be able to make a normal cat cough at least once) while the owner observes the consequence and then ask the owner if this is what is occurring. The respiratory abnormalities observed in cats with hypertrophic cardiomyopathy are due to pulmonary edema, pleural effusion, or both. Since household cats are generally sedentary, owners usually do not notice that they are having respiratory difficulty until the dyspnea is advanced. At that time, the onset of the disease commonly appears to be acute or peracute to the owner, whereas in reality the disease has been present for years and the heart failure has probably been gradually worsening over months to years. Peracute pulmonary edema can be precipitated by fever, severe anemia, fluid therapy, or anesthesia.

Cats with thromboembolic disease present most commonly because of the peracute onset of posterior paresis or paralysis and pain due to a large thromboembolus lodged at the aortic trifurcation. These cats do not have a palpable femoral artery pulse, have pale to blue-tinged pads or nail beds, and have turgid gastrocnemius muscles. Lack of flow to the rear limbs can be documented by Doppler examination or cutting a nail back to the "quick" and observing for lack of blood flow. Smaller thromboemboli may exit the aorta, causing a variety of signs. One of the more common signs due to smaller thromboemboli is right front leg lameness. This occurs when a small thromboembolus takes the first major exit off the aorta (the brachiocephalic trunk) and then the next exit, the right subclavian artery, to the leg. Renal embolization is not uncommon.

Cats with severe HCM also die suddenly, oftentimes with no prior clinical signs referable to heart failure. To the author's knowledge, an electrocardiogram has not been recorded during sudden death of any cat that had HCM. Consequently, we do not know what causes the sudden death. In humans, sudden death appears to be either due to arrhythmic or hemodynamic causes. The hemodynamic cause is usually an acutely worsening outflow tract obstruction associated with strenuous exercise (which probably ultimately leads to a terminal arrhythmia). Since cats are not usually subjected to strenuous exercise, this is a less likely scenario in cats. In the author's experience, sudden death in Maine coons is usually not associated with any type of physical stress. It is more likely that these cats die from an acute ventricular tachyarrhythmia that degenerates into ventricular fibrillation. The incidence of sudden death in feline HCM is probably underrepresented in the veterinary literature because cats that die suddenly are not examined by veterinarians and owners commonly do not report their cat's death to a veterinarian, especially if the event is unwitnessed and the cat is found dead.

## DIAGNOSIS

The diagnosis of HCM should be made using echocardiography. Angiocardiography can be used to make the diagnosis, but it is invasive and associated with complications. On echocardiography, cats with severe HCM usually have markedly thickened left ventricular walls (8 to 11 mm in diastole), papillary muscle hypertrophy, and an enlarged left atrium. The hypertrophy can be global, affecting all areas of the left ventricular wall or can be more regional. Regional forms can include involvement of the: entire length or simply a portion of the interventricular septum; the ventricular apex; or the papillary muscles (and oftentimes adjacent free wall). Because of these forms, HCM is a diagnosis that should be made by examining several different two-dimensional echocardiographic views and measuring wall thicknesses from the region or regions of thickening on the two-dimensional images. M-mode echocardiography may miss regional thickening unless it is guided by the two-dimensional view. It is emphasized that an M-mode echocardiogram, taken from immediately below the mitral valve leaflets (the standard view for measuring left ventricular wall thicknesses and chamber diameter), oftentimes misses regional wall thickening.

Color-flow Doppler echocardiography frequently demonstrates a regurgitant jet of mitral regurgitation when moderate to severe left atrial enlargement is present as described above. Systolic anterior motion of the mitral valve may be present and can sometimes be observed on an M-mode echocardiogram (Fig. 2). This appears to produce the mitral regurgitant jet and the dynamic subaortic stenosis jet (Fig. 1). Spectral Doppler can be used to determine the pressure gradient across the region of SAM. This pressure gradient probably correlates with the degree of SAM and so can be used to document whether therapy has decreased the amount of SAM.

The diagnosis of HCM is much more difficult and controversial in cats with lesser wall thickening or only regional thickening as observed by echocardiography. In human families with HCM associated with specific gene abnormalities, varying degrees of severity have been noted within the affected family members (Scott et al., 1993). In other words, in one family with a specific gene mutation, echocardiographic findings in family members with the mutation range from no abnormalities to severe HCM. This may also be true in cats so that milder forms of the disease do exist. However, distinguishing mild disease from normal or distinguishing mild to moderate HCM from hypertrophy secondary to other abnormalities may not be easy in individual cases. Even within the author's family of Maine coons, it is difficult to distinguish whether or not some cats are affected. In a clinical situation where one is examining an older cat with what appears to be mild hypertrophy, one must first decide whether hypertrophy is present or not and then determine if another disease is causing the hypertrophy before one can really make the diagnosis of feline HCM. The upper limit for normal diastolic left ventricular wall thickness is 5 to 6 mm in the cat. The author conservatively considers significant concentric hypertrophy in the cat to be anything 7 mm or greater. Once concentric hypertrophy is diagnosed, especially in an older cat, hyperthyroidism, systemic hypertension, and possibly acromegaly must be ruled out. Hyperthyroidism is usually easy to rule out. Devices to measure blood pressure in the cat, however, are not always available. The author prefers to measure systolic blood pressure using a pediatric inflatable cuff placed around the distal forelimb and then uses a Doppler flow sensing device placed on the ventral metacarpal region to detect flow (see Section 2 for details). Most cats with systemic hypertension will have an increase in systolic blood pressure, although it is theoretically possible to have just diastolic hypertension, which would be missed using this technique. The author has had difficulties with oscillometric devices in cats. The author considers a systolic blood pressure above 150 mm Hg to be abnormally high. Others have used up to 180 mm Hg as an upper limit. If systemic arterial blood pressure cannot be measured, one should at least rule out the common causes of systemic hypertension in a cat with left ventricular concentric hypertrophy (i.e., hyperthyroidism and renal failure).

## TREATMENT

### Initial Therapy

Cats presented in heart failure are almost always symptomatic because of pulmonary edema and/or pleural effusion. Consequently, therapy is generally aimed at decreasing left atrial and pulmonary vein pressures in these cats. In some cats with severe heart failure, clinical evidence of hypoperfusion (low-output heart failure) may be apparent in addition to the signs of congestive heart failure, and may be manifested as cold extremities and total body hypothermia.

The cat presented for respiratory distress that is suspected of having heart failure secondary to HCM should be initially evaluated by doing a cursory physical examination, taking care not to stress the patient. Most cats with severe HCM will have a readily audible heart murmur or an audible gallop sound (gallop rhythm). A butterfly catheter should be used to perform thoracentesis on both sides if pleural effusion is suspected. Generally, this should be done in a sternal position so that the cat does not become stressed during the procedure. If pleural fluid is identified, it should be removed. If none is identified, a lateral or a dorsoventral chest radiograph may be taken with the veterinarian in attendance to ensure that the cat is not stressed (assuming the cat is not stretched or the procedure in any way interferes with ventilation). If the patient struggles or appears stressed or fractious during or prior to radiographic examination, the procedure should be cancelled and the patient placed immediately into an oxygen-enriched environment.

Furosemide (Lasix, Hoechst-Roussel) should be administered intravenously (IV) or intramuscularly (IM). The route of administration depends on the stress level of the patient. Furosemide should be administered IM to cats that are very distressed and cannot tolerate restraint for an IV injection. Cats that can tolerate an IV injection may benefit from the more rapid onset of action (within 5 min of an IV injection versus 30 min for an IM injection). Initial furosemide dose to a cat in distress should generally be in the 1- to 2-mg/kg range. This dose may be repeated within 1 hr of an IV injection (duration of effect following IV administration is approximately 1 hr) or within 2 hr of an IM injection (duration of effect following an IM injection is approximately 2 hr). In general, the higher end of the dosage range is used for the IM injection, while the lower end of the range is administered more frequently for the IV route. Dosing must be reduced sharply once resting respiratory rate starts to decrease.

Persistent, high-dose parenteral furosemide therapy commonly produces electrolyte disturbances, dehydration, and azotemia in cats. Sick cats are precarious and may not drink or eat sufficiently even when CHF has been treated effectively. Some cats become dehydrated and electrolyte depleted because of this and continuing diuretic treatment. Judicious IV or subcutaneous (SC) fluid administration may be required to clinically improve these cats. Overzealous fluid administration will result in the return of clinical signs referable to heart failure.

Nitroglycerin cream (Nitro-Bid, Marion; Nitrol, Adria; Nitrong, Wharton; Nitrostat, P-D) may be beneficial in cats with severe edema formation secondary to feline HCM. However, no studies have examined the effects of this drug in this species. When nitroglycerin is used clinically, it is almost universally administered in conjunction with furosemide, a drug known to have profound beneficial effects in congestive heart failure. Consequently, it is generally impossible to tell if any observed beneficial effects are due to the furosemide or to the combination of furosemide and nitroglycerin. Because of this, the numerous anecdotal reports of nitroglycerin's benefits in this situation are suspect. However, nitroglycerin is safe when administered judiciously, and some benefit may occur with its administration. Consequently, the author would not dissuade anyone from administering $\frac{1}{8}$ to $\frac{1}{4}$ inch of a 2% cream to the inside of an ear every 4 to 6 hr for the first 24 hr as long as furosemide was administered concomitantly. Nitroglycerin tolerance develops rapidly in other species and probably does so in the cat, so prolonged administration is probably of no or lesser benefit.

No other drugs are proven useful for treating acute, severe congestive heart failure due to HCM. Once furosemide and nitroglycerin are administered, the cat should be left to rest quietly in an oxygen-enriched environment. Care should be taken not to distress the cat by placing catheters, taking body temperature, and so forth. A baseline measurement of respiratory rate should be taken when the cat is resting. This should be followed at 30-min intervals and furosemide administration continued until the respiratory rate starts to decrease (a consistent decrease of 10 breaths per minute over an hour is a good general guide). Once this occurs, the furosemide dose and dosage frequency should be curtailed sharply.

## Long-Term Management

Cats that have survived their respiratory crisis, or cats identified with less critical degrees of heart failure, can be started on chronic drug therapy for their heart failure. Many aspects of chronic therapy of HCM are controversial.

In cats with congestive heart failure, furosemide administration should be maintained in most cases. Occasionally, furosemide may be discontinued gradually once the cat has been stabilized. In some cases, furosemide may not be required because the administration of another drug has improved cardiac function; for example, diltiazem has improved left ventricular diastolic function or decreased the amount of mitral regurgitation sufficient to allow decreasing the dose of or discontinuing furosemide. The maintenance dose of furosemide in cats usually ranges from 6.25 ($\frac{1}{2}$ of a 12.5-mg tablet) once a day to 12.5 mg every 8 hr. The dose needs to be titrated carefully in each patient. Having the owner count the resting respiratory rate at home and keep a daily log of the respiratory rate is highly beneficial for making decisions regarding dosage adjustment in individual patients. Periodic measurements of serum creatinine and electrolytes are also useful.

In cats with severe HCM in which congestive heart failure has occurred, administration of diltiazem or a $\beta$-adrenergic blocking agent is generally indicated. Both provide symptomatic benefit in human patients. Since the idea for administering both of these drugs comes from their administration to human patients, it may be worthwhile to compare the human and the feline diseases and the therapeutic goals for each species. The pathology of HCM in humans is somewhat different than in the cat. The primary difference is the predominant septal hypertrophy that almost always occurs in humans. Despite this difference, the pathophysiology of the disease in the two species is similar (Maron et al., 1987). Human patients with severe disease also have marked hypertrophy, a smaller than normal left ventricular cavity, impaired diastolic function, and SAM of the mitral valve. These abnormalities culminate in symptoms of dyspnea, reduced exercise capability, and chest pain. The dyspnea is caused by increased left ventricular diastolic pressure (interestingly, this is rarely called "congestive heart failure" in human patients with HCM, though it is a form of CHF). The major difference between the two species from this aspect appears to be the degree of elevation in ventricular diastolic or left atrial pressure. These pressure elevations appear to be mild to moderate at rest in humans and result in mild to moderate left atrial enlargement. In cats, the increases in left ventricular diastolic or left atrial pressure are oftentimes marked, resulting in severe pulmonary edema or pleural effusion. Consequently, drug therapy only has to reduce diastolic pressure mildly to moderately in people to produce symptomatic benefit, whereas in the cat, major reductions in left ventricular filling pressure must be produced. Because of this, furosemide is required to treat cats with heart failure secondary to HCM, whereas in humans, diuretic administration is not used or is thought to be contraindicated because decreases in end-diastolic volume are thought to worsen SAM of the mitral valve. Improvement in exercise capability is an important therapeutic goal in humans. Domestic cats rarely exercise, so improvement in exercise tolerance is not a therapeutic goal. Relief of chest pain is a major goal in humans. Chest pain may occur in cats due to ischemia but, obviously, evidence is lacking. In summary, in the cat, the primary therapeutic goal is to treat or prevent moderate to severe congestive heart failure; accordingly, diuretic administration is often required along with other drugs such as diltiazem and propranolol. In human patients, the therapeutic goals are to treat mild heart failure, alleviate chest pain, and prevent sudden death. Calcium channel blockers and propanolol are commonly used alone to achieve these goals.

Diltiazem (Cardizem, Marion) is a calcium channel blocker documented to have beneficial effects in cats with HCM when dosed at 7.5 mg every 8 hr (see *CVT XI*, p 766). Beneficial effects include lessened edema formation and decreased wall thickness in some cats (Bright et al., 1991). Exactly how these beneficial effects occur is open to debate. Diltiazem appears to improve the early diastolic relaxation abnormalities seen in feline HCM. Whether this helps decrease diastolic intraventricular pressure and so decrease pulmonary edema formation is unknown. Slower myocardial relaxation can increase diastolic intraventricular pressure if the heart rate is very fast so that the myocardium does not have time to relax. Incomplete relaxation and decreased compliance, however, are more plausible explanations for increased diastolic pressure due to diastolic dysfunction in feline HCM. Diltiazem may also improve these abnormalities as well as slow heart rate. In addition, diltiazem may decrease SAM, as verapamil does in humans, thereby decreasing the amount of mitral regurgitation and left atrial pressure.

In humans, angina, dyspnea, and exercise tolerance improve one third to two thirds of patients following the administration of large doses of β-adrenergic blocking agents. β-Blockers may also decrease the incidence of sudden death, although this has not been proven. The β-blocker of choice in humans is propranolol. High-dose propranolol therapy is often recommended in people where doses exceeding 300 mg are used unless there are contraindications to its use. This means that people commonly receive more than 4 mg/kg of propanolol per day, which would be comparable to more than 1.0 to 1.5 mg/kg every 8 hr in a cat. Maximum doses in humans appear to be in the 500- to 800-mg/day range, which would be comparable to around 3 mg/kg every 8 hr in the cat. The mechanisms by which propranolol improves symptoms in people are not well understood. Original studies suggested improvement in diastolic function, but it is now suggested that this improvement is purely due to a slowing of heart rate. β-Blockers may prevent exercise-induced increase in outflow tract obstruction, but usually do not alter the degree of resting obstruction in humans. The decrease in resting or effort-induced angina is probably related to decreased myocardial oxygen consumption.

No studies of propranolol use in feline HCM have been completed. Consequently, reports of improvement or lack of improvement are anecdotal. One study has examined the effects of esmolol, a short-acting β₁-blocking drug, in six cats with HCM and obstruction to left ventricular outflow (Bonagura, Stepien, and Lehmkuhl, 1991). In this study, the degree of outflow tract obstruction decreased and heart rate slowed. If these data can be translated to propranolol's effects in cats, one might predict that propranolol might decrease SAM in cats and in so doing decrease the amount of mitral regurgitation and degree of dynamic subaortic

stenosis. Propranolol dose in the cat is generally in the 0.5- to 1.0-mg/kg range, although higher doses might be beneficial, as noted earlier. Some clinicians use the longer acting β-blocker, atenolol, dosed at one fourth of a 50-mg tablet daily. With either drug, heart rate reduction should be expected.

The author commonly uses diltiazem first and then either switches to propranolol or titrates propranolol into the therapeutic regimen if the response is suboptimal or becomes suboptimal. Other veterinary cardiologists use β-blockers first and, if the response is minimal, switch to diltiazem. Since many cats undergoing treatment for HCM are currently or have been in congestive heart failure and are receiving furosemide, response to diltiazem or propranolol therapy may be difficult to evaluate unless one takes the time and effort to tailor diuretic therapy and to reduce diuretic administration to the lowest possible level.

Treatment of asymptomatic cats is controversial. In humans, treatment of asymptomatic patients with a definite family history of HCM with either propranolol or a calcium channel blocker is sometimes recommended in the hope of slowing the progression of the disease. Similar advice might be prudent in cats. However, progression of the disease in adult humans occurs very slowly, if at all, so this recommendation may be suspect. The author owns a Maine coon cat with severe HCM that receives no therapy and that he has been following for 3 years as an adult. No progression of the hypertrophy has been noted in this cat. Consequently, this recommendation may also be suspect in cats. Diltiazem appears to produce regression of the hypertrophy in some cats. For this reason, it may be reasonable to administer diltiazem to an asymptomatic cat with moderate to severe hypertrophy for several months to see if hypertrophy regression will occur.

Treatment of the HCM case that is refractory to conventional drugs is also controversial. The angiotensin-converting enzyme (ACE) inhibitors may be beneficial or may be detrimental in this type of patient. Captopril and enalapril are efficacious drugs in congestive heart failure due to other diseases in the cat. Angiotensin-converting enzyme inhibitors are potentially contraindicated in cats with HCM. The rationale for this contraindication is that ACE inhibitors cause arteriolar dilation, and in so doing may increase the vigor of left ventricular contraction and increase the amount of SAM of the mitral valve, increasing the outflow tract gradient and potentially worsening the mitral regurgitation. Certainly this could potentially occur. However, the arteriolar dilating capabilities of the ACE inhibitors are relatively mild. Their primary benefit appears to come from their ability to decrease plasma aldosterone concentration, and in so doing decrease sodium and water retention. The author has documented increases in plasma aldosterone concentration in cats with HCM and has observed beneficial responses to ACE inhibitors in a limited number of cats with HCM. Consequently, the author does not believe that ACE inhibitor administration should be ruled out in cats with HCM that are refractory to other drugs based on theoretical concerns. Rather, they should be used judiciously in such cases.

Captopril (Capoten, Squibb) is dosed at ¼ to ½ of a 12.5-mg tablet every 8 hr. Enalapril (Vasotec, Merck) is dosed at 0.25 to 0.5 mg/kg once or twice daily. The dosing frequency of enalapril is controversial in the cat primarily because one study showed that plasma ACE activity was depressed to below 50% of control for up to 2 to 3 days after enalapril administration in normal cats. However, generally, one must suppress an enzyme system to below 10% of control activity to produce clinical effect, so instead of administering enalapril every 2 to 3 days, the author administers the drug every 12 to 24 hr.

Prevention of thromboembolic disease in cats with HCM is controversial. Aspirin (80 mg every 48 to 72 hr) is commonly prescribed to prevent the formation of intravascular thrombi in cats. Since there is little risk associated with administering this drug on this schedule to cats (other than gastric upset or erosions), the author recommends continuing this practice. One should realize, however, that aspirin administration in no way guarantees that thromboembolic disease will not occur. In a recent study of the use of tissue plasminogen activator to lyse thromboemboli in cats, most of the cats rethrombosed within months of successful thrombolysis, despite the administration of aspirin (Pion and Kittleson, 1989).

Because of the potential lack of benefit with aspirin, some veterinarians are now advocating the use of Warfarin sodium (Coumadin, DuPont) to prevent the formation of intracardiac thrombi. Warfarin is standard preventive therapy in people at risk for the formation of intracardiac thrombi. To date, however, the use of Warfarin to prevent the formation of intracardiac thrombi has not been adequately studied, so the benefit and the incidence of complications are unknown. The major risk with Warfarin is hemorrhage. The author has observed this complication in several cats on Warfarin therapy, despite appropriate monitoring of coagulation parameters. If Warfarin therapy is contemplated, the author recommends that the patient be carefully monitored using prothrombin times. (For details, see "Warfarin Therapy of the Cat at Risk of Thromboembolism," this volume, p 868).

In addition to standard antithrombotic agents, calcium channel blockers and nitrates also have antiplatelet effects. Potentially, diltiazem and nitroglycerin may do more than produce beneficial hemodynamic effects in cats with HCM.

## PROGNOSIS

Prognosis is determined by clinical presentation and echocardiographic severity of the disease. Adult cats that are asymptomatic and have mild to moderate disease and no left atrial enlargement have a good long-term prognosis. Asymptomatic cats with severe wall thickening and normal left atrial size have a guarded prognosis for developing heart failure at some point in time in the future. They should have a lower risk for developing thromboembolism but may be at risk for sudden death. Asymptomatic cats with severe wall thickening and left atrial enlargement are at risk for developing heart failure or, more likely, already have mild to moderate heart failure that has gone undetected. These cats also are at risk for developing thromboembolic disease and are at risk for sudden death. Cats that present in heart failure, in general, have a poor prognosis and in one study have had a median survival time of 3 months (Atkins et al., 1992). However, some cats (about 20% in this study) in this class stabilize and do well for prolonged periods of time for unknown reasons. Cats with HCM and aortic thromboembolism in this same study had a poor prognosis, with a median survival of 2 months.

## References and Suggested Reading

Atkins CE, Gallo AM, Kurzman ID, et al: Risk factors, clinical signs, and survival in cats with a clinical diagnosis of idiopathic hypertrophic cardiomyopathy: 74 cases (1985–1989). J Am Vet Med Assoc 201:613, 1992.
   *A retrospective study of 74 cats with hypertrophic cardiomyopathy examining clinical signs and prognosis.*
Bonagura JD, Stepien RL, and Lehmkuhl LB: Acute effects of esmolol on left ventricular outflow obstruction in cats with hypertrophic cardiomyopathy: A Doppler-echocardiographic study. Proc 19th Ann Vet Med Forum, 1991, p 879.
   *An abstract describing the effects of a β-adrenergic blocker on systolic anterior motion in cats with HCM.*
Bright JM, Golden AL, Gompf RE, et al: Evaluation of the calcium channel-blocking agents diltiazem and verapamil for treatment of feline hypertrophic cardiomyopathy. J Vet Intern Med 5:272, 1991.
   *The only study of calcium channel blocker use in cats with hypertrophic cardiomyopathy.*
Kittleson MD, Pion PD, and Mekhamer Y: Hypertrophic cardiomyopathy in a group of highly interrelated Maine coon cats. J Vet Intern Med 7:117, 1993.
   *An abstract describing the first family of cats identified with hypertrophic cardiomyopathy.*
Liu SK, Roberts WC, and Maron BJ: Comparison of morphologic findings in spontaneously occurring hypertrophic cardiomyopathy in humans, cats, and dogs. Am J Cardiol 72:944, 1993.
   *A review of the pathology identified in cats with hypertrophic cardiomyopathy, and comparison to those of humans and dogs.*
Maron BJ, Bonow RO, Cannon RO III, et al: Hypertrophic cardiomyopathy. Interrelations of clinical manifestations, pathophysiology, and therapy. N Engl J Med 316:780, 1987.
   *A review of the pathophysiology of hypertrophic cardiomyopathy in humans.*Pion PD and Kittleson MD: Therapy for feline aortic thromboembolism. In Kirk RW (ed): Current Veterinary Therapy X. Philadelphia, WB Saunders Co, 1989, p 295.
   *A book chapter describing the treatment of acute aortic thromboembolism in cats.*
Scott SD, Wolff S, Watkins H, et al: Left ventricular morphology in familial hypertrophic cardiomyopathy associated with mutations of the beta-myosin heavy chain gene. J Am Coll Cardiol 22:498, 1993.
   *A paper describing the varied echocardiographic findings in individual family members that have a gene mutation known to be associated with human familial hypertrophic cardiomyopathy.*
Seidman CE and Seidman JG: Mutations in cardiac myosin heavy chain gene cause familial hypertrophic cardiomyopathy. Mol Biol Med 8:159, 1991.
   *A review of the first human families identified with hypertrophic cardiomyopathy and point mutations on the cardiac myosin heavy chain gene.*
Thierfelder L, Watkins H, MacRae C, et al: Alpha-tropomyosin and cardiac troponin T mutations cause familial hypertrophic cardiomyopathy: A disease of the sarcomere. Cell 77:701, 1994.
   *A description of the original studies that identified mutations of genes that encode for sarcomere proteins other than myosin as causes of familial hypertrophic cardiomyopathy in man.*
Watkins H, Rosenzweig A, Hwang DS, et al: Characteristics and prognostic implications of myosin missense mutations in familial hypertrophic cardiomyopathy. N Engl J Med 326:1108, 1992.
   *A paper describing the types of myosin mutations and their detection in people with hypertrophic cardiomyopathy.*

# RESTRICTIVE CARDIOMYOPATHY

JOHN D. BONAGURA
*Columbus, Ohio*

*and* PHILIP R. FOX
*New York, New York*

Myocardial diseases are the most frequent cause of congestive heart failure (CHF) and thromboembolism in cats. These cardiomyopathies are usually characterized by echocardiographic or necropsy features. The most common of these disorders is idiopathic hypertrophic cardiomyopathy (see "*CVT* Update: Feline Hypertrophic Cardiomyopathy," this volume, p 854). Myocarditis of undetermined cause has been recognized in cats that die of congestive heart failure, thromboembolism, or arrhythmias (see "Myocarditis in the Dog and Cat," this volume, p 842). Dilated cardiomyopathy represents another form of cardiomyopathy; however, the increased concentration of taurine now added to commercial cat foods has made this disorder uncommon. Of increasing clinical importance is restrictive cardiomyopathy (RCM), an idiopathic myocardial disorder that appears to share functional abnormalities of both hypertrophic and dilated forms of cardiomyopathy. These characteristics have led to another term, "intermediate cardiomyopathy," which is often used to describe this condition (Harpster, 1986). We prefer the term "restrictive CM," which better describes the presumptive functional derangement of impaired diastolic ventricular filling consequent to fibrosis of the left ventricle. The exact pathophysiologic and diagnostic criteria of this disorder are incompletely understood; however, the practitioner should be aware of typical features of this relatively common condition.

## PATHOLOGY

Restrictive cardiomyopathy in cats does not constitute a single morphologic disorder. The most common feature observed at necropsy is striking biatrial dilation and hypertrophy. The left ventricle often displays variable degrees of hypertrophy and dilatation; however, the left ventricular wall thickness can be normal in some cases. There may be regional thinning of the left ventricular free wall or left ventricular apex interspersed with focal or regional wall hypertrophy. Prominent papillary muscle hypertrophy or fibrosis is evident in some cats. Left ventricular endomyocardial fibrosis is typical and may be patchy, multifocal, or diffuse in distribution. Extensive endocardial fibrotic scarring may be observed, and when extreme, can affect the mitral valve apparatus, lead to midventricular constriction or stenosis, or obliterate the left ventricular apex. Myocardial infarction has been recognized, most often

at the left ventricular apex. Systemic thromboemboli are common and left atrial and ventricular mural thrombi may be observed.

Histologic lesions include endocardial thickening, endomyocardial fibrosis, myocardial interstitial fibrosis, myocyte hypertrophy, and focal myocytolysis and necrosis. Arteriosclerosis of intramural coronary arteries may be recognized. Severe, diffuse, endomyocardial fibrosis of the interventricular septum, left ventricular free wall, and atria is recognized in advanced cases (Liu, 1988).

The pathogenesis of these lesions is undetermined. Antecedent myocarditis seems a likely, though unproven, initiating cause. Restrictive cardiomyopathy in some cats could represent a "late" stage of hypertrophic cardiomyopathy complicated by myocardial failure or myocardial infarction. In human patients, an underlying eosinophilic myocarditis has been recognized, though this is a rare necropsy finding in cats. A number of similar human disorders have been reported, including eosinophilic endomyocarditis, endomyocardial fibrosis, and noneosinophilic restrictive myocardial disease (Wynne and Braunwald, 1992). Some human patients demonstrate restrictive physiology with autopsy findings of left ventricular hypertrophy and fibrosis. The relevancy of these findings to the feline disease is unknown, but many features are similar to those described in affected cats.

## PATHOPHYSIOLOGY

The pathophysiology of RCM in the cat is unresolved, but the following points merit consideration. Echocardiography generally demonstrates a low-normal to mildly reduced shortening fraction (ejection fraction). When decreased ejection fraction is present, it is probably caused by a loss of functional myocardium, and the systolic dysfunction may progress over time. Regional left ventricular wall dysfunction may be observed, characterized by diminished free wall systolic thickening and excursion. Doppler studies may demonstrate mitral insufficiency, but the regurgitation is usually mild. Because the abnormalities of ejection fraction and mitral valve function do not sufficiently explain the marked left atrial dilation characteristic of this disease, it is assumed that impaired left ventricular distensibility is the principal pathophysiologic disorder. Myocardial or endomyocardial fibrosis is the most likely explanation for this diastolic dysfunction. If present, myocardial ischemia, relaxation abnormalities, cardiac arrhythmias, or ventricular dilation could further impair ventricular diastolic function. Progressive increases of left atrial pressure develop to fill the stiff left ventricle and thereby predispose the cat to elevated pulmonary venous pressure and pulmonary edema. One can also speculate that the marked left atrial dilation and fibrosis increase the resistance to right ventricular ejection (Mehta et al., 1991). These factors probably lead to chronic pulmonary hypertension and cause the progressive enlargement of the right side of the heart and the elevated central venous pressure that are so often observed in advanced cases. Pulmonary edema, pleural effusion, and hepatic congestion are typical manifestations of CHF, and can be explained by the aforementioned disorders and the neurohumoral and renal compensations activated in response to limited cardiac output. Stasis of blood in a dilated left atrium undoubtedly predisposes affected cats to atrial thrombi and systemic thromboembolism.

## CLINICAL SIGNS

### Clinical Examination

Most cats with RCM are middle aged or older (Stalis and Van Winkle, 1992), though young cats have also been recognized with this condition. Clinical signs of RCM are similar to those of other heart diseases in cats. The most frequently observed *historical problems* are tachypnea and respiratory distress caused by CHF. Sudden paresis, most often affecting the rear limbs, is typical of thromboembolic occlusion of the terminal aorta. Clients may also report decreased activity or exercise capacity, malaise, weight loss, or inappetence. Congestive heart failure may be precipitated by stress, fever, moderate to severe anemia, thyrotoxicosis, anesthesia, or fluid therapy. Some affected cats appear normal to the client; however, cardiac auscultation or thoracic radiography may indicate heart disease.

Examination of the cat with RCM can reveal a variety of *physical manifestations*. The most consistent auscultatory finding is a gallop sound, indicative of ventricular diastolic dysfunction. A soft to moderately loud systolic murmur of mitral or tricuspid regurgitation may be detected near the left or right sternal borders. Premature ventricular or atrial beats may be heard, leading to an irregular rhythm and arterial pulse. The femoral pulse is otherwise normal or slightly reduced in amplitude. Inspection of the jugular veins is quite helpful in cats with palpable hepatomegaly or pleural effusion, as elevated jugular venous pressure or prominent jugular pulsations are suggestive of concurrent right ventricular failure. Pulmonary edema or pleural effusion are most often manifested as tachypnea, though orthopnea, respiratory distress, and cyanosis may develop in severe cases of CHF. Thoracic auscultation is variable, but careful auscultation may reveal loud bronchial sounds, fine crackles, or a fluid line.

Aortic obstruction is characterized by vascular, musculoskeletal, and neurologic deficits that include paresis, pain, muscle contracture, and hyporeflexia in a limb that is cold, pale, and pulseless. The arterial blood pressure, determined by indirect measurement (Parks Medical Instruments, Aloha, OR), is usually normal. The clinician should consider fever, thyroid tumors, renal disease, systemic hypertension, and anemia during the course of the examination, as these disorders often precipitate or complicate CHF in cats with RCM.

### Radiography

The thoracic radiograph is characterized by left atrial dilation and cardiac elongation that is typical of left ventricular enlargement. The dorsoventral and ventrodorsal views are typified by a bulge at the 1- to 3-o'clock position, caused by an enlarged left auricle. The cardiac apex can be pointed or rounded. Some cats manifest astounding left atrial enlargement which, on the lateral projection, can be seen to separate the mainstream bronchi and create a convex dorsocaudal border. Generalized cardiomegaly is observed in some cases, while other cats demonstrate a "valentine-shaped" heart reminiscent of hypertrophic cardiomyopathy. Pulmonary hypertension may be evident radiographically as dilation of both lobar arteries and veins. Interstitial and alveolar infiltrates indicative of pulmonary edema or bilateral pleural effusions herald the development of CHF. Diuretic therapy usually decreases or clears these labile radiographic patterns. Left ventricular angiography is not often performed, but can delineate a number of anatomic lesions; marked left atrial dilation, mild left ventricular dilation, and irregular filling defects of the left ventricular lumen seem most characteristic of this disease. In some cases, the left ventricular cavity is distorted by fibrotic papillary muscles, endocardial plaques, or prominent moderator bands; midventricular cavity obliteration may be evident.

### Electrocardiography

The electrocardiogram (ECG) is frequently abnormal in cats with RCM. Ventricular enlargement and myocardial disease can be manifested as any of the following abnormalities: widened QRS complexes (>0.04 sec); increased amplitude R waves (>0.7 mV) in leads II, aVF, or III; intraventricular conduction disturbances including splintered R waves, right-axis deviation, or left bundle-branch block; and ventricular extrasystoles. Atrial enlargement is characterized by widened (>0.035 sec) or tall (>0.2 mV) P waves, atrial ectopic rhythms, or atrial fibrillation.

### Echocardiography

Echocardiography is especially important when there is CHF or when auscultatory signs of heart disease are supported by radiographic or ECG abnormalities. The most characteristic feature of RCM is marked left atrial or biatrial dilation. The left ventricle, in typical cases of RCM, is neither as hypertrophied nor as dynamic as that observed in most cases of hypertrophic cardiomyopathy. In contrast to cats with dilated cardiomyopathy, ventricular shortening fraction is either normal or just mildly reduced (generally >25%) and the mitral opening (E point) to septal distance is minimally increased. However, marked regional wall dysfunction may be noted, most often affecting segments of the left ventricular free wall. Two-dimensional echo examination often reveals a ventricle that is mildly dilated (>18 mm end-diastolic dimension) just below the mitral valve; yet, apically, the left ventricle may appear hypertrophied and the papillary muscles thick or rigid. Discrete thinned areas of ventricular atrophy, infarction, or scar may be imaged. Focal or diffuse, subendocardial, hyperechoic wall segments probably denote fibrosis or endomyocardial plaques. In extreme cases of endocardial fibrosis, imaging of the mid to apical left ventricular lumen may demonstrate thickened, hyperechoic, fibrous tissue bridging the septum, papillary muscles or free wall; obliterating the apical left ventricular cavity; or conferring an appearance of diminished systolic motion or restricted filling. Prominent left ventricular moderator bands (false tendons) also may span portions of the lumen. Left atrial or ventricular mural thrombi are observed infrequently. The right ventricle is often dilated in symptomatic cats, but is otherwise devoid of structural lesions. Doppler studies can indicate atrioventricular valve regurgitation, but it is rarely severe. Owing to the rapid feline heart rate, Doppler assessment of diastolic function is very difficult. When congestive heart failure has developed, pleural and pericardial effusions will usually be present. The pericardial effusion can be substantial, but decreases markedly following successful treatment of heart failure.

## Clinical Laboratory Studies

Clinical laboratory studies of cats with RCM are not specific. The complete blood count (CBC) is usually normal. Urinalysis is unremarkable unless diuretic therapy impairs tubular-interstitial concentrating ability or there is preexistent renal disease. Serum biochemistries may indicate azotemia that is usually mild; potential causes include heart failure, diuretic therapy, angiotensin-converting enzyme (ACE) inhibition, or prior renal disease. Severe azotemia may be observed in conjunction with suprarenal aortic thrombosis. Thyroxine concentration is normal unless there is concurrent hyperthyroidism. Serum potassium is usually normal but may decrease following diuretic therapy or anorexia. Aortic thrombosis causes dramatic increases in serum creatine kinase (CK), aspartate aminotransferase (AST or GOT), and alanine aminotransferase (ALT or GPT) as well as hematologic signs of disseminated intravascular coagulopathy. A plasma or whole-blood taurine should be measured, since decreased concentrations have been noted in some cats and could contribute to reduced myocardial contractility. When plasma taurine concentration is low, the dietary history should be reexplored.

Analysis of pleural effusates indicates either a transudate, modified transudate, or chyle. The predominant cells present are macrophages, mesothelial cells, and small lymphocytes unless there is chylothorax, in which case, well-preserved neutrophils may be more numerous. Chylothorax, which is most likely due to right-sided heart failure and impaired lymphatic drainage into the systemic venous system, is characterized by a high triglyceride/cholesterol ratio when compared to the serum.

## Differential Diagnosis

The differential diagnosis of RCM includes other cardiac diseases as well as primary thoracic and pulmonary disorders. Most noncardiac respiratory diseases can be identified by obtaining a good history, performing a thorough physical examination, and scrutinizing good-quality thoracic radiographs. Heartworm disease should be considered when relevant to the practice area. Pulmonary infiltrates that do not respond to diuretic therapy are unlikely to be related to congestive heart failure. Advanced thyrotoxicosis can lead to congestive heart failure and should be excluded in older cats with clinical signs of heart disease. Less frequent causes of heart failure such as congenital heart disease, bacterial endocarditis, pericardial effusion with tamponade, constrictive pericarditis, infiltrative cardiac neoplasia, and growth hormone excess (acromegaly) also should be considered. Distinguishing RCM from hypertrophic and dilated forms of cardiomyopathy is virtually impossible without an echocardiogram or angiogram. The echocardiogram is the preferred study and should be done, or obtained by referral, following initial treatment of CHF. When the diagnosis remains in doubt, it is useful to obtain a second opinion from a cardiologist or an internist with substantial experience in cardiopulmonary diseases.

## THERAPY

### Emergency Treatment

Emergency or urgent treatment of RCM is needed in cases of thromboembolism (see below) or CHF. Respiratory distress in this condition is attributed to pulmonary edema, pleural effusion, or both, and initial treatment should be directed accordingly. Clinical judgment must be exercised, as radiography initially may be inadvisable in the dyspneic cat; 1 or 2 hr of cage rest with supplemental oxygen and administration of furosemide (2 to 3 mg/kg IM or IV) may be helpful.

When *pleural effusion* is present and sufficient to cause atelectasis, thoracocentesis should be performed while the cat rests in sternal recumbency. A 23-gauge butterfly catheter is recommended. A fractious or very anxious cat will require sedation and can usually tolerate 0.1 mg/kg acetylpromazine SC, followed 30 min later by 2 to 5 mg ketamine HCl IV. Bilateral thoracocentesis may be necessary in some cases. A sample of the effusate should be retained for chemical and cytologic analysis. Thoracic radiographs obtained after thoracocentesis may be less stressful and more illustrative of any underlying heart or primary thoracic disease.

*Pulmonary edema* can be severe in some cats with RCM. Initial therapy includes supplemental oxygen, furosemide (2 to 4 mg/kg IM or IV every 8 hr), and 2% transdermal nitroglycerine paste ($\frac{1}{8}$ to $\frac{1}{4}$ inch, topically every 12 hr). Once diuresis has been observed, the diuretic dose is decreased (1 to 2 mg/kg SC every 8 to 12 hr).

Should *systemic thromboembolism* occur, the clinician faces the dilemma of a very complicated problem with no proven or best therapy. Since a substantial number of cats may clinically improve following a variety of therapies (or no therapy), sufficient time should be allotted for establishment of collateral circulation: this often requires 2 to 5 days. With little exception, an analgesic should be given for this painful condition. Torbutrol (0.15 to 0.2 mg/kg IM, in the cranial lumbar muscles or SC every 8 hr) has been effective, especially when combined with low doses of acetylpromazine (0.05 to 0.1 mg/kg SC). Pain is usually most pronounced within the first 24 to 36 hr of embolization. The clinician must balance the humane considerations of analgesia with the complication of excessive sedation that may impair monitoring of clinical status.

Supportive therapy for cats with systemic thromboembolism may be administered. This may include empiric symptomatic therapy or attempted thrombolysis. Empiric treatment includes α-adrenoceptor blockers like acetylpromazine (initial dose 0.1 mg/kg SC; up to 0.3 mg/kg every 8 hr) and sodium heparin (200 IU/kg IV followed by 150 to 200 IU/kg SC every 8 hr). These unproven treatments are designed to promote collateral vasodilation and prevent growth of the thrombus. Treatment can be given for 2 to 4 days. Complications include hypotension, hypothermia, bradycardia, and hemorrhage.

More aggressive, thrombolytic therapy might be considered when the thrombosis is suspected to be of recent origin (<8 hr) and intensive monitoring is available. Streptokinase (200,000-IU vials) can be administered as an intravenous infusion dosed at 90,000 IU for the first hour and 45,000 IU/hr thereafter, for a total of 6 to 8 hr (Killingsworth et al., 1986). This therapy should not be undertaken if the cat is heparinized, as excessive hemorrhage may occur. Moreover, thrombolytic therapy should not be attempted if anuria is evident or if serum potassium and an ECG cannot be evaluated regularly. Thrombolysis and sudden reperfusion of injured skeletal muscles can lead to severe hyperkalemia that can result in cardiac arrest. The ECG should be continuously monitored for signs of hyperkalemia during any thrombolytic therapy. Sodium bicarbonate (1 to 2 mEq/kg IV), 5% dextrose

solution, furosemide (2 mg/kg IV), and 10% calcium chloride solution (0.1 ml/kg IV over 10 min) may be used to treat severe hyperkalemia. Complications related to general thrombolysis may also be encountered and are difficult to control.

*Supportive treatment* of the seriously ill cat with RCM includes an environment that prevents hypothermia, good nursing care, and treatment of dehydration. Following initial diuresis, the cat should be given fresh water, *ad libitum*. Should water be refused or continual weight loss occur, maintenance IV or SC fluids should be given (40 to 50 ml/kg/day of 0.45% NaCl–2.5% dextrose solution; add 8 to 12 mEq KCl per 500 ml fluid). In cats with aortic thrombosis, both serum potassium and renal function should be monitored at least daily, and more often if thrombolytic therapy is given. Liquid nutritional support (e.g., Jevity, Ross Labs) given by an indwelling nasogastric tube may be considered if anorexia persists; however, one should maintain good control of CHF prior to initiating such therapy. Most cats begin to eat following effective resolution of CHF.

## Home Care

Chronic therapy of the cat with RCM is administered by the client. Asymptomatic cats with RCM are recognized infrequently, but "prophylactic" therapy with enalapril (Enacard or Vasotec, Merck, 2.5- and 5-mg tablets, 0.25 mg/kg PO, q.o.d.) may be advisable in these cases. A sodium-restricted diet such as Feline H/D (Hill's Pet Products) or Pro-vision-h (Ralston-Purina) should be dispensed if it is accepted by the patient. Aspirin (one baby aspirin every 3 days) or warfarin (see this volume, p 868) may be prescribed to inhibit thrombogenesis. The authors have attained the best results in treating CHF using a combination of furosemide, digoxin, and enalapril.

When RCM has led to CHF, *furosemide* (Lasix, Hoechst-Roussel) is prescribed. The daily dosage depends on the severity of fluid accumulation and must be individualized. Initial doses between 1 and 2 mg/kg every 12 hr are reasonable; however, doses as high as 4 mg/kg every 8 hr have been tolerated. Efficacy of diuretic therapy is monitored using respiratory rate, level of activity, and the chest radiograph. The easiest method of preventing overzealous diuresis is periodic measurement of serum blood urea nitrogen (BUN), creatinine, and electrolytes. Mild azotemia may be the necessary price of effective diuretic therapy.

*Digitalization* in cats requires caution. We most often prescribe digoxin tablets (Lanoxin, Burroughs-Wellcome; 0.125 mg) at a dose of $\frac{1}{4}$ tablet every 48 hr. A serum digoxin concentration is measured 10 to 14 days later with the blood samples drawn 10 to 12 hr after treatment. A serum concentration between 1 and 2 ng/ml is the therapeutic goal. Azotemia and hypokalemia predispose to digitalis intoxication.

Enhanced neurohumoral activity, including activation of the renin-angiotensin-aldosterone system, is known to be injurious in CHF. Inhibition of angiotensin-converting enzyme with a drug like *enalapril* has been used frequently in cats with RCM. The initial dosage is low (0.25 mg/kg PO, every 48 hr), but it can be administered daily after 1 or 2 weeks. Dosages as high as 0.5 mg/kg every 12 hr have been administered to cats with refractory CHF, but the usual maintenance dosage is lower (between 0.25 and 0.5 mg/kg/day). Enalapril therapy is monitored by measuring arterial blood pressure indirectly and with periodic monitoring of renal function and serum sodium and potassium. Angiotensin inhibition, when combined with diuretic or aspirin therapy or a sodium-restricted diet, can cause acute renal failure that is reversible with fluid therapy or discontinuation of drug therapy. If systolic blood pressure (the easiest to measure indirectly) is below 100 mm Hg, or if BUN increases significantly above pretreatment levels, the dose of enalapril, furosemide, or both should be reduced by 33 to 50% (see "Doppler Assessment of Blood Flow and Pressure in Surgical and Critical Care Patients," this volume, p 113, for details of pressure monitoring).

## Refractory Cases

Feline RCM is a very serious disease, and while the clinician may experience therapeutic initial success, complications or progressive CHF do occur. The first point to consider is the current therapy: Is it appropriate and dosed sufficiently or to excess? Can the client administer the treatments? Is it possible to improve the patient by altering the dosages or better educating the client? If CHF has progressed, it should be evident as a pleural effusion that is demonstrable by radiography, and this provides one objective measure of treatment efficacy. If anorexia has developed, even though CHF appears well controlled, consider digoxin toxicosis, renal failure, and gastric ulcers. The latter also may be related to uremia, stress, or poor splanchnic perfusion. Empiric therapy with famotidine (0.5 mg/kg/day PO) for 2 weeks may be considered. Of course, infections or moderate anemia (packed cell volume [PCV] <20%) must be dealt with promptly to prevent cardiac "decompensation."

Should progressive pleural effusion develop, despite digoxin, furosemide, and enalapril therapy, the clinician can consider performing thoracocentesis and then consider one or more of the following strategies: (1) increase the enalapril to a maximal dosage of 0.5 mg/kg every 12 hr; or (2) increase furosemide to 4 mg/kg every 8 hr; or (3) add nitroglycerine paste at a dose of ¼ inch topically every 12 hr; or (4) add a second diuretic, hydrochlorothiazide plus spironolactone (25/25-mg tablet; 2 to 3 mg/kg of the combination daily); or (5) prescribe diltiazem (7.5 mg every 8 to 12 hr; see below). The cat should be reassessed in 7 to 10 days by clinical examination and by radiography. A serum BUN and potassium also should be measured. Should each of these treatments fail, euthanasia should be considered.

The value of other treatments in RCM is unresolved. The calcium channel antagonist, diltiazem (Cardizem, Marion; 30-mg tablets), is often prescribed to improve diastolic function and coronary perfusion in feline hypertrophic cardiomyopathy. Whether such treatment is useful in the RCM heart with extensive fibrosis in uncertain. The negative inotropic effects are a source of worry, but the treatment merits consideration in refractory cases. β-Adrenergic blockers, including propranolol (10-mg tablets), are also used for treatment of hypertrophic cardiomyopathy. Again, the negative inotropic action of this class of drugs constitutes a relative contraindication. Diltiazem or a β-blocker is indicated in cases of RCM complicated by atrial fibrillation, as either drug can slow the rapid ventricular rate response that develops with this arrhythmia. When used for this purpose, the dose of propranolol (initial doses 0.1 to 0.25 mg/kg to a maximum dose of 1 to 2 mg/kg, every 8 hr) or diltiazem (⅛ to ¼ of a 30-mg tablet every 8 to 12 hr) should be increased gradually, over several days, to achieve a ventricular rate of less than 200/min.

Treatment of very frequent and recurrent ventricular extrasystoles or ventricular tachycardia in cats with RCM is problematic. Propranolol (2.5 to 5.0 mg every 8 hr) or procainamide (¼ of a 250-mg capsule mixed in the food every 8 hr) have been used, but negative inotropic effects, client and patient compliance, and lack of documented efficacy suggest that such treatments be reserved for symptomatic (i.e., syncopal) patients or those with sustained ventricular arrhythmias. Occasional ventricular extrasystoles are relatively common in this condition and are not treated.

The long-term prognosis of RCM is guarded and quite variable. Some cats have been successfully managed for CHF for over 2 years and such cases have been rewarding to clients and clinicians alike. Unfortunately, relentless CHF, refractory pleural effusion, and systemic thromboembolism present formidable obstacles to long-term survival.

## References and Suggested Reading

Harpster NK: Feline myocardial diseases. *In* Kirk RW (ed): *Current Veterinary Therapy IX.* Philadelphia, WB Saunders Co, 1986, pp 380–398.
  *An overview of feline myocardial diseases.*
Killingsworth CR, Eyster GE, Adams T, et al: Streptokinase treatment of cats with experimentally induced aortic thrombosis. Am J Vet Res 47:1351, 1986.
  *A study of the effects of streptokinase infusion on surgically induced aortic thrombosis describing variable results among cats and reviewing the relevancy to the clinical condition.*
Liu S-K: Cardiovascular pathology. *In* Fox PR (ed): *Canine and Feline Cardiology.* New York, Churchill Livingstone, 1988, pp 650–655.
  *A summary of the gross and microscopic pathology of feline myocardial diseases.*
Mehta S, Charbonneau F, Fitchett DH, et al: The clinical consequences of a stiff left atrium. Am Heart J 122:1184, 1991.
  *A description and discussion of the clinical, hemodynamic, and pathophysiologic consequences of a dilated, stiff left atrium in human patients.*
Stalis I and Van Winkle T: Feline endomyocarditis (EMC) and restrictive cardiomyopathy (RCM): Are they the same disease? (abstr). Vet Pathol 29:5, 1992.
  *Abstract summary of necropsy cases of endomyocarditis in younger cats and restrictive cardiomyopathy in older cats.*
Wynne J and Braunwald E: The cardiomyopathies and myocarditides: Toxic, chemical, and physical damage to the heart. *In* Braunwald E (ed): *Heart Disease: A Textbook of Cardiovascular Medicine.* Philadelphia, WB Saunders Co, 1992, pp 1415–1424.
  *A review of the causes, pathology, and hemodynamic abnormalities of restrictive myocardial diseases in human patients.*

# WARFARIN THERAPY OF THE CAT AT
# RISK OF THROMBOEMBOLISM

NEIL K. HARPSTER

*Boston, Massachusetts*

*and* CATHERINE J. BATY

*Raleigh, North Carolina*

Systemic thromboembolism is a well-recognized and well-reported complication of primary myocardial diseases (cardiomyopathies) in the cat. While aspirin is commonly recommended for the prevention of this serious and often life-threatening complication, one of the authors (NKH) recognized in the late 1970s that most cats that recovered from a bout of systemic thromboembolism suffered a second episode within 2 to 6 months despite the use of aspirin. Similar findings have been reported elsewhere (Atkins et al., 1991). Warfarin has been used as an alternative to aspirin for thromboembolic prophylaxis in cats that have survived a thromboembolic episode at Angell Memorial Hospital since 1984. This article summarizes our experience with and current recommendations for warfarin use.

## OVERVIEW OF ANTITHROMBOGENIC AGENTS AND ANTICOAGULANTS IN HEART DISEASE

### Antithrombogenic Drugs

Drugs that alter platelet function are used therapeutically or prophylactically in the treatment of many cardiovascular conditions in humans, including myocardial infarction, stroke, atrial fibrillation, prosthetic valve or saphenous vein bypass graft surgery, and percutaneous transluminal angioplasty (Hardin and Loscalzo, 1992).

Most drugs that alter platelet function do so by inhibiting the platelet enzyme cyclooxygenase. These drugs include aspirin, as well as the nonsteroidal anti-inflammatory drugs indomethacin, sulfinpyrazone, and ibuprofen. Of these, only aspirin irreversibly inhibits cyclooxygenase. Other drugs that alter (inhibit) platelet function by less-well-defined mechanisms include ticlopidine (Haes and Kamm, 1984), nitroglycerin (Schror et al., 1984), and the calcium channel blockers (Pumphrey et al., 1983).

The ideal antithrombogenic drug would safely prevent systemic thromboembolism without causing serious side effects such as hemorrhage. This drug does not currently exist, and several problems complicate the evaluation of the safety and efficacy of available antithrombotic therapy:

1. Lack of firm guidelines indicating which patients need therapy.

2. Paucity of prospective, controlled clinical trials establishing the safety and efficacy of any currently available drug.

3. Poor correlation between *in vitro* platelet function inhibition and clinical antithrombogenic effect.

4. Failure of available drugs to completely inhibit platelet participation in thrombus formation.

### Oral Anticoagulants

The authors believe that oral anticoagulants, which are all derivatives of the basic compound warfarin, are currently the agents of choice for the long-term prevention of thromboembolic complications of heart disease.

## PHARMACOLOGY OF WARFARIN

Warfarin produces its anticoagulant effect by interfering with the cyclic interconversion of vitamin K and vitamin K epoxide, inhibiting the formation of vitamin K–dependent clotting factors (II, VII, IX, and X) and the anticoagulant proteins C and S. The differences in half-lives among these procoagulants and anticoagulants theoretically results in a transient hypercoagulable state that is well documented in humans when warfarin therapy is first initiated. Decreases in serum concentration of factors IX and X, the changes responsible for the antithrombotic effect, first occur 4 to 6 days after the onset of warfarin therapy in human patients. Because the anticoagulant protein C concentration falls rapidly following warfarin administration, patients may be hypercoagulable for the first 3 or 4 days of treatment. Heparin (which must be given parenterally) provides its antithrombotic action independently of these mechanisms. Ideally, heparin is initially administered concurrently with warfarin for the first 2 to 5 days of therapy, although no clinical study has tested the need for this overlap.

The authors could locate no published pharmacokinetic data on warfarin in cats. In humans, warfarin is rapidly absorbed from the gastrointestinal tract and achieves peak blood concentration within 90 min. The half-life of warfarin is approximately 35 hr; steady state is reached in about 1 week. Different drug preparations vary substantially in bioavailability, and the anticoagulant response may change following a change in drug preparation. Warfarin is metabolized primarily by the liver via the cytochrome P-450 system, and liver diseases and/or drugs that either inhibit or induce this enzyme system can potentially affect warfarin pharmacokinetics (see "Effects of Hepatic Disease on Drug Disposition," this volume, p 758). No data are available addressing the metabolism of warfarin in patients with chronic liver disease, although decreased synthesis of clotting factors predisposes to increased pharmacodynamic sensitivity. Drug interactions are so numerous that they are dealt with in a separate section below. Warfarin is highly protein bound, almost entirely to albumin. Interestingly, studies have shown that the increased free drug fraction in hypoalbuminemic human patients is essentially balanced by increased drug clearance, such that no substantial change in anticoagulant response was observed.

Warfarin resistance occurs occasionally in humans, and an autosomal dominant trait has been described where the pharmacokinetics of warfarin are normal, but affected individuals require 5- to 20-fold higher doses than average to achieve an anticoagulant effect. Another cause of warfarin resistance is excessive intake of vitamin K in the diet; to the authors' knowledge, warfarin resistance has not been documented in the cat. The anticoagulant effect of warfarin can be potentiated by fat malabsorption, or by hypermetabolic states caused by fever or hyperthyroidism.

## POTENTIAL DRUG INTERACTIONS

Numerous drugs affect the response to warfarin therapy in humans, and presumably in cats as well. Most drugs that influence the anticoagulant effect of warfarin do so by either reducing intestinal absorption of the drug or altering its metabolic clearance. Other drugs may cause problems by altering coagulation factors or platelet function. Table 1 lists those drugs known to affect the anticoagulant response of warfarin

in humans that might be used by veterinarians to medicate cats. Veterinarians should be cautious when adding or withdrawing concurrent therapy in cats on warfarin, even if the drug in question is not included in this table. Increased frequency of prothrombin time (PT) monitoring is prudent in these circumstances.

## PATHOPHYSIOLOGY OF THROMBOEMBOLISM IN THE CAT

Left atrial enlargement and stasis of blood flow in the left atrium appear to be important factors initiating thrombus formation in cats with predisposing cardiovascular disease. Resistance to left atrial emptying and high left atrial pressures, which occur in cats with hypertrophic and restrictive forms of cardiomyopathy, may also contribute to stasis of blood in the left atrium and especially puts cats with these forms of heart disease at increased risk. Platelet hyperaggregability to adenosine diphosphate has been identified in some cats with cardiomyopathy and may be an additional predisposing factor to thromboembolism (Helenski and Ross, 1987).

The left atrium is the most common site for thrombus formation; less commonly, the left ventricular chamber or even the right atrium may serve as the nidus. Thrombus formation may occur in the left atrium as a large "ball" thrombus occupying the left auricular appendage, but more commonly occurs as a much smaller thrombus that breaks free and is carried via the aorta to some distal artery in the body where it causes embolic occlusion. Embolization may occur to the brain, heart, kidney(s), mesenteric artery, brachial artery, or to the terminal aorta. In the terminal aorta, embolization causes the classic signs of hindleg paresis or paralysis depending upon the severity of circulatory compromise to both the femoral arteries and collateral circulating pathways (Schaub et al., 1976). Presumably, the release of vasoactive substances by platelets or other factors within the embolus constricts the collateral circulation to the hindlegs and damages the cir-

**Table 1.**  *Drugs that Potentially Alter the Pharmacokinetics and Clinical Effects of Warfarin*

| Potentiated Anticoagulant Effect | Inhibited Anticoagulant Effect | Impaired Platelet Function/Factor Activity |
| --- | --- | --- |
| Anabolic steroids | Barbiturates | Aspirin |
| Chloramphenicol | Corticosteroids | Nonsteroidal anti-inflammatory agents |
| Cimetidine | Griseofulvin | Penicillins at high doses |
| Erythromycin | Sucralfate | Cephalosporins, second and third generation |
| Fluconazole | | Heparin |
| Ketoconazole | | Streptokinase |
| Metronidazole | | Vitamin K |
| Omeprazole | | |
| Tetracycline | | |
| Thyroxine | | |
| Trimethoprimsulfamethoxazole | | |

culation to the spinal cord, as paralysis is not observed after experimental aortic ligation.

## INDICATIONS FOR USE OF WARFARIN IN THE CAT

The high incidence of recurrent thromboembolic episodes in cats treated prophylactically with aspirin, combined with the frequently fatal nature of these recurrences, provided the impetus to investigate alternatives to aspirin prophylaxis. Initially, warfarin was offered only to cats recovering from a thromboembolic episode that had normal clotting parameters (i.e., platelet count >200,000, normal PT, and fibrin split products <10), and only to cats that would be kept indoors following discharge from the hospital. Increased experience and routine noninvasive (echocardiographic) measurement of left atrial size have led us to our current recommendation of warfarin prophylaxis for all cats with M-mode–derived left atrial/aortic ratio (LA/Ao) of 2.0 or greater even in the absence of a prior thromboembolic event.[*] Another criterion used by some clinicians is the presence of swirling, highly ech-

(*Editor's note: There are no published investigations documenting that this criterion is an independent risk factor for arterial thromboembolism)

ogenic, spontaneous contrast in the left atrium. This striking finding is thought to be a predictor of increased thrombogenesis in this setting.

Warfarin poses substantial risks that are not encountered with aspirin, as well as the expense of monitoring the drug's effect. For this reason, cats receiving warfarin at Angell Memorial are periodically restudied by echocardiography (i.e., every 4 to 6 months) to evaluate changes in their presumptive risk factors, as well as to monitor the status of the underlying cardiac disorder. In cats that have suffered a thromboembolic episode in the past, aspirin is substituted for warfarin if left atrial size becomes normal (LA/Ao ratio is $\leq 1.25$); cats started on warfarin solely because of an LA/Ao ratio of 2.0 or greater are switched from warfarin to aspirin if the LA/Ao ratio decreases to 1.5.

## RESULTS OF WARFARIN IN A CLINIC POPULATION

The vital statistics of a group of 25 cats in which warfarin was administered for the prevention of systemic thromboembolism is presented in Table 2. The sole selection criterion for this population was the administration of prophylactic warfarin therapy; these are 25 consecutive cases. Twenty-three of these cats were started on warfarin following recovery from a throm-

**Table 2.** *Vital Statistics in a Group of Cats With Systemic Thromboembolism Treated With Warfarin Following their Recovery*

| Case Number | Age | Breed | Sex | Body Weight (lb) | CHF Present | ECHO Dx | Initial LA/Ao | Survival (months) | Complications |
|---|---|---|---|---|---|---|---|---|---|
| 1 | 15 | DSH | CM | 8.5 | No | RCM | 2.00 | 8.0 | Recurrent TBE |
| 2 | 12 | DSH | CM | 18.4 | Yes | HCM | 1.77 | >9.0 | Recurrent TBE |
| 3 | 7 | DLH | CM | 12.5 | Yes | HCM | 1.60 | 6.0 | Acute CHF ? TBE |
| 4 | 13 | DSH | CM | 10.3 | Yes | RCM | 2.50 | 5.0 | Recurrent TBE |
| 5 | 17 | DSH | SF | 5.3 | No | TAG | 1.73 | 0.0 | Acute death unknown cause |
| 6 | 6 | DSH | CM | 10.0 | No | HCM | 1.62 | 18.0 | Recurrent TBE |
| 7 | 10 | DSH | SF | 8.5 | No | DCM | 1.26 | >77.0 | None |
| 8 | 4 | DSH | CM | 10.0 | No | RCM | 1.93 | >78.0 | Gingival bleeding |
| 9 | 9 | DSH | CM | 8.5 | Yes | RCM | 2.14 | 23.0 | Recurrent TBE |
| 10 | 2 | DSH | CM | 11.5 | Yes | HCM | 1.31 | 4.0 | Recurrent TBE |
| 11 | 11 | DSH | CM | 9.5 | No | TAG | 2.69 | 0.0 | Acute death no PM |
| 12 | 14 | DSH | SF | 7.5 | Yes | RCM | 2.08 | 0.0 | Acute death no PM ? DIC |
| 13 | 5 | DSH | CM | 16.0 | Yes | HCM | 2.24 | 12.5 | Sudden death LA thrombus |
| 14 | 10 | Siamese | CM | 14.0 | No | RCM | 1.56 | 18.0 | Died—severe anemia |
| 15 | 10 | DSH | CM | 12.0 | No | HCM | 1.77 | 20.0 | CHF—Died |
| 16 | 4 | DSH | SF | 14.5 | Yes | HCM | 2.14 | >14.0 | Lost to follow-up |
| 17 | 7 | DLH | CM | 12.0 | Yes | HCM | 2.29 | 6.0 | Recurrent TBE |
| 18 | 15 | DSH | CM | 8.0 | No | TAG | 1.62 | 21.0 | Recurrent TBE Bleeding |
| 19 | 19 | DSH | SF | 6.4 | Yes | RCM | 1.68 | 0.0 | Renal infarct Marked increase in waste levels |
| 20 | 1.5 | DSH | SF | 10.0 | Yes | HCM | 2.00 | >36.0 | None |
| 21 | 2 | DSH | CM | 10.5 | No | HCM | 1.44 | 7.0 | GI Signs Euthanasia |
| 22 | 9 | DSH | CM | 13.5 | Yes | RCM | 2.49 | 8.0 | Warfarin O.D. |
| 23 | 3 | DLH | CM | 11.5 | Yes | HCM | 2.43 | 6.0 | Recurrent TBE |
| 24 | 7 | DSH | CM | 8.0 | Yes | RCM | 2.29 | 4.0 | Lost to follow-up |
| 25 | 10 | DSH | CM | 11.0 | Yes | RCM | 2.03 | >5.0 | None |

Abbreviations: CHF = congestive heart failure, CM = castrated male, DCM = dilatative cardiomyopathy, DIC = disseminated intravascular coagulation, DLH = domestic longhair, DSH = domestic shorthair, ECHO Dx = echocardiographic diagnosis, GI = gastroenteric, HCM = hypertrophic cardiomyopathy, RCM = restrictive cardiomyopathy, LA = left atrial, LA/Ao = left atrial/aortic ratio, O.D. = overdose, PM = postmortem, SF = spayed female, TAG = thyroid adenomatous goiter (i.e., hyperthyroid), TBE = thromboembolic episode.

boembolic episode (TBE), with the remaining cats treated because of an LA/Ao ratio greater than 2.0.

The majority of cats presented in the table had either hypertrophic (HCM, 11 cats) or restrictive (RCM, 10 cats) cardiomyopathy. Three cats diagnosed with primary hyperthyroidism were also included. Approximately four times more male than female cats were treated. The average age of the HCM cats was 5.41, as compared to 11.0 years in cats with RCM, and 14.3 years in those with primary hyperthyroidism. The LA/Ao ratio was evaluated echocardiographically in 23 cats with thromboembolism. The left atrium was considered mildly enlarged with a LA/Ao ratio of 1.26 to 1.49, moderately enlarged with a ratio of 1.50 to 1.99, and markedly enlarged with a ratio of 2.00 or greater. Of these cats, three (13.0%) had mild left atrial enlargement, nine (39.1%) had moderate left atrial enlargement, and 11 (47.8%) had marked left atrial enlargement. Fifteen (60%) of the cats were in congestive heart failure (CHF) at the time of presentation.

No conclusions regarding the safety or efficacy of warfarin therapy can be made from this diverse group of cats of widely varying ages, differing cardiac conditions requiring different therapies, and varying levels of renal function. Except for cat number 13 (markedly prolonged PT and partial thromboplastin time [PTT] when discharged at owner's insistence) and cat number 20 (bilateral renal infarcts and impaired renal function at discharge), the rest of the cats were considered stable at discharge with normal limb pulses despite gait abnormalities. Six of the 25 cats are alive at this writing, with a survival range of 5 to 78 months (average = 35.2 months). Of the total group, the survival ranged from a few days to 78 months (average = 15.7 months), and 14 cats (56.0%) survived over 6 months.

The most common complication encountered during the management of this group of cats was recurrent thromboembolism. This was documented in 10 of 23 cats (43.5%), and two cats had at least two recurrent embolic episodes during warfarin therapy. Other complications included bleeding episodes, both minor (oral, urinary tract) and major (associated with weakness, lethargy, anemia) in five cats (20.0%), symptomatic congestive heart failure in three cats (12.0%), and sudden death of undetermined cause in three cats (12.0%). Two cats were lost to follow-up after 4 and 14 months (8.0%), and one cat died of renal failure. One cat was euthanized at 7 months when acute gastroenteric signs developed following the discontinuation of warfarin and substitution of aspirin, as the left atrial size had decreased to normal. In three cats (12.0%), no complications were reported.

It should be noted that four cats were treated with both aspirin (1.25 grains two or three times weekly) and warfarin (case numbers 5, 10, 13, and 17). Reasons for combined therapy included recurrent thromboembolism in one cat, a documented left atrial thrombus in one cat, one cat with marked left atrial enlargement, and one cat on low-dose warfarin therapy. These cats were considered at high risk for recurrent thromboembolism, and all suffered either recurrent thrombo-

embolism or sudden death within 6 months of institution of combined therapy. Bleeding complications were not felt to play a role in any of these cats' complications or deaths.

## MONITORING THE FELINE PATIENT ON WARFARIN

The large interindividual variability in dose response to warfarin coupled with the risk of hemorrhage mandate relatively careful patient monitoring. As much as 20-fold variability in dose response has been reported in humans, and significant variability has been observed by the authors and others familiar with warfarin therapy in cats. Initially, because of the perceived need to overlap heparin and warfarin therapies, hospitalization is recommended. Prior to therapy, a coagulation profile, including platelet count, is obtained to provide a baseline to gauge subsequent therapy and to rule out a preexisting coagulopathy. If the patient is already heparinized, the activated partial thromboplastin time (APTT) may be somewhat prolonged, but other values should be unchanged. If the cat is being treated with aspirin, it is recommended that it be discontinued because of the increased risk of hemorrhage.

Warfarin therapy can be commenced with a total maintenance dose of 0.5 mg (½ of a 1-mg tablet) every 24 hr PO; heparin is dosed at 100 IU/kg, three times daily SC. The time of drug administration and blood sampling should be standardized to optimize interpretation of monitoring results. Assuming warfarin absorption in cats is similar to that in humans, it is recommended that monitoring samples be obtained at least 2 hr after the drug is given. The one-stage prothrombin time test is the most common method used for monitoring oral anticoagulation therapy, and can be obtained using a commercial clinical laboratory or an inexpensive in-clinic monitoring device such as the Coumatrak. A daily blood sample to determine the patient's PT value prior to subsequent warfarin is strongly recommended. Heparin is discontinued after 3 to 4 days, and a small decrease in the patient's PT should be expected. Prothrombin time monitoring is conducted daily for a day or two more to ensure a desired response (see below) prior to discharge. Once at home, monitoring frequency is reduced to twice weekly for 2 weeks, then once a week for several weeks to 2 months, and ultimately, assuming satisfactory response, every 6 to 8 weeks. In the event of a change in brand of warfarin or any change in concurrent drug therapy, more frequent monitoring is temporarily indicated.

Previous recommendations have suggested that the dosage of warfarin be adjusted to result in a PT of 1.3 to 1.6 times normal. Because of the variability of commercial thromboplastin used in the PT assay, it is now recommended that PTs be standardized using the international normalization ratio (INR) (Hirsh et al., 1992). This ratio expresses the PT as though it was determined using the international reference preparation of standardized human brain thromboplastin. In this way, PTs (and thus warfarin dosages), can be directly compared from laboratory to laboratory, and from time to time within the same laboratory.

$$INR = (\text{patient PT} \div \text{control PT})^{ISI}$$

where ISI is the international sensitivity index of the thromboplastin used in the PT assay. The ISI reflects the responsiveness of a given thromboplastin to reduction of vitamin K–dependent coagulation factors as compared to that of the international reference preparation. Manufacturers of thromboplastin provide the ISI of each batch produced. There is significant potential for inappropriate anticoagulation if the INR is not used for monitoring, since thromboplastins used in the United States have ISIs ranging from 1.2 to 2.8. It is important to know that different batches of the same brand of thromboplastin may have different ISIs.

Extrapolating from human data, the recommended INR for prophylactic warfarin for prevention of feline thromboembolism is 2.0 to 3.0. Recent studies in humans have confirmed that low-intensity warfarin therapy with an INR of 2.0 to 3.0 is as effective in preventing thromboembolism and less likely to cause bleeding than high-intensity warfarin therapy (INR >3.0). Practically, veterinarians may have to accept INRs outside of this goal range because of the small size of our patients and limited dosage options (a 1-mg tablet is the smallest commercially available dose). For cats requiring unusually small doses or particularly accurate doses, help may be sought from pharmacists to reformulate a small dose or provide a liquid form of the drug.

### Antithrombogenic and Oral Anticoagulant Therapy

In difficult-to-control thromboembolic disease conditions, the combination of oral anticoagulant therapy with the antithrombogenic agents has been advocated. The combined use of warfarin and either dipyridamole (Sullivan, Harken, and Gorlin, 1971) or aspirin (Alexander et al., 1993) has been shown to markedly reduce the incidence of major systemic embolism following human heart valve replacement. However, the combined use of warfarin and aspirin also increased the incidence of bleeding.

## COMPLICATIONS OF WARFARIN THERAPY

The experience of the authors in the management of a group of cats with serious cardiac disease and anticoagulant therapy has made it crystal clear that warfarin is not an innocuous drug, and that it must be treated with a great deal of respect. There appears to be considerable variation in the dosage required to give the desired therapeutic response as well as how rapidly this

effect is achieved. Bleeding complications range from minor gumline or other oral lesions that ooze, to epistaxis, bleeding from a skin lesion, hematuria, or even bleeding into a body cavity with acute onset of weakness, collapse, or even sudden death. Severe crises can generally be avoided with the above monitoring protocol.

Most cats receiving a significant overdose of warfarin will have a PT of 40 to greater than 100 sec (INR >6). If the cat's condition is stable, stopping the warfarin and administering vitamin K, at 1 to 2 mg/kg/day PO or SC for 3 days, normally results in a return of the PT value to normal. If the PT value remains prolonged, then warfarin should be withheld and vitamin K continued for a longer period. In more critical situations when significant blood loss has occurred, fresh blood or plasma may be life saving along with the administration of vitamin K SC at 1 to 2 mg/kg/day. Therapy should be continued until the PT level returns to normal and the hematocrit stabilized. Warfarin can generally be reinstituted at a 50% reduction in the original dose; heparinization may once again be indicated for the first few days of therapy.

## CONCLUSIONS

Thromboembolic episodes rival congestive heart failure as a life-threatening consequence of acquired feline heart disease, contributing significantly to the morbidity and mortality of these diseases. While warfarin is clearly not the ideal solution to this serious clinical problem, our experience suggests that clinical outcomes with warfarin prophylaxis are probably substantially better than those previously observed with aspirin alone.

Accurate criteria for identifying a population at high enough risk for thromboembolism to justify the added expense and risk of warfarin prophylaxis remain to be accurately defined. While we await the results of well-controlled, prospective clinical trials addressing this issue, the authors hope that the guidelines presented here will help maximize the benefit while minimizing the risk of warfarin therapy.

### References and Suggested Reading

Alexander GC, Turpie MB, Gent M, et al: A comparison of aspirin with placebo in patients treated with warfarin after heart-valve replacement. N Engl J Med 329:524, 1993.

Atkins CE, Gallo AM, Kurman ID, and Cowen P: A retrospective study of risk factors, presenting signs, and survival in 74 cases of feline idiopathic hypertrophic cardiomyopathy. J Vet Intern Med 5:122, 1991.

Hardin RI and Loscalzo J: Hemostasis, thrombosis, fibrinolysis and cardiovascular disease. In Braunwald E (ed): Heart Disease: A Textbook of Cardiovascular Medicine, 4th edition. Philadelphia, WB Saunders Co, 1992, p 1767.

Haes WK and Kamm B: The North American Ticlopidine Aspirin Stroke Study: Structure, stratification, variables and patient characteristics. Ticlopidine: quo vadis? Agents Actions 15(suppl):273, 1984.

Helenski CA and Ross JN: Platelet aggregation in feline cardiomyopathy. JACVIM 1:24, 1987.

Hirsh J, Dalen JE, Deykin D, and Poller L: Oral anticoagulants. Mechanism of action, clinical effectiveness, and otimal therapeutic range. Chest 102(suppl):312S, 1992.

Pumphrey CW, Fuster V, Dewarjee MK, et al: Comparison of the anti thrombotic action of calcium antagonist drugs with dipyridamole in dogs. Am J Cardiol 51:591, 1983.

Schaub RG, Meyers KM, Sands RD, et al: Inhibition of feline collateral vessel development following experimental thrombotic occlusion. Circ Res 39: 736, 1976.

Schror K, Ahland B, Darius H, and Weiss P: Stimulation of vascular PGI$_2$ by organic nitrates and its significance for the antianginal effect. Scand J Lab Clin Invest 173(suppl):33, 1984.

Sullivan JM, Harken DE, and Gorlin R: Pharmacologic control of thromboembolic complications of cardiac-valve replacement. N Engl J Med 284: 1391, 1971.

# CARDIAC NEOPLASIA

WENDY A. WARE

*Ames, Iowa*

Tumors of the heart occur sporadically in small animals. A search of the Veterinary Medical Database at Purdue University from 1982 to 1993° revealed 1068 dogs with cardiac tumors from a total pool of 638,867 dogs seen. This represents an overall incidence of only 0.17% in dogs of all ages combined. The majority of animals with cardiac neoplasia are late middle-aged to geriatric. Nevertheless, occasional puppies or kittens and young adults are affected. When different age groups were evaluated, 30.3% of dogs with cardiac tumors were between the ages of 7 and 10 years and 52.6% were between 10 and 15 years of age. There was no difference between the overall number of males and females affected with cardiac tumors.

The most commonly reported cardiac tumors in dogs are located either in the right atrium/auricle or at the heart base. Some tumors are found in other intracavitary, intramural, or intrapericardial locations. The majority of tumors involving the right atrium and adjacent tissue in dogs are hemangiosarcomas (or hemangiomas), which is the most common type of cardiac tumor in dogs. Cardiac hemangiosarcomas are often associated with hemorrhagic pericardial effusion and cardiac tamponade. German shepherd dogs, and possibly golden retrievers, have an increased risk for cardiac hemangiosarcoma.

Masses at the heart base are usually neoplasms of the chemoreceptor aortic bodies (alternately named chemodectoma, aortic body tumors, or nonchromaffin paragangliomas), ectopic thyroid tissue, ectopic parathyroid tissue, or mixed cell type tumors. Heart-base tumors tend to be locally invasive around the root of the aorta and surrounding structures; metastasis to other organs has been reported but is uncommon. These tumors may be present for some time without causing clinical signs and may be an incidental finding at necropsy. Clinical signs associated with heart-base tumors are usually related to the development of pericardial effusion and cardiac tamponade. Brachycephalic breeds, such as the Boston terrier, bulldog, and boxer, have a greater tendency to develop chemodec-

tomas. Males are more commonly affected, especially in the bulldog and Boston terrier breeds.

Other types of primary tumors involving the heart are quite rare in dogs but have included myxoma, fibro(sarco)ma, rhabdomyo(sarco)ma, leiomyo(sarco)ma, chondro(sarco)ma, intracardiac ectopic thyroid tumors, pericardial mesothelioma, and others. Most cases involve right heart structures. Metastatic tumors, including lymphosarcoma, other sarcomas and various carcinomas may involve the heart as well. Mesothelioma is increasingly reported in searches of hospital data bases. Reasons for this may include (1) regional or environmental factors (e.g., asbestosis), (2) overreliance on aspiration cytology of pericardial effusates (reactive mesothelial cells may be misinterpreted), or (3) a true increase in the incidence of this neoplasm.

Cats are less likely to be affected with cardiac tumors than are dogs. A search of the Veterinary Medical Database, from 1982 to 1993, revealed 58 cats with cardiac tumors from a total of 210,388 cats seen; the overall incidence was less than 0.03% in cats of all ages combined. Fifty-three per cent of the affected cats were female, 47% were male. Age distribution was different for cats than for dogs: 27.6% of affected cats were 7 years of age or younger, 15.5% were between the ages of 7 and 10 years, 34.5% were between 10 and 15 years, and 17.2% were older than 15 years.

The most common histologic diagnosis found in cats was lymphosarcoma. Several types of tumors were represented. Cardiac lymphosarcoma accounted for 18 cases (31%) and various (mostly metastatic) carcinomas accounted for 11 cases (19%). Only five cases of hemangiosarcoma (8.6%) and two cases of aortic body tumor (3.4%) were reported; two cases (3.4%) were diagnosed with fibrosarcoma. Twenty cases in the Veterinary Medical Database (34.5%), however, were coded as "tumor heart" with no histologic diagnosis given.

## CLINICAL SIGNS

Tumors involving the heart cause varied clinical signs. In general, signs can be referable to (1) the phys-

°The author thanks Alan Warble for his assistance in this search.

ical presence of the mass causing obstruction of blood flow into or out of the heart, (2) external compression of the heart that impedes filling (if pericardial effusion and resulting cardiac tamponade are present), or (3) disruption of normal heart rhythm or contractility if myocardial infiltration occurs or ischemia develops.

Specific clinical signs that occur are dependent on the location of the tumor and resulting pathophysiology that develops in the individual animal. Signs of right-sided congestive heart failure are common with tumors that obstruct blood flow into or within the right atrium or ventricle or that cause pericardial effusion with cardiac tamponade. These signs include ascites, pleural effusion, jugular venous distention, abnormal jugular pulsations, and occasionally, subcutaneous edema. Syncope and weakness with exertion or excitement are also common signs in animals with cardiac tumors; these signs of low cardiac output can result from cardiac tamponade, blood flow obstruction, arrhythmias, or impaired myocardial function. Tachyarrhythmias of any type can occur with cardiac neoplasia. Likewise, conduction disturbances, including major bundle-branch block or atrioventricular (AV) nodal blocks can result from tumor infiltration into the conduction system. Marked lethargy or collapse can occur with bleeding from tumors (e.g., hemangiosarcoma) that may be concurrently present in extracardiac locations. Clinical signs may be absent if the tumor is small or located in an area such that cardiac function is not significantly impaired.

## DIAGNOSIS

### Physical Examination

Physical examination findings also depend on the location and hemodynamic disturbances caused by the mass. Signs of congestive or low output heart failure as described above are often present to some degree. Auscultation may reveal a murmur caused by blood flow obstruction (e.g., with an intracardiac mass lesion), a murmur of unrelated disease (e.g., degenerative mitral insufficiency in an older small breed dog), or no auscultable abnormalities at all. Muffled heart sounds accompany significant pericardial effusion.

### Thoracic Radiographs

Thoracic radiographs are an important part of the data base; yet, findings also can be quite variable. In animals with a large volume of pericardial effusion, the cardiac silhouette loses its normal contours and appears rounded ("globoid"); intrapericardial masses are obscured by the fluid. Smaller fluid accumulations allow identification of various cardiac contours, especially atrial shadows. Fluoroscopy of the cardiac shadow reveals diminished to absent motion if the heart is surrounded by fluid. Other radiographic findings, secondary to impaired cardiac filling, may include pleural effusion, pulmonary densities compatible with interstitial edema, widening of the caudal vena cava (or pulmonary veins), hepatomegaly, or ascites. Dorsal deviation of the trachea, widened cranial mediastinum, and increased perihilar opacity are seen with some heart-base tumors. Large heart-base tumors may create unusual bulges at the dorsal aspect of the heart shadow, with or without the presence of pericardial effusion. Intracardiac masses, especially those involving the right atrium, may cause enlargement or unusual contours of the affected chamber(s). Radiographic evidence of hemodynamic sequelae may be observed (e.g., obstruction of the tricuspid valve orifice by a right atrial tumor can lead to caudal vena caval distention, and signs of pleural effusion or ascites on radiographs). Some intracardiac tumors cause no noticeable radiographic abnormalities. Evidence for pulmonary metastasis may be seen with some primary or secondary (metastatic) cardiac neoplasms.

### Electrocardiography

The electrocardiogram (ECG) may be normal in patients with cardiac tumors or may show abnormalities reflective of the location and sequelae of the underlying disease. For example, the presence of pericardial effusion tends to diminish ECG complex size, often to an abnormal degree (e.g., QRS complexes <1.0 mV in dogs). This finding is inconsistent, however, and very hemorrhagic effusates may not diminish QRS amplitude. Large pericardial effusions may be associated with electrical alternans, where QRS complexes are alternately taller then shorter, as a result of the swinging motion of the heart within the pericardial sac. Elevation of the ST segment (epicardial injury current) is also seen infrequently in some cases with pericardial effusion. Sinus tachycardia is common with cardiac tamponade. Tumor invasion of atrial or ventricular myocardium may be accompanied, respectively, by atrial or ventricular arrhythmias such as premature complexes and paroxysmal tachycardias. Involvement of the AV conduction system can lead to varying degrees of AV block and symptomatic bradycardia or a major bundle-branch block pattern. Intracardiac tumors that obstruct right ventricular outflow can cause a right axis shift and right ventricular hypertrophy pattern on the ECG. Other chamber enlargement patterns may result depending on the location and hemodynamic sequelae of the mass.

### Echocardiography

Echocardiography is now a widely available, noninvasive tool for diagnosing cardiac neoplasia as well as the presence or absence of pericardial effusion. Intrapericardial or intracardiac mass lesions can be imaged and their location, size and sonographic "texture" assessed. Secondary changes in cardiac chamber size, shape, and ventricular function can also be detected.

Doppler echocardiography allows qualitative and quantitative assessment of blood flow abnormalities that may be present. Pericardial effusion appears as an echo-free space between the echogenic parietal pericardium and the epicardium, since fluid is typically sonolucent unless there is recent hemorrhage or a highly exudative intrapericardial process as might occur with secondary infection. In these cases, a "mixed" echogenic pattern is observed and echogenic blood clots may be detectable. Very large amounts of pericardial fluid allow the heart to either swing or move erratically within the pericardial sac. Cardiac tamponade is manifested by compression of the cardiac chambers; usually collapse of the right atrial and right ventricular walls is visualized during portions of the cardiac cycle. The presence of effusion dorsally aids in the identification of heart-base tumors that extend into the pericardial space. Intracardiac masses are likewise accentuated by the echolucent intracardiac blood pool that surrounds them.

Assessment of cardiac tumors includes: the location, size, attachment (pedunculated or broad-based) and extent (superficial or deeply invading adjacent myocardium). Imaging is valuable in determining whether surgical resection or biopsy may be possible. Differential diagnosis is aided by comparing echocardiographic findings to known predilection sites of various neoplasms. Hemangiosarcoma should always be suspected when a right atrial mass is identified in a dog, and these patients should undergo further ultrasonic evaluation of the spleen and liver. A thorough echocardiographic exam is important. Some cardiac tumors may not be easily visualized initially, depending on their size and location. The overall sensitivity and predictive value of this technique has not been published, though undoubtedly it is influenced by operator experience and resolution limits of the ultrasound machine and transducers used. All standard echocardiographic views (Thomas et al., 1993) should be obtained from both right and left parasternal positions; variations on these imaging planes may be needed to further evaluate individual animals. The identification of a suspected mass lesion in more than one echocardiographic plane helps the clinician to avoid overinterpretation of artifacts. Images obtained from the left cranial parasternal position and from subcostal placement can be especially helpful in evaluating the ascending aorta, right auricle, and surrounding structures.

## Other Techniques

Other techniques that have been used in the diagnosis of cardiac neoplasms include pneumopericardiography, in cases where pericardial effusion exists, and angiocardiography. The advent of echocardiography has reduced, if not replaced, the use of these tests. Pneumopericardiography uses carbon dioxide or air injected into the drained pericardial sac via a preplaced catheter. Radiographs are taken from different orientations; the left lateral and dorsoventral views are most helpful. These views allow the injected gas to contrast the areas around the right atrium and heart base, respectively, where pathologic changes are most common. While pneumopericardiography can aid in the identification of intrapericardial masses, it cannot define the extent or presence of intracardiac masses. Angiocardiography can also be useful in the diagnosis of cardiac tumors when echocardiography is not available. Increased endocardial to pericardial distance is seen with pericardial effusion. Displacement of normal structures, filling defects within a cardiac chamber, or a contrast-enhanced area of increased vascularity ("tumor blush") can be identified with neoplasms. Selective cardiac catheterization allows measurement of intravascular and intracardiac pressures to document hemodynamic disturbances caused by the tumor.

When cardiac tumors are associated with pericardial effusion, cytology of the pericardial fluid is recommended. Most pericardial effusates associated with cardiac neoplasia are very hemorrhagic; however, transudates may be recognized especially with heart-base masses that obstruct lymphatic drainage (e.g., thyroid carcinoma). However, a definitive diagnosis of neoplasia often is not reliable when based on cytology alone, as reactive mesothelial cells closely resemble neoplastic cells. Cardiac lymphosarcoma usually can be diagnosed based on cytologic examination of pericardial fluid. Hematologic and serum biochemical test results are generally nonspecific in cases of cardiac neoplasia. Cardiac enzymes may be elevated from ischemia or myocardial invasion; mild increases in serum alanine aminotransferase and azotemia can occur from congestive heart failure. Hemangiosarcoma is often associated with a regenerative anemia, increased number of nucleated red blood cells (RBCs) and shistocytes, leukocytosis, and thrombocytopenia. Pleural and peritoneal fluids, when present, are usually modified transudates caused by heart failure or vascular obstruction.

## THERAPY

If cardiac tamponade has occurred, pericardiocentesis is indicated as the initial therapeutic procedure. Thoracocentesis should be performed if there is pleural effusion. Therapy with drugs that reduce systemic arterial resistance (arteriolar vasodilators) or cardiac filling (venodilators, diuretics) are dangerous and cannot replace pericardiocentesis. These drugs can reduce ventricular filling and cause hypotension; therefore, they should either be avoided or used with caution after pericardiocentesis. Most congestive signs will resolve within 72 hr once the pericardial fluid is removed. Since cardiac tamponade primarily causes diastolic dysfunction, there is generally no indication for a positive inotropic agent such as digoxin. Hypotension can be treated with judicious fluid administration and a dopamine infusion (see "Use of Catecholamines in Critical Care Patients," this volume, p 188). Conservative therapy (pericardiocentesis as needed, possibly with a glucocorticoid to decrease inflammation) is used in some patients until episodes of cardiac tamponade become unmanageable.

Partial pericardiectomy (removal of the pericardium ventral to the phrenic nerve) can also provide temporary clinical improvement, and is indicated in patients with recurrent tamponade (see *CVT XI*, p 725). Allowing pericardial effusion to drain into the pleural space relieves the external compression on the heart and impediment to cardiac filling caused by increased intrapericardial fluid pressure and which leads to congestive and low cardiac output signs. The larger pleural surface area should facilitate reabsorption of this fluid; however, neoplastic cells (especially hemangiosarcoma and mesothelioma) present in the fluid might be expected to seed the pleural space.

Although most cardiac tumors cannot be completely excised in the live animal, some tumors are amenable to surgical resection, depending on their location and invasiveness. For example, tumors involving only the tip of the right auricular appendage or a pedunculated mass in a surgically accessible location are more likely to be resectable. Intracardiac masses within the right heart might be reached using venous inflow occlusion techniques and rapid cardiotomy; however, surgical access to left heart lesions and large or medially attached right heart masses generally require cardiopulmonary bypass.

Surgical biopsy of a nonresectable mass may be helpful if chemotherapy is contemplated. While many cardiac tumors appear to be fairly unresponsive to chemotherapy, some are treated with short-term success. The clinician should always consult an oncologist prior to embarking on a course of chemotherapy for cardiac neoplasia. Cases of cardiac hemangiosarcoma, treated with vincristine, doxyrubicin, cyclophosphamide combination chemotherapy (VAC protocol), have had increased survival time. Lymphosarcoma may also be treated according to standard protocols (see Section 6).

Other tumor types may or may not be responsive to available chemotherapy.

The prognosis for animals with cardiac tumors is generally guarded to poor. Many die or are euthanized shortly after diagnosis. However, some cases will survive for several months to more than 1 year with appropriate management. Occasionally, a case with a surgically resectable mass may live for years after initial diagnosis.

## References and Suggested Reading

Aronsohn M: Cardiac hemangiosarcoma in the dog: A review of 38 cases. J Am Anim Med Assoc 187:922, 1985.
*Clinical review article.*

Bright JM, Toal RL, and Blackford LM: Right ventricular outflow obstruction caused by primary cardiac neoplasia. J Vet Intern Med 4:12, 1990.
*Report of two unusual cardiac masses.*

Hammer AS, Couto CG, Filppi J, et al: Efficacy and toxicity of VAC chemotherapy (vincristine, doxorubicin, and cyclophosphamide) in dogs with hemangiosarcoma. J Vet Intern Med 5:160, 1991.
*Reference for chemotherapy of hemangiosarcoma.*

Krotje LJ, Ware WA, and Niyo Y: Intracardiac rhabdomyosarcoma in a dog. J Am Vet Med Assoc 197:368, 1990.
*Clinical report of an unusual cardiac tumor.*

Sisson D, Thomas WP, Ruehl WW, and Zinkl JG: Diagnostic value of pericardial fluid analysis in the dog. J Am Vet Med Assoc 184:51, 1984.
*Retrospective study concluding that cytology was not able to reliably distinguish between neoplastic and non-neoplastic pericardial effusions.*

Swartout MS, Ware WA, and Bonagura JD: Intracardiac tumors in two dogs. J Am Anim Hosp Assoc 23:533, 1987.
*Brief review and clinical report of two intracardiac cardiac tumors.*

Thomas WP: Pericardial disorders. In Ettinger SJ (ed): Textbook of Veterinary Internal Medicine, 3rd edition. Philadelphia, WB Saunders Co, 1989, p 1132.
*An overview of pericardial diseases, including neoplastic causes.*

Thomas WP, Gaber CE, Jacobs GJ, et al: Recommendations for standards in transthoracic two-dimensional echocardiography in the dog and cat. J Vet Intern Med 7:247, 1993.
*Reference for performing echocardiographic studies.*

Tilley LP, Bond B, Patnaik AK, et al: Cardiovascular tumors in the cat. J Am Anim Hosp Assoc. 17:1009, 1981.
*Overview of necropsy reports in cats.*

Ware WA, Merkley DF, and Riedesel DH: Intracardiac thyroid tumor in a dog: Diagnosis and surgical removal. J Am Anim Hosp Assoc 30:20, 1994.
*Report of the diagnosis and treatment of an unusual cardiac mass.*

# BUDD-CHIARI–LIKE SYNDROMES IN DOGS

AMY M. GROOTERS
*Columbia, Missouri*

*and* DANIEL D. SMEAK
*Columbus, Ohio*

Portal hypertension is most often caused by an increase in resistance to portal blood flow. Obstructive lesions that cause portal hypertension can be classified based on their location as prehepatic (portal vein), hepatic, or posthepatic (large hepatic veins, caudal vena cava, heart). Hepatic obstruction can be further classified as presinusoidal, sinusoidal, or postsinusoidal. This distinction is important because the protein content of the ascites produced by portal hypertension is dependent to a large degree on the location of the obstruction in relation to the hepatic sinusoid. Obstruction of portal blood flow that occurs before the sinusoid typically produces low-protein ascites. However, lesions that obstruct hepatic venous flow beyond the hepatic sinusoid (postsinusoidal obstruction) cause increased formation of hepatic lymph, which is high in protein. Leakage of this proteinaceous lymph from the surface of the liver results in high-protein ascites. Postsinusoidal causes of portal hypertension include obstructive lesions of the hepatic veins, caudal vena cava, and right heart.

In the nineteenth century, Chiari and, later, Budd described a specific hepatic lesion characterized by "endophlebitis obliterans" of the small hepatic veins, which was associated with hepatomegaly and progressive ascites in their human patients. Since that time, the use of the term "Budd-Chiari syndrome" in the medical literature has been expanded to include many different causes of hepatic venous outflow obstruction. Presently, Budd-Chiari syndrome is most commonly defined as obstruction of the hepatic veins or inferior vena cava between the liver and the right atrium. However, inconsistent application of this term in the medical literature had led to ambiguity in its definition. Some authors have included disorders of the right atrium, pericardium, and right ventricle as potential causes of this syndrome, whereas others have specifically excluded them.

Inconsistent and infrequent use of the term "Budd-Chiari syndrome" or "Budd-Chiari—like syndrome" has also contributed to its ambiguity in the veterinary literature. It has been defined as specifically including congestive heart failure, pericardial disease, and cirrhosis by one author (Miller et al., 1988), and as excluding these disorders by another (Otto et al., 1990). In our opinion, the clinical usefulness of this term lies in its ability to distinguish obstructive disease of the hepatic veins, caudal vena cava, and caudal right atrium from more common causes of postsinusoidal obstructive ascites in dogs, such as right-sided congestive heart failure and pericardial disease. In addition, because none of these disorders is identical to the lesions originally described by Budd and Chiari, it would seem more appropriate to use the term "Budd-Chiari–like" syndrome than "Budd-Chiari syndrome."

We propose that the term "Budd-Chiari–like syndrome" be used to describe the clinical manifestations of hepatic venous outflow obstruction caused by a *mechanical* obstruction between the hepatic sinusoids and the heart. *Functional* venous obstruction caused by right-sided congestive heart failure or restrictive pericardial disease probably should not be considered Budd-Chiari–like syndrome. Because the caudal right atrium functions basically as an extension of the caudal vena cava in terms of venous return, it seems logical to include obstructive lesions of the caudal right atrium within the definition of Budd-Chiari–like syndrome. This is supported by the fact that the clinical manifestations caused by obstructive lesions of the caudal right atrium are identical to those caused by obstruction of the caudal vena cava or hepatic veins, but differ from

the clinical anormalities associated with other cardiac causes of postsinusoidal ascites. Using this definition, Budd-Chiari–like syndrome would be used in a clinical setting to describe a dog with high-protein ascites and hepatomegaly but without evidence of right-sided heart failure or pericardial disease (i.e., cardiac murmur, jugular pulses, cardiomegaly).

## CLINICAL FINDINGS

The clinical findings associated with Budd-Chiari–like syndrome in dogs are the result of postsinusoidal portal hypertension. The predominant sign is progressive abdominal distention caused by ascites that is often poorly responsive to diuretic therapy. The ascites is characterized by a high protein content (>2.0 gm/dl) but fairly low cellularity, which helps to differentiate it from neoplastic or exudative abdominal effusions. Hepatomegaly secondary to passive hepatic congestion is another typical finding. Histologic examination of the liver indicates centrilobular congestion that is often severe. Hepatocellular necrosis and centrilobular fibrosis may also be present.

## ETIOLOGIES

Potential causes of Budd-Chiari–like syndrome in the dog include obstructive lesions of the caudal right atrium, caudal vena cava, and hepatic veins or venules.

### Abnormalities of the Caudal Right Atrium

#### COR TRIATRIATUM DEXTER

Cor triatriatum dexter (CTTD) is a rare congenital malformation of the right atrium in which an anomalous membrane divides the atrium into two chambers, causing obstruction of venous return to the heart (Fig. 1). Embryologically, this membrane results from persistence of all or part of the right sinus venosus valve. Nine dogs with CTTD have previously been described in the veterinary literature (van der Linde-Sipman and Stokhof, 1974; Stern et al., 1986; Miller et al., 1989; Otto et al., 1990; Malik et al., 1990; Tobias et al., 1993; Jevens et al., 1993). Anatomically, the anomalous membranes in these dogs have been of two basic types: either a midatrial membrane, or a membrane at the junction of the right atrium and caudal vena cava. Midatrial membranes originate from the area of the intervenous tubercle, and are located just caudal to the orifice of the tricuspid valve, placing the coronary sinus and fossa ovalis in the caudal atrial chamber (Fig. 1). Membranes at the cavoatrial junction are caudal to both the fossa ovalis and coronary sinus. Membranes of both types may be either perforate or imperforate. In contrast to human patients, CTTD in dogs is not usually associated with other congenital cardiac abnormalities. Of the nine reported canine cases, only two

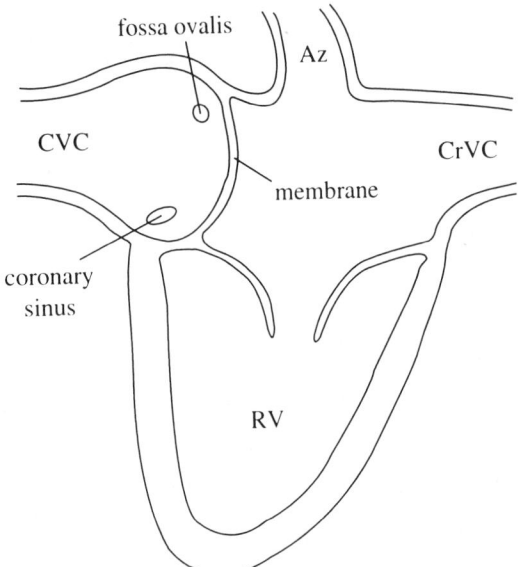

**Figure 1.** Schematic drawing of the right side of the heart indicating the location of a midatrial anomalous membrane in a dog with cor triatriatum dexter. Abbreviations: CVC = caudal vena cava, CrVC = cranial vena cava, RV = right ventricle, Az = azygous vein.

had associated defects (pericardial agenesis in one; Ebstein's type anomaly and an incomplete persistent left cranial vena cava in the other).

Dogs with CTTD are typically presented at a young age with progressive abdominal distention due to ascites, often without any other clinical signs. The diagnosis of CTTD is supported by clinical and diagnostic abnormalities suggestive of postsinusoidal portal hypertension in a dog without evidence of other cardiac abnormalities. Definitive diagnosis of CTTD is made through either echocardiography or cardiac catheterization. Echocardiographically, a membrane dividing the right atrium into two chambers is apparent. If the membrane is perforate, Doppler ultrasonography may demonstrate blood flow between the two chambers. Cardiac catheterization and selective angiography can be used to demonstrate a pressure difference between the cranial right atrium and the caudal vena cava, as well as to visualize the anomalous membrane.

Surgery is the treatment of choice for CTTD. Several techniques have been described for relief of the venous hypertension associated with this anomaly. The first is a modification of the patch-graft technique originally described for correction of pulmonic stenosis (Stern et al., 1986). A section of atrial wall over the anomalous membrane is resected, and a strip of pericardium is sutured over the defect, allowing blood to flow past the membrane. A second technique involves enlarging a central perforation in the membrane using an instrument passed through a stab incision in the right auricular appendage (Stern et al., 1986; Jevens et al., 1993). In membranes that are imperforate, an initial opening is made with a urethral catheter or mosquito forceps. A valve dilator is then passed into the perforation and used to tear the membrane and enlarge the

opening. The third technique used for treatment of CTTD is right atriotomy and membrane excision under direct visualization (Malik et al., 1990; Tobias et al., 1993). This technique necessitates temporary occlusion of venous inflow to the right heart, which can be done under either normothermic or hypothermic conditions, depending on the time required to complete the procedure. All three of these techniques have been used successfully for long term alleviation of clinical signs associated with CTTD.

### RIGHT ATRIAL TUMORS

The right atrium is the most common site for primary cardiac neoplasia in the dog. Right atrial tumors that have been reported to cause obstruction of venous return from the caudal vena cava include hemangiosarcoma, fibrosarcoma, fibroma, sarcoma, aortic body tumor, and myxoma. In addition to signs of Budd-Chiari–like syndrome, right atrial tumors can also result in signs of low cardiac output (syncope, weakness) and pericardial tamponade. Diagnosis is usually based on echocardiography for angiographic findings. Treatment of right atrial tumors is difficult. Surgical resection is sometimes successful for temporarily improving clinical signs, but recurrence is common. Chemotherapy with doxorubicin, cyclophosphamide, and vincristine has been used with very limited success for treatment of right atrial hemangiosarcoma.

## ABNORMALITIES OF THE CAUDAL VENA CAVA

Intraluminal obstruction of the caudal vena cava can be caused by thrombosis, neoplasia, fibrosis, or adult dirofilaria. Venous obstruction can also be caused by extraluminal masses that compress the caudal vena cava. Kinking of the thoracic caudal vena cava secondary to automobile-associated trauma has been reported to cause partial venous obstruction and signs of Budd-Chiari–like syndrome in dogs (Cornelius and Mahaffey, 1985). Abdominal distention due to progressive ascites developed several days following trauma. The presumed mechanism for narrowing of the caval lumen in these dogs was stretching of the vessel at the time of impact. Perivenular hemorrhage, inflammation, and scarring at the site of caval injury then resulted in narrowing of the vessel lumen. Angiography is the diagnostic method of choice for identification of caudal vena caval obstruction. Ultrasonography is a less invasive tool that may allow visualization of an intraluminal clot or tumor in the caudal vena cava, but in general it is less sensitive than angiography for the identification of venous obstruction.

Treatment options for correcting intraluminal obstruction of the caudal vena cava are limited. Alligator forceps passed down the jugular vein can be used to remove adult dirofilaria from the proximal caudal vena cava. In human patients, thrombotic and fibrotic lesions of the caudal vena cava have been treated successfully using percutaneous transluminal angioplasty. However, attempts at dilation of obstructive lesions in the caudal vena cava have not to date been described in dogs. Kinking of the caudal vena cava has been treated successfully by surgical resection of the affected portion of the vessel. An intraluminal shunt is placed through the kinked portion of the caudal vena cava via an incision in the right atrium. This shunt allows blood flow through the caudal vena cava while resection is performed.

## ABNORMALITIES OF THE LIVER AND HEPATIC VEINS

Like the caudal vena cava, obstruction of the major hepatic veins can be caused by either intraluminal lesions (thrombosis, fibrosis, or neoplasia), or extraluminal compression (hepatic neoplasia). Venous obstruction restricted to small hepatic veins and venules is rare, and is more likely to be caused by extraluminal than intraluminal lesions. Postsinusoidal obstruction secondary to progressive perivenular fibrosis has been reported in a single dog with clinical signs of Budd-Chiari–like syndrome (Cohn et al., 1991). The location of the venous lesion in this dog was similar to that associated with hepatic veno-occlusive disease, which is an important cause of Budd-Chiari syndrome in people.

Diffuse parenchymal liver diseases (such as cirrhosis) that result in portal hypertension generally cause sinusoidal and/or presinusoidal as well as postsinusoidal obstruction. Therefore, the protein content of the ascitic fluid in these animals is variable. In addition, the formation of ascites in cirrhosis is dependent on several factors other than portal hypertension, such as hypoal-buminemia and sodium and water retention. For these reasons, cirrhosis and other forms of parenchymal liver disease in which ascites is not caused strictly by postsinusoidal venous obstruction are not considered to be Budd-Chiari–like syndromes.

## References and Suggested Reading

Cohn L, Spaulding KA, Cullen JM, et al: Intrahepatic postsinusoidal venous obstruction in a dog. J Vet Intern Med 5:317, 1991.
*Case report describing a young dog with intrahepatic postsinusoidal portal hypertension.*
Cornelius L and Mahaffey M: Kinking of the intrathoracic caudal vena cava in five dogs. J Small Anim Pract 26:67, 1985.
*Description of the clinical signs, diagnostic findings, and response to treatment in five dogs with kinking of the caudal vena cava.*
Jevens DJ, Johnston SA, Jones CA, et al: Cor triatriatum dexter in two dogs. J Am Anim Hosp Assoc 29:289, 1993.
*Case report describing surgical treatment of cor triatriatum dexter using a valve dilator.*
Malik R, Hunt GB, Chard RB, and Allan GS: Congenital obstruction of the caudal vena cava in a dog. J Am Vet Med Assoc 197:880, 1990.
*Case report describing surgical treatment of cor triatriatum dexter via right atriotomy and membrane excision.*
Miller MW, Bonagura JD, DiBartola SP, and Fossum T: Budd-Chiari–like syndrome in two dogs. J Am Anim Hosp Assoc 25:277, 1989.
*Description of one dog with cor triatriatum dexter and one dog with a stenotic lesion at the cavoatrial junction.*
Otto CM, Mahaffey M, Jacobs C, and Binhazim A: Cor triatriatum dexer with Budd-Chiari syndrome and a review of ascites in young dogs. J Small Anim Pract 31:385, 1990.
*Case report describing a dog with cor triatriatum dexter.*
Stern A, Fallon RK, Aronson E, et al: Cor triatriatum dexter in a dog. Compend Cont Educ Pract Vet 8:401, 1986.
*Case report describing surgical treatment of cor triatriatum dexter using a modified patch-graft technique.*
Tobias AH, Thomas WP, Kittleson MD, and Komtebedde J: Cor triatriatum dexter in two dogs. J Am Vet Med Assoc 202:285, 1993.
*Case report describing surgical treatment of cor triatriatum dexter via right atriotomy using hypothermic venous inflow occlusion.*
van der Linde-Sipman JS and Stokhof AA: Triple atria in a pup. J Am Vet Med Assoc 165:539, 1974.
*Case report describing a dog with cor triatriatum dexter.*

# GUIDELINES FOR DIAGNOSIS AND MANAGEMENT OF HEARTWORM (*DIROFILARIA IMMITIS*) INFECTION

DAVID H. KNIGHT
*Philadelphia, Pennsylvania*

These guidelines reflect those currently recommended by the American Heartworm Society (American Heartworm Society, 1993) and focus on new information in the areas of epidemiology, diagnostic testing, chemoprophylaxis, and chemotherapy (Knight, 1993). Readers should consult other sources for a review of the pathophysiology and clinical signs of the disease. The following discussion relates primarily to the dog, with references to the cat limited to important differences in this species.

## EPIDEMIOLOGY

Mosquitoes capable of acting as intermediate hosts and vectors for *Dirofilaria immitis* are prevalent worldwide in the tropical and temperate latitudes. Therefore, wherever a reservoir of infection (microfilaremic primary host), a climate favoring development of infective heartworm larvae in the intermediate host, and mosquitoes that regularly feed on susceptible mammals coexist, it is possible for the infection to become endemic. In addition to domestic dogs, wild canids such as the coyote can become important regional reservoirs of heartworm infection.

Despite extensive, but not universal, use of chemoprophylaxis, heartworm infection continues to spread. Although completely preventable, once established in a population of dogs, it is virtually impossible to eliminate all reservoirs of infection. Therefore, the low incidence of infection detected by clinic surveys greatly underestimates the true prevalence in the general community.

## HEARTWORM TESTING

By conservative estimate, approximately 20% of dogs infected with mature heartworms do not have circulating microfilariae. The percentage of so-called occult infections more than doubles in symptomatic dogs with chronic pulmonary arterial disease, and nearly all of those exhibiting signs of the pneumonitis syndrome are microfilariae-negative. Dogs that are heavily enough infected with viable mature heartworms to develop recognizable signs of disease virtually always have a detectable antigenemia. Conversely, less than 1% of microfilaremic dogs fail to test positive for antigen (Courtney, Zeng, and MacKinnon, 1993).

### Routine Screening

Heartworm infections do not become patent (microfilaremic) or antigenemic until about 6.5 months after infection. The futility of testing during the prepatent period can be avoided by calculating the interval since the beginning of the peak period of transmission (July and August). If a negative test result is obtained more recently than 7 months since the latest possible exposure, testing should be repeated after waiting an appropriate interval of time.

The high degree of specificity and greater sensitivity of the current enzyme immunoassays for circulating heartworm antigen compared to a microfilaria examination have made these tests the primary method of prospectively identifying infection in asymptomatic dogs and in those with provocative but ambiguous clinical signs. The only exception to this general recommendation occurs when diethylcarbamazine (DEC) is used for chemoprophylaxis. In those circumstances, it is imperative that the blood also be examined for microfilariae, because potentially life-threatening side effects may develop when microfilaremic dogs are administered DEC. Any dog testing positive for heartworm antigen should also be tested for microfilariae, since the presence of microfilariae must be taken

into consideration during the subsequent management of the patient.

## Immunodiagnostic Tests for Heartworm Antigen

ENZYME-LINKED IMMUNOASSAYS. The enzyme-linked immunoassays (ELISA) are the standard for this category of heartworm test. Their greatest virtue is the ability to correctly recognize uninfected animals (i.e., not give false-positive results). Whenever a positive test result (usually a weak test reaction) is at odds with other relevant clinical information, the test should be rerun using meticulous technique. False-positive results with these tests are due to technical error in nearly all instances. Cross reactivity with *Dipetalonema reconditum*, the second most common dog filariid in the United States, is not a problem. However, in the Mediterranean and other parts of the world where *Dirofilaria repens* is found, cross-reactivity must be considered.

The sensitivity of the ELISA heartworm tests is a function of the duration of infection and the number of adult worms. Although an antigenemia may be detectable as early as 5 months after infection, it usually does not occur until the worms start producing microfilariae at about 6.5 months, and may not be found until after 7 months. Most, if not all, of the antigen shed into circulation is attributable to the female worms. Mixed-sex, mature infections consisting of 20 worms or more are nearly always antigen-positive, but antigen can be detected in only about half of infections consisting of three or fewer worms. These odds are likely to improve as refinements are made in these tests.

In most clinic populations where a high rate of chemoprophylaxis is practiced, there should be very few infected dogs. Test accuracy in these circumstances depends on a high degree of specificity. The fact that lightly infected dogs may go undetected by antigen testing is of less concern, since the health of such animals is unlikely to be threatened and periodic retesting will eventually detect these animals before they are at risk of clinical consequences should they continue to accumulate worms.

WHOLE BLOOD IMMUNOASSAYS. The most recently introduced immunologic heartworm diagnostic tests have the additional convenience of accepting whole blood. The first of these (VetRED, Rhône-Merieux, Inc) utilizes a bifunctional antibody that recognizes the canine red cell and a different epitope of the same circulating heartworm antigen incorporated in the ELISA tests. A positive reaction produces agglutination within 2 min. Speed in obtaining test results is the major advantage of this test.

In the author's experience testing matched samples, neither the sensitivity nor specificity of VetRED are as high as for the ELISA tests. Although rated as 97% specific, even if it identified every infected dog in a clinic population with a 1% prevalence of infection (which is commonly the case in many parts of the country), the predictive value of a positive test would only be 25% (i.e., one true-positive for every three false-positive test results). This example illustrates the importance of high test specificity when screening dogs that are unlikely to be infected.

The Snap (IDEXX) ELISA-based test now has been modified to also run on canine whole blood. The accuracy of this test has been preserved using whole blood, and test sensitivity with serum or plasma may have improved.

### SELECTING A HEARTWORM ANTIGEN TEST KIT

IDEXX and Synbiotics are the two primary manufacturers of ELISA-based heartworm antigen test kits. Both utilize the ELISA in several different formats. IDEXX introduced the membranous solid-phase kits, one of which can be used with whole blood and also has a microtiter well system in their product line. Synbiotics has added to their microwell system a single-tube test and a solid-phase kit. Rhône-Merieux has recently entered the heartworm testing market with a whole blood agglutination immunoassay, with which there is comparatively little performance record.

Antigen test kits can be classified as either "stat" tests, designed to be run singly or in small groups, and "batch" tests, which permit large numbers of samples to be tested concurrently. If a hospital is performing a high volume of testing and prefers to batch, a microwell system will be more efficient and economical. In addition to the format primarily used for testing, access to an alternative method that complements those features adds flexibility and quality assurance. In-hospital heartworm antigen testing is a practical procedure with the important advantage over reference laboratories of providing immediate, qualitative results. At least one of the available formats should be compatible with any hospital routine.

At the present time, the ELISA-based test kits set the standard for accuracy. All are highly specific. Small differences in reported sensitivity should not be over-interpreted, since these comparisons have generally not been based on matched samples or a uniform method of reporting adult worm burdens. Selection should also take into account the technical expertise of the person running the test, ease of operation and critical time constraints in performing different steps, clarity and stability of the end result, time required to complete a test, and unit cost.

### EXAMINATION FOR MICROFILARIAE

The probability of finding microfilariae is directly related to the severity of infection, but the number of circulating microfilariae bears no relationship to the number of adult heartworms. At every level of adult worm infection, a smaller percentage of dogs will be microfilaremic than antigenemic. Therefore, although both types of testing complement each other, testing for microfilarie has become secondary to testing for heartworm antigen when screening for infection (Courtney, Zeng, and MacKinnon, 1993).

Methods that concentrate microfilariae are superior to wet blood mounts and capillary tube techniques. The modified Knott technique is the standard. The recovery of microfilariae by this method is equivalent to filtration, larger numbers of samples can be processed efficiently, and filarial species identification by morphology is more accurate.

SCREENING FOR HEARTWORM INFECTION IN CATS. Although about half of experimentally infected cats become transiently microfilaremic for 1 to 2 months about 8 months following infection, a microfilaremia is seldom found in natural infections (McCall et al., 1993). Since cats are usually very lightly infected, they are often not antigenemic either. Therefore, testing is reserved for cats that are suspected of being infected. The ELISA antigen tests can be used on cat serum or plasma. The utility of ELISA testing for host antifilarial antibody has not been determined. Antibody tests are considered to be more sensitive in cats but lack the specificity of antigen tests. If attempted, testing for microfilariae should always be done by concentration.

## CHEMOPROPHYLAXIS

Heartworm infection is easily prevented and difficult to cure. Therefore, chemoprophylaxis should be encouraged whenever a reasonable chance of infection exists. Two alternative classes of drugs are available. The monthly administered macrolide antibiotics ivermectin (Heartgard-30 and Heartgard-30 Plus, Merck AgVet) and milbemycin oxime (Interceptor, Ciba Animal Health) are currently the most popular methods of chemoprophylaxis. These products provide the advantages of greater convenience of administration, safety, and assurance of protection, and are presently the most important filaricides for preventing heartworm infection. Heartgard-30 Plus (ivermectin and pyrantel) and Interceptor are also useful for controlling slightly different spectra of gastrointestinal helminths. Though once the mainstay of heartworm chemoprophylaxis, DEC (Filaribits and Filaribits Plus, American Cyanamid and other brands) has largely been superseded by the macrolides.

### Seasonal Transmission of Heartworm Infection

Maturation of microfilariae to the infective larval stage following ingestion by a mosquito can only occur when the ambient temperature exceeds 57° (Slocombe, Surgeoner, and Srivastava, 1989). There is no evidence that the occasional emergence of overwintering mosquitos on warm days represents a risk of infection. Development requires the accumulation of warmth applied over an extended period of time. The incubation period shortens from 29 days at an average daily temperature (maximum-minimum/2) of 64°F to about 8 days at 86°F. Higher temperatures may be lethal to the larvae.

There are probably few places in the United States where year-found heartworm transmission is possible, and studies at sites as far south as Orlando, FL have failed to document transmission between mid-December and mid-April (McTier et al., 1993). In southern Ontario, the transmission season is less than 5 months (June 1 to October 8) (Slocombe, Surgeoner, and Srivastava, 1989) and is probably limited to no more than 6 to 8 months in most of the United States. Transmission increases gradually late in the spring, reaching a peak during July and August, before declining in the fall. A conservative estimate of the duration of transmission can be calculated for a particular region from a 30-day moving accumulation of at least 234 "heartworm development units" (degrees Fahrenheit above the threshold temperature of 57°F), 30 days being the estimated maximum life expectancy of mosquitos in the wild. Guidelines based on this analysis should derive from years when the spring and fall were unseasonably warm. With the possible exception of some areas in the deep south, no scientific justification can be made for keeping dogs on heartworm chemoprophylaxis year-round. Arguments that continuous administration all year promotes client compliance are conjectural, at best.

## Pretesting

Heartworm chemoprophylaxis should not be initiated within 7 months of the latest potential exposure without first testing for infection. Antigen testing is adequate except when DEC is to be used. For those dogs, the blood also must be examined for microfilariae to avoid causing DEC-induced side reactions. Secondly, it is impossible to determine whether infection has occurred due to irregular compliance during the course of prophylaxis if infection status was not established at the onset. Chemoprophylaxis can be administered to infected dogs, but this should only be done with medical justification, not inadvertently (see "Alternative Management of Chemotherapy," below).

MACROLIDE PROPHYLAXIS.    Heartgard 30 and Interceptor provide the greatest measure of protection against heartworm infection. The prophylactic dose rates are completely safe, even in dogs with a low tolerance to ivermectin, and provide a wider margin of safety than does DEC. Monthly administration is possible despite their short half-life because the filaricidal effect on precardiac larvae is prompt and absolute and, apparently, partially extends to immature adults as well. The monthly interval of administration provides a lengthy margin of protection but should not be exceeded intentionally, since efficacy is gradually diminished with less frequent use. The efficacy of Interceptor is maintained for at least 60 days following infection if monthly administration is resumed for two doses, and recent evidence suggests that the window of protection may be even greater for Heartgard 30. In the event

several doses are omitted, administration should be resumed promptly and continued for at least two more doses.

Macrolide prophylaxis may be started in weaned puppies, if at that time they are considered to be already at risk. Ordinarily, administration should commence within 1 month of the expected onset of transmission and terminate within the same interval following the end of the transmission season. For the Philadelphia area, for example, six monthly doses from early June through early November should be adequate protection.

DIETHYLCARBAMAZINE PROPHYLAXIS.    The efficacy of prophylaxis with DEC, unlike that with the macrolides, is critically dependent on faithful adherence to a schedule of daily administration. Protection ceases following a discontinuation of only two to three doses. Also, unlike the macrolides, which provide protection retroactive to the date of infection, DEC administration should begin in anticipation of exposure and continue for an additional 2 months. Lapses in compliance can be covered by the administration of one of the macrolide prophylactics. If the dog is microfilariae-negative, DEC can then be promptly resumed or conversion to monthly macrolide prophylaxis continued.

Administration of DEC to microfilaremic dogs is hazardous and may produce signs of gastrointestinal distress, culminating in hypovolemic shock and even death. Fluid and corticosteroid therapy are the best antidotes for this complication. Diethylcarbamazine may be given safely to dogs with immunologically occult infections, but with today's alternative options, there is no reason to do so.

ACQUIRED PROTECTIVE IMMUNITY.    Protective immunity to heartworm infection can be demonstrated following the inoculation of irradiated third-stage larvae or by in situ chemical abbreviation of fourth-stage larvae (Grieve, 1989). Based on this evidence, it can be assumed that chemoprophylaxis is reinforced by some degree of protective immunity induced by continual interruption of fourth-stage larval development acquired by natural trickle infection. The level of secondarily acquired protective immunity is probably greatest in regions where the rate of transmission is highest and stimulation of natural defenses would exert the greatest benefit.

### HEARTWORM PREVENTION IN CATS

Cats are less susceptible to heartworm infection than dogs, and infection occurs more commonly in male than in female cats. Since most heartworm-infected cats are neither microfilaremic nor antigenemic, surveys based on these screening methods greatly underestimate the actual prevalence of infection in this species. Based on necropsy surveys, only about 10% as many cats are infected as dogs from the same area. This still puts a potentially large number of cats at significant risk where the prevalence of infection in dogs is high. Consequently, greater consideration needs to be given to heartworm prevention in cats.

An ivermectin formulation specifically for use in cats has been tested and may be available in 1994. The bioavailability of ivermectin is lower in cats than in dogs. Therefore, the minimum effective dose is 24 $\mu$g/kg body weight (10.9 $\mu$g/lb) PO, four times higher than for the dog. When administered at 30- to 45-day intervals, the efficacy is 100%. At this dose rate, it also effectively controls hookworms in cats.

Milbemycin oxime also effectively prevents heartworm infection at the same 0.5- to 1.0-$\mu$g/kg (0.23 to 0.45 $\mu$g/lb) PO dose rate used in dogs. Partial protection is conferred by a single dose 60 days following infection, but a second dose administered 30 days later fully restores protection.

### RETESTING

Periodic retesting monitors the efficacy of heartworm chemoprophylaxis and is an indispensable component of any serious prevention program. As with primary screening, retesting should take into account the interval of time since the last potential exposure to infection. At least 7 months should have lapsed since the end of the peak summer period of transmission. For this reason, retesting to verify prophylaxis during the preceding season should be delayed until late April or May in the Northern Hemisphere. The prepatent period of late fall infections will overlap with resumption of transmission the following year. If late seasonal infections are a primary concern, a second retest later in the summer is indicated.

An antigen test should be selected for retesting dogs that received chemoprophylaxis with ivermectin or milbemycin. Both drugs interrupt heartworm embryogenesis and are capable of gradually clearing circulating microfilariae from dogs with patent infections (Bowman et al., 1993; Lok et al., 1993). Therefore, these dogs may not become microfilaremic if monthly prophylaxis has been in nominal use since infection occurred. However, antigenemia is not affected by embryostasis or the absence of microfilariae.

Reliance on testing for heartworm antigen is inadequate protection for dogs receiving DEC. In this instance, detecting microfilariae is the main concern, since failure to do so may result in serious complications when administration of this drug is resumed. As an added precaution, testing for antigen as well as microfilariae is advised for these dogs, in order to increase the probability of detecting an infection.

### PERIODIC VERSUS ANNUAL RETESTING

It has been commonplace to annually retest for heartworms. This practice should continue to be encouraged for dogs receiving DEC. However, for most dogs on monthly prophylaxis, periodic retesting every second or third year is adequate. The key issue is compliance with administration during the transmission season. Prior to renewing medication, the pet owner should be questioned briefly concerning the pattern of administration. Based on the strength of those responses, the degree of compliance is usually evident. If there is reasonable doubt (not just an inherent mistrust) that adequate protection has not been maintained, then retesting is justified. Dogs that were initially tested less than 7 months following the end of the transmission season and those for which the dose may have been underestimated for failure to realistically anticipate the weight gain of a growing puppy should be retested the first year. In the absence of some other extenuating circumstance, retesting can be conducted less frequently.

Reconsideration of the conventional belief that annual retesting is an obligatory part of macrolide prophylaxis is supported by medical evidence. The efficacy of these drugs is extremely high. Even when administration is delayed or occasionally skipped for a month, protection remains high. Thus, with any reasonable regularity of administration, protection is high. It is also unlikely that a heavy infection would result in the event of a brief break in protection. On the other hand, light infections are commonly missed by all methods of testing. Furthermore, light infections are not life threatening and seldom, if ever, cause overt signs of illness. Upon retesting such cases, infection will either continue to be missed or eventually identified at a later date and can be treated at that time without adversely affecting the prognosis. In fact, those hospitals that distribute their heartworm retesting throughout the year already are, in some instances, inadvertently testing on a nearly alternate-year basis. For example, if a dog became infected in June and was scheduled for annual testing in December, the current year infection could be missed due to the length of the prepatent period and, at the earliest, would not be detected until 18 months following infection. The delay in detecting light infections is not critical, and more heavily infected dogs usually provide clues that testing should be pursued. As a practical matter, the increasing number of dogs being put on chemoprophylaxis requires conservation of resources and targeting retesting for maximum efficiency and benefit.

## PREADULTICIDE EVALUATION

The choice of clinical laboratory tests and other methods of evaluation should be purposeful, based on a thorough history and physical examination. Therefore, the extent of the preadulticide evaluation will differ among cases depending on whether there are reasons to suspect secondary organ dysfunction or concurrent primary problems. A complete blood count (CBC), blood chemistry profile, and urinalysis are not automatically prerequisites to adulticide treatment in young and middle-aged healthy dogs. The negative results from such tests can be predicted based on the physical findings. Elevated liver enzymes are expected in more heavily infected dogs and provide no assessment of liver function or the likelihood of acute hepatic necrosis during the course of adulticide administration. Similarly, dipstick evidence of protein in the urine of dogs without clinical signs suggestive of renal disease are also inconsequential. Indiscriminate testing more often needlessly raises concerns than uncovers unrecognized problems.

Some degree of pulmonary thromboembolism is inevitable whenever adult heartworms are destroyed *in situ*. The two most important variables affecting the prognosis for postadulticide thromboembolic complications are the number of heartworms and the severity of the pulmonary vascular disease they have already caused. An antigen test and radiographs of the chest complement each other by providing information about the severity of infection and disease, respectively. The heavier the infection and the more severe the pulmonary end-arteritis and obstructive fibrosis, the greater the risk of fever, cough, respiratory distress, hemoptysis, or death during convalescence from adulticide therapy.

SEMIQUANTITATIVE ANTIGENEMIA. The intensity of a positive reaction in any of the enzyme-linked immunoassays is directly related to the amount of antigen in circulation and, indirectly, the biomass of adult (primarily the larger female) heartworms. This relationship is not precisely linear and only serves as a guide for identifying dogs that probably are either relatively lightly or heavily infected. Antigen levels may underestimate the infection when male worms predominate or the infection is still immature, and can be disproportionately high during the transient rise associated with the recent death of some worms.

RADIOGRAPHIC SIGNS OF PULMONARY VASCULAR AND PARENCHYMAL DISEASE. The earliest signs of heartworm-induced pulmonary vascular disease are found in the periphery of the caudal lung lobes. As heartworm disease worsens, the larger, more proximal lobar arteries become enlarged, nontapering, tortuous, and truncated. Right-sided cardiomegaly and diffuse interstitial and patchy consolidated lung disease are secondary signs indicative of severe underlying vascular disease. When respiratory signs and pulmonary infiltrates are severe, diminishing doses of prednisolone (starting at 0.5 mg/kg/day) prior to adulticide therapy usually reduce these clinical and radiographic signs. The 7 to 10 day course of prednisolone should not be administered concomitantly with the adulticide. Often, the signs of large-vessel disease will persist following recovery from spontaneous or adulticide-induced elimination of heartworms, but the parenchymal signs will diminish and may eventually disappear.

## ELIMINATION OF ADULT HEARTWORMS

The health consequences of heartworm infection range from negligible to serious, depending on the severity of infection. Treatment for adult heartworms should be elected only after a firm diagnosis of infection has been made. Ambiguous antigen test results in the absence of either confirming evidence or a high probability of exposure do not justify treatment, considering the potential for direct drug-related side effects, in addition to the time, effort, and cost of the undertaking. Deferred action in lightly infected dogs will not jeopardize a successful resolution. When infection is certain, its severity and the inherent risks associated with treatment can be determined based on the patient's general health, radiographic evidence of disease, and antigen assessment of infection. Clinical signs are more likely to develop in a dog that is very active or used for a high-performance sport than in one that is comparably infected but has a limited opportunity for exercise.

## Adulticide Chemotherapy

### SODIUM THIACETARSAMIDE

This organoarsenical (Caparsolate, CEVA Laboratories) is the only heartworm adulticide currently available in the United States. Though useful, it does not dependably kill all the worms. It is also potentially hepatotoxic, and must be administered intravenously with extreme care to avoid causing severe local inflammation and necrosis at the injection site. Given these shortcomings, adulticide treatment with this drug should not be started or repeated unless the infection is considered heavy enough to pose a risk to health or interfere with performance.

The intravenous (IV) dose of Caparsolate is 1 ml of a 1% solution per 10 lb body weight (2.2 mg/kg) twice daily for 2 days. Efficacy is critically dependent on maintaining an effective blood level. Doses administered at 6- to 8-hr intervals maintain blood levels longer than those given at 12-hr intervals. The most efficient protocol for administrating Caparsolate is to pair the daily doses within 8 hr starting late in the morning of the first day, and resuming first thing on the second morning, with the overnight interval limited to 16 hr or less.

In addition to the dose and interval of administration, the age and sex of the parasites also affect the efficacy of thiacetarsemide. Precardiac larvae are most susceptible and recent arrivals in the lungs are most resistent. Worms that survive treatment are nearly always female. Since there is very little difference between the therapeutic and toxic thresholds, the dose should be calculated on the basis of gross body weight. Anything less than a full dose produces totally undependable results.

When biliary excretion of thiacetarsamide is reduced due to compromised liver function in dogs with heartworm disease, filaricide efficacy, secondary thromboemboli, and the risk of toxicity are increased. Conversely, worms are more likely to survive treatment in healthy dogs because the drug is eliminated more rapidly. However, extending treatment to a third day does not dependably improve efficacy.

Acute hepatotoxicosis occasionally occurs during the course of Caparsolate administration. If total anorexia, recurrent vomiting, and especially icterus develop, the treatment should be discontinued. Most dogs will recover spontaneously, without having to resort to supportive fluid therapy, and the treatment can be restarted from the beginning in 4 to 6 weeks.

If clinical signs of worm embolization (fever, cough, occasional hemoptysis) develop, they usually occur between 5 and 10 days after treatment. To prevent and minimize these signs, exercise should be limited for a month. Anti-inflammatory doses of glucocorticosteriods are useful after the fact, but are not recommended prospectively, since they may reduce filaricide efficacy. The American Heartworm Society has never endorsed the use of aspirin as either a preadulticide or postadulticide treatment.

Perivascular infiltration of thiacetarsamide causes clinicians more apprehension than the unavoidable risk of pulmonary emboli. The pain, swelling and, in the worst accidents, sloughing of skin over the injection site provide troubling evidence of failure to manage the one variable we control. If there is leakage, swelling will be evident within an hour. At the first sign of swelling (or immediately if the venipuncture was not well executed), hot pack the site and apply dimethyl sulfoxide (DMSO) liberally. This should be repeated every 4 to 6 hr until the swelling begins to subside. Infiltrating the area with saline and anti-inflammatory steroids is ineffective and may exacerbate the situation.

### MELARSOMINE HYDROCHLORIDE

Melarsomine hydrochloride (RM-340) (Immiticide, Rhone-Merieux, Inc) is a new organoarsenical adulticide that is currently available in some parts of Europe and is expected to be licensed in the United States by some time in 1995. The efficacy of melarsomine is superior to thiacetarsamide. It also possesses several other advantages, not the least of which is greater ease of administration by deep intramuscular (IM) rather than IV injection. Some muscle swelling and a few days of mild soreness may develop. However, this is generally barely noticeable compared to the intense periphlebitis that develops when even a small amount of thiacetarsamide is injected or leaks at the injection site.

The filaricide efficacy of melarsomine, unlike that of thiacetarsamide, can be graded by dose. For the first time, this makes it possible to eliminate worms from heavily infected dogs in stages, thereby distributing the impact of worm emboli. Standard administration consists of two 2.5-mg/kg (1.1 mg/lb) IM doses 24 hr apart and repeated in 4 months. With this regimen, all male and nearly all female worms are eliminated by the first two doses. Melarsomine also differs from thiacetarsamide by not causing any hepatic necrosis.

### ADULTICIDE THERAPY FOR CATS

The dog dose of thiacetarsamide has been successfully used in cats. However, cats are less durable patients and the possibility of sudden death following treatment is a definite concern. The life span of heartworms in cats is much shorter than in dogs and generally does not exceed 2 to 3 years (McCall et al., 1993). Since heartworm infections in cats tend to be self-limiting, it is prudent to allow time for the infection to run its course. Cats symptomatic for heartworm disease can be treated with anti-inflammatory doses of prednisolone, which may be associated with improvement in clinical signs.

### SURGICAL EXTRACTION OF HEARTWORMS

Extraction of heartworms from the pulmonary arteries, heart, and venae cavae by fluoroscopic guidance of flexible alligator forceps (Fujinon Inc) is an effective and commonly used technique in Japan. Forceps extraction is the only way to save dogs that have developed the caval syndrome (dirofilarial hemoglobinuria). These dogs become acutely ill and may die within hours if the entangled worms are not removed promptly from the orifice of the tricuspid valve. Heavily infected dogs exhibiting signs of pulmonary hypertension and severe cor pulmonale also benefit from removal of worms, which reduces postadulticide embolization. Although the recovery rate of worms is high, some usually remain and may justify the subsequent use of chemotherapy.

Surgery rather than chemotherapy was made a matter of necessity in Japan where thiacetarsemide has been difficult to obtain. In the United States, where adulticide therapy is an easy alternative, this invasive procedure requiring general anesthesia and fluoroscopy is neither cost-effective nor medically superior for treating cases of mild heartworm infection.

## CONFIRMATION OF ADULTICIDE EFFICACY

Clinical improvement of symtomatic dogs is the most meaningful evidence of at least partial adulticide efficacy. However, although thiacetarsemide may kill most of the worms, infection is completely eliminated less than half the time. Future management decisions depend on making a distinction between a postadulticide residual infection and subsequent reinfection, if it occurs. Heartworm antigenemia disappears within 12 weeks following adulticide treatment if all, or in some cases, nearly all the worms are eliminated. Therefore, an antigen test should be repeated after this interval of time as part of the adulticide protocol. Ordinarily, if an antigen test is still positive, it is much weaker, indicating a partial elimination of the infection. The membrane on which the reaction takes place in the solid-phase tests can be removed, dried, and retained as a permanent visual record. If a cat is antigenemic prior to treatment, the same practice should be followed.

Residual infections invariably consist entirely of female worms. Female unisex infections cease producing and releasing microfilariae after several weeks, and once circulating microfilariae are cleared with a microfilaricide, they do not return unless a dog acquires a new patent infection. Consequently, permanent disappearance of circulating microfilariae is not a reliable indicator of adulticide efficacy. However, recrudescence of microfilariae after 3 to 4 months would be indicative of reinfection.

## MICROFILARICIDE CHEMOTHERAPY

Ordinarily, microfilariae are the last life cycle stage to be eliminated, because complete clearance is usually a slow process prior to treating for the adult heartworms; 3 to 4 weeks after administering the adulticide, the microfilaricide treatment can begin. This final step should be taken so adulticide-treated dogs do not remain effective reservoirs of infection. Also, treatment with a microfilaricide must precede DEC chemoprophylaxis.

No Food and Drug Administration (FDA)–approved microfilaricide is available in the United States. Extralabel use of ivermectin or milbemycin oxime are the only alternatives that are sufficiently safe and efficient to justify consideration.

### MILBEMYCIN OXIME

Interceptor is a potent microfilaricide at the prophylactic dose and easily doubles in this capacity. In adulticide-pretreated dogs, one dose is usually sufficient to eliminate the microfilariae. The dose can be repeated in 2 weeks if necessary. If the heartworm transmission season has already begun, a regular monthly schedule of administration should be continued.

Side effects related to the rapid, first-dose reduction in microfilaremia include transient weakness, pale membranes, intestinal hyperperistalsis, and tachypnea (Kitagawa et al., 1993). Although these signs are common, they are usually overlooked because they are mild and seldom require supportive therapy with fluids or glucocorticosteroids. However, the higher the microfilaria count, the greater the chance of encountering noticeable side effects. A reasonable precaution when treating dogs with high counts (on the order of 15,000/ ml or greater) is to keep them under observation for 8 to 10 hr following milbemycin dosing.

### IVERMECTIN

Ivermectin is weakly microfilaricidal at the 6 to 12 $\mu$g/kg body weight (2.7 to 5.5 $\mu$g/lb) prophylactic dosage. In dogs with untreated patent infections, it may require 6 to 10 monthly doses to clear all the microfilariae (Bowman et al., 1993). Presumably, clearance is more rapid in adulticide-treated dogs, but this has yet to be investigated.

To effect a rapid reduction of microfilariae with ivermectin, the "microfilaricidal" dose of 50 $\mu$g/kg body weight (23 $\mu$g/lb), which is eight times the low end of the prophylactic dose range, is required. The cattle anthelmintic Ivomec (Merck AgVET) has been used commonly as an extralabel source for large oral doses of ivermectin. Side effects following the use of Ivomec are usually due to miscalculation of the correct volume of this highly concentrated (10 mg/ml) formulation. As with milbemycin, microfilaricidal reactions also may occur at this high dose and are managed in a similar manner. The microfilaricidal dose of ivermectin is half the threshold at which the mildest signs of toxicosis develop in the most sensitive collie dogs and, when properly administered, provides an acceptable margin of safety. Rather than risk miscalculating the dose of Ivomec, consideration should be given to using the appropriate multiple of the larger sized Heartgard-30 tablets or chewables as a microfilaricide for small dogs or the standard prophylactic dose of Interceptor.

### ALTERNATIVE MANAGEMENT OF CHEMOTHERAPY

The conventional life cycle stage specific sequence of heartworm chemotherapy (adults, microfilariae, and precardiac larvae) should be considered, but need not always be followed. Certain medical management and utilitarian scenarios may be handled effectively without first initiating the adulticide phase of the treatment. The rationale for such an approach is based upon the following facts. Lightly infected dogs (low antigenemia) with no appreciable radiographic signs of disease are unlikely to become functionally compromised or exhibit clinical signs. Heartworms in peripheral branches of the pulmonary arteries ordinarily remain fixed *in situ*. The intimal lesions they cause mature rapidly, and any obstruction to blood flow in those branches usually has already occurred by the time the infection is recognized. Therefore, assuming such a dog does not continue to acquire more heartworms, the pulmonary vascular disease remains essentially static.

Balanced against this low probability of significant consequence of disease in lightly infected dogs is the equally low probability that adulticide treatment will improve their health. Considering the expense of treatment, the cost/benefit ratio is very high. In fact, morbidity of treatment may be higher than for the disease in such cases. There is always the chance of accidental perivascular infiltration of thiacetarsamide, and there is no way to avoid causing acute hepatic swelling and necrosis in some dogs. Furthermore, even if the treatment of a clinically healthy dog progresses without complication, there is at least a 50% chance that some worms will survive. Unlike heavily infected dogs in which significant clinical improvement may follow partial elimination of infection, lightly infected dogs are not much better off following an equivalent percentage reduction in the number of worms. The future availability of melarsomine will diminish many of these reservations and may shift the cost/benefit ratio in favor of adulticide treatment for more asymptomatic dogs.

An alternative approach is to provide ivermectin or milbemycin chemoprophylaxis during the transmission season and live with the adult heartworms. If a microfilaremia is present, it will gradually decline and eventually disappear over 6 to 10 months. If not reinfected, these dogs will remain microfilariae-negative despite discontinuation of chemoprophylaxis in the off-season. Such an approach should be considered rather than doing nothing when, for whatever reason, a client declines the adulticide treatment. Furthermore, it is a legitimate option to propose for dogs that have been chronically but lightly infected and show little or no signs of disease. The older the dog, the more consideration should be given to maintaining the status quo. Electing this restrained approach assumes that there will be periodic physical check-ups and antigen retesting to ensure that good health is maintained.

## References and Suggested Reading

American Heartworm Society: Recommended procedures for the diagnosis and management of heartworm (*Dirofilaria immitis*) infection. *In* Soll MD (ed): *Proceedings of the Heartworm Symposium '92.* Batavia, IL: American Heartworm Society, 1993, p 289.
*The latest guidelines established by the American Heartworm Society.*

Bowman DD, Johnson RC, Ulrich ME, et al: Effects of long-term administration of ivermectin and milbemycin oxime on circulating microfilariae and parasite antigenemia in dogs with patent heartworm infections. *In* Soll MD (ed): *Proceedings of the Heartworm Symposium '92.* Batavia, IL, American Heartworm Society, 1993, p 151.
*Longitudinal study of naturally infected dogs.*

Courtney CH, Zeng Q-Y, and MacKinnon BR: Comparison of two antigen tests and the modified Knott test for detection of canine heartworm at different worm burdens. Canine Pract 18:5, 1993.
*A nonmatched evaluation of the DiroCHEK and CITE Semi-Quant antigen tests based on a large bank of sera from dogs of known infection status.*

Grieve RB: Potential for immunoprophylaxis against heartworm (*Dirofilaria immitis*) infection. *In* Otto GF (ed): *Proceedings of the Heartworm Symposium '89.* Washington, DC, American Heartworm Society, 1989, p 187.
*Review of progress toward developing a vaccine against heartworms.*

Kitagawa H, Sasaki Y, Kumasaka J, et al: Clinical and laboratory changes after administration of milbemycin oxime in heartworm-free and heartworm-infected dogs. Am J Vet Res 54:520, 1993.
*Detailed examination of hematologic, blood chemical, and quantitative microfilarial counts during 24 hr after treatment.*

Knight DH: How current knowledge has affected the diagnosis, prevention, and treatment of heartworm infection. *In* Soll MD (ed): *Proceedings of the Heartworm Symposium '92.* Batavia, IL, American Heartworm Society, 1993, p 253.
*A perspective on recent developments affecting the management of heartworm infection.*

Lok JB, Knight DH, LePaugh DA, et al: Kinetics of microfilaremia suppression in *Dirofilaria immitis*–infected dogs during and after a prophylactic regimen of milbemycin oxime. *In* Soll MD (ed): *Proceedings of the Heartworm Symposium '92.* Batavia, IL, American Heartworm Society, 1993, p 143.
*Discussion of the pathogenesis of drug-induced occult dirofilariasis in experimentally infected dogs and its clinical implications.*

McCall JW, Dzimianski MT, McTier TL, et al: Biology of experimental heartworm infections in cats. *In* Soll MD (ed): *Proceedings of the Heartworm Symposium '92.* Batavia, IL, American Heartworm Society, 1993, p 71.
*Comprehensive description of the unique features of infection in this species.*

McTier TL, McCall JW, Dzimianski MT, et al: Epidemiology of heartworm infection in beagles naturally exposed to infection in three southeastern states. *In* Soll MD (ed): *Proceedings of the Heartworm Symposium '92.* Batavia, IL: American Heartworm Society, 1993, p 47.
*A controlled study documenting seasonal heartworm transmission.*

Slocombe JOD, Surgeoner GA, and Srivastava B: Determination of heartworm transmission period and its use in diagnosis and control. *In* Otto GF (ed): *Proceedings of the Heartworm Symposium '89.* Washington, DC, American Heartworm Society, 1989, p 19.
*Model described for calculating when heartworm transmission occurs, based on climatologic records in Canada.*

# RECOGNITION AND TREATMENT OF PULMONARY HYPERTENSION

LYNELLE R. JOHNSON
*Fort Collins, Colorado*

*and* ROBERT L. HAMLIN
*Columbus, Ohio*

Pulmonary hypertension (PH) in human patients is defined by a mean pulmonary artery pressure exceeding 25 mm Hg at the time of cardiac catheterization. This value has been used as a criterion for definitive diagnosis in veterinary medicine (Perry, Dillon, and Bowers, 1991), although pulmonary hypertension may also be diagnosed with an accumulation of less invasive clinical information. Pulmonary hypertension has been well characterized in human medicine, and it represents a significant cause of mortality in patients with cardiopulmonary disease. Primary pulmonary hypertension is a rare, idiopathic form of the disease seen in people, and while suspected, it has not yet been definitively described in the dog or cat. Pulmonary hypertension may also occur secondary to pulmonary, cardiac, and systemic diseases. Little data have been

collected on the incidence of pulmonary hypertension in veterinary medicine, except for that associated with canine heartworm disease or left-sided heart failure.

In the University of Illinois Veterinary Medical Teaching Hospital medical records data base, only 22 cases (two cats) with pulmonary hypertension unrelated to heartworm disease have been documented in the last 10 years. The overall incidence of pulmonary hypertension is not well known; however, the frequency of diagnosis at this institution has increased during the last several years due to an increased awareness of the condition. The purpose of this discussion is to define the clinical syndrome of pulmonary hypertension as it is known in human medicine, and to alert the veterinary clinician to the recognition of animal diseases that may secondarily result in pulmonary hypertension. Pulmonary hypertension, unrelated to heartworm disease (see "Guidelines for Diagnosis and Management of Heartworm [*Dirofiliaria immitis*] Infection," this volume, p 879) or left-sided heart failure, is the focus of this review.

## MAINTENANCE OF NORMAL PULMONARY ARTERY PRESSURE

The pulmonary circulation normally maintains low perfusion pressures despite the large volume of blood delivered to the lungs by the right ventricle. The tremendous surface area of the pulmonary capillary bed lowers pulmonary vascular resistance through recruitment of additional blood vessels and distention of thin-walled pulmonary arteries. The pulmonary circulation maintains low resistance and low pressure in the system, which is essential for efficient gas exchange. The highly compliant right ventricle is closely dependent on pulmonary hemodynamics. Low pulmonary pressures are necessary to minimize the workload on the right heart and to maintain myocardial blood flow to the right ventricle (Klinger and Hill, 1991). Physical characteristics of the lung such as dynamic compliance and airway resistance are also important in maintaining normal pulmonary arterial pressures because the vasculature and lung parenchyma are highly interdependent. Negative intrathoracic pressures exert radial traction on the blood vessels to increase luminal diameter and lower pulmonary vascular resistance (West, 1992). Conditions that affect pulmonary compliance or resistance cause a change in patterns of respiration and pressure gradients within the lung. This can result in alterations of vascular tone, structure, and function.

## PATHOPHYSIOLOGY AND DISEASE ASSOCIATION

Normal pulmonary pressures are approximately 25 mm Hg in systole and 8 mm Hg in diastole, with a mean pressure between 12 and 15 mm Hg (Brown, 1991; Perry, Dillon, and Bowers, 1991). Three mechanisms may lead to the generation of increased pulmonary arterial pressures. These are: increased left atrial pressure, increased pulmonary blood flow, and increased pulmonary vascular resistance (Brown, 1991; Perry, Dillon, and Bowers, 1991; Tancredi, 1992).

Cardiac conditions such as mitral stenosis, chronic mitral insufficiency, and cardiomyopathy can cause chronic elevations of left atrial pressure and lead to pulmonary venous and subsequent pulmonary arterial hypertension. Pulmonary dysfunction caused by pulmonary edema or chronic congestion could further predispose to increased pulmonary vascular resistance. Pulmonary function testing in dogs with experimentally induced mitral regurgitation has demonstrated a decrease in compliance of the lung and increased resistance to airflow, changes that would be expected to precede the development of pulmonary hypertension.

Pulmonary artery pressures were not assessed in these dogs, and the overall incidence of pulmonary hypertension secondary to heart failure has not been reported, though it has clearly been recognized in some patients.

Increased pulmonary blood flow following lung lobectomy may cause pulmonary hypertension in people; however, clinical observations and experimental studies in dogs following pneumonectomy have not shown an increase in blood flow sufficient to result in pulmonary hypertension. This is probably related to species differences in pulmonary capacitance. Congenital cardiac shunts often result in cardiac hypertrophy or dilatation and subsequent heart failure. Shunting of increased volumes of blood into the pulmonary circulation causes high perfusion pressures, which can damage pulmonary vessels and lead to pulmonary hypertension. Uncorrected patent ductus arteriosus can lead to pulmonary hypertension secondary to severe congestive heart failure complicated by left-to-right shunting. Marked elevation of pulmonary arterial resistance also can cause reverse shunting of blood (right-to-left) through a patent ductus arteriosus, ventricular septal defect, or atrial septal defect. In a recent report, a family of Pembroke Welsh corgis with a high incidence of patent ductus arteriosus in the line was shown to have an early onset of pulmonary hypertension and reversed shunting of blood (Oswald and Orton, 1993). Such documented cases of Eisenmenger's physiology virtually always occur prior to 6 months of age and are attributed to flow-induced pulmonary vascular injury.

Elevated pulmonary arterial pressures commonly develop in association with an increase in pulmonary vascular resistance, which may occur with primary pulmonary diseases or various systemic conditions. A common cause of increased pulmonary vascular resistance in people with chronic obstructive pulmonary disease is hypoxic vasoconstriction, which is a natural phenomenon induced by a fall in the partial pressure of alveolar oxygen. By increasing vascular resistance in a region of low oxygen availability, perfusion is better matched to ventilation and overall gas exchange is improved (West, 1992). Regional hypoxia is sufficient to initiate this pulmonary response, and intermittent hypoxia causes sustained increases in vascular tone in humans (Schulman and Matthay, 1992).

The degree of hypoxia that might result in pulmonary hypertension could be expected in a large number of dogs with both upper and lower airway obstructive disease. Conditions such as chronic bronchitis, bronchiectasis, laryngeal paralysis, and tracheal collapse are associated with sustained or intermittent hypoxia; however, the prevalence of pulmonary hypertension in these conditions is unknown. Restrictive pulmonary conditions such as idiopathic pulmonary fibrosis or fibrosing pleuritis also have the potential to elevate pressure in the pulmonary circulation. In these diseases, pulmonary hypertension can develop due to mechanical stresses placed on the lung parenchyma, increased respiratory effort at high lung volumes, and hypoxic conditions within the alveoli (West, 1992). Because the dog has a relatively poor vasoconstrictive response to hypoxia, pulmonary hypertension may occur only in very advanced lung disease or when animals are affected with other predisposing conditions. Examples of these predisposing disorders would include pulmonary thromboembolism, conditions that predispose to hypercoagulability or hyperviscosity, and septic shock.

Obstructive pulmonary vascular disease occurs with pulmonary thromboembolization or with widespread tumor emboli, and evidence of embolic disease is commonly found in humans with pulmonary hypertension (Tancredi, 1992). Emboli may directly cause pulmonary hypertension through mechanical obstruction and hypoxic vasoconstriction, or clots may form *in situ* as a result of the abnormal endothelial environment in the pulmonary circulation. By reducing the cross-sectional area available for perfusion, an increase in pulmonary arterial pressure develops, with subsequent intimal proliferation and medial hypertrophy within the vasculature. Abnormal blood flow and endothelial perturbation increase platelet adherence and aggregation, causing additional obstruction to blood flow and activation of the clotting cascade. Circulating inflammatory mediators released from platelets, such as histamine, serotonin, and thromboxane $A_2$, are potent vasoactive agents that enhance vascular reactions throughout the lung. Endothelial disruption causes elaboration of endothelin, a very potent vasoconstrictor, and may also cause a reduction in endothelial-derived relaxant factor (nitric oxide). These conditions would favor increased vascular reactivity. Exposure of the major histocompatibility complex due to endothelial interruption is also thought to perpetuate humoral mechanisms responsible for increases in pulmonary vascular resistance in humans.

Diseases associated with pulmonary embolization in companion animals include hyperadrenocorticism, nephrotic syndrome, immune-mediated hemolytic anemia, and pancreatitis (see *CVT XI*, p 137). Polycythemia and hyperviscosity associated with hyperadrenocorticism increase sludging of blood in the microvasculature, increase platelet adhesion and activation, and enhance endothelial disruption. Panting due to obesity or steroid excess increases shearing stresses within the lung parenchyma, increases the likelihood of pulmonary thromboembolus or hypertension, and increases right ventricular workload. Nephrotic syndrome is characterized by hypercoagulability due to loss of antithrombin III in the urine. This feature coincident with the primary disease that led to nephrotic syndrome may result in thromboembolus and the sudden development of increased pulmonary pressures, tachypnea, and heart failure. Pancreatitis is associated with hypercoagulability and release of various cytokines and inflammatory mediators that potentiate vascular reactivity.

Immune-mediated disorders such as systemic lupus erythematosis, rheumatoid arthritis, and polyarteritis are commonly implicated as causes of pulmonary hypertension in people, but the incidence in veterinary patients is unknown. Thromboembolic disease has been associated with immune-mediated hemolytic anemia in dogs, and investigation into the incidence of pulmonary hypertension in these cases would seem warranted, since prognosis worsens in dogs with thromboembolus.

Septic conditions activate multiple mediator systems and lead to the generation of adult respiratory distress syndrome (ARD) with severe pulmonary hypertension. Recognition of elevated pulmonary arterial pressure could be crucial in the management of septic shock patients because the onset of right ventricular dysfunction heralds a worsening prognosis.

## DIAGNOSIS OF PULMONARY HYPERTENSION

### History

The diagnosis of pulmonary hypertension that is unrelated to left-sided heart failure, congenital heart disease, or heartworm disease is the focus of this section.

The primary complaint noted in humans with pulmonary hypertension is dyspnea, and over half of our veterinary patients with pulmonary hypertension developed acute onset of severe dyspnea. Pulmonary thromboembolism should be considered in any patient with sudden onset of dyspnea. Cough, cyanosis, or exercise intolerance were reported in approximately one third of our veterinary patients. Syncope is not uncommon. Syncope with exercise is reported in humans when the patient is unable to increase cardiac output in response to exercise-induced peripheral vasodilation (Tancredi, 1992).

### Physical Examination

Auscultation of the patient with pulmonary hypertension often reveals underlying pulmonary disease; characterized by the presence of crackles or wheezes throughout the lung fields. An end-expiratory snap indicates collapse of the intrathoracic trachea, and increased end-expiratory effort is a classic finding in chronic bronchitis. Hyperresonance in the thoracic cage suggests air trapping. This results in an increase in intrathoracic pressure, compression of the pulmonary vessels, and subsequent increases in right ventricular afterload. Accentuation or splitting of the second heart sound may be detected due to increased pulmonary artery pressures (Tancredi, 1992). Cardiac filling increases during inspiration due to a fall in intrapleural pressure, and detection of a gallop or murmur that increases on inspiration is an early indicator of right ventricular dysfunction. Murmurs of tricuspid or possibly pulmonic insufficiency can be detected when right ventricular dilatation occurs, and an $S_3$ (ventricular) gallop may also be auscultated due to increased diastolic pressures in the right ventricle (Klinger and Hill, 1991; Tancredi, 1992). Jugular venous distention would support a diagnosis of right heart failure.

## Laboratory Data

Laboratory evaluation should include a complete blood count (CBC), chemistry profile, and urinalysis to identify underlying disease conditions that may be associated with pulmonary hypertension or thromboembolism. Immunologic testing should be performed if immune-mediated hemolytic anemia or systemic lupus is suspected. Caution is recommended when interpreting these tests, since a positive antinuclear antibody titer has been reported in 29% of human patients with pulmonary hypertension (Tancredi, 1992). This finding may reflect an immunologic basis for this condition, or it may indicate exposure of self-antigens due to endothelial disruption.

Hypoxemia is expected in pulmonary hypertension regardless of cause and arterial blood gas evaluation should be performed when possible. This analysis provides useful information on the degree of pulmonary dysfunction, will help guide therapy, and will aid in determining prognosis. Hypercarbia, if present, should be corrected when possible, since increased carbon dioxide concentrations may be associated with sodium retention, hypervolemia, increased end-diastolic pressures, and increased cardiac work load. Retention of carbon dioxide also causes acidosis and increases the likelihood of pulmonary vasoconstriction.

## Other Studies

*Chest radiographs* can be normal; indicate right heart enlargement and right heart failure; or show radiographic patterns consistent with chronic bronchitis, bronchiectasis, pulmonary fibrosis, pulmonary embolism, or tracheobronchial collapse. Upper airway obstruction due to tracheal collapse or collapse of the mainstem bronchus are other potential lesions that may be observed in some dogs with pulmonary hypertension. Prominent hilar arteries are supportive of pulmonary hypertension.

An electrocardiogram (ECG) in severe PH may reveal a right-axis deviation characterized by deep S waves in leads I, II, III, aVF, and $V_3$ if right ventricular enlargement is severe (Miller, Tilley, and Calvert, 1986). It has been reported that this occurs in a minority of veterinary patients with pulmonary hypertension; however, most of the dogs seen at the University of Illinois showed an ECG pattern consistent with right ventricular enlargement.

Echocardiography of the patient with pulmonary hypertension reveals right-sided pressure and often volume overload as indicated by right ventricular hypertrophy, increased right ventricular dimension, and flat or paradoxic septal motion. The pulmonary artery may be dilated, and the pulmonic valve closes early in midsystole when pulmonary arterial pressures are elevated (Tancredi, 1992). Large pulmonary thrombi have been recognized echocardiographically. Doppler echocardiography may reveal the presence of high-velocity tricuspid regurgitation even in the absence of a murmur.

Pulsed Doppler evaluation has been recognized as a noninvasive predictor of pulmonary artery pressure in humans. In humans with pulmonary hypertension, these studies have shown a characteristic flow velocity curve typified by an early onset of right ventricular ejection followed by a rapid decrease in flow as increased resistance is encountered. The time to peak velocity of right ventricular ejection is typically shortened in patients with pumonary hypertension (Marchandise et al., 1987). Similar findings were present in some of the dogs at the University of Illinois in which Doppler echocardiography was performed. When present, the velocity of a pulmonic valve insufficiency jet can provide direct evidence of diastolic pulmonary hypertension. Thus, when available, this procedure provides very useful diagnostic and clinical information.

Ancillary diagnostic testing may be performed at a referral institution. Radionuclide angiography may be used to evaluate right ventricular ejection fraction and can diagnose moderate to severe pulmonary hypertension. Pulmonary angiography will show dilated or tortuous pulmonary arteries. Both nuclear scintigraphy and pulmonary angiography may be used to outline patchy perfusion deficits suggestive of pulmonary thromboembolism.

## Cardiac Catheterization

Definitive diagnosis of pulmonary hypertension requires cardiac catheterization. Right heart catheterization should be performed with a Swan-Ganz–type catheter. The inflatable balloon tip will follow the flow of blood through the venous system into the pulmonary artery. The position of the balloon tip may be determined through fluoroscopy or by monitoring the pulse pressure trace. Inflation of the balloon should produce a wedge pressure—an estimate of left atrial pressure. An elevated wedge pressure indicates PH is secondary to left-sided heart disease. When PH is a consequence of bronchopulmonary or pulmonary vascular disease, the pulmonary arterial diastolic pressure is substantially greater than the wedge pressure. This procedure provides accurate measurements of pulmonary artery pressures, will rule out left-to-right shunts and left-sided heart failure, and allows evaluation of response to therapeutic intervention. Intravenous aminophylline (10 mg/kg) should be administered to assess the effect on pulmonary artery pressures, cardiac output, and pulmonary vascular resistance. Within 5 to 10 min, similar measurements should be obtained following administration of intravenous terbutaline (0.01 mg/kg). Further testing with intravenous vasodilators such as hydralazine (1 mg/kg), verapamil (0.05 mg/kg), or nifedipine (<0.1 mg/kg) could also be attempted (Perry, Dillon, and Bowers, 1991; Schulman and Matthay, 1992). Caution should be employed when using the latter drugs, and the patient should be monitored very carefully for systemic hypotension.

## THERAPY

The only therapy shown to improve survivability in humans with pulmonary hypertension is long-term oxygen therapy. Supplemental oxygen dilates pulmonary vessels and improves hemodynamics, reduces acidosis and ischemia, and improves right ventricular function (Klinger and Hill, 1991; Schulman and Matthay, 1992; Tancredi, 1992). This therapy should be instituted immediately in veterinary patients when pulmonary hypertension is suspected. Human patients are also treated with judicious doses of diuretics to achieve volume reduction and phlebotomy is considered if the hematocrit is above 55%. This treatment has not been evaluated in veterinary patients and is not recommended because of the risk of depleting electrolytes, worsening acid-base status, or decreasing cardiac output due to a reduction in preload. Patients with chronic obstructive pulmonary disease may suffer a worsening of gas exchange when diuretics are employed due to inspissation of bronchial secretions and mucus plugging of the airways.

Bronchodilators can be helpful in the treatment of pulmonary hypertension (see *CVT XI*, p 660, for a discussion of bronchodilators). Theophylline, a methylxanthine bronchodilator, has positive inotropic effects on the cardiopulmonary system. Theophylline produces sustained pulmonary vasodilatation and long-term improvement in right ventricular function in humans with chronic obstructive pulmonary disease and pulmonary hypertension (Klinger and Hill, 1991; Schulman and Matthay, 1992). In dogs, theophylline has been proven to improve diaphragmatic contractility and to lessen fatigue of respiratory muscles through calcium-dependent mechanisms. This is beneficial in extremely dyspneic or tachypneic animals in whom muscle fatigue leads to respiratory failure. Data on the efficacy of theophylline as a bronchodilator in dogs has not yet been reported; however, theophylline is commonly used to bronchodilate animals with chronic pulmonary disease and to improve intrathoracic pressure gradients in animals with bronchiectasis or tracheal collapse, thus lessening the tendency for airway collapse. The recommended dosage for sustained-release theophylline (Slo-bid, Rorer; Theo-Dur, Key Pharmaceuticals) is 20 mg/kg every 12 hr (Some dogs cannot tolerate this dose and develop sympathomimetic side effects). $\beta_2$-Agonists, such as terbutaline (Brethine, Ciba-Geigy), also improve pulmonary hemodynamics; however, long-term beneficial effects in treatment of pulmonary hypertension have not been reported in people (Klinger and Hill, 1992; Schulman and Matthay, 1992). This drug is administered at 1.25 to 5 mg/kg every 8 to 12 hr and 1.25 mg/cat every 12 hr.

Digoxin is occasionally used in pulmonary hypertension since it acts as a positive inotrope and may improve right ventricular function. The risks and benefits of digoxin should be carefully considered. Although digoxin will decrease cardiac filling pressure, it will also increase cardiac output and pulmonary artery pressures. It might result in acute vasoconstriction in the pulmonary bed (Schulman and Matthay, 1992). In addition, animals, like people with pulmonary disease, might have an increased susceptibility to digoxin-associated arrhythmias due to concurrent hypoxia or acidosis (Miller, Tilley, and Calvert, 1986). Therefore, digoxin is not routinely recommended in treatment of dogs with chronic obstructive pulmonary disease or pulmonary hypertension.

Vasodilators are used in human medicine as indicated by response to therapeutic trials during cardiac catheterization. Selected patients may respond to hydralazine, high doses of calcium channel blockers, angiotensin-converting enzyme (ACE) inhibitors, or prostacyclin. No clinical data are available to predict response to these medications in the individual patient. Significant side effects can be associated with the use of vasodilators because of systemic hypotension. Dogs with pulmonary hypertension secondary to heartworm disease have an unpredictable response to the direct-acting vasodilator hydralazine; therefore, unless direct provocative testing with a vasodilator agent during pulmonary artery catheterization has shown a reduction in pulmonary artery pressure, trial therapies are not recommended.

Anticoagulant therapy should be employed when thromboembolus is diagnosed, or when disseminated intravascular coagulation (DIC) complicates the clinical presentation. Because a large percentage of human patients with pulmonary hypertension show evidence of embolic disease, mini- or low-dose heparin therapy should be considered for veterinary patients in which pulmonary hypertension is likely.

Clinically detectable pulmonary hypertension is associated with a grave prognosis in human medicine, with predicted survival times of less than 3 years. Prognosis is probably similar in veterinary medicine. Most of the animals treated at the University of Illinois died or were euthanized within 4 months of diagnosis, although two dogs seemed to improve clinically with theophylline therapy.

An increased awareness of conditions that predispose to elevated pulmonary arterial pressures will hopefully forestall the onset of serious pulmonary hypertension and subsequent cardiac disease. In particular, appropriate treatment and monitoring of animals with serious pulmonary or tracheobronchial disorders and those at risk for thromboembolus is warranted.

Further investigation into the causes of pulmonary hypertension is needed in veterinary medicine in order to establish incidence rates with various clinical disorders, to develop a reliable means of early diagnosis, and to establish methods for determining therapeutic efficacy. In all species, preventive measures are more likely to prolong survival and improve quality of life than treatments instituted after diagnosis.

## References and Suggested Reading

Brown G: Pharmacologic treatment of primary and secondary pulmonary hypertension. Pharmacotherapy 11:137, 1991.

*An excellent review of pathophysiology and treatment recommendations in the human literature.*

Klinger JR and Hill NS: Right ventricular dysfunction in chronic obstructive pulmonary disease. Evaluation and management. Chest 99:715, 1991.

*A concise discussion of cardiopulmonary interactions in lung disease, stressing clinical evaluation of the patient and management of cor pulmonale.*

Marchandise B, De Bruyne, Delaunois L, and Kremmer R: Noninvasive prediction of pulmonary hypertension in chronic obstructive pulmonary disease by Doppler echocardiography. Chest 91:361, 1987.

*The procedure for Doppler evaluation of human patients with pulmonary disease is presented.*

Miller MS, Tilley LP, and Calvert CA: Electrocardiographic correlations in pulmonary heart disease. Semin Vet Med Surg 1:331, 1986.

*A complete analysis of the ECG patterns and arrhythmias associated with pulmonary disease along with a discussion of pathophysiology, clinical findings, and disease association in cor pulmonale.*

Oswald GOP and Orton EC: Patent ductus arteriosus and pulmonary hypertension in related Pembroke Welsh corgis. J Am Vet Med Assoc 202:761, 1993.

*An interesting presentation of a family of dogs affected with early-onset pulmonary hypertension and a congenital cardiac defect.*

Perry LA, Dillon AR, and Bowers TL: Pulmonary hypertension. Compend Cont Educ 13:226, 1991.

*An excellent veterinary-oriented review of pulmonary hypertension with additional information on potential therapy for pulmonary hypertension.*

Schulman DS and Matthay: The right ventricle in pulmonary disease. Cardiol Clin 10:111, 1992.

*An additional review of cardiopulmonary interactions, stressing pathophysiology of disease and therapy.*

Tancredi RG: Pulmonary vascular disease: Primary pulmonary hypertension. Cardiovasc Clin 22:113, 1992.

*A textbook discussion of disorders of pulmonary vasculature, including physiology, pathogenesis of diseases, clinical and laboratory studies, and treatment options.*

West JB: Pulmonary pathophysiology—the essentials. Baltimore, Williams & Wilkins, 1992.

*The classic reference book for an understanding of respiratory physiology in health and disease.*

# RECOGNITION AND TREATMENT OF CONGENITAL RESPIRATORY TRACT DEFECTS IN BRACHYCEPHALICS

Joan C. Hendricks

*Philadelphia, Pennsylvania*

The most common congenital respiratory disorders result from breeding practices that select for shortened facial appearance. English bulldogs appear to be the most compromised, but other brachycephalic breeds such as English pugs, Shar-Peis, French bulldogs and Boston bull terriers, Pekinese, Shih Tzus, and Lhasa apsos are also affected to some degree. Short-faced cats (Persians and Persian crosses such as Himalayans) do not appear to suffer from the same degree of upper airway obstruction as brachycephalic dogs.

The syndrome is the result of anatomic abnormalities that narrow the airway in multiple locations: stenotic nares; tortuous, compressed turbinates; caudally displaced maxillae with a resulting caudal displacement of the soft palate ("overlong soft palate"); everted laryngeal saccules; and hypoplastic trachea. Although not all dogs suffer obvious clinical signs from these features, it seems likely that all brachycephalic dogs have subclinically increased upper airway resistance. For example, tracheal diameter can be measured from a lateral thoracic radiograph. When the size of the tracheal diameter is compared to the size of the thoracic inlet (the distance from the ventral surface of T1 to the sternum), the ratio in bulldogs is significantly below this same ratio in normal dogs. Despite this evidence that anatomical narrowing can be shown objectively in all bulldogs, many of these dogs are thought to be normal by their owner. No correlation between the size of the ratio and the onset or degree of clinical signs has been demonstrated.

From the foregoing discussion, it should be apparent that brachycephalic anatomy chronically increases the workload of the respiratory system. Although compensation for this chronic respiratory difficulty is remarkable, what would normally be minor perturbations commonly lead to the sudden onset of overt respiratory distress.

The precarious situation of respiration in bulldogs can be illustrated by studies of breathing during sleep. During sleep, the upper airway muscles normally relax, and control of respiration is altered in a number of ways that tend to compromise ventilation, especially during the rapid-eye-movement (REM) sleep stage. Thus, numerous syndromes of "sleep-disordered breathing" have been documented in humans. In such syndromes, normal respiration is maintained during waking, but sleep onset is followed by repeated episodes of decreased or absent respiration, with decrements of oxygen saturation ($SaO_2$) of greater than 4%. The $SaO_2$ nadirs commonly fall below 70% (equivalent to a $PO_2$ of approximately 40 mm Hg). A similar study of respiration during sleep was undertaken in English bulldogs. Twenty dogs have been studied to date, ranging in age from newborn to 7 years. During waking, these animals generally had normal arterial blood gas measurements and were considered normal by their owners. However, every dog over 2 weeks of age exhibited repeated episodes of sleep-disordered breathing (i.e., pauses in breathing and drops in $SaO_2$). The frequency of these episodes was the greatest, by far, during REM sleep, with an occurrence rate of up to 52 events per hour during REM sleep. The SaO$_2$ nadirs dropped as low as 69%. Even thin, active adults and pups aged 5 weeks of age had frequent (>20 events per hour) sleep disordered breathing. Further studies, recently completed, show that bulldogs require compensatory hyperactivity of the upper airway dilating muscles to maintain upper airway patency. Upper airway dilating muscles in bulldogs have recently been shown to exhibit damage, including fibrosis. This is thought to be a consequence of the chronically increased workload imposed by the brachycephalic anatomy. This damage, accumulated over time, could lead eventually to inability to dilate the airway. When the muscles relax in the normal fashion during REM sleep, hypoxia results immediately. Thus, a normal change in respiratory function, superimposed on the abnormal anatomy, is all that is required to cause a significant decrease in SaO$_2$.

## DIAGNOSIS

### History

.Because of the predisposing anatomic features, the question of diagnosis is actually a question of degree of abnormality, rather than a question of distinguishing normal from abnormal. The appropriate approach to a brachycephalic is to assume that the potential for clinical upper airway obstruction is present. If the animal has presented with acute signs, the aim is to elicit information about triggering factors such as overheating, excitement, or increased exercise. A simple walk in humid weather can lead to a crisis. Heat is especially dangerous, because the thermal polypnea (panting) necessary for heat dissipation in dogs often produces some edema and further airway narrowing; this in turn allows the body temperature to rise further, produces anxiety, and initiates a vicious cycle. Even minimal stimuli may produce hyperthermia: an apparently normal bulldog's temperature rose to 103.8°F after walking approximately 100 yards in 75°F ambient temperature.

An important group of triggering causes includes manipulations performed by veterinarians such as restraint in lateral recumbency or supine posture (e.g., for radiographs); endotracheal intubation; and sedation or general anesthesia relaxing the respiratory muscles. Virtually all sedative or anesthetic agents relax the upper airway dilating muscles while allowing the diaphragm to continue its contractions. This combination allows the upper airway to collapse, and the collapse is worsened by the negative inspiratory pressure that sucks the pharyngeal walls shut. Thus, anesthesia or sedation carries an extreme risk in brachycephalic animals.

It should also be noted that problems with ingestion are commonly part of extreme respiratory distress. The dogs may have trouble swallowing, because the necessary occlusion of the respiratory system compromises ventilation. Aspiration pneumonia can result from in-coordinated swallowing. Distention of the gastrointestinal system with air often occurs, and vomition and diarrhea accompany extreme hyperthermia, struggling to relieve airway obstruction or severe aerophagia. Thus, questions regarding the gastrointestinal system can be helpful.

### Diagnostic Tests

A lateral head and neck radiograph is often helpful to evaluate the extent of the upper airway obstruction. Most bulldogs will have a very thick, long palate. The view must be precisely lateral, as slight obliquity will dramatically increase the apparent thickness of the palate. The overlong soft palate is dramatically different from the normal anatomy of the pharynx. If available, fluoroscopy of the upper airway while the dog is in lateral recumbency can aid in the assessment of the degree of obstruction.

An assessment of the degree of palatal elongation and of laryngeal cartilage collapse is best carried out under general anesthesia. Because of the risks of anesthetizing a brachycephalic dog, this assessment should ideally be carried out when the owners are also ready to proceed with surgical treatment, as necessary. The presence of a hypoplastic trachea may complicate the surgery, as it will be more difficult to place a tracheostomy, and the dog may have more difficulty recovering from any pneumonia that occurs. However, as bulldogs all have relatively narrow tracheas, a hypoplastic trachea is not an absolute contraindication to performing surgery. Furthermore, several anecdotal reports document that a trachea that is severely hypoplastic in a young pup may actually increase in diameter as the animal matures.

## TREATMENT

Management and eventual treatment of the brachycephalic syndrome has to be directed at relieving the upper airway obstruction. Oxygen treatment can theoretically remove the hypoxic drive to breathe, though it often seems to improve the patient. On a more practical level, hyperthermia commonly develops when dogs are in oxygen cages or tents, and this will exacerbate the respiratory distress. Both obvious upper airway obstruction and consequent pulmonary edema can occur. Sedation without intubation will relax the upper airway muscles, and can cause obstruction. Thus, these measures must be undertaken with appropriately cautious monitoring.

In very mild cases of obstruction, or when the owners do not wish to pursue surgery, treatment of any exacerbating factors should be carried out. A single steroid treatment (e.g., 0.5 to 2.0 mg/kg prednisolone IV or IM) to reduce pharyngeal or laryngeal edema or inflammation can relieve temporary swelling. Cooling the animal and providing oxygen while it calms down can return it to a stable state. The use of sedatives to reduce anxiety is problematic, since most sedatives also relax upper airway dilating muscles. The most prudent course is to soothe the animal or leave it alone while monitoring its respiratory rate and pattern closely. If available, noninvasive monitoring of $SaO_2$ (ear oximetry) can be helpful during this period (see "Pulse Oximetry," this volume, p 117), and during management of brachycephalics in the hospital. Owners, of course, must be aware that the animal could have another crisis if the anatomy is not surgically altered. However, if the dog returns to its stable compensated state it may survive months or years before the condition again becomes overt.

If the owner wishes to pursue surgery, and the dog is a good surgical candidate, an examination of the oropharynx under general anesthesia is indicated. The induction of anesthesia will usually be accompanied by complete upper airway obstruction, so intubation should be carried out promptly. However, the conformation and patency of the laryngeal aperture should be assessed quickly before intubation. The presence of laryngeal collapse will lead to a worse prognosis; indeed, if severe laryngeal collapse is present, a chronic tracheostomy should be considered rather than, or in addition to, resection of obstructing upper airway tissue. The mucosal lining of the laryngeal ventricles will often be everted into the airway; these are easily removed and should be. The palate and nares should be resected. These techniques have previously been described by Harvey and others and will not be described in detail. Readers should consult appropriate textbooks of veterinary surgery. As a general rule, once surgery has been undertaken, all resectable tissue should be removed, as the airway will still be narrowed by the distorted facial and pharyngeal anatomy. If the veterinarian does not feel confident in performing these surgeries, a temporary tracheostomy can be performed to allow temporary relief while the dog is referred to a specialist.

Postoperative concerns include care of a tracheostomy, if present; reobstruction of the pharynx due to swelling; and infections. We have also found that some bulldogs require intermittent positive-pressure ventilation for up to a week after surgery. This is apparently due to respiratory muscle fatigue as a consequence of the chronic overload.

Most surgeons will administer steroids for 1 to 2 days postoperatively to minimize swelling. Food and water are withheld to prevent trauma to the pharyngeal tissues and reduce the risk of aspiration for at least 1 to 2 days. Intravenous fluid support must therefore be provided throughout this period. Pulmonary edema or aspiration pneumonia may become apparent during this period, so an increase in respiratory effort or signs of pneumonia should be pursued with chest radiographs. An airway aspirate through the tracheostomy is a trivial procedure, and this sample should be evaluated by cytology and culture and sensitivity. When the animal is sufficiently recovered, small amounts of water are provided and the animal's behavior and respiration monitored closely for several hours. If no problems occur, small amounts of semifluid or wet dog food can be provided.

While retrospective studies have shown that 90% of owners feel their pets are improved by these surgical procedures, it is clear that surgery can only partly correct the abnormal anatomy. These dogs remain partly obstructed, and the workload of their respiratory muscles is still increased.

The anatomy typical of short-faced breeds leads to increased upper airway resistance, and to clinical signs of upper airway obstruction in some individuals. The repertoire of management and treatment approaches open to veterinarians is limited, but can often improve the lives of individual dogs. The improvement of these breeds is a challenge to the breeders that veterinarians can only encourage.

## References and Suggested Reading

Harvey CE and Fink EA: Tracheal diameter: Analysis of radiographic measurements in brachycephalic and non-brachycephalic dogs. J Am Anim Hosp Assoc 18:571, 1982.

Harvey CE: Everted laryngeal saccule surgery in brachycephalic dogs. J Am Anim Hosp Assoc 18:538, 1982.

Harvey CE: Stenotic nares surgery in brachycephalic dogs. J Am Anim Hosp Assoc 18:535, 1982.

Harvey CE: Soft palate resection of brachycephalic dogs. J Am Anim Hosp Assoc 18:533, 1982.

Hendricks JC: State-related changes in breathing: Are we missing sleep-disordered breathing syndromes in veterinary patients? Probl Vet Med 4:265, 1992.

Knecht CD: Upper airway obstruction in brachycephalic dogs. Compend Cont Educ 1:35, 1979.

Leonard HC: Collapse of the larynx and adjacent structures in the dog. J Am Vet Med Assoc 360:137, 1960.

# PARASITES OF THE RESPIRATORY SYSTEM

CRAIG R. REINEMEYER

*Knoxville, Tennessee*

It is uncommon for dogs and cats to be presented for clinical problems that are ultimately attributed to respiratory parasitism. In many instances, respiratory parasites are only detected serendipitously when their reproductive products are discovered during fecal examination. This circumstance results because the respiratory and gastrointestinal tracts are contiguous in the pharynx, and the reproductive products of respiratory parasites are routinely swallowed and passed with feces.

The eggs and larvae of respiratory parasites are not described in detail in this article, and other sources (Georgi and Georgi, 1990; Sloss, Kemp, and Zajac, 1994) are recommended for information about the definitive identification of reproductive products.

The few primary parasites of the respiratory tracts of domestic dogs and cats belong to three major phyla of organisms: nematodes, trematodes, and arthropods.

## NEMATODES

The parasitic group with the greatest number of representatives in the respiratory tract is the nematode superfamily Metastrongyloidea. Female metastrongyloids typically produce thin-shelled eggs that hatch quickly to liberate first-stage larvae (L1). The L1 stage is found in feces, and many species have a unique, S-shaped tail that is useful for identification. Metastrongyloid life cycles often require intermediate or paratenic hosts, but some species are transmitted directly.

In most prior publications, three of the metastrongyloid species of dogs were grouped together in the genus *Filaroides*, but taxonomic evidence suggests that each should be assigned to a separate genus.

### Oslerus osleri

*Oslerus osleri* occurs in feral canids such as wolves, coyotes, dingoes, and foxes, and is only rarely reported as a parasite of the domestic dog.

*Oslerus osleri* adults live within subepithelial, fibrous nodules in the major airways, and are most commonly located near the bifurcation of the trachea. Thin-shelled eggs or first-stage larvae are coughed up and swallowed, and L1s appear in the feces. The L1 is the infective stage of *O. osleri*. This capacity is biologically unique because most other parasitic nematodes require additional larval development in the environment to become infective.

Transmission of *O. osleri* occurs primarily from dam to offspring via regurgitative feeding or through salivary contamination during grooming activities. Horizontal transmission, even among dogs sharing the same pen, occurs rarely. The prepatent period of *O. osleri* ranges from 10 to 18 weeks (Clayton and Lindsay, 1979).

CLINICAL SIGNS AND DIAGNOSIS. Although some dogs with *O. osleri* infection are asymptomatic, most exhibit a chronic cough that can be elicited by tracheal palpation and that worsens with exercise. Heavy infections may result in dyspnea, exercise intolerance, emaciation, and death. The majority of clinical cases occur in young dogs in the first year of life.

The most accurate method of diagnosis is bronchoscopy and direct visualization of parasitic nodules in the major airways. Alternatively, metastrongyloid eggs or larvae may be recovered by tracheal washes or swabs, and tracheal nodules occasionally can be visualized by radiography.

The least invasive method of diagnosis is fecal examination by the Baermann technique or zinc sulfate (sg 1.18) flotation. The sensitivity of these tests is limited, however, because *O. osleri* larvae may be few in number and are shed only intermittently. Multiple fecal samples should be examined in suspected cases, but negative results are inconclusive.

TREATMENT. Despite reported successes with a variety of regimens (Table 1), some authorities consider that no currently available treatment for *O. osleri* is consistently effective (Georgi and Georgi, 1990).

PREVENTION. The preceding caveat suggests that it may be impossible to eradicate *O. osleri* from a breeding kennel. One option is to breed only bitches that have been screened intensively by bronchoscopy. Alternatively, infected bitches can be bred, but pups should be removed at birth and placed with an *Oslerus*-negative foster mother or raised by hand.

Although frequent removal of feces and routine hygiene are good general recommendations for parasite control, horizontal transmission is not considered a major route of infection for *O. osleri*.

### Filaroides hirthi

*Filaroides hirthi* apparently infects only dogs and has not been reported from other carnivores. This nematode occurs most frequently in commercial breeding colonies, but infections have also been reported in privately owned pets.

***Table 1.*** *Parasiticides for Treatment of Respiratory Parasitisms of Dogs and Cats*

| Drug | Spectrum of Activity | Regimen |
|---|---|---|
| Albendazole (Valbazen, SmithKline Beecham) | Fh, Oo | 25 mg/kg q12h × 5 days, PO; may repeat in 2 wk |
| | Pk | 25 mg/kg q12h × 14 days, PO |
| Fenbendazole (Panacur, Hoescht-Roussel) | Cv | 50 mg/kg q24h × 3 days, PO |
| | Ca, Eb, Fh, Pk | 50 mg/kg q24h × 10–14 days, PO |
| | Aa | 20 mg/kg q24h × 5 days, PO; repeat in 5 days |
| Ivermectin (Ivomec, MSD AgVet) | Eb | 0.2 mg/kg, PO |
| | Aa, Oo | 0.4 mg/kg, SC |
| | Pc | 0.2 mg/kg, SC |
| Levamisole (Levasole, Mallinckrodt) | Ca | 10 mg/kg q24h × 5 days, PO; repeat in 9 days |
| Oxfendazole (Synanthic, Syntex) | Oo | 10 mg/kg q24h × 28 days, PO |
| Praziquantel (Droncit, Miles) | Pk | 23 mg/kg q8h × 3 days, PO |

Abbreviations: Aa = *Aelurostrongylus abstrusus*; Ca = *Capillaria aerophila*; Cv = *Crenosoma vulpis*; Eb = *Eucoleus boehmi*; Fh = *Filaroides hirthi*; Oo = *Oslerus osleri*; Pc = *Pneumonyssoides caninum*; Pk = *Paragonimus kellicotti*.

Adult *F. hirthi* live in the pulmonary parenchyma and alveoli, and produce thin-shelled eggs or larvae that are carried up the airways and swallowed. First-stage larvae are infective, and transmission occurs by ingestion of feces or objects contaminated by feces. Horizontal transmission of *F. hirthi* occurs readily among dogs housed together, and some may acquire massive burdens by autoinfection. The prepatent period is approximately 5 weeks.

CLINICAL SIGNS AND DIAGNOSIS. Most infected dogs are asymptomatic, but fatal pulmonary disease attributable to *F. hirthi* has been reported. It should be noted that immunosuppression with corticosteroids and toy-breed status were potential risk factors in some fatalities. Clinical signs may be precipitated or exacerbated by specific treatment for *F. hirthi* infection. This is consistent with the observation of surprisingly little reaction to living worms in the pulmonary parenchyma, but a severe inflammatory response to dead or dying nematodes.

Diagnosis is achieved by demonstration of first-stage larvae in feces using zinc sulfate (sg 1.18) flotation. The sensitivity of other fecal examination techniques (e.g., Baermann, saline smear) is inconsistent for diagnosing *F. hirthi*.

Radiographic lesions of *F. hirthi* infection include linear and nodular interstital infiltrates, with occasional peribronchial and alveolar involvement. Focal granulomatous reaction were observed subsequent to successful anthelmintic therapy.

TREATMENT. Alleviation of clinical signs and termination of larval shedding can be accomplished with albendazole (Valbazen, SmithKline Beecham) or fenbendazole (Panacur, Hoechst-Roussel) (Table 1).

PREVENTION. The most likely sites for endemic *F. hirthi* transmission are breeding colonies and kennels. In these venues, all dogs should be screened by zinc sulfate flotation. If any are found to be infected, it is advisable to administer specific treatment to all males and all nonpregnant, nonlactating females intended for breeding (Erb and Georgi, 1982). Treated dogs should be rigidly segregated from untreated dogs of undetermined infection status. Because L1 stages in fresh feces are immediately infective, hygiene alone cannot totally prevent infection.

It is essential to eliminate *F. hirthi* infections from colonies of dogs used for scientific experimentation because lungworm lesions can be misinterpreted histopathologically as a primary effect of drugs being tested in toxicology or carcinogenicity studies.

### Andersonstrongylus milksi

This metastrongyloid nematode has been recorded only rarely from dogs in North America, and some reports apparently involved misidentifications of *F. hirthi*. Details of the life cycle, pathogenicity, and chemotherapy of *A. milksi* are unknown.

### Aelurostrongylus abstrusus

*Aelurostrongylus abstrusus* is the most common metastrongyloid nematode that uses cats as definitive hosts. Adults reside in the pulmonary parenchyma, and first-stage larvae are swallowed and passed in the feces.

*Aelurostrongylus abstrusus* has an indirect life cycle with a molluscan intermediate host (e.g., terrestrial snails or slugs). Cats are infected by eating molluscs or by ingesting birds or rodents (i.e., paratenic hosts) that feed on snails or slugs. The prepatent period is approximately 4 to 6 weeks (Georgi and Georgi, 1990).

CLINICAL SIGNS AND DIAGNOSIS The majority of *Aelurostrongylus* infections are asymptomatic. When present, clinical signs consist of coughing, sneezing, lethargy, anorexia, and weight loss, and are more apparent in younger cats. Pleural effusion and death have been reported as infrequent sequelae of aelurostrongylosis.

Infections are readily diagnosed by demonstration of first-stage larvae in feces using the Baermann technique. *Aelurostrongylus abstrusus* L1s display an additional spine at the base of the typical S-shaped, metastrongyloid tail. Eosinophilia is an inconsistent feature of *Aelurostrongylus* infection. Accompanying radiographic changes include bronchial thickening, alveolar infiltrates, and increased interstitial opacity.

TREATMENT. Many cases of aelurostrongylosis are self-limiting, with regression of clinical signs within 2 to 3 months of onset. Specific therapy with fenbendazole or ivermectin (Ivomec, Merck Sharp & Dohme) (Table 1) usually alleviates symptoms and disrupts patency within 1 week of treatment.

PREVENTION. *Aelurostrongylus* infections can be prevented by confining cats to preclude predation on birds and rodents, and by protecting outdoor food and water dishes from invasion by slugs or snails.

### *Crenosoma vulpis*

*Crenosoma vulpis* is a parasite of wolves, foxes, and raccoons, and is rarely reported in the dog. The life cycle is similar to that of *Aelurostrongylus abstrusus*, with a molluscan intermediate host and vertebrate paratenic hosts.

CLINICAL SIGNS AND DIAGNOSIS. In a recently reported case, an infected dog had a chronic cough and abnormal lung sounds. Radiography revealed bronchial patterns with some interstitial component throughout the parenchyma.

*Crenosoma* infection can be diagnosed by demonstrating the characteristic first-stage larvae in feces, either with the Baermann technique or by zinc sulfate flotation.

TREATMENT. In the case mentioned previously, a regimen of fenbendazole (Table 1) alleviated clinical signs and stopped larvae shedding for at least 6 weeks (Peterson et al., 1993).

PREVENTION. *Crenosoma* infections in dogs presumably can be prevented by the same prophylactic measures recommended for *A. abstrusus* in cats.

### *Capillaria aerophila*

*Capillaria aerophila*, also known as *Eucoleus aerophilus*, is not a metastrongyloid nematode; it is more closely related to the common intestinal whipworm of dogs. Adult *Capillaria* are embedded in the epithelial lining of the large airways of dogs and cats. Eggs are expelled from the respiratory passages, passed in the feces, and become infective in about 40 days.

The life cycle is not clearly known, but dogs and cats probably become infected with *C. aerophila* by ingesting embryonated eggs or earthworm paratenic hosts. The prepatent period is approximately 3 to 5 weeks.

CLINICAL SIGNS AND DIAGNOSIS. *Capillaria aerophila* infection is fairly common but rarely causes any symptoms. Clinical signs that have been attributed to respiratory capillariasis include wheezing, chronic cough, loss of weight and poor body condition (Campbell, 1991).

Diagnosis is easily accomplished by demonstrating the characteristic eggs with various fecal flotation techniques. It is probably a common occurrence for examiners to misidentify *C. aerophila* eggs as those of *Trichuris vulpis*.

Radiographic signs of capillariasis are consistent with general pulmonary inflammation and are not pathognomonic.

TREATMENT. Therapy is probably unnecessary in asymptomatic animals, but specific treatment (Table 1) reduces environmental contamination with eggs and decreases the risk of future reinfection. Fenbendazole appears to disrupt egg shedding, but it is unknown whether this reflects primary adulticidal activity or the general sterilizing effect of benzimidazole anthelmintics on female worms.

Several reports of anthelmintic efficacy against *C. aerophila* in the dog apparently have involved misidentified infections with *Eucoleus boehmi* (see below).

PREVENTION. Embryonated *Capillaria* eggs are likely to persist in the environment, so cats and dogs should be confined or denied access to contaminated soil or infected earthworms.

### *Eucoleus boehmi*

This nematode, which has frequently been misidentified as *C. aerophila*, is normally found in the mucosa of the nasal passages and associated sinuses. *Eucoleus* eggs enter the environment with nasal discharges or are swallowed and passed with feces. The life cycle of *E. boehmi* is unknown, but is assumed to be direct.

CLINICAL SIGNS AND DIAGNOSIS. *Eucoleus* infections may be asymptomatic, but when present, clinical signs include chronic sneezing or nasal discharge, epistaxis, face rubbing, and other signs of nasal irritation (Campbell, 1991).

Infection can be diagnosed by demonstration of the typical eggs in nasal discharges, swabs, or flushes; eggs are also easily recovered by fecal flotation. *Eucoleus boehmi* infection can be diagnosed histopathologically in biopsies of the nasal mucosa.

TREATMENT. Regimens of ivermectin or fenbendazole alleviate clinical signs and disrupt patency, but improvement may be only temporary (King et al., 1990). Relapses are attributable either to reinfection or to a suppressive rather than nematocidal effect of therapy. Long-term, post-treatment monitoring is indicated for clinical cases.

PREVENTION. The same measures for prevention of *C. aerophila* are assumed to be applicable for *Eucoleus boehmi* infections as well.

## TREMATODES

The trematodes, or flukes, are hermaphroditic parasites with obligatory, indirect life cycles involving one or more intermediate hosts.

### *Paragonimus kellicotti*

*Paragonimus kellicotti* normally occurs in mink and other carnivores, and is found occasionally in the lungs of dogs and cats. Pairs of adult flukes reside in subpleural cysts that communicate directly with a bronchiole. Fluke eggs are produced within the cyst, pass into the bronchiole, and are swept up the airways and swallowed.

The life cycle of *Paragonimus* requires two intermediate hosts: the first is an aquatic snail and the second is a crayfish. Carnivores are infected by ingesting crayfish. Pulmonary cysts are present and egg production begins within 4 to 5 weeks after infection.

CLINICAL SIGNS AND DIAGNOSIS. Most pets with paragonimiasis are presented for a chronic cough that has not responded to various therapies. Spontaneous pneumothorax is an occasional clinical feature of *Paragonimus* infection.

Diagnosis is accomplished by demonstrating the large, operculated eggs in fecal samples. The technique of choice for demonstrating intact trematode eggs is fecal sedimentation, but centrifugal flotation using saturated sucrose (sg 1.275) or zinc sulfate (sg 1.18) solutions recovers identifiable eggs or shells. Typical eggs also can be identified in the rust-colored phlegm that is often present in the pharynx of an infected animal. Thoracic radiography reveals multiloculated cysts in dogs and interstitial nodules in cats; evidence of pneumothorax also may be present.

TREATMENT. Clinical paragonimiasis has been treated successfully with fenbendazole, albendazole, or praziquantel (Droncit, Miles) (Table 1). Efficacy can be documented by the cessation of coughing, disappearance of eggs in the feces, and radiographic regression of cystic lesions within a few weeks of therapy (Dubey, Miller, and Sharma, 1979).

PREVENTION. Paragonimiasis can be prevented by confining predatory or scavenging dogs and cats to preclude ingestion of infected crayfish.

## ARTHROPODS

### *Pneumonyssoides caninum*

*Pneumonyssoides caninum*, the nasal mite, is found in the nasal cavity and associated sinuses of dogs and cats. Transmission is assumed to occur by direct contact with infected animals.

CLINICAL SIGNS AND DIAGNOSIS. Nasal mites cause sneezing, epistaxis, and chronic nasal discharges. An affected animal may show signs of nasal irritation by pawing at its face or rubbing its nose on the ground.

The presence of mites can be detected by direct visualization with a rhinoscope (i.e., an otoscope inserted into the nares), or by finding mites and eggs in the material recovered with nasal swabs or flushes.

TREATMENT. Parenteral ivermectin provided prompt relief for the few dogs in which this regimen has been tested (Table 1).

PREVENTION. Treatment of all affected and in-contact pets should be sufficient for control. Other reservoirs of infection are unlikely because the mites probably do not survive well in the environment.

## Miscellaneous Parasites

Due to space limitations, this article does not address parasitic infections in which pulmonary disease can be an important component of systemic infection (e.g., *Toxoplasma gondii*). Similarly, the parasites of dogs and cats that migrate through pulmonary tissues in the course of normal development (e.g., *Toxocara canis* and *Ancylostoma caninum*) are not discussed.

## References and Suggested Reading

Campbell BG: *Trichuris* and other trichinelloid nematodes of dogs and cats in the United States. Compend Cont Educ Pract Vet 13:769, 1991.
*A review of the biology of* Capillaria, Eucoleus, *and closely related nematodes.*

Clayton HM and Lindsay FEF: *Filaroides osleri* infection in the dog. J Small Anim Pract 20:773, 1979.
*A review of the biology, diagnosis, and management of* Filaroides osleri *infections.*

Dubey JP, Miller TB, and Sharma SP: Fenbendazole for treatment of *Paragonimus kellicotti* infection in dogs. J Am Vet Med Assoc 174:835, 1979.
*A report of the anthelmintic efficacy of fenbendazole against induced* Paragonimus kellicotti *infections.*

Erb HN and Georgi JR: Control of *Filaroides hirthi* in commercially reared beagle dogs. Lab Anim Sci 32:394, 1982.
*A report of successful management of endemic* Filaroides hirthi *infections in large breeding colonies.*

Georgi JR and Georgi ME: *Parasitology for Veterinarians*, 5th edition. Philadelphia, WB Saunders Co, 1990, p 412.
*A textbook presenting fairly complete information on the biology, diagnosis, and management of parasitic infections of domestic animals.*

King RR, Greiner EC, Ackerman N, and Woodard JC: Nasal capillariasis in a dog. J Am Anim Hosp Assoc 26:381, 1990.
*A case report of the presentation, diagnosis, and management of* Eucoleus boehmi *infection in a dog.*

Peterson EN, Barr SC, Gould WJ, et al: Use of fenbendazole for treatment of *Crenosoma vulpis* infection in a dog. J Am Vet Med Assoc 202:1483, 1993.
*A caes report of the presentation, diagnosis, and management of* Crenosoma vulpis *infection in a dog.*

Sloss MW, Kemp RL, and Zajac AM: *Veterinary Clinical Parasitology*, 6th edition. Ames, IA, Iowa State University Press, 1994, pp 198.
*A manual of parasitologic diagnostic techniques with numerous photomicrographs for identification of common parasitisms of domestic animals.*

# TREATMENT OF NASAL ASPERGILLOSIS WITH TOPICAL CLOTRIMAZOLE

AUTUMN P. DAVIDSON
*and* DEMOSTHENES PAPPAGIANIS
*Davis, California*

## ETIOLOGY AND PATHOGENESIS

Canine nasal aspergillosis is characterized by a colonization and invasion of the nasal passages and frontal sinuses, most commonly by *Aspergillus fumigatus*, a ubiquitous, saprophytic species of filamentous fungus. Destruction and necrosis of the nasal mucosa and underlying turbinate bones result, often accompanied by frontal sinus osteomyelitis. *Aspergillus* is regarded as an opportunistic pathogen, suggesting that some preexisting immunologic defect allowed its establishment (Washburn, 1988). Human cancer patients with chemotherapy-induced neutropenia are at significant risk for invasive aspergillus rhinosinusitis (Talbot, Huang, and Provencher, 1991). Alternatively, an *in vitro* inhibition of B- and T-lymphocyte transformation by *A. fumigatus* products is described, suggesting that immunosuppression may result from infection (Sharp, Harvey, and Sullivan, 1991). The clinical signs, diagnosis, and management of nasal aspergillosis are well reviewed (Sharp, 1989). The condition must be distinguished from nasal mites infestation, neoplasia, lymphacytic-plasmacytic rhinitis, and other causes of rhinitis-sinusitis.

## PREVIOUS THERAPIES

Therapeutic recommendations for nasal aspergillosis have included surgery as well as systemic and topical antimycotic medications. Rhinotomy and turbinectomy with perioperative thiabendazole administration results in improvement in less than or equal to 50% of cases. Oral ketoconazole administration is efficacious in 47% of cases, oral fluconazole in 60%, and oral intraconazole in 60 to 70%. Enilconazole applied topically through frontal sinus tubes, twice daily for 7 to 10 days, is efficacious in 80 to 90% of cases, but is not readily available in the United States (Sharp, 1989). Invasive surgical exposure of the nasal passages and frontal sinuses, topical 10% povidone-iodine application, and delayed closure 6 to 8 weeks postoperatively is recommended for refractory cases, but has poor client acceptance (Pavletic and Clark, 1991).

## CLOTRIMAZOLE THERAPY

Clotrimazole is a synthetic imidazole derivative. At concentrations achieved during systemic use, imidazoles impair the biosynthesis of ergosterol, the major component of fungal cell membranes, resulting in interference with certain membrane-bound enzyme systems and fungistatic inhibition of growth (Bodey, 1992). Clotrimazole is fungicidal at certain higher concentrations ($1.5 \times 10^{-4}$ mol/L). Electron microscopic observations indicate clotrimazole causes alteration in the cell membrane with consequent changes in permeability and leakage of cellular constituents in a manner similar to the effect of polyene antifungal antibiotics (Iwata, Yamaguchi, and Hiratani, 1973).

Clotrimazole is available as human topical preparations for cutaneous, oral, or vaginal applications. Clotrimazole has been employed successfully topically in the management of refractory human ophthalmic aspergillosis. Clotrimazole adminstered orally is poorly absorbed; what small amount is absorbed undergoes hepatic metabolism and biliary excretion. Gastrointestinal irritation and cutaneous pruritus are reported human side effects. Absorption of clotrimazole from human vaginal application is low. Fungicidal concentrations remain in the vagina up to 3 days after a single topical application. The 80% or higher cure rate for vaginal candidiasis treated with topical clotrimazole is the same with a dosage of 100 mg applied every 24 hr for 7 days, 200 mg applied every 24 hr for 3 days, or 500 mg applied once (Milsom and Forssman, 1982). Treatment of canine nasal aspergillosis by a 1-hr continuous topical clotrimazole infusion, maximizing exposure of the affected mucosa, was modeled after these findings (Davidson et al., 1992).

Therapy consists of bilateral infusion of a total of 1 gm clotrimazole, dissolved in 1 dl polyethylene glycol 200 into the frontal sinuses and nasal passages. The 1% clotrimazole solution has moderate viscosity, enabling coating of mucous membranes, yet passes through infant feeding tubes without difficulty. The 1-hr infusion is performed under inhalational anesthesia. Ideally, diagnostics (radiology, rhinoscopy, biopsies, and cultures) are performed during the same period of anesthesia as the therapy. Rhinoscopic evidence of fungal plaques and turbinate destruction lends strong clinical support for the diagnosis of nasal aspergillosis. Mycologic, histologic, and serologic studies provide confirmation of aspergillosis (Sharp, Harvey, and Sullivan, 1991).

Clotrimazole is infused through infant feeding tubes placed into the frontal sinuses by trephination as described previously (Sharp, 1989). One tube is placed into each frontal sinus, and an additional tube is passed through the sinus into the ipsilateral caudal nasal passage. The size of the trephine hole into the sinuses

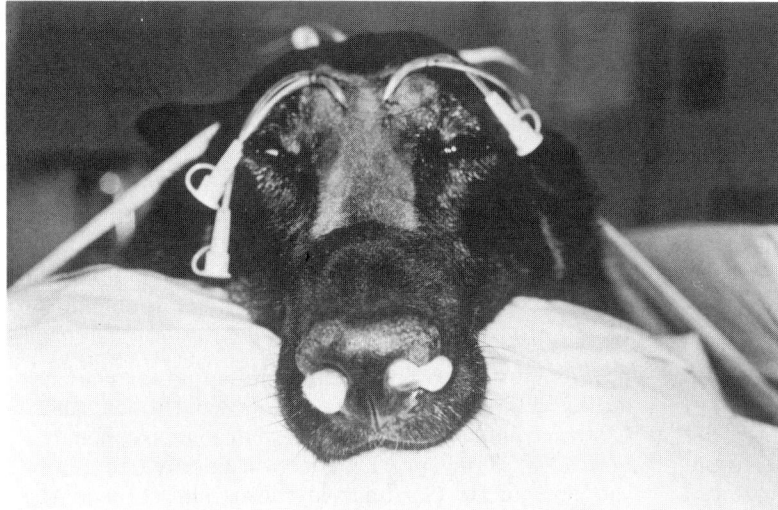

**Figure 1.** Two infant feeding tubes are placed for infusion bilaterally, one into the frontal sinus and one through the frontal sinus into the caudal nasal passage. The nostrils are occluded with dental sponges; cotton-tipped applicators have not yet been added.

should be small, minimizing leakage. Bilateral treatment is always indicated, even in the absence of bilaterally evident disease, as the gross and radiographic changes appear to lag behind infection. The lower airways and esophagus should be protected during the infusion, by placing the dog's nose lower than the nasopharynx, and packing the caudal pharynx and larynx with a laparotomy sponge. Obstruction of the nares with dental sponges or tampons, filling in gaps with cotton-tipped applicators, permits maximal contact of the clotrimazole solution with the entire mucosa (Fig. 1).

Initially, approximately 30 ml of the total solution is used to fill the sinuses and nasal passages, infused by means of 60-ml syringes attached to each feeding tube. The remainder of the solution is then slowly infused over 60 min, keeping the sinuses and nasal passages filled maximally (Fig. 2). The infusion should not require force; if great resistance is met, the patency of the tubes should be evaluated. Clotrimazole should drip *very slowly* from both nares, at a rate of approximately one drop every 3 to 5 sec. Mild manual pressure with a surgical sponge placed over the trephina-

tion sites may be necessary during the infusion to avoid subcutaneous leakage of clotrimazole. At the conclusion of therapy, any clotrimazole remaining in the infusion tubes is emptied into the frontal sinuses and nasal passages by injecting a small amount of air through the tubes, which are then removed. Skin closure over the trephination sites should not be complete, allowing air to escape through the incision, to avoid significant subcutaneous emphysema.

Clotrimazole therapy has been generally well tolerated, with minimal side effects. Mild subcutaneous emphysema and cutaneous inflammation associated with the incisions can occur. Antibiotics are indicated only if significant secondary bacterial infection is present. Mild analgesia may be needed postoperatively (see *CVT XI*, p 82). Overnight hospitalization for observation following the procedure is advised. The majority of epistaxis and subcutaneous emphysema should resolve in 24 hr. A favorable response to clotrimazole therapy is reflected by resolution of the signs of nasal aspergillosis, and can be confirmed rhinoscopically and histologically. Nasal discharge, depigmentation, facial

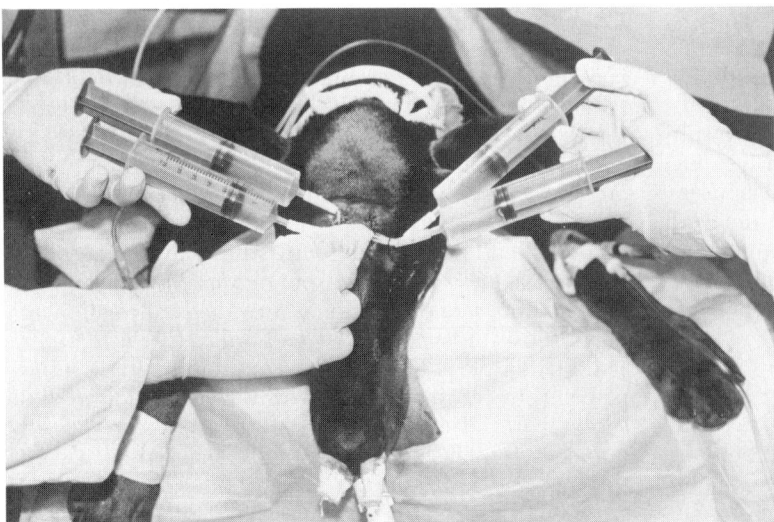

**Figure 2.** After filling the sinuses and nasal passages, a 1-hr continuous infusion is performed simultaneously through all four feeding tubes.

pain, and sneezing diminish markedly from 1 to 2 weeks after therapy. As compared to twice-daily infusion of an antimycotic solution, patient discomfort is minimized, the contact of clotrimazole with the affected mucosal surfaces is maximized, and hospitalization time and expense are markedly reduced. Concurrent systemic antifungal therapy has not been found to be advantageous, and may interfere with the proposed fungicidal effect of the drug. In severe cases complicated by chronicity or immunosuppression, a second treatment performed 3 to 4 weeks later may be indicated. Cases selected for topical clotrimazole therapy should have aspergillosis limited to the frontal sinuses and nasal passages.

### References and Suggested Reading

Bodey GP: Azole antifungal agents. Clin Infect Dis 14 (suppl 1):S161, 1992.
  *A review of the azole antifungal compounds' mechanism of action, spectrum of activity, pharmacokinetics, adverse effects, and clinical efficacy.*
Davidson AP, Komtebedde J, Pappagianis D, et al: Treatment of nasal aspergillosis with topical clotrimazole. *In* Proc 10th Ann Vet Med Forum, 1992, p 307.
  *Results of topical therapy for nasal aspergillosis evaluated in 21 dogs.*

Iwata K, Yamaguchi H, and Hiratani T: Mode of action of clotrimazole. Sabouraudia 11:158, 1973.
  *Describes studies showing that clotrimazole is fungicidal at high concentrations, its lethal effect secondary to membrane damage allowing leakage of cellular constituents of susceptible fungi.*
Milsom I and Forssman L: Treatment of vaginal candidosis with a single 500-mg clotrimazole pessary. Br J Vener Dis 58:124, 1982.
  *Reports the results of a double-blind study of the therapeutic efficacy of a single 500-mg topical clotrimazole application for vaginal candidiasis.*
Pavletic MM and Clark GN: Open nasal cavity and frontal sinus treatment of chronic canine aspergillosis. Vet Surg 20:43, 1991.
  *The potential clinical application of surgery with delayed closure of the nasal cavity and frontal sinus in nasal aspergillosis.*
Sharp NJ: Nasal aspergillosis. *In* Kirk RW (ed): *Current Veterinary Therapy X.* Philadelphia, WB Saunders Co, 1989, p 1106.
  *A review of the clinical signs, etiology, diagnosis, and management of nasal aspergillosis, using systemic and/or topical therapy.*
Sharp NJ, Harvey CE, and Sullivan M: Canine nasal aspergillosis and penicilliosis. Compend Cont Educ Vet 13:41, 1991.
  *A review of the causative factors, pathogenesis, epidemiology, therapy, and prognosis of canine nasal aspergillosis.*
Talbot GH, Huang A, and Provencher M: Invasive aspergillus rhinosinusitis in patients with acute leukemia. Rev Infect Dis 13:219, 1991.
  *A summary of the potentially lethal complication of invasive aspergillosis in neutropenic cancer patients, reviewing therapy and preventative measures.*
Washburn RG, Kennedy DWW, Begley MG, et al: Chronic fungal sinusitis in apparently normal hosts. Medicine (Baltimore) 67:231, 1988.
  *A discussion of noninvasive fungal sinusitis in immunocompetent patients unresponsive to antibiotic therapy.*

# LARYNGEAL PARALYSIS

DALE E. BJORLING

*Madison, Wisconsin*

Laryngeal paralysis is characterized by failure of the vocal folds and arytenoid cartilages to abduct during inspiration. This is due to loss of innervation of the intrinsic musculature of the larynx. The intrinsic muscles of the larynx receive motor innervation through the recurrent laryngeal nerves. Motor neurons that supply the intrinsic muscles of the larynx arise in the brainstem and accompany the vagi to the level of the thoracic inlet, at which point they separate into the recurrent laryngeal nerves. The right recurrent laryngeal nerve passes around the right subclavian artery, and the left around the arch of the aorta, before returning to the larynx.

Laryngeal paralysis has been reported in both dogs and cats. Laryngeal paralysis can occur unilaterally, but this seldom results in clinically apparent disease in dogs and cats. Failure of the vocal folds and arytenoid cartilages to abduct during inspiration due to bilateral laryngeal paralysis results in marked inspiratory dyspnea.

## ETIOLOGY

The causes of laryngeal paralysis can be generally grouped into congenital, systemic neuromuscular or metabolic diseases, trauma, inflammation, and idiopathic. Congenital laryngeal paralysis appears to be inheritable and has been reported to affect Siberian huskies, bouvier des Flandres, English bulldogs, and possibly bull terriers, before 18 months of age (Aron, 1989; *CVT XI*, p 343). Laryngeal paralysis has been observed as one manifestation of various peripheral neuropathies, including myasthenia gravis (Braund et al., 1989). Hypothyroidism alone or in conjunction with peripheral neuropathy has been associated with laryngeal paralysis (Braund et al., 1989). However, a consistent relationship between hypothyroidism and laryngeal paralysis has not been established.

Laryngeal paralysis has also been reported in dogs and cats due to traumatic injury of the recurrent laryngeal nerves during surgery and as a result of animal bites or blunt trauma. Less common causes of loss of function of the recurrent laryngeal nerves include inflammation due to local abscessation, parasitic infiltration, or neoplasia.

Without question, the vast majority of cases of laryngeal paralysis in dogs and cats are due to unknown (idiopathic) causes (Aron, 1989; White, 1989). In dogs, this is most commonly observed in large-breed animals (Labrador retrievers, Saint Bernards, golden retrievers,

Siberian huskies) older than 7 years. Other causes of laryngeal paralysis should be eliminated to establish a diagnosis of idiopathic laryngeal paralysis.

## DIAGNOSIS

### History and Clinical Signs

Owners commonly seek veterinary care for animals with laryngeal paralysis because of exercise intolerance; increased effort and noise associated with inspiration (laryngeal stridor); altered vocalization; and gagging, retching, or coughing associated with swallowing food or water. Affected animals are often hypoxemic and may be in obvious respiratory distress, and syncope may occur (LaHue, 1989; Love, Waterman, and Lang, 1987). Airway obstruction due to laryngeal paralysis in dogs has resulted in pulmonary edema (Kerr, 1989), and this can contribute to respiratory distress. Laryngeal paralysis should be considered in animals that exhibit these clinical signs.

Laryngeal stridor and inspiratory respiratory distress are the direct result of an inability of the animal to increase inspiratory airflow upon demand. The animal is unable to increase inspiratory airflow because the diameter of the larynx is fixed due to failure of the arytenoid cartilages and vocal folds to abduct. Coughing and gagging while eating or drinking is due to aspiration of food or water. It is unclear whether aspiration is due to incomplete adduction of the arytenoid cartilages and vocal folds or incoordinated swallowing as a result of altered pharyngeal innervation associated with laryngeal paralysis.

### Electromyography

Function of the intrinsic muscles of the larynx has been evaluated by electromyography in some animals to confirm the presence of laryngeal paralysis (Braund et al., 1989). Results of electromyography have not always been consistent with clinically apparent laryngeal paralysis. This is in part due to difficulties associated with accurate placement of electrodes into the intrinsic muscles of the larynx. This procedure is infrequently used to diagnose laryngeal paralysis because of the need for specialized equipment and uncertainty of accurate electrode placement.

### Radiography

Radiographic evaluation of the larynx may identify the presence of cervical or intralaryngeal masses but is seldom useful in diagnosing laryngeal paralysis. Thoracic radiographs should be made of severely dyspneic animals to evaluate the lungs for the presence of pulmonary edema, pneumonia, or other intrathoracic causes of dyspnea. Aspiration pneumonia is uncommon but occasionally accompanies laryngeal paralysis. Thoracic radiographs should be interpreted with caution. Airway obstruction due to laryngeal paralysis can cause radiographically apparent atelectasis that may be confused with parenchymal disease (Fig. 1).

### Laryngoscopic Examination

A diagnosis of laryngeal paralysis is suggested by a history and clinical signs consistent with this disorder. The diagnosis is confirmed in these animals by direct laryngoscopic examination while the animal is lightly anesthetized. A short-acting thiobarbiturate (thiamylal sodium or sodium pentothal) is given intravenously to allow examination of the larynx while the animal is spontaneously breathing. The barbiturate is administered slowly in 2 to 4 mg/kg boluses, and the total dose should not usually exceed 6 to 10 mg/kg. This will usually provide adequate restraint for laryngeal examination but not suppress spontaneous breathing. Additional boluses may be given if needed, but laryngeal function cannot be evaluated if the animal is not breathing spontaneously.

The larynx should be examined during several respiratory cycles. It is often useful to have an assistant watch the animal and inform the person performing the examination each time the animal makes an obvious inspiratory effort. The arytenoid cartilages and vocal folds normally abduct in a coordinated manner at the onset of each inspiration. In the presence of laryngeal paralysis, the arytenoid cartilages and vocal folds are neither completely adducted or abducted, but rather remain in a neutral position (Fig. 2A). Weak, fluttering movements or nearly complete adduction of the arytenoid cartilages and vocal folds may be observed due to changes in airway pressure and airflow. Occasionally, spastic, twitching movements of the arytenoid cartilages and vocal folds may be observed. Passive or spastic movement of the arytenoid cartilages and vocal folds should not be confused with normal, purposeful abduction. Sudden expiratory openings related to coughing should not be confused with inspiratory abduction. It is useful to examine unaffected animals while similarly anesthetized to gain an appreciation for normal laryngeal function.

## TREATMENT

Laryngeal paralysis can cause respiratory distress, which requires emergency treatment. Initial therapy for these animals should include supplemental oxygen, steroids (dexamethasone 2 to 4 mg/kg IV) and, if pulmonary edema is present, diuretics (furosemide 2 mg/kg IV). (For a more complete discussion of treatment of respiratory distress, please see *CVT X*, p 195.) Performance of a tracheostomy is very rarely needed but should be considered for animals that do not respond to supportive care (see "Temporary Tracheostomy, this volume, p 179).

Conservative treatment of laryngeal paralysis (reduced activity, stress avoidance, tranquilization) is seldom effective in preventing intermittent or continuous inspiratory stridor or respiratory distress and will have no effect on coughing or gagging while the animal is eating or drinking. The primary goal of surgery is to increase the fixed diameter of the larynx to a size that allows airflow compatible with the animal's activity pattern. It is not necessary to create a fixed diameter of the larynx equivalent to that normally attained during inspiration, and this in fact will predispose the animal to aspiration of food, water, and saliva. Surgical procedures used to treat laryngeal paralysis include partial laryngectomy, castellated laryngofissure combined with vocal fold resection, and fixing one of the arytenoid cartilages in an abducted position (arytenoid lateralization).

## Partial Laryngectomy

Partial laryngectomy consists of removal of one or both vocal folds and/or removal of a portion of the dorsolateral aspect of the corniculate process of one of the arytenoid cartilages. Removal of the vocal folds alone

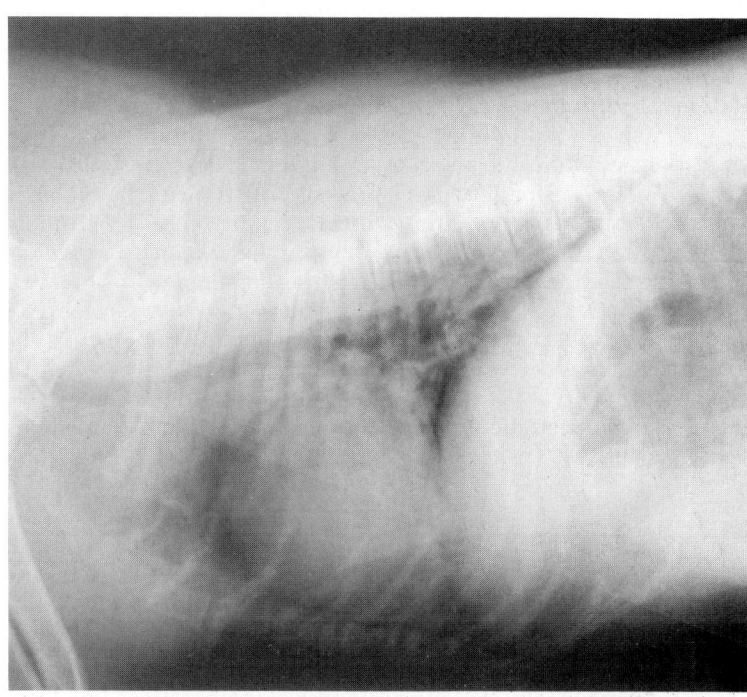

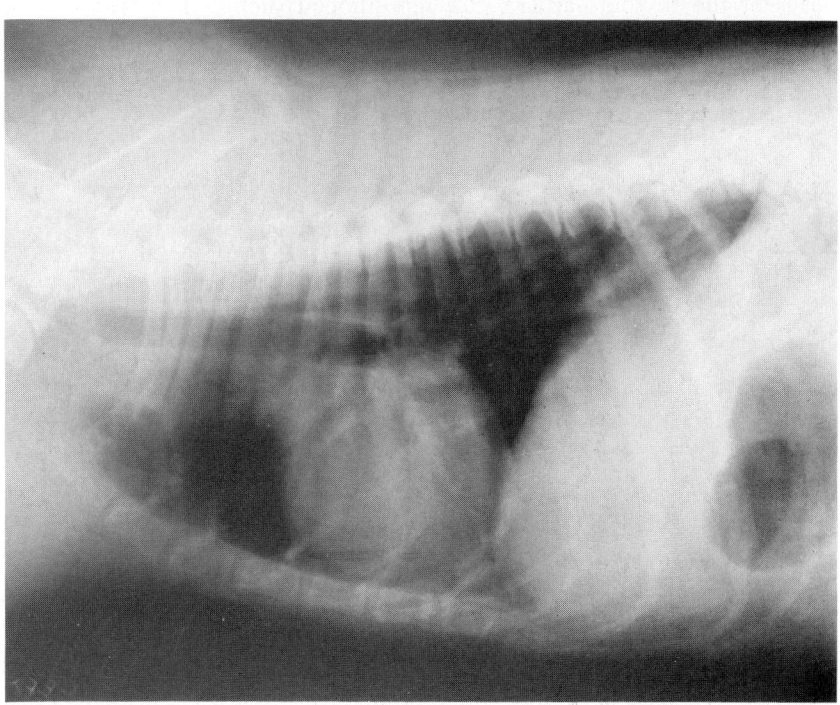

**Figure 1.** Lateral thoracic radiographs of a Labrador retriever with laryngeal paralysis. Initial radiograph (A) demonstrates increased radiodensity of the parenchyma suggestive of lung disease. The animal was anesthetized, ventilated with positive pressure, and a subsequent radiograph was made 1 hr later (B). This demonstrates that the changes apparent in the initial radiograph were due to atelectasis associated with upper airway obstruction.

will alleviate symptoms in some animals. However, the opening created is often insufficient, and signs may recur if scar tissue forms (Ross et al., 1991).

Removal of the vocal folds may be performed through an oral approach or via a ventral laryngotomy. The oral approach necessitates that the mucosal defects be left open, and postoperative formation of scar tissue can result in laryngeal obstruction. Removal of the vocal folds through a ventral laryngotomy allows more complete removal of the vocal folds and vocalis muscle and primary closure of the mucosa with sutures. Formation of scar tissue that obstructs the larynx has not been reported after ventral laryngotomy in dogs or cats. The ventral laryngotomy approach can also be used to treat formation of scar tissue after vocal fold removal through the mouth (Matushek and Bjorling, 1988).

Removal of part of the arytenoid cartilage is most commonly performed through the mouth using cutting forceps. Care must be taken to avoid removing too much of the arytenoid cartilage, predisposing the animal to aspiration of food and water. Partial arytenoidectomy should not be performed bilaterally. Aspiration of food and water and subsequent development of aspiration pneumonia is a relatively common occurrence after partial arytenoidectomy, and bilateral partial arytenoidectomy increases the potential for aspiration (Ross et al., 1991). The author does not recommend partial arytenoidectomy for treatment of laryngeal paralysis because of the relatively high complication rate.

### Castellated Laryngofissure

The goal of castellated laryngofissure is to increase laryngeal circumference (Gourley, Paul, and Gregory, 1983). A castellated, or stepped, incision, is made in the ventral aspect of the thyroid cartilage. The two halves of the thyroid cartilage are repositioned such that the length of the flap created by the stepped incision is added to the circumference of the larynx. It is recommended that the vocal folds be resected during

this procedure to further increase the diameter of the laryngeal opening.

Although good functional results have been reported after this procedure, it does not appear to be superior to arytenoid lateralization (Burbidge, Goulden, and Jones, 1991). This procedure is technically more difficult and is therefore performed less often than arytenoid lateralization.

### Arytenoid Lateralization

Arytenoid lateralization entails a ventrolateral approach to the larynx, disarticulation of the arytenoid cartilage from the rest of the larynx, and placement of one or more sutures between the muscular process of the arytenoid cartilage and the cricoid or thyroid cartilage (LaHue, 1989; White, 1989). This fixes the arytenoid cartilage and associated vocal fold in a lateral position, increasing the diameter of the laryngeal opening (Fig. 2B). Placement of sutures between the muscular process of the arytenoid cartilage and either the thyroid or cricoid cartilage has been described; however, better results are more consistently achieved when the sutures are placed through the cricoid cartilage (LaHue, 1989), and the author prefers this technique.

When first reported, it was recommended that arytenoid lateralization be performed bilaterally. It has subsequently been found that unilateral arytenoid lateralization provides similar clinical improvement, with a lower incidence of aspiration. Bilateral arytenoid lateralization should be reserved for those animals that fail to improve satisfactorily after unilateral arytenoid lateralization. Unilateral arytenoid lateralization has been shown to significantly increase arterial oxygen tensions in dogs with laryngeal paralysis (Love, Waterman, and Lane, 1987) and is currently the most commonly performed surgical procedure for treatment of laryngeal paralysis in dogs and cats.

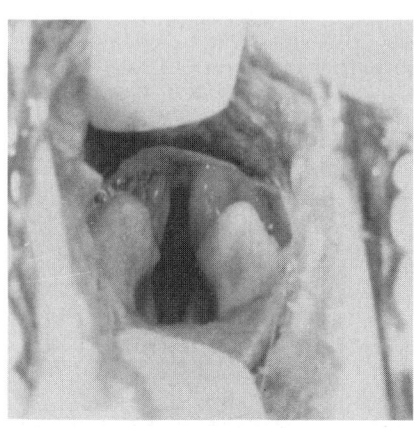

A

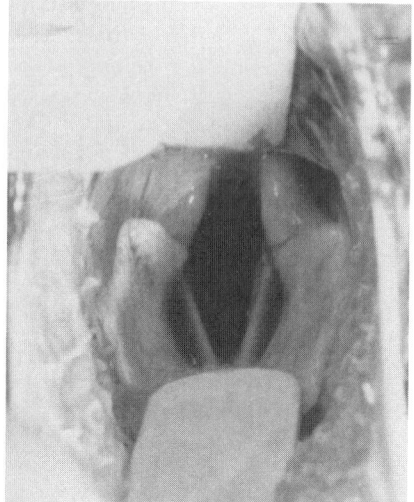

B

**Figure 2.** *A*, Laryngeal examination of dog with laryngeal paralysis. The arytenoid cartilages and vocal folds are in a neutral position, neither adducted or abducted. *B*, Laryngeal examination of same dog after lateralization of the right arytenoid cartilage demonstrates abduction of the arytenoid cartilage and vocal fold.

## PROGNOSIS

Arytenoid lateralization appears to provide satisfactory functional improvement in as many as 90% of treated animals (LaHue, 1989; White, 1989). Many of the animals affected by laryngeal paralysis are Labrador retrievers used for hunting, and these animals can commonly resume moderately strenuous activity after surgery. Increased inspiratory sounds often continue to be heard after surgery, but these should be less harsh and lower pitched. Vocalization is altered after this procedure, and many animals will occasionally cough while eating and drinking. Interestingly, the incidence of aspiration pneumonia after this procedure appears to be quite low.

Pneumonia is obviously a serious and life-threatening complication of this disorder. Transtracheal aspiration should be performed to identify the causative organisms, and appropriate antibiotic therapy instituted. If aspiration of food persists postoperatively, a variety of consistencies of food should be tried in an attempt to determine whether a particular consistency of food will diminish aspiration.

The most common complications of treatment of laryngeal paralysis are lack of improvement in the animal's clinical signs or recurrence of signs. It must be assumed until proven otherwise that surgery has failed to provide an adequate laryngeal opening or that scar tissue or swelling (possibly due to infection) is obstructing the airway. In any event, failure of the animal to improve or recurrence of signs should be evaluated by repeated laryngeal examination and consideration of treatment alternatives.

### References and Suggested Reading

Aron DN: Laryngeal paralysis. *In* Kirk RW (ed): *Current Veterinary Therapy X.* Philadelphia, WB Saunders Co, 1989, p. 343.

Braund KG, Steinberg, S, Shores A, et al: Laryngeal paralysis in immature and mature dogs as one sign of a more diffuse polyneuropathy. J Am Vet Med Assoc 194:1753, 1989.

Burbidge HM, Goulden BE, and Jones RR: An experimental evaluation of castellated laryngofissure and bilateral lateralisation for the relief of laryngeal paralysis in dogs. Aust Vet J 68:268, 1991.

Gourley IM, Paul H, and Gregory C: Castellated laryngofissure and vocal fold resection for the treatment of laryngeal paralysis in the dog. J Am Vet Med Assoc 182:1084, 1983.

Kerr LY: Pulmonary edema secondary to upper airway obstruction in the dog: A review of nine cases. J Am Anim Hosp Assoc 25:207, 1989.

LaHue TR: Treatment of laryngeal paralysis in dogs by unilateral cricoarytenoid laryngoplasty. J Am Anim Hosp Assoc 25:317, 1989.

Love S, Waterman AE, and Lane JG: The assessment of corrective surgery for canine laryngeal paralysis by blood gas analysis: A review of thirty-five cases. J Small Anim Pract 28:597, 1987.

Matushek KJ and Bjorling DE: A mucosal flap technique for correction of laryngeal webbing: Results in four dogs. Vet Surg 17:318, 1988.

Ross JT, Matthiesen DT, Noone KE, et al: Complications and long-term results after partial laryngectomy for the treatment of idiopathic laryngeal paralysis in 45 dogs. Vet Surg 20:169, 1991.

White RAS: Unilateral arytenoid lateralization: An assessment of technique and long term results in 61 dogs with laryngeal paralysis. J Small Anim Pract 30:543, 1989.

# INFECTIOUS TRACHEOBRONCHITIS

RICHARD B. FORD
*Raleigh, North Carolina*

Infectious tracheobronchitis (ITB)—also called kennel cough, bordetellosis, and canine cough—is the most common infectious respiratory infection of dogs. Affecting the larynx, tachea, bronchi, and occasionally the pulmonary interstitium, this highly contagious disease has worldwide distribution. The clinical disease is characterized by an acute-onset, high-pitched "honking" cough lasting from 1 to 2 weeks. Respiratory complications associated with secondary bacterial infection and airway collapse are occasionally encountered, and may substantially prolong the clinical course. Several organisms have been implicated in the cause of ITB, and most infections are likely to be associated with multiple agents. *Bordetella bronchiseptica* is the most common bacteria recovered from affected dogs, while canine parainfluenza virus is the most common viral isolate. Although the majority of infections are self-limiting, antimicrobial and supportive antitussive therapy are indicated.

## CAUSATIVE ORGANISMS

Multiple bacteria and viruses have been implicated in the etiopathogenesis of ITB. However, since some of the causative organisms can be isolated from healthy dogs, a direct cause-and-effect relationship is difficult to establish. Clinical ITB is generally recognized as occurring subsequent to two or more organisms acting synergistically on respiratory epithelium in the larynx, trachea, and bronchi.

*Bordetella bronchiseptica* is still recognized as the most common bacteria isolated from dogs with ITB. The ability of *B. bronchiseptica* to adhere to respiratory cilia and to colonize in the respiratory tract may lead to complete ciliostasis within 3 hr following attachment. *Bordetella bronchiseptica* may also compromise local immune responses within the respiratory tract by secreting adenylate cyclase, impairing the ability of alveolar macrophages to kill phagocytized bacteria. Of particular significance is the fact that *B. bronchiseptica* may facilitate colonization of respiratory epithelium by other organisms, a critical factor during natural infections (Bemis, 1988).

The canine parainfluenza virus is a primary respiratory pathogen. Although a parainfluenza virus is isolated in up to 50% of children with viral croup (Thomsen and Edmonds, 1991), the canine strain of parainfluenza associated with ITB in dogs is not regarded as zoonotic (Ford and Vaden, 1990). Infection may involve the epithelium from the nasal cavity to the bronchioli and peribronchial lymph nodes. Although clinical signs develop at about 9 days following exposure and last less than 1 week, viral shedding may last for up to 9 days. Persistent infections have not been documented.

Mycoplasmas have been recovered from the respiratory tract in 20 to 25% of the healthy dog population and in only 34% of dogs with documented pulmonary disease, including ITB (Randolph et al., 1993). The role of mycoplasms in causing clinical signs of ITB appears to be one of facilitation.

Other organisms occasionally recovered from dogs with ITB include canine adenovirus type 1 and canine adenovirus type 2; canine herpesvirus; reovirus types 1, 2, and 3; as well as the canine distemper virus. Although ureaplasmas have been isolated from tracheobronchial specimens of a dog with pulmonary disease, their role in ITB is not considered significant.

## CLINICAL SIGNS

Dogs with uncomplicated ITB are characteristically presented for a paroxysmal, high-pitched cough described as a "goose-honk" or "seal-bark." This characteristic cough is attributable to laryngitis and swelling of the vocal folds. At presentation, the history typically includes the complaint of episodic, severe coughing, particularly manifest during periods of excitement or increased activity. Affected dogs will generally maintain a normal appetite and are free of other clinical signs. There is no age, breed, or sex predisposition. Frequently, there is a history of recent (within 2 to 10 days) exposure to other dogs. Since clinical signs cannot be uniformly linked to infection by a single organism, knowledge of the affected dog's vaccination status is generally not useful in ruling a diagnosis in or out. Clinical signs may resolve spontaneously within 2 weeks from the time of onset.

Affected dogs will produce excess secretions from the trachea and bronchi. Attempting to expel these secretions following an episode of cough, the dog may arch its back, open its mouth, retch or gag, and ultimately discharge a small volume of white, mucoid liquid. Owners frequently misinterpret this behavior as vomiting. In practice, there is little value in attempting to define the cough as "productive" versus "nonproductive," since the volume of secretions is highly variable from one case to another and dogs are likely to swallow secretions after expectoration.

Physical examination is unremarkable with the exception that a cough may be elicited in most, but not all, dogs by manipulating the trachea. On occasion, dogs will present with mild rhinitis and a serous to mucopurulent nasal discharge.

Complications secondary to ITB in otherwise healthy dogs are rare, the most serious being bacterial bronchopneumonia, usually associated with *B. bronchiseptica*, in untreated dogs. The occurrence of ITB in dogs with underlying respiratory disease, particularly chronic airway disease, may lead to airway collapse, obstruction and, ultimately, death. Miniature and toy-breed dogs with congenital airway collapse, dogs with chronic bronchitis, and dogs with immotile cilia syndrome (ciliary dyskinesia) should be considered at increased risk of developing life-threatening complications subsequent to ITB.

## DIFFERENTIAL DIAGNOSIS

Infectious tracheobronchitis is the primary cause of acute-onset, uncomplicated cough in dogs. Since most infections are self-limiting, with or without treatment, spontaneous resolution of signs within 2 weeks of onset is an important consideration in ruling out other causes of cough. Table 1 lists the differential diagnoses for dogs presented for acute cough (Ford and Roudebush, 1988).

## DIAGNOSIS

A clinical diagnosis of ITB is made on the basis of the history, physical examination, and clinical signs. Results of laboratory testing are expected to be within normal limits unless underlying complications are present. A complete blood count (CBC), biochemical profile, heartworm antigen test, and thoracic radiographs are indicated in the presence of fever, lethargy, inappetence, or when evidence of respiratory distress or airway obstruction exists. Dogs with combined *B. bronchiseptica* and parainfluenza virus infection may have radiographic evidence of lobar consolidation. Transtracheal aspiration from dogs with complicated ITB typically reveals a neutrophilic exudate and a mixture of gram-negative and gram-positive bacteria.

Diagnostic confirmation of ITB is seldom pursued in clinical practice, since attempts to isolate *B. bronchiseptica* and one or more viruses are required and will require several days to complete. Serologic studies for the presence of antibody (IgG) to *B. bronchiseptica* and parainfluenza virus are not recommended, since secretory IgA is the predominant antibody elicited during an infection. A negative serum IgG titer does not rule out infection.

## THERAPY

Despite the role of viruses in ITB, antimicrobial therapy is still recommended as empiric therapy against

**Table 1.** *Differential Diagnoses for Acute-Onset Cough in Dogs*

| Airway Disease | Pulmonary Vascular Disease | Pulmonary Parenchymal Disease |
|---|---|---|
| Tonsillitis | Heartworm disease | Pneumonia (bacterial or viral) |
| Pharyngitis | Pulmonary edema | |
| Laryngitis | Congestive heart failure | |
| Laryngeal paralysis | | |
| Tracheobronchitis | | |
| Tracheitis | | |
| Tracheal collapse | | |
|    Acquired or | | |
|    Congenital | | |
| Tracheal neoplasia | | |
| Tracheal osteochondral dysplasia | | |
| Foreign body | | |
| Aspiration | | |
| Respiratory parasites | | |
|    *Filaroides osleri* | | |

*B. bronchiseptica.* Orally administered tetracycline, 22 mg/kg every 8 hr for a minimum of 7 days, is an inexpensive, highly effective treatment for *B. bronchiseptica.* To avoid tooth discoloration in puppies, tetracycline should be avoided in pregnant females during the last 3 weeks of pregnancies and during the first 2 months of life. As an alternative, trimethoprim-sulfonamide may be administered orally at 15 mg/kg twice daily for 7 to 14 days. However, there is no evidence that antimicrobial treatment will significantly decrease the duration of clinical signs, nor is it known to decrease the transmissibility of either *B. bronchiseptica* or associated viruses. In mild, uncomplicated cases, antimicrobial therapy is optional.

Short-term administration of prednisolone at anti-inflammatory doses (0.25 to 0.5 mg/kg, every 12 hr) orally for 5 to 7 days is justified. Corticosteroids rapidly diminish the intensity of cough; are safe to administer in dogs with active, uncomplicated ITB; and may even reduce the volume of respiratory secretions produced. Like antimicrobials, corticosteroids are not likely to shorten the course of infection nor alter the period of active shedding for either bacteria or viruses. Furthermore, short-term administration of corticosteroids does not put the infected dog at risk of developing a complicated infection (Ford, 1984). Direct intratracheal administration of either antimicrobials or corticosteroids offers no advantage over oral administration.

Aerosol therapy is seldom required in the treatment of dogs with ITB and is generally reserved for those with complicated infections. Nebulization of saline with and without antibiotics has been shown to benefit patients with excessive accumulation of respiratory secretions and those with *B. bronchiseptica* infection. Four to 6 ml of sterile saline can be nebulized in 15 to 20 min up to four times daily. Nebulization of antimicrobials is reserved for dogs with bronchopneumonia when orally administered antimicrobials have not been effective. Gentamicin, kanamycin, and polymyxin B have been shown to reduce the population of *B. bronchiseptica* in the trachea and bronchi of affected dogs for up to 3 days following discontinuation of drug (Bemis and

Appel, 1977). Nebulization of mucolytic agents, such as acetylcysteine, is not recommended, since these compounds are irritating and act to liquify respiratory secretions, making expectoration difficult.

Several other products have been used to treat canine ITB with little or no success. The use of over-the-counter antitussives is discouraged, since they have little or no anti-inflammatory activity and are usually ineffective at suppressing cough in dogs with ITB. Narcotic antitussives, while moderately effective cough suppressants, may compromise ventilation and lead to the accumulation of secretions in the lower airways. In complicated ITB, suppression of cough with narcotic antitussives is not recommended. The therapeutic efficacy of saline expectorants, guaifenesin, inhaled volatile oils, and bronchodilators in treating respiratory infections in dogs has not been established. As such, these products are not currently recommended in the treatment of canine ITB.

## PREVENTION AND CONTROL

A comprehensive vaccination program is still regarded as the most important factor in reducing the prevalence and severity of ITB in the individual animal as well as among animals subjected to confinement within a kennel environment. Despite the fact that ITB is a localized, self-limiting infection, the prevalence of outbreaks, especially within kennels, and the effectiveness of the airborne route of transmission, is strong justification for routine vaccination of all dogs.

When selecting a vaccine that will provide protection against ITB, vaccination with the following antigens is indicated: *B. bronchiseptica*, canine parainfluenza virus, canine adenovirus type 2, and canine distemper virus. Each of these antigens may be administered parenterally as commercially available vaccines. Alternatively, two products containing a combination of avirulent live *B. bronchiseptica* and modified live canine parainfluenza virus are available for intranasal administration.

Vaccines administered by injection are vulnerable to

neutralization by maternal antibody; dogs vaccinated prior to 4 months of age should be boostered at 4 months of age to ensure effective immunization. Two injections are required initially, 2 to 4 weeks apart, usually beginning at 3 months of age. Parenteral vaccines produce high agglutinating titers (IgG) lasting at least 12 months. Exposure following immunization by the parenteral route is expected to lessen the severity of signs but may not completely prevent respiratory infection. Annual boosters are recommended.

Intranasal vaccines appear to be capable of stimulating the production of both secretory IgA and IgG following a single inoculation. A protective local immune response occurs within 4 days, a potential advantage in boarding kennel and shelter management. Although puppies may be vaccinated as early as 2 weeks of age, the duration of immunity following intranasal vaccination may last only 10 to 12 months. Annual boosters or vaccination 7 days prior to kennel confinement is recommended. A small percentage of dogs are reported to develop postvaccinal cough or nasal discharge for 3 to 10 days following intranasal vaccination. Some dogs may require antimicrobial treatment.

Combined canine parainfluenza virus and *B. bronchiseptica* vaccines are associated with higher serum antibody titers than those following vaccination with monovalent vaccines. Furthermore, clinical signs following postvaccinal challenge are less severe suggesting a bacterial-viral vaccinal synergism (Konter, Wegrzyn, and Goodnow, 1981). There is currently no approved mycoplasma bacterin available for use in dogs.

The incidence of ITB outbreaks within confined environments (e.g., veterinary hospitals, boarding kennels, shelters) can be reduced by minimizing population density and maximizing ventilation to more than 12 air changes per hour. Strict segregation of dogs believed to have been exposed to ITB and dogs suspected of having ITB is critical in decreasing the likelihood of transmission. When handling infected dogs, the use of disposable dishware in kennels is strongly recommended. Kennel personnel can further decrease the risk of transmitting infectious organisms by wearing clean, disposable gloves when handling coughing dogs. Household bleach (5.6% sodium hypochlorite) diluted with water by adding 1 part bleach to 32 parts water is an effective, inexpensive virucidal solution recommended for use in contaminated facilities.

## References and Suggested Reading

Bemis DA and Appel MJG: Aerosol, parenteral and oral antibiotic treatment of *Bordetella bronchiseptica* infections in dogs. J Am Vet Med Assoc 170: 1082, 1977.
  *Compares efficacy of aerosol therapy with parenteral and oral antibiotic preparations.*
Bemis DA: Current strategies for the control of canine infectious tracheobronchitis. *Proceedings from the Symposium on Chronic Cough.* Eastern States Veterinary Conference. Orlando, FL, 1988, p 22.
  *Reviews the role of B. bronchiseptica in canine tracheobronchitis and addresses control measures, including intranasal vaccination.*
Ford RB: Concurrent use of corticosteroids and antimicrobial drugs in the treatment of infectious diseases in small animals. J Am Vet Med Assoc 185: 1142, 1984.
  *Reviews both indications and contraindications for the use of corticosteroids therapy in animals with confirmed infections.*
Ford RB and Roudebush P: Chronic cough. *In* Ford RB (ed): *Clinical Signs and Diagnosis in Small Animal Practice.* New York, Churchill Livingstone, 1988, p 203.
  *Outlines the diagnostic approach to the small animal patient presented for chronic cough.*
Ford RB and Vaden SL: Canine infectious tracheobronchitis. *In* Greene CE (ed): *Infectious Diseases of the Dog and Cat.* Philadelphia, WB Saunders Co, 1990, p 259.
  *A review of the agents involved in canine tracheobronchitis, treatment, and control measures.*
Konter EJ, Wegrzyn RJ, and Goodnow RA: Canine infectious tracheobronchitis: Effects of an intranasal live canine parainfluenza–*Bordetella bronchiseptica* vaccine on viral shedding and clinical tracheobronchitis (kennel cough). Am J Vet Res 42:1694, 1981.
  *A scientific study that addresses the efficacy of combined intranasal vaccination against the parainfluenza virus and B. bronchiseptica.*
Randolph JF, Moise NS, Scarlett JM, et al: Prevalence of mycoplasmal and ureaplasmal recovery from tracheobronchial lavages and prevalence of mycoplasmal recovery from pharyngeal swab specimens in dogs with or without pulmonary disease. Am J Vet Res 54:387, 1993.
  *A prospective study on the prevalence of mycoplasmas and ureaplasmas in healthy dogs and in dogs with respiratory disease.*
Thomsen JR and Edmonds C: Croup. Postgrad Med 90:97, 1991.
  *A basic review article on human croup.*

# DIAGNOSIS AND THERAPY OF CANINE CHRONIC BRONCHITIS

PHILIP PADRID
*Chicago, Illinois*

Chronic bronchitis (CB) is an inflammatory airway disease which, in association with tracheobronchial collapse, is arguably the most common chronic canine airway disorder. Although the etiology of most cases of CB in dogs remains obscure, the result is chronic airway inflammation, chronic cough, and excessive mucus production. Because dogs do not expectorate, the production of excessive mucus may be difficult to recognize. Therefore, the diagnosis of CB is usually based on a history of chronic cough alone. It should be emphasized that because the diagnosis of CB can reasonably be based on clinical criteria (cough), the diagnosis should not be made until it has been determined that other causes of chronic cough (e.g., heart failure, heartworm infestation, pneumonia, lung tumor) have been ruled out. Complicating matters is the finding that dogs with CB may have any of these other, coexisting disorders, which can by themselves cause cough. Additionally, certain drugs used to treat CB in dogs may be inappropriate and even contraindicated for disorders other than CB that cause chronic cough. It is important, then, that the diagnosis of CB be made with some degree of certainty to avoid potential complications related to therapy. The purposes of this article are to (1) summarize the main clinical features of canine CB, (2) highlight the most important tests used to confirm the diagnosis of canine CB, and (3) emphasize practical treatment principles and specific treatment strategies. Every effort will be made to distinguish what has been *proven* to be true in dogs from what has been *assumed* to be true, so that rational diagnostic and therapeutic choices may be made.

## CLINICAL FINDINGS IN DOGS WITH CHRONIC BRONCHITIS

Precise actuarial data regarding the typical age, breed(s), and sex of dogs with CB are lacking. Despite the seemingly high prevalence of this disease in the aging canine population, most of the available information regarding dogs with CB has been based upon relatively few, isolated case reports and one retrospective postmortem evaluation of 24 dogs with histories compatible with CB (Wheeldon et al., 1974). More recently, the clinical presentation, pathophysiology, and efficacy of treatment for 18 dogs with confirmed CB was reviewed (Padrid et al., 1990). Information from these published reviews, case reports, anecdotal reports from practitioners across the country, and the experience of the author form the basis for the following.

### Signalment

Dogs diagnosed with CB are generally 8 years of age or older. There does not seem to be a clear sex or breed predilection, although a disproportionate number of small and toy breeds such as poodles and pomeranians have been clinically diagnosed with CB. It is possible that many of these dogs cough because of extrathoracic tracheal collapse that is not associated with CB. Alternately, these cases may reflect a true increased incidence of CB in these breeds of dogs.

### History

By definition, dogs with CB have a chronic cough. The quality of this cough is generally deeper and "throatier" than the high-pitched "honking" cough caused by extrathoracic tracheal collapse, and yet harsher than the "soft moist" cough caused by pneu-

monia. Careful history-taking from clients will often elicit the information that the cough terminates in gagging or retching, reflecting the production and swallowing of coughed-up mucus. Some dogs with CB may be otherwise normal, while others will be severely exercise limited by their disease. Although easily fatigued, these animals are bright, alert, and in all other respects systemically well. The clinical signs of depression, lethargy, anorexia or weight loss, and so forth are not consistent with the diagnosis of isolated CB and should alert the practitioner to the presence of other significant medical problems.

### Physical Examination

*Inspection* is usually unremarkable. In more advanced cases, the alert clinician may notice a prolonged expiratory phase accompanied by an increased expiratory effort. This would be a significant finding, as CB is the only common chronic respiratory disorder of dogs that causes an increase in respiratory effort predominantly during the expiratory phase of breathing. However, it is rare for dogs with even advanced CB to show signs of severe respiratory distress at rest. *Palpation* of the chest wall is unremarkable. Although deep palpation of the trachea will often cause the dog to cough, this finding is common to most dogs with cough from any cause and is not by itself a marker for CB. Chest *percussion* may theoretically reveal hyperresonance consistent with air trapping. In practice, though, chest percussion only infrequently provides significant diagnostic information during the physical examination of dogs with CB. Thoracic *auscultation* may be normal or reveal diffuse crackles in all lung fields. Because the dog at rest is breathing at tidal volume, these adventitious lung sounds are not always easily appreciated. Holding one nostril (of the dog) closed for 15 sec will usually cause the dog to inhale deeply when the nostril is released. Auscultation at this time may reveal previously occult crackles, especially at the lung bases (ventrally). Conversely, crackles may disappear for a few breaths immediately following a cough, and this would not be an appropriate time to determine whether abnormal lung sounds are present.

### Diagnostic Tests

Because the diagnosis of CB is based on a history of chronic cough, it is only necessary to perform those diagnostic tests that are required to rule out the presence of other disorders that cause cough. Still, results of certain common examinations can significantly raise the index of suspicion for the presence of CB.

#### THORACIC RADIOGRAPHS

Thoracic radiographs of dogs with CB may appear normal. This finding alone should not cause the practitioner to abandon the diagnosis of CB. More commonly, however, thoracic radiographs reveal the presence of "doughnuts" or "tram lines," which are prominent and thickened bronchial walls seen on end or in parallel, respectively. Historically, it has been taught that a mild to moderate peribronchial pattern in the chest radiograph of an older dog is "compatible with age." Interestingly, these changes in the chest radiograph of an aging human would almost certainly be considered a sign of significant peribronchial pathology. Additionally, it was documented three decades ago (Reif and Rhodes, 1966) that peribronchial and interstitial densities in the radiographs of older dogs correspond to multiple and significant histologic abnormalities found on necropsy examination. It is the opinion of the author that mild to moderate peribronchial infiltrates found on examination of chest radiographs of older dogs most likely represent significant airway pathology. If this is correct, then clinical signs of airway disease that could be attributable to CB in these animals are mistakenly assumed to be signs of "old age," "arthritis," or other-activity-limiting disorders.

Perhaps the most important reason to obtain chest radiographs in suspected cases of CB is to confirm or deny radiographic evidence for other potential causes of chronic cough besides CB.

### BRONCHOPULMONARY CYTOLOGY

In contrast to the cellular analyses of other body fluids such as blood, cerebrospinal fluid, joint fluid, or urine, total and differential cell counting of tracheobronchial cells is generally not performed, and is in any case very difficult to interpret when the sample is mixed with mucus. Additionally, tracheobronchial cells may be obtained by many techniques including tracheal wash, bronchial wash, bronchial brushing, and bronchoalveolar lavage. Consequently, the clinical pathologist's interpretation of tracheobronchial secretions is usually offered in general rather than specific terms (i.e., relatively large number of neutrophils, lesser numbers of lymphocytes, and so forth). As might be expected then, the interpretation of bronchopulmonary cytology is to some degree dependent upon the manner in which the material was collected and analyzed. Additionally, it should be recalled that cytologic analysis of bronchopulmonary secretions in clinical veterinary medicine was based on the use of transtracheal wash (TTW) in human medicine to collect samples for bacterial culture only. Despite many book chapters to the contrary, the cytologic interpretation of bronchopulmonary secretions in noninfectious, noncancerous respiratory disease remains largely arbitrary.

Neutrophils are usually the predominant cell recovered from specimens taken by tracheal wash; these cells do not independently indicate current or past infection. Intracellular bacteria or a toxic appearance of neutrophils would of course suggest the presence of bacterial infection. Mucus is generally abundant even when a relatively small volume of fluid is recovered. Lesser numbers of lymphocytes, eosinophils, and epithelial cells are recovered in most samples.

Recovery of large numbers of eosinophils in airway washings from dogs with CB has led to the use of the term "allergic" bronchitis, a clinical diagnosis that is meant to be distinguished from "idiopathic" bronchitis. The underlying assumption for the adoption of this term is that eosinophils reflect or represent a "hypersensitivity" or "allergic reaction" to some unknown antigenic stimulus. Clearly, pulmonary parasitism and inhaled fungal spores (for example) will incite an intense eosinophilic response. However, this interpretation is not foolproof, as increased numbers of eosinophils may be recovered from tracheobronchial secretions of dogs with flea allergy dermatitis and an otherwise normal respiratory tract. While the appropriateness of the term "allergic" for any case in which increased eosinophils are recovered is questionable, the author has found that some dogs with CB and large numbers of eosinophils in airway secretions can be distinguished in two ways from bronchitic dogs without this finding: (1) "allergic" dogs are frequently symptomatic on a seasonal basis only (suggesting an environmental source of the offending antigen and cause for the subsequent cough), and (2) these cases also seem to respond most dramatically to anti-inflammatory therapy (see "Glucocorticoid Therapy," below).

Alveolar macrophages may be found in various morphologic stages, from relatively quiescent to "activated" in all normal animals as well as dogs with CB. Techniques such as bronchoalveolar lavage allow the wash fluid to come into contact with the lung surface and result in retrieval of a higher percentage of alveolar macrophages compared to tracheal washing. Regardless of the techniques used, the alveolar macrophage is an absolutely normal finding and should not be interpreted as a sign of bronchopulmonary inflammation or pathology.

### TRACHEOBRONCHIAL CULTURE

A presumptive diagnosis of "bacterial" bronchitis is most commonly made on the finding of small numbers of a mixed population of aerobic bacteria in cultures of tracheobronchial secretions recovered from dogs with CB. It is tempting to assume that the recovered bacteria are a primary source of airway inflammation and cause of clinical signs. However, the airways and lungs of healthy dogs, cats, horses, and humans are frequently inhabited by a broad range of inhaled bacterial flora (McKiernan, Smith, and Kissil, 1984; Padrid et al., 1991; Lindsey and Pierce, 1978). Said in other terms, neither the airways nor the lungs of healthy dogs are continuously sterile. It is the opinion of the author that, in most cases, bacteria recovered from the airways of bronchitic dogs reflects innocuous colonization rather than infection. Nevertheless, the author suggests two situations in which aerobic culture and sensitivity testing should be done on airway secretions from dogs with CB: (1) newly diagnosed CB with radiographic or bronchoscopic evidence of concurrent bronchiectasis, and (2) an acute exacerbation of signs in a dog with previously stable CB (see "Antibiotic Therapy" below). Fever, mucopurulent nasal discharge, or a lobar consolidation would be other indications that a dog with CB has developed a respiratory infection.

## BRONCHOSCOPY

The airways of dogs with CB are universally erythematous and usually have a roughened or granular appearance. The mucosa is often thickened, irregular, and edematous. Excessive and viscid mucus may be seen to span the lumen of an airway or gather together as a mucus plug, which can occlude smaller airways. Collapse of the dorsal tracheal membrane into the lumen of the airway is common in dogs with CB. This finding does not rule out CB, but instead reflects concurrent tracheal collapse in association with CB. A striking finding in some dogs with CB is the collapse of intrathoracic airways during passive tidal exhalation. This may not be apparent on thoracic radiographs and in any case is much more dramatic when visualized endoscopically in dynamic motion. In the author's experience, dogs with intrathoracic airway collapse respond only marginally to therapy and in general have a less fortunate prognosis than dogs whose intrathoracic airways are unaffected by passive expiration. Clearly then, while the diagnosis of CB does not require bronchoscopy, endoscopic evaluation of the airways of dogs with CB can reveal a great deal of information regarding the severity of the disease and potential response to therapy.

Bronchoscopic evaluation of the airways is a critically valuable tool when the diagnosis of CB is confounded by the presence of concurrent heart failure with left atrial enlargement. Dogs with chronic cough due to heart failure and enlarged left atrium have, in most respects, normal appearing airways. This is an important distinguishing feature. However, at the carina in the area of the left mainstem bronchus, the airways may show signs of chronic inflammation similar to bronchitic airways, including erythema, excessive mucus secretion, and irregular and roughened mucosa. The critical finding is a left mainstem bronchus that can be seen to narrow with each heartbeat, as the ventral floor of the bronchus is raised upward by the enlarged atrium (also see "Mitral Valve Disease in Cavalier King Charles Spaniels," this volume, p 837).

## BIOPSY AND HISTOPATHOLOGY

Chronic bronchitis is a clinical diagnosis and does not require tissue biopsy for confirmation. Nevertheless, certain histologic features of chronic bronchial disease are characteristic of the chronic inflammatory nature of the syndrome, including goblet cell hypertrophy and hyperplasia, and mononuclear cell infiltration and increased connective tissue within the lamina propria. These changes may be demonstrated in tissue taken by bronchoscopically guided pinch biopsy.

## ANCILLARY PROCEDURES

Additional studies more commonly performed in specialty practice or university settings include arterial blood gas analysis, tidal breathing flow volume loops, and radioaerosol ventilation scanning. These tests are valuable to better understand the pathophysiology of the disorder and may be helpful in evaluating response to medical therapy, but are not required examinations to diagnose or treat most dogs with CB.

## THERAPEUTIC OPTIONS IN THE TREATMENT OF CANINE CHRONIC BRONCHITIS

Although the primary cause of CB in humans is known to be an addiction to inhaled tobacco smoke, the etiology of most cases of CB in dogs remains obscure, and may include environmental pollutants; antigen-induced hypersensitivity reactions; bacterial or fungal invasion; and/or inherited or acquired defects in ciliary, immunoglobulin, or cellular structure or function. Documented cases of parasitic infestation, for example, can usually be effectively treated by eradication of the offending organism. However, in most cases of canine CB, the cause is never identified. As a result, *the primary treatment of CB is based on controlling airway inflammation.* Chronic bronchial inflammation, regardless of cause, will result in variable mucosal and airway wall thickening, mucus hypersecretion, and some degree of airway smooth muscle constriction. The clinical signs that result from these pathologic changes in airway structure and function are the defining features of canine CB, and include chronic cough and exercise intolerance. Unfortunately, the primary treatment goal of decreasing airway inflammation is not always attainable and in any case may take weeks to months to accomplish. Therefore, *a secondary goal of therapy is to minimize clinical signs of chronic bronchial disease without adversely affecting the body's normal defense mechanisms.* Three additional points are worthy of special mention:

1. Bronchiectasis, or destruction and dilation of airway walls, is an important complicating factor in some cases of CB. Bronchiectatic airway segments do not by themselves affect pulmonary function. However, bronchiectasis is commonly caused by bacterial infection and subsequent disruption of the integrity of the airway wall. These dilated airway wall segments may serve as a bacterial reservoir and act as a nidus for chronic bacterial infections.

2. Specific drug dosage recommendations are intended as a guide for the clinician when initiating therapy. However, the optimal dosage and frequency of administration can only be determined by frequent evaluation of the patient's response to therapy.

3. The guiding principle of any therapy must always be "if in doubt, do no harm."

## Corticosteroids

Glucocorticoids (GC) have been used to treat human patients with bronchial disease for over 50 years. They are clearly the single most effective means of ameliorating the symptoms of CB in people, although potentially debilitating side effects limit their use in this clinical setting to transient administration only (see "Corticosteroid Withdrawal Syndrome," this volume, p 413). Even though GC have no primary antitussive activity, by decreasing inflammation they may decrease stimulation of airway sensory nerves responsible for initiating cough in canine CB. Additionally, GC markedly decrease the volume of mucus produced by bronchitic airways. In the author's experience, GC are the most effective drugs available to treat dogs with CB, and should be considered the mainstay of chronic therapy.

Glucocorticoids may be administered parenterally, orally, or by inhalation. Very few studies in any species have been carried out to determine the specific bioavailability of the various steroid preparations for lung tissue. In humans, *hydrocortisone* appears to have the greatest penetrability for lung, followed by *methylprednisolone* and *prednisone*. Although only 10% of inhaled steroids reach the small airways, they are rapidly absorbed into the lung and, therefore, bioavailability is assumed to be high. Additionally, direct absorption into the lung greatly diminishes the side effects of systemically administered corticosteroids. Unfortunately, this route of administration is not presently feasible for veterinary patients.

The author begins treatment of dogs with CB by administering prednisone, 1 mg/kg PO every 12 hr for 5 days, followed by 0.5 mg/kg PO every 12 hr for 5 additional days. At this point, the clinical signs will have greatly improved for the vast majority of dogs with CB. The owner should continue to give the drug on an alternate-day basis, while the dose is gradually decreased over the ensuing 2 months to the least amount of drug needed to adequately, if not completely, control clinical signs. A maintenance dose of prednisone, 0.1 to 0.25 mg/kg PO every 12 hr every other or every third day, is frequently sufficient to minimize cough and significantly improve exercise tolerance in these cases. Additionally, after an additional 2 to 4 months, an attempt can be made to gradually stop the drug entirely. Commonly, signs may not worsen for months afterward, at which time prednisone may be reinstituted using the schedule described above.

The many adverse side effects associated with chronic alternate-day GC therapy in dogs have been documented (also see "Clinical Applications or Glucocorticoid Therapy in Nonendocrine Disease," this volume, p 406). Both the owner and attending veterinarian must reach a consensus opinion regarding the relative benefits of chronic GC therapy versus the frequency and magnitude of side effects encountered. In some cases of CB, glucocorticosteroids and $\beta_2$-agonists (see "Bronchodilator Therapy," below) are best administered together, in which case the dose of each drug can be lowered while maintaining an acceptable therapeutic result.

## Bronchodilators

The rational use of bronchodilators to treat dogs with CB is based on two assumptions: (1) some degree of bronchoconstriction exists, and (2) this bronchoconstriction causes clinical signs. Until recently, there was no objective evidence that either of these two assumptions was true. Recently, a positive therapeutic response to orally administered albuterol was demonstrated in a small percentage of dogs with documented CB (Padrid et al., 1990). Tidal breathing flow volume loops demonstrated an increase in expiratory airflow, thoracic radiographs were improved, chest auscultation showed a decrease in wheezing, and owners reported an increase in their dogs' tolerance for exercise. Based upon these limited data and personal experience, the author recommends, for dogs with exercise intolerance and/or wheeze on chest auscultation, a trial of albuterol syrup at 0.02 mg/kg PO every 12 hr for 5 days. The volume of syrup required is minimal, and the flavor is well tolerated by most dogs. Common side effects include skeletal muscle tremors and restlessness, which usually subside within a 2- to 5-day time frame. This information should always be shared with the owner, so that noncompliance with the medical plan is avoided. After 5 days the dose may be increased to 0.05 mg/kg PO every 8 to 12 hr **ONLY IF:** (1) the dog is tolerating the drug, and (2) a positive therapeutic response is not yet appreciated. If a positive response is not seen within 2 weeks of initiating albuterol therapy, further bronchodilator treatment will probably not be effective. If, on the other hand, a positive response is noted, the drug dose and frequency of administration should be decreased until the lowest effective dose that minimizes cough and increases exercise tolerance is found. The best results may be obtained when the drug is given on an "as-needed" basis.

It should be emphasized that only a relatively few dogs with CB have reversible bronchoconstriction, and they are suitable candidates for continued bronchodilator therapy. In *this subset* of dogs, the combination of $\beta_2$-agonists and corticosteroids acts synergistically and only may provide the most effective therapy. Additionally, using both classes of drugs may allow the practitioner to minimize the dose and frequency of administration of each. It is tempting in these animals to withhold the corticosteroids completely and rely solely on the beneficial effects of the bronchodilator. This is probably a mistake, because the inflammatory nature of CB is chronic and progressive. Use of bronchodilators alone may temporarily minimize clinical signs but does not stop the progression of airway inflammation. When the inflammatory nature of the disease progresses past a certain point, the resulting clinical signs may be unmanageable with any combination of drugs.

Other bronchodilator drugs that are anecdotally reported to be occasionally effective for dogs with CB include *terbutaline* and the methylxanthines, including *aminophylline* and *theophylline* (see *CVT XI*, p 660). Terbutaline is another $\beta_2$-selective agonist whose mode of action is very similar to albuterol. The dose of terbutaline for dogs with CB is based upon empiric data only. Approximately 1 mg/kg PO every 12 hr has been recommended (Boothe and McKiernan, 1992). Theophylline, in addition to relaxation of bronchial smooth muscle, may improve airway function in dogs with bronchial disease by increasing mucociliary transport rates, stabilizing mast cell membranes, and decreasing bronchovascular leak. A recent observation that theophylline increases contractility of fatigued diaphragmatic muscle has revived interest in this drug for the chronic treatment of dogs with CB. However, the clinical relevance of diaphragmatic muscle fatigue in veterinary medicine is unclear. Importantly, the pharmacokinetics of theophylline in dogs have been well described. The preferred theophylline preparation for dogs is a slow-release tablet (Theo-Dur, Key Pharmaceuticals), given at a dosage of 20 mg/kg PO every 12 hr (Booth and McKiernan, 1992; McKiernan et al., 1981); however, some dogs develop adverse effects (excitement, restlessness) at this dose.

Natural or synthetic catecholamines such as *isoproterenol* or *epinephrine* are nonselective $\beta$ (isoproterenol) or mixed $\alpha$ and $\beta$ (epinephrine) agonists. They produce undesirable and untoward cardiovascular side effects, and are no less expensive, easier to administer, or easier to obtain than previously mentioned bronchodilators. There is no reason to use these drugs to treat dogs with CB.

## Antibiotics

It has already been mentioned that a mixed population of aerobic bacteria resides commensally in the canine airway. There is no objective evidence that bacterial infection plays a significant role in the cause or perturbation of the majority of cases of canine CB. Similarly, there is no objective evidence that antibiotic therapy has any effect on the duration or intensity of signs displayed by the dog with CB. It is important to recognize that the signs of bronchial disease in dogs frequently wax and wane in severity as well as in frequency of occurrence. Anecdotal reports describing the therapeutic effect of antibiotics in controlling chronic cough are consistent with the "waxing and waning" nature of the symptom in nontreated cases. A positive culture result obtained from a tracheobronchial wash does not necessarily imply the presence of a clinically significant airway infection, and should not automatically indicate antibiotic therapy. In the author's opinion, antibiotics are indicated for dogs with signs caused by CB when there is other clinical or radiographic evidence of superimposed airway infection or when a culture of tracheobronchial secretions results in the growth of a pure bacterial culture on a primary culture plate. This is based on the finding that the concentration of aerobic bacteria recovered from the airways of

healthy cats and humans does not exceed $5 \times 10^3$ organisms/ml (Padrid et al., 1991). In contrast, growth of a single organism recovered without the use of enrichment broth implies more than $10^5$ organisms/ml, and this is consistent with an "infected" airway.

The author does not routinely collect tracheobronchial washings or prescribe antibiotics for dogs with newly diagnosed CB. This is because, in the author's experience, dogs with newly diagnosed CB have a more favorable response to corticosteroids than to antibiotics, and because these dogs do not have a better therapeutic response when antibiotics are given concurrently with corticosteroids. Additionally, the author has never recognized the development of bacterial pneumonia in dogs with CB who were given corticosteroids and not antibiotics. On the other hand, collection, cytologic analysis, and bacterial culture of tracheobronchial washings *are* indicated (1) when a dog with newly diagnosed CB has evidence of bronchiectasis on chest radiographs or bronchoscopy, (2) when a dog with newly diagnosed CB lives in or has been exposed to an environment favorable to parasitic infestation of the airways (the work-up of suspected cases of parasitic bronchitis should also include routine and Baermann evaluation of feces), and (3) when a previously stable bronchitic dog has an acute exacerbation of symptoms.° When culture results reflect a true bacterial infection, the choice of antibiotics should be based on the effectiveness of the drug against the bacteria identified (sensitivity) *and* the ability of the drug to reach the affected tissue. There exists a "blood-bronchus" barrier that effectively limits the concentration of many blood-borne antibiotics in bronchial tissue. Many antibiotics that reach bactericidal levels in lung parenchyma do not reach similar levels in the airway. Chloramphenicol is lipid soluble, reaches relatively high concentrations in bronchial tissues, and has a spectrum of activity against a wide range of bacteria most commonly recovered from airways of dogs with CB. For these reasons, chloramphenicol, 50 mg/kg PO every 8 hr for 7 to 10 days, is the author's antibiotic of choice when bacterial infection is believed to play a role in the clinical signs of canine CB. Prophylactic or long-term therapy using any antibiotic should be avoided unless there is documentation of a chronic airway infection, as may be the case with concurrent bronchiectasis.

## Cough Suppressants

Chronic inflammatory disorders of the lower airway often result in the production of excessive viscid mucoid secretions. Coughing serves to clear these secretions, and thus may be viewed as a protective physiologic reflex. However, there are many cases in which the cough is dry and nonproductive. In these situations, the cough is not protective, and serves to further irri-

---

°Fever, muco-purulent nasal discharge, signs of systemic disease, or lobar lung consolidation should also prompt consideration of complicating bacterial infection.

tate the airway, leading to a vicious cycle of "cough-irritation-cough." In addition, some dogs with chronic cough are unable to sleep, and may awake their owners at night. Occasionally, some dogs with chronic cough may become syncopal. In each of these clinical settings, cough suppression may be indicated. The author's preference for antitussive therapy for dogs with CB (who fit the criteria listed above) is *hydrocodone bitartrate*, 0.22 mg/kg PO every 6 to 12 hr as needed. Although in theory any morphine-like drug can induce respiratory depression, in practice the most common side effects of overadministration of hydrocodone in dogs are drowsiness and constipation. Given at night, the side effect of drowsiness may be a welcome advantage to both the dog and the owner.

Although the antitussive effect of *dextromethorphan* is reportedly 50% that of codeine, it is a non-narcotic and can be prescribed without a narcotic license. Anecdotal reports suggest that *dextromethorphan* is occasionally effective in controlling cough in some dogs with CB. In the author's experience, *dextromethorphan* is much less effective than hydrocodone. Its primary advantage compared to hydrocodone is its availability "over the counter."

## Anticholinergics

Anticholinergic drugs have been used to treat respiratory disorders in humans at least since the seventeenth century. The classic drug in this category is *atropine*. Chronic airway inflammation increases vagus nerve (cholinergic) transmission to airway cells and smooth muscle. This causes epithelial goblet cells and submucosal glands to produce and release excessive quantities of thick and tenacious mucus, and causes smooth muscle to contract. In theory, therefore, these drugs have a role in the management of CB by relaxing smooth muscle and decreasing mucus production. Additionally, anticholinergics are effective bronchodilators for dogs with experimentally (allergen) induced bronchoconstriction. In practice, atropine is not an effective bronchodilator for dogs with CB. One reason for this finding is that increased vagal tone is only one of the (minor) contributing factors causing airway narrowing in dogs with CB. As a result, anticholinergic therapy is not indicated for the treatment of canine CB.

Newer drugs in this class such as *ipratroprium bromide* are effective in the treatment of CB in humans. This drug is administered by inhalation. The benefits of this route of administration include fewer adverse effects on ciliary function and mucus secretion. However, administration of any drug by inhalation limits the drug's veterinary application; therefore, *ipratroprium* is not at present a practical alternative in clinical veterinary practice.

## Nonsteroidal Anti-inflammatory Drugs

Commonly used drugs in this category include *acetylsalicylic acid* and *ibuprofen*. The basic mechanism of action of these drugs is inhibition of synthesis of prostaglandins (PG), prostacyclins, and thromboxane (TX) by inhibition of the enzyme cyclooxygenase. While certain of these compounds, notably $TXA_2$, $PGF_2$, and $PGD_2$, cause bronchoconstriction under experimental conditions, they are not currently thought to play an important role in the pathogenesis of bronchoconstriction in humans or dogs. There is little experimental or anecdotal evidence to support the use of nonsteroidal anti-inflammatory drugs in the treatment of dogs with CB.

## Other Drugs

Drugs such as *cromolyn sodium*, generally considered "mast cell stabilizing" agents, are useful in the treatment of humans with certain chronic bronchial disorders such as asthma, and have occasionally been recommended for the treatment of CB in dogs. Interestingly, cromolyn has been shown to inhibit the release of substance P from stimulated C fibers in the dog; this mechanism of action is thought to be of potential importance in the generation of cough and bronchoconstriction in humans. However, there is no evidence that excessive C-fiber discharge plays a prominent role in canine CB. Additionally, aerosolization of cromolyn (to cats) has resulted in significant airway irritation in one clinical trial.

Mucolytics have been suggested as a form of therapy for dogs with airway disease associated with excessive secretion of mucus. While drugs such as *acetylcysteine* are capable of breaking the disulphide bonds that are partially responsible for the particularly viscid nature of airway mucus, in practice, aerosolized *acetylcysteine* is irritating to airway epithelium and can promote significant bronchoconstriction. The potential beneficial effects of other classes of drugs, such as calcium channel blockers, antihistamines, and specific blockers of leukotrienes and platelet activating factor, await discovery.

## PROGNOSIS

Canine CB is a common, progressive, and chronic airway disorder in which patient signs can often be ameliorated but almost never eradicated. Establishment of excellent client communications is critical so that client expectations are realistic, and so that the therapeutic regimen established by the clinician is adhered to. There is a great deal left to learn about canine CB, including etiology, exacerbating factors, role of bacterial infection, prognosis, and optimal course of therapy. As veterinary clinicians and researchers continue to diligently report their observations, many of these questions will no doubt soon be answered.

## References and Suggested Reading

Boothe DM and McKiernan BC: Respiratory therapeutics. Vet Clin North Am 22:1239, 1992.

*A comprehensive discussion of common and not so common treatment options for dogs and cats with respiratory disease.*
Lindsey JO and Pierce AK: An examination of the microbiologic flora of normal lung of the dog. Am Rev Respir Dis 117:501, 1978.
*Documents the presence of commensal bacteria in the lung parenchyma of healthy dogs.*
McKiernan BC, Smith AR, and Kissil M: Bacteria isolated from the lower trachea of clinically healthy dogs. J Am Anim Hosp Assoc 20:139, 1984.
*Documents the presence of commensal bacteria in the trachea of healthy dogs.*
McKiernan BC, Neff-Davis CA, Kortiz GD, et al: Pharmacokinetic studies of theophylline in dogs. J Vet Pharmacol Ther 4:103, 1981.
*Determines the half-life and bioavailability of various theophylline preparations in the dog.*
Padrid PA, Hornof W, Kurpershoek C, and Cross CE: Canine chronic bronchitis: A pathophysiologic evaluation of 18 cases. J Vet Intern Med 4:172, 1990.

*A thorough evaluation of dogs with chronic bronchitis, including chest radiographs, blood gases, tracheobronchial cytology and culture, bronchoscopy, pulmonary function testing, histology, and response to bronchodilator therapy.*
Padrid PA, Feldman BF, Funk K, et al: Cytologic, microbiologic and biochemical analysis of bronchoalveolar lavage fluid obtained from 24 healthy cats. Am J Vet Res 52:1300, 1991.
*Documents and quantifies the amount of bacteria in healthy cat airways.*
Reif JS and Rhodes WH: The lungs of aged dogs: A radiographic-morphologic correlation. J Am Vet Radiol Soc 7:5, 1966.
*Documents the presence of histologic abnormalities in the lungs of aging dogs, and correlates this with abnormalities found on thoracic radiographs.*
Wheeldon EB, Pirie HM, Fisher EW, et al: Chronic bronchitis in the dog. Vet Rec 94:466, 1974.
*A retrospective histologic evaluation of the airways of 24 dogs with historical evidence of chronic bronchitis.*

# ASPIRATION PNEUMONIA

ELEANOR C. HAWKINS
*Raleigh, North Carolina*

Aspiration pneumonia refers to pulmonary inflammation resulting from the inhalation of liquid or particulate matter. Examples of material that can be aspirated into the lungs include food and gastric contents, fresh and salt water (near-drowning), mineral oil (lipid pneumonia), hydrocarbons (e.g., kerosene or petroleum distillates), and foreign bodies. In people, aspiration pneumonia is sometimes used more specifically to describe bacterial infection (bronchopneumonia) secondary to organisms originating in the oropharynx, even in the absence of overt aspiration.

This article addresses the management of aspiration pneumonia occurring from inhalation of food or gastric contents. Aspiration pneumonia is a serious and potentially fatal disease, and successful management must consist of three components: (1) immediate management, (2) identification and therapy of any underlying etiology, and (3) diagnosis and treatment of secondary complications.

## IMMEDIATE MANAGEMENT

### Pathophysiology

Rational management of aspiration pneumonia requires an understanding of the mechanisms resulting in pulmonary dysfunction. Significant damage to the lung occurs from gastric acid, food particles, and bacteria. Resulting pathology depends on which of these factors are involved, as well as the quantity of material aspirated and its distribution within the lung. Signs may be acute or chronic, mild or severe; however, profound hypoxemia, with or without hypercapnia, is common. Aspiration of acidic gastric contents (pH <2.5) causes collapse of alveoli, bronchoconstriction, pulmonary edema, and systemic hypotension. Alveolar collapse occurs due to the denaturation and dilution of surfactant, leading to atelectasis and ventilation/perfusion mismatching (low $\dot{V}/\dot{Q}$ regions and intrapulmonary shunts). Pulmonary compliance is decreased, increasing the work of ventilation. Alveolar ventilation is further impeded by bronchoconstriction and pulmonary edema.

Pulmonary edema can be fulminant. The acid causes epithelial necrosis and increased capillary permeability. High-protein fluid, and sometimes blood, leaks from the capillaries into the interstitium and alveoli. The edema is consistent with that of adult respiratory distress syndrome (ARDS). Pulmonary arterial pressure is not elevated, although pulmonary vascular resistance is increased due to vasoconstriction. Neutrophilic infiltration occurs rapidly. Systemic hypotension, partly as a result of the extravascular redistribution of fluid, contributes to poor tissue oxygenation.

Particulate matter causes airway obstruction. Tracheal obstruction with large particles is associated with acute ventilatory failure. More often, smaller airways are blocked. Further obstruction occurs from bronchospasm and inflammation, including hemorrhage and edema. Particulate matter induces a marked granulomatous inflammatory response.

Infection can occur immediately, due to the aspiration of contaminated material, or at some later time, due to compromise of normal pulmonary defense mechanisms by aspiration damage or therapy (e.g., tracheal tube placement). Risk factors for immediate infection in people include intestinal obstruction, use of antacids, and periodontal disease. Use of antacids promotes the growth of bacteria in the stomach by interfering with the bactericidal effect of an acidic pH. The relatively high incidence of megaesophagus as an underlying cause for aspiration (without gastric acid to inhibit bacterial growth of ingesta), and the frequent presence of periodontal disease, may make immediate infection more common in small animals than in people. A reivew of the records of 32 dogs with final clinical diagnoses of aspiration pneumonia and megaesophagus at North Carolina State University showed that aerobic bacterial cultures of transtracheal wash fluid were positive in 20 of the 22 dogs (91%) in which the procedure was performed.

## Clinical Diagnosis

Diagnosis of aspiration pneumonia is made by the identification of signs of bronchopneumonia or ARDS in combination with signs of a condition known to predispose to aspiration (Table 1). In many cases the relationship is obvious, with acute respiratory distress developing within hours of known vomiting or regurgitation. In animals with mild or chronic signs, the diagnosis may be more difficult. Although the dependent lung lobes (right middle, and left and right cranial) are classically involved in aspiration pneumonia, this distribution is not pathognomonic. Bacterial bronchopneumonia frequently involves the dependent lung lobes in the absence of overt aspiration of food or gastric contents. Aspiration pneumonia may involve other lobes due to position of the animal during aspiration, distribution of material throughout the lungs by cough, and development of ARDS. Careful attention must be paid to the history and physical examination to identify predisposing conditions.

**Table 1.**   *Conditions Predisposing to Aspiration Pneumonia*

Esophageal disease
  Megaesophagus
  Myesthenia gravis
  Esophageal obstruction
  Reflux esophagitis
  Cricopharyngeal motor dysfunction (achalasia)
Anatomic defects
  Cleft palate
  Bronchoesophageal fistulae
Pharyngeal dysfunction
  Laryngoplasty
  Polyneuropathy
  Polymyopathy
Vomiting*
Iatrogenic causes
  Aggressive force-feeding
  Pharyngostomy, nasogastric, or stomach tube†
Decreased consciousness
  Postictus
  Head trauma
  Metabolic derangement
  General anesthesia
  Sedation

*Usually severe, protracted vomiting, or vomiting in conjunction with debilitation, sedation, or other predisposing factors.
†Due to incorrect placement or decreased competence of lower esophageal sphincter from presence of tube.

Bronchoscopic findings can provide support for a diagnosis of aspiration pneumonia, but the need for general anesthesia precludes routine bronchoscopic examination. If performed immediately after aspiration, gastric contents or food particles can be seen. Later, severe tracheobronchitis with hemorrhage and edema, and possibly food particles, are present. Cytologic specimens collected from the lung may contain macrophages with lipid-filled vacuoles, free fat globules, or vegetable material.

## Therapeutic Considerations

Animals with aspiration pneumonia can develop severe respiratory distress with extensive pulmonary injury. Shock may occur. Because the mechanisms of pulmonary dysfunction are varied, each animal must be managed as an individual, and careful patient monitoring is essential to determine effectiveness of therapy. Serial arterial blood gas determinations are ideal for monitoring pulmonary function. Arterial specimens are sufficiently stable on ice to allow transport to a diagnostic laboratory. Thoracic radiography is helpful for initial diagnosis, evaluation for underlying causes, and early detection of secondary complications. Radiographs are of limited use in the early monitoring of response to therapy because there may be a time delay of up to 36 hr for the full development of lesions. Radiographic lesions in humans do not correlate well with degree of hypoxemia or prognosis. Central venous pressure measurements are valuable for guiding the rapid treatment of hypovolemia and shock, while decreasing the risk of overhydration.

### AIRWAY PATENCY

Animals in severe distress are quickly assessed for a patent airway. The character of respiration is noted. Marked inspiratory efforts and stridor suggests a possible tracheal obstruction. The oral cavity is examined. Neck radiographs are rarely useful; animals are usually not sufficiently stable to undergo the procedure, and soft tissue dense foreign material is rarely visible. Unconscious animals should be examined endoscopically. If an endoscope is not available, a laryngoscope can be used to visualize the larynx and proximal trachea while holding the laryngeal cartilages open with a cotton swab or instrument. The majority of dogs and cats who have aspirated food or gastric contents do not have tracheal obstruction, so convincing evidence for obstruction should be present prior to anesthetizing a conscious animal for examination. Obstructing material is removed with alligator forceps or endoscopic foreign body retrievers. It is rarely necessary to place a tracheal tube to bypass an obstruction.

### AIRWAY SUCTION AND LAVAGE

Airway suctioning for primary treatment is useful only if the incident is observed (e.g., aspiration following extubation from an anesthetic procedure), because aspirated liquid quickly disperses from the large airways. Suction and postural drainage is indicated in intubated animals with fulminant edema. Suction should be intermittent, followed by several "sighs" with an anesthesia or ambu bag to minimize further alveolar collapse.

Bronchial or bronchoalveolar lavage is not recommended. Acid is quickly neutralized by the body without intervention, and further instillation of liquid can worsen the animal's respiratory status. Small particles may be pushed further out in the lungs and become lodged, rather than being carried out of the lungs by the mucociliary apparatus and coughing. The fluid may also add to obstruction and decreased compliance.

### OXYGEN SUPPLEMENTATION AND VENTILATORY SUPPORT

Oxygen supplementation or ventilatory support can be crucial for the management of hypoxemic animals. Ventilation/perfusion mismatching can be severe. Oxygen supplementation is administered by mask, nasal tube, or cage. Placement of a tracheal or endotracheal tube and administration of 100% oxygen may be necessary. In some animals, oxygen supplementation alone is inadequate. Perfusion of regions of lung with no ventilation (due to atelectasis; airway obstruction; and flooding of alveoli with edema, blood, and inflammatory cells) results in actual shunting of blood. Increasing the inspired oxygen concentration will not improve blood oxygenation because none of the enriched air can reach these regions. Oxygen supplementation also does not promote expansion of collapsed alveoli, and may actually contribute to their further collapse.

Ventilatory support is indicated for animals that do not respond favorably to supplemental oxygen (persistent hypoxemia, hypercarbia, or dyspnea), or that cannot be maintained on concentrations of inspired oxygen of less than 40%. In these instances, intermittent positive-pressure ventilation should be initiated (see *CVT XI*, p 98). In experimental dogs, the initiation of positive-pressure ventilation for 6 hr immediately following aspiration has been associated with improved survival. The beneficial effect is not seen when ventilation is delayed for 24 hr. Therefore, the clinician should not hesitate to begin positive-pressure ventilation early in the treatment of aspiration pneumonia. The addition of positive end-expiratory pressure (PEEP) may be necessary in some animals, to combat alveolar collapse and to treat ARDS or hypoxemia. Alternatively, continuous positive airway pressure (CPAP) can be used. Whenever positive-pressure ventilation, PEEP, or CPAP are used, extensive nursing care and patient monitoring are essential. Pulse oximetry and end-tidal carbon dioxide monitoring may be useful (see this volume, pp 117 and 119).

Recumbent animals should not be permitted to lie on the same side for longer than 2 hr. Animals with diffuse lung involvement should be kept in sternal recumbency at all times. Animals on ventilators should be maintained in sternal recumbency or, if lateral, with the more severely affected side up. Supplemental oxygen should be humidified prior to delivery to the animal.

### FLUID THERAPY

The edema associated with aspiration pneumonia is not cardiogenic in origin and should not be treated with diuretics. Affected animals are often hypovolemic. Administration of diuretics further decreases cardiac output and the delivery of oxygen to tissues. Dehydration also interferes with normal mucociliary clearance. Maintenance of hydration and expansion of blood volume are actually required. Crystalloids are recommended, because no improvement in survival has been identified with the use of colloids. Ideally, if severe pulmonary edema is suspected, a Swan-Ganz catheter should be placed in order to monitor pulmonary arterial pressures and cardiac output by thermodilution. Although pulmonary edema is not cardiogenic in origin, maintenance of the minimum pulmonary capillary pressures necessary to support adequate cardiac output ($\geq 3.5$ L/min/m$^2$) will reduce the leakage of fluid through the damaged pulmonary capillary endothelium. If pulmonary artery catheterization is unavailable, a jugular catheter should be placed to allow for monitoring of central venous pressure. Adequate hydration is essential; however, overhydration is avoided to prevent additional edema formation. Weight gain is a sign of fluid retention and excessive weight gains in people is related to increased pulmonary edema.

Management of edema due to ARDS consists primarily of oxygen-therapy and positive-pressure ventilation. To date, no other therapies have produced consistently beneficial effects.

### BRONCHODILATORS

Bronchodilators may be useful immediately following aspiration to counter bronchospasm. Theophylline derivatives (e.g., aminophylline) or $\beta$-agonists (e.g., terbutaline) can be used. Treatment with bronchodilators after the first 24 to 48 hr following aspiration is controversial. Potential benefits include bronchodilation, decreased ventilatory muscle fatigue, and mild anti-inflammatory effects. Potential negative effects include anti-inflammatory effects (possibly enhancing infection) and contribution to $\dot{V}/\dot{Q}$ mismatching.

### CORTICOSTEROIDS

Corticosteroids are indicated for initial treatment of shock. No benefit has been demonstrated for the routine use of corticosteroids following aspiration. They decrease inflammation, but also interfere with the beneficial response to foreign matter and promote the development of infection. If corticosteroids are used, only short-acting products should be administered. They should be discontinued within 24 hr.

### ANTIBIOTICS

Antibiotic administration immediately following aspiration is controversial. In most people, aspiration of gastric contents does not result in primary infection. However, damage to the lungs from aspiration predisposes the patient to secondary infection. The preventative use of antibiotics can promote the development of secondary infection with resistant organisms, rather than preventing infection. The usual recommendation for people is to withhold antibiotics unless signs of secondary infection occur. However, in animals, aspiration of contaminated material may be more frequent than in people (see "Pathophysiology" above), and the routine use of antibiotics may be justified.

Prior to initiating antibiotics, tracheal wash is indicated for cytologic and microbiologic evaluation. Culture and sensitivity information is valuable for the management of these cases. Prolonged treatment may be required, and it can be impossible to differentiate clinical signs due to infection from the marked inflammatory response that occurs from acid and particulate aspiration. Aspiration occurring in the hospital (e.g., during recovery from anesthesia) can result in infection with highly resistant organisms. Tracheal wash can be readily performed in unconscious or relatively stable animals. In conscious but fragile animals with recent aspiration, it may be advisable to withhold antibiotics until the animal has been stabilized and tracheal wash can be safely performed. Such delay may not be prudent in animals with a chronic history of aspiration, whose clinical signs may largely be the result of advanced infection. Based on common organisms isolated from people, anaerobic cultures should be considered in addition to aerobic cultures. The role of anaerobic bacteria in aspiration pneumonia of small animal patients is not known.

Pending results of culture, broad-spectrum antibiotics are selected. Parenteral administration is recommended for initial treatment. Reasonable choices include trimethoprim-sulfas, cephalosporins, or chloramphenicol. Monitoring for secondary infection is necessary regardless of whether or not antibiotics are administered initially.

## UNDERLYING ETIOLOGIES

Aspiration of small amounts of saliva and bacteria into the airways can occur in clinically normal animals. Protective mechanisms such as pharyngeal reflexes, mucociliary clearance, and cough normally prevent the development of pneumonia. Aspiration pneumonia occurs when these protective mechanisms are compromised or overwhelmed. In order to prevent reoccurrence, the situation or combination of situations that allowed for aspiration to occur must be identified and managed. Potential underlying etiologies are listed in Table 1. Careful history and physical examination are performed, including thorough neurologic examination. As indicated by these initial evaluations, other tests are selected, such as contrast radiography (barium swallow if the esophagus is not obviously dilated), complete oral and pharyngeal examination, upper gastrointestinal endoscopy, and tests of neuromuscular function (e.g., electromyography, acetylcholine antibody titer).

Nothing should be administered orally until the animal is stabilized and potential underlying abnormalities have been addressed. Animals with respiratory distress are particularly likely to reaspirate. Placement of a nasoesophageal tube in animals with megaesophagus and respiratory distress is useful for removing esophageal contents by suction and preventing continued aspiration.

## COMPLICATIONS

Infection is the most common complication of aspiration pneumonia. Aspiration of gastric acid decreases the lungs' ability to clear bacteria. Even if antibiotics have been initiated prophylactically, secondary infection with organisms resistant to those antibiotics is possible. Lung abscessation can also occur. Frequent monitoring of animals following initial stabilization is essential for at least 2 weeks. Measurements of body temperature, thoracic radiographs, and complete blood counts (CBC) are routinely performed. Monitoring frequency depends on patient status. In severely ill animals, laboratory and radiographic monitoring is indicated at least every 48 hr. The interval is extended for animals that are improving or that have mild signs. It is necessary to detect deterioration in these parameters to differentiate secondary infection from profound inflammation secondary to acid and particulate aspiration. The development of fever in a previously normothermic animal, increasing neutrophil count in conjunction with a left shift and increasing neutrophil toxicity, and increased pulmonary densities on radiographs 36 hr or longer after aspiration are suggestive of secondary infection. Tracheal wash is indicated to confirm suspected infection and to provide material for culture and sensitivity testing.

Antibiotics are continued for 1 week beyond the complete resolution of clinical signs (body temperature, thoracic radiographs, and CBC should be normal before discontinuation is considered). A minimum antibiotic course of 3 to 4 weeks should be anticipated. It is prudent to reevaluate radiographs 5 to 7 days following discontinuation of antibiotics for the detection of localized densities that might indicate the presence of persistent foreign material and for the early identification of recurrence of infection due to incomplete elimination of bacteria.

Saline nebulization followed by coupage and postural drainage can be useful for facilitating mucociliary clearance in animals with consolidation of peripheral lung regions. Initiation should be delayed until the animal is stabilized and edema has largely resolved.

Localized pulmonary densities following appropriate therapy, unresolved atelectasis, or recurrent pneumonia in spite of elimination of predisposing causes suggests the possibility of persistent foreign material. Complete bronchoscopic examination is indicated. Rarely, exploratory thoracotomy is required.

## References and Suggested Reading

Broe PJ, Toung TJ, and Cameron JL: Aspiration pneumonia. Surg Clin North Am 60:1551, 1980.
*A well-referenced review of pathophysiology, clinical findings, and treatment of aspiration pneumonia in people.*

Bynum LJ and Pierce AK: Pulmonary aspiration of gastric contents. Rev Respir Dis 114:1129, 1976.
*Retrospective study of 50 human patients, including discussion of clinical course, response to therapy, and prognostic indicators.*

Khawaja IT, Buffa SD, and Brandstetter RD: Aspiration pneumonia. Postgrad Med 92:165, 1992.
*Recent review of aspiration pneumonia in people, including management recommendations.*

Orton EC and Wheeler SL: Continuous positive airway pressure therapy for aspiration pneumonia in a dog. J Am Vet Med Assoc 188:1437, 1986.
*Case report describing use of continuous positive airway pressure in the management of aspiration pneumonia in the dog.*

Tams TR: Aspiration pneumonia and complications of smoke inhalation. Vet Clin North Am [Small Anim Pract] 15:971, 1985.
*Clinical review of pulmonary injury in dogs and cats secondary to aspiration.*

Wynne JW and Modell JH: Respiratory aspiration of stomach contents. Ann Intern Med 87:466, 1977.
*Detailed review of pathophysiology of aspiration with discussion of experimental canine studies.*

# LUNG LOBE TORSION

MARTHA MOON
*Blacksburg, Virginia*

and THERESA W. FOSSUM
*College Station, Texas*

Lung lobe torsion is defined as a rotation of the lung lobe along its long axis, with twisting of the bronchus and pulmonary vessels at the hilus. Torsion causes venous congestion of the affected lobe; however, the arteries remain at least partially patent, allowing blood to enter the lobe. Fluid and blood enter the alveoli, resulting in lung consolidation, transforming the lobe into a dark, firm, "liver-like" mass. The shape of the affected lobe may be altered, and the lobe appears displaced from its normal location within the thorax on thoracic radiographs. Pleural fluid accumulates with continued venous congestion. Spontaneous correction of torsion is rare due to swelling of the affected lobe and rapid formation of adhesions. Recurrence has been reported in dogs following lobectomy for earlier lung lobe torsion.

## MECHANISMS

Lung lobe torsions have been reported in dogs, cats, and human beings (Felson, 1987; Brown and Zontine, 1976; Lord et al., 1973). Mechanisms are poorly understood, but situations that result in increased mobility of a lobe seem to favor development of torsion (Felson, 1987). Partial collapse frees the lung lobe from normal spatial relationships with the thoracic wall, mediastinum, and adjacent lung lobes, destabilizing the lobe and enhancing mobility. Trauma may result in sudden compression of a lung lobe, altering anatomic relationships with adjacent lung lobes and thoracic wall. Rotation of the lobe occurs, followed by reexpansion. Pleural effusion or pneumothorax, along with subsequent atelectasis of the lung lobe, can result in increased freedom of movement, predisposing the lobe to torsion. In many cases, it is impossible to determine whether pleural fluid occurred first, with secondary lung lobe torsion, or whether pleural effusion occurred secondary to a spontaneous torsion. It is likely that in many animals (particularly those with chylothorax), chronic pleural effusion predisposes to lung lobe torsion. Lung lobe torsion has been reported secondary to previous thoracic surgery, where lung lobes may be partially collapsed or manipulated. Primary pulmonary disease such as pneumonia or a mass lesion may also predispose to torsion of the affected lobe.

Breed conformation appears to play a role in lung lobe torsion in that deep-chested large-breed dogs, especially Afghan hounds, are more commonly affected (Lord et al., 1973; Feeney et al., 1984). It is interesting to note that Afghan hounds are also predisposed to chylothorax, and the combination of lung lobe torsion and chylothorax has been reported in this breed. In large breeds, lung lobe torsion has been reported to occur spontaneously, without previous history of disease or trauma. Lung lobe torsion can also occur in small breeds such as poodles, but is usually secondary to primary pleural effusion, thoracic surgery, or trauma.

The right middle lung lobe is the most frequently affected by torsion, probably due to its long narrow shape and small pedicle, features which enhance mobility. Less frequently, torsion has been reported in the entire left cranial lobe, the caudal part of the left cranial lobe, the right cranial lobe, the right cranial and right middle lobes simultaneously, and the left caudal lobe.

## CLINICAL AND DIAGNOSTIC FEATURES

Clinical signs of lung lobe torsion are variable, but usually include some degree of respiratory distress (Su-

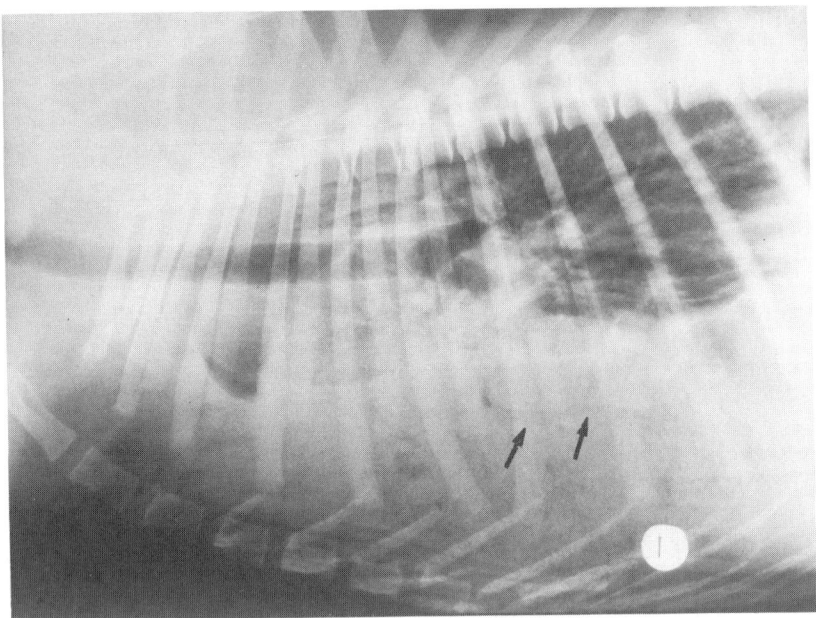

**Figure 1.** Lateral thoracic radiographic of a 6-year-old coonhound presented for respiratory distress of 24-hr duration. Pleural fluid obscures the cardiac silhouette. An air bronchogram originating from the torsed right middle lung lobe can be seen extending caudally in an abnormal direction (*arrow*).

ter, 1984; Lord et al., 1973). Coughing and hemoptysis can also occur, and may be chronic. Systemic signs include depression, anorexia, fever, and occasional vomiting. Clinical signs may be due to a preexisting condition, such as trauma, pleural effusion, pneumothorax, or pneumonia, making signs attributable to lung lobe torsion difficult to discern.

Pleural effusion is a consistent finding in animals with lung lobe torsion. Fluid analysis may reveal a sterile, inflammatory effusion; chyle; or may be quite bloody. However, pleural effusion of any etiology can initiate a secondary lung lobe torsion, making pleural fluid analysis variable and confusing in the diagnosis of lung lobe torsion. The appearance of blood in a previously nonhemorrhagic pleural fluid may indicate the occurrence of lung lobe torsion. An inflammatory leukogram may be present, but again, changes in the leukogram may reflect the initial disease process rather than the lung lobe torsion.

Thoracic radiography is an important tool in the diagnosis of lung lobe torsion; however, radiographic changes are variable depending on the volume of pleural fluid, presence or absence of preexisting disease, and the duration of the torsion. The most consistent finding is the presence of pleural effusion accompanied by an opacified lung lobe. Initially, air bronchograms will be present in the torsive lobe, and can be seen extending in an abnormal direction (Fig. 1). Eventually, air bronchograms disappear as fluid and blood fill the bronchial lumen. The presence of a noninflated, radiopaque lung lobe that persists after removal of pleural fluid should increase suspicion for lung lobe torsion (Fig. 2). Positional radiographs, using horizontal beam x-rays (lateral decubitus or upright ventrodorsal), are often helpful. Pleural fluid secondary to lung tor-

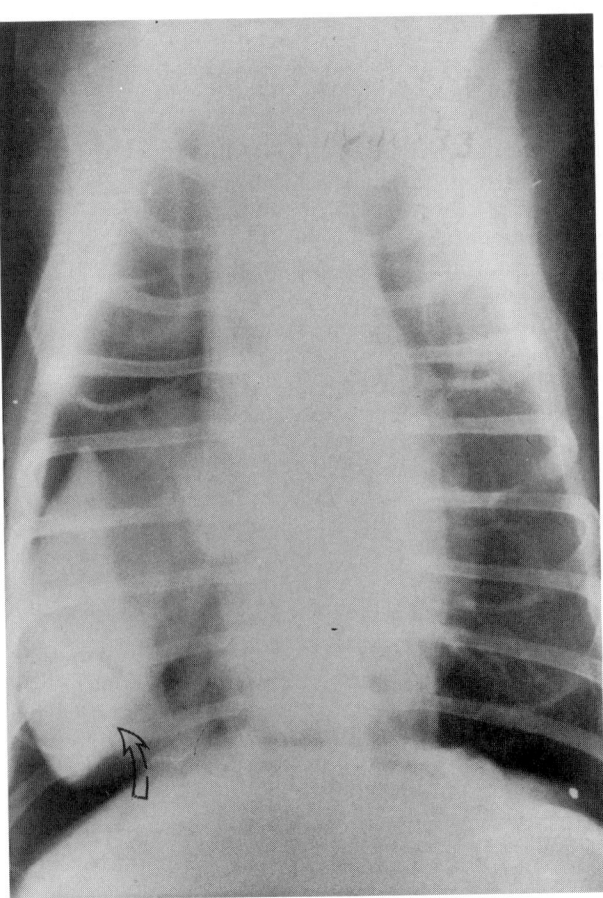

**Figure 2.** Ventrodorsal radiograph of a 7-year-old Doberman pinscher presented for evaluation of pleural effusion. After thoracocentesis, radiographs were taken. The right middle lung lobe remains collapsed despite removal of pleural fluid (*arrow*).

sion may persist around the affected lobe rather than fall to the dependent site. Failure of the lobe to reinflate in the "up," or nondependent, hemithorax is another indication of lung lobe torsion. Diseases such as pneumonia, pulmonary thromboembolism, contusions, neoplasia, atelectasis, pleural hemorrhage, diaphragmatic hernia, and pyothorax can mimic radiographic changes seen with lung lobe torsion, and should be included in the differential diagnosis.

Diagnosis of lung lobe torsion can be aided by bronchoscopy where partial or complete occlusion of the affected bronchus may be visualized. The bronchial mucosa at the site of the obstruction may appear folded and edematous. Demonstration of lung lobe torsion at surgery provides the definitive diagnosis.

## TREATMENT

Initial therapy is aimed at stabilizing the animal and alleviating respiratory distress, prior to surgical intervention. Thoracentesis should be performed to remove pleural fluid and should be done prior to radiographic procedures in animals that are extremely dyspneic. Persistent or massive pleural effusion may require placement of a chest tube. Oxygen therapy given by oxygen cage or nasal intubation is beneficial in some animals. Underlying diseases such as pneumonia should be treated with appropriate antibiotic therapy, and antibiotics should be administered to animals undergoing surgical correction of this condition. Intravenous fluid therapy is beneficial preoperatively and during surgery to maintain hydration.

The treatment of choice for lung lobe torsion is lobectomy of the affected lobe. Unless diagnosed very quickly (i.e., immediately after a surgical procedure), the damage to the pulmonary parenchyma is generally severe enough that attempts to salvage the lobe are not warranted. The pedicle should be clamped with a non-crushing forceps to prevent release of toxins into the bloodstream, prior to any attempts to derotate it. Untwisting the lobe prior to its removal may facilitate identification of the vascular structures and bronchus for ligation; however, in some cases, the lobe cannot be easily returned to its normal position due to extensive adhesions. The remaining lobes should be carefully checked for positioning and normal expansion. Culture of the pulmonary parenchyma following removal may help discern secondary bacterial infections. Histopathologic examination of tissues is rarely beneficial, but may occasionally help define underlying conditions such as neoplasia or infection.

Following removal of the affected lobe, a chest tube should be placed to monitor for continued pleural fluid production. Most effusions will resolve following lobectomy; however, chylous effusions may continue and require additional treatment (see *CVT X*, p 393). Antibiotics should be continued postoperatively if there is evidence of infection.

### References and Suggested Reading

Brown NO and Zontine W: Lung lobe torsion in the cat. Vet Radiol 17:219, 1976.
  *A review of clinical and radiographic aspects of lung lobe torsion in the cat.*
Feeney DA, O'Brien TD, Klausner JS, et al: Recurring lung lobe torsion in three Afghan hounds. J Am Vet Med Assoc 7:842, 1984.
  *A description of recurring lung lobe torsion in Afghan hounds after lobectomy for earlier lung lobe torsion.*
Felson B: Lung torsion: Radiographic findings in nine cases. Radiology 162:631, 1987.
  *A description of mechanisms and radiographic changes of lung lobe torsions in humans.*
Lord PF, Greiner TP, Greene RW, et al: Lung lobe torsion in the dog. J Am Anim Hosp Assoc 9:473, 1973.
  *A description of the clinical, radiographic, and surgical aspects of lung lobe torsion in 14 dogs.*
Suter PF: Lower airway and pulmonary parenchymal diseases. *In* Suter PF (ed): Thoracic Radiography: Thoracic Diseases of the Dog and Cat. Wettswil, Switzerland, Peter F. Suter, 1984, p 517.
  *A review of mechanisms, clinical signs, and radiographic changes of lung lobe torsion in dogs and cats.*

# MANAGEMENT OF FELINE CHYLOTHORAX

DANIEL D. SMEAK
and STEPHEN J. KERPSACK
*Columbus, Ohio*

Chylothorax is an uncommon but potentially fatal disease characterized by the accumulation of chyle in the pleural cavity. Chyle is composed of lymphatic fluid principally derived from the abdominal organs and contains chylomicrons and other suspended lipid by-products of digestion. A tentative diagnosis of chylothorax is made upon aspiration of a characteristic pink to milky white (fat-laden) fluid from the pleural cavity. In patients with anorexia or those fed a reduced-fat diet, the diagnosis may be less obvious. As the fat content of chyle is reduced, the appearance of the effusion becomes less opaque and more serous in character.

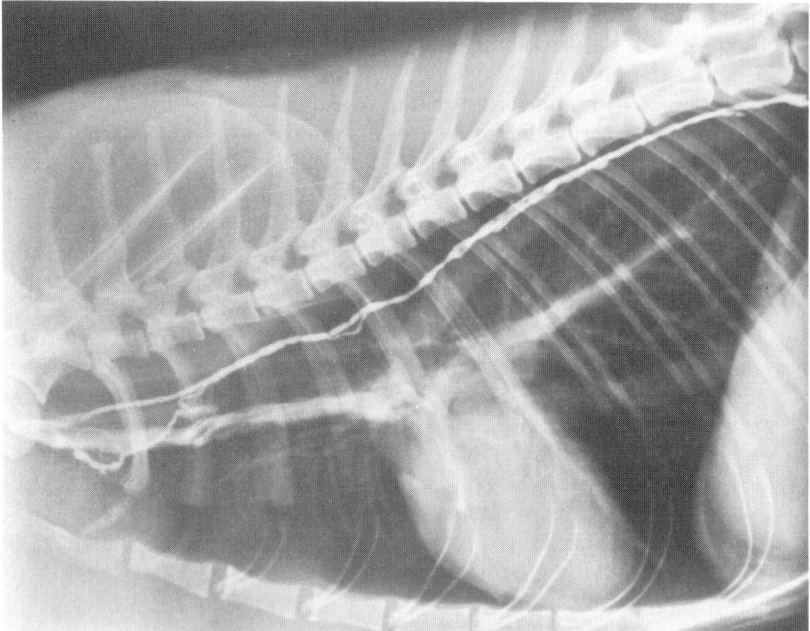

**Figure 1.** Mesenteric lymphangiogram in a normal cat.

Although a number of diseases have been associated with this condition in dogs and cats, the underlying cause in most cases remains an enigma (Fossum, 1989). When a cause for chylothorax is identified in the cat, it is usually related to significant heart failure or thoracic neoplasia (Kerpsack et al., in press). Most normal cats possess one or a few interconnected terminal thoracic duct branches on mesenteric lymphangiograms (Birchard and Fossum, 1987) (Fig. 1); lymphangiograms of cats with chylothorax consistently show numerous dilated lymphatics in the cranial mediastinum, a condition called thoracic lymphangiectasia (Fig. 2). Seldom is leakage detected through a thoracic duct ruptured from trauma, as this disease was originally described. Instead, seepage (extravasation) apparently occurs through the walls of these intact, thin-walled vessels.

Signs of respiratory compromise secondary to chyle accumulation eventually prompt owners to seek veterinary care for their pet. Medical management, such as intermittent pleural evacuation and dietary therapy, is rarely successful, but has been recommended before more invasive treatment (thoracic duct ligation) is considered. Such a medical strategy may be ill-advised for a number of reasons: it delays more successful therapy; increases costs to the owner; extended loss of chyle can

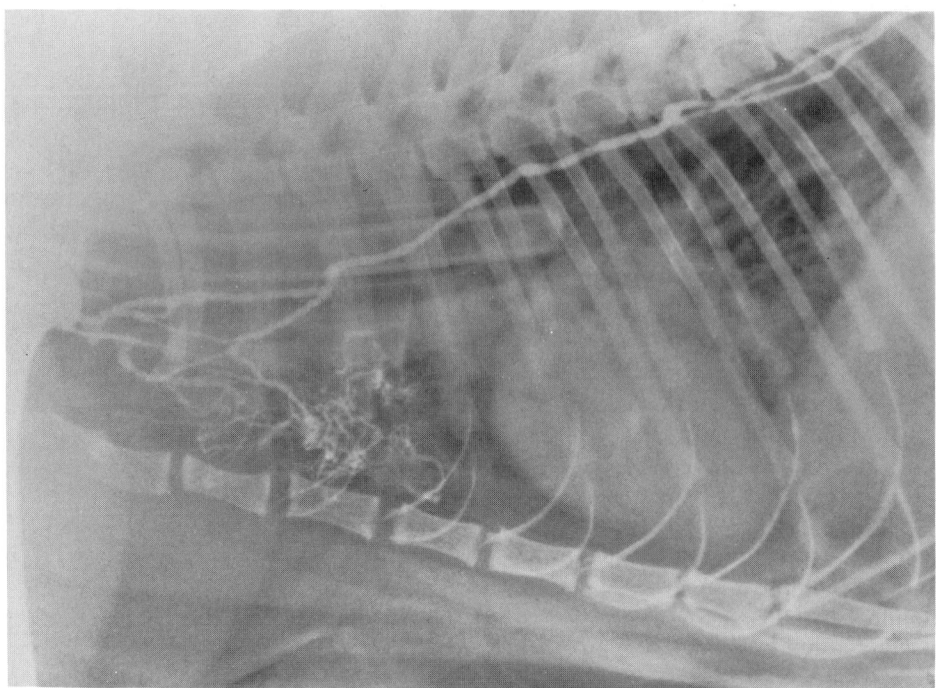

**Figure 2.** Preoperative mesenteric lymphangiogram showing lymphangiectasia in the cranial mediastinum.

cause malnutrition and immunocompromise; and prolonged contact of chyle with pleural surfaces induces an inflammatory reaction that may lead to incurable pleural fibrosis. Thus, delayed surgery may result in a poor clinical response. Early detection, proper patient selection, and aggressive surgical treatment are the primary management goals in cats.

## PATHOPHYSIOLOGY

Patients afflicted with chylothorax often become debilitated due to chronic loss of chyle subsequent to thoracocentesis. Most cats develop respiratory compromise from pleural fluid accumulation or chylofibrosis. Depending to some extent on diet and hydration, the basal rate of lymph flow through the thoracic duct has been estimated at 2 ml/kg/hr (Birchard and Fossum, 1987). Respiratory compromise may develop rapidly because up to several hundred milliliters of chyle can be produced in a cat daily. Expansion of the pleural space compresses functional lung tissue, which may lead to acute ventilatory failure due to alveolar atelectasis and reduced vital capacity.

Nearly two thirds of all ingested fats are delivered to the bloodstream by way of the thoracic duct. In addition, this duct is the main transportation pathway of proteins from the interstitium back to the venous system. Removal of large volumes of chyle from the pleural space may cause water and electrolyte losses sufficient to induce significant dehydration and electrolyte imbalance (Fossum et al., 1991). Loss of lipid, fat-soluble vitamins, and protein leads to protein-calorie malnutrition and hypoproteinemia. Immunocompetence may be impaired if malnutrition and the loss of lymphocytes and antibodies are protracted (Orton, 1993). Prevention of these pathophysiologic effects must address the goals of adequate pleural evacuation and reduction in the loss or production of chyle. Proper measures are undertaken to stabilize the patient's nutritional, fluid, and electrolyte imbalance before contemplating surgery.

## ETIOLOGY

The etiology of chylothorax remains poorly understood. Chylothorax has been associated with induced and naturally occurring dirofilariasis, traumatic leakage, diaphragmatic hernia, lymphosarcoma, cranial mediastinal masses (thymoma, lymphoma, lymphangiosarcoma) cardiomyopathy, severe right-sided heart failure, and pulmonary neoplasia. In most cats with chylothorax, a cause is not discovered; this is termed "idiopathic chylothorax" (Fossum et al., 1994).

Development of lymphangiectasia in the cranial mediastinum appears to be the most common anatomic lesion identified in cats with experimental or naturally occurring chylothorax. Experimental and clinical evidence suggests that cranial mediastinal lymphangiectasia is produced by either a functional or mechanical obstruction to thoracic duct flow (Fossum, 1989). Obstruction of cranial vena caval blood flow to the heart or direct duct obstruction from, for example, a caval thrombosis or mass may restrict thoracic duct flow. Increased lymph flow from right-sided congestive heart failure or heartworm disease may result in a functional obstruction caused by an inability of the lymphaticovenous junction to dilate to accommodate these flows as well as obstructed drainage caused by elevated central venous pressure. Lymphangiectasia could be a result of the lymphatic system's attempt to bypass an obstruction. Congenital abnormalities of the thoracic duct itself or its terminal lymphaticovenous junction resulting in chylothorax have been documented in humans, and this has been a proposed etiology in Afghans and purebred cats (Fossum, 1989). Idiopathic chylothorax that develops later in life in cats and dogs does not suggest a congenital condition, although a predisposing genetic factor may be involved. Rupture of the thoracic duct could result from blunt or penetrating trauma, inadvertent surgical disruption, venous catheterization or direct neoplastic invasion, although this is uncommon (Orton, 1993).

## CLINICAL MANIFESTATIONS

Most cats with chylothorax are middle-aged (average 8 years); however, affected cats may present as early as 6 months or greater than 15 years of age. There appears to be no sex predilection and purebred cats may be overrepresented (Fossum et al., 1991).

Cats with chylothorax present with a variety of historical problems ranging from depression and lethargy to overt dyspnea. Nearly half of cats have clinical signs for more than 1 month, suggesting that they can compensate for prolonged periods of time to slow pleural fluid accumulation. Dyspnea or tachypnea and coughing are the most common historical findings. The character of the ventilation is typical of restrictive pleural disease. Cats attempt to compensate by increasing the frequency of respiration with pronounced inspiration and delayed expiration phases. Coughing is thought to result from pleural irritation induced by the effusion rather than being a cause of the disease.

Cats presenting with only vague clinical signs are known to decompensate rapidly due to the stress of examination. In this instance, complete examination should be delayed until measures are taken to improve respiratory function. On physical examination, dyspnea, dorsally increased bronchovesicular sounds, muffled heart sounds, a dull (hyporesonant) thoracic percussion note, and depression are the most common abnormalities found. Even historically fractious cats seem to be more passive than expected and often prefer to stand or sit rather than lay down (orthopnea). Depending on the chronicity of the disease, amount of pleural effusion, and prior treatment attempts, cats may be emaciated, dehydrated, and cyanotic (Fossum et al., 1991).

## DIAGNOSTIC APPROACH

If the cat with suspected chylothorax is not overtly dyspneic, thoracic radiographs are taken to confirm the presence of pleural effusion. Otherwise, supplemental oxygen is provided via mask or cage and thoracentesis is best performed before radiography. To minimize the stress of handling, only a single dorsoventral radiographic view is required initially.

Once pleural effusion is verified by physical or radiographic examination, thoracentesis is performed. If the cranial mediastinum is not adequately visualized due to the effusion, thoracic ultrasonagraphy, if available, should be performed before massive amounts of fluid are removed. Air present in the pleural space or in expanded lung lobes produces a highly reflective barrier to the ultrasound beam, obscuring structures deep to the air interface, and inhibiting adequate evaluation of the thorax. Thoracentesis is best performed with a 21-gauge butterfly needle attached to a three-way stopcock and large syringe. The needle is placed through the eighth intercostal space (centered around the costochondral junction), and as much fluid as possible is aspirated with the cat in sternal recumbency. As the cat's breathing becomes more stable during chest aspiration, various body positions and needle locations are tried to improve fluid evacuation. Once both hemithoraces are evacuated, thoracic radiographs are repeated to allow more complete evaluation of the thoracic viscera. Fluid collected should be placed in an ethylenediaminetetraacetic acid (EDTA) tube (for cytologic analysis), and sterile vial for culture and susceptibility. Paired samples of serum and pleural fluid should be submitted for triglyceride and cholesterol content. A complete cell blood count, biochemical, and serologic (enzyme-linked immunosorbent assay [ELISA], feline leukemia virus [FeLV], feline immunodeficiency virus [FIV], heartworm) evaluation usually do not reveal any abnormalities but should be performed to rule out concurrent disease.

The presence of pleural fluid is detected on lateral thoracic radiographs as a diffuse hazy ventral density causing indistinct cardiac borders. Small rounded lung lobes, blunting of costophrenic angles, and interlobar fissures are seen, depending on the amount of effusion. Elevation of the trachea or persistent soft tissue density within the cranial mediastinum is suggestive of a cranial mediastinal mass. Presence of a mass in this area is confirmed via thoracic ultrasonography when available. An enlarged heart shadow with signs of pulmonary venous congestion signals cardiac disease. Fractured ribs, diaphragmatic hernia, and other signs of trauma may be seen in rare cases. More often, no specific radiographic signs are present other than those for pleural effusion.

A definitive diagnosis is made if the effusion is determined to be chyle. Chylous effusions are typically opaque, milky white to pink in appearance. A cream layer will usually form when the fluid is left to stand. When centrifuged, chylous fluid will not separate as would an exudate with a high cellular content (pyothorax). Other characteristics typical of chylous effu-

sions are listed in Table 1. Fluid indices may be classified as a modified transudate to exudate depending on the chronicity and prior drainage attempts; as the duration of chylothorax increases, the protein, specific gravity, and cellular content also tend to increase. Lymphocytes comprise the majority of cells seen on examination of most chylous effusions in cats, though in some cats, the neutrophil count is relatively high. A chylous effusion with a high neutrophil count and a positive Gram stain for intracellular bacteria may indicate a secondary infection from repeated attempts at thoracic aspiration. Fluid is also evaluated cytologically for evidence of neoplasia. The most definitive and consistent method to diagnose chylothorax is to detect higher triglyceride and lower cholesterol concentrations in the effusion than in the serum (Fossum, Jacobs, and Birchard, 1986). Alternately, if a serum sample is not available, a cholesterol/triglyceride concentration ratio of the pleural effusion of less than 1 is diagnostic for chyle. A pseudochylous effusion is defined as having a similar gross appearance as chylous effusions but the cholesterol content of the effusion is more and the triglyceride content is less than the serum. There is no compelling evidence that pseudochylous effusions have ever been documented in the cat.

A complete cardiac work-up, including echocardiography and occult heartworm testing, should be performed on all cats with confirmed chylothorax.

## TREATMENT

Treatment of chylothorax varies considerably, depending on the underlying cause; therefore, proper patient work-up is critical to developing an appropriate therapeutic plan (Fig. 3). If a cause of chylothorax is determined, primary treatment is usually directed at the underlying cause. Besides a handful of case reports, little information is available on whether successful treatment of these associated diseases resolves the chylous effusion. Successful management of chylothorax secondary to cardiac disease has been observed following effective treatment of heart failure.

The goal of medical management is to support the metabolic and nutritional needs of the patient until the

***Table 1.*** *Feline Chylothorax Effusion Characteristics**

| | |
|---|---|
| Color/clarity | Pink to white |
| Specific gravity | 1.019–1.038 (mean = 1.030) |
| Total protein | 3.5–7.8 (mean = 5.32 g/dl) |
| Chylomicrons | Present |
| Total WBC µl | 1.6–60,800 (mean = 11,919) |
| Predominant cell type | Lymphocyte or neutrophils |
| Triglyceride content | > Serum |
| Cholesterol content | < Serum |
| Ether clearance test | Clears |
| Cholesterol/triglyceride ratio | <1 |

*From Fossum TW, Forrester SD, Swenson CL, et al: Chylothorax in cats: 37 cases (1969–1989). J Am Vet Med Assoc 198:672, 1991, with permission.

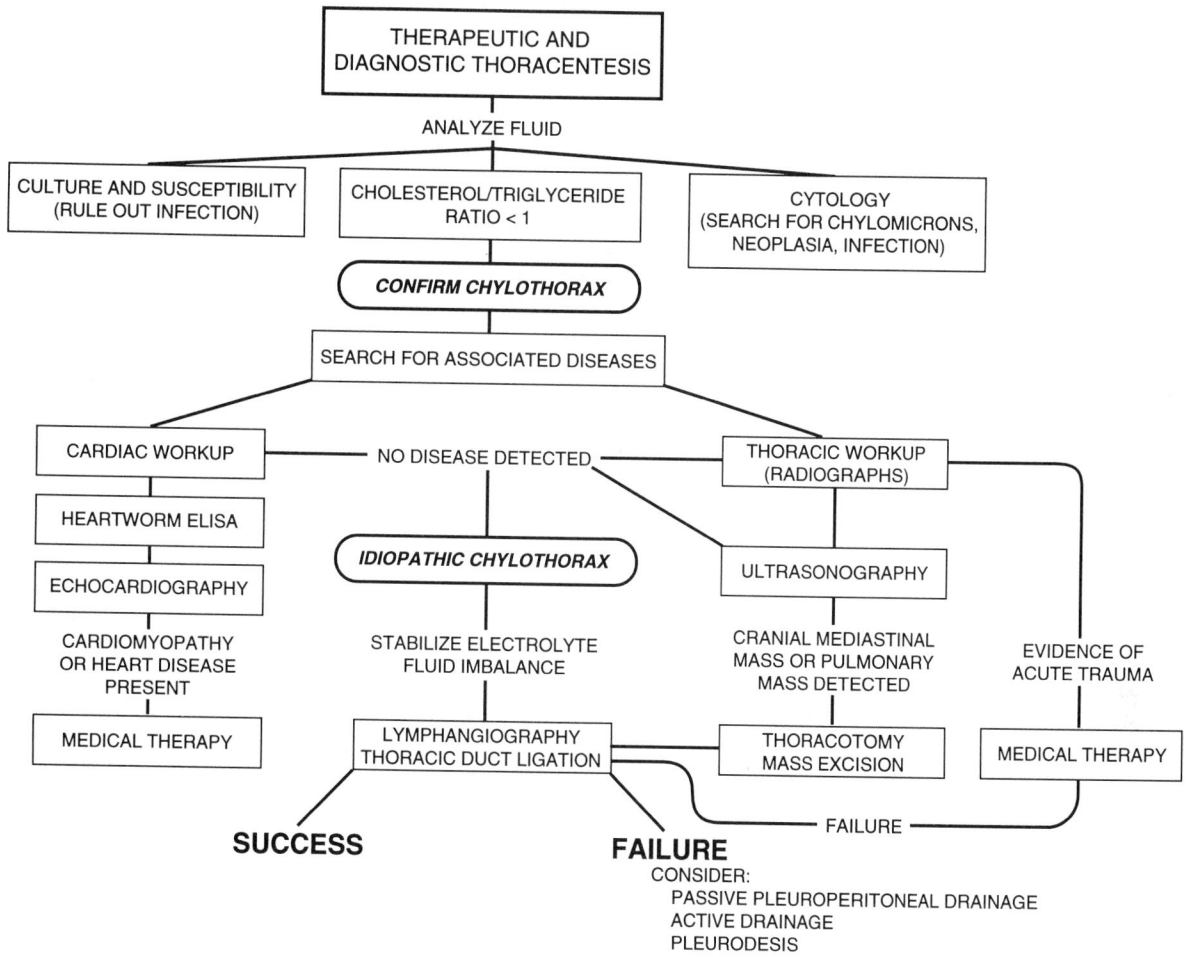

**Figure 3.** Management algorithm for cats with chylothorax.

effusion spontaneously resolves. Evacuation of the thorax by means of thoracostomy tube or thoracentesis and dietary management are the mainstays of medical therapy. Intermittent thoracentesis is attempted first; if this is unsuccessful in alleviating clinical signs, a thoracostomy tube is implanted. Optimally, intravenous alimentation is instituted, since this is a proven way to reduce the quantity of lymph flow through the thoracic duct in humans. Because this is costly and impractical in most cases, the patient's caloric needs are met by feeding a reduced-fat diet (r/d Prescription Diet, Hill's Pet Products, or, alternately, a homemade tuna and rice diet supplemented with vitamins may be acceptable). Medium-chain triglycerides (MCT oil, Mead Johnson) may be used to supplement the above diets. Short- or medium-chain triglyceride supplementation has been recommended because these fats are thought to be absorbed directly into the portal system, bypassing the thoracic duct. Recent research suggests that MCT oil may contribute to thoracic duct flow in dogs, and alterations in fat content in diet causes little change in overall thoracic duct flow. Until more information is available, the primary goal of dietary therapy is to satisfy the nutritional needs of the patient first, rather than focusing on dietary changes designed to reduce chyle

production. We consider medical management as a *temporary* means to support our patients with idiopathic chylothorax before surgery; less than 20% of cats with idiopathic chylothorax respond long term to the aforementioned medical regimen (Fossum, 1991; Harpster, 1986).

Cats that have concrete evidence of recent trauma, but otherwise have no detectable cause for chylothorax, may respond to medical therapy alone. Cats that do not require surgery for the trauma (e.g., fractured ribs, pulmonary contusion) may be treated conservatively for several weeks to determine if the effusion resolves spontaneously. This approach is supported by a report of two cats with traumatic chylothorax that had resolution of the effusion after surgical correction of a diaphragmatic hernia alone (Meineke, Hobbie, and Barto, 1969). Our experience has been less rewarding. We currently recommend surgical ligation of the thoracic duct in addition to correction of a diaphragmatic hernia, since both can be achieved through a ventral midline approach (Martin et al., 1988).

Specific therapy (i.e., chemotherapy, radiation, surgical resection) should be instituted following definitive diagnosis of a cranial mediastinal or thoracic mass. Medical management for chylothorax is instituted while specific therapy is undertaken to treat the cause. If the patient responds to therapy and the effusion resolves, no further therapy is instituted; otherwise (depending on the prognosis for the specific cause of the chylothorax), thoracic duct ligation may be advisable. If lung lobe torsion or neoplasia is detected, lobectomy is performed and, in addition, thoracic duct ligation is recommended if these procedures can be completed through the same approach. Otherwise, attempt to remove the intrathoracic mass first; thoracic duct ligation is considered if the effusion fails to resolve.

Treatment of cats with evidence of cardiomyopathy or congenital heart disease and concurrent chylothorax is directed at standard medical therapy for chylothorax and improving cardiac function with appropriate drug therapy (see elsewhere in this section). Adulticide treatment is not recommended for cats with dirofilariasis. Thoracic duct ligation was successful in alleviating the chylous effusion in a cat with dirofilariasis.

### Thoracic Duct Ligation

Early thoracic duct ligation is recommended in cats with idiopathic chylothorax because no other alternative available today has superior results (Kerpsack et al., in press). The standard surgical approach for thoracic duct ligation in the cat is a left intercostal thoracotomy; however, we prefer to perform a median sternotomy and ventral midline abdominal approach if another surgical disorder such as thymoma, lung lobe torsion, or diaphragmatic hernia is present in a cat with chylothorax. This approach allows both correction of the underlying disorder and thoracic duct ligation (Martin et al., 1988).

Prior to anesthesia, all electrolyte and fluid imbalances are corrected and the pleural space is fully evacuated. No food is given for 12 hr before surgery, 30 ml of heavy cream is administered orally 4 to 6 hr before surgery to dilate and accentuate the intestinal lymphatics. The left lateral thorax and abdomen are prepared and draped for aseptic surgery. A 6- to 8-cm left paracostal incision is created with the cat in right lateral recumbency. The distal portion of the small intestine is exteriorized to expose the cecal area. If lymphatics are not readily apparent, 0.10 ml of methylene blue is injected with a 25-gauge tuberculin needle in a mesenteric lymph node in the cecal area. Gently squeeze the lymph node to distribute blue dye into the lymphatic trunks. A 22- or 24-gauge over-the-needle catheter (Surflo, The Burrows Co, Wheeling, IL) is placed in a mesenteric lymphatic adjacent to the cecum and secured to adjacent bowel serosa. A mesenteric lymphangiogram is performed utilizing 1 ml/kg of a water-soluble iodinated contrast agent (Diatrizoate meglumine). The agent is slowly infused through the lymphatic catheter and a right lateral thoracic radiograph is taken as the last milliliter of contrast agent is infused. The cat is repositioned in dorsal recumbency and the procedure is repeated to obtain a ventrodorsal lymphangiogram if this is possible.

Using the lymphangiogram as a guide, an appropriate intercostal space is entered for thoracic duct ligation. Preferably, the thoracotomy is centered in the caudal thorax over an area of the thoracic duct with the fewest branches; usually the left ninth or tenth space is chosen. After the chest is open, the caudal lung lobe is retracted cranially and the mediastinal pleura is incised just dorsal to the aorta. If the lymphatic trunk(s) is not readily apparent within the mediastinal fat, 0.25 ml of methylene blue diluted in 1 ml of saline is injected in the mesenteric catheter until the lymphatics are visible. The thoracic duct branches are ligated with 3-0 silk or hemostatic clips (Versaclips, Ethicon Inc, Somerville, NJ). If no duct can be definitively isolated, all mediastinal fat and periadventitial tissues are mass ligated from the dorsal and left lateral aspects of the aorta while avoiding the sympathetic trunk.

Theoretically, postligation lymphangiograms should help detect branches that may not have been included in the ligature. This procedure has been recommended to ensure complete occlusion of thoracic duct flow. However, the value of this study is questionable, since we have not demonstrated collateral thoracic duct branches after ligation in any of the cats we have surgically treated; several cats have had persistent chylous effusion after surgery despite documentation of no collaterals after ligation (Kerpsack et al., in press). In support of this observation, Martin et al. (1988) demonstrated that surgical manipulation of mediastinal tissues alone, without attempting ligation, blocks contrast flow through the thoracic duct and results in a negative lymphangiogram in cats.

Once ligation is complete, closure is begun. We make no attempt to suture the mediastinum over the ligation area. A fenestrated 14-Fr. thoracostomy tube is inserted at the eighth or ninth intercostal space. The mesenteric catheter is removed and the abdominal and thoracotomy incisions are closed routinely.

Cats are given intravenous balanced electrolyte solution at maintenance rates to support hydration after surgery. The thoracostomy tube is aspirated as indicated and the amount of fluid removed is recorded. Cats are fed whatever diet they choose after surgery. Anorexic cats may require nasogastric or gastrostomy tube feeding to maintain an appropriate nutritional status. Thoracostomy tubes are removed when less than 1 ml/kg of pleural fluid is withdrawn daily and minimal pleural fluid is demonstrated radiographically.

If sufficient amounts of pleural fluid remain after the seventh postoperative day, pleural fluid is examined cytologically and cholesterol/triglyceride concentrations are obtained. Septic nonchylous effusions are treated with appropriate antibiotics. Passive or active pleuroperitoneal drainage techniques may be considered in cats that have persistent sterile effusions following thoracic duct ligation (Fossum, 1989), although we have had minimal long-term success with these methods. The passive drainage technique described is accomplished by the use of a fenestrated Silastic sheet and tubes placed in the diaphragm. Pleural fluid flows through this sheet and is apparently absorbed via the peritoneum. While two cats were successfully managed with this technique for more than 1 year in one report, these implants are occluded by peritoneal adhesions within months following implantation in experimental cats. An implanted, manually activated pump has also been used to shunt pleural fluid into the peritoneal cavity similar to the passive technique. We have used two-valve Denver shunt catheters for this purpose in four cats. The catheters became obstructed within 2 weeks in two cats and the shunts were removed due to infection in the remaining cats. Pleurodesis with tetracycline hydrochloride may also be considered, but our results and those of others (Fossum et al., 1991) suggest that this is also rarely successful in eliminating pleural effusion.

Cats that exhibit signs of respiratory difficulty but have minimal pleural fluid present may be suffering from restrictive pleuritis ("Chylofibrosis"). In chronic cases, lung lobes become encased in a thick white membrane that restricts pulmonary expansion. If this capsule is removed surgically, more complete lung expansion may improve ventilation. Only a few anecdotal reports of cats with restrictive pleuritis have been successfully managed this way. Presence of severe pleural fibrosis and collapse of more than half the total lung volume is generally a poor prognostic sign.

## PROGNOSIS AND POSTOPERATIVE COMPLICATIONS

Thoracic duct ligation is less successful in eliminating chylous effusion in cats when compared to dogs (Fossum et al., 1991; Harpster, 1986). Fossum stated in a retrospective study of 37 cats with chylothorax that only 20% of cats treated by thoracic duct ligation had resolution of the effusion. This success rate was not significantly different than cats treated with conservative medical therapy alone. A recent retrospective study conducted at The Ohio State University suggests that the prognosis after surgical therapy may be more favorable than previously documented. Thoracic duct ligation resulted in complete resolution of the effusion between 3 and 7 days after surgery and long-term survival in 53% of cats with idiopathic chylothorax. Chylous effusion persisting for more than 7 days following thoracic duct ligation is unlikely to resolve and other surgical procedures such as passive or active drainage techniques or pleurodesis may be considered if owners want to pursue further treatment. Continued effusion following thoracic duct ligation occurs in approximately 30% of cats. Postoperative deaths are usually attributed to restrictive pleural disease or complications of nutritional support. In our experience, chronically affected cats that are malnourished or those that exhibit signs of respiratory compromise despite adequate evacuation of the pleural space appear to be at greater risk for these complications.

## References and Suggested Reading

Birchard SJ and Fossum TW: Chylothorax in the dog and cat. Vet Clin North Am [Small Anim Pract] 17:271, 1987.
*A review of the anatomy, physiology, etiologies, diagnosis, and treatments of chylothorax in dogs.*

Fossum TW, Jacobs RM, and Birchard SJ: Evaluation of cholesterol and triglyceride concentrations in differentiating chylous and nonchylous pleural effusions in dogs and cats. J Am Vet Med Assoc 188:49, 1986.
*A study demonstrating the value of pleural and serum cholesterol and triglyceride concentrations in a series of animals with effusions of chylous and nonchylous origin.*

Fossum TW: Chylothorax: Recent advances and new perspectives. Semin Vet Med 1:300, 1989.
*A historical review of chylothorax and discussion of controversial contemporary treatment issues.*

Fossum TW, Forrester SD, Swenson CL, et al: Chylothorax in cats: 37 cases (1969–1989). J Am Vet Med Assoc 198:672, 1991.
*A retrospective review detailing the results of medical and surgical therapy of cats with chylothorax.*

Fossum TW, Miller MW, Rogers KS, et al: Chylothorax associated with right-sided heart failure in five cats. J Am Vet Med Assoc 204:84, 1994.
*A case series demonstrating that jugular distention and results of echocardiography may be important in the diagnosis of right-sided heart failure in cats with chylothorax.*

Harpster NK: Chylothorax. In Kirk RW (ed): Current Veterinary Therapy IX. Small Animal Practice. Philadelphia, WB Saunders Co, 1986, p 295.
*A review of current medical and surgical treatments for chylothorax in dogs and cats.*

Kerpsack SJ, McLoughlin MA, Birchard SJ, Smeak DD, et al: Results of mesenteric lymphangiography and thoracic duct ligation in cats with chylothorax: 19 cases (1987–1992). Personal observations, 1993.
*A retrospective study describing the postoperative results of a series of cats treated by thoracic duct ligation.*

Martin RA, Richards DLS, Barber DL, et al: Transdiaphragmatic approach to thoracic duct in the cat. Vet Surg 17:22, 1988.
*A study demonstrating the ability to ligate the thoracic duct through a ventral midline abdominal approach.*

Meineke JE, Hobbie WV, and Barto LR: Traumatic chylothorax with associated diaphragmatic hernias in the cat. J Am Vet Med Assoc 155:15, 1969.
*A case report showing successful resolution of chylothorax in two cases after repair of traumatic diaphragmatic hernias.*

Orton EC: Pleura and pleural space. In Slatter DH (ed): Textbook of Small Animal Surgery. Philadelphia, WB Saunders Co, 1993, p 381.
*A summary of the pathophysiology, diagnosis, and treatment of pleural space disorders in the dog and cat.*

# Section

# 10

# URINARY
# DISORDERS

JEANNE A. BARSANTI
*Consulting Editor*

***Still Current Information Found in Current Veterinary Therapy XI:***

Finco DR, Barsanti JA, and Brown SA: Solute Fractional Excretion Rates, p 818.
Dow SW and Fettman MJ: Renal Disease in Cats: The Potassium Connection, p 820.
DiBartola SP: Renal Amyloidosis in Dogs and Cats, p 823.
Relford RL and Green RA: Coagulation Disorders in Glomerular Diseases, p 827.
Forrester SD and Lees GE: Acute Renal Failure Associated With Systemic Infectious Disease, p 829.
Brown SA, Barsanti JA, and Finco DR: Effects of Vasoactive Agents on Kidney Function, p 832.
Podell M: Use of Blood Pressure Monitors, p 834.
Littman MP: Update: Treatment of Hypertension in Dogs and Cats, p 838.
Brown SA, Barsanti JA, and Finco DR: Medical Management of Canine Chronic Renal Failure, p 842.
Polzin DJ, Osborne CA, Adams LG, and Lulich JP: Medical Management of Feline Chronic Renal Failure, p 848.
Chew DJ, DiBartola SP, Nagode LA, and Starkey RJ: Phosphorus Restriction in the Treatment of Chronic Renal Failure (CRF), p 853.
Chew DJ and Nagode LA: Calcitriol in the Treatment of Chronic Renal Failure, p 857.
Vaden SL and Grauder GF: Medical Management of Canine Glomerulonephritis, p 861.
Lane IF, Carter LJ, and Lappin MR: Peritoneal Dialysis: An Update on Methods and Usefulness, p 865.
Gregory CR and Gourley IM: Renal Transplantation in Clinical Veterinary Medicine, p 870.
Arnold S: Relationship of Incontinence to Neutering, p 875.
Senior DF: Use of Cystoscopy, p 878.
Senior DF: Urethral Dilation, p 880.
Barsanti JA, Finco DR, and Brown SA: Feline Urethral Obstruction: Medical Management, p 883.
Osborne CA, Lulich JP, and Unger LK: Nonsurgical Retrieval of Uroliths for Mineral Analysis, p 886.
Dieringer TM and Lees GE: Nephroliths: Approach to Therapy, p 889.
Lulich JP, Osborne CA, and Smith CL: Canine Calcium Oxalate Urolithiasis: Risk Factor Management, p 892.
Bartges JW, Osborne CA, and Felice LJ: Canine Xanthine Uroliths Risk Factor Management, p 900.
Osborne CA, Lulich JP, Bartges JW, and Polzin DJ: Feline Metabolic Uroliths Risk Factor Management, p 905.
Lees GE and Forrester SD: Update: Bacterial Urinary Tract Infections, p 909.
Lulich JP and Osborne CA: Fungal Urinary Tract Infections, p 914.
Rogers KS and Walker MA: Therapy of Transitional Cell Carcinoma of the Canine Bladder, p 919.
Gilson SD and Stone EA: Tumor Markers for Diagnosis of Urinary Tract Neoplasms, p 922.

***Elsewhere in Current Veterinary Therapy XII:***

# WHEN AND HOW TO MEASURE GLOMERULAR FILTRATION RATE AND EFFECTIVE RENAL PLASMA FLOW

DONALD R. KRAWIEC
*and* RANDALL J. ITKIN
*Urbana, Illinois*

Renal failure remains an important cause of morbidity in small animals. The most common renal syndrome in small animals is chronic renal failure. Unfortunately, chronic renal failure is largely an idiopathic problem; consequently, the veterinarian's role in the management of this disease is largely directed to early detection and slowing disease progression. Renal failure can be diagnosed by both qualitative and quantitative methods. Qualitative methods identify renal failure but poorly describe the magnitude of dysfunction. Qualitative diagnosis of primary renal failure is based on finding azotemia along with the inability to concentrate urine. In many instances, this qualitative assessment is the end point of the diagnostic process and the beginning of the therapeutic process. In certain instances, it is important to further pursue the case diagnostically by performing a quantitative renal function assay. Glomerular filtration rate (GFR) and effective renal plasma flow (ERPF) are the two most common parameters used to quantify renal function. This article will describe the indications and techniques for performing quantitative renal function assays.

## GLOMERULAR FILTRATION RATE

### Indications

The kidney performs a number of important functions to maintain normal physiologic homeostasis. These functions include the elimination and conservation of water, the removal and elimination of waste products from blood, the conservation of essential constituents of blood, and the regulation of acid-base balance. The kidney has a number of endocrine functions as well. However, determination of the rate of glomerular filtration is the "gold standard" of tests of renal function. Glomerular filtration rate measures the rate at which the kidneys remove and excrete waste from the blood. Great emphasis is placed on this assay because GFR determinations will usually have a direct correlation to total functional renal mass and, therefore, provide an indirect evaluation of all the functions of the kidney.

Evaluations of GFR provide information that can be valuable to the care of any patient with renal failure, but because they tend to be time consuming and somewhat invasive they are usually only performed on a select group of patients. A retrospective study identified the ultimate diagnosis of patients evaluated for GFR at the University of Illinois Teaching Hospital. The most common diagnoses in dogs that were assessed for GFR in descending order were chronic renal failure, glomerulonephritis, renal calculi, acute renal failure, and pyelonephritis. Other diagnoses included ectopic ureter, renal neoplasia, renal cyst, and hydronephrosis. The most common diagnoses in cats were chronic renal failure, renal calculi, acute renal failure, and pyelonephritis. These patients were critically evaluated for specific indications for measuring GFR and were summarized to provide the following general recommendations.

Patients with chronic renal failure, glomerulonephritis, and acute renal failure should be evaluated for GFR in order to (1) diagnose renal failure in the nonazotemic, polyuric animal; (2) provide owners with a more accurate prognosis of animals with renal failure; and (3) provide veterinarians with more precise guidelines for optimizing the dose rates of renal-excreted drugs in patients with renal failure. In addition to these general recommendations, serial quantitative assessments of renal failure can provide the clinician an accurate assessment of response to therapy and progression of disease.

Recommendations for measuring GFR of patients with renal calculi, ectopic ureter, renal neoplasia, renal cyst, and hydronephrosis include all those listed above. In addition, GFR assays that provide individual kidney function determinations are important if a unilateral surgical nephrotomy or nephrectomy is planned. In these instances, it is important to assess the contralateral kidney independently to be sure it can sustain life, if there is appreciable loss of function due to the procedure performed on the affected kidney.

### Techniques

Glomerular filtration rates are classically determined by performing creatinine or inulin clearances. Endogenous creatinine clearance is the most common method performed in practice and has been described

931

in detail in *CVT IX* (Ross, 1986). This procedure requires the quantitative collection of a 24-hr urine sample, which often requires multiple urethral catheterizations. Due to the intrinsic limitations of the assay, endogenous creatinine clearance only provides an estimate of GFR. Exogenous creatinine clearance also has been used to measure GFR in small animal medicine (Finco, Coulter, and Barsanti, 1981). It is more accurate than endogenous clearances and is not much more difficult to perform. Inulin clearance for the determination of GFR is the standard against which the accuracy of all other methods to assess renal function are compared. Unfortunately, inulin clearance requires physical restraint for long periods of time or general anesthesia as well as indwelling urinary catheterization. Inulin clearance is thus invasive and stressful, making it less desirable for use on client-owned animals.

The above methods evaluate the sum of function of both kidneys and cannot evaluate individual kidney function. Renal scintigraphy can be used to assess kidney structure and function of clinically normal dogs and cats or animals in renal failure. Renal imaging and dynamic radionuclide evaluations using $^{99m}$Tc-diethylenetriaminepentaacetic acid to determine GFR in dogs and cats have been described and are noninvasive, accurate and reproducible (Krawiec et al., 1988; Uribe et al., 1992). Scintigraphic measurement of GFR offers several advantages over conventional renal function tests. They provide rapid and accurate assessment of individual kidney function, require only one intravenous administration, eliminate serial blood and urine sampling, and do not further compromise critical patients. Unfortunately, equipment necessary to measure GFR in this way is expensive and at present limited mostly to academic teaching hospitals.

## EFFECTIVE RENAL BLOOD FLOW

### Indications

Renal blood flow determinations have been shown to provide valuable information concerning the nature and progression of renal failure in experimentally induced renal failure in dogs and other species (Duarte et al., 1980). However, due to the stressful nature of the assay, ERPF is not often assessed in spontaneous canine or feline renal failure. Information concerning the effect of various therapeutic modalities used to treat renal disease on renal blood flow in animals with spontaneously occurring renal disease is, therefore, not available.

Current theories on the progression of chronic renal failure in humans and animals centers on the "hyperfiltration theory" (Brenner et al., 1982). After a reduction in kidney function, the remaining nephrons are subject to increases in GFR and ERBF, leading to glomerular hyperfiltration and renal compensatory hypertrophy. These increases were thought to be beneficial and part of the healing process, but it has recently

been hypothesized that chronic increases in renal plasma flow may cause glomerular capillary hypertension. Glomerular hypertension perpetuates and accelerates renal failure by causing damage to mesangial cells and inducing mesangial cell proliferation, which leads to glomerulosclerosis. This theory has been developed from studies performed in rats and may or may not apply to dogs. Most current information regarding renal plasma flow in dogs was obtained by research utilizing animals with experimentally induced renal failure (remnant kidney model), and conclusions from these studies also might not be applicable to naturally occurring renal failure. Nevertheless, many therapeutic recommendations made for dogs and cats to slow the progression of mild chronic renal failure, including restricting dietary protein and salt, are aimed at reducing glomerular hyperfiltration. We currently have no easy, nonstressful way of evaluating the effect of these recommendations on individual dogs with chronic renal failure. If a renal blood flow assay became available that could be used on client-owned animals, we would be able to evaluate the hemodyamic effect of therapeutic modalities and adapt an individual's therapy accordingly.

### Techniques

Classically, renal plasma flow measurement is confined to research laboratories studying dogs with experimentally induced renal failure. Client-owned animals are not used to study renal hemodynamics due to the invasiveness of the techniques required. *Para*-aminohippuric acid (PAH) clearance is a standard method of assessing ERPF (Duarte et al., 1980). Briefly, dogs are either anesthetized or placed in a restraint sling. An intravenous priming dosage of PAH is administered, followed by a maintenance infusion of PAH. This infusion phase lasts approximately 120 min. During the first 60 min, the plasma concentration of PAH is allowed to equilibrate. The second 60 min is divided into three 20-min collection intervals when heparinized blood and urine specimens are obtained. Plasma and urine PAH concentrations are assayed using standardized techniques and the values will be used to determine renal plasma flow.

We are currently evaluating a scintigraphy technique using $^{99m}$Tc-mercaptoacetyltriglycine to validate the quantitation of ERPF. This technique has the noninvasive characteristics of scintigraphic GFR determinations and thus will allow us to study the hemodynamics of spontaneously occurring canine renal failure and the effect of various therapeutic modalities (e.g., diet, converting enzyme inhibitors) on renal perfusion.

## References and Suggested Reading

Brenner BM, et al: Dietary protein intake and the progressive nature of renal disease: The role of hemodynamically mediated glomerular sclerosis in ag-

ing, renal ablation, and intrinsic renal disease. N Engl J Med 307:652, 1982.
*An in-depth discussion of the hyperfiltration theory.*

Duarte G, et al: Glomerular filtration rate and renal plasma flow. *In* Duarte CG (ed): *Renal Function Tests.* Boston, Little, Brown & Co, 1980, p 29.
*A general discussion of indications, techniques, and interpretation of renal blood flow and glomerular filtration rate assays.*

Finco DR, Coulter DB, and Barsanti JA: Simple accurate method for clinical estimation of glomerular filtration rate in the dog. Am J Vet Res 42:1874, 1981.
*An in-depth discussion of how to perform exogenous creatinine clearances.*

Krawiec DR, et al: Use of ⁹⁹ᵐTc-diethylenetriaminepentaacetic acid for assessment of renal function in dogs with suspected renal disease. J Am Vet Med Assoc 192:1077, 1988.

*Discusses the effectiveness of scintigraphic GFR for assessing renal function in dogs.*

Ross LA: Assessment of renal function in the dog and cat. *In* Kirk RW (ed): *Current Veterinary Therapy IX.* Philadelphia, WB Saunders Co, 1986, p 1103.
*An in-depth discussion of how to perform various renal function assays.*

Uribe D, et al: Quantitative renal scintigraphic determination of the glomerular filtration rate in cats with normal and abnormal kidney function, using ⁹⁹ᵐTc-diethylenetriaminepentaacetic acid. Am J Vet Res 53:1101, 1992.
*Discusses the effectiveness of scintigraphic GFR for assessing renal function in cats.*

# ULTRASONOGRAPHIC FINDINGS IN RENAL DISEASE

AMY M. GROOTERS

*Columbia, Missouri*

*and* DAVID S. BILLER

*Manhattan, Kansas*

Ultrasonography has become a valuable tool for the evaluation of renal disease in small animals. It offers several advantages over radiography for examination of the kidneys. Ultrasound is easy, noninvasive, and requires little patient preparation. It is not associated with adverse effects and, unlike intravenous urography, can be performed regardless of renal function. In the assessment of renomegaly, ultrasound is more specific than contrast radiology because it can differentiate cavitary lesions from solid masses. The major disadvantages of ultrasound are lack of specificity and inability to quantify functional loss in patients with diffuse renal parenchymal disease (see "Renal Biopsy Using an Automated Biopsy Device," this volume, p 940). For this reason, in the evaluation of renal disease, ultrasound is best used to complement, and not to replace, other diagnostic tools.

## NORMAL APPEARANCE

Ultrasonographic evaluation of the kidney involves measurement of renal size; assessment of cortical and medullary echogenicity; and examination of the architecture of the cortex, medulla, and pelvis. The echogenicity of the normal renal cortex is less than that of the spleen, and is less than or equal to that of the liver. Cortical echogenicity is more variable in cats than in dogs, likely due to the variable amount of fat in feline proximal tubular cells. Similarly, the fat within the normal renal sinus makes it very echogenic.

## DIFFUSE PARENCHYMAL ABNORMALITIES

Hyperechogenicity of the renal cortex is the most common ultrasonographic finding in diffuse parenchymal disease. Unfortunately, this finding is nonspecific; it has been associated with a number of infiltrative, inflammatory, and degenerative renal disorders in small animals, and can also be produced artifactually (Table 1). A second sonographic finding in diffuse parenchymal disease is the renal medullary rim sign, which is characterized by an echogenic line at the corticomedullary junction. The rim sign has been observed in animals with ethylene glycol toxicosis, hypercalcemic ne-

***Table 1.*** *Causes of Increased Renal Cortical Echogenicity in Small Animals*

Renal diseases
  Ethylene glycol toxicosis
  Nephrocalcinosis
  Hypercalcemic nephropathy
  Renal lymphoma
  Acute tubular nephrosis
  Interstitial nephritis
  Pyogranulomatous nephritis secondary to feline infectious peritonitis
  End-stage renal disease
  Glomerulonephritis
  Amyloidosis
  Pyelonephritis
Artifactual causes
  Improper time-gain compensation settings
  Decreased echogenicity of reference organs
  Ascites

phropathy, pyogranulomatous nephritis secondary to feline infectious peritonitis, acute tubular necrosis, and severe chronic interstitial nephritis, and may also be a normal finding in some cats (Biller, Bradley, and Partington, 1992). Several diffuse parenchymal diseases in which ultrasound plays an important diagnostic role are discussed in more detail below.

## Ethylene Glycol Toxicosis

Ultrasonographic abnormalities associated with ethylene glycol intoxication in dogs and cats include severe hyperechogenicity of the renal cortex and medulla and, in some animals, the presence of a hypoechoic "halo" at the corticomedullary junction (Fig. 1). The severe increase in cortical and medullary echogenicity is thought to be caused by the presence of calcium oxalate crystals (Adams, Toal, and Breider, 1991) and can develop within hours of injection (Adams et al., 1989). The relative hypoechogenicity at the corticomedullary junction (halo sign) corresponds histologically to an area of relatively low crystal deposition. Sonographic detection of the halo sign may be a poor prognostic indicator because its appearance coincided with the onset of anuria in 10 of 13 animals (Adams, Toal, and Breider, 1991).

## Hypercalcemic Nephropathy

Renal ultrasonographic findings in dogs with hypercalcemic nephropathy include increased cortical echogenicity and the presence of a hyperechoic rim at the corticomedullary junction (Fig. 2). Histologically, these changes correlate with calcification of the tubular epithelium and basement membranes, which is especially severe at the corticomedullary junction (Barr et al., 1989). The renal calcification associated with hypercal-

cemic nephropathy is usually not radiographically apparent; ultrasound, which can detect relatively smaller amounts of calcification, is a more sensitive tool for the identification of these lesions. Because hypercalcemia can cause significant tubular damage before renal calcification is histologically apparent, the absence of sonographic abnormalities does not preclude the possibility of renal disease.

## Renal Lymphoma

Lymphoma of the kidney has a variable sonographic appearance. In cats, renal lymphoma causes either diffuse cortical hyperechogenicity, or multiple hypoechoic nodules within the renal parenchyma (Walter et al., 1988). Ultrasonographic findings in canine renal lymphoma include single or multiple anechoic to hypoechoic masses involving the cortex, medulla, or pelvis (Walter et al., 1987). The hypoechoic lesions of renal lymphoma can be differentiated from fluid-filled lesions, such as renal cysts or hydronephrosis, because lymphoma causes little or no through transmission (enhancement of echoes distal to a fluid-filled structure). Renomegaly and irregularity of the renal margins are other common findings in both dogs and cats.

## Interstitial Nephritis and Glomerulonephritis

Ultrasonographic abnormalities associated with glomerulo/interstitial nephritis include mild to moderate cortical hyperechogenicity and decreased corticomedullary demarcation (Fig. 3). Renal size is often small in animals with chronic interstitial nephritis. Unfortunately, the severity of ultrasonographic abnormalities does not correlate with the type or severity of inflammatory disease. Furthermore, normal renal

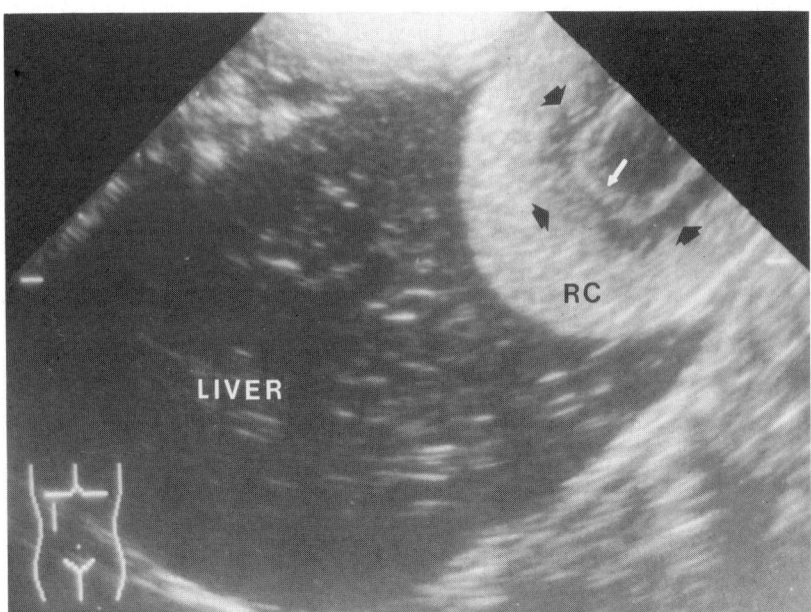

**Figure 1.** Longitudinal sonogram of the cranial pole of the right kidney and the adjacent liver in a dog with ethylene glycol intoxication. Note the severe hyperechogenicity of the renal cortex (RC) in comparison to the hepatic parenchyma. There is an echogenic line (renal medullary rim sign, *white arrow*) surrounded by a hypoechoic halo (*black arrows*) at the corticomedullary junction.

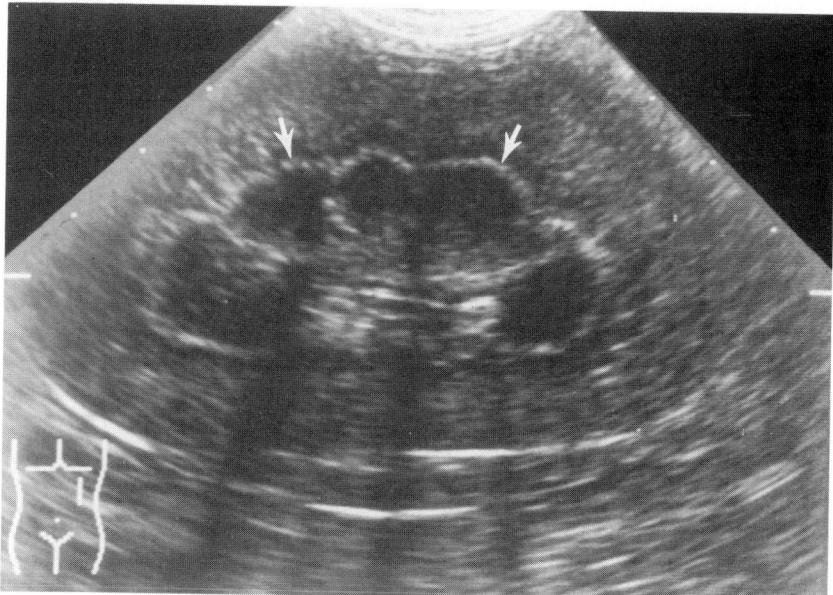

**Figure 2.** Longitudinal sonogram of the left kidney of a 6-year-old male Chesapeake Bay retriever with hypercalcemia secondary to lymphoma. An echogenic rim (*arrows*) is present at the corticomedullary junction. Moderate cortical hyperechogenicity is present.

sonograms are common, especially in animals with acute lesions and those with glomerulopathies.

## FOCAL PARENCHYMAL ABNORMALITIES

Focal renal parenchymal abnormalities include cysts, neoplasia, infarcts, hematomas, abscesses, and nephrocalcinosis. Cysts are round, sharply marginated, anechoic structures that cause considerable through transmission. Single or multiple renal cysts are a fairly common incidental sonographic finding in small animals, and are not routinely associated with renal dysfunction. However, renal cysts may also be a manifestation of polycystic kidney disease (PKD), which is characterized by progressive displacement of func-

tional renal tissue by multiple enlarging cysts. The sonographic appearance of focal or multifocal renal neoplasia is variable. Most renal masses are invasive and expansile, disrupting the normal architecture. The echogenicity of renal masses is usually heterogenous, reflecting secondary necrosis, edema, and hemorrhage within the neoplastic tissue. Renal infarcts appear sonographically as wedge-shaped lesions in the cortex that are initially hypoechoic, but become hyperechoic after approximately 7 days. Depression of the cortical surface over the infarcted area may also be observed. Renal hematomas and abscesses are focal hypoechoic or anechoic lesions that may contain mixed echoes, depending on their cellularity. Nephrocalcinosis can be detected using ultrasonography even when it is not radiographically apparent. It is identified as multifocal hyperechoic areas in the renal parenchyma that typi-

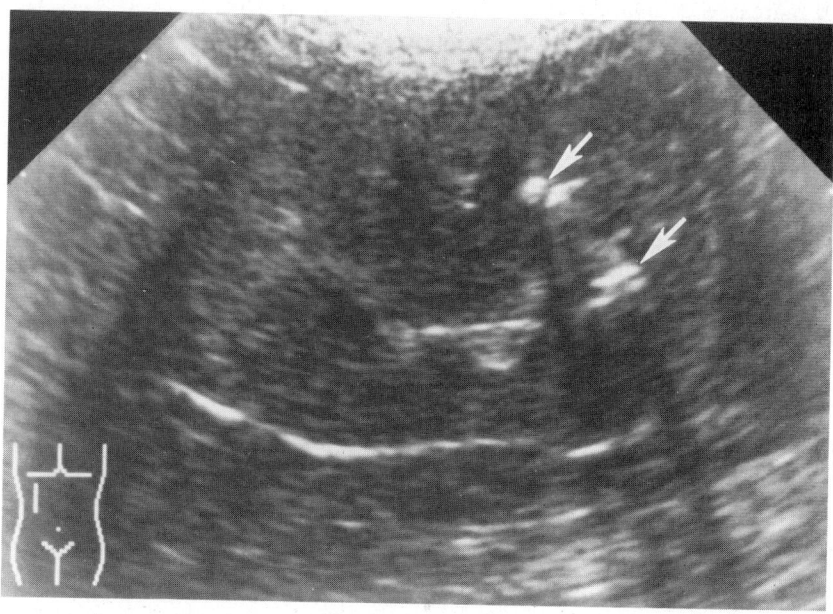

**Figure 3.** Longitudinal sonogram of the right kidney of a dog with chronic interstitial nephritis and nephrocalcinosis. Note the lack of a clear demarcation between the renal cortex and medulla. The nephrocalcinosis appears as two highly echogenic areas (*arrows*) that produce an anechoic acoustic shadow.

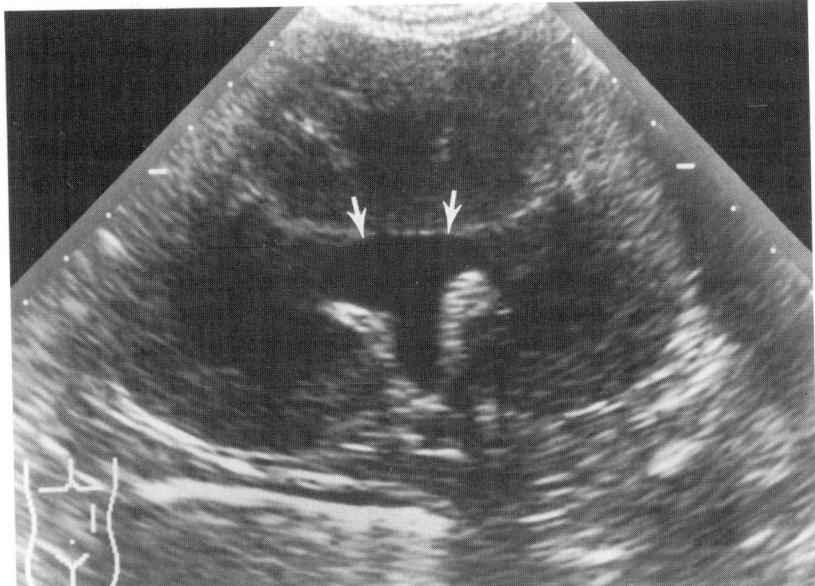

**Figure 4.** Longitudinal sonogram of the left kidney of a 7-year-old female Rottweiler with hydronephrosis. The renal pelvis (*arrows*) is dilated and filled with anechoic fluid.

cally produce an anechoic acoustic shadow (Fig. 3). Diffuse microscopic nephrocalcinosis causes a generalized increase in renal cortical echogenicity.

## ABNORMALITIES OF THE COLLECTING SYSTEM

Hydronephrosis is characterized sonographically by dilation of the renal pelvis, which appears as an anechoic area at the center of the medulla (Fig. 4). Blunting of the pelvic recesses may be present, and the dilated pelvis can often be followed to a dilated proximal ureter at the renal hilus. A severely hydronephrotic kidney appears as an anechoic sac surrounded by a rim of cortical tissue. Pyelonephritis also causes renal pelvic dilation, but can often be differentiated from hydronephrosis because the pelvis contains mixed echoes due to increased cellularity and inflammatory debris in the urine. Cortical hyperechogenicity and decreased corticomedullary definition are often present in chronic cases. Unfortunately, because renal pelvic dilation is not always present in pyelonephritis, ultrasound is a fairly insensitive diagnostic tool for this disease. Nephroliths appear sonographically as highly echogenic structures at the renal pelvis that cause acoustic shadowing. One of the advantages of using ultrasound to evaluate nephrolithiasis is the ability to determine whether or not the urolith is causing secondary hydronephrosis.

## References and Suggested Reading

Adams WH, Toal RL, Walker MA, and Breider MA: Early renal ultrasonographic findings in dogs with experimentally induced ethylene glycol nephrosis. Am J Vet Res 50:1370, 1989.
*A study of the ultrasonographic renal changes associated with experimentally induced ethylene glycol toxicosis.*

Adams WH, Toal RL, and Breider MA: Ultrasonographic findings in dogs and cats with oxalate nephrosis attributed to ethylene glycol intoxication: 15 cases (1984–1988). J Am Vet Med Assoc 199:492, 1991.
*A retrospective study of renal ultrasound findings in 12 dogs and three cats with ethylene glycol toxicosis.*

Barr FJ, Patteson MW, Lucke VM, and Gibbs C: Hypercalcemic nephropathy in three dogs: Sonographic appearance. Vet Radiol 30:169, 1989.
*A description of the ultrasound findings in three dogs with hypercalcemic nephropathy.*

Barr FJ, Holt PE, and Gibbs C: Ultrasonographic measurement of normal renal parameters. J Small Anim Pract 31:180, 1990.
*Study of normal values for renal length and volume in dogs.*

Biller DS, Bradley GA, and Partington BP: Renal medullary rim sign: Ultrasonographic evidence of renal disease. Vet Radiol 33:286, 1992.
*Description of the clinical and ultrasonographic findings in four dogs and two cats with a renal medullary rim.*

Walter PA, Feeney DA, Johnston GR, and O'Leary TP: Ultrasonographic evaluation of renal parenchymal diseases in dogs: 32 cases (1981–1986). J Am Vet Med Assoc 191:999, 1987.
*Retrospective evaluation of ultrasound findings in canine parenchymal renal disease.*

Walter PA, Johnston GR, Feeney DA, and O'Brien TD: Applications of ultrasonography in the diagnosis of parenchymal kidney disease in cats: 24 cases (1981–1986). J Am Vet Med Assoc 192:92, 1988.
*Retrospective evaluation of ultrasound findings in feline parenchymal renal disease.*

# PROTEINURIA IN DOGS AND CATS: A DIAGNOSTIC APPROACH

KARYL J. HURLEY
*and* SHELLY L. VADEN
*Raleigh, North Carolina*

Proteinuria occurs with a variety of systemic, renal, and urogenital diseases. An understanding of normal mechanisms of glomerular filtration, potential sources of protein loss, and methodologies of urine protein detection is helpful in the development of a systematic approach to localizing the source of urinary protein excretion and implementing appropriate management.

## NORMAL SOURCES OF URINE PROTEIN

The glomerular filtration barrier acts to selectively restrict passage of individual proteins. The pores of the filtration barrier have a size limitation of approximately 65,000 daltons, restricting large molecules such as immunoglobulins, fibrinogen, and albumin. However, the concentration of low-molecular-weight proteins, such as lysozyme, myoglobin, and amylase, that appears in the urine is dependent on their concentration in the plasma. The fixed negative charge of the glomerulus facilitates the passage of cations and impedes the passage of anions. Albumin, a negatively charged protein with a molecular weight that approximates glomerular pore sizes, may constitute 40 to 60% of normal urinary proteins. Tubular and lower urinary tract epithelial cell secretion of immunoglobulins, enzymes, and other proteins contribute to the small amount of protein found in normal urine samples.

## ABNORMAL SOURCES OF URINE PROTEIN

Proteinuria can result from preglomerular, glomerular, or postglomerular abnormalities (Table 1). Physiologic preglomerular causes of proteinuria such as fever, seizures, stress, extreme temperatures, or exercise (Table 1) are usually transient and rarely of clinical significance. Overload proteinuria may occur in hyperproteinemic states (total protein >9 gm/dl) due to a reversible increase in permeability of the filtration barrier, or with excessive production of low-molecular-weight proteins including hemoglobin, myoglobin, and paraproteins. Postglomerular proteinurias usually result from protein exudation into the urogenital tract via infection, inflammation, hemorrhage, or neoplasia. Primary tubular dysfunction (familial, inflammatory, or toxic) often induces a mild proteinuria. Glomerular proteinuria is a result of the disruption of the normal filtration barrier. Glomerulonephritis, amyloidosis, and glomerulosclerosis constitute the three primary differentials for marked protein loss.

## DIAGNOSTIC TESTS SPECIFIC FOR DETECTION OF URINARY PROTEIN

The most readily available method of urinary protein detection is the urine dipstick. Proteinuria induces a rapid color change at protein concentrations of 20 mg/dl and above. This test is more sensitive to albumins than to globulins and does not detect Bence Jones proteins. False-positives can occur when urine is highly alkaline (pH >8 to 9) or has been contaminated with quaternary ammonium or chlorhexidine solutions.

The sulfosalicylic acid test (SSA; Bumintest) is a semiquantitative method available at most laboratories that can detect protein concentrations of 5 mg/dl. This test is commonly used in conjunction with the dipstick to increase the probability and accuracy of protein detection. The sulfosalicylic acid test has a high sensitivity to albumin, but also detects globulins and Bence Jones proteins (see "Syndromes of Hyperglobulinemia: Diagnosis and Therapy," this volume, p 523). Test results may be falsely decreased by very alkaline urine and falsely increased by radiographic contrast media, penicillins, cephalothins, sulfa drugs, and uncentrifuged urine.

These are valuable screening tests in that they are quick and inexpensive, but must be interpreted in light of the urine specific gravity. A low-level protein reaction (trace or 1+) may be normal in a concentrated sample. However, in a dilute sample, significant quantities of protein may not be detected. Urine protein should be quantified in dogs that are hypoalbuminemic or that have repeatedly positive urine dipstick or SSA tests in the absence of lower urinary tract hemorrhage or inflammation.

Quantitative measurement of urinary protein content to 2 mg/dl is available at most reference laboratories. These tests are equally sensitive to albumin and globulins and also detect Bence Jones proteins and glycoproteins. Urine samples obtained via 24-hr collection or for determination of urine protein/creatinine ratios (UP/C) are analyzed by this method. The "gold standard" of protein quantification remains the 24-hr urine protein content. The value is derived by multiplying the protein concentration in a well-mixed aliquot of urine

**Table 1.** *Differential Diagnosis of Proteinuria*

*Preglomerular*
  Physiologic
    Stress
    Extreme temperatures
    Strenuous exercise
    Renal venous congestion
  Overload
    Hyperproteinemia (total protein >9 gm/dl)
    Hemoglobinemia
    Myoglobinemia
    Paraproteinemia

*Glomerular*
  Glomerulonephritis
    Infectious
      Dirofilariasis
      *Ehrlichia canis*
      Chronic bacterial infections
      Bacterial endocarditis
      Brucellosis
      Leishmaniasis
      Borrelliosis
      Septicemia
    Inflammatory
      Systemic lupus erythematosus
    Neoplastic
    Familial
    Idiopathic
  Amyloidosis
    Familial
    Inflammatory
      Systemic lupus erythematosus
    Neoplastic
    Idiopathic
  Glomerulosclerosis
    Diabetes mellitus
    Hyperfiltratoin
    Hypertension

*Postglomerular*
  Tubular dysfunction
    Fanconi's syndrome
    Acute tubular necrosis
  Hemorrhage
  Urinary tract infection
  Urolithiasis
  Trauma
  Neoplasia

collected over 24 hr by the volume produced in 24 hr. This number is then divided by the animal's weight, and the value is expressed in milligrams per kilogram per day. Normal protein excretion is less than 20 mg/kg/day in the dog and less than 10 mg/kg/day in cats fed a normal diet (Adams, Polzin, and Osborne, 1992). Endogenous creatinine clearance can be determined simultaneously to allow for assessment of renal function. Frequent catheterization or use of a metabolic cage is necessary, albeit inconvenient, and calculations are prone to error if *all* urine produced is not collected.

Alternatively, a UP/C is a sensitive, convenient tool for quantifying protein loss and requires a single random urine sample obtained by cystocentesis or uncontaminated catheterization or a midstream catch. Dividing the urine protein concentration by the urine creatinine concentration negates the effect of urine concentration on the interpretation of urine protein content. Values have been shown to correlate well with 24-hr urine protein content in both dogs and cats under normal urinary protein losses; however, as the UP/C exceeds an estimated value of 5.0 in the dog and 2.0 in the cat (Adams, Polzin, and Osborne, 1992), the correlation between the two methodologies is less consistent and 24-hr urine protein content may be the more reliable and accurate indicator of protein loss. General guidelines have been established for the interpretation of UP/Cs in the dog. A UP/C less than 0.5 is normal. Values greater than 0.5 but less than 1.0 are of questionable significance, and repeat measurements and monitoring is recommended. The majority of preglomerular and postglomerular disorders including tubular dysfunction cause a mild proteinuria, with UP/Cs in the range of 1.0 to 5.0; mild or early glomerular lesions may fall in this range as well. The magnitude of glomerular proteinuria may be an indicator of the degree of damage to the filtration barrier, with increasing UP/Cs suggestive of increasing severity of disease. Progressive glomerulonephritis and glomerulosclerosis commonly have UP/Cs in the 5.0 to 13.0 range, and severe proteinuria with a UP/C greater than 13.0 is most often associated with amyloidosis or, less commonly, severe glomerulonephritis. Lower urinary tract inflammation will substantially increase urinary protein content and should not be mistaken for glomerular disease. Although microscopic hematuria may cause persistently positive protein reactions on qualitative tests, blood contamination in the urine must be significant in order to cause a considerable increase in the UP/C (Bagley, 1991).

## DIAGNOSTIC APPROACH OF PERSISTENT PROTEINURIA

When a positive reaction is detected on a routine screening urinalysis, the urine sediment should be evaluated (Fig. 1). A urine sample should be submitted for bacterial culture if pyuria is present. Hematuria necessitates evaluation for causes of urinary tract hemorrhage. Occult blood positivity without intact red cells in the sediment could indicate hemolysis in an untimely processed sample; specific tests for detection of hemoglobinuria or myoglobinuria should be performed if indicated. In samples with inactive sediments, the urine protein content should be quantified with a 24-hr urine protein quantification or UP/C. Finding granular or hyaline casts is suggestive of renal disease. Once proteinuria is confirmed, a complete blood count (CBC) and biochemical profile should be evaluated for evidence of inflammatory, infectious, or neoplastic diseases.

Glomerular disease should be suspected when hypoalbuminemia is detected and there is little evidence of preglomerular disease or postglomerular conditions. In dogs with suspected glomerular disease, an aggressive search for an underlying systemic disease that may result in immune complex deposition within the glomerular capillary walls is indicated. Chest radiographs should be made to evaluate for metastatic, fungal, par-

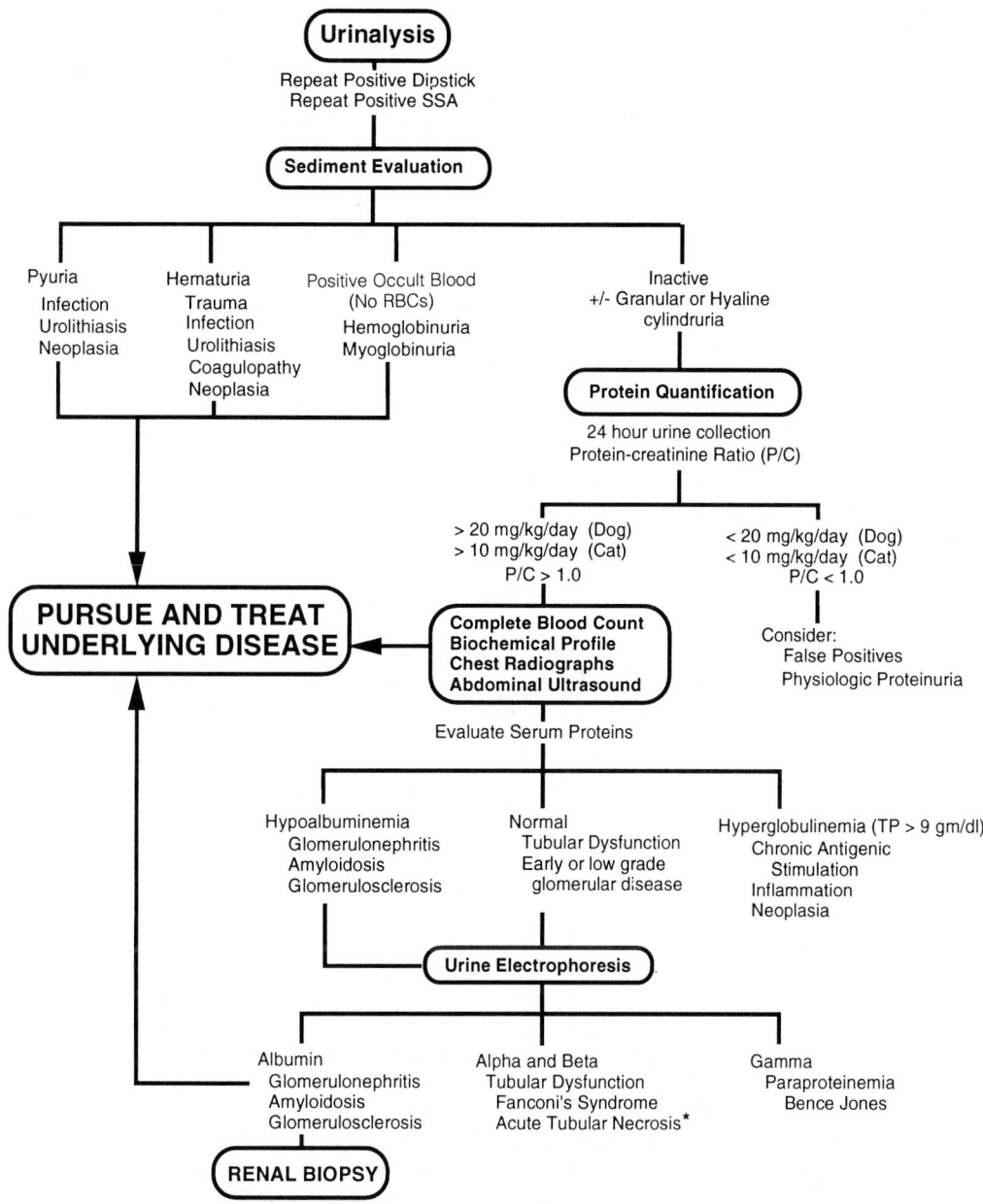

**Figure 1.** Algorithm of a diagnostic approach to proteinuria. This algorithm is meant to be used as a guideline in the assessment of persistent proteinuria. Potential diagnostic tests should be pursued in light of the historical and clinical findings of each patient. ° = Diagnosis may require renal biopsy.

asitic, or bacterial disease. Abdominal radiographs and/or ultrasound may be an invaluable tool in assessing the size, shape, and relative echogenicity of the kidneys and other abdominal structures in pursuit of occult disease. Infectious disease, heartworm, and antinuclear antibody (ANA) serologies may also be indicated. Renal amyloidosis can also be associated with an underlying infectious, inflammatory, or neoplastic disorder, but as with glomerulonephritis, very often a predisposing factor is not found.

Urine protein electrophoresis may aid in localization of the cause of proteinuria. Both early glomerular disease and hemorrhage have electrophoretic patterns that resemble normal serum protein electrophoresis

(see "Syndromes of Hyperglobulinemia: Diagnosis and Therapy," this volume, p 523), with albumin representing the major fraction of protein lost. This so-called selective proteinuria occurs when glomeruli have lost their fixed negative charges and albumin freely penetrates the filtration barrier while higher molecular weight proteins are retained. As glomerular disease progresses, larger molecules are lost, including immunoglobulins, resulting in nonselective proteinuria that is characterized electrophoretically by a larger proportion of proteins in the gamma region. Low-molecular-weight proteinuria, as occurs in tubular proteinuria, is associated with increased α and β fractions.

In animals with idiopathic glomerular proteinuria

that persists or progresses in spite of attempted therapeutic intervention, a renal biopsy is necessary to define the glomerular lesions, form a prognosis, and direct treatment options (see "Renal Biopsy Using an Automated Biopsy Device," this volume, p 940).

Once the source of proteinuria has been localized to the glomerulus, protein quantification can be used to monitor progression of renal disease and response to therapy. Urine specific gravity and serum creatinine should be monitored simultaneously, since the decreased glomerular filtration rate accompanying deterioration of renal function can also reduce renal protein losses, resulting in declining UP/Cs. The stability of this ratio from day to day in individual patients with stable renal function has yet to be evaluated, but UP/Cs are not appropriate for monitoring progression in animals with rapidly changing glomerular filtration rates (e.g., acute renal failure). Until further data are available, assessment of disease progression and subsequent therapeutic changes should be made on the basis of 24-hr urine protein content or trends noted in repeat sampling of the UP/C ratio rather than on the basis of one or two data points.

## References and Suggested Reading

Adams LG, Polzin DJ, and Osborne CA: Correlation of urine protein/creatinine ratio and twenty-four hour urinary protein excretion in normal cats and cats with surgically induced chronic renal failure. J Vet Intern Med 6:36, 1992.

Bagley RS, Center SA, and Lewis RM: The effect of experimental cystitis and iatrogenic blood contamination on the urine protein/creatinine ratio in the dog. J Vet Intern Med 5:66, 1991.

Barsanti JA and Finco DR: Protein concentration in urine or normal dogs. Am J Vet Res 40:1583, 1979.

Grauer GF: Glomerulonephritis. Semin Vet Med Surg 7:187, 1992.

Lulich JP and Osborne CA: Interpretation of urine protein-creatinine ratios in dogs with glomerular and nonglomerular disorders. Compend Cont Educ Pract Vet 12:59, 1990.

White JV: Diagnostic approach to proteinuria. *In* Kirk RW (ed): *Current Veterinary Therapy X.* Philadelphia, WB Saunders Co, 1989, pp 1139–1142.

# RENAL BIOPSY USING AN AUTOMATED BIOPSY DEVICE

LINDA A. ROSS
*and* DOMINIQUE PENNINCK
*North Grafton, Massachusetts*

Renal biopsy in dogs and cats is indicated when there is a need to obtain more specific information about the cause, duration, and severity of renal disease or renal failure than can be obtained by noninvasive diagnostic tests, and when the information so obtained may alter management of the case. Perhaps the most common reason for performing a renal biopsy is to differentiate acute from chronic renal failure; other indications include determining a specific cause for renal disease such as pyelonephritis or ethylene glycol toxicity, and characterization of glomerular lesions causing protein-losing nephropathy. It must be noted, however, that renal pathology does not necessarily correlate with renal function.

The objective of performing a renal biopsy is to obtain a diagnostic tissue sample from the kidney while minimizing risk to the animal from anesthesia, hemorrhage, or biopsy-induced renal damage. A variety of techniques have been described, although none fulfills all of the objectives (Chew and DiBartola, 1989). Surgical biopsy during laparotomy can be performed by excising a wedge of kidney tissue, or with a biopsy instrument such as the Franklin-modified Vim-Silverman or Tru-Cut biopsy needle. These biopsy instruments are also used to biopsy the kidney during laparoscopy, with the keyhole technique, using ultrasonographic guidance (Smith, 1985), or in cats, percutaneously. Hemorrhage is the most common complication of renal biopsy. The keyhole, ultrasound-guided, and blind percutaneous techniques have the disadvantage of lack of direct observation of the kidney and hemorrhage. All of these techniques have the disadvantage of requiring general anesthesia, both for analgesia and because the kidney must be manually immobilized so that the biopsy needle will enter the kidney instead of pushing it away. In addition, although some of the techniques allow the operator to observe the entrance of the biopsy needle into the kidney, the entire path of the needle can be seen only with ultrasonography (Hager, Nyland, and Fuher, 1985).

## AUTOMATED BIOPSY INSTRUMENT

Recently, new biopsy instruments have been introduced that have improved both the safety and efficacy of performing renal biopsies (Hoppe et al., 1986; Pokieser et al., 1993). One such instrument is a spring-loaded automated biopsy device (Biopty Biopsy Gun, Bard Radiology) (Figs. 1 and 2) that uses a dis-

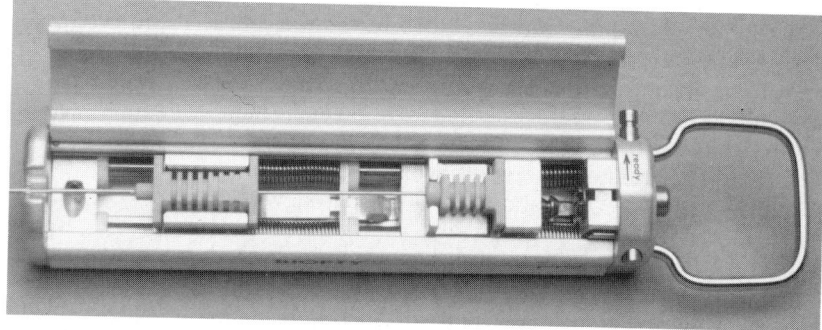

**Figure 1.** An automated biopsy instrument with a biopsy needle loaded (Biopty Biopsy System, Bard Radiology).

posable cutting needle to obtain a core of tissue. The needle has the same mechanics as the Tru-Cut needle. However, rather than manually thrusting the needle into the kidney and advancing the outer cutting sheath, the biopsy gun performs both of these maneuvers in a fraction of a second after being "fired." This rapid procedure allows a core of tissue to be obtained with minimal displacement of the kidney. Therefore, manual immobilization of the kidney prior to biopsy is unnecessary. The rapid biopsy and small diameter of the biopsy needle also minimize pain associated with the procedure.

Automated biopsy guns are available with various lengths of needle penetration, ranging from 3 to 23 mm. The choice of length is based upon the size of the kidney to be biopsied. An adjustable automated biopsy device (3 to 19 mm core length) has been recently described. This device can adjust the core length in relation to kidney size (Jorulf and Von Bennett, 1992). Biopsy needles (Biopty-Cut Needle, Bard Radiology) (Figs. 1 and 2) can be obtained in a variety of diameters and lengths ranging from 14-gauge, 10 cm to 20-gauge, 20 cm. For comparison, the traditional Tru-Cut needle has an outside diameter of 2.0 mm or 14-gauge. For most dogs and cats, an 18-gauge, 20-cm needle provides an appropriate core with the least probability of complications; for very small animals, a 20-gauge needle is used.

Numerous studies have been conducted in people (Cozens et al., 1992; Hanas et al., 1992; Komaiko et al., 1989; Kumar et al., 1992; Mahoney et al., 1993; Tartini, Hood, and Rimmer, 1990) and animals (Hoppe et al., 1986) describing the benefits of obtaining ultrasound-guided renal biopsies with an automated biopsy system, as compared to standard manual techniques. These include greater reliability in obtaining an adequate specimen for histologic examination and fewer postbiopsy complications. In dogs and cats, the system has been used at our institution for several years, and similar benefits have been noted. In addition, biopsies using the automated device can be performed under intravenous anesthesia in most animals. This improves the safety of the procedure for the animal as well as reduces costs for the owner.

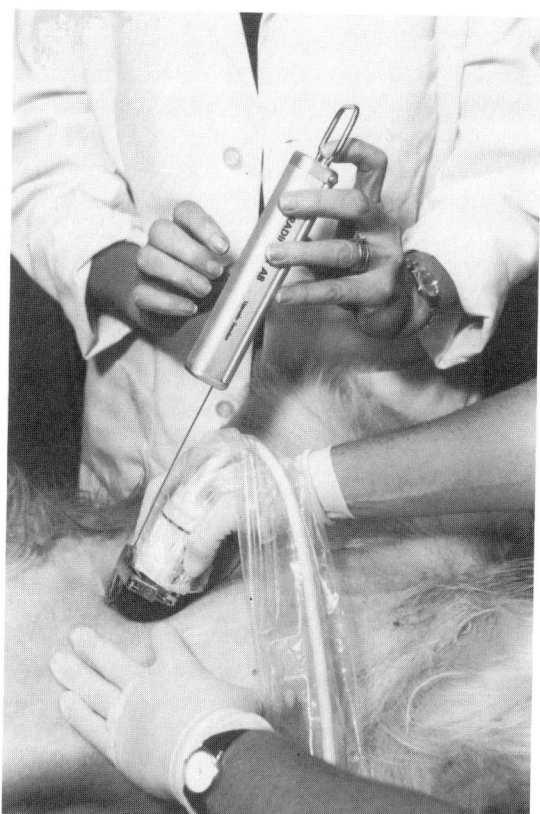

**Figure 2.** A renal biopsy being performed using ultrasonography and an automated biopsy gun (Biopty Biopsy System, Bard Radiology).

## TECHNIQUE

Prior to renal biopsy, the animal's coagulation ability is evaluated with an activated clotting time and bleeding time, at a minimum; a platelet count and other coagulation assays are performed if indicated. Measurement of arterial blood pressure is also helpful in evaluating bleeding tendencies.

The animal is placed in dorsal recumbancy and the ventral surface of the abdomen is clipped. Ultrasonography of the kidneys is performed prior to biopsy to characterize architectural abnormalities. The presence of some abnormalities, such as hydronephrosis, cysts, or abscesses may be a contraindication to performing a biopsy. The animal is then given intravenous anesthesia. At our hospital, we have found that a ketamine-diazepam combination provides good restraint in most dogs and cats. Ketamine (Vetalar, Fort

Dodge) and diazepam (Valium, Roche Products) in a 1:1 ratio by volume are drawn into one syringe and administered slowly IV to effect, up to a maximum dose of 1 ml/9 kg body weight. Because of the small diameter of the biopsy needle (18-gauge) and the rapid process of obtaining the core, additional analgesia is usually not necessary. The abdomen is prepared with a surgical scrub, and the ultrasound probe is covered with a sterile gel and sleeve. The biopsy gun is loaded with the appropriate needle. A biopsy guide is clamped to the probe and is used to maintain the alignment of the needle (Fig. 2). The biopsy can be safely performed with only one hand while the other maneuvers the transducer. The kidney is located by ultrasound, and the needle is advanced to contact the renal cortex. The caudal pole of the left kidney is usually the easiest to target. However, interposition of other organs (bowel, spleen) or the presence of a focal renal lesion can necessitate a different biopsy location. The needle is then directed so that the trajectory will avoid the renal medulla and pelvis. The gun is fired, the gun and needle are immediately withdrawn as a unit, and the biopsy specimen is removed. Two to three biopsies are taken, depending upon the size of the kidney, types of diagnostic tests planned for the tissue, and degree of satisfaction with the samples. After completion of the biopsy procedure, the biopsy site is carefully evaluated by ultrasound for evidence of excessive hemorrhage (subcapsular or retroperitoneal fluid accumulation). It has not been found necessary to apply pressure to the kidney for purposes of hemostasis after the biopsy is performed; because of the small size of the biopsy needle, hemorrhage from the biopsy site is usually minimal.

Postbiopsy management of the animal is the same as for any renal biopsy. Diuresis to minimize blood clot formation in the renal pelvis or ureter is accomplished by administering intravenous fluids for 12 to 24 hr. The presence of excess hemorrhage is determined by evaluating mucous membrane color, capillary refill time, and hematocrit and total solids hourly for the first 4 hr, then every 4 hr until 24 hr after biopsy. In the rare instance where excess hemorrhage has occurred, a single whole blood transfusion has been successful in stabilizing the animal; exploratory laparotomy for hemostasis as yet has not been necessary.

Clinicians at our hospital are now performing substantially more biopsies and at an earlier point in case management than previously because of the ease, reduced patient risk, and reduced cost of performing renal biopsies with the automated biopsy device. The cost of the instrument is rapidly recouped by the number of biopsies performed. Use of an automated biopsy device should be considered by any practice that has ultrasound capability.

## References and Suggested Reading

Chew DJ and DiBartola S: Diagnosis and pathophysiology of renal disease. *In* Ettinger SJ (ed): Textbook of Veterinary Internal Medicine, 3rd edition. Philadelphia, WB Saunders Co, 1989, p 1893.
*This chapter contains a section covering indications, techniques, and complications of renal biopsy in the dog and cat.*

Cozens NJ, Murchison JT, Allan PL, and Winney RJ: Conventional 15 G needle technique for renal biopsy compared with ultrasound-guided spring-loaded 18 G needle biopsy. Br J Radiol 65:594, 1992.
*More reliable procurement of specimens, fewer complications, and a shorter hospital stay were reported for renal biopsies performed with the automated device than with a conventional manual technique.*

Hager D, Nyland T, and Fuher P: Ultrasound-guided biopsy of the canine liver, kidney and prostate. Vet Radiol 26:82, 1985.
*Techniques for ultrasound-guided biopsies of various organs are described.*

Hanas E, Larsson E, Fellstrom B, et al: Safety aspects and diagnostic findings of serial renal allograft biopsies, obtained by an automatic technique with a midsize needle. Scand J Urol Nephrol 26:413, 1992.
*Biopsies of human renal allografts were performed using an automated device; adequate tissue specimens were obtained and few complications were observed.*

Hoppe FE, Hager DA, Poulos PW, Ekman S, and Lindgren PG: A comparison of manual and automatic ultrasound-guided biopsy techniques. Vet Radiol 27:99, 1986.
*Larger and higher quality samples of the kidney were obtained from dogs using an automated biopsy device than with a manual technique.*

Jorulf H and Von Bennett L: Adjustable automated biopsy device. Radiology 185:897, 1992.
*A new adjustable automated biopsy device is described.*

Komaiko MS, Jordan SC, Querfeld U, and Goodman MD: A new percutaneous renal biopsy device for pediatric patients. Pediatr Nephrol 3:191, 1989.
*A preliminary report discussing the successful use of an automated biopsy device in children.*

Kumar A, Mitchell MJ, Aggarwal S, et al: Ultrasonography-directed native renal biopsy: Comparison of an automated biopsy device with a needle system. Can Assoc Radiol J 43:359, 1992.
*The results reported here of renal biopsies in people indicated that the automated device delivered a higher quality tissue core with a lower frequency of minor complications than the Tru-Cut needle system.*

Mahoney MC, Racadio JM, Merhar GL, and First MR: Safety and efficacy of kidney transplant biopsy: Tru-Cut needle vs sonographically guided Biopty gun. Am J Roentgenol 160:325, 1993.
*Performing biopsies of renal allografts in people was as accurate and safer than biopsy with the Tru-Cut needle.*

Pokieser P, Kain R, Helbich T, Mallek R, et al: Renal biopsy: In vitro and in vivo comparison of a new automatic biopsy device and conventional biopsy system. Radiology 186:573, 1993.
*A new type of automated biopsy device using a full-cut needle produced larger and better quality tissue cores than a Tru-Cut–type biopsy gun.*

Smith S: Ultrasound-guided biopsy. Vet Clin North Am [Small Anim Pract] 15:1249, 1985.
*A description of the techniques for performing ultrasound-guided biopsies of organs using standard biopsy needles.*

Tartini A, Hood V, and Rimmer J: Use of the Biopty instrument in percutaneous needle biopsy of the native kidney [comment]. J Am Soc Nephrol 1:219, 1990.
*One of the first descriptions of advantages of this technique.*

# PREVENTION OF HOSPITAL-ACQUIRED ACUTE RENAL FAILURE

GREGORY F. GRAUER

*Fort Collins, Colorado*

Acute renal failure (ARF) is frequently caused by an ischemic or toxic insult to the kidneys. In general, this injury damages tubular epithelial cells, causing impaired regulation of water and solute balance. Ischemia-induced ARF is frequently iatrogenic (e.g., hypovolemia or hypotension associated with anesthesia and surgery or overzealous use of vasodilators). Likewise, toxicant-induced ARF frequently occurs in the hospital setting associated with the use of therapeutic agents (e.g., gentamicin, nonsteroidal anti-inflammatory drugs [NSAIDs], amphotericin B, and cisplatin). Nephron damage associated with ARF is not always reversible; animals that do recover adequate renal function usually do so only after prolonged and expensive intensive care. While similar statistics are not available in veterinary medicine, toxicant and ischemia-induced acute renal failure in human beings is associated with a mortality rate of 50 to 60%, despite the widespread availability of hemodialysis. Prevention is truly the best therapy for either ischemia- or toxicant-induced renal failure.

## RISK FACTORS FOR ACUTE RENAL FAILURE

Prevention of hospital-acquired ARF is aided by the identification of patients at increased risk. Many studies assessing risk factors associated with ARF, as well as prevention of ARF, have dealt with gentamicin-induced nephrotoxicity, which is a well-established model in many species. Several risk factors have been identified that predispose dogs to gentamicin-induced ARF (Table 1) (Brown, Barsanti, and Crowell, 1985); however, it is likely that many of these risk factors also predispose dogs and cats to other types of toxicant-induced ARF as well as ARF induced by ischemia.

Poor renal perfusion increases the risk of toxic and

ischemic damage to the kidney, and dehydration and volume depletion are perhaps the most common factors that decrease renal perfusion. Studies in human beings indicate that volume depletion increases a patient's risk of developing ARF by a factor of ten. Renal hypoperfusion is also associated with decreased cardiac output, decreased plasma oncotic pressure, increased blood viscosity, systemic vasodilatation, and decreased renal prostaglandin formation (e.g., administration of NSAIDs). In addition to poor renal perfusion, hypovolemia decreases the volume of distribution of nephrotoxic drugs and decreases the flow rate of glomerular filtrate through the tubules, which may enhance tubular absorption of toxicants.

Preexisting renal disease and advanced age, which is often associated with some degree of decreased renal function, can increase the potential for nephrotoxicity by several mechanisms. For example, the pharmacokinetics of potentially nephrotoxic drugs can be altered in the face of decreased renal function. Gentamicin clearance has been shown to be decreased in dogs with subclinical renal dysfunction (Frazier, Aucoin, and Riviere, 1988). Animals with renal insufficiency may also have reduced urine concentrating ability and, therefore, decreased ability to compensate for prerenal influences. Renal disease may also compromise production of prostaglandins that help maintain renal vasodilation and blood flow. Additionally, the hyperphosphatemia that can occur in patients with renal insufficiency is thought to increase the risk of ARF (Zager, 1982).

Plasma concentrations of several electrolytes can affect the development of ARF. Hyponatremia exacerbates gentamicin nephrotoxicity in rats and potentiates contrast media–induced ARF in dogs; therefore, sodium depletion and hyponatremia should be corrected in patients that are to receive potential nephrotoxicants or undergo elective anesthetic procedures. As a prophylactic measure, oral sodium loading reduces renal cortical gentamicin concentrations and nephrotoxicity in rats treated with gentamicin. Similarly, establishing a natriuresis with saline fluid therapy prior to a potential renal insult may be important in preventing ARF. Saline diuresis is beneficial in dogs prior to administration of cisplatin and amphotericin B (Ogilvie et al., 1993). The benefits of saline diuresis may be due to suppression of intrarenal and plasma renin activity and attenuation of early renin-angiotensin responses or an increased volume of distribution of nephrotoxic drugs.

Hypocalcemia, hypomagnesemia, and hypokalemia

***Table 1.*** *Risk Factors for Gentamicin-Induced ARF in Dogs*

| | |
|---|---|
| Preexisting renal disease | Dehydration° |
| Advanced age | Decreased cardiac output° |
| Fever | Hypotension° |
| Sepsis | Electrolyte imbalances° |
| Liver disease | Acidosis° |
| Multiple organ involvement | Concurrent use of potentially nephrotoxic drugs° |
| Trauma | |
| Diabetes mellitus | Hyperviscosity syndromes° |
| Hypoalbuminemia | Dietary protein level° |

°Potentially correctable risk factors, see text.

are additional electrolyte abnormalities that may potentiate nephrotoxicity. Calcium and magnesium compete with gentamicin for anionic phospholipid membrane binding sites so that attachment, binding, and uptake of gentamicin in various tissues are inversely proportional to local divalent cation concentrations. These cations also tend to suppress parathyroid hormone production and release, leading to decreased production of membrane phospholipid and, therefore, gentamicin binding to tissues. Indeed, dietary supplementation of calcium and magnesium protects against gentamicin-induced nephrotoxicity in rats because there is less tubular cell absorption of gentamicin. Studies in dogs have demonstrated that dietary potassium restriction exacerbates gentamicin nephrotoxicity, possibly because potassium-depleted cells are more susceptible to necrosis (Brinker et al., 1981). It is important to note that gentamicin administration in dogs is associated with increased urinary excretion of potassium (Brinker et al., 1981). This increased urinary excretion of potassium could result in potassium depletion and increase the risk of gentamicin nephrotoxicity in clinical patients. Therefore, serum electrolyte concentrations should be monitored closely in patients receiving nephrotoxic drugs, especially if these patients are anorectic, vomiting, or have diarrhea.

Administration of potentially nephrotoxic drugs or drugs that may enhance nephrotoxicity obviously increases the risk of ARF. For example, concurrent use of furosemide and gentamicin in dogs is associated with increased risk and severity of ARF (Adelman et al., 1979). Furosemide probably potentiates gentamicin-induced nephrotoxicity by causing dehydration, reducing the volume of distribution of gentamicin, and increasing the renal tubular absorption of gentamicin. Fluid repletion minimizes, but does not avoid, the potentiating effect of furosemide on gentamicin nephrotoxicity in the dog, because furosemide facilitates cellular uptake of gentamicin independent of hemodynamic changes. By similar mechanisms, furosemide has been shown to enhance radiocontrast-induced nephrotoxicity in human beings. Use of NSAIDs can also increase the risk of ARF. Anesthesia, sodium and/or volume depletion, sepsis, congestive heart failure, nephrotic syndrome, and hepatic disease are conditions in which prostaglandin-induced renal vasodilatation becomes important and the susceptibility to NSAIDs is increased. Dogs are particularly sensitive to newer NSAIDs such as ibuprofen and naproxen which, in addition to ARF, may cause vomiting and gastrointestinal ulceration.

Recent evidence in dogs suggests that the quantity of protein fed prior to a nephrotoxic insult can significantly affect the subsequent renal damage and dysfunction. Feeding high dietary protein prior to and during gentamicin administration reduces nephrotoxicity, enhances gentamicin clearance, and results in a larger volume of distribution compared with feeding medium or low protein (Behrend et al., 1992; Grauer et al., 1992). The beneficial effects of high dietary protein are likely associated with increased glomerular filtration and, therefore, improved toxicant excretion. High dietary protein also results in increased urinary excretion of protein that may compete for nephrotoxicant reabsorption by tubular epithelial cells. Further research in the area of dietary protein conditioning is needed; if dietary protein conditioning can be shown to have renal protective effects, it may have important clinical implications. Once renal damage has occurred, however, high dietary protein would likely result in increased serum urea nitrogen and phosphorus concentrations and, therefore, would not be recommended.

Risk factors are additive and any complication occurring in high-risk patients increases the potential for ARF. Patients with shock, acidosis, sepsis, and major organ system failure are at increased risk for ARF, and these are the patients that are likely to require aggressive treatment including prolonged anesthesia, surgery, or chemotherapeutics, which are potentially damaging to the kidneys. For example, ARF is common in dogs with pyometra and *Escherichia coli* endotoxin-induced urine concentrating defects, especially if fluid therapy is inadequate during anesthesia for ovariohysterectomy or during the recovery period. Trauma, extensive burns, vasculitis, pancreatitis, fever, diabetes mellitus, and multiple myeloma are additional conditions associated with a high incidence of ARF in veterinary medicine. Knowledge of these predisposing risk factors allow the clinician to assess the risk/benefit ratio in individual cases in which an elective anesthetic procedure is considered or the use of potentially nephrotoxic drugs is indicated.

## POTENTIAL PROTECTIVE MEASURES

Methods designed to protect the kidneys from acute insults attempt to prevent or interrupt the pathophysiologic events that result in ARF. Goals of protective maneuvers are to: (1) preserve or restore renal hemodynamics; (2) increase solute excretion and minimize intratubular obstruction; and (3) reduce the toxicity of nephrotoxic agents.

Fluid therapy sufficient to cause volume expansion and diuresis is frequently used prior to administration of amphotericin B and cisplatin (see *CVT XI*, p 395) to decrease the nephrotoxicity of these compounds. Several protocols for saline diuresis have been described; the protocol currently recommended for cisplatin adminstration calls for 0.9% saline to be administered IV for 3 hr at a rate of 25 ml/kg/hr followed by an additional hour of saline administration at the same rate after the cisplatin is given (Ogilvie et al., 1993). In a similar fashion, the prophylactic administration of diuretics and vasodilators may be protective against potential renal insults. Mannitol (1 gm/kg of a 5 to 25% solution IV) has been used to increase intravascular volume and tubular flow rates and to prevent tubular obstruction prior to potential ischemic or toxic insults. Mannitol also has weak vasodilatory effects mediated via prostaglandins or by the release of atrial natriuretic peptide and may improve renal blood flow and glomerular filtration if given early in ARF. Administration of constant-rate IV infusion of dopamine (1 to 3 µg/kg/min) is also effective in increasing glomerular filtration and inducing diuresis in dogs, especially when administered before or soon after the induction of ARF. Diuretics and vasodilators, however, should only be used in well-hydrated patients. Prophylactic treatment with furosemide is usually not recommended, since it is a potent diuretic agent that may result in volume depletion, which would potentiate an ischemic or toxic insult.

Specific alterations in the dosage of medications that have nephrotoxic potential may aid in minimizing side effects. In dogs with apparently normal renal function, frequent dosing of gentamicin (every 8 hr) may be less efficacious and potentially more nephrotoxic than an equivalent total daily dosage given at 12-hr intervals (Frazier and Riviere, 1987). When treatment with an aminoglycoside is necessary, monitoring serum drug concentrations allows the clinician to tailor individual dosage regimens. Nephrotoxicity increases with elevated serum trough concentrations (>2 µg/ml for gentamicin, >5 µg/ml for amikacin). Trough serum antibiotic concentrations can be reduced by decreasing the dosage or increasing the dosage interval. Recent investigations indicate that increasing the dosage interval of gentamicin by a factor related to serum creatinine or creatinine clearance is the most effective means of reducing nephrotoxicity (e.g., if the serum creatinine concentration is 5 mg/dl, the dosing interval should be 40 hr [8 hr multiplied by 5] rather than 8 hr) (Frazier and Riviere, 1987). When treatment with cisplatin is indicated, the time of administration may be important. Pharmacokinetics and nephrotoxicity of cisplatin in dogs vary between 8:00-AM and 4:00-PM administration; reduced toxicity is observed with 4:00-PM dosing

(Hardie et al., 1991). Lastly, intravenous radiographic contrast medium administration causes renal vasoconstriction and has been associated with ARF in the dog. Low-osmolar contrast agents (e.g., iopamidol and ioxaglate) produce less vasoconstriction in dogs than do high-osmolar contrast agents (e.g., diatrizoate) and, therefore, low-osmolar contrast agents should be used in high-risk patients (Deray et al., 1991).

## References and Suggested Reading

Adelman RD, Spangler WL, Beasom F, et al: Furosemide enhancement of experimental gentamicin nephrotoxicity: Comparison of functional and morphological changes with activities of urinary enzymes. J Infect Dis 140: 342, 1979.

Behrend EN, Grauer GF, Greco DS, et al: Effects of dietary protein conditioning on gentamicin pharmacokinetics in dogs. J Am Soc Nephrol 3:720, 1992.

Brinker KR, Bulger RE, Dolgan DC, et al: Effect of potassium depletion on gentamicin nephrotoxicity. J Lab Clin Med 98:292, 1981.

Brown SA, Barsanti JA, and Crowell WA: Gentamicin-associated acute renal failure in the dog. J Am Vet Med Assoc 186:686, 1985.

Deray G, Baumelou B, Martinez F, et al: Renal vasoconstriction after low and high osmolar contrast agents in ischemic and non ischemic canine kidney. Clin Nephrol 36:93, 1991.

Frazier DL, Aucoin DP, and Riviere JE: Gentamicin pharmacokinetics and nephrotoxicity in naturally acquired and experimentally induced disease in dogs. J Am Vet Med Assoc 192:57, 1988.

Frazier DL and Riviere JE: Gentamicin dosing strategies for dogs with subclinical renal dysfunction. Antimicrob Agents Chemother 31:1929, 1987.

Grauer GF, Behrend EN, Greco DS, et al: Effects of dietary protein conditioning on gentamicin-induced nephrotoxicity in healthy male dogs. Am J Vet Res 55:90, 1994.

Hardie EM, Page RL, Williams PL, and Fischer WD: Effect of time of cisplatin administration on its toxicity and pharmacokinetics in dogs. Am J Vet Res 52:1821, 1991.

Ogilvie GK, Straw RC, Jameson VJ, et al: Prevalence of nephrotoxicosis associated with a four-hour saline solution diuresis protocol for the administration of cisplatin to dogs with naturally developing neoplasms. J Am Vet Med Assoc 202:1845, 1993.

Zager RA: Hyperphosphatemia: a factor that provokes severe acute renal failure. J Lab Clin Med 100:230, 1982.

# IMMUNE FUNCTION IN RENAL FAILURE

LAINE A. COWAN
*and* SCOTT MCVEY
*Manhattan, Kansas*

Humoral and cell-mediated immunity protects normal animals from microbial pathogens. Because bacterial infections often contribute to morbidity in human beings and animals with decreased renal function, immune function has been investigated in naturally occurring and experimentally induced renal failure. The specific etiopathogensis of renal failure–associated immunocompromise is not completely understood. The most likely etiologies include malnutrition, uremic tox-

ins, or alterations in parathyroid hormone (PTH) and vitamin D concentrations. In addition, decreased immune responsiveness in human beings with chronic renal failure is influenced by the patient's age, duration and degree of decreased renal function, and the type and duration of dialysis therapy. The applicability of the immunologic results of human dialysis patients to veterinary medicine is not known, since dialysis (and blood transfusions that may accompany dialysis) is also immunosuppressive. In interpretation of the immune function literature, one must distinguish the results obtained during acute versus chronic renal failure, as the responses often differ. In human beings, the underlying etiology of the renal insufficiency, however, does not influence the immunologic outcome.

## NEUTROPHILS

Most studies have demonstrated abnormal neutrophilic chemotaxis, normal phagocytosis, and impaired intracellular bactericidal activity associated with uremia. Decreased neutrophilic phagocytosis has been reported by some investigators. In one study of peritoneal dialysis patients, increased bacterial infection rate was present in only the patients with decreased neutrophil phagocytosis. This suggests neutrophil phagocytic function is important in protection against bacterial peritonitis.

In addition to the resultant increased susceptibility to bacterial infection, decreased neutrophil mobilization may be an important consideration in the diagnoses of a urinary tract infection in animals with renal insufficiency. Pyuria may be absent in these animals despite the presence of a urinary tract infection. Therefore, urine should be cultured for bacteria in animals with impaired renal function regardless of the number of urine leukocytes present.

## IMMUNOGLOBULIN RESPONSES

Although total blood immunoglobulin concentrations are in the normal range, antigen-specific immunoglobulin production and vaccine response are impaired in uremia. The clinical consequences of these immunologic impairments include increased susceptibility to bacterial infections and decreased vaccination-induced protection.

The exact mechanism of the decreased B-lymphocyte response is unknown, but may be in part due to adverse effects of hyperparathyroidism resulting in increased cyclic adenosine monophosphate (cAMP) production and increased intracellular calcium concentration in the B lymphocyte (Gaciong et al., 1991). Investigators have found a dose response suppressive effect of parathyroid hormone (PTH) on B-lymphocyte proliferation. Also, parathyroidectomy returned the serum antibody response to near normal concentrations in rats with chronic renal failure.

When human dialysis patients treated with recombinant erythropoietin were compared to a similar group of patients with no erythropoietin therapy, those treated had a greater antibody response to a viral vaccine (Sennesael, Van der Niepen, and Verbeelen, 1991). The mechanism of the beneficial response to erythropoietin is unknown. The influence of PTH or erythropoietin on the immunoglobulin response in dogs or cats with chronic renal failure has not been investigated.

## T-LYMPHOCYTE RESPONSES

Diminished cell-mediated immunity associated with renal failure is in part due to decreased circulating T-lymphocyte numbers and function. The suppression of T-lymphocyte function resulted in prolonged graft survival (Mannick et al., 1960). Early studies investigating the mechanism of extended graft survival noted a dramatic lymphopenia in nondialyzed renal failure patients and in experimental animal models of uremia. The lymphopenia in this situation is not due only to stress mediated by corticosteroids, since lymphopenia also occurs in adrenalectomzied, uremic animals.

Decreased function is probably more important than lymphopenia associated with renal failure. When assessed by in vitro lymphocyte blastogenesis, dogs with chronic but not acute renal failure have a decreased T-lymphocyte response. In human beings, a portion of the decreased proliferation is due to a serum factor, since uremic serum suppresses blastogenesis of normal, heterologous lymphocytes.

When compared to healthy controls, human beings with end-stage renal failure maintained on hemodialysis have increased T suppressor/cytotoxic lymphocyte ($T_s$) activity. T-helper lymphocyte ($T_h$)/$T_s$ ratio is often used as an index of T-cell activity in vitro. In some studies involving chronic hemodialysis patients, the $T_h$/$T_s$ ratio has been reported as normal, and others have reported a ratio of less than the $T_h$/$T_s$ ratios of healthy controls. In unpublished studies, when dogs with chronic renal insufficiency were compared to normal dogs, the azotemic dogs had increased peripheral blood $T_s$ cell numbers and decreased $T_h$/$T_s$ ratios.

Lymphocytes have PTH receptors, and since patients with chronic renal failure have increased PTH production and impaired lymphocyte function, PTH was evaluated as an immunosuppressive mediator in uremia. Incubation of normal peripheral blood lymphocytes with increasing concentrations of PTH resulted in a decreased blastogenesis and $T_h$/$T_s$ ratios (Shasha et al., 1988). Collaborating support of an immunosuppressive role of PTH was found in a preliminary investigation of primary hyperparathyroidism (Shasha et al., 1989). In these human patients, the $T_h$/$T_s$ ratios were decreased but returned to normal following the decrease in serum PTH concentration after parathyroidectomy.

The mechanism of the suppressive effect of uremia on lymphocyte function is unclear. Recently, the role of interleukins on immunologic function in uremia has been investigated. Interleukin-2 (IL-2) production is impaired in T lymphocytes from renal failure patients. Addition of uremic serum to peripheral blood lymphocytes from healthy controls impairs IL-2 production. In addition, the decreased IL-2 production may cause the abnormal state of lymphoblast activation present in uremia (Donati et al., 1992). These combined events are likely responsible for the decreased lymphocyte response in chronic renal failure. Other interleukins are being investigated in the immunosuppression of uremia.

## POTENTIAL THERAPY

Unfortunately, evidence of the incidence of abnormal immune function and subsequent adverse effects is lacking in dogs and cats with chronic renal failure. Similarly, objective responses to treatment are absent in the veterinary literature. Therapy to relieve other adverse consequences of renal insufficiency may concomitantly improve the animal's immune function.

The malnutrition and chronic blood loss which may occur with chronic renal failure should be addressed, since negative nitrogen balance and iron deficiency compromise immune function. Nutritional support, management of gastric ulcers (cimetidine, sucralfate), and iron replacement therapy, if needed, are indicated and may have the added beneficial effect of improving the host's immune status.

Since hyperparathyroidism is immunosuppressive, normalizing serum PTH concentrations may be beneficial in restoring the immune response is dogs and cats with renal failure. This may be accomplished in some animals by restricting phosphorus intake and absorption. In some animals, supplemental vitamin $D_3$ may be needed. Although the effect of vitamin D administration on the immune status of dogs with renal failure has not been investigated, it may be beneficial, since treating human chronic renal failure patients (including three patients not using dialysis) with oral vitamin D resulted in increased numbers of $T_h$ cells, decreased $T_s$ cells, and a dramatic increased the $T_h/T_s$ ratio. Modifying the immune response may be an added beneficial effect of using erythropoietin in managing the anemia of chronic renal failure.

Preliminary investigations have evaluated the effects of anabolic or androgenic hormones on the immune response. These hormones may have a direct effect on the immune system or, by stimulating appetite and a positive nitrogen balance, may have an indirect beneficial effect on animals with chronic renal failure. Administration of dehydroepiandrosterone increased IL-2 production in young and aged mice (Daynes, Dudley, and Araneo, 1990), and increased the antibody response to vaccination in aged mice. Whether the androgen metabolite has similar beneficial affects in uremia is unknown. Administration of stanozolol, an anabolic hormone, to dogs with chronic renal insufficiency has been beneficial in decreasing the number of circulating $T_s$ cells.

## References and Suggested Reading

Daynes RA, Dudley DJ, and Araneo BA: Regulation of murine lymphokine production *in vivo* II. Dehydroepiandrosterone is a natural enhancer of interleukin 2 synthesis by helper T cells. Eur J Immunol 20:793, 1990.
*The effect of steroid hormones on IL-2 and IL-4 production by murine T cells is described.*

Donati D, Degiannis D, Raskova J, et al: Uremic serum effects on peripheral blood mononuclear cell and purified T lymphocyte responses. Kidney Int 42:681, 1992.
*The effect of human uremic serum on in vitro T cell proliferation, IL-2 production, and IL-2 response is discussed.*

Gaciong Z, Alexiewicz JM, Linker-Israeli M, et al: Inhibition of immunoglobulin production by parathyroid hormone. Implications in chronic renal failure. Kidney Int 40:96, 1991.
*A prospective study examining the effect of parathyroid hormone on antibody production by lymphocytes obtained from healthy and hemodialysis human patients.*

Mannick JA, Powers JH, Mithoefer J, et al: Renal transplantation in azotemic dogs. Surgery 47:340, 1960
*Results of renal transplantation in an experimental model of renal failure in dogs is described.*

Shasha SM, Kristal B, Barzilai M, et al: In vitro effect of PTH on normal T cell functions. Nephron 50:212, 1988.
*Using lymphocytes from healthy human donors, the effects of three different concentrations of glucagon, and human and bovine PTH on in vitro lymphocyte blastogenesis and T-cell numbers were investigated.*

Shasha SM, Kristal B, Steinbeg O, et al: Effect of parathyroidectomy on T cell functions in patients with primary hyperparathyroidism. Am J Nephrol 9:25, 1989.
*This study evaluated the effect of parathyroidectomy on T-lymphocyte function in three human beings with primary hyperparathyroidism.*

Sennesael JJ, Van der Niepen P, and Verbeelen DL: Treatment with recombinant human erythropoietin increases antibody titers after hepatitis B vaccination in dialysis patients. Kidney Int 40:121, 1991.
*Antibody response to hepatitis B vaccine was evaluated in 50 human hemodialysis patients.*

# CHRONIC RENAL FAILURE: IMPROVING THERAPEUTIC RESPONSE WITH PATIENT MONITORING

DAVID J. POLZIN

*St. Paul, Minnesota*

## THE BENEFITS OF PATIENT MONITORING

While the goal of conservative medical management is to ameliorate the clinical and metabolic consequences of chronic renal failure (CRF), treatments vary in efficacy and may have unintended effects. Unfortunately, the safety and therapeutic efficacy of many treatments currently advocated for dogs and cats with CRF have not yet been confirmed by controlled clinical trials. Even for those forms of therapy where data are available, individual patient responses appear to vary greatly and appropriate therapeutic monitoring is recommended. In addition, many medications for patients with CRF are administered "to effect" and thus it is necessary to monitor patient response and adjust dosages accordingly.

Therapeutic safety and efficacy may be optimized by: (1) determining the pretreatment status of the patient; (2) establishing specific, measurable goals for therapy; and (3) monitoring patient response to therapy. Monitoring patient response guides the clinician in modifying treatments to better achieve the specified therapeutic goals. It further allows the clinician to recognize new complications or changes in the course of the patient's disease that may mandate changes in therapy.

Frequent patient monitoring may improve owner compliance. Discussing the patient's response to treatment with the owner provides encouragement to follow through with therapy as recommended. Monitoring also provides important feedback to the veterinarian when therapeutic problems develop. For example, owners may discontinue treatments they find difficult or unacceptable without consulting the veterinarian. By detecting therapeutic problems or client dissatisfaction, alternative treatments acceptable to the owner and the pet may be sought. Patients with more advanced renal dysfunction typically require multiple medications, often leading to confusion and errors on the part of the owner. Patient monitoring provides a means of recognizing and correcting therapeutic errors.

It has been recognized in many studies with human patients that clinical response appears to improve with increased patient monitoring (a placebo or clinic effect). Although unproved, this "clinic effect" may also occur in dogs and cats. While this potential benefit may or may not occur, it is clear that failure to monitor response to treatment can have adverse consequences

in some patients. Treatments for which monitoring is an essential component of therapy include administration of recombinant human erythropoietin (r-HuEPO), calcitriol, and antihypertensive medications (see elsewhere in this volume). Failure to monitor the response to these therapies may have dire consequences. Other treatments, such as sodium bicarbonate administration, potassium supplementation, and intestinal phosphate-binding agents, may prove ineffective if response to therapy is not determined so that dosages can be adjusted. Potential complications of therapy and specific recommendations for monitoring therapy are summarized in Table 1.

## RECOMMENDATIONS FOR MONITORING

### Data Base for Patient Monitoring

The clinician should focus on the goals of therapy and changes occurring since the previous examination. During each visit, the owner's impression of response to therapy and new problems or complications should be sought. Drug and diet histories should be obtained. The owner should be asked to list all medications the pet is receiving. Dosage and timing of administration (particularly the relationship to feeding) should be established for each medication. The relationship between medication administration and feeding is important because food ingestion often affects drug efficacy (e.g., calcium acetate is a phosphate-binding agent when administered with food, but a calcium supplement when administered between meals). The owner should be asked whether there have been any problems or difficulties related to medications. Diet history should include a listing of all foods, treats, and supplements the pet is receiving. The appetite and quantity of food consumed and specific food preferences should be determined. Treatment-specific questions are appropriate for some medications to detect response to therapy or drug-related complications (e.g., the owner of a dog receiving intestinal phosphate-binding agents may be asked if the dog is experiencing difficulty defecating or with constipation).

A physical examination should be performed with particular emphasis placed on hydration status, nutri-

***Table 1.***  *Potential Therapeutic Complications and Recommendations for Monitoring*

| Therapy | Therapeutic goals | Potential Complications | Recommended Monitoring |
|---|---|---|---|
| Dietary protein restriction | Ameliorate clinical signs of uremia; maintain adequate nutrition (as established by physical examination, body weight, serum albumin concentrations, and packed cell volumes) | Protein malnutrition, poor dietary acceptance, poor dietary compliance, failure to ameliorate signs of uremia | Physical examination, body weight, strength and activity, serum albumin concentrations, and packed cell volumes; obtain diet history from owner, blood urea nitrogen and creatinine concentrations, clinical response to therapy |
| Dietary salt restriction | Limit systemic hypertension and polyuria | Volume depletion | Body weight, hydration status, blood pressure |
| Dietary phosphorus restriction | Normalize serum phosphorus concentration, limit hyperparathyroidism | Failure to normalize serum phosphorus concentration | Serum phosphorus concentrations |
| Aluminum-based intestinal phosphate-binding agents | Normalize serum phosphorus concentration, limit hyperparathyroidism | Inadequate therapy, hypophosphatemia, constipation, adverse effect on appetite | Serum phosphorus concentrations, question owner about pet's bowel habits, physical examination, obtain diet history from owner |
| Calcium-based intestinal phosphate-binding agents | Normalize serum phosphorus concentration, limit hyperparathyroidism | Inadequate therapy, hypercalcemia, hypophosphatemia, adverse effect on appetite | Serum phosphorus and calcium concentrations, obtain diet history from owner |
| Sodium bicarbonate therapy for metabolic acidosis | Correct metabolic acidosis | Inadequate therapy, excessive alkalization, sodium/fluid overload, systemic hypertension, poor patient acceptance | Serum bicarbonate or total carbon dioxide ($TcO_2$) concentration, body weight, blood pressure, obtain medication history from owner and determine effect of therapy on food intake |
| Potassium supplementation | Prevent or correct hypokalemia | Inadequate therapy, hyperkalemia, alkalosis due to associated anion (e.g., citrate) | Serum potassium and bicarbonate or $TcO_2$ concentrations |
| Antihypertensive medications | Ameliorate systemic hypertension | Inadequate response to therapy, hypotension, adverse drug events | Measure systemic blood pressure, fundic examination for hypertensive retinopathy, consult drug insert or reference texts for possible adverse drug events |
| Recombinant human erythropoietin therapy | Normalize packed cell volumes | Polycythemia, inadequate response to therapy, development of antibodies to erythropoietin, iron deficiency, adverse drug event, induction of systemic hypertension | Hematocrit, bone marrow examination (if indicated), serum iron levels (if indicated), consult references concerning possible drug reactions in dogs and cats, measure blood pressure, fundic examinations for hypertensive retinopathy |
| Calcitriol therapy | Correct renal secondary hyperparathyroidism | Hypercalcemia, failure to correct hyperparathyroidism | Serum calcium and phosphorus concentrations, serum intact parathyroid hormone activities |
| Drug therapy | Drug/diagnosis specific | Adverse drug events, nephrotoxicity | Maintain accurate record of drugs patient is receiving, review drug inserts for possible adverse drug events or nephrotoxicity, monitor renal function to determine need to adjust dosages |

tional status, and general well-being of the patient. Nutritional status may be subjectively assessed by examining body condition, muscle mass and strength, activity, and hair coat qualities such as shedding and gloss. A fundic examination should be performed to detect hypertensive retinopathy and blood pressure should be measured (see Section 2). An accurate body weight should always be obtained. Because changes or trends in values are often more revealing than the values themselves, it is recommended that a flow sheet be established for serially monitored quantities such as body weight and hematologic and biochemical parameters.

Essential laboratory evaluations for patients with CRF include packed cell volumes; urinalyses; and serum (or plasma) urea nitrogen, creatinine, phosphorus, potassium, bicarbonate (or total carbon dioxide), and albumin concentrations (Table 2). Ideally, serum calcium, sodium, and chloride concentrations and urine cultures (if indicated) will also be performed. In proteinuric patients, urine protein/creatinine ratios should be monitored. If previous radiographs have indicated the presence of nephrolithiasis or renal mineralization, survey abdominal radiographs may also be indicated.

## Frequency of Patient Monitoring

As a rule, dogs and cats with CRF should be reexamined within 2 to 4 weeks of initiating therapy, and

**Table 2.** *Guidelines for Monitoring Patients with Chronic Renal Failure*

| Test | Purpose |
|------|---------|
| History | To assess response to therapy; to ascertain compliance with recommendations and owner-perceived problems with therapy; to detect communication problems with the client; to detect new problems or complications; to encourage client compliance |
| Physical examination | To detect new problems or complications; to assess hydration; to assess nutritional status and well-being of the animal |
| Body weight | To assess nutritional and hydration status |
| Serum creatinine concentration | To assess severity and progression of renal dysfunction; to detect concomitant prerenal and post-renal azotemia |
| BUN concentration | To assess compliance with dietary recommendations; to detect concomitant prerenal and post-renal azotemia |
| Urinalysis | To detect urinary tract infection; to detect changes in urine sediment or urine chemistries that may suggest active or changing renal lesions which may warrant specific therapy or changes in therapy; to monitor proteinuria |
| Serum phosphorus concentration | To determine success of dietary phosphorus restriction and to adjust dosages of intestinal phosphate binders |
| Serum calcium concentration | To assess need for and to adjust dosage of calcium supplements and vitamin D |
| Serum albumin concentration | To assess nutritional status; important for monitoring impact of urinary protein loss in patients with glomerulopathies; necessary for interpretation of serum calcium values and assess influence on protein-bound drugs |
| Blood bicarbonate or TCO$_2$ concentration | To assess need for alkalization therapy; necessary for adjusting dosage of alkalization therapy |
| PCV or CBC | To assess response to therapy for anemia; may also be useful for assessing nutritional status |
| Urine culture | Indicated: (1) if urinalysis supports possible UTI, (2) to confirm that previously detected and treated UTI have been successfully eradicated, and (3) as routine part of follow-up studies in patients with recurrent UTI and CRF. |
| Blood pressure | To assess development of systemic hypertension or hypotension; to monitor antihypertensive therapy |

Abbreviations: BUN = blood urea nitrogen, CO$_2$ = carbon dioxide, PCV = packed cell volume, CBC = complete blood count, UTI = urinary tract infection, CRF = chronic renal failure, TCO$_2$ = total carbon dioxide.

three to four times yearly thereafter. The severity of renal dysfunction and types of therapy provided will influence the frequency of follow-up examination. Dogs and cats with more advanced CRF should probably be examined at least every 2 to 3 months. In addition, recheck examinations should be scheduled whenever therapy is changed in order to assess the response to the change. For most medications, follow-up examinations should be scheduled about 2 to 4 weeks after medication changes.

Some medications require more frequent monitoring. Patients receiving antihypertensive drugs should have their blood pressure monitored every 1 to 2 weeks until pressures decline into the target range. Once blood pressure has been stabilized in the target range, blood pressure may be monitored monthly for several months, and every other month thereafter in well-controlled patients. Patients receiving r-HuEPO for anemia of CRF should have their packed cell volumes

monitored weekly until the appropriate maintenance dosage has been established (see "*CVT* Update: Use of Recombinant Human Erythropoietin," this volume, p 961). During the maintenance phase of r-HuEPO therapy, packed cell volumes should be monitored monthly. Serum calcium, phosphorus, urea nitrogen, and creatinine should be monitored 1 week and 1 month after initiating low-dose calcitriol therapy, and monthly thereafter.

## References and Suggested Reading

Cowgill L: Pathophysiology and management of anemia in chronic progressive renal failure. Semin Vet Med Surg [Small Anim Pract] 7:175, 1992.
   *A review of the pathophysiology, diagnosis, and treatment (with erythropoietin) of anemia of chronic renal failure in dogs and cats.*
Littman M: Update: Treatment of hypertension in dogs and cats. *In* Kirk R and Bonagura J (eds): *Current Veterinary Therapy XI.* Philadelphia, WB Saunders Co, 1992, p 838.

*A summary of the diagnosis and treatment of systemic hypertension in dogs and cats.*
Nagode L and Chew D: Nephrocalcinosis caused by hyperparathyroidism in progression of renal failure: Treatment with calcitriol. Semin Vet Med Surg [Small Anim Pract] 7:202, 1992.

*A review of the pathophysiology and consequences of renal secondary hyperparathyroidism and its treatment with calcitriol.*
Polzin DJ, Osborne CA, and O'Brien TD: Diseases of the kidneys and ureters. *In* Ettinger SJ (ed): *Textbook of Veterinary Internal Medicine.* Philadelphia, WB Saunders Co, 1989, p 1963.

# MANAGEMENT OF FLUID AND ELECTROLYTE DISORDERS IN UREMIA

STANLEY I. RUBIN

*Saskatoon, Saskatchewan, Canada*

Uremia is the constellation of clinical signs and biochemical abnormalities associated with a critical loss of functional nephrons. It is a toxic disorder caused by the combined effects of a variety of metabolites retained due to loss of renal excretory function. The uremic syndrome also includes many metabolic and endocrinologic disturbances that arise thorough loss of homeostatic, synthetic, and catabolic functions of the kidney, as well as abnormalities arising from renal compensatory mechanisms and therapeutic intervention. The presence of extrarenal manifestations (e.g., hemorrhagic gastroenteritis, anemia, osteodystrophy, coagulopathies) is usually implied when a patient is described as being uremic.

The most important therapy in the initial management of a uremic patient is parenteral fluid administration. Initial goals include restoration and expansion of extracellular fluid (ECF) volume, correction of serious electrolyte and acid-base disturbances, and reduction in the magnitude of the azotemia through intensive replacement and maintenance therapy.

The purpose of this article is to discuss specific details of fluid management and electrolyte disorders in uremic dogs and cats. Please see other articles in this volume for further discussion of treatment of uremia (also see *CVT XI*, p 842 and p 848).

## CAUSES OF UREMIA

Reversible or irreversible loss of at least 75% of renal excretory function must occur before azotemia (elevated serum urea or serum creatinine concentrations) is detected. Although uremia usually occurs as a result of primary renal disease (e.g., acute and chronic renal failure), it may also occur from prerenal or postrenal causes. Prerenal disorders result from disease processes that reduce renal perfusion such as hypovolemic shock, severe ECF volume depletion, hypoadrenocorticism, heart failure, and any other disorder that reduces effective circulating blood volume. In prerenal azotemia,

the kidneys are structurally normal and can resume normal function when adequate perfusion is restored. Prerenal disorders are usually characterized by a physiologic oliguria. The kidneys reduce urine production by making a highly concentrated, small volume of urine in order to maintain ECF volume. Protracted renal hypoperfusion, however, can result in the development of primary renal lesions.

Postrenal azotemia and uremia result when elimination of urine from the body is impaired. Urine accumulation may result either from obstruction to urine flow or rupture of the excretory pathway. The kidneys are usually morphologically normal in acute postrenal disorders and can excrete retained nonprotein nitrogenous wastes following relief of obstruction or repair of urinary tract discontinuity. Chronic partial obstruction, however, may result in primary renal lesions such as hydronephrosis.

Primary renal failure occurs in cats and dogs with comparable frequency, with chronic renal failure (CRF) being more common than acute renal failure (ARF) (Chew, 1992). Both ARF and CRF may be classified as oliguric or nonoliguric. Chronic renal failure is usually polyuric; however, affected animals may become oliguric when ECF volume is depleted or during terminal decompensation.

The relative proportion of oliguric versus nonoliguric forms of ARF are not documented in dogs and cats (Chew and DiBartola, 1989). Patients with ARF tend to be more severely affected based on history, clinical signs, and laboratory evaluation compared to those patients with compensated CRF. Animals with decompensated CRF, however, may be as severely affected as those with ARF.

## DIAGNOSTIC APPROACH

Because of the urgency in management of the patient in uremic crisis, treatment and diagnostic testing are often performed simultaneously. A specific diagnosis is paramount, not only for treatment of prerenal and postrenal causes, but also for prognosis and therapeutic adjustments in the patient with primary renal failure. In many cases, approach to therapy for the patient with primary renal failure is similar regardless of specific histologic diagnosis. Although diagnosis may not be apparent at the time of initiation of therapy for uremia, the clinician should ensure that as many tests are performed, and samples collected, prior to the initiation of therapy in order to ultimately establish a definitive diagnosis. Table 1 presents a recommended diagnostic and therapeutic approach.

## THERAPY

### Disorders of Water and Sodium

Extracellular fluid volume is the volume of water held outside cells by the osmotic force of sodium ($Na^+$) and its attendant anions, chloride ($Cl^-$) and bicarbonate ($HCO_3^-$). $Na^+$ content determines ECF volume; with $Na^+$ deficit there is ECF volume contraction. Patients with uremia typically have large deficits in ECF volume due to combined loss of water and $Na^+$ through obligatory polyuria (e.g., CRF, polyuric phase of ARF), gastrointestinal loss (e.g., vomiting, diarrhea), or loss of blood or protein.

Serum $Na^+$ and $Cl^-$ concentrations are usually normal in dogs and cats with uremia and ECF volume depletion (Chew, 1992). This is the result of isotonic losses of NaCl and water in urine or gastrointestinal fluids. Hypernatremia may result when loss of free water exceeds $Na^+$ loss. Hyponatremia occurs less commonly and is the result of continued water consumption and impaired water excretion that may occur with ECF-volume depletion due to NaCl loss or to inappropriate or marked antidiuretic hormone (ADH) secretion. (Chew, 1992).

#### DEFICIT THERAPY

Restoration of ECF volume with parenteral fluid therapy facilitates correction of prerenal factors contributing to uremia. Adequate ECF volume will increase renal blood flow (RBF) and glomerular filtration rate (GFR) to prevent further renal injury.

Fluid requirements for restoration of deficits can be calculated [estimated deficit (%) × body weight in kilograms = liters required] (Table 2). The author prefers to consider fluid deficits in terms of ECF volume rather than water deficits, hydration deficits or percentage dehydration. Pure water deficits are unusual; most patients have both water and electrolyte deficits as a result of combined loss from the disease process.

The intravenous route of fluid administration is necessary during initial treatment of the uremic patient with severe ECF volume deficits, ongoing fluid loss (e.g., vomiting, diarrhea, polyuria), or serious electrolyte and acid-base derangements. An indwelling jugular venous catheter is favored for the management of the uremic patient in order that large volumes of fluids be

**Table 1.** *Recommended Diagnostic and Therapeutic Approach for the Uremic Patient*

1. Collect baseline data prior to treatment:
    Physical examination
    Complete blood count
    Serum biochemistry
    Urine analysis including urine specific gravity
    Consider urine culture
    Consider measurement of blood gases
    Measure blood pressure
2. Rule out prerenal and postrenal azotemia/uremia
3. Calculate/estimate fluid deficits
4. Begin intravenous administration of replacement type fluid (lactated Ringer's solution, normal saline)
5. Assess response to fluid challenge
6. Replace fluid deficits, correct electrolyte, and acid-base abnormalities identified in step 1
7. Continue diagnostic work-up to rule out potentially reversible causes of decreased glomerular filtration rate or determine the cause of intrinsic renal failure
    Urine culture
    Urine protein/creatinine ratio
    Abdominal radiographs
    Contrast radiography
        Intravenous urography
        Contrast cystography
    Ultrasonography
    Renal biopsy
8. Continue maintenance therapy with maintenance-type fluid
9. Monitor response to therapy—tailor according to needs of patient:
    Serial assessment of physical factors
        Body weight
        Skin turgor
    Repeat baseline laboratory data
        Packed cell volume and total protein
        Serum biochemistry including electrolytes, serum urea, and serum creatinine
        Blood gas analysis
        Measurement of fluid "ins-and-outs"

given rapidly and central venous pressure (CVP) monitored during aggressive fluid administration. Fluids should be administered at a rate calculated to correct the ECF deficit over a 4- to 6-hr period in order to facilitate restoration of renal function. Some authors recommend a fluid challenge of 20 ml/kg over 10 min

**Table 2.** *Estimation of Extracellular Fluid Volume Deficit*

| % | Clinical Signs |
|---|---|
| <5 | Not detectable |
| 5–6 | Subtle loss of skin elasticity |
| 6–8 | Definite delay in return of skin to normal position<br>Slight prolongation of capillary refill time<br>Possibly eyes sunken in orbits<br>Possibly dry mucous membranes |
| 10–12 | Tented skin stands in place<br>Definite prolongation of capillary refill time<br>Eyes sunken in orbits<br>Dry mucous membranes<br>Possibly signs of shock (tachycardia, cool extremities, rapid and weak pulse) |
| 12–15 | Definite signs of shock<br>Death imminent |

while measuring CVP to assess the likelihood of subsequent volume overload. The CVP should not rise more than 2 cm $H_2O$ if cardiopulmonary function is normal (Chew, 1992).

In most cases, either normal (0.9%) saline or lactated Ringer's solution is the fluid of choice for deficit therapy because they have the same tonicity and a similar concentration of $Na^+$ as normal plasma. Normal saline is devoid of $K^+$ and anions other than $Cl^-$; lactated Ringer's solution contains only 4 mmol/L of $K^+$. Care should be taken in choice of fluid and overly rapid correction when the uremic animal is either hypernatremic or hyponatremic.

Hypernatremic patients usually have both an ECF volume deficit and a pure water deficit. These patients should initially receive isotonic fluids, either normal (0.9%) saline or lactated Ringer's solution to correct ECF volume deficits. Hypotonic solutions such as half normal (0.45%) saline, dextrose in saline (2/3 $D_5W$ + 1/3 normal saline), or $D_5W$ are then administered to correct the water deficiency. Guidelines for rates of correction have not been established for the dog and cat; in people, the aim is to lower the serum $Na^+$ by 0.5 to 1.0 mmol/L/hr. More aggressive therapy should be employed for patients with central nervous signs (e.g., convulsion) as a result of hypernatremia; serum $Na^+$ is rapidly lowered by 3 to 4 mmol/L, an amount usually sufficient to stop the seizures.

Hyponatremic patients should receive isotonic fluids, either normal (0.9%) saline or lactated Ringer's solution to restore ECF deficits. Hypertonic saline solution (3.0%) should only be used when the patient has neurologic signs associated with severe hyponatremia. Serum $Na^+$ should be raised slowly, at a rate of 0.5 to 1.0 mmol/L/hr.

Urine output will vary depending on the cause of the uremic crisis. It is important to recognize oliguria (defined as production of less than 1 ml/kg/hr), as it will dictate the volume of fluid that can be safely administered. An indwelling urinary catheter is recommended for critical patients and those suspected of being oliguric to monitor urine output and facilitate fluid therapy over the first 24 to 48 hr. Under these circumstances, fluid administration can be matched with urine output and previous fluid loss; both urinary and calculated sensible losses can be given to the patient. Previously calculated deficits in ECF volume are replaced first and then the "in's-and-out's" method of fluid monitoring is carried out. Alternatives to bladder catheterization include collecting urine in a metabolic cage, sequentially weighing a cat's litter pan, or weighing absorbent pads used to collect urine from recumbent animals who spontaneously void. Less reliable methods for assessing urine production include observation of urinations and serial palpation of bladder filling. Oliguria at the beginning of therapy may be physiologic, secondary to ECF volume depletion (e.g., hypodipsia, vomiting, diarrhea), or from severe renal damage. Development of oliguria at any stage of fluid therapy necessitates careful attention to further fluid input to avoid overexpansion of the ECF and its consequences (e.g., pulmonary edema in dogs, hydrothorax in cats).

## MAINTENANCE THERAPY

Maintenance therapy is instituted following correction of ECF volume deficits and provides for sensible and insensible water losses. Water requirements for most animals over a 24-hr period range from 44 to 110 ml/kg, with lighter animals requiring a proportionately higher volume. The author prefers to use 60 ml/kg/day for most animals; however, adjustments in volume may be necessary for animals with very small or very large body weights. Volume of ongoing fluid losses, in diarrhea or vomitus, should be estimated and included in the volume of fluid to be administered.

Although normal saline is the fluid of choice for deficit therapy, it is unsuitable for maintenance therapy. It contains excessive $Na^+$ relative to maintenance needs, which may contribute to ECF volume overload and hypernatremia if administered in excess over several days. Several fluid types are appropriate for maintenance therapy. These include half-normal (0.45%) saline ($Na^+$=76 mmol/L); a mixture comprising 2/3 $D_5W$ + 1/3 normal saline; 1/3 normal (0.3%) saline; and half-normal (0.45%) saline in 2.5% dextrose. Each of these fluids serves to expand both ECF and also intracellular fluid (ICF) volumes. However, all these fluids are devoid of $K^+$. KCl should be added to maintenance fluids (20 mmol/L) to maintain homeostasis, as long as the animal is not hyperkalemic. $K^+$ supplementation of fluids should be monitored by serial measurement of serum $K^+$.

## DIURESIS

Intensive diuresis with vigorous fluid therapy and diuretics has been recommended to facilitate loss of some substances that have accumulated during the uremic state and may have contributed to clinical illness associated with uremia. Any resultant increase in RBF, GFR, and urine production, however, may be independent of each other. Volume expansion may increase GFR, but an increase in urine production due to diuretics is not usually accompanied by an increase in GFR. Therefore, an increase in urine production should not be equated with improved renal function. In some cases, it is not possible to increase urine production. It has not been established whether intensive diuresis, with vigorous fluid therapy or diuretic agents, actually changes the clinical course of an animal in uremic crisis. One could argue that following restoration of ECF volume deficits and mild expansion of the ECF volume, any additional fluid administration (over and above maintenance needs) or augmentation of urine flow with diuretics makes little sense. In human patients, loop diuretics have been recommended for converting oliguric ARF to nonoliguric forms (Russo, Memoli, and Andreucci, 1992). It is accepted, however, that this therapy does little to alter the clinical course of illness.

In light of the above, it seems reasonable to question the value of intensive diuresis in the treatment of chronic renal failure. Diuretics such as mannitol, glucose, furosemide, and dopamine have been commonly used to convert oliguric to nonoliguric acute renal failure, although their merit appears to be marginal at best. The merits of using diuretic agents, over ECF deficit therapy and volume expansion, have dubious theoretical basis, and no solid experimental justification. The author prefers achieving diuresis by first correcting ECF volume deficits, followed by the administration of maintenance fluids at 1.5 to 3.0 times the volume required for maintenance. This method achieves adequate replacement of deficits and ongoing losses. The reader may refer to previous articles for other modes of inducing diuresis and converting oliguria to nonoliguria (Cornelius, 1983; Chew, 1992).

## Disorders of Potassium

### HYPERKALEMIA

Hyperkalemia is most commonly recognized with hypoadrenocorticism, ARF, and postrenal failure. It is most often seen in severely oliguric patients, particularly those with severe metabolic acidosis. Recognition and therapy of hyperkalemia is essential because even moderate increases in the serum $K^+$ can contribute to life-threatening cardiac arrhythmias. In these instances, serial or continuous electrocardiographic (ECG) monitoring is recommended to detect the physiologic effects of hyperkalemia on the heart. An ECG is essential, and should be performed when results of serum $K^+$ measurement are not immediately available. Electrocardiographic changes often become apparent when serum $K^+$ concentration exceeds 7.0 mmol/L, although there is a considerable amount of variation among animals with respect to what changes are seen and at what concentration. Characteristic features, in approximate order of the severity of the hyperkalemia, consist of a tall peaked T wave (greater than 50% of the height of the R wave; however, an inconsistent finding in animals), bradycardia, diminished amplitude of P waves, absence of P waves (atrial standstill—the most consistent feature of moderate to severe hyperkalemia), or widening of the QRS complex. The presence of any of these changes, or a serum $K^+$ greater than 6.0 mmol/L, indicates the need for therapy to reduce the serum $K^+$ concentration.

The most important step in the therapy of hyperkalemia is restoration of ECF deficits to ensure urine production and excretion. Volume expansion of the ECF with normal saline will eliminate any prerenal factors, if present, and restore GFR and urine production. This will allow the excretion of excess $K^+$. Urethral obstruction, or tears in the urine-collecting system, should be rectified as soon as possible. Sodium bicarbonate ($NaHCO_3$) may be administered when the above maneuvers fail to correct the arrhythmias. $NaHCO_3$ may be administered to shift $K^+$ from the ECF space to the ICF space. The recommended dose of $NaHCO_3$ is 1 to 2 mmol/kg IV over 5 to 15 min. If $NaHCO_3$ fails to work, calcium gluconate may be given to counteract toxic effects of hyperkalemia on the myocardium. The recommended dose is 0.5 ml/kg of a 10% solution administered slowly over 5 to 10 min, while monitoring the ECG or heart rate. Infusion of calcium gluconate is stopped when heart rate increases or the ECG becomes more normal. Calcium salts do not lower the serum $K^+$ concentration and have the disadvantage of promoting soft tissue mineralization if hyperphosphatemia is present. Calcium salts, however, may be beneficial in a patient with symptomatic hypocalcemia. Other measures advocated for the treatment of hyperkalemia include administration of glucose and insulin to cause intracellular shift $K^+$. In the author's opinion, glucose and insulin infusions are rarely required. Atropine sulfate may increase the heart rate in some patients with hyperkalemia and sinoventricular rhythm.

### HYPOKALEMIA

Hypokalemia is a more common abnormality than hyperkalemia and often exists in anorectic patients with polyuric renal failure. It may also develop following deficit therapy with $K^+$-deficient fluids, during periods of intensive therapeutic diuresis, or during periods of spontaneous diuresis. Hypokalemia may be a cause or consequence of chronic renal failure, particularly in cats (Dow and Fettman, 1992).

The most common clinical signs of hypokalemia are gastric atony, ileus, and skeletal muscle weakness. Therapy is indicated if serum $K^+$ is below the reference range, although clinical signs are not usually apparent until serum concentrations fall below 2.5 mmol/L. Serum $K^+$ concentrations less than 2.0 mmol/L may be life threatening due to respiratory paralysis and cardiac arrhythmias.

In most cases, hypokalemia can be corrected by the addition of KCl to intravenous fluids. The dose delivered is dependent on the severity of the hypokalemia (Table 3). It has been recommended to calculate the infusion rate so that not more than 0.5 mmol/kg/hr of $K^+$ is delivered. Oral therapy using potassium salts has been administered to cats with severe hypokalemia (*CVT XI*, p 820), but this is not well tolerated in uremic patients already affected by vomiting.

**Table 3.** *Guidelines for Potassium Supplementation of Intravenous Fluids*

| Serum Potassium | Add KCl/L of Fluid | Maximum Infusion Rate |
|---|---|---|
| <2.0 mmol/L | 80 mmol/L | 6 ml/kg/hr |
| 2.0–2.5 mmol/L | 60 mmol/L | 8 ml/kg/hr |
| 2.5–3.0 mmol/L | 40 mmol/L | 12 ml/kg/hr |
| 3.0–3.5 mmol/L | 28 mmol/L | 16 ml/kg/hr |

## Acid-Base Disorders

Metabolic acidosis is common when there is a severe reduction in GFR. Treatment is required when acidosis is severe (pH <7.2). In the absence of blood gas measurements, a total carbon dioxide ($Tco_2$) concentration less than 15 mmol/L usually indicates acidosis severe enough to require alkali administration. Ideally, bicarbonate should be administered to replace the bicarbonate deficit:

0.3 × body weight (kg)

× (normal serum bicarbonate

− measured serum bicarbonate)

= mmol bicarbonate needed

This method of deficit correction requires serial monitoring with blood gas measurements. Therapy may need to be adjusted based on the results. Alternatively, $NaHCO_3$ may empirically be added to calcium-free IV fluids at a dosage of 1 to 5 mmol/kg, depending on the severity of the acidosis (Chew, 1992).

## Monitoring Therapy

A systematic plan for monitoring therapy is essential to formulating the appropriate strategy and assessing adequacy of response to initial therapy. The amount of data collected and intensity of monitoring is dependent on the severity of the patient's condition. Data collected should be recorded on flow charts to facilitate easy retrieval and analysis. The minimum data recorded on a daily basis includes clinical assessment of ECF volume status, body weight, capillary refill time, packed cell volume, total serum protein, and volume of fluid administered and lost. Thoracic ausculation and careful observation for signs of respiratory distress should be routine, particularly in animals receiving aggressive fluid therapy or in those with questionable cardiovascular function (Cornelius, 1978). Body weight should be measured, on an accurate scale, at least twice daily, as it is one of the most accurate determinants of changes in fluid balance. A gain or loss of 1 kg in body weight represents a gain or loss of 1 L of fluid. Other data that may be useful include CVP, serum analytes (urea, creatinine, $Na^+$, $K^+$, $Cl^-$), blood gas analysis, or $Tco_2$ and serum osmolality.

## Duration of Fluid Therapy

Fluid therapy is continued until one of the following outcomes is apparent: (1) serum creatinine and urea return to normal, (2) clinical signs of uremia abate with concomitant reduction and stabilization of urea and serum creatinine, or (3) signs of uremia persist with continued elevation of urea and creatinine (Ross, 1989). The first outcome is compatible with either ARF or prerenal uremia. The second outcome suggests either the presence of ARF with residual renal dysfunction or compensated CRF with superimposed prerenal factors. The third situation is a consequence of nonresponsive ARF or end-stage renal disease.

Intravenous fluids should be continued in the face of declining serum creatinine and urea nitrogen concentrations. Fluid therapy should never be terminated abruptly in a patient that has been in renal failure; fluid volume should be reduced by approximately 25% daily for 2 to 3 days prior to discontinuing fluid therapy (Chew, 1992). It is essential to monitor the patient during this period to ensure volume status remains positive (based on parameters used to assess ECF volume; see Table 2) and the magnitude of azotemia either stabilizes or decreases. Subcutaneous fluid therapy may be substituted for IV therapy when signs of uremia abate and the patient is able to tolerate oral food and water.

## References and Suggested Reading

Brown SA, Barsanti JA, and Finco DR: Medical management of canine chronic renal failure. *In* Kirk RW and Bonagura JD (eds): *Current Veterinary Therapy XI.* Philadelphia, WB Saunders Co, 1992, p 842.
*A review of the medical management of chronic renal failure in the dog.*
Chew DJ: Fluid therapy during intrinsic renal failure. *In* DiBartola SJ (ed): *Fluid Therapy in Small Animal Practice.* Philadelphia, WB Saunders Co, 1992. p 554.
*An in-depth approach to fluid therapy for the patient with renal failure.*
Chew DJ and DiBartola S: Diagnosis and pathophysiology of renal disease. *In* Ettinger S (ed): *Textbook of Veterinary Internal Medicine,* 3rd edition. Philadelphia, WB Saunders Co, 1989, p 1893.
*A review on the principles of diagnosis and the pathophysiology of renal disease.*
Cornelius LM: Fluid therapy in the uremic patient. *In* Kirk RW (ed): *Current Veterinary Therapy VIII.* Phildelphia, WB Saunders Co, 1983, p 989.
*A review of fluid therapy in the uremic patient.*
Cornelius LM, Finco DR, and Culver DH: Physiologic effects of rapid infusion of Ringer's lactate solution into dogs. Am J Vet Res 39:1185, 1978.
*Reults of a study of various infusion rates of intravenous fluids in the dog.*
Dow SW and Fettman MJ: Renal disease in cats: The potassium connection. *In* Kirk RW and Bonagura JD (eds): *Current Veterinary Therapy XI.* Philadelphia, WB Saunders Co, 1992, p 820.
*A review of the relationships between hypokalemia and chronic renal disease in cats.*
Polzin DJ, Osborne CA, Adams LG, et al: Medical management of feline chronic renal failure. *In* Kirk RW and Bonagura JD (eds): *Current Veterinary Therapy XI.* Philadelphia, WB Saunders Co, 1992, p 848.
*A review of the medical management of chronic renal failure in the cat.*
Ross LA: Fluid therapy for acute and chronic renal failure. Vet Clin North Am 19:343, 1989.
*A review of fluid therapy for acute and chronic renal failure in the dog and cat.*
Russo D, Memoli B, and Andreucci VE: The place of loop diuretics in the treatment of acute and chronic renal failure. Clin Nephrol 38 (suppl 1): S69, 1992.
*A review on the use of loop diuretics in acute and chronic renal failure in people.*

# METABOLIC ACIDOSIS IN RENAL FAILURE: CONSEQUENCES, DIAGNOSIS, AND TREATMENT

DAVID J. POLZIN,
KATHERINE M. JAMES,
*and* CARL A. OSBORNE
*St. Paul, Minnesota*

Metabolic acidosis has long been known to accompany chronic renal failure (CRF). In a retrospective case series of cats with renal failure, approximately 80% had metabolic acidosis based on decreased venous blood pH values and bicarbonate concentrations (Lulich et al., 1992). In renal failure, metabolic acidosis results primarily from the limited ability of failing kidneys to excrete hydrogen ions, particularly as ammonium. The pathophysiology of uremic acidosis has recently been reviewed (Berlyne et al., 1992; Giovannetti, Cupisti, and Barsotti, 1992).

## CONSEQUENCES OF METABOLIC ACIDOSIS

### Nutritional Effects of Acidosis in Renal Failure

Chronic acidosis may accelerate protein catabolism and promote protein malnutrition in patients with CRF. This protein catabolism provides a source of nitrogen for hepatic glutamine synthesis, glutamine being the substrate for renal ammoniagenesis (Mitch, Jurkovitz, and England, 1993). Current evidence suggests that uremia directly impairs insulin-stimulated protein synthesis. Metabolic acidosis stimulates protein degradation, even in nonuremic states. The combined effects of reduced protein synthesis due to uremia and accelerated proteolysis due to acidosis promotes azotemia, increased nitrogen excretion, and the negative nitrogen balance typical of uremic acidosis. Alkalization therapy effectively reverses acidosis-associated protein breakdown.

Acidosis poses an additional risk for CRF patients consuming protein-restricted diets. Dietary protein requirements appear to be similar for normal humans and humans with CRF unless uremic acidosis is present. When acid-base status is normal, adaptive reductions in skeletal muscle protein degradation protect patients consuming low-protein diets from losses in lean body mass. In rats and humans, these adaptive responses may be overridden even by mild acidosis. Thus, acidosis may limit the ability of patients to adapt to dietary protein restriction. These findings have not yet been confirmed in dogs and cats.

## Clinical Manifestations of Metabolic Acidosis

Chronic metabolic acidosis promotes a variety of adverse clinical effects including anorexia, nausea, vomiting, lethargy, weakness, muscle wasting, and weight loss. Correcting acidosis appears to ameliorate these signs. In addition, chronic mineral acid feeding to dogs has been shown to increase urinary calcium excretion and progressive bone demineralization, the magnitude of which depends on age and dietary calcium levels. Studies on the effects of dietary acidification in cats have revealed that chronic metabolic acidosis can cause negative calcium balance and bone demineralization or negative potassium balance that may in turn promote hypokalemia, renal dysfunction, and taurine depletion (Fettman et al., 1992).

When blood pH values decline below 7.20, acidemia may directly depress cardiac contractility. Furthermore, severe acidemia promotes peripheral arterial vasodilatation and central venoconstriction. Decreases in central and pulmonary vascular compliance may predispose patients to pulmonary edema during fluid administration. This effect may be particularly important in patients with acute uremic crises requiring intensive fluid therapy.

## Acidosis and Progressive Renal Injury

Metabolic acidosis is hypothesized to play a role in progression of renal failure because it promotes increased renal ammoniagenesis. Elevated renal parenchymal ammonia concentrations may be one of the common pathways whereby diverse renal insults result in similar pathologic manifestations of renal injury (Nath, Hostetter, and Hostetter, 1991). Renal ammoniagenesis is augmented by chronic metabolic acidosis, hypokalemia, subtotal renal ablation, feeding high-protein diets, diabetic nephropathy, and antioxidant (vitamin E or selenium) deficiency. All of these states are associated with the induction or progression of renal failure in an experimental model or clinical disease state. High tissue ammonium concentrations activate the third component of complement by the alternative pathway. Complement-mediated renal inflammation results in tubulointerstitial damage, which may in turn promote progression of renal disease. Preventing metabolic acidosis using sodium bicarbonate supplementation prevents the development of tubulointerstitial lesions in rats with induced CRF.

## DIAGNOSIS OF METABOLIC ACIDOSIS

Because even mildly reduced plasma bicarbonate concentrations may promote some of the adverse effects of chronic metabolic acidosis, oral alkalization therapy is indicated when serum bicarbonate concentration declines below normal. Thus, a reliable measure of metabolic acidosis is necessary for diagnosis and treatment. Ideally, the acid-base status of the patient will be determined by blood gas analysis on a properly collected arterial or venous blood sample. A somewhat less reliable alternative is determination of serum or plasma total carbon dioxide concentration. However, a word of caution is necessary regarding the use of serum total carbon dioxide ($TCO_2$) concentrations determined on chemical autoanalyzers as a method to monitor metabolic acidosis and therapy. When blood collection tubes are not fully filled or left exposed to air while awaiting analysis, the vacuum or air above the tube can draw carbon dioxide out of the serum, falsely lowering carbon dioxide concentrations. This may result in a falsely low $TCO_2$ reading and an incorrect conclusion that the patient has metabolic acidosis (James et al., 1993). In addition, there may be a substantial systematic difference between blood bicarbonate concentrations determined by blood gas analysis and serum $TCO_2$ concentrations determined on autoanalyzers due to inherent differences in the analysis methods. Appropriate reference ranges are equipment and method specific; therefore, published ranges for therapeutic goals must be extrapolated with caution. Appropriate reference ranges should be determined for each hospital and laboratory. It is possible that problems associated with clinical determination of acid-base status may have resulted in artifactually expanded reference ranges and clinician mistrust of the accuracy of $TCO_2$ determinations, resulting in an underappreciation of the true prevalence of metabolic acidosis in CRF.

## TREATMENT OF METABOLIC ACIDOSIS

### Eliminating Factors Promoting Acidosis

Extrarenal factors may exacerbate uremic acidosis and should be identified and corrected. Unexpectedly severe metabolic acidosis should prompt consideration of possible extrarenal acidosis superimposed on uremic acidosis. Factors that may promote metabolic acidosis in patients with renal failure include: (1) administration of certain drugs, including urinary acidifiers, salicylates, and hyperalimentation solutions; (2) feeding high protein diets or diets designed to produce acid urine; (3) dehydration; (4) severe diarrhea; (5) conditions that may promote catabolism, including infections and glucocorticoid administration; (6) hypokalemia; and (7) hyporeninemic hypoaldosteronism. The need for alkalization therapy should be reevaluated after eliminating extrarenal causes for acidosis.

### Alkalization Therapy

Alkalization therapy designed to correct metabolic acidosis is an important part of the overall management of patients with CRF. Potential benefits of alkalization therapy in patients with CRF include: (1) improving signs of anorexia, lethargy, nausea, vomiting, muscle weakness, and weight loss; (2) limiting the catabolic effects of metabolic acidosis on protein metabolism; (3) minimizing the potential adverse effects of increased renal ammoniagenesis on self-perpetuation of progressive renal failure; (4) enhancing the patient's capacity to adapt to additional acid stress resulting from such factors as diarrhea, dehydration, or respiratory acidosis; (5) limiting skeletal damage; and (6) rectifying the adverse effects of severe acidosis on the cardiovascular system.

#### PARENTERAL ALKALIZATION THERAPY

Parenteral alkalization therapy is indicated when blood pH values decline below 7.20. Blood bicarbonate or total carbon dioxide concentrations of about 10 mEq/L or lower suggest that blood pH may be below 7.20. However, blood pH and $PCO_2$ should be determined to confirm metabolic acidosis. The immediate goal of therapy with severe acidosis is to administer sodium bicarbonate solution intravenously in a dose sufficient to elevate blood pH above 7.20, which will minimize the adverse cardiovascular effects of acidemia. The dosage of sodium bicarbonate may be estimated from the following equation (with the assumption being that elevating serum bicarbonate to 11 mEq/L will increase blood pH above 7.20):

$$\text{Bicarbonate dose (mEq)} = (\text{body weight in kg}) \times (0.5) \times (11\text{-measured serum bicarbonate concentration})$$

This quantity of sodium bicarbonate is small and may be administered over 30 to 60 min. These recommendations assume a simple metabolic acidosis is present. Therapy of mixed acid-base disorders requires blood gas analysis to determine the need for treatment and establish therapeutic response (see "Strong Ions and Acid-Base Disorders," this volume, p 121).

#### ORAL ALKALIZATION THERAPY

Sodium bicarbonate is the most commonly used alkalinizing agent. Because the interaction between gastric acid and ingested sodium bicarbonate is quantitatively unpredictable, the dosage should be individualized for each patient. The suggested initial dose of sodium bicarbonate is 8 to 12 mg/kg body weight given every 8 to 12 hr. A particularly convenient method of measuring and administering sodium bicarbonate is to prepare a solution containing approximately 80 mg of sodium bicarbonate per milliliter of solution (about 1 mEq/ml) by adding one third of an 8-ounce box (76 gm) of sodium bicarbonate to 1 quart (946 ml) of water. This solution may be stored capped and refrigerated for several months. Initially, this solution is administered at a dose of 1 to 1.5 ml/10 kg of body weight. The solution is most acceptable when mixed with the food, but can be directly administered orally. However, some dogs and cats find oral sodium bicarbonate solutions very unpalatable.

Potassium citrate is a particularly attractive alternative alkalization agent. Potassium citrate may offer the advantage, at least in cats, of allowing for the simultaneous treatment of both hypokalemia and acidosis with a single drug. Metabolic acidosis when accompanied by potassium depletion or magnesium depletion may respond poorly to alkali therapy alone. There is a risk for overalkalization, however, in that potassium doses required for adequate correction of hypokalemia may exceed the citrate dose required to correct acidosis. Starting doses of 0.3 to 0.5 mEq/kg of potassium every 12 hr are recommended (Lulich et al., 1992).

Regardless of the alkalinizing agent chosen, administration of several smaller doses is preferred to a single large dose in order to minimize fluctuations in blood pH. The patient's response to therapy should be determined by measuring blood bicarbonate or serum (plasma) $TCO_2$ concentrations 10 to 14 days after initiating therapy. Ideally, blood should be collected just prior to administration of the drug. Dosage should be adjusted with the goal to maintain blood bicarbonate concentrations within the normal range. Urine pH is insensitive as a means of assessing the need for or response to treatment and is not routinely recommended for this purpose.

### References and Suggested Reading

Berlyne G, Adler A, Barth R, et al: Perspectives in acid-base balance in advanced chronic renal failure. Contrib Nephrol 100:105, 1992.
   *A review of current theories on acid-base metabolism in chronic renal failure.*
Fettman M, Coble J, Hamar D, et al: Effect of dietary phosphoric acid supplementation on acid-base balance and mineral and bone metabolism in adult cats. Am J Vet Res 53:2125, 1992.
   *A study exploring the effects of chronic acidification therapy on normal cats.*
Giovannetti S, Cupisti A, and Barsotti G: The metabolic acidosis of chronic renal failure: pathophysiology and treatment. Contrib Nephrol 100:48, 1992.
   *A recent review of the pathophysiology and treatment of chronic renal failure in humans.*
Lulich J, Osborne C, O'Brien T, et al: Feline renal failure: Questions, answers, questions. Compend Cont Educ Pract Vet 14:127, 1992.
   *A retrospective survey and review of renal failure in cats.*
Mitch W, Jurkovitz C, and England B: Mechanisms that cause protein and amino acid catabolism in uremia. Am J Kidney Dis 21:91, 1993.
   *A review of the factors affecting protein nutrition in renal failure.*
Nath K, Hostetter M, and Hostetter T: Increased ammoniagenesis as a determinant of progressive renal injury. Am J Kidney Dis 17:654, 1991.
   *A review of the possible role for acidosis and renal ammoniagenesis in progressive renal injury.*

# INAPPROPRIATE DIETARY PROTEIN AND MINERAL RESTRICTION IN DOGS AND CATS

DELMAR R. FINCO
*and* SCOTT A. BROWN
*Athens, Georgia*

Several food manufacturers sell protein- and mineral-restricted diets for use as recommended by veterinarians. By labeling these products for use as directed by veterinarians, legal responsibility for adverse responses to a product may be shared by or shifted to the veterinarian. Thus, both legal and professional responsibilities dictate that members of the veterinary profession advise use of these diets appropriately. A recent survey indicated that diets were being recommended by veterinarians for circumstances for which they may not be indicated (Finco, 1992). It is desirable that veterinarians reexamine the principles that form the basis for use of nutrient-restricted diets and consider recent research findings that have led to modification of older ideas. With newer information, the indications for use of nutrient-restricted diets seem substantially reduced.

## PROTEIN RESTRICTION, PROTEIN DEPLETION

In this discussion, protein restriction refers to use of diets containing less protein than foods commercially available for maintenance of young adult dogs and cats.

Protein restriction, if indicated, should limit dietary intake of protein to the smallest amount still adequate for normal body functions. Normal catabolism of body components requires ingestion and digestion of proteins with appropriate basal quantities of essential amino acids. Additional quantities of appropriate amino acids are required for growth, reproduction, lactation, or tissue repair following injury. If inadequate protein is ingested to provide the amino acids required for body functions, protein restriction may lead to protein depletion. With protein depletion, body protein components are catabolized and used for energy and the animal may be compromised by loss of needed, functional proteins.

The amount of food that an individual patient must ingest to avoid protein depletion depends on a large number of factors. These include "quality" and "digestibility" of protein, caloric density of the food, and body size of the patient. Body weight or body surface area is used to assist in individualizing estimates of the amount of protein needed.

## PROTEIN EXCESS

There is no major body storehouse for proteins as there is for fats, although muscle may serve as a modest storehouse for labile proteins. Amino acids ingested in excess of body needs for anabolism are degraded. Metabolism of the carbon skeleton of the amino acids provides energy (roughly 4 cal/gm of protein). The nitrogen of the amino acids is converted to urea and other nitrogenous wastes, which are excreted by the kidneys. As subsequently discussed, misconceptions may exist regarding the risk associated with consuming protein in excess of body needs for anabolism.

Theoretically, feeding excess protein would be unappealing economically, because protein is more expensive than fat or carbohydrates. Ironically, some manufacturers charge more for protein-restricted diets than for regular or high-protein diets.

## DETECTING PROTEIN DEPLETION

If protein restriction but not protein depletion is desired for a patient, some way of differentiating the states is necessary. Unfortunately, no simple test is available for detecting subtle protein depletion. Classically, nitrogen balance studies are done during research procedures, and protein depletion is indicated by negative nitrogen balance. However, this procedure is too expensive for clinical application on individual patients. In addition, there is some suggestion that even nitrogen balance studies are not as sensitive as desired, being unable to detect depletion of labile protein stores found in the muscle of dogs (Wannemacker and McCoy, 1966).

Severe protein depletion is associated with hypoalbuminemia and loss of muscle mass. An important unanswered question is whether patients in a constant state of suboptimal protein intake suffer damage from protein depletion prior to the development of hypoalbuminemia. Clinically, loss of muscle mass or body weight, or hypoalbuminemia in animals consuming protein-restricted diets, should be considered indicative of protein depletion.

## CRITICAL EVALUATION OF INDICATIONS FOR PROTEIN RESTRICTION

### Prevention of Renal Damage

#### NORMAL DOGS AND CATS

Studies that demonstrate an adverse effect of high levels of dietary protein on kidneys of normal dogs and cats are conspicuously absent. The hypothesis of kidney damage from dietary protein was borrowed from studies on rats. Rats are not small dogs or cats. Considering the results of dietary studies on dogs with reduced renal mass (subsequently discussed), there is no basis for using protein-restricted diets in normal adult dogs.

#### GERIATRIC PATIENTS

An older hypothesis advocated protein restriction based on the presumption that renal function deteriorated in association with aging. However, a controlled study in dogs failed to demonstrate a progressive loss of renal function between the age of 7 and 11 years (Finco et al., 1994). These geriatric dogs had renal mass reduced by uninephrectomy to increase risk of renal damage, and then half were fed an 18% protein (3.5 gm protein/kg/day) diet, while the other half received a 34% protein (6.1 gm protein/kg/day) diet for the 4 years. No decline in glomerular filtration rate (GFR) occurred with either diet. Thus, neither aging itself nor feeding a high-protein diet to aging dogs with only one kidney adversely affected renal function.

Since there are no data documenting adverse effects from high-protein diets in old, otherwise healthy dogs, there is no rational basis for dietary protein restriction. Studies are needed in geriatric cats to determine whether they respond the same or differently than dogs.

### Preventing Progression of Renal Failure

Renal failure may be diagnosed prior to onset of azotemia, based primarily on the presence of proteinuria or polyuria. Since many nonrenal causes of both proteinuria and polyuria exist, these nonrenal causes must be eliminated before a diagnosis of primary renal failure is justified. Empiric restriction of dietary protein intake based only on detection of proteinuria or polyuria is not defensible.

Dogs presented with azotemia may have a prerenal, renal, postrenal, or mixed cause of the azotemia. Prerenal and postrenal causes of azotemia usually require no dietary management, since the azotemia resolves when the primary abnormality is corrected.

Mild elevation in blood urea nitrogen (BUN) by routine screening procedures does not warrant restricting dietary protein intake for two reasons. First, the azotemia may be prerenal or extrarenal (e.g., BUN mildly increased because of blood sampling postprandially).

Second, there is no scientific basis for dietary restriction of protein in dogs with mild azotemia, even when the azotemia is renal in cause. The theory of protein restriction to prevent self-perpetuating renal damage was developed based on studies in rats. Studies in dogs have not demonstrated a beneficial effect of protein restriction on development of renal lesions in dogs with induced renal failure, even when renal mass was reduced by as much as 15/16 (Finco et al., 1992a; Polzin et al., 1993). No studies have been reported in dogs with common forms of naturally occurring renal failure that document that protein restriction has slowed progression of renal damage.

### Reducing Signs of Uremia

When moderate to severe azotemia is caused by primary renal disease, studies have demonstrated a clinical benefit from protein restriction (Barsanti and Finco, 1985; Polzin et al., 1983). The benefit appears to be extrarenal rather than renal, resulting in relief of signs of uremia. Many dogs and cats presented with azotemia have primary renal disease, with azotemia due to both renal dysfunction and secondary prerenal factors (dehydration, hypovolemia). The magnitude of azotemia often decreases markedly when prerenal factors are resolved with fluid therapy. Once stabilized, a decision on the need for a protein-restricted diet can be made. Empirically, protein restriction seems rational when BUN values from primary renal failure exceed 75 mg/dl.

### CRITICAL EVALUATION OF INDICATIONS FOR MINERAL RESTRICTIONS

Previous National Research Council advisements for mineral composition of diets for normal dogs and cats were liberal, but were used for years without known adverse effects of mineral excess. Of pets consuming diets based on these older recommendations, a low percentage developed certain disease states that benefited from dietary restriction of certain minerals (i.e., sodium restriction in overt congestive heart failure).

An important but largely unanswered question is whether any relationship exists between liberal mineral intake, and development of a disease that benefits from mineral restriction. If restricted mineral intake prevents disease without causing mineral depletion, it is rational to feed all dogs and cats mineral-restricted diets. On the other hand, if mineral restriction does not address the cause of disease but merely ameliorates

signs once disease develops, then there is no rational basis for imposing dietary mineral restriction on normal dogs and cats.

Restriction of dietary phosphorus intake has been advocated to prevent renal damage in normal dogs, presumably by preventing renal mineralization. In the uninephrectomized geriatric dogs previously described, a phosphorus-replete diet failed to result in an increase in renal mineral concentration between the 7th and 11th years of life (Finco, Brown, and Barsanti, 1994). Studies of dogs with induced renal failure and moderate to marked azotemia indicated that phosporus restriction reduced mortality and prolonged life (Brown et al., 1991; Finco et al., 1992b), but renal mineralization was not alleviated.

Results of these studies do not support the theory that normal dogs benefit from phosphorus and calcium restriction, but indicate that dogs with moderate to severe azotemia should have dietary phosphorus restricted. Unfortunately, nutrient-restricted diets presently available are not adequately restricted in phosphorus to prevent the development of renal secondary hyperparathyroidism in patients with even moderate renal failure.

### SUMMARY OF RECOMMENDATIONS

Adequate proof of efficacy has not been provided by food manufacturers, or by independent studies, to support advertised claims for nutrient-restricted diets. Data available at present do not support routine use of protein- or mineral-restricted diets in either normal adult dogs or cats, or in geriatric dogs.

Dietary protein restriction does not prevent progression of renal lesions in dogs with induced chronic renal failure. From information available at present, protein restriction is indicated therapeutically, but not prophylactically. Therapeutically, the value of protein restriction is due to extrarenal rather than renal benefits. We recommend that dietary protein restoration be implemented only in patients with primary renal failure with BUN values in excess of 75 mg/dl.

Dietary phosphorus restriction was found beneficial in dogs when implemented once azotemia was moderate, but not in uninephrectomized geriatric dogs. Thus, no data have shown a beneficial effect from routine phosphorus restriction.

Diets restricted in one or more nutrients provide potential for adverse effects associated with depletion of that dietary component. Veterinarians have professional as well as legal reasons for not misusing these diets.

### References and Suggested Reading

Barsanti JA and Finco DR: Dietary management of chronic renal failure in dogs. J Am Anim Hosp Assoc 21:371, 1985.
*Experience with commercially available diets in dogs with chronic renal failure.*
Brown SA, Crowell WA, Barsanti JA, et al: Beneficial effects of dietary mineral restriction in dogs with marked reduction of functional renal mass. J Am Soc Nephrol 1:1169, 1991.

*Effects of phosphorus-restricted versus phosphorus-replete 16% protein diets on dogs with induced, chronic renal failure.*

Finco DR: Effects of dietary protein and phosphorus on the kidneys of dogs. *The 16th Waltham/OSU Symposium.* 1992, pp 39–41.
*Information on a survey of veterinarians' perception of diet effects on kidney function and renal failure.*

Finco DR, Brown SA, and Barsanti JA: Diet effects on renal mineral concentration in geriatric dogs. *Proc 11th Ann Vet Med Forum.* 1993, p 935.
*Effects of phosphate-replete diets on kidney mineral concentration of uninephrectomized geriatric dogs.*

Finco DR, Brown SA, Crowell WA, et al: Effects of dietary protein intake on geriatric dogs with reduced renal mass. Am J Vet Res 55:867, 1994.
*Effects of low-protein and high-protein diets on kidney function of uninephrectomized geriatric dogs.*

Finco DR, Brown SA, Crowell WA, et al: Effects of dietary phosphorus and protein in dogs with chronic renal failure. Am. J. Vet Res 53:2264, 1992a.
*Effects of four diets representing combinations of phosphorus and protein levels on dogs with induced, chronic renal failure.*

Finco DR, Brown SA, Crowell WA, et al: Effects of phosphorus/calcium-restricted and phosphorus/calcium-replete 32% protein diets in dogs with chronic renal failure. Am. J. Vet Res, 53:157, 1992b.
*Effects of low- and high-protein, phosphorus-replete 32% protein diets on dogs with induced chronic renal failure.*

Polzin DJ, Osborne CA, O'Brien TD, et al: Effects of protein intake on progression of canine chronic renal failure (CRF). *Proc 11th Ann Vet Med Forum,* 1993, p. 938.
*Effects of dietary protein intake on development of renal lesions in dogs with induced renal failure.*

Polzin DJ, Osborne CA, Stevens JB, et al: Influence of modified protein diets on the nutritional status of dogs with induced chronic renal failure. Am J. Vet Res 44:1694, 1983.
*Effects of commercially available diets on dogs with induced renal failure.*

Wannemacher RW and McCoy JR: Determination of optimal dietary protein requirements of young and old dogs. J. Nutr 88:66, 1966.
*Limitations of nitrogen balance in determining protein depletion in young and old dogs.*

# *CVT* UPDATE: USE OF RECOMBINANT HUMAN ERYTHROPOIETIN

LARRY D. COWGILL
*Davis, California*

Anemia secondary to erythropoietin deficiency is an invariable consequence of chronic renal failure in companion animals, but its significance remained poorly characterized and its management was ignored until the recent development of recombinant human erythropoietin (see *CVT XI*, p 484; Cowgill, 1992; Cowgill, 1992a; King et al., 1992). Recombinant human erythropoietin (r-HuEPO) is a genetically engineered replica of native human erythropoietin, and in preliminary trials, it effectively corrected the anemia and improved well-being in dogs and cats analogously to its effects in human patients (Cowgill, 1992; Cowgill, 1992b). Since its availability, r-HuEPO has been used with increased frequency in animal patients, and accumulating anecdotal and documented experiences with the drug have generated the proverbial "good news" and "bad news" accounts of its actions.

## CLINICAL USE OF r-HuEPO—THE "GOOD NEWS"

### Effects on Hematopoiesis

Recombinant human erythropoietin produces a rapid and effective erythroid proliferative response in virtually every dog and cat with naturally occurring renal failure. Significant increases in hematocrit, red blood cell count, and hemoglobin concentration can be detected within weeks of starting therapy (Cowgill, 1992;

Cowgill, 1992a). With adequate doses, the erythron in the majority of animals can be normalized in the first month of therapy and sustained indefinitely. The proliferative response is signaled by an initial reticulocytosis and increases in hematocrit of 0.5 to 1.0% per day. Generally, there are no effects of r-HuEPO on leukocyte production or distribution, but transient increases in platelet count may be recognized.

### Effect on Clinical Well-Being

Improvements in appetite, energy, and weight gain, and increased alertness are seen in most patients. Changes in physical strength and playfulness are noted commonly in dogs, while weight gain, increased vocalization, and restoration of behavior and personality traits are observed frequently in cats. Hypokalemia seen commonly in uremic cats will normalize with r-HuEPO administration and likely reflects improved dietary intake of potassium. The improvements in well-being facilitate the concurrent dietary and conservative medical management and bolster owner satisfaction and commitment to therapy. These changes also affirm the significance of anemia in the clinical expression of uremia in animals. The efficacy of erythropoietin replacement to improve clinical well-being is unequaled by any other therapy and reinforces the necessity to resolve the anemia as part of the therapeutic approach to renal failure in companion animals.

## CLINICAL USE OF r-HuEPO—THE "BAD NEWS"

### Development of Anti–r-HuEPO Antibodies

Development of anti–r-HuEPO antibodies and progressive decreases in hematocrit, red blood cell count, and hemoglobin concentration are the most problematic consequence of r-HuEPO therapy in animals. Figure 1 illustrates the typical effect of anti–r-HuEPO antibodies on hematocrit in a uremic cat. The development of antibodies is variable, but current experience predicts the incidence may approach 25 to 30% of treated animals. The binding of antibody to both r-HuEPO and native erythropoietin nullifies their physiologic actions on erythroid progenitor cells, causing bone marrow failure and refractory anemia. Anti–r-HuEPO antibodies dissipate after discontinuation of r-HuEPO therapy, and the anemia resolves in time to pretreatment hematocrit values; but further therapeutic use of r-HuEPO is prohibited (Fig. 1). Assays to document the production of anti–r-HuEPO antibodies are not available for clinical assessment, but their presence can be predicted by myeloid/erythroid cell ratios greater than 8 in bone marrow aspirates of animals receiving r-HuEPO.

### Miscellaneous Adverse Events

Seizures, systemic hypertension, and iron depletion may be associated with r-HuEPO therapy and develop from pathophysiologic adaptations to the increased red cell volume in animals acclimated to the anemic state and to the stimulation of erythropoiesis per se. Seizures occur infrequently during r-HuEPO therapy in animals with profound azotemia or severe hypertension. It is unknown if rheogenic or hemodynamic changes associated with r-HuEPO therapy contribute to the seizures or whether they are consequences of preexisting uremia and hypertension. Systemic hypertension may develop or worsen during r-HuEPO therapy. Increased peripheral vascular resistance secondary to reversal of the vasodilatation induced by the anemic state is the major contributing factor. The intensive erythropoiesis induced by r-HuEPO imposes heavy demands on endogenous iron stores. In patients with preexisting iron deficiency or inadequately supplemented with iron, the requirement for iron may exceed available supplies and impair the erythropoietic response.

## RECOMMENDATIONS FOR r-HuEPO ADMINISTRATION IN UREMIC ANIMALS

Erythropoietin-replacement is indicated in animals symptomatic for the hypoproliferative anemia of renal failure. The clinical consequences of anemia become apparent as the hematocrit falls below 30% and become more profound as the anemia progresses. The benefits from correction of even mild degrees of anemia can be dramatic, but the projected clinical gains of r-HuEPO administration must justify its attendant risks. For animals with moderate anemia and minimal disability, the use of r-HuEPO should be reserved. In animals with moderate to severe anemia (hematocrit <25%), the risks of treatment usually are overshadowed by the improvements in clinical well-being.

Recombinant human erythropoietin* should be used with informed consent of the client and the understanding that it is not licensed for use in dogs or cats. To activate the erythropoietic response, an initial dose of 100 U/kg body weight subcutaneously three times weekly is administered until the target hematocrit of 37 to 45% for dogs or 30 to 40% for cats is achieved. As the target range is reached, the dosage interval is decreased to twice weekly to prevent overshooting the target range. A lower initial dose (50 to 75 U/kg thrice weekly) may be used if a slower erythropoietic response is acceptable or appropriate. If the target hematocrit is

---

*Epoetin alfa (Epogen, Amgen Inc, Thousand Oaks, CA; Procrit, Ortho Biotech, Raritan, NJ); epoetin beta (Marogen, Chugai-Upjohn, Inc, Rosemont, IL).

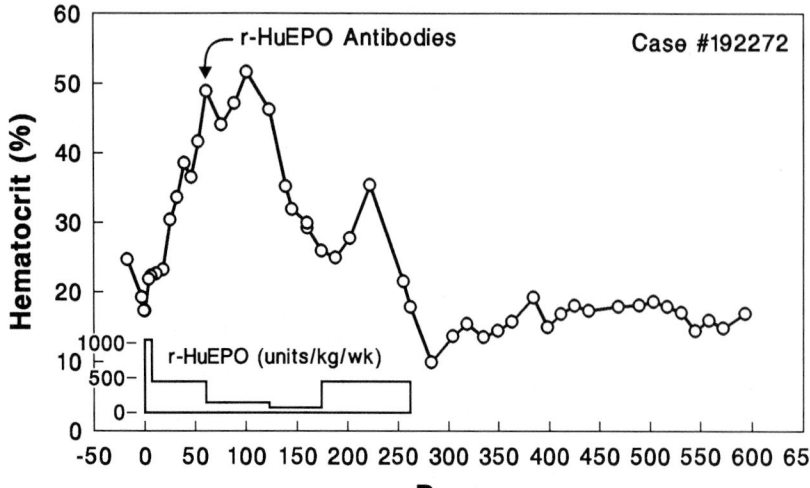

**Figure 1.** Changes in hematocrit following r-HuEPO administration and anti–r-HuEPO antibody formation in a uremic cat. Erythropoietin administration promoted an initial increase in hematocrit. With development of anti–r-HuEPO antibodies, the hematocrit declined rapidly but returned to pretreatment values with cessation of r-HuEPO therapy and dissipation of the antibodies. (From Cowgill LD: Management of anemia associated with renal failure. In August JR (ed): Consultations in Feline Internal Medicine 2. Philadelphia, WB Saunders Co, 1993, p 337, with permission.)

not achieved within 8 to 12 weeks, the initial dose may be incremented progressively by 25 to 50 U/kg. The maintenance dosage to sustain the hematocrit within the target range must be established individually according to the patient's own response. Generally, a dose of 75 to 100 U/kg subcutaneously one to two times weekly is sufficient. Treatment should be withheld temporarily if the hematocrit exceeds normal limits until it is reestablished within the target range.

Iron deficiency, external blood loss, hemolytic disease, concurrent infectious, inflammatory or neoplastic diseases, or the development of anti–r-HuEPO antibodies should be investigated in animals who respond inadequately or become unresponsive to r-HuEPO. The development of anti–r-HuEPO antibodies contraindicates further r-HuEPO administration. Most patients require oral or parenteral iron supplementation to prevent iron depletion and foster the erythropoietic response. Weekly or biweekly assessments of hematocrit and the clinical response are advisable during the first 2 to 3 months of therapy until the hematocrit stabilizes within the target range. Treatment should be started cautiously or withheld from patients with moderate to severe hypertension or iron deficiency until these conditions have been controlled.

Erythropoietin replacement with r-HuEPO affords an unprecedented ability to correct the anemia and improve clinical well-being in uremic animals. However, this therapy imposes the responsibility for close supervision of the patient and threatens therapeutic complications that must be confronted realistically and conscientiously figured in risk-versus-benefits decisions.

## References and Suggested Reading

Cowgill LD: Application of recombinant human erythropoietin (r-HuEPO) in dogs and cats: In Kirk RW (ed): *Current Veterinary Therapy XI: Small Animal Practice.* Philadelphia, WB Saunders Co, 1992, p 484.
*Discussion of the pathophysiologic basis for the anemia of chronic renal failure, development of r-HuEPO, and its application in uremic dogs and cats.*
Cowgill LD: Pathophysiology and management of anemia in chronic progressive renal failure. Semin Vet Med Surg 7:175, 1992a.
*Review of the pathogenesis of the anemia of chronic renal failure and a comprehensive discussion of its management including use of r-HuEPO.*
Cowgill LD: Erythropoietin: Its use in the treatment of chronic renal failure in dogs and cats. *Proc 1991 Waltham/OSU Symposium for the Treatment of Small Animal Diseases.* 1992b, p 65.
*Discussion of the clinical significance of the anemia of chronic renal failure and initial clinical experiences and recommendations for the use of r-HuEPO in uremic dogs and cats.*
King LG, Giger U, Diserens D, et al: Anemia of chronic renal failure in dogs. J Vet Intern Med 6:264, 1992.
*Clinical investigation of the causes of anemia of chronic renal failure in dogs. Includes measurement of serum erythropoietin concentrations in normal and uremic dogs.*

# REASSESSMENT OF THE USE OF CALCITRIOL IN CHRONIC RENAL FAILURE

SCOTT A. BROWN
*and* DELMAR R. FINCO
*Athens, Georgia*

Calcitriol is 1,25-dihydroxycholecalciferol, the biologically activated form of vitamin D. In the normal animal, the production of calcitriol is precisely regulated at the level of the $1\alpha$-hydroxylase enzyme in the kidney, with parathyroid hormone (PTH) and hypophosphatemia enhancing the activity of this enzyme. Calcitriol has a variety of important functions in the body, most being related to the regulation of calcium and phosphorous metabolism:

- Increases gut absorption of calcium (and possibly phosphorus)
- Enhances bone release of calcium and phosphorus
- Enhances renal reabsorption of calcium and phosphorus
- Suppresses the production of PTH

These first three biologic effects of calcitriol will enhance plasma calcium and phosphate concentrations, maintaining an adequate calcium-phosphate product to allow mineralization of bone. The fourth effect acts as a negative feedback loop by reducing plasma PTH concentration, thereby limiting the production of calcitriol by the kidney.

## RENAL SECONDARY HYPERPARATHYROIDISM

In animals with renal failure, enhanced PTH secretion is frequently (but not always) observed. This is termed "renal secondary hyperparathyroidism" and has generally been attributed to one of two central mechanisms:

1. Renal retention of phosphate leading to a reduction in plasma calcium concentration by a "mass action" effect (i.e., calcium × phosphate = constant value).
2. Inadequate functioning renal tissue to adequately convert 25-hydroxycholecalciferol to 1,25-dihydroxycholecalciferol (calcitriol) leading to:
   a. Impaired intestinal absorption of calcium and a consequent reduction in plasma calcium, which stimulates PTH secretion.
   b. Loss of direct inhibitory effects of calcitriol on PTH production and secretion.

Data to support an independent role for both phosphate retention and reduced production of calcitriol in the genesis of renal secondary hyperparathyroidism have accumulated over the past two decades. In addition, since hyperphosphatemia directly inhibits renal conversion of 25-hydroxycholecalciferol to calcitriol, there is an interaction between these mechanisms.

## RATIONALE FOR PTH SUPPRESSION

It has been proposed (Massry, 1989) that renal secondary hyperparathyroidism is responsible for a variety of uremic signs and for the progression of chronic renal disease (Table 1). While hyperparathyroidism may contribute to these clinical abnormalities, some of them are primarily attributable to mechanisms unrelated to PTH (e.g., the anemia of chronic renal failure is primarily caused by a lack of erythropoietin). Renal osteodystrophy, evidenced by radiographic changes in bone density, bone pain, and pathologic fractures, has historically been the primary indication for calcitriol administration in animals. Since there is currently no clear evidence that the suppression of renal secondary hyperparathyroidism by calcitriol ameliorates other signs in dogs and cats, calcitriol remains an experimental therapy at this time.

In dogs with renal failure that do not exhibit signs of uremia, the sole rationale for calcitriol therapy is to slow the progression of renal failure. Such an effect would be important, since dogs with chronic renal failure frequently have a poor prognosis, succumbing to progressive deterioration of renal function when end-stage uremia develops. A variety of therapies aimed at slowing the progression of renal failure have been recommended, including dietary restriction of protein and phosphorus (see "Inappropriate Dietary and Mineral Restriction in Dogs and Cats," this volume, p 958) and recently, the administration of calcitriol. While these or related therapies may ultimately prove efficacious, they do not replace the careful medical care of animals with renal failure. Treatment of the primary renal disease, correction of metabolic acidosis, elimination of secondary urinary tract infections, selective use of antiemetics, limiting physical and emotional stress, use of effective therapy for intercurrent diseases, adjustment of dose to avoid toxicity when drug administration becomes necessary, and provision of adequate fresh water and a palatable diet are critical considerations for these animals that should be provided by the veterinarian.

Recent evidence does support the contention that renal secondary hyperparathyroidism contributes to the progression of chronic renal failure in rats (Shigematsu, Aversasio, and Bonjour, 1993). However, this hypothesis was not supported by a study in dogs with reduced renal mass (Finco et al., 1994). Further studies will be necessary to determine whether or not renal secondary hyperparathyroidism contributes to the progression of renal disease in dogs or cats. At this time, calcitriol may be employed as an experimental therapy with a goal of slowing the progression of renal failure. This should be attempted only if the existence and rate of progression of chronic renal failure have been documented. This is feasible clinically, with some compromises in accuracy, by sequential ($\geq$3) plasma creatinine determinations and a graphical depiction of creatinine concentration ($y$ axis) versus time (months or weeks; $x$ axis) or the inverse of plasma creatinine concentration ($y$ axis) versus time (months or weeks; $x$ axis). If progression is documented and the veterinary practitioner desires to use calcitriol in an attempt to slow the progression of renal failure, then sequential plasma creatinine determinations should be utilized to assess the efficacy of suppression of PTH secretion to achieve this purpose. If there is no apparent effect of PTH suppression on the rate of progression within 6 months, there is little rationale for continuing calcitriol therapy aimed solely at slowing the progression of renal failure in the individual animal being treated.

## EFFICACY/TOXICITY OF CALCITRIOL

Recent studies in our laboratory have indicated that calcitriol suppresses PTH secretion within 30 days in most dogs with experimentally induced renal secondary hyperparathyroidism at an oral dose of 6.6 ng/kg given in one daily dose. Others have recommended a lower dose of 1.5 to 3.5 ng/kg given orally in one daily dose (Chew and Nagode, 1992 in *CVT XI*, p 857). Calcitriol

**Table 1.** *Hypothesized Effects of Renal Secondary Hyperparathyroidism*°

Uremic abnormalities
  Anemia
  Arthritis
  Cardiomyopathy
  Encephalopathy
  Glucose intolerance
  Hyperlipidemia
  Immunosuppression
  Myopathy
  Pancreatitis
  Pruritis
  Skin ulcerations
  Soft tissue calcification
Progression of chronic renal disease

°Adapted from Massry SG: Parathyroid hormone as a uremic toxin. *In* Massry SG and Glassock RJ (eds): Textbook of Nephrology. Baltimore, Williams & Wilkins, 1989, p 1126, with permission.

will not lower plasma PTH concentration in all animals at 6.6 ng/kg/day and higher doses may be required. Similar to human beings with renal secondary hyperparathyroidism (Gallieni et al., 1992), frequent dose adjustments are required in individual dogs. In some dogs, calcitriol will not be effective at any dose. At doses of 11 to 22 ng/kg every 24 hr, hypercalcemia is observed in some dogs and daily doses exceeding 6.6 ng/kg should be attempted only if ionized calcium measurements are available.

Calcitriol (Rocaltrol, Hoffmann-La Roche, Nutley, NJ) is available in 250- and 500-ng capsules. At a dose of 6.6 ng/kg, these represent the appropriate daily dose for a dog weighing 38 and 76 kg, respectively. The capsules cannot be readily divided and, for smaller animals, it has been recommended (Chew and Nagode, 1992) that veterinarians contact a pharmacist to reformulate these products to a size that is appropriate for the individual pet (Island Pharmacy Services, PO Box 23124, Hilton Head Island, SC, Telephone 800-328-7060).

To document the efficacy of calcitriol in individual animals, it is necessary that plasma PTH measurements be obtained. Since considerable day-to-day variation in plasma PTH may occur, it is preferable to pool equal volumes from sequential samples obtained on 2 to 3 consecutive days to obtain a value that is more representative of the secretory status of the parathyroid gland. Assays utilized should measure the intact hormone or the N-terminal portion of the molecule. Results of different assays or different laboratories are not directly comparable.

Calcitriol may increase plasma calcium and phosphate concentrations by increasing the contribution of bone, kidney, and intestine to plasma pools of these minerals. To avoid a dangerous elevation of the plasma calcium-phosphate product, calcitriol should be administered only in normophosphatemic animals. This will usually require the use of a low phosphorus diet and phosphorus binders. Calcitriol should be given several hours before a meal and should generally not be administered in conjunction with calcium containing phosphorus binders.

In animals receiving calcitriol, frequent measurement of plasma PTH and calcium concentrations are critical. Since ionized calcium measurements are not routinely available to veterinary practitioners, total calcium measurements must be relied upon. In animals with renal failure, acid-base disturbance, hypoalbuminemia, and increased concentration of complexed calcium cause considerable unpredictability in the relationship between total calcium and ionized calcium. The correlation between these two parameters may be less than 0.8 in these animals, indicating that only about 60% of the variations in ionized calcium in dogs with renal failure are reflected as changes in total calcium. In addition, many dogs with renal failure and normal plasma ionized calcium concentrations actually have an elevated total calcium concentration. Calcitriol therapy should be considered in animals with an elevated plasma total calcium concentration only if ionized calcium measurements are available.

## CURRENT RECOMMENDATIONS

### Dogs

Since most of the hypothesized effects of renal secondary hyperparathyroidism are chronic in nature, the utilization of calcitriol in animals with acute renal failure is not recommended. Currently, we do not recommend the routine use of calcitriol in all animals with renal failure. The following represents a plan for the judicious use of calcitriol to suppress renal secondary hyperparathyroidism in selected azotemic or uremic dogs. The use of calcitriol for this purpose remains experimental and thus the veterinarian must establish efficacy in each patient treated. The plan is sequential and a veterinarian should proceed to a step only after satisfying the conditions of the preceding step:

*Step 1.* Establish a normal plasma phosphate concentration.
  A. Low phosphorus diet.
  B. Aluminum containing phosphorous binders to effect with an initial dose of 100 mg/kg/day administered with meals.

*Step 2.* After 2 weeks or more of stable plasma phosphate concentration, document the presence of renal secondary hyperparathyroidism.
  A. Considerable day-to-day variation in plasma PTH concentration may be present and it is best to submit a pooled sample drawn from two to three samples obtained on consecutive days.
  B. Radioimmunoassay: intact hormone or N-terminal.

*Step 3.* Develop a rationale for use of calcitriol in this individual animal.
  A. Document a rate of progression of renal failure in the animal.
  B. Document the presence of one or more abnormalities hypothetically attributable to renal secondary hyperparathyroidism (Table 1).

*Step 4.* Administer calcitriol to normophosphatemic, normocalcemic animal.
  A. Initial dose of 6.6 ng/kg in one daily dose apart from meals.
  B. Assess plasma calcium concentration 7 and 14 days later and then at least every month for the first 6 months of therapy. Discontinue medication if hypercalcemia develops, and consider reinstitution of calcitriol at a lower dose only after normocalcemia is documented.
  C. Document efficacy 4 to 6 weeks later by reassessment of plasma PTH concentration.
  D. If calcitriol does not suppress plasma PTH by 4 to 6 weeks, either increase the dose or discontinue therapy.
  E. Unless ionized calcium measurements are available, do not exceed 6.6 ng/kg/day.

*Step 5.* Determine the benefit to the animal.
  A. Document a slowing of the rate of progression of renal failure with serial plasma creatinine measurements.

B. Document an improvement in one or more abnormalities that were attributed to renal secondary hyperparathyroidism.

C. If renal osteodystrophy is present, continue calcitriol therapy as long as azotemia is present.

D. If renal osteodystrophy is not evident and calcitriol does not provide a verifiable benefit within 3 to 6 months, discontinue therapy.

## Cats

Although the authors do not have experience with the use of calcitriol in cats with renal secondary hyperparathyroidism, a dose of 1.5 to 3.5 ng/kg/day has been recommended (Chew and Nagode, 1992). It seems reasonable to conclude that an ordered sequence of patient selection and therapy similar to that recommended above for dogs should be employed in affected cats and that calcitriol will not replace careful monitoring and appropriate medical therapy.

## References and Suggested Reading

Brown SA, Crowell WA, Barsanti JA, et al: Beneficial effects of dietary mineral restriction in dogs with marked reduction of functional renal mass. J Am Soc Nephrol 1:1169, 1991.
*An experimental study of the role of dietary phosphorus intake in the chronic course of renal disease in dogs.*
Chew DJ and Nagode LA: Calcitriol in the treatment of chronic renal failure. *In* Kirk RW and Bonagura JD (eds): *Current Veterinary Therapy XI.* Philadelphia, WB Saunders Co, 1992, p 857.
*A review of the pathogenesis and management of renal secondary hyperparathyroidism with calcitriol.*
Finco DR, Brown SA, Cooper T, et al: Effects of parathyroid hormone depletion on dogs with reduced renal mass. Am J Vet Res 55:867, 1994.
*An experimental study of the effects of selective parathyroidectomy in dogs with renal failure.*
Gallieni M, Brancaccio D, Padovese P, et al: Low-dose intravenous calcitriol treatment of secondary hyperparathyroidism in hemodialysis patients. Kidney Int 42:1191, 1992.
*A discussion of the use of calcitriol (15 ng/kg IV thrice weekly) to suppress renal secondary hyperparathyroidism in people emphasizing that while generally efficacious, approximately one in four patients did not respond to calcitriol administration and one in three patients had to undergo a dosage reduction due to an elevation in the calcium-phosphate product.*
Massry SG: Parathyroid hormone as a uremic toxin. *In* Massry SG and Glassock RJ (eds): *Textbook of Nephrology.* Baltimore, Williams & Wilkins, 1989, p 1126.
*A review of the possible toxic effects of PTH in animals with renal failure.*
Shigematsu T, Caverzasio J, and Bonjour J: Parathyroid removal prevents the progression of chronic renal failure by high protein diet. Kidney Int 22:173, 1993.
*An experimental study of the effects of parathyroidectomy implicating PTH in the progression of renal failure observed in rats fed a high-protein diet.*
Slatopolsky E, Caglar S, Pernnell J, et al: On the pathogenesis of hyperparathyroidism in chronic experimental renal insufficiency in the dog. J Clin Invest 50:498, 1971.
*A study of the pathogenesis of renal secondary hyperparathyroidism in dogs with an emphasis on the role of dietary phosphorus and the effectiveness of dietary phosphorus restriction in preventing the development of elevated PTH levels.*

# TREATMENT OF UREMIC ANOREXIA

CARL A. OSBORNE,
JODY P. LULICH,
SHERRY L. SANDERSON,
*and* DAVID J. POLZIN
*St. Paul, Minnesota*

## PATHOPHYSIOLOGY OF ANOREXIA ASSOCIATED WITH RENAL FAILURE

Modification of diets so that they contain reduced quantities of protein, phosphorus, sodium, and acid metabolites is a cornerstone of therapeutic regimens for renal failure. However, many patients with renal failure may refuse to eat some or all of such diets offered to them. Reduction in the palatability of renal failure diets is commonly incriminated as a major factor leading to inappetence. Reduced palatability is often attributed to reduction in dietary protein, sodium, and phosphorus. That unpalatability of diets is not the only factor involved can be surmised by the fact that patients with renal failure may selectively eat diets containing unrestricted quantities of these ingredients. In fact, anorexia may be the primary abnormality prompting owners of dogs and cats with renal failure to seek the assistance of veterinarians. In a retrospective study of clinical manifestations of renal failure in 132 cats performed at the University of Minnesota, anorexia was observed by owners in 80% of the patients (Lulich et al., 1992). Weight loss was the second most common clinical sign (72%) observed by owners, followed by depression (68%), vomiting (52%), and weakness (47%). Polyuria and polydipsia were observed in only 40% of affected cats.

Anorexia associated with renal dysfunction is not directly caused by renal lesions, but rather develops as a result of multiple metabolic deficits and excesses that develop as a result of decreased renal function caused by renal lesions. Anorexia, nausea, and vomiting are manifestations of an interaction between: (1) autointoxication caused by reduction of glomerular filtration and tubular secretion below that required to clear plasma of metabolic waste products; (2) impaired tu-

**Table 1.** *Examples of Some Metabolic Deficits and Excesses Contributing to Anorexia, Nausea, and Vomiting in Patients with Renal Failure*

| Metabolic Abnormality | Cause | Sequela |
|---|---|---|
| Polyuria associated with impaired polydipsia | Impaired tubular reabsorption of water; nausea, vomiting | Dehydration, anorexia, others |
| Hypokalemia | Impaired tubular reabsorption of potassium; inadequate intake of potassium | Anorexia, muscle weakness, chronic vomiting, nephropathy, others |
| Metabolic acidosis | Impaired glomerular filtration of acid catabolites; impaired tubular secretion of hydrogen ion; impaired tubular reabsorption of bicarbonate | Anorexia, nausea, vomiting, hypokalemia, bone demineralization, others |
| Nonregenerative anemia | Impaired renal production of erythropoietin; others | Anorexia, weakness, cold intolerance |
| Hypergastinemia | Impaired renal clearance of gastrin from blood | Anorexia, nausea, and vomiting due to gastric hyperacidity |
| Hyperparathormonemia | Renal secondary hyperparathyroidism causing PTH-mediated interference of insulin release | Mild hyperglycemia leading to inappetance |
| Retention of catabolic wastes such as guanidines | Stimulation of medullary emetic chemoreceptor trigger zone | Anorexia, nausea, and vomiting |
| Retention of urea | Impaired glomerular filtration; degradation of urea to ammonia by urease-producing bacteria in the mouth (especially in tartar) | Caustic stomatitis |

Abbreviation: PTH = parathyroid hormone.

bular reabsorption of vital metabolites in glomerular filtrate; (3) impaired renal production of some hormones; and (4) impaired renal degradation and elimination of some hormones (Table 1).

Because nutritional support is a cornerstone of long-term management of patients with renal failure, management must encompass a plan to minimize inappetance. If catabolic patients with renal failure do not consume their daily requirements of dietary nutrients, further catabolism characterized by metabolism of endogenous proteins for energy will follow. Catabolism of endogenous proteins will in turn augment production of protein catabolic wastes, which further contribute to anorexia.

How can veterinarians and clients enhance the desire of uremic dogs and cats to consume diets modified to minimize metabolic deficits and excesses associated with renal failure? In addition to strategies designed to enhance the palatability of renal failure diets, our approach to this question places emphasis on recognition and treatment of the underlying causes of uremic anorexia (Table 1; Fig. 1).

## CORRECTION OF UNDERLYING ABNORMALITIES

### Dehydration

Dehydration of patients with oliguric, nonoliguric, and polyuric renal failure is typically associated with multiple deficits and excesses in electrolyte and acid-base balance. It is not surprising that various combinations of these abnormalities would contribute to anorexia, nausea, and vomiting. Recommendations about

deficit, maintenance, and continuous components of fluid therapy are found elsewhere in this section (see "Management of Fluid and Electrolyte Disorders in Uremia," this volume, p 951).

Care must be used not to induce electrolyte disturbances by inappropriate use of replacement and maintenance fluids. Maintenance fluids differ from replacement fluids in that they generally have a much lower sodium concentration (40 mEq/L versus 130 mEq/L in lactated Ringer's solution), and a higher potassium concentration (13 mEq/L versus 4 mEq/L). The reason for this difference is that daily maintenance requirements of sodium and potassium are not directly related to the serum concentration of sodium and potassium. Inappropriate use of replacement fluids for maintenance

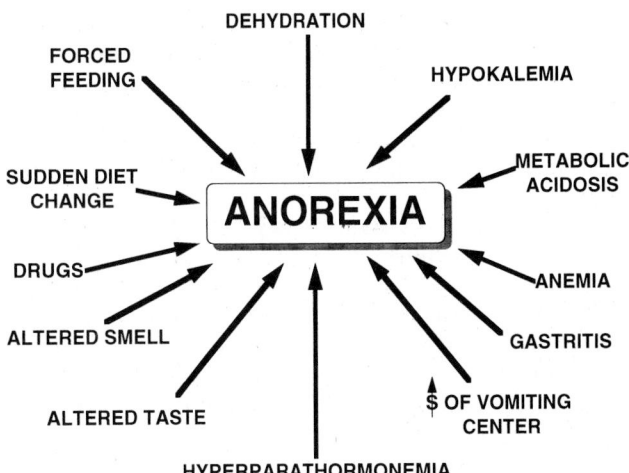

**Figure 1.** Schematic illustration of multiple interacting factors that may contribute to anorexia in patients with renal failure.

fluids could lead to hypokalemia and hypernatremia, which in turn could contribute to anorexia.

## Hypokalemia

In a retrospective study of 132 cats with renal failure performed at the University of Minnesota, 19% were hypokalemic (serum potassium <3.5 mEq/L) (Lulich et al., 1992). A predisposition of cats with polyuric renal failure to hypokalemia has been observed by several groups of investigators (Dow and Fettman, 1992; Lulich et al., 1992). Dietary factors incriminated in the development of hypokalemia in uremic cats include inadequate potassium in the diet (it should be 0.5% dry matter), diets with acidifying metabolites, and diets designed to contain reduced magnesium (Dow and Fettman, 1992; Zawada et al., 1988; Whang et al., 1985). Dietary protein may also be a factor, since dietary potassium requirement increases as dietary protein content increases. In our experience, hypokalemia is an uncommon manifestation of renal failure in dogs, except as an iatrogenic complication of fluid therapy. Irrespective of underlying causes, hypokalemia may be associated with anorexia, vomiting, weight loss, lethargy, hypokalemic nephropathy, muscle weakness, and mild cardiac arrhythmias.

Potassium gluconate as an elixir (Kaon elixir, Adria) or powder (Tumil-K, Daniels) is commonly used as a potassium supplement for uremic cats with hypokalemia. Oral potassium chloride is not recommended, since it may contribute to metabolic acidosis, and is less palatable. Initial dosages range from 2 to 6 mEq per cat per day, depending on the size of the patient and magnitude of hypokalemia (Dow and Fettman, 1992). The maintenance dosage should be titrated on the basis of serially monitored serum potassium concentration.

## Metabolic Acidosis

Metabolic acidosis is estimated to occur in two thirds to three fourths of dogs and cats with renal failure. It is caused by limited ability of surviving nephrons to excrete hydrogen ions. Consequences of metabolic acidosis associated with renal failure include anorexia, nausea, vomiting, weight loss, lethargy, intolerance to dietary acids, hypokalemia, muscle weakness, bone demineralization, and possibly progression of renal failure.

Oral sodium bicarbonate has been the most commonly used alkalinizing drug to correct metabolic acidosis caused by renal failure. Because the effect of gastric acid on orally administered sodium bicarbonate is unpredictable, the dosage must be individualized. A commonly used initial dosage is 8 to 12 mg/kg body weight given every 8 to 12 hr. The patient's response should be monitored by serially monitoring blood bicarbonate or serum total carbon dioxide ($TCO_2$) concentrations. Potassium citrate (Polycitra-K, Willen; Urocit-K, Mission Pharmacal) may be used for hypokalemic acidemic cats (40 to 60 mg/kg every 12 hr). Other alkalinizing agents that may be considered for sodium-intolerant patients include calcium carbonate and calcium acetate.

## Hypoproliferative Anemia

Hypoproliferative anemia is a common sequela to chronic progressive renal failure in dogs and cats. In the retrospective survey of 132 cats previously cited, 35% were anemic (Lulich et al., 1992). Because 70% of the cats were clinically dehydrated, it is probable that anemia occurred with greater frequency than detected. The primary cause of hypoproliferative anemia in dogs and cats with renal failure is impaired renal production of erythropoietin. Factors that contribute to the magnitude of the anemia include blood loss, decreased red blood cell survival time, and nutritional deficiencies. The consequences of anemia include anorexia, weight loss, weakness, and intolerance to cold.

Treatment of anemia associated with renal failure encompasses correction of nutritional deficiencies (protein, calories, vitamins $B_6$ and $B_{12}$, folic acid, niacin, and iron), control of gastrointestinal hemorrhage (with $H_2$-receptor antagonists and/or sucralfate), and parenteral administration of recombinant human erythropoietin (Epogen, Amgen, Inc.) (also see "CVT Update: Use of Recombinant Human Erythropoietin," this volume, p 961) (Cowgill, 1991).

## Hyperparathormonemia

A PTH-mediated interference with the response of pancreatic insulin-secreting islet cells to dietary glucose has been incriminated as a mechanism of carbohydrate intolerance on uremic patients. Inadequate insulin to facilitate reduction of blood glucose in uremic patients may contribute to inappetance. Lowering PTH in uremic dogs and cats by administration of calcitriol has been reported to minimize anorexia (Rocaltrol, Roche) (Nagode et al., 1991).

## Nausea and Vomiting

Uremic vomiting is mediated by local and central factors. Local factors include gastritis, forced foods and fluids, and intolerance to some medications. Central factors consist of stimulation of the medullary emetic chemoreceptor trigger zone by circulating uremic toxins (such as methylguanidine) and intolerance to some medications (Borison and Hebertson, 1959; Grovannetti et al., 1969).

Anorexia, nausea, and vomiting associated with renal failure are in part related to gastric hyperacidity induced by hypergastrinemia. Normally, gastrin stimulates receptors located on parietal cells in the stomach mucosa to produce and secrete hydrogen ions. Because up to 40% of the circulating gastrin is metabolized by the kidneys, reduction in renal function results in increased and more prolonged stimulation of parietal cells to produce hydrogen ions by retained gastrin (Clendinnen et al., 1971). The resultant gastric hyperacidity leads to mucosal irritation, ulceration, and hemorrhage. Back-diffusion of hydrochloric acid and pepsin into the stomach wall leads to further hemorrhage, inflammation, and the release of histamine from mast cells. Thus, the cycle is perpetuated, as mast-cell–derived histamine causes further stimulation of parietal cells to produce hydrogen ions. The cycle of hypergastrinemia-induced anorexia, nausea, and vomiting may be interrupted by administration of $H_2$-receptor antagonists such as cimetidine (Tagamet, SmithKline Beecham) or ranitidine (Zantac, Roche). For dogs, cimetadine is commonly administered intravenously or orally at a dosage of 5 mg/kg every 8 to 12 hr. After 2 to 4 weeks of oral therapy at this dosage, 5 mg/kg is given once daily for 2 to 3 weeks prior to withdrawal. In cats, an initial dosage of 2.5 to 5.0 mg/kg body weight given every 8 to 12 hr is commonly used. If cimetidine is given intravenously, it may be diluted with saline and slowly given over a 2-min period to minimize potential bradycardia. Because cimetidine may interfere with the hepatic metabolism of drugs (such as diazepam and propanolol) by P-450 enzymes, ranitidine is sometimes chosen as an alternative. Ranitidine is more potent than cimetidine, and has less effect on hepatic P-450 enzymes. Ranitidine is commonly given orally or intravenously at a dosage of 2 to 4 mg/kg every 12 hr. Because cimetidine and ranitidine are dependent on renal excretion for elimination, the lower end of the dosage ranges should be considered. As an alternative to $H_2$-receptor antagonists, sucralfate (Carafate, Marion Merrell Dow) may be given to create a protective layer over the gastric mucosal surface. In an acid environment, sucralfate becomes charged and binds to gastric proteins of the opposite charge, thereby minimizing back-diffusion of hydrochloric acid and pepsin into the stomach wall. An empirically established dosage of sucralfate for dogs is 0.25 to 1.0 gm every 8 to 12 hr. Because sucralfate may interfere with the action of other orally administered drugs, they should be given approximately 30 min prior to the administration of sucralfate. Caution should also be used if consideration is being given to using sucralfate for extended periods, since significant elevations in serum aluminum concentration may occur (Burgess et al., 1992).

As an alternative or supplement to $H_2$-receptor antagonists and sucralfate, metoclopramide (Reglan, Robbins) may be given to minimize the action of uremic toxins on the medullary emetic chemoreceptor trigger zone. An empirically established oral dose of metoclopramide is 0.2 to 0.4 mg every 6 to 8 hr. Injectable metoclopramide may be given at a dosage of 1.0 to 2.0 mg/kg every 24 hr. The lower dosages are preferred because metoclopramide is eliminated by the kidneys. Signs of metoclopramide overdosage include drowsiness, disorientation, tremors, muscle hypertonia, and reduction in seizure thresholds.

## Drug-Induced Anorexia, Nausea, and Vomiting

Patients in renal failure commonly are intolerant to side effects of many drugs. Examples include captopril, enalopril, trimethoprim-sulfa, digoxin, and tetracyclines. In addition, some drugs may contribute to anorexia by impairing taste or smell (Schiffman, 1983). They include ampicillin, sulfas, tetracyclines, aminoglycosides, allopurinol, D-penicillamine, and captopril. The manufacturer's recommendations and description of side effects should be reviewed before giving any drug to a patient in renal failure. Because many renal failure patients are intolerant to drugs, they should not be routinely given with the philosophy that they might help but will do no harm.

## B-Vitamin Deficiency

Deficiencies of thiamine and niacin may result in anorexia. Patients with renal failure are at risk for B-vitamin deficiency as a result of decreased appetites, vomiting, diarrhea, and perhaps losses associated with polyuria. In these circumstances, administration of supplemental B vitamins is logical. The daily B-vitamin requirement of normal cats is estimated to be six to eight times greater than that of dogs. If multiple vitamin supplements are used, caution must be used not to give excessive quantities of fat-soluble vitamins. There are no data to support the notion that consumption of B vitamins in excess of daily requirement stimulates appetite. More is not necessarily better.

## ENHANCING DIET PALATABILITY

### Changes in Diet

Because preference for new flavors and textures of food may be a learned response for some dogs and cats, it is advisable to make diet changes gradually over a period of 1 to 2 weeks. When obtaining the medical history, special emphasis should be placed on the diet history, especially in relation to the preferred foods of the patient. If the patient is hospitalized, it may be preferable to continue with these foods, rather than making a sudden diet change.

In addition to making gradual dietary changes at the appropriate time, it may be beneficial to choose new diets with the same texture and flavor as preferred diets. Warming food to just below body temperature may improve its palatability. If dry foods are selected, addition of warm water may be of benefit. Offering fresh aromatic food is sometimes helpful. Be sure that the patient's nasal passages are open.

### Food Aversion

The possibility that food aversion may develop should also be considered. If a nauseated or vomiting uremic patient is given a diet designed for long-term management of renal failure, aversion to that food may develop. Food aversion is most likely to occur if nauseated patients are force-fed, or if painful sample collection or drug administration are associated with feeding. In general, unpalatable drugs should not be mixed with the primary source of food or water. To minimize the possibility of the patient's aversion to renal failure diets designed for long-term use, they should not be offered to renal failure patients until the underlying causes contributing to anorexia, nausea, and vomiting are minimized or eliminated.

### Flavoring Agents

A variety of agents may be used to enhance the palatability of diets. They include animal fat, butter, dehydrated cottage cheese, garlic, bullion, clam juice, brewer's yeast, and carnitine. Enteral nutrition liquids designed for renal failure may also be used as flavoring agents.

## MODIFYING FEEDING PATTERNS AND ENVIRONMENT

When patients with renal failure are anorexic or nauseated, it is generally best to provide small quantities of food several times each day. Minimizing distention of the stomach may minimize gastric secretions and the feeling of nausea. Likewise, consumption of smaller quantities of food will minimize postprandial elevation of absorbed nutrients, including protein catabolites.

Placing small quantities of palatable food in the mouth or on the patient's paws may stimulate a licking response. This, in turn, may stimulate neural and humoral mechanisms that normally stimulate appetite (Morley, 1987).

The feeding environment should also be considered when managing renal patients with anorexia. Timid animals should not be hospitalized in noisy wards with heavy traffic. Loud and persistent barking may be especially stressful to cats. Food should be placed in wide bowls or flat saucers so that tactile whiskers are not adversely stimulated. A comfortable environmental temperature should be maintained.

Rewarding patients at the time of feeding may be helpful. Owners may play an important role by providing a reassuring voice and gentle hand. Partially anorexic cats may begin to eat if gently stroked at the time a meal is offered.

## PHARMACOLOGIC APPETITE STIMULANTS

### Anabolic Steroids

Although manufacturers of veterinary anabolic agents state that these drugs will improve appetite, there are no data to support this claim in dogs or cats with renal failure. In one six-week study in moderately azotemic dogs with induced renal failure, anabolic agents had no beneficial effect on food intake, body weight, nitrogen balance, or lean body mass (Finco et al., 1984).

### Corticosteroids

There are no data to support a long-term beneficial effect of glucocorticoids in uremic dogs or cats. To the contrary, glucocorticoids enhance catabolism, impair the repair of gastric mucosa, and enhance glomerular hyperfiltration. Although they may enhance appetite, this effect does not translate into weight gain.

### Benzodiazepines

Benzodiazepine derivatives such as diazepam and oxazepam are known to stimulate appetite in a variety of species. They have been most effective in patients with partial anorexia. The objective is to simulate the appetite of the patient in a "jump-start" fashion, so that licking and chewing will stimulate normal and humoral and neural appetite mechanisms. Diazepam (Valium, Roche) may be given orally, intramuscularly, or intravenously, but is most effective when given at an intravenous dose of 0.2 mg/kg with a maximum dose of 5 mg per patient. Diazepam may be given twice per day. Oxazepam (Serax, Wyeth-Ayerst) is available only for oral administration. It is commonly given at a dosage of 2.5 mg per cat. Care must be used to not use excessive dosages of these drugs in depressed patients.

### Other Agents

Propofol (Diprivan, Stuart), a rapidly acting anesthetic, has been observed to have antiemetic effects in humans given chemotherapeutic agents (Scher et al., 1992). We have observed an appetite-stimulating effect of propofol in dogs and cats following propofol anesthesia.

Megestrol acetate has been reported to increase appetite and promote weight gain in animals and humans. We have had no experience with the use of this drug to stimulate appetite in dogs or cats with renal failure.

### References and Suggested Reading

Borison HL and Herbertson LM: Role of medullary emetic chemoreceptor trigger zone in post-nephrectomy vomiting in dogs. Am J Physiol 197:850, 1959.
Burgess E, et al: Aluminum absorption and excretion following sucralfate therapy in chronic renal insufficiency. Am J Med 92:471, 1992.
Clendinnen BG, et al: Renal uptake and excretion of gastrin in the dog. Surg Gynecol Obstet 132:1039, 1971.
Cowgill LD: Erythropoitein: Its use in treatment of chronic renal failure in dogs and cats. In Proceedings 15th Annual Waltham Symposium For Treat-

ment of Small Animal Diseases: Endocrinology. Columbus, OH, 1991, pp 65–71.

Dow SW and Fettman MS: Renal disease in cats: The potassium connection. In Kirk RW and Bonagura JD (eds): Current Veterinary Therapy XI. Philadephia, WB Saunders Co, 1992, pp 820–822.

Finco DR, et al: Effect of an anabolic steroid on acute uremia in the dog. Am J Vet Res 45:2285, 1984.

Grovannetti S, et al: Uremia-like syndrome in dogs chronically intoxicated with methylguanidine and creatinine. Clin Sci 36:445, 1969.

Lulich JP, et al: Feline renal failure: Questions, answers, questions. Compend Cont Educ 14:127, 1992.

Morley JE: Neuropeptide regulation of appetite and weight. Endoc Rev 8:256, 1987.

Nagode LA, et al: The use of low doses of calcitriol in the treatment of renal secondary hyperparathyroidism. In Proceedings 15th Annual Waltham Symposium for Treatment of Small Animal Diseases: Endocrinology. Columbus, OH, 1991, pp 49–63.

Scher CS, et al: Use of propofol for the prevention of chemotherapy-induced nausea and emesis in oncology patients. Can J Anesthesiol 39:170, 1992.

Schiffman SS: Taste and smell in disease. N Engl J Med 308:1275, 1337, 1983.

Whang R, et al: Magnesium depletion as a cause of refractory potassium depletion. Arch Intern Med 145:1686, 1985.

Zawada ET, et al: Canine renal and systemic hemodynamic measurements after 4 weeks of a magnesium deficient diet. Nephron 50:253, 1988.

# NUTRITIONAL SUPPORT IN UREMIA

### MARY ANNA LABATO
*North Grafton, Massachusetts*

Uremia is a polysystemic toxic syndrome that occurs as a result of decreased renal function. Uremia may result from acute or chronic renal failure. The onset and degree of clinical signs of uremia vary depending on the nature, severity, duration, and rate of progression of the underlying disease.

## ACUTE RENAL FAILURE

Acute renal failure (ARF) is a syndrome characterized by abrupt deterioration of renal function and an inability to regulate solute and water balance adequately. It is a tenuously reversible state, which must be quickly diagnosed and aggressively treated. Acute renal failure may be due to prerenal, postrenal, or primary renal problems.

The primary reason for prerenal ARF is inadequate renal perfusion resulting from a variety of causes, including intravascular depletion (hemorrhage) or translocation of intravascular fluids (peritonitis, pancreatitis, burns), marked reductions in cardiac output (myocardial, valvular, or pericardial disease), or an abrupt decline in peripheral vascular resistance (vasodilation, sepsis).

Interference with urine flow caused by a variety of traumatic, inflammatory, or neoplastic processes in the upper or lower urinary tract may result in postrenal ARF.

Acute tubular necrosis is a syndrome of abrupt and sustained reduction in glomerular filtration rate (GFR) resulting from an ischemic or toxic renal insult and accounts for the majority of cases of primary (intrinsic) ARF.

## NUTRITION IN UREMIA

Critically ill animals are frequently unable or unwilling to take in food in the presence of diseases that produce significant increases in their protein and energy requirements. The importance of nutritional support as a means of decreasing the morbidity and mortality associated with many diseases has only recently been recognized in veterinary medicine.

There are three goals in the nutritional therapy of ARF: (1) amelioration of the consequences of uremia, (2) improvement of the overall nutritional status of the patient, and (3) reduction of the high mortality. In human medicine, the mortality of patients with ARF, particularly those who have had surgery and/or septicemia, has not changed substantially in the past 30 years. Since dialytic therapy can adequately correct azotemia and many of the electrolyte disturbances in most patients, it seems likely that the associated illnesses are responsible for the high mortality (Feinstein and Massry, 1988). One important factor that contributes to poor survival of patients with ARF is their increased protein catabolism. In veterinary medicine, there is also a very high mortality associated with ARF. The need to adequately support our patients nutritionally is equally as important.

## METABOLIC DISTURBANCES

The consequences of malnutrition and the relationship between protein and energy requirements have been discussed in detail elsewhere (Donoghue, 1992; Labato, 1992). When dogs are fasted, glycogen stores are exhausted in approximately 2 to 3 days. Fatty acids and amino acids are mobilized from adipose and lean tissue, respectively. Fat is used for about 70 to 85% of caloric needs, including up to 15% from ketones. Hepatic and renal gluconeogenesis converts certain amino acids to glucose to supply cells with an obligatory glucose need. Overall, protein provides up to 25% of calories and carbohydrate is used for less than 10%.

Metabolic stress in the sick animal imposes hypermetabolism, which is characterized by peripheral insulin resistance, marked protein catabolism, and negative nitrogen balance.

## Energy

A study performed in humans (Schneeweiss et al., 1990) concluded that renal failure has no influence on energy expenditure as long as septicemia is absent. The increased utilization of fat and decreased oxidation of glucose and protein as energy sources in patients with severe untreated azotemia is similar to the metabolic pattern of starvation. Both hypometabolic and hypermetabolic states have been recognized in ARF.

A rising blood urea nitrogen (BUN) is a clinical hallmark of ARF, reflecting the loss of renal excretory function. Studies have demonstrated that nitrogen retention was greatly exaggerated by coexisting catabolic processes in ARF. This hypercatabolic state is related to the underlying primary disease such as sepsis or severe trauma. The implicating factors in the pathologic process can be classified into three categories: (1) circulating proteolytic enzymes, (2) hormonal disturbances, and (3) nitrogen and calorie deficiency (Li, 1991).

## Nitrogen Balance

Nitrogen balance may be neutral, positive, or negative. Neutral nitrogen balance indicates that protein synthesis is equal to protein degradation. Positive nitrogen balance indicates that protein synthesis exceeds protein degradation. This occurrence usually suggests tissue growth or rebuilding. Negative nitrogen balance is a sign of protein degradation exceeding protein synthesis. The most likely cause of this catabolic state is carbohydrate and lipid intake insufficient to meet the animal's energy requirements, which results in the diversion of protein from structural uses to energy supply. In addition, inadequate protein ingestion may arise from dietary problems and further contribute to a negative balance (Labato, 1992). Studies suggest that muscle protein turnover is abnormal in uremia and more specifically that protein degradation is accelerated. Amino acid uptake by muscle is apparently depressed in ARF. Nitrogen arising from degradation of amino acid is converted almost completely to urea. Negative nitrogen balance can be recognized in animals by noting weight loss; muscle wasting; and lowered serum levels of total protein, albumin, and transferrin.

## Water and Mineral Balance

The excretion of water, electrolytes and other minerals is often impaired in ARF. When renal failure occurs in patients with diseases that are associated with accelerated catabolism (sepsis, trauma, and burns), release of substances such as potassium and phosphate into the extracellular fluid occurs. When the rate of release exceeds the capacity of the kidney to excrete these ions, hyperkalemia and hyperphosphatemia result.

The acute onset of renal failure does not allow time for the animal to adapt to changes in the internal environment. Animals with ARF are at risk for developing edema and hyponatremia even when salt and water are limited. In animals with ARF, frequent monitoring of serum electrolytes and careful adjustment of intake to match output of water and electrolytes are a critical aspect of management. An important part of the management of a patient with ARF should be daily weight, measured using the same scale.

## Acid-Base Balance

Metabolic acidosis occurs commonly in patients with ARF not only because hydrogen ion excretion is diminished, but also because in some patients the production of hydrogen ions is increased. Feeding patients large amounts of protein to provide amino acids necessary to induce anabolism may aggravate the tendency to develop metabolic acidosis because of the phosphates, sulfates, and other products contained in proteinaceous foods. Amino acid mixtures for intravenous feedings also contain acid that must be excreted. A potential acid-base complication of administering synthetic diets is the development of respiratory acidosis. This can occur when large quantities of glucose are administered, because the respiratory exchange ratio (RQ) is increased; and in patients with an inadequate respiratory reserve, the marked increase in respiratory quotient can lead to respiratory acidosis. This can be corrected by substituting fats as the calorie source in place of carbohydrates (Wesson, Mitch, and Wilmore, 1983).

## Carbohydrate Metabolism

Carbohydrate metabolism may be abnormal in patients with ARF. Studies in animals with experimentally induced ARF indicate that there is a diminished response of muscle to the hypoglycemic action of insulin. In humans with ARF associated with trauma, sepsis, or other hypermetabolic conditions, there may be enhanced hepatic glucose production and altered glucose disposal (Wesson, Mitch, and Wilmore, 1983). Hyperglycemia is fairly common after the initiation of total parenteral nutrition in patients with ARF. This may be related to underlying disease, such as diabetes mellitus, pancreatitis, sepsis, or concomitant peritoneal dialysis utilizing glucose as the osmotic agent. Above all, insulin resistance may be caused by ARF itself. As ARF varies from mild to marked, so the glucose intolerance may also be mild to severe.

## DETERMINATION OF ENERGY REQUIREMENTS

A number of different methods have been used to determine the energy needs of animals. As a general rule, the basal caloric requirements estimated for dogs is 40 to 60 kcal/kg/day, depending upon size; and for cats, 70 kcal/kg/day. Energy needs can also be based on the basal energy requirement (BER). The BER is the number of calories expended by an animal while awake and resting in a thermoneutral environment. The BER is determined using the following formula:

$$BER \text{ (kcal/24 hr)} = 70 \times BW \text{ (kg)}^{0.75}$$

This formula is based on two parameters: 70 is a K factor for placental animals that is derived from specific core body temperature set points; and body weight (BW) raised to the power of 0.75 is an estimation of biologic size derived from the rate of oxygen consumption in relation to body size. The energy needs for an animal experiencing illness or stress is referred to as the illness energy requirement (IER). The value for IER of hospitalized animals is approximately 25% greater than their BER values. The IER can be determined using the formula:

$$IER = BER \times stress factor$$

Stress factors are cage rest (1.25), postoperative periods (1.25 to 1.35), trauma or cancer (1.35 to 1.50), sepsis (1.50 to 1.70), and burns (1.70 to 2.0). In general, for an adult hospitalized cat, 1.4 should be employed as a stress factor. Maintaining adequate nutritional intake in patients on peritoneal dialysis is compounded by the anorexia and vomiting that are often present in uremic patients, as well as by protein loss in the dialysate. A stress factor of 2.0 should be used when animals are being treated with peritoneal dialysis to account for severe catabolic needs and protein loss. Dextrose present in the dialysate supplies approximately 8 kcal/kg/day in energy sources toward this total (Lane, Carter, and Lappin, 1992).

## NUTRITIONAL STRATEGIES IN ACUTE RENAL FAILURE

Which animal needs nutritional intervention? The decision to initiate nutritional support is influenced by the nutritional status of the animal as well as the type of underlying illness and the degree of accompanying catabolism. If the animal shows evidence of malnutrition (e.g., low serum albumin, weight loss, muscle wasting), nutritional therapy should be used. If a well-nourished animal will be able to resume a normal diet within 3 to 5 days, no specialized support is necessary. However, in animals with diseases associated with excess protein catabolism, nutritional support should be initiated early in the course of hospitalization.

When should nutrition be started? During the acute phase of ARF (within the first 24 to 48 hr), nutritional support should be avoided. Infusion of large quantities of amino acids or glucose during this phase can increase renal oxygen requirements and may aggravate tubular damage and the degree of renal functional loss. Animal experiments have shown that protein synthesis in muscle is decreased when renal function falls below 30% of normal (Druml, 1993).

In all animals who can tolerate them, oral feedings should be used. Calories should be provided by simple carbohydrates and fats at regular intervals. Initially, dogs should be provided between 0.6 and 2.0 gm/kg/day of dietary protein. Cats have a significantly higher requirement for dietary protein than dogs. The higher protein requirement for cats is apparently not solely the result of a higher requirement for one or more essential amino acids. Cats have a limited ability to adapt to extremes in dietary protein because of limited capacity to appropriately modify hepatic enzyme activity. Cats should receive between 1.7 and 3.0 gm/kg/day of protein.

## ROUTES OF NUTRITIONAL SUPPORT

The two main routes of nutritional support are the enteral and parenteral routes. Whenever possible it is best to employ the enteral route. It is both physiologic and economic, and it entails few complications. It can easily be used in a busy clinical setting.

The various types of enteral routes have been discussed in detail elsewhere (see *CVT XI*; Abood, Dimski, and Buffington, 1992). In ARF the most important limiting factor for enteral feedings is vomiting. Once vomiting is brought under control, then enteral feedings should be instituted. Also, in situations where peritoneal dialysis is being employed, the surgical placement of gastrostomy or jejunostomy tubes may result in compromised dialysis catheter function and leakage. Nasoesophageal and pharyngostomy tubes are enteral feeding methods that may be used as alternatives that do not require entry into the peritoneum when parenteral support is not feasible.

There are standardized tube feeding formulas for animals with normal renal function. Unfortunately, the fixed compositions of nutrients and the high content of proteins and electrolytes (especially potassium and phosphate) limit their use in ARF patients (Druml, 1993). Certain products are high in protein in terms of human requirements, but may be suitable for animal use (Ensure, Ross Laboratories; Peptamen, Clintec; Osmolite, Ross Laboratories; Vivonex T.E.N., Sandoz). The only liquid diet formulated for renal failure in dogs and cats is Renal Care (PetAg, Inc). Other alternatives are to use a low-protein renal failure formulation (Hill's Prescription Diet k/d) or a homemade low-protein diet and blenderize the meal into a slurry that can be easily passed through feeding tubes.

To avoid problems with abdominal cramping, vomiting, and diarrhea when using enteral products, the total requirement should not be administered on the first day. Feed only room-temperature or warmed solutions through feeding tubes. The total daily feeding volume should be divided and fed in four to six daily feedings.

Total parenteral nutrition (TPN) entails providing all necessary nutrients via administration through a central, peripheral, or portal vein. If nutrient requirements cannot be met by the enteral route, TPN should be used. Because fluids are usually restricted for ARF patients in the oliguric stage, the administration of TPN should be closely monitored.

Although the BER and IER are calculated as previously described, the administration of nutrients by the parenteral route requires certain modifications. When dogs are treated in our hospital, it is customary to supply the IER as nonprotein calories: 50 to 60% of the IER is supported by 20% lipid solution (2 kcal/ml), and the remainder is supplied by 50% dextrose solution (1.7 kcal/ml). The daily protein requirement is compounded into the TPN solution and supplies 0.6 to 2.0 gm/kg/day for dogs in ARF. Cats with ARF are supplied 1.7 to 3.0 gm/kg/day. Cats are particularly sensitive to overfeeding, so an adjustment is made in formulating the nutritional requirement to avoid problems with overfeeding, such as glucose intolerance, lipidosis, and hyperammonemia. Thus, the calories supplied by protein (4 kcal/gm) are subtracted from the total calories needed, and the balance is provided as a 50:50 mixture of dextrose and lipid.

Amino acid formulations are available for patients in renal failure (RenAmin, Clintec; Aminess, Clintec; NephrAmine, Kendall McGaw). There is considerable debate as to whether essential only or mixed amino acid solutions should be used. Essential amino acid solutions are probably sufficient for noncatabolic patients; however, patients who are hypercatabolic should receive both essential and nonessential amino acids (Druml, 1993). Most standard formulations will use a mixture of essential and nonessential amino acids.

Technical problems and infectious complications are similar in ARF patients and in nonuremic subjects. Most complications are related to excess infusion of substrates (hyperglycemia, hepatic lipidosis, increased carbon dioxide production, hypertriglyceridemia, hyperkalemia, accelerated increase in BUN). Additional common complications are often catheter related and include thrombophlebitis, edema, cellulitis, thrombembolism, sepsis, catheter occlusion, line disconnection or breakage, and an inability to recatheterize the animal (see *CVT XI*, p 117). Complications that are at increased risk with ARF are fluid overload, worsening of metabolic acidosis, electrolyte imbalances, and hyperglycemia. Since ARF impairs glucose tolerance, insulin administration is frequently necessary to maintain normoglycemia.

## CONCLUSIONS

In ARF, it is not renal insufficiency per se that determines the need for nutritional support, but the type and severity of the underlying disease and the degree of associated hypercatabolism. The optimal nutritional protocol has not been defined in veterinary medicine, nor has nutritional support convincingly reduced morbidity and mortality in ARF in humans. The poor prognosis in ARF is related to the severity of the underlying illness and the difficulty of providing long-term dialytic therapy as a routine economical procedure. Nutritional therapy, like dialysis, should be viewed as a means of supporting the animal until renal repair has occurred to the point that the animal can be self-sustaining. The supply of calories helps decrease the catabolic response, lessening the degree of protein breakdown products requiring renal excretion. Additionally, regeneration of renal tubular cells requires an extensive supply of energy and protein. By considering the demands in the initial treatment of animals with ARF, complications (weight loss, infection, and decubital ulcers) may be avoided.

## References and Suggested Reading

Abood SK, Dimski DS, Buffington CAT, et al: Enteral nutrition. *In* DiBartola SP (ed): *Fluid Therapy in Small Animal Practice*. Philadelphia, WB Saunders Co, 1992, p 419.
*A detailed review of enteral nutritional techniques in dogs and cats.*

Donoghue S: Dietary Management of Sick and Postoperative Dogs and Cats—A Monograph. Waltham, 1992.
*A review of dietary management principles in the dog and cat.*

Druml W: Nutritional support in acute renal failure. *In* Mitch WE and Klahr S (eds): *Nutrition and the Kidney*, 2nd edition. Boston, Little, Brown & Co, 1993, p 314.
*An up-to-date review of nutritional therapy in acute renal failure.*

Feinstein EJ and Massry SG: Nutritional therapy in acute renal failure. *In* Mitch WE and Klahr S (eds): *Nutrition and Kidney*. Boston, Little, Brown & Co, 1988, p 80.
*An overview of the pathophysiology of acute renal failure, its metabolic consequences, and how to supply nutritional therapy.*

Labato MA: Nutritional management of the critical care patient. *In* Kirk RW and Bonagura JD (eds): *Current Veterinary Therapy XI: Small Animal Practice*. Philadelphia, WB Saunders Co, 1992, p 117.
*A discussion of enteral and parenteral feeding techniques.*

Labato MA: Urologic emergencies. *In* Murtaugh RJ and Kaplan PM (eds): *Veterinary Emergency and Critical Care Medicine*. St. Louis, Mosby Year Book, 1992, p 295.
*An overview of acute renal failure; its pathophysiology, diagnosis, and treatments.*

Lane IF, Carter LJ, and Lappin MR: Peritoneal dialysis: An update on methods and usefulness. *In* Kirk RW and Bonagura JD (eds): *Current Veterinary Therapy XI: Small Animal Practice*. Philadelphia, WB Saunders Co, 1992, p 865.
*A discussion on the use of peritoneal dialysis.*

Li S: Acute renal failure. *In* Fischer JE (ed): *Total Parenteral Nutrition*. Boston, Little, Brown & Co, 1991, p 191.
*A review of the application of total parenteral nutrition in acute renal failure.*

Lippert AC: The metabolic response to injury: Enteral and parenteral nutritional support. *In* Murtaugh RJ and Kaplan PM (eds): *Veterinary Emergency and Critical Care Medicine*. St. Louis, Mosby Year Book, 1992, p 593.
*A review of the metabolic response to injury and illness and how to nutritionally support a critical animal.*

Lippert AC and Buffington CAT: Parenteral nutrition. *In* DiBartola SP (ed): *Fluid Therapy in Small Animal Practice*. Philadelphia, WB Saunders Co, 1992, p 384.
*A discussion of the indications and application of TPN.*

Schneeweiss B, Graninger W, et al: Energy metabolism in acute and chronic renal failure. Am J Clin Nutr 52:596, 1990.
*A prospective study evaluating energy metabolism in acute and chronic renal failure in humans..*

Wesson DE, Mitch WE, and Wilmore DS: Nutritional considerations in the treatment of acute renal failure. *In* Brenner BM and Lazarus JM (eds): *Acute Renal Failure*. Philadelphia, WB Saunders Co, 1983, p 618.
*An overview of nutritional support in acute renal failure.*

# *CVT* UPDATE: VETERINARY APPLICATIONS OF HEMODIALYSIS

LARRY D. COWGILL
*and* CRAIG H. MARETZKI

*Davis, California*

Hemodialysis is a therapy in which an artificial kidney is used to correct the fluid, acid-base, and electrolyte imbalances and uremic toxicity induced by failure of the natural kidneys. The principles and techniques to perform hemodialysis in dogs have been described sporadically since 1968 but, in contrast to its application in human medicine, only isolated clinical usage has been reported in veterinary medicine (Cowgill, 1980; Dhein, 1981; Thornhill, 1984). Recent improvements in hemodialysis delivery have extended its feasibility and indications in veterinary therapeutics to both acute and chronic renal failure (Table 1). Hemodialysis procedures suitable for cats suffering from acute and chronic renal failure have also been established. The ultrafiltration and diffusive properties of hemodialysis make it applicable also for the rapid correction of life-threatening fluid overload and dialytic removal of toxins in acute poisoning or drug overdoses.

## TECHNICAL IMPROVEMENTS IN THE DELIVERY OF HEMODIALYSIS

Hemodialysis remains technically demanding because of the intricacies of dialysis delivery equipment, complex interactions with the patient, and the unstable clinical status of uremic animals. Although little has changed to alter patient variables, the technical demands and adverse interactions of hemodialysis delivery have lessened. Delivery of hemodialysis requires (1) repeated access to the patient's blood, (2) a hemodialyzer (artificial kidney), and (3) a dialysis delivery system that formulates and monitors the dialysate and regulates the flow of blood in the extracorporeal circuit.

### Vascular Access

Arteriovenous shunts composed of exteriorized silicone tubes and Teflon vessel cannulas have been the mainstay for vascular access in veterinary hemodialysis (Dhein, 1981; Thornhill, 1984). However, transcutaneous (double lumen) venous dialysis catheters* are a recent and more desirable choice for either short-term or long-term vascular access in dogs and in cats and have generally replaced arteriovenous shunts. The catheters are placed percutaneously in the external jugular vein via a subcutaneous tunnel that exits the skin in the cranial cervical area of the neck. The vascular portals are located in the right atrium or cranial vena cava, and a subcutaneous Dacron felt cuff stabilizes its positioning and prevents accidental displacement from the vessel. Transcutaneous venous catheters obviate the extensive surgery required for arteriovenous shunts and can be inserted in minutes. They are easier to use, impose less risk of damage and dislocation, and are easier to maintain than shunts.

### Hemodialyzer (Artificial Kidney)

The hemodialyzer must have a high capacity to remove small- and middle-molecular weight solutes from blood, selectively retain plasma proteins and cellular components of blood, regulate water removal independently of solute flux, and be nontoxic and free of adverse biologic interactions with the animal. Modern dialyzers are generally of hollow fiber design and composed of chemically altered cellulosic membrane materials (Cupraphane, regenerated cellulose, cellulose acetate, cellulose triacetate) or thermoplastic synthetic polymers (polycarbonate, polyacrylonitrile, polysulfone). Synthetic membrane dialyzers possess superior diffusion and ultrafiltration characteristics, mechanical strength, low thrombogenicity, and biocompatibility.

***Table 1.*** *Indications for Hemodialysis*

Acute renal failure
  Failure of conservative Rx to control the biochemical and clinical manifestations of uremia
  Failure of conservative Rx to promote adequate urine formation —severe oliguria or anuria
  Life-threatening fluid overload
  Life-threatening electrolyte or acid-base disturbances
  BUN ≥ 100 mg/dl; Serum creatinine ≥10 mg/dl
  Clinical course refractory to conservative therapy for more than 24 hr
Chronic renal failure
  Azotemia and uremic signs unresponsive to medical therapy
  BUN ≥90 mg/dl; serum creatinine ≥8 mg/dl
Miscellaneous
  Severe pulmonary edema
  Acute poisoning/drug overdose

---

*Permcath, Quinton Instruments Co, Seattle, WA. The Duo-Flow Internal Jugular Catheter, Medcomp, Harleysville, PA.

However, synthetic membrane dialyzers are less economical than newer cellulosic dialyzers that are disposable and provide high diffusion and ultrafiltration rates, low priming volumes, and lower cost.[†]

## Dialysis Delivery Systems

The dialysis delivery system proportions the dialysate from commercial concentrates and continuously monitors the composition, temperature, and pH of the final fluid. It also controls the extracorporeal flow of blood, regulates the rate of ultrafiltration, and regulates delivery of anticoagulant. A recent and significant advance is the ability to formulate bicarbonate-based dialysate in lieu of traditional acetate-based formulations. The substitution of bicarbonate permits use of highly permeable hemodialyzers, high-flux dialysis prescriptions, and alleviates the hemodynamic instability and acetate intolerance associated with acetate dialysis. Variable sodium proportioning is an additional feature that automatically formulates the dialysate with sodium concentrations more suited to dogs and cats and permits "sodium modeling" wherein the dialysate sodium concentration is changed during the course of the dialysis treatment. Sodium modeling improves hemodynamic stability by increasing dialysate sodium at the beginning of the dialysis treatment when solute transfer (primarily urea) from the extracellular fluid is greatest. Later in the treatment, when solute transfer is slower, the dialysate sodium concentration is automatically "stepped down" to prevent sodium expansion and hypernatremia at the end of dialysis. Ultrafiltration controllers are new design features that precisely and accurately regulate the rate of ultrafiltration. With precise ultrafiltration, fluid removal on small animals becomes less problematic and dangerous.

## USE OF HEMODIALYSIS IN ACUTE RENAL FAILURE

Acute renal failure continues to be the primary indication for hemodialysis in veterinary medicine. Dialytic therapy should be started immediately if initial therapy fails to promote an adequate diuresis or alleviate the azotemia and metabolic disturbances of renal failure. Hemodialysis is 10 to 20 times more efficient than peritoneal dialysis and will more rapidly correct the uremic state. Initial dialysis prescriptions need only correct life-threatening fluid overload and electrolyte abnormalities and moderate the severity of the azotemia (Fig. 1). Hemodialysis treatments should be repeated daily for 3 to 4 days until the predialysis blood urea nitrogen (BUN) is less than 90 mg/dl. Thereafter, maintenance treatments are performed every 48 to 72

[†]Cobe Centrysystem 100 HG or 200 HG, CGH Medical, Inc, Cobe, Lakewood, CO.

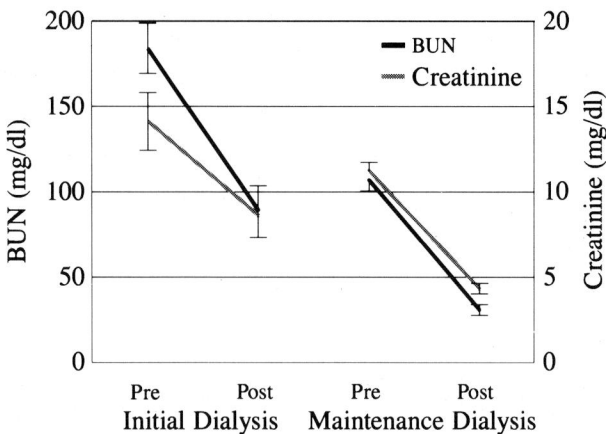

**Figure 1.** Effects of initial (dialysis time <180 min; blood flow <150 ml/min; *n*=12) or maintenance (dialysis time >180 min; blood blow >150 ml/min; *n*=64) hemodialysis treatments to decrease the azotemia in 15 dogs with severe acute renal failure. Abbreviations: Pre = prehemodialysis values, Post = posthemodialysis values. Data are presented as the mean ± standard error of the mean.

hr and the dialysis prescription intensified to more fully resolve the uremia (Fig. 1). Initial dialysis treatments that are too aggressive can predispose the patient to dialysis disequilibrium, which is characterized in its early stages by restlessness, vocalization, depression, vomiting, tremors or focal muscle twitching, and by generalized seizures and coma when severe. Recovery of renal function can be expected in as little as 15% of animals presenting with severe uremia refractory to conservative therapy. Nevertheless, hemodialysis affords the life support, clinical stability, and additional longevity these patients must have to achieve their full potential to repair the renal damage and recover from the excretory failure.

## USE OF HEMODIALYSIS IN CHRONIC RENAL FAILURE

A new and provocative use of hemodialysis is to supplement the medical management of chronic, end-stage kidney disease in animals. Hemodialysis provides an "excretory boost" that lessens their azotemia and urea exposure. This concept is illustrated conceptually in Figure 2 from the results of 12 dogs with end-stage renal disease treated with intermittent hemodialysis at the University of California. With medical management alone, the BUN was sustained and unremitting at 158 mg/dl for the group of dogs. Institution of intermittent hemodialysis for 5 hr every 5 days lowered the maximum (predialysis) BUN from 158 mg/dl to 115 mg/dl; and, more importantly, the "time-averaged" BUN concentration during the interdialysis interval was decreased to 65 mg/dl. The time-averaged BUN concentration is a kinetically modeled value that reflects the effective urea exposure of the animal over the dialysis cycle and represents a considerable reduction

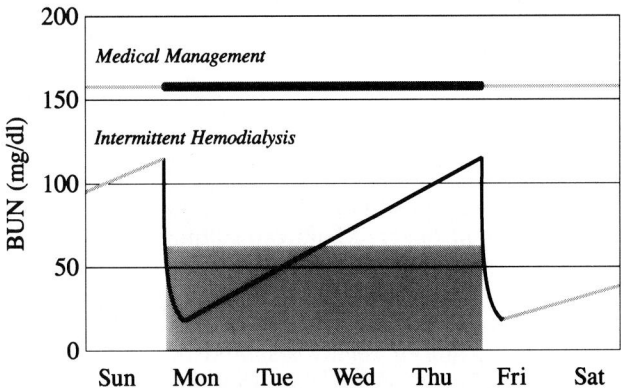

**Figure 2.** Conceptualized daily changes in BUN before (Medical Management) and following (Intermittent Hemodialysis) the initiation of hemodialysis treatments in animals with end-stage renal disease. The solid segment of the lower curve reflects the change in BUN during sequential hemodialysis treatments and the intervening interdialysis period. The shaded insert on this curve depicts the kinetically modeled "time-averaged" urea concentration or the effective urea exposure of the patient during this dialysis cycle. The expanded segment on the upper curve depicts the corresponding urea exposure in the animals before starting hemodialysis. The data reflect the mean values from 12 dogs with chronic renal failure in response to 85 hemodialysis treatments.

from the equivalent urea exposure (158 mg/dl) without dialysis. Ultimately, intermittent hemodialysis can provide the difference between an animal that can be treated and one that cannot be effectively managed or survive.

## COMPLICATIONS OF HEMODIALYSIS

Complications associated with hemodialysis reflect its technical complexities and the clinical compromises of the dialysis patient. The most common intradialytic complications include transient hypotension, vomiting, tremors, seizures, and clotting in the extracorporeal circuit. The incidence and frequency of these complications are influenced by the underlying condition of the patient and are more common with dialysis for acute renal failure. Major complications during the interdialytic period include sepsis, bleeding, clotting in the vascular access, thromboembolism, and inadequate dialysis. Clearly, it is impossible to eliminate all risks associated with hemodialysis, but meticulous patient supervision and the improvements in dialysis delivery minimize many of these hazards.

## References and Suggested Reading

Cowgill LD: Current status of veterinary hemodialysis. *In* Kirk RW (ed): *Current Veterinary Therapy VII.* Philadelphia, WB Saunders Co, 1980, p 1111.
  *A review of the indications, procedures, and clinical experience with hemodialysis in veterinary medicine.*
Dhein CRM: Hemodialysis in the dog. Compend Cont Educ Pract Vet 3: 1031, 1981.
  *This article describes the theory of hemodialysis and its application for dogs.*
Thornhill JA: Hemodialysis. *In* Bovee KC (ed): *Canine Nephrology.* Harwal Publishing Co, 1984, p 755.
  *Comprehensive discussion of the theory, principles, and procedures of dialysis delivery to dogs.*

# FAMILIAL RENAL DISEASE IN CATS

DAVID S. BILLER
*Manhattan, Kansas*

*and* STEPHEN P. DIBARTOLA
*Columbus, Ohio*

A *familial* renal disease is one that occurs in related animals with a higher frequency than would be expected by chance. Familial renal diseases are less commonly recognized in cats than in dogs. Increasing use of diagnostic ultrasound in veterinary medicine will allow more accurate diagnosis of PKD in cats.

## POLYCYSTIC KIDNEY DISEASE IN PERSIAN CATS

Polycystic kidney disease (PKD) is inherited as an autosomal dominant trait in Persian cats (Biller et al., 1991). Autosomal dominant polycystic kidney disease is a slowly progressive, irreversible disease that may lead to chronic renal failure. It is characterized by development and growth of cysts in both kidneys and occasionally in the liver. The kidneys become enlarged and may contain hundreds of fluid-filled cysts of widely differing sizes. Compression of normal renal parenchyma by enlarging cysts is thought to be the most important factor in the development of chronic renal failure.

No single hypothesis completely explains development of PKD in any species (Evan, 1987). One hypothesis is that hyperplastic epithelial cells form polyps that cause potential obstruction and dilatation of renal tubules. Another hypothesis is that the tubular basement membrane itself is defective, weakening the renal tubule and causing secondary dilatation. Both factors may play a role in the pathogenesis of PKD. Failure of nephron segments to fuse has not yet been excluded as a cause of cyst formation in cats, but this mechanism has not been determined to cause cyst formation in other species.

## Clinical Findings

Sporadic cases of PKD have been described in cats since 1967. Related and unrelated cats of varying ages have been affected. Six of nine reported cats with PKD have been Persian or Persian crosses (Biller, Chew, and DiBartola, 1990; Lulich et al., 1988; Stebbins, 1989).

The period of the time before onset of renal failure is variable in Persian cats with PKD. Clinical signs are those of chronic renal failure, including lethargy, anorexia, polydipsia, polyuria, and weight loss. Neither physical examination findings nor routine laboratory tests are sufficient to establish or exclude a diagnosis of early PKD. The laboratory findings in Persian cats with renal failure due to PKD are similar to those observed in cats with chronic renal failure of any cause. Diagnostic ultrasound is required for definitive diagnosis early in the course of the disease.

Survey abdominal radiographs are normal early in the course of the disease because cysts are small and few in number. As the disease progresses, bilateral renomegaly and irregular renal contours are observed. Excretory urography is helpful in the diagnosis of PKD and its differentiation from other causes of renomegaly in cats. The nephrogram is characterized by numerous sharply marginated radiolucencies throughout the parenchyma of both kidneys because the cysts do not fill with contrast. The renal contour appears irregular. The renal collecting system may be distorted by expanding cysts.

Ultrasound is an excellent noninvasive technique for the early diagnosis of PKD (also see "Ultrasonographic Findings in Renal Disease," this volume, p 933). Cysts as small as 2 mm may be seen with a high-frequency (7.5 to 10 mHz) transducer. Diagnosis by ultrasound can be made in cats prior to the development of clinical disease. Ultrasonographically, cysts are round, smooth, anechoic structures that demonstrate through-transmission. Diagnosis should be based on the finding of multiple cysts in both kidneys or the finding of a few cysts in at least one kidney in a cat from a family of cats previously diagnosed with PKD. Variation in the size of the cysts is common.

## Pathologic Findings

Cyst formation almost always affects both kidneys. Grossly, the kidneys are enlarged and irregular. Cysts vary in size (<1 mm to >1 cm) depending upon the age of the animal, with older cats having larger and more numerous cysts. Renal involvement can be slightly to extremely asymmetric. Cysts have been found in the cortex, medulla, and renal papilla (Biller et al., 1991). Cysts also have been found in the liver of affected Persian cats (Lulich et al., 1988; Stebbins,

1989). Uncomplicated cysts contain clear or straw-colored fluid. Complicated cysts may contain blood or purulent material.

## Treatment

There is no specific therapy for polycystic kidney disease. Treatment of renal failure resulting from PKD is similar to that of chronic renal failure of any cause (see elsewhere in this section). A Persian cat with PKD should be considered to have an inherited disease. If possible, offspring or relatives should be examined by ultrasound. Owners should be informed that this is a heritable disease and that if the animal is bred, 50% of the offspring are likely to be affected. It is important to emphasize to an owner that this is a late-onset disease. Thus, an affected cat may live many years before demonstrating clinical disease, and breeding of affected cats has great potential to produce PKD-affected offspring. Simple ultrasound screening and neutering of all affected cats could eliminate this disease from the at-risk population.

## FAMILIAL AMYLOIDOSIS IN ABYSSINIAN CATS

Spontaneous systemic amyloidosis is uncommon in mixed-breed cats but has been observed in young Abyssinian cats (Chew et al., 1982). Affected Abyssinian cats usually are presented between 1 and 5 years of age, and there is no sex predilection. Systemic amyloidosis also has been reported in young Oriental shorthaired and Siamese cats (Zuber, 1993).

Amyloid deposits usually appear in the kidneys of affected Abyssinian cats between 9 and 24 months of age. In some of these cats, amyloid deposition is rapid and severe, and renal failure develops within 1 year of diagnosis. In others, amyloid deposition in the kidney is mild, and affected cats may live to an advanced age without detection of their amyloid deposits.

Difficulty in determining the mode of inheritance arises from variability in severity and progression of amyloidosis among affected Abyssinian cats. Amyloidosis has been observed in one offspring of an affected Abyssinian male and a female Persian cat. Occurrence of amyloidosis in the first generation of an out-cross is suggestive of a dominant inheritance pattern. The disease is variably penetrant, and amyloid deposition has been observed at necropsy in the kidneys of some older Abyssinian cats that were normal clinically yet had produced affected offspring.

Characterization of the amyloid protein from the kidneys of affected Abyssinian cats has demonstrated that this disease is an example of reactive systemic amyloidosis based on the presence of amyloid protein AA (DiBartola et al., 1985). The amyloid deposits in young Oriental shorthaired and Siamese cats are resistant to permanganate oxidation, suggesting that they may contain a protein other than amyloid AA (Zuber, 1993).

## Clinical Findings

Abyssinian cats with amyloidosis usually are presented for poor hair coat, weight loss, polydipsia, polyuria, lethargy, and anorexia. Physical examination findings include dehydration; pallor of mucous membranes; rough hair coat; and kidneys that are small, firm, and irregular on palpation. Oriental shorthaired and Siamese cats may present for spontaneous hepatic hemorrhage leading to acute collapse, severe pallor, and hemoabdomen (Zuber, 1993). Affected cats that survive acute hemorrhage later may develop chronic renal failure as a result of amyloid deposition in their kidneys.

Laboratory evaluation of Abyssinian cats with amyloidosis reveals evidence of chronic renal failure including azotemia, hyperphosphatemia, metabolic acidosis, nonregenerative anemia, and low urine specific gravity. Proteinuria is a variable finding and reflects the severity of glomerular involvement.

## Pathologic Findings

Amyloid deposits may be detected in biopsy or necropsy specimens. Tissue deposits of amyloid stained with alkaline Congo red and viewed under polarized light demonstrate birefringence and a characteristic green color. Amyloid deposits that lose their Congo red affinity after permanganate oxidation usually contain amyloid A protein, whereas amyloid deposits containing other proteins retain the Congo red stain after permanganate oxidation.

The principal pathologic lesions in cats with amyloidosis include medullary amyloid deposits, papillary necrosis, chronic tubulointerstitial nephritis characterized by lymphoplasmacytic infiltration and fibrosis, and variable glomerular amyloid deposits (Boyce et al., 1984). Glomerular amyloidosis is mild and often difficult to detect in many affected cats, but occasionally can be severe, resulting in marked proteinuria. Medullary amyloid deposition was found in all affected Abyssinians, whereas glomerular deposits were found in 75% (DiBartola, Tarr, and Benson, 1986). Medullary interstitial amyloid deposits are believed to interfere with blood flow to the renal papilla through the vasa recta, resulting in papillary necrosis and secondary interstitial medullary fibrosis and mononuclear inflammation.

Amyloid deposition is not restricted to the kidneys in Abyssinian cats with familial amyloidosis. Deposits are frequently found in other organs including adrenal glands, thyroid glands, spleen, gastrointestinal tract, heart, liver, and pancreas (DiBartola, Tarr, and Benson, 1986). Amyloid deposits in these other organs usually do not make an important contribution to the clinical syndrome, which typically is that of chronic renal failure. A notable exception is a syndrome observed in Oriental shorthaired, Siamese, and some domestic shorthaired cats in which potentially fatal acute hepatic hemorrhage has been observed (Zuber, 1993; Blunden and Smith, 1992). The liver in these cats is very friable and usually contains extensive amyloid deposits (Zuber, 1993; Blunden and Smith, 1992).

## Treatment

The goals of treatment for amyloidosis are (1) to provide supportive medical management of renal failure if present; (2) to identify and treat any underlying disease that may be predisposing the patient to amyloidosis; and (3) to consider therapy to inhibit deposition or to increase mobilization of amyloid itself. Concomitant infections should be treated with appropriate chemotherapeutic agents.

Dimethyl sulfoxide (DMSO) and colchicine are drugs that may have specific effects in patients with reactive amyloidosis. Any value of DMSO in treatment of amyloidosis probably is due to its anti-inflammatory effects. Prompt reduction in serum amyloid A protein concentrations may further reduce amyloid AA deposition and allow mobilization of existing deposits by the host's degradative systems. Administration of DMSO would most likely be beneficial in reactive amyloidosis early in the course of renal disease. Later, when renal failure has been established and fibrosis is severe, only stabilization of renal function may be anticipated. In cats, the usefulness of DMSO probably is limited. Decreased appetite and water consumption, accompanying nausea and bad odor, may cause dehydration that could worsen prerenal azotemia.

Colchicine impairs the release of serum amyloid A protein from hepatocytes by binding to microtubules and preventing secretion. Its role is primarily in the prevention of reactive amyloidosis in human patients with high risk for development of reactive amyloidosis. It is less useful in patients with established nephrotic syndrome because its role lies primarily in prevention of amyloidosis. Colchicine has not yet been evaluated in the treatment of feline amyloidosis.

## References and Suggested Reading

Biller DS, Chew DJ, and DiBartola SP: Polycystic kidney disease in a family of Persian cats. J Am Vet Med Assoc 196:1288, 1990.

Biller DS, Pflueger SMV, Miller LM, et al: Autosomal dominant polycystic kidney disease in cats (abstr). *Proceedings of the American Society of Nephrology.* Baltimore, MD, 1991.

Blunden AS and Smith KC: Generalized amyloidosis and acute liver hemorrhage in four cats. J Small Anim Pract 33:566, 1992.

Boyce JT, DiBartola SP, Chew DJ, et al: Familial renal amyloidosis in Abyssinian cats. Vet Pathol 21:33, 1984.

Chew DJ, DiBartola SP, Boyce JT, et al: Renal amyloidosis in related Abyssinian cats. J Am Vet Med Assoc 181:139, 1982.

DiBartola SP, Benson MD, Dwulet FE, et al: Isolation and characterization of amyloid protein AA in the Abyssinian cat. Lab Invest 52:485, 1985.

DiBartola SP, Tarr MJ, and Benson MD: Tissue distribution of amyloid deposits in Abyssinian cats with familial amyloidosis. J Comp Pathol 96:387, 1986.

Evan AP: Cyst formation and growth in autosomal dominant polycystic kidney disease. Kidney Int 31:1145, 1987.

Lulich JP, Osborne CA, Walter PA, et al: Feline idiopathic polycystic kidney disease. Compend Cont Educ Pract Vet 10:1029, 1988.

Stebbins KE: Polycystic disease of the kidney and liver in an adult Persian cat. J Comp Pathol 100:327, 1989.

Zuber RM: Systemic amyloidosis in Oriental and Siamese cats. Aust Vet Pract 23:66, 1993.

# NEPHROLITHIASIS: PREVALENCE OF MINERAL TYPE

GERALD V. LING

*Davis, California*

In only a small percentage of all cases of urinary stone disease in dogs and cats are calculi located in the renal pelves. Most are located in the urinary bladder, the urethra (males), or are passed in the urine. The opposite situation occurs in human beings with urinary stone disease, about 97% of whom have renal calculi.

The pertinent history, clinical signs, radiographic and ultrasonographic findings, and therapy in dogs and cats with renal calculi have been reviewed recently (see *CVT XI*, p 889). The purpose of this article is to provide information regarding the breed and gender distribution, and mineral composition of canine and feline renal calculi. Consideration must be given to the mineralogic composition of calculi of renal origin when therapeutic and preventive management strategies are planned.

## RENAL CALCULI IN DOGS

A total of 284 specimens of canine urinary calculi of renal origin (renal pelves and ureters) were analyzed at the University of California between 1981 and the end of December 1992. One hundred ninety-six (69%) specimens were from female dogs (average age 8.3 years), including 33 purebreds and a crossbred group; 88 (31%) specimens were from male dogs (average age 7.9 years), including 27 purebreds and a crossbred group. These calculi represented approximately 4% of all canine calculus specimens submitted for analysis from female dogs and 2% of those submitted for analysis from male dogs. Approximately 25% of the specimens from either gender were from both kidneys, approximately 37% were from left kidneys, and approximately 30% were removed from right kidneys (in about 8% of the specimens, the kidney(s) of origin was not indicated). Forty-seven per cent of the male dogs with renal calculi also had calculi in the bladder and/or urethra, whereas only 23% of the female dogs represented had concurrent calculi in the lower urinary tract. Thus, when renal calculi occurred in dogs, they were located only in kidney(s) ≥50% of the time in males and ≥75% of the time in females.

Although breed differences occurred within each gender, among male dogs, approximately 38% of the specimens of renal calculi were at least partially composed of struvite ($MgNH_4PO_4.6H_2O$), 33% contained urate, 33% contained calcium oxalate, 32% contained calcium phosphate (apatite and/or brushite), 9% were partially composed of silica, and 1% were composed of cystine. Forty-one per cent of the specimens were composed of mixtures of two or more mineral substances (e.g., struvite and apatite), and 50% were composed of two or more mineralogically different layers (i.e., layers of differing percentages of the same minerals or different minerals in each layer). Among female dogs, approximately 58% of the specimens were at least partially composed of struvite, 38% contained calcium phosphate, 35% contained calcium oxalate, 12% contained urate, and 5% contained silica. Fifty-five per cent of the specimens were composed of mixtures of two or more mineral substances, and 60% were composed of two or more mineralogically different layers.

## RENAL CALCULI IN CATS

A total of 62 specimens of feline calculi of renal origin were analyzed between 1981 and the end of 1992. Thirty-four (55%) specimens were from females and 28 (45%) were from males. The average age of both males and females was 8.6 years. Eleven purebreds and a crossbred group were represented. These calculi represented about 5% of all feline calculus specimens submitted for analysis. Approximately 15% of cats of either gender with renal calculi also had calculi in the urinary bladder. About 12% of specimens were from both kidneys, 57% were from left kidneys, and 31% were removed from right kidneys. Fifteen per cent of the cats had calculi concurrently in the lower tract.

The mineral composition of the renal calculi was very similar for both genders. Approximately 73% of the calculi from both females and males were at least partially composed of calcium oxalate, 34% contained calcium phosphate, 6% contained struvite, and 1% contained urate. Eighteen per cent of the specimens were composed of mixtures of two or more mineral substances. Seventy-one per cent of the specimens were composed of a single mineral layer; 19% contained two distinct mineralogic layers; and 10% were composed of three or more mineralogically different layers.

## References and Suggested Reading

Dieringer TM and Lees GE: Nephroliths: Approach to therapy. *In* Kirk RW and Bonagura JD (eds): *Current Veterinary Therapy XI*. Philadelphia, WB Saunders Co, 1992, p 889.
*A short review of history, clinical signs, laboratory, radiographic, and ultrasonographic findings and therapeutic options in dogs and cats with nephrolithiasis.*

# CANINE AND FELINE NEPHROLITHS

CARL A. OSBORNE,
LISA K. UNGER,
*and* JODY P. LULICH
*St. Paul, Minnesota*

## EPIDEMIOLOGY

Knowledge of the epidemiology of canine and feline nephroliths is of clinical significance in identifying underlying risk factors, and in predicting the mineral composition of nephroliths prior to formulating therapeutic plans to manage them. Whereas the majority of canine and feline urocystoliths are composed of struvite, naturally occurring nephroliths in these species most commonly are composed of calcium salts (oxalate and phosphate) (see "Nephrolithiasis: Prevalence of Mineral Type," this volume, p 980). This observation is of importance when considering the feasibility of medical dissolution of nephroliths.

## Canine Nephroliths

During a 12-year period, 17,610 uroliths from dogs were analyzed by quantitative methods at the Minnesota Urolith Center. Of these, 226 (1.3%) were nephroliths. Urolithiasis only affected the kidneys in 154/226 cases, whereas 72/226 affected the kidneys and other portions of the tract. Nephroliths composed of calcium salts comprised 43% of the total (Table 1).

### CALCIUM OXALATE

Thirty-nine per cent of the canine nephroliths were predominantly composed of calcium oxalate (CaOx). They affected males (54%) more commonly than females (44%). The gender of 2% of the patients with CaOx nephroliths was not specified. The mean age of dogs with CaOx nephroliths was $9.4 \pm 2.4$ years (range = 3.8 months to 14 years). Twenty-four different breeds had CaOx nephroliths. The most commonly affected breeds were: miniature schnauzer (18.2%), Lhasa apso (12.5%), Yorkshire terrier (11.4%), miniature poodle (11.4%), and Shih Tzu (10.2%). These breeds are apparently predisposed to calcium oxalate urolithiasis. Of 4509 dogs with CaOx uroliths, 91.5% were located in the bladder and urethra, 3.1% affected the kidneys and ureters, and 1% were voided. The location of 4.4% of CaOx uroliths removed from dogs was not specified.

**Table 1.** *Mineral Composition of 226 Canine Nephroliths Evaluated by Quantitative Methods*

| Predominant Mineral Type | Proportion of Predominant Mineral (%) | Number | % |
|---|---|---|---|
| Calcium oxalate | | 88 | 39 |
|   Calcium oxalate·1H$_2$O | 70–100° | (70) | (31) |
|   Calcium oxalate·2H$_2$O | 70–100 | (13) | (6) |
|   Calcium oxalate·1H$_2$O & 2H$_2$O | 70–100 | (5) | (2) |
| Calcium phosphate | | 9 | 4 |
|   Calcium apatite | 70–100 | (8) | (4) |
|   Calcium hydrogen phosphate 2H$_2$O | 70–100 | (1) | (<1) |
| Magnesium ammonium phosphate 6H$_2$O | 70–100 | 79 | 35 |
| Purines | | 18 | 8 |
|   Ammonium acid urate | 70–100 | (16) | (7) |
|   Sodium acid urate | 70–100 | (1) | (<1) |
|   Xanthine | 70–100 | (1) | (<1) |
| Silica | 70–100 | 1 | <1 |
| Mixed† | | 17 | 8 |
| Compound‡ | | 9 | 4 |
| Matrix | | 5 | 2 |
| TOTAL | | 226 | 100 |

°Uroliths composed of at least 70% of mineral type listed; no nucleus or shell was detected.
†Uroliths contained less than 70% of predominant mineral; no nucleus or shell was detected.
‡Uroliths contained an identifiable nucleus and one or more surrounding layers of a different mineral.

### STRUVITE

Thirty-four per cent of the canine nephroliths were composed of struvite. In contrast to calcium oxalate, struvite affected females (76%) more commonly than males (19%). The gender of 5% of the dogs with struvite nephroliths was not recorded. The higher prevalence of struvite urolithiasis in female dogs is likely associated with the higher prevalence of bacterial urinary tract infection (UTI) in females. The mean age of dogs with struvite nephroliths was 7 ± 3 years (range = 17 months to 15 years). Twenty-two different breeds had struvite nephroliths. The most commonly affected breeds were: miniature schnauzer (17.7%), *bichon frise* (10.1%), Shih Tzu (7.6%), Yorkshire terrier (6.3%), Lhasa apso (6.3%), cocker spaniel (6.3%), and miniature poodle (6.3%). Of 9927 dogs with struvite uroliths, 89.4% were located in the bladder and urethra, 4.6% were voided, and 1.2% were located in the kidneys and ureters. The location of 4.9% of the struvite uroliths removed from dogs was not specified.

### PURINES

Eight per cent of the canine nephroliths were composed of ammonium urate, sodium urate, or xanthine. Purine nephroliths affected males (56%) more frequently than females (28%). The gender of 16% of the dogs with purine nephroliths was not specified. The mean age of dogs with purine nephroliths was 4.8 ± 3.5 years (range = 3 months to 12 years). Twelve different breeds had purine nephroliths. The most commonly affected were: Dalmation (18%), Yorkshire terrier (18%), and English bulldog (12%). Of 1078 dogs with purine uroliths, 86% were located in the bladder and urethra, 7.1% were voided, and 2.1% affected the kidneys and ureters. The location of 4.8% of the purine uroliths removed from dogs was not specified.

## Feline Nephroliths

During a 12-year period, 3989 feline uroliths were analyzed by quantitative methods at the Minnesota Urolith Center. Of these, 113 (2.8%) were nephroliths. Urolithiasis in 95/113 cases only affected the kidneys, while 18/113 affected the kidneys and other portions of the urinary tract. Nephroliths composed of calcium salts comprised 58% of the total (Table 2).

### CALCIUM OXALATE

Forty-three per cent of the feline nephroliths were composed of CaOx. Calcium oxalate affected males (54%) more commonly than females (42%). The gender of 4% of the patients with calcium oxalate nephroliths was not specified. The mean age of cats with calcium oxalate nephroliths was 7.9 years ± 3.9 (range = 2 to 18 years). Five different breeds had calcium oxalate nephroliths. The affected breeds were: domestic shorthair (DSH) (52%), domestic longhair (DLH) (15%), Siamese (6%), Persian (8%), and unknown (19%). Of 1004 cats with CaOx uroliths, 85.7% were located in the bladder and urethra, 6.6% affected the kidneys and the ureters, and 3.5% were voided. The location of 3.9% of the CaOx uroliths removed from cats was not specified.

### STRUVITE

Surprisingly, only 5% of the feline nephroliths were composed of magnesium ammonium phosphate. Struvite nephroliths affected males (83%) more commonly than females (17%). The mean age of cats with struvite nephroliths was 6 ± 3.8 years (range = 2 months to 11 years). Four breeds had struvite nephroliths. The most affected breeds were: DSH (33%), DLH (17%), and unknown (33%). Of 2467 cats with struvite uroliths,

***Table 2.*** *Mineral Composition of 113 Feline Nephroliths Evaluated by Quantitative Methods*

| Predominant Mineral Type | Proportion of Predominant Mineral (%) | Number | % |
|---|---|---|---|
| Calcium oxalate | | 48 | 43 |
|   Calcium oxalate·1H$_2$O | 70–100° | (45) | (40) |
|   Calcium oxalate·2H$_2$O | 70–100 | (1) | (1) |
|   Calcium oxalate·1H$_2$O & 2H$_2$O | 70–100 | (2) | (2) |
| Calcium phosphate | | 17 | 15 |
|   Calcium apatite | 70–100 | (16) | (14) |
|   Tricalcium phosphate | 70–100 | (1) | (1) |
| Magnesium ammonium phosphate 6H$_2$O | 70–100 | 6 | 5 |
| Mixed[†] | | 13 | 12 |
| Compound[‡] | | 1 | <1 |
| Matrix | | 28 | 25 |
| TOTAL | | 113 | 100 |

° Uroliths composed of at least 70% of mineral type listed; no nucleus or shell was detected.
† Uroliths contained less than 70% of predominant mineral; no nucleus or shell was detected.
‡ Uroliths contained an identifiable nucleus and one or more surrounding layers of a different mineral.

90% were located in the bladder and urethra, 4% were voided, and 0.3% were located in the kidneys and ureter. The location of 5.4% of the struvite uroliths removed from dogs was not specified.

## BIOLOGIC BEHAVIOR

Clinical and experimental studies performed at the University of Minnesota revealed that struvite uroliths can form within 2 to 8 weeks following infection of the urinary tract with urease-producing staphylococci (Osborne et al., 1993). Struvite uroliths associated with UTI caused by staphylococci or *Proteus* species have been detected in puppies and kittens as young as 5 weeks of age. We have also observed formation of struvite renoliths in dogs within weeks of developing staphylococci-induced struvite urocystoliths. The pathophysiology appeared to be related to secondary vesicoureteral reflux and ascending urinary tract infection. The rates of formation and growth of nonstruvite uroliths are less well defined.

Infection-induced struvite nephroliths are associated with increased risk of persistent or progressive bacterial pyelonephritis, especially if urinary tract obstruction occurs. Complete obstruction to urine outflow associated with bacterial infection may result in destruction of renal parenchyma and septicemia within days. However, sterile nonobstructive nephroliths may persist for years without substantial change in urinary tract function.

Although spontaneous dissolution of nephroliths appears to be uncommon, it can occur. We have observed two cases of struvite renoliths in dogs in which uroliths underwent spontaneous dissolution. Spontaneous dissolution of canine nephroliths has also been reported by others. It is likely that spontaneous dissolution of infection-induced struvite uroliths is associated with abatement of the infection, rapid formation of large volumes of urine, or reduction in urine area concentration.

## DIAGNOSIS

Formation of nephroliths from less-soluble urine crystalloids is the result of congenital and/or acquired physiologic and pathologic processes. Proper management of nephrolithiasis requires a careful diagnostic work-up including urinalysis, urine culture, serum and urine chemistry evaluation, radiography and/or ultrasonography, and determination of the composition of the uroliths (Tables 3, 4, and 5). An understanding of the specific etiopathogenesis of each case is essential to proper management.

## MEDICAL MANAGEMENT

Although surgery may play an important role in therapy of nephrolithiasis, detection of nephroliths is not,

**Table 3.** *Problem-Specific Data Base for Nephrolithiasis*

1. Obtain appropriate history and perform physical examination, including rectal examination of urethra.
2. Perform complete urinalysis. If necessary, evaluate ability of the kidneys to concentrate urine. Save aliquot of urine for possible determination of mineral concentration.°
3. Perform complete blood cell count.
4. Perform serum biochemical profile with special emphasis on urea nitrogen, creatinine, calcium, phosphorus, uric acid, bicarbonate ($Tco_2$), and chloride concentrations.
5. Obtain quantitiative urine culture and determine urine urease activity; obtain antimicrobial susceptibility if bacterial pathogens are identified. Consider attempts to isolate ureaplasmas if urease-positive urine is bacteriologically sterile.
6. Obtain radiographs
   a. Take survey radiographs of entire urinary system.
   b. Consider IV urography for patients with renal or ureteral uroliths.
      1) Evaluate size and shape of kidneys.
      2) Evaluate patency of excretory pathway.
      3) Compare size of nephroliths detected by intravenous urography to size detected by survey radiography.
   c. Ultrasonography is recommended if equipment is available.
7. "Guesstimate" nephrolith composition (Table 5).
8. Initiate therapy to promote dissolution or arrested growth of uroliths, if necessary.
9. Initiate therapy to eradicate urinary tract infection, if present.
10. Remove kidney biopsy specimens for microscopic examination if nephrotomy is performed.
11. If irreversible anatomic defects are present, correct them during surgical procedure performed to remove uroliths.
12. Compare number of uroliths removed during surgery with number of uroliths identified by radiography; postsurgical radiographs should be obtained to evaluate completeness of urolith removal, if necessary.
13. Save all uroliths for quantitative analysis.
14. Initiate therapy to prevent recurrence of uroliths.
15. Formulate follow-up protocol with clients.

°The patient should be consuming food utilized at time of urolith formation. Alternately, a standardized diet designed to promote reproducible excretion of minerals in the urine of normal animals may be used.

in itself, an indication for surgery. Specific cases may be managed by medical therapy alone. All cases that require surgical intervention also require medical management. Persistent urinary tract disease and recurrence of urolithiasis may occur if surgical removal of nephroliths is the only form of therapy.

### Precautions

Nephroliths and/or ureteroliths causing outflow obstruction and substantial impairment of the function of

**Table 4.** *Radiodense Structures that May Resemble Nephroliths*

Mineralization of renal parenchyma
Radiodense intestinal ingesta
Radiodense medications in the intestinal tract
Large abdominal thela
Calcified lymph nodes
Osseous metaplasia of transitional epithelium
Cholecystoliths

**Table 5.** *Checklist of Factors that Suggest the Probable Mineral Composition of Canine and Feline Nephroliths*

1. Urine pH.
   a. Struvite and calcium apatite nephroliths—usually alkaline. Sterile struvite nephroliths may be observed when urine pH is 6.5 or higher.
   b. Ammonium urate nephroliths—acid to neutral.
   c. Cystine nephroliths—acid.°
   d. Calcium oxalate nephroliths—often acid to neutral.°
   e. Silica, nephroliths, acid to neutral° (only in dogs).
2. Identification of crystals in uncontaminated fresh urine sediment, preferably at body temperature.
3. Type of bacteria, if any, isolated from urine.
   a. Urease-producing bacterial especially staphylococci and less frequently *Proteus* spp. are typically associated with canine struvite nephroliths. Ureaplasmas may cause struvite nephroliths in dogs.
   b. UTI often are absent in patients with calcium oxalate, cystine, ammonium urate, and silica nephroliths.
   c. Calcium oxalate, cystine, ammonium urate, or silica nephroliths may predispose to UTI; if infections are caused by urease-producing bacteria, struvite may precipitate around metabolic nephroliths.
4. Radiographic density and physical characteristics of nephroliths.
   a. Nephroliths that are very large are commonly composed of infection-induced struvite.
   b. Nephroliths containing calcium salts are more radiodense than those containing other mineral types.
5. Serum chemistry evaluation.
   a. Hypercalcemia may be associated with calcium-containing nephroliths.
   b. Hyperuricemia may be associated with uric acid or urate nephroliths.
   c. Hyperchloremia, hypokalemia, and acidemia may be associated with distal renal tubular acidosis and calcium phosphate or struvite nephroliths.
6. Urine chemistry evaluation.
   a. Patient should be consuming a standardized diagnostic diet, or the diet consumed when uroliths formed.
   b. Excessive quantities of one or more minerals contained in the urolith are expected. The concentration of crystallization inhibitors may be decreased.
7. Breed of dog or cat and history of uroliths in patient's ancestors or littermates.
8. Quantitative analysis of uroliths fortuitously passed during micturition, or collected via catheter technique or voiding urohydropropulsion.

°Concomitant infection with urease-producing microbes may result in formation of an alkaline urine.

the associated kidney should be managed by surgical intervention, especially if associated with concomitant bacterial infection. Medical therapy designed to induce urolith dissolution over a period of several weeks is unlikely to be effective in patients with poorly functioning kidneys, since the urolith(s) will not be continually bathed with newly formed urine modified to induce litholysis.

### Struvite Nephroliths

We have successfully induced dissolution of nephroliths presumed to be composed of infection-induced struvite in six dogs. The mean time required for dissolution was $184 \pm 99$ days (range = 67 to 300 days). Although the dogs had varying degrees of impaired ca-

pacity to concentrate urine as a result of pyelonephritis, none had primary renal azotemia at the time therapy with calculolytic diet and antimicrobial agents was initiated. This point is emphasized because dogs with moderate to severe primary renal failure require a greater quantity of protein for anabolism than normal. The calculolytic diet (Prescription Diet Canine s/d, Hill's) used in our studies could induce or aggravate protein malnutrition if given for prolonged periods to dogs with moderate azotemic primary renal failure, or other concomitant disorders associated with protein malnutrition.

In general, we would not expect dietary and antimicrobial therapy to be effective in dissolving struvite ureteroliths causing partial outflow obstruction. To be dissolved, uroliths must be completely surrounded by urine that is undersaturated with struvite for prolonged periods. Intermittent passage of urine through a partially obstructed ureter would logically preclude dissolution of struvite ureteroliths.

### Calcium Oxalate Nephroliths

Medical protocols that will induce dissolution of calcium oxalate uroliths are a goal for the future. However, increases in the size and number of nonobstructing calcium oxalate nephroliths unassociated with urinary tract infection may be prevented by dietary and/or pharmacologic therapy. In our ongoing series, the size and number of nonobstructing calcium oxalate nephroliths did not increase in six dogs fed a diet restricted in sodium and protein and formulated to alkalinize urine for 5 to 8 months (Prescription Diet Canine u/d or similar prototype diets).

### Calcium Phosphate Nephroliths

Nephroliths composed of blood clots mineralized with calcium phosphate have been found in the renal pelvis and renal pelvic diverticula of cats. The formation of small quantities of highly concentrated urine may favor formation of blood clots in cats with renal hemorrhage. In our experience, such nephroliths often remain inactive for months to years. Consumption of a protein-restricted, sodium-restricted, alkalinizing diet may minimize hypercalciuria (also see "Canine and Feline Calcium Phosphate Urolithiasis," this volume, p 996).

### NEPHROTOMY

Recent observations in our veterinary teaching hospital indicate that the long-term consequences of nephrotomy on renal function should be evaluated in normal dogs and cats. We observed progressive reduction in the size of the right kidney of an 8-year-old female domestic shorthair cat during the 3-year period following nephrotomy to remove multiple calcium phosphate nephroliths. Although a similar number of calcium phosphate nephroliths in the left kidney were not removed, the left kidney did not change in size or morphology during the 3-year period of study. There has apparently been only one short-term (6 weeks) study of the effect of nephrotomy in normal dogs (Gahring et al., 1977). Results of that study revealed a 20 to 40% decline in glomerular filtration rate compared to presurgical values. Would further decline have been observed if dogs had been evaluated longer?

Surgical procedures that may be considered for removal of renoliths in dogs and cats include nephrolithotomy, pyelolithotomy, and nephrectomy (Osborne et al., 1993). Techniques utilized in humans that may have application for selected cases of nephrolithiasis in dogs and cats include percutaneous nephropyelostomy and autotransplantation (McCullogh and Ehrhart, 1974). The procedure of choice is determined principally by the likelihood of complete removal of the uroliths, and depends on their locations, size, and shape. Other important factors include the structural and functional integrity of affected and unaffected kidneys, the presence of concomitant but unrelated disorders that affect anesthetic and surgical risks, and the skill of the surgeon.

Nephroliths may be bilateral, forcing the surgeon to choose between simultaneous procedures and staged unilateral procedures. This decision should be based on the following factors: (1) renal function of the patient, (2) whether the renoliths are causing partial or complete obstruction to urine flow, (3) whether one kidney has severe infection resulting in systemic signs, and (4) the overall condition of the patient.

If staged unilateral procedures are necessary and urine flow is not obstructed, the choice of which kidney to repair first is a personal judgment. However, the surgeon should attempt to choose the kidney most likely to sustain the patient and least likely to be compromised by surgical intervention. If, after the first surgery, the second kidney is considered unsalvageable, it may be removed with the knowledge that the first kidney is more likely to provide adequate function.

Staged unilateral procedures should be separated by several weeks in patients with renal dysfunction. Nephrotomy further compromises the patient because of the irreversible loss of nephrons caused directly by the incision and indirectly by damage to transected vessels. The patient's renal function is assessed after the first surgery; plans for the second procedure are based on results of this reevaluation. There are two reports of spontaneous dissolution of struvite nephroliths in dogs with bilateral nephrolithiasis a few weeks after nephrotomy to remove stones from one kidney. Radiographs should be repeated prior to the second surgery to be sure the nephroliths are persistent.

## References and Suggested Reading

Gahring DR, et al: Comparative renal function studies of nephrectomy closure with and without sutures in dogs. J Am Vet Med Assoc 171:537, 1977.

Gregory JG, Park KY, and Burns TC: Effect of alkalinizing agents on calcium oxalate stone formation in a rat model. Urol Res 12:48, 1984.

Groen J: An experimental syndrome of fatty liver, uric acid, kidney stones, and acute pancreatitis produced in dogs by exclusive feeding of bacon. Science 107:425, 1948.

McCullogh KG and Ehrhart LA: Silica urolithiasis in laboratory dogs fed semisynthetic diets. J Am Vet Med Assoc 164:712, 1974.

Osborne CA, Lulich JP, Unger LK, Bartges JW, and Felice LJ: Canine and feline urolithiasis: Relationship of etiopathogenesis with treatment and prevention. *In* Bojrab MJ (eds): *Disease Mechanisms in Small Animal Surgery*, 2nd edition. Malvern, PA, Lea & Febiger, 1993, pp 464–511.

# *CVT* UPDATE: MANAGEMENT AND PREVENTION OF URATE UROLITHIASIS

GERALD V. LING
*and* JULIE L. SORENSON
*Davis, California*

## INTRODUCTION

Most cases of urate urolithiasis are in Dalmatians. Dalmatians are unique among dogs in that the principal urinary end-products of purine metabolism in this breed are sparingly soluble salts of uric acid, rather than allantoin which is very soluble. Dalmatians have a defective urate transport system within hepatocytes, the result of which is greatly decreased hepatic conversion of urate to allantoin. Also, a membrane transport defect is present in the kidneys of Dalmatians that results in reduced reabsorption of filtered urate in the renal tubules. Active renal tubular secretion of urate occurs as well. The result of these inherited abnormalities in Dalmatians is a urinary urate excretion of 200 to 800 mg (or more)/24 hr, as compared to a urinary urate excretion of about 50 mg/24 hours in other breeds of dogs that eliminate most of their purine breakdown products in the urine as allantoin.

Dalmatians that excrete more than 550 mg of urate

per 24 hr are at increased risk for urate urolithiasis because urate begins to precipitate at about this value. For unknown reasons, male Dalmatians are at much greater risk for urate stone disease than are female Dalmatians. In a recently published report of 275 stone-forming Dalmatians, the gender ratio encountered was 261 males/14 females (Case et al., 1993). However, reports of genetic studies that were conducted during the 1920s and 1930s indicated that the hyperuricosuric trait is not sex linked. Rather, it resided on a single pair of somatic, completely recessive genes (Sorenson and Ling, 1993a). Data from studies at the University of California suggest that male Dalmatians older than 5 years that have not formed calculi excrete more urinary urate on average than do non–stone-forming females of comparable age. Moreover, male Dalmatians that are stone formers excrete more urate than do non–stone formers of either gender. These data do not support the findings of earlier investigators who have reported that male and female Dalmatians have hyperuricosuria of equal magnitude. It is safe to say that the nature of the inheritance of hyperuricosuria and the gender influence as it relates to urate urolithiasis in Dalmatians are incompletely understood and that additional studies are needed.

Dogs and cats of any breed and either gender that have congenital or acquired portosystemic vascular shunts may have constant or intermittent urate crystalluria, urate calculi, or both. These animals typically are young adults up to about 4 years old, and the diagnosis of a shunt usually is made after, and indirectly as a result of, recognition of the urate crystals or calculi. Little is known regarding the mechanism by which urate calculi form in these animals except that it is related to the shunting of hepatic portal blood around the liver. Stones usually do not form again after a surgical procedure, such as ligation or banding of the shunt(s), that results in significantly increased portal blood flow through the liver.

Some dogs and cats of either gender form calculi that are composed of urate in combination with one or more other minerals such as struvite or (less commonly) silica. The urate is found during a layer-by-layer quantitative analysis of the calculi and usually is confined to a single layer of a multilayered specimen. In our experience, these animals very rarely test positive for portalsystemic shunts. At this time, it is not known for certain what the presence of urate in these "mixed" calculi signify or what, if anything, should be recommended as prevention.

## DIAGNOSIS AND MANAGEMENT

Urate calculi usually are multiple, small (range <1 mm to about 1.5 cm), smooth, green, and ovoid. Although they can form in dogs of any age, they form most commonly at about 4 to 5 years of age in male Dalmatians. Urate calculi are most often found in the urinary bladder or urethra (97%); only 3% occur in the kidneys or ureters. Stones that form in the urinary bladder often pass into the urethra in male dogs and may cause signs of partial or complete urinary obstruction such as stranguria, hematuria, and diminished or absent urine stream.

The diagnosis of urate urolithiasis can be difficult because urate calculi may be relatively or completely radiolucent. The radiopacity increases with increasing calculus size and when other minerals (e.g., calcium salts) are present in the calculi. Plain radiographs of the abdomen, contrast urethrocystography, abdominal ultrasonography, and/or intravenous pyelography may be used to diagnose and/or localize urate calculi.

The conventional approach to management of urate urolithiasis in Dalmatians, other canine breeds, and cats is surgical removal of all calculi. The obvious advantage of surgical intervention is that the patient is cured of its clinical problem, at least temporarily. Hydropropulsion of urethral calculi in male dogs back into the urinary bladder may be used in an attempt to temporarily relieve signs of urinary obstruction and gain time with which to prepare the patient for surgery. Hydropropulsion is not an alternative to surgery, however, because dogs that have obstructed once usually will do so again unless the offending concretions are removed. A disadvantage of surgery is that it may be difficult to remove all of the calculi because they are small, numerous, and radiolucent. Dissolution of urate calculi has been described in dogs (Osborne et al., 1989) but, for a variety of reasons including, but not limited to, poor results, we do not utilize it in most patients at this time.

Accurate quantitative analysis of urinary calculi is very important in the selection of management strategies to prevent recurrence of urolithiasis, even in Dalmatians. Dalmatians, especially females, can and do form calculi composed of minerals other than urate as well as mixtures of urate and other minerals (e.g., struvite). The presence of minerals other than urate must be taken into account whenever treatment and preventive management plans are formulated.

## PREVENTION

The cornerstone in the prevention of recurrence of urate stone disease in Dalmatians involves lowering the urate concentration of the urine. This is accomplished by (1) increasing water consumption; (2) feeding a low purine diet; (3) alkalinizing the urine; (4) control of urinary tract infections; and, most importantly, (5) partial blockade of the purine degradation pathway above the level of uric acid (see Fig. 1) by administration of a specific enzyme inhibitor, allopurinol (Table 1).

Maintaining dilute urine as a result of increased water consumption is recommended as a general means of decreasing crystalloid supersaturation in the urine. When the crystalloid concentration is low as a result of increased water consumption, calculus formation is less likely, in part because urinary volume and frequency of urinations are increased, resulting in quicker elimination of crystalloids before they can aggregate into larger

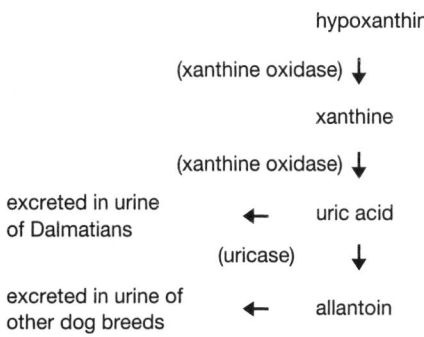

**Figure 1.** Pathway of purine metabolism.

concretions. The goal of this strategy is to achieve a repeatable urine specific gravity of about 1.018 in dogs and about 1.025 in cats. Our preferred method to increase water consumption is by giving an oral salt load in the form of KCl (light salt). KCl is available for pur-

**Table 1.** *Summary of Management and Prevention Steps for Urate Urolithiasis*

**Dalmatians**
1. Surgical removal of all calculi.
2. Increase water consumption to an amount that results in a repeatable specific gravity of about 1.018. Give encapsulated light salt (KCl) to effect.
3. Change the diet to one that has a high-quality, low-purine, plant-based protein source (e.g., Prescription Diet Canine k/d dry, u/d dry, or u/d canned, Hill's Pet Products).
4. Maintain the fasting urinary pH at a repeatable 7.0–7.5. Usually changing the diet (as in #3 above) will be sufficient to accomplish this. If not, use oral potassium citrate (initial dosage 100 mg/kg/day in two divided doses); adjust as needed to achieve the desired result.
5. Give allopurinol (initial dosage 10 mg/kg/day) orally; adjust the dose to achieve a urinary urate excretion of 300 mg/day (±25 mg) based upon determinations of urinary urate concentration conducted as per the protocol outlined below.
6. Remember that this therapy is lifelong. The compliance of even the most dedicated owners will "slip" a little unless continuing support and a stimulus to continue it are provided by the veterinarian. It is recommended that this support and stimulus be in the form of patient examinations twice each year and determination of 24-hr urinary urate excretion once each year.

**Cats and Non-Dalmatian Dogs**
1. Surgical removal of all calculi.
2. Increase water consumption to an amount that results in a repeatable specific gravity of about 1.018 for dogs and about 1.025 for cats. Give encapsulated light salt (KCl) to effect.
3. Maintain the fasting urinary pH at a repeatable 7.0–7.5. Usually changing the diet (see #4 below) will be sufficient to accomplish this. If not, use oral potassium citrate (initial dosage 100 mg/kg/day in two divided doses); adjust as needed to achieve the desired result.
4. Change the diet for dogs to one that has a high-quality, low-purine, plant-based protein source (e.g., Prescription Diet Canine k/d dry, u/d dry, or u/d canned, Hill's Pet Products). Change the diet for cats to one that is low in purine and low in magnesium (e.g., Purina Cat Chow dry). Commercial "acidified diets" should not be fed to these animals.
5. Since the majority of these animals have portal vascular anomalies, a decision to initiate a complete diagnostic work-up should be made if there is an intent to attempt surgical correction if a vascular anomaly is found.

chase only in granular form, but it can easily be capsulized by owners who have a supply of empty gelatin capsules of the appropriate size. Empty gelatin capsules are available from veterinary drug supply houses in a variety of sizes. Number 4 capsules usually are appropriate for cats, whereas number 2 or number 1 capsules are appropriate for Dalmatian-size dogs. Give one capsule filled with KCl twice daily, determine the urinary specific gravity after 4 to 7 days, and adjust the daily amount of salt administered to achieve the desired result.

Feeding a low-purine diet also can result in reduction of urinary urate. Diets containing lean meat and glandular organs have a high purine content, whereas diets composed of vegetable protein usually are much lower in purines. Alkalinization of the urine by administration of potassium citrate or sodium bicarbonate, or by feeding a diet that is high in vegetable protein, acts to decrease production of ammonia and ammonium ion by the kidneys. Moreover, urate is more soluble in urine pH at or above 7.0. The goal of urinary alkalinization is to achieve and maintain a fasting urine pH of 7.0 to 7.5. The fact that ammonium ion plays a role in the precipitation of urate in dogs emphasizes the importance of examining for and properly treating urinary tract infections in these patients. Infections with urease-producing bacteria result in urease-mediated hydrolysis of urea and production of ammonium ion as well as precipitation of struvite ($NH_4PO_4.6H_2O$).

Lowering the urinary urate excretion is most easily and dramatically achieved with the use of allopurinol. Allopurinol is an inhibitor of xanthine oxidase, the enzyme responsible for catalyzing the conversion of hypoxanthine and xanthine to uric acid (see Fig. 1). During treatment with allopurinol, hypoxanthine, xanthine and urate all are excreted in the urine. Each of these purine metabolites has a different urinary solubility; hypoxanthine is very soluble in urine, whereas xanthine and urate are only sparingly soluble. The goal of allopurinol therapy is to reduce (but not stop) the oxidation of xanthine to urate as a result of partial inhibition of the action of xanthine oxidase. As a result of inhibiting the action of xanthine oxidase, the xanthine concentration in the urine is allowed to increase. It is noteworthy that administration of excessive doses of allopurinol can cause hyperxanthinuria and formation of xanthine calculi (Ling et al., 1991). To minimize the possibility of excessive production of urinary xanthine, the dose of allopurinol must be adjusted to the needs of each patient. It is adjusted based upon the urate excretion value, since urate is easier to measure in the laboratory than is xanthine. In successfully treated Dalmatians, the goal is to achieve and maintain a 24-hr urate excretion of about 300 mg (± about 25 mg) (Table 2). At this rate of urate excretion, both urate and xanthine are below urinary supersaturation levels.

Evaluation of urinary urate excretion includes collection of all of the patient's urine for 24 hr. The urine must be kept at refrigerated temperatures during and after collection in order to minimize destruction of the urate by heat and bacterial action. The quantity of

**Table 2.** *Protocol for 24-Hr Urine Collection and Calculation of Urate Excretion*

1. Begin the collection period with the bladder empty. Catheterize male dogs to empty the bladder; allow female dogs to void. Discard this urine.
2. Maintain the patient in a cage during the collection period. Catheterize to empty the bladder (both sexes) as often as necessary to keep the patient comfortable during the collection period (usually three or four times).
3. During the collection period, give water, feed normal diet, and give allopurinol at the usual dose and dosing intervals. (**NOTE:** This is a critical step; it is very important that the patient consume the normal amount of food during the collection period. Failure to do so will result in a falsely low urate value. If problems enticing the patient to eat are anticipated, one successful strategy is to have the owner come to the hospital to feed the patient).
4. Catheterize to empty the bladder (both sexes) at the end of the 24-hr collection period. Dispense a broad-spectrum antimicrobial agent (e.g., trimethoprim-sulfa, cefadroxil, or amoxicillin-clavulanate) for 3 days to kill any bacterial pathogens that may have been introduced during the catheterization procedures.
5. Store all urine obtained in a large, clean, covered container in a refrigerator to minimize destruction of urate by heat and bacterial action.
6. Measure the total volume of urine collected as accurately as possible (in milliliters) and record this volume for use in subsequent calculations.
7. Mix the urine thoroughly to suspend any precipitate that formed in the bottom of the container; immediately fill a 10-ml clean, dry test tube with the well-mixed urine. (**NOTE:** This is a critical step; failure to achieve complete suspension of the precipitate during the decantation procedure will result in a falsely low urate value). Send the filled tube to a commercial laboratory for determination of urate concentration.
8. The laboratory will report the urate concentration in mg/dl (or mg % or mg/100 ml). Multiply this concentration by the total number of milliliters of urine that were collected during the 24-hr period divided by 100 (the number of 100s of ml that were collected). The product is the amount of urate excreted by the patient expressed in mg/24 hr.
9. The amount of excreted urate in successfully treated Dalmatians should be 300 mg/24 hr (± about 25 mg). Adjust the dosage of allopurinol as needed (down if the result is <300 mg/24 hr, up if the result is >300 mg/24 hr) and repeat the collection procedure every 2 to 3 weeks until the desired result is obtained.
10. Therapy will be lifelong. Repeat the collection procedure at least once each year throughout the life of the dog.

urine collected should be measured to the nearest 1 ml and this value recorded so that it may be referred to during subsequent calculations of urate excretion. Thorough mixing of the urine should immediately precede decantation of 5 to 10 ml into a clean, dry test tube that is sent to a commercial laboratory for urate determination. The laboratory will report the urine urate result in mg/100 ml (or mg/dl or mg %). This value must be multiplied by the number of deciliters of urine collected in order to determine the urinary urate excretion per 24 hr (see below for details).

A "spot" test of urine, the result of which is calculated from the ratio of urinary urate/urinary creatinine concentrations determined on a random sample of urine, has been recommended for use in diagnosis and assessment of effectiveness of management strategies in Dalmatians (Senior, 1989). Currently, we believe that postprandial excretion of urinary urate in Dalmatians increases relative to the amount of purine in the meal, the amount of food consumed, and the genetics of the patient in question. This increase is variable for approximately an 8-hr period following ingestion of food. After about 8 hr, the urate excretion curve becomes more or less horizontal. Theoretically, in order to avoid this variability, this test must be conducted on urine from animals that have undergone at least an 8-hr fast and that have voided completely at least once after the fast. However, preliminary results at the University of California indicate that, even from this part of the curve, results of the spot test are too variable to be used accurately for monitoring of treatment in Dalmatians. Unfortunately, this may leave no alternative but to conduct 24-hr urine collections and urate determinations (Table 2).

As indicated above, prevention of urate stone disease in dogs and cats with shunts is best affected by surgical repair of the vascular anomaly. If this is not possible, the patient may be managed using the same basic medical and dietary strategies used in stone-forming Dalmatians, with the exception of allopurinol. Allopurinol should not be given to urate stone-forming, shunt patients for the following reasons.

1. The genetic abnormalities that result in hyperuricosuria in Dalmatians are not present in these animals.

2. The magnitude of urinary urate excretion in these animals has not been documented adequately but it may be substantially less than the 600 to 900 mg urate/24 hr that is commonly seen in stone-forming Dalmatians.

3. The therapeutic half-life of allopurinol, which is relatively short in normal dogs, may be greatly prolonged in shunt patients with impaired liver function. This may cause unrecognized but prolonged overdosing of allopurinol if it is used at the same dose and dosing interval recommended for stone-forming Dalmatians. Overdosing will increase the degree of inhibition of xanthine oxidase and may increase the likelihood of xanthine stone disease.

## References and Suggested Reading

Case LC, Ling GV, Ruby AL, et al: Urolithiasis in dalmatians: 275 cases (1981–1990). J Am Vet Med Assoc 203:96, 1993.
   *Presentation of the results of calculus analyses, bacterial isolations, age and gender distributions, and estimation of relative risk of contracting stone disease in 275 stone-forming Dalmatians.*
Ling GV, Ruby AL, Harrold DR, et al: Xanthine-containing urinary calculi in dogs given allopurinol. J Am Vet Med Assoc 198:1935, 1991.
   *Presentation of the clinical features and laboratory findings in 10 dogs that formed xanthine uroliths while receiving allopurinol.*
Osborne CA, Polzin DJ, Johnston GR, et al: Canine urolithiasis. In Ettinger SJ (ed): Textbook of Veterinary Internal Medicine, 3rd edition. Philadelphia, WB Saunders Co, 1989, p 2083.
   *A review of the diagnosis and management of the various types of uroliths formed by dogs.*
Senior DF: Medical management of urate urolithiasis. In Kirk RW (ed): Current Veterinary Therapy X. Philadelphia, WB Saunders Co, 1989, p 1178.
   *A review of diagnosis and management, including dietary dissolution strategies, of urate urolithiasis in dogs.*

Sorenson JL and Ling GV: Metabolic and genetic aspects of urate urolithiasis in Dalmatians. J Am Vet Med Assoc 203:857, 1993a.
*A literature review of metabolic aspects and genetics of urate urolithiasis in dogs.*

Sorenson JL and Ling GV: Diagnosis, prevention and treatment of urate urolithiasis in Dalmatians. J Am Vet Med Assoc 203:863, 1993b.
*A literature review of diagnosis, treatment, and prevention of urate urolithiasis in Dalmatians.*

# FELINE CALCIUM OXALATE UROLITHS

CARL A. OSBORNE,
JODY P. LULICH,
*and* ROSAMA THUMCHAI
*St. Paul, Minnesota*

## CLINICAL AND EXPERIMENTAL OBSERVATIONS RELATED TO DIAGNOSIS AND TREATMENT

In our most recent series, calcium oxalate comprised 27% (1278/4800) of feline uroliths analyzed by quantitative methods at the Minnesota Urolith Center (Tables 1 and 2). They were detected more commonly in the lower than the upper urinary tract. Male cats (57%) were affected more than females (43%). Neutered males (51%) and neutered females (39%) were affected more often than intact males (6%) and intact females (4%). The mean age of affected cats was 7.2 ± 3.5 years (range = 3 months to 22 years). Case control epidemiologic studies performed at the University of Minnesota indicate a higher prevalence of calcium oxalate uroliths in Burmese, Himalayan, and Persian breeds (Table 2).

In most cases with calcium oxalate uroliths, serum concentrations of minerals, including calcium, have been normal. However, mild hypercalcemia (11.1 to 13.5 mg/dl) has been observed with sufficient frequency to warrant routine evaluation of serum calcium concentrations in affected patients. Hypercalcemia promotes urinary calcium excretion, and may result in precipitation of calcium oxalate crystals. Although primary hyperparathyroidism has been recognized as a cause of hypercalcemia and calcium oxalate uroliths in cats, the underlying cause of hypercalcemia in most cats with calcium oxalate uroliths has not been determined. The relationship between hypercalcemia, parathormone secretion, vitamin D homeostasis, and calcium oxalate urolith formation is deserving of further study.

Cats with calcium oxalate urolithiasis typically have concentrated (mean pretreatment urine specific gravity of about 1.040) and acid (urine pH of 6.3 to 6.7) urine. Pretreatment blood pH is often reduced (pH = 7.3). The association between aciduria, acidemia, and calcium oxalate urolithiasis may be that acidemia promotes mobilization of carbonate and phosphorus from bones to buffer hydrogen ions. Concomitant mobilization of bone calcium may result in hypercalciuria.

It is noteworthy that magnesium has been reported to be a calcium oxalate inhibitor in rats and humans (Osborne et al., 1986). For this reason, orally administered magnesium was at one time recommended to prevent recurrence of calcium oxalate uroliths. It also is of interest that use of urine acidifiers and/or supplemental sodium (usually sodium chloride) has been associated with hypercalciuria in some species. Because therapy of feline struvite uroliths often encompasses restriction of magnesium, sodium chloride–induced diuresis, and acidification of urine, the relationship of these factors to feline calcium oxalate uroliths deserves further study.

## TREATMENT AND PREVENTION

Medical protocols that will promote dissolution of calcium oxalate uroliths in cats are unavailable. Urocystoliths small enough to pass through the urethra may be removed by voiding urohydropropulsion (Lulich et al., 1993). Very small urocystoliths may be retrieved with the aid of a urinary catheter (Lulich and Osborne, 1992). Surgery is the only practical alternative for removal of larger calcium oxalate uroliths. However, some calcium oxalate uroliths, especially those located

**Table 1.** *Location of 1278 Feline Calcium Oxalate Uroliths*

| Site | Number | % |
|------|--------|---|
| Kidney | 39 | 3 |
| Ureter | 22 | 2 |
| Kidney and ureter | 7 | <1 |
| Kidney and bladder | 8 | <1 |
| Ureter and bladder | 5 | <1 |
| Ureter, bladder, and urethra | 1 | <1 |
| Ureter and urethra | 1 | <1 |
| Urinary bladder | 884 | 70 |
| Urethra | 100 | 8 |
| Urinary bladder and urethra | 108 | 8 |
| Kidney, ureter, bladder, and urethra | 1 | <1 |
| Voided | 52 | 4 |
| Unknown | 50 | 4 |
| TOTAL | 1278 | 100 |

**Table 2.** *Common Characteristics of Feline Calcium Oxalate Uroliths*

| Chemical Name | Formula | Crystal Name |
|---|---|---|
| Calcium oxalate monohydrate | $CaC_2O_4 \cdot H_2O$ | Whewellite |
| Calcium oxalate dihydrate | $CaC_2O_4 \cdot 2H_2O$ | Weddellite |

**Variations in Composition**
  Calcium oxalate monohydrate only
  Calcium oxalate dihydrate only
  Combinations of calcium oxalate monohydrate and dihydrate
  Calcium oxalate (monohydrate and/or dihydrate) mixed with variable quantities of calcium phosphate; variable quantities of struvite or ammonium acid urate may also be present
  Calcium oxalate (monohydrate and/or dihydrate) nucleus surrounded by other minerals, especially infection-induced struvite

**Physical Characteristics**
  Color:
    Calcium oxalate monohydrate uroliths are usually tan or brown
    Calcium oxalate dihydrate uroliths are usually white or cream colored. Their surfaces may be red to black if they are coated with blood
  Shape: Variable
    Calcium oxalate monohydrate uroliths are usually round or elliptical and have a smooth, polished surface; on occasion, they may develop a jackstone or mulberry shape
    Calcium oxalate dihydrate uroliths and mixed calcium oxalate monohydrate-calcium oxalate dihydrate uroliths are usually round to ovoid and have an irregular surface caused by protrusion of sharp-edged crystals; on occasion they may develop a jackstone shape.
  Nuclei: Nuclei, radial striations, and concentric laminations may occur
  Density: Very dense and brittle; survey radiographs reveal that they are radiodense compared with soft tissue
  Number: Single or multiple
  Location: May be located in renal pelves, ureters, urinary bladder (most common), and/or urethra
  Size: Subvisual to several centimeters

**Prevalence**
  30 to 40% of uroliths
  May be recurrent

**Characteristics of Affected Feline Patients**
  More common in males, 56%, than females, 44%
  Mean age of diagnosis is about 7 years (range = <1 to >20 yr)
  Most commonly observed in Burmese, Himalayan, and Persian breeds

in the kidneys, may remain clinically silent for months to years. Because of the unavoidable destruction of nephrons during nephrectomy, this procedure is not recommended unless it can be established that the stones are a cause of clinically significant disease. Serially performed urinalyses, renal function tests, serum electrolyte evaluations, and ultrasonographic and/or radiographic studies may be indicated to determine whether calcium oxalate nephrolits are clinically active.

Following urolith removal, medical protocols should be considered to minimize urolith recurrence or to prevent further growth of uroliths remaining in the urinary tract. In general, medical therapy should be formulated in a stepwise fashion, with the initial goal of reducing urine concentration of calculogenic substances. Medications that have the potential to induce a sustained alteration in body composition of metabolites, in addition to urine concentration of metabolites, should be reserved for patients with active or frequently recurrent calcium oxalate uroliths. Caution must be used so that side effects of treatment are not more detrimental than the effects of uroliths. In cats with hypercalcemia, the cause of hypercalcemia (e.g., primary hyperparathyroidism) should be corrected. Whether calcium oxalate uroliths remaining in the patient following parathyroidectomy will subsequently dissolve is unknown; however, calcium oxalate urolith growth or recurrence is less likely. In patients with normal serum calcium concentrations, an attempt should be made to identify risk factors for urolith formation. Amelioration or control of the consequences of risk factors should minimize urolith growth and recurrence.

## Dietary Considerations

Although reduction of urine calcium and oxalic acid concentrations by reduction of dietary calcium and oxalic acid appears to be a logical therapeutic goal, it is not necessarily harmless. Reducing consumption of only one of these constituents (such as calcium) may increase the availability of the other (such as oxalic acid) for intestinal absorption and subsequent urinary excretion. In general, reduction in dietary calcium should be accompanied by an appropriate reduction in dietary oxalic acid.

Humans with calcium oxalate uroliths are often advised to avoid milk and milk products because the carbohydrate component (lactose) of these products may augment intestinal absorption of calcium from any dietary source (Osborne et al., 1986). Likewise, they are often discouraged from consuming foods containing relatively high quantities of oxalic acid (chocolate, nuts, beans, sweet potatoes, wheat germ, spinach, and rhubarb).

Consumption of high levels of sodium may augment renal excretion of calcium; 24-hr urinary calcium excretion of normal dogs consuming diets with 0.8% sodium (dry weight analysis) was comparable to calcium excretion observed in dogs with naturally occurring calcium oxalate uroliths. If similar results occur in cats, moderate dietary restriction of sodium would be a logical recommendation for active calcium oxalate urolith formers.

Dietary phosphorus should not be restricted in patients with calcium oxalate urolithiasis because reduction in dietary phosphorus may be associated with activation of vitamin D, which in turn promotes intestinal calcium absorption and subsequent urinary calcium excretion. In addition, pyrophosphate is an inhibitor of calcium oxalate urolith formation. If calcium oxalate urolithiasis is associated with hypophosphatemia and normal serum calcium concentration, oral phosphorus supplementation may be considered (Neutra-Phos, Willen Drug Company, Baltimore, MD). Caution must be used, however, since excessive dietary phosphorus may predispose to formation of calcium phosphate uroliths (also see "Canine and Feline Calcium Phosphate Urolithiasis," this volume, p 996).

Increased urine magnesium concentration reduces formation of calcium oxalate crystals *in vitro*. For this reason, supplemental magnesium has been used to minimize recurrence of calcium oxalate uroliths in humans. However, supplemental dietary magnesium may contribute to formation of magnesium ammonium phosphate uroliths and hypercalciuria. Pending further studies, we do not recommend dietary magnesium restriction or supplementation for treatment of calcium oxalate uroliths in cats.

Ingestion of foods that contain high quantities of animal protein may contribute to calcium oxalate urolithiasis by increasing urinary calcium and oxalic acid excretion, and by decreasing urinary citric acid excretion. Some of these consequences result from obligatory acid excretion associated with protein metabolism.

A diet with reduced quantities of protein, calcium, and sodium and one that does not promote formation of acidic urine (such as Prescription Diet Feline k/d, Hill's Pet Products, Topeka, KS) should be considered to help minimize recurrence of active calcium oxalate uroliths in cats. We have had success in reducing mild hypercalcemia in some calcium oxalate urolith–forming cats by feeding a high-fiber reducing diet (Prescription Diet Feline w/d, Hill's). Ideally, diets should not be restricted or supplemented with phosphorus or magnesium. Excessive levels of vitamin D (which promotes intestinal absorption of calcium) and ascorbic acid (a precursor of oxalate) should also be avoided. The diet should be adequately fortified with vitamin $B_6$, since vitamin $B_6$ deficiency promotes endogenous production and subsequent urinary excretion of oxalic acid.

The relationship of water content in the diet and formation of uroliths has also been studied in cats by several investigators. Factors involved include dietary moisture, drinking behavior, digestibility of food and its relationship to fecal water loss, and the quantity of sodium chloride in the diet. Because of numerous variables, a cause-and-effect relationship between dietary moisture, urine volume, and urolithiasis has not been clearly established. Pending further studies, it is logical to recommend consideration of highly digestible, high-moisture diets to minimize recurrence of uroliths.

### Citrate

Citric acid inhibits calcium oxalate crystal formation because of its ability to form soluble salts with calcium. This may explain why some humans with abnormally low quantities of urine citric acid are at risk for development of calcium oxalate uroliths (Pak et al., 1984). Oral administration of potassium citrate (approximately 90 mg/kg/day) to human patients has been associated with marked increases in urinary citric acid excretion. Potassium citrate also may be beneficial in the management of calcium oxalate because of its alkalinizing effects. In dogs, chronic metabolic acidosis inhibits renal tubular reabsorption of calcium, whereas metabolic

alkalosis enhances tubular reabsorption of calcium (Marone et al., 1983). Potassium citrate (Urocit-K, Mission Pharmacal; Polycitra-K, Willen) is preferred to sodium bicarbonate as an alkalinizing agent because oral administration of sodium may enhance urinary calcium excretion. We currently recommend a dose of 80 to 120 mg/kg/day (divided into two or three subdoses).

### Vitamin $B_6$

Vitamin $B_6$ increases the transamination of glyoxylate, an important precursor of oxalic acid, to glycine. Although experimentally induced vitamin $B_6$ deficiency resulted in renal precipitation of calcium oxalate and hyperoxaluria in kittens (Bai et al., 1989), a naturally occurring form of this syndrome has not been observed. In our hospital, administration of vitamin $B_6$ (10 mg/kg/day) to a normal cat for 10 days was not associated with decreased urine oxalic acid concentration ($1.13 \pm 0.11$ mmol/L prior to vitamin $B_6$ supplementation compared to $1.39 \pm 0.19$ mmol/L during vitamin $B_6$ administration) (Lulich et al., in press). Although additional vitamin $B_6$ was associated with decreased oxalic acid excretion in cats consuming diets deficient in vitamin $B_6$, the ability of supplemental vitamin $B_6$ to reduce urinary oxalic acid excretion in cats with calcium oxalate uroliths consuming diets with adequate quantities of vitamin $B_6$ is unknown.

### Thiazide Diuretics

Thiazide diuretics have been recommended to reduce recurrence of calcium-containing uroliths in humans because of their ability to reduce urine calcium excretion (also see "Canine Calcium Oxalate Urolithiasis," this volume, p 992). Although hydrochlorothiazide diuretics may be beneficial in minimizing urinary calcium excretion in humans and dogs, no data have been provided to indicate their efficacy in cats with calcium oxalate uroliths. Because thiazide diuretic administration can be associated with adverse affects (dehydration, hyopkalemia, hypercalcemia), we do not recommend their use, pending further evaluation.

### Recurrent Struvite and Calcium Oxalate Uroliths

In those situations where cats have documented occurrences of both calcium oxalate and struvite urolithiasis, uncontrollable risk factors (defective inhibitors of crystal aggregation) may be present. If struvite urolithiasis is associated with urease-positive urinary tract infections, appropriate therapy should be devised to eradicate the urinary tract infection (UTI) and prevent its recurrence.

When considering dietary management, we recommend that emphasis be placed on minimizing recurrence of calcium oxalate uroliths, since this type of urolith cannot be dissolved by medical management. Should struvite uroliths recur, they often can be dissolved by dietary management (Prescription Diet Feline s/d, Hill's) and, if necessary, antimicrobial agents. This strategy tends to minimize the need for repeated surgical intervention.

### Follow-up Evaluation

Regardless of the type of preventive management selected to minimize recurrent urolithiasis, periodic reevaluation of the patient to determine efficacy of treatment is highly recommended. Special emphasis should be placed on evaluation of urine specific gravity, urine pH, crystalluria, and evidence of UTI. If risk factors for a type of urolith other than one being managed are discovered, appropriate adjustments in management should be made.

In our experience, a commonly encountered problem associated with recurrent urolithiasis has been the lack of owner or patient compliance. Giving the patient a variety of treats is especially noteworthy. To eliminate this problem, we advise owners to give treats comprised of the preventive diet being utilized.

### References and Suggested Reading

Bai SC, Sampson DA, Morris JG, et al: Vitamin B-6 requirement of growing kittens. J Nutr 119:1020, 1989.

Lulich JP, et al: Nonsurgical removal of urocystoliths in dogs and cats by voiding urohydropropulsion. J Am Vet Med Assoc 202:660, 1993.

Lulich JP, et al: Feline calcium oxalate urolithiasis: Cause, detection, control. In August JR (ed): Consultations in Feline Internal Medicine 2. Philadelphia, WB Saunders Co, pp 343–349, 1994.

Lulich JP and Osborne CA: Catheter assisted retrieval of urocystoliths from dogs and cats. J Am Vet Med Assoc 201:111, 1992.

Marone CC, et al: Effects of metabolic alkalosis on calcium excretion in the conscious dog. J Lab Clin Med 101:264, 1983.

McKerrell RE, et al: Primary hyperoxaluria (L-glyceric aciduria) in the cat: A newly recognized inherited disease. Vet Res 125:31, 1989.

Osborne CA, et al: Etiopathogenesis, clinical manifestations and management of canine calcium oxalate urolithiasis. Vet Clin North Am 16:133, 1986.

Pak CYC, et al: Augmentation of renal citrate excretion by oral potassium citrate administration: Time course, dose frequency schedule, and dose-response relationship. J Clin Pharmacol 24:19, 1984.

# CANINE CALCIUM OXALATE UROLITHS

JODY P. LULICH
and CARL A. OSBORNE
St. Paul, Minnesota

Struvite, urate, and cystine uroliths dissolve when supersaturation of urine with calculogenic substances is abolished. Unfortunately, we have not been able to dissolve calcium oxalate uroliths in dogs and cats. Physically removing calcium oxalate uroliths remains the only method to resolve clinically active disease. Surgery is a relatively easy method to remove calcium oxalate uroliths from the urinary tract; however, because of the small size and irregular contour of many calcium oxalate uroliths, complete surgical removal of all uroliths may be difficult. Small urocystoliths can be removed by voiding urohydropropulsion or (see elsewhere in this section) transurethral catheterization and aspiration instead of cystotomy. In patients with clinically silent calcium oxalate uroliths, surgical intervention may not be necessary. With clinically silent uroliths that are not removed, the clinical status of the patient should be assessed by urinalyses, renal function tests, and/or radiography at appropriate intervals.

## PREVENTING UROLITH RECURRENCE

Most dogs who have formed calcium oxalate uroliths are likely to form them again. In one study, uroliths recurred following surgery in 3% of dogs by 3 months, 9% by 6 months, 36% by 1 year, and 48% by 2 years (Lulich et al., 1992). These results emphasize the need for medical protocols to minimize urolith recurrence following urolith removal.

Medical therapy should be formulated in a stepwise fashion, with the initial goal of reducing urine concentration of calculogenic substances. Caution must be used so that side effects of treatment are not more detrimental than the effects of uroliths. In order to prevent urolith recurrence, we use the following chronological sequence: (1) obtain baseline data, (2) eliminate iatrogenic risk factors, (3) provide dietary modification, (4) consider pharmacologic intervention, and (5) monitor urolith recurrence (Fig. 1).

### Baseline Data

In order to assess the effectiveness of therapy, the current status of the patient must be determined. For example, if all uroliths were not completely removed by surgery and radiographs were not immediately obtained following surgery, it would be impossible to distinguish surgical failure from medical failure as the cause of uroliths detected at a later date. Flushing the urinary bladder and urethra at the time of surgery is

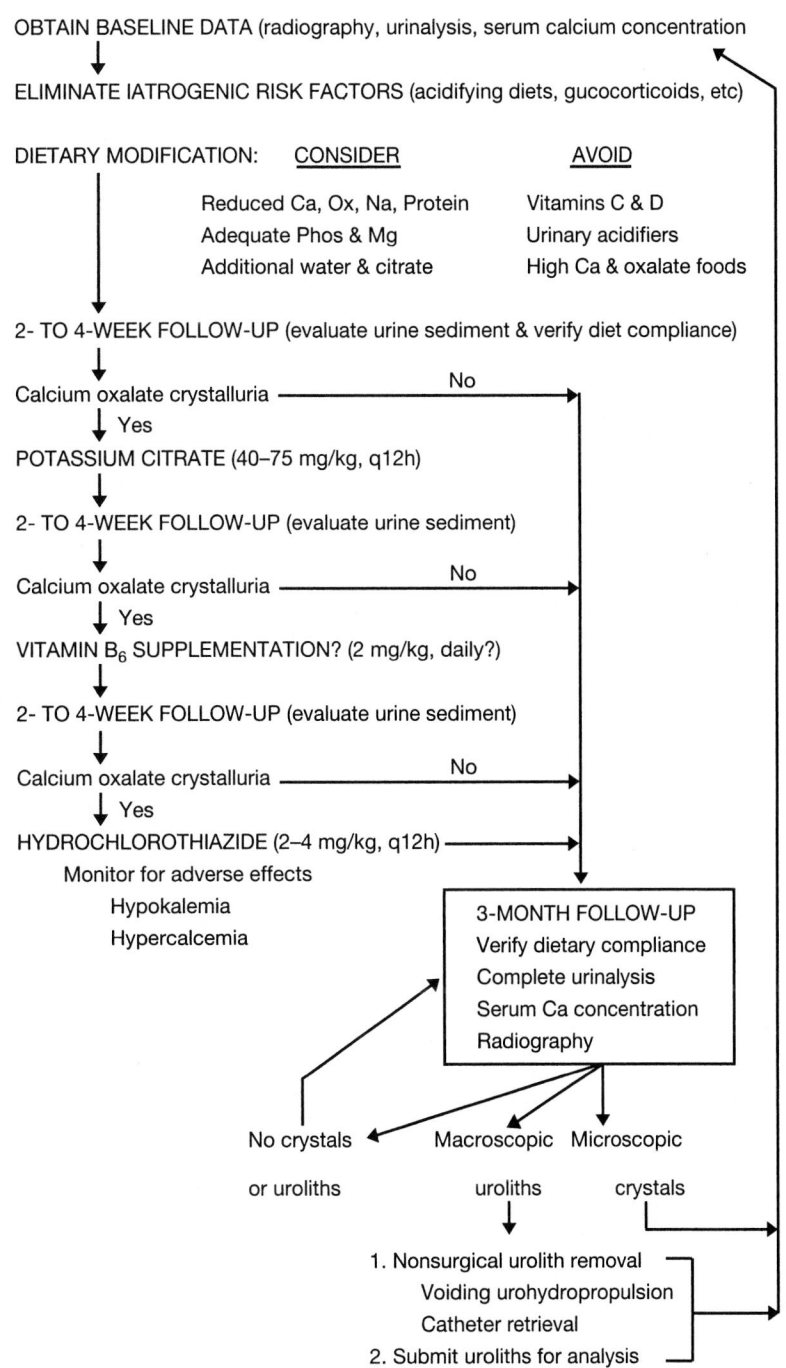

OBTAIN BASELINE DATA (radiography, urinalysis, serum calcium concentration

ELIMINATE IATROGENIC RISK FACTORS (acidifying diets, gucocorticoids, etc)

DIETARY MODIFICATION:  CONSIDER  AVOID

Reduced Ca, Ox, Na, Protein  Vitamins C & D
Adequate Phos & Mg  Urinary acidifiers
Additional water & citrate  High Ca & oxalate foods

2- TO 4-WEEK FOLLOW-UP (evaluate urine sediment & verify diet compliance)

Calcium oxalate crystalluria ——— No

Yes

POTASSIUM CITRATE (40–75 mg/kg, q12h)

2- TO 4-WEEK FOLLOW-UP (evaluate urine sediment)

Calcium oxalate crystalluria ——— No

Yes

VITAMIN $B_6$ SUPPLEMENTATION? (2 mg/kg, daily?)

2- TO 4-WEEK FOLLOW-UP (evaluate urine sediment)

Calcium oxalate crystalluria ——— No

Yes

HYDROCHLOROTHIAZIDE (2–4 mg/kg, q12h) ———

Monitor for adverse effects
Hypokalemia
Hypercalcemia

3-MONTH FOLLOW-UP
Verify dietary compliance
Complete urinalysis
Serum Ca concentration
Radiography

No crystals  Macroscopic  Microscopic

or uroliths  uroliths  crystals

1. Nonsurgical urolith removal
Voiding urohydropropulsion
Catheter retrieval
2. Submit uroliths for analysis

**Figure 1.** Algorithmic approach to the management of canine calcium oxalate urolithiasis.

not a reliable method to ensure complete urolith removal. In a retrospective study, uroliths were not completely removed from the urinary bladder in one of every seven dogs and one of every five cats following cystotomy (Lulich et al., 1993). Therefore, prior to initiating medical therapy, radiography should be performed to verify urolith status. Rectal palpation may be helpful in detecting uroliths lodged in the pelvic urethra.

A urinalysis should be used to screen for crystalluria and bacteriuria. If calcium oxalate crystals are detected, therapy should be designed and monitored to ensure that crystals no longer form. Bacteriuria mandates treatment with appropriate antimicrobials selected on the basis of culture and susceptibility results.

It is also helpful to assess serum calcium concentration. Hypercalcemia warrants further evaluation of the underlying cause. If the underlying cause can be determined and corrected, further therapy for calcium oxalate urolithiasis is usually unnecessary. In dogs with normal serum calcium concentrations, risk factors for urolith formation should be identified and controlled. This may require lifelong therapy.

## Eliminate Iatrogenic Risk Factors

Several commonly used medications augment excretion of calcium and oxalate and therefore promote calcium oxalate urolith formation. Diets that promote formation of acidic urine are beneficial in preventing struvite urolith formation; however, acidosis is a risk factor for calcium oxalate urolith formation. To neutralize acidifying metabolites in diets, phosphate and carbonate are mobilized from bone. Calcium mobilized during this process is subsequently excreted in urine. Metabolic acidosis also inhibits renal tubular reabsorption of calcium. Therefore, acidifying diets as well as urine acidifiers (ammonium chloride and methionine) should be avoided in dogs predisposed to calcium oxalate urolith formation.

Glucocorticoids enhance bone resorption and increase urine calcium excretion. Therefore, these compounds should also be avoided in dogs with calcium oxalate uroliths. Likewise, affected dogs with concomitant hyperadrenocorticism should be appropriately treated to minimize excessive endogenous glucocorticoid release.

Diuretics have been recommended for dogs with uroliths to dilute the concentrations of minerals in urine. However, the success of diuretic therapy depends on the type administered. After an initial natriuresis, thiazide diuretics promote sodium reabsorption and subsequently calcium reabsorption. However, loop diuretics (furosemide) promote sodium and calcium excretion and therefore should not be used to treat dogs with calcium oxalate uroliths. Alternatives to diuretics to promote dilution of urine include provision of canned instead of dry diets, or addition of water to food.

Supplements containing vitamin D and vitamin C should be discontinued in dogs with calcium oxalate uroliths. Vitamin D promotes intestinal calcium absorption and subsequent urinary calcium excretion. Vitamin C is a precursor of oxalate.

## Diet Modification

Increased gastrointestinal absorption of calcium has been recognized in dogs with calcium oxalate urolithiasis (Lulich et al., 1991). Based on this finding, reduction of dietary calcium appears to be a logical recommendation. However, this is not necessarily a harmless maneuver. Reducing the consumption of calcium may increase the bioavailability of oxalate for intestinal absorption and subsequent urinary excretion. In general, reduction of dietary calcium should be accompanied by an appropriate reduction in dietary oxalate.

Humans with calcium oxalate uroliths are often cautioned to avoid milk and milk products because their carbohydrate component (lactose) may augment intestinal absorption of calcium from any dietary source. Likewise, they are often discouraged from consuming foods containing relatively high quantities of oxalic acid (chocolate, nuts, beans, sweet potatoes, wheat germ, spinach, and rhubarb).

Consumption of high levels of sodium increases renal excretion of calcium. The 24-hr urinary calcium excretion by normal dogs consuming diets with 0.8% sodium (dry weight analysis) was comparable to calcium excretion observed in dogs with naturally occurring calcium oxalate uroliths. Therefore, moderate dietary restriction of sodium (0.30% dry weight or less) is recommended for active calcium oxalate urolith formers.

Dietary phosphorus should not be restricted in patients with calcium oxalate urolithiasis because reduction in dietary phosphorus may be associated with activation of vitamin D. Activation of vitamin D in turn promotes intestinal calcium absorption and subsequent urinary calcium excretion. In addition, pyrophosphates are inhibitors of calcium oxalate urolith formation. If calcium oxalate urolithiasis is associated with hypophosphatemia and normal serum calcium concentration, oral phosphorus supplementation may be considered (Neutra-Phos, Willen Drug Company, Baltimore, MD) to achieve normal blood concentrations of phosphorus.

Increased urine magnesium concentration reduces formation of calcium oxalate crystals *in vitro*. For this reason, supplemental magnesium has been recommended to minimize recurrence of calcium oxalate uroliths in man. However, supplemental dietary magnesium may contribute to formation of magnesium ammonium phosphate uroliths and hypercalciuria in dogs. Pending further studies, we do not recommend dietary magnesium restriction or supplementation for treatment of calcium oxalate uroliths.

Ingestion of foods that contain high quantities of animal protein may contribute to calcium oxalate urolithiasis by increasing urinary calcium and oxalic acid excretion, and by decreasing urinary citric acid excretion (Goldfarb, 1988). Some of these diet-mediated effects result from obligatory acid excretion associated with protein metabolism.

A diet moderately restricted in protein, calcium, oxalate, and sodium (i.e., Prescription Diet Canine u/d, Hill's, Topeka KS) may be considered to help prevent recurrence of active calcium oxalate uroliths in dogs. Additional benefits of this diet are that it contains potassium citrate, a urine alkalinizing agent. Other diets that may also be beneficial include Prescription Diet Canine w/d (Hill's, Topeka KS) and Prescription Diet Canine k/d (Hill's, Topeka KS). Ideally, diets should not be restricted or supplemented with phosphorus or magnesium.

## Pharmacologic Treatment

The decision to institute pharmacologic therapy is based on detection of persistent calcium oxalate crystalluria or recurrence of uroliths despite diet modification. If pharmacologic therapy is needed, it should be initiated in a stepwise fashion, evaluating urinalyses before selecting additional medications.

Citric acid inhibits calcium oxalate crystal formation because of its ability to form soluble salts with calcium.

This may explain why some people with abnormally low quantities of urine citrate are at risk for development of calcium oxalate uroliths. Oral administration of potassium citrate (approximately 90 mg/kg/day) to people has been associated with marked increases in urinary citrate excretion. However, administration of up to 150 mg/kg/day of potassium citrate to normal dogs was not associated with a consistent increase in urine citrate concentration. Nonetheless, a dose-dependent rise in urine pH did occur. These results suggest that metabolism and excretion of potassium citrate in dogs differ from that in humans. While 10 to 35% of filtered citrate is excreted in urine by humans, only 1 to 3% of filtered citrate is excreted by dogs (Simpson, 1983).

Even though administration of potassium citrate orally may not be associated with a sustained increase in urine citrate concentration, potassium citrate may be beneficial in management of calcium oxalate because of its alkalinizing effect. In dogs, chronic metabolic acidosis inhibits renal tubular reabsorption of calcium, whereas metabolic alkalosis enhances tubular reabsorption of calcium. Potassium citrate is preferred to sodium bicarbonate as an alkalinizing agent because oral administration of sodium enhances urine calcium excretion. A commercially available diet (Prescription Diet Canine u/d) contains potassium citrate. If hypocitrituria is recognized in dogs (mean and median urinary citrate excretion of 33 normal beagles was 2.57 ± 2.31 mg/kg/24 hr, and 1.88 mg/kg/24 hr, respectively), wax matrix tablets of potassium citrate (Urocit-K, Mission Pharmacal) may be considered. Potassium citrate can also be initiated if urine remains persistently acidic. We currently recommend a dose of 50 to 75 mg/kg every 12 hr; tablets can be broken into smaller pieces and then mixed with food.

### VITAMIN B6

Vitamin $B_6$ increases the transamination of glyoxylate, an important precursor of oxalic acid, to glycine. Although experimentally induced vitamin $B_6$ deficiency resulted in renal precipitation of calcium oxalate and hyperoxaluria in kittens (Bai et al., 1989), a naturally occurring form of this syndrome has not been observed. In our hospital, administration of vitamin $B_6$ (10 mg/kg/day) to a normal cat for 10 days was not associated with decreased urine oxalic acid concentration (1.13 ± 0.11 mmol/L prior to vitamin $B_6$ supplementation compared to 1.39 ± 0.19 mmol/L during vitamin $B_6$ administration). Although additional vitamin $B_6$ was associated with decreased oxalic acid excretion in cats consuming diets deficient in vitamin $B_6$, the ability of supplemental vitamin $B_6$ to reduce urinary oxalic acid excretion in cats or dogs with calcium oxalate uroliths consuming diets with adequate quantities of vitamin $B_6$ is unknown.

### THIAZIDE DIURETICS

Thiazide diuretics have been recommended to reduce recurrence of calcium-containing uroliths in humans because of their ability to reduce urine calcium excretion. The exact mechanism(s) by which thiazide diuretics reduce urinary calcium excretion is unknown; however, several factors appear to be involved. For instance, studies in rats revealed that thiazide diuretics directly stimulated distal renal tubular resorption of calcium. Although results of studies in humans suggest that thiazide diuretics potentiate the action of parathyroid hormone, effects of thiazide diuretics on urinary calcium excretion were not altered in parathyroidectomized rats or dogs. Because the hypocalciuric response to thiazide diuretics was blocked when volume depletion was prevented by sodium chloride administration in humans, it was hypothesized that thiazide diuretics promote mild extracellular volume contraction, thereby promoting proximal tubular reabsorption of several solutes, including sodium and calcium.

In dogs, urinary calcium excretion may increase, decrease, or remain unchanged following thiazide diuretic administration. In one canine study, fractional clearance of calcium increased following intravenous administration of chlorothiazide. In contrast, infusion of thiazide diuretics into left renal arteries of dogs resulted in a significant reduction in calcium clearance compared to calcium clearance by right kidneys. In another canine study, distal tubular concentrations of calcium did not change following intravenous administration of chlorothiazide. These results suggest that the effect of thiazide diuretics on urinary excretion of calcium in dogs is variable. When we evaluated the effect of chlorothiazide (21, 42, and 65 mg/kg every 12 hr) in six normal dogs, a hypocalciuric effect was not observed. However, hydrochlorothiazide (2 mg/kg every 12 hr) decreased urinary calcium excretion in eight dogs with naturally occurring calcium oxalate urolithiasis fed diets providing maintenance requirements, or fed a diet designed to minimize calcium oxalate recurrence. Because thiazide diuretic administration can be associated with adverse effects (dehydration, hypokalemia, hypercalcemia), chronic therapy should be appropriately monitored.

## Monitor Urolith Recurrence

For most dogs, treatment of calcium oxalate uroliths rarely corrects the underlying cause. Therefore, complete elimination of all urolith recurrences may be too great of an expectation. It is likely that therapy will eliminate recurrence for some dogs and delay urolith recurrence for others. Whatever the outcome, by monitoring the biologic behavior of uroliths, therapy can be implemented such that future surgeries to remove urocystoliths can be avoided. However, if the decision to monitor patients is based on recurrence of clinical signs, uroliths may be too large by this time to remove by nonsurgical procedures. We recommend that a complete urinalysis and radiography of the urinary tract be performed every 3 months. If after 1 year urolith recurrence is controlled, evaluations can be performed less frequently. If uroliths are detected, they can be removed by voiding urohydropropulsion or retrieved with a catheter.

## References and Suggested Reading

Bai SC, Sampson DA, Morris JG, et al: Vitamin B6 requirements of growing kittens. J Nutr 119:1020, 1989.

Goldfarb S: Dietary factors in the pathogenesis and prophylaxis of calcium nephrolithiasis. Kidney Int 34:544, 1988.
   *Review of dietary factors important in human calcium oxalate urolithiasis.*
Lulich JP, Perrine L, Osborne CA, et al: Postsurgical recurrence of calcium oxalate uroliths in dogs. J Vet Intern Med 6:119, 1992.
Lulich JP, Osborne CA, Polzin DP, et al: Incomplete removal of canine and feline urocystoliths by cystotomy. J Vet Intern Med 7:124, 1993.
Lulich JP, Osborne CA, Parker ML, et al: Evaluation of urine and serum analytes in miniature schnauzers with calcium oxalate urolithiasis. Am J Vet Res 52:1583, 1991.
Simpson DP: Citrate excretion: A window on renal metabolism. Am J Physiol 244:F223, 1983.
   *Review of citrate metabolism in many species including dogs.*

# CANINE AND FELINE CALCIUM PHOSPHATE UROLITHIASIS

CARL A. OSBORNE,
JEFFREY S. KLAUSNER,
*and* JODY P. LULICH
*St. Paul, Minnesota*

Uroliths composed predominantly of calcium phosphate have been infrequently identified in dogs or cats. However, calcium phosphate is commonly found as a minor component in naturally occurring struvite and calcium oxalate uroliths. Occasionally, a shell of calcium phosphate will form around a urolith composed primarily of struvite.

Identification of calcium phosphate as a major component in uroliths should prompt consideration of metabolic abnormalities that affect calcium metabolism and urine pH. Therapy to prevent recurrent calcium phosphate uroliths should be designed to control or eliminate any underlying metabolic disorders.

## EPIDEMIOLOGY

### Canine Calcium Phosphate

Of 22,810 canine uroliths analyzed by polarizing light microscopy, infrared spectroscopy, and x-ray diffraction at the Minnesota Urolith Center, 195 (0.85%) were composed primarily (70 to 100%) of calcium phosphate. Of the 195 canine calcium phosphate uroliths, 99 were hydroxyapatite, 77 were brushite, 18 were carbonate apatite, and one was tricalcium phosphate (Table 1). More than one crystalline form of calcium phosphate may be present in a single urolith. In alkaline urine, Brushite is readily transformed to apatite; it is possible that some apatite identified in uroliths originated from brushite (Pak et al., 1971). In addition, mixtures of calcium phosphate and calcium oxalate often occur.

### HYDROXYAPATITE

Of 99 canine hydroxyapatite uroliths, 46 were composed entirely (100%) of calcium phosphate, and 53 were composed of at least 70% of this mineral. The mean age of dogs at the time of urolith retrieval was 7 $\pm$ 3.8 years (range = 1 month to 16 years). Males were affected (62%) more commonly than females (31%; the gender of 7% of the dogs was not recorded). Thirty five different breeds were affected, including cocker spaniels (10%), mixed breed (10%), miniature schnauzers (8%), Yorkshire terriers (8%), German shepherd dogs (6%), miniature poodles (5%), and springer spaniels

**Table 1.**   *Glossary of Calcium Phosphate Crystals that May Occur in Uroliths*

| Chemical Name | Crystal Name | Formula |
| --- | --- | --- |
| β-Tricalcium phosphate (calcium orthophosphate) | Whitlockite | $\beta\text{-}CA_2(PO_4)_2$ |
| Carbonate apatite | Carbonate apatite | $Ca_{10}(PO_4CO_3OH)_6(OH)_2$ |
| Calcium hydrogen phosphate dihydrate | Brushite | $CaHPO_4 2H_2O$ |
| Calcium phosphate | Hydroxyapatite or calcium apatite | $Ca_{10}(PO_4)_6(OH)_2$ |

(5%). Hydroxyapatite uroliths were more commonly removed from the lower urinary tract (77%) than the upper urinary tract (7%) (the location of 16% of the hydroxyapatite uroliths was not specified).

### BRUSHITE

Of 77 calcium hydrogen phosphate dihydrate uroliths, 40 were composed entirely (100%) of this mineral, and 37 were composed of at least 70% of this mineral. The mean age of dogs at the time of urolith retrieval was 7.5 ± 2.8 years (range = 1 month to 16 years). Males were affected (77%) more commonly than females (16%; the gender of 7% of affected dogs was not recorded). Twenty-seven breeds were affected, including Yorkshire terriers (10%), *bichon frise* (7%), miniature poodles (7%), Shih Tzus (7%), and mixed (5%). Brushite uroliths were more commonly retrieved from the lower urinary tract (94%) than the upper urinary tract (3%; the location of 3% of the brushite uroliths was not recorded).

### CARBONATE APATITE

Of 18 carbonate apatite uroliths, 3 were composed entirely (100%) of this mineral, and 15 were composed of at least 70% of this mineral. The mean age of dogs at the time of urolith retrieval was 8 ± 4 years (range = 1 month to 12 years). Thirteen different breeds were affected. Females were affected (72%) more commonly than males (28%). Calcium carbonate were more commonly retrieved from the lower urinary tract (72%) than the upper urinary tract (28%).

## Feline Calcium Phosphate

Of 4800 feline uroliths analyzed by quantitative methods at the Minnesota Urolith Center, 59 (1.2%) were composed primarily (70 to 100%) of calcium phosphate. Of the 59 feline calcium phosphate uroliths, 44 were composed of hydroxyapatite, 13 were composed of brushite, and 2 were composed of tricalcium phosphate.

Feline calcium phosphate uroliths were located in the kidneys (n = 17), ureters (n = 3), the urinary bladder (n = 27), urethra and bladder (n = 3), and urethra (n = 1). Two calcium phosphate uroliths were voided (the location of six uroliths was not recorded). Calcium phosphate uroliths occurred more commonly in females (n = 31) than in males (n = 23). The mean age of affected cats was 8 ± 5 years (range = 5 months to 19 years).

## Solubility of Calcium Phosphates in Urine

The solubility of calcium phosphates in urine is dependent on the following: (1) urine pH, (2) urine calcium ion concentration, (3) total urine inorganic phosphate concentration, (4) urine concentration of inhibitors of calcium crystallization, and (5) urine concentration of potentiators of crystallization. Factors that decrease calcium phosphate solubility predispose to urolith formation.

### URINE pH

Urine pH has a profound effect on the solubility of some forms of calcium phosphate. With the exception of brushite, calcium phosphate solubility markedly decreases in alkaline urine and increases in acid urine. Increased urine pH increases the availability of ionic $PO_4$ and $HPO_4$, which are available for incorporation into calcium phosphates (Coe and Flavus, 1991). In contrast to carbonate apatite and hydroxyl apatite, the solubility of brushite decreases in acid urine.

## Hypercalciuria

Hypercalciuria decreases calcium phosphate solubility and may result in oversaturation with calcium phosphate (Pak, 1978). Hypercalciuria may result from excessive resorption of calcium from bone, enhanced intestinal absorption of calcium, impaired renal tubular reabsorption of calcium, or combinations of these factors. Urine specimens obtained from human patients with hypercalciuria and calcium uroliths are usually supersaturated with brushite.

Controversy exists as to the relative importance of urine pH and hypercalciuria as determinants of calcium phosphate solubility *in vivo*. Some believe that calcium phosphate crystallization is primarily governed by changes in urine pH; they minimize the importance of hypercalciuria (Elliot, 1968). However, it has been suggested that persistent hypercalciuria tends to raise the calcium phosphate saturation of urine so that small increases in urine pH will result in calcium phosphate crystalluria. There have been no studies on the relative effect of hypercalciuria and urine pH on the solubility of different types of calcium phosphate in canine and feline urine.

### CRYSTALLIZATION INHIBITORS

Normally, urine contains calcium phosphate crystal inhibitors. One mechanism by which inhibitors prevent urolith formation is by chelating with stone constituents, making them unavailable for nidus formation or crystal growth. In addition, crystallization inhibitors may alter crystalline structure in such a way that crystal growth and aggregation are prevented. Inhibitors of calcium phosphate crystallization include inorganic pyrophosphates, citrate, and magnesium ions (Bisaz et al., 1978). These inhibitors provide 30 to 40% of the inhibitory capacity of normal human urine to calcium phosphate crystallization. The remaining 60 to 70% is provided by as yet unidentified low-molecular-weight inhibitors.

**Table 2.**  *Disorders that May Predispose to the Formation of Calcium Phosphate Uroliths*

Primary hyperparathyroidism
Other hypercalcemic disorders
    Neoplasia
    Vitamin D intoxication
    Excessive calcium intake
    Thyrotoxicosis
    Hyperadrenocorticism
    Immobilization
Distal renal tubular acidosis
Normocalcemic hypercalciuria
    Intestinal hyperabsorption
    Renal leak

### CRYSTALLIZATION PROMOTERS

Formation of calcium phosphate uroliths may be promoted by epitaxy. Epitaxy is the process by which crystals of one salt induce the formation of crystals of another salt. Epitactic induction occurs between crystals having similar lattice dimensions. Calcium phosphate precipitation has been reported to be stimulated by calcium oxalate and monosodium urate crystals (Fleisch, 1978).

## DISORDERS ASSOCIATED WITH FORMATION OF CALCIUM PHOSPHATE UROLITHS

Calcium phosphate uroliths may occur in patients with primary hyperparathyroidism, other hypercalcemic disorders, distal renal tubular acidosis, and idiopathic hypercalciuria (Table 2). Because the prevalence of calcium phosphate uroliths in dogs and cats is low, and because appropriate metabolic studies have rarely been performed in affected cases, the association of calcium phosphate uroliths with other canine and feline metabolic disorders has not been as well established as it has been in humans (Table 3).

### Primary Hyperparathyroidism

In one study of 21 dogs with primary hyperparathyroidism, 4 (20%) had uroliths (Berger and Feldman, 1987). We have encountered a 9-year-old neutered male domestic shorthair cat with a parathyroid adenocarcinoma and calcium oxalate urolithiasis. Uroliths

from patients with primary hyperparathyroidism are typically composed of calcium phosphate, calcium oxalate, or mixtures of the two. Uroliths composed predominantly of calcium phosphate are more commonly identified in human patients and dogs with primary hyperparathyroidism; uroliths composed predominantly of calcium oxalate are more commonly identified in human patients and dogs with normocalcemic hypercalciuria. Bladder uroliths composed primarily of calcium phosphate have been experimentally induced in dogs following injections of parathyroid hormone (Klausner and Osborne, 1986).

Factors that predispose patients with primary hyperparathyroidism to calcium phosphate urolith formation include the following: hypercalciuria, increased urine pH, and increased renal excretion of a substance that promotes spontaneous precipitation of calcium salts. Hypercalcemia results from parathyroid hormone–induced bone resorption and renal tubular reabsorption of calcium. In addition, increased intestinal absorption of calcium results from parathyroid hormone–stimulated conversion of 25-hydroxycholecalciferol to 1,25-dihydroxycholecalciferol (Pak, 1978). Hypercalcemia results in increased glomerular filtration of calcium and hypercalciuria, which in turn enhances the likelihood of urolith formation by increasing urine saturation with brushite and calcium oxalate (Pak, 1978). The urine of most hypercalciuric human patients with primary hyperparathyrodisim is supersaturated with brushite and calcium oxalate. Hypercalciuria has been documented in dogs with primary hyperparathyroidism and calcium uroliths (Klausner et al., 1987; Klausner and Osborne, 1986).

Persistent elevation in urine pH may predispose some patients with primary hyperparathyroidism to calcium phosphate urolithiasis. Urine pH is elevated in these patients because of impaired renal tubular reabsorption of bicarbonate (Rasmussen et al., 1974). This abnormality may explain, at least in part, the increased incidence of calcium phosphate uroliths in patients with primary hyperparathyroidism compared with patients with other hypercalciuric disorders.

### Other Hypercalcemic Disorders

In addition to primary hyperparathyroidism, other hypercalcemic disorders are occasionally associated with formation of calcium phosphate uroliths. Uroliths

**Table 3.**  *Differential Diagnostic Features of Disorders that Predispose to Formation of Calcium Phosphate Uroliths*

| Diagnostic Test | Renal Leak Hypercalciuria | Absorptive Hypercalciuria | Primary Hyperparathyroidism |
|---|---|---|---|
| Serum calcium concentration | Normal | Normal | Increased |
| Serum parathormone concentration | Increased | Normal to decreased | Increased |
| Serum 1,25-vitamin D concentration | Increased | Variable | Increased |
| Serum $PO_4$ concentration | Normal | Normal to decreased | Normal to decreased |
| Fasting urine calcium concentration | Increased | Normal | Increased |

have been identified in human patients with hypervitaminosis D, neoplastic disorders, Cushing's syndrome, and in patients who are immobilized for long periods (Smith, 1979). Although calcium phosphate is the most frequently identified mineral in uroliths obtained from these patients, calcium oxalate may also be present. Because the frequency of occurrences of uroliths in patients with these hypercalcemic disorders is low, it is likely that factors other than hypercalcemia are involved.

## Distal Renal Tubular Acidosis

Nephrolithiasis is a common manifestation of hereditary distal renal tubular acidosis (type I) in humans (Konnak et al., 1982). Uroliths are typically composed entirely of calcium phosphate, although calcium oxalate and struvite stones have also been identified (Konnak et al., 1982). Urolith formation has not been observed in patients with acquired distal renal tubular acidosis or proximal renal tubular acidosis (type II).

Distal renal tubular acidosis results from functional inability of the distal nephron to establish a hydrogen ion gradient between blood and tubular fluid, regardless of the severity of acidemia. The disorder in humans is characterized by inability to lower urine pH below 5.4, hypokalemia, hyperchloremia, hypophosphatemia, hypocalcemia, metabolic acidosis, osteomalacia, nephrocalcinosis, and urolithiasis (DeFronzo and Their, 1981).

Hypercalciuria, alkaline urine, low urine citrate concentration, and excessive urinary phosphate excretion contribute to formation of calcium phosphate uroliths observed in patients with distal renal tubular acidosis. Acidosis increases calcium mobilization from bone, causing an increase in the quantity of calcium excreted in urine. In addition, acidosis decreases renal tubular fractional reabsorption of calcium and further increases calcium excretion (Klausner and Osborne, 1986). Acidosis may alter renal tubular calcium transport, the response of tubules to parathyroid hormone, or both.

Patients with distal renal tubular acidosis excrete decreased amounts of citrate in their urine. Citrate is reabsorbed more avidly in proximal convoluted tubules as a consequence of intracellular acidosis. Recall that because citrate is a major chelator of calcium, decreased citrate concentration decreases calcium solubility.

In humans, distal renal tubular acidosis sometimes occurs as an incomplete form in which urolith formation occurs without systemic acidosis (Konnak et al., 1982). Urolithiasis may be the only clinical manifestation of this disorder. The tubular defect can only be recognized by abnormal response to the ammonium chloride loading test.

## Normocalcemic Hypercalciuria

Normocalcemic hypercalciuria is a syndrome characterized by normal serum calcium concentration, increased urinary excretion of calcium, absence of systemic disease, and increased tendency for formation of calcium phosphate or calcium oxalate uroliths. Normocalcemic hypercalciuria has been recognized in the dog. It has not been documented in cats, primarily because there has been little effort to detect it.

Two types of normocalcemic hypercalciuria have been recognized in dogs (Lulich et al., 1991). One type, called absorptive hypercalciuria, is associated with increased intestinal absorption of calcium. The subsequent increase in serum calcium concentration suppresses parathyroid hormone secretion, resulting in decreased tubular reabsorption of calcium and hypercalciuria. Hyperabsorption of calcium from the intestinal tract may result from a primary intestinal disturbance in calcium transport. It is also possible that increased calcium absorption results from increased synthesis of 1,25-dihydrocholecalciferol.

The second type of normocalcemic hypercalciuria, termed "renal leak" hypercalciuria, is thought to result from impaired ability of the proximal tubules to reabsorb filtered calcium (Lulich et al., 1991). A defect in reabsorption of magnesium may also be present. Renal calcium loss stimulates 1,25-dihydrocholecalciferol and parathyroid hormone synthesis, resulting in an increase in intestinal absorption of calcium. Unlike absorptive hypercalciuria, renal leak hypercalciuria is not affected by food fasting.

Hypercalciuria is probably not the only factor involved in urolith formation in patients with normocalcemic hypercalciuria, because many hypercalciuric patients do not form stones. Interaction of crystallization inhibitors and promoters are important contributing factors.

The diagnosis of idiopathic hypercalciuria is established by demonstrating an increase in 24-hr urine calcium excretion and by eliminating other nonhypercalcemic, hypercalciuric disorders such as renal tubular acidosis.

## Mineralization of Blood Clots

We have observed nephroliths, urocystoliths, and urethroliths composed of blood clots mineralized with calcium phosphate on numerous occasions. They occur primarily in cats, and are most commonly found in the renal pelvis and renal pelvic diverticula. Formation of highly concentrated urine in patients with gross hematuria may favor formation of blood clots in patients with hematuria. Contrary to one theory, these black-colored uroliths are not composed of bile metabolites.

## EVALUATION OF DOGS WITH CALCIUM PHOSPHATE UROLITHS

History and physical examination may reveal etiologic factors that predispose to formation of calcium phosphate uroliths. Primary hyperparathyroidism may be associated with generalized weakness, polyuria, polydipsia, weight loss, or bone pain. An enlarged parathyroid gland may be palpable in the ventral region of the neck. Pathologic fractures have been infrequently noted, probably because they represent an advanced stage of primary hyperparathyroidism. Vitamin D intoxication is suggested by excessive intake of the vitamin. Because hypercalciuria has a hereditary tendency in humans, questions should be asked regarding the occurrence of calcium uroliths in related dogs and cats.

## Radiographic and Ultrasonographic Evaluation

Radiographic and ultrasonographic evaluation is useful in identifying and localizing uroliths within the urinary tract and may be of some benefit in helping to differentiate between urolith types. Uroliths containing calcium are much more radiodense than cystine or ammonium urate uroliths of comparable size. In our experience, with the exception of Brushite, calcium phosphate uroliths do not have a characteristic shape. Brushite uroliths are typically round and smooth; on cross section, they are often laminated. All forms of calcium phosphate uroliths tend to be multiple, and vary in size, with smaller sizes being more common.

## Laboratory Evaluation

All retrieved uroliths should be evaluated by quantitative methods. A problem-specific data base (Table 4) should be evaluated on dogs and cats with calcium phosphate uroliths to aid in identification of factors that predispose to formation of uroliths and to detect concomitant disease. Detection of hypercalcemia should

**Table 4.** *Problem-Specific Data Base for Dogs and Cats with Calcium Phosphate Uroliths*

Blood tests
   SUN and/or serum creatinine
   Calcium
   Phosphorus
   Sodium
   Chloride
   Potassium
   Blood gas or $TCO_2$
   Intact PTH (if serum Ca is elevated)
   1,25-hydroxyvitamin D
   Magnesium (if possible)
   Uric acid (if possible)
Complete urinalysis including careful evaluation of pH and crystals
Bacterial culture of urine
Consider 24-hr urine collection°
   Volume
   Creatinine
   Calcium
   Phosphorus
   Magnesium
   Citrate (if possible)
   Oxalate (if possible)

°A standardized diet should be fed as described in the text.
Abbreviations: SUN = serum urea nitrogen, $TCO_2$ = total carbon dioxide, PTH = parathyroid hormone, Ca = calcium.

prompt a search for primary hyperparathyroidism or other hypercalcemic disorders (Tables 2 and 3). Serum parathyroid hormone determination or exploratory surgery of the neck may be necessary to document primary hyperparathyroidism.

Detection of hypercalciuria in the absence of hypercalcemia suggests the possibility of renal tubular acidosis or normocalcemic hypercalciuria. Hypercalciuria may be documented by evaluating calcium concentration in at least two 24-hr urine samples. The animal should be fed a diet of known composition during test periods to eliminate variation caused by differences in the mineral content and composition of dog foods. Mean 24-hr urine calcium excretion in 33 normal beagles was $0.32 \pm 0.2$ mg/kg/24 hr during fasting, and $0.51 \pm 0.3$ mg/kg/24 hr when dogs consumed a standard diet (Prescription Diet Canine u/d, Hill's) (Lulich et al., 1991).

## MEDICAL THERAPY OF PATIENTS WITH CALCIUM PHOSPHATE STONES

Surgery remains the most reliable way to remove active calcium phosphate uroliths from the urinary tract. However, we emphasize that surgery may be unnecessary for clinically inactive calcium phosphate uroliths.

The likelihood of recurrence of calcium phosphate uroliths following removal is not well established. Therefore, patients should be periodically monitored by urinalysis, appropriate radiographic procedures and, if indicated, laboratory tests on blood and urine (Table 4). If recurrent urocystoliths are detected when they are small, they may be nonsurgically removed by voiding urohydropropulsion or by aspiration through a urinary catheter (Lulich et al., 1993). Medical therapy of patients with recurrent calcium phosphate uroliths should then be directed at removing or minimizing risk factors that contribute to supersaturation of urine with calcium phosphate.

### Primary Hyperparathyroidism

Patients with primary hyperparathyroidism usually require surgery (Berger and Feldman, 1987). Parathyroidectomy may result in dissolution of uroliths and generally prevents their recurrence. In a dog with primary hyperparathyroidism and recurrent calcium phosphate uroliths, parathyroidectomy resulted in decreased urinary calcium excretion and prevention of new urolith formation (Klausner et al., 1987).

### Distal Renal Tubular Acidosis

To our knowledge, medical dissolution of calcium phosphate uroliths has not been attempted in dogs with distal renal tubular acidosis (RTA). Diets designed to dissolve struvite uroliths would not be expected to promote dissolution of calcium phosphate uroliths, because they may tend to promote acidemia and aciduria, thus potentially enhancing hypercalciuria and hypocitraturia. However, correction of hypercalciuria, hyperphosphaturia, and hypocitraturia by alkalinization therapy with potassium citrate might promote dissolution of these uroliths in patients with complete or incomplete distal RTA.

Chronic alkalinization therapy appears to be beneficial in preventing calcium phosphate urolith formation in humans with distal RTA. Such therapy has been advocated for patients with complete or incomplete forms of distal RTA because it decreases urolith formation and nephrocalcinosis, and increases urine citrate concentration.

## Normocalcemic Hypercalciuria

Several different medical protocols have been reported to be of value in humans with normocalcemic hypercalciuria (Coe and Flavus, 1991). Ideally, the choice of therapy should be based on the cause of idiopathic hypercalciuria. There has been little clinical experience in the use of drugs in dogs and cats with calcium phosphate uroliths. However, medications that can enhance calcium excretion such as glucocorticoids, furosemide, and those containing large quantities of sodium should be avoided if possible.

### DIETARY MODIFICATION

Diets designed to avoid excessive protein, calcium, and vitamin D may be of benefit. Excessive restriction or supplementation of dietary phosphorus should probably be avoided. Enhancement of urine volume by feeding a canned diet (and/or a protein-restricted diet to dogs to reduce renal medullary urea) and encouraging water consumption may also be of benefit. In humans, high-fiber diets have been shown to reduce intestinal absorption and urinary excretion of calcium. Oral administration of sodium chloride, long recommended for all forms of urolithiasis, may promote hypercalciuria and calcium phosphate urolith formation. Therefore, oral salt therapy is not recommended to promote diuresis in dogs with uroliths containing calcium salts.

### URINE ACIDIFIERS

With the exception of brushite, calcium phosphates tend to be less soluble in alkaline urine. Whether or not such patients would benefit by use of appropriate dosages of acidifiers is unknown. Acidification tends to enhance urine calcium excretion, and is a risk factor for calcium oxalate urolith formation. Pending further studies, we do not recommend the routine use of urine acidifiers for patients with calcium phosphate urolithiasis.

Because calcium hydrogen phosphate dihydrate (brushite) is less soluble in acid urine, it might seem logical to promote formulation of alkaline urine by patients with brushite uroliths. However, brushite may be converted to other insoluble forms of calcium phosphate in alkaline urine. Use of potassium citrate, an alkalinizing agent, might be rationalized on the basis of minimizing acidosis-induced hypercalciuria, and formation of the soluble calcium citrate rather than insoluble calcium phosphate in urine. We emphasize that the beneficial and/or detrimental effects of orally administered potassium citrate to dogs and cats with calcium phosphate urolithiasis has not been carefully evaluated. Consult the article, "Canine Calcium Oxalate Urolithiasis," this volume, p 992 for additional therapeutic information about potassium citrate.

### THIAZIDE DIURETICS

Because thiazide diuretics decrease renal calcium excretion, they may be considered to minimize renal leak hypercalciuria. Hydrochlorothiazide may be given on a trial basis to dogs with recurrent calcium phosphate urolithiasis at a dosage of 2 to 4 mg/kg every 12 hr. Because administration of thiazide diuretics may be associated with unwanted side effects (dehydration, hypercalcemia, hypokalemia, and magnesium depletion), patients should be appropriately monitored during therapy. Thiazide therapy is not recommended to treat absorptive hypercalciuria because it does not correct the hyperabsorptive state and may promote positive systemic calcium balance with possible soft-tissue calcification.

## References and Suggested Reading

Berger B and Feldman EC: Primary hyperparathyroidism in dogs: 21 cases (1976–1986). J Am Vet Med Assoc 191:350, 1987.

Bisaz S, Felix R, Newman WF, et al: Quantitative determination of inhibitors of calcium phosphate precipitation in whole urine. Miner Electrolyte Metab 1:74, 1978.

Coe FL and Flavus MJ: Nephrolithiasis. In Brenner BM and Rector FC (eds): The Kidney, 4th edition, volume 12. Philadelphia, WB Saunders Co, 1991, pp 1728–1767.

DeFronzo RA and Their SO: Inherited disorders of renal function. In Brenner BM and Rector FC Jr (eds): The Kidney. Philadelphia, WB Saunders Co, 1981, pp 1816–1971.

Elliot JS: Solubility and crystallization in urinary stone disease. In Hodgkinson A and Nordin BEC (eds): Proceedings of the Renal Stone Research Symposium, London, J & A Churchill Ltd, 1968, pp 199–207.

Fleisch H: Inhibitors and promoters of stone formation. Kidney Int 13:361, 1978.

Klausner JS, et al: Calcium urolithiasis in two dogs with parathyroid adenomas. J Am Vet Med Assoc 191:1423, 1987.

Klausner JS and Osborne CA: Calcium phosphate urolithiasis. Vet Clin North Am 16:171, 1986.

Konnak JW, et al: Renal calculi associated with incomplete renal tubular acidosis. J Urol 128:900, 1982.

Lulich JP, et al: Evaluation of urine and serum metabolites in miniature schnauzers with calcium oxalate urolithiasis. Am J Vet Res 52:1583, 1991.

Lulich JP, et al: Urine metabolite values in fed and nonfed clinically normal beagles. Am J Vet Res 52:1573, 1991.

Lulich JP, et al: Nonsurgical removal of urocystoliths in dogs and cats by voiding urohydropropulsion. J Am Vet Med Assoc 203:660, 1993.

Pak CYC, et al: Spontaneous precipitation of brushite in urine: Evidence that brushite is the nidus of renal stones originating as calcium phosphate. Proc Natl Acad Sci USA 68:1456, 1971.

Pak CYC: Primary hyperparathyroidism and other causes of hypercalciuria. In Pak CYC (ed): Calcium Urolithiasis: Pathogenesis, Diagnosis, and Management. New York, Plenum Medical Books Co, 1978, pp 81–117.

Rasmussen E, et al: Hormonal control of skeletal and mineral homeostasis. Am J Vet Med 56:751, 1974.

# LITHOTRIPSY IN COMPANION ANIMALS

DAVID F. SENIOR

*Baton Rouge, Louisiana*

Clients frequently confront veterinarians with questions concerning the differences between human and veterinary treatment for patients with urolithiasis. The prospect of an instant nonsurgical treatment for their pets is understandably appealing, and clients frequently question why the options available to themselves are not available for companion animals. The following information may assist veterinarians to answer questions concerning lithotripsy and appropriately support more conventional treatment strategies.

Lithotripsy literally means stone breakup or fragmentation. The main methods of lithotripsy used in human medicine are mechanical lithotripsy—usually confined to treatment of bladder uroliths—and shock-wave lithotripsy, which can be delivered either internally or externally.

## MECHANICAL LITHOTRIPSY

Mechanical lithotrites were initially developed and are still used in human medicine to fragment uroliths in the urinary bladder. Typical devices have jaws between which the urolith is positioned. The jaws are mechanically pulled together to crush the urolith, and the resulting fragments are flushed out of the bladder. Access to the urolith requires urethral passage of the instrument into the urinary bladder. Currently available instruments are designed for use in humans and are relatively large in diameter (24-Fr.). This excessive size severely limits use of such instruments in veterinary medicine, and at this time there have been no reports of mechanial lithotripsy being performed in animals.

## ULTRASONIC LITHOTRIPSY

Ultrasonic lithotriptors are long rigid instruments that can be passed per urethra into the bladder. Currently available models have an ultrasound generator at one end and an ultrasonically vibrating tip at the other. The ultrasonic lithotripsy (USL) device is passed via a cystoscope per urethra into the bladder, then the tip is held against the surface of the urolith and activated. In one model, a suction device carries particles fragmented from the surface of the urolith through the core of the lithotriptor into a container outside the body. The device is relatively expensive (over $11,000). In tests performed on canine uroliths *in vitro* by the author, one commercial unit was found to lack the power necessary to cause urolith fragmentation. There are currently no reports of USL in veterinary medicine.

## ELECTROHYDRAULIC SHOCK-WAVE LITHOTRIPSY

Elecrohydraulic shock-wave lithotripsy (EHL) is based on the premise that the generation of a spark in a fluid medium causes the development of a shock wave. Shock waves pass through the body of a urolith and are reflected back from the distant border to pass once again through the body of the particle. The passage of many primary and reflected shock waves through a urolith causes the development of shearing forces that destroy the crystal lattice.

In EHL, the shock wave is generated at the tip of a wire that can be passed into the bladder through a cystoscope placed in the urethra. The wire consists of a central electrode separated from a surrounding coaxial electrode by an insulating layer. Typical shock-wave generators develop a spark between the central electrode and the coaxial electrode at approximately 100 times per second. The shock waves are generated in a fluid medium next to the surface of the stone urolith to be fragmented. Usually, only 1 to 3 sec of activation are required to cause major fragmentation of a large urolith. Some of the sub fragments may require further lithotripsy to allow passage through the urethra.

The spark probes for EHL are sufficiently small (1.6-, 3-, 4.5-, and 7-Fr.) to be passed through a rigid cystoscope. Use of EHL to break up bladder uroliths has been reported in veterinary medicine (Senior, 1984). Although this technique is possible for all animals in which a cystoscope can be passed per urethra into the bladder (i.e., female dogs >5 kg), the equipment is expensive. A cystoscope set usually costs about $5000 without a light source. The spark generator costs an additional $10,000, and spark probes are $550 for a box of four. After both mechanical lithotripsy and EHL, urolith fragments are readily rinsed out of the bladder (Lulich et al., 1993).

## EXTRACORPOREAL SHOCK-WAVE LITHOTRYPSY

The original extracorporeal shock-wave lithotrypsy (ESWL) units have a large tub filled with water into which the patient is lowered. The base of the tub contains a metallic ellipsoid cup. Using a dual fluoroscope system, the urolith to be fragmented (usually a nephrolith) is positioned at the secondary focus of the ellipse. At the primary focus of the ellipsoid cup, a spark between two electrodes develops a high-energy shock wave. Shock waves generated at the primary focus of the ellipse are reflected from the surface of the ellipsoid cup and refocused again at the secondary focus of the ellipse. The electrical spark is initiated by the R wave of the patient's electrocardiogram (ECG). Shock waves pass relatively unimpeded through soft tissue; however, where they concentrate at solid material, such as the urolith, most of their energy is absorbed, and the absorbed energy causes urolith fragmentation. Although more recent devices use piezoelectric generation of the shock waves and the fluid medium through which the shock waves pass before entering the body is now much smaller than in the original ESWL, the basic principle of focusing shock waves from a wide area onto a small area inside the body (i.e., the urolith) remains the same.

Several animal studies have been performed using ESWL, and there is one report describing the number of shock waves necessary to destroy canine renal tissue; however, reports of veterinary patients treated with the ESWL are rare (Newman et al., 1987; Adams et al., 1994).

Because uroliths tend to move as shock waves pass through them, the method is most applicable to uroliths in the kidney where they are likely to remain fixed

in position. The mobility of ureteral and bladder uroliths tends to preclude ESWL. Furthermore, the number of shocks required to reduce human nephroliths to a particle size capable of passing through the ureter is quite close to the number of shock waves that will destroy renal tissue. In smaller patients, such as dogs or cats, the number of shock waves necessary to fragment the nephrolith to even smaller particles so they may pass through the ureter requires an even larger number of shocks. Finally, shock waves damage lung tissue and ESWL causes pulmonary edema and hemorrhage. Patients must be positioned so that pulmonary trauma is minimized.

The expense of purchase and maintenance of ESWL devices is currently beyond the reach of most situations in veterinary medicine and even rental of instrument time is prohibitively expensive.

## References and Suggested Reading

Adams LG, Block G, Widmer WR, et al: Extracorporeal shock-wave lithotripsy for treatment of canine uroliths. Proceedings 12th ACVIM Forum, San Francisco, CA, 1994, pp 478–479.

Lulich JP, Osborne CA, Carlson M, et al: Non surgical removal of urocystoliths in dogs and cats by voiding urohydropropulsion. J Am Vet Med Assoc 203:660, 1993.

Newman RC, Hackett RL, Senior DF, et al: Pathological effects of ESWL on canine renal tissue. Urology 29:194, 1987.

Senior DF: Electrohydraulic shock-wave lithotripsy in experimental canine struvite bladder stone disease. Vet Surg 13:143, 1984.

# VOIDING UROHYDROPROPULSION: A NONSURGICAL TECHNIQUE FOR REMOVAL OF UROCYSTOLITHS

JODY P. LULICH
and CARL A. OSBORNE
St. Paul, Minnesota

## WHAT IS VOIDING UROHYDROPROPULSION?

Cystotomy has been considered an effective method of removing all types of uroliths from the urinary bladder. However, we have developed a nonsurgical alternative called voiding urohydropropulsion (Lulich et al., 1993a). Voiding urohydropropulsion permits safe and rapid removal of small to moderately sized urocystoliths of any mineral composition from dogs and cats. This procedure does not require special equipment; in some patients, uroliths can be removed without anesthesia.

## HOW IS VOIDING UROHYDROPROPULSION PERFORMED?

The effectiveness of voiding urohydropropulsion is dependent on altering the patient's body position prior to micturition so as to take advantage of gravitational force to assist urolith repositioning and expulsion. To enhance movement of urocystoliths by gravity, the urinary bladder should be moderately distended. If the urinary bladder is not distended with urine, it can be moderately distended with physiologic saline (0.9% NaCl) solution injected through a transurethral catheter. As a general guideline, the normal empty canine or feline urinary bladder can be moderately distended by injecting 4 to 6 ml of fluid per kilogram of body weight. In order to minimize overdistention of the bladder, its size should be assessed by abdominal palpation during infusion. After the bladder is distended, the catheter is removed. Next, the dog or cat should be positioned so that the vertebral column is approximately vertical (Fig. 1). The urinary bladder is then gently agitated by palpation to promote gravitational movement of all urocystoliths into the bladder neck. By applying steady digital pressure to the urinary bladder to induce micturition, urine and uroliths are voided through the urethra and into a cup (Fig. 1, *inset*). If the number of uroliths voided is less than that previously detected by radiography, the procedure can be repeated. If uroliths detected by radiography were too numerous to count, voiding urohydropropulsion should be repeated until uroliths are no longer voided by induced micturition. Before discontinuing voiding urohydropropulsion, double-contrast cystography should be performed to ensure that all urocystoliths have been removed.

## SHOULD PATIENTS BE ANESTHETIZED?

Anesthesia is not necessary to perform voiding urohydropropulsion in all patients. However, sedation facilitates positioning of the patient and palpation of the urinary bladder. The advantage of performing voiding urohydropropulsion without anesthesia is that micturition is not affected by pharmacologic agents. As a result, voiding is facilitated by contraction of bladder smooth muscle and relaxation of urethral smooth muscle. However, greater force is often required to initiate voiding in conscious animals compared to those anesthetized. We have not been able to determine if increased digital pressure applied to the urinary bladder of conscious animals is associated with a greater degree of hematuria and dysuria immediately following the procedure.

When anesthetics are used, we recommend agents that provide analgesia and muscle relaxation. In dogs, a combination of intramuscularly administered oxymorphone (0.1 to 0.2 mg/kg) followed by intravenously administered propofol titrated to effect has provided the proper degree and duration of anesthesia. In cats, oxymorphone (0.05 to 0.1 mg/kg) and a tranquilizer (midazolam, 0.05 to 0.1 mg/kg) are intramuscularly administered prior to propofol titration. Because these drugs depress respiration, patients should be appropriately monitored. Once uroliths have been removed, the effects of oxymorphone can be antagonized with nalbuphine HCl (0.03 to 0.1 mg/kg IV) if continued analgesia is desired, or naloxone (0.002 to 0.02 mg/kg IV) if respiratory depression is of greater concern. For small urocystoliths unlikely to induce urethral discomfort, we typically use propofol as the sole anesthetic agent. Propofol-induced anesthesia is easily titrated,

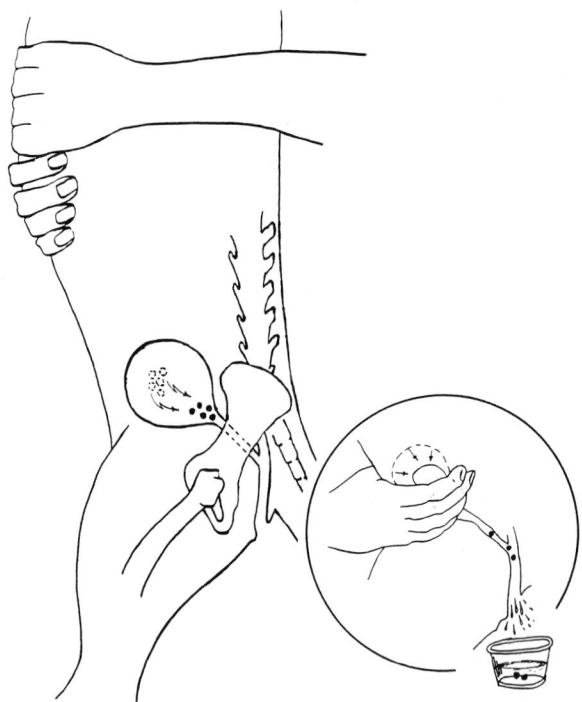

**Figure 1.** To remove urocystoliths by voiding urohydropropulsion, the patient is positioned so that the vertebral column is approximately vertical. The urinary bladder is then gently agitated in an effort to promote gravitational movement of urocystoliths into the bladder neck. To expel urocystoliths, voiding is induced by applying steady pressure to the urinary bladder (*inset*). (Adapted from Lulich JP, Osborne CA, Carlson M, et al: Nonsurgical removal of uroliths in dogs and cats by voiding urohydropropulsion. J Am Vet Med Assoc 203:660–663, 1993, with permission.)

and recovery is rapid and smooth (Ilkiw, 1992) (see "Propofol: A New Sedative-Hypnotic Anesthetic Agent," this volume, p 77). Inhalation anesthetics (isoflurane or halothane) also provide good analgesia and muscle relaxation.

## WHAT COMPLICATIONS HAVE BEEN ASSOCIATED WITH VOIDING UROHYDROPROPULSION?

Visible hematuria is a common complication of voiding urohydropropulsion, and is probably induced by manual compression of inflamed urinary bladders. In our experience, visible hematuria resolved within 4 hr in dogs; dysuria has not been observed in dogs (Lulich et al., 1993a). In cats, however, hematuria and dysuria can persist for up to 2 days. Urethral obstruction with uroliths is a potential complication, especially when dysuria persists in animals with uroliths remaining in the urinary bladder. Use of urinary catheters has been associated with urinary tract infection. Catheter-induced infection can be minimized by providing antimicrobials 4 to 8 hr prior to and for 2 to 5 days immediately following catheter use.

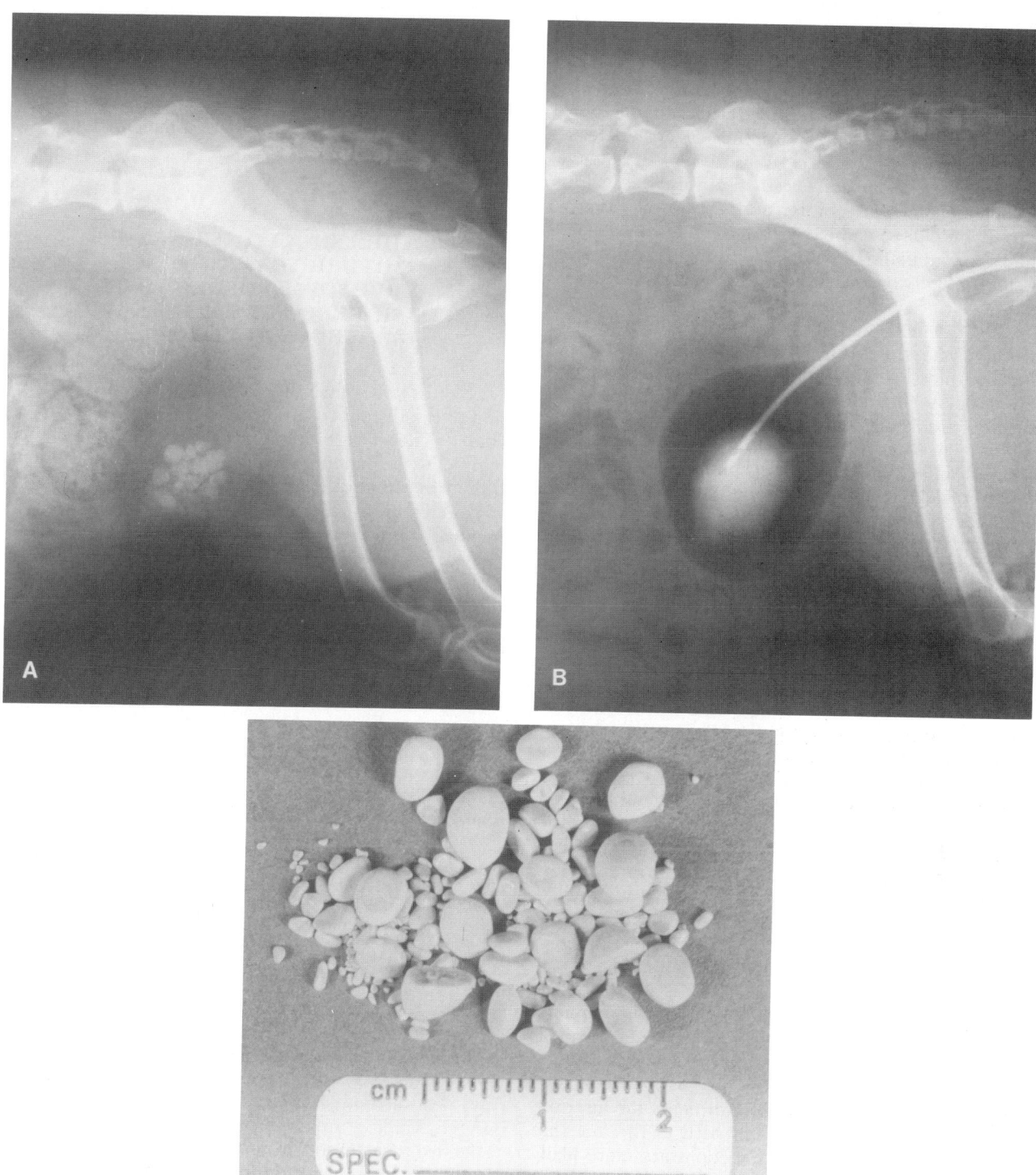

**Figure 2.** Lateral survey abdominal radiograph of a 13-year-old female miniature schnauzer with multiple urocystoliths before voiding urohydropropulsion (A), and double-contrast cystogram immediately after voiding urohydropropulsion (B). Four hundred seventeen calcium oxalate monohydrate urocystoliths, ranging in size up to 7mm in diameter, were voided (C).

## WHAT CARE IS NEEDED FOLLOWING VOIDING UROHYDROPROPULSION?

Following voiding urohydropropulsion, we routinely perform double-contrast cystography to determine if any uroliths remain in the bladder. Survey radiography or ultrasonography can also be used to determine the success of voiding urohydropropulsion. If the presence or absence of urocystoliths is not verified immediately following completion of the procedure, it will be impossible to distinguish between urolith recurrence or incomplete urolith removal at a later date.

For patients with urocystoliths unassociated with bacterial urinary tract infection (UTI), antimicrobials are not needed, provided that normal host defenses have not been disrupted by transurethral catheterization. In most of our cases, catheters were used either during the procedure or for postprocedural radiography. To minimize catheter-induced UTI, consider administering therapeutic doses of antimicrobial drugs excreted in high concentrations in urine 4 to 8 hr before and for 2 to 5 days following catheterization (Osborne, 1993). Urine collected by cystocentesis 3 to 7 days later can be cultured to verify that the urinary tract has not become infected.

If urocystoliths persist despite voiding urohydropropulsion, urethral obstruction may occur, especially if the patient is dysuric. If urethral obstruction occurs, uroliths can be easily moved back into the urinary bladder by retrograde urohydropropulsion. They can then be dissolved with medical management or surgically removed.

## WHEN SHOULD VOIDING UROHYDROPROPULSION BE CONSIDERED?

Proper selection of patients for voiding urohydropropulsion will enhance removal of urocystoliths. The relationship of the size, shape, and surface contour of urocystoliths to the luminal diameter of the urethra are important factors. Uroliths that are larger than the smallest diameter of any portion of the distended urethral lumen are unlikely to be voided. In our clinical case series, diameters of the largest uroliths expelled from the urinary bladder were 7 mm from a 7.4-kg female dog (Fig. 2), 5 mm from a 9-kg male dog, 5 mm from a 4.6-kg female cat, and 1 mm from a 6.6-kg male cat (Lulich et al., 1993a). It is logical to hypothesize that uroliths greater than 1 mm in diameter could be voided from a male cat with a perineal urethrostomy.

Compared to uroliths with an irregular contour, smooth uroliths readily passed through the urethra. This may be related, at least in part, to the fact that uroliths with sharp surface projections are more likely to adhere to the urethral mucosa. In addition, contact of the surface of smooth uroliths with the urethral mucosa may form a continuous seal that would prevent voiding of saline solution without concomitant advancement of the urolith. However, fluids may pass by a urolith with an irregular contour and projections without forcing it through the urethral lumen.

Because uroliths can be removed in conscious animals, voiding urohydropropulsion may be considered for patients at high risk for anesthesia-related morbidity and mortality. Even if anesthesia is needed for patient restraint, it is often of shorter duration than that required for cystotomy. The mean time required to complete voiding urohydropropulsion and postvoiding double-contrast cystography in 15 patients from which all uroliths were completely removed was 22 min (Lulich et al., 1993a). In one female dog, it took 7 min to remove a solitary urolith and complete follow-up cystography.

## WHEN SHOULD STRATEGIES OTHER THAN VOIDING UROHYDROPROPULSION BE CONSIDERED FOR ANIMALS WITH UROCYSTOLITHS?

Uroliths larger than the smallest diameter of any portion of the distended urethral lumen are unlikely to be voided. Therefore, voiding urohydropropulsion may be ineffective in patients with uroliths lodged in the urethra at the time of diagnosis.

Voiding urohydropropulsion should not be used if manual compression of the urinary bladder is likely to cause extravasation of urine into the peritoneal cavity. Consequently, this procedure should not be used during the period of healing after urinary bladder surgery.

Manual compression of the urinary bladder to induce voiding is not without risk in patients with urinary tract infections. If excessive pressure is applied to the urinary bladder, vesicoureteral reflux of urine and bacteria can occur (Feeney, Osborne, and Johnston, 1983). Therefore, urinary tract infections should be controlled prior to voiding urohydropropulsion. By reducing inflammation, the severity of hematuria and dysuria induced by urinary bladder palpation should be lessened.

## WHY SHOULD VOIDING UROHYDROPROPULSION BE CONSIDERED BEFORE CYSTOTOMY IS PERFORMED?

Compared to cystotomy, voiding urohydropropulsion offers several advantages. Because a surgical incision is unnecessary, the time required for healing is reduced, and post-technique dysuria and hematuria may be less severe. Voiding urohydropropulsion also may be more effective than surgery in removing small uroliths. Small uroliths often remain in the lower urinary tract following cystotomy (Lulich et al., 1993b). In some cases, voiding urohydropropulsion can be performed without anesthesia. Even if needed, the anesthetic period is typically of much shorter duration than that required for cystotomy. Cystotomy does provide the advantage of removing uroliths larger than the dilated urethral lumen. However, if the size of urocystoliths can be reduced by medical therapy (Osborne et al, 1989) or electrohydraulic shock-wave lithotripsy (Senior, 1984; see elsewhere in this section), voiding urohydropropulsion can be used to facilitate their removal from the urinary bladder.

## References and Suggested Reading

Feeney DA, Osborne CA, and Johnston GR: Vesicoureteral reflux induced by manual compression of the urinary bladder. J Am Vet Med Assoc 182: 795, 1983.

Ilkiw JE: Other potentially useful new injectable agents. Vet Clin North Am [Small Anim Pract] 22:281, 1992
*Discusses use of proprofol and other anesthetics.*

Lulich JP, Osborne CA, Carlson M, et al: Nonsurgical removal of uroliths in dogs and cats by voiding urohydropropulsion. J Am Vet Med Assoc 203:660, 1993a.
*Prospective study on the effectiveness of voiding urohydropropulsion.*

Lulich JP, Osborne CA, Polzin DJ, et al: Incomplete removal of canine and feline urocystoliths by cystotomy (abstr). J Vet Intern Med 7:124, 1993.

Osborne CA: Bacterial infections of the canine and feline urinary tract: Cause, cure, and control. In Bojrab MJ (ed): *Disease Mechanisms in Small Animal Surgery,* 2nd edition. Philadelphia, Lea & Febiger, 1993, p 458.
*Review chapter discussing treatment and prevention of UTI.*

Osborne CA, Polzin DJ, Lulich JP, et al: Relationship of nutritional factors to the cause, dissolution, and prevention of canine uroliths. Vet Clin North Am [Small Anim Pract]. 19:583, 1989.

Senior DF: Electrohydraulic shock-wave lithotripsy in experimental canine struvite bladder stone disease. Vet Surg 13:143, 1984.

# ULTRASONOGRAPHIC FINDINGS IN FELINE LOWER URINARY TRACT DISEASES

### BARBARA A. SELCER
*Athens, Georgia*

Ultrasonography is a safe, noninvasive means of examining the urinary bladder. The urethra is usually not visualized ultrasonically because of its course through the pelvic canal. Ultrasound alone can be used to examine the bladder, but is more frequently combined with radiography (Mahaffey and Barber, 1992). Pneumocystography or double-contrast cystography should be performed after sonographic evaluation. The air introduced into the urinary bladder during these procedures interferes with transmission of the ultrasound beam. Sonographic evaluation can, however, be performed following positive-contrast cystography (Barr, 1990). The sonographic examination is best performed when the urinary bladder is full and should, therefore, be performed prior to catherization.

## TECHNIQUE

Preparation for sonographic examination is simple. The hair over the caudal half of the ventral abdomen is clipped. Air trapped between hairs creates artifacts and degrades the sonographic image. Since the urinary bladder is located just dorsal to the ventral abdominal wall, minimal depth penetration by the sound beam is required. A high-frequency (e.g., 7.5 mHz) transducer is recommended. The higher frequency transducers allow greater resolution of the sonographic image. Little attenuation of the sound beam occurs in the urinary bladder. Acoustic coupling gel is recommended as an interface between the transducer and the abdominal wall. Scans of the urinary bladder can be made in multiple planes. Most commonly, transverse and sagittal planes are used. The examination is easily performed with the cat in dorsal recumbency; however, lateral recumbency or prone positioning may be beneficial, par-

ticularly when trying to distinguish between adherent mural masses and free intraluminal masses such as blood clots or calculi (Fig. 1).

## SONOGRAPHIC FINDINGS

A normal full bladder appears as a well-defined, smoothly outlined, sonolucent structure directly dorsal to the abdominal wall. The individual layers of the bladder wall usually cannot be differentiated. Generally, urine within the bladder is free of internal echoes and is therefore highly anechoic. Acoustic enhancement is seen dorsal to the bladder image. It is important to properly adjust gain settings, particularly within the near field. High gain settings in the near field will increase the intensity of the returning echoes and obscure evaluation of the ventral urinary bladder wall. A gas- and/or feces-filled colon can also artifactually create echoes over the bladder image that can degrade the quality of the image and even mimic bladder lesions (Fig. 2). Shifting the position of the transducer or the urinary bladder can often eliminate such examination artifacts. The overall size of the urinary bladder is dependent upon its degree of distention.

Many common feline lower urinary tract diseases are readily sonographically recognizable. Both radiolucent and radiopaque cystic calculi can be detected. Calculi are hyperechoic, located in the gravity-dependent portion of the bladder, and may exhibit posterior acoustic shadowing (Fig. 3).

Urinary bladder wall thickening can also be sonographically detected. In the normal patient, the urinary bladder wall is thin and its margins are poorly distinguished. Cats with chronic cystitis can show prominent thickening of the bladder wall (Fig. 3). Mucosal irreg-

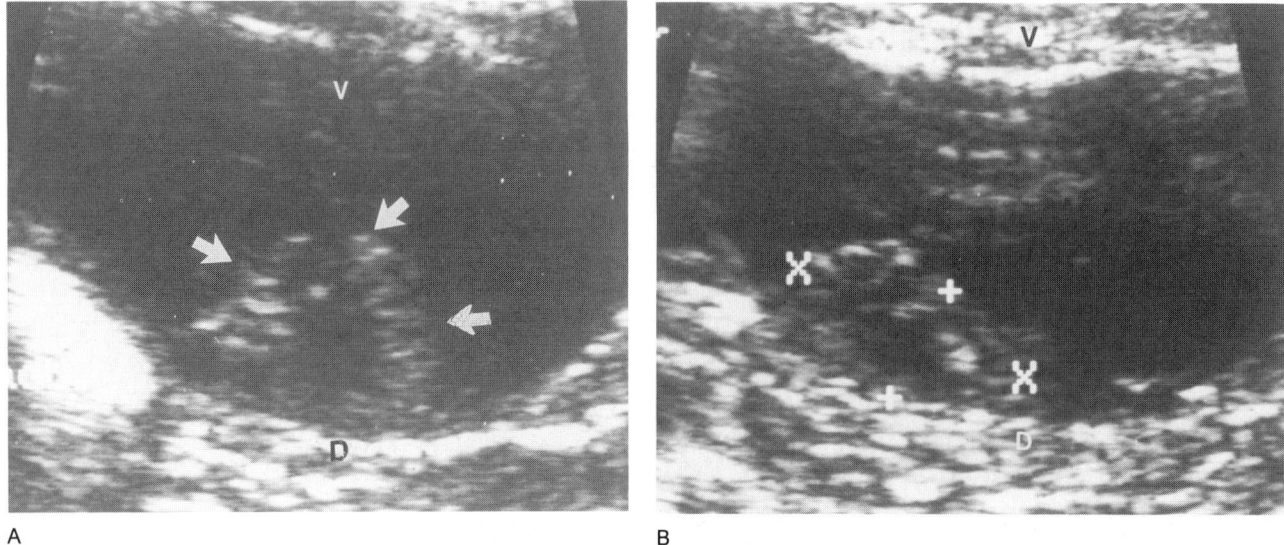

A                                                        B

**Figure 1.** *A,* Sagittal sonogram of the urinary bladder made with the cat in dorsal recumbency. A medium-level echoic mass (*arrows*) is identified adjacent to the dorsal bladder wall. *B,* Sagittal sonogram of the same cat as Figure 1*A,* but made with the cat in sternal recumbency. The echogenic mass is adherent to the dorsal bladder wall and did not gravitate to the dependent side, suggesting a fixed mural or mucosal lesion, which in this cat was felt to represent an adherent blood clot. Abbreviations: V = ventral, D = dorsal, "x"'s outline clot.

ularity can also be apparent. In some cats, as in those with polypoid cystitis, irregular protrusions of the mural/mucosal surface into the bladder lumen may be seen.

Urinary bladder sand is a prominent feature in many cats with hematuria and/or dysuria. Urinary bladder sand can be sonographically detected if it is present in sufficient quantity. The sand is usually hyperechoic and gravitates to the dependent bladder wall (Fig. 4). Depending upon the volume of sand present and its mineral content, there is variable associated acoustic shad-

owing. If the sand is unsettled or somewhat dispersed within the urine, the normal anechoic urine appearance may change to an overall increased echogenicity with small scattered areas of specular reflection.

Blood clots are identified as irregular echogenic masses either adherent to the bladder wall or free within the lumen. Adherent blood clots can be difficult to distinguish from intramural bladder masses. Urinary bladder disease can lead to secondary upper urinary tract lesions. When significant lower urinary tract dis-

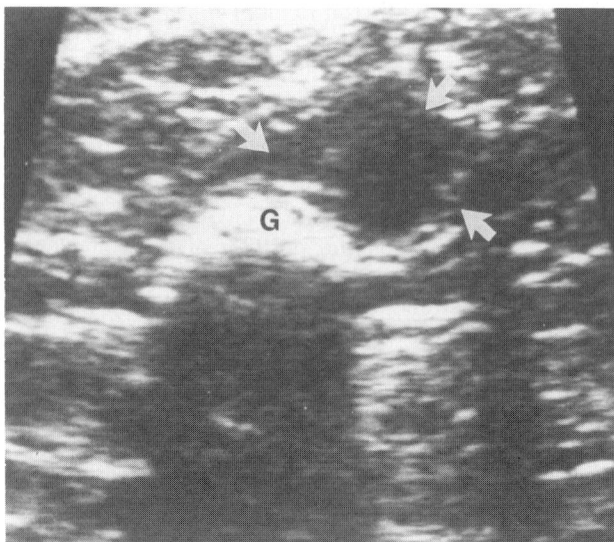

**Figure 2.** Transverse sonogram of the urinary bladder in a cat. The curvilinear hyperechoic "mass" (G) impinging upon the bladder (*arrows*) is an artifact created by colon gas. Repositioning the transducer or patient can alleviate this problem.

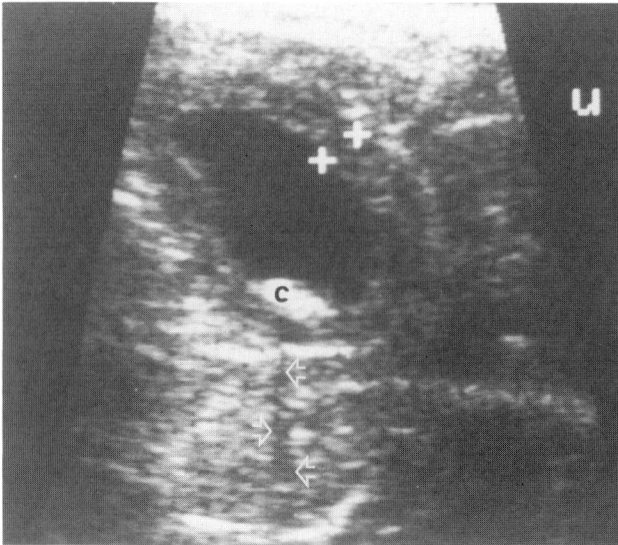

**Figure 3.** Transverse sonogram of the urinary bladder of a cat with chronic cystitis and urinary calculi (C). The bladder wall is thick (measured space between the two "+" caliper markers). Posterior acoustic shadowing (*arrows*) is seen dorsal to the calculi.

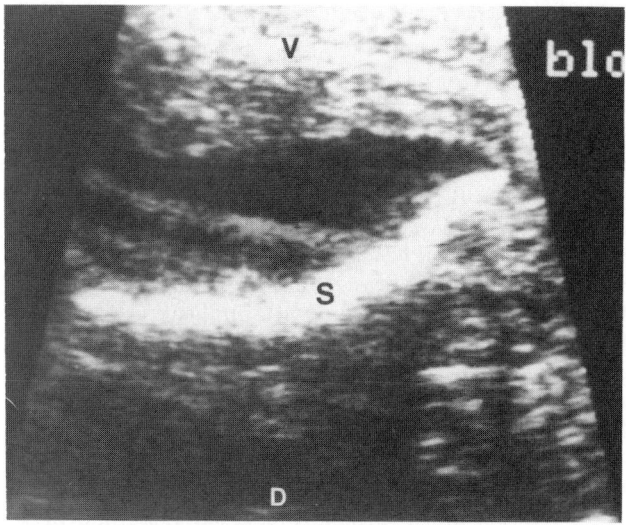

**Figure 4.** Sagittal sonogram of the urinary bladder of a cat with finely granular hyperechoic "sand" (S) along the dependent dorsal bladder wall. Abbreviations: V = ventral, D = dorsal.

ease is present, examination of the kidneys and ureter is warranted. In many instances, associated hydronephrosis or hydroureter can be detected.

Urinary bladder ultrasound should not be used to diagnose bladder rupture or tear. Free intra-abdominal fluid can be sonographically detected; however, the origin or nature of the fluid is not likely to be determined sonographically. Actual bladder wall ruptures or tears cannot definitively be sonographically identified. The sonographic visualization of a distended urinary bladder does not preclude the presence of lower urinary tract trauma.

### References and Suggested Reading

Barr F: Imaging of the urinary tract. *In* Barr F (ed): *Diagnostic Ultrasound in the Dog and Cat.* Oxford, Blackwell Scientific Publication, 1990, p 46.
   *A review of general sonographic principles pertinent to urinary tract ultrasonography.*
Mahaffey M and Barber D: Radiographic and ultrasonographic evaluation of the urinary tract. *In* Stone EA and Barsanti JA (ed): *Urologic Surgery of the Dog and Cat.* Philadelphia, Lea & Febiger, 1992, p 53.
   *A comprehensive review of radiographic and sonographic procedures valuable in the diagnostic work-up of urinary tract disease.*

# DOES INTERSTITIAL CYSTITIS OCCUR IN CATS?

C.A. TONY BUFFINGTON
*and* DENNIS J. CHEW
*Columbus, Ohio*

Lower urinary tract disease (LUTD) has long been one of the more common ailments of cats. Hamilton Kirk, in his 1925 book, *"The Diseases of the Cat,"* described blood in the urine, inflammation of the bladder, and retention of urine and urinary deposits as very common conditions of cats. Signs of LUTD do not imply an etiology: they may be caused by urolithiasis, urinary tract infection, neoplasia, congenital anomalies, or inflammation. For many years, LUTD was thought to be caused most commonly by struvite (magnesium ammonium phosphate) urolithiasis, because of the typical finding of struvite crystals in the urine and urethral plugs of afflicted cats. Struvite crystals occur commonly in the urine sediment of normal cats, however, because of their dietary habits. A comparison of the intake of protein, phosphorus, and magnesium of humans and cats, and the resulting supersaturation of urine for struvite, is presented in Table 1.

The oversaturation of struvite in cat urine, and the presence of struvite crystals in normal urine, suggests that struvite may be associated with signs of LUTD without causing them. Moreover, urine stasis and inappetence could promote struvite crystallization in the urine of obstructed patients (Buffington, 1994).

Recent evidence suggests that struvite urolithiasis is a minor cause of LUTD. Of 141 cats presented to the University of Minnesota Veterinary Hospital between 1982 and 1985 with signs of LUTD (Kruger, Osborne, and Goyal 1991), only 23% had struvite urolithiasis. No diagnosis could be made in 58% of female and 79% of unobstructed male cats, based on absence of evidence of infection (bacterial, mycoplasmal, or viral), urolithiasis, neoplasia, or congenital abnormality.

**Table 1.** *Approximate Intakes per $kg^{0.75}$ of Constitutents of Struvite by Women (50 kg) and Cats (4 kg), and the Resulting Relative Supersaturation (RSS) of Urine With Respect to Struvite*

| Nutrient | Unit | Approximate Intake | |
|---|---|---|---|
| | | **Woman** | **Cat** |
| Protein | gm | 3.5 | 8.5 |
| Phosphorus | mg | 65 | 250 |
| Magnesium | mg | 10 | 30 |
| Struvite RSS | | 1 | 8 |

The inability to make a diagnosis in such a high percentage of cases, despite diagnostic efforts of urinalysis, urine culture, and radiography, suggests the presence of another cause of LUTD. Recently, Clasper (1990) suggested that some cases of idiopathic LUTD (iLUTD) may be similar to interstitial cystitis in women. Interstitial cystitis (IC) is a lower urinary tract syndrome of humans characterized by difficult, painful, and frequent urination in the absence of a diagnosable cause. Messing (1992) states that, "The syndrome is defined by chronic irritative voiding symptoms, sterile and cytologically negative urine, and characteristic cystoscopic findings. Documentation of all three, along with failure to find a more objective cause for this clinical picture, must be present before a diagnosis of IC can be established." The "characteristic cystoscopic findings" Messing refers to is the observation of submucosal petechial hemorrhages (glomerulations) in the bladder wall after the bladder has been distended to approximately 80 cm $H_2O$ via a cystoscope.

Descriptions of iLUTD and IC presented in the veterinary and human urology literature are surprisingly comparable in their description of patient signalment, clinical signs, and diagnostic features. We recently have identified additional similarities suggesting that the pathophysiology of the two diseases may be similar. Patients afflicted with these diseases usually present as adults with signs of variable severity that appear to be exacerbated by stress. Spontaneous remission also occurs in both species. One potential species difference is that both genders of cats are affected, whereas the incidence of the disease is much higher in women than in men. Recently, however, sterile prostatitis has been recognized to be sufficiently similar to IC that it may be reclassified to "male IC." If this occurs, the gender difference will not be as large.

Patients with iLUTD and IC both present with variable combinations of increased frequency of urination, pain, and urgency. And in both species, the diagnosis is based upon history and presenting signs, bacteriologically sterile urine, and exclusion of other causes. As mentioned above, the diagnosis in women also requires observation of "glomerulations" during cystoscopic evaluation. Lesions in cat bladders are indistinguishable from glomerulations, and we commonly observe them during cystoscopic evaluation of our patients. In addition to glomerulations, increased vascularity and denuding of the superficial layer overlying the epithelium with crystal adherence to the exposed epithelium have been observed in some patients, both during periods of active disease and at time when clinical signs have abated. Careful attention to manipulation of the cystoscope is essential to clearly differentiate pathologic findings from artifacts of cystoscope-induced trauma.

As with iLUTD, evaluation of bladder biopsy specimens from patients with IC is unrewarding if they are stained with hematoxylin and eosin. What usually is observed is increased vascularity, edema, and an unremarkable inflammatory infiltrate. Using special stains however, increased numbers of mast cells have been demonstrated in the bladder submucosa of some iLUTD and IC patients. Mast cells can be activated by a number of stimuli, including antigens, cold, drugs, neurotransmitters, stress, and trauma. Once activated, mast cells release a variety of mediators that could be responsible for the observed inflammation. There are arguments both for and against the involvement of mast cells in IC. In agreement is that 30 to 50% of cases have increases in mast cells in the bladder wall, urine, or both, and that mast cell numbers correlate with concentrations of mast cell–released chemicals in the urine. A major problem with implicating mast cells in the pathophysiology of IC has been the difficulty encountered in accurately identifying the different mast cell subtypes, particularly after they have released their contents, by conventional methods of fixation and staining. Moreover, increased numbers of mast cells have been found in tissue samples of humans with other types of lower urinary tract disease, so their presence probably is not specific for IC. Nevertheless, they may mediate some of the symptoms of IC, and some drugs known to act on mast cells (hydroxyzine) have recently shown promise in treatment of some patients with IC. Although results are preliminary, we have found increased numbers of mast cells in the bladder, and increased histamine concentrations in cystoscopy effluent after hydrodistention, of some afflicted cats.

A defect in the glycosaminoglycan (GAG) layer that coats the bladder epithelium also has been found in some patients with IC. Such a defect might permit urine to penetrate the urothelium and induce inflammation. Studies have found that urinary GAG excretion in IC patients is lower than it is in normal humans, which was attributed to increased binding of GAG to the damaged urothelium. Some qualitative differences in GAG composition also have been reported. We also have found decreased GAG excretion in cats with iLUTD, further suggesting that the diseases may be similar.

The defective GAG layer, and/or epithelial damage, results in increased bladder permeability in women with IC. We recently have compared the bladder permeability of normal cats with that of cats with iLUTD. We instilled sodium salicylate, a small molecule known to diffuse out of the bladder into the bloodstream in the presence of epithelial damage, into the bladder of cats and measured the concentration of salicylate in the blood during the following 3 days. In normal cats, salicylate absorption was much lower than it was in cats with iLUTD, and it was cleared from the blood much more quickly. We are now investigating the possibility that bladder permeability differences could be used diagnostically, or to evaluate potential therapies.

Finally, many nondietary therapies used in people, such as corticosteroids, dimethyl sulfoxide (DMSO), and bladder stripping (with hypochlorous acid or silver nitrate in women), have been tried in cats, with similar disappointing results. In humans, none of the generally recommended therapies has been more effective than one would expect from a placebo.

Recent reports in the human urology literature have suggested that increased sensory afferent neuron

(SAN) density in the bladder may play a significant role in IC. Sensory afferent neurons are small-diameter fibers that conduct pain signals to the central nervous system and release neuropeptides locally, the so-called axon reflex (Maggi, 1991). They are stimulated by a variety of inputs, including distention, high concentrations of potassium or hydrogen ion, and a number of chemicals. For example, the burning sensation felt during ingestion of chili peppers is the result of stimulation of SAN in the mouth by capsaicin in the peppers. Enhanced conduction of pain and axon reflex activity would explain a number of the signs of iLUTD and IC: neuropeptide receptors are present on blood vessels, mast cells, and detrusor muscle cells, where they stimulate vascular leakage, histamine release, and contraction, respectively. Vascular leakage would appear as glomerulations during cytoscopy, histamine release would explain the inconsistency of mast cell identification (because they no longer stain after release of granules), and increased detrusor contractions could increase frequency and urgency of urination. Research on SAN has been conducted in cats, and we have tentatively identified SAN involvement in iLUTD by measuring increased concentrations of substance P, a neuropeptide released from SAN, in the hydrodistention effluent of cats with iLUTD.

To return to the question of the title, interstitial cystitis clearly does exist in cats; iLUTD meets all of the applicable diagnostic criteria promulgated by the National Institutes of Health, and probably should be renamed feline interstitial cystitis (FIC). Recent observations suggest that both FIC and IC result from neurogenic inflammation, which would add the bladder to the list of epithelia, including skin, lung, intestine, and joint, that react to some noxious stimuli by increasing SAN activity. Even if the pathogenetic mechanisms are similar, however, the etiologies still are unknown, and may or may not be similar between species, or even between patients. Identification of parallels between FIC and IC should improve our understanding of inflammatory bladder disease; the more similar the diseases, the more likely cats with FIC will be able to be used as a naturally occurring disease model to study the etiology of IC in humans, and the more likely cats are to benefit from research progress in IC.

## References and Suggested Reading

Buffington CAT: Lower urinary tract disease in cats; new problems, new paradigms. J Nutr in press.
  *Review of the nutritional aspects of urolithiasis, the dangers presented by acidified cat foods, and why nutrition no longer is a significant cause of signs of LUTD.*

Clasper M: A case of interstitial cystitis and Hunner's ulcer in a domestic shorthaired cat. NZ Vet J 38:158, 1990.
  *Case report suggesting similarities between iLUTD and IC.*

Kruger JM, Osborne CA, and Goyal SM: Clinical evaluation of cats with lower urinary tract disease. J Am Vet Med Assoc 199:211, 1991.
  *Presentation of data from 1982–85 that show that the majority of cases of LUTD are idiopathic.*

Maggi CA: The role of peptides in the regulation of the micturition reflex: An update. Gen Pharmacol 22:1, 1991.
  *Explanation of the axon reflex as it applies to the urinary system.*

Messing EM: Interstitial cystitis and related syndromes. *In Campbell's Urology*, 3rd edition. Philadelphia, WB Saunders Co, 1992, p 982.
  *Current, comprehensive review of IC in humans.*

---

# THE ROLE OF DIMETHYL SULFOXIDE AND GLUCOCORTICOIDS IN LOWER URINARY TRACT DISEASES

JEANNE A. BARSANTI,
DELMAR R. FINCO,
*and* SCOTT A. BROWN

*Athens, Georgia*

Anti-inflammatory drugs are rarely the primary mode of therapy in lower urinary tract diseases. Recently, a nonsteroidal anti-inflammatory drug, piroxicam, has been found useful in improving quality of life in dogs with transitional cell carcinoma (see "Medical Therapy of Canine Transitional Cell Carcinoma of the Urinary Bladder," this volume, p 1016). This article will focus on the use of glucocorticoids and dimethyl sulfoxide (DMSO) in non-neoplastic diseases of the lower urinary tract. An overview of glucocorticoids, including mechanism of action, indications, and adverse effects, can be found in *CVT X* (Papich and Davis, 1989) and elsewhere in this volume.

## INDICATIONS

### Granulomatous Urethritis

The only disease currently recognized for which glucocorticoids are the primary therapy is granulomatous urethritis in dogs (Matthiesen and Moroff 1989; Moroff et al., 1991). This disease affects the same population (older, females) and produces the same clinical signs (dysuria, hematuria, partial urethral obstruction) as transitional cell carcinoma of the bladder neck and urethra, which is more common. Abdominal, rectal, and vaginal palpation, contrast urethrography; or urethrocystoscopy are necessary to document urethral obstruction. Biopsy via a urethral catheter, cystoscopy, or surgery is essential to confirm a diagnosis of granulomatous urethritis and to exclude transitional cell carcinoma. The cause of granulomatous urethritis is unknown. Affected dogs often have a bacterial urinary tract infection (UTI), but whether this is secondary to inability to empty the bladder or causative of the inflammatory response is unknown. Most bacterial UTIs in dogs are not associated with such a severe inflammatory response in the urethra.

Immunosuppressive doses of glucocorticoids (1.1 mg/kg PO every 12 hr of prednisolone) have been recommended as initial therapy of granulomatous urethritis. If the response is favorable, the dose is gradually decreased by 50% every 7 to 14 days until the dosage reaches approximately 0.14 mg/kg/day. After 7 to 14 days at this low dose, glucocorticoids are discontinued. If glucocorticoids alone are unsuccessful, addition of cyclophosphamide at 2.2 mg/kg PO every 24 hr for 4 consecutive days has been recommended. Cyclophosphamide is used for 4 days each week until clinical signs have resolved for at least 7 days and then discontinued.

If an affected dog has urethral obstruction, the bladder must be kept empty with an indwelling catheter (Stone and Barsanti, 1992) until ability to urinate returns. Since affected dogs often have UTI, a urine culture should be performed to identify the causative organism and its antibiotic sensitivity. The UTI should be treated with appropriate antibiotics during immunosuppressive therapy and urinalyses should be carefully monitored to be sure the infection is controlled and does not worsen with immunosuppressive therapy. Antibiotic therapy should be continued at least 3 weeks beyond immunosuppressive therapy. Urine cultures should be obtained at the end of therapy and every month thereafter for 2 to 3 months to be sure infection does not recur.

### Idiopathic Feline Lower Urinary Tract Disease

Both DMSO and glucocorticoids have been advocated for therapy of idiopathic lower urinary tract disease of cats (feline urologic syndrome). These drugs should be considered only after identifiable causes of hematuria and dysuria in cats (such as urolithiasis, UTI, neoplasia, and traumatic injuries) have been excluded by survey radiographs, contrast radiography or ultrasonography, urinalysis, and urine culture. These drugs should not be used in cats with urethral obstruction, especially those which require urethral catheterization (see "Contraindications," below).

An anti-inflammatory dose of glucocorticoids (0.5 to 1 mg/kg PO every 12 to 24 hr of prednisolone) has been most frequently used in cats with nonobstructive, idiopathic, lower urinary tract disease. However, limited studies of this population of cats have not shown any increased rate of resolution of signs with glucocorticoids, as compared to placebo (Osborne et al., 1994). Such cats generally improve to normal within 5 days without any therapy (Barsanti et al., 1982; Osborne et al., 1994).

The use of DMSO has been suggested because of some similarities between cases of idiopathic feline lower urinary tract disease and interstitial cystitis in women (see "Does Interstitial Cystitis Occur in Cats?" this volume, p 1009). Dimethyl sulfoxide has mainly been used in cases that do not spontaneously resolve without therapy within 7 days and which are found on radiography or ultrasonography to have markedly thickened bladder walls. The recommended regimen is to place the cat under general anesthesia, catheterize and empty the bladder, infuse 10 to 20 ml of a 10% solution of DMSO, and leave this in the bladder for 10 min (Ross, 1990). Efficacy of this therapy is unknown.

## CONTRAINDICATIONS

The major contraindications to the use of glucocorticoids are the presence of a urinary tract infection or the necessity for urethral catheterization, especially indwelling catheterization. The only exception to these contraindications would be biopsy-proven granulomatous urethritis as described above. Glucocorticoids are also contraindicated in cats with urethral obstruction and postrenal azotemia because of their catabolic effects.

Most urinary tract infections are bacterial in origin, although fungal infections occur occasionally. Bacterial infections generally respond well to appropriate antibiotic therapy so that anti-inflammatory therapy is unnecessary. Glucocorticoid therapy in the face of infection may be harmful through its immunosuppressive effects. Dimethyl sulfoxide therapy may be harmful, since administration is usually intravesicular, requiring urethral catheterization, which in itself can lead to infection.

In cats with indwelling urethral catheters, the administration of glucocorticoids at anti-inflammatory doses led to a high incidence of bacterial pyelonephritis in experimental cats (Barsanti et al., 1992). This occurred even if the cats were receiving antibiotics, due to the development of antibiotic-resistant infections. The administration of glucocorticoids to these cats did not diminish catheter-induced inflammation, perhaps because of the development of bacterial infection. Thus, glucocorticoids were not beneficial, and probably were harmful in cats with indwelling urethral catheters. One would assume that similar results would occur in dogs, since dogs are at least as prone to the development of catheter-induced infection as are cats (Barsanti, Blue, and Edmunds, 1985).

Use of 45% DMSO, infused intravesicularly, in cats with indwelling urethral catheters also was not beneficial and may have been harmful (Barsanti et al., 1992). The DMSO did not diminish catheter-induced inflammation. The cats treated with DMSO seemed to be uncomfortable when the drug was infused and had a higher incidence of renal injury, although the relationship of the DMSO therapy to renal lesions could not be determined.

## ADVERSE EFFECTS

Use of glucocorticoids has been shown to predispose to bacterial urinary tract infections (Ihrke et al., 1985). Urinary tract infections in animals on glucocorticoids are often asymptomatic, requiring urinalysis and urine culture for diagnosis. Because of the frequency with which glucocorticoids are used to treat allergic dermatitis in dogs, glucocorticoids are probably a frequent cause of lower urinary tract infections in dogs. To detect these infections, it is important to perform urinalysis and/or urine culture when glucocorticoid therapy is discontinued at the end of the animal's allergy season or two to four times a year if the animal requires constant glucocorticoid therapy for allergic or immune-mediated diseases. Glucocorticoids are also a proposed risk factor for the development of calcium oxalate urolithiasis due to production of hypercalciuria (Lulich, Osborne, and Smith, 1992).

The primary adverse effect of DMSO is irritation, producing mucosal edema and hemorrhage, especially at high concentrations (>50%). Dimethyl sulfoxide produces heat when mixed with water for dilution. This exothermic reaction should be allowed to subside before intravesicular administration. There is a risk of introducing bacteria into the lower urinary tract during DMSO infusion.

## References and Suggested Reading

Barsanti JA, Finco DR, Shotts EB, et al: Feline urologic syndrome: Further investigation into therapy. J Am Anim Hosp Assoc 18:387, 1982.
*This prospective study of cats with hematuria and dysuria found that most cats became normal within 5 days whether they were treated with antibiotics, antispasmotics, fluid diuresis, or no therapy.*

Barsanti JA, Blue J, and Edmunds J: Urinary tract infection due to indwelling bladder catheters in dogs and cats. J Am Vet Med Assoc 187:384, 1985.
*A prospective study which showed that most animals with indwelling urinary catheters for more than 2 or 3 days developed urinary tract infections, whether or not they received antibiotics.*

Barsanti JA, Shotts EB, Crowell WA, et al: Effect of therapy on susceptibility to urinary tract infection in male cats with indwelling urethral catheters. J Vet Intern Med 6:64, 1992.
*This paper reports an experimental study of cats with cystitis and indwelling urethral catheters, which found a high incidence of pyelonephritis in cats that received anti-inflammatory doses of prednisolone.*

Ihrke PJ, Norton AL, Ling GV, et al: Urinary tract infection associated with long-term corticosteroid administration in dogs with chronic skin diseases. J Am Vet Med Assoc 186:43, 1985.
*This prospective study found a high incidence of urinary tract infections in dogs receiving anti-inflammatory doses of glucocorticoids for treatment of allergic dermatitis.*

Lulich JP, Osborne CA, and Smith CL: Canine calcium oxalate urolithiasis: Risk factor management. *In* Kirk RW (ed): *Current Veterinary Therapy XI.* Philadelphia, WB Saunders Co, 1992, p 892.
*This article is a review of risk factors, diagnosis, and therapy of calcium oxalate urolithiasis in dogs.*

Matthiesen DT and Moroff SD: Infiltrative urethral diseases in the dog. *In* Kirk RW (ed): *Current Veterinary Therapy X.* Philadelphia, WB Saunders Co, 1989, p 1161.
*This article reviews the diagnosis and therapy of infiltrative diseases of the urethra, focusing on transitional cell carcinoma and granulomatous urethritis.*

Moroff SD, Brown BA, Matthiesen DT, et al: Infiltrative urethral disease in female dogs: 41 cases (1980–1987). J Am Vet Med Assoc 199:247, 1991.
*This paper is a retrospective review of cases of urethral obstruction in female dogs due to neoplasia or granulomatous urethritis.*

Osborne CA, Kruger JM, Lulich JP, et al: Disorders of the Feline Lower Urinary Tract. *In* Osborne CA and Finco DR (eds): *Canine and Feline Nephrology/Urology.* Philadelphia, Lea & Febiger, 1994 (in press).
*This chapter reviews all the causes of hematuria and dysuria in cats and reports on a placebo-controlled study of prednisolone in cats with idiopathic, nonobstructive disease.*

Papich MG and Davis LE: Glucocorticoid therapy. *In* Kirk RW (ed): *Current Veterinary Therapy X.* Philadelphia, WB Saunders Co, 1989, p 54.
*This article reviews the mechanisms of action, the indications, and the potential adverse effects of glucocorticoid therapy in small animals.*

Ross LA: Treating FUS in unobstructed cats and preventing its recurrence. Vet Med 85:1218, 1990.
*This paper reviews possible modes of treatment and prevention of recurrence of idiopathic lower urinary tract disease in cats without urethral obstruction.*

Stone EA and Barsanti JA: *Urologic Surgery of the Dog and Cat.* Philadelphia, Lea & Febiger, 1992, p 149.
*This book is a general review of urinary tract problems with special emphasis on those requiring surgical therapy. The placement and care of urethral and bladder catheters is covered in detail.*

# TRANSITIONAL CELL CARCINOMA: SURGICAL LIMITATIONS

ELIZABETH A. STONE
*Raleigh, North Carolina*

*and* STEPHEN D. GILSON
*Scottsdale, Arizona*

Surgical excision of transitional cell carcinoma of the urinary bladder offers the potential for a complete cure. As with most neoplasias, early diagnosis is the key to successful surgical treatment because complete resection is only possible when a localized tumor has sufficient surrounding normal tissue to allow complete removal. Unfortunately, dogs and cats often have had clinical signs for up to 6 months before a definitive diagnosis of neoplasia. Many have had prolonged antibiotic therapy for presumed urinary tract infection.

The most commonly performed surgical procedure for bladder cancer is partial cystectomy. Complete cystectomy with ureterocolonic anastomosis allows excision of the entire bladder with maintenance of urinary continence. This procedure is performed much less frequently than partial cystectomy. Placement of a permanent cystostomy catheter may be palliative for dogs with urinary outflow obstruction. Each procedure has different indications and limitations.

## PARTIAL CYSTECTOMY

Partial cystectomy has been recommended for dogs with localized neoplasia of the urinary bladder in which adequate (1 to 2 cm) normal tissue margins can be excised with the tumor, and the bladder can be reconstructed following excision (Stone and Barsanti, 1992). Owners should be forewarned that until the bladder expands, the dogs may be pollakiuric for several weeks after surgery. The primary advantage of partial cystectomy is the preservation of urinary tract continuity.

Unfortunately, bladder neoplasia often recurs locally after partial cystectomy (Schwartz et al., 1985). Local recurrence may result from technical errors during the partial cystectomy, such as incomplete resection of the original tumor or implantation of tumor cells into normal tissue (tumor seeding). Incomplete resection may not be apparent at the time of surgery. In one report, all grossly visible tumor was excised from eight dogs, but in four of the dogs, histopathologic evaluation revealed neoplastic tissue in the surgical margins (Stone* et al., 1994). Thus, tumor-free margins should be verified at the time of resection by intraoperative cytologic or histologic (frozen-section) examination. After surgery, histologic examination of formalin-fixed tissues provides further confirmation of complete excision. To facilitate evaluation by the pathologist, the excised specimen should be pinned out flat to a corkboard and the tissue margins marked with India ink before immersion in formalin solution. Measurements are made between the cut edge of the fresh specimen and the first evidence of gross tumor around the entire circumference of the specimen. The clinician should request that the pathologist examine all of the margins.

Tumor seeding is a documented hazard of partial cystectomy for transitional cell carcinoma (Gilson et al., 1990). Precautions to prevent tumor seeding include using drapes to protect the abdominal wall from tumor implantation and using laparotomy pads to isolate the tumor from the peritoneal cavity. The incision in the bladder should not penetrate the tumor. After the excision is completed, gloves and drapes are changed, and new instruments are used to close the bladder and abdominal incisions. Flushing the wound with distilled water may help kill exfoliated cells.

Tumor recurrence after partial cystectomy also may be caused by *de novo* tumors arising from the remaining bladder mucosa, which is exposed to the same conditions that caused the original tumor. To help detect multifocal tumors during the initial surgery, any abnormal looking mucosa should be biopsied during the partial cystectomy. As cystoscopy becomes more widely available, cystoscopic examination may help in the early detection of multifocal and recurrent tumors.

Although partial cystectomy can provide a complete cure of bladder neoplasia, it is only recommended when metastasis has not occurred, intraoperative diagnosis enables a complete resection, and tumor seeding of the wound is prevented.

## COMPLETE CYSTECTOMY AND URETEROCOLONIC ANASTOMOSIS

Surgical excision of multiple bladder tumors or tumors that extend into the bladder neck necessitates total cystectomy and permanent urinary diversion. With ureterocolonic anastomosis, dogs maintain continence without the use of an external collecting bag or inter-

---

*Stone EA, George TF, Gilson SD, and Page RL: Partial cystectomy for urinary bladder neoplasia: Surgical technique and outcome in nine dogs. Personal observations.

mittent catheterization. The procedure is not recommended for dogs with hydroureter, renal disease, or liver disease. After ureterocolonic anastomosis, dogs void a watery mixture of feces and urine that has a pungent odor. The dogs must be allowed to urinate-defecate every 3 to 4 hr to prevent accumulation of urine in the colon and excessive absorption of urea and electrolytes from the colon. Dogs must be monitored for metabolic acidosis, hyperammonemia, and electrolyte abnormalities for the remainder of their lives.

Compared to partial cystectomy, the risk of tumor seeding may be less with complete cystectomy because the bladder is removed intact. Unfortunately, in our experience, complete cystectomy and urinary diversion has not been curative because of the advanced stage of the disease at the time of surgery (Stone et al., 1988). Clinicians should consider performing complete cystectomy earlier in the course of the disease, particularly in those dogs that would currently be treated with partial cystectomy. For both partial and complete cystectomy, additional evaluation is needed to determine the role of adjuvant chemotherapy or radiation therapy for residual microscopic or metastatic neoplasia.

## PERMANENT CYSTOSTOMY CATHETER

Placement of a permanent cystostomy catheter is a minimally invasive method for palliating dogs with urinary outflow obstruction from a bladder tumor. A mushroom catheter is placed into the bladder and exited through the abdominal wall (Stone and Barsanti, 1992). A collapsible basket catheter is not suitable because the basket may collapse and pull out of the bladder. Owners find the cystostomy catheter easy to manage, draining the urine with a syringe three to four times a day. In seven dogs with advanced bladder neoplasms, a permanent cystostomy catheter allowed dogs to survive for similar lengths of time (median survival = 97 days) as dogs treated with chemotherapy or radiotherapy (Smith et al., 1994).

Placement of a cystostomy catheter is indicated when (1) imaging studies indicate a trigonal mass and owners do not want a complete cystectomy and ureterocolonic anastomosis; (2) metastasis is evident, so complete cystectomy will not be curative; (3) an exploratory laparotomy reveals a nonresectable tumor; (4) the specific diagnosis of a bladder mass is uncertain (i.e., potential for polypoid cystitis, granulomatous urethritis) and the owners will not allow an open biopsy; or (5) for complete obstruction or severe stranguria while awaiting a response to adjuvant therapy. Most dogs with transitional cell carcinoma are relatively healthy, except for the urinary tract signs associated with the neoplasm. Placement of a permanent cystostomy catheter gives the owners time to understand the severity of their dog's disease and to consider further treatment or euthanasia.

## References and Suggested Reading

Gilson SD and Stone EA: Surgically induced tumor seeding in eight dogs and two cats. J Am Vet Med Assoc 11:1811, 1990.
*A review of the mechanism of tumor seeding and a report on tumor seeding in ten animals.*
Norris AM, Lanig EJ, Valli VEO, et al: Canine bladder and urethral tumors: A retrospective study of 115 cases (1980–1985). J Vet Intern Med 6:145, 1992.
*A multicenter retrospective study of bladder and urethral tumors that compares the results following surgery, chemotherapy, and/or radiation therapy.*
Smith JD, Stone EA, and Gilson SD: Permanent cystostomy catheter as a palliative treatment for urine outflow obstruction from presumed transitional cell carcinoma. J Am Vet Med Assoc (in press) 1995.
*A description of the indications and results of the use of permanent cystostomy catheters in dogs with transitional cell carcinoma.*
Stone EA: Temporary bypass of urethral obstruction. In Stone EA and Barsanti JA (eds): *Urologic Surgery of the Dog and Cat.* Philadelphia, Lea & Febiger, 1992, p 152.
*Describes the technique for placement of a cystostomy catheter.*
Stone EA, Withrow SJ, Page RL, et al: Ureterocolonic anastomosis in ten dogs with transitional cell carcinoma. Vet Surg 17:147, 1988.
*Describes the postoperative course, including management of hyperchloremic acidosis, hyperammonemia, and colitis in dogs following ureterocolonic anastomosis.*

# MEDICAL THERAPY OF CANINE TRANSITIONAL CELL CARCINOMA OF THE URINARY BLADDER

DEBORAH W. KNAPP

*West Lafayette, Indiana*

Transitional cell carcinoma (TCC) is the most common neoplasm of the canine urinary bladder (Withrow, 1989; Norris et al., 1992). It is an uncommon tumor, occurring as less than 1% of all reported canine malignancies (Withrow, 1989). The diagnosis, treatment, and biologic behavior of TCC has been reviewed (Withrow, 1989; Norris et al., 1992). Briefly, TCC is a locally infiltrative and invasive tumor. This form of cancer presents a therapeutic challenge because it is often advanced at the time of diagnosis, is usually not amenable to complete surgical resection, and can result in partial or complete urinary tract obstruction. Norris et al. (1992) reported that 37% of dogs with TCC had metastasis at the time of tumor diagnosis. Although the prognosis is guarded to poor in most dogs with TCC, some patients may benefit from medical therapy, with long-term tumor control being possible.

## DIAGNOSIS AND CLINICAL STAGING

Clinical signs of TCC of the bladder commonly include hematuria, dysuria, and pollakiuria (Norris et al., 1992). Signs may have been present for weeks to months, and may have temporarily improved with antibiotic therapy. Occasionally, dogs with TCC present with lameness due to hypertrophic osteopathy or bone metastasis.

Physical examination including a thorough rectal examination, may reveal thickening of the urethra and trigone region of the bladder and enlargement of sublumbar (illiac) lymph nodes. In advanced cases of TCC, abdominal palpation may reveal a mass in the bladder or a distended urinary bladder if urinary tract obstruction is present. In female dogs, vaginal examination may aid in localization of urethral masses. Thirty per cent of dogs with urethral and bladder tumors are reported to have normal physical examination (Norris et al., 1992).

Transitional cell carcinoma should be included in the differential diagnosis list for dogs with chronic or recurrent urinary tract infection, chronic hematuria or dysuria, abnormal epithelial cells detected by urinalysis, and thickening or mass lesions of the urethra or bladder wall. Evaluation of these dogs should include complete blood count (CBC), serum biochemistry profile, urinalysis, urine culture, contrast cystography, urethrography where appropriate, and ultrasonography. In one study, contrast cystography demonstrated a mass or filling defect in 96% of dogs with TCC of the bladder or urethra (Norris et al., 1992). Care must be taken when passing a urinary catheter during diagnostic procedures because tumor infiltration increases the risk of catheter penetration through a weakened urethral or bladder wall.

The diagnosis of TCC requires histologic confirmation. Although neoplastic cells may be present in the urine of 30% of dogs with TCC, neoplastic cells are often indistinguishable from reactive epithelial cells associated with inflammation. Methods of obtaining tissue for histpathologic examination include laparotomy and cystotomy, cystoscopy, and traumatic catheterization.

Once a diagnosis of TCC has been confirmed, clinical staging should be completed. Abdominal and thoracic radiography should be performed to detect gross metastasis in lymph nodes, abdominal organs, and the lungs. Abdominal ultrasonography is also useful in searching for metastatic disease in the abdomen.

## TREATMENT

Surgical excision with wide margins is the treatment of choice for localized TCC that does not involve the urethra or trigone region of the bladder. Surgery may also be considered as an emergency, palliative procedure to debulk nonresectable tumors in dogs with urinary tract obstruction. Medical management of TCC is indicated in dogs with nonresectable or metastatic tumors.

### Cisplatin Therapy

Cisplatin (*cis*-diamminedichloroplatinum) (Platinol, Bristol Laboratories) has been the most extensively studied chemotherapeutic agent against canine TCC (also see *CVT XI*, p 395).

In a retrospective study, 18 dogs with measurable, histopathologically confirmed TCC of the bladder were treated with cisplatin at the Purdue University Veterinary Teaching Hospital between 1983 and 1993. Cisplatin was administered at a dosage of 60 mg/m$^2$ IV once every 3 weeks (Knapp et al., 1988) for one to six treatments. In this series of cases, there were no complete remissions, two partial remissions (≥50% decrease in tumor volume with no new tumor lesions), and three dogs with stable disease (<50% change in tumor volume with no new tumor lesions at 42 days on therapy). Cisplatin toxicity occurred in the form of acute seizures and death in one dog, and progressive azotemia in two dogs.

Similar results were reported by Moore et al. (1990) in a retrospective study of 15 dogs with TCC of the bladder or urethra treated with one to nine doses of cisplatin (40 to 50 mg/m$^2$). Of 12 tumors evaluable following therapy, there were no complete remissions, three partial remissions, and six dogs had stable disease. The median survival of these 15 dogs was 114 days. Six dogs developed increased serum creatinine concentrations during therapy. Similar results were noted by Shapiro et al. (1988) in a retrospective study including eight dogs with TCC treated with 25 to 50 mg/m$^2$ cisplatin.

Although these studies demonstrate activity of cisplatin in canine TCC, the remission rate appears low, and renal toxicity is a possible complication of therapy.

## Carboplatin Therapy

Carboplatin (Paraplatin, Bristol Laboratories) at a dosage of 300 mg/m$^2$ IV every 21 days has been proposed as a method of treating canine transitional cell carcinoma. Carboplatin, a cisplatin analog, is usually not associated with renal toxicity, and appears to have a different spectrum of antitumor activity than cisplatin in human tumors (Christian, 1992). Preliminary results of a pilot study conducted by investigators in the Purdue Comparative Oncology Program has shown no renal toxicity or severe vomiting, but tumor response has been disappointing. No partial or complete remissions were obtained in the first seven dogs entered into the study.

## Piroxicam Therapy

Piroxicam (Feldene, Pfizer Laboratories), a nonsteroidal anti-inflammatory drug (NSAID) and cyclooxygenase inhibitor, has shown antitumor activity against canine TCC of the urinary bladder (Knapp et al., 1992; Knapp et al., 1994). The antitumor activity does not appear to be a direct cytotoxic effect, and immunomodulation is thought to play a role (Knapp et al., 1994). Piroxicam (0.3 mg/kg PO every 24 hr) was given to 34 dogs with TCC of the bladder. Responses included two dogs with complete remission (disappearance of all clinical and radiographic evidence of tumor for a minimum of 30 days), four dogs with partial remission (≥50% reduction in tumor volume and no new lesions), 18 dogs with stable disease (<50% change in tumor volume at 56 days of therapy), and ten dogs with progressive disease (≥50% increase in tumor volume

or the appearance of new lesions). The median survival of all dogs was 181 days.

Piroxicam therapy was generally well tolerated. Many (29 of 34) pet owners reported increased activity level and improved mental alertness in their dogs. Gastrointestinal irritation occurred in 6 of 34 dogs as characterized by anorexia, melena, and vomiting. Signs of gastrointestinal irritation resolved with discontinuation of piroxicam and administration of cimetidine (Tagamet, SmithKline Beecham) and sucralfate (Carafate, Marion Merrell Dow). In two of the six dogs, reinstitution of piroxicam therapy was attempted and was successful when given with misoprostol (Cytotec, Searle) (see "Gastrointestinal Ulcer Therapy," this volume, p 706). As with all NSAIDs, if signs of gastrointestinal irritation occur, it is important to discontinue piroxicam therapy to prevent more advanced gastrointestinal ulceration and potential perforation.

Renal papillary necrosis, which is considered a form of NSAID toxicity, was detected on postmortem examination in 2 of 25 dogs. These two dogs died of tumor progression and the clinical significance of the renal pathology could not be determined.

## Supportive Care

Due to the disruption of the normal urinary epithelium, dogs with TCC frequently develop urinary tract infections. Urinalyses should be performed regularly to detect secondary infection. Urine culture and sensitivity testing should be used to select appropriate antibiotic therapy. Improvement in clinical signs will often occur with appropriate antibiotic therapy. Long-term or repeated antibiotic therapy is often necessary.

Urination in dogs with TCC should be monitored closely to detect possible urinary tract obstruction. If urinary tract obstruction occurs, temporary catheterization, definitive therapy aimed at the TCC, antibiotics to reduce inflammation associated with a secondary bacterial infection, or surgical debulking could be considered.

## References and Suggested Reading

Christian MC: The current status of new platinum analogs. Semin Oncol 19: 720, 1992.
    *A review of platinum analogs in human cancer medicine.*
Knapp DW, Richardson RC, Bonney PL, et al: Cisplatin therapy in 41 dogs with malignant tumors. J Vet Intern Med 2:41, 1988.
    *A retrospective study describing treatment protocol, toxicity, and tumor response of cisplatin therapy in 41 tumor-bearing dogs.*
Knapp DW, Richardson RC, Bottoms GD, et al: Phase I trial of piroxicam in 62 dogs bearing naturally occurring tumors. Cancer Chemother Pharmacol 29:214, 1992.
    *A phase I trial (dose escalation study) of piroxicam in 62 tumor-bearing dogs.*
Knapp DW, Richardson RC, Chan TCK, et al: Piroxicam therapy in 34 dogs with transitional cell carcinoma of the urinary bladder. J Vet Intern Med 8:273, 1994.
    *Report of the antitumor activity of piroxicam in 34 dogs with transitional cell carcinoma.*
Moore AS, Cardona A, Shapiro W, et al: Cisplatin (cisdiamminedichloroplatinum) for treatment of transitional cell carcinoma of the urinary bladder or urethra. A retrospective study of 15 dogs. J Vet Intern Med 4:148, 1990.

*Retrospective study of tumor response, survival, and toxicity associated with cisplatin therapy in dogs with transitional cell carcinoma.*

Norris AM, Laing EJ, Valli VEO, et al: Canine bladder and urethral tumors: A retrospective study of 115 cases (1980–1985). J Vet Intern Med 6:145, 1992.

*A retrospective study of histologic type, diagnosis, staging, and treatment of bladder and urethral tumors in 115 dogs.*

Shapiro W, Kitchell BE, Fossum TW, et al: Cisplatin for treatment of tran-

sitional cell and squamous cell carcinomas in dogs. J Am Vet Med Assoc 193:1530, 1988.

*A retrospective study of cisplatin therapy in eight dogs with transitional cell carcinoma and five dogs with squamous cell carcinoma.*

Withrow SJ: Tumors of the urinary system. *In* Withrow SJ and MacEwen EG (eds): *Clinical Veterinary Oncology.* Philadelphia, JB Lippincott Co, 1989, p 312.

*Review of canine and feline urinary tract tumors.*

# FELINE URINARY INCONTINENCE

PETER E. HOLT

*Bristol, Avon, United Kingdom*

Compared to the dog the cat has a low incidence of urinary incontinence. Urinary incontinence is defined as involuntary leakage of urine, as distinct from inappropriate micturition.

## NORMAL CONTROL OF URINARY CONTINENCE

As in other species, feline urinary continence is achieved by means of a low intravesical pressure that is exceeded by urethral resistance. A low pressure in the bladder reservoir is maintained by $\beta$-adrenergic innervation (via the hypogastric nerve) and lack of parasympathetic activity (from the pelvic nerve). The hypogastric nerve also supplies $\alpha$-adrenergic innervation to urethral smooth and, in the cat, striated muscle. The latter is also under voluntary control via the pudendal nerve. Passive elasticity also contributes to urethral tone, but the proportion of urethral sphincter function due to such elasticity compared to neuromuscular function is unknown.

## INVESTIGATION OF INCONTINENT CATS

Physical examination of the incontinent cat is frequently unrewarding and ancillary investigations are mandatory. These should include intravenous urography, vaginourethrography, urethrocystography, urine laboratory examinations (particularly bacteriology and cytology) and, in some cases, ultrasonography and urodynamics.

## CAUSES OF URINARY INCONTINENCE

### Congenital Abnormalities

These include ureteral ectopia, urethral sphincter mechanism incompetence, pervious urachus, bladder

hypoplasia, urethrorectal fistula, and congenital paralysis.

### URETERAL ECTOPIA

Only 23 cases of feline ureteral ectopia have been described in the literature (Holt and Gibbs, 1992). Affected kittens are usually incontinent, but occasionally ectopic ureters may be detected in continent cats undergoing contrast radiographic examinations for recurring urinary tract infections. Domestic shorthaired cats are commonly affected, and exotic species such as Siamese, Persian, and Burmese do not appear to be overrepresented. The condition can be uni- or bilateral, with most ectopic ureters terminating in the urethra (Figs. 1 and 2) or, occasionally, the vagina. Complications such as hydroureter/hydronephrosis (Fig. 1) and pyelonephritis are frequently present. Cats with gross unilateral hydronephrosis or severe pyelonephritis are best treated by ureteronephrectomy (as long as a functional second kidney is present!), but milder degrees of hydronephrosis may reduce following successful ureteral transplantation. An intravesical transplantation technique is not usually possible since, unlike the situation in the dog, feline ectopic ureters usually completely bypass the bladder without entering the bladder wall (Fig. 2). Bladder wall tunneling techniques (e.g., Robins and Presnell, 1974) can be used, but the small size of feline ureters makes transplantation technically difficult. The use of an operating microscope allows more accurate and less traumatic suture placement by means of fine ophthalmic instruments and sutures. The prognosis after treatment (ureteral transplantation or ureteronephrectomy) is usually good unless concomitant problems such as congenital urethral sphincter mechanism incompetence or bladder hypoplasia are present.

### CONGENITAL URETHRAL SPHINCTER MECHANISM INCOMPETENCE

This condition has been reported recently (Holt and Gibbs, 1992). Most affected animals are domestic

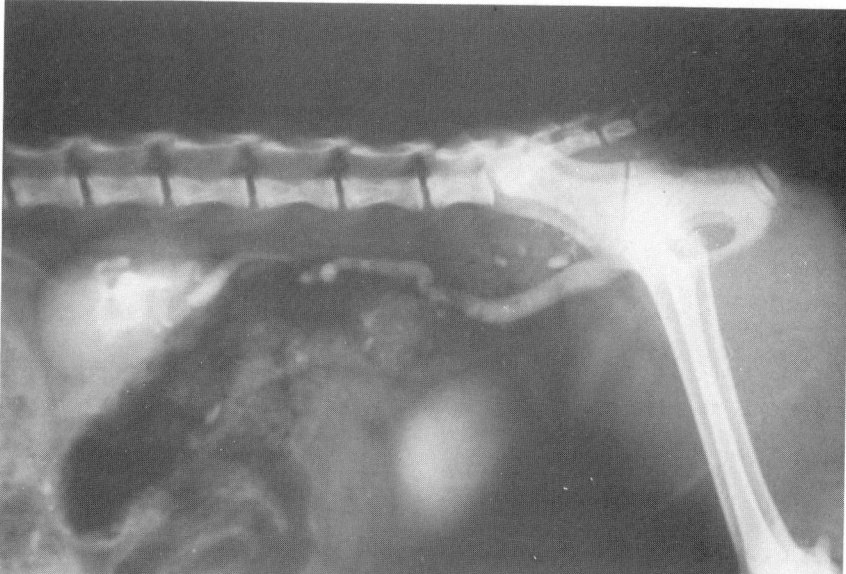

**Figure 1.** Ureteral ectopia, renal pelvic dilatation and hydroureter demonstrated by intravenous urography in a neutered male domestic shorthaired cat. Both ureters were ectopic in this cat, terminating in the urethra. (From Holt PE and Gibbs C: Congenital urinary incontinence in cats: A review of 19 cases. Vet Rec 130: 437, 1992, with permission.)

shorthaired cats and all are female. Incontinence in these cats is more copious than in those with ureteral ectopia and is worse when the animal is recumbent. Contrast radiography demonstrates marked urethral hypoplasia, with a urethral tube virtually absent in some cats (Fig. 3). Concomitant abnormalities are common. Vaginal aplasia is often present and the uterine horns insert into the dorsal bladder wall, resulting in bladder "diverticula" if the lumena are continuous and leading to recurring cystitis. Other associated abnormalities include bladder hypoplasia, ureteral ectopia, and unilateral renal aplasia. An attempt has been made to treat these cases (Holt, 1993) by creation of a longer urethra using bladder neck reconstruction techniques. The degree of incontinence is greatly reduced in most

animals and almost half of affected cats are cured by these procedures.

### PERVIOUS URACHUS

Pervious urachus is an extremely rare congenital abnormality, resulting in urine leakage from the umbilicus. The diagnosis can be confirmed by positive contrast cystography. Surgical excision of the urachus will cure the incontinence.

### BLADDER HYPOPLASIA

Bladder hypoplasia is a subjective diagnosis. The author has not diagnosed bladder hypoplasia alone in cats.

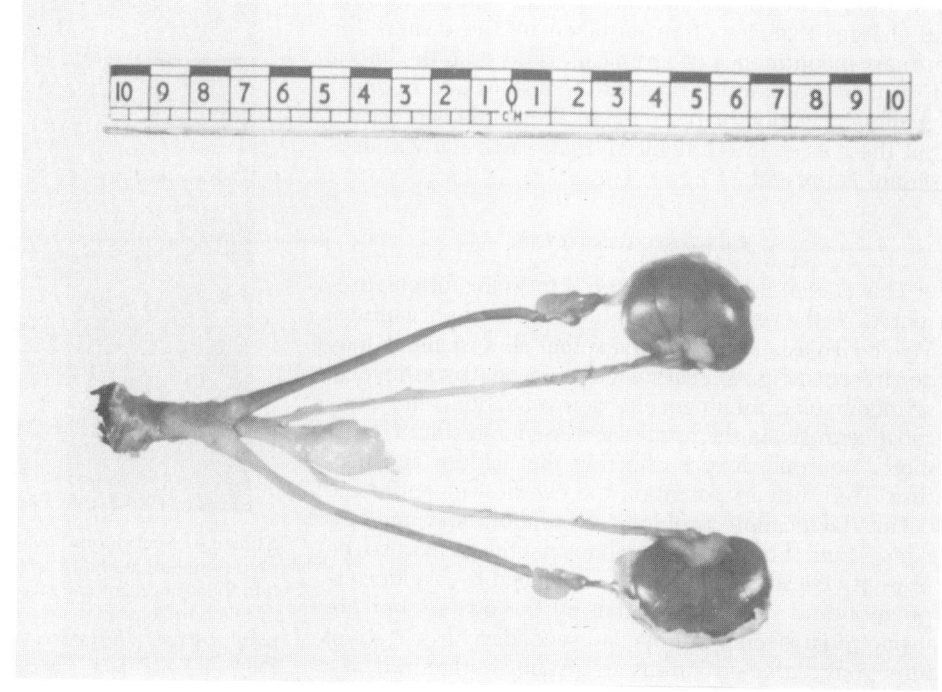

**Figure 2.** *Postmortem* specimen from a 3-month-old female domestic shorthaired cat. Note the bilateral ureteral ectopia into the short urethra. There had also been embryonic failure of the müllerian ducts to unite to form a vagina in this cat and thus the uterine horns open directly into the vestibule. (From Holt PE and Gibbs C: Congenital urinary incontinence in cats: A review of 19 cases. Vet Rec 130:439, 1992, with permission.)

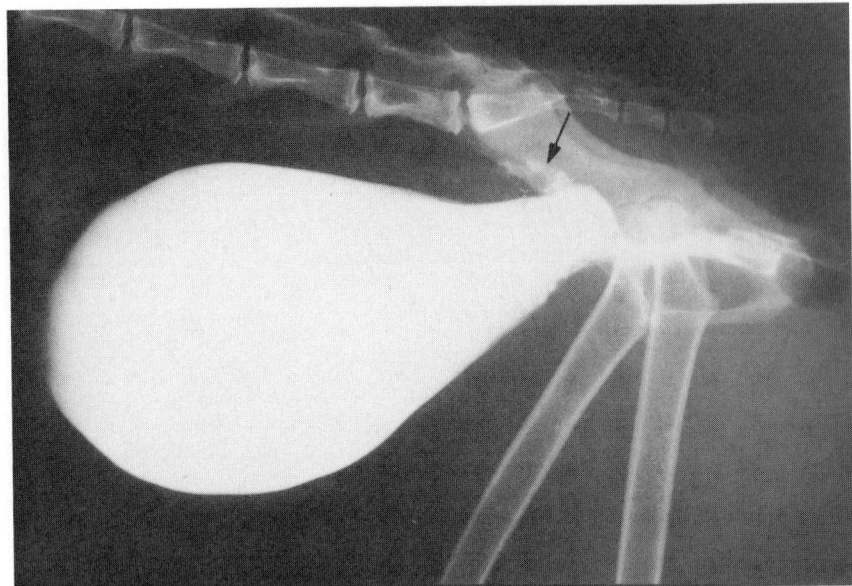

**Figure 3.** Marked urethral hypoplasia (compare with Fig. 5) in a 1-year-old neutered female domestic shorthaired cat. No vagina can be seen, but there is reflux of contrast medium from the caudodorsal bladder into uterine horn remnants (*arrowed*), the lumena of which are confluent with that of the bladder. These may form "diverticula," predisposing to recurring urinary tract infection (as does the short urethra). (From Holt PE: Urinary incontinence in dogs and cats. Vet Rec 127:348, 1990, with permission.)

It has always accompanied other congenital conditions such as ureteral ectopia or/and urethral sphincter mechanism incompetence (Fig. 2). Although its presence may adversely affect the prognosis in incontinent cats, experience suggests that the hypoplastic bladder usually develops a normal capacity after successful treatment of the primary cause of incontinence.

### URETHRORECTAL FISTULA

This is due to an embryonic failure of the urorectal fold to completely divide the primitive hind gut (the cloaca) into a dorsal (rectal) portion and a ventral urogenital sinus that in the male will give rise to the pelvic urethra. It is extremely rare and is often associated with atresia ani. Kittens present with recurring urinary tract infections and discolored urine or fecal-stained urethral discharges that are often mistaken by the owners for urinary incontinence. If atresia ani is present, the kitten is usually presented earlier with tenesmus and perineal swelling. Ligation or resection of the fistula is possible, but these cases are difficult to treat, particularly if atresia ani is present.

### CONGENITAL PARALYSIS

This is commonly encountered in Manx kittens presented with vesicourethral functional abnormalities. Myelodysplasia and vertebral spinal abnormalities may be present (Fig. 4). Pathologic changes (hydromyelia, syringomyelia, meningocele, demyelination, and neuronal necrosis) in the lumbosacral region result in lower motor neurone disease affecting the bladder and urethra. Thus, urinary retention and overflow incontinence occur. Defecation problems (retention and incontinence) and hindlimb gait abnormalities may also be present. These animals can be managed by bladder expression and rectal evacuation by the owners but are prone to iatrogenic trauma and secondary urinary tract infections. Affected kittens are usually euthanized.

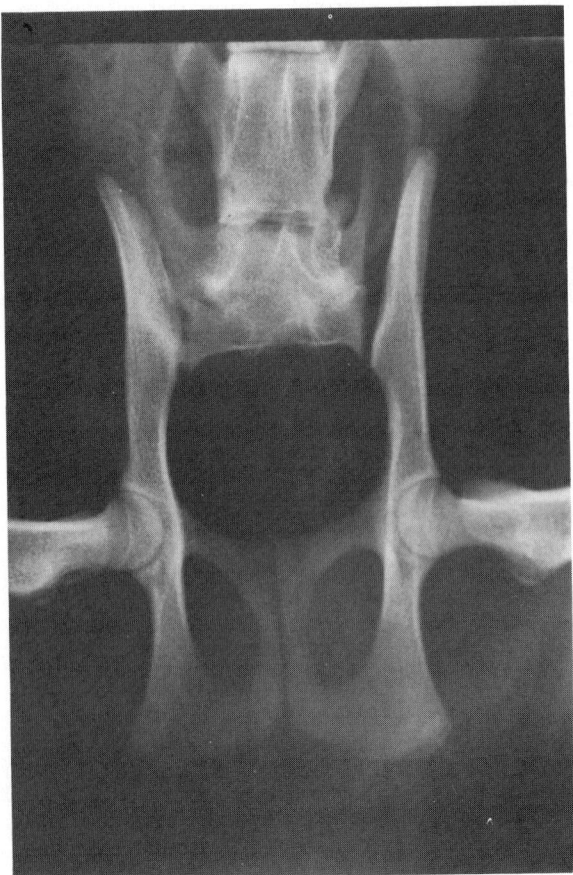

**Figure 4.** Ventrodorsal pelvic radiograph of a young Manx cat with urinary retention and overflow incontinence. There is a lack of vertebral development caudal to the sacrum. (From Holt PE: Aspects of feline urology. *In* Raw M-E and Parkinson TJ (eds): *The Veterinary Annual. Thirty-Second Issue.* Oxford, Blackwell Scientific Publications, 1992, p 20, with permission.)

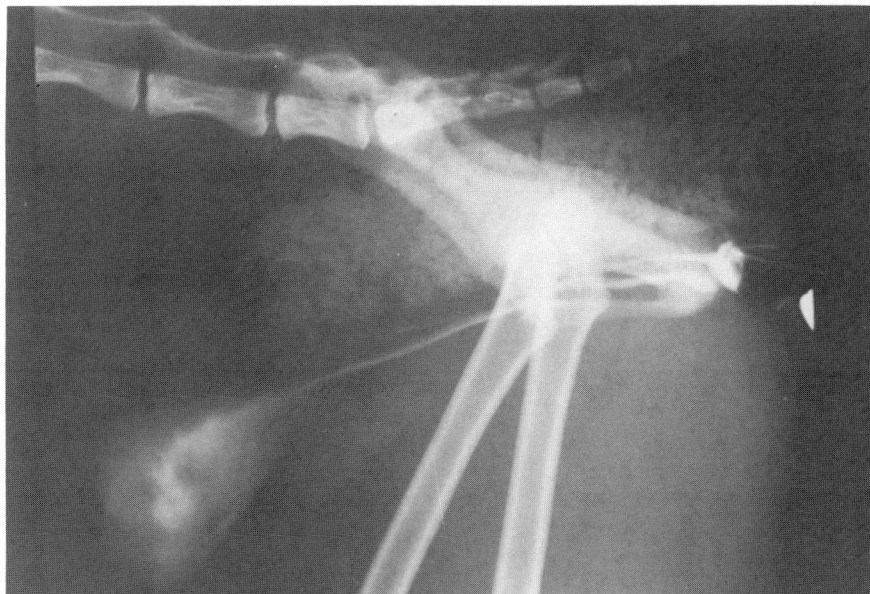

**Figure 5.** Normal feline vaginoureth-rogram. Note the wide vestibule leading into the much narrower vagina and the (normally) long urethra. (From Holt PE: Surgical management of congenital urethral sphincter mechanism incompetence in eight female cats and a bitch. Vet Surg 22:100, 1993, with permission.)

## Acquired Conditions

These include urethral sphincter mechanism incompetence, neoplasia, ureterovaginal fistula, and acquired neurogenic problems.

### URETHRAL SPHINCTER MECHANISM INCOMPETENCE

This is extremely rare in the adult cat, probably because, for its size, the cat has a long urethra (compared to a dog of similar size) and thus, presumably, an efficient urethral sphincter mechanism (Fig. 5).

### NEOPLASIA

Neoplasia of the feline lower urinary tract is also rare. The bladder is usually affected. The signs are hematuria, frequency/tenesmus, and dysuria, but occasionally urge incontinence may be exhibited. Most tumors are malignant carcinomas (transitional cell carcinomas, squamous cell carcinomas, and adenocarcinomas). Local lymphatic and distant pulmonary metastasis may have occurred by the time the condition is diagnosed, and the prognosis is usually hopeless.

### URETEROVAGINAL FISTULA

This is a rare complication of abdominal genital surgery (ovariohysterectomy or caesarian section) in cats and results in acquired ureteral ectopia into the vagina. The history is of continuous postoperative incontinence. The treatment is ureteral transplantation or ureteronephrectomy, depending on the presence and degree of secondary ureteral and renal problems.

### ACQUIRED NEUROGENIC PROBLEMS

Bladder and urethral function can be affected by central, upper, or lower motor neuron disease. The most common cause is trauma to the spine. Caudal lumbar and sacral injuries may result in lower motor neuron vesicourethral dysfunction, manifest as urinary retention with overflow incontinence. Often, the degree of vertebral fracture displacement or dislocation detected radiographically bears little relationship to the severity of the clinical signs associated with trauma/avulsion of sacral nerve roots. Affected cats may have complete paralysis of the bladder, urethra, rectum, and tail, with loss of perineal and tail sensation. The prognosis is guarded and bladder expression or catheterization/centesis may be required for several weeks until an improvement (or lack of) can be appreciated. In cases that regain vesicourethral function, amputation of the paralyzed tail may be required.

## References and Suggested Reading

Allen WE and Webbon PM: Two cases of urinary incontinence in cats associated with acquired vagino-ureteral fistula. J Small Anim Pract 21:367, 1980.
*The first case reports of this unusual cause of feline incontinence.*
Barsanti JA and Downey R: Urinary incontinence in cats. J Am Anim Hosp Assoc 20:979, 1984.
*Urinary incontinence in cats associated with feline leukemia virus infection.*
Holt PE: Positive contrast vagino-urethrography for diagnosis of lower urinary tract disease. In Kirk RW (ed): Current Veterinary Therapy X. Small Animal Practice. Philadelphia, WB Saunders Co, 1989, p 1142.
*A description of the technique and application of vaginourethrography in bitches that is equally useful in cats.*
Holt PE: Aspects of feline urology. In Raw M-E and Parkinson TJ (eds): The Veterinary Annual. Thirty-Second Issue. Oxford, Blackwell Scientific Publications, 1992, p 13.
*A review of feline urologic disorders, excluding the feline urologic syndrome.*
Holt PE and Gibbs C: Congenital urinary incontinence in cats: A review of 19 cases. Vet Rec 130:437, 1992.
*A review of ureteral ectopia and descriptions of the clinical and radiographic features of congenital urethral sphincter mechanism incompetence.*
Holt PE: Surgical management of congenital urethral sphincter mechanism incompetence in eight female cats and a bitch. Vet Surg 22:98, 1993.
*Descriptions of bladder neck reconstruction techniques and the results obtained.*
Holt PE: A Color Atlas of Small Animal Urology. London, Mosby Year Book Europe, 1994.

*Pictorial descriptions of diagnostic methods, surgical indications, and urologic techniques.*
Robins GM and Presnell KR: Ureteroneocystostomy in the dog. J Small Anim Pract 15:185, 1974.
*A description of a bladder wall tunneling technique for ureteral transplantation, suitable for use in the cat.*

Stone EA and Barsanti JA: *Urologic Surgery of the Dog and Cat.* Philadelphia, Lea & Febiger, 1992.
*Descriptions of pathophysiology, diagnostic methods, and surgical treatments with excellent line drawings.*

# URINARY INCONTINENCE AND CONGENITAL UROGENITAL ANOMALIES IN SMALL ANIMALS

INDIA F. LANE

*Charlottetown, Prince Edward Island, Canada*

*and* MICHAEL R. LAPPIN

*Fort Collins, Colorado*

Causes of urinary incontinence in small animals include neurogenic, anatomic, and functional abnormalities of the lower urinary tract. In juvenile animals, urinary incontinence is frequently attributed to anatomic anomalies, but may be complicated by urinary bladder or urethral dysfunction. Congenital anatomic anomalies in which urinary incontinence may be observed include urethral or urinary bladder hypoplasia, ectopic ureters, vaginal anomalies, pseudohermaphroditism, urinary bladder exstrophy, ureteroceles, and urethral fistulae. Multiple anomalies are frequently observed in affected individuals, which is not unexpected in light of the complex embryologic development involved. It follows that functional abnormalities of the urinary tract also may be expected in animals with anatomic urogenital abnormalities. The most common functional abnormality contributing to urinary incontinence is urethral incompetence (or urethral sphincter mechanism incompetence), in which reduced urethral resistance during urine storage allows urine leakage. Less commonly, urinary bladder dysfunction resulting in poor storage ability creates urinary incontinence. Anatomic and functional factors contributing to urinary incontinence in small animals with ectopic ureters, congenital urethral hypoplasia, and vaginal anomalies will be discussed in this article.

## Ectopic Ureters

Ectopic ureters are congenital urogenital malformations in which one or both ureters terminate in an aberrant position, usually the distal urethra or vagina. Ectopic ureters are the most common cause of urinary incontinence in young female dogs, and are diagnosed sporadically in cats and male dogs. Anatomic urinary

incontinence is easily explained, as the ectopic ureteral termination bypasses the normal storage mechanisms of the urinary bladder, bladder neck, and urethra. Surgical intervention may successfully correct the anatomic abnormality, but persistent urinary incontinence is frequently observed. The problem of postoperative urinary incontinence is significant in dogs, with incidences as high as 50 to 67% (Dean and Constantinescu, 1988; Mason et al., 1990; McLaughlin and Miller, 1991). Persistent urinary incontinence has been attributed to concurrent anatomic abnormalities, urinary tract infection, recanalization of ureteral branches, and concurrent urinary bladder or urethral dysfunction.

Urethral dysfunction in dogs with ectopic ureters may result from mechanical interference with urethral function by ureteral branches or ureteral remnants, acquired urethral sphincter incompetence (reproductive hormone–responsive urinary incontinence), or concurrent congenital urethral abnormalities. Radiographic findings supportive of urethral dysfunction were described in several early reports of dogs with persistent incontinence following surgical repair of ectopic ureters, and postoperative incontinence was considered more likely if the ureter terminated in the urethra than in the uterus or vagina. In a prospective series of 18 dogs, dogs with nonpatent intramural ectopic ureters, ureteral troughs, or double ureteral openings (ureteral branching) were more likely to exhibit postoperative urinary incontinence than were dogs with patent intramural ectopic ureters, suggesting a link between anatomic variation of the ureteral termination and disruption of urethral continence mechanisms (Stone and Mason, 1990). Reports of reduction or resolution of postoperative urinary incontinence following the administration of estrogens or $\alpha$-agonists further supported the role of urethral incompetence (Rigg, Zenoble, and Riedesel, 1988; Dean and Constantinescu, 1988; McLaughlin and Miller, 1991). α-Adrenergic agents act at receptors in the bladder neck and urethra to increase urethral smooth muscle contractility; reproductive hormones have multiple effects on the urethra, including enhanced responsiveness of α-receptors and improved urethral tone. However, clinical responses to pharmacologic agents are inconsistent in dogs with postoperative urinary incontinence (Stone and Mason, 1990; McLaughlin and Miller, 1991), and a prognosis for postoperative success has been difficult to generate for individual animals.

Urinary bladder and urethral function were assessed preoperatively in nine dogs with ectopic ureters evaluated by the authors at the Colorado State University Veterinary Teaching Hospital. Functional abnormalities were common, with urethral incompetence docu-

mented by urethral pressure profile (UPP) measurements in six of the nine dogs. The UPP response to phenylpropanolamine (PPA) (generic, Rugby) administration was recorded in these dogs prior to surgical intervention (Fig. 1). Measurements suggesting a good response to PPA were observed in three dogs, all of which remained continent postoperatively with continued PPA administration. Minimal improvement in maximum urethral closure pressures following PPA administration was observed in three dogs that later exhibited postoperative urinary incontinence. Reduced frequency and severity of urinary incontinence was obtained in two of these dogs when the PPA dosage was increased. One dog with normal UPP findings remained incontinent following attempted repair of a ureteral trough; the incontinence was attributed to poor urinary bladder compliance or persistent anatomic anomaly. Preopera-

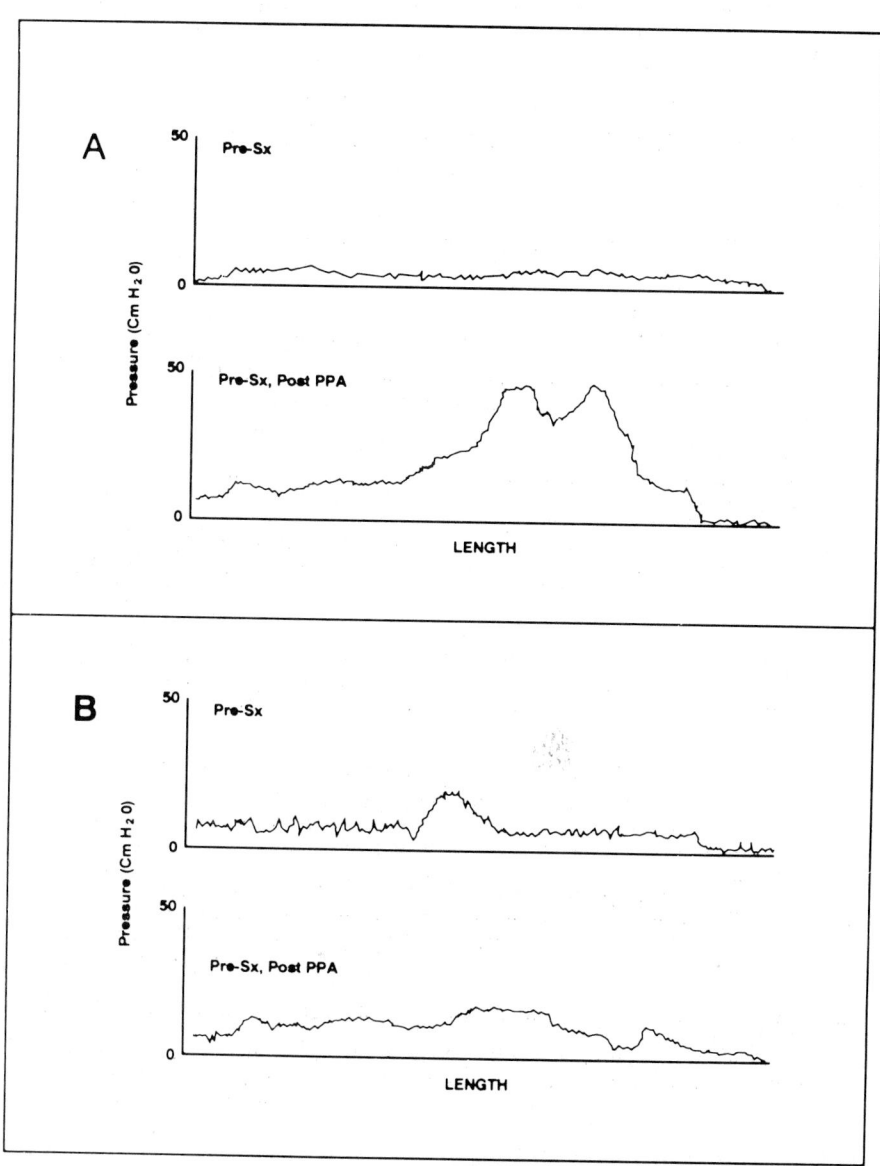

**Figure 1.** Preoperative (Pre Sx) urethral pressure profiles (UPP) from two dogs with ectopic ureters and urethral incompetence. *A*, A good UPP response to phenypropanolamine (PPA) administration is observed. *B*, A poor UPP response to PPA administration is observed.

tive measurements correlated well with postoperative outcome in this series; predicted postoperative outcomes were accurate in eight of the nine dogs overall. These findings support a major role for urethral incompetence in the problem of postoperative urinary incontinence in dogs with ectopic ureters, and emphasize the value of urodynamic measurements in their preoperative evaluation.

Urinary bladder storage function also may be compromised in dogs with ectopic ureters. It has been suggested that the urinary bladder that does not receive the entire urine volume, particularly with bilateral ectopic ureters, fails to develop appropriate compliance and storage function. In theory, if urinary bladder structure is normal, accommodation may improve following surgical repair and restoration of normal urine flow. Subjectively "hypoplastic" urinary bladders have been described in selected cases. Radiographically observable abnormalities of urinary bladder size, shape, or location were observed in 7 of 18 dogs with ectopic ureters in one series (Mason et al., 1990). Reduced urinary bladder capacity and poor bladder accommodation was documented by cystometrographic measurements in four of the nine dogs (44.4%) in our series. Postoperative urinary incontinence was observed in all four of these dogs; however, urethral incompetence was also demonstrated in three dogs. Cystometrographic alterations were persistent in two dogs that were reevaluated several months following surgery. The administration of anticholinergic agents may improve urinary bladder storage function and alleviate urinary incontinence. We have observed clinical improvement in dogs with reduced storage function following the administration of oxybutynin (Ditropan, Marion), an anticholinergic agent with antispasmodic and local anesthetic effects on the urinary bladder. Administration of oxybutynin was helpful in reducing the degree of urinary incontinence in two of the dogs with ectopic ureters and persistent incontinence, but was not curative. The influence of urinary bladder dysfunction on postoperative urinary incontinence remains unclear; further studies investigating bladder storage capacity in dogs with ectopic ureters are in progress.

### Congenital Urethral Incompetence

Urinary incontinence attributable to urethral dysfunction also may be observed as a congenital anomaly in dogs and cats without ectopic ureters. In both disorders, urine leakage is marked, and may appear continuous or intermittent in frequency. In dogs, large to medium breeds are most frequently affected, with springer spaniels overrepresented in one study (Holt, 1985a). Contrast radiographic studies may demonstrate a grossly short, wide, or absent urethra in cats and female dogs (Fig. 2), or urethral dilation in males. Urinary bladder hypoplasia is a common concurrent finding. Congenital urethral dysfunction also may be encountered in animals with normal urethral confor-

mation, as suggested by findings in dogs with ectopic ureters.

### Vaginal Anomalies

Vaginal anomalies, including vestibulovaginal stenoses and vaginal bands, have been variably associated with urinary incontinence in juvenile and adult female dogs. The most frequent clinical findings in dogs with vaginal anomalies include chronic vaginitis, vaginal discharge, recurrent urinary tract infections, and difficulty in mating. Urinary incontinence, however, was observed in 12 of 22 dogs (55%) with vestibulovaginal stenoses in one series (Holt and Sayle, 1981), and vestibulovaginal stenoses were observed in 11 of 42 (26%) dogs presented for the problem of urinary incontinence in another study (Holt, 1985b). A similar incidence of anomalies was observed in a group of continent dogs, however (Holt, 1985b). Urinary incontinence has been attributed to pooling of urine in the cranial vagina, resulting in intermittent urine loss that appears as incontinence. Surgical repair of the anatomic defect or complete vaginectomy has been recommended to alleviate incontinence. However, as observed with surgical correction of ectopic ureters, persistent urinary incontinence is common and concurrent functional abnormalities are suspected.

Retrospective and prospective analyses were completed in order to further characterize the association between vaginal anomalies and urinary incontinence. Urinary incontinence was a presenting complaint in 15 of 34 (44%) dogs with annular vestibulovaginal strictures or dorsoventral vaginal bands evaluated at Colo-

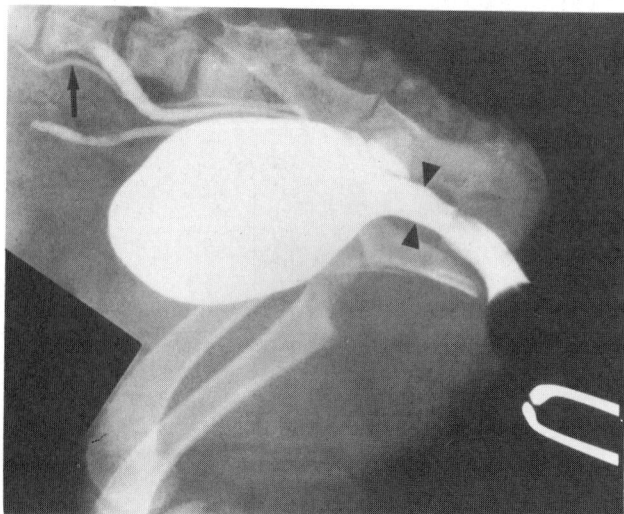

**Figure 2.** Retrograde vaginourethrogram from a 14-week-old miniature poodle with severe urinary incontinence. Urethral hypoplasia is demonstrated by the short, wide urethra (*arrowheads*), which is difficult to differentiate from bladder neck and vestibule. Retrograde filling of the uterine horns and one ureter (*arrow*) is also observed; however, the ureteral termination was not ectopic. Urethral incompetence and reduced bladder storage capacity were confirmed by urodynamic measurements.

rado State University over a 10-year period. Urinary incontinence persisted following surgical intervention in four of six dogs managed surgically, whereas six of eight dogs managed medically with $\alpha$-agonists or diethylstilbestrol administration exhibited significant reduction or resolution of urinary incontinence, supporting urethral incompetence. In a prospective evaluation of 32 female dogs with urinary incontinence attributable to urethral incompetence, vaginal anomalies were identified in 11. Clinical features and urodynamic measurements in dogs with vaginal anomalies were compared to those in dogs without significant vaginal anomalies. Although urodynamic variables and response to PPA administration were not remarkably different between the groups, clinical characteristics suggested that the presence of the vaginal anomaly may influence urethral function. The age at presentation in dogs with vaginal anomalies was younger than in dogs without vaginal anomalies. In those dogs in which the time of onset of urinary incontinence was known, dogs with vaginal anomalies were again younger than dogs without vaginal anomalies, and incontinence developed more rapidly following ovariohysterectomy. Clinical responses to phenylpropanolamine administration were slightly less favorable in dogs with vaginal anomalies, with excellent responses (complete continence) recorded in only 5 of 11 (45.5%), as opposed to 13 of the 21 (61.9%) dogs without vaginal anomalies.

The nature and progression of acquired urethral incompetence appears to differ in dogs with significant vaginal anomalies; a propensity for early urethral dysfunction may be another manifestation of aberrant urogenital development. Recurrent cystitis/urethritis associated with vaginal anomalies may contribute to the development of urethral incompetence in some cases. Alternatively, preexisting subnormal urethral resistance may predispose these dogs to urinary tract infection. We have also observed a phenomenon of "subclinical" urinary incontinence in dogs with vaginal anomalies that exhibit clinical signs primarily of vaginitis, including vaginal discharge and vaginal licking. Overt urinary incontinence is not observed, but poor urethral tone can be demonstrated by UPP measurements, and improvement is observed following $\alpha$-agonist administration.

## DIAGNOSIS AND MANAGEMENT

The evaluation of juvenile animals exhibiting urinary incontinence should include a complete physical examination, vaginal examination, neurologic evaluation, urinalysis, and urine culture. Contrast radiographic procedures that demonstrate upper and lower urinary tract anatomy should be completed. Excretory urography is employed for the evaluation of the upper urinary tract and the identification of ectopic ureters. Visualization of the ureteral termination may be improved by simultaneous pneumocystography. Retrograde vaginourethrography is valuable in the characterization of the urinary bladder, urethra, and reproductive tract, and

may be more sensitive than excretory urography for detecting ectopic ureters in some animals (see *CVT X*, p 1142). A complete vaginoscopic examination should be performed in dogs with vaginal anomalies. Urodynamic techniques, if available, provide objective information regarding urinary bladder capacity, compliance, and urethral tone, and are particularly valuable in the diagnostic evaluation of juvenile dogs with multiple anomalies (see *CVT X*, p 1145).

Management of dogs with ectopic ureters exhibiting postrepair urinary incontinence should initially include appropriate identification and management of urinary tract inflammation or infection. Pollakiuria and urinary incontinence associated with surgical trauma should resolve over 7 to 14 days. Dogs with persistent postoperative urinary incontinence should undergo a complete reevaluation, which may include additional contrast radiographic procedures, vaginoscopy, and urodynamic measurements. In the absence of demonstrable anatomic causes of urinary incontinence, trial administration of $\alpha$-agonists or reproductive hormones for possible urethral incompetence is appropriate. Phenylpropanolamine (generic, Rugby) is administered at an initial dosage of 1.5 mg/kg every 8 hr PO. If the clinical response to $\alpha$-agonist administration is poor, an increased dosage (2.0 to 3.0 mg/kg) may be administered, provided adverse effects are minimal. Following good clinical response, dosages are then reduced to the minimum amount and frequency required to maintain acceptable continence. $\alpha$-Adrenergic agents should be avoided in animals with underlying cardiovascular or hypertensive disease, including those with renal insufficiency. Diethylstilbestrol (DES) (Eli Lilly) or stilbesterol (Stilbestrol, A & H) is an alternative medication that may increase urethral resistance in females. A total dose of 0.5 to 1.0 mg/day DES is administered for 5 to 7 days, followed by an equivalent dose administered once every 5 to 14 days. Prolonged reproductive hormone administration in intact animals is not recommended. The activity of reproductive hormones and $\alpha$-agonists may be synergistic when used in combination. Anticholinergic agents may be valuable in some dogs with postoperative urinary incontinence. Oxybutynin is administered at an approximate dosage of 0.2 mg/kg every 8 to 12 hr. Potential side effects of oxybutynin administration include vomiting, ileus, constipation, and urine retention, which are usually dose related (see also *CVT X*, p 1214). Spontaneous resolution of urinary incontinence may be observed in some animals months to years following surgery.

In some female dogs with congenital urethral incompetence, improvement may be observed following the first estrous cycle. In others, pharmacologic manipulation of urethral tone may be attempted with $\alpha$-adrenergic agonists or reproductive hormones. In our experience, medical management has been unrewarding in dogs with congenital urethral incompetence and gross abnormalities of the bladder neck and urethra. Bladder neck reconstruction has been successful in reducing the severity and frequency of incontinence in several cats and a dog with congenital urethral hypoplasia (Holt, 1993). Surgical techniques are designed to increase urethral length and to create an intra-abdominally located bladder neck. Colposuspension or cystourethropexy techniques may provide some improvement in animals with congenital incompetence in which the urethra is grossly normal.

In juvenile dogs with vaginal anomalies and urinary incontinence, the response to pharmacologic manipulation of urethral tone should be evaluated prior to considering surgical intervention. Surgical management of vaginal anomalies is frequently successful in alleviating clinical signs in dogs without urinary incontinence, and may be indicated in a small subset of dogs with vaginal anomalies and urinary incontinence. These cases are likely to be dogs with markedly constricted vestibulovaginal canals and vaginal urine pooling demonstrated by vaginoscopy. Management of dogs with adult-onset urinary incontinence in which a vaginal abnormality is found is similar to that employed for other dogs with acquired urethral incompetence; identification and management of concurrent urinary tract infection is especially important. A guarded long-term prognosis may be warranted in these dogs, however, and the use of more aggressive medical regimens or surgical options may be required in refractory cases.

## References and Suggested Reading

Dean PW and Constantinescu GM: Canine ectopic ureter. Compend Cont Ed Pract Vet 10:146, 1988.
  *Review of developmental anatomy, diagnosis, and management of ectopic ureters in dogs; includes a review of clinical findings and outcome in 11 cases.*
Holt PE: Urinary incontinence in the bitch due to sphincter mechanism incompetence: Prevalence in referred dogs and retrospective analysis of sixty cases. J Small Anim Pract 26:181, 1985a.
  *A review of urinary incontinence in 174 juvenile and adult dogs, focusing on clinical features of 60 females with suspected urethral sphincter mechanism incompetence.*
Holt PE: Importance of urethral length, bladder neck position and vestibulovaginal stenosis in sphincter mechanism incompetence in the incontinent bitch. Res Vet Sci 39:364, 1985b.
  *Selected anatomic findings in 57 female dogs with urethral incompetence are compared to those in 42 continent females.*
Holt PE: Surgical management of congenital urethral sphincter mechanism incompetence in eight female cats and a bitch. Vet Surg 22:98, 1993.
  *A description of bladder neck reconstructive techniques in the management of congenital urethral hypoplasia in small animals.*
Holt PE and Sayle B: Congenital vestibulo-vaginal stenosis in the bitch. J Small Anim Pract 22:67, 1981.
  *A review of the clinical findings, methods of correction, and results of treatment in 22 dogs with vestibulovaginal stenosis.*
Lane IF, Lappin MR, and Seim HB: Predictive value of urodynamic measurements in the management of dogs with ectopic ureters (abstr). J Vet Intern Med 6:119, 1992.
  *Abstract describing preoperative urodynamic evaluation and postoperative outcome in nine dogs with ectopic ureters.*
Mason LK, Stone EA, Biery DN, et al: Surgery of ectopic ureters; pre- and postoperative radiographic morphology. J Am Anim Hosp Assoc 26:73, 1990.
  *A review of radiographic findings, concurrent urogenital abnormalities, and postoperative outcome in a series of 18 dogs with ectopic ureters.*
McLaughlin R and Miller CW: Urinary incontinence after surgical repair of ureteral ectopia in dogs. Vet Surg 20:100, 1991.
  *A retrospective study of 20 dogs with ectopic ureters, focusing on features of 11 dogs with persistent urinary incontinence following surgical repair.*
Richter KP: Use of urodynamics in micturition disorders in dogs and cats. In Kirk RW (ed): Current Veterinary Therapy X: Small Animal Practice. Philadelphia, WB Saunders Co, 1989, p 1145.
  *A review of the methods, interpretation, and applications of urodynamic procedures in small animals.*
Rigg DL, Zenoble RD, and Riedesel EA: Neoureterostomy and phenylpropanolamine therapy for incontinence due to ectopic ureter in a dog. J Am Anim Hosp Assoc 19:237, 1983.
  *Case report describing resolution of postoperative urinary incontinence in a dog with a surgically repaired ectopic ureter following administration of an α-agonist.*
Stone EA and Mason LK: Surgery of ectopic ureters: Types, method of correction, and post-operative results. J Am Anim Hosp Assoc 26:81, 1990.
  *The relationship between anatomic type of ectopic ureter, method of correction, and postoperative outcome is examined in 18 dogs.*

# MEDICAL MANAGEMENT OF URETHRAL PROLAPSE IN MALE DOGS

CARL A. OSBORNE
*and* SHERRY L. SANDERSON
*St. Paul, Minnesota*

## ETIOLOGY

Prolapse of the mucosal lining of the distal portion of the urethra through the external urethral orifice occurs primarily in young male dogs (Fig. 1). Of seven cases reported in the literature, and ten cases retrieved from medical records at the University of Minnesota Veterinary Teaching Hospital, 11 were male English bulldogs and two were male Boston terriers. Urethral prolapse also affected a male Yorkshire terrier, a male cocker spaniel, a male Alaskan malamute, and a male springer spaniel. The mean age of affected dogs at the time of diagnosis of urethral prolapse was 18 months (median age = 11 months; age range = 4 months to 5 years). Ten of the 17 dogs were less than 1 year of age.

In humans, urethral prolapse occurs primarily in prepuberal girls and postmenopausal women. The disorder in girls is thought to be related to a congenital defect. Poor attachment between the longitudinal and circular-oblique smooth muscle layers of the urethra in association with superimposed episodes of increased intra-abdominal pressure have been hypothesized as etiopathogenic events. Concomitant diseases associated with increased intra-abdominal pressure include epilepsy, respiratory disorders, and dysuria.

We hypothesize that the predilection of brachycephalic Boston terriers and English bulldogs to urethral prolapse may be related to abnormal development of the urethra with superimposed increased intra-abdominal pressure as a consequence of labored breathing, dysuria, or sexual activity. Increased intra-abdominal pressure could impair venous return of blood through the pudendal veins, predisposing susceptible dogs to engorgement of the corpus spongiosum surrounding the distal urethra. The observation that English bulldogs are predisposed to congenital urethrorectal fistulas supports the hypothesis that maldevelopment of the urethra may be involved. Increased intra-abdominal pressure secondary to stertorous breathing caused by stenotic nares and abnormal elongation of the soft palate may impair venous return from the penis. Detection of urocystoliths and vesicourachal diverticula in some affected dogs suggests that increased intra-abdominal pressure secondary to dysuria may also be a predisposing factor. The observation that urethral prolapse is more severe when male dogs are sexually active may be linked to distention of submucosal vascular channels located in the penis.

Acquired urethral prolapse in postmenopausal women does not appear to have a well-recognized counterpart in other species. Diseases incriminated as underlying causes of acquired urethral prolapse include all forms of increased intra-abdominal pressure, urinary tract infections, debility, malnutrition, and estrogen deficiency.

## BIOLOGIC BEHAVIOR

The biologic behavior of untreated urethral prolapses has not been evaluated in a large number of cases. This may be related to the fact that most textbooks recommend some form of surgery to treat prolapsed urethras. Cases reported in the literature have all been managed by manual reduction of the prolapse combined with a purse-string suture, or surgical excision at the prolapsed portion of the urethra. We had the opportunity to follow an untreated urethral prolapse affecting a 4-year-old intact male English bulldog over a 3-year period. The urethral prolapse was first noted 1 year earlier by a referring veterinarian who was managing the dog for recurrent cystine urocystoliths. During a 4-year span, the urethral prolapse was not associated with any clinical signs. It did not change in size, shape, or color (Fig. 1). The clinical course of this patient with urethral prolapse indicates that surgical excision is not always necessary. This point may be especially relevant to patients that are poor anesthetic risks.

Of five bulldogs with prolapsed urethras treated by surgical excision at the University of Minnesota, varying degrees of urethral prolapse recurred in four 1 week to 18 months following surgery. In three dogs, further surgery was not performed. In these dogs, recurrent episodic bleeding was observed by the owners. One dog was subsequently euthanized because of the owner's concern about episodic bleeding.

## DIAGNOSTIC CONSIDERATIONS

The primary concerns of clients have been bleeding from the prolapsed urethra independent of micturition, and their dogs' intermittent or persistent licking of the penis. Signs related to urinary tract infection or uroliths affecting the lower urinary tract may also be present. Physical examination usually reveals a red to purple, pea-sized, doughnut-shaped mass protruding from the

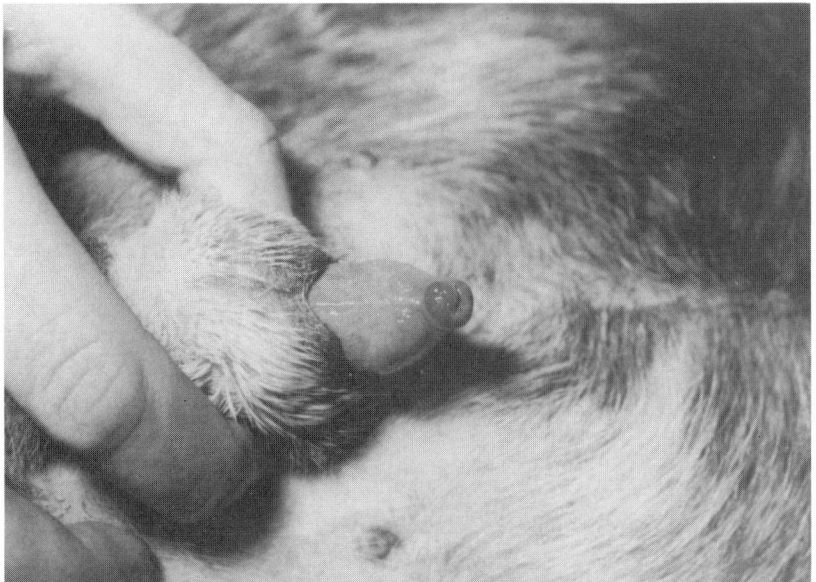

**Figure 1.** Photograph of a urethral prolapse of a 7-year-old intact male English bulldog. The urethral prolapse was first detected 4 years previously.

distal end of the penis (Fig. 1). Uroliths may be palpated in the urinary bladder or urethra.

Prior to formulating a treatment plan, the initial portion of a voided urine sample and a urine sample subsequently collected by cystocentesis should be analyzed and compared. Comparison of results of urine samples collected in this fashion may aid in localization of hematuria or inflammation. If the results of urinalysis indicate an inflammatory process, appropriate urine samples should be collected for quantitative bacterial culture and antimicrobial susceptibility tests. Survey abdominal radiography and contrast urethrocystography should be considered to evaluate the anatomic integrity of the lower urinary tract, and to look for evidence of uroliths. In our limited experience, additional anatomic abnormalities of the urethra have not been associated with urethral prolapse. However, we have detected concomitant uroliths in the urinary bladder or urethra, and vesicourachal diverticula.

If the prolapsed portion of the urethra is surgically excised, it should be processed for examination with a light microscope. Lack of deep-seated inflammation and scarring may suggest that recurrence is less likely. In contrast, mucosal ulceration, extensive inflammation, necrosis, and scarring may indicate that problems are more likely to recur.

## MANAGEMENT

If our hypothesis is valid that increased intra-abdominal pressure is a contributing factor to urethral prolapse in dogs predisposed to this abnormality, consideration should be given to minimizing this problem. This may include eliminating underlying causes of dysuria, castration to prevent sexual activity, and correction of stenotic nares or elongated soft palates. We emphasize that these recommendations are based on a theory, and should be considered in this light.

In those situations where a prolapsed urethra is asymptomatic, or when episodic bleeding is no more than an inconvenience, therapy may not be required. We do not recommend use of glucocorticoids, since they are unlikely to provide any beneficial effect, but are likely to increase the risk for ascending bacterial urinary tract infection. If excessive licking contributes to trauma of the prolapsed urethra, Elizabethan collars or similar types of restraint devices may help to break the licking cycle.

If the urethral prolapse is small, and if further treatment is deemed necessary, manual reduction may be considered. Manual reduction of the prolapsed segment is facilitated by using general anesthesia and a urinary catheter. The catheter should be as large as it can be without its use causing further damage to the urethra. Alternatively, a Swan-Ganz balloon catheter may aid in reducing the prolapse. Following correction of the problem, a purse-string suture of nonabsorbable material should be placed at the external urethral orifice. The urinary catheter should then be removed. The purse-string suture should be removed in approximately 5 days. Appropriate antibiotics should be given if urethritis is a cause or result of the prolapse. The owners should be advised that urethral prolapse may recur, especially if an underlying predisposing cause has not been identified and eliminated or controlled.

Surgery should be considered for patients with excessive bleeding, pain, or extensive ulceration and/or necrosis of the prolapsed tissue. Two procedures for resecting the prolapsed portion of the urethra have been described. In both, the distal edge of the transected mucosa is reunited to the external surface of the penis. The primary difference between these procedures is the method used to prevent retraction of the urethral mucosa into the penis after the prolapse is amputated. In one technique, two straight intestinal surgical needles are inserted at right angles to each other through the nonprolapsed portion of the distal urethral lumen through the external surface of the penis. The prolapsed portion of the urethral mucosa is then excised, and the urethra is reunited to the external surface of the penis with simple interrupted sutures (4-0 to 5-0 absorbable suture).

In the other procedure, stay sutures are placed in the mucosa of the prolapsed portion of the urethra to facilitate manipulation. After inserting a sterile catheter into the urethral lumen, an incision is then made approximately 0.5 cm caudal to the prolapsed portion of the urethra and completely encircling the penis. The initial incision is carried down to the urethral mucosa. After dissecting penile tissue away from the urethral mucosa, the ventral portion of the mucosa is incised halfway around its circumference. By incising only half of the urethral circumference, stay sutures are not required to prevent the mucosa from retracting back into the penis. After ventral portions of the urethral mucosa are sutured to the external surface of the penis with 4-0 to 5-0 absorbable suture, the remaining portion of the urethra is excised and reunited to the penis. A "purse-string" effect should be avoided by not pulling the suture material too tight during closure. Electrosurgery (not electrocautery) has been recommended to reduce hemorrhage during surgery. An Elizabethan collar may be used to prevent licking-induced trauma to the anastomosis site. Appropriate antibiotics should be given if urethritis is a cause or result of the prolapse.

### References and Suggested Reading

Golomb J, Merimsky E, and Braf Z: Strangulated prolapse of the urethra in the elderly female. Int J Gynecol Obstet 23:61, 1985.

Hobson HP and Heller RA: Surgical correction of prolapse of the male urethra. Vet Med Small Anim Clin 66:1177, 1971.

Jerkins GR, Verheeck K, and Noe HN: Treatment of girls with urethral prolapse. J Urol 132:732, 1984.

Lowe FC, Hill GS, Jeffs RD, and Brendler CB: Urethral prolapse in children: Insights into etiology and management. J Urol 135:100, 1986.

McDonald RK: Urethral prolapse in a Yorkshire terrier. Compend Cont Educ 11:682, 1989.

Mitre A, Nahas W, Gilbert A, et al: Urethral prolapse in girls: Familial case. J Urol 137:115, 1987.

Osborne CA, Engen MH, Yano BL, et al: Congenital urethrorectal fistula in two dogs. J Am Vet Med Assoc 166:999, 1975.

Richardson DA, Hojj SN, and Herbst AL: Medical treatment of urethral prolapse in children. Obstet Gynecol 59:69, 1982.

Sinibaldi KR and Green RW: Surgical correction of prolapse of the male urethra in three English bulldogs. J Am Anim Hosp Assoc 9:450, 1973.

# CVT UPDATE: TREATMENT OF CANINE BACTERIAL PROSTATITIS

MARK DORFMAN

*Roswell, Georgia*

*and* JEANNE A. BARSANTI

*Athens, Georgia*

Bacterial prostatic infections are common among sexually mature male dogs and may be acute or chronic (see "Canine Prostatic Disorders," this volume, p 1103). Both acute and chronic bacterial prostatitis are usually due to bacteria ascending the urethra, although hematogenous spread and extension from the testes, epididymus, or peritoneal cavity is possible. In approximately 70% of dogs with bacterial prostatitis, a single organism is isolated, primarily Enterobacteriaceae, especially *Escherichia coli*, but gram-positive infections with *Staphylococcus* or *Streptococcus* occur. *Mycoplasma* spp. have been cultured from dogs with prostatitis from which no other bacteria were cultured, but mycoplasmas have been also isolated from the ejaculates of clinically normal dogs. *Brucella canis* can cause prostatitis experimentally.

The development and persistence of an infection within the prostate gland depends upon a complex interaction between normal host defense mechanisms and bacterial pathogenicity. Conditions that increase bacterial numbers in the periprostatic urethra or urinary bladder, or which compromise local or systemic resistance of the host, will increase the likelihood that an infection will develop. Diseases of other segments of the urinary tract predispose to development of bacterial prostatitis. Examples include urolithiasis, renal failure, neoplasia, and incontinence. Conditions that alter the normal secretion of prostatic fluid such as squamous metaplasia can also predispose the prostate to infection.

Antimicrobial therapy is the mainstay of treatment for bacterial prostatitis, but factors predisposing the dog to infection should also be identified and eliminated whenever possible. Specific antibiotic features, along with patient characteristics and the severity of illness, should be considered in the selection of an antimicrobial agent for bacterial prostatitis. The preferred method for evaluating an organism's susceptibility to a particular antimicrobial requires determination of the drug's minimum inhibitory concentration (MIC) (see *CVT X*, p 1206 and *CVT XI*, p 912). Successful regimens for treatment of bacterial prostatitis should provide prostatic tissue and prostatic fluid concentrations in excess of the MICs for the pathogens. Finally, the safety profile and cost of therapy may impact on anti-microbial selection.

## ACUTE BACTERIAL PROSTATITIS

### Diagnostic Evaluation

Acute bacterial prostatitis is easier to diagnose and treat than chronic bacterial prostatitis. A diagnosis of acute bacterial prostatitis should be based on history, physical examination findings, hematology, urinalysis, and urine culture. Patients with acute prostatic infections often present with signs and symptoms of an acute septic process including fever, anorexia, lethargy, and inflammatory leukograms with or without a left shift. In addition, a urethral discharge and a prostate gland that is painful to very gentle palpation are often present in patients with acute infections. Urinalysis usually reveals pyuria, hematuria, and bacteriuria. Urinary tract infections in sexually mature, noncastrated male dogs should always be presumed to involve the prostate gland, and an effort must be made to determine if any complicating factors exist such as hyperplasia, abscess, or neoplasia. If the urinalysis shows evidence of an infection within the urinary tract, a urine culture and sensitivity should be done on a sample obtained by cytstocentesis. Because dogs with acute bacterial prostatitis are usually painful, obtaining prostatic fluid from an ejaculate is usually not possible and prostatic massage or vigorous palpation may be contraindicated because of the risk of bacteremia.

### Treatment

Because of disruption of the blood-prostatic barrier by acute inflammation, most antimicrobial drugs will reach the site of infection in dogs with acute bacterial prostatitis. Therefore, therapy should be based on results of urine culture and *in vitro* sensitivity testing. If the infection is severe, an antimicrobial agent with low resistance potential and adequate tissue/urine concentrations is critical (Table 1). The initial route of administration should be dictated by the severity of the dog's clinical signs. Dogs with acute bacterial prostatitis may also require supportive care with intravenous fluids. A minimum of 3 to 4 weeks of oral antimicrobial therapy

should follow to prevent the infection from becoming chronic. Because resolution of clinical signs does not provide assurance that the infection has been eliminated, the dog should be reevaluated and urine cultures repeated 7 to 10 days after antimicrobial therapy is discontinued. Prostatic fluid cultures are also important to evaluate when these dogs are reexamined.

## CHRONIC BACTERIAL PROSTATITIS

### Diagnosis

The diagnosis of chronic bacterial prostatitis should be based on history, physical examination findings, and analysis of prostatic fluid. Dogs with chronic bacterial prostatitis may be clinically asymptomatic or may present with signs of lower urinary tract disease including a constant or intermittent hemorrhagic, purulent, or clear urethral discharge. Because of the continuous reflux of prostatic fluid into the proximal urethra and bladder, prostatic infections often lead to secondary lower urinary tract infections with clinical signs such as dysuria, hematuria, and pollakiuria. With chronic bacterial prostatitis, the prostate gland is usually not painful and its size is variable depending on the amount of hyperplasia or fibrosis present. Chronic infection alone does not cause an increase in prostatic size.

Complete blood counts (CBC), serum chemistry profiles, and radiologic procedures including survey radiographs, contrast procedures, and two-dimensional ultrasound can be helpful in determining if concurrent prostatic disease such as abscessation or neoplasia is present. These tests are usually normal in dogs with primary chronic bacterial prostatitis. However, radiographic changes such as granular parenchymal mineralization or ultrasonographic changes such as diffuse, multifocal, hypoechoic lesions may be present in dogs with chronic bacterial prostatitis. Urinalysis findings such as bacteriuria, hematuria, or pyuria may or may not be present. Diagnosis should be based on culture and cytology of prostatic fluid collected from an ejaculate. Prostatic fluid is usually sampled from the third and largest fraction of the ejaculate. A quantitative culture is necessary because there is a normal bacterial flora in the distal urethra of dogs. If an ejaculate cannot be collected, a prostatic massage sample should be obtained (see *CVT X*, p 1244). If cystitis is not present,

***Table 1.*** *Antimicrobial Characteristics of Commonly Used Agents in the Treatment of Urinary Tract Infections*

| Parameter | Trimethoprim-Sulfa | Ampicillin | Amoxicillin/Clavulanate | Enrofloxacin | Cephalothin |
|---|---|---|---|---|---|
| Frequency of resistance[*] | 20%[t] | 44%[t] | 9%[§] | <2%[t] | 40%[§] |
| Urine concentration | High | High | High | High | High |
| Half-life in urine | Long | Moderate | Moderate | Long | Moderate |
| Side effects | Moderate/high | Low | Low | Low/moderate | Low/moderate |
| Relative cost | Low | Low | Moderate | High | Moderate/high |

[*]Based on susceptibility patterns to veterinary isolates of *E. coli.*
[t]Ling et al., 1986.
[t]Berg et al., 1987.
[§]Kilgore et al., 1986.

comparison of a preprostatic massage sample obtained after flushing the bladder with physiologic saline with a postprostatic massage sample may help localize an infection to the prostate gland. When cystitis is present, sterilization of the urine with an antibiotic that reaches high concentrations in urine but not prostatic fluid (e.g., ampicillin) may be necessary to obtain reliable results.

Normal dogs will have occasional white blood cells (WBCs), red blood cells (RBCs), and positive bacterial cultures in prostatic fluid obtained by ejaculation. The number of WBCs is low and the bacteria are gram-positive and found in concentrations of less than $10^5$/ml. Large numbers of gram-negative organisms ($>10^5$/ml) and high WBC numbers indicate infection. Large numbers of gram-positive organisms and WBCs probably also indicate infection. Fewer numbers of either gram-positive or gram-negative organisms need to be interpreted in light of the dog's clinical signs, cytologic findings of the prostatic fluid, and cultures of urine.

A biopsy sample is usually not necessary to make a diagnosis of chronic bacterial prostatitis unless it is obtained to rule out concurrent prostatic disease. However, a definitive diagnosis of prostatitis can be made by culture of prostatic tissue. Histologically, the presence of inflammation with or without the presence of macrophages is necessary to support a diagnosis of chronic bacterial prostatitis.

## Treatment

In the treatment of chronic bacterial prostatitis, antimicrobials should be chosen based on results of culture and sensitivity testing of the organism isolated and the pharmacologic properties of the specific drug. In chronic bacterial infections, many antimicrobials do not penetrate prostatic acini. The prostatic epithelium's bi-lipid membrane serves as a structural and functional barrier, limiting the penetration of antimicrobials from plasma into prostatic secretions. Because the passage of an antimicrobial agent across the prostatic epithelium occurs by passive diffusion, its lipid solubility plays a key role in determining its ability to diffuse across this barrier. Drugs with low lipid solubility such as ampicillin, cephalosporins, oxytetracycline, and the aminoglycosides are unable to readily cross the prostatic epithelium and enter prostatic fluid. Chloramphenicol, erythromycin, trimethoprim, ciprofloxacin, enrofloxacin, and carbenicillin are some examples of antimicrobials that are relatively lipid soluble and may cross the prostatic epithelium more readily.

A drug's lipid solubility at any given time depends on the $pK_a$ of the drug and the pH of the body fluid in which the drug is present. The $pK_a$ is the pH at which a drug exists equally in its ionized and un-ionized form. Since most antimicrobial drugs are either weak acids or bases, their $pK_a$ will determine how much ionization occurs at the pH of the body fluid containing the antimicrobial. The un-ionized form crosses membranes readily, while the ionized form does not. The pH of blood and prostatic interstitium is 7.4, whereas the pH of normal and infected prostatic fluid in dogs has been shown to be more acidic. This pH difference allows ion trapping to occur on the side of the membrane where most drug ionization occurs. Antimicrobials with higher $pK_a$s ($>7$) cross the canine prostatic epithelium and then become ionized in the more acidic environment. These antimicrobials are theoretically "trapped" within prostatic acini and should reach concentrations in prostatic fluid equal to or greater than those attained in plasma. Examples of antimicrobials with high $pK_a$s include trimethoprim, clindamycin, and erythromycin. It is important to remember that chronic bacterial prostatitis is most frequently caused by *E. coli*. Because of its spectrum of activity, trimethoprim has traditionally been the antibiotic of choice for the treatment of gram-negative chronic prostatic infections. Clindamycin or erythromycin may be used to treat gram-positive chronic prostatic infections if prostatic fluid cultures indicate appropriate susceptibility (Table 2).

The fluoroquinolones, a new class of orally potent antimicrobial agents, have an antibacterial spectrum that covers most of the bacteria causing chronic bacterial prostatitis, attaining serum and tissue concentrations above the MICs for most susceptible pathogens. In addition, because they are zwitterions possessing two $pK_a$ values, they may exhibit favorable acid-base properties that would allow concentration in prostatic fluid and tissue. Several different fluoroquinolone derivatives have demonstrated the ability to penetrate into the canine prostate gland, but only enrofloxacin and enoxacin have been shown to achieve prostatic interstial fluid/plasma ratios and prostatic tissue/plasma ratios greater than 1.0. This would indicate that both enrofloxacin and enoxacin concentrate within the prostate gland (Table 3). Not all quinolone derivatives may be equally effective in treating chronic bacterial prostatitis in the dog. Enrofloxacin, which is approved for use in veterinary medicine, may become clinically valuable in the treatment of chronic bacterial prostatitis.

Once an antimicrobial is selected, therapy should be continued for at least 4 to 6 weeks. If a positive urine

**Table 2.** *Recommended Antimicrobials for Canine Chronic Bacterial Prostatitis (Based on Culture and Sensitivities)*

| | |
|---|---|
| *Staphylococcus, Streptococcus* | Clindamycin, chloramphenicol, trimethoprim-sulfa, erythromycin, carbenicillin |
| Enterobacteriaceae (*E. coli, Klebsiella*) | Enrofloxacin, ciprofloxacin, trimethoprim-sulfa, chloramphenicol |

**Table 3.** *Tissue Concentration and Tissue/Plasma Concentration Ratio of Seven Quinolone Derivatives in the Clinically Healthy Canine Prostate Gland*

| Drug | Tissue Concentration (Median) | Tissue/Plasma Ratio (Median) |
|---|---|---|
| Cinoxacin° | 2.8 µg/gm | 0.1 |
| Norfloxacin° | 3.2 µg/gm | 0.8 |
| Rosoxacin° | 3.7 µg/gm | 0.3 |
| Ciprofloxacin° | 4.0 µg/gm | 0.7 |
| Amifloxacin° | 9.4 µg/gm | 0.7 |
| Enoxacin° | 5.8 µg/gm | 2.1 |
| Enrofloxacin[†] | 0.9 µg/gm | 1.3 |

°Data from Dorflinger et al., 1986.
[†]Data from Dorfman et al., 1993.

culture was found during the initial examination, a urinalysis should be reexamined for bacteriuria 3 to 4 days after beginning therapy. Urine and prostatic fluid should be cultured at 4 to 7 days and again at 30 days after the completion of therapy because initial negative cultures may not correlate with resolution of the infection. If the infection has not been eliminated, a 3-month course of antibiotics should be given. If adjunctive therapy has not been included in the treatment regimen, it should be at this time. If two prolonged treatments with antimicrobials fail to eradicate the infection, two options exist: chronic low-dose antimicrobial therapy (see *CVT X*, p 1208) or prostatectomy.

## Adjunctive Therapy

Adjunctive therapy is performed to reduce the size of the prostate gland and to decrease its secretions. Hormonal manipulation is the most common treatment used to decrease prostatic mass. Castration is the most common and most effectively used method to decrease the size of the prostate gland in dogs. Experimentally, castration has been shown to increase the speed of resolution of infections in dogs with chronic prostatic infections.

## Conclusion

The prognosis for dogs with acute bacterial prostatitis is usually good if treated aggressively with appropriate antimicrobials and fluids as needed. Follow-up cultures are important to ensure eradication of the infection. Based on studies in men, the prognosis for curing chronic bacterial prostatitis with antimicrobial therapy alone is fair. Efficient therapies for this disease still do not exist and a high rate of relapse is common. The quinolones have many pharmacologic properties that may prove to be beneficial in treating patients with chronic bacterial prostatitis. Castration is effective at reducing the size and secretions of the prostate gland and should help resolve bacterial infections.

## References and Suggested Reading

Barsanti JA and Finco R: Canine prostatic diseases. *In* Ettinger (ed): *Textbook of Veterinary Medicine*, 3rd edition. Philadelphia, WB Saunders Co, 1989, pp 1859–1880.
  *A general review of prostatic diseases, their diagnosis, and treatment.*
Berg JN, Ling GV, et al: Susceptibility of bacterial isolates to a new quinolone antimicrobial, BAY Vp 2674. Abstracts 23rd World Veterinary Congress: 7.4.2, 1987.
  *A report on the inhibition of bacteria by enrofloxacin and a comparison of susceptibility patterns of several antimicrobials to enrofloxacin.*
Cowan LA, Barsanti JA, et al: Effects of castration on chronic bacterial prostatitis. J Am Vet Med Assoc 199:346, 1991.
  *A report on the effects of castration on the resolution of infection in dogs with experimentally induced chronic bacterial prostatitis.*
Cowan LA and Barsanti JA: Chronic bacterial prostatitis in the dog. *In* Kirk RW (ed): *Current Veterinary Therapy X*. Philadelphia, WB Saunders Co, 1989, pp 1243–1247.
  *A general review of the diagnosis and treatment of chronic bacterial prostatitis.*
Dorflinger T, Larsen TC, et al: The concentration of various quinolone derivatives in the dog prostate. *In* Weidner (ed): *Therapy of Prostatitis, Experimental and Clinical Data*. Munchen, Bern, Wien, W. Zuckschwerdt, 1986, pp 35–39.
  *A report on the penetration of six quinolone carboxylic acids under steady-state conditions into the dog prostate gland in an experimental model.*
Dorfman MI, Barsanti JA, et al: Enrofloxacin concentrations in the normal prostate gland and in chronic bacterial prostatitis in the dog (abstr): ACVIM Scientific Proceedings, 1993, p 935.
  *A report on the penetration of enrofloxacin into canine prostatic fluid and prostatic tissue in clinically healthy dogs and dogs with an experimentally induced chronic bacterial prostatic infection.*
Kilgore WR, Simmons RD, et al: Beta-lactamase inhibition: A new approach in overcoming bacterial resistance. Compend Cont Educ 8:325, 1986.
  *A review on the clavulanate-potentiated antibiotics.*
Lees GE and Forrester SD: Update: Bacterial urinary tract infections. *In* Kirk RW and Bonagura JD (eds): *Current Veterinary Therapy XI*. Philadelphia, WB Saunders Co, 1992, pp 909–914.
  *A review of the diagnosis of urinary tract infections and specific guidelines for their treatment.*
Ling GV: Management of urinary tract infections. *In* Kirk RW (ed): *Current Veterinary Therapy IX*. Philadelphia, WB Saunders Co, 1986, p 1175.
  *A review of diagnosis and treatment of urinary tract infections in dogs and cats.*
Rogers KS and Lees GE: Management of urinary tract infections. *In* Kirk RW (ed): *Current Veterinary Therapy X*. Philadelphia, WB Saunders Co, 1989, pp 1204–1209.
  *An overview of the principles of diagnosis and treatment of urinary tract infections in dogs and cats.*

# MEDICAL MANAGEMENT OF CANINE PROSTATIC HYPERPLASIA

JEANNE A. BARSANTI
*and* DELMAR R. FINCO

*Athens, Georgia*

Benign prostatic hyperplasia is an aging change of intact male dogs (Barsanti and Finco, 1994). Development of prostatic hyperplasia is associated with an altered androgen/estrogen ratio, and requires the presence of the testes. The hyperplastic process is facilitated by estrogens that may enhance androgen receptors. Thus, even in the face of declining androgen production with age, with increasing estrogen production, hyperplasia develops. Dihydrotestosterone (DHT) within the gland probably serves as the main hormonal mediator for hyperplasia. Dihydrotestosterone is produced from testosterone via the enzyme 5-$\alpha$-reductase.

Benign prostatic hyperplasia in the dog begins as glandular hyperplasia, as early as 2.5 years of age in some dogs (see "Canine Prostatic Disorders," this volume, p 1103). After 4 years of age, a tendency to cystic hyperplasia begins. Although size increases with hyperplasia, prostatic secretory function decreases (decreased seminal volume). The vascularity of the prostate is increased in hyperplasia and the gland has a tendency to bleed. Histologic evidence of mild chronic interstitial inflammation is also common.

## CLINICAL SIGNS OF PROSTATIC HYPERPLASIA

Most dogs with prostatic hyperplasia have no clinical signs. When signs occur, tenesmus associated with defecation may be present because of encroachment on the pelvic canal by the enlarged prostate. An intermittent hemorrhagic or clear light yellow urethral discharge or intermittent or persistent hematuria occurs in some dogs. Hyperplasia is not associated with any systemic signs of illness. On physical examination, the prostate gland is nonpainful and symmetrically enlarged. Consistency varies from normal to mild irregularity.

Hematologic findings and serum biochemical parameters are unaffected by hyperplasia. Urinalysis may be normal or contain blood. If a urethral discharge is present, the discharge is hemorrhagic or clear but not purulent. Semen and postprostatic massage samples may be normal or hemorrhagic.

Survey abdominal radiographs confirm mild to moderate prostatic enlargement with dorsal displacement of the colon and cranial displacement of the bladder. The prostate appears otherwise normal. On ultrasonography, the prostate is often normal, but it may also be diffusely hyperechoic with parenchymal cavities if intraparenchymal cysts have developed. The prostatic capsule is smooth and the gland is symmetrically enlarged (Peter and Jakovljevic, 1992). The degree of enlargement is often mild (Johnston et al., 1989). The cavitary areas are typically well defined and smoothly marginated.

## DIAGNOSIS OF PROSTATIC HYPERPLASIA

Definitive diagnosis is only possible by biopsy. A presumptive diagnosis can be made by history and physical examination with support from hematology, urinalysis, and prostatic fluid analysis, depending on the severity of the presenting complaint.

## TREATMENT OF PROSTATIC HYPERPLASIA

Treatment is only required if related abnormal signs are present. The most effective and standard treatment is castration. If castration of the dog is refused by the owner, various medical options are available, but none is currently recognized to be as safe or effective as castration.

### Estrogens

Estrogens have been the most frequently utilized medical therapy. Estrogens cause prostatic atrophy by reducing androgen concentrations by depressing gonadotropin secretion by the pituitary gland. Estrogens primarily act to decrease prostatic size by decreasing cellular mass; there may be no effect on intraparenchymal cysts. Effective doses of estrogens have not been determined, but diethylstilbestrol administered orally at 0.2 to 1 mg/day for 5 days is the usual recommended dose. Short courses of estrogen therapy have been shown to markedly reduce prostatic secretory capability for 2 months. The potential side effects of estrogens must be compared to their potential clinical benefit in each case before a decision is made to administer them. With toxicity, an initial leukocytosis with a left shift is followed by severe bone marrow depression with resultant anemia, thrombocytopenia, and leukopenia. These effects have been noticed with overdosage, with repeated administration, and at the recommended dose as an idiosyncratic reaction. The dose and duration of estrogen therapy that will produce toxicity varies with the presence or absence of other factors that modify bone marrow function.

Although low doses of estrogens decrease prostatic size, repeated administration and overdosage can also cause growth of the fibromuscular stroma of the prostate, metaplasia of prostatic glandular epithelium, and secretory stasis. These changes can result in further prostatic enlargement and a predisposition to cyst formation, bacterial infection, and abscessation.

### Dihydrotestosterone Receptor Blockers

A drug that avoids the side effects of estrogens is the antiandrogen flutamide (Neri, 1989). This drug specifically blocks DHT activity in the prostate by competing for DHT receptors. Thus, it has few effects on testicular function. This drug was administered to research dogs at 5 mg/kg/day orally for 1 year. Within 6 weeks, prostatic size decreased, with no change in libido, sperm production, or apparent fertility. In another study, a significant decrease in prostatic size as detected by ultrasonography was evident within 10 days (Cartee et al., 1990). Prostatic hyperplasia recurs within 2 months of drug discontinuation. The drug is not approved for veterinary use and is expensive.

### Progestins

Megestrol acetate also has antiandrogenic properties. Megestrol reduces serum testosterone concentrations, competitively inhibits binding of DHT to intracellular receptors, decreases DHT concentrations by inhibiting 5-$\alpha$-reductase, and decreases the number of androgen receptors in the prostate. An oral dose of 0.55 mg/kg/day for 4 weeks has been recommended in dogs (Olson et al., 1987). This therapy caused no decrease in sperm numbers in seven of seven dogs (one of these dogs sired puppies) and resulted in resolution of clinical signs of hyperplasia in 20 of 20 dogs. A dose of 0.55 mg/kg once a week has been used in a few dogs, but effects of prolonged use have not been studied (Olson et al., 1987). A single subcutaneous injection of medroxyprogesterone acetate (3 mg/kg) relieved clinical signs in 16 of 19 dogs, with relapse of signs occurring in 10 to 24 months (Bamberg-Thalen and Linde-Forsberg, 1993). Breeding soundness was not reported. These drugs are not approved for use in male dogs and the oral drug is not approved for use longer than 32 days in female dogs. Therefore, the primary use would be to maintain a short period of breeding soundness in dogs prior to neutering.

### 5-$\alpha$-Reductase Inhibitors

Finasteride is a 5-$\alpha$-reductase inhibitor that was approved in 1992 for oral use in prostatic hyperplasia in men. The drug caused an approximately 20 to 30% decrease in prostatic size in men in 6 to 12 months (Gormley et al., 1992). Although the drug has little effect on libido, it can cause fetal anomalies and is present in semen (Medical Letter, 1992). If the same adverse effects occur in dogs, the drug would not be useful as an alternative to castration for owners who wish to maintain the dog's breeding soundness. Also, owners may be at risk using a potentially teratogenic drug to treat their dog.

### Other

The antifungal drug ketoconazole and gonadotropin-releasing hormone analogs (which block the release of luteinizing hormone) are also antiandrogenic. However, these drugs are essentially chemical castrators. Thus, they have no advantage over surgical castration in dogs.

### References and Suggested Reading

Bamberg-Thalen B and Linde-Forsberg C: Treatment of canine benign prostatic hyperplasia with medroxyprogesterone acetate. J Am Anim Hosp Assoc 29:211, 1993.
  *This paper reports the results of using medroxyprogesterone acetate to treat prostatic hyperplasia in dogs.*
Barsanti JA and Finco DR: Prostatic Diseases. *In* Ettinger SJ and Feldman EC (eds): *Textbook of Veterinary Internal Medicine*, 4th edition. Philadelphia, WB Saunders Co, 1994 pp 1162–1685.
  *This chapter is a review of the pathophysiology, diagnosis, and therapy of prostatic diseases in dogs and cats.*
Cartee RE, Rumph PF, Kenter DC, et al: Evaluation of drug-induced prostatic involution in dogs by transabdominal B-mode ultrasonography. Am J Vet Res 51:1773, 1990.
  *This paper reports on the use of flutamide in dogs as monitored by ultrasonography.*
Gormley GJ, Stoner E, Bruskewitz RC, et al: The effect of finasteride in men with benign prostatic hyperplasia. N Engl J Med 327:1185, 1992.
  *This paper reports on the efficacy of finasteride in men.*
Johnston GR, Feeney DA, Rivers B, et al: Diagnostic imaging of the male canine reproductive organs. Vet Clin North Am [Small Anim Pract] 21:553, 1991.
  *This paper reviews the radiographic and ultrasonographic findings of the prostate gland in health and disease, as well as the testicles and epididymes.*
Medical Letter: Finasteride for benign prostatic hypertrophy. Med Lett Drugs Ther 34:83, 1992.
  *This paper reviews the use, efficacy, and potential adverse effects of finasteride in humans.*
Neri R: Pharmacology and pharmacokinetics of flutamide. Urology 34 (suppl): 19, 1989.
  *This paper reviews the use of flutamide in dogs.*
Olson PN, Wrigley RH, Thrall MA, et al: Disorders of the canine prostate gland: Pathogenesis, diagnosis, and medical therapy. Compend Cont Educ Pract Vet 9:613, 1987.
  *This paper is a general review of prostatic diseases in dogs and reports on the use of megestrol acetate to treat prostatic hyperplasia.*
Peter AT and Jakovljevic S: Real-time ultrasonography of the small animal reproductive organs. Compend Cont Educ Vet Med 14:739, 1992.
  *This paper reviews the ultrasonographic characteristics of the prostate gland, testicles, and epididymes.*

# Section

# 11

# REPRODUCTIVE DISORDERS

VICKI N. MEYERS-WALLEN
*Consulting Editor*

*Still Current Information Found in Current Veterinary Therapy XI:*

# EARLY NEUTERING OF THE DOG AND CAT

W. PRESTON STUBBS,
*Gainesville, Florida*

KATHARINE R. SALMERI,
*Red Bank, New Jersey*

*and* MARK S. BLOOMBERG
*Gainesville, Florida*

Pet overpopulation continues to be a leading cause of death in dogs and cats in the United States, with millions of animals being euthanatized each year despite current population control programs. Surgical sterilization is the most common and reliable means of pet population control, leading most animal shelter/control facilities to employ mandatory neuter policies. However, because surgery is usually delayed until dogs and cats are at least 6 months of age (Stone, Cantrell, and Sharp, 1993), many animals adopted from shelters remain sexually intact and are never neutered. Prepubertal gonadectomy or early age neutering (6 to 14 weeks) is being advocated by animal shelter and humane organizations as a means of enhancing the efficacy of sterilization programs. As the terminology suggests, surgical sterilization is performed prior to the onset of sexual maturity, and hence reproductive capability, which may occur as early as 6 months of age in dogs and 4 months of age in cats.

Although it is one of the oldest surgical procedures performed on domestic animals, few objective scientific data exist to suggest an optimal age for elective gonadectomy in the dog and cat (Salmeri, Olson, and Bloomberg, 1991). In the United States, dogs and cats are routinely neutered between 5 and 8 months of age. Most veterinarians are comfortable performing elective gonadectomy on animals of this age group because untoward effects are minimal. A more rational basis for this policy is lacking, however.

The safety of early neutering has been questioned by veterinarians because of their unfamiliarity with surgery and anesthesia on pediatric patients. Other concerns about prepubertal neutering of dogs and cats include stunted growth, obesity, perivulvar dermatitis, vaginitis, behavioral changes, urinary incontinence, increased morbidity/mortality during surgery and anesthesia, and impaired immunocompetence (Salmeri, Olson, and Bloomberg, 1991). In the cat, urethral obstruction (males) and defective formation of the preputial cavity (Herron, 1971) have been cited as potential problems. Mounting clinical and research data, however, would suggest that most concerns regarding prepubertal gonadectomy are unfounded (Aronsohn

and Faggella, 1993; Theran, 1993; Salmeri et al., 1991). In fact, several studies have found that early neutering affects skeletal and physical development, behavior, and urethral function in much the same manner as more traditionally timed gonadectomy.

## CLINICAL AND RESEARCH DATA

The aforementioned concerns were addressed in two separate but parallel studies conducted at the University of Florida. The effects of prepubertal gonadectomy on skeletal growth, weight gain, food intake, body fat, secondary sex characteristics, urethral function, and behavioral development were investigated in both dogs (Salmeri et al., 1991) and cats. Both studies divided animals into three treatment groups: animals neutered at 7 weeks of age (I), 7 months of age (II), and those which remained sexually intact as a control population (III).

Gonadectomy (groups I and II) delayed closure of the distal radial growth plate in both dogs and cats as compared with sexually intact controls. This allowed for an extended period of growth and greater radial/ulnar length in all neutered male dogs and group I bitches. Although delayed physeal closure was observed in neutered cats, there was no significant difference in mature radius/ulna length amongst the three treatment groups. Thus, rather than causing stunted growth, prepubertal gonadectomy may actually result in normal or greater stature. This delay in physeal closure probably occurs because gonadal hormones facilitate physeal cartilage maturation; in their absence the growth plate remains open for a longer period of time. Some investigators have suggested that this may increase the risk of physeal fractures (Houlton and McGlennon, 1992).

In dogs, gonadectomy did not affect growth rate, food intake, weight gain, or back-fat depth (body fat). Body weight and body fat were similar among neutered (group I and II) cats; however, sexually intact cats weighed less and had less body fat than their neutered counterparts. Prepubertal gonadectomy had no adverse effect on urethral function in the dog or cat as determined by urethral pressure profilometry. Male cats of all three groups had similar urethral diameters.

The external genitalia of prepubertally neutered animals of both sexes and species remained infantile in appearance. Male cats neutered at 7 weeks of age had a virtual absence of penile spines, but the penis could be fully exteriorized, indicating separation of the balanopreputial fold. This is contrary to results describing persistent preputial adhesions in four of ten male cats neutered at 5 months of age (Herron, 1971). The penis, prepuce, and os penis of group I dogs were infantile, as were the vulvas of early neutered bitches and queens. No problems with vaginitis or perivulvar dermatitis were noted, however. Behavioral characteristics were similar amongst all groups with the exception of greater intraspecies aggression and fewer demonstrations of affection in sexually intact cats. Neutering did not result in lethargy or inactivity in either dogs or cats.

The safety of early neutering in a clinical setting has been well established (Aronsohn and Faggella, 1993; Theran, 1993). In the Massachusetts SPCA study (Theran, 1993), gonadectomies were performed on over 350 6- to 14-week-old dogs and cats without serious complications or mortality. The authors have had similar experience with a smaller group of research animals.

## SURGICAL TECHNIQUES

### Ovariohysterectomy

Methods for prepubertal ovariohysterectomy are similar to those routinely used in more mature animals and have been described in detail (Salmeri et al., 1991; Aronsohn and Faggella, 1993; Theran, 1993). Because of the small amount of abdominal fat present in young animals, visualization of the ovarian pedicle is excellent. This, coupled with the small vessel size, allows for precise hemostasis and shortens operative time. Fine (3-0 or 4-0) absorbable suture material such as chromic gut (chromic gut, Ethicon), polyglyconate (Maxon, Davis and Geck) or stainless steel hemostatic clips may be used for ligation of the ovarian pedicles and uterine body. The linea alba can be closed using either fine (3-0 or 4-0) absorbable or nonabsorbable suture material in an interrupted or continuous pattern. Closure of the subcutaneous layer is optional if skin sutures are to be used. The use of subcuticular sutures without skin sutures has been suggested (Aronsohn and Faggella, 1993) to decrease the patient's interest in the incision.

### Orchidectomy

In dogs and cats, the testicles are usually descended at birth and are easily palpable in the immature scrotum by 6 to 8 weeks of age. Orchidectomy in the kitten is similar to the procedure performed in adult cats. The spermatic cord may be ligated in a closed or open fashion with fine absorbable suture material, stainless steel

hemostatic clips, or by tying the cord upon itself using a hemostat. The scrotal incisions are left to heal by second intention. A scrotal (rather than prescrotal) approach to the testicles is also used in 6- to 8-week old puppies. The procedure can be performed in an open or closed fashion, using absorbable suture material or hemostatic clips for ligatures. Fine subcuticular sutures can be used to close the scrotal incisions or they can be left to heal by second intention.

## Pediatric Considerations

The potential for hypothermia and hypoglycemia, a relatively small blood volume, and delicate tissues are factors that must be considered when performing surgery on pediatric patients.

Hypothermia can be minimized by placing patients on recirculating warm water blankets during surgery and by administering warm balanced electrolyte solutions intravenously (ovariohysterectomy). The animal should also be kept from getting excessively wet during preparation of the surgical site. Neonates are also more susceptible to hypoglycemia than adults; therefore, food should be withheld no longer than 8 hr prior to surgery, with 3 to 4 hr being optimal in the youngest patients. If necessary, oral or intravenous 50% dextrose or oral corn syrup can be administered perioperatively and animals should be fed within a few hours of recovery. If not yet weaned, neonates should be returned to their dam and littermates as soon as they have recovered sufficiently from anesthesia. Handling of the animals should be minimized and they should be housed in a quiet environment preoperatively and postoperatively. Friable pediatric tissues necessitate gentle handling, with special attention given to careful hemostasis in light of the relatively small blood volume of these patients.

## ANESTHETIC TECHNIQUES

Although concerns are often expressed regarding the risks and feasibility of pediatric anesthesia, it can be performed safely using a number of different techniques. Special considerations in the pediatric patient include differences in drug uptake, distribution, and action as compared to adults as well as immature hepatorenal, respiratory, and cardiovascular system function (Grandy and Dunlop, 1991; Theran, 1993).

Neonates have a larger percentage of total body water, lower albumin concentration and body fat levels, and relatively high cardiac output to vessel-rich organs. All of these factors affect drug pharmacokinetics. A heightened sensitivity to protein-bound drugs may be seen and, in general, dosages of parenterally administered anesthetic agents should be reduced (Grandy and Dunlop, 1991). Pediatric patients have immature hepatic enzyme systems responsible for drug metabolism; therefore, anesthetics metabolized in this manner may have a longer duration of action. Glomerular filtration and tubular function are also incompletely developed, delaying renal excretion of certain drugs.

The high rate of oxygen consumption in neonates necessitates a greater respiratory rate; therefore, anesthetic-induced respiratory depression and subsequent hypoventilation should be avoided by careful monitoring. Because of differences in respiratory dynamics, atelectasis is also of concern (Grandy and Dunlop, 1991). Cardiac output in young animals is mainly rate dependent and baroresponses are immature; therefore, bradycardia and hypotension should be avoided.

Various anesthetic combinations have been used successfully in pediatric patients. The preanesthetic administration of anticholinergics (atropine or glycopyrrolate) has been advocated by some authors to stabilize heart rate and thus cardiac output, and to decrease respiratory secretions (Grandy and Dunlop, 1991). We have not found this to be necessary, however.

General anesthesia can be rapidly induced and maintained with isoflurane (AErrane, Anaquest) or halothane (Halocarbon Labs) administered by mask or tank infusion. Most young animals (6 to 14 weeks) will tolerate the required restraint with minimal excitement or struggling. A tight-fitting mask will serve well throughout the short duration of an orchidectomy procedure. Endotracheal intubation should be performed in animals undergoing ovariohysterectomy. A 2.0- to 3.5-mm Cole or Magill endotracheal tube is recommended in kittens (Aronsohn and Faggella, 1993). Intubation should be gentle to avoid airway trauma and edema and the tube should be suctioned at 30-min intervals to prevent obstruction by respiratory secretions, a potential problem with tubes of such small diameter (Grandy and Dunlop, 1991). It is also vitally important to select a tube of proper length to minimize dead space and avoid endobronchial intubation. Isoflurane is probably the preferred inhalant agent in young animals due to its rapid induction and recovery characteristics (low solubility), decreased need for metabolism, and diminished cardiovascular depression as compared with halothane (Grandy and Dunlop, 1991). A nonrebreathing anesthetic circuit should be used for neonatal patients weighing less than 5 kg (Ayres T-piece, Bain circuit, Norman elbow). Fresh gas flow rates of 200 ml/kg/min are recommended.

Several injectable anesthetics are suitable for premedication or anesthetic induction for longer procedures (ovariohysterectomy) or as sole agents for a shorter procedure (orchidectomy). In kittens, benzodiazepine/dissociative combinations such as tiletamine/zolazepam (Telazol, AH Robins) and midazolam (Versed, Hoffman-LaRoche)/ ketamine (Ketaset, Fort Dodge Laboratories) are very safe and effective. Tiletamine/zolazepam at 11 mg/kg IM (2 to 4 mg/kg IV) has been recommended for orchidectomy in young kittens (Faggella and Aronsohn, 1993; Theran, 1993). If necessary, supplemental inhalational anesthetic can be provided by mask. This combination can also be used in puppies.

Midazolam (0.22 mg/kg IM)/ketamine (11 mg/kg IM) followed by intubation and administration of an inhalant agent is recommended for feline ovariohysterectomy (Faggella and Aronsohn, 1993; Theran, 1993). The authors have successfully used an intravenous combination of 0.2 mg/kg diazepam (Valium, Hoffman-LaRoche) and 5 to 7 mg/kg ketamine for anesthetic induction. Xylazine (Rompun, Miles) and phenothiazine tranquilizers (such as acepromazine) should be avoided in animals less than 3 months old because of their potential to cause bradycardia (decreased cardiac output) and hypotension, respectively. The use of barbiturates in animals less than 3 months of age is also discouraged.

Opioids provide analgesia and sedation as premedicants but should be administered with anticholinergics to prevent bradycardia. An advantage to their use is the potential for reversal with antagonists or agonist/antagonist agents.

Another option for intravenous anesthetic induction is propofol (Diprivan, Stuart Pharmaceuticals). This drug produces a rapid, smooth induction and recovery. It is given at a dose of 4 to 6 mg/kg following premedications and 8 to 12 mg/kg as a sole agent. It has been used successfully for early neutering in pups (Theran, 1993).

Monitoring during anesthesia is similar to that performed in adults, with care being taken to prevent bradycardia, hypotension, and hypothermia. A Doppler ultrasound device (Ultrasonic Doppler Flow Detector Model 811-AL, Parks Medical Electronics) is useful to monitor blood pressure.

## SUMMARY

Early neutering in dogs and cats is a safe and effective means of pet population control. The risks associated with surgery and anesthesia of pediatric patients are minimal, with the advantages being a shorter operative time, better visualization, rapid recovery, and decreased morbidity. The effects of prepubertal gonadectomy on skeletal, physical, and behavioral development are similar to those seen in animals that are neutered at a more traditional age.

## References and Suggested Reading

Aronsohn MG and Faggella AM: Surgical techniques for neutering 6- to 14-week-old kittens. J Am Vet Med Assoc 202:53, 1993.
   *A study describing the surgical techniques and considerations for early neutering in 96 kittens.*
Faggella AM and Aronsohn MG: Anesthetic techniques for neutering 6 to 14 week-old kittens. J Am Vet Med Assoc 202:56, 1993.
   *A study comparing four anesthetic protocols used for early neutering in kittens.*
Grandy JL and Dunlop CI: Anesthesia of pups and kittens. J Am Vet Med Assoc 198:1244, 1991.
   *An article reviewing physiology, pharmacokinetics, and anesthetics used in pediatric patients.*
Herron MA: A potential consequence of prepubertal feline castration. Feline Pract 1:17, 1971.
   *Research article describing preputial adhesions in cats castrated at 5 months of age.*

Houlton JEF and McGlennon NJ: Castration and physeal closure in the cat. Vet Rec 131:466, 1992.
  *A pilot study describing delayed physeal closure in two cats castrated at 28 weeks of age.*
Salmeri KR, Olson PN, and Bloomberg MS: Elective gonadectomy in the dog: A review. J Am Vet Med Assoc 198:1183, 1991.
  *A review of the physiology of puberty and the current knowledge and potential effects of gonadectomy.*
Salmeri KR, Bloomberg MS, Scruggs SL, et al: Gonadectomy in immature dogs: Effects on skeletal, physical, and behavioral development. J Am Vet Med Assoc 198:1193, 1991.
  *Results of a study investigating the developmental effects of early neutering in dogs.*
Stone EA, Cantrell CG, and Sharp NJH: Ovary and uterus. *In* Slatter D (ed): Textbook of Small Animal Surgery. Volume 2. Philadelphia, WB Saunders Co, 1993, p 1293.
  *Description of surgical diseases and techniques of the ovaries and uterus.*
Theran P: Early-age neutering of dogs and cats. J Am Vet Med Assoc 202: 914, 1993.
  *A review of surgical and anesthetic techniques for neutering 6- to 14-week-old puppies and kittens.*

# ULTRASONOGRAPHY OF THE REPRODUCTIVE TRACT OF THE FEMALE DOG AND CAT

AMY E. YEAGER
*and* PATRICK W. CONCANNON
*Ithaca, New York*

## INDICATIONS, EQUIPMENT, AND PATIENT PREPARATION FOR ULTRASOUND EXAMINATION

There are multiple indications for ultrasonographic examination of the female reproductive tract of the dog and cat. The most common use is during pregnancy for detection of fetal number, determination of fetal well-being, and estimation of stage of gestation. In addition, ultrasonography is very useful for detection of pyometra in bitches and queens with vaginal discharge, fever, lethargy, or depression and for evaluation of mass lesions palpated in intact females. Other indications for ultrasonographic examination include infertility, persistent estrus, complications of the postpartum uterus, and complications following ovariohysterectomy.

The same real-time B-mode ultrasound equipment that is commonly used for cardiac and abdominal examination of dog and cat is appropriate for examination of the reproductive tract. Sector or linear probes of 10, 7.5, and 5.0 MHz are useful. In this range, the higher frequencies are used for examination of the ovary, nonpregnant uterus, and early pregnancy. A 5.0-MHz probe is most useful for examination of late pregnancy and masses in animals weighing 10 to 20 kg or more.

Preparation of the dog or cat for ultrasonographic examination of the reproductive tract is the same as for examination of the other abdominal viscera. To obtain high-quality images, position the animal in dorsal or lateral recumbency, clip the hair coat with a No. 40 blade, clean the skin, and apply ultrasonographic coupling gel. A full urinary bladder is helpful but not essential for examination of the cervix, uterine body, and caudal parts of the uterine horns. Fasting the dog or cat for 12 hr before examination improves detection of the ovaries, nonpregnant uterine horns, and early pregnancy, because intestinal gas can obscure these small structures.

## OVARY

### Technique for Examination and Appearance of the Normal Ovary

The caudal poles of the kidneys are used as landmarks to find the ovaries. The ultrasound transducer is positioned in a longitudinal scan plane just caudal to a kidney. To locate an ovary, the transducer is then swept medially and laterally, applying varying degrees of abdominal compression. Detection of the anestrus ovary is variable depending on the experience of the sonographer and the age, body weight, skin quality, and demeanor of the dog or cat. Detection is more likely in mature, thin animals that range from approximately 10 to 25 kg body weight; have thin, smooth skin with few hair follicles; and have a quiet, relaxed demeanor. Canine ovaries are easier to visualize around the time of ovulation because they are enlarged and contain anechoic follicles or corpora lutea.

From the ultrasonographic appearance, it is possible to categorize the canine ovary as typical of anestrus or early proestrus, a few days before or after ovulation, late estrus, or mid-diestrus (Table 1; Fig. 1). However, evaluation of ovaries for precise determination or prediction of the day of ovulation is difficult at best, even when serial daily examinations are performed. This difficulty is due to multiple factors. Ovaries are not nec-

**Table 1.** *Ultrasonographic Appearance of Canine Ovaries Throughout the Estrous Cycle*

| Time of the Estrous Cycle | Appearance of the Ovary |
|---|---|
| Anestrus and early proestrus | Small (mean length = 1.2 cm)<br>Oval shape with a smooth contour<br>Uniform echogenicity (no follicles, CLs, or other structures) |
| Proestrus | Gradual increase in size, becomes a plumper oval shape, and contour usually remains smooth<br>Follicles appear as round or oval-shaped anechoic fluid cavities with thin wall or no apparent wall<br>Mean follicle number 4 (range-0–10)<br>Follicle diameter is breed dependent; on the day prior to ovulation, mean diameter ranges from 5 mm in beagles to 8 mm in retrievers; maximum diameter of preovulatory follicles may be as large as 11 mm. |
| Day of ovulation | Follicle number usually decreases to 0 or 2 follicles per ovary<br>The follicles that do not "disappear" tend to decrease in diameter but the ovary does not decrease in size<br>Contour may appear bumpy<br>Solid, hypoechoic CLs may appear<br>A scant amount of fluid is occasionally detected adjacent to the ovary |
| Estrus | Maximum ovarian size is reached 5–6 days after ovulation (300–400% of anestrus volume)<br>Bumpy contour<br>Fluid-filled CLs have anechoic centers:<br>Mean of 3 fluid-filled CLs per ovary<br>May be indistinguishable from follicles<br>Tend to be several millimeters larger, thicker walled, and more variable shape than follicles<br>Solid CLs are 5–9 mm diameter |
| Diestrus | Bumpy contour<br>Fluid filled CLs gradually decrease in size and increase in echogenicity to become 6-mm solid CLs between 10 and 14 days after ovulation<br>Ovarian size decreases somewhat (200–300% of anestrous volume) as fluid-filled CLs regress<br>Solid CLs persist through most of diestrus |

Abbreviation: CL = corpora lutea

essarily bilaterally symmetric. The maximal diameter of the preovulatory follicle just prior to ovulation may vary with dog breed. Frequently, the change in the appearance of the ovary at the time of ovulation is not dramatic. Although apparent follicle number and size tend to decrease, follicles do not necessarily completely disappear from view on the day of ovulation. Lastly, it is possible to identify corpora lutea and follicles incorrectly because both can appear as fluid cavity structures around the time of ovulation. Characteristics that are associated with ovaries after ovulation are a bumpy contour, one or more solid corpora lutea, and fluid cavity structures which, if present, may have a large diameter (≥10 mm) or have thick, irregular walls.

For detection of the feline ovary, use a transducer with excellent imaging characteristics in the near field. This is important because the cat's ovary is small and may be located less than 1 cm from the transducer surface. A built-in stand-off is recommended for sector probes. Ovulation in the feline is marked by the disappearance of anechoic follicles at 24 hr after breeding (Fig. 2).

In some species, ultrasonography is useful for monitoring estrus induction protocols and retrieving oocytes for *in vitro* fertilization. At present, there are no routinely successful methods of estrus induction in the dog. Ultrasonographic detection of hyperstimulation or hypostimulation of the ovary (Fig. 3) might aid in the development of improved protocols for estrus induction. Aspiration of canine follicles for oocyte retrieval is technically difficult because of their small size.

## Lesions of the Ovary

Ultrasonography is useful for detection of ovarian cysts, neoplasms, and other mass lesions. The characteristic features of benign cystic lesions are: oval shape, thin smooth wall, anechoic fluid-filled lumen with no internal echoes, and acoustic enhancement artifact (tissues are increased in echogenicity) deep to the cystic structure (Fig. 4). It is not possible to differentiate functional from nonfunctional ovarian cysts by ultrasonographic appearance. Ovarian masses that are cystic but lack benign characteristics or have solid components are potentially neoplastic. Mineralization may be detected (intensely hyperechoic foci that cast acoustic shadows) in ovarian carcinomas and teratomas. Ovarian carcinoma can be highly malignant, and metastasis to the peritoneal cavity can occur. This may appear as peritoneal fluid, thickening and adhesions of the omentum and mesentery, or small nodules on peritoneal surfaces.

## UTERUS

### Technique for Examination and Appearance of Normal Nonpregnant Uterus

The uterus is most reliably located dorsal or lateral to the urinary bladder. The caudal poles of the kidneys and the ovaries can also be landmarks for the detection of the uterus because the cranial parts of the uterine horns are located immediately caudal to the ovaries. Segments of the midportions of the uterine horns appear along a "V"-shaped line drawn between the caudal poles of the kidneys and the midline of the caudal abdomen. It is possible to incorrectly identify the uterus as empty small intestine because both are tubular struc-

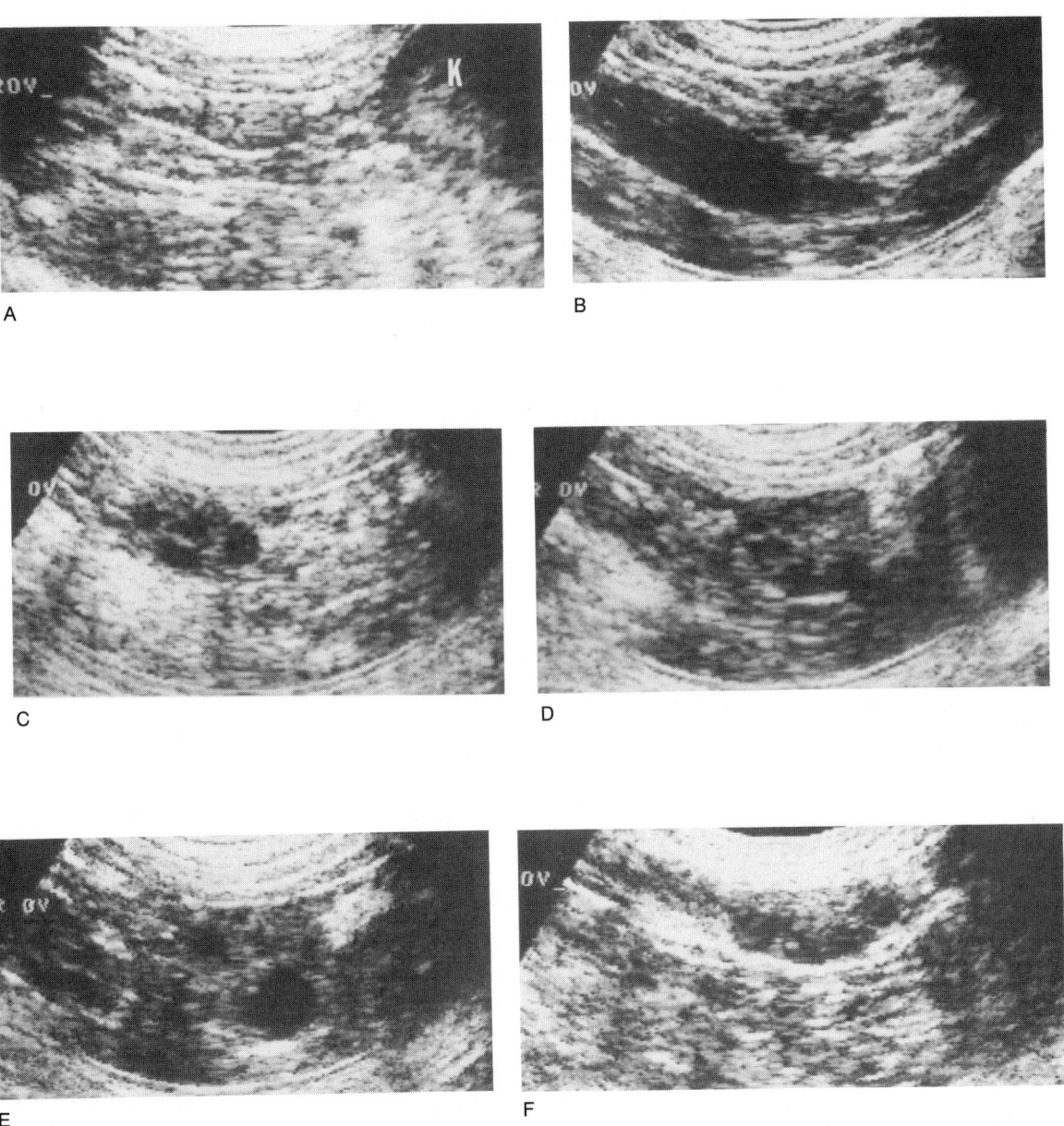

**Figure 1.** Ultrasonograms made in the longitudinal plane showing beagle ovaries at various times of the estrus cycle. *A,* This anestrus ovary is small (1 cm length), has a smooth contour, and appears uniformly hypoechoic compared to the surrounding fat. The caudal pole of the kidney is marked (K). Figures 1*B, C, D,* and *E* are from the same bitch. *B,* The proestrus ovary (3 days before the luteinizing hormone peak) is filled with seven small (1- to 2-mm) follicles. *C,* The day before ovulation (1 day after the luteinizing hormone peak), the ovary is slightly larger than the proestrus ovary and is filled with four follicles that have increased to 3 to 5 mm in diameter. *D,* On the day of ovulation, the ovary is mainly hypoechoic. *It contains three less defined structures that are either echogenic follicles or corpora lutea.* *E,* six days after the luteinizing hormone peak, the ovary has continued to increase in size, has a bumpy contour, and contains three hypoechoic corpora lutea and one fluid cavity (5 × 7 mm). *F,* This diestrus ovary (20 days after the luteinizing hormone peak) shows four hypoechoic, 5-mm diameter corpora lutea.

tures of similar diameter. However, empty small intestine characteristically has a central echo that is the lumen and its wall has multiple layers (the serosal interface, muscularis, submucosa, and mucosa) (Fig. 5). The small intestine is easy to correctly identify when there is peristalsis or gas in the lumen.

During late diestrus and anestrus, the uterus is uniformly hypoechoic compared to background fat. It has neither a layered wall nor a luminal echo (Fig. 5). In

bitches, uterine diameter ranges from 3 mm in toy and miniature breeds to 8 mm in large and giant breeds. During anestrus, the uterus is difficult to detect, except at the level of the bladder, and the vagina and cervix are difficult to distinguish from the uterine body.

Throughout proestrus, estrus, and early diestrus, a 1-mm hyperechoic luminal echo and a hypoechoic inner layer of the uterine wall are variably present (Fig. 5). Detection of the uterus is easier at these times com-

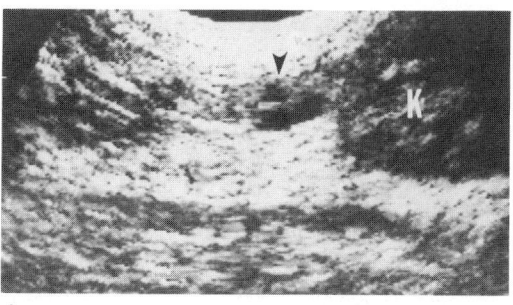 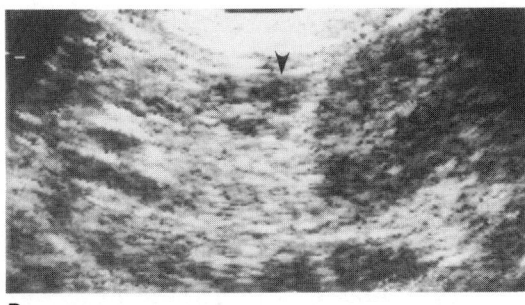

A   B

**Figure 2.** Serial ultrasonograms made in the longitudinal plane showing a queen's ovary before and after ovulation. A, On the day of first coitus, the 1-cm-length ovary (*arrowhead*) located just caudal to the kidney (K) shows three follicles. B, Two days later, no follicles are apparent in the ovary (*arrowhead*).

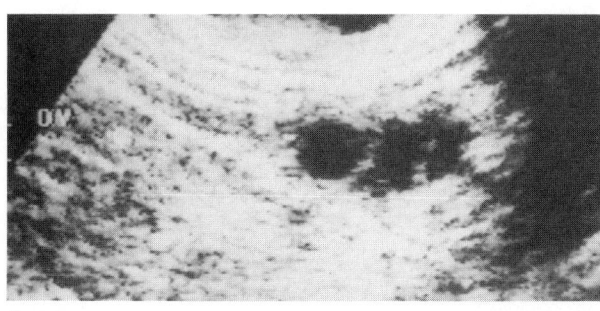 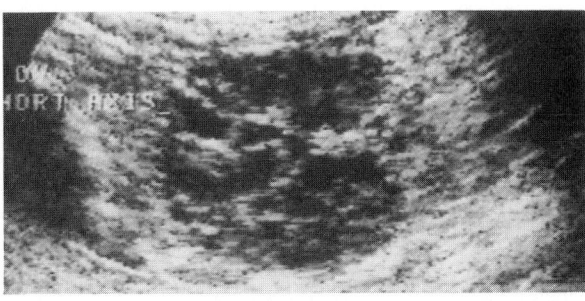

A   B

**Figure 3.** Ultrasonograms of the ovaries of two beagles that underwent estrus induction. A, The appearance of this ovary is typical of 1 to 3 days prior to ovulation because it is filled with follicles that measure 4 to 6 mm in diameter and has a smooth contour. The ultrasonogram was obtained at the end of 2 weeks of gonadotropin-releasing hormone pump therapy, close to the time of a fertile ovulation. B, This image shows an enlarged ovary of a bitch treated with pregnant mare serum gonadotropin. It contains many more follicles than a normal proestrus ovary.

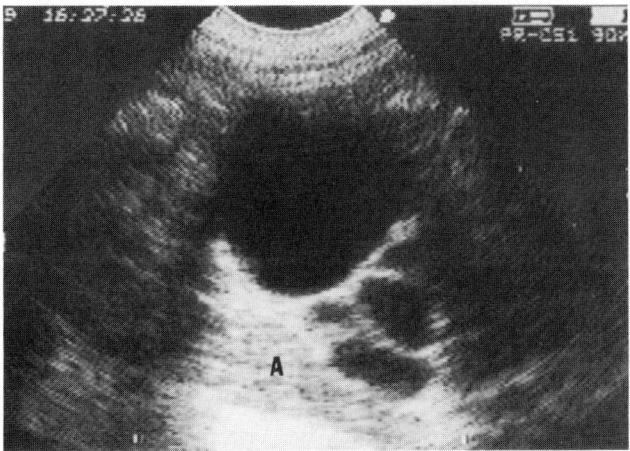

**Figure 4.** Ultrasonogram of the ovary of a fertile 7-year-old German shepherd bitch. The ovary appears abnormally large (2.8 × 3.8 cm) and multicystic. The cysts appear to be benign because they are anechoic, have thin smooth walls, and exhibit acoustic enhancement artifact (A).

pared to anestrus because it is turgid and 1 to 3 mm larger in diameter. There is also obvious, focal enlargement of the canine cervix. It has multiple layers that give it a "bull's-eye" appearance in cross-section (Fig. 6). The uterus may appear coiled during the first and second weeks of diestrus. Its appearance is the same for pregnant and nonpregnant bitches before detection of the gestational sac.

## Pregnancy

### PREGNANCY DETECTION AND ESTIMATION OF GESTATION LENGTH

Ultrasonography is a more accurate method of pregnancy detection than palpation and it can be used to diagnose pregnancy much earlier than radiography. The gestational sac is the earliest evidence of pregnancy. These can be detected as 1- to 2-mm spherical anechoic structures in the lumen of the uterus as early as

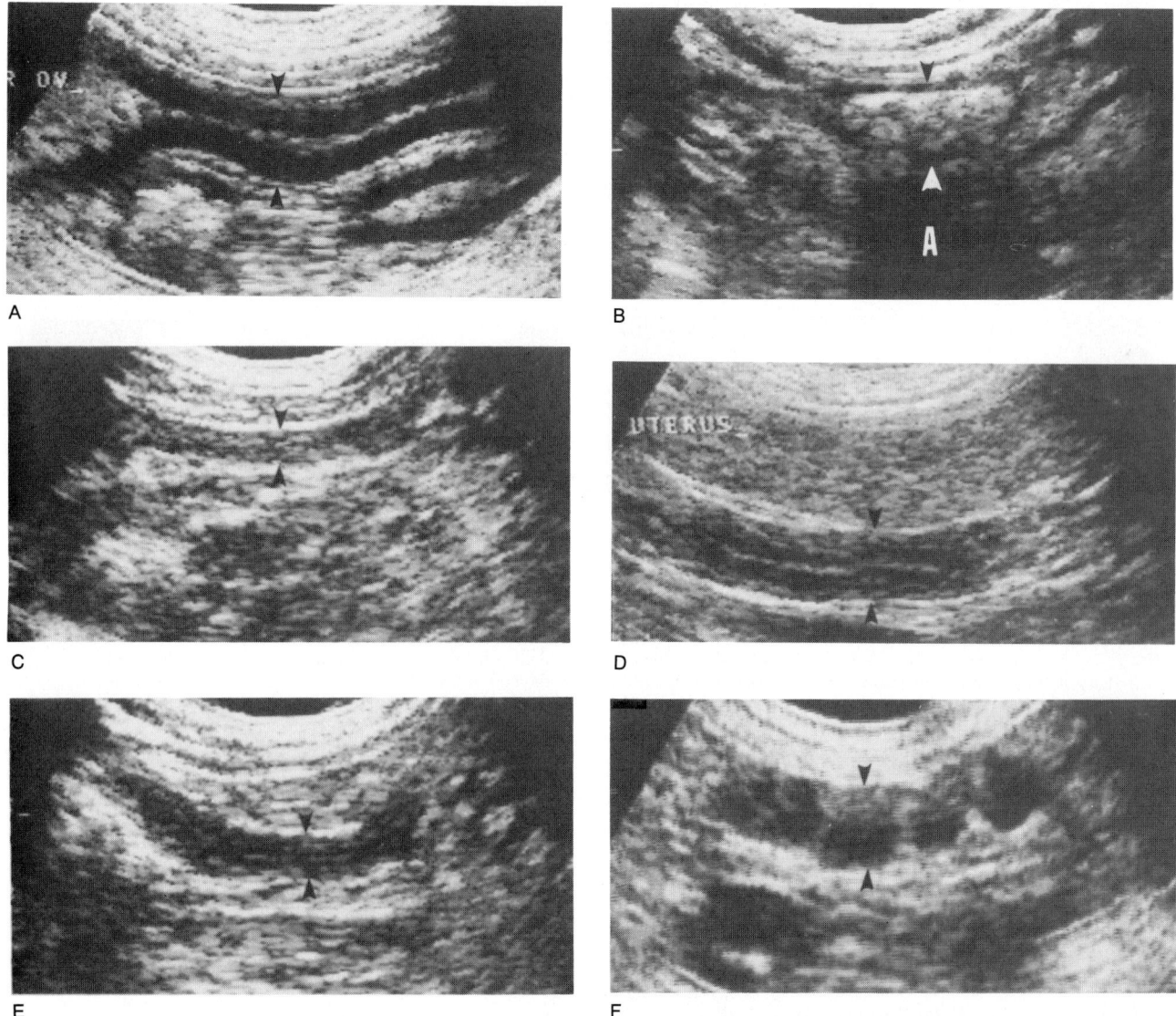

**Figure 5.** Ultrasonograms showing longitudinal segments of small intestine and anestrus, proestrus, and diestrus uterine horn. Arrows mark the serosal margins of these structures. *A*, Empty small intestine. The intestinal wall is composed of multiple layers. Typically, the thickest is the mucosa, which is very hypoechoic. The empty lumen appears as a thin (1 mm) central echo. *B*, Gas-filled segments of small intestine. The intestinal wall is stretched thin (1 to 2 mm) and the lumen is wide (7 mm), hyperechoic, and casts an acoustic shadow (A). *C*, Uterine horn of an anestrus beagle. The uterine horn is uniformly hypoechoic compared to surrounding fat and is 4 mm in diameter. *D*, Uterine horn of a proestrus beagle. This uterine horn is 7 mm in diameter, the wall is composed of layers, and there is a luminal echo. *E*, Uterine horn of a diestrus shorthaired queen. The 4-mm-diameter uterine horn is uniformly hypoechoic compared to background fat. *F*, Uterine horn of a diestrus beagle. The uterine horn is uniformly hypoechoic compared to surrounding fat (perhaps it is more hypoechoic than during anestrus) and it has a coiled contour.

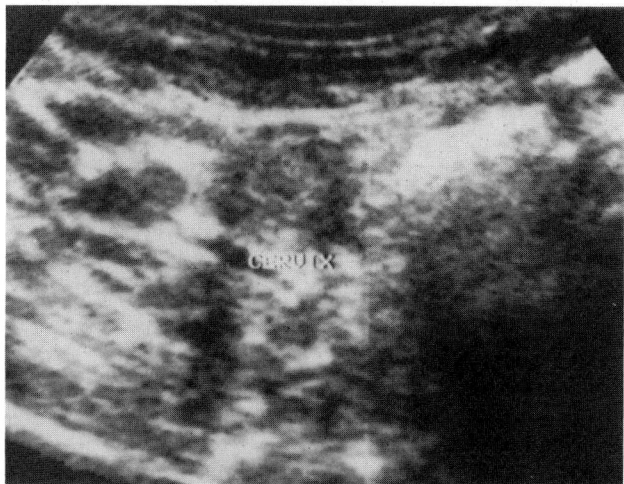

**Figure 6.** Ultrasonogram made in the transverse plane of the cervix of a beagle bitch that is in estrus. The cervix is enlarged (1.3 cm diameter) and is composed of multiple layers, creating a "bull's-eye" appearance.

**Table 2.** *Estimation of Gestation Length Based on Pregnancy Size*

| Pregnancy Size (cm) | Gestation Length (Days) | | |
|---|---|---|---|
| | Beagles° | Retrieverst | Domestic Cats† |
| Body diameter | | | |
| 0.2 | 24–27 | | |
| 0.5 | 27–32 | | |
| 1.0 | 33–36 | | 32–36 |
| 1.5 | 39–41 | | 37–41 |
| 2.0 | 41–45 | 40–49 | 43–47 |
| 2.5 | 43–45 | 43–52 | 48–52 |
| 3.0 | 47–49 | 46–55 | 53–57 |
| 3.5 | 49–54 | 49–58 | 57–61 |
| 4.0 | 56–59 | 52–61 | ≥64 |
| 5.0 | ≥59 | ≥55 | |
| Biparietal diameter | | | |
| 1.0 | 34–38 | | 27–31 |
| 1.5 | 41–45 | | 40–44 |
| 2.0 | 50–53 | 46–56 | 52–56 |
| 2.5 | 56–60 | 53–64 | ≥64 |
| 3.0 | ≥62 | ≥57 | |
| Gestational sac diameter | | | |
| 0.2 | 19–22 | | |
| 0.5 | 22–25 | | |
| 1.0 | 25–28 | | |
| 1.5 | 28–31 | | |
| 2.0 | 31–34 | | |
| 2.5 | 34–38 | | |
| 3.0 | 38–42 | 25–40 | |
| Fetal length | | | |
| 0.2 | 23–25 | | |
| 1.0 | 27–31 | | |
| 1.5 | 31–33 | | |
| 2.0 | 33–35 | | |
| 2.5 | 34–36 | | |
| 3.0 | 36–37 | | |
| 4.0 | 38–39 | | |
| 5.0 | 39–40 | | |
| 7.0 | 43–45 | | |
| 9.0 | 47–48 | | |

°Day 0 of gestation is the day of the luteinizing hormone peak (LHP) (Yeager et al., 1992) (also see "The Elective Cesarean Section," this volume, p 1085).

†Day 0 of gestation is the estimated day of the LHP (65 days minus the estimated number of days prior to whelping) (England, Allen, and Porter, 1990).

‡Day 0 of gestation is the estimated day of coitus (66 days minus the estimated days prior to queening) (Beck, Baldwin, and Bosu, 1990).

17 to 20 days after luteinizing hormone peak (LHP) in the bitch and 11 to 14 days after coitus in the queen. An embryo with a heartbeat is earliest definite evidence of viable pregnancy. These are apparent as early as 23 to 25 days after the canine LHP and 16 to 20 days after coitus in the queen. Both anatomic appearance and pregnancy size are useful for estimation of gestation length (Tables 2 and 3; Fig. 7). A recommended time for reliable, early pregnancy detection in the bitch is 25 days after the last breeding, which can range from 23 to 33 days after the LHP. At this time, the gestational sac of a viable pregnancy is likely to be large enough to reliably detect (it will be at least 8 mm diameter on day 25 after the LHP) and more likely than not it will contain an embryo with a heartbeat. Day 16 after coitus is recommended for early pregnancy detection in the queen.

### ESTIMATION OF FETAL NUMBER

Approximate fetal number can be determined from ultrasonography. The count is more accurate if litter size is four or fewer. In large litters, fetal number is often greatly underestimated. It is best to obtain this information between 25 and 35 days after the last breeding (Fig. 8). After this time, fetuses are more difficult to count because they become confluent, are surrounded by relatively little fetal fluid, and crown-rump length may exceed the width of the ultrasound image depending upon the configuration and size of the ultrasound transducer.

### PROBLEMS OF FETAL WELL-BEING

From 20 to 30 days after the LHP, it is not uncommon to detect the death of one or two embryos. Ultrasonographic signs of distress or death of the embryo include: aberrant (usually smaller) size of the gestational sac or embryo compared to others in the litter, thickened or irregular placenta, echogenic fluid within the gestational sac, and absent or abnormally slow heartbeat (Fig. 9). Usually, dead embryos resorb or mummify. In the bitch, they commonly resorb. When there is fetal resorption, the implantation site may be detected as a focal thickening of the uterine horn that persists to the end of gestation. In the queen, dead embryos frequently mummify (Fig. 10). Mummified embryos progressively decrease in size, but the yolk sac, allantoic membranes, and fetal fluid may increase in volume until the end of gestation. When the

**Table 3.** *Estimation of Gestational Age Based on Anatomic Appearance of the Pregnancy*

| Gestation Length (Days) | | Anatomic Appearance of the Pregnancy |
| Dog° | Cat† | |
| --- | --- | --- |
| 17–24 | 11–17 | Small gestational sac and no visible embryo |
| 23–27 | 15–23 | Small embryo directly attached to uterine wall |
| 25–30 | 21–30 | Bipolar-shaped embryo attached to the yolk sac membrane, which appears to be a single-strand structure |
| 27–35 | ≥26 | Early in this time period, the yolk sac membrane changes from a single strand to a tubular structure (2 strands in the longitudinal plane and a circular or folded structure in the transverse plane); the allantoic membrane and ventricles in the fetal head may also be detected |
| | | Later in this time period, the bipolar-shaped embryo develops a few additional features such as limb buds, faintly hyperechoic axial skeleton (mandible and maxilla mineralize first), and fetal movement; the zonary placenta is distinct |
| 35–47 | | The majority of fetal anatomy is detected, such as fetal bladder, stomach, lung, liver (hypoechoic compared to lung and hypoechoic compared to rest of the abdomen), kidney, rib shadows, hyperechoic appendicular skeleton |
| | | Body diameter ≤50% of the outer uterine diameter |
| 38–42 | | Body diameter 2 mm >biparietal diameter and fetal crown-rump length = length of the zonary placenta |
| ≥48 | | Gallbladder, pulmonary vessels detected |
| | | Body diameter >50% outer uterine diameter |
| ≥57 | | Intestinal motility |

°Day 0 of gestation is the day of the luteinizing hormone peak (Yeager et al., 1992) (also see "The Elective Cesarean Section," this volume, p 1085).

†Day 0 of gestation is the day of first coitus (Davidson, Nyland, and Tsutsui, 1986).

majority of embryos in a litter die, a fertility disorder is likely. A differential diagnosis includes metritis, cystic endometrial hyperplasia, maternal systemic disease (endocrinopathy, organ failure, viral infection, toxicity), failure to maintain adequate progesterone levels, improper diet, or fatal genetic defects (inbreeding).

When fetal death occurs in the third trimester, it may trigger early whelping or spontaneous abortion of the entire litter. Within 24 to 48 hr, the organs of a dead fetus appear hypoechoic and less defined due to autolysis (Fig. 11). There is rapid resorption of fetal fluid and the body of the dead fetus decreases in size. After several days, only skeletal structures may be recognized (Fig. 11).

Ultrasonographic evaluation of fetal viability is valuable for planning the timing of a cesarean section when there are complications around the time of parturition. (see "The Elective Cesarean Section," this volume, p 1085). If the fetal heart rate is less than 150 bpm and stimulation of the fetus (gently ballot it with the transducer) fails to elevate the heart rate, there is fetal distress and reason to consider performing a cesarean section without delay. Radiography is more accurate than ultrasonography to determine whether or not the fetus is full term and to compare fetal size to the size of the maternal pelvis.

Although ultrasonography is an excellent method for evaluating fetal malformation, ultrasonographic detection of fetal malformation is rare in the dog and cat. The veterinary literature includes one case of hydrops fetalis in a dog. In contrast, the human literature abounds with descriptions of a variety of malformations. Detection of dog and cat fetal malformations may be infrequent because many pregnancy examinations occur too early in gestation for optimal visualization of fetal malformation, and evaluation of individual fetuses may be brief when there are multiple fetuses in the litter.

## Uterine Involution

Immediately postpartum, uterine structure appears distorted because it is markedly hypertrophied, flaccid, and the lumen contains multifocal accumulations of fluid, clotted blood, and necrotic debris. After several days, the structure of the uterus becomes recognizable (Fig. 12). The endometrium appears as a thick hyperechoic inner layer. Placental sites appear as focal hypoechoic enlargements in the endometrial layer. Three layers are initially detected in the myometrium (the circular and longitudinal muscle layers and a vascular layer in between them). Small foci of fluid may persist in the lumen for as long as 11 weeks postpartum. Overall uterine size rapidly decreases during the first week after parturition. At 1 week postpartum, the placental sites are generally no larger than 2 to 3 cm in diameter. Those located caudally in the uterus tend to be smaller than those located cranially. By 5 to 6 weeks postpartum, placental sites are minimally larger than the rest of the uterine horn, which is 1 cm or less in diameter. Ultrasonography may be useful for the detection of retained placenta, subinvolution of placental sites, and postpartum metritis; however, studies of such evaluations have not been published.

## Lesions of the Uterus

In cases of pyometra, the uterus appears as a tubular viscus with fluid in the lumen (Fig. 13). Uterine shape varies from straight to convoluted and the fluid is either anechoic or echogenic. Ultrasonographic diagnosis of mucometra or pyometra is very accurate because it is

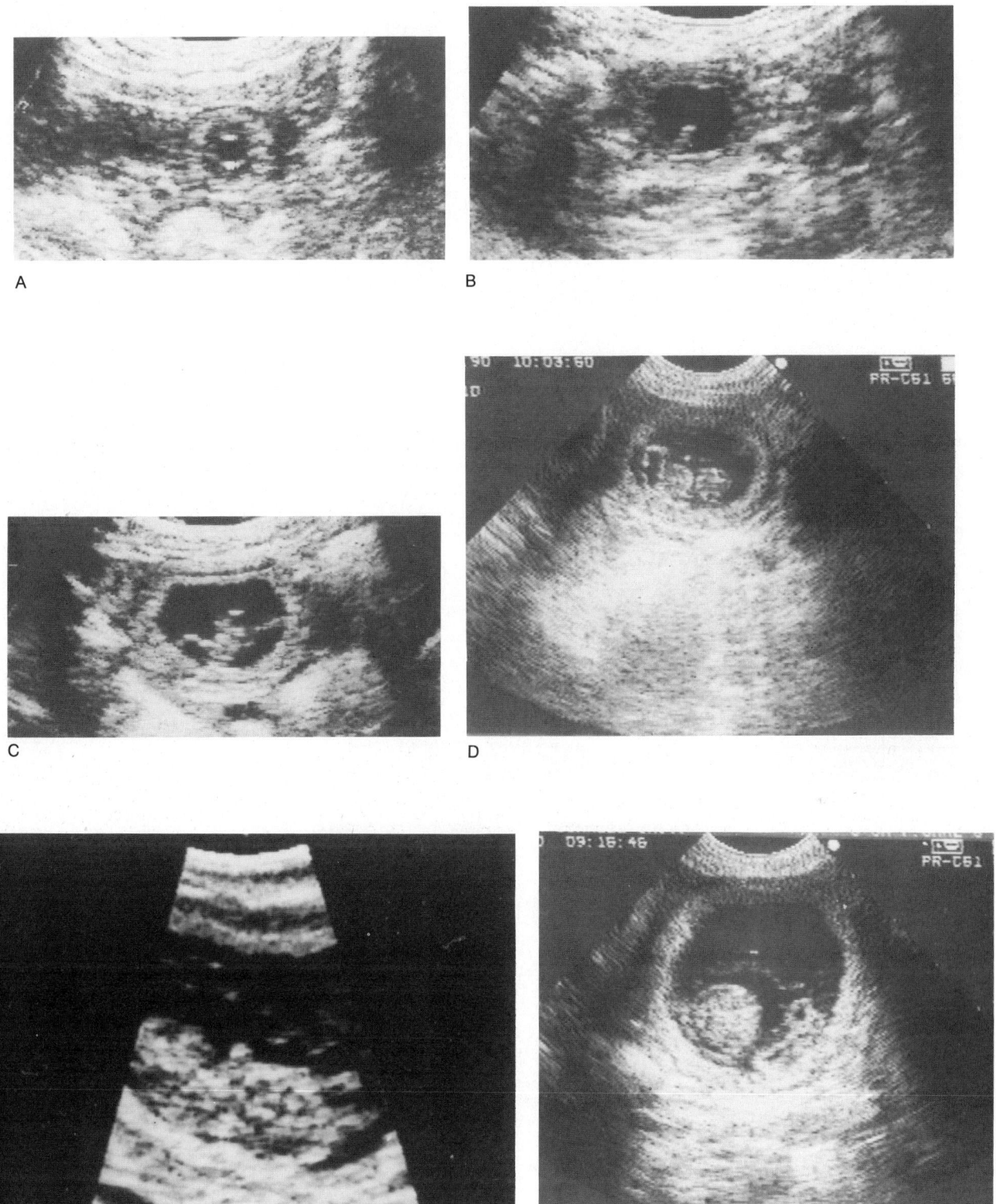

**Figure 7.** Ultrasonograms of beagle pregnancy at known times after the luteinizing hormone peak. *A*, 21 days. Uterus with focal swelling at the location of a 4-mm-diameter gestational sac. *B*, 25 days. The gestational sac is 8 mm in diameter and an embryo is directly attached to the uterus. *C*, 27 days. Bipolar-shaped embryo attached to yolk sac membrane. *D*, 30 days. The 1.2-cm-length fetus has two distinct poles. In this image, it has no other distinguishing features (although there would be obvious cardiac contractions in the real-time image). The yolk sac is the oval membrane to the left of the fetus. *E*, 35 days. Limb buds are apparent in this longitudinal image of the fetus. The thorax is not yet distinct from the abdomen and the abdominal viscera are not detectable. The thin folded membrane is the allantois. *F*, 35 days. A transverse image through the fetal body shows the thin allantoic membrane encircling the fetus and a thick folded yolk sac membrane to the right of the fetus. *Illustration continued on following page*

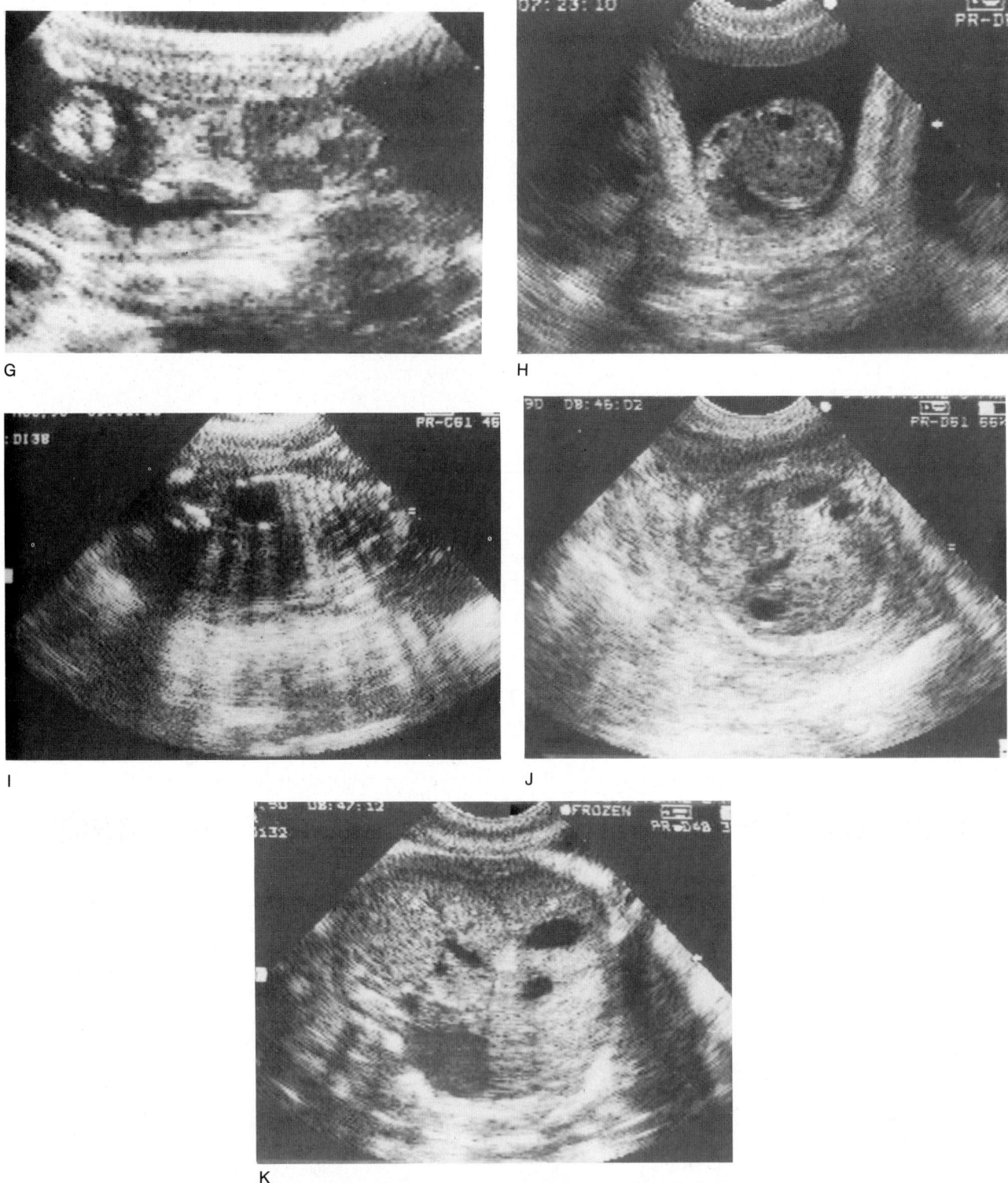

**Figure 7.** (*Continued*) *G*, 43 days. Various viscera are distinguishable in this 6.3-cm-length fetus. The hyperechoic lung surrounding the heart, hypoechoic liver, hyperechoic caudal abdomen, anechoic bladder, head with mineralized skeletal structures, and cranial limbs are apparent. The fetus is slightly longer than the zonary placenta. *H*, 43 days. The round anechoic stomach and surrounding liver are apparent in the transverse image of the 2-cm-diameter fetal body. The thick folded yolk sac membrane is to the left of the fetus. Notice that fetal diameter is less than half of the outer uterine diameter. *I*, 54 days. Lung, heart, liver, stomach, and ribs casting obvious acoustic shadows are apparent in this longitudinal image of a fetus. *J*, 54 days. The 3.5-cm body diameter of this fetus is obviously greater than half the outer diameter of the uterus. The anechoic structures are the aorta, stomach, a large vein in liver, and gallbladder. *K*, 61 days. This is a transverse image of the fetal body made at the liver. Except for larger diameter (5 cm), it has the same appearance and the same anechoic structures as the image of the 54-day fetus (Fig. 7*J*). In the final 2 weeks of pregnancy, there is very little change in the anatomic appearance of the fetus.

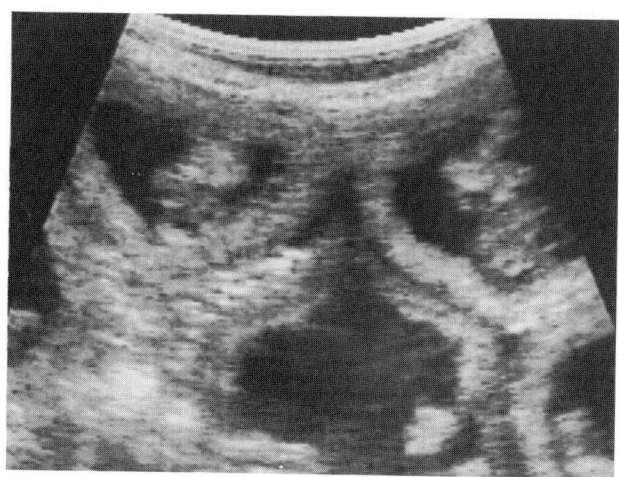

**Figure 8.** Ultrasonogram showing portions of five confluent gestational sacs. This border terrier pregnancy is 40 days after the estimated luteinizing hormone peak and 33 days after the last breeding. Once the gestational sacs are confluent, counting fetuses becomes increasingly difficult as the pregnancy progresses to term.

easy to detect small accumulations (≥5 mm) of fluid, and there should be no confusion between uterine enlargement caused by pregnancy and pyometra. Although the clinical signs of a bitch with pyometra are usually quite different from those of a dog with a primary gastrointestinal disorder, it may be necessary to distinguish pyometra from fluid-filled segments of small intestine. The uterus can be identified by absence of peristalsis and its characteristic location in the caudal abdomen.

Ultrasonographic diagnosis of metritis and endometrial hyperplasia is not very accurate because the changes caused by these conditions are often subtle and inconsistent. Either of these conditions may enlarge uterine diameter (usually by only several millimeters) and in some cases the uterus may have "blotchy" echogenicity, multiple 1- to 5-mm cysts, or a central echogenic layer (Fig. 14). This layer could represent thickened endometrium or a small accumulation of bloody discharge, exudate, mucus, or necrotic debris. It is not uncommon to detect a few endometrial cysts

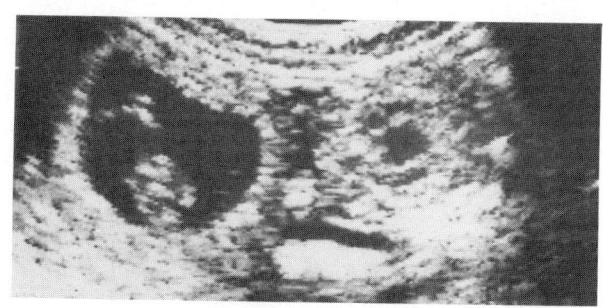

A

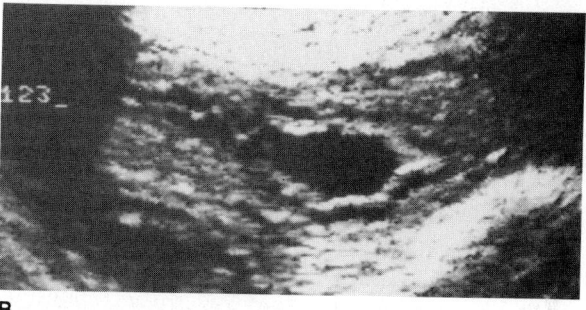

B

**Figure 9.** Ultrasonograms of beagle embryo resorption. *A,* Two gestational sacs imaged at 30 days after the luteinizing hormone peak show an obvious discrepancy in diameter. The larger sac contains a live, 7-mm-diameter embryo. The smaller sac does not contain an embryo. *B,* This image of a gestational sac made in the longitudinal plane at 28 days after the luteinizing hormone peak is smaller (6 mm diameter) than expected, contains no embryo, and has an irregular contour.

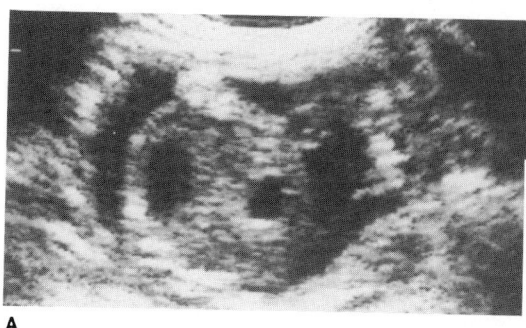

A

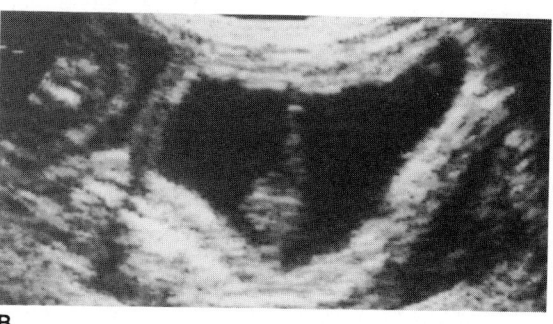

B

**Figure 10.** Ultrasonograms of a feline pregnancy made during the final trimester. *A,* This is a transverse image of a live, 2-cm-diameter fetus showing liver and stomach. *B,* This image from the same pregnancy shows a small featureless mummified embryo and associated membranes contained in a 3.2 × 1.8–cm gestational sac.

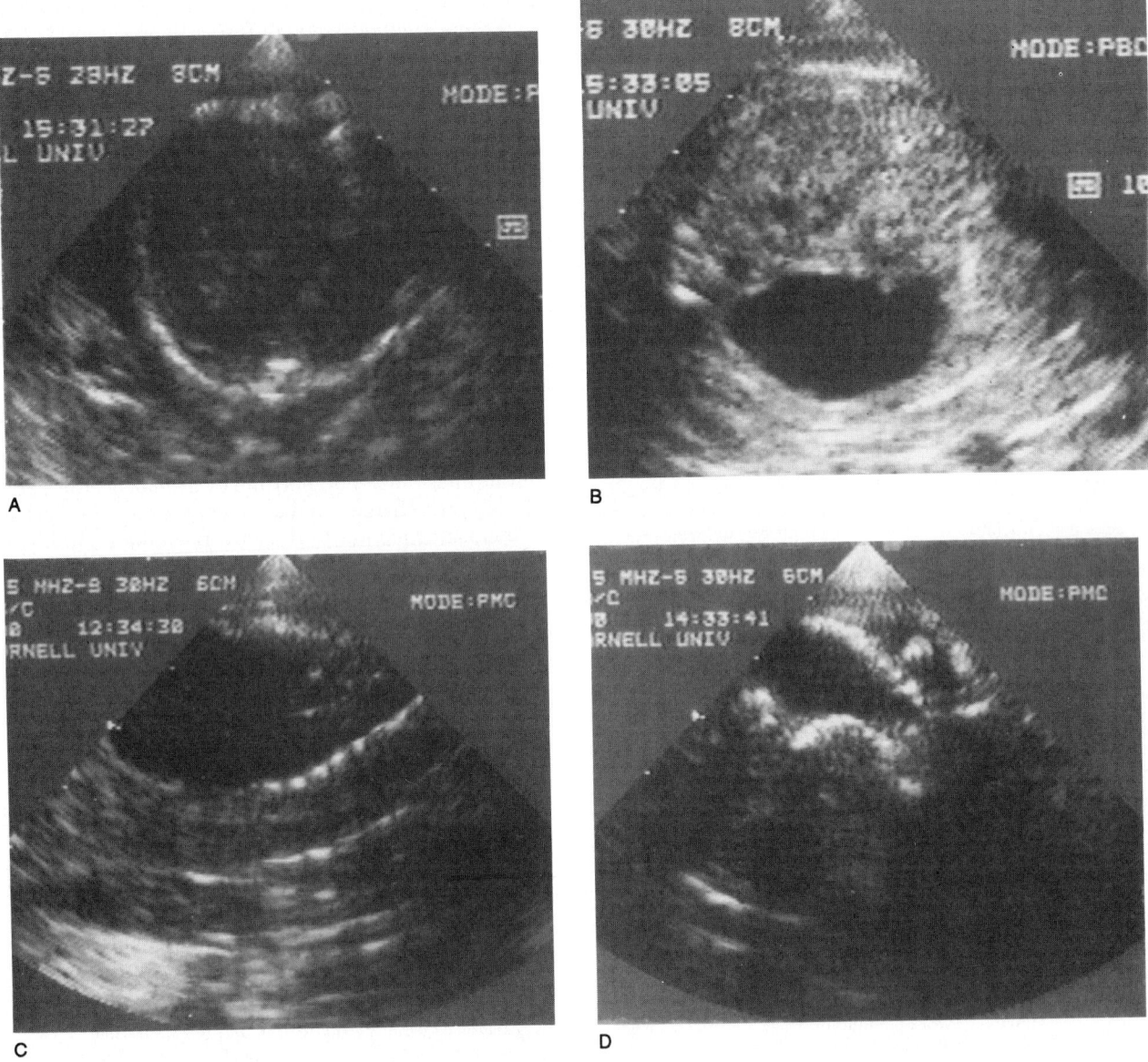

**Figure 11.** Ultrasonograms demonstrating fetal autolysis. *A*, This is a transverse image through the body of fetus that has been dead for 1 day. Its body is the same size (4.8 cm diameter) but obviously more hypoechoic than (*B*) a live fetus from the same pregnancy (61 days after the luteinizing hormone peak). *C*, This longitudinal image of a fetus that has been dead for 1 day shows markedly hypoechoic soft tissues. It is difficult to distinguish the viscera. The hyperechoic ribs, however, are obvious. Gestation length is 59 days after the luteinizing hormone peak. *D*, A longitudinal image of the same dead fetus made 4 days later shows that the fetus has decreased in size and has a flexed position, and that the ribs are still detectable.

in fertile bitches. Typically, infertile bitches with histologically proven cystic endometrial hyperplasia have numerous cysts and the majority of these are less than 1 mm in diameter and therefore not readily detectable by ultrasonography. During diestrus, some bitches with presumptive endometrial hyperplasia may accumulate small amounts of anechoic or hypoechoic fluid (≥1 cm diameter) in the lumen of the uterus. This has not been observed in the gravid uterus, and may be associated with or cause infertility.

Mass lesions of the uterus are readily detected by ultrasonography. A uterine stump hematoma or abscess characteristically appears as a unilocular or multilocular fluid cavity surrounded by a wall. The fluid is either anechoic or echogenic and may contain strands of fibrin or focal irregular accumulations of necrotic debris. Granulomas are more apt to be solid masses. Scar tissue and necrotic fat are usually hyperechoic and poorly marginated in appearance (Fig. 15). Uterine polyps can appear as multicystic uterine masses (Fig. 16). Uterine neoplasms are rare in the bitch and queen and their ultrasonographic appearance is not well described. Depending on the composition of the neoplasm, the ul-

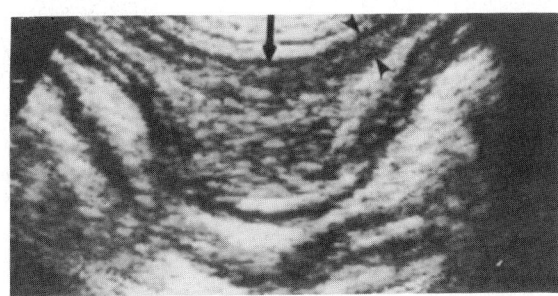

**Figure 12.** A longitudinal ultrasonogram of beagle uterus made 1 week postpartum. Note the 1.5-cm-thick focal hypoechoic placental site (*arrow*), hyperechoic endometrium cranial and caudal to the placental site, and the myometrium (*arrowheads*) that is composed of three layers.

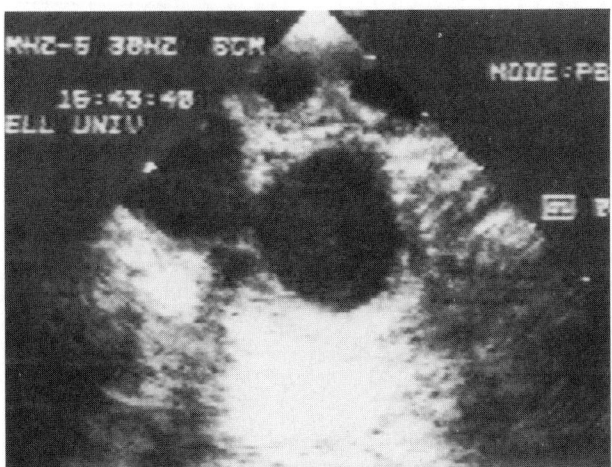

**Figure 13.** Ultrasonogram of canine uterus demonstrating pyometra. The uterus is enlarged (ranging up to 2.5 cm thick) because the lumen is distended with anechoic fluid.

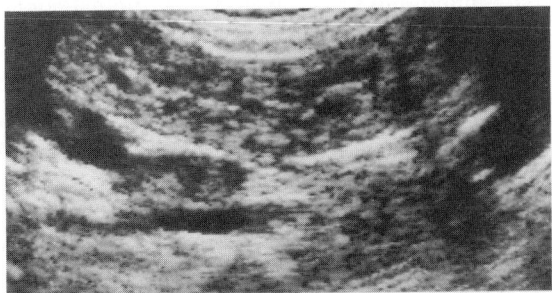

**Figure 14.** An ultrasonogram made in the longitudinal plane of a uterine horn of an aged diestrus Brittany spaniel with vaginal discharge. The uterine horn is mildly thickened (1.3 cm diameter) and has abnormal echogenicity including multiple 1-mm or smaller cysts and a fragmented central linear echo. The histologic diagnosis was extensive cystic endometrial hyperplasia and septic endometritis.

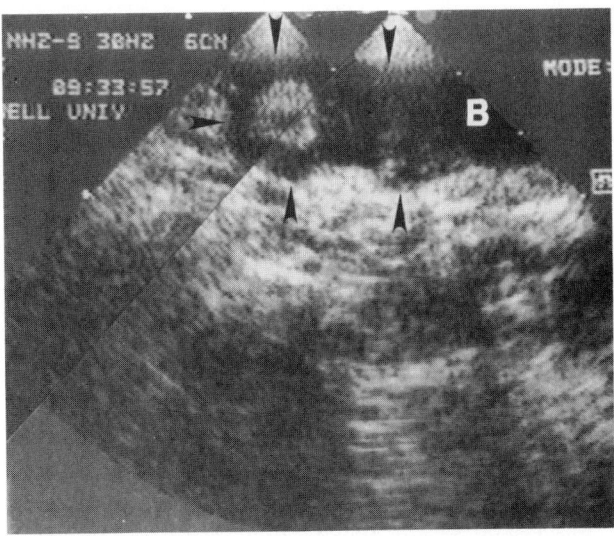

**Figure 15.** Combined ultrasonograms made in the transverse plane at the bladder neck of a recently ovariohysterectomized Shih Tzu with a palpable caudal abdominal mass. The mass (*arrowheads*) appears to have a hyperechoic lumen and is surrounded by hyperechoic tissue. It is adhered to the bladder serosa but does not extend into the bladder lumen (B). Grossly and histologically, the mass was a uterine stump granuloma that was surrounded by scar tissue and adhered to the bladder trigone.

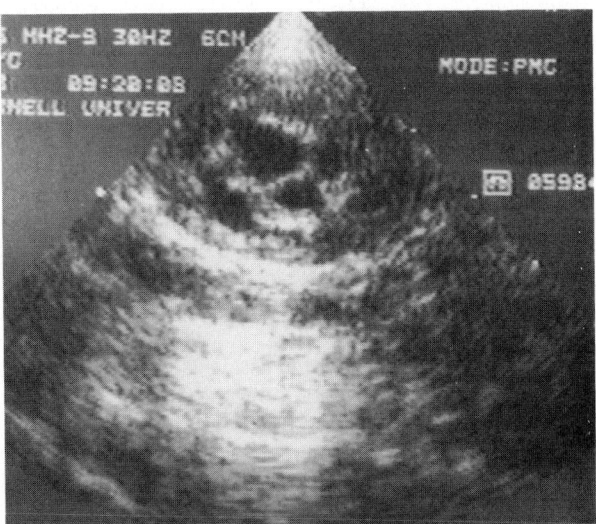

**Figure 16.** Ultrasonogram of the uterine horn of an 8-year-old beagle showing a 2.5-cm multicystic mass in the lumen of the uterus. Acoustic enhancement artifact is present deep to the mass. Gross and histologic diagnosis was uterine polyp composed of cystic endometrium.

trasonographic appearance may be uniform or complex as is the case with neoplasms of other organs.

## References and Suggested Reading

Beck KA, Baldwin CJ, and Bosu WT: Ultrasound prediction of parturition in queens. Vet Radial 31:32, 1990.

*Results of serial ultrasound examination of eight pregnancies in five queens deriving growth curves for head and body diameters relative to the day of parturition.*

Davidson AP, Nyland TG, and Tsutsui T: Pregnancy diagnosis with ultrasound in the domestic cat. Vet Radiol 27:109, 1986.
*Results of serial ultrasound examination describing the anatomic appearance of pregnancy in seven cats from day 1 to day 30 after breeding.*

England GCW, Allen WE, and Porter DJ: Studies on canine pregnancy using B-mode ultrasound: Development of the conceptus and determination of gestational age. J Small Anim Pract 31:324, 1990.
*Results of serial examination of pregnant retriever dogs describing the anatomic appearance of pregnancy and predicting whelping date based on head and body diameter.*

England GCW and Yeager AE: Ultrasonographic appearance of the ovary and uterus of the bitch during oestrus, ovulation and pregnancy. J Reprod Fertil 47:107, 1993.
*Results of serial ultrasound examination of the ovaries and uterus of ten pregnant bitches from 10 days before the preovulatory luteinizing hormone surge to 30 days after this surge.*

Rivers B and Johnston GR: Diagnostic imaging of the reproductive organs of the bitch. Vet Clin North Am [Small Anim Pract] 21:437, 1991.
*A review of radiography and ultrasonography of dog ovary, uterus (gravid and nongravid), and vagina with discussion of the normal appearance and the appearance of lesions of these structures.*

Spaulding K: Ultrasound evaluation of the gravid uterus in the bitch. *Syllabus 2nd Annual Am Institute Ultrasound Med*, 1990, p 67.
*A review of ultrasonographic appearance of dog pregnancy relative to gestation length based on the onset of diestrus.*

Wallace SS, Mahaffey MB, Miller DM, et al: Ultrasonographic appearance of the ovaries of dogs during follicular and luteal phases of the estrous cycle. Am J Vet Res 53:209, 1992.
*Results of serial ultrasound examination of ovaries of ten bitches from proestrus through diestrus describing the appearance of follicles, corpora lutea, and ovulation.*

Yeager AE, Mohammed HO, Meyers-Wallen V, et al: Ultrasonographic appearance of the uterus, placenta, fetus, and fetal membranes throughout accurately timed pregnancy in beagles. Am J Vet Res 53:342, 1992.
*Results of serial ultrasound examination of pregnant beagles describing the anatomic appearance and deriving growth curves for gestational sac diameter, head diameter, body diameter, and crown-rump diameter relative to the day of the preovulatory luteinizing hormone peak.*

Yeager AE and Concannon PW: Serial ultrasonographic appearance of postpartum uterine involution in beagle dogs. Theriogenology 34:523, 1990.
*Results of serial ultrasound examination of involuting beagle uterus describing the appearance and size of the uterus from the day of parturition to the beginning of anestrus.*

# IMAGING THE REPRODUCTIVE TRACT IN THE MALE DOG

RALPH C. WEICHSELBAUM,
GARY R. JOHNSTON,
DANIEL A. FEENEY,
*and* PATRICIA A. WALTER

St. Paul, Minnesota

The reproductive tract of the male dog includes the testicles, spermatic cord (epididymis, arteries, and veins), prostate gland, and urethra. Evaluation of the reproductive tract begins with a thorough physical examination and observation of the dog's behavior. Other procedures such as hormonal assays, semen evaluation, and prostatic massage for culture and cytology are often indicated. Further valuable information can also be obtained from survey abdominal radiography, positive contrast urethrocystography, and ultrasonography. This article will summarize the strengths and weaknesses of survey and contrast radiography and ultrasonography and describe some observable variations of normal and abnormal radiographic and sonographic anatomy.

## SURVEY RADIOGRAPHY

Survey radiography should precede ultrasonography, but should follow the initial physical examination when evaluating the reproductive tract of the male dog. Survey radiography is valuable for determining the location, shape, size, and radiographic density of the prostate gland relative to other caudal abdominal organs.

The location of the prostate gland varies. Factors that may influence the position of the prostate gland are bladder distention, age, other contiguous organs, intrapelvic diseases, or prostatomegaly. When the urinary bladder is fully distended, the prostate gland may take on a partially or totally intra-abdominal location, cranioventral to the pubis as viewed on lateral radiographs. The cranioventral margin of the prostate gland may be identified by a triangular fat pad that is bordered by the ventral abdominal wall and the urinary bladder. The dorsal border of the prostate gland may not be defined due to masking by the luminal contents of the descending colon. With the urinary bladder empty, the prostate gland may assume a partially or totally intrapelvic location.

The age of the dog may affect the position of the prostate gland. In the fetus, the prostate gland is pulled cranioventrally due to the presence of the urachus, which holds the urinary bladder and associated structures in an intra-abdominal location. With atrophy of the urachus in the young dog, the bladder and the prostate gland assume a more intrapelvic position. With sexual maturity, the prostate gland may move, once again, to a partially or totally intra-abdominal location, depending on the degree of urinary bladder distention. Castration and subsequent atrophy of the prostate gland may allow reversion to a pelvic location (Lattimer, 1994).

Intrapelvic or caudal abdominal diseases not directly involving the prostate gland may alter its normal position. Perineal hernias, abdominal hernias, colonic impaction, iliac lymphadenopathies, or urinary bladder masses may change the expected location of the prostate gland. In addition, prostatic diseases such as benign hypertrophy, paraprostatic cysts, and neoplasia may alter its normal location.

On radiographs, the density of the prostate gland is that of soft tissue. The normal prostate gland should not contain opacities or gas. Presence of mineralization within the prostate gland mandates the need for further evaluation (Fig. 1A). The presence of gas within the prostate gland may be iatrogenic from prior urinary bladder catheterization or indicative of an abscess.

Survey radiography is usually the best means of measuring prostatic size. Normal measurements have been debated. We define the normal prostate gland as

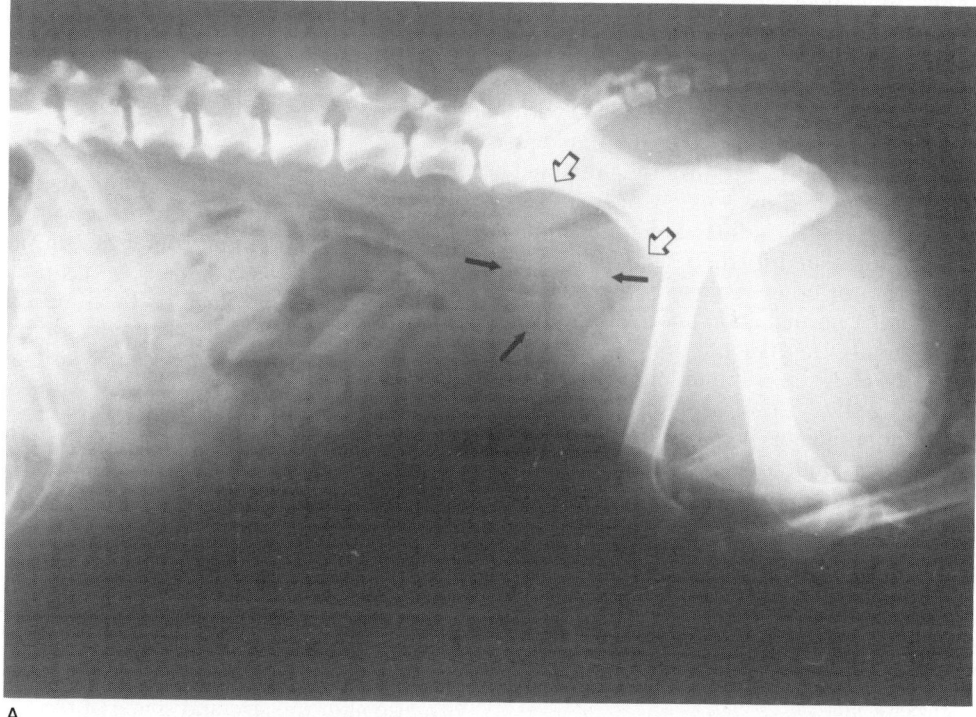

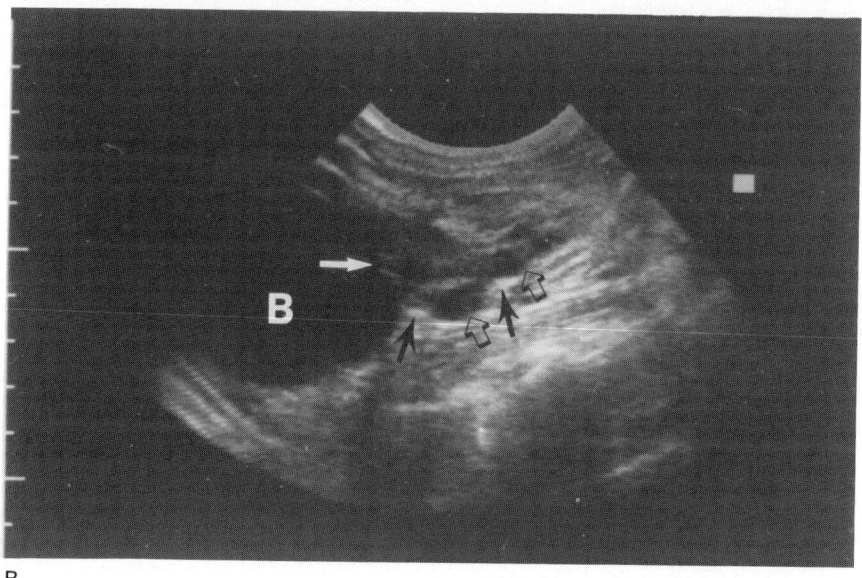

**Figure 1.** *A,* Lateral survey abdominal radiograph. Note the distance from the sacral promontory to the pubis (*open arrows*) relative to the size of the prostate gland (*solid arrows*). Also note the subtle diffuse mineralization of the prostatic parenchyma. *B,* Ultrasonogram of the same dog. Note the relationship of the prostate gland to the urinary bladder (B). The prostate gland has a mixed echogenicity with hyperechoic (*solid arrows*) and hypoechoic regions (*open arrows*). Note the streaking acoustic shadowing in areas of mineralization seen on Figure 1A. Also note the extension of a mass into the urinary bladder (*white arrow*). (Dx = prostatic adenocarcinoma.)

being less than or equal to 70% of the distance from the sacral promontory to the pubis as viewed on the lateral radiograph (Fig. 1A). Normal size alone does not rule out the presence of prostatic disease. The physical examination and laboratory, clinical, and radiographic findings must all be considered. A measurement of greater than 70% of this distance is defined as prostatomegaly, but is of unknown etiology. To further define the structural changes associated with prostatomegaly (e.g., hypertrophy, inflammation, neoplasia), contrast urethrocystography, ultrasonography, and biopsies are needed.

Radiographs can define the spread of disease by identifying contiguous tissues that may be involved with the prostate gland. Care should be taken to rule out the presence of urocystoliths, urethroliths, regional lymph node enlargement, and osseous changes in the lumbar vertebrae or pelvis. These may help determine if the clinical signs are related to the urinary bladder, urethra, prostate gland, or other regional involvement. A listing of radiographic normal and abnormal findings and possible differentials are presented in Table 1.

Survey radiography does have limitations. Differentiating among hypertrophy, abscessation, cystic disease, or neoplasia is frequently not possible. Radiographs may not demonstrate asymmetric conditions found on physical examination. Radiographs cannot demonstrate

**Table 1.** *Canine Prostate: Normal and Abnormal Survey Radiographic Findings*

**Location**
　Abdominal or intrapelvic prostate
　　Cranial displacement of urinary bladder = prostatomegaly
　　Dorsal displacement of colon = prostatomegaly

*Size*
　≤70% of the sacral promontory to pubis distance = normal or abnormal
　>70% of the sacral promontory to pubis distance = prostatomegaly
　　Hypertrophy
　　Inflammation
　　Abscesses
　　Tumor

**Radiodensity**
　Soft tissue = urinary bladder = normal
　Mineralization = abnormal
　　Uroliths
　　Dystrophic
　　　Neoplasia
　　　Chronic inflammation
　　Paraprostatic cysts = "egg shell"
　Gas = abnormal
　　Artifact due to catheterization
　　Abscess = *Escherichia coli*?

**Contour**
　Smooth = normal or diffuse disease such as hypertrophy or prostatitis
　Irregular = abnormal
　　Focal enlargement (asymmetric)
　　　Cysts
　　　Abscesses
　　　Neoplasia

the urethra or intraprostatic cavitations and may not provide a prostatic silhouette in cases of patient emaciation or ascites.

## CONTRAST URETHROCYSTOGRAPHY

Contrast urethrocystography should follow survey radiography in the evaluation of the prostate gland. This procedure allows assessment of the prostate gland and its relationship to adjacent structures. Additionally, it can define urethral morphology and help localize concurrent diseases in the lower urinary tract.

The dog's urethra is divided into prostatic, membranous, and penile regions. The prostatic urethra is spindle shaped, with its widest dimension in the midprostatic region. The normal prostatic urethra has smooth borders and is wider than the membranous or penile regions (Pechman, 1994). Narrowing of the prostatic urethral lumen indicates disease. A narrowed prostatic urethral lumen and smooth prostatic urethral mucosa may be seen with benign prostatic hypertrophy or an intraprostatic mass that compresses but does not invade the urethra. A narrowed prostatic urethral lumen with an undulant urethral mucosa is more often indicative of infection, bacterial prostatitis, or possible neoplasia. A jagged or irregular prostatic urethral mucosa usually indicates neoplasia.

Mucosal changes in the prostatic urethra can be caused by mural disease or by parenchymal disease of the prostate gland. Mucosal irregularity is frequently encountered with mural disease such as transitional cell carcinoma and may be associated with diminished distensibility. Benign prostatic hypertrophy, abscessation, prostatic cysts, paraprostatic cysts, or prostatic neoplasia can also alter the size and shape of the prostatic urethra. By demonstrating urethroprostatic reflux, prostatic urethrocystography can illustrate that cystic lesions or abscesses communicate with the prostatic urethra.

Urethroprostatic reflux gives an assessment of the distribution of lesions in the prostate gland (Fig. 2A). Some degree of urethroprostatic reflux seen as thin, finger-like projections into the prostatic parenchyma is normal. Urethroprostatic reflux is usually less than or equal to the diameter of the midprostatic urethra. Urethroprostatic reflux greater than the diameter of the prostatic urethra with coalescent accumulations is a nonspecific indicator of prostate disease. The amount and character of the urethroprostatic reflux may aid in differentiating diseases of the prostate gland. Reflux that is greater than the diameter of the prostatic urethra, but uniform in distribution, is seen often with abscessation or nonbacterial prostatitis. Large accumulations of refluxed contrast media with an irregular distribution within the prostate gland usually result from neoplastic disease.

## TECHNIQUES OF CONTRAST URETHROCYSTOGRAPHY

Like survey radiography, contrast urethrocystography has limitations. Contrast urethrocystography cannot

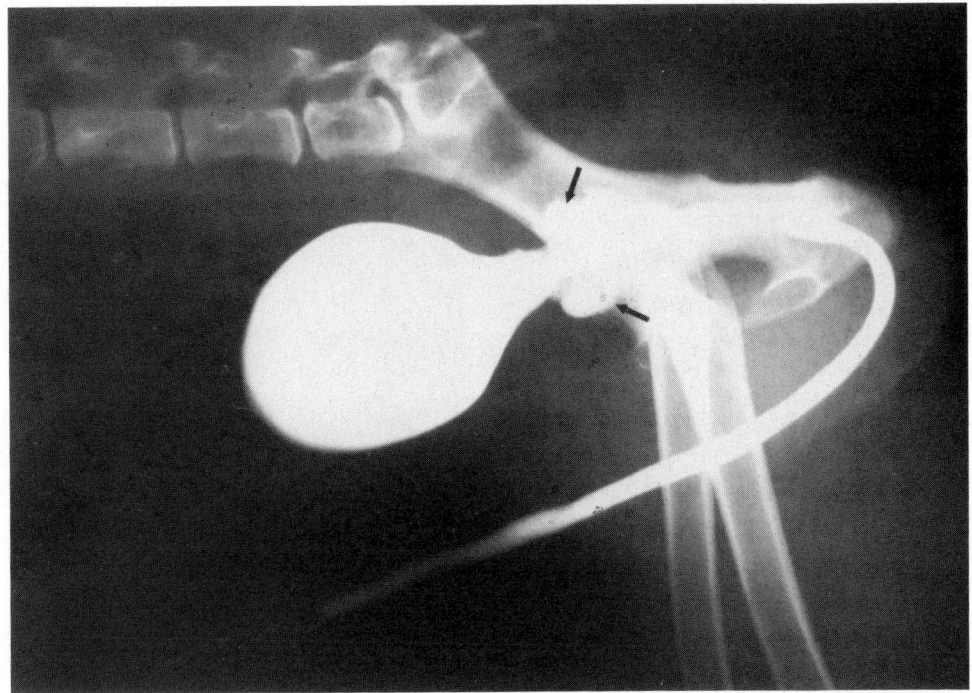

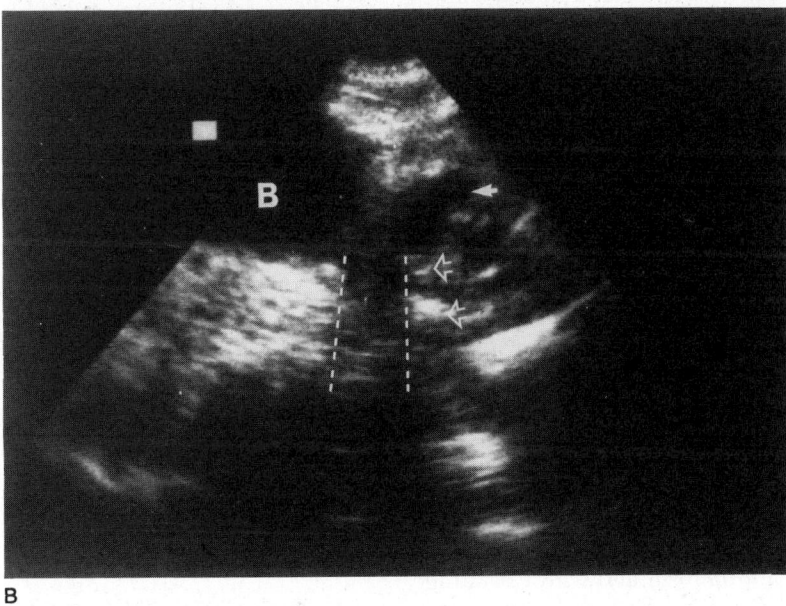

**Figure 2.** *A*, Lateral radiograph of a positive contrast urethrocystogram. Note the distention of the urinary bladder and urethra as well as the marked reflux of contrast media into the parenchyma of the prostate gland (*solid arrows*). This indicates that the cavitations communicate with the prostatic urethra. Communicating cavitations are nonspecific indicators and may be found in infectious and noninfectious conditions. *B*, Ultrasonogram of the same patient. Note the hypoechoic area (*solid arrow*) and far enhancement (*open arrows*) indicating that this is a fluid-filled (versus solid mass) lesion. Additionally, there is some shadowing (*dashed lines*) that indicates mineralization, probably due to chronic inflammatory changes. (Dx = prostatic alveolar adenocarcinoma.)

rule out diseases of the prostate gland that do not affect the urethral lumen by direct communication, luminal compression, or asymmetric parenchymal distribution around the prostatic urethra. Contrast urethrocystography may require sedation of the dog. Because aqueous iodinated contrast agents used for contrast urethrocystography are bacteriostatic, samples for urinalysis and culture should be taken prior to the procedure. Maximum distention techniques require filling the urinary bladder with diluted contrast media until it is turgid by palpation (Feeney et al., 1987). Caution must be used so as not to rupture the urinary bladder. In our experience, this is rare. Since the technique requires maximum distention of the bladder, a transient macroscopic hematuria may occur, but should resolve within 72 hr. Vesicoureteral reflux may occur secondary to maximum bladder distention and can potentially result in an ascending urinary tract infection. In our experience, iatrogenic urinary tract infections secondary to contrast urethrocystography are rare.

## PROSTATIC ULTRASOUND

Although prostatic ultrasound will not provide information regarding the function of the prostate, it complements contrast urethrocystography by providing valuable morphologic information that is especially helpful in determining the size, shape, and internal architecture of the prostate gland. There have been no proven safety concerns with ultrasound. Ultrasound does not require the use of ionizing radiation, avoids the use of contrast agents and, unless the animal is particularly uncooperative or unless biopsies are needed, sedation is usually not required.

Ultrasound is helpful in staging prostatic disease. Regional lymph node involvement may be detected earlier in the course of disease by ultrasound than by radiography. Ultrasound is also helpful in defining contiguous masses associated with the prostate gland to determine if surgical removal of the mass is feasible.

Prostatic ultrasonographic findings have been described in the human and veterinary literature (Feeney et al., 1989). We have separated prostatic disease into classes based on overall echotexture. The normal prostatic echotexture has been described as being uniformly coarse, inhomogeneous echogenicity. The normal prostate gland is symmetric, smooth, and may contain an area in the cranial midsagittal region of the gland referred to as a hilar echo that represents the wall of the prostatic urethra. This area is often slightly hyperechoic in relation to the rest of the prostatic parenchyma, but its presence in the normal dog is quite variable.

The echogenicity of prostatic disease can be further classified into two divisions based on intraparenchymal cavitations. The first category describes a relatively uniform prostatic echotexture, but with cavitations less than 1.5 cm in diameter. The second category describes an echotexture that is not uniform and with cavitating lesions greater than 1.5 cm in diameter (Finn and Wrigley, 1989). These two main divisions of prostatic disease can be subdivided into six areas based on etiology, and include: noncavitating bacterial prostatic disease, noncavitating nonbacterial prostatic disease (Fig. 3), cavitating bacterial prostatic disease, cavitating nonbacterial prostatic disease, neoplastic disease, and paraprostatic disease (Johnston et al., 1989). The ultrasonographic findings, differential diagnoses, and further diagnostic recommendations are shown in Figure 4.

Intraparenchymal architectural changes are best identified with ultrasound. In particular, ultrasound allows discrimination between solid masses and fluid-filled cavitations by the far enhancement characteristic of the latter (Fig. 2B). Mineralization and gas within

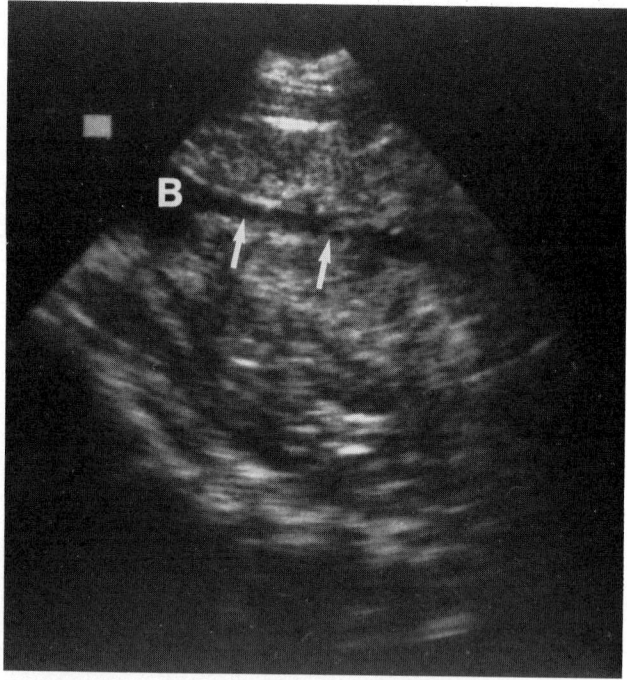

**Figure 3.** Midsagittal prostatic ultrasound. The prostatic urethra (*white arrows*) and urinary bladder (B) are identified. The prostate gland has a coarsely homogeneous echotexture. This represents the category of noncavitating bacterial or noncavitating nonbacterial prostatic disease. (Dx = prostatic hyperplasia.)

the prostate gland cause acoustic shadowing, which is characterized sonographically by the absence of ultrasound transmission deep to the gas or mineralized area (Figs. 1B and 2B). Differentiation of cavitating versus solid noncavitating intraprostatic lesions and mineralization or gas are important factors in reaching a differential diagnosis and in determining the type of biopsy needed. For example, with a far enhancing fluid-filled lesion, abscessation would be a primary differential diagnosis and would necessitate fine-needle aspiration of the lesion to minimize the possibility of contamination of the peritoneal cavity. On the other hand, nonenhancing solid mass lesions are more likely candidates for core biopsy.

## TECHNIQUE OF ULTRASOUND-GUIDED PROSTATIC BIOPSY

Preparation for ultrasound-guided prostatic biopsy begins with clipping hair of the caudoventral abdomen and a surgical scrub of the biopsy site. The transducer head also needs to be cleaned and disinfected. The sterile biopsy guide should be attached to the transducer. Finally, a mild sedative-analgesic is recommended to avoid discomfort to the animal and to obtain the biopsy sample with minimal trauma to the prostate and surrounding structures.

Begin the biopsy process by applying sterile surgical lubricant over the biopsy site. Locate the area(s) within the prostate gland to be biopsied and align the biopsy

## Prostatic Ultrasonography

Prostatic Ultrasonography → Uniform | Not uniform

### Uniform

**Noncavitating non-bacterial disease**

U/S Findings
- hyperechoic
- +/- hilar echo
- smooth reg. margins, shape, and size

Differential Dx.
- BPH
- bact. prostatitis

Further Dx. Tests
- fine needle aspirate
- ejaculate

**Noncavitating bacterial disease**

U/S Findings
- hyperechoic
- +/- hilar echo
- usually symmetr. intact capsule
- inc. size early
- dec. size later
- shadowing (mineral or gas)

Differential Dx.
- acute prostatitis
- chronic prostatitis
- BPH

Further Dx. Tests
- fine needle aspirate
- ejaculate

**Cavitating non-bacterial disease ( > 1.5 cm lesions)**

U/S Findings
- hyperechoic
- +/- hilar echo
- cavitations w/ irr. margins

Differential Dx.
- non-bact. prostatitis
- cystic hyperplasia
- hematocysts
- hematomas
- sterile abscesses

Further Dx. Tests
- * fine needle aspirate
- ejaculate

### Not uniform

**Cavitating bacterial disease ( > 1.5 cm lesions)**

U/S Findings
- hyperechoic
- +/- hilar echo
- smooth or irr. capsule
- asymmetrical peripheral lesions
- hypoechoic w/ far enhancement

Differential Dx.
- cysts
- abscesses
- focal edema
- hematomas

Further Dx. Tests
- * fine needle aspirate
- ejaculate

**Neoplastic Disease**

U/S Findings
- hypertrophy
- irr. margins
- shadowing (mineral)
- coalescing lesions
- mixed echogenicity
- uneven distribution
- rare caviations

Differential Dx.
- carcinoma
- transitional cell carcinoma

Further Dx. Tests
- fine needle aspirate
- core biopsy

**Paraprostatic Disease**

U/S Findings
- smooth margins
- anechoic
- similar to urinary bladder
- CU reflux rare

Differential Dx.
- retention cyst
- Mullerian Duct remnant
- pyometra of utriculus masculinus

Further Dx. Tests
- fine needle aspirate

* Be aware of the risk of leakage of purulent material and possible contamination of the peritoneal cavity.

**Figure 4.** Prostatic ultrasonography.

guide lines on the screen with the site to be sampled. Pass the biopsy instrument through the transducer biopsy guide holes and through the skin. The skin may require a small incision if the biopsy instrument is of large diameter. Using the television monitor of the ultrasound unit, visualize the hyperechoic biopsy instrument over the area to be sampled. Estimate the depth that the biopsy instrument will travel and pass the instrument deeper or retract it as needed. Avoid vessels, colon, and urethra. Core biopsies should avoid cavitating lesions. Obtain the sample and withdraw the instrument immediately. Check for any evidence of hemorrhage or other complications by ultrasound examination.

## TESTICULAR RADIOGRAPHY

Survey radiography usually provides limited information regarding intrascrotal testes, since the scrotum, testes, and related structures are all soft tissue densities. Additionally, exposure of the germinal cells to ionization radiation in a breeding animal is not without risks to future fertility and should be minimized.

Survey radiographs may assist in managing testicular disease by ruling out evidence of intra-abdominal masses (testicular tumors secondary to cryptorchidism), iliac lymphadenopathies (secondary to metastasis or inflammation), and related bony changes such as discospondylitis or osteomyelitis from *Brucella canis* or other infectious agents.

## TESTICULAR ULTRASONOGRAPHY

Intrascrotal testicular ultrasound requires minimal clipping of hair and usually does not require sedation. Aqueous acoustic coupling gel should be applied to the scrotum and the transducer head. A 5.0- or 7.5-MHz transducer with a gel standoff pad or fluid offset help place the intrascrotal structures in the focal zone of the transducer for best imaging.

The normal testis has a coarsely homogeneous echotexture with a hyperechoic midsagittal area corresponding to the mediastinum testes (Fig. 5). The testicular capsule is composed of a hyperechoic peritoneum consisting of two layers that cannot be differentiated sonographically: the parietal (outside) layer and the visceral (inside) layer, which is firmly adhered to the testis and epididymis. The epididymis consists of cranial (head), middle (body), and caudal (tail) segments. The epididymis lies dorsally and somewhat laterally on the normally positioned testicle. The epididymis is a hypoechoic to anechoic convoluted tubular structure. Scanning should be done in sagittal, parasagittal, and transverse planes. The scrotum itself is divided into two cavities by an external raphe and an internal median septum.

Testicular lesions can be categorized as intratesticular and extratesticular diseases (Fig. 6). Ultrasound features can help localize the disease, but differentiation

may require semen collection, aspiration biopsy, serology, blood cultures, and other diagnostic procedures. Normal and abnormal testicular ultrasound findings and differential diagnoses are listed in Figure 7.

## References and Suggested Reading

Feeney DA, Johnston GR, Klausner JS, et al: Canine prostatic disease—comparison of radiographic appearance with morphological and microbio-

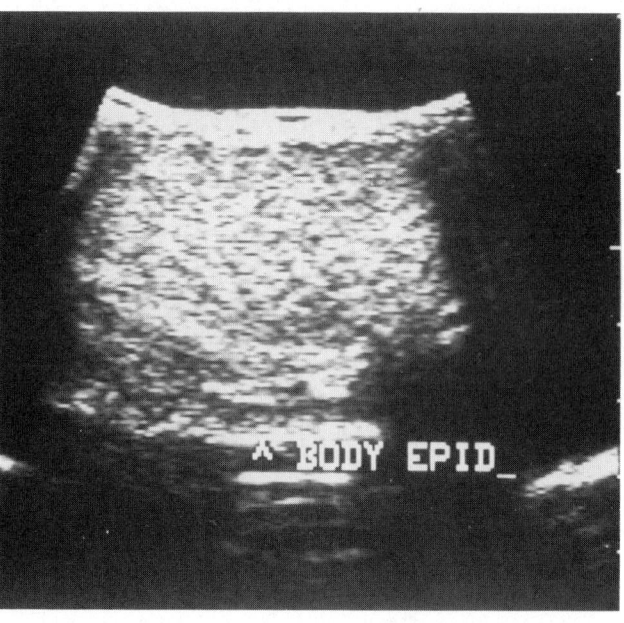

**Figure 5.** Sagittal ultrasonography of a normal testis and epididymis. The normal testis has a coarsely homogeneous echotexture. The epididymis is slightly lateral to the midsagittal plane and is hypoechoic relative to the testes. (Dx = normal testes.)

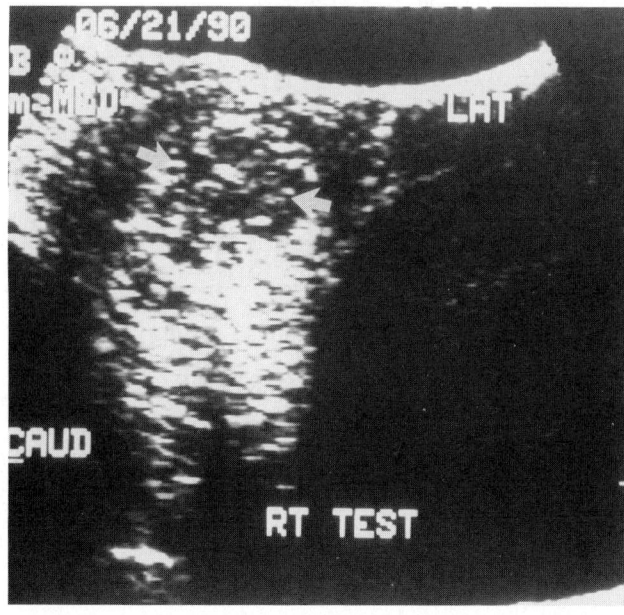

**Figure 6.** Testicular mass. The mass (*arrows*) is generally hypoechoic with a mixed echotexture relative to the more normal testicular tissue deep to it. The changes seen are consistent with orchitis secondary to epididymitis. (Dx = severe epididymitis.)

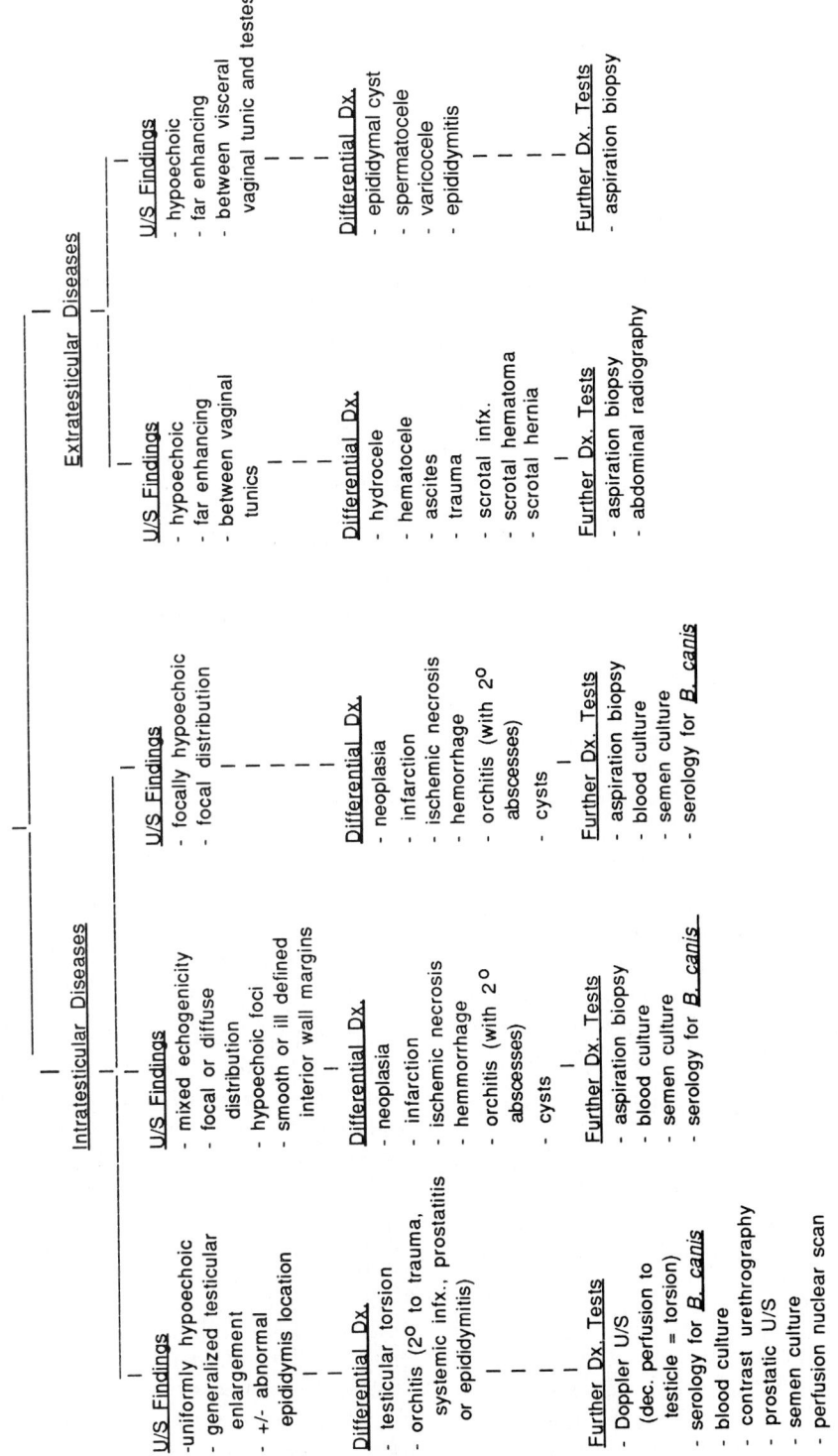

**Figure 7.** Intrascrotal testicular ultrasonography (U/S).

logical findings: 30 Cases (1981–1985). J Am Vet Med Assoc 190:1018, 1987.
  *A retrospective analysis identifying the survey and contrast radiographic appearances associated with various spontaneous prostatic diseases. Illustrated.*

Feeney DA, Johnston GR, Klausner JS, and Bell FW: Canine prostatic ultrasonography—1989. Semin Vet Med Surg [Small Anim] 4:44, 1989.
  *An illustrated summary of the ultrasonographic findings in various canine prostatic diseases.*

Finn ST and Wrigley RH: Ultrasonography and ultrasound-guided biopsy of the canine prostate. Current Veterinary Therapy X: Small Animal Practice. Philadelphia, WB Saunders Co, 1989, pp 1227–1239.
  *A discussion of the indications, scanning procedures, and normal and abnormal findings of the canine prostate as seen on ultrasound. A description of ultrasound-guided biopsy technique is also included. Illustrated.*

Johnston GR, Feeney DA, Rivers B, and Walter PA: Diagnostic imaging of the male canine reproductive organs. Vet Clin North Am [Small Anim Pract] 21:553, 1991.
  *A description of indications, techniques, and limitations of the radiographic and sonographic examination of the canine prostate and testes. Illustrated.*

Lattimer JC: The prostate. In Thrall DE (ed): Textbook of Veterinary Diagnostic Radiology. Philadelphia, WB Saunders Co, 1994, pp 479–493.
  *An illustrated discussion of the normal anatomy, various diseases, clinical signs, and radiographic changes associated with the canine prostate.*

Pechman RD, Jr: The urethra. In Thrall DE (ed): Textbook of Veterinary Diagnostic Radiology. Philadelphia, WB Saunders Co, 1994, pp 475–478.
  *An illustrated discussion of the anatomy, survey radiography, and contrast radiography of the canine urethra.*

# SPERM ABNORMALITIES AND FERTILITY IN THE DOG

E. E. OETTLÉ

*Wellington, South Africa*

The assessment of sperm morphology provides valuable information about the reproductive status of an individual. Unfortunately, it is an approach that is often neglected by practicing veterinarians. A certain amount of skill is required to ensure that high-quality preparations are consistently produced, and experience is needed for their interpretation. Two commonly available stains can be used for sperm smears. However, Diff Quik (Baxter Healthcare, McGaw Park, IL) does not stain the acrosomal area of sperm. Eosin nigrosin (Morphology stain, Society for Theriogenology, Hastings, NE), like India ink, is a background stain that merely outlines the sperm. It is not very practical. Of all the stains available for spermatozoa, Spermac stain (Oettlé, 1993) is currently the stain of choice for morphology due to its wide species applicability, speed of application, and differential qualities. The sperm nucleus stains red, and the acrosome, midpiece, and tail are stained green. The equatorial region of the acrosome stains pale green. Background staining is very faint. A semiquantitative assessment of staining of cell organelles is obtained with the stain, which makes it particularly useful for the identification of sperm defects. Spermac stain may be used on diluted (extended) semen, since constituents such as egg yolk, serum, or milk commonly included in diluents do not interfere with the staining. Unfavorable processing conditions or techniques may damage the acrosome, which is a labile organelle. Such damage is related to the integrity of the acrosome, a parameter that is in turn related to fertility (Foote, 1975). This staining technique thus provides a useful method for the assessment and monitoring of acrosome integrity (Oettlé, 1986a,b; Oettlé and Soley, 1988). This has specific application in the field of cryopreservation.

## SAMPLE PREPARATION

Evenly spread thin smears are air dried, fixed as soon as possible (within 5 min of making the smear) and stained with Spermac stain (Fertility Technologies Inc., Natick, MA). Smears are examined unmounted under oil immersion. At least 100 sperm must be evaluated per slide to ensure a representative assessment of the samples.

## NORMAL MORPHOLOGY

The classification of dog sperm abnormalities is based on Blom's classification for the bull spermiogram (1972). It provides a systematic morphologic description of the abnormality based on comparison of light and electron microscopic findings, with the defect categories being further functionally divided into major and minor defects. Major defects are more liable to influence sperm function, and they usually arise during spermatogenesis. Minor defects tend to occur after sperm are formed and may be secondary to trauma, heat, aging, and so forth. A normal dog sperm is shown in Figures 1A and 5. Under the electron microscope, the nucleus of the mature dog spermatozoon stains very deeply and appears dense and homogeneous (Fig. 5A, B). The acrosome of dog sperm is a cap-like structure covering slightly more than the anterior half of the head (Fig. 5A, B). The equatorial segment, which is thinner and thus stains paler, has the shape of an ellipse. This is most easily seen when viewed under the light microscope (Fig. 1A). The mitochondrial sheath of the midpiece in the dog is approximately 1.5 times

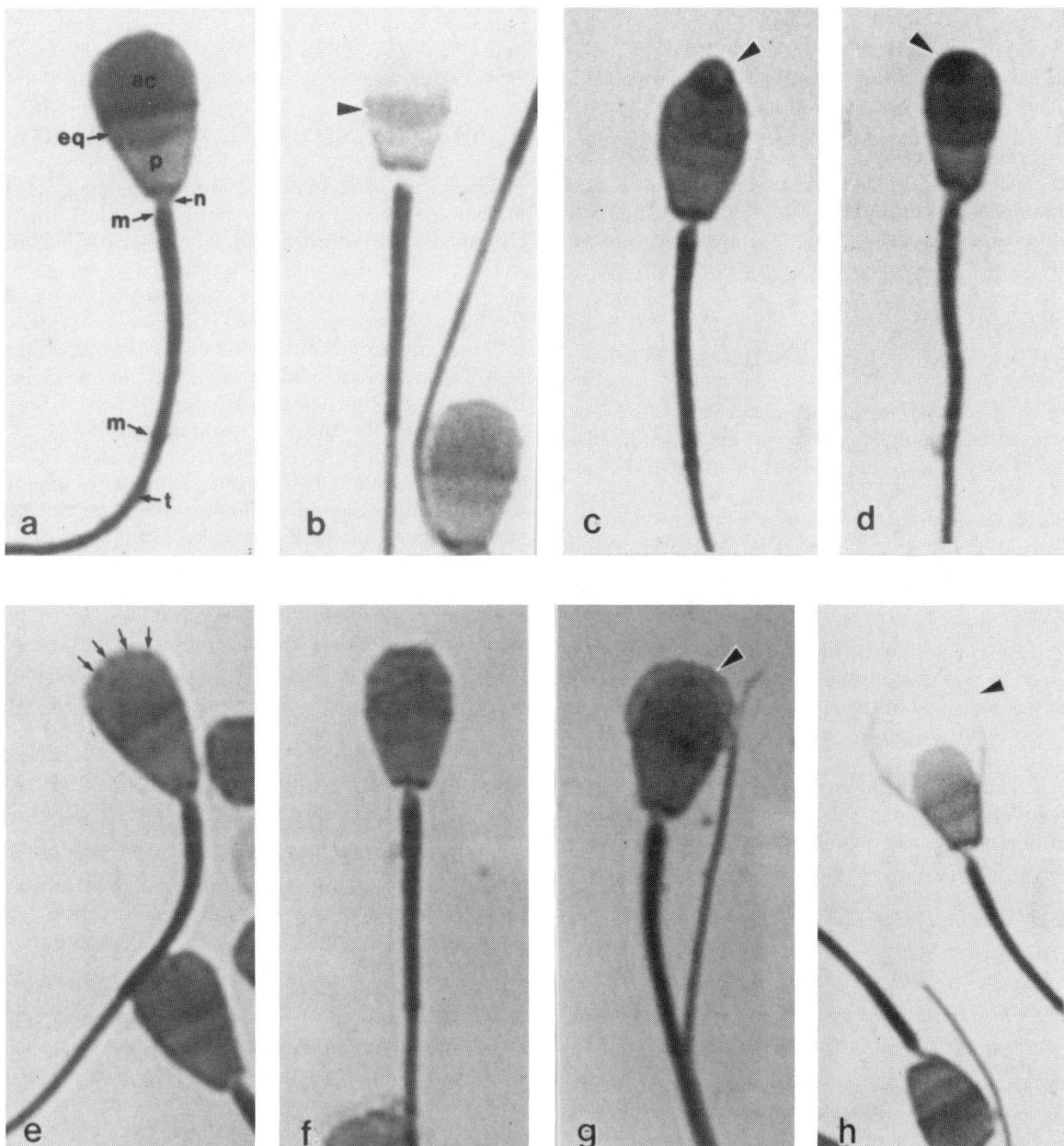

**Figure 1.** Normal dog sperm, acrosomal loss, major acrosomal abnormalities, and minor acrosomal abnormalities. A, Normal dog sperm. Acrosome (ac), equatorial region of the acrosome (eq), postacrosomal region of the head (p). The midpiece (m,m) connects to the base of the head at the neck (n). The latter does not possess mitochondria, and may be seen as a paler staining area immediately below the head base. Where the mitochondria end distally, the principal piece of the tail (t) continues as a thinner axoneme (compare with Fig. 5A,B). B, Acrosome loss, not involving the equatorial region. Note pale staining of the area that used to be covered by the acrosome, while the equatorial region (*arrowhead*) still stains normally. C, Acrosome cyst, apical and partially filled with acrosomal material. Note the round appearance of the cyst and the more intense staining circumferentially. D, Acrosome lipping. The acrosome has folded back on itself, resulting in extra-acrosomal material in the region of the lip (*arrowhead*). The head is also narrow. E, Start of the acrosome reaction. At this stage, all that is visible under the light microscope is irregular staining of the acrosome (*arrows*). This extends, as may be seen in F, where the irregular staining is obvious over the acrosome excluding the equatorial region. G, Moderately severe acrosomal swelling (*arrowhead*). More acrosomal contents have been lost, with consequent further loss of staining affinity. H, Severe acrosomal swelling. The ballooned membrane (*arrowhead*) is clearly visible as a pale halo around the head. There is almost no staining in the acrosome, indicating that most of the acrosomal contents have been lost.

the length of the head. That part of the midpiece which does not possess mitochondria is seen as a paler staining area immediately below the base of the head. The mitochondria are helically arranged (Fig. 5C); distally, the mitochondria end at the annulus, and the principal piece of the tail continues as a thinner axoneme. The flagellum possesses the same basic pattern of microtubules and matrix components that have been observed throughout most of the animal kingdom; nine evenly spaced pairs of microtubules around a central pair of single microtubules (Fig. 5C, D). The cell membrane of the mature spermatozoon has the usual trilaminar unit membrane structure throughout.

## MAJOR ACROSOMAL ABNORMALITIES

Major acrosomal abnormalities occur in the form of acrosomal cysts, lipping, ridging, and an irregular distribution of acrosomal material. Most commonly, acrosomal cysts occur apically, where they are sometimes referred to as "nipple acrosomes." They are usually filled with cytoplasmic material (Fig. 1C). Acrosomal lipping is seen under the light microscope as a distinct increase in acrosomal density, and typically occurs apically. The acrosome folds back on itself, resulting in extra-acrosomal material in the region of the lip (Fig. 1D). There is also a wide range of other abnormalities that may be observed in the acrosome; however, all are various combinations of lips, cysts, and irregular distribution. Acrosome abnormalities have been well documented as causes of sterility in the bull, boar, and ram (Andersen, 1974; Blom, 1972; Savage, 1984). They are commonly encountered in dogs, but are often associated with other head abnormalities. They occur alone in much lower frequency. In humans, both primary and secondary acrosomal defects have been shown to es-

**Table 1.** *Morphologic Classification of Dog Sperm**

**Normal Morphology**

**Acrosome Abnormalities**
  Major—lipped, cysts, abnormal distribution
  Minor—acrosome reaction, swelling, severe damage, loss

**Head Abnormalities**
  Major—macrocephalic, microcephalic, pyriform, diadem defects, other nuclear vacuoles, ridged sperm, double forms, severe pleiomorphism or bizarre forms
  Minor—narrow heads, head-base defects, detached heads, nuclear decondensation

**Midpiece Abnormalities**
  Major—retained cytoplasmic droplets, ruptured midpiece, pseudodroplet defect, kinked midpiece
  Minor—distal droplets

**Tail Abnormalities**
  Major—the "Dag" defect, double tails
  Minor—simple bent or coiled tail, terminally coiled tail

**Sperm Agglutination**
  Head to head, head to tail to tail, or attachment to other cells

*From Oettlé EE: Sperm morphology and fertility in the dog. J Reprod Fertil 47(suppl): 257–260, 1993, with permission.

cape selection due to the filtering imposed by the "swim-up" technique (see *CVT XI*, p 933 for details), and thus these abnormal sperm are in a position to compete with normal sperm for fertilization (Oettlé and Wiswedel, 1989).

## MINOR ACROSOMAL ABNORMALITIES

These are secondary acrosomal changes, and are known to arise after the sperm have left the testis (Blom, 1972; Bedford, 1970). They may be divided into the acrosome reaction and pathologic damage to the acrosome. Since membrane detail is not visible under the light microscope, the two conditions are difficult to differentiate accurately, especially in cases of mild damage. The acrosome reaction is a physiologic change in the acrosome that leads eventually to loss of both the contents and the outer acrosomal membrane. It normally only occurs on contact with the zona pellucida. The reaction starts as a slight irregularity of staining of the acrosome (Fig. 1E). This extends, and the irregularity becomes obvious over most of the acrosome, but excludes the equatorial region (Fig. 1F). The end of the reaction occurs with loss of the apical part of the acrosome (Fig. 1B). The acrosome reaction of dog sperm appears to follow the same basic pattern as that of most mammals (Bedford, 1970). In its early stages, acrosome damage is seen under the light microscope as a decrease in acrosomal staining; this indicates a loss of acrosomal contents. As the damage progresses, the acrosome takes on a ruffled appearance; the acrosome then swells (Fig. 1G, H), and thereafter ruptures and the contents are lost. Aging of dog sperm, either as a result of extended epididymal transit time or from prolonged postejaculation incubation of semen, and semen processing techniques (e.g., cryopreservation) causes damage to the apical portion of the acrosome. The equatorial region appears to be relatively resistant to damage, and severely damaged acrosomes are often noted with normal, intact equatorial regions (Oettlé, 1986b; Zalewski and Andersen-Berg, 1983).

## MAJOR HEAD ABNORMALITIES

In *macrocephalic* sperm, the proportions of acrosome and nucleus may be normal (Fig. 2A) or abnormal. Macrocephalic sperm are most often associated with other defects, usually with double tails and abnormal acrosomes. Bizarre forms of macrocephalic sperm were among the severe multiple sperm abnormalities found in a bulldog that had suffered from a derangement of testicular thermoregulation (Oettlé and Soley, 1986). Despite the grossly abnormal appearance of a high percentage of the sperm, the dog recovered over a period of 5 months, and regained full fertility. In the bull, macrocephalic sperm are usually diploid (Bertschinger, 1975). *Microcephalic* sperm have a severe reduction in head size. It is usually accompanied by an increased intensity of nuclear staining (Fig.

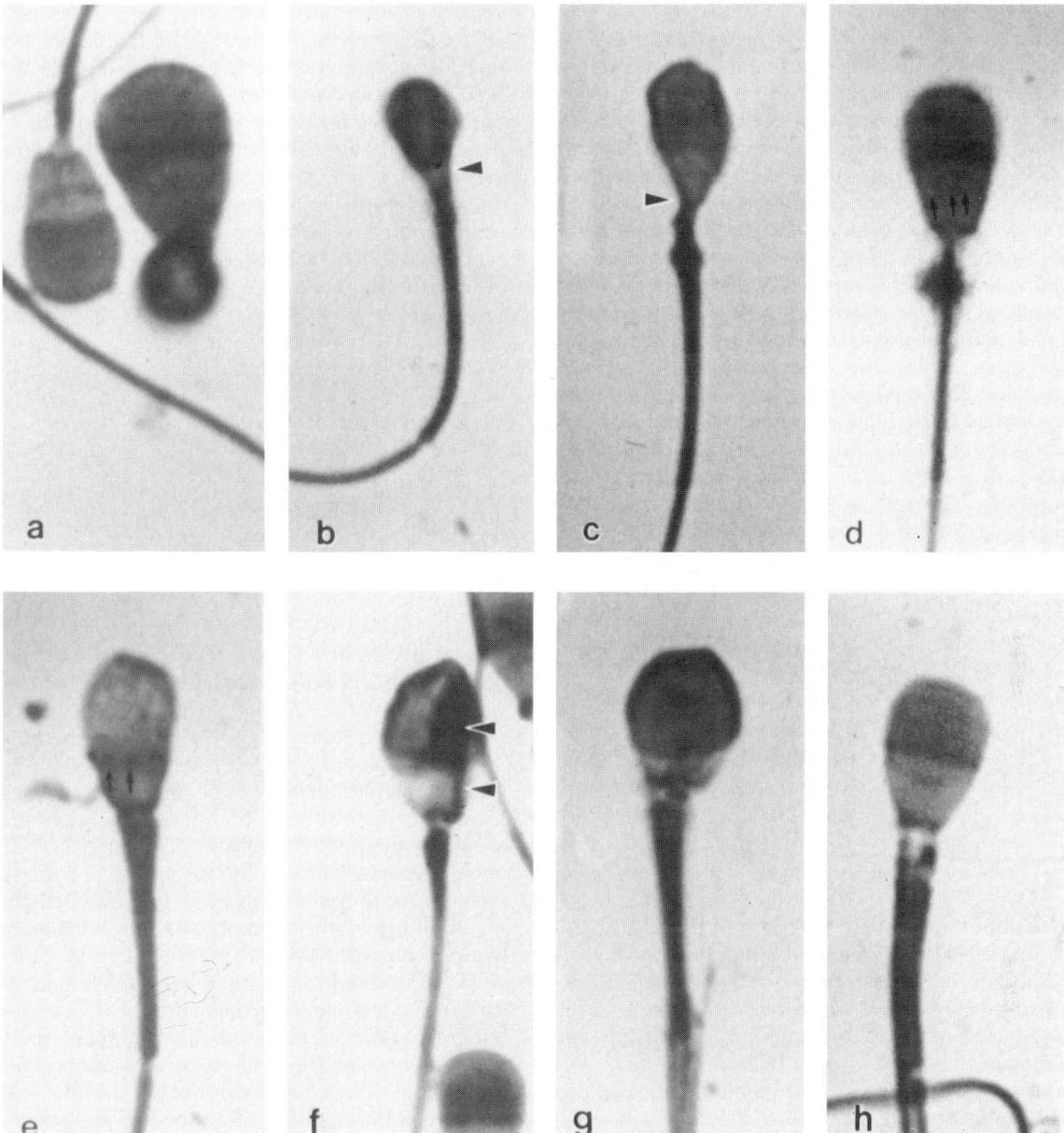

**Figure 2.** Major head abnormalities. *A*, Macrocephalic. The large head with the coiled tail may be compared with the normal head alongside. *B*, Microcephalic. This small head also shows an abnormal acrosomal arrangement. Note the increased intensity of the staining at the head base (*arrowhead*), possibly due to the condensation of chromosomal material. *C*, Pyriform head. The severely narrowed head base typical of these pear-shaped sperm heads is clearly visible (*arrowhead*). There is also a greater intensity of staining, but not to the degree seen in microcephalic heads. This is a fairly constant finding for pyriform heads, and is immediately seen by comparison with normal sperm. *D*, *E*, Diadem defect. This is also known as the crater defect, and is caused by nuclear vacuoles (*arrows*). Due to the limited depth of field of the light microscope, it is not possible to show the complete defect in one picture. In one focal plane, the defect appears as a row of light dots (*D*); at a lower focal plane, these dots become dark ridged sperm (*E*). *F*, In this sperm, the ridged portion is seen to run centrally and has an acrosomal region (*upper arrowhead*) as well as a postacrosomal region (*lower arrowhead*). *G*, Macrocephalic, with a double midpiece and tail. *H*, Relatively normal heads with double tails are also encountered, as is shown in this figure.

2*B*), as a result of hypercondensation of the chromatin. In humans, a form of microcephalic sperm, called "pinhead" sperm, occurs; these are often highly motile (Chemes et al., 1987). *Pyriform head* ("*pear-shaped head*") is characterized by a greater intensity of staining in the narrowed portion of the head, due to the increased nuclear condensation in this area (Fig. 2*C*).

The *diadem*, or crater defect, is the term given to single or multiple nuclear vacuoles that typically occur in the equatorial region of the head. Due to the depth of field of the light microscope being less than the depth of the sperm head, it is not possible to visualize the complete defect in one focal plane. In one focal plane, the defect appears as a row of white dots, while on a lower focal plane, these dots appear black (Fig. 2D, E). The diadem defect has been described in many species (Ploen, 1973). It is an unusual defect in that it is a major defect that is usually transient in nature, and thus carries a good prognosis (Heath and Ott, 1982; Oettlé and Soley, 1985b). Many causes have been implicated in its production, notably frostbite, increased testicular temperature, stress, and the administration of corticosteroids (Coulter, 1976). The presence of the defect indicates that the animal has undergone some form of transient testicular degeneration, and recovery should occur within a few months. Gross nuclear invaginations by acrosomal material are occasionally noted. These are clearly visible under the light microscope as large deeply stained areas displacing the nuclear material, and are typically irregular in appearance and distribution. *Ridged sperm* are usually binucleate (Bertschinger, 1975), the "extra" nucleus that forms the ridge being positioned at right angles to the other nucleus. Varying degrees of this abnormality occur, depending on the orientation and the degree of separation of the two nuclei. The ridge may be partial or complete, and aligned laterally, centrally, or horizontally. Photographic reproduction of this defect encounters similar problems to that of the diadem defect, and so it is difficult to get both head and ridge in focus (Fig. 2F). Double tails are often encountered in ridged sperm. Multiple ridges with corresponding bizarre shapes are occasionally noted.

### Double Forms

In this abnormality, the separation of the spermatids is incomplete. Double heads always possess double tails, although the reverse does not hold true. The degree of separation of the two components varies, from almost none to complete separation of the heads and the midpieces, with only the tails still joined. The sperm usually share a common plasma membrane over the area of fusion (Fig. 2G, H). *Bizarre forms* are severe multiple head abnormalities that do not allow classification into any other category (Fig. 3H).

### MINOR HEAD ABNORMALITIES

*Narrow heads* show a mild degree of uniform narrowing of the head, while showing normal staining characteristics. *Small, normal heads* are occasionally encountered. *Head-base defects* include mildly narrowed head bases, abaxial implantation of the midpiece, skew head bases, and broad and concave head bases (Fig. 3A, B, C). *Detached heads* are associated with aging of sperm, and it is thus not surprising that they often show degenerating or lost acrosomes. In these instances, repeat collections of semen at short time intervals causes a reduction in the number of detached heads and an improvement in acrosomal integrity. However, in the bull and in humans, a major defect

associated with loose heads has been reported (Blom, 1972; Chemes et al., 1987). In the latter instances, there is no reduction in the number of loose heads on repeated semen collections, and the tails are often motile. On very rare occasions, separated motile tails are noted in the dog. *Nuclear decondensation* and *nuclear degeneration* may be noted in the semen of dogs with defective testicular thermoregulation and in dogs suffering from heat stress to the scrotal contents and in aged sperm. This has also been noted in the rabbit and in humans (Bartoov et al., 1980; Ploen, 1973).

### MAJOR MIDPIECE ABNORMALITIES

*Retained cytoplasmic droplets* are seen in the neck region and are usually associated with failure of sperm to mature fully (as seen in prepubertal or overused stud dogs), but are also caused by epididymal malfunction. Under the light microscope, a normal midpiece is usually discernible running through the droplet (Fig. 3E). In humans, retained cytoplasmic droplets of less than half the size of the head are considered normal (Bartoov et al., 1980). *Ruptured midpieces* are manifestations of mitochondrial damage and disorganization, as well as axonemal damage, which usually occurs with concomitant retention of cytoplasmic material (Fig. 3D). The *pseudodroplet defect* is due to disruption of the mitochondrial helix. The mitochondria aggregate proximally or proximally and distally, leaving part of the axoneme denuded (Fig. 3H). The presence of a denuded axoneme differentiates this defect from retained cytoplasmic droplets. The *kinked midpiece* abnormality was found to be the predominant abnormality in sperm from a sterile Maltese poodle (Oettlé and Soley, 1985a). This defect has not been described in other species. A relatively normal midpiece is seen distally, but proximally at the point of attachment to the segmented columns there is rupture of fibers, kinking of the midpiece, and loose disorientated fibrils (Fig. 3G). Midpiece abnormalities often involve defects of the axoneme, which partially reduces or entirely eliminates motility. In most species, midpiece abnormalities are frequently associated with infertility and are often associated with retained cytoplasmic droplets (Blom and Birch-Andersen, 1966; Blom, 1972; Oettlé and Soley, 1985a; Plummer, Watson, and Allen, 1987).

### MINOR MIDPIECE ABNORMALITIES

Where the retained cytoplasmic droplets are caused by sperm immaturity, the droplets are classified as minor defects and designated *proximal droplets*. Differentiation between this minor defect and the major defect described in the previous section, which appears morphologically identical, is based on retesting the dog after a period of sexual rest. If the percentage of droplets is significantly reduced, the defect is classified as a minor defect. *Distal droplets* have the same structure

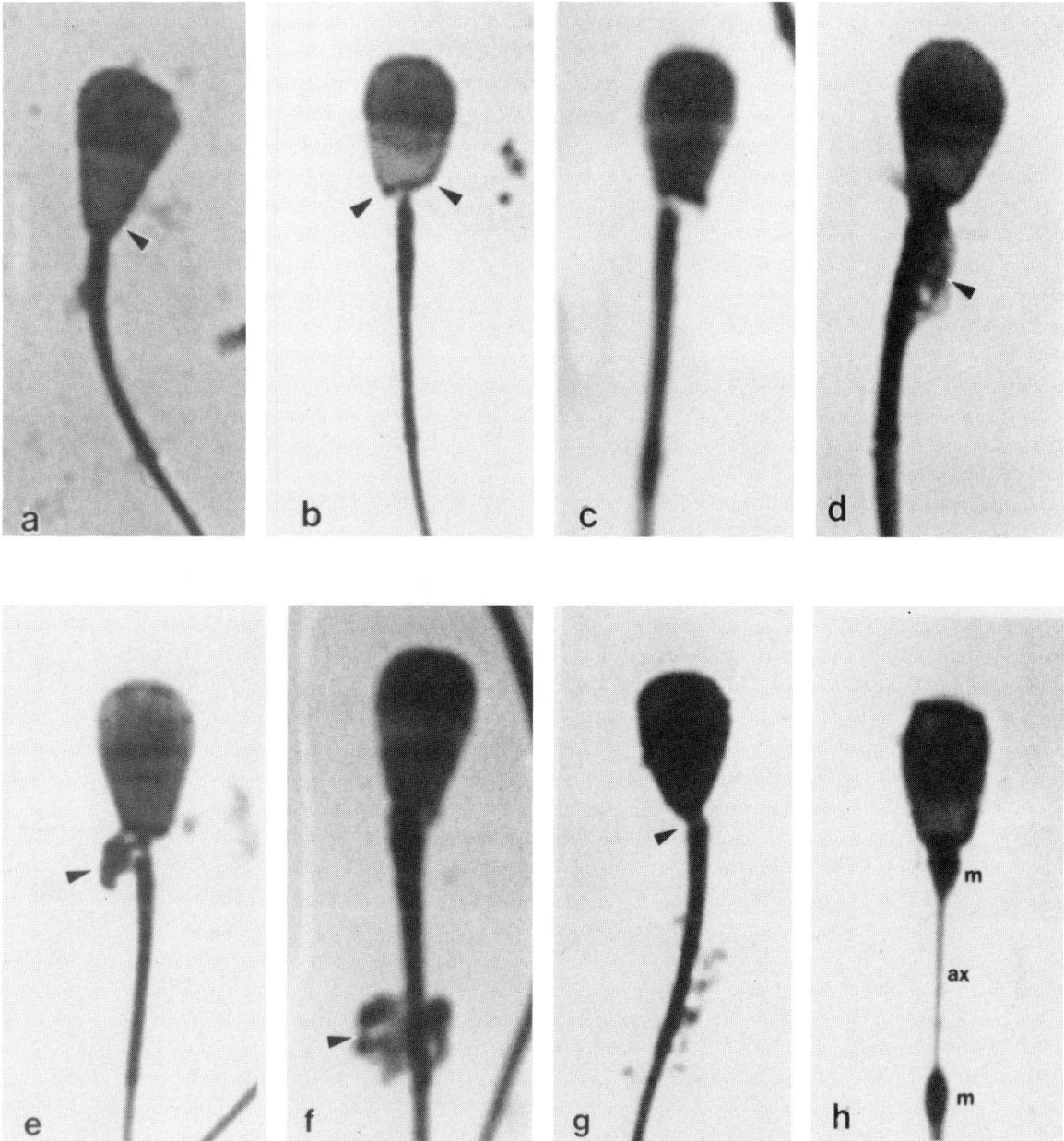

**Figure 3.** Minor head abnormalities, midpiece abnormalities. *A*, Narrow based head. The head is narrowed at the base only (*arrowhead*). *B*, Skew head base of normal width (*arrowheads*). *C*, Abaxial implantation of the midpiece. The midpiece is attached to the left lateral portion of the head base. *D*, Ruptured midpiece. Note that the rupture is located proximal (*arrowhead*), and that the double midpiece seems relatively normal distally. This defect should not be confused with a protoplasmic droplet (*E*), where the normal midpiece can usually be distinguished running through the droplet. *E*, Proximal protoplasmic droplet (*arrowhead*). *F*, Distal protoplasmic droplet (*arrowhead*). *G*, Kinked neck (*arrowhead*). *H*, Pseudodroplet defect. Here the mitochondrial spiral has ruptured and has been drawn proximally and distally into two pseudodroplets containing the aggregation of mitochondria (m,m); the denuded axoneme (ax) may be seen between the pseudodroplets.

as the proximal droplets, but occur at the junction between the midpiece and the principal piece of the tail (Fig. 3*F*). These probably represent a milder degree of sperm immaturity, and are only occasionally noted.

## MAJOR TAIL ABNORMALITIES

By far the most common tail abnormality is the *"Dag" defect*, which often is overall the predominant defect in the semen. It manifests as various degrees of coiling of the tail within an intact plasma membrane. The coiling varies from quite loosely to extremely tightly coiled, the latter often virtually obliterating the head. The tail may or may not be coiled around the

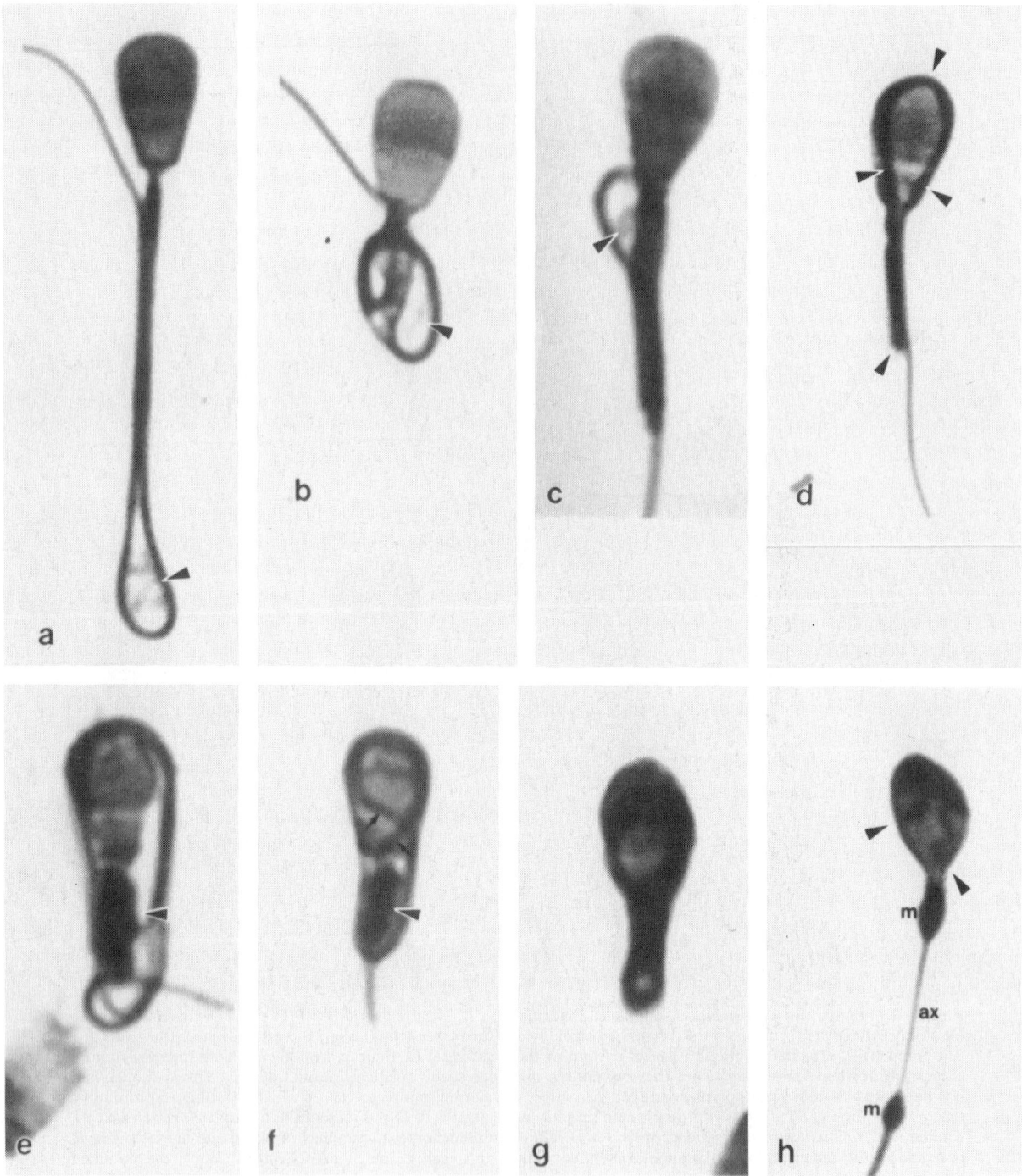

**Figure 4.** Major tail abnormalities, multiple abnormalities. *A,* Tail folded back on itself, around a distal droplet (*arrowhead*). This may be the simplest form of the "Dag" defect, shown in *B* to *G.* Note that the recurved portion of the tail is situated next to the midpiece. *B* to *G,* "Dag" defect of the tail. This defect is associated with various degrees of coiling of the tail within an intact plasma membrane. In *B,* the tail is coiled fairly loosely, tighter in *C:* the arrowheads show cytoplasmic material within the defect that appears fibrillar in *B,* and diffuse in *C.* In *D,* the tail coils around the head (follow the coil around with the arrowheads). The greatest degree of coiling is seen in *G.* *H,* Multiple abnormalities. Note the irregular distribution of the acrosome (*arrowheads*), which extends on the right side into the pyriform head base. There is also a pseudodroplet defect, as seen by the proximal and distal accumulations of mitochondria (m,m) and the denuded axoneme (ax).

head (Fig. 4 A–G). The "Dag" defect was first described in a bull of that name, where it was associated with epididymal malfunction. The defect has been described in many species, in all the ultrastructure of the defect being similar (Coubrough and Soley, 1982). In a bulldog that had suffered from deranged testicular thermoregulation, numerous sperm with "Dag" defects were noted. These abnormalities gradually reduced as the dog returned to normal over a period of 5 months (Oettlé and Soley, 1986). Thus, in this case, when the cause of the epididymal derangement had been removed, the sperm morphology returned to normal. *Double tails* are seen on sperm with normal and abnormal heads, the abnormal heads usually being macrocephalic or ridged. Sometimes double-tailed sperm share common central mitochondria; two base plates are always associated with the defect.

## MINOR TAIL ABNORMALITIES

### Simple Coiling of the Tail

This defect is differentiated from the "Dag" defect by the loose coiling and movement of the tail. The tail coils are not contained within a common plasma membrane, and the axonemes are normal. Terminal coiling of the tail is seen occasionally, usually as an incidental finding. When dogs are kept under tropical conditions, minor tail defects such as looped and bent tails, as well as bent midpieces and detached heads, were reported to comprise the majority of abnormalities encountered in their semen (Wong and Dhaliwal, 1985).

### Sperm Agglutination

Sperm agglutination may occur as tail to tail, tail to head, or head to head agglutination. It is differentiated from incomplete separation of spermatids by the large numbers of sperm involved and by the random alignment of the sperm. Sperm agglutination has been reported in dogs with *Brucella canis* infection; in these cases, there is production of antibodies to sperm with a high affinity for the acrosome (Christiansen, 1984). Immunologic causes of infertility in humans are associated with sperm agglutination. Immunologic infertility has not yet been clearly identified as a clinical entity in dogs (Burke, 1986).

## FOREIGN CELLS

### Macrophages and Phagocytosis of Sperm

Both normal and abnormal sperm are seen to be phagocytosed by macrophages. When normal sperm are phagocytosed, they usually have damaged acrosomes; it is not known whether this damage occurs before or after phagocytosis. *Sperm precursors* and *leukocytes* do not stain differentially with Spermac stain. The intense green staining of the cytoplasm obscures nuclear detail, except in spermatids, where a degree of nuclear differentiation is obtained. In Diff-Quick–stained samples, however, cytologic detail is sufficient to identify the cell types seen. Leukocytes are noted in cases of epididymitis, orchitis, and contamination of semen by preputial secretions. In the latter, the semen often contains a large number of *epithelial cells* as well. A preputial wash with physiologic saline should be performed prior to collecting semen the following day; in cases of preputial contamination, a dramatic reduction in the number of contaminating cells is noted on the subsequent evaluation.

## SEMEN QUALITY AND FERTILITY

The ultimate test for the quality of semen is the evaluation of fertility data from controlled breeding trials, but this is a lengthy and involved process. The long cycle interval of the bitch makes the collection of sufficient results from fertility trials for significant statistical analysis an even more protracted and costly affair than in other domestic species (Fig. 5).

Various suggestions regarding the influence of sperm abnormalities on fertility have been offered in the literature. Rosenthal (1983) suggested that total head and midpiece abnormalities in excess of 40% of sperm in an ejaculate is associated with infertility, while 20% head, acrosome, and retained cytoplasmic droplets may be associated with decreased conception rates. According to Seager (1986), the fertile dog should not have more than 20 to 30% abnormal forms present in the ejaculate. Krause (1965) reported on the fertility of seven dogs with abnormal spermiograms. Only occasional litters were produced when sperm showed normal morphology less than 57%. Oettlé (1993) found that fertility of dogs was statistically reduced when the percentage normal sperm fell below 60%. By use of the strength of association ($\Phi$ coefficients) of the $\chi^2$ values, dogs were divided into normal and subnormal groups, taking 60% normal morphology as the cut-off point. A marked difference in fertility was noted between the two groups (61% versus 13% fertility, respectively). Until further data become available, this figure may be used as a convenient "rule of thumb" when evaluating a dog for genital soundness. Since no significant difference was found between the ages of the normal and subnormal groups, subfertility may affect dogs of any age from puberty to reproductive senescence. From a practical point of view, the best means of ensuring subsequent fertility and availability of valuable sires would be the cryopreservation and storage of sufficient quantities of semen early in the sire's career, as soon as he is proved fertile.

Normal dogs usually have relatively uniform spermiograms, but when there is a disturbance in the spermatogenic environment, there is much variation in sperm morphology, and a wide range of sperm abnormalities is encountered. Conditions that induce pathognomonically unique abnormalities in sperm are uncommon.

Collection of semen from dogs more than once every second day caused a reduction in sperm output and an increase in retained cytoplasmic droplets (Boucher, Foote, and Kirk, 1958). Total azoospermia resulted in one dog from which semen was collected four times weekly for 4 months; the dog made a subsequent recovery after 3 months of sexual rest (Evans and Renton, 1973). For purposes of artificial insemination, it may be necessary to collect semen daily for a few days, but epididymal reserves are usually sufficient to cope with the required short-term increase in sperm output.

## ASSESSMENT OF DOGS FOR GENITAL SOUNDNESS

The evaluation of a dog for breeding is usually based on an assessment of his genital soundness; this concept encompasses the ability of the animal to produce a normal semen sample, and to perform normal copulatory behavior. In assessing an animal, the concept of optimum fertility as opposed to the ability to fertilize

should always be borne in mind. While a single offspring may well be sufficient to satisfy an owner, optimum fertility is obviously preferable. A prognosis is often difficult to give on a single consultation, since the examination gives only the current status of the animal. The spermiograms of a dog may vary quite markedly over a period of time. Sperm in an ejaculate may be at varying stages of their life histories (Cohen, 1971), and this should be taken into account when assessing the potential fertility of a sire. This is particularly important when confronted with a spermiogram indicating sperm immaturity, aging, or induced morphologic changes. The potential of the dog testis to recover should not be underestimated (Bane, 1970; Evans and Renton, 1973; Larsen, 1980; Oettlé and Soley, 1986), and retesting subnormal dogs at suitable intervals is essential. The frequency of subsequent examinations will vary, depending on the spermiogram and the type, cause, and duration of the condition that caused the disturbance to spermatogenesis. If after 3 months there is still a poor spermiogram, the prognosis is guarded. If there is no improvement after 6 months, the prognosis may be regarded as poor. If there is still no improvement after 12 months, the prognosis is virtually hopeless. The final assessment of genital soundness is thus

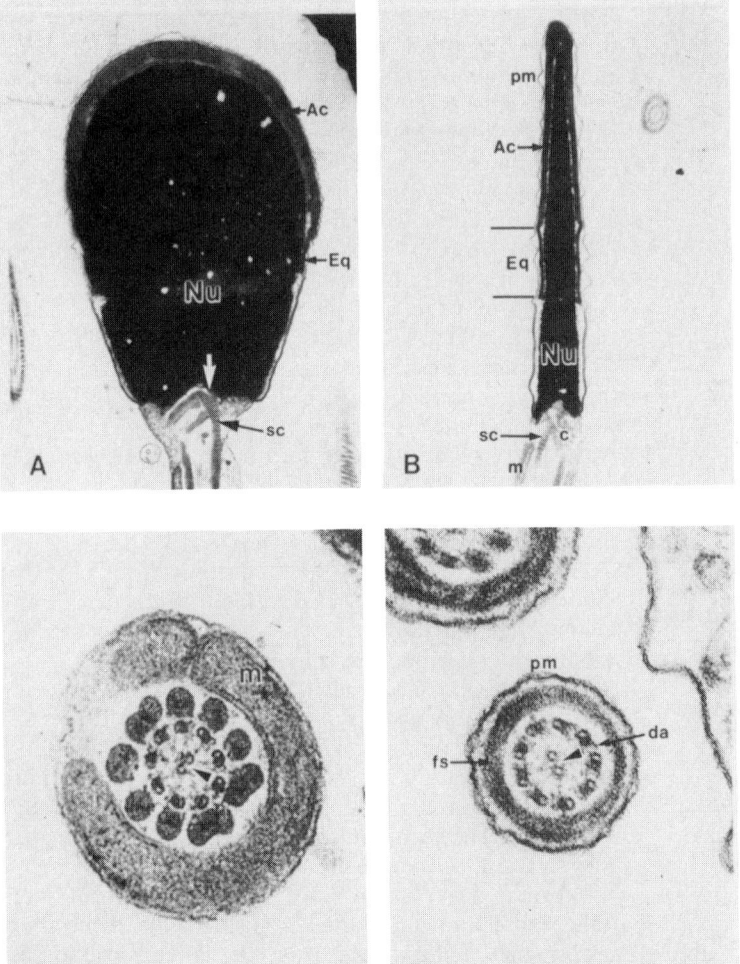

**Figure 5.** Electron micrographs: normal dog sperm. *A,* Planar section. The acrosome cap (Ac) enclosing the apical portion of the nucleus (Nu) may clearly be seen at the perimeter, but the thinning of the acrosome at the equatorial region (Eq) is better seen in the following sagital section (*B*). Note the base plate (*white arrow*) and the segmented columns (sc) of the midpiece (X14,400). *B,* Sagital section. Note the plasma membrane (pm), the thinning of the acrosome (Ac) at the equatorial region (Eq), the centriole (c), segmented columns (sc), and the mitochondria (m) of the midpiece (X15,800). *C,* Transverse section through a midpiece. Note the spirally arranged mitochondria (m) surrounding the nine coarse fibrils, the nine fine fibrils, and the two central fibrils (*arrowhead*) of the axoneme (X42,500). *D,* Transverse section through a tail. Note that the coarse fibrils have coalesced into the fibrous sheath (fs), surrounded by the plasma membrane (pm). The dynein arms (da) may be seen on the nine fine fibrils, and the central two fibrils are designated by the arrowhead (X48,500).

a synthesis of the information obtained from all the tests performed into a comprehensive picture of the potential fertility of the dog.

## References and Supplemental Reading

Aitken RJ, Ross A, Hargreave T, Richardson D, and Best F: Analysis of human sperm function following exposure to the Ionophore A23187. J Androl 5, 321, 1984.

Andersen K: Morphological abnormalities in the acrosome and nucleus of boar sperm. Nord Vet Med 26:215, 1974.

Bane A: Sterility in male dogs. Nord Vet Med 22:561, 1970.

Bartoov B, Eltes F, Weissenberg R, and Lunenfeld B: Morphological characterization of abnormal human spermatozoa using transmission electron microscopy. Arch Androl 5:305, 1980.

Bedford JM: Sperm capacitation and fertilization in mammals. Biol Reprod 2 (suppl):128, 1970.

Bertschinger HJ: The hereditary occurrence of diploid spermatozoa in the semen of brown Swiss bulls. DVM Thesis, University of Zurich 1975, pp 1–47.

Blom E: The ultrastructure of some characteristic sperm defects and a proposal for a new classification of the bull spermiogram. In Atti del VII Symposio Internationale de Zootechia, Milano, 1972, pp 125–129.

Blom E and Birch-Andersen A: Ultrastructure of the decapitated sperm defect in Guernsey bulls. J Reprod Fertil 23:67, 1966.

Boucher JH, Foote RH, and Kirk RW: The evaluation of semen quality in the dog and the effects of frequency of ejaculation upon semen quality, libido and depletion of sperm reserves. Cornell Vet 48:67, 1958.

Burke TJ: Small Animal Reproduction and Infertility: A Clinical Approach to Diagnosis and Treatment. Philadelphia, Lea & Febiger, 1986, pp 207–217.

Chemes HE, Carizza C, Scarinci F, et al: Lack of a head in human spermatozoa from sterile patients: A syndrome associated with impaired fertilization. Fertil Steril 47:310, 1987.

Christiansen J II: Reproduction in the Dog and Cat. London, Bailliere Tindall, 1984, pp 80–109.

Cohen J: The comparative physiology of male gametes. In Lowenstein O (ed): Advances in Comparative Physiology and Biochemistry. London, Academic Press, 1971, pp 267–380.

Coubrough RI and Soley JT: The "Dag defect" in mammalian spermatozoa. Proc Electron Microsc Soc So Afr 12:75, 1982.

Coulter GH: Effect of dexamethasone on the incidence of the "crater" defect of bovine sperm. VII International Congress on Animal Reproduction and Artificial Insemination, Cracow, 1976, pp 694–697.

Evans J and Renton JP: A case of azoospermia in a previously fertile dog with subsequent recovery. Vet Rec 92:198, 1973.

Foote RH: Semen quality from the bull to the freezer: An assessment. Theriogenology 3:219, 1975.

Heath E and Ott RS: Diadem/crater defect in spermatozoa of a bull. Vet Rec 110:5, 1982.

Krause D II: Zur Fertilitatsuntersuchung beim Hund. DTW 72:3, 1965.

Larsen RE: Infertility in the male dog. In Morrow DA (ed): Current Therapy in Theriogenology. Philadelphia, WB Saunders Co, 1980, pp 646–654.

Oettlé EE: An improved sperm staining technique which facilitates sequential monitoring of the acrosome state Develop Growth Different 28(suppl):96, 1986a.

Oettlé EE: Changes in acrosome morphology during cooling and freezing of dog semen. Anim Reprod Sci 12:145, 1986b.

Oettlé EE: Sperm morphology and fertility in the dog. J Reprod Fertil 47 (suppl): 47:257, 1993.

Oettlé EE and Soley JT: Infertility in a Maltese poodle as a result of a sperm midpiece defect. J S Afr Vet Assn 56:103, 1985a.

Oettlé EE and Soley JT: The diadem defect in dog spermatozoa. Proc Electron Microsc Soc S Afr 15:159, 1985b.

Oettlé EE and Soley JT: Severe sperm abnormalities with subsequent recovery following on scrotal oedema and posthitis in a bulldog. J Small Anim Pract 27:477, 1986.

Oettlé EE and Soley JT: Sperm abnormalities in the dog: A light and electron microscopic study. Vet Med Rev 59:28, 1988.

Oettlé EE and Wiswedel K: Influence of the swim-up procedure on acrosome damage induced by freezing human semen. S Afr Med J 75:23, 1989.

Ploen L: An electron microscope study of the delayed effects on rabbit spermateleosis following experimental cryptorchidism for twenty four hours. Arch [B] 14:159, 1973.

Plummer JM, Watson PF, and Allen WE: A spermatozoal midpiece abnormality associated with infertility in a Llasa apso dog. J Small Anim Pract 28:743, 1987.

Rosenthal RC: Infertility in the male dog. Compend Cont Educ Pract Vet 5: 983, 1983.

Savage NC: Infertility in a ram associated with a knobbed acrosome abnormality of the spermatozoa. Can Vet J 25:126, 1984.

Seager SWJ: Artificial insemination in dogs. In Burke TJ (ed): Small Animal Reproduction and Infertility: A Clinical Approach to Diagnosis and Treatment. Philadelphia, Lea & Febiger, 1986, pp 207–217.

Wong WT and Dhaliwal GK: Observations on semen quality of dogs in the tropics. Vet Rec 116:313, 1985.

Zalewski W and Andersen-Berg K: Acrosomal damage caused by processing frozen semen from the silver fox (Vulpes argenteus) and the blue fox (Alopex lagopus). Zuchthyg 18:22, 1983.

# THE USE AND MISUSE OF REPRODUCTIVE HORMONES IN CANINE REPRODUCTION

JANICE L. CAIN

San Ramon, California

Naturally produced and synthetically prepared reproductive hormones are frequently used as pharmaceuticals in canine reproduction. Specific indications for the use of these preparations are few; too often hormonal therapies are used incorrectly and at times deleteriously. Appropriate uses of reproductive hormones are based on known physiologic mechanisms in order to improve reproductive efficiency or to treat specific disorders.

## FUNCTIONS OF REPRODUCTIVE HORMONES

### Gonadotropin-Releasing Hormone and Its Analogs

After isolation and identification of the gonadotropin-releasing hormone (GnRH) decapeptide structure that is common to all mammals, there were great expectations for its use to treat human infertility. The physiology of GnRH and its pulsatile release from the hypothalamus provided some problems with administration, however. Gonadotropin-releasing hormone is rapidly deactivated and cleared after traversing the hypothalamic-hypophyseal portal system to stimulate anterior pituitary gonadotrophs. The goal of pharmacologic administration of GnRH is to simulate its natural secretion pattern and thereby induce secretion of endogenous luteinizing hormone (LH) and follicle-stimulating hormone (FSH). Administration of GnRH in 60- 120-min pulses can restore gonadotropin release in humans with hypothalamic amenorrhea or hypothalamic hypogonadism. Administration of GnRH can induce folliculogenesis and fertile ovulation in women, mares, and bitches when delivered by an infusion pump that provides pulsatile delivery over a period of several days. Infusion pumps are small enough to attach to a harness in a bitch, but their use is often cumbersome and they are expensive.

Gonadotropin-releasing hormone analogs are synthetically prepared substances that differ from native GnRH structure by various amino acid substitutions in the decapeptide sequence. Analogs with minor substitutions (i.e., one to three amino acids) generally act as GnRH agonists due to increased binding affinity and decreased clearance. This results in a prolonged duration of effect such that agonists require less frequent administration than the native GnRH hormone to induce the same effect. Heavily substituted analogs result in antagonists with extreme potency such that their pharmacologic use results in down-regulation and consequent decreased LH and FSH secretion. Prolonged use of a GnRH agonist will also lead to down-regulation, which is a major consideration when developing a protocol using a GnRH agonist to stimulate increased LH and FSH secretion.

Lack of availability is the major hindrance to widespread use of GnRH analogs to control reproduction in humans and animals. Whereas native GnRH is readily available (Cystorelin, Abbott Laboratories, North Chicago, IL), analogs are very expensive or are available only to those individuals associated with research institutions. Some specific uses of GnRH for canine reproduction have been identified (see below). Additional uses of GnRH analogs are under investigation and may be practical should the drug become commercially available.

## Gonadotropins

The pituitary gonadotropins, FSH, and LH are glycoproteins consisting of two nonidentical $\alpha$ and $\beta$ subunits. The $\alpha$ subunit is similar between species and is identical in both LH and FSH. The $\beta$ subunit is species specific and different for each gonadotropin, thus providing the functional specificity of each hormone. After stimulation by GnRH, LH release from the anterior pituitary is pulsatile, whereas FSH release is slow and more sustained.

Some species also produce placental gonadotropins. Human placenta syncytial trophoblasts produce the luteotropic hormone human chorionic gonadotropin (HCG). In most species, HCG has potent LH activity with little to no FSH effects. Administration of HCG results in prolonged LH effects when compared to administration of either LH directly or GnRH. In the pregnant mare, placental trophoblasts produce equine chorionic gonadotropin (eCG), which is also identified as pregnant mare serum gonadotropin (PMSG). Administration of eCG results in a mixed FSH and LH effect, although FSH activity predominates. Since the structure of gonadotropins is species specific, the administration of either HCG or eCG to dogs is potentially antigenic, and repeat administration may result in decreased response to the hormone because of neutralizing antibody production.

The use of gonadotropins to manipulate or enhance canine reproduction has been attempted; however, the availability of some hormones is limited. Both FSH (FSH-P, Schering-Plough, Kenilworth NJ) and HCG (Chorionic gonadotropin, Rugby Laboratories, Long Island, NY) are readily available. In the United States, eCG is not commercially available and LH is not available in a purified form. A preparation consisting of equal amounts of FSH and LH (Menotropin-Pergonal, Serono Laboratories, Randolph, MA) is used to treat human infertility, but is generally cost-prohibitive for use in veterinary medicine (in Canada, eCG is available: Equinex, Ayerst Laboratories, Quebec; PMSG can be obtained in some European countries).

## Gonadal Steroids

Serum estrogen, produced by developing ovarian follicles, increases throughout proestrus and typically peaks in concentration 1 to 2 days prior to the end of proestrus. While the signs of proestrus are due to estrogen-mediated effects, sexual receptivity is triggered by declining estrogen and rising progesterone serum concentrations. At that phase, progesterone is produced from preovulatory luteinization of follicles. After ovulation and production of corpora lutea, ovarian progesterone production continues until parturition or termination of the luteal phase in a nonpregnant bitch (i.e., 70 or more days).

Testosterone, released from the testicular interstitial cells in response to LH stimulation, is necessary for spermatogenesis and normal libido in the stud dog. The normal function of Sertoli cells is dependent on an intratesticular testosterone concentration that greatly exceeds circulatory levels. The administration of exogenous testosterone will inhibit further production of testosterone, due to inhibition of LH and possibly other factors, and lead to a decrease in the intratesticular testosterone concentration. A decrease in spermatogenesis is the likely sequela to testosterone administration. The prostate is dependent on the trophic effects of dihydrotestosterone, which is produced by an intraprostatic conversion of testosterone.

Gonadal steroid preparations are readily available for use in veterinary medicine, but while indications for their use are few, the potential for misuse is great. In addition to the diminution of fertility associated with imbalancing sensitive negative feedback mechanisms of the hypothalamic-pituitary-gonadal axis, administration of gonadal steroids may be systemically toxic to the patient. Estrogen toxicity has been well documented with the administration of all commercially available estrogen preparations, and progesterone administration during pregnancy can be teratogenic.

## CONDITIONS FOR WHICH REPRODUCTIVE HORMONES ARE USED

### Estrus Induction

Reliable fertile estrus induction protocols have been difficult to devise in the bitch because of a lack of understanding of the hormonal events necessary for folliculogenesis. The natural cause for termination of anestrus and onset of a new cycle (i.e., folliculogenesis) is not clearly understood. Serum concentrations of FSH remain relatively high in the bitch during the late anestrus period and then decrease during proestrus. Why the bitch fails to respond to FSH during anestrus and what triggers eventual response and folliculogenesis is speculative. It has been theorized that either an increase in LH release or a change in basal serum estradiol concentration, or perhaps both events, trigger the onset of a new follicular phase in the bitch. What causes this increase in LH pulse frequency and amplitude prior to proestrus is also unknown.

Clinical applications of an estrus induction protocol include treatment of infertility due to primary anestrus and stimulation of estrous cyclicity in bitches previously treated with androgens to prevent estrus (e.g., racing greyhound bitches given testosterone). It is important to thoroughly evaluate all apparent causes of reproductive failure before attempting estrus induction and realize that protocols are designed and tested in bitches that are reproductively normal.

Pulsatile administration of GnRH using a programmable pump (Pulsamat, Ferring Laboratories, Ridgewood, NJ) induced fertile estrus in seven of eight beagle bitches in one study (Cain et al., 1988). Bitches received 140 ng of GnRH/kg/pulse every 90 min for 11 to 13 days. All bitches had signs of behavioral estrus and were mated. Seven bitches conceived and whelped normal litters. The major drawback to this protocol is the need for the infusion pump to deliver a precise dose every 90 min. Continuous infusions of GnRH and a GnRH agonist were thus investigated. The advantage of continuous drug delivery is that an inexpensive mini-osmotic pump temporarily implanted subcutaneously can be used. The disadvantage of continuous delivery of GnRH is that down-regulation may occur because of digression from the pulsatile pattern of endogenous secretion. In one study evaluating continuous infusion of GnRH, varying dose regimens and duration of treatment were attempted (Cain et al., 1989). Overall, the response to treatment was poor and only two of eight bitches treated had signs of estrus and ovulated. In another continuous infusion study, bitches received a GnRH agonist ([D-Trp$^6$NmeLeu$^7$Pro$^9$NEt]GnRH)* at 1.7 to 2.5 $\mu$g/kg/day for 14 days (Concannon, 1989). Nine of 24 bitches ovulated and whelped litters and another four bitches may have ovulated (i.e., serum progesterone concentration >2 ng/ml) but had a short luteal phase and return of serum progesterone concentrations to basal levels within 46 to 55 days.

Intermittent injections of a GnRH agonist are currently under investigation for the purpose of estrus induction. In a preliminary report, the use of [D-Trp-$^6$Pro$^9$NEt]GnRH(GnRH-A)* was administered to bitches of various breeds with the following protocol: GnRH-A (1 $\mu$g/kg every 8 hr SC) until the observation of behavioral estrus, at which time the dose was decreased to 0.5 $\mu$g/kg and continued for another 3 days (Cain et al., 1990). In five of six bitches, behavioral estrus was apparent by day 9 or 10 of treatment. Mating resulted in pregnancy in all five bitches bred and four litters were whelped. A single pup litter was evidently resorbed in one bitch that was treated with GnRH-A during late diestrus.

In the bitch, gonadotropin protocols have been unreliable for induction of fertile estrus that results in term pregnancy. Most protocols use either eCG (i.e., PMSG) or FSH to stimulate folliculogenesis, and use HCG to cause ovulation. The failure of these protocols may be due to the high levels of endogenous serum FSH normally present in bitches prior to folliculogenesis. Some protocols utilize administration of estrogen prior to gonadotropin administration, since estrogen can increase ovarian response to gonadotropins.

One estrus induction protocol was based on an inversion of the routine sequence of gonadotropin injections. After a treatment period with diethylstilbestrol (DES), LH injections were administered prior to FSH administration: 5 mg DES/bitch/day until day 3 of proestrus (vaginal bleeding); 5 mg LH/bitch IM on day 5; and 10 mg FSH/bitch IM on days 9 and 11 (Moses and Shille, 1988). Using this protocol, all seven treated bitches conceived and produced litters. Since LH is no longer commercially available, this protocol was reevaluated using HCG in place of LH, or administering FSH on days 5, 9, and 11. Results using these substitutions have been disappointing.

Another protocol used a combination of DES and FSH to attempt estrus induction. Bitches were given 5 mg DES PO until 2 days after the onset of vaginal bleeding (day 3 where day 1 = first day of vaginal bleeding); and 10 mg FSH/bitch was administered IM on days 5, 9, and 11 (Bouchard et al., 1991). Eight bitches were treated with this protocol in late anestrus of which six came into estrus and three bitches conceived. An additional five bitches were treated with this protocol during mid anestrus; three came into estrus

---

*These forms of GnRH are not commercially available at the time of writing.

and only one bitch conceived. An overall pregnancy rate of 30% (4/13) was attained with this method, which underscores the unreliability of a gonadotropin protocol to induce fertile estrus in the bitch.

In a preliminary report, DES was used alone to induce fertile estrus in mongrel bitches with great success (Bouchard et al., 1992). Bitches received 5 mg of DES PO daily until day 3 of the induced proestrus. All bitches treated ($n = 5$) came into estrus, were bred, and conceived. Average litter sizes were within the normal range. Estrogens are folliculotropic, but the exact mechanism of how estrogen administration alone can induce folliculogenesis is unknown. The average weight of the bitches treated in this study was not reported and care should be given when considering the administration of DES at the dose of 5 mg/day/bitch because of potential estrogen toxicity. Further investigation into this method of estrus induction should be conducted before treating client-owned animals.

## Induction of Ovulation

Preovulatory luteinization of follicles normally occurs in the bitch causing serum progesterone concentration to rise significantly prior to ovulation. During the ensuing diestrus, which is the luteal phase of both pregnant and nonpregnant bitches, corpora lutea produce progesterone for approximately 63 or up to 90 days, respectively. If serum progesterone concentration fails to rise above 2 ng/ml during estrus or falls below this level in the few weeks following estrus, either ovulation did not occur or the luteal phase was abnormally short (i.e., luteal insufficiency). A bitch with ovulation failure may have a seemingly normal proestrus and estrus phase but would fail to conceive after breeding. It is difficult to clinically determine the difference between ovulation failure and luteal insufficiency based on a basal progesterone level obtained several weeks after breeding when it is determined that the bitch is not pregnant. Successive estrous cycles may need to be monitored to determine that a bitch continuously fails to ovulate.

Prior to instituting therapy to induce ovulation, it is prudent to determine that infertility would likely otherwise result and that intervention is therefore indicated. True ovulation failure is rare in the bitch. Hormonal therapies may be inappropriately recommended for use in bitches that have an atypically long estrous period or have produced small litter sizes. Bitches that are sexually receptive for up to 21 days are still considered normal and are usually fertile. Bitches may consistently produce single pup litters or uncharacteristically small litters for the breed for a wide variety of reasons. Partial litter resorption or male subfertility should be considered. Also, some young bitches will have a "split heat," a condition in which proestrus and estrus are evident, but ovulation does not occur. The bitch then undergoes a 2- to 4-week period of anestrus and then another, usually ovulatory, estrous cycle.

A single injection of native GnRH may induce ovu-

lation of mature follicles. In a bitch with apparent ovulation failure, GnRH (50 μg/bitch IM) can be administered during the next spontaneous estrus. Alternatively, mature follicles can be induced to ovulate with IM administration of 500 to 1000 IU of HCG. Knowing when to administer the GnRH or HCG is difficult; treatment too early or late will most likely be unsuccessful. Treatment should be considered when more than 90% of the exfoliative vaginal cells appear cornified for a least 3 days. Success rates using GnRH or HCG in such cases have not been reported.

## Luteal Insufficiency

Luteal insufficiency, a condition in which corpora lutea do not produce adequate progesterone to support pregnancy to term, is not well documented in the bitch. Owners may erroneously conclude that fetuses were resorbed in bitches that were misdiagnosed pregnant by palpation. Owners may be subsequently fooled by physical changes in the bitch associated with pseudopregnancy and then are surprised when no litter is produced. The minimum serum progesterone concentration necessary to support pregnancy in the bitch is unknown. Serum progesterone concentrations above 5 ng/ml appear adequate, but some bitches can sustain pregnancy with serum progesterone concentrations in the 2- to 5-ng/ml range. Serum progesterone concentration 2 ng/ml or lower is considered insufficient to support pregnancy; however, transient decreases in progesterone to the 2-ng/ml level do not produce spontaneous abortion in all dogs. The finding of decreased serum progesterone concentration immediately prior to spontaneous abortion may be the result of fetal death rather than the cause, making the diagnosis of luteal insufficiency extremely difficult to confirm.

In bitches with a documented history of fetal resorption or spontaneous abortion for which an underlying cause cannot be determined, serum progesterone concentrations should be evaluated throughout the next pregnancy. If serum progesterone falls below 5 ng/ml, and pregnancy is documented by ultrasonography, progesterone supplementation is recommended. Excessive progesterone supplementation can cause masculinization of female fetuses and may prevent parturition. Supplementation with progesterone in oil (3 mg/kg/day IM) will maintain serum progesterone concentration at 10 ng/ml or higher (Scott-Moncrieff et al., 1990). Progesterone supplementation should be discontinued 3 days prior to the expected date of parturition to allow progesterone to fall to basal levels; otherwise, delayed parturition may occur.

## Luteinization of Follicular Cysts

Ovarian cysts are often incidental findings at ovariohysterectomy in older bitches, but they can be an infrequent cause of reproductive failure. Follicular cysts that produce estrogens may cause prolonged proestrus, nymphomania, and possibly estrogen toxicity with bone marrow aplasia. Follicular cysts that have become luteinized spontaneously may be nonfunctional (i.e., no excessive hormone production) or they may cause persistent anestrus possibly associated with excessive progesterone or other hormone secretion. Follicular cysts can be medically treated by administering a hormone that will induce luteinization of the cyst. Before attempting treatment of follicular cysts, the diagnosis must be confirmed by ultrasonography and measurement of serum estradiol and progesterone concentrations. Also, measurement of these hormone concentrations from percutaneously aspirated cystic fluid (i.e., with ultrasound guidance) may aid the diagnosis. It is possible that an ovarian neoplasm is the underlying cause of a cystic structure and accurate diagnosis may only be possible by biopsy.

Luteinization of a follicular cyst may be attempted by injecting GnRH 50 μg/bitch IM. A single injection or repeated injections once daily for up to 3 days have been recommended. The IM administration of 500 to 1000 IU of HCG may also luteinize a follicular cyst. Response to therapy can be seen as termination of estrous behavior or by detection of decreasing estrogen and increasing progesterone serum concentrations.

## Cryptorchidism

Although the precise mechanism for inheritance is unknown, unilateral or bilateral cryptorchidism is considered a heritable trait. Recommended treatment is bilateral orchidectomy. Ideally, the parents of the affected pup and any littermates should be removed from future breeding programs. Treatment of cryptorchidism by surgical or medical methods is considered unethical for the purpose of producing show or breeding animals. One ethical indication for the medical resolution of cryptorchidism is to induce descent of retained testicles such that a routine prescrotal castration could be performed. The use of GnRH to induce descent of retained testicles has been reported, but no information on efficacy, other than anecdotal, has been provided. One protocol uses GnRH (50 to 100 μg/pup SC or IM) with the dose repeated after 4 to 6 days if no effect is observed. Another protocol is to administer HCG at 100 to 1000 IU/dog IM four times over a 2-week period (i.e., on days 1, 5, 10, and 15). Success with this protocol has been observed more often when treatment is initiated in dogs under 16 weeks of age (Feldman and Nelson, 1987).

## Challenge Testing

To evaluate the functional integrity of the hypothalamic-pituitary-gonadal axis, GnRH can be administered, and gonadotropin and gonadal steroid production measured in response. In normal male dogs, 2.2 μg GnRH/kg IM will evoke an increase in serum testosterone concentrations detected 60 min after GnRH administration. Serum LH concentrations increase 10 min after IV injection of GnRH at 250 ng/kg (see *CVT X*, p 1282).

To aid in the diagnosis of ovarian remnant syndrome, bitches with signs of estrus after ovariohysterectomy can be given GnRH (50 to 100 μg/bitch IM) to induce luteinization of retained ovarian follicles. Serum progesterone concentration greater than 1 ng/ml 5 to 7 days after GnRH injection indicates the presence of functional luteal tissue and is an indication for exploratory surgery. An injection of 500 to 1000 IU of HCG can also be used for this purpose (see *CVT XI*, p 966).

To evaluate testosterone production in dogs that are suspected of having retained testicular tissue or in bitches that are suspected of having an intersex condition such as ovotestes, an HCG challenge test can be performed. An IM injection of 44 μg HCG/kg will result in increased serum testosterone concentration in 4 hr. Poststimulation testosterone concentrations were 4.6 to 7.5 ng/ml in normal intact male dogs in one report (Johnston, 1987).

## Androgen-Dependent Disorders

Since administration of a GnRH analog will cause eventual or immediate down-regulation, these analogs may be used to treat androgen-dependent disorders. A GnRH antagonist (Luprolide, TAP Pharmaceuticals, North Chicago, IL) has been evaluated as an agent to aid the treatment of prostate cancer in men. Factors including cost, lack of appropriate dosing information, and the routine acceptance of surgical castration in the dog make treatment with GnRH analogs for such cases impractical. Prostatic carcinoma reportedly occurs with equal frequency in previously castrated dogs, so it is unclear whether removal of testosterone influence would have a beneficial effect in the dog. It is unknown whether down-regulation therapy can be effective to treat other conditions such as benign prostatic hyperplasia and perianal adenoma in dogs. One major consideration with this method of treatment is that infertility (i.e., oligospermia) would also occur. Whether or not fertility could be restored with cessation of therapy is unknown. The original condition most likely would recur after drug withdrawal.

The use of estrogens to treat androgen-dependent disorders is not recommended. In addition to the potential toxicity of estrogen therapy, estrogen-induced squamous metaplasia of the prostate may increase the risk of bacterial prostatitis.

## Idiopathic Infertility

In the stud dog, idiopathic oligospermia is most frequently a primary gonadal disorder and not due to lack of pituitary hormone stimulation. In fact, serum FSH and LH concentrations may be significantly elevated in these cases, probably due to lack of negative feedback inhibition. Administration of pituitary hormones (i.e.,

LH or FSH) is therefore unwarranted and administration of GnRH with the purpose of increasing LH and FSH levels is inappropriate. In addition, while bolus injections of native GnRH will cause transient gonadotropin response, GnRH half-life is relatively short; thus, frequent administration (i.e., pulsatile) would be necessary to provide constant gonadotropin stimulation. Acquired infertility secondary to pituitary dysfunction due to invasive effects of a neoplasm is possible but uncommon. The following protocol has been suggested to treat such cases: HCG 500 IU/dog biweekly SC and FSH dosed either 1 mg/kg IM every 48 hr or 25 mg/dog SC once a week. Because spermatogenesis and spermatozoal maturation require approximately 77 days, therapy must be continued for at least 3 months before response to therapy can be expected.

The use of testosterone to improve libido or augment fertility in the male dog is contraindicated. Exogenous androgens will decrease spermatogenesis because of negative feedback inhibition of LH secretion by the pituitary. Even though serum testosterone concentration may be elevated with exogenous supplementation, the intratesticular testosterone concentration will be inadequate to support spermatogenesis, and oligospermia can result. If a stud dog has poor libido, treatment of an underlying cause (i.e., prostatic disease) or behavior modification (i.e., increase exposure to estrous bitches) should be attempted.

For treatment of bitches with apparent infertility but normal estrous cyclicity, a thorough understanding of the complex ovarian cycle is necessary. There is no indication that FSH administration will augment follicular development in infertile bitches. Also, because of normal hormonal physiology, intermittent injections of GnRH to augment fertility would be predictably unsuccessful. Proper identification and treatment directed at the cause of infertility should be attempted whenever possible.

### Estrus Suppression

Megestrol acetate (Ovaban, Schering-Plough, Kenilworth, NJ) is a progestogen compound approved for use in the bitch for estrus suppression and prevention of ovulation (also see "Use of Progesterone-Suppressing Drugs for Termination of Unwanted Pregnancy in Dogs," this volume, p 1075). Adverse effects of progestogen administration include inhibition of local uterine immunity and endometrial gland proliferation, both of which can increase the incidence of pyometra. The use of progestogens as contraceptives is *not recommended for bitches intended for future breeding*.

Mibolerone (Cheque, Upjohn, Kalamazoo, MI), a compound with androgenic and anabolic activity, is approved for use as a contraceptive in the bitch. Dosing information is provided on the product insert and is based on body weight in all but German shepherd bitches, which receive the maximum dose regardless of body weight. Folliculogenesis will be prevented if mibolerone is administered daily to bitches beginning no fewer than 30 days prior to the expected onset of the next proestrus. Because of teratogenic potential, bitches should not be bred if estrus occurs during mibolerone administration (breakthrough estrus). Androgens do not exert a trophic effect on endometrial glands and, therefore, increased incidence of pyometra is not expected. Adverse effects on the reproductive tract include clitoral hypertrophy, mucoid vaginal discharge, and atrophy of the glandular endometrium. Although mibolerone has fewer adverse effects than progestogens as contraceptives, the product package insert states it is *not recommended for use in bitches intended for future breeding*.

One clinical indication for the purposeful delay of estrus is to treat infertility in bitches that have ovulatory cycles with less than a 4.5-month interestrous interval. Frequent estrous cycles may not allow sufficient time for the endometrium to recover from the trophic influences of progesterone during a nonpregnant diestrus. Mibolerone suppression of ovarian activity for a period of 6 to 9 months has been recommended after ruling out other causes of infertility in bitches with short interestrous intervals. Success rates using mibolerone for this purpose have not been reported.

Testosterone injections are often administered to racing greyhound bitches to prevent estrous cyclicity. A major problem after retirement from the track and testosterone withdrawal is prolonged anestrus for which there is no successful treatment. The advantage of track performance must be evaluated versus the potential sequela to later reproductive performance in these cases.

### Pregnancy Prevention

The use of either estradiol cypionate (ECP) or DES as a treatment to prevent pregnancy in cases of misalliance (mismating) is unsafe. Not only is there a high chance of fatal estrogen-induced bone marrow suppression, but bitches that survive treatment with estrogens for this purpose may be rendered infertile due to estrogen-induced endometritis and pyometra. Whereas most cases of bone marrow toxicity have been associated with ECP administered at high doses (i.e., >1.0 mg total or >22 μg/kg), aplastic anemia has occurred in bitches treated at lower doses; thus one should consider less deleterious techniques to prevent unwanted pregnancy (see "Use of Progesterone-Suppressing Drugs for Termination of Unwanted Pregnancy in Dogs," this volume, p 1075).

### Reducing the Signs of Pseudocyesis

Mibolerone can be used to alleviate clinical signs of pseudocyesis. While signs of pseudocyesis such as nesting and galactorrhea are not considered abnormal and in general pose no health problem, some bitches can become aggressive and agitated. In one study, 17 of 22 bitches treated with 16 μg mibolerone/kg PO for 5 days had improvement in the signs of pseudocyesis (Brown, 1984).

## References and Suggested Reading

Bouchard G: Estrus induction in the bitch with the synthetic estrogen diethylstilbestrol. In Proc 2nd Inter Symp Canine and Feline Reprod 1992, p 160.
*A preliminary report of the administration of DES (5 mg/bitch/day for 6 to 9 days) to induce estrus in five mongrel bitches.*

Bouchard G, Youngquist RS, Clark B, et al: Estrus induction in the bitch using a combination diethylstilbestrol and FSH-P. Theriogenology 36:51, 1991.
*Estrus induction was attempted in eight bitches using a protocol of oral DES followed by injections of FSH.*

Brown JM: Efficacy and dosage titration study of mibolerone for the treatment of pseudopregnancy in the bitch. J Am Vet Med Assoc 184:14667, 1984.
*Report of 22 bitches treated with mibolerone (16 μg/kg/day for 5 days PO) to alleviate signs of pseudopregnancy.*

Cain JL, Cain GR, Feldman EC, et al: Use of pulsatile intravenous administration of gonadotropin-releasing hormone to induce fertile estrus in bitches. Am J Vet Res 49:1993, 1988.
*An estrus induction method using GnRH administered IV via a pulsatile infusion pump in eight beagle bitches.*

Cain JL, Davidson AD, Cain GR, et al: Induction of ovulation in bitches using subcutaneous injections of gonadotropin-releasing hormone analog (abstr). In Proc 8th Ann Vet Med Forum, ACVIM, 1990, p 1126.
*A preliminary report of the use of a GnRH agonist administered subcutaneously every 8 hr to induce fertile estrus in six bitches of various breeds.*

Cain JL, Lasley BL, Cain GR, et al: Induction of ovulation in bitches with pulsatile or continuous infusion of GnRH. J Reprod Fertil 39(suppl):143, 1989.
*Various doses of GnRH administered by continuous infusion to attempt estrus induction in eight beagle bitches.*

Concannon PW: Induction of fertile oestrus in anoestrous dog by constant infusion of GnRH agonist. J Reprod Fertil 39(suppl):149, 1989.
*A GnRH agonist was administered by constant infusion via a miniosmotic pump to 24 beagle bitches to attempt estrus induction.*

Feldman EC and Nelson RW: Disorders of the canine male reproductive tract. In Canine and Feline Endocrinology and Reproduction. Philadelphia, WB Saunders Co, 1987, p 493.
*Description of a protocol to treat cryptorchidism in dogs using injections of HCG.*

Johnston SD: Reproductive disorders: Diagnostic endocrinology. Proc 54th Ann Meeting Am Anim Hosp Assoc, Phoenix, AZ, 1987, p 184.
*Report of serum testosterone concentrations in dogs after an injection of HCG.*

Moses DL and Shille VM: Induction of estrus in greyhound bitches with prolonged idiopathic anestrus or with suppression of estrus after testosterone administration. J Am Vet Med Assoc 192:1541, 1988.
*Seven bitches induced into fertile estrus with oral DES followed by an injection of LH and two injections of FSH.*

Scott-Moncrieff JC, Nelson RW, Bill RL, et al: Serum disposition of exogenous progesterone after intramuscular administration in bitches. Am J Vet Res 51:893, 1990.
*Injections of progesterone in oil (3 mg/kg IM every 24 hr) will maintain serum progesterone concentration at ≥10 ng/ml.*

# USE OF PROGESTERONE-SUPPRESSING DRUGS FOR TERMINATION OF UNWANTED PREGNANCY IN DOGS

PATRICK W. CONCANNON

*Ithaca, New York*

For the majority of bitches, the most appropriate means to prevent the birth of an unwanted litter following an unplanned mating is to perform an ovariohysterectomy following the diagnosis of pregnancy by ultrasound or by palpation around 3 to 4 weeks after mating. However, for some bitches there is a real or perceived need to maintain the potential for future reproduction, and a pharmacologic means of pregnancy termination is requested. The administration of high doses of estrogen in the form to estradiol cypionate (ECP) has become common, but is no longer recommended because of potential side effects of uterine disease and blood dyscrasias, and because there is no dose that routinely can be considered to be both safe and effective (Bowen et al., 1985). Ethical and legal concerns regarding the use of ECP should also be considered. Other estrogens have not been adequately studied for efficacy and safety. The alternative experimental methods reviewed here all act by removing the normal progesterone support of the uteroplacental unit and the normal progesterone blockade of uterine contraction, both of which are required for the maintenance of normal pregnancy.

## PROSTAGLANDINS

### Prostaglandin $F_{2\alpha}$

Prostaglandin $F_{2\alpha}$ (PGF) is luteolytic in pregnant and nonpregnant dogs (Concannon et al., 1989) if given repeatedly. Dinoprost tromethamine, a veterinary preparation of naturally occurring PGF (Prostin-F or Lutalyse, Upjohn) is currently used for the termination of pregnancy at mid gestation (Wichtel et al., 1990; Concannon et al., 1989; Feldman et al., 1993) and even earlier, around the time of implantation (Oettlé et al., 1988; Romagnoli, Cela, and Camillo, 1991) (also see "Pregnancy Termination in the Bitch Using Prostaglandin $F_{2\alpha}$," this volume, p 1079). In the United States, these preparations are not Food and Drug Administration (FDA) approved for use in dogs. As outlined in

Table 1, PGF is effective at doses of 30 to 250 $\mu$g/kg, only if given two or more times a day, for 4 or more days or "to effect." Doses, side effects, and efficacy have been reviewed extensively (Concannon and Meyers-Wallen, 1991; Concannon et al., 1989; Feldman et al., 1993) and are considered in detail elsewhere in this volume (also see "Pregnancy Termination in the Bitch Using Prostaglandin $F_{2\alpha}$," this volume, p 1079). Administration three times a day may be more effective than twice a day. Delaying treatment until after diagnosis of pregnancy avoids the treatment of nonpregnant bitches. In one study, 62% of bitches claimed to be mismated were not actually pregnant (Feldman et al., 1993).

## Synthetic Analogs of PGF

Only the synthetic form of native PGF has been recommended because there have been no studies of either safety or efficacy using a sufficient range of doses of any of the more potent PGF analogs. The only readily available PGF analog reported to terminate pregnancy in dogs with acceptable side effects is cloprostenol; however, this preparation is *not* FDA approved for use in dogs. Cloprostenol can terminate pregnancy in dogs at doses of 2.5 $\mu$g/kg given subcutaneously three times at 48-hr intervals (see Fieni et al. in Concannon et al., 1989). In that study, side effects were reduced by fasting, or by administration of additional drugs including the anticholinergic atropine, prior to PGF administration.

## DOPAMINE AGONISTS

### Bromocriptine

Pituitary prolactin is a required luteotropin in dogs. Prolactin secretion is normally regulated in part by the

**Table 1.** *Effective Experimental, Proposed, and Nonapproved Methods Reported for Termination of Pregnancy in Dogs Following Unwanted Matings*

| Drug | Day of Cycle | Day of Diestrus | Dose (Frequency and Route) | Days | Efficacy[°] | Side Effects[†] | References[‡] |
|---|---|---|---|---|---|---|---|
| **Prostaglandins** | | | | | | | |
| Prostaglandin $F_{2\alpha}$ | 25–49 | (DD 17–41) | 30–250 $\mu$g/kg ($\geq$b.i.d.; IM, SC) | 4–11 | 80–100%[°] | Yes[†] | 1,2,3 |
| | 30–40 | (DD 22–32) | 100, 200 $\mu$g/kg (q8h; IM, SC) | 3–9 | 100% | Yes[†] | 4 |
| | 13–27 | (DD 5–19) | 250 $\mu$g/kg (b.i.d.; IM, SC) | 4–6 | 80–100%[°] | Yes[†] | 5 |
| | 6–11 | (DD 1) | 250 $\mu$g/kg (b.i.d.; IM, SC) | 5 | 0% | Yes[†] | 1,2 |
| Cloprostenol | 30–40 | (DD 22–32) | 2.5 $\mu$g/kg (q48h; IM, SC) | 4 | 100% | Yes[†] | 1 |
| **Dopamine Agonists** | | | | | | | |
| Bromocriptine | 42 | (DD 34) | 100 $\mu$g/kg (b.i.d.; IM, PO) | 6 | 100% | Yes[†] | 6 |
| | 35–45 | (DD 28–38) | 30–60 $\mu$g/kg (b.i.d.; PO) | 4–6 | 50% | Yes[†] | 3 |
| | 35–45 | (DD 28–38) | 100 $\mu$g/kg (b.i.d.; IM, PO) | $\geq$7 | 100% | Yes[†] | 7 |
| Cabergoline | 30–40 | (DD 22–32) | 1.7 $\mu$g/kg (daily; SC) | 6 | 70–100%[°] | Yes? | 8 |
| | 25 | (DD 17) | 15 $\mu$g/kg (daily; PO) | 5 | 0% | Yes? | 9 |
| | 45 | (DD 37) | 5 $\mu$g/kg (daily; PO) | 5 | 100% | No? | 9 |
| **Other Drugs** | | | | | | | |
| Mifepristone | 32 | (DD 24) | 2.5 mg/kg (b.i.d.) | 4 | 100% | No? | 10 |
| | 20–35 | (DD 12–28) | 10–20 mg/kg (once) | 1 | 100% | No? | 11 |
| Epostane | 10 | (DD 1) | 3–7 mg/kg (daily) | 7 | 100% | No? | 1,2 |

[°]Efficacy is increased to 100% by continuing treatment to effect; that is, treating until verification of complete pregnancy termination based on palpation or on ultrasound examination after day 25 of cycle when fetal heartbeats are normally detectable (also see "Ultrasonography of the Reproductive Tract of the Female Dog and Cat," this volume, p 1040).
[†]Predictable nonlethal side effects considered preferable to potentially lethal side effect of depoestrogen treatment.
[‡]Sources include:

1. Concannon, Morton, and Weir: J Reprod Fertil 139 (suppl):350, 1988.
2. Concannon and Myers-Wallen: J Am Vet Med Assoc 198(7):1214, 1991.
3. Wichtel et al: Theriogenology 33(4):829, 1990.
4. Feldman et al: J Am Vet Med Assoc 202:1855, 1993.
5. Romagnoli, Cela, and Camillo: Vet Clin North Am [Small Anim Pract] 21(3):487, 1991.
6. Concannon et al: J Reprod Fertil 81:175, 1987.
7. Unpublished protocol.
8. Onclin et al: J Reprod Fertil 47(suppl):403, 1993.
9. Post, Evans, and Jochle: Theriogenology 29:1233, 1988.
10. Concannon et al: J Reprod Fertil 88:99, 1990.
11. Sankai: et al: J Vet Med Sci 53(6):1069, 1991.

inhibitory action of hypothalamic dopamine. Prolactin levels are routinely elevated after day 30 of pregnancy. Administration of a dopamine agonist can terminate pregnancy during mid or late gestation by suppressing prolactin secretion and, thus, progesterone secretion. Tolerated doses given systemically or orally before day 25 only cause slight or transient reductions in progesterone (Concannon et al., 1987) and termination of pregnancy has only been reported for dopamine-agonist administration after day 25. In the United States, the dopamine agonist bromocriptine (Parlodel, Sandoz) is available for treatment of hyperprolactinemia in humans.[*] Presumably, oral doses of 100 $\mu$g/kg, twice daily, would be reliable in terminating pregnancy if given to effect, which in some dogs could be 7 days or more, but the necessary testing has not been reported. Emesis is a common side effect and retention of oral doses has not been studied in dogs. Side effects of emesis and of inappetence can be of considerable concern if owners and staff are not forewarned. As with prostaglandins or other methods, treatment after days 35 to 40 is likely to result in some expulsion of uterine contents (abortion) rather than complete resorption.

## Cabergoline

The dopamine agonist cabergoline, available in Europe, is effective at much lower doses and is claimed to have fewer and less severe side effects (see Jochle et al. in Concannon et al., 1989). Cabergoline doses of 1.7 $\mu$g/kg injected every 2 days over 6 days terminated pregnancy in 25%, 67%, and 100% of bitches first treated on days 25, 30, and 40 of pregnancy, respectively (Onclin et al., 1993). An oral dose of 15 $\mu$g/kg daily for 5 days was not effective at day 25, but a dose of 5 $\mu$g/kg daily for 5 days was routinely effective at day 45. At publication, this drug was not available in the United States.

## OTHER HORMONAL INTERCEPTIVES

### Epostane

Epostane is a steroid-shaped molecule that inhibits steroid synthesis because it is a competitive inhibitor of the hydroxysteroid-dehydrogenase-isomerase enzyme system, which converts pregnenolone to progesterone. Oral or parenteral administration results in a decrease in the production of progesterone. In many species the effect appears to be more prominent in the ovaries and/or placenta than in the adrenals. Epostane has been shown to terminate pregnancy in dogs when give orally (50 mg/dog/day) for 7 days starting on the first day of diestrus (metestrus) as determined by vaginal cytology (see Keister et al. in Concannon et al., 1989). It will also terminate pregnancy when administered later in gestation. No adverse side effects have been reported. Efficacy is associated with a decline in progesterone to low levels during treatment, and a rise in progesterone after the end of treatment. Interest in marketing epostane as a treatment for mismating in dogs has been significant in recent years. However, additional trials on safety, efficacy, and dose requirements in dogs of various sizes and breeds are still needed, and it is not commercially available in the United States.

### Gonadotropin-Releasing Hormone Antagonists

Antagonists of gonadotropin-releasing hormone (GnRH) act by competitive binding to GnRH receptors, rapid inhibition of GnRH action, and suppression of the secretion of luteinizing hormone (LH) and follicle-stimulating hormone (FSH), with a resulting decline in ovarian steroid secretion. Luteinizing hormone is a required luteotrophin in dogs. A single injection of a potent GnRH antagonist suppressed luteal function and terminated pregnancy in bitches when administered at mid gestation (see Vickery et al. in Concannon et al., 1989). Efficacy was reduced when administered only once earlier in pregnancy. Administration of a PGF analog along with the GnRH antagonist in early pregnancy resulted in a more protracted, albeit transient, luteolysis and greater anticonceptive efficacy. Treatment was effective as early as day 2 of diestrus in some dogs but not others. Use of multiple doses of a GnRH antagonist in early pregnancy has not been reported. Gonadotropin-releasing hormone antagonists are relatively expensive to manufacture, and commercial availability for veterinary use is unlikely in the near future.

### Antiprogestin Therapy

Administration of a progesterone antagonist at effective doses will prevent establishment of pregnancy or terminate pregnancy in several species if administered before implantation. The most extensively studied antiprogestin, mifepristone (RU 486), has been shown to bind to the progesterone receptor with high affinity and to prevent progesterone-directed changes in deoxyribonucleic acid (DNA) transcription in progesterone target tissues. Mifepristone can also act as a glucocorticoid antagonist. Doses that have strong antiprogesterone action and little anticorticoid action in dogs have been determined. Administration of mifepristone orally at a dose of 2.5 mg/kg twice daily for 4.5 days starting at day 32 of pregnancy resulted in complete fetal resorption in all bitches tested (Concannon et al., 1990).

---

[*]Fractions of original tablets, or portions of pulverized tablets placed in gelatin capsules, can yield body weight–adjusted doses for dogs of approximately 0.1 mg/kg/day or 0.05–0.1 mg/kg (i.e., 50 to 100 $\mu$g/kg) per 12 hr. Treatment for 4 to 7 days, or to effect, will terminate pregnancy after day 30 (Concannon et al., 1987) at systemic doses of 100 $\mu$g/kg once or twice a day, and in some cases at oral doses of 30 $\mu$g/kg twice daily (see Concannon and Meyers-Wallen, 1991). However, use of oral doses of 62.5 $\mu$g/kg, twice daily, for 6 days was ineffective in some dogs (Wichtel et al., 1990).

Based on ultrasound observations, pregnancy termination (resorption) occurred by 3.5 to 4 days of treatment, and was without adverse clinical side effects. Single injections of mifepristone at doses of 20 mg/kg have also terminated pregnancy as early as days 20 to 25 of gestation in dogs (Sankai et al., 1991). No commercial effort to develop or test an antiprogestin for veterinary application has been reported, perhaps due to the controversy surrounding the potential use of such compounds (e.g., RU 486) for human fertility regulation.

## GLUCOCORTICOIDS

### Dexamethasone

Serial injections of dexamethasone can terminate pregnancy in dogs. Successful termination of pregnancy was reported for doses of 5 mg/dog IM, every 12 hr, administered for 10 days, starting at day 30 or 45 of pregnancy (Austad, Lunde, and Sjaastad, 1976). Treatment caused a decline in progesterone. Intrauterine death and resorptions or abortions occurred within a few days of the end of treatment. Recent unpublished studies by Zone and Wanke and colleagues at the University of Buenos Aires suggest that orally administered dexamethasone doses of 0.1 to 0.2 mg/kg, administered twice daily for 8 days beginning around day 35 of pregnancy will also terminate pregnancy. The mechanism of action may involve the release of luteolytic amounts of endogenous PGF, as occurs at normal parturition, but PGF has not been measured in these studies. Furthermore, additional studies are needed to determine if the corticoid side effects seen during treatment are clinically acceptable. Therefore, the use of glucocorticoids for the termination of pregnancy in dogs cannot be recommended until further information on efficacy and side effects is published.

## References and Suggested Reading

Austad R, Lunde A, and Sjaastad OV: Peripheral plasma levels of oestradiol-17β and progesterone in the bitch during the oestrus cycle, in normal pregnancy and after dexamethasone treatment. J Reprod Fertil 46:129, 1976.
*Reports the resorption or abortion of fetuses in bitches treated with dexamethasone every 12 hr for 10 days beginning at day 30 or 45 of pregnancy, and associated changes in progesterone and estrogen.*

Bowen RA, Olson PN, Behrendt MD, et al: Efficacy and toxicity of estrogens commonly used to terminate canine pregnancy. J Am Vet Med Assoc 186:783, 1985.
*Reports the efficacy of pregnancy prevention and the incidence of pyometra in dogs administered oral DES, and in dogs administered a single injection of estradiol cypionate in proestrus, estrus, or after end of estrus.*

Concannon PW and Meyers-Wallen VN: Current and proposed methods for contraception and termination of pregnancy in dogs and cats. J Am Vet Med Assoc 198:1214, 1991.
*Reviews the use of ovariohysterectomy and the use of progestins and androgens as methods to prevent or curtail estrous cycles, and the use of estrogens, prostaglandins, steroidogenesis inhibitors, antiprogestins, and dopamine agonists to prevent or terminate pregnancy following unwanted matings (76 references).*

Concannon PW, Morton DB, and Weir BJ: Dog and Cat Reproduction, Contraception and Artificial Insemination. Proc 1st Int Symp Canine and Feline Reprod. Cambridge, The Journals of Reproduction and Fertility Ltd, 1989, p 350.
*Monograph with 40 review papers and research reports on canine and feline reproduction topics including pregnancy termination by prostaglandin, dopamine agonists, and epostane.*

Concannon PW, Weinstein R, Whaley S, et al: Suppression of luteal function in dogs by luteinizing hormone anti-serum and by bromocriptine. J Reprod Fertil 81:175, 1987.
*Reports the termination of pregnancy in bitches treated with the dopamine agonist bromocriptine at day 42 of gestation, but not at day 8 or 22 of gestation.*

Concannon PW, Yeager A, Frank D, et al: Termination of pregnancy and induction of premature luteolysis by the antiprogestagen, mifepristone, in dogs. J Reprod Fertil 88:99, 1990.
*Reports termination of pregnancy in dogs administered the antiprogestin orally twice a day for 4.5 days starting at day 32 of gestation.*

Feldman EC, Davidson AP, Nelson WN, et al: Prostaglandin induction of abortion in pregnant bitches after misalliance. J Am Vet Med Assoc 202:1855, 1993.
*Reports that 62% of bitches presented for prevention of unwanted pregnancy were actually nonpregnant. Reports 100% efficacy and various side effects for PGF$_{2\alpha}$ administered every 8 to 12 hr at doses of 0.1 to 0.25 mg/kg for 9 days or less for termination of day 30 to 35 pregnancies following unwanted matings.*

Onclin K, Silva LDM, Donnay I, et al: Luteotrophic function of prolactin in dogs and the effects of a dopamine agonist, cabergoline. J Reprod Fertil 47(suppl):403, 1993.
*Reports pregnancy termination as a result of cabergoline administration in four of six dogs treated at day 30 of pregnancy and five of five dogs treated at day 40 of pregnancy, but only one of four dogs treated at day 25 of pregnancy.*

Post K, Evans LE, and Jochle W: Effects of prolactin suppression with cabergoline on the pregnancy of the bitch. Theriogenology 29:1233, 1988.
*Reports efficacy of pregnancy termination for cabergoline at doses of 5 to 15 μg/kg/day for 5 to 28 days, including failure in early and mid gestation and success when initiated around day 45 of pregnancy.*

Romagnoli SE, Cela M, and Camillo F: Use of prostaglandin F2a for early pregnancy termination in the mismatched bitch. Vet Clin North Am [Small Anim Pract] 21(3):487, 1991.
*Reports 80% efficacy in termination of early pregnancy by administration of PGF$_{2\alpha}$ ( (250 μg/kg, b.i.d.) for 4 days beginning 5 or more days after end of cytologic estrus.*

Sankai T, Endo T, Kanayama K, et al: Antiprogesterone compound, RU486 administration to terminate pregnancy in dogs and cats. J Vet Med Sci 53:1069, 1991.
*Reports termination of pregnancy in dogs by administering the antiprogestin mifepristone at a dose of 10–20 mg/kg once at 11–35 days after mating.*

Wichtel JJ, Whitacre MD, Yates DJ, et al: Comparison of the effects of PGF2a and bromocryptine in pregnant beagle bitches. Theriogenology 33:829, 1990.
*Reports termination of pregnancy after mid gestation in dogs, including use of PGF$_{2\alpha}$ (125 μg/kg, b.i.d., SC) with 100% efficacy and use of bromocriptine (62.5 μg/kg, b.i.d., PO) with only 50% efficacy.*

# PREGNANCY TERMINATION IN THE BITCH USING PROSTAGLANDIN $F_{2\alpha}$

MARGARET V. ROOT
*and* SHIRLEY D. JOHNSTON
*St. Paul, Minnesota*

Prostaglandin $F_{2\alpha}$ ($PGF_{2\alpha}$) is an agent that can be used for pregnancy termination at any stage of gestation in the bitch. It has no life-threatening side effects, and does not adversely affect future fertility.

## MECHANISM OF ACTION

Prostaglandin $F_{2\alpha}$ is a luteolytic agent produced by the uterus, which may cause decline in ovarian progesterone secretion at the end of diestrus. Close apposition of the uterine and ovarian vessels in mammals allows local diffusion of endogenous $PGF_{2\alpha}$ from the uterine veins to the ovarian arteries, allowing a large dose of $PGF_{2\alpha}$ to reach the ovary in domestic ruminants, swine, and horses. In the ovary, $PGF_{2\alpha}$ acts indirectly, causing decreased luteal blood flow and subsequent hypoxia of the corpus luteum (CL), and directly, causing luteal cell death and decreased progesterone production. The end result is regression of the CL and cessation of progesterone production. In both pregnant and nonpregnant bitches, this phenomenon probably occurs naturally at the end of diestrus.

All domestic mammals are dependent on progesterone throughout gestation for pregnancy maintenance. In bitches, abortion usually will occur if serum progesterone concentrations fall below 2 ng/ml for 36 to 48 hr. The CL is the primary source of gestational progesterone in the bitch. Therefore, any compound that causes luteolysis will cause a decrease in progesterone production, and subsequent abortion.

In the bitch, the CL is not uniformly responsive to the luteolytic action of $PGF_{2\alpha}$ throughout diestrus. Day one of diestrus is the first day after estrus on which vaginal cytology consists of predominantly noncornified cells. Serum progesterone concentrations do not decline in dogs treated with $PGF_{2\alpha}$ before day five of diestrus. The CL is responsive to high doses of $PGF_{2\alpha}$ after day five of diestrus, and responsiveness appears to increase as diestrus progresses, allowing the use of lower doses of $PGF_{2\alpha}$ later in gestation.

Prostaglandin $F_{2\alpha}$ also acts as an ecbolic agent, causing contraction of the smooth muscle of the uterus. This may contribute to its efficacy as an abortifacient.

## PROTOCOL

Dosage recommendations made here refer *only* to use of the THAM salt of the native compound, $PGF_{2\alpha}$

(Lutalyse, Upjohn, Kalamazoo, MI). Prostaglandin analogues have been used experimentally to induce abortion in the bitch, but the various compounds differ greatly in potency, and doses are not interchangeable between native and analogue compounds.

The appropriate treatment regimen may vary, depending on the stage of gestation at which the bitch is presented (Fig. 1). There is no accurate early pregnancy test in the dog, making it difficult to determine efficacy of the protocol by monitoring fetal loss during the first 25 to 28 days of gestation. Treatment response is monitored, therefore, by measurement of serum progesterone concentrations. If luteolysis is induced, serum progesterone concentrations will decrease to less than 2 ng/ml. Successful pregnancy termination usually requires that serum progesterone concentrations remain less than 2 ng/ml for 36 to 48 hr.

The currently recommended regimen for $PGF_{2\alpha}$ pregnancy termination in the first half of gestation is 250 $\mu$g/kg $PGF_{2\alpha}$ every 12 hr SC for 4 days, starting at least 5 days after onset of cytologic diestrus. After the eighth injection of $PGF_{2\alpha}$, a blood sample should be drawn for measurement of serum progesterone concentrations. Because treatment failures have been reported in the literature using this regimen, the bitch should be examined several weeks after treatment to verify pregnancy termination.

In the second half of gestation, pregnancy should be verified by palpation and/or ultrasound before therapy is instituted. Treatment response is determined by monitoring completeness of pregnancy termination.

The currently recommended regimen for $PGF_{2\alpha}$ pregnancy termination in the second half of gestation is 250 $\mu$g/kg $PGF_{2\alpha}$ every 12 hr SC until abortion is complete. Duration of therapy is determined by length of time required for abortion to be complete as monitored by serial radiographic or ultrasonographic examinations. The bitch will pass aborted tissues vaginally. Serum progesterone concentrations should be measured at the time of the final treatment to monitor completeness of luteolysis, and the bitch should be examined, ultrasonographically if possible, after treatment to verify completeness of pregnancy termination.

Lower doses of $PGF_{2\alpha}$ have been demonstrated to successfully induce luteolysis and abortion in the latter half of gestation in the dog, but more treatment failures were reported at these lower doses.

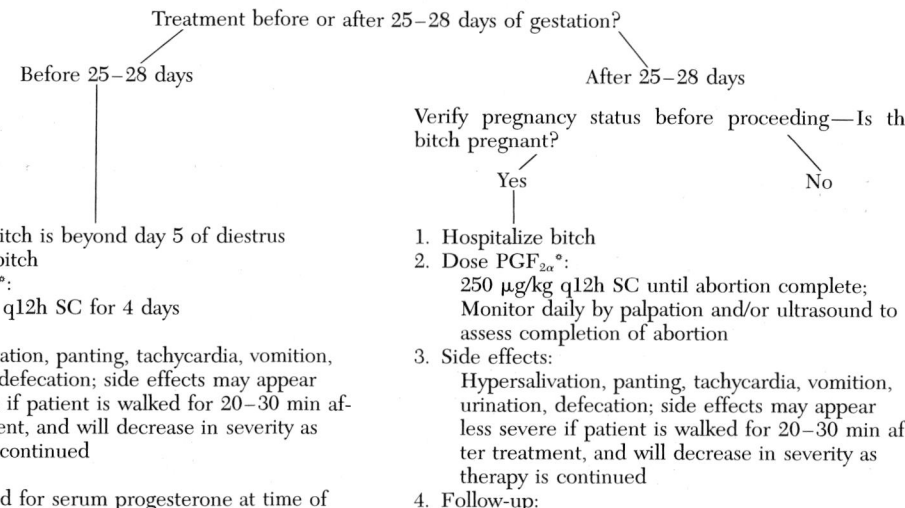

Treatment before or after 25–28 days of gestation?

Before 25–28 days

After 25–28 days

Verify pregnancy status before proceeding—Is the bitch pregnant?

Yes                                        No

1. Verify that bitch is beyond day 5 of diestrus
2. Hospitalize bitch
3. Dose PGF$_{2\alpha}$°:
   250 µg/kg q12h SC for 4 days
4. Side effects:
   Hypersalivation, panting, tachycardia, vomition, urination, defecation; side effects may appear less severe if patient is walked for 20–30 min after treatment, and will decrease in severity as therapy is continued
5. Follow-up:
   Draw blood for serum progesterone at time of last injection of PGF$_{2\alpha}$; progesterone <2 ng/ml is indicative of luteolysis
   Check pregnancy status 4 weeks later by palpation, ultrasound, and/or radiology
   Bitch may show earlier return to estrus than expected

1. Hospitalize bitch
2. Dose PGF$_{2\alpha}$°:
   250 µg/kg q12h SC until abortion complete;
   Monitor daily by palpation and/or ultrasound to assess completion of abortion
3. Side effects:
   Hypersalivation, panting, tachycardia, vomition, urination, defecation; side effects may appear less severe if patient is walked for 20–30 min after treatment, and will decrease in severity as therapy is continued
4. Follow-up:
   Draw blood for serum progesterone at end of therapy; progesterone <2 ng/ml is indicative of luteolysis
   Verify completeness of pregnancy termination at end of therapy by palpation, ultrasound, and/or radiology
   Bitch may show earlier return to estrus than expected

°Lutalyse, The Upjohn Company, Kalamazoo, MI, 49001.

**Figure 1.** Algorithm for PGF$_{2\alpha}$ pregnancy termination in the dog

## PRECAUTIONS

The side effects of PGF$_{2\alpha}$ are referable to its action on smooth muscle. While the effect of causing uterine smooth muscle contraction may contribute to the efficacy of PGF$_{2\alpha}$ as an abortifacient, it also causes a dose-dependent stimulation of gastrointestinal smooth muscle contraction. Reported side effects of PGF$_{2\alpha}$ administration include hypersalivation, panting, tachycardia, vomition, urination, defecation, and transient hypothermia. Locomotor incoordination and mild central nervous system signs have been reported in dogs treated with doses that approached the LD$_{50}$ of PGF$_{2\alpha}$ (5.13 mg/kg). Side effects usually will diminish within 30 min of administration of the drug, and will decrease in severity over the treatment course. Side effects may be minimized by walking the bitch for 20 to 30 min after injection of PGF$_{2\alpha}$. Preliminary studies suggest that concurrent administration of atropine may also decrease severity of side effects. Reported doses of atropine range from 100 to 500 µg/kg SC given at the time of PGF$_{2\alpha}$ injection.

Prostaglandin F$_{2\alpha}$ treatment has not been shown to adversely affect fertility in the bitch. Induction of luteolysis causes premature termination of diestrus, and the owner should be aware that the bitch may come back into estrus earlier than expected. The shortening of the interestrous interval is dependent on the degree to which early termination of the diestrus occurred.

## References and Suggested Reading

Concannon PW and Meyers-Wallen VN: Current and proposed methods for contraception and termination of pregnancy in dogs and cats. J Am Vet Med Assoc 198:1214, 1991.
   *A review of the mechanism of action, efficacy, side-effects, and availability of abortifacients and contraceptives for dogs and cats.*
Concannon PW and Hansel W: Prostaglandin F2 alpha induced luteolysis, hypothermia, and abortions in beagle bitches. Prostaglandins 13:533, 1977.
   *A study of the effect of treatment with 20 to 30 µg/kg PGF$_{2\alpha}$ every 8 to 12 hr SC during mid gestation on serum progesterone concentrations, and pregnancy maintenance.*
Feldman EC, Davidson AP, Nelson RW, et al: Effect of prostaglandin F2 alpha THAM in the bitch. J Am Vet Med Assoc 202:1855, 1993.
   *A study of the effect of treatment with 100 to 250 µg/kg PGF$_{2\alpha}$ every 8 to 12 hr SC on serum progesterone concentrations and pregnancy maintenance.*
Johnston SD: Canine pregnancy termination with prostaglandin F2 alpha. Society for Theriogenology Proceedings, Annual Meeting, Toronto, Ontario, 1990, p 264.
   *A review of experimental protocols for pregnancy termination with PGF$_{2\alpha}$ and recommendations for best protocol.*
Lein DH, Concannon PW, Hornbuckle WE, et al: Termination of pregnancy in bitches by administration of prostaglandin F2 alpha. J Reprod Fertil 39(suppl):231, 1989.
   *A review of normal physiology in the pregnant bitch, and experimental protocols for pregnancy termination with PGF$_{2\alpha}$.*
Oettlé EE, Bertschinger HJ, Botha AE, et al: Luteolysis in early diestrous beagle bitches. Theriogenology 29:757, 1988.
   *A study of the effect of treatment with 250 µg/kg PGF$_{2\alpha}$ every 12 hr SC during early diestrus on pregnancy maintenance.*
Paradis M, Post K, and Mapletoft RJ: Effects of prostaglandin F2 alpha on corpora lutea formation and function in mated bitches. Can Vet J 24:239, 1983.
   *A study of the effect of treatment with 250 µg/kg PGF$_{2\alpha}$ every 12 hr IM during early or mid diestrus on serum progesterone concentrations, and pregnancy maintenance.*
Sokolowski JH: The effect of ovariectomy on pregnancy maintenance in the bitch. Lab Anim Sci 21:696, 1971.
   *A study proving that the dog is dependent on luteal progesterone for pregnancy maintenance throughout gestation.*

# MEDICAL TREATMENT OF PYOMETRA WITH PROSTAGLANDIN F$_{2\alpha}$ IN THE DOG AND CAT

AUTUMN P. DAVIDSON

*Davis, California*

## ETIOPATHOGENESIS

The cystic endometrial hyperplasia-pyometra complex is a progesterone-mediated uterine disorder. During the luteal phase of the estrous cycle, progesterone suppresses intrauterine leukocyte response to foreign stimuli, decreases myometrial contractility, and stimulates endometrial gland development and activity. The resultant uterine quiescence is a prerequisite for normal pregnancy. The nongravid diestrual uterus is flaccid and contains endometrial gland secretions, previously elaborated in response to estrogen elevated earlier during the estrous cycle. These secretions are a potential growth medium for bacteria. Bacteria can reach the uterus via ascension of normal flora from the distal portion of the genitourinary tract or, less frequently, by hematogenous spread. *Escherichia coli* is most commonly isolated from both bitches and queens with pyometra. A strong correlation exists between the onset of clinical signs of pyometra and recent diestrus. The incidence of pyometra is thought to be greater in the bitch than in the queen, presumably because the former is a spontaneous ovulator, found under the influence of elevated progesterone concentrations more frequently. The incidence of cystic endometrial hyperplasia, however, in the older queen is significant, thought due to repeated cycles of estrogen elaboration with or without progesterone elevation (see "Complications of Noncopulatory Ovulation in Queens," this volume, p 1083). An increased incidence of pyometra occurs with exogenous estrogen administration in the bitch; estrogen potentiates the effects of progesterone.

Administration of exogenous progesterone to queens can also precipitate pyometra (Shille, 1989; Johnson, 1989).

## CLINICAL SYNDROME

Pyometra can occur with or without purulent vaginal discharge, depending on the patency of the cervix. Closed-cervix pyometra is more serious, due to the potential for uterine rupture and septic peritonitis. The classic clinical signs of pyometra include copious vaginal discharge, partial to complete anorexia, lethargy, weight loss, an unkempt appearance, and polydipsia/polyuria. Most pets are considered ill (lethargic, ano-

rexic) by their owners at the time of examination. Abnormalities detected most frequently by physical examination include a mucopurulent to hemorrhagic vaginal discharge, palpable uterus, and pyrexia. Some bitches and queens have no physical signs of disease other than an abnormal vaginal discharge (Nelson, Feldman, and Stabenfeldt, 1982; Davidson, Feldman, and Nelson, 1990).

Clinicopathologic evaluation most commonly demonstrates neutrophilic leukocytosis, hyperfibrinogenemia, and hyperglobulinemia. Azotemia and low urinary specific gravity can reflect nephrogenic diabetes insipidus secondary to endotoxin elaboration by *E. coli*. Vaginal cytology shows septic inflammation. Plasma progesterone concentration is typically greater than or equal to 5 ng/ml, typical of diestrus.

Abdominal radiography can demonstrate a large, tubular, soft tissue density compatible with uterine enlargement. Ultrasonography is indicated to differentiate the enlarged, fluid-filled uterus of pyometra from early pregnancy. Pyometra can occur in one uterine horn, with viable pregnancy in the other (Nelson, Feldman, and Stabenfeldt, 1982; Davidson, Feldman, and Nelson, 1990).

## THERAPEUTIC OPTIONS

The treatment of choice for pyometra, following stabilization of the patient with intravenous fluids and antibiotics, is ovariohysterectomy, an undesirable option for valuable breeding bitches or queens. A salvage surgical treatment utilizing hysterotomy with placement of uterine drainage tubes has been reported (Vasseur and Feldman, 1982). Systemic antibiotic treatment alone, with or without antiseptic vaginal douching, is ineffective in resolving clinical signs. Medical management of open-cervix pyometra, using prostaglandin F$_{2\alpha}$ (PGF$_{2\alpha}$), has been successfully employed in both the bitch and queen (Nelson, Feldman, and Stabenfeldt, 1982; Davidson, Feldman, and Nelson, 1990).

## PROSTAGLANDIN TREATMENT

Successful treatment of pyometra by use of PGF$_{2\alpha}$ results from its effect on the uterine myometrium, cervix, and corpora lutea. $PGF_{2\alpha}$ stimulates uterine motility in bitches and, presumably, in queens. This myotonic effect increases intrauterine pressure. In women, a progressive decrease is observed in the concentration of endometrial prostaglandin receptor sites and myometrial smooth muscle closer to the cervix. Administration of $PGF_{2\alpha}$ should thus cause movement of uterine contents toward the cervix (Nelson, Feldman, and Stabenfeldt, 1982; Davidson, Feldman, and Nelson, 1990).

Although prostaglandin E has a relaxant effect on the rabbit and human cervix, reports on the effect of prostaglandin F on the cervix are inconsistent, restricting the recommended use of $PGF_{2\alpha}$ to treatment of patients with open-cervix pyometra (Davidson, Feldman, and Nelson, 1990). Complications related to the expulsion of septic uterine contents into the peritoneal cavity following myometrial contraction are infrequent with open-cervix pyometra, but are more likely with contraction against a closed cervix.

The luteolytic effect of $PGF_{2\alpha}$ has been observed in several domestic species. A decrease in plasma progesterone concentration occurs after $PGF_{2\alpha}$ administration to bitches and queens in diestrus, and is attributable to luteolysis or to an inhibition of steroidogenesis via depletion of intracellular free cholesterol. The luteolytic effect of $PGF_{2\alpha}$ is most reliable in late diestrus (Nelson, Feldman, and Stabenfeldt, 1982; Davidson, Feldman, and Nelson, 1990). The presence of live fetuses should be ruled out by use of ultrasonography prior to $PGF_{2\alpha}$ administration, because of the drug's abortifacient potential. Administration of $PGF_{2\alpha}$ causes abortion reliably in bitches after 30 days gestation, by causing luteolysis. Administration of $PGF_{2\alpha}$ causes abortion in queens after the 40th gestational day, presumably because of myometrial contraction and expulsion of uterine contents (i.e., fetuses). The $PGF_{2\alpha}$-induced decrease in luteal function should not induce abortion during late gestation because of concurrent placental production of progesterone in the queen (Davidson, Feldman, and Nelson, 1990). However, Vestegen et al. suggest that placental progesterone alone may not be sufficient to maintain pregnancy after 45 days of gestation.

Bitches and queens may be hospitalized for the duration of $PGF_{2\alpha}$ treatment as warranted by their clinical condition, to enable administration of adjunct supportive care, such as IV fluids and antibiotics; and to permit monitoring of adverse effects and outcome of treatment. Some could be treated on an outpatient basis. Concurrent administration of a broad-spectrum bactericidal antimicrobial is advised. The drug (Prostin F2 Alpha or Lutalyse [dinoprost tromethamine], Upjohn), 0.10 to 0.25 mg/kg of body weight, is administered SC every 24 hr for 3 to 5 days. Predictable physical reactions occur after SC injection of $PGF_{2\alpha}$ and include restlessness; panting; salivation; emesis; tenesmus; diarrhea; urination and mydriasis (bitch and queen); and grooming, lordosis, and kneading (queens). These reactions resolve within 1 hr after $PGF_{2\alpha}$ injection. After each subsequent $PGF_{2\alpha}$ administration, reactions diminish in severity and duration. Reactions are rarely considered severe enough to warrant discontinuation of

the drug (Nelson, Feldman, and Stabenfeldt, 1982; Davidson, Feldman, and Nelson, 1990). Adverse reactions observed after $PGF_{2\alpha}$ administration reflect the physiologic effects of endogenous prostaglandins. Endogenous prostaglandins are derived from dietary arachidonic acid by the action of cyclooxygenase, and mediate many normal physiologic processes, including vasodilation, hemostasis, pulmonary vasoconstriction and bronchodilation, gastrointestinal tract secretion, renal blood flow and glomerular filtration rate, inflammation, hyperalgesia, and fever. Prostaglandins regulate intracellular synthesis of cyclic adenosine monophosphate (cAMP) to induce alterations in cellular protein kinases, and ultimately cell function. The contractile effect of $PGF_{2\alpha}$ on the myometrial, gastrointestinal, tracheobronchial, and bladder smooth musculature accounts for the clinical responses observed (Boothe, 1984).

Successful short-term response, defined as resolution of the signs of pyometra, should be evident at the completion of $PGF_{2\alpha}$ treatment. At the time of release from the hospital, bitches and queens should have an improved appetite, normal rectal temperature, and diminished or no vaginal discharge. Initial reexamination should be scheduled within 2 weeks of $PGF_{2\alpha}$ administration, at which time little or no vaginal discharge, and no palpable evidence of uterine enlargement is expected. Abdominal radiography or ultrasonography can be used to evaluate reduction in uterine size, compared with that of previous examinations. Persistence of clinical signs warrants retreatment; sequential treatment of recurrent pyometra can be successful and could be considered if the bitch or queen's condition permits. Resolution of the immediate clinical signs of open pyometra following therapy varies from 82 to 100% (Johnson, 1989; Davidson, Feldman, and Nelson, 1990).

Successful long-term response is defined as a return to normal estrous cycles and, if bred, conception and carrying a litter to term. Breeding at the next estrus is recommended, to avoid the potential complications following progesterone's effects on a nongravid uterus. Prostaglandins do not resolve underlying cystic endometrial hyperplasia. The onset of proestrus in the bitch following $PGF_{2\alpha}$ therapy is variable. The onset of proestrus following $PGF_{2\alpha}$ treatment in queens varies from 0.5 to 12 months, suggesting the influence of day length on this seasonally polyestrous species. The overall conception rate following $PGF_{2\alpha}$ treatment has been reported as 40 to 82% in bitches and 85% in queens (Johnson, 1989; Davidson, Feldman, and Nelson, 1990).

Candidates for $PGF_{2\alpha}$ treatment should be young and otherwise healthy, with evidence of a patent cervix (i.e., vaginal discharge). Potential contraindications to the use of prostaglandins include planned pregnancy, sepsis, peritonitis, significant organic disease, or the presence of mummified fetal remains.

The response to $PGF_{2\alpha}$ therapy most likely depends on the degree of underlying uterine pathology rather than the dosage of $PGF_{2\alpha}$ (dinoprost tromethamine, Prostin F2 Alpha or Lutalyse, Upjohn). The lower dosage (0.10 mg/kg every 24 hr) is recommended, although the minimal effective dose of $PGF_{2\alpha}$ has not been established. *This dosage should only be used for natural $PGF_{2\alpha}$.* Synthetic $PGF_{2\alpha}$ is more potent in its actions than is natural $PGF_{2\alpha}$. The use of synthetic $PGF_{2\alpha}$ at the dosage recommended for natural $PGF_{2\alpha}$ could result in a *fatal outcome*. A safe and effective dosage of synthetic $PGF_{2\alpha}$ has not yet been established. Because prostaglandins are not approved for use in dogs or cats, informed consent must be obtained prior to their use (Boothe, 1984).

### References and Suggested Reading

Boothe DM: Prostaglandins: Physiology and clinical implications. Compend Contin Educ Pract Vet 6:1010, 1984.
  *Discussion of the pharmacology and physiology of prostaglandins.*

Davidson AP, Feldman EC, and Nelson RW: Treatment of feline pyometra with prostaglandin F2-alpha. Proc ACVIM Forum 8:1126, 1990.
  *Review of 20 feline pyometra cases successfully treated with $PGF_{2\alpha}$.*
Johnson CA: Uterine diseases. *In* Ettinger SJ (ed): *Textbook of Veterinary Internal Medicine.* Philadelphia, WB Saunders Co, 1989, p 1797.
  *Review of uterine disease in the bitch and queen.*
Nelson RW, Feldman EC, and Stabenfeldt GH: Treatment of canine pyometra and endometritis with prostaglandin $F_{2\alpha}$. J Am Vet Med Assoc 181:899, 1982.
  *Review of canine pyometra cases treated with $PGF_{2\alpha}$.*
Shille VM: Reproductive physiology and endocrinology of the female and male. *In* Ettinger SJ (ed): *Textbook of Veterinary Internal Medicine.* Philadelphia, WB Saunders Co, 1989, p 1777.
  *An overview of the physiology and endocrinology of reproduction.*
Vasseur PB and Feldman EC: Pyometra associated with extrauterine pregnancy in a cat. J Am Anim Hosp Assoc 18:872, 1982.
  *Description of surgical management of pyometra using uterine drainage and cannulation.*
Verstegen J, Onclin K, Donnay I, et al: Progesterone and Pregnancy Regulation in the Cat. *Proc 2nd Internat Symp Canine and Feline Reproduction,* Univ. of Liege, Faculty of Veterinary Medicine, Liege, Belgium, 1992.

# COMPLICATIONS OF NONCOPULATORY OVULATION IN QUEENS

DENNIS F. LAWLER
*St. Louis, Missouri*

*and* SHIRLEY D. JOHNSTON
*St. Paul, Minnesota*

The domestic cat is reported to be an induced ovulator, requiring copulation or mechanical stimulation of the cervix or vagina for release of luteinizing hormone (LH) and subsequent ovulation (Paape et al., 1975). Release of LH from the anterior pituitary follows copulation within minutes (Johnson and Gay, 1981), with maximum serum LH concentration occurring about 4 hr later (Goodrowe et al., 1989). Ovulation occurs 30 to 50 hr after copulation (Goodrowe et al., 1989). An increase in the number of copulations results in greater magnitude and duration of LH release (Concannon, Hodgson, and Lein, 1980) and greater likelihood of successful ovulation than occurs with a single copulation. Return to estrus occurs approximately 14 to 19 days after nonovulatory estrus (Paape et al., 1975; Shille, Lundstrom, and Stabenfeldt, 1979a).

Review of the literature provides evidence that the classically accepted sequence of events and mechanisms of ovulation in domestic cats may not occur universally or exclusively. Ovulation without cervical stimulation has been suggested occasionally from indirect evidence. The subjects of these reports frequently were household pet cats with an unknown history of social contact with male cats. Observational and prospective studies of female cats in a controlled environment have confirmed anecdotal reports of ovulation in domestic queens in the absence of copulation, although the mechanisms of these events remain to be elucidated.

## SUMMARY OF RECENT RESEARCH

One report described 44 intact female American shorthair cats with uterine disease (Lawler et al., 1991). Histopathologic examination of reproductive tissues revealed 19 (43.2%) queens with active or cystic follicles, and 25 (56.8%) queens with luteal-phase ovaries. Anatomic data were supported by endocrine assays demonstrating mean serum progesterone concentration of 3.79 ng/ml ($n=17$) for subjects with luteal-phase ovaries, and 0.33 ng/ml ($n=14$) for subjects with follicular-phase ovaries. The study population was divided into two groups, by ovarian phase, for further evaluation.

Histopathologic lesions in uterine tissue were compared between the two ovarian groups. Adenomatous hyperplasia of the superficial and glandular epithelium were prominent features of uterine tissue under luteal but not follicular influence. Myometrial hyperplasia also was prominent in uterine tissue under luteal influence. Histopathologic lesions that did not differ between the two groups included polyp formation, cystic hyperplasia of glandular epithelium, atrophy, and cuboidal or stratifying hyperplasia of superficial or glandular epithelium. Cystic hyperplasia of the endometrium, often with moderate to severe polyp formation, occurs frequently in virgin queens over age 3 years, regardless of ovarian phase. These lesions create chronic and palpable firm enlargement of the uterus, and are the most common cause of infertility in young to middle-aged queens.

Inflammatory changes, including endometritis, metritis, and pyometra, did not differ between the two ovarian groups in frequency or overall severity. *Escherichia coli* was the organism most frequently isolated from uterine contents, in agreement with previous studies (Dow, 1962; Kenney et al., 1987). Other organisms isolated occasionally may include *Streptococcus* spp., *Staphylococcus* spp., *Klebsiella oxytoca, Pseudomonas aeruginosa, Pasteurella multocida,* and mixed bacterial isolates (Lawler et al., 1991).

Initial uterine lesions (hyperplasia) result from luteal ovarian activity (progesterone), which is a predisposing factor for clinical endometritis, metritis, and pyometra, as a usual consequence of secondary infection (Dow, 1962). Therefore, functional classification of the disease complex based on ovarian phase (Lawler et al., 1991) may be more appropriate than classification based on the inflammatory component (Dow, 1962).

Epidemiologic evaluation of these two groups of cats revealed that the mean age of all cats in the study ($n=44$) was 4.3 (range = 1 to 10) years. Mean age of cats with luteal-phase ovaries was 3.4 years, compared to 5.5 years for cats with follicular-phase ovaries. History of reproductive performance of 27 cats varied from poor to excellent. Fourteen cats had no history of pregnancy (history unknown for three cats).

Thirteen of the 44 affected cats had been housed with other breeding queens, with no male present, for periods ranging from 1.0 to 13.0 (mean 4.7) months. Ten of these 13 cats had weaned litters 1.0 to 3.5 months prior to diagnosis (mean=2.5 months). Eleven of these 13 cats had luteal-phase ovaries.

Twenty-two of the 44 affected cats had been housed separately, in rooms of individually maintained sexually intact female cats, continuously for up to 84 months (mean=36.8 months). Nine of these cats had luteal-phase ovaries.

Therefore, 35 of the 44 cats studied had no recent exposure to male cats, or had borne, nursed, and weaned litters without subsequent exposure to male cats. Nevertheless, 20 of these 35 cats had a histologic diagnosis of luteal-phase ovaries.

An important question raised by studies of feline inflammatory uterine disease is whether normal intact queens, without uterine disease (subclinical or clinical) exhibit similarly unexpected ovarian activity. A second study was conducted to examine this question (Lawler et al., 1993). Twenty normal intact adult queens and four spayed controls were caged individually, in sight and hearing of other male and female cats. The cats ranged from 2.5 to 11.0 (mean=7.4) years of age. At approximately monthly intervals for 9 months (April to December), blood samples were obtained by jugular venipuncture from each cat for assay of serum proges-

terone. Evidence of ovulation was defined by serum progesterone concentrations above 2.0 ng/ml. Serum progesterone concentrations above 1.5 ng/ml have been reported as indicative of luteal function in previous studies (Shille and Stabenfeldt, 1979). A higher reference value was chosen for this study to avoid the possibility of incorrect assignment of positive responses. Seven of 20 queens (35%) had serum progesterone concentration exceeding 2.0 ng/ml in a total of 13 monthly serum samples, while unspayed controls continued to have very low values.

## DISCUSSION

In both of these studies, the age range and average age of the subjects was greater than in some earlier investigations. Whether age is a factor in response thresholds of queens to one or more stimuli for ovulation has not been investigated, and cannot be deduced from these data. Likewise, it is not clear whether population size or density, and possibly associated visual, olfactory, or auditory cues, may influence ovulatory stimuli. Characterization of these findings in the context of historical knowledge likely will require considerable further study.

The pathogenesis of the cystic endometrial hyperplasia-pyometra complex in cats and dogs appears to be similar, and very probably is initially endocrine in nature. Alternate progression and regression, possibly associated with successive ovarian cycles and apparently associated at times with noncopulatory ovulation and subsequent progesterone exposure, seems likely.

Cats traditionally are described as requiring fertile, sterile, or sham coitus to stimulate the neuroendocrine reflexes that lead to ovulation. The findings discussed here raise questions relative to the mechanisms of induced ovulation in this species, an issue that had been raised by previous investigators (Dow, 1962). Some investigators have suggested that arbitrary classification of mammals as exclusively induced or exclusively spontaneous ovulators may not be entirely precise, and have noted the importance of external stimuli in influencing ovulation in both groups (Milligan, 1982).

From a clinical perspective, if anesthetic risk is acceptable, surgery remains the treatment of choice for chronic or inflammatory uterine disease in cats not destined for reproductive service. For cats having reproductive value and potential, medical treatment of pyometra using prostaglandin $F_{2\alpha}$ has been suggested (Feldman and Nelson, 1989). Knowledge of the ovarian state (presence or absence of luteal function) at the time of diagnosis of uterine disease may influence management decisions for some individuals. Likewise, ovarian state may influence therapeutic trials with new pharmacologic agents, such as prostaglandin analogues or RU486. Veterinary recommendations for management of breeding catteries may be influenced by the pattern of endocrine, pathologic, and clinical events. Therefore, veterinarians and cattery operators must learn to keep current, complete, and detailed records of reproductive performance and possible environmental influences.

## References and Suggested Reading

Concannon P, Hodgson B, and Lein D: Reflex LH release in estrous cats following single and multiple copulations. Biol Reprod 23:111, 1980.
*Single copulations in the estrous queen cause lower serum concentrations of luteinizing hormone and lower likelihood of ovulation than do multiple copulations, suggesting that copulation induction is difficult in this species.*

Dow C: The cystic hyperplasia-pyometra complex in the cat. Vet Rec 74:141, 1962.
*A survey of 91 cases of feline pyometra, with classification of histologic appearance of the uterus, uterine culture, and clinical signs; some queens with corpora lutea were reported to have been unmated.*

Goodrowe KL, Howard JG, Schmidt PM, et al: Reproductive biology of the domestic cat with special reference to endocrinology, sperm functioning, and in-vitro fertilization. J Reprod Fertil 39 (suppl):1989.
*A discussion of various aspects of feline reproduction.*

Johnson LM and Gay VL: Luteinizing hormone in the cat. II. Mating-induced secretion. Endocrinology 109:247, 1981.
*Repeated matings of the estrous queen trigger GnRH release and cumulative increased increments of plasma LH concentrations.*

Kenney KJ, Matthiesen DT, Brown NO, et al: Pyometra in cats: 183 cases (1979–1984). J Am Vet Med Assoc 191:1130, 1987.
*A description of clinical appearance, laboratory findings, histopathology, and response to treatment of 183 cases of feline pyometra.*

Lawler DF, Evans RH, Reimers TJ, et al: Histologic features, environmental factors, and serum estrogen, progesterone, and prolactin values associated with ovarian phase and inflammatory uterine disease in cats. Am J Vet Res 52:1747, 1991.
*A characterization of inflammatory uterine disease in the cat, classified by ovarian phase; some queens without opportunity for coitus had luteal phase ovaries.*

Lawler DF, Johnston SD, Hegstad RL, et al: Ovulation without cervical stimulation in domestic cats. J Reprod Fertil Suppl 47 (suppl): 1993.
*Up to one third of normal adult female intact cats housed alone, but maintained in populations, may experience ovulation and subsequent luteal function.*

Milligan SR: Induced ovulation in mammals. Oxford Rev Reprod Biol 4:1, 1982.
*A review of reflex ovulation in mammals, as defined by acute increase in luteinizing hormone secretion following sexual stimuli.*

Paape SR, Shille VM, Seto H, et al: Luteal activity in the pseudopregnant cat. Biol Reprod 13:470, 1975.
*Induction of ovulation and pseudopregnancy in the domestic cat by copulation with a vasectomized male, and measurement of interestrual intervals in the presence or absence of ovulation.*

Shille VM, Lundstrom KE, Stabenfeldt GH: Follicular function in the domestic cat as determined by estradiol 17-B concentrations in plasma: Relation to estrous behavior and cornification of exfoliated vaginal epithelium. Biol Reprod 21:953, 1979.
*Characterization of ovarian follicular function in the domestic cat, using serum estradiol concentrations, vaginal cytology, and behavioral estrus.*

Shille VM and Stabenfeldt GH: Luteal function in the domestic cat during pseudopregnancy and after treatment with prostaglandin F2 alpha. Biol Reprod 21:1217, 1979.
*Characterization of ovarian luteal function in domestic cats, using queens with pseudopregnancy established by sterile coitus, and subsequent attempted luteolysis using prostaglandin $F_{2\alpha}$.*

# THE ELECTIVE CESAREAN SECTION

VICKI N. MEYERS-WALLEN

*Ithaca, New York*

## INDICATIONS

In this article, the term "elective cesarean section" is used to imply that a cesarean section is planned as a pregnancy outcome, even before the bitch is bred. Such a course may be anticipated when the history or prebreeding physical examination findings indicate that there is a reasonable expectation of difficult or abnormal parturition. In such cases, prompt and careful intervention with cesarean section in a full-term pregnancy can be the alternative with the highest probability of a favorable outcome for the dam and pups.

The following are examples of conditions in which elective cesarean section may be indicated. Clearly, bitches are likely candidates that have a history of obstructive dystocia due to production of relatively large pups for the size of the dam's pelvic outlet. There are breeds where this is more likely to occur, due to selection for a small pelvis and large head size. Bitches that have a small pelvic outlet due to pelvic fracture are also candidates for elective cesarean section. Vaginal strictures or soft tissue bands in the vagina (Wykes, 1986) may cause difficulty in delivery. Some vaginal strictures relax sufficiently in the last few days of gestation to allow vaginal delivery. Vaginal bands and strictures that do not relax can be a cause of obstructive dystocia. Although the inheritance of such vaginal abnormalities is unknown, the breeder should consider the possible implications before breeding these bitches. The less obvious cases where elective cesarean may be planned include bitches that have a history of failing to initiate true labor (no second stage) or that were "overdue" and then delivered dead, autolyzed pups. In such cases, it is often unclear whether gestation was full term or actually longer than normal. Another reason to plan for surgical intervention would be a history of secondary uterine inertia, long labor, or large litters with delivery of dead or weak pups, and obvious stress to the bitch. Valuable bitches that historically do not exhibit obvious signs of impending parturition, such as a decrease in rectal temperature, can also benefit from careful calculation of gestation length and tentative scheduling of cesarean section as a precautionary measure. In bitches in which parenteral progesterone supplementation for insufficient luteal phase (Scott-Moncrieff, Nelson, and Bill, 1990; Purswell, 1991) is anticipated, careful calculation of gestation length is essential for proper timing of progesterone withdrawal (Concannon et al.,

1977) and, if labor fails to proceed normally at term, is helpful in determining when to intervene surgically.

## TIMING OF GESTATION

An accurate method of timing gestation must be used in order to determine whether the bitch is full term. If she is not full term at the time of surgery, premature pups may be delivered. Alternatively, if a bitch is truly overdue, pups are likely to die *in utero* if parturition is considerably delayed (Concannon et al., 1977). Previous methods of estimating gestation have relied upon imaging techniques. Radiographic examinations are helpful in pregnancy diagnosis and in determining the number, size, and position of the pups. First evidence of skeletal calcification can be used to determine that the pregnancy is at least 44 days' gestational age (Concannon and Rendano, 1983). Ultrasound is useful in determining fetal viability, but it is rarely used to predict whether a pregnancy is full term. A formula has been reported for estimating gestational age from fetal measurements obtained by ultrasound of beagle pregnancies (Yeager et al., 1992). Although it has not been tested in other breeds, it may be helpful in combination with other methods.

To accurately predict when a pregnancy will be full term, data should be collected beginning in *proestrus*, as discussed below. The gestational age of the embryo is closely linked to the time of ovulation rather than the time of insemination. Sperm can be deposited before or after ovulation and still be successful in fertilization, but the time of insemination does not alter the actual length of gestation (Concannon et al., 1983). The exact time of ovulation is not easily determined. However, the length of gestation can be timed most accurately from the hormonal stimulus for ovulation: the preovulatory luteinizing hormone (LH) peak (Concannon et al., 1983). A full-term gestation is 65 days $\pm 1$ day, counting from the day of the serum LH peak (Table 1) (Concannon et al., 1983).

Timing gestation by vaginal cytology is a less accurate but practical method of retrospectively estimating the day of ovulation (Holst and Phemister, 1974). The first day of diestrus occurs approximately 8 days *after* the serum LH peak (Fig. 1). Counting from the first day of diestrus vaginal smear (D1), a full-term gestation is 57 days, with a range of 51 to 60 days (Table 1). Finally, timing gestation from insemination or breeding dates is not recommended for the purposes of elective cesarean section, since the apparent gestation length can range from 57 to 72 days from any one breeding date (Concannon, 1983).

### Estimation from Serum Progesterone Concentrations

Measurement of serum canine LH is performed at only a few reference laboratories, and the delay in obtaining results is sufficient to preclude its use as a

**Table 1.** *Methods of Estimating Parturition Date in the Bitch*

| Method | Time from | Parturition |
|---|---|---|
| Serum progesterone | Abrupt rise (day 0) | Day 65$\pm$1° |
| Vaginal cytology | First day of diestrus (D1) | D57[†] Range = D51–D60 |
| Breeding date | Days of mating | Range = 57–72 days[‡] |

°Data derived from Concannon P, Hansel W, and McEntee: Changes in LH, progesterone and sexual behavior associated with preovulatory luteinization in the bitch. Biol Reprod 17:604–613, 1977.
[†]Data derived from Holst PA and Phemister RD: Onset of diestrus in the beagle bitch: Definition and significance. Am J Vet Res 35:401–406, 1974.
[‡]Data derived from Concannon P, Whaley S, Lein D, and Wissler R: Canine gestation length: Variation related to time of mating and fertile life of sperm. Am J Vet Res 44:1819–1821, 1983.

practical method of timing gestation. However, in the bitch, serum progesterone is used to estimate the day of the LH peak (day 0) because progesterone increases abruptly on the same day (Concannon, Hansel, and McEntee, 1977) (Fig. 1). Enzyme-linked immunosorbent assay (ELISA) tests for qualitative assessment of serum progesterone concentration (Target and Status Pro, International Canine Genetics, Malvern, PA; Estruchek, Synbiotics Corporation, San Diego, CA) are very practical for this purpose, as well as for determining the ideal time to perform insemination (also see *CVT XI*, p 943). For purposes of timing cesarean section, the qualitative estimate of progesterone concentration provided by the ELISA tests should be confirmed later by progesterone radioimmunoassay (RIA), which is readily available at most reference laboratories. This author recommends vaginal cytology in addition to measurement of progesterone, as described below, particularly in bitches that have a history of infertility or a history of an unusual or abnormal estrus (e.g., long, short, variable standing). The plan below should be discussed in detail with the owner prior to proestrus, so that all parties are prepared in advance. All serum and cytology samples are retained until pregnancy is confirmed. Serum samples are dated and stored frozen. Stained vaginal cytology slides are stored in a dry, closed box.

The owner begins by examining the bitch's vulvar area at least twice weekly to detect the first signs of proestrus: vulvar swelling and/or sanguinous discharge. Within 1 to 2 days of these signs, samples for vaginal cytology and serum progesterone are obtained from the bitch. Usually the bitch will be in early proestrus at this time, but it is not uncommon for the bitch to be presented in late proestrus or even estrus, as determined by vaginal cytology. If sampling is begun sufficiently early, the progesterone ELISA test should indicate that progesterone is less than 2 ng/ml; that is, that the preovulatory rise in serum progesterone has not yet begun. Samples for vaginal cytology and serum progesterone are taken every other day to monitor the transition from proestrus to estrus, and to estimate the day of the preovulatory serum LH peak (day 0) (Fig. 1).

Of the ELISA tests mentioned, the author has had most experience with the Status Pro kit (International Canine Genetics, Malvern, PA) and will use it in examples hereafter. This test has the potential to display three blue dots in a triangular pattern (Fig. 1). The apex of the triangle is the control spot, which should always appear blue if the test is working properly. Looking at the test well with the control spot as the apex of the triangle, the spot at the lower right corner of the triangle fades to white when serum progesterone is greater than 2 ng/ml (low spot). The spot at the lower left corner of the triangle fades to white when the serum progesterone concentration is above 7.5 ng/ml (high spot). As the bitch progresses through proestrus to the LH peak and ovulation, this test should show three blue spots prior to the LH peak, then two blue spots as the progesterone concentration rises, then only one blue spot (the control) when progesterone concentration are high (Fig. 1). Although the manufacturer suggests that fading of the low spot from blue to light blue occurs coincident with the LH peak (day 0), it is the author's experience that the low spot may appear to be light blue for several days even in normal bitches. Thus, it is important to continue testing serum samples every other day until the low spot is observed to be completely white while the control and high spots remain blue (progesterone is >2 ng/ml but <7.5 ng/ml). The first day that this is observed is designated day 1.

It is recommended that insemination be performed on days 3 and 5 or on days 4 and 6 when natural mating or artificial insemination with fresh or chilled semen is used. On the day of the second breeding (day 5 or 6), vaginal cytology and the serum ELISA test are repeated. If the cycle has progressed as expected, cytologic estrus will be observed and only the control spot will be blue on the progesterone ELISA test (Fig. 1). If the high spot is still blue on the day of the second breeding, it is possible that the LH peak was later than originally estimated, or that there is a problem with the

ovulation process (anovulation) or formation of the corpora lutea (shortened luteal phase). Another breeding should be planned, and serum progesterone should be reevaluated on that day. Cytology is continued every other day, and the first day of diestrus smear should be observed *approximately* 8 days after day 0, the estimated day of serum LH peak (Holst and Phemister, 1974) (Fig. 1).

Using this method of timing gestation, pregnancy can be confirmed at day 28 to 30 by ultrasound examination. Once pregnancy is confirmed, the frozen serum samples from the estimated day of serum LH peak (day 0), 2 days prior to LH peak, and 2 days after LH peak should be sent to a reference laboratory for quantitative confirmation (progesterone RIA) of the qualitative ELISA test. On the day of the LH peak, progesterone usually abruptly rises at least two times above the baseline concentration (Concannon, Hansel, and McEntee, 1977). In the reference laboratory we use, baseline progesterone RIA values are usually less than 1.0 ng/ml, and on the day of LH peak range between 1.0 and 2.5 ng/ml (Table 2). The date of parturition is estimated from the progesterone RIA measurements as day 65 from the LH peak, ±1 day. The tentative date for elective cesarean section is day 65.

## Estimation from Vaginal Cytology

This method of timing gestation is less expensive than measuring serum progesterone, but is also less accurate. It may be most useful in targeting a 3-day period during which the bitch will be full term and elective cesarean section can be performed. In those bitches that have a history of an appropriate decrease in rectal temperature occurring 24 to 48 hr before whelping, this information can be used to further narrow the time period in which cesarean section can be performed, as discussed below.

Again, these plans should be discussed with the owner of the bitch prior to the expected time of pro-

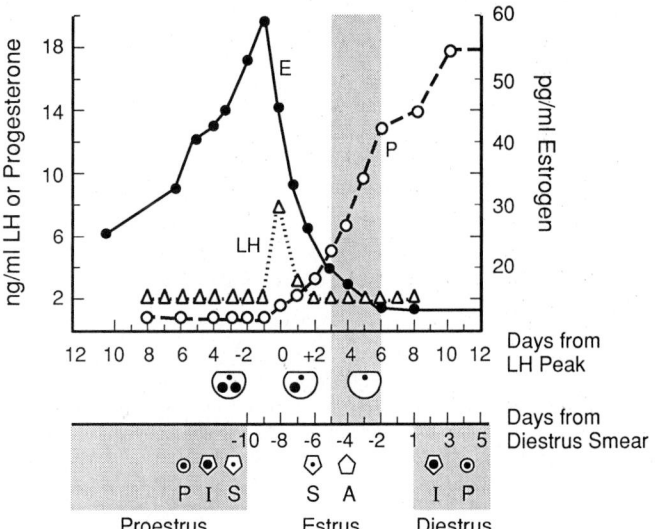

**Figure 1.** Hormonal and cytologic changes occurring during proestrus, estrus, and early diestrus in the bitch. Serum progesterone increases abruptly on the day of the serum LH peak (day 0), and is measured qualitatively by an ELISA test (Status Pro, International Canine Genetics, Malvern, PA). Ovulation occurs on day 2, the eggs mature during an approximately 3-day period, and breeding is recommended on days 3 and 5 or 4 and 6 (*shaded area*). Using vaginal cytology, noncornified epithelial cells (P = parabasal, I = intermediate) decrease and cornified cells (S = superficial, A = anuclear squames) increase during proestrus. Cytologic estrus is defined by 90% or more cornified epithelial cells in the vaginal smear. The first day of diestrus (D1) is determined by vaginal cytology as the first day that cornified cells decrease to 50% or less. (Adapted from Concannon PW, et al: The ovarian cycle of the bitch: Plasma estrogen, LH and progesterone. Biol Reprod 13:118, 1975, with permission.)

**Table 2.** *Examples of Serum Progesterone (RIA) and Serum LH (RIA) Concentrations in Individual Estrus Bitches*

|        | Serum LH (ng/ml) | Serum Progesterone (ng/ml) |        |
| ------ | ---------------- | -------------------------- | ------ |
| Dog #1 | 0.32             | 0.41                       |        |
|        | 0.51             | 0.40                       |        |
|        | 9.18             | 1.96                       | day 0  |
|        |                  |                            |        |
|        | 0.32             | 5.58                       |        |
|        | 1.09             | 2.12                       |        |
|        | 0.86             | 2.82                       |        |
|        | 0.53             | 7.17                       |        |
| Dog #2 | 0.5              | 0.2                        |        |
|        | 11.12            | 0.51                       |        |
|        | 12.5             | 1.4                        | day 0  |
|        |                  |                            |        |
|        | 1.87             | 2.03                       |        |
|        | 0.46             | 2.06                       |        |
| Dog #3 | 0.84             | 0.6                        |        |
|        | 4.74             | 1.0                        |        |
|        | 7.4              | 1.2                        | day 0  |
|        |                  |                            |        |
|        | 1.14             | 1.2                        |        |
|        | 1.07             | 2.97                       |        |
|        | 0.98             | 9.82                       |        |

estrus. As soon as the bitch shows evidence of proestrus, the first vaginal smear is obtained and sampling is continued every other day. With this method, it is recommended that breeding begin as soon as the first day of estrus is identified: 90% or more of the vaginal epithelial cells are cornified cells (superficial cells or anuclear squames; Fig. 1). Breeding is usually continued every other day during the period of cytologic estrus. Although the average length of estrus is 9 days, there is considerable variation between bitches. Normal estrus as short as 4 days and as long as 21 days has been reported (also see *CVT X*, p 1269). The end of estrus is marked by the first day of diestrus vaginal smear (D1). This is identified as the first day that cornified cells are 50% or less of the vaginal epithelial cells (Fig. 1). The first day of diestrus frequently occurs very suddenly; that is, an estrous smear is followed the next day by a diestrous smear (Holst and Phemister, 1974). When cytology is obtained every other day, it is not uncommon to observe 90% cornified epithelial cells in the vaginal smear obtained on one day, and then 90% *non*cornified cells in the smear obtained on the next day. In that case, the day in between, in which no sample was actually obtained, can be estimated as the first day of diestrus (D1). If a decrease in cornified cells is observed, but is not clearly below 50%, another smear should be obtained in 2 days to confirm passage into diestrus.

Ultrasound confirmation of pregnancy can be performed at 21 days from the first day of diestrus smear (D1). The date of parturition is estimated as the 57th day (D57), counting from the first day of diestrus (D1). Approximately 74% of bitches studied by this method

were found to whelp between D56 and D58, but parturition ranged from D51 to D60 for all bitches studied (Table 1) (Holst and Phemister, 1974). Therefore, this method of timing gestation for planning elective cesarean section is most useful in bitches that reliably exhibit other signs of impending parturition, such as a decrease in rectal temperature.

## TIMING SURGICAL INTERVENTION

The veterinarian has confirmed that the dog is pregnant and has planned an elective cesarean section for the estimated date of parturition (65 days from the estimated LH peak, or 57 days estimated from the first day of diestrus vaginal smear). One week before the date of parturition, the client begins to record the bitch's rectal temperature twice daily. Serum progesterone ELISA tests should also be performed every other day if the bitch does not have a history of rectal temperature decrease prior to parturition.

Although serum progesterone concentrations gradually decrease after midgestation, the actual value varies widely between dogs, and may vary within a dog throughout the day (Steinetz et al., 1990). A decrease in serum progesterone below 2 ng/ml for several hours is necessary for the initiation of parturition (Concannon et al., 1983). In association with a serum progesterone decrease below 2 ng/ml, the rectal temperature should decrease below 100°F, and may be as low as 98°F, within 24 hr of parturition (Concannon and Hansel, 1977) (Fig. 2). A sustained temperature decrease, observed at 56 to 58 days from the first day of diestrus vaginal smear (D1), is good evidence of a full-term gestation.

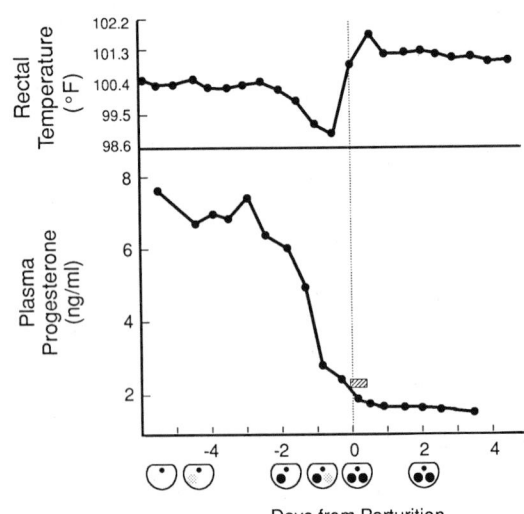

**Figure 2.** An abrupt decrease in serum progesterone (<2 ng/ml) and rectal temperature usually occurs 24 hr prior to parturition in normal bitches. The progesterone decrease can be detected by the reappearance of the blue spot in the lower right hand corner of the ELISA test well (Status Pro, International Canine Genetics, Malvern, PA). (Reproduced from Concannon PW, Powers ME, Holder W, et al: Pregnancy and parturition in the bitch. Biol Reprod 16: 523, 1977, with permission.)

However, if the bitch does not exhibit a decrease in rectal temperature by D57, an ELISA test should be performed to determine whether the expected prepartum decrease in serum progesterone has occurred. On the Status Pro test, for example, all three spots—the control, the high, and the low spot—should be blue within 24 to 48 hr of parturition. The combination of a decrease in serum progesterone (<2 ng/ml) and/or rectal temperature (<100°F) with confirmation that the bitch is 57 days from the first day of diestrus vaginal smear, or 65 days from the estimated day of LH peak, is sufficient to conclude that gestation is full term. An elective cesarean section can be performed within 24 hr of the observed decrease in rectal temperature or serum progesterone.

However, if the bitch fails to exhibit a decrease in rectal temperature or serum progesterone, it is possible that she has an abnormality in initiation of parturition, such as a failure of progesterone to decrease even though the gestation is full term. In such cases, timing gestation from the first day of diestrus vaginal smear is not recommended. Bitches that have this history, and have gestational age timed from the day of LH peak, can still have elective cesarean section planned for day 65±1 day. Should the bitch fail to show signs of impending parturition, an ultrasound examination can be helpful in assessing fetal viability. Heart rates in term fetuses that we have observed have been in the range of 150 to 250 bpm. In a bitch of this type that is known to be full term and has no evidence of labor, cesarean section should not be delayed if fetal heart rates are consistently below 100 bpm or if heart beats are absent in some fetuses, and slow heart rates are observed in others.

## References and Suggested Reading

Concannon PW and Hansel W: Prostaglandin F2 alpha induced luteolysis, hypothermia and abortions in beagle bitches. Prostaglandins 13:533, 1977.
*An experimental study describing luteolysis as a consequence of prostaglandin administration. When luteolysis was achieved and serum progesterone concentrations remained below 2 ng/ml for a period of time, abortions resulted.*

Concannon PW, Hansel W, and McEntee K: Changes in LH, progesterone and sexual behavior associated with preovulatory luteinization in the bitch. Biol Reprod 17:604, 1977.
*An experimental study describing preovulatory luteinization of the ovarian follicles and the coincidental preovulatory rise in serum progesterone and luteinizing hormone in the bitch.*

Concannon PW, Powers ME, Holder W, et al: Pregnancy and parturition in the bitch. Biol Reprod 16:517, 1977.
*A study describing the normal endocrine characteristics of the pregnant and nonpregnant bitch. In particular, the prepartum decrease in serum progesterone concentrations and coincident decrease in rectal temperature are described. The effects of exogenous estradiol or progesterone administration on pregnancy and parturition are explored.*

Concannon P and Rendano V: Radiographic diagnosis of canine pregnancy: Onset of fetal skeletal radiopacity in relation to times of breeding, preovulatory luteinizing hormone release, and parturition. Am J Vet Res 44:1506, 1983.
*A study describing the radiographic features of canine pregnancy in which gestational age was timed from the preovulatory serum LH peak.*

Concannon PW, Whaley S, Lein D, et al: Canine gestation length: Variation related to time of mating and fertile life of sperm. Am J Vet Res 44:1819, 1983.
*A study in 290 beagles that demonstrated that the actual length of gestation is very consistent between bitches, when computed from the day of the preovulatory rise in serum luteinizing hormone. Apparent differences in gestation length between bitches when computed from breeding date was related to variation in time of estrus onset and in the time that canine sperm remain viable within the female reproductive tract.*

Holst PA and Phemister RD: Onset of diestrus in the beagle bitch: Definition and significance. Am J Vet Res 35:401, 1974.
*A study demonstrating that the first day of diestrus vaginal smear can be used to retrospectively determine the time of ovulation in bitches and to predict the day of parturition.*

Purswell BJ: Management of apparent luteal insufficiency in a bitch. J Am Vet Med Assoc 199:902, 1991.
*A case report describing the use of progesterone injection for treatment of suspected insufficient luteal phase in a bitch.*

Scott-Moncrieff JC, Nelson RW, and Bill RL: Serum disposition of exogenous progesterone after intramuscular administration in bitches. Am J Vet Res 51:893, 1990.
*An experimental study in which progesterone injections were administered to anestrus bitches to determine the dosage which would maintain serum progesterone concentrations in the range of normal diestrus.*

Steinetz BG, Goldsmith LT, Hasan SH, et al: Diurnal variation of serum progesterone, but not relaxin, prolactin, or estradiol-17β in the pregnant bitch. Endocrinology 127:1057, 1990.
*A study describing variation in serum progesterone concentrations within 24-hr periods in the bitch.*

Wykes PM: Diseases of the vagina and vulva in the bitch. *In* Morrow DA (ed): *Current Therapy in Theriogenology*, 2nd edition. Philadelphia, WB Saunders Co, 1986, pp 476–481.
*A review of the types of anatomic abnormalities found in the vagina and vulva of the bitch.*

Yeager AE, Mohammed HO, Meyers-Wallen VN, et al: Ultrasonographic appearance of the uterus, placenta, fetal membranes throughout accurately timed pregnancy in beagles. Am J Vet Res 53:342, 1992.
*An ultrasonographic study of eight bitches in which gestation was timed from the preovulatory serum LH peak. First ultrasonographic detection; appearance; and sizes of certain features of the embryo, placenta, and uterus are described. A formula for calculating gestational age is included.*

# CANINE GENITAL MYCOPLASMAS AND UREAPLASMAS

CATHARINA LINDE-FORSBERG
*and* GÖRAN BÖLSKE
*Uppsala, Sweden*

## ETIOLOGY

Mycoplasmas and ureaplasmas are the smallest free-living organisms known. They belong to the class *Mollicutes*, which means "soft skin," and their closest relatives are certain gram-positive bacteria. These organisms and bacteria share many of the same characteristics, but the former are smaller and lack the rigid cell wall of the latter. Their deoxyribonucleic acid (DNA) contains only about half as many genes as that of bacteria. Consequently, their metabolic and synthetic capacities are limited, and they depend on their environment or on a host organism for nourishment and protection. In nature, mycoplasmas within the genera *Mycoplasma*, *Acholeplasma*, and *Ureaplasma* often inhabit the moist mucosal membranes of respiratory and genital tracts of animals. Although the absence of a rigid cell wall renders them fragile outside the host, it is advantageous in that they are resistant to cell wall–inhibiting antibiotics, such as the penicillins and cephalosporins. Most mycoplasma and ureaplasma species are host specific, and there are few reports of canine mycoplasmas being isolated from man, or vice versa.

More than 12 species of mycoplasmas have been isolated from dogs. The most common ones are *Mycoplasma canis*, *M. edwardii*, *M. gateae*, *M. spumans*, *M. cynos*, *M. bovigenitalium*, and four serologic groups of *Ureaplasma* (formerly called T-mycoplasmas). Several studies have clearly shown that they are part of the normal flora in both the upper respiratory tract and lower genital tract. Species less common, but also found in healthy animals, are *M. maculosum*, *Acholeplasma laidlawii*, *M. opalescens*, *M. arginini*, *M. molare*, *M. feliminutum* and the unclassified *Mycoplasma* strain HRC689. Several of these species have been isolated from dogs with pneumonia, vaginitis, balanoposthitis, infertility, inflammation of the urinary tract, colitis, and endocarditis. However, there is little published evidence documenting their pathogenicity, and it has not been possible to implicate mycoplasmas as the primary causative agent in any single important disease of dogs (Rosendal, 1982).

Mycoplasmas usually cause slowly developing, chronic disease, often of multifactorial origin. Expression of the disease is considered to depend more on environmental conditions and on the genetic predisposition of the host than on the nature of the infecting microbe (also see p 301).

## GENITAL MYCOPLASMAS AND UREAPLASMAS IN OTHER SPECIES

Mycoplasmas have long been recognized as pathogens of the respiratory tract and joints in a variety of animal species (cattle, humans, mice, poultry, rats, and swine). Although some mycoplasmas have also been proven to be pathogenic in the urogenital tract, their role in this site has been subject to considerable debate.

In humans, *M. pneumoniae*, *M. hominis*, and *Ureaplasma urealyticum* are considered to possess pathogenic properties. A correlation between colonization by *M. hominis* and/or ureaplasmas during pregnancy, and low birth weight of the infant, has been postulated. Experimental inoculations of *U. urealyticum* in humans proved that it could cause urethritis and suggested that it plays a role in acute urethroprostatitis. Patients harboring ureaplasmas showed significantly decreased sperm motility and an increased proportion of morphologically aberrant spermatozoa. Thus, *U. urealyticum* can elicit an inflammatory response in the human male genital tract and has also been isolated directly from testicular biopsies of infertile men. If *U. urealyticum* affects spermatogenesis and/or motility, however, it does so only in a small percentage of infected individuals, which could explain why studies involving small numbers of poorly characterized patients showed no significant differences between infected and uninfected groups.

In cattle, *M. bovigenitalium* has been incriminated in cases of seminal vesiculitis, decreased sperm motility, and reduced post-thaw motility. *Ureaplasma diversum* has been isolated from field cases of bovine granular vulvitis, endometritis, salpingitis, abortion, and seminal vesiculitis, and the disease was reproduced following experimental inoculation (Doig and Ruhnke, 1986).

In rats, a naturally occurring, chronic genital tract disease that results in reproductive failure has been proven to be due to *M. pulmonis*. The disease progresses slowly, with colonization limited to cell surfaces, and mycoplasmas do not penetrate into the submucosa. Colonization of the vagina and cervix was common, but colonization of the uterus and fallopian tubes only occurred in 25% of the infected females. In many cases, minimal or no microscopic changes were evident; however, cervicitis, vaginitis, endometritis, salpingitis, and perioophoritis occurred sporadically. Although uteri often appeared normal histologically, organisms lined the entire epithelial surface. *Mycoplasma pulmonis* was isolated from the urethra, vas deferens, and epididymis in association with chronic inflammation in 5% of males bred with infected females. The disease can be reproduced in female rats by intranasal, intravaginal, or intravenous inoculation, and progresses slowly for up to 8 months. However, it produces very mild lesions. Distinct differences in response to challenge between strains of rats indicate that genetic factors are important determinants of susceptibility to the disease. Reduced fertility was found in 50% of the infected animals. Acute inflammation of the placental disks was observed, with *M. pulmonis* being found at the fetomaternal junction. Recent experimental studies with *M. pulmonis* in specific pathogen-free rats and mice gave similar results.

## WHAT DO WE KNOW ABOUT THE CANINE GENITAL MYCOPLASMAS AND UREAPLASMAS?

The first isolation of mycoplasmas and ureaplasmas from the canine genital tract was reported in 1951 and 1971, respectively. However, after more than 40 years, considerable disagreement still exists concerning their role in canine infertility and neonatal deaths.

Most studies aimed at evaluating their pathogenicity have used one of three approaches: (1) isolation from clinical cases of genital disease, (2) comparisons of isolation rates of the organisms from the genital tracts of fertile dogs with corresponding rates in infertile dogs, and (3) experimental inoculations.

When it comes to the mere isolation of mycoplasmas from clinical cases, several studies have shown that samples from the vagina, prepuce, and semen submitted because of infertility problems often are positive for mycoplasmas and ureaplasmas. However, since they may occur in the normal flora at these sites, their presence may be incidental. Some of these studies were biased in that no attempts were made at culturing aerobic and anaerobic bacteria. Lein (1986) mentioned a syndrome characterized by poor conception, early embryonic death, embryonal or fetal resorption, abortion, stillborn pups, weak newborns, and neonatal death from which mycoplasmas or ureaplasmas or both were isolated, but no further details were given.

A survey of infertile dogs and normal dogs showed that the former had mycoplasmas and ureaplasmas in vaginal and preputial samples more often than the latter. For ureaplasmas, this difference was statistically significant in male dogs with balanoposthitis, semen abnormalities (subnormal motility, low sperm counts, and/or a high percentage of midpiece and tail abnormalities), and infertility, but no significant differences were found in female dogs (Doig, Ruhnke, and Bosu, 1981). However, since only single samples were obtained from each animal, permanent colonization with mycoplasmas was not proven, and no attempts to isolate possible coexisting aerobic or anaerobic bacteria were made; thus the connection between the ureaplasmas and infertility remains unclear. In a more recent

preliminary report (Zöldag et al., 1992), mycoplasmas were also found more often in dogs with genital disorders than in healthy animals, and a comparison of the breeding results before and after natural infection indicated that the mycoplasmas had a harmful effect. No mention was made of whether bacterial culturing was done, and not all the results were reported; thus again the importance of the mycoplasmas is difficult to assess. This kind of study can be biased due to a failure to match the two groups for factors known to influence mycoplasma and ureaplasma colonization, to an inadequate diagnostic evaluation of the infertility cases, or to the possible involvement of other infectious agents. Another reason for bias would be that the dogs in the infertile group were, or recently had been, on antibiotic treatment, since antibiotics to which mycoplasmas are insensitive (e.g., ampicillin and trimethoprim-sulfamethoxazole) can disturb the normal genital flora and allow the mycoplasmas, as well as other resistant pathogens, to multiply and spread (Ström and Linde-Forsberg, 1993).

The only experimental studies involving genital mycoplasmas in dogs are those by Laber and Holzmann (1977) and Holzmann, Laber and Walzl (1979), who induced epididymitis, orchitis, and scrotal edema in two dogs out of four, 3 to 4 weeks after inoculating two strains of *M. canis* into a ductus deferens fistula. The mycoplasmas were, however, only recovered from one of the male dogs, while *Staphylococcus aureus* was isolated from one of the other dogs. Using the same two strains of *M. canis* isolated from bitches with pathologic findings in the genital tract, they also induced a purulent endometritis, intramural phlegmon, and cystic glandular endometritis in four bitches out of ten after intrauterine inoculation by laparotomy. The mycoplasmas were recovered from the cervix and vagina of eight of the 10 bitches, but not from the uterus at postmortem examination, 10 to 26 days after inoculation. Thus, by strict definition, Koch's postulates were not fulfilled even in these experimental studies.

### Ways of Spreading the Infection

As dogs harbor essentially the same mycoplasma flora in the respiratory and in the genital tracts, transmission of mycoplasmas and ureaplasmas between dogs can occur not only at mating but also via the airborne route or by nose contact. Thus, isolation of infected dogs is necessary to prevent spread of the organisms, and since mycoplasmas do not survive in the environment, this is also an effective preventive measure. Intrauterine spread to developing fetuses probably also occurs. In addition, pups can acquire the mycoplasmas when passing through the birth canal. It has been observed that at kennels where a large number of dogs are kept close together, the colonization and spread of mycoplasmas and ureaplasmas are greatly facilitated. However, when the occurrence of mycoplasmas in those kennels coincides with reproductive problems, it must be kept in mind that the same circumstances also facilitate the spread of other infectious agents.

## Clinical Signs of Infection

Fertility problems, rather than overt signs of disease, generally draw attention to the possibility of a mycoplasma infection, since most dogs and bitches harbor mycoplasmas and ureaplasmas without showing any obvious clinical signs. Bitches with vulvovaginitis may, however, show a mucopurulent vulvar discharge (Doig, Ruhnke, and Bosu, 1981), and mycoplasma-infected stud dogs may have balanoposthitis, prostatitis, epididymo-orchitis, and scrotal edema (Laber and Holzmann, 1977; Lein, 1986).

## Possible Mode of Action

Inflammatory reactions in the genital tract may create an abnormal environment for the ova and the spermatozoa, thereby reducing the fertility of the host. In cattle, ureaplasmas introduced into the uterus at breeding seldom persist for more than 7 days, but this has been shown to be sufficient time to severely reduce the conception rate.

Scanning electron microscopy studies have shown that there is a close physical association between spermatozoa and ureaplasmas in human and bovine infertility cases. Ureaplasma has been shown to induce ciliostasis in bull spermatozoa. In addition to altering motility, the adsorption of ureaplasmas to sperm could impair spermatozoal function by interfering with the normal metabolism of the spermatozoa, by masking sperm membrane receptor sites involved in sperm-egg recognition, by impairing ova-penetrating ability, or by mediating damage by immunologic mechanisms (e.g., by inducing autoantibody formation).

*Mycoplasma pulmonis* in rats causes acute inflammation of the placental disks, which may lead to nutrient deprivation of the fetuses and result in lower birth weight or fetal death.

## Diagnostic Techniques

Samples for mycoplasma and ureaplasma isolation should be submitted to a laboratory that can perform the special techniques for culturing and preferably also for typing these organisms. Specimens from vagina, prepuce, or semen are taken on plain, sterile cotton wool swabs or on one of the commercially available swabs (e.g., Culturette, Baxter Healthcare, McGaw Park, IL). To facilitate recovery of organisms from the mucous membranes, it is recommended that the swab be moistened in saline or special culture media, or by breaking the culture media capsule of the commercial swab before sampling.

When collecting the specimen, care should be taken to avoid contact with antiseptic solutions. The vulva or

preputial opening should preferably be disinfected using 70% ethanol, which is allowed to evaporate before the swab is introduced. To avoid contamination from the surrounding skin surfaces, a speculum should be used for the vaginal sampling, and the preputial sampling can be performed in connection with semen collection, directly from the erect pars longa glandis or from the junction between the preputial sheath and the penile mucous membrane. Specimens are collected by firmly stroking the swab over the mucous membrane. Semen samples should be collected in a sterile vial, avoiding the first fraction of the ejaculate to minimize contamination by bacteria colonizing the distal urethra. It is also important to avoid any contact with the preputial mucous membrane. The swab is dipped into the semen sample, carefully avoiding contact with the possibly contaminated vial opening. The swabs should be immediately transferred to a vial containing a transport medium, which can be a specialized mycoplasma culture medium (obtainable from the laboratory), phosphate buffered saline, Amies medium (Difco, Molesey, Surrey, United Kingdom) (without charcoal) or modified Stuarts medium (Baxter Healthcare, McGaw Park, IL). Samples should be transported to the laboratory as quickly as possible, particularly if the specific mycoplasma media, which prevent overgrowth of bacteria, are not used. Samples should be shipped refrigerated and preferably reach the laboratory within 24 hr. As mycoplasmas and ureaplasmas have different growth requirements, the laboratory should be notified if both cultures are desired. In most cases, it would also be relevant to culture for aerobic, and possibly anaerobic, bacteria.

Of greatest diagnostic value would be the isolation of mycoplasmas or ureaplasmas from inner organs, where they never occur as normal flora. This means that, when possible, samples should be obtained from the uterus, oviducts, gonads, or the prostate at laparotomy or by biopsy, strictly avoiding contamination by the normal flora of the skin and outer genitals. Isolation of these organisms from inner organs (stomach contents, spleen, liver) of aborted fetuses or stillborn pups is a significant finding. Isolation from fetal membranes or placenta is of less value because contamination can occur during their passage through the birth canal.

In clinical cases, specimen collection usually has to be restricted to the vagina, prepuce, and semen. The culturing of mycoplasmas or ureaplasmas from the anterior vagina or cervix or from uterine pus at the cervix in bitches with clinical symptoms may be significant in the absence of other organisms. However, the neutrophilic granulocytes of the pus may inhibit growth of bacteria and could give false-negative cultures, or false pure cultures of mycoplasmas. Seminal plasma is also known to possess antibacterial activity; thus a two- or three-fold dilution of the ejaculate might improve culture results.

Serology is not useful for diagnostic purposes in clinical cases because antibody detection normally can only be performed for one or a few mycoplasma species at one time; thus it is not possible to screen for all the known species. Also, all the canine mycoplasmas occur as normal flora in healthy animals and may stimulate antibody production to some degree. Furthermore, infections of mucous membranes sometimes only give rise to low antibody levels or very slowly rising titers.

## Treatment

Tests of susceptibility to antimicrobial agents are not available for mycoplasmas on a routine basis. Kato et al. (1972), who tested the sensitivities of 103 canine strains of mycoplasmas (55 strains of *M. canis*, 11 of *M. spumans*, seven of *M. maculosum*, and 30 unclassified strains) to 22 antibiotics, found a wide range of variation in sensitivity among the species of mycoplasmas studied, especially to erythromycin (E-mycin) and oleandomycin (not available in the United States). Thus, these antibiotics should be avoided. For all mycoplasma strains tested, tylosin (Tylan)* was the most effective antibiotic. To some degree, the strains were all sensitive to the other macrolides (spiramycin, leucomycin, and josamycin; Baxter Healthcare), to two of the tetracyclines (tetracycline and methacycline; Baxter Healthcare) and to chloramphenicol (Chloromycetin) and lincomycin (Lincocin). Recent studies indicate that resistance of human genital mycoplasmas to tetracyclines is increasing. For *M. hominis*, trospectomycin was the most active agent; spectinomycin (Baxter Healthcare), tetracycline (Sumycin), and doxycycline (Vibramycin) had comparable antimycoplasmatic activity, and the macrolides were ineffective. Against *U. urealyticum*, spectinomycin and trospectinomycin were the most active drugs, being at least twice as active as the macrolides and tetracyclines (Echaniz-Aviles et al., 1992). The newer quinolones (ciprofloxacin, Cipro; enrofloxacin, Baytril) have been shown to be effective against most mycoplasmas, but may be ineffective against ureaplasmas. Erythromycin, although not active against some of the mycoplasmas, often is active against the ureaplasmas.

Treatment should be continued for at least 10 to 14 days, and repeated culturings should be made to confirm eradication of the mycoplasmas. Suspected carriers should be tested and treated *before* being mated, since most of the suggested antibiotics are detrimental to the developing fetuses and should be avoided during pregnancy (Papich, 1989).

To prevent spread of the infection, the carriers, or suspected carriers, should be kept isolated from other dogs. Visiting bitches with undiagnosed reproductive problems should be artificially inseminated.

## CONCLUSIONS

Infertility on a kennel basis usually has a multifactorial background. Anatomic as well as hormonal, ge-

netic, immunologic, infectious, parasitic, toxic, management, and nutritional factors all may play an important role in this complex problem. Based on present knowledge, it seems unlikely that mycoplasmas and ureaplasmas play a primary role in canine infertility and neonatal deaths although, as is the case with other species, it seems reasonable to assume that some species, or strains, of mycoplasma or ureaplasma may cause disease under certain circumstances and in certain individuals. Environmental factors and genetic predisposition of the host, or a compromised immune system, rather than microbial virulence, have been shown to be of importance for the development of disease in other species. Mixed infections also occur. In such cases, it is difficult to assess the relative importance of the mycoplasmas or ureaplasmas and the various bacteria, or if synergistic effects exist among them. It is understandable that breeders want to find a quick and simple answer to their problems and want their veterinarian to provide a quick and simple remedy. No one who was in practice 15 to 20 years ago will have forgotten the β-hemolytic streptococci (BHS) scare that prevailed among breeders during that time. Since then, several studies have proved that the BHS, like the mycoplasmas and ureaplasmas, constitute a part of the normal genital flora of healthy bitches and dogs. At the same time, these agents are known to be "opportunistic pathogens" and may cause disease given the right circumstances. Samplings from dogs and bitches without obvious clinical symptoms of disease are of little value, since there is no way of knowing whether the presence of bacteria or mycoplasmas is incidental rather than a sign of disease.

Until more conclusive knowledge is gained about the role of mycoplasmas and ureaplasmas, cases of canine infertility and neonatal deaths should be approached from a wide perspective, taking into consideration all possible causes of disease. This can be time consuming and requires close cooperation between the breeders and the veterinary profession, but is probably the only way breeders can be helped on a long-term basis. Breeders should also be made aware that misuse of antibiotics actually may worsen the situation by disturbing the normal genital flora and thus giving opportunistic pathogens a chance to multiply and spread.

More research is clearly needed to reveal the true importance of mycoplasmas and ureaplasmas in canine genital disease. Unfortunately, they are difficult to study because of their low-grade pathogenicity (usually only about half the number of experimentally inoculated animals become infected), their subtle host-parasite relation, and their slow mode of inducing disease. Studies in other species indicate that mycoplasmas and ureaplasmas can vary in pathogenicity at both the species and strain level. This means that to get conclusive results a large number of animals have to be used, which always is a problem in canine studies. If available at all, dogs for research are expensive to obtain and maintain. This may be one explanation for why so few studies have been published within this field in spite of the great interest created by early reports.

---

*Only dosage form available in the United States is powder for turkey medication.

## References and Suggested Reading

Doig PA, Ruhnke HL, and Bosu WTK: The genital mycoplasma and ureaplasma flora of healthy and diseased dogs. Can J Comp Med 45:233, 1981.
 *A study of the genital mycoplasma and ureaplasma flora in 136 dogs, some of which were healthy and others had various reproductive problems.*
Doig PA and Ruhnke HL: Effects of ureaplasma infection on bovine reproduction. *In* Morrow DA (ed): *Current Therapy in Theriogenology 2.* Philadelphia, WB Saunders Co, 1986, p 282.
 *A review of all aspects pertaining to the effects of bovine genital ureaplasma infection, including diagnosis and treatment.*
Echaniz-Aviles G, Conde-Gonzales C, Juarez-Figueroa L, et al: In vitro activity of several antimicrobial agents against genital mycoplasmas. Clin Ther 14:688, 1992.
 *An in-vitro study of the susceptibility of* Mycoplasma hominis *and* Ureaplasma urealyticum *to macrolides, tetracyclines, spectinomycin, and trospectinomycin.*
Holzman A, Laber G, and Walzl H: Experimentally induced mycoplasmal infection in the genital tract of the female dog. Theriogenology 12:355, 1979.
 *An experimental study of the effects of two strains of* Mycoplasma canis *on the uterus in the bitch.*
Kato H, Murakami T, Takase S, and Ono K: *Sensitivities* in vitro *to antibiotics of mycoplasma isolated from canine sources.* Jpn J Vet Sci 34:197, 1972.
 *An in vitro study of the sensitivity of 103 canine strains of mycoplasmas to 22 antibiotics.*
Laber G and Holzmann A: Experimentally induced mycoplasmal infection in the genital tract of the male dog. Theriogenology 7:177, 1977.
 *An experimental study of the effects of two strains of* Mycoplasma canis, *injected through a vas deferens fistula, on the reproductive tract in male dogs.*
Lein DH: Canine mycoplasma, ureaplasma, and bacterial infertility. *In* Kirk RW (ed): *Current Veterinary Therapy IX.* Philadelphia, WB Saunders Co, 1986, p 1240.
 *A review of the possible significance of the mycoplasmas, ureaplasmas, and various bacteria in canine infertility, including diagnosis and treatment.*
Papich MG: Effects of drugs on pregnancy. *In* Kirk RW (ed): *Current Veterinary Therapy X.* Philadelphia, WB Saunders Co, 1989, p 1291.
 *A review of the safety of various drugs during canine pregnancy, including lists of the most common drugs and their possible effects on fetuses.*
Rosendal S: Canine mycoplasmas: Their ecologic niche and role in disease. J Am Vet Med Assoc 180:1212, 1982.
 *A review of the possible significance of the mycoplasmas in canine disease.*
Ström B and Linde-Forsberg C: Effects of ampicillin and trimethoprim-sulfamethoxazole on the vaginal bacterial flora of bitches. Am J Vet Res 54:891, 1993.
 *An experimental study of the effects of two commonly used antibiotics on the vaginal flora in healthy bitches.*
Zöldag L, Stipkovits L, Thuróczy J, and Balogh L: Mycoplasma isolation from genital tract of healthy dogs and of animals with genital disorders. *Proc 12th Int Congr Anim Reprod,* Haag, 1992, p 1832.
 *A clinical study of the prevalence and effects of mycoplasmas in breeding dogs.*

# MANAGEMENT OF *BRUCELLA CANIS* OUTBREAKS IN BREEDING KENNELS

CHERI A. JOHNSON
*East Lansing, Michigan*

The diagnosis of *Brucella canis* should be considered in a kennel when reproductive performance is less than expected in otherwise normal, healthy animals. The most common signs of *B. canis* infection are sudden abortion in bitches and infertility in stud dogs. Most often, abortion occurs during the third trimester in an otherwise healthy bitch. Fetal death due to *B. canis* infection can occur at any stage of gestation. When it occurs during the first trimester, there are no overt signs of pregnancy loss. Therefore, the kennel manager may assume that conception never occurred and that the bitch is infertile. Puppies born to infected bitches are usually weak and do not survive to weaning age.

The most commonly recognized sign of *B. canis* infection in males is infertility. Orchitis is not as prominent a feature of *B. canis* infection as is epididymitis. Although epididymal swelling routinely occurs 3 to 5 weeks after infection, it is often not detected because affected dogs are not ill, they are afebrile, and show no signs of discomfort unless the scrotal contents are palpated. Teratozoospermia (morphologic abnormalities of spermatozoa), neutrophils, and macrophages are found in semen of infected dogs as early as 5 weeks after infection. Testicular atrophy occurs in chronically infected dogs.

In addition to the classic signs of abortion in females and infertility in males, *B. canis* may be suspected in a kennel when positive serologic tests for *B. canis* are found during routine, prebreeding evaluation of asymptomatic animals. The approach to suspected *B. canis* infection in a kennel should include confirmation of the diagnosis, quarantine of the kennel, determination of the source of infection, elimination of the mode of transmission within the kennel, identification and elimination of infected animals, and initiation of practices to prevent future outbreaks. These procedures should be initiated as soon as *B. canis* infection is suspected and vigorously continued until the infection is eradicated from the colony. Failure to act promptly and aggressively will result in significant additional losses, which often do not become apparent for several months after the index case is recognized.

## CONFIRMATION OF THE DIAGNOSIS

The diagnosis is confirmed by isolation and identification of the causative organism, *B. canis*, from at least one colony member. Specimens for *Brucella* culture should be collected using proper technique and promptly transported to the laboratory. *Brucella canis* grows slowly, so it may be easily overgrown by other organisms contaminating the specimen. Because of the zoonotic potential, it is important to avoid direct contact with infected material and to alert laboratory personnel of the possibility of *B. canis* infection. Successful recovery of the organism depends primarily on the number of organisms present in the material submitted. Therefore, it is important to submit material that is expected to contain large numbers of organisms and is most likely to yield positive results. These include postabortion discharge, semen from dogs infected for 3 to 11 weeks, and blood during weeks 5 to 52 after infection (Table 1). Previous treatment with antibiotics may cause negative culture results. Bacterial cultures provide the definitive diagnosis when *B. canis* is isolated; however, they are time-consuming and may yield false-negative results. Bacterial cultures are therefore not convenient for colony-wide testing and screening of asymptomatic animals.

Serologic tests for *B. canis* have advantages over bacterial isolation in that they are rapid and easy to perform, and have wide commercial availability. The disadvantage of serologic tests is that, to some extent, most of the tests are nonspecific for *B. canis* and can give false-positive results. Nonprotective antibodies are produced against cell wall antigens and cytoplasmic antigens of *B. canis*. They become detectable 8 to 12 weeks after infection. Antibody titers remain high (e.g., 1:400 to 1:3200) as long as bacteremia persists. When bacteremia becomes intermittent or subsides, as it does with chronic (30 to 60 weeks) infection, antibody titers decline and may become equivocal (e.g., 1:50 to 1:200) or negative; however, the organism still persists in infected tissues (Carmichael, Zoha, and Flores-Castro, 1984; Carmichael and Greene, 1990). In some animals, there are fluctuations in titers in the presence or absence of bacteremia. Therefore, the magnitude of the titer does not necessarily reflect the stage of the disease, nor do declining titers indicate recovery from infection.

*Brucella canis* has cell wall antigens common to other bacterial organisms including *Bordetella bronchiseptica*, *Pseudomonas aeruginosa*, mucoid *Staphylococcus* species, and *B. ovis* and *B. abortus*. Therefore, the results of serologic tests for *B. canis* that utilize cell wall antigens are not specific for *B. canis* infection. Antibodies produced against common antigens of these other organisms can cross-react with the *B. canis* test, generating a false-positive result. Identification of the causative organism(s) of false-positive reactions is usually not of clinical importance, but *Pseudomonas* and *Staphylococcus* have been most commonly incriminated. The rapid slide agglutination test (Canine Brucellosis Antibody Test Kit, Pitman-Moore, Washington Crossing, NJ) and tube agglutination tests detect antibodies to cell wall antigens. Positive results must be confirmed by other methods. Cytoplasmic or internal antigens of *B. canis* are unique to the genus *Brucella*. Cytoplasmic antigens are used in certain agar gel immunodiffusion (AGID) tests for *B. canis*. The AGID test using cytoplasmic antigens is the most specific serologic test currently available for detection of *B. canis* infection. Positive reactions will occur with infections by *Brucella* species other than *B. canis*. Previous antibiotic therapy can cause serologic tests to become negative for an unknown period of time.

Because the results of bacterial isolation and serologic tests are related to the quality of the specimen submitted and to the chronicity of infection, which may be unknown in the kennel, test results must be carefully interpreted in conjunction with the history and clinical signs. For example, a vaginal culture for *B. canis* is an excellent diagnostic choice for a bitch that

***Table 1.*** *Confirmation of* Brucella canis *Infection*[°]

| Material to Culture | Time to Culture | Expected Results |
|---|---|---|
| Postabortion discharge | When present | Positive |
| Placenta | When present | Positive |
| Abortus | When present | May be negative |
| Semen | 3–11 weeks after infection | Positive |
| | 12–60 weeks after infection | Positive but few organisms are shed |
| | >60 weeks after infection | Negative |
| Blood[†] | 5–30 weeks after infection | "100%" positive |
| Blood[†] | 6–12 months after infection | >80% positive |
| | 28–48 months after infection | 50%–80% positive |
| | 48–58 months after infection | 25%–50% positive |
| | >58 months after infection | <25% positive |
| Epididymis | 35–60 weeks after infection | 50–100% positive |
| | >100 weeks after infection | Negative |
| Urine | 8–30 weeks after infection | Usually positive; more organisms shed by male than by female |
| Prostate | Until 64 weeks after infection | Usually positive |
| Lymph node, spleen, and bone marrow | When animal is bacteremic | Usually positive |
| | When animal is abacteremic | Positive or negative |
| Eye | When uveitis is present | Usually positive |
| Intervertebral disk | When discospondylitis is present | Positive or negative |

[°]From Johnson CA and Walker RD: Clinical signs and diagnosis of *Brucella canis* infection. Compend Cont Educ 14:767, 1992, with permission.
[†]Blood cultures are intermittently positive 30 weeks after infection.

has just experienced a third-trimester abortion. If *B. canis* is the cause of the abortion, the vaginal culture should be positive. Conversely, a vaginal culture is a poor diagnostic test for an asymptomatic bitch during the normal anestrus phase of her cycle because the results are likely to be negative in the presence or absence of *B. canis* infection. The results of the common diagnostic tests (culture and serology) are usually negative when the animal has been infected for less than 4 weeks, as well as when an animal is chronically infected (>2 years), or when the animal has received antibiotic therapy.

## QUARANTINE OF THE KENNEL

The kennel should be quarantined as soon as the diagnosis of *B. canis* is confirmed. In kennel situations where the clinical signs are classic for *B. canis* infection, it may be prudent to quarantine the colony as soon as the disease is suspected, while the diagnosis is being confirmed. No animals should be admitted to or released from the kennel until the disease is known to be eradicated. New additions are not only at risk of becoming infected, they increase the number of animals needing to be tested during the eradication procedures. This is an unnecessary increase in risk and expense. Animals should not be released from the kennel for sale or for performance purposes because they may transmit the infection directly or indirectly by contaminating the environment. It is important to remember that the most common mode of transmission of *B. canis* is by ingestion of the organism. Some kennel managers mistakenly believe their animals to be safe from infection as long as coitus does not occur. Movement of animals within the colony should be restricted to prevent additional exposure while the source of infection and the mode of transmission are being investigated.

## SOURCE OF INFECTION AND MODE OF TRANSMISSION

The index case is the first animal in the group in which the disease is recognized. Being the first animal recognized does not necessarily mean that it is also the first animal in the colony to be infected with *B. canis*. If the index case was infected before entering the colony, it could be the source of infection for the entire colony. On the other hand, if the index case was infected after entering the colony, the source of infection remains unidentified, but is presumed to still exist within the kennel. Testing of the entire colony should begin immediately after the diagnosis is confirmed. Animals known to have been in close contact with the index case should be tested first because one of them may be the source of infection, or conversely, any of them may have been infected by the index case. The type of test chosen to screen animals with known exposure depends upon the suspected duration of infection (Tables 1 and 2). Animals infected for less than 4 to 8 weeks usually have negative serologic tests because the antibody response is not yet sufficient to be detected. A search for the mode of transmission within the kennel should proceed simultaneously with the search for the source of infection.

All possible modes of transmission should be considered. Infection by *B. canis* occurs through oral, nasal, conjunctival, and genital mucous membranes. The oral route is considered to be the most common. *Brucella canis* can survive for an extended period in the environment under the proper conditions. Because post-abortion vaginal discharge, aborted material, semen of recently infected males, and urine of infected males contain the largest numbers of organisms, contact with or contamination by these materials should receive close attention. The organism is also present in salivary, nasal, and nonestrous vaginal secretions and in milk of infected animals, but the importance of these body fluids in transmission of the disease is uncertain. *In utero* infection also occurs. Unfortunately, the potential role

***Table 2.*** *Serologic Tests for* Brucella canis*

| Serologic Test | Antigen | Time Frame for Positive Results | Comments |
|---|---|---|---|
| 2-ME–RSAT | Cell wall | 8–12 weeks after infection to 3 months after the animal is abacteremic | Very sensitive; false-positive results are common; few (1%) false-negative results are reported; easy and fast |
| 2-ME–TAT | Cell wall | 10–12 weeks after infection to 3 months after the animal is abacteremic | Semiquantitative; false-positive results are possible |
| AGID test | Cell wall | 12 weeks after infection to 4 months after the animal is abacteremic | Test procedure is complex; more specific than 2-ME–RSAT |
| AGID test | Cytoplasmic | 12 weeks after infection to 36 months after the animal is abacteremic | Most specific serologic test but not sensitive; detects chronic cases when other tests give negative results |
| ELISA | Cell wall | Unknown (expect time to be similar to that observed with the TAT) | Very specific; less sensitive than TAT; limited availability |

*Modified from Carmichael LE and Green CE: Comparison of serologic procedures for canine brucellosis. *In* Greene CE (ed): *Infectious Diseases of the Dog and Cat.* Philadelphia, WB Saunders Co, 1990, p 579, with permission.
Abbreviations: RSAT = rapid slide agglutination test, 2-ME = 2 mercaptoethanol, TAT = tube agglutination test, AGID = agar gel immunodiffusion, ELISA = enzyme-linked immunosorbent assay.

of puppies in the maintenance of infection within the colony and in the spread of infection has not been evaluated.

The organism can be transmitted throughout the colony via fomites. Methods by which cages and equipment are disinfected, and all sanitation practices of the colony, should be reviewed. Hygiene of the animal caretakers should receive special attention because of the zoonotic potential of *B. canis* and because of the possibility that the caretakers may unknowingly be the mode of transmission. Although it has been reported that *B. canis* is killed by iodophors, in the presence of organic material it may survive exposure to povidone-iodine (Johnson and Walker, 1992).

## IDENTIFICATION AND ELIMINATION OF INFECTED ANIMALS

After the confirmation of *Brucella canis* infection in a kennel, testing of every member of the colony should be done on a monthly basis until the infection has been eradicated. Testing and elimination of infected animals is the only proven method of eradication of *B. canis* infection from a kennel. To date, no therapeutic regimen for *B. canis* has shown 100% efficacy (Nicoletti, 1989). Antibiotic regimens that are less that 100% effective are unacceptable in a kennel situation because infection will persist in the colony. Dogs that are unsuccessfully treated, no matter how few in number, remain a source of infection for the entire colony. Even those dogs that are "successfully" treated remain at risk because they are readily susceptible to reinfection (Flores-Castro and Carmichael, 1977). Strict isolation of infected dogs coupled with stringent sanitation procedures have failed to protect uninfected animals in the kennel (Johnson and Walker, 1992).

Because of the insidious nature of *B. canis*, the kennel manager often has no reason to suspect infection exists, even in the index case, until sudden abortion or infertility occur. Therefore, the clinician must assume that many colony members have had chance exposure and are in various stages of incubation at the time the index case is recognized. Animals that have recently been infected will not immediately be identifiable because antibodies usually do not reach detectable levels for 8 to 12 weeks after infection. Even blood cultures may be negative during the first 4 weeks of infection. Although these recently infected animals may not be detectable, they are capable of transmitting the infection to others.

During the monthly testing, all the animals in the colony are tested, including those that were negative on previous tests. All positive animals are immediately eliminated as they are identified. Additional positive animals can be expected to be identified for the next 4 to 5 months, which represents the length of time from infection until antibodies are detected by serologic testing in animals exposed initially and those exposed to infected but serologically unrecognized animals during the first rounds of colony testing. Monthly testing of all remaining colony members should continue until a minimum of three consecutive monthly tests fail to identify any positive animals. If the colony is closed (i.e., no animals entering or leaving) and the entire colony is tested monthly and all positive animals are eliminated, monthly testing is likely to continue for 7 to 8 months. This would represent 4 to 5 months during which new positive animals will probably be identified, followed by 3 consecutive months of negative test results. Thereafter, quarterly or biannual testing may be sufficient to ensure that the disease remains eradicated. If the colony is not closed, monthly testing may continue indefinitely as former colony members return.

## PREVENTION OF FUTURE OUTBREAKS

There is no vaccine for *B. canis*. Future outbreaks are averted by preventing exposure to the organism. This is accomplished by strict quarantine of all new acquisitions until monthly testing during an 8- to 12-week period indicates negative results. Animals known to have been exposed to *B. canis* and animals with any of the clinical signs of *B.canis*, including infertility, should not be considered for acquisition by a breeding kennel. Additional procedures should be tailored to the individual kennel. The most important determinant will be whether the kennel remains closed. In kennels that are not closed, animals that are temporarily housed on the premises, such as animals to be bred, should be certified to be negative for *B. canis* before being admitted, and should not be allowed access to permanent colony members. To ensure that they have not become infected, studs that breed noncolony members should be tested before they are allowed to breed colony members. Bitches should be tested before breeding. Colony members that temporarily leave the kennel should be tested before being readmitted.

## References and Suggested Reading

Carmichael LE and Greene CE: Canine brucellosis. *In* Greene CE (ed): *Infectious Diseases of the Dog and Cat.* Philadelphia, WB Saunders Co, 1990, p 573.
*A review of the pathophysiology, diagnosis, and treatment of* Brucella canis *infection.*
Carmichael LE, Zoha SJ, and Flores-Castro R: Problems with the serodiagnosis of canine brucellosis: Dog responses to cell-wall and internal antigens of *Brucella canis.* Dev Biol Standards 56:371, 1984.
*A review of results of various serologic tests with respect to chronicity of infection and results of hemoculture and tissue cultures for* B. canis.
Flores-Castro R and Carmichael LE: Canine brucellosis: Current status for diagnosis and treatment. Gaines Symposium, College Station, TX, Texas A & M University, 1977, p 17.
*The classic comprehensive review of responses to antibiotic therapy for* B. canis *infection. Some of the information in this paper is summarized by Nicoletti in* Current Veterinary Therapy X.
Johnson CA and Walker RD: Clinical signs and diagnosis of *Brucella canis* infection. Compend Contin Educ 14:763, 1992.
*A review of diagnostic and treatment approaches for canine brucellosis, with emphasis on control programs for kennels.*
Nicoletti P: Diagnosis and treatment of canine brucellosis. *In* Kirk RW (ed): *Current Veterinary Therapy X.* Philadelphia, WB Saunders Co, 1989, p 317.
*Overview of diagnostic and therapeutic procedures for* Brucella canis *with emphasis on antibiotic therapy.*

# MAMMARY TUMORS

BARBARA E. KITCHELL

*Urbana, Illinois*

Little progress has been made in the clinical management of mammary carcinoma in recent years. This fact is surprising, because these tumors are common in veterinary practice. Breast tumors represent 25 to 50% of all neoplasms of female dogs, and are the second most frequent neoplasm seen in dogs after skin tumors. The incidence of breast cancer in the dog is approximately three times that seen in women, with an incidence rate of 199/100,000 female dogs. In the cat, mammary glands are the third most common site of cancer after hematopoietic and skin tumors, and will be discussed separately (Madewell and Theilen, 1987).

Of all dogs presented with mammary masses in veterinary practice, about 50% will have benign disease that is easily eliminated by surgery. Of the 50% with mammary malignancy, a further one half are cured by adequate surgery. Thus, 75% of dogs with mammary masses are managed straightforwardly. The challenge facing veterinary oncologists and general practitioners today is twofold. First, criteria must be established and accepted that identify the 25% of dogs at risk of death from malignant mammary disease, so that more intensive therapy can be used to improve survival for this group. Progress has been made in this area, and several studies identifying prognostic factors will be summarized here. The second challenge is to develop better treatments for aggressive mammary cancer in the dog; few studies of treatments beyond surgery have been published. Several rational approaches to the management of dogs with microscopic and gross metastatic mammary tumors will be discussed. (For additional information and approaches, see "Mammary Tumors in the Dog," this volume, p 518.)

## EPIDEMIOLOGY

### Age, Breed, and Sex Factors

The median age of dogs with mammary tumors is 10 to 11 years. The tumor is rare in dogs less than 2 years of age, with a sharp increase beginning at approximately 6 years. Female sex is a strong predilection factor. Mammary tumors are rarely seen in male dogs (approximately 1% of malignant mammary tumors in one study were seen in males), and when mammary tumors occur in males they tend to be highly malignant.

Breed predisposition has been reported in several studies but no consensus has been established. The fact that different studies cite different breed predisposi-

tions may be confounded by early ovariectomy, which is the leading preventive factor. Spaying practices may vary in different countries or in different regions of the United States. A higher incidence of mammary tumors is expected when estrus cycle control is accomplished pharmaceutically rather than surgically, as occurs in some of the European countries from which epidemiologic studies have been published. Age at time of neutering may also be affected by folklore propagated among fanciers of the various breeds. Familial predisposition, a known risk factor in humans, has not been well studied in dogs.

### Reproductive Hormone Factors

The most widely accepted risk factor for developing mammary carcinoma in the dog is the number of estrous cycles in bitches before spaying. The risk in neutered bitches for developing mammary tumors is only 12% of the mammary cancer risk for intact bitches. Bitches spayed before the first heat cycle had a relative risk of 0.05% for mammary cancer, while those with one heat cycle had 8%, and those with two or more cycles had 26% relative risk. After 2.5 years of age or four estrus cycles, the sparing effect of ovariohysterectomy is lost.

Other reproductive factors that may play an etiologic role but which are less clearly defined include nulliparous whelping status or small numbers of litters as compared to dogs with large numbers of litters. Pseudopregnancy, irregular estrus cycles, ovarian follicular cysts, persistent corpora lutea, and fecundity may also be involved in onset of breast cancer in dogs, although statistical association of these factors and breast cancer has been disputed. Long-term administration of progesterone derivatives is associated with increased risk in laboratory beagles. Elevated growth hormone levels and acromegalic changes may be found in dogs with mammary tumors (Madewell and Theilen, 1987).

Dogs that are obese may have poorer survival when surgically treated, but the risk of developing breast cancer in obese versus thin dogs was not clearly different, as happens in women. However, one study suggested that dogs fed low-fat diets (<39% of dietary calories derived from fat) had a significantly better prognosis for 1 year survival after surgical removal of mammary tumors, particularly if also on a high-protein diet, than those dogs fed higher fat diets regardless of protein content (Shofer et al., 1989).

## CLINICAL CHARACTERISTICS

Clinical signs associated with canine mammary tumors are usually limited to the physical presence of the mass or masses. The typical pattern of metastasis is to regional nodes through lymphatics and to lung by way of lymphatic and venous spread. Less common sites of metastasis include liver, kidneys, bone, heart, adrenal gland, brain, skin or subcutis, and eyes. Physical examination of regional nodes and thoracic radiographs (three views, including a dorsoventral or ventrodorsal and both lateral projections) are required for pretreatment staging. Abdominal ultrasound may also be helpful. Patients may become emaciated if the cancer elaborates paraneoplastic factors, or if lymphokines from anticancer immune response (cachetin, tumor necrosis factors) are released. Hypercalcemia is rarely seen in association with mammary carcinoma.

The caudal two mammary glands are most commonly affected, possibly because of their growth rate, weight, lobularity, and secretion as compared to cranial glands. Location of the tumor is not important to prognosis, however. Fifty to 65% of dogs with mammary neoplasia have multiple tumors at presentation. Number of masses at presentation is not prognostic. Mammary masses in dogs are highly heterogeneous; a given individual may have benign and malignant masses simultaneously.

Careful history can identify the rate of growth and duration of mammary tumors. Rapid growth or regrowth usually indicates aggressive malignancy. Physical examination should be performed to identify *negative* correlates for survival, including infiltrative growth with fixation to underlying tissues or ulceration of the skin, lymph node enlargement, and lymphedema of the legs or vulva. Tumor size is of prognostic significance. In a study of 253 dogs with mammary tumors, there was significant difference in survival between groups of dogs when primary tumors were classed as less than 5 cm, 5 to 10 cm, 11 to 15 cm, and greater than 15 cm in diameter (Misdorp and Hart, 1976). A more recent study confirmed this finding, with tumors of less than 3 cm diameter having significantly better prognosis than tumors greater in size. This size effect was lost if the primary tumor was associated with lymph node metastasis or vessel invasion, however (Kurzman and Gilbertson, 1986).

Inflammatory carcinoma carries the worst prognosis of all the histologic subtypes of mammary cancer, and is generally metastatic at presentation. Dogs with inflammatory carcinoma have warm, painful tumors often associated with thickened, ulcerated skin and lymphedema in the nearest limb. This condition can mimic mastitis, and dogs may be clinically depressed with nonspecific signs of illness when affected by inflammatory carcinoma. Biopsy is warranted to distinguish infectious from neoplastic cause of this condition, but mastectomy is rarely curative in inflammatory carcinoma. If surgical resection of the primary lesion is attempted, it is common to see tumor nodules recurrent in the incision line at the time of suture removal (Loar, 1989).

## HISTOPATHOLOGIC CHARACTERISTICS

Fine needle aspiration cytology of masses, scraping of ulcerating lesions, or expression of fluid from affected glands may be diagnostic of mammary cancer. However, because of the heterogeneous nature of the tumors, a benign cytologic evaluation *does not rule out* malignant disease. Excisional or incisional biopsy is needed to make a definitive diagnosis. Excisional biopsy is a rational approach for smaller (<2.5 cm diameter) lesions, in that such excision of benign and some malignant lesions will be curative, provided adequate tumor margins are obtained (see "Definitive Surgical Treatment of Cancer," this volume, p 462). For larger lesions, an incisional biopsy can confirm the diagnosis and facilitate planning for definitive surgical therapy.

Several histopathology classification systems have been developed to define the mammary malignancies of dogs, but none is universally accepted. The aim of all these classification systems is to provide a more accurate prognosis. Because the pathology of these tumors is complex and tumors are heterogeneous, pathologists may disagree as to the placement of an individual tumor between classification systems, and potentially even within the criteria of a given classification system. In most studies, epithelial tumors that are more highly differentiated (those with acinus and tubule formation) and tumors with few mitotic figures and more regular nuclear size and shape are associated with a more favorable prognosis.

The most recently published classification system (Kurzman and Gilbertson, 1986), is based on a system developed for human epithelial mammary neoplasms that correlates well with biologic behavior of tumors. Using this system, the degree of cellular atypia correlates with degree of tumor aggressiveness. If tumors were classified as benign with moderate to marked cellular atypia, dogs had a ninefold higher risk of later developing invasive carcinoma than those with benign mastopathy without atypia. Also, this system allows for histologic staging of tumors based on extent of disease. This histologic staging proved to be of prognostic value (Table 1). Degree of nuclear differentiation within these histologic stages further helped to identify subsets of patients. More aggressive tumors were associated with less nuclear differentiation, and tumors with better overall prognosis tended to be those with well-differentiated nuclei. This effect of nuclear differentiation was most apparent in dogs with histologic stage I disease, in that recurrence rates within 2 years of mastectomy were 77%, 63%, and 40% for poorly, moderately, and well-differentiated stage I tumors, respectively.

Furthermore, this classification system identified lymphoid cellular reactivity as a positive correlate for prognosis, in that dogs with tumors infiltrated with lym-

**Table 1.** *Histologic Stage Correlated With Disease-Free Interval After Mastectomy in 233 Dogs With Mammary Cancer*

| Histologic Stage | Definition | % Recurrence 2 Years After Mastectomy |
|---|---|---|
| 0 | Carcinoma *in situ* | 19% |
| I | Invasive carcinoma without lymphatic or venous invasion | 60% |
| II | Invasive carcinoma with vascular or lymphatic invasion or metastasis to regional nodes | 97% |
| III | Evidence of distant metastasis | 100% |

**Table 2.** *Histologic Grading System and Correlates With Survival in 320 Dogs With Mammary Carcinoma*

| Histologic Description | Median Survival Time (Weeks) | |
|---|---|---|
| | *Invasive* | *Noninvasive* |
| Papillary carcinoma | 65 | 128 |
| Tubular carcinoma | 38 | 110 |
| Solid carcinoma | 26 | 82 |
| Anaplastic carcinoma | 11 | Not applicable |

phoid cells had a threefold decreased risk of recurrence or metastasis within 2 years of surgery, as compared to dogs whose tumors failed to elicit such an immune response. The final correlate with prognosis in this study was presence or absence of lymph node involvement with carcinoma; dogs with metastasis to regional nodes had a poor prognosis, regardless of other factors.

Another classification system (Misdorp and Hart, 1976), based on descriptive morphology of tumors in 253 surgically treated dogs, refers to "complex" tumors (mixed tumors with both secretory and myoepithelial components) and "simple" tumors (only one cell type present). These subclasses were correlated with prognosis. Patients with complex carcinomas survived better than those with simple carcinomas or sarcomas. In this study, 63% of bitches with malignant mammary tumors died or were euthanatized because of recurrent or metastatic tumors within 2 years of surgery.

A large series of surgically treated dogs (320 bitches) in Great Britain (Bostock, 1975) was subjected to classification by histopathologic morphology, and correlates with survival time were reported. Dogs with benign tumors had a median survival time of 114 weeks as compared to 70 weeks for those with carcinoma. More than half the dogs with mammary carcinoma were surgically cured, and those that were destined to die of their malignancy did so within 1 year of surgery. Of the dogs that died of cancer, the pathologic description of the tumor and degree of invasiveness were correlated with length of survival (Table 2).

### Investigational Diagnostics

In human oncologic practice, several other criteria to establish the extent of malignancy of mammary tumors are routinely used. Some of these assays have been used on a limited basis in veterinary medicine. The most common of these assays in human medicine detects the level of hormone receptors for estrogen and progesterone in breast tumors. In women, these tests are used to establish prognosis. Tumors with high levels of cellular hormone receptors tend to be better differentiated and therefore to carry a better prognosis. Also, patients with hormone receptors present on their tu-

mors are more likely to respond to hormone therapy as an adjuvant to other forms of treatment or as single-agent therapy. Assays for estrogen and progesterone receptors can be technically demanding and have not been routinely available in veterinary medicine. In the dog, limited studies have revealed that 50 to 60% of canine mammary tumors are positive for estrogen and progesterone receptors; as is the case in women, the better-differentiated tumors are more likely to be receptor-positive. A recent limited study suggests that survival time is correlated with hormone receptor status in the dog, in that dogs whose tumors expressed estrogen or a combination of estrogen and progesterone receptors had longer survivals than those dogs whose tumors expressed progesterone receptors alone. Dogs that failed to express detectable hormone receptors on their mammary tumor cells had the poorest survival.

Other investigational diagnostics that may prove useful in classifying mammary carcinomas in the future include: flow cytometry to determine the degree of aneuploidy in deoxyribonucleic acid (DNA) content; monoclonal antibody studies for determination of intermediate filaments and cytoplasmic proteins such as cathepsin D; determination of circulating immune complex levels as a correlate with metastatic behavior; and analysis of oncogenes and cytogenetic analysis, which is thought to correlate with outcome in human patients (Hahn, Richardson, and Knapp, 1992).

### THERAPY

#### Surgery

Surgical excision is the most curative modality for treatment of local breast neoplasia (see "Definitive Surgical Treatment of Cancer," this volume, p 462). Some controversy exists as to the best form of surgical therapy. Most large surveys of dogs treated with surgical excision demonstrate that approximately 50% of patients are cured. Most tumors that cause death of the animal do so within 1 year of surgery.

Traditionally in veterinary medicine, five surgical approaches have been used for canine mammary neoplasia: (1) mass excision ("lumpectomy"); (2) removal of the affected gland (simple mastectomy); (3) removal of the tumor, gland, intervening lymphatics, and regional nodes (*en bloc* resection); (4) removal of the gland and adjacent glands plus lymphatics (half chain resection);

and (5) removal of the entire chain of glands plus regional nodes (unilateral mastectomy). As happens in women, radical or whole-chain excision has been demonstrated to provide no survival advantage over excisional biopsy with 2-cm margins in the dog (Allen and Mahaffey, 1989). Different surgeons advocate different approaches, however. Less extensive surgery is associated with less morbidity and more rapid recovery. More extensive surgery may prevent the onset of *de novo* tumors by reducing remaining glandular tissue and thus may be more cost-effective in the long term. More extensive surgery also allows for more thorough evaluation to detect lymphatic and venous invasion, multicentric carcinoma *in situ*, and the regional lymph nodes for metastatic disease (also see "Mammary Tumors in the Dog," this volume, p 518).

Ovariohysterectomy has been advocated at the time of mastectomy. Most studies have demonstrated no advantage in terms of duration of survival, local recurrence rates, or distant metastasis in dogs spayed at the time of mastectomy. However, since 50 to 60% of canine mammary malignancies have receptors for hormones (estrogen or progesterone), removal of the hormone source may be helpful for a subpopulation of cases. Ovariohysterectomy also prevents other reproductive tract diseases such as pyometra and ovarian neoplasia.

## Adjunctive and Palliative Therapy

### RADIATION THERAPY

Radiation therapy to facilitate local control of breast cancer in women is well established. No published studies demonstrate the efficacy of radiotherapy in prolonging survival or preventing local recurrence for canine mammary malignancy. It is very likely that local radiotherapy would prove helpful in a palliative setting for select cases. Further studies are indicated to evaluate the benefits of adjuvant radiotherapy in canine patients.

### CHEMOTHERAPY

In human medicine, the value of chemotherapy for patients with mammary carcinoma has been established. Drugs that have the greatest proven efficacy in women are cyclophosphamide (Cytoxan, Bristol-Myers Oncology), doxorubicin (Adriamycin, Adria Laboratories), methotrexate (Methotrexate, Lederle Laboratories), and fluorouracil (Fluorouracil, Roche Laboratories). In the dog, very limited information has been published to support the use of chemotherapy. Doxorubicin (30 mg/M$^2$ body surface area [BSA] IV every 21 days, maximum eight cycles of therapy) and mitoxantrone (Novantrone, Lederle Laboratories, 5.5 mg/M$^2$ BSA IV every 21 days) have shown efficacy in inducing remission in dogs with advanced mammary cancer (see *CVT XI*, p 389). The author has also found cisplatin (Platinol, Bristol-Myers Oncology, 50 to 70 mg/M$^2$ BSA

IV every 21 days, administered with 6-hr 0.9% saline diureses; see *CVT XI*, p 395) and a combination of fluorouracil, doxorubicin, and cyclophosphamide (FAC protocol) to be useful in palliating canine patients with metastatic mammary carcinoma. Little information is available regarding the use of chemotherapy in an adjuvant (micrometastatic disease) setting in dogs. The FAC protocol consists of: doxorubicin (30 mg/M$^2$ BSA IV day 1); fluorouracil (150 mg/M$^2$ BSA IV days 8 and 15); cyclophosphamide (100 to 200 mg/M$^2$ BSA IV day 1 *or* 50 mg/M$^2$ BSA PO days 3, 4, 5, and 6 of week 1 only); and monitoring with weekly complete blood count (CBC) throughout protocol. This protocol is typically repeated six times for patients with gross metastatic disease if evidence of efficacy is seen. Note that if the IV administration of cyclophosphamide is chosen over the oral route, leukopenia is expected and patients should start sulfa-trimethoprim at 15 mg/kg PO twice daily at the outset of therapy to avoid potential septic complications.

It is difficult to counsel clients about the advisability of adjuvant therapy after surgery because little information is published to support the use of chemotherapy or hormone therapy for these patients. Therefore, careful discussion of the potential benefits and risks of such therapy should take place before any treatment is started; some advise the use of an informed consent form prior to therapy as well. Certainly, for dogs with pulmonary or visceral metastasis or nonresectable tumor, chemotherapy may prove palliative. Palliation can be noble and worthwhile if the treatment goals of relieving discomfort, controlling symptoms, and potentially prolonging the life of the patient are clearly articulated at the outset. However, dogs with aggressive or metastatic mammary carcinoma cannot currently be considered candidates for curative therapy. The issue of treatment of micrometastatic disease in an adjuvant setting, which might ultimately lead to cures for some patients, cannot be adequately addressed until better clinical trials of chemotherapy for gross disease have been carried out for canine and feline patients. The author's guidelines for clinical indications for the consideration of adjunctive chemotherapy and/or hormone therapy are given in Table 3.

### IMMUNE THERAPY

Because mammary tumors induce lymphoid cellular infiltrates detectable on histopathology, stimulation of the immune system has been attempted as an adjuvant to surgical therapy. Immune stimulation approaches that have been tried include levamisole, *Corynebacterium parvum*, and bacilles Calmette-Guérin (BCG). Removal of circulating immune complexes by plasmapheresis or selective immunoabsorption have been attempted in an effort to remove inhibition to the host's native immune reaction to mammary tumors. Thus far, all of these immune treatment approaches remain investigational. Antitumor responses and prolongation of disease-free interval and survival have been reported, but results have not been universally confirmed. Fur-

**Table 3.** *Guidelines for Consideration of Therapy in Dogs With Mammary Cancer*

| Prognostic Factor | Treatment Course |
| --- | --- |
| Any mammary mass | Surgical therapy with 2-cm margins and staging evaluation of regional nodes |
| Malignant mammary mass any size | Baseline therapy is surgical resection with 2-cm margins and staging evaluation of regional nodes, thoracic radiographs |
| Malignant masses >3 cm diameter | As above, followed by monthly physical examination for local relapse and biomonthly thoracic radiographs for 1 year ("tumor watch") |
| Malignant masses, any size, with lymphatic or venous invasion, or lymph node metastasis | As above, plus consider adjuvant chemotherapy with FAC or single-agent therapy with doxorubicin or mitoxantrone; tamoxifen may be helpful for spayed females (pyometra risk) |
| Metastatic disease | Surgery not indicated except as palliation for infected or draining masses; chemotherapy and/or hormone therapy as above |
| Inflammatory carcinoma | Surgery not indicated; palliation with chemotherapy and/or hormone therapy as above; local radiotherapy might be considered |

Abbreviation: FAC = fluorouracil, doxorubicin (Adriamycin), and cyclophosphamide.

ther studies are warranted in academic centers to prove or disprove the utility of immunotherapy for mammary carcinoma in veterinary medicine (Loar, 1989).

### HORMONE THERAPY

The drug tamoxifen (Nolvadex, ICI Pharma) is useful in an adjuvant or advanced disease setting in human patients. Tamoxifen is a nonsteroidal antiestrogenic compound, capable of binding tightly to cytoplasmic estrogen receptors. The drug has estrogenic effects in some tissues, as well as antiestrogenic effects. The anticancer effect of tamoxifen in treating mammary malignancy may be mediated by other mechanisms as well. A subpopulation of women with estrogen receptor–negative tumors have been found to undergo remission when treated with the drug.

Because of difficulty of performing routine estrogen and progesterone receptor assays in dog tissue, hormone therapy has not been established for treatment of canine mammary tumors. The author recently conducted a study of tamoxifen for treatment of mammary carcinoma in 16 dogs (Kitchell and Fidel, 1992). Nine dogs were treated in an adjuvant setting with mammary tumors considered at high risk of relapse based on histologic criteria, and seven dogs had nonresectable or metastatic disease. In our pilot study, tamoxifen (2.5 to 10 mg, mean dose 0.42 mg/kg b.i.d. PO) was shown to be effective in reducing tumor burden in five of seven dogs with nonresectable or metastatic mammary carcinoma. Side effects seen in these 16 dogs included the

relatively minor complaints of vulvar swelling, vaginal discharge, urinary incontinence, urinary tract infection, clinical signs of estrus, mental "dullness," and partial alopecia in less than 40% of these 16 dogs. The most significant side effect seen was pyometra; one intact female had a closed-cervix pyometra that required surgical intervention, and three recently spayed bitches had stump pyometras that were managed medically. The potential for pyometra induction by tamoxifen had been previously reported to occur in 5 of 20 bitches given 1 mg/kg tamoxifen twice daily orally for 10 days, for prevention and termination of pregnancy (Bowen et al., 1988). Our limited study indicates a possible role for tamoxifen therapy in the management of canine mammary carcinoma; however, the practitioner is cautioned to consult an oncologist before considering this therapy (see "Mammary Gland Tumors in the Dog," this volume, p 518, for an alternative view of tamoxifen). The practical considerations of daily oral tamoxifen administration are attractive, given the potential benefits of cancer management over the risk of side effects, which seemed manageable in this preliminary study. Additional studies are needed to establish the potential benefit of hormone therapy for canine mammary carcinoma patients, particularly when coupled with hormone receptor assays.

### FELINE MAMMARY CARCINOMA

Feline mammary tumors present with an overall more aggressive biologic behavior than the disease seen in dogs. When a mammary mass develops in a feline patient, it is 80 to 90% likely to be malignant, with the majority being adenocarcinomas. Median age at onset is 10 to 12 years. Siamese cats have an increased risk of mammary tumor development, with an earlier age at onset than other breeds. Association with age at spaying has not been made for the disease in cats. Mammary carcinoma cells from cats are more likely to express progesterone receptors, and cats treated with progestational drugs are more likely to develop mammary carcinoma.

Most feline mammary cancers are locally invasive and have lymphatic infiltration. Size of tumor is prognostic, in that cats with smaller tumors have longer disease-free intervals and survival times. Surgical excision is the treatment of choice for local control. Uni- or bilateral radical mastectomy has been demonstrated to lead to longer disease-free intervals but not necessarily to longer overall survival times. Cats frequently develop local recurrence after mastectomy; it is not uncommon to manage these by multiple surgeries before eventual metastasis. Doxorubicin and cyclophosphamide have been demonstrated to be effective as an adjuvant therapy to palliate advanced mammary carcinoma in cats. Note that fluorouracil is contraindicated for use in cats because of fatal neurotoxicity; the FAC protocol is indicated for *canine use only* (Loar, 1989).

## References and Suggested Reading

Allen SW and Mahaffey EA: Canine mammary neoplasia: Prognostic indicators and response to surgical therapy. J Am Anim Hosp Assoc 25:540, 1989.
*A review of surgical therapy that demonstrates that simple lumpectomy with adequate margins is the optimum treatment for canine mammary carcinoma.*

Bostock DE: The prognosis following surgical excision of canine mammary tumors. Eur J Cancer 11:389, 1975.
*A large series of surgically treated mammary tumors in dogs revealed histologic correlates for survival that could be useful for practitioners in giving owners an accurate prognosis and help to determine the appropriateness of adjuvant therapy.*

Bowen RA, Olson PN, Young S, et al: Efficacy and toxicity of tamoxifen citrate for prevention and termination of pregnancy in bitches. Am J Vet Res 49:27, 1988.
*The only published discussion of tamoxifen use in the dog, which recommends against the use of this antiestrogen drug for fertility control due to the relatively high incidence of pyometra as an adverse effect.*

Hahn KA, Richardson RC, and Knapp DW: Canine malignant mammary neoplasia: Biological behavior, diagnosis, and treatment alternatives. J Am Anim Hosp Assoc 28:251, 1992.
*A good review of the state of our understanding of mammary carcinoma in dogs follows two brief case reports demonstrating the efficacy of doxorubicin as a single agent in the treatment of metastatic mammary tumors.*

Kitchell BE and Fidel JL: Tamoxifen as a potential therapy for canine mammary carcinoma. Proc Vet Cancer Soc Annual Forum 12:91, 1992.
*Sixteen dogs with mammary carcinoma were treated with tamoxifen; observed toxicities and efficacy rates are reported.*

Kurzman ID and Gilbertson SR: Prognostic factors in canine mammary tumors. Semin Vet Med Surg (Small Anim) 1:25, 1986.
*An excellent review of a large series of cases evaluated for several clinical and histologic criteria to determine prognosis in canine mammary tumors.*

Loar AS: Tumors of the genital system and mammary glands. *In* Ettinger SJ (ed): *Textbook of Veterinary Internal Medicine*, 3rd edition. Philadelphia, WB Saunders Co, 1989, p 1820.
*An overview of mammary tumors in the dog and cat.*

Madewell BR and Theilen GH: Tumors of the mammary gland. *In* Theilen GH and Madewell BR (eds): *Veterinary Cancer Medicine*, 2nd edition. Philadelphia, Lea & Febiger, 1987, p 327.
*The definitive overview of mammary cancer in dogs and cats; a must for practitioners seeking an understanding of this disease.*

Misdorp W and Hart AAM: Prognostic factors in canine mammary cancer. J Natl Cancer Inst 56:779, 1976.
*A large series of cases is reviewed correlating histologic type of malignancy with survival time.*

Shofer FS, Sonnenschein EG, Goldschmidt MH, et al: Histopathologic and dietary prognostic factors for canine mammary carcinoma. Breast Cancer Res Treat 13:49, 1989.
*An interesting epidemiologic and histologic study correlating several prognostic factors including dietary fat content with eventual outcome of dogs with mammary cancer.*

# CANINE PROSTATIC DISORDERS

JEFFREY S. KLAUSNER,
SHIRLEY D. JOHNSTON,
*and* FORD W. BELL
*St. Paul, Minnesota*

Prostatic disease is common in the male dog. Prostatic disorders comprise approximately 2.5% of canine cases referred to veterinary teaching hospitals, but the prevalence is probably much greater in the general practice population, since many dogs with prostatitis and benign prostatic hyperplasia are not referred. Doberman pinschers are reported to be at increased risk for prostatic disease.

## BENIGN PROSTATIC HYPERPLASIA

Benign prostatic hyperplasia (BPH) is an extremely common aging change in the male dog (see "Medical Management of Canine Prostatic Hyperplasia, this volume, p 1033). Benign prostatic hyperplasia is observed initially in intact male dogs between 1 and 2 years of age, with the prevalence increasing linearly so that 60% of intact male dogs are affected by age 6. By 9 years of age, the prevalence of BPH in intact male dogs is 95%.

### Pathology

Canine BPH occurs in two phases: glandular and complex (Coffey and Walsh, 1990). In dogs less than 5 years of age, BPH is primarily glandular. Glandular hyperplasia is characterized by symmetric enlargement of the prostate; secretory cells are increased in number and size. Proliferation is primarily epithelial, with minimal stromal involvement. Complex hyperplasia, typically observed in dogs greater than 5 years of age, is characterized by asymmetric enlargement of the prostate, with areas of glandular hyperplasia intermingled with areas of atrophy. Stromal elements are prominent, especially in atrophic areas. Alveoli frequently are dilated, cystic, and filled with eosinophilic material. Chronic inflammation and squamous metaplasia of the epithelium may be present.

### Etiology

Although the exact cause of BPH has not been determined, aging and testicular hormones are important prerequisites. Castration results in rapid involution of affected prostates. Androgen and estrogen administration to intact or castrated dogs results in pathologic changes similar to spontaneously occurring BPH. Administration of androgen results in orderly proliferation of prostatic epithelial cells, while estrogen administration results in atrophy of glandular epithelial cells, proliferation of prostatic basal cells, and squamous metaplasia of epithelial ducts.

Circulating testosterone is converted to $5\alpha$-dihydrotestosterone (DHT) by $5\alpha$-reductase within prostatic epithelial cells. DHT, the active metabolite of testosterone, regulates prostatic growth by binding to specific nuclear androgen receptors. Prostates of dogs with BPH do not contain more DHT than normal dogs, but increased DHT receptors are present.

Stromal elements within the prostate also may contribute to the pathogenesis of BPH. Extensive connections exist between the prostatic stroma, basement membrane, epithelial cell cytoskeleton, and nucleus. Prostatic stroma has embryonic-like inductive properties, and stromal alterations have been demonstrated to stimulate basal cell proliferation. Prostatic stroma also may contribute to the genesis of BPH by altering the differentiation of epithelial cells. Although BPH is typically associated with stimulation of epithelial cell proliferation, prostatic enlargement also could result from a decrease in normal cell loss. Prostatic cells normally proliferate, differentiate, and then die. If terminal differentiation were blocked, a decrease in cell death would follow. In support of this theory, it has been noted that deoxyribonucleic acid (DNA) synthesis and cell turnover rates are decreased in dogs with experimental BPH.

Estrogens also contribute to the development of BPH. As intact male dogs age, serum estrogen levels remain constant, while serum testosterone and prostatic DHT levels fall. Estrogens induce nuclear DHT receptors and thus may increase the sensitivity of the prostate to DHT. Estrogens have also been reported to alter the rate of prostatic cell death.

### Clinical Findings and Diagnosis

Most dogs with BPH are asymptomatic. Clinical signs, when present, may include bloody urethral discharge, blood in the urine or ejaculate, and straining to defecate. Dysuria rarely is noted unless concurrent urinary tract infection is present. Occasionally, ribbon-like stools and dyschezia are observed if the enlarged prostate compresses the descending colon. Cause-and-effect relationships between BPH and bacterial prostatitis have not been definitely established, but clinical evidence suggests that BPH is a likely risk factor in prostatitis.

Physical examination in dogs with BPH typically reveals symmetric or nonsymmetric prostatic enlargement with normal prostatic consistency. The prostate is not painful to palpation unless bacterial infection also is present. Because the signs of BPH are similar to other prostatic disorders, laboratory and radiographic evaluations are typically required to confirm the diagnosis.

Samples for cytologic analysis and culture can be obtained by ejaculation, prostatic massage, or aspiration biopsy of the prostate. Prostatic fluid is the last portion of the ejaculate and follows the sperm-rich fraction.

Prior to ejaculation, the dog should be allowed to urinate to remove urethral contents. Prostatic massage is performed by removing urine from the bladder, placing the tip of a urinary catheter in the prostatic urethra using rectal palpation as a guide, gently massaging the prostate per rectum or per abdomen for 1 to 2 min, and aspirating material into the catheter.

In dogs with BPH, prostatic fluid and prostatic massage samples may be clear or hemorrhagic. Epithelial cells are similar in appearance to those obtained from normal prostates. Red blood cell numbers vary from none to too numerous to count. Inflammatory cells are absent or present in low number unless bacterial prostatitis is present. Culture of prostatic fluid from dogs with BPH reveals less than 10,000 bacteria per milliter of semen if bacterial infection is not present.

Prostatomegaly is the most frequent abnormality noted on survey abdominal radiographs (Feeney et al., 1987a). Retrograde urethrocystography may reveal narrowing of the prostatic urethra or reflux of contrast media into the hyperplastic gland. Reflux is considered abnormal if it extends more than one urethral diameter into the prostatic parenchyma and/or has a jagged, irregular appearance. Ultrasonographic evaluation reveals prostatic enlargement with uniform parenchymal echogenicity. Small fluid-filled cysts may be noted. Radiographic and ultrasonographic changes are nonspecific, and similar changes may be observed in dogs with bacterial prostatitis or prostatic neoplasia (see "Imaging the Reproductive Tract in the Male Dog," this volume, p 1052).

A serum test may be available soon to aid in the diagnosis of BPH. The major protein in canine seminal plasma is canine secretory prostatic esterase (CPSE) (Isaccs and Sharper, 1985). CPSE is produced by prostatic epithelial cells under the influence of testosterone, and in studies performed at the University of Minnesota, serum CPSE concentration was significantly elevated in dogs with BPH compared to normal dogs, dogs with bacterial prostatitis, and dogs with prostatic carcinoma.

Clinical evaluation, laboratory findings, evaluation of prostatic fluid, and imaging studies usually provide a presumptive diagnosis of BPH. If required, definitive diagnosis of BPH can be established by needle or surgical biopsy of the prostate. Biopsy with ultrasound guidance is a safe and effective means of obtaining prostatic tissue (see "Imaging the Reproductive Tract in the Male Dog," this volume, p 1052).

### Therapy

Treatment of BPH may be necessary in dogs with clinical signs. Castration is the most effective therapy, resulting in rapid involution of the enlarged prostate. If castration is not acceptable, medical methods of reducing androgenic stimulation of the prostate may be considered. A decrease in prostatic size was noted in dogs with BPH following treatment with megestrol acetate (Ovaban, Schering) at a dose of 0.11 mg/kg orally daily for 3 weeks. Megestrol inhibits luteinizing hormone (LH) release and decreases 5α-reductase activity without adversely affecting semen quality. Medroxyprogesterone (Gestapuran vet; 25mg/ml) at a dose of 3 mg/kg subcutaneously resulted in a decrease in clinical signs in 84% and a decrease in prostatic size in 53% of dogs with BPH. Finasteride (Proscar, Merck Sharp & Dohme), a 5α-reductase inhibitor, decreases intraprostatic DHT concentration without affecting serum testosterone levels and should not affect semen production. Finasteride, at 5 mg/kg per os once daily, reduced prostatic size by one third in dogs with BPH (Cohen et al., 1991). This dose is high in comparison to the human dose of 5 mg/day, and a lower canine dose may be effective, but dose-response studies in the dog have not been reported. Other agents that might be of benefit in treating dogs with BPH include antiandrogens and luteinizing hormone releasing hormone (LHRH) agonists.

## PROSTATITIS

Prostatitis has been described as the most common of the diagnosed prostatic diseases identified in intact male dogs (Krawiec and Heflin, 1992). It may occur as acute or chronic prostatitis, with or without abscessation (see "CVT Update: Treatment of Canine Bacterial Prostatitis," this volume, p 1029). The disorder usually is associated with bacterial infection of a hyperplastic prostate gland. Prostatic abscessation, which usually occurs in dogs older than age 5 years, is associated with relatively high mortality, due to rupture of abscesses and resulting peritonitis. Prostatitis is rare in dogs castrated more than 1 year prior to presentation.

### Pathology

Suppurative or chronic active prostatitis is the most common histologic characterization of prostate tissue from affected dogs, with pyogranulomatous prostatitis occurring rarely in fungal infections. Exfoliative cytology of the prostate reveals presence of prostatic epithelial cells, degenerate neutrophils, macrophages, and free or phagocytized gram-negative rods or gram-positive cocci. Lymphocytes and plasma cells are observed infrequently. Benign prostatic hyperplasia often is present concurrently. Prostatic abscesses may occur in either lobe of the prostate, and may drain into the urethra; abscess rupture may be associated with acute peritonitis.

### Etiology

Canine prostatitis usually is caused by ascending bacterial or mycoplasmal infection of the canine prostate by organisms that comprise normal urethral flora. *Escherichia coli* is the most common bacterial organism identified in dogs with bacterial prostatitis, followed by *Staphylococcus aureus*, *Klebsiella spp.*, *Proteus mirabilis*, *Mycoplasma canis*, *Pseudomonas aeruginosa*, *Enterobacter spp.*, *Streptococcus spp.*, *Pasteurella spp.*, and *Haemophilus spp.* *Brucella canis* may infect the canine prostate, but is more commonly associated with testicular infection and clinical signs referable to the testes. Anaerobic bacteria occasionally are isolated from the prostatic fluid of dogs with bacterial prostatitis. Rarely, *Blastomyces dermatitidis*, *Cryptococcus neoformans*, or *Coccidioides immitis* may cause fungal infection of the canine prostate by ascending infection, systemic infection or, in the case of *Blastomyces*, penetration of the scrotal skin and descending prostatic infection from a testicular source. The presence of benign prostatic cystic hyperplasia may predispose to ascending infection of the prostate.

### Clinical Findings and Diagnosis

Clinical signs in dogs with acute prostatitis include fever, depression, straining to urinate or defecate, pain on rectal palpation of the prostate, abnormal texture or contour to the prostate palpated per rectum, stiff-legged gait, hematuria, scrotal/preputial/hindlimb edema, and pollakiuria; one, some, or all of these signs may be present. Dogs with prostatic abscessation and/or peritonitis may, in addition, show signs of sepsis and shock (tachycardia, delayed capillary refill time, pale or muddy mucous membranes, weak pulses, vomition). Laboratory findings in most affected dogs include leukocytosis with regenerative left shift; a small number of dogs may show leukopenia. Dogs with prostatic abscessation also have been reported to have elevated serum alkaline phosphatase (47%), hypoglycemia (40%), elevated serum alanine transaminase (13%), hyperglobulinemia (12%), and azotemia (11%) (Mullen, Matthiesen, and Scavelli, 1990). Urine collected by cystocentesis may contain blood, bacteria, and leukocytes, because prostatic fluid constantly drips retrograde from the prostatic urethra into the urinary bladder in the intact male dog.

Chronic prostatitis may occur following acute infection, or may develop unnoticed. Clinical signs in dogs with chronic prostatitis may be absent, or may consist of poor semen quality (decreased percentage of motile or morphologically normal sperm in the ejaculate) or decreased libido if prostatic contraction is painful. Urine may contain blood, bacteria, and leukocytes as with acute prostatitis, and dogs with chronic prostatitis may be presented to the veterinarian for suspected lower urinary tract infection.

Presumptive diagnosis of acute prostatitis is based on presence of clinical signs in an intact or recently castrated male dog. Definitive diagnosis is made by detecting inflammatory exudate in prostatic fluid collected by ejaculation, prostatic massage, or ultrasound-directed needle aspiration of prostatic cysts. Needle aspiration of an infected prostate or prostatic abscess should be avoided, when possible, so as to prevent seeding of the needle track with bacteria. The exudate should be characterized cytologically and microbiologically, which permits diagnosis of bacterial and fungal disease as well as determination of bacterial sensitivity to antibiotics. Normal canine semen and/or prostatic fluid should contain less than 10,000 bacteria per milliter, and sediment should not contain significant numbers of inflammatory cells. Prostatic ultrasonography is recommended for all dogs with prostatic disease because, diagnostically, this procedure can detect more than one type of prostatic disease in a single prostate, and because, therapeutically, presence of cysts/abscesses may indicate need for surgical drainage (see "Imaging the Reproductive Tract in the Male Dog," this volume, p 1052). Alternatively, radiographic imaging with retrograde cystourethrography may permit detection of increased prostatic size and presence of intraprostatic cysts or abscesses. *Brucella canis* serology is indicated in male dogs with prostatitis, to rule out canine brucellosis.

## Therapy

The three treatment strategies that should be considered for canine prostatitis include specific antimicrobial therapy, drainage of abscesses, if present, and consideration of castration or antiandrogen therapy to cause decrease in prostate size. Supportive fluid and/or shock therapy also may be indicated in dogs with severe compromise due to acute prostatitis.

Antibacterial therapy should be selected based on sensitivity of bacteria cultured from inflammatory exudates and on ability of the antibiotic to diffuse into prostatic fluid in therapeutic concentrations. The blood-prostate barrier in the normal dog prevents diffusion of drugs with low lipid solubility or those that are highly protein bound in plasma from entering the prostatic fluid in therapeutic concentration. In addition, pH gradients between blood and prostatic fluid may influence ionized drug trapping in prostatic fluid. In general, antibiotics known to diffuse into prostatic fluid of the normal dog in therapeutic concentrations include trimethoprim-sulfa, chloramphenicol, and enrofloxacin, all of which are effective in treating most aerobic bacterial infections of the canine prostate. Enrofloxacin is effective against mycoplasma infections. Trimethoprim-sulfa and enrofloxacin are not effective against anaerobic infections; chloramphenicol is indicated if anaerobes are present. Inflammatory compromise of the blood-prostate barrier in acute and chronic prostatitis, which might permit therapeutic concentrations of other antibiotics to reach the site of infection, has not been well studied. Fungal prostatitis usually is a part of systemic fungal infection in the dog, which should be treated with systemic antifungal regimens.

Drainage of the prostate is indicated if abscessation is present, as antibiotic therapy alone or that therapy used with castration will not cure the abscessation. Surgical drainage of prostatic abscesses has been accomplished by needle aspirate, surgical application of multiple Penrose drains drawn through and fixed to the ventral lateral abdominal wall, partial prostatectomy, and marsupialization. Complications may occur with all methods. In one study of 92 dogs treated with multiple Penrose drain application for prostatic abscessation, three dogs died during surgery, and 19 died or were euthanized in the immediate postoperative period because of sepsis, shock, and peritonitis (Mullen, Matthiesen, and Scavelli, 1990). Long-term follow-up of 56 dogs was associated with good to excellent results in 33, fair results in 14, and poor results in nine. Postoperative complications included painful abdomen, scrotal/preputial/hindlimb edema, hyoproteinemia, hypoglycemia, anemia, sepsis/shock, hypokalemia, and urine leakage from Penrose drains.

Castration should be considered in dogs with prostatitis if the disorder is a recurrent one, if infection is associated with a hyperplastic gland, or if reproductive potential is unimportant to the client. Castration will result in prostatic atrophy, even of the hyperplastic gland, and has been shown to reduce duration of chronic bacterial prostatitis and number of bacterial colony-forming units per milliliter of urine in experimentally infected dogs (Cowan et al., 1991). Castration is not recommended in the presence of acute infection, as such surgery may result in presence of scirrhous spermatic cords. Therapy with the antiandrogens megestrol acetate (0.11 mg/kg PO once daily) or finasteride (5 mg/kg PO once daily) may be used to accomplish decrease in prostate size temporarily, until infection is controlled with antibiotics and castration or breeding, if desired, can be accomplished.

## PROSTATIC ADENOCARCINOMA

Prostatic adenocarcinoma (PAC) is an uncommon, highly malignant disease of intact and castrated male dogs. Because clinical signs and laboratory and radiographic findings are similar among the different forms of prostatic disease, a definitive diagnosis of prostatic adenocarcinoma usually is made when the disease is at an advanced stage. The disease is most frequent in 8- to 10-year-old dogs (Bell et al., 1991). The prevalence of PAC in dogs castrated at a young age is at least equal to, and may be greater than, the prevalence in intact dogs (Obradovich, Walshaw, and Goullaud, 1987).

## Pathology

Five histopathologic grades of PAC have been described ranging from well-differentiated to anaplastic, poorly differentiated tumors. Neutered dogs are most likely to have poorly differentiated tumors, although well-differentiated tumors, with evidence of gland formation, also occur in neutered dogs. Prostatic hyperplasia and resultant prostatomegaly occur commonly with PAC in intact dogs, and may aggravate clinical signs. Other secondary histopathologic findings in dogs with PAC include inflammatory cell infiltrates (lymphocytes and/or plasma cells most commonly), intratumoral necrosis, fibrous connective tissue proliferation (scirrhous reaction), and mineralization.

## Etiology

The etiology of PAC has not been determined, although androgens have been proposed as an etiologic factor in human prostatic carcinomas, which often respond to antiandrogen therapy. Canine PAC does not appear to be androgen responsive, as androgen deprivation (orchiectomy, estrogen therapy) has not been of benefit in management of canine PAC. Testosterone may exert an etiologic influence at a very early age, which could explain why intact and neutered dogs are both at risk. Androgen-independent basal cells, which persist after neutering, may provide the cell of origin for development of PAC in both neutered and intact dogs. Nontesticular androgens (adrenal origin) may have a role in the development of the disease in neutered dogs.

## Clinical Findings and Diagnosis

Lower gastrointestinal signs (tenesmus, dyschezia, constipation) predominate in dogs with PAC. Anorexia and weight loss were the second most common complaints in one series of cases. Urinary tract signs (hematuria, stranguria, pollakiuria) occur more frequently in neutered dogs with PAC. Presumably, the absence of concurrent hyperplastic change in neutered dogs results in a smaller prostatic mass, thus delaying or preventing manifestation of gastrointestinal signs. With time, continued tumor growth results in progressive invasion and compromise of the urinary tract. Signs referable to extensive tumor burden or metastatic disease may result in severe cachexia and bone pain, especially in the lumbosacral area.

Prostatomegaly is the most common finding on physical examination. Enlargement is often asymmetric; palpation may be painful. The gland often feels indurated and irregular on digital exam. The prostate may become so enlarged that it drops over the pelvic brim and cannot be palpated rectally, creating a palpable mass in the caudal abdomen. It is important to note that prostatomegaly is relative in a neutered patient. Neutered dogs should have no detectable prostatic tissue, and a "normal size prostate" in a neutered dog is highly suggestive of malignancy. The only exceptions to this would be dogs who have an unsuspected cryptorchid testicle, who are receiving estrogen therapy, or who have been neutered because of severe inflammatory disease or complex (cystic) BPH. In the latter group, persistence of cystic prostatic tissue after castration may result in palpable remnant tissue in the area of the prostate.

Exfoliative cytology is the simplest and most consistently successful means of diagnosing PAC. Transrectal aspiration biopsy of the prostate can be done without sedation or prior bowel preparation, and complications

are extremely rare. Bleeding following biopsy occurs occasionally, but virtually always resolves without complication or need for therapy. Transrectal biopsy is best done using the Franzen needle guide (Precision Dynamics, Burbank, CA). Transrectal aspiration may be difficult or impossible in very large dogs, or when the prostatic mass has dropped over the pelvic brim and is not accessible per rectum. Transabdominal prostatic aspiration often is possible, especially with very large prostatic masses. Ultrasound-guided aspiration allows sonographic visualization of the area to be sampled, and may increase the likelihood of obtaining a diagnostic aspiration. Urethral catheter biopsy also may be used to obtain cytologic samples. A rigid (polypropylene) catheter is advanced into the bladder, and then pulled back slightly, to the level of the prostatic urethra. The catheter is then advanced and retracted several times, rapidly, for a short distance, while aspirating. Care should be taken to avoid diluting the sample with urine; the aspirated sample should be expressed onto slides to make appropriate cytologic preparations.

Needle core biopsy (Tru-Cut Biopsy Needle, Travenol Laboratories, Deerfield, IL) of the prostate usually is performed by a transabdominal approach. The procedure is very simple in those cases where the prostatic mass is easily palpated abdominally, and can be immobilized during the procedure. The skin should be shaved and surgically prepared prior to biopsy; a small stab incision is made with a No. 11 scalpel blade to permit passage of the biopsy instrument. Ultrasound-guided biopsy greatly enhances the accuracy of needle core biopsy, increases the likelihood of a diagnostic procedure, and minimizes the risks of postbiopsy complications.

The combination of ultrasonography and distention retrograde urethrography is helpful in the diagnosis and staging of PAC (Feeney et al., 1987b) (see "Imaging the Reproductive Tract in the Male Dog," this volume, p 1052). Ultrasonography allows assessment of prostatic contour as well as texture of prostatic parenchymal tissue. Focal to multifocal areas of echogenicity (a "mottled" pattern) is very characteristic of PAC. The presence of mineralization may be detected by prostatic ultrasonography (manifested as echodense foci with resultant acoustic shadowing), and is highly correlated with the presence of PAC, although mineralization also can occur with chronic prostatitis. Intraprostatic cysts or cavities also are observed occasionally in dogs with PAC. The most common abnormalities seen with distention retrograde urethrography in dogs with PAC include compression of the prostatic urethra and abnormal prostatic reflux. Reflux is considered abnormal if it extends more than 1 urethral diameter into the prostatic parenchyma and/or has a jagged, irregular appearance. In normal dogs, prostatic reflux usually has a symmetrical, smoothly marginated appearance. Urethral mucosal irregularity and/or urethral obstruction also may be evident.

In contrast to human patients with prostatic adenocarcinomas, serum markers (prostatic alkaline phosphatase and prostate-specific antigen) have not been shown to be of benefit in the diagnosis and/or staging of PAC in dogs. Canine prostate-specific esterase is the major protein in canine prostatic fluid. Although it appears to be of benefit in the diagnosis of benign prostatic hyperplasia, significant elevations have not been documented in dogs with PAC. Studies on the potential usefulness of CPSE in the diagnosis and staging of canine PAC are in progress at the University of Minnesota.

## Therapy

Therapeutic options for canine PAC are limited. Surgical resection of prostatic tumors generally is not an option because the disease is rarely diagnosed at an early stage. Prostatic surgery is difficult, and urinary incontinence is a common sequela.

Chemotherapy is of limited value in the treatment of prostatic malignancy in men. Similarly, chemotherapy has not shown promise in the treatment of canine PAC.

Prostatic adenocarcinoma in dogs does not respond to androgen deprivation therapy (e.g., castration, estrogens) as does PAC in men. However, intact dogs with PAC may benefit from surgical or pharmacologic castration, as regression of the hyperplastic component of the prostatic mass can result in symptomatic relief. Megestrol acetate or finasteride, at dosages noted above, may be of benefit.

External beam radiation therapy has been of some benefit in the treatment of PAC. Shrinkage of tumor, with relief of urinary outflow obstruction and/or obstipation, occurred in dogs treated with $^{60}$Co teletherapy. Unfortunately, survival times remain short. At the University of Minnesota, maximum survival following radiation therapy has been 5 months. In one report of ten dogs treated with intraoperative radiation therapy (in some cases in conjunction with chemotherapy), five of the dogs showed no response. The median survival for all dogs was 114 days (Turrel, 1987).

Dogs with PAC may benefit from stool softeners, if obstipation is present. Dogs with signs arising from the urinary tract may benefit from control of secondary bacterial cystitis, a common complication in dogs with PAC. Continuous antibiotic therapy may reduce pollakiuria and stranguria, and improve quality of life.

The prognosis for dogs with PAC is grave. It is unknown whether earlier diagnosis and aggressive early therapy will result in better quality of life and longer survival times for dogs with this disease.

## References and Suggested Reading

Bell FW, Klausner JS, Hayden DW, et al: Clinical and pathologic features of prostatic adenocarcinoma in sexually intact and castrated dogs: 31 cases (1970–1987). J Am Vet Med Assoc 199:1623, 1991.
*A retrospective study comparing the clinical manifestations of prostatic adenocarcinoma in intact and castrated dogs.*

Cohen SM, Taber KH, Malatesta PF, et al: Magnetic resonance imaging of the efficacy of specific inhibition of 5 alpha reductase in canine spontaneous benign prostatic hyperplasia. Magn Reson I Med 21:55, 1991.
*An experimental study of six male beagles and five controls that demonstrated a significant reduction in prostate volume with oral administration of finasteride (5 mg/kg/day) over a 12-week period.*

Coffey DS and Walsh PC: Clinical and experimental studies of benign prostatic hyperplasia. Urol Clin 17:461, 1990.
*A review of experimental studies of dogs with benign prostatic hyperplasia.*

Cowan LA, Barsanti JA, Crowell W, et al: Effects of castration on chronic bacterial prostatitis in dogs. J Am Vet Med Assoc 199:346, 1991.
*Experimental study providing support for the use of castration in the therapy of bacterial prostatitis in the dog.*

Feeney DA, Johnston GR, Klausner JS, et al: Canine prostatic disease—comparison of radiographic appearance with morphologic and microbiologic findings: 30 cases (1981–1985). J Am Vet Med Assoc 190:1018, 1987a.
*A retrospective study describing the radiographic appearance of canine prostatic disorders.*

Feeney DA, Johnston GR, Klausner JS, et al: Canine prostatic disease—comparison of ultrasonographic appearance with morphologic and microbiologic findings: 30 cases (1981–1985). J Am Vet Med Assoc 190:1027, 1987b.
*A restrospective study describing the ultrasonographic appearance of canine prostatic disorders.*

Isaacs WB and Shaper JH: Immunological localization and quantitation of the androgen-dependent secretory protease of the canine prostate. Endocrinology 117:1512, 1985.
*An experimental study characterizing canine prostatic secretory esterase.*

Krawiec DR and Heflin D: Study of prostatic disease in dogs: 177 cases (1981–1986). J Am Vet Med Assoc 200:1119, 1992.
*A restrospective study describing the clinical manifestions of canine prostatic disorders.*

Mullen HS, Matthiesen NDT, and Scavelli TD: Results of surgery and postopertive complications in 92 dogs treated for prostatic abscessation by a multiple Penrose drain technique. J Am Anim Hosp Assoc 26:369, 1990.
*A clinical study describing the results of surgical treatment of prostatic abscesses in 92 dogs.*

Obradovich J, Walshaw R, and Goullaud E: The influence of castration on the development of prostatic carcinoma in the dog. J Vet Intern Med 1:183, 1987.
*A retrospective study emphasizing the occurrence of prostatic carcinoma in castrated dogs.*

Turrel J: Intraoperative radiotherapy of carcinoma of the prostate gland in ten dogs. J Am Vet Med Assoc 190:48, 1987.
*A clinical study describing the results of intraoperative radiation therapy on survival in dogs with prostatic adenocarcinoma.*

# Section

# 12

# NEUROLOGIC AND MUSCULOSKELETAL DISORDERS

KYLE G. BRAUND
*and* STEVEN C. SCHRADER
*Consulting Editors*

# CONGENITAL AND INHERITED NEUROLOGIC DISORDERS IN DOGS AND CATS

JOAN R. COATES
*Athens, Georgia*
*and* KAREN L. KLINE
*Columbia, Missouri*

Many neurologic diseases constitute an inherited or congenital defect. Signalment is an important consideration for identifying inherited or congenital disorders (Braund, 1994). Inherited disorders often show clinical signs through chronic degenerative processes. The congenital disorders are static or result in secondary degenerative processes. Paroxysmal or episodic disorders can have a breed predisposition or an inherited basis. This article will categorize these disorders in tabular form: degenerative conditions clinically manifesting central nervous system, neuropathic, or myopathic diseases (Tables 1, 2, and 3); congenital malformations (Table 4); and paroxysmal disorders (Table 5).

Clinical signs can serve as a basis for the initial identification of these disorders; however, neuropathology is usually necessary for a definitive diagnosis. Degenerative diseases of the central nervous system (CNS) represent a variety of clinical signs, depending upon the neuronal structure afflicted and the location of the lesion (Duncan, 1987; Evans, 1989; Vandevelde, 1980). Localization is considered multifocal or diffuse in many instances. *Abiotrophy* is a general term describing the neuropathologic features of these degenerative disorders (de Lahunta, 1990). Neuropathology may only show selective involvement of certain columns, tracts, and/or nuclei. Neuromuscular diseases often show

***Table 1.*** *CNS Degenerative Disorders*

| Disorder | Breeds | Age | Inheritance |
|---|---|---|---|
| **Afghan Hound Myelopathy** | Afghan hound | 3–13 mo | AR |
| Myelinolytic disorder of white matter with cavitation and necrosis extending from the caudal cervical regions to midlumbar region; most severely affecting the midthoracic region | | | |
| **Calcinosis Circumscripta** | English springer spaniel | <1 yr | Unknown |
| Single or multiple calcium deposits which may originate from vertebral bodies and cause spinal cord impingement | German shepherd | | Suspect |
| | Great Dane | | Suspect |
| | Rottweiler | | Unknown |
| | Vizsla | | Suspect |
| **Cerebellar Abiotrophies** | | | |
| Purkinje neuron degeneration | Airedale | <6 mo | Familial |
| Purkinje and granule cell degeneration | Australian kelpies | 6–12 wk | AR |
| Purkinje and granule cell degeneration | Beagles | 3 wk | Familial? |
| Purkinje neuron degeneration | Bern running dog | <6 mo | Suspect |
| Purkinje neuron degeneration | Bernese mountain dog | <6 mo | Familial |
| Loss of granule and Purkinje neurons of rostral vermis | Border collies | 6–8 wk | Familial? |
| Purkinje neuron degeneration of vermis | Brittany spaniels | 7–13 yr | Suspect |
| Vacuolation, gliosis, spheroids around cerebellar peduncle, vestibular nuclei and caudal colliculus | Bull mastiffs | 4–9 wk | AR |
| Purkinje neuron degeneration | Bull terrier | <3 mo | Unknown |
| Purkinje neuron degeneration | English springer spaniel | 6–16 wk | Unknown |

*Table continued on following page*

1111

**Table 1.** *Continued*

| Disorder | Breeds | Age | Inheritance |
|---|---|---|---|
| Purkinje neuron degeneration | Finnish harrier | <6 mo | Familial |
| Purkinje neuron degeneration | German shepherd | 6–16 wk | Unknown |
| Degeneration of Purkinje neurons in cortex; loss of granule neurons | Gordon setter | 6 mo–3 yr | AR |
| Purkinje neuron degeneration | Irish setter | <3 mo | Unknown |
| Degeneration of cortical nuclei, Purkinje cells olivary nuclei, substantia nigra, caudate nuclei | Kerry blue terrier | 9–12 wk | AR |
| Purkinje and granule cell degeneration all regions | Labrador retriever | 12 wk | Familial |
| Purkinje neuron degeneration; diffuse degeneration in cerebral cortex | Miniature poodle | 3–4 wk | Familial |
| Degeneration of cortex, nuclei in cerebellum and brain stem (olivary and vestibular nuclei), lateral and ventral funiculi | Rough coated collie | 4–12 wk | AR |
| Purkinje neuron degeneration | Samoyed | <6 mo | Suspect |
| Purkinje neuron degeneration | Schnauzer-beagle X | 4.5–6 mo | Unknown |
| ***Dalmatian Leukodystrophy*** <br> Brain atrophy, cavitation of white matter of cerebral hemispheres, ventricular dilatation | Dalmatian | 3–6 mo | AR? |
| ***Degenerative Myelopathy*** | Chesapeake Bay retriever | | Unknown |
| | Domestic shorthair cat | | Unknown |
| Degeneration of white matter in dorsolateral and ventromedial funiculi; dorsal root and neuronal loss in dorsal gray matter | German shepherd | >5 yr | Suspected |
| | Kerry blue terrier | | Unknown |
| | Rough coated collie | | Unknown |
| | Siberian husky | | Unknown |
| ***Demyelinating Myelopathy*** <br> Diffuse demyelination of all white matter tracts of spinal cord; focal areas of demyelination in cerebellum, midbrain, and cerebrum | Miniature poodles | 2–4 mo | Unknown |
| ***Fibrinoid Encephalomyelopathy*** <br> Alexander's disease; accumulation of Rosenthal fibers in midbrain and pons | Labrador retriever | 8 mo | Unknown |
| | Miniature poodle | 9 mo | Unknown |
| | Scottish terrier | 6 mo | Unknown |
| ***Hereditary Ataxia*** <br> Focal wallerian degeneration in dorsolateral and ventromedial white matter of cervical and thoracic spinal cord; including central auditory pathway and peripheral nerves in Jack Russel terrier | Jack Russell terrier | 2–6 mo | AR? |
| | Smooth fox terrier | 2–6 mo | AR |
| ***Hound Ataxia*** <br> Wallerian degeneration of all spinal tracts except dorsal columns and lateral funiculi in cervical region | Beagle | 2–7 yr | Unknown |
| | Fox hound | 2–7 yr | Unknown |
| | Harrier hound | 2–7 yr | Unknown |
| ***Hypomyelinogenesis CNS*** <br> Spinal cord; no brain involvement | Bernese mountain dog | 2–8 wk | AR? |
| Generalized in CNS; especially cerebellum | Chow chow | 2–4 wk | Familial? |
| No myelin in CNS | Dalmatian | 2–4 wk | Unknown |
| Generalized in CNS | Lurcher hound | 2–4 wk | Unknown |
| Generalized in CNS | Samoyed | 2–4 wk | Familial? |
| Especially in cerebrum and optic nerve | Springer spaniel | 2–4 wk | X-linked |
| Generalized in CNS | Weimaraner | 1–3 wk | Familial? |

*Table continued on opposite page*

**Table 1.** *Continued*

| Disorder | Breeds | Age | Inheritance |
|---|---|---|---|
| ***Irish Setter Quadriplegia and Amblyopia*** | Irish setter | Birth | AR |
| ***Intervertebral Disk Disease*** | | | |
| | Basset hounds | 3–7 yr | Suspected |
| | Beagles | 3–7 yr | Suspected |
| | Cocker spaniels | 3–7 yr | Suspected |
| | Dachshund | 3–7 yr | Suspected |
| | French bulldog | 3–7 yr | Suspected |
| | Lhasa apso | 3–7 yr | Suspected |
| | Shih Tzu | 3–7 yr | Suspected |
| | Welsh corgi | 3–7 yr | Suspected |
| ***Leukoencephalomyelopathy*** Bilateral symmetric lesions in dorsal and lateral funiculi, brain stem, trigeminal nerve, caudal cerebellar peduncle, pyramidal tracts, and medial lemniscus | Rottweiler | 1.5–4 yr | AR |
| ***Meningitis/Vasculitis*** Fibrinoid necrosis of vessel walls and periartertitis in meninges; suppurative leptomeningitis | Beagle | <1 yr | Unknown |
| | Bernese mountain dog | <1 yr | Unknown |
| | German shorthair | <1 yr | Unknown |
| Cerebral white and gray matter, asymmetric, nonsuppurative meningoencephalitis | Pug dog | 6 mo–7 hr | Unknown |
| ***Multisystem Neuronal Degenerations*** Chromatolysis in brain stem and spinal cord | Cairn terrier | 4–7 mo | Familial |
| Neuronal degeneration in brain; no spinal cord lesions; symmetric neuronal loss, gliosis and dystrophic axons of cortical, subcortical, and brain stem regions | Cocker spaniels | 10–14 mo | AR? |
| ***Neuroaxonal Dystrophy*** Spheroids in internal capsule and cerebellar white matter | Chihuahua | 7 wk | Unknown |
| Spheroids with mild wallerian degeneration in cerebellar peduncle, folia white matter, vestibular nuclei | Collie sheepdog | 2–4 mo | AR? |
| Spheroids in granular layer cerebellum, vestibular nuclei, nuclei gracilis and cuneatus, dorsal horn spinal cord | Rottweiler | 10 wk–6 yr | AR |
| Spheroids in nuclear groups of thalamus to medulla, cerebellar vermis | Domestic tricolored | 5–6 wk | AR |
| ***Shaker Dog Disease*** | | 9 mo–2 yr | |
| | Beagle | | Unknown |
| | Bichon frise | | Unknown |
| | Maltese | | Unknown |
| | Samoyed | | Unknown |
| | Spitz | | Unknown |
| | West Highland white terrier | | Unknown |
| | Yorkshire terrier | | |
| ***Spongiform degenerations*** Vacuolation of white and gray matter of brain, spinal cord, and cerebellum | Egyptian Mau | 7 wk | Unknown |
| Spongiform degeneration in CNS cerebellar peduncle and cerebral white matter, PNS | Labrador retriever | 4–6 mo | Unknown |
| Spongiform degeneration of gray matter in brain and spinal cord | Malinois X | 3 wk | Unknown |
| Vacuolation of white matter brain and spinal cord most severe in cerebellum | Samoyed | 12 day | Unknown |
| Vacuolation of cerebrum and cerebellum | Silky terrier | | Unknown |

*Table continued on following page*

**Table 1.** *Continued*

| Disorder | Breeds | Age | Inheritance |
|---|---|---|---|
| **Storage Diseases** | | | |
| **Glycogen Storage Diseases** | | | |
| *Type 2 Glycogen Storage Disease* α-Glucosidase deficiency (Pompe's disease) | Swedish Lapland dog | 12–18 mo | AR |
| *Type 3 Glycogen Storage Disease* Amylo-1,6-glucosidase deficiency (Cori's disease) | German shepherd | 2 mo | AR |
| *Type 4 Glycogen Storage Disease* Branching enzyme deficiency (amylopectinosis) | Norwegian forest cat | 5–9 mo | AR |
| *Type 7 Glycogen Storage Disease* Phosphofructose kinase deficiency | English springer spaniel | 8–12 mo | AR |
| **Glycoproteinosis** | | | |
| α-*Glucosidase deficiency* (Lafora's disease) | Beagle | 5–9 mo | AR |
| | Basset hound | 3 yr | AR? |
| | Poodle | 9–12 yr | Unknown |
| **Lysosomal Storage Diseases** | | | |
| *Ceroid Lipofuscinosis* (Batten's disease) | | | |
| Accumulation of lipofuscin pigment in many organs | Australian cattle dog | 1–2 yr | Unknown |
| | Australian blue heeler | 18 mo | Unknown |
| | Border collie | 2 yr | AR |
| | Chihuahua | 2 yr | Unknown |
| | Cocker spaniel | 1.5 yr | Unknown |
| | Dalmatian | 5–6 mo | Unknown |
| | English setter | 2 yr | AR |
| | Japanese retriever | 3 yr | Unknown |
| | Saluki | 2 yr | Unknown |
| | Siamese cat | 2 yr | Unknown |
| | Terrier X | 4 mo | Unknown |
| | Tibetan terriers | 3–6 yr | AR |
| | Wirehaired dachshund | 4.5 yr | Unknown |
| | Yugoslavian sheepdog | >1 yr | Unknown |
| *Fucosidosis* (α-L-Fucosidase Deficiency) | English springer spaniel | 6 mo–3 yr | AR |
| *Gangliosidosis GM₁* (β-Galactosidase Deficiency) | | | |
| Type 1 (Norman-Landing disease) | Beagle X | 4–7 mo | AR |
| | Domestic shorthair | 2–3 mo | AR? |
| | English springer spaniel | 4–5 mo | AR |
| | Portuguese water dog | 4.5–5 mo | AR |
| Type 2 (Derry's disease) | Domestic short-haired | 2–3 mo | AR? |
| | Korat cat | 2–3 mo | AR |
| | Siamese cat | 2–3 mo | AR |
| *Gangliosidosis GM₂* Hexosaminidase deficiency (A, B) | | | |
| Type B (Tay-Sachs disease) | German shorthair | 6–12 mo | Unknown |
| Type B⁻¹ (deficient activatory protein) | | | |
| Type AB (Bernheimer-Seitelberger disease) | Japanese spaniel | 18 mo | AR |
| | Mixed breed dog | 1.5 yr | Unknown |
| Type O (Sandhoff's disease) | Domestic cats | 2–3 mo | AR? |
| *Glucocerebrosidosis* β-*Glucosidase deficiency* (Gaucher's disease) | Australian silky terrier | 6–8 mo | AR? |
| *Globoid Cell Leukodystrophy* β-*Galactosidase deficiency* (Krabbe's disease) | Bassett hound | 1.5–2 yr | Unknown |
| | Beagle | 4 mo | Unknown |
| | Blue tick hound | 4 mo | Unknown |
| | Cairn terrier | 2–5 mo | AR |
| | Domestic shorthair | 5–6 wk | Unknown |
| | Pomeranian | 1.5 yr | Unknown |
| | Poodle | 2 yr | Unknown |
| | West Highland terrier | 2–5 mo | AR |

*Table continued on opposite page*

***Table 1.*** *Continued*

| Disorder | Breeds | Age | Inheritance |
|---|---|---|---|
| *Mannosidosis* | | | |
| α-Mannosidase deficiency | Domestic longhair | 7–10 mo | AR |
| (mannosidosis) | Domestic shorthair | 4–7 mo | AR |
| | Persian | Birth–6 mo | AR |
| *Metachromatic Leukodystrophy* | Domestic cat | 2 wk | Unknown |
| Arylsulfatase deficiency | | | |
| *Mucopolysaccharidosis* | | | |
| Type 1—α-L-iduronidase deficiency | Domestic shorthair | 10 mo | AR |
| (Hurler's syndrome) | Mixed breed | 4–6 mo | AR |
| | Plott hound | 3–6 mo | AR |
| Type VI—arylsulfatase B deficiency | Siamese | 4–7 mo | AR |
| (Maroteaux-Lamy disease) | Domestic shorthair | 4–7 mo | AR |
| | Miniature pinscher | 6 mo | Unknown |
| *Sphingomyelinosis* | Balinese cat | 2–4 mo | Unknown |
| Sphingomyelinase deficiency | Domestic shorthair | 2–4 mo | Unknown |
| (Niemann-Pick disease) | Miniature poodle | 5 mo | Unknown |
| | Siamese | 2–4 mo | AR |

Abbreviations: AR = autosomal recessive, CNS = central nervous system, PNS = peripheral nervous system.

***Table 2.*** *Degenerative Conditions With Clinical Signs of Neuropathic Disease*

| Disorder | Breeds | Age | Inheritance |
|---|---|---|---|
| **Deafness** | | Birth | Congenital |
| May have partial agenesis of the organ of corti, the spiral ganglion, and cochlear nuclei | Australian heeler | | |
| | Australian shepherd | | |
| | Catahoula | | |
| | Dalmatian | | |
| | English setter | | |
| | White cat | | AD |
| | Many other breeds | | |
| **Distal Sensorimotor Polyneuropathy** | Rottweiler | 1.5–4 yr | Unknown |
| Myelinoaxonal necrosis | | | |
| **Distal Central-Peripheral Axonopathy** | Birman cat | 8–10 wk | Recessive |
| Involvement of distal portions of CNS and PNS | | | |
| Diffuse loss of myelinated fibers in pyramidal tracts of lumbar spinal cord, fasciculi gracilus in cervical spinal cord, cerebellar vermian white matter, and sciatic nerves | | | |
| **Giant Axonal Neuropathy** | German shepherd | 14–16 mo | AR |
| Loss of myelinated nerve fibers; swollen axons containing masses of neurofilaments | | | |
| **Hyperchylomicronemia** | Feline | 8 mo | AR? |
| Peripheral nerves susceptible to compression from xanthomas near foramina and bony prominences | | | |
| **Hyperoxaluria** | Domestic shorthair | 5–9 mo | AR? |
| Associated peripheral neuropathies; accumulation of neurofilaments in ventral root, and proximal axons | | | |
| **Hypomyelinogenesis PNS** | Golden retriever | 7 wk | Unknown |
| **Inherited Hypertrophic Neuropathy** | Tibetan mastiff | 7–12 wk | AR |
| Widespread demyelination with little axonal degeneration; suspect inborn defect of Schwann cells | | | |
| **Laryngeal paralysis** | | | |
| | Bouvier des Flandres | 4–6 mo | AD |
| | Siberian husky | | Suspected |
| | Bull terrier | | Suspected |
| | Dalmatian | | AR? |

*Table continued on following page*

***Table 2.***  *Continued*

| Disorder | Breeds | Age | Inheritance |
|---|---|---|---|
| **Motor Neuronopathies** (Degeneration of motor neurons in the gray matter of the spinal cord) | | | |
|   ***Muscular Atrophy*** | | | |
|     Atrophy of proximal spinal and pelvic muscles | Brittany spaniel | 6–8 wk | AD |
|     Concurrent chromatolysis of certain brain stem nuclei; axonal swelling in spinal cord and proximal ventral roots | | | |
|     Focal degeneration of motor neurons in brachial plexus | German shepherd | 2 wk–5 mo | Unknown |
|     Similar to Brittany spaniels; axonal degeneration in peripheral nerves, concurrent chromatolysis of hypoglossal and spinal accessory nuclei | English pointer | 5 mo | AR |
|     Similar to Brittany spaniels; concurrent chromatolysis of brain stem nuclei (red, oculomotor, trigeminal, ambiguous nuclei) | Rottweiler | 4–8 wk | Unknown |
|   ***Hereditary Neuronal Abiotrophy*** | Swedish Lapland dog | 5–7 wk | AR? |
|     Atrophy of pelvic limbs and distal muscles; chromatolysis primarily at cervical and lumbar intumescences and dorsal root ganglia; marked degeneration of Purkinje neurons; axonal degeneration in dorsal funiculus, spinocerebellar tracts, trigeminal, optic and vestibular nerves | | | |
|   ***Stockard's Paralysis*** | Great Dane-Bloodhound | 11–14 wk | Suspected |
|     Atrophy of pelvic limb and distal muscles; chromatolysis of motor and preganglionic sympathetic neurons | Great Dane-Saint Bernard | 11–14 wk | Suspected |
|   ***Sensory Ganglioradiculitis*** | Brittany spaniel | 9 yr | Unknown |
|     Degeneration and loss of neurons in the dorsal root ganglion cells and in cranial sensory ganglia; ventral roots are spared | Doberman pinscher | 2 yr | Unknown |
| | Golden retriever | 2 yr | Unknown |
| | Scotch collie | 2.5 yr | Unknown |
| | Scottish terrier | 6 yr | Unknown |
| | Siberian husky | 4 yr | Unknown |
| | Welsh corgi | 1.5 yr | Unknown |
|   ***Sensory Neuronopathies*** | | | |
|     In PNS small paranodal axonal swellings in the dorsal and ventral nerve roots and axonal degeneration in distal nerves; large axonal swellings in brain stem nuclei; spheroids in the lateral and ventral funiculi | Boxer | 2 mo–1 yr | AR |
| | Pyrenean mountain dog | 5 mo | |
|     Degeneration in dorsal root and peripheral nerves; decrease numbers of cell bodies in spinal ganglia | English pointer | 3–8 mo | AR |
|     Nerve biopsy of sensory nerve showed absence of myelinated fibers with preservation of unmyelinated fibers | Jack Russell terrier | ?–6 yr | Unknown |
|     Distal sensory nerves show degenerative changes with concurrent degeneration in the fasciculus gracilus | Long haired dachshund | 8–12 wk | AR? |
| | Border collie | 2 mo | Unknown |
|     Loss of nerve fibers primarily in sensory branches of trigeminal nerve | Rough coated collie | 2 yr | Unknown |
|   ***Walker Hound Mononeuropathy*** | Walker hound | 2 wk | Acquired? |
|     Restricted to tibial and peroneal nerves; nerve fiber loss with scattered demyelination | | | |

Abbreviations: AD = autosomal dominant, CNS = central nervous system, PNS = peripheral nervous system, AR = autosomal recessive.

**Table 3.** *Degenerative Conditions with Clinical Signs of Myopathic Disease*

| Disorder | Breeds | Age | Inheritance |
|---|---|---|---|
| **Bouvier des Flandres Myopathy** | Bouvier des Flandres | 2 yr | Unknown |
| **Core-like Myopathy** | Great Dane | 6 mo | Unknown |
| **Dancing Doberman Disease** Primary myopathy? affecting gastrocnemius; multifocal atrophy and hypertrophy | Doberman pinscher | 6 mo–7 yr | Unknown |
| **Dermatomyositis** | | | |
| | Australian cattle dog | 3 mo | Unknown |
| | Rough coated collie | 13–19 wk | AD |
| | Shetland sheepdog | 13–19 wk | AD |
| **Esophageal Hypomotility** | | | |
| | Bouvier des Flandres | 6 mo–9 yr | Suspected |
| | Great Dane | | Congenital |
| | German shepherd | | Congenital |
| | Greyhound | | Congenital |
| | Irish setter | | Congenital |
| | Wirehaired fox terrier | 2–8 wk | AR |
| | Miniature schnauzer | 3 wk | AD or 60% AR |
| | Newfoundland | | Congenital |
| | Shar-Pei | | Congenital |
| | Siamese cat | | Congenital |
| **Fibrotic Myopathy** | German shepherd | 2–7 yr | Unknown |
| **Malignant Hyperthermia** | | Any age | |
| | Border collie | | Unknown |
| | Domestic shorthair | | Unknown |
| | German shepherd/ Doberman pinscher X | | Unknown |
| | Greyhound | | Unknown |
| | Pointer | | Unknown |
| | Spaniel | | Unknown |
| | Saint Bernard | | Unknown |
| **Mitochondrial Myopathies** Pyruvate dehydrogenase deficiency | Clumber spaniel | 3 mo | Suspected |
| | Old English sheepdog | 3 mo | Unknown |
| | Sussex spaniel | 3 mo | Suspected |
| **Muscular Dystrophies** | Devon rex cat | 3–23 wk | AR |
| | Domestic shorthair | 5–6 mo | X-linked |
| | European shorthair | 5–6 mo | X-linked |
| | Golden retriever | 6–8 wk | X-linked |
| | Irish terrier | 8–13 wk | X-linked |
| | Labrador retriever | 6–8 wk 3–7 mo | AR |
| | Rottweiler | <6 mo | X-linked |
| | Samoyed | <6 mo | X-linked |
| **Myasthenia Gravis** | | | |
| | Domestic shorthair | 4 mo | Congenital |
| | Gammel Dansk honsehund | 6–9 wk | AR |
| | Jack Russell terriers | 6–9 wk | AR |
| | Siamese cat | 5 mo | Congenital |
| | Samoyed | 6–9 wk | Congenital |
| | Smooth fox terriers | 6–9 wk | AR |
| | Springer spaniel | 6–9 wk | AR |
| **Reflex Myoclonus** | Labrador retriever | 3 wk | Familial |
| **Myotonic Myopathies** | Chow chow | 8–10 wk | AR? |
| | Great Dane | 8–10 wk | Suspected |
| | Rhodesian ridgeback | | Acquired? |
| | Staffordshire terrier | 8–10 wk | Suspected |
| | West Highland white terrier | 8–10 wk | Unknown |
| **Nemaline Myopathy** Nemaline rods within myofibers | Feline | 6–18 mo | Familial |
| **Ossifying Myositis** | Domestic shorthair | 2 yr | Unknown |

Abbreviations: AD = autosomal dominant, AR = autosomal recessive.

***Table 4.*** *Congenital Malformations*

| Disorder | Breeds | Age | Inheritance |
|---|---|---|---|
| ***Atlantoaxial Luxation*** | | | |
| | Australian silky terrier | <1 yr | Congenital |
| | Bichon frise | <1 yr | Congenital |
| | Cavalier King Charles spaniel | <1 yr | Congenital |
| | Chihuahua | <1 yr | Congenital |
| Congenital absence of dens | Doberman pinscher | | Congenital |
| | German shepherd | | Congenital |
| | Japanese chin | <1 yr | Congenital |
| | Pekinese | <1 yr | Congenital |
| | Pomeranian | <1 yr | Congenital |
| | Poodle | <1 yr | Congenital |
| Congenital absence of dens | Rottweiler | | Congenital |
| | Schipperke | <1 yr | Congenital |
| | Schnauzer | <1 yr | Congenital |
| Congenital absence of tranverse ligament | Shih Tzu | <1 yr | Congenital |
| Congenital absence of dens | Weimaraner | | Congenital |
| | Yorkshire terrier | <1 yr | Congenital |
| ***Atlanto-occipital Malformation*** | Domestic shorthaired cat | | Congenital |
| ***Arachnoid Cyst*** | | | |
| | Beagle | 4 yr | Congenital? |
| | Chow chow | | Congenital? |
| | Pekinese | 15 mo | Congenital? |
| | Toy poodle | 6 yr | Congenital? |
| | Weimaraner | 10 yr | Congenital? |
| ***Cerebellar Hypoplasia*** | Chow chow | Birth | AR? |
| ***Dandy-Walker Syndrome*** | Irish setter | Birth | Congenital |
| | Wirehaired fox terrier | Birth | Congenital |
| ***Cerebellar Vermal Hypoplasia*** | Boston terrier | Birth | Congenital |
| | Bull terrier | Birth | Congenital |
| ***Cervical Vertebral Malformation/ Malarticulation*** | | | |
| Lesions at C5–C7 | Borzoi | 5–8 yr | Recessive? |
| | Great Dane | <2 yr | Suspected |
| | Doberman pinscher | >2 yr | Unknown |
| | Rottweiler | >2yr | Unknown |
| Lesions at C2–3 and/or C2–3 | Boxer | | Unknown |
| | Chow chow | | Unknown |
| | Fox terrier | | Unknown |
| | German shepherd | | Unknown |
| | Golden retriever | | Unknown |
| | Irish setter | | Unknown |
| | Irish wolfhound | | Unknown |
| | Labrador retriever | | Unknown |
| | Old English sheepdog | | Unknown |
| | Pyrenean mountain dog | | Unknown |
| | Rhodesian ridgeback | | Unknown |
| | Weimaraner | | Unknown |
| Lesions at C2–3 | Basset hound | <8 mo | Suspected |
| | Beagle | | |
| ***Dermoid Cysts*** | | | |
| | Boxer | Birth | Unknown |
| | Rhodesian ridgeback | Birth | AR? |
| | Shih Tzu | Birth | Unknown |
| ***Hemivertebrate*** | | | |
| | Boston terrier | Birth | Congenital |
| | Chinese pug | Birth | Congenital |
| | Doberman pinscher | Birth | Congenital |
| | English bulldog | Birth | Congenital |
| | French bulldog | Birth | Congenital |
| | German shepherd | Birth | AR |
| | German shorthaired pointer | Birth | AR |
| | Rottweiler | Birth | Congenital |

*Table continued on opposite page*

**Table 4.** *Continued*

| Disorder | Breeds | Age | Inheritance |
|---|---|---|---|
| *Hydrocephalus* | Boston terrier | Birth | Congenital |
| | Cairn terrier | Birth | Congenital |
| | Chihuahua | Birth | Congenital |
| | English bulldog | Birth | Congenital |
| | Lhasa apso | Birth | Congenital |
| | Maltese | Birth | Congenital |
| | Pekinese | Birth | Congenital |
| | Pomeranian | Birth | Congenital |
| | Shih Tzu | Birth | Congenital |
| | Toy poodle | Birth | Congenital |
| | Yorkshire terrier | Birth | Congenital |
| *Lissencephaly* | Lhasa apso | Birth | Congenital |
| | Wirehaired fox terrier | Birth | Congenital |
| | Irish setter | Birth | Congenital |
| | Domestic shorthair | Birth | Congenital |
| *Meningoencephalocele* | Burmese cat | Birth | AR |
| *Occipital Dysplasia* | Beagle | Birth | Congenital |
| | Chihuahua | Birth | Congenital |
| | Lhasa apso | Birth | Congenital |
| | Maltese | Birth | Congenital |
| | Miniature poodle | Birth | Congenital |
| | Pomeranian | Birth | Congenital |
| | Shih Tzu | Birth | Congenital |
| | Toy poodle | Birth | Congenital |
| | Yorkshire terrier | Birth | Congenital |
| *Optic Nerve Hypoplasia* | Beagle | Birth | Congenital |
| | Collie | Birth | Congenital |
| | Dachshund | Birth | Congenital |
| | German shepherd | Birth | Congenital |
| | Miniature poodle | Birth | AR |
| | Russian wolfhound | Birth | Congenital |
| | Saint Bernard | Birth | Congenital |
| *Sacrocaudal Dysgenesis* | Maltese kitten | Birth | Congenital |
| | Manx cat | Birth | AD |
| *Spina Bifida* | Beagle | Birth | Congenital |
| | Boston terrier | Birth | Congenital |
| | Chihuahua | Birth | Congenital |
| | Dalmatian | Birth | Congenital |
| | English bulldog | Birth | Congenital |
| | Manx cat | Birth | Congenital |
| | Samoyed | Birth | Congenital |
| | Siamese cat | Birth | Congenital |
| *Spinal Dysraphism* | Chihuahua | Birth | Congenital |
| | Dalmatian | Birth | Congenital |
| | Siberian husky | Birth | Congenital |
| | Labrador retriever | Birth | Congenital |
| | Rottweiler | Birth | Congenital |
| | Weimaraner | Birth | Dominant lethal |
| *Spinal Stenosis* | | | |
| Thoracic spinal cord segments | Doberman pinscher | Birth | Congenital |
| Lumbosacral stenosis | Beagle | 5 yr | Congenital? |
| | Lhasa apso | 5 yr | Congenital? |
| | Mixed breed | 3–8 yr | Congenital? |
| | Toy poodle | 4–8 yr | Congenital? |
| *Vestibular Syndromes* | | Birth–4 mo | |
| Concurrent deafness | Akita | | Congenital |
| | Beagle | | Congenital |
| | Burmese cat | | Congenital |
| | Cocker spaniel | | Congenital |
| Concurrent deafness | Doberman pinscher | | AR |
| | German shepherd | | Congenital |
| | Smooth fox terrier | | Congenital |
| Concurrent deafness | Siamese cat | | Congenital |
| | Tibetan terrier | | Congenital |
| | Tonkanese cat | | Congenital |

Abbreviations: AR = autosomal recessive, AD = autosomal dominant.

**Table 5.** *Paroxysmal Disorders*

| Disorder | Breeds | Age | Inheritance |
|---|---|---|---|
| **Muscle Cramping** | | | |
| *Episodic Falling*<br>? Muscular dystrophy | Cavalier King Charles spaniel | 3–4 mo | Unknown |
| *Scotty Cramp* | | | |
| Serotonin disorder | Scottish terrier | <6 mo | AR |
| | Dalmatian | <1 yr | Unknown |
| | Norwich terrier | <1 yr | Unknown |
| **Idiopathic Epilepsy** | | 1–4 yr | |
| | Beagles | | Suspected |
| | Belgian tervurens | | Suspected |
| | Cocker spaniels | | Suspected |
| | German shepherds | | Suspected |
| | Golden retrievers | | Suspected |
| | Irish setters | | Suspected |
| | Keeshonds | | Suspected |
| | Labrador retrievers | | Suspected |
| | Poodles | | Suspected |
| | Saint Bernards | | Suspected |
| | Wirehaired fox terrier | | Suspected |
| **Narcolepsy** | Dachshund | 3–5 mo | Suspected |
| | Doberman pinscher | <6 mo | AR |
| | Labrador retriever | 3–5 mo | AR? |
| | Miniature poodle | 4–18 mo | Suspected |
| | Many other breeds | | |

Abbreviation: AR = autosomal recessive.

weakness as the major clinical sign (Shelton et al., 1987; Amann, 1987; Cuddon, 1992). There are some myopathic disorders that do not exhibit weakness as a major clinical sign (Kortz, 1989). Inherited peripheral neuropathies can show selective involvement of sensory or motor nerves (Duncan, 1980). Congenital disorders are usually manifested as malformations within the CNS as a result of inborn errors during development (Bailey et al., 1992). Clinical signs are varied, depending upon lesion location. Animals with paroxysmal diseases are usually normal neurologically between episodes of showing clinical signs of the disease (Berry, 1990).

Inherited diseases can be a significant problem in the genetic management of some breeds. Many neurologic disorders have an unknown inherited status and are represented as single case reports. Inherited neurologic disorders usually have been identified as autosomal recessive. Some muscular dystrophies are unique by having X-linked characteristics (Kornegay, 1992). Identification of an inherited status is important in detecting carriers of the recessive traits using biochemical tests or molecular genetic methods. This is important for the pet owner and the medical profession because many of these neurologic diseases can serve as animal models for human-related diseases. Gene therapy is on the horizon, and treatment of these disorders prior to development of clinical signs relies heavily upon these animal models as a basis for developing molecular genetic therapies.

## References and Suggested Reading

Amann JF: Congenital and acquired neuromuscular disease of young dogs and cats. Vet Clin North Am [Small Anim Pract] 17:617, 1989.

*Concepts and pathoanatomic classification of neuromuscular diseases in dogs and cats.*

Bailey CS and Morgan JP: Congenital spinal malformations. Vet Clin North Am [Small Ani Pract] 22:985, 1992.

*A review of congenital spinal disorders in dog and cats with discussions of clinical signs, diagnosis, and treatment.*

Berry WL: Episodic weakness in dogs. Compend Cont Educ Pract Vet 12: 141, 1990.

*A review of episodic conditions in dogs.*

Braund KG: *Clinical Syndromes in Veterinary Neurology*, 2nd edition. St. Louis, Mosby, 1994, p 81.

*A comprehensive compilation of neurologic disorders in dogs and cats emphasizing signalment, clinical signs, and diagnostic findings.*

Cuddon PA: Feline neuromuscular diseases. In Kirk RW (ed): *Kirk's Current Veterinary Therapy XI*. Philadelphia, WB Saunders Co, 1992, p 1024.

*A review of inherited and acquired feline neuromuscular disorders.*

De Lahunta A: Abiotrophy in domestic animals: A review. Can J Vet Res 54: 65, 1990.

*A comprehensive review and classification of abiotrophies in domestic animals.*

Duncan ID: Peripheral nerve disease in the dog and cat. Vet Clin North Am [Small Anim Pract] 10:177, 1980.

*Concepts and discussions of neuropathic disorders.*

Duncan ID: Abnormalities of myelination of the central nervous system associated with congenital tremor. J Vetern Intern Med 1:10, 1987.

*A pathophysiologic review of myelin and myelin-related disorders of the CNS.*

Evans RJ: Lysosomal storage diseases in dogs and cats. J Small Anim Pract 30:144, 1989.

*An overview of lysosomal storage diseases.*

Kortz G: Canine myotonia. Semin Vet Med Surg (Small Anim) 4:141, 1989.

*A review of clinical signs and diagnostic features associated with myotonic disorders.*

Kornegay JE: The X-linked muscular dystrophies. In Kirk RW (ed): *Kirk's Current Veterinary Therapy XI*. Philadelphia, WB Saunders Co, 1992, p 1042.

*A review of muscular dystrophies emphasizing animal models for human disease with discussions of clinical signs and pathologic findings.*

Shelton GD and Cardinet GH: Pathophysiologic basis of canine muscle disorders. J Vetern Intern Med 1:36, 1987.

*Pathophysiologic concepts and discussion of myopathic disorders.*

Vandevelde M: Degenerative diseases of the spinal cord. Vet Clin North Am 10:147, 1980.

*Concepts and descriptions of degenerative diseases of the spinal cord.*

# THE ANALYSIS OF CEREBROSPINAL FLUID IN CATS

JACQUELINE S. RAND

*St. Lucia, Queensland, Australia*

The composition of cerebrospinal fluid (CSF) provides a glimpse at pathologic events occurring in the central nervous system (CNS). Cerebrospinal fluid analysis can help to differentiate between inflammatory, degenerative, and neoplastic disease processes. For maximum diagnostic value, the results of CSF analysis must be interpreted with knowledge of the patient's signalment, history, general clinical examination, and neurologic examination findings.

## TO COLLECT CEREBROSPINAL FLUID

Induce anesthesia using gas or a short-acting injectable agent such as thiamyl, and maintain with gas. Do not use ketamine, because of its potential for inducing seizures. Always place an endotracheal tube to maintain airway patency during CSF collection. Cerebrospinal fluid should be collected before corticosteroids are administered, as these drugs can alter the CSF composition.

For CSF collection, position the cat on the edge of a flat, rimless table, in right lateral recumbency for the right-handed operator. Clip and surgically prepare the skin over the cerebellomedullary cistern. Have an assistant place one hand on the shoulder of the cat to stabilize its position, and use the other hand to gently pull the head forward and flex it. Maximum flexion is unnecessary and dangerous, as it may occlude the endotracheal tube. Ensure that the spine is not flexed laterally or the head rotated, so that the dorsal midline, from the occipital crest to the dorsal process of the axis, is horizontal.

The clinician sits or squats so the clipped area of the neck is at eye level. For the right-handed operator, position the left hand with the thumb on the lower anterior border of the wing of the atlas and the major finger on the upper wing (Fig. 1). Use the index finger to mark the point of entry. The site for needle entry is the intersection of a line joining the anterior borders of the wings of the atlas, with a line from the occipital crest to the dorsal process of the axis. Confirm the correct location by palpating the underlying depression formed by the attachments of the ligamentum nuchae to the caudal surface of the calvaria.

Use a 22-gauge, $1\frac{1}{2}$ inch spinal needle for CSF collection in cats (Becton, Dickinson and Company, Rutherford, NJ). Control the skin insertion, so the needle is not driven deeply once the skin resistance is overcome. In thick-skinned cats, puncture the skin first with an 18-gauge needle, or with a scalpel blade. Use the table edge to support the hand holding the needle and slowly advance the spinal needle with the stylet in place. In the majority of cats, a distinct "pop," or sudden decrease in resistance, is felt as the needle penetrates the subarachnoid space. With experience, this sensation can be readily appreciated and the average insertion distance to the subarachnoid space recognized.

If the operator is inexperienced, or a "pop" is not detected at the expected insertion distance, remove the stylet and check for flow of CSF. If no CSF flow occurs, replace the stylet and advance the needle a millimeter at a time, checking after each advancement for CSF flow. If no flow of CSF occurs when the needle is advanced past the usual depth for CSF collection, withdraw the needle slowly, checking for CSF flow every millimeter. Avoid passing through the spinal cord to the underlying bone. This can cause clinical damage to the spinal cord and a severely blood-contaminated CSF sample. Abandon the procedure in a patient after three unsuccessful attempts at CSF collection, as repeated penetration of the cord may result in serious complications and even death. It is strongly recommended that the clinician initially uses fresh cadavers to develop competence in the procedure.

Collect 1 to 1.5 ml of CSF by free flow into a plain

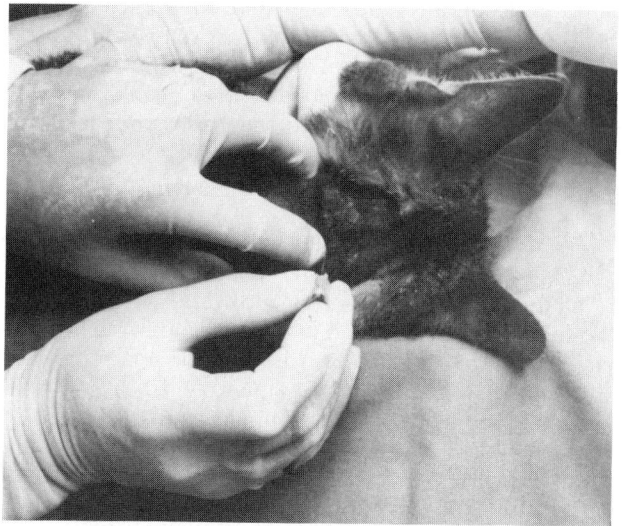

**Figure 1.** The site for needle entry is the intersection of the line joining the anterior borders of the wings of the atlas with a line extended caudally from the occipital crest to the dorsal process of the axis.

**Table 1.** *Reference Intervals for Feline CSF (n=33)**

| | Low | | High | |
|---|---|---|---|---|
| **Cell Counts†** | | | | |
| Red cells | 0 cells/$\mu$l | | 30 cells/$\mu$l | |
| White cells | 0 cells/$\mu$l | | 2 cells/$\mu$l | |
| **Differential Cell Counts†** | | | | |
| Neutrophils | 0 cells/$\mu$l | (0%) | 0.18 cells/$\mu$l | (9%) |
| Lymphocytes | 0 cells/$\mu$l | (0%) | 0.54 cells/$\mu$l | (27%) |
| Monocytes | <1 cells/$\mu$l | (69%) | 2.00 cells/$\mu$l | (100%) |
| Macrophages | 0 cells/$\mu$l | (0%) | 0.06 cells/$\mu$l | (3%) |
| Eosinophils | 0 cells/$\mu$l | (0%) | 0.02 cells/$\mu$l | (<1%) |
| **Biochemistry** | | | | |
| Total protein | 6 mg/dl | | 36 mg/dl | |
| Glucose | 18 mg/dl | | 130 mg/dl | |
| CK | 2 U/L | | 236 U/L | |
| LDH | 0 U/L | | 24 U/L | |
| AST | 0 U/L | | 34 U/L | |

*Data derived from Rand et al., 1990a,b.
†Values for white and differential cell counts are only valid for CSF with ≤30 red cells/$\mu$l. For CSF with >30 red cells/$\mu$l, add 1 white cell/$\mu$l for every 100 red cells/$\mu$l and 1 mg/dl protein for every 1200 red cells/$\mu$l.

tube. Do not aspirate CSF with a syringe, as this greatly increases the risk of a nondiagnostic blood-contaminated sample. One milliliter of CSF is sufficient for all routine tests and is readily collected in most cats. Less than 0.5 ml will limit the number of tests possible. Cell counts and cytologic preparations must be made within 30 to 60 min of CSF collection, because cells rapidly deteriorate in the low-protein environment of CSF. If the sample cannot be processed by an external laboratory within this time, the total cell count and differential cell count preparation must be made in the practice laboratory.

## TO ANALYZE CEREBROSPINAL FLUID

If the volume of CSF is limited, the most useful diagnostic tests, in decreasing order, are white and red cell count, sedimentation cytology, protein concentration, and cytocentrifuge cytology.

Normal CSF is clear and colorless. Visible turbidity occurs when there are more than 200 white cells or 700 red cells/$\mu$l.

### Red and White Cell Counts

Determine the erythrocyte and white cell counts using a hemocytometer. Fill both chambers with unstained CSF. After allowing 10 min for settling, count the cells in the nine largest squares on both sides of the chamber. Calculate the average number of cells in the 18 squares and multiply by 10 to determine the number of cells/$\mu$l (cells/$\mu$l = total cells in 18 squares/ $18 \times 10$). Some experience is required to accurately count white and red cells in unstained samples, but most technicians quickly develop this skill.

The normal feline CSF has 0 to 2 white cells/$\mu$l ($2 \times 10^6$/L), and less than 31 red cells/$\mu$l ($31 \times 10^6$/L)

(Table 1). Always obtain a red cell count, because blood contamination greater than 30 red cells/$\mu$l will have a profound effect on the total and differential cell counts.

### Cytologic Preparations

When the CSF white cell count is less than 500 cells/ $\mu$l, the CSF must be concentrated to obtain sufficient cells for cytologic assessment. Cytocentrifuge and sedimentation procedures are used for concentration of CSF. However, cytocentrifuge equipment may not be available in many private practices, and the time delay involved in submission of a CSF sample to a commercial laboratory usually results in significant cellular deterioration. Therefore, it is highly recommended that a sedimentation preparation be made at the practice. This is a simple procedure that requires no special equipment and has negligible cost (Sörnäs, 1967). Although sedimentation requires 0.5 ml of CSF, the supernatant can be used for protein estimation.

### Sedimentation Preparation

For the sedimentation preparation, make a well-slide (Fig. 2). Construct this using a glass slide, Vaseline, strong scissors or scalpel blade, and a 16-mm-diameter plastic tube, such as a urine or bacteriology tube. Cut the plastic tube 1.5 to 2 cm from the open end using the scissors or, for a more elegant finish, a flame-heated scalpel blade. Place the original open end of the tube on a glass slide and make a water-tight seal around the tube by applying Vaseline at room temperature. A thermometer is useful to apply the Vaseline. For a smoother finish, dip the original open end of the tube into melted Vaseline and quickly press it to the slide to form a seal. Place a 0.5-ml aliquot of CSF in the well-slide and leave to sediment for 30 to 40 min. It is very

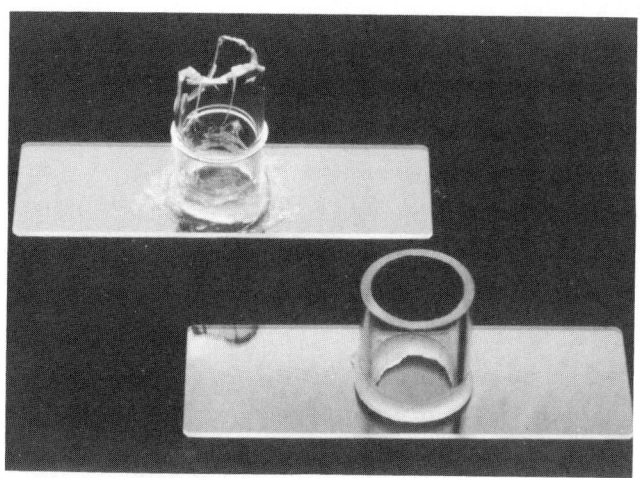

**Figure 2.** Two slide-wells constructed using a glass slide, Vaseline, strong scissors (*left*) or flame-heated scalpel blade (*right*), and a 16-mm-diameter plastic tube, such as a urine or bacteriology tube.

important not to disturb the preparation during this settling period.

After sedimentation, aspirate the supernatant using a pipette or 1.5-inch, 18-gauge needle attached to a 2-ml syringe. Keep the tip of the needle or pipette just beneath the fluid level, and take great care not to disturb the settled cells. When most of the supernatant has been removed, gently tilt the slide to allow better access to the remaining fluid.

Complete the next steps quickly, as delayed drying of the cells results in poor morphology. Detach the cylinder from the slide and quickly remove excess Vaseline with a scalpel blade. Wick away the remaining fluid on the slide using a corner of tissue or blotting paper applied to the fluid edge. Wave the slide very vigorously in the air to rapidly dry the cells. This takes about 2 min, and is complete when a barely visible white film covers the sedimentation area on the slide. If the film is incomplete, more rapid waving is required. The cells are easily damaged by excess heat and moisture, and the use of hair dryers for drying can produce disap-

pointing results. Once the slide is dry, scrape and wipe away the remaining Vaseline. After drying the slide, leave it for 15 to 30 min before staining.

The differential cell count is best performed by an experienced cytologist in a commercial laboratory, as differentiation between monocytoid and lymphoid cells can be difficult. If the preparation will not reach a commercial laboratory within a few hours, fix the slide at the practice, or stain it with Diff-Quik (Diff-Quik Differential StainSet, American Scientific Products), Wright's, or Giemsa stain. The cell quality can deteriorate if the unfixed slide is sent by post or overnight courier. During transport, it is important to protect the unfixed slide from heat and humidity.

### CYTOCENTRIFUGE PREPARATION

Most commercial laboratories and institutions use cytocentrifuge concentration for CSF. This technique requires a smaller CSF volume than the sedimentation preparation, and the cell morphology is usually better. However, the total number of cells per slide is smaller than the cytocentrifuge preparation, and when the total cell count is low, insufficient cells may be present for a meaningful differential cell count. Therefore, it is strongly recommended that a sedimentation preparation also be made at the practice, even when the CSF sample can be quickly delivered to a commercial laboratory for processing.

## Normal Cytology

Always make a differential cell count, as it may be abnormal, even when the total white cell count is normal. Most cells in normal feline CSF are monocytoid cells and, in the sedimentation preparation, comprise 69 to 100% of the white cells (Table 1) (Rand et al., 1990a). The nucleus is usually eccentrically placed and oval, horseshoe, reniform, or irregularly shaped (Fig. 3). The nuclear diameter is usually equal or greater than two erythrocytes, and the nuclear/cytoplasmic ratio is low.

**Figure 3.** Typical monocytoid cells. Note the eccentrically placed, irregularly shaped nuclei and low nuclear/cytoplasmic ratio. Small cytoplasmic vacuoles are more frequent in cytocentrifuged cells.

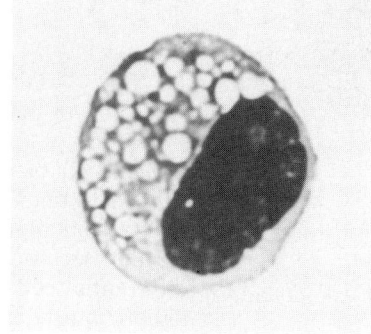
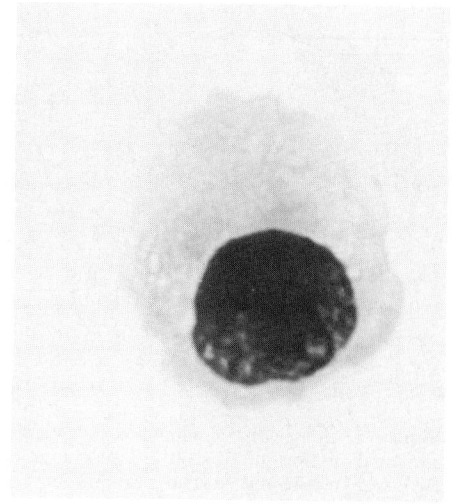

Because monocytoid cells can transform within minutes of contact with glass to cytoplasmic rich cells, only classify mononuclear cells as macrophages if ingested material is visible in the cytoplasm. Normally, they comprise no more than 3% of cells. Cells with voluminous foamy vacuolated cytoplasm are abnormal and are seen in association with a number of disease processes, especially those involving necrosis, including bacterial emboli, toxoplasmosis, and ischemic encephalopathy (Fig. 4).

Lymphocytes comprise up to 27% of the white cell population, and consist predominantly of large lymphocytes with prominent pale-staining cytoplasm and a loose nuclear chromatin pattern. An occasional neutrophil or eosinophil is normal, but these cells should not comprise over 10% or 1%, respectively, of the total white cell population. Even low levels of blood contamination (>500 red cells/μl) will dramatically change the differential cell count and increase the percentage of neutrophils and eosinophils. Occasionally, a clump of choroid plexus cells (Fig. 5) or mitotic figure is found in normal CSF.

## Protein Concentration

The concentration of protein in normal CSF is much lower than blood and therefore requires special techniques for analysis. Because CSF protein concentration is similar to that found in urine, urinary dipsticks can be used to obtain a rough estimate of protein concentration. It is important to estimate the protein concentration from the dipstick at the correct time. Normal CSF protein concentration in cats is less than or equal to 36 mg/dl (0.36 gm/L) (Rand et al., 1990b), and most normal cats will test negative or trace (<30 mg/dl) using a urine dipstick (e.g., N-Multistix SG, Bayer, Miles, Di-

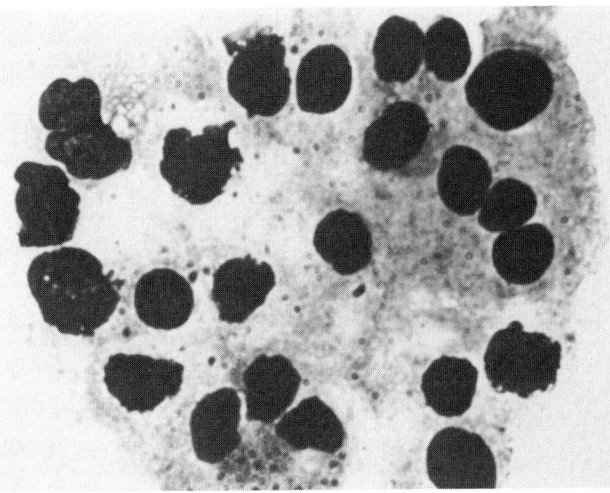

**Figure 5.** Clump of choroid plexus cells with round to oval eccentric nuclei and abundant cytoplasm.

agnostic Division, Elkhart, IN). Cats that test +1 (30 to 100 mg/dl) may be normal, or more likely have elevated protein concentration, and precise measurement of protein is required for differentiation. Cats with +2 or higher (≥100 mg/dl) have moderately to markedly elevated CSF protein concentration. Cats with greater than 200 mg/dl usually have the CNS form of feline infectious peritonitis (FIP).

Accurate measurement of CSF protein is usually only available in commercial laboratories. Various methods are used including trichloroacetic acid (TCA), Ponceau S dye binding, and ultraviolet spectrophotometry.

## Other CSF Parameters

Although the CSF activities of creatine kinase, aspartate transferase, and lactate dehydrogenase have been shown to markedly increase after experimentally induced acute brain injury in cats, they do not appear in practice to be useful indicators of CNS disease in cats (Rand et al., 1994a). Glucose concentration has also not been found to be useful, and on a cost-versus-value basis, none of these tests can be recommended. The diagnostic usefulness of protein electrophoresis of CSF has yet to be fully evaluated in cats. It can only be performed in certain laboratories and requires microconcentration techniques to minimize the volume of CSF used.

## TO INTERPRET BLOOD-CONTAMINATED CSF

Blood contamination with greater than 30 red cells/μl is a frequent problem in cats, and will affect the CSF results before a visible increase in turbidity is observed. Because of its dramatic effect on the total and differential cell counts, the degree of blood contamination must always be evaluated before deciding

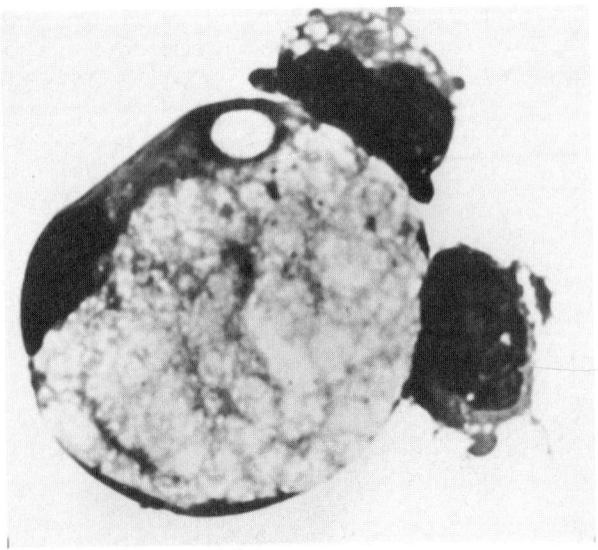

**Figure 4.** Cells with voluminous foamy vacuolated cytoplasm are abnormal, and are often seen in diseases associated with necrosis. Two large monocytoid cells are also present.

whether the CSF results are abnormal. The total white cell count has been shown to increase as much as one white cell/$\mu$l per 100 red cells/$\mu$l (Rand et al., 1990a). When the increase in white cell count is greater than that predicted by this formula, the increase is likely due to disease. However, when it is increased above two white cells/$\mu$l, but less than that predicted by the formula, then the increase may be due to blood contamination or disease. Protein concentration is much less affected by blood contamination, and a correction factor of 1 mg/dl protein per 1200 red cells/$\mu$l can be used. Both of these correction factors are based on the maximum increase observed with blood contamination, and in many cases overestimate the effect of blood contamination on CSF parameters.

Blood contamination has a marked effect on the differential cell count, with the maximum percentage of neutrophils increasing from 9% in feline CSF with less than 31 red cells/$\mu$l to 55% in CSF with greater than 500 red cells/$\mu$l. Interpretation of differential cell counts when blood contamination is greater than 30 red cells/$\mu$l is very difficult. However, even in heavily blood-contaminated samples, "foamy" cells with copious vacuolated cytoplasm are abnormal and indicate CNS necrosis.

## TO INTERPRET CSF RESULTS

The maximum benefit from feline CSF analysis will be gained only if the results are interpreted together with the patient's signalment, history, systemic physical examination, and neurologic examination data.

The most frequent CNS diseases found in a study of 61 Canadian cats were neoplasia (20%), FIP (18%), non-FIP viral encephalitis (16%), and ischemic encephalopathy (7%) (Rand et al., 1994a). These diseases, except FIP and non-FIP encephalitis, can usually be separated on the basis of the age, acuteness of onset, focal or multifocal disease, CNS location, and progression of clinical signs.

### Feline Infectious Peritonitis

Feline infectious peritonitis is the most likely diagnosis when a cat is less than 4 years of age and has progressive clinical signs of 5 or more weeks duration. Neurologic signs are usually multifocal and referable to the thalamocortex, brain stem, cerebellum, and/or spinal cord. Typically, CSF has a protein concentration of greater than 200 mg/dl (2 gm/l), a white cell count of greater than 100 cells/$\mu$l, and more than 70% neutrophils in the differential cell count (Fig. 6) (Rand et al., 1994a,b).

### Non-FIP Viral Encephalitis

Non-FIP viral encephalitis is the most likely disease when a cat is 2 years of age or younger, and presents with progressive clinical signs of less than 5 weeks' duration. Neurologic signs, usually focal and referable to the thalamocortex, brain stem, or cerebellum, are present. Usually, CSF protein concentration is less than 100 mg/dl, and the total cell count is less than 50 cells/$\mu$l. The differential cell count may be normal or abnormal with an increased percentage of neutrophils or lymphocytes (Rand et al., 1994b).

Clinically, FIP and non-FIP viral encephalitis may be similar, but the CSF protein concentration is invaluable in separating these two diseases. As cats with non-FIP disease often recover, in contrast to the almost universally fatal nature of FIP, it is very important to differentiate these two common causes of feline CNS disease. Although the etiology of non-FIP viral encephalitis is unknown, arboviruses or feline immunodeficiency virus could be involved. Histologically, these cats have only

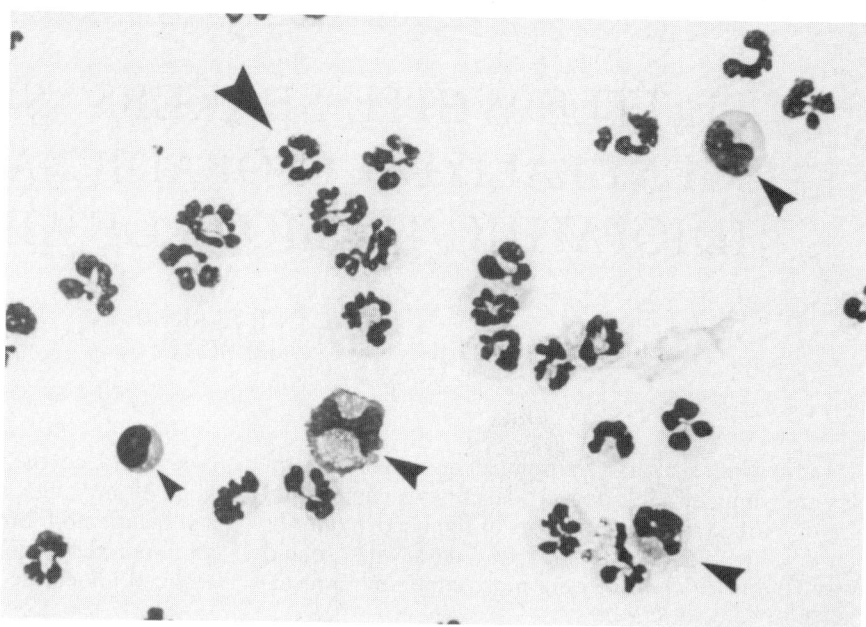

**Figure 6.** Typical CSF from a cat with feline infectious peritonitis. Note nontoxic neutrophils (*large arrow*), large monocytoid cells (*medium arrows*), and small monocytoid cell (*small arrow*).

perivascular cuffs and mild mononuclear meningitis, and do not have the pyogranulomatous lesions in the CNS and peripheral tissues characteristic of FIP.

## Neoplasia

Neoplasia is the most likely diagnosis when a cat 7 years of age or older has progressive clinical signs of over 4 weeks duration. Usually, neurologic signs are focal and CSF total protein is less than 100 mg/dl (Rand et al., 1994a).

## Protozoan Disease

*Toxoplasma gondii* appears to be a very uncommon cause of CNS disease in the cat. Clinical signs and CSF findings may mimic those of neoplasia. Typically, cats are old (>10 years) and neurologic signs associated with the granulomatous lesion are often focal. The CSF may have only mild changes with a mild to moderate increase in protein concentration (<100 mg/dl) and normal total white cell count, but abnormal differential cell count (Rand et al., 1994b). The presence of many voluminous mononuclear cells with "foamy" cytoplasm is suggestive of extensive necrosis, which may occur in toxoplasmosis.

## Ischemic Encephalopathy

Ischemic encephalopathy is the most likely diagnosis when a cat 4 years of age or younger develops acute nonprogressive neurologic signs that are confined to the thalamocortex. Typically, CSF total protein is less than 100 mg/dl (Rand et al., 1994a).

## Miscellaneous Degeneration

Although a wide variety of diseases can cause a primarily degenerate lesion in the CNS, these cats are generally less than 3 years old and have a long duration of clinical signs. Neurologic signs are usually focal and clues to the diagnosis are often evident in the history or physical examination. The CSF protein is often normal, and when increased is usually less than 100 mg/dl (Rand et al., 1994a). The white cell count may be normal or increased, and the differential count is often abnormal. Because the age and CSF findings may be indistinguishable from non-FIP viral encephalitis, the history or physical examination data may provide a clue to the diagnosis.

## References and Suggested Reading

Rand JS, Parent J, Jacobs R, et al: Reference intervals for feline CSF: Cell counts and cytologic features. Am J Vet Res 51:1044, 1990a.
*Normal values for CSF for total and differential cell counts in cytocentrifuge and sedimentation preparations; includes pictures of typical cells.*
Rand JS, Parent J, Jacobs R, et al: Reference intervals for feline CSF: Biochemical and serologic variables, IgG concentration, and electrophoretic fractionation. Am J Vet Res 51:1049, 1990b.
*Normal values for CK, AST and lactate dehydrogenase, glucose, total protein, antibodies to* Toxoplasma gondii *and coronavirus, IgG concentration, and protein electrophoresis.*
Rand JS, Parent J, Percy D, and Jacobs R: Clinical, cerebrospinal fluid and histologic data from 34 cats with non-inflammatory CNS disease. Can Vet J 35:174, 1994a.
*Retrospective study of 34 cats with primary degenerative and neoplastic CNS disease.*
Rand JS, Parent J, Percy D, and Jacobs R: Clinical, cerebrospinal fluid and histologic data from 27 cats with inflammatory central nervous system disease. Can Vet J 35:103, 1994b.
*Retrospective study of 27 cats with FIP, non-FIP viral encephalitis, toxoplasmosis, and other inflammatory diseases.*
Rand JS: Cerebrospinal fluid in the cat (DVSc dissertation). Guelph, Ontario, University of Guelph, 1987.
*Detailed clinical, CSF, and histologic data from 58 clinically normal cats and 61 cats with CNS disease.*
Sörnäs R: A new method for the cytological examination of the cerebrospinal fluid. J Neurol Neurosurg Psychiatry 30:568, 1967.
*Original description of sedimentation technique.*

# "LITTLE WHITE SHAKERS" SYNDROME: GENERALIZED, SPORADIC, ACQUIRED, IDIOPATHIC TREMORS OF ADULT DOGS

ALAN J. PARKER
*Urbana, Illinois*

"Little white shakers" syndrome is seen in older puppies and younger adult dogs. It describes a clinical picture of marked intention tremors of the head and limbs that develop over a period of 1 to 3 days. Maltese and West Highland white terriers most commonly are affected (hence the name of the syndrome). However, dogs of any color, size, or breed (including mongrels) can be affected. More accurate terms for this syndrome are "sporadic, acquired tremors of adult dogs," or "generalized idiopathic tremors of adult dogs."

## PATHOGENESIS AND ETIOLOGY

There have been no large surveys to document the relative breed incidences of this syndrome. Anecdotally, there seems to be a varying breed incidence within the United States, around the world, and even seasonally. The apparent preponderance of this condition in two breeds of small white dogs, combined with our limited knowledge of its histopathology, has stimulated some interesting speculation about the etiology and pathogenesis of this syndrome. Does it have a genetic or a partially genetic component allowing an infectious agent or immune mechanism to affect these patients? How important is inflammation in the pathogenesis? Is it immune mediated or virally precipitated? How is it (or is it) related to white color? Is there a neurotransmitter block or delay? Does tyrosine metabolism play a role (Bagley et al., 1993; Cuddon, 1990; Chrisman, 1991; de Lahunta, 1983)? Tyrosine is metabolized to melanin by melanocytes (which are derived from embryonic neural crest cells). In the nervous system, tyrosine is metabolized to form various catecholamine neurotransmitters (epinephrine and dopamine). Affected white dogs are not albinos; they do produce melanin. The drugs we use to usually rapidly and successfully treat this syndrome (corticosteroids and benzodiazepines) fuel this speculation. The first is an anti-inflammatory agent that might affect neurosteroids and the latter is GABAergic (Parker, 1981).

## SIGNALMENT AND SIGNS

The syndrome most commonly is seen in young adult dogs (5 months to 3 years of age) of either sex. Its onset has not been consistently associated with any event, disease, laboratory result, or other clinical sign. Cerebrospinal fluid examination may demonstrate mild elevation of cell numbers (mostly lymphocytes) and of protein. There is no evidence the syndrome is spread by contact; cases are sporadic even in kennel situations. An abnormal incidence in one breeding line of dogs has not been reported, although Maltese terriers and West Highland white terriers seem to make up the bulk of the cases. Signs are progressive over 1 to 3 days and then usually remain static until treatment is initiated or, in a few cases, there is spontaneous clinical improvement months later. All four limbs and the head are affected by mild to severe intention tremors. Sometimes, these tremors are violent and the eyes may be affected with bilateral fast nystagmus or disconjugate movements. The menace response may be lost. There is mild to moderate hypermetria and body swaying. Mild to marked ataxia of all four limbs (pelvic limbs worse) may be present. Occasionally there is a head tilt. Conscious proprioception, spinal and higher reflexes, cranial nerves, personality, and voluntary motor functions are not affected. Paraparesis or tetraparesis may occur. Seizures rarely occur. There is no circling or sign of pain exhibited. Signs are bilaterally symmetric.

A "cerebellar" lesion is usually diagnosed, but the limb tremors are more typical of puppies with a generalized process such as dysmyelinogenesis, rather than a purely cerebellar lesion. Even cats with cerebellar hypoplasia do not exhibit such marked limb tremors, just the head tremors. Histology of the few cases that have been autopsied usually revealed a mild nonsuppurative encephalomyelitis with some perivascular cuffing; no dramatic lesions were detected. The lesions were not confined to the cerebellum (de Lahunta, 1983). Thus, this syndrome appears to be a diffuse, central nervous system process, affecting the cerebellum and cerebellar tracts more than the conscious proprioceptive or voluntary motor tracts.

## THERAPY

Corticosteroids or benzodiazepines (diazepam, mostly) have been described as the treatment of choice, but neither alone is rapidly and consistently effective (Bagley et al., 1993; Chrisman, 1991). The use of both types of drug simultaneously has been more effective and reliable in the author's experience. The duration of therapy is critical; premature cessation of therapy usually leads to a relapse. Simultaneous use of oral prednisolone (1 to 2 [rarely 4] mg/kg every 24 hr for 4 weeks, then 1/2 to 1 mg/kg every 24 hr for 2 weeks, then 1/2 to 1 mg/kg every 48 hr for 2 weeks, and then 1/2 to 1 mg/kg every 72 hr for 4 weeks) with oral diazepam (1/2 to 1 mg/kg every 8 hr for 4 weeks, then 1/2 to 1 mg/kg every 12 hr for 4 weeks, and then 1/2 to 1 mg/kg every 24 hr for 4 weeks) is preferable.

Clinical signs usually decrease during the second day and the dogs are usually 80% normal by the fifth day. Some dogs never become 100% normal and a few dogs relapse at the end of treatment, requiring titration of dosage versus clinical signs for an additional 1 to 3 months.

A few dogs have relapses months or years later or within a month of routine vaccination. Retreatment is effective.

### References and Suggested Reading

Bagley RS, Kornegay JN, Wheeler SJ, et al: Generalized tremors in Maltese. J Am Anim Hosp Assoc 29:141, 1993.

Chrisman C: *Problems in Small Animal Neurology*, 2nd edition. Philadelphia, Lea & Febiger, 1991, p 314.

Cuddon PA: Tremor syndromes. Prog Vet Neurol 1:285, 1990.

de Lahunta A: *Veterinary Neuroanatomy and Clinical Neurology*, 2nd edition Philadelphia, WB Saunders Co, 1983, p 150.

Parker AJ: Hypermetria and tremors. Mod Vet Prac 62:919, 1981.

# OTITIS MEDIA AND INTERNA

LINDA SHELL

*Blacksburg, Virginia*

## ANATOMIC CONSIDERATIONS

Middle ear structures include the tympanic membrane, the tympanic cavity, the tympanic nerve, the auditory tube, and the three auditory ossicles (malleus, incus, stapes) and their associated muscles and ligaments. Separating the horizontal portion of the external auditory canal from the middle ear cavity is the thin, semitransparent tympanic membrane.

The external aspect of the tympanic membrane, as observed on otoscopic examination, is somewhat concave because of the traction on the medial surface by the malleus, one of the three auditory ossicles. These three tiny bones form a chain from the tympanic membrane to the inner ear where the base of the stapes attaches to the vestibular or oval window.

Most of the middle ear is composed of the air-filled tympanic cavity, the ventral portion of which is within the tympanic bulla, part of the temporal bone. Within the cavity is the opening to the auditory or eustachian tube, a short canal connecting the nasopharynx to the middle ear. The facial nerve courses near the middle ear and a small branch, the tympanic nerve, passes through the tympanic cavity near the malleus. Other structures in or adjacent to the middle ear include the vagus nerve and the carotid and lingual arteries.

The inner ear structures include the cochlea, vestibule, and semicircular canals, which are housed within a membranous labyrinth contained within an osseous labyrinth. The middle and inner ears are connected via the oval and round windows (Fig. 1).

## INCIDENCE

The incidence of otitis media secondary to otitis externa is relatively high, varying from 16% of early otitis externa cases to about 52% of chronic cases (Spruell, 1964). But many cases of otitis media are apparently overlooked because they may have signs similar to otitis

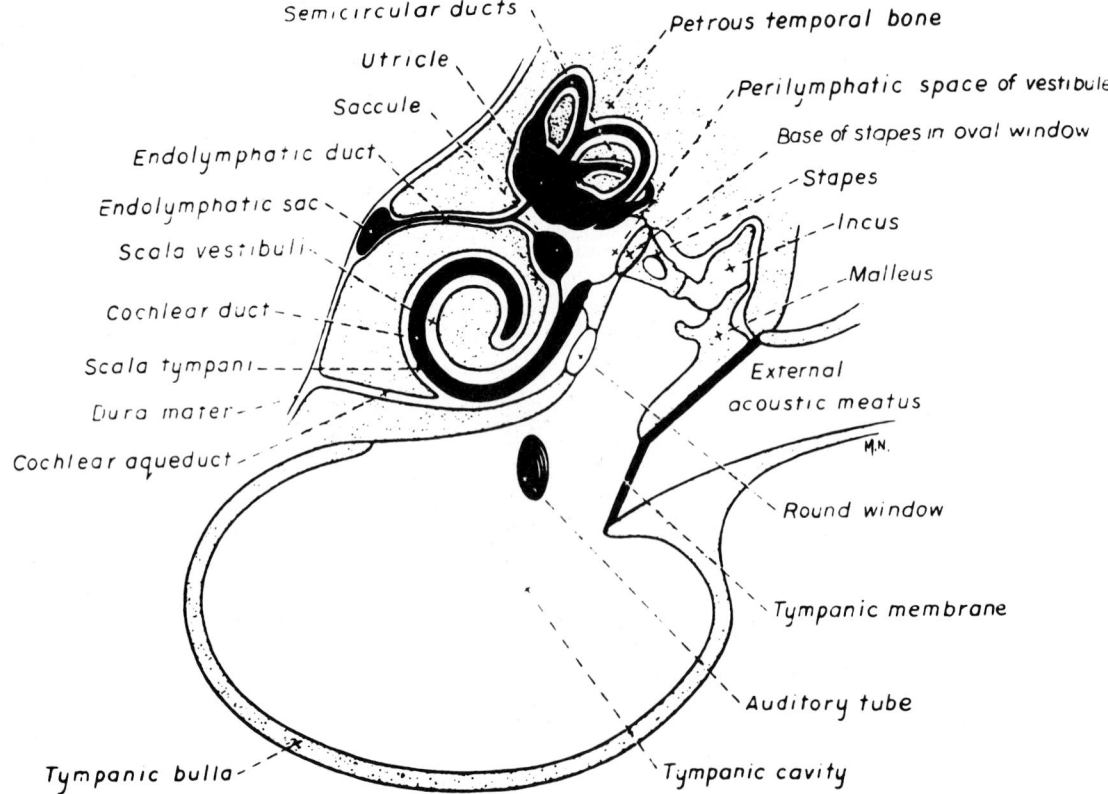

**Figure 1.** A diagram of the structures contained within the middle and inner ears of the dog. (From Getty R, Foust HL, Presley ET, et al: Macroscopic anatomy of the ear of the dog. Am J Vet Res 17:364–375, 1956, with permission.)

externa. Debris or proliferative changes in the ear canal and lack of patient cooperation often impede a thorough otic examination.

Otitis interna accounts for about one half of the acute peripheral vestibular signs in dogs (Schunk and Averill, 1983). Its incidence may appear to be falsely higher than that of otitis media because the clinical signs of vestibular dysfunction are so drastic.

## ROUTE OF INFECTION

The middle ear can become inflamed via three routes:

- *Across the tympanic membrane.* Debris, hair, foreign bodies, and exudate associated with external ear canal disease can cause inflammation, necrosis, and rupture of the tympanic membrane, allowing extension of infection to the tympanic cavity. This is the most common route.
- *Through the auditory tube.* Since the auditory tube connects the nasopharynx to the middle ear cavity, a pharyngeal infection can extend to the middle ear cavity. Cats especially may develop otitis media by this route as a sequela to upper respiratory disease.
- *By hematogenous spread.* Blood-borne pathogens may invade the middle ear, but this route of infection appears to be uncommon.

One study has supported a strong association between otitis externa and/or an abnormal tympanic membrane and the development of otitis interna (Schunk and Averill, 1983). Thus, the most common route of infection to the inner ear is most likely an extension of an external ear infection, across the tympanic membrane to the middle ear, and then to the inner ear. It is possible that cases of otitis interna have a concurrent otitis media and that the signs of otitis media are clinically or radiographically silent or are obscured by clinical signs of otitis externa.

## ETIOLOGIES

Data that compare the organisms isolated from the external, middle, and inner ears of dogs with otitis interna are not available; and because inner ear cultures are not anatomically feasible, it is not known what organisms are most commonly involved in otitis interna. It is presumed that the same bacterial organisms associated with otitis externa and otitis media are responsible for otitis interna.

It is generally agreed that most cases of otitis media are caused by bacteria. *Staphylococcus* and *Streptococcus* spp. and *Escherichia coli* are among the most commonly isolated organisms. Other agents include *Pseudomonas* and *Proteus* spp., *Clostridium* spp., *Candida* spp., and *Malassezia canis*. *Otodectes cynotis*, a ubiquitous psoroptid mite, will occasionally damage the tympanic membrane and invade the middle and inner

ears, especially in cats. Trauma, polyps, neoplasms, and foreign bodies (such as plant awns) can initiate inflammation and signs of middle ear disease. Because of expansive or invasive growth, neoplasms may also invade the middle or inner ears.

## CLINICAL SIGNS

### Otitis Media

Signs of otitis media may include discharge from the external ear canal, pawing or rubbing of the affected ear, head shaking, auditory deficits, or pain when the head is touched. These signs are indistinguishable from those observed with otitis externa. Occasionally, animals will tilt their head because of discomfort rather than because of abnormal vestibular function. Lethargy, depressed appetite, or fever can develop. Because the facial and sympathetic nerves course near the middle ear, a facial nerve palsy or Horner's syndrome may occur on the same side as the otitis media. Signs of facial nerve injury include drooping of or inability to move the ear or lip, drooling of saliva, and a decreased or absent palpebral reflex. Horner's syndrome is characterized by ptosis, miosis, enophthalmus, or protrusion of the nictitating membrane.

### Otitis Interna

The most commonly observed clinical signs of otitis interna are a head tilt to the affected side, spontaneous horizontal or rotary nystagmus, and an asymmetric limb ataxia with preservation of strength. In the acute stage, the pet may be so severely disoriented that it may circle, fall, or even roll to the affected side; ambulation is difficult or even impossible. These signs usually become less pronounced within several days. Vomiting is sometimes observed because of the vestibular connections to the emetic center in the brain stem. A reduction in hearing ability has also been occasionally observed.

## DIAGNOSIS

A thorough history and physical examination will help to establish systemic signs of disease or localized infections, which may suggest hematogenous spread of infection. Swelling, lumps, or pain may be found on careful palpation of the temporomandibular joints and base of the ears. The pharyngeal area should be visualized for signs of inflammation or masses that may have spread to the middle ear via the auditory tube.

### Neurologic Examination

It is important to perform a neurologic examination on all those cases that present with vestibular signs in order to distinguish peripheral vestibular signs from central vestibular signs. Disorders that affect the vestibulocochlear nerve or the inner ear include otitis interna, idiopathic vestibular syndrome in cats and geriatric dogs, ototoxic drugs, trauma, neoplasia, or metabolic polyneuropathies. Disorders that affect the vestibular nuclei in the brain stem (central vestibular) include neoplasia; trauma; ischemia; granulomatous meningoencephalitis; and infections such as canine distemper, feline infectious peritonitis, Rocky Mountain spotted fever, and ehrlichiosis. Central vestibular disorders are frequently progressive in nature with the exception of trauma and ischemia.

### Tympanic Membrane Examination

Heavy sedation or general anesthesia is necessary in most cases to thoroughly examine the external ear canal and the tympanic membrane. Even under anesthesia, the presence of ulcerations, masses, debris, or hyperkeratosis or hyperplasia of the surrounding tissues may hamper visualization of the tympanic membrane. Removal of debris may be accomplished by lavage of the ear canal with warm normal saline. A number of antiseptic agents, even in dilute solutions, have been incriminated in causing irreversible inner ear damage if the tympanic membrane is perforated. Thus, these agents should be avoided. Swabs for cytologic evaluation and culture and sensitivity should always be taken prior to the cleaning.

A normal tympanic membrane consists of a smaller triangular portion called the pars flaccida and a larger portion called the pars tensa (Fig. 2). The pars flaccida is an opaque white or pink loose membrane with small branching vessels. The pars tensa is a glistening transparent or pearl gray translucent membrane through

which the crescent-shaped malleus can be observed. Opaque radiating strands or radiating branches of blood vessels can also be observed. Middle ear pathology should be suspected if the tympanic membrane is absent, torn, bulging, cloudy, opaque, or discolored. In one report, perforations were rarely found, but the membrane appeared thickened (Little, Lane, and Pearson, 1991). Thickened cloudy areas may represent scars or adhesions from previous inflammation.

### Radiologic Evaluation

Oblique lateral, open-mouth, and ventrodorsal views of the skull are recommended for adequate radiographic evaluation of the tympanic bullae; general anesthesia is usually required to obtain quality radiographs. In cases of chronic otitis externa, narrowing of the external ear canal and/or ossification of the annular cartilages may be found on the ventrodorsal skull radiographs. The oblique lateral and open-mouth views are particularly useful for evaluating the air-filled tympanic cavity. If fluid, granulation tissue, or neoplasia fill this cavity, a soft tissue density becomes apparent. In cases of chronic otitis media, the wall of the tympanic bulla may appear thickened or sclerotic. In advanced disease, bony proliferation may extend to the rest of the petrous temporal bone, the temporomandibular joint, or both. Destruction of the bulla may be observed in some cases. Radiographic changes may not be present for several weeks in acute cases of otitis media, and chronic cases may only show sclerosis of the bulla. A recent retrospective study indicated that positive radiographic findings are highly sensitive in the diagnosis of otitis media, but negative findings do not rule it out (Remedios, Fowler, and Pharr, 1991).

Otitis interna does not produce readily apparent radiographic changes in the petrous temporal bone. However, radiographs of the tympanic bullae are indicated in suspected cases of otitis interna because of the close anatomic association between the inner and middle ears. Since an infection of the middle ear cavity can be clinically silent and yet spread to the inner ear, radiographic evidence of otitis media may help to support the diagnosis of otitis interna in a dog with peripheral vestibular signs.

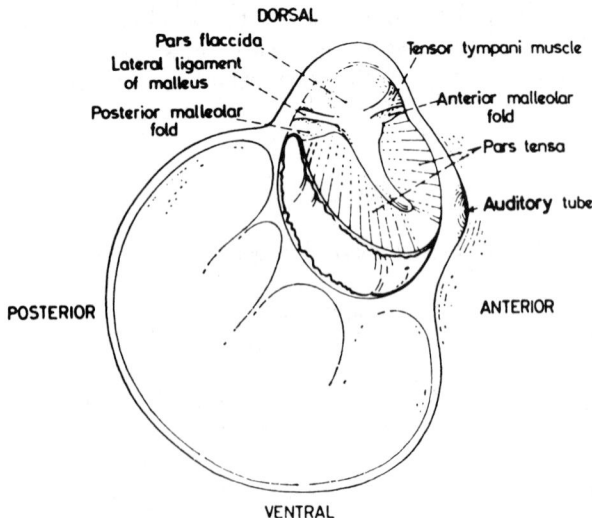

**Figure 2.** Diagram of the medial face of the lateral wall of the left tympanic cavity of the dog. (From Spreull JSA: Otitis media in the dog. *In* Kirk RW (ed): *Current Veterinary Therapy* V. Philadelphia, WB Saunders Co, 1974, with permission.)

### TREATMENT

The goals of treatment of otitis media and otitis interna are to remove inflammatory, infected, or foreign material and to provide ventilation and drainage. These goals can be accomplished by medical or surgical means or both, depending upon the chronicity, the results of otoscopic examination, and the radiographic changes.

## Myringotomy

If there is otoscopic or radiographic evidence of increased middle ear density or fluid, the tympanic membrane can be incised (myringotomy) to obtain samples for cytology and culture and to drain fluid from the middle ear cavity. A myringotomy may also relieve pressure and pain caused by the fluid or inflammatory material within the middle ear.

Several types of myringotomy have been described. The type most commonly used in veterinary medicine is a simple paracentesis procedure (Neer and Howard, 1982). Using an otoscope and a clean cone, the tympanic membrane should be visualized. A blunt probe is then directed through the otoscope cone to perforate the tympanic membrane caudal to the malleus. The probe is then removed and a 20-gauge spinal needle of adequate length is passed through the perforated membrane. A syringe is attached to the spinal needle and fluid or material from the middle ear cavity is aspirated. Disadvantages to this technique include inadequate otoscopic visualization of the procedure and obstruction of the aspiration needle with thick exudate.

The middle ear contains many nerve endings and the smallest and most delicate bones in the body, all of which can be easily damaged. The myringotomy should always be made caudal to the malleus, in the posteroinferior quadrant of the tympanic membrane. If otitis externa is present, the ear canal should be thoroughly cleaned before the myringotomy is performed, to decrease the likelihood of spreading infection to the middle ear cavity. Harsh chemicals and disinfectants should never be placed into the middle ear cavity. Warm saline is recommended for flushing the middle ear cavity as well as the external ear canal.

To flush the middle ear cavity, a suction cannula with a metal tip is used to perforate the tympanic membrane caudal to the malleus (Harvey, 1985). A 20-gauge spinal needle of adequate length, attached to a 20-cc syringe of warm water, is also inserted through the tympanic membrane caudal to the malleus. Warm water is flushed into the tympanic cavity and gently suctioned. The flushing and aspiration should be directed toward the tympanic bulla (posterior to and downward from the cochlea and ossicles) to avoid damage to the ossicles and cochlea. Because too much pressure during flushing could damage the ossicles, this procedure is only recommended when medical treatment has failed and surgery is not an option.

## Antibiotics

Systemic antibiotics are administered for 3 to 6 weeks, keeping in mind any potential side effect of administering the chosen antibiotic for this duration of time. Ideally, the antibiotic should be selected based upon the cytology and/or culture and sensitivity results of the exudate obtained from the external ear canal or the middle ear. If culture results are not available, one of the following broad-spectrum antibiotics can be chosen:

Cefadroxil, 22 mg/kg every 12 hr PO.
Cefalexin, 22 mg/kg every 8 hr PO.
Chloramphenicol, 50 mg/kg every 8 hr (every 12 hr in cat) PO, IV, IM.
Trimethoprim-sulfadiazine (Tribrissen) 15 mg/kg every 12 hr PO, SC.

## Topical Treatments

If otitis externa is present, the etiology or predisposing factors should be explored and treatment should be initiated. However, topically applied disinfectants and therapeutic agents should be used cautiously if the tympanic membrane is not intact. Some of these preparations (such as aminoglycosides, chloramphenicol, iodine, iodophor, cetrimide, and chlorhexidine) can cause ototoxicity if they are inadvertently introduced into the middle ear through a perforation in the tympanic membrane.

There are no specific treatments for facial nerve paralysis or Horner's syndrome. Artificial tears can be used to alleviate the signs associated with keratitis sicca.

## Surgical Intervention

If there is radiographic or otoscopic evidence of fluid or soft tissue in the tympanic bullae, a bulla osteotomy is recommended followed by appropriate antibiotic treatment. Some cases of otitis media and interna will have negative findings on otoscopic and radiologic evaluations and yet will have significant middle ear inflammation when a surgical exploration is performed (Remedios, Fowler, and Pharr, 1991). Thus, if there is inadequate response to systemic antibiotics, surgical options should be considered. Total ear canal ablation and bulla osteotomy and curettage is a standard surgical treatment in dogs that have chronic nonresponsive otitis externa and media (Beckman, Henry, and Cechner, 1990).

## PROGNOSIS

If the inflammatory process is identified early and treated with appropriate antibiotics or surgery, the prognosis for recovery is good. Minor residual vestibular deficits, such as a head tilt or mild ataxia, may persist in cases of otitis interna. Keratitis sicca, facial nerve paralysis, or Horner's syndrome may persist in cases of otitis media. Some cases develop osteomyelitis of the osseous bulla and petrous temporal bone. Occasionally, the infection ascends the vestibulocochlear and facial nerves to the brain stem, resulting in a brain stem abscess or meningitis and central vestibular signs. Central vestibular infections can progress rapidly and cause death despite appropriate and aggressive treatments and intensive monitoring.

## References and Suggested Reading

Beckman SL, Henry WB, and Cechner P: Total ear canal ablation combining bulla osteotomy and curettage in dogs with chronic otitis externa and media. J Am Vet Med Assoc 196:84, 1990.
*A description of the total ear canal ablation technique and the results of the procedure in 44 dogs with chronic otitis externa and media.*
Harvey CE: Disease of the middle ear. *In* Slatter DH (ed): *Textbook of Small Animal Surgery.* Philadelphia, WB Saunders Co, 1985, p 1915.
*A review of the anatomy and surgical management of middle ear disorders.*
Little CJL, Lane JG, and Pearson GR: Inflammatory middle ear disease of the dog: The pathology of otitis media. Vet Rec 128:293, 1991.
*A prospective study of the clinical and pathologic findings of otitis media in 42 dogs.*

Neer TM and Howard PE: Otitis media. Compend Cont Educ Pract Vet 4: 410, 1982.
*A review of the causes and treatment of otitis media.*
Remedios AM, Fowler JD, and Pharr JW: A comparison of radiographic versus surgical diagnosis of otitis media. J Am Anim Hosp Assoc 27:183, 1991.
*A retrospective study of the radiographic and surgical findings in 19 cases of middle ear disease.*
Schunk KL and Averill DR: Peripheral vestibular syndrome in the dog: A review of 83 cases. J Am Vet Med Assoc 182:1354, 1983.
*A review of the clinical records and follow-up evaluations on 83 cases of peripheral vestibular syndrome.*
Shell LG: Otitis media and otitis interna. Vet Clin North Am 18:885, 1988.
*A review of the etiology, diagnosis, and medical management.*
Spreull JS: Treatment of otitis media in the dog. J Small Anim Pract 5:107, 1964.
*A review of the causes and treatment of otitis media.*

# CANINE NEURODEGENERATIVE DISEASES INVOLVING MOTOR NEURONS

JOHN F. CUMMINGS
*and* ALEXANDER DE LAHUNTA
*Ithaca, New York*

The degenerative diseases affecting the motor neurons of dogs may vary considerably in their clinical and pathologic findings. The earlier recognized and more thoroughly studied of these disorders have established inherited bases. These diseases include: hereditary neuronal abiotrophy in Swedish Lapland dogs, hereditary spinal muscular atrophy in Brittany spaniels, and hereditary progressive neurogenic muscular atrophy in pointer dogs. In this section, we will not review these conditions, since they have been thoroughly described in the past (see *CVT XI*). Instead, we will focus on more recently identified, breed-associated disorders with presumed but unconfirmed hereditary bases.

## CLINICAL FINDINGS

Motor neuron disease is characterized clinically by progressive weakness with difficulty supporting weight, hyporeflexia, and muscle atrophy. Ventral horn cell loss in puppies often results in malpositioned immovable joints due to denervation muscle atrophy in a growing animal. Electromyography typically reveals spontaneous denervation potentials in the form of fibrillations and positive sharp waves. Fasciculations are not usually seen or recorded in dogs. Motor nerve conduction velocities may be normal or slightly delayed. Muscle biopsy samples typically will contain angular atrophied fibers of mixed type. Scattered hypertrophied fibers may also be seen. Subterminal sprouting of unaffected motor axons and reinnervation of muscle fibers lead to

the fiber type grouping that may be encountered on biopsy specimens taken later in the course of the disease.

## CLASSIFICATION

The term "spinal muscular atrophy" is applied to most of the inherited motor neuron diseases in humans including Werdnig-Hoffmann disease, which is designated as type 1 or the acute infantile form. In Werdnig-Hoffmann disease and similar diseases of animals, the degeneration may involve motor neurons preponderantly but not exclusively. Postmortem studies, in fact, may reveal that the degenerative process is widespread in the nervous system, as in the case of the Lapland dogs, but the rapidly evolving tetraplegia essentially masks clinical expression of wider involvement. Thus, a spinal muscular atrophy or motor neuron disease may include but not clinically reflect substantial multisystemic involvement. In classifying these disorders, it can be very difficult to make a clear distinction between motor neuron and multisystemic neurodegenerative disease. In this regard, the four diseases presented here form a clinical and pathologic continuum starting with a focal degeneration of spinal motor neurons in German shepherds and ending with a multisystem degeneration in cairn terriers. Only in the relatively benign disorder of the German shepherds was treatment attempted and survival possible with minimal residual disabilities. Despite their low prevalence, these disorders merit consideration because they may pose larger problems to breeders in the future and they can be easily confused clinically with other diseases that are better known.

## Focal Spinal Muscular Atrophy in German Shepherd Pups

Two 4-week-old German shepherd pups, a male and a female, were presented with a valgus deformity of the right carpus that was fixed in flexion due to shortened atrophic flexor muscles. The two pups were from a litter of six. The sire had produced many normal litters but this was the dam's first litter. The maternal grandsire had produced a litter of four in which one pup was similarly affected.

Weakness was noted at 2 weeks in one forelimb in the female, but asymmetric bilateral forelimb involvement was observed in the male. At 4 weeks, a tenotomy of the right flexor carpi ulnaris was performed on the female pup. Postoperatively, the owner continued to splint the carpus to gradually reduce the flexion deformity. At 15 months, forelimb muscle atrophy was no longer obvious and slight weakness was seen only with prolonged exercise.

Surgical correction was not attempted on the male and, by 8 weeks, forelimb paresis had worsened so that the pup was unable to rise and relied on hindlimb propulsion or swimming movements to slither forward on the floor. Electromyography revealed denervation potentials bilaterally in the muscles of the shoulder, arm, and forearm.

The male pup was euthanatized. Our postmortem studies revealed asymmetric loss and degeneration of motor neurons in the cervical intumescence of the spinal cord. Changes were more severe on the right. Motor neuron depletion was most marked in the C7 and 8 segments, where small glial scars marked the sites of neuron loss. Of the motor neurons that remained, many were degenerating. Some were undergoing peripheral chromatolysis with loss and dispersion of ribosomes that had formed the peripheral Nissl bodies. Other cell bodies were vacuolated and some necrotic neurons were undergoing neuronophagia. Cell body degeneration resulted in fragmentation and loss of motor axons in the small fascicles that traverse the ventral funiculus en route to enter the ventral roots.

This focal spinal motor disease differs from the other neurodegenerative diseases considered in this section in that the degenerative process is confined to motor neurons and only those of the cervical intumescence. It contrasts with other canine motor neuron diseases because it is more benign and even treatable. In some ways, this neuronopathy resembles the asymmetric and unilateral benign spinal muscular atrophies described in the upper extremities of humans. In the latter, however, onset is later, progression is slower, and there is no indication of familial incidence. Without more pedigree information, the inherited nature of this canine disorder is only presumptive. In its clinical presentation, this illness easily could be confused with canine protozoan radiculomyelitis.

## Motor Neuron Disease in Doberman Pinscher Pups

Recently, we observed two male Doberman Pinscher pups from a litter of eight that developed hindlimb weakness at 4 weeks of age. By 5 weeks, the forelimbs were involved and the pups were unable to walk. When referred to this teaching hospital at 6 weeks, they were in lateral recumbency with their forelimbs in rigid extension. When their trunks were supported, their heads dropped due to cervical muscle weakness. Their hindlimbs were paretic but they were still capable of short strides and delayed hopping reactions. Forelimb muscle atrophy was marked. The elbows were fixed in extension due to the coincidence of the wasting and fibrosis of the triceps muscles and the rapid growth of the long bones of the forelimb. Hindlimb muscle atrophy was less advanced and the patellar and withdrawal reflexes remained intact. Electrical studies revealed widespread denervation potentials and motor nerve conduction velocities were reduced.

The lower motor neuron signs in these young pups were judged to be consistent with protozoan radiculomyelitis (see *CVT XI*, p 265) or spinal muscular atrophy. Postmortem studies confirmed the latter diagnosis. Diffuse spinal motor neuron degeneration was accompanied by degenerative changes in the hypoglossal and facial nuclei and nucleus ambiguus. A few affected neurons occurred also in the reticular, pontine, and vestibular nuclei. Some degenerating neurons were swollen and chromatolytic with eccentric nuclei and eosinophilic cytoplasm. Other cell bodies had vacuolated cytoplasm and were more greatly enlarged (Fig. 1). Ultrastructurally, the vesicles appear to be derived largely from distended endoplasmic reticulum; however, swollen Golgi and mitochondrial profiles were also observed. Occasional glial scars marked the sites of neuron loss. Degenerating axons in the ventral rootlets were fewer than anticipated based on the extent of cell body involvement. Although a genetic basis is suspected, it is well to recall that retroviral infections in rodents have been associated with vacuolar degeneration of motor neurons.

## Familial Motor Neuron Disease in Rottweiler Pups

This disease was first described by Shell, Jortner, and Leib (1987b) in two 6-week-old female Rottweiler pups in a litter of seven. These two pups regurgitated milk soon after birth and were smaller and clumsier than the others. By 6 weeks, one was quadriparetic, wasted in the hindlimb muscles, and recumbent; the other was paraparetic and tired quickly when walking. Megaesophagus was confirmed radiographically in both. The

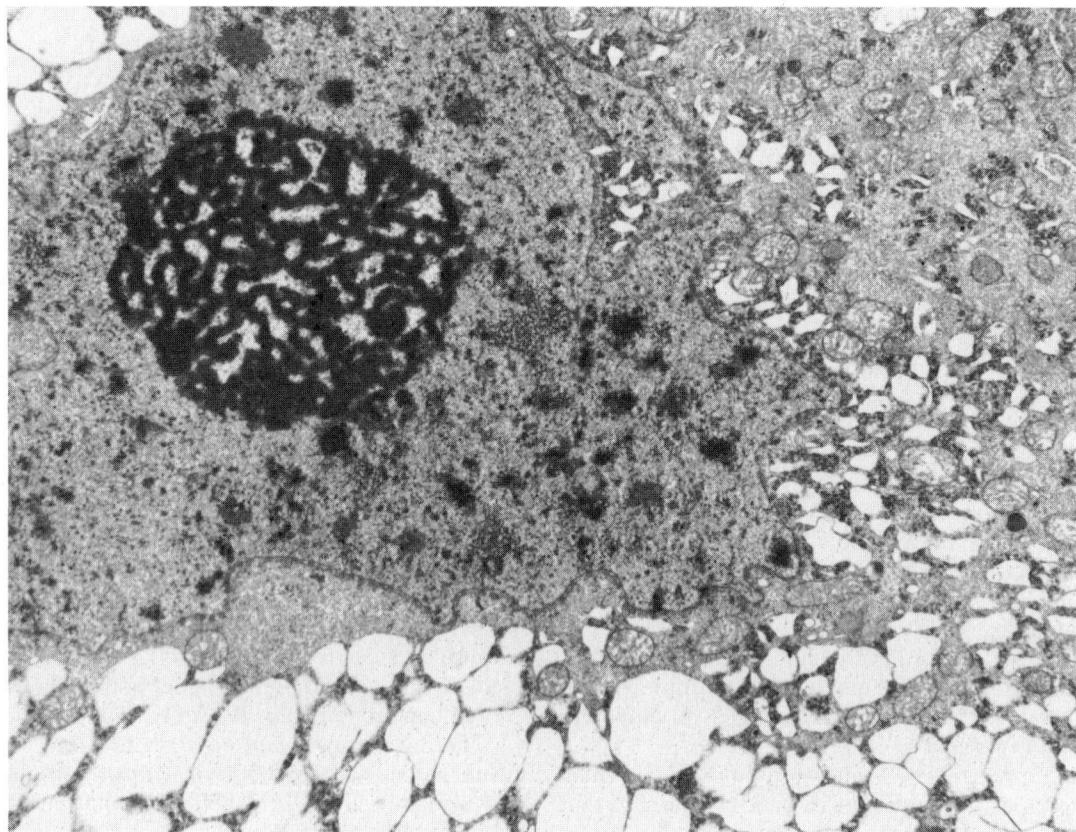

**Figure 1.** Vacuolated spinal motor neuron. (X8400.)

quadriparetic pup was euthanatized at 6 weeks. Weakness had increased and denervation atrophy had resulted in hindlimb extension when the second pup was euthanatized at 8 weeks.

Postmortem studies revealed swollen, centrally chromatolytic spinal and bulbar motor neurons including neurons in the nucleus ambiguus. Increased neurofilaments were found within the affected cell bodies and swollen axons in the spinal ventral horns. The peripheral nerves and dorsal and ventral roots contained degenerating axons. Chromatolytic neuronal changes also were noted in the red nucleus.

More recently, we studied one of two pups from a litter of six with signs similar to those reported by Shell et al. This 2-month-old male had survived a more severely affected female that had been euthanatized. He was presented because he tired easily, had difficulty walking, would fall on his hindlimbs, and had begun to "bunny hop." On arrival, the pup was in sternal recumbency and moved by swimming movements of the forelimbs. The pup's limbs were weak and hypotonic. The patellar relfexes were absent and the withdrawal reflexes were depressed in the hindlimbs. Although muscle atrophy was not apparent, electrodiagnostic testing revealed denervation potentials and delayed motor nerve conduction with depressed evoked responses. During 3 weeks of hospitalization, the pup's condition deteriorated slightly before euthanasia.

Despite this pup's less severe clinical course, on nec-

ropsy the degenerative changes were more widespread and varied than those reported in the initial cases. In addition to the bulbospinal motor neurons, the affected population included cell bodies in the zona intermedia; the nucleus of the dorsal spinocerebellar tract; the spinal ganglia; and the cochlear, vestibular, and cerebellar nuclei. Besides central chromatolysis, a less extensive, patchy loss of Nissl substance occurred in some neurons. Although pale swollen cell bodies with accumulations of neurofilaments were common, extensively vacuolated and necrotic neurons were also encountered. Neurons in the earlier stages of degeneration often contained enlarged eccentric nuclei with large, irregular, open nucleoli. Neurofilament-distended axonal spheroids were found in the ventral horns (Fig. 2). Wallerian-type degeneration, however, appeared in both the sensory and motor roots, the peripheral nerves as well as in spinal funiculi, especially the dorsal one.

## Multisystemic Chromatolytic Neuronal Degeneration in Cairn Terriers

In 1988, Palmer and Blakemore described this neuronopathy in pups from the United Kingdom and Australia and at the same time we reported this neurodegenerative condition in the United States in a single pup. The clinical manifestations of this disease, which

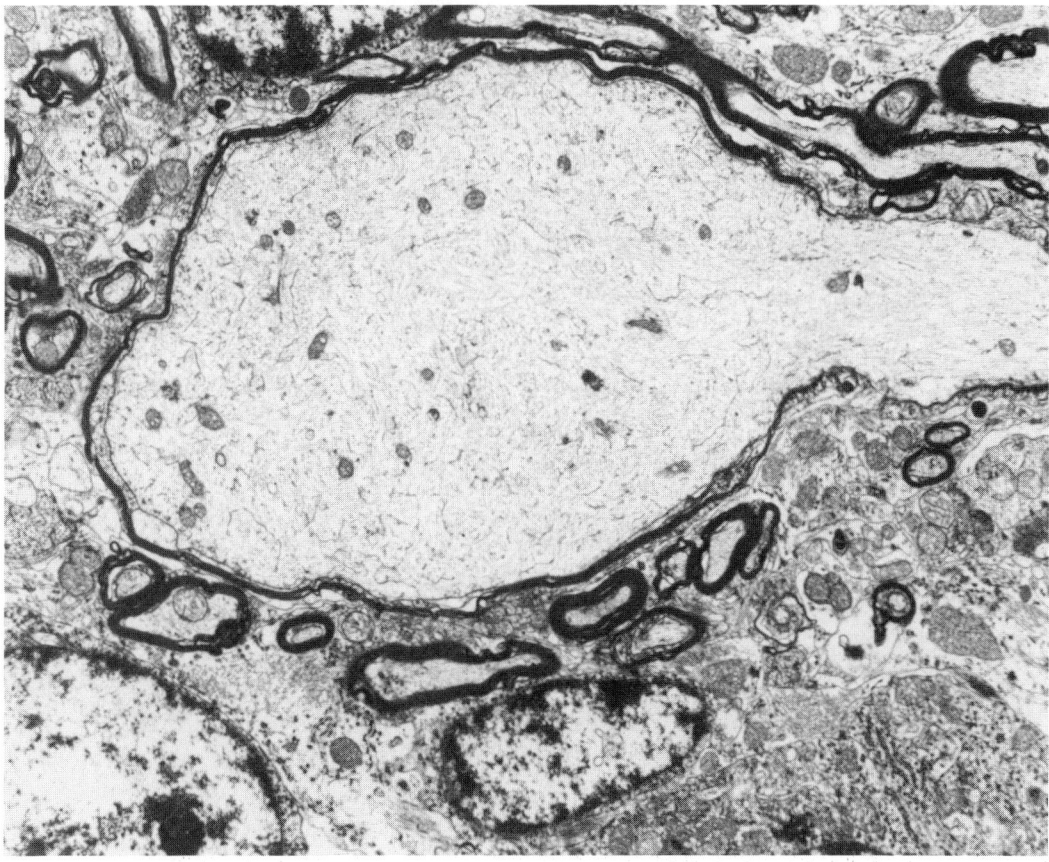

**Figure 2.** Swollen axon in spinal ventral horn. (X7350.)

have been confused with those of globoid cell leuko-dystrophy, have varied among the reported cases. The three puppies, both male and female, studied at Cambridge at 5 to 7 months exhibited paraparesis, quadriparesis, ataxia, loss of spinal reflexes, and head tremor. The affected cairn terrier female pup, first referred to us for pathology studies at 4½ months of age, was the only one in a litter of four to exhibit mild paraparesis with infrequent episodes of hindlimb collapse. A second female pup from a litter of three by the same dam and a brother of the sire of the first litter was noted at 10 weeks to fall frequently while playing and seemed to have a head tilt. When referred to us at 12 weeks, the pup had difficulty standing and head tremors developed when the pup attempted to stand. When fully supported, the pup would try to walk, but limb movements were spastic and hypermetric. When supported, the pup at 30- to 45-sec intervals experienced recurrent 5- to 15-sec episodes of generalized hypotonia in which she became limp. Electrical studies revealed a cessation or reduction in cervical muscle potentials during episodes of collapse and a concurrent shift in the electroencephalogram (EEG) to faster, lower amplitude activity. True rapid eye movement (REM) patterns, however, were not recorded. During a cataplectic episode, intravenous injection of 1 mg of imipramine produced prompt and prolonged arousal. The earlier and more overt signs in the second pup contrasted with those in the first, yet the infrequent bouts of hindlimb collapse in the first pup were probably a milder form of the cataplectic episodes observed in the second.

Palmer and Blakemore (1989) relied on signs of lower motor neuron paralysis and the absence of clinical evidence of severe brain involvement to distinguish this disease in cairn terriers from globoid cell leuko-dystrophy. Our experience with two pups would suggest that the cataplectic bouts may prove reliable in distinguishing these two diseases.

Postmortem studies of affected pups revealed that chromatolytic degenerative changes involved diverse neuron populations throughout the brain and spinal cord and also included cell bodies in sensory and autonomic ganglia. Central, peripheral, and patchy forms of chromatolysis were encountered in affected neurons. The chromatolytic changes were most striking in large cell bodies (e.g., bulbospinal motor neurons). Perikaryal lesions were clearly in excess of the associated axon degeneration. In our second pup, we found that the chromatolytic degeneration was accompanied by myelomalacia symmetrically localized to the dorsal horn region in thoracolumbar segments. The lesion triggering the cataplectic attacks could not be localized because chromatolytic involvement occurred diffusely among the brain stem nuclei.

## References and Suggested Reading

Cummings JF, de Lahunta A, and Moore JJ: Multisystemic chromatolytic neuronal degeneration in a Cairn terrier pup. Cornell Vet 78:301, 1988.
*A case with mild and episodic weakness but extensive pathologic changes.*

Cummings JF, de Lahunta A, and Gasteiger EL: Multisystemic chromatolytic neuronal degeneration in Cairn terriers. A case with generalized cataplectic episodes. J Vet Intern Med 5:91, 1991.
*References all earlier published reports on this disease and discusses cataplectic episodes and spinal malacia.*

Cummings JF, George C, de Lahunta A, et al: Focal spinal muscular atrophy in two German shepherd pups. Acta Neuropathol 79:113, 1989.
*Initial report on this relatively benign motor neuron disease.*

de Lahunta A: Abiotrophy in domestic animals: A review. Can J Vet Res 54:65, 1990.
*A review of abiotrophies including motor neuron and multisystem degenerations.*

Palmer AC and Blakemore WF: A progressive neuronopathy in the young Cairn terrier. J Small Anim Pract 30:101, 1989.
*Clinical and pathologic studies on three cases.*

Shell LG, Jortner BS, and Leib MS: Familial lower motor neuron disease in Rottweiler dogs: Neuropathological studies. Vet Pathol 24:139, 1987a.
*Initial report on motor disease in this breed.*

Shell LG, Jortner BS, and Leib MS: Spinal muscular atrophy in two Rottweiler littermates. J Am Vet Med Assoc 190:878, 1987b.

Towfighi J, Young RSK, and Ward RM: Is Werdnig-Hoffmann disease a pure lower motor neuron disorder? Acta Neuropathol 65:270, 1985.
*A report on four cases in which multiple neuronal systems were involved.*

Virmani V and Mohan PK: Non-familial, spinal segmental muscular atrophy in juvenile and young subjects. Acta Neurol Scand 72:336, 1985.
*Presents 32 cases of nonfamilial spinal segmental muscular atrophy with insidious progression.*

# LARYNGEAL PARALYSIS-POLYNEUROPATHY COMPLEX IN YOUNG DALMATIAN DOGS

KYLE G. BRAUND

*Auburn, Alabama*

Hereditary, acquired, and idiopathic forms of laryngeal paralysis have been reported in dogs and cats. An hereditary form has been documented in young bouvier des Flandres, either as unilateral or bilateral disease. A presumed hereditary form has been reported in young Siberian huskies and young husky crossbreds. The idiopathic form has been reported mostly in middle-aged and older large and giant-breed dogs, such as Saint Bernard, Chesapeake Bay retriever, and Irish setter; but medium, small, and toy breeds also may be affected. Acquired laryngeal paralysis in dogs and cats has been reported sporadically as a result of lymphomatous infiltration of the vagus nerve, as a complication of lead poisoning, as a result of a foreign body penetrating the wall of the esophagus, and as a postoperative complication of carotid body tumors. Laryngeal paralysis may be one of several signs seen in animals with rabies and is sporadically observed in animals with idiopathic polyradiculoneuritis. Several years ago, we reported laryngeal paralysis in immature and mature dogs as one sign of a more diffuse polyneuropathy (Braund et al., 1989). Three of the young dogs in that report were dalmatians, a breed that had not previously been associated with laryngeal paralysis. Since that time, we have seen an additional 13 young dalmatian dogs with laryngeal paralysis (Braund et al., 1994). An overview of the present knowledge about dalmatians with laryngeal paralysis-polyneuropathy complex is summarized below.

## CLINICAL FINDINGS

To date, we are aware of 16 young Dalmatian dogs (eight males and eight females; mean [± SD] age 4.6 ± 2.7 months) from 13 litters (12 in the United States, one in Canada) with laryngeal paralysis. Muscle and nerve biopsy samples from the majority of these dogs[*] have been processed for histochemistry, single nerve fiber teasing, semithin, and thin nerve section preparations.

Onset of clinical signs in most dogs is from 2 to 6 months of age; however, in one dog, signs were first noted at 12 months of age. The mean observation period between onset of signs and euthanasia or death was 3.7 months (range = 1 to 18 months). All dogs had signs of acute respiratory distress. These included inspiratory/expiratory stridor (which was accentuated by exercise), cyanosis, syncopal episodes, dysphonia/aphonia, coughing or gagging when eating or after exercise, exercise intolerance, tachycardia, prolonged capillary refill times, and regurgitation. The laryngeal paralysis was episodic in some dogs and was associated with visible spasmodic contractions of the laryngeal muscles. Laryngeal paralysis was diagnosed in all dogs by direct visual or endoscopic inspection of the larynx, usually with animals under light sedation or anesthesia. Impaired abduction of the arytenoid cartilages (vocal

---

[*]Mailed via an overnight delivery service to the Neuromuscular Laboratory, Scott-Ritchey Research Center, Auburn University.

folds) was typically bilateral, but not always symmetric. Megaesophagus was present in 9 of 16 dogs. Other neurologic deficits also were noted in 12 of 16 dogs. Neurologic signs preceded respiratory signs in three dogs, occurred simultaneously with respiratory signs in six dogs, and developed after respiratory signs in three other dogs. Neurologic signs included hyporeflexia, paresis, proprioceptive deficits, muscle atrophy, muscle fasciculations, limb hyperextension, facial/lingual paralysis, and hypermetria. To date, no dogs have had hearing deficits. Several dogs euthanatized at 3 to 4 months of age had respiratory signs and megaesophagus without definitive evidence of other neurologic deficits; however, these dogs had evidence of peripheral neuropathy (see below).

## LABORATORY FINDINGS

Electromyographic testing reveals a moderate number of fibrillation potentials and positive sharp waves primarily in muscles below the elbow and stifle joints, and in laryngeal, esophageal, and facial muscles. Motor nerve conduction velocity studies are frequently slow—ranging from 24 to 46 m/sec in the sciatic-tibial nerves. Sensory nerve conduction velocities have been slow in one of two dogs tested. Results of routine hematologic and blood biochemical analyses and thyroid-stimulating hormone (TSH) response testing, blood lead concentration, serum cholinesterase activity, and immunologic function are normal. No abnormalities have been noted in cerebrospinal fluid (CSF).

## PATHOLOGIC FINDINGS

In cross-sectional preparations of peripheral nerves from Dalmatians with laryngeal paralysis, abnormal findings include focal or diffuse loss of myelinated nerve fibers, axonal degeneration, and increased endoneurial fibrosis (Fig. 1). Small groups of regenerating clusters are observed infrequently. These changes are more severe in distal parts of nerves compared to more proximal regions. Inflammation has not been observed in any nerve. The predominant abnormality in teased nerve fibers is axonal necrosis (graded lesion E), characterized by linear rows of myelin ovoids and balls (Table 1). Demyelination, remyelination, or both involving the same fiber are observed infrequently. The percentage of abnormalities is higher in distal portions of nerve samples (e.g., distal tibial versus proximal sciatic nerve, and distal recurrent laryngeal versus proximal recurrent laryngeal nerve). Diameter measurements of myelinated nerve fibers in distal nerves reveal a unimodal distribution and marked loss of medium (5.5 to 8 $\mu$m) and large-caliber (8.5 to 12 $\mu$m) fibers compared to more proximal portions of nerves.

Ultrastructurally, peripheral nerves from affected dogs are characterized by loss of myelinated fibers, marked increase in endoneurial collagen, variable ovoid presence, numerous Büngner bands, multifocal macrophage infiltration, and presence of dark endoneurial fibroblasts. Myelin debris, membranous bodies, and prominent organelles, especially mitochondria, sometimes are observed in axons and Schwann cell cytoplasm. In unmyelinated fibers, there is multifocal presence of collagen pockets; flattened axons and empty Schwann cell subunits; intra-axonal membranous accumulations; and swollen, watery axons. Vessels appear normal. Demyelinating fibers are seen only rarely, and there is no evidence of "onion-bulb" formation.

Appendicular and intrinsic laryngeal skeletal muscle changes are characterized by marked fiber size variation associated with atrophic and hypertrophic fibers. Atrophic fibers are angular and sometimes form small and large groups in a disseminated random distribution. Most of the atrophic fibers are type II, while hypertrophic fibers are both type I and type II. Fiber type grouping is often present. In some areas, there is a relative increase in perimysial and, sometimes, endomysial connective tissue. Depletion of myelinated fibers is noted in some intramuscular nerves. Muscle changes are more prominent in distal muscles (such as lateral head of gastrocnemius and cranial tibial muscle) compared to more proximal muscles (such as biceps femoris). There is no evidence of necrosis, phagocytosis, or inflammation in any muscle sample examined.

To date, there has been no evidence of degeneration or loss of neurons in spinal cord gray matter, brain stem nuclei or spinal ganglia. Dorsal and ventral nerve roots appear normal.

## ETIOLOGY

The cause remains uncertain—no dog has had any evidence of metabolic, toxic, or autoimmune disease. The widespread peripheral and cranial nerve involvement, without visible neuronal degeneration or loss, strongly suggests that laryngeal paralysis in Dalmatians represents one sign of a more diffuse primary polyneuropathy. Accordingly, we have proposed the term "laryngeal paralysis-polyneuropathy" (LPP) complex for animals with this disease. The fact that the condition has occurred in 12 of 14 dogs under 6 months of age indicates it is congenital, and possibly hereditary. Although detailed pedigree data are not available to us, an autosomal recessive mode of inheritance is suggested by the occurrence of this disorder in approximately 25% of littermates. Laryngeal paralysis is reportedly inherited as an autosomal dominant trait in bouvier des Flandres, while inheritance, as yet undefined, is presumed in young Siberian huskies and Husky crossbreds. A "roaring" disorder, which may be laryngeal paralysis, has been reported as a congenital condition in bull terrier puppies.

## DIFFERENTIAL DIAGNOSIS

Laryngeal paralysis in Dalmatians appears to be clinically and pathologically different from a respiratory

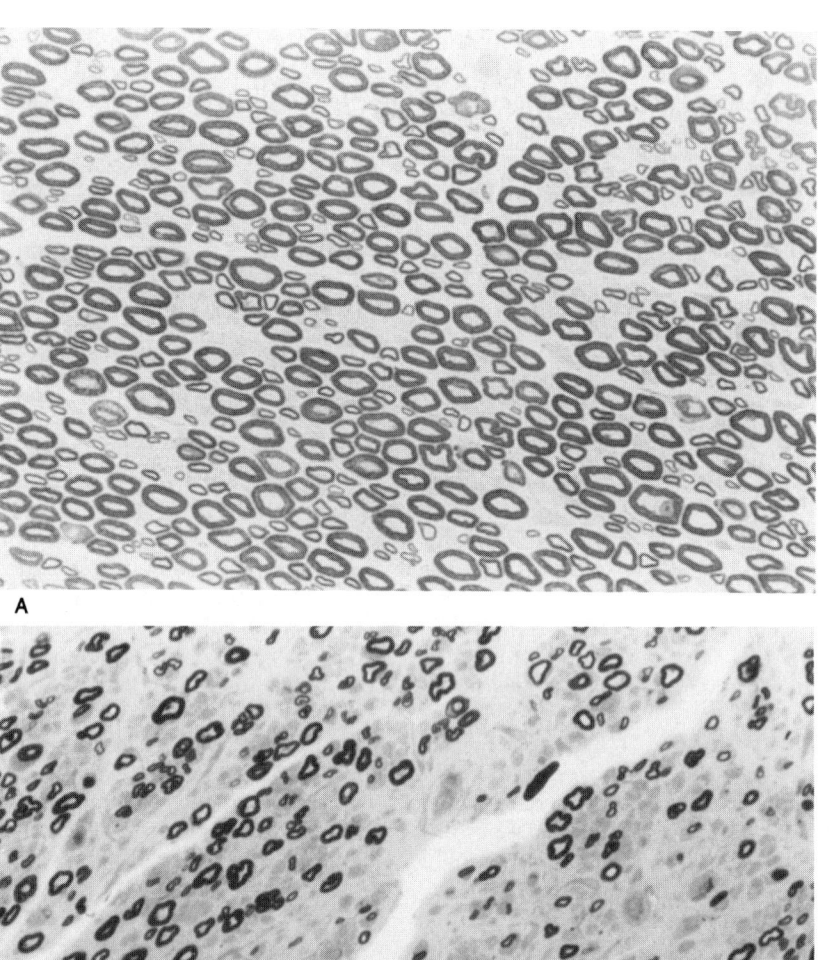

**Figure 1.** Section of the distal tibial nerve from (A) control dog showing a normal distribution of small- and large-caliber fibers; and (B) a Dalmatian with laryngeal paralysis-polyneuropathy complex showing multifocal loss of myelinated nerve fibers. (Paraphenylene diamine stain, ×132.)

distress syndrome recently reported (Jarvinen, Saario, and Happonen, 1992) in young Dalmatians (average age = 6.5 months). Signs of this presumably inherited disease included progressive dyspnea, tachypnea, and noisy respiration, leading to severe respiratory distress and cyanosis. The average time between onset of signs and death/euthanasia is reported to be 3 weeks. There is radiographic evidence of alveolar, interstitial, and peribronchial densities throughout the lungfield. Histopathologic changes in the lungs were typical for adult respiratory distress syndrome.

## TREATMENT

No definitive treatment is presently available. Occasional dogs respond to corticosteroid treatment (e.g., prednisolone, 0.5 mg/kg PO every 48 hr). Various surgical procedures including castellated laryngofissure,

arytenoid cartilage lateralization, permanent tracheostomy, and unilateral cricoarytenoid laryngoplasty may prove to be beneficial for a short time period (e.g., 6 to 9 months) (see "Laryngeal Paralysis," this volume, p 901).

## PROGNOSIS

Prognosis for Dalmatians with LPP complex is guarded to poor since, in our experience, most dogs either die or are euthanatized within a month or two of medical or surgical management because of inhalation pneumonia. One dog has survived to 30 months of age.

## CONCLUSIONS

The results of the present study reinforce the observation made previously that the Dalmatian breed is sus-

**Table 1.** *Percentage of Abnormalities in Teased Nerve Fibers from Dalmatians With Laryngeal Paralysis-Polyneuropathy Complex*

| Dog No. | Age (mo) First Signs/Death | Nerve | Histologic Classification[*] | | | | | Percentage of Abnormal Fibers[†] |
|---------|------------|-------|---|---|---|---|---|----------|
| | | | C | D | E | F | G | |
| 1 | 4/5 | Ulnar | 0 | 0 | 25 | 1 | 0 | 26(0) |
| | | Sciatic | 0 | 0 | 25 | 1 | 0 | 26(0) |
| | | Tibial | 0 | 0 | 41 | 0 | 0 | 41(0) |
| 2 | 8/9 | Tibial | 3 | 0 | 19 | 1 | 0 | 23(0) |
| 3 | 2/9 | Tibial | 0 | 0 | 20 | 0 | 0 | 20(0) |
| | | CPN[†] | 0 | 0 | 23 | 0 | 0 | 23(0) |
| 4 | 6/11 | Tibial | 0 | 0 | 35 | 2 | 0 | 37(0) |
| 5 | 12/30 | Tibial | 6 | 2 | 14 | 14 | 0 | 36(0) |
| 7 | 4/6 | Tibial | 0 | 0 | 36 | 0 | 0 | 36(0) |
| 8 | 3/16 | Prox Sci | 1 | 0 | 10 | 1 | 0 | 12(0) |
| | | CPN | 1 | 0 | 17 | 1 | 0 | 19(0) |
| | | Tibial | 0 | 0 | 29 | 0 | 0 | 29(0) |
| 10 | 4/5 | Prox Sci | 2 | 0 | 6 | 3 | 0 | 11(0) |
| | | Tibial | 0 | 0 | 25 | 0 | 0 | 25(0) |
| | | Prox RLN | 0 | 0 | 11 | 0 | 0 | 11(0) |
| | | Distal RLN | 0 | 0 | 18 | 0 | 0 | 18(0) |
| 15 | 3/4 | CPN | 0 | 0 | 27 | 0 | 0 | 27(0) |
| 16 | 5/still alive | CPN | 3 | 0 | 40 | 0 | 0 | 43(0) |

[*]A = normal appearance, B = excessive irregularity of myelin not attributable to preparative artifacts, C = single or multiple regions of nodal lengthening or internodal myelin absence, D = single or multiple C and F abnormalities combined, E = linear rows of myelin ovoids and balls, F = 50% or more difference in myelin thickness between internodes, G = thickening or reduplication of myelin to form globules within internodes.

[†]Figures in parentheses refer to range of abnormalities reported in comparable nerves from age-matched control dogs.

Abbreviations: CPN = common peroneal nerve, Prox Sci = proximal sciatic nerve, Prox RLN = proximal recurrent laryngeal nerve.

ceptible to laryngeal paralysis. In affected Dalmatians, the nature and distribution of electrophysiologic findings are indicative of a distal polyneuropathy. These data are supported by (1) the quantitative teased nerve fiber studies indicating more severe involvement in distal parts of nerves (e.g., distal tibial versus proximal sciatic nerve; and distal recurrent laryngeal nerve versus proximal recurrent laryngeal nerve), (2) more severe loss/degeneration of myelinated nerve fibers in semithin cross-sectional nerve preparations of distal nerves, and (3) morphometric histographic data showing preferential loss of medium and larger caliber myelinated fibers in distal nerves. Axonal degeneration that selectively involves the distal parts of long and larger diameter fibers, with a slow proximal spread of nerve fiber breakdown with time, has been termed "dying-back neuropathy." Laryngeal paralysis in horses also is associated with preferential involvement of the distal parts of the recurrent laryngeal nerves, as well as multiple limb nerves. This equine LPP complex is now considered to represent a dying-back disorder.

Laryngeal paralysis-polyneuropathy complex in Dalmatians appears to be different from laryngeal paralysis in bouviers (Venker-van Haagen, Hartman, and Goedegebuure, 1978) and Siberian huskies (O'Brien and Hendriks, 1986) based on (1) clinical signs (e.g., megaesophagus and other signs of a generalized polyneuropathy have been reported only in Dalmatians), (2) pathologic mechanisms (e.g., wallerian degeneration of the recurrent laryngeal nerves secondary to neuronal changes in bouviers and Siberian huskies contrasts with

distal dying-back disease affecting multiple cranial and appendicular nerves in Dalmatians), (3) electrophysiologic findings (e.g., the distal, generalized distribution of abnormal spontaneous potentials observed in Dalmatians has not been reported in bouviers and Siberian huskies), and (4) probable genetic differences (e.g., autosomal dominant inheritance in bouviers versus suspected recessive inheritance in Dalmatians).

Motor nerve conduction velocities have been slow in several Dalmatians with LPP complex. Since demyelination is not a dominant feature in peripheral nerves from affected dogs, this slowing of nerve conduction is most likely associated with loss of the large-diameter myelinated fibers. It is well established that motor nerve conduction velocity is based on the fastest conducting fibers, which are those with the largest diameters. Future studies are needed to substantiate sensory nerve involvement in affected Dalmatians. Proprioceptive deficits have been noted in at least one Dalmatian puppy, and a decrease in sensory nerve conduction velocity has been recorded in one dog.

Pedigree analysis is needed also to confirm the suspected autosomal recessive hereditary nature of LPP complex in Dalmatians. Molecular biologic studies may help in the development of a neonatal antemortem screening test that will identify affected animals early in life as well as clinically normal carriers.

ACKNOWLEDGMENTS I wish to thank Dr. Joane Parent, Dr. Linda Shell, Dr. Andy Shores, Dr. Nina Di Pinto, Dr. Susan Cochrane, Dr. Dru Forrester, Dr. Jacek M. Kwiecien, Dr. Mike Podell, Dr. Craig Martin, and Dr. Janet E. Steiss for providing additional clinical, electrophysiologic, and pathologic data; and Mrs. Karen Amling and Dr. Maria Toivio-Kinnucan for technical assistance.

## References and Suggested Reading

Braund KG, Steinberg HS, Shores A, et al: Laryngeal paralysis in immature and mature dogs: One manifestation of an underlying more diffuse distal polyneuropathy. J Am Vet Med Assoc 194:1735, 1989.
*A clinical and pathologic report on the association between laryngeal paralysis and polyneuropathy in six dogs (four immature, two mature).*

Braund KG, Shores S, Cochrane S, et al: Laryngeal paralysis-polyneuropathy complex in young Dalmatian dogs. Am J Vet Res 55:534, 1994.
*A clinical and pathologic report on laryngeal paralysis and polyneuropathy in 14 young Dalmatian dogs.*

Jarvinen A-K, Saario E, and Happonen I: Respiratory distress syndrome in young Dalmatian dogs. In Proc Am Coll Vet Intern Med 1992, p 799.
*An abstract describing a respiratory distress syndrome in young Dalmatian dogs.*

O'Brien JA and Hendriks J: Inherited laryngeal paralysis. Analysis in the Husky cross. Vet Q 8:301, 1986.
*A clinical and pathologic review on laryngeal paralysis in young husky and husky cross dogs.*

Venker-van Haagen AJ, Hartman W, and Goedegebuure SA: Spontaneous laryngeal paralysis in young bouviers. J Am Anim Hosp Assoc 14:714, 1978.
*A clinical and pathologic review on laryngeal paralysis in young bouvier des Flandres.*

# NEUROTOXIC DRUGS IN DOGS AND CATS

DAVID C. DORMAN

*Research Triangle Park, North Carolina*

Neurotoxicology is the study of adverse effects of chemical, biologic, and certain physical agents on the nervous system. There are a wide range of agents that may induce neurotoxicity, including metals; pesticides; solvents and other chemicals; bacterial, animal, and plant-derived toxins; as well as therapeutic agents. Drug-induced neurotoxicity is usually dose dependent and often represents an extension of the pharmacologic action (e.g., excessive central nervous system [CNS] depression observed with barbiturate ingestion). Neurotoxicity may represent an undesired drug side effect following its administration at normal therapeutic doses. For other therapeutic agents (e.g., anesthetics), altered CNS function may represent a desirable, beneficial change and such effects would generally not be referred to as a neurotoxic response (e.g., CNS depression). For almost all drugs, extreme overdoses as may occur following accidental, iatrogenic, or intentional poisoning will result in some neurotoxic effect.

Several neurotoxic insecticides used on companion animals (e.g., organophosphorus, carbamates, pyrethroids, pyrethrins, and lindane) are involved in a significant number of poisonings each year. Although relevant, a discussion of these agents is beyond the scope of this article and the reader is referred to recent editions of this text and Section 3 of this volume for more information. This article will primarily focus on selected drug-induced neurotoxicities in the dog and cat. A brief description of diagnosis and treatment of drug-induced neurotoxicosis will be given initially. The remainder of the article will discuss individual neurotoxic drugs, with emphasis placed on their source, toxicity, mechanism of action, clinical signs, and treatment.

The careful interpretation of data collected from the history, clinical and neurologic examinations, neurodiagnostic tests, chemical analyses, and other supportive diagnostic tests, as well as postmortem findings, can be used to form a presumptive *diagnosis* of neurotoxicosis. Establishing a history of drug use in an affected animal is often a first step in identifying a drug-induced neurotoxicosis. For example, an acute onset of salivation, lacrimation, urination, defecation, diarrhea, muscle tremors, and pulmonary edema is commonly associated with exposure to insecticidal preparations that inhibit acetylcholinesterase activity (e.g., organophosphorus and carbamate insecticides). The sudden onset of neurologic signs in a previously normal animal receiving a therapeutic agent is strong putative evidence that a drug-induced neurotoxicosis may have occurred. However, in spite of seemingly strong exposure or temporal associations, nontoxicologic differentials should always be considered. Chemical analysis of blood and other tissues for the suspected drug (or its metabolites) often provides the strongest evidence that a drug-induced toxicosis has occurred. However, few veterinary toxicology laboratories are equipped to either analyze or interpret results of these chemical analyses.

There are only three strategies for the *treatment* of drug-induced neurotoxicosis, namely (1) initiation of life support, (2) modification of toxicokinetics (i.e., alteration of drug absorption, distribution, metabolism, or excretion), and (3) antagonism of the drug's pharmacologic effects. The reader is referred to "Emergency Treatment of Toxicoses," this volume, p 211 for complimentary treatment recommendations.

Neurotoxic drugs can be *classified* by their drug class, cellular target sites, mode of action, or by the toxic syndrome they induce. These classification schemes can be misleading; for example, the clinician may only observe one particular phase of the neurotoxic syndrome. Animals exposed to toxicants that affect other body systems early in the clinical course could also present terminally with signs of depression, coma, and seizures. In all cases, the clinician must consider atypical presentations for a neurotoxicant as well as other nontoxicologic rule-outs.

## DRUGS THAT INDUCE CNS OVERSTIMULATION AND SEIZURES

### Amphetamine

Amphetamine poisoning is most common in dogs and may occur as the result of the accidental ingestion of amphetamine-based stimulants ("speed," "uppers," "bennies"). Prescribed forms of amphetamine include tablets, capsules, and sustained-release capsule forms. Although amphetamine (and cocaine) poisoning is rarely recognized in animals, the true incidence may be higher because of the reluctance of owners to admit to illegal drug use. The estimated acute oral $LD_{50}$ of amphetamine in rodents ranges from 10 to 30 mg/kg. Amphetamine is rapidly absorbed from the gastrointestinal tract and, once absorbed, significant amphetamine concentrations may be detected in the cerebrospinal fluid. Amphetamines stimulate the release of catecholamines (e.g., norepinephrine) from the adrenals as well as the cerebral cortex, medullary respiratory center, and reticular activating system.

Amphetamine poisoning may result in both cardiac and CNS effects similar to those induced by cocaine. Clinical signs may include hyperactivity, mydriasis, hyperthermia, tachycardia, lactic acidosis, hypertension and, infrequently, seizures. The treatment of amphetamine toxicosis is primarily supportive. In addition to oral decontamination therapy, amphetamine elimination may be enhanced by ion trapping with urine acidification. Urine acidification is, however, contraindicated if the animal is in renal failure for any reason or if severe myoglobinuria from muscle damage is occurring. Chlorpromazine (10 to 18 mg/kg IV) or haloperidol (1 mg/kg IV) given after administration of a lethal intravenous dose of amphetamine sulfate (10 mg/kg) experimentally reduced the severity of hyperthermia and also increased survival rates in amphetamine-poisoned dogs. Diazepam may also be used to control seizures and may assist in calming the affected animal.

### Caffeine

Caffeine is a methylated xanthine present in human stimulant preparations and chocolate, as well as coffee, tea, and other cola beverages. Although caffeine toxicosis in animals most commonly occurs following the ingestion of chocolate, accidental poisonings may also occur from the ingestion of caffeine-based tablets or elixirs. The approximate oral $LD_{50}$ of caffeine in the

dog is 140 mg/kg. The plasma half-life of caffeine in the dog is approximately 4.5 hr. The exact toxicologic mechanism of action of caffeine is not known but may include inhibition of phosphodiesterase, enhanced catecholamine release, adenosine antagonism, or increased calcium entry into the cell. Gaps in information exist with regard to the relationship between mechanisms of action *in vivo* and those identified in studies performed *in vitro*.

The primary organ systems affected in cases of caffeine toxicosis include the central nervous, peripheral nervous, and the cardiovascular systems. Clinical signs of caffeine toxicosis in the dog and cat generally develop within several hours of ingestion and may include vomiting (often the first sign), restlessness, hyperactivity, ataxia, muscle tremors, tachycardia, cardiac arhythmias, seizures, polyuria/polydipsia, hyperthermia, cyanosis, and coma. There are usually no histologic lesions in the brain or spinal cord. The treatment of caffeine toxicosis in animals is usually symptomatic and supportive. Anticonvulsant, antiarrhythmic, and repeated activated charcoal administration, as well as fluid therapy to enhance diuresis, are generally recommended. $\beta$-Blockers have been used with caution to reduce some of the sympathomimetic cardiovascular effects.

### Cocaine

Cocaine is a natural alkaloid obtained from the coca plant (*Erythroxylon coca* and *E. monogynum*). Historically, cocaine has been used in both veterinary and human medicine as both a topical and local anesthetic, and as a mydriatic. In addition to its hydrochloride or salt form ("coke," "snow," "blow," "nose-candy"), cocaine also exists in the cocaine alkaloid or free-base form ("crack," "rock," "flake"). Cocaine is commonly diluted or cut with adulterants before its illegal sale. Adulterants may include sugar, local anesthetics, phencyclidine, amphetamine, caffeine, and quinine. Animal toxicosis most commonly results from the deliberate poisoning or accidental ingestion of this illicit drug.

The acute $LD_{50}$ of intravenously administered cocaine hydrochloride in dogs and cats is reported to be 13 to 15 mg/kg. The oral $LD_{50}$ may be two to four times this intravenous dose. Cocaine is rapidly absorbed from mucous membranes, the gastrointestinal tract, and all parenteral routes. The mechanism by which cocaine induces CNS stimulation is unknown. Depression of cortical inhibitory pathways has been postulated as a possible mechanism for cocaine-induced neurotoxicity. Catecholamine (e.g., dopamine) depletion through both inhibition of reuptake as well as increased release by cocaine may contribute to its neurotoxicity. Central nervous system and cardiovascular stimulation is the predominant effect of cocaine overdose in humans and animals. Dogs given lethal intravenous infusions of cocaine develop seizures, hyperesthesia, hyperthermia, tachycardia, and lactic acidosis. Accidental poisonings in dogs and cats result in similar clinical signs, which may include hyperactivity, erratic behavior, depression, coma, seizures, vomiting, increased salivation, tachycardia, dyspnea, and pulmonary edema. Treatment for cocaine poisoning is primarily supportive (gastrointestinal tract decontamination, seizure control with diazepam, antiarrhythmic therapy).

## 5-Fluorouracil (5-FU)

5-Fluorouracil (Efudex, Fluoroplex) –containing solutions and creams are used topically in human patients for the treatment of solar and actinic keratoses, and some superficial skin tumors (e.g., basal carcinoma). 5-Fluorouracil is also used in veterinary medicine for the treatment of some cancers. Animal poisonings may occur following its accidental ingestion or as a side effect of therapy following its absorption through intact skin. Toxic and lethal 5-FU oral doses in the dog have been reported to be 6 and 43 mg/kg, respectively. The exact mechanism of neurotoxicity is unknown; however, limited studies conducted in cats suggest that neurotoxicity may be related to the metabolism of 5-FU to the potent neurotoxicant, fluorocitrate.

The toxicity of 5-FU is most pronounced on rapidly dividing cell lines (e.g., bone marrow stem cells and epithelial cells of the intestinal crypts). Central nervous system effects, however, may also occur in 5-FU–poisoned animals. Adverse reactions from intravenous 5-FU therapy or accidental ingestion by dogs and cats include seizures, hyperesthesia, hyperexcitability, nervousness, muscle tremors, and cerebellar ataxia. Other commonly observed clinical signs may include vomiting, diarrhea (occasionally bloody), pulmonary edema, respiratory failure, cardiac arhythmias, cardiac failure, and death. Treatment of 5-FU poisoning is primarily supportive. In addition to oral or dermal decontamination, fluid therapy, anticonvulsants, and gastrointestinal protectants are often indicated. Blood transfusions may be required in animals with excessive gastrointestinal blood loss. Antiemetics may be indicated for the control of protracted vomiting. Metoclopramide given intravenously or orally at 0.1 to 0.3 mg/kg three times daily may also be considered. Animals receiving metoclopramide should be monitored closely for the development of additional neurologic signs, since metoclopramide may produce extrapyramidal reactions.

## DRUGS THAT INDUCE CNS DEPRESSION OR COMA

### Barbiturates

Barbiturate use in human medicine has decreased significantly in recent years, but they are still widely used in veterinary medicine. Barbiturates are commonly classified according to their duration of effect into long, intermediate, short, and ultrashort acting. Animal poisoning may be the result of the ingestion of barbiturate-based drugs, ingestion of barbiturate-eu-thanized animals, ingestion of illicit street preparations ("downers," "reds," "Christmas trees," and "dolls"), or from iatrogenic overdose.

Clinically, short- and ultrashort-acting barbiturates are typically given intravenously to effect. By this technique, 50 to 70% of the $LD_{50}$ is needed to achieve anesthesia, so barbiturates have relatively narrow margins of safety. When given orally, short-acting agents produce their effect within 10 to 30 min of ingestion, while long-acting agents take up to 1 hr to produce initial effects. Barbiturates are rapidly distributed throughout the body, with distribution influenced by their lipid solubility. Barbiturates inhibit calcium accumulation in neural tissue and thereby inhibit the release of neurotransmitters. Barbiturate anesthetics also have a $\gamma$-aminobutyric acid (GABA) mimetic action within the CNS. Profound respiratory and CNS depression, general anesthesia, hypothermia, hypotension, shock, cyanosis, and coma are the predominant clinical signs observed. Death is usually caused by respiratory arrest. Treatment of barbiturate poisoning involves gastrointestinal tract decontamination (e.g., emetics, repeated administration of activated charcoal, gastric lavage) and the initiation of life-supportive measures (e.g., ventilation support, fluid therapy). Forced alkaline diuresis may also be of benefit in phenobarbital toxicoses. Hemodialysis and hemoperfusion are also employed in severely affected human patients. Redistribution of these drugs from fat back to the plasma may cause prolonged depression; therefore, continued patient monitoring is required.

### Ivermectin

Ivermectin is a naturally occurring combination of the polycyclic lactones 22,23-dihydro avermectin $B_1a$ and $B_1b$. Ivermectin is used as an anthelmintic in cattle, horses, and swine, and has also been approved for the prevention of canine heartworm infection (6 $\mu g$/kg, monthly). In general, the blood-brain barrier of mammals excludes ivermectin such that the host animal is unaffected by reasonable doses. In collies and perhaps in other related breeds, however, the blood-brain barrier is relatively ineffective as an ivermectin barrier. In any breed or species, sufficiently high doses can overcome the ability of the blood-brain barrier to exclude ivermectin from the CNS, resulting in neurotoxicosis. Ivermectin toxicosis in dogs and cats often follows the inappropriate administration of ivermectin-based equine anthelmintic by owners.

Ivermectin is only poorly absorbed from the gastrointestinal tract. Ivermectin undergoes only limited liver metabolism and is primarily excreted unchanged in the feces. Peak plasma concentrations are reached within 3 hr after oral administration, and the plasma half-life in non–collie breed dogs has been reported to be 2 to 3 days. Ivermectin has a wide oral margin of safety in non–collie dogs. In these studies, a single oral dose of ivermectin at 2500 $\mu g$/kg produced only mydriasis. Likewise, no treatment-related toxic effects were observed in dogs given oral ivermectin (500 μg/kg/day) for 14 weeks. Conversely, ivermectin has been reported to be neurotoxic in collies and related breeds following single oral doses of approximately 100 to 500 μg/kg. Some individuals (*but not all*) in these breeds, are, therefore, extremely susceptible to ivermectin. There has also been a single report in which an Old English sheepdog developed clinical signs compatible with ivermectin toxicosis following ingestion of 150 μg/kg.

Ivermectin neurotoxicity is related to its effects at the γ-aminobutyric acid (GABA) –chloride channel. The normally inhibitory neurotransmitter, GABA, is only found in the central nervous system of mammals (cerebellum, cerebral and limbic cortices, extrapyramidal system, and horizontal layer of the retina), whereas GABA acts peripherally in invertebrates. Ivermectin and other avermectins increase the activity of GABA receptors in three ways: (1) by potentiating synaptic GABA effects by enhancing its presynaptic release; (2) by enhancing the binding of GABA to its postsynaptic receptors; and (3) through direct GABA agonist effects. Ivermectin neurotoxicosis results in excessive GABA-mediated effects, resulting in ataxia, muscle tremors, seizures (rarely observed), disorientation, mild to severe CNS depression, and sometimes coma, which may be prolonged or proceed to cause death. Some dogs develop mydriasis, decreased menace response, and apparent blindness, which with time is reversible. Vomiting, diarrhea, hyperthermia, bradycardia, and sinus arrhythmia have also been reported. Experimentally, dogs that develop clinical signs within 4 to 6 hr of ingestion often go on to develop severe CNS depression and coma. In contrast, dogs that did not develop clinical signs until 10 to 12 hr after ingestion developed a more mild toxic syndrome. There are no characteristic lesions in ivermectin-poisoned animals. Ivermectin reactions related to microfilaricide therapy often evokes a shock-like reaction in affected dogs.

Activated charcoal and a saline cathartic are suggested if an animal has been recently exposed to ivermectin by the oral route. The treatment of ivermectin toxicosis in companion animals is also largely dependent on the delivery of supportive nursing care. Dogs with severe signs require intensive supportive therapy (fluids, shock doses of corticosteroids) but usually recover; however, full recovery may take up to several weeks. Picrotoxin and physostigmine have been advocated as possible antidotes for ivermectin toxicosis; however, these agents should be used only if life-threatening signs (e.g., coma) are present.

## Methionine

Methionine (DL-methionine) is an essential amino acid, and is incorporated into some urinary acidifiers. Although poisonings are uncommon, ingestion of excessive amounts of methionine can result in neurotoxicity and metabolic acidosis. Animals with preexisting liver disease are especially predisposed to methionine

toxicosis. Methionine is degraded by gut flora to a group of metabolites, collectively termed mercaptans (methanethiol, ethanethiol, and dimethylsulfide). The toxicity of methionine is related to its metabolism (in part by the gastrointestinal flora) to ammonia and other metabolites. Elevated blood ammonia levels are commonly reported to occur during methionine toxicosis.

Naturally occurring preexistent hepatic disease (e.g., portosystemic shunt) is an important factor in methionine-induced hepatic encephalopathy (see "Medical Management of Chronic Hepatic Encephalopathy," this volume, p 1153). The longer hepatic disease has been present, the less methionine, methanethiol, or ammonia is required to induce coma. After high doses in any animal, effects most often include ataxia, depression, lethargy, excessive salivation, and vomiting. Other clinical signs may include circling, head pressing, aimless pacing, abnormal aggression, somnolence, blindness, seizures, and stupor, leading to coma. Cats experimentally given DL-methionine at 0.5 to 1 gm/kg also developed severe hemolytic anemia with increased Heinz body formation and increased methemoglobin concentrations. Treatment of methionine toxicosis is primarily supportive. Emetics, as well as activated charcoal and a saline cathartic, may be used if not contraindicated. Fluids containing bicarbonate may be needed for the control of acidosis. The use of methionine should be ceased in animals that develop signs consistent with hepatic encephalopathy and treatment for hepatic encephalopathy initiated.

## Opiates

Opiates include opium, drugs semisynthesized from opium, and totally synthetic agents. Morphine is an important opiate precursor that is chemically altered to form methylmorphine (codeine), hydromorphone, diacetylmorphine (heroin), and oxymorphone. The opiates are used in veterinary medicine as analgesics, sedatives, and hypnotic agents. Animal poisonings most often occur following the ingestion of human prescription medications, consumption of illicit drugs, or from iatrogenic causes.

The toxicity of opiates is highly variable; in the dog, 100 to 220 mg/kg of morphine subcutaneously or intravenously represents a potentially lethal dose. Opiate neurotoxicity is primarily mediated through a variety of receptor binding sites, including the opiate receptors. Species variation in opiate effects may be related to differences in the distribution of opiate receptors in the brain. Clinical signs of opiate toxicosis in dogs initially include vomiting and increased salivation, defecation, increased respiration, and urination. Central nervous system depression, ataxia, respiratory depression, stupor, coma, hyperactivity or seizures, and cyanosis with peripheral vasodilation and hypotension often develops later. In contrast, CNS stimulatory effects are seen in cats. Miosis is observed initially, but as the hypoxia worsens, mydriasis is seen. Hypothermia is observed in dogs, while hyperthermia is commonly observed in cats. Naloxone hydrochloride (Narcan, EI DuPont de Nemours, Wilmington, DE) is antidotal (0.01 to 0.02 mg/kg IV, IM, or SC) and is the drug of choice in the cat or dog for opiate neurotoxicosis. Gastrointestinal decontamination (emetics, activated charcoal) and supportive therapy are also indicated.

## DRUGS THAT INDUCE PARALYSIS

### Hexachlorophene

Hexachlorophene-induced toxicosis is occasionally reported in dogs and cats following its overzealous dermal use or from accidental ingestion of hexachlorophene-based surgical scrubs or soil fungicides. Dogs (especially neonatal animals) are most susceptible; however, cats and other species may also be poisoned. The estimated oral $LD_{50}$ in the rat is reported to be 60 mg/kg. Hexachlorophene is rapidly absorbed from both the skin and the gastrointestinal tract. Excessive exposure to hexachlorophene may result in severe myelin damage and secondary axonal degeneration. Hexachlorophene neurotoxicity results from the uncoupling of oxidative phosphorylation and reduced adenosine triphosphate synthesis. Clinical signs of hexachlorophene toxicosis may include hyperthermia, muscle tremors, apparent blindness, CNS excitation or depression, seizures, ataxia, hypermetria, and paralysis. Other clinical signs may include bradycardia, diarrhea, anorexia, salivation, and death secondary to cardiopulmonary arrest. Treatment of hexachlorophene poisoning involves the initiation of life-supportive measures (e.g., seizure control, ventilation support), skin and gastrointestinal tract decontamination (e.g., bathing, repeated administration of activated charcoal, gastric lavage), and the intravenous use of mannitol and dexamethasone for cerebral edema.

### Levamisole

Levamisole (1-2,3,5,6-tetrahydro-6-phenylimidazo-[2,1-b]-thiazole monohydrochloride) is a white, water-soluble crystalline powder used in veterinary medicine as an anthelmintic, microfilaricide, and immunostimulant. Levamisole is a nicotine-like ganglionic stimulant, inducing both nicotinic and muscarinic effects at cholinergic receptors, as well as depolarization of nerve cell membranes. The therapeutic dose of levamisole in dogs is 10 to 11 mg/kg. Clinical signs of neurotoxicity may occur at approximately four times this dose rate. Clinical signs of levamisole toxicity in dogs may include vomiting, hypersalivation, depression, diarrhea, anorexia, cardiac arrhythmias, dyspnea, behavioral changes, pulmonary edema, tachypnea, ataxia, muscle tremors, seizures, paralysis, and death due to respiratory failure. Hemolytic anemia has also been reported in some dogs due to repeated levamisole administration. Treatment of toxicosis is largely supportive (gas-trointestinal tract decontamination, seizure control, fluids, oxygen, and respiration support).

## DRUGS THAT INDUCE MIXED CNS EFFECTS

### Chlorhexidine

Chlorhexidine (Hibitane, Ayerst; Nolvasan, Fort Dodge Laboratories) is a commonly used antiseptic and disinfectant with veterinary application in the management of pyodermas, abrasions, superficial wounds, dermatophytosis, and otitis externa. Chlorhexidine has a low degree of oral toxicity, and is only poorly absorbed following either dermal or oral exposure. Chlorhexidine neurotoxicosis can occur, however, following accidental injection into the cerebrospinal fluid. Permanent deafness may also be observed following the application of chlorhexidine-based otic preparations in animals with a ruptured tympanum. The sensory cell nerve ending complex is the main target for chlorhexidine auditory toxicity and may result in degeneration of the afferent nerve terminals and the hair cells in the organ of Corti. There is no specific treatment for chlorhexidine toxicosis, although immediate flushing with saline of an ear with a known tympanum rupture may be of some benefit.

### Metoclopramide

Metoclopramide (Reglan, AH Robins) is a gastrointestinal prokinetic used in animals for the treatment of gastric dysfunction, vomiting, nausea, and reflux esophagitis. Use of metoclopramide tablets, syrup, or injectable formulations may occasionally result in neurotoxicity. The mechanism of action of metoclopramide is poorly understood; it is a dopaminergic agonist and will also sensitize tissues to the effect of acetylcholine. Neurotoxicity may be observed at therapeutic levels, resulting in extrapyramidal effects manifested by movement disorders characterized as slow to rapid twisting movements involving the face, neck, trunk, or limbs as well as CNS depression, nervousness or restlessness. Treatment is supportive, and diphenhydramine (4 mg/kg t.i.d.) administration may decrease the extrapyramidal signs. Clinical signs generally resolve within 2 to 3 days after stopping metoclopramide medication.

### Metronidazole

Metronidazole (Flagyl, Searle) is used in dogs for the treatment of giardiasis, trichomoniasis, and certain anaerobic infections. Most neurotoxicoses with this drug are associated with its longer term administration at high dose rates, as occurs for the treatment of bacterial infections. Metronidazole is well absorbed orally, and plasma half-life ranges from 3 to 13 hr. Effective metronidazole concentrations are reached in the cerebrospinal fluid and brain parenchyma. Clinical signs have been associated with oral doses greater than 66 mg/kg/day. Neurologic signs develop acutely, and often begin 7 to 12 days following induction of therapy. Clinical signs include severe ataxia, vertical or rotatory nystagmus, seizures (occasionally), stomatitis, and glossitis. An increase in cerebrospinal fluid protein may be observed in some dogs. Histopathologic lesions have been observed in the central vestibular system and brain stem of dogs. Recovery usually occurs within 1 to 2 weeks after cessation of metronidazole therapy. Treatment is purely supportive.

## Toluene and Dichlorophen-Based Anthelmintics

Toluene and diclorophen-based anthelmintics are effective against ascarids, hookworms, and some tapeworms of dogs and cats. This combination is available over the counter under a wide variety of trade names and strengths. The recommended single oral dose for the combination product in dogs and cats is 220 mg of dichlorophen and 264 mg of toluene per kilogram body weight, and a dose of only 1.5 times this recommended dose may result in signs of neurotoxicity. Common clinical signs reported in suspected toluene/dichlorophen poisoning include ataxia, aberrant behavior mydriasis, vomiting, CNS depression, tremors, hypersalivation, seizures, weakness and, rarely, death. Clinical signs commonly develop within 6 hr of ingestion of the combination product, while in most cases of suspected toluene/dichlorophen toxicosis, clinical signs resolve within 24 hr after ingestion with just supportive care. The mechanism of action of neurotoxicity for this combination product is unknown.

## Tricyclic Antidepressants

The tricyclic antidepressant (TCA) medications represent a commonly used class of human psychotherapeutic medications used for the treatment of endogenous depression, childhood enuresis, and certain phobic disorders. The TCAs have also found limited use in veterinary medicine for the treatment of canine narcoleptic hypersomnia syndrome, canine narcoleptic cataplexy syndrome, and canine separation anxiety. Poisonings with the TCAs represent the most common life-threatening drug ingestion in human patients. Although infrequently encountered in veterinary medicine, the incidence of accidental animal poisonings is apparently rising. Commonly encountered TCAs include amitryptyline, nortryptyline, protryptyline, amoxapine, desipramine, imipramine, and trimipramine.

Depending on the specific TCA, the typical therapeutic TCA dose in animals and humans falls in the range of 2 to 4 mg/kg. In general, 15 to 20 mg/kg is thought to be a potentially lethal dose of TCAs in both human and veterinary patients. At therapeutic oral doses, the TCAs are rapidly absorbed. Massive inges-

tions may result in prolonged gastrointestinal absorption due to TCA-induced anticholinergic effects that result in decreased intestinal motility. In humans, the TCAs have somewhat variable elimination half-lives ranging from 10 to 21 hr.

The TCAs have pronounced toxic effects on the central nervous, parasympathetic, and cardiovascular systems. In addition to their atropine-like anticholinergic effects, TCAs also inhibit biogenic amine (serotonin, norepinephrine) uptake. Clinical signs of TCA poisoning in animals include hyperexcitability, vomiting, depression, ataxia, mydriasis, muscle tremors, pulmonary edema and, occasionally, seizures. Cardiac abnormalities should also be anticipated to occur and may include hypotension, cardiac arrhythmias (e.g., sinus tachycardia, ventricular tachyarrhythmias), cardiac arrest, and death. Treatment of TCA poisoning involves the initiation of life-supportive measures (e.g., seizure control, ventilation support), gastrointestinal tract decontamination (e.g., repeated administration of activated charcoal, gastric lavage; note: emetics are generally not recommended), the intravenous use of sodium bicarbonate (2 to 3 mEq/kg) to control signs of acidosis, and antiarrhythmic drugs to treat tachycardia, bradycardia, and other cardiac conductance abnormalities.

## References and Suggested Reading

Dorman DC, Coddington KA, and Richardson RC: 5-Fluorouracil toxicosis in the dog. J Vet Intern Med 4:254, 1990.
*A case report describing several cases of spontaneous 5-fluorouracil poisonings in dogs. Estimates of the oral toxicity of 5-FU–based ointments is provided.*

Dow SW, LeCouteur RA, Poss ML, and Beadleston D: Central nervous system toxicosis associated with metronidazole treatment of dogs: Five cases (1984–1987). J Am Vet Med Assoc 195:365, 1989.
*A report of several cases of spontaneous metronidazole toxicosis in dogs.*

Hooser SB and Beasley VR: Methylxanthine poisoning (chocolate and caffeine) toxicosis. *In* Kirk RW (ed): *Current Veterinary Therapy IX.* Philadelphia, WB Saunders Co, 1986, p 191.
*A useful summary of poisonings due to common methylxanthine (e.g., caffeine).*

Johnson LR: Tricyclic antidepressant toxicosis. Vet Clin North Am [Small Anim Pract] 20:393, 1990.
*A recent review of the diagnosis and management of the tricyclic antidepressants. A summary of the clinical findings from spontaneous cases of tricyclic antidepressant toxicosis is also presented.*

Kisseberth WC and Trammel HL: Illicit and abused drugs. Vet Clin North Am [Small Anim Pract] 20:405, 1990.
*A good review of the available forms, toxicity and pharmacokinetics, mechanism of action, clinical signs, and treatment of toxicoses from amphetamine, caffeine, cocaine, marijuana, and other common illicit drugs.*

Lovell RA, Trammel HL, Beasley VR, and Buck WB: A review of 83 reports of suspected toluene/dichlorophen toxicoses in cats and dogs. J Am Anim Hosp Assoc 26:652, 1990.
*A review of 83 spontaneous cases of poisonings in companion animals from the administration of toluene and dichlorophen anthelmintics. Estimates of oral toxicity are also provided.*

Maede Y, Hoshino T, Jaaba M, and Namioka S: Methionine toxicosis in cats. Am J Vet Res 48:289, 1987.
*An experimental study examining the oral toxicity of methionine in cats.*

Montgomery RD and Pidgeon GL: Levamisole toxicosis in a dog. J Am Vet Med Assoc 189:684, 1986.
*A case report describing the neurotoxicity of levamisole in a dog following its oral administration.*

Neer TM: Drug-induced neurologic disorders. Proc 11th ACVIM Forum, 1993, p 861.
*A useful review in outline form of neurotoxic syndromes associated with metoclopramide, hydroxyzine, phenobarbital, amitraz, metronidazole, pyrethrin insecticides, tricyclic antidepressants, ivermectin, and other veterinary drugs.*

# TREATMENT OF CANINE INTERVERTEBRAL DISK DISEASE: RECOMMENDATIONS AND CONTROVERSIES

JAMES M. FINGEROTH
*Rochester, New York*

## TERMINOLOGY AND PATHOPHYSIOLOGY

The terms "type I" and "type II" disk degeneration, as described by Hansen, are clinically useful but have led to some confusion. Hansen used type I disk degeneration to describe a rupture of the disk whereby a large mass of disk material (mainly nucleus pulposus) was found within the vertebral canal and compressed the spinal cord. A type II lesion was defined as a degeneration with primarily annular protrusion and associated spinal cord compression at one or more sites. Over the years, it has become somewhat common to see an association made between the Hansen type I lesion and the type of intervertebral disk (IVD) disease seen in chondrodystrophoid dogs. Likewise, type II lesions have been associated with IVD disease in nonchondrodystrophoid dogs, particularly large-breed dogs. This is not always the case. It is important for the practitioner to recognize that many chondrodystrophoid dogs are found to have type II disk lesions (which may or may not cause clinical signs), while acute, massive, paralyzing type I disk injuries occasionally are diagnosed in large, nonchondrodystrophoid dogs. In addition, what has been called a type III or "gunshot" disk lesion has also been described wherein a very small fragment of nucleus pulposus is ejected into the vertebral canal at very high velocity; this type of disk displacement results in an acute or peracute onset of rapidly progressive paralysis, frequently with loss of sensation. Examination of dogs with type III lesions usually reveals minimal extradural compression, but severe swelling of the spinal cord, often with focal hemorrhagic necrosis and myelomalacia. This is often the result of direct penetration of the spinal cord by the disk material, and the tremendous bolus of kinetic energy transmitted to the cord. Surgery in these dogs is usually unrewarding.

Various terms are used to describe disk displacement, such as "bulging," "protrusion," "prolapse," "rupture," "herniation," and "extrusion." These descriptive terms mean different things to different people, and no universally accepted lexicon exists to distinguish them. Rather than getting bogged down in terminology, it is more useful to keep in mind the potential effects of disk degeneration and displacement.

Occasionally, signs of pain develop in the absence of myelographically detectable disk displacement (i.e., no apparent spinal cord or nerve root attenuation). These animals may be suffering from a lateral disk displacement or from so-called discogenic pain. In humans, and possibly dogs, the annulus fibrosus is innervated by small branches of the sinuvertebral nerve. Presumably, degeneration and internal deformation of the disk can result in signs of pain. Based on a recent study (Morgan, Parent, and Holmberg, 1993), discogenic pain may have been the cause of pain in 3 (6%) of 53 dogs with cervical hyperpathia. The remaining 50 (94%) dogs with signs of neck pain alone (no neurologic deficits) had myelographic evidence of disk material in the vertebral canal, usually with significant compression of the dural tube. From these data, it appears that the clinical signs of pain and paralysis seen in dogs with disk disease are usually due to a mass effect (i.e., compression of the spinal nerves [radiculopathy] and spinal cord [myelopathy]). The degree of radiculopathy and myelopathy in a given patient is related not only to the compressive effect, but also to the amount of kinetic energy absorbed by the neural elements. It is important to bear in mind that, since kinetic energy is more a function of velocity than mass ($KE = 1/2mv^2$), the rate at which a disk displaces against the spinal cord may be more important than how much spinal cord displacement (compression) persists (Prata, 1983). This explains why some dogs with severe spinal cord compression might recover quickly after decompressive surgery, and others, with minimal compression, can have a severely contused spinal cord and recover more slowly, if at all. Also, often there is no direct correlation between severity of signs and amount of compression, explaining why dogs may have significant disk displacement and only mild clinical signs (e.g., pain alone).

## INITIAL TREATMENT AND DIAGNOSIS

### General Recommendations

The key to clinical management of IVD disease is accurate determination of the degree of spinal cord injury and careful monitoring of the progression of the clinical signs. Signs in patients with a history of acute onset and rapidly progressive neurologic deterioration are likely to worsen over a short period of time. Such patients should be hospitalized (even if ambulatory at the time of presentation), carefully monitored (reexamined), and given appropriate medication. If it becomes apparent that medical therapy is not altering the trend towards loss of function, the patient should be considered a possible surgical candidate and further diagnostics should be pursued. In such situations, the veterinarian should not wait until the dog becomes paraplegic before surgery is contemplated. Conversely, dogs with a history of a gradual loss of motor function over a period of days or those having pain alone may be treated medically and as an outpatient. Owners should be instructed to return immediately if any progression of signs is observed. Dogs having recurrent signs over recent months should probably be evaluated more aggressively (and considered possible surgical candidates) than those suffering a single episode of pain or paresis. This harkens back to pathophysiology, and the conclusion that dogs may have mild signs and yet have massive amounts of compression. It also touches on the subject of recurrent disk disease, which will be addressed later in this article. Mental construction of a time-sign graph (Fig. 1) helps the veterinarian determine the best course of therapy. An accurate history and serial reevaluations are necessary in order to properly construct this mental picture of the course of the condition.

## Serial Physical Examinations

Regardless of whether the dog is treated on an inpatient or outpatient basis, it is imperative that the veterinarian monitor the response to therapy. Patients responding to medical treatment may be continued on this course. However, those who fail to improve or whose neurologic status continues to decline in spite of medical therapy need revised treatment plans and possibly surgery.

Serial assessment is obviously most critical for patients with severe neurologic deficits such as motor weakness or paralysis. These signs imply the presence of a substantial amount of compression (mass effect) or spinal cord injury (kinetic energy effect). If the veterinarian is unable to provide careful monitoring, the patient should be referred to a facility where constant supervision is available.

## Use of Corticosteroids

Although many drugs have been used in the treatment of spinal cord injury, only the corticosteroids have gained widespread acceptance. Even so, a great deal of controversy exists regarding which corticosteroid preparation is most effective and how the drugs should be used (dosage). Most recommendations have been based on clinical experience. The beneficial effects of

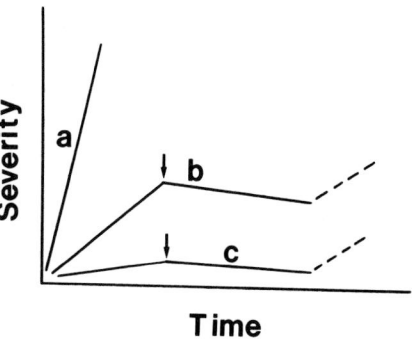

**Figure 1.** Time-sign graph used to help determine the urgency and type of treatment for dogs with intervertebral disk disease. Dogs with rapid deterioration (a) are emergencies and, if not responding promptly to aggressive medical treatment, should be considered possible surgical candidates. Dogs with neurologic deficits (paresis) that respond to treatment (*arrow*, b) should be hospitalized and closely monitored. Medical treatment can be continued so long as the neurologic status is stable or improving. Dogs with mild clinical signs (pain and/or mild paresis) who are responsive to treatment (*arrow*, c) can be managed as outpatients. Neurologic status may deteriorate (*dashed lines*, b and c) during the course of medical treatment or after medical treatment has been discontinued; serial examinations should be done to monitor neurologic status. Dogs with pain and little or no paresis (c) who have had multiple bouts of similar clinical signs usually have a single disk that is displacing over time. Surgical intervention is often indicated is dogs with recurrent signs.

high-dose corticosteroid therapy in spinal cord injury appear to range far beyond the glucocorticoid-based anti-inflammatory effect. Glucocorticoids appear to counter the secondary injury phenomenon of self-perpetuating necrosis by inhibition of lipid peroxidation by free radicals, normalization of extracellular calcium, support of blood flow, normalization of metabolism, enhancing neuronal excitability, and preservation of neurofilament proteins. A study on humans and experimental animals with spinal cord injury evaluated the use of methylprednisolone sodium succinate (Solu-Medrol, Upjohn). Initial doses of 30 mg/kg IV of the drug significantly improved the outcome after spinal cord injury. This benefit was greater than that achieved with closely related drugs such as prednisolone sodium succinate (Solu-Delta-Cortef, Upjohn), which is more commonly found in veterinary hospitals. This study also found a sharp, biphasic dose-response curve: at 15 mg/kg, there was a suboptimal response, but at 60 mg/kg, there were deleterious effects owing to decreased spinal cord blood flow. The positive results seen in this study should be interpreted with caution; methylprednisolone did not, for example, restore the ability to walk in tetraplegic patients. Moreover, chronic studies show that the positive effects of the drug may not be sustained for all patients. Thus, the advantages of methylprednisolone observed in humans may not be relevant to dogs.

Dexamethasone also appears to be effective in the treatment of spinal cord injury. Some believe this particular corticosteroid is more valuable in the treatment of central nervous system injuries than prednisone or other glucocorticoids. However, the dose of dexamethasone is open to debate. It is known that prolonged use of dexamethasone at high dosages in dogs with spinal cord injury is associated with a risk of severe gastrointestinal complications, including colonic perforation, which may result in death (Toombs et al., 1980). Some veterinarians routinely treat the acutely paralyzed animal with dexamethasone at a dose of 2.2 mg/kg IV. This is probably acceptable, as long as this dose is only used once or twice. Thereafter, I think it is critical to reduce the dose, probably in the range of 0.1 mg/kg IV, or less, every 8 hr to every 12 hr. Because of its long half-life, alternate-day therapy with dexamethasone is not indicated.

In general, corticosteroid therapy is most effective in the first 12 to 24 hr after injury; the beneficial effects seem to wane thereafter. It seems prudent to use the lowest dose possible that will produce or maintain the desired effect, while minimizing adverse reactions. There is probably not a linear relationship between dose and patient body weight; as such, large dogs may require a lower dose, on a milligram-per-kilogram basis, than smaller dogs. A protocol for the use of dexamethasone has been reported (Table 1) (Scavelli and Schoen, 1989). I recommend use of this protocol as the guideline for veterinarians treating the dog with IVD disease.

## Use of Other Drugs

Many dogs with IVD disease also have clinical signs owing to spasm of neck or back muscles. In some cases, particularly with cervical disk disease, muscle spasms and the pain that accompanies them can cause as much or more incapacitation as spinal cord compression. It is helpful to treat these dogs with muscle relaxants in addition to corticosteroids. The most commonly used agents are methocarbamol (Robaxin-V, AH Robins) and diazepam (Valium, Roche Laboratories). Diazepam is probably more effective than methocarbamol. However, orally administered diazepam is inconsistently absorbed by dogs and may undergo extensive elimination after first pass through the liver. In addition, its scheduling as a controlled substance makes diazepam an inconvenient drug to dispense or prescribe for home use. For the hospitalized dog, diazepam can be adminis-

tered by intramuscular injection (0.2 to 0.5 mg/kg divided every 12 hr), with the dose titrated to the individual patient. Methocarbamol seems to be effective for some patients and is administered orally (Table 1). Some dogs will exhibit clinical signs of sedation, lethargy, or ataxia while receiving this drug.

Some controversy exists regarding the management of urinary incontinence (specifically, the means of maintaining an empty bladder) and the use of antibiotics in dogs having urinary retention. Theoretical considerations aside, the choice between manual bladder expression, intermittent catheterization, or indwelling catheterization with a closed collection system should be based on what is most practical for the situation at hand, emphasizing the goal rather than the means. Dogs with urinary incontinence, even with upper motor neuron lesions and increased sphincter tone, appear likely to develop some infectious cystitis regardless of how urine retention is managed. I use broad-spectrum antibiotics in patients whenever urine retention is likely to occur, though there is an added risk of selecting for resistant microorganisms.

## Radiographic Evaluation

The goal of spinal radiography is to determine whether the dog's pain/paralysis is disk-related or due to some other pathologic process. Whenever the signalment and history strongly suggest that the clinical signs are due to IVD disease, there is little to be gained from plain radiography as long as the patient is going to be managed medically (i.e., is not considered a surgical candidate). There is little value in knowing, for example, that disk displacement occurred at T12–13 versus L1–2 if that knowledge does not alter the treatment plan. Obviously, radiographs should be made if disk disease is not as likely (the diagnosis is in doubt) or if the clinical signs suggest that the animal is a surgical candidate and the veterinarian needs to confirm the presence and location of the "mass effect."

Unfortunately, there are limitations associated with spinal radiography in the diagnosis of intervertebral disk disease. Without proper positioning and immobilization of the patient, only gross abnormalities will be detected, some of which may be misleading. Chief among these is the presence of calcified disks. Mineralization of the nucleus pulposus, especially in the chondrodystrophoid dog, can be widespread without the presence of any clinical signs. Most calcified disks seen on radiographs are not responsible for the development of pain or paresis. Only when the calcified material is located within the vertebral canal or it is in the intervertebral disk space but is incomplete or fragmented should it be incriminated as the possible cause of clinical signs (Fig. 2).

Spinal radiography usually requires general anesthesia. In addition, because noncalcified disk material is inapparent and narrowing of the intervertebral joint spaces and foramina may be absent or subtle, contrast

**Table 1.** *Drug Protocols for the Management of Intervertebral Disk Disease in the Dog*

| Drug | Dosage |
| --- | --- |
| Dexamethasone° | <3-kg dog; 0.125 mg (total dose) q8h PO |
| | 3- to 15-kg dog; 0.25 mg (total dose) q8h PO |
| | 15- to 35-kg dog; 0.5–1.5 mg (total dose) q8h PO |
| | >35-kg dog; 0.75–3.0 mg (total dose) q8h PO |
| Methocarbamol | <6-kg dog; 125 mg (total dose) q8–12h PO |
| | 6- to 15-kg dog; 250 mg (total dose) q8–12h PO |
| | >15-kg dog; 500 mg (total dose) q8–12h PO |

°All dexamethasone dosages are initial dosages; thereafter, the recommended dose is decreased over 1 to 2 weeks.

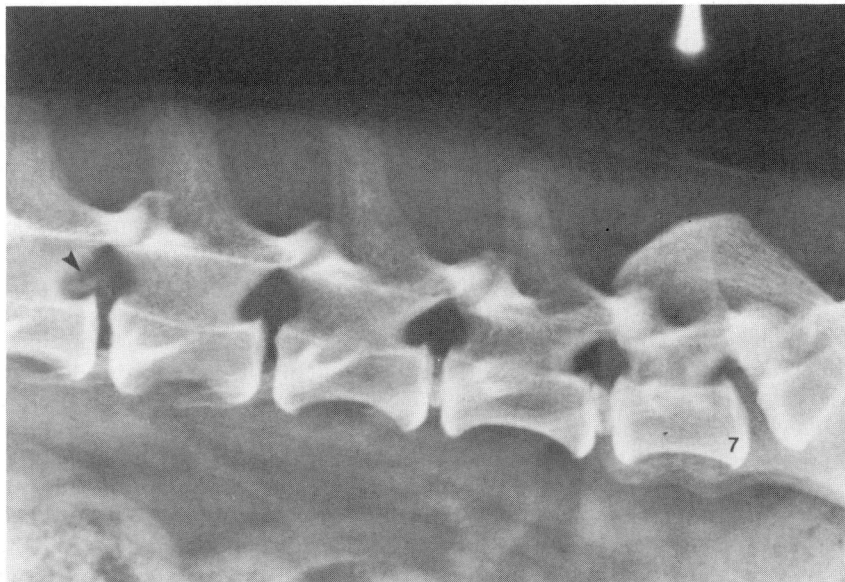

**Figure 2.** Radiograph of the lumbar spine of a 5-year-old dog. Note the presence of mineralized disks at L5–6 and L6–7. Such findings are especially common in chondrodystrophoid dogs; there are usually no clinical signs associated with such lesions. Unless there is calcified disk material in the vertebral canal at a level that matches the dog's clinical signs, the finding of "mineralized" disks is of little significance. This dog was paraparetic and seemed painful when digital pressure was applied to the midlumbar region. There appears to be calcified disk material in the vertebral canal at the L3–4 level (*arrowhead*). Myelography is indicated whenever the cause of clinical signs remains in doubt.

radiography (myelography) is often necessary to delineate the lesion. The clinical implication of the above is that there is little to be gained by obtaining radiographs of the spine, even good quality ones, only to have to refer the patient elsewhere for definitive diagnostic imaging and surgery. When one considers costs, anesthesia time, and the value of the information derived, it is my opinion that spinal radiography should not be done for suspected disk disease unless the veterinarian is also able to perform myelography and is capable of performing surgery immediately thereafter. Obviously, there are instances when obtaining spinal radiographs, even on unanesthetized patients, is warranted. For example, if one suspects that the clinical signs might be due to a vertebral tumor or fracture, radiographs obtained without the benefit of anesthesia are indicated.

## Management of the Sensorimotor Plegic Patient

There is considerable controversy concerning the management of the dog who has lost all sensory and motor function caudal to the level of spinal cord injury (sensorimotor plegia). So-called deep pain is nociception transmitted to the brain via small unmyelinated nerves (called C-fibers) in the spinal cord. The presumption is that loss of deep pain perception (nociception) occurs due to disruption of these fibers. The relative invulnerability of these fibers to all but the most severe spinal cord injuries is based on their small size, location deep within the spinal cord white matter, and nonreliance on myelin for nerve transmission. Since the C-fibers are relatively resistant to injury, loss of nociception implies a severe and probably irreversible injury to the spinal cord. The inference then is that the sensorimotor plegic patient (i.e., the dog with "no deep pain") will not recover. It is important to remember that, at our current level of clinical treatment, the spinal cord has a poor, almost absent, reparative capability.

A major problem that the veterinarian faces is determining whether the animal has actually lost all sensation caudal to the level of spinal cord injury. Nociceptive testing, such as closing the jaws of a hemostat on the digits, is subjective and depends upon a conscious reaction by the patient. One might conclude that the patient is plegic when there is no apparent conscious response to a noxious stimulus. This can be erroneous. Some animals with normal spinal cord function, and certainly animals that have decreased sensory function (hypalgesia), may fail to respond appropriately to a noxious stimulus. We are using a crude test to make a critical decision. This is the most likely explanation of how recovery of ambulatory function has occurred in dogs who were diagnosed as being sensorimotor plegic.

When we examine a dog that appears to have lost deep pain perception, the most that can be said is just that the patient *appears* to be plegic. This puts the patient in a "gray zone" for which the therapeutic decisions are less than clear. If the dog is truly plegic and one accepts this as an indicator of severe spinal cord injury, the patient is doomed no matter what or how soon treatment is delivered. Fortunately, many dogs who are initially determined to have "no deep pain" are, in fact, in the gray zone; they are severely hypalgesic but might subsequently recover.

Because determination of nociceptive ability is so critical, other methods of evaluation have been tried, such as electrical evoked response measurement. The basic concept is to place a stimulating electrode caudal to the level of injury and a recording electrode in the scalp to measure a cortical or thalamic reaction to the stimulus. In principle, this seems a good idea; unfortunately, it has thus far proven to be unreliable in the clinical setting.

Another way of assessing spinal cord integrity is by direct examination (i.e., via laminectomy and durotomy). Dogs with loss of deep pain are presumed to have an irreversible spinal cord injury, which would imply anatomic derangement such as transection or myelomalacia. Unfortunately, gross appearance does not always allow one to predict whether or not recovery is possible. I have had patients with what appeared to be a malacic spinal cord (not quite liquified but extremely soft and disrupted in appearance), who eventually recovered. Therefore, unless the spinal cord is transected, or literally oozes through the durotomy site, one cannot conclude with absolute confidence that recovery is impossible.

Because of the problem in distinguishing the sensorimotor plegic dog from the gray-zone hypalgesic patient, any extreme position concerning the value of surgery in this patient would seem unwise. Some surgeons believe that they can accurately make this distinction and refuse to operate on any dog who they conclude is sensorimotor plegic. Certainly, a consistent lack of a conscious response to noxious stimulation with serial examination strongly suggests a loss of deep pain; operating on these dogs will result in a high rate of failure. A number of texts have attempted to provide guidelines concerning surgery for the plegic patient that are based on duration; that is, decompression must be achieved in "X" hours or surgery is not warranted ("X" has been variously reported to be 12, 24, 36, or 48 hr). There are few data to support any of these recommendations, and the information that is available leads to further confusion. These inconsistencies are better understood when we classify dogs who appear to be sensorimotor plegic as gray-zone dogs and recognize that some plegic dogs may recover following surgery. The gray-zone concept does imply, however, that the earlier the surgery the greater the likelihood of a successful outcome, since at some point the patient may slip from what may be hypalgesia to true and irreversible analgesia.

Finally, one should consider other potential diagnostic and therapeutic benefits yielded by exploration and durotomy in the plegic patient. If the spinal cord is grossly transected, severely malacic, or riddled with hemorrhage, and this information will determine whether the client continues treatment or elects euthanasia, then surgery can be utilized independent of any expected therapeutic benefit. In addition, surgical intervention may result in pain relief. Some dogs who are sensorimotor plegic caudal to the lesion are extremely painful at the site of the injury. If the client is prepared to manage the dog, even if it will be permanently paralyzed, surgery to relieve compression and ischemia of nerve roots may be warranted.

## SURGICAL CONTROVERSIES

### Durotomy and Myelotomy

Some surgeons believe that durotomy has potential therapeutic value in addition to the diagnostic value that has been described above. This is debatable. Durotomy and piotomy have been shown to sometimes result in a temporary slowing of the progression of clinical signs in patients with intramedullary masses, where there is outward growth of the tumor against the restrictive dura mater. However, in a patient that is plegic due to spinal cord trauma, opening the dura or performing a myelotomy seems to result in little difference with regard to recovery. Functional disruption of the spinal cord appears to be largely related to the self-perpetuating necrotizing process (see "Use of Corticosteroids," above). Durotomy and myelotomy do not appear to alter or interrupt this self-destructive autolysis once it has begun.

In addition to the above, the decompressive effect of durotomy and myelotomy is probably negligible. Spinal cord decompression is predicated on mass removal. In the case of IVD disease, this demands removing the disk material that has entered the vertebral canal. By themselves, neither laminectomy nor laminectomy with durotomy will result in spinal cord decompression. Because the spinal cord is "held" to the floor of the vertebral canal by the nerve roots, it will not simply "move out of harm's way" when the overlying bone has been removed or dura mater opened. Moreover, durotomy or myelotomy might result in further structural injury or hemorrhage that would hamper recovery of spinal cord function. Therefore, if the dog has pain perception going into surgery, I believe that durotomy and myelotomy are contraindicated.

### Therapeutic Fenestration

Intervertebral disk fenestration does not remove disk material from the vertebral canal, and as such, fenestration is not a decompressive procedure. It is reasonable to consider that dogs with "discogenic" pain (see "Terminology and Pathophysiology," above), might be helped by this procedure. However, since it appears that clinical signs are usually associated with a compressive or "mass" effect and not discogenic pain, the use of fenestration as the primary treatment of IVD disease is rarely indicated.

When first described, fenestration was thought to have several therapeutic effects. There was a presumption that disk material within the vertebral canal created signs of radiculopathy or myelopathy because of the inflammation that it incited. The theory held that removal of the remaining nucleus pulposus from the intervertebral disk space would prevent further displacement of nucleus pulposus and reduce the stimulation of any further inflammation. The disk material already within the vertebral canal would eventually be resorbed and recovery would follow. While it *may* be true that disk material within the vertebral canal can incite inflammation, it is generally accepted that myeloradiculopathy is due to spinal cord or nerve root compression (mass effect) and not due to an inflammatory response to the disk. It was also once believed that fenestration of the disk space induced an inflammatory reaction in the intervertebral disk space, bringing phagocytic cells to the area. The presumption was that this encouraged, over time, the resorption of additional disk material. This theory has been disproved (Shores et al.,

1985). When a fenestration is performed, there is a minimal to absent inflammatory response in the intervertebral disk space. Therefore, since fenestration seemingly does nothing to alleviate mass effect within the vertebral canal, and it has no effect that promotes additional resorption of remaining disk, it would not appear very useful as sole treatment of canine IVD disease (Fingeroth, 1989). Nonetheless, anecdotes abound about paralyzed dogs who recover function with fenestration alone. The basis for this recovery is unexplained.

There is an implicit argument found in some texts that fenestration should be used as a "first-attempt" surgical treatment of IVD disease; that is, that laminectomy or ventral slotting procedures (decompressive surgery) should be "held in reserve" for more seriously incapacitated patients or for those patients with pain alone that fail to recover following fenestration. I disagree with this reasoning. First, it presupposes that the severity of signs is directly correlated with the volume of displaced disk material (i.e., dogs with pain alone or with mild deficits probably have "small disk prolapses," while dogs who are paraplegic or tetraplegic must have "massive extrusions"). As has already been stated, this may not be true. Only through proper diagnostic imaging (myelography, magnetic resonance imaging [MRI]) can one determine the degree of cord compression. Fenestration may be an inappropriate treatment, even for the animal whose only clinical sign is pain, because it fails to treat the compressive mass (which may be considerable). Second, fenestration is not without its complications. There is trauma from muscle dissection to expose the disk (which may equal or exceed that required for laminectomy) and a possibility of causing more disk to be displaced into the vertebral canal as the disk space is fenestrated. Finally, while in humans it may make sense to perform a less invasive surgery first, with the idea that, if it fails, the patient will accede to a second, more invasive approach, the same logic may not apply in veterinary medicine. Most pet owners have emotional and financial limits regarding care of their pets; they often stipulate that they are likely to pursue surgical treatment only once. Since fenestration requires similar anesthesia, operating costs, and hospital care as decompressive surgery, the patient who fails to respond adequately to fenestration may not be given a second chance for a more "definitive" surgery. Furthermore, the concept that laminectomy and ventral slotting are more difficult and dangerous than fenestration is irrelevant and probably wrong (Fry et al., 1993).

## Prophylactic Fenestration

While the use of primary therapeutic fenestration is becoming less popular, fenestration is still widely employed as an adjunct to decompressive surgery for prevention of future disk herniation at other levels. The basis for doing this rests on the assumption that dogs with IVD disease are likely to have multiple disk herniations during their lifetime. This assumption may not be correct.

When we consider the chondrodystrophoid breeds, for whom prophylactic fenestration is advocated, it is apparent that only a relatively small number of these dogs are ever presented to a veterinarian with clinical signs referrable to IVD disease. Even though many of these dogs have degenerating disks, the vast majority live a life that is apparently free of neck pain, back pain, or paresis. To me this implies a relatively low risk for a degenerating disk to displace and cause clinical signs that would necessitate surgical intervention. Therefore, when confronted with the patient who has clinical signs of IVD disease, and who (not unexpectedly) has radiographic evidence of diffuse disk degeneration (multiple calcified disks), there may not be logical justification for the belief that those disks will cause problems in the future.

Certain other facts must be considered when measuring the value of prophylactic fenestration. When dogs that have never had surgery are examined because they have "recurrent disk disease," one usually finds that with myelography there is only a single compressive lesion. Thus, most dogs with a history of "multiple disk problems" are probably having recurrent herniation at the same site, rather than displacement at multiple sites. One disk is usually causing the repeated problem, even though the veterinarian may find that several disks are calcified or showing signs of degeneration on the radiographs (Fig. 2). Retrospective studies of dogs who have undergone decompressive surgery (with or without "prophylactic" fenestration) have been done to determine the risk of recurrence. When evaluating such studies, it becomes apparent that one must be very careful to define what is meant by "recurrence." Recurrence of clinical signs following decompressive surgery is fairly common, ranging between 10 and 25% of dogs that have had surgery. However, most recurrences happen only once, are not proven to be disk-related, and usually resolve with short courses of medical therapy. In a study of 187 cases, the percentage of dogs with thoracolumbar disk disease who have had proven new lesions that warranted a second decompressive surgery was only about 3% (Brown, Helphrey, and Prata, 1977). In the cervical region, the percentage of dogs needing second surgeries is considered the same or lower. Moreover, when new level herniations do develop, they sometimes occur in disks remote from the levels where prophylactic fenestration has or would have been performed. Based on this information, it is doubtful that fenestration of intervertebral disks adjacent to the site of decompressive surgery is of significant prophylactic value in most patients. Some surgeons, however, feel that the prophylactic benefit of fenestration, even if small, is still enough to justify fenestration of adjacent disks during a decompressive procedure. Given what has been said about the need to perform the most effective operation the first time, this argument may have merit.

Regardless of its use at other sites, fenestration of the disk at the same site as the decompression is logical. There is usually some nuclear material left in the intervertebral disk space even when a massive amount is found in the vertebral canal. Completing the discectomy via fenestration may prevent displacement of any remaining nucleus pulposus through the damaged annulus. Since recurrences often involve the same site repeatedly, this use of fenestration is appropriate.

### "Chemical Fenestration" (Chemonucleolyis)

Over the last few years, there has been a flurry of research into the use of drugs such as chymopapain and collagenase to "dissolve" disks (see *CVT XI*, p 1018). There are a number of inherent problems with the extrapolation of this technique from people to dogs. First, in people, the disk lesion in question is usually "contained," (i.e., the nucleus is causing a bulge in the overlying annulus but is not displaced into the vertebral canal). The opposite is usually true in dogs, even those with signs of pain alone. The entrance of chymopapain into the epidural space, or worse, inadvertent passage into the intrathecal space, may be associated with severe complications. Chemonucleolysis was not designed to treat the ruptured/displaced disk lesion that is most often encountered in dogs. In people, chemonucleolysis is virtually limited to the lumbar spine, and since the spinal cord ends at about T12–L1 in humans, there is minimal risk to the cord itself. However, its use in dogs carries a much greater inherent risk, since we are almost always injecting in an area where the spinal cord itself is present. One of the advantages of this procedure in people is the avoidance of general anesthesia and major surgery. However, in the studies reported in dogs, general anesthesia is employed and, even where fluoroscopy is available, the disks are usually exposed surgically before needle placement. Thus, chemonucleolysis seems to be just another way of accomplishing virtually the same goals as routine surgical fenestration, possibly with increased risks, and with all the potential shortcomings alluded to.

### OTHER TREATMENTS

Some dogs with presumed spinal cord compression are effectively treated with *acupuncture*, particularly if their signs are moderate (i.e., not paralyzed), or if other factors are present that mitigate against surgery. For the patient with signs of chronic pain, acupuncture may be a reasonable treatment to try prior to more invasive procedures (Scavelli and Schoen, 1989).

*Chiropractic manipulation* is another modality that some have attempted to use on dogs with IVD disease. I have no experience with this, nor are there objective studies to cite. However, I have strong reservations about the safety, efficacy, and ethics of this unconventional form of therapy. As there is almost always a compressive mass effect in dogs having signs of "disk disease," spinal manipulation could have serious con-

sequences (i.e., cause further spinal cord compression or injury) in our patients.

### RECOMMENDATIONS

Understanding how disk displacement produces clinical signs of spinal cord injury via compression (mass effect), and velocity at impact (kinetic energy), is much more important than having a consensus on such terms as prolapse, protrusion, herniation, rupture, or extrusion. When confronted with a dog that is painful, paretic, or plegic, it is important that the veterinarian bring a calm, rational, and well-informed approach to the situation. The veterinarian should, at the very least, be able to distinguish upper motor neuron signs (reflexes preserved) from lower motor neuron signs (decreased muscle tone and reflexes) and be capable of detecting spinal hyperpathia (extradural lesions such as disk herniation tend to result in spinal pain). Although it may be difficult or impossible to distinguish severe hypalgesia from sensorimotor plegia, one should never equate reflex withdrawal of the tested limb with conscious perception of pain (nociception). Careful serial examination is important to determine the location, severity, and progression of the spinal cord injury.

If the neurologic status of the patient dictates potential surgical intervention, radiographs are indicated to confirm the presence and location of the compression. When the results of the neurologic examination and survey radiography are in conflict or when plain films fail to clearly disclose the lesion, myelography or MRI is indicated.

Since the severity of the mass effect cannot always be predicted from clinical signs alone and a compressive effect is usually present in animals with disk displacement, surgery is often indicated for the patient that has signs of persistent or recurrent pain even when there are no other neurologic deficits. Likewise, decompression of the spinal cord may be indicated whenever the neurologic status of the patient is static or continues to decline despite proper medical therapy. Delayed referral of the patient with rapidly diminishing function and apparent loss of sensation could mean the difference between success and failure of treatment.

Decompressive surgery is far more likely to be of benefit than fenestration alone regardless of the severity of clinical signs. However, decompressive surgery means more than just performing a laminectomy or ventral slot. There is a pervasive belief that when disk material enters the vertebral canal, it causes compression by "squeezing" the spinal cord against the overlying bone. No doubt, some compression of this type does occur, and it is readily evident at the time of surgery. However, even after the adjacent bone has been removed via dorsal laminectomy or hemilaminectomy, the cord is still seen to be deformed or displaced by the disk itself. Dorsal laminectomy, hemilaminectomy, and ventral slotting procedures are primarily bone-removal procedures. They allow access to the vertebral canal, but complete decompression is not achieved until the offending mass of disk material has been removed (Thatcher, 1989). This has been proven in numerous studies, and the concept has been summarized in the neurosurgical literature by the observation that laminectomy alone is akin to "taking the roof off the house to eliminate the flood in the basement."

Veterinarians treating dogs with presumed IVD disease need to keep the above points in mind as they formulate their treatment plans and counsel owners. Appropriate assessment of patients, understanding pathophysiology, and timely referral (when indicated) will result in better outcomes for patients and owners alike.

## References and Suggested Reading

Brown NO, Helphrey ML, and Prata RG: Thoracolumbar disc disease in the dog. A retrospective analysis of 187 cases. J Am Anim Hosp Assoc 13:665, 1977.
*A large-scale study that defines the true incidence of recurrent disk disease.*
Fingeroth JM: Fenestration. Pros and cons. Probl Vet Med (Intervertebral Disc Disease) 1:445, 1989.
*A more detailed review of the history and controversy surrounding the use of fenestration for intervertebral disk disease in dogs.*
Fry TR, Johnson AL, Hungerford L, et al: Surgical treatment of cervical disc herniations in ambulatory dogs. Ventral decompression vs fenestration. 111 cases (1980–1988). Prog Vet Neurol 2:165, 1993.
*A direct comparison of the surgical results from fenestration versus decompression in a similar population of ambulatory tetraparetic dogs with cervical disk disease.*
Morgan PW, Parent J, and Holmberg DL: Cervical pain secondary to intervertebral disc disease in dogs; Radiographic findings and surgical implications. Prog Vet Neurol 4:76, 1993.
*An analysis of dogs with signs of neck pain alone using myelography to define the nature of the underlying disk lesion.*
Prata RG: Cervical and thoracolumbar disc disease in the dog. In Kirk RW (ed): *Current Veterinary Therapy VIII.* Philadelphia, WB Saunders Co, 1983, p 708.
*A review of pathophysiology and clinical management of intervertebral disk disease in dogs.*
Scavelli TD and Schoen A: Problems and complications associated with the nonsurgical management of intervertebral disc disease. Prob Vet Med 1: 402, 1989.
*A review of ancillary and alternative treatments for intervertebral disk disease, including drug use and acupuncture.*
Shores A, Cechner PE, Cantwell HD, et al: Structural changes in thoracolumbar discs following lateral fenestration. A study of the radiographic, histologic, and histochemical changes in the chondrodystrophoid dog. Vet Surg 14:117, 1985.
*An analysis of the true short- and long-term effects of fenestration on the intervertebral disk.*
Thatcher C: Neuroanatomic and pathophysiologic aspects of intervertebral disc disease in the dog. Prob Vet Med 1:337, 1989.
*A review of surgical and functional anatomy of the spine, spinal cord, and nerve roots, and their relationship to the pathophysiogy of intervertebral disk disease.*
Toombs JB, Caywood DD, Lipowitz AJ, et al: Colonic perforation following neurosurgical procedures and corticosteroid therapy in four dogs. J Am Vet Med Assoc 177:68, 1980.
*A description of potential consequences of high-dose steroid therapy.*

# MEDICAL MANAGEMENT OF CHRONIC HEPATIC ENCEPHALOPATHY

JILL E. MADDISON
*Sydney, New South Wales, Australia*

Hepatic encephalopathy (HE) is a neurologic syndrome that results from acute or chronic liver failure. The most common cause of HE in dogs and cats is the presence of congenital portacaval shunts that allow mesenteric blood to bypass the liver and directly enter the systemic circulation. Acquired portosystemic shunting also occurs in dogs and cats as a consequence of diseases that induce portal hypertension such as cirrhosis, arteriovenous fistula, and hepatoportal fibrosis. A small number of animals may develop HE without shunting after acute hepatic destruction induced by drugs, toxins, or infection.

## CLINICAL SIGNS

The clinical signs of HE in dogs and cats have been well described (for review, see Center and Magne, 1990). There are many similarities in the clinical signs observed in the two species; however, there are also differences. Seizures appear to occur more frequently in cats than in dogs with HE. Seizures are reported in approximately 50% of feline cases but are not a common feature in dogs. Bizarre behavior (particularly aggression) is also observed more commonly in cats than in dogs. Neurologic signs such as disorientation, ataxia, and stupor are common in both species.

Dogs with congenital HE are usually poorly grown and experience episodes of anorexia, vomiting, and other gastrointestinal signs. In contrast, cats are often well grown and in good body condition. Vomiting, diarrhea, and anorexia are reported less frequently in cats than in dogs. The most marked species difference in the clinical presentation of HE is hypersalivation, which is very common in affected cats but uncommon in dogs.

Polyuria and polydipsia occur in approximately one third of dogs with HE, but are less frequently reported in cats. Occasional animals present with signs referable only to the urinary tract, caused by development of urate cystic calculi.

## ANATOMY

Most congenital shunts in dogs are single large intrahepatic or extrahepatic conduits. A variety of shunt types have been recognized, including patent ductus venosus, portal vein atresia with development of multiple collateral portal systemic communications (rare), drainage of the portal vein into the caudal vena cava (portacaval shunt), drainage of the portal vein into the azygous vein (porta-azygous shunt), drainage of the portal vein and caudal vena cava into the azygous vein with discontinuation of the prerenal segment of the caudal vena cava, drainage of the left gastric vein into the caudal vena cava, and intrahepatic arterioportal fistula.

Intrahepatic shunts occur most commonly in large breeds such as the Doberman pinscher, Labrador retriever, golden retriever, Old English sheepdog, and Irish wolfhound. In contrast, extrahepatic shunts predominate in the smaller breeds such as Yorkshire terrier, Maltese terrier and miniature schnauzer. Single extrahepatic shunts predominate in cats, although intrahepatic shunts have been reported.

## PATHOGENESIS

The neurochemical basis for the neurologic dysfunction that occurs in HE is incompletely understood. The encephalopathy that occurs in acute or chronic hepatic failure is in most cases reversible with amelioration of the underlying liver disease. The potential for structural and functional reversal of the neurologic abnormalities in HE is consistent with a metabolic encephalopathy.

Hepatic encephalopathy is a complex pathophysiologic state that is probably multifactorial in origin. It is generally accepted that gut-derived substances of bacterial and protein metabolism are important in the pathogenesis. The evidence for this includes the observation that therapeutic agents that reduce gut bacterial flora or dietary protein often result in improvement of neurologic function, without altering the underlying liver disease.

Current theories of the pathogenesis of HE essentially fall into four major areas (for review, see Maddison, 1992). The four theories are:

1.  Ammonia as the putative neurotoxin ± other synergistic toxins.
2.  Alteration in monoamine or catecholamine neurotransmitters as a result of perturbed aromatic amino acid metabolism.
3.  Alteration in amino acid neurotransmitters, brain γ-aminobutyric acid (GABA), and/or glutamate.
4.  Increased cerebral levels of an endogenous benzodiazepine-like substance.

Other theories that have been proposed but which are no longer believed to be tenable include lack of a brain protective factor, decreased cerebral energy, alterations in the blood-brain barrier, increased GABA concentrations, and increased brain GABA-receptor density.

### Ammonia

It is not the purpose of this article to review current concepts of the pathogenesis of HE, but it is pertinent to consider the role of ammonia, as most medical treatments used in the management of HE alter blood and/or central nervous system (CNS) ammonia levels.

Evidence for a central role for ammonia in the pathogenesis of HE includes the observations that: encephalopathy can be precipitated in cirrhotic patients by ingestion of ammonia-generating substances such as protein, urea, and ammonium salts; congenital hyperammonemia caused by urea cycle disorders results in encephalopathy and coma in children and dogs; and therapeutic measures that result in decreased intestinal production and absorption of ammonia, such as low-protein diet, lactulose administration, and reduction of gut bacteria by antibiotics, usually result in improvement of clinical signs. In addition, metabolic derangements that increase movement of ammonia across cell membranes or increase ammonia production can precipitate encephalopathy in susceptible patients. Such derangements include alkalosis, which facilitates brain uptake of ammonia by increasing the concentration of ammonia base ($NH_3$), and profound hypokalemia. Hypokalemia potentiates alkalosis and also increases renal ammonia production.

Further evidence of the role of ammonia are studies where administration of sodium benzoate to human patients with chronic HE induced clinical and electroencephalographic (EEG) improvements that paralleled reductions in blood ammonia (Butterworth, 1992). Sodium benzoate decreases blood ammonia concentrations by promoting its excretion in the form of hippurate. Other treatments that enhance ammonia excretion, such as levodopa (which increases renal blood flow and hence renal ammonia excretion), have also been reported to ameliorate encephalopathy in human patients.

However, although blood ammonia concentrations are increased in most patients with HE, the correlation between blood ammonia and degree of encephalopathy is poor and some patients are encephalopathic without hyperammonemia. In addition, some medications may influence the severity of HE in human patients without altering blood ammonia concentrations. Conversely, treatment of human patients with a monoamine oxidase inhibitor decreased blood ammonia concentrations, but failed to improve the encephalopathy.

On balance, there is good evidence that ammonia plays a role in the pathogenesis of HE and that limiting ammonia absorption from the gut can benefit many patients by reducing clinical signs of encephalopathy. However, there continues to be controversy regarding the importance of ammonia in the pathogenesis of HE because its precise effect on cerebral function is unknown.

## Endogenous Benzodiazepines

It has been suggested that there may be increased concentrations of benzodiazepine-like compounds in brains of patients with HE and that these may contribute to the pathogenesis by facilitating inhibitory neurotransmission (Basile, Jones, and Skolnick, 1992). It is appropriate to consider the evidence for this hypothesis, as some human patients are being treated with benzodiazepine antagonists and it has been suggested that benzodiazepine antagonists may be useful in veterinary patients. The issue has attracted heated debate and is unresolved (Basile, Jones, and Skolnick, 1992; Butterworth, 1992).

Benzodiazepine-like compounds have been detected in plasma, cerebrospinal fluid (CSF), and brain of animals and human patients with HE. Plasma concentrations of benzodiazepine-like activity have been reported to correlate with the degree of encephalopathy in human patients with hepatic cirrhosis and chronic HE. In addition, administration of benzodiazepine antagonists such as flumazenil (Ro 15-1788) has been reported in some studies to improve, although often only transiently, the neurologic status of human patients with HE, particularly in the earlier stages of encephalopathy. Most of these studies were not controlled and other randomized double-blind crossover studies have not found benzodiazepine antagonists to be beneficial in the treatment of HE (Butterworth, 1992).

The origin of these endogenous benzodiazepine-like compounds has not been determined, and as yet there is little or no evidence that they are related to gut bacterial metabolism. While it would be of great benefit to patients with HE to receive effective treatment that ameliorated signs of encephalopathy without requiring protein restriction, the evidence that benzodiazepine antagonists are useful for long-term management of HE is lacking.

## TREATMENT

Ideally, treatment of any disorder is based on current knowledge and understanding of the pathogenesis of the clinical signs and abnormalities observed. Surgical correction of congenital portosystemic shunts is an example of rational treatment that directly addresses the specific anatomic abnormality that causes HE in patients.

However, not all animals with HE have a surgically correctable problem. For example, acute hepatic failure, acquired portosystemic shunting secondary to chronic liver disease, and multiple congenital shunts are conditions not amenable to surgical correction. Surgical correction of single congenital shunts is not always possible because of lack of access to appropriate surgical expertise or economic factors. In addition, patients may need medical management prior to undergoing surgical correction to optimize their condition for surgery. In all of these instances, medical management may be instituted. However, medical management of HE is at best empiric, because the pathogenesis of HE is uncertain.

## Surgical Treatment

Both intrahepatic and extrahepatic shunts can be ligated (Lawrence, Bellah, and Diaz, 1992) and this treatment option is becoming more widely available with the increasing number of specialist veterinary surgeons. Extrahepatic shunts are more amenable to surgical correction than intrahepatic shunts and a reasonable prognosis can be given for this surgery. The difficulty with surgery for intrahepatic shunts lies with their relative inaccessibility. However, they can be ligated successfully (Breznock et al., 1983).

A good to excellent clinical outcome after surgery has been reported in most cases (Johnson, Armstrong, and Hauptman, 1987; Lawrence, Bellah, and Diaz, 1992) although, unfortunately, most retrospective reviews do not clearly identify the relative success of surgery for intrahepatic versus extrahepatic shunts. Fasting serum bile acids have been shown to decrease significantly after shunt ligation, but they may not return to the reference range. Postprandial serum bile acids did not significantly decrease after shunt ligation in one study, suggesting that liver function is not completely normal postoperatively (Lawrence, Bellah, and Diaz, 1992). Blood ammonia concentrations may be a more sensitive measure of the outcome of ligation, although concentrations postoperatively have been reported to be above the reference range in dogs without signs of encephalopathy (Johnson, Armstrong, and Hauptman, 1987).

Complete attenuation of the shunt is often not possible because of unacceptable increases in portal vein pressure that develop as the shunt is ligated. However, long-term amelioration of clinical signs is often achieved even with partial attenuation. Lawrence and colleagues (1992) reported no statistically significant difference in clinical result after complete or partial shunt occlusion in 20 dogs. Others found continued medical management with low-protein diets was needed in some dogs with partial ligation and occasionally there was no clinical improvement after partial ligation (Johnson, Armstrong, and Hauptman, 1987). Partial ligation of portosystemic shunts in cats has been reported to result in a satisfactory clinical outcome, although clinical relapse has been documented in several cases. Clinical outcome was significantly worse in dogs older than 2 years at the time of surgery (Lawrence, Bellah, and Diaz, 1992).

Mortality associated with shunt ligation ranges from 10 to 30%. Postsurgical deaths can occur due to several causes, including anesthetic complications, excessive postligation portal pressure, and blood loss. An uncommon postsurgical sequela in both dogs and cats is the development of intractable seizures several hours to several days after shunt ligation (Matushek, Bjorling, and Mathews, 1990). There are reports of successful management of this problem; however, management is unsuccessful in many cases. Neurologic deficits such as blindness and ataxia persisted in several cases after seizures were controlled with anticonvulsants. The pathogenesis of this unusual and uncommon syndrome has not been determined. An obvious metabolic cause such as hypoglycemia, hyperammonemia, or hypocalcemia was not evident in most cases.

## Medical Management

Medical management may be attempted if surgical correction is not feasible. However, it is important to recognize that such treatment is palliative and commonly results in only temporary alleviation of clinical signs. Medical treatment will not ameliorate portacaval shunting (either congenital or acquired), hence the liver will continue to be deprived of portal blood. As a result there will be continued hepatic atrophy and progressive failure of hepatic function, particularly protein synthesis. In acute hepatic failure, recovery of liver function is possible if the patient survives. However, acute hepatic failure carries a poor prognosis and, in human medicine, the treatment of choice is hepatic transplantation.

The most successful medical treatment is based on reducing gut bacterial protein metabolism. This is achieved by: (1) decreasing dietary protein intake and (2) suppressing urease-producing gut bacteria. In addition, limiting the absorption of ammonia from the colon may also be beneficial.

### RESTRICTED-PROTEIN DIET

A restricted-protein diet is the cornerstone of medical management of chronic HE. Excessive fat intake should be avoided and a good quality vitamin supplement (without methionine) should be provided, as vitamin metabolism is often perturbed in patients with liver dysfunction.

Unfortunately, the consequences of prolonged protein restriction will usually be deleterious for the patient, and intractable ascites and other complications of hypoproteinemia may eventually result. It is therefore advisable to restrict protein only as needed to ameliorate encephalopathic signs and to use antibiotic therapy and lactulose to permit the maximum dietary protein intake possible without precipitating encephalopathy.

The source of dietary protein should also be considered. Studies in human medicine suggest that dairy proteins are better tolerated than meat proteins in chronic HE and are associated with lower blood ammonia concentration. Cottage cheese is therefore suitable for dogs and cats, as it has a high biologic value and is easily digested. Recent attention has focused in human medicine on the benefits of vegetable protein diets compared with diets based on animal protein. Vegetable protein diets appear to result in improved nitrogen balance, which is particularly important in patients with muscle wasting and cachexia and at risk of worsening encephalopathy if dietary protein is in-creased. Commercial or homemade diets based on vegetable proteins may prove beneficial in the management of chronic HE in dogs and cats if difficulties with palatability can be overcome. Controlled clinical studies are required to determine the optimal dietary protein source for cats and dogs with HE.

### ANTIMICROBIAL AGENTS

Bacterial protein metabolism can also be reduced by the use of gut active antibiotics. Neomycin has been used for many years in human and veterinary medicine. Occasional problems associated with ototoxicity, bacterial resistance, and malabsorption have been reported in humans. As a result, neomycin is usually used in humans to treat acute exacerbations of encephalopathy rather than for chronic therapy, and this recommendation is reasonable for veterinary patients as well.

Metronidazole has also been used successfully in both human and veterinary medicine to reduce gut flora. Acute CNS dysfunction has been reported in dogs associated with use of relatively high doses of metronidazole. It is therefore recommended that a conservative dose not exceeding 30 mg/kg/day be used in the management of patients with HE. Metronidazole treatment should also primarily be used if possible to treat acute exacerbations of encephalopathy rather than as chronic therapy.

Other antimicrobial agents that have been used to ameliorate acute signs of encephalopathy include ampicillin and vancomycin.

### LACTULOSE

Lactulose (1-4-β-galactosidofructose) is a synthetic disaccharide that is neither hydrolyzed nor absorbed by the small intestine. Although its mode of action is uncertain, it has been shown to be beneficial in portosystemic encephalopathy and to reduce ammonia absorption from the gut. Daily protein intake can often be increased while lactulose treatment continues without resulting in mental deterioration.

The therapeutic effect of lactulose cannot be attributed only to its cathartic effect because sorbitol, which also induces an osmotic diarrhea but without altering stool pH, has little effect on clinical signs of HE in humans. Presumed modes of action of lactulose include (1) an effect of lowered colonic pH on bacterial flora, (2) decreased ammonia absorption from the colon due to reduced relative concentration of $NH_3$ (to which the colonic mucosa is more permeable than $NH_4^+$), and (3) increased bacterial assimilation of ammonia or decreased ammonia generation by bacteria.

The therapeutic goal is to administer sufficient lactulose orally to result in the passage of two to three soft stools per day. The precise dose rate has not been determined for dogs, but is approximately 2.5 to 25 ml given two or three times daily. Cats usually require 2.5 to 5.0 ml two or three times daily. Lactulose may also be administered as an enema in acute hepatic coma.

Recent studies in humans have suggested that another disaccharide, lactitol (β-galactosidosorbitol), is as effective as lactulose in controlling HE and is associated with fewer adverse effects, such as flatulence. The use of lactitol has not been reported in veterinary medicine but may be considered as an alternative if lactulose-induced flatulence in canine or feline patients is unacceptable to the owner.

### PRECIPITATING FACTORS

Several factors can induce encephalopathy in susceptible patients and must be controlled for optimum patient management.

ALKALOSIS. As discussed previously, alkalosis can increase cerebral $NH_3$ uptake and is therefore potentially detrimental to HE patients. Most veterinary patients with acid-base disorders are acidotic rather than alkalotic. Metabolic alkalosis is uncommon in veterinary patients even after sustained vomiting, as loss of gastric acid is usually accompanied by loss of bicarbonate-rich intestinal fluid. Respiratory alkalosis is even less common. Sodium bicarbonate should be administered with extreme caution (and preferably not at all) to patients with HE, due to the risk of inducing alkalosis.

HYPOKALEMIA. A more common exacerbating factor is hypokalemia. Hypokalemia may result from profuse vomiting or diarrhea or from excessive diuretic therapy with furosemide or other loop diuretics. Diuretics are often prescribed to reduce ascites in patients with hepatic cirrhosis. These patients are at risk of developing hypokalemia if diuretic therapy is overzealous, particularly if the patient has a poor appetite and hence reduced dietary intake of potassium. Hypokalemia can be exacerbated in a dehydrated patient when aldosterone release promotes renal sodium retention at the expense of potassium.

The major mechanism by which hypokalemia may induce or exacerbate encephalopathy is probably related to increased renal ammonia production. In addition, in the alkalotic patient, hypokalemia potentiates alkalosis, which in turn increases CNS uptake of $NH_3$. Hypokalemia is accompanied by intracellular acidosis which may trap ammonium ion ($NH_4^+$) and thus impair CNS cellular function.

SEDATIVES AND ANESTHETICS. A relatively common feature of the history of a patient with HE is markedly delayed recovery from barbiturate anesthesia or prolonged sedation following tranquilization. Increased sensitivity to sedative drugs is also a feature in human HE and has been attributed to increased cerebral sensitivity to the drugs and to impaired drug elimination, the latter probably being more important.

Use of barbiturates and tranquilizers such as acepromazine should be avoided in dogs and cats with HE. However, benzodiazepines such as diazepam and midazolam appear to cause few problems in animals with HE even when used at normal dose rates as premedicants or anticonvulsants. The half-life of these drugs is quite short in the dog and cat, and even if recovery is prolonged in a patient with HE, the risk of serious adverse consequences is small.

GASTROINTESTINAL HEMORRHAGE. Hepatic disease is one of the most common medical disorders associated with gastroduodenal ulceration in dogs (Stanton and Bright, 1989). The reason is unknown but may involve decreased hepatic degradation of gastrin or histamine. The coma-producing potential of digested blood proteins is believed to be markedly greater than any other type of protein in humans. Gastrointestinal hemorrhage is a common precipitating cause of encephalopathy in both human and veterinary patients with chronic liver disease. Hence prompt treatment and preferably prevention of gastroduodenal ulceration is essential in patients with chronic HE. The value of prophylaxis with antiulcer drugs such as $H_2$-receptor antagonists (cimetidine, rantidine), sucralfate, omeprazole, or misoprostol has not been evaluated in veterinary or human medicine (see "Gastrointestinal Ulcer Therapy," this volume, p 706).

MISCELLANEOUS. Stored blood may contain high concentrations of ammonia; therefore, patients with HE who require transfusion should receive fresh blood products if possible.

Constipation can increase colonic absorption of neurotoxic products of bacterial protein digestion and hence precipitate or exacerbate encephalopathy in susceptible patients.

Administration of methionine to cirrhotic human patients can precipitate coma. Methionine is presumed to be metabolized to mercaptans by gut bacteria. Although there is no conclusive evidence for a primary role for mercaptans in the pathogenesis of HE, patients with severe liver disease should not be given methionine or supplements containing methionine because of the risk of exacerbating encephalopathic signs.

## References and Suggested Reading

Basile AS, Jones EA, and Skolnick P: The pathogenesis and treatment of hepatic encephalopathy: Evidence for the involvement of benzodiazepine receptor ligands. Pharmacol Rev 43:27, 1992.
*Comprehensive review of the clinical manifestations, neuropathology, pathogenesis, and treatment of HE in humans, with emphasis on the endogenous benzodiazepine theory.*

Breznock EM, Berger B, Pendray D, et al: Surgical manipulation of intrahepatic portocaval shunts in dogs. J Am Vet Med Assoc 182:798, 1983.
*Review of surgical procedures and outcome in 12 dogs with intrahepatic shunts.*

Butterworth RF: Pathogenesis and treatment of portal-systemic encephalopathy: An update. Dig Dis Sci 37:321, 1992.
*Excellent balanced review of the current concepts regarding the pathogenesis of HE in humans.*

Center SA and Magne ML: Historical, physical examination, and clinicopathologic features of portosystemic vascular anomalies in the dog and cat. Semin Vet Med Surg 5:83, 1990.
*Review of the literature and case records of cats and dogs with congenital portosystemic encephalopathy.*

Johnson CA, Armstrong PJ, and Hauptman JG: Congenital portosystemic shunts in dogs: 46 cases (1979–1986). J Am Vet Med Assoc 191:1478, 1987.
*Signalment, clinical signs, and surgical outcome in 46 dogs with congenital portosystemic shunts.*

Lawrence D, Bellah JR, and Diaz R: Results of surgical management of portosystemic shunts in dogs: 20 cases (1985–1990). J Am Vet Med Assoc 201:1750, 1992.
*Serum bile acid concentrations monitored before and after surgical correction of portosystemic shunts in 20 dogs.*

Maddison JE: Current concepts of hepatic encephalopathy. J Vet Intern Med 6:341, 1992.

*Comprehensive review of current knowledge of the pathogenesis of HE.*
Matushek KJ, Bjorling D, and Mathews K: Generalized motor seizures after portosystemic shunt in dogs: Five cases (1981–1988). J Am Vet Med Assoc 196:2014, 1990.

*Description of clinical signs, pathology, and outcome in five dogs with postshunt ligation seizures.*
Stanton ME and Bright RM: Gastroduodenal ulceration in dogs. J Vet Intern Med 3: 238, 1989.
*Retrospective study of 43 cases of gastroduodenal ulceration in dogs.*

# UREMIC ENCEPHALOPATHY

WILLIAM R. FENNER
*Columbus, Ohio*

Increasingly, evidence of nervous system (NS) dysfunction is recognized in patients with renal failure. This probably reflects two factors. First, patients with neurologic diseases are being evaluated more completely, thus increasing the likelihood of recognizing a metabolic disorder. Second, patients with renal disease are surviving longer, increasing the potential for complications of renal failure. Although both the central nervous system (CNS) and peripheral nervous system (PNS) may become abnormal in renal failure, most patients develop signs of CNS disease (Arieff, 1986; Lockwood, 1989). As with most metabolic encephalopathies, the most prominent signs involve seizures, altered mental states, and weakness. The signs are quite variable, often changing dramatically over the course of a 24-hr period. The clinical signs probably occur through several mechanisms. To best understand the implications of neurologic signs and the treatment of patients with uremic encephalopathy (UE), it is best to first review cerebral metabolism, then the pathophysiology of signs, the clinical presentation of patients, and finally the diagnostic and therapeutic approach.

## CEREBRAL METABOLISM

Cerebral energy requirements are the highest of all body tissues. These requirements are met by hydrolysis of high-energy phosphate bonds, especially adenosine triphosphate (ATP), which are dependent on oxidative phosphorylation. The primary fuel for cerebral metabolism is glucose, which enters the CNS using an insulin-independent, facilitated transport across the blood-brain barrier (BBB). Cerebral metabolic systems have a limited ability to utilize glycogen and ketoacids; therefore, they are uniquely susceptible to the effects of both hypoxia and hypoglycemia. Metabolites produced by cerebral metabolism include biosynthetic neurotransmitter precursors (e.g., acetyl coenzyme A [CoA]), as well as neurotransmitters themselves (e.g., acetylcholine, aspartate, glutamate, and γ-aminobutyric acid [GABA]). The end result of these anabolic and catabolic cerebral functions include: active transport of molecules and ions, membrane potential maintenance, neurotransmitter production, and storage and information transmission through neurotransmitter release.

Normal CNS neuronal activity relies on a stable extracellular environment that provides a constant source of essential fuel substrates; is controlled with respect to osmotic, acid-base, and ionic balance; and is safeguarded from potential toxins. In normal animals, the BBB and cerebral circulation maintain this required environment. Many metabolic illnesses (e.g., renal failure) affect the biochemical composition of blood or the brain's blood supply. In chronic uremic patients, low-grade anemia may result in chronic CNS hypoxia, diminishing neural function (Nissenson, 1992). Additionally, in uremia, critical homeostatic processes may be overwhelmed (hypernatremia), endogenous toxins may circulate (e.g., uremia), exogenous neurotoxins may be ingested (e.g., ethylene glycol poisoning), or cerebral perfusion may be compromised (e.g., hyperviscosity syndromes or vasculitis). In some patients, the drugs used to correct the underlying metabolic abnormalities (e.g., aluminum hydroxide) may result in secondary neurologic dysfunction (Lockwood, 1989). These changes may disturb neuronal metabolic activity, resulting in clinically detectable neurologic abnormalities. The dysfunction may represent subcellular biochemical alterations that alter cellular physiologic activity or specific neuronal behavior.

## PATHOPHYSIOLOGY

In most metabolic encephalopathies, brain energy metabolism is normal (Arieff, 1986; Biasioli et al., 1986; Lockwood, 1989). Dysfunction results from altered ion balances, altered membrane charges, altered neurotransmission, or altered neurotransmitter levels. Uremic encephalopathy may alter neurotransmitter biosynthesis, storage, release, or their interaction with the postsynaptic receptor that results in termination of the transmitter's effect. The question in uremic encephalopathy is, which of these mechanisms can be invoked to explain the patient's signs?

Anatomically and clinically, the signs are bilateral and diffuse. Certain neuronal populations have differences in sensitivity to metabolic diseases, a phenomenon referred to as selective vulnerability. For example, in thiamine deficiency, there is a difference in sensitivity of certain regions of CNS, with the cerebrum most sensitive (cortex and basal nuclei), the brain stem second in sensitivity, and the spinal cord third. Similar sensitivity to the effects of parathyroid hormone (PTH) and aluminum intoxication may account for the predominance of cerebral signs in uremic encephalopathy.

Evidence of focal CNS injury is seen in some patients with uremic encephalopathy. These focal abnormalities tend to be nonfixed deficits, meaning they change frequently over time. They may reflect prior structural injuries to the NS that have been unmasked by the uremia or they may reflect selective vulnerability, such as the cortical blindness seen following hypoxia. In uremic patients with vasculitis, the signs may reflect a true structural injury (e.g., CNS infarction); in those patients, the deficits will be fixed rather than changing.

Proposed explanations for the specific signs in UE include arterial hypertension, elevated brain calcium (with neural mineralization), elevated PTH levels, abnormal serum ionized calcium levels, abnormal magnesium homeostasis, acid-base disturbances, uremic vasculitis, osmolar changes, anemia, and other electrolyte derangements. In addition, therapy may play a role in initiating some clinical signs, such as the pontine myelinolysis seen with overrapid correction of hyponatremia or aluminum intoxication (secondary to aluminum hydroxide therapy) (O'Brien, 1992).

In patients with UE, cerebral blood flow is reduced, yet there are normal levels of energy metabolic byproducts. This suggests that energy failure is not involved in the pathogenesis of UE. In at least some studies, CSF acid-base values are normal. The osmotic activity of urea suggests that altered osmolality and water balance may play a role, yet most uremic patients have normal brain osmolality. It is possible that osmotically active substances crucial to the pathogenesis of UE remain to be identified. Abnormal neurotransmitter production or release may be significant in the pathogenesis of UE (Biasioli et al., 1986). Transmitters of greatest interest include glutamine, glycine, and amino acids. The GABA neurotransmitters play a role in hepatic encephalopathy; however, no role for these has been found in the pathogenesis of the clinical signs in UE (Steindl et al., 1991).

There is decreased ATP turnover in uremia, which leads to decreased ion turnover, which affects membrane threshold. This has the potential for affecting neural activity. Urea also may act directly on the brain stem. These findings suggest that there are direct effects of uremia on the CNS.

Electrolytes are abnormal in most patients with uremia, and abnormal electrolyte levels or homeostasis are of particular interest. Abnormalities of sodium, potassium, calcium, and phosphorous may play a significant role in the pathogenesis of UE, as may abnormal PTH levels. Uremic patients have been found to have both elevated brain calcium and brain PTH levels. Parathy-

roid hormone not only regulates serum and soft tissue calcium and phosphorous levels, but plays a role in abnormal aluminum levels as well. Parathyroid hormone may also directly affect neural function. Exogenous administration of PTH can produce electroencephalographic (EEG) changes in dogs that mimic those seen in uremic patients. Phosphorous levels appear unrelated to clinical signs in both acute and chronic renal failure patients. Calcium levels have been elevated in brain tissues of uremic patients, but the significance of that finding is unclear. Those same patients also had significantly elevated PTH levels (Arieff, 1986).

Although the pathogenesis of UE remains uncertain, its reality is clear. The encephalopathy produced in renal failure is often both an important and a frequent sign of the underlying renal failure. In some cases, it may be the only clinical sign seen of the underlying disturbance. In most patients, if the underlying disorder is corrected, neurologic function will be completely restored with no residual histopathologic evidence of neuronal injury.

## CLINICAL PRESENTATION

The most common complaints in patients with UE are seizures and mental changes. Other common signs include weakness of limbs, ataxia, and tremors (Fenner and Mandel, 1992; Wolf, 1980). At The Ohio State University, neurologic manifestations are seen in as many as 65% of patients with primary renal failure. The most common clinical signs are altered consciousness, especially depression or stupor (31% of patients); and seizures (29% of patients). Other, less commonly seen signs included muscle fasciculations, twitching, weakness, and dementia. The patients with chronic renal failure are more likely to have mentational changes, while patients with acute renal failure are more likely to develop seizures; however, all signs may be seen in all patients without regard to the duration of the renal failure (Fenner and Mandel, 1992). Patients with UE usually present with an acute confusional state and nonfixed focal deficits. There is no correlation between the severity of the clinical signs and the degree of azotemia. Many patients will display what is known at the "twitch-convulsive" state, where there is a combination of tremor, myoclonus, and seizures all in the same patient at the same time.

There are four major clinical signs that alert the clinician to examine a patient for a metabolic encephalopathy: (1) altered consciousness, (2) normal ocular motility, (3) abnormal muscle tone, and (4) abnormal ventilation. Finding this combination in any patient should start a vigorous search for a metabolic cause for the signs.

### Altered Consciousness

Most metabolic encephalopathies alter a patient's consciousness. You may see confusion, delirium, obtundation, stupor, or coma, depending on the severity of the clinical condition. Many patients with UE will be agitated or restless and have exaggerated responses to stimulation.

## Oculomotor Responses

Ocular motility and pupillary responsiveness are rarely affected by metabolic brain diseases. The corneal reflexes and oculovestibular reflexes (OVR) should remain intact in most patients with metabolic encephalopathies. Although random, roving eye movements are seen in patients with metabolic encephalopathies, these patients will still have normal OVRs. Normal pupillary reflexes and ocular motility in the presence of abnormal consciousness should immediately start you looking for a metabolic encephalopathy.

## Abnormal Motor Responses

Many patients with metabolic abnormalities will have nonspecific motor abnormalities that center around abnormal tone, including spasms of rigidity, tremors, paratonia, flaccidity, and seizures. Paratonia is a fluctuating resistance to passive movement. In my experience, both focal myoclonus and focal seizures are seen in patients with UE, especially patients with acute renal failure. You may also see generalized myoclonus in alkalotic and hypocalcemic patients. Patients with ethylene glycol intoxication frequently have direct neural intoxication, acid-base abnormalities, electrolyte disturbances, and UE all concurrently. These patients often have a confusing neurologic examination.

## Abnormal Ventilation (Respiration)

In humans, metabolic encephalopathies almost always alter respiratory patterns, frequently in a characteristic manner. These alterations have not been reported in veterinary medicine, possibly because we have not looked carefully enough. Many patients with UE have ataxic respiration. This respiratory pattern is characterized by slow, shallow, irregular respirations that are not increased by hypoxia or hypercapnia. Ataxic respiration appears to reflect a hyposensitivity of the brain stem to chemoreceptor stimulation. Uremia itself may also cause abnormal respiration, especially hyperventilation. Hyperventilation may also be seen in UE patients secondary to acid-base disturbances.

## DIAGNOSTIC APPROACH

Uremic encephalopathy usually presents as an acute confusional state with nonfixed focal deficits. There is no correlation between the severity of the signs and the degree of uremia. Many patients display the twitch-convulsive state, manifested by a combination of tremor, myoclonus, and seizures all at the same time. Serum biochemistries will document renal failure. In some cases, there may be severe associated electrolyte, osmolality, and acid-base disturbances. The anemia of chronic renal failure may also contribute to many of the observed clinical signs, inasmuch as human patients treated with erythropoietin improved in parallel with the change in hematocrit levels (Nissenson, 1992) (see "CVT Update: Use of Recombinant Human Erythropoietin," this volume, p 961).

Electrodiagnostic studies are used extensively in humans with renal failure and could be used in veterinary practice to document this condition. Quantitative electroencephalography and sensory-evoked potentials have shown that as many as 37% of human renal failure patients have abnormal neural function (Nissenson, 1992). Routine electroencephalography has often been used as a screening tool for patients with metabolic encephalopathy. In patients with renal failure, the presence of triphasic waves is considered a reliable indicator of CNS dysfunction. Especially in patients with persistent focal deficits, magnetic resonance imaging (MRI) or computed tomography (CT) is indicated to rule out the presence of mass effects or vascular injury to the CNS. Even in patients with systemic neoplasms, onset of neurologic signs may be related to concurrent metabolic encephalopathy rather than to brain metastases. Reversible abnormalities, especially in white matter, have been seen on CT and MRI of patients with UE. These changes have been symmetric, suggesting they were metabolic in nature (Okada et al., 1991).

In short, the diagnosis of UE is based on serum biochemistries supporting a diagnosis of renal failure and a neurologic examination consistent with a diffuse cerebral encephalopathy. When clinical signs persist despite successful management of renal failure, additional studies or referral is appropriate.

## TREATMENT

The principal therapy is to treat the underlying condition (see Section 10). If a patient has severe electrolyte disturbances, they should be corrected, as they may contribute directly to the encephalopathy (O'Brien, 1992). Both sodium excess and deficiency are detrimental to the CNS; however, rapid correction of hyponatremia may induce severe, long-term consequences including myelinolysis of CNS.

Correction of moderate to severe anemia is critical in renal failure patients (see "Approach to the Anemic Patient," this volume, p 447), as is correction of calcium and phosphorus abnormalities. Hyperphosphatemia should be treated with magnesium hydroxide rather than aluminum hydroxide oral suspensions, to prevent the development of aluminum intoxication.

Supportive therapy, including treatment of seizures, may be necessary in the short term. Acute renal failure patients are more likely to seizure due to the effects of the uremia. Use of short-acting anticonvulsants such as diazepam are preferred. Careful serum monitoring of anticonvulsant levels is essential, as the excretion of anticonvulsants is diminished in patients with UE.

The long-term prognosis in these patients is determined by the reversible nature of the renal failure. In acute renal failure patients with a reversible condition, the UE may be completely reversed. In chronic renal failure patients, the long-term prognosis is poor and daily management is the key to success.

## References and Suggested Reading

Arieff AI: Neurologic manifestations of uremia. *In* Brenner BR and Rector FC (eds): *The Kidney*, 3rd edition. Philadelphia, WB Saunders Co, 1986, p 1731.
*A review of the clinical manifestations of uremic encephalopathy with a brief review of pathophysiology.*
Biasioli S, D'Andrea G, Ferianin M, et al: Uremic encephalopathy: An updating. Clin Nephrol 25:57, 1986.
*A review of the pathophysiology, clinical presentation, and proposed treatment of uremic encephalopathy.*
De DP, Saxena VK, Abts H, et al: Clinical and pathophysiological aspects of neurological complications in renal failure. Acta Neurol Belg 92: 191, 1992.
*A review and historical overview of the pathophysiology and clinical presentation of uremic encephalopathy and neuropathies.*
Fenner WR and Mandel W: Uremic encephalopathy. *In Proc 10th Ann ACVIM Forum*, San Diego, CA, 1992, p 745.
*A review of the clinical presentation of uremic encephalopathy in dogs, with an emphasis on proposed mechanisms of injury.*
Lockwood AH: Neurologic complications of renal disease. *In* Riggs JE (ed): *Neurologic Manifestations of Systemic Disease*. Philadelphia, WB Saunders Co, 1989, p 617.
*A review of the pathophysiology, clinical presentation, and proposed treatment of uremic encephalopathy.*
Nissenson AR: Epoetin and cognitive function. Am J Kidney Dis 20(suppl 1): 21, 1992.
*A review of the effects of anemia on cognitive function in uremic encephalopathy and research results using erythropoietin to reverse the anemia.*
O'Brien D: The CNS effects of sodium imbalances. Proc 10th Ann ACVIM Forum, San Diego, CA, 1992, p 741.
*A review of the clinical presentation of electrolyte imbalances in dogs, with an emphasis on proposed mechanisms of injury.*
Okada J, Yoshikawa K, Matsuo H, et al: Reversible MRI and CT findings in uremic encephalopathy. Neuroradiology 33:524, 1991.
*A case presentation of MRI and CT findings in a human patient with uremic encephalopathy.*
Steindl P, Puspok A, Druml W, et al: Beneficial effect of pharmacological modulation of the GABA a-benzodiazepine receptor on hepatic encephalopathy in the rat: Comparison with uremic encephalopathy. Hepatology 14:963, 1991.
*A research discussion of the attempts to elucidate the neurotransmitters involved in metabolic encephalopathies.*
Wolf AM: Canine uremic encephalopathy. J Am Anim Hosp Assoc 16:735, 1980.
*A case presentation and discussion of uremic encephalopathy in the dog.*

# CANINE LIPID STORAGE MYOPATHIES

## G. DIANE SHELTON
*La Jolla, California*

A lipid storage myopathy can be defined as one in which abnormal amounts of lipid accumulate in muscle and the lipid accumulation represents the predominant, or a predominant, pathologic alteration (Engel, 1986). In humans, most lipid storage myopathies recognized to date are associated with a derangement of carnitine metabolism (either primary or secondary), with mitochondrial abnormalities, or with disorders of fatty acid oxidation involving β-oxidation. Findings of a vacuolar myopathy with increased intramyofiber lipid within a fresh frozen muscle biopsy specimen should provide a clue to an underlying metabolic abnormality and a stimulus for further metabolic and biochemical studies.

## FATTY ACID OXIDATION IN NORMAL SKELETAL MUSCLE

Fatty acid oxidation is the preferred energy source in the heart and skeletal muscle and is important in the smooth functioning of these organs. Adequate muscle carnitine concentrations are essential for this process. Carnitine is a carrier for long-chain fatty acids from the sarcoplasma across mitochondrial membranes. With inadequate concentrations of carnitine, triglycerides accumulate within the cytoplasm and may be demonstrated as lipid droplets within a muscle biopsy section. Once inside mitochondria, fatty acids are uncoupled from carnitine and react with coenzyme A (CoA) to form acyl-CoAs. During the process of β-oxidation, each molecule of acyl-CoA (carbon chains of greater than two atoms in length) is cleaved to form one molecule of acetyl-CoA (carbon chain of two atoms) and a new acyl-CoA (shortened by two carbon atoms). Resulting acetyl-CoA then enters the citric acid cycle and electron transport chain for generation of adenosine triphosphate (ATP).

Carnitine also functions to remove toxic acyl compounds that build up when the metabolic system malfunctions or is overloaded by rejoining with the acyl group and forming an acylcarnitine ester. This scavenging function is important, since high concentrations of acyl-CoA compounds are mitochondrial toxins resulting in inhibition of oxidative phosphorylation.

A derangement in one or more steps in the above scheme may result in impaired oxidation of fatty acid, diversion of fatty acids for triglyceride synthesis, and symptoms related to lack of energy utilization from fatty acids.

## CLINICAL PRESENTATIONS

The most common presenting clinical signs in a large group of dogs studied at the Comparative Neuromuscular Laboratory at the University of California, San Diego were poorly localizable muscle pain (acute and chronic), muscle atrophy, and weakness (Shelton, 1993). Less frequently reported clinical presentations included stiffness, lameness, cramping, exercise intolerance, and tremors. Cardiomyopathy was reported in only two cases. In most cases, a diagnosis was not reached after extensive clinical and laboratory evaluations. The majority of the dogs were adult, without a sex or breed predilection.

## DIAGNOSIS

A diagnosis of a lipid storage myopathy is based upon the light microscopic demonstration of accumulation of lipid droplets within myofibers in fresh-frozen muscle biopsy sections (Fig. 1). Normally, there is very little if any lipid within a muscle biopsy section using the oil red O or Sudan black stains. The abnormal lipid deposits in humans have consisted predominantly of triglycerides. Since triglyceride accumulation may result from an abnormality in any of the several steps involved with oxidative energy production in muscle, extensive metabolic and biochemical analyses must be performed for further definition of the disorder(s) (Carroll, 1988; Haas and Nyhan, 1992). In humans, ischemia and obesity have also been reported to increase the muscle fiber lipid content. The diagnostic pathway used at the Comparative Neuromuscular Laboratory for investigating these patients is shown in Figure 2.

Evaluation of lactate and pyruvate levels within plasma and urine has been valuable in differentiating these disorders and providing a preliminary subclassification. Lactic acidemia and aciduria may be physiologic or pathologic and it is important to differentiate

these disorders, as some are treatable. Comprehensive quantitative organic acid analysis in the urine is the major tool for differentiating the pathologic causes of lactic acidemia (Haas, 1992). Carnitine quantitation in muscle, plasma, and urine (total, free, and esterified) should also be performed, since some primary and secondary disorders with low muscle carnitine can be successfully treated with carnitine supplementation. While these testing procedures are expensive and performed only in very specialized laboratories studying metabolic disorders, an ongoing study is currently underway at the Comparative Neuromuscular Laboratory on dogs with confirmed lipid storage myopathy that subsidizes these further studies.

As in human medicine, it is clear from preliminary studies in dogs that defects in many areas of oxidative metabolism may result in increased intramyofiber lipid and muscle weakness (Shelton, 1993). It is important that these disorders are defined so that specific therapies can be formulated.

## TREATMENT

If low levels of muscle carnitine are documented, a trial course of oral L-carnitine (Sigma-Tau Pharmaceuticals, Gaithersburg, MD) should be instituted at 50 mg/kg twice daily. This has resulted in a dramatic improvement in muscle mass and strength in some dogs (Shelton, unpublished observation). Response to therapy has not been as dramatic in dogs with significant lactic and pyruvic aciduria and secondary low muscle carnitine; however, some improvement may be noted.

A number of other therapeutic modalities have been suggested for human patients such as supplementation with riboflavin (50 to 100 mg daily), vitamin C (50 mg/kg daily), or coenzyme Q (1 mg/kg daily); however, their efficacy is not clear. Dietary manipulations such as a low-fat, high-carbohydrate, high-protein diet and supplementation with medium-chain triglycerides may be

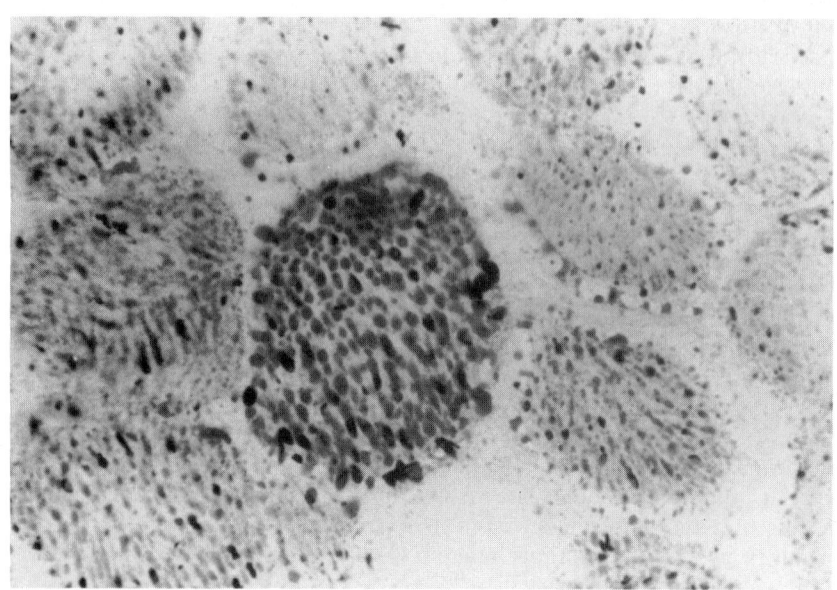

**Figure 1.** Oil red O stain of a fresh frozen muscle biopsy from a dog with secondary muscle carnitine deficiency. Triglyceride droplets characteristic of a lipid storage myopathy are present within the myofibers. X400.

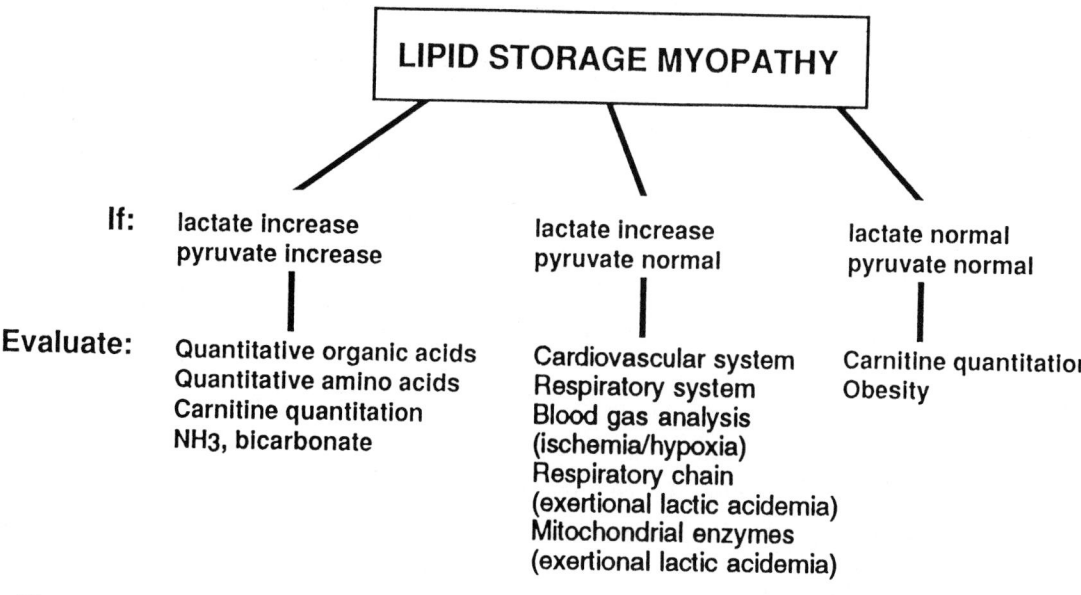

**Figure 2.** Diagnostic pathway used by the Comparative Neuromuscular Laboratory, University of California, San Diego for the investigation of lipid storage myopathies.

helpful in some cases. In humans, corticosteroid-responsive lipid myopathies have also been reported (Carroll, 1988).

## References and Suggested Reading

Carroll JE: Myopathies caused by disorders of lipid metabolism. *In Neurologic Clinics.* Philadelphia, WB Saunders Co, 1988, p 563.

*A general discussion of clinical presentations and diagnosis of lipid storage myopathies in human patients.*
Engel AG: Carnitine deficiency syndromes and lipid storage myopathies. *In* Engel AG and Banker BQ (eds): *Myology.* New York, McGraw-Hill Book Company, 1986, p 1663.
*In-depth discussion of myopathology and known biochemical pathways involved in lipid storage in humans.*
Haas RH and Nyhan WL: Disorders of organic acids. *In* Berg B (ed): *Neurologic Aspects of Pediatrics.* Boston, Butterworth-Heinemann, 1992, p 47.
*In-depth discussion of lactic acidemias and organic acid disorders in humans.*
Shelton GD: Canine lipid storage myopathies. *In Proc 11th ACVIM Forum,* Washington, DC, 1993, p 707.
*General discussion of what is known about lipid storage disorders in dogs.*

# HYPERCHYLOMICRONEMIA IN THE CAT

BOYD R. JONES
*Palmerston North, New Zealand*

Hyperchylomicronemia is the presence of excess concentrations of chylomicrons (CM) in plasma resulting from a decrease in clearance of this lipoprotein from plasma. Chylomicrons transport dietary lipids from the intestine, delivering triglyceride (TG) to the extrahepatic tissues and cholesterol to the liver. Chylomicrons and the very-low-density lipoproteins (VLDLs) are predominantly involved in triglyceride transport. Low-density lipoproteins (LDLs) and high-density-lipoproteins (HDLs) are involved predominantly in cholesterol transport. Lipoprotein metabolism and hyperlipidemia in the dog and cat have been reviewed recently (Watson and Barrie, 1993).

The enzyme lipoprotein lipase (LPL), which is located in the vascular endothelium, is responsible for hydrolysing the TG of CM and VLDL, releasing free fatty acids and monoglycerides. The activity of LPL is dependent on apolipoprotein C-II as a cofactor, which is transferred from HDL to the surface of CM as they enter circulation. The removal of TG from the core of CM leaves a cholesterol-rich remnant particle that is rapidly cleared from circulation by the liver. Another lipase enzyme located in the liver, hepatic lipase (HL), also has a function in the hydrolysis of TG.

Both primary and secondary disorders of lipid metabolism that result in hyperchylomicronemia have

**Table 1.** *Clinical Features of Idiopathic or Primary Hyperchylomicronemia in the Cat (after Watson et al., 1992)*[*]

| Author | Breed | Age | Sex | Presenting Signs | Triglyceride | Other Findings |
|---|---|---|---|---|---|---|
| Jones et al. (1983) | Domestic shorthair | 8 mo | M | Hindlimb lameness Horner's syndrome | 90 | Lipemia retinalis Cutaneous xanthomas One half brother affected |
| Bauer and Verlander (1984) | Himalayan | 3 wk | M | Poor growth Xantholesma | 143 | Lipemia retinalis Anemia One sibling affected |
| Jones et al. (1986) | Domestic shorthair (20 cats) | | M/F | Peripheral nerve paralyses | 10.02 (mean) | Lipemia retinalis Splenic rupture Xanthomas in abdominal organs Cutaneous xanthomas |
| Sottiaux (1986) Brooks (1989) | European Persian | 9 yr 2 yr | MN FN | Xantholesma Iridocyclitis | 17 2.5 | Lipid in aqueous humor Lipemia retinalis Xanthogranulomata skin |
| Smerdon (1990) | Siamese | 4 wk | M | Hindlimb paralysis | Not reported | Two siblings affected |
| Grieshaber et al. (1991) | Domestic shorthair long hair | 2 yr 5 yr | MN | Eruptive xanthomas skin | 63 and 146 | |
| Watson et al. (1992) | Siamese | 4–8 wk | M/F | Lethargy Inappetance ataxia | 14.9–72.0 | Severe anemia |

[*]From Jones BR: Hyperchylomicronaemia in the cat. J Small Anim Pract 34:493, 1993, with permission.

been described in cats (Whitney, 1992). The most common secondary disorder is diabetes mellitus, most often induced by megestrol acetate administration. The activity of LPL is reduced in insulin deficiency.

Primary inherited disorders of lipoprotein metabolism resulting in hyperchylomicronemia are uncommon but have been reported in cats in the United States, United Kingdom, France, and New Zealand (Table 1) (Jones, 1993). The family of affected cats in New Zealand has been investigated in some depth, with the genetic and molecular basis of the defect in CM metabolism being known.

## CLINICAL SIGNS

The clinical signs of hyperchylomicronemia are shown in Table 2. The clinical signs are associated with an excessive concentration of TG due to increased numbers of CM and, to a lesser extent, VLDL, in the plasma. For unexplained reasons, some cats can have massive hyperchylomicronemia but show no or few clinical signs, whereas cats with much lower CM and TG concentrations develop significant clinical signs. The most common signs detected are lipemia retinalis and the formation of xanthomas. Lipemia retinalis occurs when the plasma TG concentration is greater than 1300 mg/dl, and can be detected by examination of the ocular fundus. The retinal arterioles and veins develop a pale pink color due to scattering of light by the large CM. Vision is not affected and there appear to be no clinical sequelae. Other ocular consequences of hyperchylomicronemia may be seen in some cats: xantholesma, lipid keratopathy, and lipid in the anterior chamber have been reported. In these cases, the lipid has

accumulated due to ocular inflammation from another cause.

Xanthomas are deposits of lipid in the skin or other tissues. Trauma and damage to small blood vessels predisposes to their formation. In the 20 cases reported by Jones et al. (1986), xanthomas occurred in areas of the body subjected to trauma. Common sites included those where nerves emerged through a vertebral foramina, at the ischiatic notch, or over bony prominences. The presence of xanthomas at these sites resulted in pressure on the nerves with loss of conscious proprioception and motor paralysis. Sensation to painful stimuli was retained when mixed motor and sensory nerves were affected. Horner's syndrome and tibial and radial nerve paralyses were the most frequently detected neuropathies. Xanthomas occurred at other sites, in the skin where they were observed or palpable as firm nodules or eruptive plaques. The liver, spleen,

**Table 2.** *Clinical Signs of Hyperchylomicronemia*

**Common Signs**
Fasting hyperlipidemia
 CM and VLDL elevation
Lipemia retinalis
Xanthomas
 Cutaneous and other tissues
Peripheral nerve paralysis
 Horner's syndrome
 Tibial nerve
 Radial nerve
 Other neuropathies

**Less Common Signs**
Splenomegaly
Xantholesma
Lipid keratopathy
Anemia

kidney, and intestinal mesentery may contain xanthomas, where they may be palpable if large enough.

Severe anemia may be found in young (<4 weeks) hyperlipidemic kittens. The kittens are weak and lethargic, usually in the suckling period, and some may die. It appears that there may be factors common to the pathogenesis of the hyperlipidemia and the anemia, but this possible association needs further investigation (Watson et al., 1992).

## INHERITANCE

Hyperchylomicronemia has a familial incidence. The affected cats in New Zealand were all related and the disease inherited as an autosomal recessive trait. The heterozygous cats may appear healthy, but they have reduced LPL activity (a gene dosage effect) and can become hyperlipidemic if fed a high-fat diet. Related animals should be investigated if a primary hyperlipidemia is suspected.

## LABORATORY EVALUATION

Most affected cats show fasting (>24 hr) hyperchylomicronemia. The blood has the appearance of "cream-of-tomato" soup. The plasma is lactescent. A minimum of laboratory data (complete blood count [CBC], biochemistry panel, urinalysis) will eliminate or confirm secondary causes of hyperlipidemia (e.g., diabetes mellitus). Confirmation of a primary cause of hyperlipidemia requires elimination of the secondary causes and then detailed apolipoprotein analysis, measurement of LPL activity, and so forth. These latter tests are usually only completed at lipid research laboratories and are *not* routinely available at veterinary clinical laboratories. The most basic tests include measurement of plasma cholesterol and triglyceride concentrations. Some individual animals may have massive elevation of plasma TG (6000 to 12000 mg/dl) but most are lower. The mean cholesterol and TG concentrations of 24 affected cats were 250 mg/dl and 900 mg/dl. The plasma usually becomes lactescent when the TG concentration is greater than 500 mg/dl. These basic measurements allow confirmation of hyperchylomicronemia and hypertriglyceridemia, measure the severity of the problem, and also give a baseline for the success or otherwise of management and therapy.

Lipoprotein electrophoresis identifies altered distribution of the different classes of apolipoprotein, but the patterns are not disease specific. In inherited hyperchylomicronemia, there is an increased CM concentration and a more marked VLDL band in the pre-$\beta$ position. Ultracentrifugation studies have shown that the major proportion of TG and cholesterol is contained in CM and, although HDL is still the predominant cholesterol carrier, its concentration is decreased in the plasma of hyperchylomicronemic cats. This finding is expected with reduced LPL activity. Ultracentrifugation studies provide a quantitative method of measurement of cholesterol TG and apolipoprotein in the different lipoprotein classes.

## LIPOPROTEIN LIPASE ACTIVITY

Defective LPL function and the delayed clearance of CM from circulation is the main cause of hyperchylomicronemia. Determination of the activity of this enzyme is sometimes warranted, but assays are not readily available to veterinarians in practice. If LPL assays are required, special assistance should be sought from a lipid research laboratory. Some lipid research laboratories have the ability to measure not only LPL enzyme activity but also enzyme mass. Because of the close homology of structure between the human and cat LPL enzyme, enzyme-linked immunosorbent assay (ELISA) technology has allowed the determination of the mass of enzyme in circulation (Peritz et al., 1990).

Lipoprotein lipase activity can be measured indirectly by collecting plasma before and 10 min after the intravenous administration of heparin (40 to 90 IU/kg), which activates the enzyme *in vivo*. The concentration of lipoprotein can be measured before and afterwards. No change in the pattern suggests defective LPL activity. Alternatively, if special laboratories are used, lipase activity and lipase mass can be measured in both samples. Lipoprotein lipase activity can also be differentiated from HL activity.

Peritz et al. (1990) showed that the family of cats from New Zealand had large quantities of LPL protein in circulation in the presence and absence of heparin, but no LPL activity. The defect in this family of cats is an inactive LPL protein with a point mutation of the LPL gene at a site that codes for the heparin-binding domain of the protein. Subsequent studies have identified a base-pair mutation (arginine for glycine) at the human equivalent of amino acid codon 409 (Ginzinger, personal communication, 1993). Despite definition of the molecular defect in one family of cats, other affected cats might have different defects in LPL structure and function. The presence of plasma factors that inhibit LPL function and the absence of the activator (apolipoprotein C-II) have been identified in humans with inherited hyperchylomicronemia.

## MANAGEMENT

All of the clinical signs of hyperchylomicronemia are reversible if the plasma TG concentrations are reduced. The presence of excess CM in plasma is directly proportional to the fat content in the diet. Cats with a fasting plasma TG concentration of greater than 500 mg/dl should be treated. In cats with secondary hyperlipidemia, treating the primary disease will usually return the lipid concentrations to the reference range. The main thrust of management must be directed towards treating the cause of the hypertriglyceridemia.

In primary hyperchylomicronemia, a low-fat, high-fiber diet will result in a reduction in plasma lipid concentrations. Affected kittens that are still suckling should be weaned. Prescription diets (Hill's r/d, Hill's Pet Nutrition, Topeka, KS), or a homemade low-fat diet, are effective in reducing plasma TG concentrations close to the reference range. Measurement of plasma TG and cholesterol concentrations each month is recommended to assess the response to dietary therapy.

Often, dietary management is unsuccessful, and drugs used to decrease plasma TG concentrations in human patients must be prescribed. Most of these drugs have not been evaluated in cats, but this author has found Gemfibrozil (Parke-Davis; 7.5 mg/kg every 12 hr PO) to be effective in some patients.

## References and Suggested Reading

Jones BR, Johnstone AC, Cahill JI, et al: Peripheral neuropathy in cats with inherited primary hyperchylomicronaemia. Vet Rec 119:268, 1986.
*Results of investigation of 20 cases of inherited hyperchylomicronemia with description of the nervous signs caused by xanthomata.*
Jones BR: Hyperchylomicronaemia in the cat. J Small Anim Pract 34:493, 1993.
*A review of hyperchylomicronemia in the cat.*
Peritz LN, Brunzell JH, Harvey-Clark C, et al: Characterisation of a lipoprotein lipase Class III type defect in hypertriglyceridemic cats. Clin Invest Med 13:259, 1990.
*An investigation of the molecular basis of lipoprotein lipase deficiency in a family of cats.*
Watson TDG, Gaffrey D, Mooney CT, et al: Inherited hyperchylomicronaemia in the cat. Lipoprotein lipase function and gene structure. J Small Anim Pract 33:207, 1992.
*An investigation of the molecular basis of lipoprotein lipase deficiency in a family of cats.*
Watson TDG and Barrie J: Lipoprotein metabolism and hyperlipidaemia in the dog and cat: A review. J Small Anim Pract 34:479, 1993.
*A review of lipoprotein metabolism and hyperlipidemia in the dog and cat.*
Whitney MS: Evaluation of hyperlipidemias in dogs and cats. Semin Vet Med Surg 7:292, 1992.
*A review of lipid metabolism in the dog and cat and evaluation of the lipidemic patient.*

# THE USE OF THE LABORATORY IN THE DIAGNOSIS OF JOINT DISORDERS OF DOGS AND CATS

STEVEN C. SCHRADER
*Columbus, Ohio*

Veterinarians can usually determine the cause of lameness without radiologic evaluation or laboratory testing if they have an accurate history, are knowledgeable of the clinical features of the various disorders that cause lameness, and have the ability to perform and interpret the physical examination. Radiologic evaluation may help to further define the problem or to confirm or deny the clinical diagnosis or supposition. Unfortunately, radiographic abnormalities are usually subtle and nonspecific in the early stages of many joint disorders. The radiographic changes remain so even in the later stages of the nonerosive inflammatory disorders (i.e., idiopathic immune-mediated arthritis and systemic lupus erythematosus).

Laboratory testing is indicated whenever the cause or nature of the joint disorder remains in doubt. Knowledge of sensitivity and specificity of a particular test provides the veterinarian with an insight concerning the value of the test in the diagnostic process. As there are limitations associated with most methods of laboratory evaluation, it is always prudent to consider the results of serologic, microbiologic, and histopathologic evaluations within the context established by the historical and physical examinations. Although there are few hematologic, serum biochemical, or urine tests that are specifically indicated in animals having joint disease, some joint disorders are a manifestation of systemic illness and such tests are indicated. Systemic lupus erythematosus (SLE) provides a good example. Anemia, thrombocytopenia, leukopenia, hypoproteinemia, and proteinuria are common with this disease.

## ARTHROCENTESIS AND JOINT FLUID ANALYSIS

Joint fluid (synovia) analysis provides more clinically useful information than any other laboratory test used in the diagnosis of joint disease in dogs and cats. It is illogical to perform tests for rheumatoid factor, antinuclear antibodies, and the antibodies to *Borrelia burgdorferi* without prior or concurrent examination of joint fluid.

Joint fluid collection and analysis is especially useful in differentiating inflammatory from noninflammatory joint disease and in determining the presence of bacterial infection (Table 1). Even though polymorphonuclear cells are the predominate cells in most of the inflammatory joint disorders, the numbers and relative proportions of nucleated cells can have diagnostic significance. Joint fluid analysis also provides information that can help the veterinarian determine the diagnosis

**Table 1.** *Classification of Joint Disease Based on Joint Fluid Analysis*\*

| | Noninflammatory | | | Inflammatory | |
| | Degenerative | Hemarthrosis (Trauma) | Neoplastic | Infectious | Noninfectious |
|---|---|---|---|---|---|
| Color | Pale yellow | Red | Yellow to blood-tinged | Yellow to sanguineous | Yellow to sanguineous |
| Turbidity | Clear-slight | Blood-tinged | Slight to moderate | Turbid to purulent | Slight to turbid |
| Viscosity | Normal | Reduced | Reduced | Reduced | Reduced |
| Mucin clot | Normal | Fair | Normal | Poor | Poor to fair |
| Red cells | Few | Many | Few to moderate | Moderate | Few to moderate |
| White cells | Few | Moderate | Moderate | Many | Many |
| Neutrophils | Few | Moderate | Moderate | Many | Moderate to many |
| Toxic change | None | None | None | Mild to prominent | None to mild |
| Neoplastic cells | — | — | +† | | — |
| Microorganisms | — | — | — | +‡ | — |
| Fluid blood/ glucose ratio | Normal (0.8–1) | Normal (1.0) | Low (0.5–0.8) | Very low (<0.5) | Low (0.5–0.8) |

\*Modified from Wilkins RJ: Joint serology. *In* Bojrab MJ (ed): *Pathophysiology in Small Animal Surgery.* Philadelphia, Lea & Febiger, 1981, p 553, with permission.
†Neoplastic cells not always detected.
‡Microorganisms not always detected.

when radiographic changes have not had time to develop or when the changes are subtle or nonspecific. Joint fluid analysis is more sensitive than palpation for detecting the presence of joint inflammation. Analysis of joint fluid often suggests continuation of the inflammatory process even though joint swelling and lameness appear to have resolved.

One must also consider the diagnostic limitations associated with joint fluid analysis. Based on joint fluid analysis alone, it may not be possible to differentiate one inflammatory or noninflammatory disorder from another. All of the various inflammatory disorders are characterized by high nucleated cell counts; these cells directly or indirectly affect clarity, color, and viscosity of the fluid (Table 1). White blood cell (WBC) counts of 50,000/cm³ or greater are commonplace with septic arthritis, SLE, and idiopathic immune-mediated joint disease. Septic arthritis may be difficult to confirm when no degenerative neutrophils or bacteria are seen and when culturing techniques fail. As such, the results of joint fluid analysis should always be considered in concert with clinical, radiographic, and other findings. Knowledge of the clinical features of the various joint disorders allows the veterinarian to properly interpret the analysis.

## Collection

The methods used for collection of joint fluid are similar in the dog and cat. The procedure is relatively simple and complications are rare. Some of the sites used for arthrocentesis are illustrated in Figure 1. Arthrocentesis can usually be performed without chemical restraint or local anesthesia. The hair is clipped from the arthrocentesis site(s) and the exposed skin is cleansed. It is not necessary to perform a surgical scrub or to wear sterile gloves in order to safely collect joint fluid. I prefer to use a 21-gauge needle attached to a 3-cc syringe to collect the fluid; it is difficult to obtain

inspissated fluid when a needle of smaller bore is employed. Once the joint is entered, gentle suction is applied until fluid is no longer obtained or if blood appears in the syringe.

Once the fluid has been collected, the color, clarity, viscosity, and amount of fluid are noted and recorded. A drop of fluid is used to make a smear for cytologic examination and a portion of the sample submitted for culture and sensitivity testing. Inoculation of some type of enriched media such as trypticase soy or thioglycollate broth is recommended. Any remaining fluid is placed in a tube containing ethylenediaminetetraacetic acid (EDTA) anticoagulant and submitted for cell count and biochemical evaluation.

As the amount of joint fluid obtained is often insufficient for complete analysis, priorities must be established for the analysis to yield the most information. Cytologic evaluation and microbiologic testing are of utmost importance. When only one or two drops of fluid have been obtained, a small drop of fluid is transferred to a glass slide (without touching the needle to the slide) and a smear is made; the needle and syringe are then flushed with enrichment broth to allow culture and sensitivity testing.

## Gross Examination

Joint fluid analysis should begin at the very moment that the fluid is withdrawn from the joint. Normal joint fluid is clear (acellular) and is light straw colored or colorless, it has a sticky viscid character due to the presence of hyaluronate and will not clot, because of a lack of prothrombin, fibrinogen, factor V, factor VII, and tissue thromboplastin. Only a small amount of fluid is normally present; no more than a few tenths of a milliliter of joint fluid can be collected from most normal joints.

Bloody fluid may be obtained when the arthrocentesis is traumatic; iatrogenic blood is usually incom-

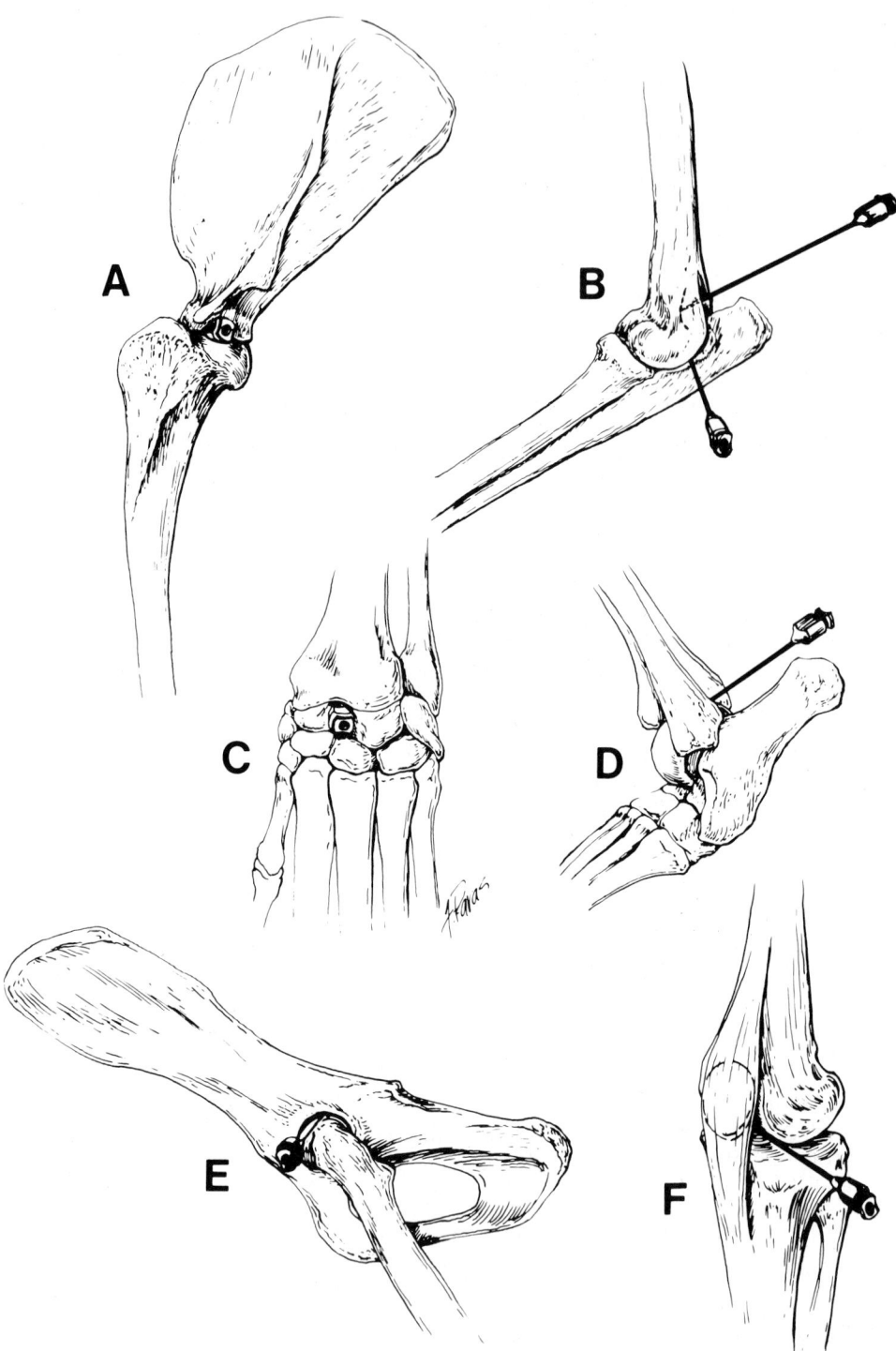

**Figure 1.** Schematic representation of sites recommended for arthrocentesis of various joints of the cat and dog. *A*, Lateral view of the shoulder joint. The needle is advanced from lateral to medial just caudodistal to the distal tip of the acromion. *B*, Lateral view of the elbow joint. The needle is advanced in a craniomedial direction through the anconeus muscle and into the joint. Alternatively, the needle is directed medial to the lateral epicondylar ridge and into the olecranon fossa while the elbow is held in a moderate degree of flexion. *C*, Cranial view of the carpus. The needle is advanced between the tendons of insertion of the extensor carpi radialis and common digital extensor muscles and into the radiocarpal joint. *D*, Lateral view of the tarsal joint. The needle is inserted into the caudal portion of the joint immediately medial to the lateral malleolus or immediately lateral to the medial malleolus. The joint is held in slight flexion to facilitate entry into the joint. *E*, Lateral view of the hip joint. The needle is advanced in a medial direction into the craniodorsal portion of the joint. The greater trochanter is used for orientation. *F*, Craniolateral view of the stifle joint. The needle is advanced in a caudomedial direction to enter the joint immediately lateral and distal to the distal tip of the patella. (From Schrader SC and Sherding RG: Disorders of the skeletal system. *In* Sherding RG (ed): *The Cat; Diseases and Clinical Management.* New York, Churchill Livingstone, 1989, p 1251, with permission.)

pletely mixed with the joint fluid and is usually bright red or pink. The presence of blood in joint fluid may allow a clot to develop. High numbers of nucleated cells increase joint fluid turbidity; viscosity of joint fluid may decrease because of destruction, dilution, or insufficient production of hyaluronate. Synovitis may result in excessive production of fluid. If joint fluid is discolored, turbid, lacks viscosity, or is excessive in amount, joint disease is present. Viscosity can be estimated by placing a drop of fluid on the fingertip, touching the drop with the pulp of the thumb, and then withdrawing the thumb. Normal fluid will form a 1- to 2-inch-long continuous strand between the apposing digits. Viscosity can also be estimated by observing a drop of the fluid fall to the slide that is used to prepare a smear. Because the aforementioned abnormalities are characteristic of inflammatory joint disease (Table 1), gross evaluation alone can help the veterinarian distinguish between inflammatory and noninflammatory joint disease. Correlation of the gross characteristics of joint fluid with the clinical scenario can help the veterinarian begin to make diagnostic and therapeutic decisions while cytologic and microbiologic analyses are pending.

## Cytologic and Microbiologic Examinations

Joint fluid analysis should always include microscopic examination of a smear preparation. Such examination allows the veterinarian to determine the number and relative proportions of various cell types. It allows the detection of toxic change in polymorphonuclear cells and may allow the detection of microorganisms. Culture and sensitivity testing should always be performed because it is crucial to differentiate septic from immune-mediated joint disease; such differentiation is not usually possible by gross or cytologic examinations alone.

Normal joint fluid contains less than 2500 to 3000 WBC/cm$^3$ and very few red blood cells; mononuclear cells predominate. Elevation of WBC count indicates inflammatory joint disease. The WBC count can be estimated by comparing blood and joint fluid smears. For example, if an average of ten cells are found per high-power field (HPF) on the blood smear of a dog having a WBC count of 20,000/cm$^3$ and there is an average of 20 cells per HPF on the joint fluid smear, the joint fluid would contain about 40,000 WBC/cm$^3$. With very little practice, one can accurately determine that the joint fluid WBC count is elevated and establish the relative proportions of nucleated cells that are present.

There is tremendous variation in WBC count with each of the inflammatory joint disorders and considerable overlap between disorders. Polymorphonuclear cells are the principal cell type of most inflammatory joint disorders; however, mononuclear cells may predominate in animals having rheumatoid arthritis and plasmacytic-lymphocytic arthritis. The WBC count rarely exceeds 40,000/cm$^3$ with these diseases, whereas the WBC count may easily surpass this number with SLE, idiopathic immune-mediated arthritis, and septic

arthritis (also see "Treatment of the Immune-Based Inflammatory Arthropathies of the Dog and Cat," this volume, p 1188).

In addition to culture and sensitivity testing, detecting neutrophils with toxic changes and observing microorganisms on microscopic examination of joint fluid will help one distinguish infectious from noninfectious inflammatory disorders. Unfortunately, culture and sensitivity testing of joint fluid has failed to document the presence of bacteria in known cases of infection, not all infections cause such changes in neutrophils, and organisms may not be detected on examination of the smear even if they are present. The veterinarian will have to rely on the clinical scenario and their own good judgment when analysis of joint fluid has failed to distinguish between septic and noninfectious inflammatory joint disease.

## Other Joint Fluid Examinations

Once enough fluid has been collected for cytologic and microbiologic evaluations of joint fluid, very little additional information of diagnostic significance can be gained by determination of biochemical values and mucin clot test. Assays for antibody or immune complexes might become more practical and meaningful in the future.

## RHEUMATOID FACTOR(S)

A number of antibodies have been detected in the blood and joint fluid of humans with an erosive or destructive form of arthritis known as rheumatoid arthritis. Collectively, these antibodies have been deemed the rheumatoid factors (RFs); their presence suggests that immunologic processes may, in some way, be associated with the pathogenesis of the disease. The exact role that these immunoglobulins play in the pathogenesis of the disease is unknown.

An IgM class immunoglobulin is generally considered the rheumatoid factor in dogs. Modified Waaler-Rose and latex agglutination tests are most frequently used to detect its presence. There is controversy over what constitutes a positive titer with the Waaler-Rose test. Bennett and Kirkham (1987a) suggest the test is positive with titers of 1:40 or greater; others have considered a titer as low as 1:8 to be positive (Halliwell, 1978; Newton, 1976). Rheumatoid factor has been detected in dogs having septic arthritis and SLE. In addition, it has been detected in apparently healthy dogs and in dogs with nonarticular diseases. Of 141 apparently healthy dogs, 57 had detectable rheumatoid factor using the Waaler-Rose test (Bennett and Kirkham, 1987a). Fourteen of these dogs had a titer of 1:20 and three had a titer of 1:40. In the same report, 11.7% of dogs with disease other than polyarthritis were significantly positive for rheumatoid factor; 6.4% of dogs having degenerative joint disease had a titer of 1:40.

It is obvious that it would be imprudent to make a diagnosis of rheumatoid arthritis or to eliminate it from the list of differential diagnoses solely on the basis of a positive or negative RF test. The rheumatoid factor test is only one of several criteria used to make a diagnosis of rheumatoid arthritis (see "Treatment of the Immune-Based Inflammatory Arthropathies of the Dog and Cat," this volume, p 1188). In one report (Bennett, 1987a), only 22 (73%) of 30 dogs with rheumatoid arthritis had a positive titer, and six of these had tested negative on one or more occasions. Thus, it is reasonable to repeat the test in dogs having negative or insignificant titers when the clinical and radiographic features of the disease suggest that rheumatoid arthritis is the diagnosis.

## ANTINUCLEAR ANTIBODIES

A variety of antinuclear antibodies have been detected in the serum of humans having SLE. The presence of these autoantibodies suggests that immunologic processes play a role in the pathogenesis of this disease.

Antinuclear antibodies (ANA) are detected in a variety of ways; no method of detection is ideal. Indirect immunofluorescence testing (FANA) is considered the most reliable. Detection of neutrophils and other white blood cells that have phagocytized nuclear material *in vitro*, so-called lupus erythematosus (LE) cells, is another means of determining the presence of antinuclear antibodies. Unfortunately, the LE cell test can be difficult to interpret because of confusion of nondiagnostic nucleophagocytic cells with true LE cells. The test is laborious and reliability depends on the experience and diligence of the technician performing the test (Grindem and Johnson, 1983). In addition, the LE cell test is considered insensitive; formation of LE cells seems to depend on the concentration of antibody, and many human hospitals require a high-positive FANA as a prerequisite to performing the LE cell test.

The indirect immunofluorescence test for ANA is considered a sensitive indicator of SLE. There is, however, some controversy over what constitutes a significant titer. Titers of 1:20 or greater were considered significant by Grindem and Johnson (1983). Bennett and Kirkham (1987b) suggest that a titer of 1:32 or greater is abnormal. Halliwell (1981, 1982) found that it is not unusual for normal dogs and dogs having other diseases to have a titer of 1:40 or less. Positive ANA titers have been documented in dogs having autoimmune skin disease, rheumatoid arthritis, and bacterial endocarditis and in dogs receiving the antiarrhythmic drug procainamide. Positive titers have been documented in dogs receiving hydralazine.

The definitive diagnosis of SLE is based on fulfillment of certain clinical and clinicopathologic criteria, including presence of ANA. Some feel that a diagnosis of "suspected" SLE may be justified even when ANA has not been detected. Halliwell (1981, 1982) reported 267 cases of *suspected* canine SLE; only 31 had an ANA titer of 1:40 or greater, and 146 were completely negative. Even though a positive titer does not necessarily mean that the animal has the disease, many authorities feel that definitive diagnosis of SLE rests on detection of ANA at appreciable levels (Halliwell, 1981; Bennett, 1897b). Bennett (1987b) has described 13 cases of *definitive* SLE in dogs; all had a positive ANA titer. Since the criteria established for SLE in humans have been used as a model for the disease in dogs and cats, emphasizing the importance of detecting antinuclear antibodies in making a diagnosis of SLE would seem reasonable. Over 80% of human patients with SLE have a positive ANA titer.

## LYME DISEASE TITER

Exposure to the spirochete *Borrelia burgdorferi* causes an antibody response that can be documented with indirect immunofluorescent antibody testing. The organism causes Lyme disease, a systemic illness that often has articular manifestations (see "CVT Update: Canine Lyme Disease," this volume, p 303, for a full discussion).

A positive titer to *B. burgdorferi* is important in the diagnosis of Lyme disease because the causative spirochete is difficult to culture or otherwise identify in dogs suspected of having borreliosis. Unfortunately, many apparently normal dogs in endemic areas have positive titers as well. Levy and Magnarelli (1992) have found that the presence of antibodies does not necessarily indicate active disease or that clinical signs are likely to ensue. They found that seropositive dogs were no more likely than seronegative dogs to develop signs typical of borreliosis. Because the clinical signs of Lyme disease are varied, nonspecific, and similar to those seen with other inflammatory joint disorders, the significance of a positive titer to *B. burgdorferi* must be carefully considered. Confusion over what constitutes a positive titer as well as public and commercial pressures generated by an enormous amount of publicity have probably adversely influenced the diagnostic process and increased the likelihood of overdiagnosis.

## SYNOVIAL MEMBRANE EXAMINATION

Histopathologic and microbiologic examinations of the synovial membrane are sometimes useful in the diagnosis of joint disease even though joint fluid analysis usually mirrors synovial membrane pathology. Histopathologic examination is especially valuable in diagnosis of joint neoplasia (synovial cell sarcoma, fibrosarcoma) and may help confirm or deny the clinical diagnosis of noninflammatory or inflammatory joint disease. When coupled with microbiologic examination, synovial membrane analysis may help differentiate infectious arthritis from other inflammatory disorders.

Synovial membrane analysis is warranted when the cause of joint disease remains undetermined or when symptomatic treatment has proven ineffective. Histopathologic and microbiologic examinations of the synovial membrane should be performed anytime exploration of a joint has failed to uncover the cause of lameness or when an apparent cause has been found but the synovial membrane appears uncharacteristically thick, hyperemic, discolored, and so forth. Rupture of the cranial cruciate ligament may be the sequela of a number of inflammatory joint diseases. In such cases, the synovial membrane usually appears more hyperemic and thickened than one would normally expect with cruciate ligament rupture alone. Failure to examine the synovial membrane might preclude an accurate diagnosis and lead to inappropriate and unsuccessful treatment.

Percutaneous needle biopsy of the synovial membrane has been described, but the sample size is small. Biopsy via surgical arthrotomy has the advantages of allowing complete exploration of the joint, selective sampling of the synovial membrane, and collection of larger samples. In addition, treatments such as synovectomy or stabilization procedures can be performed at the same time. Samples should include the synovial membrane and the fibrous capsule and should be atraumatically harvested. Routine histopathologic and microbiologic methods are utilized.

## OTHER TESTS

Other testing methods for *Rickettsia* or *Rickettsia*-like organisms and for mycotic infections are indicated when the clinical findings suggest that they may be the cause of lameness. Such tests are especially indicated when the affected animal lives in or has traveled to an area where the organism is endemic. Blood cultures and echocardiography are indicated when bacterial endocarditis is suspected.

Measurement of immune complexes and other so-called acute-phase proteins might be of benefit in diagnosis and management of inflammatory joint disorders. There are numerous methods for documenting their presence; however, since the result of such testing is usually nonspecific, these tests are not routinely used in diagnosis or management of joint disease in dogs or cats.

Coombs' testing is not usually indicated or of diagnostic value in animals with joint disease; it is indicated for use when there is a hemolytic event. The test is sometimes positive in animals with SLE.

## References and Suggested Reading

Bennett D: Immune-based erosive inflammatory joint disease of the dog: Canine rheumatoid arthritis. 1. Clinical, radiological and laboratory investigations. J Small Anim Pract 28:779, 1987a.

Bennett D: Immune-based non-erosive inflammatory joint disease of the dog. 1. Canine systemic lupus erythematosus. J Small Anim Pract 28:871, 1987b.

Bennett D and Kirkham D: The laboratory identification of serum rheumatoid factor in the dog. J Comp Pathol 97:541, 1987a.

Bennett D and Kirkham D: The laboratory identification of serum antinuclear antibody in the dog. J Comp Pathol 97:523, 1987b.

Grindem CB and Johnson KH: Systemic lupus erythematosus: Literature review and report of 42 new canine cases. J Am Anim Hosp Assoc 19:489, 1983.

Halliwell REW: Autoimmune disease in the dog. Adv Vet Sci Comp Med 22: 221, 1978.
*Forty-page review of the various autoimmune disorders of dogs; includes descriptions of systemic lupus erythematosus and rheumatoid arthritis.*

Halliwell REW: Skin disease associated with autoimmunity. The nonbullous autoimmune skin diseases. Compend Cont Educ Pract Vet 3:156, 1981.
*Contains results of antinuclear antibody testing on normal dogs, dogs hospitalized with other problems, and dogs with suspected systemic lupus erythematosus.*

Halliwell REW: Autoimmune disease in domestic animals. J Am Vet Med Assoc 181:1088, 1982.
*Review of the clinicopathologic features of the major autoimmune diseases of domestic animals; includes description of systemic lupus erythematosus.*

Levy SA and Magnarelli LA: Relationship between development of antibodies to *Borrelia burgdorferi* in dogs and the subsequent development of limb/joint borreliosis. J Am Vet Med Assoc 220:344, 1992.

Newton CD, et al: Rheumatoid arthritis in dogs. J Am Vet Med Assoc 168: 113, 1976.

# DIFFERENTIAL DIAGNOSIS OF NONTRAUMATIC CAUSES OF LAMENESS IN YOUNG GROWING DOGS

STEVEN C. SCHRADER
*Columbus, Ohio*

"The first step toward the cure is to know the disease" (a Latin proverb). Differentiating one cause of lameness from another depends on a knowledge of the clinical features of the various disorders that result in lameness, and on careful physical examination (i.e., accurate localization of pain, swelling, and muscle atrophy). It is crucial that the veterinarian be able to detect or elicit pain; pain and lameness are one in the same. Radiographic examination and, occasionally, laboratory testing are indicated after the affected part has been found. Accurate interpretation of the historical, physical, and radiographic findings is essential; it is important to remember that pups can have coexisting conditions (e.g., hip dysplasia and panosteitis), and that many structural lesions remain asymptomatic.

The causes of lameness in young skeletally immature dogs are many and varied. Traumatic injuries probably account for the majority of lameness cases seen in veterinary practice. The clinical and radiographic features of several important nontraumatic causes of lameness in young dogs are described in this article.

## CLINICAL AND RADIOGRAPHIC FEATURES

### Panosteitis

Panosteitis is a poorly understood inflammatory condition that is a common cause of lameness in large-breed dogs (German shepherd dog, Doberman pinscher, retrievers) that are between 5 and 18 months old. Males are more often affected than females.

Lameness usually begins between 5 and 10 months of age. The onset of lameness is usually acute, often developing after periods of strenuous activity or play. Classically, the disorder affects more than one limb or bone, causing the lameness to wax and wane and shift from one limb to another. However, clinically evident involvement of multiple limbs (i.e., shifting limb lameness) is not a consistent feature of the disorder. Lethargy and anorexia may accompany the lameness in some animals; these animals are often quite painful (lame).

The lameness associated with panosteitis may vary from subtle to non–weight-bearing; it is usually quite apparent that the dog is limping and which limb is affected. As the long bones of the proximal portions of the limb are most commonly affected, pain is detected on palpation of the shaft of the humerus, femur, or proximal ulna. Some muscle atrophy may be evident. The veterinarian should be careful to avoid being bitten during the examination, as many dogs with panosteitis are quite painful.

Radiographic evidence of panosteitis consists of one or more poorly defined irregular areas of increased density in the medullary cavity of affected bone(s). These areas may coalesce to produce larger areas of increased radiopacity (Fig. 1). In addition, slight periosteal new-bone formation is seen in 15 to 20% of the cases. No radiographic abnormalities may be seen in the early stages of the disorder or in dogs that are mildly affected.

### Hip Dysplasia

Hip dysplasia is a common cause of lameness in young growing large-breed dogs; it especially common in dogs having endomorphic features (i.e., Rottweiler and Saint Bernard versus Doberman pinscher and Great Dane). There is no apparent sex predisposition.

Disturbance of gait may become evident as early as 5 to 6 months of age. The onset of gait abnormality is usually insidious and the course is usually slowly progressive. Both hindlimbs are usually affected. There are no signs of systemic illness in dogs with hip dysplasia.

The functional disturbance associated with hip dysplasia is of variable intensity; many pups appear to be normal. Hip dysplasia rarely causes severe or non–weight-bearing lameness in the young dog. Instead, clinically affected pups appear to have hindlimb weakness. The rump sways from side to side as they walk and the hindlimb gait or stance is narrow based. Some dogs move the hindlimbs in unison (i.e., "bunny hop") when running. Affected dogs may have difficulty climbing stairs and fatigue rapidly; their body weight may be shifted to the forelimbs so that the elbows are abducted, the back is arched, and the dog appears to stand "tip-toed" on the hindlimbs. Despite bilateral involvement, lameness is often more pronounced on one side than the other.

The hindlimbs and gluteal regions of clinically affected individuals may appear poorly developed. The dogs appear painful when the hips are abducted or hyperextended and hip instability (Ortolani, Barden signs) may be detected. Sedation or anesthesia may be required to detect hip joint laxity.

The radiographic abnormalities associated with hip dysplasia in young dogs include subluxation of the femoral heads, shallow acetabula, irregular subchondral outlines, and mild periarticular osteophyte formation (Fig. 1). No radiographic abnormalities can be seen in certain dogs; in such cases, stress radiographic methods may be needed to document hip joint subluxation. Radiographic signs of degenerative joint disease become more evident as time passes.

### Patellar Luxation

Patellar luxation is a common cause of lameness in young large- and small-breed dogs; it is usually considered a congenital problem. This condition is especially common in small dogs such as the toy and miniature poodle, Yorkshire terrier, and dogs of the chondrodystrophoid breeds. Clinical signs are rarely evident before 6 months of age unless the patella is completely and persistently luxated. Undoubtedly, many dogs with patellar instability remain asymptomatic. There is no apparent sex predisposition.

The onset of lameness with congenital patellar instability is usually insidious; onset of lameness is acute when the luxation is the result of a traumatic incident. In very young pups, slowly progressive limb deformity may develop as the result of persistent (grade III or IV) luxation. Intermittent medial or lateral luxation of the patella results in episodic lameness; dogs so affected walk normally when the patella is reduced. Persistent luxation with or without deformity results in continuous lameness. There are no systemic signs of illness in animals with this condition.

Medial or lateral luxation of the patella results in lameness that is easily recognized. Intermittent luxation

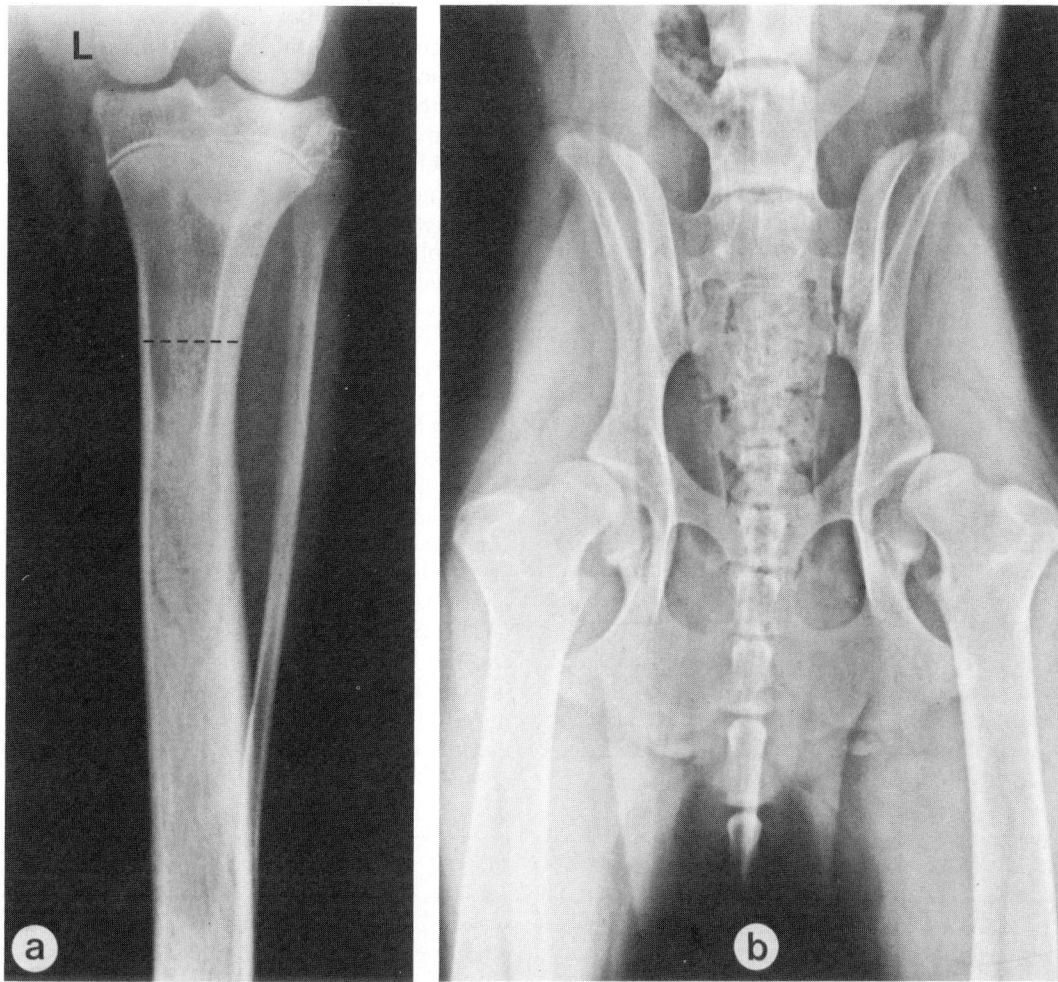

**Figure 1.** Radiographs of a young German shepherd dog having intermittent left hindlimb lameness. There is increased radiopacity of the medullary canal of the left tibia (*a*, distal to the level of the dashed line). This is consistent with a diagnosis of panosteitis. In addition, the dog has hip dysplasia (i.e., both femoral heads are subluxated) (*b*). In this case, lameness was attributed to panosteitis because a painful response was easily elicited on palpation of the left tibia but could not be elicited by abduction or hyperextension of the hip. Radiographic findings must always be interpreted within the clinical context.

results in brief periods of non–weight-bearing or otherwise overt lameness followed by variable periods of normal ambulation. Persistent luxation causes persistent lameness, but the animal usually bears weight on the limb while walking or running. Both limbs are usually affected unless there is a traumatic cause. Medial luxation is more common than lateral luxation. Patellar instability is usually easy to detect. Digital pressure on the medial (lateral luxation) or lateral (medial luxation) aspect of the patella with the stifle in various positions will cause displacement of the bone. There is usually little or no swelling or deformity of the joint unless the luxation is chronic and persistent. The animal may or may not respond as the patella is manually luxated or reduced. Deformity of the distal femur and proximal tibia may be seen when persistent luxation developed at an early age.

Radiographic evaluation is usually not essential for diagnosis. Associated bony changes are minimal when luxation is intermittent (grades I and II) and may remain so as the dog ages. The patella may be spontaneously reduced as the dog is being positioned for the study. Radiographic abnormalities may be quite dramatic when there has been disturbance of growth secondary to persistent luxation.

## Osteochondritis Dissecans

Osteochondritis dissecans (OCD) is a developmental disorder whereby a flap of articular cartilage becomes partially or totally detached from the underlying subchondral bone. Osteochondritis dissecans is a common cause of lameness in young large-breed dogs. The most common site of involvement is the caudomedial surface of the humeral head (many breeds) and the medial trochlear ridge of the talus (Rottweiler, retriever). Occasionally, OCD lesions develop on the lateral trochlear ridge of the talus (Rottweiler), the medial portion of the humeral condyle, and the lateral condyle of the femur. Males are affected more commonly than females.

Lameness starts insidiously between 7 and 10 months of age. Lameness is usually constant (present every day) and can be slowly progressive. The degree of lameness is mild to moderate; it may be most obvious when the dog first gets up to walk or run. Bilateral involvement is common, but clinical signs tend to predominate on one side. The lesions on the opposite side will often remain asymptomatic. There are no signs of systemic illness associated with OCD.

Pain can usually be elicited by hyperextending the affected joint(s). Mild to moderate muscle atrophy is present in chronic cases. Palpation of the elbow, tarsus, or stifle may reveal the presence of joint capsular thickening or effusion; such abnormalities are inconsistently found and cannot usually be detected when the joint is deeply situated (shoulder).

Radiography is consistently helpful in the diagnosis of OCD. Routine craniocaudal and mediolateral views are sufficient except with lesions of the lateral trochlear ridge of the talus where, on the craniocaudal view, the lesion becomes superimposed on the calcaneus. Making the craniocaudal projection with the tarsus in a flexed position will overcome this problem (Miyabayashi et al., 1991). Radiographs reveal subchondral de-

fects or irregularities that may result in apparent widening and irregularity of the "joint space" at the site of the lesion (Fig. 2). There is sclerosis of the underlying bone. It is usually not possible to see the cartilage flap on plain radiographs unless it contains a small portion of subchondral bone. The flap may mineralize if an attachment to synovial membrane develops. Soft tissue swelling may be evident with lesions of the talus. Radiographic signs of degenerative joint disease become more evident as time passes.

## Fragmented (Medial) Coronoid Process

Fragmented coronoid process (ulna) is probably a more common cause of lameness in growing large-breed dogs (Rottweiler, retriever, Bernese mountain dog) than many currently believe. Clinical signs usually become evident between 6 and 10 months of age or later in life as the result of progressive degenerative joint disease. There is no apparent sex predisposition.

The onset of lameness associated with fragmented coronoid process is usually insidious; lameness may be intermittent in the early stages but, with time, becomes more continuous. Lameness is usually unilateral even though many dogs are bilaterally affected. There are

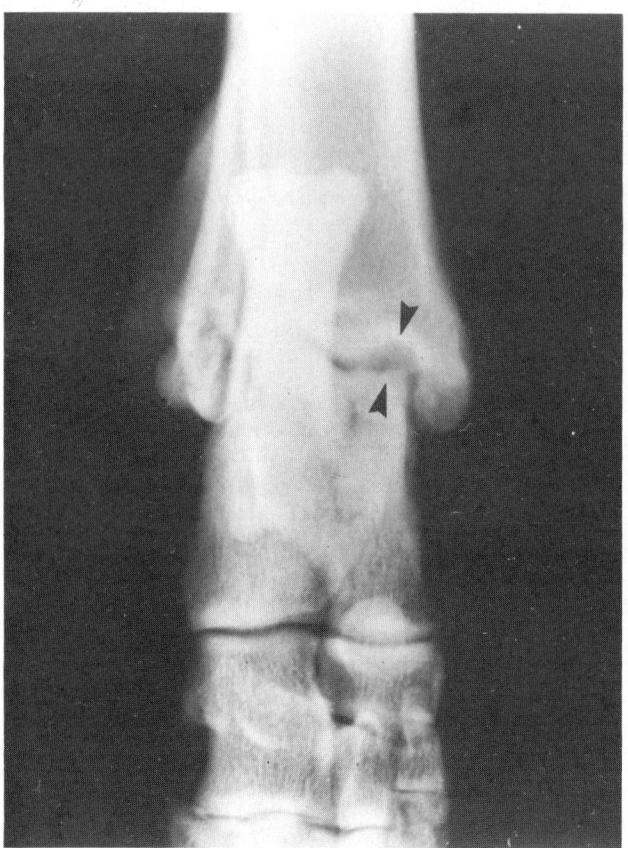 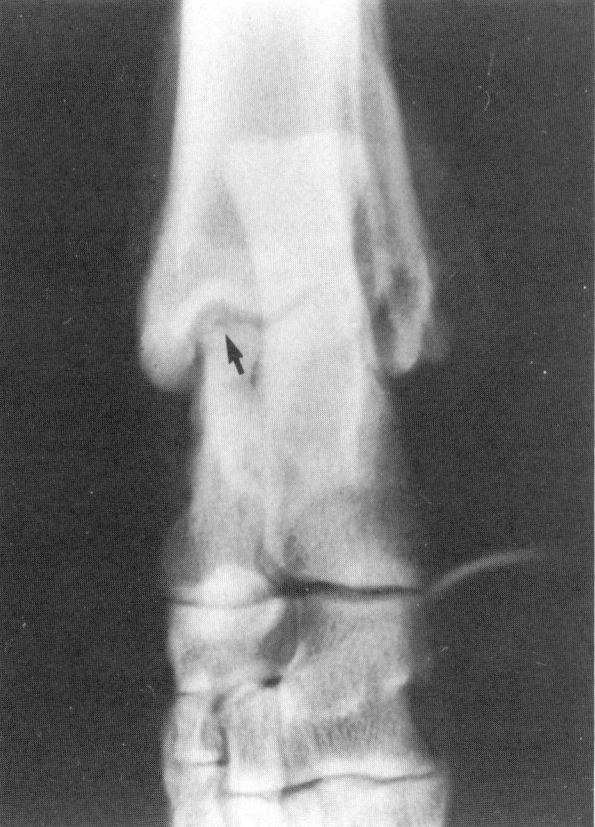

**Figure 2.** Craniocaudal radiographs of the tibiotarsal joints of a young Labrador retriever having bilateral osteochondritis dissecans of the medial trochlear ridge of the talus. There is loss of the medial trochlear ridge of the talus and secondary widening of the joint space (*left, arrowheads*). On the opposite side (*right*), the subchondral bone of the medial trochlear ridge is irregular and a detached fragment of bone can be seen (*arrow*).

no signs of systemic illness in dogs having this condition.

The lameness associated with fragmented coronoid process is usually subtle. In the early stages, it may be difficult to document that the animal is indeed lame, and considerable time may pass before the diagnosis is considered or made. There is usually little or no detectable muscle atrophy or restriction in elbow movement. Affected dogs usually resist hyperextension of the elbow as well as alternate pronation and supination of the antibrachium and paw with the elbow positioned in 90 degrees of flexion. They generally respond to direct digital pressure applied over the medial aspect of the joint (Fig. 3). Joint effusion can be considerable; however, effusion is an inconsistent finding.

In the early stages, radiographic changes associated with fragmented coronoid process can be subtle or absent. The cleavage plane between the detached fragment and the parent bone is usually oblique to the radiographic beam. In addition, the detached portion of the coronoid process is superimposed on the radial head and minimally displaced. Thus, the detached fragment of bone is rarely apparent and the veterinarian needs to identify the secondary changes associated with this condition in order to make the correct diagnosis.

The early secondary changes that are associated with fragmented coronoid process include sclerosis of the adjacent ulna and the presence of periarticular osteophytes along the ulna and medial portion of the humeral condyle. In the ulna, subchondral sclerosis obliterates the normal trabecular pattern of the bone and the adjacent medullary cavity may appear to narrow at this site (Fig. 4). Comparing mediolateral views of the elbows is helpful, especially if the opposite side is unaffected. In some cases, radiographs reveal the presence of a radiopaque mass adjacent to the medial portion of the coronoid process. This is usually an enthesiophyte or osteophyte, not the detached piece of coronoid process. The radiographic signs of degenerative joint disease become more evident as time passes.

## Hypertrophic Osteodystrophy

Hypertrophic osteodystrophy (HOD) is a condition of unproven etiology that occasionally affects large-breed dogs (Great Dane, setters, retrievers, German shepherd dog, Doberman pinscher, Weimaraner). Clinical signs begin early in life, usually between 3 and 6 months of age. There is no apparent sex predisposition.

The onset of lameness associated with HOD is acute; clinical dysfunction is overt and often cyclic. Affected pups spend most of their time laying down and often resist the owner's efforts to make them walk. As all limbs are usually affected, the gait is stiff and deliberate. The dog may stand with the back arched and all four limbs tucked under the body; they appear to be painful. There is usually firm painful symmetric swelling or enlargement at the level of the distal metaphysis of the radius, ulna, and tibia. Conformational abnormalities such as hyperextension of the carpi and angular deformities of the lower limbs may develop as the disorder becomes chronic (giant breeds). Dogs with HOD appear lethargic and are often anorectic; rectal temperature may exceed 104°F. Fever is an inconsistent clinical feature of the disease, and is often cyclic in nature. Some affected pups will die as the result of the disease process. Frustrated owners sometimes elect euthanasia in persistent cases or when the pup is especially painful.

There are two very different radiographic pictures that have been associated with HOD. In one, the abnormalities resemble those associated with hematogenous osteomyelitis of young dogs. There is widening of the metaphyses with associated irregular periosteal new-bone formation and soft tissue swelling; the trabecular pattern of the metaphyseal bone appears distorted (Fig. 5). In the other, there is a radiolucent band parallel and adjacent to but separated from the physeal cartilage (Fig. 6). The clinical and radiographic features of HOD are fairly unique; however, hematogenous osteomyelitis should be considered a differential diagnosis whenever the clinical and radiographic features suggest the presence of infection. There is some evidence to support an infectious (bacterial or viral) etiology for this condition.

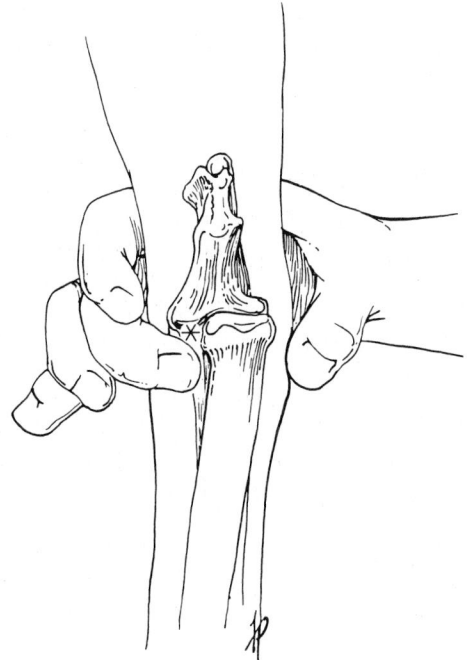

**Figure 3.** Schematic representation of the elbow of a dog. Dogs having fragmented medial coronoid process will usually seem painful when digital pressure is applied to the area defined by the asterisk.

## Aseptic Necrosis of the Femoral Head

Aseptic necrosis of the femoral head (avascular necrosis, Legg-Calvé-Perthes disease) is an occasional cause of lameness in young small-breed dogs (poodle,

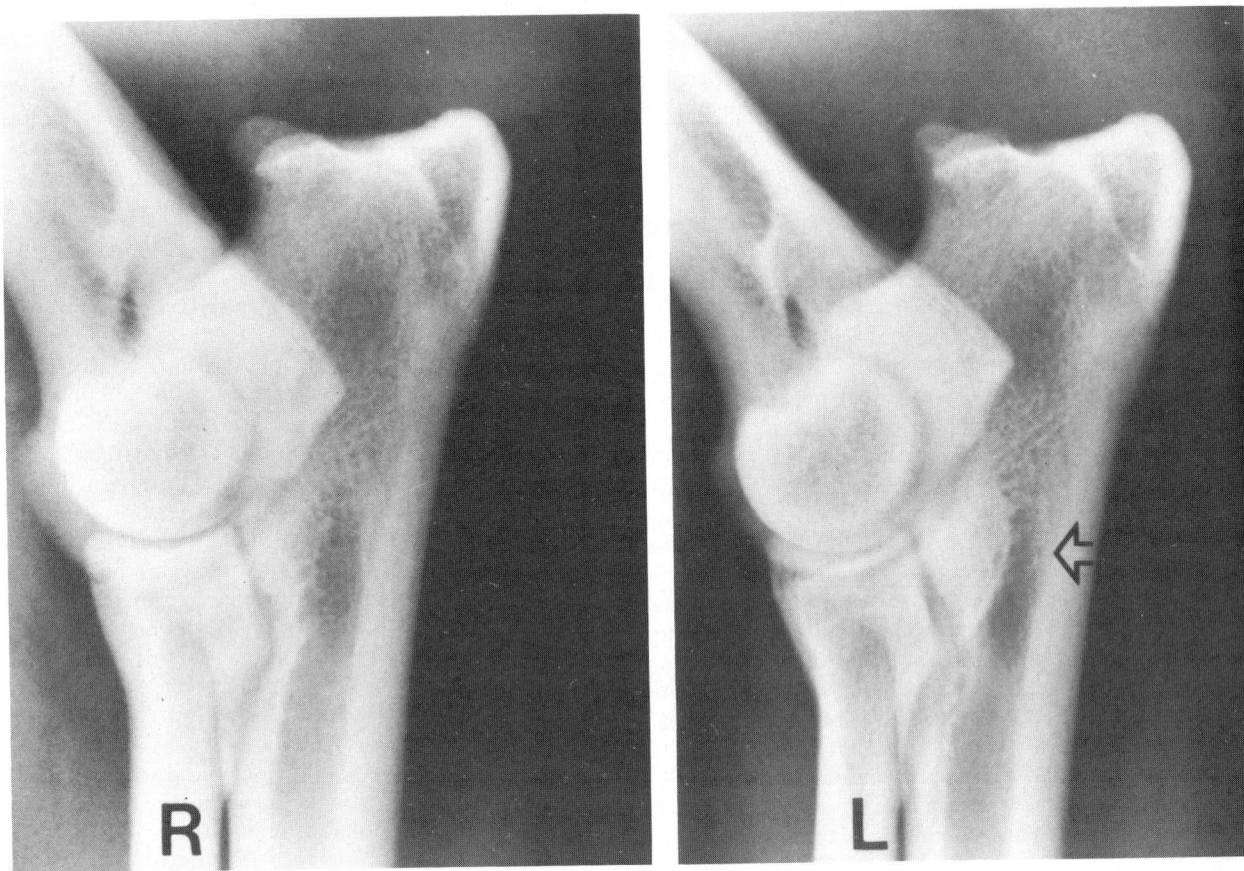

**Figure 4.** Mediolateral radiographs of the elbows of a young Rottweiler. The right elbow appears normal (*R*). Comparatively, there is increased radiopacity, loss of trabecular pattern, and apparent narrowing of the medullary canal adjacent to the distal portion of the trochlear notch of the left ulna (*L*, *arrow*). Such changes are suggestive of fragmented medial coronoid process; the detached portion of the coronoid process is rarely seen on radiographs regardless of the projection. In this case, the diagnosis was confirmed by surgical exploration of the joint.

terriers, miniature pinscher) between 6 and 10 months of age. There is no apparent sex predisposition.

Lameness associated with this condition usually begins insidiously and is gradually progressive over 3 to 5 weeks. Occasionally, the onset of lameness may coincide with a traumatic event. The lameness associated with this condition is usually obvious and muscle atrophy can become evident within 2 to 3 weeks of the onset. A painful response is easily elicited by abduction and extension of the hip. The condition is bilateral in 10 to 15% of dogs. There are no signs of systemic illness associated with avascular necrosis of the femoral head.

Radiographic changes may be subtle in the early stages of this condition. Widening of the joint space occurs early, but the bony changes that represent revascularization and remodeling of the affected bone may take some time to develop. If the veterinarian suspects this diagnosis and there are no radiographic changes to support it, repeating the radiographic procedure in 2 to 3 weeks is recommended. Radiographic abnormalities are consistently present in the later stages of the disease (after 3 weeks). The hip joint space appears widened and incongruent and the femoral epiphysis becomes flattened, irregularly radiolu-

cent, or otherwise distorted (Fig. 7). Muscle atrophy is often apparent on the radiograph.

## Ununited/Fragmented Anconeal Process

Ununited anconeal process is an occasional cause of lameness in young large-breed dogs. A disproportionate number of cases have been reported in the German shepherd dog and males are more commonly affected than females. Although the etiology may differ from the above, this condition also develops in chondrodystrophoid breeds, particularly the basset hound. The lameness that is associated with ununited anconeal process may be subtle or overt; both sides may be affected. A painful response can usually be elicited by hyperextension of the elbow. The affected joint is usually thickened and crepitus can often be detected; an effusion may be present. In the chondrodystrophoid dog, there may be associated angular limb deformities. There are no other signs of illness in dogs having this condition.

Radiographic evaluation is straightforward (i.e., the diagnosis is confirmed whenever the anconeal process is detached from its parent bone) (Fig. 8). Abnormalities are particularly evident on a mediolateral projec-

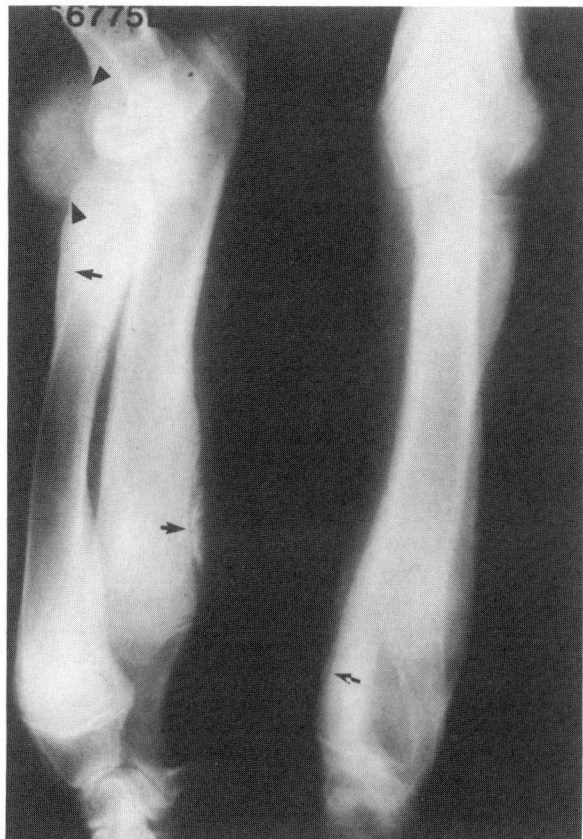

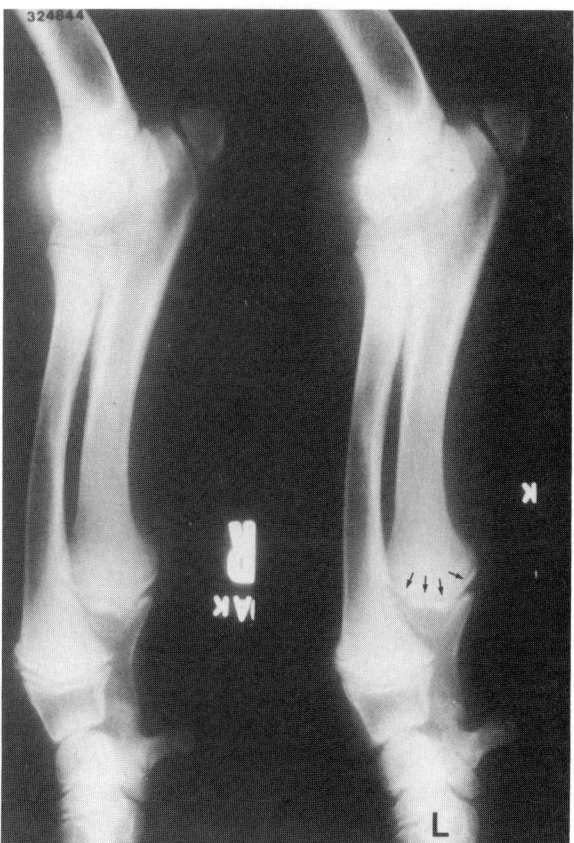

**Figure 5.** Radiographs of the left radius and ulna of a young Great Dane dog having hypertrophic osteodystrophy. There is increased radiopacity at the level of the proximal and distal metaphyses of the radius and the distal metaphysis of the ulna. There is periosteal new-bone formation at these sites (*arrows*). Similar radiographic abnormalities were present on the opposite limb and the tibiae. This dog also had several focal areas of subcutaneous mineralization; one such area was located cranial to the left elbow (*arrowheads*).

**Figure 6.** Mediolateral radiographs of the left and right antebrachial regions of a young Irish setter having hypertrophic osteodystrophy. There is a linear radiolucency that runs parallel and proximal to the distal physis of the radius and ulna of both limbs. This radiolucency is most evident in the left ulna (*L, arrows*).

tion of the flexed elbow. Radiographic signs of degenerative joint disease become more evident as time passes.

### Carpal Instability/Flexion Syndrome

This condition develops in pups between the ages of 8 and 16 weeks. It has been documented in several breeds, but there appears to be a breed predisposition in the Doberman pinscher and shar pei. There is no sex predisposition.

Clinical signs usually develop quite quickly. Affected pups stand with the carpi in a flexed position. The paws are inwardly deviated. When weight is placed on the limb, the carpi appear to buckle over and the pup appears to walk on the lateral or outside aspect of the digits and forepaws (Fig. 9). The carpi are not swollen, painful, or palpably unstable. Occasionally, the condition is unilateral. There are usually no radiographic abnormalities associated with this condition.

The etiology of this problem is not known. Vaughan (1992) has suggested that there is an excessive tautness

of the flexor carpi ulnaris muscle in affected pups. Spontaneous recovery occurs within 2 to 4 weeks in the majority of dogs. When the problem persists or appears to be worsening, a lightweight splint can be applied to hold the carpus in a slightly extended position. The splint is applied at 3- to 5-day intervals for 5 to 7 days at a time until the deformity resolves. Vaughan (1992) transected portions of the tendon of insertion of the flexor carpi unlaris muscle in two dogs that failed to spontaneously recover. Both dogs improved. Radiographic evaluation is indicated whenever the condition fails to improve by itself.

### Septic Arthritis

Septic arthritis, unrelated to trauma or surgery, is an occasional cause of lameness in young dogs. One or more joints can be affected; large-breed dogs seem to be predisposed. There is no sex predisposition.

The onset of the clinical signs of septic arthritis are both sudden and overt and the condition can develop in very young pups (6 to 8 weeks old). Although some dogs are apparently healthy, there may be previous or concurrent illness. Affected dogs are often lethargic and anorectic and may be febrile. Local or generalized

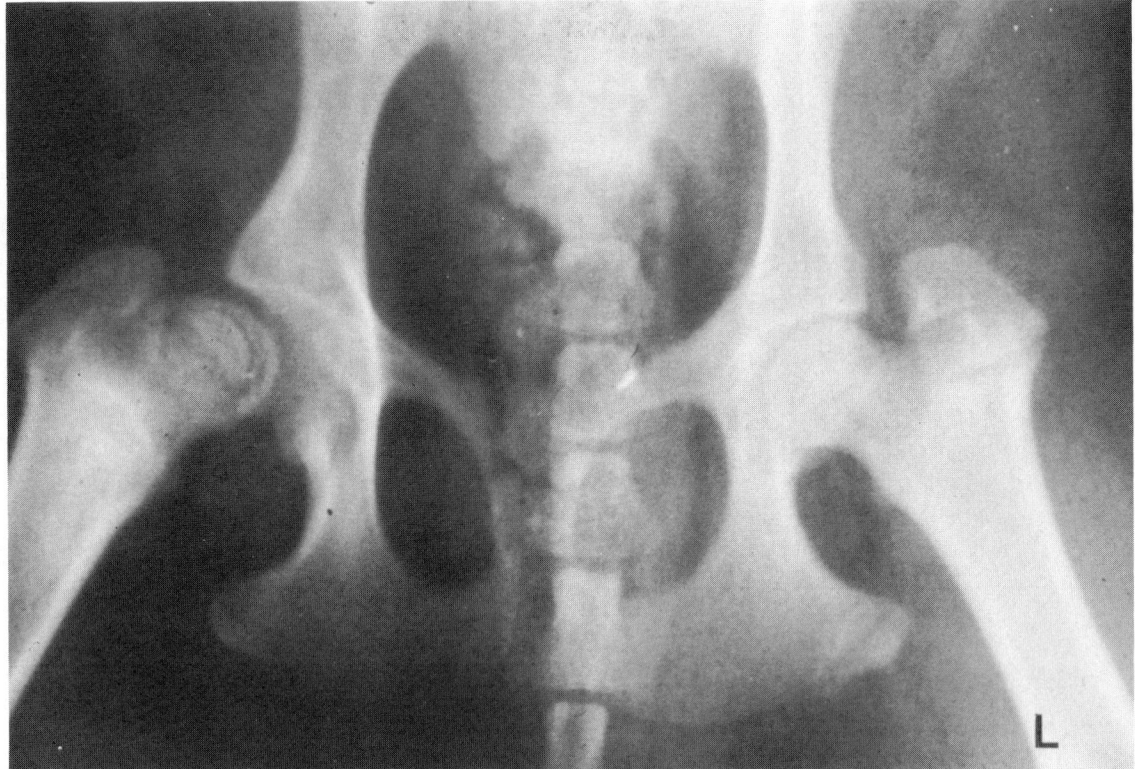

**Figure 7.** Radiograph of the pelvis of a young miniature poodle having aseptic necrosis of the right femoral head. When compared with the opposite (*left*) side, there is subluxation of the hip and radiolucency and flattening of the epiphysis.

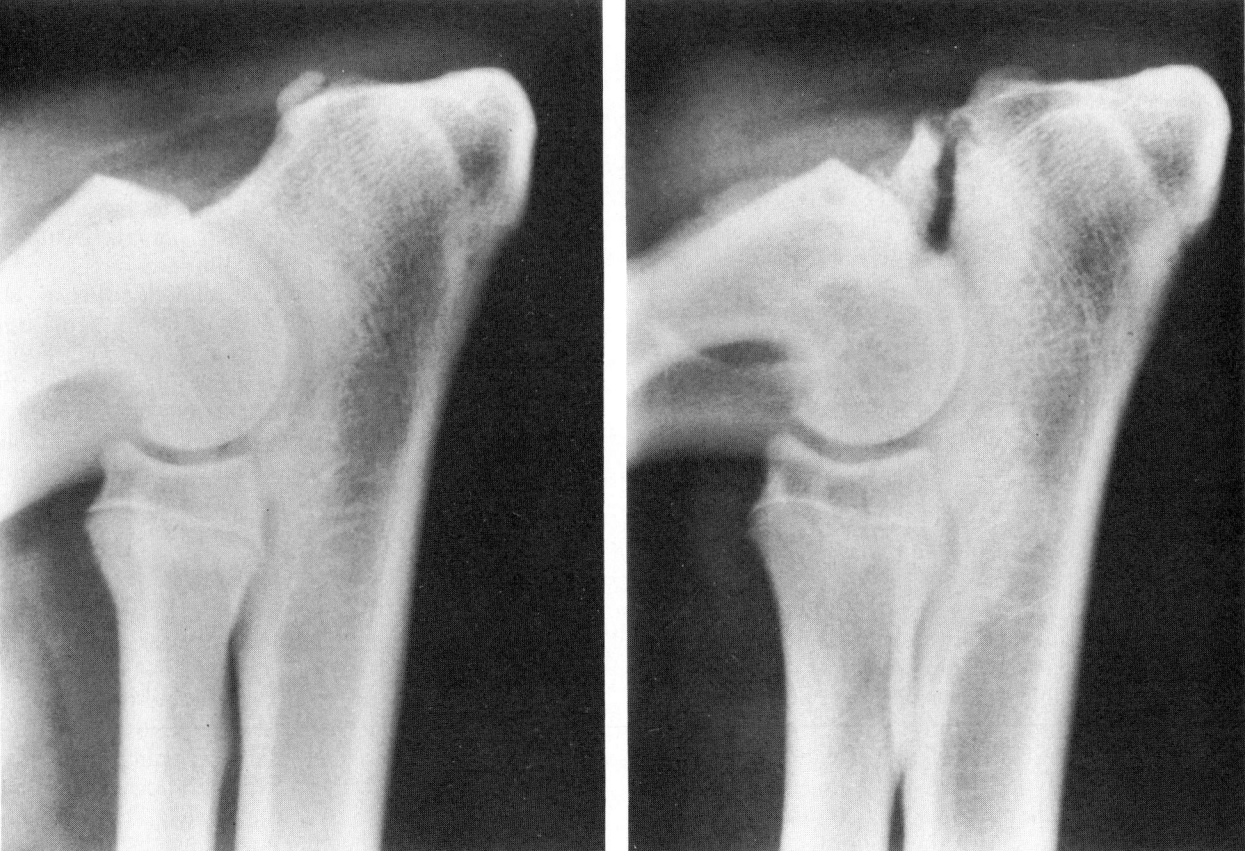

**Figure 8.** Mediolateral radiographs of the left (*left*) and right (*right*) elbows of a young German shepherd dog having right ununited anconeal process.

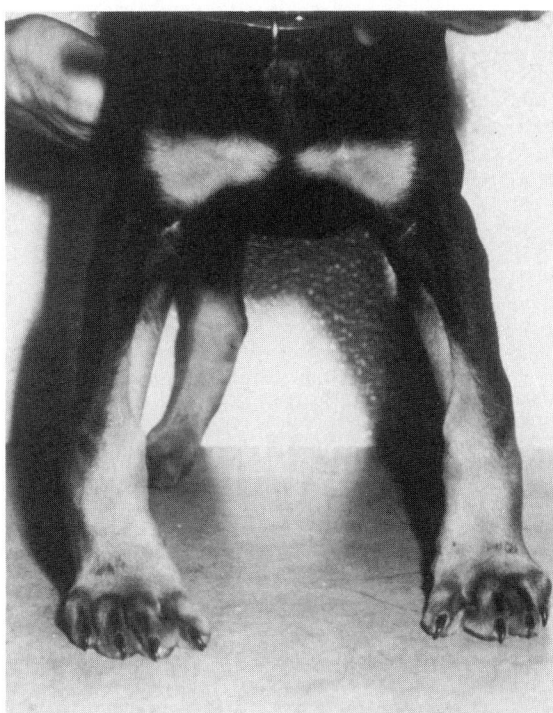

**Figure 9.** Photograph of the forelimbs of a 14-week-old Doberman pinscher having so-called carpal instability syndrome. The carpi tend to buckle forward, and affected dogs appear somewhat "bow-legged." Affected pups appear to walk on the lateral aspect of the digits (paws).

lymph node enlargement may be present. Lameness is usually severe. When multiple joints are affected, the dog may be reluctant to walk. Infected joints are swollen and painful.

In the early stages of joint infection, radiographic abnormalities are limited to soft tissue swelling; bony changes are not usually visible during the first 2 weeks. Because early treatment is important, arthrocentesis and joint fluid analysis are usually of greater diagnostic value than radiographs.

## CASE EXAMPLES

The veterinarian should be able to list the most likely *nontraumatic* causes of lameness in each of the following self-evaluation cases. These case examples should underscore the importance of knowing the clinical features of the various causes of lameness and the importance of careful physical examination.

### Case 1.

A 10-month-old female Doberman pinscher. Waxing/waning right hindlimb lameness of 10 weeks' duration. Resists palpation of the limb. Seems painful as the femur is palpated.
*Response*: The breed, vacillating nature of the lameness, and presence of bone pain suggest that this dog has panosteitis. Another reason to consider this diagnosis highly is that panosteitis is a common condition.

### Case 2.

An 8-month-old cairn terrier; 1-month progressive left hindlimb lameness. Muscle atrophy is present in the affected limb. Seems painful on abduction of the right hip.
*Response*: The progressive nature of this *small* dog's hip problem is a classic presentation for aseptic necrosis of the femoral head. At 1 month, there should be radiographic changes present to support this clinical conclusion.

### Case 3.

An 11-month-old female Labrador retriever. Seems somewhat weak on the hindlimbs, stiff gait, reluctant to climb stairs. Poor muscling of the right hindlimb; "sloppy" base narrow hindlimb gait.
*Response*: All of the features of this scenario are consistent with the diagnosis of hip dysplasia. A slight change in history to include intermittent alternating hindlimb lameness would change the character of the case (i.e., it would be important to determine if the dog had a painful response to palpation of the long bones of the limbs. Panosteitis and hip dysplasia can occur in the same animal (Fig. 1) and hip dysplasia does not always result in clinical dysfunction.

### Case 4.

A 7-month-old Irish setter; 1-month subtle but persistent right forelimb lameness. Resistance felt when right shoulder is hyperextended.
*Response*: Osteochondritis dissecans of the humeral head. It is good practice to evaluate the other shoulder, as the condition is frequently bilateral.

### Case 5.

A 7-month-old Chihuahua. Intermittently lifts right hindlimb off the floor when running. Growls and tries to bite you during the physical examination.
*Response*: Although complete physical examination is not always possible, every attempt should be made to perform as much of the examination as possible before sedating the dog or pursuing radiographic evaluation. Fortunately, in this case, the breed and character of the lameness strongly suggest a diagnosis of patellar luxation and we can, at least initially, discuss this with the owner and avoid undue stress for the dog, the client, and ourselves.

### Case 6.

A 9-month-old German shepherd dog. Bilateral forelimb lameness of 8 weeks' duration. Crepitus on manipulation of the right elbow; both elbows are "thickened."
*Response*: This probably represents a case of bilateral ununited anconeal process. Fragmented coronoid process is not as likely because of the breed and because joint changes associated with fragmented coronoid process are usually not this evident so early in life.

### Case 7.

A 5-month-old male Great Dane dog. Poor appetite and "stiff" gait. Back appears arched and dog seems painful to owner. Reluctant to walk; limbs are swollen and painful near the carpal and tarsal joints.

*Response*: The early onset, multiple limb involvement, presence of systemic signs and swelling *near* joints, and the painful nature of this *Great Dane's* problem point to hypertrophic osteodystrophy as the diagnosis. Septic polyarthritis could create a similar clinical picture. Joint swelling and periarticular swelling are not always easily differentiated by palpation. Arthrocentesis would be indicated in such cases.

### Case 8.

A 7-month-old male Rottweiler. Subtle but persistent "favoring" of the left forelimb of 6 weeks' duration. Dog is mildly lame but no other abnormalities are found.

*Response*: Many of the nontraumatic causes of lameness (osteochondritis dissecans, panosteitis, fragmented coronoid process, and ununited anconeal process) are possible in this case. If we assume that the physical examination was properly performed, FCP should be moved to the beginning of the list. This condition is quite common in the Rottweiler, and its clinical features are usually more subtle than those associated with the other possibilities. Heightened awareness of this condition will ensure that it is not overlooked. Both elbows should be radiographed and compared. If nothing is found on radiographic examination of the elbows (FCP, OCD, UAP), making radiographs of the shoulder to rule out OCD of the humeral head would seem a rational next step. A combination of elbow and shoulder radiographs would also allow evaluation of the humeral shaft and proximal radius and ulna (i.e., examination for bony changes associated with panosteitis).

### References and Suggested Reading

Newton CD and Nunamaker DM: *Textbook of Small Animal Orthopaedics.* Philadelphia, JB Lippincott Co, 1985.
  *Excellent comprehensive review of the various bone and joint disorders of dogs.*
Newton CD and Biery DN: Skeletal diseases. *In* Ettinger SJ (ed): *Textbook of Veterinary Internal Medicine,* 3rd edition. Philadelphia, WB Saunders Co, 1985, p 2378.
Miyabayashi T, Biller DS, Manley PA, and Matushek KJ: Use of a flexed dorsoplantar radiographic view of the talocrural joint to evaluate lameness in two dogs. J Am Vet Med Assoc 199:598, 1991.
Pedersen NC, Wind A, Morgan JP, and Pool RR: Joint diseases of dogs and cats. *In* Ettinger SJ (ed): *Textbook of Veterinary Internal Medicine,* 3rd edition. Philadelphia, WB Saunders Co, 1985, p 2329.
Vaughan LC: Flexural deformity of the carpus in puppies. J Small Anim Pract 33:381, 1992.

# CURRENT CONCEPTS IN THE DIAGNOSIS OF CANINE HIP DYSPLASIA

GAIL K. SMITH
*Philadelphia, Pennsylvania*

*and* PAMELA J. McKELVIE
*Havertown, Pennsylvania*

Canine hip dysplasia (CHD) was first described by Schnelle in the mid 1930s. Originally termed "bilateral congenital subluxation of the coxofemoral joints," it was thought to be rare. Today we recognize that CHD is the most common inherited orthopedic disease in large- and giant-breed dogs. Since its first description, CHD, its diagnosis, and particularly its treatment have been the source of considerable debate, controversy, and conjecture among veterinarians, dog breeders, and dog owners. While clearly our understanding of CHD has evolved over the years, progress has been more a result of empiricism than well-planned scientific investigation.

From Latin, the definition of hip dysplasia is "faulty development of the hip." A more descriptive definition is one introduced by Henricson, Norberg, and Olssen in 1966; hip dysplasia is "a varying degree of laxity of the hip joint permitting subluxation during early life, giving rise to varying degrees of shallow acetabulum and flattening of the femoral head, finally inevitably leading to osteoarthritis." Therefore the connection was recognized early between *joint laxity* and *radiographic subluxation* in young dogs and the subsequent development of osteoarthritis later in life. It is the purpose of this article to provide background information on the topic of CHD, to review popular methods of CHD diagnosis, and to elaborate on a newly introduced diagnostic method.

## PREVALENCE, ETIOLOGY, AND PATHOGENESIS

Canine hip dysplasia can affect all breeds of dogs; however, it has highest prevalence in the large and giant breeds. Prevalence estimates published by the Orthopedic Foundation for Animals (OFA) fall between 10% and 50% for many of the popular breeds of dogs (Corley, 1992). It is generally recognized, however, that such figures are biased toward normality owing largely to preselection by owners and veterinarians who submit only those hip radiographs with the greatest likelihood of being certified as normal. A review of records at the Veterinary Hospital of the University of Pennsylvania (VHUP) indicated that approximately 50% of the clients who requested OFA hip radiographs actually submitted them to the OFA for official interpretation. Regarding CHD prevalence, a clinical survey of popular large-breed dogs presenting to VHUP for routine hip evaluation showed breed-specific CHD prevalence figures, as determined by board-certified veterinary radiologists, to be two to three times higher than those published by the OFA.

Canine hip dysplasia is thought to have a genetic basis, being polygenic and multifactorial. It is a quantitative or metric trait, with estimates of heritability ranging from 0.2 to 0.6. Clearly, nongenetic factors also play a role in the expression of CHD. Some factors studied include dog size, growth rate, hypernutrition, level of dietary anion gap, *in utero* endocrine influences, and muscle mass. In spite of research efforts to date, however, the precise cause of CHD remains unknown.

## CLINICAL SIGNS

The clinical presentation of CHD can be divided into two forms; a severe form typically appearing between 5 and 12 months of age (range = 4 to 36 months) producing marked debilitating lameness in the dog; or a milder chronic form with more subtle, often variable, signs presenting at any age but usually appearing later in life. The severe form is associated with a noticeably abnormal gait, pain, low exercise tolerance, reluctance to rise or climb stairs, thigh muscle atrophy, occasionally an audible click when walking and, sometimes, if very severe, an obviously increased intertrochanteric (rump) width. The chronic form, on the other hand, comprises the vast majority of cases with CHD. Dogs affected with this form are either functionally asymptomatic or only mildly painful, particularly after periods of rest following excessive exercise or unaccustomed activity. In its mildest form, chronic CHD is frequently detectable only by careful orthopedic examination or hip radiography. The chronic condition typically becomes evident in the geriatric years and is characterized by mild pain, stiffness, and slowness or hesitation to rise. There may be mildly restricted range of joint motion or pain and crepitus upon palpation at extremes of range of motion. Though less acute and debilitating than severe CHD, the chronic form can progress in some cases to marked disuse and muscular wasting requiring medical or surgical treatment. The clinical signs in chronic CHD are due to progression of degenerative joint disease.

Other conditions may present with clinical signs resembling those of CHD, and very often CHD is an incidental finding (see "Differential Diagnosis of Nontraumatic Causes of Lameness in Young, Growing Dogs," this volume, p 1171). Panosteitis in the young dog and cranial cruciate ligament rupture in older dogs are examples. Other problems must be ruled out before

concluding that the observed signs are attributable solely to CHD. For example, in the German shepherd breed of dog, it is very common for spinal degenerative myelopathy in its early stages to be confused with progression of the chronic form of CHD. Therefore, in addition to a complete orthopaedic evaluation, a thorough neurologic examination is warranted.

## DIAGNOSIS

Tentative diagnosis of CHD can be made on the basis of history, clinical signs, and palpation. By convention, however, a definitive diagnosis can be made only if the hips show characteristic radiographic signs of CHD. Radiography is traditionally performed with the dog, preferably sedated, in a supine position, the legs fully extended and the stifles internally rotated. This is the position promulgated by the AVMA Panel on Hip Dysplasia in 1961, adapted by the Orthopedic Foundation for Animals (OFA) in 1966 and in common use for more than 30 years (Fig. 1). Radiographic diagnosis is based on the appearance of hip subluxation (a radiologist's term for joint laxity), evidence of degenerative joint disease (DJD), or both.

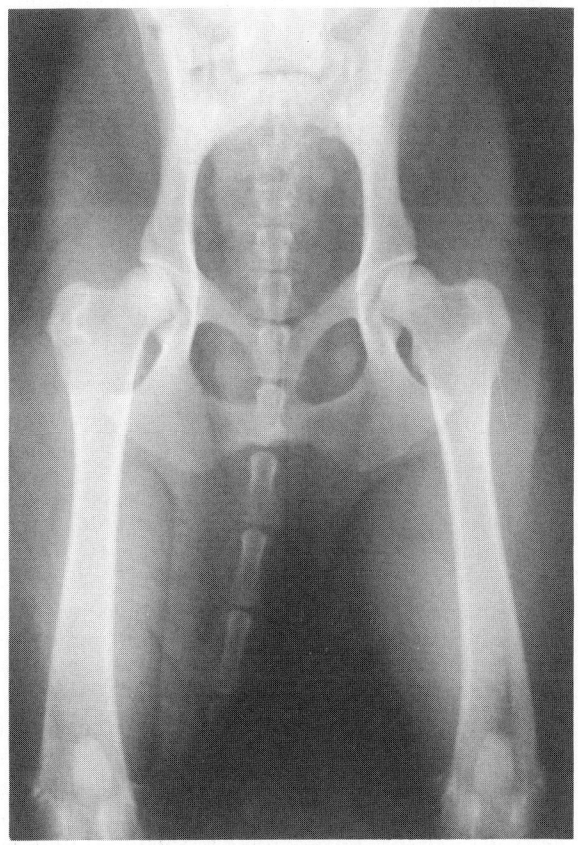

**Figure 1.** Standard ventrodorsal radiographic projection of the pelvis and hips of a 2.5-year-old female golden retriever demonstrating proper radiographic technique with the hips fully extended and the stifles internally rotated. Based on this radiograph, the dog was judged to have "fair normal" hips by the Orthopedic Foundation for Animals and was approved for breeding.

Because CHD is such a common disease afflicting many breeds of dogs, it is not surprising that many scoring schemes, whether subjective, objective, or semiquantitative, have evolved in an attempt to characterize the radiographic changes associated with this disease. All popular scoring methods have adopted the ventrodorsal hip-extended radiograph from which to derive a diagnosis (Fig. 1).

## Subjective Method of Diagnosis

Subjective criteria for CHD diagnosis as applied to the hip-extended radiographic view have gained international acceptance and, though different in detail, all methods have in common two basic diagnostic criteria: the relative degree of joint laxity (subluxation) and/or the magnitude of DJD. We have shown that the subjective method of hip evaluation used in North America by the OFA is fraught with problems associated with wide variation in interpretation among radiologists (Smith et al., 1992).

In a study conducted at the University of Pennsylvania, hip radiographs from a sample of 65 large- and giant-breed dogs were evaluated by three radiologists (all board-certified and one of whom regularly provided hip interpretations for the OFA) and by the OFA itself. Based on the OFA 7-point scoring scheme (Excellent, Good, Fair, Borderline, Mild HD, Moderate HD, Severe HD) the two non-OFA readers agreed with the OFA in fewer than 50% of the cases. The radiologist who regularly interprets for the OFA compared somewhat more favorably with official 7-point OFA score (overall agreement on score = 61%). When each radiologist was compared with himself for repeatability of hip score using the same pool of dogs at two different times (within-examiner variability), agreement ranged between 48% and 75%. Therefore, there was considerable disagreement on hip score, not only between radiologists but within the same radiologist at two different times.

The above radiographs were analyzed for the presence or absence of CHD by evaluating agreement among radiologists using a 3-point scoring scale (Normal, Borderline, or Dysplastic). As expected, agreement improved. Nevertheless, the two non-OFA readers disagreed with the OFA more than 25% of the time, representing an agreement only slightly better than chance. In contrast, the OFA-affiliated radiologist agreed with the OFA 95% of the time, supporting the OFA's published data that there is a high level of overall agreement among the OFA radiologists who provide hip scores (Corley, 1992). Of concern was the finding that of the 65 dogs comprising the study sample, ten dogs were determined to be dysplastic by the OFA (and 11 dogs were dysplastic according to the OFA-affiliated radiologist) while, notably, the two non-OFA radiologists diagnosed 25 and 29 dogs to be dysplastic, respectively.

This small study indicated a troubling amount of variability among board-certified radiologists regarding subjective hip interpretation, not only when the 7-point OFA scoring scale was used, but even when only 3-point scoring was performed. As reported, OFA consensus was very uniform for the presence or absence of hip disease. This was interpreted to mean that either the OFA selected for radiologists who read alike or alternatively that OFA radiologists have conformed to a common standard. It should be understood, however, that consistent scoring by a group of radiologists, while seemingly desirable, is only of value if the hip phenotypes identified (OFA scores) can be shown to have acceptably high heritability. The most reliable estimates of heritability of CHD range in the German Shepherd dog breed from a low of 0.22 (Leighton et al., 1977) to a high of 0.43 (Hedhammar et al., 1979). While these figures were thought to be high enough to expect a lowering of disease frequency by selective breeding, they were calculated for German shepherd dogs more than 15 years ago when, presumably, variation in disease phenotypes was greater than today. In the mathematical calculation of heritability, it is an unavoidable phenomenon that when the phenotypic variability of a quantitative genetic trait diminishes, the estimate of heritability also diminishes. Though not yet tested, it is conceivable that if present-day German shepherd pedigrees were analyzed for variation in subjective hip phenotype, heritability of CHD as determined by the OFA method may be too low to expect significant further change by applying the current method of hip evaluation as a selection criterion.

## Quantitative Methods of Diagnosis

Because of the inherent problems with subjective scoring, physical and radiographic techniques have been proposed or practiced in an attempt to provide more reliable CHD diagnosis. Few techniques, however, have experienced widespread acceptance or have found strong scientific support. Diagnostic methods such as those of Ortolani, Barden, and Barlow have used palpation of the hip to provide semiquantitative information regarding joint laxity and associated CHD susceptibility.

Of the radiographic methods to quantitate joint laxity (subluxation), the Norberg angle (NA) method has been used primarily in Europe and applied sporadically over the years in the United States, but usually as an investigational rather than clinical tool. The Norberg angle quantitates joint laxity from the standard hip-extended radiographic projection. It is the numerical representation of subjective joint laxity (subluxation) seen on the hip-extended radiograph (Fig. 2). Norberg angle scores typically range between a low of 55 degrees to a high of 115 degrees. Smaller numbers in the NA scale indicate greater hip laxity. No studies have been conducted to document the range of NA associated with normal hip laxity; however, one report suggests that above 105 degrees is normal.

Norberg angle scores derived from a sample population of 113 dogs radiographed at the VHUP and

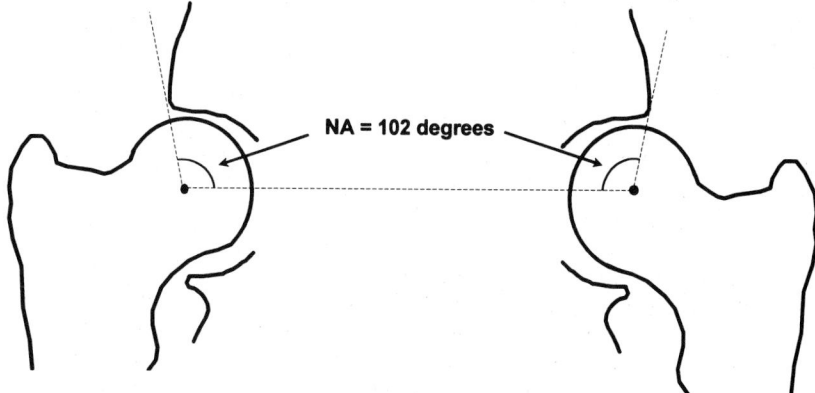

**Figure 2.** The Norberg angle is the included angle between a line connecting the femoral head center and a line from the center of the femoral head to the craniodorsal acetabular rim.

scored subjectively by the OFA ranged between 87 degrees and 115 degrees. Mean NA score of the 99 dogs graded "normal" by the OFA was 104.2 degrees, and for the 14 dogs graded "dysplastic," mean NA was 96 degrees. Interestingly, hips judged to be normal by the OFA had Norberg angles as low as 89 degrees and 46 of the 99 OFA normal dogs had hip laxity less than 105 NA degrees. While the OFA does not measure NA as part of its evaluation, it is clear from this study that many dogs with NA less than 105 degrees are being certified for breeding. It is likely that the criterion of 105 degrees is too stringent to be practical, particularly since its diagnostic utility has not been definitively demonstrated. Likely this explains the poor acceptance of the NA method as a CHD diagnostic tool.

## COMPRESSION/DISTRACTION METHOD

A new stress-radiographic diagnostic method was introduced into the veterinary literature in 1990, culminating 7 years of development and testing at the University of Pennsylvania School of Veterinary Medicine (Smith, Biery, and Gregor, 1990). Studies were initiated in 1983 with an investigation of the role of passive hip laxity in the development of DJD. As previously mentioned, it had been generally accepted that joint laxity (subluxation) appearing on the standard hip-extended radiograph portended the development of DJD, yet there was no good scientific evidence that supported this. It was clear that prevalence of CHD was very high even in the face of concerted efforts on the part of dog breeders and veterinarians to reduce CHD incidence by selective breeding using the OFA method. Also, it was becoming increasingly clear that while hip dysplasia was thought to be a quantitative genetic trait, the adherence to OFA guidelines for breeding normal to normal dogs was still yielding a disappointingly high incidence of CHD in the offspring. For example, in the German shepherd breed, normal to normal matings were shown to produce only 27% (Jessen and Spurrell, 1972) to 81% (Snavely, 1959) normal offspring. Furthermore, the 2-year age requirement for determining definitive hip status by the OFA method was of marginal value to breeders wishing to select at the youngest possible age the puppies to keep as potential breeding candidates. In the face of this uncertainty, breeders

were compelled to follow their instincts in puppy selection or forced to invest substantial time and money in feeding and maintaining many animals with good breeding potential until 2 years of age.

Improvements, therefore, in the method of hip evaluation and, indeed, in the understanding of hip dysplasia as a disease were clearly warranted. Our initial studies began by looking at the hip from an anatomic/mechanical perspective. From studies of cadaver hips, it was observed that the standard hip-extended radiographic view masked hip laxity by a winding up of the

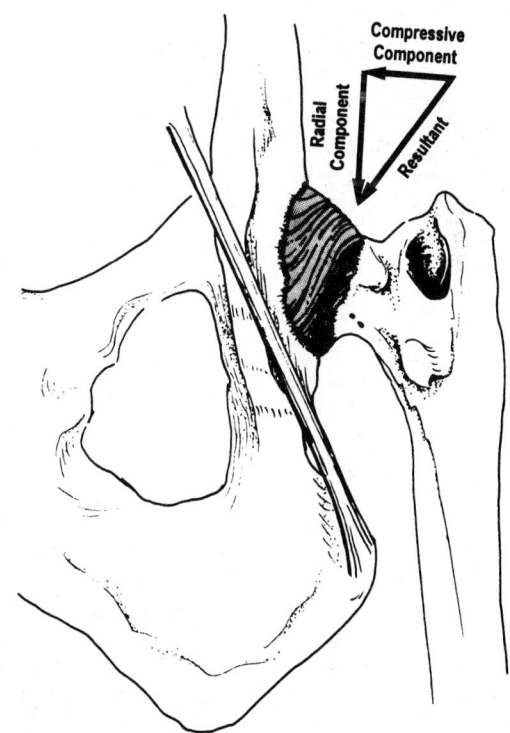

**Figure 3.** Dorsal view drawing of an extended hip, showing the orientation of lines of stress in the fibrous elements of the joint capsule as the hip is extended and internally rotated. Note that a "compressive" component of force is generated that acts to mask the true passive laxity of the hip. (Adapted from Smith GK, Biery DN, and Gregor TP: New concepts of coxofemoral joint stability and the development of a clinical stress-radiographic method for quantitating hip joint laxity in the dog. J Am Vet Med Assoc 196:63, 1990, with permission.)

tensile elements in the joint capsule (Smith, Biery, and Gregor, 1990) (Fig. 3). Also, a hydrostatic (vacuum-like) mechanism was discovered that critically influenced hip joint stability (Smith, Biery, and Gregor, 1990). We conjectured, with support from the literature (Lust et al., 1980), that increased synovial fluid volume acted to negate the effect of the hydrostatic mechanism in its function to passively stabilize the hip. Although at the time the clinical significance of our findings were unclear, the discovery led to the development and investigation of a new stress-radiographic positioning method to quantitate hip laxity in the dog. Mechanical testing instrumentation was designed and machined to evaluate the biomechanics of the newly discovered hydrostatic phenomenon and to explore the role of passive hip laxity in overall hip stability (Heyman, Smith, and Cofone, 1993). The first part of the study involved mechanical testing of cadaver canine hips to reveal the range of flexion/extension, adduction/abduction, and internal/external rotation associated with maximal passive laxity of the hip joint. This information was critical for optimizing the new distraction method and maintaining quality assurance and repeatability from one examiner to another. Relative to the plane of the pelvis, the optimal range of hip position was found to be between 10 degrees of flexion and 30

degrees of extension, between 10 degrees of abduction and 30 degrees of abduction, and between 0 and 10 degrees of external rotation. Any deviation out of this range was observed to cause a precipitous decrease in lateral displacement of the femoral head from the acetabulum. In fact, mechanical data from cadaver hips oriented in the standard hip-extended, internally rotated, OFA position demonstrated a minimum 50% reduction in measurable hip laxity, corroborating earlier necropsy observations that the winding up of the joint capsule (Fig. 3) had a profound effect on reducing apparent hip laxity.

The new stress-radiographic method required the dog to be under deep sedation or general anesthesia and incorporated two views with the dog in supine position and hips at neutral (standing or stance phase) flexion/extension angle—a compression view with the femoral heads fully seated in the acetabula, and a distraction view obtained by levering a custom-designed device between the legs at the level of the ventral pelvis, creating maximal lateral displacement of the femoral heads (Smith, Biery, and Gregor, 1990) (Fig. 4). Additionally, a new measurement method was developed to quantitate the relative degree of femoral head displacement from the acetabulum visible in either the compression view (not shown) or distraction views (Fig.

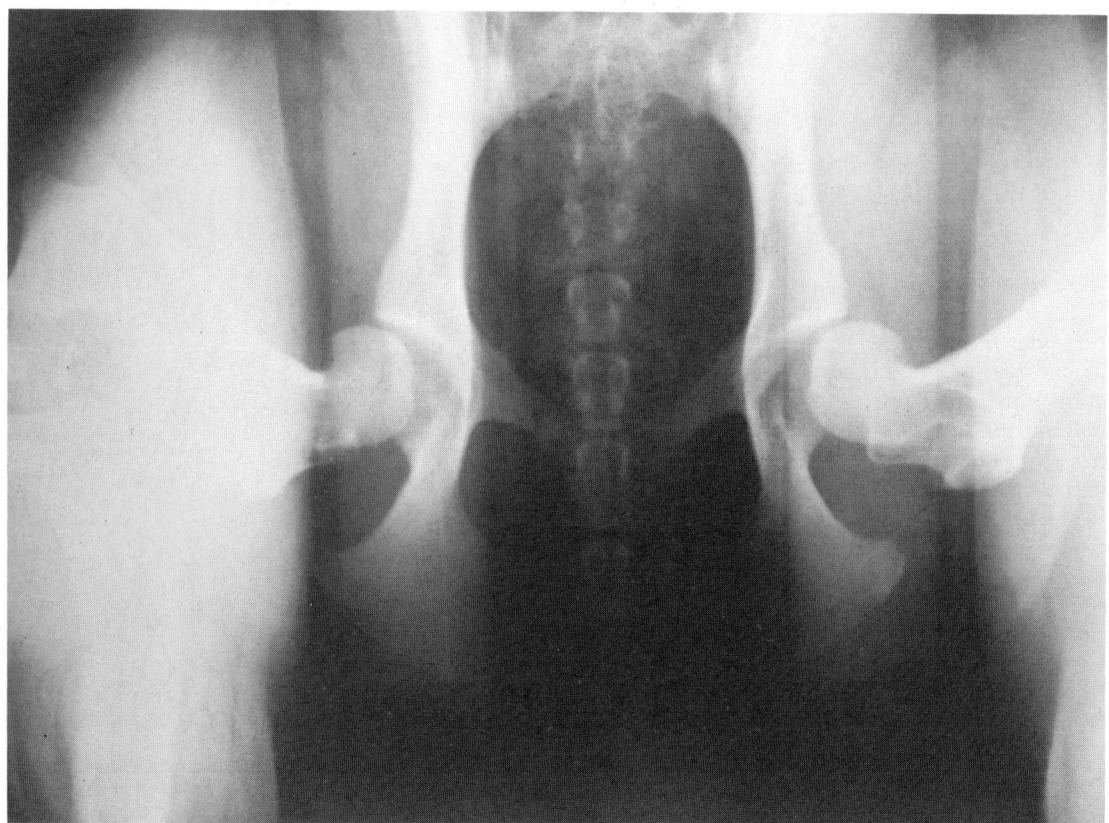

**Figure 4.** New "distraction" stress-radiograph of the dog previously shown in Figure 1 illustrating the orientation of the coxofemoral joints associated with maximal lateral displacement. Note the marked passive laxity apparent in the hip (DI = 0.53 bilateral) in contrast to that in the standard hip-extended radiograph of Figure 1 (NA = 99 degrees). This golden retriever would be judged to have hip hyperlaxity and therefore would be considered CHD susceptible and not a particularly good candidate for breeding.

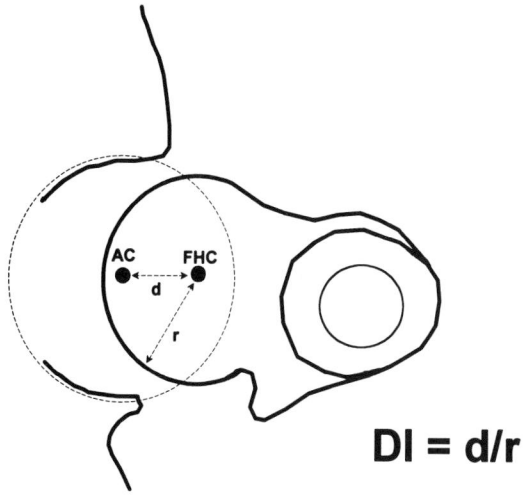

$$DI = d/r$$

**Figure 5.** The distraction index is determined by measuring the separation distance, *d*, of the femoral head center (FHC) from the acetabular center (AC) and dividing by the radius of the femoral head (DI = *d/r*). In the schematic above DI = 0.72.

5). The new measurement method utilized an *index* from 0 to 1, with 0 being a congruent hip, as seen in the compression radiographic view and 1 representing the most extreme joint laxity as might be seen in the distraction view of hips that are virtually luxated. The distraction index (DI) is a ratio scale, meaning a hip with a DI of 0.6 shows twice the laxity of a hip with a DI of 0.3. The femoral head of a hip with an index of 0.6 can be considered 60% subluxated from the acetabulum. The OFA scoring method is an ordinal scale and the Norberg angle is an interval scale, neither of which is similarly proportional. Also, the DI is more intuitive than NA score; i.e., a hip 60% luxated is more easily envisaged than one with NA of 85 degrees.

## PERTINENT RESEARCH FINDINGS

The remainder of this article will summarize pertinent research findings and attempt to put into perspective the new stress-radiographic diagnostic method relative to OFA scoring and the NA method, both of which are derived from the standard hip-extended radiographic position.

### Hip Laxity Comparisons

In a population of purebred dogs (*n* = 142), hip laxity (subluxation) in the standard OFA radiographic view was compared with hip laxity from the distraction view. The distraction radiograph was found on average to reveal 2.5 times more joint laxity than the standard hip-extended radiograph (Smith, Biery, and Gregor, 1990). For a specific hip, the distraction view always revealed more laxity than the hip-extended view and often showed obvious measurable laxity when the hip-extended view showed none (Smith et al., 1993). Joint

laxity on the distraction view was found to correlate positively with laxity from palpation of the hip joint (Ortolani and Bardens signs); however, not highly enough to be predictive. None of the dogs in the study were clinically symptomatic of CHD and therefore no correlations could be made between clinical signs and DI score.

### Correlation of Laxity to DJD

An analysis of hip laxity and the coexistence of DJD in large- and giant-breed dogs (mean age = 28 months; *n* = 227), showed hip laxity from the distraction radiographic view to be more highly correlated with the radiographic appearance of DJD than was laxity (subluxation) from the hip-extended view. Particularly striking was the observation that hips showing very low laxity, so-called tight hips, were highly unlikely to have evidence of DJD. As laxity increased, there was an associated increase in the probability for hip DJD. Interestingly, no hip with a distraction index less than 0.3 had radiographic evidence of DJD. However, the converse was not true (i.e., not all dogs having hip laxity greater than 0.3 ["loose hips"] demonstrated evidence of DJD within the age range of the sample population [1 to 5 years of age]).

In the same sample of 227 dogs, the correlation of Norberg angle with hip DJD from the standard hip-extended radiograph also yielded a statistically significant, though weaker, correlation. Unlike the distraction method, however, there was no recognizable threshold of joint laxity below which no dogs were found to have hip DJD. That is, although DJD susceptibility clearly decreased as laxity (subluxation) decreased on the standard radiographic view, there was no practical range of joint laxity at which hips could be considered nonsusceptible to DJD. Similar to patterns observed for the distraction method, not all dogs demonstrating obvious hip subluxation showed radiographic evidence of DJD even though the mean age of this population was 28 months.

From these data, it was theorized that hip laxity was divisible into two forms; *passive hip laxity*, which is the relative looseness of the hip joint as measured in the sedated dog absent of active muscle contracture or weight bearing; and *functional hip laxity*, the pathologic form of hip laxity, occurring during weight bearing resulting in wear of the joint cartilage, ultimately leading to DJD. While functional hip laxity is clearly of greatest diagnostic interest, there currently are no means to measure it. Passive hip laxity, on the other hand, is a readily measurable quantity and, since it was shown in this study to be a prerequisite for functional laxity, it appeared to represent a risk factor for DJD or, loosely defined, perhaps a carrier state. In other words, passive hip laxity was necessary for DJD but not by itself sufficient to cause DJD. Importantly, however, dogs having hip distraction index less than 0.3 were true-negatives for CHD within the span of the study. Dogs with DI greater than 0.3 were considered to have hip *hyperlaxity*, and were DJD *susceptible* even though often appearing phenotypically normal on the standard hip-extended radiograph (Smith et al., 1993).

## Breed-Specific Passive Hip Laxity and Susceptibility to DJD

Breeds of dogs known to have very low frequency of hip dysplasia (<1%) were found to have uniformly tight hip joints (i.e., extremely low laxities) on distraction radiography. In fact, the mean passive laxity for racing greyhounds and performance-bred borzois was significantly tighter than breeds of dogs commonly afflicted with CHD, such as German shepherd dogs, golden retrievers, and Rottweilers ($p < .0001$). Greater than 98% of all borzois and greyhounds had distraction index less than 0.3, with some being as low as 0.08 (Smith et al., 1992). All dogs were phenotypically normal by OFA scoring. This finding supported the hypothesis mentioned above that 0.3 was a biologic threshold separating normal, disease-free hips from hips susceptible to DJD. In contrast, using the standard hip-extended procedure to determine joint laxity (NA), there were no statistically significant differences in breed-specific joint laxity, nor was a disease threshold identified.

## Repeatability of Distraction Index Over Time and the Prediction of DJD

In a 3-year longitudinal evaluation of more than 140 dogs followed from 4 months of age, the distraction index was shown to be clearly more repeatable over time than either the Norberg angle or the OFA score (Smith et al., 1993). Four-month DI correlated highly with 6-month, 12-month, and 24-month DI ($r_i = .82$ to .87). The ranges of correlation coefficients for NA and OFA score over the same interval were much lower. Early distraction index was shown to correlate better with the development of DJD than Norberg angle or OFA score. A subsequent analysis confirmed that of the variables measured, DI at an age as young as 4 months was the best predictor of DJD probability and that the strength of the prediction improved when the analysis was done at 6 months or 1 year (Smith, Popovitch, and Gregor, 1993). Specifically, German shepherd dogs were found to have a 6.3 times higher probability to show DJD than the other dogs in the sample. Furthermore, each 0.1 increase in DI was associated with a 4.1-fold increase in the risk of DJD, supporting the hypothesis that "tighter hips are better hips." A subsequent study of Rottweilers confirmed the patterns of DJD found in German shepherd dogs, where again distraction index was the only significant predictor of the risk for hip DJD. In Rottweilers, however, each 0.1 increase in distraction index was associated with a 2.9-fold increase in DJD risk, a risk factor lower than that for GSDs. Accordingly, in a direct comparison of DJD susceptibility in Rottweilers with GSDs, the latter had 6.4 times more risk of developing DJD. This might sug-

gest either that the German shepherd breed is more sensitive to passive hip laxity or, alternatively, that Rottweilers are laxity tolerant and therefore relatively DJD resistant (Popovitch et al., 1993). These data emphasized the need to develop similar logistic regression curves for all popular breeds of dogs to permit valid application of the distraction index as a selection criterion. Such a need underscores the importance of a nationwide data base to study the relationship of passive hip laxity to DJD on a breed by breed basis.

Our results in GSDs and Rottweilers have recently received support from Lust and coworkers in independent investigations invoking a similar logistic regression model to hip laxity data derived from a small population of Labrador retrievers followed longitudinally. Hip laxity on the distraction radiographic view at 4 and 8 months of age was shown to significantly correlate with later development of DJD determined at necropsy. Each 0.1 increase in DI at 8 months of age corresponded to a 3.1 fold increase in the risk of developing DJD by 2 years of age (Lust et al., 1993).

## Distraction Radiography Before 16 Weeks of Age

A study of 39 8-week-old German shepherd puppies was conducted to learn whether hip laxity at an age younger than 16 weeks would also be predictive of disease susceptibility. Results in this sample of puppies revealed that hip laxity at 8 weeks of age is not sufficiently reliable to use in a predictive sense. Preliminary evidence, however, from other collaborative centers, suggests that some breeds of dogs may demonstrate joint laxity and disease susceptibility at an age earlier than 16 weeks. For the present, however, it is recommended that dogs should not be evaluated before 16 weeks of age and that follow-up radiography to confirm the 16-week laxity should be done at 6 months or 1 year of age.

## Relationship of OFA Score to DI

Hips were evaluated in a population of 65 large-breed dogs both by the official OFA radiographic process and by the compression/distraction stress-radiographic method (Smith et al., 1992). An analysis of the distribution of DI scores corresponding to the seven OFA scoring categories revealed several interesting findings. All dogs graded to have mild, moderate, or severe hip dysplasia by the OFA had corresponding distraction index scores above 0.3 (mean DI = 0.55), indicating excellent agreement of the two scoring methods relative to disease phenotypes. That is, all dogs that the OFA judged to be dysplastic were clearly in the hip hyperlaxity (DJD susceptible) category as judged by the distraction method. The converse, however, was not true. Of the dogs having hips judged excellent by the OFA, 50% had DI scores in the DJD-susceptible category, above 0.3 (mean DI = 0.3). Furthermore, 66%

of the dogs judged to be good and 100% of the dogs judged fair by the OFA had DI scores greater than 0.3 (mean DI = 0.35 and 0.50, respectively). Therefore, a high percentage of dogs (71%) officially certified for breeding by OFA had hip laxities corresponding to DJD susceptibility according to distraction data. Whether the dogs with hip hyperlaxity actually express DJD within their lifetimes or not may be of little importance if in their genetic makeup they carry or have the potential to transmit the susceptibility for DJD to their offspring. It is this fundamental association between hip laxity and the susceptibility for DJD that we feel is not addressed by the current OFA diagnostic method and which perhaps explains the poor progress in reducing CHD frequency after 27 years of application of OFA score as a selection criterion.

## Heritability of Passive Hip Laxity

Studies of CHD heritability, or more specifically of passive hip laxity heritability, are ongoing. All estimates of heritability to date are presently limited to the German shepherd and the Labrador retriever breeds. Heritability of passive laxity is a property of the population under study; therefore, heritability of passive hip laxity must be calculated for each breed. An upper limit of a trait's heritability is the intraclass correlation coefficient of repeatability over time, and this correlation coefficient for German shepherd dogs in the sample mentioned above was between 0.67 and 0.74, an extremely high upper limit. Heritability can also be estimated by analyzing the resemblance of parent to offspring relative to passive hip laxity. Regression analysis of litter DI mean plotted against midparent DI mean has yielded estimates of laxity heritability for the German shepherd breed from 0.42 to 0.65 and an upper limit for the Labrador retriever breed of 0.85. Although heritability analyses are still incomplete, these early results are promising that the heritability of passive laxity (and therefore the likelihood for DJD) will be much higher than the low heritability estimate of 0.22 for CHD as diagnosed by the standard hip-extended method (Leighton et al., 1977). If so, the use of the distraction index as a selection criterion can be expected to result in more rapid progress in reducing the incidence and severity of CHD.

## CONCLUSIONS

It is our belief that sufficient research on safety and efficacy of the new CHD diagnostic technology has been accomplished to warrant initiating multicenter clinical trials. Of paramount importance in the transfer of the new diagnostic technology for widespread utilization is the need for optimal quality assurance and repeatability among centers. By design, the introduction of the new method into the ever-expanding arsenal of diagnostic techniques has followed (and will follow) a cautious path. In the spring of 1993, the University of Pennsylvania Hip Improvement Program (PennHIP) was established as a collaborative effort of academic and private-practice veterinarians to facilitate the controlled transfer of technology to multiple centers. The program was designed to fulfill many objectives, the primary one being to reduce the frequency of hip dysplasia in all breeds of dogs. Approximately 100 veterinarians, mostly surgery or radiology specialists, were trained as "collaborators" in the new distraction radiographic procedure. Training consisted of a full-day seminar, where the rapidly expanding body of scientific information on canine hip dysplasia was covered in great detail. In addition, a set of quality assurance exercises were specified for each participant to perform in their respective practices prior to being officially certified in the method. The seminar attempted to provide a full understanding of the strengths and weaknesses of the new method in an effort to avoid misinterpretation and, particularly, misuse of the technology. As of the writing of this article, there are approximately 100 certified collaborators in the United States and Canada.

Data from collaborators will be compiled in a large medical data base at PennHIP and will be used to investigate genetic aspects of passive hip laxity by breed. The approximately 2000 dogs evaluated thus far as part of the research effort must be expanded manyfold to address the numerous breed-specific questions and concerns of breeders. Specific emphasis will be placed on means to optimally control or eliminate CHD by mass selection and on monitoring the progress of the PennHIP system on a regular basis. The process entails hip evaluation of large populations of dogs with respect to many parameters including age, sex, body weight, and breed, and appropriate utilization of statistical/mathematical methodology to discern relationships between passive hip laxity and the expression of DJD, both within generation and across generations. By periodic monitoring and reporting of the success of this method as it becomes more widely available, we hope that it will retain its scientific integrity and that those performing it will benefit from the associated scientific credibility. Conversely, if after a reasonable trial period the method proves ineffective in reducing the frequency of hip dysplasia, our protocol of regular analyses will ensure that the technique will not be dogmatically misapplied for decades to come.

For pet owners or dog breeders desiring to have their animals evaluated by the PennHIP system, practitioners are requested to refer them to one of the collaborative centers. We are encouraged by the enthusiasm and feedback from PennHIP collaborators and from the positive response of the public. If current trends continue, we plan in 1994 and 1995 to expand the network of PennHIP collaborators to grow the data base at a faster rate and to make the new diagnostic technology more available to the public. For veterinarians interested in training and participating in PennHIP, the current minimum recommended requirements include a 300-mA radiographic unit and an automatic film processor. PennHIP information including training programs or an updated list of certified collaborators may be obtained by writing [International Canine Genetics, Inc., 271 Great Valley Parkway, Malvern, PA 19355], telephone [800-248-8099], or fax [610-640-5754].

ACKNOWLEDGMENTS: This work was supported by the University of Pennsylvania Research Fund; the National Institutes of Health; the Morris Animal Foundation; The Seeing Eye, Inc.; Ralston Purina, Co; and the PennHIP collaborative effort.

## References and Suggested Reading

Corley EA: Role of the Orthopedic Foundation for Animals in the control of canine hip dysplasia. Vet Clin North Am 22:579, 1992.
*Beyond its title, this paper gives a summary of compiled data regarding the frequency of CHD for most popular breeds of dogs, with tabulation of the efficacy of the OFA method over a 16-year period.*

Hedhammar A, Olsson SE, Andersson SA, et al: Canine hip dysplasia: A study of heritability in 401 litters of German shepherd dogs. J Am Vet Med Assoc 174:1012, 1979.
*An analysis of 401 matings of German shepherd dogs revealing a heritability for CHD of 0.43 as diagnosed by the standard hip-extended method.*

Henricson B, Norberg I, and Olsson S-E: On the etiology and pathogenesis of hip dysplasia: A comparative review. J Small Anim Pract 7:673, 1966.
*A review of the similarities and differences of CHD in dogs, and humans.*

Heyman SJ, Smith GK, and Cofone MA: A biomechanical study of the effect of coxofemoral positioning on passive hip joint laxity in the dog, Am J Vet Res 54:210, 1993.
*A biomechanical study of cadaver dogs identifying the range of motion of the hip joint where maximum passive laxity can be measured.*

Jessen CR and Spurrell FA: Radiographic detection of canine hip dysplasia in known age groups. In Proc AVMA Symposium on Hip Dysplasia, 1972, p 93.
*A longitudinal study of large populations of German shepherd dogs and vizslas relative to the age and frequency of radiographic expression of CHD.*

Leighton EA, Linn JM, Willham RL, et al: A genetic study of canine hip dysplasia. Am J Vet Res 38:241, 1977.
*A study of generations of a large population of German shepherd army working dogs yielding an estimate of heritability for CHD of 0.22 using the standard hip-extended radiographic method.*

Lust G, Beilman WT, Dueland DJ, and Farrell PW: Intra-articular volume and hip joint instability in dogs with hip dysplasia. J Bone Joint Surg 62-A:576, 1980.
*A study of Labrador retriever puppies from dysplastic parents identifying an association between susceptibility for CHD and increased synovial fluid volume.*

Lust G, Williams AJ, Burton-Wurster N, et al. Joint laxity and its association with hip dysplasia in Labrador retrievers. Am J Vet Res 54:1990, 1993.
*A longitudinal study of a small population of Labrador retrievers invoking a logistic regression model and showing that hip laxity on the distraction radiograph at 4 and 8 months of age significantly correlated with later DJD determined at necropsy.*

Smith GK, Biery DN, and Gregor TP: New concepts of coxofemoral joint stability and the development of a clinical stress-radiographic method for quantitating hip joint laxity in the dog. J Am Vet Med Assoc 196:59, 1990.
*Introduction of a new stress-radiographic method and measurement procedure to quantitate passive hip laxity in dogs from 16 weeks of age.*

Smith GK, Gregor TP, Biery DN, Rhodes WH, and Reid CF: Hip dysplasia diagnosis: A comparison of diagnostic methods and diagnosticians. Proc 1992 Ann Scientific Meeting of the Veterinary Orthopedic Society, Keystone, CO, 1992, p 20.
*A study of the variation among board-certified veterinary radiologists in subjective interpretation of hip radiographs in the extended position and a comparison of these interpretations with distraction index from the same hips.*

Smith GK, Gregor TP, Rhodes WH, and Biery DN: Coxofemoral joint laxity from distraction radiography and its contemporaneous and prospective correlation with laxity, subjective score, and evidence of degenerative joint disease from conventional hip-extended radiography in dogs. Am J Vet Res 54:102, 1993.
*A longitudinal study of the variation and accuracy of various hip scoring methods relative to DJD as an outcome.*

Snavely JG: Genetic aspects of hip dysplasia in dogs. J Am Vet Med Assoc 135:201, 1959.
*A study of 32 German shepherd dogs showing that the frequency of CHD in offspring of normal to normal matings was 19%.*

# TREATMENT OF THE IMMUNE-BASED INFLAMMATORY ARTHROPATHIES OF THE DOG AND CAT

DAVID BENNETT

*Liverpool, United Kingdom*

The immune-based inflammatory arthropathies are a group of arthritides characterized by an active synovitis of unknown etiology, usually affecting several joints in a bilaterally symmetric fashion. The histologic and laboratory features of these conditions supports the view that the immune system is involved in their pathogenesis. High levels of immune complexes are found within the joints and autoantibodies are common (Carter et al., 1989). Systemic involvement is common with these disorders.

Although the immunologic stimuli are unknown, it is thought that in many cases microbial infections are involved. It is possible that an initial joint infection occurs and the microorganism is destroyed but antigens persist within the joint cavity or synovial membrane. Alternatively, distant infection may create circulating immune complexes that are then deposited in the joint, or microbial antigens may be transported to joints by an "inappropriate" antigen-processing mechanism. Other possible sources of antigens include tumor-related antigens. Some immune-based joint disorders in humans are associated with genetic susceptibilities and immune-based arthritis is seen more commonly in certain breeds such as spaniels, German shepherd dogs, collies, boxers, and setters, and there are certain breed-specific conditions seen in the Akita and Shar-Pei. Examples of viral antigens localizing to joints include calicivirus in cats (Bennett et al., 1989) and distemper virus in dogs (Bell, Carter, and Bennett, 1990).

The clinical features of the various immune-based arthritides are similar (Bennett, 1987a,b,c,d; Bennett and Kelly, 1987; Bennett and Nash, 1988). With few exceptions, affected animals have a bilaterally symmetric polyarthritis (involving six or more joints); or a pauciarthritis (affecting two to five joints). Very rarely, only a single joint may be affected. A polyarthritis or pauciarthritis will be characterized by a generalized stiffness, although an obvious limp can be apparent. Some animals are so severely affected that they are unable to walk. Many cases have systemic illness (fever, inappetence, and lethargy) and, indeed, immune-based arthritis is a common cause of "fever of unknown origin." Affected joints are often palpably swollen and painful on manipulation; however, it may not be possible to detect affected joints by palpation alone. Many of these diseases can affect other body systems and produce multisystemic disease (e.g., dermatitis, hemolytic anemia, thrombocytopenia, myositis, meningitis, glomerulonephritis). A diagnosis of inflammatory joint disease can be confirmed by arthrocentesis and synovial fluid examination. Multiple joints should be aspirated under aseptic conditions and total and differential white blood cell (WBC) counts performed. Immune-based arthropathies are generally characterized by high WBC counts (>5000/mm$^3$) most of which are polymorphonuclear cells. Bacterial infections of joints may result in similar changes in the synovial fluid, but infections usually involve only a single joint.

There are a number of different immune-based arthropathies (Table 1). The criteria used to diagnose these different arthropathies are listed in Table 2. It is important to be able to differentiate erosive from non-

erosive disorders (i.e., whether or not there is bony destruction within one or more affected joints as assessed by radiography). The erosive (destructive) types of arthritis generally have a poorer prognosis. Continual assessment of animals is important because the true nature of the disease may only become apparent as it progresses. This probably reflects the fact that many of these conditions have a similar etiopathogenesis and certain individual factors will decide how the disease will be manifested.

## GENERAL PRINCIPLES OF TREATMENT

Dogs and cats with immune-based arthropathies need strict rest, especially initially. Once there is a positive response to treatment, gentle restricted exercise can be given. Exercise should always be regular, the amount and time of day when exercised should be kept constant. Animals should receive good quality diets. Special diets may be indicated in some cases, as in animals with severe kidney damage (see this volume, p 958). Weight control is especially important. Weight gain is likely because affected dogs are often sedentary and may have increased appetite as a result of corticosteroid therapy. Dietary supplementation with essential fatty acids (e.g., evening primrose oil and fish liver oils) may help to reduce the inflammatory load within the joints and aid anti-inflammatory drug therapy. These supplements are often used unless cost is a factor. Dogs and cats that are being immunosuppressed should be protected from possible infection as much as possible, especially if being hospitalized where nosocomial infections are a risk. Animals receiving immunosuppressive drugs should be regularly checked and particular attention paid to the possibility of secondary infections; these are particularly likely to occur in the urinary and respiratory tracts. Appropriate therapy should be given if secondary infections have developed. When deciding to use immunosuppressive doses of drugs, it is best to delay therapy for a few days if biopsies have been taken, in order that some degree of wound healing can occur. Antibiotics for a few days are sometimes given after surgical biopsy. Otherwise, antibiotics are not used in the treatment of immune-based arthritis unless secondary bacterial infections occur (but see idiopathic type I). Low doses of steroids can be used during this initial period, since they will not significantly affect healing.

Vaccination should probably not be given if the animal is receiving immunosuppressive drugs. However, routine vaccination is desirable in animals with immune-based arthritis to reduce the risk of serious infections. It may be possible to suspend or reduce drug administration so that vaccination can be performed. The possible involvement of distemper virus in the etiopathogenesis of the immune-based arthropathies (Bell, Carter, and Bennett, 1990) suggests that distemper vaccination might be better avoided.

There are two objectives of drug therapy: reduction and control of articular inflammation and immunosup-

---

**Table 1.** *Classification of Immune-Based Arthritis*

**Erosive**
  Rheumatoid arthritis
  Periosteal proliferative polyarthritis
  Polyarthritis of greyhounds

**Non-erosive**
  Systemic lupus erythematosus
  Polyarthritis/polymyositis
  Polyarthritis/meningitis
  Arthritis of Akita
  Amyloidosis of Shar-Pei
  Polyarteritis nodosa
  Idiopathic
    Type I (uncomplicated)
    Type II (reactive)
    Type III (enteropathic)
    Type IV (malignancy)

**Miscellaneous**
  Vaccination "reactions"
  Plasmacytic/lymphocytic synovitis
  Drug-induced

**Table 2.** *Criteria for the Diagnosis of Immune-Based Arthropathies*

**Erosive**

***Canine (Feline) Rheumatoid Arthritis***°

1. Stiffness after rest
2. Pain or tenderness on motion of at least one joint
3. Swelling of at least one joint
4. Swelling of one other joint within 3 mo
5. Symmetric joint swelling
6. Subcutaneous nodules
7. Erosive changes on joint radiographs
8. Serologic test positive for rheumatoid factor
9. Abnormal synovial fluid
10. Histopathology of synovium
11. Histopathology of subcutaneous nodules

°Seven criteria must be fulfilled, including at least two of criteria 7, 8, and 10. Criteria 1, 2, 3, 4, and 5 should be present for at least 6 wk. More common in the dog.

***Feline (Canine) Periosteal Proliferative Polyarthritis***†

1. At least four joints affected
2. Periosteal articular new bone on radiographs
3. Erosive changes on joint radiographs
4. Enthesiopathies

†Criteria 1, 2, and 3 must be satisfied. More common in the cat, especially males.

***Polyarthritis of Greyhounds***

1. Breed specific
2. Erosive polyarthritis
   (possible *Mycoplasma* infection)

**Nonerosive**

***Systemic Lupus Erythematosus***†

1. Multisystem disease; most common manifestations include polyarthritis, skin disease, anemia, glomerulonephritis
2. Antinuclear antibody present in blood
3. Immunopathologic features consistent with clinical involvement should be present (e.g., antibodies should be shown against RBC in hemolytic anemia, platelets in thrombocytopenia; and immunoglobulin/complement deposits shown in tissue biopsies in cases of glomerulonephritis, dermatitis, arthritis)

†Criteria 1 and 2 must always be satisfied.

***Polyarthritis/Polymyositis Syndrome***

1. Nonerosive polyarthritis
2. Chronic active myositis in at least two muscle biopsies
3. Negative for antinuclear antibody

***Polyarthritis/Meningitis Syndrome***

1. Nonerosive polyarthritis
2. Clinical signs of neck pain
3. Abnormal CSF-increased protein content, increased WBC count, increased CPK levels
4. Negative for antinuclear antibody

***Familial Renal Amyloidosis in Shar-Pei Dogs***

1. Breed specific
2. Swollen hock or carpus (or other joints)
3. Pyrexia (lethargy and inappetence)
4. Other organ involvement (renal failure due to amyloidosis)
5. Enthesiopathies
6. Negative for antinuclear antibody

***Heritable Polyarthritis of the Adolescent Akita***

1. Breed specific
2. Young dogs—<1 year of age
3. Other organ involvement (e.g., meningitis)
4. Negative for antinuclear antibody

***Polyarteritis Nodosa***

1. Symmetric polyarthritis
2. Necrosis and inflammation of blood vessels seen on biopsy of synovium, and other tissues
3. Negative for antinuclear antibody

***Idiopathic***

Includes all cases of polyarthritis that do not satisfy criteria for the above

Type I:    No associations
Type II:   Arthritis associated with infection elsewhere in body (reactive arthritis)
Type III:  Arthritis associated with gastrointestinal disease (enteropathic arthritis)
Type IV:   Arthritis associated with neoplastic disease
Some cases originally classified as IP may require reclassification as the disease process progresses

**Miscellaneous**

**"Vaccination Reactions"**

Arthritis develops within 5–7 days of inoculation
Arthritis normally resolves within 1–3 days
Mainly associated with calicivirus vaccination in the cat

***Plasmacytic/Lymphocytic Synovitis***

Often present as cranial cruciate ligament failure

***Drug-Induced***

Arthritis associated with drug administration
Usually antibiotic
Previous exposure to drug
Arthritis resolves within 5–7 days of stopping drug
Challenge studies can confirm diagnosis

pression. The rationale of the latter is to control or even stop the immune response occurring within the joints (and other areas of the body). The most commonly used drugs and drug protocols are listed in Table 3. Careful serial evaluation is essential because immune-based arthritis may be associated with systemic disease. Because there are toxic side effects associated with the various therapeutic agents, it may be difficult to differentiate between toxic drug effect and systemic effects of the disease. Efficacy of individual drugs may be difficult to assess because combination therapy is common. A number of different therapeutic regimens are used. They vary not only between the different types of arthropathy, but also between different individuals where one particular regimen may be successful in one case, but not in another. Joint fluid analysis is the best

method for assessing efficacy of drug therapy; serial synovianalysis is indicated in dogs with immune-based arthritis.

## Corticosteroid (Glucocorticoid) Therapy

Corticosteroids are the most useful drugs used to treat the immune-based arthropathies. They can be used at an anti-inflammatory dose or at an immunosuppressive dose. Ideally, the drug should have potent anti-inflammatory actions, minimal mineralocortical potency, and a predictable half-life. Some of the very potent anti-inflammatory glucocorticoids have very long half-lives and it is difficult to accurately assess the dosing interval. For these reasons, prednisolone is the

**Table 3.** *Drugs Used to Treat Immune-Based Polyarthritis*

| Drug | Trade Name | Recommendations for Use |
|---|---|---|
| Prednisolone (prednisone) | Precortisyl (Decortisyl) | Immunosuppressive dose (1–2 mg/kg q8h PO) for "acute" cases; this dose continued for 2–3 wk and then gradually reduced over 3–4 mo<br>Anti-inflammatory dose (e.g., 0.25 mg/kg q8h PO); smallest dose that provides clinical improvement for "chronic" cases |
| Cyclophosphamide | Cytoxan | 1.5 mg/kg in dogs >30 kg<br>2.0 mg/kg in dogs 15–30 kg<br>2.5 mg/kg in dogs <15 kg and cats<br>Given on 4 consecutive days each week for up to 16 wk<br>Given in conjunction with anti-inflammatory dose of prednisolone each day; hematology every 7–14 days; if WBC <6000/mm$^3$, or platelets count <125,000/mm$^3$, reduce cyclophosphamide by 25%, if WBC <4000/mm$^3$ or platelets count <100,000/mm$^3$ discontinue for 2 wk, then recommence at 50% original dose |
| Azathioprine | Imuran | 2.0 mg/kg EOD, PO; used as an alternative to cyclophosphamide; given with prednisolone (each drug given on different days); not to be used for cats; hematology every 7–14 days (see cyclophosphamide) |
| Sulfasalazine | Salazopyrin | 25 mg/kg q12h PO |
| Sodium aurothiomalate | Myochrysine | 0.5 mg/kg by intramuscular injection once a week for 6 wk; usually given with daily oral prednisolone (anti-inflammatory doses); can be repeated after 2–3 mo; give small test dose first; hematology every 7–14 days |
| Auranofin | Ridaura | 0.05–2.0 mg/kg b.i.d. PO (maximum 9 mg/day); can be given with prednisolone; can be given as continuous regime; hematology every 7–14 days |
| Colchicine | Colchicine | 0.03 mg/kg b.i.d. PO |
| Dimethyl sulfoxide | DMSO | Up to 250 mg/kg; can be given PO, IV, SC, topically, or intra-articularly |
| Levamisole | Levacide | 3–7 mg/kg EOD, PO; maximum dose of 150 mg/day; used for up to 4 mo; anti-inflammatory dose of prednisolone used initially |

most common drug used, although methylprednisolone is a useful alternative.

The most commonly encountered side effects of corticosteroid therapy are polydipsia/polyuria and polyphagia, and these can be minimized by using low doses. Animals on steroid therapy must always have access to water, although food intake should be controlled. Long-term steroid therapy can cause atrophy of skin and hair loss and steroid-induced hepatopathy. Steroids can also induce muscle weakness, which may reduce the animal's functional capability, and very occasionally, untoward behavioral changes may occur (i.e., aggression, lethargy, and disorientation) (see "Clinical Applications of Glucocorticoid Therapy in Nonendocrine Disease," this volume, p 406).

The anti-inflammatory dose of prednisolone used by the author is 0.25 mg/kg every 8 hr PO, whereas the immunosuppressive dose is at least 3 to 6 mg/kg daily (initially divided into three daily doses PO). The anti-inflammatory dose is often used to treat the erosive arthropathies (rheumatoid arthritis, periosteal proliferative polyarthritis), since immunosuppression is unlikely to induce remission of the disease. The anti-inflammatory dose will certainly improve the quality of life and ambulation, and the risks associated with immunosuppression are avoided. In these cases, the drug should preferably be used only when the disease is particularly active and the lowest possible dose given consistent with an acceptable clinical improvement. If continuous therapy is necessary, it can often be used on an alternate-day basis or even less frequently. With continuous maintenance therapy, glucocorticoids are best given in a single dose at approximately 10 AM. This will minimize suppression of the endogenous adrenocorticotrophic hormone (ACTH) production, although this may not be true for cats.

Immunosuppressive doses of prednisolone can be used in the treatment of erosive arthropathies, although immunosuppressive therapy is better suited to treatment of the nonerosive disorders, where the chances of achieving disease remission are greater. The immunosuppressive dose is, of course, also anti-inflammatory. Prednisolone at 3 to 6 mg/kg daily (in divided doses PO) should be given for at least 2 to 3 weeks even though clinical improvement usually occurs within 2 to 3 days. After 2 weeks of therapy, repeat synovianalysis is helpful for assessing the efficacy of treatment. If the WBC count has fallen below 4000/mm$^3$ and most of the cells are mononuclear, the inflammatory reaction has subsided. If the WBC count is still high and most cells are polymorphonuclear, the prognosis for remission is poor. In the latter case, the immunosuppressive dose of steroid should be continued for another 2 weeks and the joint fluid analysis repeated. If the cell count has fallen, the dose of prednisolone can be gradually reduced over a period of 3 months. Continual clinical assessment is essential during this period. If there is any suspicion that the disease is becoming active again, arthrocentesis and synovianalysis should be performed. If the disease symptoms recur while the glucocorticoid dose is being reduced, the dose should be increased and therapy continued for a longer time. If relapse occurs again when the dose is reduced, immunosuppression by the use of cytotoxic drugs is recommended. If relapse occurs some time after the initial therapy has been completed, then further treatment with steroids using the same dose regimen is justified. However, if continual relapses occur after therapy has finished, particularly within a few weeks, then immunosuppression with cytotoxic drugs should again be tried.

## Cytotoxic Drugs

### CYCLOPHOSPHAMIDE

The cytotoxic drug of choice is the alkylating agent, cyclophosphamide (Cytoxan). The dose ranges from 1.5 to 2.5 mg/kg (every 24 hr PO) depending upon the size of the animal (Table 3). The drug is given for only 4 consecutive days of each week and is always combined with an anti-inflammatory dose of prednisolone. As remission with the cytotoxic drugs can take up to 16 weeks, concurrent glucocorticoid therapy is needed to relieve inflammation (pain) and improve the animal's quality of life. Because of their slow action, cyclophosphamide and other cytotoxic agents are often referred to as slow-acting antirheumatic drugs (SAARDs).

Cyclophosphamide is continued for up to 4 months, although it can be discontinued after 2 to 3 months if remission has been achieved and maintained. Routine hematology should be performed on animals receiving any cytotoxic drug to check for bone marrow suppression. If the WBC count falls below 6000/mm$^3$, or the platelet count falls below 125,000/mm$^3$, the drug should be reduced by 25%; if the WBC count falls below 4000/mm$^3$, or the platelet count below 100,000/mm$^3$, the drug is stopped for 2 weeks and then recommenced at half the original dose. The hematologic examination should be carried out every 7 to 14 days. Hemorrhagic cystitis is another side effect of cyclophosphamide therapy; it is advisable to monitor the urine on a weekly basis for the presence of blood. If hematuria occurs, the drug should be stopped. Cyclophosphamide should never be continued for more than 4 months, because of the possibility of bladder toxicity (i.e., protracted cystitis and carcinoma development).

### AZATHIOPRINE

If cytotoxic therapy is needed for more than 4 months, azathioprine (a purine antagonist) is used. This drug *should not* be given to the feline patient. The dose of azathioprine is approximately 2.0 mg/kg PO every other day; this dose can be alternated with an anti-inflammatory dose of prednisolone. Bone marrow suppression is more likely when using the thiopurines than cyclophosphamide; it can occur within 4 to 6 weeks as compared to several months. Routine hematologic monitoring is thus essential when using azathioprine (see "Cyclophosphamide," above). Azathioprine can cause hepatitis and regular biochemical assessment of liver damage is thus indicated. Synovial fluid analysis should also be carried out to check the efficacy of treatment.

If relapse occurs after using cytotoxic drugs and prednisolone, it is always worth trying a second course of cytotoxic therapy, perhaps using one of the alternatives (i.e., azathioprine if cyclophosphamide has been used). Otherwise, continuous steroid therapy is necessary. In refractory cases, the lowest effective anti-inflammatory dose of prednisolone should be used, based on an acceptable clinical response and quality of life. Euthanasia has to be considered in those cases that cannot be controlled by drug therapy or where the doses of steroid required are causing unacceptable side effects.

### CHRYSOTHERAPY

The use of gold compounds is mainly indicated in rheumatoid arthritis and should always be tried first in treating this particular disease. The mode of action of gold is unknown, although it does cause immunosuppression (e.g., reduces immune complex and immunoglobulin levels in the blood, reduces lymphocyte responsiveness to mitogens), inhibits certain connective tissue enzymes (e.g., elastase, collagenase, hyaluronidase) and has certain anti-inflammatory properties (e.g., protection against free oxygen radicals).

Gold can be given either by intramuscular injection as sodium aurothiomalate (Myochrysine) or orally as auranofin (Ridaura). Chrysotherapy is generally combined with low-dose (anti-inflammatory) glucocorticoid treatment. The intramuscular injection is given weekly for 6 to 8 weeks at an approximate dose of 0.5 mg/kg. A small test dose should be given first to ensure there are no sensitivities to the drug such as skin reactions or postinjection flares of joint inflammation. The injections themselves can be painful for the animal; incorporation of local anesthetic (e.g., lidocaine) is used by some clinicians. Toxic side effects of gold therapy include stomatitis, dermatitis, thrombocytopenia, leukopenia, and renal damage. Routine hematologic examination should be done and urine should be regularly tested for the presence of protein. If proteinuria develops or progresses or any other adverse effects are noted, gold therapy should immediately be discontinued. Once a course of intramuscular gold has been given, it can be repeated every 2 to 3 months as a maintenance therapy or repeated if a disease flare-up occurs.

The oral preparation (auranofin) is less toxic but is also less effective, and is more expensive than the injectable form. Although auranofin can produce the same side effects as sodium aurothiomalate, diarrhea is the most troublesome. Reducing the dose and using dietary additives to absorb intestinal fluid can help. The oral preparation should be used for at least 1 month to attempt remission; if remission occurs, the drug can be stopped and reinstated if relapse occurs. Alternatively, low-dose maintenance therapy can be tried where the drug is given once or twice weekly. Complete remission is not likely with the erosive arthropathies; however, clinical improvement will occur in many cases.

## Other Therapies

### SULFASALAZINE

Sulfasalazine (Salazopyrin) has been used to treat immune-based polyarthritis, particularly idiopathic type III and occasionally erosive (rheumatoid) arthritis. It is a drug that is mainly used to treat gastrointestinal disorders, in particular ulcerative colitis, and hence its indications in enteropathic (type III) polyarthropathy. The drug has antibacterial properties and local and systemic anti-inflammatory properties. It also causes immunosuppression. Adverse side effects include vomiting, hemolytic anaemia, stomatitis, jaundice, dermatitis, and leukopenia, but the most common in the dog is keratitis sicca (see "Keratoconjunctivitis Sicca," this volume, p 1231). Regular monitoring (once weekly) of the tear flow by the Schirmer test is advisable if this drug is to be used in the dog. The drug should be stopped if tear flow is substantially reduced or other adverse side effects develop. Sulfasalazine is another SAARD and has to be used for 2 to 4 months to be of benefit.

### LEVAMISOLE

Levamisole at a dose of 3 to 7 mg/kg PO every other day can be tried in cases of systemic lupus erythematosus that do not respond to conventional immunosuppressive therapy, or show frequent relapses. Prednisolone is used initially (at an anti-inflammatory dose) in combination with the levamisole until clinical improvement has occurred. The drug is used for up to 4 months depending upon the clinical response.

### COLCHICINE/DIMETHYL SULFOXIDE

Some cases of polyarthritis are complicated by amyloidosis; for example, rheumatoid arthritis (Bennett, 1987a) and familial renal amyloidosis of the Chinese shar pei (May, Hammill, and Bennett, 1992). These cases are difficult to treat, although dimethylsulfoxide and colchicine have the potential to reduce amyloid deposition. These drugs have been used but with no clear evidence of efficacy.

### NONSTEROIDAL ANTI-INFLAMMATORY DRUGS

The nonsteroidal anti-inflammatory drugs (NSAIDs) are generally not very effective in treating the immune-based arthropathies. They are mainly used to treat the animal while awaiting the results of investigations to establish a diagnosis. Very mild cases, particularly those likely to spontaneously recover (e.g., vaccination reactions), can be treated with NSAIDs.

### INTRA-ARTICULAR AND TOPICAL THERAPY

Local medical treatment of joints is seldom indicated. However, if one particular joint is causing a major clinical problem, local intra-articular steroids can be tried. Injectable triamcinolone or methylprednisolone can be used. Repeated injection is not advisable. Local NSAID creams can also help if rubbed into the skin over a joint. The hair needs to be clipped in order to facilitate penetration. Piroxicam gel (Feldene), which is a human formulation, can be used; the drug is absorbed through the skin and into the joints.

### SURGERY

Surgical treatment of diseased joints is seldom indicated in the immune-based arthropathies. Excision arthroplasties (femoral head excision, patellectomy) have been done to relieve pain. Arthrodesis of a badly damaged joint might be used if the disease is in remission. Synovectomy may help to reduce the inflammatory load in one particular joint.

## TREATMENT AND PROGNOSIS OF SPECIFIC IMMUNE-BASED ARTHROPATHIES

### Erosive (Destructive) Arthropathies

#### CANINE (FELINE) RHEUMATOID ARTHRITIS

The prognosis associated with rheumatoid arthritis (RA) is generally poor but in some cases the disease will eventually resolve, although residual joint damage is generally severe and lameness and deformity persist (Bennett, 1987a). Chrysotherapy with low-dose glucocorticoid treatment is often helpful in ameliorating clinical signs. Otherwise, anti-inflammatory doses of prednisolone can be used either when the disease is particularly active or as a continuous maintenance therapy in order to preserve a reasonably good quality of life. Amyloidosis can occur as a complication to rheumatoid arthritis and further worsens the prognosis.

#### FELINE (CANINE) PERIOSTEAL PROLIFERATIVE POLYARTHRITIS

This is mainly seen in the feline patient and more commonly affects males. The disease is best treated by low-dose prednisolone given for 2 to 3 weeks when the clinical signs are particularly severe. Chrysotherapy can be used in these cats, but toxicity is more likely than in the dog. Although the disease progresses, many animals can cope for considerable periods of time.

#### POLYARTHRITIS OF GREYHOUNDS

This erosive disease has been reported principally in Australia and there is some evidence to support that it is associated with *Mycoplasma spumans* infection. The prognosis is poor and such cases are perhaps best treated with antimycoplasma agents such as tylosin (Tylan) rather than steroid drugs. As greyhounds can suffer many of the other nonerosive polyarthropathies, careful evaluation is necessary.

## Nonerosive Arthropathies

### SYSTEMIC LUPUS ERYTHEMATOSUS

Systemic lupus erythematosus (SLE) is a multisystemic disease. Animals with SLE should be immunosuppressed using high doses of prednisolone; if relapses occur, which are common, cytotoxic drugs (cyclophosphamide and/or azathioprine) should be used. The prognosis is always guarded, since relapses are common and multiorgan involvement is present. In some cases, special therapy may be indicated; for example, with hemolytic anemia, a blood transfusion may be necessary; with thrombocytopenia, transfusion with platelet-rich plasma may be indicated. Single intravenous injections of vincristine (Oncovin) (0.015 mg/kg) have been used to treat thrombocytopenia. Levamisole (Levacide) (3 to 7 mg/kg EOD PO) can be used as an alternative treatment if steroid immunosuppression is unsuccessful.

### POLYARTHRITIS/POLYMYOSITIS SYNDROME

This disorder is most often seen in the spaniel breeds and produces marked stiffness. Muscle fibrosis can be a permanent feature of this disease. Treatment involves immunosuppression with glucocorticoids or cytotoxic drugs. Complete recovery is possible, but residual stiffness is likely.

### POLYARTHRITIS/MENINGITIS SYNDROME

This syndrome has been seen in several breeds including the Weimaraner, German shorthaired pointer, boxer, Bernese mountain dog, and also in the cat. Neck pain is the main feature of a meningitis. Immunosuppressive doses of glucocorticoids are generally successful in treating this syndrome.

### ARTHRITIS OF JAPANESE AKITAS

This syndrome generally affects dogs of less than 1 year of age. As meningitis is sometimes present, this disease may appear similar to the polyarthritis/meningitis syndrome; however, the prognosis with this disease is very poor. Other signs such as anorexia and pyrexia can also occur. Immunosuppression with corticosteroids is advisable. Cytotoxic drugs are probably best avoided in immature dogs. Euthanasia is often a common outcome.

### FAMILIAL RENAL AMYLOIDOSIS IN SHAR PEI DOGS

These dogs generally present with episodes of fever and swelling of one or both hock joints, so-called shar pei fever or shar pei hock. The joint inflammation and fever spontaneously resolve in a few days and generally do not require specific therapy. Amyloidosis is an important feature of this disease and the prognosis is poor because it eventually leads to renal and/or hepatic failure. Steroid therapy is of no value in amyloidosis and may actually enhance the deposition of amyloid. The disease can start in growing pups or adults and the attacks of fever and arthritis are episodic and sometimes very regular (e.g., every month). Colchicine and dimethyl sulfoxide have been used in an attempt to control the amyloidosis. It is difficult to know if the drugs have any beneficial effect; they certainly do not stop the episodic fever and articular inflammatory attacks. Monitoring the levels of urinary protein will help to assess the renal damage and any response to treatment.

### POLYARTERITIS NODOSA

Polyarteritis nodosa is a histologic diagnosis. Generally, affected dogs have multisystemic disease such as polyarthritis, meningitis, and polymyositis. Response to immunosuppressive doses of steroids or cytotoxic drugs is often good. In some cases, the polyarteritis is confined only to the cervical meninges, where neck pain is the only feature; this is common in immature beagles. There is an obvious overlap here with the Akita disease and the polyarthritis/meningitis syndrome.

### IDIOPATHIC DISEASE

Cases of idiopathic polyarthritis include all those that cannot be classified into any other type. This group, particularly the type I form, is the most prevalent group of immune-based polyarthritis. Some cases of idiopathic polyarthropathy can be reclassified into other types, as the disease progresses.

TYPE I—UNCOMPLICATED IDIOPATHIC ARTHRITIS. Most of these respond well to high doses of glucocorticoids. Relapses can occur, where cytotoxic drugs should be used. Some of these cases can later be classified as rheumatoid arthritis.

TYPE II (REACTIVE) ARTHRITIS. These cases of polyarthritis are associated with infections elsewhere in the body, remote from the joints. The common infections are respiratory tract (viral and bacterial), ocular infection (e.g., chlamydial conjunctivitis in cats), urinary tract infections, uterine infections, skin infections, anal furunculosis, oral cavity infections, *Leishmania* infection, and *Ehrlichia* infection (Bennett, 1987d). Treatment is directed towards controlling the infection by the use of drugs (antibiotics) or surgery (removing infected organs or tissues). If the infection is cleared, the arthritis will generally resolve. Low-dose glucocorticoids may be necessary to reduce joint inflammation while the infection is being treated. Immunosuppressive therapy is contraindicated as long as the infection is present.

TYPE III (ENTEROPATHIC) ARTHRITIS. Polyarthritis is sometimes associated with gastrointestinal disease (e.g., gastroenteritis, ulcerative colitis, bacterial overgrowth, with diarrhea). Treatment of the gastrointestinal problem is indicated, and once this has resolved, the arthritis will resolve. Low doses of glucocorticoids can help reduce the joint problem and may also be appropriate therapy for the gastrointestinal problem. Sulphasalazine can help, especially in cases of ulcerative colitis.

TYPE IV (ARTHRITIS OF MALIGNANCY). Arthritis can be associated with neoplastic processes remote from the joints. Examples have included squamous cell carcinoma, mammary adenocarcinoma, leiomyomas, and heart-base tumors (Bennett, 1987d). In the cat, myeloproliferative disease is the most common association with polyarthritis (Bennett and Nash, 1988), and cats with nonerosive polyarthritis should always have a bone marrow biopsy taken for histopathologic examination. The prognosis depends on the neoplastic process. If the neoplasm can be removed or treated, the joint problem will improve. Low-dose steroid therapy can help control the joint inflammation, which is usually only mild. Cytotoxic drug therapy for a neoplasm may also help relieve joint inflammation.

### MISCELLANEOUS IMMUNE-BASED ARTHRITIDES

DRUG-INDUCED ARTHRITIS. Drug-induced vasculitides are becoming increasingly more common in dogs. The most commonly incriminated drugs are antibiotics, particularly the sulpha drugs, lincomycin, erythromycin, cephalosporins, and penicillins. The Dobermann breed appears particularly sensitive to sulphadiazine-trimethroprin. Polyarthritis may be only one feature of these syndromes. Other lesions are common (i.e., glomerulonephritis, retinitis, polymyositis, skin rash, fever, anemia, leukopenia, and thrombocytopenia). An SLE-like syndrome has been reported in cats treated with propylthiouracil. These arthropathies are generally diagnosed on the basis of worsening clinical signs while the animal is on drug therapy and rapid improvement (within 2 to 7 days) after the drug is stopped. Challenge studies can be done to prove the diagnosis.

VACCINATION REACTIONS. Occasionally, inflammatory arthropathy develops after vaccination. Such reactions are most likely to occur following the first injection of the vaccine. Generally, the lameness occurs within 5 to 7 days of the inoculation and only lasts for 1 to 3 days; the arthritis does not require therapy, although low doses of glucocorticoids can be given if the pain is severe. Generally, if an animal has an episode of lameness after one vaccination, there is little chance of further episodes and thus a routine vaccination program can be continued. Some dogs will develop a typical persistent nonerosive polyarthritis after a vaccine inoculation and require immunosuppressive treatment. Canine distemper virus has been incriminated as a cause of immune-based polyarthritis of the dog. In cats, the calicivirus component of vaccines may result in arthropathy as part of a vaccine reaction (Bennett et al., 1989). Calicivirus can also be involved in a true viral infective arthritis.

PLASMACYTIC-LYMPHOCYTIC SYNOVITIS. This is reported in the United States, but is not recognized in the United Kingdom. This immune-based synovitis of the stifle joints may lead to cranial cruciate ligament failure. It is suggested that the joint inflammation must first be controlled by immunosuppressive drugs before surgical stabilization of the joint is attempted.

## TREATMENT IN THE FUTURE

Treatment of the immune-based arthropathies is, at the present time, crude and restricted. The symptoms are treated by anti-inflammatory and immunosuppressive drugs, but there are no controlled studies that support the use of one drug protocol over another. Further advances are unlikely until the etiopathogenesis of these diseases is better understood. If the role of microbial agents can be elucidated, then therapeutic measures such as specific T-cell vaccination might be possible. Many of the cytokines are involved in joint inflammation, in particular interleukins-1 and -6 and tumor necrosis factor. Therapy against these cytokines is possible (e.g., by the use of monoclonal antibodies against the cytokine or the use of soluble cytokine receptor protein or the use of specific cytokine inhibitors as exists for interleukin-1 (see CVT XI, p 461). Unfortunately, such therapy has not yet proved very successful. The nonspecific control of T cells, especially helper T cells, which are involved in driving the immune response within the synovium, is also possible. This has been attempted by the use of monoclonal antibodies (e.g., against T-cell activation antigen, or interleukin-2 receptors). Monoclonal antibodies linked to cytotoxic drugs (e.g., ricin) have also been used to attempt T-cell destruction. Inhibition of T-cell migration by monoclonal antibodies against lymphocyte function associated molecule is another possibility. Because the joint inflammation probably involves inappropriate antigen presentation within the synovium, monoclonal antibodies against the antigen peptides or major histocompatability molecules may be used to block this process.

## References and Suggested Reading

Bell SC, Carter SD, and Bennett D: Canine distemper viral antigens and antibodies in dogs with rheumatoid arthritis. Res Vet Sci 50:64, 1990.

Bennett D: Immune-based erosive inflammatory joint disease of the dog. Canine rheumatoid arthritis. 1. Clinical, radiological and laboratory investigation. J Small Anim Pract 28:779, 1987a.

Bennett D: Immune-based erosive inflammatory joint disease of the dog. Canine rheumatoid arthritis. 2. Pathological investigations. J Small Anim Pract 28:799, 1987b.

Bennett D: Immune-based non-erosive inflammatory joint disease of the dog. Systemic lupus erythematosus. J Small Anim Pract 28:871, 1987c.

Bennett D: Immune-based non-erosive inflammatory joint disease of the dog. 3. Idiopathic polyarthritis. J Small Anim Pract 28:909, 1987d.

Bennett D, Gaskell RM, Mills A, et al: Detection of feline calicivirus antigens in the joints of infected cats. Vet Rec 124:329, 1989.

Bennett D and Kelly DF: Immune-based non-erosive inflammatory joint disease of the dog. 2. Polyarthritis/polymyositis syndrome. J Small Anim Pract 28:891, 1987.

Bennett D and Nash A: Feline immune-based polyarthritis; a study of 31 cases. J Small Anim Pract 29:501, 1988.

Carter SD, Bell SC, Bari ASM, and Bennett D: Immune-complexes and rheumatoid factors in canine joint disease. Ann Rheum 48:986, 1989.

May C, Hammill J, and Bennett D: Shar pei fever syndrome: A preliminary report. Vet Rec 131:586, 1992.

# TREATMENT OF DEGENERATIVE JOINT DISEASE

PAUL A. MANLEY

*Madison, Wisconsin*

Degenerative joint disease (DJD), or osteoarthritis (OA), is a chronic progressive disorder principally affecting diarthrodial joints. Pathologically, DJD is characterized by articular cartilage destruction, and by alterations in the subchondral bone and synovial fluid. Clinically, DJD is characterized by a decreased range of joint motion, pain and crepitation or both on flexion and extension of the joint, and joint effusion. The loss of joint function due to fibrosis and pain leads to decreased exercise tolerance, lameness after exercise, and a variable degree of muscle atrophy. Treatment of DJD has traditionally focused on drugs that decrease pain.

## ANATOMY OF ARTICULAR CARTILAGE

Articular cartilage has a unique structure to enhance load transmission and motion across the joint surface. Articular cartilage is composed of hyaline cartilage consisting of an extracellular matrix produced and assembled by a relatively small number of cells called chondrocytes. The chondrocytes maintain the matrix integrity despite normal wear and tear and a lack of vascular and neural connections between adjacent cells. The major molecular components of the extracellular matrix are collagen and proteoglycan. Type II collagen is the predominant collagen of articular cartilage. Collagen provides tensile strength for the matrix by forming a framework to contain the proteoglycan macromolecules (Kuettner et al., 1991).

The proteoglycan molecule is composed of a central core of protein with numerous (in excess of 100) attached disaccharide chains (mainly chondroitin sulfate and keratan sulfate). The proteoglycan molecule is relatively mobile within the articular cartilage matrix until it attaches to a hyaluronan molecule via a link protein to become an aggrecan macromolecule. The chondroitin sulfate and keratan sulfate chains have negative charges at their terminal ends and they repel other chondroitin sulfate and keratan sulfate chains. This results in an expansion of the aggrecan macromolecule and an increase in osmotic pressure that attracts water into the matrix. The collagen fibrils act as a mechanical constraint to contain and stabilize the swollen aggrecan macromolecule. In this way, proteoglycans provide resistance to compressive loads across the joint surface (Kuettner et al., 1991). If a substance is introduced into the joint to alter the collagenous structure, unabated swelling of the aggrecan macromolecules occurs, increasing matrix water content, and softening the matrix.

## PATHOLOGY OF DEGENERATIVE JOINT DISEASE

The majority of cases of degenerative joint disease are caused by biomechanical or biochemical alterations in the joint environment. Disruption of the normal articular surface or joint instability results in changes in the normal load pattern of the joint that will lead to areas of increased wear and tear with accelerated turnover of the articular matrix. Although chondrocytes increase synthesis in response to loss of extracellular matrix, they cannot keep up with the rate of depletion. Degradation of the matrix is mediated by cytokines (interleukin-1, catabolin) and prostaglandins released by synovial cells into the joint in response to alterations in the biomechanical or biochemical environment. The inflammatory mediators may directly inhibit production of proteoglycans and indirectly increase breakdown of proteoglycans by stimulating the release of metallo and serine proteinases (cathepsin, stromelysin, collagenase, elastase, plasmin, and gelatinase) and oxygen-derived free radicals from chondrocytes and synovial cells (Burkhardt and Ghosh, 1987). As degradation of the extracellular matrix continues, the chondrocytes and the subchondral bone are subjected to increased biomechanical loads. The chondrocytes appear in clusters at the site of increased load; however, even the increased number of chondrocytes are unable to sustain production of proteoglycans and collagen, and the balance tips in favor of matrix depletion. This process of matrix loss progresses relentlessly until the joint surface is denuded of articular cartilage and the subchondral bone is exposed.

## TREATMENT OF DEGENERATIVE JOINT DISEASE

Current medical therapy for DJD has been directed towards decreasing further degradation of the extracellular matrix by inhibiting the release of inflammatory mediators and controlling pain associated with the inflammatory process. Treatment of DJD is often separated into medical and surgical management. Medical management (Table 1) is directed towards providing symptomatic relief of joint pain and slowing the degradative process; surgical treatment is aimed at correcting the underlying cause of the DJD or altering the articular environment.

***Table 1.*** *Drug Therapy for DJD in Dogs\**

| Drug | Dose Rate and Route | Drug Effects | Precautions | References |
|---|---|---|---|---|
| Aspirin | 10–20 mg/kg PO q8h<br>20–40 mg/kg PO q12h | Analgesic, antipyretic<br>Anti-inflammatory | Gastric ulceration, increased bleeding | Jenkins, 1987<br>Lipowitz et al., 1986 |
| Phenylbutazone | 10–15 mg/kg PO q8h (maximum dose = 800 mg) | Analgesic, antipyretic, anti-inflammatory | Gastric ulceration, blood dyscrasia | Jenkins, 1987 |
| Acetaminophen | 15 mg/kg PO q8h | Analgesic, antipyretic | Gastric ulceration, hepatic and renal dysfunction | Jenkins, 1987 |
| Ibuprofen | 10 mg/kg PO q24–48h | Analgesic, antipyretic, anti-inflammatory | Gastric ulceration, slow elimination | Jenkins, 1987 |
| Banamine | 0.5–2.2 mg/kg IM or IV, 1–2 mg/kg PO for a maximum of 3 days | Analgesic, antipyretic, anti-inflammatory | Gastric ulceration; not for long-term therapy | Jenkins, 1987; Johnson and Davis, 1993 |
| Misoprostol | 2–5 $\mu$g/kg PO q8h | Decreases gastric ulceration | | Murtaugh et al., 1993 |
| Prednisolone | 1–2 mg/kg PO q12–24h | Anti-inflammatory | Gastric ulceration; articular cartilage matrix degradation | Johnson and Davis, 1993 |
| Adequan | 1–2 mg/kg IM, SC q4days for 7 injections; periodically as needed | Anti-inflammatory | Increased bleeding | Altman et al., 1989 |

\*This table refers to use in *dogs only.*

## Weight and Exercise Control

An arthritic joint may be unable to endure the loads associated with normal activity. Certainly, the load and joint stresses are exacerbated if the animal is overweight; so, regardless of the specific treatment, weight loss is recommended in the overweight animal. Ideal weight is calculated based on the physical examination, assessment of body type, and determination of the animal's activity level. Either a prescribed reduction diet or a decrease in food intake of the animal's normal food is recommended.

The animal's activity level is modified and is dependent on the degree of degenerative joint disease and the level of discomfort. High-impact exercise is discouraged (off-leash running, jumping), whereas low-impact exercise (swimming, leash walking) is encouraged to provide positive physiotherapy and weight control.

## Surgical Treatment

Surgical correction of an underlying injury may return the joint to normal biomechanical function (i.e., repair of a ruptured cranial cruciate ligament); however, this will not eradicate existent DJD. At best, surgical intervention may help slow down an inevitable degenerative process. More aggressive surgical procedures, such as joint arthrodesis, joint excision, and joint replacement, are often reserved for patients that are unresponsive to initial surgery or to medical management.

## Nonsteroidal Anti-inflammatory Drug Therapy

Various drugs have been recommended for the medical therapy of DJD. The most common are the nonsteroidal anti-inflammatory drugs (NSAIDs). NSAIDs suppress the synthesis of prostaglandins by inhibiting the transformation of arachidonic acid to prostaglandins via blockage of the enzyme cyclooxygenase. The NSAIDs also exert an inhibitory effect on neutrophil activation (Abramson and Weissmann, 1989). NSAIDs are often prescribed for their effects as antipyretic, analgesic, and anti-inflammatory agents; however, not all NSAIDs exert all of these effects (Abramson and Weissmann, 1989).

One of the most common side effects associated with the NSAIDs is gastric and/or intestinal ulceration. Local irritation and inhibition of prostaglandin E ($PGE_1$ and $PGE_2$) synthesis in the gastric mucosa are believed to be responsible for gastric irritation. Prostaglandin $E_1$ and $PGE_2$ normally inhibit gastric secretion and stimulate the production of mucus from the gastric mucosa (Jenkins, 1987). Cimetidine (Tagamet), an $H_2$ antagonist, has been shown to inhibit gastric acid secretion. Cimetidine does not appear to be effective in dogs in decreasing the tendency towards gastrointestinal ulceration. Misoprostol (Cytotec) has demonstrated effectiveness in decreasing gastrointestinal hemorrhage when combined with an NSAID in dogs (Murtaugh et al., 1993). Misoprostol (Cytotec) is a $PGE_1$ analogue and, at a dose of 2 to 5 $\mu$g/kg every 8 hr PO, suppresses gastric acid secretion, demonstrating a protective effect on the gastric mucosa (also see "Gastrointestinal Ulcer Therapy," this volume, p 706).

Increased bleeding tendency noted with NSAID use is due to prevention of thromboxane $A_2$ formation in platelets, which decreases platelet adhesion (Jenkins, 1987). A more specific side effect for articular cartilage is the ability of NSAIDs to inhibit enzymes required for chondrocyte replication and biosynthesis of proteoglycans (Burkhardt and Ghosh, 1987). It should also be apparent that any analgesic effect may result in more patient comfort, with a subsequent increase in patient activity. This increased activity may exacerbate cartilage degradation.

### ASPIRIN

Aspirin, a salicylate, is the most commonly used NSAID for canine DJD. The recommended dosage in dogs is 10 to 40 mg/kg every 8 hr PO, and in cats is 10 mg/kg every 52 hr PO. In dogs, at the lower dose (10 mg/kg every 8 hr) aspirin offers analgesic and antipyretic effects. Higher doses (20 to 40 mg/kg every 8 h) are recommended to obtain anti-inflammatory effects. At higher dosages, toxic side effects are likely so that only short-term therapy is advised. Gastrointestinal bleeding is decreased by addition of misoprostol and the presence of food in the stomach. Buffered or enteric coated aspirin is often recommended to further decrease the tendency towards gastrointestinal hemorrhage and ulceration (Lipowitz, Boulay, and Klausner, 1986).

### PHENYLBUTAZONE

Another NSAID, phenylbutazone (Butazolidin), a pyrazolon derivative, is also approved for use in dogs but not in cats. The recommended dose is 10 to 15 mg/kg every 8 hr PO, with a maximum of 800 mg/day. Phenylbutazone may cause gastric irritation; a less common side effect with chronic therapy is increased bleeding, agranulocytosis, and thrombocytopenia.

### ACETAMINOPHEN

Acetaminophen (Tylenol), a *para*-aminophenol derivative, is an NSAID with only analgesic and antipyretic actions. Unlike aspirin and phenylbutazone, acetaminophen has no anti-inflammatory activity. Although acetaminophen may be used in the treatment of DJD, its clinical effect is often negligible. The recommended dose is 15 mg/kg every 8 hr PO in dogs, and it should not be used in cats due to severe toxic side effects in this species. Toxic side effects may include cyanosis, dose-dependent hepatic necrosis, renal dysfunction, respiratory depression, and gastrointestinal upset.

### IBUPROFEN

Ibuprofen (Motrin, Advil), an arylpropionic acid derivative, has been recommended for use in dogs. Other drugs in the same family include ketoprofen, naproxen, fenoprofen, and carprofen. The recommended dose for ibuprofen is 10 mg/kg every 24 to 48 hr PO (Jenkins, 1987). Toxic side effects include vomiting, diarrhea, gastrointestinal bleeding and ulceration, and renal dysfunction. The therapeutic and toxic doses of ibuprofen are very close so that caution should be exercised in its use in dogs (see *CVT XI*, p 191). Ibuprofen is not recommended in cats. Carprofen (Rimadyl-V) has been used in dogs in the treatment of DJD (Holtsinger et al., 1992). It appears to be a potent anti-inflammatory, analgesic, and antipyretic agent without the ulcerogenic side effects of other NSAIDs. Unlike some of the other arylpropionic acid derivatives, carprofen has only mild inhibitory effects on $PGE_2$ biosynthesis. Carprofen probably maintains its anti-inflammatory activity by inhibiting neutrophil migration. At this writing, carprofen is not licensed for use in the United States.

### FLUNIXIN MEGLUMINE

Flunixin meglumine (Banamine) has been recommended in dogs at a dose of 0.5 to 2.2 mg/kg IM or IV or 1 to 2 mg/kg daily PO for a maximum of 3 days. It is not recommended in cats nor for long-term therapy in dogs due to its toxic side effects.

## Corticosteroid Drug Therapy

Corticosteroids, specifically the glucocorticoids, have been used intra-articularly and systemically for DJD. These are potent anti-inflammatory agents, inhibiting release of degradative enzymes from chondrocytes and synovial cells. However, they are not widely recommended for DJD because they also inhibit chondrocyte synthesis of proteoglycans and collagen resulting in matrix depletion (steroid arthropathy). Corticosteroids have also been shown to suppress production of hyaluronan in the joint fluid. In animals with end-stage DJD, corticosteroids may be used with the realization that the short-term anti-inflammatory benefits outweigh the degradative effects of the drug.

## Chondroprotective Drug Therapy

Chondroprotective drugs are agents that protect articular cartilage from matrix degradation normally associated with DJD. Presumably, they work by either increasing matrix production or decreasing matrix degradation.

### ADEQUAN

Adequan (polysulfated glycosaminoglycan) is an extract of bovine lung and tracheal tissue that has been sulfated, purified, and buffered to physiologic pH. Adequan has received anecdotal endorsements for use in dogs as an analgesic, anti-inflammatory, and potential chondroprotective agent in the treatment of DJD. Adequan is currently used by intramuscular, intra-articular, and subcutaneous routes of injection in the horse, but it is not licensed for use in dogs. Adequan has been shown to decrease synthesis of neutral proteases, proteinases, and $PGE_2$ associated with matrix degradation, and to increase the synthesis of proteoglygans, collagen, and hyaluronan in rabbits, mice, and dogs in *in vitro* and *in vivo* experiments. However, these results have not been substantiated by clinical trials. Based on experimental work in dogs, Adequan has been recommended at a dose of 1 to 2 mg/kg IM at 4-day intervals for a total of seven injections (Altman et al., 1989). In the horse, Adequan has been shown to potentiate the infectivity of *Staphylococcus aureus* in a septic arthritis model. This may present a potential hazard for the intra-articular route of injection. Toxic side effects in dogs include a dose-dependent inhibition of coagulation and primary hemostasis in dogs (Johnson and Davis, 1993).

### HYALURONATE

Hyaluronate (HA) is a normal component of joint fluid, contributing viscosity to the fluid and facilitating boundary lubrication of the joint. Hyaluronate is also structurally important to the extracellular matrix, providing stability to the proteoglycan molecules. Exogenous HA injected intra-articularly has been used in horses, for the treatment of lameness associated with DJD. Experimentally, intra-articular HA has demonstrated some chondroprotective effects on extracellular matrix in a canine model of DJD. The drug is rapidly cleared from the joint, so that any effect of HA is likely very transitory.

## RECOMMENDATIONS

When a dog is presented with early clinical signs of DJD, an attempt is made to evaluate the cause of the degenerative process. If DJD is secondary to a biomechanical abnormality (ruptured cranial cruciate ligament), surgical correction of the underlying condition is recommended. As well, I recommend as part of the long-term treatment weight reduction (if appropriate), exercise control, and periodic use of NSAID for pain management. Buffered or enteric coated aspirin are my drugs of choice at 10 mg/kg every 8 hr as necessary for discomfort. If this dose is ineffective, I will increase the dose up to 25 mg/kg every 8 hr. However, at this higher dose, I will combine the aspirin with misoprostol at 2 to 5 $\mu$g/kg every 8 hr. For chronic DJD or end-stage DJD, I recommend a similar regime of "as-necessary" drug therapy.

## References and Suggested Reading

Abramson SB and Weissmann G: The mechanism of action of nonsteroidal antiinflammtory drugs. Arthritis Rheum 32:1, 1989.
*This is an excellent review of the use of NSAIDs in human beings. The authors discuss the pathogenesis of osteoarthritis and specific mechanisms of action of commonly used drugs.*

Altman RD, Dean DD, Muniz OE, and Howell DS: Therapeutic treatment of canine osteoarthritis with glycosaminoglycan polysulfuric acid ester. Arthritis Rheum 32:1300, 1989.
*This is an experimental study of the effect of polysulfated glycosaminoglycans (PSGAG) on an experimental model of DJD in dogs. The authors demonstrated a positive effect of PSGAG on histologic and biochemical analysis of articular cartilage.*

Burkhardt D and Ghosh P: Laboratory evaluation of antiarthritic drugs as potential chondroprotective agents. Semin Arthritis Rheum 17:3, 1987.
*This is a good review of arthritis and the use of several experimental and clinically available drugs. The authors site evidence for drug use in several experimental animals including dogs.*

Holtsinger RH, Parker RB, Beale BS, and Friedman RL: The therapeutic efficacy of carprofen (Rimadyl-V™) in 209 clinical cases of canine degenerative joint disease. Vet Comp Orthop Trauma 5:140, 1992.
*This paper documents the use of carprofen (an arylpropionic acid derivative) in a placebo-controlled, blinded clinical trial. The drug proved to be safe and effective in alleviating discomfort associated with DJD.*

Jenkins WL: Pharmacologic aspects of analgesic drugs in animals: an overview. J Am Vet Med Assoc 191:1231, 1987.
*This paper is an excellent review of the use of analgesics in animals. The author discusses mode of action of the commonly used analgesics and lists appropriate dosages in a variety of species.*

Johnson KA and Davis PE: Drug therapy in surgical musculoskeletal disease. In Bojrab MJ (ed): *Disease Mechanisms In Small Animal Surgery*. Philadelphia, Lea & Febiger, 1993, p 1105.
*This is a book chapter that discusses the pathogenesis of DJD in small animals and a variety of drugs that have been used for treatment.*

Kuettner KE, Schleeyerbach R, Peyron J, and Hascall VC: *Articular Cartilage and Osteoarthritis*. New York, Raven Press, 1991.
*This is an excellent book that is actually a compilation of articles presented at a symposium bearing the above title. Many of the most noted researchers in arthritis and articular cartilage are represented in this text. It is a must read for anyone interested in pathogenesis of osteoarthritis and the biochemistry of articular cartilage.*

Lipowitz AL, Boulay JP, and Klausner JS: Serum salicylate concentrations and endoscopic evaluation of the gastric mucosa in dogs after oral administration of aspirin-containing products. Am J Vet Res 47:1586, 1986.
*This paper represents an experimental study investigating the effects of different dosages and types of aspirin. Therapeutic serum salicylate concentrations were achieved with doses of 25 mg/kg every 8 hr. Buffered and enteric coated aspirin were less irritating to the gastric mucosa than plain aspirin.*

Murtaugh RJ, Matz ME, Labato MA, and Boudrieau RJ: Use of synthetic prostaglandin $E_1$ (misoprostol) for prevention of aspirin-induced gastroduodenal ulceration in arthritic dogs. J Am Vet Med Assoc 202:251, 1993.
*This paper documents the use of misoprostol with aspirin in clinical patients with DJD. This combination was less likely to cause gastrointestinal hemorrhage than aspirin alone.*

# TREATMENT OF OSTEOMYELITIS, DISCOSPONDYLITIS, AND SEPTIC ARTHRITIS

KENNETH A. JOHNSON

*Madison, Wisconsin*

Infections involving bone, intervertebral disks, or diarthrodial joints can be difficult to treat because of the refractoriness of certain infections, the long duration of therapy necessary, the expense, and the frustration of recurrence. Contrary to long-held beliefs, most antimicrobial drugs penetrate infected bone well (Esterhai, Gristina, and Poss, 1992). More critical factors contributing to the contumacy of bone infection are compromise of host defense mechanisms and blood supply in tissues around the infection, and the clever adaptive mechanisms of microorganisms that ensure their adhesion, persistence, and virulence. Therefore, in management of these infections, alterations of the local environment in the infected tissues by surgical débridement, sequestrectomy, open drainage, irrigation, and fracture stabilization are just as important as antimicrobial drug therapy.

## SOURCES AND TYPES OF INFECTION

The three routes by which microorganisms reach bone, intervertebral disks, or joints are direct inoculation, extension from contiguous soft tissue, and hematogenously. Most orthopedic infections in dogs and cats are bacterial, and *Staphylococcus* spp. are isolated from approximately 50% of cases of osteomyelitis, discospondylitis, and septic arthritis (Bennett and Taylor, 1988). In dogs, isolates are predominately *S. intermedius* that are penicillin resistant due to β-lactamase production. Polymicrobial infections may contain mixtures of *Streptococcus* spp. and gram-negative aerobes, and sometimes anaerobic bacteria. Until recently, the contribution of anaerobic bacteria to osteomyelitis went unrecognized, but anaerobes can be involved in up to 70% of bone infections (Muir and Johnson, 1992). Anaerobic infections usually contain several anaerobes, or a mixture of anaerobes and aerobes. Some proliferative bone diseases may be viral in origin, as recent findings suggest canine distemper virus is involved in the etiopathogenesis of metaphyseal osteopathy (hypertrophic osteodystrophy) (Mee et al., 1993).

Mycotic agents that cause osteomyelitis (*Coccidioides immitis*, *Blastomyces dermatitidis*, *Histoplasma capsulatum*, and *Cryptococcus neoformans*) are acquired via ingestion, inhalation or skin penetration, and are disseminated hematogenously. German shepherd dogs seem predisposed to disseminated aspergillosis (*Aspergillus terreus*, *A. deflectus*, and *A. fumigatus*) that causes osteomyelitis, discospondylitis, and multiorgan pyogranulomatous abscesses (Day et al., 1986).

## TREATMENT

### Osteomyelitis

#### ACUTE HEMATOGENOUS OSTEOMYELITIS

Young animals with acute hematogenous osteomyelitis (AHO) exhibit signs of systemic illness with pyrexia, anorexia, dehydration, and generalized limb pain. Fluid therapy, nutritional support, and analgesic drugs are indicated, aside from treatment of the bone infection. Localization of bacteria in the metaphyses in AHO was classically attributed to sluggish blood flow in capillary loops adjacent to the physis. Actually, capillary endothelium in this region is discontinuous, allowing extravasation of erythrocytes and possibly bacteria. When local tissue defenses are compromised, osteomyelitis develops, apparently through the incompetence of tissue-based phagocytes (Esterhai, Gristina, and Poss, 1992). Mechanisms responsible for altered local defenses are not well defined, but in each patient, immunodeficiency disorders, malnutrition, and concurrent diseases should be eliminated. The primary focus of infection in AHO is not always apparent.

Provided there is minimal bone necrosis seen radiographically, antibiotic therapy alone may be effective in resolution of AHO. Since penicillin resistant, β-lactamase–producing *Staphylococci* spp. are often involved in this type of infection, treatment with intravenous cefazolin (Table 1) is initiated immediately and continued until results of bone and blood cultures are known. Identification of microorganisms and determination of drug susceptibility are desirable because *Clostridium* spp. and gram-negative aerobes have also been isolated from AHO (Dunn, Dennis, and Houlton, 1992). After clinical improvement has been observed, antimicrobial therapy is continued orally for at least another 4 weeks. Cage confinement is recommended, but limb bandaging is contraindicated due to its deleterious effects on joint cartilage. Complications of AHO are extension to adjacent joint, subperiosteal extension of infection resulting in sequestration of the diaphyseal cortex, and development of chronic infection. With resolution of AHO, physeal growth seems to continue normally, without limb shortening or deformity (Dunn, Dennis, and Houlton, 1992).

Metaphyseal osteopathy (hypertrophic osteodystrophy) has signs similar to AHO, but there is no specific therapy, as it is probably viral in etiology (Mee et al., 1993).

### ACUTE POST-TRAUMATIC OSTEOMYELITIS

The principal causes of acute post-traumatic osteomyelitis are contamination during open fractures and open reduction for internal fixation of fractures. Early clinical signs may include anorexia, lethargy, depression, limb swelling, excessive tenderness on palpation, and exudation from wounds. Pyrexia that persists beyond 48 hr after surgery, and increasing severity of lameness are also signs of impending infection. Smears of fluid obtained by sterile aspiration that contain toxic neutrophils and phagocytosed bacteria are indicative of infection. Aerobic and anaerobic microbiologic culturing of samples provides confirmation. Deep postoperative wound infection cannot be readily differentiated from acute post-traumatic osteomyelitis because there is no radiographic change in bone structure. However, treatment of each is similar and must be early and aggressive, because progression to chronic osteomyelitis is potentially devastating. Under aseptic conditions, surgical wounds are reopened completely, as are traumatic wounds associated with open fracture, to allow complete débridement of necrotic tissues. Bone blood supply is carefully preserved. Specimens of necrotic tissue adjacent to the bone are collected for aerobic and anaerobic microbiologic testing.

Fractures must be stable for union to occur in the presence of infection. Fixation devices such as plates, pins, and screws that contribute to fracture stability are retained. In unstable fractures, all loose implants are removed and fracture stability obtained by another means, usually an external fixator. The wound is copiously lavaged with sterile saline solution. Even if implants are exposed, the wound is usually left open and covered by sterile dressing. Only when there is no gross evidence of tissue necrosis or exudation can the wound be closed primarily, usually over a suction drainage system (mini-Snyder Hemovac, Zimmer, Dover, OH).

However, immediate wound closure carries inherent risk of abscessation and progression to chronic osteomyelitis.

Dressing are changed at least every 24 hr and the wound aseptically débrided and lavaged using sterile saline, with the animal sedated or anesthetized. Drains are removed within 48 hr. Once granulation tissue forms, healing by secondary intention invariably occurs, and delayed primary closure is rarely necessary. Delayed cancellous bone grafting of fractures and bone defects can safely be done after granulation tissue has formed. Antimicrobial drugs are administered for at least 4 weeks. The drug regimen chosen will depend on the microbiology results, but initial broad-spectrum activity is obtained with amoxicillin-clavulanate or metronidazole, combined with ciprofloxacin or enrofloxacin (Table 1). Physical therapy and hot packing for 30 min twice daily aids recovery.

### CHRONIC OSTEOMYELITIS

Chronic osteomyelitis can be caused by progression of acute post-traumatic osteomyelitis. Other causes are bite wounds, extension from soft tissue infection, and foreign body penetration that are initially unrecognized. Lameness, tracts that periodically discharge purulent exudate, and soft tissue atrophy are consistent signs. Radiographic signs include periosteal new bone, cortical resorption, sclerosis, and sequestration (Fig. 1). Aerobic and anaerobic culturing of samples collected from close to the bone allows identification of microorganisms and determination of in vitro drug susceptibility. Signs of systemic illness (pyrexia and neutrophilic leukocytosis) are rare. Chronic osteomyelitis may be accompanied by joint stiffness, muscle contracture, and compromised vascularity and innervation. Limb amputation is indicated if any of these pre-existing complications would significantly preclude adequate limb function subsequent to resolution of chronic osteomyelitis. Localized chronic osteomyelitis of phalanges, tail, sternum, or mandible can also be managed by an en bloc resection.

Principles of treatment of chronic bacterial osteomyelitis are similar to treatment of acute post-traumatic osteomyelitis, with the following additions. A careful search is made for sequestra. At least two radiographic

***Table 1.*** *Antimicrobial Drugs Recommended for Treatment of Bone Infections*

| Generic Drug (Trade) | Dosage Regimen | | |
| --- | --- | --- | --- |
| | Rate | Route | Frequency |
| Amoxicillin-clavulanate (Clavamox) | 20–25 mg/kg | PO | q8h |
| Cephalexin (Keflex) | 30 mg/kg | PO | q12h |
| Cefazolin (Kefzol) | 20 mg/kg | IV, IM, SC | q6h |
| Clindamycin (Antirobe) | 11 mg/kg | IV, IM, PO | q8–12h |
| Ciprofloxacin (Cipro) | 5.5–11 mg/kg | PO | q12h |
| Enrofloxacin (Baytril) | 15 mg/kg | PO | q12h |
| Amikacin (Amiglyde-V) | 15 mg/kg | IV, IM, SC | q24h |
| Gentamicin (Gentocin) | 6 mg/kg | IV, IM, SC | q24h |
| Metronidazole (Flagyl) | 15 mg/kg | PO, IV | q12h |
| Itraconazole (Sporanox) | 5–10 mg/kg | PO | q12h |

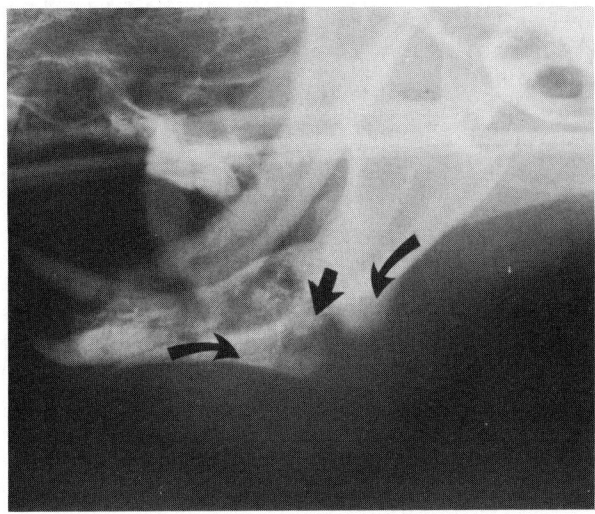

**Figure 1.** Chronic osteomyelitis due to anaerobic bacteria in the mandible of a cat. A localized area of lysis containing a sequestrum (*straight arrow*) is surrounded by new periosteal bone (*curved arrows*) in the body of the mandible. Overlying soft tissues are swollen. (Reproduced from Johnson KA, et al: Osteomyelitis in dogs and cats caused by anaerobic bacteria. Aust Vet J 61:57, 1984, with permission.)

In chronic osteomyelitis, a wide variety of gram-positive and gram-negative aerobes and anaerobes may be isolated. Therefore, it is essential that the chosen antimicrobial drug regimen be based on the *in vitro* susceptibility of microorganisms isolated, and that these drugs be given for at least 6 weeks (Table 1).

Bone defects and fractures are grafted with autogenous cancellous bone once infection has abated and granulation tissue fills the wound. Bone graft can be inserted by elevation of the granulation tissue, or via separate surgical approach through healthy tissue. Massive diaphyseal cortical deficits can be bridged using Ilizarov technique of bone transport. A transverse osteotomy is made in one metaphysis, and the intermediate segment is advanced at a rate of 1 mm/day towards the deficit until it is bridged. The resultant osteotomy gap fills with new bone by the process of distraction osteogenesis (Lesser, 1993).

Recurrence of chronic osteomyelitis may occur months or years after an apparent resolution. Additional courses of antimicrobial drugs may produce a transient remission, but complete cure is unlikely unless many of the aforementioned steps of treatment are repeated.

views are necessary to get a three-dimensional appreciation of their location in relation to other anatomic landmarks. Sequestra can harbor infection and perpetuate chronic draining tracts because some bacteria have receptors that bind to exposed collagen of damaged cortical bone. A standard surgical approach is made to the bone for sequestrectomy and wound débridement. To get access to sequestra, overlying periosteal new bone of the involucrum may need to be removed with an osteotome or rongeur. Following débridement, transposition of adjacent muscle over exposed cortical bone enhances local bone blood supply during the healing process. Otherwise, débrided wounds are left open but covered with sterile dressings, to facilitate drainage, daily wound irrigation, and débridement until healing by second intention occurs.

Fractures complicated by chronic osteomyelitis are invariably unstable and have a tendency to proceed to nonunion. Loose and functionless implants are removed and the fracture is stabilized by an alternate means. Stabilization with an external fixator has the advantage that the device can be applied with minimal intrusion into the region of infected bone. Implants placed within infected bone can contribute to bacterial persistence because they become coated with serum proteins, fibronectin, and other material. *Staphylococcus* spp. and other bacteria bind to fibronectin in this coating and produce a bacterial slime. Slime combined with the implant coating forms biofilm (Esterhai, Gristina, and Poss, 1992). Biofilm is a virulence factor that ensures bacterial adhesion and persistence. It protects bacteria from phagocytes and antibodies, and also induces phenotypic transformation of bacteria to more virulent strains. Therefore, once fractures have healed, all implants are removed to aid elimination of biofilm.

## Discospondylitis

Discospondylitis is caused by bacterial or fungal infection of intervertebral disk and adjacent vertebral body end plates (Fig. 2). Most infections are acquired hematogenously. Multiple disks are frequently affected, and common sites of involvement are midthoracic and L7–S1 disks. Clinical signs can include systemic illness, back pain, difficulty with locomotion, paresis, or paralysis.

Discospondylitis causing pain without neurologic deficit is treated with rest and antimicrobial drugs for at least 6 weeks, and up to 6 months if necessary. Ideally, isolation of microorganisms from blood, urine, or aspirated disk material is performed prior to initiating therapy. Unfortunately, cultures are negative in approximately 50% of cases. In culture-negative cases, amoxicillin-clavulanate is administered, as most infections are β-lactamase, penicillin-resistant *Staphylococci* spp. Buffered aspirin (10 to 15 mg/kg every 12 hr PO) is given to alleviate pain. Positive response to therapy is indicated by clinical improvement and radiographic signs of progressive ankylosis of vertebrae. Lack of clinical improvement after 2 to 4 weeks indicates the need to repeat radiographic and microbiologic evaluations, and possibly to change antibiotic regimen and consider surgery.

In dogs with persistent severe pain or neurologic deficits, cerebrospinal fluid (CSF) examination and myelography can be performed to rule out meningitis and spinal cord compression, respectively. Electromyography may be useful for detecting cauda equina compression. If there is no clinical or myelographic evidence of spinal cord or nerve root compression, refractory discospondylitis lesions are curetted and

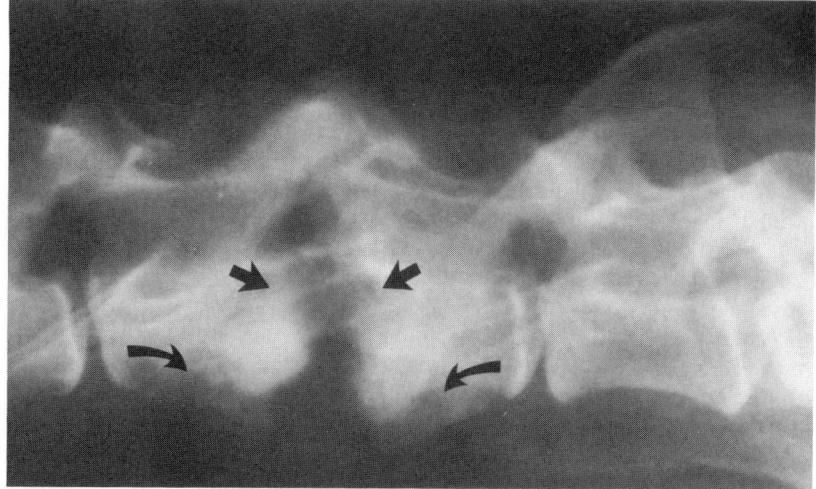

**Figure 2.** Bacterial discospondylitis at L5–6 in a 9-year-old golden retriever presented with signs of hindlimb lameness and back pain. Extensive lysis of vertebral body end plates (*straight arrows*) is seen in combination with sclerosis and new bone proliferation (*curved arrows*).

grafted with autogenous cancellous bone to promote ankylosis, via a lateral or ventral approach. If there is evidence of spinal cord or nerve root compression, hemilaminectomy or laminectomy is performed in addition to the above to allow decompression of cord or nerve root. Internal fixation of the spine to promote ankylosis may be indicated. Dogs that have discospondylitis causing neurologic deficits have a poor prognosis.

Discospondylitis and lumbar vertebrae osteomyelitis caused by migrating grass awns commonly have infections with *Actinomyces* spp. and draining tracts from the retroperitoneal space. Surgical drainage from a lateral approach, removal of awns and infected tissue, and antimicrobial drug therapy are the ideal treatment. Complications are intraoperative hemorrhage and recurrence of draining tracts associated with failure to control infection and remove foreign bodies.

Treatment of discospondylitis due to disseminated aspergillosis by continuous administration of itraconazole may control the disease for 1 to 2 years, but affected dogs ultimately succumb with multifocal pyogranulomatous abscesses (Dr. PR Watt, personal communication, 1993).

## Septic Arthritis

Most joint infections are secondary to wounds or hematogenous dissemination through the synovial membrane. *Staphylococcus* spp. and other bacteria bind to articular cartilage, provoking interleukin-1 release from synovial membrane that in turn initiates an inflammatory cascade and joint effusion. Bacterial- and interleukin-1–mediated responses may produce loss of cartilage glycosaminoglycan (2 to 5 days), cartilage fibrillation (7 days), and complete joint destruction (1 to 2 months) (Esterhai, Gristina, and Poss, 1992). Early diagnosis of septic arthritis and effective therapy are essential to prevent loss of the joint.

Young animals with acute septic arthritis may have monoarticular or polyarticular infections. The primary source of infection is not always apparent but it should

be sought out and, if possible, treated. Clinical signs include joint swelling and severe pain. The only radiographic sign of acute joint infection is effusion. Joints are decompressed (evacuated) immediately by arthrocentesis, and synovia is submitted for analysis and microbiology. Synovial fluids with 50,000 to 200,000 leukocytes/mm$^3$, protein greater than 4 gm/dl, and bacteria are consistent with joint infection. Microbiologic culturing of synovial membrane biopsies may be more successful than synovial fluid cultures, which are often negative. Cefazolin is administered intravenously, until there is a response, then oral antimicrobial drugs are continued for 4 weeks.

In most cases of septic arthritis arthrotomy, débride-

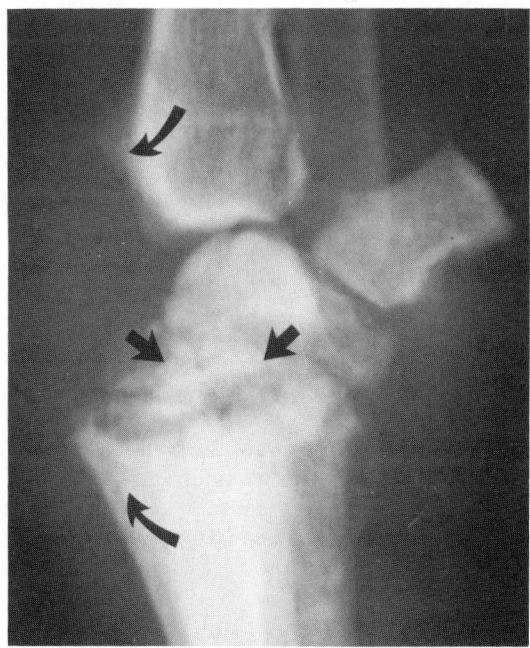

**Figure 3.** Destruction of middle carpal and carpometacarpal joints as a sequela to chronic septic arthritis. Note the extensive lysis of the distal row of carpal bones (*straight arrows*), collapse of carpal joints, new bone formation (*curved arrows*), and soft tissue swelling. Carpal arthrodesis is indicated.

ment, synovectomy, culture, and joint lavage are indicated, especially if there is (1) no response of acute septic arthritis by 48 hr, (2) postsurgical infection, (3) chronic septic arthritis, or (4) penetrating and open joint wound or foreign body. Joints are lavaged with sterile isotonic saline, without any added antiseptic or antibiotic. Joint lavage and drainage systems are difficult to maintain in animals, and open wound management with sterile dressing is an acceptable alternative. Prognosis in pups and kittens with acute septic arthritis is usually poor.

In adults, septic arthritis is usually monoarticular and may be secondary to chronic osteoarthritis (e.g., hip dysplasia, elbow arthritis, chronic sprain injury). After resolution of infection by arthrotomy and open wound lavage, arthrodesis or excision arthroplasty may be indicated (Fig. 3). Open shearing injuries of carpus and tarsus with loss of soft tissue and exposure of articular cartilage may require some form of fixation or coaptation.

### References and Suggested Reading

Bennett D and Taylor DJ: Bacterial infective arthritis in the dog. J Small Anim Pract 29:207, 1988.

Staphylococcus intermedius *was the predominant isolate in 58 dogs with septic arthritis, and 32 dogs completely recovered with antibiotic therapy.*
Day MJ, Penhale WJ, Eger CE, et al: Disseminated aspergillosis in dogs. Aust Vet J 63:55, 1986.
*Clinical and pathologic features of disseminated aspergillosis affecting 11 German shepherd dogs and one Dalmatian are reported.*
Dunn JK, Dennis R, and Houlton JEF: Successful treatment of two cases of metaphyseal osteomyelitis in the dog. J Small Anim Pract 33:85, 1992.
*Report of acute hematogenous osteomyelitis of metaphyses that responded to amoxicillin-clavulanate and metronidazole in two dogs, together with literature review.*
Esterhai JL, Gristina AG, and Poss R (eds): Musculoskeletal Infection. Park Ridge, American Academy of Orthopaedic Surgeons, 1992.
*Compilation of workshop reports on microbiology, pathogenesis, and therapy of osteomyelitis.*
Johnson KA: Osteomyelitis. *In* Birchard SJ and Sherding RG (eds): *Saunders Manual of Small Animal Practice.* Philadelphia, WB Saunders Co, 1993, p 1091.
*A review of diagnosis and treatment of osteomyelitis in dogs and cats.*
Lesser AS: Segmental bone transport for the treatment of bone deficits. J Am Anim Hosp Assoc 30:322, 1994.
*Ilizarov technique of bone segment transport used to bridge massive tibial diaphyseal defects that were the result of infected nonunion in two animals.*
Mee AP, Gordon MT, May C, et al: Canine distemper virus transcripts detected in the bone cells of dogs with metaphyseal osteopathy. Bone 14:59, 1993.
*Detection of canine distemper virus RNA within metaphyseal bone cells of dogs affected with metaphyseal osteopathy, suggests virus may cause this disease.*
Moore MP: Discospondylitis. Vet Clin North Am [Small Anim Pract] 22:1027, 1992.
*Review of clinical signs, diagnosis, and therapy of discospondylitis in dogs.*
Muir P and Johnson KA: Anaerobic bacteria isolated from osteomyelitis in dogs and cats. J Vet Surg 21:463, 1992.
*Anaerobic bacteria were isolated from 18/24 osteomyelitic lesions that frequently resulted from fight wounds or abscesses.*

# THE ROLES OF THE VETERINARIAN AND THE VETERINARY SPECIALIST IN THE MANAGEMENT OF NEUROLOGIC AND MUSCULOSKELETAL PROBLEMS

WILLIAM D. LISKA
*and* WAYNE O. WHITNEY
*Houston, Texas*

Disorders of the nervous and musculoskeletal systems are common in dogs and cats. A wide variety of problems can arise, but some of the more common are seizures, paresis, fractures, ligament injuries, and lameness. Each veterinarian (practitioner or specialist) must determine their level of competence in the diagnosis and treatment of these problems. Patients with these problems are frequently referred to a veterinary specialist. In fact, the treatment of neurologic and musculoskeletal disease may account for most, if not all, of the case load of some specialists.

Reasons for referral include the need for a specialist's clinical or surgical expertise, advanced diagnostic capabilities, special equipment, and a staff in facilities to support intensive nursing care. Upon accepting a patient from a referring veterinarian, the responsibility for the diagnosis, treatment, and communication is transferred to the veterinary specialist.

A specialist is defined by the Principles of Veterinary Medical Ethics as a veterinarian who is a diplomate of a specialty organization recognized by the American Veterinary Medical Association (AVMA). Solicitation claims as a specialist by a nondiplomate, either stated or implied, are considered false, deceptive, or misleading.

The relationship between the referring veterinarian and the veterinary specialist should be based on mutual respect, which will ultimately benefit both the patient and the client. The relationship ideally is noncompetitive. Fees for services should always be collected separately with no financial gain, or kickbacks, for either resulting directly from the recommendation for, or acceptance of, the referral.

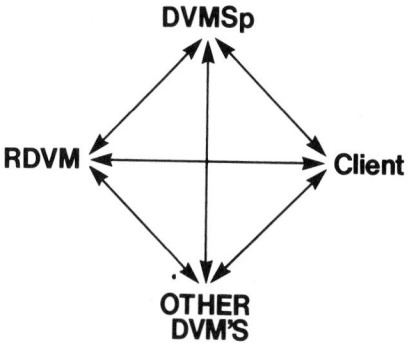

**Figure 1.** Multiple lines of communication are necessary in the development and maintenance of the client–referring veterinarian–veterinary specialist relationship.

## CLIENT–REFERRING VETERINARIAN–VETERINARY SPECIALIST RELATIONSHIP (MEASURING SUCCESS)

The client, referring veterinarian, and veterinary specialist each have a stake in the outcome of treatment. The relationship that develops between these individuals may be either positive or negative. The client's opinion of patient care and well-being is based on service, what they see, what they hear, their perception of the specialist's level of expertise, and results of treatment. Obviously, the client's opinion may or may not be justified. The perception of success or failure is often determined by the client's expectations. The client should have a thorough understanding of the problem, treatment, and potential complications so that their expectations are reasonable and appropriate. Sometimes, less than optimal methods of treatment must be discussed due to a client's limited financial resources. Honest, open communication is crucial in such situations.

The referring veterinarian judges the veterinary specialist from another perspective. The referring veterinarian is not only concerned about their client's opinion of patient care, but also the client's opinion of the veterinary specialist. Client's *expect* the referring veterinarian not only to decide *when* a referral is indicated, but also *who* can provide the kind of care that is needed. The client's opinion of the veterinary specialist is a reflection on the referring veterinarian's ability or inability to find expertise and service. A client's negative opinion of the veterinary specialist, justified or not, can undermine the referring veterinarian–client relationship and translate into loss of a client, or worse yet, the threat of litigation.

With this in mind, it is essential to understand the importance of good communication and to understand the responsibilities of the referring veterinarian and the veterinary specialist to each other and to the client.

## COMMUNICATION RESPONSIBILITIES

Timely communication must become an accepted way of life for the veterinary specialist who is actively engaged in a specialty practice. A significant portion of each day must be devoted to verbal and written communication. The veterinary specialist must maintain close contact with both the referring veterinarian and the client (Fig. 1).

Cases are ideally discussed between the referring veterinarian and the veterinary specialist prior to presentation to the referral hospital. The client should be informed by the veterinary specialist about certain as-

pects of treatment and their financial responsibility at patient presentation. The veterinary specialist should discuss diagnostic results and pretreatment findings with both the referring veterinarian and the client. This is especially important if the information alters the diagnosis, treatment, or prognosis that was previously described. Contact should be made with the client and referring veterinarian as soon as important information is received and as soon as possible after procedures or surgery. Client contact with the veterinary specialist should occur daily. There should be a thorough explanation of aftercare given at the time of discharge. Communication after release from hospitalization and prior to recheck may be initiated by the client, the veterinary specialist, or the referring veterinarian. All findings, treatment, aftercare, and long-term follow up information should be summarized by the veterinary specialist at or near resolution of the case. This case summary becomes part of the permanent medical records of the veterinary specialist and the referring veterinarian.

The veterinary specialist should be accessible to discuss possible referrals during regular business hours. Some provisions should be made for accessibility or alternative care in cases of emergency for the referring veterinarian and the client.

Case complexity or multidisciplinary problems may dictate other specialist's consultation or active involvement. The veterinary specialist should seek the client's and referring veterinarian's consent before additional consultations are requested. Also, more than one referring veterinarian may have been involved prior to the referral. Each referring veterinarian should receive follow-up communication.

## RESPONSIBILITY OF THE VETERINARY SPECIALIST TO THE REFERRING VETERINARIAN AND THE CLIENT

"Locality rule" at one time effectively set standards of professional expertise based on the professional level of care provided in a particular region, state, county, and so forth. Today, veterinarians have access to an abundance of publications, videos, continuing education programs, lecturers and consultants. Therefore, locality rule is no longer valid and a national "same or similar" standard of practice is in force. Neither the referring veterinarian nor the veterinary specialist is protected from liability based on where they live or practice.

The veterinary specialist is held responsible for maintaining a higher standard of expertise than the accepted norm of general practice. Diagnostic and surgical capability, equipment and supply availability, and patient care staff with advanced training are implied to accompany the higher standard. In addition, because competence is essential to maintain and sustain longevity in a clinical setting, self-imposed standards of excellence are usually followed.

Nondiplomates accepting referrals are held to the same standards as the veterinary specialist when questions of professional liability arise. The AVMA's Principles of Veterinary Medical Ethics Advertising Guidelines should be followed by those who solicit or encourage referrals and by those who refer clients.

The veterinary specialist should always make an effort to minimize professional liability exposure of the referring veterinarian. It is never in the veterinary specialist's best interest to belittle any actions or behavioral characteristics of the referring veterinarian. In many instances, the tone of communications between the client and the veterinary specialist concerning prior treatment of the patient can either calm or inflame the client. Diplomacy alone can promulgate a win-win or a no-win situation. The scenario can be particularly sensitive when the veterinary specialist accepts a patient already treated by a nondiplomate "specialist" who treated the patient on a referral basis. In that instance, liability could exist for the nondiplomate and the referring veterinarian.

The veterinary specialist should exercise good judgment when making recommendations. Proven indications should always be the motivators over financial gain. Occasionally, the veterinary specialist may delay surgery or refer the client to yet another veterinary specialist. Examples include: lack of proper equipment, lack of technical support, inadequate aftercare availability, more expertise by another veterinary specialist, or inability to accept another patient for whatever reason.

Services provided by the veterinary specialist should be limited to those problems prompting the referral. The veterinary specialist should consult the referring veterinarian if other services are indicated or are requested by the client. Once the presenting problems are resolved, the client should be urged to return to the referring veterinarian for continuing primary care. The services provided by the veterinary specialist can be perceived by the client as an extension of the services the referring veterinarian has to offer. However, it is inappropriate for the referring veterinarian to request and collect fees for veterinary specialist services, especially if the client is not fully informed of the arrangement.

As already discussed, timely detailed follow-up reports should be transmitted from the veterinary specialist to the referring veterinarian(s). The report should contain information regarding diagnosis, treatment, aftercare, progress, complications, and prognosis. Appropriate methods of communication vary, but they include direct contact, telephone, letter, fax, and direct computer access. If the veterinary specialist observes evidence of professional incompetence or negligence, colleagues involved should be contacted and informed of methods that could be employed to improve their expertise or conduct.

## RESPONSIBILITY OF THE REFERRING VETERINARIAN TO THE VETERINARY SPECIALIST AND THE CLIENT

The referring veterinarian should inform clients about the availability of additional diagnostic or treatment options that specialists have to offer whenever such services would benefit the patient or otherwise enhance the quality of veterinary care. If consultations or referrals are appropriate, they should be done in a timely manner relative to the health of the patient. If for any reason a client requests a referral to another veterinarian or veterinary institution, the attending veterinarian should be willing to honor the request and facilitate the necessary arrangements.

It is not necessary for the referring veterinarian to judge which clients are able or will be willing to pay for specialty veterinary care. Nor is it necessary for the referring veterinarian to judge whether a referral will be "worth the trouble" for the client (be it distance traveled, frequency of visits, emotional stress, or time away from family and work). The referring veterinarian should, however, be available for consultation on these problems upon the client's request, provided the referring veterinarian has a *thorough* understanding of the subject matter.

Pertinent information including history, treatments, radiographs, and laboratory results should be transmitted to the veterinary specialist before or at the time of the veterinary specialist's first contact with the client. Telephone calls, couriers, and clients carrying documents are practical, effective methods. Occasionally, the referring veterinarian will bring the patient to the veterinary specialist as a service or convenience for the client. From the veterinary specialist's perspective, this action is usually undesirable and should *only* be done after obtaining the client's and specialist's consent. Even in this situation, the client and the veterinary specialist must communicate directly prior to any treatment.

The referring veterinarian is free to refer to whomever they deem appropriate for the situation, but a cavalier decision must be avoided. Ideally, the referring veterinarian should take time to personally inspect facilities, observe surgery in progress, and examine equipment used in the referral hospital. They should meet receptionists that will greet the client and the nursing staff that will provide care for the patient. The referring veterinarian should also inquire about after-hours patient care. They should have a mental image of how to easily direct clients to the referral hospital. The referring veterinarian should read literature the veterinary specialist makes available to clients and to the other referring veterinarians in the community. All of the above information will help the referring veterinarian to determine who will provide the *best* patient care and the *best* client service. Patient care and service should always have priority over low fees. Clients should have the opportunity to use whatever veterinary services they need (but might not know about).

It is best that the referring veterinarian provide a general, but not a detailed, description of what the veterinary specialist will do. Decisions relative to diagnostics or treatments are best left to the veterinary specialist with the consent and understanding of the client. In some cases, a patient is referred for a specific procedure. While the proposed procedure often is indicated, in other cases, a different study or therapy may be best. Clients with a preconceived notion of exactly what "will be done" can have difficulty understanding why something else "was done." In this instance, the referring veterinarian and veterinary specialist may not appear to be in agreement, and further explanation can easily leave one or the other (or both) embarrassed.

The fee for veterinary specialist services, other than the basic office visit charges, are also best *not* discussed by the referring veterinarian. It is best for the veterinary specialist or designated office staff to provide the client a fee estimate, preferably at the time that the animal is examined. Referring clients with no financial resources is acceptable, especially if the veterinary specialist is advised in advance. If the client requests a fee estimate prior to accepting the referral, the referring veterinarian should discuss this with the veterinary specialist so a range of fees may be given for dealing with that specific problem. Both the referring veterinarian and veterinary specialist must remember that accurately estimating fees is extremely difficult in some situations. Accurate fee quotes, except for the most routine problems, are usually impossible if a system of fees for services and reasonable compensation is implemented. Most clients, when considering referral options, anticipate that the fees for veterinary specialist services at secondary or tertiary care facilities are relatively high. This in fact might not, and often is not, true.

The range of veterinary specialty services available has dramatically increased over the past 10 years. It is becoming increasingly challenging for both the referring veterinarian and veterinary specialist to keep abreast of new techniques and services available. Veterinarians must be lifelong learners. They should strive to broaden their own knowledge in various ways. Referring veterinarians should take advantage of the veterinary specialist's expertise through personal and telephone contact.

Finally, the referring veterinarian should inform the veterinary specialist when problems pertaining to pa-tient care or communication occur. Constructive criticism is welcomed, much appreciated, and nurtures a good working relationship.

Referring veterinarian perception that a problem is in some way insignificant should be avoided. Problems detected early are generally easier to resolve and less expensive to treat. Early detection of problems by the referring veterinarian fosters client confidence in the primary care provider (i.e., the referring veterinarian).

## SITUATIONS THAT JEOPARDIZE THE CLIENT–REFERRING VETERINARIAN–VETERINARY SPECIALIST RELATIONSHIP

Situations arise in which the client–referring veterinarian–veterinary specialist relationship becomes strained. One or more individuals involved may be responsible. The relationship can be jeopardized over apparently trivial issues. Some clinical examples of how stressful situations develop are listed below. It is not within the scope of this article to present every possible scenario. The examples are intended not to place blame but rather to provoke thought.

1. *Untimely referral*: The acutely paretic nonambulatory dachshund with deteriorating neurologic status that is treated medically is not referred until 48 hr after sensory perception is lost. The client asks the veterinary specialist, "would it have made a difference if I had been referred sooner?"

2. *Complications*: A 50-kg aggressive dog with a far undersized, migrating, single intramedullary pin used 2 weeks ago to repair a now collapsed, infected, comminuted midshaft humerus fracture is referred for surgery. The client expects his guard dog to have normal function of the leg!

3. *Incorrect information given to the client*: A 10-month-old, 40-kg dog with hip pain, hip subluxation, and minimal to no radiographic evidence of degenerative joint disease is presented to the veterinary specialist for a second opinion. The dog belongs to a client who has just agreed to have a bilateral femoral head ostectomy performed by another veterinarian after being told "nothing else can be done." The client was not informed about other options such as triple pelvic osteotomy or total hip replacement.

4. *Contraindicated medication*: There is continued concurrent administration of high levels of corticosteroids and aspirin to the nonambulatory paretic patient with hemorrhagic enteritis. The dog is then tranquilized and referred for a neurologic examination and surgery as soon as possible.

5. *Inadequate emergency or primary care*: A bandage is applied to a dog's grade III open distal tibia fracture. The dog cannot be transported for at least 36 hr. Oral antibiotic therapy is begun but the wound is not thoroughly cleaned, lavaged, and the limb is not rigidly supported.

6. *Overzealous emergency management*: A grade I

open noncomminuted femur fracture is referred and transported immediately after recovery from anesthesia induced for aggressive lavage of the wound by the referring veterinarian. Open reduction and internal fixation is planned by the veterinary specialist for the same day.

7. *Improper or incomplete diagnostics that must be repeated*: A 6-year-old cocker spaniel with severe neck pain that has become refractory to medical therapy is referred for "cervical disk surgery." The accompanying noncontrast radiographs are poorly positioned and poorly produced. The client asks why more money must be spent for additional radiographs and a myelogram.

8. *Undiagnosed concurrent problem*: A cat is referred for repair of a mandibular symphyseal fracture. The fracture repair is successful, but the cat died during the immediate postoperative period. A necropsy revealed that a diaphragmatic hernia and a ruptured urinary bladder were present.

9. *Underestimated fees*: A client presents a dog with a fracture and has been given an unrealistic low fee quote that had not been previously discussed by the referring veterinarian and veterinary specialist. The client wants to be billed, take 15 months to pay, and has no deposit money.

10. *Overestimated fees*: A client with a large dog that has a torn cranial cruciate ligament seeks a third opinion from the veterinary specialist recommended by referring veterinarian #2. The client states that money is not a factor and inquires why referring veterinarian #1 estimated the veterinary specialist fees would be two to three times greater than what the veterinary specialist actually charges.

11. *Poor communication with possible misrepresentation*: A dog has been a patient of the referring veterinarian for several years. The dog became lame and the client decided to go directly to the veterinary specialist for surgery, bypassing the referring veterinarian. The client indicated to the veterinary specialist that a referral had been made. The veterinary specialist did not provide follow-up information to the referring veterinarian. Six weeks later, complications arise. The now unhappy client presents the dog to the referring veterinarian and wants the dog "taken care of."

12. *Poor follow-up communication*: A client was referred by the referring veterinarian to a veterinary specialist with a dog that had periodic neck pain and seizures. The diagnosis was made, treatment was initially successful, and the veterinary specialist communicated with the referring veterinarian concerning patient care. Ten months later, the patient is presented to the referring veterinarian in status epilepticus. The veterinary specialist has been managing the seizure disorder but has not communicated with the referring veterinarian over the past 10 months.

All of the mentioned problems can usually be avoided by proper communication. Other scenarios can arise that are client management problems that are unrelated to the patient's medical or surgical problems. All veterinarians should adhere to the Veterinary Oath, abide by ethical principles, and try to sustain a lifelong effort to fulfill their responsibilities in a professional manner.

The client, specialist, referring veterinarian, and patient all benefit from a timely referral. The client receives appropriate treatment for a loved pet. The specialist is given the opportunity to provide the level of care for which he or she is trained. The referring veterinarian is content fulfilling the obligation to provide care that clients desire and deserve. Above all, animals are the beneficiaries of teamwork to enhance health and quality of life.

## References and Suggested Reading

Dinsmore JR: Veterinary lawsuits. Vet Clin North Am [Small Anim Pract] 23:1019, 1993.

Fessler JF, Burt JK, and Brown RR: Specialization in veterinary medicine: Where we've been and where we're going. J Am Vet Med Assoc 197:328, 1990.

Geyer LL: Malpractice and liability. Vet Clin North Am [Small Anim Pract] 23:1027, 1993.

La Frana J (ed): AVMA Membership Dierctory and Resources Manual, Principles of Veterinary Medical Ethics, 1992, p 536.

La Frana J (ed): AVMA Membership Directory and Resources Manual, Guidelines to Referrals, 1992, p 565.

Stiff ME: Adding value to your practice: Using a board certified specialist. Am Anim Hosp Assoc, Trends, Feb. 1991, p 31.

Tannenbaum J: Ethics: The why and wherefore of veterinary law. Vet Clin North Am [Small Anim Pract] 23:921, 1993.

Wilson JF: Professional liability and the duty to refer to a specialist. Am Anim Hosp Assoc, Trends, Feb. 1991, p 37.

# Section

# 13

# OPHTHALMOLOGIC DISEASES

THOMAS J. KERN
*Consulting Editor*

***Still Current Information Found in Current Veterinary Therapy XI:***

Davidson M: Ocular Therapeutics, p 1049.
Glaze MB: Ocular Manifestations of Systemic Disease, p 1061.
Kern TJ: Feline Ophthalmic Disorders, p 1070.
Smedes SL: Geriatric Ophthalmic Disorders, 1077.
Lindley DM: Disorders of the Orbit, p 1081.
Kirschner SE: Diseases of the Eyelids and Conjunctiva, p 1085.
Kaswan RL: Diagnosis and Management of Tear Film Disorders, p 1092.
Murphy CJ: Disorders of the Cornea and Sclera, p 1101.
Wilkie DA: Disorders of the Uvea, p 1112.
Riis RC: Disorders of the Lens, p 1119.
Scherlie PH, Jr: Glaucoma, p 1125.

***Elsewhere in Current Veterinary Therapy XII:***

Reptile Ophthalmology, p 1361.

# ANTIBIOTIC THERAPY OF THE EYE

KIMBERLY M. STANZ

*Madison, Wisconsin*

In order to determine appropriate antibiotic therapy for the various infectious diseases of the eye, the veterinarian needs to address five basic questions: When? Who? Where? How? and What? It is this chapter's intent to help direct and simplify decision making concerning antibiotic therapy for the eye. This will begin with a brief review of the basic fundamental concepts of antibiotic selection in light of the more specific concerns that pertain to the target organ, the eye or the adnexae. To make recalling this information easier, it has been organized under subheadings that correspond to the "basic five" questions that you should ask yourself before walking into your pharmacy.

## WHEN?

*When is antibiotic therapy appropriate?* The objective of antibiotic therapy is to eliminate or reduce the number of pathogenic organisms. Antibiotics can be used prophylactically, empirically, or specifically. Prophylactically, antibiotics are often employed in preoperative and postoperative situations. Normal skin and conjunctival flora have the potential to become pathogenic. *Staphylococci* spp. are most likely to be encountered, and so a parenteral antibiotic with activity against gram-positive cocci, such as a first-generation cephalosporin, is administered intravenously immediately before and then subcutaneously or intramuscularly 6 hours postoperatively. Often, surgical procedures that involve extensive tissue dissection, removal of heavily contaminated tissues, or the implantation of an orbital prosthesis require the continuation of antibiotics for a longer period postoperatively, usually orally. Prophylactic systemic antibiotics are also indicated in penetrating injuries or in the case of a descemetocele where corneal perforation is impending. Topical antibiotics are used prophylactically in superficial, uninfected lesions of the cornea such as corneal abrasion, indolent ulcer in the dog, and herpesvirus keratitis in the cat.

Specific antibiotic therapy is instituted when the causative organism is identified by culture, the results of which are usually available 48 to 72 hr later. Empiric therapy is instituted immediately after history taking, examination, and sample collection, and is based on both cytology and an educated guess of the most likely pathogen involved. This is done because therapy must be instituted before culture results are available, as in the case of a melting corneal ulcer where delay may lead to perforation. Often, one or two antibiotics are employed to ensure broad-spectrum coverage. This therapeutic approach and specific recommendations are covered in more detail in the following sections.

## WHO?

*Get a diagnosis or at least know "who" you expect to be there.* Imperative in the clinician's decision regarding antibiotic selection is knowing which organism(s) are most likely responsible for the pathology observed. This is especially important in the case of bacterial keratitis. All corneal ulcers with evidence of an infectious process should be cultured and a cytologic examination performed (see "Bacterial Keratitis," this volume, p 1239). The immediate information gained with cytology is invaluable and guides empiric therapy before culture and sensitivity results are available. This is especially important in the case where antibiotic therapy already has been instituted and the chance of a "no growth" culture is very high. Also, cytology is helpful in instances in which a culture is not done because of client financial concerns. Cytologic specimens can also be collected from the conjunctiva and lid lesions and then stained with either Dif-Quick, Wright-Giemsa, or Gram's stain. Ideally, enough material should be collected to be able to use the Gram's and one of the other stains in order to assess the staining and morphologic characteristics of the organism(s) involved.

Generally, the organisms most commonly associated with external ocular disease are similar to the indigenous flora of the eyelids and conjunctiva. Table 1 lists the most common pathogens isolated at the University of Wisconsin-Madison from dogs that had evidence of an infectious process of the cornea or conjunctiva. The

**Table 1.** *Common Isolates From Dogs With Evidence of an Infectious Disease of the Conjunctiva or Cornea at the University of Wisconsin-Madison Between 1/1/92 and 7/1/93.* *

| Conjunctivitis (n = 114) | Corneal Ulcer (n = 17) |
|---|---|
| Coagulase-positive *Staphylococcus* spp. (42.9%) | β-Hemolytic *Streptococcus canis* (22.2%) |
| β-Hemolytic *Streptococcus* spp. (21.9%) | Coagulase-positive *Staphylococcus* spp. (16.7%) |
| *Escherichia coli* (4.4%) | *Escherichia coli* (16.7%) |
| Coagulase-negative *Staphylococcus* spp. (4.4%) | *Pasteurella multocida* (11.1%) |
| *Proteus mirabilis* (2.6%) | α-Hemolytic *Streptococcus* spp. (5.6%) |
| *Propionibacterium* spp. (2.6%) | *Pseudomonas aeruginosa* (5.6%) |
| α-Hemolytic *Streptococcus* spp. (1.8%) | *Enterococcus* spp. (5.6%) |
| Others (11.4%) | Others (16.5%) |

*The author is very thankful to Faye Hartmann MT ASCP, Section Head of Microbiology, for providing the data presented in this table.

data presented in this table closely represent what is reported for other geographic regions; however, it is important to understand that the identity and frequency of isolated organisms can vary with location.

## WHERE?

*Where is the organism located and will the chosen antibiotic get there?* The location of the pathogen may be obvious, but to be able to adequately determine whether an antibiotic will get there relies on basic understanding of drug pharmacodynamics and the ocular physical and physiologic barriers (also see *CVT XI*, p 1049). This leads us into considering the next question, "How should I administer the antibiotic?"

## HOW?

*How can the antibiotic be administered to get it to where it's needed?* This requires an understanding of different routes of administration and their indications:

### Topical

Generally, superficial infections involving the conjunctiva and cornea are treated topically with antibiotic solutions and ointments. The conjunctival and corneal epithelium constitute a significant barrier (the conjunctiva less so) to drug penetration across the tight junctions that exist between cells. This should be kept in mind when deeper penetration is desired, as water-soluble substances do not readily pass into the corneal stroma unless there is a break in the epithelium. Since most indications for topical therapy for the cornea involve an ulcerative process, most antibiotics have adequate access to the corneal stroma. Even so, intraocular penetration is poor regardless of the state of the epithelium and should not be the route of choice for intraocular or periocular infections involving the lids and retrobulbar tissues. The relative impermeability of the epithelium is taken advantage of in that some bactericidal drugs can be used in the eye without much risk of causing systemic toxicity. It does remain a concern, however, when the conjunctiva is inflamed; the epithelium is less resistant to drug penetration and the engorged conjunctival vessels are leakier and more capable of carrying the drug into general circulation. This is a more important consideration in smaller patients or the older animal with renal or hepatic insufficiency receiving the topical medication at a high frequency.

Topical antibiotics generally come in two forms, solution or ointment. Most are available as commercial human ophthalmic preparations, although a few veterinary products exist (see Table 2). The decision as to which form to use depends on several practical consid-

***Table 2.*** *Commercially Available Ophthalmic Antibiotic Preparations.*

| Antibiotic | Supplied as | Sources |
|---|---|---|
| ***Individual Drug Preparations*** | | |
| Chloramphenicol | 0.5% solution<br>1% ointment | H: Allergan, Akorn, Parke-Davis, Pharmafair, Rugby, Schein<br>V: Aveco, Evsco, Pharmaderm, Pitman-Moore, Schering-Plough |
| Chlortetracycline | 1% ointment | H: Lederle |
| Ciprofloxacin | 0.3% solution | H: Alcon |
| Gentamicin | 0.3% solution<br>0.3% ointment | H: Allergan, Akorn, Bausch & Lomb, Iolab, Major, Parke-Davis, Pharmafair, Rugby, Schein, Schering<br>V: Schering-Plough |
| Tetracycline | 1% solution<br>1% solution | H: Lederle |
| Tobramycin | 0.3% solution<br>0.3% ointment | H: Alcon |
| ***Combination Preparations*** | | |
| Neomycin–polymyxin B | Solution | H: Alcon<br>V: AgriLabs, Syntex |
| Neomycin–polymyxin B–gramicidin | Solution | H: Akorn, Bausch & Lomb, Burroughs Wellcome, Major, Rugby |
| Neomycin–polymyxin B–bacitracin | Ointment | H: Akorn, Bausch & Lomb, Burroughs Wellcome, Upjohn<br>V Pharmaderm, Pitman-Moore, Schering-Plough, SmithKline Beecham, Upjohn |
| Oxytetracycline–polymyxin B | Ointment | H: Roerig<br>V: Pfizer |

Abbreviations: *H* = human, *V* = veterinary.

erations. To start, is the antibiotic of choice available in either form? The decision will also depend on the frequency of administration. A solution would be less desirable when a high frequency of application is necessary but cannot be practically done. Contact time of solutions is relatively short compared to ointments. Epiphora significantly decreases the duration of an antibiotic solution even more, as it is rapidly carried away in the tear film. In such instances, an ointment or a fortified antibiotic solution may be more appropriate. Antibiotic solutions are "fortified" by adding the parenteral form of the drug to increase the concentration. This allows delivery of a higher concentration of antibiotic per application to the site of infection. Studies suggest that the concentration of antibiotic in commercial ophthalmic solutions may not be very effective in the face of severe bacterial keratitis. Therefore, antibiotic solutions of commercial concentration tend to be used for prophylactic purposes and conjunctival infections, whereas the fortified solutions are reserved for and used routinely in corneal infections. Other indications for solutions can include: concurrent use of a therapeutic soft contact lens, and relative ease of application for some owners with animals that are more resistant to receiving topical medication. Ointments are preferred when longer contact time is necessary and in situations that would benefit from the lubrication and added protection that an ointment can provide (e.g., keratoconjunctivitis sicca, trichiasis, distichiasis). The use of ointments in very dry eyes, however, may create a thick tenacious tear film and then a solution would be preferred, at least intermittently, in these animals. Ointments should be avoided with corneal epithelial healing disorders and prior to intraocular surgery, penetrating wounds, or a descemetocele (impending perforation), as some ointments may elicit a severe granulomatous reaction if there is direct contact with intraocular structures.

The application rate of topical medications will depend on the nature of the ocular disease. Three to four times daily is usually sufficient for prophylactic treatment of corneal abrasions and most cases of bacterial conjunctivitis, although severe cases may require up to six applications daily. Infected corneal ulcers need to be treated much more aggressively, frequently requiring hourly application of one or more topical antibiotics. To rapidly obtain a high corneal concentration of an antibiotic, a loading dose consisting of one drop of a fortified antibiotic solution every minute for 5 min, which is repeated again in an hour, is given initially and then the rate is reduced to one drop hourly. Few owners are able to treat at this frequency (which initially may need to be continued through the night), and if facilities are not readily available to provide around-the-clock treatment, provisions should be made to provide necessary therapy or referral should be strongly considered. Treatment is usually kept up at this rate until progression of the infectious process has halted and the ulcer has begun to epithelialize. Application of certain topical antibiotics at a high frequency, though necessary to combat the infection, may cause epithelial

toxicity (see "Ocular Drug Reactions and Toxicities," this volume, p 1223). Clinically, this can be manifested by the presence of a superficial punctate keratitis, which creates a stippled, fluorescein-positive staining pattern on the cornea. The use of a cobalt filter light source helps to highlight this lesion, which may not be otherwise appreciated. This should also be suspected when signs of infection have resolved but the ulcer has not re-epithelialized. Aminoglycoside antibiotics are the most likely to be toxic in this way; however, some of the preservatives present in commercial antibiotic preparations have similar potential for injury. Tapering of the application frequency should be done slowly and the cornea watched for signs indicating return of the infectious process. A topical hypersensitivity, manifested by an increase in conjunctival irritation several days to weeks after starting therapy with a topical aminoglycoside (particularly neomycin), is not uncommon and rapid improvement occurs when the aminoglycoside is discontinued and a different effective antibiotic is used.

The use of various drug delivery systems designed for humans has been attempted in veterinary patients. Antibiotic-soaked collagen shields generally do not work well in animals due to differences in tear-flow dynamics. As a result, they do not last as long as they do in people. There probably is no advantage in their use over frequent topical medication and subconjunctival injections. Subpalpebral and nasolacrimal lavage systems usually are not well tolerated in small animal patients and their use is more practical in the equine patient.

## Subconjunctival

Injection of a systemic antibiotic into the subconjunctival space directly bypasses the epithelial barrier to obtain a rapidly higher concentration of drug in the tissues of the anterior segment of the eye. The injected fluid reaches the ocular tissues in two ways: it dissects circumferentially under Tenon's fascia to diffuse into the sclera and cornea, and leaks from the puncture hole into the precorneal tear film allow for transcorneal absorption. Therapeutic drug levels are usually maintained for approximately 3 to 6 hr after injection and then tend to slowly taper off over the following 24 hr. Subconjunctival injection is reserved for severe bacterial infections of the cornea. This method is losing favor, since similar drug concentrations can be obtained by the very frequent application of a topical, fortified antibiotic solution. Subconjunctival injections are indicated if frequent dosing cannot be done, topical fortified antibiotic drops are not readily available, or client compliance is a concern. This method of administration is not, however, meant to be a substitute for topical antibiotic therapy. Injections will need to be repeated every 12 to 24 hr if the desired frequency of topical medication cannot be met. In these instances, severe conjunctival irritation is to be expected.

Subconjunctival injections can be performed fairly

easily in the awake animal with the application of topical anesthesia. Firm restraint is essential to avoid penetrating the globe. In some animals, sedation may be required to safely perform the procedure. After instilling several drops of a topical anesthetic solution, anesthesia at the site of injection can be further enhanced by retracting the upper eyelid and directly applying the anesthetic to the dorsal bulbar conjunctiva with a sterile cotton-tip applicator soaked with topical anesthetic. A 27-gauge needle on a tuberculin syringe is held so that the injection can be performed without the need to reposition your hand once the needle is properly placed. The needle is positioned parallel to the surface of the globe, 4 to 5 mm behind the limbus, with the bevel up so that the tip of the needle just engages the conjunctiva. Then a short, swift controlled movement is used to insert it under the conjunctiva. Without aspirating, a volume of fluid up to 1.0 ml is injected slowly and proper placement is confirmed by the formation of a bleb. Table 3 lists recommended dosages of antibiotics for subconjunctival injection.

## Systemic

This route usually provides therapeutic levels of antibiotic to the periocular and retrobulbar tissues. The ability of systemically administered antibiotics to reach the various structures of the eye is more variable. Very low concentrations are delivered to the cornea; therefore, systemic antibiotics generally are not useful for most corneal infections. The passage of a given antibiotic into intraocular structures is impaired by the blood-eye barriers. Concentrations of systemic antibiotics in the aqueous often parallel those of the central nervous system (CNS) due to the physiologic similarity of the blood-ocular and blood-brain barriers. Vitreal levels often are not significant, which makes endophthalmitis difficult to treat. Inflammation, which disrupts the blood-ocular barriers, enhances ocular penetration of drugs administered by any systemic route. Lipophilic antibiotics (e.g., chloramphenicol and tetracyclines) can cross the intact barrier. However, because these antibiotics are bacteriostatic, other antibiotics are preferable, as some degree of barrier breakdown usually is present with the intraocular conditions that require systemic antibiotics. In general, peak plasma levels promote the passage of antibiotics into the eye. Therefore, intravenously administered drugs are superior in achieving therapeutic levels in tissues over the subcutaneous, intramuscular, and oral routes. Systemic antibiotics are indicated in infections of the lids, lacrimal system, orbit, and whenever there exists a high risk or there is actual intraocular contamination or infection.

## Intravitreal

Generally, this route is not recommended. Intravitreal injections are used in the management of endophthalmitis. Although safe and appropriate levels of antibiotics are known, the potential hazards in performing this procedure limit its use. It is frequently employed as a salvage procedure in general practice, since animals are often presented when the endophthalmitis is so severe that destruction of intraocular structures is likely to be permanent.

## Retrobulbar

Retrobulbar injections are not recommended, since systemically administered antibiotics can reach therapeutic levels in the tissues surrounding the eye. This method does not offer any advantage over subconjunc-

**Table 3.**  *Recommended Dosages for Subconjunctival Antibiotics*

| Drug | Dose° | Concentration of Preparation | Volume to Inject |
|---|---|---|---|
| Amikacin (Amikin, Bristol) | 75–100 mg | 125 mg/ml (dilute 250 mg/ml, 1:1) | 0.6–0.8 ml |
| Ampicillin sodium (Ampicillin Sodium, Lilly) | 50 mg | 125-mg vial, add 1 ml sterile water | 0.4 ml |
| Cefazolin (Kefzol, Lilly) | 50–100 mg | 250-mg vial, add 2.5 ml sterile water | 0.5–1.0 ml |
| Cephalothin (Keflin, Lilly) | 50–100 mg | 1-gm vial, add 10 ml sterile water | 0.5–1.0 ml |
| Gentamicin (Gentocin, Schering) | 10–20 mg | 50 mg/ml | 0.2–0.4 ml |
| Penicillin G (aqueous, many name brands) | 500,000 U | 1 million–U vial, add 1 ml sterile water | 0.5 ml |
| Tobramycin (Nebcin, Lilly) | 10–20 mg | 80 mg/2 ml | 0.25–0.35 ml |
| Vancomycin (Vancocin, Lilly) | 15–25 mg | 500-mg vial, add 9.7 ml sterile water | 0.3–0.5 ml |

°May consider reducing the dosage at the lower end of the range given by 50% in very small animals. A good rule of thumb is to make sure the subconjunctival dose does not exceed the calculated systemic dose that could be safely administered in that patient.

tival injections for penetration of antibiotics into the posterior segment (e.g., vitreous) when the eye is inflamed. This route should also be avoided in the proptosed globe, where it may be tempting to administer in the exposed retrobulbar tissues before replacement.

## WHAT?

*What is the most appropriate antibiotic?* Obviously, the answer to this question relies heavily on the factors considered above. Familiarity with the characteristics and properties of the various classes of antibiotics is essential but will not be reviewed in detail here, as there are several excellent references available (Pavan-Langston and Dunkel 1991a,b; Slatter, 1990; Steinert, 1991; Wyman, 1986). It is also important to be familiar with what antibiotics are available and in what form (see Table 2). However, instead of trying to master this vast amount of information, a more reasonable approach would be to use it to select a few antibiotics in various forms to keep in your pharmacy and become familiar with their use and limitations.

To select the appropriate antibiotic, it is essential to know which organism you are dealing with and its sensitivity profile (see Table 4). Occasionally, for economic reasons, culture and sensitivity is not performed and so therapy is empiric and based on the most likely organism to be present. This is usually based on cytology, which is then considered in light of the frequency and sensitivity data reported in the literature. Since this can vary according to the geographic area and among different hospitals, some caution is advised when interpreting these data. Unless a culture and sensitivity has been done, or while waiting for the results, the rule is to use broad-spectrum coverage initially. Topical ophthalmic preparations that are a combination of several antibiotics are available (Table 2) and are an adequate and economic way to provide broad-spectrum coverage. These products (e.g., neomycin–polymyxin B–bacitracin, or "triple antibiotic") are a good choice for the initial treatment of most uncomplicated superficial diseases of the conjunctiva and cornea. The use of a fortified aminoglycoside eyedrop, to cover the gram-negative bacilli, along with a cephalosporin or a penicillin eyedrop, to cover the gram-positive cocci, is "in vogue" for the initial treatment of severe bacterial keratitis. The aminoglycoside, gentamicin (tobramycin and amikacin to a lesser extent), is synergistic with cephalosporins and penicillins. Cephalosporin and penicillin eyedrops are not commercially available and need to be prepared with the parenteral form and artificial tear solutions. Recipes for making these eyedrops can be found in Table 5. Recently, ciprofloxacin has become commercially available as a topical ophthalmic solution. This drug may be useful as a single agent that would be comparable to combination therapy with two or more antibiotics in the treatment of bacterial keratitis (Leibowitz, 1991). No controlled veterinary clinical trials have been performed, but in humans, ciprofloxacin has good efficacy against corneal infections involving most *Pseudomonas* spp., although some *Staphylococcus* and *Streptococcus* spp. may be resistant. Indiscriminate use of fortified antibiotics, ciprofloxacin, and the aminoglycosides such as tobramycin and amikacin not only increases the cost of treatment to clients unnecessarily,

**Table 4.** *Susceptibility Patterns for Bacterial Eye Isolates at the University of Wisconsin-Madison for January–December 1992.*[°†]

| Antibiotic | Organisms (% Susceptible by Kirby-Bauer Disk Diffusion) | | | | | | | |
|---|---|---|---|---|---|---|---|---|
| | Staphylococcus (Coagulase Positive)[‡] | Staphylococcus (Coagulase Negative)[§] | β-Hemolytic Streptococcus[⁎] | Enterococcus[¶] | Escherichia coli | Pseudomonas aeruginosa | Proteus mirabilis | Corynebacterium |
| Amoxi/clavulanic acid | 100 | 100 | 100 | 50 | 100 | NT | 100 | 100 |
| Bacitracin | 86 | 100 | 100 | 50 | 0 | 0 | 0 | 50 |
| Cefazolin[#] | 100 | NT | 100 | NT | 100 | NT | 100 | NT |
| Cephalothin | 100 | 100 | 100 | 0 | 83 | NT | 100 | 50 |
| Ciprofloxacin | 100 | 100 | 100 | 50 | 100 | 100 | 100 | 100 |
| Chloramphenicol | 97 | 100 | 100 | 100 | 100 | NT | 0 | 100 |
| Gentamicin | 92 | 100 | 79 | 0 | 100 | 100 | 100 | 100 |
| Neomycin | 73 | 100 | 29 | 0 | 83 | 0 | 100 | 100 |
| Oxacillin | 100 | 100 | NT | NT | NT | NT | NT | NT |
| Polymyxin B | 95 | 83 | 8 | 0 | 100 | 100 | 0 | 50 |
| Tetracycline | 35 | 50 | 21 | 50 | 83 | NT | 0 | 100 |
| Tobramycin | 92 | 100 | 58 | 50 | 100 | 100 | 100 | 100 |

°Data from the University of Wisconsin-Madison Veterinary Medical Teaching Hospital, Clinical Pathology Laboratory, Section of Microbiology (n = 121).
†The author is very thankful to Faye Hartmann MT ASCP, Section Head of Microbiology, for providing the data presented in this table.
‡Includes *Staphylococcus aureus*, *S. intermedius*.
§Includes *Staphylococcus epidermidis*.
⁎Includes *Streptococcus canis*, *S. zooepidemicus*.
¶An α-hemolytic *Streptococcus*.
#Information is based on few isolates; this antibiotic was only recently added to the antibiotics routinely tested.

***Table 5.***   *Compounding Fortified and Noncommercial Topical Antibiotic Solutions.*[*]

**Amikacin**
1.  Remove 2 ml from a 15-ml squeeze bottle of artificial tear solution[†] and discard.
2.  Add 2 ml of injectable amikacin (50 mg/ml [Amikin, Bristol]).
    Final concentration = 6.7 mg/ml (0.67% solution).
    Shelf life[‡] = 30 days.

**Cefazolin**
1.  Remove 2 ml from a 15-ml squeeze bottle of artificial tear solution and discard.
2.  Reconstitute a 500-mg vial of cefazolin (Kefzol, Lilly) with 2 ml of sterile water.
3.  Add entire 500 mg of the reconstituted cefazolin (2.4 ml) to the bottle of artificial tear solution.
    Final concentration = 33 mg/ml (3.3% solution).
    Shelf life[§] = 14 days.
    Keep the solution refrigerated.

**Cephalothin**
1.  Remove 6 ml from a 15-ml squeeze bottle of artificial tear solution and save.
2.  Add the 6 ml of tear solution to a 1-gm vial of cephalothin (Keflin, Lilly).
3.  Add the entire 1 gm of the reconstituted cephalothin (6.4 ml) to the bottle of artificial tear solution.
    Final concentration = 65 mg/ml (6.5% solution).
    Shelf life[‖] = 14 days.
    Keep the solution refrigerated.

**Gentamicin (Fortified)**
1.  Add 2 ml of injectable gentamicin (50 mg/ml [Gentocin, Schering]) to the 5-ml bottle of commercial ophthalmic gentamicin solution (0.3%).
    Final concentration = 14 mg/ml (1.4% solution).
    Shelf life[‡] = 30 days.

**Ticarcillin**
1.  Reconstitute a 1-gm vial of ticarcillin (Ticar, Beecham) with 9.4 ml of sterile water.
2.  Add 1.0 ml (100 mg) of this solution to a 15-ml squeeze bottle of artificial tears.
    Final concentration = 6.3 mg/ml (0.63% solution).
    Shelf life[‡] = 4 days.
    Keep the solution refrigerated.

**Tobramycin (Fortified)**
1.  Add 1.0 ml of injectable tobramycin (40 mg/ml [Nebcin, Lilly]) to a 5-ml bottle of commercial ophthalmic tobramycin solution (0.3%).
    Final concentration = 9.2 mg/ml (0.92% solution).
    Shelf life[‡] = 30 days.

**Vancomycin**
1.  Remove 9 ml from a 15-ml squeeze bottle of artificial tear solution and discard.
2.  Reconstitute a 500-mg vial of vancomycin (Vancocin, Lilly) with 10 ml of sterile water.
3.  Add the entire 500 mg of reconstituted vancomycin (10.2 ml) to the bottle of artificial tear solution.
    Final concentration = 31 mg/ml (3.1% solution).
    Shelf life[‡] = 4 days.
    Keep the solution refrigerated.

[*]Adapted from Baum JL: Antibiotic use in ophthalmology. *In* Tasmen W and Jaeger EA (eds): *Duane's Clinical Ophthalmology,* volume 4. Philadelphia, JB Lippincott Co, 1988, p 4, with permission.
[†]Recommended artificial tear solutions are Isopto Alkaline (Alcon), which contains 1% hydroxypropyl methylcellulose; and Adapt (Alcon), which contains polyvinyl alcohol. These solutions are a little more viscous than others, which helps to increase the contact time.
[‡]Data derived from Glasser DB and Hyndiuk RA: Antibiotics. *In* Lamberts DW and Potter DE (eds): *Clinical Ophthalmic Pharmacology.* Boston, Little, Brown & Co, 1987, p 73.
[§]Shelf life for cefazolin is a conservative estimate based on data from Bowe BE, Snyder JW, and Eiferman RA: An in vitro study of the potency and stability of fortified ophthalmic antibiotic preparations. Am J Ophthalmol 111:686, 1991.
[‖]Data derived from Osborne E, Baum JL, Ernst C, and Koch P: The stability of ten antibiotics in artificial tear solutions. Am J Ophthalmol 82(5):775, 1976.

but can lead to development of resistant organisms. To have another antibiotic in reserve, the use of these newer or higher generation antibiotics should be restricted to severe bacterial keratitis that has not responded to your initial therapy or as indicated by culture and sensitivity results. Culturing is strongly recommended and is actually a very cost-effective procedure in that it can save the client the unnecessary cost associated with the use of a very expensive ophthalmic antibiotic if a more economical one is found to be just as effective.

An important point needs to be made regarding interpretation of sensitivity profiles. Most sensitivity profiles are performed using the Kirby-Bauer method. This is based on therapeutic antibiotic levels that can be achieved in the serum and, therefore, in most tissue fluids in the body other than the eye and tears. Since markedly higher levels can be obtained in the cornea and tears via the topical administration of an antibiotic, a "resistant" organism may actually be sensitive under these circumstances. Clinical improvement of an infectious process despite sensitivity results that indicate resistance to the chosen antibiotic may not warrant a change. Likewise, a poor response to therapy that is deemed appropriate by the culture and sensitivity may represent a misdiagnosis or persistence of the underlying cause of the disease.

The clinician must be careful to avoid treating nonbacterial intraocular inflammatory diseases such as uveitis with topical and systemic antibiotics. Antibiotic therapy is not indicated in most cases of uveitis in the dog or cat, because the majority tend to be idiopathic or secondary to cataracts or fungal disease; rarely is it bacterial in nature (see "Canine Uveitis," this volume, p 1248). In cats, uveitis can be associated with toxoplasmosis infection. Often, however, affected cats are not actively infected with toxoplasmosis and systemic antibiotic therapy is reserved for cats with serologic tests supportive of an active infection (see "Feline Uveitis" and "Feline Toxoplasmosis," this volume, pp 1253 and 309, respectively). It can be difficult to differentiate a severe uveitis with a sterile hypopyon from an endophthalmitis. Referral to a veterinary ophthalmologist should be considered if a decision cannot be made between anti-inflammatory or antibiotic therapy. The "shotgun" approach of using a combination of both in such cases is inappropriate and may lead to disastrous consequences.

## GUIDELINES FOR ANTIBIOTIC SELECTION IN OCULAR DISEASE

### Staphylococcal Blepharitis

MOST LIKELY ORGANISM(S).   *Staphylococcus intermedius* and *S. epidermidis.*

ANTIBIOTIC THERAPY

*Systemic.*   Amoxicillin trihydrate/clavulanate potassium (Clavamox, Beecham): 15 mg/kg PO three times daily.

Cephalexin (Cefa-Tabs, Fort Dodge) or cefadroxil (Keflex, Dista): 22 mg/kg PO three times daily.

Oxacillin sodium (Prostaphlin, Bristol; Bactocill, Beecham): 22 mg/kg PO three times daily.

*For a minimum of 3 weeks for acute infections, up to 6 to 8 weeks if chronic.

*Topical.* Neomycin–polymyxin B–bacitracin (or gramicidin) ointment, three to four times daily.

### OTHER CONSIDERATIONS

Corticosteroids and immunostimulants may be indicated in complicated and chronic cases (see *CVT XI*, p 1087).

## Bacterial Conjunctivitis

#### CANINE

MOST LIKELY ORGANISM(S): See Table 1.

### ANTIBIOTIC THERAPY

*Topical.* For acute uncomplicated infections, neomycin–polymyxin B–bacitracin (or gramicidin) solution/ointment, three or four times daily. Otherwise, chronic or recurrent infections warrant culture and sensitivity. Cytology should be performed in such cases and initial topical antibiotic therapy is started according to these "rules of thumb":

Cocci: neomycin–polymyxin B–bacitracin (gramicidin) or chloramphenicol ointment/solution, four times daily, up to six times daily initially if severe.

Bacilli: gentamicin ointment/solution, four times daily, up to six times daily initially if severe.

Mixed: neomycin–polymyxin B–bacitracin (gramicidin) or gentamicin ointment/solution, four times daily, up to six times daily initially if severe.

No bacteria seen: neomycin–polymyxin B–bacitracin (gramicidin) ointment/solution, four times daily, up to six times daily initially if severe.

OTHER CONSIDERATIONS. Rule out keratoconjunctivitis sicca, allergy, and dacryocystitis, as the latter can re-seed the conjunctiva and be the source of the recurrent disease.

#### FELINE

MOST LIKELY ORGANISM: *Chlamydia psittaci* (felis)

### ANTIBIOTIC THERAPY

*Topical.* Chloramphenicol or oxytetracycline ointment, four times daily for 3 weeks minimum (or 2 weeks past resolution of clinical signs).

*Systemic.* (May be indicated only if showing systemic signs or if recurrent). Doxycycline (Vibramycin, Pfizer): 5 mg/kg PO twice daily for 3 to 4 weeks.

OTHER CONSIDERATIONS: For infections with *Mycoplasma felis*, topical therapy as for chlamydia. Herpesvirus infection is also very common and usually does not require antibiotic therapy unless a secondary bacterial infection is present or as a prophylactic measure for keratitis. Cytology, culture, and immunofluorescent antibody tests can help to differentiate among these feline pathogens and direct therapy (see "Feline Keratoconjunctivitis," this volume, p 1227).

## Dacryocystitis

MOST LIKELY ORGANISM(S). Same as for conjunctivitis.

### ANTIBIOTIC THERAPY

*Topical.* Same rationale as for conjunctivitis except solutions are preferred, as generally they achieve better access to the nasolacrimal system.

*Systemic.* If culture and sensitivity are not available, a broad-spectrum antibiotic with good skin/soft tissue penetration characteristics is beneficial.

## Bacterial Keratitis

MOST LIKELY ORGANISM(S). See Table 1.

ANTIBIOTIC THERAPY. The following recommendations are for the initial therapy until culture and sensitivity results are known, or for continuous therapy based on clinical response if a culture was not performed. Although an approach of using two antibiotics is recommended initially to provide broad-spectrum coverage, cytology and culture should still be performed to help guide therapeutic decisions during the course of treatment.

*Topical.* See Table 5 for recipes.

*Combination gram-positive and -negative bactericidal therapy (for broad-spectrum coverage):* cephalosporin drops and fortified gentamicin (tobramycin) drops, each hourly until progression of stromal loss has halted and infiltrates are decreasing, then taper very slowly. Ideally, the drops are alternated with one given every half-hour. If this is not possible, wait at least 10 min between drops; this avoids a dilution effect created by following one drop immediately with another. Consider performing the "loading technique" as described above in the section "How?"

*Other combinations to consider if no clinical improvement:* a fortified aminoglycoside along with ticarcillin drops (for some resistant *Pseudomonas* spp.), or vancomycin drops (great for resistant gram-positive cocci). Don't hesitate to perform another cytologic examination and consider reculturing.

*Single agent therapy:* ciprofloxacin ophthalmic solution, hourly initially and then taper slowly when indicated. Provides broad-spectrum coverage, although some *Pseudomonas*, *Staphylococcus*, and *Streptococcus* spp. may be resistant.

*Subconjunctival.* See Table 3 for recommended dosages and the section "How?" for a description on technique.

• Consider using when topical antibiotics cannot be given as frequently as needed.

- Two antibiotics can be given at the same time, each in a separate site.

## Bacterial Endophthalmitis

MOST LIKELY ORGANISM. Depends on inciting cause, usually gram-positive cocci in postoperative complications, and gram-negative bacilli in the case of a penetrating foreign body, or either when the result of a ruptured descemetocele.

ANTIBIOTIC THERAPY. Prognosis is very poor and often enucleation is the end result. Can attempt broad-spectrum systemic antibiotic therapy, subconjunctival injections, and intravitreal injections. Most antibiotics given systemically and subconjunctivally will be able to gain access to the inflamed intraocular structures but will not be able to penetrate exudate if abundant. Therefore, one must focus on systemic prophylactic therapy, which needs to be administered soon after intraocular contamination has occurred.

PROPHYLACTIC THERAPY

*Systemic.*

Perioperative: cephalothin (Keflin, Lilly) or cefazolin (Kefzol, Lilly), 22 mg/kg IV, IM, or SC (two doses, one given just prior to surgery; the second follows 6 hr later).

Postoperative: cephalexin or cefadroxil, 22 mg/kg PO three times daily for 7 to 10 days (Ultracy, Bristol Laboratories).

Actual or impending perforations/penetrating injuries: amoxicillin trihydrate/clavulanate potassium, 15 mg/kg PO three times daily; enrofloxacin (Baytril, Haver/Mobay) or ciprofloxacin (Cipro, Miles), 5 to 10 mg/kg PO twice daily (or per culture and sensitivity results).

ACUTE BACTERIAL ENDOPHTHALMITIS

*Intravitreal.* Contact a specialist when considering this for treatment of an active endophthalmitis.

*Subconjunctival.* Per culture and sensitivity results or use a combination of a cephalosporin and an aminoglycoside for broad-spectrum coverage. May need to administer every 12 to 24 hr.

*Topical.* Same recommendations as for subconjunctival administration, but topical antibiotics need to be administered at a high frequency. This route is not recommended to be the sole method of administration of antibiotics in the face of an active endophthalmitis.

*Systemic.* Often broad-spectrum antibiotics are administered intravenously; however, there is some debate as to the effectiveness of this route of administration in the treatment of bacterial endophthalmitis.

OTHER CONSIDERATIONS. Rule out fungal, protozoal, or a sterile uveitis with hypopyon.

## References and Suggested Reading

Leibowitz HM: Clinical evaluation of ciprofloxacin 0.3% ophthalmic solution for treatment of bacterial keratitis. Am J Ophthalmol 112:34S, 1991.
  *A prospective study comparing topical ciprofloxacin as a single therapeutic agent with standard therapy regimens for bacterial keratitis in people.*
Pavan-Langston D and Dunkel EC: Antibiotics. *In Handbook of Ocular Drug Therapy and Ocular Side Effects of Systemic Drugs.* Boston, Little, Brown & Co, 1991a, p 22.
  *A concise synopsis of the spectrum of activity, mechanism of action, routes of administration, and adverse side effects of various antimicrobial agents used in treating ocular infections.*
Pavan-Langston D and Dunkel EC: Pharmacokinetics of ophthalmic drug administration. *In Handbook of Ocular Drug Therapy and Ocular Side Effects of Systemic Drugs.* Boston, Little, Brown & Co, 1991b, p 3.
  *A brief and practical review of the pharmacokinetics of ocular drug therapy.*
Slatter D: Ocular pharmacology and therapeutics. *In Fundamentals of Veterinary Ophthalmology,* 2nd edition. Philadelphia, W.B. Saunders Co, 1990, p 32.
  *An overview of veterinary ocular pharmacology and therapeutics.*
Steinert RF: Current therapy for bacterial keratitis and bacterial conjunctivitis. Am J Ophthalmol 112:10S, 1991.
  *A review of the current concepts behind the use of fortified topical antibiotics and topical preparations made from parenteral forms for the treatment of bacterial keratitis and conjunctivitis in people.*
Wyman M: Contemporary ocular therapeutics. *In Kirk RW (ed): Current Veterinary Therapy IX.* Philadelphia, W.B. Saunders Co, 1986, p 684.
  *An overview of veterinary ocular therapeutics with an emphasis on antimicrobial agents.*

# ANTI-INFLAMMATORY THERAPY OF THE EYE

THOMAS R. MILLER
*Largo, Florida*

Corticosteroids and other anti-inflammatory drugs stabilize blood-ocular barriers, reduce the production of intraocular fibrin and exudates, and limit collagen formation that can lead to scarring. Anti-inflammatory therapy is indicated for the treatment or prevention of chemosis or other periocular swelling; corneal infiltrates or pigmentation; and complications of intraocular inflammation such as synechia formation, glaucoma, or retinal detachments. Because of the potentially devastating effect of inflammation on ocular function, it is frequently desirable, and often essential, to use anti-inflammatory agents to preserve vision. This is particularly true in immune-mediated or traumatic ocular disease, but can also apply to the judicious use of anti-inflammatory agents in selected cases of infectious disease. Care must be taken in these cases not to potentiate the effect the primary pathogen.

## ROUTES OF ADMINISTRATION

As important as the choice of drug is the route of administration. This choice will be influenced by the target site of inflammation, as well as by the drug itself. Topical administration is appropriate in cases of eyelid or conjunctival disease, as well as in corneal or anterior segment inflammation. This route has the advantage of providing a high drug level in a localized area, with a low systemic drug level (Leibowitz and Kupferman, 1980). It may be limited by rapid drug clearance from the ocular surface, as well as by the ability of the drug to penetrate the ocular tissues. These factors can be influenced by the vehicle, the drug formulation, and the severity of inflammation present. In general, solutions provide the most rapid uptake and highest peak tissue levels. However, contact time can be improved by using suspensions, viscous vehicles, soluble gels, or ointments, thus prolonging the drug effects, reducing systemic uptake, and achieving a greater therapeutic effect. A notable exception to this rule is dexamethasone phosphate prepared in an ointment base; the vehicle apparently slows the release of the drug into the tear film, reducing its effect (Leibowitz and Kupferman, 1980). Contact time may also be improved by the use of various delivery systems, such as extended-wear contact lenses or corneal collagen shields.

Topical corticosteroid therapy can have significant systemic side effects, affecting glucose metabolism, serum enzymes levels, and the adrenocortical axis (Eichenbaum et al., 1988).

The formulation of the drug can significantly influence intraocular penetration. In general, drugs in an acetate form have the best corneal penetration, followed by alcohol-based, then phosphate-based drugs.

Subconjunctival injections have the advantage of establishing high tissue levels of drug by avoiding the epithelial barrier to drug penetration. A maximum volume of 0.25 to 0.5 ml should be used in small animals. This route is probably best reserved for the use of repositol corticosteroids, where a therapeutic drug level can be maintained for days to weeks. Triamcinolone or betamethasone are preferred over methylprednisolone, as the latter is associated with a higher frequency of plaque or granuloma formation at the injection site. As in topical administration, this route provides high drug levels in the anterior segment, but may fail to achieve adequate levels in the posterior segment.

Orbital or retrobulbar injections of anti-inflammatory agents offer little added drug penetration over subconjunctival injections, and may contribute to discomfort and swelling in an already compromised orbit. When high levels of drug are required in the posterior segment of the eye, or in the orbit, systemic administration is the route of choice.

Systemic administration of medication can deliver large quantities of drug to the eyelids, orbit, and eye. Intraocular penetration may be limited by the blood-ocular barrier, although in an inflamed eye, these barriers are frequently compromised. Direct intraocular injections of anti-inflammatory drugs are seldom indicated, as the trauma of the injection and potential local toxicity of the drug usually far outweigh the advantage of drug delivery.

Agents available for the treatment of ocular inflammation can be divided into three main groups: corticosteroids, nonsteroidal anti-inflammatory drugs (NSAIDs), and immunosuppressive agents.

## CORTICOSTEROIDS

Corticosteroids are the most commonly used anti-inflammatory agents in veterinary ophthalmology and are in many cases the most effective choice. In addition to being immunosuppressive if used at adequate doses, corticosteroids are more complete anti-inflammatory agents than most NSAIDs because of their effect of blocking arachidonic acid formation, preventing the formation of both prostaglandins and leukotrienes. Corticosteroids in particular should be used with great discretion in infectious disease.

Commonly used corticosteroids include, in increasing order of anti-inflammatory potency, hydrocortisone (Table 1), prednisolone, triamcinolone, betamethasone, and dexamethasone. In addition to potency, one must consider the duration of action, as well as the bioavailability of the drug of choice. For example, although betamethasone is more potent, prednisolone acetate has much better intraocular penetration, and would therefore be a superior choice for uveitis or nonulcerative keratitis. Newer generations of corticosteroids, such as fluoromet  halone, may be more potent than some of the standard choices, but in many cases they are short acting or have limited intraocular penetration (Polansky and Weinreb, 1984). These properties have advantages in human patients, where the risk of corticosteroid-

**Table 1.** *Anti-inflammatory Potency of Corticosteroids*

| Corticosteroid | Relative Anti-inflammatory Potency |
|---|---|
| Hydrocortisone | 1 |
| Prednisone | 4 |
| Prednisolone | 4 |
| Methylprednisolone | 5 |
| Triamcinolone | 5 |
| Dexamethasone | 25 |
| Betamethasone | 25 |

induced side effects such as ocular hypertension is common, but the reduction in anti-inflammatory effect limits their usefulness in veterinary medicine.

## Indications

### CONJUNCTIVITIS

In conjunctivitis resulting from allergic or immune-mediated mechanisms, or from contact irritants, corticosteroids can reduce or resolve chemosis and hyperemia. The choice of corticosteroid is not important in most cases, as even hydrocortisone is frequently adequate to control the inflammation. Concurrent therapy with a broad-spectrum antibiotic is often useful to control secondary bacterial overgrowth.

LIMITATIONS. Specific causes for conjunctivitis, such as keratoconjunctivitis sicca, foreign body, or concurrent uveitis, should be ruled out. The prolonged use of antibiotic-corticosteroid combinations may predispose to superinfections. Conjunctivitis in cats is most frequently caused by primary infectious agents that are potentiated by corticosteroid therapy.

### DACRYOCYSTITIS

Nasolacrimal duct infections and obstruction frequently have an inflammatory component that contributes to the problem by narrowing or occluding the duct lumen. Corticosteroids can be used along with antibiotic therapy to reduce swelling within the duct to help restore patency. Solutions may be more beneficial than ointments because they drain through the duct more effectively.

LIMITATIONS. The nasolacrimal duct should be cannulated and flushed to aid in the restoration of patency. Cannulating the entire duct with a nylon suture may aid in maintaining patency during initial therapy.

### KERATITIS

In cases of nonspecific keratitis, as well as specific inflammations such as chronic superficial keratitis (pannus), eosinophilic keratitis, and nodular granulomatous episclerokeratitis (NGE), corticosteroids can be used to reduce or prevent corneal vascularization and pigmentation and may also reduce lipid and mineral deposits within the cornea, thereby maintaining corneal clarity. Therapy may be topical or subconjunctival, depending on the severity and the chronicity of the disease. For stromal keratitis associated with feline herpes virus, concurrent antiviral and corticosteroid therapy may be required for control.

LIMITATIONS. As a rule, corticosteroids are *contraindicated* for ulcerative keratitis and active corneal infections because they delay corneal healing and potentiate infectious agents.

### ANTERIOR UVEITIS

Corticosteroids are indicated in anterior uveitis in an effort to minimize synechia formation and secondary glaucoma. Reduction of lymphocytic infiltrates may reduce the chronicity or recurrence of the inflammation. Intraocular penetration is important; prednisolone acetate is frequently the drug of choice. Systemic or subconjunctival therapy (prednisone 1 mg/kg every 12 hr PO, or triamcinolone 1 to 2 mg subconjunctival) should be considered in severe cases to supplement topical therapy.

LIMITATIONS. Animals with uveitis from infectious causes, such as blastomycosis, should be treated with caution to avoid exacerbating the primary infection.

### POSTERIOR UVEITIS

Corticosteroids are indicated to control choroidal effusions, retinal detachments, and retinal degenerations secondary to inflammation. Systemic therapy is the most effective route of administration. Prednisone (1 mg/kg every 12 hr) is my drug of choice. The same precautions as for anterior uveitis apply.

### OPTIC NEURITIS

Optic neuritis may result in optic atrophy and demyelination, which may be prevented or reduced by corticosteroid therapy in the early stages. Prednisone (1 mg/kg every 12 hr) is recommended after infectious causes of meningitis have been ruled out.

LIMITATIONS. Optic neuritis may be recurrent or chronic, especially in diseases such as granulomatous meningoencephalitis, necessitating long-term corticosteroid therapy to preserve vision. Damage to the nerve may be severe enough in acute cases to result in demyelination even after the resolution of the active inflammation.

## NONSTEROIDAL ANTI-INFLAMMATORY DRUGS

NSAIDs are in general less potent than corticosteroids. In most cases, NSAIDs specifically block cyclooxygenase, preventing prostaglandin formation. However, inflammatory precursors may be shunted to form leukotrienes, with a resulting increase in inflammation. Because of this relatively specific anti-inflammatory effect, NSAIDs may be most useful in the prevention of inflammation rather than the treatment of inflammation already in progress (Flach, 1992). Therefore, NSAIDs are frequently recommended as presurgical medication. Because of the effect of inflammatory mediators in creating miosis, topical NSAIDs are frequently touted for their effect of maintaining mydriasis intraoperatively during cataract surgery, rather than for specific anti-inflammatory effects. NSAIDs are useful in situations where corticosteroids are contraindicated, such as infectious diseases and diabetes mellitus. Topical NSAIDs delay corneal wound healing, but do not potentiate collagenase, and may have some use in the treatment of ulcerative keratitis.

Topical NSAIDs are now available, with suprofen 1%

(Profenal, Alcon Laboratories), flurbiprofen 0.03% (Ocufen, Allergan), and diclofenac 0.1% (Voltaren Ophthalmic, Burroughs Wellcome) in common use in the United States. Indomethacin is used in many other countries but is not available as an ophthalmic preparation in the United States. Dosage of topical NSAIDs is four times daily, with a preoperative loading dose of 1 drop every 30 min for 2 hr before surgery often recommended. Systemic absorption of topical NSAIDs is minimal, making their use in cats relatively safe.

## Limitations

### TOPICAL

NSAIDs probably have limited usefulness in routine cases of conjunctivitis and keratitis. Their use may potentiate keratitis associated with feline herpesvirus (Collins and Moore, 1991). The use of topical NSAIDs may result in increased intraocular pressure following surgery in dogs (Millichamp and Dziezyc, 1991). Wound healing is delayed by topical NSAIDs, although this effect may be as pronounced as that caused by corticosteroids (Flach, 1992).

NSAIDs commonly used systemically in veterinary medicine are flunixin meglumine (Banamine, Schering), phenylbutazone, and acetylsalicylic acid. Although all three are useful in both anterior and posterior uveitis, flunixin use is restricted to acute therapy, at a dose of 0.25 to 0.5 mg/kg IV daily for 2 to 3 days in the dog. Acetylsalicylic acid is a better choice for chronic therapy, at a dose of 10 to 25 mg/kg PO twice daily in dogs and a dose of 80 mg PO every 48 to 72 hr in cats (Wilkie, 1992).

### SYSTEMIC

Systemic NSAID therapy can result in side effects including gastrointestinal ulceration and hemorrhage, acute renal papillary necrosis, and decreased platelet function (Rubin and Papich, 1990). Concurrent use of corticosteroids may potentiate the gastrointestinal side effects (Collins and Moore, 1991). The use of flunixin in cases receiving methoxyflurane anesthesia can result in acute renal tubular necrosis (Mathews et al., 1990).

**Table 2.** *Anti-inflammatory Drug Therapy*

| Drug Classification | Brand Name | Dose |
|---|---|---|
| **Topicals** | | |
| Corticosteroid | Multiple preparations, | q6–24h |
| Short-acting | in combination with | |
| Hydrocortisone | triple antibiotic | |
| Intermediate-acting | Econopred Plus (Alcon) or Pred Forte (Allergan) | q6–24h, up to q1h |
| Prednisolone acetate 1% suspension | | |
| Long-acting | Maxidex (Alcon) or Decadron (Merck Sharpe & Dohme) | q6–24h |
| Dexamethasone 0.1% solution | | |
| Dexamethasone 0.05% ointment | | q6–24h |
| NSAIDs | | |
| Flurbiprofen 0.03% | Ocufen (Allergan) | q6h |
| Suprofen 1.0% | Profenal (Alcon) | q6h |
| Diclofenac 0.1% | Voltaren Ophthalmic (CIBA) | q6h |
| Immunosuppressants | Not yet commercially available | q12h |
| Cyclosporine 2% | | |
| **Subconjunctival Corticosteroids** | | |
| Triamcinolone acetonide | Vetalog (Solvay) | 1–2 mg q1–4wk |
| Methylprednisolone acetate | Depo-Medrol (Upjohn) | 4–12 mg q1–3wk |
| Betamethasone | Betasone (Schering) | 0.75–1 mg q1–3wk |
| **Systemic** | | |
| Corticosteroids | | 1 mg/kg q12h PO for 7 days, then taper |
| Prednisone | | |
| NSAIDs | | *Dog:* 10–25 mg/kg q12h |
| Acetylsalicylic acid | | *Cat:* 10 mg/kg q48–72 h |
| Flunixin meglumine | Banamine (Schering) | *Dog:* 0.25–0.5 mg/kg IV q24h for 2–3 days |
| Immunosuppressant | Imuran (Burroughs Wellcome) | *Dog:* 2.2 mg/kg q12h PO then reduce |
| Azathioprine | | |

## IMMUNOSUPPRESSANTS

The third class of anti-inflammatory drugs is the immunosuppressive agents. Two of these drugs used most often in veterinary ophthalmology are cyclosporine and azathioprine. Cyclosporine is frequently used for its lacrimomimetic effect in keratoconjunctivitis sicca (KCS) (see "Cyclosporine," this volume, p 74). Although an ophthalmic preparation is not currently available, oral cyclosporine solutions are diluted to 1 to 2% solution in corn oil or light mineral oil for veterinary ophthalmic use. In addition to the effect on tear production, cyclosporine may be useful in controlling the secondary inflammatory changes seen in KCS, such as corneal pigmentation (see "Keratoconjunctivitis Sicca," this volume, p 1231). This anti-inflammatory effect may also be beneficial in treatment of immune-mediated ocular diseases, such as chronic superficial keratitis (pannus) (see "Pannus," this volume, p 1245).

### Limitations

Cyclosporine therapy may potentiate ocular herpes infections in cats. Few treated animals develop blepharoconjunctivitis from contact with the eyelids. This is usually avoided using corn oil or mineral oil as a diluent, rather than olive oil.

Azathioprine (Imuran, Buroughs Wellcome) is not available as an ophthalmic preparation, but is used parenterally in the control of nodular granulomatous episclerokeratitis (fibrous histiocytoma) and immune-mediated uveitis, such as cases of uveodermatologic syndrome (Vogt-Koyanagi-Harada syndrome). Although these cases may be managed with corticosteroid therapy, chronic or refractory cases usually respond to azathioprine given at an initial dose of 2 mg/kg PO, and reduced over time to minimize side effects (Paulsen et al., 1987). Animals on therapy should be monitored for leukopenia.

The concurrent use of multiple classes of anti-inflammatory drugs may be beneficial in that, because of differing mechanisms of activity, a synergistic effect may be achieved. As a result of this increase in activity, the total dose of an individual drug may be reduced, lessening the possibility of side effects.

Table 2 summarizes the durations of action and dosages of commonly used ocular anti-inflammatory agents.

### References and Suggested Reading

Collins BK and Moore CP: Canine anterior Uvea. *In* Gelatt KN (ed): *Veterinary Ophthalmology, 2nd edition.* Philadelphia, Lea & Febiger, 1991, p 357.
*A review of the therapy of anterior uveitis in small animal practice.*
Eichenbaum JD, Macy DW, Severin GA, and Paulsen ME: Effect in large dogs of ophthalmic prednisolone acetate on adrenal gland and hepatic function. J Am Anim Hosp Assoc 24:705, 1988.
*A prospective study evaluating topical prednisolone and its effect on glucagon tolerance and ACTH stimulation tests.*
Flach AJ: Cyclo-oxygenase inhibitors in ophthalmology. Surv Ophthalmol 36:259, 1992.
*A review of the indications, pharmacodynamics, and side effects of ophthalmic cyclooxygenase inhibitors.*
Leibowitz HM and Kupferman A: Anti-inflammatory medications. Int Ophthalmol Clin 20:117, 1980.
*A review of the indications, pharmacodynamics, and clinical usage of ophthalmic corticosteroids.*
Mathews KA, Doherty T, Dyson DH, et al: Nephrotoxicity in dogs associated with methoxyflurane anesthesia and flunixin meglumine analgesia. A retrospective study of acute tubular necrosis resulting from the concurrent use of these drugs. Can Vet J 31:766, 1990.
Millichamp NJ and Dziezyc J: Comparison of flunixin meglumine and flurbiprofen for control of ocular irritative response in dogs. Am J Vet Res 52:1452, 1991.
*A prospective trial comparing the effects of flunixin and flurbiprofen or intraocular pressure, and pupil diameter.*
Paulsen ME, Lavach JD, Snyder SP, et al: Nodular granulomatous episclerokeratitis in dogs: 19 cases (1973–1985). J Am Vet Med Assoc 190:1581, 1987.
*A retrospective study on the prevalence and treatment of NGE.*
Polansky JR and Weinreb RN: Anti-inflammatory agents: Steroids as anti-inflammatory agents. *In* Sears ML (ed): *Handbook of Experimental Pharmacology,* volume 69. Berlin, Springer-Verlag, 1984, p 459.
*A review of the pharmacodynamics, clinical indications, and administration of ophthalmic corticosteroids.*
Rubin S and Papich MG: Clinical uses of nonsteroidal anti-inflammatory drugs in companion animals. Part II: Drugs, therapeutic uses and adverse effects. Canine Pract 15:27, 1990.
*A review of classes, indications, and side effects of systemic NSAIDs.*
Wilkie DA: Disorders of the uvea. *In* Kirk RW and Bonagura JD (eds): *Current Veterinary Therapy XI: Small Animal Practice.* Philadelphia, WB Saunders Co, 1992, p 1112.
*A review of uveal disease in general, emphasizing the treatment of uveitis.*

# OCULAR DRUG REACTIONS AND TOXICITIES

KENNETH L. ABRAMS

*Warwick, Rhode Island*

Some pharmacologic proverb reminds us that there is a fine distinction between the therapeutic and toxic effects of medications. The beneficial effects of the drugs presented in this article can be found in many references. The purpose of this article is to discuss the most common toxicities of medications used to treat eye disease, both topically and systemically administered, as well as drugs used for other purposes that may have deleterious effects on the eye. Many ophthalmic medications are marketed as combination drugs and, therefore, the practitioner must use forensic skills in order to determine the actual cause of an adverse effect (i.e., was the problem caused by one of the active ingredients or by the preservative?).

Drugs that may cause adverse effects on the eye may be classified by their use or therapeutic effects: ocular diagnostic drugs, antimicrobials, anti-inflammatory agents, antiglaucoma drugs, drugs for systemic diseases, and preservatives and surgical preparation agents.

## OCULAR DIAGNOSTIC AGENTS

Drugs used during a complete ophthalmic examination may have toxic effects on the eye. Most of these effects occur on the ocular surface, the cornea and conjunctiva. Often it is difficult to determine which medication caused the problem, since the drugs are used in rapid sequence during the examination and the eye often shows a problem toward the end of the exam.

### Topical Anesthetic Agents

These medications are used prior to performance of tonometry, examination of the third eyelid, removal of surface foreign bodies, corneal and conjunctival scrapings for cytology, and débridement of corneal ulcers. All topical anesthetics are toxic to the corneal epithelium and retard healing by affecting cell mitosis and migration. They should NEVER be prescribed or dispensed for treatment! Abuse of topical anesthetics has been reported to cause blindness by promoting corneal perforation. In one report, a veterinary technician who had been applying topical anesthetics to her own painful eye developed stromal keratitis and subsequent perforation and iris prolapse resulting in blindness (Rosenwasser et al., 1990). Often the subtle effects of topical anesthesia can be seen with slit-lamp biomicroscopy, where irregularities in the corneal surface occur after a single drop of anesthetic. Corneal irregularities also result in a blurred view of the fundus.

Proparacaine (Alcaine, Alcon) is the most commonly used topical anesthetic, but tetracaine (Tetracaine, Pharmafair) is also available. Tetracaine appears to be more painful upon application to the cornea, but both drugs have similar effects on the cornea. Benoxinate is combined with fluorescein solution (Fluress-Sola, Barns Hind) and also produces a stinging sensation, but less than that of tetracaine. All anesthetics may be associated with hypersensitivity reactions causing pain, corneal edema, and epithelial slough.

### Dilating Agents

Three medications are most often used in veterinary ophthalmology to dilate the pupil for examination of the lens, vitreous, and fundus or for therapeutic reasons. All of the dilating agents should be used with caution in eyes with narrow angles and predisposition to glaucoma, since the drugs can cause elevation of intraocular pressure (Regnier and Toutain, 1991). In addition, all dilating agents can cause photophobia, simply due to the large amount of light that is allowed to contact the retina.

Tropicamide (Tropicacyl, Akorn) is most commonly used for diagnostic purposes, since the duration of action is only about 6 hr in dogs and cats. Application of this drug can cause a stinging sensation and the patient might temporarily become startled or rub at the treated eye.

Atropine (Atropisol 1%, Iolab), a long-lasting dilating agent, should not be used for diagnostic examination because the duration of action is at least several days. My suggestion is to never keep atropine in the examination room, to reduce the risk of inadvertent use. Cats are particularly sensitive to the bitter taste of atropine, especially to the solution. The drug travels to the nose and mouth through the nasolacrimal duct, causing severe salivation and head shaking! Therefore, atropine ointment should be used therapeutically. Atropine also decreases tear production and, therefore, should be used with caution in patients with dry eye syndrome, lagophthalmos, or exposure keratitis (Glaze, 1988). Mentation changes occur in people with systemic absorption, and some clients report that their pet's behavior has changed while receiving atropine. Systemic absorption can also result in urinary, gastrointestinal, and cardiac changes.

Phenylephrine (Ak-Dilate, Akorn) is often used as an adjunct to dilation for examination in combination with tropicamide. Corneal edema may occur, which is thought to be secondary to pH changes. A vasoconstrictor, phenylephrine causes the conjunctival vessels to blanch upon application.

## ANTIMICROBIAL DRUGS

Antibiotic, antiviral, and antifungal drugs potentially cause a wide range of toxicities when applied topically to the eye.

### Antibiotics

These drugs are often marketed as combinations of an aminoglycoside, polymyxin, and bacitracin or gramicidin. The aminoglycosides (gentamicin, neomycin, tobramycin) can cause reactions such as toxic conjunctivitis consisting of hyperemia, chemosis, and a superficial keratopathy, which appears as multiple punctate corneal lesions. Higher concentrations of these drugs (8 to 10 mg/ml) have been shown to inhibit corneal re-epithelialization, but the commercially available concentrations (3 mg/ml) are nontoxic (Petroutsos et al., 1983). Bacitracin, gramicidin, and polymyxin usually do not cause irritation.

Chloramphenicol is available as an ophthalmic preparation, but because of the risk of non–dose-dependent fatal aplastic anemia in humans, I usually do not recommend this drug simply for the legal implications. However, if dispensed, it is recommended that owners wear gloves when handling the container. Tetracycline has a similar spectrum of activity against *Chlamydia* and *Mycoplasma* and is recommended for these specific infections.

### Antiviral Drugs

Idoxuridine (Herplex, Allergan), trifluridine (Viroptic, Burroughs Wellcome), and vidarabine (Vira-A, Parke-Davis) are the topical antiviral drugs available for treatment of feline herpetic keratitis. All of these DNA base analogs sting on application, but trifluridine seems to be tolerated best by cats. This drug has been shown to be most effective *in vitro* against feline herpesvirus and, therefore, should be the first choice for treatment after laboratory confirmation of infection (Regnier and Toutain, 1991).

### Antifungal Drugs

Fungal keratitis is rare in small animals. When it occurs, it may be treated with a specific ophthalmic antifungal medication (natamycin [Natacyn, Alcon] or preparations compounded from antifungal drugs intended for systemic use (e.g., 1% ketoconazole [Nizoral, Janssen]; 1% miconazole [Monistat, Ortho]).

Topical administration of the antifungal drugs may cause adverse effects on the cornea, with pain, superficial punctate keratopathy (natamycin), and delayed corneal epithelialization (ketoconazole). Miconazole is often used topically without delayed healing or significant side effects.

## ANTI-INFLAMMATORY AGENTS

Steroidal and nonsteroidal drugs are administered topically and systemically in order to control intraocular inflammation. Traditionally, topical corticosteroids have been used alone or in combination with antibiotics to control inflammation, but topical nonsteroidal medications have been available for the past 6 years.

### Corticosteroids

Both topical and systemic administration of corticosteroids delay corneal wound healing and increase the risk of infection (Schuman, 1994), especially fungal disease, by the following mechanisms:

1. Delayed stromal healing—decreased keratocyte proliferation and collagen deposition. Stromal melting occurs by increased collagenase activity.
2. Decreased epithelial healing rates.
3. Impaired host defenses—decreased monocyte/macrophage ingestive capability. Therefore, corticosteroids should not be used with fluorescein-positive corneal ulcers, infections, or when stromal melting is evident.

Use of corticosteroids in human beings carries the risk of glaucoma and cataracts and these side effects are clearly listed in package inserts. Glaucoma has not been documented in pets with use of steroids, but the author has observed some correlation between cataract formation and regular use of systemic corticosteroids.

Topical administration of corticosteroids has been shown to cause adrenal suppression and hepatopathy in small and large dogs with application frequency similar to clinical usage (Eichenbaum et al., 1988). Some animals have polydipsia, polyuria, and polyphagia during ophthalmic corticosteroid use (also see "Corticosteroid Withdrawal Syndrome," this volume, p 413).

### Nonsteroidal Medications

The well-described gastrointestinal, hemorrhagic, renal, and hepatic effects of systemically administered NSAIDs are mentioned here, but more complete references are found elsewhere.

#### TOPICAL NSAIDs

Available drugs include flurbiprofen (Ocufen, Allergan), suprofen (Profenal, Alcon), diclofenac (Voltaren,

Ciba), and ketorolac (Acular, Allergan), and are used most frequently prior to surgery to prevent intraoperative miosis (profenal, suprofen), but there is some interest in the use of these drugs for treatment of uveitis (diclofenac) and allergic conjunctivitis (ketorolac). All of the topical NSAIDs currently approved for use on the eye may cause stinging upon instillation, and there is some evidence that they may promote intraocular bleeding in patients with underlying bleeding disorders (Schuman, 1994). The effects of these agents on corneal wound healing are controversial.

## GLAUCOMA MEDICATIONS

There are many types of medication used for treatment of glaucoma, and various drugs, strengths, and concentrations of oral, intravenous, and topical formulations can be prescribed. Therefore, the types of reactions are varied.

### Carbonic Anhydrase Inhibitors

These systemically administered drugs decrease intraocular pressure by reducing formation of aqueous humor. Although they do not produce ocular effects, their potential systemic effects are common. Three drugs are available and are commonly prescribed, including dichlorphenamide (Daranide, Merck), methazolamide (Neptazane, Storz), and acetazolamide (Diamox, Storz). Acetazolamide is most commonly prescribed for people with glaucoma and, therefore, is most readily available at pharmacies, but this drug causes frequent side effects in dogs and cats. Dichlorphenamide and methazolamide produce notably fewer side effects in our patients (Regnier and Toutain, 1991); methazolamide is now available as a convenient 25-mg tablet for use in smaller patients. Common side effects of this class of medications include diuresis, anorexia, vomiting, diarrhea, panting, hypokalemia, and lethargy. Less commonly, some dogs develop neurologic signs, including unilateral circling and confusion. Most signs resolve quickly when the dose is lowered or the drug is discontinued, but dogs that develop circling may continue this behavior for several weeks after discontinuing the drug. Cutaneous drug eruptions have been observed rarely. Oral potassium supplementation should be considered for animals receiving carbonic anhydrase inhibitors chronically (see "Glaucoma," this volume, p 1265).

### Miotic Drugs

Drugs that constrict the pupil and improve aqueous outflow act either directly on the receptors or indirectly by blocking acetylcholinesterase. Pilocarpine is a direct-acting miotic that causes local irritation and conjunctival hyperemia. In addition, impairment of vision may occur with any of the miotics due to the small pupil

and change in lenticular accommodation. Pilocarpine gel may cause corneal edema with resultant corneal haze. Systemic effects may occur due to its parasympathomimetic effects, including vomiting, diarrhea, sweating, and bradycardia. Pilocarpine administered topically or orally has also been used as a lacrimogenic agent in pets with keratoconjunctivitis sicca (KCS), but the development of topical cyclosporine has superseded this prior use (see "Keratoconjunctivitis Sicca," this volume, p 1231).

Demecarium bromide (Humorsol, Merck) and echothiophate (Phospholine Iodide, Wyeth-Ayers) are indirect-acting miotics and have similar gastrointestinal and cardiac side effects to pilocarpine. All miotics may exacerbate uveitis by promoting anterior uveal vasodilatation. There is some evidence associating miotics with retinal detachment, cataracts, and iris cyst formation in human beings, but these associations have not been reported in small animals. Animals receiving these drugs should not be treated with other cholinesterase inhibitors (e.g., flea dips).

### β-Blockers

These topical drugs reduce intraocular pressure by reducing aqueous humor formation and are classified as either nonselective ($B_1$ and $B_2$) or selective β-adrenergic receptor blocking agents. Timolol (Timoptic, Merck), the original drug in this class, has been available for 15 years and now several others are available, including betaxolol (Betoptic, Alcon), levobunolol (Betagan, Allergan), and OptiPranolol (metipranolol, Bausch & Lomb). Topical β-blockers have ocular side effects including irritation and dry eye syndrome (possible $B_2$-blockade) and, depending on the type of receptor blockade, can cause cardiac and pulmonary problems in people. We have found a similar number of dogs that develop KCS (10%) after a 5-day treatment period but no decrease in heart rate or blood pressure in these normal dogs (Abrams et al., 1991).

### Osmotic Drugs

Hypertonic drugs such as 20% mannitol (USP) and 50% glycerin (Osmoglyn, Alcon) reduce intraocular pressure by dehydrating the vitreous. They can cause volume overload in patients with cardiac insufficiency. Mannitol, given intravenously, is safe for diabetic animals, whereas glycerin, administered orally, should not be given to diabetics because it is converted to glucose. Failure to use a filter for intravenous mannitol administration may result in widespread vascular embolization.

Although hypertonic saline (Ak-NaCl, Akorn) is available for topical use, its indications are for corneal and conjunctival edema rather than glaucoma. This 5% saline solution or ointment is nontoxic to the corneal epithelium, but may be irritating when applied to the eye.

## SYSTEMIC MEDICATIONS AFFECTING THE EYE

Sulfonamide drugs, including sulfasalazine, sulfadiazine, sulfisoxazole, and trimethoprim, have been shown to cause KCS in dogs (Morgan and Bachrach, 1982). This toxicity appears to be related to the nitrogen-containing rings and is not dose related. The prognosis for restoration of normal tear function is poor.

Dimethyl sulfoxide administration has been associated experimentally with development of severe myopia in dogs, rabbits, and swine due to refractive changes in the lens (Jaanus, 1989).

Chemotherapeutic agents such as cyclophosphamide (Cytoxan, Mead-Johnson), cisplatin (Platinol, Bristol), and mitomycin C (Mutamycin, Bristol) result in blurred vision in humans, but this change would be difficult to detect in small animals. Cardiac drugs such as propranolol and digitalis have resulted in KCS and electroretinographic changes, respectively, in humans (Schuman, 1994). The antiarrhythmic drug, tocainide, has been associated with development of corneal dystrophy in Doberman pinchers.

## PRESERVATIVES AND SURGICAL PREPARATION AGENTS

Preservatives are used in most ophthalmic solutions to prevent microbial growth. Commonly used preservatives include: benzalkonium chloride, thimerosal, chlorobutanol, ethylenediaminetetraacetic acid (EDTA), and boric acid. These agents are toxic to the corneal epithelium, causing loss of superficial cells, inhibition of cell adhesion, and retardation of healing, which may result in potentially severe corneal edema. One must try to differentiate a toxic effect of the preservative from a toxic effect of the active ingredient by selectively eliminating either an active ingredient or by changing the preservative.

Povidone-iodine solution (not soap) (Betadine, Purdue) is commonly used as a presurgical preparation on the eyelids. Dilutions of 1:2 or less cause corneal edema; a dilution of 1:50 is advised to prevent reactions and still destroy bacteria (Roberts, Severin, and Lavach, 1986). Alcohol should never be applied to the eye because it causes epithelial sloughing and corneal edema.

## MISCELLANEOUS COMMENTS

Although ophthalmic ointments once were considered to delay wound healing, contemporary, nonemulsive products do not. They should not be used, however, in the presence of unsealed penetrating corneal wounds or incisions because they may cause uveitis if present in the anterior chamber.

Acetylcysteine (Mucosil, Dey) is often used as an antiprotease in melting ulcers. This drug does not delay corneal re-epithelialization but can be irritating if used at concentrations greater than 5%.

The toxicities and reactions described in this aticle represent common side effects of frequently prescribed medications. The clinician must be attentive to the owner's concerns and the patient's clinical signs in order to detect an adverse drug effect before it causes major problems. A quick review of the package insert or *Physician's Desk Reference* will aid the clinician in the search for ophthalmic drug reactions and toxicities!

## References and Suggested Reading

Abrams KL, Brooks DE, Laratta LJ, et al: Angiotensin converting enzyme system in the normal canine eye: Pharmacological and physiological aspects. J Ocular Pharm 7:41, 1991.
  *Evaluation of ophthalmic and physiologic effects of timolol and an experimental angiotensin-converting enzyme inhibitor.*
Eichenbaum JD, Macy DW, Severin GA, et al: Effect in large dogs of ophthalmic prednisolone acetate on adrenal gland and hepatic function. J Am Anim Hosp Assoc 24:705, 1988.
  *The results of this study indicated that topical prednisolone acetate can suppress normal adrenal gland function and carbohydrate metabolism in large-breed dogs.*
Glaze MB: Contemporary pharmacology in veterinary ophthalmology. Semin Vet Med Surg 3:40, 1988.
  *Review of ophthalmic medications used in veterinary ophthalmology.*
Jaanus SD: Anti-inflammatory drugs. In Bartlett JD and Jaanus SD (eds): *Clinical Ocular Pharmacology*, 2nd edition. Boston, Butterworth's, 1989, p 163.
  *Ocular pharmacology text includes chapter on anti-inflammatory drugs.*
Morgan RV and Bachrach A: Keratoconjunctivitis sicca associated with sulfonamide therapy in dogs. J Am Vet Med Assoc 180:432, 1982.
  *Systemic administration of sulfa-containing drugs decreased tear secretion in 14 dogs.*
Petroutsos G, Guimaraes R, Giraud J, et al: Antibiotics and corneal epithelial wound healing. Arch Ophthalmol 101:1775, 1983.
  *Healing of de-epithelialized cornea was measured by photography after treatment with various antibiotics.*
Regnier A and Toutain PL: Ocular pharmacology and therapeutic modalities. In Gelatt KN (ed): *Veterinary Ophthalmology*, 2nd edition. Philadelphia, Lea & Febiger, 1991, p 162.
  *Contemporary discussion of drug therapy in veterinary ophthalmology.*
Roberts SM, Severin GA, and Lavach JD: Antibacterial activity of dilute povidone-iodine solutions used for ocular surface disinfection in dogs. Am J Vet Res 47:1207, 1986.
  *Prospective study of different concentrations of povidone-iodine to compare efficacy and side effects.*
Rosenwasser GO, Holland S, Pflugfelder SC, et al: Topical anesthesia abuse. Ophthalmology 97:967, 1990.
  *Case reports of people that developed topical anesthesia-induced keratitis.*
Schuman JS: Toxicology. In Albert DM and Jakobiec FA (eds): *Principles and Practice of Ophthalmology. Basic Sciences.* Philadelphia, WB Saunders Co, 1994, p 1119.
  *Discussion of toxicologic aspects of ophthalmic practice.*

# INFECTIOUS FELINE KERATOCONJUNCTIVITIS

DEBORAH S. FRIEDMAN

*Fremont, California*

Infectious keratoconjunctivitis is a common condition in the cat, but determination of a specific etiology can be frustrating. Presenting signs include serous, mucoid, or mucopurulent ocular discharge; chemosis; blepharospasm; and hyperemia. If the cornea is involved, ulceration, edema, neovascularization, or stromal infiltration with inflammatory cells may be evident. The most common causes of feline infectious keratoconjunctivitis (FIK) include feline herpesvirus (FHV), chlamydia, and mycoplasma. Other viruses, bacteria, fungi, and parasites have also been implicated though less commonly. Noninfectious causes of conjunctivitis may mimic FIK, including allergy, eosinophilic conjunctivitis, sensitivity to medications, environmental irritants, neoplasia, and trauma. Chronic conjunctivitis of various causes can be complicated by secondary infection, inappropriate medication, and self-trauma. In the diagnostic process, it is necessary to exclude other ophthalmic problems, such as glaucoma, uveitis, or orbital cellulitis, which cause secondary corneal and conjunctival inflammation (also see *CVT XI*, pp 1070 and 1085).

## VIRUSES

Feline herpesvirus, or feline rhinotracheitis, can cause a wide range of signs. In kittens, the disease manifests as acute, purulent conjunctivitis with severe upper respiratory infection. Corneal ulceration progressing to corneal rupture may also occur. In adult cats, FHV infection usually represents reactivation of latent virus. Conjunctivitis is milder, corneal disease is more common, and respiratory disease is rare.

The virus stimulates a poor immune response and can persist in a latent form with reactivation following stresses such as general anesthesia, lactation, surgery, or corticosteroid therapy. The virus evades the immune system by living within epithelial cells with minimal antibody contact. Therefore, although antibodies may be detected in serum for up to 5 months following infection, their presence does not confer immunity, and the cat may continue to shed virus during that period. Cell-mediated immunity and local production of secretory IgA play a larger role and may help to prevent recurrence of herpesvirus infection.

Feline herpesvirus can cause superficial ulcerative keratitis as well as stromal keratitis accompanied by edema and deep vessels. The typical superficial lesion is initially dendritic, linear, or punctate, the result of direct destruction of epithelial cells by the virus. Deep stromal ulcers and descemetoceles are also seen but are most likely due to secondary bacterial infection of superficial lesions.

Severe keratoconjunctivitis can cause secondary entropion and symblepharon. In the latter condition, the conjunctiva becomes permanently adherent to the cornea and to other conjunctival surfaces. A large proportion of cats with entropion and symblepharon, as well as corneal sequestrum formation, eosinophilic keratitis, and keratoconjunctivitis sicca (KCS), test positive for FHV by the immunofluorescent antibody test (IFA). However, a specific causation has not been established and FHV may be only one of several causes of these conditions. Treatment of eosinophilic keratitis is complicated by the association with herpesvirus, as corticosteroids (important in treatment of eosinophilic keratitis) should usually be avoided in the face of FHV.

Calicivirus and reovirus cause conjunctivitis in cats, but are much less prevalent than FHV. Feline immunodeficiency virus (FIV) also causes conjunctivitis as a component of an upper respiratory infection (Gardner, 1991).

## CHLAMYDIA

*Chlamydia psittaci* is an obligate intracellular bacteria that initially infects and reproduces in the epithelial cells lining mucous membranes. Infection usually begins with marked unilateral chemosis and purulent discharge, becoming bilateral within 10 days. Upper respiratory signs may be present, but the cornea is not involved. Definitive diagnosis is more likely in the acute stages and involves identification of intracytoplasmic inclusions in epithelial cells or a positive conjunctival immunofluorescent antibody test. Follicular lymphoid hyperplasia of the conjunctiva is common in chronic cases. Immunity is temporary and the disease recurs after reexposure to infected cats. Untreated, the signs may persist for several months. Vaccination with modified live *C. psittaci* reduces severity of conjunctivitis but has no effect on shedding of organism. An asymptomatic carrier state is common and makes control difficult (Pointon et al., 1991). Transmission is by direct contact with infected secretions.

*Chlamydia psittaci* is a cause of conjunctivitis and respiratory disease in humans. Although there is no conclusive evidence that feline strains can infect humans, owners should be cautioned to wash their hands after handling an infected cat.

## MYCOPLASMA

Although mycoplasma has been considered to be a major cause of feline infectious conjunctivitis, its role is controversial. It is occasionally found in conjunction with other infectious processes, and may be more important as a secondary pathogen following damage to conjunctival epithelium by herpesvirus, chlamydia, or other organisms. Some studies have found mycoplasma to be present in the normal feline conjunctiva. However, in a recent study, *M. felis* were cultured from 25% of cats affected with conjunctivitis but none were cultured from conjunctivitis-free cats (Gerding, et al., 1993). In another study, no *Mycoplasma* spp. were recovered from culture of 91 cats with chronic conjunctivitis (Nasisse et al., 1993).

Cats that have been inoculated with *M. felis* develop bilateral conjunctival hyperemia, but cats must be young and the inoculum large. Signs of acute disease include epiphora, blepharospasm, severe hyperemia, and papillary hypertrophy (tiny projections of epithelium surrounding a capillary). These signs usually fade after several weeks and the conjunctiva becomes pale and thickened. Pseudomembrane formation has been reported. The cornea is not involved.

## BACTERIA

Primary bacterial conjunctivitis (other than that due to chlamydia) is rare in the cat. Clinical signs include chemosis, hyperemia, and mucopurulent ocular discharge. Bacterial conjunctivitis may occur secondary to orbital abscess, eyelid infection, corneal infection, dacryocystitis, or panophthalmitis. In addition, immunosuppression due to stress, disease, or chronic use of

topical medications may result in bacterial conjunctivitis.

Keratoconjunctivitis sicca may be a predisposing factor. The most likely pathogen is *Staphylococcus* spp., but infections due to *Salmonella* and *Moraxella*, though rare, have also been reported. Diagnosis is made by bacterial culture, cytology, and rapid response to an appropriate antibiotic (see "Antibiotic Therapy of the Eye," this volume, p 1211). Because dacryocystitis may be a contributing factor in recurrent bacterial conjunctivitis, lavage of the nasolacrimal duct can be an important aspect of diagnosis and therapy. Lavage of the duct with isotonic buffered saline through a 30-gauge lacrimal cannula (Sontec Surgical Instruments) may result in drainage of mucopurulent material from the other puncta or nares. This material can be submitted for culture and sensitivity. The lavage will facilitate access of topical medications to the duct. Further diagnostic, medical, and surgical procedures may be necessary to treat dacryocystitis.

## PARASITES

A variety of parasites have been implicated in the etiology of feline conjunctivitis. Some reside directly in the conjunctiva, while others cause pruritus resulting in periorbital self-trauma, inflammation, and secondary bacterial infection. *Thelazia californiensis*, which causes mild conjunctivitis, can be found in the conjunctival fornix. Manual removal of the worms under topical anesthesia (0.5% proparacaine [Ophthetic, Allergan Pharmaceuticals]), followed by application of 0.03% echothiophate (Phospholine Iodide, Ayerst) once daily for several days, should be curative. *Cuterebra* larvae may burrow in the conjunctiva of kittens, causing granulomatous conjunctivitis. Surgical removal should be followed by topical treatment with broad-spectrum antibiotics such as neomycin–bacitracin–polymyxin B (Ak-Spore, Akorn) three to four times daily for 10 days. Other parasites such as fleas, lice, and mites may inhabit the haired skin around the eye or migrate to the conjunctival fornix or nasolacrimal duct. The conjunctivitis that results is due to a combination of a foreign body reaction, allergic reaction, and self-trauma. Usually, these parasites cause generalized dermatitis, but occasionally conjunctivitis will be a primary sign. Careful examination of conjunctival surfaces, flushing the nasolacrimal ducts, and examination of skin and nares with magnification are necessary for diagnosis. Two injections of ivermectin (Ivomec, Merck), 200 $\mu$g/kg SC, 2 to 3 weeks apart are effective for lice and mites. Standard flea-control measures should be implemented when indicated.

## FUNGUS

Fungal conjunctivitis and keratitis, rare in the cat, are unlikely without alteration of the normal conjunctival defense mechanisms by chronic topical medica-

***Table 1.*** *Conjunctival Cytology*

General guidelines
    Erythrocytes may be seen on any conjunctival scrape
    Most cellular composition is highly dependant on the duration
        of infection and the presence of secondary infections
Feline herpesvirus
    Predominantly lymphocytes in acute disease
    Predominantly neutrophils in chronic
    Multinucleated giant cells
Chlamydia
    Large basophilic intracytoplasmic inclusions (seen only in acute
        disease) in epithelial cell or neutrophil
    Neutrophils
    More lymphocytes later in disease
Mycoplasma
    Small basophilic inclusions on cell membrane (rarely observed
        and only in acute disease)
    Many neutrophils
Bacteria and fungi
    Mostly neutrophils
    Few lymphocytes in acute, many in chronic infection
    Many bacteria, fungal elements, or yeast in acute infection, may
        or may not be present in chronic infection

°Adapted from Murphy JM: Exfoliative cytologic examination as an aid in diagnosing ocular diseases in the dog and cat. Semin Vet Med Surg (Small Anim) 3:12, 1988, with permission.

tion, especially with corticosteroids. One case of *Cladosporium* keratitis has been reported following chronic topical corticosteroid usage.

## NEONATAL CONJUNCTIVITIS

Acute conjunctival inflammation, characterized by severe mucopurulent ocular discharge, commonly affects neonatal kittens ("neonatal ophthalmia"). The etiologic agent may be herpes, chlamydia, mycoplasma, or other bacteria and is acquired either during birth (from genital infections of the queen) or soon after, by exposure to carrier animals in the household. The discharge distends the eyelids if it develops prior to eyelid opening at 10 to 14 days. If the eyelids are closed, they should be opened manually starting at the medial canthus with small blunt scissors inserted under the eyelid margins. The discharge should be flushed out and the cornea stained with fluorescein dye to check for ulcers. An antibiotic ointment such as oxytetracycline–polymyxin B (Terramycin, Pfizer) should be applied every 6 hr for 2 to 3 weeks. Response to treatment is good if the conjunctivitis is caused by bacteria and poor if virus is involved. Corneal involvement would suggest viral involvement and appropriate diagnostic tests to be discussed later should be instituted. Treatment with an antiviral medication such as 3% vidarabine ointment (Vira-A, Parke-Davis) five to six times daily may be indicated. If not treated, symblepharon, corneal opacification, scarring, and blindness may result.

## DIAGNOSIS

Etiologic diagnosis of feline conjunctivitis is facilitated by assessment of clinical signs combined with results of specific laboratory tests. Differentiation between acute chlamydial and FHV infections can be difficult based on clinical signs alone. In general, however, the following trends are helpful: FHV is more likely to cause respiratory disease than chlamydial infection, chlamydial infection is usually unilateral and FHV bilateral, chemosis is more marked in chlamydial infection, hyperemia is more pronounced in FHV infection, and corneal disease is not caused by chlamydia but by FHV. Determination of the cause of conjunctivitis is easier in the acute stage, when inclusions may be present and disease is uncomplicated by medication and secondary infection. A recent study (Nasisse et al., 1993) reported that the most commonly used diagnostic tests for feline conjunctivitis would not confirm etiology in most cats with chronic conjunctivitis. These tests included cytology and immunofluorescent assay of conjunctival scrapings; culturing for aerobic bacteria, mycoplasma, and virus; and serologic evaluation for FHV-neutralizing antibody. The study also identified cats with chronic conjunctivitis as being more likely to be positive for feline leukemia virus (FeLV) and FIV than the general feline hospital population. Results of cytologic examination of conjunctival scrapes did not correlate well with other diagnostic tests. Although impractical in most cases, virus isolation is the most sensitive diagnostic test for feline herpesvirus. Immunofluorescent antibody tests are readily available in clinical practice for detection of herpesvirus and chlamydia on conjunctival scrapings. However, false-negatives are common. Serologic evaluation may have limited value in identification of FHV carrier cats that have not been vaccinated.

A thorough history and physical examination should precede ocular evaluation. An inflamed conjunctiva is a nonspecific sign of many ocular disorders, not just conjunctivitis. Therefore, an essential preliminary step to investigation into specific etiology of conjunctivitis is to be sure that the conjunctiva is inflamed due to conjunctivitis and not secondarily from intraocular inflammation or glaucoma. Examination of the eye should be conducted with a bright light, such as a Finnoff ocular transilluminator (Welch Allyn) and magnifying head loupes (Optivisor, Donegan Optical). Evaluate pupil size. With uncomplicated conjunctivitis without corneal involvement, the pupils should be of equal size. If one pupil is smaller, it may be due to a problem such as uveitis, Horner's syndrome, or corneal ulceration on that side. A large pupil could indicate either glaucoma or a problem with the retina or optic nerve. The intraocular pressure, taken with either an indentation type (Schiøtz) tonometer (Optequip) or applanation tonometer (Tonopen, Oculab), will be useful. A high intraocular pressure indicates glaucoma, and a low pressure indicates anterior uveitis. The intraocular pressure should be done after application of topical anesthetic, in the sequence of tests described below. Dilation of the pupils with 1% tropicamide (Mydriacyl, Alcon Laboratories) is useful for examination of the posterior aspects of the eye. If problems are found in areas of the eye other than the conjunctiva and cornea, serious consideration must be given to an intraocular condition.

A sample for bacterial culture and sensitivity should be obtained if conjunctivitis is recurrent or nonresponsive to medications. It must be obtained prior to applications of topical anesthetic or medication. Minitip culturettes (Becton Dickinson Microbiology Systems) are well tolerated without topical anesthesia. The tip should be rolled in the conjunctival fornix without contact with skin or hair. However, bacteria identified by culture are not likely to be the primary cause of feline conjunctivitis. *Mycoplasma* and *Chlamydia* will not grow with routine culturing techniques, but may be isolated by diagnostic laboratories if special transport and culture media are used.

A Schirmer tear test (STT) should be performed after culture but before topical anesthesia. The strips should remain in the upper or lower conjunctival fornix for 1 min. Normal STT values for cats range from 11 to 23 mm/min. However, unlike dogs, many apparently normal cats have tear production less than 10 mm/min. Herpesvirus is the most common cause of dry eye in cats.

After the STT, the eye should be irrigated with eyewash to remove all discharge. Then, following application of a topical anesthetic, forceps and cotton swabs are used to retract the third eyelid and inspect the conjunctival surfaces for lymphoid follicles, parasites, and foreign bodies. The nares should be examined for discharge, foreign material, and parasites.

Obtain samples for IFA tests and cytology by scraping the inferior conjunctiva with a platinum spatula (Kimura spatula, Storz Instrument Company) or the blunt end of a scalpel blade. Scrape firmly and place the cells obtained onto a glass slide. It is important to obtain a sufficient quantity of epithelial cells rather than just mucopurulent debris. Save several slides for cytologic examination with a modified Wright-Giemsa stain (Diff-Quik, Harleco) and Gram's stain (Harleco) and several to be sent for IFA tests for herpes and chlamydia. False-positive tests are rare, but can be associated with recent use of topical fluorescein dye. Wait at least 24 hr (and preferably several days) after application of fluorescein dye before obtaining samples for IFA tests or collect samples before fluorescein stain application. If corneal lesions are present, it is useful to scrape the edge of the lesion gently with a Kimura spatula to obtain a sample. However, if a deep stromal or melting ulcer is present, use extreme care to avoid further corneal damage.

A conjunctival biopsy is useful to rule out squamous cell carcinoma, which can mimic chronic conjunctivitis. A biopsy should be obtained in cases of chronic conjunctivitis poorly responsive to medical therapy. Instill topical anesthetic, pull up a small amount of conjunctiva from the affected area with forceps, and snip with small, sharp scissors.

After the conjunctival scraping is obtained, fluorescein and/or rose bengal stain can be applied to the eye. Visualization of corneal ulcers, which are often very small, is greatly aided by use of a cobalt filter (Welch Allyn) to detect fluorescein dye uptake. Fluorescein dye is retained by defects in the corneal epithelium. Rose bengal stains intact but devitalized epithelium, and may be useful in the diagnosis of herpetic keratitis before corneal ulceration is evident. Examine the nares for fluorescein passage through the nasolacrimal duct.

If general anesthesia is required for these procedures, note that anesthetic agents can decrease tear production and alter intraocular pressure.

## TREATMENT

The treatment of feline conjunctivitis involves cleaning discharge, prevention of self-trauma, and treatment of specific infectious agents where possible. Topical medications should be used sparingly to avoid exacerbation of signs from sensitivity to medications.

Because mucopurulent conjunctival discharge is impervious to medications and could render them ineffective, treatment should be preceded by cleaning with eyewash (Ak-Rinse, Akorn). Warm compresses are helpful to soften dried discharge.

Self-trauma can exacerbate any conjunctival inflammation and cause secondary infections by transfer of skin and ear pathogens to the eye and by creation of corneal ulceration. To prevent this, use of an Elizabethan collar is recommended.

Topical medications can be irritating and even toxic to the conjunctival epithelium. Chronic use can also predispose the conjunctiva to secondary infection. The bacterial flora that normally resides in the conjunctiva is thought to exert a protective effect and prevent the growth of pathogens. Topical antibiotic therapy can predispose to bacterial and fungal overgrowth by ridding the conjunctiva of its normal inhabitants and promoting growth of resistant organisms.

Treatment of feline conjunctivitis must often be initiated without knowledge of the specific etiologic agent. The initial treatment of choice for conjunctivitis without corneal involvement is tetracycline–polymyxin B or chloramphenicol (Ak-Chlor, Akorn) ointment. These are effective against both chlamydia and mycoplasma and should be used every 6 hr for 4 weeks to ensure elimination of all stages of the organism. Both eyes should be treated even if conjunctivitis is unilateral. If recurrence occurs, consider treatment of other cats in the household, as they may be asymptomatic carriers. In some cases, systemic therapy with tetracycline (Panmycin, Upjohn), 5 to 15 mg/kg every 8 hr, is helpful.

Because the antiviral medications are frequently irritating, treatment of FHV is recommended only if there is corneal involvement or if herpesvirus has been confirmed as the cause of conjunctivitis. Three are currently available: idoxuridine solution (Herplex, Allergan Pharmaceuticals), adenine arabinoside ointment (Vira-A, Parke-Davis), and trifluorothymidine solution (Viroptic, Burroughs Wellcome). Trifluridine is the drug of choice due to its ability to penetrate the cornea and efficacy against FHV. It should be used hourly for the first 24 hr, then every 4 hr thereafter. Many cats become irritated by this medication. Vidarabine ointment, which is usually less irritating, should be substituted every 4 hr if irritation is significant. Idoxuridine solution should be applied every 2 hr. Topical antiviral therapy should be continued until corneal ulcerations are healed. Acyclovir (Zovirax, Burroughs Wellcome), while effective against human herpes simplex virus, is much less effective than trifluridine for FHV, according to *in vitro* studies. Its effectiveness is increased when used in combination with interferon (Nasisse, 1990).

Use of topical corticosteroids is contraindicated in feline conjunctivitis, unless specific infectious agents have been ruled out. This is especially true for FHV infections. Not only do corticosteroids delay healing of epithelial wounds, but they suppress immune function, may cause prolonged virus shedding, and may worsen clinical signs. They may also promote progression of superficial infections to deep stromal ones. Infections that have been treated with topical steroids often will become much more difficult to treat later on.

Cyclosporin A (Sandimmune, Sandoz Pharmaceuticals) has been used topically to treat KCS and pannus in dogs. Unfortunately, although it might be helpful in the restoration of tear function reduced by FHV, cyclosporine should be avoided in cats with viral conjunctivitis because its immunosuppressive characteristics have the potential to exacerbate infection (see "Keratoconjunctivitis Sicca," this volume, p 1231).

Infection with many of the agents that cause feline keratoconjunctivitis can result in an asymptomatic carrier state that facilitates dissemination within a cattery. Optimal control is achieved by reduction of contact among cats, solid partitions between cats, increasing ventilation, decreasing humidity, and use of cage fronts that are at least 4 feet apart. All affected animals should be isolated. Hands and instruments should be washed and disinfected between animals. The best disinfectants are bleach at a 1:32 dilution and povidone-iodine (Betadine Solution, Purdue Frederick).

## References and Suggested Reading

Arnett BD and Greene CE: Feline respiratory disease. *In* Greene CE (ed): *Clinical Microbiology and Infectious Diseases of the Dog and Cat.* Philadelphia, WB Saunders Co, 1984, p 527.
*A summary of the respiratory diseases that affect cats, including a section on control of infection within catteries.*

Gardner SA: Current concepts of feline immunodeficiency virus infection. Vet Med, 300, 1991.
*A review of the characteristics, diagnosis, and prevention of FIV infection.*

Gerding PA, Jr, Cormany K, Weisiger R, and Kakoma I: Survey and topographic distribution of bacterial and fungal microorganisms in eyes of clinically normal cats. Feline Pract 21:20, 1993.
*A study of the microbial inhabitants of the normal feline conjunctiva.*

Haesebrouck F, Devriese LA, van Rijssen B, and Cox E: Incidence and significance of isolation of *Mycoplasma felis* from conjunctival swabs of cats. Vet Microbiol 26:95, 1991.
*A study attempting to determine the role of mycoplasma as a pathogen.*

Murphy JM: Exfoliative cytologic examination as an aid in diagnosing ocular diseases in the dog and cat. Semin Vet Med Surg (Small Anim) 3:10, 1988.
*An illustrated guide to conjunctival cytology.*

Nasisse MP: Feline herpesvirus ocular disease. Vet Clin North Am 29:667, 1990.
*A review of the current wisdom concerning feline herpesvirus.*

Nasisse MP, Guy JS, Stevens JB, et al: Clinical and labaoratory findings in chronic conjunctivitis in cats: 91 cases (1983–1991). J Am Vet Med Assoc 203:834, 1993.
*A study of the usefulness of diagnostic testing in feline conjunctivitis.*

Nasisse MP: Feline ophthalmology. *In* Gelatt KN (ed): *Veterinary Ophthalmology.* Philadelphia, Lea & Febiger, 1991, p 534.
*A review of the ophthalmic diseases in cats.*

Pointon AM, Nicholls JM, Neville S, et al: Chlamydia infection among breeding catteries in South Australia. Aust Vet Pract. 21: 58, 1991.
*A study of diagnosis and treatment of chlamydia in catteries.*

Szymanski C: The eye. *In* Holzworth J (ed): *Diseases of the Cat, Medicine and Surgery,* volume 1. Philadelphia, WB Saunders Co, 1987, p 692.
*A review of ophthalmic diseases and ophthalmic surgery in cats.*

# KERATOCONJUNCTIVITIS SICCA

M-A SALISBURY

*Sarasota, Florida*

Keratoconjunctivitis sicca (KCS), xerophthalmia, or dry eye are synonyms for an ocular disease due to a quantitative deficiency of the precorneal tear film. KCS is a potentially vision-threatening disease that is often misdiagnosed as bacterial or allergic conjunctivitis or overlooked as the cause of corneal ulceration. When these conditions are recognized, KCS should always be considered as a possible initiating and perpetuating ocular problem. Addressing the primary problem, by proper diagnosis and appropriate therapy, is important for optimal long-term ocular care and comfort. Early diagnosis and therapy to replace deficient tear components prevents further corneal injury and may result in regression of existing related pathology. Keratoconjunctivitis sicca may be acute or chronic, transient or permanent, unilateral or bilateral. Most often, KCS is a progressive inflammatory and degenerative ocular disease requiring lifelong therapy. The recent introduction of topical dilute cyclosporine as a tear stimulant for canine KCS has dramatically improved the success of long-term management and has decreased the need for surgery.

Tears are taken for granted until the destructive effects on ocular tissues lacking sufficient precorneal tear film are recognized. Continuous production and distribution of tears are essential for the corneal health and transparency. Tears have cleansing, lubricating, nutritional, bacteriostatic, immunologic, and healing functions.

The tear film is a trilaminar wetting complex composed of lipid, aqueous, and mucous layers. The thin outermost lipid portion is secreted by the meibomian (tarsal) glands of the eyelid margins. Lipids retard evaporation and aid in tear film stabilization and distribution across the ocular surface. Qualitative changes in the lipid content of tears may result from inflammation of the meibomian glands. The middle aqueous layer constitutes the bulk of the tear film. This aqueous portion is secreted by the lacrimal glands. A deficiency or obstruction of aqueous component secretion accounts for the typical type of KCS seen in small animals. The aqueous layer is a vehicle for immunoglobulins, enzymes, glucose, urea, proteins, ions, and inorganic salts. In canine KCS tears appear to have equal or higher protein concentrations than normal tears due to evaporation and lack of aqueous secretion. When tear secretion rate and concentration are considered, the absolute protein amount in KCS tears is greatly reduced (Kaswan, Zhou, and Fullard, 1993). Studies need to be age matched because the proteins in dog tears become more concentrated with increasing age. The mucus or innermost layer of the precorneal tear film is secreted primarily by conjunctival goblet cells. Mucin adheres to the hydrophobic corneal surface and modifies the surface to a more hydrophilic environment to which the overlying tear layer adheres. Mucin tear deficiencies, described in dogs and humans, are characterized by rapid tear breakup time, a normal Schirmer tear test (STT), and a diagnostic conjunctival biopsy (Moore, 1990). Canine mucin deficiency may be difficult to diagnose, but important clues include abnormal tear distribution, reduced corneal wetability, and dryness of the ocular surface. Tears normally leave the conjunctival sac by evaporation and through the nasolacrimal excretory duct system.

Dogs and cats have two lacrimal glands per eye: one in the orbit (like humans) located in a periorbital fold beneath the orbital ligament; and one superficial lacrimal gland at the base of the T-shaped cartilage within the third eyelid or nictitans. Secretory ductules of the nictitans lacrimal gland are located on the bulbar side of the third eyelid (Moore, Frappier, and Linton, 1992); their preservation may be important during surgical replacement of prolapsed nictitans glands.

In the dog, orbital lacrimal glands contribute approximately 70% of the tear volume measured by the STT, and the nictitans lacrimal gland contributes 30% (Gelatt, 1991). Excision or destruction of either lacrimal gland may result in lower measurable aqueous tear production, although if normal functional glandular tissue is present, the remaining glands may hypertrophy to compensate for the loss. Loss of both glands produces KCS.

With chronic KCS, lacrimal gland degeneration is obvious histologically. Findings include variable degrees of multifocal chronic adenitis characterized by fibrosis, atrophy, hypertrophy, acini and ductule dilation, loss of secretory granules, and inflammatory cell infiltrates (Kaswan, Martin, and Chapman, 1984). Plasma cells, lymphocytes, and neutrophils are associated with the lacrimal adenitis in KCS. The relative ratio of lymphocyte subtypes present in KCS lacrimal tissue is under study. Atrophied lacrimal glands are unable to secrete tears, resulting in severe xerosis; affected glands remain unresponsive to tear stimulant therapy.

## CAUSES

Identification of a specific cause for KCS in clinical cases is not always possible, but a careful history and physical examination may be helpful. Causes of KCS include viral infections, congenital anomalies, breed predisposition, neurologic and inflammatory lesions, drug-related toxicity, immune-mediated disease, iatrogenic (surgical or drug-related), and radiation; however, most cases are idiopathic (Table 1).

Distemper virus in the dog and herpesvirus in the cat may cause transient acute KCS. Conjunctivitis or acute lacrimal gland adenitis may be associated with

**Table 1.**　*Causes of Keratoconjunctivitis (KCS)*

Breed predisposition
Congenital anomaly
Drug-induced toxicity
Iatrogenic
　Surgical or drug related
Idiopathic
Immune-mediated
Infectious agents
　Canine distemper virus
　Feline herpesvirus
Neurogenic
Radiation therapy for nasal or intracranial neoplasms
Trauma to orbit or eye

these epitheliotropic viruses. Keratoconjunctivitis sicca due to distemper virus may be concurrent with other systemic signs of distemper or may occur weeks after cessation of symptoms (Gelatt, 1991). Congenital anomalies leading to KCS are rare. Congenital KCS is usually unilateral and found in toy breeds, especially the Chinese pug and Yorkshire terrier. Lacrimal gland hypoplasia or aplasia may be the cause.

Cholinergic innervation of the lacrimal gland is required for aqueous production, while mucus-secreting cells are autonomous. A unilateral facial (cranial nerve VII) or trigeminal (cranial nerve V) nerve lesion near their respective proximities with the parasympathetic lacrimal nerve may result in KCS on the ipsilateral side. Trauma, ear infections, and brain stem damage may result in neurogenic KCS. With damage to either cranial nerve V or VII, tear production should be evaluated.

Several drugs have been identified as potential causes of acute KCS in the dog. Systemic treatment with sulfonamides—sulfasalazine (Azulfidine, Pharmacia), sulfadiazines (Tribrissen, Cooper's Animal Health), and sulfisoxazole (Azo Gantrisin, Roche), as well as 5-aminosalicylic acid and phenazopyridine (Azo Gantrisin, Roche)—may cause transient or permanent KCS. A history of urinary tract infections or colitis should elicit questions on drug treatment. Recommended drug dosages or overdosages may result in drug-related KCS. The incidence of iatrogenic KCS secondary to trimethoprim-sulfadiazine (Tribrissen, Pitman-Moore) therapy in dogs was 15.2% in a recent study, developing within 7 days to 7 months after initiation of the drug (Berger and Scagliotti, 1992). Clinicians are advised to use these drugs judiciously, perform STTs before and during treatment, and advise clients of potential risks and signs of KCS. Alternative drugs should be chosen when KCS is already present. Cessation of lacrimotoxic therapy and commencement of medical tear supplementation or stimulation therapy should be prescribed when developing KCS is identified. Reevaluation of tear production over time should indicate if KCS was transient and if therapy is no longer needed. The period of temporary tear deficiency after withdrawal of the drug may vary from less than a week to over a month.

Systemic or topical atropine treatment and anesthetic protocols may result in transient KCS. Atropine-induced ocular dryness may last 5 weeks (Hollingsworth et al., 1992). The dryness may affect an atropine-treated eye and/or the contralateral untreated eye. Use of atropine is not advised for dogs and cats with ulcers secondary to KCS, since it may further exacerbate the primary cause of the ulceration and slow healing.

Immune-mediated lacrimal gland destruction, KCS with other concurrent immunologic disorders, and KCS with circulating antilacrimal gland antibodies and hypergammaglobulinemia have been reported in dogs (Kaswan and Salisbury, 1990). Immune-mediated KCS in dogs has been associated with concurrent atopy, endocrinopathies (hypothyroidism, hypo- or hyperadrenocorticism, diabetes mellitus), rheumatoid arthritis, chronic active hepatitis, autoimmune hemolytic anemia, systemic lupus erythematosus, and pemphigoid disorders. Sjögren's syndrome is a human autoimmune disease that includes KCS, xerostomia, and various connective tissue disorders.

Irradiation of the head for malignant nasal cavity or intracranial neoplasms resulted in KCS in 35.1% of the dogs, acutely or months later (Jamieson et al., 1991). Radiation-associated KCS ultimately may be unresponsive to tear stimulants, since the lacrimal secretory tissues have been destroyed.

The relationship between excision of the nictitans lacrimal gland (rather than replacement or leaving the gland prolapsed) and KCS is still being clarified. Short-term studies in normal dogs and cats have failed to demonstrate development of KCS after excision of the nictitans lacrimal gland. However, in both breeds predisposed to KCS and in less susceptible breeds, a dry eye may develop then or years later when remaining lacrimal tissue can no longer compensate for the loss.

Breeds commonly associated with nictitans gland prolapse are also predisposed to KCS. Keratoconjunctivitis sicca developed in 37.5% of canine eyes with a prior prolapsed gland in contrast to only 5.56% of eyes without a history of cherry eye; the onset of KCS usually was delayed 0.5 to 6 years after diagnosis of the prolapsed gland of the third eyelid (Morgan, Duddy, and McClurg, 1993). Partial or complete excision of lacrimal tissue also greatly limits the ability to treat subsequent KCS with a tear gland stimulant such as cyclosporine or pilocarpine. Excision of the third eyelid or its glandular tissue should be limited to rare cases of carcinoma. Restrained excision should lower the number of iatrogenically accelerated cases of KCS. Surgical replacement of prolapsed nictitans lacrimal glands may also lower the incidence of KCS; KCS reportedly developed in 48.1% of eyes treated with gland excision and in 42.8% of eyes where the gland remained prolapsed, compared to only 14.2% of eyes treated with surgical replacement (Morgan, Duddy, and McClurg, 1993). Figures 1 and 2 illustrate a surgical technique described by Morgan et al. (1993) to easily correct cherry eye without sacrificing lacrimal gland tissue. This surgery has a higher success rate of 94.1% compared to techniques tacking the gland to the periosteum of the orbital rim (Kaswan and Martin, 1983) or sclera. Unlike other approaches, Morgan's protocol has no permanent buried sutures and has less risk of perforating the eye, since it requires no scleral sutures.

## INCIDENCE

The incidence of KCS in the general dog and cat population is unknown. KCS is more commonly diagnosed in the dog than in the cat. Both purebred and mixed heritage dogs and cats can have KCS. However,

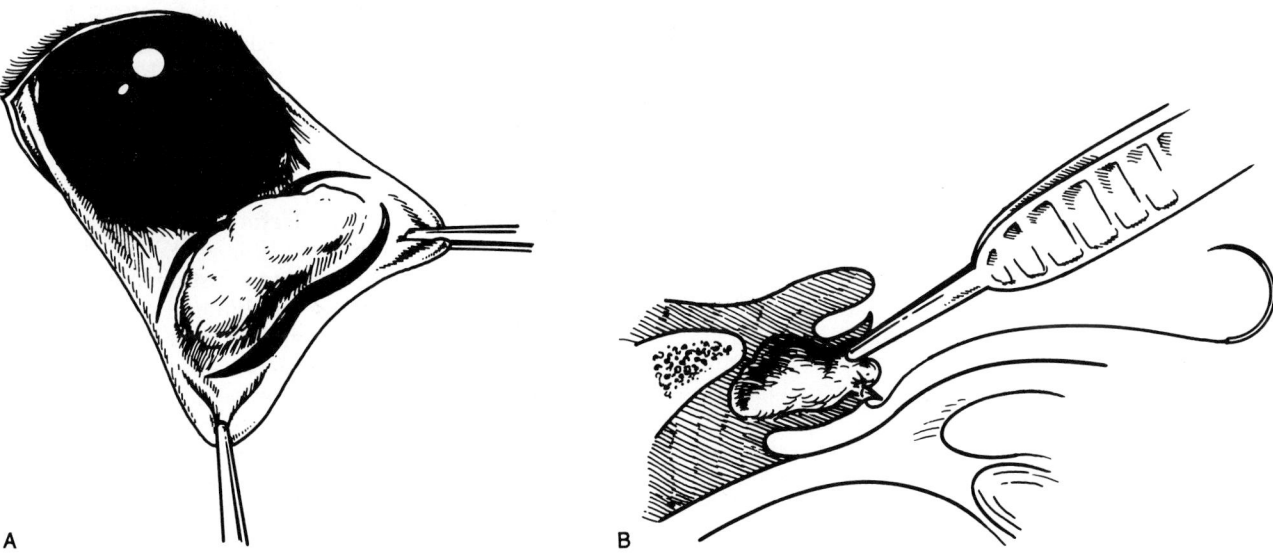

**Figure 1.** Two parallel incisions are made through the conjunctiva of the posterior surface of the third eyelid to either side of the gland. *A*, Anterior view. *B*, Side view. (From Morgan RV, Duddy JM, and McClurg K: Prolapse of the gland of the third eyelid in dogs: A retrospective study of 89 cases (1980–1990). J Am Anim Hosp Assoc 29:56, 1993, with permission.)

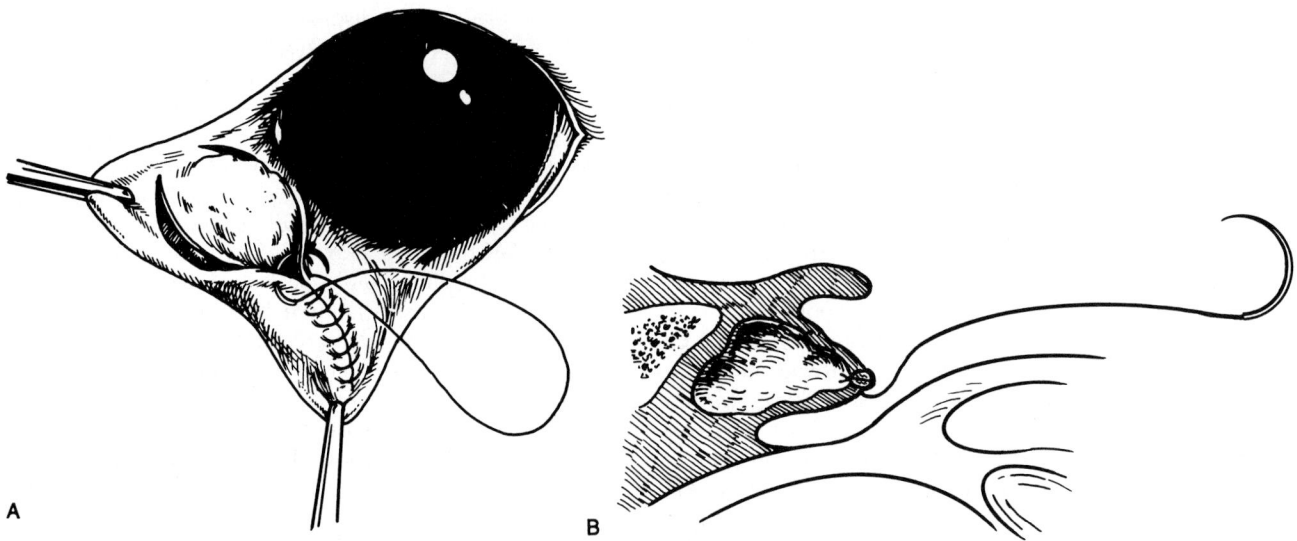

**Figure 2.** The prolapsed gland returned to a more normal position by suturing the two incisions together with absorbable suture. *A*, Anterior view. *B*, Side view. (From Morgan RV, Duddy JM, and McClurg K: Prolapse of the gland of the third eyelid in dogs: A retrospective study of 89 cases (1980–1990). J Am Anim Hosp Assoc 29:56, 1993, with permission.)

***Table 2.*** *Breed Predisposition to Keratoconjunctivitis Sicca (KCS)**

| Breed | Relative Risk of KCS[†] |
|---|---|
| **Canine** | |
| Lhasa apso | 18.7 |
| Chinese pug | 12.3 |
| English bulldog | 10.8 |
| West Highland white terrier | 7.1 |
| Pekingese | 6.0 |
| Shih Tzu | 5.7 |
| Bloodhound | 5.0 |
| English cocker spaniel | 4.9 |
| American cocker spaniel | 4.4 |
| Miniature poodle | 2.1 |
| Miniature schnauzer | 2.0 |
| All canine breeds | 1.6 |
| Boston terrier | 1.6 |
| Shar pei | 1.5 |
| Yorkshire terrier | 1.2 |
| Basset hound | 1.0 |
| Chow chow | 1.0 |
| Doberman pinscher | 0.6 |
| Boxer | 0.4 |
| Old English sheepdog | 0.4 |
| Labrador retriever | 0.3 |
| Golden retriever | 0.3 |
| German shepherd | 0.1 |
| **Feline** | |
| Burmese | 1.9 |
| Himalayan | 0.8 |
| Persian | 0.6 |
| Domestic shorthair | 0.1 |
| All feline breeds | 0.1 |

*Data from the American Veterinary Data Program, Inc. 1983–October 1993.
†The estimate relative risk is the ratio of KCS-affected animals to the general hospital population for the specified breed.

certain breeds of dogs and cats appear to be more predisposed to KCS, suggesting a possible genetic predisposition. Table 2 lists dog and cat breeds in order of their observed relative risk of KCS. The West Highland white terrier female is reported more likely to develop KCS than the male (Gelatt, 1991). A recent survey on canine KCS examined male versus female, spayed versus neutered, and age interactions, and found that neutered animals of either gender are predisposed to KCS as their age increases (Kaswan, Salisbury, and Lothrop, 1991). Loss of either male or female sex hormones appears to predispose aged dogs to develop KCS. Previous reports of female predisposition for KCS in aged dogs may represent an iatrogenic artifact because most older females are neutered compared to a minority of older male dogs. A new theory proposes that testosterone and female ovarian hormones (possibly female androgens) may inhibit pituitary secretion of endogenous tear suppressors such as prolactin or enkephalin (Kaswan, Salisbury, and Lothrop, 1991). Prolactin inhibits lacrimal secretion and is an immunostimulant promoting lymphocyte proliferation and immunoreactivity. Cyclosporine, a canine tear stimulant, is also a prolactin receptor antagonist. Prolactin receptors have been identified on lacrimal tissue from some species. This is a current area of ongoing KCS research.

Animals of any age may be diagnosed with KCS, but the incidence of KCS increases with age in all sex groups. KCS in cats and dogs is most common between 4 and 10 years of age, especially 7 years and older. Young KCS patients may have a congenital form due to maldevelopment of lacrimal tissue in one eye.

## CLINICAL SIGNS

Signs of KCS are variable depending on severity and duration of the tear deficiency and accompanying eyelid conformation. Clinical onset may be acute or chronic, unilateral or bilateral; and when bilateral, asymmetry may be evident. When first diagnosed, the condition often appears unilateral and months later develops into a bilateral problem. Dogs with KCS present primarily for marked recurrent conjunctivitis, recurrent corneal ulcers, keratitis, and often blindness. A thick tenacious mucoid or mucopurulent ocular discharge coating the cornea, tucked into the conjunctival fornices, and on periocular tissues is the most common presenting sign of canine KCS. A mucoid discharge accumulating at the medial canthus with increasing regularity or blepharospasm should suggest KCS as a possible cause. A green or yellow coloration of the ocular discharge indicates suppurative inflammation due to abnormal bacterial composition or overgrowth; a clear or off-white hue suggests a more normal ocular flora. In feline KCS, excessive mucoid ocular discharge is less prevalent.

Cornea and conjunctiva deprived of sufficient tears appear dull, dry, and irregular. Inflamed conjunctiva may be hyperemic, chemotic, or have keratinized plaques. Corneal edema, ulceration, and/or superficial vascularization may be present. Ulceration may be recurrent, superficial, deep, or absent. Corneal ulceration with KCS is more common in early or acute cases and is at risk to deepen and perforate quickly with desiccation and inadequate tear distribution. Melting ulcers may be accelerated by *Pseudomonas,* a pathogenic bacteria that releases proteolytic enzymes or by endogenous proteases from neutrophils attracted to the area. Perforation of the cornea due to ulceration seriously jeopardizes vision, necessitating surgery and therapy for KCS.

With chronic KCS, the normal transparent cornea transforms into an opaque, thickened, scarred, fibrotic, vascularized surface. These conditions change the corneal refractive index and can result in blindness. Breeds with periocular pigmentation and exophthalmic globes are prone to pigmentary keratitis. The irritation of a dry eye exacerbates corneal melanosis that often results in permanent vision loss. Corneal sensation may be diminished or lost with chronic KCS. Some dogs develop crusting and dryness of the external nares, often with mucopurulent nasal discharge.

Signs of discomfort observed in acute or chronic tear-deficient states include blepharospasm, third eyelid elevation, photophobia, and rubbing of periocular tissues. People with KCS liken the irritative sensation to sand paper under their eyelids felt with every blink.

## DIAGNOSIS OF TEAR DEFICIENCY

An STT (CooperVision or IOLAB Pharmaceuticals) should be performed routinely before instillation of any eyedrops or ointments in all patients with ocular discharge, irritation, or corneal lesions. KCS is diagnosed when consistent clinical signs and a low STT value are documented. Normal STT values in small animals are 15 to 25 mm/min in the dog, and 11 to 23 mm/min in the cat. Eyelid conformation and function may modify the range of STT values needed to remain asymptomatic. Dogs with loose fitting eyelids, macropalpebral fissures, exophthalmos, or lagophthalmos normally require a greater tear flow. Exposed corneas facilitate tear evaporation and often suffer from inadequate tear distribution. Such anatomic features should be taken into account when evaluating the STT results. Affected individuals may show signs of early KCS with equivocal or marginal tear deficiencies.

Prior to instillation of diagnostic eyedrops or eyewash, the STT is performed by placing a standardized test strip with the short rounded end, creased at the notch, and bent over the inferior eyelid margin into the conjunctival sac. The strip is left in place for 1 min to imbibe tear secretions; the STT is performed for 5 min in humans. Immediately, the moistened area of the strip is measured by placing it against the millimeter ruler on the STT package. Results are reported as millimeters per minute. Dogs with KCS consistently have STT values less than 15 mm/min and severely affected patients have STT values less than 5 mm/min on repeated trials.

Corneal fluorescein dye staining should be performed to diagnose corneal ulceration. A cobalt-blue filtered light aids in illuminating the fluorescein. Deep ulcerations or descemetoceles have a fluorescein ring with a dark, often protruding center. A subtle dappled appearance with fluorescein dye testing often is observed in chronic KCS. Mucus debris may stain with fluorescein.

Rose bengal dye stains devitalized conjunctival or corneal epithelial cells and mucus strands. This test is not specific for KCS; recurrent corneal erosions and lesions due to exposure keratitis may also retain stain. Even healthy cells may stain under certain circumstances and light may enhance rose bengal's cytotoxic effects. Routine use of rose bengal stain is NOT recommended.

## THERAPEUTIC OPTIONS

Goals of KCS treatment include restoring moisture to desiccated ocular tissues and treatment of secondary conditions such as bacterial conjunctivitis, corneal ulcers, and keratitis. Medical and surgical approaches to the problem can be cited. Medical therapy should be exhausted prior to surgical considerations. Sufficient time is required to evaluate medical treatment efficacy, its practicality, and the permanent versus transient nature of KCS.

Tear stimulants and artificial tear replacements are the mainstay of KCS treatment. Natural tears with their cleansing, lubricating, nutritional, bacteriostatic, immunologic, and healing properties remain superior to man-made products. Tear stimulants, when effective, are preferable to artificial tear replacement for long-term dry eye treatment. Often tear replacement schedules are arduous and owners are unable to treat frequently enough on a long-term basis to alleviate clinical signs. In severe cases, tear stimulants alone may not be able to increase tear production sufficiently. A combination of tear-stimulant and tear-replacement products may be most efficacious in severe cases to curb KCS-induced pathologic changes and keep the patient comfortable.

A plethora of tear-replacement solutions and ointments to add moisture to a dry ocular surface are commercially available (Table 3). Because solutions drain quickly from the eye, they have only a transient (1/2 to 2 hr) effect and require frequent applications for continued comfort. Ointments remain on the eye longer, permitting fewer applications for a similar effect. Preservatives in solution and ointment preparations can be irritating and disruptive to the outer oil layer. Preservative-free medications are available for the most sensitive patients. Hypotears

**Table 3.** *Artificial Tear Solutions and Ointments*°

| Product Name | Source | Principal Ingredients | Preservative |
|---|---|---|---|
| **Solutions** | | | |
| Adsorbotear | Alcon | HEC, adsorbobase, povidone | Thimerosal, EDTA |
| Artificial Tears | Varies | PVA | Benzalkonium Cl, EDTA |
| Aqua Site | Ciba | DEX, PEG-400 | EDTA |
| Bion Tears | Alcon | DEX 0.1%, HPMC 0.3% | **No preservative** |
| Cellufresh | Allergan | CMC | **No preservative** |
| Celluvisc | Allergan | CMC 1% | **No preservative** |
| Comfort Tears | Barnes-Hind | HEC | Benzalkonium Cl, EDTA |
| Dakrina | Dakryon | Povidone, PVA 0.6%, vitamin A, vitamin C | EDTA |
| Dry Eye Therapy | B & L | Glycerin | **No preservative** |
| Dry Eyes | B & L | PVA 1.4% | Benzalkonium Cl, EDTA |
| Dwelle | Dakryon | PVA, poly N-glucose | EDTA |
| Eye-Lube-A | Optopics | Glycerin | Benzalkonium Cl, EDTA |
| Hypo Tears | Iolab | PVA 1%, HEC, DEX | Benzalkonium Cl, EDTA |
| Hypo Tears PF | Iolab | PVA 1%, HEC, DEX | **No preservative** |
| Isopto Alkaline | Alcon | HPMC 1% | Benzalkonium Cl |
| Isopto Tears Plain | Alcon | HPMC 0.5% | Benzalkonium Cl, EDTA |
| Just Tears | Blairex | Saline | Benzalkonium Cl, EDTA |
| Lacril | Allergan | HPMC 0.5%, GEL, PSB | Chlorobutanol |
| Lacri-Lube-NP | Allergan | Petrolatum, lanolin | **No preservative** |
| Liquifilm Forte | Allergan | PVA 3% | Thimerosal, EDTA |
| Liquifilm Tears | Allergan | PVA 1.4% | Chlorobutanol |
| Lubri Tears | B & L | HPMC 0.3%, DEX | Benzalkonium Cl, EDTA |
| Murocel | B & L | MC 1%, PEG | Parabens |
| Murine | Ross | PVA 0.5%, povidone | Benzalkonium Cl, EDTA |
| Moisture Drops | B & L | HPMC 0.5%, DEX | Benzalkonium Cl, EDTA |
| Nature's Tears | Rugby | HPMC 0.3%, DEX | EDTA |
| Nutra Tear | Dakryon | Vit B$_{12}$, PVA | Benzalkonium Cl, EDTA |
| Refresh | Allergan | PVA 1.4%, povidone | **No preservative** |
| Refresh plus | Allergan | CMC 0.5% | **No preservative** |
| TearGard | Med Tech | HPMC 0.5% | EDTA, Sorbic acid |
| Tearisol | Iolab | HPMC 1.0% | Benzalkonium Cl, EDTA |
| Tears Naturale | Alcon | HPMC 0.3%, DEX | Benzalkonium Cl, EDTA |
| Tears Naturale II | Alcon | HPMC 0.3%, DEX | Polyquaterium-1 |
| Tears Naturale Free | Alcon | HPMC 0.3%, DEX | **No preservative** |
| Tears Naturale Free | Alcon | HPMC 3.0%, DEX | **No preservative** |
| Tears Plus | Allergan | PVA 1.4%, povidone | Chlorobutanol |
| Vit-A-Drops | Vision | PSB, vitamin A | EDTA |
| **Ointments** | | | |
| Duo-lube | B & L | Petrolatum, MO | **No preservative** |
| Dry Eyes | B & L | Petrolatum, MO | **No preservative** |
| Duratears Naturale | Alcon | Petrolatum, lanolin, MO | **No preservative** |
| Hypo Tears | Iolab | Petrolatum, lanolin, MO | **No preservative** |
| Lacri-lube | Allergan | Petrolatum, lanolin, MO | Chlorobutanol |
| Lacri-lube NP | Allergan | Petrolatum, lanolin | **No preservative** |
| Lacri-lube S.O.P. | Allergan | Petrolatum, MO, lanolin | Chlorobutanol |
| Lubri Tears | B & L | Petrolatum, mineral oil, lanolin | Chlorobutanol |
| Puralube | Fougera | Petrolatum, MO, lanolin | **No preservative** |
| Refresh PM | Allergan | Petrolatum, MO, lanolin | **No preservative** |
| Puralube | Fougera | Petrolatum, MO, lanolin | **No preservative** |

°Special thanks to Dr. RL Kaswan, University of Georgia, Athens, GA, for compilation of this table.
Abbreviations: CMC = carboxymethyl cellulose, DEX = dextran, GEL = gelatine, HEC = hydroxyethyl cellulose, HPMC = hydroxypropyl methyl cellulose, MC = methyl cellulose, PSB = polysorbate 80, PVA = polyvinyl alcohol, B & L = Bausch & Lomb, MO = mineral oil, PEG = propylene glycol, EDTA = ethylenediametetraacetic acid.

(Coopervision) and Tears Naturale (Alcon) are well tolerated by dogs. They replace the mucin and aqueous layers of the tear film. A petrolatum ophthalmic ointment like Duratears (Alcon), Lacrilube (Allergan), or Duolube (Bausch & Lomb) ideally should be applied after liquid tears to protect against evaporation. When cost is a concern and only a few daily treatments can be applied, sterile ophthalmic ointments without solutions may provide and hold moisture on the cornea. Bedtime use of artificial tear ointment is recommended in patients with insufficient eyelid closure.

Ocular inserts with slow-release hydropropylmethylcellulose (Lacriserts, Merck Sharp & Dohme) have been tried in dogs to prevent desiccation. Difficulties with insertion of the product by the owner and retention of the insert within the conjunctival sac were encountered. Financial factors also prevent their popularity in canine and feline KCS therapy. Lacriserts, at this printing, are not readily available due to manufacturing delays.

Sodium hyaluronic acid solutions in artificial tears have been reported to be effective in dogs and humans with refractory KCS. Many different concentrations and preparations have been recommended for their palliative effect. These products are not commercially available and must be formulated by compounding pharmacists or veterinarians.

Tear stimulants include dilute topical cyclosporine (Optimmune, Schering-Plough; Sandimmune, Sandoz) and oral or topical ophthalmic pilocarpine. Oral pilocarpine for KCS requires administration of one to two drops of 2% pilocarpine for a 20 to 25 pound dog in food twice daily. A major disadvantage of oral pilocarpine is the systemic effects of an overdose. Salivation, vomiting, diarrhea, and bradycardia are undesirable signs of pilocarpine toxicity. Pilocarpine's maximal effect as a tear stimulant starts 45 to 60 min after application and is maintained for only a few hours. To determine the optimal oral pilocarpine dose, one additional drop is administered per day until signs of toxicity are observed; then the dose is decreased to a slightly subtoxic level for long-term maintenance. Using 0.5% topical pilocarpine solution may avoid ocular irritation and systemic side effects and increase tear production. Pilocarpine use is contraindicated if cardiac failure, pancreatitis, or chronic diarrhea is present. Many dogs do not respond to pilocarpine, and its effects may diminish as the disease progresses.

Cyclosporine is the first-choice tear stimulant, since it offers distinct advantages over pilocarpine. Cyclosporine is a noncytotoxic natural cyclic polypeptide isolated from the fungus *Tolypocladium inflatum;* its pharmacologic mechanism of action is only partly understood (Hess, 1993). Both immunosuppressive and neurohormonal theories have been proposed for cyclosporine's ability to increase tear production in the dog.

Therapeutic trials of topical 1 and 2% cyclosporine in corn oil and olive oil substrates (compounded using the oral form of cyclosporine) demonstrated increased STT values in dogs with KCS when applied once, twice, or three times daily (Salisbury et al., 1990; Olivero et al., 1991; Morgan and Abrams, 1991). The severity of the KCS and the response to therapy dictate the number of daily applications required to stimulate a normal level of tears. Ophthalmic cyclosporine in a more dilute ointment form will soon be commercially available (Optimmune, Schering-Plough).

In severely dry eyes (STT < 5 mm/min), response to cyclosporine may not become evident for 3 to 4 weeks or longer. Supplemental tear replacement is advised until sufficient tear production is established. The lag phase is thought to be consistent with an immunosuppressive mechanism.

Failure of cyclosporine therapy to increase tear production in the dog is associated with end-stage lacrimal gland fibrosis and atrophy. Four months of treatment with one drop applied every 8 hr is considered the maximum time and dose needed to determine if the patient will respond to topical cyclosporine with increased tears. Usually, a favorable response is elicited after only a few weeks, even in dogs starting with minimal tear production.

Consistent evaluation of the STT 3 hr after cyclosporine treatment is recommended to optimally assess results and to compare subsequent STT values. Reevaluation on a 3- to 4-week basis is advised until sufficient tear secretion is established. At reexamination 6 months after treatment initiation, the tear production is often still improving on the same dose. If tear overflow or STT values are in the high 20s with minimal corneal changes, a decrease in the daily application frequency to once daily (or rarely, once every 2 days) may maintain efficacy. Long-term cyclosporine therapy is needed to maintain increased tear production in patients with permanent KCS. When therapy is discontinued, recurrence of typical clinical signs over time is observed.

Systemic toxic effects have not been observed with ophthalmic cyclosporine. The dog is resistant to the renal toxicity observed in some people receiving oral 10% cyclosporine. An estimated 2 to 5% of dogs may develop a hyperemic conjunctival response with chronic topical usage. This is more commonly seen in dogs with sensitive skin, often those with white hair and little pigmentation around the eyelid margin. Stopping the drug reverses the irritation. The irritative or atopic response in these few individuals may be due to (1) failure to remove the alcohol by evaporation when formulated from the parent product or (2) the vehicle used to dilute the cyclosporine. Reinstitution of cyclosporine therapy in a different vehicle often does not result in irritation, suggesting the substrate may be the cause of the hyperemic response. Anecdotal reports have rarely suggested that topical 2% cyclosporine may have activated latent ocular herpesvirus infection in cats. Therefore, clinicians should monitor treated cats carefully.

Cyclosporine is NOT a cure for KCS but rather a therapy to successfully manage what otherwise is a frustrating, progressive, and potentially blinding disease. Clients must be made aware of this to enlist their attention to regular continued daily treatments even after increased lacrimation is evident. Topical cyclosporine is the treatment of choice for canine KCS due to its high efficacy at increasing tear production, need for fewer daily applications, and lack of undesirable systemic side effects compared to conventional therapies for KCS.

Besides increasing lacrimation in most dogs with KCS, long-term use of cyclosporine also improves corneal pathologic changes induced by low tear production. Corneal vascularization and pigmentation may slowly diminish, restoring the transparency of the cornea and increasing vision. Topical cyclosporine also is used successfully in canine chronic superficial keratitis (see "Pannus," this volume, p 1245).

Short-term topical broad-spectrum antibiotic therapy is indicated in conjunction with KCS tear stimulant or replacement therapy when bacterial conjunctivitis is evident. Use of a topical antibiotic alone for bacterial conjunctivitis without tear stimulant or replacement therapy in dogs with KCS results in recurrence of the infection and purulent ocular discharge after cessation of therapy. This is a common sequela of inadequate investigation of the primary problem that resulted in the bacterial overgrowth. Flora commonly cultured from affected dogs include: *Staphylococcus* spp. (usually coagulase-positive), and *Streptococcus* spp., with β-*Streptococcus* isolated more often than α or nonhemolytic γ species (Salisbury, Kaswan, and Brown, 1994). The frequency of corneal bacterial isolation is decreased significantly in dogs that respond to chronic cyclosporine tear stimulation, and the flora resembles that of normal dogs (Salisbury, Kaswan, and Brown, 1994). Increased tear production induced by cyclosporine is believed to be the primary reason for the improved microbial environment.

Corticosteroids are sometimes judiciously used to reduce inflammation and swelling of conjunctiva that may retard tear secretion or to suppress corneal neovascularization and scarring. Corticosteroids should never be used if ulcers are present.

Mucolytic agents such as dilute (5 to 8%) acetylcysteine (Mucomyst, Bristol-Myers Company) in artificial tear solutions may be formulated to break up the thick tenacious ocular secretions of KCS. According to the package insert, the shelf life of dilute acetylcysteine is 5 days; refrigeration may extend this.

Nasal dryness and related discharge should be alleviated with regular cleaning and application of lubricants like petrolatum as needed.

Agents contraindicated for KCS patients include: anticholinergics like atropine, topical anesthetics to decrease discomfort, and sulfonamides and other drugs reported to decrease tear secretion. Contact lenses are contraindicated for use in dry eyes, since they tend to imbibe fluid from their surroundings. Dry eyes may be more sensitive to preservatives in ocular medications than eyes with normal lacrimal function, in which they are diluted and flushed away. If conjunctival hyperemia and ocular discomfort persist despite apparently appropriate treatment, the use of preservative-free tear replacements and medications should be considered.

Surgical considerations in KCS patients include conjunctival or nictitans flaps for corneal ulcers, blepharoplasty to reduce exposure keratitis, and parotid duct transportation (PDT) as an alternative source of moisture in medically refractory cases. Only PDT offers a substitute for the lack of tear secretion. The high efficacy of cyclosporine therapy has dramatically decreased the need for this surgery in the past few years. Sufficient time to evaluate the response to cyclosporine therapy should be allowed prior to PDT surgery. "Natural" tears stimulated by cyclosporine are superior to saliva to bathe and nourish the cornea and conjunctiva. A recent study comparing immunoglobulins of canine tears and parotid saliva concluded parotid secretion appears to be a valid substitute for tears based on immunologic components (Barrera et al., 1991). Parotid gland secretions are usually not irritating to the eye.

Parotid gland function must be tested before surgery to ensure sufficient saliva is produced. This gland can be stimulated by a drop of 1% atropine ophthalmic solution applied caudally on the patient's tongue on the side to be transposed. Profuse salivation in response to atropine's bitter taste is a normal response. The parotid duct papilla is caudal to the carnassial tooth; saliva may be seen flowing from the site. A few dogs with KCS have xerostomia; they are not candidates for this surgery. The gland and duct should be palpated for abnormalities.

The surgery is delicate, and accidental cutting or twisting of the duct when relocating it to the inferior conjunctival sac can result in failure. Postoperative fibrosis or stenosis of the parotid duct inhibits flow of the saliva to the eye. Surgical procedures for a lateral skin or an oral approach have been described for the dog and the cat (Gelatt, 1991; Gwin, Gelatt, and Peiffer, 1977).

Clients should be well informed of possible postoperative complications of PDT. Crystal-like white mineral deposits may precipitate on the cornea, conjunctiva, or periocular skin. Topical 0.5 to 3% ethylenediaminetetraacetic acid formulations may help to dissolve or chelate the precipitates. Calcium carbonate, phosphate, oxalate, or combinations are believed to be the offending precipitates, which may be irritating and obstruct vision if profuse, giving a frosted appearance to affected tissues. Saliva overflow onto the face is another undesirable sequela seen in some cases.

## PROGNOSIS

The prognosis for resolution of KCS remains guarded. When early identification and removal or correction of the cause is possible, restoration to normal tear secretion may be possible, provided lacrimal tissue is still functional. KCS related to distemper virus, herpesvirus, iatrogenic drug toxicities, and minor neurologic lesions may resolve with time and supplemental protective therapy. An estimated 15 to 20% of KCS patients may exhibit remission with spontaneous improvement in tear production (Gelatt, 1991). Xerophthalmia has the poorest prognosis, but therapy should be attempted. Cases that fail to respond to tear stimulants over a sufficient time interval probably have atrophied glandular tissue.

Most animals with KCS require chronic therapy to alleviate clinical signs and preserve vision. Clients should be advised that KCS is a serious, often progressive, non–life-threatening disease limited to corneal and conjunctival tissues. Adequate long-term therapy is necessary to preserve vision and comfort.

## References and Suggested Reading

Barrera AJ, Mane MC, Andres S, et al: Immunoglobulins of tears and parotid saliva in the dog. Prog Vet Comp Ophthalmol 2:55, 1991.
*A comparison between canine tears and saliva immunoglobulin content.*
Berger S and Scagliotti R: A quantitative study of the effects of Tribrissen on canine tear production. Vet Pathol 29:474, 1992.
*An abstract reporting a study of iatrogenic KCS secondary to Tribrissen therapy.*
Gelatt KN: Canine lacrimal and nasolacrimal diseases. *In* Gelatt KN (ed): *Veterinary Ophthalmology*, 2nd edition. Philadelphia, Lea & Febiger, 1991, p 281.
*A general review of KCS in the latest edition of this classic textbook.*
Gwin RM, Gelatt KN, and Peiffer RL: Parotid duct transposition in a cat with keratoconjunctivitis sicca. J Am Anim Hosp Assoc 13:42, 1977.
*Description and illustrations of PDT in a cat with severe KCS.*
Hess AD: Mechanisms of action of cyclosporine: Considerations for the treatment of autoimmune diseases. Clin Immunol Immunopathol 68:220, 1993.
*A review of cyclosporine's known therapeutic mechanisms of action.*
Hollingsworth SR, Canton DD, Buyukmihci NC, et al: Effect of topically administered atropine on tear production in dogs. J Am Vet Med Assoc 200:1481, 1992.
*A study on the effects of topical atropine on canine tear production in treated and untreated fellow eyes.*
Jamieson VE, Davidson MG, Nasisse MP, et al: Ocular complications following cobalt 60 radiotherapy of neoplasms in the canine head region. J Am Anim Hosp Assoc 27:51, 1991.
*KCS is one potential side effect of radiation therapy to the head reported in this paper.*
Kaswan RL, Martin CL and Chapman WL: Keratoconjunctivitis sicca: Histopathologic study of nictitating membrane and lacrimal glands from 28 dogs. Am J Vet Res 45:112, 1984.
*Histologic examination of lacrimal tissue from 28 dogs diagnosed with KCS due to several causes.*

Kaswan RL and Martin CL: Diseases of the lacrimal apparatus. *In* Kirk RW (ed): *Current Veterinary Therapy VIII.* Philadelphia, WB Saunders Co, 1983, p 549.
*A review of medical and surgical management of lacrimal system disorders.*
Kaswan RL and Salisbury MA: A new perspective on canine keratoconjunctivitis sicca. Treatment with ophthalmic cyclosporine. Vet Clin North Am Small Anim Pract 20:583, 1990.
*A review of canine KCS, its causes, and treatments.*
Kaswan RL, Salisbury MA, and Lothrop CD: Interaction of age and gender on occurrence of canine keratoconjunctivitis sicca. Prog Vet Comp Ophthalmol 1:93, 1991.
*A new approach and evaluation of KCS in the dog examining age and sex incidence.*
Kaswan RL, Zhou DH, and Fullard RJ: Components in normal dog tears and tears from dogs with KCS treated with cyclosporine. Invest Ophthalmol Vis Sci 34:1468, 1993.
*An abstract on a study using gel electrophoresis to study tears from normal and KCS-affected dogs under cyclosporine therapy to stimulate tear production.*
Moore CP: Qualitative tear film disease. *In* Millichamp NJ and Dziezyc J (eds) Small Animal Ophthalmology. Vet Clin North Am [Small Anim Pract] 20:583, 1990.
*A review of mucin-deficient canine tear deficiencies.*
Moore CP, Frappier B, and Linton L: Distribution and course of secretory ducts of the canine third eyelid gland. Vet Pathol 29:5, 1992.
*An abstract describing the location and course of the secretory ducts of the lacrimal gland of the nictatans.*
Morgan RV and Abrams KL: Topical administration of cyclosporine for treatment of keratoconjunctivitis sicca in dogs. J Am Vet Med Assoc 199:1043, 1991.
*A controlled study evaluating the use of cyclosporine for canine KCS to increase tear production.*
Morgan RV, Duddy JM, and McClurg K: Prolapse of the gland of the third eyelid in dogs: A retrospective study of 89 cases (1980–1990). J Am Anim Hosp Assoc 29:56, 1993.
*This retrospective study evaluates different surgical approaches and the consequences of surgery versus no surgery for nictatans gland prolapse.*
Olivero, DK, Davidson MG, English RV, et al: Clinical evaluation of 1% cyclosporine for topical treatment of keratoconjunctivitis sicca in dogs. J Am Vet Med Assoc 199:1039, 1991.
*This study reports that topical 1% cyclosporine is effective in increasing tear production in dogs with KCS.*
Salisbury MA, Kaswan RL, Ward DA, et al: Topical application of cyclosporine in the management of keratoconjunctivitis sicca in dogs. J Am Anim Hosp Assoc 26:269, 1990.
*An early report on topical 2% cyclosporine treatment for idiopathic canine KCS.*
Salisbury MA, Kaswan RL, and Brown J: Ocular micro-organisms before and during topical cyclosporine therapy. Am J Vet Res (in press), 1995.
*A 12-month study of corneal cultures taken before and during 2% cyclosporine therapy for KCS in dogs.*

# BACTERIAL KERATITIS

HARRIET J. DAVIDSON
*Fayetteville, North Carolina*

Bacterial keratitis most commonly presents as a corneal ulcer. It is a fairly common clinical problem that requires immediate evaluation, accurate diagnosis, and careful therapy and follow-up to ensure resolution.

## PATHOGENESIS

Several surveys of conjunctival flora of the dog and cat have been completed (Gerding and Kakoma, 1990). Bacteria found in the normal eye include *Staphyloccus*

spp., *Streptococcus* spp. with $\alpha$ more common than $\beta$, *Corynebacterium*, *Bacillus*, *Neisseria*, and *Pseudomonas*. Anaerobic organisms are not frequently recovered. Fungi have been isolated from conjunctival swabs in up to 22% of dogs and 40% of cats (Samuelson, Andresen, and Gwin, 1984). Bacterial or fungal organisms do not normally cause clinical problems, because of normal ocular protective mechanisms. These include the tight junctions of the corneal epithelial cells, the normal cellular sloughing of epithelial cells, and antimicrobial actions of the tear film. Corneal ulcers are most commonly caused by abrasions, usually traumatic, mechanical, or less commonly chemical, in origin. After the corneal epithelial surface has been abraded, as in an ulcer, organisms can adhere to the stroma or remaining epithelial cells and cause an infection. Following a corneal abrasion, these same bacteria are those most commonly found in an infected ulcer: *Staphylococcus aureus*, *Staphylococcus epidermidis*, β-*Streptococcus*, and α-*Streptococcus* (also see "Antibiotic Therapy of the Eye," this volume, p 1211). Bacterial organisms colonize the corneal ulcer and release both chemotactic substances, which attract leukocytes; and exotoxins such as collagenase, proteases, and peptidases, which result in corneal destruction. Corneal cells and leukocytes also release collagenolytic enzymes. As the corneal ulcer progresses, the cornea may melt, resulting in perforation of the eye. Corneal perforation is usually accompanied by leakage of the aqueous and iris prolapse. Secondary intraocular infection, endophthalmitis, can then occur.

## DIAGNOSIS

Corneal ulceration is usually painful. The animal may have blepharospasm, epiphora or a mucoid discharge, photophobia, or "redness." Initial examination of the animal should include: (1) a detailed history of the eye problem, including previous treatments; (2) a complete physical examination to rule out concurrent physical abnormalities; and (3) a complete ophthalmic examination. Ophthalmic examination should begin with examination of the lids for entropion, ectropion, distichiasis, trichiasis, ectopic cilia, and foreign bodies. Foreign bodies are commonly found behind the third eyelid. If lid abnormalities or foreign bodies are detected, they need to be surgically corrected at the time therapy is initiated for the corneal ulcer. The normal cornea is clear, with a smooth, regular surface. An ulcer appears as an imperfection in the corneal surface. If the ulcer has been present for longer than 24 hr, blood vessels may be present. Superficial vessels are few in number, may extend to the center of the cornea, and branch in a tree-like pattern. Deep blood vessels may be numerous, appear around the limbus, and extend only a few millimeters with little branching; these indicate a deeper infection or inflammation. The cornea surrounding the ulcer may be slightly swollen or opaque, which indicates edema. Infiltration of neutrophils lends a white to yellow color to the surrounding stroma. The anterior chamber is evaluated for evidence of intraocular infection or inflammation. Leukocytes in the anterior chamber, hypopyon, appear as white fluffy material; this may indicate corneal infection but does not confirm extension of the infection into the anterior chamber. An increase in the aqueous protein, flare, indicates inflammation. Aqueous flare gives the anterior chamber a hazy appearance. Pupil size and shape are evaluated; miosis suggests concurrent iridocyclitis. Special diagnostic procedures should be considered: (1) bacterial culture collection; (2) Schirmer tear test

(STT); (3) fluorescein stain; and (4) corneal cytology. Tonometry is generally contraindicated in severe ulceration because of the possibility of rupturing the cornea.

Corneal infection should be suspected when the history indicates a rapid progression of the ulcer, the surrounding cornea is markedly opaque and has a swollen appearance, the cornea is soft and melting, or intense miosis accompanies a small or superficial ulcer. If infection is suspected, a culture sample should be taken. This can be done with a standard or mini culture swab (Culturette, Scientific Products). The mini swab allows for accurate sample collection from small areas without contamination from the surrounding structures such as lids and conjunctiva. The culture swab should be moistened prior to obtaining the sample by breaking the transport media container provided. The eyelids are retracted and the edges of the corneal ulcer are swabbed. If possible, culture collection should be performed before instillation of eye washes, topical anesthetics, or mydriatics because these things contain preservatives that might impair recovery of organisms.

An STT should be completed to rule out concurrent keratoconjunctivitis sicca (KCS). If KCS is detected, it should be treated appropriately at the same time the bacterial keratitis is being treated (see "Keratoconjunctivitis Sicca," this volume, p 1231).

Fluorescein stain should be used to confirm the presence of an ulcer and assess the size and depth of the lesion. The flat surface of a premoistened dye strip should be touched to the bulbar conjunctiva, not cornea, to prevent an inadvertent paper cut of the corneal surface. Excess fluorescein is rinsed from the eye with sterile eye wash. A positive stain will appear green when viewed with a penlight; it will fluoresce brilliant green if viewed with a Wood's lamp or penlight with a cobalt blue filter. Fluorescein will not penetrate intact epithelium but will be absorbed by the stroma. Descemet's membrane does not retain stain; the stromal edges of the ulcer do stain and give the ulcer a "bullseye" appearance.

Cytology samples may be obtained after the other diagnostic tests have been completed. A topical anesthetic is applied to the corneal surface. A Kimura spatula or the butt end of a scalpel blade is used to gently scrape the corneal surface. The sample is smeared on a glass slide. Several scrapings and subsequent slides are made. Slides may be stained with Wright's, Diff-Quik, or Gram's stain to evaluate the cell types and demonstrate bacteria present.

## THERAPY

Ophthalmic drops or ointments are appropriate in most ulcers (for details, see "Antibiotic Therapy of the Eye," this volume, p 1211). In cases of deep ulceration, where there is danger of corneal perforation, drops are preferable. Ointments can cause severe intraocular inflammation if they gain access to the anterior chamber. Topical ophthalmic antibiotics are used prophylactically for simple corneal ulcers. The antibiotic used should have a broad spectrum (such as bacitracin, chloramphenicol) or combination preparation (such as bacitracin-neomycin-polymyxin). When a corneal infection is suspected or confirmed, an antibiotic is used to kill the organisms. The choice of antibiotic is selected based on the sensitivity of the organism (see "Antibiotic Therapy of the Eye," this volume, p 1215). When the identity of the organism is unknown, a broad-spectrum antibiotic is used. Ulcers that appear quickly or are progressing rapidly and have a melting appearance are suspected of being a *Pseudomonas* infection; an aminoglycoside (such as gentamicin [Gentocin] or tobramycin) should be used.

Anterior uveitis commonly accompanies corneal ulceration, stimulated by an axonal reflex mediated by the ophthalmic branch of the trigeminal nerve. The corneal nerves are stimulated and cause ciliary muscle spasm. The uveitis is usually treated with a cycloplegic agent (e.g., 1% atropine). Other forms of uveitis therapy are only necessary if the inflammation is severe enough to threaten vision (see "Feline Uveitis," and "Canine Uveitis," this volume, pp 1253 and 1248, respectively).

## Simple Ulcers

A typical, simple ulcer appears as a divot in the corneal surface with the surrounding cornea being slightly swollen. Therapy should include: (1) cleaning the eye one or two times daily (a sterile eye rinse is best; however, a clean cloth or cotton balls soaked in warm water are effective); (2) application of a broad-spectrum topical ophthalmic antibiotic drop or ointment three to four times daily; (3) application of 1% atropine solution or ointment one to two times daily; and (4) reevaluation of the animal in 5 to 7 days. Owners should be instructed how to clean the eye and to examine the eye daily. If the eye becomes painful or increasingly white or red in color, the animal should be reevaluated immediately. Uncomplicated ulcers heal at a rate of approximately 1 mm/day. This is a general rule of thumb to assess the progress of the ulcer. Ulcers heal in a typical manner; the process is well described elsewhere (Nasisse, 1985). If the ulcer is healing normally, no changes in treatment are needed; antibiotic therapy is continued 1 week after the cornea is fluorescein stain–negative. At the time of reexamination, ulcers that have enlarged in size or that have an increased opacity, swollen appearance, or appear melting should be suspected of being infected.

## Infected Ulcers

A corneal ulcer is suspected of infection when the cornea surrounding the ulcer is soft in appearance and to touch, is markedly swollen in comparison to the normal cornea, or is yellowish-white in color. Suspected infected ulcers should be cultured at the time of initial diagnosis. A complete ophthalmic examination should be completed to include: STT, fluorescein stain, and corneal cytology. Examination of all ocular structures, STT, and stain should be repeated with each subsequent examination. Once a diagnosis of corneal infection has been made, the aim of therapy is to eliminate the organism and support the cornea through its normal healing process.

In general, the deeper and larger the ulcer, the more intensive the therapy. Initial treatment should include the following:

1. The eye should be cleaned one or two times daily with a sterile eye wash, or clean cloth or cotton balls soaked in water, to remove mucoid or purulent discharge.

2. A topical ophthalmic antibiotic is applied six or more times daily. In severely infected ulcers, antibiotics can be applied every 1 to 2 hr for the first 24 hr. As the ulcer becomes smaller, the frequency of medications can be decreased.

3. Topical 1% atropine should be used two or three times daily to relieve pain through cycloplegia.

Infected ulcers can change rapidly and need to be monitored closely to assess adequacy of treatment.

Hospitalization may be necessary to ensure adequate cleaning, medication, and evaluation. If the animal is discharged, the owners need to be instructed how to clean the eye and what to evaluate in the eye. If the eye changes color, if there is an increase in opacity or redness, if there is excess fluid drainage from the eye, or if the animal appears acutely painful, reexamination should be performed immediately. If no problems are noted, reexamination should be done in 1 or 2 days. Culture and sensitivity results are usually returned in 48 hr. A change in antibiotics may be made if dictated by antibiotic sensitivity test results. If the ulcer is becoming deeper or larger or if the cornea is melting, surgical intervention should be recommended.

Fungal keratitis is not very common in dogs and cats. Keratomycosis is often characterized historically by a long insidious course and chronic topical corticosteroid therapy. The cornea may appear opaque, swollen, and soft. Assessment of suspected fungal keratitis requires close ocular examination, corneal cytology, and fungal culture. Intensive treatment for fungal infection should be directed at elimination of the fungal organisms. This usually requires surgical intervention such as a keratectomy to remove as many of the organisms as possible. Antifungal medications include: natamycin 5% suspension (Natacyn, Alcon Laboratories), which is the only commercially available ophthalmic preparation; 1% miconazole (Miconazole IV preparation, Janssen Pharmaceutica); and amphotericin B (Fungizone, Squibb). Antifungal medications can be used initially every 4 hr, with the frequency of medication being decreased as the cornea begins to clear. Topical ophthalmic antibiotics should be used concurrently to prevent secondary bacterial infection.

## ADJUNCTIVE AND SURGICAL THERAPY

Several forms of adjunctive therapy are available: contact lenses, collagen shields, nictitans flap, and temporary tarsorrhaphy. Soft contact lenses can be used to protect the cornea from irritating structures, such as distichiasis or ectopic cilia, until surgical correction is completed. Contact lenses are best avoided in cases of infected ulcers. Collagen shields (Bio-Cor, Bausch & Lomb) can be used in infected ulcers for corneal support, to provide a matrix for keratocytes, and to augment antibiotic therapy. Collagen shields come in a desiccated form; they can be rehydrated with an ophthalmic antibiotic, which is then slowly released. They will dissolve over a period of 72 hr. Third-eyelid flaps and temporary tarsorrhaphies have been used in corneal ulcer therapy. They do not increase the healing time and may in fact impede the penetration of ophthalmic preparations. They should not be used for infected corneal ulcers because they provide a good environment for organism growth and impede treatment and evaluation of the healing process.

Surgical intervention for treatment of an ulcer should be recommended when the cornea is in danger of rupturing or the ulcer worsens despite intensive medical therapy. Very deep corneal ulcers can rupture if too much pressure is exerted on or around the eye during examination or treatment. Deep ulcers and descemetoceles can be recognized by their slightly clear centers. Surgical intervention should be recommended in cases of severe corneal infection. Severe corneal infection is recognized on cytology by numerous polymorphonuclear cells with intracytoplasmic bacteria.

Surgical alternatives include keratectomy, conjunctival flaps, conjunctival island grafts, autogenous corneal advancement grafts, and corneal allografts. The goals of surgical intervention are to: remove as much infected tissue as possible, supply healthy tissue to fill in the defect, and increase the vascular supply to the healing ulcer bed. Ophthalmic procedures of this type require delicate instrumentation and surgical magnification and are well described in surgical texts (Slatter and Hakanson, 1993). In many cases, these procedures are best completed through referral to a veterinary ophthalmologist. Medical therapy following surgical intervention is the same as for an infected corneal ulcer. Reexamination is recommended 2 to 7 days following surgery.

### References and Suggested Reading

Gerding PA and Kakoma I: Microbiology of the canine and feline eye. Vet Clin North Am 20:615, 1990.
  *A review of the microbial organisms found in dogs and cats from both normal and diseased eyes.*
Kern TJ: Ulcerative keratitis. Vet Clin North Am 20:643, 1990.
  *A detailed review of the pathogenisis, diagnosis, and medical and surgical treatment of ulcerative keratitis.*
Nasisse MP: Canine ulcerative keratitis. Compend Cont Educ 7:686, 1985.
  *A review of the pathogenesis, including normal healing process, of corneal ulcers.*
Samuelson DA, Andresen TL, and Gwin RM: Conjunctival fungal flora in horses, cattle, dogs and cats. J Am Vet Med Assoc 184:1940, 1984.
  *Results of a survey of normal fungal flora from the conjunctival sac.*
Slatter D and Hakanson N: Cornea and sclera. *In* Slatter D (ed): *Textbook of Small Animal Surgery.* Philadelphia, WB Saunders Co, 1993, p 1211.
  *A detailed description of the techniques for corneal surgical repair.*

---

# INDOLENT CORNEAL EROSIONS

MICHELLE M. TAYLOR
*Guelph, Ontario, Canada*

Indolent corneal erosions (ICEs) are epithelial defects that often occur spontaneously or following minor trauma and tend to persist beyond the expected time of healing. They are characterized by a nonadherent lip of epithelium and little if any stromal involvement. Originally described in the boxer, this condition has since been reported in many breeds. These ICEs have also been called persistent corneal ulcers, refractory epithelial erosions, indolent ulcers, boxer ulcers, and rodent ulcers. They are a common and often frustrating problem in veterinary ophthalmology and many treatments have been recommended, with variable success.

## DIAGNOSIS

Affected dogs are usually middle-aged or older and have an acute onset of ocular pain manifested by blepharospasm, photophobia, and epiphora, which tend to decrease with chronicity. Typical findings on ophthalmic examination include a paracentral epithelial defect with either normal stroma or variable corneal edema. Corneal vascularization and inflammation are absent, although with chronicity, significant neovascularization may develop. The ulcer margin has a lip of nonadherent epithelium that can be easily stripped away with a cotton-tipped swab. After application of fluorescein stain, a central area of bright fluorescence is surrounded by an area of dull fluorescence that represents seepage of dye under the loose epithelial lip.

A thorough examination should be performed to rule out other causes of prolonged corneal healing such as foreign bodies, ectopic cilia, entropion, distichiasis, trichiasis, keratoconjunctivitis sicca, goblet cell deficiency, infection, or corneal dystrophy (e.g., Shetland sheepdogs). In cats, feline herpesvirus (FHV) has been implicated as a cause of recurrent erosions.

## PATHOGENESIS

Indolent corneal erosions are thought to be the result of: (1) a primary epithelial dystrophy involving abnormalities of the basement membrane/basal epithelial cells, or (2) chronic stromal edema. Uncomplicated corneal erosions heal by the flattening of adjacent basal epithelial cells that then slide across the denuded surface to cover the defect. Mitosis of the migrated cells reestablishes normal corneal thickness. Such an erosion would be expected to reepithelialize in 7 to 10 days. If the epithelial basement membrane has been damaged, a new basement membrane must be secreted and full adhesion may take 6 to 8 weeks.

Normal attachment of the basal epithelial cells to the underlying stroma is dependent upon the epithelial basement membrane, anchoring fibrils, and hemidesmosomes. Both the basement membrane and the hemidesmosomes are secreted by the basal epithelial cells. These structures comprise the basement membrane adhesion complex and are essential for tight epithelial-stromal adhesion.

Indolent corneal erosions appear to have two histologic variations. One group is characterized by basal epithelial cell or basement membrane lesions and the other by diffuse corneal edema but minimal cellular or membrane alteration. The initial studies in boxers showed decreased numbers of hemidesmosomes and marked ultrastructural alterations of the basement membrane. Other breeds have shown flattening of the basal epithelial cells with pyknosis of their nuclei, abnormal thickening of the basement membrane, and accumulations of basement membrane material. The basal epithelial cells are usually separated from the basement membrane, which tends to remain on the stromal surface. The cause of these abnormalities may be a change in the biochemical composition of the basement membrane. Human patients with bullous keratopathy show an absence of three important extracellular matrix proteins (laminin, type IV collagen, and fibronectin) that make up the basement membrane and presumably enhance adhesion. Absence of these proteins may be important in the development of poor epithelial adhesion and secondary corneal erosions.

The second group has essentially normal basal epithelial cells and few basement membrane changes but varying degrees of stromal edema. Some of the basal epithelial cells have intracellular and intercellular edema. Stromal edema may impair epithelial adherence, resulting in subepithelial bullae and secondary erosions. Causes of chronic stromal edema include glaucoma, uveitis, and primary endothelial degeneration or dystrophy.

## CLINICAL MANAGEMENT

The standard therapy for superficial corneal ulcers includes topical antibiotics to prevent secondary infections and cycloplegics to decrease painful ciliary muscle spasm. Antiviral medications should be used in FHV-positive cats (see "Infectious Feline Kerataconjunctivitis," this volume, p 1227). Although these treatments are certainly recommended in the management of ICE, when used alone they are seldom effective. Additional goals in the therapy of ICE include stimulating epithelial attachment and preventing self-trauma that may disrupt the fragile new epithelium. As healing of these erosions may take weeks, it is important that the owner be well informed of the progression, expected healing time, and possibility of recurrence to increase compliance and reduce dissatisfaction.

To address these goals, many treatments have been developed, including débridement of loose epithelium with or without chemical agents, bandage soft contact lenses or collagen shields, multiple punctate keratotomies or grid keratotomies, topical hyperosmotics, topical growth factors (epidermal growth factor, insulin) or fibronectin, cyanoacrylate tissue glue, nictitans flaps, temporary tarsorrhaphies, superficial keratectomies, conjunctival flaps, and corneal epithelial transplantation. First I will outline our current treatment protocol and then discuss the advantages and disadvantages of others.

My initial management of an ICE includes débridement of the nonadherent epithelium with a dry cotton-tipped swab followed by a multiple punctate keratotomy (MPK). A topical broad-spectrum antibiotic solution is administered every 8 hr and topical 1% atropine is applied every 12 to 24 hr if painful.

Débridement of the corneal epithelium will often greatly enlarge the erosion. Removal of the nonadherent cells back to the normal margins may allow for multiplication of the adjacent epithelium and production of a new basement membrane. As débridement alone is frequently not satisfactory, some have advocated the use of chemical agents for débridement (e.g., tincture of iodine). Such agents may remove abnormal basement membrane and alter the underlying stroma enough to encourage adhesion. They also can enhance potentially troublesome neovascularization.

The MPK (Fig. 1) involves making a series of anterior stromal punctures with a 25-gauge needle held perpendicular to the corneal surface. Puncture depth is adequate when the cornea begins to indent. The punctures are placed 0.5 to 1.0 mm apart across the entire affected area and 1 to 2 mm into normal cornea.

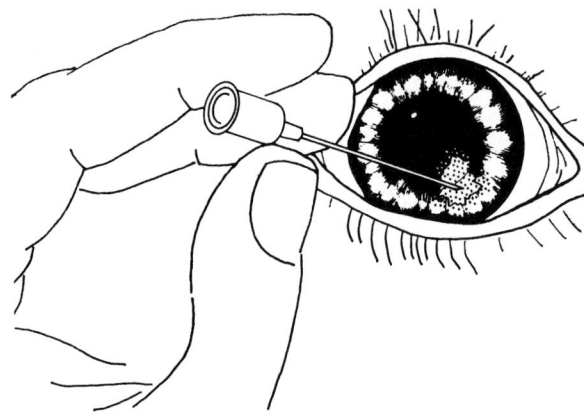

**Figure 1.** Multiple punctate keratotomy. (From Champagne ES and Munger RJ: Multiple punctate keratotomy for the treatment of recurrent epithelial erosions in dogs. J Am Anim Hosp Assoc 28: 213, 1992, with permission.)

Alternatively, a grid pattern of superficial crosshatches can be used. The procedure can be performed with topical anesthesia and sedation. The enhanced contact between the epithelium and stroma is thought to permit a more secure bond. MPK may also increase adhesion by stimulating production of important extracellular matrix proteins and enhancing subepithelial fibrosis. The procedure is simple to perform and seems to be highly effective. In one study, 16 of 18 erosions healed in an average of 1.75 weeks without the need for further therapy (Champagne and Munger, 1992). In another study, 72% of erosions had healed within 25 days using this technique (Morgan, 1994). This procedure should not be used on infected corneas. In cases in which the erosion has not healed within 2 weeks, the MPK can be repeated or used in combination with a nictitans flap or bandage soft contact lens (CL) (Canis I & II, The Cutting Edge) to protect the ingrowing epithelium from eyelid trauma.

Nictitans flaps can be easily performed with minimal anesthesia and should be combined with débridement and MPK, as they are usually unsuccessful used alone. Bandage soft contact lenses may also help to protect the new epithelium and maintain close apposition between the epithelium and stroma. Use of a CL after débridement allowed successful healing in 61 to 73% of cases (Morgan, 1994; Morgan, Bachrach, and Ogilvie, 1984). The major disadvantage of this technique is premature loss of the CL. Poor retention is likely due to poor fit, conformational exophthalmos, and movement of the nictitans. Use of a partial temporary tarsorrhaphy may help prevent early loss. Contact lenses should be removed for cleaning every 7 to 10 days.

Conjunctival flaps and superficial keratectomies have been shown to be effective in promoting healing of ICE. The former provides a direct blood supply and a source of fibrous connective tissue, but has the disadvantages of requiring general anesthesia and increased time and expense. It may also result in a greater degree of scarring. Superficial keratectomies will remove all abnormal epithelium and basement membrane but again require general anesthesia, special instruments, and experience.

Topical hyperosmotic agents such as 5% sodium chloride (5% Sodium Chloride, Akorn) may be useful in ICE secondary to chronic stromal edema. By reducing subepithelial edema, they may improve epithelial adhesion. One disadvantage is that they can be quite irritating.

Various topical growth factors have been used in the treatment of ICE. Epidermal growth factor (EGF) is a polypeptide found in tears that is thought to function in the normal growth and metabolism of the corneal epithelium. It stimulates epithelial cell mitosis and protein synthesis, and its effectiveness in treatment of ICE may be by enhancing synthesis of structural and attachment proteins that promote adhesion and migration of epithelial cells. In one study, 8 of 10 dogs with ICE treated with EGF healed in 2 weeks compared to 2 of 10 treated with a placebo (Kirschner et al., 1991). No such controlled studies have been performed using insulin, and clinical response has been variable. Fibronectin, a plasma glycoprotein, promotes epithelial attachment in rabbits, but again, studies of its efficacy in dogs are lacking. It is also not readily available, although autogenous serum could be used.

Cyanoacrylate tissue glue (Vetbond, 3M Animal Care Products) can be applied as a very thin layer through a small gauge needle to protect the cornea. The glue is sloughed when the new epithelium has grown underneath it. The major disadvantage is the difficulty in technique.

In conclusion, successful management of this common and difficult problem is dependent on early recognition, treatment aimed at promoting epithelial adhesion, and client communication.

### References and Suggested Reading

Champagne ES and Munger RJ: Multiple punctate keratotomy for the treatment of recurrent epithelial erosions in dogs. J Am Anim Hosp Assoc 28: 213, 1992.
*A study of the healing of corneal erosions in response to MPK.*

Gelatt KN and Samuelson DA: Recurrent corneal erosions and epithelial dystrophy in the boxer dog. J Am Anim Hosp Assoc 18:453, 1982.
*A description of the clinical and histologic findings of a series of boxers with indolent corneal erosions.*

Hsu JKW, Rubinfeld RS, Barry P, et al: Anterior stromal puncture. Immunohistochemical studies in human corneas. Arch Ophthalmol 111:1057, 1993.
*A study investigating the mechanism of action of anterior stromal punctures in nine patients with erosions secondary to bullous keratopathy.*

Kern TJ: Ulcerative keratitis. Vet Clin N Am [Small Anim Pract] 20:643, 1990.
*A current review of ulcerative keratitis in dogs and cats.*

Kirschner SG, Brazzell RK, Stern ME, et al: The use of topical epidermal growth factor for treatment of nonhealing corneal erosions in dogs. J Am Anim Hosp Assoc 27:449, 1991.
*A clinical trial studying the effect of EGF on healing of indolent erosions.*

Kirschner SG, Niyo Y, and Betts DM: Idiopathic persistent corneal erosions: Clinical and pathological findings in 18 dogs. J Am Anim Hosp Assoc 25: 84, 1989.
*A study of the clinical, histopathologic, and ultrastructural findings in 18 dogs other than boxers with persistent corneal erosions.*

Morgan RV and Abrams KL: A comparison of six different therapies for persistent corneal erosions in dogs and cats. Prog Vet Comp Ophthalmol 4:38, 1994.

Morgan RV, Bachrach A, and Ogilvie GK: An evaluation of soft contact lens usage in the dog and cat. J Am Anim Hosp Assoc 20:885, 1984.
*A review of soft contact lens use in 169 animals with chronic erosions or corneal irritation secondary to eyelid abnormalities.*

Whitley RD: Canine cornea. *In* Gelatt KN (ed): *Vet Ophthalmology.* Philadelphia, Lea & Febiger, 1991, p 312.
*A discussion of the pathophysiology, clinical signs, histopathology, and treatment of corneal diseases in dogs.*

# PANNUS

STEVEN M. ROBERTS

*Fort Collins, Colorado*

Numerous corneal disorders occur in the dog but, despite the diversity of specific clinical conditions, this tissue responds to insult in a limited fashion. Basic tissue responses include edema, vascularization, pigmentation, accumulation of cellular or metabolic infiltrates, stromal fibrosis, and loss of tissue (ulceration). These may occur singly or in combination. The generic term "pannus" (Bedford and Longstaffe, 1979) refers to superficial corneal vascularization and infiltration of granulation tissue. Pannus is frequently used to describe the specific clinical syndrome of chronic superficial keratitis (CSK) (Austad and Øen, 1978). This condition is also referred to as chronic superficial pigmentary keratitis, degenerative pannus, German shepherd pannus, superficial stromal keratitis (Stanley, 1988), chronic immune-mediated keratoconjunctivitis sicca, and historically as Überreiter's syndrome. The specific syndrome of CSK is intriguing and challenging because it may involve simultaneous occurrence of most of the previously mentioned corneal responses to insult.

Chronic superficial keratitis appropriately describes this progressive, usually bilateral, degenerative, and potentially blinding condition of dogs. Lesions begin at the limbus and consist of subepithelial corneal infiltration with blood vessels, lymphocytes, plasma cells, and melanocytes. The initial stages of CSK have subtle limbal corneal changes that frequently go unrecognized. Longstanding cases often develop corneal stromal accumulations of cholesterol. Corneal ulceration is also possible. The rate of progression varies from slow, requiring months to years for an increase in the area of corneal involvement, to those cases developing pancorneal involvement within a few months. Vascularized lesions are noticed sooner than pigmented lesions. Some CSK cases have nictitating membrane and nasal canthus involvement and exhibit thickening, depigmentation, and ulceration of the tissues. These lesions consist of a lymphocytic-plasmacytic infiltrate.

The etiopathogenesis of CSK is unknown, but histopathology and responsiveness to local ocular immunosuppressive treatments suggest an immune-mediated basis (Cambell et al., 1975; Eichenbaum et al., 1986). The disorder has a positive correlation to increased altitude and levels of ultraviolet radiation (Slatter et al., 1977). Many dog breeds develop this disorder, but most

CSK occurs in purebred and crossbred German shepherd dogs. Epidemiologic evaluation of CSK cases using odds ratios and 95% confidence intervals demonstrates the magnitudes of breed, altitude, and age association with this disorder (Table 1) (Chavkin, 1994). Such data reveal the Belgian Tervuren to be at greater risk of developing CSK than the German shepherd dog. Dogs living at elevations greater than 5000 feet are more likely to develop CSK and this risk increases with increasing altitude. Middle-aged dogs are more likely to develop CSK than young or old dogs. Other risk factors implicated in CSK include low humidity (Slatter et al., 1977), ultraviolet radiation (Campbell et al., 1975), and gender (Bedford and Longstaffe, 1979).

Clinical diagnosis is based on the signalment and presence of bilateral lesions composed primarily of vascularization, pigmentation, or a combination of both. Lesions involve the temporal corneal quadrant in greater than 95% of cases. The inferior, nasal, and superior corneal quadrants are involved in 88, 77, and 59% of CSK cases, respectively. Other ocular abnor-

**Table 1.** *Breed, Altitude, and Age-Related Risk of Developing Chronic Superficial Keratitis (Pannus)*

| Variable | Odds Ratio[†] | 95% Confidence Interval |
|---|---|---|
| Breed | | |
| Belgian Tervuren | 62.2 | 25.3, 148.2 |
| German shepherd dog | 43.2 | 30.1, 62.3 |
| Border collie | 8.1 | 3.0, 20.2 |
| Greyhound | 6.4 | 3.0, 13.1 |
| Siberian husky | 4.4 | 2.0, 9.3 |
| Australian shepherd | 3.8 | 1.8, 8.0 |
| Altitude (feet) | | |
| >7000 | 7.8 | 5.8, 10.4 |
| 5001–7000 | 2.9 | 2.3, 3.5 |
| 3001–5000 | 1.0 | — |
| Age (years) | | |
| ≥7 | 0.9 | 0.72, 1.11 |
| 4 to <7 | 2.4 | 2.0, 2.8 |
| <4 | 1.0 | — |

*Modified from Chavkin MJ, Roberts SM, Salman MD, et al. Epidemiologic characteristics of chronic superficial keratitis (pannus) in dogs: A national and regional retrospective study. J Am Vet Med Assoc (in press), with permission.

[†]The odds ratio indicates how many times more likely the variable is to be associated with the disorder.

malities associated with CSK include corneal stromal crystalline cholesterol deposits; nictitating membrane thickening and depigmentation; and corneal ulceration in up to 25, 15, and 9% of CSK cases, respectively. Diagnosis may be facilitated by collection of a tissue scraping from the cornea, nictitating membrane, or nasal canthus for cytologic evaluation. A lymphocytic and plasmacytic inflammatory cell population is typically observed. Chronic CSK must be differentiated from other disorders capable of causing pigmentary and vascular keratitis.

## TREATMENT

Once diagnosed, CSK requires lifelong consistent treatment for lesion regression or control. Cure of this disorder is improbable. The goal of treatment is to prevent visual loss or return as much lost vision as possible. Table 2 lists corticosteroid drugs, dosages, and frequencies of administration for treatment of CSK. The treatment cornerstone consists of topical anti-inflammatory agents such as potent corticosteroids and cyclosporin A (CSA) (Sandimmune, Sandoz Pharmaceutical Corp) either alone or in combination (Jackson et al., 1991; Chavkin et al., 1994). Specific treatment recommendations depend on lesion severity. Initial topical treatment should be administered four times a day. As lesion size decreases, the lowest frequency of treatment that maintains lesion control should be utilized. Potent topical corticosteroids are used for severe cases. Corticosteroid preparations commonly distributed to veterinarians often do not have sufficient corneal anti-inflammatory activity to control the problem. Recommended potent topical corticosteroid eye drops include 1% prednisolone acetate, 1% prednisolone sodium phosphate, and 0.1% dexamethasone. Overtreatment with topical corticosteroids may cause iatrogenic adrenal axis suppression (Roberts et al., 1984). Cyclosporin A is a relative newcomer in the ophthalmic armamentarium and is effective in managing CSK. When used topically in combination with topical corticosteroids, the overall anti-inflammatory effect on the cornea appears enhanced. Thus, combination treatment allows reduced frequency of topical administration and does not sacrifice control of the clinical disease. Many mild cases, especially those with predominantly vascular keratitis, respond to CSA alone. Topical corticosteroids are contraindicated if corneal ulceration is present, but CSA treatment appears relatively safe.

Cyclosporin A, although not commercially available as an ophthalmic preparation as of late 1994, is formulated for topical use by mixing the commercial oral solution (100 mg/ml) with food grade corn oil using a 1:10 or 1:5 ratio to achieve a 1 or 2% solution, respectively. The preparation should be dispensed in amber glass eye dropper bottles. The oral solution is available in 50-ml multiple-use vials and has an unopened bottle expiration date of approximately 12 to 18 months from the date of purchase. Once the bottle is opened, the solution should be used within 2 months. Dilution of CSA with corn oil does not improve the stability and solutions should be discarded after 2 months. Capsules containing either 100 mg or 25 mg CSA are available and typically have an expiration date 18 to 24 months from the date of purchase. However, when this form is used to formulate a dilute solution for topical use, a white precipitate often collects at the bottom of the eye dropper bottle. This may be due to the red iron oxide and titanium dioxide contained in the capsule.

Topical treatment controls CSK in most dogs. Severe corneal vascularization and pigmentation lesions or those responding slowly to topical treatment may be augmented with subconjunctival corticosteroid injections. Periodic injections may be necessary, and a variety of preparations are available with different durations of action (Table 2). If an excessive dose is administered, systemic corticosteroid side effects will occur. If CSK obscures vision or responds poorly to topical and subconjunctival anti-inflammatory agents, $\beta$ irradiation with a strontium-90 medical applicator to deliver an empiric dose of 45 to 75 Gy helps induce lesion regression. After irradiation, much of the superficial corneal pigmentation dissipates in 3 to 6 weeks, leaving only a patchy or punctate pigment distribution. No discomfort is associated with $\beta$ irradiation and subsequent lesion regression. Anti-inflammatory and $\beta$ irradiation treatment will not improve corneal stromal fibrosis or cholesterol deposition. If these latter disorders are extensive and cause visual loss, a superficial keratectomy is indicated, but should be reserved for those cases nonresponsive to other treatment modalities. After a superficial keratectomy, the corneal stroma will not regenerate to a normal thickness and subsequent surgeries will be difficult or detrimental to overall ocular function. $\beta$ Irradiation performed in combination with a superficial keratectomy allows for optimal surgical control.

Cryosurgery with liquid nitrogen (Holmberg, Scheifer, and Parent, 1986) or nitrous oxide is an alternative to an excisional keratectomy. Careful freezing of the cornea results in depigmentation of the superficial cornea. Dogs are uncomfortable for several days after corneal cryosurgery and should be treated with topical antibiotics, atropine, and cyclosporin A. Systemic treatment with a nonsteroidal anti-inflammatory agent such as aspirin is warranted. Corneal depigmentation occurs in 2 to 3 weeks and has a patchy or punctate distribution pattern similar to cases treated with $\beta$ irradiation.

Reexamination of CSK cases is imperative. Initial reevaluation should occur 30 days after starting or changing treatment. As the condition improves, the topical treatment frequency should be gradually decreased to determine the minimal frequency that controls the disorder. Annual reevaluation is important to monitor lesion progression and encourage the owners to continue the lifelong treatment. Lesion severity may worsen during periods of increased environmental irritation, ultraviolet light exposure, or as a result of poor owner treatment compliance. Sporadic treatment allows slow lesion progression and corneal degeneration. A small percentage of CSK cases may eventually de-

***Table 2.*** *Corticosteroid Treatment Options Available for Chronic Superficial Keratitis (Pannus)**

| Route and Potency | Preparation (Generic and Trade Name) | Source | Initial Frequency or Dose and Duration |
|---|---|---|---|
| Topical | | | |
| 1 | Prednisolone acetate 1% suspension | | Two to four times daily |
| | AK-Tate | Akorn | |
| | Econopred Plus | Alcon Laboratories | |
| | Ocu-Pred-A | Ocumed | |
| | Pred Forte | Allergan Pharmaceuticals | |
| | Pred-G | Allergan Pharmaceuticals | |
| | Dexamethasone 0.1% suspension | | Two to four times daily |
| | AK-Trol | Akorn | |
| | Dexacidin | IOLAB Corp. Pharmaceuticals | |
| | Dexasporin | Bausch & Lomb Pharmaceutical | |
| | Maxidex | Allergan Pharmaceuticals | |
| | Maxitrol | Allergan Pharmaceuticals | |
| | Ocu-Trol | Ocumed | |
| 2 | Dexamethasone sodium phosphate 0.1% solution | | Three to six times daily |
| | AK-Dex | Akorn | |
| | Decadron | Merck & Co | |
| | Dexamethasone sodium phosphate | Bausch & Lomb Pharmaceutical | |
| | Prednisolone sodium phosphate 1% solution | | Three to six times daily |
| | AK-Pred | Akorn | |
| | Inflammase Forte | Alcon Laboratories | |
| | Ocu-Pred Forte | Ocumed | |
| | Prednisolone sodium phosphate | Allergan Pharmaceuticals | |
| | Cyclosporin A 1% to 2% | | One to two times daily |
| | Sandimmune | Sandoz Pharmaceuticals | |
| 3 | Isoflupredone 0.1% ointment | | Three to four times daily |
| | Neo-predef | Upjohn | |
| 4 | Flumethasone 0.01% solution | | Three to six times daily |
| | Anaprime† | Syntex Animal Health | |
| | Betamethasone 0.1% solution | | Three to six times daily |
| | Gentocin Durafilm | Schering-Plough Animal Health | |
| 5 | Prednisolone acetate 0.25% ointment | | Four to six times daily |
| | Cetapred | Alcon Laboratories | |
| | Chlorosone | Evsco Pharmaceuticals | |
| 6 | Prednisolone acetate 0.2% ointment | | Four to six times daily |
| | Blephamide | Allergan Pharmaceuticals | |
| | Optisone | Evsco Pharmaceuticals | |
| 7 | Hydrocortisone 1% ointment | | Four to eight times daily |
| | Bacitracin–neomycin–polymyxin B | Pharmaderm | |
| | Neobacimyx-H | Schering-Plough Animal Health | |
| | Trioptic-S | SmithKline Beecham Animal Health | |
| | Vetropolycin HC | Pitman-Moore | |
| Subconjunctival injection | | | |
| 1 | Betamethasone acetate and sodium phosphate (3 mg/ml each) | | 0.2 ml; 4 wk |
| | Celestone Soluspan | Schering Corporation | |
| 2 | Isoflupredone acetate (2 mg/ml each) | | 0.05 ml; 2 wk |
| | Predef 2X | Upjohn | |
| | Triamcinolone acetonide | | 0.1 ml; 2 wk |
| | Vetalog Parenteral | Solvay | |
| | Triamcinolone acetonide injection | Various generic sources | |
| 3 | Methylprednisolone acetate (20 mg/ml) | | |
| | Depo-Medrol | Upjohn | 0.2 ml; 3 wk |
| | Methylprednisolone acetate injection | Various generic sources | |
| 4 | Prednisolone acetate (50 mg/ml) | Various generic sources | 0.5 ml; 24 hr |

*Preparations are listed in order of ocular anti-inflammatory potency from greatest to least.
†This drug is on indefinite backorder; check with the manufacturer regarding availability.

velop corneal degeneration that includes persistent edema, fibrosis, subepithelial bulla formation, and ulceration. These cases are poorly responsive to medical or surgical treatment and salvage procedures such as enucleation may be necessary. This is especially true for dogs living at elevations greater than 6000 feet. Conversely, many cases respond dramatically to treatment and will appear nearly normal for long periods of time with minimal medical care. However, all CSK cases require lifelong management.

## References and Suggested Reading

Austad R and Øen EO: Chronic superficial keratitis (keratitis superficialis chronica) in the dog. I. A review of the literature. J Small Anim Pract 19: 197, 1978.
*A review describing clinical features, pathologic changes, and treatment options of dogs with chronic superficial keratitis.*
Bedford PGC and Longstaffe JA: Corneal pannus (chronic superficial keratitis) in the German shepherd dog. J Small Anim Pract 20:41, 1979.
*A retrospective description of the clinical features, pathologic changes, and response to treatment of 84 German shepherd dogs with chronic superficial keratitis.*
Campbell LH, Okuda HK, Lipton DE, and Reed C: Chronic superficial keratitis in dogs: Detection of cellular hypersensitivity. Am J Vet Res 36:669, 1975.
*An experimental study of clinical chronic superficial keratitis cases, suggesting that cell-mediated immunity may be contributing to the corneal lesions.*
Chavkin MJ, Roberts SM, Salman MD, et al: Epidemiologic characteristics of chronic superficial keratitis (pannus) in dogs: A national and regional retrospective study. J Am Vet Med Assoc 204:1630, 1994.
*A retrospective statistical analysis of the odds ratios associated with chronic superficial keratitis and various associated variables.*
Eichenbaum JD, Lavach JD, Gould DH, et al: Immunohistochemical staining pattern of canine eyes affected with chronic superficial keratitis. Am J Vet Res 47:1952, 1986.
*An experimental study of chronic superficial keratitis indicating that this disease is not due to autoimmunity against epithelial structures, but possible due to alteration in the function of conjunctival-associated lymphoid tissue and Langerhans cells.*
Holmberg DL, Scheifer HB, and Parent J: The cryosurgical treatment of pigmentary keratitis in dogs: an experimental and clinical study. Vet Surg 15:1, 1986.
*A description of an experimental technique and clinical case study using corneal cryosurgery with liquid nitrogen to treat pigmentary keratitis.*
Jackson PA, Kaswan RL, Merideth RE, and Barrett PM: Chronic superficial keratitis in dogs: A placebo-controlled trial of topical cyclosporine treatment. Prog Vet Compar Ophthalmol 1:269, 1991.
*A prospective clinical study demonstrating the effectiveness of topical cyclosporin A as a treatment of chronic superficial keratitis.*
Roberts SM, Lavach JD, Macy DW, and Severin GA: Effect of ophthalmic prednisolone acetate on the canine adrenal gland and hepatic function. Am J Vet Res 45:1711, 1984.
*An experimental study documenting the potential adrenal axis and hepatic carbohydrate metabolic abnormalities as a result of the use of topical prednisolone acetate eye drops.*
Slatter DH, Lavach JD, Severin GA, and Young S: Überreiter's syndrome (chronic superficial keratitis) in dogs in Rocky Mountain area. J Small Anim Pract 18:757, 1977.
*A retrospective study of 463 cases of chronic superficial keratitis in the Rocky Mountain area describing breed, age, and sex variables in addition to lesion distribution, treatment, and syndrome prognosis.*
Stanley RG: Superficial stromal keratitis in the dog. Aust Vet J 65:321, 1988.
*A concise review of chronic superficial keratitis describing medical and surgical treatment, and discussing prognosis, breeding recommendations, and potential sequela.*

# CANINE UVEITIS

## THOMAS J. KERN
*Ithaca, New York*

Inflammation of the iris, ciliary body, and choroid is one of the most uncomfortable and visually destructive conditions to befall the eye. A complex entity, uveitis often presents a mystery to clinicians. The clinical signs may seem nonspecific, even subtle. Recognition and accurate assessment require familiarity and dexterity with intraocular examination techniques. Etiologic diagnoses may be difficult and expensive to discover and confirm. Therapy is often challenging and follow-up often necessarily long term. Associations with systemic diseases are frequent (see *CVT XI*, p 1061). Despite these potentially intimidating characteristics, clinicians can develop an approach to ocular examination and assessment by which uveitis can be consistently recognized and satisfactorily managed.

## CLINICAL SIGNS

Most eyes with uveitis are at least minimally hyperemic. The most common causes of red eyes in dogs include *keratoconjunctivitis, uveitis,* and *glaucoma.* Successful ophthalmic diagnosis requires that the clinician perform a *complete* ocular examination *every time* that one is indicated. Complete ocular examination should include a Schirmer tear test (STT) (if mucoid or mucopurulent discharge is present), conjunctival cytology, fluorescein dye application to the cornea, tonometry, and pupillary dilatation with 1% tropicamide (Tropicacyl, Akorn) prior to funduscopy if intraocular pressure is not elevated in either eye. Evaluation of the external eye and anterior segment should be made using a bright light source in a darkened room and a source of magnification (Optivisor, Donegal). The normally clear ocular media (tear film, cornea, aqueous humor, lens, and vitreous) may be best evaluated using retroillumination from the tapetum through a dilated pupil; significant lesions are usually identified easily as shadows or imperfections in the reflection. Posterior segment evaluation is best performed by indirect ophthalmoscopy, using a bright light source and a 20 diopter or 2.2 indirect condensing lens (Volk). Direct ophthalmoscopy is a less satisfactory alternative, owing to the limitations of viewing small areas of the central fundus under high magnification.

## Anterior Uveitis

The signs of acute iris and ciliary body inflammation include epiphora, ciliary injection, general conjunctival hyperemia, corneal edema, aqueous flare (often with floating inflammatory and pigment cells), miosis, hyphema, dyscoria, anterior vitreous opacity, vision loss, photophobia, and hypotony. Ciliary injection is subtle and almost pathognomonic for uveitis. It appears as either a purple-red flush in the perilimbal sclera or as multiple short radial dark red intrascleral vessels at the limbus. Diffuse conjunctival capillary hyperemia and vessel engorgement often overshadow ciliary injection, which is subtle at best. Ciliary injection may be made more obvious if conjunctival hyperemia is dampened by topical application of very dilute (1:1000) epinephrine or 2.5% phenylephrine (Ak-Dilate Solution 2.5%, Akorn). Intraocular pressure is typically low due to reduced aqueous production and increased outflow.

With chronicity, other signs may predominate. Ciliary neovascularization of the cornea is comprised of deep vessels originating from the limbal ciliary vessels around the complete circumference of the cornea in a "paintbrush" pattern. The cornea may become completely covered by this neovascularization, resembling granulation tissue. Keratic precipitates represent multifocal inflammatory cell aggregations on the ventral endothelium. With death of corneal endothelial cells, permanent diffuse corneal edema results. Anterior, peripheral, and/or posterior synechiae may result in corneal opacities, iridocorneal angle closure with or without iris bombe, and secondary glaucoma. The iris may become atrophic, hyperpigmented, or covered by neovascularization (rubeosis). Focal to diffuse anterior capsular and cortical cataract may develop. If ciliary body atrophy occurs, aqueous production is greatly reduced and phthisis bulbi results. The degree and permanence of vision loss varies with the severity and duration of intraocular inflammation.

## Posterior Uveitis

The signs of acute choroiditis without marked iridocyclitis are often very subtle. Unilateral or bilateral vision loss is rarely detected until choroiditis has caused widespread retinal dysfunction. Retinal edema, degeneration, and often detachment usually result. Active chorioretinitis in the tapetal area appears as areas of reduced reflectivity with indistinct borders; in the nontapetal area, foci of inflammation appear lighter in color than the brown background with indistinct borders. Retinal vessels may appear elevated or deviated from their normal course. Focal to diffuse or complete retinal detachment is common. The degree of vision loss varies with the extent of retinal dysfunction.

Chronic choroiditis is often characterized by retinal detachment with or without disinsertion from the ora ciliaris retinae. Granulomatous lesions give the appearance of solid tissue and are often dark. Inactive nongranulomatous tapetal lesions are frequently hyperreflective and hyperpigmented with distinct borders. Inactive nontapetal lesions may be hyperpigmented or hypopigmented with distinct margins.

Although posterior uveitis may predominate, slight anterior uveitis usually is present, manifest by mild ciliary and conjunctival vessel injection, hypotony, and relative miosis.

## Panuveitis

Concurrent anterior and posterior uveitis commonly occur. If anterior uveitis is severe, examination of the posterior segment may be impeded. Clinicians should entertain the possibility that any anterior uveitis may involve the choroid and retina until proven otherwise.

## ETIOLOGY

The pathophysiology of uveitis is complex, involving mechanisms that trigger, modulate, and promote inflammation. These mechanisms include: (1) replication of organisms within or near the uvea; (2) local immune sensitization to ocular and other antigens; (3) local manifestations of immune complex disease; and (4) alteration of native ocular antigens to increase their antigenicity. Prostaglandins, leukotrienes, histamine, kinins, neutrophils, monocytes, macrophages, eosinophils, basophils, mast cells, lymphocytes, plasma cells, and platelets may all contribute to ocular inflammation (Hakanson and Forrester, 1990). This multifactorial causation and promotion of uveitis may ultimately explain its sometimes intractable and recurrent nature.

The major causes of uveitis in dogs include *infections, nonseptic inflammation, neoplasia and pseudoneoplastic disorders*, and *trauma* (Hakanson and Forrester, 1990; Slatter, 1990).

### Infections

#### BACTERIA

Bacteremia or septicemia from any generalized or localized infections may cause uveitis (e.g., pyometra, prostatitis, neonatal umbilical infections, abscesses, bacterial endocarditis, dental and oral infections, pyelonephritis). *Brucella canis* infection is occasionally manifest as uveitis.

#### SPIROCHETES

Fulminant leptospirosis in dogs is sometimes accompanied by anterior uveitis. In dogs with uveitis but not systemically ill, index of suspicion for this disease should be low; confirmed diagnosis is rare in such instances.

Lyme disease, caused by *Borrelia burgdorferi*, probably causes uveitis in dogs. The frequently presumptive nature of this diagnosis in dogs and the difficulty of confirmation cloud the certainty of this diagnosis. In humans with borreliosis, many ocular disorders have been reported, including uveitis.

### RICKETTSIA

*Ehrlichia canis* and *E. platys* may cause anterior or posterior uveitis; secondary glaucoma, retinal detachment, chorioretinitis, and papilledema have been reported (Martin, 1990). Orbital, conjunctival, uveal, and retinal hemorrhages may develop.

Rocky Mountain spotted fever, caused by *Rickettsia rickettsii*, has produced ocular signs that are similar to but milder than those caused by ehrlichiosis (Martin, 1990).

### VIRUSES

In addition to causing conjunctivitis, keratoconjunctivitis sicca, and optic nerve and central nervous system lesions, canine distemper virus may cause multifocal nongranulomatous chorioretinitis.

Canine adenovirus-1 (CAV-1), the cause of infectious canine hepatitis, has been estimated to cause anterior uveitis in up to 20% of naturally infected dogs; prevalence of uveitis following vaccination with the previously used modified live CAV-1 vaccines was estimated to be 0.4% or less. The iridocyclitis, caused by an immune complex Arthus reaction, occurs 10 to 21 days after infection or first vaccination. Usually unilateral, uveitis is bilateral in up to one quarter of cases. The Afghan and other sight hounds and Siberian huskies may be at increased risk of uveitis as well as serious complications such as secondary glaucoma. In most dogs, the uveitis is sudden in onset and short lived. The most visible lesion is corneal edema caused by endothelial destruction. Prognosis for most affected dogs is good; especially in young dogs, corneal edema usually resolves over several weeks or months (Martin, 1990). Secondary glaucoma is manifest in pups by early buphthalmos, before increased intraocular pressure can be documented. Fortunately, the current widespread use of vaccines substituting CAV-2 for CAV-1 has virtually eliminated postvaccinal reactions of this type.

Neonatal canine herpesvirus infection may cause bilateral panuveitis with keratitis, synechiae, cataract, retinal necrosis and atrophy, retinal dysplasia, and optic neuritis or atrophy (Martin, 1990).

### MYCOSES

The North American systemic mycoses cause granulomatous anterior and posterior uveitis and panuveitis in their endemic areas. Of these, blastomycosis seems most commonly reported. Coccidioidomycosis and cryptococcosis are predominantly posterior segment infections. Histoplasmosis and cryptococcosis seem relatively uncommon in the dog. Systemic infection with other opportunistic fungi may also involve the eye.

### PROTOZOA

Toxoplasmosis causes nongranulomatous multifocal retinochoroiditis, more common in cats than dogs. Anterior uveitis may be present. Ocular leishmaniasis, rare in the United States, may afflict dogs originating from endemic areas of Europe, Africa, Asia, and Central and South America.

### ALGAE

Protothecosis, caused by an algae ubiquitous in soil and water, is rare in dogs but more than 50% of affected animals have granulomatous posterior uveitis or panuveitis (Martin 1990).

### OTHER PARASITES

Ocular invasion by adult *Dirofilaria immitis* or larvae of *Diptera* spp., *Toxocara*, *Baylisascaris*, and others may cause uveitis in dogs.

## Nonseptic Inflammation

In the uveodermatologic syndrome (Vogt-Koyanagi-Harada–like syndrome) dogs develop anterior, posterior, or panuveitis prior to or in association with predominantly facial poliosis, vitiligo, and mucocutaneous ulceration. Arctic dog breeds, including the Akita, husky, and Samoyed, are at increased risk, although dogs of many breeds have become affected. The cause is an acquired, immune-mediated destruction of melanin-containing tissues. Uveitis is rarely associated with other immune-mediated dermatoses.

Lens-associated anterior uveitis commonly develops in association with hypermature cataracts (phacolytic) and following penetrating lens injuries (phacoclastic). The normal ocular tolerance of low levels of circulating lens proteins is breached, inciting a chronic inflammatory response. Typical long-term sequelae of uveitis may be caused by hypermature cataracts; retinal detachment is common. Fulminant lens-associated uveitis sometimes occurs in diabetic dogs with rapidly developing osmotic cataracts. Presumably, sudden leakage of lens protein associated with lens swelling is the cause. Secondary glaucoma is common, due to mechanical iridocorneal angle closure from the intumescent cataractous lens. The panuveitis that may follow lens injury typically is not immediate; rather, it develops 2 to 4 weeks following injury.

In many instances of idiopathic uveitis, immune-mediated inflammation may be responsible but difficult or impossible to prove.

Proliferative keratoconjunctivitis or episclerokeratitis, an unusual nodular inflammatory disorder of the sclera and mucocutaneous junctions with a predilection for collies, rarely infiltrates the iris and ciliary body. Commonly, bilaterally symmetric lesions predominate at the nasal and temporal limbus, appearing as pink nodules.

For unknown reasons, some dogs with hyperlipidemia develop dramatic acute unilateral or bilateral anterior uveitis with lipid aqueous effusion. The anterior chamber contains a lactescent flare that may initially be mistaken for severe corneal edema.

Some dogs with systemic hypertension develop unilateral or bilateral hyphema, uveitis, and vitreous hemorrhage, often with retinal detachment (Davidson, 1992).

## Neoplasia

Primary ocular neoplasia in dogs sometimes causes significant uveitis. Anterior uveal melanomas, epibulbar melanomas, ciliary body adenomas, adenocarcinomas, medulloepitheliomas, and the rare choroidal melanomas are usually identifiable as mass lesions, but may be inapparent if marked inflammation results from their infiltration.

Metastatic or multicentric neoplasia commonly causes uveitis, probably associated with its aggressive and destructive growth. Signs of uveitis commonly mask mass lesions that may be present. Although lymphosarcoma, hemangiosarcoma, and other widely disseminated neoplasms commonly cause uveitis, metastases of any malignant neoplasm may target the uveal tract.

## Pseudoneoplastic and Paraneoplastic Conditions

The ocular form of granulomatous meningoencephalitis includes optic neuritis, peripapillary retinitis, diffuse chorioretinitis, scleritis, retinal detachment and, very rarely, solitary uveitis (Collins and Moore, 1991).

Systemic histiocytosis of Bernese mountain dogs has been associated with blepharoconjunctivitis and anterior uveitis (Collins and Moore, 1991).

## Trauma

Both blunt and perforating trauma may incite uveitis. Blunt trauma may cause shearing injury. Perforating injury may lacerate the lens and/or inoculate bacteria or fungi into the eye.

Reflex neurogenic anterior uveitis frequently results from injury of the ocular adnexa, cornea, and conjunctiva. The ophthalmic and other branches of the trigeminal nerve provide sensation to the eye and periocular tissues; stimulation of these branches often causes an axon reflex within the iris and ciliary body, whereby mild to moderate inflammation is stimulated. Thus, corneal ulceration and adnexal injury often cause secondary anterior uveitis that requires treatment.

## DIAGNOSTIC EVALUATION

In addition to complete ocular examination, diagnostic evaluation of dogs with uveitis should include a detailed specific history (especially regarding travel, vaccination status, and other clinical signs and illnesses) and careful complete physical examination. This may suffice for dogs with mild unilateral uveitis at first presentation. For dogs with moderate, severe, or recurrent unilateral or bilateral uveitis, selective laboratory investigation is warranted in addition. A hemogram, serum biochemistry panel, urinalysis, and serologic tests dictated by geographic location and travel history are recommended. The limitations and presumptions inherent in interpretation of serologic results should be reviewed (see "Oculomycoses," this volume, p 1257, and other articles in Section 4 that describe specific infectious diseases). Despite complete (and costly) diagnostic pursuit, the cause of uveitis often eludes detection, especially initially. This pursuit is justifiable, however, on the premise that if detected, the cause is usually an important one (e.g., a treatable infectious disease or lymphosarcoma).

Aqueous or vitreous paracentesis may be considered for severe uveitis. Such aspirates are most helpful in documenting oculomycosis and diffuse intraocular neoplasia (e.g., lymphosarcoma); vitreous aspirates have higher diagnostic yield than aqueous samples.

If initial diagnostic pursuit is inconclusive, the clinician should be alert for the development of other nonocular clinical signs (e.g., respiratory or gastrointestinal abnormalities, lameness, neurologic signs). Thorough diagnostic work-up of these signs commonly yields the etiology of the uveitis as well.

## THERAPY

The objectives of treatment of uveitis are to: (1) eliminate or specifically treat the cause; (2) reduce inflammation; (3) preserve the pupil; (4) control pain; and (5) prevent or treat secondary glaucoma. Infectious diseases for which there are specific and effective treatments should be treated appropriately while addressing the other objectives (see "Oculomycoses," this volume, p 1257, and other articles in Section 4 that describe specific infectious diseases). Dogs with ocular lymphosarcoma may benefit from chemotherapy.

Ocular inflammation may be treated with topical and systemic corticosteroids and nonsteroidal anti-inflammatory drugs (NSAIDs) well as with systemic immunosuppressants.

## Corticosteroids

Corticosteroids are the foundation of ocular anti-inflammatory therapy. For mild or moderately severe anterior uveitis, topical dexamethasone with (Maxitrol, Alcon) or without (Maxidex, Alcon) antibiotic applied six or more times daily (solution) or four times daily (ointment) may be effective. Topical 1% prednisolone acetate suspension (Econopred, Alcon) penetrates the eye better than other corticosteroids; its use every 4 hr or more frequently is recommended if uveitis is poorly responsive to other topical therapy. If topical treatment alone is incompletely effective, subconjunctival or oral corticosteroid administration may be indicated in addition in conjunction (see "Anti-inflammatory Therapy of the Eye," this volume, p 1218). Oral prednisone or prednisolone (1.1 to 2.2 mg/kg PO every 24 hr or divided every 12 hr) may be administered to effect for 1 or more weeks, then tapered to the lowest effective dose every other day or less. Oral corticosteroid therapy is superior to subconjunctival administration because it may be readily discontinued or modified if ocular or other side effects become serious (e.g., corneal ulceration, exacerbation of uveitis associated with fungal infection).

Corticosteroids administered orally at high doses (1.1 to 2.2 mg/kg/day) are the treatment of choice for generalized posterior uveitis associated with complete or extensive multifocal retinal detachment *if* the possibility of infection is unlikely or has been ruled out.

## Nonsteroidal Anti-inflammatory Drugs

Topical NSAIDs are available and are approved for use in humans for ocular premedication prior to (suprofen [Profenal 1% Sterile Ophthalmic Solution, Alcon Surgical]; flurbiprofen [Ocufen, Allergan Medical Optics]) and after cataract surgery (diclofenac [Voltaren, CIBA Vision Ophthalmics]). They are used up to four times daily commonly for canine cataract surgery patients to prevent and treat associated uveitis. Less effective than corticosteroids, topical NSAIDs may be useful in conjunction with them to treat intractable anterior uveitis or alone in patients at risk when treated with corticosteroids (e.g., diabetic dogs). (NOTE: increased intraocular bleeding tendencies and increased intraocular pressure have been noted in some dogs and humans treated with topical NSAIDs.)

Systemic NSAIDs available for veterinary use include flunixin meglumine (Banamine, Schering-Plough), phenylbutazone (Butazolidin, Geigy), and aspirin. Short-term administration of flunixin meglumine (0.11 to 0.22 mg/kg IV every 24 hr for up to three consecutive treatments) may be effective as adjunctive therapy with topical or systemic corticosteroids for severe anterior or posterior uveitis. Ulcerative gastroenteritis may occur but is more likely if the recommended dosage or frequency is exceeded. (NOTE: flunixin meglumine is not approved for use in dogs and cats.) Phenylbutazone may be used instead of corticosteroids (15 to 22 mg/kg every 8 to 12 hr PO—maximum dose, 800 mg); gastrointestinal ulceration is an important potential complication. Aspirin is much less potent than corticosteroids and other NSAIDs but may be effective when used for mild uveitis or chronically to suppress uveitis recurrence (10 to 25 mg/kg PO every 12 hr).

## Immunosuppressants

Azathioprine (Imuran, Burroughs Wellcome) (2.2 mg/kg PO every 24 hr to 48 hr) may be effective for control of severe uveitis incompletely responsive to corticosteroids or in place of them in patients intolerant to them. As with other immunosuppressants, patients receiving them must be regularly monitored for serious side effects (e.g., leukopenia).

## Mydriatic/Cycloplegic Drugs

Pupil preservation and pain control are achieved by the topical use of 1% atropine to effect (i.e., mydriasis). Relaxation of the ciliary muscle, an effect independent of mydriasis, abolishes ciliary spasm, improving comfort. Anticholinergic drugs alone may not optimally dilate an inflamed iris; concurrent use of topical sympathomimetic drugs (e.g., 2.5% phenylephrine [Ak-Dilate Solution 2.5%, Akorn]) synergistically promotes mydriasis. (NOTE: excessive topical administration of anticholinergics and sympathomimetics may cause systemic and local side effects, including ileus, reduced lacrimation, tachycardia, and epithelial toxicity.) Initial application frequency should be four times daily or less, then reduced to the minimal effective frequency.

## Re-Evaluation

Tonometry should be performed initially, then at every follow-up visit. If pressure is elevated or even in the high normal range, treatment with hyperosmotics, carbonic anhydrase inhibitors, topical β-blockers, and/or topical sympathomimetics should be instituted and maintained (see "Glaucoma," this volume, p 1265). The parasympathomimetic miotic drugs are *contraindicated* for uveitic glaucoma because they intensify the inflammation.

If medical therapy for uveitis fails to preserve vision and comfort and cannot be terminated, limited surgical options are available. For eyes with uveitis of unknown cause, enucleation *with histopathologic examination* should be recommended. For blind painful eyes with uveitis from certain known causes (trauma, lens-associated inflammation, uveodermatologic syndrome), evisceration with silicone prosthesis *may* be recommended with reservation.

## PROGNOSIS

The prognosis for response to therapy and vision preservation depends upon the location, extent, and duration of inflammation; its underlying cause; the occurrence and extent of secondary complication such as glaucoma, cataract, phthisis bulbi, and so forth; and the timeliness and adequacy of treatment. Prognosis is better when inflammation is mild to moderate, rapidly responsive to reasonable therapy, and when the underlying cause is discovered and treatable. Severe or recurrent uveitis typically has a poor long-term prognosis. Prognosis is potentially good for systemic spirochete, rickettsial, and adenoviral infections treated early with specific antibiotic and anti-inflammatory agents and for judiciously treated hyperlipidemic and phacolytic uveitis. Prognosis is guarded to poor for systemic bacterial, protozoal, mycotic, and algal infections, as well as the uveodermatologic syndrome. Prognosis for intraocular neoplasia is grave if metastatic or multicentric. Most primary intraocular neoplasms in the dog are benign; if they cause intractable uveitis, however, enucleation should be recommended.

## References and Suggested Reading

Collins BK and Moore CP: Canine anterior uvea. *In* Gelatt KN (ed): *Veterinary Ophthalmology*, 2nd edition. Philadelphia, Lea & Febiger, 1991, p 357.
   *A comprehensive review of anterior uveal disorders of the dog.*
Davidson MG: Diseases of the anterior uveal tract. *In* Morgan RV (ed): *Handbook of Small Animal Practice*, 2nd edition. New York, Churchill Livingstone, 1992, p 1077.
   *An outline of the developmental, degenerative, inflammatory, and neoplastic conditions of the anterior uvea, their assessment and treatment.*
Hakanson N and Forrester SD: Uveitis in the dog and cat. *In* Millichamp NJ and Dziezyc J (eds): Small animal ophthalmology. *Vet Clin North Am [Small Anim Pract]*. Philadelphia, WB Saunders Co, 1990, p 715.
   *A contemporary review of the causes, signs, and therapy of uveitis in dogs and cats.*
Martin CL: Ocular infections. *In* Greene CE (ed): *Infectious Diseases of the Dog and Cat*. Philadelphia, WB Saunders Co, 1990, p 197.
   *A review of infectious causes of external and intraocular diseases of the dog and cat.*
Slatter D: *Fundamentals of Veterinary Ophthalmology*, 2nd edition. Philadelphia, WB Saunders Co, 1990, p 304.
   *An introduction to the anatomy, physiology, and medical and surgical disorders of the uvea.*
Wilkie DA: Uvea. *In* Birchard SJ and Sherding RG (eds): *Saunders Manual of Small Animal Practice*, Philadelphia, WB Saunders Co, 1994, p 1213.
   *A brief review of uveal disorders of the dog and cat.*

# FELINE UVEITIS

MATTHEW J. CHAVKIN
*Denver, Colorado*

*and* GLENN A. SEVERIN
*Fort Collins, Colorado*

Uveitis is inflammation of the uveal tract (iris, ciliary body, and choroid) of the eye. Anterior uveitis is inflammation of the iris and ciliary body; posterior uveitis is inflammation of the choroid and ciliary body. More specific terms such as iritis, iridocyclitis, pars planitis (ciliary body), choroiditis, and panuveitis (iris, ciliary body, choroid) are also used.

Uveitis is common in cats and potentially may lead to blindness. Approximately 1% of all cats examined at Colorado State University and 6% of cats examined by the Ophthalmology Service have uveitis. The prevalence of uveitis in the general feline population is unknown, but increased age and gender (male) are risk factors. Approximately 50% of cases are bilateral. The insidious nature of the disease and the stoicism of cats makes early diagnosis and treatment of feline uveitis difficult.

## CLINICAL SIGNS

The blood-ocular barriers are tight junctions between nonpigmented ciliary body epithelial cells, retinal pigment epithelial (RPE) cells, and vascular endothelial cells in the iris and retina. Uveitis begins with local tissue injury that compromises the blood-ocular barrier. Plasma proteins and cells normally excluded from the aqueous humor accumulate to produce a cloudy anterior chamber known as aqueous flare (Table 1). A sharply focused bright light directed through aqueous flare will be scattered by the suspended particles (Tyndall effect), producing a track of light in the normally clear anterior chamber. Keratic precipitates are focal accumulations of inflammatory cells and protein on the corneal endothelium. Gravitation of inflammatory cells to the ventral anterior chamber is termed hypopyon.

Acute anterior uveal inflammation is painful as evidenced by blepharospasm, photophobia, excessive lacrimation, and globe retraction (enophthalmos) with passive and active third eyelid protrusion. Chronic an-

***Table 1.*** *Clinical Signs of Feline Uveitis*

| Anterior Segment | Posterior Segment | Sequelae |
|---|---|---|
| Aqueous flare | Vitreal infiltrate | Synechiae |
| Hypopyon | Chorioretinitis | Glaucoma |
| Keratic precipitates | Retinal hemorrhage | Lens luxation |
| Miosis | Retinal detachment | Cataract |
| Rubeosis iridis | | Blindness |
| Iris thickening | | |
| Corneal edema | | |
| Ciliary flush | | |
| Conjunctival/episcleral hyperemia | | |
| Low intraocular pressure | | |

terior uveitis is usually less painful. Deep perilimbal blood vessels invade the cornea (ciliary flush), leak fluid into the stroma, and produce corneal edema. Alternatively, diffuse corneal edema may result from corneal endothelial dysfunction induced by inflammatory mediators present in the aqueous humor. Decreased aqueous humor production or increased uveoscleral outflow causes low intraocular pressure. Conjunctival and episcleral vessels may be engorged.

Posterior uveitis is usually accompanied by concurrent retinal and anterior uveal involvement. Active chorioretinitis is characterized by cellular infiltration and edema and appears as light-absorbing grayish foci on ophthalmoscopy. Altered RPE and retinal vascular permeability produces retinal edema and detachment, perivascular cuffing, and hemorrhage. Inactive chorioretinitis appears as altered tapetal coloration, RPE hyperpigmentation or hypopigmentation, and tapetal hyperreflectivity caused by retinal thinning.

Several sequelae of feline uveitis that can lead to blindness occur commonly. The iris may adhere to the cornea (anterior synechia) or lens (posterior synechia) with subsequent pupillary distortion or occlusion. Secondary glaucoma occurs after obliteration of the trabecular meshwork by preiridal fibrovascular membranes (rubeosis iridis), iridoscleral adhesion, or inflammatory cell infiltration. Altered lens metabolism produces cataract, and zonular rupture causes lens luxation.

## ETIOLOGY AND DIAGNOSIS

Uveitis may result from exogenous or endogenous causes (Table 2) (Nasisse, 1991). Exogenous causes (e.g., ocular trauma and corneal ulceration) arise outside the eye and are easily diagnosed with a complete history and examination. Endogenous causes arise within the eye or may be manifestations of systemic diseases. For this reason, determination of the underlying etiology of endogenous uveitis requires evaluation for systemic infectious and neoplastic conditions that have known ocular tropism. Additionally, intermittent bacterial antigen or toxin release from isolated chronic infections (e.g., pyelonephritis) may induce uveitis. Histopathologic studies suggest that the majority of feline uveitis cases are idiopathic (Peiffer and Wilcock, 1991). However, recent serologic studies indicate that infectious etiologies (especially toxoplasmosis) may be more important considerations than previously suspected (Chavkin et al., 1992).

**Table 2.**  *Conditions Associated With Feline Uveitis*

| Exogenous | Endogenous |
| --- | --- |
| Trauma | Feline infectious peritonitis |
| Corneal ulcer | *Toxoplasma gondii* |
| Perforating wound | Feline immunodeficiency virus associated |
| | Various mycoses |
| | Neoplasia (especially lymphoma) |
| | Lens rupture |
| | Idiopathic |

## Feline Infectious Peritonitis

The coronavirus feline infectious peritonitis (FIP) causes systemic vasculitis often manifested as uveitis. Antigen-antibody complexes are deposited perivascularly in the uvea, where they are chemotactic for neutrophils and macrophages. The ensuing pyogranulomatous perivasculitis appears as nonspecific anterior segment changes such as aqueous flare, hypopyon, and keratic precipitates. In the posterior segment, retinal perivascular exudates ("cuffing") precede choroidal exudation and retinal detachment.

A diagnosis of FIP is supported by the presence of characteristic polysystemic signs and laboratory test results. Lymphopenia and polyclonal hyperglobulinemia are common. Current serologic tests cannot distinguish infection with the FIP coronavirus from the relatively benign feline enteric coronavirus. Although many cats with FIP have high coronaviral antibody titers (>1:1600), some cats with FIP have negative coronaviral antibody titers. Thus, histopathologic examination of affected organs is often necessary to confirm FIP. Glucocorticoids and cytotoxic agents have been used to suppress the severe immune-mediated systemic signs of FIP, but long-term prognosis is grave.

## Feline Immunodeficiency Virus

The feline immunodeficiency virus (FIV) is associated with anterior uveitis in cats (English et al., 1990). Although the pathogenesis of FIV-induced uveitis is unknown and direct causation has not been conclusively proven, some FIV-seropositive cats with uveitis have no other apparent cause for their disease. Ocular lesions are nonspecific and include aqueous flare, iridal hyperemia, posterior synechiae, and cataracts. Pars planitis was present in nearly half of the reported cases. Topical glucocorticoids are administered to control inflammation, but systemic glucocorticoids should not be used in a potentially immunocompromised patient. Other opportunistic infections including *Toxoplasma gondii* may cause clinical disease in FIV infected cats.

## Systemic Mycoses

Systemic fungal infections capable of ocular involvement include the regionally restricted *Blastomyces dermatitidis*, *Coccidioides immitis*, *Histoplasma capsulatum*, and the ubiquitous *Cryptococcus neoformans*. These environmentally derived fungi initially colonize the respiratory tract and spread hematogenously with a potential for uveal infiltration. Posterior segment changes including granulomatous chorioretinitis predominate, although anterior segment inflammation also occurs. Positive serologic test results document exposure. Diagnosis is confirmed by identification of organisms in cytologic preparations of aqueous humor, vitreous humor, cerebrospinal fluid, lymph node, or bone marrow aspirates. Early systemic antifungal treatment is indicated (see "Oculomycoses," this volume, p 1257 for specific antifungal treatment).

## Toxoplasmosis

*Toxoplasma gondii* is an obligate intracellular protozoan parasite that replicates in all tissues of vertebrates, including the eye. Ocular disease due to toxoplasmosis often occurs without polysystemic signs and is associated with either recent infection, or more commonly, reactivation of a latent infection.

The mechanism by which *T. gondii* causes uveitis in cats is poorly understood. It is only rarely the result of intraocular replication with rupture of infected cells in the uvea and retina. Indirect immunologic phenomena are more important. *Toxoplasma gondii*–specific antigens and *T. gondii*–containing immune complexes are present in the bloodstream of cats for years after primary infection. Uveal immune complex deposition may incite a type-III hypersensitivity reaction, and circulating antigen may stimulate *T. gondii*–specific intraocular lymphocytes to induce inflammation. Nonspecific anterior and posterior segment disease may occur. Lens luxation and glaucoma are common in cats with toxoplasmosis.

The diagnosis of *Toxoplasma*-induced uveitis is complicated by the high seroprevalence of *T. gondii* infection in healthy cats and the absence of specific ocular or systemic signs. The presence in the serum of *T. gondii*–specific immunoglobulin M (IgM), antigen, increasing sequential immunoglobulin G (IgG) titer, or immune complexes without immunoglobulins is supportive of recent or active infection. While cats with uveitis are more likely to have *T. gondii*–specific IgM, IgG, antigen, or immune complexes in the serum than healthy cats, such generalizations are not helpful in the diagnosis of an individual cat with uveitis. *Toxoplasma gondii*–specific antibodies are detectable in the aqueous humor of many cats with uveitis (Lappin et al., 1992). A Goldman-Witmer coefficient (C-value) is calculated to distinguish intraocularly produced antibody from antibody that leaked from the serum into the aqueous humor through a blood-aqueous barrier compromised by any cause of uveitis.* For each immunoglobulin class, the ratio of *T. gondii*–specific immunoglobulin in serum (S) and aqueous humor (A) is compared to the total immunoglobulin concentration in the serum (S) and aqueous humor (A):

IgM C-value = *T. gondii* IgM-A/S X total IgM-S/A

IgG C-value = *T. gondii* IgG-A/S X total IgG-S/A

A C-value less than 1 indicates antibody leakage; a C-value 1 to 8 suggests intraocular antibody production; and a C-value greater than 8 is definitive evidence of intraocular antibody production. A C-value greater than 1 in a clinically affected cat appears to support a diagnosis of *Toxoplasma*-induced uveitis.

*Colorado State University Diagnostic Laboratory, Fort Collins, CO 80523, (303) 491–1281.

The diagnosis of *Toxoplasma*-induced uveitis is supported by the exclusion of other likely etiologies, aqueous humor or serologic evidence of recent or active infection, and response to an anti-*Toxoplasma* drug. Most cats with uveitis with humorally produced and especially intraocularly produced *T. gondii*–specific antibody have a significant reduction in inflammation after treatment with an anti-*Toxoplasma* antibiotic, clindamycin HCl (Antirobe, Upjohn) at 12.5 mg/kg PO every 12 hr for 21 days. Since clindamycin only destroys actively replicating organisms, post-treatment toxoplasmosis is possible. A reduction in ocular inflammation due to ocular and nonocular *T. gondii* replication is anticipated with clindamycin therapy. Cats with suspected *Toxoplasma*-induced uveitis should also be treated with topical and systemic glucocorticoids to suppress the immune-mediated components of this infectious disease and to help prevent secondary glaucoma and lens luxation (also see "Feline Toxoplasmosis," this volume, p 309).

## Neoplasia

Any metastatic neoplasm can involve the eye, but lymphoma is the most common type to do so. Although many dogs with lymphoma have ocular lesions, ocular involvement in feline lymphoma is uncommon. Ocular disease is referable to neoplastic uveal infiltration. The few reported cases had locally extensive iris masses that invaded the trabecular meshwork and distorted the pupil with and without detectable systemic lymphoma. Diagnosis is based upon identification of characteristic neoplastic lymphocytes on cytologic examination of aqueous humor, vitreous humor, or lymph node aspirate. Histopathologic examination of enucleated globes or other involved organs may be necessary. Cats with lymphoma may or may not have serologic evidence of feline leukemia virus infection. Feline ocular lymphoma should be assumed to be a manifestation of systemic lymphoma and treated accordingly.

## DIAGNOSTIC PROCEDURES

Every case of nontraumatic feline uveitis requires a systemic evaluation that includes a complete blood count, serum chemistry profile, and urinalysis (Table 3). Serologic and aqueous humor immunoglobulin and antigen assays for infectious agents are often helpful in identifying an etiologic diagnosis. However, serologic

**Table 3.** *Diagnostic Tests in Endogenous Feline Uveitis*

Complete blood count
Serum chemistry profile
Urinalysis
Serologic titers (*T. gondii*, FIV, FeLV, FIP, mycoses)
Aqueous paracentesis (cytology, immunoglobulin assays)
Vitreous paracentesis (cytology)
Ocular ultrasonography

evidence of coronavirus, retrovirus, *T. gondii*, or mycotic infection does not indicate a definitive diagnosis.

## Aqueous Paracentesis

Collection of aqueous humor is indicated for the diagnosis of endogenous uveitis with anterior segment involvement (Fig 1). The patient must be anesthetized; intravenous administration of ketamine (Ketaset, Fort Dodge Laboratories, 2 to 4 mg/kg) and diazepam (Lederle, 0.1 to 0.2 mg/kg) provides an adequate duration of sedation. Accumulated debris is irrigated from the conjunctival sac with 0.2% povidone-iodine solution (Betadine, Purdue Frederick). The conjunctiva 2 mm from the temporal limbus is grasped with a fine-toothed thumb forceps to immobilize the globe. A 27-gauge needle attached to a 1-ml syringe is directed subconjunctivally 4 to 5 mm, prior to penetrating the anterior chamber at the temporal limbus. Care is taken not to traumatize the corneal endothelium, iris, or lens. The feline anterior chamber contains 0.6 to 0.9 ml of aqueous humor; 0.2 to 0.3 ml may be safely withdrawn. Rapid and excessive ocular decompression will aggravate the temporary breakdown of the blood-aqueous barrier induced by paracentesis and may produce retinal detachment in an eye with extensive choroidal inflammation. Aqueous humor will leak subconjunctivally from the limbal puncture for several minutes; the an-

terior chamber will reform within 60 min. Hyphema that lasts 24 to 36 hr occurs commonly after aqueous humor collection from eyes with rubeosis iridis. Aqueous humor samples may be examined cytologically for neoplastic cells and infectious agents, cultured, and analyzed for specific immunoglobulins and antigens. Samples not immediately analyzed should be refrigerated in a 2-ml ethylenediaminetetraacetic acid (EDTA) tube.

## TREATMENT

The treatment of feline uveitis is directed toward eliminating the inciting cause. Additionally, anti-inflammatory therapy is instituted to suppress intraocular inflammation and minimize the potential for blinding sequelae.

### Corticosteroids

Corticosteroids remain the backbone of uveitis treatment. Primary beneficial effects include accelerated reestablishment of the blood-ocular barriers, inhibition of leukocyte chemotaxis and pro-inflammatory mediator release, inhibition of fibroblast formation and function, and inhibition of eicosanoid production (prostaglandins and leukotrienes). Interference with host defenses warrants judicious use of corticosteroids in potentially immunocompromised patients (e.g., FIV, FeLV-infected) and in cases with an infectious etiology (e.g., mycotic). Systemic corticosteroids are beneficial in *Toxoplasma*-induced uveitis when used concurrently with an anti-*Toxoplasma* drug, and at standard doses will not lead to oocyst shedding or fulminant toxoplasmosis.

In general, topical preparations containing 1% prednisolone (e.g., 1% Econopred Plus, Alcon) or 0.1% dexamethasone (e.g., Maxidex, Alcon) will suppress anterior segment inflammation. Treatment efficacy is enhanced by frequent instillation (every 2 to 3 hr) and may be augmented by subconjunctival injection of a repositol corticosteroid formulation (e.g., 4 mg triamcinolone acetonide, [Kenalog-40, Westwood Squibb]). Prednisolone (1.1 to 2.2 mg/kg every 12 hr) is indicated in cases that are severe or involve the posterior segment (see "Anti-inflammatory Therapy of the Eye," this volume, p 1218).

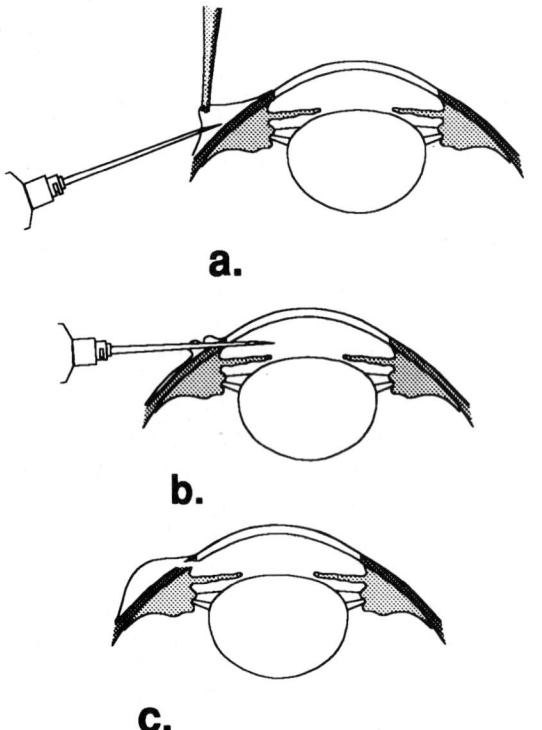

**a.**

**b.**

**c.**

**Figure 1.** Aqueous paracentesis. *A,* A 25- to 27-gauge needle is advanced subconjunctivally 4 mm to the limbus. *B,* The needle is inserted parallel to the iris and 0.2 ml of aqueous humor is slowly aspirated. *C,* Aqueous humor may leak subconjunctivally for 24 to 48 hr.

### Cycloplegics

Topical 1% atropine may be instilled every 12 to 24 hr to control parasympathetically mediated painful ciliary muscle spasm during the acute phase of disease. Cats may salivate profusely after administration. Cycloplegics should be used with caution, given their potential to compromise aqueous humor outflow.

## Glaucoma Therapy

When uveitis is complicated by elevated intraocular pressure (>30 mm Hg), therapy is indicated. Methazolamide (Neptazane, Storz Ophthalmic Pharmaceuticals), a carbonic anhydrase inhibitor, may be given at 2.2 to 4.4 mg/kg every 12 hr PO. The most common side effects are anorexia and lethargy. A topical $\beta$-blocker, 0.5% timolol maleate (Timoptic, Merck Sharp & Dohme) or 0.1% dipivefrin HCl (Propine, Allergan America) may be instilled twice daily. Blind painful eyes that do not respond to medical treatment should be enucleated.

## References and Suggested Reading

Chavkin MJ, Lappin MR, Powell CC, et al: Seroepidemiologic and clinical observations of 93 cases of uveitis in cats. Prog Vet Compar Ophthalmol 2:29, 1992.
  *A retrospective study describing the serologic prevalence of selected infectious diseases in feline uveitis and the treatment response of* T. gondii–*seropositive cats.*
Davidson MG, Nasisse MP, English RV, et al: Feline anterior uveitis: a study of 53 cases. J Am Anim Hosp Assoc 27:77, 1991.
  *A retrospective study detailing clinical, clinicopathologic, serologic, and histopathologic findings in feline uveitis.*
English RV, Davidson MG, Nasisse MP, et al: Intraocular disease associated with feline immunodeficiency virus infection in cats. J Am Vet Med Asoc 196:1116, 1990.
  *A detailed description of ophthalmic lesions in a series of FIV-infected cats.*
Gelatt KN: Ophthalmic examination and diagnostic procedures. In Gelatt KN (ed): Veterinary Ophthalmology. Philadelphia, Lea & Febiger, 1991, p 195.
  *A comprehensive text detailing ophthalmic examination and diagnostic procedures for veterinary patients.*
Lappin MR, Roberts SM, Davidson MG, et al: Enzyme-linked immunosorbent assays for the detection of Toxoplasma gondii–specific antibodies and antigens in the aqueous humor of cats. J Am Vet Med Assoc 201:1010, 1992.
  *A retrospective study illustrating the use of Goldman-Witmer C-values in the diagnosis of* Toxoplasma-*induced uveitis.*
Nasisse MP: Feline ophthalmology. In Gelatt KN (ed): Veterinary Ophthalmology. Philadelphia, Lea & Febiger, 1991, p 547.
  *A well-referenced review of manifestations, diagnosis, and treatment of feline uveitis.*
Peiffer RL and Wilcock BP: Histopathologic study of uveitis in cats: 139 cases (1978–1988). J Am Vet Med Assoc 198:135, 1991.
  *An extensive histopathologic description of feline uveitis.*

# OCULOMYCOSIS

## DANIEL A. WARD
### Knoxville, Tennessee

Oculomycosis refers to fungal infection of the eye, adnexa, orbit, or periorbital tissues. This article focuses on ocular infections resulting from dissemination of systemic ("deep") mycoses, as they account for the vast majority of oculomycoses. Mycotic keratitis resulting from direct inoculation of the cornea from the environment occurs rarely in dogs and cats, and will be discussed briefly.

## SYSTEMIC MYCOSES

### Epidemiology, Pathogenesis, and Clinical Findings

Blastomycosis, coccidioidomycosis, cryptococcosis, and histoplasmosis cause over 95% of all systemic mycoses with ocular involvement. Less commonly, aspergillosis, candidiasis, geotrichosis, paecilomycosis, penicilliosis, protothecosis,° pseudallescheriasis, pythiosis, and sporotrichosis invade the eye. *Blastomyces*, *Coccidioides*, and *Histoplasma* have distinct geographic distributions based on their respective environmental requirements for survival (Table 1). While dogs and cats can be infected with any of these organisms, blastomycosis and coccidioidomycosis occur predominately in dogs, and cryptococcosis occurs primarily in cats. Histoplasmosis is somewhat more common in dogs than in cats. The principal route of infection for all four of these fungi is inhalation. Initially, *Blastomyces*, *Coccidioides*, and *Histoplasma* infect the lungs, causing pneumonia. *Cryptococcus* usually lodges in the upper airways, causing nasal granulomas and swelling over the bridge of the nose. It is suspected that primary pulmonary disease is sometimes self-limiting and does not disseminate. Veterinary care is only sought for animals that have overt respiratory disease or dissemination beyond the pulmonary system. Dissemination is lymphohematogenous, although nasal cryptococcosis may invade through the cribriform plate, producing meningitis and optic neuritis. Systemic fungi may cause a local infection following entry into a skin wound, but these cases are rare and usually don't disseminate.

While animals with disseminated mycoses may be seen because of ocular disease, history or physical examination will usually identify nonocular infection as well (Table 2). Pulmonary blastomycosis, coccidioidomycosis, and histoplasmosis usually cause dyspnea, harsh lung sounds, and occasionally coughing. Radio-

---

°The causative agents of protothecosis, *Prototheca zopfii* and *Prototheca wickerhamii*, are actually blue-green algae. Protothecosis is included in this discussion because its clinical behavior and ocular manifestations are essentially identical to those of the fungi discussed.

**Table 1.** *Characteristics of Organisms Causing Systemic Mycoses*

| Mycosis | Causative Agent | Type of Fungus | Geographic Distribution | Reservoir |
|---|---|---|---|---|
| Blastomycosis | *Blastomyces dermatitidis* | Dimorphic fungus | Mississippi, Missouri, and Ohio river valleys, mid-Atlantic states | Soil |
| Coccidioidomycosis | *Cocidioides immitis* | Dimorphic fungus | Southwestern United States | Soil |
| Cryptococcosis | *Cryptococcus neoformans* | Yeast-like fungus | None | Soil, pigeon excreta |
| Histoplasmosis | *Histoplasma capsulatum* | Dimorphic fungus | Mississippi, Missouri, and Ohio river valleys | Soil, avian and bat excreta |

graphically, these pneumonias produce a nodular interstitial pattern with varying degrees of hilar lymphadenopathy. Fungi typically produce draining skin lesions, although cats with cutaneous cryptococcosis may have nonulcerated, erythematous nodules on the face and trunk. Fungal osteomyelitis causes lameness, with or without draining tracts. Cryptococcosis of the central nervous system causes meningitis, seizures, and ataxia. Histoplasmosis in dogs frequently affects the intestinal tract, resulting in tenesmus, large- or small-bowel diarrhea, and hematochezia.

## Ocular Disease

Ocular manifestations of all disseminated mycoses are similar and most frequently include anterior uveitis, posterior uveitis (i.e., chorioretinitis), endophthalmitis (i.e., concurrent anterior and posterior uveitis), and optic neuritis. Most animals have unilateral involvement. Secondary glaucoma accompanies anterior uveitis and endophthalmitis in a large percentage of cases. Less frequent manifestations include keratitis, conjunctivitis, and orbital cellulitis.

Anterior uveitis is the most common ocular disorder associated with systemic mycosis, and is characterized by photophobia, aqueous flare, injected episcleral and conjunctival vessels, miosis, and (in the early stages) subnormal intraocular pressure. Keratic precipitates, corneal edema, hyphema, and intraocular fibrin are sometimes present. Secondary keratitis may develop with chronicity, resulting in corneal neovascularization, pigmentation, and granulation tissue. Iris adhesions can

**Table 2.** *Sites of Infection of Systemic Mycoses*

| Mycosis | Most Common Nonocular Sites of Infection |
|---|---|
| Blastomycosis | Lung, skin, bone, lymph nodes |
| Coccidioidomycosis | Lung, bone, skin, pericardium |
| Cryptococcosis | *Cat:* Upper respiratory tract, skin, CNS<br>*Dog:* CNS, skin, lymph nodes |
| Histoplasmosis | *Cat:* Lung, bone<br>*Dog:* Lung, gastrointestinal tract |

occur in chronic cases, disrupting aqueous humor flow and leading to elevated intraocular pressure (i.e., secondary glaucoma). The presenting complaint is ocular pain and redness. If secondary glaucoma has developed, the presenting complaint is an enlarged or cloudy eye.

Chorioretinal inflammation appears as dull, poorly demarcated, grayish white masses beneath the retina. These "subretinal granulomas" usually contain fungal organisms and a pyogranulomatous inflammatory reaction. Large retinal detachments caused by extensive exudation between the neurosensory retina and retinal pigment epithelium are common. In some cases, the retinal vessels appear engorged and tortuous. As chorioretinitis presents no outwardly visible signs, owners seek veterinary care only when the retinal disease progresses to blindness. Therefore, if chorioretinitis is the only ocular change present, the owner will probably not notice it unless it is extensive and bilateral.

Endophthalmitis indicates that both anterior uveitis and chorioretinitis are present. Since severe anterior uveitis produces cloudy ocular media, the posterior segment may not be visible. Thus, many cases diagnosed as anterior uveitis *in vivo* are designated endophthalmitis on histopathology.

Optic neuritis occurs secondary to hematogenous dissemination of fungal organisms or local invasion along the meningeal covering of the optic nerve. The latter mechanism occurs most frequently in cryptococcosis. Optic neuritis may occur singly or in conjunction with anterior uveitis, chorioretinitis, or endophthalmitis. If the rostral portion of the optic nerve is involved the optic disk will appear swollen and hyperemic. If only the middle or caudal portions are inflamed (i.e., retrobulbar optic neuritis), the optic disk will appear normal. When optic neuritis is the only lesion present, the presenting complaint is sudden blindness. As with chorioretinitis, if anterior uveitis is also present, haziness of the cornea and aqueous humor may preclude detection of optic neuritis.

Keratitis occurs most frequently secondary to chronic anterior uveitis or glaucoma. Actual corneal infection and granulomatous keratitis from disseminated cryptococcosis sometimes occurs in dogs. Similarly, conjunctivitis is usually present due to extension of uveal tract inflammation. Occasionally, however, conjunctivitis and large subconjunctival granulomas are seen in the absence of intraocular disease. Infection of retrobulbar tissues is seen on rare occasions with all of

**Table 3.** *Cytologic Characteristics of Organisms Causing Systemic Mycoses*

| Organism | Cytologic Characteristics |
|---|---|
| *Blastomyces dermatitidis* | 5–30 μm diameter; broad-based budding; thick (0.5–0.75 μm), refractile, double-contoured capsule; organisms almost never found phagocytized within leukocytes |
| *Coccidioides immitis* | 25–100 μm diameter spherules containing numerous 5–7 μm endospores; birefringent capsule |
| *Cryptococcus neoformans* | 3.5–7 μm diameter yeast; narrow-based budding; very thick capsule (up to 30 μm) |
| *Histoplasma capsulatum* | 2–4 μm diameter; thin capsule; organisms usually found phagocytized within macrophages, sometimes neutrophils |

the oculomycoses, resulting in varying degrees of exophthalmia.

## Diagnosis

The diagnosis of systemic fungal infection is best made by finding the organism on cytology or histopathology (Table 3). Common sites for collection of cytologic samples include enlarged lymph nodes, nodular or draining skin lesions, osseous lesions and, in animals with chorioretinitis, vitreous humor. Transtracheal washes may identify organisms in animals without more accessible lesions. Bone marrow aspirates or rectal scrapings may yield organisms in animals with histoplasmosis. Aqueous humor paracentesis samples *rarely* yield organisms, even in cases with severe anterior uveitis. Fungal culture is also accurate, but caution must be exercised with most organisms to prevent infection of laboratory personnel. A variety of serodiagnostic tests are available and serve as useful adjuncts to cytology (Table 4). Clinical signs and serologic tests con-

sistent with systemic mycotic infection warrant treatment even if cytology does not yield a definitive diagnosis. In areas endemic for blastomycosis, characteristic nodular interstitial lung changes are adequate evidence of the disease if clinical signs suggest a high index of suspicion.

## Treatment

Therapy for oculomycosis associated with disseminated fungal disease should address both the systemic infection and the ocular disease present. The most successful therapies for systemic infection employ ketoconazole (Nizoral, Janssen), itraconazole (Sporanox, Janssen), fluconazole (Diflucan, Roerig), amphotericin B (Fungizone, Apothecon), or combinations thereof (details of systemic therapy are discussed in "Antimycotic Drug Therapy," this volume, p 327).

### OCULAR THERAPY

Symptomatic treatment of anterior uveitis is important to prevent the development of intraocular adhesions and secondary glaucoma. Topical corticosteroids are applied every 3 to 4 hours. Prednisolone acetate is the best choice due to its superior ocular penetrability, but dexamethasone alcohol or dexamethasone sodium phosphate are also effective. If corneal ulceration is present, topical corticosteroids are contraindicated, and should be replaced with topical nonsteroidal antiinflammatory drugs (NSAIDs). Flurbiprofen (Ocufen, Allergan Pharmaceuticals) and diclofenac (Voltaren, CIBA Vision Ophthalmics) are the most effective topical NSAIDs in dogs, with suprofen (Profenal, Alcon Surgical) being somewhat less effective. In dogs, frequency of administration is the same as corticosteroids,

**Table 4.** *Serodiagnostics for Systemic Mycoses*

| Mycosis | Test | Quantitation | Interpretation | Source |
|---|---|---|---|---|
| Blastomycosis | Agar gel immunodiffusion | Nonquantitative | Pos result confirms exposure and strongly suggests active infection. | (1,2) |
| Coccidioidomycosis | CF titer (3) | ≤1:4 Neg<br>1:8 Suspicious<br>≥1:16 Pos | Neg PPT and CF: No infection, early disease, or fulminating disease in immunocompromised patient. Pos PPT, Neg CF: Exposure, subclinical infection, or early disease. Pos PPT and CF: Active disease. Neg PPT, Pos CF: Past exposure or disease, late infection. | (2,4) |
|  | PPT test | Nonquantitative |  |  |
| Cryptococcosis | Cryptococcal antigen titer | ≥1:1 Pos | Pos result confirms active infection. | (2,5) |
| Histoplasmosis | No reliable serodiagnostic test available |  |  |  |

1. Many veterinary diagnostic laboratories offer this test.
2. Kits for in-office use available from Meridian Diagnostics, Inc, Cincinnati OH 45244, (800)543-1980, (513)271-3700 (in Ohio).
3. Approximately 25% of dogs have anticomplementary factors that will render the CF titer inaccurate.
4. Southwest Veterinary Diagnostics, Inc, 13633 North Cave Creek Rd, Phoenix AZ 85022, (602)971-4110, (602)275-7460.
5. Department of Environmental Practice, Virology Lab, 2407 River Dr, Room A239, Knoxville TN 37996-4500.
Abbreviations: Pos = positive, Neg = negative, CF = complement fixation, PPT = precipitin.

but these drugs must be used with caution in cats, since systemic absorption may be sufficient to result in NSAID toxicitiy. Short-term administration (no more than 24 hr) at 3 to 6 hr intervals should be safe, but frequency should be decreased after that. One per cent atropine sulfate should be used in an attempt to dilate the pupil and relieve painful ciliary spasm. However, if the inflammation is severe or adhesions are present, dilation may not occur.

There is no good anti-inflammatory therapy for chorioretinal lesions, since topical anti-inflammatories do not reach the posterior segment in appreciable concentrations and systemic corticosteroids are contraindicated. Systemic NSAIDs such as aspirin or flunixin meglumine (Banamine, Schering) may be used but are of limited benefit. Animals receiving systemic NSAIDs should be monitored closely for signs of toxicity.

Secondary glaucoma is treated with osmotic diuretics, oral carbonic anhydrase inhibitors, and topical beta blockers (see "Glaucoma," in this volume, p 1265). Topical miotics are not recommended in these cases, since they predispose to pupillary block and may exacerbate intraocular pressure elevation.

Enucleation should be considered in many animals with systemic mycoses. The eye is particularly difficult to clear of fungal organisms using most treatment protocols, and therefore may serve as a nidus of reinfection in animals that have otherwise responded to systemic therapy. Anterior uveitis associated with fungal infections often persists following successful systemic therapy, underscoring the immunologic component of the inflammation that probably exists in these cases. This inflammation is often unresponsive to the anti-inflammatory therapy described above, and may warrant enucleation. Eyes that are permanently blind and painful from secondary glaucoma should always be enucleated as soon as the animal's systemic condition will allow general anesthesia. If focal chorioretinitis is the only ocular change present, enucleation can be delayed and the lesions monitored at weekly intervals. These lesions may resolve with systemic therapy (particularly itraconazole therapy for blastomycosis), resulting in retinal scars but an otherwise healthy, visual eye. However, expansion of these lesions or the appearance of new lesions justifies enucleation.

## Prognosis

The prognosis for life in animals with systemic mycoses depends on the organism involved, the species of animal, and the degree of dissemination. Blastomycosis in dogs carries a favorable prognosis, with approximately 80% of itraconazole-treated cases recovering fully. The prognosis in cats is more difficult to gauge due to the limited number of cases reported, but it appears to be good. The percentage of dogs recovering from coccidioidomycosis is somewhat difficult to assess since long-term relapses (>1 year) are common, but overall recovery is estimated at about 60%. A larger number may be controlled with maintenance antifungal

therapy. As with blastomycosis, predicting prognosis in cats is hampered by the low infection rate in that species. Histoplasmosis in cats responds well to treatment. Histoplasmosis in dogs, especially the intestinal form, responds less favorably. Cryptococcosis in cats often responds well to treatment, especially if the skin is the only extrapulmonary site affected. In dogs, successful therapy is less common, especially if central nervous system disease is present.

The ocular prognosis depends on the degree of involvement at the time of presentation. Resolution of focal chorioretinal lesions results in "blind spots" due to irreparable photoreceptor destruction, but functional vision may be maintained if enough of the retina is uninvolved. Prompt institution of systemic therapy is critical in preventing enlargement of existing chorioretinal lesions and development of new ones. Visual retention in dogs with blastomycosis is more likely in dogs treated with itraconazole than in dogs treated with amphotericin B or amphotericin B plus ketoconazole. Animals with extensive chorioretinitis are unlikely to regain vision, especially if large areas of retinal detachment are present. Chorioretinal lesions should be reevaluated within 1 week of institution of systemic therapy. If, at this time, new lesions are present or if the initial lesions are expanding, it is unlikely that the chorioretinitis will resolve, and enucleation should be considered. If anterior uveal involvement is present (i.e., anterior uveitis or endophthalmitis), the ocular prognosis is poor. Secondary glaucoma in these cases is common and is often refractory to treatment. Animals with pain and/or vision loss due to secondary glaucoma should be enucleated as soon as they can tolerate general anesthesia.

## MYCOTIC KERATITIS

The cornea may become infected with fungi by direct inoculation with organisms from the environment. These infections are common in horses, but are very rare in dogs and cats. Filamentous fungi such as *Aspergillus* and *Fusarium* are the most common isolates. The corneal changes associated with mycotic keratitis are not pathognomonic, and include corneal edema, neovascularization, pigmentation, and varying degrees of ulceration. A dense white plaque may be present. These cases often have a history of prolonged topical corticosteroid or antibiotic usage. Diagnosis is achieved by cytology and/or culture of corneal scrapings, which should be pursued in cases of chronic active keratitis that don't respond to conventional therapies. Topical antifungals are required, with additional therapy for corneal ulceration if necessary. Optimally, antifungal treatment should be guided by sensitivity testing, but sensitivity testing for fungal agents is expensive and not widely available. The only antifungal approved for topical use is natamycin (Natacyn, Alcon), but the intravenous formulation of miconazole (Monistat, Janssen) can be used topically and is more effective. Initial treatment should be aggressive (every 2 to 4 hr), decreasing every 2 to 4 days if a favorable response occurs. Total duration of therapy should be 4 to 8 weeks. The paucity of reported cases of mycotic keratitis in small animals makes it difficult to gauge prognosis, but if experience in horses can be extrapolated, a guarded prognosis should be given.

## References and Suggested Reading

Angell JA, Merideth RE, Shively JN, et al: Ocular lesions associated with coccidioidomycosis in dogs: 35 cases (1980–1985). J Am Vet Med Assoc 190:1319, 1987.
*A discussion of the clinical and ocular findings, diagnosis, and treatment in 35 dogs with coccidioidomycosis seen in ophthalmic referral practices in Arizona.*
Buyukmihci N: Ocular lesions of blastomycosis in the dog. J Am Vet Med Assoc 180:426, 1982.
*A summary of the clinical and ocular findings in 21 dogs with blastomycosis presented to The University of Tennessee, including detailed descriptions of seven representative cases.*
Clinkenbeard KD, Cowell RL, and Tyler RD: Disseminated histoplasmosis in cats: 12 cases (1981–1986). J Am Vet Med Assoc 190:1445, 1987.
*A summary of the signalment, clinical, laboratory, and histopathologic findings, and treatment results of 12 cats diagnosed with histoplasmosis at Oklahoma State University.*
Fischer CA: Intraocular cryptococcosis in two cats. J Am Vet Med Assoc 158:191, 1971.
*A detailed clinical and histopathologic description of two cats with cryptococcosis that had ocular involvement.*
Legendre AM, Walker M, Buyukmihci N, et al: Canine blastomycosis: A review of 47 clinical cases. J Am Vet Med Assoc 178:1163, 1981.
*A comprehensive review of the signalment, clinical, laboratory, and radiographic findings, diagnostic procedures, and therapy in 47 dogs with blastomycosis presented to The University of Tennessee.*
Medleau L and Barsanti JA: Cryptococcosis. In Greene CE (ed): Infectious Diseases of the Dog and Cat. Philadelphia, WB Saunders Co, 1990, p 687.
*A review of the etiology, pathogenesis, clinical findings, diagnosis, and therapy of cryptococcosis in dogs and cats.*
Wolf AM: Histoplasmosis. In Greene CE (ed): Infectious Diseases of the Dog and Cat. Philadelphia, WB Saunders Co, 1990, p 679.
*A review of the etiology, pathogenesis, clinical findings, diagnosis, and therapy of histoplasmosis in dogs and cats.*

# INNOVATIONS IN CATARACT SURGERY

MARK P. NASISSE

*Raleigh, North Carolina*

## HISTORY OF CANINE CATARACT SURGERY

There is no disease of dogs whose management has changed as dramatically over the preceding 5 years as that of cataracts. What makes the history of this transition interesting is the logarithmic sequence of events to which it is attributable. Lens extraction has been routinely performed on dogs for more than 30 years, and the roots of the procedure can be found in the efforts of William Magrane and other pioneering veterinary ophthalmologists (Magrane, 1969). Although the subtleties of the procedure varied between surgeons, the general approach of lifting the lens nucleus from the eye through a large anterior capsulectomy and corneal incision (open sky extracapsular extraction [ECCE]) remained unchanged for many years. The reported success of this procedure is somewhere between 60 and 80% (Magrane, 1969; Rooks et al., 1985), a level considerably below that enjoyed by our counterparts in the medical profession. It has been known for many years that there are conspicuous differences in the uveal response of different animal species to surgical trauma, and it is to these differences that the relatively poor success of canine lens extraction has been historically attributed. Most of us who received our ophthalmic training prior to 1985 were exposed to the dogma that canine eyes just responded poorly to intraocular surgery. The implicit assumption was that there was no reason to try improving the success of canine cataract extraction, because it wouldn't do any good anyway. In my opinion, the science of canine lens extraction took its biggest leap forward when veterinary ophthalmologists began to accept responsibility for the outcome of the surgery, rather than blaming it exclusively on the patient. The result of this change in philosophy has been the refinement of the technique of cataract surgery such that the procedure now has a success rate of approximately 90% (Davidson et al., 1991).

The single most important event in the improved success following canine lens extraction has been the evolution of phacoemulsification (phacofragmentation). Consider that the canine species possesses a blood-ocular barrier that is comparatively fragile. As a result, any prolonged collapse of the anterior chamber results in a drop in intraocular pressure that is accompanied by leakage of protein, including fibrin, into the anterior chamber. The failure of many ECCE procedures is attributable to closure (seclusion) of the pupil as the fibrin to which it is attached contracts and organizes. During phacoemulsification, however, because continuous irrigation through the phacoemulsification needle keeps the globe inflated during most of the procedure, intraocular pressure rarely drops, and fibrin exudation does not occur. Another leading cause of failure after lens extraction is the retention of lens cortical material, which often causes chronic postoperative uveitis. Because lens material can be efficiently and atraumatically removed with the automated irrigation and aspiration technology that is inherent to phacoemulsification, chronic uveitis is uncommon. The advent of viscoelastic materials and intraocular lenses (IOL) designed for the canine eye, and a growing appreciation for optimum patient selection, have further contributed to the success of this procedure.

## PATIENT SELECTION

In view of the anticipated poor result following canine extracapsular cataract extraction, and the fact that dogs with monocular vision function adequately, it is not surprising that veterinary ophthalmologists have traditionally recommended waiting until the patient was completely blind before surgically intervening. Although the outcome of such a primitive approach is often disastrous, the psychological benefit to the owner is substantial; if the dog was blind anyway, there was nothing to lose! There are some compelling reasons, however, why a dog should not be allowed to become blind before electing to pursue surgery. First, bilateral cataracts rarely progress at a symmetric rate. In most cases, by the time the more slowly progressing cataract becomes complete, the contralateral cataract has progressed to hypermaturity. Because hypermature cataracts are associated with lens-induced uveitis and retinal detachment, the prognosis for successful surgery is at least 20 to 30% below what would have been feasible earlier in the course of the disease. Hypermature cataracts are also likely to be associated with capsular opacification, a complication that can add great complexity to the technique required to remove them. Because of these potential complicating factors, the only prerequisite for considering cataract extraction is *the probability that the patient will eventually be blinded by the condition*, and this can usually be predicted by the animal's age, and the location of the cataract. For example, a 2-year-old cocker spaniel with cataracts that are only 30% complete, given that there is virtually a 100% probability that the cataracts will progress, should be viewed as an ideal candidate. Conversely, a 12-year-old poodle with a unilateral cataract involving less than 50% of the lens should probably be observed for progression. Because the decision to recommend lens extraction is often based on subtle clinical and historical findings, *the appropriate time to refer a dog for evaluation for lens extraction is when the cataracts are first detected.*

## SURGICAL TECHNIQUE

### Preoperative Considerations

Preoperative patient assessment should include a thorough ophthalmic examination that includes gonioscopy and slit lamp biomicroscopy. Retinal function should be assessed by electroretinography, and if the cataract is hypermature, B-mode ultrasonography should be done to rule out retinal detachment. It is imperative that lens-induced uveitis be controlled with 1% prednisolone acetate (Econopred, Alcon) or 0.1% dexamethasone (Ak-Dex 0.1% solution, Akorn) applied

every 6 hr to the affected eye for 1 to 2 weeks prior to surgery. Atropine therapy should be avoided unless absolutely necessary, as chronic atropinization results in parasympathetic receptor hyperplasia that may contribute to intraoperative miosis. In routine cases, no topical treatment is initiated until the day before surgery, when topical antibiotic solution is applied every 8 hr. Beginning 2 hr prior to surgery, 1% atropine solution and 10% phenylephrine (Ak-Dilate 10% solution) are applied every 30 min to induce mydriasis. The preoperative application of flurbiprofen (Ocufen, Allergan America) further helps to maintain intraoperative mydriasis (Heinrichs and Leith, 1990).

### Unilateral versus Bilateral Surgery

It has been conventionally held by both human and veterinary ophthalmologists that only one eye should be operated at a time. It has been demonstrated, however, that surgical outcome is identical after unilateral versus bilateral procedures (Davidson et al., 1990). The advantage of doing surgery on both eyes is that the cost to the owner can be reduced substantially, the patient is subjected to the risk of only one anesthetic episode, and should surgery not be successful in one eye, the patient will still have functional vision. In any event, from the perspective of the owner, the decision of whether to operate on one or both eyes should be strictly an economic one.

### Phacoemulsification

Phacoemulsification is the process by which a lens is simultaneously fragmented and aspirated from the eye (Miller et al., 1987; Nasisse et al., 1991). Although canine cataracts have been removed by phacoemulsification for more than 20 years, the assumption that only the soft lenses of young dogs were amenable to this technique limited its application. Currently, however, machines possess sufficient fragmenting power to allow removal of lenses from dogs of all ages. The basic components of a phacoemulsification machine are a power source, a fluid pump, and two handpieces that allow for the simultaneous infusion and aspiration of fluid from the eye; one ultrasonically vibrates (fragmenting handpiece), and one does not (irrigation-aspiration [IA] handpiece). The vibration source in most contemporary (piezoelectric) fragmentation handpieces is a crystal that causes a titanium needle mounted at its end to move backward and forward at ultrasonic frequencies (30,000 to 50,000 cycles per second). Aspirated fluid pulls cataract material into the needle, where it is *emulsified* and removed from the eye. The IA handpiece is used to remove soft cortical material from the periphery of the lens capsule after the harder portions have been fragmented.

In a standard procedure, the patient is positioned in dorsal recumbency with the globe directed upward into the operating microscope. After an incision is made at the dorsal corneal limbus, the anterior chamber is entered with either a cystotome or hypodermic needle that is used either to make a hole in (capsulotomy), or remove (capsulectomy) the anterior capsule. The size and shape of the capsulectomy depends on surgeon preference, and whether or not a lens is to be implanted. The current trend in cataract surgery is to make capsulectomies that are circular and continuous, because they resist inadvertent tearing during phacoemulsification, and provide optimum support of the implanted IOL. After the capsulotomy is completed, the fragmenting needle is inserted into the anterior chamber and moved in a dorsal to ventral direction across the exposed lens to *sculpt* the cataract (Fig. 1). When most of the lens has been removed, one of a variety of maneuvers is used to break the posterior remnants into pieces so that they may be moved away from the posterior lens capsule for fragmenting. When the brittle lens fragments have been removed, the IA handpiece is used to aspirate the pliable cortical remnants from the peripheral portions of the capsule (Fig. 2).

Phacoemulsification is a considerably more complex surgical procedure than ECCE, and numerous intraoperative complications can occur. Because corneal endothelial damage may result in permanent postoperative corneal edema, its protection during surgery is essential. To this end, it is critical that the lens be fragmented within the capsular bag, and not in the anterior chamber. If a vibrating needle should contact uveal tissue, inflammation or hemorrhage can result. More devastating, however, are the effects of damage to the posterior lens capsule during phacoemulsification; the lens nucleus may luxate into the vitreous humor, or the vitreous humor may become displaced into the capsular bag, both conditions often necessitating vitrectomy or conversion to extracapsular extraction. Also, damage to the posterior lens capsule makes it difficult or impossible to implant the intraocular lens. The prevention of

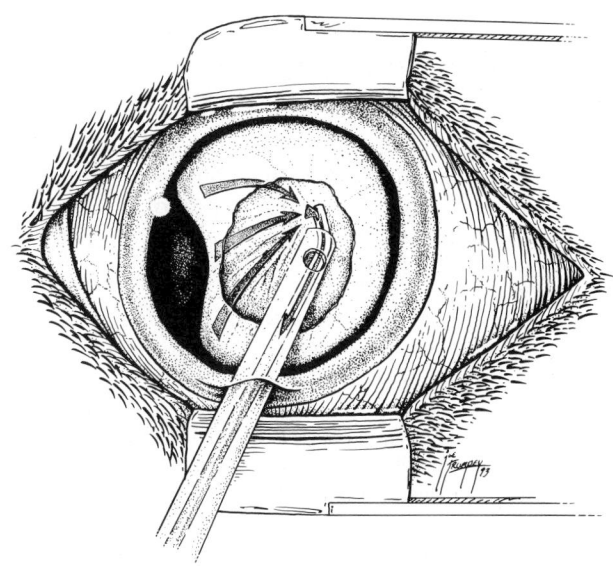

**Figure 2.** Illustration of the soft peripheral cortical material being aspirated from the capsular bag. In contrast to the phacoemulsification needle, the cannula used in IA is blunt, and does not vibrate.

these, as well as a myriad of other possible complications, requires the surgeon have considerable experience with, and a thorough theoretical understanding of, the procedure.

## Intraocular Lens Implantation

In the normal dog, the lens provides approximately 14.5 diopters of refractive power (Davidson et al., 1993). Its removal, therefore, renders them extremely farsighted (hyperopic). Although it is well known that aphakic dogs can function very well in many instances, a nearly normal postoperative refractive state can be achieved by implanting a prosthetic lens. Prosthetic lenses for dogs are now available from a variety of manufacturers (The Cutting Edge; Domilens; Surgidev; Eye Care Distributors). Most are lathe-cut from polymethylmethacrylate, after which they are polished and sterilized. In the most common designs, IOLs consist of a central refractive disk (optic) that is supported by two arms (haptics) (Fig. 3). In contrast to the proce-

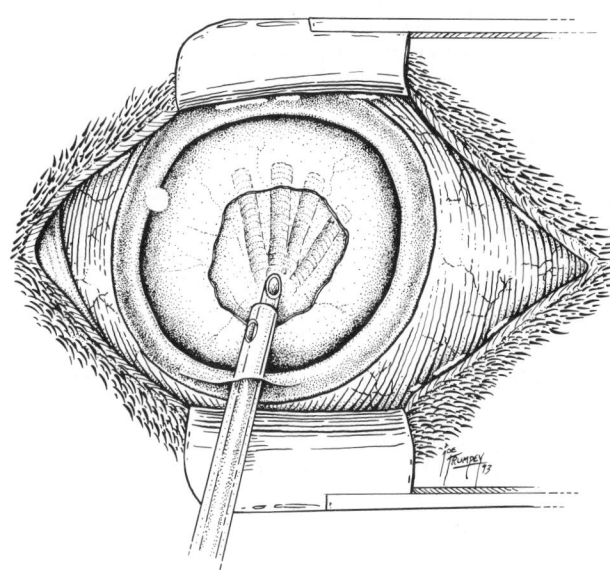

**Figure 1.** Illustration of a phacoemulsification needle in the process of sculpting the anterior lens nucleus.

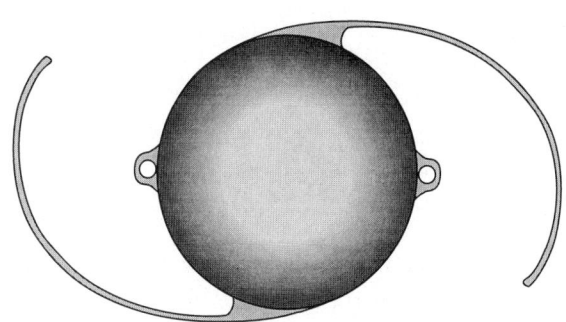

**Figure 3.** Illustration of a typical intraocular lens. The central optic is supported by arms termed "haptics."

dure performed on humans, in which the IOL power is calculated for each patient with a formula that takes into account variations in radius of corneal curvature, axial length of the eye, and anterior chamber depth, a standard power of 42 diopters has been shown to correct the vast majority of dogs to within several diopters of emmetropia. The IOL is inserted into the capsular bag following the aspiration of cortical material (Fig. 4).

## Use of Viscoelastic Materials

The term "viscoelastic material" describes a diverse group of highly viscous, transparent substances that are used to lubricate the anterior chamber of the eye in order to minimize the trauma associated with intraocular surgery. Sodium hyaluronate, a polysaccharide that is extracted from rooster combs, was the first such material to be marketed, and is considered by many to be superior to others on the basis of its consistency and handling characteristics. Due to its expense (>$100.00/ 0.5 ml), it is rarely used by veterinary ophthalmologists. Other less expensive products are various combinations of chondroitin sulfate and methylcellulose (Keragel, Cutting Edge; Phalon, Surgidev). Viscoelastic material is nearly always used to fill the capsular bag to facilitate atraumatic IOL insertion, and is often used to keep the anterior chamber inflated during the capsulectomy. Filling the anterior chamber prior to phacoemulsification also helps to minimize corneal endothelial cell trauma. The viscoelastic material is usually aspirated from the eye at the conclusion of the surgery. Except for causing a transient increase in intraocular pressure, complications are rarely associated with its usage. Due to the fragility of the blood-ocular barrier in dogs, viscoelastic materials have a particularly important role to play in veterinary ophthalmic surgery.

## ANTICIPATED OUTCOME OF PHACOEMULSIFICATION AND IOL IMPLANTATION

If the cataracts have not been allowed to progress to hypermaturity, and if no concurrent ocular diseases are present, phacoemulsification should be successful in more than 90% of patients. In most cases, owners will notice an improvement in their dog's vision within 48 hr of surgery, and if an IOL is implanted, within several weeks most clients perceive their dog's vision to be as good as it was prior the development of the cataracts.

Because IA so effectively removes all potentially antigenic lens cortex, chronic uveitis and therefore secondary glaucoma is relatively uncommon following phacoemulsification. Because the incision is at most only 9 mm in length, wound dehiscence is also uncommon. For yet unexplained reasons, however, phacoemulsification is associated with a higher postoperative rate of retinal detachment (approximately 4%) than is ECCE. Most occur within 2 to 6 weeks of surgery and eventually cause blindness. Bacterial endophthalmitis is a rare complication of cataract surgery, but when it does occur, it usually results in loss of vision. The most common complication of cataract extraction is a condition called *secondary cataracts*. Regardless of how meticulously the procedure is performed, some lens epithelial cells remain adhered to the anterior lens capsule. These cells subsequently migrate across the posterior capsule and attempt to produce new lens material. They also undergo fibrous metaplasia, and in the process of contracting cause wrinkling of the posterior lens capsule. These *secondary cataracts* can be treated by making holes in the opacified posterior capsule with an ophthalmic neodymium:yttrium-aluminum-garnet (Nd:YAG) laser (Nasisse et al., 1990). The presence of an IOL, however, sufficiently inhibits capsular opacification so that it is rarely necessary (Nasisse and Cobo, 1992).

Although IOLs are not by themselves causes of postoperative complications, problems can occur if they are improperly made, cleaned, sterilized, or implanted. Foreign particulate matter, particularly polishing compound, is a potent stimulus of postoperative uveitis, that usually manifests as severe flare or hypopyon within several days of surgery. Severe uveitis may also develop if ethylene oxide used to sterilize the IOL is not allowed to adequately diffuse from the polymer prior to implanting. Fortunately, the quality control methods used in currently manufactured canine IOLs are sufficiently good that these problems are uncommon. Otherwise, IOLs only contribute to postoperative problems if they fail to remain securely positioned in the capsular bag; IOL luxation, however, is a function of suboptimum surgical technique, and is a rare sequela to procedures done by experienced surgeons.

## THE FUTURE OF CANINE CATARACT SURGERY

Veterinary ophthalmology has come a long way since the era when IOLs were not implanted into the eyes of dogs simply because it was assumed that it could not be done. As veterinarians become accustomed to referring cataract patients earlier in the course of the disease, and as veterinary ophthalmologists perfect their surgical skills, the rate of success will further increase.

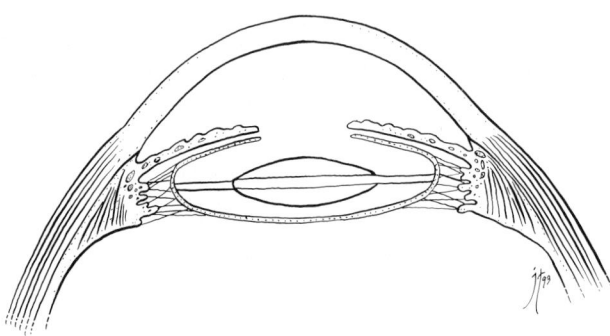

**Figure 4.** Cross section of the anterior segment of an eye showing the relationship of the IOL within the capsular bag.

As the outcome of cataract surgery becomes more predictable, the hesitance of veterinarians to refer dogs for this procedure will progressively diminish. The inevitable consequence of these trends can only be that more dogs will experience a better quality of life, and more pet owners will benefit from the services veterinarians have to offer.

## References and Suggested Reading

Davidson MG, Nasisse MP, Jamieson VE, et al: Phacoemulsification and intraocular lens implantation: A study of results in 182 dogs. Prog Vet Comp Ophthalmol 1:233, 1991.
*A summary of the complications seen following phacoemulsification and IOL implantation in dogs.*
Davidson MG, Nasisse MP, Rusnak IM, et al: Success rates of unilateral versus bilateral cataract extraction in dogs. Vet Surg 19:232, 1990.
*A retrospective study demonstrating that lens extraction can safely be done on both eyes of dogs during the same anesthetic episode.*
Davidson MG, Murphy CJ, Nasisse MP, et al: Refractive state of aphakic and pseudophakic eye of dogs. Am J Vet Res 54:174, 1993.
*A prospective study describing the effects of IOL implantation on the refractive error of dogs.*
Heinrichs DA and Leith AB: Effect of flurbiprofen on the maintenance of pupillary dilation during cataract surgery. Can J Ophthalmol 25:239, 1990.
*An original study demonstrating that topically applied flurbiprofen helps to maintain mydriasis during cataract surgery.*
Magrane WG: Cataract extraction: A follow-up study (429 cases). J Small Anim Pract 10:454, 1969.
*One of the first retrospective studies demonstrating the efficacy of lens extraction in dogs.*
Miller TR, Whitley RD, Meek LA, et al: Phacofragmentation and aspiration for cataracts in dogs: 56 cases (1980–1984). J Am Vet Med Assoc 190: 1577, 1987.
*A retrospective study demonstrating the efficacy of phacoemulsification in removing canine cataracts.*
Nasisse MP, Davidson MG, Jamieson VE, et al: Phacoemulsification and intraocular lens implantation: A study of technique in 182 dogs. Prog Vet Comp Ophthalmol 1:225, 1991.
*A retrospective study describing phacoemulsification techniques used in dogs.*
Nasisse MP, Davidson MG, English RV, et al: Neodymium:YAG laser treatment of lens extraction-induced pupillary opacification in dogs. J Am Anim Hosp Assoc 26:275, 1990.
*A retrospective study demonstrating the efficacy of Nd:YAG laser therapy to treat pupillary opacification in dogs.*
Nasisse MP and Cobo M: Effects of intraocular lens implantation on secondary cataracts. Invest Ophthalmol Vis Sci 31(suppl):1168, 1992.
*An experimental study demonstrating the features of secondary cataract formation in aphakic and pseudophakic eyes of dogs.*
Rooks RL, Brightman AH, Musselman EE, et al: Extracapsular cataract extraction: An analysis of 240 operations in dogs. J Am Vet Med Assoc 187: 1013, 1985.
*A retrospective study addressing the efficacy of extracapsular lens extraction in dogs.*

# GLAUCOMA

PAUL E. MILLER
*Madison, Wisconsin*

Elevations in intraocular pressure (IOP) are one of the most frequent causes of irreversible blindness in dogs and cats. According to the Veterinary Medical Data Base, approximately 1 in every 119 dogs and 1 in 367 cats over the last 20 years were blinded by this disease. To hope to maintain vision or a pain-free eye in animals with elevated IOP, the clinician must be constantly aware of the circumstances in which alterations in IOP occur, use a tonometer to accurately measure IOP, and have a working understanding of both the pharmacologic agents and surgical modalities currently available for glaucoma therapy. Vision is more likely to be preserved if high-risk patients are prophylactically medicated, and if overtly glaucomatous eyes are aggressively treated with a combination of medical and surgical therapy early in the course of the disease before vision is substantially impaired.

Numerous ophthalmic disorders can produce elevated IOP, and it is more appropriate to think of glaucoma as a *group* of diseases each with a specific etiology and therapy rather than as a single disease entity. Indeed, the only unifying theme in this diverse group of disorders is that IOP is too high to permit the optic nerve to function normally. Although some glaucomatous animals may exhibit optic nerve damage at IOPs generally regarded as within the normal range, most demonstrate clinical visual loss only when IOP exceeds high normal values (Table 1). Generally, the rate of vision loss is proportional to the magnitude of IOP elevation, with complete blindness resulting in as little as 24 to 48 hr if IOP is massively elevated (60 to 70 mm Hg), and more slowly (weeks to months) if the increase is mild.

## PATHOGENESIS

The mechanisms of normal aqueous humor production and outflow have been reviewed (Scherlie, 1992; Gelatt, 1991; Brooks, 1990). Most forms of glaucoma result when egress of aqueous humor from the eye is impaired and aqueous production continues at a relatively excessive (although less than normal) rate. Common mechanisms of outflow impairment in the dog include: (1) narrowing of the drainage angle secondary to an anteriorly positioned lens or increased axial length of the lens or vitreous; (2) developmental abnormalities of the pectinate ligaments; (3) peripheral iridocorneal adhesions or drainage apparatus neovascularization; (4) overt anterior lens luxations/subluxations; and (5) intraocular neoplasia. Continued aqueous humor production despite high IOP may initially appear to be phys-

**Table 1.** *Normal IOP for Dogs and Cats as Determined With Two Applanation Tonometers and the Schiøtz Tonometer (Using the 5.5-gm Weight) and 3 Conversion Tables\**

| | Applanation Tonometry | | | Schiøtz Tonometry | | |
| | Tono-Pen | MacKay-Marg | Scale | 1955 Human Table[†] | 1977 Dog Table[‡] | 1988 Dog Table[§] |
|---|---|---|---|---|---|---|
| Dog X̄ ± SD | 16.8 ± 4.0 | 17.1 ± 3.9 | 4.9 ± 1.5 | 18.0 ± 4.1 | 30.9 ± 4.7 | 19.7 ± 3.7 |
| Range | 9–24 | 9–25 | 2–8 | 10–26 | 21–40 | 12–27 |
| Cat X̄ ± SD | 20.2 ± 5.5 | 22.2 ± 5.2 | 3.9 ± 1.4 | 21.6 ± 5.0 | 35.0 ± 5.8 | 27.1 ± 5.9 |
| Range | 9–31 | 12–32 | 1–7 | 12–32 | 23–49 | 15–39 |

\*Ranges reflect 95% confidence intervals.
[†]The human calibration table is supplied with the tonometer.
[‡]Data derived from Peiffer RL, Gelatt KN, Jessen CR, et al: Calibration of the Schiøtz tonometer for the normal canine eye. Am J Vet Res 38:1881, 1977.
[§]Data derived from Morgan R: Calibration tables for the Schiøtz tonometer. In Morgan RV (ed): *Handbook of Small Animal Practice,* 2nd edition. New York, Churchill Livingstone 1992, pp 1389–1390.
Abbreviations: X̄ = mean, SD = standard deviation.

iologically nonadaptive, but probably reflects the eye opting to maintain a major source of nutrition over IOP control.

## DIAGNOSIS

In general, *glaucoma can only be accurately diagnosed by measuring IOP with a tonometer.* Glaucoma should be suspected in all red eyes in which the cause of the vascular injection is not obvious (e.g., simple corneal ulcer, foreign body), and in eyes with unexplained corneal edema, pupillary abnormalities, chronic anterior uveitis, lens positional abnormalities, or visual impairment. Because one of the greatest impediments to the timely diagnosis of glaucoma is the clinician's index of suspicion, the above clinical signs, especially in a breed predisposed to glaucoma (Table 2), should prompt the clinician to immediately measure IOP.

It is important to note that the normal range of IOP varies with tonometerist, tonometer, conversion table, breed, age (IOP may be lower in older dogs), and species. The latter is of particular significance, as cats probably have higher normal IOP limits than dogs (Table 1) and often manifest more subtle clinical signs of glaucoma. Unlike dogs, cats typically exhibit relatively little ocular injection, and often mydriasis and progressive buphthalmia are the only overt clinical signs of feline glaucoma.

## Schiøtz Tonometry

Quantitative measurement of IOP has been the standard of care for over 75 years in human medicine, and *clinicians lacking a tonometer should probably refer every glaucoma suspect to a colleague or specialist for tonometry.* Failure to definitively diagnose glaucoma on initial presentation, or mistaking it for less visually threatening conditions such as conjunctivitis or uveitis, has devastating consequences for both vision and patient comfort. Manually estimating IOP by assessing the compressibility of the globe through the upper eyelid (so-called digital tonometry) is notoriously inaccurate—and usually permits the diagnosis to only be made in end-stage glaucomatous eyes where all hope of preserving vision is lost.

The inexpensive Schiøtz tonometer can attain a level of accuracy equal to that of the much more expensive and reliable applanation tonometers if a clean instrument and good technique are carefully employed (Miller and Pickett, 1992a,b). Following topical anesthesia, IOP is measured in either the sitting or dorsal recumbency positions by vertically applying the instrument

**Table 2.** *Dog Breeds Most Commonly Affected With Glaucoma (in Descending Order) as Recorded by the Veterinary Medical Data Base for the Years 1972 to 1992*

| Primary Open Angle | Narrow/Closed Angle | Secondary |
|---|---|---|
| Mixed breeds | American cocker spaniel | Mixed breeds |
| American cocker spaniel | Mixed breeds | American cocker spaniel |
| Basset hound | Basset hound | Wire fox terrier |
| Boston terrier | Samoyed | Toy poodle |
| Miniature schnauzer | Beagle | Boston terrier |
| Beagle | Siberian husky | Miniature poodle |
| | Chow chow | Labrador retriever |
| | Wire fox terrier | Siberian husky |
| | Toy poodle | Basset hound |
| | Standard poodle | Beagle |

(with the 5.5-gm weight attached) to the center of the cornea and averaging three readings. Ideally, each reading should take 1 to 2 sec to perform, and all three readings should be within 1 to 1.5 scale units of each other. If IOP is elevated, or one wishes to verify the accuracy of the 5.5-gm weight readings, the 7.5- or 10.0-gm weights are added individually to the 5.5-gm base weight (all three weights are never used simultaneously). In general, estimates of IOP with the 7.5-gm weight should be within 6 mm Hg of those with the 5.5-gm weight.

Erroneous readings with a Schiøtz tonometer are usually the result of faulty technique and include: compressing the globe by retracting the lids at the lid margin rather than over the bony orbital rim (IOP too high); occluding the jugular veins during restraint (IOP too high); application of the tonometer off from vertical, to the sclera or third eyelid (IOP too high or too low); not resting the footplate completely on the cornea (IOP too low); and prolonged application (subsequent IOPs will be lower and corneal ulceration is possible). Corneal scarring, infiltrates, or thinning may also render the readings inaccurate, as corneal resistance to indentation is altered.

## Schiøtz Calibration Tables

A potential source of confusion with the Schiøtz tonometer is that several different calibration tables have been advocated for converting Schiøtz scale readings to estimates of IOP in mm Hg for dogs and cats. Given the same Schiøtz scale readings, dog-specific conversion tables yield a higher estimate of IOP than either the human calibration table (which is provided with the tonometer) or the more reliable applanation tonometers (Table 1). Dog-specific conversion tables can result in approximately 65% of *normal* dogs and 75% of *normal* cats having an IOP greater than the previously published normal limits of 25 to 30 mm Hg. This is not surprising because the published normal limits for dogs and cats were determined with either the Schiøtz and the human calibration table, or applanation tonometers. Clearly, canine-specific conversion tables require a substantial redefinition of the normal range for IOP if they are to be clinically useful.

Although canine-specific conversion tables may have minor theoretical advantages in a research setting, *the human conversion table is the preferred table for conversion of Schiøtz scale readings to estimates of IOP in mm Hg in clinical practice.* In contrast to using canine-specific conversion tables or even just raw scale readings to define normal, the human table results in measurements that are not significantly different from those obtained with the most widely used applanation tonometers, and eliminates the need to radically redefine normal canine and feline IOP. Additionally, reliance solely on raw scale readings to define normal can be confusing because IOP is inversely related to scale readings (lower scale readings mean higher IOP), and the measurements are in units (mm of indentation) that

are not directly comparable to the units (mm Hg) used by other tonometers.

### APPLANATION TONOMETRY

Applanation tonometers such as the discontinued MacKay-Marg and the commercially available Tono-Pen (Oculab) are accurate, very fast, and easy to use. They permit IOP to be measured in almost any position, and the smaller tip allows precise, atraumatic corneal placement. The Tono-Pen automatically averages three to six readings and displays the mean IOP with the percentage variance from the high to low reading. Its expense, however, has generally limited its use to ophthalmic referral practices and to private practitioners frustrated by Schiøtz tonometry in uncooperative patients.

## THERAPY

Glaucoma therapy is driven by four questions (Fig. 1):

1. *Is IOP elevated?* Tonometry confirms the diagnosis and allows the response to treatment to be accurately assessed.
2. *Is the eye potentially sighted or irreversibly blind?* Aggressive medical therapy is usually indicated only if vision is still present or has just recently been lost, or if there is uncertainty as to the eye's visual status. Seldom is the use of potentially toxic and expensive antiglaucoma drugs worthwhile in irreversibly blind eyes in which the battle has already been lost. For irretrievably blind eyes, the author prefers enucleation (with histopathology); or a globe salvage procedure such as evisceration and prosthesis or cyclocryosurgery, depending on the etiology of the glaucoma. In the author's experience, intravitreal injections with gentamicin (Moller et al., 1986) in an effort to destroy the ciliary body and lower IOP frequently yields less than satisfactory long-term results. Although a blind, buphthalmic globe with a IOP of 60 mm Hg may not seem painful to the animal (humans with identical elevations may complain of pain similar to a migraine headache), most owners will comment that the pet is "more like its old self" once IOP is effectively reduced surgically. It is critical, however, that in the course of treating the blind eye, the risk to the remaining visual eye be carefully determined and preventative therapy begun if indicated.
3. *Is the glaucoma primary or secondary?* Primary drainage angle abnormalities (primary glaucoma) are generally treated differently than glaucoma that is secondary to other intraocular disorders such as chronic uveitis, lens luxation, neoplasia, and so forth. Primary glaucoma in dogs has two morphologic forms: primary open-angle glaucoma (POAG) and primary narrow/closed-angle glaucoma (CAG). POAG is the least common though most extensively investigated form in dogs. The onset is typically relatively slow and characterized

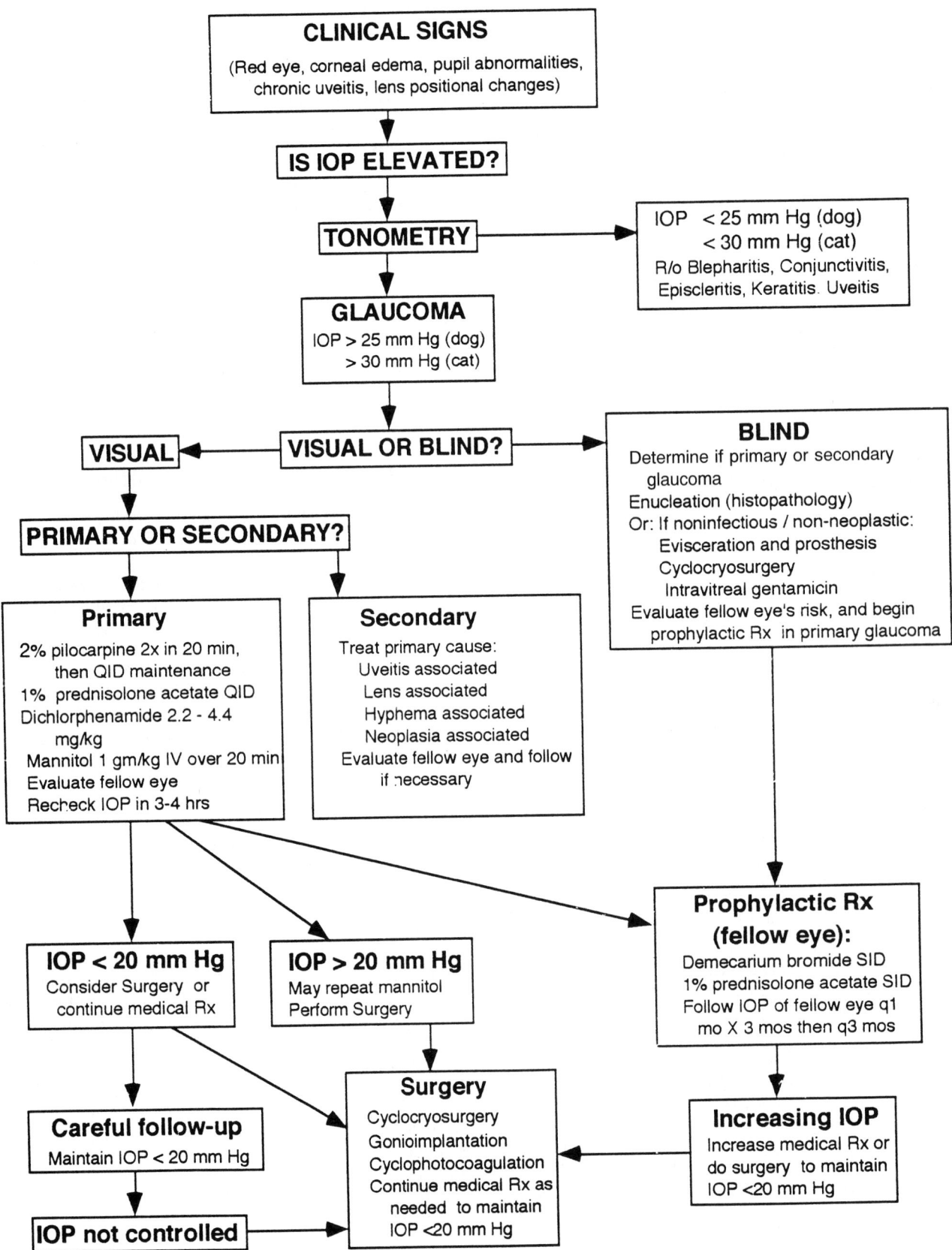

**Figure 1.** A flow-chart for the treatment of dogs and cats with glaucoma.

by an initially insidious, mild to moderately elevated IOP (10 to 15 mm Hg increase). These small elevations suggest that POAG may, at least initially, be controllable by medical therapy alone in some cases. Narrow/closed-angle glaucoma is at least eight times more common than POAG in dogs, and tends to be characterized by an initially unilateral, sometimes episodic, acute elevation in IOP that either spontaneously resolves or persists at very high levels (50 to 80 mm Hg). CAG almost always requires immediate surgical intervention to preserve vision.

4. *Can medical therapy control IOP and ocular pain, or is surgery needed?* In general, most forms of glaucoma are surgical diseases and antiglaucoma drugs generally are only used as a bridge to surgery or as a surgical adjunct when additional minor IOP reductions are needed postoperatively. Existing antiglaucoma drugs alone, or even in combination, are rarely capable of maintaining more than a 10 to 15 mm Hg reduction in IOP, and therefore seldom prevent progressive visual loss. The apparent efficacy of many of these drugs also diminishes over a few weeks to months, either as a result of tachyphylaxis or progressive angle closure. Finally, because virtually every evaluation of antiglaucoma drug efficacy in dogs has been performed in either normal animals or dogs with POAG, the effectiveness of these drugs in dogs with the more common closed-angle glaucoma is unclear.

## Visual Eyes

In general, given the heterogeneous causes of elevated IOP, no single therapeutic regimen can be advocated for all cases of glaucoma in which vision is still present. The principal goal of therapy for either primary or secondary glaucoma is the reduction of IOP to a "safe" level (i.e., a pressure at which progressive visual impairment and optic nerve damage no longer occurs). It is probable that for the vast majority of dogs and cats this target IOP is substantially lower than the high normal limit of 25 to 30 mm Hg, and may be in the low teens or even single digits in some animals. Unfortunately, this numerical level varies by animal, disease state, tonometer, and tonometerist; and a method for clinically determining the safe upper limit of IOP for dogs and cats with glaucoma is not yet available. When treating glaucomatous patients, the author tries to maintain IOP below an arbitrarily set target of 20 mm Hg (as measured by applanation tonometry or the Schiøtz using the human conversion table).

### ACUTE PRIMARY GLAUCOMA: INITIAL THERAPY

Figure 1 outlines the initial regimen the author uses in acute primary glaucoma affecting a potentially visual eye. In an acute attack in which IOP is very high, antiglaucoma drugs are usually used aggressively and in combination to try to quickly reduce IOP to as low a level as possible (Table 3). Attempts to slowly titrate IOP down over time by sequentially adding drugs usually only results in more severe optic nerve damage. Suboptimal therapy (e.g., using only 2% pilocarpine in an eye with an IOP of 60 mm Hg) only ensures blindness and must be avoided. Once IOP is reduced, surgery is usually performed, as it is uncommon to be able to maintain the target IOP of 20 mm Hg or less with medication alone. Generally, if IOP is less than 40 to 45 mm Hg and the pupil is still reactive to light or a miotic, the author will attempt to control IOP with only

**Table 3.** *Dosages of Drugs for Antiglaucoma Therapy*

**Hyperosmotics**
  Mannitol (20%) (Mannitol 20% injection, Abbott)—1 gm/kg IV (heat or filter); give over 20 min; withhold water for 2 hr; repeat in 4 hr if needed
  Glycerol (50%) (Osmoglyn, Alcon)—1–2 ml/kg PO; repeat in 8 hr if needed

**Carbonic Anhydrase Inhibitors (Oral)**
  Dichlorphenamide (Daranide, Merck Sharp & Dohme)—2.2–4.4 mg/kg q8–12h (dogs); (1–2 mg/kg q8–12h in cats)
  Methazolamide (Neptazane, Lederle)—2.2–4.4 mg/kg q8–12h

**Parasympathomimetic Miotics (Topical)**
  Pilocarpine solution 2%—q6–12h
  Demecarium bromide (Humorsol, Merck Sharp & Dohme)—0.125% (dogs ≤10 kg) or 0.25% (dogs >10 kg); q12h in overt glaucoma, or q24h as prophylaxis
  Echothiophate iodide (Phospholine Iodide, Wyeth-Ayerst)—0.06% (dogs ≤10 kg) or 0.25% (dogs >10 kg); q12h in overt glaucoma, or q24h as prophylaxis

**β-Blocking Agents (Topical)**
  Timolol maleate (Timoptic, Merck Sharp & Dohme)—0.5% q12h; monitor heart rate in small dogs/cats.
  Betaxolol HCL (Betoptic, Alcon)—0.5% q12h; a cardioselective (β-1) blocker.
  Metipranolol HCL (OptiPranolol, Bausch & Lomb)—0.3% q12h (less expensive than timolol)

**Mydriatic Adrenergics**
  Epinephrine (1 or 2%) (Epifrin, Allergan)—q8–12h
  Dipivefrin HCL (0.1%) (Propine, Allergan)—q8–12h; a less irritating but more expensive proepinephrine compound

**Potassium Supplementation**
  Potassium chloride (Slow-K, Summit)—600-mg tablet/50 lb PO q24h

a topical miotic and an oral carbonic anhydrase inhibitor (CAI). If IOP is greater than 45 mm Hg or the pupil is nonresponsive to a miotic, then a hyperosmotic such as mannitol is added as well.

TOPICAL AGENTS. Concentrations of pilocarpine greater than 2% are generally not initially used because they are more irritating, marginally more effective, and rarely permit surgery to be avoided. Some authors prefer a mydriatic adrenergic or β-blocker to pilocarpine if surgery is contemplated because of the potential for breakdown of the blood-aqueous barrier by miotics, but pilocarpine is the most effective topical antiglaucoma agent currently available. Organophosphate miotics such as echothiophate iodide and demecarium bromide may have a longer duration of action than pilocarpine, but their potential toxicity limits their use to an every 12- to 24-hr schedule.

The author often uses topical 1% prednisolone acetate at the same frequency as pilocarpine during an acute attack of glaucoma in an effort to reduce miotic-induced breakdown in the blood-aqueous barrier, and address any low-grade uveitis associated with severely elevated IOP. Topical corticosteroids are also usually continued postoperatively to treat the uveitis that results from surgical intervention. Corticosteroids may need to be used with caution in patients with glaucoma, however, as dogs receiving topical 0.1% dexamethasone for 6 months demonstrated a 5 mm Hg rise in IOP (Keates et al., 1991). A similar study in a select population of cats demonstrated a 3 to 6 mm Hg increase with 1% prednisolone acetate twice daily after 22 days (Zhan, Miranda, and Bito, 1992). Clinical cases of steroid-induced glaucoma, however, have not been reported in dogs or cats to the author's knowledge.

CARBONIC ANHYDRASE INHIBITORS. In contrast to most topical agents, the carbonic anhydrase inhibitors generally maintain their pressure-lowering abilities over time. The author prefers dichlorphenamide or methazolamide over acetazolamide. Clinically apparent adverse effects of these drugs may include: hypokalemia, metabolic acidosis, panting, anorexia, fatigue, depression, confusion, polyuria/polydypsia, vomiting and diarrhea, thrombocytopenia, blood dyscrasias, and nephrolithiasis. Although dichlorphenamide and methazolamide are less likely to induce hypokalemia than acetazolamide, it recently has been demonstrated in normal dogs that continuous administration of dichlorphenamide at 4.4 mg/kg twice daily resulted in continuously decreasing serum potassium levels over the 43-day duration of the study (Pickett and Champagne, 1993). Although the clinical significance of this is unclear, it would seem reasonable to follow serum potassium in animals receiving CAIs and supplement potassium if necessary. In the near future, topical CAIs will become commercially available, although their efficacy probably will be less than systemic CAIs.

HYPEROSMOTICS. Mannitol more reliably reduces IOP than oral glycerol, but it should be heated or filtered (Arygle 5 micron filters, Sherwood Medical) to remove crystals prior to slow IV administration over 20 min. Mannitol can reduce IOP from 60 to 80 mm Hg

to within normal limits in a few hours, although its clinical effects last only 12 to 48 hr. The 1-gm/kg dose can be repeated one time if necessary. Side effects include headache; osmotic diuresis; and worsening of dehydration, renal failure, or preexisting cardiovascular disease. Fatalities have been reported following IV administration of crystals and from pulmonary edema in animals anesthetized with methoxyflurane. Additionally, if the blood-aqueous barrier is incompetent as is common in uveitis-induced glaucoma, IOP may increase (less likely with mannitol than glycerol) as water is drawn into the eye. Glycerol may exacerbate hyperglycemia in diabetes mellitus.

FOLLOW-UP. IOP is closely monitored whether surgery was performed or not (Fig. 1), and medications may be slowly adjusted downwards over several days to weeks as long as IOP is maintained at 20 mm Hg or less. If surgery was not performed, and a miotic and CAI come very close (2 to 3 mm Hg) to achieving the target IOP, a topical adrenergic mydriatic (1.0% epinephrine or dipivefrin) or a topical β-blocker (timolol, metipranolol, or betaxolol) can be added. These drugs may also be used in place of a miotic if the postoperative uveitis is significant. Topical adrenergic mydriatics and β-blockers in the commercially available concentrations are typically less potent IOP-reducing agents than miotics and the clinician should realistically expect to achieve only a few mm Hg (if any) additional reduction in IOP with these drugs. β-Blockers may be more effective at reducing IOP in cats with glaucoma than in dogs, although this remains to be experimentally verified.

The exact mechanism by which mydriatic adrenergics and β-blockers lower IOP in dogs and cats is unclear, and probably differs from that in primates. It is believed that mydriatic adrenergics act by reducing aqueous production and improving outflow facility. β-Blockers have been postulated to lower IOP by reducing aqueous humor production, although they also appear to have a miotic effect in dogs and cats (unlike in humans). Timolol may act systemically and can result in significant bradycardia in small dogs and cats.

## PRIMARY GLAUCOMA: SURGICAL THERAPY

Surgery is indicated if medical therapy is likely to fail to maintain IOP within the safe range over the entire 24-hr period, or if the owners are unwilling to bear the cost of drug therapy or frequently medicate the eye. Given the limited ability of the retina and optic nerve to tolerate high IOP, surgery is often performed immediately once the eye is softened by the initial medical regimen. Medical antiglaucoma therapy may then continue as an adjunct to surgery or prophylactically for the fellow eye.

Although a complete description of the surgical procedures used in the management of primary glaucoma is beyond the scope of this article (see Gelatt, 1991); surgical intervention in primary glaucoma has two general thrusts: the reduction of aqueous humor production, or improvements to aqueous outflow. Because the natural role of aqueous humor is to maintain ocular health, procedures that control IOP solely by altering aqueous production either by freezing the ciliary body (cyclocryosurgery) or lasing with a neodymium: yttrium-aluminum-garnet (Nd:YAG) laser (cyclophotocoagulation), may ultimately result in cataract formation and corneal degeneration. Theoretically, procedures that address the underlying problem by improving outflow and allowing production to continue (and hence continued intraocular nutrition and waste removal) would be preferable.

FILTERING PROCEDURES. A variety of procedures that create new outflow routes by making holes in the sclera, or by disinserting part of the ciliary body, have been attempted in dogs. The success of these filtering surgeries, however, is usually shortlived (1 to 6 months) primarily because of postoperative fibrosis, and a cyclodestructive procedure may become necessary. Recent advances in microsurgical technique, and antiproliferative agents such as 5-FU (Fluorouracil, Roche) or mitomycin C (Mitomycin, Bristol-Myers Oncology), however, may rekindle interest in filtering procedures.

GONIOIMPLANT DEVICES. Gonioimplantation seeks to enhance outflow by placing a small tube into the anterior chamber, thereby permitting aqueous to drain subconjunctivally into a larger filtering "bleb" that is maintained by the implant body. Gonioimplants made of silicone, Silastic, or nylon, in both valved and free-flowing shunt models, have recently become commercially available for dogs. Pressure-sensitive valves prohibit aqueous drainage in the event IOP becomes too low, thereby avoiding a flat anterior chamber. Current devices are improved from those tried and abandoned in the 1970s, but encapsulation of the filtering bleb by nonabsorptive fibrous connective tissue, closure of the tube orifice or lumen by scar tissue, and tube migration remain formidable problems. In humans, antiproliferative agents such as mitomycin C recently have been shown to improve the ability of gonioimplants to achieve and maintain target pressures—probably by reducing filtering bleb encapsulation. Tissue plasminogen activator is also a potent addition to the glaucoma surgeon's armamentarium, as it lyses intraocular fibrin clots and potentially reduces the matrix for future fibrosis.

The author's preference for glaucomatous eyes that have the potential for vision is to use a gonioimplant with a pressure-sensitive valve (Ahmed glaucoma valve, models S-1 or S-2, New World Medical) in combination with limited cyclocryosurgery. If this insufficiently controls IOP, then a topical mydriatic adrenergic or $\beta$-blocker is added. If even further reduction in IOP is required to achieve target pressures, dichlorphenamide is added, or additional surgery performed. Combination therapy such as this has proven to be, in the author's experience, the most effective method of controlling IOP and maintaining vision for extended periods of time; it is more effective than either medical therapy alone or a single surgical procedure alone.

### PROPHYLACTIC THERAPY FOR PRIMARY GLAUCOMA

Although primary glaucoma typically presents as a unilateral disease, the initially normotensive fellow eye usually becomes overtly glaucomatous in a short period of time (median = 5 months). A retrospective study has suggested that preventative medication for the fellow normotensive eye in dogs with primary glaucoma could significantly reduce the risk of developing glaucoma in the fellow eye, or prevent it entirely (Slater and Erb, 1986). The efficacy of any specific protocol, however, is unproven, and a survey of veterinary ophthalmologists demonstrated that although 89% of the respondents advocated prophylactic therapy, over 20 separate treatment regimens were used. Only a small percentage of ophthalmologists would advocate preventative therapy for a dog that has never experienced glaucoma in either eye but has abnormal drainage angles. A miotic (demecarium bromide) or a $\beta$-blocker (timolol or betaxolol) are among the most widely used drugs, and a national multicenter clinical trial is underway to clarify the efficacy of these two drug classes in glaucoma prevention.

Currently, the author uses a long-acting miotic such as demecarium bromide (Humorsol, Merck Sharp & Dohme) 0.125 to 0.25% once daily at bedtime. In certain breeds such as basset hounds in which a low-grade inflammation of the ciliary body has been postulated to aid in occluding a congenitally compromised drainage angle, 1% prednisolone acetate once daily is also given at bedtime. IOP is measured monthly for the first 3 months following an attack in the first eye, and then at 3-month intervals thereafter. Progressively rising IOPs on follow-up exams, IOPs exceeding 20 mm Hg, changes in the appearance of the retina or optic nerve head, or an episode of acute glaucoma warrants an increase in the frequency of the topical drugs, adding a CAI, or performing surgery. It is the author's perception that a consistently applied protocol can maintain vision for a longer period of time in the second eye than previously thought, and that the eye on preventative therapy is also more responsive than the first eye to therapeutic intervention should it become overtly glaucomatous.

## SECONDARY GLAUCOMA IN VISUAL EYES

Secondary glaucoma is increased in IOP occurring as a sequela of other intraocular diseases. It is at least twice as common as primary glaucoma in dogs, and seven times more common in cats. Although therapy is directed at the primary disease in these cases, the IOP elevation cannot be ignored if pressure-induced destruction of the optic nerve head is to be avoided. The diagnostic and therapeutic protocols for these primary conditions are discussed in detail in most ophthalmic textbooks. Blind eyes with secondary glaucoma are probably best treated by enucleation if IOP is not readily controllable.

### Glaucoma Associated With Uveitis

Aggressive use of systemic or topical corticosteroids, once infectious etiologies of the uveitis have been ruled out, form the cornerstone of therapy for glaucoma that is the sequela of anterior uveitis. Intravenous corticosteroids or flunixin meglumine can rapidly reduce IOP in acute uveitis-induced glaucoma. Without a history of trauma or lens-induced uveitis, a thorough uveitis work-up is usually indicated in these animals.

Since topical miotics such as pilocarpine risk iris bombe and may exacerbate anterior uveitis by further breaking down the blood-aqueous barrier, a topical adrenergic mydriatic (epinephrine or dipivefrin), every 6 to 12 hr, or β-blocker (timolol) are better choices in mildly (5 to 10 mm Hg increase) glaucomatous inflamed eyes. Carbonic anhydrase inhibitors are useful if the IOP elevation is greater, but hyperosmotic agents such as mannitol should be reserved for last-ditch efforts, as they may cross an incompetent blood-aqueous barrier and further raise IOP. Atropine usually should be avoided in uveitis-induced glaucoma. Because aqueous humor production is typically lower than normal in anterior uveitis, patients with normotensive but inflamed eyes deserve very careful IOP monitoring, as their outflow capacity is likely to be impaired. With subsequent control of intraocular inflammation in these patients, aqueous production may return to normal levels and produce glaucoma by overwhelming a still compromised outflow system.

## Glaucoma Associated With the Lens

Glaucoma secondary to lens luxation is common in terriers and is best treated by immediate lens extraction if the eye is still visual. Attempts to trap a posteriorly luxated lens behind the pupil with miotics are often unsuccessful, and can result in acute glaucoma if the drug is administered when the lens is in the pupillary plane or anterior chamber. Markedly intumescent (swollen) lenses, especially in diabetics, can also lead to glaucoma by moving the iris base anteriorly and occluding the drainage angle. Again, immediate lensectomy usually breaks the attack in these dogs. The treatment of glaucoma secondary to chronic lens-induced uveitis is similar to that of other forms of uveitis-induced glaucoma. Lens removal in these animals, however, typically has a high complication rate and often fails to preserve vision over the long term.

## Glaucoma Associated With Hyphema

IOP needs to be carefully monitored in patients with a significant anterior chamber hemorrhage as glaucoma is often a sequela of red blood cells (RBCs) occluding the drainage apparatus. If a coagulopathy is the cause of the hyphema and inflammation is minimal, topical 2% pilocarpine may help control IOP and facilitate RBC outflow from the eye. If inflammation is suspected to be the underlying cause, and the IOP elevation is mild, topical and/or systemic corticosteroids and topical 1% epinephrine may control IOP. Hyperosmotic agents probably should be avoided in the hyphema-associated glaucomas, but carbonic anhydrase inhibitors often are useful in controlling more substantial rises. Anterior chamber drainage generally is to be avoided, as it can reinitiate bleeding and create additional inflammation. Intraocular neoplasia should always be considered in patients with glaucoma and unexplained hyphema.

## Glaucoma Associated With Neoplasia

Primary intraocular tumors such as melanoma or ciliary body adenoma/adenocarcinoma frequently result in glaucoma. Lymphosarcoma or metastasis to the eye by numerous other malignant tumors also have been reported to cause glaucoma. Although systemic chemotherapy may resolve the IOP rise in some intraocular neoplastic processes (e.g., lymphosarcoma), enucleation is often the best route.

## References and Suggested Reading

Brooks DE: Glaucoma in the dog and cat. Vet Clin North Am [Small Anim Pract] 20:775, 1990.
  *A review of glaucoma diagnosis and therapy in dogs and cats.*
Gelatt KN: The canine glaucomas. *In* Gelatt KN (ed): *Veterinary Ophthalmology*, 2nd edition. Philadelphia, Lea & Febiger, 1991, p 396.
  *A good description of glaucoma surgical techniques.*
Miller PE and Pickett JP: Comparison of the human and canine Schiøtz tonometry conversion tables in clinically normal dogs. J Am Vet Med Assoc 201:1021, 1992a.
  *A comparison of Schiøtz tonometry conversion tables to applanation tonometers in normal dogs.*
Miller PE and Pickett JP: Comparison of the human and canine Schiøtz tonometry conversion tables in clinically normal cats. J Am Vet Med Assoc 201:1017, 1992b.
  *A comparison of Schiøtz tonometry conversion tables to applanation tonometers in normal cats.*
Moller I, Cook CS, Peiffer RL, et al: Indications for and complications of pharmacological ablation of the ciliary body for the treatment of chronic glaucoma in the dog. J Am Anim Hosp Assoc 22:319, 1986.
  *A description of the technique for intravitreal gentamicin injections for the treatment of end-stage primary glaucoma.*
Pickett JP and Champagne ES: Effects of chronic administration of an oral carbonic anhydrase inhibitor (dichlorphenamide) on intraocular pressure and serum potassium levels in the normal canine. *Proc 24th Ann Meet Am Coll Vet Ophthalmol.* 24:125, 1993.
  *An experimental study that demonstrated continually declining serum potassium levels when dichlorphenamide was given at 4.4 mg/kg PO for 43 days.*
Keates EU, Druzgala PD, Howes JF, and Reaves TA: Loteprednol etabonate: A new steroid without ocular hypertensive effect. Invest Ophthalmol Vis Sci 32 (suppl):947, 1991.
  *An experimental study using dogs in which topical 0.1% dexamethasone over 6 months increased IOP 5.5 mm Hg.*
Scherlie PH: Glaucoma. *In* Kirk RW and Bonagura JD (eds): *Current Veterinary Therapy XI.* Philadelphia, WB Saunders Co, 1992, p 1125.
  *A discussion of aqueous humor dynamics, glaucoma classification, and treatment.*
Slater MR and Erb HN: Effects of risk factors and prophylactic treatment of primary glaucoma in the dog. J Am Vet Med Assoc 188:1028, 1986.
  *A retrospective study of medical antiglaucoma prophylaxis therapy.*
Zhan GL, Miranda OC, and Bito LZ: Steroid glaucoma: Corticosteroid-induced ocular hypertension in cats. Exp Eye Res 54:211, 1992.
  *A description of steroid-induced intraocular pressure elevations in cats following administration of 1% prednisolone acetate at clinically relevant intervals.*

# Section

# 14

# DISEASES OF
# BIRDS
# AND EXOTIC PETS

R. ERIC MILLER
*Consulting Editor*

*Still Current Information Found in Current Veterinary Therapy XI:*

Redig PT: Management of Medical Emergencies in Raptors, p 1134.
Kuehler CM and Loomis MR: Artificial Incubation of Nondomestic Bird Eggs, p 1138.
Clubb SL: Psittacine Neonatology, p 1142.
Gould WJ: Liver Disease in Psittacines, p 1145.
Flammer K: An Update on the Diagnosis and Treatment of Avian Chlamydosis, p 1150.
Abou-Madi N and Kollias GV: Avian Fluid Therapy, p 1154.
Quesenberry K: Avian Nutritional Support, p 1160.
McCluggage DM: Application of Splints, Bandages, and Collars, p 1163.
Burke TJ: Skin Disorders of Rodents, Rabbits and Ferrets, p 1170.
Fish RE and Besch-Williford C: Reproductive Disorders in the Rabbit and Guinea Pig, p 1175.
Finkler MR: Ferret Colitis, p 1180.
Palley LS and Fox JG: Eosinophilic Gastroenteritis in the Ferret, p 1182.
Hillyer EV: Ferret Endocrinology, p 1185.
Fowler ME: Feeding Llamas and Alpacas, p 1189.
Johnson LW: Llama Neurology, p 1193.
Citino SB: Water Quality and the Marine Aquarium, p 1199.
Noga EJ: Important Problems in Marine Aquarium Fishes, p 1202.
Jacobson ER: Reptile Dermatology, p 1204.
Junge RE and Miller RE: Reptile Respiratory Diseases, p 1210.
Bush M: An Update of Antibiotic Therapy in Reptiles, p 1214.
Brannian RE: Reptile Surgical Procedures, p 1215.
Crawshaw GJ: Amphibian Medicine, p 1219.

*Elsewhere in Current Veterinary Therapy XII:*

Immunization of Wild Animal Species Against Common Diseases, Appendix, p 1427.

# NONSURGICAL MEANS OF SEX DETERMINATION IN PSITTACINE BIRDS

SUSAN L. CLUBB

*Miami, Florida*

Most psittacine species are monomorphic or show very slight or indistinct dimorphic traits. For successful aviculture, a number of sex determination techniques have been developed utilizing surgical sexing techniques ranging from endoscopy to karyotyping and deoxyribonucleic acid (DNA) probes.

The most common means for sex determination in monomorphic psittacines is by endoscopic examination or surgical sexing. Surgical sexing in the hands of an experienced veterinarian is safe, rapid, and reliable. Surgical sexing has the advantages of (1) visualization of the gonads as well as other organs, and (2) of being a hands-on assessment of health and fitness for breeding. In addition, the birds are typically tattooed at the time of sexing to avoid later confusion. It does, however, carry with it some surgical and anesthetic risk and is not universally available. Laboratory methods (chromosomal and DNA probe sexing techniques) are commercially available and accessible nationwide.

## CHROMOSOMAL ANALYSIS

Male birds are homogametic (have two Z chromosomes), while females are heterogametic (have one Z and one W chromosome). The Z and W chromosomes differ in size and shape and can be differentiated by microscopy. For chromosomal analysis, a blood feather is submitted to the laboratory.[*] The pulp tissue is grown in cell culture for 7 to 9 days. A squash preparation is stained and karyotypic evaluation is accomplished by matching chromosomes based on gross morphologic characteristics such as length, shape, centromeric position, and specific staining qualities.

Chromosomal analysis has the additional potential to identify chromosomal defects that may result in embryonic mortality. Some chromosomal abnormalities that have been identified include inversions, translocations, and triploidy. An inversion occurs when a segment of a chromosome is removed, rotated 180 degrees, and reunited with the chromosome. Such a bird may look normal but have poor breeding performance. Chromosome translocations occur when two segments of two different chromosomes are exchanged, resulting in two different abnormal chromosomes. Such birds will exhibit approximately 50% reduction in fertility. In triploidy, the chick receives the normal one set of chromosomes from one parent, while receiving two sets of chromosomes from the other, resulting in three sets of chromosomes. Invariably, triploid parrots are infertile.

## SEXING BY DNA PROBE

DNA probes have been developed that can accurately distinguish the DNA in the sex chromosomes of male and female birds.[†] The DNA probe is a labeled DNA fragment cloned from the sex chromosomes. This fragment tags similar sequences in the DNA samples of many bird species and gives characteristic and sex-specific patterns for each taxonomic group. The examination of both sex chromosomes and the internal controls implicit in the method (species-specific patterns and DNA quality cross-checks) make this method extremely accurate.

Samples for DNA sexing are stable and can be stored for years; therefore, in questions of accuracy or identity, stored samples can be referred to. These samples are also suitable for DNA fingerprinting as a means of individual identification.

## HORMONAL SEXING METHODS

Measurement of sex steroid hormones in feces, egg wastes, or plasma has been used for sex determination as well as for assessment of functional activity of reproductive organs. Fecal steroid analysis was extensively researched at San Diego Zoo but is not currently commercially available due to the inability to sex immature birds or birds with low gonadal activity.

## VENT SEXING

Palpation, examination, or eversion of the vent is used for sexing avian species such as newly hatched poultry, mature waterfowl, and ratites. A rudimentary copulatory organ is present in males of these species.

---

[*]Avian Genetic Sexing Laboratory, Marc Valentine, Call ahead for test kit: (901) 388–9548.

[†]Zoogen, Inc, 1105 Kennedy Place, Suite 4, Davis CA 95616, (916) 756–8089.

**Table 1.** *Sexual Dimorphism in Psittacines*

**Parrots of Australian and Pacific Distribution**

***Loridae***—Most species are monomorphic. The head is usually larger in male birds.

    Monomorphic genera

        *Pseudeos*—**dusky lory**

        *Chalcopsitta*—**black lory, duivenbode's lory**

        *Eos*—**red lories**

        *Lorius*—**chattering lories**

        *Vini*—**blue lories**

        Most *Trichoglossus* spp.—**rainbow lories**

    Dimorphic genera (species)

        *Charmosyna*—**Stella lory** (*Charmosyna papou*)—The female has a yellow patch on the rump and lower back that is absent in the male. Apparent in red and black color morphs.

        —**Red-flanked lory** (*Charmosyna placentis*)—The male has bright red patches on the flank that are absent in the female. The male has bright blue cheek patches, while the female has yellow-streaked cheek patches. Other less common members of the genus are also dimorphic.

        *Trichoglossus* (*T. flavoviridis meyeri*)—**Meyer's lorikeet**—The male has a larger and brighter yellow ear patch than the female.

***Cacatuidae***—Psittaci-formes

    Cacatuinae

    Monomorphic genera

        *Probosciger*—**palm cockatoo**—Male is usually larger and has a larger beak. Size also varies geographically and with subspecies.

    Dimorphic genera

        *Calyptorhynchus*—**black cockatoos**—Dimorphism is striking in some species and barely noticeable in others. In the Banksian cockatoo (*C. Magnificus*), the male plumage is black except for bands of red in the tail, whereas the female is dotted and barred with orange yellow.

        *Callocephalon*—**gang gang cockatoo**—The male is slate grey with a red head and crest. The female has a gray head and crest and plumage that is barred with yellow orange.

        *Cacatua* and *Eolophus*—**white and pink cockatoos**—Adult birds, except for the bare-eyed cockatoo (*C. sanguinea*), can usually be sexed by eye color. The female has a red iris, whereas the iris of the male is dark brown to black. A bright light may be needed to determine eye color in some species such as the moluccan cockatoo (*C. moluccensis*). The female of most species is smaller than the male. Red-eyed males and dark-eyed females have been reported and are more common in captive reared birds. The iris is brown in immature birds of both sexes.

    Nymphicinae

        *Nymphicus*—**Cockatiel**—Sex is easily determined in the wild type (gray), as the male has a large yellow facial patch and crest that is gray in the female. The primary flight feathers and tail feathers of the female are diagonally barred with white. Immature birds resemble females. Cinnamon, lutino and fallow cockatiels can be sexed by the faint diagonal barring of the primary flight feathers in the females and in cinnamons a faint yellow mask in the male. Pied cockatiels can be sexed as grays unless heavily pied and these areas are white. Pearl cockatiel males loose their pearling when mature. White-faced cockatiels are sexed as grays.

***Psittacidae***

    Psittacinae

    Monomorphic genera

        *Cyanoramphus*—**Kakarikis**

    Dimorphic genera

        *Melopsittacus*—**Budgerigar**—In the normal green variety, the cere of the adult male is blue, whereas the cere of the adult female in pinkish brown. This is not dependable in color mutations such as lutino, blue, or white birds.

        *Platycercus*—**rosellas**—The male of most rosella species is slightly brighter than the female or immature. Female and young of several species have a row of white spots on the ventral surface of seven or eight primary and secondary flight feathers. These are lost by the male at the time they reach sexual maturity. Wing spots are retained in adult female yellow rosellas (*P. flaveolus*), golden-mantled rosellas (*P. eximius*), mealy rosellas (*P. adscitus*) and Stanley's rosellas (*P. icterotis*). Male Stanley's rosellas have red heads and bright yellow cheek patches, while females have green heads and dull cheek patches.

        *Psephotus*—**red rumped parakeet** (*P. haematonotus*)—Most species in the genus exhibit sexual dimorphism. The male red-rumpted parakeet has a red patch on the rump, while the female is drab. Other species are uncommon in aviculture.

        *Neophema*—**grass parakeets**—Sexual dimorphism varies from a slight variation in the Bourke's parakeet (*N. bourkii*) (the male has more blue and pink on the breast) to extreme sexual dimorphism in the scarlet-chested parakeet (*N. splendida*) (the chest is red in the male, green in the female).

        *Polytelis*—**Barraband's, rock pebblars (P. anthopeplus)**—The males of this genus are typically larger and brighter in color than females and young birds. Female Barraband's parakeets (*P. swainsonii*) lack the yellow feathers of the male. In rock pebblars, the ventral surface of the male's tail is black, while tail feathers of the female are margined and tipped in pink. The male Princess of Wales (*P. alexandrae*) is brighter in color and the bill is deeper red than the female. In many species, the male has an elongated spatula tip on the third primary.

        *Aprosmictus*—**crimson-winged parakeet**—The male has a black mantle.

        *Alisterus*—**king parrots**—Sexual dimorphism is present in plumage and beak color of some species. Some subspecies of green-winged king parrots (*A. chloropterus*) show dimorphism in the green patch on the wing which is absent in the female, but some subspecies are monomorphic. In Australian king parakeets (*A. scapularis*), the male is red and the female's head is green.

        *Roratus*—**eclectus parrots**—The male is brilliant emerald green with a yellow-orange beak. The female is red-maroon and purple with a black beak. The color difference is evident at the time of emergence of the first tail and contour feathers in chicks. The down of both sexes is black.

        *Tanygnathus*—**great bills, blue napes, and Muller's parrots**—The beak of the male Muller's parrot (*T. mulleri*) is red, and the beak of the female is white. The beak of the male great billed parrot (*T. megalorynchos*) is much larger than the female's.

        *Psittaculirostris*—**fig parrots**—Most species are obviously dimorphic in plumage.

        *Psittrichas*—**Pesquet's parrot**—Male has a red line behind the eye that is absent in the female.

**Parrots of Afro-Asian Distribution**

***Psittacidae***

    Psittacinae

    Monomorphic genera

        *Coracopis*—**Vasa** or **black parrots**—Monomorphic in plumage, however the tissues of the vent in males is hypertrophied especially in breeding season.

        *Agapornis*—**lovebirds**—Commonly available species are monomorphic. Some species show definitive dimorphism such as the Abyssinian lovebird (*A. taranta*) in which the male has a red patch on the forehead and lores that is absent in the female. The male Madagascar lovebird (*A. cana*) has a gray head, while the female has a green head.

        *Psittacus*—**African gray parrots**—Very slight dimorphism is evident on close examination but should not be considered definitive. Females (*P. erithacus erithacus*) tend to be lighter gray than males and have red edging on the under tail coverts caudal to the vent. Tinmeh grays (*P. e. timneh*) are monomorphic.

*Table continued on opposite page*

**Table 1.** *Continued*

| | |
|---|---|
| Dimorphic genera | Nandayus—**Nanday conure.** |
| *Psittacula*—**ringnecks**—All male birds in the genus have a ring encircling the neck or a wide black moustache ring. In some species, this is lacking in the female and young, while in some it is less prominent. Adult male plumage may not be evident until 1 1/2 to 2 1/2 years of age. In some species, the beak color is different. The male derbyan parakeet (*P. derbyana*) and some subspecies of the moustache parakeet (*P. alexandri*) have a red beak, while the female's beak is black. | *Enidognathus*—**slender-billed and Austral conures.** |
| | *Cyanoliseus*—**Patagonian conure.** |
| | *Deroptyus*—**hawkhead parrots.** |
| | *Myiopsitta*—**Quaker parakeets.** |
| | *Rhynchopsitta*—**thick-billed parrots.** |
| | *Brotogeris*—**bee-bee parakeets.** |
| | *Pionus*—**pionus parrots.** |
| | *Pionites*—**caiques.** |
| | *Amazona*—**Amazon parrots**—Most species are monomorphic. In the spectacled Amazon (*A. albifrons*), the male has red marking on the cranial edge of the carpus and adjacent upper wing coverts on the dorsal side of the wing that are absent or reduced in the female. In the yellow-lored Amazon (*A. xantholora*), the female is duller and lacks white on the head and red facial markings that are found in the male. The adult male yellow-faced Amazon (*A. xanthops*) has a patch of yellow-orange on the breast and abdomen that is reduced or absent in the female. |
| *Loriculus*—**hanging parrots**—Adult birds are dimorphic in plumage and in some species in eye color. In most species, the forehead and/or crown of the male is blue or red and is green in the female. | |
| *Poicephalus*—**Senegal parrots and related species**—Some members of the genus show marked sexual dimorphism, whereas other are monomorphic. The male red-bellied parrot (*P. rufiventralis*) has a deep red-orange breast and abdomen, whereas the female's breast is greenish brown. The female Rüppell's parrot (*P. rueppellii*) is more brightly colored than the male, having a bright blue rump patch that is absent in the male. The Senegal parrot (*P. senegalus*) shows slight but unreliable dimorphism. The undertail coverts of the male are yellow or orange, while the female's are greenish yellow to greenish orange. | |
| | *Bolborhynchus*—**mountain parakeets**—Only one species, the golden-fronted mountain parakeet (*B. aurifrons*) is dimorphic. The male has yellow markings on the lores, forehead, throat, and part of the cheek; whereas the female is predominantly green. |
| **Parrots of South American Distribution** | Dimorphic genera |
| **Psittacidae** | *Pionopsitta*—**pileated parrot**—The male has a red head and the female has a green head. Dimorphism is evident in immataure plumage. Other members of the genus are monomorphic and very rare in aviculture. |
| Psittacinae | |
| Monomorphic genera | |
| *Ara*—**macaws.** | |
| *Anodorhynchus*—**hyacinth macaw.** | *Forpus*—**parrotlets**—All species are dimorphic. In most species, the male will have coloration on the rump or wings, while the females are usually predominantly green. |
| *Aratinga*—**conures.** | |
| *Pyrrhura*—**conures.** | |

## SEXUAL DIMORPHISM IN PSITTACINES

A few physical characteristics can be helpful in determining gender in monomorphic birds. For most species, these traits cannot be relied upon totally for pairing. Sexual dimorphism is reliable and definitive in some species. Eclectus parrots (*Eclectus* spp.) are an example of striking sexual dimorphism in which the female is deep red and purple with a black beak, while the male is a brilliant emerald green with a yellow-orange beak. For many years the sexes were mistaken for separate species with obvious difficulties in captive propagation (Table 1).

Size and shape of the head and beak may be an indication of sex. The male bird usually has a larger, broader head and heavier beak than the female. Males of some species, such as cockatoos, are often significantly larger than females.

Behavioral differences can be helpful in gender determination. Male birds will often sing a courting song and dance while the female observes. This is more common in passerines than in psittacines and is the most reliable way of sexing society finches. The characteristic courting song of a male cockatiel is usually apparent before chicks moult to adult plumage. A parrot that spends excessive time rooting around on the cage floor and shredding paper is likely to be a female attempting to build a nest. Male birds of many species tend to be more aggressive than females, with some

notable exceptions such as eclectus parrots and Buffon's macaws. Females tend to be more likely to bite and protest more loudly when restrained.

Observation of copulation does not assure that birds are properly paired. Homosexual pairing is uncommon if birds are allowed to choose their mates. Groups of large psittacines that are allowed to pair up in a group cage must be watched carefully, especially macaws. If one pair decides to breed, they may become very aggressive toward other birds in the cage.

Palpation of the pelvic bones is commonly used by aviculturists for sexing birds. The pelvic bones are located slightly caudal to the vent and can be palpated with the bird restrained in dorsal recumbency or in a standing position grasping a perch. The pelvic bones of the mature female are supposedly farther apart to allow her to lay eggs. In addition, the pelvic bones of the female are supposedly more pointed, while in the male they are more rounded and directed medially. When performed on known-sex birds, it has been highly inaccurate.

Sexual dimorphism is often found in Australian and Asian psittacine species, whereas neotropical (Central and South American) and African species are typically monomorphic. Birds that inhabit arid climates show a higher incidence of sexual dimorphism than jungle or forest species, which may indicate more dependence on sight identification among species in arid climates. Intensive observation of a species may reveal slight dimorphic traits. If African gray parrots from the same region are observed, the females will appear lighter in color than males. Many birds (not typically psittacines) molt into a prenuptual plumage prior to the breeding season.

In most species that exhibit sexual dimorphism, immature birds resemble females. Some species such as

Asian parakeet species, which have ringed necks, do not exhibit adult dimorphic plumage until 1.5 to 2.5 years of age after reaching sexual maturity. Surgical or laboratory sex determination techniques are the logical alternative to excessive holding time prior to accurate gender determination by dimorphic traits.

# ANTIMICROBIALS IN PET BIRDS

HEIDI L. HOEFER
*New York, New York*

Antimicrobials are commonly used in pet avian practices. While many antibiotic regimens have been derived empirically for use in avian species, recent advances in pharmocokinetic research is changing our approach to therapeutics in the avian patient. It is becoming increasingly evident that drug disposition and metabolism differs significantly between mammals and birds and, in some cases, between different species of birds. Simple extrapolation of mammalian therapeutic protocols is not an effective means of drug application in birds.

There are several factors that need to be considered when treating the avian patient. The normal bacterial flora of healthy avian species is predominately grampositive, with *Lactobacillus* spp., *Streptococcus* spp., *Bacillus* spp., and *Corynebacterium* spp. common isolates. Small numbers of gram-negative bacteria may be seen occasionally. The normal microflora provides natural protection and, when suppressed, may facilitate the overgrowth of opportunistic bacteria. Colonization with gram-negative bacteria, especially of the family Enterobacteriaceae, indicates a disturbance in the normal balance and may represent the initiation of disease. Chronic stress and prolonged antibiotic therapy can result in microflora upsets and may predispose opportunistic bacterial overgrowths.

Pet birds often suffer from an entirely different set of disease-causing factors than small companion animals. Inappropriate management and husbandry techniques (e.g., inadequate diets, overcrowding, and poor hygiene) adversely affect the immune system. Onset of disease can appear insidious and many birds actually present in the final stages of illness. Specific diagnoses can be difficult, especially in the debilitated or very small patient. Therapy must be rapid and effective and is often done in a "shotgun" manner until the patient is stabilized. It is therefore critical that antibiotic selection be rational and administered appropriately. Hospitalization and supportive care of the sick patient improves the immune response and enhances the effectiveness of antibiotic therapy.

## ANTIBIOTIC SELECTION CRITERIA

The ideal therapeutic protocol would include the early recognition of disease; identification and antibiotic sensitivity of the causative agent, and the administration of appropriate antimicrobials utilizing the most effective routes of drug delivery. In treating the avian patient, additional factors to consider include: type and size of bird, flock versus individual treatment, and temperament (Table 1).

### Antibiotic Spectrum and Minimum Inhibitory Concentration

Many avian pathogens are becoming increasingly resistant to antibiotic therapy. Indiscriminant use of antibiotics and prolonged antibiotic use in quarantine stations have played a significant role in the development of drug resistance. For optimal effectiveness, an antimicrobial agent should maintain tissue levels at the site of infection that is equal to or above the minimum inhibitory concentration (MIC) for that particular organism. Differences in bioavailability, drug half-lives, and attainable drug blood levels between avian species and mammals are not represented by standard disk sensitivity assays (Kirby-Bauer). Antimicrobial sensitivity tests are based on attainable serum levels of drug in humans and may not adequately represent the interaction that will occur in avian species *in vivo*. Ineffective treatment of a "sensitive" organism might therefore be related to the inadequacy of the antibiotic regimen.

### Drug Dosages

Substantial differences in drug metabolism between mammals and birds make extrapolation of drug doses based on weight alone difficult and clinically inadequate. For example, the $\beta$-lactam antibiotics are generally dosed more frequently and at a much higher dosage in psittacines than in companion mammals. The use of allometric scaling based on metabolic rate and weight may provide a more technical approach to drug extrapolation across species (Dorrestein, 1991). Specific pharmocokinetic data on commonly used antibiotics in different avian species are continually being generated and will result in more effective protocols.

## Route and Frequency of Administration

One of the first decisions a clinician must make is which route of administration can be successfully delivered to the bird. Drug administration techniques vary considerably between small mammals and birds. It is very difficult to "pill" a bird and many drugs are not available in a palatable and concentrated liquid form. Route of administration will depend on the preparation available, the number and size of the species being dosed, and the tenacity of the individual bird. It may be easier to dose a large parrot parenterally, but some owners are unable to adequately restrain their birds or may be uncomfortable handling hypodermic needles. It can be equally as disconcerting to force a liquid antibiotic into the biting mouth of an untamed parrot. The clinician must also consider the amount of stress involved; the value of a frequently administered drug must be weighed against the stress of frequent handling.

### PARENTERAL ADMINISTRATION

Antibiotics can be given intravenously (IV), intraosseously (IO), subcutaneously (SC), or intramuscularly (IM). It is difficult to repeatedly administer intravenous or intraosseous injections without an indwelling catheter. Catheter placement requires a fair amount of dexterity and is usually reserved for the larger species that require parenteral fluid administration. Most injections are delivered subcutaneously or intramuscularly. Many

**Table 1.** *Antibiotics for Use in Birds*[*]

| Drug | Form and Route | Dosage |
|------|----------------|--------|
| Amikacin[†] | Inj, SC, IM | 15 mg/kg q12h |
| Amoxicillin | Inj, SC, IM | 100 mg/kg q8h |
| | Oral susp, PO | 100 mg/kg q8h |
| Amoxicillin/Clavulanic acid | Oral susp, PO | 50–100 mg/kg q6–8h |
| Ampicillin | Inj, IM, IV | 100 mg/kg q8h |
| Carbenicillin | Inj, IM, IV | 100 mg/kg q6–8h |
| Cephalothin | Inj, IM, IV | 10 mg/kg q6–8h |
| Cefotaxime | Inj, IM, IV | 75–100 mg/kg q6–8h |
| Cephalexin | Oral susp, PO | 40–100 mg/kg q6h |
| Chloramphenicol | Inj (succinate), IM, IV | 50 mg/kg q8h |
| | Oral susp (palmitate), PO | 75 mg/kg q8h |
| Chlortetracycline | Medicated feed | 1% in large birds, 45 days |
| | Impregnated millet seed | 0.5% in small birds, 30 days |
| Ciprofloxacin | Tablets (crush or suspend) | 10–15 mg/kg q12h |
| Doxycycline | Oral susp, PO | 25–50 mg/kg q24h (low dose in macaws) |
| | Medicated feed | 1 gm/kg of feed |
| | Inj, IM (Vibravenos, not available in United States) | 75 mg/kg q7d (macaws, lovebirds) |
| | | 100 mg/kg q7d |
| Enrofloxacin | Tablets (crush or suspend) | 15 mg/kg q12h |
| | Inj, PO, IM, IV (dilute) | 15 mg/kg q12h |
| | 10% liquid (not in United States) | 250 mg/L drinking water |
| Erythromycin | Oral susp, PO | 60 mg/kg q12h |
| Ethambutol[‡] | Oral | 15–25 mg/kg q24h |
| Gentamicin[†] | Inj, IM, IV | 10 mg/kg q24h |
| Metronidazole | Tablets (crush or suspend) | 50 mg/kg q24h |
| Oxytetracycline[†] | Inj, SC, IM (long-acting prep) | 50–100 mg/kg q2–3d |
| Piperacillin | Inj, IM, IV | 100–150 mg/kg q8h |
| Rifampin[‡] | Oral | 15 mg/kg q12h |
| Streptomycin[‡] | Inj, IM | 30 mg/kg q12h |
| Ticarcillin | Inj, IM, IV | 200 mg/kg q8h |
| Tobramycin[†] | Inj, IM | 5–10 mg/kg q12h |
| Trimethoprim-sulfadiazined or sulfamethoxazole | Inj, SC, IM Oral susp | 50–100 mg/kg q12h (of combined drug) 50–100 mg/kg q12h |
| Tylosin | Inj, IM | 30 mg/kg q12h |

[*]Not all drug doses are based on pharmocokinetic data, values represent a review of the literature and the author's clinical experience.
[†]Use with caution; potential toxicity or muscle necrosis.
[‡]Combination treatment for avian tuberculosis.
Abbreviations: Inj = injection, oral susp = oral suspension.

intravenous antibiotics can be safely administered in the muscle, while some products can result in extensive muscle necrosis. For example, the intravenous preparation of doxycycline manufactured in the United States cannot be given IM, while the European counterpart (Vibravenos SF, Pfizer, Germany) is safe for IM use. Product inquiries should be made prior to use if unfamiliar with the appropriate administration of the drug.

The recommended site for IM injections is in the pectoral muscle mass. Care must be taken in cachexic or juvenile birds, as they have a limited amount of muscle in this area. Because birds have a renal portal system (similar to reptiles), injections should never be given in the legs. Repeated injections of muscle necrotizing agents should be avoided. For example, enrofloxacin (Baytril, Miles, Elkhart, Indiana) can result in extensive bruising of the pectoral muscle mass and should only be given IM in the initial phase of treatment. Small-gauge hypodermic needles (27- to 28-gauge) are recommended for IM injections and large volumes can be given in divided sites.

### ORAL ADMINISTRATION

Oral medications can be a reliable and effective means of dosing avian patients. Many antibiotics are available in a flavored suspension that can be administered directly into the oral cavity. Antibiotics only available in tablet form can be crushed and mixed with a sticky or viscous food for home administration (peanut butter, fruit jelly, and coconut syrup work well). Injectable enrofloxacin can be given orally at the same parenteral dose but is very unpalatable and may need to be sweetened. Water administration is the least reliable route of drug administration. Most birds will not drink enough water to maintain therapeutic blood levels of a drug. Some species like the budgerigar and zebra finch are desert dwellers in their native habitat and can go for several days without drinking. Sick birds are especially reluctant to take water that has been medicated, and this may further compromise the patient. It is also difficult to predict the stability of a therapeutic agent once it is dissolved in water. Oral administration of therapeutics is not recommended in birds with gastrointestinal mobility impairment (e.g., crop stasis).

### MEDICATED FEEDS

The administration of antibiotics in the feed is used most frequently in aviaries where large groups of birds

need to be treated. Some individual pet birds may accept the medicated diet, but the majority of birds (especially sick ones) are reluctant to accept an unfamiliar food. Treatment for chlamydiosis is often attempted through the administration of medicated feed because of the lengthy duration of treatment (28 to 45 days). Several medicated food products are commercially available for use in birds (Table 2).

### TOPICAL MEDICATIONS

Topical preparations should be used sparingly in treating avian patients. Greasy ointments result in matting of the feathers and can interfere with thermoregulation in the bird. Whenever possible, nontoxic water-soluble agents should be used. In treating skin lesions, the feathers surrounding the affected areas should be gently plucked or trimmed back. Liquid ophthalmic preparations are easier to administer than ointments.

### NEBULIZATION

Nebulization is an effective way to deliver antibiotics into the respiratory system. Because the blood supply to the avian sinuses and airsacs is limited, the use of nebulized particles can be considered a form of topical therapy for the airways. The size of the nebulized particles must be less than 3 $\mu$m to be able to reach the level of the airsacs and lungs. The author uses an ultrasonic unit (Ultra Neb, Devilbiss) to nebulize sterile saline and a parenteral antibiotic preparation. A sample protocol might consist of 50 ml of sterile saline plus 100 mg cefotaxime (Claforan, Hoechst-Roussel, Somerville, New Jersey) or 50 mg of amikacin sulfate (Amiglyde-V, Aveco); antimicrobial selection varies according to sensitivity testing results.

## ANTIBIOTIC CLASSES

### Aminoglycosides

Aminoglycoside antibiotics are bactericidal agents that interfere with bacterial protein synthesis. Commonly used drugs are gentamicin, amikacin, and tobramycin. Streptomycin, neomycin, and kanamycin have a limited spectrum of activity and increased toxicity and are seldom used in avian medicine. Aminoglycosides must penetrate the bacterial cell wall to interfere with synthetic activities. This requires an oxygen-rich environment, making aminoglycosides ineffective in low-oxygen sites (abscesses and exudates). They are poorly

***Table 2.*** *Manufacturers of Medicated Feed for Psittacine Birds*

| Company | Product | Address |
| --- | --- | --- |
| Bird Life | 1% CTC medicated pellets | Box 745, Poway, CA 92064 |
| Hartz Mountain | 0.5% CTC millet (Keet Life) | Harrison, NJ 07029 |
| Lafeber Co | 1% CTC medicated pellets | RR 2, Odell, IL 60460 |
| Zeigler Brothers | 1% CTC medicated pellets | Box 95, Gardners, PA 17342 |

effective against anaerobic organisms and, because they are lipid insoluble, have poor penetration into the central nervous system (CNS) and the eye. Aminoglycosides are not fully absorbed from the gastrointestinal tract and must be administered parenterally. They are eliminated almost exclusively by glomerular filtration. There is a moderate toxicity potential with aminoglycoside use; nephrotoxicity, ototoxicity, and neuromuscular blockade have been reported. Toxic side effects reported in avian species includes polyuria, polydipsia, weakness, and apnea from neuromuscular blockade. Aminoglycosides should not be used in dehydrated patients or in those with suspected renal disease.

Aminoglycosides are broad-spectrum antibiotics with particularly good efficacy against common gram-negative pathogens. Pharmocokinetic studies using amikacin in psittacine birds has shown that it has good activity against many gram-negative bacteria and has fewer toxic side effects than gentamicin and tobramycin. Amikacin is the aminoglycoside of choice in avian species. This group of antibiotics may reach maximal effectiveness when combined with a penicillin-derived β-lactam antibiotic.

## Cephalosporins

Cephalosporins are a class of β-lactam antibiotics that are similar in mode of action to the penicillins. The β-lactam moiety confers antimicrobial activity against the β-lactamase–producing bacteria. As a class, the β-lactams are bactericidal agents that inhibit the formation of the bacterial cell wall. The antimicrobial spectrum of activity of the cephalosporins includes most gram-positive cocci, many gram-negatives, and some anaerobes. The newer products have an increased activity against gram-negatives. The distribution of the cephalosporins is limited to the extracellular space with poor distribution to the CNS and eye. They are well absorbed after oral or parenteral administration but have a short half-life and may require multiple daily dosing to maintain therapeutic blood levels. Cephalosporins are rapidly eliminated by the kidneys. They are considered to be relatively nontoxic.

Cephalosporins are broadly classified into first-, second-, or third-generation products. First-generation antibiotics (cephalothin, cephalexin) have good activity against most gram-positive cocci, many gram-negatives, and some anaerobes. Second-generation products (cefoxitin) have increased spectrum against gram-negatives. Third-generation cephalosporins (cefotaxime) have the best activity against gram-negatives, including many *Pseudomonas* spp. and variable activity against gram-positive bacteria. Cefotaxime may penetrate the CNS more effectively than other cephalosporins. The author uses cefotaxime to nebulize birds with lower airway disease. The majority of second- and third-generation products are only available in parenteral preparations and have a short shelf life following reconstitution. The cephalosporins are well suited for avian use; however, they must be dosed three or four times daily and may not be recommended in birds that are too stressed or too difficult to handle frequently.

## Penicillins

The penicillins are β-lactam antibiotics derived from 6-aminopenicillanic acid. The pharmocology is similar to the cephalosporins: they are bactericidal agents that inhibit the formation of the bacterial cell wall. In mammals, the penicillins are excreted primarily through the kidneys by tubular secretion and glomerular filtration. They are considered to be relatively nontoxic; however, anaphylactic reactions have been reported. The penicillins have a wide extracellular distribution, especially in inflamed tissues, but poor penetration into the CNS. They are potentially synergistic with aminoglycosides and, in severe infections, especially with *Pseudomonas*, penicillins are more effective in combination.

The various penicillins have a similar pharmacology but vary in antimicrobial spectrum. The earlier generation products (penicillin, amoxicillin, ampicillin) have a predominantly gram-positive spectrum and are not used as much in avian medicine due to the availability of more effective drugs. The later generation semisynthetic penicillin derivatives (ticarcillin, pipericillin, carbenicillin) have increased spectrum against gram-negative bacteria and are very good for use in avian species. These products are only available in parenteral preparations and require frequent dosing to maintain therapeutic concentrations (at least three times daily). An effective protocol for severe bacterial infections in hospitalized avian patients might include ticarcillin or pipericillin used in combination with parenteral amikacin. Potentiation of amoxicillin with clavulinic acid increases activity against the β-lactamase–producing bacteria and is available in a palatable oral preparation (Clavamox, SmithKline Beecham Laboratories, Pittsburgh, Pennsylvania) that many birds will accept. The combination works well for the treatment of chronic dermatitis in birds.

## Chloramphenicol

Chloramphenicol is a synthetic broad-spectrum antimicrobial agent. It is a bacteriostatic drug that interferes with bacterial protein synthesis. Chloramphenicol is highly lipid soluble and has good tissue and cellular penetration, including the CNS and eye. Tissue concentrations may exceed serum levels. Elimination of the drug is through metabolism by the liver. There is a toxicity potential associated with the use of chloramphenicol that may vary with species. Possible side effects in mammals include bone marrow suppression, decreased immunoglobulin synthesis, and decreased wound healing due to its action as a protein synthesis inhibitor. Some mammalian species may become anorexic when on the drug, but this is not a common side effect in birds. Because of potential toxicity in humans, chloramphenicol should be handled carefully.

The antimicrobial spectrum of chloramphenicol includes both gram-positive and gram-negative oganisms; however, many avian gram-negative pathogens are resistant. Chloramphenicol has some activity against mycoplasma, chlamydia, and some protozoa. It is a popular drug for use in avian pediatrics and in the treatment of neurologic and gastrointestinal disorders. Chloramphenicol is not recommended in the "shotgun" treatment of severe bacterial infections in birds because of its limited spectrum and its static activity. It should not be combined with a bactericidal drug.

Chloramphenicol is available in two forms. The palmitate ester is a tasteless oral suspension that is rapidly absorbed, but it may result in erratic blood concentrations, and may no longer be commercially available. The sodium succinate ester can be administered SC, IM, or IV and results in more predictable serum levels of drug. The oral suspension may work well in the outpatient treatment of a stable avian patient while waiting for sensitivity testing results. Suspensions can be made from the tablets.

## Tetracyclines

The tetracyclines are bacteriostatic antibiotics that interfere with bacterial protein synthesis. The natural tetracyclines include chlortetracycline and oxytetracycline and the semisynthetic drugs include tetracycline, doxycycline, and minocycline. All tetracyclines are amphoteric, with doxycycline and minocycline being the most lipid soluble of the group. This results in wide tissue distribution and penetration. Drug excretion is either by the liver or kidneys; doxycycline is excreted as an inactive conjugate in the feces. Because dietary calcium interferes with the absorption of the tetracyclines from the gastrointestinal tract; mineral blocks and cuttlebones must be removed from the bird cage during treatment. Care must also be taken with long-term oral tetracycline use in juvenile birds because of the calcium chelation effect. Prolonged treatment can also alter gastrointestinal flora and result in bacterial or yeast (Candida) overgrowths. Periodic Gram staining of the feces during treatment is recommended to monitor gut flora.

The tetracyclines have a limited antimicrobial spectrum and have poor activity against most gram-negative avian isolates. They are primarily used for the treatment of chlamydiosis in birds. Because tetracyclines are only effective when the chlamydiae are actively replicating, prolonged treatment periods of 30 to 45 days are required to successfully clear the infection.

Chlortetracycline (CTC) is commonly recommended for the treatment of chlamydiosis. It is usually administered in medicated feed because the drug's short elimination half-life makes oral or parenteral dosing impractical. The medicated diet must contain less than 0.7% calcium and be the sole food source for the duration of treatment. Small birds (canaries, budgerigars) can be treated for 30 days with a medicated seed diet containing 0.05% CTC (Keet Life, Hartz Mountain,

Harrison, New Jersey). Larger psittacines require 0.1% CTC diet and need to be treated for 45 days. Medicated seeds and pellets are commercially available (Table 2) or the bird can be placed on a home-cooked mash to which the CTC powder can be added after cooking.

Doxycycline is considered to be the clinical drug of choice in treating chlamydiosis in avian species, although it is not specifically labeled for this use. Doxycycline is more lipophilic, achieves greater tissue concentrations, and has less gastrointestinal side effects than the other tetracyclines. The bioavailability of doxycycline in birds is higher than that of CTC. Doxycycline can be administered directly into the mouth or administered parenterally. The half-life following oral dosing varies with the species: macaws and cockatoos have a longer drug half-life and may therefore require a lower dose of doxycycline. It is available in a raspberry-flavored syrup (Vibramycin, Pfizer, New York, New York) that is palatable but is not concentrated enough for use in the larger species. Some species (e.g., macaws) may regurgitate following administration of the oral suspension. Doxycycline tablets or capsules do not suspend well in solution but can be mixed into small amounts of food and administered to the bird. This method will only be effective in those species that will accept a variety of table foods. Alternatively, a corn, rice, and bean mash diet can be medicated with doxycyline at a dose of 1 gm/kg of feed for treating larger psittacines. Commercially prepared doxycycline-medicated feeds are not available. A parenteral doxycycline formulation appropriate for intramuscular treatment of chlamydiosis is available in Canada and Europe (Vibravenos, Pfizer, Germany). This preparation can effectively maintain therapeutic blood levels of doxycycline for 5 to 7 days following a single IM injection. A similar product is not available in the United States. An intravenous preparation is available in the United States (Doxycycline hyclate, Pfizer) but cannot be administered IM due to the extensive muscle necrosis that results from its use. The other tetracyclines are not extensively used in avian medicine.

## Quinolones

Common quinolones used in avian medicine include enrofloxacin and ciprofloxacin (Cipro, Miles Laboratories). The quinolones are bactericidal antimicrobial agents that are targeted against bacterial gyrase. This enzyme is responsible for coiling bacterial deoxyribonucleic acid (DNA), a unique mode of action that does not result in cross-resistance with other antibiotics. The quinolones are widely distributed, and tissue concentrations may exceed serum levels of the drug. They are primarily excreted by the kidneys following metabolism by the liver. Potential toxic side effects of quinolone includes gastrointestinal upset, muscle necrosis with multiple IM injections, and articular defects in young mammals. Although this has not been reported in juvenile psittacines, joint lesions have been induced in pigeon nestlings with high doses of enrofloxacin.

The antimicrobial spectrum of the quinolones includes most avian gram-negative pathogens, some gram-positive bacteria, and mycoplasmas. Chlamydial organisms show some sensitivity to enrofloxacin, but it is not known if the drug can eliminate the carrier state. Quinolones have poor activity against anaerobes and some streptococcal organisms. Both enrofloxacin and ciprofloxacin are excellent for use in most avian species. Ciprofloxacin is a human drug that is metabolized by the liver into enrofloxacin. It is available in oral tablets that do not suspend very well. Enrofloxacin is available in coated tablets of varying strengths and in a parenteral formulation, and in other countries, a 10% liquid is available for use in the drinking water. Enrofloxacin is the only quinolone labeled for veterinary use. The injectable form can be used orally at the same dose and volume; however, it is malodorous and unpalatable and must be disguised before most birds will accept it. Repeated IM injections of enrofloxacin can cause extensive pectoral muscle necrosis; oral dosing should be considered after the initial stages of therapy.

## Trimethoprim-Sulfa Combinations

Trimethoprim may be combined with a sulfonamide to enhance antibacterial activity. Both drugs work synergistically to interfere with microbial folic acid synthesis. Trimethoprim-sulfa (TMS) drugs are bactericidal *in vitro* but may be static *in vivo* at the doses used in birds. They have a wide extracellular distribution and are effective in treating infections involving the skin, respiratory tract, and urinary tract. Elimination is primarily renal following biotransformation by the liver. Potential side effects include gastrointestinal upset, and the possibility of crystal formation in the glomeruli. The use of TMS should be restricted in birds with elevated plasma uric acid levels. Some birds, especially macaws, will regurgitate following oral administration. Several other side effects have been reported to occur with TMS use in mammals but have not been reported in birds.

TMS is a broad-spectrum antibiotic with activity against many gram-positive and gram-negative bacteria. Some gram-negative pathogens are resistant to TMS, including some *Pseudomonas* spp. and Enterobacteriaceae (*Escherichia coli, Klebsiella, Enterobacter*). TMS is useful as a broad-spectrum antibiotic for use in stable avian outpatients while pending sensitivity results. It has been available as a injectable product for IM or SC use (Ditrim, Syntex Animal Health, West Des Moines, Iowa) or as a palatable fruit-flavored suspension (Septra, Burroughs Wellcome, Research Triangle Park, North Carolina).

## Macrolides

Macrolides are bacteriostatic antibiotics that include tylosin, erythromycin, and clindamycin. They have a predominantly gram-positive spectrum with little activity against gram-negative pathogens and are not frequently used in avian medicine. Tylosin had been advocated for the treatment of mycoplasma upper respiratory infections before the advent of the quinolones. Erythromycin opthalmic ointment is useful for the treatment of mycoplasmal conjunctivitis seen in canaries and cockatiels.

## References and Suggested Reading

Bauck L and Hoefer HL: Avian antimicrobial therapy. Semin Avian Exotic Pet Med 2:17, 1993.
 *A review of commonly used antibiotics in pet birds.*
Dorrestein GM: The pharmacokinetics of avian therapeutics. *In* Rosskopf WJ and Woerpel RW (eds): *The Veterinary Clinics of North America Small Animal Practice.* Philadelphia, WB Saunders Co, 1991, p 1241.
 *Drug disposition and metabolism in various avian species with a review of allometric scaling for dose extrapolation.*
Flammer K: An update on the diagnosis and treatment of avian chlamydiosis. *In* Kirk RW (ed): *Current Veterinary Therapy XI.* Philadelphia, WB Saunders Co, 1991, p 1150.
 *A review of available laboratory tests for the diagnosis of chlamydiosis and treatment considerations.*
Flammer K: An update on psittacine antimicrobial pharmacokinetics. *Proc Ann Meet Assoc Avian Vet,* Phoenix, AR, 1990, p 218.
 *Brief report on pharmacokinetic investigations on the use of quinolones and β-lactam antibiotics in psittacines.*
Quesenberry KE: Avian antimicrobial therapeutics. *In* Jacobson ER and Kollias GV (eds): *Exotic Animals.* New York, Churchill Livingstone, 1988, p 177.
 *Article presents antimicrobial pharmacokinetics in various avian species including a review of the literature.*

# AVIAN POLYOMAVIRUS

BRANSON W. RITCHIE
*and* KENNETH S. LATIMER
*Athens, Georgia*

The Papovaviridae family of viruses consists of two genera which vary in virion and genome size. These two genera are *Papillomavirus*, characterized by a 55-nm-diameter nonenveloped icosahedral virion with a 7.5- to 8-kb circular ds DNA genome; and *Polyomavirus*, characterized by a 40- to 50-nm-diameter nonenveloped icosahedral virion with a 4.8- to 5.5-kb circular ds DNA genome.

Papillomaviruses generally are associated with the formation of benign skin tumors (warts). In contrast, the polyomaviruses usually induce persistent infections that become active following stressful events.

The first acute, generalized infection associated with an avian polyomavirus was described in young budgerigars and was called budgerigar fledgling disease (BFD) (Bozeman et al., 1981). A similar polyomavirus has been shown to be associated with morbidity and mortality in some passerines and various genera of larger psittacine birds.

Polyomaviruses from various avian hosts appear to be morphologically and antigenically similar. However, the clinical presentation, distribution of lesions, and epidemiology of these viruses are dramatically different among susceptible species.

## CLINICAL FEATURES

### Clinical Features in Budgerigars

The type of clinical disease induced by polyomavirus in budgerigars appears to depend on the age and condition of the bird when exposed to the virus. Neonates from infected flocks may develop normally for 10 to 15 days and then die suddenly with no premonitory signs. Other infected hatchlings may develop clinical signs including abdominal distention, subcutaneous hemorrhage, tremors of the head and neck, ataxia, and reduced formation of down and contour feathers (Bozeman et al., 1981; Hirai et al., 1984). Infections also have been associated with decreased hatchability and embryonic deaths (Gough, 1989).

Infected budgerigars may die rapidly once clinical signs develop, with 30 to 100% mortality in affected hatchlings (Bozeman et al., 1981; Hirai et al., 1984; Gough, 1989). Mortality rates are highest in budgerigars less than 15 days of age. Survivors may exhibit symmetric feather abnormalities characterized by dys-

trophic primary and tail feathers, lack of down feathers on the back and abdomen, and lack of filoplumes on the head and neck (Bozeman et al., 1981; Hirai et al., 1984; Gough, 1989). Birds with dystrophic flight feathers are unable to fly and have been called "runners." Progressive feather changes in these birds may be referred to as French molt.

It has been speculated that French molt may represent a nonfatal form of BFD (Bozeman et al., 1981; Hirai et al., 1984; Krautwald and Kaleta, 1985); however, budgerigars with classic French molt lesions are often seronegative for polyomavirus antibodies (Krautwald and Kaleta, 1985). In North America and Europe, lesions attributable to French molt are thought to be caused either by avian polyomavirus or by the psittacine beak and feather disease (PBFD) virus. Investigations in Australian budgerigars have demonstrated that clinical signs associated with French molt are associated with the PBFD virus and not with avian polyomavirus (Bozeman et al., 1981; Hirai et al., 1984; Krautwald and Kaleta, 1985). Staining of infected tissues with viral-specific DNA probes may be required to differentiate intranuclear inclusion bodies caused by polyomavirus from those caused by PBFD virus.

### Clinical Features in Other Psittacine Birds

In larger psittacine birds, polyomavirus infections may cause peracute death with no premonitory signs. Death also may occur following a brief period of depression, anorexia, weight loss, delayed crop emptying, regurgitation, diarrhea, dehydration, subcutaneous hemorrhages, dyspnea, polyuria, or posterior paresis and paralysis. The feather abnormalities that are commonly observed with polyomavirus infections in budgerigars are seen less frequently in other psittacine species. Clinical signs of disease develop commonly at the time of weaning, and infected fledglings typically die within 12 to 48 hr. Infections may occur in both parent-raised and hand-raised birds (Clubb and Davis, 1984; Jacobson et al., 1984; Graham and Calnek, 1986; Gaskin, 1989). Infected birds that recover are thought to become asymptomatic virus carriers.

In addition to disease in neonates, polyomavirus infections also may cause sporadic acute deaths in fully-fledged juveniles and adults. An outbreak of polyomavirus in an aviary with numerous psittacine species resulted in the deaths of an adult eclectus parrot, a painted conure, and 3 of 11 adult white-bellied caiques in the collection. The affected birds were 2 to 2.5 years

Reprinted in part, with permission, from Journal Association of Avian Veterinarians.

old and had lesions similar to those described with polyomavirus infections in psittacine neonates (Ritchie et al., 1991).

## Clinical Features in Passeriformes

Lesions suggestive of a polyomavirus infection have been described as a cause of acute mortality in finches and seed-crackers. Disease has been reported in fledgling, young adult, and mature birds. The clinical progression of disease is similar to that described with larger psittacine birds in which affected individuals may die with no premonitory signs (Marshall, 1989; Garcia et al., 1993). Finch fledglings that survive an infection have been found to have poor feather development and long, tubular misshapen beaks (Marshall, 1989).

## PATHOLOGY/PATHOGENESIS

### Lesions

Neonates presented for necropsy are usually in excellent overall condition and may have full crops and gastrointestinal tracts, indicating that an avian polyomavirus infection can be rapidly fatal. Enlarged clear basophilic or amphophilic nuclear inclusions in various tissues, hepatic necrosis, and hemorrhages are the most consistent histologic lesions in larger psittacine birds (Clubb and Davis, 1984; Graham and Calnek, 1986). Inclusions suggestive of polyomavirus infections are most commonly demonstrated in spleen, kidney, and liver (Bozeman et al., 1981; Clubb and Davis, 1984; Hirai et al., 1984; Jacobson et al., 1984; Graham and Calnek, 1986). Viral antigen present within inclusion bodies from some infected psittacine and passerine birds has been confirmed to be antigenically related to the polyomavirus isolated from budgerigars through the use of fluorescent-antibody staining techniques (Hirai et al., 1984; Graham and Calnek, 1986; Wainwright et al., 1987; Garcia et al., 1993). However, the genome of the polyomavirus that infects seed-crackers is not identical to the genome of the polyomavirus that infects budgerigars (Garcia et al., 1993).

### Pathogenesis

As a group, polyomaviruses typically reside in a latent state and infections become patent following periods of excessive stress. The acute nature of avian polyomavirus infections is most unusual for members of the Papovaviridae family, which classically are associated with nonpathogenic subclinical infections and chronic diseases characterized by tumor formation in mammals. The age of a bird at the time of viral exposure may be a major factor in the pathogenesis of polyomavirus infections. Budgerigars that die shortly after birth have more severe and widespread lesions than do birds in which the morbid state is more prolonged. When 11-

to 12-day-old chicken embryos are experimentally infected with polyomavirus, the hatched chicks remain normal and produce detectable antibodies by 2 weeks of age. In contrast, chicken embryos infected at 10 days of age are susceptible to the virus and develop pansystemic lesions (Lynch et al., 1984). It is theorized that persistently infected birds may become infected before immunocompetence is achieved (Wainwright et al., 1987; Gaskin, 1989).

The pathogenesis of polyomavirus infections in larger psittacine birds has not been investigated in detail. The clinical incubation period of the virus has been estimated at less than 14 days, but this period has not been confirmed experimentally (Clubb and Davis, 1984; Graham and Calnek, 1986; Gaskin, 1989). In a study to evaluate the efficacy of an inactivated polyomavirus vaccine, virus-neutralizing (VN) antibodies were first demonstrated 21 days after initial exposure of naive chicks to live virus by oral and intracloacal inoculation. This finding suggests that infection can occur by the oral or intracloacal routes. Virus neutralizing antibodies were detected in naive chicks within 7 days of intramuscular inoculation. This observation suggests that the virus is capable of infecting a host and inducing a detectable antibody response in less than 7 days following exposure to an infectious dose of virus by this route.

Some mammalian polyomavirus infections are known to persist by incorporating viral genome into host cell DNA. It has not been proven that avian polyomavirus uses a similar method of inducing a persistent infection. Polyomaviruses in mammals are natural tumor inducers. Thus far, there has been no correlation between polyomavirus infections in birds and an increased incidence of tumors, although in-depth studies are needed.

## DIAGNOSIS AND CONTROL

### Serology/Diagnosis

Immunodiffusion and virus-neutralization techniques have been used to demonstrate polyomavirus antibodies in exposed birds (Clubb and Davis, 1984; Jacobson et al., 1984; Lynch et al., 1984; Wainwright et al., 1987; Gaskin, 1989). During outbreaks in mixed psittacine bird collections, virus-infected survivors and some asymptomatic birds exposed to them have been shown to develop anti-BFD neutralizing antibodies (Clubb and Davis, 1984; Jacobson et al., 1984). The prevalence of VN antibody titers against BFD in aviaries containing cockatoos, macaws, Amazon parrots, and conures was found to range from 11 to 45%. Titers in these birds were found to decrease within a 2-month period after exposure. The demonstration of waning antibody titers suggests a transient serologic response in many exposed birds (Wainwright et al., 1987).

Subclinical virus carriers that intermittently shed polyomavirus have been thought to maintain high antibody titers in serial serologic assays (Wainwright et al.,

1987; Gaskin, 1989). Based on these suppositions, the demonstration of sustained high antibody titers was suspected to be an indicator of a polyomavirus carrier state (Clubb and Davis, 1984; Wainwright et al., 1987; Gaskin 1989). However, viral-specific DNA probe testing has indicated that there is no correlation between active shedding of polyomavirus in excrement and the titers of neutralizing antibody in the blood of large psittacine birds (Niagro et al., 1991).

A DNA probe test has been used to demonstrate polyomavirus nucleic acid in various tissues including liver, spleen, kidney, cloacal secretions, intestinal secretions, serum, and blood. Viral nucleic acid occasionally can be detected in the blood or serum of some infected birds, particularly budgerigars (Phalen, Wilson, and Graham, 1991; Ritchie et al., 1991). However, cloacal swabs appear to provide the most reliable samples for detecting the viral infection in larger psittacines. The DNA probe test also can be used to detect subclinical shedders of avian polyomavirus° (Niagro et al., 1991; Ritchie et al., 1991).

In a study to evaluate the efficacy of an inactivated polyomavirus vaccine, viral nucleic acid was not detected by DNA probe analysis of blood collected from vaccinated or unvaccinated chicks following challenge with live virus. This may reflect a transient period of viremia, inopportune collection of blood samples, an absence of viremia, or a lack of sufficient quantity of circulating virus to be detected by the DNA detection procedures used.

Demonstration of large, clear basophilic or amphophilic intranuclear inclusion bodies is considered suggestive of a polyomavirus infection. Definitive diagnosis may require immunohistochemical staining of suspected lesions using viral specific antibodies or the detection of viral nucleic acid using polyomavirus-specific DNA probes, especially when inclusions are absent or infected cells are not grossly enlarged.°

## Epidemiology

Avian polyomavirus causes disease in a number of different species of companion and aviary birds in the United States, Europe, Canada, Asia, and Australia. Experimental data and observations with natural disease suggest that polyomavirus transmission may occur by both horizontal and vertical routes (Clubb and Davis, 1984; Jacobson et al., 1984; Gaskin, 1989). Findings that support vertical transmission include the identification of intranuclear inclusion bodies in day-old budgerigars and the occurrence of polyomavirus infection when eggs from parents that consistently produce diseased neonates are cross-fostered to parents producing normal young (Gough, 1989).

Asymptomatic adults that intermittently shed the virus are thought to be responsible for the persistence, transmission, and spread of the virus through various

avian populations (Bozeman et al., 1981; Gaskin, 1989; Niagro et al., 1991). Seronegative young adults will seroconvert when housed adjacent to seropositive breeding adults, implicating indirect transmission of the virus (Clubb and Davis, 1984; Jacobson et al., 1984; Wainwright et al., 1987). The presence of viral particles in crop epithelium suggests that virus may be transmitted to neonates by parenteral feeding via regurgitation of exfoliated crop epithelium. The demonstration of viral particles in lung tissue suggests that contaminated respiratory secretions also may be involved in disease transmission (Gaskin, 1989).

Demonstration of polyomavirus inclusions in follicular and renal tissue from persistently infected clinically normal adults suggests that feather dander and excrement may also serve as sources of virus exposure. Localization of polyomavirus in renal epithelium where the virus may be protected from antibodies could account for viral persistence (Bozeman et al., 1981; Hirai et al., 1984; Graham and Calnek, 1986; Gaskin, 1989). The polyomavirus genome can be detected in cloacal swabs taken from birds during polyomavirus outbreaks. The recovery of viral DNA from the cloaca and colon in some birds suggests that the virus can be shed from gastrointestinal, renal, or reproductive tissues (Niagro et al., 1991; Ritchie et al., 1991).

Theoretically, a persistently infected hen could pass maternally derived antibodies, virus, or both to her young (Gaskin, 1989). The clinical status of the chick would then depend on the level of maternally derived antibodies, the stage of immunocompetency when viral exposure occurs, and the presence of provirus in gametes or other maternally derived tissues. Chicks that have protective levels of maternal antibodies as well as infections derived from the parents may subsequently infect susceptible neonates in the psittacine nursery (Gaskin, 1989). Persistent infections with intermittent viral shedding and vertical transmission are also suspected to occur in Passeriformes, resulting in early embryonic deaths (Garcia et al., 1993).

## Control

Polyomavirus virions are small, nonenveloped particles that are resistant to severe environmental conditions and a variety of disinfectants. Avian polyomavirus previously has been shown to be resistant to organic solvents, to freezing and thawing, and to heating at 56°C for 2 hr (Bozeman et al., 1981). The stability of avian polyomavirus causes a considerable problem in the aviary because persistently infected birds can shed virus in their feather dander or excrement (Bozeman et al., 1981; Hirai et al., 1984; Graham and Calnek, 1986). The environmental stability of avian polyomavirus and predisposition to infection in susceptible birds underscores the importance of choosing an effective disinfectant. This is particularly true in a veterinary hospital, where infected birds can contaminate the hospital environment, creating the potential for nosocomial infections. Manual removal of any organic material, followed

---

°Avian Research Associates, 100 Techne Center, Milford, OH 45150.

by the use of an appropriate disinfectant, is required to prevent or interrupt a disease outbreak.

The results of a study to determine the efficacy of various disinfectants against avian polyomavirus are listed in Table 1. The results of this study suggest that sodium hypochlorite is the most inexpensive disinfectant tested that would inactivate avian polyomavirus. However, this compound produces fumes that can be irritating to mucous membranes, and must be used in areas with sufficient ventilation. In addition, sodium hypochlorite is irritating to skin and is corrosive to metals.

Stabilized chlorine dioxide[†] also has been found to inactivate polyomavirus. At working dilutions, this disinfectant is considered safe for humans and animals and has been used by many municipalities as the principal agent to eliminate potential pathogens from drinking water. In Europe, chlorine dioxide is used to treat drinking water because, unlike chlorine, it does not form carcinogenic compounds when oxidized.

In contrast, chlorhexidine[‡] did not completely inactivate avian polyomavirus, which may explain why nurseries that use this product to cleanse syringes between feedings may still experience polyomavirus outbreaks.

With the highly infectious nature of the polyomavirus, particularly to young psittacine birds, closed breeding operations that do not allow visitors should be encouraged. A cloacal swab of any bird that is being added to a collection should be analyzed during the quarantine period to determine whether a bird is shedding polyomavirus (Niagro et al., 1991; Ritchie et al., 1991). During an epornitic, birds that are actively shedding the virus can be identified by using the DNA probe test to screen cloacal swabs for presence of virus nucleic acid. Birds that are shedding the polyomavirus should be isolated, not euthanatized. These intermittent viral shedders are likely to be of no further concern when an effective vaccine is available. Birds that are subclinically infected with avian polyomavirus can be managed by maintaining them in restricted environments where they do not directly or indirectly (i.e., through contaminated excrement, secretions, bedding, or enclosures) expose susceptible birds. Nosocomial or iatrogenic transmission of the virus can be reduced by strict hygiene and appropriate use of disinfectants.

## Vaccination

Immunodiffusion and virus neutralization techniques have been used to demonstrate antipolyomavirus antibodies in psittacine birds (Clubb and Davis, 1984; Jacobson et al., 1984; Lynch et al., 1984; Wainwright et al., 1987; Gaskin, 1989). During epornitics in mixed psittacine bird collections, infected survivors and asymptomatic birds exposed to them have been shown to develop antipolyomavirus neutralizing antibodies (Clubb and Davis, 1984; Jacobson et al., 1984; Wainwright et al., 1987). Seronegative young adult birds will

**Table 1.** TCID$_{50}$ of Avian Polyomavirus Following Exposure to Disinfectants.[*]

| Agent | 1-Min Exposure | 5-Min Exposure |
|---|---|---|
| Avinol-3 | $<10^1$ | $<10^1$ |
| Clorox | $<10^1$ | $<10^1$ |
| Dent-A-Gene | $<10^1$ | $<10^1$ |
| Ethanol | $<10^1$ | $<10^1$ |
| Mikroklene | $10^2$ | $10^2$ |
| Nolvasan solution | $10^4$ | $10^4$ |
| Orange Power | $10^4$ | $10^4$ |
| Roccal-D | $10^2$ | $10^2$ |

[*]The initial infectivity titer of the virus preparation was $10^5$ TCID$_{50}$/ml.
Abbreviation: TCID$_{50}$ = median tissue culture infective dose.

seroconvert when housed adjacent to seropositive breeding adults, indicating that an antibody response does occur following natural exposure to the virus (Clubb and Davis, 1984; Jacobson et al., 1984).

An inactivated avian polyomavirus vaccine has been found to induce an immunologic response that can be measured by detecting an increase in the level of VN antibodies following vaccination. This experimental vaccine appears to be efficacious because it is able to protect vaccinates from subsequent challenge with live virus. Acemannan was found to be a safe adjuvant to use in conjunction with the inactivated avian polyomavirus, and this vaccine is being tested in preparation for commercial release.

Vaccinates that were seropositive due to a previous or sustained infection have not been found to react adversely to vaccination. Given the seroprevalence of the disease in companion birds and the frequency of subclinical carriers, the fact that an inactivated vaccine intended for commercial release does not cause adverse reactions in vaccinates that were seropositive prior to vaccination is noteworthy.

## References and Suggested Reading

Bozeman LH, Davis RB, Gaudry D, et al: Characterization of a papovavirus isolated from fledgling budgerigars. Avian Dis 25:972, 1981.
  *Description of polyomavirus infection in budgerigars and characteristics of the virus.*

Clubb SL and Davis RB: Outbreak of papova-like viral infection in a psittacine nursery—a retrospective view. Proc Assoc Avian Vet, 1984, p 121.
  *Epidemiology of a polyomavirus outbreak in a psittacine breeding facility.*

Garcia AP, Latimer KS, Niagro FD, et al: Diagnosis of polyomavirus infection in seedcrackers (Pyrenestes sp.) and blue bills (Spermophaga haematina) using DNA in situ hybridization. Avian Pathol 23:525, 1994.
  *Review of avian polyomavirus in passerine birds and a description of current diagnostic methodologies.*

Gaskin JM: Psittacine viral disease: A perspective. J Zoo Wildl Med 20:249, 1989.
  *A review of avian polyomavirus up to 1989.*

Gough JF: Outbreaks of budgerigar fledgling disease in three aviaries in Ontario. Can Vet J 30:672, 1989.
  *Epidemiology and management of a polyomavirus outbreak in a group of budgerigar breeding facilities.*

Graham DL and Calnek BW: Papovavirus infection in hand-fed parrots: Virus isolation and pathology. Avian Dis 31:398, 1986.
  *Description of the pathologic changes caused by polyomavirus in naturally infected psittacine birds.*

Hirai K, Nonaka H, Fukushi H, et al: Isolation of a papova-like agent from young budgerigars with feather abnormalities. Jpn J Vet Sci 46:577, 1984.
  *Description of polyomavirus infection in budgerigars and characteristics of the virus.*

---

[†]Dent-A-Gene, 4029 Brookfield Avenue, Louisville, KY 40207.
[‡]Nolvasan, Fort Dodge, PO Box 518, Fort Dodge, IA 50501.

Jacobson ER, Hines SA, Quesenberry K, et al: Epornitic of papova-like virus-associated disease in a psittacine nursery. J Am Vet Med Assoc 185:1337, 1984.
*Epidemiology of a polyomavirus outbreak in a psittacine breeding facility.*

Krautwald M-E and Kaleta EF: Relationship of French moult and early virus induced mortality in nestling budgerigars. Proc 8th Intl Cong World Vet Poult Assoc, 1985, p 115.
*Description of the relationship between French moult and avian polyomavirus.*

Lynch J, Swinton J, Pettit J, et al: Isolation and experimental chicken-embryo-inoculation studies with budgerigar papovavirus. Avian Dis 28:1135, 1984.
*Characteristics of avian polyomavirus.*

Marshall R: Papova-like virus in a finch aviary. Proc Assoc Avian Vet, 1989, p 203.
*Description of the clinical appearance of polyomavirus in finches.*

Niagro FD, Ritchie BW, Lukert PD, et al: Avian polyomavirus. Discordance between neutralizing antibody titers and viral shedding in an aviary. Proc Assoc Avian Vet, 1991, p 22.
*Comparison of diagnostic techniques available for detecting large psittacine birds that are subclinically infected with avian polyomavirus.*

Phalen DN, Wilson VG, and Graham DL: Polymerase chain reaction assay for avian polyomavirus. J Clin Microbiol 29:1030, 1991.
*Use of the polymerase chain reaction for detection of polyomavirus nucleic acid in infected budgerigars.*

Ritchie BW, Niagro FD, Latimer KS, et al: Polyomavirus infections in adult psittacine birds. J Assoc Avian Vet 5:202, 1991.
*Epidemiology of a polyomavirus outbreak in a psittacine breeding facility.*

Wainwright PO, Lukert PD, Davis RB, et al: Serological evaluation of some psittaciformes for budgerigar fledgling disease virus. Avian Dis 31:673, 1987.
*A description of the serologic response that occurs during an outbreak of polyomavirus in a psittacine aviary.*

# PSITTACINE BEAK AND FEATHER DISEASE VIRUS

BRANSON W. RITCHIE
*and* KENNETH S. LATIMER
*Athens, Georgia*

## HISTORY AND CLASSIFICATION

A chronic disease characterized by symmetric feather dystrophy and loss, development of beak deformities, and eventual death was first described in various species of Australian cockatoos in the early 1970s. Subsequently, this syndrome was named psittacine beak and feather disease (PBFD) by Perry in 1981. In the late 1800s, free-ranging red-rumped parrots that are indigenous to South Australia were described with feather abnormalities suggestive of PBFD. In retrospect, these birds may have been the first to be described with this disease.

Psittacine beak and feather disease is caused by a 14- to 17-nm icosahedral nonenveloped virion with a 1.7- to 2.0-kb single-stranded circular DNA molecule. The virion size and nucleic acid characteristics described for the PBFD virus are similar to those of the chicken anemia virus (CAV), porcine circovirus (PCV), and of a virus recovered from pigeons and doves (Todd et al., 1991; Pass, 1993; Woods et al., 1993). Based on the unique characteristics of these viruses, they have been tentatively placed in the Circoviridae family and are the smallest pathogenic DNA animal viruses that have been described. The PBFD virus infecting different psittacine birds is antigenetically similar and has sufficiently conserved nucleic acid sequences to allow detection of the virus using viral-specific DNA probes.

Histologic or clinically suggestive lesions of PBFD have been described in 42 species of psittacine birds. Historically, PBFD was thought to be restricted to Old

World and South Pacific psittacine birds, with the white and pink cockatoos being particularly susceptible. However, the disease has been documented in several black cockatoos as well as New World psittacine birds including Amazon parrots, macaws, and pionus parrots. A similar virus recently has been reported to be the cause of dystrophic feathers in doves in Australia (Pass, 1993). A virus that morphologically resembles the PBFD virus has been associated with poor growth and death in pigeons. However, the virus that causes disease in pigeons differs antigenically and genomically from the PBFD virus (Woods et al., 1993).

The PBFD virus appears to be endemic in free-ranging populations of sulphur-crested cockatoos, galahs, little corellas, Major Mitchell's cockatoos, crimson rosellas, budgerigars, and rainbow lorikeets (Pass and Perry, 1985; McOrist, 1989). Some populations of free-ranging doves from Australia have also been shown to be naturally infected (Pass, 1993). It is postulated that PBFD has historically been endemic in free-ranging populations of Old World and South Pacific psittacine birds, and that the virus has been introduced to other susceptible populations of birds through the worldwide movement of birds for the pet market.

## CLINICAL DISEASE

The first sign of PBFD is the appearance of necrotic, abnormally formed feathers. The type of feathers that are initially involved depends on the stage of molt when the clinical signs of disease are manifested. In young birds, all of the feather tracts may be affected during a 1-week period; whereas in older birds, the disease is more prolonged, with progressive feather changes during ensuing molts. If beak lesions develop, they may include palatine necrosis, progressive elongation, and transverse or longitudinal fractures (Pass and Perry, 1984; Jacobson et al., 1986; Ritchie et al., 1989). Peracute, acute, and chronic disease syndromes may be caused by PBFD virus infection. These syndromes differ markedly in clinical presentation as detailed below.

## Peracute Disease

Peracute disease is suspected in neonatal psittacines that show signs of septicemia accompanied by pneumonia, enteritis, rapid weight loss, and death (Pass and Perry, 1984). Histologic lesions in these cases may be limited to edema in follicular epithelium and severe necrosis of the bursa and thymus. The peracute syndrome appears to be particularly common in young cockatoos and African gray parrots. Peracute cases of PBFD may be missed if a complete necropsy and thorough histologic examination are not performed on birds that die with suspicious clinical signs.

## Acute Disease

Acute disease (commonly called French molt in Australia) is most frequently reported in young or fledgling birds during their first feather formation after replacement of the neonatal down. Chicks as young as 28 to 32 days of age have been described with classic lesions (Pass and Perry, 1985). Acute infections are characterized by several days of depression followed by sudden changes in developing feathers, including necrosis, fractures, bending, bleeding, or premature shedding of diseased feathers. In some acute cases of PBFD, birds with minimal feather changes may be depressed, develop crop stasis and diarrhea, and die within 1 to 2 weeks. Gross feather lesions in the acute form of the disease can be quite subtle, with only a few feathers showing dystrophic changes. This clinical picture is particularly common in young sulphur-crested cockatoos and lovebirds (Pass and Perry, 1985).

Experimentally infected galah, umbrella cockatoo, and African gray parrot neonates generally develop an acute-type infection characterized by a rapid onset of depression followed in 24 to 48 hr by the appearance of abnormal feathers (Wylie and Pass, 1987; Ritchie et al., 1992). Chicks that develop clinical lesions while the majority of feathers are still in a developmental stage exhibit the most severe feather pathology. These birds may appear totally normal one day and exhibit 80 to 100% feather dystrophy within a week (Ritchie et al., 1992). The clinical progression of disease is less dramatic in neonates that develop clinical signs after body contour feathers are mature. In these birds, feather changes may be limited to the still developing flight and tail feathers (Pass and Perry, 1985).

## Chronic Disease

Chronic disease is characterized by the progressive appearance of abnormal feathers during successive molts. Gross changes include retention of feather sheaths, hemorrhage within the pulp cavity, fractures of the proximal rachis, and failure of developing feathers to exsheathe. Short clubbed feathers, deformed curled feathers, stress lines within vanes, and circumferential constrictions may also be present. Replacement feathers become increasingly abnormal. If birds live long enough, they will eventually develop baldness as the feather follicles become inactive (Pass and Perry, 1985; Jacobson et al., 1986; Ritchie et al., 1989).

## Feather Lesions

The distribution of dystrophic feathers within individual pterylae is variable, and depends upon the stage of molt when the bird begins to develop clinical signs. In older birds, the first sign of PBFD is the replacement of normal powder down and contour feathers with dystrophic, necrotic, nonviable feathers that stop growing shortly after emerging from the follicle. The disease then progresses to involve the contour feathers in most tracts, followed by dystrophic changes in the primary, secondary, tail, and crest feathers. Primary feathers are usually the last to manifest abnormalities. It has been assumed that the susceptibility of the powder down feathers is based on their consistent molt pattern, compared to the seasonal loss found in other feather tracts. Alternatively, some birds have substantial involvement of the flight, tail, and crest feathers, with only minimal changes in the powder down feathers (Pass and Perry, 1985; Jacobson et al., 1986; Ritchie et al., 1989).

## Beak Lesions

Depending on the avian species involved, and other factors that remain unresolved, beak changes may or may not be present in birds with PBFD. In one study involving 22 cockatoos of mixed Asian origin, birds greater than 1 year of age had a lower incidence of beak lesions than did birds that were under 1 year of age (Jacobson et al., 1986). Beak pathology does not routinely occur with some affected species, while with others, such as the sulphur-crested cockatoos, galahs, little corellas, and Moluccan cockatoos, beak lesions are relatively common (Pass and Perry, 1985; Jacobson et al., 1986; Ritchie et al., 1989).

If present, changes in the beak and oral mucosa of clinically affected birds include progressive beak elongation with transverse or longitudinal fractures, palatine necrosis, and oral ulceration (Pass and Perry, 1985; Jacobson et al., 1986; Ritchie et al., 1989). The upper beak is generally more severely affected than is the lower beak (Jacobson et al., 1986). If the powder down feathers are dystrophic, the beak may appear to be semigloss or gloss black, instead of its normal gray color (Pass and Perry, 1985).

Classically, beak deformities develop in birds following a protracted course of PBFD where substantial feather changes have occurred. However, some individuals develop severe beak lesions with relatively minor feather pathology, and cracking of the hard corneum at the distal portion of the beak may be the initial complaint requiring veterinary attention (Pass and Perry, 1985; Jacobson et al., 1986).

## TRANSMISSION

Susceptible birds can be experimentally infected with the PBFD virus through the combined oral, intracloacal, and intranasal routes (Wylie and Pass, 1987; Ritchie et al., 1992). Psittacine beak and feather disease virus was recovered in the feces and crop washings from various species of psittacine birds diagnosed with PBFD. During a test period, 26% (8 of 31) of the birds screened were found to be excreting PBFD virus in their feces, and 21% (3 of 14) of crop washings were positive for the PBFD virus. While the concentration of PBFD virus demonstrated in the crops of positive birds was low, the possibility of an adult transmitting the virus to neonates during feeding activities that involve the regurgitation of food and exfoliated crop epithelium deserves consideration. Virus that was recovered from the crop may have originated from infected cells located in the crop or esophageal epithelium, or may have been deposited in the crop after swallowing of exfoliated epithelium from beak or oral mucosal lesions. High concentrations of the virus also can be demonstrated in feather dust collected from a room where birds with active cases of PBFD are being housed (Ritchie et al., 1991). It has been postulated that the frequent demonstration of PBFD inclusions in tissues of the palate, esophagus, crop, intestines, bursa, and liver probably account for viral shedding in the feces (Latimer et al., 1991).

The demonstration of high concentrations of virus recovered from a room where PBFD birds were being maintained implicates contaminated dust from any source as a major vehicle for the environmental persistence and natural transmission of the virus (Ritchie et al., 1991). Artificially incubated chicks from a PBFD-infected hen consistently develop PBFD, suggesting that vertical transmission of the virus occurs.

An age-related susceptibility to the virus has been suggested by previous experimental transmission studies. Neonatal budgerigars infected at less than 7 days of age were found to develop severe disease, while birds infected at 10 to 14 days were reported to experience lower levels of morbidity and some remained asymptomatic (Wylie and Pass, 1987). Other transmission studies have indicated that the apparent age-related resistance to the virus was due to the birds not being followed through an appropriate incubation period and may have had nothing to do with an age-related resistance. Older birds that develop clinical signs later in life may have been infected at a younger age and remained latently infected (Ritchie et al., 1992).

Several reports suggest the possibility of asymptomatic adults producing progeny with clinical signs of PBFD in successive breeding seasons. These findings suggest a carrier state may exist with vertical or horizontal transmission of PBFD virus from parent to offspring and/or a genetic predisposition to the disease. However, in most suspected cases of parent-to-offspring transmission, epidemiologic investigations indicate probable exposure to the PBFD virus occurring through sources other than the parents. The widespread use of DNA probes[*] to detect subclinically infected birds may provide more information on what role, if any, subclinically infected birds play in transmitting the virus.

## INCUBATION PERIOD

Infected chicks and fledglings may show the first signs of disease during the initial molt (Ritchie et al., 1992). Galah chicks experimentally infected with PBFD virus have been reported to develop clinical signs of PBFD approximately 4 weeks after infection (Wylie and Pass, 1987). African gray parrot chicks infected at 3 to 8 days of age became depressed by 30 days of age and developed progressive feather dystrophy by 33 to 44 days of age. Umbrella cockatoo chicks infected at 3 to 8 days of age became depressed by 40 days of age and developed progressive feather dystrophy from 42 to 47 days of age. The time variance in developing clinical signs associated with PBFD among different psittacine chicks may be attributed to differences in concentrations of maternally transmitted antibodies, titer of virus in the inoculum, or host responses to the virus (Ritchie et al., 1992).

These experimental infection studies suggest that the minimum incubation period is 22 to 25 days (Ritchie et al., 1992). DNA probe testing of blood for the presence of PBFD virus nucleic acid has been used to demonstrate that the incubation period can be months (18 months documented), and clinical experience suggests that the incubation period can be years.

## PATHOLOGY

Gross feather and beak changes associated with PBFD are described in the section "Clinical Disease," above. Predominant histologic lesions have been described in the feather shaft, where necrosis and ballooning degeneration of epithelial cells in the epidermal collar and epidermal basal and intermediate zones of the developing rachis are seen (Pass and Perry, 1985; Jacobson et al., 1986; Latimer et al., 1991). The PBFD virus appears to target feather epithelial cells more fre-

---

[*]Avian Research Associates, 100 Techne Center, Milford OH 45150.

quently than follicular epithelial cells (Latimer et al., 1991). Feather sheath hyperkeratosis prevents the feather from exsheathing, and results in the terminal clubbing and midshaft constrictions of the developing feather, which are clinically evident (Jacobson et al., 1986). Feather pulp lesions are characterized by non-suppurative inflammation, including perivascular accumulation of plasma cells, lymphocytes, macrophages, and heterophils (Pass and Perry, 1985; Jacobson et al., 1986; Latimer et al., 1991).

In peracute cases, PBFD virus may infect and destroy bursal or thymic tissue without inducing detectable inclusion bodies within macrophages. Feather pathology in such cases may be minimal edema in the follicular epithelium or absent (Pass and Perry, 1985; Jacobson et al., 1986; Latimer et al., 1991).

## Inclusion Bodies

Psittacine beak and feather disease virus may cause basophilic intranuclear or intracytoplasmic inclusion bodies as observed in hematoxylin and eosin–stained sections of feathers, beak, thymus, and bursa taken from birds with clinical signs of PBFD (Pass and Perry, 1985; Jacobson et al., 1986; Latimer et al., 1991). Immunohistochemical staining with viral-specific antibodies was used to confirm that intracytoplasmic basophilic inclusion bodies and some intranuclear inclusion bodies observed in hematoxylin and eosin–stained tissue sections contain PBFD viral antigen (Latimer et al., 1991).

Both intranuclear and intracytoplasmic inclusion bodies were identified in 23 of 32 birds examined in one study. In this group, intranuclear inclusion bodies were restricted to epithelial cells and intracytoplasmic inclusion bodies were found only within macrophages (Latimer et al., 1991).

In addition to being localized in the feather and follicle epithelium and lymphoid tissues, PBFD viral inclusion bodies have also been demonstrated by viral-specific antibody staining in the beak and hard palate, bursa, thymus, tongue, parathyroid gland, crop, esophagus, spleen, intestines, bone marrow, liver, thyroid, testis, ovary, and adrenal glands (Latimer et al., 1991).

Intracytoplasmic inclusions are thought to originate in epidermal cells, and attain their greatest size within macrophages that engulf these infected cells (Pass and Perry, 1985; Jacobson et al., 1986; Latimer et al., 1991). It has been postulated that PBFD virus replicates in the nuclei of infected epidermal cells, and inclusions are then released when necrotic cells are phagocytized by macrophage-like cells in the pulp and epidermis (Pass and Perry, 1985; Jacobson et al., 1986; Latimer et al., 1991). However, the occurrence of viral antigen within macrophages in the bone marrow and within circulating monocytes suggest that these cells may be infected directly.

## PATHOGENESIS/IMMUNITY

Except for reported recoveries in budgerigars, lorikeets, and lovebirds, the chronic form of PBFD is con-sidered fatal in birds originating from the Old World (Pass and Perry, 1985; Ritchie et al., 1989). Most clinically affected birds survive less than 6 months to 1 year after the onset of clinical signs, although some birds have been known to live over 10 years in a featherless state. Death usually occurs either from changes induced by secondary bacterial, chlamydial, fungal, other viral agents, or from terminal changes that necessitate euthanasia (Pass and Perry, 1985; Jacobson et al., 1986; Latimer et al., 1991). Cockatoos with PBFD have been diagnosed with severe cryptosporidiosis infections that are generally considered to occur only in patients with immunodeficiencies (Latimer et al., 1991).

PBFD-positive birds with inclusion bodies located only within the nucleus of infected epithelial cells have been found to spontaneously recover. Larger Old World psittacine birds with intracytoplasmic inclusion bodies located in macrophages have been considered to be fatally infected. Recently, however, *Pionus* spp. and scarlet macaw chicks have been shown to recover from active infections in which intracytoplasmic inclusion bodies were demonstrated in macrophages. This finding would suggest that these species are capable of responding to an infection in a manner different from that demonstrated by larger Old World Psittaciformes.

Most birds exposed to the PBFD virus remain clinically normal and develop hemagglutination-inhibition (HI) and precipitating antibody titers to the virus. These findings suggest that many infected birds develop subclinical infections that result in the development of protective antibodies. The factors that determine whether a bird mounts an immune response or is fatally infected could depend on the age of virus exposure, the presence and levels of maternal antibodies, the route of viral exposure, and the titer or the infecting virus.

## DIAGNOSIS

PBFD should be suspected in any psittacine bird with progressive feather loss involving malformed feathers. A tentative diagnosis of PBFD involves the identification of basophilic intracytoplasmic or intra-nuclear inclusion bodies in the feather pulp or follicular epithelium from birds with clinical signs of dystrophic, nonviable feathers (Pass and Perry, 1985; Jacobson et al., 1986; Latimer et al., 1991). Basophilic intracytoplasmic inclusion bodies are considered diagnostic. Because several viruses may result in similar appearing intranuclear inclusion bodies, a confirmatory diagnosis of PBFD requires the use of viral-specific antibodies to demonstrate PBFD virus antigen or the use of DNA probes to detect PBFD virus nucleic acid (Latimer et al., 1991). Viral-specific DNA probes are the most sensitive test for detecting PBFD virus. These probes can be used on biopsy samples of suspect feathers by DNA *in situ* hybridization to confirm an infection or on a blood sample by DNA amplification and dot-blotting to demonstrate viral nucleic acid sequence in circulating white blood cells.

## DNA Probe Testing

The latter DNA probe test can be used to detect PBFD viral nucleic acid in the white blood cells of infected birds before clinical changes in the feathers are apparent (Table 1). This test is now commercially available in the United States and in several European countries.[°] A positive test in a bird that has feather abnormalities suggests that the bird has an active PBFD viral infection. A positive blood test in a bird that does not have feather abnormalities may indicate that the bird is latently infected or that it recently has been exposed to the PBFD virus and is viremic. A bird that tests positive and has no feather abnormalities should be retested in 90 days. If the bird is still positive, then it should be considered to be latently infected or is continuously being exposed to the virus. A negative test result indicates that viral nucleic acid was not detected in the submitted sample.

All breeding birds of a susceptible species should be tested to determine if they are latently infected with the PBFD virus. In addition, neonates should be tested before they leave the aviary and patients should be tested during prepurchase or postpurchase examinations. The DNA probe test can also be used to screen walls, enclosures, air circulating ducts, and equipment in the home or hospital to determine if PBFD virus is contaminating these surfaces. The appropriate sample for testing for environmental contamination is a swab collected from the premises in question.

**Table 1.** *Diagnostic Flow Chart for PBFD Virus*

**Bird Has Dystrophic, Necrotic Feathers**
***Test Blood for PBFD Virus Using DNA Probes[°]***
- *If positive:* Suggests active infection.
  Management:
    If bird is from a breeding aviary: Bird should be removed and all areas that could be contaminated with feather dust from the infected bird should be repeatedly cleaned.
    If companion bird: Bird should not be exposed to other birds outside of the household and one should be aware that the virus can be transported to other locations on one's clothes or in one's hair. Be courteous of other birds and do not expose them. It should be noted that, occasionally, some PBFD infected Psittaciformes of South American descent have spontaneously recovered from the disease.
- *If negative:* A feather biopsy (including the feather follicle) should be submitted for histopathologic examination.

**Bird Has Normal Appearing Feathers**
***Test Blood for PBFD Virus Using DNA Probes[°]***
- *If positive:* Indicates that the bird has been exposed to PBFD virus and that the virus is present in the blood. The bird must be retested in 90 days. If the bird is negative when retested, it indicates that the virus was not detected in the blood cells. If the bird is still positive, it indicates that the bird is either subclinically infected or that the bird is being repeatedly exposed to the virus. It should be noted that most birds that are exposed to the PBFD virus develop a transient viremia followed by an appropriate immune response that results in the bird clearing the infection.
- *If negative:* Indicates that PBFD virus was not detected in the blood.

[°]Avian Research Associates, 100 Techne Center, Milford, OH 45150.

## HA and HI Testing

PBFD virus has hemagglutination (HA) activity for cockatoo and some guinea pig erythrocytes but not for chicken or sheep erythrocytes. The HA test can be used to demonstrate and quantify the amount of virus recovered from PBFD positive birds. The HI test provides a rapid, specific technique to assess the immunologic response of psittacine birds to the PBFD virus. Precipitating antibodies can be demonstrated using an agar-gel immunodiffusion test (Ritchie et al., 1991).

Many birds of a susceptible species have some detectable anti-PBFD virus antibodies, indicating previous exposure to the virus. Antibody titer surveys in the United States would suggest that most birds of a susceptible species are exposed to the virus at some time in their life and are able to mount an effective immune response; 41 to 94% of clinically normal free-ranging cockatoos tested in Australia were found to have antibodies to PBFD virus. Titers in tested flocks ranged from 0 to 1:512 (Raidal et al., 1993). These findings suggest that the detection of antibodies is common in free-ranging birds as well.

In six flocks of free-ranging cockatoos tested in Australia, the mean HI antibody titers ranged from less than 1:4 to 1:16, depending on the flock (Raidal et al., 1993). Both clinically affected birds and those that have not recently been exposed to the virus can have low HI antibody titers (Ritchie et al., 1991; Raidal et al., 1993). Because these low HI antibody titers can suggest that a bird is infected or susceptible, HI antibody titers would not be expected to provide clinically relevant information in a field situation. The susceptibility of a bird with a low antibody titer would depend on the age and condition of the bird and the amount of virus to which it is exposed (Ritchie et al., 1992).

As a general screening tool, DNA probes remain the most informative diagnostic technique. In contrast to the DNA probe test, HI antibody titers provide no information that would suggest if a bird is subclinically infected. When necessary, the HI test can be used in combination with the DNA probe test to determine the immunologic status of a bird that has been recently exposed to the virus.[†] Paired serum samples in which a fourfold increase in antibody titer occurs indicates that the bird has recently been exposed to the virus. If the blood from a bird with no feather abnormalities is positive for PBFD virus using the DNA probe test and is then negative when retested 90 days later, an increase in HI titer would suggest that the bird has mounted a successful immunologic response and eliminated the virus. A paired titer that does not change would indicate that the bird's immune system is not being stimulated.

Without the use of the DNA probe test, a single-point HI antibody titer rarely provides diagnostic information, and paired serum samples provide limited information unless the titer is extremely high (>1:1280)

[†]Avian Research Associates, 100 Techne Center, Milford OH, 45150.

or extremely low (<1:32) (Ritchie et al., 1991). A high HI antibody titer (>1280) has been shown to be suggestive of a protective immunologic response. Neonates from hens with HI antibody titers greater than 1280 were shown to be protected from viral challenge, while neonates from hens with HI antibody titers less than 320 were shown to be susceptible to virus challenge (Ritchie et al., 1992).

## CONTROL

The chicken anemia virus (CAV), which is similar in ultrastructure and DNA composition to the PBFD virus, has been found to be environmentally stable, and infectivity remains unchanged when the virus is heated to 80°C for 30 min and following treatment with detergents, enzymes, and many commercial disinfectants (Yuasa, 1992). A 1% iodine disinfectant and sodium hypochlorite were effective in inactivating CAV derived from cell culture. A 10% concentration of these same disinfectants was necessary to inactivate virus that was present in liver tissue. While the environmental stability of the PBFD virus is unknown, it would be prudent to consider its stability to be similar to that described for CAV. Psittacine neonates, which seem to be most susceptible to the PBFD virus, should definitely not be exposed to areas that may have been contaminated by feces or feather dust from a PBFD-positive bird (Wylie and Pass, 1987; Ritchie et al., 1991).

## EXPERIMENTAL VACCINATION

β-Propiolactone–treated PBFD virus was used to inoculate a group of 30- to 45-day-old and adult psittacine birds. All the adult and neonate vaccinates had increased concentrations of HI antibodies by day 21 postinoculation. Precipitating antibodies to the PBFD virus were detected by the agar-gel diffusion test in serum from experimentally vaccinated adult birds. Chicks from vaccinated and unvaccinated African gray parrot and umbrella cockatoo hens were exposed to purified PBFD virus by the combined oral, intracloacal, and subcutaneous routes. The chicks from vaccinated hens remained clinically normal throughout the 50-day test period. The chicks from the unvaccinated hens developed gross and histologic lesions consistent with PBFD following viral challenge.

The fact that all of the chicks from the vaccinated hens were temporally resistant to infection, whereas the control chicks from unvaccinated hens developed clinical disease, suggests that maternally transmitted immunologic factors can protect neonates from virus challenge. Determining the level and type of antibodies that are needed to protect a bird from infection and the critical period when these antibodies provide protection from infection will require further investigation.

Because PBFD virus is extremely difficult to completely inactivate, is extremely infectious to susceptible birds, and has not been grown in cell culture, any inactivated vaccine that contains whole virus derived from the tissues of infected birds should be considered too dangerous for use in companion birds. Growth of the virus in cell culture or the development of a subunit vaccine that contains only the immunogenic proteins from the virus is necessary to ensure that PBFD can be safely prevented through vaccination. Batch testing of a virus preparation that has been exposed to an inactivating agent is not possible because it has been found that portions of a virus preparation may be inactivated, while other portions of the same sample have not been inactivated and are capable of inducing disease. The β-propiolactone–treated PBFD virus vaccine that has been developed and evaluated should provide a model vaccine by which a commercially feasible product can be produced and tested (Ritchie et al., 1992).

## References and Suggested Reading

Jacobson ER, Clubb S, Simpson C, et al: Feather and beak dystrophy and necrosis in cockatoos. Clinicopathologic evaluations. J Am Vet Med Assoc 189:999, 1986.
*Description of the gross and clincopathologic changes associated with PBFD.*

Latimer KS, Rakich PM, Niagro FD, et al: An updated review of psittacine beak and feather disease. J Assoc Avian Vet 5:211, 1991.
*A review of research findings associated with PBFD virus, with particular emphasis on diagnostic techniques.*

McOrist S: Some diseases of free-living Australian birds. ICBP Tech Publ 16: 13, 1989.
*A description of the type of lesions and problems associated with PBFD virus in free-ranging birds from Australia.*

Pass DA: Natural infection of wild doves (*Streptopelia senegalensis*) with the virus of psittacine beak and feather disease. *Xth World Vet Poul Assoc Congress*, 1993, p 165.
*A description of PBFD virus infection in free-ranging doves.*

Pass DA and Perry RA: The pathology of psittacine beak and feather disease. Aust Vet J 61:69, 1984.
*A description of the pathology associated with PBFD.*

Pass DA and Perry RA: Psittacine beak and feather disease. An update. Aust Vet Pract 15:55, 1985.
*A review of the clinical and pathologic features of PBFD as they occur in Australia.*

Raidal SR, McElnea CL, and Cross GM: Seroprevalence of psittacine beak and feather disease in wild psittacine birds in New South Wales. Aust Vet J 70:137, 1993.
*A description of the seroprevalence of PBFD in free-ranging psittacine birds from New South Wales.*

Ritchie BW, Niagro FD, Latimer KS, et al: Hemagglutination by psittacine beak and feather disease virus and use of hemagglutination-inhibition for detection of antibodies against the virus. Am J Vet Res 52:1810, 1991.
*Description of the HA and HI characteristics of the PBFD virus and methodology for performing these tests.*

Ritchie BW, Niagro FD, Latimer KS, et al: Routes and prevalence of shedding of psittacine beak and feather disease virus. Am J Vet Res 52:1804, 1991.
*Description of the routes by which PBFD virus may be excreted from an infected host.*

Ritchie BW, Niagro FD, Latimer KS, et al: Antibody response to and maternal immunity from an experimental PBFD virus vaccine. Am J Vet Res 53: 1512, 1992.
*Description of the progression of experimentally induced disease and demonstration of the efficacy of an inactivated PBFD virus vaccine.*

Ritchie BW, Niagro FD, Lukert PD, et al: A review of psittacine beak and feather disease. J Assoc Avian Vet 3:143, 1989.
*A review of psittacine beak and feather disease.*

Todd D, Niagro FD, Ritchie BW, et al: Comparison of three animal viruses with circular single-stranded DNA. Arch Virol 117:129, 1991.
*Comparison of the structural, antigenic, and genomic characteristics of PBFD virus, porcine circovirus, and chicken anemia virus.*

Woods LW, Latimer KS, Niagro FD, et al: Circovirus infection in pigeons. *Assoc Avian Vet*, 1993, p 156.
*Pathologic findings associated with and characteristics of a circovirus described in pigeons.*
Wylie SL and Pass DA: Experimental reproduction of psittacine beak and feather disease/French molt. Avian Pathol 16:269, 1987.

*Experimental reproduction of PBFD in budgerigars and galahs using tissues from affected birds.*
Yuasa N: Effect of chemicals on the infectivity of chicken anemia virus. Avian Pathol 21:315, 1992.
*A description of the effect of disinfectants on chicken anemia virus derived from tissues and from cell culture.*

# DIAGNOSIS AND TREATMENT OF AVIAN ASPERGILLOSIS

ROBERTO F. AGUILAR

*New Orleans, Louisiana*

*and* PATRICK T. REDIG

*St. Paul, Minnesota*

Aspergillosis is the most frequently occurring debilitating disease among nondomestic birds held in captivity (Redig, 1993). It is a fungal disease of the respiratory system, caused principally by the monomorphic thermophilic fungus *Aspergillus fumigatus*. Its onset is characteristically insidious, and its outcome is usually fatal. The infective spores of the agent are ubiquitous. Damp feed, moldy hay, contaminated bedding, accumulated fecal material, and poor ventilation may increase the number of spores in the immediate environment. Wood shavings used as bedding material have been frequently implicated in outbreaks of the disease. Multiple clinical presentations, a slow and insidious course, and expression in immunocompromised hosts make aspergillosis one of the most difficult avian diseases to treat.

Several unique structural and functional aspects of the avian respiratory system make it both the portal of entry and the target system for the disease. Dissemination to other systems is possible, but generally depends on the immune status of the animal. Most avian species possess nasal choanae, infraorbital sinuses, and upper respiratory diverticula. Communication between the oral and nasal cavities through the choanal slit facilitates fungal colonization of the oral cavity. Unlike most other avian orders, psittacines possess only two openings to the sinuses, both in the dorsal sinus wall. One opening exists into the caudal nasal concha and the other into the nasal cavity. Nutritional or environmental factors may compromise epithelial linings. Parrots then develop localized abscessation of bacterial and/or fungal etiology due to poor sinus drainage (Fudge, 1993). The syringeal bifurcation is a frequent site for localized aspergillomas in raptors, psittacines, and most waterfowl. In most species, the syrinx is a tracheal, intrathoracic structure, and is responsible for sound production. It is a paired bronchial structure in owls, herons, and storks. In birds with a tracheal syrinx, primary bronchi branch from each caudal termination,

giving it a Y-shape. A voice change or the inability to vocalize is strongly suggestive of this form of aspergillosis. Fungal colonization of air sacs and their osseous extensions may also occur. Most avian species have seven or more air sacs. The cervical and clavicular air sacs are single structures, while the cranial thoracic, caudal thoracic, and abdominal air sacs are paired. Psittacines also have a cervicocephalic air sac system arising from the infraorbital sinuses. Diverticula of various air sacs connect to pneumatic bones; notably the humerus, the coracoid, and the femur. Thus, fungal colonies may also occur in any of these structures. In birds with neopulmonic parabronchi, inspired air goes from the trachea directly to the abdominal air sac before recirculation. Most fungal air sac lesions are found in the cranial part of the abdominal air sac, next to the lungs. Anecdotal findings point to a higher frequency in the left air sac in raptors, and this site should be carefully scrutinized during radiographic (Fig. 1) and endoscopic exams.

Stress seems to be the major predisposing factor in the development of aspergillosis. Birds that have been recently captured, have undergone changes in management, or have had a change of ownership are thought to experience stress-related immunosuppression. Transportation and heat stress of even a short duration have caused outbreaks of aspergillosis in penguins. Trauma, concurrent disease, and inadequate nutrition may also predispose birds to the development of the infection.

## ACUTE ASPERGILLOSIS

An acute form of aspergillosis occurs when birds are exposed to an overwhelming dose of spores. This form is relatively independent of the physiologic state of the host. Anecdotal reports indicate that apparently healthy raptors exposed to moldy hay have died within 48 hr. Similar cases where the birds present with dyspnea,

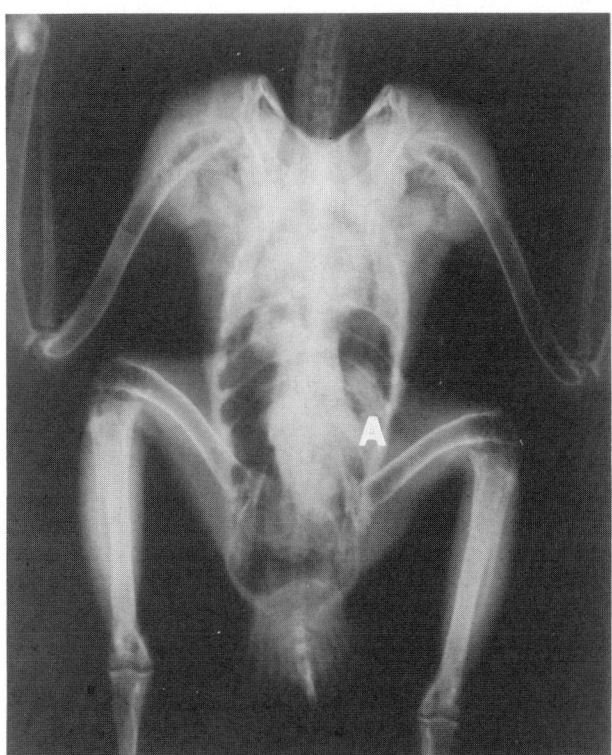

**Figure 1.** Characteristic radiographic lesions of generalized air sac granulomatous aspergillosis, as found in a gyrfalcon (*Falco rusticolis*) on a ventrodorsal view. Note the absence of visible lesions in the lungs. There is extensive accumulation of granulomatous exudate in the left abdominal air sac (A).

polyuria, anorexia, and acute death have been noted in psittacine chicks (VanDerHeyden, 1993). At necropsy, the lungs are found to be covered with numerous punctate inflammatory lesions (microgranulomas) associated to fungal spores. *Aspergillus* can be isolated from most tissues, including liver, spleen, and blood.

## CHRONIC ASPERGILLOSIS

Chronic aspergillosis is the most commonly observed form of the disease. Clinical presentations can be grouped into two classes: focal and generalized. Each class has two distinguishable forms. Combined forms of localized and generalized presentation are possible. Focal aspergillosis is more amenable to treatment, while treatment of the generalized forms tends to be prolonged and unrewarding. It is speculated that focal forms of the disease indicate an active immune response, while the generalized forms may overwhelm the immune system. The clinical presentations, diagnosis, and treatment vary between species. The following are generalities and treatment protocols for all birds. Species variations and caveats are addressed in separate sections.

## Focal Forms

### Nasal Aspergillosis

The nasal form of aspergillosis usually presents as a solid mycotic plug (aspergilloma) localized in the nares or choana. It is frequent in psittacines, particularly African gray parrots (*Psittacus erithacus*) and amazons (*Amazona* spp.). Combined infections of gram-negative bacteria and *Aspergillus* are frequent, and may be misleading if diagnosis is based on bacterial culture alone. Open-mouth breathing is a common sign. The presenting complaint is usually one of blocked nares. Exudative rhinitis is frequently the only sign of infection.

DIAGNOSIS. Diagnosis depends on strong clinical suspicion, history, presenting signs, culture characteristics, and cytology of the extracted material. Serology is usually unrewarding.

TREATMENT. Treatment depends on successful plug removal or dissolution by nasal, choanal, and sinus lavage. Systemic fungistatic treatment should be initiated immediately and continued until total remission. Vigorous flushing with saline solution under isoflurane anesthesia is sufficient to initiate breakdown of the plug. Surgical excision by trephination should be considered if mechanical breakdown fails. Once partial patency to the choana is established, a combined fungicidal/proteolytic solution can be used to flush the nares. The solution is made by combining 0.2 to 0.4 ml of a commercial neomycin-chymotrypsin-trypsin-hydrocortisone ointment (Kymar soluble ointment, Schering-Plough Animal Health, Kenilworth, NJ) with 1.0 mg/kg amphotericin B and then diluting the mix in 20 ml of saline solution. The resulting combination has proven to be effective in dissolving and dislodging the caseous plug; 10 ml should be flushed vigorously but in small amounts through each naris. Patency through the upper respiratory tract should be verified by observation of drainage through the choana. Anesthesia and tracheal intubation are seldom necessary once patency to the oral cavity is established. After the third or fourth sinus flush, the plug usually becomes dislodged, and is seen to appear through the choana. Flushes should be continued using only physical restraint. Maintaining the unsedated bird in a vertical position is critical to preventing aspiration. If the solution enters the lower airway, it can cause severe tissue damage. Daily topical treatment of the nares and sinuses should continue until the lesion and signs disappear. Treatment by sinus lavage rarely exceeds 7 days.

Fungistatic protocols for this form vary. Itraconazole (5 mg/kg PO s.i.d.) is effective. The compound has good fungistatic qualities, but seems to have a relatively narrow safety margin, so its use must be discontinued if emesis or anorexia occur. Fluconazole (15 mg/kg PO b.i.d.), although less effective as a fungistatic drug, has fewer adverse effects at a therapeutic dose, and can be used as an alternative treatment. Parenteral fungistatic treatment must be maintained for at least 1 month after clinical signs resolve to prevent recurrence. Nasal and choanal saline flushes should be cultured monthly until three successive samples are negative to fungal or gram-negative bacterial growth. Cytology should remain negative for the presence of hyphae using standard staining techniques.

### TRACHEAL OR SYRINGEAL ASPERGILLOSIS

The tracheal focal form is characterized by the presence of mycotic colonies above the syrinx or at the bifurcation. The lesions reduce air movement through the lower airway, so inspiratory dyspnea and voice changes are cardinal signs of this form of the disease. In spite of the severity of the signs, treatment can be successful if dyspnea is alleviated and localized treatment is initiated immediately.

DIAGNOSIS.    Diagnosis should be based on visualization of the lesion by endoscopy, although serology and tracheal culture on Sabouraud dextrose agar may strengthen clinical suspicion of infection. Occasionally, fungal colonies can be found below the syringeal bifurcation. These lower lesions are difficult to visualize using endoscopy or radiography. In most cases, lesions are single and appear as a nodular, elevated and caseated mass partially obstructing the airway. More than one nodule can be present, but this is rare. The location or degree of obstruction will determine the severity of dyspnea. The lungs and air sacs are initially unaffected and remain fully functional. If left untreated, however, fungal hyphae from the tracheal lesion may shower the lungs and air sacs, seeding colonies for the disseminated form of the disease.

TREATMENT.    Treatment may be successful if the lesion can be removed surgically without destruction of the syrinx, or if its growth is controlled by pharmacologic means. Air sac cannulation is indicated in birds presenting with open-mouth breathing, noticeable neck extension and discomfort, or in acute respiratory crisis. The bird should also be placed in an oxygen cage if dyspnea is severe. Air sacs can be cannulized as described by Rosskopf and Woerpel (1990), or simply by securing a large-bore (18-gauge or larger) flexible Teflon intravenous catheter in one of the abdominal air sacs. Dyspnea will be relieved by extratracheal airflow. Intratracheal injection of amphotericin B (1.0 to 1.5 mg/kg ITR s.i.d.) has proven to be extremely effective. Volumes should not exceed 0.25 ml in birds weighing less than 300 gm and 2.0 ml in birds weighing 1 kg or more. Amphotericin B is truly fungicidal, and direct contact over the lesion usually breaks down the granuloma. An alternative is the use of 2 to 3 ml of 1% clotrimazole (Clotrimazole, Island Pharmacy Services, Woodruff, WI) nebulized for periods of 1 hr once daily in a Devilbiss chamber (Betamist Sub-2 Medication Nebulizer, Professional Medical Products, Greenwood, SC). Its neutral pH makes it less irritating than other preparations. The granuloma may become larger until it bursts at the center, giving it the appearance of a rosette. The lesion will then rapidly decrease in size and become dislodged. The debris falls as a plug into the syrinx or one of the bronchi. Total obstruction of the lower airway may initiate an acute respiratory crisis. Extratracheal respiration through an air sac cannula prevents asphyxia. Complete blockage, if it occurs, is fatal. Once endoscopy reveals no visible lesion, the air sac cannula can be removed. Most tracheal lesions resolve after 7 to 10 days of intratracheal amphotericin B treatment. Favorable results have been achieved by long-term fungistatic treatment with 5-flucytosine (60 mg/kg PO b.i.d. in birds weighing >500 gm; 150 mg/kg PO b.i.d. in birds weighing <500 gm). Although the fungus can develop resistance to this compound, it has fewer negative side effects. An alternative long-term fungistatic protocol can involve the daily use of itraconazole (5 mg/kg PO s.i.d.). Oral fungistatic administration should continue for 90 to 120 days. Treatment should be discontinued if signs of depression or anorexia develop.

## Generalized Forms

### PULMONARY ASPERGILLOSIS

The pulmonary form appears as myceliated colonies (granulomas) disseminated throughout the pulmonary tissue. Lesions may also appear in the air sacs and their extensions, but the vast majority are pulmonary (Fig. 2). Characteristic lung lesions include a granuloma that is evidently larger and more diffuse than the rest. This is the site of implantation, and indicates the primary nidus of infection. Granulomatous lesions become caseated as the disease progresses. This is the most common presentation of aspergillosis in nondomestic birds, and is considered the classic form of the disease. Clinical signs are usually progressive and include nonspecific depression or inappropriate tameness, a reluctance towards physical exertion, polyuria, anorexia, and mild to severe expiratory dyspnea. In contrast to the localized tracheal form, where dyspnea is primarily inspiratory, in both of the generalized forms, the expiratory component is noticeably increased. Clinicians will frequently initiate diagnostic testing and presumptive treatment simultaneously upon observing this characteristic respiratory pattern. Posterior paresis is possible, and is associated with cavitating lesions in the lung and kidney, causing secondary damage to the sacral plexus and ischiatic nerve (Greenacre, Latimer, and Ritchie 1992). Aspergillosis should be suspected in any bird showing general malaise, depression, dyspnea, or lower motor neurologic signs.

DIAGNOSIS.    Diagnosis by any single method has proven daunting. For the time being, a combination of methods is preferred when establishing a diagnosis. Most clinicians initiate treatment based on clinical evidence and use more than one method to assess the impact of the selected protocol. Diagnosis is based on (1) species susceptibility (Table 1); (2) clinical signs; (3) elevated estimated total white cell count (15,000 to 30,000 cells/mm$^3$ typical), with moderate to severe monocytosis (>4%); (4) deep tracheal culture; (5) endoscopic examination of visible lung margins and abdominal air sacs; (6) radiology; and (7) serology.

The Raptor Center has a successful *Aspergillus*-reduction program based on an enzyme-linked immu-

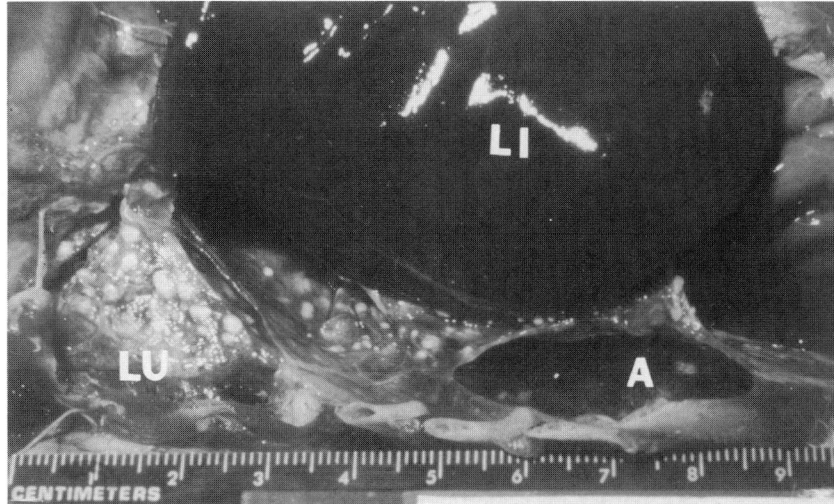

**Figure 2.** Characteristic lesions of generalized pulmonary aspergillosis, as found in a golden eagle (*Aquila crysaetos*). Note the extensive development of mycelomas within the parenchyma of the lung (LU). In this case, the air sacs also contain well-developed lesions (A). The liver (LI) was unaffected.

nosorbent assay (ELISA) test that is used to screen most raptors admitted for rehabilitation. The test is conducted in microtiter plates that have been coated with *Aspergillus* antigen. Specificity has been obtained by development of antisera systems for raptors, psittacines, penguins, swans, and other avian species. The test is estimated to have a 95% sensitivity and an 80% specificity. False-negatives result from a lack of antibody production associated with immunosuppression. This test is currently available commercially (c/o The Raptor Center at the University of Minnesota, 1920 Fitch Ave, St. Paul, MN 55108).

Species with known susceptibility (Table 1) should receive prophylactic treatment for the first 2 weeks after admission and test negative by ELISA before discontinuing medication. ELISA-negative individuals of other species should be treated if they yield a positive result on any two of the other parameters used in assessment. In practice, total white cell count and deep tracheal culture have the highest clinical relevance,

while endoscopy and radiography are used to evaluate and confirm disease in suspicious cases. A clinical example would be a 10-week-old red-tailed hawk that is slightly underweight, has an ELISA of 0.350, an estimated white cell count of 15,000 cells/mm$^3$, and yields a recovery of two *Aspergillus* colonies on a fungal plate. Even without the positive tracheal culture, this bird would be regarded as aspergillus-positive and treated accordingly until the ELISA and estimated white cell count had returned to acceptable levels.

TREATMENT. Treatment varies greatly. Most regimens are based on: (1) removal of lesions that restrict flow of air through major airways, (2) elimination of the fungal organism, and (3) providing supportive care (Redig, 1993). Itraconazole (5 mg/kg PO b.i.d.) can be effective. However, its use must be discontinued if emesis or anorexia occur. Fluconazole (15 mg/kg PO b.i.d.), although less effective as a fungistatic drug, has fewer adverse effects at a therapeutic dose, and can be used as an alternative treatment. Amphotericin B (1.0 to 1.5 mg/kg IV t.i.d.) has serious adverse effects. Parenteral use should probably be avoided unless the clinician feels the fungicidal activity outweighs the negative side effects. Careful patient monitorization and maintenance is indispensable if this protocol is elected. Parenteral fungistatic treatment must be maintained for at least 1 month after clinical signs resolve to prevent recurrence. Clotrimazole can be used as an alternative agent. Recent cases have shown excellent results in resolution of radiographic and clinical signs, but a small case number and lack of long-term follow-up make it difficult to recommend this as the protocol of choice. Good results have been obtained if 2 to 3 ml of a 1% clotrimazole solution are aerosolized for periods of 1 hr once daily in a Devilbiss chamber. Nebulization should be continued for up to 5 months in the most severe cases. Simultaneous oral itraconazole (5 mg/kg PO b.i.d.) therapy for the first 4 weeks of treatment is extremely beneficial if tolerated. Periodic radiography should demonstrate the slow disappearance of lesions in the lung and associated air sacs. Long-term fungistatic treatment with 5-flucytosine (60 mg/kg PO

**Table 1.** *Nondomestic Bird Species With Observed Higher Incidence of Aspergillosis*

**Raptors**
Gyrfalcon (*Falco rusticolis*)
Snowy owl (*Nyctea scandiaca*)
Goshawk (*Accipiter gentilis*)
Rough-legged hawk (*Buteo lagopus*)
Red-tailed hawk (*Buteo jamaicensis*)—in immature birds
Golden eagle (*Aquila crysatoes*)
Bald eagle (*Haliaeetus leucocephalus*)—in lead-poisoned birds

**Psittacines**
African gray parrot (*psittacus erithacus*)
Amazon parrot (*Amazona* spp.)
Pionus parrot (*Pionus* spp.)

**Other Nondomestic Birds**
Penguins
    Gentoo (*Pygoscelis papua*)
    Adelie (*Pygoscelis adelaie*)
    Blackfoot (*Sphenicus demersus*)
    Antarctic species
Ostrich (*Strutio camelus*)
Trumpeter Swan (*Cygnus buccinator*)

b.i.d. in birds weighing >500 gm; 150 mg/kg PO b.i.d. in birds weighing <500 gm) is recommended. Severely caseated lesions that occupy an entire air sac may require surgical curretage. Air sac removal affects flight capability, so lesion removal should be attempted only when indispensable in flighted birds.

Immunostimulation is considered an essential part of the treatment protocol by many clinicians. Treatment with levamisole at standard mammalian doses has yielded poor or equivocal results. The use of nontraditional supplements in psittacines has been recently advocated. Kaprycidin-A (calcium, magnesium, and zinc caprylates), a homeopathic preparation, is used as an oral adjunct to serial 5-day treatments with intralesional amphotericin B (1.5 mg/kg s.i.d.), oral ketoconazole (25 mg/kg b.i.d. PO) and 5-flucytosine (250 mg/kg PO b.i.d.). The protocol is repeated after 3 weeks. One quarter capsule of Kapricydin-A (Ecological Formulas, Concord, CA) is given daily PO for every 400 gm of the bird's weight, along with a gavaged maintenance formula. A β-carotene–rich diet also seems to improve clinical response in psittacines.

### AIR SAC ASPERGILLOSIS

The air sac form is characterized by few pulmonary lesions. Abundant, caseated, necrotic debris fills most of the visceral air sacs. This is the most chronic and debilitating form of the disease, and is the least responsive to treatment. Clinical signs are the same as the pulmonary form, but tend to be extremely chronic in development. While signs of pulmonary aspergillosis take days to weeks to develop, it is not uncommon for air sac granulomas to develop over the course of several months. Since the lungs remain functional, the birds are capable of surviving for a long time.

DIAGNOSIS. Diagnosis is made using the same methods and techniques described in the pulmonary form. Abundant caseated granulomas in the abdominal air sacs are characteristic lesions, and are visible by endoscopy and radiography (Fig. 1).

TREATMENT. Treatment is also the same, with the exception of surgical removal of the lesions. Since air sacs are surgically accessible, granuloma removal is sometimes necessary to attempt to debulk the lesions. Debulking of air sac lesions and partial lung amputations can be performed by midline abdominal approach. While success has been achieved in a few cases, most have proven to be intractable. Spontaneous death or euthanasia following protracted courses of treatment has been the usual outcome. Nebulization therapy with 2 to 3 ml of 1% clotrimazole for periods of 1 hr once daily in a Devilbiss chamber has been successful in some cases. If the bird succumbs, necropsy reveals extensive infiltration and filling of the air sacs with heavy masses of necrotic material. There is little or no involvement of the lungs.

## PREVENTION

Prevention is predicated upon good environmental hygiene, reduction of stress, and a species-specific approach to evaluation and prophylactic treatment. Vaccination for aspergillosis looms on the horizon as a better means of controlling and treating this problem. At present, various preparations are being tested in raptors, penguins, and other species of birds particularly prone to the disease. It is hoped that they will lead to programs of prevention through regular vaccination.

## RAPTORS

Most raptors present with the chronic disseminated forms of aspergillosis. The course of the disease is usually short in red-tailed hawks (*Buteo jamaicensis*), goshawks (*Accipiter gentilis*), golden eagles (*Aquila chrysaetos*), and bald eagles (*Haliaeetus leucocephalus*); usually between 4 and 6 weeks after the onset of clinical signs. Gyrfalcons (*Falco rusticolus*) and Saker falcons (*Falco cherrug*) present with the chronic air sac form, exhibiting a protracted course that may extend over several months. Peregrine falcons (*Falco peregrinus*) and prairie falcons (*Falco mexicanus*) are much more resistant to infection, but present with air sac aspergillosis similar to that seen in gyrfalcons. Aspergillosis rarely occurs in owls and the usual form is an acute or subacute syndrome related to exposure to a large number of spores.

## PSITTACINES

As noted previously, African gray parrots (*Psittacus erithacus*) and amazons (*Amazona* spp.) are particularly susceptible to focal nasal aspergillosis. The same two species present, at least subjectively, with the generalized pulmonary forms more often than other psittacines. Acute aspergillosis is an important disease in psittacine chicks. Mortality due to adverse environmental conditions may be higher than was previously suspected. Contaminated bedding material or food and inadequate nutrition play an important part in the development of the disease. Serum γ-globulins have proven effective as prognostic indicators. Failure to increase γ-globulins after treatment indicates immunosuppression, and a poor prognosis for recovery.

## RATITES

Ostriches (*Strutio camelus*) seem prone to aspergillosis. The incidence is higher in Australia, due mainly to environmental conditions. Chicks under 6 months of age present with the acute form, while older birds usually have the chronic air sac form. Clinically, dyspnea, tachypnea, and mucous tracheitis are apparent. Most protocols attempted to date have failed. Drug combinations and fumigation or nebulization have not yielded positive results. Two treatment protocols hold some promise, based on limited results. Itraconazole (5 mg/kg s.i.d. PO) has been used with success, and is the drug of choice. Sodium iodide (50 ml of 20% solution/100 kg IV by slow administration or with IV fluids every 5 days times three treatments), followed by ethyodide (Vet-A-Mix, Shenandoah, IO) granules, added at $\frac{1}{4}$ ounce once daily to feed, seem to have good degranulating and antifungal capabilities. Simultaneous fungistatic therapy with ketoconazole (25 mg/kg b.i.d. PO) should be maintained for 2 to 3 weeks. In cases that are diagnosed early, the combination has been successful.

## OTHER BIRDS

Penguins present with the chronic forms, and air sac aspergillosis is particularly prevalent. Antarctic birds are extremely susceptible, and defrosting exhibit areas for cleaning may be sufficient stress to start an outbreak. Contaminated air filters have also been implicated. Granulomas form readily in the interclavicular air sac. Laparoscopy is not recommended, since it is of high risk, difficult, and frequently unrewarding. Radiographic signs are usually present. Dyspnea is due to tracheal compression by the growing granuloma. The mass grows until it obliterates the tracheal lumen or compresses the heart. Surgical excision of the air sac is extremely difficult. Nebulization and fungistatic or fungicidal treatment is rarely successful. Clotrimazole nebulization may hold some promise.

Swans and some gallinaceous birds (pheasants) present with chronic forms that are usually lethal. Birds admitted for treatment should receive preventive treatment with itraconazole (5 mg/kg s.i.d.) or 5-flucytosine (60 mg/kg PO b.i.d. in birds weighing >500 gm; 150 mg/kg PO b.i.d. in birds weighing <500 gm) while hospitalized or until negative on ELISA.

**Acknowledgments:** The authors are grateful for the assistance and comments of Drs. Brian Speer, Jeff Jenkins, Jim Jensen, Greg Harrison, Susan Orosz, Terry Campbell, Doug Black, Tom Reardson, and Sam Dover.

## References and Suggested Reading

Flammer K: An overview of antifungal therapy in birds. *Proc Ann Conf Assoc Avian Vet*, Nashville, TN, 1993, p 1.
  *A comprehensive description of available antifungal pharmaceuticals and their recommended use in birds.*
Fudge AM, Reaviu DR, and Rosskopf WV: Diagnosis and management of avian dyspnea: A review. Proc Ann Conf Assoc Avian Vet, Nashville, TN, 1993, p 187.
Greenacre CB, Latimer KS, and Ritchie BW: Leg paresis in a black palm cockatoo (*Probosciger aterrimus*) caused by aspergillosis. J Zoo Wild Anim Med 23:122, 1992.
  *A description of the association of a pulmonary fungal granuloma to posterior leg paresis in a cockatoo.*
Redig PT: Avian aspergillosis. *In* Fowler ME (ed): *Zoo and Wild Animal Medicine, Current Therapy 3.* Philadelphia, WB Saunders Co, 1993, p 178.
  *A description of the clinical presentations of aspergillosis in raptors, as well as recent therapeutic modalities.*
Redig PT: Pharmacokinetics of antifungal drugs in domestic turkeys, red-tailed hawks, broad-winged hawks, and great-horned owls. Avian Dis 29: 649, 1985.
  *A comparison of antifungal pharmacokinetics in domestic and nondomestic birds.*
Rosskopf WJ and Woerpel RW: Abdominal air sac breathing tube placement in psittacine birds and raptors: Its use as an emergency airway in cases of tracheal obstruction. *Proc Ann Conf Assoc Avian Vet*, Phoenix, AZ, 1990, p 215.
  *A description of the technique of abdominal air sac cannulation in birds to relieve respiratory distress caused by tracheal obstruction.*
VanDerHeyden N: Aspergillosis in psittacine chicks. Proc Ann Conf Assoc Avian Vet, Nashville, TN, 1993, p 207.
  *Fourteen cases of avian aspergillosis in psittacine chicks, as well as an account of successful and failed therapy.*

---

# HOUSEHOLD POISONINGS IN CAGED BIRDS

JERRY LABONDE
*Englewood, Colorado*

Household poisonings of caged birds are usually a result of the bird owner being unaware of what is potentially toxic to their pets or from unsupervised activity of the bird. Most pet birds have a curious nature and commonly chew on foreign materials. Avian species are much more susceptible to gaseous fumes than mammals, owing to their small size and unique respiratory system. The most frequent reports of household toxicity cases are heavy metal, gaseous, and pesticide exposures. The most common toxicity questions from bird owners include exposures to plants (see Section 3), pesticides, Teflon, and miscellaneous household chemicals. Inquiries about heavy metal exposures, such as lead, are infrequent, most likely due to increased awareness of the experienced bird owner or total lack of awareness of the novice bird owner.

## DIAGNOSIS AND MANAGEMENT OF TOXICOSES

There are no pathognomonic signs for a specific toxicity and very few specific physiologic antagonists (antidotes) available for treatment. The clinical signs of a toxic bird can mimic many different metabolic or infectious disorders. However, because of the unique physiology of birds and the life-threatening nature of most toxicities, prompt and well-informed action is necessary. It is important to focus on treating the patient, not the toxin, in the management of a toxic bird. Specific diagnostic tests and therapies will be discussed with each specific toxin.

## Diagnosis

Most cases of toxicity present acutely ill, and the pet owner is unaware of any toxin exposure. A thorough history from the owner is the most important information obtained in a fundamental diagnostic approach to rule in or out a potential toxin exposure. Based on the bird's clinical signs and duration of illness, the owner should be questioned regarding common household toxins and their routes of exposure. The primary routes by which toxins are absorbed are ingestion, cutaneous absorption, and inhalation. Therefore, any history involving the use of, or exposure to, gaseous fumes or household chemicals as well as any changes in, or quality of, the bird's environment, diet, and state of health is helpful. Toxicities can be aggravated by age or preexisting illness. There can be some cases of low-dose chronic exposure to a toxin. These birds will show a lack of response to traditional therapies, such as antibiotics, requiring a review of the bird's environment and potential exposure to toxins.

## Management

Emergency medical treatment to stabilize the patient may preclude getting a thorough history from the owner. This may include fluid therapy, anticonvulsants, oxygen, or other treatments as indicated. Physiologic antagonists can have potential toxic effects, and their use based on an incorrect diagnosis can be detrimental. Once the bird is stabilized, diagnostic samples can be taken for later analysis.

There are numerous household items that, if used inappropriately or if a bird accidentally exposes itself to one, can be toxic. At this time, if a specific household toxin is suspected, it may be helpful to contact one of the animal poison information centers or a local certified regional poison control center. Regional poison control centers may not have specific data on avian toxicities, but can supply information on many household chemicals and suggested therapies.

Preventing further exposure and delaying absorption of a toxin is the first step in managing any toxicity. If gaseous fumes are suspected, the bird should be removed from the area and ventilation provided. Ocular exposures should be lavaged frequently with saline. Contact of a toxin to the skin or feathers can be treated by flushing with water or bathing the bird with a mild detergent. Acid corrosive exposures can be treated by flushing with water and a sodium bicarbonate paste externally or a small amount of Milk of Magnesia if internal ingestion is suspected. Alkali caustic exposures should be treated by flushing with water and applying vinegar externally or giving lemon juice or dilute egg whites followed by a cathartic with internal exposure (Beasley and Dorman, 1990).

To delay further absorption of a toxicant in acute cases of ingestion requires an igluviotomy or aggressive crop gavaging. This may require placing the bird under anesthesia with an endotracheal tube in place to avoid aspiration. Saline or activated charcoal can be used by flushing the crop until it is slightly distended and aspirating the contents. This should be repeated three or four times. A small amount of activated charcoal should be left in the crop as an absorbent for the lower intestinal tract.

To hasten the elimination of an ingested toxin that has passed through the proventriculus, absorbents, cathartics, and bulk diets are helpful. Products such as activated charcoal (1 gm/5 to 10 ml water), high-fiber psyllium laxatives (1/2 tsp/60-ml gruel mix), magnesium sulfate (5% solution), and mineral oil (0.3 ml/35-gm body weight) can be used. These products are generally tube fed with a baby food gruel mix. Activated charcoal should always be given first in a slurry mix.

Birds that have suffered a toxicity can be in a severely compromised condition. Instituting aggressive supportive therapy can oftentimes mean the difference between the success or failure of a case. Fluid and electrolyte replacement is important, as gastrointestinal disturbances may be the primary clinical signs. Subcutaneous routes are often combined with intravenous bolus therapy. Severely compromised birds should have a jugular or interosseous catheter for intermittent fluid administration. Anticonvulsants such as diazepam (0.6 mg/kg) can be given intramuscularly as needed.

Dyspneic or hypoxic birds, especially in cases of gaseous inhalation, will benefit from oxygen therapy as well as heat and humidity. Severely anemic birds may necessitate homologous transfusions in a few cases of chronic heavy metal exposures. Oral electrolyte and nutritional therapy is indicated once regurgitation has ceased.

The final step in the management of any toxicity case is client education. Counseling of the pet owner should include discussion of the more common household toxins and methods of prevention. Most toxicities have an initial guarded prognosis, and the potential for relapses should be communicated to the owner.

## HOUSEHOLD TOXINS

### Inhalant Toxins

Birds are the first to suffer the toxic effects of gasses or fumes in the household and often results in acute death. Many exposures occur in the kitchen, due to fumes emitted from burning food or cleaning. Most stove top ventilators and filters are inadequate protection for birds. There are numerous fumes or gasses that can be potentially toxic at the right concentration (Table 1). Any strong odor from any household product should be considered as potentially toxic. If there is any suspicion of toxic fumes present in the home, the birds

**Table 1.** *Inhalant Household Toxins*

Most nonstick cooking surfaces (e.g., pots, pans, woks, and drip pans)
Hair dryer fumes (primarily from new hair dryers)
Smoke (tobacco or any other source)
Automobile exhaust/carbon monoxide
Leaded gasoline fumes
Self-cleaning ovens
Bug bombs, pesticide strips and sprays
Hair permanents and hair sprays
Chemical sprays (e.g., disinfectants, deodorizers, and furniture polish)
Glues, paints, and nail polish and remover
Ammonia and strong bleach
Mothballs (naphthalene, paradichlorobenzene)
Fluoropolymers from spray starch
Burning foods and cooking oils

should be removed from the house and windows opened for ventilation.

Polytetrafluoroethylene (PTFE) poisoning is the most lethal inhalant toxicity reported in birds. Common sources of household items are Teflon and Silverstone nonstick cookware, drip pans, and some sprays. With proper use of the cookware, there are no reported toxicities, except for the drip pans. When pans are left to boil dry or are preheated, the Teflon surface undergoes pyrolysis at 280°C (536°F) resulting in polymer fume fever. Acute death is the common history, but mild exposures exhibit dyspnea, ataxia, moist rales, and frantic behavior. Humans experience flu-like symptoms. At necropsy, airsacculitis, pulmonary congestion, and hemorrhagic and necrotizing pneumonitis are common (LaBonde, 1991).

With all toxic inhalants, prevention is the best therapy. If the bird survives, oxygen, diuretics, and supportive therapy are recommended.

## Pesticides

Pesticide toxicities result from inappropriate application of rodenticides, herbicides, and insecticides. Indoor environments increase the chance of toxic exposures due to limited ventilation in the home. Open windows can be a source of exposure to indoor birds from inappropriate use of pesticides in the yard. Bird owners should be warned that their pets can be more sensitive to pesticides than are mammals, as in the case with certain organophophates.

Organophosphates (OP) and carbamates such as dursban (chlorpyriphos), carbaryl (Sevin Dust), diazinon, malathion, dichlorvos, and dieldrin are found in many insecticides or fertilizers. Clinical signs observed in birds are due to inhibition of acetylcholinesterase. Gastrointestinal signs include anorexia, diarrhea, and crop stasis. Neurologic dysfunctions include ataxia tremors, seizures, and paralysis. Other clinical signs may include dyspnea with moist rales and bradycardia. Young and small birds are more susceptible to OP toxins. Chronic low-level exposure can result in decreases in egg production, hatchability, and hatchling size (Mohan, 1990).

Recent history of use or exposure to these products along with supporting clinical signs is the basis for diagnosis. Cholinesterase analysis of whole blood or brain tissue may establish exposure, but paired samples from birds not exposed may be required for comparative analysis. Normal avian cholinesterase levels have been reported as greater than 2000 IU/L. Acute toxicoses can have no detectable cholinesterase levels and chronic low-grade exposures can be below 50% of normal. The analytic laboratory should be consulted before submission of samples. Histopathology may give some suggestion of exposure but is not consistent. Insecticide identification can be made from suspected food or container sources, gastrointestinal contents, liver, body fat, and skin.

The physiologic antagonists used to treat organophosphate and carbamate toxicoses are atropine (0.2 mg/kg IM every 3 to 4 hr as needed until cessation of clinical signs) and praladoxime chloride (2-PAM, Ayerst Labs; 10 to 100 mg/kg IM every 8 to 12 hr as needed). 2-PAM is of benefit within the first 24 hr of exposure and can be used in conjunction with atropine at the lower dose of 10 to 20 mg/kg. Both drugs are used until the patient is asymptomatic, then as needed up to 48 hr after presentation. The use of 2-PAM in carbamate toxicities is controversial due to reports indicating a reduction in the protective effects of atropine in carbaryl toxicities (LaBonde, 1991).

Rodenticides such as warfarin, brodifacoum, and indadione derivatives are anticoagulants that interfere with the recycling of vitamin K. Brodifacoums are 40 to 200 times as toxic as warfarin and have a much longer half-life. Poisonings can occur by primary ingestion or from contaminated food or water.

Clinical signs vary from depression, anorexia, diarrhea, and crop stasis, to subcutaneous hemorrhage, bleeding from the nares, and oral petechiation. At necropsy, hemorrhage can be observed in the lungs and other parynchymatous organs.

Diagnosis is based on history of exposure and clinical signs. Coagulation profiles are technically possible in birds but are not readily available or reliable at this time.

Vitamin $K_1$ is the treatment of choice at a dose of 0.2 to 2.2 mg/kg IM every 4 to 8 hr until stable, then daily. Duration of treatment depends on clinical signs and type of toxin, extending up to 2 weeks if needed.

Other rodenticides that have been reported causing toxicities are crimidine (Castrix), zinc phosphide, and alphachoralose (Humphreys, 1988). Zinc phosphide is treated with supportive therapy and a 5% sodium bicarbonate gavaging solution.

Paradichlorobenzene is an insecticide used in avian mite protectors that are hung on the bird's cage. Toxicities occur from the bird chewing through the protective cover and ingesting the product. Clinical signs include gastrointestinal signs, tremors, and seizures.

Herbicide and fungicide toxicities usually result from bedding or grain contamination. Organomercurial compounds (thiram) are used as grain fungicides and can cause abnormal egg production as well as leg deformities in young birds. Mortalities have been observed from chlorophenol-contaminated bedding. Chlorophenols have been used for termite control and as a herbicide or fungicide (Fowler, 1983).

## Heavy Metals

Lead poisoning in psittacine birds is addressed in *CVT IX* (McDonald, 1986), but a brief update for lead and zinc toxicoses will be included. There are many household items that contain lead that a curious bird that chews can ingest (Table 2). Common sources of zinc are galvanized wire or containers, hardware cloth, zinc phosphate, metal fasteners, and pennies. Zinc is soluble in soft water and organic acids, which can result in food or water contamination.

Clinical signs for heavy metal exposures are usually multisystemic. Gastrointestinal and neurologic signs are the common signs present in clinically affected birds. Anorexia, diarrhea, weight loss, crop stasis, and regurgitation are often reported. Head tremors and seizures are common in acute highly toxic cases. Premature destruction and decreased production of erythrocytes results in anemia and hematuria or hemaglobinuria that is often seen in Amazon parrots. Polyuria and polydypsia can also be observed. Combinations of lead and zinc toxicities can occur.

Diagnosis is based on history, clinical signs, radiographic demonstration of metallic particles in the gastrointestinal tract, and blood levels of lead or zinc. The lack of heavy metal densities on radiographs does not rule out a heavy metal toxicity. Blood lead levels above 20 $\mu$g/dl (0.2 ppm) are suggestive and levels above 50 $\mu$g/dl are diagnostic of toxicity. Tissue lead levels (liver, kidney, or brain) greater than 6 ppm (wet weight) are significant. Whole blood for lead analysis should be collected in heparinized or sodium citrate tubes. Zinc levels are more difficult to interpret. Blood and tissue levels in macaws suffering from zinc toxicoses have been reported as greater than 200 $\mu$g/dl and 75 ppm, respectively. Serum should be submitted in plastic containers for zinc analysis because rubber stoppers leach out the zinc from the serum.

Treatment involves stabilizing the patient, removal of metal particles (bulk cathartic diets, gavaging, endoscopy, or surgery), and chelation therapy. Chelating agents are available in both injectable and oral forms. Calcium EDTA (calcium versonate, Riker) can be given at 35 mg/kg twice daily for 5 to 7 days with a rest period between additional courses if needed for both lead and zinc. Continued treatment is based on blood lead or zinc levels and the presence or absence of metal fragments on radiographs. Oral treatment with D-penicillamine (55 mg/kg b.i.d.) can be used after the bird is stabilized with calcium EDTA. This is usually made into a suspension and refrigerated for use when injectable calcium EDTA is too difficult for owner compliance or for long-term chelation.

## Miscellaneous Household Toxins

### OIL TOXICOSIS

Common medical problems associated with household oils or petroleum products are burns from cooking oils, hypothermia, diarrhea, dehydration, regurgitation, and pneumonia. All except skin burns and hypothermia involve ingestion or absorption of the oil, which can occur after the bird gets the oil product on the feathers and subsequently preens. Activated charcoal is indicated if ingestion has occurred but hypothermia is the primary concern. Burns most commonly occur on the feet, and aggressive supportive therapy should be initiated.

If the bird is weak and stressed, an absorbent towel can be used to soak oil from the feathers while the bird is being warmed and stabilized. Once the bird is stable, baths in a mild 4 to 15% solution of a mild detergent are indicated. The detergent solution is applied over the feathers and stroked gently in the direction of the feather. Then the bird is rinsed with warm water and dried. This should be repeated as needed.

### CHOCOLATE TOXICITY

The tendency of owners to feed chocolate treats and the bird's ability to eat considerable amounts compared to their body size can result in a toxic condition. The reaction to the alkaloid theobromine found in chocolate can cause depression and regurgitation. In severe cases, convulsions and death can occur. Treatment is directed toward gastrointestinal protectants, cathartics, and supportive therapy.

### CHLORINE

Inappropriate use of concentrated chlorine compounds near birds can result in photophobia, conjunctivitis, and dyspnea. Eye lavages followed by protective ophthalmic medications and supportive therapy are indicated.

***Table 2.*** *Sources of Lead (Pb) and Zinc (Zn)*

| | |
|---|---|
| Lead shot (Pb) | Galvanized wire and fasteners (Pb, Zn) |
| Lead-based paints (Pb) | Plaster impregnated with lead (Pb) |
| Lead putty (Pb) | Solder (Pb) |
| Galvanized containers/dishes (Pb, Zn) | Hardware cloth (Pb, Zn) |
| Foil from some champagne and wine bottles (Pb) | Linoleum (Pb) |
| Some welds on older cages (Pb) | Contaminated feed and bone meal (Pb) |
| Curtain or fishing weights (Pb) | Bells with lead clappers (Pb) |
| Stained glass seams (Pb) | Improperly glazed ceramics (Pb) |
| US pennies since 1982 (Zn) | Batteries (Pb) |
| Costume jewelry (Pb) | Backs of mirrors (Pb) |
| Bird toys with lead weights (Pb) | Leaded gasoline fumes (Pb) |

### HEXACHLOROPHENE

Sources include soaps and deodorants. Blindness is the primary clinical sign that may be temporary or permanent. Supportive therapy is critical, as well as absorbents.

### SODIUM CHLORIDE

Salt toxicities in household birds have been observed from ingestion of contaminated water or ingestion of large amounts of salty foods. Clinical signs include polydypsia, depression, hemoglobinuria, excitement, tremors, torticolis, opisthotonus ataxia, and death. At necropsy, cerebral edema and hemorrhage are observed. Treatment involves diuretics and fluids such as 5% dextrose in water or 2 1/2% dextrose in 0.45% saline.

### ALCOHOL

Depending on the type and amount of alcohol ingested, clinical signs include lethargy, ataxia, anorexia, regurgitation, and death. Therapy would include fluids and placing the bird in a quiet dark incubator.

### NICOTINE

Birds have been presented after chewing and ingesting tobacco products with depression, cyanosis, and dyspnea. Treatment involves absorbents and cathartics, as well as supportive therapy.

There are numerous household products that a bird could potentially get into for which there is no specific therapy. If a toxic exposure is suspected, treat the patient, not the toxin.

## References and Suggested Reading

Beasley V and Dorman D: Management of toxicoses. Vet Clin North Am 20: 307, 1990.

Fowler M: Disinfectant and insecticide usage around birds and reptiles. *In* Kirk RW (ed): *Current Veterinary Therapy VIII.* Philadelphia, WB Saunders Co, 1983, pp 606–611.

Humphreys DJ: Veterinary Toxicology, 3rd edition. London, Balliere Tindal, 1988.

LaBonde J: Avian toxicology. Vet Clin North Am 21:1329, 1991.

McDonald S: Lead poisoning in psittacine birds. *In* Kirk RW (ed): *Current Veterinary Therapy IX.* Philadelphia, WB Saunders Co, 1986, pp 713–718.

Mohan R: Dursban toxicosis in a pet bird breeding operation. *Proc Assoc of Avian Vet Conf,* Phoenix, AZ, 1990, pp 112–114.

# CURRENT APPROACHES TO FEATHER PICKING

NANCY P. LUNG

*Fort Worth, Texas*

*and* APRIL ROMAGNANO

*Raleigh, North Carolina*

Progress in avian medicine this past decade has brought a better understanding of the feather-picking bird. A syndrome which 10 years ago was attributed solely to "behavior problems" or "mental disorders" has since been associated with many treatable medical conditions. The skin and feathers of a bird mirror the body as do the skin and coat of a mammal. Therefore, as in the mammal, a systematic dermatologic work-up of any avian skin disorder is warranted.

Despite medical advances, the feather picking bird can remain an enigma to conscientious veterinarians and compliant clients. Many cases are still attributable to behavioral abnormalities, either as the primary cause or as a learned behavior left over from a previous medical condition. Therefore, a complete medical work-up must be coupled with thorough behavioral counseling of clients with affected birds. As diagnostic and therapeutic regimens can be expensive and labor intensive, open communication with clients regarding the clinical approach and possible outcomes will reduce frustration and disillusionment. It will also encourage clients to play an integral role in the work-up and treatment of their pet.

There are numerous approaches to the feather-picking patient. This article will present a practical three-visit protocol that systematically rules out the known medical causes of feather picking while simultaneously addressing nutritional and behavioral causes at home.

## DIAGNOSTIC APPROACH

### First Visit

#### FIRST-VISIT HISTORY

When presented with a feather-picking bird, ample time should be allotted for in-depth discussion and physical examination as well as for preliminary diagnostic tests. Thorough history taking is essential and sometimes alone can lead to a diagnosis. First, focus on the species presented. Due to their highly intelligent nature, African gray parrots are commonly affected by psychological or "boredom" feather picking. The high emotional state of cockatoos predisposes them to sexual and psychological feather picking. These birds will often mutilate the keel and breast muscles. In contrast, Amazon parrots are not known for psychological picking. However, they have been associated with a cyclic self-mutilation syndrome that can occur every 3 to 6 months, sometimes for years. Giardiasis is a common cause of pruritus in cockatiels. Budgerigars are rarely associated with psychological feather picking. Look for a medical cause in these cases.

Second, make sure the owner is not confusing normal seasonal molts or preening behavior with feather picking. Education of clients on normal psittacine physiology and behavior may be useful. Differentiate feather loss from feather picking. Many systemic diseases can result in loss of feathers or abnormal molt without actual picking. Next, discuss at length the diet of the bird, not only what is fed but what is actually eaten, in what amounts, and at what time of the day. A useful tool to help elucidate behavior and nutritional problems is to review "24 hr in the life of the bird." Ask the owner to keep a detailed log of the bird's activities for 1 to 2 days. From this you can determine the patient's sleep cycles, play time, feeding time, amount of interaction with the owner, bonds to other birds or specific family members, aberrant behaviors, signals associated with feather picking, and stresses in the house such as another pet or excessive exposure to energetic children. Determine cage size, location, availability of toys and stimuli, and any recent changes in these things. Also inquire about home remedies or therapies attempted by other veterinarians for this problem. Home remedies and misinformation abound and can make the problem worse!

### First Visit Physical Exam

A thorough physical exam of the feather-picking bird is essential and rewarding. Evaluate overall health status based on alertness, fecal and urine quality, respiratory rate and pattern, body condition, and weight. Upon examination of the integument, determine if the problem affects both skin and feathers. Feather loss on the head where the bird cannot reach may indicate a feather loss condition. Note evidence of pruritus such as the bird picking throughout the visit. Are the feathers damaged and chewed or are they dysplastic as occurs with some viral diseases. Look for evidence of dermatitis, folliculitis, cutaneous neoplasia, feather cysts, xanthomas, external parasites, and any indication of systemic disease. Such findings can help direct your diagnostic approach.

### First-Visit Diagnostic Tests

The following diagnostic approach for the first visit is noninvasive, inexpensive, and provides a tremendous amount of information. This approach has been particularly useful for those cases in which financial constraints exist. Note that all or any combination of the following diagnostic tests will be employed based on history and physical exam findings. They can all be done in house and, with practice, interpretation can be very rewarding.

*Skin scrape*—parasite and cytologic exam.

*Feather squash prep*—pluck new feather from affected area, cut shaft longitudinally and smear contents on slide for cytologic exam (e.g., bacteria, yeast, inflammatory cells).

*Feather exam*—gross and microscopic for barbering, breaking, clubbing, ectoparasites.

*Cloacal swab*—gram stain and cytology plus culture and sensitivity.

*Fecal direct, trichrome, and IFA*—for *Giardia*, other flagellates.

*Fecal gross exam and floatation*—for cestodes and nematodes.

For those cases in which a medical cause of picking is highly suspected, a complete blood count, serum chemistry, chlamydia, and viral screens should be considered at the time of the first visit.

### First-Visit Therapeutics

Any or all of the following treatments may be recommended at the first visit based on history, physical exam and diagnostic findings.

*Systemic antibiotics*—for bacterial dermatitis, folliculitis, enteritis.

*Systemic antifungals*—for yeast or fungal dermatitis, folliculitis, or enteritis.

*Paraciticides*—for external (mites, lice) and intestinal (nematodes, cestodes) parasites.

*Nitroimidazoles*—(e.g., metronidazole) for gastrointestinal flagellates such as *Giardia*.

*Vitamin A, E, B complex, injection*—for specific nutritional deficiencies, particularly hypovitaminosis A.

*Improve diet*—educate client and begin diet modification.

*Behavior modification*—begin to modify the daily routine of the bird with specific recommendations based on history.

### Second Visit

If the results of the first visit did not lead directly to a diagnosis and if the therapeutic plan did not lead to clinical improvement, a second visit is recommended from 1 week to several months after the first. History taking at this visit is geared at evaluating client compliance with therapeutic recommendations and evaluating success with dietary and behavior modifications. Obtain specific information. Repeat the physical exam to note improvement/regression and compare this with the owner's perception of change. Diagnostic tests conducted at this visit are more expensive but give a more thorough evaluation of the health status of the patient. These include any or all of the following:

*Complete blood count*—heterophilia with bacterial infections, eosinophilia with parasites and giardiasis, anemia with systemic disease, hemoparasites, and so forth.

*Serum chemistry*—hepatic/renal disease, electrolyte imbalance, diabetes, hypoproteinemia, and so forth.

*Radiographs*—focal lesions such as orthopedic fractures, organomegaly, and airsacculitis can lead to focal picking. Spinal injuries/metabolic bone disease can lead to inability to preen normally. Look for evidence of systemic disease or masses.

*Skin/follicle biopsy*—histopathology and culture for viral, bacterial, fungal, mycobacterial infections; hypersensitivity; follicle dysplasia; parasitic infections; hypovitaminosis A.

*Chlamydia*—serum antibody titer or antigen capture test.

*Culture and sensitivity*—of cloaca or skin lesions based on abnormal cytology.

*Psittacine beak and feather disease virus*—DNA probe analysis of whole blood (retest in 90 days if positive).

*Polyoma virus*—DNA probe analysis of cloacal swab.

The therapeutic plan following the second visit may include several of those items used after the first visit. However, the treatment will be geared specifically to the results of the diagnostic tests. See "Therapeutic Options," below, for specific treatment. If the diagnostic tests performed in the second visit are normal, you may be getting closer to a diagnosis of behavioral feather picking. Pay attention to the history and continue to work closely with the owner on behavioral and dietary modifications.

### Third Visit

If the diagnostic tests of the second visit suggest a systemic disease problem, hospitalization for a more thorough evaluation of the bird may be warranted. Diagnostic tests appropriate at this time may include:

*Surgery*—for removal of tumors, cysts, xanthomas for histopathology.

*Laparoscopy*—for evaluation of liver, kidneys, reproductive tract, air sacs, spleen, intestinal serosa. Biopsies, cytology, and culture can be taken at this time.

*TSH stimulation test*—for diagnosis of hypothyroidism (rare).

Treatment is geared specifically to the diagnosis and clinical signs. For example, xanthomas may respond well to surgical excision. See "Therapeutic Options," below.

The diagnosis of behavioral feather picking can be strongly suspected based on species predisposition and history. If after the third visit no evidence for a medical illness exists, behavioral feather picking, a diagnosis of exclusion, should be strongly considered. Once diagnosed, aggressive treatment of behavioral picking should be undertaken. Mild cases with a recent onset may respond to behavior modification alone. Prognosis for permanent cure in chronic pickers is guarded and treatment will require strong dedication from the owner. The management of chronic feather pickers will likely involve combinations of behavior modification, physical barriers such as collars, and short-term tranquilization. Feather follicles may no longer be viable. Management of the behavioral feather picker requires a tremendous investment of time and expertise by the veterinarian. Utilizing the services of a qualified avian behaviorist can be an invaluable tool to the veterinarian and the client (Davis, 1991). Behaviorists work in the home one-on-one with families of affected birds, or provide professional telephone consultations.

### THERAPEUTIC OPTIONS

Few pharmacokinetic studies have been performed on psittacine birds. Drug doses included in the following section are based on the clinical impressions of avian practitioners and may not fall within optimal therapeutic protocols.

#### Cutaneous Bacterial Infections

Systemic antibiotics are useful for primary bacterial infections as well as for infections secondary to stress and mutilation. For gram-positive skin infections such as *Staphyloccus* spp. and *Streptococcus* spp., trimethoprim-sulfa, injectable first-generation cephalosporins, and penicillins are useful. For gram-negative infections, aminoglycosides, quinolones, third-generation cephalosporins, and potentiated penicillins are recommended. Severe cases may need extended course of treatment. Watch for overgrowth of opportunistic yeast and bacteria.

#### Yeast/Fungal Infections

Nystatin (300,000 U/kg PO b.i.d.) is useful for enteric *candida* infections. For resistant *candida* or systemic yeast and fungal infections, use ketoconazole (10 to 30 mg/kg PO b.i.d.), fluconazole (5 mg/kg PO once daily), or itraconazole (10 mg/kg PO b.i.d.; 5 mg/kg OD in African Greys).

## Giardiasis

The nitroimidazoles have provided the most effective treatment, although complete cure is difficult. Metronidazole is effective both orally (10-30 mg/kg PO b.i.d. for 7 days) and by injection (20 mg/kg s.i.d. for 2-5 days). It can be crushed into the water or juice or compounded by your local pharmacist into an oral suspension. Dimetridazole is no longer available in the United States and has a narrow margin of safety.

## Sexual Feather Picking

This will occur in both sexes and often coincides with the age of sexual maturity. It can manifest as "brood patch" picking or frustration from improper outlets for species-typical behaviors. Diagnosis should be made based on the patient's age, the time of the year, and knowledge of species-typical behaviors. Medroxyprogesterone acetate and megestrol acetate have been used to halt sexual cycles. However, side effects including diabetes mellitus, hepatopathy, and obesity can be devastating. Use of hormonal compounds should be undertaken only after other causes of picking have been ruled out and when the history supports the diagnosis.

## Parasites

External skin and feather mites can be treated with 5% topical carbaryl powder. Ivermectin at a dose of 200 $\mu$g/kg PO or IM is effective against *Knemidokoptes* and some intestinal nematodes. Fenbendazole should be used for ascarids (10 to 50 mg/kg PO; repeat in 10 to 14 days), and praziquantel for treatment of cestodes (10-20 mg/kg PO; repeat in 10 to 14 days).

## Endocrine Imbalances

Levothyroxine sodium is used in the treatment of primary hypothyroidism. Clinicians also use it short term to induce a molt in conjunction with feather-picking treatment. This use is somewhat controversial. Levothyroxine sodium should be used at 0.05 to 0.2 mg/120 ml drinking water. Start low and increase the dose to therapeutic levels while monitoring blood $T_3$ and $T_4$ levels. Weight loss can be a dangerous side effect of oversupplementation.

## Hypersensitivity

Due to our poor understanding of the psittacine immune system and lack of diagnostic tools in this area, hypersensitivity is probably an underdiagnosed entity in avian medicine. Treatment of suspected hypersensitivity cases with anti-inflammatory and antihistamine drugs has been unrewarding. Steroidal anti-inflammatory therapy, as is used with atopy in small animal medicine, can be tried but should be used with caution, as use of these products is poorly documented in avian medicine and may lead to secondary infections by opportunistic pathogens.

## Viral Infections

Psittacine beak and feather disease and polyoma virus infections can result in feather loss that mimics feather picking. However, other signs of systemic illness combined with new diagnostic modalities will aid in accurate diagnosis. Antiviral drugs are not routinely used for these conditions. Supportive care for the individual pet bird is warranted, as cures are not available at this time. The infectious nature of these viruses should be considered in multibird households.

## Chemical Behavior Modification

As with any behavior modification program of domestic animals, tranquilizers can be a valuable tool in a balanced approach to change. However, these products do *not* serve as a substitute to appropriate medical and behavioral therapies. Their use should be discontinued once directed treatment has been achieved. Diazepam and phenobarbital are the most commonly used products. Recent reports on the use of tricyclic antidepressants such as clomipramine (Johnson, 1987) and the long-acting neuroleptic haloperidol are available (Lennox and VanDerHeyden, 1993).

## Elizabethan Collars

As with tranquilizers, collars can be an important tool in the management of a feather picker, but should not substitute for appropriate diagnosis and treatment. Collars can be used as a diagnostic tool to see if the follicles are still viable. They can also be used in the early stages of behavior modification programs. For severe mutilators such as cockatoos and Amazons, the collar may be necessary to protect the health of the bird. Some birds will stop picking when the collar is removed. Others will start again as soon as they can reach the area of interest. Hospitalization for 24 hr following placement of the collar is recommended, as the acclimation period can be violent and adjustments may need to be made to the collar. Most birds will acclimate to the collar and clients can be instructed as to their placement and management. For a review of the use and design of collars, see Galvin (1983).

## Behavior Modification

Behavioral feather picking can be a displacement behavior resulting from boredom, fear, frustration, sudden change (e.g., new family schedule, favorite family member moved away, new bird or pet, new cage location), or anxiety. It can also be an escalation of a normal behavior such as grooming or sexual courtship. Identification of the underlying cause can be time consuming, but is essential to successful treatment. "Tricks of the trade" include more varied diet, cage design, and toy selection; more healthy interaction between bird and owner (e.g., do not reinforce bad behavior with more attention); leaving on a television or radio when not home; assuring adequate nutrition and day/night cycle; routine spritzing with water to stimulate normal preening; and acquiring a mate or eliminating an incompatible mate. There is inadequate space for comprehensive coverage of this topic here. Readers are referred to Davis (1991).

## Over-the-Counter Preparations

Many clients will have approached the pet store or breeder for advice before seeking help from the veterinarian. Feather-picking remedies available to the client include topical and systemic "cures." Topical feather-picking remedies are designed to give the feathers an unpleasant taste with such products as bitter apple or bitter orange. These products can leave the feathers sticky and do very little to dissuade the motivated picker. Systemic remedies come in liquids and powders that are mixed with the drinking water. Read the labels carefully. Most contain promazine derivatives or herbal tranquilizers such as valarian. Because of their mood-modifying action, these products can stop feather picking. However, indiscriminant use by uninformed clients can be dangerous due to inaccurate dosing and prolonged use.

## Alternative Medicine

Practices such as acupuncture and homeopathy are becoming popular with some clinicians. Preliminary re-

ports are encouraging. However, controlled scientific evaluation of such treatments is needed. For more information, see Lennox and VanDerHeyden (1993).

Unfortunately, there are no quick fixes for feather picking. If you educate your clients about the problem, conduct a systematic medical and behavioral work-up, and scrutinize response to therapy carefully, you will have rewarding cases and satisfied clients. Don't be discouraged that there will be a small percentage of cases for which a solution will not be achieved. The key is to understand the problem well enough that these cases can be identified accurately.

### References and Suggested Reading

Davis CS: Parrot psychology and behavior problems. In Rosskopf WJ and Woerpel RW (eds): Pet Avian Medicine. Veterinary Clinics of North America. Philadelphia, WB Saunders Co, 1991, p 1281.
  Provides a practical approach to pet parrot behavior modification and insight into parrot psychology.
Fudge AM and McEntee L: Avian giardiasis: Syndromes, diagnosis and therapy. Proc Assoc Avian Vet, Miami, FL, 1986, p 155.
  Discusses giardiasis as a cause of pruritis in cockatiel feather syndrome.
Galvin C: The feather picking bird. In Kirk RW (ed): Current Veterinary Therapy VIII. Philadelphia, WB Saunders Co, 1983, p 646.
  Describes construction and management of Elizabethan collars in psittacine birds.
Hillyer EV, Quesenberry KE, and Baer K: Basic avian dermatology. Proc Assoc Avian Vet, Miami, FL, 1989, p 101.
  This is a well-referenced review of avian skin and feather physiology and dermatology.
Johnson CA: Chronic feather picking: A different approach to treatment. Proc Joint Meeting Am Assoc Zoo Vet Assoc Avian Vet, Hawaii, 1987, p 125.
  Discusses the use of antidepressant medications in feather-picking birds.
Lennox AM and VanDerHeyden N: Haloperidol for use in treatment of psittacine self mutilation and feather plucking. Proc Assoc Avian Vet, Nashville, TN, 1993, p 119.
  Discusses the use of neuroleptic medications in feather-picking birds.
Ritchie BW, Harrison GJ, and Harrison LR: Avian Medicine: Principles and Applications. Lake Worth, Wingers Publishing, Inc, 1994.
  Provides a comprehensive avian drug formulary as well as updates on psittacine viral diseases such as PBFD and polyoma virus.
Rosskopf WJ and Woerpel RW: Feather picking in psittacine birds: A clinician's approach to diagnosis and treatment. Proc Assoc Avian Vet, Miami, FL, 1986, p 265.
  A practical and comprehensive clinician's approach to the feather-picking patient.

# OSTRICH MANAGEMENT

KAREN HICKS-ALLDREDGE

*Sweetwater, Texas*

Ostriches have been raised domestically in South Africa since the 1850s. Ostrich farming is rapidly increasing in various countries around the world, including the United States. The world demand for ostrich meat, leather, and feathers far exceeds current production levels. The growth of the ostrich industry has resulted in a demand for veterinary services including management programs and preventative medicine. Veterinarians offering services to ostrich producers need to have

a basic understanding of management techniques as well as medicine and surgery.

## ANATOMY

Ostriches are large flightless birds belonging to the ratite group. The major anatomic differences between ostriches and other birds include rudimentary wings, a digestive system modified for grazing, and the loss of three phalanges as an adaption for running.

Mature ostriches may stand 2.4 to 2.8 m tall and weigh 160 kg. Males are black and white, females are brown. There are three recognized subspecies of ostrich in the United States: the red neck, the blue neck, and a hybrid African black. It is important to recognize the breeds for insurance claims and prepurchase exams. The red neck is the largest of the subspecies, originating in the northern regions of Africa. The male has a red neck, red legs, and a bald spot on the top of his head. The male also has a white ring of feathers on the neck where the long feather line ends. The blue neck originated from the middle to the southern part of the African continent, and the male has a blue pigmentation of the neck and legs. However, the beak and shins are red. It is intermediate in size, and its head is feathered on top. The "African black" is a term that has been designated to the hybrid that is domestically raised in South Africa. This bird was selected for feather quality. It is the shortest of the subspecies and its body type is distinguished by shorter legs and a "boat-shaped" body. The male has a very dark blue to black pigmentation to the skin on the neck and legs, and again, a red beak and shin scales comparable to the blue subspecies. They are difficult to differentiate by color alone. The hens of all subspecies are brown and can only be differentiated by size and body type. South Africa has selected some birds for white feather color over their bodies and these birds are showing up in the United States.

The ostrich keel is flattened; the birds do not have pectoral (breast) muscles. A detailed description of the anatomy of ratites has been published (Fowler, 1991). The ostrich has several anatomic adaptations of the gastrointestinal tract that allows grazing with other ungulates in its native habitat.

The ostrich has a large sac-like proventriculus with a defined area of secretory glands. The ventriculus (gizzard) is a large bivalved structure lying just caudal to the keel bone on the standing bird.

Ostriches are hindgut fermenters and rely on microflora for digestion of their highly fibrous diet. The colon comprises 60% of the length of the intestinal tract compared to 6% in the domestic chicken. The microflora of the intestinal tract is similar to that of the rumen of other grazing animals.

Other important anatomic considerations for the veterinary practitioner include the location of venipuncture sites. The cutaneous ulnar veins on the ventral side of the wings and the medial metatarsal veins are good venipuncture and catheterization sites in all age birds. Venipuncture and catheterization of the jugular vein should be avoided if possible, as hematomas form easily and sudden movement by the bird can result in lacerations and exsanguination. The right jugular vein is more developed than the left.

Cocks lack the accessory reproductive organs present in mammals. Paired testes are located dorsal to the abdominal air sacs and ventral to the cephalic end of the kidneys, deep in the body cavity. The simple epididymis lies on the dorsomedial surface of the testes, the ductus deferens leaves the epididymis as a fairly straight tube parallel to the ureter near the midline. The ductus deferens has a sac-like ampulla proximal to the ejaculatory ducts which projects into the dorsal part of the urodeum. They are palpable on physical exam. The terminal proctodeum contains the phallus.

The phallus in the mature cock is approximately 20 cm in diameter at the proximal end and 34 cm in length. There is a prominent dorsal groove with erectile tissue on either side. When the phallus is erect and engorged with lymph, the groove is essentially tubular and acts to transport ejaculated semen from the urodeum to the hen's cloaca.

Hens have a single left ovary and oviduct. The ovary lies dorsal to the abdominal air sacs and ventral to the cephalic end of the left kidney. The ovary consists of a stroma and follicles of varying sizes.

The oviduct lies on the left side of the abdominal cavity and consists of the infundibulum, where fertilization occurs within the first 15 min after ovulation; the magnum; the isthmus; the uterus or shell gland; the uterovaginal sphincter, which separates the uterus from the vagina; and the vagina, which opens into the urodeum at about the 10 o'clock position. The presence of sperm host glands has not been verified, although they are thought to exist.

## PHYSIOLOGY

The ostrich becomes sexually mature at 2 to 4 years of age. Factors affecting the onset of maturity include: (1) subspecies (the smaller African-black subspecies mature earlier than larger red necks), (2) the season of hatch (birds that hatch during a period of increasing day length mature faster than those hatched during a period of decreasing day length), (3) the nutritional status of the bird, and (4) the environmental conditions under which it is kept.

Ostrich reproduction is dependent on the photoperiod. In the United States, the breeding season varies from north to south. Birds in the northern United States have a defined laying season of May to September, and birds in the southern United States may produce all year. The effect of temperature on the season is unknown; however, extremes in temperature stop production.

### Males

With increasing day length, testosterone production increases. The testes increase in size 200 to 400% during the breeding season and secondary sexual characteristics such as reddening of beak and legs, vocalization (booming), and territorialistic displays (kanteling) appear. Spermatozoa production, which is initiated by increasing levels of follicle-stimulating hormone (FSH), as in mammals, starts at the same time. Cocks do not produce spermatozoa during the nonbreeding season.

Avian semen is collected by one of three techniques: electroejaculation, forced massage, or voluntary ejaculation. None of these methods has worked well with the ostrich because of its physical size, demeanor, and lack of sexual imprinting response. The ostrich semen that has been collected by a combination of forced massage and voluntary response has been heavily contaminated with urine, making assessments of concentrations, volume, and pH unreliable. Emu semen is easily collected by voluntary ejaculation, as this species does sexually imprint on humans.

### Females

Follicular maturation is controlled by increasing circulating levels of FSH. The ovary contains approximately 200,000 immature follicles at hatch. As sexual maturity approaches, gonadotropin stimulation of the ovary results in a hierarchy of follicular development being established. Each maturing follicle is steroidogenically active, as is the postovulatory follicle. This hierarchy of follicles F1, F2, F3, and postovulatory follicles must be maintained for ovulation to occur. In other avian species, the administration of exogenous gonadotropins results in a preponderance of F2 follicles and ovulation is blocked. Ovulation is controlled by luteinizing hormone (LH) as it is in mammals; however, avian species have three LH peaks in a 24-hr period rather than two in a 21-day cycle. Ostrich hens are indeterminate layers; they will continue to lay as long as eggs are removed from the nest. In the wild, an average clutch is 20 to 22 eggs. In the United States, hens average 42 eggs per year. Ostrich hens lay every other day during the breeding season. Oviposition occurs late afternoon to early evening, with the time of lay becoming a few minutes later each day.

### RESTRAINT AND PHYSICAL EXAMINATION

Ostriches are intimidating because of their size and sometimes threatening demeanor during the breeding season. Fortunately, their range of motion is limited. They kick forward and down and have a large claw that is dangerous. When restrained, they attempt to flip over backward, which requires being able to climb with their legs against a restraint while lowering their pelvis or rear end. Therefore, the safest place to be is behind the bird supporting its pelvis upward. Any attempts to hold the bird down by applying pressure to its back will result in struggling by the bird.

If the ostrich cannot see, it will usually stand calmly for physical exams, venipuncture, cultures, radiographs, and ultrasound without tranquilization. The less handling and physical restraint used, the calmer the ostrich will remain. The ostrich is curious by nature and can frequently be hooded by the veterinarian or owner when approached with a feed bucket. A hood (sweat shirt sleeve works well) is placed on the restrainer's arm. The beak is grasped with the hand with the hood and the head pulled to chest level as the hood is slipped over the bird's head with the free hand. It is helpful to have someone step behind the bird to lift up on the pelvis if the bird is backing away. The head can be turned loose and the bird moved with one person gently holding a wing and one person on the tail. Occasionally, a bird reacts negatively to a hood, in which case it should be removed immediately before the bird is turned loose. If the bird is reluctant to move with the hood on, the back of the head can be held at chest level and the bird led rather than pushed. The person behind the bird should remember when the bird's leg comes up the hock is level with the human groin!

Having the bird in an enclosed area with at least two and preferably three solid walls will enable capture of a bird that will not approach feed. The bird can be pushed by two people into a corner with the head held over the back while the hood is applied. Holding the bird in the corner lifting up on its pelvis when no enclosure is available allows limited physical exam. Shepherd's hooks are commonly used in South Africa to select birds out of a group by catching the head with the hook and bringing the head to chest level. It is commonly misused in this country to hook the head of a bird that is at a full run down the fence line. Cervical dislocations and fractures occur even when performed by experienced handlers.

Once captured, the adult bird should be placed in a small solid confined area or in a trailer where it will stand calmly. Birds with leg injuries should be secured in a sitting position to a pallet, and the pallet loaded into the trailer if at all possible.

Juvenile birds from 4 months to yearlings are best handled by slowly and calmly herding them into an enclosed barn. If they cannot see out and are crowded into a corner, they will usually sit. They can easily be sexed, banded, blood drawn, dewormed, and so forth. Several people can hold them in the group while the veterinarian moves from individual to individual. If there is no enclosed area, portable panels with plywood applied can be used to crowd them into a small area.

There are several commercially available restraint devices that I do not recommend. A simple V-shaped restraint can be used placing the bird with its chest in the narrowest part of the "V" and holding it from behind.

### Physical Examination

Before the animal has been restrained, it should be examined moving in its enclosure for conformation, gait, body condition, respiration rate and character, and behavior-related problems.

The enclosure should be examined for fresh droppings and urine, and their characteristics noted. An orange to red pigmentation in the urine is generally from a porphyrin pigment in the diet and is noticed when environmental changes result in urine concentration. Green urates may indicate muscle disease or liver disease. The droppings should be observed for tapeworm segments and collected for fecal flotation.

The eyes and sinuses should be examined for any discharge or swelling. The beak and oral cavity should be examined for any lesions. The neck should be palpated, especially in the area of the thoracic inlet for any swellings. The overall condition of the body should be observed and a body score assigned based on fat percentage. The feathers and skin should be examined for lesions or parasites. The thorax should be auscultated. The abdomen should be palpated from the ventriculus, which lies immediately caudal to the breast plate, to the proventriculus, which is palpated between the legs. The caudal abdomen should be palpated and blotted for any evidence of fluid build-up or retained eggs. Finally, a cloacal exam should be performed to verify normal anatomy. A general physical exam should include cultures of the trachea and vagina when indicated. Blood should be drawn for a complete blood count (CBC) and chemistry panel. Sodium heparin and sodium fluoride are preferred anticoagulants. Blood hemolyzes very rapidly in calcium ethylenediaminetetraacetic acid (EDTA) tubes. A coverslip smear should be prepared immediately for cytologic evaluation. Cellular morphology is extremely important and should be interpreted by an experienced technician.

Serology for viral and bacterial antibodies is an enigma at this time. Requirements for interstate transport may be the only real significance the tests have. No relationships for positive antibody tests to disease states of the ostrich exist.

If the bird is an adult hen, an abdominal radiograph or ultrasound is recommended, especially if the bird is being examined prior to purchase. A metal detector can be used to determine the presence of hardware in the ventriculus or proventriculus if radiology is not practical.

## ANESTHESIA

There are many protocols for induction and maintenance of anesthesia in the ostrich. The protocol the author prefers is: birds under 18.18 kg are masked down with 5% isoflurane and maintained on 2% isoflurane. Halothane and methoxyflurane can also be used; however, the recovery is not as smooth. Birds over 18.18 kg are premedicated with azeperone-Stesnil (Pitman-Moore, Mundalein, IL) 0.3 to 0.4 mg/kg IM. When the bird is relaxed (about 5 to 10 min)—which means nictitating membrane up, head down, and wings forward—a combination of ketamine 8 to 10 mg/kg mixed with an equal volume of diazepam or 0.2 to 0.4 mg/kg is administered intravenously. The bird is hooded, and the only support given is lightly lifting up on the pelvis as the bird sits down. Induction and recovery are generally smooth with this protocol. If the bird struggles on recovery, an additional 0.1 to 0.2 mg/kg of diazepam can be administered intramuscularly. Underdosing the bird for induction makes the whole anesthetic episode more difficult. In wild-captured adults, the induction dose may need to be doubled. The bird

is intubated and maintained on 2 to 5% isoflurane through the surgical procedure.

Other induction protocols include xylazine as a tranquilizer at 2 to 4 mg/kg IM followed in 5 min by ketamine 8 to 10 mg/kg IV. A combination of xylazine 1 to 2 mg/kg and ketamine 8 to 10 mg/kg can be given intravenously. After induction, maintenance on isoflurane, halothane, or methoxyflurane is possible.

Telazol (AH Robins, Richmond, VA) tiletamine-zolazepam 4 to 6 mg/kg provides a very smooth induction. A true surgical plane of anesthesia is not reached, and multiple dosing is required to prevent sudden movement. The recovery is prolonged and very difficult, and the bird is difficult to maintain in sternal recumbency and thrashes violently.

Positioning for surgery and recovery is important. A quiet, padded surgical suit is ideal but not always available. If the bird is in lateral recumbency, pad the down leg to prevent myositis and neuritis. If a temporary paralysis is present on recovery, figure-of-8 bandage the foot in a normal standing position for 72 to 96 hr following surgery. In dorsal recumbency, the bird must be well padded and the legs extended caudally to prevent neuritis and paralysis. In both positions, the head should be elevated above the proventriculus to prevent refluxing of fluid.

Recovery should be in a dark, quiet place with the bird in sternal recumbency and its head elevated. If recovering a bird in a location that is considered hazardous to the bird, a soft cotton rope can be tied from one ankle, over the back as far forward as possible, which is just under the attachment of the wings, to the other ankle. This prevents the bird from flipping over backwards. Tying the ankles together in the sitting position will add further security. Birds should not be placed in slings to recover (they may prevent normal air flow and lead to suffocation).

## REPRODUCTIVE BEHAVIOR

The scrape (nest) consists of a shallow depression in the ground that is formed and protected by the male. Ostriches lay every other day in the evening. If left to parental care, the eggs are incubated by the male at night and the female during the day. In free-ranging groups, the dominant hen will incubate the eggs during the day. The dominant hen recognizes her eggs, and if the nest is overcrowded (20 to 25 eggs), the hen will remove the eggs laid by other females. Nondominant hens may lay in several nests and be bred by several males. Both adults brood the chicks.

The cock displays to the hen during breeding season by dropping to his hocks, fanning his wings, and striking the back of his head on either side of his back. In captivity, males frequently display and make a booming noise to any visitor that approaches the enclosure. The hen flutters her wings, drops her head, and makes a snapping motion with her beak. She will drop to the ground with her head extended. The male mounts from the left placing his right foot on the hen's back. He drops to his hocks and intromission occurs. During copulation, the male will strike his back with his head. When ejaculation occurs, the male extends his neck forward and makes a guttural sound.

## REPRODUCTIVE FAILURE

In the United States, infertile eggs average from 40 to 50%, representing a significant economic loss. Eggs are candled at 7 to 10 days of age to determine fertility and eliminate the possibility of early embryonic death. The embryonic disk floats up (that is why it is called "polar") and can be examined for development. This is best performed during the incubation cycle, since early dead embryos will not be seen after 40 days of incubation. Early embryonic death has many causes, including poor nutrition in the hen, toxins, improper egg storage, and improper incubation (Stewart, 1994).

Infertility may result from behavioral problems that result in failure to copulate. Although ostriches are gregarious in nature, with one male breeding several hens, they do have preferences and incompatible pairs are common when the birds are not allowed to select their mates. Environmental conditions may also result in behavioral infertility. High-voltage power lines overhead, predators in the area, the presence of oil field equipment, and movement of the ostrich form pen to pen have interfered with normal breeding behavior. Extreme environmental temperatures may also adversely affect fertility.

The effects of group size on fertility have been investigated with conflicting results. Further investigation is necessary to determine if pairs or trios have fertility rates different from larger numbers in a group or colony breeding.

Seasonal infertility is common early in the breeding season when the hen comes into production before the cook has mature spermatozoa, and late in the season, nutritional influences may also play a role. Ostriches in the United States tend to be overfed, with obesity being more of problem than deficiency diseases. Obese poultry hens have a higher incidence of infertile eggs as well as lower lifetime egg production. In other avian species, deficiencies of vitamins A, E, and selenium have been linked to infertility.

Anatomic causes of infertility include anomalies in the cock's phallus that prevent copulation, such as a deviation or lack of a seminal groove. The black pigment of the male's feathers is a result of the lack of estrogen. A mature black bird that sexes cloacally as a hen may be an intersex, have portions of the reproductive tract missing, or have the ability to lay eggs, even though the male does not recognize her as a hen and will not breed her. Some young hens 18 to 24 months old may be very dark brown or even have black feathers; however, these hens should not be confused with mature "black hens" because, as the hen matures, the feathers turn brown due to increasing estrogen.

Proper hatchery management is essential to the success of any ostrich production operation. Producers frequently request veterinary evaluation of their farm management. This requires working knowledge of egg collection and handling techniques, incubation, hatching, and chick management during the first 24 hr of life. Medical therapy cannot correct problems caused by improper hatchery management.

Eggs should be collected as soon as possible after oviposition occurs. They can be picked up with paper towels or gloved hands; bare hand collections should be avoided. For best results, eggs should be laid in a clean, dry environment and any eggs that are wet or muddy should not be set. Providing shelters or sand in the scrape (nest) may be necessary in some geographic locations. Eggs are laid with several natural defense mechanisms against infectious agents. The first line of defense is the cuticle or mucin coating on the egg; however, mucin is water soluble; therefore, wet and overwashed eggs lose this first line of defense. Washing setting eggs is a very controversial procedure even in the commercial poultry industry. If eggs are to be washed, they can be washed in a number of disinfectants including chlorhexadene, sodium hypochlorite, quaternary ammonia, as well as other compounds. The wash solution should be at least 10°F warmer than the egg to avoid cooling the egg and drawing contamination in through the pores. If eggs are going to be washed, they should be washed before cool storage. All eggs have pores in the shell that allow for transfer of gases and water. Once bacteria get through these pores, the next line of defense is the shell membranes. Infectious agents must be able to digest holes in these membranes to gain access to the albumin. The role of maternal immunoglobulins passing from the yolk to the embryo has not been defined in the ostrich.

Eggs can be stored safely for up to 7 days at 55° to 60°F. Below 45°F, embryo death occurs. Above 70°F (physiologic zero), the embryonic cells start dividing asynchronously. Cooling and storing eggs increases hatchability about 0.5% by ensuring cell synchrony. However, the benefit of storing eggs comes from allowing batch hatches. One advantage of having a batch hatch is allowing time for proper hatcher sanitation. Eggs should be stored at a relative humidity of 60 to 75%. No weight loss or gain should be obtained during storage, and moisture should not condense on the eggs. Increasing storage time decreases albumin quality, which increases evaporative water loss through the egg shell; therefore, if the eggs from a particular hen are not losing enough weight, the storage time may be increased beyond 7 days. Any eggs stored over 7 days should be turned 2 to 3 times daily.

## INCUBATION

Although many farmers in South Africa allow adult ostriches to incubate their eggs in the scrape (nest), this is not done in the United States. The commercial incubators available to producers vary widely in quality. They should be stainless steel for ease of cleaning, have proper airflow, and maintain a consistent temperature throughout the incubator.

## Temperature

The incubation temperature determines the rate of embryo development. The optimum incubation temperature for ostrich eggs has not been determined. Genetic selection for uniformity of egg size and shell quality will help a producer maximize hatchability. Incubation parameters will vary from farm to farm based on the type of incubator used, the predominant egg size, and the porosity of the shell characteristic for each hen.

Temperature should be set so that an egg loses 13 to 15% of its initial weight during a 42-day incubation period. Ostrich eggs vary in weight from 800 to 2100 gm; however, most will be in the 1300- to 1600-gm range. Eggs should be weighed weekly, thus allowing adjustment of temperature and humidity settings throughout the incubation cycle. Most producers set ostrich eggs between 97.5° and 98.8°F. Larger eggs require lower temperatures and may take a day or two longer to hatch.

Excessive heat during incubation results in an early hatch, increased rate of embryo mortality at any stage of development, and an increased incidence of head and limb deformities. Yolk sacs may be pinched off at the navel with yolk remaining externalized. Temperatures in excess of 100°F for over 8 hr have resulted in death of all embryos in the incubator. Temperatures that are too low result in a delayed hatch, increased embryonic mortality, and soft, weak chicks at hatch. The yolk sac may not be internalized and chicks may fail to pip.

## Humidity

Humidity settings in the incubator are set to maintain a 13 to 15% egg weight loss during the incubation period. In general, this will range from 20 to 35% relative humidity. Approximately 75 to 80% of the calcium in the chick's body is absorbed from the shell and the absorption is humidity dependent. Therefore, it is desirable to maintain the highest relative humidity possible, while maintaining the 13 to 15% evaporative water loss. Rotational leg deviations have been linked to low humidity in the incubator (Perelman, 1991).

Ostrich eggs that lose less than 12% of the initial weight during incubation have poor hatchability without assistance, the chicks are edematous, and have poor survival the first week. Although those that lose in excess of 16% may have good hatchability, early chick mortality from 2 to 3 weeks of age will be high.

Eggs should not be incubated in relative humidity less than 20%. Eggs that are incubated in excessively low relative humidity will have a thick jelly-like substance (which is dehydrated albumin) literally gluing the chick to the shell membranes. To increase evaporative water loss, increase the storage time rather than having humidity below 20%. Eggs have been successfully stored up to 14 days without a significant decrease in hatchability. Eggs that are stored over 7 days must be turned two or three times daily. If the producer has a wide range of egg sizes, multiple incubators allowing different relative humidity settings will be beneficial.

## Ventilation

Proper temperature, humidity, and ventilation in the room housing the incubator are essential for its function. Fresh air flow into the incubator is required to supply an adequate amount of oxygen to the embryo and to exhaust carbon dioxide from the incubator. Air flow within the incubator is important in maintaining uniform temperature, humidity, and oxygen levels circulating within the incubator.

## Position

Ostrich eggs should be incubated with the air cell up. The air cell end of the egg is more porous, allowing an increased gaseous transfer in this area, and in early stages of incubation, before the circulatory system has formed, this allows the embryo to be closest to its oxygen supply. Incubating with the air cell up also helps decrease the incidence of embryonic malposition in which the chick's head is opposite the air cell end at hatch and the chick is unable to pip into the air cell. Ostrich chicks develop with their head between their legs at the end opposite the air cell. Shortly before hatching, the head moves toward the air cell.

Ostrich eggs should be turned through a 90-degree angle; 45 degrees from vertical in two directions, at least three times a day. Most commercial incubators available turn the eggs every 2 hr. Turning the egg prevents the embryo from sticking to the shell membranes during early formation and the nutrients and waste products surrounding the early embryo are also circulated.

Ostrich veterinarians should be familiar with candling techniques. Eggs should be candled weekly so that infertile and nonviable eggs can be removed from the incubator. Eggs are generally candled by removing them from the incubator and illuminating them by using a bright light behind a small aperture. In large operations, this is not practical and a small bright flashlight may be used to illuminate the eggs from the ventral surface as they sit in the incubator. Slide projectors make excellent candlers.

## Hatching

Ostrich eggs are transferred from the incubator to the hatcher either at 40 days of incubation or when the chick pips into the air cell. The temperature and humidity setting in the hatcher should be the same as the incubator. This is a controversial issue even within the commercial poultry industry, with some people advocating a cooler hatcher with a higher humidity and others recommending a warmer hatcher with a lower humidity.

Hatching should be a gradual process and, although assisting the hatch is common in the industry, this practice is undesirable. It results in higher chick mortality from yolk sacculitis and other complications than chicks that are allowed to hatch naturally. Producers want all their chicks to hatch at day 42, when in reality, normal egg variability will result in hatches from 39 days to 46 days. If allowed to hatch on their own, ostrich chicks should have dry navels that require no treatment; however, many producers will use iodine or bandages on the navels. Bandages tend to keep the navel wet, therefore increasing the possibility of infections.

Chicks should be removed from the hatcher when they can stand, generally at 4 to 12 hr after hatch. Leaving them in the hatcher too long can result in dehydration. If footing is not adequate in the hatcher, the chicks may be unable to stand and splay legs may result. Taping the legs together will help these chicks.

## REPRODUCTIVE DISEASES

Many diseases may result in reproductive failure, either through failure to produce eggs or through production of abnormal or contaminated eggs.

### Bacterial

Bacterial salpingitis/mertritis is common in the ostrich. The etiologic agents vary, as does the severity of the infection. Common isolates on culture are *Escherichia coli*, *Pseudomonas*, *Acinetobacter*, and other gram-negative bacteria as well as *Streptococcus* and *Staphylococcus*. *Mycoplasma* spp. have been isolated; however, the subspecies is not typable to known poultry pathogens and significance is unknown. In mild cases, only the uterus or shell gland is affected (metritis) and clinical symptoms range from abnormal shells to no egg production at all. There may be an associated salpingitis and/or peritonitis, depending on the duration of the disease process and the route of infection. Infection may result from retrograde bacterial infection from breeding or uterine fatigue, an extension of an air sacculitis, or a perforation of the abdominal cavity by a foreign body.

Affected hens generally present with a history of erratic egg production, malformed or odoriferous eggs, or a sudden stop in production. A hen that flutters and accepts the male should be producing eggs. On physical examination, temperature and respiration are variable, there may be a discharge below the cloaca, and hens may have a peculiar odor. Affected hens often have white blood cell counts ranging from 8000 to more than 100,000. The differential ranges from a pronounced heterophilia in acute cases to lymphocytosis

and toxic heterophilia in cases of longer duration. Serum chemistries are frequently unremarkable. Ultrasonography and radiology are useful in assessing the amount and consistency of exudate in the oviduct. Abdominocentesis may be indicated to assess the nature of the abdominal fluid.

Treatment should be based on culture and sensitivity. When large amounts of exudate are present in the oviduct, lavaging of the oviduct is indicated. This may be accomplished by surgical placement of a Foley catheter in the magnum or isthmus and normograde flushing of debris from the oviduct. This is the method of choice when large amounts of exudate are present. A Foley catheter (size varies with the size of the bird) may also be placed in the vagina or uterus and a retrograde lavage with a 1% povidone-iodine solution or buffered solution with gentamicin performed.

The hen should also be treated with systemic antibiotics. Ciprofloxacin hydrochloride 20 mg/kg PO twice daily or doxycycline 10 mg/kg PO twice daily for 14 days are effective, although the adverse effects of these antibiotics on any eggs produced during the period of treatment has not been determined.

Cocks may develop ascending infections of the seminiferous tubules. Gram-negative organisms are generally isolated; treatment should be based on culture and sensitivity. The prognosis is guarded. The role of the male in transmitting diseases from hen to hen has not been established.

### Viral

Although papillomavirus has been isolated from the reproductive tracts of both cocks and hens, its pathogenicity has not been determined. However, most avian species are also affected by other viruses that can affect the reproductive tract or be transmitted transovarially.

### Egg Binding

Egg binding is a frequently encountered problem in ostrich hens. It is thought that egg binding may be genetically predisposed and complicated by poor nutrition, obesity, metritis, or environmental factors. Although some hens may present with a history of straining or with a vaginal prolapse, most hens exhibit no clinical signs. The egg may be palpable in the caudal abdomen in thin hens. Radiology and/or ultrasonography are generally required for diagnosis.

Medical treatment consists of injections of multivitamins A, D, and E; calcium; and oxytocin. The decision to treat medically versus surgically is based on age, assurance that no infectious process is involved, and history of the individual hen. Breaking the egg in the uterus is dangerous due to the risk of lacerations from shell fragments. Surgical intervention is generally required. If the vagina has prolapsed, the egg may have to be broken to allow replacement of the vagina before extraction of the egg.

## Cystic Ovaries

Cystic ovarian follicles occur infrequently in very high producing hens that have been laying eggs year-round for several years. Diagnosis is based on sonographic appearance. It can be difficult to differentiate cystic lesions on the infundibulum caused by bacterial infections from a cystic follicle. The cystic ovary may fill the entire abdominal cavity. The cystic follicles contain a serous tan fluid that cultures negative. Treatment with human chorionic gonadotropin has not resulted in regression of the cystic follicles in the dose range tried by the author.

## Tumors

Ovarian tumors ranging from granulosa cell tumors to adenocarcinomas have been reported in other avian species. A recent case of lymphoid leukemia affecting the reproductive tract, the abdominal viscera, and cranial mediastinal lymph nodes has been seen in an ostrich. Attempts at viral isolation are under way at this time. Lipomas affecting the caudal abdomen intraperitoneally, extraperitoneally, and subcutaneously around the vent have been seen in both sexes. The role of thyroid hormone imbalances in these birds is being investigated. Tumors of the male reproductive tract have yet to be reported.

## Prolapse

Prolapses are frequently secondary, and a complete physical exam is necessary to determine underlying causes. Prolapsed phalluses are seen in birds that are debilitated from other diseases, such as hardware disease, peritoneal hernias, and sand impaction. Cocks nearing the end of breeding season that have been subjected to extreme weather fluctuations or are simply fatigued may also prolapse. Frostbite, necrotizing dermatitis, or both are frequent sequela to prolapse of the phallus. The prognosis is good for return to normal function if the damage is not too extensive and the condition is treated promptly.

After culturing the phallus, treatment consists of cleaning and replacing it within the vent three times a day until the bird can retain it in the cloaca. If this is not successful after 72 hr, a pursestring suture can be placed in the cloaca. On the dorsal aspect of the cloaca there is a pocket that the tip of the phallus stays in which the phallus is in the vent. Some males lack this pocket-like structure and their phallus is always prolapsed a few inches. Prognosis in these males is poor. The phallus is chronically infected and serves as a vehicle for transmitting disease to the hen. When placing suture material in the vent, avoid placing it through this pocket. Systemic antibiotics and nonsteroidal anti-inflammatory agents are indicated. Corticosteroids are contraindicated, as they can interfere with gonadotropin release in avian species and are not recommended

in birds that may be reproductively active after the prolapse has been treated. Treatment for 5 to 7 days is generally adequate. Males should be separated from females during treatment and for 10 days after resolution of the condition.

Prolapse of the vagina may occur without egg laying; it has been seen in hens as young as 1 year of age. Vaginal prolapse can be associated with cold weather stress, and can be seen in young hens as they mature. In young hens, the prolapse consists of a fluid-filled sac (persistent membrane); lancing it resolves the problem.

Peritoneal hernias may occur in the caudal abdominal cavity, allowing the intestines and uterus to prolapse into the pericloacal region; this condition is usually secondary to egg peritonitis or internal ovulation. The hen appears to have a large swelling around the vent. Ultrasound examination is diagnostic; surgical repair is required.

## Abnormal Eggs

Eggs with rough textured surfaces, ridges, a lack of mucin coat, or soft shells may be an indication of metritis. Soft shells may also occur as a result of dietary deficiencies. Yolkless eggs may be caused by metritis, deposition of yolk into the peritoneal cavity, or abnormalities of the ovary. Double yolks are postulated to be related to abnormal egg passage and high-energy diets.

If metritis is suspected, appropriate antimicrobial therapy should be instituted. Nutritional inadequacies may be treated with multiple vitamin and calcium injections while dietary corrections are instituted.

## CHICK MANAGEMENT/PEDIATRICS

The three basic principles inherent to successful ostrich production are an "all-in, all-out" system of management, biosecurity of the flock and facility, and a stress-free environment for the birds. These concepts are basic to animal husbandry and aviary management; however, they are frequently overlooked aspects of ostrich production.

When a practitioner is presented a sick chick(s), the term "fading chick syndrome" has been adopted in the lay literature to describe any chick that is losing weight, and the individual chick is often just a symptom of management problems. When considering the sick chick, it is important to evaluate the population at risk and take appropriate steps to prevent the other chicks from developing the problem. This often means elimination of clinically ill chicks from the production by appropriate quarantine or euthanasia. If an infectious disease is involved, then treating the individual animal in its environment places all the chicks at risk.

The second major consideration when presented with a chick(s) that is abnormal is to realize that for the most part there is generally a low level of infectious or contagious disease and most clinical symptoms are produced by stress factors such as poor ventilation, overcrowding, excessively high ambient temperatures, overuse of antibiotics, improper incubation and/or hatching, improper nutrition, and other management-related disease.

Management systems that allow groups of chicks that hatch together (e.g., 1 week's hatch) to be placed in a clean pen and kept in that pen until 3 months of age with no additions to the group are the most successful. The pen is then cleaned, disinfected, and left empty for 30 days before more birds are put in the pen. Moving chicks from pen to pen within a barn should be avoided to decrease stress and pathogen spread.

Ostrich chicks do well on a wide range of substrates, including sand grass, alfalfa, or native pasture, if they are introduced to the substrate at hatch, have adequate space, and have enough feeders and waterers available. Ostrich chicks up to 3 months of age grow best and have the fewest management-related diseases such as proventricular impaction, leg problems, and feather picking, if they have 100 to 133 square feet of pen space per bird. Ostrich chicks do not do well when confined to concrete floored housing. Exercise is a very important consideration in ostrich chicks for normal leg growth and digestive function.

Ventilation is the most commonly overlooked management aspect of ostrich production. In an attempt to keep chicks warm, producers may eliminate ventilation in barns and brooder areas. Additionally, keeping ostrich chicks too hot for extended periods of time may interfere with the chicks' development of a normal immune system as it does in the other avian species. Keeping the barn or brooder 70° to 72°F with additional heat from overhead sources is adequate. By observing the chick's behavior, the producer can tell if the chick is too hot (wings extended and panting) or too cold (huddling near the heat source).

Producers and veterinarians alike must recognize normal behavior patterns in chicks. They should be gregarious, curious, and active. Chicks that are frightened and scatter when approached are frequently stressed chicks, often a result of excessive handling by the producer. The amount of feed consumed daily by young chicks is also a good indicator of their health. They decrease feed consumption before they lose weight. Weighing the food consumed daily is a better management tool than handling and weighing individual chicks.

Traffic flow in chick-rearing areas should also be monitored closely because most infectious diseases are spread by humans. Traffic movement on any farm should be unidirectional from the youngest birds to the oldest. The closed flock concept is essential for disease prevention and control.

## Identification

Electronic microchips implanted in the pipping muscle at hatch are the industry standard. Various leg bands are available for visual identification. Sterile equipment should be used to avoid cervical abscesses.

## Sexing

DNA sexing is available commercially, although it is quite expensive at this time. Vent sexing is approximately 90 to 95% accurate at 3 months of age, although it can be done at any age. The male ostrich chick has a phallus that is conical in cross section, contains a palpable core of fibroelastic tissue, and is characterized by the presence of a seminal groove. In the hen, the clitoris is laterally compressed, soft, small, and may have a dorsal groove.

## Nutrition

There has been little research on ostrich nutrition. the formulatins of commercial diets available are based on extrapolations from the available poultry information. They are either high-protein, high-energy diets extrapolated from turkey and game bird formulations; or low-protein, low-energy diets extrapolated from chicken formulations.

The most common practice is to start chicks on high-protein starter (28 to 30%) for the first 10 to 14 days and then switch to a diet that is 21% protein until the chick reaches 3 months of age. This is generally supplemented with some form of roughage, such as chopped greens, although this may imbalance the diet and should be done with caution. Current trends are to feed 23% protein from the time they hatch to 3 months of age, reducing the protein level after 3 months of age.

The ostrich is a hindgut fermenter, as are many herbivorous mammals. When an ostrich is between 3 and 6 weeks old, the microflora of the cecum and large intestine are like those of the rumen. Therefore, the ostrich has the ability to digest fiber from a young age, and diets will change to reflect this as research continues.

## Infectious Disease

Infective agents associated with disease in ostrich chicks include bacterial, fungal, viral, and parasitic agents. However, the isolation of disease agents in a sick chick must be done in conjunction with a review of nutritional, environmental, management, and genetic factors. These factors, compounded by the lack of understanding of the pathogenesis of frequently isolated infective agents, make a clear-cut diagnosis difficult to obtain.

### CONJUNCTIVITIS

Conjunctivitis frequently results when a primary irritant, such as dust, alfalfa, or flies, is present. *Staphylococcus Haemophilus* spp. and the nematode *Philophthalmus gralli* are often secondary invaders that further complicate the conjunctivitis. Treatment includes topical antibiotics for the bacterial infections and, if the irritation is from nematodes, topical 5% carbamate powder (Sevin Dust, Rhône-Poulenc, Research Triangle Park, NC) placed in the conjunctival sac.

### RHINITIS/SINUSITIS

Rhinitis/sinusitis is observed most commonly when chicks are confined in poorly ventilated areas. The organisms causing the diseases are highly transmissible, and disease spread in the flock is rapid.

Bacteria such as *Pseudomonas*, *E. coli*, and *Haemophilus* and *Bordetella* spp. are common isolates. Antibiotic therapy is based on culture results and route of administration. In refractory cases, it may be necessary to surgically drain the sinuses.

*Chlamydia psittaci* has been isolated from ostrich chicks after periods of stress. Treatment with chlortetracycline or doxycycline alleviates clinical signs in chicks. Transmission and pathogenesis of the organism in the ostrich has not been documented; however, it is possible that a carrier state exists. Although clinically associated with conjunctivitis, rhinitis, sinusitis, and generalized depression, the disease is systemic, and the organism can be found in the feces.

Avian influenza has been isolated and is characterized by sinusitis, neurologic signs, and green urates. The disease has produced high mortality in chicks in South Africa. There have been no isolations from ostrich chicks in the United States at this time. Newcastle disease has also been reported in the ostrich.

### PNEUMONIA/AIR SACCULITIS

Pneumonia and air sacculitis is associated with poor ventilation, stress caused by shipping, and environmental change, especially exposure to cold wet climates. Systemic infections may also present with clinical symptoms of pneumonia.

Causative agents may be *Staphylococcus*, *E. coli*, *Pseudomonas*, *Haemophilus* spp., and the fungal agents *Aspergillus* and *Cryptococcus*. Viral diseases associated with pneumonia have not been documented at this time. Treatment based on culture and sensitivity from tracheal wash is indicated for bacterial infections. Aspergillosis has reportedly been associated with acute death and high mortality in ostrich chicks (Black, 1993). Itraconazol (Sporanox, Janssen Pharmaceuticals, Goirle, Holland) is the drug of choice for treatment. Fumigation of the premises to decrease contamination with the organism is also indicated.

The lung worm *Paronchoceca struthionus* has been reported in ostrich chicks. The filariid parasite is transmitted by an insect vector. This parasite may be found in the heart, lungs, body cavity, and subcutaneous tissues of the affected ostrich. Ivermectin 0.2 mg/kg is effective against larval stages.

### ENTERITIS

Diarrhea is the most frequently observed clinical symptom in ostrich chicks. Many chicks will experience diarrhea when the yolk sac is absorbed and the chick starts eating well, at 8 to 12 days of age. If the chicks are alert and active they should not be medicated unless further symptoms develop. However, in pathogenic cases, diarrhea also often presents as a flock problem because few owners isolate symptomatic chicks. Chicks are notoriously coprophagic; therefore, transmission is rapid (Table 1).

### OMPHALITIS/YOLK SACCULITIS

The incidence of yolk sacculitis generally is low in naturally hatched chicks. However, owners often assist the chick in hatching or tie off the omphalomesenteric vessels, using a variety of techniques and bandage the abdomen. These practices often result in yolk sacculitis.

Improper storage and handling of eggs also contributes to yolk sacculitis. As discussed, washing eggs before setting is a controversial area in management. Various techniques for washing eggs, dipping eggs in antibiotic solutions, and injecting eggs with antibiotics have been described. These techniques often enhance the penetration of bacteria into the egg.

The yolk sac may also be contaminated through the ostium at the ileal opening when absorption of the yolk material by the vitelline membrane (yolk sac lining) is delayed.

Bacteria commonly isolated from the yolk sac are gram-negative; however, yolk sac retention secondary to noninfectious causes also exists. The rate of yolk sac absorption is determined by the temperature of incubation. Starving chicks after hatch does not increase yolk absorption.

Treatment includes surgical removal of the yolk sac, replacement fluids, and appropriate antibiotic therapy. Injecting the yolk sac with antibiotics has been advocated in the lay literature, but it is a dangerous technique that may result in a yolk peritonitis. Positive results from this technique have not been reported.

### CENTRAL NERVOUS SYSTEM DISEASES

Cental nervous system (CNS) diseases can be caused by bacterial, viral, or parasitic agents. Encephalitis may occur as an extension of a rhinitis/sinusitis or septicemia. A variety of bacteria have been cultured from these cases.

Newcastle disease or paramyxovirus causes neurologic signs and mortality in chicks. Experimental infection of 3- to 4-month-old chicks with a viscerotropic velogenic Newcastle disease (VVND) strain virus resulted in an 80% mortality. Endemic forms of Newcastle disease produce milder symptoms. Vaccination for VVND using a modified live vaccine is practiced in other countries.

Parasitic encephalitis caused by *Chandlurella quiscali* has been reported in emu chicks as an aberrant nematode host relationship. A young ostrich was necropsied at Iowa State University with a verminous encephalitis; however, the parasite was unidentified.

The CNS symptoms can also be observed with toxins

**Table 1.** *Common Causes of Diarrhea and their Management*

| Cause | Treatment | Prevention |
|---|---|---|
| Sudden change in diet | Correct diet, Pepto-Bismol (Proctor & Gamble, Cincinnati, OH) | Always acclimate to a new diet slowly |
| Bacterial diseases<br>*Escherichia*<br>*Salmonella*<br>*Pseudomonas*<br>*Campylobacter jejuni*<br>*Klebsiella*<br>*Clostridium perfringens*<br>*Clostridium colinum*<br>*Mycobacterium* (adults)<br>*Streptococcus*<br>*Staphylococcus* | The appropriate antibiotic is determined by culture/sensitivity testing | The source of the bacteria must be identified (i.e., barn, hatcher, hygene, airborne vectors such as flies) |
| Viral diseases (suspected pathogens)<br>Paramyxovirus<br>Reovirus<br>Herpesvirus<br>Birna-like virus<br>Enterovirus<br>Adenovirus<br>Coronavirus | There is no treatment; symptomatic treatment for the diarrhea only | Eliminate source (i.e., wild birds, infected hens, people) |
| Gastrointestinal obstruction | Surgical | Make environmental and feed changes slowly |
| Fungal candidiasis | Stop antibiotics | Keep environment dry |
| Protozoal | Flagyl | Pathogenecity questionable |

such as nicotine, insect bites, and the overconsumption of water with electrolytes, resulting in sodium toxicity.

### ARTHRITIS/TENOSYNOVITIS

Bacterial and probably viral infections of the joints and tendon sheaths occur either as primary lesions or secondary to septicemia. Treatment should be based on culture and sensitivity testing. Osteochondritis dessicans–type lesions are a frequent finding at necropsy of apparently healthy birds and may be secondary to previous infections.

### DERMATITIS

Poxvirus infections in young chicks produce typical pox lesions on the face, ears, and neck of the young ostrich. The poxvirus is transmitted by insects. Mortality is low with the infection. Vaccination of a flock during an outbreak with fowlpox vaccine may stop the spead of the disease. Staphylococcal dermatitis occurs as a secondary problem in debilitate chicks, especially when external parasites are a problem.

Vitamin B deficiencies can also result in dermatitis around the head and neck. This is usually observed secondary to long-term antibiotic therapy, which has interfered with vitamin B production by normal intestinal microflora, or when fed a home-made diet that is deficient in vitamin B.

## Parasitic Diseases

PROTOZOA. A number of intestinal protozoa including *Hexamita*, *Giardia*, *Trichomonas*, *Cryptospor-* *idium*, and *Toxoplasma* have been isolated from ostrich chicks. Their pathogenicity is unknown; development of disease from these organisms may require immune suppression. When isolated, most people treat with metronidazole at the rate of 10 mg/kg PO. Coccidiosis is a common finding, and although not believed to be pathogenic, it is usually treated with sulfa drugs.

CESTODES. The tapeworm *Houttuynia struthionis* is seen only sporadically in the United States, although it is common in Africa. The intermediate host is not known. Diagnosis is made by observing tapeworm segments in the feces. Treatment is fenbendazole 15 mg/kg PO used at regular intervals.

NEMATODES. The wireworm *Libostrongylus douglassii* is the most economically significant gastrointestinal parasite of the ostrich. The mature worm and late larval stages live in the crypts of the glandular portion of the stomach. Diagnosis is based on finding trichostrongyloid-type eggs in the feces. Treatment is ivermectin 0.2 mg/kg, fenbendazole 15 mg/kg, or levamisole hydrochloride 30 mg/kg. Another nematode with clinical significance is *Baylisascaris*, which is transmitted from skunks or raccoons through feed to the ostrich. It is a neurotropic parasite resulting in CNS lesions and symptoms. Restricting exposure to raccoon and skunk feces is the best prevention.

ARTHROPODS. Three types of arthropods affect ostrich—lice, ticks, and quill mites. Biting lice, *Struthioliperurus struthionis*, result in skin and feather damage. The mites can be seen on the feather shaft. Treatment is 5% carbaryl dust at 14-day intervals. A number of ticks affect the ostrich, their main significance being the possibility of vectoring diseases. The feather mites that ostrichs have live in the vein on the underside of the feather and feed on blood. They can be visualized as small, reddish, dust-like particles. Treatment for ticks and mites is ivermectin 0.2 mg/kg at 30-day intervals.

## Toxicities

Many different toxicities have been documented in the ostrich. They include acute selenium toxicity from exogenously administered selenium, resulting in pulmonary edema and congestion. The feed additives furazolidone and monesin have been associated with myositis and malabsorption syndromes. Gossypol in commercial feed contaminated with cattle feed resulted in a malabsorption syndrome. Cathardin from blister beetles results in hemorrhagic gastritis and enteritis. Nicotine from cigarette butts results in CNS symptoms. Toxic plants containing solanine, such as silverleaf nightshade, result in vomiting and diarrhea. Plants containing high levels of nitrates result in dyspnea and CNS symptoms. Ammonia toxicity is seen in poorly ventilated barns, resulting in corneal edema, epiphora, and dyspnea.

## Capture Myopathy Myositis

Myositis results in all aged birds from capture, transport, attack by predators, or fighting. Reports of degenerative myopathy from vitamin E or selenium deficiencies are in the literature. Borderline nutritional deficiencies may exacerbate stress-related myositis. Clinically, the birds are often presented because they are unable to stand. Fluid therapy to correct metabolic acidosis and to effect diuresis, combined with anti-inflammatory therapy and prophylactic antibiotics to prevent clostridial disease are indicated. The administration of vitamin E 5.0 mg/kg with or without selenium at 0.06 mg/kg is recommended. If nutritional deficiencies are expected, correcting the diet by adding oral formulas of vitamin E to the diet or drinking water is indicated.

When myositis is secondary to overexertion or trauma, slinging the bird to exercise the legs has been used by practioners in the past as well as swimming. The stress of handling a bird in this manner outweighs the benefits of allowing the bird to sit until it can rise. If the bird is alert and has a good appetite, the prognosis for it recovering is good. It may take as long as 90 days for the bird to stand. Measuring uric levels in the blood helps determine prognosis.

Deficiencies in vitamin E and selenium have been reported in chicks, causing muscular degeneration, leading to leg weakness and the inability to stand. Treatment is the administration of parenteral vitamin E at the dose of 200 to 300 IU per bird.

## Iron Storage Disease (Hemochromatosis)

Clinical signs of hemochromatosis include emaciation and dyspnea. Diagnosis is generally made at necropsy by histopathology and determining liver iron concentrations. Antemortem diagnosis is made with liver biopsies. Other avian species, such as toucans, can have a genetic predisposition to the disease. In the ostrich, the disease appears to be secondary to exposure to toxic levels of iron.

## Diabetes

Idiopathic diabetes mellitus has been diagnosed in the ostrich. Clinical symptoms include weight loss, polyuria, polydipsia, glycosuria, and hyperglycemia (600 to 1000 mg/dl often occur). A dietary relationship has not been determined at this time. Diabetes mellitus has been reported secondary to pancreatic islet cell tumors. Therapy has not been attempted by this author, although protamine zinc insulin (0.1 to 0.5 U b.i.d.) has been suggested as a possible treatment.

## Gout

Visceral gout and articular gout are both seen in the ostrich. Males are affected more frequently than females. Clinical signs of lameness with or without swelling of the affected joints and tendons occur. Blood uric acid levels are elevated and crystals can be demonstrated on cytology of the synovial fluid or peritoneal fluid. Allopurinol (Zyloprim, Burroughs Wellcome) is used in other avian species along with a restricted-protein diet. There appears to be a genetic predisposition, so treatment in food-producing animals is questionable.

## Cataracts

Unilateral and bilateral cataracts occur in young chicks at hatch or in the first few weeks of life and may be congenital, heritable, or from septicemia. Cataracts may also develop at 2 to 3 years of age. Surgical removal will result in the bird's ability to be put back with the group and reproduce again. Some birds adapt to the vision loss better than others. No documentation of hereditability has been done.

## Aortic Rupture

Spontaneous rupture of the aorta is most common at the aortic arch; however, it can be located anywhere along the abdominal aorta. It can be seen as a flock problem generally in obese birds under 1 year of age. The role of a possible copper deficiency is unknown but should be considered. Traumatic rupture of the cervical aorta is common from capturing birds with a hook, fence and trailering injuries, or holding the neck with excessive force while the bird is struggling.

## Megaesophagus

Persistent right fourth aortic arch and tetralogy of Fallot are seen in the ostrich. Although encountered in young chicks, most producers notice the bird refluxing fluids when it approaches sexual maturity and they are observing the birds more closely. The esophagus will be distended at the base of the neck. When the bird lowers its head, ingesta will reflux out the beak. A heart murmur is usually present. Feeding and watering the birds from an elevated position rather than on the ground decreases clinical signs. Hereditability is unknown; therefore, attempts at surgical repair may not be justified.

## Musculoskeletal Disorders

Noninfectious problems in chicks include developmental musculoskeletal defects. Clinical signs of rickets include enlarged joints and epiphyses, lameness, and pathologic fractures. Rickets is caused by a lack of calcium and phosphorous, or vitamin $D_3$, or a calcium and phosphorous imbalance. Oversupplementation with calcium is common, resulting in a phosphorous deficiency. Rickets can be induced in young chicks by housing them with inappropriate light for 10 days.

The etiology of tibiotarsal rotation (rotated leg) seems to be multifactorial. Although not documented, a strong genetic predisposition is suspected. When reviewing records from large farms producing more than 100 chicks annually, the leg deviations can usually be traced back to one or two hens. A genetic predisposition coupled with inadequate exercise, floor heating, and improper nutrition (primarily oversupplementation) may contribute to the disease process. There is an avascular necrosis of the cartilage core in the tibiotarsus, resulting in rotational deformity of some birds. Soft tissue injury resulting in unequal weight bearing has also been implicated as causitive. There are several procedures that have been tried on a rotated tibiotarsus. These include derotational osteotomies, periosteal stripping, and various splinting and casting techniques. Derotational osteotomies of the tiobiotarsus are performed just proximal to the hock, either using plates or Kirschner apparatus for fixation. Periosteal stripping of the distal tibiotarsus and the splinting and casting techniques have been used with or without calcium and vitamin injections. Approximately 20% of the chicks will survive the surgery or splinting and appear to heal. The author is not aware of any chicks that have had this procedure that have matured to normal adults. There is a high recurrence of the rotation postsurgically, because the underlying pathology is not changed by rotating the leg with an osteotomy. Euthanasia is indicated.

Curled toes are common and unlikely to be related to riboflavin deficiency, which produces curly toe paralysis in chickens. In ostriches, it is usually a problem of individual birds rather than a flock problem. Splinting the toes when the chick is less than 10 days old corrects most cases of curled toes. Surgical correction may be indicated on older chicks with severe deviations.

Pathologic fractures of the tibiotarsus and tarsometatarsus are common in young chicks. Internal fixation using plating techniques, Kirschner techniques, and intramedullary pinning can all be successful on the tibiotarsus. On the tarsometatarsus, in addition to the previously mentioned procedures, cast application is often all that is required.

Slipped tendon occurs in all aged ostrichs and is more common in chicks than in adults; however, the term "slipped tendon" refers to the gastrocnemius tendon slipping from the caudal aspect of the hock. The retinacular sheath that is holding the tendons in place generally tears on the medial aspect of the hock. When a bird presents with one tendon slipped, the conformation of that bird also allows the tendon on the opposite leg to slip easily; therefore, both legs are generally repaired at the same time. These chicks generally do quite well. When a bird presents with slipped tendons and open wounds over the hocks, the prognosis is guarded because the cruciates and the lateral collateral ligaments are likely also to have ruptured. Surgical repair in adults has been successful.

## Digestive Tract Disorders

Impaction of the proventriculus and ingestion of foreign bodies are management-related problems. Often, the stress associated with the new environment, with or without a change in substrate or diet, places the chick in a high-risk category for impaction the first 2 weeks after movement. Proventricular impactions are also observed as sequela to diseases creating ileus in the gastrointestinal tract. Impactions with sand and concentrated feed can be managed medically with psyllium laxatives and supportive therapy. Proventriculotomy is indicated for removal of foreign material such as hardware, rocks, and jewelry from the proventriculus or impaction of the proventriculus with forages.

Cloacal prolapses are common in young chicks. When presented with a cloacal prolapse, the possible causes should be considered and treated and the prolapse corrected. Frequently, the chick has diarrhea or an impaction within the intestinal tract, causing it to strain and prolapse the cloaca. The cloaca is easily replaced, and a pursestring suture is applied for 24 to 48 hr.

Intestinal torsion or volvulus, primarily involving the colon, occurs in all age birds. It can be seen as a flock problem when the diet is suddenly changed, especially if the new diet has a high fiber content. Birds present clinically with scant to no feces, slight diarrhea, abdominal enlargement, and vomiting. Abdominocentesis and radiology are diagnostic. When diagnosed early, surgical intervention is corrective.

## Vaccination Protocols

Some people advocate the use of clostridial vaccines in the ostrich; the efficacy of the vaccine is not known. Although the use of killed vaccines for equine encephalomyelitis virus is also advocated by some veterinarians based on the isolation of the virus from ostrichs, Kochs postulates have not been fulfilled in determining the role of encephalitis viruses in production of disease. The author uses autogenous bacterins for *Salmonella*, *E. coli*, and clostridial diseases when indicated in a specific flock.

## Surgical Procedures

Proventriculotomy is indicated for removal of foreign material from the proventriculus such as hardware, rocks, jewelry, and so forth, or impaction of the proventriculus with forages. Position the bird in right lateral recumbency with the down stifle well padded and the left leg abducted. An incision is made caudal to the ribs, dorsal to the feather line, cranial to the caudal abdominal air sac, and ventral to the caudal thoracic air sac. Incise through the skin, abdominal wall, and peritoneum, exercising care in young birds, as the abdominal wall is very thin. The left lateral wall of the proventriculus will be visible. Retracting the proventriculus with Allis tissue forceps, make a stab incision into the proventriculus, and elongate the incision with scissors. The incised margins of the proventriculus may be held in position with Allis tissue forceps or sutured to the skin to minimize contamination. Remove proventricular contents, being careful to check the esophageal and ventricular openings.

To close, appose the incised margins of the proventriculus. Suture through the serosal and muscular layers using a continuous horizontal mattress pattern of suitably sized absorbable suture material, inverting the incised margins. Place a second layer of continuous vertical mattress sutures over the previous suture line. Suture the abdominal wall with absorbable suture in a simple interrupted pattern incorporating the peritoneum. The skin may be sutured with absorbable or nonabsorbable suture.

The procedure for proventriculotomy was published by Honnas et al. (1991).

Yolk sac removal in chicks from hatch to 6 weeks of age is a common if not controversial procedure. Position the chick in dorsal recumbency with the legs tied caudally. Make a paramedian elliptical incision 1/2 cm lateral to the umbilicus through the skin and a *very* thin abdominal wall. Evert the yolk sac from the abdomen by applying gentle pressure to the lateral abdominal wall. Place a hemostat across the vitelline vessels and ligate the umbilical stalk with absorbable suture. Suture the abdominal wall with absorbable su-

ture (4-0 Vicryl in continuous pattern). The skin may be sutured with absorbable or nonabsorbable suture.

A common sequelae to impaction is an intussusception of a portion of the duodenum of the ostrich chick. The intussusception can occur anywhere in the intestinal tract and is not restricted to impacted chicks, but is most common at the ileocecal junctions. Surgical correction of an intussusception involves resecting the affected bowel and an anastomosis of the intestinal tract. The same procedures for anastomosis that are used in small animals will work, although the ostrich intestine is much more friable and difficult to suture. Diagnosis is often difficult and may require an exploratory laparotomy.

Pathologic fractures of the tibiotarsus and tarsometatarsus are common in young chicks. Internal fixation using plating techniques, Kirschner techniques, and intramedullary pinning can all be successful on the tibiotarsus. On the tarso metatarsus, in addition to the above-mentioned procedures, cast application is often all that is required.

A common surgical procedure on adult birds is exploratory laparotomy. Laparotomies may be done for cases of foreign body ingestion, intestinal torsion, or reproductive tract evaluation. The approach for the removal of most foreign bodies is the same as described previously for the proventriculotomy. Metal foreign bodies will be lodged in the ventriculus itself; however, an approach to the proventriculus has fewer complications than an approach through the ventriculus. Depending upon the radiographic diagnosis and the location of the foreign body, a ventral midline incision and approach to the foreign body through the ventriculus may be indicated, occasionally a thoracotomy may be required. The surgical approach is mandated by the location of the foreign body.

Resuturing the ventriculus is difficult due to eversion of the incised margins and the vascularity of the organ. To close, use a large absorbable suture material. A three-layer closing technique is recommended.

The approach for correction of an intestinal torsion is a caudal abdominal midline incision. Resection of the affected bowel can be accomplished as in other species. The surgical procedure carries a very poor prognosis due to the condition of the bird before the diagnosis is made.

Exploratory laparotomy is indicated in cases of oviduct infection both for diagnosis and evaluation of the reproductive tract and to perform a normograde oviductal flush in cases of salpingitis and egg peritonitis. Place the hen in right lateral recumbency with the left leg abducted. The surgical approach is approximately 10 cm caudal to the normal standing position of the thigh and 10 cm ventral to the pubis. If the laparotomy is to flush the oviduct itself, the incision is made through skin, muscle wall, and peritoneum. The oviduct is isolated and a Foley catheter placed in the magnum portion of the oviduct. The size Foley catheter will vary with the size of the bird and her reproductive status at the time of the flush. A normograde flush using 2 L of 1% povidone-iodine (Betadine) solution and/

or a gentamicin (Gentocin) solution can be accomplished in this way. There will frequently be a large amount of exudate in the uterus itself. Manipulating the oviduct will generally break this loose so that it can be flushed free. After removal of the Foley, the oviduct is sutured with 3-0 absorbable suture. A three-layer closure, closing peritoneum abdominal musculature, and skin is used for the abdomen. In cases of overt peritonitis with a large volume of exudate, placement of a drain for peritoneal lavage is indicated. A perforated tubing is placed from the most proximal portion of the incision exiting through the ventral abdominal wall and sutured in place. Lavage with 6 L of a 1% Betadine solution per day for 3 days, then pull the drain. The incidence of adhesions appears to be minimal.

The laparotomy approach to relieve egg binding is directly over the uterine portion of the oviduct, which is caudal to the incision described above. The oviduct is isolated, the uterine portion of the oviduct externalized through the abdominal incision, and the uterus incised over the egg. After the egg is removed, close with a double inverting suture pattern, the first layer horizontal mattress, the second layer vertical mattress of 3-0 absorbable suture. The abdominal wall will be closed as described earlier.

## Trauma

Wing luxations and fractures result from hauling or breeding accidents. Most birds that are diagnosed as having a wing luxation actually have a radial paralysis rather than a true luxation of the joint itself. Simply taping the wings up over the back for a period of 2 or 3 weeks generally alleviates the condition. Fractured wings, depending upon the location of the fracture, can be repaired with a half-Kirschner apparatus and/or splints. Occasionally, intramedullary pinning is required. Avian surgery texts can be consulted for further descriptions of those procedures.

Lacerations of the neck involving the trachea and esophagus are common fence injuries. Primary closure of the trachea is required. Primary closure of the esophagus in fresh injuries is successful; if the injury is old, the esophagus will granulate. An esophagostomy tube placed in the distal third of the cervical portion of the esophagus may be required for alimentation with severe injuries.

Lower leg injuries due to cable fencing are also common in the ostrich; débriding and bandaging the wound and standard wound management techniques work well. If bone is exposed in a lower leg injury, radiographing the bird at weekly intervals is recommended as stress fractures occur. It is not uncommon for a bird to be presented with the soft tissues healing normally 3 weeks after trauma and have the tarsometatarsus fracture through. Luxation of the phalanges is common, especially in areas that have ice and mud. If not compounded and treated soon after the luxation occurs, casting the foot in a normal flexed position for 5 to 6 weeks generally allows enough soft tissue fibrosis and repair to hold the luxated joint in place. When casting alone is unsuccessful, arthrodesis of the joint following standard equine procedures is successful.

## References and Suggested Reading

Black D: *Proc Aust Ost Assoc* University of Syndey, 1993.
  *Aspergillosis, diagnosis, and treatment.*
Fowler ME: Comparative clinical anatomy of ratites. J Zoo Wildl Med 22: 204, 1991.
  *A description of ratite anatomy.*
Honnas C, et al: Proventriculotomy to relieve foreign body impaction in ostriches. J Am Vet Med Assoc 199:461, 1991.
  *The surgical procedure for proventriculotomies.*
Perelman B: *Proc 3rd Ann Conf Ostrich Med Surgery*, College Station, TX, Texas A&M University, 1991.
  *A description of pediatic problems in the ostrich.*
Stewart JS: Ostriches. *In* Ritchie et al. (eds): *Avian Medicine: Principles and Applications.* Lake Worth, FL, Wingers Publishing, 1994.
  *Principles of incubation and hatching.*

# ANESTHESIA AND POSTOPERATIVE MANAGEMENT OF RABBITS AND POCKET PETS

MICHAEL J. HUERKAMP
*Atlanta, Georgia*

Although the medical care of rabbits and pocket pets (guinea pigs, hamsters, gerbils, rats, and mice) is uncommon for most veterinarians, these pets may present to veterinary clinics for routine or emergency medical care. In many cases, anesthesia will be needed to permit exploratory surgery, abscess drainage, nodule resection, tissue biopsy, nail or teeth clipping, ovariohysterectomy, and orchiectomy. Chemical restraint may also be needed to facilitate a thorough diagnostic evaluation, especially for procedures such as radiography and blood collection. Because of their relatively small size, timid or intractable demeanor, and unique biologic characteristics, rabbits and rodents present an anesthetic challenge to unfamiliar practitioners. However, the means to safely and humanely anesthetize rabbits and small rodents is available in any modern veterinary practice (Table 1).

## PREANESTHETIC CONSIDERATIONS

As with other companion animals, obtaining a thorough history and a preanesthetic physical examination is important in detecting underlying medical conditions, such as rabbit pasteurellosis and murine mycoplasmosis, that can complicate anesthesia. For rabbits, examination of the nares for rhinorrhea suggestive of respiratory disease, careful auscultation of the thorax for evidence of cardiac or pulmonary disease, and determination of the rectal temperature should be done. Physical examination of rodents is more difficult due to their small size, generally uncooperative nature, and high heart and respiratory rates. Once admitted to the clinic, rabbits and rodents should be kept in escape-proof cages in a quiet area. If aromatic wood shavings (i.e., cedar, pine) have been used for contact bedding, the duration of anesthesia may be shortened due to the enhanced metabolism of anesthetics associated with increased hepatic microsomal enzyme activity. Rabbits and rodents have high metabolic energy requirements and are unable to vomit. Consequently, with the exception of adult rabbits and guinea pigs, preanesthetic fasting is not recommended. Mature rabbits and guinea pigs should be fasted for 12 hr to decrease the amount of ingesta in the cecum and stomach that may result in anesthetic overdosages due to overestimating the real body weight. Since rabbits breathe primarily by dia-phragmatic movement, fasting to increase stomach volume will enhance respiration during anesthesia. Fasting in excess of 12 hr is contraindicated, as it may promote hypoglycemia and metabolic acidosis.

Preanesthetic medications are not recommended, with the exception of anticholinergic drugs, because single-injection anesthesia techniques have been developed that minimize the handling stress and eliminate the discomfort associated with multiple injections. Serum and tissue atropinesterases found in many rabbits and rats render atropine sulfate ineffective; therefore, 0.01 to 0.02 mg/kg subcutaneous (SC) administration of glycopyrrolate (Robinul, AH Robins, Richmond, VA), a quaternary ammonium parasympatholytic, should be given to reduce salivary and bronchial secretions and prevent vagal bradycardia.

Interscapular SC injections are preferred for rabbits, provided the administered agent is not excessively irritating. Because of the stress of restraint, relatively low muscle mass, risk of accidental sciatic nerve injection, inflammation, and prolonged recovery times, intramuscular (IM) injection of anesthetics to rodents is not recommended. Intraperitoneal (IP) injection is better tolerated than IM and is recommended. Injections by the IP route should be given lateral to the umbilicus in order to avoid injection of the cecum. Properly restrained rabbits will tolerate IM injections into the semimembranosus, semitendinosus, and epaxial muscles.

## ANESTHESIA

Historically, injectable drugs have been popularly used for anesthesia of rabbits and rodents because they are inexpensive; avoid the technical demands of gas anesthesia; and have been generally safe, effective, and easy to administer. However, disadvantages attendant to anesthesia by injection include the lack of precision in controlling anesthetic depth; prolonged recovery time; and physiologic changes such as hypotension, hypercarbemia, and hypoxemia. For uncomplicated procedures involving healthy animals, these drawbacks may not be of consequence, but their safety and predictability when used in ill animals is not known, because injectable anesthetic techniques are largely developed for use in healthy experimental animals.

***Table 1.***  *Anesthetic Agents for Rabbits and Pocket Pets*

| Drug | Dose (mg/kg) | Time Interval | Route | Comments |
|---|---|---|---|---|
| Acepromazine maleate | *Rabbit*: 0.75 | Once | SC, IM | For surgical procedures, give in combination with ketamin-xylazine |
| Acetaminophen (Children's Tylenol) | *Rabbit, rodent*: 1–2 mg/ml in the drinking water | | | Effective in controlling low-grade nociception |
| Buprenorphine (Buprenex) | *Rabbit*: 0.02–0.05 | q6–12 h | Sc, IM | For the control of acute or chronic visceral pain |
| | 0.50 | q12 h | Per Rectum | |
| | *Rodent*: 0.1–3.0 | q6–12 h | Sc, IM | |
| Butorphanol tartrate (Torbutrol) | *Rabbit*: 0.1 | Once | SC, IM | For surgical procedures, give in combination with ketamine-xylazine |
| | *Rabbit* 0.4 | q4–6 h | SC | Used as a postoperative analgesic |
| Diazepam (Valium) | *Rabbit*: 1.0 | As needed | IV | Given to increase relaxation of lightly anesthetized animals and permit endotracheal intubation |
| Doxapram (Dopram-V) | *Rabbit*: 2–5 | q15 min | IV, SC | For treatment of respiratory depression |
| | *Rodent*: 2–5 | q15 min | SC | |
| Droperidol (Inapsine) | *Rat, Mouse*: 7.0 | Once | IP, SC | Combination with fentanyl and midazolam provides neuroleptanesthesia |
| Fentanyl (Sublimaze) | *Rat, Mouse*: 0.1 | Once | IP, SC | Combination with droperidol and midazolam provides neuroleptanesthia |
| Fentanyl-fluanisone (Hypnorm) | *Gerbil*: 2 ml/kg | Once | IP, SC | A neuroleptanalgesic that, in combination with midazolam, will provide neuroleptanesthesia; to prolong anesthesia, 5–10% increments of the induction dose can be given as needed |
| | *Guinea pig*: 2 ml/kg | Once | IP, SC | |
| | *Hamster*: 1 ml/kg | Once | IP, SC | |
| | *Mouse*: 2.5 ml/kg | Once | IP, SC | |
| | *Rat*: 0.75 ml/kg | Once | IP, SC | |
| Flunixin meglumine (Banamine) | *Rabbit*: 1.1 | q12 h | SC, IM | |
| | *Rodent*: 2.5 | q12 h | SC, IM | |
| Glycopyrrolate (Robinul) | *Rabbit*: 0.01–0.02 | As needed | SC | Given as an adjunct to prevent vagal bradycardia and reduce salivary and bronchial secretions |
| | *Rodent*: 0.01–0.02 | | | |
| Halothane (Fluothane) | *Rabbit*: 1.5–2.5% | As needed | Inhalation | For maintenance following induction using injectable agents |
| Isoflurane (Aerrane) | *Rabbit*: 2–4% | As needed | Inhalation | For maintenance following induction using injectable agents |
| Ketamine (Ketaset) | *Hamster*: 200.0 | Once | IP | *Rabbits*: In combination with xylazine, useful for minimally invasive procedures lasting less than 30–45 min |
| | *Guinea pig*: 60.0 | Once | IP | |
| | *Mouse*: 87.0 | Once | IP | |
| | *Rabbit*: 35.0 | Once | SC, IM | *Hamster, guinea pig, mouse, rat*: General anesthetic in combination with xylazine |
| | *Rat*: 87.0 | Once | IP | |
| Lidocaine (Xylocaine) | *Rabbit*: 10% | As needed | Topical | 10% oral spray for application on the glottis to prevent laryngospasm and facilitate intubation |
| Meperidine HCl (Demerol Hydrochloride Syrup) | *Rabbit, Rodent*: 0.2 mg/ml in the drinking water | | | Patient-administered moderate pain relief |
| Midazolam (Versed) | *Rabbit*: 1.0 | As needed | IV | *Rabbit*: Given to increase relaxation of lightly anesthetized animals and permit endotracheal intubation |
| | *Rodent*: 5.0 | | | *Rodent*: Given in combination with fentanyl-fluanisone or fentanyl-droperidol for neuroleptanesthesia |
| Nalbuphine (Nubain) | *Rabbit*: 1–2 | q4–8 h | SC, IM | For the control of acute or chronic visceral pain |
| | *Rodent*: 1–4 | q4–8 h | SC, IM | |
| Naloxone (Narcan) | *Rodent*: 0.01–0.1 | As needed | SC, IP | Reversal of the sedative and respiratory depressive effects of narcotics |
| Tiletamine-Solazepam (Telazol) | *Gerbil*: 60.0 (alone) | Once | SC, IP | *Rabbits*: contraindicated |
| | 20.0 (with xylazine) | | | *Gerbils*: Recovery is smoother, shorter and safer if used in combination with xylazine; do not redose |
| Xylazine (Rompun) | *Hamster*: 8.0–10.0 | Once | IP | *Rabbit*: In combination with ketamine; useful for minimally invasive procedures lasting less than 30–45 min |
| | *Gerbil*: 10.0 | Once | IP | |
| | *Guinea pig*: 8.0–10.0 | Once | IP | |
| | *Mouse*: 13.0 | Once | SC, IM | *Hamster, guinea pig, mouse, rat*: General anesthetic in combination with ketamine |
| | *Rabbit*: 5.0 | Once | IP | |
| | *Rat*: 13.0 | Once | | *Gerbil*: General anesthetic in combination with Talazol |
| Yohimbine HCL (Yobine) | *Mouse*: 0.2 | As needed | IP | Will reverse the effects of xylazine and partially antagonize the effects of ketamine and acepromazine |
| | *Rabbit*: 0.2 | As needed | IV | |
| | *Rat*: 0.2 | As needed | IP | |

## Inhalation Anesthesia

For rabbits, inhalation anesthesia is preferred because it is technically feasible, precise, rapidly adjustable, and is safe and effective for procedures lasting 2 hr or more. Postoperative recovery is rapid and less complicated than with injectable anesthetics. Inhalation anesthesia, with the exception of mask systems, is generally impractical for rodents in the clinical setting. For brief anesthesia, to permit IP injections, blood collection, or nail and incisor trimming, rodents can be placed in an induction chamber and exposed to inhalation agents delivered from a precision vaporizer or, alternatively, from cotton balls or gauze sponges in a chamber constructed to prevent physical contact of the animal with the anesthetic liquid. Disadvantages of the latter procedure include the exposure of personnel to anesthetic vapors if scavenging is not adequate; prolonged excitement during induction if methoxyflurane (Metofane, Pitman-Moore, Mundelein, IL), a gas with a low vapor pressure, is used; and the potentially rapidly fatal effects of excessive concentrations of isoflurane (Aerrane, Anaquest, Madison, WI) or halothane (Fluothane, Wyeth-Ayerst Laboratories, Philadelphia, PA). Although 5% halothane or isoflurane is sufficient to induce anesthesia in a chamber, lethal concentrations of these gases (in excess of 30%) are rapidly reached at room temperature. Because direct intubation of rodents requires either a tracheostomy or specialized endotracheal tube and laryngoscopic equipment, gas anesthesia is most easily maintained using a semiclosed mask system with a means of waste gas scavenging. Typically, 1 to 3% halothane and 2 to 4% isoflurane are adequate for anesthesia maintenance, provided system leaks are minimal. Inhalant agents may also be used to supplement the anesthesia of rodents recovering prematurely from injectable agents.

For anesthetic induction of rabbits, an SC or IM injection of xylazine HCl (Rompun, Miles, Shawnee Mission, KS) and ketamine HCl (Ketaset, Aveco, Fort Dodge, IA), as described in the section "Injection Anesthesia" below, is preferred over IV infusion, which is too time consuming; and inhalation induction, using a mask or induction chamber, which may result in struggling, distress vocalization, and breath-holding. Xylazine-ketamine induction is also preferred over intravenous injection of ultra–short-acting thiobarbiturates, which have a narrow margin of safety, are slowly eliminated in obese animals, and may cause marked respiratory depression or fatal apnea if intubation is not done immediately.

The narrow oral cavity, limited range of mandibular abduction, large incisors and cheek teeth, dorsal protrusion of the tongue, and ventral sloping of the larynx all combine to obscure visualization and access to the glottis and make endotracheal intubation of the rabbit challenging. The key to intubation is to bring the mouth, larynx, and trachea into linear alignmment by positioning the rabbit in dorsal recumbency and hyperextending the head by placing a rolled towel under the cervical spine or permitting the head to overhang a table edge. The tongue should be retracted laterally through one of the diastema, the bilateral spaces between the incisors and premolars, to prevent laceration on the incisors and an inverted laryngoscope with a #1 Miller blade (Baxter Health Care, McGaw Park, IL) should be inserted into the contralateral diastema and maintained either between the incisors in alignment with the midline or lateral to the incisors at a slight angle to the sagittal plane of the body. Gentle pressure should be directed ventrally with the blade tip while slight rostrodorsal traction is placed on the head until the epiglottis and arytenoid cartilages are seen. At this point, lidocaine 10% oral spray (Xylocaine, Astra Pharmaceutical Products, Westborough, MA) should be judiciously misted on the glottis to prevent laryngospasm and to facilitate intubation. Topical benzocaine should not be used, because it may cause methemoglobinemia. In cases where relaxation of the musculature is not sufficient to permit intubation, 1 mg/kg slow boluses of either diazepam (Valium, Roche Products, Manati, PR) or midazolam (Versed, Roche Laboratoaries, Nutley, NJ) can be given IV to effect. Intubation should be done with a transparent, cuffed, 14-cm-long 3.0- to 4.0-mm internal diameter endotracheal tube (CT Cuffed Tracheal Tube Murphy Eye, Sheridan Catheter, Argyle, NY) for rabbits weighing 3 to 6 kg or an uncuffed 1.0- to 2.5-mm endotracheal tube for rabbits weighing less than 3 kg. Using a metal dowel or cotton-tipped applicator as a stylet to prevent bending of the tube, intubation should be done by advancing the endotracheal tube through the diastema until it is immediately rostral to the epiglottis. As the tip of the endotracheal tube approaches the epiglottis, visualization will be impaired and the final passage must be done blindly during inspiration when the vocal cords are abducted. If a 1 3.0-mm or larger internal diameter endotracheal tube is used, intubation can be done using the polypropylene guide technique (Gilroy, 1981). A 56-cm, 8-Fr. polypropylene catheter (Sovereign Urinary Catheter, Sherwood Medical, St. Louis, MO) should be passed through the endotracheal tube lumen from the connector to the distal end until the blunt catheter tip extends 15 to 20 cm past the bevel. Under direct visualization, the tip of the catheter should be cautiously advanced through diastema, past the vocal folds, and into the trachea. Once the guide is in the trachea, the laryngoscope can be removed and the endotracheal tube advanced as a sheath over the stationary catheter into the trachea.

If a sufficiently small laryngoscope blade is not available, intubation can be attemped blindly. After anesthesia is deepened by delivery of gas from a mask until the rabbit is completely relaxed and areflexic, it should be placed in sternal recumbency with the head extended dorsally such that the alignment of mouth, larynx, and trachea is perpendicular to the table surface. An endotracheal tube should then be advanced to the proximal aspect of the larynx. This can be confirmed by listening for respiratory sounds through the endotracheal tube and adjusting position until the sounds are at maximal intensity. At this point, the endotracheal tube should be gently advanced into the trachea. A cough reflex often confirms correct insertion. This blind technique carries a high risk of trauma and should be abandoned in favor of injection anesthesia if intubation is not successful after several gentle attempts. Regardless of the intubation technique, intubation should never be forced, because the trachea, tracheal bifurcation, and tissues of the oropharynx are easily damaged and the vagus nerve may be stimulated. Following intubation, the stylet or guide should be immediately removed and the endotracheal tube secured. Correct placement in the trachea should be further confirmed by visualizing the respiration-associated condensation of water vapor on the internal surface of the endotracheal tube or by auscultation in conjunction with manual respiration using an Ambu bag.

The intubated rabbit should be connected to a gas anesthesia machine with a closed breathing circuit for ventilation with a mechanical respirator at a rate of 30 to 40 breaths per minute and a tidal volume of 11 to 15 ml/kg. The inspiration/expiration ratio should be 1:2 or 1:3 and airway pressures should not be permitted to exceed 20 cm $H_2O$. Mechanical ventilation should not be done until intubation is confirmed, because overzealous ventilation into the stomach can lead to acute dilatation and rupture. If mechanical ventilation is not available, spontaneous ventilation should be accommodated with a semiclosed pediatric breathing circuit. Spontaneous respirations should be regular and deep and occur at a rate of 15 or more breaths per minute. Anesthesia should be maintained with 2 to 3% isoflurane or 1.5 to 2.5% halothane in 100% oxygen. Balanced gas anesthesia with nitrous oxide is contraindicated, as it contributes to operating room pollution and may accumulate in the gastrointestinal tract, causing life-threatening gastric dilatation.

### Injection Anesthesia

For minimally invasive diagnostic procedures requiring immobilization; surgical procedures of moderate intensity (i.e., wound suturing, tissue biopsies) lasting less than 30 to 45 min; or anesthesia permitting preparation of a surgical field, placement of intravascular catheters, and intubation for subsequent administration of gas anesthetics, rabbits should be given 5 mg/kg xylazine with 35 mg/kg ketamine SC or IM. For procedures with intense sympathetic stimulation (i.e., laparotomy) or for anesthesia lasting 60 to 90 min, 0.1 mg/kg butorphanol tartrate (Torbutrol, Aveco, Fort Dodge, IA) or 0.75 mg/kg acepromazine maleate (Promace, Aveco, Fort Dodge, IA) should be given at the time of anesthesia induction with xylazine and ketamine. If it is necessary to further extend anesthesia, incremental doses of one half the original ketamine dose can be given.

The combination of ketamine and xylazine has been popular for the anesthesia of a wide variety of rodent species, with the effective dose varying widely among species and between strains of the same species. While there may be genetic variability in response to anes-

thesia within rodent species, as a general rule, surgical anesthesia can be maintained for 45 to 60 min in rats and mice with a single injection of xylazine (13 mg/kg) and ketamine (87 mg/kg) IP. Additional ketamine can be given to increase the plane of anesthesia. The combination can also be given to guinea pigs and hamsters at 60 mg/kg or 200 mg/kg ketamine, respectively, with 8 to 10 mg/kg xylazine IP. Because xylazine-ketamine doses have not been established for gerbils, 20 mg/kg tiletamine-zolazepam (Telazol, Aveco, Fort Dodge, IA) given in balance with xylazine (10 mg/kg) IP or SC is recommended for 40 to 50 min of surgical anesthesia. Tiletamine-zolazepam (60 mg/kg) can be given alone as a single dose, but the postanesthetic recovery period may last several hours. Redosing of tiletamine-zolazepam has been associated with fatal apnea in rodents, and it should not be used in rabbits for which tiletamine is nephrotoxic.

A combination of fentanyl and fluanisone (Hypnorm, Janssen Pharmaceutica, Beerse, Belgium) is marketed in Europe, where it is commonly used in conjunction with the water-soluble benzodiazepine, midazolam, for neuroleptanesthesia. This combination can be given by IP or SC injection and best preserves cardiac output and peripheral tissue perfusion. One part Hypnorm (fentanyl citrate 0.316 mg/ml, fluanisone 10 mg/ml) mixed with one part midazolam (5 mg/ml) and two parts sterile water gives a stable solution that can be given to rats (3.0 ml/kg), hamsters (4.0 ml/kg), gerbils and guinea pigs (8 ml/kg), and mice (10 ml/kg) to induce and maintain neuroleptanesthesia for 30 to 60 min. To prolong anesthesia, 5 to 10% increments of the induction dose can be given as needed. Although fentanyl-fluanisone is currently unavailable, efforts are underway to market it in the United States. Until that time, a nonproprietary equivalent can be made by combining 5 ml fentanyl citrate (Sublimaze, Janssen Pharmaceutica, Piscataway, NJ), 7 ml droperidol (Inapsine, Janssen Pharmaceutica, Piscataway, NJ), 2.5 ml midazolam (5 mg/ml), and 10.5 ml sterile water to give a stable solution containing 0.01 mg/ml fentanyl, 0.7 mg/ml droperidol, and 0.5 mg/ml midazolam. This combination is given IP or SC to rats or mice at a dose of 0.1 ml/10 gm body weight to obtain 90 min of surgical anesthesia.

## PERIOPERATIVE CONSIDERATIONS

While anesthetized, rabbits and rodents should have bland ophthalmic ointment placed in the eyes to prevent exposure keratitis and should be maintained on a water-circulated heating pad to prevent hypothermia. Other means of promoting euthermia include using warmed solutions for irrigation and, where inhalation anesthesia is done, humidifying inspired gases. The marginal lateral ear vein of rabbits should be catheterized with a 22-gauge, 25-mm catheter (Jelco catheter, Critikon, Tampa, FL) for administration of warmed lactated Ringer's solution at a rate of 5 to 10 ml/kg/hr via a 60 drop/ml intravenous fluid administration set. To facilitate venous access for catheterization, vasodilation can be induced by topical application of ethanol or methylsalicylate (oil of wintergreen) on the skin overlying the blood vessel. Once a patent catheter is established, it should be secured to the convex surface of the ear by taping in butterfly fashion. A roll of 4-5 gauze 4×4 inch sponges should be placed in the concave pinna, and the IV line should be secured with a circumferential wrap of tape. If it is desirable to gain arterial access for blood gas analysis or blood pressure monitoring, a 22-gauge catheter can be placed in the central auricular artery and secured with a heparin-lock (for blood gases) or connected to a transducer (for continuous arterial pressure monitoring). Because controlled ventilation may increase mean intrathoracic pressure, decrease venous return, compromise cardiac output, and cause hypotension, blood and airway pressure monitoring should be done. The systolic/diastolic arterial pressure of an anesthetized rabbit is approximately 95/75 mmHg. As a rule, arterial pressures should not be permitted to decrease below 80/60. Intubated animals undergoing lengthy procedures should have cuffed tubes deflated, rotated, and reinflated hourly, while those that are not intubated should be positioned to maintain an open airway. Alterations in heart rate and blood pressure are the most reliable indicators of anesthetic depth, with changes of 20% or more from baseline dictating modifications in anesthetic management. The monitoring of heart rate and rhythm can be done with an esophageal stethoscope (rabbits) or by electrocardiography (all species). In addition to direct blood pressure monitoring via the central auricular artery of the rabbit, indirect monitoring can be done with cuffs placed on the tail (rat, mouse, gerbil) or a limb (rabbit, hamster, guinea pig). Capnography (end-tidal carbon dioxide determination) and pulse oximetry are useful in evaluating the adequacy of ventilation. Ventilation-perfusion efficiency can also be assessed through observation of mucous membrane color and capillary refill time. Unlike rabbits, rodents present difficulties in comprehensive monitoring because visualization can be obstructed by surgical drapes, peripheral pulses are not easily detected, respiratory and heart rates are rapid, and changes are difficult to detect.

Where sophisticated cardiovascular monitoring is not practical, reflex assessment is the most accurate determinant of adequate anesthesia. In rabbits, a lack of response to pinching the pinna of the ear (pinna reflex) is the best indicator of adequate depth followed by the hindlimb pedal withdrawal and abdominal pinch reflexes. Other indicators, such as jaw tone and purposeful movements in response to surgical stimuli, may also be used as measures of anesthetic depth. In rodents, unfortunately, movement in response to painful stimuli is the most dependable indicator of light anesthesia, because the tail pinch and pedal withdrawal reflexes may persist in some deeply anesthetized rodents. In all of these species, ocular position and the corneal and palpebral reflexes are inconsistent and unreliable indicators of anesthetic depth and are often preserved until dangerously deep levels of anesthesia are reached. Guinea pigs, hamsters, and gerbils may show an idiosyncratic writhing before entering a surgical plane of anesthesia that should not be confused with light anesthesia. When reflex assessment is used as the sole determinant of anesthetic depth, more than one reflex should be monitored to ensure adequate anesthesia.

## POSTANESTHETIC RECOVERY

The most likely causes of delayed or complicated recovery from general anesthesia are hypothermia, anesthetic overdosage, hypoglycemia, and dehydration. Anesthetic agents directly affect central and peripheral thermoregulatory mechanisms, and rodents and rabbits are highly prone to radiative and conductive heat losses because of their high body surface area/body weight ratio. Because the pharmacokinetics of anesthetic metabolism are partially temperature-dependent, maintaining euthermia is critical to recovery from anesthesia. Ideally, recovering animals should be kept in an escape-proof incubator on a clean, dry towel or blanket. The use of an incubator permits careful control of the ambient temperature and enables oxygen administration. Recovery should not be done on metal flooring or in suspended wire cages, because heat loss will be accelerated. Small-particle contact beddings will stick to the eyes, nose, and mouth of recovering animals; may be aspirated; and are contraindicated in recovery cages. Where an incubator is not available, supplemental heating can be provided with a water-circulated heating pad or a heat lamp judiciously placed outside of the cage. It is important to remember that rabbits and rodents are gnawing species that, left unattended following recovery, may mutilate heating pads or wiring. The ambient temperature in the recovery area should be 29° to 32°C for rabbits, rats, and guinea pigs, and 32° to 35°C for smaller species. Temperature monitoring of the animal and the recovery area should be done regularly.

Animals slow to recover from anesthesia should be turned every 30 to 60 min, to prevent hypostatic lung congestion and should be given warmed, parenteral fluids to compensate for metabolic needs and for losses during surgery. Extubation should be done only when chewing begins or coughing is elicited. Yohimbine (Yobine, Lloyd Laboratories, Shenandoah, IA) can be given at 0.2 mg/kg IV to rabbits or IP to rodents to reverse the effects of xylazine and partially antagonize the effects of ketamine and acepromazine. The sedative and respiratory depressive effects of narcotics can be reversed by the injection of 0.01 to 0.1 mg/kg naloxone (Narcan, Dupont Pharmaceuticals, Marati, PR). Where reversal is not possible, respiratory depression can be treated with 2 to 5 mg/kg doxapram (Dopram-V, Aveco, Fort Dodge, IA) given SC or IV every 15 min.

Analgesics are generally underutilized in veterinary medicine, but well-established studies have shown repeatedly that effective analgesia enhances locomotion, increases appetite, and reduces the time of postoperative recovery. Rabbits, in particular, benefit from pain-killing medication because they are sensitive to pain due to inflammation at the site of a surgical wound. This pain can lead to self-mutilation and distress that may also result in cecal hyperacidity precipitating a syndrome of anorexia, ileus, dysbiosis, and impaction. To preclude these effects, the use of a 12-inch Elizabethan collar (Ejay International, Glendora, CA) to prevent self-mutilation in conjunction with administration of analgesics for discomfort is recommended. As a general rule, analgesics should be first administered before the animal is fully recovered from anesthesia and should be continued for the next 48 to 72 hr.

Nonsteroidal anti-inflammatory drugs (NSAIDs) inhibit the production mediators that activate peripheral nociceptors and are sufficiently potent to treat musculoskeletal, incisional, and acute mild visceral pain. Cherry- or grape-flavored formulations of acetaminophen (Children's Tylenol, McNeil Consumer Products Company, Fort Washington, PA) mixed into the drinking water to provide a solution containing 1 to 2 mg/ml are palatable to rabbits and rodents and often effective in controlling low-grade nociception. For enhanced analgesia, an elixir of acetaminophen-codeine phosphate (Tylenol with codeine, McNeil Pharmaceuticals, Spring House, PA) can be added to the drinking water with 2.5 to 5.0% dextrose to provide a palatable solution of 1 to 2 mg/ml acetaminophen and 0.1 to 0.2 mg/ml codeine. Where water consumption may not be adequate or where an analgesic with anti-inflammatory properties may be desirable, flunixin meglumine (Banamine, Schering, Kenilworth, NJ) should be given by IM or SC injection every 12 hr at a dose of 1.1 mg/kg to rabbits and 2.5 mg/kg to rodents.

For the control of acute or chronic visceral pain, opioids are the most powerful and effective analgesics. However, the use of traditional, parenterally administered opioid analgesics such as morphine, meperidine, and pentazocine are impractical in rabbits and rodents because of their high metabolic rate, which necessitates intensive dosing schedules to maintain therapeutic blood concentrations. Morphine also carries the risk of inducing ileus and nausea/anorexia. Moderate pain relief can be obtained by giving a banana-flavored preparation of meperidine HCl (Demerol Hydrochloride Syrup, Winthrop Pharmaceuticals, New York, NY) in the drinking water at a concentration of 0.2 mg/ml. Opioid agonist-antagonists, such as nalbuphine (Nubain, Dupont Pharmaceuticals, Marati, PR), butorphanol, or buprenorphine (Buprenex, Reckitt and Colman Pharmaceuticals, Richmond, VA), have relatively long half-lives and offer the advantage of attenuating or ablating visceral pain while minimizing the undesirable respiratory and cardiovascular side effects associated with opioids. Buprenorphine, a class V controlled

substance, should be given by injection every 6 to 12 hr to rabbits (0.02 to 0.05 mg/kg IM, SC) and rodents (0.1 to 3.0 mg/kg SC). Administration of buprenorphine per rectum (0.5 mg/kg) will diminish the degree of analgesia but extend the duration of effect to a minimum of 12 hr. Nalbuphine and butorphanol offer the advantage of not being controlled drugs, but must be given by parenteral injection. Nalbuphine should be given every 4 to 8 hr to rabbits (1 to 2 mg/kg) and rodents (1 to 4 mg/kg), and butorphanol (0.4 mg/kg) must be given every 4 to 6 hr. An effective analgesic regimen for uncomplicated cases is to administer parenteral opioid agonist-antagonists the evening of and next morning following surgery while providing acetaminophen in the drinking water for 3 days.

Following recovery from anesthesia, the most reliable indicator of postoperative well-being, including the effectiveness of analgesia, is the daily assessment of body weight and food and water consumption. A nutritious pelleted diet should be provided as soon after surgery as feasible, because rabbits and rodents are prone to hypoglycemia due to high metabolic rates and, in juvenile animals, limited fat reserves. Inappetant animals can be offered supplements such as hay, dandelion leaves, or clover or be given 50% dextrose solution orally or through a stomach tube. In the case of chronic anorexia and ileus, bacteriotherapy may be useful in recolonizing the gastrointestinal tract. Unfortunately, the use of yogurt or probiotics containing *Lactobacillus* are of little value in treating this syndrome, because rabbits are not normally colonized with lactobacilli. The only effective means of bacterial recolonization is to administer a fecal cocktail made from the soft night feces collected from the cage of a donor rabbit that has been outfitted with an Elizabethan collar to prevent coprophagy. Fresh night feces should be mixed with warmed saline, strained through gauze, and administered with a stomach tube.

## References and Suggested Reading

Flecknell, PA: *Laboratory Animal Anaesthesia: An Introduction for Research Workers and Technicians.* London, Academic Press, 1987.
*The European perspective of laboratory animal anesthesia by a pioneer in laboratory animal analgesic management.*
Gilroy, BA: Endotracheal intubation of rabbits and rodents. J Am Vet Med Assoc 179:1295, 1981.
*A description of the polypropylene catheter intubation guide technique.*
Green CJ: *Animal Anaesthesia.* London, Laboratory Animals Limited, 1982.
*A good general overview of laboratory animal anesthesia and considerations such as handling for injection.*
Kohn DF, Wixson SK, and White WJ: *Anesthesia and Analgesia in Laboratory Animals.* Orlando, Academic Press, 1995.
*The authoritative source of state-of-the-art rabbit and rodent anesthesia.*
Wixson SK: Anesthesia and analgesia for rabbits. *In* Manning PJ, Ringler DH, and Newcomer CE (eds) *The Biology of the Laboratory Rabbit 2nd edition.* Orlando, Academic Press, p 87, 1994.
*A comprehensive review of rabbit anesthesia and analgesia.*

# EMERGENCY MEDICINE FOR POCKET PETS

BARBARA L. OGLESBEE

*Columbus, Ohio*

Guinea pigs, rats, mice, gerbils, and hamsters, commonly called pocket pets, constitute a small but significant proportion of cases in most small animal practices. These animals may present as an emergency due to a variety of causes, but trauma, neoplasia and debility from chronic or geriatric disease predominate. Deficiencies in nutrition and husbandry are often significant contributing factors. The life expectancies of these species are considerably shorter than those of a cat or dog: hamsters, mice, and rats live approximately 2 to 4 years; whereas guinea pigs and gerbils often live to be 3 to 6 years old. Because of this short life expectancy, a large percentage of small pets seen in an emergency situation are in the later stages of geriatric or chronic disease. Due to the small size of the animal, and frequently, to financial limitations imposed by the owner, the performance of diagnostic testing may be limited. Allowing for these differences, emergency care for pocket pets is similar to that of other, more familiar mammalian pets.

## HISTORY

A thorough history should include the age and sex of the animal, and onset, duration, and progression of the presenting complaint. Information pertaining to husbandry is extremely important when dealing with these animals, since many diseases seen in pocket pets can be directly related to poor husbandry. A dietary history should include the type, quantity, frequency, and method of feeding, as well as the availability of clean, fresh water. This history will aid one in identifying nutritional diseases, such as hypovitaminosis C in guinea pigs. Rancid food is a common problem in pets fed off of the floor of the cage, especially when cage sanitation is poor. The owner should be questioned about the type of litter used in the cage, and the frequency of cage cleaning and disinfection. The accumulation of ammonia from animal waste and bacteria from improper disinfection are often contributing factors in the development of respiratory disease in these pets.

The owner should also be questioned as to the presence or absence of cage mates, as well as the amount of time spent outside of the cage, the amount of handling the pet receives from children, and the presence of other (predatory) pets, especially if trauma is suspected. Information regarding the owner's previous experience with pocket pets and any previous illness in these pets should also be obtained.

## PHYSICAL EXAMINATION

Whenever possible, the physical examination is begun by observing the animal in its cage. The cage contents are examined for the degree of sanitation, type and method of feeding, and the quantity and quality of fecal pellets. The animal should be observed while at rest for posture, activity level, level of mentation, quality of haircoat, and respiratory rate. Dyspnea and/or a blue discoloration of the ears or tail (cyanosis) carry a poor prognosis. These animals should be placed in oxygen prior to handling (see "Oxygen Therapy," below).

Nondyspneic animals should then be restrained for a full physical examination. Rats and mice may be captured by grasping the base of the tail with one hand, then scruffing the neck with the opposite hand. A towel can be used to capture hamsters, guinea pigs, and gerbils. Rats, mice, hamsters, and gerbils should be restrained by grasping the scruff, the remainder of the body being restrained by holding the *base* of the tail between the examiner's third and fourth digits. The thorax should be held loosely to allow for unencumbered breathing. Always hold the tail by the base only, as restraint at the tip may cause degloving injuries, especially when handling gerbils. Guinea pigs should be held about the thorax, with one hand under the axillary region and the other supporting the hindquarters.

The physical examination is continued by examining the head for the presence of nasal or ocular discharges, swellings, or ptyalism. In gerbils, rats, and mice, red tears (chromodacryorrhea), a pigment often mistaken for hemorrhage, is a common finding in stressed or diseased animals. Cranial nerves are assessed as they would be in other mammals. A thorough examination of the mouth is essential, as malocclusion, oral abscesses and, in hamsters, impacted cheek pouches frequently cause anorexia and/or ptyalism. An otoscope is extremely useful to examine the interior of the mouth in these pets. The color, texture, and hydration of the oral mucosa should be examined; a blue discoloration indicates cyanosis, whereas red, injected mucous membranes may indicate septicemia. Similar discolorations can be seen in hairless areas, such as the ears and tail.

Due to the small size of these pets, abdominal masses and organomegaly are easily palpable. Irregularities in renal size and shape are frequently palpated in geriatric mice, rats, and hamsters, because end-stage renal disease is common in these animals. Benign cysts arising from the liver, pancreas, epididymis, or seminal vesicles are often palpated in geriatric hamsters. Abscesses and mammary tumors may be palpated as subcutaneous masses, particularly in mice and rats. The perineal area should be examined for pasty stools, urine scalding, or vaginal discharges. It is also important to carefully examine the feet, since lameness due to abscesses or cellulitis are common causes of debility in these species.

The thorax should be auscultated for the presence of crackles and rales, and to assess the heart rate. The normal heart rate is generally quite rapid, ranging from 150 to 780 bpm, the smaller animals having higher rates. Due to this rapid rate, arrhythmias and murmurs are difficult to hear. An electrocardiogram (ECG) may be performed utilizing the same leads as in the dog or cat. In smaller rodents, however, it is often necessary to attach the alligator clips to the hubs of metal 27-gauge needles that have been pierced through the skin.

## DIAGNOSTIC TESTING

Obtaining blood samples for complete blood count and serum biochemical analysis may be challenging in pocket pets due to their small size. Most debilitated animals can safely withstand the collection of blood volumes up to 1% of body weight. In animals weighing over 100 gm, the lateral saphenous vein may be cannulated with a 25- to 27-gauge needle, and the blood collected into microhematocrit tubes directly from the hub of the needle. Hair should be clipped from the leg prior to venipuncture to allow adequate visualization of the vessel. In guinea pigs, this technique also works well when collecting blood from the cephalic vein. Blood may be collected using the same technique from the dorsal tail vein in rats. The tail should be soaked in warm water to dilate the vessel prior to cannulization with a 27-gauge needle. In thin animals, blood may be collected from the jugular veins in a manner similar to that used for jugular venipuncture in cats. These animals tend to struggle when restrained for jugular venipuncture, so sedation is recommended in all but severely debilitated animals. Liberal clipping of the area is needed to visualize the vein.

In animals weighing less than 100 gm, the skin overlying the lateral saphenous vein may be coated with petroleum jelly and a small stab incision made into the vessel. Blood is then collected directly from the incision into a microhematocrit tube. Blood may also be collected in a similar fashion using a toenail clip; however, the yield from this method is usually very low. In mice, a much better yield is obtained when the distal 1 to 2 mm of the tail is clipped. Hemorrhage is then controlled by direct pressure and the application of chemical cautery agents. Blood can also be obtained via the orbital sinuses in mice, however, this method is often unacceptable to owners.

In animals weighing over 100 gm, urine is collected via cystocentesis using a 25- to 27-gauge needle. Smaller animals should be confined in a cage with a wire mesh bottom with plastic wrap underneath, and urine collected from the cage bottom. Feces should be collected over a period of several hours. Fecal flotation may reveal the presence of nematode and possibly trematode and cestode ova. Oxyurid ova may be detected by pressing cellophane tape to the perineal area, then examining the tape under low (10X) magnification. Protozoal parasites can be detected by direct saline fecal smears.

Radiography is often an essential diagnostic tool when used to evaluate critically ill small mammals. Restraint may be accomplished either by chemical sedation or manually. Manual restraint for positioning may be accomplished by placing slip-knotted loops of string proximal to the elbows and hocks, with masking tape placed over the thorax and pelvis. Some animals may struggle excessively during restraint, causing undue stress or making proper positioning impossible. In these cases, sedation is advised. For critically ill small animals, isoflurane is the anesthetic of choice. Mask induction may be achieved by either placing the cone over the animal's face or, for small rodents, by placing the entire rodent inside the cone and placing the cone on end. Induction rates vary from 2% to 4%, and maintenance rates vary from 0.25% to 2%. If isoflurane is not available, ketamine hydrochloride at 22 mg/kg IM in rats and mice, 22 to 30 mg/kg IM in guinea pigs, and 40 mg/kg IM in hamsters and gerbils, combined with diazepam (1 to 2 mg/kg), will provide light sedation.

## SUPPORTIVE CARE

In some cases, the patient may be too severely debilitated to initiate diagnostic testing until its condition has stabilized. The emergency treatment of these animals would follow that of larger mammals (i.e., establish and maintain respiratory function, maintain circulatory volume, arrest hemorrhage, manage fractures or luxations, and pursue a definitive diagnosis).

### Oxygen Therapy

Animals that are dyspneic or cyanotic (as described above) should receive immediate administration of oxygen. An oxygen-delivery mask may be either held over the patient's face or, if the animal is small enough, the entire animal may be placed within the cone, as described above. Minimal restraint is essential. If the patient becomes stressed when held for oxygen administration, it should be placed in an oxygen cage. As respiratory efforts or mucous membrane color improve, these animals may again be restrained. Often, diagnostic or therapeutic measures must be taken in stages, returning the animal to oxygen when struggling ensues. A poor to grave prognosis should be given to any animals whose color and/or respiratory efforts do not improve with oxygen therapy.

## Fluid Therapy

Most critically ill small mammals are clinically dehydrated upon presentation and require fluid replacement therapy. Maintenance therapy is estimated at 50 to 100 ml/kg/day, the larger volumes to be given to smaller rodents. As in larger mammals, the fluid deficit volume, determined by multiplying the percent of dehydration by body weight in grams, should be added to the maintenance volume. The choice of fluids and degree of dehydration is assessed in the same manner as larger mammals. If the state of hydration cannot be determined, critically ill small mammals should generally be estimated to be 5 to 10% dehydrated when calculating fluid therapy doses. Fluids should be warmed to 37°C prior to administration.

Rapid access to circulation is imperative in the treatment of critically ill small mammals. The small size of these patients makes intravenous catheterization difficult, if not impossible, especially if peripheral circulatory volume is compromised, as in cases of shock. Therefore, the route of choice for fluid replacement therapy is via interosseous catheter administration (see "Intraosseous Fluid Therapy in Small Exotic Animals," this volume, p 1331). If accessible, intravenous fluids may be given utilizing any of the veins previously mentioned. If an intravenous catheter cannot be maintained, fluids may be given by intravenous bolus injection at a rate of 10 to 25 ml/kg, given slowly over a 5- to 10-min period. Patients should be monitored closely while receiving bolus therapy to prevent circulatory and respiratory collapse. Once dehydration has been corrected, maintenance fluids may be given subcutaneously over the shoulder area. Subcutaneous fluid administration will not be effective in severely dehydrated patients, as vasoconstriction of peripheral vessels will retard fluid absorption.

Intraperitoneal injections should be used only if attempts at administration by all other routes have failed. The bladder should be expressed and the abdomen aseptically prepared prior to administration. The animal should be restrained with its head down to move abdominal organs cranially, and fluids injected 0.5 to 2 cm from the midline in the lower left quadrant of the abdomen.

## Nutritional Support

Protein-calorie malnutrition is a common exacerbating factor among critically ill pocket pets. Anorexia is one of the leading reasons for presentation and subsequent hospitalization of these animals. As in other mammals, adequate nutritional support is essential to prevent exacerbation of the detrimental effects of most disease processes.

The maintenance caloric requirement for healthy, mature rodents ranges from 150 to 350 kcal/kg/day, the smaller rodents having the highest requirements. The requirement for critically ill animals can be as much as twice maintenance, approximately 300 to 700 kcal/kg/day. Due to their high metabolic rate, small mammals should be force-fed if anoretic for longer than 12 hr. If the gastrointestinal tract is functioning and fresh feces are being produced, the animal can be fed a slurry of pelleted food, water, and a nutritional supplement such as Nutrical (Evsco Pharmaceuticals, Buena, NJ) prepared in a blender. Other options include slurries of prepared avian hand-rearing formulas, or a mixture of vegetable, cereal, and meat baby foods. For guinea pigs, 200 mg of ascorbic acid should be added per 500 ml of slurry. If the function of the gastrointestinal tract is in question, isotonic electrolyte or dextrose solutions, or commercial human oral electrolyte solutions such as Pedialyte (Ross Laboratories, Columbus, OH) may be fed at first, gradually adding solids to form a slurry.

Stronger animals may readily accept these slurries when offered via a dosing syringe. The syringe should be placed in the mouth over the tongue, and not into the cheek pouches of hamsters, or the animal may simply store, rather than swallow, the slurry. If the food is not accepted, it should be administered via a stomach tube. In animals weighing less than 100 gm, a ball-tipped metal feeding tube is preferred, as these rigid tubes pass easily, and the ball is usually of sufficient size to prevent entry into the trachea. For larger animals, a soft rubber Brunswick catheter or infant feeding tube can be used. A speculum is required in order to pass these flexible catheters. An avian speculum, small otoscope head, or tongue depressor with a hole drilled through its center all work well.

Sedation is not required or recommended for gastric intubation. Prior to insertion, the gastric tube, regardless of type, should be measured and marked from the tip of the nose to the last rib and lubricated. The speculum (if a flexible tube is used) is placed in the mouth and the tube placed through the center. The animal's head should be slightly ventroflexed and the tube passed to the premeasured length. If the tube will not pass easily, the tube should be gently manipulated and repositioned, not forced forward. If it will still not advance, a smaller diameter tube may be necessary. The tube should be palpated within the esophagus, alongside the trachea, and a small amount of sterile saline injected to ensure that the tube is not within the trachea. If the tube is positioned properly, the slurry is injected. Up to 3 ml/100 gm of body weight may be administered per feeding.

## Antibiotics

Primary or secondary bacterial respiratory or enteric infections are commonly encountered in critically ill pocket pets. If signs of bacterial infection are seen— such as elevations in the total white blood cell count, the presence of mucopurulent discharges, or evidence present in cytologic preparations and Gram stains— antibiotic treatment is warranted. Whenever possible, the choice of antibiotic should be based on the results of culture and susceptibility testing. Antibiotics that may be safely initiated empirically include chloramphenicol palmitate at 50 mg/kg every 8 hr PO; chloramphenicol succinate at 30 mg/kg every 8 hr IV or IM; trimethoprim-sulfamethizole at 15 to 30 mg/kg every 12 hr PO; or gentamycin at 5 mg/kg every 24 hr IM or SC. Enrofloxacin tablets may be crushed and made into a solution by mixing with simple syrup, dosed at 5 to 15 mg/kg every 12 hr PO.

Although the small size of these pets may make them more difficult to work with, emergency care procedures are often efficacious when employing the same principles used in treating larger, more familiar mammals.

## References and Suggested Reading

Anderson NL: Basic husbandry and medicine of pocket pets. *In* Birchard S and Sherding R (eds): *Saunder's Manual of Small Animal Medicine and Surgery.* Philadelphia, WB Saunders Co, 1993.

*Emergency Medicine and Critical Care in Practice.* The Compendium Collection, Trenton, Veterinary Learning Systems, 1992.

Harkness JE and Wagner JE: *The Biology and Medicine of Rabbits and Rodents.* Philadelphia, Lea & Febiger, 1977.

Jacobson ER and Kollias GV: *Contempory Issues in Small Animal Practice: Exotic Animals.* New York, Churchill Livingstone, 1988.

Schuchman SM: Individual care and treatment of rabbits, mice, rats, guinea pigs, hamsters, and gerbils. *In* Kirk RW (ed): *Current Veterinary Therapy X.* Philadelphia, WB Saunders Co, 1980.

# INTRAOSSEOUS FLUID THERAPY IN SMALL EXOTIC ANIMALS

NANCY L. ANDERSON
*Columbus, Ohio*

Intraosseous (IO) fluid therapy introduces fluids and drugs directly into the bone marrow cavity. Intraosseous catheters are now used extensively in pediatric emergencies where traditional venous access is difficult to obtain. This technique is extremely useful to veterinarians treating small exotic animals for the same reasons.

## GENERAL PRINCIPLES

With a few exceptions, IO catheters are utilized in the same fashion as intravenous (IV) catheters. Intraosseous catheters function similarly to IV catheters because bone marrow is another component of the circulatory system. Drugs placed in the bone marrow cavity eventually drain into the central venous system. Drugs, blood products, and colloids given intraosseously are safely administered at the same rate and dose as products given intravenously (Spivey et al., 1985). Hypertonic and caustic solutions only cause mild necrosis and inflammation, which resolve. Studies in multiple species of animals have proven that fluids administered intraosseously distribute within the body at the same rate as IV fluids.

One study suggested that some drugs may be metabolized by the bone marrow. In this study, chloramphenicol sodium succinate, vancomycin, and tobramycin failed to achieve therapeutic levels when standard IV dosages were administered through IO catheters. A separate study showed that phenobarbital achieved therapeutic levels, whereas phenytoin did not (Jaimovich, 1989). It is advisable for practitioners to use proven medications whenever possible and to run drug serum levels when possible to ensure that a therapeutic dose is being administered.

## Advantages

Intraosseous catheters have several advantages over IV catheters in small patients.

1. Placement is independent of vascular collapse.
2. A peripheral route for venous access is available when veins are too small or fragile for cannulization.
3. Vascular access is readily available in animals that would otherwise require a cut-down technique to utilize a peripheral vein (i.e., lizards, many pocket pets).
4. Intraosseous catheters are often easier to secure and maintain than IV catheters because of the stabilizing effects of the surrounding bone. Intraosseous catheters are tolerated by animals as well if not better than IV catheters. Discomfort is minimal unless fluids are administered under pressure.

## Disadvantages and Contraindications

There are a few disadvantages and contraindications associated with using IO catheters when compared to IV catheters (Table 1).

1. Complications from use of IO catheters were 0.6% in a study performed on more than 4000 people compared to a complication rate of 3.7% for IV catheters. Osteomyelitis is the most common problem associated with IO catheters. Infection is easily managed in most cases by removal of the catheter and use of antibiotics based on culture and sensitivity. It can be avoided by using aseptic technique, bandaging catheters, and changing catheter sites every 72 hr. Do not place catheters through cellulitis or into traumatized or osteomyelitic bones. Intravenous catheters are preferable to IO catheters in septicemic individuals. However, the author successfully uses IO fluids in septic animals when vascular access is not available.

2. The most significant disadvantage is limited flow rate. The maximum flow rates of colloids through 20-gauge, 2.5-inch spinal needles placed in puppy tibias were 11 ml/min gravity flow and 24 ml/min at 300 mmHg pressure. Assuming a shock dose of colloids to be 90 ml/kg/hr, gravity flow through this size catheter only provides shock doses of fluids for animals up to 7.3 kg (16 lb). Using fluids under 300 mmHg provides enough fluids for an animal weighing up to 16.4 kg (36 lb) (Hodge, Delagado-Paredes, and Fleisher, 1987).

Smaller diameter and/or longer length catheters produce lower flow rates, as can blockage of the catheter tip. Limited flow rates can be overcome by using the largest appropriate catheter size, a stylet, multiple catheters, and hypertonic saline.

3. Both IO and IV catheters can share the problem of extravasation of fluids or pharmaceuticals. Necrosis secondary to compartmentalization syndrome or caustic drugs occurs with both types of catheters and can have severe consequences. Extravasation of fluids from IO catheters may be more difficult to detect than that from IV catheters. This is because peripheral IV catheters leak close to the injection site, whereas IO catheters, if misplaced or if the cortical bone is not intact, leak away from the insertion site. Extravasation can also occur at the site of insertion.

Extravasation can be avoided by closely following instructions for placement (aspirate bone marrow, use radiology, limit attempts to one per bone within a 72-hr period, use 90-degree catheter placement, avoid bones with previous or current defects, check entire limb for signs of extravasation).

**Table 1.** *Contraindications to IO Fluid Therapy*

Current or previous fracture to bone intended for catheter placement
Congenital/developmental orthopedic defect
Cellulitis over site of catheter placement
Existing osteomyelitis
Pneumatic bones in birds
Bone marrow toxic drugs

4. Intraosseous catheters are not useful for the administration of bone marrow suppressive agents.

5. Pneumatic bones *cannot* be used for IO catheters. These bones are directly connected to the respiratory tract. Use of these bones can cause iatrogenic drowning. The humerus and femur in most bird species are pneumatic bones.

6. Avoid placement of IO catheters through active growth plates even though some studies indicate that catheters did not cause recognizable growth abnormalities (Brickman et al., 1988; Dedrick et al., 1992).

7. A study conducted in rabbits showed mild alterations of red and white cell counts and morphology after IO fluids. If possible, draw blood for baseline hematology prior to initiating IO infusions (Ros, McMannis, and Kowal-Vern, 1991).

## EQUIPMENT

The gauge of the spinal needle should be between 33% and 67% of the diameter of the marrow cavity at its thinnest point. The length of the needle should be between 33% and 67% of the length of the bone. Animals less than 300 gm usually require 23-gauge needles or smaller; 22-gauge needles usually work well for animals between 300 and 750 gm. For most animals up to 3 kg, 20-gauge needles are adequate. Pediatric IO catheters or bone marrow aspirate needles are appropriate for individuals greater than 3 kg.

If a spinal needle is not available, a regular hypodermic needle may be used. However, these needles *frequently* plug with cortex upon insertion. The plugs can sometimes be pushed out the tip of the needle into the marrow cavity by inserting a longer, but smaller, gauge hypodermic needle or Kirschner wire.

Other required equipment includes tissue cement/suture material, bandaging material, antiseptic cream/ointment, IV catheter plug, extension tubing or T-piece, heparinized saline in syringe, and sterile gloves.

## TECHNIQUE

### Tibia

Pluck feathers or shave fur from the proximal tibia. Perform a surgical scrub and use sterile technique. Locate the tibial crest. If the patient is conscious, infuse a small amount of 0.2% lidocaine around the catheter site. Standard lidocaine (2.0%) can be diluted 1:10 with sterile saline or water.

Advance the tip of the needle through the skin and tibial crest at a 45- to 90-degree angle until the tip of the needle is through the cortex. A nick incision with a surgical blade may be required in patients with tough skin (Fig. 1). It is *extremely* important to keep the needle straight while boring through the cortex. If the needle is rotated at different angles as it is drilled into the bone, the diameter of the entrance hole will be

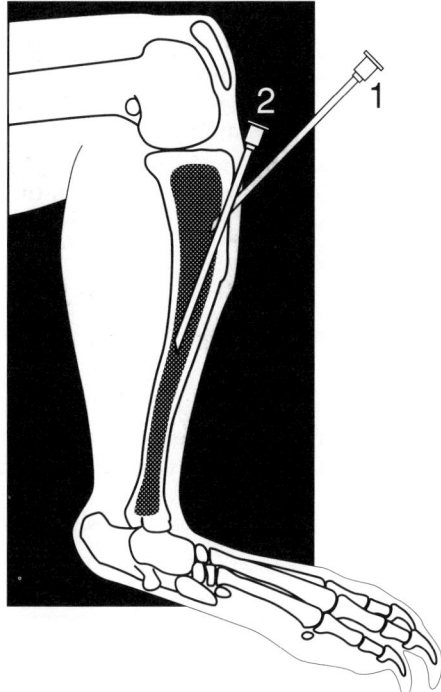

**Figure 1.** Placement of an intraosseous catheter in the tibia. *Step 1:* Introduce the catheter through the cortex at a 45- to 90-degree angle. *Step 2:* After the cortex has been penetrated, angle the catheter distally until the hub touches the skin.

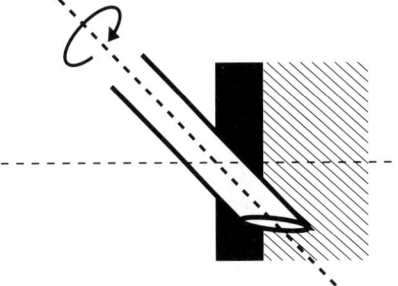

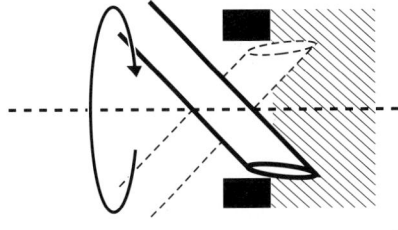

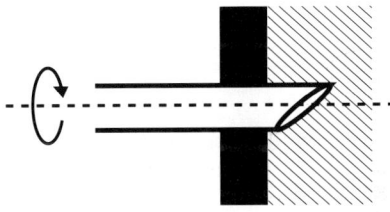

**Figure 2.** Extravasation of fluids is avoided by minimizing the size of entry hole in the cortex by keeping the length of the pin in alignment with the angle at which the pin is being driven into the bone.

larger than the needle and fluids will leak around the base of the catheter (Fig. 2).

Expect to feel a sudden lack of resistance once the tip of the needle reaches the marrow cavity. At this point, angle the needle distally and insert it down the marrow cavity until the hub of the needle is seated against the skin. The needle normally advances *easily*. If it does not, the tip of the needle may be against a distal portion of the cortex. If this happens, withdraw the needle slightly (leaving the tip in the marrow cavity) and reposition. If the needle is advanced against resistance, the tip of the needle may penetrate the opposite cortex and cause extravasation of fluids.

Remove the stylet and attach a syringe and aspirate. In most mammals, young birds, and reptiles, bone marrow is aspirated. Perform cytology on the fluid to differentiate between hemorrhage and bone marrow. If it is bone marrow, proceed to the next step. If blood or nothing is aspirated, radiograph the limb (two views) to ensure the location of the tip of the catheter. If the tip of the needle is not in the marrow cavity, select a *new* bone for catheter placement.

Attach an IV catheter plug to the end of the needle. Flush the needle with heparinized saline. The resistance encountered while injecting the saline feels like injecting into a vein. Excessive resistance indicates a clot or cortical plug in the needle, intracortical or extramarrow placement of the tip of the catheter, or structural defect in the bone.

Check the soft tissues around the tibia for extrava-

sation of fluids. If present, select another bone for catheter placement.

Suture or glue the hub of the needle to the surrounding skin. Apply an antiseptic ointment to the entrance site and place a light bandage. The purpose of the bandage is to keep the infusion site clean and give additional support to the catheter. If a patient actively resents a bandage, but does not mind a stable catheter, the catheter can be left in place by itself. Lightweight self-adherent dressings such as Tegaderm (3M Medical-Surgical Division, St. Paul, MN) are tolerated well by these patients and still work well to protect the infusion site from contamination.

When administering a continuous infusion, attach extension tubing or a T-piece to the hub of the needle. Tape the tubing to the leg to prevent excess torque on the needle at the infusion site. Attach the free end of the extension tubing to a fluid administration set or pump. For bolus administration, inject the drug or fluids through the plug and then flush catheter with

**Table 2.** *Helpful Rules of Thumb for Fluid Therapy in Small Exotics*

Assume 10% dehydration for debilitated animals
Replace 50% of the fluid deficit in 12 hr
Replace the entire deficit plus maintenance plus current losses in 48 to 72 hr
Maintenance fluids for normal small exotics is 40 to 60 ml/kg/day
Animals experiencing continuing fluid losses (i.e., diarrhea, vomiting, thermal burns) need more than standard maintenance fluids
In emergency situations of hypovolemia, bolus volumes of one blood volume, approximately 100 ml/kg, can be administered over 20 min without observable signs of volume overload

**Table 3.** *Clinical Signs of Dehydration in Small Exotics*

| Percent Dehydration | Clinical Signs |
|---|---|
| <5 | None observable |
| 5–7 | Lack of luster in eyes <br> Slight loss of skin turgor |
| 10 | Eyes "sunken" <br> Skin tents <br> Tacky mucous membranes <br> Extremities cool to touch |
| >12 | Shock <br> Death |

heparinized saline. Flush IO catheters with heparinized saline at least every 4 to 6 hr. *Caution:* incorporate the volume of fluid used for flushing catheters into fluid needs for patients weighing less than 250 gm to avoid iatrogenic overhydration (Tables 2 and 3).

Change IO catheter sites at least every 72 hr. Catheters are removed by simply withdrawing the needle. Cover the infusion site with an antiseptic ointment and bandage for 48 hr.

### EMERGENCY TECHNIQUE

In an emergency situation, the tip of IO catheters can be placed into the bone marrow at 90 degrees anywhere along the craniomedial aspect of the tibia (Fig. 3). These catheters are only for temporary use, because they are unstable. They are easy to place and work extremely well for cardiopulmonary resuscitation.

### Femur

Although this technique works extremely well for lizards, it is not recommended for use in birds. Follow the same steps as for tibia except for catheter placement.

Insert needle at 45 degrees on the dorsal midline into the distal femur just proximal to the condyles until the tip of the needle enters the marrow cavity. Retrograde the needle up the femur (Fig. 4).

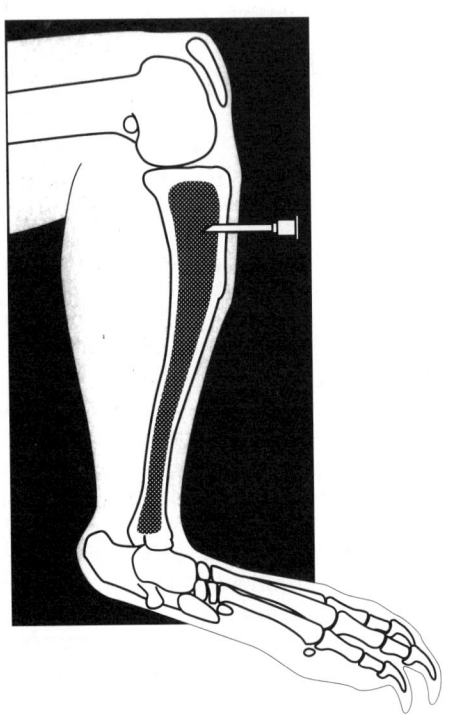

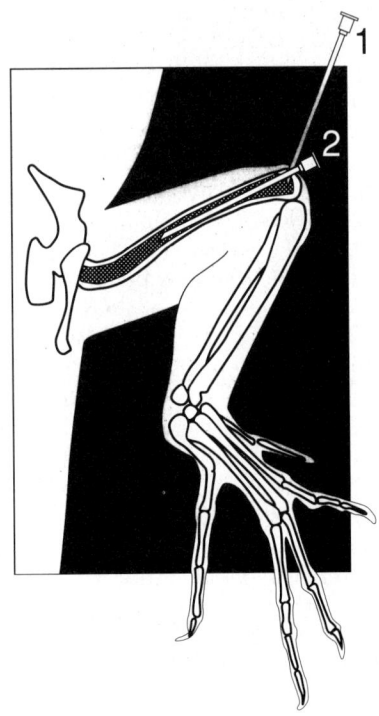

**Figure 3.** Placement of a temporary intraosseous catheter in the tibia for emergency use. Drive the catheter through the craniomedial aspect of the tibia at a 90-degree angle until the tip of the needle has penetrated the cortex.

**Figure 4.** Placement of an intraosseous catheter in the distal femur. *Step 1*: Insert needle at 45 degrees on the dorsal midline into the distal femur just proximal to the condyles. *Step 2*: Retrograde the needle up the femur.

## Ulna

Recommended for use in birds only. Follow the same steps as for tibia except for catheter placement.

Locate the distal ulna at the carpus. When the carpus is held in flexion, the distal end of the ulna can be felt as a flat "plateau" surface on the lateral aspect of the joint. If in doubt, palpate the shaft of the ulna and follow it along its length to its end. Introduce the tip of the needle at 90 degrees to the "plateau." No redirection of the needle is required (Fig. 5). It naturally follows the shaft of the bone. It is advisable but not necessary to immobilize the wing with a figure-of-8 bandage (Ritchie et al., 1990).

## Other Bones

If the above bones are unavailable, the humerus may be used in reptiles and mammals, but *not* in birds. The catheter is introduced as an antegrade intramedullary pin. If the pelvis is large enough, a bone marrow aspirate needle can be placed into the ileum using standard bone marrow aspiration technique and utilized as a temporary IO catheter.

## References and Suggested Reading

Brickman KR, Rega P, Koltz M, et al: Analysis of growth plate abnormalities following intraosseous infusion through the proximal tibial epiphysis in pigs. Ann Emerg Med 17:121, 1988.
  *Scientific paper showing minimal effects of intraosseous infusion on active growth plates.*
Dedrick DK, Mase C, Ronger W, et al: The effects of intraosseous infusion on the growth plate in a nestling rabbit model. Ann Emerg Med 21:494, 1992.
  *Scientific paper showing minimal effects of intraosseous infusion on growth plates.*
Hodge D, Delagado-Paredes C, and Fleisher G: Intraosseous infusion flow rates in hypovolemic "pediatric" dogs. Ann Emerg Med 16:305, 1987.
  *Scientific paper investigating maximal flow rates through intraosseous catheters.*
Jaimovich DG: Comparison of intraosseous and intravenous routes of anticonvulsant administration in a porcine model. Ann Emerg Med 18:842, 1989.
  *Scientific paper comparing the effects of route of administration on blood levels of anticonvulsants.*
Jaimovich DG: Evaluation of intraosseous versus intravenous antibiotic levels in a porcine model. Am J Dis Child 8:946, 1991.
  *Scientific paper comparing effects of route of administration (intraosseous versus intravenous) on antibiotic blood levels.*
Otto CM, Kaufman GM, and Crowe DT: Intraosseous infusion of fluids and therapeutics. Comp Clin Educ (SA Pract) 11:421, 1989.
  *Practical overview of the use of intraosseous catheters in small animals.*
Redig PT: Fluid therapy and acid-base balance in the critically ill avian patient. Proc Assoc Avian Vet, Toronto, Canada, 1984, p 59.
  *A review of evaluation of dehydration and use of fluid therapy in birds.*
Ritchie B, Otto CM, Latimer K, et al: A technique for intraosseous cannulation for intravenous therapy in birds. Compend Cont Educ 12:55, 1990.
  *Excellent, practical explanation of placing ulnar intraosseous catheters in birds.*
Ros SP, McMannis SI, and Kowal-Vern A: Effect of intraosseous saline infusion on hematologic parameters. Ann Emerg Med 20:243, 1991.
  *A study showing intraosseous fluids creating mild changes in hematologic parameters of New Zealand white rabbits.*
Spivey WH, Lathers CM, Malone DR, et al: Comparison of intraosseous, central, and peripheral routes of NaHCO$_3$ administration during CPR in pigs. Ann Emerg Med 14:1135, 1985.
  *A comparison of the efficacy of intraosseous catheters versus traditional routes of vascular access for CPR with postinfusion histopathology of the bone marrow.*

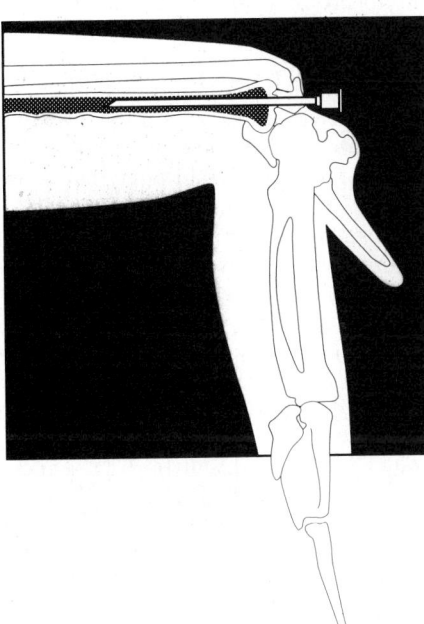

**Figure 5.** Placement of an intraosseous catheter in the ulna of a bird. Introduce the tip of the catheter 90 degrees to the "plateau" formed by the distal end of the ulna. Advance the catheter until the hub touches the skin.

# "WET TAIL" IN HAMSTERS AND OTHER DIARRHEAS OF SMALL RODENTS

THOMAS J. BURKE

*Urbana, Illinois*

As with other animals, diarrhea in small rodents is a common primary complaint. One survey of laboratory animal veterinarians listed it as the most common clinical sign of hamsters. Also as in other animals kept as pets, diarrhea is seen most frequently in the very young and very old (for the species). For our discussion here, we will not adhere to the strict definition of diarrhea (increased frequency, liquidity, and volume of stools), as most owners are unable to make sufficiently accurate observations of all three of these factors in their pet rodents. Usually they only notice that the stools are loose or watery and assume that this is diarrhea. Furthermore, it is not uncommon to have a patient presented for other reasons (see below) whose physical examination reveals evidence of loose or watery stools and we also conclude that it has had or is having "diarrhea."

## "WET TAIL" OF HAMSTERS

Wet tail of hamsters is also known as proliferative ileitis, regional enteritis, terminal ileitis, and transmissible ileal hyperplasia.

The term "hamsters" in this article refers to the Syrian or gold hamster (*Mesocricetus auratus*), as it is the one most commonly sold and kept as a pet. The Chinese or striped back (*Cricetus griseus*), Armenian or gray (*Cricetulus migratorius*), and European (*Cricetus cricetus*) hamsters are infrequent pets but are commonly used as laboratory animals. A recent introduction to the pet market, the Siberian or dwarf hamster (*Phodopus sengoris*) is increasing its popularity because of its gentle nature. It is listed as not prone to "wet tail."

Proliferative ileitis (PI) is the most common spontaneous disease of hamsters. It is most common in animals 3 to 8 weeks of age. It may, however, be seen in older animals who have undergone stressful events such as overcrowding and fights, severe environmental temperature fluctuations, malnutrition, and geriatric-associated disease.

The disease gets its common name "wet tail" from the appearance of wet matted hair in the perineum. Most owners, however, do not notice this, but instead present the animal with vague primary complaints of sick, not eating, matted eyes, rough fur, not moving, and so forth. These observations indicate an advanced stage of the disease, signaling that sepsis and/or enterotoxemia have occurred.

The etiology is as yet undefined. *Compylobacter fetus jejuni* has been incriminated, but pure cultures of this organism from clinical cases have failed to reproduce the clinical syndrome when given per os to weanling hamsters, although organism shedding and microscopic lesions were observed in some. The disease can, however, be reproduced by per os administration of ileal contents from sick hamsters. It thus appears that *Campylobacter* plays a synergistic role in the development of PI. Other bacteria (especially *Escherichia coli*) and environmental stressors must also be incriminated. Furthermore, asymptomatic random source hamsters may have microscopic lesions consistent with PI containing visible *C. jejuni*. Others may have, and presumably shed, only *C. jejuni* organisms.

Thus transmission appears to be by the fecal-oral route. Direct contact may also spread the disease.

Physical findings depend on the stage of the disease. As already stated, most animals are presented in an advanced state of illness. The hallmark is finding a wet, matted perineum. Abdominal palpation usually reveals thickened, turgid bowel loops (not unlike those of cats with panleukopenia) alternating with gas-filled segments. Any stool passed will be liquid and frequently bubbly. Other common findings are hunched posture, unkempt hair coat, rapid respiration, loss of muscle mass, and palpebral matting with the lids held shut. Death during the initial physical examination of patients so presented is frequent. Warn the owner prior to beginning your examination.

Hamsters with chronic PI may present with rectal prolapses. Here the stool is often bloody and the owner may have only noticed blood on the bedding material, or they may have noticed the prolapse when examining their pet for the source of the blood.

Gram stains of rectal smears and fecal cultures, especially for *C. jejuni*, are helpful in diagnosis. The differential diagnosis should include Tyzzer's disease, salmonellosis, and antibiotic-associated enteritis. Antemortem diagnosis is seldom possible, but precise diagnosis is advisable for several reasons including prevention in future pets and the threat of zoonotic disease.

Treatment is usually unrewarding. Virtually all of those presented by owners will be so ill that they will die in spite of our best efforts. I usually try warm (37°C) subcutaneous lactated Ringer's solution, intramuscular aminoglycoside plus carbenicillin antibiotics, and hospitalization in an incubator at 35° to 38°C. While intraperitoneal fluids should be more readily absorbed, the distended bowel loops make this route of administration very risky.

A grave prognosis should always be given. Although there have been no documented cases of *C. jejuni* infection in people from hamsters, the threat remains. Because of the association of this disease with *C. jejuni*, the owner should be warned to handle the cage with care and dispose of all bedding, food, and other porous materials in a sanitary manner. I write the name of the organism on paper, give it to the owner, and suggest that they contact their physician, especially if young children or immunosuppressed individuals have been in contact with the hamster. Practitioners and their staff should also keep this in mind when handling ill hamsters and during necropsy. *Campylobacter jejuni* will survive for fairly long periods at 4°C—3 weeks in feces and milk, 4 weeks in water, and 5 weeks in urine.

Prevention involves the source of the animal. Most hamsters are purchased from pet shops. They obtain their animals from commercial wholesalers and/or breeders. In the former case, the animal is shipped from the breeder to the wholesaler to the pet shop and then to the consumer all within a short time. This means that the average buyer (pet owner) receives an animal that has been shipped and handled "from pillar to post" with frequent changes in the source and quality of water and food and with wide temperature fluctuations. All are stressors.

Since many pet shops replace ill or dying animals within a reasonable time of the purchase, this disease represents an economic loss to them as well. My attempts at prevention are thus twofold: (1) to the owner and (2) to the pet shop.

For the owner, I recommend that they clean the cage thoroughly, discarding any porous items. Water bottles and feed dishes must be thoroughly cleaned and disinfected (sodium hypochlorite with multiple rinses). Replacement hamsters should be obtained from another pet shop if possible. In some instances, the original shop will only replace the hamster and will not offer a cash refund. In either case, the new hamster must have been kept in quarantine (no direct contact with other rodents) for at least 7 days at the shop. Furthermore, the owner is strongly advised to clean the cage daily and observe the droppings for the next 2 weeks. These simple steps have greatly reduced the incidence of a second pet dying of PI.

For pet shops, I also recommend that they change their source of supply and that hamsters be held in quarantine for 7 days prior to any retail sale. During this time, the bedding, food, and water are changed daily. If outbreaks continue, then newly acquired hamsters are treated with oral neomycin (two to three drops of a 200 mg/ml solution b.i.d.) plus per os commercial preparation of live *Lactobacillus acidophilus* for 5 days and not sold for another 7 days.

Control of outbreaks has also been achieved with tetracycline hydrochloride (400 mg/L) in the drinking water for 10 days or erythromycin phosphate (0.5 gm/gallon) given continuously in the drinking water. The dose of erythromycin for individual animals is 20 mg/kg PO twice daily. Erythromycin may cause fatal alterations in gastrointestinal flora and should be administered with caution. I always supplement antibiotic therapy in rodents with a *Lactobacillus acidophilus* preparation during and several days beyond cessation of treatment.

## OTHER DIARRHEAS OF SMALL RODENTS

The general approach is the same regardless of species: obtain a history and perform a physical. Signalment (especially age), source of the pet, length of time owned, diet, and housing are very important. Also determine if the pet is on any other therapy (are you sure you didn't pick something up at the pet shop?). The latter is a common cause of antibiotic-associated enteritis/clostridial enterotoxemia. Physical examination is usually limited to observation and palpation. The mouth should be carefully examined with an otoscope, rinsing with water via dental (anal sac) syringe as necessary.

Commonly employed diagnostic aids are Gram stain of rectal swab smears, fecal flotation and direct smear, fecal culture, and "Scotch tape" exams for pinworm ova. If the patient succumbs—and many will—necropsy and histopathology are mandatory if there is concern for other exposed animals, small colonies, or replacement animals.

The major cause of diarrhea in rodents kept as pets is dietary indiscretion. Especially the feeding of relatively large quantities of high-fiber, high-water-content vegetables and fruits. These are treated with oral protectants such as barium or kaolin-pectin compounds and feeding of fresh, good quality, block-type commercial diet designed for the species.

### Viruses

The viral diarrheas of rodents are usually seen in the suckling-weanling age group. Unless the client is raising their own—usually as a food source for other animals such as reptiles or birds of prey—the practitioner is not apt to encounter these diseases. These include mouse hepatitis virus (a coronavirus), reovirus type 3 and epizootic diarrhea of infant mice (a rotavirus), and a similar syndrome of rats. Diagnosis is made by various studies of necropsy-derived tissues. There is no treatment. Prevention is to depopulate, disinfect, and repopulate. Check with a laboratory animal veterinarian to assist your client in choosing a source for replacement animals free of the disease in question.

### Bacteria

Tyzzer's disease is caused by *Bacillus piliformis*, a gram-negative pleomorphic rod that is an obligate intracellular organism. It causes a variety of clinical signs including diarrhea and wasting. This is most common in mice, hamsters, guinea pigs, and gerbils. Diarrhea is not a feature of this disease in rats. The onset of signs is often predisposed by stress, especially high temperature and humidity, and immunosuppression. Fecal-oral transmission is probably the most common route of spread, with spores remaining viable in the environment for up to a year. Antemortem diagnosis is extremely difficult. It infects most mammals and may be zoonotic. Tetracycline hydrochloride is the antibiotic of choice in animals exposed to a known positive case.

Very young (2 to 4-week-old) mice are susceptible to infection with *Citrobacter freundii* variant 4280. Infection causes a syndrome termed "transmissible murine colonic hyperplasia," with clinical signs of diarrhea and/or rectal prolapse. Treatment is usually futile, but oral aminoglycosides may be tried combined with symptomatic therapy.

Enteritis and clinical diarrhea have been associated with *Salmonella* infection, particularly *S. typhimurium* and *S. enteritidis*. Guinea pigs, mice, and rats are most commonly involved, with hamsters and gerbils only occasionally being infected. Diagnosis is based on fecal cultures. Treatment is unwise, since human infection is likely and reservoirs, even in so-called treated animals, exist. Euthanasia is recommended.

Clostridial-associated disease may take either of two forms: invasion by *Clostridium perfringens* type D producing severe enteritis with high mortality or antibiotic-associated clostridial enterotoxemia (AACE). The latter is caused by toxins from *C. difficile*, *C. sordellii*, and *C. histolyticum*. *Clostridium perfringens* infections appear to be of little clinical significance in individual pets, but the AACE is, unfortunately, quite common. Those antibiotics with a primary gram-positive spectrum (especially penicillin, erythromycin, and clindamycin) suppress competing microflora of the gut and allow for clostridial proliferation and toxin elaboration. Affected animals usually die. Prevention is the key. Rodents should be treated with broad-spectrum antibiotics, and I always prescribe a commercial live *Lactobacillus acidophilus* preparation for concomitant use.

*Campylobacter* infection has been discussed in the section "Wet Tail of Hamsters," above. It has been associated with enteritis in other rodents with varying degrees of implication. However, one should note that pregnant guinea pigs are very susceptible to infection. Tetracyclines or chloramphenicol are the best choice for therapy.

Mice exposed to wild rats or (rarely) domestic rats may develop diarrhea from *Streptobacillus moniliformis* infection. This is asymptomatic in the rat. It is also the organism responsible for rat bite or Haverhill fever in humans. Antemortem diagnosis is most difficult and requires organism isolation. There is no reliable treatment.

Bacterial diarrhea may also be caused by *E. coli* (colibacillosis), *Proteus mirabilis*, and other enterobacteria. Predisposing causes include malnutrition, contaminated feed, environmental stressors, and antibacterial therapy. Diagnosis is based on Gram stain and fecal culture. Treatment is protectants plus oral and/or parenteral antibiotics that have a gram-negative spectrum and good management.

## Protozoan Infections

Chronic diarrhea and/or rectal prolapse have been associated with protozoal infection with *Coccidia* (mouse and guinea pig), cryptosporidia (several species), *Giardia muris* (rat, no diarrhea in mouse), and *Spironucleus muris* (*Hexamita*) (mouse, rat, and hamster). Diagnosis is based on fecal examination for protozoa.

*Coccidia* are treated with coccidiostats until host resistance can establish itself: sulfaquinoxaline 0.1% daily in the drinking water; sulfamethazine 0.2% in the drinking water–both for several weeks–or sulfadimethoxine PO at 75 mg/kg once daily for 7 to 14 days.

*Giardia* and *Spironucleus* are treated with 14 days of dimetridazole 0.1% in the drinking water. Fenbendazole (50 mg/kg/day PO for 5 days) also is effective for *Giardia* in most mammals.

Daily bedding changes and cage cleaning will prevent reinfection.

## Metazoan Infections

Both *Hymenolepis nana* and *diminuta* may infect rats, mice, and gerbils. Most often there are no symptoms, but heavy parasite burdens may cause diarrhea and unthriftiness. *Hymenolepis nana* can have a direct life cycle. Insects are the intermediate hosts for both. Both also are zoonotic, with *H. nana* posing the greatest threat because of its direct life cycle. Diagnosis is made by fecal flotation. Treatment is praziquantel at 30 mg/kg PO, three doses at 2-week intervals. Cages should be insect proof.

Mice, rats, hamsters, and gerbils may have pinworms of the genus *Syphacia*. *Aspiculuris* occurs in mice only. Heavy parasite burdens can produce diarrhea. Diagnosis is by Scotch tape testing. Treatment is piperazine adipate at 0.5 gm/L of drinking water for 3 days or fenbendazole at 50 mg/kg PO daily for 3 days. Repeat both in 2 and 4 weeks. Also improve sanitation and cage cleaning.

Guinea pigs may harbor the cecal worm *Paraspidodera uncinata*. It is not known to cause clinical disease. Its egg does resemble that of an ascarid and may be confusing on fecal flotation. (See Fox, Cohen, and Loew [1984] for an excellent picture.) If found in association with diarrhea, I would treat with ivermectin at 200 μg/kg PO or SC but look elsewhere for the cause of the diarrhea. Frequent bedding changes and cage cleaning prevent reinfection.

## Miscellaneous Causes

Dental malocclusion frequently causes inability to utilize pelleted food. Affected animals will, seemingly compensatorily, increase water consumption, which may lead to loose stools. They will lose body condition from decreased food intake, and without an adequate oral examination, one can be fooled into making a diagnosis of chronic intestinal disease. This is especially true in guinea pigs where molar malocclusion predominates. *Always do a thorough physical*!

Hamsters are prone to ingestion of bedding material, especially chlorophyll-scented wood shavings. This has led to gastrointestinal impactions. Severe ones are routinely fatal, but mild episodes can lead to straining with rectal prolapse and/or staining of the perineum with blood or serum that resembles wet tail. I have yet to have an owner permit a retrograde barium series for diagnosis, but necropsy is helpful in establishing an etiology and preventing future mistakes. Avoid chlorophyll-scented bedding.

## References and Suggested Reading

Fox JG: Campylobacteriosis—a "new" disease in laboratory animals. Lab Anim Sci 32:625, 1982
*An excellent review of the history, culture requirements, taxonomy, and disease syndromes associated with Campylobacter in rodents, rabbits, ferrets, dogs, cats, lower primates, and humans.*

Fox JG, Cohen BJ, and Loew FM: *Laboratory Animals Medicine.* Orlando, FL, Academic Press, 1984.
*A general text covering most species used as laboratory animals including rodents, rabbits, ferrets, dogs, cats, ungulates, primates, birds, fish, amphibians, and reptiles.*

Harkness JE and Wagner JE: *The Biology and Medicine of Rabbits and Rodents,* 3rd edition. Philadelphia, Lea & Febiger, 1989.
*A very useful, well-organized text on the management and diseases of rodents and rabbits.*

# *DESULFOVIBRIO*-ASSOCIATED PROLIFERATIVE COLITIS IN FERRETS

JAMES G. FOX
*Cambridge, Massachusetts*

Gastrointestinal diseases manifested as diarrhea are one of the most frequently encountered clinical entities in the domestic ferret. Proliferative colitis was first reported in research ferrets in 1983. Since then it has become a commonly recognized clinical syndrome in pet ferrets. A similar proliferative intestinal disease has been recognized for decades in swine and hamsters and more recently in rabbits.

## DIAGNOSIS

### History and Presentation

The disease has been identified in both research and pet ferrets in several geographic areas in the United States. The disease is most commonly diagnosed in young ferrets less than 1 year of age and often less than 6 months old. Clinically, ferrets have watery to mucoid blood-tinged diarrhea; are dehydrated, lethargic, and anorexic; and unless given supportive and antimicrobial therapy, rapidly lose weight. Tenesmus is often evident and rectal prolapses are noted, particularly if the segmental hyperplasia is present in the terminal colon. Abdominal palpation will reveal a segmentally thickened colon and enlarged mesenteric lymph nodes. Infre-

quently, the disease can produce inflammation, fibrosis, and calcification in extraintestinal abdominal organs that can be detected radiographically or by abdominal palpation. Culture for *Salmonella* and *Campylobacter jejuni* as well as fecal examination for *Coccidia*, *Giardia*, and *Cryptosporidium* should be performed to rule out these potential intestinal pathogens. A definitive diagnosis of proliferative colitis, however, requires a colonic biopsy.

### Histopathologic Findings

The histologic features are distinctive and consist of epithelial hyperplasia, glandular irregularity, multiple foci of epithelial necrosis, crypt abscesses, and inflammatory infiltrate in the lamina propria. A universal feature of the disease is the presence of comma-shaped intracellular organisms demonstrated by Warthin-Starry silver stain within the apical portion of columnar epithelial cells. These organisms have been referred to as intracellular *Campylobacter*-like organisms (ICLO). Fluorescent-labeled monoclonal and polyclonal antibodies, directed against the ICLO isolated from pigs and hamsters, also recognize ICLO present in infected epithelia of ferrets. We have recently identified the ICLO obtained from ferrets with proliferative colitis by using polymerase chain reaction (PCR) and 16S rRNA sequence analysis. In the index ferret, proliferative bowel tissue containing the ICLO had translocated to the mesenteric lymph nodes, omentum, and liver.

Comparison of the RNA sequence of the ICLO with those of over 400 bacteria in our data base indicated that the ICLO was most closely related to that of *Desulfovibrio desulfuricans* (87.5% similarity). Phylogenetic analysis using 12 *Desulfovibrio* species and 20 species from related genera placed the ICLO in a subcluster within the genus *Desulfovibrio* with *D. desulfuricans* and five other *Desulfovibrio* species. Thus, the organism is now referred to as the intracellular *Desulfovibrio* organism (IDO). Specific primers have also demonstrated the IDO from other cases of proliferative colitis in ferrets as well as hamsters with proliferative ileitis, but not from intestinal tissue samples from animals without the proliferative bowel. Recent publications indicate that the same intracellular organism has been identified in proliferative intestinal tissues of swine and that the organism has been successfully maintained in tissue culture.

### Differential Diagnosis

Proliferative colitis must be differentiated from acute colitis caused by *Campylobacter jejuni*, intestinal lymphoma, eosinophilic gastroenteritis, *Helicobacter mustelae*–associated gastroduodenal ulcers, intestinal foreign bodies, intestinal mycobacterial infection, salmonellosis, and Aleutian disease. The presence of IDO in hyperplastic colonic epithelial cells will differentiate proliferative colitis from these other ferret diseases, which can have signs referable to the gastrointestinal tract. A differential diagnosis must also include a "new" disease manifested as acute episodes of diarrhea that has been diagnosed recently in ferrets residing in the eastern coastal states. Though the disease has some features of a parvovirus-like syndrome, an etiologic agent has not been identified.

### THERAPY

Fortunately, proliferative colitis responds to oral chloramphenicol therapy at a dose of 10 to 40 mg/kg every 8 hr PO for 2 weeks, or 50 mg/kg every 12 hr PO for 10 days. If the animal is hospitalized, chloramphenicol can be more easily administered to the ferret orally. Relapses are infrequently observed. Gentamicin (2 mg/kg) every 12 hr PO has been recommended as an alternate antibiotic therapy. This drug, however, has been shown to be particularly nephrotoxic and ototoxic to ferrets. This is especially true when the animal is dehydrated. Therefore, gentamicin probably should not be prescribed.

Supportive parenteral or oral electrolyte fluids are given during the treatment course as well as nutritional supplements such as Nutri-Cal (Evsco Pharmaceuticals, Buena, NJ). Rectal prolapses usually respond to the antimicrobial therapy and are reduced manually. A purse-string suture can be placed in ferrets in which the prolapse is large or likely to reprolapse. Prompt and diligent antibiotic therapy is necessary because untreated ferrets, in our experience, have a poor prognosis.

### CONCLUSIONS

The *Desulfovibrio* species have been proposed in the pathogenesis of ulcerative colitis in humans. In patients with ulcerative colitis, 96% harbor sulfate-reducing bacteria (SRB), with the majority of human gut SRB belonging to the genus *Desulfovibrio*. Because hydrogen sulfide produced by these bacteria is toxic to intestinal tissue, mucin, a highly sulfated mucoprotein, stimulates growth of SRB at the expense of methanogens. Ulcerative colitis and intestinal adenomas and carcinomas in rodent and rabbits can be produced by feeding these animals sulfate-containing polysaccharides such as dextran sulfate, sulfated pectin, or degraded carrageenan. Thus, the intracellular *Desulfovibrio* organism associated with proliferative bowel disease falls within a group of bacteria already implicated in lower bowel disease.

The intracellular *Desulfovibrio* organism in ferrets, hamsters, and pigs appears to be the previously unclassified ICLO that reacts with Warthin-Starry silver stain and omega antiserum. These intracellular organisms grown in tissue culture produce proliferative lesions in conventional pigs but not in germ-free pigs; in addition, the organism could not be reisolated from the intestine of germ-free animals. Thus, while IDO is associated with disease, it may not have the ability without other microbial agents or insults to produce the proliferative intestinal lesions. The availability of molecular techniques for detection of the intracellular *Desulfovibrio* organism *in vivo* and ability to grow the bacteria in tissue culture should facilitate further studies of the role of this organism in the pathogenesis, epidemiology, and treatment of ferret proliferative bowel disease. In addition, it is now possible to carefully assess how modulation of diet and indigenous gut flora influence the ability of *Desulfovibrio* to evade the host's immune defenses and thereby initiate and sustain a hyperplastic response in the infected colonic epithelium.

### References and Suggested Reading

Finkler MR: Ferret colitis. *In* Kirk RW and Bonagura JD (eds): *Current Veterinary Therapy XI.* Philadelphia, WB Saunders Co, 1992, pp 1180–1181.
*Discusses acute colitis versus chronic proliferative colitis and treatment strategies for each clinical condition.*
Fox JG, Dewhirst FE, Fraser GJ, et al: The intracellular *Campylobacter*-like organism from ferrets and hamsters with proliferative bowel disease is a *Desulfovibrio* sp. J Clin Microbiol 32:1229, 1994.
*Describes molecular characterization of the ICLO associated with proliferative colitis and ileitis in the ferret and hamster, respectively, as an intracellular* Desulfovibrio *spp.*
Fox JG, Ackerman JI, Taylor NS, Claps M, and Murphy JC: *Campylobacter jejuni* infection in the ferret: An animal model of human campylobacteriosis. Am J Vet Res 48:85, 1987.

*An experimental study demonstrating that oral inoculation with* C. jejuni *produces diarrhea and acute colitis in weanling ferrets.*

Fox JG and Lawson GHK: *Campylobacter*-like omega intracellular antigen in proliferative colitis of ferrets. Lab Anim Sci 38:34, 1988.
  *Demonstrates that ICLO reacts to* Campylobacter *omega antigen with the same specificity as ICLOs in proliferative bowel disease of swine and hamsters.*

Fox JG, Murphy JC, Ackerman JI, et al: Proliferative colitis in ferrets. Am J Vet Res 43:858, 1982.
  *Initial description of clinical and histopathologic features of ICLO associated proliferative colitis in ferrets.*

Fox JG, Murphy JC, Otto G, et al: Proliferative colitis in ferrets: Epithelial dysplasia and translocation. Vet Pathol 26:515, 1989.
  *Describes ability of ICLO to translocate to extraintestinal sites and present clinically and pathologically as an "abdominal mass."*

Gebhart CJ, Barns SM, McOrist S, Lin GF, and Lawson GHK: Ileal symbiont intracellularis, an obligate intracellular bacterium of porcine intestines showing a relationship to *Desulfovibrio* species. Int J Syst Bacteriol 43:533, 1993.
  *Utilizes molecular techniques to describe the ICLO observed in proliferative ileitis in pigs as a* Desulfovibrio *species.*

Kruger KL, Murphy JC, and Fox JG. Treatment of proliferative colitis in ferrets. J Am Vet Med Assoc 194:1435, 1989.
  *A study describing the successful treatment of proliferative colitis with chloramphenicol versus palliative but not curative supportive treatment.*

# BLOOD COLLECTION AND TRANSFUSION IN FERRETS

ELIZABETH V. HILLYER

*Oldwick, New Jersey*

Domestic ferrets are carnivores and share many anatomic and physiologic features with dogs and cats. However, the challenge of blood collection from ferrets prevents some clinicians from working with this species. A knowledge of restraint and venipuncture techniques and the use of appropriate equipment make blood collection a routine procedure. Indeed, obtaining larger volumes for transfusion purposes can also be accomplished relatively easily and often without tranquilization.

## PREPARATION

A routine history and physical examination should be performed before collecting blood. In particular, the color of the oral mucosa should be assessed. If the mucous membranes appear pale, a few drops of blood can be taken to measure the packed cell volume (PCV) before taking a larger sample.

Most laboratories can run a complete blood count (CBC) and biochemistry analysis on a relatively small volume of blood if the appropriate specimen containers and handling techniques are used. Each laboratory has a preferred protocol, which should be followed. Because the hematocrit of ferrets is relatively high (45 to 60%), the blood volume drawn should be three times the desired volume of serum or plasma. If the ferret is difficult to bleed or anemic and only a small sample is obtained, the blood for biochemical analysis should be placed in a *heparinized* tube, rather than in a tube without anticoagulant. This is because the harvested plasma sample will be larger than a serum sample from an equivalent volume of whole blood. Most laboratories can perform the biochemistry analysis on plasma rather than serum.

The blood volume of ferrets is about 5 to 7% of body weight, or 50 to 70 ml/kg body weight (23 to 32 ml/pound). From a healthy, nonanemic animal, up to 20% of blood volume can be removed without danger, which translates to roughly 10 to 12 ml/kg (4.5 to 5.5 ml/pound). The average ferret weighs about 2 pounds (900 gm), with a range of 1 to 3 pounds (440 to 1320 gm).

## Equipment

The equipment needed for venipuncture and transfusion will be available at most small animal hospitals (Table 1). The appropriate small-gauge needles and butterfly catheters facilitate blood collection in this small species. Moreover, use of the smallest possible syringe, such as an insulin or 3-cc syringe, is less likely to cause collapse of the vein during phlebotomy.

## Restraint

Most ferrets are docile and easy to handle, and the physical examination can be performed with minimal

**Table 1.** *Equipment Needed for Blood Collection and Transfusion in Ferrets*

Lo-Dose U-100 insulin syringes°
Syringes: tuberculin to 12-ml
Needles: 20- to 27-gauge
Butterfly catheters: 20- to 25-gauge
Spinal needles: 20- and 22-gauge
Blood containers (serum, heparinized, and EDTA): 0.7 ml capacity
Acid-citrate-dextrose (ACD) solution

°Becton Dickinson, Rutherford, NJ.
Abbreviation: EDTA = ethylenediaminetetraacetic acid.

restraint. However, total immobility is required for venipuncture. This is achieved using firm physical restraint, a distraction such as a food treat, or chemical restraint.

### PHYSICAL RESTRAINT

A neck scruff hold has a calming effect on most ferrets. Moreover, a firm grasp, rather than a light touch, seems to give better immobilization in this species. Depending on the venipuncture site, the ferret can be restrained in dorsal or ventral recumbancy with the neck scruff hold. The hindquarters should be restrained around the hips without pulling on the hindlegs, because pulling the legs back causes most ferrets to struggle. Specific positioning is discussed further below.

A food treat, such as Nutri-Cal (Evsco Pharmaceuticals, Buena, NJ), is a good tool to distract a ferret. A small amount of Nutri-Cal is placed on the ferret's tongue or nose before restraining it; then the ferret will usually continue eating during restraint and venipuncture, seemingly oblivious to the procedure. However, blood for glucose determination or other fasting samples should be drawn before offering any food.

### CHEMICAL RESTRAINT

Some ferrets are best immobilized with chemical restraint for venipuncture, including the uncommon aggressive ferret and the occasional one, typically younger animals, that may struggle when manually restrained. Chemical restraint may also be preferable for inexperienced clinicians or if reliable assistance is not available.

Inhalational anesthesia with isoflurane (AErrane, Anaquest, Madison, WI) is ideal for a short immobilization because of the rapid induction and recovery with this agent. In addition, isoflurane is relatively safe and can be used if the stress of physical restraint might present undue risk to a ferret in poor physical condition, such as one with severe anemia or dyspnea. For a short immobilization, the anesthetic gas is administered by facemask or by placing the ferret in an induction box. Isoflurane has a strong irritating odor; ferrets tend to offer less resistance if the concentration is gradually increased by 0.5% increments, starting at 0.5% and stopping when the ferret relaxes, typically at a concentration of 2 to 2.5%.

Injectable agents can also be used; however, the level of tranquilization and muscle relaxation is unreliable, and recovery is considerably longer than with isoflurane. A combination of ketamine (10 mg/kg IM) and acepromazine (0.1 mg/kg IM) is one option. Alternatively, tiletamine-zolazepam (Telazol, AH Robins, Richmond, VA) is dosed at 1.5 to 5 mg/kg IM.

## VENIPUNCTURE

Practical sites for venipuncture in pet ferrets include the jugular vein, cranial vena cava, ventral tail artery, cephalic vein, and lateral saphenous vein. In ferrets used for laboratory research purposes, blood may be taken from the retro-orbital sinus or via cardiac puncture; however, neither of these techniques is appropriate for pet ferrets.

Each clinician will develop preferred techniques for blood sampling. The author utilizes the cephalic vein for collection of small volumes and the jugular vein or cranial vena cava for collection of larger volumes. The jugular vein is probably the best site for obtaining a large volume of blood for transfusion purposes. The cephalic and lateral saphenous veins are probably the best sites for repeated sampling. For example, in an intensive care setting when repeat glucose determinations are necessary, a few drops of blood can be obtained multiple times from the cephalic vein without hematoma formation using a Lo-Dose U-100 insulin syringe with 28-gauge needle (Becton Dickinson, Rutherford, NJ).

### Jugular Vein

A 20- to 22-gauge needle is appropriate for jugular venipuncture. A needle and 3-cc syringe can be used to draw a sample for CBC and blood biochemistry analysis, while a butterfly catheter attached to a larger syringe can be used for larger sample volumes. Shaving the area over the vein facilitates visualization.

Two restraint positions are used for jugular venipuncture: dorsal recumbancy or ventral recumbancy at the edge of a table. For the table edge technique, the ferret is held with the forelegs pulled down and the chin held up vertically. A second assistant may be needed to restrain the hindquarters. The jugular vein is occluded at the thoracic inlet and venipuncture is performed routinely. With this positioning, care must be taken not to apply excessive suction, which readily collapses the vein. Moreover, blood flow may be rapid at first and then become frustratingly slow.

Positioning in dorsal recumbancy is used by some clinicians and is better for sedated ferrets. The ferret's head is extended, restrained around the angle of the jaw, and the forelegs are pulled caudally. Depending on the ferret's size and positioning and the preferences of the phlebotomist, the needle can be bent at a 30-degree angle to better access the vein. Alternatively, nonsedated ferrets can be held by the neck scruff, wrapped tightly in a towel with just the head and neck exposed, distracted with a food treat, and then placed on their dorsum for venipuncture (Otto, Rosenblad, and Fox, 1993). With a ferret in dorsal recumbancy, the jugular vein has a tendency to roll; applying tension to the overlying skin helps to stabilize the vein.

### Cranial Vena Cava

Phlebotomy of the cranial vena cava is performed to draw up to 3 ml of blood using a 25-gauge needle and 3-cc syringe. The advantages of this technique are that it is easy to learn and blood flow is rapid, allowing blood collection in a few seconds. The obvious disadvantage is that it is a "blind" technique with no way to "hold off" the vein after removing the needle. The author has drawn blood from this site from dozens of ferrets without morbidity. Nonetheless, *phlebotomy of the cranial vena cava should be performed only if the ferret is immobile and restraint is secure and only if there is no possibility of cranial thoracic disease*, such as megaesophagus or a cranial mediastinal mass.

Manual restraint is usually sufficient, particularly if the ferret is distracted with a food treat. The ferret is placed in dorsal recumbency with its head restrained around the mandibles or by the neck scruff. Its forelegs are pulled caudally. Positioning must be precise and symmetric, with the hindquarters firmly restrained. Standing at the ferret's head, the phlebotomist directs the needle caudally through the skin to either side of the midline in the notch between the manubrium and the first rib. The needle is placed at a shallow angle to the skin, aiming toward the opposite hip. Gentle suction is applied as the needle is advanced in this orientation; when blood enters the hub, the sample is collected and the needle is withdrawn. Alternatively, the needle is first advanced in the same orientation and then withdrawn while applying gentle suction.

## Ventral Tail Artery

The tail artery is used by some clinicians to collect blood samples from ferrets; 1 to 3 ml of blood, or sometimes more, can be collected from this site. A 22- to 25-gauge needle is used with the appropriate size syringe. With the ferret restrained in dorsal recumbancy, and possibly distracted with Nutri-Cal, the needle is inserted into the ventral aspect of the tail at a distance of about 2 to 3 cm from the anus. The needle is oriented toward the head at a 30-degree angle to the skin and is advanced to bone and then withdrawn while applying gentle suction.

## Cephalic and Lateral Saphenous Veins

The cephalic and lateral saphenous veins are readily accessible sites for collecting up to 0.5 ml of blood. These veins are small but easily visualized when they are occluded, particularly if the fur is shaved from the overlying area. Recommended equipment is a tuberculin syringe with 25- to 27-gauge needle or a Lo-Dose insulin syringe. The author prefers the latter because the needles are relatively atraumatic and back-pressure on the small syringe is unlikely to collapse the vein. However, the needles are preattached and not easily removed from the syringes. To avoid injecting the blood back out through the 28-gauge needle into a specimen container, with a bit of practice the needle can be removed using a hemostat and a gentle rotating motion. An alternative technique is to place a 25- to 27-gauge needle in the vein and allow the blood to flow out from the hub into a hematocrit tube, small blood tube, or onto a reagent strip.

For cephalic venipuncture, the ferret is restrained by the neck scruff and held either suspended in the air or in ventral recumbancy on a table top. Similarly, as for dogs and cats, the assistant can hold off the vein by rolling it outward with a thumb. Alternatively, a small tourniquet can be constructed from a section of rubber band and an alligator clip or bulldog clamp (Otto, Rosenblad, and Fox, 1993).

For lateral saphenous venipuncture, the ferret is positioned in ventral recumbancy. The assistant uses one hand to "scruff" the ferret by the neck skin and places the other hand around the femoral area of the uppermost leg, simultaneously causing the leg to extend and occluding the vein. The vein runs very superficially just proximal to the hock.

## Toenail Clip

Clipping a toenail to obtain one or two drops of blood is painful for the ferret and should be reserved for use in emergencies when phlebotomy is unsuccessful. The technique is the same as for dogs and cats.

## BLOOD TRANSFUSION TECHNIQUES

The need for a blood transfusion in an anemic ferret, as for other species, is based on clinical status of the animal and measurement of PCV. The required transfusion volume is calculated using the canine formula (O'Rourke, 1983).

## Blood Donors

Ideal blood donors are healthy ferrets in early maturity. Male ferrets tend to be larger than females and are therefore preferred because a larger volume of blood can be obtained. Ideally, donor ferrets should be vaccinated routinely and screened periodically with a CBC, biochemistry profile, and microfilaria test. (Microfilaremia from dirofilariasis is very uncommon; nonetheless, routine screening is advisable for blood donors, particularly in endemic areas.)

Most veterinary hospitals are not equipped to house a ferret solely for the purpose of donating blood. Therefore, a list should be maintained of clients willing to allow their pet to serve as a blood donor. Many owners have multiple ferrets and will allow one pet to serve as blood donor for another.

Transfusions are relatively safe, and crossmatching is not necessary in ferrets because blood groups have not been identified in this species. Indeed, repeated attempts were unsuccessful to identify naturally occurring erythrocyte antibodies or to experimentally induce erythrocyte antibodies (Manning and Bell, 1990). These findings suggest the safety of three transfusions, and probably more, from the same unrelated donor ferret.

## Obtaining Blood for Transfusions

Blood is collected from the jugular vein of the donor ferret using a 20- to 22-gauge butterfly catheter with a 12-cc syringe. The techniques for blood collection and safe volumes to collect have been discussed above. Aseptic technique should be used. Before drawing blood, an anticoagulant is flushed forward and back through the catheter and syringe. Acid citrate-dextrose (ACD) is the preferred anticoagulant and is used at 1 ml/6 ml of donor blood.

## Administering Blood Transfusions

Ferret blood is not stored but is administered immediately to the recipient ferret. The blood can be administered by the intravenous, intraosseous, or intraperitoneal route. The first two are preferred because of more rapid entry into the circulation.

### INTRAVENOUS ADMINISTRATION

Blood transfusions are administered through a butterfly catheter in the jugular vein or through a pre-placed IV catheter. A short indwelling IV catheter in the cephalic vein is tolerated relatively well by most ferrets. Ferret skin is tough; therefore, a small skin hole is made for catheter insertion by tenting the skin over the vein and inserting a 20-gauge needle through it (taking care not to pierce the vein). The catheter is then placed, taped into position, and maintained routinely.

### INTRAOSSEOUS ADMINISTRATION

If venous access is unavailable, the intraosseus route can be used. The recipient ferret, unless very weak, should probably be sedated for this technique (isoflurane by face mask works well). A 20-gauge, 1.5-inch spinal needle flushed with anticoagulant is inserted into the femur using aseptic technique in the same manner as for dogs and cats (Otto and Crowe, 1992; Palley et al., 1990). A 22-gauge spinal needle can be used for juvenile or small adult ferrets. The blood transfusion is then administered slowly through the spinal needle.

## References and Suggested Reading

Hillyer EV and Brown SA: Ferrets. *In* Birchard SJ and Sherding RG (eds): *Manual of Small Animal Practice.* Philadelphia, WB Saunders Co, 1993, p 1317.
   *An overview of pet ferret medicine and surgery, including preventive medicine, clinical techniques, basic physiologic values, and causes and treatment of anemia.*
Hoefer HL: Transfusions in exotic species. Probl Vet Med 4:625, 1992.
   *A description of blood collection and administration of blood transfusions in ferrets, including the care of blood donor ferrets.*
Manning DD and Bell JA: Lack of detectable blood groups in domestic ferrets: Implications for transfusion. J Am Vet Med Assoc 197:84, 1990.
   *A research study failed to detect erythrocyte antibodies in ferrets, suggesting that multiple transfusions can be given from the same donor to the same recipient ferret.*
O'Rourke LG: Practical blood transfusions. *In* Kirk RW (ed): *Current Veterinary Therapy VIII.* Philadelphia, WB Saunders Co, 1983, p 408.
   *The basic principles of collecting blood and administering blood transfusions in dogs and cats.*
Otto CM and Crowe DT Jr. Intraosseous resuscitation techniques and applications. *In* Kirk RW and Bonagura JD (eds): *Current Veterinary Therapy XI.* Philadelphia, WB Saunders Co, 1992, p 107.
   *A comprehensive review of the indications, complications, and techniques for placement of intraosseous catheters.*
Otto G, Rosenblad WD, and Fox JG: Practical venipuncture techniques for the ferret. Lab Anim 27:26, 1993.
   *A detailed description of a jugular venipuncture technique and a technique for intravascular injection into the cephalic vein in ferrets.*
Palley LS, Marini RP, Rosenblad WD, and Fox JG: A technique for femoral bone marrow collection in the ferret. Lab Anim Sci 40:654, 1990.
   *Description of the equipment and technique used to obtain bone marrow from the femur in anesthetized ferrets.*

# BLOOD COLLECTION TECHNIQUES IN AMPHIBIANS AND REPTILES

MICHELLE WILLETTE-FRAHM
*Brownsville, Texas*

Numerous venipuncture sites have been described in amphibians and reptiles. Each has its own advantages and disadvantages, and every clinician has his or her own personal preferences (Barten, 1993; Jacobson, 1988, 1992, 1993; Mautino and Page, 1993; Raphael, 1993). In addition, the size and health status of the patient will have a bearing on which site is chosen; some sites require immobilization in certain species.

In general, veterinarians should choose those sites with which he or she is most familiar and skilled. Necropsy specimens can be utilized to learn the anatomy

The author acknowledges the medical illustrations of Marina Peñalver.

of novel sites. In a healthy herptile, a maximum of 1% of the patient's body weight can be safely withdrawn at one setting (1 ml from a 100-gm specimen); lesser amounts should be removed from diseased patients over a longer period of time. Microtainer blood collection tubes (Becton Dickinson, Rutherford, NJ) are useful for handling small samples.

Herptile veins seem to collapse easily, so it is important to choose an appropriately sized needle and syringe, commonly a 1- or 3-cc syringe with a 25- or 22-gauge needle; larger syringes can be used with large patients and may require 1 1/2-inch, 20-gauge needles to reach deeper veins and to prevent bending of the needle. Avoid excessive negative pressure on the syringe to decrease the possibility of cell lysis. Herptile blood can coagulate rapidly and blood flow into the syringe may not be rapid or steady; additionally, it often results in very low serum yields. For these reasons, it may be helpful to coat the syringe and needle with an anticoagulant. Ethylenediaminetetraacetic acid (EDTA) can affect the morphology of some herptile blood cells and should not be used for complete blood count (CBC) samples. Heparin is a superior cell protectant and permits chemistries to be run off of the same sample. Remove all excess liquid heparin from the syringe and needle to avoid dilution of small samples, and place the sample into a serum tube, not into another heparinized container. An anticoagulant is neither required nor preferred when bleeding only for blood smears.

All locations should be aseptically prepared to prevent the introduction of pathogens. Clear fluid is frequently obtained initially and must be discarded or it will cause hemodilution. This is fluid from the lymphatic system that runs adjacent to the blood vessels, or pericardial fluid if performing cardiocentesis. When sufficient blood has been obtained, withdraw the needle and hold light pressure over the sight if accessible.

Once the sample is obtained, it should be processed rapidly. Herptile blood cells are very fragile, and making coverslip slides can result in fewer smudge cells and artifacts. Slides should be made immediately, as thin as possible, and quickly air dried. Some authors recommend fixing slides with absolute methanol (Frye, 1991) to preserve morphology, hemoparasites, and so forth, but enquire first with your reference laboratory, as some prefer unfixed slides. Techniques developed for avian hematology can be utilized; however, Crawshaw (1991) states that the eosinophil Unopette (Becton Dickinson, Rutherford, NJ) method is unsuitable for amphibian blood.

The hematologic and plasma biochemical values for numerous species have been published over the years, with a wide range of values cited. Differences in sample collection, processing, and analytic methodology make comparisons difficult. Many values are based on very small sample sizes. In addition, differences related to age, sex, reproductive state, season of the year, ambient temperature, disease processes, nutritional condition, and so forth occur and have been very poorly characterized.

In all aspects of amphibian and reptile clinical pathology, consistency is the key. Develop expertise with a few sites, always use the same technique, handle samples in an identical manner, utilize the same diagnostic laboratory (if not processed in house), and build a data base of normative blood values for those species commonly seen.

## TECHNIQUES FOR SELECTED SITES

### Cardiocentesis

This is one of the preferred sites of venipuncture in snakes and amphibians. Snakes should be securely restrained in dorsal recumbency (Fig. 1). The heart can be located by visualizing the beating organ or by palpation. Once pinpointed, the heart must be stabilized between the thumb and forefinger. Insert the needle under the posterior edge of a ventral scale overlying the apex of the heart. Advance the needle from the apex to the base of the heart under gentle negative pressure. Usually, blood will fill the syringe with each beat of the heart. Avoid multiple punctures.

Amphibians are also placed in dorsal recumbency (Fig. 2). The needle is directed under the xiphoid process at a 10- to 15-degree angle from the ventrum of the body. Cardiocentesis in chelonians requires penetration and subsequent repair of the plastron and is not recommended.

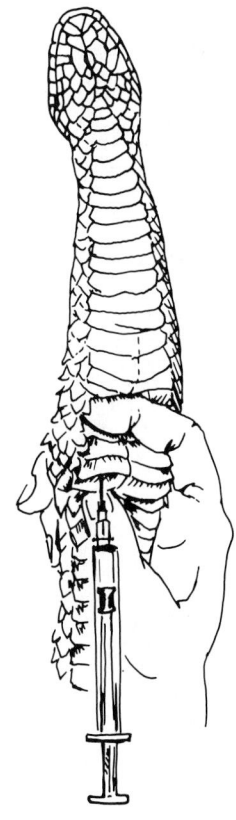

**Figure 1.** Restraint and positioning for cardiocentesis in snakes.

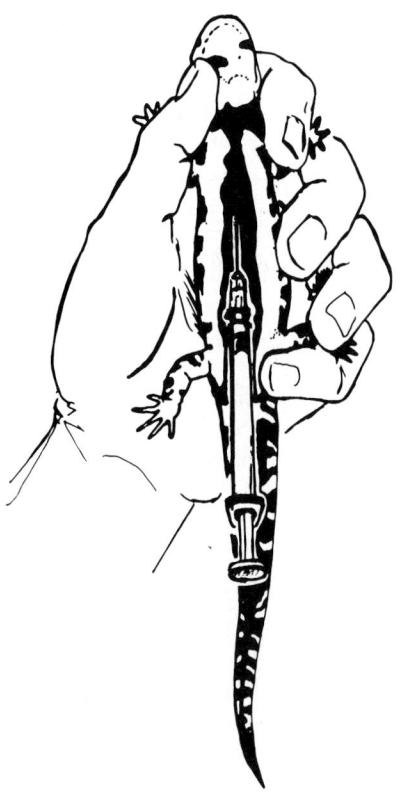

**Figure 2.** Restraint and positioning for cardiocentesis in amphibians.

## Coccygeal Vein

The ventral coccygeal vein is one of the preferred sites of venipuncture in snakes, lizards, and crocodilians, and the dorsal coccygeal vein is frequently successful in chelonians. For ventral coccygeal vein venipuncture, the animal is placed in dorsal recumbency and the tail is stabilized (Fig. 3). The needle is inserted on the midline (under the posterior edge of a ventral scale, if present), perpendicular to the long axis of the tail, and advanced until the tip touches the ventral surface of the vertebrae. The needle is then withdrawn slightly while under negative pressure until the sample is obtained. With small vessels, the needle may need to be redirected down to 45 degrees; some species of snakes have tails that are too small for venipuncture. In lizards, one third the distance between the vent and the tail tip is an optimum insertion point (Fig. 4). In large crocodilians, it is necessary to go further down the tail in order to reach the vessel. In male snakes and lizards, care must be taken to avoid the hemipenes, which are found on the lateral aspects of the cloaca (except in crocodilians, which have no hemipenes).

The dorsal coccygeal vein can be utilized for small amounts of blood in midsized or larger chelonians (Fig. 5). The procedure is identical except that the vein is approached on the dorsal midline close to where the vertebrae joins the carapace. Pulling the tail ventrally

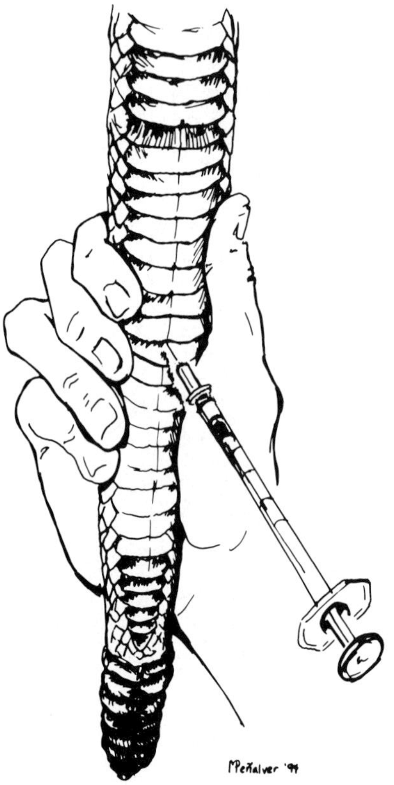

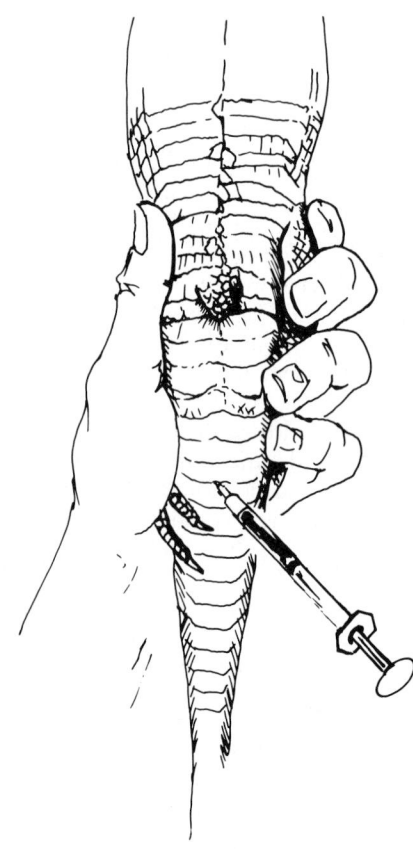

**Figure 3.** Restraint and positioning for venipuncture of the ventral coccygeal vein in snakes.

**Figure 4.** Restraint and positioning for venipuncture of the ventral coccygeal vein in lizards.

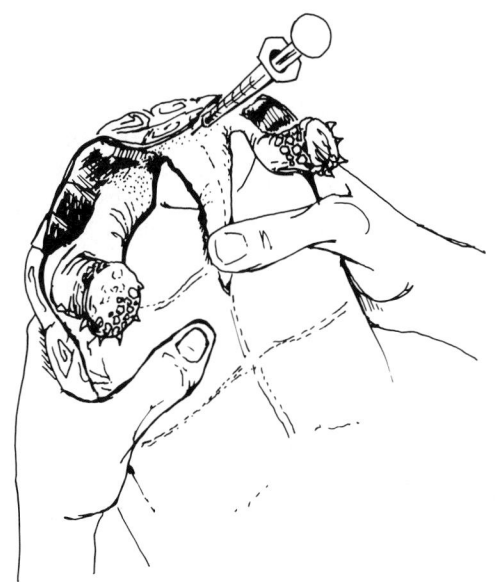

**Figure 5.** Restraint and positioning for venipuncture of the dorsal coccygeal vein in chelonians.

and putting a slight bend in the needle facilitates the process. If the animal thrashes the base of the tail, the attempt will be futile. Release the tail, and once still, locate the midline by palpation (appearances can be deceiving) and proceed again.

## Jugular Vein

The jugular vein is one of the preferred sites for venipuncture in chelonians, although it may require immobilization due to the strength, disposition, and anatomy of the animal (Fig. 6). Once restrained with the head and neck extended, the jugular vein can occasionally been seen; if not, it can be located at the 10 o'clock and 2 o'clock positions coursing from the area of the tympanic membrane ventrally to the thoracic inlet. It is approached rostrally in much the same manner as any jugular venipuncture.

## Brachial Vein

The brachial vein is frequently used for venipuncture in chelonians although, as with the above site, accessibility can be a problem (Fig. 7). Pushing the hindlimbs into the shell can sometimes force the forelimbs out, allowing them to be grasped and restrained. It is a blind approach on the ventromedial aspect of the forelimb just proximal to the carpal joint. The needle is held between 45 and 90 degrees perpendicular to the long access of the limb. It can require multiple attempts due to lymph contamination and inability to locate the vessel. Overextension of the limb can hinder procurement of the sample.

## Postoccipital Venous Sinus

This site is frequently used in some species of chelonians, primarily sea turtles and crocodilians. In sea turtles, the paired sinuses lie on either side of the midline in a concavity located in the curvature of the skull extending from the occiput laterally (Fig. 8). It is a blind approach, with the needle perpendicular to the long axis of the head and neck. It is stated that these sinuses are present in other species of chelonians (Frye, 1991).

In crocodilians, the site is more accurately described as a supravertebral vessel on the dorsal midline just distal to the occiput. The animal can be pithed at this site if the needle is advanced too deeply.

## Other Venipuncture Sites

The ventral abdominal vein can be used for venipuncture in lizards and amphibians. This vein lies on the midline just deep to the abdominal muscles. Caveats include internal bleeding and damage to adjacent vital organs. Small amounts of blood can be obtained from most species from the medial canthus of the orbit using microhematocrit tubes. It is frequently contami-

**Figure 6.** Restraint and positioning for venipuncture of the jugular vein in chelonians.

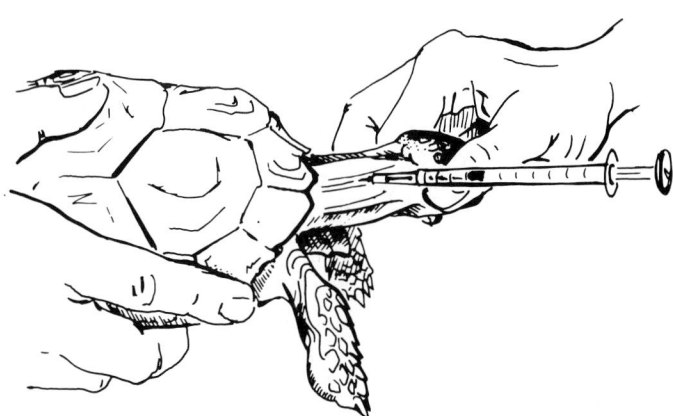

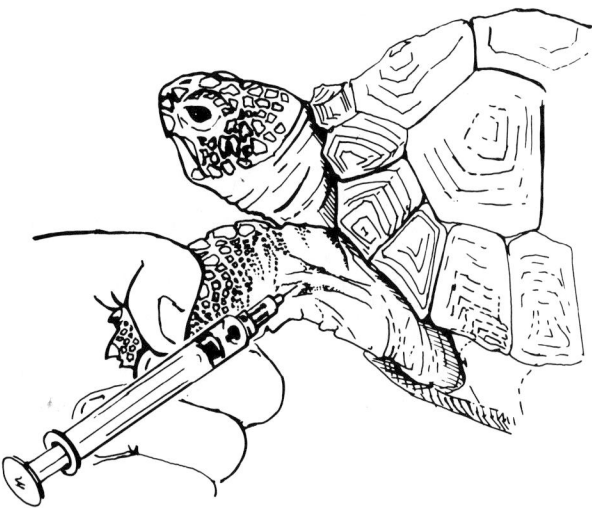

**Figure 7.** Restraint and positioning for venipuncture of the brachial vein in chelonians.

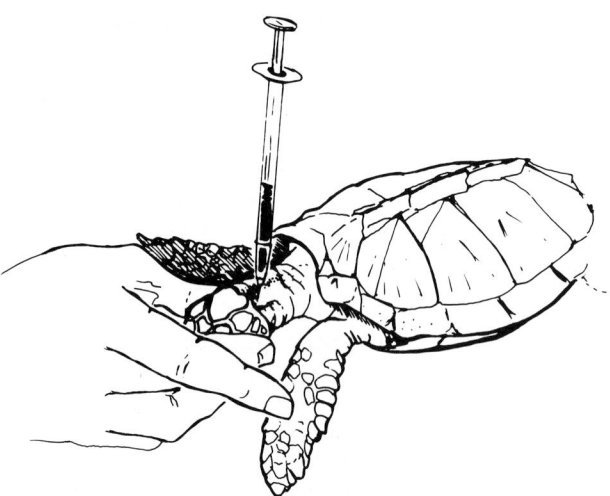

**Figure 8.** Restraint and positioning for venipuncture of the postoccipital sinus in chelonians.

nated with other ocular fluids; the cornea or spectacle may be damaged if overzealous. The palatine vein is located on the lateral aspects of the roof of the mouth; frequently, one side is larger than the other. Problems include those obvious to working inside the mouth. Other sites listed include the axillary plexus and the popliteal vein. The final and most accessible site for small amounts of blood in those animals with nails is to clip the toenail.

## References and Suggested Reading

Barten SL: The medical care of iguanas and other common pet lizards. *In* Quesenberry KE and Hillyer EV (eds): *The Veterinary Clinics of North America.* volume 23. *Exotic Pet Medicine I.* Philadelphia, WB Saunders Co, 1993, pp 1227–1229.
*An excellent overview of the most pertinent aspects of iguana and other common pet lizard husbandry, medicine and disease.*
Crawshaw GJ: Amphibian medicine. *In* Kirk RW and Bonagura JD (eds): *Current Veterinary Therapy XI.* Philadelphia, WB Saunders Co, 1992, p 1223.
*An excellent overview of amphibian physiology, husbandry, medicine, and disease.*
Frye FL: *Reptile Care—An Atlas of Diseases and Treatments.* Neptune City, NJ, TFH Publications, 1991.
*An extensive, well-illustrated text on reptile medicine.*
Jacobson ER: Evaluation of the reptile patient. *In* Jacobson ER and Kollias GV (eds): *Contemporary Issues in Small Animal Practice,* volume 9. *Exotic Animals.* New York, Churchill Livingstone, 1988, pp 8–9.
*An experienced review of the medical evaluation of reptile patients.*
Jacobson ER: Laboratory investigations. *In* Beynon PH, Lawton MPC, and Cooper JE (eds): *Manual of Reptiles.* Gloucestershire, British Small Animal Veterinary Association, 1992, pp 50–52.
*A British publication that presents a concise review of diagnostic and laboratory procedures involving reptiles.*
Jacobson ER: Snakes. *In* Quesenberry KE and Hillyer EV (eds): *The Veterinary Clinics of North America,* volume 23. *Exotic Pet Medicine I.* Philadelphia, WB Saunders Co, 1993, pp 1185, 1193.
*An excellent overview of the most pertinent aspects of snake medicine and disease.*
Mautino M and Page CD: Biology and medicine of turtles and tortoises. *In* Quesenberry KE and Hillyer EV (eds): *The Veterinary Clinics of North America,* volume 23. *Exotic Pet Medicine I.* Philadelphia, WB Saunders Co, 1993, pp 1256–1257.
*An excellent overview of the most pertinent aspects of chelonian medicine and disease.*
Raphael BL: Amphibians. *In* Quesenberry KE and Hillyer EV (eds): *The Veterinary Clinics of North America.* Volume 23. *Exotic Pet Medicine I.* Philadelphia: WB Saunders Co, 1993, p. 1276.
*An excellent overview of the most pertinent aspects of amphibian medicine and disease.*

# REPTILE ANESTHESIA

R. AVERY BENNETT

*Gainesville, Florida*

Veterinarians who treat reptiles are frequently faced with situations requiring chemical restraint or anesthesia. In chelonians able to retreat into their shell, or in large and intractable reptiles, even a physical examination or sampling for diagnostic evaluation may require sedation. The respiratory anatomy and physiology of reptiles and their unique response to many of the commonly used anesthetic agents can present a significant challenge. Methods used for immobilizing reptiles in the past such as hypothermia and ether have been shown to cause serious metabolic consequences and, in the case of hypothermia, may be considered inhumane. Recently, both inhalant and injectable agents have been used clinically with a wide margin of safety, making it possible to perform a variety of surgical procedures.

## RESPIRATORY ANATOMY AND PHYSIOLOGY

The trachea of squamate reptiles (lizards and snakes) is composed of incomplete, C-shaped tracheal rings with a dorsal tracheal membrane connecting the ends of each ring (Bennett, 1991). The tracheas of crocodilians and chelonians (turtles and tortoises) are composed of complete tracheal rings. Chelonians have a relatively short trachea and care must be taken when placing an endotracheal tube to avoid intubation of a single lung. Compared with the lungs of mammals, those of reptiles are structurally much simpler with a larger tidal volume but smaller surface area for gas exchange. In some reptiles, they are simple endothelium-lined sacs that are attached to the main bronchi. However, there is variation in the complexity of the lungs, with those of crocodilians approaching that of mammalian lungs. In some species, the sac-like lungs have ridges on the surface, creating a reticular pattern that increases the surface area for gas exchange. In others, there are invaginations or folding of the lung wall, creating partitions within the lung and air chambers that further increase the surface area of the lung. The left lung is absent or vestigial in most snakes; it is most developed in the boids (boas and pythons). The right lung extends very far caudally in snakes, approaching the level of the vent. Here, the lung becomes thin and loses the reticular pattern on its surface to become an air sac. Some lizards also have air sacs, the function of which remains speculative. The lungs of reptiles are very fragile and care must be taken when positive-pressure ventilation is performed to avoid rupture of the lung.

The glottis of reptiles remains closed between breaths, but opens for respiration through the function of a glottis dilator muscle. The larynx is generally located rostrally in the mouth at the base of the tongue, making it easy to locate and intubate. In chelonians, the tongue is thick and fleshy, making it more difficult to identify the glottis. Crocodilians have a well-developed epiglottis (basihyal valve) on the ventral floor of the pharynx. This allows them to open their mouth while underwater without aspirating. This valve must be depressed in order to identify the glottis for intubation.

There are two mechanisms by which reptiles create pressure changes within the lungs to establish air movement. Since they do not have a functional muscular diaphragm, they have a combined pleuroperitoneum or coelomic cavity. Chelonians have a membranous separation between the abdominal and thoracic viscera, while crocodilians have the most developed pseudodiaphragm. In most reptiles, the muscles of the abdomen and trunk augment the function of the intercostal muscles to generate negative pressure. In chelonians, which do not have intercostal muscles, changes in the position of the abdominal viscera, limbs, and pelvic girdle are responsible for creating pressure differences within the lungs. At a surgical plane of anesthesia, the function of the skeletal muscles may be lost, making it necessary to assist ventilation. Furthermore, when the patient is positioned in dorsal recumbency, the viscera may compress the lungs, reducing their tidal volume and making assistance of ventilation even more important. The second mechanism used for ventilation in reptiles relies on smooth muscle present within the lung wall. This muscle contracts and relaxes, changing the volume of the lung and moving air. This mechanism allows reptiles to breathe even when there is a defect in the body wall as occurs in chelonians missing a portion of their shell or during celiotomy.

In addition to alveolar ventilation, reptiles may employ other surfaces for gas exchange, such as cloacal and pharyngeal mucosa. Cutaneous gas exchange is also a mechanism for respiration in some reptiles. Many reptiles are capable of converting to anaerobic metabolism when they "breath-hold." Turtles of the genus *Pseudemys* have been shown to be able to survive in an environment of 100% nitrogen for up to 27 hr, and green iguanas (*Iguana iguana*) for up to 4.5 hr.

## PREANESTHETIC MEDICATIONS

If the patient's condition permits, preanesthetic fasting is recommended. Aspiration is not common in reptiles because the glottis is closed at rest; however, because the tidal volume is affected by visceral volume, fasting may allow for improved ventilation. Supplemental heat should be provided to ensure that the patient's body systems are functioning efficiently. It is best to try to maintain the patient within its preferred temperature range (approximately 29.5°C [85°F]). Balanced electrolyte solutions may be administered at a rate of 5 ml/kg/hr IV, IP, or SC and are especially indicated for procedures of more than 1 hr duration.

### Anticholinergics

Information on the efficacy of anticholinergics in reptiles is anecdotal; however, atropine sulfate at 0.01 to 0.04 mg/kg IM or IP or glycopyrrolate at 0.01 mg/kg IM or SC should be given 10 to 15 min prior to induction of anesthesia to decrease oral secretions and reduce the risk of inducing profound bradycardia (Boyer, 1992). These complications have not been observed in most studies regardless of the use of anticholinergics. Their use may be most appropriate for small reptiles, where even a small amount of oral secretion may plug an endotracheal tube.

### Tranquilizers

Tranquilizers given as preanesthetic medications may decrease the amount of induction and maintenance agent required during anesthesia. They are also beneficial for reducing patient excitement and smoothing induction and recovery.

PHENOTHIAZINES. Acepromazine at 0.1 to 0.5 mg/kg IM approximately 1 hr prior to induction of anesthesia has been reported to smooth induction and reduce the amount of induction agent required. Chlorpromazine has shown similar effects in chelonians (10 mg/kg IM).

BENZODIAZEPINES. Diazepam at 0.22 to 0.62 mg/kg 20 min prior to the administration of succinylcholine to American alligators (*Alligator mississippiensis*) resulted in sedation of the animals for smoother induction and also lowered the required dose of succinylcholine for immobilization. Midazolam at 2 mg/kg also augmented the effects of ketamine in snapping turtles (*Chelydra serpentina*) but failed to sedate painted turtles (*Chrysemys picta*). Zolazepam is a benzodiazepine used in combination with tiletamine to eliminate the seizures and muscle rigidity associated with tiletamine.

## INJECTABLE ANESTHETICS

These anesthetics require little equipment but, once given, the effects and depth of anesthesia cannot be controlled. Many are most effective when given by the IV route, which may not be feasible with some reptile patients. The effects of most injectable agents in reptiles are often unpredictable. The same dose given to two different animals may yield no effect in one while producing profound anesthesia in the other. Reptiles have a relatively slow metabolism and the effects of injectable agents are usually prolonged, with induction requiring hours and recovery up to several days.

### Narcotics

Reptiles seem to require unusually high doses of narcotics to produce sedative or anesthetic effects, making them of little value in reptile anesthesia. It is unknown why reptiles are refractory to opiates or whether these agents produce analgesia.

### Barbiturates

Barbiturates generally have a long and unpredictable induction time and a very long recovery period. Size, condition, nutritional status, temperature, handling, and physiology of the individual animal may influence the effects of barbiturates, making their use in reptiles questionable. The mechanism of elimination of these agents in reptiles is unknown; however, the duration of effect of thiobarbiturates is similar to that of longer acting agents, indicating that reptiles rely on metabolism of these agents rather than redistribution to nonnervous tissue for termination of their effect. Increasing the environmental temperature may speed recovery by increasing the metabolic rate and the efficiency of enzyme systems. Doses for various barbiturates have been reported (Bennett, 1991).

In mammals, methohexital is an ultra–short-acting barbiturate anesthetic that is rapidly detoxified rather than being metabolized or redistributed to non-nervous tissues. Its action in reptiles appears to be similar, being three times more potent and having an onset of action three times faster than thiopental sodium. There is a significant variation in response to this agent at the recommended dose of 5 to 20 mg/kg SC. A 0.125% solution should be used for patients weighing less than 5 gm, 0.25% for lizards 4.5 to 39 gm, 0.5% solution for snakes 5 to 100 gm, and a 1.0% solution for animals more than 100 gm. Some species appear to be especially sensitive to this agent and the dose should be reduced when working with young animals (Bennett, 1991).

### Dissociative Anesthetics

KETAMINE. Ketamine has been successfully used in all orders of reptiles. The response is dose dependent, but also varies with the species and individual. It is most useful for sedation or for induction of anesthesia for intubation, especially in "breath-holding" species. A dose of 22 to 44 mg/kg IM or SC has been recommended for sedation and 55 to 88 mg/kg for surgical anesthesia. It appears that, consistent with concepts of metabolic scaling, larger reptiles require a smaller per-kilogram dosage than smaller patients (Boyer, 1992). Generally, at doses above 110 mg/kg, respiratory arrest and decreased heart rate make ventilatory support essential. Induction usually occurs in 10 to 30 min and recovery from 24 to 96 hr. Additional doses of 10 mg/kg may be administered at 30-min intervals to maintain anesthesia. Even at surgical anesthesia, some animals will exhibit serpentine movement. Ketamine may be a satisfactory injectable anesthetic, but when used in debilitated or compromised patients, recovery may be dangerously prolonged (up to 6 days). The mechanism for elimination of ketamine in reptiles is unknown. It is excreted unchanged by the kidneys in cats but must be metabolized by the liver prior to excretion in dogs. Reptiles have a renal portal system, so the majority of blood from the caudal half of the reptile passes through the kidney prior to reaching the systemic circulation. If ketamine is excreted unchanged by the kidney, injection in the caudal half of the body may diminish the effect of the drug.

TILETAMINE-ZOLAZEPAM (TELAZOL). Tiletamine's action is similar to that of ketamine but is two to three times more potent, which makes the volume of administration smaller. Tiletamine alone causes seizures and severe muscle rigidity; however, in combination with zolazepam, with which it is synergistic, it produces anesthesia, analgesia, and muscle relaxation with anticonvulsant and antianxiety effects. There is great species variation in response to this agent. In early studies with this agent, doses as high as 88 mg/kg were used to produce anesthesia. At such doses, the animals were anesthetized for up to 16 hr, with a recovery time of more than 22 hr. Because of the rapid onset of effect, Telazol may be most useful as a tranquilizing agent or an induction agent for maintenance with inhalant anesthetics. A dose of 4 to 5 mg/kg IM will provide sedation adequate for performing diagnostic procedures or for intubation. At most doses, animals are sensitive to stimulation, resulting in excessive movement. Because of this, it is not acceptable as the sole agent for anesthesia in reptiles.

## Neuromuscular Blocking Agents

Neuromuscular blockers have primarily been used for restraint of large crocodilians and chelonians. Depolarizing blockers mimic the effect of acetylcholine at the neuromuscular end plates, but bind more tightly, so the end plates are depolarized for a longer period of time. They are metabolized by cholinesterases freeing the end-plate receptors, allowing normal neuromuscular function. Nondepolarizing blockers block the acetylcholine receptors. Their effects are reversible with agents such as neostigmine. Succinylcholine is a depolarizing agent and is the neuromuscular blocking agent used most commonly in reptiles. The dosage appears to be variable among species and sizes. For chelonians, 0.5 to 1.0 mg/kg is recommended; 0.75 to 1.0 mg/kg for large lizards such as monitors; and 0.5 to 2.0 mg/kg for crocodilians (Boyer, 1992; Johnson, 1991). Paralysis occurs 5 to 30 min following injection. It is very important to administer this agent intramuscularly

because the drug may not be absorbed rapidly enough to be effective when administered subcutaneously. Because of the risk of prolonged respiratory paralysis requiring assisted ventilation, the lack of analgesic properties, and the relatively narrow margin of safety, neuromuscular blocking agents are not commonly used.

Other neuromuscular blockers have been used with variable success, including nondepolarizing agents such as gallamine triethiodide and d-tubocurarine chloride (Bennett, 1991). All of these agents may cause respiratory paralysis, requiring that the patient be intubated and ventilated until spontaneous breathing resumes.

## INHALANT ANESTHETICS

Inhalant anesthesia has become the standard of practice for many species, including reptiles. These agents offer several advantages over injectable agents and many can be used without a precision vaporizer in reptile patients. When the patient is intubated and a precision vaporizer is used, anesthetic depth can be controlled, the patient is receiving supplemental oxygen and may be ventilated, recovery is usually quick once the anesthetic gas is discontinued, and an accurate patient weight is not critical.

Endotracheal intubation and assisted ventilation are recommended. The normal respiratory rate for most reptiles is 10 to 20 breaths per minute. Because the inspired concentration of oxygen will be higher than that of room air, an assisted ventilation rate of 2 to 4 breaths per minute and a pressure of less than 20 cm $H_2O$ are adequate during assisted ventilation. Ventilating to excessive inspiratory pressures may result in pulmonary rupture. In chelonians and crocodilians with complete tracheal rings that do not expand, care should be taken to not overinflate a cuffed tube which could result in tracheal damage.

A nonrebreathing system is indicated for patients less than 5 kg with an oxygen flow rate of twice the minute volume (flow rate = 300 to 500 ml/kg/min). Larger reptiles may be maintained using a circle system with 2 to 4 L/min oxygen for induction and 1 to 2 L/min for maintenance because the flow rate required for a nonrebreathing system is prohibitively high.

When using an open drop technique, the concentration of anesthetic gas within the container cannot be accurately controlled and varies with the volume of the container, the volume that the patient displaces, the amount of gas taken up by the patient, and the environmental temperature. Some agents may reach concentrations that would be dangerous for anesthetizing mammals; however, some species of reptiles may not be affected by concentrations achieved using a precision vaporizer. Finally, it may not be possible to induce some breath-holding species with inhalant anesthetics.

## Methoxyflurane

Methoxyflurane (MOF) has a slow induction and recovery when compared with other fluorinated hydrocarbon volatile anesthetics. At 20°C, MOF reaches a maximum concentration of 3%. The open drop technique can be used placing 10 ml MOF in a 42,800-cm³ box. A single exposure provides 10 to 30 min of surgical anesthesia. If more time is needed, the patient should be intubated and maintained using a precision vaporizer. In mammals, approximately 50% of the drug is metabolized by the liver, making its use in patients with liver disease inappropriate. Elapids and some pythons may be especially sensitive to this agent.

### Halothane

Halothane may be used for induction using a precision vaporizer or the open drop method. With the vaporizer, induction may be achieved using 2.0 to 5.5% halothane in oxygen and maintenance using 1.5 to 2.5%. The concentration should be gradually increased to minimize irritation, which may induce breath-holding. There is generally an excitement phase just prior to complete relaxation during induction with halothane. Recovery usually occurs approximately 10 min after the anesthetic is discontinued. At 20°C, the maximum attainable concentration that can be reached with halothane is 32%. For the open drop technique, 5 ml halothane is placed in a 2840-cm³ (1 cu ft) box. Induction with this technique occurs in 5 to 33 min and has a duration of 5 to 20 min following a single exposure. These times are prolonged when the environmental temperature is outside the range of 24 to 30°C (Boyer, 1992). Venomous species appear to require a higher concentration of halothane than nonvenomous species and viperids require more than elapids. In mammals, only 12% is metabolized by the liver, the remainder being eliminated by the respiratory system.

### Isoflurane

Isoflurane is eliminated almost exclusively by the lungs in mammals and, therefore, causes minimal metabolic compromise, making it the agent of choice for use in debilitated or compromised patients. A concentration of 4 to 5% isoflurane in 3 to 4 L/min oxygen has been used to induce anesthesia in 6 to 20 min. Maintenance at 1.5 to 4% isoflurane results in recovery in 30 to 60 min. In common snapping turtles administered isoflurane at 5% for 90 min, the level of anesthesia was less than that achieved with ketamine and midazolam. Because it has a vapor pressure and maximum concentration similar to halothane, the open drop method of induction should be as effective for isoflurane as for halothane, though controlled studies are lacking.

### ANESTHETIC MONITORING

As reptiles become anesthetized, relaxation progresses from cranial to caudal, and during recovery motor function returns in the opposite direction. The righting reflex (turning over when placed in dorsal recumbency) is lost early during anesthetic induction but is a useful indicator of recovery. Failure to elevate the ribs when a finger is run down the back or failure to move the tail when the vent (in snakes) or foot is squeezed indicates loss of spinal reflexes and a surgical plane of anesthesia. This reflex may be slow but not lost in crocodilians at a plane of surgical anesthesia. In chelonians, the head withdrawal reflex (retracting the head when it is gently pulled from within the shell borders) is also useful. The corneal reflex (except in snakes and some lizards with spectacles) should be present at a surgical plane and when absent the patient is excessively deep. Tongue withdrawal in snakes (retracting the tongue when it is pulled from the sheath) is present at a surgical plane and lost if the patient is too deep. At a surgical plane of anesthesia, many patients will lose motor function, including the ability to ventilate spontaneously. Assisted ventilation will help maintain a proper acid-base balance and prevent the patient from converting to anaerobic metabolism.

Often an anesthetized reptile will suddenly go from a state of surgical anesthesia to appearing to be fully awake. This is probably because of the tendency to keep the patient as light as possible, but also because it is more difficult to accurately evaluate the depth of anesthesia in reptiles.

It is somewhat difficult to monitor vital signs during anesthesia in reptiles because it can be difficult to visualize respiratory and cardiac movements. The three-chambered heart of most reptiles does not produce readily auscultable sounds, making stethoscopy difficult. In snakes, it may be possible to visualize cardiac movement; however, patient draping and movements caused by the surgeon may inhibit accurate assessment of heart rate. An electrocardiographic (ECG) monitor is very valuable in monitoring the anesthetized reptile patient. The presence of electrical cardiac activity is reassuring; however, the QRS patterns of reptiles are generally inverted and slurred. The heart rate should remain steady throughout the procedure, and a decrease in rate indicates the patient is excessively deep.

A Doppler blood flow monitor provides an audible signal that monitors blood flow. A small amount of contact gel should be utilized and the crystal placed over the heart. The sounds of blood flowing through the heart confirm proper placement and it may then be taped in place for the duration of the procedure. This device also works for chelonians; however, the creptal must be placed in the thoracic ineto.

Recovery should occur in a quiet environment with the temperature and humidity at the upper end of the optimum range. Excessive warmth may be deleterious by excessively increasing the patient's metabolic activity, which increases tissue oxygen demand. During recovery, the patient may be stimulated by pinching a toe or the tail, causing the animal to move and take a breath. Doxapram at 5 mg/kg IV may be used to stimulate respiration (Boyer, 1992).

In some cases, it is possible to revive patients that

demonstrate apnea and apparent cardiac arrest. Because reptiles are capable of converting to anaerobic metabolism, the tissues are capable of surviving even several hours of hypoxia. The patient must be ventilated at least once per minute to make oxygen available when cardiopulmonary function returns and, if inhalant anesthetics were used, to aid in the elimination of the agent. Cardiac function may be supported by intermittent external cardiac compression. There are numerous anecdotal reports of reptiles surviving several hours of cardiopulmonary arrest.

There is still much to be learned regarding chemical immobilization in reptiles. The following key points should be emphasized when approaching anesthesia in reptiles. The patient should be maintained within its optimum temperature during the entire experience for proper metabolic function. During general anesthesia, the patient should be intubated and ventilation assisted

if possible. The low end of the dosage range should be used until the clinician is comfortable with the agent and the effects produced in reptile patients. Based on metabolic scaling, larger patients require a smaller per-kilogram dosage. The patient's depth of anesthesia and vital signs must be constantly and carefully monitored. Anesthesia is an important part of clinical reptile medicine and surgery but can be challenging.

### References and Suggested Reading

Bennett RA: A review of anesthesia and chemical restraint in reptiles. J Zoo Wildl Med 22:282, 1991.
   *General review of reptile anesthesia.*
Boyer TH: Clinical anesthesia of reptiles. Bull Assoc Rept Amph Vet 2:10, 1992.
   *Review of reptile anesthesia.*
Johnson JH: Anesthesia, analgesia and euthanasia of reptiles and amphibians. *Proc Am Assoc Zoo Vet*, Calgary, Canada, 1991, pp 132–138.
   *Review of reptile anesthesia and euthanasia.*

# CLINICAL REPTILIAN MICROBIOLOGY

THOMAS H. BOYER

*Fort Collins, Colorado*

Mammalian veterinarians may question why cultures and sensitivities are crucial for treating bacterial infections in reptiles. The answer is twofold. First, reptiles respond very slowly to antibiotic treatment. The author typically treats bacterial infections in reptiles for a minimum of 3 weeks and often longer, and sensitivity results can be available within a week, well before the patient shows any clinical response. Second, many bacterial infections in reptiles yield several bacteria, each with different sensitivity patterns. Thus, culture and sensitivity ensure proper antibiotic selection and improve clinical efficacy.

## CULTURE COLLECTION, TRANSPORT, AND SUBMISSION

Specimens for culture should be collected prior to antibiotic treatment so that bacterial growth is not inhibited. Standard sterile swabs can be used for sampling a variety of lesions. After sampling, the swab should be immediately placed in a commercial anaerobic, facultative, and aerobic transport medium, such as the BBL Port-A-Cul tubes (Beckton Dickinson, Cockeysville, MD). One study found that more than half of reptilian bacterial cultures with growth yielded anaerobes (Stewart, 1990). Thus, bacterial culture of reptiles should routinely include anaerobic culture. Chlamydial, mycobacterial, mycloplasmal, and fungal infections are

sufficiently rare and difficult to culture that routine culture for them is not recommended unless histopathology or cytology indicates otherwise (Jacobson, 1992).

Skin lesions should be swabbed at the periphery. Abscesses may be filled with solid cellular debris or, less commonly, liquid cellular debris. Disinfect the surface of the abscess and débride it with a sterile blade, then take a culture from deep within. Gloves should be worn, as reptilian abscesses may contain acid-fast bacteria and many potentially pathogenic gram-negative organisms (Needham, 1981; Frye, 1991). Abscesses in close proximity to bone should be radiographed before débridement to ascertain bone involvement (Cooper, 1981). Likewise, in cases of infectious stomatitis, cultures should be collected from within the infected tissue, rather than swabbing the gingival surfaces (Mader, 1993).

Respiratory tract infections are common in snakes and chelonians and should also be cultured. Tracheal washes are one method of sampling lung bacteria. An appropriately sized sterile urinary catheter is carefully inserted through the open glottis and down to the respiratory portion of the lung. In large chelonians, this procedure may be facilitated by the administration of 50 mg/kg ketamine SC. In boid and colubrid snakes, the respiratory porton of the lung lies caudal to the heart and cranial to the liver; in viperids, the respiratory portion of the lung is cranial to the heart. Sterile saline (approximately 1% of the reptile's body weight) can be infused into the lung field, withdrawn, and examined for parasites, cytology, and bacterial culture. Do not be concerned if all the saline is not retrieved; the lungs will absorb it.

A practical, and medically reasonable, alternative to tracheal wash is glottal culture, especially if cost or large snake size is a limiting factor. Once the reptile's mouth is open, a swab is passed through the glottis during inhalation to sample the glottal rimb, or exudate within the glottus. Once again, avoid oral mucosa. Although more studies are necessary, in four boids, Hilif, Wagner, and Yu (1990) found the results of glottal cultures to be similar to tracheal wash cultures.

Cloacal cultures are indicated in reptiles with diarrhea if fecal examinations and cloacal or colonic washes are negative, especially as regards protozoans (Mader, 1993).

Bacterial culture at necropsy is also useful. Obvious lesions can be incised and cultured. If no lesions are grossly discernable, atrial blood cultures can be performed. Remove the pericardial sac and proceed with sterile preparation of the atrial surface. A swab can easily be inserted through a small atrial incision or blood collected with a syringe and needle for blood culture. Eggs can be cultured, after sterile preparation of the egg shell, in a similar manner.

The author utilizes commercial laboratories because the time, expense, and expertise required for small-scale aerobic and anaerobic microbiology is not cost-effective. The sealed culture should be enclosed in a Zip-Loc bag and mailed, or delivered, to the laboratory for appropriate culture and sensitivity.

Appropriate incubation temperature for reptilian cultures are uncertain. Standard incubation temperatures for isolation of pathogenic bacteria is 37°C; however, most reptiles prefer temperatures well below this. Needham (1981) noted that in many cases more organisms were isolated from reptilian cultures grown at 25°C.

Combined oral/cloacal cultures (culture of the oral cavity followed by culture of the cloaca with the same swab) grow a myriad of potential pathogens, but are not recommended (Mader, 1993) because interpretation is haphazard. It is much more meaningful to sample specific sites. It is important to note that "normal" reptilian flora contains many potential pathogens, yet prophylactic treatment is generally not recommended.

## COMMON BACTERIAL ISOLATES IN REPTILES

### Normal Bacterial Flora

Only a few studies have examined what constitutes normal flora in reptiles. Oral cultures of healthy snakes have revealed gram-positive bacteria (coagulase-negative *Staphyloccus*, *Corynebacterium* spp.), gram-negative bacteria (*Providencia rettgeri*, *Pseudomonas* spp., and a wide variety of other coccobacilli and rods), anaerobes (*Clostridium* spp. and *Bacteroides*), and also no growth

(Hilif, Wagner, and Yu, 1990; Draper, Walker, and Lawler, 1981; Soveri and Seuna, 1986). Cloacal cultures reveal similar results except that *Arizona* and *Salmonella* are much more common (Draper, Walker, and Lawler, 1981). One study (Hilif, Wagner, and Yu, 1990) examined serial samples and noted that bacterial species isolated varied over time. Others concluded that the presence of common environmental bacteria, wide variation between snakes, and bacteriologically negative samples indicated a lack of specific oral autochthonous flora (Soveri and Seuna, 1986). Rather, oral bacteria in snakes may represent transient environmental bacteria. The type of food did not have any effect on the flora. Cloacal cultures are rarely without growth; this could indicate that the lower intestinal tract is persistently colonized. Perhaps these bacteria are one source of environmental bacteria for snakes (Soveri and Seuna, 1986).

Another study compared the bacterial flora of healthy captive and free-ranging tortoises, as well as clinical and necropsy samples from tortoises with respiratory illness. Major differences were not observed in bacterial flora from the mouth, nares, trachea, lungs, and cloaca of the different groups. Overall, bacteria were similar to those seen in snakes except for the conspicuous absence of *Pseudomonas* and *Aeromonas*, and the presence of *Pasteurella*.

*Aeromonas hydrophila* was frequently isolated from the oral cavity, external jaw area, and internal tissues of American alligators in different localities. *Aeromonas* should be considered part of the normal flora of alligators, but can be pathogenic under adverse conditions.

An obvious conclusion from these studies is that many potential pathogens are present in healthy reptiles. Cooper (1981) noted a predominance of gram-negative bacteria (*Escherichia coli*, *Proteus* spp., *Aeromonas* spp., and *Pseudomonas aeruginosa*) from feces, cloacal swabs, gut contents, skin, and external orifices of snakes, lizards, and chelonians in captivity. Under suboptimal environmental conditions, these bacteria may become opportunistic pathogens. A common predisposing condition is too cool environmental temperature.

### Opportunistic Pathogens

The following is a list of the most common bacteria, in the author's experience, cultured from diseased reptiles. They are listed in rough estimate of frequency. Many of these bacteria are found in mixed culture, making interpretation of individual pathogenicity difficult. As noted, many of these same bacteria can be present in healthy animals. Once again, it is important to treat patients, not lab results.

#### PSEUDOMONAS

*Pseudomonas aeruginosa* is perhaps the most common bacterial cause of disease, although a wide variety of other species (*P. maltophida*, *P. fluorescans*, *P. ce-*

*pacia*) also cause infectious disease. *Pseudomonas spp.* are frequently isolated from infectious stomatitis, hepatic and respiratory tract infections, skin infections (especially burns), septicemias, necrotizing enteritis, and abscesses of snakes, lizards, and crocodilians.

### ESCHERICHIA

*Escherichia coli* is a common gram-negative pathogen. It can be associated with infectious stomatitis, respiratory and hepatic disease, skin infections, abscesses, bone and joint infections, and conjunctivitis.

### ANAEROBIC BACTERIA

Anaerobic bacteria are common pathogens in reptiles but are often missed because anaerobic culture is not performed. Many different species have been isolated from the following genera: *Clostridium, Bacteroides, Fusobacterium, Propionibacterium,* and *Peptostreptococcus.* Anaerobic bacteria are frequently encountered in abscesses located in subcutaneous tissues, liver, bone, or the middle ear of chelonians and with respiratory tract infections.

### MORGANELLA

Another common aerobic reptile pathogen, *Morganella morgani,* can cause septicemia, abscesses, respiratory and hepatic disease, conjunctivitis, infectious stomatitis, and skin infections.

### SALMONELLA AND ARIZONA

Many different serotypes of *Salmonella* and *Arizona* can be cultured from reptiles. For expediency, the rest of this discussion will refer to both simply as *Salmonella.* Two surveys of large zoologic reptile collections commonly found *Salmonella.* Snakes and lizards had the highest carriage rate (one fourth to one half of snakes, and one third of lizards). Interestingly, chelonians had very low rates (11% and 3%). Amphibians generally failed to culture positive for *Salmonella,* although wild amphibian populations in close association with humans may culture positive.

All reptiles, except perhaps crocodilians, should be considered potential asymptomatic carriers of *Salmonella.* A single negative fecal culture does not mean the reptile is not a carrier. To better determine the absence of *Salmonella,* fecal cultures should be repeated one or two more times at 2-week intervals (Mader, 1993). Treatment of healthy reptiles for *Salmonella* may not eliminate it, but instead may select for antibiotic resistance. Given this, and the expense of repeated fecal cultures, the author does not recommend routine screening of reptiles for *Salmonella.* Rather, the owners are advised *Salmonella* is common in reptiles, and the following precautions (Mader, 1993) should be observed:

1. Do not eat or put anything in your mouth while working with reptiles.

2. Do not clean cages in the kitchen or food preparation areas.

3. Wash your hands with iodine-based soaps (Betadine, Wescondyne, Prepodyne) after working with reptiles.

4. Clean cages and water bowls on a regular basis or whenever soiled.

5. Have your veterinarian perform necropsies on reptiles that die suddenly and check for *Salmonella.*

6. Infants, people under medical care from their physician (such as antibiotic or immunosuppressive therapy), or people with immunodeficiencies should not handle reptiles or their cages.

7. Notify your physician if you have symptoms of salmonellosis (acute enterocolitis, headache, abdominal pain, diarrhea, nausea, vomiting, fever).

Although *Salmonella* has been associated with septicemia, hepatic and respiratory disease, enterocolitis, abscesses, and infectious stomatitis, it most often is asymptomatic. In snakes, *Salmonella* septicemias are often associated with protozoal infections (Jacobson, 1988). Cooper (1981) and Mader (1993) suggest euthanasia of clinically affected reptiles. This seems reasonable for high-risk humans (infants <1 year of age, immunosuppressed individuals).

### PROTEUS

*Proteus mirablis* and *P. vulgaris* are frequent gram-negative pathogens encountered in infectious stomatitis, respiratory disease, abscesses, wounds, and conjunctivitis. It also is normally found in lizards and snakes. It was found more frequently in fecal cultures of diseased tortoises compared to healthy tortoises.

### STREPTOCOCCUS

*Streptococcus spp.* have been isolated from respiratory tract infections, infectious stomatitis, and skin infections. Their significance is unknown but should be considered as capable of causing disease.

### KLEBSIELLA

*Klebsiella* pathogens in reptiles include *K. pneumoniae* and *K. oxytoca.* It is common in lizards, snakes, and turtles as a cause of infectious stomatitis, respiratory disease, abscesses, and skin and ocular infections.

### CITROBACTER

*Citrobacter freundii* is a common isolate from abscesses, infectious stomatitis, respiratory tract infections, and septicemias. At one time, *C. freundii* was thought to be the causative agent of septicemic cutaneous ulcerative disease (SCUD). This disease causes necrotic ulcers on the shell and skin of aquatic turtles, particularly soft-shelled turtles. However, other gram-negative pathogens cause similar lesions (Frye, 1991).

## PROVIDENCIA

*Providencia rettgeri* is a common isolate from healthy boids (Hilif, Wagner, and Yu, 1990) but not colubrids or viperids (Draper, Walker, and Lawler, 1981). It has also been recovered from infectious stomatitis and respiratory tract infections. Its presence should be evaluated with respect to other isolates and the condition of the animal.

## AEROMONAS

In the past, *Aeromonas hydrophila* had been classified as a pseudomonad. Veterinary literature frequently implies *Aeromonas* is as common a pathogen as *Pseudomonas*. In the author's experience it is much less common than *Pseudomonas* except in those animals housed in aquatic environments, such as amphibians and crocodilians. *Aeromonas* has frequently been implicated in "red-leg" and cutaneous ulcerative diseases of amphibians. It can also cause peripheral, necrotizing, hemorrhagic skin lesions in alligators under adverse environmental conditions. *Aeromonas* has also been found commonly in abscesses, respiratory tract infections, infectious stomatitis, and septicemias in other reptiles. Proper water quality control is essential in outbreaks of aeromoniasis. Affected reptiles should be checked for ectoparasites, as *Aeromonas* can be spread by snake mites (Mader, 1993).

## ENTEROBACTER

*Enterobacter cloacae* is most often recovered from oral and cloacal cultures and abscesses.

## CORYNEBACTERIUM

Several studies have found the prevalence of this gram-positive bacteria to vary from common to rare. However, it can be an opportunistic pathogen. It has been isolated from infectious stomatitis and abscesses.

## PASTEURELLA

*Pasteurella* is most commonly encountered in chelonians. One study found *Pasteurella* spp. more frequently in sick tortoises compared to healthy tortoises. Another study consistently isolated *Pasteurella* from ill tortoises that also had a *Mycoplasma*-like agent present in the surface membranes of the upper respiratory tract (Jacobson, 1993). Although Koch's postulates have not been fulfilled, it appears that *Mycoplasma* may be the etiologic agent of upper respiratory disease in tortoises, and that other gram-negative bacteria, such as *Pasteurella*, may exacerbate the disease (Jacobson, 1993).

## SERRATIA

*Serratia marscescens* and *S. liquefaciens* are primarily a problem in lizards, especially iguanas. It can cause subcutaneous abscesses, joint and bone infections, and may be transmitted by bites. It has also been isolated from snakes and turtles with SCUD.

## DERMATOPHILUS

*Dermatophilus congolensis* causes cutaneous streptothricosis in lizards and snakes and is relatively uncommon. Affected reptiles have subcutaneous, hyperkeratotic nodules in the ventral skin that can progress to visceral abscessation, septicemia, and death (Frye, 1991). Dermatophilus can cause pustular dermatitis in humans.

## MYCOBACTERIUM

Mycobacteria are not common in reptiles. The most frequent isolates are *M. marinum, M. chelonei*, and *M. thamnopheos*. Granulomata can develop in the lungs, liver, spleen, central nervous system, gonads, bone, alimentary tract, and subcutaneous tissue (Frye, 1991). Treatment is not recommended because these bacteria are generally resistant to common antibiotic regimens and are potentially zoonotic. Furthermore, pharmacokinetics on potentially toxic antituberculosis drugs are lacking in reptiles.

## Interpretation

Interpretation of bacterial cultures and sensitivities derived from diseased reptiles and amphibians is fairly straightforward. Some general rules include:

1. Look for opportunistic reptile pathogens in heavy growth and their common antibiotic sensitivities. Select bactericidal antibiotics. Aminoglycosides and quinolones are effective against most aerobic pathogens and there is little bacterial resistance to them. The author prefers quinolones because they have less potential for renal toxicity. Enrofloxacin (Baytril, Haver/Mobay) at 5 mg/kg every 24 hr SC, IM, or PO has proven efficacious. Ciprofloxacin (Cipro, Miles) at 11 mg/kg every 48 to 72 hr PO is more practical in large reptiles.
2. The isolation of pathogenic anaerobes dictates different antibiotics. In lieu of sensitivity testing, carbenicillin (400 mg/kg every 24 hr for snakes, every 48 hr for snakes, SC, IM) or ceftazidime (20 mg/kg every 72 hr SC, IM) are good broad-spectrum antibiotics useful against anaerobes as well as most gram-negative pathogens. If *Pseudomonas* spp. and anaerobes are present, ceftazidime is the best choice. For an extensive reviews of antibiotic usage in reptiles, see Jacobson (1988) or Mader (1991).

It is crucial to isolate and maintain patients at the upper range of their preferred optimum temperature during treatment to ensure consistent pharmacokinetics and immune response. For most reptiles, 27°C (80°F) to 32°C (90°F) is optimal.

## References and Suggested Reading

Cooper JE: Bacteria. *In* Cooper JE and Jackson OF (eds): *Diseases of the Reptilia*, volume 1. London, Academic Press, 1981, pp 165–191.
*An overview of normal flora, pathogenicity, types of bacterial disease, zoonoses, equipment, disinfection, disposal, hygiene, stains, reagents, collection of specimens, bacterial cultivation and identification, and sensitivity tests.*

Draper CS, Walker RD, and Lawler HE: Patterns of oral bacterial infection in captive snakes. J Am Vet Med Assoc 179:1223, 1981.
*Bacterial isolates from oral and cloacal cultures in healthy boids, viperids, and colubrids were compared to isolates from snakes with infectious stomatitis.*

Frye FL: Infectious diseases. *In Biomedical and Surgical Aspects of Captive Reptile Husbandry*, 2nd edition. Malabar, FL, Kreiger Publishing Co, 1991, pp 101–157.
*A review of algal, fungal, bacterial, rickettsial, and viral diseases, as well as specific bacterial infections, approach to treatment, metabolic scaling and antibiotic dosages.*

Hilif M, Wagner RA, and Yu VL: A prospective study of upper airway flora in healthy boid snakes and snakes with pneumonia. J Zoo Anim Med 21:318, 1990.
*Glottal cultures were taken from eight boids twice a month for 1 year, one of which developed pneumonia and died.*

Jacobson ER: Use of chemotherapeutics in reptile medicine. *In* Jacobson ER and Kollias GV (eds): *Exotic Animals*. New York, Churchill Livingstone, 1988, pp 35–48.
*A review of routes of administration and chemotherapeutics for bacterial, mycotic, and parasitic pathogens in reptiles.*

Jacobson ER: Laboratory investigations. *In* Beynon PH, Lawton MPC, and

Cooper JE (eds): *Manual of Reptiles*. Gloucestershire, British Small Animal Veterinary Association, 1992, p 58.
*A chapter on blood evaluations; biopsies; cytodiagnostics; negative-staining electron microscopy; microbiology; fecal examinations; and urine, blood, and spinal fluid collection.*

Mader DR: Antibiotic therapy in reptile medicine. *In Biomedical and Surgical Aspects of Captive Reptile Husbandry*, 2nd edition. Malabar, FL, Kreiger Publishing Co, 1991, pp. 101–157.
*A review of algal, fungal, bacterial, rickettsial, and viral diseases, as well as specific bacterial infections, approach to treatment, metabolic scaling, and antibiotic dosages.*

Mader DR: Clinical reptilian microbiology. Salmonellosis in reptiles. Vet Proc NA Vet Conf, volume 7. Orlando, FL, 1993, pp 773–774, 779–780.
*A short review of collection of samples for bacterial culture and review of common bacteria isolated and an in-depth discussion on Salmonella.*

Needham FR: Microbiology and laboratory techniques. *In* Cooper JE and Jackson OF (eds): *Diseases of the Reptilia*, volume 1. London, Academic Press, 1981, pp 93–132.
*An overview of normal flora, pathogenicity, types of bacterial disease, zoonoses, equipment, disinfection, disposal, hygiene, stains, reagents, collection of specimens, bacterial cultivation and identification, and sensitivity tests.*

Soveri T and Seuna ER: Aerobic oral bacteria in healthy captive snakes. Acta Vet Scand 27:172, 1986.
*Twenty-three snakes were cultured from the ventral mouth and proximal esophagus and compared.*

Stewart JS: Anaerobic bacterial infections in reptiles. J Zoo Wildl Med 21:180, 1990.
*A retrospective study of 65 reptile cultures submitted to the California Veterinary Medical Teaching Hospital over a 2-year period to determine the prevalence, species, and antibiotic sensitivities of anaerobic bacteria present.*

# NON-NUTRITIONAL BONE DISEASES IN REPTILES

RAMIRO ISAZA
*and* ELLIOTT R. JACOBSON
*Gainesville, Florida*

Reptiles are susceptible to a wide range of non-nutritional bone diseases, and there are even several published accounts of bone disease in dinosaurs (Rothschild, 1987; Rothschild and Berman, 1991). In clinical practice, the most important causes of bone disease in reptiles are related to poor nutrition and husbandry. The presentation, pathogenesis, and treatment of these nutritional diseases have previously been reviewed (Jackson and Cooper, 1981). This article focuses on the bone diseases in reptiles that are common in clinical practice but not thought to be directly related to nutrition.

An accurate diagnosis is important for the successful treatment of the reptile patient with bone disease. A complete history, including husbandry practices and complete physical examination, should be obtained at the initial stages of patient evaluation. The animal should be allowed to ambulate so that any gait abnormalities may be observed. A compete blood count (CBC) and serum or plasma chemistries are also help-ful in assessing the reptile patient. Radiographic imaging is a useful diagnostic tool for evaluation of bone in reptiles (Silverman, 1989). Most reptiles can be radiographed without anesthesia by gentle restraint using tape. However, anesthesia or sedation should be used when radiographing uncooperative animals or when handler safety is a consideration. Alternate imaging techniques such as nuclear imaging, magnetic resonance imaging (MRI), or fluoroscopy are potentially valuable for examination of reptile bones but are not commonly available to most veterinary clinicians.

## TRAUMATIC DISEASES

### Long Bone Fractures

Reptiles may be presented for traumatic long bone fractures. Pet lizards allowed to roam free in the house are commonly seen with limb fractures caused by falls, crushing injuries, or dog and cat bites. In chelonia, limb fractures are much less common than shell fractures; however, such injuries can be caused by cars, dog bites, and forceful extraction of the limbs. Adult crocodilians kept in multiple animal enclosures are commonly presented with fractures of the limbs due to intraspecies aggression.

Diagnosis of long bone fractures in reptiles is usually made by physical examination and radiography. Because fractures in captive reptiles are commonly secondary to a nutritional metabolic bone disease, all radiographs should be evaluated for bone density. Therapy for simple, closed fractures in small reptiles usually consists of cage confinement with minimal handling, and an adequate diet that provides an appropriate calcium/phosphorus ratio. If the fracture is very displaced or unstable, external fixation using tape and rigid splints can be considered. If presented with an unstable closed fracture, internal fixation techniques similar to those used in mammals can be attempted. However, the bones must have both large enough and sufficiently mineralized to accept the internal fixation devices.

### Spinal Fractures

Chelonia with shell fractures that cross the dorsal midline of the carapace may have spinal fractures and should therefore be assessed for neurologic deficits. Spinal fractures can occur in lizards, crocodiles, and snakes that are dropped during manipulation or handled in a way that fails to support the back. Neurologic examination and radiography often help in confirmation of the diagnosis. Many reptiles with spinal fractures in the distal portion of the body are often able to ambulate despite a partial neurologic deficit. These animals are often presented for examination with a history of anorexia or constipation (rather than paralysis). As in other vertebrates, the prognosis for full recovery of neurologic function after spinal cord transection is poor. However, in cases with partial paresis, extended periods of cage rest may eventually result in return of function.

### Traumatic Shell Injuries in Turtles and Tortoises

Crushing injuries of the shell caused by cars, lawn mowers, and dog bites are common in chelonian species. These animals are often submitted for examination with open fractures of the carapace and plastron that may extend into the coelomic cavity. Initial treatment of shell fractures should focus on supportive care with an emphasis on restoring proper hydration and control of hemorrhage. After stabilization, the turtle should be radiographed to assess the extent of the injuries. It is important to treat these fractures as open, contaminated wounds, providing aggressive débridement and cleansing of the wounds before any repair is attempted. Cultures of infected or contaminated tissue and the subsequent use of appropriate antibiotics are recommended in most turtles with shell fractures.

The management of shell injuries has been previously reviewed (Rosskopf, 1986). Application of epoxy patches using fiberglass cloth and epoxy resin to cover shell defects has also been described (Harwell, 1989). In our experience, epoxy patches used in this manner have been associated with the development of osteomyelitis and coelomitis beneath the patch. For this reason, we prefer to use a combination of cerclage wire and small epoxy patches used only to stabilize shell fragments, thus leaving the majority of the shell deficit uncovered. After stabilization of the fracture, wet to dry bandages applied to the open wound and changed daily allows for débridement of necrotic tissue. This usually results in the formation of granulation tissue and subsequent healing of the shell without the need for complete epoxy patches. The major disadvantage of this method of shell repair is that it often takes weeks to months of wound care.

In the past, turtles sold in the pet trade developed shell deformities caused by thick layers of paint applied to the carapace. Although less common today, overzealous application of epoxy resins used for repair of shell fractures in growing turtles may result in similar deformities. If presented with a growing turtle in need of shell repair, the size of the epoxy patch should be minimized and the epoxy should be filed away at the suture margins to allow for shell growth. Additionally, the patch should be examined frequently and replaced if needed.

### Thermal Shell Injuries

Free-ranging tortoises and terrapins surviving forest fires often have burns on the carapace and plastron with exposure of the underling bone. Burn injuries to the shell should be treated with gentle débridement and antiseptic salves. Animals with these injuries are often able to heal by epithelization under the affected area with subsequent extrusion of the dried segments of sequestered bone.

### Rodent Bite Trauma

Snakes fed live rodents may sustain bite wounds to their body. These lesions may range from a single bite to an extensive area of exposed muscle and bone where the rodent has mutilated a significant amount of tissue. Since bite wounds involving bone may develop into osteomyelitis, management is more complicated than just simple débridement. Efforts should be made to thoroughly clean the wounds, prevent further contamination by bandaging, and fight bacterial infection with antibiotic therapy. These injuries are best prevented by recommending that all snakes be offered only dead prey. If live prey must be used, the owners should be given specific instructions to never leave live rodents unattended inside snake cages.

## OSTEOMYELITIS

Bacterial osteomyelitis secondary to shell fractures can occur in chelonia. Crocodiles and lizards commonly have osteomyelitis of the toes, stifles, skull, and spine. Snakes are often presented with a severe, disseminated form of vertebral osteomyelitis that is grossly and radiographically very similar to a disease described as osteitis deformans (see below).

Radiographs, bone cultures, and histopathology are necessary for initial assessment of any reptile with proliferative or lytic lesions involving bone. Radiographs of the affected bone provide the most valuable information in the initial assessment of these cases (Fig. 1). Radiographs of the whole body are helpful to determine the extent and distribution of the osteomyelitis in areas that are not evident on physical examination. Additionally, radiographs taken periodically throughout the treatment process help document the effect of treatment.

Bacterial cultures, both aerobic and anaerobic, should ideally be collected and submitted prior to beginning antibiotic therapy. In our hospital population, gram-negative organisms including *Salmonella* spp., *Aeromonus* spp., *Pseudomous* spp., *Escherichia* spp., and *Morganella* spp. are the most commonly isolated bacteria from reptiles with osteomyelitis. However, gram-positive bacteria (*Streptococcus* spp., *Staphylococcus* spp., and *Corynebacterium* spp.) and anaerobic organisms (*Clostridium* spp. and *Bacteroides* spp.) are occasionally cultured from infected reptile bone.

Septicemia appears to be common in reptiles with osteomyelitis. In these cases, we have found blood cultures to be useful in isolating bacteria that are responsible for septicemia. Blood samples for culture can be collected from the heart or any vessel that can provide a large blood sample with a single venipuncture attempt. For meaningful culture results, strict attention must be given to aseptic technique during collection of the blood culture sample.

Osteomyelitis in a reptile should be considered a life-threatening condition that has potential for recurrence despite aggressive therapy. Therapy should begin with careful débridement of the affected bone and adjacent soft tissues. Consideration must be given to amputation of affected limbs where bone has been severely affected.

The results of bone cultures are the best guides for the selection of antibiotic therapy. Only a limited number of pharmacokinetic studies have been reported in reptiles, making selection of antibiotic dosages for an individual reptile species difficult without extrapolation (Bush, 1992). Table 1 lists several antibiotics used by the authors for treatment of osteomyelitis. Because osteomyelitis may be caused by multiple bacteria species, combinations of antibiotics are often selected to provide a broad spectrum of bactericidal activity. In our experience, resolution of osteomyelitis in reptiles requires prolonged antibiotic treatment of at least 2 or 6 months. In some cases, complete resolution has not been achieved and the animal was euthanatized a year after initial therapy was started. Because of the necessity for a long-term treatment period, nephrotoxic drugs such as aminoglycosides should be used with caution. If these drugs are selected, they should be combined with less nephrotoxic drugs so that the aminoglycoside therapy is only given for the first six to nine doses with the second antibiotic continued for the duration of the treatment period.

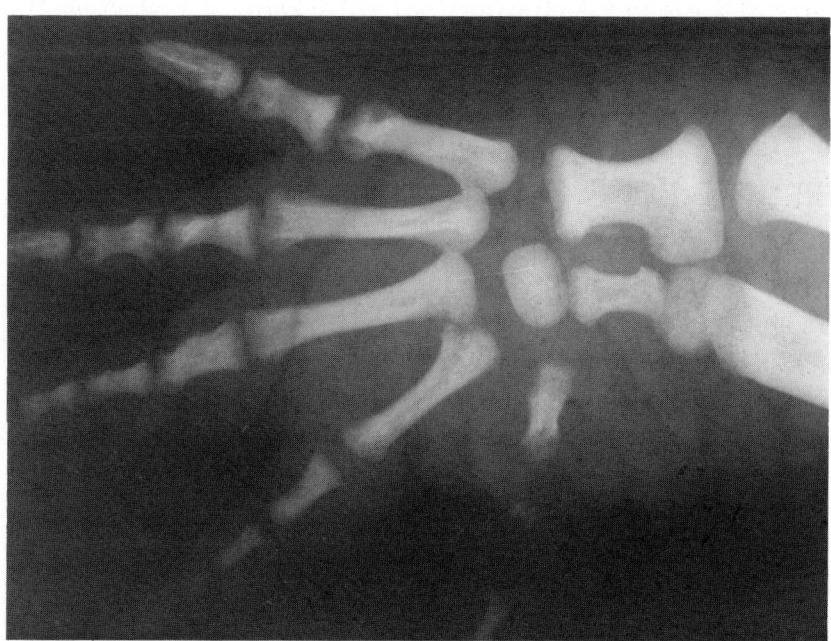

**Figure 1.** Radiograph of the right forelimb of a siamese crocodile (*Crocodylis siamensis*) with evidence of osteomyelitis in P1 and P2 of the fifth digit.

**Table 1.** *Selected Antibiotics and Doses for Use in Reptiles With Bacterial Osteomyelitis\**

| Antibiotic | Dosage (mg/kg) | Route | Frequency |
|---|---|---|---|
| Amikacin | 5 (first dose), 2.5 (subsequent doses) | IM | q72h |
| Ampicillin | 20 | IM | q24h |
| Carbenicillin | 400 | IM | q24h |
| Cephalothin | 30 | IM | q12h |
| Ceftiofur | 4 | IM | q24h |
| Ceftazidime | 20 | IM | q72h |
| Enrofloxacin | 5 | IM | q48h |
| Metronidazole | 20 | PO | q24h |
| Piperacillin | 100 | IM | q24h |
| Trimethoprim/sulfadiazine | 30 | IM | q24h |

\*Compiled from various sources. Many of the dosages and frequencies presented here are not based on pharmacokinetic data. These dosages are extrapolations from selected reptile or mammalian pharmacokinetic data and used by the authors for the treatment of osteomyelitis.

### Bacterial Stomatitis

Bacterial stomatitis of lizards and snakes can progress from a simple localized soft tissue infection to osteomyelitis. In the initial assessment of even mild cases of stomatitis, radiographs should be taken to determine if there is any evidence of osteomyelitis in bones of the skull or jaw. Therapy for bacterial stomatitis needs to be instigated early and consists minimally of local treatment of the mouth with flushes of dilute iodine or chlorhexidine solutions and application of topical salves. Systemic antibiotics are indicated in animals that have necrotic or infected tissue deep into the gingiva or with any radiographic evidence of osteomyelitis.

## MISCELLANEOUS BONE DISEASES

### Osteitis Deformans

Osteitis deformans or Paget's disease appears to be common in captive snakes (Frye, 1991). The condition is characterized clinically by a diffuse, segmental spondylosis that results in the loss of mobility of the spine. Gentle palpation of the spine during physical examination is often diagnostic. In severe cases, kyphosis and ankylosis can be easily observed on physical examina-

tion. Overzealous manipulation of the affected segments of spine during physical examination can result in iatrogenic vertebral fractures. Because this disease is usually multifocal and segmental, radiographs are needed to both confirm the diagnosis and document the extent of the lesions.

This disease in snakes was originally described as an idiopathic, noninflammatory metabolic disease similar to osteitis deformans or Paget's disease in humans (Frye, 1991). However, we have seen several cases of proliferative spinal disease in snakes which, while grossly and radiographically similar to osteitis deformans, were subsequently diagnosed as osteomyelitis (Fig. 2). These diagnoses were based on histologic evidence of granulomatous inflammation associated with bacterial colonies, along with positive bacterial cultures of the bone. It remains unclear if osteitis deformans in snakes is actually a chronic, quiescent form of osteomyelitis, or if two distinctly different diseases result in similar gross and radiographic lesions.

For the clinician presented with a snake with proliferative spinal lesions, it is important to determine the underlying cause before treatment recommendations can be made. Diagnostic tests such as bacterial cultures (from blood and bone) and histopathology of bone biopsies can be used to identify the etiology. In cases with evidence of bacterial osteomyelitis, antibiotic therapy should be started. If no evidence of osteomyelitis is

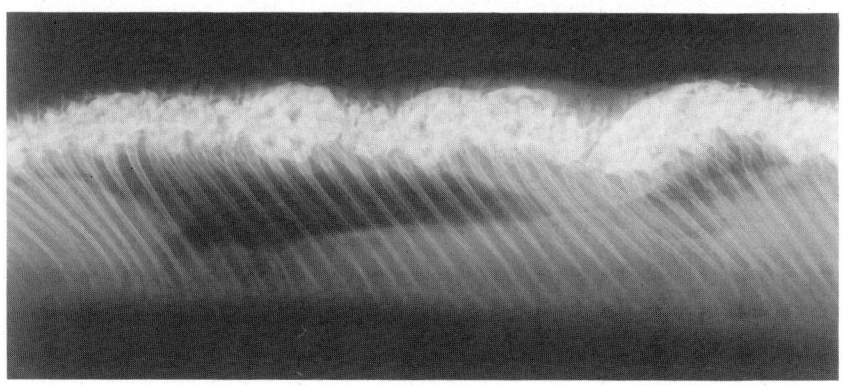

**Figure 2.** Radiograph of a boa constrictor with proliferative lesions in the spine. This animal had histologic evidence of multifocal bacterial osteomyelitis and cultured positive for *Salmonella* spp.

found, then treatment should consist of cage rest with limited handling. Because of limitation in the ability of these snakes to prehend food, affected animals should be offered only small, dead prey items that limit the need for constriction prior to consumption. Unfortunately, most snakes with either form of this disease become progressively worse despite attempts at treatment.

## Degenerative Diseases

Degenerative lesions of the bone and joints in reptiles can be observed in older animals or as a sequelae to trauma. As an example, arthritis can be observed in the feet and limbs of lizards and tortoises chronically housed on hard flooring.

## Neoplastic Diseases

Although cases of osteochondrosarcomas, chondrosarcomas, and chondro-osteofibromas have been reported in lizards and snakes (Machotka, 1984), neoplasia involving bone and joint tissues apparently are uncommon in reptiles.

## Congenital Malformations

Many cases of congenital malformations involving bone have been reported and reviewed (Frye, 1991). Captive born corn snakes and related species occasionally have multiple malformations of the vertebrae that result in the spine forming a series of kinks (Frye, 1991). One of the authors (E.R.J.) has observed hemi-

vertebrae resulting in cervical curvatures in neonate gharials (*Gavialis gangeticus*). Treatment options for congenital deformities are limited and reptiles with extensive lesions may need to be euthanatized.

## References and Suggested Reading

Bush M: An update of antibiotic therapy in reptiles. *In* Kirk RW (ed): *Current Veterinary Therapy XI: Small Animal Practice.* Philadelphia, WB Saunders Co, 1989, p 789.
   *A review of antibiotic dosages derived from pharmacokinetic data in reptiles.*
Frye FL: *Biomedical and Surgical Aspects of Captive Reptile Husbandry,* volume 2, 2nd edition. Malabar, FL, Krieger Publishing Company, 1991, p 540.
   *A description of osteitis deformans in snakes.*
Frye FL: *Biomedical and Surgical Aspects of Captive Reptile Husbandry,* volume 2, 2nd edition. Malabar, FL, Krieger Publishing Company, 1991, p 393.
   *A review of congenital and developmental anomalies in reptiles.*
Harwell G: Repair of injuries to the chelonian plastron and carapace. *In* Kirk RW (ed): *Current Veterinary Therapy X: Small Animal Practice.* Philadelphia, WB Saunders Co, 1989, p 789.
   *A more detailed description of shell repair in chelonian species.*
Jackson JO and Cooper JE: Nutritional diseases. *In Diseases of the Reptilia,* volume 2. London, Academic Press, 1981, p 409.
   *A review of nutritional diseases in reptiles.*
Machotka SV: Neoplasia in reptiles. *In* Hoff GL, Frye FL, and Jacobson ER (eds): *Diseases of Amphibians and Reptiles.* New York, Plenum Press, 1984, p 519.
   *A detailed review of reported cases of neoplasia in reptiles.*
Rosskopf WJ: Shell disease in turtles and tortoises. *In* Kirk RW (ed): *Current Veterinary Therapy IX: Small Animal Practice.* Philadelphia, WB Saunders Co, 1986, p 751.
   *A review of the management of shell diseases in chelonian species.*
Rothschild BM and Berman DS: Fusion of caudal vertebrae in late Jurassic sauropods. J Vert Paleo 11:29, 1991.
   *A report of fusion of caudal vertebrae in dinosaurs.*
Rothschild BM: Decompression syndrome in fossil marine turtles. Ann Carnegie Mus 54:253, 1987.
   *A report of multiple cases of a vascular bone necrosis in fossil turtles.*
Silverman S: Advances in avian and reptilian imaging. *In* Kirk RW (ed): *Current Veterinary Therapy X: Small Animal Practice.* Philadelphia, WB Saunders Co, 1989, p 786.
   *A discussion of radiographic imaging in reptiles.*

# REPTILE OPHTHALMOLOGY

NICHOLAS J. MILLICHAMP
*College Station, Texas*

## CLINICAL ANATOMY

Reptile eyes are similar in general morphology to those of domestic species. The most significant difference in most of the reptiles presented with ocular disease is the smaller size, which can make examination a challenge. Although the eyes of snakes differ from the general morphology seen in the other reptile orders, for the most part, the variation is minor.

The lower eyelids of lizards are best developed with more excursion over the cornea. In crocodilians, the upper lid is better developed, containing a bony tarsus.

Strong closure of the upper lid in crocodilians often hinders ocular examination. In some geckos and skinks and all snakes, the upper and lower eyelids are fused to form a transparent tertiary spectacle. This structure normally lies in close apposition with the cornea. A very narrow tear-filled space, the subspectacular or corneospectacular space lies between the two structures. The corneospectacular space communicates with the roof of the mouth via the lacrimal duct. The duct opens adjacent to the base of the vomeronasal organ or farther rostrally on the palate. Since the spectacle is continuous with the adjacent periocular skin, it may be affected by generalized skin disease. The corneospectacular space may be involved in disease of the globe itself or disease involving the lacrimal duct and roof of the mouth. The spectacle normally contains fine capillary sized blood vessels that may become engorged in cutaneous or ocular disease involving the spectacle and should always be differentiated from corneal neovascularization and, in some species, normal vascular patterns in the anterior iris stroma.

Orbital glands are developed to variable degrees in different reptile orders. They are most developed in chelonians, which explains the prevalence of hypovitaminosis A–induced ocular disease in this order. Chelonians lack a nasolacrimal duct. Excessive production of tears results in epiphora.

The sclera of lizards, chelonians, and crocodilians contains an outer layer of hyaline cartilage. Bony scleral ossicles continue the scleral cartilage in the ciliary region in lizards and chelonians. Although of limited significance clinically, these tissues need to undergo decalcification if eyes are submitted for histopathology.

The iris shows considerable diversity of surface features in different lizard species due to variations in the appearance of the pupil (especially in geckos) and vascular patterns. In all reptiles, the iris sphincter is comprised of striated muscle. For this reason, muscarinic receptor–blocking drugs do not cause mydriasis in reptiles.

The retina is avascular in all reptiles, although various vascular structures do exist in the posterior segment of some species that may provide nutrition to the inner retina. In lizards, a vascular conus papillaris arises from the optic nerve and may project across the vitreous nearly to the posterior lens capsule in some species. Analogous to the pecten in birds, this structure may provide retinal nutrition. In snakes, a network of blood vessels radiates from the optic nerve into the peripheral fundus. This structure, the membrana vasculosa retinae, lies in the posterior vitreous and presumably acts as a blood supply for the inner retina.

Ecdysis, or shedding of the outer layers of epidermis, is a normal occurrence in reptiles. It is most obvious in snakes and lizards, where the entire skin including the spectacle is shed over a period of a few days. The skin becomes dull as shedding approaches. The spectacle becomes a hazy white or blue color during this time. This opacification lasts a few days and then clears just before ecdysis.

## OCULAR EXAMINATION

Adequate restraint is essential when examining large or fractious reptiles. In many instances, anesthesia is the most appropriate means available for thorough examination. Magnification is needed for most ocular examinations. Ideally, a slit-lamp biomicroscope provides both magnification and diffuse or focal lighting that facilitates observation of ocular lesions. Alternatively, a direct ophthalmoscope can be used with a +15-D or +20-D lens or a 20-D plano convex lens used with a focal halogen light source. The adnexal tissues should be examined carefully—in particular, the folds of skin at the eyelid canthi or where the spectacle joins the periocular scales. This is a site that may harbor external parasites such as mites or ticks.

In alligators, nerve blocks may be needed in conscious animals to prevent closure of the upper lid. Mydriasis is achieved either under general anesthesia or in crocodilians by intracameral injections of 0.05 to 0.1 ml *d*-tubocurarine (Bristol-Myers Squibb, Princeton NJ, 20 U/ml) with a 27-gauge needle at the limbus. The fundus is best examined with a focal light source and 25-D lens.

The roof of the mouth adjacent to the vomeronasal organ should always be examined for evidence of inflammatory disease in snakes and lizards with any disease involving the corneospectacular space.

## EYELIDS AND ADNEXA

The eyelids may be involved in any generalized skin disease. Self-limiting poxvirus infections in crocodilians present with white, raised plaques often involving the eyelids. Papilloma-like lesions occur in green sea turtles and lacertid lizards and may have a viral etiology. Fungal infections of the skin can affect the eyelids or spectacle, forming white, yellow, or brown plaques and discolored areas within the scales. If untreated, these lesions may progress to involve orbital tissues and destroy the eye. Fungal skin disease has also been seen associated with systemic fungal infections (e.g., pneumonia). Parasites (in particular, mites or ticks) are often found in the fold of thin vascular skin between the spectacle and periocular scales or at the lateral canthi of the eyelids. Damage caused by these parasites when feeding may cause scarring that interferes with normal ecdysis. Inflammatory eyelid lesions may cause corneal irritation and subsequent keratitis with or without ulceration.

Culture or biopsy of periocular lesions may reveal pathogens and suggest appropriate therapy. Topical medications include broad-spectrum ophthalmic ointments containing neomycin, polymixin, and gramicidin (Neosporin, Burroughs Wellcome, Research Triangle Park, NC) applied to the eye and periocular tissues. Cleansing of periocular skin lesions is effected with dilute chlorhexidine (Hibistal, Stuart Pharmaceuticals, Wilmington, DE) (0.26 ml/L of water). Fungal infections may respond to topical antifungal agents (2% miconazole nitrate cream, Monsistat 7, Ortho Pharmaceuticals, Raritan, NJ; or 1% tolnaftate cream, Tinactin, Schering-Plough Healthcare, Kenilworth, NJ). For systemic infections with dermatologic involvement, systemic therapy with ketaconazole may be attempted. No pharmacologic data are available for the use of this drug in reptiles, although I have used ketoconazole by stomach tube (30 mg/kg every 2 to 3 days) in king snakes with fungal infections of the skin.

## SPECTACLE AND CORNEOSPECTACULAR SPACE

One of the most common ocular problems encountered in snakes is a failure to shed the spectacle at ecdysis. The spectacle may be retained alone or other parts of the head or body skin may also fail to shed. Common causes include inadequate environmental humidity coupled with malnutrition, dehydration, or ectoparasitic infestation in some cases. Environmental factors alone are, however, the single most common cause of this problem.

The clinical appearance of a single retained spectacle may be difficult to diagnose, since the spectacle may not differ significantly in appearance from normal. If several sheds occur and succeeding layers of spectacle are retained each time, the spectacle becomes thickened and opacified. The lesion appears to cause limited discomfort in the absence of other inflammatory disease, but can eventually limit vision if not treated.

It is inadvisable to remove the retained spectacle with forceps, since underlying healthy layers may also be damaged or even completely lifted away from the eye. Attempts to moisten the spectacle with topical ophthalmic artificial tears and petrolatum ointment (Tears Naturale II, Alcon Laboratories, Fort Worth, TX; Major Tears, Major Pharmaceuticals, Chicago, IL) should be attempted. The animal can also be soaked for a few hours in water at the animal's normal ambient temperature, taking precautions to prevent drowning. Topically applied mucolytic agents such as acetylcysteine (Mucomyst, Mead Johnson Pharmaceuticals, Princeton, NJ) may help loosen the attached layers. Alternately, the retained layers may be left *in situ* until the next shed and an attempt made to correct environmental factors in the intervening period. Increasing the cage humidity as the snake nears the time of shedding will often allow the retained layers to be shed successfully. If the spectacle is still retained, it should be removed by gently rubbing the peripheral region where it attaches to the periocular scales with a cotton-tipped applicator after applying ophthalmic tear replacement solutions and ointments to moisten the adherent layers. Retained layers of spectacles that still remain attached despite any of these attempts at therapy should be carefully removed surgically using adequate magnification to ensure that the deepest layers are left undisturbed. Occasionally, the entire spectacle may be inadvertently removed. Although keratitis may result, loss of the eye is not an inevitable consequence. Ectoparasites predisposing to spectacle retention are treated either by exposure to a small piece of dichlorvos placed in a perforated container in the cage for 24 hr or by treatment with ivermectin (MSD, Agvet, Rahwey, NJ) (200 $\mu$g/kg IM).

Infections of the corneospectacular space occur with some frequency in snakes and geckos. These may arise secondary to bacterial infections of the mouth (necrotic stomatitis) with infection ascending in the lacrimal duct, perforating injuries of the spectacle (e.g., bites from rodents), and possibly from hematogenous spread of pathogens in animals with bacteremia.

A variety of pathogens have been isolated from eyes with infections of the corneospectacular space. Bacteria, and particularly gram-negative species including *Pseudomonas* and *Proteus*, have been cultured from animals with concurrent infections (necrotic stomatitis, respiratory infections). Various protozoa have been found on cytology; examination of corneospectacular space exudate from several snakes and lizards has revealed protozoan species, including debris from trypanosomes or large numbers of flagellated trichomonad species (including *Tritrichomonas* and *Monocercomonas* spp.). The exact role of these various organisms in causing clinical disease in the corneospectacular space has not yet been determined.

The clinical appearance of animals with infections of the corneospectacular space is one of distention, opacification, and vascularization of the spectacle. Large volumes of flocculent fluid or inspissated pus accumulate in the space due to obstruction of the lacrimal duct. In animals with gram-negative bacterial infections, inspissated pus forms in large quantities that will often obscure the eye below. In animals with large numbers of protozoa present, the corneospectacular space is distended with hazy serous fluid, and flocculent deposits may be seen on the posterior surface of the spectacle and the anterior surface of the cornea. The swelling of the corneospectacular space often extends into the periocular region, with marked distention appearing around the eye. This may be associated with diffuse cellulitis or focal accumulations of tear secretions or exudate.

Diagnosis is based upon clinical appearance and aspirates of the exudate for cytology and culture. With adequate restraint, which may necessitate general anesthesia in some animals, exudate can be aspirated from the corneospectacular space with a 25- or 23-gauge needle and immediately examined for the presence of protozoa in wet preparations using polarized lighting, and submitted for bacterial and fungal culture. Inspissated pus in the corneospectacular space can be removed for culture through a 30- to 40-degree wedge excised from the ventral spectacle. The differential considerations in eyes with spectacle distention would include uveitis with glaucoma, although in my experience this occurs with far less frequency than corneospectacular space infections. Aspirates or biopsies of the corneospectacular space can usually be made with little risk of damaging the underlying globe. Usually, contrary to first impressions, the globe is not severely involved in these infections, although some degree of keratitis may be present. The large quantitiy of fluid accumulated in the corneospectacular space distends the spectacle away from the globe so that damage to the cornea is unlikely when apsirating the exudate or incising the spectacle.

After culture and sensitivity have been performed, the abscess should be drained via the wedge excised in the ventral part of the spectacle. Inspissated pus should be flushed from the space with sterile saline or a dilute povidone-iodine solution (Betadine Solution, Purdue Frederick, Norwalk, CT) (one part povidone-iodine to three parts sterile saline). Subsequently, topical antibiotic solutions or ointments are applied to the opening in the spectacle. Gentamicin ophthalmic ointment (Allergan Pharmaceuticals, Irvine, CA) is appropriate in cases of Pseudomonas infection coupled with systemic therapy with amikacin sulfate (Amiglyde-V, Fort Dodge Laboratories, Fort Dodge IA) (2.5 mg/kg IM every 72 hr) or other antibiotics based upon culture and sensitivity results. In cases where protozoa are found in the aspirate, systemic therapy with oral metronidazole (Goldline Laboratories, Fort Lauderdale, FL) (50 to 100 mg/kg PO, repeated in 14 days) is indicated.

Blockage of the nasolacrimal duct may also occur congenitally or associated with noninfectious scarring or pressure on the lacrimal duct from adjacent structures. In some of these cases, swelling of the spectacle with clear fluid will persist for long periods of time. In other cases, the fluid beneath the spectacle may become turbid, resembling an infection of the corneospectacular space. In large snakes, lacrimal drainage may be reestablished by surgically inserting fine-diameter Silastic tubing from the inferior corneospectacular space to the roof of the mouth for several weeks. Scarring of the duct may, however, occur after the Silastic is removed.

## CONJUNCTIVA AND CORNEA

Conjunctivitis is rarely reported in reptiles, with the exception of chelonians. Conjunctivitis has been reported in groups of reptiles occasionally associated with various bacterial pathogens. Topical broad-spectrum antibiotics are indicated combined with systemic antibacterial therapy if associated with systemic disease. Chelonians emerging from hibernation may present with a serous or mucopurulent ocular discharge and blepharoedema. Usually this resolves spontaneously, although in some animals the problem may be exacerbated by vitamin A deficiency or infectious disease. Oral or parenteral vitamin supplementation and antibacterial therapy are indicated in severe cases. Conjunctivitis is seen in tortoises affected with upper respiratory tract infections. Some of these are associated with *Mycoplasma* infections. Systemic and topical antibacterial drugs should be used for these infections.

Corneal ulcers may occur in traumatized eyes, often associated with injuries during shipping. Superficial ulcers respond well in most cases to broad-spectrum antibiotics (gentamicin sulfate or neomycin, polymixin, gramicidin). Parasympatholytics are not indicated due to the absence of smooth muscle in the iris or ciliary body. Ulcerative keratitis may progress to corneal perforation requiring microsurgical repair or enucleation.

Lipid deposits are occasionally seen in the corneal stroma—in most cases the etiology is unknown and therapy is rarely required.

## UVEITIS AND PANOPHTHALMITIS

Uveitis is observed sporadically in reptiles, usually associated with infectious and particularly bacterial septicemia, although it may occasionally occur secondary to corneal ulceration or ocular trauma. Affected animals may present with various signs including conjunctival injection and aqueous flare. Hypopyon is the most easily diagnosed feature if present, due to the difficulty in examining the anterior chamber of small reptiles. Attempts should be made to determine an underlying systemic etiology prior to therapy with topical and systemic antibiotics. Therapy is limited to systemic antibacterial agents in reptiles with a spectacle, since the latter effectively prevents topically applied drugs reaching the cornea or intraocular structures. No information is available regarding the inflammatory mediators in reptile eyes, although topical nonsteroidal anti-inflammatory drugs such as flurbiprofen (Ocufen, Allergan Medical Optics, Irvine, CA) every 6 hr may be used empirically to reduce intraocular inflammation. Corticosteroids should be used with caution, since many cases of uveitis are associated with systemic infectious disease.

Panophthalmitis may develop as an extension of uveitis or infectious disease affecting the cornea or adnexal structures. Enucleation is the most appropriate therapy.

## LENS AND POSTERIOR SEGMENT

Cataracts are seen with some frequency in older reptiles or associated with uveitis or hibernation in chelonians. In larger reptiles, the eye size may lend itself to effective surgical therapy, although in most cases the affected animals function quite well with compromised vision. Retinal degeneration and detachment are the most commonly detected lesions in the posterior segment. These are usually associated with inflammatory disease. Often the diagnosis is made of chronic lesions at a stage when therapy is not required.

## ORBIT

The epithelia of the orbital glands and their ducts in chelonians undergo squamous metaplasia due to hypovitaminosis A. The eyelids become edematous and crusted and eventually closed. Conjunctivitis also develops, and secondary bacterial infections may occur. Affected animals cease feeding and eventually die. Squamous metaplasia of visceral epithelia is usually diagnosed postmortem. The disease may occur in terrestrial as well as aquatic chelonia, and particularly in young rapidly growing animals maintained on a diet low in carotene. Initially, a single injection of vitamin A (1000 to 5000 IU) is given. Improvement is often rapid, with eyelid swelling subsiding in the first week after vitamin A therapy. Subsequently, the animal should be induced to feed and vitamin A supplementation given orally. Feeding plant material or fish provides ample vitamin A. Care should be taken not to oversupplement with parenteral vitamin A at this stage, since so doing may have fatal consequences. Conjunctivitis is treated with a topical broad-spectrum antibiotic ointment applied for several days that helps to lubricate the lids.

Orbital abscesses involving periocular and retrobulbar tissues are seen occasionally in snakes and lizards, not uncommonly in chameleons kept in captivity. Such infections may arise from trauma, hematogenous spread of bacteria from other sites, and parasitic infestations. Drainage and flushing of pus from the orbital spaces with dilute povidone-iodine with curettage of inspissated material is necessary. Topical applications of antibiotics alone are rarely effective. Systemic antibacterial therapy should be used after culture and sensitivity results are obtained.

## CONGENITAL ABNORMALITIES

Congenital defects are relatively common in reptiles both in the wild and in captivity. Microphthalmia, anophthalmia, and cyclopia have all been described. Microphthalmia is the most frequently reported condition, often associated with other craniofacial or skeletal anomalies. The etiologies are unknown, although inbreeding in captivity or unsuitable gestational or incubation temperatures are possible causes. With these possible etiologies in mind, avoiding breeding close relatives and using established effective methods for reptile breeding, gestation, and egg incubation are ways of preventing these problems.

## References and Suggested Reading

Frye FL: *Biomedical and Surgical Aspects of Captive Reptile Husbandry*, volume 2, Malabar, FL, Krieger Publishing Co, 1991, p 329.
  *A general review of eye diseases in reptiles, with many illustrations.*
Millichamp NJ: Exotic animal ophthalmology. *In*: Gelatt KN (ed): *Veterinary Ophthalmology*, 2nd edition. Philadelphia, Lea & Febiger, 1991, p 680.
  *A general review of reptile eye disease.*
Millichamp NJ, Jacobson ER, and Wolf ED: Diseases of the eye and ocular adnexa in reptiles. J Am Vet Med Assoc, 183:1205, 1983.
  *A review and report of reptile ophthalmic cases seen by the authors.*
Walls GL: *The Vertebrate Eye and its Adaptive Radiation*. Bloomfield Hills, MI, Cranbrook Institute of Science, 1942, p 607.
  *An excellent, readable text about reptile ocular anatomy and histology*

# ANESTHESIA OF PET FISHES

MICHAEL K. STOSKOPF

*Raleigh, North Carolina*

Medical treatment of pet fishes is an important, growing area of companion animal practice. Pet fish owners are beginning to understand the value of veterinary care for their investment, and advances in diagnostic and therapeutic methods make it possible for veterinarians to provide improved service. Most diagnostic and many therapeutic procedures for pet fish are greatly facilitated by the safe and effective use of anesthesia. An immobile and nonreactive patient allows faster, more precise and less traumatic intervention in any procedure performed on a live fish. Companion animal practitioners need to become familiar with anesthetic management in pet fishes. Fortunately, the margins of safety of the commonly used agents are wide and the procedures and concerns in fish anesthesia are very similar to those in mammalian anesthesia.

## ANESTHETIC TECHNIQUES

### Induction

The most commonly used method for inducing anesthesia in fishes involves immersion of the fish in a drug solution. Regardless of the anesthetic used, it is important to reduce stresses on the fish prior to anesthesia by eliminating environmental stressors. Induction containers (tanks or bags) should be prepared ahead of time and filled with water that is closely matched to the habitat of the patient (pH, temperature, salinity, or hardness). An excellent way to do this is to have your client bring a sufficient volume of water with the fish when it is brought to your clinic. This water can serve as induction and recovery water.

Handle the fish as little as possible. Avoid damaging its epithelium and generating a stress response that will increase the anesthetic dose and reduce the margin of safety of the drug. For a single fish, it is best to place the patient in the induction tank and slowly add the anesthetic to the induction dose. When many fish are being anesthetized sequentially, fish can be added directly to anesthetic-laden water. It is always a good idea when working with a new species of fish, or fish held under unusual conditions, to anesthetize one fish first, watching induction and recovery closely, before proceeding to a second fish. Start with a relatively low induction dose in these cases.

For short procedures (3 to 5 min), fish can be handled directly from the induction solution and returned to it when the depth of anesthesia becomes light or the fish needs to breathe. For longer procedures, anesthetized fish should be transferred to a lower dose maintenance solution. As you induce anesthesia in a fish, observe it closely. It will usually pass through planes of anesthesia very similar to those observed in mammals (Table 1). Some fish go through the stages so rapidly that it can appear that stages and planes are completely bypassed.

The individual and species variations in susceptibility to anesthetic agents are similar to those seen in mammals. These can be due to differences in metabolic rate (including those due to water temperature), physical condition (particularly related to the amount of body fat), and other factors. One general rule to remember, though, is that fish in poor condition or suffering from disease usually require much less drug to achieve a given plane of anesthesia than fish in good condition.

Hypoxia is an important problem during immersion induction of anesthesia and during maintenance. Aerate the induction and maintenance solutions throughout the anesthesia. This is even more critical when several fish are passed through the same induction water. Be sure to have a recovery tank prepared and available with undrugged water. If a fish becomes too deeply anesthetized, it can easily be moved to water free of drug.

### Recovery

Throughout anesthesia and during recovery, observe the patient carefully for opercular movements. When opercular movements are extremely weak or absent, assistance is required. During a procedure, this involves increasing the flow of water with a lower dose, or water free of drug, past the gills. Near the end of a procedure, the fish should be moved directly to recovery water free of drug.

The mouths of larger fishes can be opened in the recovery water, checking for jaw tone. Jaw tone will return before opercular movements. Opening the mouth alternately and propelling the fish forward in the water can help ram water over the gills of a large fish that is too deeply anesthetized. This increases the exchange drug and keeps the fish oxygenated, much like bagging a mammalian patient with oxygen. When jaw tone returns, and the fish begins to breathe on its own, allow it to recover further without manipulation. This is usually less stressful for the fish. Opercular rate and strength of opercular movement are good indicators of whether a fish is continuing to recover or has relapsed into a deeper stage of anesthesia.

For smaller fish where manipulation of the mouth is not feasible and could damage the delicate jaws of the fish, make sure the recovery water is well aerated and place the fish in the water so that flow takes water over its face and mouth. Watch for opercular motion. Do not be too hasty in pronouncing a failed recovery. Fish can recover after fairly long periods of no respiratory movement (10 min or more) if they are in well-oxygenated water.

Fish that have been anesthetized and recovered

**Table 1.** *Stages of Anesthesia in Fishes**

| Stage | Plane | Category | Behavioral Response of Fish |
|-------|-------|----------|------------------------------|
| 0 | | Normal | Swimming actively, reactive to external stimuli, equilibrium normal, muscle tone normal |
| I | 1 | Light sedation | Voluntary swimming continues, slight loss of reactivity to visual and tactile stimuli, respiratory rate normal, equilibrium normal, muscle tone normal |
| I | 2 | Deep sedation | Voluntary swimming stopped, total loss of reactivity to visual and tactile stimuli, slight decrease in respiratory rate, equilibrium normal, muscle tone slightly decreased, still responds to positional changes |
| II | 1 | Light narcosis | Excitement phase may precede increase in respiratory rate, loss of equilibrium, efforts to right itself, muscle tone decreased, still responds to positional changes weakly |
| II | 2 | Deep narcosis | Ceases to respond to positional changes, decrease in respiratory rate to near normal, total loss of equilibrium, no effort to right itself, muscle tone decreased, some reactivity to strong tactile and vibrational stimuli; suitable for external sampling, fin and gill biopsies |
| III | 1 | Light anesthesia | Total loss of muscle tone, responds to deep pressure, further decrease in respiratory rate; suitable for minor surgery |
| III | 2 | Surgical anesthesia | Total loss of reactivity, respiratory rate very low, heart rate slow |
| IV | | Medullary collapse | Total loss of gill movement, followed in several minutes by cardiac arrest |

*Adapted from Stoskopf MK: *Manual for the Aquatic Animal Workshop*. Washington, DC, AALAS National Capital Area Branch, 1985.

should be observed periodically for the first 4 hr and again 24 hr later to avoid occasional unexpected delayed reactions. These are extremely rare.

## COMMONLY USED IMMERSION ANESTHETICS

### Tricaine

Tricaine methane sulfonate, more commonly referred to as MS-222 (Finquel, Argent Laboratories, Redmond, WA), is a highly water-soluble sulfonated analog of benzocaine. It is the fish anesthetic most commonly used in North America. Tricaine is supplied as a crystalline powder that is stable when kept cool and dry. Standard stock solutions are made by adding 10 gm tricaine to 1 L of water.

Solutions of tricaine should be stored in dark or opaque containers because they are unstable in sunlight and will turn brown from the formation of a methyl sulfate compound. This does not affect the potency of the solution significantly, but it is still advisable to change stock solutions once a month. The shelf life of stock solutions can be extended by refrigeration or freezing.

Solutions of tricaine are acidic due to methane sulfonic acid formation, and require buffering prior to administration to freshwater fishes or applications directly to the gills. Many practitioners buffer their stock solutions by adding sodium bicarbonate to saturation. This effectively stabilizes the pH of a 10 gm/L stock solution between 7 and 7.5. Buffering highly concentrated stock solutions can result in excessive desulfonation, forming amino benzoate ethyl ester, which comes out of solution and forms oil droplets on the surface of the solution. This does reduce the potency of the solution, and solutions with an oily film on top should be discarded.

If necessary, 1-gm/L solutions of tricaine can be autoclaved without loss of anesthetic properties or increase in toxicity. This is not necessary for routine procedures. Topical exposure to tricaine stock and induction solutions is not toxic to mammals at concentrations used in fish anesthesia, and tricaine is not mutagenic.

Although tricaine is thought of as a relatively safe drug, its toxicity varies considerably depending upon fish species, fish size, water temperature, and water hardness. It has a narrow margin of safety for some species and particularly for young fish. It is more toxic in warm, soft waters. It is also important to remember that tricaine is hydrolyzed to *para*-aminobenzoic acid and caution should be exercised when administering this anesthetic to patients being treated with sulfonamides.

A good starting concentration for tricaine anesthesia of adult fish of an unfamiliar species in unknown water conditions is 50 to 100 mg/L. This can be achieved by adding 5 to 10 ml of a 10-gm/L stock solution to every liter of water being used for the induction bath. More drug is required to anesthetize some species of fish in colder water, and induction times are longer; however, safety tends to increase. This cold water effect does not hold across all species. When working with young fish or fish in relatively warm water, it is advisable to begin with a 50-mg/L induction solution. Remember that drug is absorbed and actual exposure concentrations are reduced for each successive fish. Induction solutions need to be replenished when induction times become prolonged.

Strong aeration of the induction solutions throughout induction and anesthesia is important. Throughout tri-

***Table 2.*** *Anesthetics for Pet Fishes*

| Drug | Stock Solution | Induction Dose | Maintenance Dose | Comments |
|------|----------------|----------------|------------------|----------|
| Tricaine° | 10 gm/L | 50–100 mg/L (5–10 ml stock/L) | 50–60 mg/L (5–6 ml stock/L) | Aerate water |
| Quinaldine[†] | 10 gm/L | 50–100 mg/L (5–10 ml stock/L) | 50–60 mg/L (5–6 ml stock/L) | Aerate water |
| Quinaldine:tricaine 1:10 mixture | 1 gm/L:10 gm/L | 2.5–3.0 mg/L quinaldine and 25–30 mg/ml tricaine (2.5–3.0 ml of each stock) | | |
| Metomidate[‡] | 10 gm/L | 2.5–5 mg/L 1.0–10 mg/L | 0.2–0.3 mg/L 0.1–1.0 mg/L | Marine fish Freshwater fish |
| Ketamine HCl[§] | | 66–88 mg/kg | (6.6–8.8 mg/100 gm) | IM |
| Ketamine HCl + demetomidine[‖] | | 1–2 mg/kg ketamine | | IM |
| | | 50–100 µg/kg demetomidine | | Reverse with atipamizole 200 µg/kg IM |

°Available as Finquel from Argent Chemical Laboratories, 8702 152nd Ave NE, Redmond, WA 98052 (1-800-426-6258).
[†]Available from Current Research Chemicals, 4331 E Western Star Blvd, Phoenix, AZ 85044 (1-602-893-9234).
[‡]Available from Wildlife Pharmaceuticals, 1401 Duff Dr, Suite 600, Fort Collins, CO 80524.
[§]Available as Ketoset from Fort Dodge Laboratories, 800 5th Street NW, PO Box 518, Fort Dodge, IA 50501.
[‖]Available as Dormosedan from SmithKline Beecham Animal Health, Whiteland Business Park, 812 Springdale Dr, Exton PA, 19341-2803 (1-800-366-5288).

caine anesthesia, blood lactate levels tend to increase, supporting the view that the drug may have asphyxiant properties. It is not clear whether this is a direct drug effect or due to decreased opercular activity in the anesthetized fish. Blood lactate levels increase to much higher levels in fish that have not been held off feed for at least 24 hr prior to anesthesia. Blood glucose levels remain stable throughout routine anesthesia with tricaine.

Tricaine diffuses rapidly across the gills, providing rapid recovery times that vary according to the concentration used and the duration of exposure. Blood levels of free drug reach about 75% of the concentration of the immersion solution, and are cleared in about 8 hr. In short procedures, recovery times longer than 10 min generally mean too high a final concentration of drug is being used, and doses should be adjusted downward. In longer procedures, tricaine distributes through tissues, and complete recovery can take up to 6 hr. A maintenance solution of 60 mg/L (6 ml stock per liter) is routinely used in longer procedures, after induction is achieved. Absorbed tricaine is excreted in the urine for about 24 hr after exposure. Tissue residues decline to less than detectable limits (0.1 mg/kg in fish flesh) in about 24 hr, but regulatory withdrawal time in the United States for food fishes is 21 days because of a lack of mammalian safety data.

## Quinaldine Sulfate

Quinaldine sulfate is also referred to as Quinate, or 2-methylquinoline sulfate (Argent has decided not to sell this drug in the United States and only sells it internationally now. Current Research Chemicals, Phoenix, AZ). This drug is seeing increasing use in fish anesthesia, despite being more expensive than tricaine. The drug is supplied as a highly water-soluble, light yellow crystalline powder. It should not be confused with the parent compound, quinaldine, which is nearly insoluble in water.

Quinaldine stock solutions are acidic and should be buffered with sodium bicarbonate as described for tricaine stock solutions. Stock solutions should be protected from light and kept in a tightly sealed container. A stock solution of 10 gm/L is most frequently used.

When used alone, quinaldine sulfate offers the advantages of rapid induction and recovery. Fish anesthetized with quinaldine sulfate retain a strong touch response after losing equilibrium, but this seems to extinguish after about 20 sec of contact. Most procedures are readily performed after the touch response extinguishes. The avoidance and coughing responses seen when the nonsulfated form of quinaldine is administered in alcohol or acetone are not seen with the water-soluble quinaldine sulfate.

In warm water species, induction solutions of 15 to 60 mg/L (1.5 to 6 ml stock solution per liter) are usually employed. Species vary in susceptibility to the drug. Largemouth bass are particularly sensitive, while goldfish are relatively insensitive. Quinaldine sulfate is less toxic in very soft water than in hard water. Warm water increases the toxicity of quinaldine sulfate, probably by driving the equilibrium toward the ionized form of the drug.

Quinaldine sulfate is apparently not metabolized by fishes, but is excreted entirely unchanged. Muscle residues are essentially nill at 24 hr following exposure. There is no evidence quinaldine sulfate has any carcinogenic properties.

Quinaldine sulfate is sometimes used in combination with tricaine in a ratio of 1:10 (quinaldine sulfate/tricaine). This mixture achieves faster induction than either drug alone. A common induction solution for this mixture has 25 to 30 mg/L tricaine and 2.5 to 3.0 mg/L quinaldine sulfate.

## Metomidate

Metomidate is available in Canada, marketed as *Marinil* (Wildlife Pharmaceuticals, Fort Collins, CO) and hopefully will soon be available in the United States. This drug has been used very successfully for anesthesia of many species of fishes. It is an imidazole-based nonbarbiturate hypnotic closely related to etomidate. Metomidate received a lot of attention in the 1980s because fish anesthetized with it were found to not have the spikes in serum cortisol seen when other anesthetic agents were employed. The drug was referred to as the "stressless" anesthetic. Unfortunately, the lack of a cortisol peak is more likely related to a metabolic blockade of cortisol synthesis than a lack of stress. Nevertheless, metomidate is a useful and effective fish anesthetic. The drug is supplied as a powder. Stock solutions of 1 gm/L and 10 gm/L are useful. The doses are generally so low with this drug that stock solutions are not routinely buffered.

The dose of metomidate varies somewhat with the species of fish, and the need for muscle relaxation. Fish anesthetized at lower doses commonly show muscle fasciculations. Marine tropical fishes and sharks are readily anesthetized with solutions of 2.5 to 5 mg/L. Freshwater tropical fishes can be successfully anesthetized with doses between 1 and 10 mg/L. Very low doses of 0.06 to 0.20 mg/L are used for transport sedation.

As with tricaine and quinaldine, long anesthesia times under metomidate result in long recovery times. Induction with metomidate is rapid, and fish should be removed from induction solution soon after losing equilibrium, which may occur within 1 or 2 min of exposure. If this is done, recovery from metomidate will be more rapid than from tricaine. However, if patients are allowed to remain in metomidate induction solutions after loss of equilibrium, recovery times can be very prolonged. The duration of recovery appears to be directly related in a log function to how long the fish are in the induction solution.

When some species and individuals are anesthetized with metomidate, they turn very dark. This may be related to the metabolic blockade of cortisol production, which also effectively blocks the negative feedback loop on adrenocorticotropic hormone (ACTH) production. Since ACTH and melanocyte-stimulating hormone synthesis are linked, the lack of cortisol causes melanophore responses. The effect is rapidly reversed when the fish is allowed to recover from anesthetic.

## INJECTABLE ANESTHETICS

Recent work has shown that ketamine HCl alone (Ketoset, Fort Dodge Laboratories, Fort Dodge, IA) or in combination with medetomidine (Dormosedan, SmithKline Beecham Animal Health, Exton, PA) can be used to successfully immobilize fishes for clinical procedures. So far, these drugs have been used primarily in larger marine fishes, but the technique has considerable promise for pet fish practice. Injections are delivered IM or IP, often with a remote delivery device such as a Hawaiian sling outfitted with a syringe tip. For pet fish that can be hand injected, this method of anesthesia may prove very useful.

The use of ketamine alone at a dose of 66 to 88 mg/kg (6.6 to 8.8 mg/100 gm) offers the advantage of using a drug commonly stocked in veterinary practices. It provides immobilization suitable for most short procedures and, although complete recovery can take an hour or more, it is fairly safe.

The combination of ketamine and demetomidine has the great advantage of reversibility as well as not requiring a portion of the water to be adulterated with anesthetic. Anesthetized fish are maintained on a clearwater breathing system until reversal. Demetomidine is given at a dose of 50 to 100 $\mu$g/kg combined with ketamine HCl at 1 to 2 mg/kg IM. Reversal is accomplished with 200 $\mu$g/kg atipamizole IM.

## HYPOTHERMIA

Although fishes become torpid and immobile when rapidly cooled from their acclimation temperature, hypothermia is *not* an appropriate method of anesthesia for pet fishes. The degree of analgesia is not well controlled and thermal injuries can occur. A syndrome called "cold shock" can result in death. Generalized hypothermia also causes major osmoregulatory alteration, with dramatic shifts in ionic balance as well as hematologic perturbations such as increased clotting time.

## EUTHANASIA

At some time, every practitioner is faced with the need to euthanize patients humanely. This is also true for pet fish practice. The literature and data available on euthanasia of these animals are scanty and incomplete. Overdose with anesthetic is the most appropriate method for euthanasia of these animals. Immersion in tricaine, quinaldine sulfate, or metomidate solutions; or IM or IP injection of ketamine with or without meditomidine can be used. Anesthetized fish can be exsanguinated through the caudal vessels or cardiac puncture, or be partially or completely decapitated to ensure death.

### References and Suggested Reading

Brown LA: Anesthesia and restraint. *In* Stoskopf MK (ed): *Fish Medicine.* Philadelphia, WB Saunders Co, 1993, pp 79–90.
*General review chapter with information on the pharcologic and physical properties of the drugs covered here and some additional, less frequently used anesthetics.*
Stoskopf MK and Arnold J: Metomidate anesthesia of ornamental freshwater fish. Proc Int Assoc Aquatic Anim Med 16:12–21, 1985.
*Short article providing data on induction and recovery times in several species of freshwater fishes including gouramies.*
Summerfelt RC and Smith LS: Anesthesia, surgery and related techniques. *In* Schreck CB and Moyle PB (eds): *Methods for Fish Biology.* Bethesda, MD, American Fisheries Society, 1990, pp 213–272.
*Basic coverage of field anesthesia techniques in wild and aquacultural fishes.*
Williams TD, Christiansen J, and Nygren S: A comparison of intramuscular anesthetics in teleosts and elasmobranchs. Proc Inter Assoc Aquatic Anim Med 24:6, 1993.
*Short article giving data on new initramuscular anesthetics being used experimentally with promising success.*

# EMERGENCY PET FISH MEDICINE

GREGORY A. LEWBART
*Raleigh, North Carolina*

Pet fish warrant the serious attention of veterinarians. It has been estimated that 25% of American households keep pet fish. Traditionally, pet fish disease problems have been dealt with by pet store clerks or aquarium maintenance companies. As our knowledge of fish diseases, therapeutics, and water quality increases, more and more veterinarians will be qualified to work responsibly with these animals. All veterinarians, even if they have never worked on a fish, have a broad understanding of disease processes, diagnostics, animal husbandry, and chemotherapeutics. The opportunity to apply this knowledge to a client's pet fish problem can be a very rewarding experience. This article focuses on handling and treating acute problems of pet fish where veterinary intervention is required within an emergency time frame.

## HISTORY

Pet fish are commonly presented in emergency situations arising from changes in their aquatic environment that can quickly and adversely affect fish. An accurate and concise history is essential when working up a pet fish emergency. A good history can help the clinician narrow the differential list and usually gives some clues as to the origin of the problem. Table 1 contains a list of pertinent questions to include in a pet fish history. The first question can help the clinician evaluate clients. For example, are they an experienced hobbyist with numerous aquariums and a good understanding of water quality or are they novices trying to learn about fish keeping? Frequently, novices have problems because they fail to dechlorinate the water or they overload a tank prior to establishment of the biologic filter. The second question is obvious and the third helps formulate a diagnostic plan, since duration of a problem is very important. Fish that are poisoned with chlorine or chloramine usually die quickly (within a matter of hours), while fish affected with external parasites usually go through some period of morbidity before succumbing. Questions 4 and 5 address the source of the fishes and duration of ownership as well as the status of other fishes that may be sharing the same aquarium or pond. This type of information is valuable when making the diagnosis and designing a treatment plan. Questions 6 and 7 deal with the actual aquarium or pond system and what (if any) water quality parameters have been tested. Most pet fishes can go days or even weeks without food. Anorexia usually indicates the presence of an external stressor such as poor water quality or the presence of a pathogen. Feeding questions are important because occasionally

an owner is simply feeding a food that the pet fish does not or cannot consume. Many pet fishes have already been treated by the time they reach the veterinarian and this information is an important part of the history (question 9). The final question centers on the environment outside of the aquatic system. Toxic compounds from an exterminator or other source can adversely affect pet fishes. Air pumps used to aerate the aquarium literally draw toxic compounds into the water if the compounds are in close proximity to the pump. Outdoor koi and goldfish ponds are at risk from pesticides as well as herbicides that have been introduced into the immediate environment.

## TANK-MATE AGGRESSION

Before beginning time-consuming water quality and diagnostic procedures, tank-mate aggression must be ruled out. This is a leading cause of acute mortality and morbidity in an aquarium, is usually diagnosed on the history, and is readily solved. Injuries sustained as a result of an incompability problem commonly lead to life-threatening bacterial, fungal, and parasitic disease. The solution usually requires physically separating the aggressive and submissive fishes. Many hobbyists, especially beginners, want variety in their new aquarium. All too frequently, fish that are attractive (but tanked separately) in the pet store do not get along in the same aquarium or outdoor pond (larger koi will commonly injure or even kill smaller goldfish). Members of the same species may even kill and eat smaller or weaker conspecifics. Intimidated fish that manage to survive attacks by a dominant individual may go without food if they spend all of their time hiding in the corner of the aquarium. Responsible pet store clerks advise the client on what fish are compatible.

## DIAGNOSTICS

Since this article focuses on emergency fish medicine, the emphasis of this section is placed on tests that can be performed in the clinic and yield immediate results. Several companies manufacture inexpensive kits that accurately test the appropriate water quality parameters (Hach Company, PO Box 389, Loveland, CO; Gilford Instrument Labs, Ovelin, OH; La Motte Chemicals, PO Box 329, Chestertown, MD; Orion Research, 840 Memorial Drive, Cambridge, MA). The basic pet fish diagnostic laboratory must be equipped to test for temperature, ammonia, nitrite, nitrate, pH, dissolved oxygen, and total alkalinity (buffering capacity of the water). Kits that measure copper and chlorine are desirable but not necessary.

Once the history has been taken and the water tested, biopsy and/or necropsy procedures may be necessary. Antemortem biopsy samples can be obtained with a sterile scalpel blade, scissors, and forceps. Suspect areas of skin and fins can be scraped or removed and placed on a glass slide containing a drop of water.

***Table 1.***   *Important Questions for the Client*

1.  How long have you been keeping pet fish?
2.  What are the problems with the fish(es) today?
3.  When did you first notice these problems?
4.  How long have you owned the sick fish and where did they come from?
5.  Are there other fish in the same tank or pond with the sick fish and if so, how are they doing?
6.  What is the size (volume) of the pond or aquarium and how is it heated, filtered, lighted, and aerated?
7.  Do you have a water test kit and if so, how often do you test the water? What are your most current results?
8.  What and how often do you feed your fish.
9.  Have the fish already been treated? If so, by whom, and with what medications?
10. Is there a possibility that the fish were exposed either directly or indirectly to some type of toxin?

Once a coverslip has been applied, the sample can be examined under the microscope for the presence of pathogens. A small gill biopsy can usually be safely taken by removing a few millimeters of gill lamellae from a single gill arch. Fish may be restrained manually for these procedures or tranquilized with an anesthetic agent such as tricaine methanesulfonate (MS-222, Finquel) at a dose of between 75 and 150 mg/L water (see "Anesthesia of Pet Fishes," this volume, p 1365).

Larger fishes (>10 cm in length) usually yield a blood sample large enough to run a complete blood count (CBC), packed cell volume (PCV), total protein, Gram stain, and blood culture. Very few data are published on normal ornamental fish blood parameters, but PCV values below 20% usually indicate anemia and a septic condition is frequently evident on a Gram-stained blood smear. To obtain a blood sample, locate the lateral line on the fish. Direct the needle (size and gauge will vary with the size of the fish) at a 90-degree angle to the ventral margin of the thin lateral line caudal to the vent but cranial to the tail and caudal peduncle. The needle should be inserted until resistance from the spinal column is felt. The needle should then be gently "walked" ventrally until the needle slips into the venous sinus located just ventral to the spine. An alternative method is to enter the caudal venous sinus by placing the fish in dorsal recumbency and using a midventral approach. Insert the needle at a point midway between the anal fin and tail. When resistance is felt from the vertebral bodies, withdraw the needle very slightly and obtain the blood sample. Fish blood clots quickly, so the syringe and needle should be coated with heparin before the sample is taken.

Another informative diagnostic tool is the radiograph. Pet fishes with swim bladder disorders, gastrointestinal impactions, and foreign bodies can be accurately diagnosed with a radiograph. This procedure can frequently be done without anesthesia, since many fish do not struggle for the first few seconds after they have been removed from the water. The film cassette is covered with a plastic bag and the fish is laid directly atop the cassette. Small fish can be radiographed using dental films. Most fish lie in lateral recumbency, which means the best way to obtain a dorsoventral view is by rotating the radiograph machine and sending a horizontal beam through the dorsoventral axis of the fish. Specific techniques vary with the machine and the species and size of the fish. Record all successful kilovolt peak and milliampere second values along with the size and species of the fish for future reference.

## WATER QUALITY PROBLEMS

Poor water quality is a leading killer of pet fishes. Good, clean water is the first step in keeping both freshwater and marine fishes healthy. Oxygen is the most important element dissolved in water. Tropical fishes generally require between 5 and 10 ppm dissolved oxygen to survive. When functioning properly, commercially available air pumps and filters usually provide adequate oxygen for fish. Hypoxia is more commonly a problem in outdoor ponds during the warm summer months. Hypoxia is generally exacerbated at night. During the daylight hours, plants and algae in the pond undergo photosynthesis and provide oxygen for the pond, while most plants utilize oxygen at night. If the pond is heavily planted, shallow, and warm, it becomes hypoxic and the fish will be affected. If a problem is suspected, the water should be tested at dawn when dissolved oxygen levels are at their lowest.

Adequate water temperature is critical to fish health and is an easy parameter to control. Most freshwater tropical fishes should be kept between 24° and 27°C (76° and 80°F). Tropical marine fishes require slightly higher temperatures as a rule (26° to 29°C [79° to 84°F]). Most home aquariums contain a heater equipped with a thermostat to maintain a constant environmental temperature. An accurate thermometer is necessary to properly regulate the temperature of the system. Several groups of fishes, including guppies, goldfish, and koi, thrive at room temperature and do not require supplemental heat. Fishes that are too cold may congregate at the bottom of the aquarium and refuse food. Very warm water contains less oxygen and the fish may appear at the water's surface gulping or "piping" for air.

The actual pH value is not as important as its relationship to other water chemistry parameters (e.g., ammonia is much less toxic to fish when the pH is more acidic). The ideal pH level of freshwater aquariums and ponds is between 6.5 and 7.6 and most species can tolerate a range of pH values as long as the changes are gradual. Abrupt changes must be avoided. Marine tropical fishes thrive at a pH of between 8.0 and 8.3. This leaves them particularly vulnerable to even slight elevations in ammonia concentrations. Established aquariums that do not experience frequent water changes tend to become acidic as organic acids build up in the aquarium. The author has observed freshwater fishes surviving in water with a pH as low as 3.5 (more acidic than vinegar). Nitrifying bacteria in a biologic filter usually do not break down ammonia efficiently at pH levels below 5.0. The best advice in such a situation is to gradually change water, perhaps 25% a week until the pH approaches a normal level. Routine water changes of 10% every 7 to 10 days usually prevent this problem. It is difficult to maintain a stable pH in very soft water with a low total alkalinity (buffering capacity). Dolomite or crushed coral may be added to the aquarium to solve this problem. Other pH-regulating compounds are readily available at most pet stores.

In water, ammonia occurs in the toxic un-ionized form and the relatively nontoxic ionized form. The total ammonia concentration is a measurement of both types of ammonia. As the pH increases, ammonia becomes more un-ionized and hence more toxic. An ammonia reading of 1.0 ppm at a pH of 8.5 is much more serious than at a pH of 6.5. In cases of high ammonia (>1.0 ppm), a 30 to 50% water change with dechlorinated water should be performed as soon as possible. This emergency procedure should be repeated every 12 to 24 hr until the cause of the problem is determined.

**Table 2.**  *Emergency Conditions of Pet Fish and Treatments*

| Problem | Solution |
|---|---|
| ***Hypoxia*** | Common when fish have been inappropriately transported to clinic. Place affected fish(es) in plastic bag containing 1/3 volume of water and fill rest of bag with 100% oxygen from anesthesia machine. Close bag tightly with rubber band or surgical tape. Keep fish(es) in bag until they have resumed normal swimming and respiratory behavior. |
| ***Elevated Ammonia or Nitrite*** | Water changes. Examine filtration, biologic load, and feeding practices. Measure pH to help determine how toxic the total ammonia is in the aquarium or pond. |
| ***Abnormal pH*** | Gradual water changes to bring pH back into normal range. Measure total alkalinity (buffering capacity). If low (below 50 ppm), add crushed coral or dolomite to the system to increase buffering capacity. Some fishes require very soft water, so frequent water changes may be best method of regulating pH. |
| ***Chlorine/Chloramine Toxicity*** | Water containing the fish(es) should be immediately treated with a dechlorinating agent (use commercially available compounds as directed) or the fish should be removed to an aquarium, bucket, or cooler containing clean dechlorinated water. Chlorine causes gill necrosis resulting in decreased respiratory surface area. Use ice packs in water to lower temperature which will increase the amount of dissolved oxygen (DO) in the water. Tropical fishes may be lowered to 70°F, goldfish and koi to 55°F. In addition, an oxygen bottle may be used to bubble 100% oxygen into the water to help increase DO levels. Attach an aquarium airstone to end of air tube connected to oxygen bottle. Artificial sea salt at a dose of 1 gram/liter of water should be added to treatment tank as well. This treatment may be necessary for several days or more depending on the severity of the toxicity. IP or IV dexamethasone at a dose of 2 mg/kg q24h for 3 days may also increase chance of survival. |
| ***Anorexia/Starvation*** | Most species of fishes can be tube fed. See text. A viscous food can be made by adding small amounts of water to flake or pelleted feed. Other options would be a high-calorie/protein feline or canine canned diet. Learn the gastric anatomy of the patient first if at all possible to prevent complications like perforation. Goldfish and koi lack a reservoir stomach, so amounts of food should be small. |
| ***External Bacterial Disease*** | Apply *Panalog* or *Silvadene* cream directly to wound q12h. Allow affected area to remain out of water for 30–60 sec while medication is absorbed. Gills should remain submerged. Parenteral antibiotic therapy may be warranted (see below). |
| ***Systemic Bacterial Disease*** | Injectable antibiotic therapy options: *Enrofloxacin*, 5 mg/kg given IM or IP q24h for 7–10 days; 5 mg/kg given PO for 10–14 days or 0.1% in food and feed to fish for 10–14 days. *Chloramphenicol*, 50 mg/kg given IM or IP q24h for 10 days; 50 mg/kg PO q24h for 10–14 days or 0.2% in food and feed to fish for 10–14 days. *Trimethoprim-sulfamethoxazole*, 30 mg/kg PO q24h for 10–14 days or 0.2% in food and feed to fish for 10–14 days. Culture and sensitivity results may indicate a more appropriate antibiotic. As a guideline these drugs can be blended with food at a concentration of 0.2%. As a last resort, some antibiotics can be effective as a bath treatment. Most can be dissolved in water at a concentration of between 10 and 20 mg/L. Treatment should last for 6–12 hr and should be followed by a 50% water change. Discontinue carbon filtration and water flow through biologic filter during bath treatment. Keep water well aerated. Repeat bath treatments at least 3–5 times, longer if necessary. |

*Table continued on opposite page*

Tank overstocking, overfeeding, and inadequate filtration are the most common causes of elevated aquarium ammonia levels.

Nitrite is an intermediate compound in the nitrogen cycle and is converted to relatively nontoxic nitrate by a healthy biologic filter. However, in the freshwater aquarium, nitrite levels above 0.5 ppm should be considered serious. As in terrestrial animals, nitrite causes the formation of methemoglobin in the blood and results in respiratory compromise. Daily 30 to 50% water

**Table 2.** *Continued*

| Problem | Solution |
|---|---|
| ***Protozoal Disease*** | Ectoparasitic protozoans must be treated with a dip or bath. *Options*: Many freshwater species will tolerate a 4 to 5 min dip in full strength (30–35 gm/L) *seawater*. Marine fishes can be placed in a *freshwater* dip for 4–5 min. Aerate well and monitor very closely. Certain smaller fishes may not survive this treatment. If possible, test treatment on one fish first. *Formaldehyde*, 20–25 mg/L for 12 to 24 hr followed by a 50% water change. Encysted parasites like *Ichthyophthirius* and *Cryptocaryon* will require several treatments. Always change water between treatments. *Metronidazole*, as a bath treatment will kill some external flagellates, 400 mg/L q24h for 3 consecutive days, 50% water changes between treatments; for internal flagellates use in food at 0.2% (20 mg/gm food) and feed for 10 days. |
| ***Trematode Disease*** | Ectoparasitic monogeneans can be serious. Found on skin and gills. *Options*: *Praziquantel*, 5–10 mg/L as a 3 to 6 hr bath, repeat in 7 days. Remove fish to treatment tank if possible and aerate water well. Some marine species may be sensitive. Aquarium may still be infected, so treated fish should be moved to new aquarium if possible. May not kill all species of monogeneans. This treatment will kill most internal cestodes. *Seawater/freshwater* dips may be effective against some parasites. See protozoal protocol above. *Acetic acid*, 2 ml/L glacial acetic acid as a 30 to 45-sec dip, safe for goldfish, but smaller tropicals may not tolerate this treatment. |
| ***Nematode Disease*** | Rarely an emergency. *Fenbendazole*, combine in food at a concentration of 0.2% and feed for 3 days and repeat in 14–21 days. |
| ***Cestode Disease*** | Rarely an emergency. *Praziquantel*, bath treatment (see trematode protocol above); 5 mg/kg fish PO in food, repeat in 14–21 days; 5 mg/kg given IP, repeat in 14–21 days. Injectable treatment may also work for internal digenean trematodes. |
| ***Crustacean Disease*** | Common ectoparasites of goldfish and koi (fish louse, anchorworm). More common in ponds than in aquarium. *Dimethyl phosphonate*, 0.5 mg/L, 3 treatments 10 days apart, 20–30% water change 24–48 hr following treatment. Use extreme caution when handling these organophosphate compounds. Liquid form commonly used to kill cattle grubs is easy to handle, measure, and dispense. *Acetic acid*, dip procedure described above for trematodes is effective for treating new arrivals to a pond for crustacean parasites. Always test with one fish first, if possible. Seawater dips may be effective, see above protocols. |

changes in the freshwater aquarium should help the fish until the primary cause can be determined. An alternative is to simply move the fish to a new aquarium. In the marine aquarium, high nitrite levels are less of a problem, since nitrite ions must compete with chloride ions for uptake by the gill epithelium.

Chlorine and chloramine (chlorine combined with ammonia) are added to most municipal drinking water supplies as a means of sterilization. Chlorine is deadly to pet fish and the amount of chlorine in tap water is usually between 0.5 and 2.0 ppm. Most pet stores stock commercially prepared compounds containing sodium thiosulfate, which neutralizes chlorine by forming sodium chloride. Sodium thiosulfate will still neutralize the chlorine in chloramines but the ammonia will persist. A properly functioning biologic or chemical filter is necessary to remove this ammonia, which usually measures between 0.5 and 1.0 ppm.

## BACTERIAL DISEASES

Most bacterial pathogens of fishes are gram-negative rods and include such genera as *Aeromonas*, *Pseudomonas*, *Vibrio*, and *Flexibacter*. Infections can be severe and lethal bacteremias and septicemias are not uncommon. Antemortem blood cultures can be diagnostic, and if a necropsy is performed, the kidney and/or spleen should be sampled for culture and sensitivity. Many infections are secondary to environmental or transportation stress, poor water quality, or another primary pathogen such as a protozoan or metazoan parasite.

Once a diagnosis of bacterial disease has been made or suspected on the basis of clinical signs, a treatment plan should be formulated. Larger pet fishes may be injected intraperitoneally or intramuscularly with antibiotics that are effective against gram-negative pathogens (see Table 2). Once culture and sensitivity results have been obtained, the antibiotic regimen may be altered.

An alternative to injectable antibiotic therapy is utilizing the oral route. Antibiotics may be mixed into a gelatinized food (Table 3) or given as a bolus via a gastric tube if the fish is refusing food. Fish are quite easy to force-feed, since there is no risk of aspiration (no trachea or lungs). A flexible blunt tube such as a red rubber catheter can be used to administer a gruel that should be fairly viscous. Commercial flake or pelleted food can be mixed with small amounts of water to formulate the tube feeding gruel. Special care should be taken when passing the gastric tube to avoid perforation of the gastric lining. The clinician will benefit by being familiar with the general anatomy of the particular fish patient.

A third and less desirable approach to antibacterial chemotherapy is to administer the treatment as a bath. Antibiotics and other compounds can be added directly to the water the fish is in, although this type of treatment is more appropriate for ectoparasite infections. Fish treated in this manner should be removed from the display aquarium and placed in a hospital tank. The treatment tank should be well aerated and any carbon filtration should be discontinued. Table 2 contains suggested medications, doses, and duration of treatment.

## FUNGAL DISEASES

Fungal diseases are usually external and are most always secondary to a break in the integrity of the epidermis and its mucous coating. Common pathogens include *Saprolegnia* and *Fusarium*. Fungal hyphae and spores can be observed in a skin or fin biopsy sample under the microscope. If the infection is not severe, many fish will heal with supportive care. The fungal colony can be gently removed with a cotton swab and the underlying wound may be treated topically with Panalog ointment. Silvadene cream has also been found to be helpful as a topical antimicrobial.

## PROTOZOAL DISEASES

An overwhelming protozoal disease can constitute an emergency situation for a tank of pet fish. A skin scraping and gill biopsy help identify the specific parasite or parasites. Some protozoans such as *Ichthyophthirius* ("Ich") and *Cryptocaryon* (saltwater "Ich") have an encysted stage that is resistant to chemotherapeutic treatment. When faced with a protozoal outbreak, the clinician must look for a source. Most commonly, it is the addition of an unquarantined animal to the aquarium or the presence of a stressor such as overcrowding or poor water quality. Several antiprotozoal compounds appear in Table 2.

Adding salt to the water in the right quantities will kill some protozoans and can help reduce stress on freshwater fishes by decreasing the osmotic gradient that they face. Since freshwater fishes are hyperosmotic to their environment, water tends to "leak" into them. The kidneys and gills remove this excess water, but de-

### Table 3. Gelatinized Food Recipe

This recipe yields approximately 750 gm of food. Recipe may be halved or doubled depending on amount of feed desired. Final product should be stored cold or frozen. Will keep for about 7 days in the refrigerator.

1. Weigh 125 gm of flake or pelleted fish food and place into a blender. Add 250 ml of clean water and mix well.
2. To this slurry add one can of sardines (with oil) and a half jar of baby food or some fresh spinach. Blend well.
3. Add any medications at this time.
4. In a separate pan, heat 250 ml of clean water to near boiling. Add two packets (7 gm each) of gelatin and stir well. Allow the gelatin mixture to cool for about 10–15 min and then add the food/medication mixture. If a firmer food is desired, more gelatin can be added.
5. Stir the mixture well and pour into ice cube trays or small bags to make feeding easier. Place in refrigerator.
6. The food should set in several hours and can be fed at that time.

bilitated fishes have a special problem if their normal water-removing mechanisms are working poorly. Most freshwater fishes tolerate between 0.1 and 0.3% salt in their water (i.e., between 1 and 3 gm of salt [artificial sea salt is best] per liter of water).

## METAZOAN PARASITES

This broad group of parasites includes the skin and gill flukes (monogeneans), cestodes, nematodes, trematodes, and crustacean parasites. With the exception of a severe monogenean skin and gill infestation, the presence of these parasites usually does not constitute an emergency. Antemortem fecal examination or a thorough necropsy can diagnose an internal helminth problem. Crustacean parasites such as the fish louse (*Argulus*) and the anchorworm (*Laernea*) can be observed with the naked eye. Monogeneans like *Gyrodactylus* and *Dactylogyrus* usually require microscopic examination to be seen.

## References and Suggested Reading

Blasiola GC: *The New Saltwater Aquarium Handbook.* Hauppauge, NY, Barron's Educational Series, 1991
   *General reference focusing on the marine aquarium and keeping saltwater tropical fish healthy.*
Gratzek JB: *Aquariology: The Science of Fish Health Management.* Morris Plains, NJ, Tetra Press, 1992.
   *General up-to-date reference with an emphasis on the health and maintenance of freshwater pet fishes.*
Lewbart GA: Medical management of disorders of freshwater tropical fish. Compend Cont Educ 13:969, 1991.
   *Review article on common medical problems and treatments of freshwater pet fishes.*
Roberts RJ: *Fish Pathology.* London, Baillere Tindall, 1989.
   *Well illustrated text covering all aspects of fish pathology.*
Spotte S: *Captive Seawater Fishes.* New York, John Wiley & Sons, 1992.
   *A comprehensive reference on all aspects of keeping marine fishes in captivity.*
Stoskopf MK: *Fish Medicine.* Philadelphia, WB Saunders Co, 1993.
   *A comprehensive reference text on all aspects of ornamental and food fish medicine written with the veterinarian in mind.*
Whitaker BR: Common disorders of marine fish. Compend Cont Educ 13:960, 1991.
   *Review article on common medical problems and treatments of captive marine fishes.*

# AMPHIBIAN DERMATOLOGY

DAVID L. WILLIAMS

*London, England*

An adequate understanding of amphibian dermatology rests on a clear understanding of the basic biology of the amphibian skin, its anatomy, and its physiology (Elkan and Cooper, 1980). Several unique characteristics of amphibian skin render it liable to damage through insults, both infectious and chemical. The many roles played by the amphibian integument, including such diverse functions as respiration and pH regulation, render skin disease in these animals a significant systemic problem. The amphibian skin appears to have a limited repertoire of reactions to differing insults. For example, dermal hyperemia, ulceration, and nodule formation occur in a variety of differing conditions, rendering the determination of the specific cause of a particular lesion a challenge. The use of laboratory diagnostic tests is an important part of the study of amphibian skin lesions. A large proportion of pathologic changes in the amphibian skin may also be a reflection of systemic disease, particularly septicemia with attendant dermal hyperemia. Thus changes in the skin of an amphibian can be not only a sign of localized insult, but also a window on the systemic condition of the animal. Amphibian dermatology is therefore a key part of amphibian medicine and is worth considerable attention.

## BIOLOGY OF THE AMPHIBIAN INTEGUMENT

The amphibian integument differs markedly from that of other vertebrates (Duellman and Trueb, 1986). It lacks the protective barriers found in the skin of other orders: scales in fish and reptiles or thick keratinized epidermis in birds and mammals. Although the skin of most amphibian species is covered by layers of keratin and mucus, these layers are thin and provide relatively little protection for the animal. Also, unlike most vertebrates, the epidermis of amphibians is only a few cells thick. These features render amphibians particularly susceptible to a wide range of pathogenic agents, both infectious and noninfectious, affecting the skin. The diversity of amphibian habitats results in a wide spectrum of integumental anatomy and physiology: while a totally aquatic amphibian will have an epidermis only a few cell layers thick, a mainly terrestrial amphibian will have a thicker, more highly keratinized epidermis. Such variations are also seen at different stages in the animal's life: a tadpole, being entirely aquatic, has a markedly different integumental anatomy from that of an adult frog (Fox, 1977).

The morphologic peculiarities of amphibian skin are related to its function. Not only does the amphibian skin "keep the outside out and the inside in" in common with the skin of all animals, but in many amphibian species it plays an important role in respiration and in water and pH homeostasis.

Mucus, produced by the mucous glands and ordinary epithelial cells, is important both for maintaining the oxygen permeability of the skin and as a waterproofing agent. In addition, many species of anuran have a layer of mucopolysaccharide in the dermis that is believed to be involved in the prevention of desiccation of terrestrial species. The importance of the moist integument in the amphibians must be taken into account when handling them: the use of plastic disposable gloves thoroughly wetted prevents any damage to the skin during handling.

The amphibian skin undergoes a molting process similar to that of reptiles. In terrestrial amphibians, the cornified cell layer is sloughed in one piece and is usually eaten by the animal immediately following the molt. Once an animal has started to molt, the whole process should take only a matter of minutes. The intermolt period is variable, ranging from 1 day to several weeks and is dependent upon species, age, physiologic status, and ambient temperature. The epidermal influences of endocrinologic changes related to metamorphosis and molting are complex, involving hormones such as thyroxine and aldosterone, and are incompletely understood. Aestivating amphibians may become encased in cocoons of multiple sloughs.

A knowledge of the anatomic peculiarities of the amphibian integument is important in understanding the diseases affecting the skin. The paucity of epidermal protection contributes to the prevalence of infectious dermatopathies covered below. The high skin permeability that allows paradermal respiration to occur also allows entry of noxious agents from the environment. Thus the amphibian skin is readily breached by both infectious and noninfectious agents. Once these features are understood, the importance of hygiene measures in captive amphibian housing and of environmental precautions, such as pH monitoring and meticulous attention to removal of agents such as detergents from the environment, are evident.

## RESPONSES TO DISEASE

One of the main problems with clinical amphibian dermatology is that a number of infectious agents give similar gross changes. Edema, erythema, petechiation, and dermal hyperemia are seen associated with a number of agents, but most particularly with bacterial disease, both local and generalized. The occurrence of white dermal nodules occurs in fungal infection and in mycobacteriosis, while ulceration can be found associated with infectious and parasitic disease together with environmentally related lesions. These similarities in the clinical picture of diseases with varying etiologies underline the importance of diagnostic tests relating both to the lesions themselves and to the environment in which the animals are held.

## INFECTIOUS DISEASE

### Viruses

The lack of information available concerning viral amphibian skin disease reflects the infancy of amphibian virology rather than necessarily a low incidence of dermal lesions associated with viral infections. Tadpole edema virus (TEV) is an iridovirus found to cause generalized edema and diffuse hemorrhage on the ventral skin surfaces of metamorphosing tadpoles of the American bullfrog *Rana catesbeiana*. The virus has also been isolated from normal adult and larval bullfrogs. Death, edema, and diffuse hemorrhaging on the ventral surfaces of the hindlimbs were reported following inoculation of TEV into adults of three other species: Great Basin spadefoot toads (*Scaphiopus hammondii intermontanus*), American toads (*Bufo americanus*), and Fowler's toads (*Bufo woodhousii fowleri*).

An unidentified virus has been reported causing a generalized hemorrhagic disease termed viral hemorrhagic septicemia of frogs (VHSF). Dermatologic lesions included white nodules and petechial bleeding with subsequent lethargy and death. Recently, a poxvirus-like particle has been found in the skin of common frogs (*Rana temporaria*) taken from sites of unusually high mortality in England. The frogs died with either a generalized hemorrhagic syndrome, skin ulceration with or without ectromelia, or a combination of the two findings.

The problem with definitively linking dermal lesions with a viral etiology is that viral identification necessitates electron microscopy and viral culture requires the maintenance of amphibian cell lines, neither of these being generally available to the practitioner. Hence a diagnosis of viral disease remains, unfortunately, one of exclusion. Treatment can be merely symptomatic, and vaccines have yet to be produced to any amphibian viral disease. Isolation of affected individuals is mandatory.

### Bacteria

Bacterial septicemia in amphibians is usually manifest by a reddening of the skin, particularly that of the ventral body and hindlegs. The descriptive term "red-leg" has been adopted for this condition, although it should be understood that this term is related to a clinical finding rather than a specific etiologic agent. The hindlimb flexor surfaces are typically most severely affected, but the skin over the entire body can be reddened. Skin ulceration, subcutaneous edema, or a combination of these findings may also be a feature.

Red-leg usually occurs as an epizootic, and morbidity and mortality are high. It is the most commonly reported and important disease of amphibians, first reported in the 1890s. Red-leg has been subsequently recorded in a large number of adult and larval amphibian species, both in captivity and in the wild. Most reports involve anurans and some outbreaks have resulted in the deaths of many hundreds of animals. Red-leg has been implicated in the local extinctions of some species (Bradford, 1991).

Affected skin is erythematous, hemorrhagic, or both of these, but in peracute cases congestion of the skin vasculature may be the only visible lesion. At postmortem examination, multiple hemorrhages may also be found in limb musculature and visceral organs such as the gastrointestinal tract. Histologic examination reveals focal necrosis and microscopic hemorrhages. Inflammatory cell infiltrate may be found in visceral tissues as well as the epidermis and dermis.

A large number of species of gram-negative bacteria have been recorded as causing red-leg, with *Aeromonas hydrophila* being the most frequently isolated (Glorioso et al., 1974; Hubbard, 1981). While the majority of integumental lesions seen in amphibians relate to systemic bacterial infection and septicemia, local bacterial infections have been reported to give similar hyperemic and ulcerative dermal lesions. This emphasizes the importance of local bacteriologic investigation as well as blood culture from animals with dermal hyperemia. In either local or systemic infection, systemic antibiosis is required, with the drug chosen after culture and sensitivity results are available.

The complication associated with finding such agents associated with a skin lesion is that bacteria such as *Aeromonas hydrophila* are commonly found as saprophytes in aquatic and semiaquatic conditions. Some have been described as normal flora of the amphibian gut. The interpretation of skin surface bacteriologic examination can thus be difficult. Isolation of an organism from the skin surface should not be considered to directly imply a causative role in skin lesions. Isolation as a pure rather than mixed culture, or from blood or subcutaneous fluids, is more convincing proof of a pathogenic role.

The reason for occurrence of outbreaks of disease is not known, but red-leg may in some cases be secondary to factors such as stress due to adverse environmental conditions. Infection of the skin with a primary pathogen such as *Pseudocapillaroides xenopi* may allow the entry of opportunistic bacteria. In some cases, erosive skin lesions are seen at points of contact where trauma may occur, especially in captive amphibians at high stocking density.

Various antibacterial agents may be utilized in the treatment of red-leg. Ideally, treatment should be based on the results of bacteriologic findings and sensitivity testing. It is recommended that a sick individual be sacrificed in order to carry out a postmortem examination and microbiologic testing, as the internal bacterial flora changes rapidly following death. Parenteral antibiotics are preferable to bathing the animals in antibiotic solution, although the latter may be the only practical method for treating a large number of affected and in-contact animals. Indeed, using antibiotic in solution can be highly effective in reducing environmental contamination in captive situations.

Captive amphibians are particularly at risk from the build-up of bacterial contamination in poorly maintained tanks. Adequate and frequent environmental cleaning is important, and if cases of red-leg occur, in-contact animals should be moved to a clean environment while the contaminated enclosure is thoroughly cleaned and disinfected. Once clinical signs of red-leg appear, treatment is unlikely to succeed and may be useful only prophylactically to prevent in-contact animals from succumbing to the disease. Environmental conditions should be improved and the possibility of other predisposing factors should be investigated.

## Chlamydia

Infection with *Chlamydia psittaci* has been reported in colonies of African clawed toads (*Xenopus laevis*) showing lethargy, skin sloughing, and hemorrhage. Differentiation from other bacterial infections is by histologic demonstration of basophylic intracyctoplasmic inclusion bodies. Treatment relies on parenteral doxycycline.

## Mycobacteria

Cutaneous lesions associated with mycobacteriosis are generally nodular in appearance, but ulceration may also be involved. Here, the main differential diagnosis is that of fungal disease. While impression smears can be diagnostic, skin scrapings are more likely to provide sufficient tissue for a positive diagnosis. A modified Ziehl-Neelson stain shows mycobacteria, while hyphae are to be seen with methylene blue staining in fungal disease. Culture of organisms is difficult, since many saprophytic strains are slow growing and contaminants are a frequent problem. Treatment with antitubercular drugs is rarely, if ever, effective. Control relies on removal of organisms from the environment. Mechanical removal of slimes and organic films is much more effective than disinfection, as mycobacteria are resistant to most commonly used agents except glutaraldehyde.

Several acid-fast organisms have been associated with mycobacteriosis in amphibians. While none of the primary mycobacterial pathogens of homeotherms has been linked with amphibian disease, mycobacteria cultured from poikilotherms have been shown to cause lesions in humans. Given this zoonotic potential, care should be taken when handling affected or in-contact animals. Organisms such as *Mycobacterium xenopi* are

predominantly saprophytic species that can be isolated from the environment and thus, as with *Aeromonas hydrophila* in red-leg, care has to be taken in the interpretation of their isolation from amphibian lesions.

Amphibian resistance to mycobacterial infection is considered to be high; thus lowering of host defenses as well as adequate exposure to the organism are required to allow the disease to become established. Disruption of the integument may result in a portal of entry for organisms from contaminated water and localized or disseminated mycobacteriosis may result. Other routes of entry are through ingestion with ascending biliary infection resulting in hepatic disease.

## Fungi

Of the several fungal dermatoses of amphibia, the most important is chromomycosis caused by fungi of the family *Dematiaceae* such as *Phialophora*, *Fonsecaea*, and *Cladosporium* (Schmidt, 1984). These fungi, which produce simple conidiophores with darkly pigmented conidia, are found in soil, and transmission is presumed to be through small skin lesions allowing the entry of spores. Stressed animals appear to be more susceptible to disease. Clinical characteristics include papular and ulcerative skin lesions in otherwise normal animals. Later, wasting and debilitation leading to death occur as a result of systemic spread. Skin lesions may also present as vesicles or tumor-like nodules. Ulceration is well circumscribed, and soft tissue infiltration with bone destruction may occur in some cases. The tumor-like nodules represent an inflammatory response around a dense knot of fungal mycelium. Diagnosis is by skin scrapings or biopsy in which black or brown sclerotic fungal cells can easily be identified without resorting to special stains. Although treatment of small ulcerative dermal lesions with topical ketoconazole has been reported as being beneficial in the short term, it is not curative, and no cases of long-term recovery from the condition have been reported in amphibians. Amputation in early stages of involvement of an appendage has been suggested by some workers. Control relies on management practices and strict quarantine of in-contact animals. The disease is a zoonosis, thus handlers of sick animals should wear gloves and take precautions when coming into contact with the environment in which the amphibians are kept.

Phycomycosis, associated with *Basidiobolus* infection, can cause subcutaneous granulomatous lesions in amphibians and humans. *Saprolegnia*, a common fungal organism in fish, can cause dermal ulceration in aquatic amphibia kept in highly contaminated environments. Therapeutic agents such as benzalkonium chloride (2 mg/L), mercurochrome (4 mg/L), or methylene blue (4 mg/L) should be used as baths for 1 hr daily rather than adding the drugs at lower concentrations to the captive environment. Treatment where large mats of fungal mycelia occur should include mechanical débridement.

## PARASITIC DISEASE

### Protozoa

A number of protozoa cause lesions in the amphibian skin, but diagnosis must take into account that, as with any water-dwelling animal, large numbers of purely commensal organisms can be found in scrapings from the superficial integument. Nevertheless, the finding of large numbers of organisms associated with lesions is significant. The dinoflaggelate *Ichthyosporidium* is a parasite not only of fish but also of axolotls and in tadpoles. It can parasitize the host to such an extent that a clinically apparent gray film covers the animal. *Dermocystidium* species may be found as sporozoan parasites causing small dermal masses in newts and in South American tree frogs. Among the ciliates, *Trichodina*, a common parasite of the fish integument, is also found on axolotls, and the ciliate *Tetrahymena pyriformis* has been reported causing epidermal swellings in larval salamanders *Amblystoma maculatum*, with subsequent death. Other ciliates such as *Costia* and *Vorticella* may also be noted on examination of skin scrapings, and treatment by immersion in dilute saline, formalin, or copper sulphate solutions may be used as in the case with infections in fish.

### Metazoan Parasites

*Pseudocapillaroides xenopi*, a capillariid nematode that parasitizes the epidermis of the *Xenopus laevis*, is an important pathogen of this species: there are several reports of verminous dermatitis, with high rates of morbidity and mortality in captive colonies. The larval and adult stages of *P. capillaroides* live in tunnels within the thin epidermal layer. The life cycle is direct and, as the parasite eggs are present in the epidermis, autoinfection occurs when the frog molts. Even with such reinfection ongoing in a colony, it can take up to 18 months before disease becomes apparent. Clinical signs of infection include roughening of the skin and ulceration, particularly over the dorsum with systemic signs of weight loss and lethargy occurring later in the disease. Diagnosis can be made either by histologic detection of the epidermis nematodes following biopsy or postmortem skin sampling, or by direct microscopic examination of desquamated skin or of skin scrapings. Treatment with thiabendazole at 0.1 gm/L in the water is successful. Repeated thiabendazole treatment 2 weeks after the initial dose prevents problems with reinfestation (Cohen et al., 1984).

Microfilarial infestations can cause ischemic necrosis of areas of integument by blocking vessels supplying these tissues, but more commonly in amphibians they give rise to dermal masses. While trematode infestation in amphibians most commonly affects the intestine, urinary bladder, or lungs, a number do involve the skin. Larval metacercariae occur as pigmented cysts generally around the neuromasts, giving a striking appearance. Although generally nonpathogenic, massive metacercarial infestations can be deleterious to the host.

## NEOPLASIA

Neoplasia of the integument in amphibians is not commonly reported, but this may be more a reflection of the lack of attention paid to these species rather than a low prevalence of the condition. A few cases of squamous cell carcinoma have been reported in frogs, and lesions resembling adenomas of skin glands, fibromas, papillomas, and even chondromas in the integument have been observed. Dermal neoplasia, including squamous cell carcinomas, has been reported in salamanders from a sewage lagoon contaminated with jet fuel.

## ENVIRONMENTAL INFLUENCES

The anatomy of the amphibian skin together with the close association between the aquatic environment and the integument render environmental influences an extremely important factor in amphibian skin disease. The pH of the water supply is critical: an adversely acidic or alkaline environment will cause excess production of mucus, irritation and ulceration of the skin and, in severe cases, systemic effects leading to death. Local toxic effects may occur from a number of causes ranging from traces of detergents used to clean aquaria to the irritant effects of toxic secretions from other amphibia kept in mixed exhibits. Chlorine has particularly severe noxious effects, as do chemicals such as ammonia and nitrates. Effects from chlorine may be seen if animals are housed in newly disinfected tanks, while problems with nitrates are particularly important in fertilizer-contaminated run-off from agricultural land, affecting wild populations. The influence of such agents in the environment serves to emphasize the importance of a complete history and investigation of the environment as well as clinical examination of the individual animals.

## CONCLUSION

Three problems occur in the investigation of amphibian skin disease. The first is that a number of different etiologic routes lead to the same integumental appearance—hyperemia, ulceration, or nodule formation. Thus, defining the cause of a given lesion can be difficult and may require bacteriologic, mycologic, cytologic, and histologic examination of appropriate samples. The second problem is that in many cases the skin pathology reflects systemic disease, particularly septicemia, in the affected animal and thus clinical investigation should never be confined to the skin alone. The third problem, as will have been noted from this review, is that treatment of skin disease in amphibians is rarely curative. The important steps to be taken in the face of integumental lesions are the improvement of the environment in which the amphibian is kept and the control of the disease by isolation of the affected animal, should an infectious cause be defined.

## References and Suggested Reading

Bradford DF: Mass mortality and extinction in a high-elevation population of *Rana muscosa*. J Herpetol 25:174, 1991.
*Description of a massive "die-off" from red-leg in a frog population.*

Cohen N, Effrige NJ, Parsons SV, et al: Identification and treatment of a lethal nematode (*Capillaria xenopodis*) infestation in the South African frog *Xenopus laevis*. Dev Comp Immunol 8:739, 1984.
*Paper reporting diagnosis and treatment of capillariasis in Xenopus laevis.*

Duellman WE and Trueb L: *Biology of Amphibians.* New York, McGraw-Hill, 1986, p 367.
*General biology and physiologic reference for amphibians.*

Elkan E and Cooper JE: Skin biology of reptiles and amphibians. Proc R Soc Edinb 79B:115, 1980.
*General reference article on the biology of amphibian skin.*

Fox H: The anuran tadpole skin: Changes occurring in it during metamorphosis and some comparisons with that of the adult. Symp Zool Soc Lond 39:269, 1977.
*Review detailing amphibian skin anatomy and physiology before, during, and after metamorphosis.*

Glorioso JC, Amborski RL, Amborski GL, and Culley DD: Microbiological studies on septicemic bullfrogs (*Rana catesbeiana*). Am J Vet Res 35:1241, 1974.

Hubbard GB: *Aeromonas hydrophila* infection in *Xenopus laevis*. Lab Anim Sci 31:297, 1981.
*Papers detailing Aeromonas infection and red-leg in wild and captive amphibians.*

Schmidt RE: Amphibian chromomycosis. *In* Hoff GL, Frye FL, and Jacobson ER (eds): *Diseases of Amphibians and Reptiles.* New York, Plenum Press, 1984, p 169.
*Review of chromomycosis with details of the biology of the pathogen together with diagnosis and control.*

# EUTHANASIA METHODS FOR ECTOTHERMIC VERTEBRATES

ROY B. BURNS
*and* WILLIAM MCMAHAN
*Louisville, Kentucky*

Reptiles, amphibians, and fish rely on environmental temperature to regulate their body temperature and can be collectively referred to as ectothermic vertebrates. The same basic pathways that process nociceptive information are present in all vertebrate animals. Although the perception of pain can be difficult to measure, it is reasonable to assume that reptiles, amphibians, and fish experience pain, distress, or anxiety when exposed to noxious stimuli to a similar degree as homeothermic vertebrates (mammals and birds).

Euthanasia is an important means of ending animal suffering. Euthanasia techniques should result in rapid unconsciousness followed by cardiac or respiratory arrest and ultimate loss of brain function (i.e., death). Any pain, distress, or anxiety experienced should be minimized prior to unconsciousness (Andrews, Bennett, and Clark, 1993). Some traditional methods of ending the life of ectothermic vertebrates (e.g., freezing) do not meet these requirements.

An anesthetic agent may be indicated for restraint or alleviation of pain prior to some euthanasia methods for certain species or individuals. Reviews of anesthesia for reptiles, amphibians, and fish are published (Crawshaw, 1993; Page, 1993; Brown, 1993) (also see "Reptile Anesthesia" and "Anesthesia of Pet Fishes," this volume, pp 1349 and 1365, respectively).

There are many situations outside the practice of veterinary medicine in which reptiles, amphibians, and fish are killed. This review of euthanasia methods for ectothermic vertebrates is limited to those the authors consider practical in private veterinary practice.

Safety is of special concern when working with large or poisonous ectotherms. Poisonous species should be handled by trained professionals with appropriate equipment and only when appropriate medical care for poisoning (e.g., appropriate antivenin) is readily available.

## REPTILES

For most reptiles, sodium pentobarbital (60 to 100 mg/kg) or other barbituric acid derivatives, administered intravenously or into the pleuroperitoneal cavity, are effective means of euthanasia (Andrews, Bennett, and Clark, 1993; National Research Council, 1992). Since venous access for injection is limited for most species of reptiles, injection into the pleuroperitoneal cavity serves as a good alternative route of administration. Intrapleuroperitoneal injection is performed by needle insertion lateral to the ventral midline and in the caudal one-third of the body of snakes, anterior to the hindlegs or caudoventral to the forelegs of tortoises, and lateral to the ventral midline in the abdominal region of lizards and crocodilians. Time to effect may be variable, but usually an effect is noticed within a few minutes and death occurs within 30 min.

Halothane or isoflurane can be used as euthanasia agents in reptiles. Using inhalants as a sole means of euthanasia is less satisfactory than other methods because high concentrations (near saturation) and long exposure times are required to ensure death. Modifying the reptile's enclosure into an induction chamber and using a cotton swab soaked with a volatile agent can provide a means of delivering these agents to venomous or aggressive individuals.

For small reptiles, a single blow to the head causing concussion and destruction of the brain and skull is a satisfactory method of euthanasia. Complete destruction of the brain and skull can be difficult to accomplish. The blow should at least result in unconsciousness. If the brain is not completely destroyed by the blow, this method should be followed by killing via exsanguination or double pithing (Andrews et al., 1993). For large reptiles (crocodilians, large tortoises, and turtles), gunshot to the brain is acceptable but must be performed by trained and skilled personnel. The brain of reptiles is small compared to mammals and birds and lies along the midline of the head halfway between the eyes and the occipital condyles. The cranium of some reptiles has two well-developed bony encasements.

The central nervous system of reptiles is extremely tolerant to anoxia. Some species of turtles and tortoises can survive more than 15 hr in an atmosphere of nitrogen. Therefore, methods of euthanasia that induce unconsciousness by interruption of blood supply to the head (e.g., decapitation, cervical dislocation, and exsanguination) are inappropriate for reptiles when used alone, since rapid unconsciousness does not occur (National Research Council, 1992; Cooper et al., 1989). These methods should be performed on reptiles that are unconscious either by an anesthetic agent or concussion. Decapitation is practical for small reptiles in which size allows for rapid decapitation with a large shears at the level of the first cervical vertebrae. Decapitation should be followed by double pithing (National Research Council, 1992) or freezing in liquid nitrogen (K Storey, personal communication) or dry ice to ensure death.

Pithing is generally considered as an adjunct to other methods of euthanasia. Because of variation in size and anatomy of reptiles, skill and training are required to perform pithing appropriately. Pithing should be performed after an anesthetic agent has been administered. When performed, both the brain and spinal cord should be pithed (double pithing). An appropriately sized needle is placed through the foramen magnum and directed cranially into the brain and rotated. The needle is then redirected caudally into the spinal cord and again rotated.

Although hypothermia will make reptiles and amphibians torpid, there is no evidence that it raises the pain threshold. Freezing at normal household freezer temperatures is contraindicated as a means of euthanasia, since formation of ice crystals on the skin and in the tissues is likely to cause pain or distress (Cooper et al., 1989; National Research Council, 1992). Cooling by brief exposure to subfreezing temperatures can be used as a means of restraint prior to an acceptable method of euthanasia, provided the animal does not come into direct contact with frozen surfaces and freezing of any body part does not occur.

## AMPHIBIANS

Sodium pentobarbital, 60 mg/kg intravenously or intrapleuroperitoneally, will humanely euthanize amphibians (Andrews, Bennett, and Clark, 1993; National Research Council, 1992). As with reptiles, intrapleuroperitoneal injection is preferred and is performed similarly to the method described for reptiles. In frogs and toads, the subcutaneous lymph spaces serve as alternative injection sites. The lymph spaces lie just under the skin over the back on both sides of the urostyle.

Administration of a chemical agent by immersion and absorption through the skin and gills is a simple and nonstressful means of delivering anesthetic and euthanasia agents. The depth of immersion should not result in covering the nares.

Tricaine methanesulfonate (ethyl-m-aminobenzoate, MS-222) is available in a Food and Drug Administration (FDA)–approved preparation for anesthesia and tranquilization of fish and other ectothermic animals (Finquel, Argent Chemical Laboratories, Redmond, WA), and as a chemical reagent product (MS-222, Sigma Chemicals, St. Louis, MO). Tricaine has a mechanism of action similar to other local anesthetics that decrease excitability and block impulse conduction in nervous and cardiac tissue. Tricaine is water soluble, nonflammable, and nonvolatile. Tricaine is acidic in solution (pH approximately 1.75) and can be buffered by addition of baking soda, 3 gm/L. Euthanasia of amphibians occurs in several minutes when immersed in a 10-gm/L solution of tricaine (Canadian Council on Animal Care, 1984).

Additional routes of administration of tricaine are injection into the pleuroperitoneal cavity and lymph spaces. Tricaine rapidly desensitizes exposed serosal tissues, making intrapleuroperitoneal injection essentially painless except for the initial needle passage (Letcher, 1992).

Benzocaine is similar to tricaine but is relatively insoluble in water. It must be dissolved in acetone prior to being placed in aqueous solution. The final solution has a neutral pH. Immersion in a 100-mg/L solution of benzocaine can be used to induce anesthesia in amphibians (Arena and Richardson, 1990).

An induction chamber and near saturation concentrations of halothane or isoflurane via an open drop technique will cause euthanasia in terrestrial amphibians.

As for small reptiles, concussion with destruction of the brain, concussion followed by double pithing, and decapitation immediately followed by a method to ensure death are acceptable euthanasia methods for small amphibians.

Pithing is preferably performed on anesthetized amphibians. The location of the foramen magnum of most amphibians may be readily identified by a slight depression in the skin on the dorsal midline just posterior to the eyes when the animal is restrained so the neck is flexed. If not evident visually, the tip of a needle may be placed on the skull and slid caudally along the midline. The depression of the foramen magnum is evident as the needle slides over the junction between the skull and first vertebrae. As for reptiles, both the brain and spinal cord should be pithed.

Hypothermia is an unacceptable method of euthanasia of amphibians for the same reasons as described for reptiles.

## FISH

Sodium pentobarbital (60 mg/kg) administered intraperitoneally will cause euthanasia in small fish or anesthesia in large fish (Andrews, Bennett, and Clark, 1993; National Research Council, 1992). Intraperitoneal injection in fish is accomplished by entering at the ventral midline with the needle pointing rostrodorsally.

Immersion solutions are easy to use for fish anesthesia or euthanasia. For euthanasia, immersion in tricaine solutions of 300 mg/L for 10 to 20 min is required. Benzocaine solutions of 50 mg/L will induce surgical anesthesia in a few minutes. To make a 50-mg/L solution, dissolve 200 mg benzocaine in 5 ml acetone and add this to 4 L seasoned water (Arena and Richardson, 1990). To avoid recovery in using immersion solutions for euthanasia, keep fish immersed for 10 min after opercular movements cease.

Halothane, 2 to 3 ml/L, in seasoned water at 24° to 26°C or bubbled into an induction tank from a vaporizer will induce anesthesia in fish (Arena and Richardson, 1990).

As described for small reptiles, decapitation of unconscious fish is an acceptable method for euthanasia of fish. The spinal cord is severed with a sharp shears placed at the level of the caudal margin of the operculum.

Stunning produced by a sharp blow to the head followed by killing with another method can also be used for euthanasia of fish (National Research Council, 1992).

## CONFIRMATION OF DEATH

Distinguishing between deep anesthesia or temporary unconsciousness and death in ectothermic vertebrates can be difficult but is important to avoid recovery of consciousness. It is common for the heart to continue beating after these animals appear to be dead. Electrocardiography or opening the body cavity can be used to confirm cardiac arrest.

### References and Suggested Reading

Andrews EJ, Bennett BT, and Clark JD: Report of the AVMA panel on euthanasia. J Am Vet Med Assoc 202:230, 1993.
  *A review that defines and describes acceptable, conditionally acceptable, and unacceptable methods of euthanasia.*
Arena PC and Richardson KC: The relief of pain in cold-blooded vertebrates. Aust Council Care Anim Res Teach (ACCART) News 3:1, 1990.
  *A review of anesthesia assessment and methods for reptiles, fish and amphibians.*
Brown LA: Anesthesia and restraint. *In* Stoskopf MK (ed): *Fish Medicine.* Philadelphia, WB Saunders Co, 1993, p 79.
  *A review of anesthesia and restraint for fish.*
Canadian Council on Animal Care: *Guide to the Care and Use of Experimental Animals.* Association of Universities and Colleges of Canada, volume 1, 1984, p 103.
  *A review and evaluation of euthanasia techniques for laboratory animals.*
Cooper JE, Ewbank R, Platt C, and Warwick, C: *Euthanasia of Amphibians and Reptiles.* London, Universities Federation for Animal Welfare and World Society for the Protection of Animals, 1989, p 6.
  *Description of euthanasia techniques for amphibians and reptiles.*
Crawshaw GJ: Amphibian medicine. *In* Fowler ME (ed): *Zoo and Wild Animal Medicine.* Philadelphia, WB Saunders Co, 1993, p 131.
  *A summary of amphibian medicine.*
Letcher J: Intracelomic use of tricaine methanesulfonate for anesthesia of bullfrogs (*Rana catesbeiana*) and leopard frogs (*Rana pipens*). Zoo Biol 11: 243, 1992.
  *Results of dose response trials in two species of frogs using tricaine methane sulfonamide by intracelomic administration.*
National Research Council Committee on Pain and Distress in Laboratory Animals: Recognition of Pain and Distress in Laboratory Animals. Washington, DC: National Academy Press, 1992, p 102.
  *A report on pain, stress, pain and stress control, and euthanasia in laboratory animals.*
Page CD: Current Reptilian Anesthesia Procedures. *In* Fowler ME (ed): *Zoo and Wild Animal Medicine.* Philadelphia, WB Saunders Co, 1993, p 140.
  *A review of anesthesia in reptiles.*

# PREVENTIVE MEDICINE IN LLAMAS

PETER D CONSTABLE
*Urbana, Illinois*

Llamas are native to the mountainous regions of South America, where they were domesticated around 5000 BC and used as a source of meat, transportation, and fiber. Three other New World camelids (alpaca, guanaco, and vicuna) are also found in South America, but of these only the alpaca has been domesticated. The alpaca is smaller than the llama and has been imported into North America, but is primarily used for fiber production. Llamas have recently become very popular in North America as pets or for trekking activities. In general, llamas are placid and healthy animals.

Phylogenetically, the order Artiodactyla (split toe, forestomach fermentation, and rumination) contains two suborders: Ruminantia (cud chewers, consisting of true ruminants such as cattle, sheep, antelope, deer, and so forth) and Tylopoda (padded foot). The only family in the suborder Tylopoda is Camelidae, which consists of three genera: *Camelus* (containing bactrian and dromedary camels, usually referred to as Old World camels), *Lama* (containing *Lama glama* [llama], *Lama pacos* [alpaca], and *Lama guanicoe* [guanaco]), and *Vicuna* (containing *Vicugna vicugna* [vicuña]. Llamas are therefore closely related to camels and more distantly related to ruminants and are best characterized as pseudoruminants. Important anatomic features of llamas include a split labial cleft, a dental pad, esophageal groove, glandular secretions into the pregastric fermentation chambers (called compartments), fimbriated liver lying on the right side of the abdomen, no gallbladder, a spiral colon, pelleted feces, a sigmoid flexure to the penis, a urethral recess, four nipples on the mammary gland, fusion of the distal ulnar and distal radial epiphysis, and a padded foot with a "toenail" on each claw. Important physiologic features of llamas include induced ovulation, pregnancy predominantly occurring in the left uterine horn, and a metabolism that appears to be midway between ruminants and horses, in that the plasma glucose concentration of the llama is similar to the horse but higher than ruminants, while llamas can experience both ketosis and hyperlipemia (Anderson et al., 1994).

Because there are currently no vaccines and anthelmintics approved for use in llamas and other New World camelids, veterinarians must use all products in an extralabel fashion, often by extrapolating knowledge obtained from cattle and sheep.

## VACCINATION PROGRAMS

Infectious disease appears to be uncommon in llamas. This may be due to the innate resistance of llamas or the low stocking density and small herd sizes in which most llamas are kept.

Tetanus is not a common problem in camelids, but reports exist of the disease in llamas and alpacas (Paul-Murphy et al., 1989). Tetanus toxoid should therefore be administered as part of the routine vaccination program for llamas. Commercial tetanus toxoid vaccines have been shown to produce a protective response in llamas, particularly when boosted on a yearly basis. Tetanus antibodies also appear to be transferred through the colostrum, thereby providing protection for the neonate (Paul-Murphy et al., 1989). The recommended vaccination program is two initial injections (2 to 4 weeks apart) of tetanus toxoid starting at 3 to 6 months of age followed by a yearly booster. Tetanus toxoid should be administered intramuscularly or subcutaneously to adult llamas at the dose rate recommended for horses and cattle, while llamas less than 6 months of age would be vaccinated at the sheep dose rate. It is not clear as to whether tetanus antitoxin should be routinely administered to adult llamas with necrotic wounds or neonates, as the incidence of tetanus is extremely low and anaphylactic reactions to equine proteins, although rare, can occur. When in-

dicated, tetanus antitoxin should be administered subcutaneously or intramuscularly at 500 IU (neonates) to 1500 IU (adults). The author prefers to administer tetanus antitoxin only to llamas with documented necrotic wounds and questionable or unknown tetanus toxoid vaccination history.

Enterotoxemia (due to *Clostridium perfringens* Types C and D) has been rarely diagnosed in North American camelids, although anecdotal reports exist (Thredford and Johnson, 1989). Type C enterotoxemia is characterized by sudden death and hemorrhagic enteritis, particularly in neonatal calves, lambs, pigs, and foals, and is likely to occur in milk-fed llamas. Type D enterotoxemia is characterized by sudden death, pericardial effusion, pulmonary edema, hyperglycemia, and neurologic signs. The recommended vaccination program for *Clostridium perfringens* types C and D is two injections (2 to 4 weeks apart) of a combined bacterin starting at 3 to 6 months of age, followed by a yearly booster in the last 2 months of pregnancy. Adults are vaccinated intramuscularly or subcutaneously at the cattle dose rate. Vaccination of females in late pregnancy will provide protection for the neonate. Antiserum against *Clostridium perfringens* types C and D is available, but should only be administered to neonatal llamas located on premises with documented disease occurrence, because of the risk of fatal anaphylactic reactions. Commercial vaccines combining tetanus toxoid with *Clostridium perfringens* types C and D are readily available. The adjuvant in multiway clostridial vaccines has been anecdotally associated with injection site reactions.

Although other infectious bacterial agents (*Leptospira interrogans* **serovars**, *Bacillus anthracis*, *Listeria monocytogenes*, *Clostridium septicum*, *Campylobacter* spp., and *Chlamydia psittaci*) have been isolated from diseased llamas, the author does not recommend routine vaccination for any of these agents. Specific vaccination programs should be considered for these bacteria when the disease is endemic to the geographic region or has been previously diagnosed on the property.

Viral infections also are uncommon in llamas. Vaccination against rabies should be considered in llama herds located in endemic areas. A killed rabies vaccine should be administered intramuscularly to llamas older than 3 months and repeated annually. It should be noted that the efficacy of these vaccines in llamas is unknown. Equine rhinopneumonitis virus (EHV-1) infection has been documented in llamas and alpacas with neurologic disease and blindness (Rebhun et al., 1988); however, the disease remains uncommon to rare. Although some authors have advocated vaccination with killed vaccines to prevent clinical disease in New World camelids, the efficacy of vaccination has not been proven. Moreover, experience with the neurologic form of EHV-1 in horses indicates that killed vaccines are not fully protective against the neurologic form of the disease, suggesting that vaccination may not prevent EHV-1 neurologic disease in camelids. The author, therefore, does not recommend routine vaccination against EHV-1.

## PARASITE CONTROL

Internal and external parasitism occur commonly in llamas. Unfortunately, little is currently known regarding the species involved, and it is generally assumed that the parasites are similar, if not identical, to those infecting ruminants. At least 11 different species of nematodes, one cestode species, and four protozoal species have been identified in the gastrointestinal tract of North American llamas (Rickard, 1992): *Camelostrongylus* spp., *Ostertagia* spp., *Marshallagia* spp., *Haemonchus* spp. (third compartment), *Trichostrongylus* spp. (third compartment and small intestine), *Nematodirus* spp., *Capillaria* spp., *Cooperia* spp., *Strongyloides* spp., *Moniezia* spp. (small intestine), *Trichuris* spp., *Oesophagostomum* spp., *Eimeria punoensis*, *E. alpacae*, *E. lamae*, and *E. macusaniensis* (large intestine). Heavy intestinal parasite loads will produce wasting, diarrhea, inappetence, and eventually death. Effective parasite control programs are therefore required for all llamas.

Broad-spectrum anthelmintics recommended for intestinal nematode control include ivermectin 200 μg/kg SC or PO; albendazole 10 mg/kg PO; and fenbendazole 10 mg/kg PO. These agents are preferred over other anthelmintics because of their high safety margin and broad spectrum of activity. Some owners prefer injectable ivermectin because llamas may spit out orally administered drugs and oral treatment can be difficult. In geographic regions with a cold winter, anthelmintics should be administered at least 5 days before turn out on pasture in the spring (early April), then at 8-week intervals until a final treatment immediately after the first frost (usually early November). The same anthelmintic should be administered for the duration of each year, with anthelmintic rotation occurring on an annual basis. In geographic regions with a warm winter, anthelmintics should be administered approximately every 2 months, with an additional treatment 1 month after the onset of spring pasture growth. These treatment regimens are safe, relatively economic, simple to remember, and minimize pasture contamination.

Coccidiosis rarely causes clinical disease in llamas because most young animals graze pasture and are therefore not confined to a heavily contaminated environment. When coccidiosis is suspected in young llamas, feeding a coccidostat such as amprolium (5 mg/kg PO daily) or decoquinate (0.5 mg/kg PO daily) for 21 to 28 days may control clinical signs of disease. Probably of greater importance than feeding coccidiostats is decreasing the stocking density and ensuring that feed and water troughs are located so that fecal contamination cannot occur (Rickard, 1992).

Llamas can be infected with both the common liver fluke *Fasciola hepatica* (Southern and Northwestern United States) and the large American liver fluke *Fascioloides magna* (Northern United States). Migrating and adult flukes can cause severe liver damage and death in llamas. Adult liver flukes can be killed by treatment with albendazole (15 mg/kg PO) or clorsulon (7 mg/kg PO). Note that a higher albendazole dose rate is required to kill adult *F. magna* than intestinal nematodes, clorsulon is effective against 8-week and older *F. hepatica* flukes but not *F. magna* flukes, and that ivermectin is ineffective against liver flukes.

Tapeworm infections are common in llamas and are considered nonpathogenic. Some owners appear very concerned over the presence of tapeworm segments in the feces and request treatment. Albendazole (10 mg/kg PO) and fenbendazole (10 mg/kg PO) are effective in treating cestode infections in ruminants and are likely to be effective in llamas.

Llamas can also act as aberrant hosts for the meningeal worm *Parelaphostrongylus tenuis*, for which white-tailed deer are the normal host. Migrating *P. tenuis* larvae in llamas produce neurologic signs of ataxia, incoordination, weakness, head tremors, circling, and recumbency (Lunn and Hinchcliff, 1989). Presence of eosinophils in cerebrospinal fluid of llamas with neurologic disease is highly suggestive of cerebrospinal nematodiasis with *P. tenuis*. Treatment consists of fenbendazole (50 mg/kg PO daily for 5 days), diethylcarbamazine (20 to 100 mg/kg PO daily for 2 to 10 days), and ivermectin (200 μg/kg, PO or SC once only) (Lunn and Hinchcliff, 1989). Ivermectin will only kill migrating *P. tenuis* larvae located outside the spinal cord, and will therefore not have any effect on the neurologic disease associated with larvae migrating within the central nervous system. The administration of high doses of ivermectin will not change this situation, as ivermectin neurotoxicity signs will be induced whenever central nervous system concentrations of ivermectin are adequate to kill nematodes. Prevention of additional cases of cerebrospinal nematodiasis requires deer-proof fencing and controlling the habitat of the snail that acts as an intermediate host. Administration of ivermectin at 2-weekly intervals from summer to early winter or the continuous feeding of pyrantel (dose undetermined) may provide additional protection in areas where white-tailed deer cannot be adequately controlled.

The major ectoparasites of llamas are biting lice (*Damalinia breviceps*); sucking lice (*Microthorcis cameli*); and *Sarcoptes*, *Chorioptes*, and *Psoroptes* mites (Cheney and Allen, 1989). Sucking lice, *Sarcoptes* mites, and *Psoroptes* mites can be successfully treated with ivermectin (200 μg/kg SC, two doses 2 weeks apart), whereas *Chorioptes* mites are difficult to kill with conventional antiparasitic agents. Biting lice are more common than sucking lice and reportedly are best treated with a pour-on organophosphate agent such as fenthion, administered as a 3% solution at 0.3 ml/kg directly onto the skin of the dorsum and not through the wool.

## References and Suggested Reading

Anderson DE, Constable PD, Yvorchuk-St Jean KE, et al: Hyperlipemia and ketonuria in an alpaca and a llama. J Vet Intern Med 1994, 8:207, 1994. *Discussion of metabolism and response to inadequate energy intake in New World camelids.*

Cheney JM and Allen GT: Parasitism in llamas. *In* Vet Clin North Am [Food Anim Pract] 5:217, 1989.
    *A brief review of internal and external parasites in llamas.*
Lunn DP and Hinchcliff KW: Cerebrospinal fluid eosinophilia and ataxia in five llamas. Vet Rec 124:302, 1989.
    *A retrospective study of P. tenuis meningitis in llamas describing clinical signs, treatment, and outcome.*
Paul-Murphy J, Gershwin, LJ, Thatcher EF, et al: Immune response of the llama (*Lama glama*) to tetanus toxoid vaccination. Am J Vet Res 50:1279, 1989.
    *A research paper detailing tetanus toxoid response in llamas.*

Rebhun WC, Jenkins, DH, Riis RC, et al: An epizootic of blindness and encephalitis associated with a herpesvirus indistinguishable from equine herpesvirus 1 in a herd of alpacas and llamas. J Am Vet Med Assoc 192:953, 1988.
    *A detailed description of EHV-1 infection in New World camelids.*
Rickard L: Llama parasites: Large Anim Vet 6:1992.
    *A review of internal and external parasitism in New World camelids.*
Thredford TR and Johnson LW: Infectious diseases of New World camelids. *In* Vet Clin North Am [Food Anim Pract] 5:145, 1989.
    *A review of infectious diseases in New World camelids and a brief discussion of vaccination programs.*

# REPRODUCTIVE PHYSIOLOGY OF SOUTH AMERICAN CAMELIDS

P. WALTER BRAVO
*Davis, California*

South American camelids, also known as lamoids, are comprised of four species: two are domesticated (llama [*Lama glama*] and alpaca [*Lama pacos*]), and two are wild (guanaco [*Lama guanicoe*] and vicuña [*Lama vicugna*]). They are related to the Old World camels, the dromedary (*Camelus dromedarius*) and the bactrian camel (*Camelus bactrianus*). All camelids share the same number of chromosomes (37 pairs), and intercrosses between camels and between lamoids are possible and fertile.

This article includes the basic reproductive physiology of the female and male South American camelid. Although less is known about the guanaco and vicuna, this section is also applicable to them, with some differences attributed to behavior. Guanacos and vicunas reproduce seasonally. After the breeding season, the male guanaco separate himself from females and joins a male herd. In contrast, the male vicuna lives in continuous association with a small group of four or five females.

## PUBERTY

The term "puberty" (first estrus accompanied with ovulation) as applied to livestock species is not valid for camelids. Since camelids are induced ovulators and do not show clear signs of estrus, it is difficult to assess when they attain puberty. Nonetheless, yearlings, depending on their growth and nutrition, are able to reproduce. One of the most common and reliable indicators used in livestock species to correlate with puberty is live body weight. Alpacas with 35 kg and llamas with 60 kg at 12 months of age are ready to reproduce. Under South American management and nutrition, based entirely on native pastures, 60% of yearling alpacas reach 35 kg. Furthermore, 70% of

yearlings bred become pregnant and carry out pregnancy without any harmful effect on the growth of the female and the survival of the cria. The proportion of yearlings for breeding can improve if nutrition and management are better, as occurs in the United States and other countries.

The ovarian follicular activity in yearlings is similar to adult females. Laparoscopic observation of ovaries from yearlings and adults reveals no difference in the number of follicles grown. The onset of sexual behavior in yearlings is first noted as submission to the male. At the beginning of the breeding season, a great proportion of yearlings adopt the copulatory position immediately. Some females, though, are scared and escape from the male. However, most young females observe attentively the pair copulating, quickly learning to adopt the copulatory position.

## OVARIAN CYCLE OF CAMELIDS

The ovaries of llamas and alpacas are oval in shape, weigh approximately 2.5 gm, are 1.5 × 0.3 cm in length and width, respectively, and change in shape according to the presence of follicles. The ovarian cycle of camelids is divided into follicular and luteal phases, with the follicular phase present when females are open, and luteal phase when females ovulated after copulation.

Ovaries from llamas and alpacas always have follicles, even in the presence of a corpus luteum. Ovarian follicles grow in waves that tend to overlap; in other words, follicles grow and regress without ovulation. The interval between follicle waves is 11.1 days, and ovaries alternate in 81 to 85% of the cases in the follicle growth. This means that while one ovary presents one large antral follicle, the contralateral ovary is maintained in a relatively quiescent state. The process of follicle dominance is unknown. Follicles grow up to 6 mm without showing dominance; beyond this size, only one follicle becomes dominant. Follicle dominance is maintained over the follicles from the same cohort, in the ipsilateral and contralateral ovary as well. The succession of dominant follicles is repeated back and forth between ovaries until copulation and ovulation. The follicle wave is divided into three stages: growing, mature, and regressing. The period of time for each state is on average 4 days, and it seems that the reproductive stage of the female affects the length of follicle waves. Early lactating females appear to have 19 day's follicle wave in contrast to 12 day's in open females with more than a month after parturition.

Estrogen production also occurs in "waves." Levels of estradiol 17-$\beta$, estrone sulfate in plasma, and urinary estrone sulfate correlate with follicle waves. Concentrations of 10 to 15 pg/ml of estradiol and 20 to 30 ng/mg of creatinine of urinary estrone sulfate are associated with follicles of 8 to 12 mm. The presence of urinary estrone sulfate may be a clinically useful way to monitor ovarian activity, especially in small females where rectal palpation and ultrasonography are not possible. Progesterone is present only in basal concentrations (0.5 ng/ml), during the occurrence of follicle waves.

## COPULATION AND OVULATION

Camelid copulation is different for the female assumes a unique position, known as copulatory or recumbent position. The time of copulation ranges between 5 and 50 min, and lasts on average 18 and 20 min for the alpaca and llama, respectively. During copulation, the behavior of the female is calm and quiet, and some females may lie down in lateral position. The deposition of semen is intracornual (i.e., in the uterine horns), and it is unknown when ejaculation occurs.

Ovulation is induced by copulation as well as the administration of hormones with luteinizing hormone (LH) activity. Neural stimuli in the cervix, uterine horns, and rump at time of copulation cause the hypothalamus to secrete gonadotropin-releasing hormone that stimulates the pituitary gland to release LH. Concentrations of LH are evaluated 2 to 4 hr after copulation and return to basal levels by 6 hr after copulation. Ovulation may also occur spontaneously. In South America, where breeding is seasonal and large numbers of females are bred in a short period of time, up to 5% of females can ovulate spontaneously.

Ovulation occurs 26 to 40 hr after copulation or hormone application. The endocrine events immediately before ovulation are (1) a rapid decrease in concentrations of estradiol starting at 24 hr after copulation, and (2) disappearance of the follicle previously observed by ultrasonography. The proportion of females ovulating depends on management conditions. Under ideal circumstances, when breeding takes place with 7-mm or larger follicles, up to 90% of llamas and alpacas can ovulate. On the other hand, the proportion of females ovulating in field conditions is lower, especially if only one copulatory period is permitted. In this last condition, approximately 60% of the females ovulate within 24 to 30 hr. Delayed ovulation occurs in 30%, and absence of ovulation occurs in 10% of females.

The size of the follicle plays a role in the induction of ovulation. Breeding of a female with small follicles (3 to 6 mm) does not provoke ovulation, nor are follicle waves interrupted. Females bred when follicles are regressing luteinize the follicle with a short (5 to 7 days) luteal phase. The best time to induce ovulation is breeding when follicles are greater than or equal to 7 mm and in the growing phase or in the mature phase. A follicle is considered mature when it reaches 8 to 12 mm in size.

## CORPUS LUTEUM FORMATION

The corpus luteum is formed as a result of ovulation after breeding to a male or the administration of hormones with LH activity. The corpus luteum secretes progesterone, necessary to maintain pregnancy, and grows rapidly to 10 to 13 mm at day 7 or 8 after breeding. The corpus luteum can be detected by rectal palpation and ultrasonography, and indirectly by the presence of progesterone in blood. Concentrations of progesterone in blood reflect corpus luteum function. Progesterone appears in blood 2 to 3 days after ovulation or 3 to 4 days after breeding and ovulation. Elevated levels of progesterone (>1 ng/ml), at 7 days after breeding, are used to determine ovulation and luteal activity; however, this is not an indication of pregnancy. High progesterone at day 15 after breeding is an indirect indication of pregnancy. Camelids depend on the corpus luteum and progesterone to carry out pregnancy. Ablation of the corpus luteum or ovariectomy of the ovary containing the corpus luteum in pregnant females terminates pregnancy in 24 hr.

Prostaglandins secreted by the uterus cause corpus luteum regression at approximately 10 to 11 days if the female was bred to a vasectomized male or when she is not pregnant. Repeated and successive surges of 15-keto-13,14-dihydro-PGF$_{2\alpha}$ (the main metabolite of PGF$_{2\alpha}$) occur at around days 10 to 12 after breeding to a vasectomized male, indicating that only ovulation was induced and fertilization did not happen.

## SEXUAL BEHAVIOR OF THE FEMALE

Females, when approached by the male for breeding purposes, show two states of sexual behavior: acceptance or refusal. At the beginning of the breeding season, 90% of females show positive sexual behavior. Some females even adopt the copulatory position when they observe a pair copulating, and others after a minute of courting for the male. Acceptance is generally an indication of nonpregnancy; however, some females refuse the males even when they are open. Females may also exhibit sexual acceptance when a corpus luteum is present. This last behavior is accompanied by presence of large and ovulatory follicles in the contralateral ovary. A rule that should be remembered is that females adopt recumbency or copulate at any time of the follicular phase of the ovarian cycle.

## PREGNANCY

The length of gestation in llamas and alpacas is 342 to 350 days. Ninety-eight per cent of pregnancies are carried out in the left uterine horn; reasons for this predilection are unknown. Although the precise time of implantation is unknown, recent studies using ultrasonography and estrone sulfate suggest that implantation occurs at 21 to 27 days after breeding. Concomitantly, analysis of estrone sulfate in blood and urine also reveals marked elevations of this metabolite (10- to 20-fold) over what is normal for an open female. Appearance of an embryonic heart beat at this time also suggests the occurrence of implantation.

It appears that the first 30 days of gestation are crucial. Up to 50% of the embryo mortality occurs during the early embryo development and supposedly previous to implantation. Abortions (2%) are observed in the remaining period of gestation.

The prenatal growth has been defined for the alpaca. Sexual differentiation is clear macroscopically at day 60 of pregnancy. The weight of the fetus increases rapidly during the last 4 months of gestation, from 240 gm at 7 months of pregnancy to 7.2 kg at birth. Hair is present on the body at 7 months, the fetal eye opens at 8 months. In general, the equations of prediction for body growth such as crown-rump length, and length of the spinal cord follow a quadratic model.

The endocrinology of pregnancy as regards progesterone and estrogen concentrations has been reported recently. Progesterone is elevated throughout pregnancy and starts to decline 3 days before parturition, and similar (5 days) decline is observed in urinary pregnanediol glucuronide. Estrone sulfate in urine is elevated up to the onset of the second stage of parturition, suggesting a fetal or placental secretion. Since estrone sulfate is maintained elevated, it has a diagnostic value to diagnose fetal viability in overdue females, or when breeding records are lost.

## PARTURITION

Parturition in camelids occurs mainly during the morning hours. This is an adaptation to high altitude and cold environment; however, it is not rare to observe birthing during the afternoon. Females approaching delivery separate themselves from the rest of animals and tend to hum, urinate frequently, and lie down and get up repetitively. The whole process last approximately 2 to 3 hr. The prodromic stage lasts 1.5 hr, the expulsion of the fetus, 8 to 24 min; and the placenta is expelled within 1.5 hr. Normal presentation of the fetus is with the forelimbs extended and the head towards the vulva in dorsosacral position. Crias are delivered most of the time when the female is standing, and they are not licked as occurs in lambs and calves.

The occurrence of dystocia is rare—1.6% of births in Peru, and 25% of these numbers were attributed to first-time mothers. The most common presentation of dystocia (70%) was cranial longitudinal presentation, with the forelimbs and neck bent backwards, and the remaining 30% was caudal presentation.

## POSTPARTUM PERIOD

The postpartum period as defined in other livestock is not applicable to camelids, because of induced ovulation and absence of estrous cycles. Rather, it is the length of time from parturition to the next pregnancy. Analysis of estrone sulfate in llamas indicates that the ovarian follicular activity is resumed 5 days after parturition, and they may ovulate as soon as 15 days after parturition. Field observations in Peru reveal that females are able to copulate even the day following parturition; however, full involution of the uterus occurs at 21 days after parturition. Consequently, 20 days is the length of time given to the female as resting period before the initiation of the next pregnancy.

## REPRODUCTIVE PHYSIOLOGY OF THE MALE CAMELID

The male is often used to breed many females, and the selection of a male as a sire is usually more rigorous and demanding than a female. Many characteristics are considered for llamas and alpacas, including the size of the male, conformation, quality and color of fiber, shape of ears, and so forth. In addition, a male must have normal genitalia.

The testicles are located beneath the anus and within the scrotum whose location and orientation resembles that of the boar and the dog. Its muscular structure allows it to contract during cold weather and relax during warm weather. The testicles in a mature alpaca weigh about 18 gm, and vary in size from 4 to 5 cm in length and 2.5 to 3 cm in width.

The tail of the epididymis is not well pronounced, the vas deferens has a diameter of approximately 2 to 3 mm and a length of 40 cm. One striking feature of male llamas and alpacas is a lack of well-defined thickening of the ampulla. This may contribute to the poor response to electroejaculation.

The accessory glands include the prostate and bulbourethral glands. The prostate lies dorsolateral to the urethra. The bulbourethral glands are located lateral to the base of the penis. Male camelids do not have seminal vesicles.

The penis is fibroelastic, and the length varies from 35 to 40 cm. The glans penis presents a rather unique cartilaginous urethral process that has a clockwise orientation and guides the penis through the cervix of the female during copulation. The end of the urethra is located at the base of this cartilaginous process, and not at the tip. The prepuce has a posterior orientation, which is the reason male llamas and alpacas urinate backwards.

## GROWTH AND TESTICULAR FUNCTION

The growth of testicles in the llama is slow, reaching a plateau at approximately 30 months of age. The weight, length, and width of the testicles measured every 6 months appear in Table 1.

The androgenic function of the llama testicle has been defined recently. Concentrations of testosterone are low during the first 19 months of age (35 to 90 pg/ml), start to increase rapidly at 21 months of age (300 pg/ml), and reach a plateau at 30 months of age (650 pg/ml). The spermatogenic function of the camelid testicle is difficult to assess. The length of copulation and dribble ejaculation complicate semen collection. Semen collected by electroejaculation is not consistent; however, semen collection using an artificial vagina provides the most natural sample. The volume of the ejaculate is 1.7 ml (range = 0.4 to 4.3 ml), and liquefaction of the viscous material occurs as early as 8 hr. Semen consistency is viscous and progressive motility is slow if compared to ram semen. Semen represents 12% of the total ejaculated and there is no difference in most of the biochemical components between adult and 3-year-old males (first-time breeders). Sperm concentration varies from 350 to 600,000/ml.

The prepuce is attached to the penis in the newborn male and remains as such until 12 months of age. The detachment of the penis starts from the tip, and is initiated between 12 and 15 months. A third to a half of the glans penis is free at 18 months, and the glans is completely free at 22 months (range = 21 to 26 months). This process of detachment is related to testosterone concentrations. One practical point is that males should be used as sires only when they have two testicles and the glans penis is free from any attachment to the prepuce.

**Table 1.** *Development of Llama Testicles*

| Age (months) | Weight (gm) | Length (cm) | Width (cm) |
|---|---|---|---|
| 6 | ° | 2.1 | 1.1 |
| 12 | 5.1 | 2.5 | 1.5 |
| 18 | 14.0 | 3.4 | 2.3 |
| 24 | 17.4 | 4.0 | 2.5 |
| 30 | 17.8 | 4.4 | 2.5 |
| 36 | 18.2 | 4.5 | 2.7 |
| Sires | ° | 5.9 | 3.8 |

°Not available.

## SEXUAL BEHAVIOR OF THE MALE

Yearling males may show some sexual interest in females, and may attempt to breed; however, intromission of the penis is not successful because of the natural adherence between the penis and prepuce. Two-year-old males show more interest in females, and some of them could be successful because the penis may be totally free from the prepuce. Adult males make a characteristic guttural sound, called "orgling" in the United States, during copulation.

The length of copulation varies from 5 to 55 min, and is dictated by the male. Field observations in Peru also indicate that a male can copulate up to 18 times per day, especially during the first 3 days of the breeding season; however, there are no reports between fertility of the male and number of copulatory periods.

## References and Suggested Reading

Adams GP, Sumar J, and Ginther OJ: Form and function of the corpus luteum in llamas. Anim Reprod Sci 24:127, 1991.
*The growth and progesterone secretion of the corpus luteum in the llama is reported.*

Bravo PW, Fowler ME, Stabenfeldt GH, and Lasley BL: Ovarian follicular dynamics in the llama. Biol Reprod 43:579, 1990.
*A study of the ovarian follicle dynamics in nonpregnant llamas using ultrasonography and hormone analysis.*

Bravo PW, Stabenfeldt GH, Fowler ME, and Lasley BL: The effect of ovarian follicle size on pituitary and ovarian responses to copulation in domesticated South American camelids. Biol Reprod 45:553, 1991.
*A study of ovulation after copulation in presence of different follicle sizes.*

Bravo PW, Stabenfeldt GH, Fowler ME, and Lasley BL: Pituitary response to repeated copulation and/or gonadotropin-releasing hormone administration in llamas and alpacas. Biol Reprod 47:884, 1992.
*A study of the release of LH after single or repeated copulation and/or GnRH stimulation.*

Bravo PW, Stabenfeldt GH, Fowler ME, Lasley BL, and Frey RE: Testes development and testosterone concentrations in the llama (*Lama glama*). Proc 12th Int Cong Anim Reprod 4:1698, 1992.
*A report of testis growth accompanied by testosterone concentrations from birth to sexual maturity.*

England BG, Foote WC, Matthews DH, Cardozo AG, and Riera S: Ovulation and corpus luteum function in the llama (*Lama glama*). J Endocrinol 45:505, 1969.
*A description of ovulation and corpus luteum development in the llama.*

Fernandez-Baca S, Hansel W, and Novoa C: Corpus luteum function in the alpaca. Biol Reprod 3:252, 1970.
*An analysis of corpus luteum growth in alpacas.*

Garnica J, Achata R, and Bravo PW: Physical and biochemical characteristics of alpaca semen. Anim Reprod Sci (in press), 1995.
*A study of some biochemical characteristics of alpaca semen collected by artificial vagina.*

Leon JB, Smith BB, Timm KI, and LeCren G: Endocrine changes during pregnancy, parturition and the early post-partum in the llama (*Lama glama*). J Reprod Fertil 88:503, 1990.
*A report of different hormones throughout pregnancy in the llama.*

Sumar J, Fredriksson G, Alarcon V, Kindahl H, and Edqvist L: Levels of 15-keto-13,14-dihydro-PGF$_{2\alpha}$, progesterone and oestradiol-17β after induced ovulations in llamas and alpacas. Acta Vet Scand 29:339, 1988.
*A report of concentrations of prostaglandins after copulation to a vasectomized male.*

# POTBELLIED PIGS: GENERAL MEDICAL CARE

WILLIAM F. BRAUN, JR.

*Columbia, Missouri*

The pig, in the form of the potbellied pig, has made the transition of late from the farm to the city. It is not unusual for small animal practitioners to be presented with a pet potbellied pig for examination and veterinary care. This may be quite a noisy experience, as the potbellied pig can be very vocal in its objection to handling and examination. For the owner, these pets are different than the more common dog or cat, but that is part of their allure as a pet and the source of some confusion in their husbandry and care. The intact male pig is a boar, the castrated male is a barrow, a young female is a gilt, and the older female is known as a sow.

Potbellied pigs are described as miniature pigs, but this reference must be placed in proper context. As baby pigs, these miniature pigs are cute and very tiny, and birth weight is generally less than 450 gm. But as they grow, they may obtain sizes of 150 to 175 pounds when fully mature. Compared to the miniature breeds of dogs, the potbellied pig is very large, but compared to regular, commercial pigs that may become 600 to 800 pounds, they are small. Ideally, these pigs will weigh less than 75 pounds and many mature potbellied pigs never attain 50 pounds.

The veterinarian may be unfamiliar with many of the medical conditions of pigs. In commercial operations, many sick or injured pigs are sacrificed and go untreated. In pet practice, however, an attempt is made to diagnose and treat sick pigs. This latter approach is a fairly recent development in swine medicine and there are still a number of unsolved problems. The geriatric pig is a prime example of this, as few commercial swine live over 5 years of age. Currently, there are large number of potbellied pigs, 5 to 9 years of age, whose owners seek veterinary attention. Until adequate information becomes available, the veterinarian should consider treating the problems of the pet pig in a manner similar to that of a dog that might be presented with the same symptoms.

This article will attempt to point out some of the species-specific conditions and procedures important to pet pig practice, and to emphasize some medical and husbandry practices that will keep the pig a healthy pet.

## HANDLING AND PHYSICAL EXAMINATION

Though the potbellied pig is docile in nature, it may prove a challenge to transport and examine. Small pigs are typically transported in an appropriate sized pet carrier and physically lifted out upon reaching their destination (i.e., the examination room). Larger pigs may be placed in large pet carriers or restrained with a leash and harness. These bigger pigs can be a challenge to extricate from the carrier, which may need to be disassembled to facilitate removal.

Handling of small or immature pigs is similar to the handling of puppies of the same size. Whole body support is provided by cradling the pig on the handler's forearm or with both hands. One or more people may be needed to grasp the torso of larger pigs to lift them onto the examination or surgery table. The larger pigs are best examined on the floor with no attempt at lifting. To facilitate examination, it may be necessary to wrap the pig in a towel or blanket to restrict its movement. Any of these handling techniques will more than likely result in considerable vocalization on the pig's part. Some veterinarians have resorted to examinations in a back room or outside to minimize the potential disturbance to other patients and clients caused by the pig. Lifting or holding the pig with just the legs should be avoided, as the leg and joint structure of these pigs may not endure this stress and lower back or joint injury may result.

Physical examination proceeds as for any other pet. Physiologic changes may occur due to the stress of handling, restraint, and the clinic environment. Observation prior to handling allows the veterinarian to assess the pig's demeanor, general condition, locomotor ability, respiratory pattern, and evidence of pruritus or other skin disorders. These observations are made prior to handling. Hands-on examination should begin by obtaining a rectal temperature first, prior to exciting the pig by restraint. Auscultation of the lungs and heart is performed in a similar manner as for other domestic animals. The lung field of the pig occupies the anterior one third to one half of the thorax. Both the lungs and heart may be difficult or impossible to auscultate in the uncooperative pig. Normal values for rectal temperature, heart rate, and respiratory rate are listed in Table 1. Beyond respiratory rate, the respiratory system should be examined, taking note of any nasal discharge and the anatomy of the snout. While a short snout and wrinkled nose are normal for these animals, atrophic rhinitis may result in an exaggeration of this snout anatomy. The eyes of older potbellied pigs are normally deepset and may be partially obscured by facial wrinkles. The corneas should be checked for abrasions or trauma and any ocular discharges noted. In many cases, there will be a slight amount of a brownish red dis-

**Table 1.** *Normal Physiologic Data for Pigs at Different Ages**

| Age | Temperature (°F) | Heart Rate (bpm) | Respiratory Rate (bpm) |
|---|---|---|---|
| Newborn | 102.2 | 200–250 | 50–60 |
| Weaned pig | 102.7 | 90–100 | 25–40 |
| 10–15 weeks | 102.3 | 80–90 | 30–40 |
| 15–26 weeks | 101.8 | 75–85 | 25–35 |
| Sows, boars | 101.4 | 70–80 | 13–18 |

*Adapted from Straw BE, Merten DJ: Physical examination. In Leman AD, et al (eds): Diseases of Swine, ed 7. Ames, IA, Iowa State University Press, 1992, pp 793–807, with permission.

**Table 2.** *Hematology of Miniature Pigs**

| Parameters | Mean | Range |
|---|---|---|
| Erythrocytes ($10^6/\mu L$) | 7.78 | 6.84–8.51 |
| Hemoglobin (gm/dL) | 15.6 | 13.7–16.9 |
| Hematocrit (%) | 44.5 | 38.1–48.8 |
| MCV (fl) | 57.3 | 52.9–61.4 |
| MCH (pg) | 20.0 | 186–21.4 |
| MCHC (%) | 34.9 | 34.0–36.3 |
| Platelets ($10^3/\mu l$) | 372.3 | 272.0–497.0 |
| Leukocytes (cells/$\mu l$) | 11,600 | 7400–18,500 |
|   Segmented neutrophils % | 45.6 | |
|   Bands % | 14.7 | |
|   Lymphocytes % | 41.3 | |
|   Monocytes % | 4.0 | |
|   Eosinopiles % | 1.6 | |
|   Basophils % | 0.01 | |

*Adapted from Parsons AH, Wells RE: Hematologic values of the Yucatan miniature pig. Vet Clin Pathol 18:90–92, 1989, with permission.
Abbreviations: MCV = mean corpuscular volume, MCH = mean corpuscular hemoglobin, MCHC = mean corpuscular hemoglobin concentration.

charge that, in the absence of other signs, is considered normal. Oral examination of the intact boar may prove dangerous, as they develop exaggerated canine teeth known as tusks. Umbilical and inguinal hernias are common. Baby pigs should be checked for a patent anus, as atresia ani is not uncommon. Gilts with atresia ani will have an accompanying rectal-vaginal fistula that allows evacuation of the rectum, but baby boars may die if relief is not surgically provided. Routine fecal examination is done as for other small animal patients.

Potential breeding animals are examined for normal external reproductive organs. The boar has a closely held scrotum positioned just ventral to the anus and its contents are palpated for the presence of two normal testicles. The underline of both the sow and boar are checked for the presence and spacing of teats; each should have five to six pairs of evenly spaced teats to be considered for breeding service.

The musculoskeletal system is examined last, as manipulation of the limbs may induce pain or discomfort that will make examination of the other systems more difficult. The foot, hock, carpus, and hip are the most common areas for lameness. Their swayback may also be a source of pain or locomotor dysfunction, especially in older, obese pigs.

Venipuncture is difficult in these pigs due to their size and their tendency to be uncooperative. The common sites for blood withdrawal are the jugular vein and anterior vena cava, both by blind sticks. The caudal auricular, cephalic, and lateral saphenous veins may be used in more cooperative patients. While blood values have not been fully evaluated in these miniature pigs, values have been established for other breeds of miniature swine (Tables 2 and 3).

## REGULATORY CONSIDERATIONS

Potbellied pig owners consider their pigs as pets, however, the USDA and the various state veterinarian offices categorize them as domestic swine. Thus potbellied pigs fall under the same federal and state regulations as other swine. Interstate movement of all swine is regulated by the various states and some even regulate intrastate movement. These measures are designed to protect the multimillion dollar swine industry and ensure safe and wholesome pork.

A veterinarian is essential before an owner can cross state lines with their pig. The transported pig needs a valid interstate health certificate and most require a recent negative serologic test for pseudorabies and swine brucellosis. A popular pastime is the showing of pigs, similar to dog shows, and these events are usually affiliated with county or state fairs. As such, the pigs entering the fairgrounds are required to have a health certificate and recent negative tests. Veterinarians should consult authorities of the state of destination for requirements to enter that state.

## VACCINATIONS

A wide range of recommendations have been made for vaccination protocols in potbellied pigs, varying from no vaccinations to extensive lists of immunizations. In most cases, the single-pig household needs vary little in the way of vaccinations. The breeder, on the other hand, would require a far greater array of vaccinations. In all cases, *pig-specific* vaccines must be

**Table 3.** *Serum Biochemistry of Miniature Pigs**

| Parameter | Mean | Range |
|---|---|---|
| Glucose (mg/dl) | 79.8 | 56–153 |
| BUN (mg/dl) | 19.2 | 10–29 |
| Total protein (g/dl) | 7.5 | 6.3–9.4 |
| Albumin (g/dl) | 4.7 | 4.1–5.6 |
| Globulin (g/dl) | 2.8 | 1.4–3.6 |
| Calcium (mg/dl) | 10.6 | 9.3–11.6 |
| Phosphorus (mg/dl) | 6.9 | 5.0–8.3 |
| Creatinine (mg/dl) | 1.6 | 1.2–2.0 |
| Total bilirubin (mg/dl) | 0.1 | 0.0–0.3 |
| Cholesterol (mg/dl) | 101.8 | 47.3–173.0 |

*Adapted from Reeves DE (ed): Guidelines for the Veterinary Practitioner: Care and Management of Miniature Pet Pigs. Santa Barbara, CA, Veterinary Practice Publishing, 1993, pp 113–114, with permission.
Abbreviation: BUN = blood urea nitrogen.

**Table 4.** *Minimum Recommended Vaccinations for Potbellied Pigs*[*][†]

| Type of Pig | Disease | Vaccination Timing |
|---|---|---|
| Pet pigs | Erysipelas | At 8 to 12 weeks of age; repeat in 3 weeks. Revaccinate semiannually or annually. |
| | Leptospirosis | At 8 to 12 weeks of age; repeat in 3 weeks. Revaccinate semiannually or annually. |
| Breeder pigs | Erysipelas | At 8 to 12 weeks of age; repeat in 3 weeks. Revaccinate 3 weeks prior to breeding.[‡] |
| | Leptospirosis | At 8 to 12 weeks of age; repeat in 3 weeks. Revaccinate 3 weeks prior to breeding.[‡] |
| | Parvovirus | At 5 to 6 months of age; repeat in 3 weeks. Revaccinate 3 to 8 weeks prior to breeding. |

[*]From Braun WF: Helping your clients raise healthy potbellied pigs. Vet Med 88:423, 1993, with permission.
[†]Always follow label directions for proper dosage, timing, and route of administration.
[‡]Boars should be revaccinated semianually.

used in order to ensure development of immunity. Dogs and pigs share some of the same infective organisms, but they are different strains and cause different diseases. *Bordetella bronchiseptica* causes kennel cough in the dog but atrophic rhinitis in the pig. Canine parvovirus causes a devastating enteric infection in young dogs, but porcine parvovirus has no ill effects on the pig other than to cause some reproductive loss and fetal mummification in gilt litters.

Table 4 lists the minimum recommended vaccinations for the pet and the breeder pig. *Erysipelothrix rhusiopathiae* causes systemic illness, skin lesions (diamond skin disease), and arthritis. It is easily treated with penicillin but just as easily prevented by vaccination. Leptospirosis is found in both dogs and pigs. Pigs have a wider range of diseases caused by the leptospires and more serovars are pathogenic to swine. The most common serovar affecting pigs is *Leptospira pomona*, but they are susceptible to *L. canicola*, *L. icterohaemorrhagiae*, *L. grippotyphosa*, and *L. hardjo*. In some areas of the United States, a sixth serovar, *L. bratislava*, is known to infect commercial swine, but no cases have as yet been reported in potbellied pigs. Porcine parvovirus plus the five-way leptospire and erysipelas are contained in a multivalent vaccine produced by several manufacturers. This means that the small animal prac-

titioner presented with only a few pigs to treat needs but one bottle of vaccine to have all of these covered.

Additional problems may call for added vaccinations. Table 5 offers some selected vaccination suggestions. Breeders with baby pigs may encounter infective diarrheas that may be prevented through vaccination. Colibacillosis is the most common diarrhea condition in pigs and often occurs within the first few days of life, too soon for vaccination of the baby. This and other diarrhea-causing organisms, including rotavirus, *Clostridium perfringens*, *Salmonella*, and transmissible gastroenteritis (TGE), are prevented by vaccinating the sow during the last 6 weeks of gestation. Colostral immunity then protects the baby pig.

Respiratory problems may be significant in some pigs and are best treated by preventative vaccination. Rhinitis caused by *B. bronchiseptica* and *Pasteurella multocida* type A and D, and pneumonias caused by *Mycoplasma hyopneumoniae* and *Actinobacillus pleuropneumoniae* are examples. To be effective, vaccination against these organisms should begin at 1 week of age.

Pseudorabies, caused by a herpes virus, is a pig disease that in many states is under intense eradication effort. For this reason, vaccination is often under the control of the state veterinarian's office. In most cases, this is a production disease that does not affect the

**Table 5.** *Vaccination for Selected Disease Prevention in Pet Pigs*[*][†]

| Disease | Causative Agent | Vaccination Timing |
|---|---|---|
| Colibacillosis | *Escherichia coli* | *Sows:* 5 and 2 weeks before farrowing, 2 weeks before subsequent farrowing |
| Other enteritides | Rotavirus, TGE virus, *Clostridium*, *Salmonella* | *Sows:* 5 and 2 weeks before farrowing |
| Atrophic rhinitis | *Bordetella bronchiseptica*, *Pasteurella multocida* (types A and D) | *Sow:* 7 and 3 weeks before farrowing; 3 weeks before each subsequent farrowing<br>*Piglets:* 1 week of age, repeat in 3 weeks<br>*Boars:* Semiannual or annual |
| Pneumonia | *Mycoplasma hyopneumoniae* | *Sows:* 5 and 2 weeks before farrowing; 3 weeks before subsequent farrowings<br>*Piglets:* 1 week of age, repeat in 2–3 weeks<br>*Boars:* Semiannual or annual |
| | *Actinobacillus peluroneumoniae* | *Sows:* 5 and 2 weeks before farrowing<br>*Piglets:* 3 to 8 weeks of age, repeat in 3 weeks |

[*]From Braun WF: Helping your clients raise healthy potbellied pigs. Vet Med 88:414–428, 1993, with permission.
[†]Always follow label directions for proper dosage, timing and route of administration.

potbellied pig; therefore, routine vaccination against pseudorabies is not recommended. Pet owners often confuse pseudorabies with rabies, caused by a rhabdovirus. While the pig may become infected with rabies, it is very resistant to infection. No approved vaccine exists in the United States for rabies in pigs.

## PARASITES

Parasitism does not pose a large problem for potbellied pigs, probably due to their semiseclusive lifestyle. The single-pig household offers few opportunities for the pig to become infected with parasites from other pigs. Cat and dog parasites do not cross over to the pig except in a very transient manner. Diagnosis of internal parasites is based on fecal examination and external parasites by observation or skin scrapings. Appropriate parasitology textbooks should be consulted to identify ova, larvae, or parasites.

Internal parasites of potbellied pigs include lungworms (*Metastrongylus* spp.), intestinal worms such as roundworms (*Ascaris suis*), stomach worms (*Hyostrongylus rubidus*), nodular worms (*Oesophagostomum dentatum*), threadworms (*Strongyloides ransomi*), and whipworms (*Trichuris suis*) as well as an intestinal coccidia (*Isospora suis*). These internal parasites cause illthrift, stunted growth, and diarrhea. Respiratory signs may be evident from lungworm infections or the larval migration stage of some of the intestinal worms. Whipworms and threadworms may result in bloody diarrhea and anemia.

The two common external parasites are lice and mites. The hog louse, *Haematopinus suis*, is a large creature and readily visible on the skin of the pig. Fortunately, few lice are found on pet pigs. Sarcoptic mange mite infestation results in pruritic condition with crusty scales around the ear, face, and axillary region. Occasionally, fleas are observed on pet pigs, but these are typically transient fleas from the resident dog or cat.

Anthelmintic treatment is based on the type of parasite infection. Ivermectin is most commonly used for both external and intestinal parasites and for lungworms. The pig dose of ivermectin is 300 μg/kg (SC or IM), given once for internal parasites or repeated in 10 to 14 days when treating external parasites. Pyrantel (6.6 mg/kg PO) is effective against ascarids and nodular worms. Whipworms are difficult to treat; ivermectin is only partially effective. In most cases of whipworms, a 3-day regimen of fenbendazole (9 mg/kg PO) is needed.

## SEDATION AND ANESTHESIA

Sedation and tranquilization may be needed in even the simplest of procedures in order to reduce vocalization and produce a more cooperative patient. It is also useful prior to IV catheterization to ensure minimal movement by the pig while making the initial needle insertion. Of the species commonly seen in practice, the pig has the least consistent response to these sedatives or preanesthetics.

The placement of catheters is facilitated by the administration of acepromazine (0.03 to 0.1 mg/kg), which at higher dosages (0.2 to 1.1 mg/kg) will produce profound tranquilization. Xylazine (0.5 to 3.0 mg/kg) administration produces sedation and tranquilization, and provides some analgesia. The pig is resistant to the effects of xylazine, and deep sedation is seldom encountered in pigs. When used in combination with ketamine or tiletamine, xylazine enhances muscle relaxation and analgesia. Other agents that may be used as tranquilizers or for minor procedures are droperidol (0.1 to 0.4 mg/kg), Innovar-Vet (1 ml/12 to 25 kg), and diazepam (0.5 to 3.0 mg/kg).

Injectable anesthesia is most frequently administered by the *IM route* to the potbellied pig. These pigs have a considerable layer of subcutaneous fat, so it is essential that these agents be given by deep injection to avoid deposition in this fat layer. Short-term anesthesia is attained by the injection of xylazine (2.2 mg/kg) IM followed by IM ketamine (12 to 20 mg/kg). Xylazine enhances muscle relaxation, provides some analgesia, and smooths recoveries when given in conjunction with ketamine. For longer anesthesia, this IM injection may be followed with the IV administration of additional ketamine (2 to 4 mg/kg) as needed. Diazepam (1 to 2 mg/kg) may be substituted for the xylazine but will not provide extra analgesia.

Xylazine (2.2 mg/kg IM) and Telazol (6 mg/kg IM) will induce a safe and rapid anesthesia. Each agent, given IV at 2 mg/kg each, will induce a rapid induction that should allow for easy intubation after about 5 min. The zolazepam fraction of Telazol has been known to prolong recoveries in pigs. A three-way mixture of Telazol, ketamine, and xylazine (TKX) has been used to bypass this problem and induce rapid, safe anesthesia. TKX is produced by reconstituting Telazol with 2.5 ml xylazine (100 mg/ml) and 2.5 ml ketamine (100 mg/ml) instead of the usual 5 ml sterile water. The resulting mix has a dissociative concentration of 100 mg/ml (ketamine 50 mg/ml and tiletamine 50 mg/ml). It is dosed IM at 2.2 to 4.4 mg/kg and maintained by supplementing IV with 2.2 mg/kg TKX.

The safest form of general anesthesia for the pig is inhalation anesthesia. Methoxyflurane, halothane, and isoflurane have all been used in these pigs. Prior to anesthesia, the pig is fasted for 24 hr and deprived of water for 4 hr. Anticholinergics, atropine (0.04 mg/kg), or glycopyrrolate (0.005 to 0.01 mg/kg) is given 30 min prior to induction. The pig is either masked down using gas anesthesia, or one of the injectables is administered to facilitate the passage of an endotracheal tube. Intubation may be very challenging, as the pig's mouth cannot be opened widely, the larynx is small and slopes ventrally with a sharp angle from the larynx to the trachea, and laryngospasm is easily induced. Iatrogenic injury can follow inexperienced attempts at intubation. Halothane is associated with the initiation of malignant hyperthermia in genetically predisposed pigs. So far, this condition has not been reported in potbellied pigs.

## SURGERY

Potbellied pig surgery is similar to surgery in any of the other common species encountered in practice. The two most commonly requested surgeries are castration and ovariohysterectomy (OHE). These surgeries should be performed with the age at puberty kept in mind. Little boars may reach puberty as early as 3 months of age and should be castrated prior to this time to eliminate offensive boar odors and behavior. Puberty in the gilt is slightly later, 3.5 to 4 months of age, so an OHE may not need be performed until after this time.

Pigs presented for castration are neutered using the same surgical technique as for a similar sized dog. Many owner-breeders will castrate their own baby boars using the farm castration technique employed in commercial pig farms. Since pigs are genetically predisposed to inguinal hernia, a careful examination of the external inguinal ring area should be performed prior to castration to rule out this defect. If an inguinal hernia is suspected, the external ring may be closed using a horizontal mattress suture at the time of castration.

An OHE is performed as in the dog, with some slight variation. The surgical site is caudal to the umbilical scar, in some cases halfway between it and the pelvic brim. The ovarian pedicle of the pig is not as strong as in the dog and will break down easier. The reproductive tract is more fragile, more like that of the rabbit, and should be handled with care. This author has many breeder clients who wish to place spayed gilts with adoptive families at 8 weeks of age. In these cases, an OHE is performed at 6 weeks, prior to puberty of the gilt. The reproductive tract is quite small at this age and may be found coiled just dorsal to the bladder. Since not much development has occurred in the tract, there is very little blood supply and hemostasis is easily accomplished. Older obese pigs have considerable fat deposited in the mesentery, omentum, and around the uterus. Since the sow is not very susceptible to pyometra, an ovariectomy instead of a complete OHE may be preferable.

The only effective treatment for dystocia in these little pigs is a cesarean section. Again this surgery is performed as in the dog. If live babies are expected, the surgical site may be moved from the ventral midline to a supramammary position. This is a site just dorsal to the mammary glands and ventral to the flank fold of the rear leg. By performing the cesarean in this position, the baby pigs will not be able to suckle against the suture line, which potentially could cause the incision line to dehisce.

Tusk removal may become a necessary procedure in some breeding boars. The tusks are the elongated canine teeth of the boar that may be used in fighting and could cause injury to the owner as well as other pigs. The tusks are not extracted but simply cut at the gum line using a wire saw or similar device. The process may require repeating in a year or so. Barrows and sows also have canines, but they do not show the extensive growth observed in the boar.

## REPRODUCTION

Reproductive physiology of the potbellied pig is the same as for commercial swine except that the potbellied pig reaches puberty at a much younger age. Baby boars reach puberty by 3 months of age and gilts by 3.5 to 4 months. Pigs are polyestrous, with estrous cycles averaging 21 days in length. Once cyclicity starts, they are interrupted only by pregnancy, pathology, and some seasonal effects. Estrus, or heat, lasts 1 to 3 days, with ovulation occurring close to the end of estrus. During estrus, the vulva will swell in size and become reddened.

Breeding should take place 12 to 24 hr after the onset of estrus. The boar will remain mounted on the sow for some 5 to 15 min. If pregnancy occurs from breeding, gestation averages 114 days. Pregnancy diagnosis is accomplished with real-time ultrasonography after 30 days of gestation. Estrone sulfate assay at 30 days will also confirm pregnancy. Most owners will diagnose pregnancy by failure to return to estrus 3 weeks after breeding. Abdominal radiographs may be used in the last trimester to determine pregnancy. Litter size ranges from 2 to 15 piglets, with six to eight the average.

In the week preceding farrowing, the mammary glands show rapid enlargement, the vulva becomes swollen and red, and the sow will show nesting behavior. Delivery of pigs usually takes only 3 to 4 hr but may last up to 10 hr. Piglets are delivered about every 15 min. If dystocia is suspected, the vaginal canal is carefully examined for the presence of a fetus. If no obstruction is encountered, the sow is given oxytocin (10 to 20 U IM) to help stimulate contractions. If this fails to deliver pigs, a cesarean section is the only practical alternative for delivery.

Baby pigs must be kept warm (95°F), allowed to suckle colostrum from the sow, and given supplemental iron (50 mg iron dextran IM) to be assured of a good start in life. Needle teeth, baby pig canines, are usually removed at the gum line to prevent injuries from fighting with littermates and damage to the sow's teats. Baby pigs are especially susceptible to hypothermia and hypoglycemia in the first 2 weeks of life.

## References and Suggested Reading

Braun WF: Helping your clients raise healthy potbellied pigs. Vet Med 88:414, 1993.

Braun WF: Reproduction in the potbellied pig. Vet Med 88:429, 1993.

Braun WF: Anesthesia and surgical techniques useful in the potbellied pig. Vet Med 88:441, 1993.

Braun WF and Casteel SW: Potbellied pigs: Miniature porcine pets., Vet Clin North Am [Small Anim Pract] 23:1149, 1993.

Ko JCH, Thurmon JC, Tranquilli WA, Benson GJ, and Olson WA: Problems encountered when anesthetizing potbellied pigs. Vet Med 88:435, 1993.

Reeves D (ed): Guidelines for the Veterinary Practitioner: Care and Management of Miniature Pet Pigs. Santa Barbara, CA; Veterinary Practice Publishing Co, 1993.

# APPENDICES

ROBERT M. JACOBS
*and* MARK A. PAPICH
*Consulting Editors*

# CANINE AND FELINE REFERENCE VALUES

ROBERT M. JACOBS,
JOHN H. LUMSDEN,
*Guelph, Ontario, Canada*

*and* WILLIAM VERNAU
*Sydney, New South Wales, Australia*

We provide the following tables as general guidelines for the interpretation of laboratory data in dogs and cats. There is wide variation in test results and reference values between laboratories for several reasons, including use of different reagents, instruments, and selection of reference animals. We have tried to specifiy methodologies in most instances so that other laboratories and users may more directly compare test results. Despite interlaboratory variation, laboratory data can be interpreted correctly if appropriately determined reference values[*] are supplied with the test results. Laboratory users should demand species' reference values developed in the laboratory to which the samples were submitted.

Laboratories strive to limit intralaboratory variation by careful attention to quality control practices. The performance of a laboratory in quality control programs determines the laboratory users' confidence in test results from that laboratory. Conscientious users should not hesitate to ask for details of quality assurance in their laboratory and for expected within-run and between-run analytic variation. This information is necessary for the laboratory user attempting to separate analytic from animal variation on sequential samples.

The tables show either ranges that include 95% of the population, ranges that extend from the minimum to maximum (min-max) observation, mean ± one or two standard deviations (1 or 2 SD), or mean ± one standard error of the mean (SE). These measurements of error or variation about the mean are specified where appropriate (see *CVT X*, p 8). Reference values should never be presented as simple means without some indication of error or variation or upper and lower limits for 95% of the population when provided for individual animal application. We have used mean values only to demonstrate simple trends in laboratory data with age.

A number of reference sources and scientific journals use Système International (SI) units. In the major tables, we have given reference values in both the traditional and SI units in the hopes of easing some of the

confusion. Tables showing the interconversion of traditional and SI units for most analytes are given.[†]

For ease of access, literature sources are provided as footnotes to each table. In an attempt to be concise, we did not always cite the primary sources for the data, but these are available in the footnoted articles. Along with the references, we have occasionally given short comments that indicate some aspect important in data interpretation.

Patient variables and sample quality will also affect test results and their interpretation. We have attempted to address some patient variables by the inclusion of tables showing the effects of age, gender, pregnancy, and body weight. Unless specified otherwise, all data are for adult animals and include different genders and breeds. In some cases, we have given literature sources so the reader may further explore these effects. To address problems of sample quality, we have included graphs showing the effects of bilirubinemia, hemolysis, and lipemia on the determination of most serum analytes.[‡] Many instrument manufacturers will provide interference data for human sera but generally not for animal sera. If nothing else, these graphs serve to remind laboratory users that interferences do occur and sometimes in a species-specific manner. The interferences due to drugs have not been adequately studied in animals, but such interferences must always be considered.[§]

Laboratory data should be used to support diagnoses. Laboratory data that are inconsistent with the clinical diagnosis should be interpreted with caution. In these instances, the laboratory user should request that the laboratory reanalyze the same sample. If the result is

---

[*]Lumsden JH and Mullen K: On establishing reference values. Can J Comp Med 42:293, 1978.

---

[†]For further information about SI units, refer to Young DS: Implementation of SI units for clinical laboratory data. Ann Intern Med 106:114–129, 1987, which was reprinted in J Nutr 120:20, 1990; and Beeler MF: SI units and the AJCP. Am J Clin Pathol 87:140,1987.

[‡]Jacobs RM, Lumsden JH, Taylor JA, and Grift E: Effects of interferents on the kinetic Jaffé reaction and an enzymatic colorimetric test for serum creatinine concentration determination in cats, cows, dogs, and horses. Can J Vet Res 55:150, 1991; Jacobs RM, Lumsden JH, and Grift E: Effects of bilirubinemia, hemolysis, and lipemia on clinical chemistry analytes in bovine, canine, equine, and feline sera. Can Vet J 33:605, 1992.

[§]An extensive review of drug interferences in human sera is found in Young DS, Pestaner LC, and Gibberman V: Effects of drugs on clinical laboratory tests. Clin Chem 21:1D, 1975.

similar, the laboratory user must consider alternatives to the initial clinical diagnosis or eliminate sample collection and handling or drug-related interferences, where possible, by resubmitting another sample. Samples taken at different times or analyzed in different laboratories are not comparable. Sequential laboratory data are often essential to render a prognosis and to determine response to therapy.

### Hematology—Coulter S Plus IV* with Manual Differential Counts[†]

| | Unit | | Canine | | Feline | |
| --- | --- | --- | --- | --- | --- | --- |
| | Traditional | SI[†] | Traditional | SI | Traditional | SI |
| Hemoglobin (Hgb) | gm/dl | gm/L | 13.2–19.2 | 132–193 | 8.0–15.0 | 80–150 |
| Hematocrit (Hct) | % | L/L | 38–57 | 0.38–0.57 | 24–45 | 0.24–0.45 |
| Erythrocytes | X $10^6$/$\mu$l | X $10^{12}$/L | 5.6–8.5 | 5.6–8.5 | 5.0–10.0 | 5.0–10.0 |
| Mean corpuscular volume (MCV) | $\mu^3$ or mm$^3$ | fl | 62–71 | 62–71 | 39–50 | 39–50 |
| Mean corpuscular Hgb (MCH) | $\mu\mu$g or pg | pg | 22–25 | 22–25 | 13–17 | 13–17 |
| Mean corpuscular Hgb concentration (MCHC) | % | gm/L | 33.7–36.5 | 337–365 | 32.0–36.0 | 320–360 |
| Red cell distribution width (RDW) | % | % | 12–15 | 12–15 | 13–17 | 13–17 |
| Reticulocytes | X $10^3$/$\mu$l | X $10^9$/L | 20–80 | 20–80 | 20–60 | 20–60 |
| Platelets | X $10^3$/$\mu$l | X $10^9$/L | 145–440 | 145–440 | 190–400 | 190–400 |
| Mean platelet volume (MPV) | $\mu^3$ or mm$^3$ | fl | 7.0–10.3 | 7.0–10.3 | — | — |
| Platelet distribution width (PDW) | % | % | 15.5–17.5 | 15.5–17.5 | — | — |
| Total nucleated cell count | X $10^3$/$\mu$l | X $10^9$/L | 6.1–17.4 | 6.1–17.4 | 5.5–15.4 | 5.5–15.4 |
| Segmented neutrophils | X $10^3$/$\mu$l | X $10^9$/L | 3.9–12.0 | 3.9–12.0 | 2.5–12.5 | 2.5–12.5 |
| Band neutrophils | X $10^3$/$\mu$l | X $10^9$/L | 0.0–1.0 | 0.0–1.0 | 0.0–0.3 | 0.0–0.3 |
| Lymphocytes | X $10^3$/$\mu$l | X $10^9$/L | 0.8–3.6 | 0.8–3.6 | 1.5–7.0 | 1.5–7.0 |
| Monocytes | X $10^3$/$\mu$l | X $10^9$/L | 0.1–1.8 | 0.1–1.8 | 0.0–0.85 | 0.0–0.85 |
| Eosinophils | X $10^3$/$\mu$l | X $10^9$/L | 0.0–1.9 | 0.0–1.9 | 0.0–0.75 | 0.0–0.75 |
| Basophils | X $10^3$/$\mu$l | X $10^9$/L | 0.0–0.2 | 0.0–0.2 | 0.0–0.2 | 0.0–0.2 |

*This automated cell counter was configured using Isoton III and Lyse S III DIFF. The mean nucleated cell aperature voltage was 94.2 and the mean red cell/platelet aperature voltage was 165.5.
[†]From Clinical Pathology Laboratory, Department of Pathology, University of Guelph. Feline leukocyte differential count is modified from Jain NC: *Schalm's Veterinary Hematology*, 4th edition. Philadelphia, Lea & Febiger, 1986, p 127.
[†]Systéme International.

### Hematology—Technicon H-1 Hematology Analyzer*

| | Unit | Canine | Feline |
| --- | --- | --- | --- |
| Hemoglobin | gm/dl | 14.1–20.0 | 9.0–15.6 |
| Hematocrit | % | 43.3–59.3 | 29.3–49.8 |
| Erythrocytes | X $10^6$/$\mu$l | 6.15–8.70 | 6.12–11.86 |
| Mean corpuscular volume | fl | 63.0–77.1 | 41.9–54.8 |
| Mean corpuscular hemoglobin | pg | 21.1–24.8 | 12.5–17.6 |
| Mean corpuscular hemoglobin concentration | gm/dl | 29.9–35.6 | 28.1–32.0 |
| Red cell distribution width | % | 11.9–14.9 | 14.0–18.1 |
| Hemoglobin distribution width | gm/dl | 1.49–2.17 | 1.89–2.73 |
| Platelets | X $10^3$/$\mu$l | 164–510 | 26[†]–470 |
| Mean platelet volume | fl | 3.9–6.1 | 4.1–8.3 |
| White blood cell count | X $10^3$/$\mu$l | 6.02–16.02 | 4.87–20.10 |
| Neutrophils | X $10^3$/$\mu$l | 3.23–10.85 | — |
| Lymphocytes | X $10^3$/$\mu$l | 0.53–3.44 | — |
| Monocytes | X $10^3$/$\mu$l | 0.00–0.43 | — |
| Eosinophils | X $10^3$/$\mu$l | 0.00–1.82 | — |
| Basophils | X $10^3$/$\mu$l | 0.01–0.54 | — |
| Large unstained cells (LUC) | X $10^3$/$\mu$l | 0.26–2.09 | — |
| Lobularity index (LI)[†] | — | 1.88–3.15 | 1.3–2.68 |
| Mean peroxidase index (MPXI)[†] | — | −19 to −7 | −47 to −16 |

*From Tvedten H: Reference values for the veterinary clinical center laboratory, Michigan State University, May 1991. These data were derived from approximately 120 dogs and 40 cats. Canine reference values include 95% of the population, whereas the feline values represent the minimum to maximum.
[†]The lower limit of feline platelets is falsely decreased due to clumping.
[†]Interpretation of these determinations is undetermined in canine and feline blood.

## Système International (SI) Units in Hematology

| Analyte | Example Values | | Conversion Factors | |
|---|---|---|---|---|
| | SI | Traditional | Traditional to SI | SI to Traditional |
| Hemoglobin (Hgb) | 15.0 gm/dl | 150 gm/L | 10 | 0.1 |
| Hematocrit (Hct) or packed cell volume (PCV) | 45% | 0.45 L/L | 0.01 | 100 |
| Erythrocytes | $6.0 \times 10^6/mm^3$ | $6.0 \times 10^{12}/L$ | $10^6$ | $10^{-6}$ |
| Mean corpuscular volume (MCV) | 75 $\mu^3$ | 75 fl | No change | No change |
| Mean corpuscular Hgb (MCH) | 25 $\mu\mu g$ | 25 pg | No change | No change |
| Mean corpuscular Hgb concentration (MCHC) | 33 gm/dl | 330 gm/L | 10 | 0.1 |
| White blood cell count | $15.0 \times 10^3/mm^3$ | $15.0 \times 10^9/L$ | $10^6$ | $10^{-6}$ |
| Platelets | $250 \times 10^3/mm^3$ | $250 \times 10^9/L$ | $10^6$ | $10^{-6}$ |

## Hematology–Manual or Semiautomated Methods[*]

| | Adult Dog | | Adult Cat | |
|---|---|---|---|---|
| | Range | Mean | Range | Mean |
| **Red Cell Determinations** | | | | |
| Erythrocytes (millions/dl) | 5.5–8.5 | 6.8 | 5.5–10.0 | 7.5 |
| Hemoglobin (gm/dl) | 12.0–18.0 | 14.9 | 8.0–14.0 | 12.0 |
| Packed cell volume (%) | 37.0–55.0 | 45.5 | 24.0–45.0 | 37.0 |
| Mean corpuscular volume (fl) | 66.0–77.0 | 69.8 | 40.0–55.0 | 45.0 |
| Mean corpuscular hemoglobin (pg) | 19.9–24.5 | 22.8 | 13.0–17.0 | 15.0 |
| Mean corpuscular hemoglobin concentration (gm/dl) | | | | |
| Wintrobe | 31.0–34.0 | 33.0 | 31.0–35.0 | 33.0 |
| Microhematocrit | 32.0–36.0 | 34.0 | 30.0–36.0 | 33.2 |
| Reticulocytes (%, excluding punctate reticulocytes) | 0.0–1.5 | 0.8 | 0.2–1.6 | 0.6 |
| Resistance to hypotonic saline (% saline solution) | | | | |
| Minimum (initial hemolysis) | 0.40–0.50 | 0.46 | 0.66–0.72 | 0.69 |
| Maximum (complete hemolysis) | 0.32–0.42 | 0.33 | 0.46–0.54 | 0.50 |
| Erythrocyte life span (days) | 100–120 | | 66–78 | |
| **White Blood Cell Determinations** | | | | |
| Leukocytes (cells/$\mu$l) | 6000–17,000 | 11,500 | 5500–19,500 | 12,500 |
| Neutrophils—bands (%) | 0–3 | 0.8 | 0–3 | 0.5 |
| Neutrophils—mature (%) | 60–77 | 70.0 | 35–75 | 59.0 |
| Lymphocytes (%) | 12–30 | 20.0 | 20–55 | 32.0 |
| Monocytes (%) | 3–10 | 5.2 | 1–4 | 3.0 |
| Eosinophils (%) | 2–10 | 4.0 | 2–12 | 5.5 |
| Basophils (%) | Rare | 0.0 | Rare | 0.0 |
| Neutrophils—bands (cells/$\mu$l) | 0–300 | 70 | 0–300 | 100 |
| Neutrophils—mature (cells/$\mu$l) | 3000–11,500 | 7000 | 2500–12,500 | 7500 |
| Lymphocytes (cells/$\mu$l) | 1000–4800 | 2800 | 1500–7000 | 4,000 |
| Monocytes (cells/$\mu$l) | 150–1350 | 750 | 0–850 | 350 |
| Eosinophils (cells/$\mu$l) | 100–1250 | 550 | 0–1500 | 650 |
| Basophils (cells/$\mu$l) | Rare | 0 | Rare | 0 |

[*]From Jain NC: *Schalm's Veterinary Hematology*, 4th edition Philadelphia, Lea & Febiger, 1986.

## Canine Hematology (Means) at Different Ages—Manual or Semiautomated Methods[*]

| Age | RBC (millions/$\mu$l) | Retic. (%)[†] | Nucl. RBC per 100 WBC[†] | Hgb (gm/dl) | PCV (%) | WBC/$\mu$l | Neut./$\mu$l | Bands/$\mu$l | Lymph./$\mu$l | Eos./$\mu$l |
|---|---|---|---|---|---|---|---|---|---|---|
| Birth | 5.75 | 7.1 | 1.8 | 16.70 | 50 | 16,500 | 1300 | 400 | 2500 | 600 |
| 2 weeks | 3.92 | 7.1 | 1.8 | 9.76 | 32 | 11,000 | 6500 | 100 | 3000 | 300 |
| 4 weeks | 4.20 | 7.1 | 1.8 | 9.60 | 33 | 13,000 | 8600 | 0 | 4000 | 40 |
| 6 weeks | 4.91 | 3.6 | 1.8 | 9.59 | 34 | 15,000 | 10,000 | 0 | 4500 | 100 |
| 8 weeks | 5.13 | 3.9 | 0.3 | 11.00 | 37 | 18,000 | 11,000 | 234 | 6000 | 270 |
| 12 weeks | 5.27 | 3.9 | Rare | 11.60 | 36 | 15,300 | 9400 | 115 | 4600 | 322 |

[*]From Andersen AC and Gee W: Normal values in the beagle. Vet Med 53:135, 156, 1958.
[†]From Ewing GO, Schalm OW, and Smith RS: Hematologic values of normal Basenji dogs. J Am Vet Med Assoc 161:1661, 1972.
Also see *CVT XI*, p 981.

*Canine Hematology (Means and Ranges) With Different Ages and Genders—Manual or Semiautomated Methods**

| | Sex | Birth to 12 Months | | 1–7 Years | | 7 Years and Older | |
|---|---|---|---|---|---|---|---|
| | | *Range* | *Mean* | *Range* | *Mean* | *Range* | *Mean* |
| Erythrocytes (millions/$\mu$l) | Male | 2.99–8.52 | 5.09 | 5.26–6.57 | 5.92 | 3.33–7.76 | 5.28 |
| | Female | 2.76–8.42 | 5.06 | 5.13–8.6 | 6.47 | 3.34–9.19 | 5.17 |
| Hemoglobin (gm/dl) | Male | 6.9–16.5 | 10.7 | 12.7–16.3 | 15.5 | 14.7–21.2 | 17.9 |
| | Female | 6.4–18.9 | 11.2 | 11.5–17.9 | 14.7 | 11.0–22.5 | 16.1 |
| Packed cell volume (%) | Male | 22.0–45.0 | 33.9 | 35.2–52.8 | 44.0 | 44.2–62.8 | 52.3 |
| | Female | 25.8–55.2 | 36.0 | 34.8–52.4 | 43.6 | 35.8–67.0 | 49.8 |
| Leukocytes (thousands/$\mu$l) | Male | 9.9–27.7 | 17.1 | 8.3–19.5 | 11.9 | 7.9–35.3 | 15.5 |
| | Female | 8.8–26.8 | 15.9 | 7.5–17.5 | 11.5 | 5.2–34.0 | 13.4 |
| Mature neutrophils (%) | Male | 63–73 | 68 | 65–73 | 69 | 55–80 | 66 |
| | Female | 64–74 | 69 | 58–76 | 67 | 40–80 | 64 |
| Lymphocytes (%) | Male | 18–30 | 24 | 9–26 | 18 | 15–40 | 29 |
| | Female | 13–28 | 21 | 11–29 | 20 | 13–45 | 29 |
| Monocytes (%) | Male | 1–10 | 6 | 2–10 | 6 | 0–4 | 1 |
| | Female | 1–10 | 7 | 0–10 | 5 | 0–4 | 1 |
| Eosinophils (%) | Male | 2–11 | 3 | 1–8 | 4 | 1–11 | 4 |
| | Female | 1–9 | 5 | 1–10 | 6 | 0–19 | 6 |

*From *Normal Blood Values for Dogs*, Ralston Purina Co, Professional Marketing Services, Checkerboard Square, St. Louis, 1975. Also see *CVT XI*, p 981.

*Canine Hematology (Means ± SD) at Different Ages**

| Age | RBC (millions/$\mu$l) | Hgb (gm/dl) | PCV (%) | MCV (fl) | MCH (pg) | MCHC (gm/dl) | WBC/$\mu$l |
|---|---|---|---|---|---|---|---|
| 0–3 days | 4.8 ± 0.8 | 15.8 ± 2.9 | 46.3 ± 8.5 | 94.2 ± 5.9 | 32.7 ± 1.8 | 34.6 ± 1.4 | 16,800 ± 5700 |
| 14–17 days | 3.5 ± 0.3 | 9.9 ± 1.1 | 28.7 ± 2.9 | 81.5 ± 3.3 | 28.0 ± 2.0 | 34.3 ± 1.6 | 13,600 ± 4400 |
| 28–31 days | 3.9 ± 0.4 | 9.6 ± 0.9 | 28.4 ± 2.5 | 71.7 ± 3.5 | 24.3 ± 1.6 | 33.5 ± 1.4 | 13,900 ± 3300 |
| 40–45 days | 4.1 ± 0.4 | 9.2 ± 0.7 | 28.3 ± 2.3 | 68.2 ± 2.6 | 22.4 ± 1.0 | 32.4 ± 1.7 | 15,300 ± 3700 |
| 56–59 days | 4.7 ± 0.4 | 10.3 ± 0.9 | 31.4 ± 2.4 | 65.8 ± 2.3 | 21.8 ± 1.2 | 32.6 ± 1.8 | 15,700 ± 4400 |

*From Jain NC: *Schalm's Veterinary Hematology*, 4th edition. Philadelphia, Lea & Febiger, 1986; derived from between 42 and 48 dogs at each time interval.

*Effects of Pregnancy and Lactation on Canine Hematology (Means)**

| | Gestation | | | | Term | Lactation | | |
|---|---|---|---|---|---|---|---|---|
| | 2 Weeks | 4 Weeks | 6 Weeks | 8 Weeks | 0 Weeks | 2 Weeks | 4 Weeks | 6 Weeks |
| RBC (millions/$\mu$l) | 8.85 | 7.48 | 6.73 | 6.26 | 4.53 | 5.13 | 5.65 | 6.15 |
| PCV (%) | 53 | 47 | 44 | 37 | 32 | 34 | 38 | 42 |
| Hgb (gm/dl) | 19.6 | 16.4 | 14.7 | 13.8 | 11.0 | 11.7 | 12.8 | 13.4 |
| WBC (thousands/$\mu$l) | 12.0 | 12.2 | 15.7 | 19.0 | 18.9 | 16.9 | 17.1 | 15.9 |

*From Andersen AC and Gee W: Normal values in the beagle. Vet Med 53:135, 156, 1958.

## Relative Distribution of Cell Types in Canine Bone Marrow[*]

| Cell Type | Range (%) | Mean (%) |
|---|---|---|
| Myeloid (granulocytic) series | | |
|   Myeloblasts | 0.7–1.1 | 0.9 |
|   Promyelocytes | 1.7–2.5 | 2.1 |
|   Neutrophil myelocytes | 5.3–7.3 | 6.3 |
|   Neutrophil bands | 9.1–13.5 | 11.3 |
|   Neutrophil segmenters | 22.2–24.8 | 23.5 |
|   Eosinophil myelocytes | 0.4–0.8 | 0.6 |
|   Eosinophil metamyelocytes | 0.4–1.0 | 0.7 |
|   Eosinophil bands | 0.8–1.6 | 1.2 |
|   Eosinophil segmenters | 0.3–1.3 | 0.8 |
|   Basophil series | 0.0–0.06 | 0.02 |
|   Total myeloid series | 49.3–61.1 | 55.2 |
| Erythrocytic series | | |
|   Rubriblasts and prorubricytes | 6.1–6.9 | 6.5 |
|   Rubricytes and metarubricytes | 23.2–32.0 | 27.6 |
|   Total erythroid series | 29.4–38.8 | 34.1 |
| Myeloid/erythroid (M/E) ratio | 1.3–2.1 | 1.7 |
| Other cells | | |
|   Lymphocytes | 5.5–10.9 | 8.2 |
|   Plasma cells | 0.4–1.0 | 0.7 |
|   Monocytes | 0.2–5.2 | 1.2 |
|   Macrophages | 0.2–0.6 | 0.4 |
|   Mitotic figures | 1.1–1.7 | 1.4 |

[*]From Latimer KS and Meyer DJ: Leukocytes in health and disease. *In* Ettinger SJ (ed): *Textbook of Veterinary Internal Medicine, Diseases of the Dog and Cat*, 3rd edition. Philadelphia, W.B. Saunders Co, 1989, pp 2185–2186. These data are based on the following citations: Prasse KW and Mahaffey EA: Hematology of normal cats and characteristic responses to disease. *In* Holzworth J (ed): *Diseases of the Cat: Medicine and Surgery*. Philadelphia, W.B. Saunders Co, 1987, p 739; Duncan JR and Prasse KW: *Veterinary Laboratory Medicine: Clinical Pathology*, 2nd ed. Ames, Iowa State University Press, 1986; Melveger BE, et al. Sternal bone marrow biopsy in the dog. Lab Anim Care 19:866, 1969; Bloom F and Meyer LM: The morphology of the bone marrow cells in normal dogs. Cornell Vet 34:13, 1944. For a comprehensive review of peripheral blood and bone marrow changes with illness, see Hoff B, Lumsden JH, and Valli VEO: An appraisal of bone marrow biopsy in assessment of sick dogs. Can J Comp Med 49:34, 1985.

## Feline Hematology (Means and Ranges) With Different Ages and Genders—Manual or Semiautomated Methods[*]

| | Sex | Birth to 12 Months | | 1–7 Years | | 7 Years and Older | |
|---|---|---|---|---|---|---|---|
| | | *Range* | *Average* | *Range* | *Average* | *Range* | *Average* |
| Erythrocytes (millions/$\mu$l) | Male | 5.43–10.22 | 6.96 | 4.48–10.27 | 7.34 | 5.26–8.89 | 6.79 |
| | Female | 4.46–11.34 | 6.90 | 4.45–9.42 | 6.17 | 4.10–7.38 | 5.84 |
| Hemoglobin (gm/dl) | Male | 6.0–12.9 | 9.9 | 8.9–17.0 | 12.9 | 9.0–14.5 | 11.8 |
| | Female | 6.0–15.0 | 9.9 | 7.9–15.5 | 10.3 | 7.5–13.7 | 10.3 |
| Packed cell volume (%) | Male | 24.0–37.5 | 31 | 26.9–48.2 | 37.6 | 28.0–43.8 | 34.6 |
| | Female | 23.0–46.8 | 31.5 | 25.3–37.5 | 31.4 | 22.5–40.5 | 30.8 |
| Leukocytes (thousands/$\mu$l) | Male | 7.8–25.0 | 15.8 | 9.1–28.2 | 15.1 | 6.4–30.4 | 17.6 |
| | Female | 11.0–26.9 | 17.7 | 13.7–23.7 | 19.9 | 5.2–30.1 | 14.8 |
|   Neutrophils—mature (%) | Male | 16–75 | 60 | 37–92 | 65 | 33–75 | 61 |
| | Female | 51–83 | 69 | 42–93 | 69 | 25–89 | 71 |
|   Lymphocytes (%) | Male | 10–81 | 30 | 7–48 | 23 | 16–54 | 30 |
| | Female | 8–37 | 23 | 12–58 | 30 | 9–63 | 22 |
|   Monocytes (%) | Male | 1–5 | 2 | 1–5 | 2 | 0–2 | 1 |
| | Female | 0–7 | 2 | 0–5 | 2 | 0–4 | 1 |
|   Eosinophils (%) | Male | 2–21 | 8 | 1–22 | 7 | 1–15 | 8 |
| | Female | 0–15 | 6 | 0–13 | 5 | 0–15 | 6 |

[*]From *Normal Blood Values for Cats*, Ralston Purina Co, Professional Marketing Services, Checkerboard Square, St. Louis, 1975. Also see *CVT XI*, p 981.

*Feline Hematology (Means) at Different Ages*[*]

| Age | RBC (millions/μl) | Hgb (gm/dl) | PCV (%) | MCV (fl) | MCH (pg) | MCHC (gm/dl) | WBC/μl |
|---|---|---|---|---|---|---|---|
| 0–6 hr | 4.95 | 12.2 | 44.7 | 90.3 | 24.6 | 27.3 | 7550 |
| 12–48 hr | 5.11 | 11.3 | 41.7 | 81.6 | 22.1 | 27.1 | 10,180 |
| 7 days | 5.19 | 10.9 | 35.7 | 68.8 | 21.0 | 30.5 | 7830 |
| 21 days | 4.99 | 9.3 | 31.3 | 62.7 | 18.6 | 29.7 | 8820 |
| 42 days | 6.75 | 9.0 | 35.4 | 52.4 | 13.3 | 25.4 | 8420 |
| 80 days | 7.69 | 10.3 | 39.0 | 50.7 | 13.4 | 26.4 | 9120 |
| Adult male | 9.02 | 12.2 | 40.6 | 45.0 | 13.5 | 30.0 | 12,400 |
| Adult female | 8.39 | 12.0 | 41.3 | 49.2 | 14.3 | 29.1 | 10,500 |

[*]From Jain NC: *Schalm's Veterinary Hematology*, 4th edition. Philadelphia, Lea & Febiger, 1986; data derived from between 18 and 26 cats at each time interval.
Also see *CVT XI*, p 981.

*Effects of Pregnancy and Lactation on Feline Hematology (Means)*[*]

| | Gestation | | | | | Term | Lactation | |
| | 1 Day Past Conception | 2 Weeks | 4 Weeks | 6 Weeks | 8 Weeks | 0 Weeks | 2 Weeks | 4 Weeks |
|---|---|---|---|---|---|---|---|---|
| RBC (millions/μl) | 8.0 | 7.9 | 7.1 | 6.7 | 6.2 | 6.2 | 7.4 | 7.4 |
| PCV (%) | 36.1 | 37.0 | 33.0 | 32.0 | 28.0 | 29.0 | 33.0 | 33.0 |
| Hgb (gm/dl) | 12.5 | 12.0 | 11.0 | 10.8 | 9.5 | 10.0 | 11.5 | 11.2 |
| Reticulocytes (%, includes punctate reticulocytes) | 9 | 11 | 9 | 10 | 20.1 | 15 | 9 | 6 |

[*]From Berman E: Hemogram of the cat during pregnancy and lactation and after lactation. Am J Vet Res 35:457, 1974.

*Relative Distribution of Cell Types in Feline Bone Marrow*[*]

| Cell Type | Range (%) | Mean (%) |
|---|---|---|
| Myeloid (granulocytic) series | | |
| Myeloblasts | 0.0–1.8 | 0.4 |
| Promyelocytes | 0.6–3.8 | 1.2 |
| Neutrophil myelocytes | 0.4–5.4 | 2.2 |
| Neutrophil metamyelocytes | 0.6–9.6 | 4.2 |
| Neutrophil bands | 5.0–19.4 | 11.0 |
| Neutrophil segmenters | 17.8–38.6 | 27.8 |
| Eosinophil series | 0.6–7.2 | 3.0 |
| Basophil series | 0.0–0.4 | 0.2 |
| Total myeloid cells | 39.4–64.4 | 52.0 |
| Erythrocytic series | | |
| Rubriblasts | 0.0–1.6 | 0.6 |
| Prorubricytes and rubricytes | — | 12.4 |
| Metarubricytes | 15.6–32.2 | 23.6 |
| Total erythroid cells | 24.0–48.8 | 36.6 |
| Myeloid/erythroid (M/E) ratio | 0.9–2.5 | 1.5 |
| Other cells | | |
| Lymphocytes | 3.2–22.6 | 11.4 |
| Plasma cells | 0.0–1.2 | 0.2 |
| Mitotic cells | 0.0–2.0 | 1.0 |

[*]From Latimer KS and Meyer DJ: Leukocytes in health and disease. *In* Ettinger SJ (ed): *Textbook of Veterinary Internal Medicine, Diseases of the Dog and Cat*, 3rd edition. Philadelphia, WB Saunders Co, 1989, pp 2185–2186. These data are based on the following citations: Prasse KW and Mahaffey EA: Hematology of normal cats and characteristic responses to disease. *In* Holzworth J (ed): *Diseases of the Cat: Medicine and Surgery*. Philadelphia, WB Saunders Co, 1987, p 739; Duncan JR and Prasse KW: *Veterinary Laboratory Medicine: Clinical Pathology*, 2nd edition. Ames, Iowa State University Press, 1986; Melveger BE, et al. Sternal bone marrow biopsy in the dog. Lab Anim Care 19: 866, 1969; Bloom F and Meyer LM: The morphology of the bone marrow cells in normal dogs. Cornell Vet 34:13, 1944.

*Clinical Chemistry—Coulter DACOS°*

| | Unit | | Canine | | Feline | |
|---|---|---|---|---|---|---|
| | *Traditional* | *SI*[†] | *Traditional* | *SI* | *Traditional* | *SI* |
| Alanine aminotransferase | IU/L | U/L | 0–130 | 0–130 | 10–75 | 10–75 |
| Albumin | gm/dl | gm/L | 2.2–3.5 | 22–35 | 2.5–3.9 | 25–39 |
| Albumin/globulin | — | — | 0.5–1.2 | 0.5–1.2 | 0.5–1.4 | 0.5–1.4 |
| Alkaline phosphatase | IU/L | U/L | 0–200 | 0–200 | 0–90 | 0–90 |
| Amylase | IU/L | U/L | 400–1800 | 400–1800 | 700–2000 | 700–2000 |
| Anion gap | mEq/L | mmol/L | 15–25 | 15–25 | — | — |
| Asparate aminotransferase | IU/L | U/L | 10–50 | 10–50 | 10–59 | 10–59 |
| Conjugated bilirubin | mg/dl | µmol/L | 0–0.18 | 0–3 | 0–0.06 | 0–1 |
| Unconjugated bilirubin | mg/dl | µmol/L | 0–0.41 | 0–7 | 0–0.23 | 0–4 |
| Total bilirubin | mg/dl | µmol/L | 0–0.41 | 0–7 | 0–0.23 | 0–4 |
| Calcium | mg/dl | mmol/L | 8.98–11.82 | 2.24–2.95 | 8.94–11.62 | 2.23–2.90 |
| Total carbon dioxide | mEq/L | mmol/L | 18–30 | 18–30 | 14–26 | 14–26 |
| Chloride | mEq/L | mmol/L | 105–122 | 105–122 | 112–129 | 112–129 |
| Cholesterol | mg/dl | mmol/L | 106.0–367.4 | 2.74–9.50 | 58.0–232.0 | 1.5–6.0 |
| Creatine kinase | IU/L | U/L | 0–460 | 0–460 | 0–580 | 0–580 |
| Creatinine | mg/dl | µmol/L | 0.62–1.64 | 55–145 | 0.84–2.04 | 75–180 |
| Globulins | gm/dl | gm/L | 2.2–4.5 | 22–45 | 2.6–5.0 | 26–50 |
| Glucose | mg/dl | mmol/L | 59.4–156.7 | 3.3–8.7 | 63.1–162.1 | 3.5–9.0 |
| Glutamate dehydrogenase | IU/L | U/L | 3–8 | 3–8 | 0–3 | 0–3 |
| γ-Glutamyl transferase | IU/L | U/L | 0–6 | 0–6 | 0–2 | 0–2 |
| Iron[‡] | µg/dl | µmol/L | 72.6–189.8 | 13–34 | 78.2–111.7 | 14–20 |
| Total iron-binding capacity | µg/dl | µmol/L | 363–475 | 65–85 | 296–318 | 53–57 |
| Transferrin saturation | % | % | 16–40 | 16–40 | 27–35 | 27–35 |
| Lipase | IU/L | U/L | 50–1000 | 50–1000 | 50–700 | 50–700 |
| Phosphorus | mg/dl | mmol/L | 1.55–8.05 | 0.50–2.60 | 3.19–8.73 | 1.03–2.82 |
| Potassium | mEq/L | mmol/L | 3.6–5.8 | 3.6–5.8 | 3.7–5.8 | 3.7–5.8 |
| Total serum protein | gm/dl | gm/L | 5.0–7.5 | 50–75 | 6.0–8.2 | 60–82 |
| Sodium | mEq/L | mmol/L | 145–158 | 145–158 | 150–165 | 150–165 |
| Urea | mg/dl | mmol/L | 5.9–27.2 | 2.1–9.7 | 14.0–28.0 | 5.0–10.0 |

°From Clinical Pathology Laboratory, Department of Pathology, University of Guelph. Trends in serum chemistry values with age and original citations concerning this topic are found in Lowseth LA, Gillett NA, Gerlach RF, and Muggenburg BA: The effects of aging on hematology and serum chemistry values in the beagle dog. Vet Clin Pathol 19:13, 1990. For temperature stability of enzymes see Kaneko JJ: Stability of serum enzymes under various storage conditions. *In* Kaneko JJ (ed): *Clinical Biochemistry of Domestic Animals*, 4th edition. San Diego, Academic Press, 1989, p 883.

[†]Système International.

[‡]Feline values derived from Fulton R, Weiser MG, Freshman JL, Gasper PW, and Fettman MJ: Electronic and morphologic characterization of erythrocytes of an adult cat with iron deficiency anemia. Vet Pathol 25:521, 1988.

Also see *CVT XI*, p 981, for pediatric values.

*Clinical Chemistry—Selected Manual Procedures°*

| Analyte | Unit | Canine | Feline |
|---|---|---|---|
| Ammonia (bromophenol blue, Kodak Ektachem, Rochester, NY) | | | |
| Resting | µmol/L | 20–80 | —[†] |
| 30 min after provocation | µmol/L | ≤140 | — |
| Anion gap | mmol/L | 15–25 | — |
| Bile acids (colorimetric, Enzabile, Nycomed, Oslo, Norway) | | | |
| Fasting | µmol/L | 0–9 | ≤2.2[‡] |
| 2 hr postprandial | µmol/L | 0–30 | ≤12.6 |
| Sulfobromophthalein retention | % at 30 min | ≤5 | ≤3[§] |
| Indocyanine green retention[§] | % at 30 min | 7.7–15.6 | 4.7–14.0 |
| Osmolality (freezing point depression) | mmol/kg | 295–315 | 301–314 |

°Data are from the Clinical Pathology Laboratory, Department of Pathology, University of Guelph unless indicated otherwise. Methods and reagent sources given in brackets where appropriate.

[†]Data for four cats with portosystemic shunts are reported in Center SA, Baldwin BH, de Lahunta A, Dietze AE, and Tennant BC: Evaluation of serum bile acid concentrations for the diagnosis of portosystemic venous anomalies in the dog and cat. J Am Vet Med Assoc 186:1090, 1985.

[‡]From Center SA, Baldwin BH, Erb H, and Tennant BC: Bile acid concentrations in the diagnosis of hepatobiliary disease in the cat. J Am Vet Med Assoc 189:891, 1986.

[§]From Center SA, Bunch SE, Baldwin BH, Hornbuckle WE, and Tennant BC: Comparison of sulfobromophthalein and indocyanine green clearances in the cat. Am J Vet Res 44:727, 1983; Center SA, Bunch SE, Baldwin BH, Hornbuckle WE, and Tennant BC: Comparison of sulfobromophthalein and indocyanine green clearances in the dog. Am J Vet Res 44:722, 1983.

*Système International (SI) Units in Clinical Chemistry*

| Analyte | Traditional Unit (with examples) | Conversion Factor | SI Unit (with examples) |
|---|---|---|---|
| Alanine aminotransferase | 0–40 U/L | 1.00 | 0–40 U/L |
| Albumin | 2.8–4.0 gm/dl | 10.0 | 28–40 gm/L |
| Alkaline phosphatase | 30–150 U/L | 1.00 | 30–150 U/L |
| Ammonia | 10–80 µg/dl | 0.5871 | 5.9–47.0 µmol/L |
| Amylase | 200–800 U/L | 1.00 | 200–800 U/L |
| Aspartate aminotransferase | 0–40 U/L | 1.00 | 0–40 U/L |
| Bile acids (total) | 0.3–2.3 µg/ml | 2.45 | 0.74–5.64 µmol/L |
| Bilirubin | 0.1–0.2 mg/dl | 17.10 | 2–4 µmol/L |
| Calcium | 8.8–10.3 mg/dl | 0.2495 | 2.20–2.58 mmol/L |
| Carbon dioxide | 22–28 mEq/L | 1.00 | 22–28 mmol/L |
| Chloride | 95–100 mEq/L | 1.00 | 95–100 mmol/L |
| Cholesterol | 100–265 mg/dl | 0.0258 | 2.58–5.85 mmol/L |
| Copper | 70–140 µg/dl | 0.1574 | 11.0–22.0 µmol/L |
| Cortisol | 2–10 µg/dl | 27.59 | 55–280 nmol/L |
| Creatine kinase | 0–130 U/L | 1.00 | 0–130 U/L |
| Creatinine | 0.6–1.2 mg/dl | 88.40 | 50–110 µmol/L |
| Fibrinogen | 200–400 mg/dl | 0.01 | 2.0–4.0 gm/L |
| Folic acid | 3.5–11.0 µg/L | 2.265 | 7.93–24.92 nmol/L |
| Glucose | 70–110 mg/dl | 0.05551 | 3.9–6.1 mmol/L |
| Iron | 80–180 µg/dl | 0.1791 | 14–32 µmol/L |
| Lactate | 5–20 mg/dl | 0.1110 | 0.5–2.0 mmol/L |
| Lead | 150 µg/dl | 0.04826 | 7.2 µmol/L |
| Lipase Sigma Tietz (37°C) | ≤1 ST U/dl | 280 | ≤280 U/L |
| Lipase Cherry Crandall (30°C) | 0–160 U/L | 1.00 | 0–160 U/L |
| Lipids (total) | 400–850 mg/dl | 0.01 | 4.0–8.5 gm/L |
| Magnesium | 1.8–3.0 mg/dl | 0.4114 | 0.80–1.20 mmol/L |
| Mercury | ≤1.0 µg/dl | 49.85 | ≤50 nmol/L |
| Osmolality | 280–300 mOsm/kg | 1.00 | 280–300 mmol/kg |
| Phosphorus | 2.5–5.0 mg/dl | 0.3229 | 0.80–1.6 mmol/L |
| Potassium | 3.5–5.0 mEq/L | 1.0 | 3.5–5.0 mmol/L |
| Protein (total) | 5–8 gm/dl | 10.0 | 50–80 gm/L |
| Sodium | 135–147 mEq/L | 1.00 | 135–147 mmol/L |
| Testosterone | 4.0–8.0 mg/ml | 3.467 | 14.0–28.0 nmol/L |
| Thyroxine | 1–4 µg/dl | 12.87 | 13–51 nmol/L |
| Triglyceride | 10–500 mg/dl | 0.0113 | 0.11–5.65 mmol/L |
| Urea nitrogen | 10–20 mg/dl | 0.3570 | 3.6–7.1 nmol/L |
| Uric acid | 3.6–7.7 mg/dl | 59.44 | 214–458 µmol/L |
| Urobilinogen | 0–4.0 mg/dl | 16.9 | 0.0–6.8 µmol/L |
| Vitamin A | 90 µg/dl | 0.03491 | 3.1 µmol/L |
| Vitamin $B_{12}$ | 300–700 ng/L | 0.738 | 221–516 pmol/L |
| Vitamin E | 5.0–20.0 mg/L | 2.32 | 11.6–46.4 µmol/L |
| D-xylose | 30–40 mg/dl | 0.06666 | 2.0–2.71 mmol/L |
| Zinc | 75–120 µg/dl | 0.1530 | 11.5–18.5 µmol/L |

## Clinical Chemistry—Test Characteristics for Analytes Determined on Coulter DACOS*

| Analyte | Reaction Type | Methodology |
|---|---|---|
| Alanine aminotransferase | Zero-order kinetic | Modified IFCC[†] (L-alanine and $\alpha$-ketoglutarate substrate) |
| Albumin | First-order kinetic | Modified Doumas (bromcresol green) |
| Alkaline phosphatase | Zero-order kinetic | Modified Bowers and McComb (p-nitrophenyl phosphate substrate) |
| Amylase | Zero-order kinetic | Modified Wallenfels (p-nitrophenylmaltohexaoside substrate) |
| Aspartate aminotransferase | Zero-order kinetic | Modified IFCC (L-aspartate and $\alpha$-ketoglutarate substrate) |
| Bilirubin | Equilibrium[‡] | Modified Walters and Gerarde (diazo) |
| Calcium | Equilibrium | Modified Connerty and Briggs (O-cresolphthalein complexone) |
| Total carbon dioxide | First-order kinetic | Enzymatic phosphoenol-pyruvate carboxylase |
| Chloride | Equilibrium | Modified Schoenfeld and Lewellen (thiocyanate) |
| Cholesterol | Equilibrium | Enzymatic (cholesterol esterase/oxidase) |
| Creatine kinase | Zero-order kinetic | Modified Oliver-Rosalki (creatine phosphate substrate) |
| Creatinine | Initial rate | Kinetic Jaffé |
| Glucose | Equilibrium | Modified hexokinase/glucose-6-phosphate dehydrogenase |
| Glutamate dehydrogenase[§] | Zero-order kinetic | $\alpha$-Oxoglutarate substrate |
| $\gamma$-Glutamyl transferase | Zero-order kinetic | Modified Szasz (L-$\gamma$-glutamyl-p-nitroanilide and glycylglycine substrate) |
| Iron[‖] | Equilibrium | Ferene |
| Lipase[§] | Zero-order kinetic | Triolene substrate and colipase excess |
| Phosphorus | Equilibrium | Modified Daly and Ertingshausen (molybdate) |
| Potassium | — | Ion-selective electrode |
| Total serum protein | Equilibrium | Modified biuret (cupric sulfate) |
| Sodium | — | Ion-selective electrode |
| Urea | First-order kinetic | Modified Talke and Schubert (urease) |

*From Clinical Pathology Laboratory, Department of Pathology, University of Guelph. Unless indicated otherwise all reagents are from Coulter Diagnostics, Hialeah, FL.
[†]International Federation of Clinical Chemistry.
[‡]Also termed *end-point reaction*.
[§]Boehringer Mannheim, Dorval, Quebec.
[‖]Diagnostic Chemicals Limited, Monroe, CT.

*Interferences Caused by Lipid, Bilirubin, and Hemoglobin for Analytes Determined on Coulter DACOS*

The following series of graphs are termed "interferograms." These interferograms show the effects of common interferents on the concentrations or activities of analytes determined on the Coulter DACOS (methods given in previous table) in canine (●) and feline (○) sera except for refractometer total protein, which was done using a Goldberg refractometer. The X axes show increasing amounts of lipid, bilirubin, or hemoglobin, and the Y axes show the percentage change (final/original X 100%) in any particular analyte. In those instances where the concentration or activity of a particular analyte was numerically small, the absolute values are given on the Y axes. These data are provided by the Clinical Pathology Laboratory, Department of Pathology, University of Guelph and were prepared with the assistance of Mr. E. Grift. The protocols for preparing these data are described in Glick MR, Ryder KW, and Jackson SA: Graphical comparisons of interferences in clinical chemistry instrumentation. Clin Chem 32:470, 1986. For a more complete discussion of interferences on creatinine, refer to Jacobs RM, Lumsden JH, Taylor JA, and Grift E: Effects of interferents on the kinetic Jaffé reaction and an enzymatic colorimetric test for serum creatinine concentration determination in cats, cows, dogs, and horses. Can J Vet Res 55:150, 1991 and Jacobs RM, Lumsden JH, and Grift E: Effects of bilirubinemia, hemolysis, and lipemia on clinical chemistry analytes in bovine, canine, equine, and feline sera. Can Vet J 33:605, 1992. Also see this volume, pp 14 and 20.

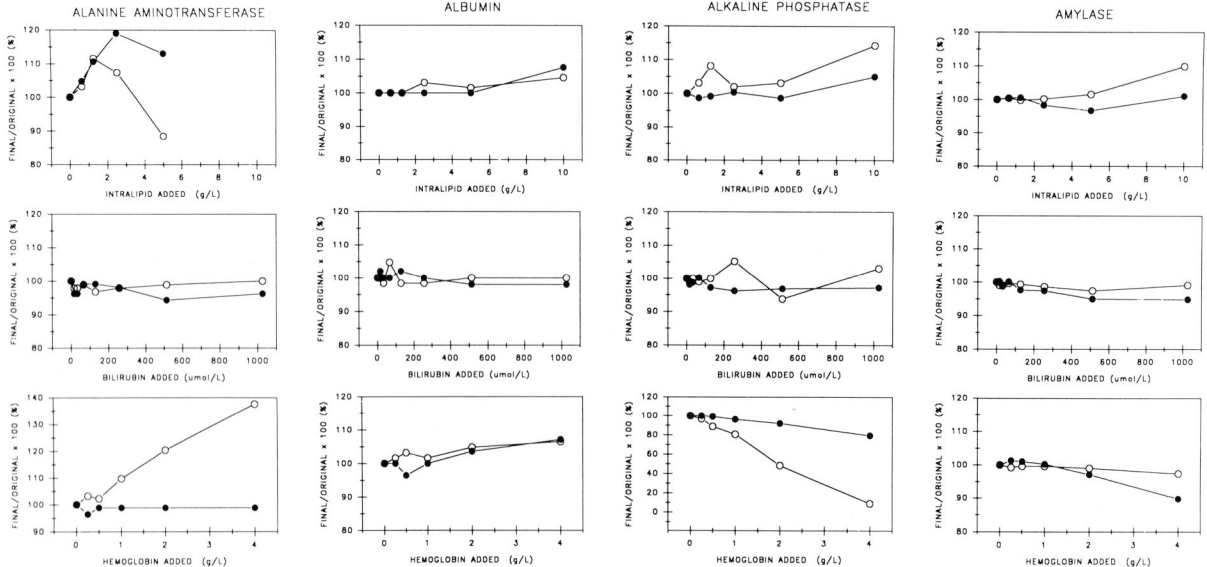

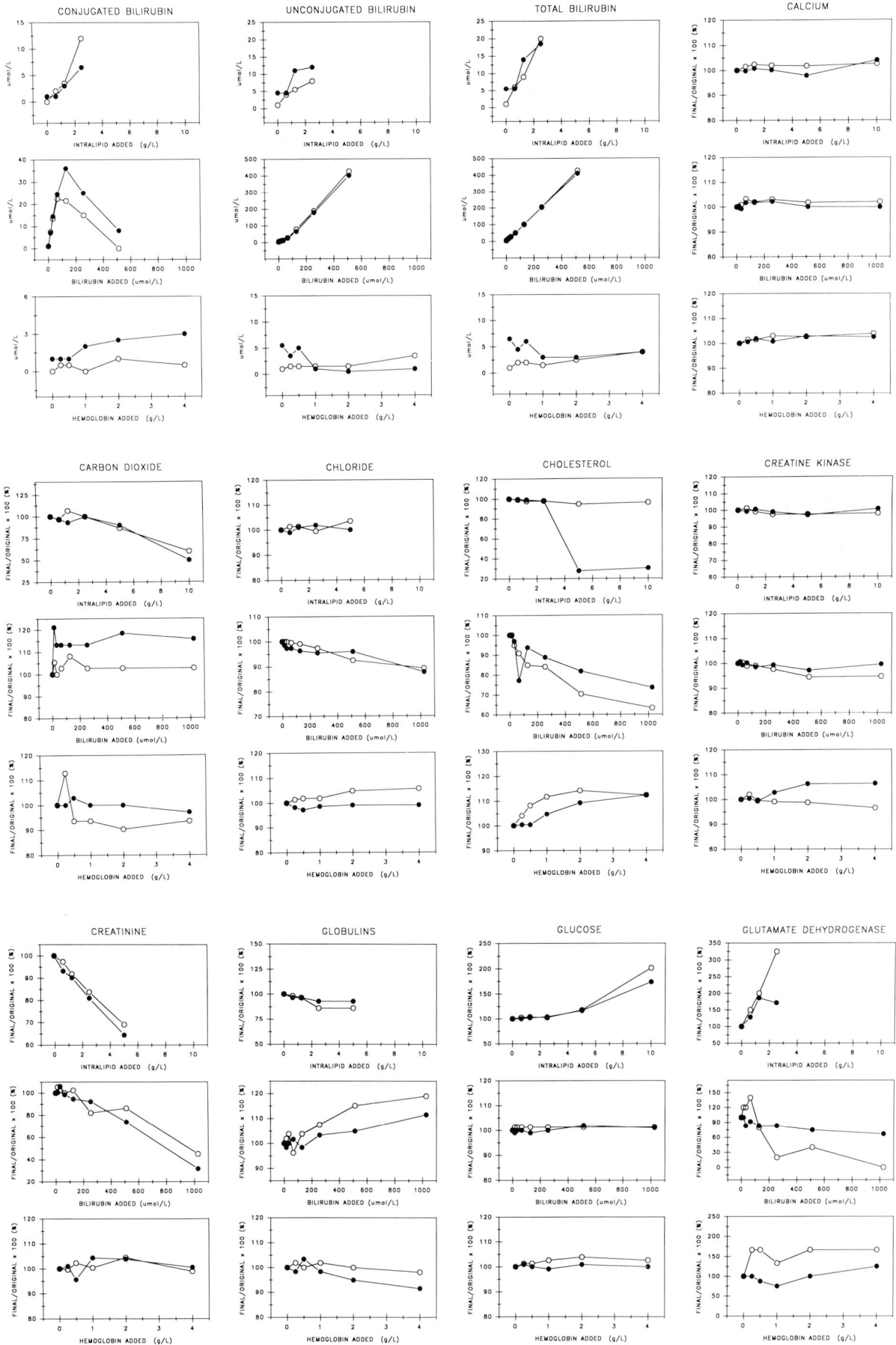

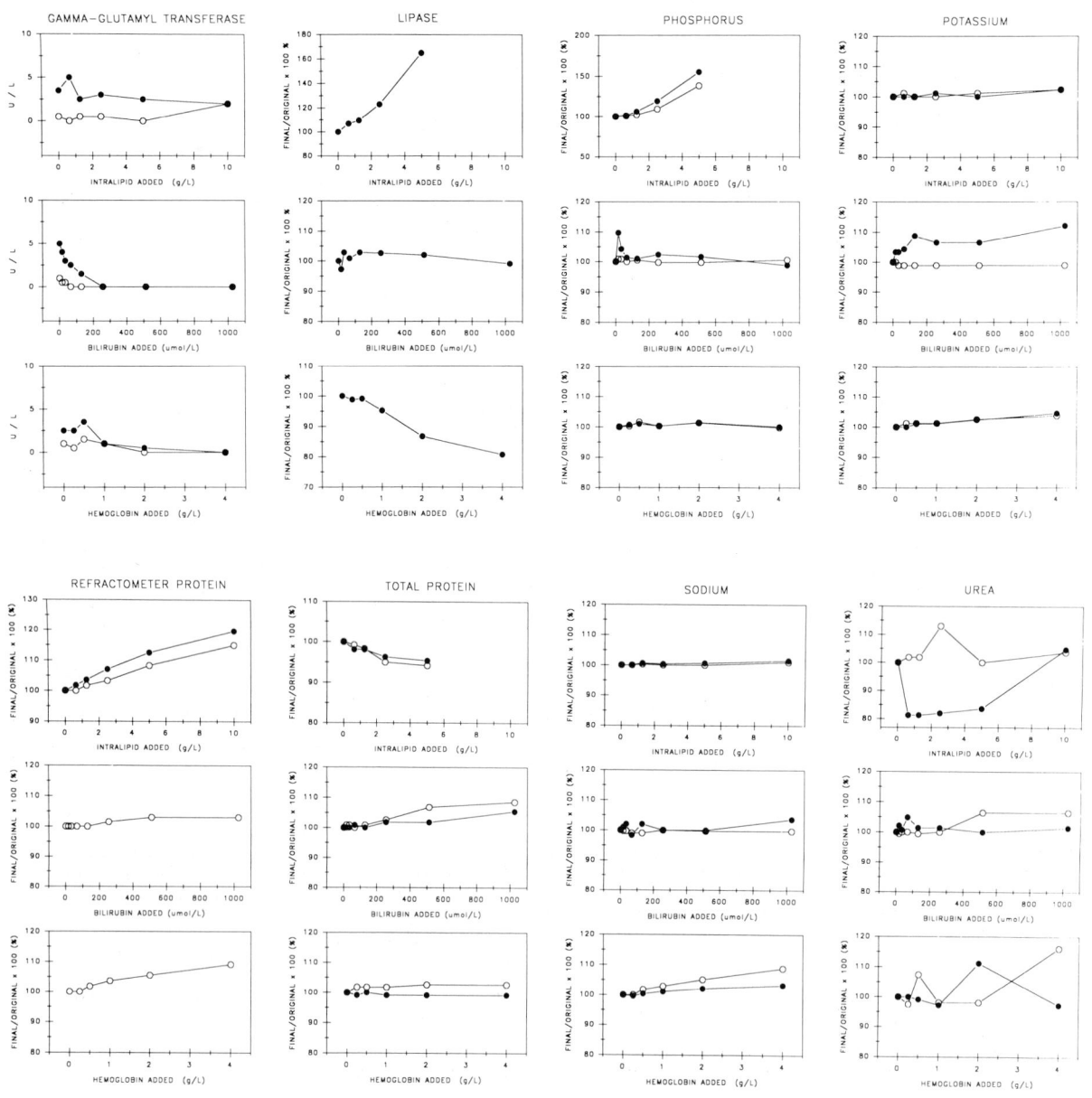

## Serum Protein Fractions°

|  | Unit | Canine | Feline |
|---|---|---|---|
| Plasma protein | gm/L | 58–76 | 60–80 |
| Serum protein | gm/L | 50–75 | 60–82 |
| Albumin | gm/L | 22–35 | 25–39 |
| Globulins | gm/L | 22–45 | 26–50 |
| A/G ratio | — | 0.50–1.20 | 0.53–1.36 |
| IgA | gm/L | 0.40–1.6 | 0.10–0.58 |
| IgM | gm/L | 1.0–2.0 | 0.06–0.39 |
| IgG | gm/L | 10.0–20.0 | 11.7–22.6 |
| Agarose gel electrophoresis: |  |  |  |
| $\alpha_1$ | gm/L | 5–8 | 2–5 |
| $\alpha_2$ | gm/L | 5–8 | 8–11 |
| $\beta_1$ | gm/L | 5–11 | 3–5 |
| $\beta_2$ | gm/L | 3–7 | 3–6 |
| $\gamma$ | gm/L | 5–18 | 12–32 |

°From Clinical Pathology Laboratory, Department of Pathology, University of Guelph. Immunoglobulin concentrations from Schultz RD and Adams LS: Immunologic methods for the detection of humoral and cellular immunity. Vet Clin North Am 8:721, 1978; Schultz RD, Scott FW, Duncan JR, et al.: Feline immunoglobulins. Infect Immun 9:391, 1974 and Barlough JE, Jacobson RH, and Scott FW: The immunoglobulins of the cat. Cornell Vet 71:397, 1981.

*Serum Iron and Iron-Binding Capacities in Iron-Deficient and Normal Dogs*[*]

| Analyte | Unit | Iron-Deficient Dogs | | Normal Dogs | |
|---|---|---|---|---|---|
| | | Mean | Range (min-max) | Mean | Range (min-max) |
| Serum iron | $\mu$mol/L | 5 | 1–11 | 27 | 15–42 |
| Total iron-binding capacity | $\mu$mol/L | 69 | 42–118 | 70 | 51–102 |
| Saturation | % | 8 | 2–19 | 39 | 19–59 |

[*]Derived from Harvey JW, French TW, and Meyer DJ: Chronic iron deficiency in dogs. J Am Animal Hosp Assoc 18:946, 1982. For a review of similar data from dogs with various hematologic changes, see Hoff B, Lumsden JH, and Valli VEO: An appraisal of bone marrow biopsy in assessment of sick dogs. Can J Comp Med 49:34, 1985.

*Serum Immunoglobulin Concentrations (mg/ml, Mean ± SD) of Normal Beagle Dogs at Various Ages*[*]

| Immunoglobulin Type | 6–12 Months (n = 10) | 1–2 Years (n = 10) | 2–3 Years (n = 10) | 3–5 Years (n = 10) | 5–7 Years (n = 10) | 7 Years (n - 6) |
|---|---|---|---|---|---|---|
| IgM | 1.24 ± 1.69 | 1.34 ± 1.43 | 1.3 ± 1.8 | 1.52 ± 0.33 | 1.67 ± 1.1 | 1.84 ± 0.35 |
| IgA | 0.64 ± 0.34 | 1.13 ± 0.42 | 1.04 ± 0.53 | 1.29 ± 0.39 | 1.77 ± 0.56 | 1.62 ± 0.61 |
| IgG$_1$ | 3.74 ± 1.44 | 3.97 ± 0.87 | 2.09 ± 0.68 | 3.16 ± 0.69 | 3.34 ± 1.3 | 2.24 ± 1.71 |
| IgG$_{2a+2b}$ | 5.0 ± 1.58 | 5.94 ± 1.16 | 6.13 ± 0.88 | 6.97 ± 0.92 | 9.05 ± 1.82 | 7.47 ± 1.68 |
| IgG$_{2c}$ | 1.25 ± 0.36 | 1.43 ± 0.21 | 1.49 ± 0.39 | 1.6 ± 0.27 | 1.88 ± 0.51 | 1.77 ± 0.58 |

[*]From Gorman NT and Halliwell REW: Immunoglobulin quantitation and clinical interpretation. *In* Halliwell REW and Gorman NT (eds): *Veterinary Clinical Immunology.* Philadelphia, WB Saunders Co, 1989, p 61.

*Acid-Base and Blood Gases (Mean ± SD)*[*]

| Analyte | Unit | Canine | | Feline | |
|---|---|---|---|---|---|
| | | Arterial | Venous | Arterial | Venous |
| pH | — | 7.407 ± 0.0097 | 7.405 ± 0.0097 | 7.386 ± 0.038 | 7.300 ± 0.087 |
| P$_{CO_2}$ | mmHg | 36.8 ± 3.0 | 36.6 ± 1.21 | 31.0 ± 2.9 | 41.8 ± 9.12 |
| P$_{O_2}$ | mmHg | 92.1 ± 5.6 | 52.1 ± 2.11 | 106.8 ± 5.7 | 38.6 ± 11.44 |
| HCO$_3$ | mmol/L | 22.2 ± 1.7 | 22.3 ± 0.43 | 18.0 ± 1.8 | 19.4 ± 4.0 |

[*]From Senior DF: Fluid therapy, electrolyte and acid-base control. *In* Ettinger SJ (ed): *Textbook of Veterinary Internal Medicine, Diseases of the Dog and Cat*, 3rd edition. Philadelphia, WB Saunders Co, 1989, p 440. These data are based on the following original citations: Haskins SC: Blood gases and acid-base balance: Clinical interpretation and therapeutic implications. *In* Kirk RW (ed): *Current Veterinary Therapy VIII.* Philadelphia, WB Saunders Co, 1980, p 201; Rodkey WG, et al.: Arterialized capillary blood used to determine the acid-base and blood gas status of dogs. Am J Vet Res 39:459, 1978; Middleton DJ, et al.: Arterial and venous blood gas tensions in clinically healthy cats. Am J Vet Res 42:1609, 1981.

## Coagulation Screening Tests°

| | | Unit | Canine | Feline |
|---|---|---|---|---|
| Buccal mucosal bleeding time (BMBT)[†] | Lip | Min | 1.7–4.2 | 1.0–3.2 |
| (Simplate, Organon Teknika) | | Min | 2.62 ± 0.49 (mean ± SD) | — |
| Cuticle bleeding time (CBT)[‡] | Nail bed | Min | 6.0 ± 3.7 (mean ± SD) | — |
| | | Min | 4.3 ± 0.3 (mean ± SEM) | — |
| Activated coagulation time (ACT)[§] | 37°C | Sec | 64–95 | ≤65 |
| | Room temperature | Sec | 60–125 | — |
| | | Sec | 83–129 | — |
| *Tests using a mechanical end point*[‖] | | | | |
| Prothrombin time (PT, Thromboplastin·C, Dade) | | Sec | 9–14 | — |
| Activated partial thromboplastin time (APTT, Actin Activated Cephaloplastin, Dade) | | Sec | ≤20 | — |
| *Tests using an electro-optical end point*[¶] | | | | |
| Prothrombin time (PT, Permaplastin, Dade) | | Sec | 13.2–22.0 | 15.5–25.9 |
| Activated partial thromboplastin time (APTT, Actin Activated Cephaloplastin, Dade) | | Sec | 21.0–35.0 | 22.8–38.0 |
| Thrombin clotting time (TCT, Thrombostat, Parke-Davis) | | Sec | 8.3–13.8 | 8.9–14.9 |
| Russell's viper venom time (RVVT) | | Sec | 10–15 | — |

°Prepared with the assistance of **Dr. I.B. Johnstone**, Hemostasis Laboratory, Department of Biomedical Sciences, University of Guelph. Abbreviations, methods, names, and sources of reagents are given in parentheses. These reference values are provided only as general guidelines. Reference values for PT, APTT, TCT, and other coagulation tests differ between laboratories depending on the type and concentration of reagents used and on the type of end-point detection (visual, mechanical, electro-optical). In interpreting patient test results, comparisons must always be made with reference values for that particular laboratory. Some laboratories may elect to run a species-specific reference plasma concurrent with patient plasma and report patient/control time. In such cases, the patient/control (P/C) ratio may be used to determine the significance of the test results. P/C ratios <0.75 or >1.25 in the PT, PTT, and TCT tests should be considered questionable or abnormal and worthy of further investigation (Johnstone IB: Classical haemophilia [haemophilia 'A'] in German shepherd dogs. Different expressions of the disease. Aust Vet Pract 17:71, 1987).

[†]From Parker MT, Collier LL, Kier AB, and Johnson GS: Oral mucosa bleeding times of normal cats and cats with Chediak-Higashi syndrome or Hageman trait (factor XII deficiency). Vet Clin Pathol 17:9, 1988; Jergens AE, Turrentine MA, Kraus KH, and Johnson GS: Buccal mucosa bleeding times of healthy dogs and of dogs in various pathologic states, including thrombocytopenia, uremia, and von Willebrand's disease. Am J Vet Res 48:1337, 1987.

[‡]From Giles AR, Tinlin S, and Greenwood R: A canine model of hemophilic (factor VIII:C deficiency) bleeding. Blood 60:727, 1982; Pijnappels MIM, Briët E, van der Zwet GTh, Huisden R, van Tilburg NH, and Eulderink F. Evaluation of the cuticle bleeding time in canine haemophilia A. Thromb Haemos 55:70, 1986.

[§]From Byars TD, Ling GV, Ferris NA, and Keeton KS: Activated coagulation time (ACT) of whole blood in normal dogs. Am J Vet Res 37: 1359, 1976; Middleton DJ and Watson ADJ: Activated coagulation times of whole blood in normal dogs and dogs with coagulopathies. J Small Anim Pract 19:417, 1978.

[‖]Fibrometer, reference values from Clinical Pathology Laboratory, Department of Pathology, University of Guelph. This APTT test uses ellagic acid and kaolin as activators.

[¶]BioData PC8, reference values from **Dr. I.B. Johnstone**, Hemostasis Laboratory, Department of Biomedical Sciences, University of Guelph. This APTT test uses ellagic acid as an activator.

## Specific Coagulation Tests°

| | Unit | Canine | Feline |
|---|---|---|---|
| Fibrinogen (fibrometer, thrombin time, TT, Thrombostat, Parke-Davis) | gm/L | 1.6–4.5 | — |
| Fibrinogen (heat precipitation) | gm/L | 1.3–4.4 | 0.8–2.9 |
| Platelets (manual, phase contrast) | X 10⁹/L | 200–600 | 190–750 |
| Fibrinogen degradation products (FDP, latex agglutination, Burroughs Wellcome) | μg/ml | ≤20 | — |
| Factor VIII coagulant (FVIII:C, one-stage differential PTT) | % of normal | 55–135 | — |
| von Willebrand factor antigen (vWF:Ag, Laurell Electroimmunoassay)[†] | % of normal | 50–178 | — |
| vWF:Ag (enzyme-linked immunosorbent assay, Diagnostica Stago)[‡] | % of normal | 60–152 | — |
| Antithrombin III (AT III, chromogenic substrate, Diagnostica Stago)[§] | % of normal | 80–136 | — |

°Prepared with the assistance of **Dr. I.B. Johnstone**, Hemostasis Laboratory, Department of Biomedical Sciences, University of Guelph. Abbreviations, methods, names, and sources of reagents are given in parentheses. Specific hemostatic factors are generally assayed by comparing test plasma to a species-specific reference plasma. The reference plasma is arbitrarily designated as having 100% activity and the activity in the patient plasma is expressed as a percentage of the "normal" plasma.

[†]From Johnstone IB and Crane S: Determination of canine factor VIII–related antigen using commercial antihuman factor VIII serum. Vet Clin Pathol 9:31, 1980.

[‡]From Johnstone IB and Crane S: Quantitation of canine plasma von Willebrand factor antigen using a commercial enzyme-linked immunosorbent assay. Can J Vet Res (in press).

[§]Johnstone IB, Petersen D, and Crane S: Antithrombin III (AT III) activity in plasmas from normal and diseased horses, and in normal canine, bovine, and human plasmas. Vet Clin Pathol 16:14, 1987.

## Quantitative Tests of Gastrointestinal Function*

*Fecal determinations*
Fecal output (gm feces/kg body weight/day, mean ± SEM)

| | | | |
|---|---|---|---|
| **Canine** | | | |
| Normal (*n* = 14) | 8.5 ± 1.1 | | |
| Malabsorption (*n* = 6) | 42.3 ± 8.0 | | |
| Colitis (*n* = 10) | 11.9 ± 1.1 | | |
| Nonsteatorrheal small intestinal diarrheal disease (*n* = 17) | 13.9 ± 2 | | |
| Exocrine pancreatic insufficiency (EPI) (*n* = 20) | 34.4 ± 4.5 | | |

Fecal fat output (g fecal fat/kg body weight/day, mean ± SEM)

| | | | |
|---|---|---|---|
| **Canine** | | **Feline** | |
| Normal (*n* = 14) | 0.24 ± 0.01 | Normal | 0.35 ± 0.23 (mean ± SD) |
| Malabsorption (*n* = 6) | 1.14 ± 0.11 | Steatorrhea | >3.5 gm fecal fat/day |
| EPI (*n* = 20) | 2.08 ± 0.36 | | |

*Note*: Values greater than 0.3 indicate steatorrhea. Fat balance in dogs with colitis and other nonmalabsorptive intestinal diseases is indistinguishable from normal dogs.

Fecal proteolytic activity (FPA) (mean of 3 samples)[†]

| | | | |
|---|---|---|---|
| **Canine** | | **Feline** | |
| Radial enzyme diffusion (mm) | | | |
| Normal | 7–15 | Normal | 6–17 |
| EPI | ≤5 | EPI | ≤5 |
| Azocasein digestion (ACU/gm feces) | | | |
| Normal | 19–122 | Normal | 29–207 |
| EPI | ≤10 | EPI | ≤10 |

*Serum concentrations of orally administered or naturally occurring substances*
Xylose (0.5 gm/kg body weight)

**Canine**

Peak at 60 min of 65 mg/dl ± 6 (mean ± SEM, *n* = 13), decreasing to 48 ± 5 at 90 min. Only 10% of dogs have 45 to 50 mg/dl at 60 min. All dogs with concentrations greater than 50 mg/dl at 60 min or 45 mg/dl at 90 min are considered normal.

*Note*: This test has poor sensitivity for detecting malabsorption in the dog and cat.

**Feline**

Peaks between 12 and 42 mg/dl

N-Benzoyl-L-tyrosyl-*para*-aminobenzoic acid (BT-PABA)

**Canine** (50 mg/kg body weight)
>400 µg/dl at 60 to 90 min

**Feline**

Peaks at 386 ± 134 µg/dl (mean ± SD, *n* = 17, 16.7 mg/kg body weight). At 50 mg/kg body weight, the peak occurred at 90 min and the range (min–max) was approximately 400–1100 µg/dl.

| | | | |
|---|---|---|---|
| Vitamin E (mg/L) | | | |
| **Canine** | >5 | **Feline** | >5 |
| Vitamin B$_{12}$ (ng/L) | | | |
| **Canine** | 225–661 | **Feline** | 200–1680 |
| Folic acid (µg/L) | | | |
| **Canine** | 6.7–17.4 | **Feline** | 13.4–38.0 |
| Trypsin-like immunoreactivity (TLI) (µg/L) | | | |
| **Canine** | | | |
| Normal | 5.0–35 | | |
| EPI | ≤2.5 | | |

*Prepared with the assistance of **Dr. D.A. Williams**. Review and original citations in Jacobs RM, Norris AM, Lumsden JH, and Valli VEO: Laboratory Diagnosis of Malassimilation. Vet Clin North Am [Small Anim Pract] 19:951, 1989.

[†]From Williams DA, Reed SD, and Perry L: Fecal proteolytic activity in clinically normal cats and in a cat with exocrine pancreatic insufficiency. J Am Vet Med Assoc 197:210, 1990; Williams DA and Reed SD: Comparison of methods for assay of fecal proteolytic activity. J Vet Clin Pathol 19:20, 1990.

## *Tests of the Endocrine System**

| Hormone | Unit | Canine | Feline |
|---|---|---|---|
| Adrenocorticotrophic hormone, basal (ACTH, plasma) | pmol/L | 2–15 | 1–20 |
| Aldosterone[†] (plasma) | | | |
|   Basal | pmol/L | 14–957 | 194–388 |
|   Post-ACTH | pmol/L | 197–2103 | 277–721 |
| Cortisol (serum or plasma, urine) | | | |
|   Basal | nmol/L | 25–125 | 15–150 |
|   Post-ACTH | nmol/L | 200–550 | 130–450 |
|   Post–**low**-dose dexamethasone (0.01 or 0.015 mg/kg) | nmol/L | ≤40 | ≤40 |
|   Post–**high**-dose dexamethasone (0.1 or 1.0 mg/kg)[‡] | nmol/L | ≤40 | ≤40 |
|   Urinary cortisol/creatinine ratio | X 10⁻⁶ | 8–24[‡], 10[§] | — |
| Insulin, basal (serum) | pmol/L | 35–200 | 35–200 |
| Intact parathormone[†] (serum) | pmol/L | 2–13 | 0–4 |
| Progesterone (serum or plasma, female) | mmol/L | ≤3.0 in anestrus, proestrus 50–220 in diestrus, pregnancy | ≤3.0 in anestrus, proestrus 50–220 in diestrus, pregnancy |
| Testosterone (serum or plasma, male) | nmol/L | 1–20 | 1–20 |
| Thyroxine (T₄, serum) | | | |
|   Basal | nmol/L | 12–50 | 10–50 |
|   Post–thyroxine-stimulating hormone (TSH) | nmol/L | >45 | >45 |
| Triiodothyronine (T₃) suppression[‖] | nmol/L | — | ≤20 |
| Triiodothyronine, basal (T₃, serum) | nmol/L | 0.7–2.3 | 0.5–2.0 |

*Prepared with the assistance of **Dr. M.E. Peterson**, The Animal Medical Center, New York, NY. Unless indicated otherwise, values in this table are adapted from Kemppainen RJ and Zerbe CA: Common endocrine diagnostic tests: Normal values and interpretations. *In* Kirk RW (ed): *Current Veterinary Therapy X.* Philadelphia, WB Saunders Co, 1989, p 961. Hormone determinations are variable between laboratories. The laboratory performing the analysis should provide reference values. Before submitting samples for hormone determinations, consult the laboratory for sample specifications, use of anticoagulants, and sample preservation. General sampling conditions are discussed in Reimers TJ: Guidelines for collection, storage, and transport of samples for hormone assay. *In* Kirk RW (ed): *Current Veterinary Therapy X.* Philadelphia, WB Saunders Co, 1989, p 968. The effects of age, gender, and size on canine serum thyroid and adrenocortical hormone concentrations are discussed in Reimers TJ, Lawler DF, Sutaria PM, Correa MT, and Erb HN: Effects of age, sex, and body size on serum concentrations of thyroid and adrenocortical hormones in dogs. Am J Vet Res 51:454, 1990.

†Provided by **Dr. R.F. Nachreiner**, Animal Health Diagnostic Laboratory, Endocrine Diagnostic Section, Michigan State University.

‡This test is used after adrenocortical hyperfunction has been confirmed. It is used to differentiate adrenal tumor (where no suppression is seen) from pituitary-dependent cases (where suppression occurs, but is variable).

§From Stolp R, Rijnberk A, Meiher JC, and Croughs RJM.: Urinary corticoids in the diagnosis of canine hyperadrenocorticism. Res Vet Sci 34:141, 1983; Rijnberk A, van Wees A, and Mol JA: Assessment of two tests for the diagnosis of canine hyperadrenocorticism. Vet Rec 122: 178, 1988.

‖From Peterson ME and Ferguson DC: Thyroid diseases. *In* Ettinger SJ (ed): *Textbook of Veterinary Internal Medicine. Diseases of the Dog and Cat,* 3rd edition. Philadelphia, WB Saunders Co, 1989, pp 1632–1675.

There are many potential drug-induced physiologic changes that can affect the results of endocrine testing; see pp 341–345, this volume.

*Système International (SI) Units for Hormone Assays*[*]

| Hormone | Unit | | Conversion Factors | |
|---|---|---|---|---|
| | *Traditional* | *SI* | *Traditional → SI* | *SI → Traditional* |
| Aldosterone | ng/dl | pmol/L | 27.7 | 0.036 |
| Corticotrophin (ACTH) | pg/ml | pmol/L | 0.22 | 4.51 |
| Cortisol | μg/dl | mmol/L | 27.59 | 0.36 |
| β-Endorphin | pg/ml | pmol/L | 0.289 | 3.43 |
| Epinephrine | pg/ml | pmol/L | 5.46 | 0.183 |
| Estrogen (estradiol) | pg/ml | pmol/L | 3.67 | 0.273 |
| Gastrin | pg/ml | ng/L | 1.00 | 1.00 |
| Glucagon | pg/ml | ng/L | 1.00 | 1.00 |
| Growth hormone (GH) | ng/ml | μg/L | 1.00 | 1.00 |
| Insulin | μU/ml | pmol/L | 7.18 | 0.139 |
| α-Melanocyte–stimulating hormone (α-MSH) | pg/ml | pmol/L | 0.601 | 1.66 |
| Norepinephrine | pg/ml | nmol/L | 0.006 | 169 |
| Pancreatic polypeptide (PP) | mg/dl | mmol/L | 0.239 | 4.18 |
| Progesterone | ng/ml | mmol/L | 3.18 | 0.315 |
| Prolactin | ng/ml | μg/L | 1.00 | 1.00 |
| Renin | ng/ml/hr | ng/L/s | 0.278 | 3.60 |
| Somatostatin | pg/ml | pmol/L | 0.611 | 1.64 |
| Testosterone | ng/ml | nmol/L | 3.47 | 0.288 |
| Thyroxine ($T_4$) | μg/dl | nmol/L | 12.87 | 0.078 |
| Triiodothyronine ($T_3$) | ng/dl | nmol/L | 0.0154 | 64.9 |
| Vasoactive intestinal polypeptide (VIP) | pg/ml | pmol/L | 0.301 | 3.33 |

[*]Contributed by **Dr. M.E. Peterson**, The Animal Medical Center, New York, NY.

*Urinary and Renal Function Tests**

| | Unit | Canine | Feline |
|---|---|---|---|
| Random specific gravity (SG) | — | 1.001–1.070 | 1.001–1.080 |
| SG after 5% dehydration | — | 1.050–1.076 | 1.047–1.087 |
| Random osmolality | mmol/kg | 50–2500 | 50–3000+ |
| Osmolality after 5% dehydration | mmol/kg | 1787–2791 | 1581–2984 |
| Urine/plasma osmolality after 5% dehydration | — | 5.7–8.9 | — |
| Volume output | ml/kg body weight/day | 24–41 | 22–30 |
| Protein—sulfosalicylic acid[†] | 0.1, 0.2, 0.3, 0.4 0.5, 0.75, and 1.0 gm/L stds. | <0.1 | |
| Protein—dipstick[‡] | Negative, trace, 0.3, 1.0, 3.0, and 20+ gm/L stds. | Negative when SG <1.035 Trace when SG >1.035 | |
| Blood—dipstick | Negative, +, ++, and +++ stds. | Negative | |
| Glucose—dipstick | Negative, 6, 14, 28, 56, and 111+ mmol/L stds. | Negative | |
| Ketones—dipstick | Negative, 0.5, 1.5, 4, 8, and 16 mmol/L stds. | Negative | |
| Bilirubin—dipstick | Negative, +, ++, and +++ stds. | + when SG >1.035 | Negative |
| Protein output[§] | mg/kg body weight/day | <22 | <30 |
| | mg/day | <200 or <600 | <115 |
| Protein/creatinine ratio[‖] | | | |
| Normal | — | <0.2 | <0.6 |
| Questionable | — | 0.2–1.0 | 0.6–1.0 |
| Abnormal | — | >1.0 | >1.0 |
| Effective renal plasma flow by clearance of | ml/min/m² body surface | 266 ± 66 | — |
| *para*-aminohippurate or | ml/min/kg body weight | 13.5 ± 3.3 | 14.1 ± 5.74 or 10.6 ± 1.7 |
| [¹³¹I]iodohippurate[¶] | | | |
| Glomerular filtration rate (GFR) by clearance | ml/min/m² body surface | 84.4 ± 19 | — |
| of [¹⁴C]inulin, [¹²⁵I]iothalamate, or other | ml/min/kg body weight | 4.2 ± 1.8 or 3.6 ± 0.1 | 5.1 ± 1.5 |
| labelled chemicals[#] | | | 3.5 ± 0.6 |
| GFR by sodium sulfanilate clearance[°°]-t₀.₅ | Min | 58 ± 13 or 66.1 ± 10.8 | 44.7 ± 5.7 |
| GFR by exogenous creatinine clearance[††] | ml/min/kg body weight | 4.0 ± 0.5 | 2.9 ± 0.3 |
| GFR by endogeneous creatinine clearance[‡‡] | ml/min/m² body surface | 60 ± 22 | — |
| | ml/min/kg body weight   20 min | 3.0 ± 1.0 | 2.7 ± 1.1 |
| | 24 hr | 3.7 ± 0.8 | 2.3 ± 0.5 |
| Fractional clearances[§§] | | | |
| Sodium | % | 0–0.7 | 0.24–0.96 |
| Chloride | % | 0–0.8 | 0.41–1.33 |
| Potassium | % | 0–20 | 6.7–23.9 |
| Calcium | % | 0–0.4 | — |
| Phosphorus | % | 3–39 | 17–73 |

*Prepared with the assistance of **Dr. J. Barsanti**, University of Georgia. Data are given in mean ± SD rounded to one decimal place. In a few instances, alternative reference values are listed. An extensive bibliography and a review of these tests can be found in Chew DJ and Dibartola SP: Diagnosis and pathophysiology of renal disease. *In* Ettinger SJ (ed): *Textbook of Veterinary Internal Medicine. Diseases of the Dog and Cat*, 3rd edition. Philadelphia, WB Saunders Co, 1989, pp 1893–1961.

[†]Albumin in Urine Test Set, Harleco, Gibbstown, NJ.

[‡]Multistix, Miles Canada Inc, Etobicoke, Ontario. Also applies for the semiquantitative analysis of blood, glucose, ketones, and bilirubin. Refer to the discussion in the package insert entitled "Ames Reagent Strips for Urinalysis" for potential interferents.

[§]From DiBartola SP, Chew DJ, and Jacobs G: Quantitative urinalysis including 24-hour protein excretion in the dog. J Am Anim Hosp Assoc 16:537, 1980; Russo EA, Lees GE, and Hightower D: Evaluation of renal function tests in cats, using quantitative urinalysis. Am J Vet Res 47:1308, 1986; Barsanti JA and Finco DR: Protein concentration in urine of normal dogs. Am J Vet Res 40:1583, 1979. Applies to urine samples with no hemorrhage or inflammation. Some differences in test results occur with different quantitative methods.

[‖]From White JV, Olivier B, Reimann K, and Johnson C: Use of protein-to-creatinine ratio in a single urine specimen for quantitative estimation of canine proteinuria. J Am Vet Med Assoc 185:882, 1984; Grauer GF, Thomas CB, and Eicker SW: Estimation of quantitative proteinuria in the dog, using the protein-to-creatinine ratio from a random, voided sample. Am J Vet Res 46:2116, 1985; Center SA, Wilkinson E, Smith CA, Erb H, and Lewis RM: 24-hour urine protein/creatinine ratio in dogs with protein-losing nephropathies. J Am Vet Med Assoc 187:820, 1985; McCaw DL, Knapp DW, and Hewett JE: Effect of collection time and exercise restriction on the prediction of urine protein excretion, using urine protein/creatinine ratio in dogs. Am J Vet Res 46:166, 1985; Jergens AE, McCaw DL, and Hewett JE: Effects of collection time and food consumption on the urine protein/creatinine ratio in dogs. Am J Vet Res 48:1106, 1987. Applies to urine samples with no hemorrhage or inflammation.

[¶]From Mercer HC, Garg RC, Powers JD, and Powers TE: Bioavailability and pharmacokinetics of several dosage forms of ampicillin in the cat. Am J Vet Res 38: 1353, 1977; Ross LA and Finco DR: Relationship of selected clinical renal function tests to glomerular filtration rate and renal blood flow in cats. Am J Vet Res 42: 1704, 1981.

[#]From Ross LA and Finco DR, 1981; Carlson GP and Kaneko JJ: Simultaneous estimation of renal function in dogs using sodium sulfanilate and sodium iodohippurate-¹³¹I. J Am Vet Med Assoc 158:1229, 1971; Maddison JE, Pascoe PJ, and Jansen BS: Clinical evaluation of sodium sulfanilate clearance for the diagnosis of renal disease in dogs. J Am Vet Med Assoc 185:961, 1984; Mercer HC, et al., 1977.

[°°]From Ross LA and Finco DR, 1981; Osborne CA, Low DG, and Finco DR: *Canine and Feline Urology*. Philadelphia, WB Saunders Co, 1972; Finco DR, Coulter DB, and Barsanti JA: Simple, accurate method for clinical estimation of glomerular filtration rate in the dog. Am J Vet Res 42:1874, 1981; Fettman MJ, Allen TA, Wilke WL, Radin MJ, and Eubank MC: Single-injection method for evaluation of renal function with ¹⁴C-inulin and ³H-tetraethylammonium bromide in dogs and cats. Am J Vet Re. 46: 482, 1985; Powers TE, Powers JD, and Garg RC: Study of the double isotope single-injection methods for estimating renal function in purebred beagle dogs. Am J Vet Res 38:1933, 1977.

[††]From Ross LA and Finco DR, 1981; Finco DR, et al., 1981. Creatinine given subcutaneously in dog and intravenously in cat.

[‡‡]From Russo EA, et al., 1986; Osborne CA, et al., 1972; Bovee KC and Joyce T: Clinical evaluation of glomerular function: 24 hour creatinine clearance in dogs. J Am Vet Med Assoc 174:488, 1979; Osbaldiston GW and Fuhrman W: The clearance of creatinine, inulin, paraamino-hippurate, and phenolsulphothalein in the cat. Can J Comp Med 24:138, 1970.

[§§]From Dibartola SP, et al., 1980; Russo EA, et al., 1986. Values vary markedly with diet.

*Bronchoalveolar Lavage Fluid Cell Populations**

| | Canine (n = 6) | Feline (n = 11) |
|---|---|---|
| Total nucleated cells/μl | ≤500 | ≤400 |
| Cell types (mean %) | | |
| Macrophages | 70 ± 11 (49–93) | 70.6 ± 9.8 |
| Lymphocytes | 7 ± 5 (1–19) | 4.6 ± 3.2 |
| Neutrophils | 5 ± 5 (1–27) | 6.7 ± 4.0 |
| Eosinophils | 6 ± 5 (1–19) | 16.1 ± 6.8 |
| Mast cells | 1 ± 1 (0–5) | NR[†] |
| Epithelial cells | 1 ± 1 (0–12) | NR |

*Canine data given as mean % ± SD (range). Feline data given as mean % ± SE. Data derived from and original citations listed in Hawkins EC, DeNicola DB, and Kuehn NF: Bronchoavelolar lavage in the evaluation of pulmonary disease in the dog and cat. J Vet Int Med 4:267, 1990.
[†]Not reported.

*Cerebrospinal Fluid (CSF)**

| | Canine | | Feline | |
|---|---|---|---|---|
| Protein (gm/L)[†] | 0.10–0.30 | | 0.04–0.32 | |
| Total nucleated cells (× 10⁹/L)[‡] | 0–0.002 | | 0–0.002 | |
| | Sediment (n = 40) | Cytospin (n = 50) | Sediment (n = 20) | Cytospin (n = 22) |
| Cell types (mean %, [range]) | | | | |
| Large foamy mononuclear | 3 (0–32) | 6 (0–46) | — | — |
| Monocytoid | — | 17 (0–50) | 87 (69–100) | 77 (25–100) |
| Small mononuclear | 26 (3–52) | 37 (0–73) | — | — |
| Large mononuclear | 38 (9–74) | 33 (0–68) | — | — |
| Small lymphocyte | 5 (0–76) | 4 (0–61) | 9 (0–27)[§] | 14 (0–50) |
| Neutrophil | 1 (0–10) | 3 (0–7) | 1 (0–9) | 2 (0–25) |
| Eosinophil | 0 | 0.3 (0–13) | 0 | 0 |
| Macrophage | 0 | 0 | 0 (0–3) | 3 (0–33) |

*Canine data adapted from Jamison EM and Lumsden JH: Cerebrospinal fluid analysis in the dog: methodology and interpretation. Semin Vet Med Surg (Small Anim) 3:122, 1988 and other unpublished data describing the CSF characteristics of histologically normal dogs. Feline data adapted from Rand JS, Parent J, Jacobs RM, and Percy D: Reference intervals for feline cerebrospinal fluid: cell counts and cytologic features. Am J Vet Res 51:1044, 1990 describing CSF characteristics in histologically normal cats. All feline CSFs had red blood cell counts between 0 and 0.030 × 10⁹/L. All data are for cerebellomedullary CSF. There are significant differences between lumbar and cerebello-medullary CSF (Bailey CS and Higgins RJ: Comparison of total white blood cell count and total protein content of lumbar and cisternal cerebrospinal fluid of healthy dogs. Am J Vet Res 46:1162, 1985); Thomson CE, Kornegay JN, and Stevens JB: Analysis of cerebrospinal fluid from the cerebellomedullary and lumbar cisterns of dogs with focal neurologic disease: 145 cases (1985–1987). J Am Vet Med Assoc 196:1841–1844, 1990.
[†]The protein concentrations here are for the Ponceau S method and the reference interval represents the range. For a comparison of Ponceau S and urine dipstick methods, see Jacobs RM, Cochrane SM, Lumsden JH, and Norris AM: Relationship of cerebrospinal fluid protein concentration determined by dye-binding and urinary dipstick methodologies. Can Vet J 31:587, 1990.
[‡]Range for hemocytometer cell counts.
[§]Includes all sizes of lymphocytes.

*Cerebrospinal Fluid Biochemical Analytes in Histologically Normal Cats**

| Analyte | Unit | Mean | Range (min-max) |
|---|---|---|---|
| Glucose | mmol/L | 4.1 | 0.5–8.1 |
| Creatine kinase | U/L | 47 | 2–236 |
| Lactate dehydrogenase | U/L | 12 | 4–30 |
| Aspartate aminotransferase | U/L | 17 | 0–39 |
| IgG | gm/L | 0.015 | 0.005–0.56 |
| [CSF IgG]/[serum IgG] | — | 0.8 | 0.3–2.1 |

*Adapted from Rand JS, Parent J, Jacobs RM, and Johnson R: Reference intervals for feline cerebrospinal fluid: Biochemical and serologic variables, IgG concentration, and electrophoretic fractionation. Am J Vet Res 51:1049, 1990. All feline CSFs had red blood cell counts between 0 and 0.030 × 10⁹/L. Also see this volume, p 1121.

## Characteristics of Body Cavity Fluids in Healthy Dogs and Cats*

| | |
|---|---|
| Volume | 0–15 ml for peritoneal cavity |
| | Approximately 3 ml in pleural cavity |
| | Approximately 0.3 ml in pericardial sac |
| Color | Colorless to slight yellow |
| Odor | None |
| Transparency | Clear, with no tissue fragments |
| Protein[†] | ≤2.5 gm/dl (≤25 gm/L) |
| | Does not coagulate |
| Specific gravity | ≤1.014 |
| Electrolytes and pH | As for plasma |
| Total nucleated cell count | ≤3000/$\mu$l (≤3.0 × 10⁹/L) |
| Cell types | Mesothelial cells |
| | Occasional well-preserved neutrophils |
| | Occasional lymphocytes and monocytes |
| | Occasional erythrocytes |

*From O'Brien PJ and Lumsden JH: The cytologic examination of body cavity fluids. Semin Vet Med Surg (Small Anim) 3:140, 1988. The original citations are listed in this review.
[†]For the Goldberg refractometer (Fisher Scientific, Toronto, Ontario), 2.5 gm protein/dl corresponds to a specific gravity of 1.014 on the plasma/serum scale. The serum/plasma specific gravity scale should be used for the estimation of protein concentration in body cavity fluids. If the urine specific gravity scale is used erroneously or unknowingly, the corresponding specific gravity is 1.020 for a protein concentration of 2.5 gm/dl.

## Cytologic Findings in Normal and Abnormal Canine Synovial Fluids*

| | Clarity | Color | Mucin Clot | Fibrin | Cell Count (× 10⁹/L) | Mononuclear Cells (%) | Neutrophils (%) |
|---|---|---|---|---|---|---|---|
| *Normal* | Clear | None to light yellow | Good | − | 0.0–3.0 | 90–100 | 0–10 |
| *Nonsuppurative inflammation* | | | | | | | |
| Degenerative | Clear | None to light yellow | Good to fair | − | 0.0–3.5 | 90–100 | 0–10 |
| Traumatic | Clear to turbid | Normal to bloody | Good | ± | 2.5–3.0 | 90–100 | 0–10 |
| Chronic hemarthrosis | Turbid | Bloody | Fair to poor | −[†] | Variably increased | Predominate | Occasional |
| *Suppurative inflammation* | | | | | | | |
| Rheumatoid-like | Turbid | Yellow to bloody | Fair to poor | + | 3.0–38 | 20–80 | 20–80 |
| SLE[‡]-like | Turbid | Yellow to bloody | Good to poor | + | 4.4–370 | 5–85 | 15–95 |
| Bacterial | Turbid | Gray to bloody | Poor to very poor | + | 110–267 | 1–10 | 90–99 |

*From Ellison RS: The cytologic examination of synovial fluid. Semin Vet Med Surg (Small Anim) 3:133, 1988. The original citations are listed in this review. The protein concentration in normal joint fluid is ≤30 gm/L.
[†]In acute hemarthrosis, fibrin clots may be present.
[‡]Systemic lupus erythematosus.
Also see this volume, p 1166.

## Canine Semen (Mean ± SEM)*

| Semen Characteristics After Sexual Rest | Unit | Body Weight (pounds) | | |
|---|---|---|---|---|
| | | *10–34* | *35–59* | *60–84* |
| Volume[†] | ml | 2.4 ± 0.3 | 3.9 ± 0.5 | 5.4 ± 1.3 |
| Sperm concentration | × 10⁶/ml | 209 ± 42 | 359 ± 72 | 228 ± 58 |
| Total sperm | × 10⁶/ml | 400 ± 110 | 1120 ± 130 | 1430 ± 460 |

*Data derived from Amann RP: Reproductive physiology and endocrinology of the dog. *In* Morrow DA (ed): *Current Therapy in Theriogenology* 2. Philadelphia, WB Saunders Co, 1986, p 536. In one study, inseminations with greater than 200 × 10⁶ morphologically normal sperm resulted in a pregnancy rate of 81% (22 of 27 bitches). As the total number of morphologically normal sperm declined, so did the pregnancy rate and litter size (Michelsen WD, Society for Theriogenology, Orlando, FL, September, 1988, p 387).
[†]The presperm and sperm-rich fractions were collected together, but ejaculation was terminated when ejaculation of the postsperm prostatic fluid was started.

### Canine Prostatic Fluid (Third Fraction)*

| | |
|---|---|
| Volume | Variable, depending on length of ejaculation |
| pH | 6.1–7.2 |
| Appearance | Clear |
| Sediment | Acellular |

*From Bartlett DJ: Studies on dog semen II. Biochemical characteristics. J Reprod Fertil 3:190, 1962.

## Electrocardiography*

It is recognized that normal and abnormal electrocardiographic measurements overlap and that the criteria for the normal electrocardiogram serve only as a guide for the clinician. Deviations from normal in an individual electrocardiogram suggest but are not always diagnostic of heart disease. As additional statistical data become available for the electrocardiograms of dogs of each breed, body type, age, and sex, the data herein may require revision and "normal" may be more precisely defined. The value of serial electrocardiograms from an individual cannot be overemphasized, since serial changes best demonstrate electrocardiographic abnormalities.

### Criteria for the Normal Canine Electrocardiogram[t]

Heart rate—60 to 160 bpm for adult dogs, up to 180 bpm in toy breeds, and 220 bpm for puppies.
Heart rhythm—Normal sinus rhythm; sinus arrhythmia; and wandering sinoatrial pacemaker.
P wave—Up to 0.4 mV in amplitude; up to 0.04 sec in duration (may be longer in giant breeds); always positive in leads II and aVF; positive or isoelectric in lead I.
P-R interval—0.06- to 0.14-sec duration.
QRS complex—Mean electric axis, frontal plane, 40 to 100 degrees.
Amplitude—Maximum amplitude of R wave 2.5 to 3.0 mV in leads II, III, and aVF. Complex positive in leads II, III, and aVF; negative in lead $V_{10}$.
Duration—To 0.05 sec (0.06/sec in dogs over 40 lb).
Q-T segment—0.15- to 0.22-sec duration.
ST segment and T wave—ST segment free of marked coving (repolarization changes).
ST segment depression not greater than 0.2 mV.
ST segment elevation not greater than 0.15 mV.
T wave negative in lead $V_{10}$.
T wave amplitude no greater than 25% of amplitude of R wave.

### Criteria for the Normal Feline Electrocardiogram[t]

Heart rate—240 bpm maximum.
Heart rhythm—Normal sinus rhythm or, infrequently, sinus arrhythmia.
P wave—Positive in leads II and aVF; may be isoelectric or positive in lead I; should not exceed 0.03 sec in duration.
P-R interval—0.04- to 0.08-sec duration (inversely related to the heart rate).
QRS complex—More variable than in the canine; the mean electric axis in the frontal plane is often insignificant. Often the QRS complex is nearly isoelectric in all frontal plane limb leads (so-called horizontal heart).
QRS amplitude—The amplitude of the R wave is usually low; marked amplitude of R wave (>0.8 mV) in the frontal plane leads may suggest ventricular hypertrophy.
QRS duration—<0.04 sec.
Q-T segment—0.16- to 0.18-sec duration.
ST segment and T wave—ST segment and T wave should be small and free of repolarization changes as well as marked depression or elevation.

*From Ettinger SJ and Suter PF: *Canine Cardiology*, Philadelphia, WB Saunders Co, 1970, pp 102–169.
[t]From Ettinger SJ: *Textbook of Veterinary Internal Medicine, Diseases of the Dog and Cat*, 3rd edition, Volume 1. Philadelphia, WB Saunders Co, 1989, p 1055.

## Système International (SI) Units Commonly Used in Biomedical Sciences

| Quantity | SI Units | Symbol |
|---|---|---|
| Length | Kilometer | km |
| | Meter | m |
| | Centimeter | cm |
| | Millimeter | mm ($10^{-3}$) |
| | Micrometer | $\mu$m ($10^{-6}$) |
| Surface area | Square centimeter | cm$^2$ |
| | Square meter | m$^2$ |
| Mass | Kilogram | kg |
| | Gram | gm |
| | Milligram | mg |
| | Microgram | $\mu$g |
| Temperature | Degree Celsius | °C |
| Time | Day | d |
| | Hour | h |
| | Minute | min |
| | Second | s |
| Volume | Liter | L |
| | Milliliter | ml |
| Concentration | Mole liter | mol/L |

## Approximate Equivalents for Degrees Fahrenheit and Celsius*

| °F | °C |
|---|---|
| 0 | −17.8 |
| 32 | 0 |
| 85 | 29.4 |
| 86 | 30 |
| 87 | 30.6 |
| 88 | 31.1 |
| 89 | 31.7 |
| 90 | 32.2 |
| 91 | 32.7 |
| 92 | 33.3 |
| 93 | 33.9 |
| 94 | 34.4 |
| 95 | 35.0 |
| 96 | 35.5 |
| 97 | 36.1 |
| 98 | 36.7 |
| 99 | 37.2 |
| 100 | 37.8 |
| 101 | 38.3 |
| 102 | 38.9 |
| 103 | 39.4 |
| 104 | 40.0 |
| 105 | 40.6 |
| 106 | 41.1 |
| 107 | 41.7 |
| 108 | 42.2 |
| 109 | 42.8 |
| 110 | 43.3 |
| 212 | 100 |

*Temperature conversion: °Celsius to °Fahrenheit, (°C)(9/5) + 32°; °Fahrenheit to °Celsius, (°F − 32°)(5/9).

## Conversion Table of Weight to Body Surface Area (in Square Meters) For Dogs*

| kg | m$^2$ | kg | m$^2$ |
|---|---|---|---|
| 0.5 | 0.06 | 26.0 | 0.88 |
| 1.0 | 0.10 | 27.0 | 0.90 |
| 2.0 | 0.15 | 28.0 | 0.92 |
| 3.0 | 0.20 | 29.0 | 0.94 |
| 4.0 | 0.25 | 30.0 | 0.96 |
| 5.0 | 0.29 | 31.0 | 0.99 |
| 6.0 | 0.33 | 32.0 | 1.01 |
| 7.0 | 0.36 | 33.0 | 1.03 |
| 8.0 | 0.40 | 34.0 | 1.05 |
| 9.0 | 0.43 | 35.0 | 1.07 |
| 10.0 | 0.46 | 36.0 | 1.09 |
| 11.0 | 0.49 | 37.0 | 1.11 |
| 12.0 | 0.52 | 38.0 | 1.13 |
| 13.0 | 0.55 | 39.0 | 1.15 |
| 14.0 | 0.58 | 40.0 | 1.17 |
| 15.0 | 0.60 | 41.0 | 1.19 |
| 16.0 | 0.63 | 42.0 | 1.21 |
| 17.0 | 0.66 | 43.0 | 1.23 |
| 18.0 | 0.69 | 44.0 | 1.25 |
| 19.0 | 0.71 | 45.0 | 1.26 |
| 20.0 | 0.74 | 46.0 | 1.28 |
| 21.0 | 0.76 | 47.0 | 1.30 |
| 22.0 | 0.78 | 48.0 | 1.32 |
| 23.0 | 0.81 | 49.0 | 1.34 |
| 24.0 | 0.83 | 50.0 | 1.36 |
| 25.0 | 0.85 | | |

*From Ettinger SJ: *Textbook of Veterinary Internal Medicine, Diseases of the Dog and Cat*, 2nd edition. Philadelphia, WB Saunders Co, 1975, p 146.

Although the above chart was compiled for dogs, it can also be used for cats. A formula for more precise values follows: BSA in m$^2$ = (K × W$^{2/3}$) × $10^{-4}$ where m$^2$ = square meters, BSA = body surface area, W = weight in gm, and K = constant of 10.1 in dogs and 10.0 in cats.

## Physical Equivalents

**Weight Equivalents**

| | | | |
|---|---|---|---|
| 1 oz = 28.350 gm | | 1 gm | = 0.0353 oz |
| 1 lb = 0.4536 kg = 16 oz | | 1 kg | = 2.205 lb |
| | | 1 μg/gm | = 1 mg/kg |
| | | 1 μg/gm | = 1 part per million |

**Volume Equivalents**

| | | | |
|---|---|---|---|
| 1 fl oz | = 29.57 ml | 1 ml | = 0.03382 fl oz |
| 1 pt | = 0.4731 L | 1 L | = 2.1134 pt |
| 1 pt | = 16 fl oz | 1 L | = 0.26417 gal |
| 1 gal | = 3.785 L | 1 μg/gm | = 1 part per million |
| 1 tbsp | = 15 ml | | |
| 1 tsp | = 5.0 ml | | |
| 1 gal (US) | = 0.833 gal (imperial) | | |

**Length Equivalents**

| | | | |
|---|---|---|---|
| 1 in | = 2.54 cm | 1 cm | = 0.3937 in |
| 1 ft | = 30.48 cm | 1 m | = 3.2808 ft |
| 1 yd | = 91.44 cm | 1 m | = 39.37 in |

**Pressure Equivalents**

| | | | |
|---|---|---|---|
| 1 cm $H_2O$ | | = 0.736 mmHg | = 0.098 kPa |
| 1 mmHg (torr) | | = 1.36 cm $H_2O$ | = 0.133 kPa |
| 1 kPa | | = 7.5 mmHg | = 10.2 cm $H_2O$ |
| 1 atm | | = 760 mmHg | = 1033.6 mm $H_2O$ |

## Weight-Unit Conversion Factors

| Units Given | Units Wanted | For Conversion Multiply by |
|---|---|---|
| lb | gm | 453.6 |
| lb | kg | 0.4536 |
| oz | gm | 28.35 |
| kg | lb | 2.2046 |
| kg | mg | 1,000,000.0 |
| kg | gm | 1000.0 |
| gm | mg | 1000.0 |
| gm | μg | 1,000,000.0 |
| mg | μg | 1000.0 |
| mg/gm | mg/lb | 453.6 |
| mg/kg | mg/lb | 0.4536 |
| μg/kg | μg/lb | 0.4536 |
| Mcal | kcal | 1000.0 |
| kcal/kg | kcal/lb | 0.4536 |
| kcal/lb | kcal/kg | 2.2046 |
| ppm | μg/gm | 1.0 |
| ppm | mg/kg | 1.0 |
| ppm | mg/lb | 0.4536 |
| mg/kg | % | 0.0001 |
| ppm | % | 0.0001 |
| mg/gm | % | 0.1 |
| gm/kg | % | 0.1 |

## Multiplication Factors and Prefixes

| Factor | Prefix | Symbol |
|---|---|---|
| $10^{18}$ | exa | E |
| $10^{15}$ | peta | P |
| $10^{12}$ | tera | T |
| $10^{9}$ | giga | G |
| $10^{6}$ | mega | M |
| $10^{3}$ | kilo° | k |
| $10^{2}$ | hecto | h |
| $10^{1}$ | deca | dk |
| $10^{-1}$ | deci | d |
| $10^{-2}$ | centi | c |
| $10^{-3}$ | milli° | m |
| $10^{-6}$ | micro° | μ |
| $10^{-9}$ | nano° | n |
| $10^{-12}$ | pico | p |
| $10^{-15}$ | femto | f |
| $10^{-18}$ | atto | a |

°Most frequently used in biomedical sciences.

# THE AAFCO DOG AND CAT FOOD NUTRIENT PROFILES

DAVID A. DZANIS

*Rockville, Maryland*

The US Food and Drug Administration (FDA) has primary federal regulatory authority over animal feeds (including pet foods) in the United States. The Association of American Feed Control Officials (AAFCO) is an advisory body comprised of representatives from the individual states. A primary function of AAFCO is the publication of a model feed bill, animal feed regulations, and ingredient definitions, all of which a state may adopt as a part of its own feed laws and regulations. Included in the model regulations are means for substantiation of nutritional adequacy for "complete and balanced" dog and cat foods. While the FDA does not have specific regulations regarding the nutritional content of pet foods, it recognizes that a label bearing a "complete and balanced" claim for a pet food that is not, in fact, nutritionally adequate is more than merely misbranded, but is also unsafe.

One means of substantiation of nutritional adequacy requires the product to be formulated so that essential nutrient levels meet a prescribed profile. Historically, AAFCO has relied on the publications of the National Research Council (NRC) as its "recognized authority on animal nutrition" with respect to the levels of nutrients that constituted a complete and balanced dog or cat food. Products that were formulated to meet all the nutrient levels as recommended by the NRC were allowed under AAFCO regulations to bear the label claim "meets or exceeds the NRC recommendations" or similar verbiage. This reliance became problematic when the NRC's most recent publication on nutrient requirements of dogs was published in 1985 and of cats in 1986. An update to reflect more recent knowledge of nutrition from its previous 1974 (dogs) and 1978 (cats) editions was fully warranted. However, the new recommendations were not in a format readily usable by AAFCO or the pet food industry. Levels were based on data using purified diets and the presumption of 100% bioavailability. There were very sound scientific reasons for presenting the data in this format. However, the new nutrient recommendations did not address the formulation of dog and cat foods based on practical, commonly used ingredients. As a result, AAFCO elected to continue to use the 1974 and 1978 recommendations until the problem could be remedied.

To address this situation, the AAFCO Canine Nutrition Expert (CNE) and Feline Nutrition Expert (FNE) subcommittees were established in 1990 and 1991, respectively. Nationally recognized experts from both ac-

ademia and industry were convened to establish updated practical profiles based on commonly used ingredients. In addition to this author, members of the CNE included: Dr. Jim Corbin, University of Illinois; Dr. Gail Czarnecki-Maulden, Westreco, Inc; Dr. Diane Hirakawa, The Iams Company; Dr. Francis Kallfelz, Cornell University; Dr. Mark Morris, Mark Morris Associates; and Dr. Ben Sheffy, Cornell University. In addition to the original members of the CNE, two new members were added to the FNE to bring additional expertise in the field of cat nutrition: Dr. Quinton Rogers, University of California-Davis; and Dr. Angele Thompson, Kal Kan Foods.

The reports of the CNE and FNE subcommittees were the bases for the AAFCO Dog and Cat Food Nutrient Profiles (Tables 1 and 2). Nutrient levels were based on the members' knowledge of published and unpublished research, as well as their personal expertise and experiences in practical formulation. Compared to the NRC recommendations, there are two separate AAFCO profiles (one for growth and reproduction, and one for adult maintenance), instead of just one for all life stages. This allows foods formulated for adult dogs or cats to contain lower amounts of some nutrients, eliminating unnecessary excesses. The new profiles also establish minimum required amounts of essential amino acids, as well as protein. This requires pet food formulators to more closely consider their sources of protein to achieve the proper complement of amino acids.

Also, maximum levels of intake of some nutrients have been established for the first time. This was done out of concern that the risk of nutrient excess, rather than deficiency, was a bigger problem with many pet foods today. Thus, maximum limits on the amounts of calcium, phosphorus, magnesium, fat-soluble vitamins, and most trace minerals in dog foods were established. Maximum levels of methionine, zinc, and vitamins A and D were also established for cat foods. While the list of maximum levels for cat foods was not as extensive as those for dog foods, it should not imply that cats are more tolerant of nutrient excesses than dogs. Rather, it reflects the paucity of information on the toxic effects of nutrients in cats. Establishing maximum levels arbitrarily might prove worse than no maximum at all. Setting a maximum level implies safety below that level, which the subcommittee could not reasonably ensure.

**Table 1.** *AAFCO Dog Food Nutrient Profiles**

| Nutrient | Units DM Basis | Growth and Reproduction Minimum | Adult Maintenance Minimum | Maximum |
|---|---|---|---|---|
| Protein | % | 22.0 | 18.0 | |
| Arginine | % | 0.62 | 0.51 | |
| Histidine | % | 0.22 | 0.18 | |
| Isoleucine | % | 0.45 | 0.37 | |
| Leucine | % | 0.72 | 0.59 | |
| Lysine | % | 0.77 | 0.63 | |
| Methionine-cystine | % | 0.53 | 0.43 | |
| Phenylalanine-tyrosine | % | 0.89 | 0.73 | |
| Threonine | % | 0.58 | 0.48 | |
| Tryptophan | % | 0.20 | 0.16 | |
| Valine | % | 0.48 | 0.39 | |
| Fat[†] | % | 8.0 | 5.0 | |
| Linoleic acid | % | 1.0 | 1.0 | |
| Minerals | | | | |
| Calcium | % | 1.0 | 0.6 | 2.5 |
| Phosphorus | % | 0.8 | 0.5 | 1.6 |
| Ca/P ratio | | 1:1 | 1:1 | 2:1 |
| Potassium | % | 0.6 | 0.6 | |
| Sodium | % | 0.3 | 0.06 | |
| Chloride | % | 0.45 | 0.09 | |
| Magnesium | % | 0.04 | 0.04 | 0.3 |
| Iron[‡] | mg/kg | 80 | 80 | 3000 |
| Copper | mg/kg | 7.3 | 7.3 | 250 |
| Manganese | mg/kg | 5.0 | 5.0 | |
| Zinc | mg/kg | 120 | 120 | 1000 |
| Iodine | mg/kg | 1.5 | 1.5 | 50 |
| Selenium | mg/kg | 0.11 | 0.11 | 2 |
| Vitamins | | | | |
| Vitamin A | IU/kg | 5000 | 5000 | 50,000 |
| Vitamin D | IU/kg | 500 | 500 | 5000 |
| Vitamin E | IU/kg | 50 | 50 | 1000 |
| Thiamin[§] | mg/kg | 1.0 | 1.0 | |
| Riboflavin | mg/kg | 2.2 | 2.2 | |
| Pantothenic acid | mg/kg | 10 | 10 | |
| Niacin | mg/kg | 11.4 | 11.4 | |
| Pyridoxine | mg/kg | 1.0 | 1.0 | |
| Folic acid | mg/kg | 0.18 | 0.18 | |
| Vitamin $B_{12}$ | mg/kg | 0.022 | 0.022 | |
| Choline | mg/kg | 1200 | 1200 | |

*Presumes an energy density of 3.5 kcal/gm metabolizable energy, based on the "modified Atwater" values of 3.5, 8.5, and 3.5 kcal/gm for protein, fat, and carbohydrate (nitrogen-free extract [NFE]), respectively. Rations greater than 4.0 kcal/gm should be corrected for energy density; rations less than 3.5 kcal/gm should *not* be corrected for energy.

[†]Although a true requirement for fat *per se* has not been established, the minimum level was based on recognition of fat as a source of essential fatty acids, as a carrier of fat-soluble vitamins, to enhance palatability, and to supply an adequate caloric density.

[‡]Because of very poor bioavailability, iron from carbonate or oxide sources that is added to the diet should not be considered as components in meeting the minimum nutrient level.

[§]Because processing may destroy up to 90% of the thiamin in the diet, allowances in formulation should be made to ensure the minimum nutrient level is met after processing.

For dog food, the new profile for growth and reproduction raises the minimum amount of fat required. Also increased in both profiles are the levels of zinc and iron. On the other hand, the levels of calcium, phosphorus, and sodium chloride (salt) are lowered, especially for adult maintenance dog foods. In addition to setting levels for amounts of calcium and phosphorus individually, minimum and maximum ranges for the calcium/phosphorus ratio have been set.

For cat foods, taurine levels were established for both extruded and canned products to account for the decreased bioavailability of taurine in canned foods. Modifications in the levels of protein, calcium, phos-

phorus, potassium, zinc, and niacin were also made. A minimum level of vitamin K activity in products containing high amounts of fish was established.

The nutritional adequacy statement found on all complete and balanced pet foods that are substantiated by this method has also changed. The required label wording for reference to the nutrient profiles is that the product is "formulated to meet the AAFCO Dog (or Cat) Food Nutrient Profile for" a given life stage. In addition to removal of the reference to NRC, the word "exceeds" must be removed because the product must also be below maximum levels of some nutrients. Products that only meet the adult maintenance profile

**Table 2.** *AAFCO Cat Food Nutrient Profiles*°

| Nutrient | Units DM Basis | Growth and Reproduction Minimum | Adult Maintenance Minimum | Maximum |
|---|---|---|---|---|
| Protein | % | 30.0 | 26.0 | |
|   Arginine | % | 1.25 | 1.04 | |
|   Histidine | % | 0.31 | 0.31 | |
|   Isoleucine | % | 0.52 | 0.52 | |
|   Leucine | % | 1.25 | 1.25 | |
|   Lysine | % | 1.20 | 0.83 | |
|   Methionine-cystine | % | 1.10 | 1.10 | |
|   Methionine | % | 0.62 | 0.62 | 1.5 |
|   Phenylalanine-tyrosine | % | 0.88 | 0.88 | |
| Phenylalanine | % | 0.42 | 0.42 | |
|   Taurine (extruded) | % | 0.10 | 0.10 | |
|   Taurine (canned) | % | 0.20 | 0.20 | |
|   Threonine | % | 0.73 | 0.73 | |
|   Tryptophan | % | 0.25 | 0.16 | |
|   Valine | % | 0.62 | 0.62 | |
| Fat[†] | % | 9.0 | 9.0 | |
|   Linoleic acid | % | 0.5 | 0.5 | |
|   Arachidonic acid | % | 0.02 | 0.02 | |
| Minerals | | | | |
|   Calcium | % | 1.0 | 0.6 | |
|   Phosphorus | % | 0.8 | 0.5 | |
|   Potassium | % | 0.6 | 0.6 | |
|   Sodium | % | 0.2 | 0.2 | |
|   Chloride | % | 0.3 | 0.3 | |
|   Magnesium[‡] | % | 0.08 | 0.04 | |
|   Iron[§] | mg/kg | 80 | 80 | |
|   Copper | mg/kg | 5 | 5 | |
|   Iodine | mg/kg | 0.35 | 0.35 | |
|   Zinc | mg/kg | 75 | 75 | 2000 |
|   Manganese | mg/kg | 7.5 | 7.5 | |
|   Selenium | mg/kg | 0.1 | 0.1 | |
| Vitamins | | | | |
|   Vitamin A | IU/kg | 9000 | 5000 | 750,000 |
|   Vitamin D | IU/kg | 750 | 500 | 10,000 |
|   Vitamin E[‖] | IU/kg | 30 | 30 | |
|   Vitamin K[¶] | mg/kg | 0.1 | 0.1 | |
|   Thiamin[#] | mg/kg | 5.0 | 5.0 | |
|   Riboflavin | mg/kg | 4.0 | 4.0 | |
|   Pyridoxine | mg/kg | 4.0 | 4.0 | |
|   Niacin | mg/kg | 60 | 60 | |
|   Pantothenic acid | mg/kg | 5.0 | 5.0 | |
|   Folic acid | mg/kg | 0.8 | 0.8 | |
|   Biotin[°°] | mg/kg | 0.07 | 0.07 | |
|   Vitamin $B_{12}$ | mg/kg | 0.02 | 0.02 | |
|   Choline[††] | mg/kg | 2400 | 2400 | |

°Presumes an energy density of 4.0 kcal/gm ME, based on the "modified Atwater" values of 3.5, 8.5, and 3.5 kcal/gm for protein, fat, and carbohydrate (nitrogen-free extract [NFE]), respectively. Rations greater than 4.5 kcal/gm should be corrected for energy density; rations less than 4.0 kcal/gm should *not* be corrected for energy.

[†]Although a true requirement for fat *per se* has not been established, the minimum level was based on recognition of fat as a source of essential fatty acids, as a carrier of fat-soluble vitamins, to enhance palatability, and to supply an adequate caloric density.

[‡]If the mean urine pH of cats fed *ad libitum* is not below 6.4, the risk of struvite urolithiasis increases as the magnesium content of the diet increases.

[§]Because of very poor bioavailability, iron from carbonate or oxide sources that is added to the diet should not be considered as components in meeting the minimum nutrient level.

[‖]Add 10 IU vitamin E above minimum level per gram of fish oil per kilogram of diet.

[¶]Vitamin K does not need to be added unless diet contains greater than 25% fish on a dry-matter basis.

[#]Because processing may destroy up to 90% of the thiamin in the diet, allowances in formulation should be made to ensure the minimum nutrient level is met after processing.

[°°]Biotin does not need to be added unless diet contains antimicrobial or antivitamin compounds.

[††]Methionine may substitute for choline as a methyl donor at a rate of 3.75 parts for 1 part choline by weight when methionine exceeds 0.62%.

should include "maintenance" as its given life stage. Products meeting the growth and reproduction profile can list its intended use as for adult maintenance, growth, reproduction, or "all life stages."

Nutrient levels in the tables are expressed on a dry matter basis. To accurately compare levels for a pet food as given in the guaranteed analysis portion of a label or elsewhere on an "as-fed" basis, values must first be corrected for moisture. For most dry pet foods (10% moisture), "as-fed" values should be multiplied by 1.1. For a 75% moisture canned product, values should be multiplied by 4.0. Products very high in ca-loric density should also be corrected for energy content before comparisons with the profiles are made.

The complete report of the CNE appeared in the 1992 edition of the *AAFCO Official Publication*, and the report of the FNE appeared in the 1993 edition. The tables and accompanying information on using the tables will be printed in subsequent editions. Inquiries about obtaining a copy of the *AAFCO Official Publication* should be addressed to: Mr. Charles Frank, Treasurer, AAFCO, Georgia Department of Agriculture, Capitol Square, Atlanta, GA 30334, (404) 656-3637.

# COMPENDIUM OF ANIMAL RABIES CONTROL, 1995

## NATIONAL ASSOCIATION OF STATE PUBLIC HEALTH VETERINARIANS, INC.

The purpose of this Compendium is to provide rabies information to veterinarians, public health officials, and others concerned with rabies control. These recommendations serve as the basis for animal rabies control programs throughout the United States and facilitate standardization of procedures among jurisdictions, thereby contributing to an effective national rabies control program. This document is reviewed annually and revised as necessary. Immunization procedure recommendations are contained in Part I; all animal rabies vaccines licensed by the United States Department of Agriculture (USDA) and marketed in the United States are listed in Part II; Part III details the principles of rabies control.

## Part I: Recommendations for Immunization Procedures

A. **VACCINE ADMINISTRATION:** All animal rabies vaccines should be restricted to use by, or under the direct supervision of, a veterinarian.

B. **VACCINE SELECTION:** In comprehensive rabies control programs, only vaccines with a 3-year duration of immunity should be used. This constitutes the most effective method of increasing the proportion of immunized dogs and cats in any population (see Part II).

C. **ROUTE OF INOCULATION:** All vaccines must be administered in accordance with the specifications of the product label or package insert. If administered intramuscularly, it must be at one site in the thigh.

D. **WILDLIFE VACCINATION:** Parenteral vaccination of captive wildlife is not recommended since the efficacy of rabies vaccines in such animals has not been established and no vaccine is licensed for wildlife. For this reason, and because virus shedding periods are unknown, wild or exotic carnivores and bats should not be kept as pets. Zoos or research institutions may establish vaccination programs which attempt to protect valuable animals, but not in lieu of appropriate public health activities that protect humans. The use of licensed oral vaccines for the mass immunization of wildlife should be considered in selected situations with the approval of the state agency responsible for animal rabies control.

E. **ACCIDENTAL HUMAN EXPOSURE TO VACCINE:** Accidental inoculation may occur during administration of animal rabies vaccine. Such exposure to inactivated vaccines constitutes no rabies hazard.

F. **IDENTIFICATION OF VACCINATED ANIMALS:** All agencies and veterinarians should adopt the standard tag system. This practice will aid the administration of local, state, national and international control procedures. Animal license tags should be distinguishable in shape and color from rabies tags. Anodized aluminum rabies tags should be no less than 0.064 inches in thickness.

1.  RABIES TAGS

| YEAR | COLOR | SHAPE |
|------|-------|-------|
| 1995 | Green | Bell |
| 1996 | Red | Heart |
| 1997 | Blue | Rosette |
| 1998 | Orange | Oval |

2.  RABIES CERTIFICATE: All agencies and veterinarians should use the NASPHV from #50 or #51, "Rabies Vaccination Certificate," which can be obtained from vaccine manufacturers. Computer-generated forms containing the same information are acceptable.

### THE NASPHV COMMITTEE

Suzanne R. Jenkins, VMD, MPH, Chair
Keith A. Clark, DVM, PhD
John G. Debbie, MS, DVM
Russell J. Martin, DVM, MPH
Grayson B. Miller, Jr., MD
F. T. Satalowich, DVM, MSPH
Faye E. Sorhage, VMD, MPH

### CONSULTANTS TO THE COMMITTEE

James E. Childs, ScD; Centers for Disease Control and Prevention (CDC)
Robert B. Miller, DVM, MPH; APHIS, USDA
Patrick Morgan, DVM, DrPH; AVMA Council on Public Health and Regulatory Veterinary Medicine
Charles E. Rupprecht, VMD, PhD; Centers for Disease Control and Prevention (CDC)
R. Keith Sikes, DVM, MPH
Richard A. Zehr; Veterinary Biologics Section, Animal Health Institute

ENDORSED BY:
American Veterinary Medical Association (AVMA)
Council of State and Territorial Epidemiologists (CSTE)

Suzanne R. Jenkins, VMD, MPH
Office of Epidemiology
Virginia State Department of Health
PO Box 2448
Richmond, VA 23218

## Part III: Rabies Control

## A. PRINCIPLES OF RABIES CONTROL

1. HUMAN RABIES PREVENTION: Rabies in humans can be prevented either by eliminating exposures to rabid animals or by providing exposed persons with prompt local treatment of wounds combined with appropriate passive and active immunization. The rationale for recommending preexposure and postexposure rabies prophylaxis and details of their administration can be found in the current recommendations of the Immunization Practices Advisory Committee (ACIP), of the Public Health Service (PHS). These recommendations, along with information concerning the current local and regional status of animal rabies and the availability of human rabies biologics, are available from state health departments.

2. DOMESTIC ANIMALS: Local governments should initiate and maintain effective programs to ensure vaccination of all dogs and cats and to remove strays and unwanted animals. Such procedures in the United States have reduced laboratory confirmed rabies cases in dogs from 6949 in 1947 to 130 in 1993. Since more rabies cases are reported annually involving cats than dogs, vaccination of cats should be required. The recommended vaccination procedures and the licensed animal vaccines are specified in Parts I and II of the Compendium.

3. RABIES IN WILDLIFE: The control of rabies among wildlife reservoirs is difficult. Selective population reduction may be useful in some situations, but the success of such procedures depends on the circumstances surrounding each rabies outbreak (see C. "Control Methods in Wild Animals").

## B. CONTROL METHODS IN DOMESTIC AND CONFINED ANIMALS

1. PREEXPOSURE VACCINATION AND MANAGEMENT

Animal rabies vaccines should be administered only by, or under the direct supervision of, a veterinarian. This is the only way to ensure that a responsible person can be held accountable to assure the public that the animal has been properly vaccinated. Within 1 month after primary vaccination, a peak rabies antibody titer is reached and the animal can be considered immunized. An animal is currently vaccinated and is considered immunized if it was vaccinated at least 30 days previously, and all vaccinations have been administered in accordance with this Compendium. Regardless of the age at initial vaccination, a second vaccination should be given 1 year later (see Parts I and II for recommended vaccines and procedures).

(a) DOGS AND CATS
All dogs and cats should be vaccinated against rabies at 3 months of age and revaccinated in accordance with Part II of this Compendium.

(b) FERRETS
Ferrets may be vaccinated against rabies at 3 months of age and revaccinated in accordance with Part II of this Compendium.

(c) LIVESTOCK
It is neither economically feasible nor justified from a public health standpoint to vaccinate all livestock against rabies. However, consideration should be given to the vaccination of livestock, especially animals which are particularly valuable and/or may have frequent contact with humans, or in areas where rabies is epizootic in terrestrial animals.

(d) OTHER ANIMALS
(1) WILD
No rabies vaccine is licensed for use in wild animals. Because of the risk of rabies in wild animals (especially raccoons, skunks, coyotes, foxes, and bats), the AVMA, the NASPHV, and the CSTE strongly recommend the enactment of state laws prohibiting the importation, distribution, relocation, or keeping of wild animals and wild animals crossbred to domestic dogs and cats as pets.

(2) MAINTAINED IN EXHIBITS AND IN ZOOLOGIC PARKS
Captive animals not completely excluded from all contact with rabies vectors can become infected. Moreover, wild animals may be incubating rabies when initially captured; therefore, wild-caught animals susceptible to rabies should be quarantined for a minimum of 180 days before exhibition. Employees who work with animals at such facilities should receive preexposure rabies immunization. The use of pre- or postexposure rabies immunizations of employees who work with animals at such facilities may reduce the need for euthanasia of captive animals.

2. STRAY ANIMALS
Stray dogs or cats should be removed from the community, especially in areas where rabies is

epizootic. Local health departments and animal control officials can enforce the removal of strays more effectively if owned animals are confined or kept on leash. Strays should be impounded for at least 3 days to give owners sufficient time to reclaim animals and to determine if human exposure has occurred.

3. QUARANTINE
   (a) INTERNATIONAL
       CDC regulates the importation of dogs and cats into the United States, but present PHS regulations (42 CFR No. 71.51) governing the importation of such animals are insufficient to prevent the introduction of rabid animals into the country. All dogs and cats imported from countries with enzootic rabies should be currently vaccinated against rabies as recommended in this Compendium. The appropriate public health official of the state of destination should be notified within 72 hours of any unvaccinated dog or cat imported into his or her jurisdiction. The conditional admission of such animals into the United States is subject to state and local laws governing rabies. Failure to comply with these requirements should be promptly reported to the director of the Division of Quarantine, CDC, (404) 639-8107.
   (b) INTERSTATE
       Prior to interstate movement, dogs and cats should be vaccinated against rabies according to the Compendium's recommendations (see B.1.). Animals in transit should be accompanied by a currently valid NASPHV Form #51, Rabies Vaccination Certificate.

4. ADJUNCT PROCEDURES
   Methods or procedures which enhance rabies control include:
   (a) LICENSURE. Registration or licensure of all dogs and cats may be used to aid in rabies control. A fee is frequently charged for such licensure and revenues collected are used to maintain rabies or animal control programs. Vaccination is an essential prerequisite to licensure.
   (b) CANVASSING OF AREA. House-to-house canvassing by animal control personnel facilities enforcement of vaccination and licensure requirements.
   (c) CITATIONS. Citations are legal summonses issued to owners for violations, including the failure to vaccinate or license their animals. The authority for officers to issue citations should be an integral part of each animal control program.
   (d) ANIMAL CONTROL. All communities should incorporate stray animal control, leash laws, and training of personnel in their programs.

5. POSTEXPOSURE MANAGEMENT
   ANY ANIMAL BITTEN OR SCRATCHED BY A WILD, CARNIVOROUS MAMMAL (OR A BAT) NOT AVAILABLE FOR TESTING SHOULD BE REGARDED AS HAVING BEEN EXPOSED TO RABIES
   (a) DOGS AND CATS
       Unvaccinated dogs and cats exposed to a rabid animal should be euthanized immediately. If the owner is unwilling to have this done, the animal should be placed in strict isolation for 6 months and vaccinated 1 month before being released. Dogs and cats that are currently vaccinated should be revaccinated immediately, kept under the owner's control, and observed for 45 days.
   (b) LIVESTOCK
       All species of livestock are susceptible to rabies; cattle and horses are among the most frequently infected of all domestic animals. Livestock exposed to a rabid animal and currently vaccinated with a vaccine approved by USDA for that species should be revaccinated immediately and observed for 45 days. Unvaccinated livestock should be slaughtered immediately. If the owner is unwilling to have this done, the animal should be kept under very close observation for 6 months. The following are recommendations for owners of unvaccinated livestock exposed to rabid animals:
       (1) If the animal is slaughtered within 7 days of being bitten, its tissues may be eaten without risk of infection, provided liberal portions of the exposed area are discarded. Federal meat inspectors must reject for slaughter any animal known to have been exposed to rabies within 8 months.
       (2) Neither tissues nor milk from a rabid animal should be used for human or animal consumption. However, since pasteurization temperatures will inactivate rabies virus, drinking pasteurized milk or eating cooked meat does not constitute a rabies exposure.
       (3) It is rare to have more than one rabid animal in a herd, or herbivore to herbivore transmission, and therefore it may not be necessary to restrict the rest of the herd if a single animal has been exposed to or infected by rabies.
   (c) OTHER ANIMALS
       Other animals bitten by a rabid animal should be euthanized immediately. Such animals currently vaccinated with a vaccine approved by USDA for that species may be revaccinated immediately and placed in strict isolation for at least 90 days.

6. MANAGEMENT OF ANIMALS THAT BITE HUMANS
   A healthy dog or cat that bites a person should be confined and observed for 10 days; it is rec-

ommended that rabies vaccine not be administered during the observation period. Such animals should be evaluated by a veterinarian at the first sign of illness during confinement. Any illness in the animal should be reported immediately to the local health department. If signs suggestive of rabies develop, the animal should be humanely killed, its head removed, and the head shipped under refrigeration for examination by a qualified laboratory designated by the local or state health department. Any stray or unwanted dog or cat that bites a person may be humanely killed immediately and the head submitted as described above for rabies examination. Other biting animals which have exposed a person to rabies should be reported immediately to the local health department. Prior vaccination of an animal may not preclude the necessity for euthanasia and testing if the period of virus shedding is unknown for that species. Management of animals other than dogs and cats depends on the species, the circumstances of the bite, and the epidemiology of rabies in the area.

## C. CONTROL METHODS IN WILDLIFE

The public should be warned not to handle wildlife. Wild mammals (as well as the offspring of wild species crossbred with domestic dogs and cats) that bite or otherwise expose people, pets, or livestock should be considered for euthanasia and rabies examination. A person bitten by any wild mammal should immediately report the incident to a physician who can evaluate the need for antirabies treatment (see current rabies prophylaxis recommendations of the ACIP).

1. TERRESTRIAL MAMMALS
   Continuous and persistent government-funded programs for trapping or poisoning wildlife are not cost effective in reducing wildlife rabies reservoirs on a statewide basis. However, limited control in high-contact areas (picnic grounds, camps, suburban areas) may be indicated for the removal of selected high-risk species of wildlife. The state wildlife agency and state health department should be consulted for coordination of any proposed population reduction programs.
2. BATS
   (a) Indigenous rabid bats have been reported from every state except Alaska and Hawaii, and have caused rabies in at least 20 humans in the United States. It is neither feasible nor desirable, however, to control rabies in bats by programs to reduce bat populations.
   (b) Bats should be excluded from houses and surrounding structures to prevent direct association with humans. Such structures should then be made bat-proof by sealing entrances used by bats.

*Part II: Vaccines Marketed in the United States and NASPHV Recommendations*

| Product Name | Produced By | Marketed By | For Use In | Dosage | Age at Primary Vaccination[1] | Booster Recommended | Route of Inoculation |
|---|---|---|---|---|---|---|---|
| **A) *Inactivated*** | | | | | | | |
| TRIMUNE | Fort Dodge License No. 112 | Fort Dodge | Dogs | 1 ml | 3 mo & | Triennially | IM[2] |
| | | | Cats | 1 ml | 1 yr later | Triennially | IM |
| ANNUMUNE | Fort Dodge License No. 112 | Fort Dodge | Dogs | 1 ml | 3 mo | Annually | IM |
| | | | Cats | 1 ml | 3 mo | Annually | IM |
| DURA-RAB 1 | ImmunoVet License No. 302-A | ImmunoVet, Vedco, Inc. | Dogs | 1 ml | 3 mo | Annually | IM |
| | | | Cats | 1 ml | 3 mo | Annually | IM |
| DURA-RAB 3 | ImmunoVet License No. 302-A | ImmunoVet, Vedco, Inc. | Dogs | 1 ml | 3 mo & | Triennially | IM |
| | | | Cats | 1 ml | 1 yr later | Triennially | IM |
| RABCINE 3 | ImmunoVet License No. 302-A | SmithKline Beecham Animal Health | Dogs | 1 ml | 3 mo & | Triennially | IM |
| | | | Cats | 1 ml | 1 yr later | Triennially | IM |
| ENDURALL-K | SmithKline Beecham License No. 189 | SmithKline Beecham Animal Health | Dogs | 1 ml | 3 mo | Annually | IM |
| | | | Cats | 1 ml | 3 mo | Annually | IM |
| ENDURALL-P | SmithKline Beecham License No. 189 | SmithKline Beecham Animal Health | Dogs | 1 ml | 3 mo | Annually | IM or SC[3] |
| | | | Cats | 1 ml | 3 mo | Annually | SC |
| RABGUARD-TC | SmithKline Beecham License No. 189 | SmithKline Beecham Animal Health | Dogs | 1 ml | 3 mo & | Triennially | IM |
| | | | Cats | 1 ml | 1 yr later | Triennially | IM |
| | | | Sheep | 1 ml | 3 mo | Annuall | IM |
| | | | Cattle | 1 ml | 3 mo | Annually | IM |
| | | | Horses | 1 ml | 3 mo | Annually | IM |
| DEFENSOR | SmithKline Beecham License No. 189 | SmithKline Beecham Animal Health | Dogs | 1 ml | 3 mo & | Triennially | IM or SC |
| | | | Cats | 1 ml | 1 yr later | Triennially | SC |
| | | | Sheep | 2 ml | 3 mo | Annually | IM |
| | | | Cattle | 2 ml | 3 mo | Annually | IM |

| | | | | | | | |
|---|---|---|---|---|---|---|---|
| RABDOMUN | SmithKline Beecham License No. 189 | Mallinckrodt Veterinary, Inc., Pitman-Moore | Dogs<br>Cats<br>Sheep<br>Cattle | 1 ml<br>1 ml<br>2 ml<br>2 ml | 3 mo &<br>1 yr later<br>3 mo<br>3 mo | Triennially<br>Triennially<br>Annually<br>Annually | IM or SC<br>SC<br>IM<br>IM |
| RABDOMUN-1 | SmithKline Beecham License No. 189 | Mallinckrodt Veterinary, Inc., Pitman-Moore | Dogs<br>Cats | 1 ml<br>1 ml | 3 mo<br>3 mo | Annually<br>Annually | IM or SC<br>SC |
| SENTRYRAB 1 | SmithKline Beecham Animal Health License No. 225 | Synbiotics Corp. | Dogs<br>Cats | 1 ml<br>1 ml | 3 mo<br>3 mo | Annually<br>Annually | IM<br>IM |
| CYTORAB | Coopers Animal Health License No. 107 | Coopers Animal Health, Inc. | Dogs<br>Cats | 1 ml<br>1 ml | 3 mo<br>3 mo | Annually<br>Annually | IM<br>IM |
| TRIRAB | Coopers Animal Health License No. 107 | Coopers Animal Health, Inc. | Dogs<br><br>Cats | 1 ml<br><br>1 ml | 3 mo &<br>1 yr later<br>3 mo | Triennially<br><br>Annually | IM<br><br>IM |
| EPIRAB | Coopers Animal Health License No. 107 | Coopers Animal Health, Inc. | Dogs<br>Cats | 1 ml<br>1 ml | 3 mo &<br>1 yr later | Triennially<br>Triennially | IM<br>IM |
| RABVAC 1 | Solvay Animal Health License No. 195-A | Solvay Animal Health, Inc. | Dogs<br>Cats | 1 ml<br>1 ml | 3 mo<br>3 mo | Annually<br>Annually | IM or SC<br>IM or SC |
| RABVAC 3 | Solvay Animal Health License No. 195-A | Solvay Animal Health, Inc. | Dogs<br>Cats<br>Horses | 1 ml<br>1 ml<br>2 ml | 3 mo &<br>1 yr later<br>3 mo | Triennially<br>Triennially<br>Annually | IM or SC<br>IM or SC<br>IM |
| PRORAB 1 | Intervet License No. 286 | Intervet, Inc. | Dogs<br>Cats<br>Sheep | 1 ml<br>1 ml<br>2 ml | 3 mo<br>3 mo<br>3 mo | Annually<br>Annually<br>Annually | IM or SC<br>IM or SC<br>IM |
| RM IMRAB 1 | Rhone Merieux, Inc. License No. 298 | Rhone Merieux, Inc. | Dogs<br>Cats | 1 ml<br>1 ml | 3 mo<br>3 mo | Annually<br>Annually | IM or SC<br>IM or SC |
| RM IMRAB 3 | Rhone Merieux, Inc. License No. 298 | Rhone Merieux, Inc. | Dogs<br>Cats<br>Sheep<br><br>Cattle<br>Horses<br>Ferrets | 1 ml<br>1 ml<br>2 ml<br><br>2 ml<br>2 ml<br>1 ml | 3 mo &<br>1 yr later<br>3 mo &<br>1 yr later<br>3 mo<br>3 mo<br>3 mo | Triennially<br>Triennially<br>Triennially<br><br>Annually<br>Annually<br>Annually | IM or SC<br>IM or SC<br>IM or SC<br><br>IM or SC<br>IM or SC<br>SC |

**B) *Combination***
***(Inactivated rabies)***

| | | | | | | | |
|---|---|---|---|---|---|---|---|
| ECLIPSE 3 KP-R | Solvay Animal Health, Inc. License No. 195-A | Solvay Animal Health, Inc. | Cats | 1 ml | 3 mo | Annually | IM |
| ECLIPSE 4 KP-R | Solvay Animal Health License No. 195-A | Solvay Animal Health, Inc. | Cats | 1 ml | 3 mo | Annually | IM |
| CYTORAB RCP | Coopers Animal Health License No. 107 | Coopers Animal Health, Inc. | Cats | 1 ml | 3 mo | Annually | IM |
| FEL-O-VAX PCT-R | Fort Dodge License No. 112 | Fort Dodge | Cats | 1 ml | 3 mo &<br>1 yr later | Triennially | IM |
| RM FELINE 4 + IMRAB 3 | Rhone Merieux License No. 298 | Rhone Merieux | Cats | 1 ml | 3 mo &<br>1 yr later | Triennially | SC |
| RM FELINE 3 + IMRAB 3 | Rhone Merieux License No. 298 | Rhone Merieux | Cats | 1 ml | 3 mo &<br>1 yr later | Triennially | SC |

[1]Three months of age (or older) and revaccinated 1 year later.
[2]Intramuscularly.
[3]Subcutaneously.
*Editors Note*: Some large animal vaccines have not been included.

# IMMUNIZATION OF WILD ANIMAL SPECIES AGAINST COMMON DISEASES

R. ERIC MILLER
*St. Louis, Missouri*

Susceptibility to disease is variable among exotic animals, sometimes even among species of the same family. Often, because thoroughly tested vaccination regimens and subsequent challenge studies are lacking, vaccination schedules for nondomestic species must be considered as recommendations. The following information on vaccination of wild species in zoologic parks is based in part on vaccination schedules found to be effective for related domestic species (see *CVT X*, p 727, for more information and a discussion of immunization of exotic carnivores). Whenever possible, inactivated vaccines should be used in preference to modified live virus (MLV) products. The use of MLV vaccines in nonapproved species carries the risk of vaccine-induced disease, possible immunosuppression, and the risk that vaccinated animals may shed virus to unvaccinated individuals.

No rabies vaccine is licensed for use in wild species, but if used, it should contain only inactivated virus. Before administering any rabies vaccine to *any* nondomestic species, always contact your local and state veterinary authorities about the legal aspects of rabies vaccination in their jurisdiction.

Further information on vaccinations may be obtained by contacting the veterinarian at your local zoo or a member of the American College of Zoo Medicine (members listed in the board specialty section of the *AVMA Directory*).

Private ownership of wild animal species as pets is strongly discouraged and in some localities may be restricted by law.

FAMILY CANIDAE. Wolf, fox, coyote, and so forth.

*Canine Distemper.* Commercial canine distemper vaccines are currently available only as MLV preparations. In nondomestic canids, it appears that the avian-origin MLV vaccine (Fromm D, Solvay Veterinary) is the safest vaccine for the widest variety of species (Montali et al., 1983). In some species (e.g., gray fox), MLV canine distemper vaccines of canine cell origin are to be carefully avoided because they are associated with a high incidence of vaccine-induced distemper (Halbrooks et al., 1981).

*Infectious Canine Hepatitis.* Inactivated vaccines are not commercially available. If performed, vaccination is recommended with canine adenovirus-2 products to reduce the risk of corneal opacity.

*Canine Parvovirus.* Infection with canine parvovirus has been reported in numerous wild canid species,

particularly South American species (maned wolf, raccoon dogs, bush dogs) (Mann et al., 1980). Vaccination with an inactivated vaccine is warranted.

*Leptospirosis.* Vaccination with a multivalent commercial bacterin is recommended.

FAMILY FELIDAE. Tiger, lion, ocelot, margay, bobcat, and so forth.

*Feline Panleukopenia.* Exotic felids appear to be particularly sensitive to this virus, so vaccination is required. Vaccination should only be performed with an inactivated virus (see later) in a regimen recommended for domestic cats.

*Feline Rhinotracheitis and Calicivirus.* Infection with feline rhinotracheitis and calicivirus has been reported in exotic felids, often with devastating consequences. All exotic felids should be vaccinated for these diseases with an inactivated vaccine (commercially available in combination with inactivated feline panleukopenia as Fel-O-Vax, Fort Dodge) (Bush et al., 1981).

*Feline Leukemia.* Reports of infection with feline leukemia virus (FeLV) in exotic felids are uncommon; however, it is advisable to test all felids for exposure. At present, FeLV vaccination is not widely practiced in zoologic parks (Citino, 1988).

FAMILY PROCYONIDAE. Raccoons, coatimundi, kinkajou.

*Canine Distemper.* Members of this family are extremely susceptible to disease caused by the canine distemper virus (Mehren, 1986). Vaccinate as for the canid family, but use great care with kinkajous. Only inactivated vaccines are safe in red pandas (Montali, 1983).

*Feline Panleukopenia.* Although reports of infection with feline panleukopenia virus are less common than those with canine distemper, most facilities currently vaccinate procyonids for this disease. Use an inactivated vaccine without components for the feline respiratory viruses (Phillips, 1989).

FAMILY MUSTELIDAE. Skunks, ferrets, mink, otter.

*Canine Distemper.* Vaccination of all mustelids for canine distemper is recommended, as for the canids. However, particular caution should be exercised with black-footed ferrets (an endangered species); they have developed vaccine-induced disease with MLV vaccines. (They are currently vaccinated with a killed CD vaccine that is not commercially available.)

*Feline Panleukopenia.* All mustelids except ferrets (Parrish et al., 1987) are susceptible to feline panleukopenia, and they should be vaccinated as for felids (but without the feline respiratory component). Mink can be vaccinated with either feline panleukopenia or mink enteritis vaccines.

*Botulism.* Mink and ferrets are susceptible to botulism induced by *Clostridium botulinum* type C toxin. Commercial mink are routinely vaccinated with the appropriate toxoid, but because of different management conditions, vaccination is not routinely practiced in pet ferrets.

*Rabies.* Recently, an inactivated rabies vaccine has been approved for use in ferrets (Imrab, Rhone Poulenc, Athens, GA).

FAMILY VIVERRIDAE. Binturong, civet, fossa.

*Canine Distemper.* Canine distemper has been reported in the binturong and civet. It is generally recommended that all captive viverrids be vaccinated (Phillips, 1989).

*Feline Panleukopenia.* Though cases of feline panleukopenia are not well documented, it is generally recommended that captive viverrids be vaccinated as for procyonids.

FAMILY URSIDAE. Bears.

*Canine Distemper and Feline Panleukopenia.* Bears are not generally considered susceptible to either of these diseases, and no vaccinations are routinely administered.

*Infectious Canine Hepatitis.* Infectious canine hepatitis has been reported from a colony of American black bears (Whetstone et al., 1988). However, vaccination of captive bears for canine adenovirus is not generally recommended.

ORDER MARSUPALIA, FAMILY DIDELPHIDAE. Opossums. Routine vaccination is not practiced.

ORDER PRIMATES.

*Tetanus.* Primates are susceptible to tetanus and should be vaccinated with human tetanus toxoid products. After two initial doses, vaccination can be practiced at more prolonged intervals (2 to 3 years) or in the interim if an injury occurs.

*Poliomyelitis.* Inoculation against poliomyelitis is advisable for great apes (chimpanzees, gorillas, orangutans). Consult with a primate center or a pediatrician for a vaccination schedule.

*Measles, Yellow Fever, Rabies.* Vaccination for all are used in certain or all primate species when circumstances warrant. Advice for these and other primate preventive medicine techniques should be sought from a primate research center.

ORDER RODENTIA. Mice, rats, hamsters, gerbils, guinea pigs, squirrels. No routine vaccinations are recommended for these animals when caged as pets.

ORDER LAGOMORPHA. Rabbits. No routine vaccinations are recommended for these animals when caged as pets.

ORDER ARTIODACTYLIA, FAMILY CAMELIDAE. Llama.

*Tetanus.* Llamas are routinely vaccinated for tetanus with a commercial toxoid (Fowler, 1989).

*Enterotoxemia.* Llamas are susceptible to enterotoxemia produced by *Clostridium perfringens* types C and D, particularly in the first 3 weeks of life. Adults should be vaccinated annually, and vaccination of pregnant dams 8 and 5 weeks prior to parturition will confer immunity on the neonate until it can respond to its own vaccination regimen (Fowler, 1989).

## References and Suggested Reading

Bush M, Povey RC, and Koonse H: Antibody response to an inactivated vaccine for rhinotracheitis, caliciviral disease, and panleukopenia in nondomestic felids. J Am Vet Med Assoc 179:1203, 1981.

Citino SB: Use of a subunit feline leukemia virus vaccine in exotic cats. J Am Vet Med Assoc 192:957, 1988.

Fowler ME: Llama basics. In Kirk RW (ed): *Current Veterinary Therapy X.* Philadelphia, WB Saunders Co, 1989, p 736.

Halbrooks RD, Swango LJ, Schnurrenberger PR, et al: Response of gray foxes to modified live virus canine distemper vaccines. J Am Vet Med Assoc 179:1170, 1981.

Mann PC, Bush M, Appel MJG, et al: Canine parvovirus infection in South American canids. J Am Vet Med Assoc 177:779, 1980.

Mehren KG: Procyonidae. In Fowler ME (ed): *Zoo and Wild Animal Medicine.* Philadelphia, WB Saunders Co, 1986, p 820.

Montali RJ, Barty CR, Teare JA, et al: Clinical trials with canine distemper vaccines in exotic carnivores. J Am Vet Med Assoc 183:1163, 1983.

Parrish CR, Leathers CW, and Pearson R: Comparisons of feline panleukopenia virus, canine parvovirus, raccoon parvovirus and mink enteritis and their pathogenicity for mink and ferrets. Am J Vet Res 48:1429, 1987.

Phillips LG: Preventive medicine in nondomestic carnivores. In Kirk RW (ed): *Current Veterinary Therapy X.* Philadelphia, WB Saunders Co, 1989, pp 728–729.

Whetstone CA, Draayer H, and Collins JE: Characterization of canine adenovirus type I isolated from American black bears. Am J Vet Res 47:778, 1988.

# TABLE OF COMMON DRUGS: APPROXIMATE DOSAGES

### MARK G. PAPICH
*Consulting Editor*

Drug doses are, in most cases, specified for use in either dogs or cats. When no designation is given, the dose is that commonly used for both dogs and cats.

| Drug Name | Brand Name(s)° | Dosage† | CVT Reference(s)‡ |
|---|---|---|---|
| Acepromazine | | Dog: 0.56–1.13 mg/kg IM, SC, IV<br>0.56–2.25 mg/kg PO q6–8h<br>Cat: 1.13–2.25 mg/kg IM, SC, IV, PO<br>(Preanesthetic dogs & cats): 0.02–0.2 mg/kg IM, SC, IV | 774, 866, 1039 |
| Acemannan | Carrisyn | Dog and cat: 2 mg intralesional; 1 mg/kg IP, weekly | 553,583 |
| Acetaminophen | Tylenol | Dog: 15 mg/kg q8h PO (see text pages)<br>Cat: do not administer | 1197 |
| Acetazolamide | Diamox | 5–10 mg/kg q8–12h PO<br>*Glaucoma:* 4–8 mg/kg q8–12 h PO | XI-1049, XI-1125 |
| Acetylcysteine (*n*-acetylcysteine) | Mucomyst | *Antidote:* 140 mg/kg (loading dose) PO, IV, then 70 mg/kg q4h for 5 doses<br>*Eye:* 2% solution topically q2h | |
| Acetylsalicylic acid (aspirin) | | *Antiflammatory:*<br>  Dog: 10–25 mg/kg q12h<br>  Cat: 10–20 mg/kg q48h<br>*Antiplatelet:*<br>  Dog: 5–10 mg/kg q24–48h<br>  Cat: 80 mg q48h | XI-27, XI-95, XI-708<br>XI-861, XI-1049<br>71t, 914, 1197<br>862 |
| ACTH | | see *Corticotropin gel (ACTH)* | |
| Actinomycin D | Cosmegen | 0.7 mg/m² IV (consult anticancer protocol for intervals) | 484, 496 |
| Activated charcoal | | see *Charcoal, activated* | 213, 250 |
| Albendazole | Valbazen | 25–50 mg/kg q12h PO | XI-228, 719, 896 |
| Albuterol syrup | Proventil, Ventolin | Dog: 0.02–0.05 mg/kg q12h up to 4 times/day PO | 912 |
| Allopurinol | Zyloprim | 10 mg/kg q8h then reduce to 10 mg/kg q24h | XI-900, 987 |
| Aluminum hydroxide gel | Amphojel | Phosphate binder: 10–30 mg/kg PO q8h (with meals) | XI-853, 708, 1160 |
| Aluminum carbonate gel | Basaljel | Phosphate binder: 10–30 mg/kg PO q8h (with meals) | |
| Amikacin | Amiglyde-V | 10 mg/kg q8h IV, IM, SC | XI-539, 1201 |
| Aminopentamide sulfate | Centrine | Dog: 0.01–0.03 mg/kg q8–12h IM, SC, PO<br>Cat: 0.02 mg/kg q8–12h IM, SC, PO | 682 |
| Aminophylline | | Dog: 10 mg/kg q8h PO, IM, IV<br>Cat: 6.6 mg/kg q12h PO<br>see *Theophylline* | XI-660, 151, 890, 912 |
| Amiodarone | Cordarone | Dog: Initial dose: 10–15 mg/kg q12h for 7 days PO; followed by: 5–7.5 mg/kg q12h for 14 days; thereafter 7.5 mg/kg once daily | 806 |
| Amitryptyline | Elavil | Dog: 1–2 mg/kg PO q12–24h | |

°The brand names included in this column are for reference purposes only and do not denote an endorsement of any specific product. Often, other proprietary products or generic products are available for a specific drug.

†Delivery methods: IC, intracardiac; IM, intramuscular; IP, intraperitoneal; IV, intravenous; PO, *per os* (oral); SC, subcutaneous. Dosages for birds, exotic pets, and zoo animals can be found in Section 1. For ocular therapeutics, also refer to Section 13 of *CVT XI* and this edition. For topical skin preparations, see "Dermatologic Diseases" Section 7 of *CVT XI* and this edition.

‡Roman numerals in this column refer to a previous *CVT* edition, and arabic numerals refer to page number of article. The letter t refers to a table reference. Previous editions: Kirk RW (ed): *Current Veterinary Therapy X: Small Animal Practice.* Philadelphia, WB Saunders Co, 1989; Kirk RW and Bonagura JD (eds): *Current Veterinary Therapy XI: Small Animal Practice.* Philadelphia, WB Saunders Co, 1992. Some drug dosages may constitute extralabel use.

*Table continued on following page*

| Drug Name | Brand Name(s) | Dosage | CVT Reference(s) |
|---|---|---|---|
| Amlodipine besylate | Norvasc | Cat: 0.625 mg (1/4 of a 2.5-mg tablet) q24h PO for treatment of systemic hypertension | |
| Ammonium chloride | | Dog: 100 mg/kg q12h PO | 216 |
| | | Cat: 800/cat mg mixed with food daily (approximately 1/4 tsp) | |
| Amoxicillin trihydrate | Amoxi-Tabs, Amoxi-Drops | 10–20 mg/kg q8–12h IM, SC, PO | 722 |
| Amoxicillin plus clavulanate | Clavamox | Dog: 12.5–25 mg/kg q12h PO° | XI-207, XI-539, 1030, 1201 |
| | | Cat: 62.5 mg q12h PO° | |
| Amphetamine | | 4.4 mg/kg IV, IM | 1141 |
| Amphotericin B | Fungizone | 0.25–0.5 mg/kg IV (slow infusion) q48h, to a cumulative dose of 4–8 mg/kg | X-1101, XI-609, XI-914, XI-1061, 327, 944 |
| Ampicillin sodium | Omnipen | 10–40 mg/kg q6–8h IV, IM, SC | X-909, XI-829, XI-969 |
| | Principen | 20–40 mg/kg q8h PO | 1030 |
| Ampicillin trihydrate | Polyflex | 6.5 mg/kg IM, SC, q12h | 1030 |
| Amprolium | Amprol | 1.25 gm of 20% amprolium powder added to daily feed, or 30 ml of 9.6% amprolium solution to 3.8 L of drinking water for 7 days. | 715 |
| | Corid | | |
| Amrinone lactate | Inocor | 1–3 mg/kg IV (loading dose) followed by 30–100 μg/kg/min IV infusion | X-247, 186 |
| Antacid drugs | | see *Aluminum* hydroxide gel, *Calcium carbonate*; *Magnesium hydroxide* | X-911 |
| Apomorphine hydrochloride | | 0.02–0.04 mg/kg IV, IM; 0.1 mg/kg SC; or instill 0.25 mg in conjunctiva of eye (dissolve 6 mg tablet in 1–2 ml of saline) | 213, 250, 681 |
| Ascorbic acid | | *Diet supplement*: 100–500 mg/day | XI-175 |
| L-Asparaginase | Elspar | see Table, p 1451 | 486 |
| Aspirin | | see *Acetylsalicylic acid* | 70 |
| Astemizole | Hismanal | Dog: 0.2 mg/kg q24h up to 1.0 mg/kg q12h PO | |
| Atenolol | Tenormin | Dog: 6.25–12.5 mg/dog q12h PO | XI-676, XI-838, 783 |
| | | Cat: 6.25–12.5 mg/cat q24h PO | |
| Atracurium besylate | Tracrium | 0.2 mg/kg IV initially, then 0.15 mg/kg q30min (or IV infusion at 3–8 μg/kg/min) | XI-98 |
| Atropine | | 0.02–0.04 mg/kg q6–8h IV, IM, SC | XI-168, XI-178, XI-183, XI-188, 164, 212, 244, 775, 914, 1039 |
| | | *Organophosphate and carbamate toxicosis*: 0.2–0.5 mg/kg (as needed) | |
| Auranofin (triethylphosphine gold) | Ridaura | 0.1–0.2 mg/kg q12h PO | X-570, 1191 |
| Aurothioglucose | Solganal | Dog <10kg: 1 mg IM first wk, 2 mg IM second wk, 1 mg/kg/wk maintenance | |
| | | Dog >10kg: 5 mg IM first wk, 10 mg IM second wk, 1 mg/kg/wk maintenance | |
| | | Cat: 0.5–1 mg/cat IM every 7 days | |
| Azathioprine | Imuran | Dog: 2 mg/kg q24h PO initially, then 0.5–1 mg/kg q48h | X-570, XI-568, XI-572, XI-660, XI-861, XI-1007, XI-1049, XI-1061, 155, 484, 558, 568, 582, 726, 750, 1191 |
| | | Cat 1.5–3.125 mg/cat q48h with great cure—see p 1192—use in cats is discouraged | |
| BAL | | see *Dimercaprol* | |
| Betamethasone | Celestone, Betasone | 0.1–0.2 mg/kg q12–24h PO | X-54, 577t |
| Bethanechol chloride | Urecholine | Dog: 5–15 mg/dog q8h PO | XI-883 |
| | | Cat: 1.25–5.0 mg/cat q8h PO | |
| Bisacodyl | Dulcolax | 5 mg/dog or cat q8–24h PO | |
| Bismuth subcarbonate | | 0.3–3.0 gm q4h PO | |
| Bismuth subsalicylate | Pepto-Bismol | 1–3 ml/kg/day (in divided doses) PO | XI-237, 704, 722 |
| Bleomycin sulfate | Blenoxane | see Table, p 1450 | 484t |
| Bromide | | see *Potassium bromide* | |
| Bromocriptine mesylate | Parlodel | 0.010 mg/kg q12h PO | 1076 |
| Bunamidine | Scolaban | 20–50 mg/kg PO | XI-626 |
| Bupivacaine hydrochloride | Marcaine | 0.22–0.3 ml epidural | XI-82, XI-96, XI-146 |
| Buprenorphine hydrochloride | Buprenex | 0.01 mg/kg IV, IM | XI-708, 166 |
| Buspirone | Buspar | Cat: (for urine spraying) 5 mg/cat q12h PO | |
| Busulfan | Myleran | see Table, p 1447 | |

°Refer to manufacturer's recommendations.

| Drug Name | Brand Name(s) | Dosage | CVT Reference(s) |
|---|---|---|---|
| Butorphanol | Torbutrol Torbugesic | *For analgesia*: Dog: 0.2–0.8 mg/kg q2–6h IV, SC Cat: 0.4 mg/kg q6h SC; 0.2 mg/kg q6h IV 0.55–1.1 mg/kg q6–12h PO° *Preanesthetic*: 0.2–0.4 mg/kg IV, IM, SC (with acepromazine)° 0.2–0.6 mg/kg SC, IM (antiemetic prior to cancer chemotherapy) | XI-27, XI-82, 166, 774, 866 |
| Cabergoline | | see text for dosing instructions | 1076, 1077 |
| Calcitriol | Rocaltrol | 0.0025–0.003 µg/kg (2.5–3 ng/kg) q24h PO (adjust dose on the basis of calcium and PTH measurement) | XI-857, 371, 949, 963 |
| Calcium carbonate | Titralac Camalox | 5–10 ml q4–6h PO 60–100 mg/kg/day (in divided doses) as phosphate binder | |
| Calcium chloride (10% solution) | | *Hypocalcemia*: 0.1–0.3 ml/kg IV (slowly) | 370, 418 |
| Calcium citrate | | Cat: 10–30 mg/kg q8h (with meals) PO | XI-853 |
| Calcium disodium EDTA | | see *Edetate calcium disodium (CaNa₂, EDTA)* | 239 |
| Calcium gluconate (10% solution) | | 0.5–1.5 ml/kg (slowly) | X-90, X-1042, 370, 954 |
| Calcium lactate | | Dog: 0.5–2.0 gm/dog/day PO (in divided doses) Cat: 0.2–0.5 gm/cat/day PO (in divided doses) | X-90, X-1042, 944 |
| Captan | | 0.25% solution topically, 2–3 times/wk | |
| Captopril | Capoten | Dog: 0.5–2.0 mg/kg q8–12h PO Cat: 3.12–6.25 mg/cat q8h PO | 782, 789 XI-700, XI-829, XI-861, 861 |
| Carbamazepine | | Dogs: not recommended | |
| Carbenicillin disodium | Geopen Pyopen | 40–50 mg/kg (up to 100 mg/kg) q6-8h IV, IM, SC | |
| Carbenicillin indanyl sodium | Geocillin | *Urinary tract infections*: 10 mg/kg q8h PO | 1031 |
| Carbimazole | Neo-Mercazole | Cat: 5 mg/cat q8h PO (induction), followed by 5 mg/cat q12h PO | XI-338 |
| Carboplatin | Paraplatin | see Table, p 1448 | XI-395 |
| Carnitine (L-carnitine) | | Dog: 50 mg/kg q12h (muscle disorders) PO; q8h (dilated cardiomyopathy) PO | 1162 |
| Cascara sagrada | | Dog: 1-4 ml/dog/day PO Cat: 0.5–1.5 ml/cat/day | |
| Castor oil | | Dog: 8–30 ml/day PO Cat: 4–10 ml/day PO | |
| Cefadroxil | Cefa-Tabs Cefa-Drops | Dog: 22 mg/kg q12h PO° Cat: 22 mg/kg q24h PO° | XI-207, XI-539, 1131 |
| Cefazolin sodium | Ancef Kefzol | 20–25 mg/kg q4–8h IV, IM | XI-829, 1200 |
| Cefixime | Suprax | 10 mg/kg q12h PO | |
| Cefmetazole sodium | Zefazone | 15 mg/kg q8h IV, IM, SC | |
| Cefotaxime sodium | Claforan | 20–80 mg/kg q6h IV, IM | |
| Cefotetan | Cefotan | 30 mg/kg q8h IV, SC | |
| Cefoxitin sodium | Mefoxin | 15–30 mg/kg q6–8h IV | XI-829 |
| Ceftiofur | Naxel Excenel | 4.4 mg/kg q12h SC (urinary tract infection) | |
| Cephalexin | Keflex | 10–30 mg/kg q6–12h PO | XI-539, XI-909, XI-969, 1030, 1131, 1201 |
| Cephalothin sodium | Keflin | 10–30 mg/kg q4–8h IV, IM | XI-829, XI-969 |
| Cephapirin sodium | Cefadyl | 10–30 mg/kg q4–8h IV, IM | |
| Cephradine | Velosef | 10–25 mg/kg q6–8h PO | |
| Charcoal, activated | Acta-Char Charcodote Toxiban | 1–4 gm/kg PO (granules) 6–12 ml/kg (suspension) | XI-173, XI-188, 213, 244, 250, 446 |
| Chlorambucil | Leukeran | see Table, p 1447 | XI-595, XI-813, 483t, 582 |
| Chloramphenicol, Chloramphenicol palmitate | Chloromycetin | Dog: 40–50 mg/kg q6–8h PO Cat: 30–50 mg/cat q12h PO | XI-539, XI-829, XI-1081, 913, 1031, 1093, 1106, 1131 |
| Chloramphenicol sodium succinate | Chloromycetin | Dog: 30–50 mg/kg q6–8h IV, IM Cat: 30–50 mg/cat q12h IV, IM | 1093, 1106, 1131 |
| Chlorothizaide | Diuril | 20–40 mg/kg q12h PO | XI-668, XI-892, 350, 995 |

| Drug Name | Brand Name(s) | Dosage | CVT Reference(s) |
|---|---|---|---|
| Chlorpheniramine maleate | Phenetron Chlor-Trimetron | Dog: 4–8 mg/dog q12h IV, IM, SC, PO (maximum recommended dose: 0.5 mg/kg q12h) Cat: 2 mg/cat q12h PO | XI-509, XI-563 |
| Chlorpromazine hydrochloride | Thorazine | 0.25–0.5 mg/kg q6–8h IM, SC, PO *Prior to cancer chemotherapy*: 2 mg/kg q3h SC | XI-395, XI-583, 251, 682, 1141 |
| Chlorpropamide | Diabinese | Dog: 10–40 mg/kg/day PO | 350 |
| Chlortetracycline hydrochloride | | 25 mg/kg q6–8h PO | |
| Cholecalciferol (vitamin D₃) | | 500–2000 U/kg/day PO (1 mg = 40,000 U) | IX-91 |
| Cholestyramine | Questran | Dog: 1–2 gm q12h PO | 434 |
| Chorionic gonadotropin | | see *Gonadotropin, Chorionic (HCG)* | |
| Cimetidine | Tagamet | 10 mg/kg q6–8h IV, IM, PO *Renal failure*: 2.5–5 mg/kg q12h IV, PO | XI-132, XI-191, XI-639, XI-848, XI-1013, 72, 198, 450, 534, 683, 707, 969, 1197 |
| Ciprofloxacin | Cipro | 5–15 mg/kg q12h PO | XI-207, XI-829, XI-909, 321, 1093, 1201 |
| Cisapride | Propulsid | Dog: 0.1–0.5 mg/kg q8–12h PO Cat: 2.5–5 mg/cat q8–12h PO | 681, 683 |
| Cisplatin | Platinol | see Table, p 1448 | XI-395, XI-919, 486, 505, 508, 944, 1016, 1101 |
| Clavamox | | see *Amoxicillin plus clavulante* | |
| Clavulanate | | see *Amoxicillin plus clavulante* | |
| Clemastine | Tavist | Dog: 0.05 mg/kg q12h PO | |
| Clindamycin | Antirobe | Dog: 11 mg/kg q12h PO, or 22 mg/kg q24h PO | XI-539, XI-1049, XI-1061, 313, 1031, 1201 |
| | Cleocin | Cat: 5.5 mg/kg q12h, or 11 mg/kg q24h (*staphylococcal infections*); 11 mg/kg q12h, or 22 mg/kg q24h (*anaerobic infections*) PO *Toxoplasmosis*: 25–50 mg/kg/day PO (in divided treatments) for 2–3 wk | |
| Clomipramine hydrochloride | Anafranil | 1 mg/kg/day PO up to a maximum dose of 3 mg/kg/ day PO | |
| Clonazepam | Klonopin | 0.5 mg/kg q8–12h PO, 50–200 µg/kg, IV once | |
| Cloprostens | | see text for dosing instructions | 1076, 1077 |
| Clorazepate dipotassium | Tranxene | 2 mg/kg q12h PO | |
| Clotrimazole | Canestran, Lotrimin | Dog: Topical use for aspergillosis: see text pages | 899 |
| Cloxacillin sodium | Cloxapen Orbenin Tegopen | 20–40 mg/kg q8h PO | |
| Cod liver oil | | 1 tsp/10 kg once daily PO | |
| Codeine | | *Analgesic*: 0.5–2 mg/kg q6–8h PO *Antitussive*: 0.1–0.3 mg/kg q6–8h PO | |
| Coenzyme Q | | see text pages for dosing instructions | 1162 |
| Colchicine | | 0.01–0.03 mg/kg q24h PO | 751, 979, 1191 |
| Colony-stimulating factor (canine) | Amgen | 5 µg/kg q24h SC | |
| Corticotropin gel (ACTH) | Acthar | *Response test*: collect pre-ACTH sample and inject 2.2 IU/kg IM; collect post-ACTH sample at 2 hr in dogs and at 1 and 2 hr in cats | X-961, 337 |
| Cosyntropin | Cortrosyn | *Response test*: collect pre-ACTH sample and inject 0.25 mg IV in dogs and 0.125 mg IV in cats; collect post-ACTH sample at 1 hr | |
| Cyanocobalamin (vitamin B₁₂) | | Dog: 100–200 µg/day PO Cat: 50–100 µg/day PO | |
| Cyclophosphamide | Cytoxan Neosar | *Anticancer therapy*: see Table, p 1447 | X-475, X-482, X-489, X-570, XI-568, XI-595, XI-813, XI-861, 155, 482, 483, 495, 501, 558, 568, 726, 1012, 1101, 1191 |
| | | *Immunosuppressive therapy*: 50 mg/m² (2.2 mg/kg q48h PO, or 2.2 mg/kg q24h for 4 days/week PO Cat: 6.25–12.5 mg/cat once daily 4 days/wk Dose listed for cats is both anticancer and immunosuppressive therapy | |

| Drug Name | Brand Name(s) | Dosage | CVT Reference(s) |
|---|---|---|---|
| Cyclosporine | Sandimmune | Dog: 10 mg/kg q12h PO q24h<br>Cat: 10 mg/kg PO q12h (adjust dose via monitoring)<br>Topical treatment for keratoconjunctivitis sicca: 1–2% solution in oil: instill 1 drop in eye q12h | X-570, XI-534, XI-861, XI-870, XI-1092, 73, 156, 569 |
| Cyclothiazide | Anhydron | 0.5–1 mg/kg q24h PO | |
| Cyproheptadine hydrochloride | Periactin | *Antihistamine:* 1.1 mg/kg q8–12h PO<br>*Appetite stimulant in cat:* mg/cat PO | 421 |
| Cytarabine (cytosine arabinoside) | Cytosar | see Table, p 1449 | X-475, X-482, XI-595, 484 |
| Dacarbazine | DTIC | see Table, p 1451 | XI-595, 484, 496 |
| Danazol | Danocrine | 5–10 mg/kg q12h PO | 155 |
| Dantrolene sodium | Dantrium | Dog: 1–5 mg/kg q8h PO<br>Cat: 0.5–2 mg/kg q12h PO | |
| Dapsone | | 1.1 mg/kg q8h PO | |
| Darbazine (prochlorperazine plus isopropamide | Darbazine | Dog and cat: 0.14–0.2 ml/kg q12h SC°<br>Dog: 2–7 kg: one #1 capsule q12h PO°<br>Dog: 7–14 kg: one #2 capsule q12h PO°<br>Dog > 14 kg: one #3 capsule q12h PO° | 704 |
| Decoquinate | Deccox | 50 mg/kg q24h PO | 715 |
| Deferoxamine mesylate | Desferal | 10 mg/kg IV, IM q2h for 2 doses, then 10 mg/kg q8h for 24 hr | 242 |
| Delta-Albaplex (novobiocin plus prednisolone plus tetracycline hydrochloride) | | Dog 3–7 kg: 1–2 tablets/day PO°<br>Dog 7–14 kg: 2–4 tablets/day PO°<br>Dog 14–27 kg: 4–6 tablets/day PO°<br>Dog >27 kg: 6–8 tablets/day PO°<br>Cat: 1 tablet q12h PO° | |
| Derm Caps (omega fatty acid) | | 1 capsule/9.1 kg daily PO | XI-563 |
| Desmopressin acetate | DDAVP (100 μg/ml) | *Diabetes insipidus:* 2–4 drops (2.0 μg/dog) q12–24h intranasally or in conjunctiva<br>*von Willebrand's disease:* 1 μg/kg (0.01 ml/kg) SC, IV† | X-973, 350 |
| Desoxycorticosterone pivalate (DOCP) | | 1.5–2.2 mg/kg q25 days IM° | XI-353, 351, 428 |
| Dexamethasone | Azium | *Anti-inflammatory:* 0.1–0.2 mg/kg q12–24h IV, IM, PO<br>*Shock or spinal injury:* 2.2–4.4 mg/kg IV | X-54, XI-509, 152, 198, 409, 427, 577t, 1078, 1147 |
| Dexamethasone sodium phosphate | | Dog and cat: 2–4 mg/kg IV | 428 |
| Dextran-70 | Gentran-70 | 10–20 ml/kg q24h to effect | 143 |
| Dextromethorphan | Benylin DM and others | 0.5–2 mg/kg q6–8h PO | 914 |
| Dextrose (5% solution) | | 40–50 ml/kg q24h IV, SC, IP | |
| Diazepam | Valium | *Preanesthetic or muscle relaxation:* 0.5 mg/kg IV<br>*Status epilepticus:* 0.25–0.5 mg/kg IV; repeat if necessary<br>*Appetite stimulant in cat:* 0.2 mg/kg IV (as needed)<br>*Urinary disorder in cat:* 1.25–2.5 mg/cat q8–12 PO | X-18, X-63, XI-27, XI-98, XI-173, XI-438, XI-655, XI-883, 197, 212, 251, 941, 970, 1039, 1127, 1141, 1148, 1160 |
| Dichlorophene | | see *Toluene* | 1145 |
| Dichlorphenamide | Daranide | 3–5 mg/kg q8–12h PO | XI-1049, XI-1125 |
| Dichlorvos | Task | Dog: 26.4–33 mg/kg PO<br>Cat: 11 mg/kg PO | XI-583, XI-626, 712 |
| Dicloxacillin | Dynapen | 11–55 mg/kg q8h | |
| Diethylcarbamazine | Caricide<br>Filaribits | *Heartworm prophylaxis:* 6.6 mg/kg q24h PO° | 712, 880 |
| Diethylstilbestrol (DES) | | *Urinary incontinence (dog):* 0.1–1.0 mg/dog q24h PO<br>*Urinary incontinence (cat):* 0.05–0.1 mg/cat q24h PO | 1023, 1033, 1071, 1451 |
| Digitoxin | Crystodigin | 0.02–0.03 mg/kg q8h PO | XI-689, 782 |
| Digoxin | Lanoxin | Dog: 0.22 mg/m² or 0.005–0.01 q12h PO (subtract 10% for elixir) | XI-689, XI-713, 782, 891 |
| | Cardoxin | Dog (*rapid digitalization*): 0.0055–0.011 mg/kg q1h IV to effect–generally inadvisable<br>Cat 2–3 kg: 0.0312 mg q48h PO<br>Cat 4–5 kg: 0.0312 mg q24–48h PO<br>Cat >6 kg: 0.0312 mg q12h PO | 866 |
| Dihydrostreptomycin sulfate | Ethamycin (Canada only) | 11–15 mg/kg q8–12h IM, SC | XI-260 |

°Refer to manufacturer's recommendations.
†IV dose diluted in 20 ml of saline and given over 10 min.

*Table continued on following page*

| Drug Name | Brand Name(s) | Dosage | CVT Reference(s) |
|---|---|---|---|
| Dihydrotachysterol (vitamin D) | Hytakerol DHT | 0.01 mg/kg/day PO; for acute treatment, 0.02 mg/kg initially, then 0.01–0.02 mg/kg q24–48h PO | XI-353, 370, 947 |
| Diltiazem hydrochloride | Cardizem | Dog: 0.5–1.5 mg/kg q8h PO<br>Cat: 1.75–2.4 mg/kg q8–12h PO | X-276, XI-684, XI-745, XI-766, 165, 783, 860 |
| Dimenhydrinate | Dramamine (US) Gravol (Canada) | 4–8 mg/kg q8h IV, IM, PO<br>Cat: 12.5 mg q8h IV, IM, PO | XI-583, 682 |
| Dimercaprol | BAL in oil | 4mg/kg q4h IM | X-159 |
| Dimethyl sulfoxide (DMSO) | | Dog and cat: 1 mg/kg of a 10–40% solution slowly IV; see text for dosing instructions | 885, 979, 1101, 1191 |
| Dinoprost tromethamine | | see *Prostaglandin $F_{2\alpha}$* | |
| Dioctyl calcium sulfosuccinate | | see *Docusate calcium* | |
| Dioctyl sodium sulfosuccinate | | see *Docusate sodium* | |
| Diphemanil methylsulfate | Diathal | 1.8 mg/kg q12h IM° | |
| Diphenhydramine hydrochloride | Benadryl | 2–4 mg/kg q6–8h IV, IM, PO<br>Dog: 25–50 mg/dog q8h IV, IM, PO | XI-583, XI-587, 227, 533, 682, 1144 |
| Diphenoxylate hydrochloride | Lomotil | Dog: 0.1–0.2 mg/kg q8–12h PO<br>Cat: 0.05–0.1 mg/kg q12h PO | XI-613, 704 |
| Diphenylhydantoin | | see *Phenytoin* | |
| Diphosphonate disodium etidronate | | see *Etidronate disodium* | |
| Dipyridamole | Persantine | 4–10 mg/kg q24h PO | XI-861 |
| Dipyrone | Novaldin | 28 mg/kg q8h IV, IM, SC | |
| Disophenol (DNP) | | 10 mg/kg SC, once° | XI-626 |
| Disopyramide phosphate | Norpace | Dog: 6–15 mg/kg q8h PO<br>Cat: none | |
| Dithiazanine iodide | Dizan | 6.6–11 mg/kg q24h PO for 7–10 days | |
| Divalproex sodium | Depakote | Equivalent to valproic acid (see *Valproic acid*) | |
| Dobutamine hydrochloride | Dobutrex | Administer 250 mg in 1 L 5% dextrose<br>Dog: 2.5–20 $\mu$g/kg/min IV infusion<br>Cat: 2.5–5 $\mu$g/kg/min IV infusion | XI-713, XI-773, 144, 185, 191 |
| Docusate calcium | Surfak Doxidan | Dog: 50–100 mg q12–24h PO<br>Cat: 50 mg q12–24h PO | XI-639 |
| Docusate sodium | Colace | Dog: 50–200 mg q8–12h PO<br>Cat: 50 mg q12–24h PO | XI-613, XI-619, XI-639 |
| Domperidone | Motilium | 2–5 mg/dog or cat PO; 0.1–0.3 mg/kg q12h IM, IV | 682 |
| Dopamine hydrochloride | Intropin | 2–10 $\mu$g/kg/min IV infusion (40 mg in 500 ml lactated Ringer's solution) | XI-191, XI-655, XI-715, 144, 151, 164, 186, 190, 945 |
| Doxapram hydrochloride | Dopram | 5–10 mg/kg IV<br>Neonate: 1–5 mg SC, sublingually, or via umbilical vein | |
| Doxorubicin | Adriamycin | see Table, p 1450 | X-475, X-482, X-489, XI-595, XI-783, 479, 484, 495, 496, 501, 504, 509, 1101 |
| Doxycycline | Vibramycin | 2.5–5 mg/kg q12h PO | XI-829, 268, 288, 292, 307, 449 |
| Edetate calcium disodium (CaNa$_2$EDTA) | Calcium disodium Versenate | 25 mg/kg q6h SC for 2–5 days | 239 |
| Edrophonium chloride | Tensilon | Dog: 0.11–0.22 mg/kg IV<br>Cat: 2.5 mg/cat IV | XI-1024, XI-1039, 557 |
| Emetine | | Dog: 1–2.5 ml/kg, up to 6.6 ml/kg PO<br>Cat: 3.3 ml/kg PO (dilute 50:50 with water) | |
| Enalapril maleate | Vasotec | Dog: 0.5 mg/kg q12–24h PO<br>Cat: 0.25–0.5 mg/kg q12–24h PO | XI-700, XI-773, XI-829, 782, 789, 861, 866 |
| Enflurane | Ethrane | 2–3% (induction); 1.5–3% (maintenance) | |
| Enilconazole | Imaverol | *Nasal aspergillosis:* 10 mg/kg q12h instilled into nasal sinus for 10–14 days (10% solution diluted 50:50 with water)°<br><br>*Dermatophytes:* solution diluted to 0.2% and lesion washed with solution 4 times at 3- to 4-day intervals.° | X-82, X-577, X-1106, 593<br><br>XI-547 |
| Enrofloxacin | Baytril | 2.5–5 mg/kg q12h PO, IM, or 5 mg/kg q24h PO, IM | XI-539, XI-829, XI-909, XI-954, 321, 449, 1030, 1093, 1106, 1201 |

°Refer to manufacturer's recommendations.

| Drug Name | Brand Name(s) | Dosage | CVT Reference(s) |
|---|---|---|---|
| Ephedrine | Many | *Urinary incontinence*: 4 mg/kg, or<br>   Dog: 12.5–50 mg/dog q8–12h PO<br>Cat: 2–4 mg/kg q8–12h PO<br>*Bronchodilator*: 1–2 mg/kg q8h PO | X-1214, XI-875 |
| Ephedrine plus<br>  phenobarbital plus<br>  potassium iodide | Quadrinal | Dog ¼ to ½ tablet q4–6h PO°<br>Cat: ¼ tablet q4–6h PO° | |
| Epinephrine | Adrenalin | 20 μg/kg, or 0.1–1.5 ml of 1:1000 (1 mg/ml)<br>  solution; or 1–5 ml of a 1:10,000 (0.1 mg/ml)<br>  solution IV, IM, SC, IC, intratracheally | X-331, XI-660, 151,<br>174, 186, 190, 227 |
| Epostane | | see text for dosing instructions | 1076, 1077 |
| Epsiprantel | Cestex | Dog: 5.5 mg/kg PO<br>Cat: 2.75 mg/kg PO | XI-626, 715 |
| Epsom salt | | see *Magnesium sulfate* | |
| Ergocalciferol (vitamin D₂) | Calciferol | 500–2000 U/kg/day PO | IX-1039 |
| Erythromycin | Many | 10–20 mg/kg q8–12h PO | XI-484, XI-539, 681,<br>1031, 1093 |
| Erythropoietin | Epogen, Amgen | 100 U/kg SC three times weekly (adjust dose to<br>  reach and maintain hematocrit of 0.30–0.34) | 450, 946, 949, 961 |
| Esmolol | Brevibloc | Dog and cat: 0.05–0.1 mg/kg slow IV boluses q5min<br>  to total cumulative dose of 0.5 mg/kg; or<br>50–200 μg/kg/min constant rate infusion | 165, 187, 849 |
| Essential fatty acids | EFA-Z-Plus | <6.7 kg: 3.7 ml/day PO°<br>6.7–22.5 kg: 7 ml/day PO°<br>>22.5 kg: 14 ml/day PO°<br>(see also *Omega fatty acids*) | |
| Estradiol cypioniate (ECP) | Depo-Estradiol | Dog: 44μg/kg (0.04 mg/kg) IM (total dose not to<br>  exceed 1.0 mg). The use of ECP for mismating is<br>  discouraged.<br>Cat: 250 μg/cat (0.25 mg/cat) IM, between 40 hr and<br>  5 days after mating | 1075 |
| Ethanol 20% solution | | *Treatment of ethylene glycol poisoning*: Dog: 5.5 ml<br>  of solution/kg q4–6 h;<br>Cat: 5 ml of solution/kg q6h; see text pages | 236 |
| Ethoxzolamide | Cardrase | *Glaucoma*: 4 mg/kg q8–12h PO | XI-1049 |
| Etidronate disodium | Didronel | Dog: 5 mg/kg/day PO<br>Cat: 10 mg/kgday PO | |
| Etretinate | Tegison | Dog: 0.75–1 mg/kg/day PO<br>Cat: 2 mg/kg/day | X-553, XI-523, 481,<br>513, 585 |
| Famotidine | Pepcid | 0.5 mg/kg q12–24h PO | XI-132, 707, 867 |
| Febantel | Rintal | 10 mg/kg q24h for 3 days PO | 712 |
| Febantel plus praziquantel | Vercom | 10 mg/kg of febantel and 1 mg/kg praziquantel q24h<br>  for 3 days PO | XI-626, 712, 715 |
| Fenbendazole | Panacur | Dog: 50 mg/kg/day for 3 days PO<br>Cat: 25–50 mg/kg q12 kg PO (lung worms); 50 mg/<br>  kg/day 3–5 days (*ascarids, hookworms, Giardia,<br>  Trichuris, or Taenia*) | XI-228, XI-626, 712,<br>715, 896 |
| Fentanyl citrate | Sublimaze | 0.02–0.04 mg/kg IV, IM, SC, or 0.01 mg/kg IV, IM,<br>  SC (with acepromazine or diazepam); 0.01 mg/kg<br>  IV, for analgesia | XI-98 |
| Fentanyl citrate plus<br>  droperidol | Innovar-Vet | These two doses are recommendation by mfr. only:<br>Dog: 0.04–0.09 ml/kg IV; 0.01–0.14 ml/kg IM<br>Cat: do not use | XI-27 |
| Ferrous sulfate | Many | Dog: 100–300 mg/dog q24h PO<br>Cat: 50–100 mg/cat q24h PO | 449 |
| Finasteride | Proscar | see text pages | 1034, 1105 |
| Fluconazole | Diflucan | Cat: 50 mg/cat q12h PO (for cryptococcosis) | 328 |
| Flucytosine | Ancobon | 25–50 mg/kg q6–8h PO (maximum dose: 100 mg/kg<br>  q12h PO) | X-1101, XI-914, XI-<br>1061 |
| Fludrocortisone acetate | Florinef Acetate | Dog: 0.2–0.8 mg (0.02 mg/kg) q24h PO<br>Cat: 0.1 mg q24h PO | 351, 428 |
| Flumazenil | Mazicon | 0.2 mg (total dose) IV, as needed | 1155 |
| Flumethasone | Flucort | Dog: 0.0625–0.25 mg/day IV, IM, SC, PO<br>Cat: 0.03–0.125 mg/day IV, IM, SC, PO<br>*Anti-inflammatory*: 0.15–0.3 mg/kg q12–24h IV, IM,<br>  SC, PO | X-54, 577t |
| Flunixin meglumine | Banamine | 1.1 mg/kg once IV, IM, SC, or 1.1 mg/kg/day 3 day/<br>  wk PO<br>*Ophthalmic*: 0.5 mg/kg once IV | X-47, XI-1049, 767,<br>1197 |

°Consult anticancer protocol for precise dosage.

*Table continued on following page*

| Drug Name | Brand Name(s) | Dosage | CVT Reference(s) |
|---|---|---|---|
| Fluorouracil | 5-Fluorouracil | see Table, p 1449 | 483, 484, 513, 1101, 1142 |
| Flutamide | Eulexin | Dog: 5 mg/kg/day PO | 1034 |
| Folic acid | Folvite | Dog and cat: 0.004–0.01 mg/kg/day (4–10 µg/kg/day) | |
| Folinic acid | | see *Leucoverin calcium* | |
| Follicle-stimulating hormone (FSH) | | see *Urofollitropin* | |
| Furazolidone | Furoxone | 4 mg/kg q12h for 7–10 days PO | XI-626, 719, 859, 866, 944 |
| Furosemide | Lasix | Dog: 2–4 mg/kg q8–12h (or as needed) IV, IM, SC, PO; adjust to lowest dose possible | XI-668, XI-713, XI-766, XI-861, 174, 198, 754 |
| Gemfibrozil | Lopid | Dog: 150–300 mg/dog q12h PO | 433, 831, 1166 |
| Gentamicin sulfate | Gentocin | Dog: 2–4 mg/kg q6–8h IV, IM, SC, or 6 mg/kg q24h<br>Cat: 3mg/kg q8h IV; q6h IM, SC | XI-539, XI-829, 767, 944, 945, 1201 |
| Glyburide (Gilbenclamide) | Diabeta<br>Micronase | 0.2 mg/kg daily PO | |
| Glipizide | Glucotrol | Cat: 2.5–5 mg/cat q12h PO | 401 |
| Glucagon | | *Tolerance test*: 0.03 mg/kg IV | |
| Glycerin | Glyrol<br>Osmoglyn | *Glaucoma*: 1–1.5 gm/kg PO initially, then 500 mg/kg q8h; or 1–2 ml of 50% solution q8h | XI-1125 |
| Glycopyrrolate | Robinul-V | 0.005–0.01 mg/kg IV, IM, SC | 164, 212, 775, 1039 |
| Gold sodium thiomalate | Myochrysine | 1–5 mg IM (first wk), then 2–10 mg IM (second wk), then 1 mg/kg once/wk IM (maintenance) | X-570 |
| Gold therapy | | see *Auranofin (triethylphosphine gold);*<br>*Aurothioglucose; Gold sodium thiomalate* | X-570 |
| Gonadorelin hydrochloride (GnRH), (LHRH) | Factrel | Dog: 50–100 µg/dog/day q24–48h IM<br>Cat: 25 µg/cat once IM | XI-947, XI-963, XI-966<br>X-2036, 1070 |
| Gonadotropin, chorionic (HCG) | Follutein | Dog: 22 U/kg q24–48h IM, or 44 U once IM | XI-947, XI-963, XI-966, 1070, 1071 |
| | Pregnyl | Cat: 250 U/cat once IM | |
| Gonadotropin-releasing hormone | | see *Gonadorelin* | |
| Griseofulvin (microsize) | Fulvicin U/F | 50 mg/kg daily (may be given in divided doses) PO (maximum dose: 110–132 mg/kg/day in divided treatments) | XI-547 |
| Griseofulvin (ultramicrosize) | Fulvicin P/G<br>Gris-PEG | 5–10 mg/kg/day PO (in divided treatments) | XI-562 |
| Growth hormone | | 0.1 U/kg 3 times/wk for 4–6 wk | X-978, 350 |
| Glipizide | Glucotrol | Cat: 2.5–5 mg/cat q12h PO with food | 402 |
| Halothane | Fluothane | 3% (induction); 0.5–1.5% (maintenance) | 1039 |
| Heparin calcium | Calciparine | Dog: 250–500 U/kg q8h SC<br>Cat: 250–375 U/kg q8h SC<br>*Low-dose therapy* (dog and cat): 70 U/kg q8–12h SC | XI-137 |
| Heparin sodium | Liquaemin (US)<br>Hepalean (Canada) | 100–200 U/kg IV, loading dose; then 100–300 U/kg q6–8h SC (adjust dose by monitoring clotting times) | XI-137, 155, 866 |
| Hetacillin potassium | Hetacin-K | 20–40 mg/kg q8h PO | |
| Human gamma globulin | Gammune | 0.5–1.5 gm/kg q12h IV | |
| Hydralazine hydrochloride | Apresoline | Dog: 0.5 mg/kg (initial dose), titrated to 0.5–2 mg/kg q12h PO<br>Cat: 2.5–5 mg/cat q12–24h | XI-700, 890 |
| Hydrochlorothiazide | HydroDiuril | 2–4 mg/kg q12h PO | X-1182, XI-838, 993, 1001 |
| Hydrocodone bitartrate | Hycodan | Dog: 0.22 mg/kg q4–8h PO<br>Cat: none | 914 |
| Hydrocortisone | Cortef | *Replacement therapy*: 1 mg/kg q12h PO<br>*Anti-inflammatory*: 2.5–5 mg/kg q12h PO | X-54, 575 |
| Hydrocortisone sodium succinate | Solu-Cortef | *Shock*: 50–150 mg/kg IV | X-54 |
| Hydrogen peroxide (3%) | | *Emetic*: 5–10 ml PO (may repeat once within 10 min) | 213, 244, 250 |
| Hydroxyethyl starch | Hetastarch | Dog: 16 ml/kg (range 10–20 ml/kg/day; use rapid IV infusion for shock therapy | 143 |
| Hydroxyurea | Hydrea | see Table, p 1451 | 450 |
| Hydroxyzine hydrochloride | Atarax | Dog: 2 mg/kg q6–8h IM, PO<br>Cat: safe dosage not established | XI-552 |
| Hyoscine | see *Scopolamine* | | |
| Hypertonic saline 7.5% solution | | Dog: 4–8 ml/kg; cat: 2–6 ml/kg; rapid IV infusion for shock therapy | |

| Drug Name | Brand Name(s) | Dosage | CVT Reference(s) |
|---|---|---|---|
| Idarubicin | Idamycin | Cat: 2 mg/kg/day for 2 days; repeat every 21 days | 501 |
| Idarubicin hydrochloride | Idamycin | 2 mg/cat for 3 consecutive days every 3 weeks PO | |
| Ibuprofen | Motrin | Safe dosage not established | X-47, XI-191, 914, 1197 |
| | Advil | | |
| | Nuprin | | |
| Imidocarb hydrochloride | | 5 mg/kg IM once | XI-829 |
| Imipenem-cilastatin sodium | Primaxin | 3–10 mg/kg q6–8h IM or slow IV infusion | |
| Indomethacin | Indocin | Safe dosage not established | X-47 |
| Insulin (NPH isophane) | | Dog <15 kg: 1 U/kg q24h SC (to effect) | X-47 |
| | | Dog >25 kg: 0.5 U/kg q24h SC (to effect) | IX-1000, XI-356, 387 |
| | | Cat: not recommended | |
| Insulin (regular crystalline) | | *Ketoacidosis:* | IX-1000, X-1008, XI-359, 387, 395 |
| | | Animals <3 kg: 1 U/animal initially, then 1 U/animal q1h | |
| | | Animals 3–10 kg: 2 U/animal initially, then 1 U/animal q1h | |
| | | Animals 3–10 kg: 2 U/animal initially, then 1 U/animal q1h | |
| | | Animals >10 kg, 0.25 U/kg initially, then 0.1 U/kg q1h IM | |
| | | (Consult *CVT* text for exact protocol) | 387 |
| Insulin, Ultralente | | Dog <15 kg: 1 U/kg q24h SC (to effect) | |
| | | Dog >25 kg: 0.5 U/kg q24h SC (to effect) | |
| | | Cat: not recommended | |
| Interferon-α 2β; HuIFN-α | Roferon (3 million IU vial) | Cat: 10,000 IU/kg SC q12h; low-dose oral administration: 30 IU Roferon PO once daily for 7 days repeated every other week (add 3 million IU to 1 liter sterile saline solution; divide stock solution into aliquots and freeze; thaw and dilute when needed to produce 30 IU/ml dispensing solution[†]) | 270, 584 |
| Iodide | | see *Potassium iodide* | |
| Ipecac syrup | | (see *Emetine*) | 213, 250 |
| | | Dog: 3–6 ml PO | |
| | | Cat: 2–6 ml PO | |
| Iron | | see *Ferrous sulfate* | |
| Isoflurane | | 5% (induction); 1.5–2.5% (maintenance) | 1039 |
| Isopropamide iodide | Darbid | Dog: 0.1–0.2 mg/kg q12h PO | 682 |
| | | Cat: 0.07 mg/cat PO q12h | |
| Isoproterenol | Isuprel | 0.04–0.08 µg/kg/min IV | 192 |
| Isosorbide dinitrate | Isordil | 2.5–5 mg/animal q12h PO | XI-700 |
| | Sorbitrate | | |
| Isotretinoin | Accutane | 1–3 mg/kg/day (maximum dose: 3–4 mg/kg/day) PO | X-553, XI-534, 481, 585, 1201 |
| Itraconazole | Sporanox | Dog: 2.5 mg/kg q12h to 5 mg/kg q24h PO | X-82, X-577, X-1101, X-1106, X-1109, XI-547, XI-609, XI-1061, 329, 592, 853 |
| | | Cat: 5 mg/kg q12h PO | |
| Ivermectin | Heartguard | *Heartworm peventative in dog:* 6 µg/kg q30d PO | X-140, X-263, X-560, XI-228, 627, 655, 881, 883, 1143 |
| | Ivomec | *Microfilaricide in dog:* 50 µg/kg PO 3 to 4 wk after adulticide therapy | |
| | | *Ectoparasite therapy:* 200–300 µg/kg IM, SC, PO (do not use in collie dogs) | XI-558, 896 |
| | | *Respiratory parasites:* 200–400 µg/kg weekly SC, PO (do not use in collie dogs) | |
| Kanamycin sulfate | Kantrim | 10 mg/kg q6–8h IV, IM, SC | |
| Kaolin plus pectin | Kaopectate | 1–2 ml/kg q2–6h PO | XI-1013 |
| Ketamine hydrochloride | Ketalar | Dog: 5.5–22 mg/kg IV, IM (adjunctive sedative or tranquilizer treatment recommended) | XI-27, XI-655, XI-929, 775, 941, 1039, 1121 |
| | Ketaset | Cat: 2–25 mg/kg IV, IM (adjunctive sedative or tranquilizer treatment recommended) | |
| Ketoconazole | Nizoral | Dog: 10–30 mg/kg/day in divided treatments PO (*Malassezia canis infection:* 10 mg/kg q24h or 5 mg/kg q12h PO) | X-82, X-577, X-1024, X-1101, X-1106, X-1109, XI-349, XI-523, XI-544, XI-547, XI-609, XI-1061, 328, 340, 421, 592, 853 |
| | | *Hyperadrenocorticism:* 15 mg/kg q12h PO (just dog) | |
| | | Cat: 5–10 mg/kg q8–12h PO | |
| Ketoprofen | Ketofen | Dog: 1.1 mg/kg once daily IV, PO for up to 5 days | |

[†]See Weiss et al.: JAVMA 199: 1477, 1991.

*Table continued on following page*

| Drug Name | Brand Name(s) | Dosage | CVT Reference(s) |
|---|---|---|---|
| Lactated Ringer's solution | Many | 40–50 ml/kg/day IV for maintenance–septic shock<br>Dog: (shock therapy) 90 ml/kg IV<br>Cat: (shock therapy) 60 ml/kg IV | 143 |
| Lactulose | Chronulac | *Constipation*: 1 ml/4.5 kg q8h PO (to effect)<br>*Hepatic encelphalopathy in dog*: 0.5 ml/kg q8h PO<br>*Hepatic encephalopathy in cat*: 2.5–5 ml/cat q8h PO | XI-613, XI-619, XI-639, 746, 754, 1156 |
| Leucovorin calcium (folinic acid) | Wellcovorin | *With methotrexate administration*: 3 mg/m$^2$ IV, IM, PO<br>*Antidote for pyrimethamine toxicosis*: 1 mg/kg q24h PO | |
| Levamisole hydrochloride | Levasole<br>Tramisol | Dog: 5–8 mg/kg PO once, up to 10 mg/kg PO for 2 days (*hookworms*); 10 mg/kg q24h PO for 6–10 days (*microfilaricide*); 0.5–2 mg/kg 3 times/wk PO (*immunostimulant*)<br>Cat: 4.4 mg/kg PO once | X-570, XI-217, XI-228, XI-539, XI-861, 583, 616, 896, 1144, 1191 |
| Levodopa (L-dopa) | Larodopa | *Hepatic encephalopathy*: 6.8 mg/kg initially, then 1.4 mg/kg q6h | XI-639 |
| Levothyroxine sodium (T$_4$) | Soloxine<br>Thyro-Tabs<br>Synthroid | Dog: 22 µg/kg q12h PO (adjust dose via monitoring)<br>Cat: 10–20 µg/kg/day PO (adjust dose via monitoring) | XI-954, 347, 364, 372, 556 |
| Lidocaine hydrochloride | Xylocaine Hydrochloride | *Antiarrhythmia in dog*: 2–4 mg/kg IV (maximum dose: 8 mg/kg over 10 min); 25–75 µg/kg/min IV infusion; 6 mg/kg q1.5h IM<br>Cat: 0.25–0.75 mg/kg IV, slowly (generally do not use as antiarrhythmic) | X-278, XI-694, 166, 187, 802, 849 |
| Lime sulfur (3% solution) | | Topically once/wk for 4–6 wk | XI-547, XI-558 |
| Lincomycin | Lincocin | 15–25 mg/kg q12h IV, IM, PO | XI-539, 337, 1093 |
| Liothyronine (T$_3$) | Cytobin or Cytomel | 4.4 µg/kg q8h PO<br>Suppression testing: collect presample for T$_4$ and T$_3$; administer 25 µg q8h PO for 7 doses; collect post samples for T$_4$ and T$_3$ after last dose | |
| Lisinopril | Prinivil | 0.25–0.5 mg/kg daily PO | 782, 789 |
| Lithium carbonate | Lithotabs | Dog: 10 mg/kg q12h PO<br>Cat: not recommended | |
| Loperamide hydrochloride | Imodium | Dog: 0.1–0.2 mg/kg q8–12h PO<br>Cat: 0.08–01.16 mg/kg q12h PO | XI-237, XI-604, XI-613, 704 |
| Luteinizing hormone | | see *Gonadorelin* | |
| Magnesium citrate | Citro-Mag (Canada)<br>Citroma, Citro-Nesia (U.S.) | 2–4 ml/kg PO | 944 |
| Magnesium hydroxide | Milk of Magnesia | *Antacid*: 5–10 ml/total dose per dog or cat<br>*Cathartic*:<br>Dog: 15–50 ml/per dog PO<br>Cat: 2–6 ml/cat q24h PO | X-911, 132, 1160 |
| Magnesium oxide | | 1–2 mEq/kg daily PO | |
| Magnesium salts | Magnesium sulfate solution; magnesium chloride solution | 0.75–1 mEq Mg$^{++}$ per kg IV over 24 hr; constant-rate infusion; thereafter, 0.3–0.5 mEq/kg/day | 132 |
| Mannitol | Osmitrol | *Diuretic*: 1 gm/kg of 5–25% solution IV to maintain urine flow<br>*Glaucoma or CNS edema*: 0.25–2 gm/kg of 15–25% solution over 15–60 min IV (repeat in 4–6 hr if necessary) | XI-173, XI-639, XI-1125, 174, 746<br><br>944 |
| Mebendazole | Telmintic | 22 mg/kg (with food) q24h for 3 days° | 712, 715 |
| Meclizine hydrochloride | Bonine | Dog: 25 mg q24h PO (*motion sickness*: administer 1 hr prior to traveling)<br>Cat: 12.5 mg q24h PO | |
| Meclofenamic acid (meclofenamate sodium) | Meclomen, Meclofen, Arquel | 1 mg/kg/day PO for 5 days | |
| Medetomidine hydrochloride | | 0.01–0.08 ml/kg IV, IM | |
| Medium-chain triglycerides (MCTs) | MCT Oil | 1–2 ml/kg daily in food | IX-909, 433 |
| Medroxyprogesterone acetate | Depo-Provera | 1.1–2.2 mg/kg q7d IM | XI-552, XI-947, 1034, 1072, 1105 |

---

°Refer to manufacturer's recommendations.

| Drug Name | Brand Name(s) | Dosage | CVT Reference(s) |
|---|---|---|---|
| Megestrol acetate | Ovaban | *Proestrus*: 2.2 mg/kg q24h PO for 8 days<br>*Anestrus*: 0.55 mg/kg q24h PO for 30 days<br>*Behavior problems*: 2–4 mg/kg q24h for 8 days (reduce dose for maintenance)<br>Cat: 2.5–5 mg/cat q24h PO for 1 wk, then reduce to 2.5–5 mg once or twice/wk (*dermatologic therapy or urine spraying*); cat (*suppress estrus*); 5 mg/cat for 3 days, then 2.5–5 mg once/wk for 10 wk[‡] | XI-509, XI-552, XI-947, XI-963, XI-966, 535, 583, 1034, 1074, 1105, 1106, 1108 |
| Melarsomine HCl (RM-340) | Immiticide | Dog: Two 2.5-mg/kg doses IM 24 hr apart; repeat in 4 months (see labeling instructions) | 885 |
| Melphalan | Alkeran | see Table, p 1447 | 479, 484, 527 |
| Meperidine hydrochloride | Demerol | Dog: 5–10 mg/kg IV, IM (as needed)<br>Cat: 3–5 mg/kg IV, IM (as needed) | XI-82, XI-631, 774 |
| Mephenytoin | Mesantoin | Dog: 10 mg/kg, q8h, PO | XI-986 |
| 6-Mercaptopurine | Purinethol | see Table, p 1448 | 485 |
| Mesalamine | Asacol<br>Mesasal<br>Pentasa | Dosage not established (human dosage is 400–500 mg q6–8h)<br>see also *Osalazine sodium*; *Sulfasalazine* | |
| Metaproterenol sulfate | Alupent<br>Metaprel | 0.325–0.65 mg/kg q4–6h PO | |
| Metaraminol bitartrate | Aramine | 0.1 mg/kg IM, SC | |
| Methazolamide | Neptazane | 2–4 mg/kg (maximum dose: 4–6 mg/kg) q8–12h PO | XI-1049 |
| Methenamine hippurate | Hiprex | Dog: 500 mg/dog q12h PO<br>Cat: 250 mg/cat q12h PO | |
| Methenamine mandelate | Mandelamine | 10–20 mg/kg q8–12h PO | VIII-1096 |
| Methimazole | Tapazole | Cat: 5 mg/cat q8–12h PO (induction), followed by 2.5–5 mg/cag q8–12h PO | X-1002, XI-334, 371 |
| Methionine (other names used are L-methionine and DL-methionine) | Uroeze<br>Methio-Form | Dog: 150–300 mg/kg/day PO[°]<br>Cat: 1–1.5 gm/cat PO (added to food each day)[°] (use in adult cats only) | |
| Methocarbamol | Robaxin-V | 44 mg/kg q8h PO on the first day, then 22–44 mg/kg q8h PO[°] | 1148 |
| Methohexital sodium | Brevital | 11 mg/kg IV (to effect) | |
| Methotrexate (MTX) | | see Table, p 1449 | 483, 485, 1101 |
| Methoxamine hydrochloride | Vasoxyl | 200–250 μg/kg IM, or 40–80 μg/kg IV | |
| Methoxyflurane | Metofane | 3% (induction); 0.5–1.5% (maintenance) | |
| Methscopolamine bromide | Pamine | 0.3–1 mg/kg q8h PO (use cautiously in cats) | |
| Methylene blue (1% solution) | | 1 mg/kg IV, slowly (beware hemolytic anemia) | 443 |
| Methylprednisolone acetate | Depo-Medrol | Dog: 1 mg/kg q1–3 wk<br>Cat: 10–20 mg/cat IM q1–3 wk | X-54, XI-509, XI-568, 409t, 406, 576 |
| Methylpyrazole (4-methylpyrazone) | 5% (compounded in polyethylene glycol) | Dog: 20 mg/kg IV, initial dose; see text for dosing instructions | 236 |
| Methylprednisolone sodium succinate | Solu-Medrol | 30 mg/kg IV (for acute spinal injury or shock) repeat at 15 mg/kg IV in 2–6 hr | 1147 |
| Methyltestosterone | | Dog: 5–25 mg/dog q24–48h PO (see also *Testosterone cypionate*; *Testosterone propionate*)[†]<br>Cat: 1–2.5 mg/cat q48h PO[†] | |
| Metoclopramide hydrochloride | Reglan<br>Maxolon<br>Maxeran (Canada) | 0.2–0.5 mg/kg q6–8h IV, IM, PO, or 1–2 mg/kg/day via continuous IV infusion | XI-191, XI-583, XI-848, 680, 969, 1142, 1144 |
| Metoprolol tartrate | Lopressor | Dog: 5–50 mg/dog q8h PO<br>Cat: 2–15 mg/cat q8h PO | XI-676, 783 |
| Metronidazole | Flagyl | Dog: 25–65 mg/kg q24h PO, 12–15 mg/kg q12h (giardiasis) or 10 mg/kg q8h (antibacterial) PO; Hepatic encephalopathy 7.5 mg/kg q12h PO; *Giardia* 22–25 mg/kg q12h for 5 days<br>Cat: 10–25 mg/kg (maximum dose: 50 mg/kg) q24h PO; *Giardia* 12–25 mg/kg q12h for 5 days | XI-568, XI-626, XI-639, XI-602, 288, 718, 722, 726, 746, 753, 1144, 1156, 1201 |
| Mexiletine hydrochloride | Mexitil | Dog: 5–8 mg/kg q8–12h PO (use cautiously) | 803 |
| Mibolerone | Cheque | Dog (2.6–5 μg/kg/day PO):<br>0.45–11.3 kg: 30 μg[°]<br>11.8–22.7 kg: 60 μg[°]<br>23–45.3 kg: 120 μg[°]<br>>45.8 kg: 180 μg[°]<br>Cat: Safe dose not established. | XI-954, XI-966, 1074 |
| Midazolam hydrochloride | Versed | 0.1–0.25 mg/kg IV, IM, or 0.1–0.3 mg/kg/hr IV infusion | XI-27, XI-98, 774, 1004, 1039 |
| Mifepristone | | see text for dosing instructions | 1076 |

[°]Refer to manufacturer's recommendations.
[†]Consult anticancer protocol for precise dosage.
[‡]Megestrol acetate not approved for use in cats.

*Table continued on following page*

| Drug Name | Brand Name(s) | Dosage | CVT Reference(s) |
|-----------|---------------|--------|------------------|
| Milbemycin oxime | Interceptor | 0.5 mg/kg q30d PO | 627, 712, 881, 883 |
| Milk of Magnesia | | see *Magnesium hydroxide* | |
| Milrinone | | 0.5–1.0 mg/kg q12h PO (not approved) | |
| Mineral oil | | Dog: 10–50 ml/dog q12h PO | |
| | | Cat: 10–25 ml/cat q12h PO | |
| Minocycline | Minocin | 5–12.5 mg/kg q12h PO | XI-1061 |
| Misoprostol | Cytotec | Dog: 2–5 μg/kg q8h PO | X-911, XI-132, 72, 709, 1017, 1197 |
| Mithramycin | | see *Plicamycin* | |
| Mitotane (o,p′-DDD) | Lysodren | For PDH: 50 mg/kg/day PO (may be given in divided doses) for 5–10 days, then 50–70 mg/kg/wk PO; *Adrenal tumor:* 50–75 mg/kg/day for 10 days PO then 75–100 mg/kg/wk PO (adjust dose based on cortisol measurements) | X-1024, X-1031, XI-345, 416, 486, 603, 1451 |
| Mitoxantrone hydrochloride | Novantrone | see Table, p 1450 | XI-399, XI-595, 484, 496, 504, 1101 |
| Morphine sulfate | | Dog: 0.2–0.6 mg/kg IV, IM, SC (as needed); 0.1 mg/kg epidrual; 0.3–3 mg/kg q4–8h PO | XI-27, XI-82, XI-95, XI-713, 774 |
| | | Cat: 0.1 mg/kg IM, SC (as needed) | |
| Nadolol | Corgard | 0.25–0.5 mg/kg q12h PO | XI-676 |
| Nafcillin sodium | Unipen | 10 mg/kg q6h IM, PO | |
| Nalbuphine HCl | | Dog: 0.03–0.1 mg/kg IV | 1004 |
| Nalorphine | Nalline | 0.44 mg/kg IV, IM, SC (1 mg for every 10 mg of morphine) | |
| Naloxone | Narcan | 0.01–0.04 mg/kg IV, IM, SC° | XI-27, XI-552, XI-995, 213, 251, 1004, 1144 |
| Naltrexone hydrochloride | Trexan | *Behavior problems*: 2.2 mg/kg q12h PO | X-18, XI-438, 535 |
| Nandrolone decanoate | Deca-Durabolin | Dog: 1–1.5 mg/kg/wk IM | |
| | | Cat: 1 mg/cat/wk IM | |
| Naproxen | Naprosyn Naxen, Aleve (OTC) | Dog: 2 mg/kg q48h (use cautiously) | X-47 |
| Neo-Darbazine (prochlorperazine plus isopropamide plus neomycin) | | Dog:° 4.5–9 kg: one #1 capsule q12h 9–13.6 kg: two #1 capsules q12h 13.6–27.3 kg: three #1 capsules or one #3 capsule q12h PO | |
| Neomycin sulfate | Biosol | 10–20 mg/kg q6–12h PO | X-829, XI-639 |
| Neostigmine bromide | Prostigmin Bromide | 2 mg/kg/day PO (in divided doses, to effect) | XI-580 |
| Neostigmine methylsulfate | Prostigmin | *Antimyasthenic*: 10 μg/kg IM, SC, as needed (atropine may be administered to counteract side effects) *Antidote for curiform block*: 40 μg/kg IM, SC (administer with atropine) *Diagnostic aid for myasthenia gravis*: 40 μg/kg IM, or 20 μg/kg IV | XI-1039 |
| Niclosamide | Yomesan | Dog: 157 mg/kg PO once[†] | |
| Nifedipine | Adalat Procardia | Dosage not established | XI-684, 890 |
| Nitrates | | see *Isosorbide dinitrate*; *Nitroglycerin ointment* | |
| Nitrofurantoin | Furadantin Macrodantin | 4 mg/kg q8h PO | |
| Nitroglycerin ointment | Nitrol Ointment | Dog: 4–12 mg (maximum of 15 mg) topically q12h | XI-700, XI-713, XI-766, 860 |
| | Nitro-Bid Ointment Nitrostat Ointment | Cat: 2–4 mg topically q12h (or 1/4 inch/cat) (1 inch of ointment is approximately 15 mg) | 860 |
| Nitroprusside sodium | Nipride | 2.5–15 μg/kg/min IV infusion | IX-329, XI-418, XI-700, XI-713, 187 |
| Nizatidine | Axid | 5 mg/kg q24h PO | XI-132 |
| Norepinephrine bitartrate | Levophed | 0.05–0.3 μg/kg/min IV | 191 |
| Norfloxacin | Noroxin | 22 mg/kg q12h PO | XI-829 |
| Novobiocin | see *Delta-Albaplex* | | |
| Omega fatty acids | see *Derm Caps* | 1 capsule q12h PO (see also *Essential fatty acids*) | X-563, XI-534 |
| Omeprazole | Prilosec | Dog: 20 mg/dog or 0.7 mg/kg q24h PO Cat: not recommended | X-911, XI-132, 72, 709, 722 |
| Ondansetron | Zofran | 0.5–1.0 mg/kg PO or 0.5 mg/kg loading dose IV followed by 0.5 mg/kg/hr infusion for 6 hr | 682 |
| o,p′-DDD | | see *Mitotane, o,p′-DDD* | |

°Refer to manufacturer's recommendations.
[†]Consult anticancer protocol for precise dosage.

| Drug Name | Brand Name(s) | Dosage | CVT Reference(s) |
|---|---|---|---|
| Orgotein | Palosein | Dog: 2.5–5 mg q24h IM, SC for 6 days, then q48h for 8 days° | |
| Ormetroprim | | see *Primor* | |
| Osalazine sodium | Dipentum | Dosage not established (human dosage is 500 mg twice daily) | |
| Oxacillin | Prostaphlin Bactocill | 22–40 mg/kg q8h PO | XI-539 |
| Oxazepam | Serax | Appetite stimulant: 2.5 mg/cat PO | X-18, XI-438, 970 |
| Oxfendazole | Synanthic | Dog: 10 mg/kg q24h PO | 896 |
| Oxtriphylline | Choledyl SA | Dog: 47 mg/kg (equivalent to 30 mg/kg theophylline) q12h PO | XI-660 |
| Oxybutynin chloride | Ditropan | 0.5 mg q8–12h PO | X-1214, 1024, 1025 |
| Oxygen | | see table | 177 |
| Oxymetholone | Anadrol | 1–5 mg/kg/day PO | |
| Oxymorphone hydrochloride | Numorphan | 0.1–0.2 mg/kg IV, SC, IM (as needed), then 0.05–0.1 mg/kg q1–2h (with acepromazine)<br>*Preanesthetic*: 0.025–0.05 mg/kg IM, SC (with acepromazine) | XI-27, XI-82, XI-95, XI-98, 774, 1004 |
| Oxytetracycline | Terramycin | 7.5–10 mg/kg q12h IV; 20 mg/kg q12h PO | 288 |
| Oxytocin | | Dog: 1–5 U IM, IV, repeat q30 min for primary inertia.<br>Cat: 0.5 U IM, IV (maximum dose: 3 U/cat) | X-1299 |
| 2-PAM | | see *Pralidoxime chloride* | |
| Pancreatic enzyme | Viokase | 2 tsp/20 kg body weight, or 1–3 tsp/0.45 kg of food, mixed with food 20 min prior to feeding | 734 |
| Pancreatic enzyme (Pancrelipase) | Festal-II | 1 tablet before, or with, meals (do not break or crush tablet) | |
| Pancreatin | | Dog: 2–10 tablets with food<br>Cat: 1–2 tablets with food | |
| Pancuronium bromide | Pavulon | 0.1 mg/kg IV | |
| Paregoric | Corrective Mixture | 0.05–0.06 mg/kg q12h PO (5 ml of paregoric corresponds to approximately 2 mg of morphine) | 704 |
| D-penicillamine | Cuprimine | 10–15 mg/kg q12h PO | X-891, X-1189, 749, 751 |
| Penicillin G benzathine | Donnazyme | Not recommended | |
| Penicillin G potassium | Many | 20,000–40,000 U/kg q6–8h IV, IM | XI-829 |
| Penicillin G procaine | Many | 20,000–40,000 U/kg q12–24 IM | XI-260 |
| Penicillin G sodium | Many | 20,000–40,000 U/kg q6–8h IV, IM | XI-829 |
| Penicillin V (previously used name is phenoxymethyl penicillin) | Many | 10 mg/kg 18h PO | |
| Pentazocine | Talwin | Dog: 1.65–3.3 mg/kg q4h IM<br>Cat: 2.2–3.3 mg/kg IV, IM, SC | XI-82 |
| Pentobarbital | | 25–30 mg/kg IV (first ½ of the dose administered rapidly, then remaining administered dose to effect) | XI-98 |
| Pentoxifyline | Trental | Dog: 400-mg tablet q24–48h (collies and Shetland sheepdogs) | 640 |
| Petrolatum, white | Vaseline Laxatone | Cat: 1–5 ml/cat q24h PO | XI-619 |
| Phenobarbital | Luminal | Dog: 2–8 mg/kg q12h PO, IM, IV<br>Cat: 1–2 mg/kg q12h PO, IM, IV<br>*Status epilepticus* (dog or cat): 15–200 mg/animal IV (to effect) | XI-986, XI-992, 47, 198, 212, 746 |
| Phenoxybenzamine hydrochloride | Dibenzyline | Dog: 0.25 mg/kg q8–12h PO, or 0.5 mg/kg q24h<br>Cat: 0.5 mg/kg q12h PO | X-1214, XI-883 |
| Phentolamine mesylate | Regitine (US) Rogitine (Canada) | 0.02–0.1 mg/kg IV (as needed to maintain blood pressure) | |
| Phenylbutazone | Butazolidin | Dog: 15–22 mg/kg q8–12h PO (maximum dose: 800 mg)°<br>Cat: not recommended | X-47, 1197 |
| Phenylephrine hydrochloride | Neo-Synephrine Hydrochloride | 0.01 mg/kg q15 min IV<br>0.1 mg/kg q15 min IM, SC | |
| Phenylpropanolamine hydrochloride | Propagest, Dexatrim | 1.5–2 mg/kg q12h PO | X-1214, XI-875, 1023, 1025 |
| Phenytoin | Dilantin | *Antiepileptic in dog*: 20–35 mg/kg q8h<br>*Antiepileptic in cat*: not recommended<br>*Antiarrhythmic in dog*: 30 mg/kg q8h PO or 10 mg/kg IV over 5 min | 341 |

°Refer to manufacturer's recommendations.

*Table continued on following page*

| Drug Name | Brand Name(s) | Dosage | CVT Reference(s) |
|---|---|---|---|
| Physostigmine salicylate | Antilirium | 0.02 mg/kg q12h IV | 1143 |
| Phytonadione | | see *Vitamin K₁* | |
| Phytomenadione | | see *Vitamin K₁* | |
| Piperazine | Many | 44–66 mg/kg PO once° | XI-626, 712 |
| Piroxicam | Feldene | Dog: 0.3 mg/kg q48h PO (use cautiously) | X-47, XI-626, 1011, |
| | | Cat: dosage not established | 1017 |
| Plicamycin | Mithracin | see Table, p 1450 | |
| Polyethylene glycol electrolyte solution | Golytely | 25 ml/kg, then repeat in 2–4 hr PO | XI-568 |
| Polysulfated glycosaminoglycan | Adequan | 1–2 mg/kg q4 days for 7 injections IM, SC | 1197 |
| Potassium bromide | | Dog: 30–40 mg/kg q24h PO (adjust dose via monitoring) | XI-986 |
| Potassium chloride | | 0.5 mEq/kg/day (do not administer at a rate faster than 0.5 mEq/kg/hr) | 35, 163, 386t, 954, 968 |
| | | 10–40 mEq/500 ml of fluids, depending on serum potassium | |
| Potassium citrate | Urocit-K | Dog: 50–75 mg/kg q12h PO | 958, 968, 991, 994 |
| Potassium gluconate | Kaon Elixir | 2.2 mEq/100 kcal of energy/day PO | XI-820, XI-842, XI- |
| | Tumil-K | Cat: 2–6 mEq daily | 848, 949, 968 |
| Potassium iodide | | 30–100 mg/cat daily (in single or divided doses) for 10–14 days | XI-301 |
| Potassium phosphate | | 0.03–0.12 mmol/kg/hr IV | 386 |
| Pralidoxime chloride (2-PAM) | Protopam Chloride | *Organophosphate toxicosis:* 20 mg/kg q8–12h (initial dose IV [slow], or IM; subsequent doses IM, SC) | XI-178, XI-188, 247 |
| Praziquantel | Droncit | Dog (PO)°: | XI-228, XI-626, 715, |
| | |   &lt;6.8 kg: 7.5 mg/kg once | 896 |
| | |   &gt;6.8 kg: 5 mg/kg once | |
| | | Dog (IM, SC)°: | |
| | |   ≤23 kg: 7.5 mg/kg once | |
| | |   2.7–4.5 kg: 6.3 mg/kg once | |
| | |   ≥5 kg: 5 mg/kg once | |
| | | Cat (PO)°: | |
| | |   &lt;1.8 kg: 6.3 mg/kg once | |
| | |   &gt;1.8 kg: 5 mg/kg once | |
| | | *Paragonimiasis:* 25 mg/kg q8h for 2 days | |
| | | Cat (IM, SC): 5 mg/kg IM, SC | |
| Prazosin hydrochloride | Minipress | 0.5–2 mg/animal q8–12h PO | XI-700, XI-840 |
| Prednisolone | Many | *Anti-inflammatory:* | X-54, XI-509, XI-539, |
| | |   Dog: 0.5–1 mg/kg q12–24h IV, IM, PO, initially, then taper to q48h | XI-568, XI-572, XI-595, XI-813, |
| | |   Cat: 2.2 mg/kg q12–24h IV, IM, PO initially, then taper to q48h | XI-1007, XI-1049, XI-1081, 155, 198, |
| | | *Immunosuppressive* (dog and cat): initially 2.2–6.6 mg/kg/day IV, IM, PO, then taper to 2–4 mg/kg q48h | 268, 288, 409t, 417, 449, 495, 558, 568, 726, 750, 884, 907, |
| | | *Shock:* see *Prednisolone sodium succinate* | 1012, 1127, 1191, |
| | | see also *Methylprednisolone acetate* | 1197, 1450 |
| Prednisolone sodium succinate | Solu-Delta-Cortef | *Shock:* 15–30 mg/kg IV, then repeat in 4–6 hr | X-54, XI-1013, 152, |
| | | *CNS trauma:* 15–30 mg/kg IV, then taper to 1–2 mg/kg q12h | 409t, 428, 1147 |
| Prednisone | Mylepsin | see *Prednisolone* | 409t |
| Primidone | Mysoline | Initial dose is 8–10 mg/kg q8–12h and then is adjusted to 10–15 mg/kg q8–12h PO | XI-992 |
| Primor (ormetoprim plus sulfadimethoxine) | | 55 mg/kg on first day, and 27.5 mg/kg/day thereafter, PO | 596 |
| Procainamide hydrochloride | Pronestyl | Dog: 10–20 mg/kg q6h PO (maximum dose: 40 mg/kg); 8–20 mg/kg IV, IM; 25–50 μg/kg/min IV infusion | 166, 187, 803, 849, 867 |
| | | Cat: 3–8 mg/kg IM, PO q6–8h | |
| Procainamide hydrochloride (extended-release tablets) | Procan-SR | Dog: 20–50 mg/kg q8h PO | |
| | | Cat: 62.5 mg/cat q8h PO | XI-694 |
| Prochlorperazine | Compazine | 0.1–0.5 mg/kg q6–8h IM, SC | XI-583, 682 |
| | | see also *Darbazine* or *Neo-Darbazine* | |
| Progesterone, repositol | | see *Medroxyprogesterone acetate* | |
| Promazine hydrochloride | Sparine | 1–2 mg/kg q6–8h IV, IM, PO | |
| Promethazine hydrochloride | Phenergan | 0.2–0.4 mg/kg q6–8h IV, IM, PO (maximum dose: 1 mg/kg) | |
| Propantheline bromide | Pro-Banthīne | 0.25–0.5 mg/kg q8–12h PO | |

°Refer to manufacturer's recommendations.

| Drug Name | Brand Name(s) | Dosage | CVT Reference(s) |
|---|---|---|---|
| *Propionibacterium acnes* bacterin | Immuno-Regulin | 0.25–2 ml, IV (see labeling instructions) | 616 |
| Propiopromazine | Tranvet | 1.1–4.4 mg/kg q12–24h° | |
| Propofol | Diprivan | 3–6 mg/kg IV; see table | 80, 775, 1004, 1039 |
| Propranolol hydrochloride | Inderal | Dog: 20–60 µg/kg over 5–10 min q8h, 0.2–1 mg/kg PO q8h | X-271, X-278, 165, 251, 783, 849 |
| | | Cat: 2.5–5 mg/cat (0.4–1.2 mg/kg) PO q8–12 | XI-338, XI-676, XI-765, XI-848, 861, 867 |
| Propylthiouracil (PTU) | | 11 mg/kg q12h PO (its use is not recommended) | 371 |
| Prostaglandin E | | see *Misoprostol* | |
| Prostaglandin F$_{2\alpha}$ | Lutalyse | *Pyometra:* | X-1305, XI-947, XI-954, XI-969 |
| | | Dog: 0.1–0.2 mg/kg, once daily for 5 days SC | |
| | | Cat: 0.1–0.25 mg/kg, once daily for 5 days SC | |
| | | *Abortion:* | 1079, 1075, 1081 |
| | | Dog: 25–50 µg/kg q12h IM | |
| | | Cat: 0.5–1 mg/kg IM for 2 injections | |
| Pseudoephedrine sulfate | Sudafed | 0.2–0.4 mg/kg q8–12h PO | |
| Psyllium | Metamucil | 1 tsp/5–10 kg (added to each meal) | XI-613 |
| Pyrantel pamoate | Nemex | Dog: 5 mg/kg PO once, then repeat in 7–10 days° | XI-626, 712 |
| | | Cat: 20 mg/kg PO once | |
| Pyridostigmine bromide | Mestinon | *Antimyasthenic:* 0.02–0.04 mg/kg q2h IV, or 0.5–3 mg/kg q8–12h PO | XI-572, XI-1024, XI-1039, 557 |
| | Regonol | *Antidote (curariform):* 0.15–0.3 mg/kg IM, IV | |
| Pyrimethamine | Daraprim | Dog: 1 mg/kg q24h PO for 14–28 days (5 days for *Neosporum caninum*) | XI-263, XI-1034, 314 |
| | | Cat: 0.5–1 mg/kg q24h PO for 14–28 days | |
| Quinacrine hydrochloride | Atabrine hydrochloride | Dog: 6.6 mg/kg q12h PO for 5 days | 719 |
| | | Cat: 11 mg/kg q24h PO for 5 days | |
| Quinidine gluconate | Quinaglute Duraquin | Dog: 6–20 mg/kg q6h IM; 6–20 mg/kg q6–8h PO (of base) | XI-694, 165, 805 |
| | | (324 mg quinidine gluconate = 202 mg quinidine base) | |
| Quinidine polygalacturonate | Cardioquin | Dog: 6–20 mg/kg q6h PO (of base) | |
| | | (275 mg quinidine polygalacturonate = 167 mg quinidine base) | |
| Quinidine sulfate | Clin-Quin | Dog: 6–20 mg/kg q6–8h PO (of base) | |
| | Quinora | (300 mg quinidine sulfate = 250 mg quinidine base) | |
| Ranitidine | Zantac | Dog: 2 mg/kg q8h IV, PO | X-911, XI-132, XI-191, XI-523, XI-639, 707, 722, 969 |
| | | Cat: 2.5 mg/kg q12h IV; 3.5 mg/kg q12h PO | |
| Retinoids | | see *Isotretinoin; Retinol; Etretinate* | X-553, 481 |
| Retinol | Aquasol A | 625–800 IU/kg q24h PO | X-553, XI-523, 481 |
| Riboflavin | | Dog: 10–20 mg/day PO | 1162 |
| | | Cat: 5–10 mg/day PO | |
| Rifampin | Rifadin | 10–20 mg/kg q24h PO | 198, 323 |
| Ringer's solution | | 40–50 ml/kg/day IV, SC, IP for maintenance | |
| Salicylate | | see *Acetylsalicylic acid* (Aspirin) | |
| Scopolamine hydrobromide (hyroscine) | | 0.03 mg/kg q6h SC, IM (not recommended for cats) | 682 |
| Senna | Senokot | Cat: 5 ml/cat q24h (syrup); ½ tsp/cat q24h with food (granules) | |
| Sodium aurothiomalate | Myochrisine | Dog: 0.5 mg/kg IM once a week for 6 weeks | 1191 |
| Sodium bicarbonate (NaHCO$_3$) | | *Acidosis:* 0.5–1 mEq/kg IV, or as guided by blood-gas analysis (8.5% solution = 1 mEq/ml of NaHCO$_3$) | X-333, XI-848, 122, 212, 385, 949 |
| | | *Renal failure:* 10 mg/kg q8–12h PO (adjust as necessary) | 954, 955, 957, 968 |
| | | *Alkalinization:* 50 mg/kg q8–12h PO (1 tsp is approximtely 2 gm) | |
| Sodium chloride (0.9%) | | 40–50 ml/kg/day IV, SC, IP | |
| Sodium chloride 7.5% (hypertonic saline) | Concentrated sodium chloride | 2–8 ml/kg IV for shock therapy | |
| Sodium iodide (20%) | | 20–40 mg/kg q8–12h PO | X-1101 |
| Sodium nitroprusside | | see *Nitroprusside sodium* | |
| Sodium thiomalate | | see *Gold sodium thiomalate* | |
| Sorbitol 70% | | 3 ml/kg PO | 244 |
| Spironolactone | Aldactone | 1–2 mg/kg q12h PO | XI-668, 755 |

°Refer to manufacturer's recommendations.

*Table continued on following page*

| Drug Name | Brand Name(s) | Dosage | CVT Reference(s) |
|---|---|---|---|
| Stanozolol | Winstrol-V | Dog: 1–4 mg/dog q12h PO; 25–50 mg/dog/wk IM° <br> Cat: 1 mg/cat q12h PO; 25 mg/cat/wk IM° | XI-438, 535, 947 |
| Styrid caricide (styrylpyridinium chloride plus diethylcarbamazine) | | 6.7 mg/kg diethylcarbamazine q24h PO and 5.5 mg/ kg styrylpyridinium chloride q24h PO° | |
| Sucralfate | Carafate (US) <br> Sulcrate (Canada) | Dog: 0.5–1 gm q8–12h PO <br> Cat: 0.25 gm q8–12h PO | X-911, XI-132, XI-191, 197, 683, 708, 754, 969 |
| Sufentanil | Sufenta | 2 $\mu$g/kg IV, up to a maximum dose of 5 $\mu$g/kg (premedicate with acetylpromazine) | |
| Sulfadiazine | | 100 mg/kg IV, PO (loading dose), followed by 50 mg/ kg q12h IV, PO (see also *Trimethoprim*) | XI-263, XI-1034 |
| Sulfadimethoxine | Albon, Bactrovet | 55 mg/kg PO (loading dose), followed by 27.5 mg/kg q12h (see also *Primor*) | XI-626, 715 |
| Sulfaguanidine | | 100–200 mg/kg q8h PO for 5 days | |
| Sulfamethazine | | 100 mg/kg PO (loading dose), followed by 50 mg/kg q12h PO | |
| Sulfamethoxazole | Gantanol | 100 mg/kg PO (loading dose), followed by 50 mg/kg q12h PO | |
| Sulfamethoxazole-trimethoprim | Bactrim <br> Septra | see dosage for *Trimethoprim-sulfadiazine* | |
| Sulfasalazine (sulfapyridine-mesalamine) | Azulfidine (US) <br> Salazopyrin (Canada) | 10–30 mg/kg q8–12h PO <br> (see also *Mesalamine, Olsalazine*) | XI-604, XI-613, 727, 1191 |
| Sulfisoxazole | Gantrisin | 50 mg/kg q8h PO (urinary tract infections) | |
| Sulfobromophthalein sodium | Bromsulphalein (BSP) (this drug's availability is limited) | 5 mg/kg IV, collect plasma or serum 30 min after BSP injection | |
| Sulfonamides | | see individual drugs | 596 |
| Tamoxifen | Nolvadex | see text | 522, 1102, 1451 |
| Taurine | | Cat: 250–500 q12h PO | X-260 |
| Telezol | | see *Tiletamine* | |
| Temaril-P (trimeprazine-prednisolone) | | 0.7–1.1 mg/kg (of trimeprazine) 12–24h PO° | |
| Terbutaline | Brethine, Bricanyl | Dog: 2.5 mg/dog q8h SC, PO <br> Cat: 0.625 mg/cat q12h SC, PO | XI-660, XI-803, 890, 891, 913 |
| Terfenadine | Seldane | 4.5–10 mg/kg q12h PO–see drug tox. file | |
| Testosterone cypionate | Andro-Cyp | 1–2 mg/kg q2–4wk IM (see also *Methyltestosterone*) | 1071, 1074 |
| Testosterone propionate | Testex, Malogen | 0.5–1 mg/kg 2–3 times/wk IM | 1071, 1074 |
| Tetanus toxoid | | 100–500 U/kg (maximum 20,000 U) | |
| Tetracycline | Panmycin, Achromycin | 15–20 mg/kg q6–8h PO <br> 4.4–11 mg/kg q8–12h IV, IM <br> (see also *Oxytetracycline, Doxycycline, Minocycline*) | 269, 292, 296, 907, 1093 |
| 2,2,2 tetramine | see *Trientine hydrochloride* | | |
| Thenium closylate | Canopar | Dogs >4.5 kg 500 mg PO, repeat in 2–3 wk° <br> Dogs 2.5–4.5 kg: 250 mg q12h for 1 day, repeat in 2–3 wk° | |
| Theophylline | | Dog: 9 mg/kg q6–8h PO <br> Cat: 4 mg/kg q8–12h PO | XI-803, 891, 917 |
| Theophylline sustained-release | Theo-Dur <br> Slo-Bid Gyrocaps <br> Choledyl-SA | Dog: 20 mg/kg q12h PO (Theo-Dur tablets only); 30 mg/kg q2h PO (Slo-Bid Gyrocaps); 47 mg/kg q12h PO (Choledyl-SA) <br> Cat: 25 mg/kg q24h PO, at night (Theo-Dur tablets and Slo-Bid Gyrocaps) <br> (see also *Aminophylline*) | |
| Thiabendazole | Omnizole, Equizole | Dog: 50 mg/kg q24h for 3 days, repeat 1 month <br> Cat (*Strongyloides*): 125 mg/kg q24h for 3 days | XI-228, XI-626, 712 |
| Thiacetarsamide sodium | Caparsolate | 2.2 mg/kg IV twice daily for 2 days | X-131, X-265, 884 |
| Thiamine (vitamin B$_1$) | | Dog: 10–100 mg/dog/day PO <br> Cat: 5–30 mg/cat/day PO (up to a maximum dose of 50 mg/cat/day) | |
| Thiamylal | Surital, Bio-Tal | Dog: 8–10 mg/kg IV, in incremental doses up to 20 mg/kg (4% solution) <br> Cat: same as dog (2% solution) | |
| Thioguanine (6-TG) | | see Table, p 1449 | |

°Consult anticancer protocol for precise dosage.

| Drug Name | Brand Name(s) | Dosage | CVT Reference(s) |
|---|---|---|---|
| Thiomalate sodium | | see *Gold sodium thiomalate* | |
| Thiopental sodium | Pentothal | Dog: 10–25 mg/kg IV (to effect)<br>Cat: 5–10 mg/kg IV (to effect) | |
| Thiotepa | | see Table, p 1448 | |
| Thyroid (desiccated) | | 15–20 mg/kg/day PO | |
| Thyroid hormone | | see *Levothyroxine, Liothyronine* | |
| Thyrotropin (TSH) | Dermathycin, Thytropar | Dog: collect baseline sample, followed by 0.1 IU/kg IV (maximum dose is 5 IU); collect post-TSH sample at 6 hr<br>Cat: collect baseline sample, followed by 2.5 IU/cat IM and collect post-TSH sample at 8–12 hr | 336 |
| Ticarcillin | Ticar | 33–50 mg/kg q4–6h IV, IM | 279 |
| Tiletamine-zolazepam | Telezol, Zoletil | 5–7 mg/kg IV, IM | XI-27, 1039 |
| Tobramycin | Nebcin | 2 mg/kg q8h IV, IM, SC | |
| Tocainide | Tonocard | Dog: 10–20 mg/kg q8h PO | XI-773, 803 |
| Toluene | Vermiplex | 267 mg/kg PO (of toluene), repeat in 2–4 wk | 1145 |
| Triamcinolone | Aristocort | *Anti-inflammatory*: 0.5–1 mg/kg q12–24h PO, taper dose to 0.5–1 mg/kg q48h PO | X-54, XI-509 |
| Triamcinolone acetonide | Vetalog | 0.1–0.2 mg/kg IM, SC, repeat in 7–10 days<br>*Intralesional*: 1.2–1.8 mg, or 1 mg for every cm diameter of tumor q2wk | 406, 577t, 637 |
| Triamterene | Dyrenium | 1–2 mg/kg q12h PO | |
| Tribrissen: see *trimethoprim-sulfadiazine* | | | |
| Trientine hydrochloride | Syprine | 10–15 mg/kg q12h PO | |
| Triethylperazine | Torecan | 0.13–0.2 mg/kg IM q8–12h | |
| Trifluoperazine | Stelezine | 0.03 mg/kg IM q12h | |
| Triflupromazine | Vesprin | 0.1–0.3 mg/kg IM, PO q8–12h | |
| Triiodothyronine | | see *Liothyronine* | |
| Trimeprazine | Panectyl | 0.5 mg/kg q12h PO (also see *Temaril-P*) | |
| Trimethobenzamide | Tigan, Trimazide | Dog: 3 mg/kg q8h IM, PO<br>Cat: not recommended | 682 |
| Trimethoprim | Proloprim | Dose not established (see *Trimethoprim-sulfadiazine*) | |
| Trimethoprim-sulfadiazine | Tribissen | 15 mg/kg q12h IM, PO, or 30 mg/kg q12–24h SC, PO (for *Toxoplasma*: 30 mg/kg q12h PO) | XI-207, XI-539, XI-626, XI-909, 313, 715, 907, 1030, 1106, 1131 |
| Tripelennamine | Pelamine | 1 mg/kg q12h PO | 596 |
| TSH (thyroid-stimulating hormone) | see *Thyrotropin* | | |
| Tylosin | Tylocine, Tylan | 7–15 mg/kg q8h PO<br>(for colitis administer 40–80 mg/kg/day with food) | XI-602, 1093 |
| Urea | | 300 mg q1h IV | |
| Urofollitropin | Metrodin | Cat: 2 mg/cat q24h IM | 1070, 1071 |
| Ursodiol (ursodeoxycholate) | Actigall | 10–15 mg/kg q24h PO | 752 |
| Valporte sodium | | see *Valproic acid* | |
| Valproic acid | Depakene | Dog: 60–200 mg/kg q8h PO; or 25–105 mg/kg/day PO when administered with phenobarbital | |
| Vanomycin | Vancocin | Dog: 15 mg/kg q6h IV | |
| Vasopressin (ADH) | Pitressin | Aqueous (20 U/mL): 10 U IV, IM<br>(see also *Desmopressin*) | X-973, 350 |
| Verapamil | Calan, Isoptin | Dog: 0.05 mg/kg q10–30 min IV (maximum cululative dose is 0.15 mg/kg); oral dose is not established<br>Cat: 1.1–2.9 mg/kg q8h PO | X-271, XI-684, XI-745, 165, 187, 890 |
| Vermiplex | | see *Toluene* | |
| Vinblastine | Velban | see Table, p 1449 | X-475, X-482, X-489, 485 |
| Vincristine | Oncovin | see Table, p 1449<br>*Thrombocytopenia*: 0.02 mg/kg IV once/wk | 485, 501, 517 |
| Viokase—see *Pancreatic enzyme* | | | X-931 |
| Vitamin A (Retinoids) | | see *Isotretinoin* (Accutane), *Retinol* (Aquasol-A), or *Etretinate* (Tegison) | |
| Vitamin B complex | | Dog: 0.5–2 ml q24h IV, IM, SC<br>Cat: 0.5–1 ml q24h IV, IM, SC | |
| Vitamin B$_1$ | | see *Thiamine* | |
| Vitamin B$_2$ | | see *Riboflavin* | |
| Vitamin B$_{12}$ | | see *Cyanocobalamin* | |
| Vitamin C | | see *Ascorbic acid* | 1162 |

| Drug Name | Brand Name(s) | Dosage | CVT Reference(s) |
|---|---|---|---|
| Vitamin D | | see *Dihydrotachysterol*; *Ergocalciferol* (oral) | 994 |
| Vitamin E (α-tocopherol) | Aquasol E | 100–400 IU q12h PO (or 400–600 IU q12h PO for immune-mediated skin disease) | X-574 |
| Vitamin K$_1$ | Aqua Mephyton, Mephyton | Short-acting rodenticides: 1 mg/kg/day SC, PO for 10–14 days; long-acting rodenticides: 3–5 mg/kg/day SC, PO for 3–4 wk; birds: 2.5–5 mg/kg q24h | X-144, 231, 445, 753 |
| Warfarin | | Dog: 0.1–0.2 mg/kg q24h PO (adjust dose by monitoring clotting time) Cat: 0.5 mg/cat q24h PO | XI-137, 868 |
| Xylazine | Rompun | Dog: 1.1 mg/kg IV, 2.2 mg/kg IM Cat: 1.1 mg/kg IM (emetic dose: 0.4–0.5 mg/kg IV) | XI-27, XI-194, 213, 680, 1039 |
| Yohimbine | Yobine | 0.11 mg/kg IV, 0.25–0.5 mg/kg q12h SC, IM | XI-194, 213, 682 |
| Zidovudine | AZT, Retrovir | Cat: 5 mg/kg q12h SQ, 5–10. mg/kg q12h PO | 270, 722 |
| Zinc acetate | | 200 mg elemental zinc q24h PO (for treatment of hepatitis) | 751, 757 |
| Zolazepam | | see *Tiletamine-zolazepam* | XI-27, 774 |

# ANTINEOPLASTIC AGENTS IN CANCER THERAPY*

J. P. THOMPSON

*Gainesville, Florida*

| Agent (Brand Name, Supplier) | Action and Cell Cycle Specificity | Indication | Dosage and Administration[†] | Toxicities | Comments |
|---|---|---|---|---|---|
| ***Alkylating Agents*** | | | | | |
| Cyclophosphamide (Cytoxan, Mead Johnson; Neosar, Adria) Tabs: 25- and 50-mg Inj: 100-, 200-, and 500-mg vials; 1- and 2-gm vials | Alkylating activity by metabolite phosphoramide mustard. Believed to cross-link DNA. Cell cycle nonspecific. | Primarily lymphoreticular neoplasms. Also mast cell, hemangiosarcoma, and mammary carcinoma. | 50 mg/m² PO once daily q48h or 4 days per week; or 150–300 mg/m² IV, PO; repeat in 21 days. | Leukopenia, gastroenteritis, and hemorrhagic cystitis. May induce transitional cell carcinoma of bladder. | Must be activated by liver. Excreted primarily by kidneys. Metabolites protein bound. |
| Chlorambucil (Leukeran, Burroughs Wellcome) Tabs: 2 mg | Bifunctional alkylation of DNA. Creates intra- and interstrand cross-links. Cell cycle nonspecific. | Lymphoreticular neoplasms, macroglobulinemia, and polycythemia vera. | 2–6 mg/m² PO q24h for 7 days; thereafter q48h; or 20 mg/m² PO q14 days. | Leukopenia. | Relatively free of gastrointestinal effects. |
| Busulfan (Myleran, Burroughs Wellcome) Tabs: 2 mg | Bifunctional alkylating agent. Interacts with cellular thiol groups. Little DNA cross-linking. Cell cycle nonspecific. | Chronic granulocytic leukemia; of no benefit in "blastic" phase. | 3–4 mg/m² PO q24h. Discontinue when total WBC is approximately 15,000. Repeat p.r.n. | Leukopenia. Rare bronchopulmonary dysplasia with pulmonary fibrosis. | May require 2 wk to observe response. Discontinue drug if rapid decline in total leukocytes is observed. |
| Melphalan (Alkeran, Burroughs Wellcome) Tabs: 2 mg | Bifunctional alkylating agent. Phenylalanine derivative of nitrogen mustard. Cell cycle nonspecific. | Multiple myeloma; some lymphoreticular neoplasms, osteosarcomas, mammary, and lung tumors. | 2 mg/m² q24h × 7–10 days, then 2–4 mg/m² PO q 48h. Alternatively, 6–8 mg/m² PO × 4–5 days and repeat q21d. | Infrequent leukopenia. | Response may be gradual over many months. |

*Table continued on following page*

| Agent (Brand Name, Supplier) | Action and Cell Cycle Specificity | Indication | Dosage and Administration† | Toxicities | Comments |
|---|---|---|---|---|---|
| Triethylenethiophosphoramide (Thiotepa, Lederle) Inj: 15-mg vial | Radiomimetic. Believed to disrupt DNA bonds by release of ethylenamine radicals. Cell cycle nonspecific. | Systemic use for carcinomas. Intravesical use for transitional cell. Intracavitary use for neoplastic effusions. | 0.2–0.5 mg/m² intracavitary or IV. | Leukopenia. | Not a vesicant. May be given intralesionally. |
| Mechlorethamine HCL (Mustargen, Merck Sharp & Dohme) Inj: 10-mg vial | Cytotoxic, mutagenic, and radiomimetic. Exact mechanism of action unknown. Cell cycle nonspecific. | Lymphoreticular neoplasms, pleural and peritoneal effusions. | 5 mg/m² PO, IV or intracavitary. Repeat p.r.n. | Leukopenia. Nausea and vomiting dose-limiting side effect. | Severe vesicant. Sloughing may occur if extravasated. |
| Lomustine (CeeNu, Bristol-Myers Oncology) Caps: 10, 40, and 100 mg | Binds DNA, alters RNA structure, and induces carbamoylation of various proteins. Cell cycle nonspecific. | Primary and metastatic brain tumors. Also active in lymphoma and multiple myeloma. | 60 mg/m² PO as single dose q6–8 wk; may increase to 80 mg/m² in absence of bone marrow suppression. | Nausea, vomiting, and anorexia. Major toxicity is delayed bone marrow suppression; toxicity is cumulative. | Highly lipid soluble. Enters CNS readily. Monitor blood counts q7–14d and do not repeat dose before 6 wk. |
| Cisplatin (Platinol, Bristol-Myers Oncology) Inj: 10- and 50-mg vials | Action similar to bifunctional alkylating agents. Produces DNA crosslinks. Cell cycle nonspecific. | Osteosarcoma, transitional cell carcinoma, and squamous cell carcinoma. | 60–70 mg/m² IV q21–28d; infuse over 20 min. Administer 0.9% saline IV for 4 hr pre- and 2 hr postinfusion. Canine only. | Nausea, vomiting, renal toxicity, and bone marrow depression. Dose-related pulmonary toxicity in cats. | Do not use aluminum-containing needles; precipitates on contact. Eliminated through kidneys. |
| Carboplatin (Paraplatin, Bristol-Myers Oncology) Inj: 50, 100, and 450-mg vials | Produces predominantly interstrand DNA crosslinks. Believed to be cell cycle nonspecific. | Anticancer spectrum believed to be similar to cisplatin; possible activity against melanoma and ovarian carcinoma. | 300 mg/m² IV q21–28d; infuse over 15–60 min. No pre- or postinfusion forced diuresis required. Canine only. | Bone marrow suppression is dose-dependent and dose-limiting. | Decreased nephro- and neurotoxicity as compared to cisplatin. Not bound to plasma proteins. Renal elimination. |
| **Antimetabolites** | | | | | |
| Mercaptopurine (Purinethol, Burroughs Wellcome) Tabs: 50 mg | Feedback enzyme inhibitor of DNA synthesis. S-phase specific. | Acute lymphocytic and granulocytic leukemias and immune-mediated disease. | 50 mg/m² PO q24h to effect, then q48h or p.r.n. | Infrequent leukopenia. | Must be activated within tumor cells; lethal synthesis. |

| Drug | Action | Indications | Dosage | Toxicity | Comments |
|---|---|---|---|---|---|
| Thioguanine (Thioguanine, Burroughs Wellcome) Tabs: 40 mg | Feedback enzyme inhibitor of DNA synthesis. S-phase specific. | Acute lymphocytic and granulocytic leukemias. | Dogs: 40 mg/m² PO q24h × 4–5 days, then q3d thereafter. Cats: 25 mg/m² PO q24h × 1–5 days, then repeat q 30d p.r.n. | Leukopenia and thrombocytopenia may be severe in cats. Hepatotoxicity. | As for mercaptopurine. Cross-resistance between thioguanine and mercaptopurine is extensive. |
| Fluorouracil (Fluorouracil, Roche; Adrucil, Adria) Inj: 500-mg vial | Inhibits enzyme thymidylate synthetase. Results in thymidine deficiency leading to inhibition of DNA synthesis. S-phase specific. | Mammary, gastrointestinal, liver, and lung carcinomas and carcinomatosis. | 150 mg/m² IV or intracavitary q7d. Canine only. | Dogs: cerebellar ataxia. Cats: neurotoxicity precludes use. | Cleared by hepatic degradation. |
| Cytosine arabinoside (Cytosar-U, Upjohn) Inj: 100- and 500-mg vials | Appears to inhibit DNA polymerase activity; mechanism incompletely understood. S-phase specific. | Lymphoreticular neoplasms, myeloproliferative disease, and CNS lymphoma. | 100 mg/m² IV or SC q24h × 2–4 days (cats: 2 days); repeat p.r.n. 20 mg/m² intrathecally × 1–5 days. | Leukopenia. | May be given intrathecally. |
| Methotrexate (Methotrexate, Lederle; Folex, Adria; Mexate, Bristol-Myers Oncology) Tabs: 2.5 mg Inj: 5-, 20-, 25-, 50-, 100-, 200-, and 250-mg vials | Competitive enzyme inhibitor of folic acid reductase. S-phase specific. | Lymphoreticular neoplasms, myeloproliferative disorders, transmissible venereal tumor, Sertoli's cell tumor, and osteosarcoma. | "Usual dose"—0.5–0.8 mg/kg IV q7–14 days; or 2.5 mg/m² PO q48h. | Leukopenia, vomiting, and renal tubular necrosis with high doses. | May be given intrathecally. Primarily excreted by kidneys. |
| **Vinca Alkaloids** | | | | | |
| Vincristine (Oncovin, Lilly) Inj: 1-, 2-, and 5-mg vials | Appears to arrest mitotic division in metaphase; mechanism incompletely understood. M-phase specific. | Lymphoreticular neoplasms, carcinomas, sarcomas, and transmissible venereal tumor. | 0.5–0.7 mg/m² IV q7–14d. | Constipation, diarrhea, and peripheral neuropathies. | Severe vesicant. Primarily excreted by liver. |
| Vinblastine (Velban, Lilly) Inj: 10-mg vial | Effects cell energy production. Exhibits antimitotic activity. Primarily M-phase specific. | Lymphoreticular neoplasms and some carcinomas. | 2 mg/m² IV q7–14 days. | Leukopenia, epilation, and peripheral neuritis. | Severe vesicant. Primarily excreted by liver. |

*Table continued on following page*

| Agent (Brand Name, Supplier) | Action and Cell Cycle Specificity | Indication | Dosage and Administration† | Toxicities | Comments |
|---|---|---|---|---|---|
| ***Antitumor Antibiotics*** | | | | | |
| Bleomycin (Blenoxane, Bristol-Myers Oncology) Inj: 15-U vial | Appears to inhibit DNA synthesis. Lesser inhibition of RNA and protein synthesis. Cell cycle nonspecific. | Squamous cell carcinoma, lymphoma, and other carcinomas. | 10 U/m² IV or SC q24h × 3–4 days, then 10 U/m² q 7d. Maximum accumulative dose 200 U/ m². | Rare interstitial pneumonia leading to pulmonary fibrosis. | Has no toxic effects on the blood-forming elements. |
| Doxorubicin (Adriamycin, Adria) Inj: 10- and 50-mg vials | Intercalates between DNA base pairs. Inhibits DNA, RNA, and protein synthesis. Cell cycle nonspecific. | Lymphoreticular neoplasms, soft-tissue and bone sarcomas, thyroid carcinoma, mammary carcinoma, and other carcinomas. | 30 mg/m² IV or intracavitary q21d or 10 mg/m² IV q 7d. Maximum accumulative dose 240 mg/m². Consider pretreatment with antihistamine. | Leukopenia, thrombocytopenia, vomiting, diarrhea, epilation, cardiomyopathy, and urticaria. | Severe vesicant. Does not cross blood-brain barrier. Primarily excreted by liver. |
| Mitoxantrone (Novantrone, Lederle) Inj: 20-, 25-, and 30-mg vials | Intercalates between DNA base pairs. Induces DNA strand breaks. Arrests cells in G2 phase. Cell cycle nonspecific. | Lymphoreticular neoplasms, some mesenchymal neoplasms, and some carcinomas. | 3–5 mg/m² IV q21–28 days. | Depression, diarrhea, vomiting, colitis, and neutropenia. Toxicities considered mild. | Myelosuppression nadir 10 days postinjection. Considered less cardiotoxic than doxorubicin. |
| Dactinomycin (Cosmegen, Merck Sharp & Dohme) Inj: 0.5-mg vial | Intercalates between DNA bases. Inhibits mRNA synthesis. Cell cycle nonspecific. | Lymphoreticular neoplasms, some carcinomas, and some sarcomas. | 0.7 mg/m² IV q7d. | Leukopenia. | Severe vesicant. Use "two-needle" technique. |
| Plicamycin (Mithracin, Miles) Inj: 2.5-mg vial | Binds DNA and inhibits mRNA and protein synthesis; exact mechanism unknown. Cell cycle nonspecific. | Malignant testicular neoplasia and hypercalcemia. | 0.015–0.025 mg/kg IV over 4–24 hr (safety of repeated doses is unknown); dilute in saline. | Hemorrhagic syndrome and gastroenteritis. | Demonstrates short-lived (24–48 hr) calcium-lowering effect unrelated to tumoricidal activity. |
| ***Hormonal Agents*** | | | | | |
| Prednisone and prednisolone (various suppliers) Tabs: 1, 2.5, 5, 10, 20, 25, and 50 mg | Penetrates to nucleus and affects RNA production. Mechanism not well understood. Cell cycle nonspecific. | Lymphoreticular neoplasms, mast cell tumors, and brain tumors. | 10–40 mg/m² PO q24h × 7 days, then 10–20 mg/m² q 24–48h. | Pancreatitis, diarrhea, and cushingoid state. | Prednisone must be activated to prednisolone by the liver. |

| Drug | Action | Indications | Dosage | Toxicity | Comments |
|---|---|---|---|---|---|
| Diethylstilbestrol (Diethylstilbestrol, Lilly) Tabs: 0.1, 0.25, 0.5, 1, and 5 mg | Enters cytoplasm and is transported to nucleus where drug affects mRNA and protein synthesis. Cell cycle nonspecific. | Perianal gland adenoma and prostatic hyperplasia. | 0.1–1 mg/dog PO q24–48h, canine dose. | Feminization and occasional bone marrow aplasia. | May cause irreversible bone marrow suppression and aplastic anemia. |
| Tamoxifen (Nolvadex, ICI Pharma) Tabs: 10 mg | Antiestrogenic properties due to competition with estrogen for binding sites in target tissues. | Primary and metastatic mammary carcinomas with estrogen receptors. | 10 mg/m² PO q12h. | Mild nausea, vomiting, and bone marrow suppression may be noted. | Competes with estradiol for estrogen receptor protein. |

### Miscellaneous Agents

| Drug | Action | Indications | Dosage | Toxicity | Comments |
|---|---|---|---|---|---|
| Mitotane (Lysodren, Bristol-Myers Oncology) Tabs: 500 mg | Adrenal cytotoxic. Primary action on adrenal cortex; biochemical mechanism unknown. | Adrenal cortical carcinoma; (functional and nonfunctional). | 50 mg/kg PO q24h for 5–10 days, then 25 mg/kg PO q 3d. | Vomiting, anorexia, diarrhea, nausea, weakness, and adrenocortical suppression. | Discontinue temporarily in shock or severe traumatic conditions. |
| Asparaginase (Elspar, Merck Sharp & Dohme) Inj: 10,000-U vial | Enzyme that hydrolyzes serum asparagine to aspartate and ammonia. Deprives tumor cells of asparagine. G1-phase specific. | Lymphoreticular neoplasia and acute lymphocytic leukemia. | 400 U/kg SC, IM q7d or p.r.n.; or 10,000 U/m² SC, IM. Consider pretreatment with antihistamine. | Pancreatitis and anaphylaxis. | Increased risk of anaphylaxis with retreatments. Only inhibits tumor cells; no effect on normal cells. |
| Dacarbazine (DTIC-Dome, Miles) Inj: 100- and 200-mg vials | Exhibits alkylating and antimetabolite activity; exact mechanism unknown. Cell cycle nonspecific. | Lymphoreticular neoplasia. Minimal activity in malignant melanoma and osteosarcoma. | 1000 mg/m² IV over 24 hr; repeat in 21 days (canine only). | Anorexia, vomiting, diarrhea, and cytopenia. | Drug extravasation may result in tissue damage and severe pain. |
| Hydroxyurea (Hydrea, Squibb) Caps: 500 mg | Inhibits DNA synthesis without interfering with mRNA and protein synthesis. S-phase specific. | Polycythemia vera and chronic granulocytic leukemia. | 50 mg/kg (feline: 25 mg/kg) PO, divided b.i.d., q24–48h (until normal CBC). | Leukopenia, anemia, occasional thrombocytopenia, vomiting, and nail slough. | Primarily excreted by kidneys. |

°Provided and updated by **Dr. J.P. Thompson,** Department of Small Animal Clinical Sciences, College of Veterinary Medicine, University of Florida.
†Consult anticancer treatment protocols for precise dose.
Abbreviations: CNS = central nervous system; p.r.n. = as needed; WBC = white blood cells.
Also see p 478 in this volume for additional dosing information; p 475 for methods of safe handling of chemotherapeutic drugs; and p 482 for drug interactions.

# INDEX

Note: Page numbers in *italics* refer to illustrations; page numbers followed by t refer to tables. Page numbers following roman numerals X and XI refer to pages in previous editions.

Procainamide (*Continued*)
  for arrhythmia, 166, 803, 804–805, 805t, 849
  for cardiomyopathy, 867
  for myoclonus, XI:1006
  stability of, 196t
Procaine, uroanalytical values and, 17t
Procarbazine
  drug interactions with, 485t
  for canine lymphoma, 496, 496t
Procardia. See *Nifedipine (Adalat, Procardia).*
Prochlorperazine (Compazine)
  action mechanism of, 682t
  as antiemetic, XI:586, 682t
  dosage of, 682t, 1442t
  for irritable bowel syndrome, XI:608
  side effects of, 682t
Prochlorperazine with isopropamide
      (Darbazine)
  for diarrhea, 704t, 705
  for irritable bowel syndrome, XI:607
Proctitis, XI:616
Profenal (suprofen)
  for uveitis, 1252, 1259
  ophthalmic, XI:1052, 1221t
Progesterone
  drug effects on, 344t
  gestation timing and, 1086–1087, 1086t, 1087, 1088t
  hormonal values and, 340
  insufficiency of, abortion and, XI:928
  laboratory values and, 18t
  luteal insufficiency and, 1072
  teratogenicity of, 1071
Progesterone ELISA, in canine breeding, XI: 943
Progestin
  endocrine effects of, 339
  for prostatic hyperplasia, 1034
  growth hormone and, 345t
Prognosis
  APACHE system for, 96
  based on organ function, 97
  blood gas analysis and, 97
  guidelines for, XI:2
  oxygen tension and, 97
  scoring systems for, 97–98
Promazine (Sparine), 1442t
Promethazine (Phenergan), 1442t
Propantheline (Pro-Banthine)
  dosage of, 1442t
  for irritable bowel syndrome, XI:607
Proparacaine (Alcaine), XI:1058
  side effects of, 1223
Propine (dipivefrin), XI:1055, XI:1129t
*Propionibacterium acnes* vaccine
  as immunoadjuvant, XI:219
  for feline infectious peritonitis, XI:219
  for pyoderma, 616
Propiopromazine (Tranvet), 1443t
Propofol (Diprivan)
  advantages of, 77–78
  anaphylactoid reactions to, 79
  anesthesia with
    for urohydropropulsion, 1004
    in cardiac patient, 775, 779
    over consecutive days, 79
    quality of, 78
    recovery from, 78, 775
    speed of, 78
  anticonvulsant/convulsant reactions to, 79
  as antiemetic, 79
  cardiovascular effects of, 78, 775, 777t
  composition of, 77

Propofol (*Continued*)
  contamination of, 77
  contraindications to, 80, 80t
  cost of, 77, 80
  dosage of, 79–80, 80t, 1442t
  drug interactions with, 78
  for anorexia, 970
  for cardiovascular sedation, 775, 777t
  for early neutering, 1039
  indications for, 79–80
  metabolism of, 78–79
  respiratory effects of, 78
  seizures and, 79
  storage of, 77, 80
Propranolol (Inderal)
  adverse effects of, 41
  dosage of, 1443t
  for atrial fibrillation, XI:778
  for cocaine intoxication, 251
  for hypertension, XI:840, XI:840t
  for hyperthyroidism, XI:344
  for restrictive cardiomyopathy, 867
  for tachycardia, 165
  for ventricular arrhythmia, 166
  growth hormone and, 345t
  hepatic blood flow and, 761t, 762
  insulin and, 345t
  laboratory values and, 18t
  stability of, 196t
  thyroid effects of, 342t–344t
Proprionibacteria, in immunotherapy, 493–494
Proptosis, XI:1084
Propulsid (cisapride)
  as antiemetic, 681, 682t, 683
  dosage of, 1432t
Propylene glycol
  for ethylene glycol poisoning, 236
  hematologic effects of, 450
Propylthiouracil
  dosage of, 1443t
  hematologic effects of, 448t
  side effects of, 371, 448t
  thyroid effects of, 340, 343t, 371
Proscar (finasteride), 1034, 1105
Prostacyclin, for pulmonary hypertension, 891
Prostaglandin(s)
  action of, XI:37
  aspirin and, 70–71
  biosynthesis of, 71
  functions of, 630t
  pain perception and, 71
  renal blood flow and, 72–73
  thyroid effects of, 342t–343t
Prostaglandin E (misoprostol)
  dosage of, 1440t
  for pyometra, 1082
Prostaglandin F2α
  adrenocortical effects of, 341t
  dosage of, 1443t
  for pyometra, 1081–1083
  progesterone and, 344t
  to terminate pregnancy, 1075–1076, 1076t, 1079–1080, 1080
Prostate gland
  adenocarcinoma of
    diagnosis of, 1107–1108
    incidence of, 1106
    pathology of, 1106–1107
    serum markers for, 1108
    therapy for, 1108
  biopsy of ultrasonic guidance of, X:1227, 1056, 1058
  disorders of, canine, 1103–1108
  hyperplasia of

Prostate gland (*Continued*)
  canine, 1033–1034
  castration for, 1033, 1104
  diagnosis of, 1033, 1104
  etiology of, 1103–1104
  medical management of, 1033–1034, 1104–1105
  pathology of, 1103
  location of, 1052–1053, 1054t
  metaplasia of, estrogen-induced, 1073
  radiography of, 1052–1054, 1053, 1054t
  ultrasound of, 1056–1057, 1056
Prostatic fluid, canine, 1415t
Prostatitis
  acute, 1030
  canine, 1029–1032, 1105–1106
  chronic, 1030–1032, 1031t–1032t
  diagnosis of, 1030–1031, 1105–1106
  estrogen therapy and, 1073
  etiology of, 1105
  fungal, canine, 1105
  pathology of, 1105
  predisposition to, 1029
  prognosis of, 1032
  therapy for
    antibiotics in, 277t, 278, 1029–1032, 1030t–1032t, 1106
    castration in, 1032, 1106
    hormonal, 1032
    megesterol in, 1106
    prostate drainage in, 1106
Protease inhibitor Z, hepatitis and, 742
Protein
  adhesive, deficiency of, XI:225t
  binding of
    hepatic disease and, 760–761
    hepatic drug clearance and, 758
  deficiency of, XI:117
  depletion of, 958–959
  dietary
    metabolic acidosis and, 956
    renal failure and, 944, 949t, 956, 958–960
    restriction of
      for hepatic encephalopathy, 1156
      indications for, 959–960
  digestibility of, 725
  drug binding to, 44–45
  energy and, XI:117
  excess of, 959
  food allergy and, 61
  functions of, 55
  ingestion of, hormonal responses to, 55t
  laboratory values and, 22–23
  metabolism of, 55, 61
    cancer cachexia and, XI:435
  serum, fractions in, 1406t
Protein-losing enteropathy, breed-associated, 696t
Proteinuria
  Bence Jones, 524
  causes of, 937
  diagnosis of, 937–940, 938t, 939
  uroanalytical values and, 17t
*Proteus* infection, in reptile, 1355
*Proteus* pyoderma, 613
Prothrombin time
  one-stage, 460
  warfarin therapy and, 871–872
Protirelin (Thypinone). See *Thyrotropin-releasing hormone (TRH).*
Proton pump inhibitor(s), for gastrointestinal ulcer, 708

ISBN 0-7216-5188-7

90071

## BUSINESS REPLY MAIL
FIRST CLASS MAIL   PERMIT NO. 7135   ORLANDO, FL

POSTAGE WILL BE PAID BY ADDRESSEE

NO POSTAGE
NECESSARY
IF MAILED
IN THE
UNITED STATES

BOOK ORDER FULFILLMENT DEPT.

## WB SAUNDERS COMPANY
*A Division of Harcourt Brace & Company*
**6277 SEA HARBOR DR
ORLANDO  FL  32821-9816**

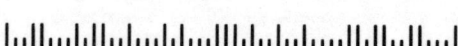

### Weight Equivalents

| | |
|---|---|
| 1 lb | = 453.6 g = 0.4536 kg = 16 oz |
| 1 oz | = 28.35 gm |
| 1 kg | = 1,000 g = 2.2046 lb |
| 1 gm | = 1,000 mg |
| 1 mg | = 1,000 $\mu$g = 0.001 gm |
| 1 $\mu$g | = 0.001 mg = 0.000001 gm |

1 $\mu$g per gm or 1 mg per kg is the same as 1 ppm

| METRIC | APOTHECARY |
|---|---|
| 0.1 milligram (mg) | = $\frac{1}{600}$ grain (gr) |
| 0.15 mg | = $\frac{1}{400}$ gr |
| 0.2 mg | = $\frac{1}{300}$ gr |
| 0.25 mg | = $\frac{1}{250}$ gr |
| 0.3 mg | = $\frac{1}{200}$ gr |
| 0.4 | = $\frac{1}{150}$ gr |
| 0.5 | = $\frac{1}{120}$ gr |
| 1.0 | = $\frac{1}{60}$ gr |
| 15.0 mg | = $\frac{1}{4}$ gr |
| 30.0 mg | = $\frac{1}{2}$ gr |
| 40.0 mg | = $\frac{2}{3}$ gr |
| 50.0 mg | = $\frac{3}{4}$ gr |
| 60.0 mg | = 1 gr (0.06 gm) |
| 1.0 gm | = 15 gr |

### Volume Equivalents

| Household | Metric |
|---|---|
| 1 drop (gt) | = 0.06 milliliter (ml) |
| 15 drops (gtt) | = 1 ml (1 cc) |
| 1 teaspoon (tsp) | = 5 (4) ml |
| 1 tablespoon (tbs) | = 15 ml |
| 2 tablesppons | = 30 ml |
| 1 ounce (oz) | = 30 ml |
| 1 teacup | = 180 ml (6 oz) |
| 1 glass | = 240 ml (8 oz) |
| 1 measuring cup | = 240 ml (1/2 pint) |
| 2 measuring cups | = 500 ml (1 pint) |

### Weight–Unit Conversion Factors

| Units Given | Units Wanted | For Conversion Multiply by |
|---|---|---|
| lb | gm | 453.6 |
| lb | kg | 0.4536 |
| oz | gm | 28.35 |
| kg | lb | 2.2046 |
| kg | mg | 1,000,000. |
| kg | gm | 1,000. |
| gm | mg | 1,000. |
| gm | $\mu$g | 1,000,000. |
| mg | $\mu$g | 1,000. |
| mg/gm | mg/lb | 453.6 |
| mg/kg | mg/lb | 0.4536 |
| $\mu$g/kg | $\mu$g/lb | 0.4536 |
| Mcal | kcal | 1,000. |
| kcal/kg | kcal/lb | 0.4536 |
| kcal/lb | kcal/kg | 2.2046 |
| ppm | $\mu$g/gm | 1. |
| ppm | mg/kg | 1. |
| ppm | mg/lb | 0.4536 |
| mg/kg | % | 0.0001 |
| ppm | % | 0.0001 |
| mg/gm | % | 0.1 |
| gm/kg | % | 0.1 |

### Temperature Conversion

°Celsius to °Fahrenheit: $(°C)\left(\dfrac{9}{5}\right) + 32°$

°Fahrenheit to °Celsius: $(°F - 32°)\left(\dfrac{5}{9}\right)$

### Conversion Factors

| | | | |
|---|---|---|---|
| 1 milligram | = 1/65 | grain | (1/60) |
| 1 gram | = 15.43 | grains | (15) |
| 1 kilogram | = 2.20 | pounds | (avoirdupois) |
| | 2.65 | pounds | (Troy) |
| 1 milliliter | = 16.23 | minims | (15) |
| 1 liter | = 1.06 | quarts | (1+) |
| | 33.80 | fluid ounces | (34) |
| 1 grain | = 0.065 | gm | (60 mg) |
| 1 dram | = 3.9 | gm | (4) |
| 1 ounce | = 31.1 | gm | (30+) |
| 1 minim | = 0.062 | ml | (0.06) |
| 1 fluid dram | = 3.7 | ml | (4) |
| 1 fluid ounce | = 29.57 | ml | (30) |
| 1 pint | = 473.2 | ml | (500−) |
| 1 quart | = 946.4 | ml | (1000−) |

Figures in parentheses are commonly employed approximate values.